ANNUAL BOOK OF ASTM STANDARDS

2001

SECTION 13

Medical Devices and Services

VOLUME 13.01

Medical Devices; Emergency Medical Services

Includes standards of the following committees:

F04 on Medical and Surgical Materials and Devices
F29 on Anesthetic and Respiratory Equipment
F30 on Emergency Medical Services
F32 on Search and Rescue

ASTM Stock Number: S130101

ASTM ■ 100 BARR HARBOR DRIVE, PO BOX C700, WEST CONSHOHOCKEN, PA 19428-2959
TEL: **610-832-9500** ■ FAX: **610-832-9555** ■ EMAIL: **service@astm.org** ■ WEBSITE: **www.astm.org**

Library of Congress Catalog Card Number: 83-641658

ISBN 0-8031-3039-2 (set)
ISBN 0-8031-3022-8 (volume)

ORDER INFORMATION: Additional copies of this book in print, on CD-ROM, or reprints (single or multiple copies) of individual standards may be obtained by contacting ASTM at the above address or at 610-832-9585 (phone), 610-832-9555 (fax), service@astm.org (email), or through www.astm.org (website).

Printed in Baltimore, MD, U.S.A.

Foreword

Organized in 1898, ASTM has grown into one of the largest voluntary standards development systems in the world. ASTM is a not-for-profit organization which provides a forum for producers, users, ultimate consumers, and those having a general interest (representatives of government and academia) to meet on common ground and write standards for materials, products, systems, and services.

From the work of 128 standards-writing committees, ASTM publishes more than 11,000 standards each year. These standards and other related technical information are sold throughout the world.

ASTM Headquarters has no technical research or testing facilities; such work is done voluntarily by 30,520 technically qualified ASTM members located throughout the world. Membership in the Society is open to all concerned with the fields in which ASTM is active. A membership application may be obtained from Member and Committee Services, ASTM, 100 Barr Harbor Drive, PO Box C700, West Conshohocken, PA 19428–2959; tel. 610-832-9694 or from the ASTM website, www.astm.org under Technical Committees/Membership Information.

2001 Annual Book of ASTM Standards

The 2001 *Annual Book of ASTM Standards* consists of 75 volumes, divided among 16 sections, of which this volume is one. It contains approved ASTM standards, provisional standards, and related material. These terms are defined as follows in the *Regulations Governing ASTM Technical Committees:*

Categories:

standard, n—as used in ASTM, a document that has been developed and established within the consensus principles of the Society and that meets the approval requirements of ASTM procedures and regulations.

standard, adj—as used in ASTM, a descriptive used in titles of test methods, specifications, and other documents to indicate consensus approval in accordance with ASTM procedures and regulations.

provisional standard—a document published for a limited period of time by the Society to meet a demand for more rapid issuance of specific documents, such as an emergency situation, regulatory requirements, or other special circumstances.
Discussion—Provisional standards are not full consensus documents because they require subcommittee consensus only. (See *Regulations Governing ASTM Technical Committees*, Section 14.)

Types:

The various types of ASTM documents are to provide a flexibility of form, communication, and usage for both the technical committees and the myriad users of ASTM documents. The type of ASTM document that is developed and titled is based on the technical content and intended use, not on the degree of consensus achieved. The two categories of ASTM documents (standard and provisional standard) can be of the following forms and types:

classification—a systematic arrangement or division of materials, products, systems, or services into groups based on similar characteristics such as origin, composition, properties, or use.

guide—a compendium of information or series of options that does not recommend a specific course of action.
Discussion—A guide increases the awareness of information and approaches in a given subject area.

practice—a definitive set of instructions for performing one or more specific operations or functions that does not produce a test result.
Discussion—Examples of practices include, but are not limited to: application, assessment, cleaning, collection,

decontamination, inspection, installation, preparation, sampling, screening, and training.

specification—an explicit set of requirements to be satisfied by a material, product, system, or service.
Discussion—Examples of specifications include, but are not limited to, requirements for: physical, mechanical, or chemical properties, and safety, quality, or performance criteria. A specification identifies the test methods for determining whether each of the requirements is satisfied.

terminology—a document comprising definitions of terms; explanations of symbols, abbreviations, or acronyms.

test method—a definitive procedure that produces a test result.
Discussion—Examples of test methods include, but are not limited to: identification, measurement, and evaluation of one or more qualities, characteristics, or properties. A precision and bias statement shall be reported at the end of a test method. (See *Form and Style for ASTM Standards*, Section A21, Precision and Bias.)

A new edition of the Book of Standards is published annually because of additions of new standards and significant revisions to existing standards. Approximately 30 % of each volume is new or revised. Each volume contains all actions approved by the Society at least six months before the publication date. New and revised standards approved by the Society between the annual editions of any given volume are made available as separate copies. Users are cautioned to follow the most current issue of a standard except when a specific edition of a standard is cited, for example, as in a contract.

Development and Use of ASTM Standards

ASTM believes that technically competent standards result when a full consensus of all concerned parties is achieved and rigorous due process procedures are followed. This philosophy and standards development system ensure technically competent standards having the highest credibility when critically examined and used as the basis for commercial, legal, or regulatory actions.

ASTM standards are developed voluntarily and used voluntarily. Standards become legally binding only when a government body references them in regulations, or when they are cited in a contract. Any item that is produced and marked as conforming to an ASTM standard must meet all applicable requirements of that standard.

ASTM standards are used by thousands of individuals, companies, and agencies. Purchasers and sellers incorporate standards into contracts; scientists and engineers use them in laboratories; architects and designers use them in plans; government agencies reference them in codes, regulations, and laws; and many others refer to standards for guidance.

Consideration of Comments on ASTM Standards

An ASTM standard is subject to revision at any time by the responsible technical committee and must be reviewed every five years and if not revised, either reapproved or withdrawn. Your comments are invited either for revision of any standard or for the development of new standards and should be addressed to ASTM Headquarters. Your comments will receive careful consideration at a meeting of the responsible technical committee, which you may attend. If you feel your comments have not received a fair hearing you should make your views known to the ASTM Committee on Standards, 100 Barr Harbor Drive, PO Box C700, West Conshohocken, PA 19428.

Using the Annual Book of ASTM Standards

The standards are assembled in each volume in alphanumeric sequence of their ASTM designation numbers. Volumes 03.06, 04.09, 05.05, and 06.03 are assembled first by committee, then in alphanumeric sequence. Each volume has a table of contents, listing the standards in alphanumeric sequence by ASTM designation; and a list by subjects, categorizing the standards according to subject. A subject index of the standards in each volume appears at the back of each volume.

Availability of Individual Standards

Each ASTM standard is available as a separate copy from ASTM. Standards can be ordered from the ASTM website at www.astm.org, in the store section. Standards can also be ordered from Customer Services at 610–832–9585, Monday through Friday, 8:30 AM to 4:30 PM Eastern Standard Time.

FOREWORD

Caveat Statements and Policies in Standards

ASTM caveat statements on Safety Hazards and Fire Hazards are required to appear in standards where appropriate. They are located in the scope section of applicable standards. The caveats on General Statement of ASTM Policy and Patents are contained in all standards and located at the end of each standard. For more information on the caveats see Section F2 of the *Form and Style for ASTM Standards.*

ANNUAL BOOK OF ASTM STANDARDS
Listed by Section and Volume

Section 1— Iron and Steel Products
Volume 01.01 Steel—Piping, Tubing, Fittings
Volume 01.02 Ferrous Castings; Ferroalloys
Volume 01.03 Steel—Plate, Sheet, Strip, Wire; Stainless Steel Bar
Volume 01.04 Steel—Structural, Reinforcing, Pressure Vessel, Railway
Volume 01.05 Steel—Bars, Forgings, Bearing, Chain, Springs
Volume 01.06 Coated Steel Products
Volume 01.07 Ships and Marine Technology
Volume 01.08 Fasteners

Section 2— Nonferrous Metal Products
Volume 02.01 Copper and Copper Alloys
Volume 02.02 Aluminum and Magnesium Alloys
Volume 02.03 Electrical Conductors
Volume 02.04 Nonferrous Metals—Nickel, Cobalt, Lead, Tin, Zinc, Cadmium, Precious, Reactive, Refractory Metals and Alloys; Materials for Thermostats, Electrical Heating and Resistance, Contacts, and Connectors
Volume 02.05 Metallic and Inorganic Coatings; Metal Powders, Sintered P/M Structural Parts

Section 3—Metals Test Methods and Analytical Procedures
Volume 03.01 Metals—Mechanical Testing; Elevated and Low-Temperature Tests; Metallography
Volume 03.02 Wear and Erosion; Metal Corrosion
Volume 03.03 Nondestructive Testing
Volume 03.04 Magnetic Properties
Volume 03.05 Analytical Chemistry for Metals, Ores, and Related Materials (I): E 32 - E 1724
Volume 03.06 Analytical Chemistry for Metals, Ores, and Related Materials (II): E 1763 - latest; Molecular Spectroscopy; Surface Analysis

Section 4—Construction
Volume 04.01 Cement; Lime; Gypsum
Volume 04.02 Concrete and Aggregates
Volume 04.03 Road and Paving Materials; Vehicle-Pavement Systems
Volume 04.04 Roofing, Waterproofing, and Bituminous Materials
Volume 04.05 Chemical-Resistant Nonmetallic Materials; Vitrified Clay Pipe, Concrete Pipe, Fiber-Reinforced Cement Products; Mortars and Grouts; Masonry
Volume 04.06 Thermal Insulation; Environmental Acoustics
Volume 04.07 Building Seals and Sealants; Fire Standards; Dimension Stone
Volume 04.08 Soil and Rock (I): D 420 - D 5779
Volume 04.09 Soil and Rock (II): D 5780 - latest; Geosynthetics
Volume 04.10 Wood
Volume 04.11 Building Constructions

Section 5—Petroleum Products, Lubricants, and Fossil Fuels
Volume 05.01 Petroleum Products and Lubricants (I): D 56 - D 2596
Volume 05.02 Petroleum Products and Lubricants (II): D 2597 - D 4927
Volume 05.03 Petroleum Products and Lubricants (III): D 4928 - D 5950
Volume 05.04 Petroleum Products and Lubricants (IV): D 5966 - latest
Volume 05.05 Test Methods for Rating Motor, Diesel, and Aviation Fuels; Manufactured Carbon and Graphite Products; Catalysts
Volume 05.06 Gaseous Fuels; Coal and Coke

Section 6—Paints, Related Coatings, and Aromatics
Volume 06.01 Paint—Tests for Chemical, Physical, and Optical Properties; Appearance

ANNUAL BOOK OF ASTM STANDARDS

Listed by Subjects

LISTED BY SUBJECTS

LISTED BY SUBJECTS

Contents

2001 ANNUAL BOOK OF ASTM STANDARDS, VOLUME 13.01

STANDARDS RELATING TO MEDICAL DEVICES; EMERGENCY MEDICAL SERVICES

A complete Subject Index appears at the end of this volume.

Listed below are those standards included in this volume(s) and those standards that have appeared previously which have been discontinued within the past three years.

In the serial designations prefixed to the following titles, the number following the dash indicates the year of original adoption as standard or, in the case of revision, the year of last revision. Thus, standards adopted or revised during the year 2001 have as their final number, 01. A letter following this number indicates more than one revision during that year, that is, 01a indicates the second revision in 2001, 01b, the third revision, etc. Standards that have been reapproved without change are indicated by the year of last reapproval in parentheses as part of the designation number, for example, (2001). A superscript epsilon indicates an editorial change since the last revision or reapproval—$^{\epsilon1}$ for the first change, $^{\epsilon2}$ for the second change, etc.

§Approved for use by agencies of the Department of Defense and, if indicated on the standard, replaces corresponding Federal or Military document. Consult the DoD Index of Specifications and Standards for the specific year of issue which has been adopted by the Department of Defense.

*Adopted by American National Standards Institute.

†Although this standard has been officially withdrawn from Society approval, a brief description is included for information only.

CONTENTS

CONTENTS

CONTENTS

CONTENTS

CONTENTS

CONTENTS

CONTENTS

RELATED MATERIAL

List by Subjects

2001 ANNUAL BOOK OF ASTM STANDARDS, VOLUME 13.01

MEDICAL DEVICES; EMERGENCY MEDICAL SERVICES

A complete Subject Index appears at the end of this volume.

Since the standards in this volume are arranged in alphanumeric sequence, no page numbers are given in this list by subjects.

ANESTHETIC AND RESPIRATORY EQUIPMENT

Airways

Specifications for:

F 1666 – 95$^{\epsilon 1}$	Adult Tracheostomy Tubes
F 1205 – 88(1999)	Anesthesia Breathing Tubes
F 1204 – 88(1998)	Anesthesia Reservoir Bags
F 1573 – 95(2000)	Anesthetic Equipment—Oropharyngeal and Nasopharyngeal Airways
§F 1242 – 96$^{\epsilon 1}$	Cuffed and Uncuffed Tracheal Tubes
F 1981 – 99	Suction Catheters for Use in the Respiratory Tract
F 1243 – 89(1995)	Tracheal Tube Connectors
F 1590 – 95	Tracheostomy Tube Connectors
F 1627 – 95	Tracheostomy Tubes-Pediatric Tracheostomy Tubes

Anesthesia Gas Machine

Specifications for:

F 1161	Minimum Performance and Safety Requirements for Components and Systems of Anesthesia Gas Machines (Discontinued 2000†)

Anesthesia Workstations

Specifications for:

F 1054 – 01	Conical Fittings
F 1208 – 89(2000)	Minimum Performance and Safety Requirements for Anesthesia Breathing Systems
F 1850 – 00	Particular Requirements for Anesthesia Workstations and Their Components
F 1101 – 90(1996)	Ventilators Intended for Use During Anesthesia

Cutaneous Gas Monitoring

Specifications for:

F 984	Cutaneous Gas Monitoring Devices for Oxygen and Carbon Dioxide (Discontinued 1999†)

Division Six on Medical Gas Supply Systems

Specifications for:

F 927	Pediatric Tracheostomy Tubes (Discontinued 1999†)

Gas Monitors

Specifications for:

F 1456 – 92	Capnometers
F 1452 – 92	Minimum Performance and Safety Requirements for Components and Systems of Anesthetic Gas Monitors
F 1462 – 93	Oxygen Analyzers
F 1415 – 92(2000)	Pulse Oximeters

Harmonization of Alarms

Specifications for:

§Approved for use by agencies of the Department of Defense and, if indicated on the standard, replaces corresponding Federal or Military document. Consult the DoD Index of Specifications and Standards for the specific year of issue which has been adopted by the Department of Defense.

*Adopted by American National Standards Institute.

†Although this standard has been officially withdrawn from Society approval, a brief description is included for information only.

F 1463 – 93(1999) Alarm Signals in Medical Equipment Used in Anesthesia and Respiratory Care

Laryngoscopes and Bronchoscopes

Specifications for:

F 1218 – 89(1999) Bronchoscopes (Rigid)
F 896 – 90(1999) Flexible Fiberoptic Bronchoscopes
F 1195 – 99 Rigid Laryngoscopes for Tracheal Intubation—Hook on Fittings for Fiberilluminated Blades and Handles
§F 965 – 99 Rigid Laryngoscopes for Tracheal Intubation—Hook-On Fittings for Laryngoscope Handles and Blades with Lamps

Medical-Surgical Suction Systems

Specifications for:

§F 960 – 86(2000) Medical and Surgical Suction and Drainage Systems

Operating Room Fire Safety

Specifications for:

F 1628 – 95(2000) Labeling and Marking of Cuffed and Uncuffed Tracheal Tubes and Related Treatments Intended for Use During Laser Surgery

Test Methods for:

F 1497 – 99a Determining Laser Resistance of the Shaft of Tracheal Tubes

Pollution Control

Specifications for:

F 1343 Anestetic Equipment-Scavenging Systems for Anesthetic Gases (Discontinued 2000†)

Terminology

Terminology for:

F 2002 – 01a Anesthesia and Respiratory Equipment

Ventilators

Specifications for:

F 1246 – 91(1999) Electrically Powered Home Care Ventilators, Part 1—Positive-Pressure Ventilators and Ventilator Circuits
F 1690 – 96 Humidifiers for Medical Use-Part 1
§F 920 – 93(1999) Minimum Performance and Safety Requirements for Resuscitators Intended for Use With Humans
F 1464 – 93(1999) Oxygen Concentrators for Domiciliary Use
F 1100 – 90(1997) Ventilators Intended for Use in Critical Care

EMERGENCY MEDICAL SERVICES

Communications

Practices for:

F 2076 – 01 Communicating an EMS Patient Report to Receiving Medical Facilities
F 1560 – 00 Emergency Medical Dispatch Management
F 1258 – 95(2001) Emergency Medical Dispatch

Guides for:

F 1220 – 95(2001) Emergency Medical Services System (EMSS) Telecommunications
F 1221 – 89(2001) Interagency Information Exchange
F 1381 – 92(1997) Planning and Developing 9-1-1 Enhanced Telephone Systems

EMS Equipment

Specifications for:

F 1274 Fixed Wing Advanced Life Support Transport Units (Discontinued 2000†)
F 1187 Fixed Wing Basic Life Support Transport Units (Discontinued 2000†)
F 1283 Fixed Wing Specialized Medical Transport Units (Discontinued 2000†)
F 1949 – 99 Medical Oxygen Delivery Systems for EMS Ground Vehicles
F 1118 – 91(1997)$^{\epsilon 1}$ National Air Medical Transport Units Resources Catalog
F 1124 Rotary Wing Advanced Life Support Transport Units (Discontinued 2000†)
F 1119 Rotary Wing Basic Life Support Transport Units (Discontinued 2000†)
F 1146 Rotary Wing Specialized Medical Transport Units (Discontinued 2000†)

LIST BY SUBJECTS

Practices for:	
F 2020 – 00	Design, Construction, and Procurement of Emergency Medical Services Systems (EMSS) Ambulances
Guides for:	
F 1558 – 94	Characteristics for Adjunct Cervical Spine Immobilization Devices (ACSID)
F 1559 – 94	Characteristics for Cervical Spine Immobilization Collar(s) (CSIC)
F 1555 – 94	Characteristics for Extremity Splints
F 1557 – 94	Full Body Spinal Immobilization Devices (FBSID) Characteristics
F 1556 – 94	Spinal Immobilization and Extrication (Spined) Device Characteristics

Organization/Management

Practices for:	
F 1149 – 93(1998)	Qualifications, Responsibilities, and Authority of Individuals and Institutions Providing Medical Direction of Emergency Medical Services
Guides for:	
F 1286 – 90(1996)$^{\epsilon 1}$	Development and Operation of Level 1 Pediatric Trauma Facilities
F 1629 – 95	Establishing Operating Emergency Medical Services and Management Information Systems, or Both
F 1268 – 90(1998)	Establishing and Operating a Public Information, Education, and Relations Program for Emergency Medical Service Systems
F 1493 – 93(1998)	Financing and Financial Accountability of Medical Transportation Systems
F 1339 – 92(1998)	Organization and Operation of Emergency Medical Services Systems
F 1288 – 90(1998)	Planning for and Response to a Multiple Casualty Incident
F 1652 – 95	Providing Essential Data Needed in Advance for Prehospital Emergency Medical Services
F 1224 – 89(1996)$^{\epsilon 1}$	Providing System Evaluation for Emergency Medical Services
F 1086 – 94	Structures and Responsibilities of Emergency Medical Services Systems Organizations

Personnel, Training and Education

Practices for:	
F 1255 – 90(1995)$^{\epsilon 1}$	Performance of Prehospital Automated Defibrillation
F 1254 – 90(2001)	Performance of Prehospital Manual Defibrillation
F 1552 – 94	Training Instructor Qualification and Certification Eligibility of Emergency Medical Dispatchers
F 1031 – 00	Training the Emergency Medical Technician (Basic)
Guides for:	
F 1229 – 00	Establishing the Qualifications, Education, and Training of EMS, Air-Medical Patient Care Providers
F 1489 – 93	Performance of Patient Assessment by the Emergency Medical Technician (Paramedic)
F 1517 – 94	Scope of Performance of Emergency Medical Services Ambulance Operations
F 1616 – 95	Scope of Performance of First Responders Who Practice in the Wilderness or Delayed or Prolonged Transport Settings
F 1287 – 90(1996)	Scope of Performance of First Responders Who Provide Emergency Medical Care
F 1653 – 95	Scope of Performance of Triage in a Prehospital Environment
F 1257 – 90(1996)$^{\epsilon 1}$	Selection and Practice of the Emergency Medical Services Instructor for Advanced Life Support/Emergency Medical Technician (ALS/EMT) Training Programs
F 1256 – 90(1996)$^{\epsilon 1}$	Selection and Practice of the Emergency Medical Services Instructor for Basic Life Support/ Emergency
F 1705 – 96	Training Emergency Medical Services Ambulance Operations
F 1328 – 00	Training Emergency Medical Technician (Basic) to Prepare Patients for Medical Transportation
F 1655 – 95	Training First Responders Who Practice in Wilderness, Delayed, or Prolonged Transport Settings
F 1453 – 92(1996)	Training and Evaluation of First Responders Who Provide Emergency Medical Care
F 1654 – 95	Training and Evaluation of Individuals Who are Responsible for or Perform Triage in a Prehospital Environment
F 1421 – 01	Training the Emergency Medical Technician (Basic) To Manage Obstetrical Emergencies
F 1419 – 00	Training the Emergency Medical Technician (Basic) To Manage Shock
F 1329 – 00	Training the Emergency Medical Technician (Basic) in Basic Anatomy and Physiology
F 1418 – 01	Training the Emergency Medical Technician (Basic) in Roles and Responsibilities
F 1285 – 90(1998)	Training the Emergency Medical Technician (Basic) to Perform Patient Examination Techniques
F 1219 – 00	Training the Emergency Medical Technician (Basic) to Perform Patient Initial and Detailed Assessment
F 1420 – 01	Training the Emergency Medical Technician (Basic) to Perform Patient Management Techniques
F 1253	Training the Emergency Medical Technician (Basic) to Perform Patient Secondary Assessment (Discontinued 1999†)

F 1651 – 95 Training the Emergency Medical Technician (Paramedic)

Terminology

Terminology for:

F 1177 – 96a Emergency Medical Services

MEDICAL AND SURGICAL MATERIALS AND DEVICES

Arthroplasty

Specifications for:

F 1357 – 99	Articulating Total Wrist Implants
F 1636 – 95$^{\epsilon 2}$	Bores and Cones for Modular Femoral Heads
F 1781 – 97	Elastomeric Flexible Hinge Finger Total Joint Implants
F 2068 – 00	Femoral Prostheses—Metallic Implants
F 370 – 94(1999)	Proximal Femoral Endoprosthesis
F 1672 – 95(2000)	Resurfacing Patellar Prosthesis
F 1378 – 00	Shoulder Prostheses
F 2033 – 00a	Total Hip Joint Prosthesis and Hip Endoprosthesis Bearing Surfaces Made of Metallic, Ceramic, and Polymeric Materials
F 2083 – 01a	Total Knee Prosthesis

Test Methods for:

F 1800 – 97	Cyclic Fatigue Testing of Metal Tibial Tray Components of Total Knee Joint Replacements
F 2009 – 00	Determining the Axial Disassembly Force of Taper Connections of Modular Prostheses
F 1820 – 97	Determining the Axial Disassembly Force of a Modular Acetabular Device
F 1829 – 98	Static Evaluation of the Glenoid Locking Mechanism in Shear
F 2028 – 00	the Dynamic Evaluation of Glenoid Loosening or Disassociation

Practices for:

F 1440 – 92(1997)	Cyclic Fatigue Testing of Metallic Stemmed Hip Arthroplasty Femoral Components Without Torsion
F 1612 – 95(2000)	Cyclic Fatigue Testing of Metallic Stemmed Hip Arthroplasty Femoral Components with Torsion
F 2025 – 00	Gravimetric Measurement of Polymeric Components for Wear Assessment

Guides for:

F 1814 – 97a	Evaluating Modular Hip and Knee Joint Components
F 1714 – 96	Gravimetric Wear Assessment of Prosthetic Hip-Designs in Simulator Devices
F 1715 – 00$^{\epsilon 1}$	Wear Assessment of Prosthetic Knee Designs in Simulator Devices

Biocompatibility Test Methods

Test Methods for:

§F 895 – 84(2001)$^{\epsilon 1}$	Agar Diffusion Cell Culture Screening for Cytotoxicity

Practices for:

F 1983 – 99	Assessment of Compatibility of Absorbable/Resorbable Biomaterials for Implant Applications
F 981 – 99	Assessment of Compatibility of Biomaterials for Surgical Implants with Respect to Effect of Materials on Muscle and Bone
F 756 – 00	Assessment of Hemolytic Properties of Materials
F 1027 – 86(1995)$^{\epsilon 1}$	Assessment of Tissue and Cell Compatibility of Orofacial Prosthetic Materials and Devices
F 1877 – 98	Characterization of Particles
F 813 – 83(1996)$^{\epsilon 1}$	Direct Contact Cell Culture Evaluation of Materials for Medical Devices
F 749 – 98	Evaluating Material Extracts by Intracutaneous Injection in the Rabbit
F 750 – 87(1996)	Evaluating Material Extracts by Systemic Injection in the Mouse
F 1906 – 98	Evaluation of Immune Responses In Biocompatibility Testing Using ELISA Tests, Lymphocyte Proliferation, and Cell Migration
*F 619 – 79(1997)$^{\epsilon 1}$	Extraction of Medical Plastics
F 748 – 98	Selecting Generic Biological Test Methods for Materials and Devices
F 1905 – 98	Selecting Tests for Determining The Propensity Of Materials To Cause Immunotoxicity
F 763 – 99	Short-Term Screening of Implant Materials
F 1408 – 97	Subcutaneous Screening Test for Implant Materials
F 719 – 81(1996)$^{\epsilon 1}$	Testing Biomaterials in Rabbits for Primary Skin Irritation
F 1903 – 98	Testing For Biological Responses to Particles In Vitro
F 720 – 81(1996)$^{\epsilon 1}$	Testing Guinea Pigs for Contact Allergens
F 2065 – 00$^{\epsilon 1}$	Testing for Alternative Pathway Complement Activation in Serum by Solid Materials
F 1984 – 99	Testing for Whole Complement Activation in Serum by Solid Materials

F 1904 – 98$^{\epsilon1}$	Testing the Biological Responses to Particles In Vivo
Guides for:	
F 1439 – 92(1996)	Performance of Lifetime Bioassay for the Tumorigenic Potential of Implant Materials

Cardiovascular Standards

Test Methods for:	
F 2079 – 01	Measuring Recoil of Balloon-Expandable Stents
Practices for:	
F 1841 – 97	Assessment of Hemolysis in Continuous Flow Blood Pumps
F 1830 – 97	Selection of Blood for In Vitro Evaluation of Blood Pumps
Guides for:	
F 2081 – 01	Characterization and Presentation of the Dimensional Attributes of Vascular Stents

Ceramic Materials

Specifications for:	
F 1088 – 87(1992)$^{\epsilon1}$	Beta-Tricalcium Phosphate for Surgical Implantation
F 1609 – 95	Calcium Phosphate Coatings for Implantable Materials
F 1581 – 99	Composition of Anorganic Bone for Surgical Implants
F 1185 – 88(1993)$^{\epsilon1}$	Composition of Ceramic Hydroxylapatite for Surgical Implants
F 1538 – 94	Glass and Glass Ceramic Biomaterials for Implantation
F 603 – 00	High-Purity Dense Aluminum Oxide for Medical Application
F 1873 – 98	High-Purity Dense Yttria Tetragonal Zirconium Oxide Polycrystal (Y-TZP) for Surgical Implant Applications
Test Methods for:	
F 1659 – 95	Bending and Shear Fatigue Testing of Calcium Phosphate Coatings on Solid Metallic Substrates
F 1926 – 99	Evaluation of the Environmental Stability of Calcium Phosphate Coatings
F 1658	Shear Testing of Calcium Phosphate Coatings (Discontinued 2000†)
F 1501	Tension Testing of Calcium Phosphate Coatings (Discontinued 2000†)
Practices for:	
F 2024 – 00	X-ray Diffraction Determination of Phase Content of Plasma-Sprayed Hydroxyapatite Coatings

Device Retrieval Analysis

Practices for:	
F 561 – 97	Retrieval and Analysis of Implanted Medical Devices, and Associated Tissues

GI Endoscopes

Practices for:	
F 1518 – 00	Cleaning and Disinfection of Flexible Fiberoptic and Video Endoscopes Used in the Examination of the Hollow Viscera
F 1992 – 99	Reprocessing of Reusable, Heat-Stable Endoscopic Accessory Instruments (EAI) Used with Flexible Endoscopes

Material Test Methods

Test Methods for:	
F 1223 – 96	Determination of Total Knee Replacement Constraint
F 2082 – 01	Determination of Transformation Temperature of Nickel-Titanium Shape Memory Alloys by Bend and Free Recovery
F 1536 – 95(1999)	Determining Strength and Setting Time of Synthetic Water-Activated Polyurethane Fiberglass Orthopaedic Casting Tape
F 1635 – 95(2000)	In Vitro Degradation Testing of Poly (L-lactic Acid) Resin and Fabricated Form for Surgical Implants
F 2052 – 00	Measurement of Magnetically Induced Displacement Force on Passive Implants in the Magnetic Resonance Environment
F 1978 – 00$^{\epsilon1}$	Measuring Abrasion Resistance of Metallic Thermal Spray Coatings by Using the Taber™ Abraser
F 897 – 84(1997)	Measuring Fretting Corrosion of Osteosynthesis Plates and Screws
F 746 – 87(1999)	Pitting or Crevice Corrosion of Metallic Surgical Implant Materials
*§F 640 – 79(2000)	Radiopacity of Plastics for Medical Use
F 1044 – 99	Shear Testing of Porous Metal Coatings
F 1160 – 00$^{\epsilon1}$	Shear and Bending Fatigue Testing of Calcium Phosphate and Metallic Medical and Composite Calcium Phosphate/Metallic Coatings

F 563 – 00	Wrought Cobalt-20Nickel-20Chromium-3.5Molybdenum-3.5Tungsten-5Iron Alloy for Surgical Implant Applications (UNS R30563)
F 1537 – 00	Wrought Cobalt-28 Chromium-6 Molybdenum Alloy for Surgical Implants
F 688 – 00	Wrought Cobalt-35 Nickel-20 Chromium-10 Molybdenum Alloy Plate, Sheet, and Foil for Surgical Implants (UNS R30035)
F 562 – 00	Wrought Cobalt-35 Nickel-20 Chromium-10 Molybdenum Alloy for Surgical Implant Applications (UNS R30035)
F 1058 – 97	Wrought Cobalt-Chromium-Nickel-Molybdenum-Iron Alloy for Surgical Implant Applications
F 2063 – 00	Wrought Nickel-Titanium Shape Memory Alloys for Medical Devices and Surgical Implants
F 1586 – 95	Wrought Nitrogen Strengthened-21 Chromium—10 Nickel—3 Manganese—2.5 Molybdenum Stainless Steel Bar for Surgical Implants
F 1314 – 95	Wrought Nitrogen Strengthened-22 Chromium-12.5 Nickel-5 Manganese-2.5 Molybdenum Stainless Steel Bar
F 1813 – $97^{\epsilon1}$	Wrought Titanium - 12 Molybdenum - 6 Zirconium - 2 Iron Alloy For Surgical Implant Applications
F 136 – $98^{\epsilon1}$	Wrought Titanium - 6Aluminum - 4Vanadium ELI (Extra Low Interstitial) Alloy (UNS R56401) for Surgical Implant Applications
F 1713 – 96	Wrought Titanium-13Niobium-13Zirconium Alloy for Surgical Implant Applications
F 2066 – 01	Wrought Titanium-15 Molybdenum Alloy for Surgical Implant Applications (UNS R58150)
F 1295 – 97a	Wrought Titanium-6 Aluminum-7 Niobium Alloy for Surgical Implant Applications
F 1472 – 00	Wrought Titanium-6Aluminum-4Vanadium Alloy (UNS R56400) for Surgical Implant Applications
§F 139 – 00	Wrought-18 Chromium-14 Nickel-2.5 Molybdenum Stainless Steel Sheet and Strip for Surgical Implants (UNS S31673)

Practices for:

F 601 – 98	Fluorescent Penetrant Inspection of Metallic Surgical Implants
F 629 – 97	Radiography of Cast Metallic Surgical Implants
§F 86 – 01	Surface Preparation and Marking of Metallic Surgical Implants

Terminology for:

F 2005 – 00	Nickel-Titanium Shape Memory Alloys

Neurosurgical Standards

Specifications for:

F 1266 – 89(1998)	Cerebral Stereotactic Instruments
F 1831 – 97	Cranial Traction Tongs and Halo External Spinal Immobilization Devices
F 982 – 86(1998)	Disclosure of Characteristics of Surgically Implanted Clamps for Carotid Occlusion
F 1719 – 96	Image-Interactive Stereotactic and Localization Systems
F 622 – 79(1998)	Preformed Cranioplasty Plates that can be Altered
*F 452 – 76(1998)	Preformed Cranioplasty Plates
F 1542 – 94(2000)	the Requirements and Disclosure of Self-Closing Aneurysm Clips

Practices for:

F 701 – 81(1998)	Care and Handling of Neurosurgical Implants and Instruments
F 647 – 94(2000)	Evaluating and Specifying Implantable Shunt Assemblies for Neurosurgical Application

Osteosynthesis

Specifications for:

F 564 – 00	Bone Staples
F 339	Cloverleaf Intramedullary Pins (Discontinued 1999†)
§F 366 – 82(2000)	Fixation Pins and Wires
F 1611 – 00	Intramedullary Reamers
F 116 – 00	Medical Screwdriver Bits
F 384 – 00	Metallic Angled Orthopedic Fracture Fixation Devices
F 382 – 99	Metallic Bone Plates
F 1839 – 97	Rigid Polyurethane Foam for Use as a Standard Material for Testing Orthopaedic Devices and Instruments
F 1350 – 01	Wrought 18 Chromium-14 Nickel-2.5 Molybdenum Stainless Steel Surgical Fixation Wire (UNS S31673)
F 1091 – 91(2000)	Wrought Cobalt-20 Chromium-15 Tungsten-10 Nickel Alloy Surgical Fixation Wire [UNS R30605]

Test Methods for:

F 1539	Consant Amplitude Bending Fatigue Tests of Metallic Bone Staples (Discontinued 2000†)
F 1691	Determining Axial Pull-Out Strength of Medical Bone Screws (Discontinued 2001†)

LIST BY SUBJECTS

F 1746	Determining In-Plane Compressive Properties of Circular Ring or Ring Segment Bridge Elements (Discontinued 1999†)
F 117	Driving Torque of Medical Bone Screws (Discontinued 2001†)
F 1660	Elastic Static Bending of Metallic Bone Staples (Discontinued 2000†)
F 1745	External Fixator Connectors (Discontinued 1999†)
F 1747	External Fixator Joints (Discontinued 1999†)
F 1748	External Fixator Subassemblies (Discontinued 1999†)
F 1541 – 01	External Skeletal Fixation Devices
F 1264 – 00	Intramedullary Fixation Devices
F 1622	Measuring the Torsional Properties of Metallic Bone Screws (Discontinued 2001†)
§F 543 – 01	Metallic Medical Bone Screws
F 1540	Pull-Out Fixation Strength of Metallic Bone Staples (Discontinued 2000†)
F 1610	Soft Tissue Fixation Strength of Metallic Bone Staples (Discontinued 2000†)

Practices for:

F 565 – 00	Care and Handling of Orthopedic Implants and Instruments
F 983 – 86(2000)	Permanent Marking of Orthopaedic Implant Components

Plastic and Reconstructive Surgery

Specifications for:

F 703 – 96	Implantable Breast Prostheses
F 2051 – 00	Implantable Saline Filled Breast Prosthesis
F 881 – 94(2000)	Silicone Elastomer Facial Implants
F 1441 – 92(1998)	Soft-Tissue Expander Devices

Polymeric Materials

Specifications for:

F 451 – 99a	Acrylic Bone Cement
F 641 – 98a	Implantable Epoxy Electronic Encapsulants
F 754 – 00	Implantable Polytetrafluoroethylene (PTFE) Polymer Fabricated in Sheet, Tube, and Rod Shapes
F 602 – 98a	Implantable Thermoset Epoxy Plastics
F 1579 – 98	Polyaryletherketone (PAEK) Resins for Surgical Implant Applications
F 997 – 98a$^{\epsilon1}$	Polycarbonate Resin for Medical Applications
F 2026 – 00	Polyetheretherketone (PEEK) Resins for Surgical Implant Applications
F 1876 – 98	Polyetherketoneetherketoneketone (PEKEKK) Resins for Surgical Implant Applications
*F 639 – 98a	Polyethylene Plastics for Medical Applications
F 1855 – 00	Polyoxymethylene (Acetal) for Medical Applications
F 702 – 98a$^{\epsilon1}$	Polysulfone Resin for Medical Applications
F 755 – 99$^{\epsilon1}$	Selection of Porous Polyethylene for Use in Surgical Implants
F 604	Silicone Elastomers Used in Medical Applications (Discontinued 2001†)
F 648 – 00	Ultra-High-Molecular-Weight Polyethylene Powder and Fabricated Form for Surgical Implants
F 1925 – 99$^{\epsilon1}$	Virgin Poly(L-Lactic Acid) Resin for Surgical Implants

Classifications:

F 665 – 98	Vinyl Chloride Plastics Used in Biomedical Application

Guides for:

F 624 – 98a$^{\epsilon1}$	Evaluation of Thermoplastic Polyurethane Solids and Solutions for Biomedical Applications
F 2038 – 00$^{\epsilon1}$	Silicone Elastomers, Gels and Foams Used in Medical Applications Part I — Formulations and Uncured Materials
F 2042 – 00$^{\epsilon1}$	Silicone Elastomers, Gels, and Foams Used in Medical Applications Part II — Crosslinking and Fabrication

Terminology for:

F 1251 – 89(1995)	Polymeric Biomaterials in Medical and Surgical Devices

Spinal Devices

Test Methods for:

F 2077 – 01	Intervertebral Body Fusion Devices
F 1717 – 96	Static and Fatigue for Spinal Implant Constructs in a Corpectomy Model

Guides for:

F 1798 – 97	Evaluating the Static and Fatigue Properties of Interconnection Mechanisms and Subassemblies Used in Spinal Arthrodesis Implants

Terminology for:

F 1582 – 98	Spinal Implants

Tissue Engineered Biomaterials

Guides for:

F 2064 – 00	Characterization and Testing of Alginates as Starting Materials Intended for Use in Biomedical and Tissue–Engineered Medical Products Application
F 2103 – 01	Characterization and Testing of Chitosan Salts as Starting Materials Intended for Use in Biomedical and Tissue-Engineered Medical Product Applications
F 2027 – 00$^{\epsilon1}$	Characterization and Testing of Substrate Materials for Tissue-Engineered Medical Products

Urological Materials and Devices

Specifications for:

§F 623 – 99	Foley Catheter
F 1828 – 97	Ureteral Stents

SEARCH AND RESCUE

Equipment, Testing, and Maintenance

Specifications for:

F 1491 – 93(1997)	An Avalanche Beacon Frequency

Guides for:

F 1764 – 97	Selection of Hardline Communication Systems for Confined-Space Rescue
F 1823 – 97	Water Rescue Personal Flotation Device (PFD)

Management and Operations

Specifications for:

F 1382 – 92(1997)	Search and Rescue Computer Software Information Exchange

Classifications:

F 1993 – 99	Human Search and Rescue Resources
F 1848 – 98	Search and Rescue Dog Crew/Teams

Practices for:

F 1583 – 95(2000)	Communications Procedures—Phonetics
F 1584 – 95	Marking Buildings During Disaster Search Operations
F 1728 – 96(2001)	Multiple Persons Cold Water Survival/Rescue Technique
F 1729 – 96(2001)	Single Person Cold Water Survival/Rescue Technique
F 1846 – 98	Symbols and Markings for Use With Land Search Maps
F 1591 – 95(2000)	Visual Signals Between Persons on the Ground and in Aircraft During Ground Emergencies
F 2047 – 00	Workers' Compensation Coverage of Emergency Services Volunteers

Guides for:

F 1847 – 98	Demonstrating Minimum Skills of Search and Rescue Dogs and Handlers
F 1879 – 98	Demonstrating Obedience and Agility in Search and Rescue Dogs
F 1767 – 98$^{\epsilon1}$	Forms Used for Search and Rescue
F 1766 – 97a	Ice Awls Self-Rescue Technique
F 1765 – 97a	Ice Staff Self-Rescue Technique
F 1633 – 97	Techniques in Land Search
F 1730 – 96	Throwing a Water Rescue Throwbag
F 2099 – 01	Use of Universal Transverse Mercator (UTM) Grids When Preparing and Using a Field Map for Land Search
F 1768 – 97	Using Whistle Signals During Rope Rescue Operations
F 1422 – 92(1999)	Using the Incident Command System Framework in Managing Civilian Search and Rescue Operations

Personnel, Training and Education

Guides for:

F 1740 – 96	Inspection of Nylon, Polyester, or Nylon/Polyester Blend, or Both Kernmantle Rope
F 1824 – 97	Performance of a Water Rescuer–Level II
F 1739 – 96	Performance of a Water Rescuer-Level I
F 1783 – 97	Performance of an Ice Rescuer—Level II

Terminology

Terminology for:

F 1490 – 96	Search and Rescue
F 1549 – 94(1999)	Underwater Search, Rescue, and Recovery Activities

Designation: F 67 – 00

Standard Specification for Unalloyed Titanium, for Surgical Implant Applications (UNS R50250, UNS R50400, UNS R50550, UNS R50700)[1,2]

This standard is issued under the fixed designation F 67; the number immediately following the designation indicates the year of original adoption or, in the case of revision, the year of last revision. A number in parentheses indicates the year of last reapproval. A superscript epsilon (ε) indicates an editorial change since the last revision or reapproval.

1. Scope

1.1 This specification covers the chemical, mechanical, and metallurgical requirements for four grades of unalloyed titanium used for the manufacture of surgical implants.

1.2 The values stated in inch-pound units are to be regarded as the standard.

2. Referenced Documents

2.1 *ASTM Standards:*

B 265 Specification for Titanium and Titanium Alloy Strip, Sheet, and Plate[3]

B 348 Specification for Titanium and Titanium Alloy Bars and Billets[3]

B 381 Specification for Titanium and Titanium Alloy Forgings[3]

E 8 Test Methods for Tension Testing of Metallic Materials[4]

E 120 Test Methods for Chemical Analysis of Titanium and Titanium Alloys[5]

E 290 Test Method for Semi-Guided Bend Test for Ductility of Metallic Materials[4]

E 527 Practice for Numbering Metals and Alloys[6]

E 1409 Test Method for Determination of Oxygen in Titanium Alloys by the Inert Gas Fusion Technique[7]

E 1447 Test Method for Determination of Hydrogen in Titanium and Titanium Alloys by the Inert Gas Fusion Thermal Conductivity Method[7]

F 981 Practice for Assessment of Compatibility of Biomaterials for Surgical Implants with Respect to Effect of Materials on Muscle and Bone[8]

F 1341 Specification for Unalloyed Titanium Wire for Surgical Implant Applications[8]

2.2 *Aerospace Material Specification:*

AMS 2249 Chemical Check Analysis Limits, Titanium and Titanium Alloys[9]

2.3 *American Society for Quality (ASQ) Standard:*

C1 Specifications of General Requirements for a Quality Program[10]

2.4 *Society of Automotive Engineers Standard:*

SAE J1086 Practice for Numbering Metals and Alloys (UNS)[9]

3. Product Classification

3.1 Product classifications are consistent with Standard Specifications B 265, B 348 and B 381.

3.1.1 *Strip*—Any product 0.1875 in. (4.75 mm) and under in thickness and less than 24 in. (610 mm) in width.

3.1.2 *Sheet*—Any product 0.1875 in. (4.75 mm) and under in thickness and 24 in. (610 mm) or more in width.

3.1.3 *Plate*—Any product 0.1875 in. (4.75 mm) in thickness and over 10 in. (254 mm) in width.

3.1.4 *Bar*—A hot rolled, forged, or cold worked semi-finished solid section product whose cross sectional area is equal to or less than 16 $in.^2$(10322 mm^2); rectangular bar must be less than or equal to 10 in. (254 mm) in width and greater than 0.1875 in. (4.75 mm) in thickness.

3.1.5 *Billet*—A solid semi-finished section hot rolled or forged from an ingot, with a cross sectional area greater than 16 in^2(10322 mm^2) whose width is less than 5 times its thickness.

3.1.6 *Forging*—Any product of work on metal formed to a desired shape by impact or pressure in hammers, forging machines, upset presses or related forming equipment.

3.1.7 *Wire*—Coiled round and non-round product with a diameter or major dimension equal to or greater than 0.3130 in.

NOTE 1—Wire less than or equal to 0.3125 in. in diameter or major dimension is covered in ASTM F 1341.

3.1.8 *Other*—Other forms and shapes, including tubing, may be provided by agreement between purchaser and supplier.

4. Ordering Information

4.1 Inquiries and orders for material under this specification

[1] This specification is under the jurisdiction of ASTM Committee F04 on Medical and Surgical Materials and Devices and is the direct responsibility of Subcommittee F04.12 on Metallurgical Materials.

Current edition approved May 10, 2000. Published August 2000. Originally published as F 67 – 66. Last previous edition F 67 – 95.

[2] New UNS designation established in accordance with E 527 and SAE J1086.

[3] *Annual Book of ASTM Standards*, Vol 02.04.

[4] *Annual Book of ASTM Standards*, Vol 03.01.

[5] *Annual Book of ASTM Standards*, Vol 03.05.

[6] *Annual Book of ASTM Standards*, Vol 1.01.

[7] *Annual Book of ASTM Standards*, Vol 3.06.

[8] *Annual Book of ASTM Standards*, Vol 13.01.

[9] Available from Society of Automotive Engineers, 400 Commonwealth Drive, Warrendale, PA 15096.

[10] Available from American Society for Quality Control, 161 W. Wisconsin Ave., Milwaukee, WI 53203.

TABLE 1 Chemical Requirements

Element	Composition[A], % (mass/mass)			
	Grade 1 UNS R50250	Grade 2 UNS R50400	Grade 3 UNS R50550	Grade 4 UNS R50700
Nitrogen, max	0.03	0.03	0.05	0.05
Carbon, max	0.08	0.08	0.08	0.08
Hydrogen, max[B]	0.015	0.015	0.015	0.015
Iron, max	0.20	0.30	0.30	0.50
Oxygen, max	0.18	0.25	0.35	0.40
Titanium	balance	balance	balance	balance

[A] Forgings are designated Grade F-1, F-2, F-3, or F-4 respectively. Forging compositions are as specified in Table 1.
[B] Maximum hydrogen content for billet is 0.0100 wt%.

shall include the following information:

4.1.1 Quantity (weight or number of pieces),

4.1.2 Grade (1, 2, 3, or 4),

4.1.3 ASTM designation,

4.1.4 Form (sheet, strip, plate, bar, billet, forging, wire or other forms),

4.1.5 Condition (5.1),

4.1.6 Mechanical properties (if applicable, for special conditions),

4.1.7 Finish (5.2),

4.1.8 Applicable dimensions and tolerances including size, thickness, width, and length (exact, random, multiples) or drawing number,

4.1.9 Special tests, and

4.1.10 Special requirements.

5. Manufacture

5.1 *Condition*—Material shall be furnished in the hot-rolled, cold-worked, forged, annealed or stress relieved condition.

5.2 *Finish*—Unalloyed titanium material shall be free of injurious external and internal imperfections of a nature that will interfere with the purpose for which it is intended. Material may be furnished as descaled, as pickled, as sand-blasted, or as ground, or combinations of these operations. The manufacturer shall be permitted to remove minor surface imperfections by spot grinding if such grinding does not reduce the dimension below the minimum permitted by the dimensional tolerance ordered.

6. Chemical Composition

6.1 The heat analysis shall conform to the requirements as to chemical composition prescribed in Table 1. Ingot analysis may be used for reporting all chemical requirements except hydrogen, samples of which shall be taken from the finished product. Supplier shall not ship material that is outside the limits specified in Table 1 for the applicable grade.

6.1.1 Requirements for the major and minor elemental constituents are listed in Table 1. Also listed are important residual elements. Analysis for elements not listed in Table 1 is not required to verify compliance with this specification.

6.2 *Product Analysis*—The product analysis is either for the purpose of verifying the composition of a heat or lot or to determine variations in the composition within the heat.

6.2.1 Acceptance or rejection of a heat or lot of material may be made by the purchaser on the basis of this product analysis.

6.2.2 Product analysis tolerances do not broaden the specified heat analysis requirements but cover variations between laboratories in the measurement of chemical content. Product analysis limits shall be as specified in Table 2

6.3 For referee purposes, Test Methods E 120, E 1409 and E 1447 shall apply.

6.3.1 Samples for chemical analysis shall be representative of the material being tested.

NOTE 2—**Precaution:** Extreme care must be taken in sampling titanium for chemical analysis because of its affinity for elements such as oxygen, nitrogen, and hydrogen. Therefore, when cutting samples for analysis, the operation should be carried out in a dust-free atmosphere, if possible. Chips should be collected from clean metal. Cutting tools should be clean and sharp. Samples for analysis should be stored in suitable containers.

7. Mechanical Requirements

7.1 Bar, billet, and forging shall conform to the mechanical property requirements prescribed in Table 3. Sheet, strip, and plate shall conform to the mechanical property requirements prescribed in Table 4. Grades may be ordered in the cold-worked condition to higher minimum tensile strength but a minimum 10 % elongation in 4*D* or 2 in. (50 mm) must be met.

7.2 For sheet and strip, the bend test specimen shall withstand being bent cold through an angle of 105° without fracture in the outside of the bent portion. The bend shall be made on a diameter equal to that shown in Table 4 for the applicable grade.

7.2.1 Supplementary bend test requirements for sheet and plate are listed in S1.

7.3 Tension testing shall be performed in accordance with Test Methods E 8. Tensile properties shall be determined using a strain rate of 0.003 to 0.007 in./in. (mm/mm)/min through the specified yield strength, and then the crosshead speed shall be increased so as to produce fracture in approximately one additional minute.

TABLE 2 Product Analysis Tolerances[A]

Element	Limit or Maximum of Specified Range %, (mass/mass)	Tolerance Under the Minimum or Over the Maximum Limit[B]
Nitrogen	up to 0.05	0.02
Carbon	0.10	0.02
Hydrogen	up to 0.015	0.0020
Iron	up to 0.25	0.10
Iron	over 0.25	0.15
Oxygen	up to 0.20	0.02
Oxygen	over 0.20	0.03

[A] Refer to AMS 2249.
[B] Under minimum limit not applicable for elements where only a maximum percentage is indicated.

TABLE 3 Mechanical Requirements: Annealed-Bar, Billet, Forging, Wire and Other Forms[A]

Grade	Tensile Strength, min		Yield Strength, 0.2 % Offset, min		Elongation in 4*D*, min, %	Reduction of Area, min, %[B]
	ksi	MPa	ksi	MPa		
1	35	240	25	170	24	30
2	50	345	40	275	20	30
3	65	450	55	380	18	30
4	80	550	70	483	15	25

[A] These properties apply to forgings having a maximum cross section area not greater than 3 in.^{2}(1935 mm ^{2}). Mechanical properties of forgings having greater cross sections shall be negotiated between the manufacturer and the purchaser.
[B]Reduction of area not required for tubing.

7.4 Any other special requirements shall be specified on the purchase order.

8. Certification

8.1 The manufacturer's certification that the material was manufactured and tested in accordance with this specification together with a report of the test results shall be furnished to the purchaser at the time of shipment.

9. Quality Program Requirements

9.1 The producer shall maintain a quality program, such as, for example, is defined in ASQ C1.

9.2 Purchaser shall be ensured of the producer's quality program conforms to the intent of ASQ C1, or other recognized program.

10. Keywords

10.1 metals (for surgical implants); orthopaedic medical devices; titanium alloys; titanium/titanium alloy; titanium/titanium alloys (for surgical implants)

TABLE 4 Mechanical Requirements: Annealed-Sheet, Strip, and Plate

Grade	Tensile Strength,[A] min		Yield Strength,[A] (0.2 % Offset)				Elongation in 2 in. or 50 mm, min,%	Bend Test[B]	
			min		max			Under 0.070 in. (1.8 mm) in Thickness	0.070 to 0.187 in. (1.8 to 4.75 mm) in Thickness
	ksi	MPa	ksi	MPa	ksi	MPa			
1	35	240	25	170	45	310	24	3*T*	4*T*
2	50	345	40	275	65	450	20	4*T*	5*T*
3	65	450	55	380	80	550	18	4*T*	5*T*
4	80	550	70	483	95	655	15	5*T*	6*T*

[A] Minimum and maximum limits apply to tests taken both longitudinal and transverse to the direction of rolling. Mechanical properties for conditions other than annealed or plate thickness over 1 in. (25 mm) may be established by agreement between the manufacturer and the purchaser.
[B] *T* equals the thickness of the bend test specimen. Bend tests are not applicable to material over 0.1875 in. (4.75 mm) in thickness.

SUPPLEMENTARY REQUIREMENTS

These requirements shall apply only when specified in the purchase order, in which event the specified tests shall be made by the manufacturer before shipment of the sheets or plates.

S1. Surface Requirements Bend Tests

S1.1 The purpose of this test is to measure the cleanliness or ductility, or both, of the metal surface.

S1.2 Two-guided or free-bend tests of sheet or plate material limited to Grades 1, 2, and 3 shall be made. Each of these bends will place opposite surfaces of the sheet or plate material in tension.

S1.3 The bends are to be made in accordance with Test Method E 290, except that the welds mentioned in these standards are not required. The bend specimen may be of less than full material thickness; however, the outer surface of the specimen must be representative of the product as supplied.

S1.4 The bend radius will be such to provide minimum elongation of the outer fibers of the bent specimen as follows:
Grade 1—20 % equivalent to 2T bend radius at 180° bend
Grade 2—20 % equivalent to 2T bend radius at 180° bend
Grade 3—16 % equivalent to 2½ T bend radius at 180° bend

S1.5 Criteria for acceptance will be the absence of any cracking or surface separations (not originating at the edge of specimen).

APPENDIXES

(Nonmandatory Information)

X1. RATIONALE

X1.1 The primary reason for this standard is to characterize composition and properties to ensure consistency in the starting material used directly or as modified by forging in the manufacture of medical devices.

X1.2 The choice of composition and mechanical properties is dependent upon the design and application of the medical device.

X1.3 Table 1 was condensed to have the same chemical requirements for flat product and bars and billet. This is consistent with current commercial practice for unalloyed titanium.

X2. BIOCOMPATIBILTY

X2.1 The unalloyed titanium compositions covered by this specification have been employed successfully in human implant applications in contact with soft tissue and bone for over a decade. Due to the well characterized level of biological response exhibited by these unalloyed titanium materials, they have been used as control materials in Practice F 981.

X2.2 No known surgical implant material has ever been shown to be completely free of adverse reactions in the human body. Long term clinical experience of the use of the materials referred to in this specification, however, has shown that an acceptable level of biological response can be expected, if the material is used in appropriate applications.

Designation: F 75 – 98

Standard Specification for Cobalt-28 Chromium-6 Molybdenum Casting Alloy and Cast Products for Surgical Implants (UNS R30075)[1]

This standard is issued under the fixed designation F 75; the number immediately following the designation indicates the year of original adoption or, in the case of revision, the year of last revision. A number in parentheses indicates the year of last reapproval. A superscript epsilon (ε) indicates an editorial change since the last revision or reapproval.

1. Scope

1.1 This specification covers the requirements for cobalt-28 chromium-6 molybdenum casting alloy in, shot, bar, or ingot form for surgical implant applications.

1.2 This specification also describes the chemical analysis requirements for investment castings produced from the alloy described in this specification. This specification is not concerned with any other specific requirements or recommendations for investment castings.

1.3 Requirements for powder produced from the alloy described in this specification are provided in Specification F 1377.

1.4 The values stated in inch-pound units are to be regarded as the standard.

2. Referenced Documents

2.1 *ASTM Standards:*

E 8 Test Methods of Tension Testing of Metallic Materials[2]

E 18 Test Methods for Rockwell Hardness and Rockwell Superficial Hardness of Metallic Materials[2]

E 354 Test Methods for Chemical Analysis of High-Temperature, Electrical, Magnetic, and Other Similar Iron, Nickel, and Cobalt Alloys[3]

F 981 Practice for Assessment of Compatibility of Biomaterials (Nonporous) for Surgical Implants with Respect to Effect of Materials in Muscle and Bone[4]

F 1377 Specification for Cobalt-28 Chromium-6 Molybdenum Powder for Coating of Orthopedic Implants (UNS-R 30075)[4]

2.2 *Aerospace Material Specification:*

AMS 2248 Chemical Check Analysis Limits, Wrought Heat, and Corrosion-Resistant Steels and Alloys[5]

AMS 2269 Chemical Check Limits, Wrought Nickel Alloys and Cobalt Alloys[5]

2.3 *American Society for Quality Standard:*

ASQ Cl General Requirements for a Quality Program[6]

3. Significance and Use

3.1 This specification characterizes the composition and properties in the starting material (for example, remelt alloy), used to investment cast cobalt-28 chromium-6 molybdenum alloy surgical implants.

4. Ordering Information

4.1 Inquiries and orders for material under this specification shall include the following information:

4.1.1 Quantity (weight),

4.1.2 ASTM designation,

4.1.3 Mechanical properties (if applicable),

4.1.4 Form (shot, bar, ingot),

4.1.5 Applicable dimensions or print number,

4.1.6 Condition,

4.1.7 Special tests, and

4.1.8 Other requirements.

5. Chemical Requirements

5.1 The heat analysis shall conform to the requirements as to chemical composition prescribed in Table 1. The product analysis tolerances shall conform to the requirements prescribed in Table 2. Product analysis tolerances do not broaden the specified heat analysis, but cover variation between laboratories in the measurement of chemical content.

5.2 Investment castings produced from alloy conforming to this specification shall also conform to the chemical requirements of Table 1.

5.3 Requirements for the major and minor elemental constituents are listed in Table 1. Also listed are important residual elements. Analysis for elements not listed in Table 1 is not required to verify compliance with this specification.

5.4 For referee purposes, Test Methods E 354 shall be used.

6. Mechanical Requirements

6.1 *Tensile Properties*:

6.1.1 Materials shall conform to the mechanical property requirements given in Table 3 when tested in accordance with Test Methods E 8.

[1] This specification is under the jurisdiction of ASTM Committee F-4 on Medical and Surgical Materials and Devices and is the direct responsibility of Subcommittee F04.12 on Metallurgical Materials.

Current edition approved Jan. 10, 1998. Published June 1998. Originally published as F 75 – 67. Last previous edition F 75 – 92.

[2] *Annual Book of ASTM Standards*, Vol 03.01.

[3] *Annual Book of ASTM Standards*, Vol 03.05.

[4] *Annual Book of ASTM Standards*, Vol 13.01.

[5] Available from Society of Automotive Engineers, 400 Commonwealth Drive, Warrendale, PA 15096.

[6] Available from American Society for Quality, 611 East Wisconsin Ave., Milwaukee, WI 53203.

TABLE 1 Chemical Requirements

Element	Composition, % min	Composition, % max
Chromium	27.0	30.00
Molybdenum	5.0	7.00
Nickel	...	1.00
Iron	...	0.75
Carbon	...	0.35
Silicon	...	1.00
Manganese	...	1.00
Tungsten	...	0.20
Phosphorous	...	0.020
Sulfur	...	0.010
Nitrogen	...	0.25
Aluminum	...	0.30
Boron	...	0.01
Cobalt	balance	balance

TABLE 2 Product Analysis Tolerances[A]

Element	Tolerance Under the Minimum Limit or Over the Maximum Limit[B]
Chromium	0.30
Molybdenum	0.15
Nickel	0.05
Iron	0.03
Carbon	0.02
Silicon	0.05
Manganese	0.03
Tungsten	0.04
Phosphorous	0.005
Sulfur	0.003
Nitrogen	0.005
Aluminum	0.02
Boron	0.002

[A]Refer to AMS Standard 2269C for Chemical Check Analysis Limits.

[B]For elements where only a maximum percentage is indicated, the "under minimum limit" is not applicable.

6.1.2 Tension specimens shall be melted and cast from the metal under casting procedures agreed upon between supplier and purchaser. The test methods shall be in accordance with the ¼-in. (6.35-mm) diameter specimen in Fig. 8 of Test Methods E 8 which may have a ground finish on the reduced section.

6.1.3 Four tension specimens shall be tested. If all results, or three of the four results, of the tension tests confrom to the requirements given in Table 3, the material is in compliance with the tensile property requirements of this standard. If two or more of the initial results do not conform to the requirements given in Table 3, an additional four tensile specimens shall be tested. For the material lot to be in compliance with the tensile property requirements of this standard, all four of the additional tensile test results must conform to the requirements given in Table 3.

TABLE 3 As-Cast Mechanical Property Requirements

Property	
Tensile strength, min, psi (MPa)	95 000 (655)
Yield strength (0.2 % offset), min, psi (MPa)	65 000 (450)
Elongation, min, %	8
Reduction of area, min, %	8

6.1.4 Tension test results for any specimen which fractures outside of the gage length shall be considered invalid and void, and a replacement shall be tested.

6.2 *Hardness*:

6.2.1 Materials conforming to this specification typically will have Rockwell C-Scale hardness of 25 to 35 HRC as in the as-cast condition. The hardness determination shall be performed in accordance with Test Methods E 18.

6.2.2 Hardness values are for guidelines only and shall not be used as a criteria for rejection.

7. Certification

7.1 A certification shall be provided by the manufacturer of the material that the material was manufactured and tested in accordance with this specification. A report of the test results shall be furnished at the time of shipment.

8. Quality Program Requirements

8.1 The producer shall maintain a quality program, for example, such as defined in ASQ C1.

9. Keywords

9.1 castings—surgical; cobalt alloys (for surgical implants); cobalt-chromium-molybdenum-metals (for surgical implants); cobalt alloys

APPENDIXES

(Nonmandatory Information)

X1. RATIONALE

X1.1 The chemical requirements in Table 1 reflect industry practice at the time of this revision. Residual element requirements are in agreement with the guidelines established by the International Organization for Standardization for surgical implant alloys.

X1.2 The mechanical properties listed in Table 3 are used to verify the capability of the alloy to produce castings of acceptable strength and ductility. For consistency of test results, it is advisable to subject test bars to the same radiographic and penetrant requirements as will be used for the castings which they represent.

X1.3 Cast microstructure and mechanical properties are dependent on cross sectional thickness. The mechanical properties measured on as-cast ¼ inch diameter test bars will not be the same as those in castings of different cross sectional thickness.

X1.4 Various heat treatments, including hot isostatic pressing, solution annealing, and sintering are used on Cobalt-28 Chromium-6 Molybdenum alloy surgical implant castings. This specification is not intended to cover the effects of such heat treatments.

X1.5 Changes made from the previous document include a change in title, addition of the UNS number, the addition of elements in Table 1; Chemical Requirements, new residual element language, new tension testing requirements, a statement that castings made from this alloy shall also conform to the chemical requirements of Table 1 and the addition of Biocompatibility language in the Appendix.

X2. BIOCOMPATIBILITY

X2.1 The alloy composition covered by this standard has been employed successfully in human implant applications in contact with soft tissue and bone for over a decade. Due to the well characterized level of biological response exhibited by this alloy, it has been used as a control material in Practice F 981.

X2.2 No known surgical implant material has ever been shown to be completely free of adverse reactions in the human body. However, long term clinical experience of the use of the material referred to in this standard has shown that an acceptable level of biological response can be expected, if the material is used in appropriate applications.

Designation: F 86 – 01

Standard Practice for
Surface Preparation and Marking of Metallic Surgical Implants[1]

This standard is issued under the fixed designation F 86; the number immediately following the designation indicates the year of original adoption or, in the case of revision, the year of last revision. A number in parentheses indicates the year of last reapproval. A superscript epsilon (ϵ) indicates an editorial change since the last revision or reapproval.

1. Scope

1.1 This practice provides a description of surface characteristics, methods of surface preparation, and methods of marking for metallic surgical implants. Marking nomenclature is not specified in this practice. Surface requirements and marking methods included in the implant specification shall take precedence over requirements listed in this practice, where appropriate.

1.2 *This standard does not purport to address all of the safety concerns, if any, associated with its use. It is the responsibility of the user of this standard to establish appropriate safety and health practices and determine the applicability of regulatory limitations prior to use.*

2. Referenced Documents

2.1 *ASTM Standards:*

A 380 Practice for Cleaning and Descaling Stainless Steel Parts, Equipment, and Systems[2]

A 967 Specification for Chemical Passivation Treatments for Stainless Steel Parts[2]

B 600 Guide for Descaling and Cleaning Titanium and Titanium Alloy Surfaces[3]

F 983 Practice for Permanent Marking of Orthopaedic Implant Components[4]

3. Significance and Use

3.1 The surface treatments documented in this specification are intended to improve the corrosion resistance of metallic surgical implants manufactured from iron, cobalt, titanium, and tantalum base materials.

3.2 Iron particles, ceramic media, and other foreign particles may become smeared over or imbedded into the surface of implants during processing operations such as forming, machining, tumbling, bead blasting, and so forth. These particles should be removed to minimize localized rust formation and superficial blemishes.

3.3 The various chemical and electrochemical surface treatments specified in this standard are intended to remove objectionable surface contaminants and to restore maximum corrosion resistance to the passive oxide film.

3.4 The need for an additional implant surface treatment such as secondary passivation in nitric acid should be evaluated for localized implant surfaces that have electrochemical or laser product markings created after the final surface treatment.

4. Description of Acceptable Surface Characteristics

4.1 Metallic implants, when inspected in accordance with this practice, shall be free of surface imperfections such as toolmarks, nicks, scratches, cracks, cavities, burrs, and other defects that would impair the serviceability of the device. The surfaces shall be cleaned to minimize the presence of foreign material.

4.2 Specific finish requirements such as texture, surface roughness, or additional surface treatments shall be included in the implant production specification.

4.3 The implants shall be given a final surface treatment according to Section 7.

5. Cleaning

5.1 The surface of the implants shall be cleaned to minimize foreign material.

5.2 The cleaning operations used shall relate to the following as appropriate:

5.2.1 A method such as organic solvent degreasing for the removal of oils, greases, and other loose surface contaminants.

NOTE 1—Anhydrous methanol and other solvents known to cause environmentally assisted cracking of titanium and its alloys should be avoided.

5.2.2 A method such as one of the following for the removal of adherent foreign material, if necessary.

5.2.2.1 Hot alkaline cleaner used as recommended.

5.2.2.2 Alkaline cleaner applied electrochemically as recommended.

NOTE 2—Avoid cathodic cleaning of metals known to be susceptible to hydrogen contamination and anodic cleaning of metals known to be susceptible to pitting. In addition, testing should be considered to confirm that acidic cleaning will not affect the mechanical properties of alloys susceptible to hydrogen contamination effects.

5.2.2.3 Ultrasonically agitated cleaning agent.

---

[1] This practice is under the jurisdiction of ASTM Committee F04 on Medical and Surgical Materials and Devices and is the direct responsibility of Subcommittee F04.12 on Metallurgical Materials.

Current edition approved Jan. 10, 2001. Published March 2001. Originally published as F 86 – 84. Last previous edition F 86 – 00.

[2] *Annual Book of ASTM Standards*, Vol. 01.03.

[3] *Annual Book of ASTM Standards*, Vol. 02.04.

[4] *Annual Book of ASTM Standards*, Vol. 13.01.

5.2.3 An acidic cleaning process may be used. For titanium, titanium alloys, and tantalum, some possible cleaning processes may be found in Practice B 600.

NOTE 3—Before an acidic cleaning, degreasing shall be considered where appropriate to make the acidic cleaning effective in a uniform manner.

5.2.3.1 If acidic cleaning methods are used, this shall be stated in the implant production specification.

5.3 A neutralizing treatment shall be carried out where appropriate.

5.4 An adequate rinsing operation shall be carried out.

5.5 An adequate drying cycle shall follow.

6. Product Marking

6.1 Markings are applied to the implant surfaces to provide traceability if the size and configuration of the implant are sufficient for such markings. To minimize potential adverse effects, it is necessary to use an appropriate marking procedure and technique and to select a suitable location for the marking of the implant.

6.1.1 Details on marking are found in Practice F 983.

6.2 Identify or label metallic implants in a manner that will minimize potential impairment of the mechanical properties or corrosion resistance and will not elicit adverse tissue response.

6.3 Locate the marking or labeling on the implant at a point of low stress in such a manner as not to intersect the edges of drilled holes, countersinks, or edges of implants. Indicate the location of the marking on the manufacturing drawing of the implant.

6.4 The marking nomenclature shall be documented.

6.5 Some methods of marking are as follows:

6.5.1 Mechanical imprinting of round-bottom and round-edge characters,

6.5.2 Chemical etching using an anodic electrolytic procedure,

6.5.3 Marking with a round rotating burr under low-contact pressure,

6.5.4 Casting of markings into the surface using round-edge and round-bottom characters,

6.5.5 Marking with vibrator-type contact,

6.5.6 Electro-pencil marking, and

6.5.7 Marking with laser beam.

6.6 Depending on the implant, its material, and the type of marking method and procedure, the marking may be applied before or after the final surface treatment. (See 7.6).

7. Final Surface Treatment

7.1 Implants shall be given a final surface treatment before they are packaged.

7.2 Final surface treatments are as follows:

7.2.1 Immerse in 20 to 45 volume % nitric acid (specific gravity 1.1197 to 1.285) at room temperature for a minimum of 30 min. For an accelerated process, a 20 to 25 % acid solution, heated at 120 to 140°F (40 to 60°C), may be used for a minimum of 20 min. (See Specification A 967 and Practice A 380).

This treatment provides passivation by surface oxidation and is able to dissolve certain foreign material that might be present from previous operations; it is therefore particularly recommended when no other treatments take place that would remove such foreign material.

7.2.2 Use a neutralizing procedure for product designs in which acidic liquid could be trapped.

7.2.3 A thorough water rinsing process and a drying process are essential.

7.3 Alternatively, for stainless steel and cobalt alloys, a final electropolishing procedure can provide passive surface conditions and cleansing from certain foreign material (see Specification A 967).

7.4 For titanium base materials, electrochemical anodizing processes can provide similar passivating and cleaning effects as the electrochemical polishing procedures have. Alternative oxidation treatments can render passive surfaces as well.

7.5 If alternative surface treatments for implants are used, these treatments should be specified in the production procedure documentation.

7.6 If marking of implants is performed after the final surface treatment, it must be evaluated whether a secondary passivation treatment is necessary or not.

8. Inspection

8.1 The surfaces of the finished implants, at least representative samples of a production lot, shall be inspected using visual examination with the unaided eye (but corrected where necessary). Other surface inspection methods may be used in addition.

9. Keywords

9.1 alkaline cleaner; cleaning; electropolishing; final inspection; marking; metal implants; passivation; surface treatment

APPENDIX

(Nonmandatory Information)

X1. RATIONALE

X1.1 The surface treatment and marking of implants can influence the following important qualities: local tissue response, bonding or lack of bonding to tissues as indicated by the application, and fatigue strength of implants.

X1.2 Local tissue response of metallic implants is affected by corrosion that, in turn, may be affected by embedded foreign particles and other factors. Foreign material on the surfaces as a result of manufacturing operations may jeopardize the compatibility even in the absence of corrosion or may affect contacting implant components. Specifications and control of surface characteristics to inhibit local undesirable tissue response are therefore required.

X1.3 The fatigue strength of implants is affected by the topography of the surfaces, residual stresses, and structure. The fatigue strength of a component may be determined experimentally. Therefore, to evaluate or test the fatigue strength of finished implants, they should have surface structures, residual stresses, surface treatments, and other characteristics that are representative of the manufacturing process by which the implant is produced.

SUMMARY OF CHANGES

(*1*) The discontinued standards (F 55, F 56, F 642, F 643, F 644, and F 666) were removed from the Referenced Documents section during the F 86-00 revision. The balance of the metallic implant material standards previously included in the Referenced Documents section have been deleted since they were not mentioned in the text and it is considered impractical to revise this document every time a new metallic implant material standard is published. Paragraph 3.1 documents that this standard is applicable for metallic surgical implants manufactured from iron, cobalt, titanium, and tantalum base materials.

(*2*) The different sections of the standard have been rearranged in a logical order, and the section on Final Surface Treatment has been slightly extended in consideration of the increased use of titanium materials.

(*3*) The passivation treatment in 7.2.1 has been adjusted to agree with the latest version of A 967.

(*4*) The information specified in 7.3 was previously changed in the F 86-00 revision to omit the nitric acid rinse required after electropolishing since it is recognized that electropolishing is a satisfactory passivation treatment.

(*5*) A Significance and Use section has been added to this standard in accordance with form and style guidelines for ASTM Practices and Guides.

(*6*) The statement "This standard has been approved for use by agencies of the Department of Defense" has been deleted.

Designation: F 90 – 97

Standard Specification for Wrought Cobalt-20 Chromium-15 Tungsten-10 Nickel Alloy for Surgical Implant Applications (UNS R30605)[1]

This standard is issued under the fixed designation F 90; the number immediately following the designation indicates the year of original adoption or, in the case of revision, the year of last revision. A number in parentheses indicates the year of last reapproval. A superscript epsilon (ϵ) indicates an editorial change since the last revision or reapproval.

1. Scope

1.1 This specification covers the requirements for wrought cobalt-20 chromium-15 tungsten-10 nickel alloy bar, wire, sheet, and strip used for the manufacture of surgical implants.

1.2 The values stated in inch-pound units are to be regarded as the standard.

2. Referenced Documents

2.1 *ASTM Standards:*

A 480/A 480M Specification for General Requirements for Flat-Rolled Stainless and Heat-Resisting Steel Plate, Sheet, and Strip[2]

A 484/A 484M Specification for General Requirements for Stainless and Heat-Resisting Bars, Billets, and Forgings[3]

A 555/A 555M Specification for General Requirements for Stainless Steel Wire and Wire Rods[2]

A 751 Test Methods, Practices, and Terminology for Chemical Analysis of Steel Products[2]

E 8 Test Method for Tension Testing of Metallic Materials[3]

E 354 Test Methods for Chemical Analysis of High-Temperature, Electrical, Magnetic, and Other Similar Iron, Nickel, and Cobalt Alloys[4]

F 981 Practice for Assessment of Compatibility of Biomaterials for Surgical Implants with Respect to Effect of Materials in Muscle and Bone[5]

F 1091 Specification for Wrought Cobalt-Chromium Alloy Surgical Fixation Wire[5]

2.2 *Aerospace Material Specification:*

AMS 2269 Chemical Check Analysis Limits, Wrought Nickel Alloys and Cobalt Alloys[5]

2.3 *American Society for Quality Control (ASQC) Standard:*

C1 Specification of General Requirements for a Quality Program[6]

3. General Requirements for Delivery

3.1 In addition to the requirements of this specification, all requirements of the current editions of Specifications A 480/A 480M, A484/A 484M, and A 555/A 555M shall apply.

3.2 In the case where a conflict exists between this specification and those listed in 2.1-2.3, this specification shall take precedence.

4. Ordering Information

4.1 Inquiries and orders for material under this specification shall include the following information:

4.1.1 Quantity (weight or number of pieces),

4.1.2 ASTM designation,

4.1.3 Form (bar, wire, sheet, strip),

4.1.4 Condition (see 6.1),

4.1.5 Finish (see 6.2),

4.1.6 Mechanical properties (if applicable, for special conditions),

4.1.7 Applicable dimensions including size, thickness, width, and length (exact, random or multiples) or print number, and

4.1.8 Other requirements.

5. Manufacture

5.1 *Condition*—Bar, wire, sheet, and strip shall be furnished to the implant manufacturer, as specified, in the annealed or cold-worked condition.

5.2 *Finish*:

5.2.1 Types of finish available for bar and wire are bright-annealed, pickled, cold-drawn, ground, ground and polished or as specified in the implant manufacturer's purchase order.

5.2.2 Types of finish available for sheet and strip are brightannealed, pickled, cold-rolled, polished or as specified in the implant manufacturer's purchase order.

6. Chemical Requirements

6.1 The heat analysis shall conform to the requirements as to chemical composition specified in Table 1.

6.1.1 Requirements for the major and minor elemental constituents are listed in Table 1. Also listed are important residual elements. Analysis for elements not listed in Table 1 is not required to certify compliance with this specification.

6.2 *Product Analysis*—Product analysis tolerances do not broaden the specified heat analysis requirements, but cover

---

[1] This specification is under the jurisdiction of ASTM Committee F-4 on Medical and Surgical Materials and Devicesand is the direct responsibility of Subcommittee F04.12 on Metallurgical Materials.

Current edition approved June 10, 1997. Published March 1998. Originally published as F 90 – 68. Last previous edition F 90 – 96.

[2] *Annual Book of ASTM Standards*, Vol 01.03.

[3] *Annual Book of ASTM Standards*, Vol 03.01.

[4] *Annual Book of ASTM Standards*, Vol 03.05.

[5] *Annual Book of ASTM Standards*, Vol 13.01.

[6] Available from American Society for Quality Control, 161 W. Wisconsin Ave., Milwaukee, WI 53203.

TABLE 1 Chemical Requirements

Element	Composition, %	
	min	max
Carbon	0.05	0.15
Manganese	1.00	2.00
Silicon	...	0.40
Phosphorus	...	0.040
Sulfur	...	0.030
Chromium	19.00	21.00
Nickel	9.00	11.00
Tungsten	14.00	16.00
Iron	...	3.00
Cobalt[A]	balance	balance

[A] Approximately equal to the difference between 100 % and the sum percentage of the other specified elements. The percentage cobalt content by difference is not required to be reported.

variations between laboratories in the measurement of chemical content. The manufacturer shall not ship material that is outside the limits specified in Table 1. Product analysis limits shall be as specified in Table 2.

6.2.1 The product analysis is either for the purpose of verifying the composition of a heat or lot or to determine variations in the composition within the heat.

TABLE 2 Product Analysis Tolerances[A]

Element	Tolerance Under the Minimum Limit or Over the Maximum Limit[B]
Carbon	0.01
Manganese	0.04
Silicon	0.03
Phosphorous	0.005
Sulfur	0.005
Chromium	0.25
Nickel	0.15 under min; 0.20 over max
Tungsten	0.25
Iron	0.07

[A] Refer to AMS 2269.
[B] Under minimum limit not applicable for elements where only a maximum percentage is indicated.

6.2.2 Acceptance or rejection of a heat or lot may be made by the purchaser on the basis of this check analysis.

6.3 For referee purposes, Test Methods E 354 shall be used.

6.4 Methods and practices relating to chemical analysis required by this specification shall be in accordance with Test Methods A 751.

7. Mechanical Requirements

7.1 The material in the annealed condition shall conform to the mechanical properties specified in Tables 3 and 4.

7.2 The level of mechanical properties for material in other than the annealed condition shall be specified in the implant manufacturer's purchase order.

7.3 Specimens for tension tests shall be machined and tested in accordance with Test Method E 8.

8. Additional Requirements

8.1 Any additional requirements shall be specified on the purchase order.

9. Certification

9.1 A certification shall be provided by the manufacturer of the material that the material was manufactured and tested in accordance with this specification. A report of the test results shall be furnished at the time of shipment.

10. Quality Program Requirements

10.1 The producer shall maintain a quality program, such as defined in ASQC C1.

10.2 The manufacturer of surgical implants may audit the producer's quality program for conformance to the intent of ASQC C1, or other recognized programs.

11. Keywords

11.1 cobalt alloys (for surgical implants); cobalt chromium; L-605 alloy; metals (for surgical implants)—cobalt alloys

TABLE 3 Mechanical Requirements, Bar and Wire[A]

Condition	Ultimate Tensile Strength, min. psi (MPa)	Yield Strength (0.2 % Offset), min., psi (MPa)	Elongation[B] in 4D or 4W, min, %
Annealed	125 000 (860)	45 000 (310)	30

[A] Annealed wire less than 0.063 in. (160 mm) diameter is covered in Specification F 1091.
[B] 4D = 4 × diameter; 4W = 4 × width.

TABLE 4 Mechanical Requirements, Sheet and Strip

Condition	Thickness, in. (mm)	Ultimate Tensile Strength, min, psi (MPa)	Yield Strength (0.2 % Offset), min, psi (MPa)	Elongation in 2 in. (50 mm), min, %
Annealed	0.010 to 0.020 (0.254 to 0.508), incl	130 000 (896)	55 000 (379)	30
	over 0.020 to 0.032 (0.508 to 0.813), incl	130 000 (896)	55 000 (379)	35
	over 0.032 to 0.043 (0.813 to 1.09), incl	130 000 (896)	55 000 (379)	40
	over 0.043 to 0.187 (1.09 to 4.75), incl	130 000 (896)	55 000 (379)	45

APPENDIXES

(Nonmandatory Information)

X1. RATIONALE

X1.1 The primary reason for this specification is to characterize composition and properties to assure consistency in the starting material used, directly or as modified by forging, casting, or shape forming, in the manufacturing of medical devices.

X1.2 This cobalt-chromium-tungsten-nickel containing alloy has the requisite mechanical and corrosion resistance properties considered necessary for certain implant applications.

X1.3 The maximum silicon content has been lowered from the value stated in Specification F 90–76, a minimum manganese limit has been included, and maximum sulfur and phosphorus limits have been specified to meet the most recent composition requirements for this alloy.

X1.4 The minimum elongation for bar and wire in the annealed condition has been increased from 10 in Specification F 90–76 to 30 % and is considered a practical limit based on manufacturing experience and published statistical data that is presently available.

X1.5 The minimum mechanical properties for sheet and strip supplied in the annealed condition are generally recognized as commercially attainable for the thickness range cited in this specification.

X1.6 Specifications A 480/A 480M, A 484/A 484M, and A 555/A 555M have been included as applicable documents to cover the general delivery requirements for Specification F 90 bar, wire, sheet, and strip manufactured for surgical implant applications. Dimensional tolerance, requirements previously specified in Paragraph 5 are covered by Specifications A 480/A 480M, A 484/A 484M, and A 555/A 555M.

X1.7 The UNS designation has been added, residual element language has been included, product analysis tolerance information has been expanded, Specification F 1091 has been included as a referenced document that replaces Specifications F 643 and F 644, and Appendix X2 Biocompatibility section has been added to the Rationale, and E 8 tension testing method has been documented.

X2. BIOCOMPATIBILITY

X2.1 The material composition covered by this standard has been employed successfully in human implant applications in contact with soft tissue and bone for over a decade. Due to the well characterized level of local biological response established by this material, it has been used as a control material in Practice F 981.

X2.2 No known surgical implant material has ever been shown to be completely free of adverse reactions in the human body. However, long term clinical experience has shown an acceptable level of biological response can be expected, if the material is used in appropriate applications.

Designation: F 116 – 00

Standard Specification for Medical Screwdriver Bits[1]

This standard is issued under the fixed designation F 116; the number immediately following the designation indicates the year of original adoption or, in the case of revision, the year of last revision. A number in parentheses indicates the year of last reapproval. A superscript epsilon (ε) indicates an editorial change since the last revision or reapproval.

1. Scope

1.1 This specification covers the acceptable dimensions and tolerances for bits of screwdrivers to insert and remove metal screws used as surgical implants.

1.2 This specification is based, in part, upon ISO 8319-1 and ISO 8319-2.

1.3 The screwdrivers with the bits described in this standard are suitable for use with screws described in F 543, ISO 5835, and ISO 9268.

1.4 *This standard does not purport to address all of the safety concerns, if any, associated with its use. It is the responsibility of the user of this standard to establish appropriate safety and health practices and determine the applicability of regulatory limitations prior to use.*

2. Referenced Documents

2.1 *ASTM Standards:*

E 18 Standard Test Methods for Rockwell Hardness and Rockwell Superficial Hardness of Metallic Materials[2]

F 90 Standard Specification for Wrought Cobalt-Chromium-Tungsten-Nickel Alloy for Surgical Implant Applications[3]

F 543 Standard Specification and Test Methods for Metallic Medical Bone Screws[3]

F 565 Standard Practice for Care and Handling of Orthopaedic Implants and Instruments[3]

F 899 Standard Specification for Stainless Steel Billet, Bar, and Wire for Surgical Instruments[3]

F 1744 Standard Practice for Care and Handling of Stainless Steel Surgical Instruments[3]

2.2 *ISO Standards:*

5832-5 Implants for Surgery—Metallic Materials—Part 5: Wrought Cobalt-Chromium-Tungsten-Nickel Alloy[4]

5835 Implants for Surgery—Metal Bone Screws with Hexagonal Driver Connection, Spherical Under Surface of Head, Asymmetrical Thread—Dimensions[4]

7153-1 Surgical Instruments—Metallic Materials—Part 1: Stainless Steel[4]

8319-1 Orthopaedic Instruments—Drive Connections—Part 1: Keys for Use with Screws with Hexagon Socket Heads[4]

8319-2 Orthopaedic Instruments—Drive Connections—Part 2: Screwdrivers for Single Slot Head Screws, screws with Cruciate Slot, and Cross-Recessed Head Screws[4]

9268 Implants for Surgery—Metal Bone Screws with Conical Under-Surface of Head—Dimensions[4]

3. Classification

3.1 This specification includes the following types of bits for medical screwdrivers:

3.1.1 *Type I*—Single-slot bit.

3.1.2 *Type II*—Cruciate-slot bit.

3.1.3 *Type III*—Cross-slot (Modified Phillips) bit.

3.1.4 *Type IV*—Hexagonal bit.

3.1.5 *Type V*—Square bit.

3.1.6 *Type VI*—Hexalobe bit.

4. Dimensions and Tolerances

4.1 Screwdriver bits conforming to this specification shall be fabricated in accordance with the dimensions and tolerances described below:

4.1.1 *Type I*—Single-slot screwdriver bits must conform to the dimensions and tolerances provided in Table 1, and described in Fig. 1.

4.1.2 *Type II*—Cruciate-slot screwdriver bits must conform to the dimensions and tolerances provided in Table 2, and described in Fig. 2.

4.1.3 *Type III*—Cross-slot (Modified Phillips) screwdriver bits must conform to the dimensions and tolerances provided in Fig. 3.

4.1.4 *Type IV*—Hexagonal screwdriver bits must conform to the dimensions and tolerances provided in Table 3, and described in Fig. 4.

4.1.5 *Type V*—Square screwdriver bits must conform to the dimensions provided in Table 4, and described in Fig. 5.

4.1.6 *Type VI*—Hexalobe screwdriver bits must conform to the dimensions provided in Table 5, and described in Fig. 6.

5. Material Requirements

5.1 The bit and shaft portion of the screwdriver should be

---

[1] This specification is under the jurisdiction of ASTM Committee F04 on Medical and Surgical Materials and Devices and is the direct responsibility of Subcommittee F04.21on Osteosynthesis.

Current edition approved Nov. 10, 2000. Published January 2001. Originally published as F 116 – 69. Last previous edition F 116 – 98.

[2] *Annual Book of ASTM Standards,* Vol 03.01.

[3] *Annual Book of ASTM Standards,* Vol 13.01.

[4] Available from American National Standards Institute, 11 W. 42nd St., 13th Floor, New York, NY 10036.

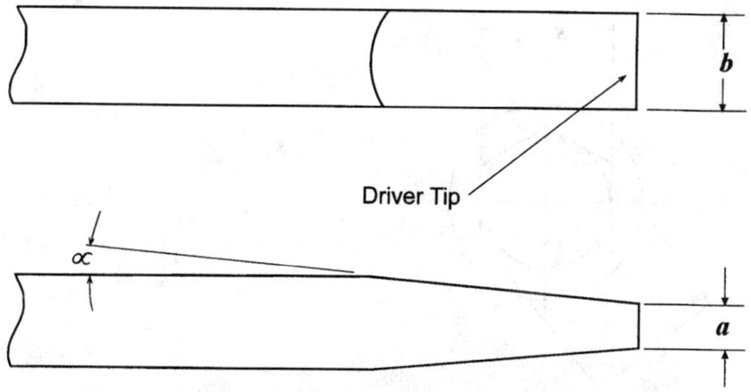

FIG. 1 Dimensions of Single-Slot Screwdriver Bit

TABLE 1 Dimensions and Tolerances of Single-Slot Screwdriver Bit

Slot Thickness, *a* (mm)		Slot Width, *b* (mm; maximum)	Slot Angle, α (degrees)	
1.10	+ 0.03 −0.07	4.8	5.0	+ 30′ − 30′
1.10	+ 0.03 −0.07	5.6	5.0	+ 30′ − 30′

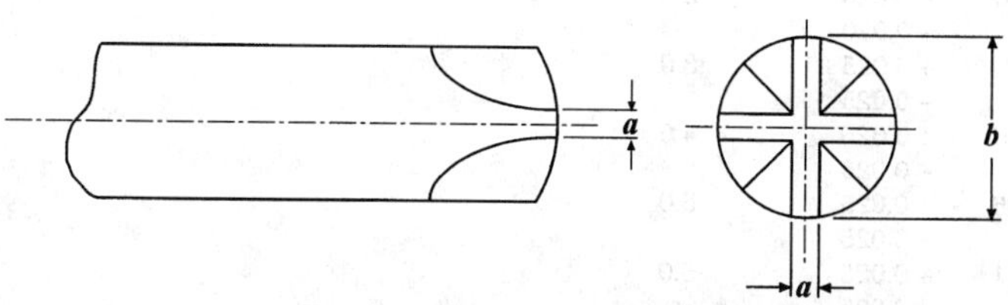

FIG. 2 Dimensions of Cruciate-Slot Screwdriver Bit

TABLE 2 Dimensions and Tolerances of Cruciate-Slot Screwdriver Bit

Slot Thickness, *a* (mm)		Slot Width, *b* (mm; maximum)
1.10	+ 0.03 − 0.07	4.8
1.10	+ 0.03 − 0.07	5.6

fabricated from one of the following materials:

5.1.1 Martensitic stainless steel (F 899 or ISO 7153-1).

5.1.2 Cold worked Cobalt-Chromium-Tungsten-Nickel alloy (F 90 or ISO 5832-5).

5.2 The hardness of the material of the bit and shaft portion shall be 45–55 (stainless steel) or 45–50 (Cobalt-Chromium-Tungsten-Nickel alloy) when measured on the Rockwell C scale according to the procedures described in E 18.

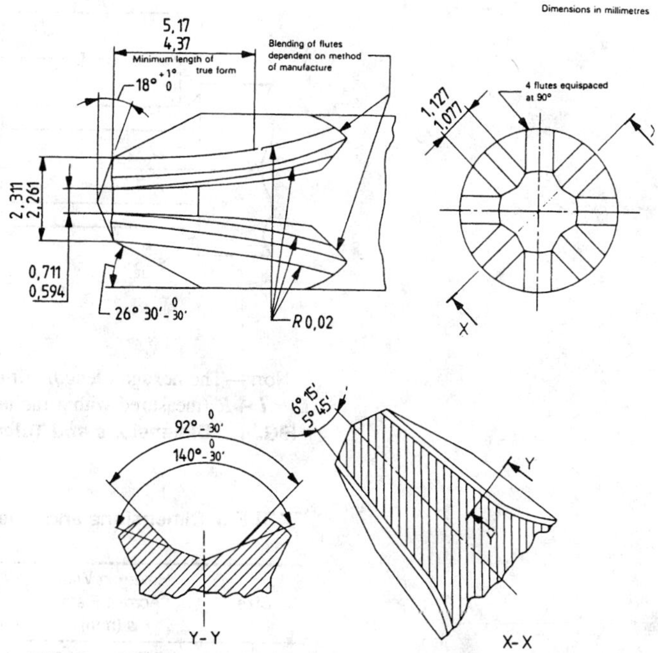

FIG. 3 Dimensions and Tolerances of Cross-Slot (Modified Phillips) Screwdriver Bit

5.3 The shaft shall be firmly fixed to a handle of appropriate material.

6. Finish and Marking

6.1 The bit portion of the screwdriver shall be free of nicks, dents, and scratches.

6.2 When size permits, the following information should be legibly marked on the shaft or handle of the screwdriver (in order of preference):

6.2.1 Manufacturer's name or logo

6.2.2 Size (for Type IV through VI screwdriver bits)

6.2.3 Catalog number

6.2.4 Manufacturing lot number

6.2.5 Material (include ASTM designation, as appropriate).

6.3 The marking should be such that the mechanical integrity of the screwdriver is not compromised.

7. Care and Handling

7.1 Screwdrivers should be handled in accordance with F 565 and F 1744, as appropriate.

8. Keywords

8.1 bone screw; orthopaedic medical devices; screwdriver; surgical instruments

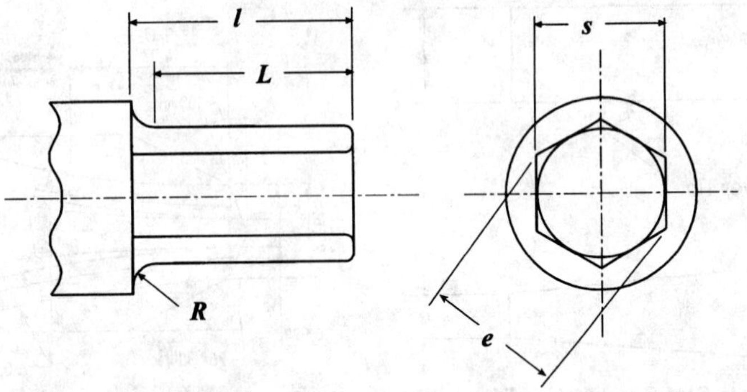

NOTE—The hexagon length (*L*) may be calculated from the following: $L \approx l - R$ (measured with a radius gage).

FIG. 4 Dimensions and Tolerances of Hexagonal Screwdriver Bit

TABLE 3 Dimensions and Tolerances of Hexagonal Screwdriver Bit

Size	Hexagon Width Across Flats, *s* (mm)		Hexagon Width Across Corners, *e* (mm)		Hexagon Length, *L* (mm; minimum)
1.5	1.500	+ 0.000 − 0.025	1.670	+ 0.020 − 0.020	2.0
2.5	2.500	+ 0.000 − 0.030	2.820	+ 0.025 − 0.025	3.0
3.5	3.500	+ 0.000 − 0.030	3.956	+ 0.025 − 0.025	4.0
4.5	4.500	+ 0.000 − 0.030	5.106	+ 0.025 − 0.025	5.0
5/32	3.950	+ 0.000 − 0.050	4.471	+ 0.025 − 0.025	5.0
3/16	4.735	+ 0.000 − 0.050	5.373	+ 0.025 − 0.025	6.0

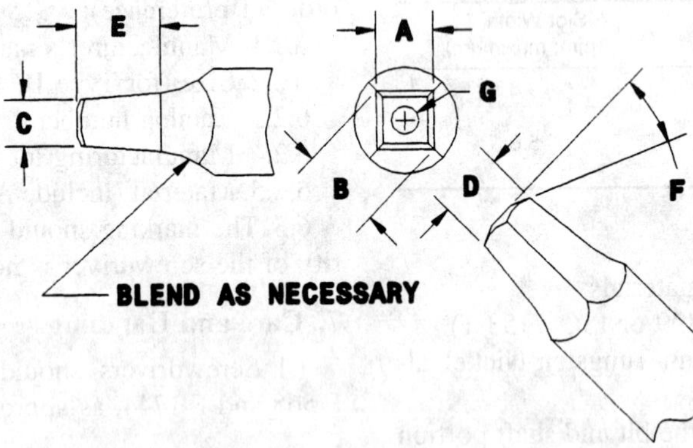

FIG. 5 Dimensions of Square Screwdriver Bits

TABLE 4 Dimensions of Square Screwdriver Bits

Screwdriver Bit Size	Width Across Flats at Radius, A (mm)	Width Across Corners at Radius, B (mm)	Width Across Flats at Chamfer, C (mm)	Width Across Corners at Chamfer, D (mm)	Length, E (mm)	Chamfer Angle, F (°)	Chamfer Diameter, G (mm)
1.0	0.84	1.19	0.67	0.95	1.25	24	0.40
1.5	1.16	1.64	0.96	1.38	1.57	28	0.48
2.0	2.03	2.87	1.20	1.70	2.69	26.5	0.76

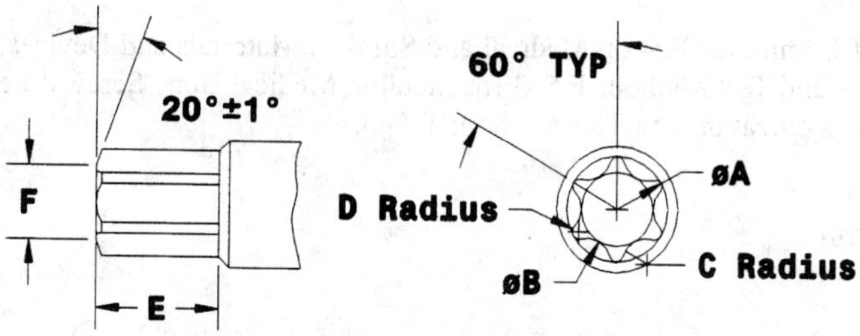

FIG. 6 Dimensions of Hexalobe Screwdriver Bits

TABLE 5 Dimensions of Hexalobe Screwdriver Bits

Screwdriver Bit Size	Major Diameter A (mm)	Minor Diameter B (mm)	Internal Radius C (mm)	External Radius D (mm)	Length E (mm)	Chamfer Diameter F (mm)
4	1.27	0.89	0.31	0.08	1.52	A
5	1.40	1.00	0.34	0.10	1.52	A
6	1.68	1.19	0.39	0.12	1.52	A
8	2.27	1.60	0.55	0.15	1.78	A
10	2.69	1.91	0.62	0.20	2.03	A
15	3.23	2.29	0.74	0.24	2.16	A
20	3.81	2.71	0.87	0.28	2.29	2.96
25	4.36	3.07	0.96	0.34	2.54	3.33
30	5.45	3.86	1.22	0.42	3.18	4.11

[A] Chamfer not necessary.

APPENDIX

(Nonmandatory Information)

X1. RATIONALE

X1.1 This standard provides dimensions and tolerances for screwdrivers used to insert and remove medical bone screws. It is intended to provide assurances to the surgical staff that the specified screwdriver will fit and perform acceptably when used with the bone screws specified in Specification F 543, ISO 5835, and ISO 9268.

The American Society for Testing and Materials takes no position respecting the validity of any patent rights asserted in connection with any item mentioned in this standard. Users of this standard are expressly advised that determination of the validity of any such patent rights, and the risk of infringement of such rights, are entirely their own responsibility.

This standard is subject to revision at any time by the responsible technical committee and must be reviewed every five years and if not revised, either reapproved or withdrawn. Your comments are invited either for revision of this standard or for additional standards and should be addressed to ASTM Headquarters. Your comments will receive careful consideration at a meeting of the responsible technical committee, which you may attend. If you feel that your comments have not received a fair hearing you should make your views known to the ASTM Committee on Standards, at the address shown below.

Last ASTM Designation: F 117 – 95 (Reapproved 1999)$^{\epsilon 1}$

Standard Test Method for Driving Torque of Medical Bone Screws

This test method establishes the recommended type of test fixtures and specimen for determining the standardized insertion torque of medical bone screws.

Formerly under the jurisdiction of Committee F04 on Medical and Surgical Materials and Devices, this test method was discontinued in 2001 and replaced by Specification and Test Methods F 543 for Metallic Medical Bone Screws[1] because the complete content of Test Method F 117 is now contained in Specification and Test Methods F 543.

[1] *Annual Book of ASTM Standards*, Vol 13.01.

Designation: F 136 – 98[ε1]

Standard Specification for Wrought Titanium - 6Aluminum - 4Vanadium ELI (Extra Low Interstitial) Alloy (UNS R56401) for Surgical Implant Applications[1]

This standard is issued under the fixed designation F 136; the number immediately following the designation indicates the year of original adoption or, in the case of revision, the year of last revision. A number in parentheses indicates the year of last reapproval. A superscript epsilon (ε) indicates an editorial change since the last revision or reapproval.

ε[1] NOTE—Editorial change was made to Table 3 in October 1999.

1. Scope

1.1 This specification covers the chemical, mechanical, and metallurgical requirements for wrought annealed titanium – 6aluminum - 4vanadium ELI (extra low interstitial) alloy (R56401) to be used in the manufacture of surgical implants.

1.2 The values stated in inch-pound units are to be regarded as the standard. The metric equivalents in parentheses are provided for information only.

1.3 *This standard does not purport to address all of the safety problems, if any, associated with its use. It is the responsibility of the user of this standard to establish appropriate safety and health practices and determine the applicability of regulatory limitations prior to use.*

2. Referenced Documents

2.1 *ASTM Standards:*

E 8 Test Methods of Tension Testing of Metallic Materials[2]

E 120 Test Methods for Chemical Analysis of Titanium and Titanium Alloys[3]

E 290 Test Method for Semi-Guided Bend Test for Ductility of Metallic Materials[2]

E 527 Practice for Numbering Metals and Alloys (UNS)[4]

E 1409 Test Methods for Determination of Oxygen in Titanium and Titanium Alloys by the Inert Gas Fusion Technique[3]

E 1447 Test Method for Determination of Hydrogen in Titanium and Titanium Alloys by the Inert Gas Fusion Thermal Conductivity Method[5]

F 981 Practice for Assessment of Compatibility of Biomaterials for Surgical Implants with Respect to Effect of Materials on Muscle and Bone.[6]

2.2 *ASQ Standard:*

C1 Specifications of General Requirements for a Quality Control Program[7]

2.3 *Aerospace Material Specifications:*[8]

AMS 2249 Chemical Check Analysis Limits, Titanium and Titanium Alloys

AMS 4930 Titanium Alloy Bars, Forgings, and Rings 6AL-4V Extra Low Interstitial Annealed

2.4 *Society of Automotive Engineers Standard:*

SAE J1086 Practice for Numbering Metals and Alloys (UNS)[9]

3. Product Classification

3.1 *Strip*—Any product under 0.1875 in. (4.75 mm) in thickness and under 24 in. (610 mm) wide.

3.2 *Sheet*—Any product under 0.1875 in. (4.75 mm) in thickness and 24 in. (610 mm) or more in width.

3.3 *Plate*—Any product 0.1875 in. (4.75 mm) thick and over and 10 in. (254 mm) wide and over, with widths greater than five times thickness. Plate up to 4.00 in. (101.60 mm), thick inclusive is covered by this specification.

3.4 *Bar*—Round bars and flats from 0.1875 in. (4.75 mm) to 4.00 in. (101.60 mm) in diameter or thickness (other sizes and shapes by special order).

3.5 *Forging bar*—Bar as described in 3.4, used for production of forgings, may be furnished in the hot rolled condition.

3.6 *Wire*—Rounds less than 0.1875 in. (4.75 mm) in diameter.

4. Ordering Information

4.1 Inquiries and orders for material under this specification shall include the following information:

4.1.1 Quantity (weight or number of pieces),

4.1.2 Applicable ASTM designation,

4.1.3 Form (sheet, strip, plate, wire, bar, or forging),

4.1.4 Condition (See 5.1),

---

[1] This specification is under the jurisdiction of ASTM Committee F-4 on Medical and Surgical Materials and Devices and is the direct responsibility of Subcommittee F04.12 on Metallurgical Materials.

Current edition approved April 10, 1998. Published September 1998. Originally published as F 136 – 84. Last previous edition F 136 – 96[ε1].

[2] *Annual Book of ASTM Standards*, Vol 03.01.

[3] *Annual Book of ASTM Standards*, Vol 03.05.

[4] *Annual Book of ASTM Standards*, Vol 01.01.

[5] *Annual Book of ASTM Standards*, Vol 03.06.

[6] *Annual Book of ASTM Standards*, Vol 13.01.

[7] Available from American Society for Quality, 161 W. Wisconsin Ave., Milwaukee, WI 53203.

[8] Available from SAE, 400 Commonwealth Drive, Warrendale, PA 15096.

[9] New designation established in accordance with E527 and SAE J1086.

4.1.5 Mechanical properties (if applicable, for special conditions),

4.1.6 Finish (See 5.2),

4.1.7 Applicable dimensions including size, thickness, width, or print number,

4.1.8 Special tests, and

4.1.9 Special requirements.

5. Materials and Manufacture

5.1 The various titanium mill products covered in this specification are normally formed with the conventional forging and rolling equipment found in primary ferrous and nonferrous plants. The ingot metal for such mill operations is usually melted in arc furnaces of a type conventionally used for reactive metals.

5.2 *Finish*—Annealed material may be furnished to the implant manufacturer as descaled or pickled, sandblasted, machined, ground, or combinations of these operations.

6. Chemical Requirements

6.1 The heat analysis shall conform to the chemical composition of Table 1. Ingot analysis may be used for reporting all chemical requirements, except hydrogen. Samples for hydrogen shall be taken from the finished mill product.

6.1.1 Requirements for the major and minor elemental constituents are listed in Table 1. Also listed are important residual elements. Analysis for elements not listed in Table 1 is not required to verify compliance with this specification.

6.2 Product analysis tolerances do not broaden the specified heat analysis requirements but cover variation between laboratories in the measurement of chemical content. The manufacturer shall not ship material that is outside the limits specified in Table 1. Product analysis limits shall be as specified in Table 2.

6.3 For referee purposes, Methods E 120, E 1409, and E 1447 shall be used.

6.4 Samples for chemical analysis shall be representative of the material being tested. The utmost care must be used in sampling titanium for chemical analysis because of its affinity for elements such as oxygen, nitrogen, and hydrogen. Therefore, in cutting samples for analysis, the operation should be carried out insofar as possible in a dust-free atmosphere. Chips should be clean and sharp. Samples for analysis should be stored in suitable containers.

7. Mechanical Requirements

7.1 Material supplied under this specification shall conform to the mechanical property requirements given in Table 3.

TABLE 1 Chemical Requirements

Element	Composition, %
Nitrogen, max	0.05
Carbon, max	0.08
Hydrogen, max	0.012[A]
Iron, max	0.25
Oxygen, max	0.13
Aluminum	5.5–6.50
Vanadium	3.5–4.5
Titanium[B]	balance

[A]Material 0.032 in. (0.813 mm) and under may have hydrogen content up to 0.0150 %.

[B]The percentage of titanium is determined by difference and need not be determined or certified.

TABLE 2 Product Analysis Tolerance[A]

Element	Tolerance Under the Minimum or Over the Maximum Limit (Composition %)[B]
Nitrogen	0.02
Carbon	0.02
Hydrogen	0.0020
Iron	0.10
Oxygen	0.02
Aluminum	0.40
Vanadium	0.15

[A] Refer to AMS 2249.

[B] Under minimum limit not applicable for elements where only a minimum percentage is indicated.

7.2 Specimens for tension tests shall be machined and tested in accordance with Test Methods E 8. Tensile properties shall be determined using a strain rate of 0.003 to 0.007 in./in. min (metric equivalent mm/mm/min) through the specified yield strength, and then the crosshead speed shall be increased so as to produce fracture in approximately one additional minute.

7.3 For sheet and strip, the bend test specimen shall withstand being bent cold through an angle of 105° without fracture in the outside surface of the bent portion. The bend shall be made on a diameter equal to that shown in Table 3. Test conditions shall conform to Test Method E 290.

8. Special Requirements

8.1 The microstructure shall be a fine dispersion of the alpha and beta phases resulting from processing in the alpha plus beta field. There shall be no continuous alpha network at prior beta grain boundaries. There shall be no coarse, elongated alpha platelets.

8.2 The beta transus temperature for each heat shall be measured by a suitable method and reported on the materials certification.

8.3 Products supplied with a machined or ground surface finish shall have no alpha case. For other products, there shall be no continuous layer of alpha case when examined at 100×.

9. Quality Program Requirements

9.1 The producer shall maintain a quality program, such as, for example, is defined in Specifications C 1.

9.2 The manufacturer of surgical implants or medical applicances shall be assured of and may audit the producer's quality program for conformance to the intent of Specifications C 1, or other recognized program.

10. Certification

10.1 A certification shall be provided by the manufacturer of the material that the material was manufactured and tested in accordance with this specification. A report of test results shall be furnished at the time of shipment.

11. Keywords

11.1 metals (for surgical implants); orthopaedic medical devices; titanium alloys; titanium/titanium alloy; titanium/titanium alloys (for surgical implants)

TABLE 3 Annealed Mechanical Properties[A]

Size in. (mm)	Tensile Strength min, psi (MPa)	Yield Strength (0.2 % offset) min, psi (MPa)	Elongation[B] in 4D or 4W min,%			Reduction of Area[C] min, %		
			L	LT	ST	L	LT	ST
Under 0.187 (4.75) thickness or diameter	125 000 (860)	115 000 (795)	10	...	...	...	...	...
0.187 (4.75) to under 1.75 (44.45), incl	125 000 (860)	115 000 (795)	10	...	...	25	...	...
1.75 (44.45) to under 2.50 (63.50), incl	120 000 (825)	110 000 (760)	8	8	...	20	15	...
2.50 (63.50) to 4.00 (101.60), incl	120 000 (825)	110 000 (760)	8	8	8	15	15	15
	Bend Test[D]							
Under 0.070 (1.778) in thickness	9 T							
0.070 (1.778) to 0.187 (4.75), incl	10 T							

[A]Mechanical properties for conditions other than those listed in this table may be established by agreement between the supplier and the implant manufacturer.
[B]Elongation of material 0.062 in. (1.575 mm) or greater in diameter or thickness shall be measured using a gage length of 2 in. or 4 D or 4 W. The gage length must be reported with the test results. Elongation of material under 0.062 in. (1.575 mm) in diameter or thickness may be obtained by negotiation. L = longitudinal; LT = long transverse; ST = short transverse.
[C]Applies to bar, plate, and forgings only. L = longitudinal; LT = long transverse; ST = short transverse. For round bar the long and short transverse are identical tests, therefore only one transverse is required.
[D]Bend test applicable to sheet and strip products; T = thickness of bend specimen in reference to diameter of bend.

APPENDIXES

(Nonmandatory Information)

X1. RATIONALE

X1.1 The purpose of this specification is to characterize the chemical, physical, mechanical, and metallurgical properties of wrought annealed titanium — 6aluminum — 4vanadium alloy to be used in the manufacture of surgical implants.

X1.2 The microstructural requirements contained in this standard represent the current general consensus of opinion with respect to optimization of mechanical properties for implant applications.

X1.3 The minimum mechanical properties specified assure a baseline of strength and ductility for the highly stressed devices for which this alloy is typically used.

X1.4 The applicable thickness range for bar and plate has been increased to 4.00 in. (101.60 mm) in accordance with AMS 4930.

X1.5 Rectangular bar and shapes, UNS designation, residual element, biocompatibility, and new alpha case requirements have been added. Size information in Table 3 has been revised.

X2. BIOCOMPATIBILITY

X2.1 The alloy composition covered by this specification has been employed successfully in human implant applications in contact with soft tissue and bone for over a decade. Due to the well characterized level of biological response exhibited by this alloy, it has been used as a control material in Practice F 981.

X2.2 No known surgical implant material has ever been shown to be completely free of adverse reactions in the human body. Longterm clinical experience of the use of the material referred to in this specification, however, has shown that an acceptable level of biological response can be expected, if the material is used in appropriate applications.

Designation: F 138 – 00

Standard Specification for Wrought 18 Chromium-14 Nickel-2.5 Molybdenum Stainless Steel Bar and Wire for Surgical Implants (UNS S31673)[1]

This standard is issued under the fixed designation F 138; the number immediately following the designation indicates the year of original adoption or, in the case of revision, the year of last revision. A number in parentheses indicates the year of last reapproval. A superscript epsilon (ϵ) indicates an editorial change since the last revision or reapproval.

This standard has been approved for use by agencies of the Department of Defense.

1. Scope

1.1 This specification covers the requirements for wrought 18 chromium-14 nickel-2.5 molybdenum stainless steel bar and wire used for the manufacture of surgical implants.

1.2 The values stated in inch-pound units are to be regarded as the standard. The SI units given in parentheses are for information only.

2. Referenced Documents

2.1 *ASTM Standards:*

A 262 Practices for Detecting Susceptibility to Intergranular Attack in Austenitic Stainless Steels[2]

A 484/A 484M Specification for General Requirements for Stainless Steel Bars, Billets, and Forgings[2]

A 555/A 555M Specification for General Requirements for Stainless Steel Wire and Wire Rods[2]

A 751 Test Methods, Practices, and Terminology for Chemical Analysis of Steel Products[2]

E 8/E 8M Test Methods for Tension Testing of Metallic Materials[3]

E 45 Test Methods for Determining the Inclusion Content of Steel[3]

E 112 Test Methods for Determining Average Grain Size[3]

F 981 Practice for Assessment of Compatibility of Biomaterials for Surgical Implants with Respect to Effect of Materials in Muscle and Bone[4]

F 1350 Specification for Stainless Steel Surgical Fixation Wire[4]

2.2 *ISO Standards:*

ISO 5832–1 Implants for Surgery—Metallic Materials—Part 1:Wrought Stainless Steel[5]

ISO 6892 Metallic Materials—Tensile Testing[5]

2.3 *ASQ Standard:*

C1 Specification of General Requirements for a Quality Program[6]

3. General Requirements for Delivery

3.1 In addition to the requirements of this specification, all requirements of the current editions of Specifications A 484/A 484M and A 555/A 555M shall apply.

3.2 In the case where a conflict exists between this specification and those listed in 2.1 and 2.2, this specification shall take precedence.

4. Ordering Information

4.1 Inquiries and orders for material under this specification shall include the following information:

4.1.1 Quantity (weight or number of pieces),

4.1.2 ASTM designation,

4.1.3 Form (bar, wire, fine wire),

4.1.4 Condition (see 5.1),

4.1.5 Mechanical properties (if applicable, for special conditions),

4.1.6 Finish (see 5.2),

4.1.7 Applicable dimensions including size, thickness, width, and length (exact, random or multiples) or print number, and

4.1.8 Special requirements.

5. Materials and Manufacture

5.1 *Condition*:

5.1.1 Bar and wire shall be furnished, as specified, in the hot-worked, annealed, cold -worked, or extra hard condition (see Table 1).

5.1.2 Fine wire shall be furnished, as specified, in the cold-drawn condition (see Table 2).

5.2 *Finish*:

5.2.1 Types of finish available for bar and wire products are cold-drawn, pickled, ground, ground and polished, or as specified in the purchase order.

5.2.2 Types of finish available for fine wire products are cold-drawn, ground, ground and polished, or as specified in the purchase order.

---

[1] This specification is under the jurisdiction of ASTM Committee F-14 on Medical and Surgical Materials and Devices and is the direct responsibility of Subcommittee F04.12 on Metallurgical Materials.

Current edition approved June 10, 2000. Published September 2000. Originally published as F 138 – 71. Last previous edition F 138 – 97.

[2] *Annual Book of ASTM Standards*, Vol 01.03.

[3] *Annual Book of ASTM Standards*, Vol 03.01.

[4] *Annual Book of ASTM Standards*, Vol 13.01.

[5] Available from American National Standards Institutite, 1430 Broadway, New York, NY 10018.

[6] Available from American Society for Quality Control, 161 W. Wisconsin Ave., Milwaukee, WI 53203.

TABLE 1 Mechanical Requirements, Wire and Bar

Condition	Diameter or Thickness, in. (mm)	Ultimate Tensile Strength, min, psi (MPa)	Yield Strength (0.2 % offset), min, psi (MPa)	Elongation[A] in 4D or 4W, min, %	Brinell[B] Hardness, max, HB
Hot-worked[C]	all	......	......	......	250
Annealed	0.063 and over (1.60)	71 000 (490)	27 500 (190)	40	...
Cold-worked	0.063 to 1.500 (1.60 to 38.1)	125 000 (860)	100 000 (690)	12	...
Extra-hard	0.063 to 0.250 (1.60 to 6.35)	196 000 (1350)	...	...	...

[A] 4D = 4 × diameter; 4W = 4 × width. Alternatively, a gage length corresponding to ISO 6892 may be used when agreed upon between supplier and purchaser.
[B] 29-kN (3000-kgf) load.
[C] Typically supplied as hot-rolled bar for forging applications.

TABLE 2 Mechanical Requirements, Fine Wire[A]

Condition[B]	Diameter, in. (mm)	Ultimate[C] Tensile Strength, psi (MPa)	Elongation in 10 in. (254 mm), min, %
Cold-drawn	under 0.063 (1.60)	125 000 to 150 000 (860 to 1035)	5

[A] Annealed fine wire requirements are covered in Specification F 1350.
[B] Recommended crosshead speed for cold-drawn fine wire is 5 in./min (2.0 mm/s).
[C] Cold-drawn wire may be ordered to tensile strengths up to 300 000 psi (2070 MPa) with lower elongation as determined by customer and supplier.

6. Chemical Composition

6.1 The heat analysis shall conform to the requirements as to chemical composition specified in Table 3.

6.1.1 The compositional requirement shall meet the following:

$$\% \text{Cr} + 3.3 \times \% \text{Mo} \geq 26.0 \quad (1)$$

6.1.2 Requirements for the major and minor elemental constituents are listed in Table 3. Also listed are important residual elements. Analysis for elements not listed in Table 3 is not required to certify compliance with this specification.

6.2 *Product Analysis*—Product analysis tolerances do not broaden the specified heat analysis requirements, but cover variations between laboratories in the measurement of chemical content. The manufacturer shall not ship material that is outside the limits specified in Table 3. Product analysis limits shall be as specified in Table 4.

6.2.1 The product analysis is either for the purpose of verifying the composition of a heat or lot or to determine variations in the composition within the heat.

6.2.2 Acceptance or rejection of a heat or lot of material may be made by the purchaser on the basis of this check analysis.

6.3 Methods and practices relating to chemical analysis required by this specification shall be in accordance with Test Methods, Practices, and Terminology A 751.

TABLE 3 Chemical Requirements, Heat Analysis

Element	Composition, %
Carbon	0.030 max
Manganese	2.00 max
Phosphorous	0.025 max
Sulfur	0.010 max
Silicon	0.75 max
Chromium[A]	17.00 to 19.00
Nickel	13.00 to 15.00
Molybdenum[A]	2.25 to 3.00
Nitrogen	0.10 max
Copper	0.50 max
Iron[B]	balance

[A] The compositional requirement shall meet the following:
$\% \text{Cr} + 3.3 \times \% \text{Mo} \geq 26.0$.
[B] Approximately equal to the difference between 100 % and the sum percentage of the other specified elements. The percentage iron content by difference is not required to be reported.

TABLE 4 Product Analysis Tolerance[A]

Element	Tolerance Under the Minimum or Over the Maximum Limit[B]
Carbon	0.005
Manganese	0.04
Phosphorous	0.005
Sulfur	0.005
Silicon	0.05
Chromium	0.20
Nickel	0.15
Molybdenum	0.10
Nitrogen	0.01
Copper	0.03

[A] Refer to Specification A 555/A 555M.
[B] Under minimum limit not applicable for elements where only a minimum percentage is indicated.

7. Metallurgical Requirements

7.1 The material shall contain no delta ferrite phase when it is examined metallographically at 100× magnification.

7.2 The microcleanliness of the steel as determined by Method A of Test Methods E 45, except using Plate I-r, on representative billet or bar samples from the heat shall not exceed the following:

Inclusion Type	A (Sulfide)	B (Alumina)	C (Silicate)	D (Globular Oxides)
Thin	1.5	1.5	1.5	1.5
Heavy	1.0	1.0	1.0	1.0

8. Mechanical Properties

8.1 Material shall conform to the appropriate requirements as to mechanical properties specified in Table 1 and Table 2. The level of mechanical properties for material in conditions other than those included in Table 1 and Table 2, shall be specified in the purchase order.

8.1.1 Bar and wire in the cold-worked condition can be supplied to a higher tensile strength and corresponding lower elongation as specified on the purchase order.

8.1.2 Fine wire in the cold-drawn condition can be supplied to a higher tensile strength and corresponding lower elongation as specified on the purchase order.

8.2 Specimens for tension tests shall be machined and tested in accordance with Test Methods E 8/E 8M.

8.3 Brinell hardness number (HB) is the preferred method of reporting the hardness of hot-worked material.

8.4 When desired, Rockwell hardness, B scale (HRB), Rockwell hardness, C scale (HRC), or other hardness limits may be specified. Hardness determination on cold-worked material shall be made on a product cross-section, midway between the center and surface, if cross-section size is adequate.

9. Special Tests

9.1 The steel shall be capable of passing the intergranular corrosion susceptibility test in accordance with Practice E of Practices A 262.

9.1.1 Samples in the hot-worked condition shall be annealed prior to Practice E of Practices A 262, sensitization heat treatment.

9.2 The grain size shall be five or finer when tested in accordance with Test Methods E 112.

9.2.1 It is preferred that samples for grain size determination be selected after the hot working operation or after the final annealing operation prior to the final cold working operation.

9.2.2 If samples are selected after a final cold working operation, specimens shall be tested in accordance with Test Methods E 112 or as agreed to between suppplier and purchaser.

9.3 Finished round bar greater than 0.250 in. (6.35 mm) diameter shall be inspected using ultrasonic or equivalent test methods. Billet shall also be ultrasonically tested prior to being hot rolled and should be free of internal defects. Acceptance criteria shall be agreed to between pruchaser and supplier.

9.4 Any other special requirements shall be specified on the purchase order.

10. Certification

10.1 The manufacturer's certification that the material was manufactured and tested in accordance with this specification together with a report of the test results, shall be furnished at the time of shipment.

11. Quality Program Requirements

11.1 The producer shall maintain a quality program, such as defined in ASQ C1.

11.2 The manufacturer of surgical implants may audit the producer's quality program for conformance to the intent of ASQ C1, or other recognized program.

12. Keywords

12.1 metals (for surgical implants); stainless steel; surgical applications wire; surgical implants

APPENDIXES

(Nonmandatory Information)

X1. RATIONALE

X1.1 The primary reason for this specification is to characterize composition and properties to ensure consistency in the starting material used directly, or as modified by forging, in the manufacturing of medical devices.

X1.2 This low carbon alloy is selected to provide an extra measure of assurance that the material will be free from susceptibility to intergranular corrosion.

X1.3 There is a general consensus that a homogeneous metallurgical structure will be superior with respect to corrosion and fatigue resistance. Based upon this, metallurgical requirements include fine-grained austenitic structure free of ferrite, with low micro-inclusion content, and capability of passing an intergranular corrosion susceptibility test.

X1.4 Acceptable metal conditions include hot-worked, annealed, and all cold-worked conditions, the choice dependent upon the implant design and application.

NOTE X1.1—Exposure to temperatures above 800°F (425°C) during fabrication may impair corrosion resistance unless such exposure is followed by a solution annealing treatment.

X1.5 Upper composition limits for nickel and lower composition limits for molybdenum have been changed in order to meet the latest requirements specified in ISO 5832–1, Composition D.

X1.6 A maximum nitrogen limit was previously added in accordance with the specified element requirements of similar austenitic stainless steels standardized by ASTM.

X1.7 The maximum copper value is considered a practical limit based on a statistical evaluation of commercially available material. Published information has shown no adverse effect for compositions containing up to 1.0 % copper content.

X1.8 The nickel range had previously been increased to ensure that compositions melted to the upper end of the molybdenum range would be free of delta ferrite.

X1.9 The title has been changed; the high carbon composition previously identified as Grade 1 has been deleted, product analysis tolerance limits have been included, UNS designation has been added, annealed fine wire was removed from Table 2, cold-drawn fine wire requirements were revised in Table 2, and Test Methods E 8/E 8M was added.

X1.10 The mechanical requirements and size ranges have been changed, the pitting resistance equivalent (PRE) and extra hard condition have been added, ISO tension test gage length requirements may be used when agreed to between supplier and purchaser, and X2.2 biocompatibility information has been added to coincide with ISO requirements.

X1.11 The pitting resistance equivalent (PRE) has been reidentified as a compositional requirement, free ferrite has been changed to delta ferrite, and grain size determination for cold-worked samples was changed to meet Test Methods E 112 or as agreed to between supplier and purchaser.

X2. BIOCOMPATIBILITY

X2.1 The material composition covered by this specification has been employed successfully in human implant applications in contact with soft tissue and bone for over a decade. Due to the well characterized level of local biological response established by this material, it has been used as a control material in Practice F 981.

X2.2 No known surgical implant material has ever been shown to be completely free of adverse reactions in the human body. However, long term clinical experience has shown an acceptable level of biological response can be expected, if the material is used in appropriate applications.

Designation: F 139 – 00

Standard Specification for Wrought-18 Chromium-14 Nickel-2.5 Molybdenum Stainless Steel Sheet and Strip for Surgical Implants (UNS S31673)[1]

This standard is issued under the fixed designation F 139; the number immediately following the designation indicates the year of original adoption or, in the case of revision, the year of last revision. A number in parentheses indicates the year of last reapproval. A superscript epsilon (ε) indicates an editorial change since the last revision or reapproval.

1. Scope

1.1 This specification covers the requirements for wrought 18 chromium-14 nickel-2.5 molybdenum stainless steel sheet and strip used for the manufacture of surgical implants.

1.2 The values stated in inch-pound units are to be regarded as the standard.

2. Referenced Documents

2.1 *ASTM Standards:*

A 262 Practices for Detecting Susceptibility to Intergranular Attack in Austenitic Stainless Steels[2]

A 480/A480M Specification for General Requirements for Flat-Rolled Stainless and Heat-Resisting Steel Plate, Sheet, and Strip[2]

A 751 Test Methods, Practices, and Terminology for Chemical Analysis of Steel Products[2]

E 45 Test Methods for Determining the Inclusion Content of Steel[3]

E 112 Test Methods for Determining the Average Grain Size[3]

F 981 Practice for Assessment of Compatibility of Biomaterials for Surgical Implants With Respect to Effect of Materials on Muscle and Bone[4]

2.2 *ISO Standard:*

ISO 5832-1 Implants for Surgery-Metallic Materials—Part 1: Wrought Stainless Steel[5]

2.3 *American Society for Quality Control (ASQC) Standard:*

C1 Specification of General Requirements for a Quality Program[6]

3. General Requirements for Delivery

3.1 In addition to the requirements of this specification, all requirements of the current edition of Specification A 480/A 480M shall apply.

3.2 In the case where a conflict exists between this specification and those listed in 2.1 and 2.2, this specification shall take precedence.

4. Ordering Information

4.1 Inquiries and orders for material under this specification shall include the following information:

4.1.1 Quantity (weight or number of pieces),

4.1.2 ASTM designation,

4.1.3 Form (sheet or strip),

4.1.4 Condition (see 5.1),

4.1.5 Mechanical properties (if applicable, for special conditions),

4.1.6 Finish (see 5.2),

4.1.7 Applicable dimensions including size, thickness, width, and length (exact, random, multiples) or print number, and

4.1.8 Special requirements.

5. Materials and Manufacture

5.1 *Condition*:

5.1.1 Sheet and strip shall be furnished as specified, in the annealed or cold-worked condition (see Table 1).

5.2 *Finish*:

5.2.1 Types of finish available in sheet and strip are dull cold rolled, bright cold rolled, intermediate polished, general-purpose polished, dull satin-finished, high luster finish, mirror finish, or as specified in the purchase order.

6. Chemical Composition

6.1 The heat analysis shall conform to the requirements as to chemical composition specified in Table 2.

6.1.1 The compositional requirement shall meet the following:

$$\% \text{Cr} + 3.3 \times \% \text{Mo} \geq 26.0 \quad (1)$$

6.1.2 Requirements for the major and minor elemental constituents are listed in Table 2. Also listed are important residual elements. Analysis for elements not listed in Table 2 is not required to certify compliance with this specification.

6.2 *Product Analysis*— Product analysis tolerances do not broaden the specified heat analysis requirements, but cover

[1] This specification is under the jurisdiction of ASTM Committee F04 on Medical and Surgical Materials and Devicesand is the direct responsibility of Subcommittee F04.12 on Metallurgical Materials.

Current edition approved June 10, 2000. Published September 2000. Originally published as F 139 – 76. Last previous edition F 139 – 96.

[2] *Annual Book of ASTM Standards*, Vol 01.03.

[3] *Annual Book of ASTM Standards*, Vol 03.01.

[4] *Annual Book of ASTM Standards*, Vol 13.01.

[5] Available from American National Standards Institute, 1430 Broadway, New York, NY 10018.

[6] Available from American Society for Quality Control, 161 W. Wisconsin Ave., Milwaukee, WI 53203.

TABLE 1 Mechanical Requirements

Condition	Ultimate Tensile Strength, min, psi (MPa)	Yield Strength (0.2 % Offset), min, psi (MPa)	Elongation in 2 in. (50 mm) min, %	Rockwell Hardness, max
Annealed	71 000 (490)	27 500 (190)	40	95 HRB
Cold-worked	125 000 (860)	100 000 (690)	10	...

TABLE 2 Chemical Requirements, Heat Analysis

Element	Composition, %
Carbon	0.030 max
Manganese	2.00 max
Phosphorus	0.025 max
Sulfur	0.010 max
Silicon	0.75 max
Chromium[A]	17.00 to 19.00
Nickel	13.00 to 15.00
Molybdenum[A]	2.25 to 3.00
Nitrogen	0.10 max
Copper	0.50 max
Iron[B]	balance

[A] The compositional requirement shall meet the following:

$$\% \text{ Cr} + 3.3 \times \% \text{ Mo} \geq 26.0$$

[B] Approximately equal to the difference between 100 % and the sum percentage of the other specified elements. The percentage iron content by difference is not required to be reported.

variations between laboratories in the measurement of chemical content. The manufacturer shall not ship material that is outside the limits specified in Table 2. Product analysis limits shall be as specified in Table 3.

6.2.1 The product analysis is either for the purpose of verifying the composition of a heat or lot or to determine variations in the composition within the heat.

6.2.2 Acceptance or rejection of a heat or lot of material may be made by the purchaser on the basis of this check analysis.

6.3 Methods and practices relating to chemical analysis required by this specification shall be in accordance with Test Methods, Practices, and Terminology A 751.

TABLE 3 Product Analysis Tolerance[A]

Element	Tolerance Under the Minimum or Over the Maximum Limit[B]
Carbon	0.005
Manganese	0.04
Phosphorus	0.005
Sulfur	0.005
Silicon	0.05
Chromium	0.20
Nickel	0.15
Molybdenum	0.10
Nitrogen	0.01
Copper	0.03

[A] Refer to Specification A 480/A 480M.

[B] Under minimum limit not applicable for elements where only a minimum percentage is indicated.

7. Metallurgical Requirements

7.1 The material shall contain no delta ferrite phase when it is examined metallographically at 100× magnification.

7.2 The microcleanliness of the steel as determined by Test Methods E 45, Method A, except using Plate I-r on representative samples from the hot-rolled band from the heat shall not exceed the following:

Inclusion Type	A (Sulfide)	B (Alumina)	C (Silicate)	D (Globular Oxide)
Thin	1.5	1.5	1.5	1.5
Heavy	1.5	1.0	1.5	1.0

8. Mechanical Properties

8.1 Material shall conform to the appropriate requirements as to mechanical properties specified in Table 1. The level of mechanical properties for material in conditions other than those included in Table 1 shall be specified in the purchase order.

8.2 When desired, Rockwell hardness, A scale (HRA), Rockwell hardness, B scale (HRB) or Rockwell hardness, C Scale (HRC), limits may be specified.

9. Special Tests

9.1 The steel shall be capable of passing the intergranular corrosion susceptibility test in accordance with Practices A 262, Practice E.

9.2 The grain size shall be five or finer when tested in accordance with Test Methods E 112.

9.2.1 It is preferred that samples for grain size determination be selected after the final annealing operation and prior to a final cold-working operation.

9.2.2 If samples are selected after a final cold-working operation, specimens shall be tested according to Test Method E112, or as agreed to between the supplier and purchaser..

9.3 Any other special requirements shall be specified on the purchase order.

10. Certification

10.1 The manufacturer's certification that the material was manufactured and tested in accordance with this specification together with a report of the test results shall be furnished at the time of shipment.

11. Quality Program Requirements

11.1 The producer shall maintain a quality program, such as defined in ASQC C1.

11.2 The manufacturer of surgical implants may audit the producer's quality program for conformance to the intent of ASQC C1, or other recognized programs.

12. Keywords

12.1 metals (for surgical implants); stainless steel; surgical implants

APPENDIXES

(Nonmandatory Information)

X1. RATIONALE

X1.1 The primary reason for this specification is to characterize composition and properties to ensure consistency in the starting material used directly, or as modified by shape forming in the manufacturing of medical devices.

X1.2 This low-carbon alloy is selected to provide an extra measure of assurance that the material will be free from susceptibility to intergranular corrosion.

X1.3 There is a general consensus that a homogeneous metallurgical structure will be superior with respect to corrosion and fatigue resistance. Based upon this, metallurgical requirements include fine-grained austenitic structure free of ferrite, with low micro-inclusion content and capability of passing an intergranular corrosion susceptibility test.

X1.4 Acceptable metal conditions include annealed and all cold-worked conditions, the choice dependent upon the particular implant design and application.

NOTE X1.1—Exposure to temperatures above 800°F (425°C) during fabrication may impair corrosion resistance unless such exposure is followed by a solution annealing treatment.

X1.5 Upper composition limits for nickel and lower composition limits for molybdenum have been changed in order to meet the latest requirements specified in ISO 5832-1, Composition D.

X1.6 A maximum nitrogen limit was previously added in accordance with the specified element requirements of similar austenitic stainless steels standardized by ASTM.

X1.7 The maximum copper value is considered a practical limit based on a statistical evaluation of commercially available material. Published information has shown no adverse effect for compositions containing up to 1.0 % copper content.

X1.8 The nickel range had previously been increased to ensure that compositions melted to the upper end of the molybdenum range would be free of delta ferrite.

X1.9 The title has been changed, the high carbon composition previously identified as Grade 1 has been deleted, product analysis tolerance limits have been included, inclusion limits have been changed in accordance with industry practice, and the UNS designation has been added.

X1.10 The mechanical requirements have been changed, the Pitting Resistance Equivalent (PRE) has been added, and X2.2 biocompatibility information has been added to coincide with ISO requirements.

X1.11 The Pitting Resistance Equivalent (PRE) has been reidentified as a compositional requirement, free ferrite has been changed to delta ferrite, and grain size determination for cold worked samples was changed to meet Test Method E112 or as agreed to between supplier and purchaser.

X2. BIOCOMPATIBILITY

X2.1 The material composition covered by this specification has been employed successfully in human implant applications in contact with soft tissue and bone for over a decade.

X2.2 No known surgical implant material has ever been shown to be completely free of adverse reactions in the human body. However, long term clinical experience has shown an acceptable level of biological response can be expected, if the material is used in appropriate applications.

Last ASTM Designation: F 339 – 71 (Reapproved 1993)$^{\epsilon 1}$

Standard Specification for Cloverleaf Intramedullary Pins

This specification covers cloverleaf-type intramedullary pins intended for internal fixation of fractures of the skeletal system. Formerly under the jurisdiction of Committee F-4 on Medical and Surgical Materials and Devices, this specification was discontined in May 1999.

Standard Specification for Fixation Pins and Wires[1]

This standard is issued under the fixed designation F 366; the number immediately following the designation indicates the year of original adoption or, in the case of revision, the year of last revision. A number in parentheses indicates the year of last reapproval. A superscript epsilon (ε) indicates an editorial change since the last revision or reapproval.

This standard has been approved for use by agencies of the Department of Defense.

1. Scope

1.1 This specification covers functional dimensions for fixation pins and wires.

1.2 In recognition of many broad and varied uses of such pins and wires, many options are included. A variety, but not necessarily all, of the options are illustrated in Figs. 1-3.

1.3 The values stated in inch-pound units are to be regarded as the standard.

1.4 The values given in parentheses are provided for information only.

2. Referenced Documents

2.1 *ASTM Standards:*

F 55 Specification for Stainless Steel Bar and Wire for Surgical Implants[2]

F 67 Specification for Unalloyed Titanium for Surgical Implant Applications[3]

F 86 Practice for Surface Preparation and Marking of Metallic Surgical Implants[3]

F 90 Specification for Wrought Cobalt-Chromium-Tungsten-Nickel Alloy for Surgical Implant Applications[3]

F 136 Specification for Wrought Titanium 6A1-4V ELI Alloy for Surgical Implant Applications[3]

F 138 Specification for Stainless Steel Bar and Wire for Surgical Implants (Special Quality)[3]

F 562 Specification for Wrought Cobalt-35 Nickel-20 Chromium-10 Molybdenum Alloy for Surgical Implant Applications[3]

F 563 Specification for Wrought Cobalt-Nickel-Chromium-Molybdenum-Tungsten-Iron Alloy for Surgical Implant Applications[3]

3. Materials

3.1 Fixation pins and wires shall be fabricated from material conforming to one of the following ASTM Specifications: F 55, F 67, F 90, F 136, F 138, F 562, or F 563.

4. Performance Requirements

4.1 Factors considered to be important, but for which values and test methods have not been established, are bending strength, fatigue strength, breaking strength (Knowles Type only), torsion strength, and ductility.

5. Dimensions and Characteristics

5.1 Fixation pins and wires shall be fabricated in accordance with the dimensions illustrated in Figs. 1-4.

5.2 Fixation pins and wires shall have surfaces prepared and marked in accordance with Practice F 86.

5.2.1 Optional marking on the fixation pins and wires shall identify the manufacturer or distributor.

6. Packaging and Labeling

6.1 Packaging shall be adequate to protect the fixation pins and wires during shipment.

6.2 Labeling for fixation pins and wires shall include:

6.2.1 Product name,

6.2.2 Size, on the immediate container,

6.2.2.1 Length,

6.2.2.2 Diameter (if round) or cross-sectional size (if square of hexagonal), that is, ¼ in. (6.4 mm) square, and

6.2.3 ASTM material specification Designation number.

7. Keywords

7.1 fixation materials; flexible surgical wire; orthopaedic medical devices; wire-surgical implants

---

[1] This specification is under the jurisdiction of ASTM Committee F-4 on Medical and Surgical Materials and Devices, and is the direct responsibility of Subcommittee F04.21 on Osteosynthesis.

Current edition approved Aug. 27, 1982. Published February 1983. Originally published as F 366-73. Last previous edition F 366-73.

[2] Discontinued—See 1991 *Annual Book of ASTM Standards*, Vol 13.01.

[3] *Annual Book of ASTM Standards*, Vol 13.01.

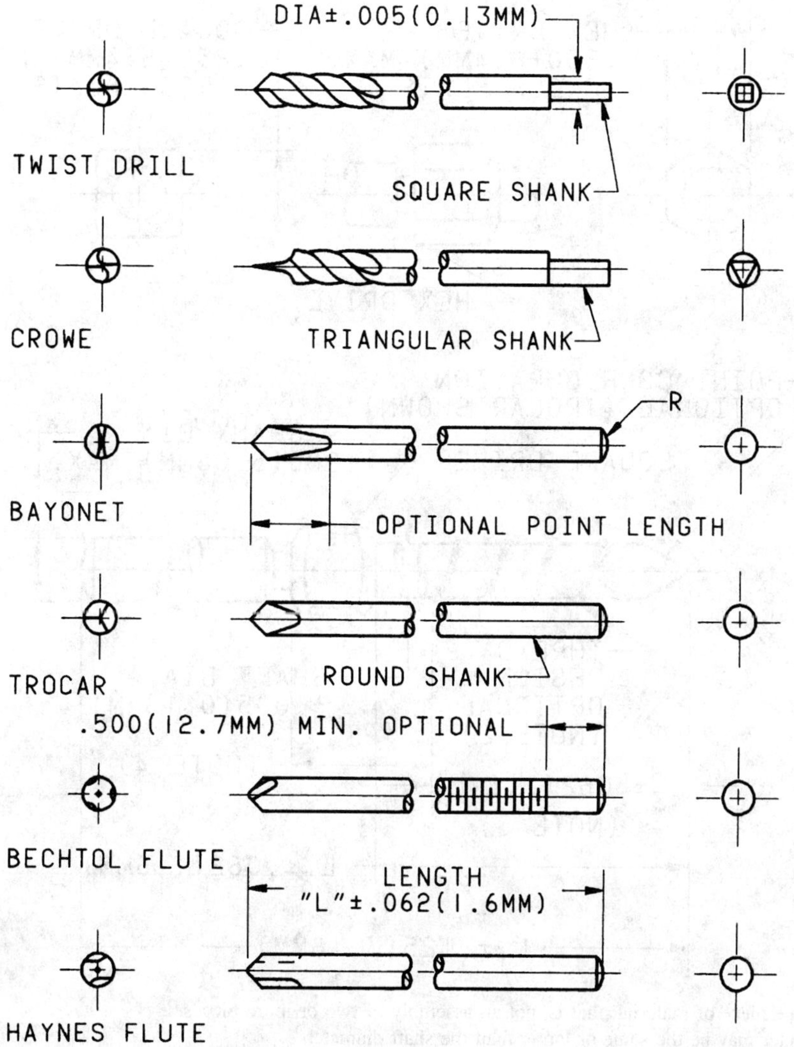

NOTE 1—Pins and wires may be smooth shank or threaded.

NOTE 2—Point angle and helix angle, where applicable, is as specified by manufacturer.

NOTE 3—On square or triangular shanks, flats are equal and corners are on the same circumference as the pin diameter. Shank diameters on pins larger than ⅛ in. (3.2 mm) may be reduced.

NOTE 4—Optional designs, both ends pointed or point with suture hole.

FIG. 1 Fixation Pins and Wires

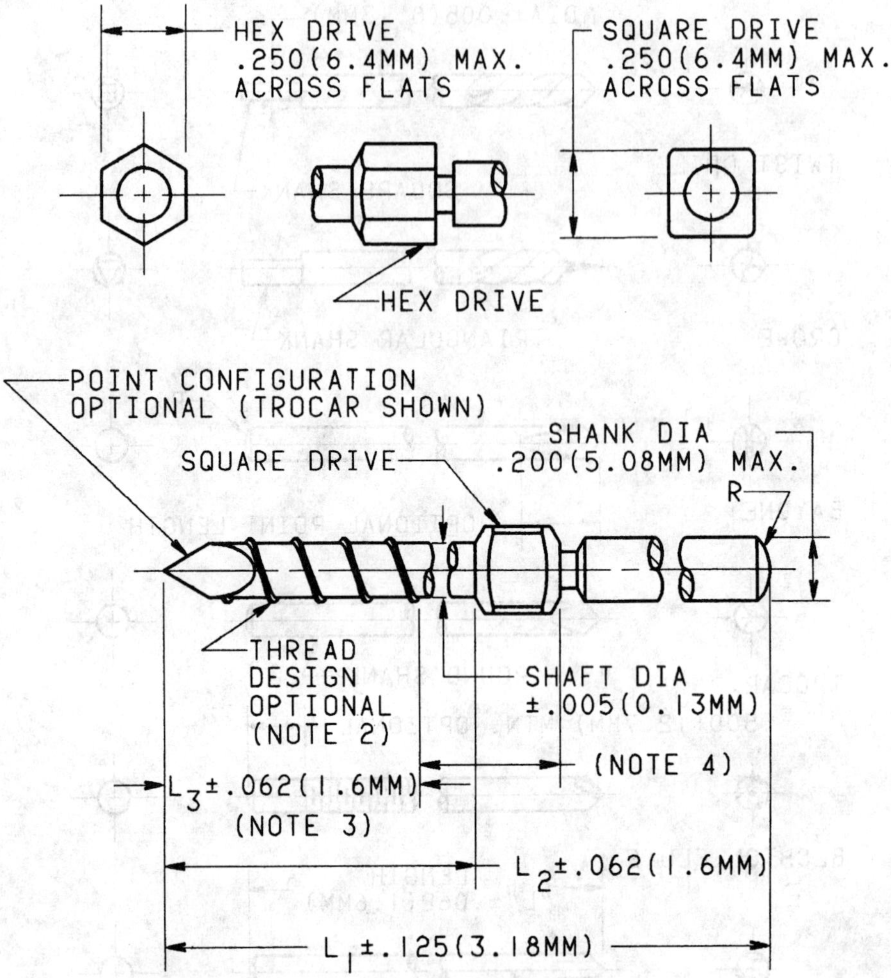

NOTE 1—Shall be made of one piece of material; that is, not an assembly of two or more pieces.
NOTE 2—Thread major diameter may be the same or larger than the shaft diameter.
NOTE 3—Thread length shall be optional to suit intended medical application.
NOTE 4—Optional marking in this location.

FIG. 2 Fixation Pin-Knowles Type

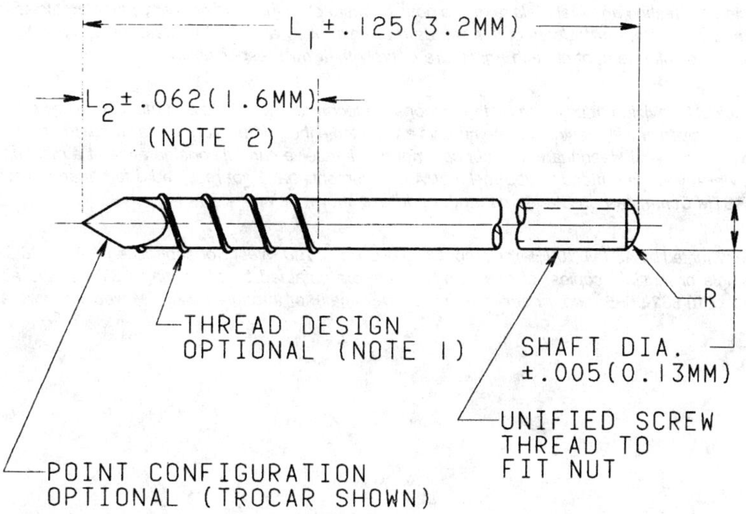

NOTE 1—Thread major diameter may be the same or larger than the shaft diameter.
NOTE 2—Thread length shall be optional to suit intended medical application.

FIG. 3 Fixation Pin-Hagie Type

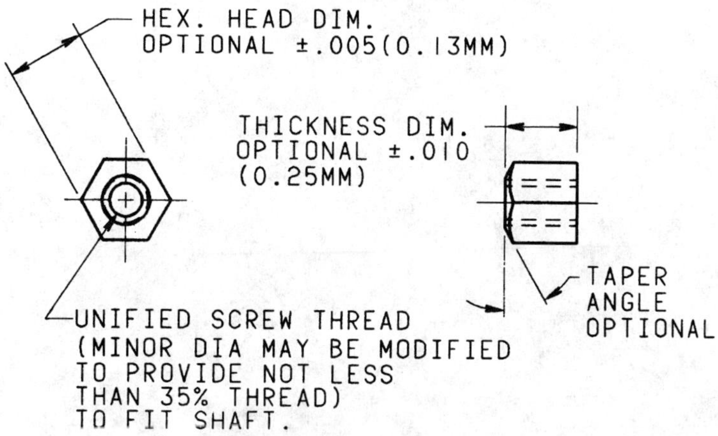

FIG. 4 Nut for Hagie Pin

APPENDIX

(Nonmandatory Information)

X1. RATIONALE

X1.1 The primary reasons for the revision of this standard are:

X1.1.1 To characterize fixation pins and wires used in the treatment of fractures or disease of the skeletal system.

X1.1.2 To incorporate fixation pins—Knowles and Hagie types (F 368).

X1.1.3 To specify marking nomenclature.

X1.1.4 To add performance requirements in accordance with Performance Section's request.

X1.1.5 To add packaging and labeling.

X1.1.6 To remove the dimensions on the Crowe since the dimensions are not essential.

X1.1.7 Specific surface finish was considered, however, not included, since test data to confirm what the requirement should be or what effect it has upon performance was not available.

X1.2 Designs listed enable the surgeon to select from a variety of fixation pins and wires.

X1.3 The materials listed represent the current usage and have demonstrated clinical acceptance in these devices.

Designation: F 370 – 94 (Reapproved 1999)

Standard Specification for Proximal Femoral Endoprosthesis[1]

This standard is issued under the fixed designation F 370; the number immediately following the designation indicates the year of original adoption or, in the case of revision, the year of last revision. A number in parentheses indicates the year of last reapproval. A superscript epsilon (ϵ) indicates an editorial change since the last revision or reapproval.

1. Scope

1.1 This specification covers the materials, functional dimensions, and tolerances for single piece, metallic proximal femoral endoprosthesis.

1.2 In recognition of many broad and varied uses of such prostheses, many options are included. A variety, but not necessarily all, of the options are illustrated in Fig. 1.

1.3 The values stated in inch-pound units are to be regarded as the standard.

2. Referenced Documents

2.1 *ASTM Standards:*

F 55 Specification for Stainless Steel Bar and Wire for Surgical Implants[2]

F 75 Specification for Cast Cobalt-Chromium-Molybdenum Alloy for Surgical Implant Applications[2]

F 86 Practice for Surface Preparation and Marking of Metallic Surgical Implants[2]

F 136 Specification for Wrought Titanium 6A1-4V ELI Alloy for Surgical Implant Applications[2]

F 138 Specification for Stainless Steel Bar and Wire for Surgical Implants (Special Quality)[2]

F 601 Practice for Fluorescent Penetrant Inspection of Metallic Surgical Implants[2]

F 620 Specification for Titanium 6A1-4V ELI Alloy Forgings for Surgical Implants[2]

F 621 Specification for Stainless Steel Forgings for Surgical Implants[2]

F 629 Practice for Radiography of Cast Metallic Surgical Implants[2]

F 983 Practice for Permanent Marking of Orthopedic Implant Components[2]

F 1108 Specification for Cast Titanium 6A1-4V Alloy for Surgical Implants[2]

2.2 *ASQC Standard:*

C1-1985 Specification of General Requirements for a Quality Control Program[3]

3. Materials

3.1 Proximal femoral endoprosthesis conforming to this specification shall be made of a material conforming to one of the following Specifications: F 55, F 75, F 136, F 138, or F 1108.

3.2 Proximal femoral endoprostheses made from stainless steel or titanium alloy forgings shall conform to one of the following, as applicable; Specifications F 620 or F 621.

4. Dimensions

4.1 Proximal femoral endoprosthesis conforming to this specification shall be fabricated in accordance with the tolerances indicated for specific dimensions illustrated in Fig. 2 of this specification. Where tolerances are not indicated for dimensions the following tolerances shall apply:

Fractional dimensions	±1⁄64 in. (0.40 mm)
Decimal dimensions	±0.005 in. (0.13 mm)
Angles	±2°
Metric dimensions	±0.5 mm (0.019 in.)

5. Finish and Marking

5.1 Proximal femoral endoprosthesis conforming to this specification shall be finished in accordance with Practice F 86.

5.2 Permanent identification marking on proximal femoral endoprostheses conforming to this specification shall be in accordance with F 983. Such markings shall include the following:

5.2.1 Head size (spherical diameter)

5.2.2 Stem length

5.2.3 Manufacturer's name and/or logo

5.2.4 Lot number or serial number

5.2.5 Catalogue number

6. Quality Program Requirements

6.1 The manufacturer shall maintain a quality program, such as, for example, is defined in the ASQC C1-1985.

6.2 Nondestructive inspection, as appropriate to the method of manufacturer, shall be used to ensure prostheses quality. Fluorescent penetrant inspection and radiography, when used, shall be in accordance with Practices F 601 and F 629 respectively.

---

[1] This specification is under the jurisdiction of ASTM Committee F-4 on Medical and Surgical Materials and Devices, and is the direct responsibility of Subcommittee F04.22 on Arthroplasty.

Current edition approved Feb. 15, 1994. Published March 1994. Originally published as F 370 – 73. Last previous edition F 370 – 73 (1991)ϵ[1].

[2] *Annual Book of ASTM Standards,* Vol 13.01.

[3] Available from American Society of Quality Control, 161 West Wisconsin Ave., Milwaukee, WI 53203.

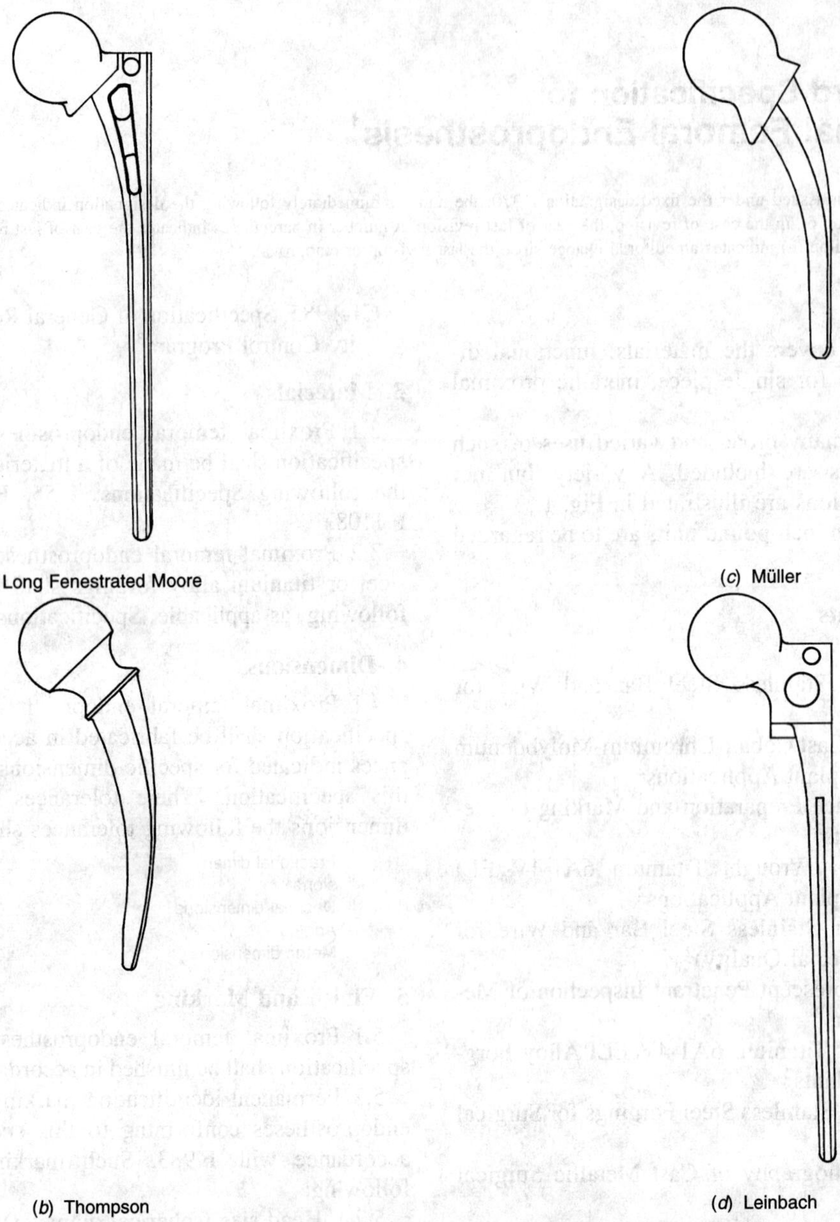

(*a*) Long Fenestrated Moore

(*b*) Thompson

(*c*) Müller

(*d*) Leinbach

FIG. 1 Proximal Femoral Endoprosthesis—Typical Examples

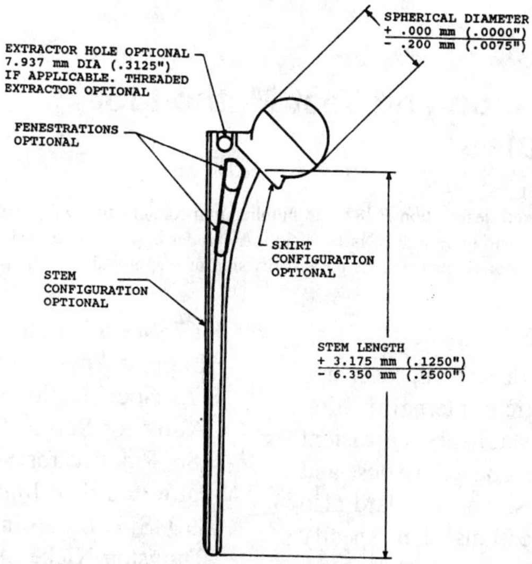

FIG. 2 Typical Features and Tolerances for Proximal Femoral Endoprostheses

APPENDIX

(Nonmandatory Information)

X1. (RATIONALE)

X1.1 This standard specification describes the basic features of classic femoral prostheses used for hemiarthroplasty of the hip (commonly termed endoprostheses). This specification applies to prostheses of fixed head construction only.

X1.2 More detailed requirements for this class of hip implant, including those of modular and bi-polar construction, are currently under development as part of comprehensive physical and performance standards for all hip prostheses. This revision of F 370 is intended to reflect current industry practice and to include reference to relevant ASTM standards passed since its last revision. In accordance with reflecting industry practice for this class of prostheses, primary dimensions are listed in inch-pound units.

X1.3 This standard is not meant to be perfect but to serve until the comprehensive standards are ready. When the comprehensive standards for hip prostheses are complete, F 370 will be balloted for withdrawal.

Designation: F 382 – 99

Standard Specification and Test Method for Metallic Bone Plates[1]

This standard is issued under the fixed designation F 382; the number immediately following the designation indicates the year of original adoption or, in the case of revision, the year of last revision. A number in parentheses indicates the year of last reapproval. A superscript epsilon (ε) indicates an editorial change since the last revision or reapproval.

1. Scope

1.1 This standard is intended to provide a comprehensive reference for bone plates used in the surgical internal fixation of the skeletal system. The standard establishes consistent methods to classify, define the geometric characteristics, and performance characteristics of bone plates. The standard also presents a catalog of standard specifications that specify material; labeling and handling requirements; and standard test methods for measuring performance related mechanical characteristics determined to be important to the *in vivo* performance of bone plates.

1.2 It is not the intention of the standard to define levels of performance or case-specific clinical performance for bone plates, as insufficient knowledge is available to predict the consequences or their use in individual patients for specific activities of daily living. Futhermore, it is not the intention of the standard to describe or specify specific designs for bone plates used in the surgical internal fixation of the skeletal system.

1.3 This standard may not be appropriate for all types of bone plates. The user is cautioned to consider the appropriateness of the standard in view of a particular bone plate and its potential application.

1.4 This standard includes the following test methods used in determining the following bone plate mechanical performance characteristics.

1.4.1 Standard Test Method for Single Cycle Bend Testing of Metallic Bone Plates - Annex A1.

1.4.2 Standard Test Method for Determining the Bending Fatigue Properties Of Metallic Bone Plates - Annex A2.

1.5 Unless otherwise indicated, the values stated in SI units shall be regarded as the standard.

1.6 *This standard does not purport to address all of the safety concerns, if any, associated with its use. It is the responsibility of the user of this standard to establish appropriate safety and health practices and determine the applicability of regulatory limitations prior to use.*

2. Referenced Documents

2.1 *ASTM Standards:*

F 67 Specification for Unalloyed Titanium for Surgical Implant Applications[2]

F 75 Specification for Cast Cobalt-Chromium-Molybdenum Alloy for Surgical Implant Applications[2]

F 86 Practice for Surface Preparation and Marking of Metallic Surgical Implants[2]

F 90 Specification for Wrought Cobalt-Chromium-Tungsten-Nickel Alloy for Surgical Implant Applications[2]

F 136 Specification for Wrought Titanium 6Al-4V ELI Alloy for Surgical Implant Applications[2]

F 138 Specification for Stainless Steel Bars and Wire for Surgical Implants (Special Quality)[2]

F 139 Specification for Stainless Steel Sheet and Strip for Surgical Implants (Special Quality)[2]

F 543 Specification for Cortical Bone Screws[2]

F 565 Practice for Care and Handling of Orthopedic Implants and Instruments[2]

F 620 Specification for Titanium 6Al-ELI Alloy Forgings for Surgical Implants[2]

F 621 Specification for Stainless Steel Forgings for Surgical Implants[2]

F 983 Practice for Permanent Marking of Orthopaedic Implant Components[2]

F 1295 Wrought Titanium - 6 Aluminum - 7 Niobium Alloy for Surgical Implant Applications[2]

F 1314 Wrought Nitrogen Strengthened - 22 Chromium - 12.5 Nickel - 5 Manganese - 2.5 Molybdenum Stainless Steel Bar and Wire for Surgical Implants[2]

F 1472 Wrought Titanium Ti-6Al-4V Alloy for Surgical Implant Applications[2]

F 1713 Standard Specification for Wrought Titanium 13Nb-13Zr Alloy for Surgical Implant Applications[2]

2.2 *ISO Standard:*[3]

FDIS 14602 Non-active surgical implants—Implants for Osteosynthesis particular requirements.

3. Terminology

3.1 *Definitions—Geometric:*

3.1.1 *auto compression*—a type of bone plate that by its design can generate a compressive force between adjacent unconnected bone fragments through the use of one or more ramped holes or another type of slot geometry. This ramp or

[1] This test method is under the jurisdiction of ASTM Committee F-4 on Medical and Surgical Materials and Devices and is the direct responsibility of Subcommittee F04.21 on Osteosynthesis.

Current edition approved October 10, 1999. Published December 1999. Originally published as F 382–73. Last previous edition F 382–98a.

[2] *Annual Book of ASTM Standards*, Vol 13.01.

[3] Available from International Standards Organization, Rue de Varembe, Case Postale 56, CH-1211, Geneva 20, Switzerland.

slot geometry contacts the underside of the screw head, and induces compressive force as the screw is inserted and tightened to the bone plate.

3.1.2 *bone plate*—a metallic device with two or more holes and/or slot(s) and a cross section that consists of at least two dimensions (width and thickness) which generally are not the same in magnitude. The device is intended to provide alignment and fixation of two or more bone sections, primarily by spanning the fracture or defect. The device is typically fixed to the bone through the use of bone screws or cerclage wire. A partial list of general types of bone plates is given in Section 4.1.

3.1.3 *bone plate length, L (mm)*—the linear dimension of the bone plate measured along the longitudinal axis as illustrated in Fig. 2.

3.1.4 *bone plate thickness, b (mm)*—the linear dimension of the bone plate measured parallel to the screw hole axis as shown in Fig. 1a, 1b, and Fig. 2. For a bone plate with a crescant section, the thickness is measured at the thickest point along the section.

3.1.5 *bone plate width, w (mm)*—the linear dimension of the bone plate measured perpendicular to both the length and thickness axes as shown in Fig. 2.

3.1.6 *contouring*—the manipulation and bending of a bone platc, either pre-operatively or intra-operatively, to match the anatomic geometry of the intended fixation location.

3.1.7 *crescent section*—a bone plate cross-section shape (perpendicular to the long axis of the bone plate) where the thickness is not constant along the section. Typically the section is thickest along the bone plate's centerline and tapers to a smaller thickness at the bone plate's edges (see Fig. 1b).

3.1.8 *uniform width*—referring to a bone plate where the width is constant along the bone plate's length.

3.2 *Definitions—Mechanical/Structural:*

3.2.1 *bending stiffness, K (N/mm)— of a bone plate*, the maximum slope of the linear elastic portion of the load versus load-point displacement curve for a bone plate when tested according to the test method of Annex A1.

3.2.2 *bending strength (N-m)— of a bone plate*, the bending moment necessary to produce a 0.2 % offset displacement in the bone plate when tested as described in Annex A1.

3.2.3 *bending structural stiffness, El (N-m²)—of a bone plate*, the bone plate's normalized effective bending stiffness that takes into consideration the effects of the test setup's configuration when tested according to the method described in Annex A1.

3.2.4 *fatigue life, n*—The number of loading cycles of a specified character that a given specimen sustains before failure of a specified nature occurs.

3.2.5 *fatigue strength at N cycles*—An estimate of the cyclic forcing parameter (for example, load, moment, torque, stress, and so on) at a given load ratio, for which 50 % of the specimens within a given sample population would be expected to survive *N* loading cycles.

4. Classification

4.1 Bone plates used in general orthopaedic surgery can be categorized into general types according to the following classifications.

4.1.1 *cloverleaf platc*—a bone plate that has one three-lobed end which contains screw holes.

4.1.2 *cobra head plate*—a bone plate that has one flared triangular or trapezoidal end which contains multiple screw holes and/or slots. This type of bone plate is often used for hip arthrodesis.

4.1.3 *reconstruction plate*—a bone plate that does not have a uniform width, but usually has a smaller cross-section between the screw holes or slots. The reduced cross-section between screw holes/slots facilitates contouring the bone plate in several planes. Reconstruction plates are often used in fractures of the pelvis and acetabulum.

4.1.4 *straight plate*—a bone plate with uniform width and a straight longitudinal axis. Straight plates are often used for fractures of the diaphysis of long bones.

4.1.5 *tubular plate*—a bone plate whose cross-section resembles a portion of a tube, and which has a constant thickness

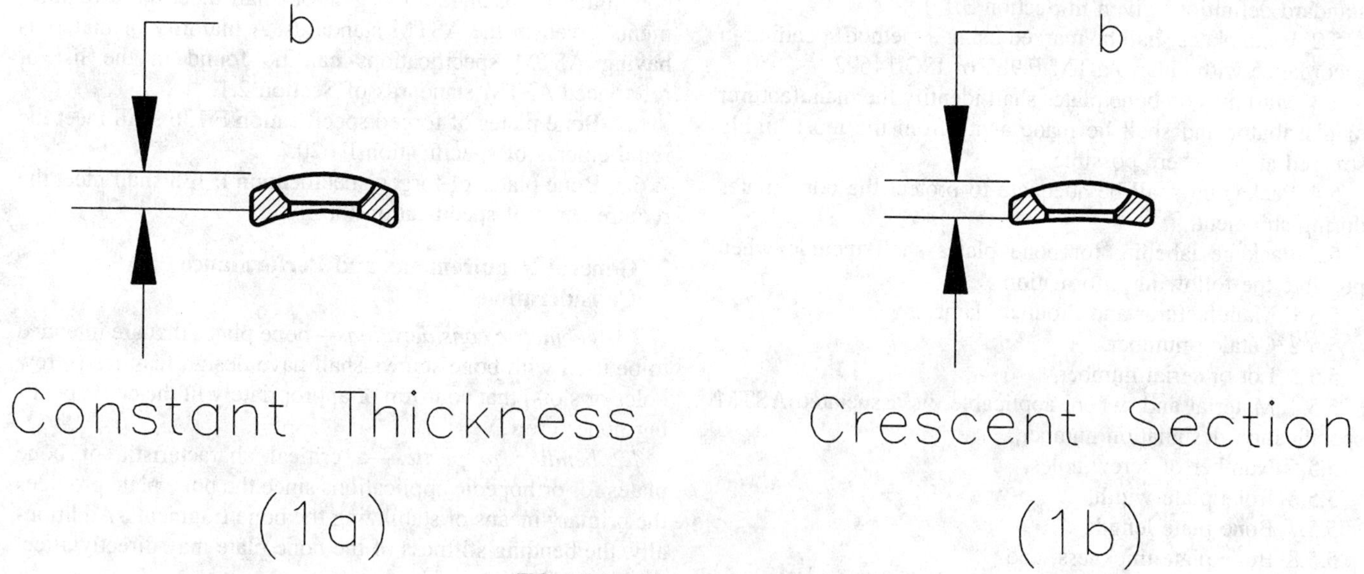

FIG. 1 Bone Plate Cross-sections

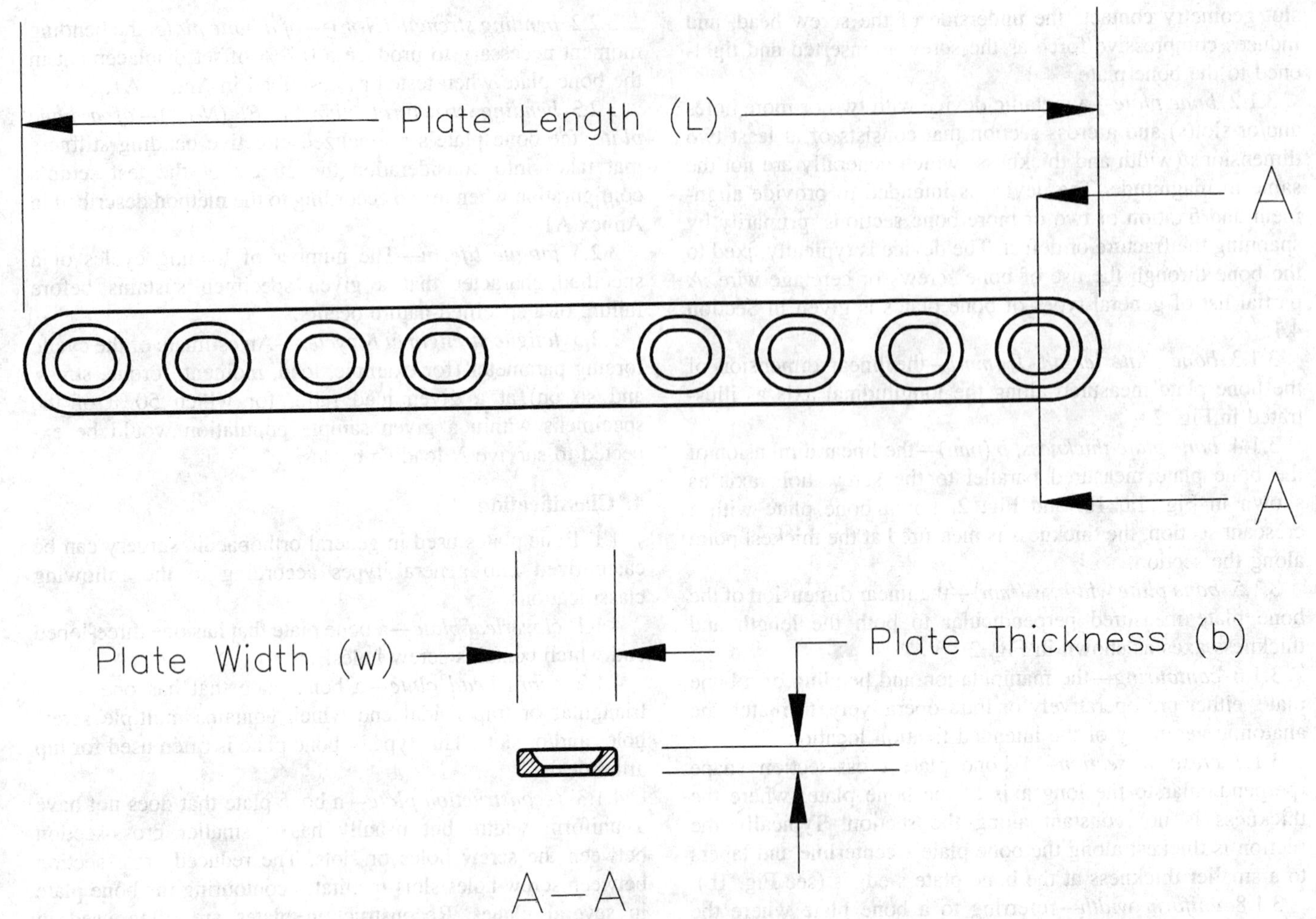

FIG. 2 Bone Plate Dimensions

or a crescent section. Tubular plates are often used for fractures of the smaller long bones (that is, radius, ulna, fibula).

5. Marking, Packaging, Labeling, and Handling

5.1 Dimensions of bone plates should be designated by the standard definitions given in Section 3.1.

5.2 Bone plates shall be marked using a method specified in accordance with either ASTM F 983 or ISO 14602.

5.3 Markings on bone plates shall identify the manufacturer or distributor and shall be made away from the most highly stressed areas, where possible.

5.4 Packaging shall be adequate to protect the bone plates during shipment.

5.5 Package labeling for bone plates shall include when possible the following information:

5.5.1 Manufacturer and Product Name,

5.5.2 Catalog number,

5.5.3 Lot or serial number,

5.5.4 Material and, where applicable, its associated ASTM specification designation number,

5.5.5 Number of screw holes,

5.5.6 Bone plate width,

5.5.7 Bone plate length,

5.5.8 Bone plate thickness, and

5.5.9 ASTM specification designation number.

5.6 Bone plates should be cared for and handled in accordance with Practice F 565, as appropriate.

6. Materials

6.1 All bone plates made of materials which have an ASTM committee F04 standard designation shall meet those requirements given in the ASTM standards. A majority of materials having ASTM specifications can be found in the list of referenced ASTM standards of Section 2.1.

6.2 Bone plates of forged specification F 136 shall meet the requirements of specification F 620.

6.3 Bone plates of forged specification F 138 shall meet the requirements of specification F 621.

7. General Requirements and Performance Considerations

7.1 *geometric considerations*—bone plates that are intended to be used with bone screws shall have design features (screw holes or slots) that conform or appropriately fit the corresponding bone screw.

7.2 *bending properties*—a critical characteristic of bone plates for orthopedic applications since the bone plate provides the primary means of stabilizing the bone fragments. Additionally, the bending stiffness of the bone plate may directly affect the rate and ability of healing.

7.2.1 The relevant bending properties (bending stiffness, bending structural stiffness, and bending strength) shall be determined using the standard test method of Annex A1.

7.2.2 Determine the relevant bending fatigue properties according to the methods described in Annex A2.

8. Keywords

8.1 bend testing - surgical implants; fatigue test; bone plate; orthopedic medical devices - bone plates; surgical devices; test methods - surgical implants

ANNEXES

A1. STANDARD TEST METHOD FOR SINGLE CYCLE BEND TESTING OF METALLIC BONE PLATES[1]

A1.1 *Scope*:

A1.1.1 This test method describes methods for single cycle bend testing in order to determine intrinsic, structural properties of metallic bone plates. The test method measures the bending stiffness, bending structural stiffness, and bending strength of bone plates.

A1.1.2 This standard is intended to provide a means of mechanically characterize different bone plate designs. It is not the intention of this standard to define levels of performance for bone plates as insufficient knowledge is available to predict the consequences of the use of particular bone plate designs.

A1.1.3 *Units*—The values stated in SI units are to be regarded as standard. No other units of measurement are included in this standard.

A1.1.4 *This standard does not purport to address all of the safety concerns, if any, associated with its use. It is the responsibility of the user of this standard to establish appropriate safety and health practices and determine the applicability of regulatory limitations prior to use.*

NOTE A1.1—There is currently an ISO standard (ISO 9585 - Implants for Surgery - Determination of Bending Strength and Stiffness of Bone Plates) that is similar, but not equivalent to this standard test method.

A1.2 Referenced Documents:

A1.2.1 *ASTM Standards*:

E 4 Practices for Load Verification of Testing Machines[4]

E 122 Practice for Choice of Sample Size to Estimate the Average Quality of a Lot or Process[5]

A1.3 *Terminology*:

A1.3.1 *Definitions:*

A1.3.1.1 *0.2 % offset displacement, q (mm)*—permanent deformation equal to 0.2 % of the center loading span distance. (point B in Fig. A1.1).

A1.3.1.2 *bending strength (N-m)—of a bone plate*, the bending moment necessary to produce a 0.2 % offset displacement in the bone plate when tested as described in Section A1.8 (the bending moment corresponding to point D in Fig. A1.1.). If the bone plate fractures before the proof point is attained the bending strength shall be defined as the bending moment at fracture.

A1.3.1.3 *bending structural stiffness, (EI_e) (N-m^2)*—of a bone plate, the bone plate's normalized effective bending stiffness that takes into consideration the effects of the test setup's configuration. For this test method the bending structural stiffness is determined from the single cycle bending response of the bone plate and the testing configuration.

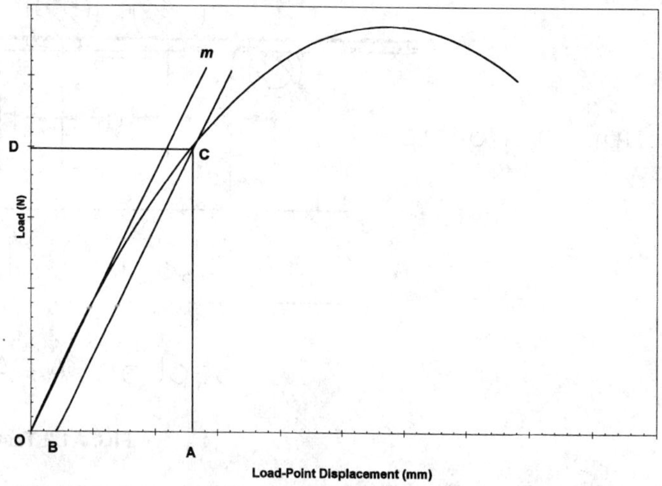

FIG. A1.1 Diagram Illustrating Methods For Determining Bending Properties of Bone Plates

A1.3.1.4 *bending stiffness, K (N/mm)—of a bone plate*, the maximum slope of the linear elastic portion of the load versus load-point curve when tested as described in section A1.8. (See the slope of line Om in Fig. A1.1).

A1.3.1.5 *bone plate width, w (mm)*—the width of the bone plate as shown in Fig. A1.3.

A1.3.1.6 *center span, a (mm)*—the distance between the two loading rollers as shown in Fig. A1.2.

A1.3.1.7 *fracture load, F_{max} (N)*—the applied load at the time when the bone plate fractures.

A1.3.1.8 *loading span, h (mm)*—the distance between the loading roller and the nearest support as shown in Fig. A1.2.

A1.3.1.9 *permanent deformation (mm)*—the vertical displacement of the point of load application remaining after the applied load has been removed.

A1.3.1.10 *proof load, P (N)*—the applied load at the intersection point of line. BC with the load versus load-point displacement curve. (See Fig. A1.1).

A1.3.1.11 *proof point displacement (mm)*—the load-point displacement associated with the bone plate's bending strength. (See point A in Fig. A1.1).

A1.3.1.12 *total deformation (mm)*—the vertical displacement of the point of application of the load when specified load is applied.

[4] *Annual Book of ASTM Standards*, Vol 03.01.

[5] *Annual Book of ASTM Standards*, Vol 14.02.

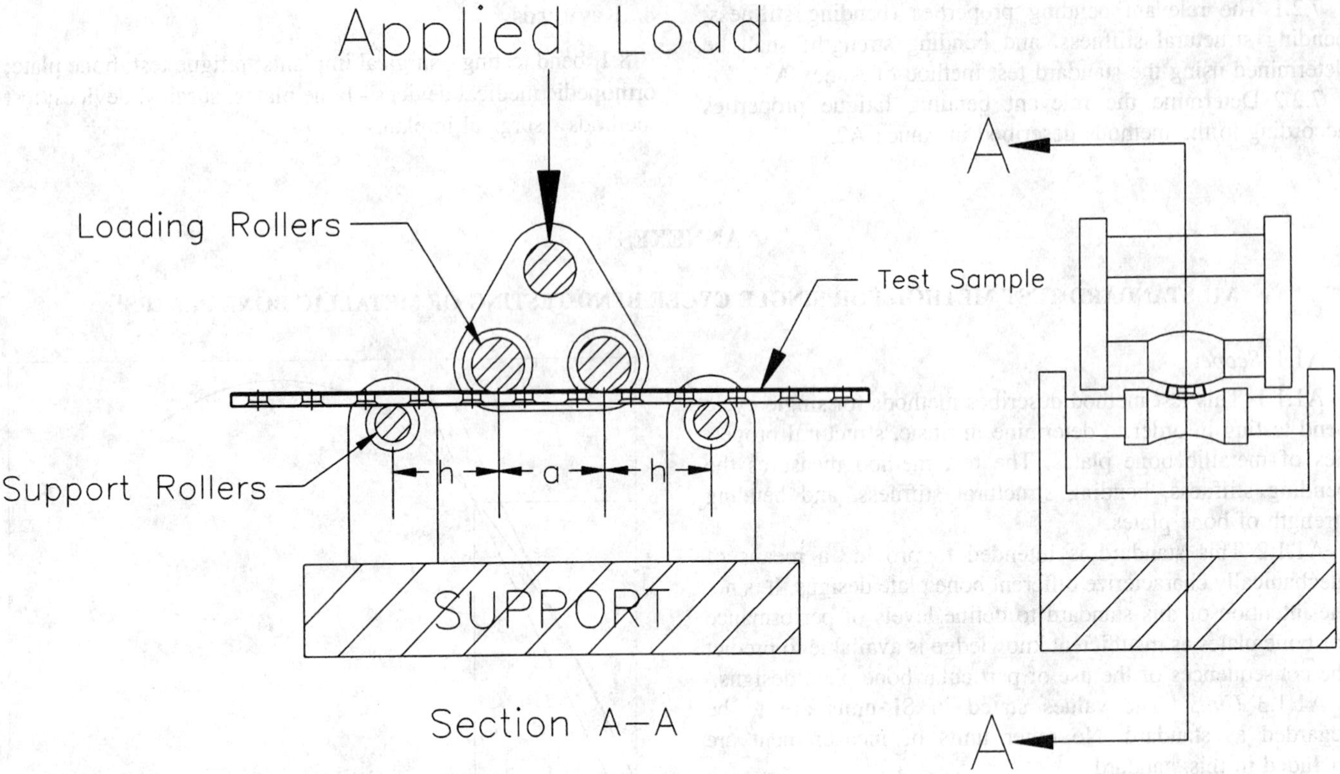

FIG. A1.2 Test Configuration

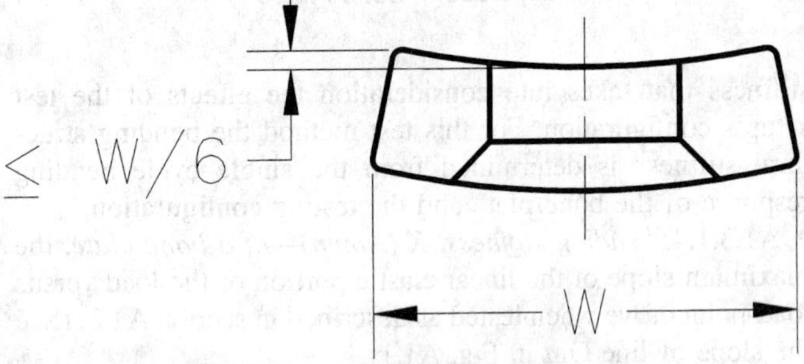

FIG. A1.3 Roller Profiling Requirements

A1.4 *Summary of Test Method*:

A1.4.1 Bone plates are subjected to a single cycle four-point bending load. The bone plate's bending stiffness, bending structural stiffness, and bending strength are then derived from the test record generated during the test and the testing configuration.

A1.5 *Significance and Use*:

A1.5.1 This bend test is used to determine values for the mechanical response of bone plates to a specific type of bending load. The information resulting from this test can give the surgeon some insight into the mechanical response of a given bone plate.

A1.5.2 Since the loading on the bone plate *in situ* will, in general differ from the loading configuration used in this method, the results obtained from this test method cannot be used directly to predict *in vivo* performance of the bone plate being tested. Such mechanical property data can be used to conduct relative comparisons of different bone plates designs.

A1.5.3 The bone plate's bending strength, as defined in Section A1.3.1.2, identifies the bending moment that must be applied to the bone plate in order to produce a specific amount a permanent deformation.

A1.5.4 The bending structural stiffness of the bone plate, as defined in Section A1.3.1.3, is an indicator of the bone plate's stiffness that is independent of the test configuration. Bending structural stiffness is simply related to the bone plate's geometry and the material used in manufacturing the bone plate.

A1.5.5 This test method assumes that linear-elastic material behavior will be observed and therefore, the method is not applicable for the testing of materials that exhibit non-linear elastic behavior.

A1.6 *Apparatus*:

A1.6.1 The typical test configuration is illustrated in Fig. A1.2.

A1.6.1.1 All loads shall be applied through rollers of equal diameters within the range of 6 to 12 mm. The selected roller diameter should not be greater than the distance between two adjacent screw holes in the bone plate to be tested.

A1.6.1.2 Cylindrical rollers shall be used to test flat bone plates and bone plates of curved cross-section, in which the deviation from flatness at the center of the bone plate does not exceed w/6. Test other bone plates using rollers of profiled form corresponding to the cross-section of the bone plate to be tested (see Fig. A1.3).

A1.6.1.3 The loading and support rollers shall be positioned as follows:

A1.6.1.3.1 The loading rollers shall be positioned so that

two screw holes will be located between the loading rollers. Record the center span distance.

A1.6.1.3.2 The support rollers shall be located equal distances away from the adjacent loading roller so that two screw holes will be located between the adjacent loading and support rollers. Record the distance between the loading roller and nearest support roller.

A1.6.1.3.3 The recommended testing configuration locates the loading rollers at approximately the one-third points between the supporting rollers.

A1.6.1.3.4 The applied load shall be shared equally by both loading rollers.

A1.6.1.4 Machines used for the bending test shall conform to the requirements of Practice E 4.

A1.6.2 The user is strongly encouraged to obtain bone plate test specimens of sufficient length that can be tested using the methods described in A1.6.1. However, alternative test configurations can be implemented to determine the single cycle bending properties of bone plates that do not lend themselves to the configuration of Sections A1.6.1 and A1.8.1. The user should bear in mind that the results obtained using the alternative method described below are not directly comparable to those obtained using the preferred method.

A1.6.2.1 Bonc plates that do not have sufficiently long section of symmetry or do not have a section of symmetry can be attached to rigid extension segments. The rigid extension segments can be used to effectively lengthen the bone plate so that the bone plate can be tested with the four point bend test method (see Fig. A1.4 for an illustration). For these tests, the following requirements apply.

A1.6.2.1.1 The rigid extension segments shall be designed so that they do not interfere with the bone plate's deformation during the single cycle bend test.

A1.6.2.1.2 The loading rollers shall contact the rigid extension segments of the test setup during the test.

A1.6.2.1.3 At the completion of the single cycle bend test, the bone plate anchor shall be examined in order to determine if the indicated permanent deformation can be related to the mechanical performance of the anchoring system.

A1.6.2.2 Alternative test configurations utilized in determining the single cycle bending properties of bone plates shall be described in the test report.

A1.7 *Sampling*:

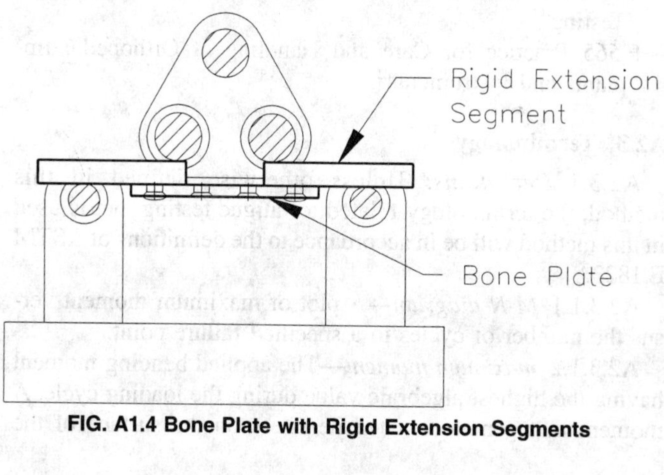

FIG. A1.4 Bone Plate with Rigid Extension Segments

A1.7.1 Determine sample size using the methods outlined in Practice E 122.

A1.7.2 Bone plates of different lengths but nominally identical cross sections, and made of the same material, may be used to constitute a sample.

A1.8 *Procedure*:

A1.8.1 Place the bone plate in the testing fixture and position it in accordance with the following:

A1.8.1.1 Place the bone plate so that the loading rollers are in contact with the surface of the bone plate intended to be in contact with the bone.

A1.8.1.2 If the bone plate is symmetrical, place it symmetrically with the two innermost screw holes between the loading rollers.

A1.8.1.3 If the bone plate has a central screw hole, place it with the central screw hole and one other screw hole symmetrically between the loading rollers.

A1.8.1.4 If the bone plate is asymmetrical, place it with two screw holes between the loading rollers so that the position of the fracture for which it is intended to be used shall be between the loading rollers.

A1.8.1.5 Ensure that the loading rollers are not in contact with parts of the bone plate where there is a screw hole. Wherever possible, the support rollers should not be in contact with parts of the bone plate which include a screw hole.

A1.8.1.6 Align the long axis of the bone plate so that it is perpendicular to the axes of the rollers.

A1.8.2 Apply loads of increasing magnitude, and generate a load versus load-point displacement diagram either autographically or from numeric data acquired during the test.

NOTE A1.2—Displacement-controlled testing is strongly preferred over load-controlled testing. The measured deformation behavior past the yield point can be different for load-controlled testing due to non-linear displacement rates.

A1.8.3 Determine the bending stiffness, bending structural stiffness, and bending strength for each tested bone plate according to the method that follows:

A1.8.3.1 A load versus load-point displacement curve (see Fig. A1.1) is produced either autographically or from numerical data acquired during the test.

A1.8.3.1.1 On the load versus load-point displacement diagram generated for the test, draw a best fit straight line (Om) through the initial (linear) portion of the load versus load-point displacement curve.

A1.8.3.1.2 Determine the bone plate's bending stiffness by calculating the slope of the line, Om, drawn in Section 8.3.1.1.

A1.8.3.1.3 Determine the bone plate's bending structural stiffness with the following expression:

$$EI_e = \frac{(2h + 3a)Kh^2}{12} \quad (A1.1)$$

where:
K = the bending stiffness,
a = the center span distance, and
h = the loading span distance.

NOTE A1.3—Since the test method requires the inclusion of screw holes the center span region, then the bone plate's bending structural stiffness really represents and average of the EI_e over the center span region.

A1.8.3.1.4 Calculate the 0.2 % offset displacement from the expression:

$$q = 0.002 \times a \quad \text{(A1.2)}$$

where:
a = the center span distance.

A1.8.3.1.5 On the load versus load-point displacement diagram lay off OB equal to q. Then draw line BC parallel to Om.

A1.8.3.1.6 Locate the proof load at the intersection point of line BC with the load versus load-point displacement curve.

A1.8.3.1.7 Calculate the bending strength of the bone plate from the expression:

$$\text{bending strength} = \frac{(Ph)}{2} \quad \text{(A1.3)}$$

where:
P = the proof load, and
h = the loading span distance.

A1.8.3.1.8 If the bone plate fractures prior to the load versus load-point displacement curve intersects the offset line BC, calculate the bending strength from the expression:

$$\text{bending strength} = \frac{F_{max} \times h}{2} \quad \text{(A1.4)}$$

where:
F_{max} = the fracture load, and
h = the loading span distance.

NOTE A1.4—It should be noted that these bending strength equations are only valid while the bone plate under test is exhibiting linear elastic behavior. The user is cautioned of this fact since this method may produce bending strength results that may not necessarily be equal to the corresponding theoretical calculations.

A1.9 *Report*:

A1.9.1 Report the following information:

A1.9.1.1 Adequate description of the test material, including the number of bone plates tested,

A1.9.1.2 Adequate description of the test configuration,

A1.9.1.2.1 The center span and loading span dimensions (*h* and *a*),

A1.9.1.3 The 0.2 % offset displacement, *q*, used to determine the bending strength,

A1.9.1.4 Mean and standard deviations of the bending stiffness values for the set of bone plates tested,

A1.9.1.5 Mean and standard deviations of the bending structural stiffness values for the set of bone plates tested,

A1.9.1.6 Mean and standard deviation of the bending strength values for the set of bone plates tested, and

A1.9.1.6.1 Number of bone plates fractured during the test.

A1.9.1.7 The method (either displacement or load) and rate utilized for controlling the test.

A1.10 *Precision and Bias*:

A1.10.1 *Precision*—Data establishing the precision of the test method have not yet been obtained.

A1.10.2 *Bias*—No statement of bias can be made, since no acceptable reference values are available, nor can they be obtained since this test is a destructive test.

A2. STANDARD TEST METHOD FOR DETERMINING THE BENDING FATIGUE PROPERTIES OF METALLIC BONE PLATES

A2.1 Scope

A2.1.1 This test method describes methods for bending fatigue testing in order to determine intrinsic, metallic bone plate structural properties. The test method may be used to determine the fatigue life at a specific or over a range of maximum bending moment levels, or to estimate the fatigue strength for a specified number of fatigue cycles of a bone plate.

A2.1.2 This standard is intended to provide a means to mechanically characterize different bone plate designs. It is not the intention of this standard to define bone plate performance levels since insufficient knowledge is available to predict the consequences of the use of a particular bone plate design.

A2.1.3 *Units*—The values stated in SI units are to be regarded as standard. No other units of measurement are included in this standard.

A2.1.4 *This standard does not purport to address all of the safety concerns, if any, associated with its use. It is the responsibility of the user of this standard to establish appropriate safety and health practices and to determine the applicability of regulatory limitations prior to use.*

NOTE A2.1—There is currently no ISO standard that is similar or equivalent to this standard test method.

A2.2 Referenced Documents

A2.2.1 *ASTM Standards:*

E 4 Practices for Load Verification of Testing Machines[4]

E 467 Standard Practice for Verification of Constant Amplitude Dynamic Forces in an Axial Fatigue Testing System[4]

E 1823 Standard Terminology Relating to Fatigue and Fracture Testing[4]

E 1942 Standard Guide for Evaluating Data Acquisition Systems Used in Cyclic Fatigue and Fracture Mechanics Testing[4]

F 565 Practice for Care and Handling of Orthopedic Implants and Instruments[2]

A2.3. Terminology

A2.3.1 *Definitions:* Unless otherwise defined in this method, the terminology related to fatigue testing that is used in this method will be in accordance to the definitions of ASTM E 1823.

A2.3.1.1 *M-N diagram*—A plot of maximum moment versus the number of cycles to a specified failure point.

A2.3.1.2 *maximum moment*—The applied bending moment having the highest algebraic value during the loading cycle. A moment that generates a tensile stress on the surface of the bone plate specimen that contacts the outer support rollers (as shown in Fig. A2.1) is considered positive. Correspondingly, a moment that generates a compressive stress is considered negative.

A2.3.1.3 *median fatigue strength at* 10^6 cycles—An estimate of the maximum moment at which 50 % of the specimens of a given sample population would be expected to survive 106 loading cycles at a given R-ratio.

A2.3.1.4 *minimum moment*—The applied bending moment having the lowest algebraic value during the loading cycle. A moment that generates a tensile stress on the surface of the bone plate specimen that contacts the outer support rollers (as shown in Fig. A2.1). is considered positive. Correspondingly, a moment that generates a compressive stress is considered negative.

A2.3.1.5 *R-ratio*—The algebraic ratio relating the minimum and maximum values of the loading parameters of a fatigue cycle. For the purposes of this test method the R-ratio is defined as:

$$R = \frac{Minimum\ Moment}{Maximum\ Moment} \tag{A2.1}$$

A2.3.1.6 *runout*—A predetermined number of cycles at which the testing on a particular specimen stopped, and no further testing on that specimen will be performed. When the intent of the fatigue test program is to determine the fatigue strength at N cycles, the runout is usually specified as N cycles.

A2.4 Summary of Test Method

A2.4.1 A bone plate is placed in a four point bending fixture and oriented in such a way so that the bone plate's section that would normally bridge the fracture site is subjected to a uniform bending moment along the length of the section length. The bone plate is subjected to a constant frequency sinusoidal cyclic load waveform in four-point bending situation. The fatigue loading is continued until the specimen fails, a limit is reached which is indicative of failure, or the runout cycle count is reached.

A2.4.2 The data generated from a series of test samples is compiled and presented in a manner that is consistent with the goals of the study. The results can either be presented in a semi-log M-N diagram that will characterize the general fatigue behavior of the bone plate over a range of applied bending moments or simply the fatigue strength determined at 10^6 cycles.

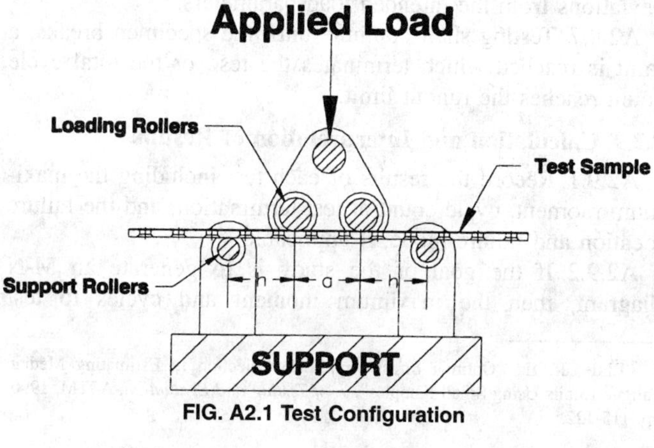

FIG. A2.1 Test Configuration

A2.5 Significance and Use

A2.5.1 The test method establishes a uniform four-point bending fatigue test to characterize and compare the fatigue performance of different bone plate designs. This method may be used to determine a bone plate's fatigue life at either a specific or over a range of maximum bending moment conditions. Additionally, the method may be alternatively used to estimate a bone plate's fatigue strength for a specified number of fatigue cycles.

A2.5.2 The test method utilizes a simplified bone plate load model that may not be exactly representative of the in-situ loading configuration. The user should note that the test results generated by this test method can not be used to directly predict the *in vivo* performance of the bone plate being tested. The data generated from this test method can be used to conduct relative comparisons of different bone plate designs.

A2.5.3 This test method may not be appropriate for all types of implant applications. The user is cautioned to consider the appropriateness of the method in view of the devices being tested and their potential application.

A2.5.4 This test method assumes that the bone plate is manufactured from a material that exhibits linear-elastic material behavior. Therefore, the method is not applicable for testing bone plates made from materials that exhibit non-linear elastic behavior.

A2.5.5 This test method is restricted to the testing of bone plates within the materials' linear-elastic range. Therefore, the method is not applicable for testing bone plates under conditions that would approach or exceed the bending strength of the bone plate being tested.

A2.6 Apparatus

A2.6.1 Test machines used for the bending fatigue test shall conform to the requirements of Practice E 4 and E 467.

A2.6.2 The suitability of any data acquisition systems used in monitoring the progress of these tests should be evaluated in accordance to the guidelines of Guide E 1942.

A2.6.3 The typical four-point bend test configuration employed for this test is illustrated in Fig. A2.1.

A2.6.3.1 The test fixture is configured in accordance to the requirements of either section A1.6.1 or A1.6.2 of Annex A1 of this standard.

A2.6.3.2 The test fixture employed should provide a means to prevent the expulsion of the test specimen during the fatigue test. Whatever means is selected, the specimen must be free to bend in response to the applied load and shall not affect the loading situation generated in the test specimen.

A2.6.4 A cycle counter is required that is capable of counting the cumulative number of loading cycles that are applied to the specimen during the course of the fatigue test.

A2.6.5 When required, a limit detector that is capable of sensing when a test parameter (for example, load, actuator displacement, DC error, and so on) reaches a limiting value and produces a signal or action that terminates the test.

A2.7 Test Specimens and Sampling

A2.7.1 All test components shall be representative of implant quality products with regard to material, cross-section, surface finish, markings, and manufacturing processes. Any deviation from this requirement must be noted in the final report.

A2.7.2 Per ASTM Practice F 565, bone plates that have been either implanted or contoured (reshaped) for implantation are not suitable for this test method and shall be excluded from the sample.

A2.7.3 Bone plates of different lengths but nominally identical cross sections, and made of the same material, may be used to constitute a sample.

A2.7.4 *M-N Diagram Testing:* The minimum sample size necessary for reporting the fatigue life of a given bone plate at a given maximum bending moment condition is three. A rudimentary M-N diagram with a corresponding fatigue curve would require three replicate tests at three load levels. Under ideal conditions, conduct five replicate tests at each of five maximum bending moment levels in order to enhance the statistical significance of the resulting information.

A2.7.5 *Fatigue Strength Testing:* No minimum sample size can be identified for this testing method since the total number of data points needed to make such a determination is dependent upon the methodology used and many other related factors. The user should be aware that such a study may require approximately twenty test specimens in order to generate statistically meaningful results.

A2.8 Procedure

A2.8.1 Prior to testing, the load level(s) for testing must be determined. To evaluate the fatigue performance of a bone plate, the user has several methodologies at their disposal whose selection is based upon the output goals of the study. Two recommended methods are as follows.

A2.8.1.1 *M-N Diagram:* The user may test a given bone plate design over a range of maximum bending moment levels to characterize the general fatigue behavior trend of the device. The user's experience is the best guide that can be used for determining the initial loading conditions. In the absence of such experience, the best recommendation would be to use initial fatigue loads corresponding to 75, 50, and 25 % of the bending strength determined in accordance to this standard's Annex A1 test method. The applied moment and the cycle to test termination data are then plotted on a semi-log M-N diagram. A curve fit may be appropriately applied to the data to develop an M-N curve.

A2.8.1.2 *Fatigue Strength Determination:* The user may also test a given bone plate design in order to determine the fatigue strength at a given number of fatigue cycles. This method recommends that the fatigue strength be determined at a 1 million loading cycles (see rationale in Appendix X3). The maximum difference between the load levels used for the fatigue strength determination shall be no greater than 10 % of the bending strength determined in accordance to this standard's Annex A1 test method. Acceptable methods which can be employed to determine the bone plate's fatigue strength include the up and down method and a modified up and down method.[6,7]

A2.8.2 Place the bone plate in the testing fixture and position it in accordance with the following:

A2.8.2.1 Place the bone plate so that the loading rollers are in contact with the surface of the bone plate intended to be in contact with the bone.

A2.8.2.2 If the bone plate is symmetrical, place it symmetrically with the two innermost screw holes between the loading rollers.

A2.8.2.3 If the bone plate has a central screw hole, place it with the central screw hole and one other screw hole symmetrically between the loading rollers.

A2.8.2.4 If the bone plate is asymmetrical (as in the case with most specialty plates), place it with two screw holes between the loading rollers so that the position of the fracture for which it is intended to be used is located between the loading rollers.

A2.8.2.5 Ensure that the loading rollers are not in contact with plate sections that contain a screw hole. If it is not possible to meet this requirement with the bone plate design being tested, then the alternative configuration recommended in section A1.6.2 of Annex A1 of this standard should be used for the fatigue test.

A2.8.2.6 Align the long axis of the bone plate so that it is perpendicular to the axes of the rollers.

A2.8.3 Ensure that the applied load is equally shared between the test specimen loading points. The magnitude of the applied load is determined from the following expression.

$$P = \frac{2M}{h} \quad \text{(A2.2)}$$

Where M is the maximum moment and h is the loading span distance (see Fig. A2.1).

A2.8.4 Load the test specimen with the test system in load control using an appropriate waveform so that the resultant time dependent bending moment generated in the test specimen is cyclic and sinusoidal in nature. Select a cyclic frequency for the tests that will not produce strain sensitive affects in the bone plate's material. Typically, a cyclic frequency of 5 Hz is more than adequate for completing the test in a timely manner and will still not affect the bone plate's material.

A2.8.5 The recommended R-ratio is 0.1. Any deviations from this should be reported and justified in the final report.

A2.8.6 The cycle counter shall record the cumulative number of cycles applied to the test specimen, and the appropriate limits should be set to indicate specimen failure and/or deviations from the intended load parameters.

A2.8.7 Testing shall continue until the specimen breaks, a limit is reached which terminates the test, or the total cycle count reaches the runout limit.

A2.9 Calculation and Interpretation of Results

A2.9.1 Record the results of each test including the maximum moment, cycle count at test termination, and the failure location and failure mode, if applicable.

A2.9.2 If the goal of the study is to generate an M-N diagram, then the maximum moment and cycles to test

[6] Little, R. E., and Jebe, E. H.: *Manual on Statistical Planning and Analysis for Fatigue Experiments*, STP 588, American Society of Testing and Materials, 100 Barr Harbor Drive, West Conshohocken, PA, 19428, 1975.

[7] Little, R. E., "Optimal Stress Amplitude Selection in Estimating Median Fatigue Limits Using Small Samples", *J. of Testing and Evaluation*, ASTM, 1990, pp. 115-122.

termination data is plotted on a semi-log graph. Various techniques may be used to estimate the mean or median fatigue lives, statistical differences between groups, curve fits to the fatigue data, probability of survival curves, etc.[8,9]

A2.9.3 If the goal of the study is to determine the fatigue strength at 10^6 cycles, it is recommended that the fatigue strength be determined as the median fatigue limit (50 % probability of survival), using acceptable techniques.[6,7]

A2.10 Report

A2.10.1 The test report will include the following information:

A2.10.1.1 Manufacturer of the bone plate specimen.

A2.10.1.2 The bone plate description and catalog number (if applicable).

A2.10.1.3 The bone plate material including applicable ASTM or ISO specifications.

A2.10.1.4 Deviations from normal implant product.

A2.10.1.5 The center and loading span dimensions (h and a).

A2.10.1.6 The loading roller diameters and profile.

A2.10.1.7 R-ratio.

A2.10.1.8 Test frequency.

A2.10.1.9 Description of the test environment.

A2.10.1.10 Deviations from recommended test method.

A2.10.1.11 Tabular listing that summarizes the maximum moment and the resulting cycles to test termination data.

A2.10.1.12 A description of the failure mode and failure location for each specimen which failed.

A2.10.1.13 If appropriate, a semi-log plot of the M-N diagram is generated. Include descriptions of any analytical or statistical techniques used when interpreting the fatigue data.

A2.10.1.14 If appropriate, an estimate of the fatigue strength should be reported. Include descriptions of any analytical or statistical techniques used for determining the fatigue strength.

A2.11 Precision and Bias

A2.11.1 *Precision*—Data establishing the precision of the test method have not yet been obtained.

A2.11.2 *Bias*—No statement of bias can be made, since no acceptable reference values are available, nor can they be obtained since this test is a destructive test.

[8] Conway, J. B., and Sjodahl, L. H.: *Analysis and Representation of Fatigue Data*, ASM International, Materials Park, OH, 1991.

[9] Collins, J. A.: *Failure of Materials in Mechanical Design*, John Wiley and Sons, New York, NY, 1981.

APPENDIXES

(Nonmandatory Information)

X1. RATIONALE FOR SPECIFICATION

X1.1 This specification is intended to provide useful and consistent information related to the terminology, performance, application of test methods, and the application of bone plates used for maintenance of alignment and fixation during the bone healing process. Bone plate geometrical definitions, classification and terminology; material specifications; and performance definitions are provided.

X1.2 The orthopaedic surgeon should be able to select the device that they feel is appropriate for the indication. In order to do this, the surgeon must have confidence that the device's designation and sizing has a specific, known meaning that is quantifiable and reliable regardless of the manufacturer or design. The mechanical behavior and material properties must also be described in a reliable, known manner which is irrespective of the manufacturer or design. In order to accomplish this uniformity of designations, the terminology, mechanical properties, material properties must be standardized.

X1.3 The subcommittee's goal is to produce a single standard identifying all pertinent information, requirements, and test methods for orthopedic bone plates. The first step in achieving this goal was to combine the current versions of F 382 and F 786. This revision of F 382 completes this first step. Additional subcommittee goals include the development of a bending fatigue and torsion test methods.

X2. RATIONALE FOR ANNEX A1

X2.1 This test method is designed to measure the mechanical properties of bone plates subjected to bending, which is the most common type of loading encountered *in vivo*. This test method addresses itself to properties of the device rather than the material from which the bone plate is made. A four-plate loading is specified since is produces a constant moment over the central span.

X2.2 The key quantities that are assessed (bending stiffness, bending structural stiffness, and bending strength) provide the user information on the bone plate's strength and stiffness.

X2.3 The previous version of this test method included an assessment of the bone plate's ductile behavior. Although this information is useful to the user, the supporting information needed to conduct this evaluation was not available. Therefore, the bone plate's ductile behavior evaluation has been eliminated from the test method.

X2.4 The offset displacement criteria used to determine the bone plate's bending strength has been reduced from 2 % to 0.2 % in the standard's current version. This was done for two reasons; (1) to establish a bending strength criteria that was minimally influenced by nonelastic bending of the bone plate, and (2) to make the test method consistent with the previous version of the F 382 standard test method. In the previous version of the standard the center span length was set at 1.57 inches with an offset displacement criteria of 0.004 in. (approximately 0.2 % of the center span length). The use of a 2 % offset displacement criteria would result in nearly eight times as much permanent deformation to occur to prior to establishing the bone plate's yield point. One typically chooses an offset that is small enough so that the elastic limit has just been reached, but large enough so that any slippage or singular behavior at the elastic limit is avoided (0.1 % and 0.2 % for the ASTM tensile test). The use of the 2 % offset displacement criteria would result in the determination of the bone plate's bending strength that has little meaning since it is located well into the plastic region. Therefore, the adoption of the 0.2 % offset criteria will satisfy both requirements.

X2.5 The test method has been adapted to accommodate the testing of smaller bone plates and/or plates that do not have enough screw holes to meet the requirements of Sections A1.6.1 and A1.8.1. In order to accommodate these tests, the option to add rigid extension segments to the bone plate being tested is allowed (see Section A1.6.2). These extension segments effectively lengthen the bone plate so that the four point bend test configuration can be used to impart a nearly constant bending moment along the section of the bone plate located in the center span of the test setup. This is the only feasible means to test bone plates that have less that six optimally located screw holes.

X3. RATIONALE FOR ANNEX A2

X3.1 Bone plate fatigue properties are an important factor when considering the surgical treatment of skeletal fractures. The bone plate may be subjected to a significant number of repetitive stress cycles during the healing process. In some situations, the bone plate may be expected to experience these conditions for several weeks until the bone healing process progresses adequately so that the bone can provide mechanical support which will reduce the stresses in the bone plate. Therefore, it is important for the surgeon to have some means to judge the fatigue performance of a given bone plate.

X3.2 Since the time frame, number of loading cycles and loading conditions are uncontrollable and unpredictable, there is no acceptable limit which can be set for the bending moment or number of cycles of load which the bone plate should withstand in any given case.

X3.3 One of the objectives of this test method is to provide a consistent methodology for determining an estimate of the bone plate fatigue strength at 10^6 cycles for comparative purposes. Bone plates are classified as temporary skeletal fixation devices since fractures and skeletal deformity corrections are generally resolved within 2-3 months (approximately 150 000 to 250 000 cycles). Even though the test method's recommendation of one million cycles for estimating the fatigue strength has been arbitrarily chosen, it still can be considered conservative since no bone plate in clinical service would normally be expected to withstand 10^6 high stress loading cycles.

X3.4 The reporting of cyclic bending fatigue strength and/or fatigue life using this standard testing technique are only suitable for comparative evaluations between devices of different sizes, designs, and materials.

Designation: F 384 – 00

Standard Specifications and Test Methods for Metallic Angled Orthopedic Fracture Fixation Devices[1]

This standard is issued under the fixed designation F 384; the number immediately following the designation indicates the year of original adoption or, in the case of revision, the year of last revision. A number in parentheses indicates the year of last reapproval. A superscript epsilon (ϵ) indicates an editorial change since the last revision or reapproval.

1. Scope

1.1 This standard is intended to provide a comprehensive reference for angled devices used in the surgical internal fixation of the skeletal system. This standard establishes consistent methods to classify and define the geometric and performance characteristics of angled devices. This standard also presents a catalog of standard specifications that specify material and labeling and handling requirements, and standard test methods for measuring performance related mechanical characteristics determined to be important to the *in vivo*performance of angled devices.

1.2 It is not the intention of this standard to define levels of performance of case-specific clinical performance for angled devices, as insufficient knowledge is available to predict the consequences of their use in individual patients for specific activities of daily living. Futhermore, it is not the intention of this standard to describe or specify specific designs for angled devices used in the surgical internal fixation of the skeletal system.

1.3 This standard may not be appropriate for all types of angled devices. The user is cautioned to consider the appropriateness of this standard in view of a particular angled device and its potential application.

1.4 This standard includes the following test methods used in determining the following angled device mechanical performance characteristics:

1.4.1 Standard test method for single cycle compression bend testing of metallic angled orthopedic fracture fixation devices (see Annex A1).

1.4.2 Standard test method for determining the bending fatigue properties of metallic angled orthopedic fracture fixation devices (see Annex A2).

1.5 Unless otherwise indicated, the values stated in SI units shall be regarded as the standard.

NOTE 1—There is currently no ISO standard that is either similar to equivalent to this standard.

2. Referenced Documents

2.1 *ASTM Standards:*

E 4 Practices for Force Verification of Testing Machines[2]

E 8 Test Methods for Tension Testing of Metallic Materials[2]

E 122 Practice for Choice of Sample Size to Estimate the Average Quality of a Lot or Process[3]

F 67 Specification for Unalloyed Titanium for Surgical Implant Applications[4]

F 75 Specification for Cobalt-28 Chromium-6 Molybdenum Casting Alloy and Cast Products for Surgical Implants (UNS R30075)[4]

F 90 Specification for Wrought Cobalt-20 Chromium 15 Tungsten-10 Nickel Alloy for Surgical Implant Applications (R30605)[4]

F 136 Specification for Wrought Titanium-6 Aluminum-4 Vanadium ELI (Extra Low Interstitial) Alloy (UNS R56401) for Surgical Implant Applications[4]

F 138 Specification for Wrought-18 Chromium-14 Nickel-2.5 Molybdenum Stainless Steel Bar and Wire for Surgical Implants (UNS S31673)

F 139 Specification for Wrought-18 Chromium-14 Nickel-2.5 Molybdenum Stainless Steel Sheet and Strip for Surgical Implants (UNS S31673)[4]

F 382 Specification and Test Methods for Metallic Bone Plates[4]

F 543 Specification for Metallic Medical Bone Screws[4]

F 565 Practice for Care and Handling of Orthopedic Implants and Instruments[4]

F 620 Specification for Titanium-6 Aluminum-4 Vanadium ELI Alloy Forgings for Surgical Implants (UNS R56401)[4]

F 621 Specification for Stainless Steel Forgings for Surgical Implants[4]

F 983 Practice for Permanent Marking of Orthopedic Implant Components[4]

F 1295 Specification for Wrought Titanium-6 Aluminum-7 Niobium Alloy for Surgical Implant Applications (UNS R56700)[4]

F 1314 Specification for Wrought Nitrogen Strengthened-22 Chromium-12.5 Nickel-5 Manganese -2.5 Molybdenum Stainless Steel Bar and Wire for Surgical Implants[4]

F 1472 Specification for Wrought Titanium-6 Aluminum-4

[1] These specifications and test methods are under the jurisdiction of ASTM Committee F04 on Medical and Surgical Materials and Devices and are the direct responsibility of Subcommittee F04.21 on Osteosynthesis.

Current edition approved Nov. 10, 2000. Published February 2001. Originally published as F 384 - 73. Last previous edition F 384 - 99.

[2] *Annual Book of ASTM Standards*. Vol 03.01.

[3] *Annual Book of ASTM Standards*. Vol 14.02.

[4] *Annual Book of ASTM Standards*. Vol 13.01.

Vanadium Alloy for Surgical Implant Applications (UNS R56400)[4]

F 1713 Specification for Wrought Titanium -13 Niobium-13 Zirconium Alloy for Surgical Implant Applications[4]

2.2 *ISO Standards:*[5]

ISO 5835 Implants for Surgery - Metal Bone Screws with Hexagonal Drive Connection - Spherical Under Surface of Head, Asymmetrical Thread

ISO 5836 Implants for Surgery - Metal Bone Plates - Holes Corresponding to Screws with Asymmetrical Thread and Spherical Under Surface

ISO 9268 Implants for Surgery - Metal Bone Screws with Conical Under-Surface of Head - Dimensions

ISO 9269 Implants for Surgery - Metal Bone Plates - Holes and Slots Corresponding to Screws with Conical Under-Surface

ISO14602 Non-active Surgical Implants– Implants for Osteosynthesis – Particular Requirements

3. Terminology

3.1 *Definitions:* Geometric

3.1.1 *angle, n*—defined at either the barrel/sideplate or blade/sideplate junction (see Fig. 1 and Fig. 2).

3.1.2 *angled device, n*—a class of orthopedic devices for the fixation of fractures in the metaphyseal areas of long bones that has a component aligned at an angle to the bone's long axis.

3.1.3 *barrel, n*—the portion of an angled device which captures the lag screw (see Fig. 1).

3.1.4 *barrel length, L_{BR}, n*— the distance from the free end of the barrel to the interior vertex of the barrel/sideplate junction (see Fig. 1).

3.1.5 *blade, n*—the portion of an angled device which transmits the off axis loading of the anatomical loading condition to the sideplate portion of the angled device (see Fig. 2).

3.1.6 *blade length, L_{BD}, n*—the distance from the free end of the blade to the interior vertex of the blade/sideplate junction (see Fig. 2).

[5] Available form American National Standards Institute, 11 W. 42nd St., New York, NY 10036.

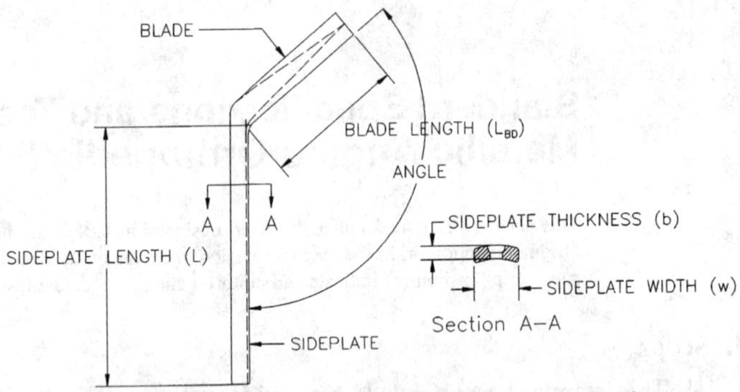

FIG. 2 Diagram Illustrating Blade Plate Angled Devices

3.1.7 *lag screw, n*—that component of a compression hip screw angled device which is threaded into the metaphyses and transmits the off axis load to the sideplate through the barrel (see Fig. 1).

3.1.8 *lag screw length, n*—the straight line distance measured between the proximal and distal ends of the lag screw (see Fig. 1).

3.1.9 *sideplate, n*—that portion of the angle device generally aligned with the bone's long axis which attaches to the bone via bone screws (see Fig. 1 and Fig. 2).

3.1.10 *sideplate length, L, n*—the distance from the free end of the sideplate to the interior vertex of the barrel/sideplate junction, shown in Fig. 1 and Fig. 2.

3.1.11 *sideplate thickness, b, n*—the thickness of the sideplate as shown in Fig. 1 and Fig. 2.

3.1.12 *sideplate width, w, n*—the width of the sideplate as shown in Fig. 1 and Fig. 2.

3.1.13 *thread diameter, n*—the maximum outside diameter of the lag screw (see Fig. 1).

3.1.14 *thread length, n*—the straight line distance measured between the tip and thread runout positions of the screw (see Fig. 1).

3.2 *Definitions:* Mechanical/Structure:

3.2.1 *bending strength, n— of the sideplate*, the bending moment necessary to produce a 0.2 % offset displacement in the sideplate when tested as described in Annex A1 of Specification and Test Methods F 382.

3.2.2 *bending structural stiffness, El_e, n—of the sideplate*, the sideplate's normalized effective bending stiffness that takes

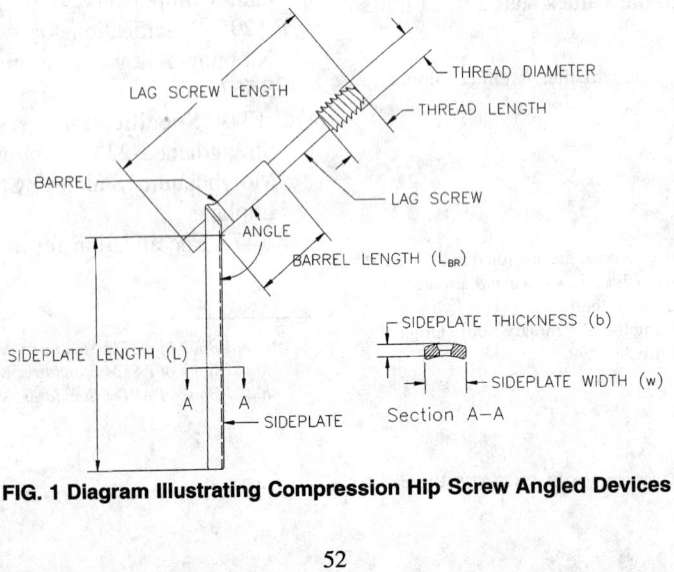

FIG. 1 Diagram Illustrating Compression Hip Screw Angled Devices

into consideration the effects of the test setup's configuration when tested according to the method described in Annex A1 of Specification and Test Methods F 382.

3.2.3 *compression bending stiffness, (K), n—of a device*, the maximum slope of the linear elastic portion of the load versus displacement curve, when tested as described in Annex A1.

3.2.4 *compression bending strength, n—of a device*, the bending moment necessary to produce a 0.2 % offset displacement in the device when tested as described in Annex A1.

3.2.5 *fatigue strength at N cycles, n*—an estimate of the cyclic forcing parameter, for example, load, moment, torque, stress, etc., at a given load ratio, for which 50 % of the specimens within a given sample population would be expected to survive *N* loading cycles.

3.2.6 *fatigue life, N, n*—the number of loading cycles of a specified character that a given specimen sustains before failure of a specified nature occurs.

4. Classification

4.1 Angled devices used in general orthopedic surgery represent a subset of bone plates. Angled devices are mainly used in the treatment of fractures in the metaphyseal areas of long bones. Angled devices can be categorized into general types according to the following classifications:

4.1.1 *Blade Plate*— an angled device where the component of the device that is oriented at an angle from the long axis of the bone is fixed relative to the sideplate; this component often is shaped like a blade to achieve fixation into the metaphyses (see Fig. 2), and

4.1.2 *Compression Hip Screw*—an angled device where the component of the device which is oriented at a angle from the long axis of the bone is free to translate relative to the sideplate through a barrel; this component often achieves fixation into the metaphyses through the use of deep threads (see Fig. 1).

5. Marking, Packaging, Labeling and Handling

5.1 Dimensions of angled devices should be designated by the standard definitions given in 3.1.

5.2 Angled devices shall be marked using a method specified in accordance with either Practice F 983 or ISO 14602.

5.3 Markings on angled devices shall identify the manufacture or distributor and shall be made away from the most highly stressed areas, where possible.

5.4 Packaging shall be adequate to protect the angled device during shipment.

5.5 Package labeling for angled devices shall include when possible the following information;

5.5.1 Manufacturer and product name,

5.5.2 Catalog number,

5.5.3 Lot or serial number,

5.5.4 Material and, where applicable, its associated ASTM specification designation number,

5.5.5 Device angle,

5.5.6 Barrel (blade) length,

5.5.7 Number of screw holes,

5.5.8 Sideplate width,

5.5.9 Sideplate length,

5.5.10 Sideplate thickness,

5.5.11 Screw hole size, and

5.5.12 ASTM specification designation number.

5.6 Bone plates should be cared for and handled in accordance with Practice F 565, as appropriate.

6. Materials

6.1 All angled devices made of materials which can be purchased to an ASTM specification shall meet those requirements given in the ASTM specification. Such specification include: F 67, F 75, F 90, F 139, F 543, F 1295, F 1314, F 1472, and F 1713.

6.2 Angled devices of forged Specification F 136 shall meet the requirements of Specification F 620.

6.3 Angled devices of forged Specification F 138 shall meet the requirements of Specification F 621.

7. General Requirements and Performance Considerations

7.1 *Geometric Considerations*—For angled devices that are intended to be used with bone screws that conform to ISO 5835 or ISO 9268, the screw holes shall correspond to the dimensions and tolerances of ISO 5836 or ISO 9269, respectively.

7.2 *Bending Properties*—Bending properties are a critical characteristic of angled devices for orthopedic applications since the plate provides the primary means of stabilizing the bone fragments. Additionally, the bending stiffness of the angled device may directly affect the rate and ability of healing.

7.2.1 The relevant compression bending properties (compression bending stiffness and compression bending strength) of the device shall be determined using Annex A1.

7.2.2 The relevant bending properties (bending stiffness, bending structural stiffness and bending strength) of the sideplate shall be determined using the Annex A1 of Specification and Test Methods F 382.

7.2.3 Determine the relevant angled device bending fatigue properties according to the methods described in Annex A2.

7.2.4 Determine the relevant side plate bending fatigue properties according to the methods described in Annex A2 of Specification and Test Methods F 382.

8. Keywords

8.1 angled devices; bend testing; blade plate; compression hip screw; fatigue test; orthopedic medical devices; surgical devices; surgical implants

ANNEXES

(Mandatory Information)

A1. STANDARD TEST METHOD FOR SINGLE CYCLE COMPRESSION BEND TESTING OF METALLIC ANGLED ORTHOPEDIC FRACTURE FIXATION DEVICES

A1.1 Scope

A1.1.1 This test method describes methods for single cycle bend testing for determining intrinsic, structural properties of metallic angled orthopedic fracture fixation devices. The test method measures the angled device's compression bending stiffness and compression bending strength.

A1.1.2 This test method is intended to provide a means to mechanically characterize different angled device designs. It is not the intention of this test method to define levels of performance for angled devices, as insufficient knowledge is available to predict the consequences of the use of particular angled device designs.

A1.1.3 This test method is designed to provide flexibility in the testing configuration so that a range of clinical failure modes for the angled fixation devices (for example, sideplate, lag screw, and barrel fractures) can be evaluated.

A1.1.4 The values stated in SI units are to be regarded as standard. No other units of measurement are included in this standard.

A1.1.5 *This standard does not purport to address all of the safety concerns, if any, associated with its use. It is the responsibility of the user of this standard to establish appropriate safety and health practices and determine the applicability of regulatory limitations prior to use.*

A1.2 Referenced Documents

A1.2.1 *ASTM Standards*:

E 4 Practices for Load Verification of Testing Machines[2]

E 122 Practice for Choice of Sample Size to Estimate the Average Quality of a Lot or Process[3]

A1.3 Terminology

A1.3.1 *Definitions:*

A1.3.1.1 *0.2 % offset displacement, q, n*—permanent deformation (mm) equal to 0.2 % of the lever arm length (see point B in Fig. A1.1).

A1.3.1.2 *compression bending stiffness, K, n—of an angled device*, the maximum slope (N/m) of the linear elastic portion of the load versus displacement curve, when tested as described in A1.8. (See the slope of line 0m in Fig. A1.1).

A1.3.1.3 *compression bending strength, n—of an angled device*, the bending moment (N - m) necessary to produce a 0.2 % offset displacement in the angled device when tested as described in A1.8 (the bending moment corresponding to point P in Fig. A1.1). If the angled device fractures before the proof load is attained, the compression bending strength shall be defined as the bending moment at fracture.

A1.3.1.4 *fracture load, F_{max}, n*— the applied load (N) at the time when the angled device fractures.

A1.3.1.5 *lever arm, L, n*—the instantaneous distance (mm) from the line of load application to the surface of the sideplate that is intended to be in contact with the bone at the most proximal location where the sideplate contacts the test fixture support (shown in Fig. A1.2); the initial unloaded angled device lever arm length shall be held constant for comparative tests.

A1.3.1.6 *permanent deformation, n*—the relative change (mm) in the load application point's position (in the direction of the applied load) remaining after the applied load has been removed.

A1.3.1.7 *potential critical stress concentrator, CSC, n*—any change in section modulus, material property, discontinuity, or other feature of an angled device design expected to cause a concentration of stress, that is located in a region of the angled device expected to be highly stressed under the normal anticipated loading conditions.

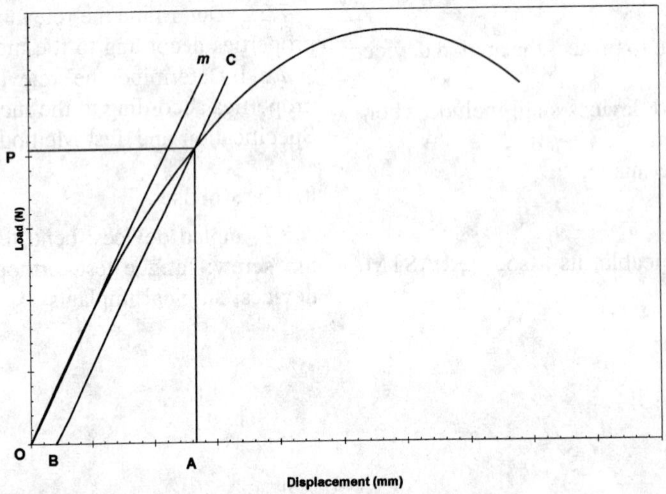

FIG. A1.1 Diagram Illustrating Methods for Determining Bending Properties of Angled Devices

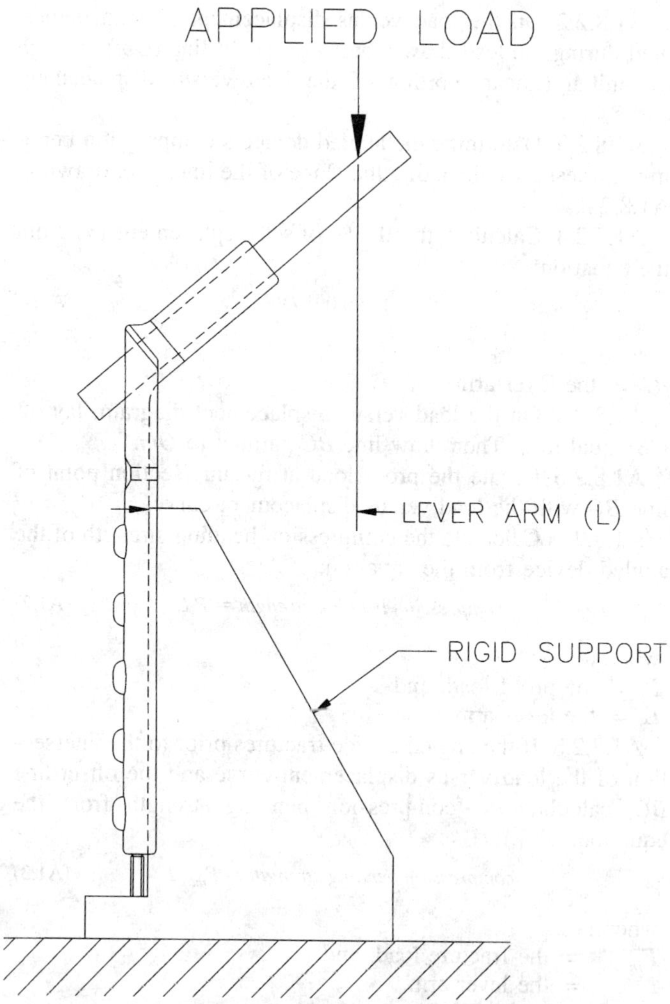

FIG. A1.2 Test Configuration

A1.3.1.8 *proof load, P, n*—the applied load (N) at the intersection point of line *BC* with the load versus total displacement curve, (see Fig. A1.1).

A1.3.1.9 *proof point displacement, n*—the total displacement associated with the angled device's compression bending strength, (see point A in Fig. A1.1).

A1.3.1.10 *total displacement, n*—the relative change (mm) in the load application point's position (in the direction of the applied load) when a specified load is applied.

A1.4 Summary of Test Method

A1.4.1 Angled devices are subjected to a single-cycle load introduced at the device's angled portion. This results in the simultaneous application of compressive and cantilever bending stresses to the device. The device's compression bending stiffness and compression bending strength are then derived from the test record generate during the test using relevant test configuration parameters.

A1.5 Significance and Use

A1.5.1 This compression bend test is used to determine values for the mechanical response of angled devices to a specific type of bending load. The information resulting from this test can give the surgeon some insight into the mechanical response of a given angled device.

A1.5.2 Since the loading on the angled device *in situ* will, in general, differ from the loading configuration used in this test method, the results obtained from this test method cannot be used directly to predict *in vivo* performance of the angled device being tested. Such mechanical property data can be used to conduct relative comparisons of different angled device designs.

A1.5.3 Since the test method provides flexibility to evaluate a variety of clinical failure modes, the user must first determine which failure mode will be evaluated. Futhermore, the user should determine the relevance of the failure mode for the angled device being evaluated.

A1.5.4 The angled device's compression bending stiffness, as defined in A1.3.1.2, is an indicator of the angled device's stiffness when subjected to a compression-bending load. This mechanical property is a comparative indicator of the stability that the user can achieve in the treatment of methaphyseal fractures with the angled device.

A1.5.5 The angled device's compression bending strength, as defined in A1.3.1.3, identifies the bending moment that must be applied to the angled device in order to produce a specific amount of permanent deformation.

A1.5.6 This test method assumes that linear-elastic material behavior will be observed and, therefore, the test method is not applicable for the testing of materials that exhibit non-linear elastic behavior.

A1.6 Apparatus

A1.6.1 A typical test configuration is illustrated in Fig. A1.2.

A1.6.2 The plate of the angled device being tested is rigidly attached to an anchor block that is fully constrained. Alternative test setups are allowed (for example, the device support is unconstrained with rollers as allowed by the previous version of this standard) as long as the following conditions are met.

A1.6.2.1 The angled device shall be loaded in such a manner to satisfy the goals or requirements of A1.4.1, A1.5.1, and X2.1.

A1.6.2.2 If the angled device's support is allowed to translate normal to the test machine's loading axis in reaction to the applied load during the test, then the lever arm distance shall be monitored during the test. This information shall then be used to correct the load versus displacement curve and the compression bending stiffness and strength values calculated in A1.8.2.1.

A1.6.2.3 If the loading adapter's contact point is allowed to translate normal to the test machine's loading axis in reaction to the applied load during the test, then the lever arm distance shall be monitored during the test. This information shall then be used to correct the load versus displacement curve and the compression bending stiffness and strength values calculated in A1.8.2.1

A1.6.3 The applied load should act only parallel to the sideplate's long axis. Apply the load at a point that will produce a lever arm length that is equivalent to 80 % of either the blade length or the longest screw. Equivalent lever arm lengths must be used for comparative tests. Deviations to this requirement shall be noted and justified in the final report. Additionally, the application of off axis loads to the load cell must be avoided since, depending on their magnitude, they can confound the determination of the device's actual loading condition.

A1.6.4 The test fixture should, in general, support the angled device in such a way to generate the failure being evaluated (sideplate, lag screw, or barrel fracture). A typical configuration that can be used to evaluate the angled device's sideplate failure characteristics is illustrated in Fig. A1.2.

A1.6.5 The device being tested should be suitably anchored to the support fixture. The intent of the test method is to evaluate the angled device and not the sideplate anchors.

A1.6.6 Displacement shall be measured as the displacement of the load application point parallel to the sideplate's long axis.

A1.6.7 Alternative loading configurations are allowed[6] but must be noted and fully described in the final report.

A1.6.8 Machines used for the bending test shall conform to the requirements of Practice E 4.

A1.6.9 The test machine and fixtures (test system) should be sufficiently stiff that their deformation under the load is negligible relative to that of the angled device being tested. The test system's machine compliance (combined test machine and fixture compliance) should be measured and reported. Typically, the test system's machine compliance should be less than 1 % of the tested angled device's compliance.

A1.7 Sampling

A1.7.1 Determine sample size using the methods outlined in Practice E 122.

A1.7.2 In those circumstances when there is insufficient information to utilize the guidance of Practice E 122, the sample size shall be no less than three.

A1.7.3 Angled devices of different lengths but nominally identical cross-sections, and made of the same material, may be used to constitute a sample.

A1.7.4 Only unused and untested angled devices are allowed for the comparative tests.

A1.8 Procedure

A1.8.1 Apply loads of increasing magnitude to the angled device at a recommended test control rate of 10 mm/min, and generate a load versus displacement diagram either autographically or from numeric data acquired during the test. Displacement-controlled testing is strongly preferred over load-controlled testing. The measured deformation behavior past the yield point can be different for load-controlled testing due to non-linear displacement rates.

A1.8.2 Determine the compression bending stiffness and compression bending strength for each tested angled device according to the following:

A1.8.2.1 Produce a load versus displacement curve (see Fig. A1.1) either autographically or from numerical data acquired during the test.

A1.8.2.2 On the load versus displacement diagram generated during the test, draw a best-fit straight line (*Om*) through the initial (linear) portion of the load versus displacement curve.

A1.8.2.3 Determine the angled device's compression bending stiffness by calculating the slope of the line, *Om*, drawn in A1.8.2.2.

A1.8.2.4 Calculate the 0.2 % offset displacement (q) from the equation:

$$q = 0.002 \cdot L \quad \text{(A1.1)}$$

where:
L = the lever arm.

A1.8.2.5 On the load versus displacement diagram, lay off *OB* equal to q. Then draw line *BC* parallel to *Om*.

A1.8.2.6 Locate the proof load at the intersection point of line *BC* with the load versus displacement curve.

A1.8.2.7 Calculate the compression bending strength of the angled device from the equation:

$$\text{compression bending strength} = P \cdot L \quad \text{(A1.2)}$$

where:
P = the proof load, and
L = the lever arm.

A1.8.2.8 If the angled device fractures prior to the intersection of the load versus displacement curve and the offset line *BC*, calculate the compression bending strength from the equation:

$$\text{compression bending strength} = F_{max} \cdot L \quad \text{(A1.3)}$$

where:
F_{max} = the fracture load, and
L = the lever arm.

A1.9 Report

A1.9.1 Report the following information:

A1.9.1.1 Adequate description of the test article, including the number of angled devices tested,

A1.9.1.2 Adequate description of the test configuration,

A1.9.1.3 The unloaded lever arm length (L),

A1.9.1.4 The 0.2 % offset displacement used to determine the compression bending strength,

A1.9.1.5 Mean and standard deviations of the compression bending stiffness values for the set of angled devices tested,

A1.9.1.6 Mean and standard deviation of the compression bending strength values for the set of angled devices tested,

A1.9.1.7 Number of angled devices fractured during the test,

A1.9.1.8 The method (either displacement or load) and rate utilized for controlling the test.

A1.10 Precision and Bias

A1.10.1 *Precision*—Data establishing the precision of this test method have not yet been obtained.

A1.10.2 *Bias*—No statement of bias can be made, since no acceptable reference values are available, nor can they be obtained in that this test is a destructive test.

[6] Peterson, R. R., Lynch, G. E., Brasher, T. W., "Cyclic Cantilever Fatigue Testing of Compression Hip Screw Plates," *ASTM STP 1217, Clinical and Laboratory Performance of Bone Plates*, pp. 72-81, 1994, American Society of Testing and Materials, West Conshohocken, PA 19428.

A2. STANDARD TEST METHOD FOR DETERMINING THE BENDING FATIGUE PROPERTIES OF METALLIC ANGLED ORTHOPEDIC FRACTURE FIXATION DEVICES

A2.1 Scope

A2.1.1 This test method describes methods for bending fatigue testing in order to determine intrinsic structural properties of metallic angled devices. The test method may be used to determine the fatigue life at a specific or over a range of maximum bending moment levels or to estimate the fatigue strength for a specified number of fatigue cycles of an angled device.

A2.1.2 This standard is intended to provide a means to mechanically characterize different angled device designs. It is not the intention of this standard to define angled device performance levels since insufficient knowledge is available to predict the consequences of the use of a particular angled device design.

A2.1.3 *Units*—The values stated in SI units are to be regarded as standard. No other units of measurement are included in this standard.

A2.1.4 *This standard does not purport to address all of the safety concerns, if any, associated with its use. It is the responsibility of the user of this standard to establish appropriate safety and health practices and to determine the applicability of regulatory limitations prior to use.*

NOTE A2.1—Currently, there is no ISO standard that is similar, or equivalent, to this test method.

A2.2 Referenced Documents

A2.2.1 *ASTM Standards:*

E 4 Practices for Force Verification of Testing Machines[2]

E 467 Practice for Verification of Constant Amplitude Dynamic Force in an Axial Fatigue Testing System[2]

E 1823 Terminology Relating to Fatigue and Fracture Testing[2]

E 1942 Guide for Evaluating Data Acquisition Systems Used in Cyclic Fatigue and Fracture Mechanics Testing[2]

F 565 Practice for Care and Handling of Orthopedic Implants and Instruments[4]

A2.3. Terminology

A2.3.1 *Definitions*—Unless otherwise defined in this test method, the terminology related to fatigue testing that is used in this test method will be in accordance to the definitions of Terminology E 1823.

A2.3.1.1 *M-N diagram, n*—a plot of maximum moment versus the number of cycles to a specified failure point.

A2.3.1.2 *maximum moment, n*—the applied bending moment having the highest algebraic value during the loading cycle. A moment that generates a tensile stress on the surface of the angled device specimen that does not come in contact with the bone when implanted is considered positive. Correspondingly, a moment that generates a compressive stress on this surface is considered negative.

A2.3.1.3 *median fatigue strength at N cycles, n*—an estimate of the maximum moment at which 50 % of the specimens of a given sample population would be expected to survive N loading cycles at a given *R*-ratio.

A2.3.1.4 *minimum moment, n*—the applied bending moment having the lowest algebraic value during the loading cycle. A moment that generates a tensile stress on the surface of the angled device specimen that does not come in contact with the bone when implanted is considered positive. Correspondingly, a moment that generates a compressive stress on this surface is considered negative.

A2.3.1.5 *R-ratio, n*—the algebraic ratio relating the minimum and maximum values of the loading parameters of a fatigue cycle. For the purposes of this test method the *R*-ratio is defined as:

$$R = \frac{Minimum\ Moment}{Maximum\ Moment} \qquad (A2.1)$$

A2.3.1.6 *runout, n*—a predetermined number of cycles at which the testing on a particular specimen stopped, and no further testing on that specimen will be performed. When the intent of the fatigue test program is to determine the fatigue strength at *N* cycles, the runout usually is specified as *N* cycles.

A2.4 Summary of Test Method

A2.4.1 The sideplate of an angled device is anchored rigidly and is loaded in cantilever bending with a load applied parallel to the long axis of the sideplate. The angled device is subjected to a constant frequency sinusoidal cyclic bending moment waveform with the cantilever bending loading configuration. The fatigue loading is continued until the specimen fails, a limit is reached which is indicative of failure, or the runout cycle count is reached.

A2.4.2 The data generated from a series of test samples is compiled and presented in a manner that is consistent with the goals of the study. The results can either be presented in a semi-log *M-N* diagram that will characterize the general fatigue behavior of the angled device over a range of applied bending moments or simply the fatigue strength determined for a specified *N* number of cycles.

A2.5 Significance and Use

A2.5.1 The test method establishes a uniform cantilever bending fatigue test to characterize and compare the fatigue performance of different angled device designs. This test method may be used to determine an angled device's fatigue life at either a specific or over a range of maximum bending moment conditions. Additionally, this test method may be alternatively used to estimate an angled device's fatigue strength for a specified number of fatigue cycles.

A2.5.2 The test method utilizes a simplified angled device cantilever bending load model that may not be exactly representative of the in-situ loading configuration. The user should note that the test results generated by this test method can not be used to directly predict the in-vivo performance of the angled device being tested. The data generated from this test method can be used to conduct relative comparisons of different angled device designs.

A2.5.3 This test method may not be appropriate for all types of implant applications. The user is cautioned to consider the appropriateness of the method in view of the devices being tested and their potential application.

A2.5.4 This test method assumes that the angled device is manufactured from a material that exhibits linear-elastic material behavior; therefore, this test method is not applicable for testing angled devices made from materials that exhibit non-linear elastic behavior.

A2.5.5 This test method is restricted to the testing of angled devices within the material's linear-elastic range; therefore, this test method is not applicable for testing angled devices under conditions that would approach or exceed the bending strength of the angled device being tested.

A2.6 Apparatus

A2.6.1 Test machines used for the bending fatigue test shall conform to the requirements of Practice E 4 and E 467.

A2.6.2 The suitability of any data acquisition systems used in monitoring the progress of these tests should be evaluated in accordance to the guidelines of Guide E 1942.

A2.6.3 The typical cantilever bend test loading conditions employed for this test is illustrated in Fig. A2.1. Suitable test fixtures for the test will meet the requirements of A1.6.

A2.6.4 A cycle counter is required that is capable of counting the cumulative number of loading cycles that are applied to the specimen during the course of the fatigue test.

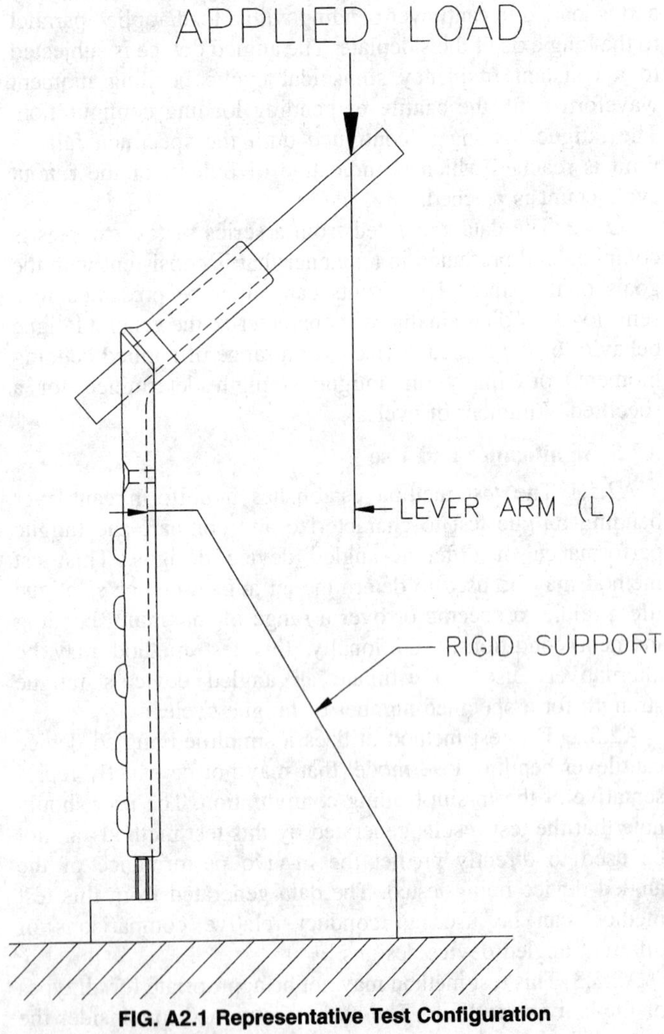

FIG. A2.1 Representative Test Configuration

A2.6.5 When required, a limit detector that is capable of sensing when a test parameter, for example, load, actuator displacement, DC error, etc., reaches a limiting value and produces a signal or action that terminates the test.

A2.7 Test Specimens and Sampling

A2.7.1 All test components shall be representative of implant quality products with regard to material, cross-section, surface finish, markings, and manufacturing processes. Any deviation from this requirement must be noted in the final report.

A2.7.2 In accordance with Practice F 565, angled devices that have been either implanted or contoured (reshaped) for implantation are not suitable for this test method and shall be excluded from the sample.

A2.7.3 Angled devices of different lengths but nominally identical cross-sections, and made of the same material, may be used to constitute a sample.

A2.7.4 *M-N Diagram Testing*—The minimum sample size necessary for reporting the fatigue life of a given angled device at a given maximum bending moment condition is three. A rudimentary *M-N* diagram with a corresponding fatigue curve would require three replicate tests at three load levels. Under ideal conditions, conduct five replicate tests at each of five maximum bending moment levels in order to enhance the statistical significance of the resulting information.

A2.7.5 *Fatigue Strength Testing*—No minimum sample size can be identified for this testing method since the total number of data points needed to make such a determination is dependent upon the methodology used and many other related factors. The user should be aware that such a study may require approximately twenty test specimens in order to generate statistically meaningful results.

A2.8 Procedure

A2.8.1 Prior to testing, the bending moment level(s) for testing must be determined. To evaluate the fatigue performance of an angled device, the user has several methodologies at their disposal whose selection is based upon the output goals of the study. Two recommended methods are as follows:

A2.8.1.1 *M-N Diagram*—The user may test a given angled device design over a range of maximum bending moment levels to characterize the general fatigue behavior trend of the device. The user's experience is the best guide that can be used for determining the initial loading conditions. In the absence of such experience, the best recommendation would be to use initial fatigue loads corresponding to 75, 50, and 25 % of the bending strength determined in accordance with Annex A1. The applied moment and the cycle to test termination data are then plotted on a semi-log *M-N* diagram. A curve fit may be applied appropriately to the data to develop an *M-N* curve.

A2.8.1.2 *Fatigue Strength Determination*—The user may also test a given angled device design in order to determine the fatigue strength at a given number of fatigue cycles. This test method recommends that the fatigue strength estimation be determined at one million loading cycles (see rationale in Appendix X3). The maximum difference between the load levels used for the fatigue strength determination shall be no greater than 10 % of the bending strength determined in accordance to this standard's Annex A1 test method. Acceptable methods, which can be employed to determine the angled device's fatigue strength, include the up and down method and a modified up and down method.[7,8]

A2.8.2 Anchor the angled device in the testing fixture and position it so that the angled device will be loaded consistent with the clinical failure mode being investigated.

A2.8.3 Ensure that the load is applied to the tested device in a manner consistent with the requirements of A1.6.3.

A2.8.4 Load the test specimen with the test system in load control using an appropriate waveform so that the resultant time dependent bending moment generated in the test specimen is cyclic and sinusoidal in nature. Select a cyclic frequency for the tests that will not produce strain sensitive effects in the angled device's material. Typically, a cyclic frequency of 5 Hz is more than adequate for completing the test in a timely manner and will still not affect the angled device's material.

A2.8.5 The recommended *R*-ratio is 0.1. Any deviations from this should be reported and justified in the final report.

A2.8.6 The cycle counter shall record the cumulative number of cycles applied to the test specimen, and the appropriate limits should be set to indicate specimen failure, or deviations, or both, from the intended load parameters.

A2.8.7 Testing shall continue until the specimen breaks, a limit is reached that terminates the test, or the total cycle count reaches the runout limit.

A2.9 Calculation or Interpretation of Results

A2.9.1 Record the results of each test including the maximum moment, cycle count at test termination, and the failure location and failure mode, if applicable.

A2.9.2 If the goal of the study is to generate an *M-N* diagram, then the maximum moment and cycles to test termination data is plotted on a semi-log graph. Various techniques may be used to estimate the mean or median fatigue lives, statistical differences between groups, curve fits to the fatigue data, probability of survival curves, etc.[9,10]

A2.9.3 If the goal of the study is to determine the fatigue strength at *N* cycles, it is recommended that the fatigue strength be determined as the median fatigue limit (50 % probability of survival), using an applicable industry accepted techniques.[7,8]

A2.10 Report

A2.10.1 The test report will include the following information:

A2.10.1.1 Manufacturer of the angled device specimen.

A2.10.1.2 The angled device's description and catalog number (if applicable).

A2.10.1.3 The angled device's material including applicable ASTM or ISO specifications.

A2.10.1.4 Deviations from normal implant product.

A2.10.1.5 The unloaded lever arm length (*L*).

A2.10.1.6 *R*-ratio.

A2.10.1.7 Test frequency.

A2.10.1.8 Description of the test environment.

A2.10.1.9 Deviations from recommended test method.

A2.10.1.10 Tabular listing that summarizes the maximum moment and the resulting cycles to test termination data.

A2.10.1.11 A description of the failure mode and failure location for each specimen that failed.

A2.10.1.12 If appropriate, a semi-log plot of the *M-N* diagram is generated. Include descriptions of any analytical or statistical techniques used when interpreting the fatigue data.

A2.10.1.13 If appropriate, an estimate of the fatigue strength should be reported. Include descriptions of any analytical or statistical techniques used for determining the fatigue strength.

A2.11 Precision and Bias

A2.11.1 *Precision*—Data establishing the precision of the test method have not yet been obtained.

A2.11.2 *Bias*—No statement of bias can be made, since no acceptable reference values are available, nor can they be obtained since this test method is a destructive test.

---

[7] Little, R. E., and Jebe, E. H., *Manual on Statistical Planning and Analysis for Fatigue Experiments*, STP 588, American Society of Testing and Materials, 100 Barr Harbor Drive, West Conshohocken, PA 19428, 1975.

[8] Little, R. E., "Optimal Stress Amplitude Selection in Estimating Median Fatigue Limits Using Small Samples," *Journal of Testing and Evaluation*, ASTM, 1990, pp. 115–122.

[9] Conway, J. B., and Sjodahl, L. H., *Analysis and Representation of Fatigue Data*, ASM International, Materials Park, OH, 1991.

[10] Collins, J. A., *Failure of Materials in Mechanical Design*, John Wiley and Sons, New York, NY, 1981.

APPENDIXES

(Nonmandatory Information)

X1. RATIONALE FOR MAIN TEXT

X1.1 This standard is intended to provide useful and consistent information related to the terminology, performance, application of test methods, and the application of angled devices used for maintenance of alignment and fixation during the bone healing process. Angled device geometrical definitions, classification and terminology, material specifications, and performance definitions are provided.

X1.2 The orthopedic surgeon should be able to select the device he/she feels is appropriate for the indication being treated. In order to do this, the surgeon must have confidence that the designation of size has a specific, known meaning that is quantifiable and reliable regardless of the manufacturer or design. The mechanical behavior and material properties must also be described in a reliable, known manner irrespective of the manufacturer or design. In order to accomplish this uniformity of designations, the terminology, mechanical properties, material properties must be standardized.

X1.3 The subcommittee's goal is to produce a single standard identifying all pertinent information, requirements, and test methods for orthopedic angled devices. The first step in achieving this goal was to combine the current versions of F 384 and F 787. This revision of F 384 completes this first step.

X2. RATIONALE FOR ANNEX A1

X2.1 This test method in Annex A1 is designed to measure the mechanical properties of angled devices subjected to a compression-bending load, which is the most common type of loading encountered *in vivo*. This test method addresses itself to properties of the device rather than the material from which the plate is made.

X2.2 The test method's intent is to specify the requirements of the loading configuration and not the design of the test fixtures needed to meet those requirements. The elimination of absence of any standardized test fixture design in the test method allows for the creative problem solving by the individual conducting the test in order to addresses the requirements of any given set of test conditions. One of the problems with the previous version of the standard was that the test configuration did not lend itself easily to the testing of angled devices in an environment.

X2.3 The offset displacement criteria used to determine the angled device's bending strength has been set at 0.2 % for two reasons; to establish a bending strength criteria that was minimally influenced by non-elastic bending of the angled device, and to make the test method consistent with the previous version. In the previous version of the test method, the lever arm length was set at 3.0 in. with an offset displacement criteria of 0.005 in. (approximately 0.2 % of the lever arm length). Additionally, the typical offset chosen is small enough that the elastic limit has just been reached, but large enough that any slippage or singular behavior at the elastic limit is avoided (0.1 % and 0.2 % for E 8).

X3. RATIONALE FOR ANNEX A2

X3.1 Angled device fatigue properties are an important factor when considering the surgical treatment of skeletal fractures. The angled device may be subjected to a significant number of repetitive stress cycles during the healing process. In some situations, the angled device may be expected to experience these conditions for several weeks until the bone healing process progresses adequately so that the bone can provide mechanical support that will reduce the stresses in the angled device. It is important, therefore, for the surgeon to have some means to judge the fatigue performance of a given angled device.

X3.2 Since the time frame, number of loading cycles and loading conditions are uncontrollable and unpredictable, there is no acceptable limit that can be set for the bending moment or number of cycles of load which the angled device should withstand in any given case.

X3.3 One of the objectives of this test method is to provide a consistent methodology for determining an estimate of the angled device fatigue strength at 10^6 cycles for comparative purposes. Angled devices are classified as temporary skeletal fixation devices since fractures and skeletal deformity corrections generally are resolved within two to three months (approximately 150 000 to 250 000 cycles). Even though the test method's recommendation of one million cycles for estimating the fatigue strength has been arbitrarily chosen, it still can be considered conservative since no angled device in clinical service would normally be expected to withstand 10^6 high stress loading cycles.

X3.4 The reporting of cyclic bending fatigue strength or fatigue life, or both, using this standard testing technique only are suitable for comparative evaluations between devices of different sizes, designs and materials.

Designation: F 451 – 99a

Standard Specification for Acrylic Bone Cement[1]

This standard is issued under the fixed designation F 451; the number immediately following the designation indicates the year of original adoption or, in the case of revision, the year of last revision. A number in parentheses indicates the year of last reapproval. A superscript epsilon (ε) indicates an editorial change since the last revision or reapproval.

1. Scope

1.1 This specification covers self-curing resins used primarily for the fixation of internal orthopedic prostheses. The mixture may be used in either the predough or dough stage in accordance with the manufacturer's recommendations.

1.2 Units of premeasured powder and liquid are supplied in a form suitable for mixing. The mixture then sets in place.

1.3 While a variety of copolymers and comonomers may be incorporated, the composition of the set cement shall contain poly(methacrylic acid esters) as its main ingredient.

1.4 This specification covers compositional, physical performance, and biocompatibility as well as packaging requirements. The biocompatibility of acrylic bone cement as it has been traditionally formulated and used has been reported in the literature (**1, 2**).[2]

1.5 *This standard does not purport to address all of the safety concerns, if any, associated with its use. It is the responsibility of the user of this standard to establish appropriate safety and health practices and determine the applicability of regulatory limitations prior to use.*

2. Referenced Documents

2.1 *ASTM Standards:*

D 695 Test Method for Compressive Properties of Rigid Plastics[3]

D 3835 Test Method for Determination of Properties of Polymeric Materials by Means of a Capillary Rheometer[4]

E 29 Practice for Using Significant Digits in Test Data to Determine Conformance With Specifications[5]

E 141 Practice for Acceptance of Evidence Based on the Results of Probability Sampling[5]

F 619 Practice for Extraction of Medical Plastics[6]

F 748 Practice for Selecting Generic Biological Test Methods for Materials and Devices[6]

F 749 Practice for Evaluating Material Extracts by Intracutaneous Injection in the Rabbit[6]

F 756 Practice for Assessment of Hemolytic Properties of Materials[6]

F 763 Practice for Short-Term Screening of Implant Materials[6]

F 813 Practice for Direct Contact Cell Culture Evaluation of Materials for Medical Devices[6]

F 895 Practice for Agar Diffusion Cell Culture Screening for Cytotoxicity[6]

F 981 Practice for Assessment of Compatibility of Biomaterials (Nonporous) for Surgical Implants with Respect to Effect of Materials on Muscle and Bone[6]

2.2 *ANSI/ADA Standard:*

No. 15 Specification for Acrylic Resin Teeth[7]

3. Terminology

3.1 *Definitions of Terms Specific to This Standard:*

3.1.1 *doughing time*—the time after commencement of mixing at which the mixture ceases to adhere to a standard probe (see 7.5).

3.1.2 *exothermic or maximum temperature*—the maximum temperature of the mixture due to self-curing in a standard mold (see 7.6).

3.1.3 *extrusion*—the rate of flow of the material through a standard orifice under load (see 7.8.1).

3.1.4 *intrusion*—the distance of flow of the mixture into a standard mold under load (see 7.8.2).

3.1.5 *setting time*—the time after commencement of mixing at which the temperature of the curing mass equals the average of the maximum and ambient temperatures (see 7.7).

3.1.6 *unit*—one package or vial of premeasured powder component and one package or vial of premeasured liquid component.

4. Physical Requirements

4.1 *Liquid:*

4.1.1 *Appearance*—The liquid shall be free of extraneous particulate matter or obvious visual contaminants in its container.

4.1.2 *Stability*—After being heated for 48 h at 60 ± 2°C, the viscosity of the liquid shall not increase by more than 10 % of its original value (see 7.3).

[1] This specification is under the jurisdiction of ASTM Committee F-4 on Medical and Surgical Materials and Devices and is the direct responsibility of Subcommittee F04.11 on Polymeric Materials.

Current edition approved May 10, 1999. Published July 1999. Originally published as F 451 – 76. Last previous edition F 451 – 95.

[2] The boldface numbers in parentheses refer to the list of references at the end of this standard.

[3] *Annual Book of ASTM Standards*, Vol 08.01.

[4] *Annual Book of ASTM Standards*, Vol 08.02.

[5] *Annual Book of ASTM Standards*, Vol 14.02.

[6] *Annual Book of ASTM Standards*, Vol 13.01.

[7] Available from American National Standards Institute, 11 W. 42nd St., 13th Floor, New York, NY 10036.

4.1.3 *Sterility*—The liquid, as poured from its container, shall pass the tests described in "Sterility Tests—Liquid and Ointments" (7.4) **(3)**.

4.2 *Powder*:

4.2.1 *Appearance*—The powder shall be pourable and free of extraneous materials, such as dirt or lint (7.2.2).

4.2.2 *Sterility*—The powder, as poured from its package, shall pass the tests described in "Sterility Tests—Solids" (7.4) **(2)**.

4.3 *Powder-Liquid Mixture*:

4.3.1 If the mixture is to be used in its predough stage, the material shall conform to the properties given in Table 1.

4.3.2 If the mixture is to be used in its dough stage, the material shall conform to the properties given in Table 1.

4.3.3 If the mixture can be used in either its predough or dough stages, separate units must be tested for compliance with 4.3.1 and 4.3.2.

4.4 *Cured Polymer*— The material after setting shall conform to the properties given in Table 2.

5. Weights and Permissible Variations

5.1 Weight and volume measurements shall be made on the respective powder and liquid components of five units (see 3.1). These units may be subsequently utilized in any of the nonsterile tests of this specification.

5.2 The weights, or volume of the powder and liquid components, or both, shall not deviate by more than 5 % from those stated on the package (9.2.2), of each of five units.

5.3 Where a radiopaque material is supplied for addition to the powder at the discretion of the surgeon, the weight or volume percent of the radiopaque material shall not deviate by more than 15 % from the value stated on the package (9.2.3).

6. Sampling

6.1 Units of powder and liquid shall be procured to provide sufficient material for all the tests of this specification. The units shall be obtained from regular retail distribution channels. Provided no repeat tests are required, this will amount to between seven and ten units.

6.2 It will only be necessary to maintain sterility in tests described in 7.4. All other tests described in this specification need not be conducted under sterile conditions.

7. Test Methods and Sample Size

7.1 Maintain all equipment, mixing surfaces, and materials at 23 ± 2°C at least 2 h prior to testing and conduct all tests at 23 ± 2°C and 50 ± 10 % relative humidity unless otherwise specified.

7.2 *Inspection*—Use visual inspection in determining compliance to the requirements outlined in 4.1.1, 4.2.1, 8.1 and 8.2.

TABLE 1 Requirements for Powder Liquid Mixture

Property	Extrusion, Viscosity Tests	Dough Usage, Intrusion Tests
Max Dough Time, min.	5.0	5.0
Setting Time Range, min.	5 to 15	5 to 15
Temperature, max., °C	90	90
Intrusion, min., mm	...	2.0

TABLE 2 Requirements for Cured Polymer After Setting

Property	Requirement
Compressive Strength, min., MPa	70

7.2.1 The liquid component of two separate units shall comply with the requirements of 4.1.1 and 8.1.

7.2.2 The powder component of two separate units shall comply with the requirements of 4.2.1 and 8.1.

7.3 *Liquid Component Viscosity*—Record the viscosity change of two separate units (4.1.2) before and after the heating exposure by timing the flow of the liquid level between the 0 and 5 mL marks of a 10 mL measuring pipet. Calculate the percent change as follows:

$$\% \text{ Change} = \frac{t_a - t_b}{t_b} \times 100 \quad (1)$$

where:

t_b = flow time before heating, and

t_a = flow time after heating exposure (4.1.2) of 60 ± 2°C for 48 h in the dark in a closed container.

7.3.1 An alternative method for viscosity may be used if it can be demonstrated to yield similar results. Both shall comply to the less than 10 % change specified (4.1.2).

7.4 The components of the two units shall be tested for sterility in accordance with the test methods described in U.S. Pharmacopoeia," Sterility Tests" **(3)**.

7.5 *Doughing Time*:

7.5.1 *Environment*— All equipment, mixing surfaces, and material (unit size) shall be maintained at 23 ± 1°C at least 2 h prior to testing and tests shall be conducted at 23 ± 1°C. The relative humidity shall be 50 ± 10 %.

7.5.2 Mix all the powder and liquid of a single unit together as directed by the manufacturer's instructions (see 8.2). Start a stop watch at the onset of combining the liquid to the powder and read all subsequent times from this stop watch. Approximately 1.5 min after the onset of mixing, gently probe the mixture with a non-powdered surgically gloved (latex) finger. Take visual notice as to the formation of fibers between the surface of the mix and the finger as it leaves the surface. Repeat this process from that time on at 15 s intervals with a clean portion of the glove until the gloved finger separates cleanly. Denote the time at which this is first observed as the doughing time. Mix the mixture between determinations to expose fresh material for each probing.

7.5.3 Determine the average doughing time from two separate units.

7.5.4 The two values found shall agree within 30 s of each other, otherwise repeat the test on two additional units. Report the average of all four tests and the range of values.

7.5.5 Report the doughing time to the nearest 15 s as the average of all determinations. Maximum and minimum values of doughing times measured shall not differ by more than ±1½ min from the average.

7.6 *Exothermic Temperature*—Within 1 min after doughing time, gently pack approximately 25 g of the dough described in 7.5 into the mold described in Fig. 1. This mold shall be made of polytetrafluoroethylene (PTFE), poly(ethyleneterephthalate), polyoxymethylene, high density polyethylene, or ultra-high molecular weight polyethylene (UHMWPE) and be

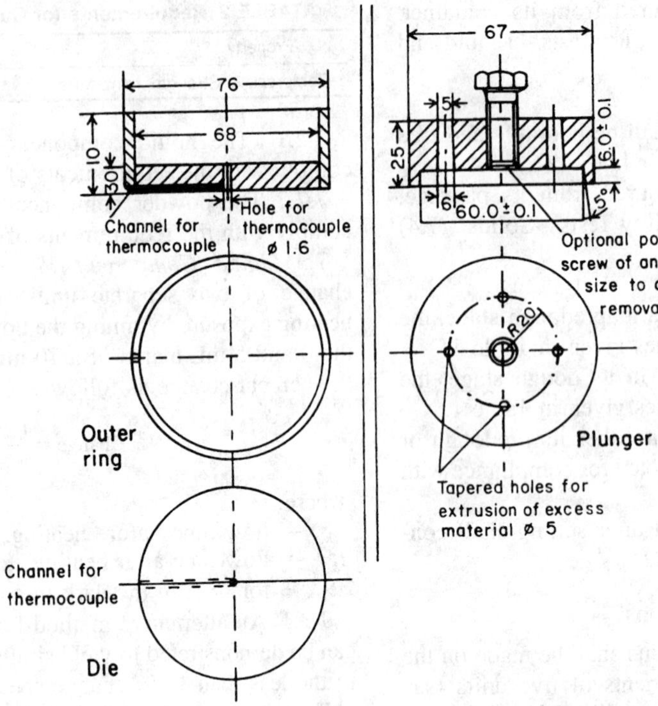

NOTE 1—Dimensions in millimetres and ±0.2 unless otherwise specified. Material for all components: Polytetrafluoroethylene, poly(ethyleneterephthalate), polyoxymethylene, high density polyethylene, or ultra-high molecular weight polyethylene (UHMWPE).

FIG. 1 Exothermic Heat Mold

equipped with a No. 24 gage wire thermocouple, or similar device, positioned with its junction in the center of the mold at a height of 3.0 mm in the internal cavity. Immediately seat the plunger with a C-clamp or suitable press to produce the 6.0 mm specimen height. Upon producing plunger seating, remove the excess material and the C-clamp or press for the remainder of the procedure. Continuously record the temperature with respect to time from the onset of mixing the liquid and the powder until cooling is observed, Fig. 2. Report the maximum temperature recorded to the nearest 1°C. This should not exceed the value given in Table 1.

7.6.1 The maximum temperature shall be the average of two separate determinations reported to the nearest 1°C.

7.6.2 If the difference between the maximum temperature for the two determinations is greater than 5.0°C, repeat the test on two additional units and report the average of all four runs to the nearest 1°C. Individual maximum and minimum values for maximum temperature shall not differ by more than ±4°C of the average value of all determinations.

7.7 *Setting Time*— From the continuous time versus temperature recording of 7.6, the setting time (T_{set}) is the time when the temperature of the polymerizing mass is as follows:

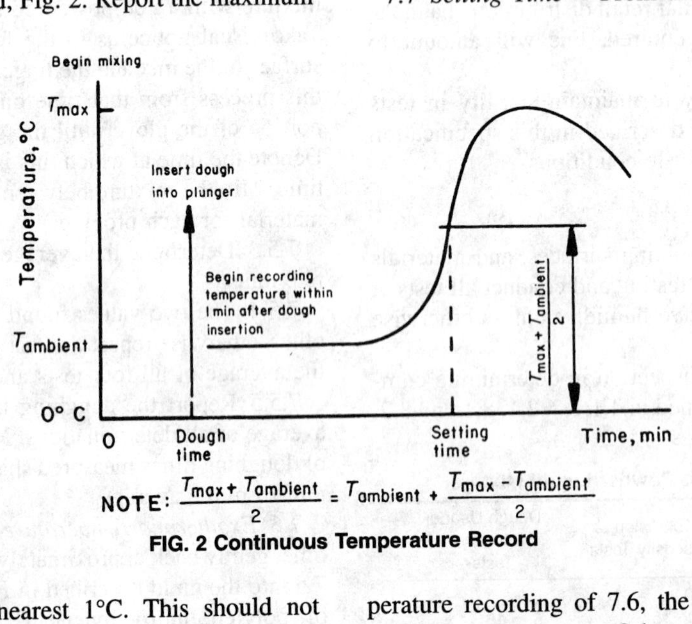

NOTE: $\frac{T_{max} + T_{ambient}}{2} = T_{ambient} + \frac{T_{max} - T_{ambient}}{2}$

FIG. 2 Continuous Temperature Record

$$(T_{max} + T_{amb})/2 \quad (2)$$

where:

T_{max} = maximum temperature, °C, and
T_{amb} = ambient temperature of 23 ± 1°C.

7.7.1 Report the setting time to the nearest 5 s.

7.7.2 Make two separate determinations of the setting time.

7.7.3 The two values should agree within 1 min of each other, otherwise repeat the test on two additional units and report the average of all runs.

7.7.4 Report the setting time to the nearest 15 s as the average of all determinations.

7.8 *Flow Properties and Viscosity Determination*—The manufacturer must specify whether the cement may be used in its pre-dough or dough state, or both. The determination of its usage dictates which of the following tests the cement should comply with. If the mixture is to be utilized in the pre-dough stage, use the extrusion, viscosity test (7.8.1) and Table 1. If the mixture is to be utilized in the dough stage, use the intrusion test (7.8.2) and Table 1. If the mixture is to be used as a dual usage cement, then both the extrusion (7.8.1) and intrusion (7.8.2) tests must be performed.

7.8.1 *Extrusion, Viscosity*:

7.8.1.1 *Apparatus*:

7.8.1.1.1 *Rheometer*—Any capillary rheometer is satisfactory in which acrylic bone cement can be forced from a reservoir through a capillary die and in which temperature, applied force, output rate, and barrel and die dimensions can be controlled and measured accurately. Equipment that provides a constant shear rate has been shown to be equally useful. The capillary die of the rheometer shall have a smooth straight bore that is held within ±0.0076 mm (±0.0003 in.) in diameter and shall be held to within ±0.025 mm (±0.001 in.) in length. The bore and its finish are critical. It shall have no visible drill or other tool marks and no detectable eccentricity.

7.8.1.1.2 Due to the extreme sensitivity of flow data to the capillary dimensions, it is important that the capillary dimensions are measured with precision and reported. The length to diameter ratio shall normally be between 20 and 40. Larger ratios and ratios less than that suggested require applying large corrections to the data **(4, 5)**. In addition, the ratio of the reservoir diameter to capillary diameter should be between 3 and 15. See Test Method D 3835 for further details of capillary rheometers.

7.8.1.2 *Calibration*—Perform the test with a certified standard viscosity fluid approximating that expected for bone cement (50 N·s/m² to 500 N·s/m²). Determine the viscosity of the standard fluid and the percent error from its specified value. Report this error along with the viscosity of the tested cements.

7.8.1.3 *Corrections*— Since bone cement is a non-Newtonian fluid, the data may be reported as corrected data. For example, true shear rates, corrected for non-Newtonian flow behavior and true shear stress corrected for end effects or kinetic energy losses, may be calculated. In such cases, the exact details of the mode of correction must be reported. Some correction factors which may apply are:

(*a*) Piston friction,
(*b*) Plunger back flow,
(*c*) Cement compressibility,
(*d*) Barrel back pressure,
(*e*) Capillary entrance effects (Bagley correction) **(6)**,
(*f*) Rabinowitsch shear rate correction **(7)**.

7.8.2 *Procedure*:

7.8.2.1 Select conditions of temperature and shear stress or shear rate in accordance with expected usage so that the flow rate will fall within desired limits.

7.8.2.2 Inspect the rheometer and clean it if necessary. Ensure that previous cleaning procedures and usage have not changed the dimensions or caused scratches or defects in the capillary or apparatus. Make the necessary measurements on the apparatus for future calculations. Prepare the apparatus for running the test.

7.8.2.3 Mix one or more complete unit(s) of powder and liquid in the recommended manner. Start a stop watch at the onset of mixing and read all subsequent times from this watch. After complete mixing, transfer the cement to the thermally equilibrated reservoir, and eject any entrapped air or excess bone cement.

7.8.2.4 Start the apparatus at a time not greater than 2½ min from the start of mixing and continue operating until the estimated dough time or the viscosity exceeds 500 N·s/m².

7.8.2.5 Disassemble the apparatus quickly before the cement sets and clean the apparatus of all remaining cement.

7.8.3 *Calculations*— Perform the calculation for viscosity of the cement at time intervals of 15 s from the start to finish of test run. Use the following equations:

$$\text{Shear Stress, Pa} = \frac{Pr}{2L} = \frac{Fr}{2\pi R^2 L} \quad (3)$$

$$\text{Shear Rate, s}^{-1} = \frac{4Q}{\pi r^3} = \frac{4V}{\pi r^3 t} \quad (4)$$

$$\text{Viscosity, Pa} \cdot \text{s} = \frac{P\pi r^4}{8LQ} = \frac{Fr^4 t}{8R^2 LV} \quad (5)$$

where:

P = pressure by ram, Pa,
F = force on ram, *N*,
r = radius of capillary, m,
R = radius of barrel, m,
L = length of capillary, m,
Q = flow rate, m³/s,
V = volume extruded, m³, and
t = extrusion time, s.

7.8.3.1 These equations yield true shear rate and true viscosity for Newtonian fluids only; for non-Newtonian fluids, such as bone cement, the apparent shear rate and viscosity are obtained.

7.8.4 *Report*—The report of the flow properties of the cement shall include:

7.8.4.1 Description of the rheometer used.

7.8.4.2 Temperature at which the data were obtained.

7.8.4.3 The capillary diameter and length to diameter ratio of the capillary.

7.8.4.4 The shear rate at which the test was performed.

7.8.4.5 Viscosity versus observation time for three runs.

7.8.4.6 Statement as to whether any correction factors (7.8.1.3) were applied.

7.8.5 *Intrusion*:

7.8.5.1 The mold necessary for this test shall be made of polytetrafluoroethylene (PTFE), poly(ethyleneterephthalate), polyoxymethylene, high density polyethylene, or ultra-high molecular weight polyethylene (UHMWPE) and is shown in Fig. 3.

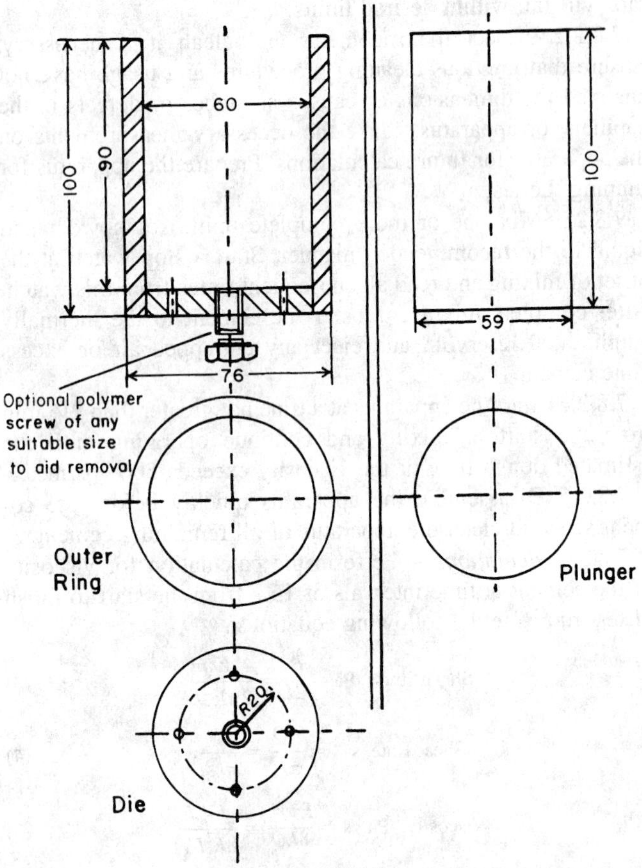

NOTE 1—Dimensions in millimetres; 4 holes in bottom to be 1.00 ± 0.05. Tolerance on all other dimensions ± 0.2.Material for all components: Polytetrafluoroethylene, poly(ethyleneterephthalate), polyoxymethylene, high density polyethylene, or ultra-high molecular weight polyethylene (UHMWPE).

FIG. 3 Intrusion Mold

7.8.5.2 Following the set, remove the specimen and measure the average height of the intrusion into all four of the 1.0-mm diameter holes of the die to the nearest 0.5 mm.

7.8.5.3 Run this test once. If the requirement is not met, it must be met so in a repeat test.

7.9 *Compressive Strength*—The test specimens shall be cylinders 12 mm high and 6 mm in diameter. The ends of the specimens shall be flat and smooth and shall be parallel to each other and at right angles to the long axis of the cylinder. An apparatus found convenient for forming these test cylinders is shown in Fig. 4. An apparatus containing more or less holes may be used as long as adequate spacing between holes is maintained. A mold release agent or silicone spray may be sparingly applied to facilitate specimen removal.

7.9.1 Place the specimen mold on a flat glass or smooth metal plate and slightly overfill using one unit of mixed cement of standard proportions at the commencement of dough time.

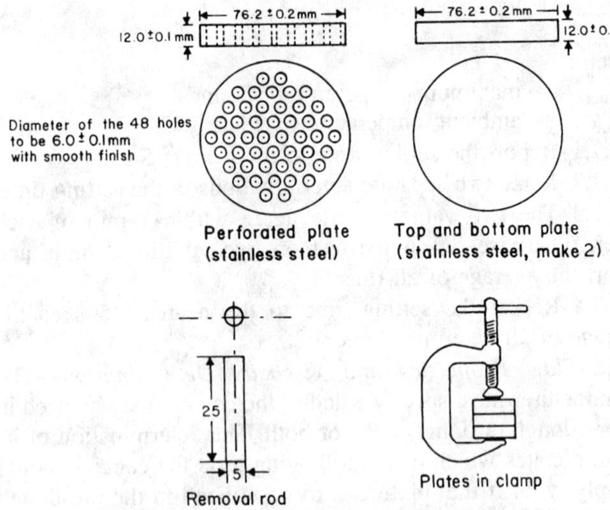

FIG. 4 Compression Specimens Mold

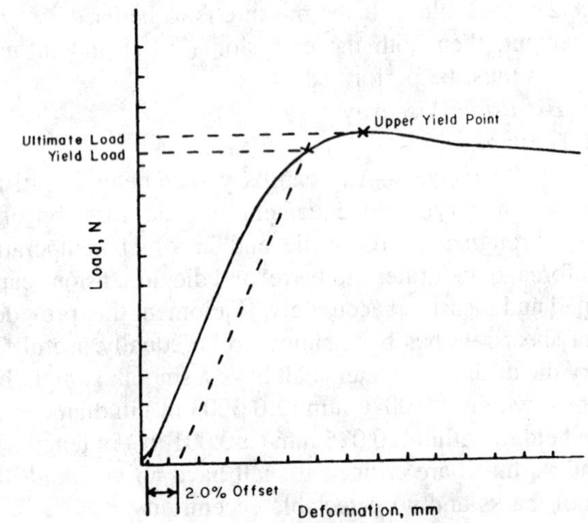

FIG. 5 Failure Load Criteria

Press a second flat glass or smooth metal plate on top of the mold. Hold the mold and plates firmly together with a small C-clamp. Then, 1 h later, surface the ends of the cylinder plane at right angles to the axis. The ends of the specimens may be ground flat to the axis by use of a small amount of 240-mesh silicon carbide powder and water. Draw the molds containing the specimens back and forth across the plate coated with the abrasive and water. After surfacing, remove the specimens from the mold. The specimens should be visually examined for surface defects. A surface defect is defined as a surface discontinuity greater than 500 microns in major diameter. Acceptable specimens for testing shall appear to be uniform and meet the dimensional requirements of 7.9. A minimum of five specimens shall be selected from the remaining acceptable specimens and tested. Report the results of all specimens tested.

7.9.2 The time lapse between the start of mixing and the measurement of the compressive strenght testing shall be 24 ± 2 h. Storage of the specimens before testing shall be at 23 ± 2 °C and 50 ± 10 % relative humidity. Run specimens on any universal testing machine equipped to record load versus deformation. Employ a deformation cross head speed of 20 to

25.4 mm/min. Test the specimens without use of any type of pad between the specimen and the platens of the machine. The failure load shall be the load at the 2.0 % offset (2.0% proof stress), upper yield point, or at fracture, whichever occurs first (Fig. 5).

7.9.2.1 The load at 2.0 % offset is the load at the intersection of the S/N curve and a straight line parallel to the Hookean portion of the S/N curve (See Fig. X1.1 in Test Method D 695) but offset along the strain axis by 2.0 % of the test's gauge length (specimen's height).

7.9.2.2 Calculate the compressive strength as the failure load divided by the calculated cross-sectional area.

7.9.2.3 Report the compressive strength of the material as the average of the compression strengths of the specimens tested in 7.9.2 to the nearest 1 MPa (145 psi). A minimum of five specimens is required.

7.10 *Precision and Bias*—Since 1976, the original Specification F 451 methodologies have reportedly been routinely utilized by the various manufacturers. With the exception of the viscosity method of 7.8.1, which is based on another accepted ASTM document (Test Method D 3835), each test methodology in Section 7 contains its own statement of reporting acceptable levels of performance, reproducibility, and precision. Therefore, no interlaboratory studies have been performed by the Committee F-4.

8. Packaging

8.1 Materials shall be supplied in properly sealed containers made of materials that shall not contaminate or permit contamination of the contents. The containers shall be packaged so as to prevent damage or leakage during shipping and storage. Materials must be packaged to permit sterile transfer of contents to the sterile field.

8.2 The contents shall be easily accessible, easy to open, and convenient to mix in the operating room. Entire package contents (both powder and liquid) must be mixed to achieve recommended proportions.

9. Labeling

9.1 Labeling on these cements must be in conformance with the Federal Food, Drug, and Cosmetic Act, Code of Federal Regulations, and other pertinent laws and regulations.

9.2 The following minimal information must appear on the container label.

9.2.1 It shall be clearly stated or color coded, or both, if the mixture is intended for usage in the pre-dough, dough, or dual usage state.

9.2.2 The weight or volume, or both, of the liquid and powder components must be stated.

9.2.3 Constituents of the powder and liquid shall be clearly stated in terms of weight or volume percent. This shall include the generic names of polymers, copolymers, chemical initiators, stabilizers, cross-linking agents, and any other ingredients, such as radiopacify agents, gels, fillers, or antibiotics.

9.2.4 A statement that the contents are sterile and that the sterility shall be guaranteed only if the containers are undamaged.

9.2.5 The following warning shall appear on the label: (*a*) Flammable liquid; (*b*) Store below 25°C, and (*c*) Protect from light.

9.2.6 A statement to the effect that federal law restricts this device for sale by or on the order of a physician should be displayed.

9.2.7 The manufacturer and distributor shall be identified.

9.2.8 Each individual component of the package unit must be clearly identified as to batch or lot number.

9.3 The following information shall appear on the product insert labeling accompanying each package.

9.3.1 Adequate and accurate instruction shall be given for handling the components and preparing the cement. Instructions shall include a directive to mix all of the powder with all the liquid of a single unit. Procedures required to mix the materials, along with recommended mixing utensils, shall be given.

9.3.2 Proper technique for administration and recommended procedures for using the cement, including any special precautions, shall be indicated.

9.3.3 Toxic, hazardous, or irritating characteristics associated with the handling and use of the components and cement shall be indicated.

9.3.4 A statement shall be included that states that high temperatures of either the ambient surroundings or material will cause shorter doughing, working, and setting times, while low temperatures of either the ambient surroundings or material will increase doughing, working, and setting times.

9.3.5 The ranges of doughing and setting times as measured at 23 ± 1°C (7.5 and 7.7) shall be clearly stated.

10. Biocompatibility

10.1 The biocompatibility of acrylic bone cement has been reported in the literature **(1, 2)**. The material has been shown to produce a well characterized level of biological response following long-term clinical use and laboratory studies. The results of these studies and the clinical history indicate an acceptable level of biological response in applications in which the material has been utilized. When new applications of the material, or significant modification to the material, or its physical forms are being contemplated, the recommendations of Practice F 748 and testing as described in Practices F 619, F 749, F 756, F 763, F 813, F 895, and F 981 should be considered.

11. Keywords

11.1 acrylic bone cement; compression strength; doughing time; exothermic temperature; extrusion; intrusion; poly(methacrylic acid esters); setting time

APPENDIX

(Nonmandatory Information)

X1. RATIONALE

X1.1 Acrylic bone cement is a powder-liquid system that is currently sold in the United States for the fixation of internal orthopedic appliances. Because it plays a key role in highly synchronized surgical procedures, such as total joint replacement, its setting characteristics must be known and consistent each time. The material must also have adequate physical properties for placement and function. To these ends, the standard is addressed.

X1.2 While many of the tests are obvious forms of good manufacturing practice, others may be slightly more subtle and require some elaboration.

X1.2.1 The stability test measures the viscosity after storing the liquid at 60°C. This is an accelerated aging test to ensure that the monomeric component of the bone cement does not readily polymerize prematurely while stored before use.

X1.2.2 The dough and set times check that the material will be ready for placement at the proper time in the surgical procedure *and that it will set* neither prematurely nor in a delayed fashion.

X1.2.3 The maximum temperature test makes sure that the mass will *not release excessive heat* during setting. This could be damaging to the patient's tissue if not properly controlled.

X1.2.4 The dough and setting times and maximum temperature test also evaluate other important parameters. These tests will only respond consistently in the required time and temperature ranges if the powder particle size distribution, the liquid to powder ratio, the complex chemical compositions of both the powder and liquid, and the catalyst amount and distribution have been properly formulated and meted out and strict quality control during all stages of manufacturing is carefully monitored.

X1.2.5 The viscosity tests of the predough material and intrusion evaluations demonstrate that the material will flow into the bony interstices and around prostheses to produce adequate mechanical interlocking upon setting of the material.

X1.2.6 The compressive strength test measures if the set material will be strong enough for clinical applications.

X1.3 Further topics presently under consideration for eventual addition to the specification are as follows:

X1.3.1 Other mechanical tests, such as tension, flexion, and fracture toughness, which may be more sensitive to internal porosity and surface defects than the current compression test.

X1.3.2 Statement of biocompatibility of the cement.

X1.3.3 Shortening the time spans of the indentation tests.

X1.3.4 Requiring doughing and setting time data to be furnished with product information.

X1.3.5 Investigating changes in physical properties when leachable additives, such as antibiotics, are purposefully added.

X1.3.6 To define the optimum conditions of the viscosity test methodology so that the performance standards can be established.

X1.4 It should be noted that this document contains both test methodology and performance standards. Currently, in the case of viscosity measurement, only the test methodology has been described. This methodology will serve as a basis for future performance standards.

REFERENCES

(1) Williams, D. F., and Roaf, R., *Implants in Surgery* , W. B. Saunders Co., Ltd., London, 1973, pp 216–218.

(2) Linder, L., *Biocompatibility of Orthopedic Implants*, Vol II, Boca Raton: CRC Series in Biocompatibility, Williams, D. F. (ed.), CRC Press, 1982, pp. 1 to 23.

(3) *U.S. Pharmacopoeia,* Revision 20, Mack Publishing Co., Easton, PA, 1980, p 880.

(4) Tordella, J. P., ed., *Transactions of the Society of Rheology*, Vol 1, 1957, p 203.

(5) Philippoff, W., and Gaskins, F. H., eds., *Transactions of the Society of Rheology*, Vol 2, 1958, p 263.

(6) Bagley, E. B., and Birk, A. M., eds., *Journal of Applied Physics*, Vol 31, 1960, p 556.

(7) Rabinowitsch, R., *Zeitschrift Fuer Physikalische Chemie*, Vol A145, 1929, p 1.

Designation: F 452 – 76 (Reapproved 1998)

An American National Standard

Standard Specification for Preformed Cranioplasty Plates[1]

This standard is issued under the fixed designation F 452; the number immediately following the designation indicates the year of original adoption or, in the case of revision, the year of last revision. A number in parentheses indicates the year of last reapproval. A superscript epsilon (ε) indicates an editorial change since the last revision or reapproval.

1. Scope

1.1 This specification covers preformed cranioplasty plates which do not require further alteration for covering skull defects. This specification covers compositional and physical performance and packaging requirements, but does not cover toxicity nor biocompatibility of the materials.

2. Referenced Documents

2.1 *ASTM Standards:*

F 56 Specification for Stainless Steel Sheet and Strip for Surgical Implants[2]

F 75 Specification for Cast Cobalt-Chromium-Molybdenum Alloy for Surgical Implant Applications[2]

F 86 Practice for Surface Preparation and Marking of Metallic Surgical Implants[2]

F 139 Specification for Stainless Steel Sheet and Strip for Surgical Implants (Special Quality)[2]

2.2 *American Society for Quality Control (ASQC) Standard:*

C1-1968 Specifications of General Requirements for a Quality Program[3,4]

3. Materials

3.1 Cranioplasty plates conforming to this specification shall be fabricated from materials described in the latest issue of Specifications F 56, Grade 2, F 75, or F 139, Grade 2. The condition of the material (such as, annealed, cold finished, etc.) should be specified in the purchase order.

4. Dimensions and Tolerances

4.1 Cranioplasty plates conforming to this specification shall be fabricated in a variety of dimensions to accommodate, without further alteration, various sized skull defects.

4.2 Shape shall be contoured so as to re-establish the normal configuration and symmetry of the skull at various anticipated sites of defect such as the parietal bosses, the inion, the brow, the linea temporalis, etc.

4.3 Plates shall contain multiple perforations (see Fig. 1).

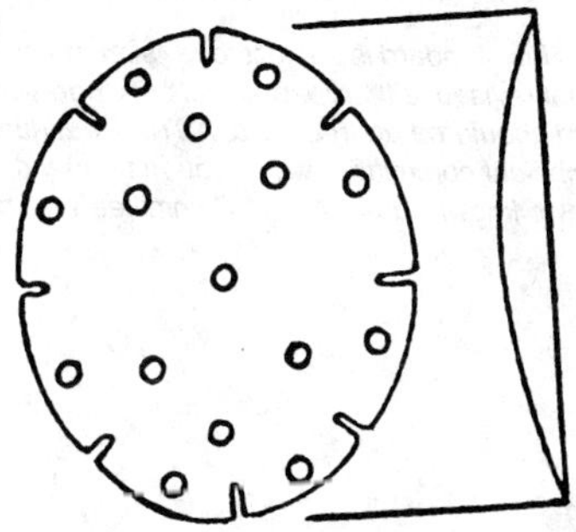

FIG. 1 Preformed Cranioplasty Plate

4.4 Thicknesses and individual shapes shall vary with need. Thickness tolerances shall be as follows:

Specified Thickness, in. (mm)	Thickness Tolerances, in. (mm)
0.005 (0.13) to 0.010 (0.25), incl	±10 %
0.010 (0.25) to 0.020 (0.51), incl	±0.0015 (0.04)
0.020 (0.51) to 0.035 (0.89), incl	±0.002 (0.05)
0.035 (0.89) to 0.050 (1.27), incl	±0.0025 (0.06)
0.050 (1.27) to 0.100 (2.54), incl	±0.003 (0.08)

5. Finish and Identification

5.1 Cranioplasty plates conforming to this specification shall have their surfaces prepared in accordance with the latest issue of Practice F 86. Specific requirements of surface finish (if any) shall be stated in the purchase order.

5.2 The method of marking the plates shall be one of those specified in Practice F 86.

6. Precautions

6.1 Cranioplasty plates covered by this specification shall *not* be reshaped in any manner after manufacture.

6.2 Material used to fasten the cranioplasty plates covered by this standard shall be the same alloy as the material used to make the specific plate being installed.

7. Packaging and Labeling

7.1 Cranioplasty plates conforming to this specification shall be supplied, packaged in accordance with the appropriate recommended practice being developed by ASTM Committee F-4. Minimum packaging and labeling for cranioplasty plates shall include the following:

7.1.1 An insert shall be included in the package for the plate showing the material from which it was fabricated and include

[1] This specification is under the jurisdiction of ASTM Committee F-4 on Medical and Surgical Materials and Devices and is the direct responsibility of Subcommittee F04.50 on Neurosurgical Standards.

Current edition approved April 5, 1976. Published June 1976.

[2] Discontinued—See 1991 *Annual Book of ASTM Standards*, Vol 13.01.

[3] *Annual Book of ASTM Standards*, Vol 13.01.

[4] Available from American Society for Quality Control, 161 West Wisconsin Ave., Milwaukee, WI 53203.

a recommendation against using fasteners other than the same material or a recommended substitute to secure the plate when implanted.

7.1.2 Labeling shall include the nominal thickness of the plate.

8. Quality Program Requirements

8.1 The manufacturer of cranioplasty plates covered by this specification shall maintain a quality program such as, for example, defined in ASQC Specifications C 1-1968.

9. Keywords

9.1 cranioplasty plates; neurosurgical medical devices/applications; orthopaedic medical devices; bone plates

Designation: F 543 – 01

Standard Specification and Test Methods for Metallic Medical Bone Screws[1]

This standard is issued under the fixed designation F 543; the number immediately following the designation indicates the year of original adoption or, in the case of revision, the year of last revision. A number in parentheses indicates the year of last reapproval. A superscript epsilon (ε) indicates an editorial change since the last revision or reapproval.

This standard has been approved for use by agencies of the Department of Defense.

1. Scope

1.1 This specification provides requirements for materials, finish and marking, care and handling, and the acceptable dimensions and tolerances for metallic bone screws that are implanted into bone. The dimensions and tolerances in this specification are applicable only to metallic bone screws described in this specification.

1.2 This specification provides performance considerations and standard test methods for measuring mechanical properties in torsion of metallic bone screws that are implanted into bone. These test methods may also be applicable to other screws besides those whose dimensions and tolerances are specified here. The following annexes are included:

1.2.1 Annex A1—Test Method for Determining the Torsional Properties of Metallic Bone Screws.

1.2.2 Annex A2—Test Method for Driving Torque of Medical Bone Screws.

1.2.3 Annex A3—Test Method for Determining the Axial Pullout Strength of Medical Bone Screws.

1.2.4 Annex A4—Specifications for Type HA and Type HB Metallic Bone Screws.

1.2.5 Annex A5—Specifications for Type HC and Type HD Metallic Bone Screws.

1.2.6 Annex A6—Specifications for Metallic Bone Screw Drive Connections.

1.3 This specification is based, in part, upon ISO 5835, ISO 6475 and ISO 9268.

1.4 Unless otherwise indicated, the values stated in SI units are to be regarded as standard. The values in parentheses are given for information only.

1.5 *This standard may involve the use of hazardous materials, operations, and equipment. This standard does not purport to address all of the safety concerns, if any, associated with its use. It is the responsibility of the user of this standard to establish appropriate safety and health practices and determine the applicability of regulatory limitations prior to use.*

2. Referenced Documents

2.1 *ASTM Standards:*

E 4 Practices for Force Verification of Testing Machines[2]

E 6 Terminology Relating to Methods of Mechanical Testing[2]

E 8 Test Methods for Tension Testing of Metallic Materials[2]

E 122 Practice for Choice of Sample Size to Estimate a Measure of Quality for a Lot or Process[3]

F 67 Specification for Unalloyed Titanium for Surgical Implant Applications[4]

F 86 Practice for Surface Preparation and Marking of Metallic Surgical Implants[4]

F 116 Specification for Medical Screwdriver Bits[4]

F 117 Test Method for Driving Torque of Medical Bone Screws[4]

F 136 Specification for Wrought Titanium – 6 Aluminum – 4 Vanadium ELI (Extra Low Interstitial) Alloy (UNS R56401) for Surgical Implant Applications[4]

F 138 Specification for Wrought 18 Chromium-14 Nickel-2.5 Molybdenum Stainless Steel Bar and Wire for Surgical Implants (UNS S31673)[4]

F 565 Practice for Care and Handling of Orthopedic Implants and Instruments[4]

F 620 Specification for Titanium-6 Aluminum 4 Vanadium ELI Alloy Forgings for Surgical Implants [UNS R56401][4]

F 799 Specification for Cobalt-28 Chromium-6 Molybdenum Alloy Forgings for Surgical Implants (UNS R31537, R31538, R31539)[4]

F 983 Practice for Permanent Marking of Orthopedic Implant Components[4]

F 1295 Specification for Wrought Titanium-6 Aluminum-7 Niobium Alloy for Surgical Implant Applications [UNS R56700][4]

F 1314 Specification for Wrought Nitrogen Strengthened-22 Chromium-12.5 Nickel-5 Manganese-2.5 Molybdenum Stainless Steel Bar and Wire for Surgical Implants[4]

F 1472 Specification for Wrought Titanium-6 Aluminum-4 Vanadium Alloy for Surgical Implant Applications (UNS R56400)[4]

---

[1] This specification is under the jurisdiction of ASTM Committee F04 on Medical and Surgical Materials and Devices and is the direct responsibility of Subcommittee F04.21 on Osteosynthesis.

Current edition approved May 10, 2001. Published May 2001. Originally published as F 543 – 77. Last previous edition F 543 – 00.

[2] *Annual Book of ASTM Standards*, Vol 03.01.

[3] *Annual Book of ASTM Standards*, Vol 14.02.

[4] *Annual Book of ASTM Standards*, Vol 13.01.

F 1537 Specification for Wrought Cobalt-28 Chromium-6 Molybdenum Alloy for Surgical Implants (UNS R31537, UNS R31538, and UNS R31539)[4]

F 1586 Specification for Wrought Nitrogen Strengthened-21 Chromium-10 Nickel-3 Manganese-2.5 Molybdenum Stainless Steel Bar for Surgical Implants[4]

F 1622 Test Method for Measuring the Torsional Properties in Metallic Bone Screws[4]

F 1691 Test Method for Determining the Axial Pull-Out Strength of Medical Bone Screws[4]

F 1713 Specification for Wrought Titanium-13 Niobium-13 Zirconium Alloy for Surgical Implant Applications[4]

F 1813 Specification for Wrought Titanium-12 Molybdenum-6 Zirconium-2 Iron Alloy for Surgical Implant Applications[4]

F 1839 Specification for Rigid Polyurethane Foam for Use As a Standard Material for Testing Orthopaedic Devices and Instruments[4]

2.2 *ISO Standards:*

5835 Implants for Surgery—Metal Bone Screws with Hexagonal Driver Connection, Spherical Under Surface of Head, Asymmetrical Thread—Dimensions[5]

6475 Implants for Surgery—Metal Bone Screws with Asymmetrical Thread and Spherical Under-Surface—Mechanical Requirements and Test Methods[5]

9268 Implants for Surgery—Metal Bone Screws with Conical Under-surface of Head—Dimensions[5]

3. Terminology

3.1 *Definitions*—Some of the terms defined in this section are shown in Fig. 1.

3.1.1 *axial pullout strength*—the tensile force required to fail or remove a bone screw from a material into which the screw has been inserted.

3.1.2 *breaking angle*—angle of rotation at which the screw demonstrates its most rapid decrease in torque.

3.1.3 *buttress thread*—an asymmetrical thread profile characterized by a pressure flank which is nearly perpendicular to the screw axis

3.1.4 *cancellous screw*—a screw designed primarily to gain purchase into cancellous bone. Cancellous screws typically have a HB thread and may or may not be fully threaded.

[5] Available from American National Standards Institute, 11 W. 42nd St., 13th Floor, New York, NY 10036.

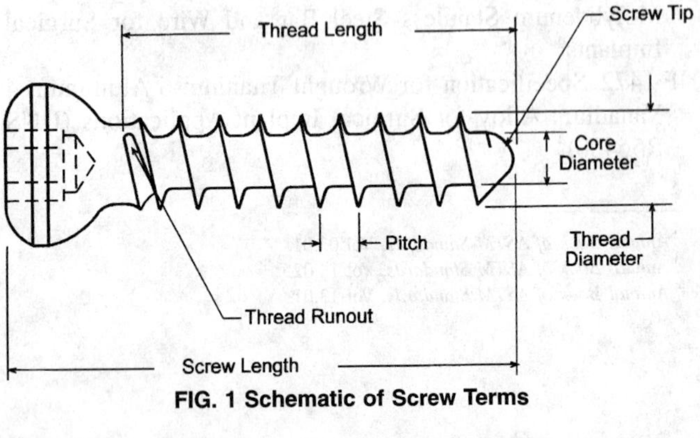

FIG. 1 Schematic of Screw Terms

3.1.5 *cortical screw*—a screw designed primarily to gain biocortical purchase into cortical bone. Cortical screws typically have a HA thread and are fully threaded.

3.1.6 *core diameter*—the smallest diameter of the threaded portion of the screw measured at the thread root. This is also known as the minor diameter or root diameter.

3.1.7 *gage length*—the distance between the holding device, for example, a split collet, and the underside of the screw head.

3.1.8 *grip length*—the length of threads held fast in the split collet or other holding mechanism.

3.1.9 *insertion depth*—the threaded length as inserted into the test block.

3.1.10 *insertion torque*—the amount of torque required to overcome the frictional force between the screw and the material used for testing while driving the screw into the material.

3.1.11 *maximum torque* (N-m)—the largest value of torque recorded during the period of rotation before screw failure in torsional shear when tested in accordance with Annex A1.

3.1.12 *nontapping screw*—a screw that has a tip that does not contain a flute. Nontapping screws usually require a tap to be inserted into the pilot hole before the insertion of the screw, when used in moderate or hard bone.

3.1.13 *partially threaded screw*—a screw whose threaded portion does not extend fully from the screw point to the screw head but instead has a smooth shaft running between the head and threads.

3.1.14 *pilot hole*—the hole drilled into the bone into which the screw tip is inserted. The pilot hole is normally slightly larger than the screw's core diameter. However, if the screw is to be used to provide compression across a fracture, a portion of the pilot hole may be larger to allow for a clearance fit.

3.1.15 *pitch*—the length between the thread crests.

3.1.16 *removal torque*—the amount of torque required to overcome the frictional force between the screw and the material used for testing while removing the screw from the material (for example, counterclockwise rotation for right-hand thread).

3.1.17 *screw head*—the end of the screw which is opposite of the tip and from which the means of inserting the screw is coupled.

3.1.18 *screw length*—the overall length of the screw measured from the screw head to the screw tip.

3.1.19 *screw thread*—a helical groove on a cylindrical or conical surface. The projecting helical ridge thus formed is called a screw thread, consisting of peaks (crests) and valleys (roots).

3.1.20 *self-tapping screw*—a screw that has any number of flutes at its tip which are intended to cut the screw's thread form into the bone upon insertion.

3.1.21 *size*—an identification of a screw based on its nominal thread diameter, as defined in Section 6.

3.1.22 *solid core*—a screw that does not contain a cannulation along its longitudinal axis.

3.1.23 *thread diameter*—the largest diameter of the threaded portion of the screw measured over the thread crests. This is also known as the major diameter.

3.1.24 *thread length*—the length of the threaded portion of the screw, measured from the thread runout to the screw tip.

3.1.25 *thread runout*—the intersection of the screw thread with either the screw shaft or screw head.

3.1.26 *torsional yield strength* (N-m)—the point at which the screw reaches its proportional limit when tested in accordance with Annex A1. This will be determined by the offset method. A 2° offset value will be used.

4. Classification

4.1 There are a large variety of medical bone screws currently in use. They may be classified by the definitions provided in Section 3. This specification currently includes information that defines the following types of screws:

4.1.1 *Type HA*—Spherical undersurface of head, shallow, asymmetrical buttress thread, and deep screw head.

4.1.2 *Type HB*—Spherical undersurface of head, deep, asymmetrical buttress thread, and shallow screw head.

4.1.3 *Type HC*—Conical undersurface of head, symmetrical thread.

4.1.4 *Type HD*—Conical undersurface of head, asymmetrical thread.

5. Material

5.1 Screws shall be fabricated from one of the following materials:

5.1.1 Stainless steel alloy (Specification F 138).

5.1.2 Nitrogen-strengthened stainless steel alloy (Specifications F 1314 and F 1586).

5.1.3 Unalloyed titanium (Specification F 67).

5.1.4 Titanium-aluminum-vanadium alloy (Specifications F 136, F 620, and F 1472).

5.1.5 Titanium-aluminum-niobium alloy (Specification F 1295).

5.1.6 Titanium-niobium-zirconium alloy (Specification F 1713).

5.1.7 Cobalt-chromium-molybdenum alloy (Specifications F 799 and F 1537).

5.1.8 Titanium-molybdenum-zirconium-iron alloy (Specification F 1813).

6. Dimensions and Tolerances

6.1 There are many types of metallic bone screw designs available, so a complete list of dimensions and tolerances for all screws covered by this specification is unfeasible. However, this specification does provide required dimensions and tolerances for four types of screws as classified in 4.1. Screws conforming to this specification, and designated HA, HB, HC, or HD screws, shall be fabricated in accordance with the dimensions and tolerances described in Annex A4 and Annex A5, respectively.

7. Finish and Marking

7.1 The screw shall be free from nicks, dents, burrs, and scratches when examined in accordance with Practice F 86.

7.2 When size permits, the following information should be legibly marked on the head of the screw (in order of preference):

7.2.1 Manufacturer's name or logo,

7.2.2 *Screw Size*—If a screw is manufactured in accordance with ASTM or ISO specifications, the ASTM or ISO designation should be provided,

7.2.3 Material,

7.2.4 Catalog number, and

7.2.5 Manufacturing lot number.

7.3 Screws shall be marked in accordance with Practice F 983, unless otherwise specified in 7.2, in a manner such that the mechanical integrity of the screw is not compromised.

8. Care and Handling

8.1 Screws should be cared for and handled in accordance with Practice F 565, as appropriate.

9. Driving Instruments

9.1 A variety of screwdrivers exist for the insertion and removal of bone screws. The classification and dimensions for various screw-drive recesses currently used in the medical industry are documented in Annex A6. Specification F 116 provides related dimensional information for several types of medical screwdrivers.

9.2 Screws conforming to this specification, and designated HA, HB, HC, or HD screws, shall be manufactured with drive recesses that conform to the requirements specified in Annex A4 and Annex A5, respectively.

10. Performance Considerations and Test Methods

10.1 The following properties may be important when determining the suitability of a screw for a particular application. However, the test methods referenced as follows may not be appropriate for all types of implant applications. The user is cautioned to consider the appropriateness of the test methods in view of the devices being tested and their potential application.

10.1.1 *Torsional Strength*—This test method is an important parameter to prevent screw breakage during insertion or removal. The torsional strength shall be determined using the test methods described in Annex A1.

10.1.2 *Breaking Angle*—This test method provides a measure of the ductility of the screw when undergoing a torsional moment. A screw with a greater breaking angle may provide an earlier tactile warning to the surgeon that the screw is reaching its maximum torsional strength. The breaking angle shall be determined using the test methods described in Annex A1.

10.1.3 *Axial Pullout Strength*—This test method may be an important parameter if the screw is subjected to axial tensile forces, or if the screw is fixed into poor quality or osteoporotic bone. The pullout strength may be determined using the test methods described in Annex A3.

10.1.4 *Insertion Torque*—This test method may be an important parameter to avoid failure of the screw during insertion and to ensure that the screw may be easily inserted by the surgeon. The insertion torque should be much less than torsional yield strength of the screw and of the appropriate screwdriver bit. The insertion torque may be determined using the test methods described in Annex A2.

10.1.5 *Removal Torque*—This test method may be an important parameter to avoid failure of the screw during removal and to ensure that the screw may be easily removed by the surgeon. The removal torque should be much less than torsional yield strength of the screw and of the appropriate screwdriver bit. The removal torque may be determined using the test methods described in Annex A2.

11. Performance Requirements

11.1 Screws shall meet the mechanical performance requirements specified in its associated specification annex.

12. Keywords

12.1 bone screw; dimensions; insertion; performance requirements; pullout; static; test methods; torsion

ANNEXES

(Mandatory Information)

A1. TEST METHOD FOR DETERMINING THE TORSIONAL PROPERTIES OF METALLIC BONE SCREWS

A1.1 Significance and Use

A1.1.1 This test method is used to measure the torsional yield strength, maximum torque, and breaking angle of the bone screw under standard conditions. The results obtained in this test method are not intended to predict the torque encountered while inserting or removing a bone screw in human or animal bone. This test method is intended only to measure the uniformity of the product tested or to compare the mechanical properties of different, yet similarly sized, products.

A1.2 Apparatus

A1.2.1 *Testing Fixture*—The torsion testing apparatus that is to be used for applying the required torque to the specimen shall be calibrated for the range of torques and rotational displacements used in the determination.[6] A suitable testing fixture for the torsional yield strength-maximum torque-breaking angle test is illustrated in Fig. A1.1.

A1.2.1.1 *Test Speed*—The torsional force shall be applied at a constant rate of 1 to 5 r/min.

A1.2.1.2 *Torque Transducer*—A transducer to translate the applied torque into an electrical signal amenable to continuous recording, calibrated over the range of torques, both in the clockwise and counterclockwise rotation, to be encountered in the test method, shall be provided.

[6] At the time that this specification was approved, no standard test method for the verification of torsion machines or transducers has been accepted. The user is urged to review Test Methods E 8 for general guidance.

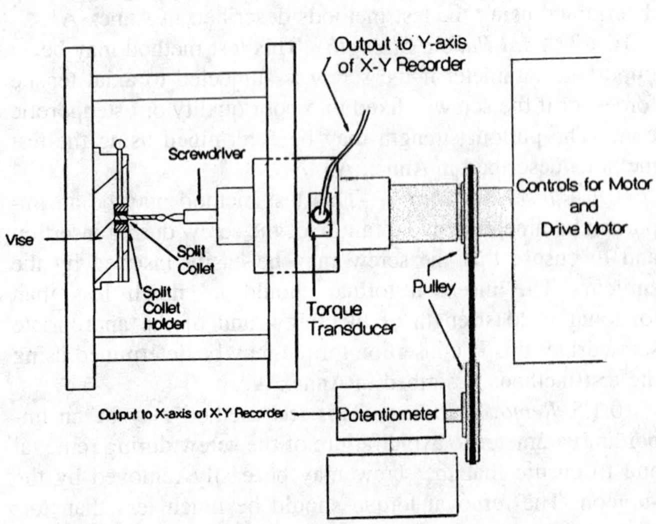

FIG. A1.1 Test Apparatus for Determination of Torsional Breaking Force and Breaking Angle

A1.2.1.3 *Torsional Displacement Transducer*—A transducer to translate the angle of twist into an electrical signal amenable to continuous recording, calibrated over the range of angles to be encountered in the test and an accuracy of ±0.3°, both in the clockwise and counterclockwise rotation, shall be provided.

A1.2.1.4 *Specimen Holder*—A mechanical device to clamp onto the bone screw to prevent its rotation while being stressed without significantly damaging its mechanical integrity shall be provided. One such method is to insert a threaded stopper into the opposite side of a test block. The test block for this holding mechanism will accommodate the insertion of a threaded stopper on the other side of the test block. The threaded stopper will prevent the screw from being completely inserted into the test block and will allow the torsional strength of the screw to be measured. This holder will be modified according to the size of the testing specimen so that the gage length of the specimen will be as outlined in A1.3.1.

A1.2.1.5 *Recorder*—The data recorder shall be suitable to continuously record torque versus angle of rotation, calibrated in units of Newton-metres for torque and degrees for angle of rotation. The value of torque shall have a resolution of 5 % of torsional yield strength. The angular displacement scale shall have a minimum sensitivity so as to enable an accurate offset measurement capability for a 2° angular displacement (see A1.3.3).

A1.2.2 *Test Specimen*—The test specimen shall be a completely fabricated and finished bone screw.

A1.3 Procedure

A1.3.1 *Torsional Yield Strength, Maximum Torque, and Breaking Angle*—Place the specimen in the holding device so that five threads, below the head of the screw, are exposed outside the holding device (for example, split collet, and so forth). If the test specimen cannot accommodate this setup because the screw is too small or is partially threaded, alternate procedures may be used. For fully threaded screws that are too small, the gage length of the specimen should represent 20 % of the threaded portion of the test specimen. For partially threaded screws, a large enough portion of the screw thread should be gripped to firmly secure the screw so that it does not rotate when under torsional load. There are no specific requirements on the gage length or the grip length in this case; however, at least one full thread shall be exposed, if possible. Since the gage length and grip length can vary for these screws, the only requirement is that both be reported.

A1.3.2 The gage length or grip length should be kept the same length for test screws of similar design. If a split collet and collet holder are used, the following test method is appropriate: place the split collet in the collet holder. Clamp the split collet and holder in the vise. The clamping force of the vise should be sufficient to prevent rotation of the screw or the split collet. Drive the specimen in the direction of insertion, using an appropriate size and configured screwdriver bit, by applying a torsional force. If an axial load is required to maintain the screwdriver bit in the screw head, its value should be noted. The torque wrench shall be driven at a rate of 1 to 5 r/min.

NOTE A1.1—The simultaneous use of two chart recorders may simplify the ability to measure torsional yield strength accurately by the offset method. One chart recorder with an angular displacement scale or sensitivity of 50°/cm is convenient for measuring maximum torque and breaking angle. A second chart recorder with an angular displacement scale or sensitivity of 10°/cm or less is suggested to provide accurate offset measurement capability for measuring a 2° angular displacement. Alternatively, one chart recorder and a digital storage oscilloscope may be used.

A1.3.3 The torsional yield strength will be determined by the offset method (Fig. A1.2), using the torque versus angle of rotation curve produced in A1.3.1 and A1.3.2.

A1.3.3.1 On the torque versus angle of rotation curve, locate Point m equal to a rotation of 2°. Draw mn parallel to OA, and locate b, the intersection of mn with the torque versus angle of rotation curve. Torque B is defined as the torsional yield strength.

A1.3.3.2 The maximum torque is determined by the largest value of torque on the torque versus angle of rotation curve.

A1.3.3.3 The breaking angle is determined from the torque versus angle plot shown in Fig. A1.3. The breaking angle is defined as the point at which the torque portion of the curve demonstrates its most rapid descent (negative slope) to total failure. The breaking angle (B.A.) is determined as the intersection of the two tangents (D and E) shown in Fig. A1.3. Line E is a tangent to the horizontal portion of the curve which represents maximum torque. Line D is drawn at the curve's most rapid descent. The intersection of these two lines is the breaking angle (B.A.) and is recorded to the nearest 10°.

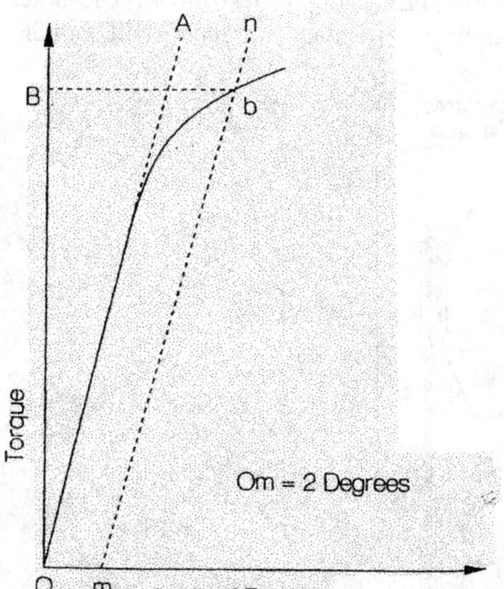

FIG. A1.2 Typical Torque Versus Angle of Rotation Curve

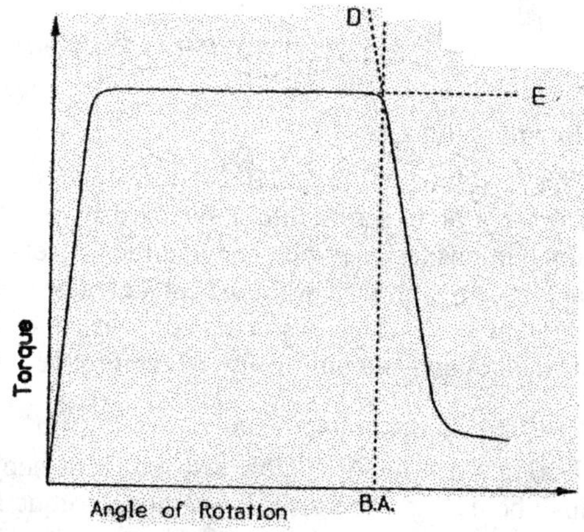

FIG. A1.3 Typical Plot of Torque Versus Torsion Angle

A1.4 Report

A1.4.1 Report the following information for each specimen tested:

A1.4.1.1 *Screw Identification*—Reference any applicable ASTM or ISO specification that may apply to the specimen. If specifications do not exist, provide head form, thread form, major and minor diameter, thread pitch, overall screw length, head and shank (unthreaded portion of the screw excluding the head) length, and type of screw point.

A1.4.1.2 Screw chemical composition.

A1.4.1.3 Surface finish.

A1.4.1.4 Gage length.

A1.4.1.5 Torsional yield strength.

A1.4.1.6 Maximum torque.

A1.4.1.7 Breaking angle.

A1.4.1.8 Torque versus angle of rotation plot.

A1.4.1.9 The size of the exposed portion of the screwdriver (that is, the length and diameter relative to the tested screw) or the angular deformation of the screwdriver assembly at maximum torque.

A1.4.1.10 *Grip Length*—Does not have to be reported for a fully threaded screw of ASTM or ISO specification whose overall length is given.

A1.4.1.11 *Fracture Location*—The location can be specified by listing the number of threads below the head at which the screw fails or by measuring the distance below the head to the approximate fracture point.

A1.5 Precision and Bias

A1.5.1 Data establishing the precision and bias to be expected from this test method have not yet been obtained.

A2. TEST METHOD FOR DRIVING TORQUE OF MEDICAL BONE SCREWS

A2.1 Significance and Use

A2.1.1 This test method is used to measure the torque required to drive a bone screw into a standard material. The results obtained in this test method bear no direct correlation to the insertion torque required to insert the subject bone screw in human or animal bone. This test method is used only for purposes of maintaining the uniformity of the product tested.

A2.2 Apparatus

A2.2.1 *Testing Fixture*—A suitable test fixture as shown in Fig. A2.1 may be used for the insertion-removal torque tests.[6] This fixture shall incorporate the test block material that conforms to Specification F 1839, test block clamp, drill bushing, and bushing support depicted. It shall be sufficiently rigid to not deflect or deform under the conditions of loading encountered during the test.

A2.2.1.1 *Torque Transducer*—A transducer to translate the applied torque into an electrical signal amenable to continuous recording, calibrated over the range of torques, both in the clockwise and counterclockwise rotation, to be encountered in the test shall be provided.

A2.2.1.2 *Torsional Displacement Transducer*—A transducer to translate the angle of twist into an electrical signal amenable to continuous recording, calibrated in a manner similar to Practices E 4 over the range of angles to be encountered in the test to an accuracy of ±0.3°, both in the clockwise and counterclockwise rotation, shall be provided.

A2.2.1.3 *Data Recorder*—The data recorder shall be suitable to record torque versus angle of rotation continuously, calibrated in units of newton-metres for torque and degrees for angle of rotation. The value of torque shall have a resolution of 10 % of the maximum measured torque. The angular displacement scale shall have sensitivity such that at least four revolutions can be recorded and displayed.

A2.2.1.4 *Bushing*—A suitable replaceable bushing, fabricated from material that conforms to Specification F 1839, shall be incorporated into the testing fixture. This bushing shall be of sufficient length and rigidity to ensure that specimens are driven into the test block normal to the top surface of the test block. The bore of the bushing shall be of such dimension as to ensure guidance of the test specimen with minimum frictional resistance between the major diameter of the test specimen and the bore of the bushing. Worn bushings shall be discarded and replaced with new bushings before conducting the test.

A2.2.1.5 *Test Block Clamp*—A clamp or holding device shall be incorporated into the testing fixture. This holding device shall maintain the drilled pilot hole in the test block in line with the test specimen. The holding device shall not deform the test block during clamping of the test block or performance of the test.

A2.2.1.6 *Test Specimen*—The test specimen shall be a completely fabricated, finished, and sterilized bone screw of sufficient length to transverse the bushing and test block.

A2.2.1.7 *Test Block*—The test block shall be fabricated from a uniform material that conforms to Specification F 1839. The top and bottom surfaces shall be flat, smooth, and parallel (within ±0.4 mm (1/64 in.)) as required to ensure that the test block will be supported in the fixture with the top surface at an angle of 90° to the centerline of the test specimen. The edges of the test block shall be of such contour or squareness as required to ensure that the test block clamp shall hold the test block free of relative motion without deformation of the test block during clamping or testing. The test block thickness shall be not less than 4.8 mm (3/16 in.).

A2.2.1.8 *Pilot Holes in Test Block*—Pilot holes shall be drilled in the test block for insertion and removal of the test specimen. The drill size used shall be that specified by the screw manufacturer, for the size screw being tested. If specified by the screw manufacturer, the specified sized tap shall be used to tap the pilot hole before testing. The holes shall be drilled at 90° to the top surface of the test block. The holes shall be drilled straight and true, free of taper, bell mouth, or barrel

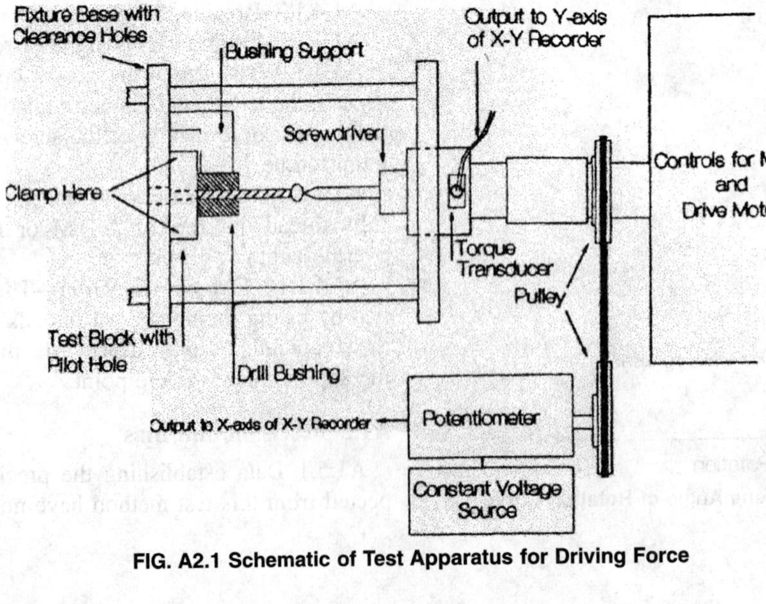

FIG. A2.1 Schematic of Test Apparatus for Driving Force

shape. If there are multiple holes in one test block, the pilot holes shall be spaced sufficiently far away from test block edges so that testing does not deform test block edges. Spacing should have as minimum distance of 5× the diameter of the screw. When the test block is inserted into the test fixture (Fig. A2.1), the pilot hole, screw, and screwdriver shall be on the same axis.

A2.3 Sampling

A2.3.1 Representative random samples may be taken from each lot or processing quantity in accordance with Practice E 122.

A2.4 Procedure

A2.4.1 *Insertion and Removal Torque*—Place the specimen in the test fixture as illustrated in Fig. A2.1. Drive the specimen into the test block, using the appropriate size and configured screwdriver bit, by applying a torsional force at a rate of 1 to 5 r/min, to the head of the specimen with the motor-driven torque wrench. The insertion torque shall be the maximum reading recorded during the initial four revolutions of the specimen. The removal torque will be measured by reversing the direction of rotation and recording the maximum torque recorded during the four revolutions required to remove the screw from the test block. Values should be reported in newton-metres. A 1.14-kgf (2.5-lbf) or less axial load should be used to maintain the screwdriver bit in the screw head during both the insertion and removal procedures. If a larger axial load is applied, this load shall be recorded on the report form. This load may be measured by any appropriate method.

A2.5 Report

A2.5.1 The report shall include the following for each specimen tested. (All standards units for reporting shall be in SI units.)

A2.5.1.1 *Screw Identification*—Reference any applicable ASTM or ISO standard specification that may apply to the specimen. If specifications do not exist, provide head form, thread form, major and minor diameter, thread pitch, overall screw length, head and shank (unthreaded portion of the screw excluding the head) length, and type of screw point.

A2.5.1.2 Screw chemical composition.

A2.5.1.3 Surface finish.

A2.5.1.4 Insertion torque.

A2.5.1.4.1 Axial load required.

A2.5.1.4.2 Insertion depth (may be calculated or measured).

A2.5.1.4.3 Specification of whether the pilot holes were or were not pretapped, if so, specifications of the tap size, tap diameter, and tap depth.

A2.5.1.4.4 Insertion test speed if outside the range specified in A2.4.1.

A2.5.1.5 Removal torque.

A2.5.1.5.1 Axial load required.

A2.5.1.5.2 Insertion test speed if outside the range specified in A2.4.1.

A2.5.1.6 *Test Block Material Description*—Specification F 1839 grade. For bushing material that does not conform to Specification F 1839, provide

A2.5.1.6.1 Trade name.

A2.5.1.6.2 Composition.

A2.5.1.6.3 Density.

A2.5.1.6.4 Tensile strength.

A2.5.1.6.5 Compression strength.

A2.5.1.6.6 Shear strength.

A2.6 Precision and Bias

A2.6.1 Data establishing the precision and accuracy to be expected from this test method have not yet been obtained.

A3. TEST METHOD FOR DETERMINING THE AXIAL PULLOUT STRENGTH OF MEDICAL BONE SCREWS

A3.1 Significance and Use

A3.1.1 This test method is used to measure the axial tensile force required to fail or remove a bone screw from a defined material. The results obtained in this test method are not intended to predict the force required to remove the subject bone screw from human or animal bone. This test method is intended only to measure the uniformity of the products tested or to compare the strength of different products.

A3.1.2 This test method may not be appropriate for all types of implant applications. The user is cautioned to consider the appropriateness of the method in view of the materials being tested and their potential application.

A3.2 Apparatus

A3.2.1 *Test Fixture*—Machines used for testing the axial pull out strength of screws shall conform to the requirements of Practices E 4. A suitable test fixture as shown in Fig. A3.1 may be used for testing. This fixture shall incorporate the test block material which conforms to Specification F 1839, test block clamp, drill bushing, and bushing support depicted in the insertion torque test method, Annex A2. In addition to these requirements, the test block clamp and bushing support should be sufficiently rigid such that deflection under the required loading conditions is negligible. The test block clamp should have a minimum grip span of five times the major diameter of the bone screw with the screw centered between the grips. The grip span should be consistent throughout testing.

A3.2.2 *Test Block*. The test block shall be fabricated from a uniform material that conforms to Specification F 1839. The top and bottom surfaces shall be flat, smooth, and parallel (within ±0.4 mm (1⁄64 in.)) as required to ensure that the test block will be supported in the fixture with the top surface at an angle of 90° to the centerline of the test specimen. The edges of the test block shall be of such contour or squareness as required to ensure that the test block clamp shall hold the test block free of relative motion without deformation of the test block during clamping or testing. The test block thickness shall be not less than 20 mm (3⁄4 in.).

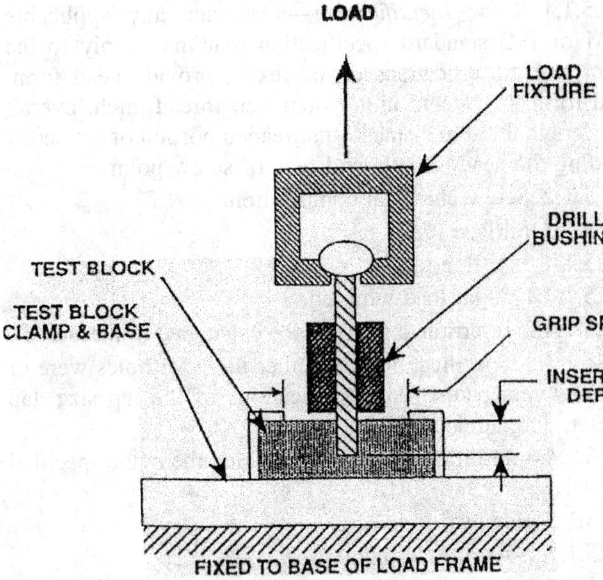

FIG. A3.1 Schematic of Test Apparatus for Pullout Strength

A3.2.3 *Data Acquisition Device*—The data recorder shall be suitable to continuously record load versus load fixture displacement.

A3.2.4 *Load Frame*—Machines used for testing shall conform to the requirements of Practices E 4. The loads used for the test method shall be within the loading range of the test machine as defined in Practices E 4.

A3.2.5 *Load Fixture*—A suitable fixture shall be used to place a tensile load on the bone screw. The load shall be transferred through the head of the screw and should be aligned with the screw's longitudinal axis. The fixture shall have a slot to capture the head of the screw without contact being made with the screw's shaft. To ensure proper alignment, the slot shall have a spherical recess into which the screw head can be seated directly under the applied load.

A3.3 Sampling, Test Specimens, and Test Units

A3.3.1 All test components shall be representative of implant quality products.

A3.4 Procedure

A3.4.1 *Insertion of the Test Specimen*—The bone screws shall be inserted into the standard material in accordance with the insertion torque test method, Annex A2. The screws shall be inserted at a rate of 3 r/min to a depth of 20 mm. For fully threaded screws with threaded lengths less than 20 mm, the insertion depth should be 60 % of the threaded length of the screw. Partially threaded bone screws should have all threads inserted into the standard material.

A3.4.2 *Axial Pullout Strength of the Test Specimen*—The test block and test block clamp depicted in Annex A2 shall be fixed to the base of the load frame so that the longitudinal axis of the screw is aligned with the direction of the applied load. The screw's head shall be placed in the slot of the load fixture and seated in the spherical recess. The load fixture shall then be attached to the load frame. A tensile load shall be applied to the test specimen at a rate of 5 mm/min until the screw fails or releases from the test block. Load (newtons) versus load fixture displacement (millimetres) shall be recorded on a data acquisition device, noting the maximum load applied and the mode of failure (screw shaft, screw threads, or material failure).

A3.5 Calculation or Interpretation of Results

A3.5.1 *Axial Pullout Strength*—Determine the axial pullout strength (newtons) of the test specimen from the load-displacement curve. The maximum load is reached during the test method.

A3.6 Report

A3.6.1 Report the following information:

A3.6.1.1 *Screw Identification*—Reference any applicable ASTM or ISO standard specification that may apply to the specimen. If specifications do not exist, provide head form, thread form, helix angle, major and minor diameter, thread pitch, overall screw length, head and shank length, length of threaded portion of shank for partially threaded screws, and type of screw point.

A3.6.1.2 Screw chemical composition.

A3.6.1.3 Surface finish.

A3.6.1.4 Axial pullout strength (as defined in 3.1.1).

A3.6.1.5 Grip span.

A3.6.1.6 Insertion depth.

A3.6.1.7 Test block thickness.

A3.6.1.8 Mode of failure.

A3.6.1.9 *Test Block Material Description*—Specification F 1839 grade or density. For materials that do not conform to F 1839, provide the following information and the appropriate test methods used to determine the properties of the test block material:

A3.6.1.9.1 Trade name,

A3.6.1.9.2 Composition,

A3.6.1.9.3 Density,

A3.6.1.9.4 Tensile strength,

A3.6.1.9.5 Compression strength, and

A3.6.1.9.6 Shear strength.

A3.7 Precision and Bias

A3.7.1 Data establishing the precision and accuracy to be expected from this test method have not yet been obtained.

A4. SPECIFICATIONS FOR HA AND HB METALLIC MEDICAL BONE SCREWS

A4.1 Screw Classification

A4.1.1 There are a large variety of medical bone screws currently in use. They may be classified by the definitions provided in Section 3. This specification includes the following types of screws with a solid head and a solid core:

A4.1.1.1 *Type HA*—Shallow, asymmetrical buttress thread, deep screw head, and spherical undersurface of head.

A4.1.1.2 *Type HB*—Deep, asymmetrical buttress thread, shallow screw head, and spherical undersurface of head.

A4.2 Screw and Thread Form Dimensions

A4.2.1 There are many types of metallic bone screw designs available, so a complete list of dimensions and tolerances for all screws covered by this specification is unfeasible. This specification specifies dimensions and tolerances for two types of screws that are classified in 4.1. Screws conforming to this specification, and designated with either the HA or HB classification shall be fabricated in accordance with the dimensions and tolerances in this Annex in accordance with the following requirements.

A4.2.1.1 *Type HA*:

(1) Screw Dimensions—The dimensions of HA screws are given in Table A4.1 and Fig. A4.1.

(2) Screw Thread—The dimensions of the threads of HA screws are given in Table A4.2 and Fig. A4.2.

A4.2.1.2 *Type HB*:

(1) Screw Dimensions—The dimensions of HB screws are given in Table A4.3 and Fig. A4.3.

(2) Screw Thread—The dimensions of the threads of HB screws are given in Table A4.4 and Fig. A4.4.

A4.3 Drive Connections

A4.3.1 Screws conforming to this specification, and designated with either the HA or HB classification shall be fabricated with the following drive connections in accordance with the dimensions and tolerances found in Annex A6.

A4.3.1.1 *Type HA*—Hexagonal recess for accepting the Specification F 116 Type IV—Hexagonal bit.

A4.3.1.2 *Type HB*—Hexagonal recess for accepting the Specification F 116 Type IV—Hexagonal bit.

A4.4 Performance Requirements

A4.4.1 Screws that meet the dimensional requirements of the HA and HB screws in A4.2 shall also meet the following mechanical performance requirements.

A4.4.1.1 *Maximum Torque*:

(1) A minimum of five screws for a particular type and size shall be tested in accordance with the test methods described in Annex A1, with five threads exposed in the gage length.

(2) The maximum torque of all screws within the sample of screws from a particular type and size of screw shall meet or exceed the requirements provided in Table A4.5.

A4.4.1.2 *Breaking Angle*:

(1) A minimum of five screws for a particular type and size shall be tested in accordance with the methods described in Annex A1, with five threads exposed in the gage length.

(2) The breaking angle of all screws within the sample of screws from a particular type and size of screw shall meet or exceed the requirements provided in Table A4.5.

TABLE A4.1 Dimensions for HA Screws (Fig. A4.1)

Screw Type and Size	Head Diameter, d_2		Head Height, k	Bottom Head Radius, r_1		Top Head Radius, r_2	Tip Radius, r_3	Screwdriver Size[A]
HA 1.5	3.00	+0.00 −0.10	1.6	1.750	+0.000 −0.075	1.5	0.3	1.5
HA 2.0	4.00	+0.00 −0.10	1.9	2.250	+0.000 −0.075	2.0	0.4	1.5
HA 2.7	5.00	+0.00 −0.15	2.3	2.750	+0.000 −0.075	2.5	0.4	2.5
HA 3.5	6.00	+0.00 −0.15	2.6	3.250	+0.000 −0.075	2.5	1.0	2.5
HA 4.0	6.00	+0.00 −0.15	2.4	3.250	+0.000 −0.075	2.5	1.0	2.5
HA 4.5	8.00	+0.00 −0.15	4.6	4.250	+0.000 −0.075	2.5	1.0	3.5
HA 5.0	8.00	+0.00 −0.15	4.6	4.250	+0.000 −0.075	2.5	1.0	3.5

[A]Type IV hexagonal screwdriver bit as specified in Specification F 116.

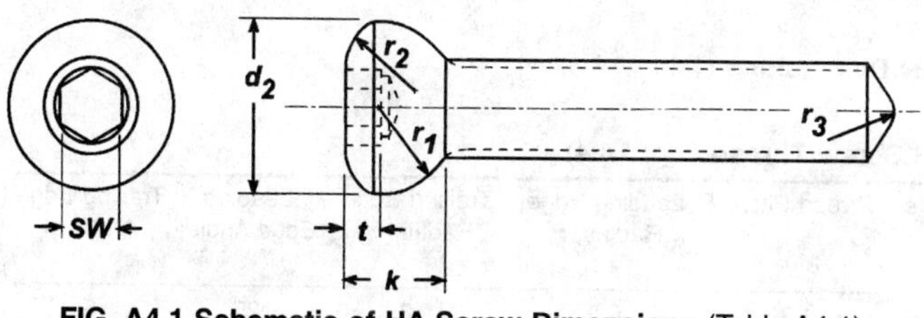

FIG. A4.1 Schematic of HA Screw Dimensions (Table A4.1)

TABLE A4.2 Dimensions for HA Screw Thread (Fig. A4.2)

Screw Type and Size	Thread Diameter, d_1		Core Diameter, d_5		Crest Width, *e*	Thread Pitch, *P*	Leading Edge Radius, r_4	Trailing Edge Radius, r_5	Leading Edge Angle, α	Trailing Edge Angle, β
HA 1.5	1.50	+0.00 −0.15	1.10	+0.00 −0.10	0.1	0.5	0.3	0.1	35	3
HA 2.0	2.00	+0.00 −0.15	1.30	+0.00 −0.10	0.1	0.6	0.4	0.1	35	3
HA 2.7	2.70	+0.00 −0.15	1.90	+0.00 −0.15	0.1	1.0	0.6	0.2	35	3
HA 3.5	3.50	+0.00 −0.15	2.40	+0.00 −0.15	0.1	1.25	0.8	0.2	35	3
HA 4.0	4.00	+0.00 −0.15	2.90	+0.00 −0.15	0.1	1.5	0.8	0.2	35	3
HA 4.5	4.50	+0.00 −0.15	3.00	+0.00 −0.15	0.1	1.75	1.0	0.3	35	3
HA 5.0	5.00	+0.00 −0.15	3.50	+0.00 −0.15	0.1	1.75	1.0	0.3	35	3

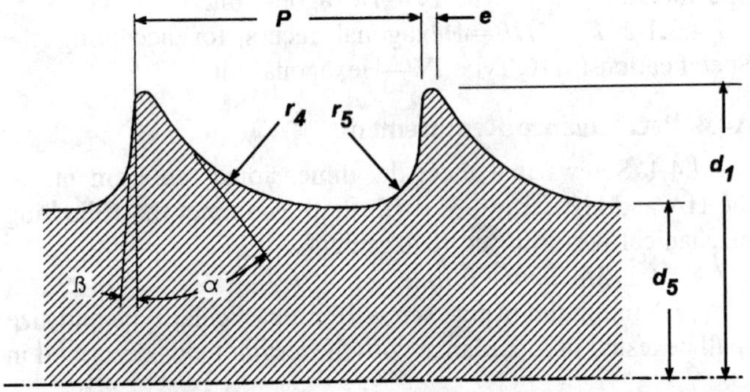

FIG. A4.2 Schematic of HA Screw Thread Dimensions (Table A4.2)

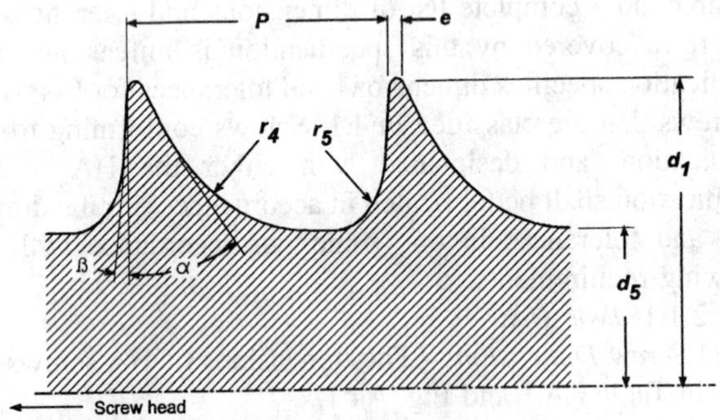

FIG. A4.4 Schematic of HB Screw Thread Dimensions (Table A4.4)

TABLE A4.3 Dimensions for HB Screws (Fig. A4.3)

Screw Type and Size	Head Diameter, d_2		Shaft Diameter, d_4		Head Height, *k*	Bottom Head Radius, r_1		Top Head Radius, r_2	Screwdriver Size[A]
HB 4.0	6.00	+0.00 −0.15	2.40	+0.00 −0.15	2.9	3.250	+0.000 −0.075	2.5	2.5
HB 6.5	8.00	+0.00 −0.15	4.50	+0.00 −0.15	4.6	4.250	+0.000 −0.075	2.5	3.5

[A]Type IV hexagonal screwdriver bit as specified in Specification F 116.

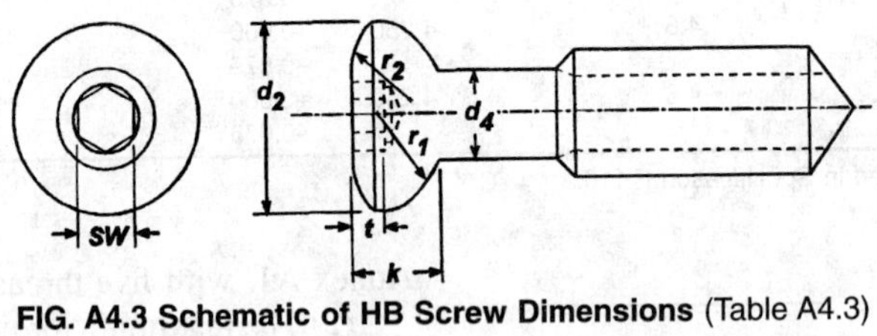

FIG. A4.3 Schematic of HB Screw Dimensions (Table A4.3)

TABLE A4.4 Dimensions for HB Screw Thread (Fig. A4.4)

Screw Type and Size	Thread Diameter, d_1		Core Diameter, d_5		Crest Width, *e*	Thread Pitch, *P*	Leading Edge Radius, r_4	Trailing Edge Radius, r_5	Leading Edge Angle, α	Trailing Edge Angle, β
HB 4.0	4.00	+0.00 −0.15	1.90	+0.00 −0.15	0.1	1.75	0.8	0.3	25	5
HB 6.5	6.50	+0.00 −0.15	3.00	+0.00 −0.15	0.2	2.75	1.2	0.8	25	5

TABLE A4.5 Torsional Strength and Breaking Angle Requirements for HA and HB Screws

Type and Size	Minimum Acceptable Values	
	Torque, νm	Breaking Angle, °, with Five Exposed Threads
HA 1.5	0.2	150
HA 2.0	0.35	150
HA 2.7	1.0	180
HA 3.5	2.3	180
HA 4	4.0	180
HA 4.5	4.4	180
HA 5	5.5	180
HB 4	1.3	90
HB 6.5	6.2	90

A5. SPECIFICATIONS FOR HC AND HD METALLIC MEDICAL BONE SCREWS

A5.1 Screw Classification

A5.1.1 There are a large variety of medical bone screws currently in use. They may be classified by the definitions provided in Section 3. This specification includes the following types of screws with a solid head and a solid core:

A5.1.1.1 *Type HC*—Conical undersurface of head, symmetrical thread.

A5.1.1.2 *Type HD*—Conical undersurface of head, asymmetrical thread.

A5.2 Screw and Thread Form Dimensions

A5.2.1 There are many types of metallic bone screw designs available, so a complete list of dimensions and tolerances for all screws covered by this specification is unfeasible. This specification specifies dimensions and tolerances for two types of screws that are classified in 4.1. Screws conforming to this specification, and designated with either the HC or HD classification shall be fabricated in accordance with the dimensions and tolerances in this Annex in accordance with the following requirements.

A5.2.1.1 *Type HC*:

(1) Screw Dimensions—The dimensions of HC screws are given in Table A5.1 and Fig. A5.1.

(2) Screw Thread—The dimensions of the threads of HC screws are given in Table A5.2 and Fig. A5.2.

A5.2.1.2 *Type HD*:

(1) Screw Dimensions—The dimensions of HD screws are given in Table A5.3 and Fig. A5.3.

(2) Screw Thread—The dimensions of the threads of HD screws are given in Table A5.4 and Fig. A5.4.

A5.3 Drive Connections

A5.3.1 Screws conforming to this specification, and designated with either the HC or HD classification shall be fabricated with the following drive connections in accordance with the dimensions and tolerances found in Annex A6.

TABLE A5.1 Dimensions for HC Screws (Fig. A5.1)

Screw Type and Size	Shaft Diameter, d_1	Head Diameter, d_2	Head Height, h	Unthreaded Length, x	Top Head Radius, r_2
HC 2.9	2.9	4.62 – 6.1	1.5 - 2	1.6	5
HC 3.5	3.5	5.8 – 6.5	1.5 - 2	1.6	6.35
HC 3.9	3.9	5.8 – 6.5	1.5 - 2	1.6	6.35
HC 4.2	4.2	5.8 – 6.5	1.5 - 2	1.6	6.35

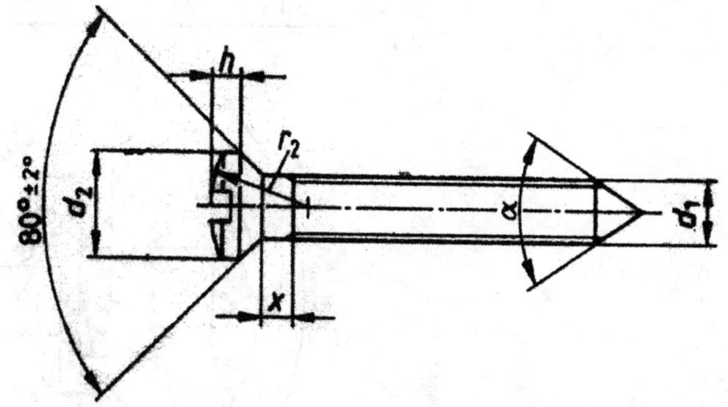

FIG. A5.1 Schematic of HC Screw Dimensions (Table A5.1)

TABLE A5.2 Dimensions for HC Screw Thread (Fig. A5.2)

Screw Type and Size	Thread Diameter, d_1	Core Diameter, d_5	Thread Pitch, P	c max
HC 2.9	2.79 – 2.90	2.03 – 2.18	1.06	0.1
HC 3.5	3.43 – 3.53	2.51 – 2.64	1.27	0.1
HC 3.9	3.78 – 3.91	2.77 – 2.92	1.27	0.1
HC 4.2	4.09 – 4.22	2.95 – 3.25	1.27	0.1

A5.3.1.1 *Type HC*:

(1) Single-slot recess for accepting the Specification F 116 Type I—single-slot bit.

(2) Cruciate recess for accepting the Specification F 116 Type II—cruciate-slot bit.

(3) Combined cruciate-slot and cross-slot recess for accepting either the Specification F 116 Type II—cruciate-slot or Type III—cross-slot (modified Phillips) bits.

A5.3.1.2 *Type HD*—Combined single-slot and cross-slot recess for accepting either the Specification F 116 Type I—single-slot or Type III—cross-slot (modified Phillips) bits.

A5.4 Performance Requirements

A5.4.1 Screws that meet the dimensional requirements of the HC or HD screws in A5.2 shall be tested to document the following mechanical performance characteristics.

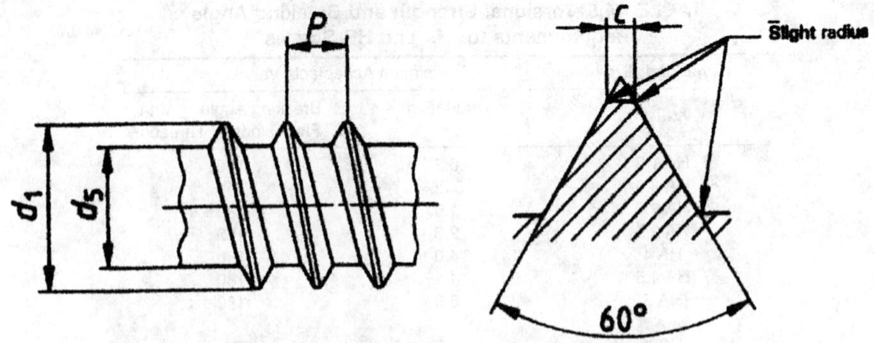

FIG. A5.2 Schematic of HC Screw Thread Dimensions (Table A5.2)

TABLE A5.3 Dimensions for HD Screws (Fig. A5.3)

Screw Type and Size	Shaft Diameter, d_4	Head Diameter, d_2	Head Height, H	Unthreaded Length, x	Head Top Radius, r_1
HD 4.0	4.0	6.75 – 7.35	1.8 – 2.1	1.6	6.35
HD 4.5	4.5	6.75 – 7.35	1.8 – 2.1	1.6	6.35

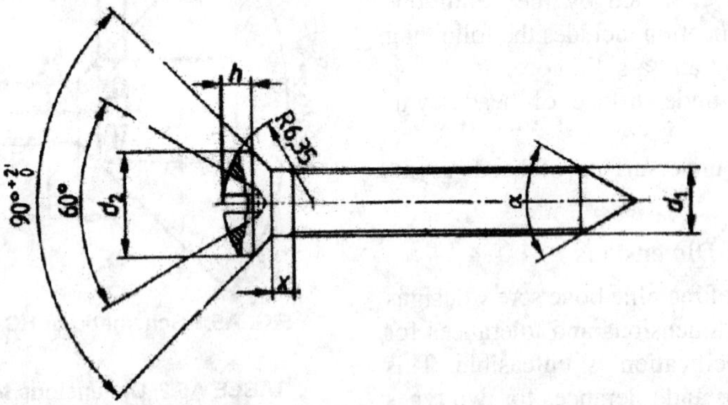

FIG. A5.3 Schematic of HD Screw Dimensions (Table A5.3)

TABLE A5.4 Dimensions for HD Screw Thread (Fig. A5.4)

Screw Type and Size	Thread Diameter, d_1	Core Diameter, d_5	Crest Width, e	Thread Pitch, P	Leading Edge Angle, α	Trailing Edge Angle, β
HD 4	3.97 – 4.03	2.89 – 2.95	0.1	1.59	45	10
HD 4.5	4.47 – 4.53	2.89 – 2.95	0.1	2.18	45	10

A5.4.1.1 *Torsional strength*—A minimum of five screws for a particular type and size shall be tested in accordance with the methods described in Annex A1, with five threads exposed in the gage length.

A5.4.1.2 *Breaking angle*—A minimum of five screws for a particular type and size shall be tested in accordance with the methods described in Annex A1, with five threads exposed in the gage length.

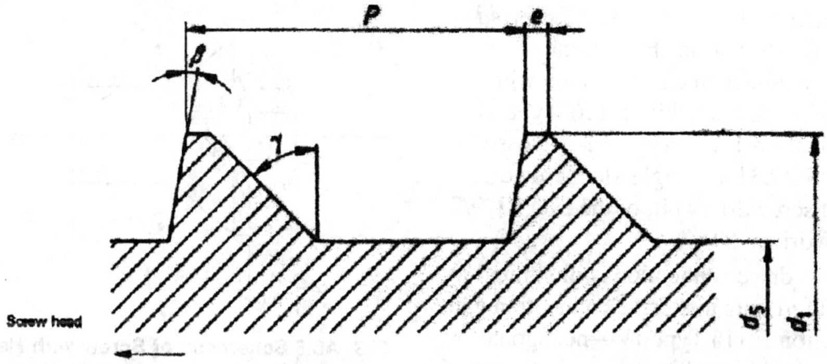

FIG. A5.4 Schematic of HD Screw Thread Dimensions (Table A5.4)

A6. SPECIFICATIONS FOR METALLIC BONE SCREW DRIVE CONNECTIONS

A6.1 Scope

A6.1.1 This annex specifies the requirements for a variety of drive connections that can be implemented in metallic medical bone screws. The screw's drive connection supplies the interconnection that is typically used in orthopedic surgery for inserting and removing bone screws.

A6.2 Classification

A6.2.1 There are many methods that can be used to classify medical bone screws. The majority of the methods currently being used in the medical industry can be found in Section 3 of this specification. An additional characteristic not covered in Section 3 is the bone screw's drive connection. This specification describes the following drive connections that are compatible with the noted screwdriver bits.

A6.2.1.1 *Single-Slot*—This drive connection is illustrated in Fig. A6.1. Screws manufactured with this drive connection can be driven with the Specification F 116 Type I—single-slot bit or the ISO 8319/2 single-slot screwdriver bit.

A6.2.1.2 *Cross-Recessed*—This drive connection is illustrated in Fig. A6.2. Screws manufactured with this drive connection can be driven with the Specification F 116 Type III—cross-slot (modified Phillips) bit or the ISO 8319/2 cross-recessed head screwdriver bit.

A6.2.1.3 *Combined Single-Slot and Cross-Recessed*—This drive connection is illustrated in Fig. A6.3. Screws manufactured with this drive connection can be driven with the F 116 Type I—single-slot bit, Specification F 116 Type III—cross-slot (modified Phillips) bit, the ISO 8319/2 single-slot screwdriver bit, or the ISO 8319/2 cross-recessed head screwdriver bit.

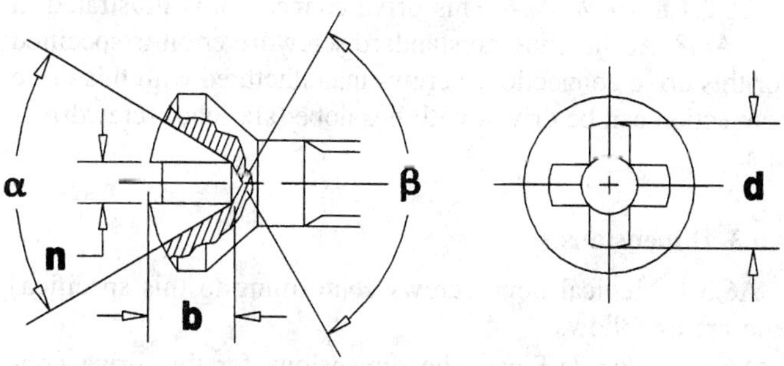

FIG. A6.2 Schematic of Screw with Cross-Recessed Drive Connection (Table A6.2)

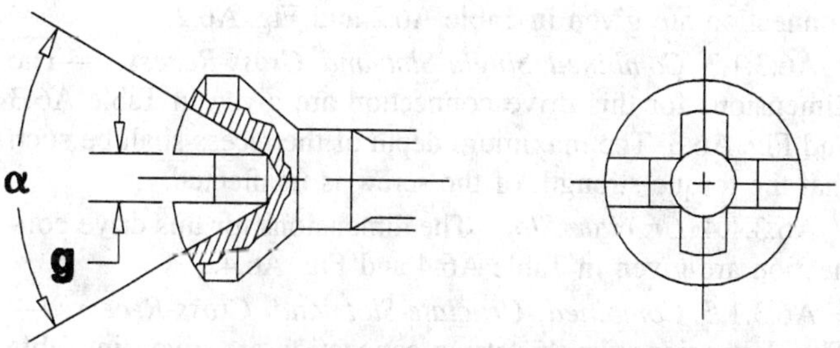

FIG. A6.3 Schematic of Screw with Combined Single-Slot and Cross-Recessed Drive Connection (Table A6.3)

A6.2.1.4 *Cruciate-Slot*—This drive connection is illustrated in Fig. A6.4. Screws manufactured with this drive connection can be driven with the Specification F 116 Type I—single-slot bit, Specification F 116 Type II—cruciate-slot bit, the ISO 8319/2 single-slot screwdriver bit, or the ISO 8319/2 cruciate-slot screwdriver bit.

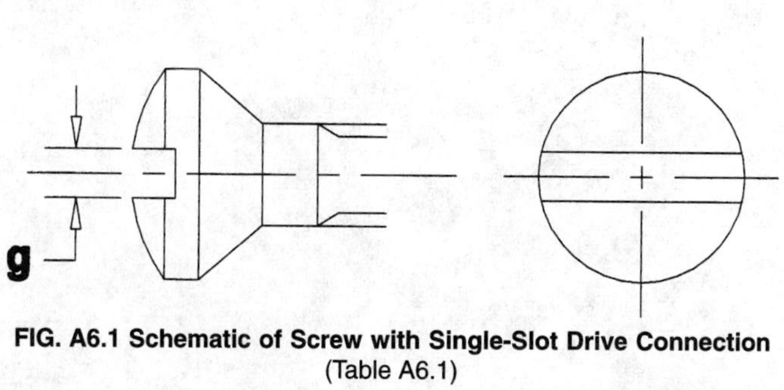

FIG. A6.1 Schematic of Screw with Single-Slot Drive Connection (Table A6.1)

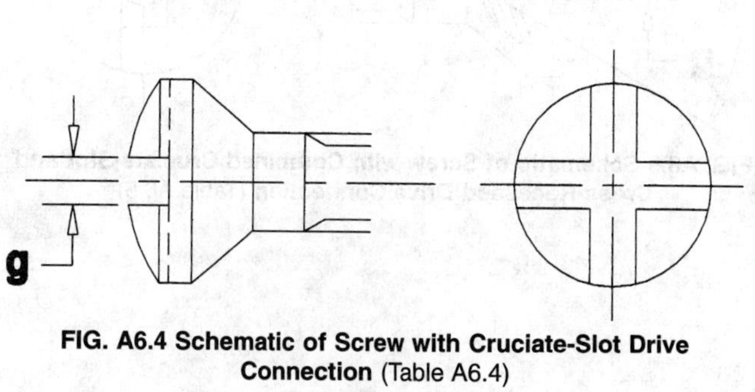

FIG. A6.4 Schematic of Screw with Cruciate-Slot Drive Connection (Table A6.4)

A6.2.1.5 *Combined Cruciate-Slot and Cross-Recessed*—This drive connection is illustrated in Fig. A6.5. Screws manufactured with this drive connection can be driven with the Specification F 116 Type I—single-slot bit, F 116 Type II—cruciate-slot bit, the Specification F 116 Type III—Cross-slot (modified Phillips) bit, the ISO 8319/2 single-slot screwdriver bit, ISO 8319/2 cruciate-slot screwdriver bit, or the ISO 8319/2 crossed-recessed head screwdriver bit.

A6.2.1.6 *Hexagonal*—This drive connection is illustrated in Fig. A6.6. Screws manufactured with this drive connection can be driven with the Specification F 116 Type IV—hexagonal or the ISO 8319/1 hexagonal screwdriver bit.

A6.2.1.7 *Square*—This drive connection is illustrated in Fig. A6.7. At this time no standard screwdriver bit is specified for this drive connection. Screws manufactured with this drive connection can be driven with square drive screwdriver bits.

A6.2.1.8 *Hexalobe*—This drive connection is illustrated in Fig. A6.8. At this time no standard screwdriver bit is specified for this drive connection. Screws manufactured with this drive connection can be driven with hexalobe (six-lobe) screwdriver bits.

A6.3 Dimensions

A6.3.1 Medical bone screws conforming to this specification are as follows:

A6.3.1.1 *Single-Slot*—The dimensions for this drive connection are given in Table A6.1 and Fig. A6.1.

A6.3.1.2 *Cross-Recessed*—The dimensions for this drive connection are given in Table A6.2 and Fig. A6.2.

A6.3.1.3 *Combined Single-Slot and Cross-Recessed*—The dimensions for this drive connection are given in Table A6.3 and Fig. A6.3. The maximum depth of the recess shall be such that the torque strength of the screw is unaffected.

A6.3.1.4 *Cruciate-Slot*—The dimensions for this drive connection are given in Table A6.4 and Fig. A6.4.

A6.3.1.5 *Combined Cruciate-Slot and Cross-Recessed*—The dimensions for this drive connection are given in Table A6.5 and Fig. A6.5. The maximum depth of the recess shall be such that the torque strength of the screw is unaffected.

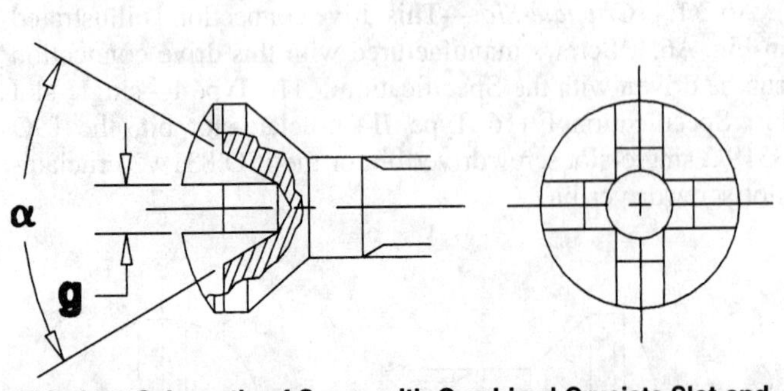

FIG. A6.5 Schematic of Screw with Combined Cruciate-Slot and Cross-Recessed Drive Connection (Table A6.5)

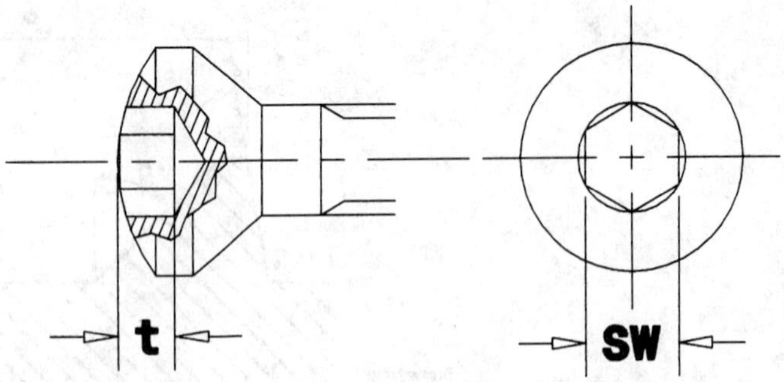

FIG. A6.6 Schematic of Screw with Hexagonal Drive Connection (Table A6.6)

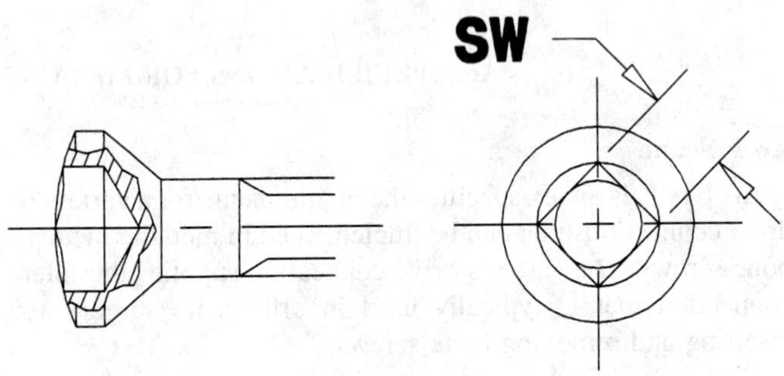

FIG. A6.7 Schematic of Screw with Square Drive Connection (Table A6.7)

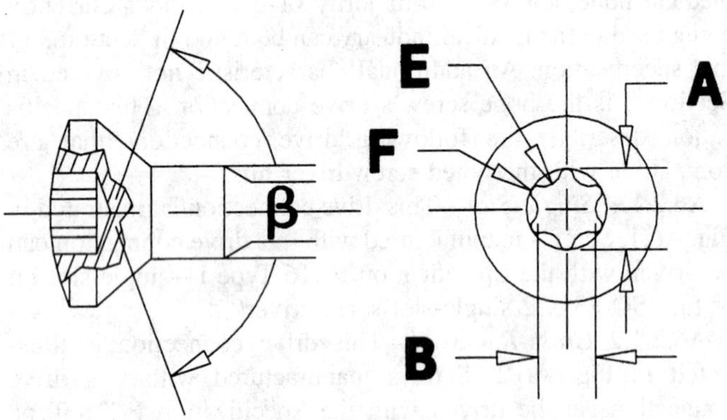

FIG. A6.8 Schematic of Screw with Hexalobe Drive Connection (Table A6.8)

TABLE A6.1 Single-Slot Drive Connection Dimensions (Fig. A6.1)

Screw Type and Size	Nominal Diameter, mm	Slot Width, *g*, mm
HC 2.9	2.9	1.25 - 1.4
HC 3.5	3.5	1.25 - 1.4
HC 3.9	3.9	1.25 - 1.4
HC 4.2	4.2	1.25 - 1.4

TABLE A6.2 Cross-Recessed Drive Connection Dimensions (Fig. A6.2)

Nominal Diameter, mm	*d*	*b* max	*n*
4.5	5	3.8	1.4

TABLE A6.3 Combined Single-Slot and Cross-Recessed Drive Connection Dimensions (Fig. A6.3)

Screw Type and Size	Slot Width, *g*, mm	Slot Angle, α, °
HD 4.0	1.25 - 1.4	60
HD 4.5	1.25 - 1.4	60

TABLE A6.4 Cruciate-Slot Drive Connection Dimensions (Fig. A6.4)

Screw Type and Size	Nominal Diameter, mm	Slot Width, *g*, mm
HC 3.5	3.5	1.25 - 1.4
HC 3.9	3.9	1.25 - 1.4
HC 4.2	4.2	1.25 - 1.4

A6.3.1.6 *Hexagonal*—The dimensions for this drive connection are given in Table A6.6 and Fig. A6.6.

A6.3.1.7 *Square:* The dimensions for this drive connection are given in Table A6.7 and Fig. A6.7. The maximum depth of the recess shall be such that the torque strength of the screw is unaffected.

A6.3.1.8 *Hexalobe*—The dimensions for this drive connection are given in Table A6.8 and Fig. A6.8. The maximum depth of the recess shall be such that the torque strength of the screw is unaffected.

TABLE A6.5 Combined Cruciate-Slot and Cross-Recessed Drive Connection Dimensions (Fig. A6.5)

Screw Type and Size	Nominal Diameter, mm	Slot Width, *g*, mm	Slot Angle, α, °
HC 3.5	3.5	1.25 - 1.4	60
HC 3.9	3.9	1.25 - 1.4	60
HC 4.2	4.2	1.25 - 1.4	60

TABLE A6.6 Hexagonal Drive Connection Dimensions (Fig. A6.6)

Screw Type and Size	Nominal Diameter, mm	Screwdriver Bit Size	*SW*, mm	*t*, mm
HA 1.5	1.5	1.5	1.507 +0.040 −0.000	0.8
HA 2.0	2.0	1.5	1.507 +0.040 −0.000	1.0
HA 2.7	2.7	2.5	2.507 +0.040 −0.000	1.2
HA 3.5	3.5	2.5	2.507 +0.040 −0.000	1.5
HA 4.0	4.0	2.5	2.507 +0.040 −0.000	1.5
HA 4.5	4.5	3.5	3.510 +0.048 −0.000	2.8
HA 5.0	4.5	3.5	3.510 +0.048 −0.000	2.8
HB 4.0	4.0	2.5	2.507 +0.040 −0.000	1.5
HB 6.5	6.5	3.5	3.510 +0.048 −0.000	2.8

TABLE A6.7 Square Drive Connection Dimensions (Fig. A6.7)

Screw Size	*SW*, mm
1.0	0.7
1.5	1.0
2.0	1.27

TABLE A6.8 Hexalobe Drive Connection Dimensions (Fig. A6.8)

Screw Size	*A*, mm	*B*, mm	*E* Radius, mm	*F* Radius, mm	β, °	Screwdriver Bit Size
1.3	1.35	0.97	0.28	0.12	140	4
1.5	1.47	1.07	0.30	0.14	140	5
2.0	1.75	1.27	0.36	0.16	140	6
2.7	2.4	1.75	0.49	0.22	140	8
3.5	2.8	2.05	0.57	0.25	140	10
4.0	3.35	2.40	0.69	0.30	140	15
4.5	3.95	2.85	0.83	0.34	140	20
5.0	4.50	3.25	0.89	0.40	140	25
6.5	5.60	4.05	1.16	0.48	140	30

APPENDIX

(Nonmandatory Information)

X1. METALLIC BONE SCREWS

X1.1 This specification is intended to provide useful and consistent information related to the performance, terminology, requirements for materials, finish and marking considerations, and care and handling of metallic bone screws. It includes the terms and requirements of Specification F 543-98. This specification also includes the test methods that were previously published separately as Specifications F 117, F 1622, and F 1691.

X1.2 Dimensional requirements are provided for four specific types of bone screws. These screws, specified here as Specification F 543 Types HA, HB, HC, and HD are dimensionally similar to those specified in ISO 5835 and ISO 9268. The dimensions and performance of these types of screws are specified because they have achieved widespread clinical use and are offered by several manufacturers. Standardization of the dimensions and tolerances of the key features of these screws is intended to allow the implants from one manufacturer to be used with the associated instruments (taps, drills, and so forth) from different manufacturers and serve as a baseline for future screw products. This may benefit the surgeon and patient by aiding the identification of the appropriate instrumentation for the implantation and removal of screws by the operating room staff.

X1.3 Performance requirements are provided for two specific types of bone screws. Those that have a solid core and a spherical head, specified here as Specification F 543 Type HA and HB, and have performance specifications developed from those specified in ISO 6475. Standardization of the performance requirements and harmonization of these requirements with the similar screws described in ISO standards is intended to facilitate the approvals to market for manufacturers declaring conformity to either or both standards.

X1.4 This specification provides minimum performance limits for the torsional properties of bone screws and a uniform test procedure by which these limits can be determined. The parameters specified in this specification are breaking torque and breaking angle.

X1.4.1 The breaking torque is intended to be a measure of the screw's strength. Torque was determined to be the critical parameter in the insertion of screws into a uniform medium. Unpublished test reports indicated that a screw could experience both torsional and tensile forces when inserted into a uniform medium. If the screw was inserted until it ruptured, then the torsional forces appear to dominate over the tensile forces. Therefore, tensile forces were neglected in analyzing screw strength.

X1.4.2 The breaking angle is a measure of the screw's ductility. For example, a screw that has a breaking angle of 360° is more ductile than one with the same design that breaks at 120° under the same test conditions. Since this parameter does not represent the point at which the screw loses its elastic properties, a torsional yield measurement was devised. This point is intended to present an approximate measure of the torque at which the screw loses its elastic properties. The task force decided that an offset method with a 2° angle offset method was considered to yield the most consistent results.

X1.4.3 The breaking force test method provides a consistent measurement method for fully threaded bone screws. For partially threaded screws, the length of the unthreaded portion of the screw and the threaded portion can vary considerably among different types of screws. Because of this variation, no exact method of fixation is required. Suggestions are made to grip enough threads to hold the screw in a fixed position with possibly one or more thread(s) exposed. If this condition is not possible, then all threads must be gripped. In any case, the experiment is required to record the gage length and the gripping length.

X1.4.4 If an axial force is necessary to engage the screwdriver in the screw head, the value of this force is to be determined by the operator. The force should be the minimum needed to engage the screwdriver bit with the screw head.

X1.5 This specification provides a uniform test procedure for measuring the insertion and removal torque of bone screws in a specified medium. This specification can thus provide a measure of the uniformity of the products tested or compare the insertion and removal torque among similar or dissimilar screws.

X1.5.1 The test method specifies that the bone screw be driven at a rate of 1 to 5 r/min into the test block. The rate specified in the original Test Method F 117 standard was selected and based upon the limitations of torsion test systems when the standard was originally developed. Faster driving rates (an order of magnitude greater at 30 r/min) can better simulate the clinical situation for hand-driven screws. Therefore, the user may choose to use higher screw-driving rates, as long as the selected rate is justified and reported. All comparative test methods must be performed at the same driving rate.

X1.5.2 During the development of this test method, the committee noted the need to test sterilized screws. *Infection Control and Sterilization Technology*, V4, No 8 p12, August 1998 reported differences in the driving torque when sterilized and unsterilized screws were tested.

X1.6 This specification provides a uniform test procedure for measuring the axial pullout strength of bone screws from a specified medium. This specification can provide a measure of the uniformity of the products tested or compare the pullout strength among similar or dissimilar screws.

Designation: F 560 – 98

Standard Specification for Unalloyed Tantalum for Surgical Implant Applications (UNS R05200, UNS R05400)[1]

This standard is issued under the fixed designation F 560; the number immediately following the designation indicates the year of original adoption or, in the case of revision, the year of last revision. A number in parentheses indicates the year of last reapproval. A superscript epsilon (ε) indicates an editorial change since the last revision or reapproval.

1. Scope

1.1 This specification covers the requirements for unalloyed tantalum sheet, rod, and wire used for the manufacture of surgical implants.

1.2 The values stated in inch-pound units are to be regarded as the standard. The metric equivalents of inch-pound units may be approximate.

2. Referenced Documents

2.1 *ASTM Standards:*

B 364 Specification for Tantalum and Tantalum Alloy Ingots[2]

B 365 Specification for Tantalum and Tantalum Alloy Rod and Wire[2]

B 708 Specification for Tantalum and Tantalum Alloy Plate, Sheet, and Strip[2]

E 8 Test Methods of Tension Testing of Metallic Materials[3]

E 29 Practice for Using Significant Digits in Test Data to Determine Conformance with Specifications[4]

F 981 Practice for Assessment of Compatibility of Biomaterials for Surgical Implants with Respect to Effect of Materials on Muscle and Bone[5]

2.2 *American Society for Quality Control Standard:*[6]

Cl Specifications of General Requirements for a Quality Program

3. General Requirements for Delivery

3.1 In addition to the requirements of this specification, all requirements of the current editions of Specifications B 364, B 365, and B 708 shall apply.

3.2 In the case where a conflict exists between this specification and those listed in 2.1 and 2.2, this specification shall take precedence.

[1] This specification is under the jurisdiction of ASTM Committee F-4 on Medical and Surgical Materials and Devices, and is the direct responsibility of Subcommittee F04.12 on Metallurgical Materials.

Current edition approved January 10, 1998. Published June 1998. Originally published as F 560 – 78. Last previous edition F 560 – 92.

[2] *Annual Book of ASTM Standards*, Vol 02.04.

[3] *Annual Book of ASTM Standards*, Vol 03.01.

[4] *Annual Book of ASTM Standards*, Vol 14.02.

[5] *Annual Book of ASTM Standards*, Vol 13.01.

[6] Available from American Society for Quality Control, 161 West Wisconsin Ave., Milwaukee, WI 53203.

TABLE 1 Chemical Requirements (Ingot)

Element	Compositions, Maximum Weight Percent Allowed[A]	
	R05200[B]	R05400[C]
Carbon	0.010	0.010
Oxygen	0.0150	0.030
Nitrogen	0.010	0.010
Hydrogen	0.0015	0.0015
Niobium	0.100	0.100
Iron	0.010	0.010
Titanium	0.010	0.010
Tungsten	0.05	0.05
Molybdenum	0.020	0.020
Silicon	0.0050	0.0050
Nickel	0.010	0.010
Tantalum	balance	balance

[A] For purposes of determining conformance with this specification, all compositional limits are absolute limits, as defined in Practice E 29.

[B] Electron beam or vacuum-arc cast tantalum.

[C] Sintered tantalum.

4. Ordering Information

4.1 Inquiries and orders under this specification shall include the following information:

4.1.1 Quantity (weight and number of pieces),

4.1.2 ASTM designation,

4.1.3 Composition designation,

4.1.4 Form (sheet, rod, wire)

4.1.5 Condition (see 5.1)

4.1.6 Applicable dimensions, including size, thickness, width, and length (random, exact, multiples), or print number,

4.1.7 Special tests, and

4.1.8 Special requirements.

5. Manufacture

5.1 *Condition:*

5.1.1 Flat mill products material shall be supplied in the cold-worked, cold-worked and stress-relieved or annealed condition.

5.1.2 Rod and wire products shall be supplied in the annealed or cold worked condition.

6. Chemical Composition

6.1 The material shall conform to the requirements as to chemical composition specified in Table 1.

6.1.1 Requirements for the major and minor elemental constituents are listed in Table 1. Also listed are important residual elements. Analysis for elements not listed in Table 1 is not required to certify compliance with this specification.

TABLE 2 Mechanical Properties, Flat Mill Products

Condition	Thickness, in. (mm)	Ulimate Tensile Strength, min, psi (MPa)	Yeild Strength, (0.2% offset) min, psi (MPa)	Elongation in 1 inch (25.4 mm), min,%
Cold worked	all	75 000 (517)	50 000 (345)	2
Stress relieved	0.0051 to 0.010 (0.13 to 0.26)	55 000 (379)	35 000 (241)	5
	over 0.010 to 0.020 (0.26 to 0.51)	55 000 (379)	35 000 (241)	10
	over 0.020(0.51)	55 000 (379)	35 000 (241)	10
Annealed	0.0051 to 0.010 (0.13 to 0.26)	30 000 (207)	20 000 (138)	20
	over 0.010 to 0.020 (0.26 to 0.51)	30 000 (207)	20 000 (138)	25
	over 0.020 (0.51)	30 000 (207)	20 000 (138)	30

TABLE 3 Mechanical Properties, Rod and Wire Products

Condition	Diameter, in. (mm)	Ultimate Tensile Strength, min, psi (MPa)	Yield Strength, (0.2% offset)min, psi (MPa)	Elongation, min, % [A]
Cold Worked	all	70 000 (482)	50 000 (345)	1
Annealed	0.005 to 0.010 (0.12 to 0.25)	35 000 (241)	. . .	8
	over 0.010 to 0.015 (0.25 to 0.38)	35 000 (241)	. . .	10
	over 0.015 to 0.025 (0.38 to 0.64)	30 500 (241)	. . .	15
	over 0.025 to 0.125 (0.64 to 0.32)	30 000 (207)	. . .	20
	over 0.125 to 2.5 (3.2 to 64)	25 000 (172)	20 000 (138)	25

[A] Use 10-in. (254-mm) gage length for 0.050 in. (1.27-mm) diameter and below, 1 or 2 in. (25.4 or 50.8 mm) gage length for diameters over 0.050 in. (1.27 mm) to 0.125 in. (3.2 mm), and 1 in. (25.4mm) gage length for diameters over 0.125 in. (3.2 mm).

7. Mechanical Properties

7.1 The material shall conform to the appropriate requirements as to mechanical properties specified in Tables 2 and 3. Mechanical properties for material in conditions other than those included in Tables 2 and 3, shall be specified in the purchase order.

7.2 Perform tension testing in accordance with Test Methods E 8. Determine tensile properties using a strain rate of 0.003 to 0.007 in./in. (mm/mm)/min through the yield point, and then increase crosshead speed to produce fracture in approximately one minute.

8. Certification

8.1 The manufacturer's certification that the material was manufactured and tested in accordance with this specification together with a report of the test results shall be furnished at the time of shipment.

9. Quality Program Requirements

9.1 The producer shall maintain a quality program, such as that defined in ASQC Cl.

9.2 The manufacturer of surgical implants may audit the producer's quality program for conformance to the intent of ASQC C1, or other recognized program.

10. Keywords

10.1 metals (for surgical implants); orthopaedic medical devices; tantalum

APPENDIXES

(Nonmandatory Information)

X1. RATIONALE

X1.1 The primary reason for this specification is to characterize composition and properties to ensure consistency in the starting material used in the manufacture of medical devices.

X1.2 The USN designation has been added to the title, residual element language has been included, the mechanical properties tables have been modified, and Biocompatibility section has been added.

X2. BIOCOMPATIBILITY

X2.1 No known surgical implant material has ever been shown to be completely free of adverse reactions in the human body. However, long term clinical experience has shown an acceptable level of biological response can be expected, if the material is used in appropriate applications.

X2.2 The material in this specification has been subjected to animal implant studies and has been shown to produce a well characterized level of biological response that is equal to or less than that produced by the reference material when tested by the procedures of Practice F 981 or the equivalent. This material has been used clinically for over a decade.[7]

[7] Black, Jonathan, " Biological Performance of Tantalum," Clinical Materials, Elsevier Science Limited, Vol 16, 1994, pp. 167–173.

Designation: F 561 – 97

Practice for Retrieval and Analysis of Implanted Medical Devices, and Associated Tissues[1]

This standard is issued under the fixed designation F 561; the number immediately following the designation indicates the year of original adoption or, in the case of revision, the year of last revision. A number in parentheses indicates the year of last reapproval. A superscript epsilon (ε) indicates an editorial change since the last revision or reapproval.

1. Scope

1.1 This practice covers recommendations for the retrieval, handling, and analysis of implantable medical devices and associated specimens which are removed from patients, during revision surgery, at postmortem, or as part of animal studies. The aim is to provide guidance in preventing damage to the associated specimens which could obscure the investigational results, and in gathering data at the proper time and circumstance to validate the study.

1.2 This practice offers guidelines for the analysis of retrieved implants to limit damage to them, and to allow comparisons between investigational results from different studies. The protocols are divided into three stages, where Stage I is the minimum non-destructive analysis, Stage II is more complete non-destructive analysis, and Stage III is destructive analysis. Standard protocols for the examination and collection of data are provided for specific types of materials in relation to their typical applications. For particular investigational programs, additional, more specific, protocols may be required. If special analytical techniques are employed, the appropriate handling procedures must be specified.

1.3 This practice recommendation should be applied in accordance with national regulations or legal requirements regarding the handling and analysis of retrieved implants and excised tissues, especially with regard to handling devices which may become involved in litigation, as per Practice E 860.

1.4 A significant portion of the information associated with a retrieved implant device is often at the device-tissue interface or in the tissues associated with the implant and related organ systems. Attention should be given to the handling of adjacent tissues, so as not to interfere with study of the particles in the adjacent tissue, a chemical analysis for the byproducts of degradation of the implant, or a study of the cellular response to the implant.

1.5 *This standard may involve hazardous materials, operations, and equipment. As a precautionary measure, removed implants should be sterilized or minimally disinfected by an appropriate means that does not adversely affect the implant or the associated tissue that may be subject to subsequent analysis. This standard does not purport to address all of the safety concerns, if any, associated with its use. It is the responsibility of the user of this standard to establish appropriate safety and health practices and determine the applicability of regulatory limitations prior to use.*

2. Referenced Documents

2.1 *ASTM Standards:*

A 262 Practices for Detecting Susceptibility to Intergranular Attack in Austenitic Stainless Steels[2]

A 751 Test Methods, Practices and Terminology for Chemical Analysis of Steel Products[2]

C 20 Test Methods for Apparent Porosity, Water Absorption, Apparent Specific Gravity and Bulk Density of Burned Refractory Brick and Shapes by Boiling Water[3]

C 158 Test Methods for Strength of Glass (Determination of Modulus of Rupture)[4]

C 169 Test Methods for Chemical Analysis of Soda-Lime and Borosilicate Glass[4]

C 573 Test Methods for Chemical Analysis of Fireclay and High-Alumina Refractories[5]

C 623 Test Method for Young's Modulus, Shear Modulus, and Poisson's ratio for Glass and Glass-Ceramics by Resonance[4]

C 633 Test Method for Adhesion or Cohesive Strength of Flame-Sprayed Coatings[6]

C 674 Test Methods for Flexural Properties of Ceramic White Ware Materials[4]

C 730 Test Method for Knoop Indentation Hardness of Glass[4]

C 849 Test Method for Knoop Indentation Hardness of Ceramic Whitewares[4]

C 1069 Test Method for Specific Surface Area of Alumina or Quartz by Nitrogen Adsorption[4]

C 1161 Test Method for Flexural Strength—Advanced Ceramics at Ambient Temperatures[3]

C 1198 Test Method for Dynamic Young's Modulus, Shear

---

[1] This practice is under the jurisdiction of ASTM Committee F-4 on Medical and Surgical Materials and Devices, and is the direct responsibility of Subcommittee F04.18 on Device Retrieval Analysis.

Current edition approved Dec. 10, 1997. Published June 1998. Originally published as F 561 – 78. Last previous edition F 561 – 87 (1994).

[2] *Annual Book of ASTM Standards*, Vol 01.03.

[3] *Annual Book of ASTM Standards*, Vol 15.01.

[4] *Annual Book of ASTM Standards*, Vol 15.02.

[5] Discontinued—See 1994 *Annual Book of ASTM Standards*, Vol 03.05.

[6] *Annual Book of ASTM Standards*, Vol 02.05.

Modulus, and Poisson's Ratio for Advanced Ceramics by Sonic Resonance[3]

D 256 Test Methods for Determining the Izod Pendulum Impact Resistance of Plastics[7]

D 412 Test Methods for Vulcanized Rubber and Thermoplastic Elastomers-Tension[7]

D 570 Test Method for Water Absorption of Plastics[7]

D 621 Test Methods for Deformation of Plastics Under Load[7]

D 624 Test methods for Tear Strength of Conventional Vulcanized Rubber and Thermoplastic Elastomers[8]

D 638 Test Method for Tensile Properties of Plastics[7]

D 671 Test Method for Flexural Fatigue of Plastics by Constant Amplitude of Force[7]

D 695 Test Method for Compressive Properties of Rigid Plastics[7]

D 732 Test Method for Shear Strength of Plastics by Punch Tool[7]

D 747 Test Method for Apparent Bending Modulus of Plastics by Means of a Cantilever Beam[7]

D 785 Test Method for Rockwell Hardness of Plastics and Electrical Insulating Materials[7]

D 790 Test Methods for Flexural Properties of Unreinforced and Reinforced Plastics and Electrical Insulating Materials[7]

D 792 Test Methods for Density and Specific Gravity (Relative Density) of Plastics by Displacement[7]

D 1004 Test Method for Initial Tear Resistance of Plastic Film and Sheeting[7]

D 1042 Test Method for Linear Dimensional Changes of Plastics Under Accelerated Service Conditions[7]

D 1238 Test Method for Flow Rates of Thermoplastics by Extrusion Plastometer[7]

D 1239 Test Method for Resistance of Plastic Films to Extraction by Chemicals[7]

D 1242 Test Methods for Resistance of Plastic Materials to Abrasion[7]

D 1505 Test Method for Density of Plastics by the Density—Gradient Technique[7]

D 1621 Test Method for Compressive Properties of Rigid Cellular Plastics[7]

D 1622 Test Method for Apparent Density of Rigid Cellular Plastics[7]

D 1623 Test Method for Tensile and Tensile Adhesion Properties of Rigid Cellular Plastics[7]

D 1708 Test Method for Tensile Properties of Plastics by Use of Micro Tensile Specimens[7]

D 2240 Test Method for Rubber Property—Durometer Hardness[7]

D 2842 Test Method for Water Absorbtion of Rigid Cellular Plastics[9]

D 2857 Test Method for Dilute Solution Viscosity of Polymers[9]

D 2873 Test Method for Interior Porosity of Poly(Vinyl Chloride) (PVC) Resins by Mercury Intrusion Porosimetry[9]

D 2990 Test Methods for Tensile, Compressive, and Flexural Creep and Creep-Rupture of Plastics[9]

D 3016 Practice for Use of Liquid Exclusion Chromatography Terms and Relationships[9]

D 3417 Test Methods for Heats of Fusion and Crystallization of Polymers by Thermal Analysis[9]

D 3418 Test Method for Transition Temperatures of Polymers by Thermal Analysis[9]

D 3835 Test Method for Determination of Properties of Polymeric Materials by Means of a Capillary Rheometer[9]

D 3919 Practice for Measuring Trace Elements in Water by Graphite Furnace Atomic Absorption Spectrophotometry[10]

D 4000 Classification System for Specifying Plastic Materials[9]

D 4001 Test Method for Determination of Weight-Average Molecular Weight by Light Scattering[11]

D 4065 Practice for Determining and Reporting Dynamic Mechanical Properties of Plastics[9]

D 4754 Test Method for Two-Sided Liquid Extraction of Plastic Materials Using FDA Migration Cell[11]

D 5152 Practice for Water Extraction of Residual Solids from Degraded Plastics for Toxicity Testing[11]

D 5227 Test Method for the Measurement of Hexane Extractable Content of Polyolefins[11]

D 5296 Test Method for Molecular Weight Averages and Molecular Weight Distribution of Polystyrenbe b Hugh Performance Size-Exclusion Chromatography[9]

E 3 Methods of Preparation of Metallographic Specimens[12]

E 7 Terminology Relating to Metallography[12]

E 8 Test Methods for Tension Testing of Metallic Materials[12]

E 10 Test Method for Brinell Hardness of Metallic Materials[12]

E 18 Test Methods for Rockwell Hardness and Rockwell Superficial Hardness of Metallic Materials[12]

E 45 Test Methods for Determining the Inclusion Content of Steel[12]

E 92 Test Method for Vickers Hardness of Metallic Materials[12]

E 112 Test Methods for Determining the Average Grain Size[12]

E 120 Test Methods for Chemical Analysis of Titanium and Titanium Alloys[13]

E 135 Terminology Relating to Analytical Chemistry for Metals, Ores, and Related Materials[13]

E 168 Practices for General Techniques of Infrared Quantitative Analysis[14]

E 204 Practices for Identification of Materials by Infrared Absorption Spectroscopy Using the ASTM Coded Band and Chemical Classification Index[12]

---

[7] *Annual Book of ASTM Standards*, Vol 08.01.

[8] *Annual Book of ASTM Standards*, Vol 09.01.

[9] *Annual Book of ASTM Standards*, Vol 08.02.

[10] *Annual Book of ASTM Standards*, Vol 11.01.

[11] *Annual Book of ASTM Standards*, Vol 08.03.

[12] *Annual Book of ASTM Standards*, Vol 03.01.

[13] *Annual Book of ASTM Standards*, Vol 03.05.

[14] *Annual Book of ASTM Standards*, Vol 03.06.

E 290 Test Method for Bend Testing of Material for Ductility[12]

E 353 Test Methods for Chemical Analysis of Stainless, Heat-Resisting, Maraging, and Other Similar Chromium-Nickel-Iron Alloys[13]

E 354 Test Methods for Chemical Analysis of High-Temperature, Electrical, Magnetic, and Other Similar Iron, Nickel, and Cobalt Alloys[13]

E 386 Practice for Data Presentation Relating to High Resolution Nuclear Magnetic Resonance (NMR) Spectroscopy[15]

E 407 Practice for Microetching of Metals and Alloys[12]

E 562 Practice for Determining Volume Fraction by Systematic Manual Point Count[12]

E 663 Practice for Flame Atomic Absorption Spectroscopy[14]

E 860 Practice for Examining and Testing Items that are or May Become Involved in Products Liability Litigation[14]

E 883 Guide for Reflected-Light Photomicrography[12]

E 986 Practice for Scanning Electron Microscope Beam Size Characterization[12]

E 1188 Practice for Collection and Preservation of Information and Physical Items by a Technical Investigator[16]

E 1452 Practice for Preparation of Calibration Solutions for Spectrophotometric and for Spectroscopic Atomic Analyses[14]

E 1479 Practice for Describing and Specifying Inductively-Coupled Plasma Optical Emission Spectrophotometers[14]

F 316 Test Method for Pore Size Characteristics of Membrane Filters for Use with Aerospace Fluids[10]

F 619 Practice for Extraction of Medical Plastics[17]

F 981 Assessment of Compatibility of Biomaterials for Surgical Implants with Respect to Effect of Materials on Muscle and Bone[17]

F 1044 Test Method for Shear Testing of Porous Metal Coatings[17]

F 1147 Test Method for Tension Testing of Porous Metal Coatings[17]

F 1501 Test Method for Tension Testing of Calcium Phosphate Coatings[17]

F 1658 Test Method for Shear Testing of Calcium Phosphate Coatings[17]

2.2 *Other Document:*

ISO/DIS 12891-1, Retrieval and Analysis of Implantable Medical Devices, Part 1: Standard Practice for Retrieval and Handling

3. Terminology

3.1 *Definition of Terms Specific to Issues of Microbial Contamination:*

3.1.1 *antiseptic*—a germicide that is used on skin or living tissue for the purposes of inhibiting or destroying microorganisms.

3.1.2 *decontamination*—a process or treatment that renders a medical device, instrument, or environmental surface safe to handle. Ranges from sterilization to cleaning with soap and water.

3.1.3 *disinfectant*—a germicide that is used solely for destroying microorganisms on inanimate objects.

3.1.4 *disinfection*—generally less lethal than sterilization. It eliminates virtually all recognized pathogenic microorganisms but not necessarily all microbial forms (e.g., bacterial endospores) on inanimate objects. It does not insure overkill.

3.1.5 *sterilization*—use of a physical or chemical procedure to destroy all microbial life; including large numbers of highly resistant bacterial endospores.

4. Summary of Practice

4.1 This practice provides recommendations for collection of clinical data, analysis of adjacent tissues and the material characterizations to be performed when an implant is retrieved as part of a clinical or an animal study.

4.2 The clinical data to be recorded include a case history review, roentgenogram reviews, tissue culture, and observations of the implant site.

4.3 Protocols are provided for the handling of the implant tissue interface, and adjacent tissues for subsequent analysis. These protocols are intended to facilitate (a) histologic and immunohistochemical examination of the tissues, (b) chemical analysis of the tissues for identification and quantification of implant corrosion or degradation products, and (c) digestion of tissues for subsequent harvesting and analysis of particulate debris.

4.4 The material characterizations include observation and description of the explanted device and adjacent tissues, determination of chemical composition, macroscopic and microscopic examinations and mechanical property determinations. The guidelines are separated in three stages. Stage I is considered to comprise an essential minimum analysis for routine examination of all types of materials. Stage II is nondestructive but provides more detail and is intended for special studies of devices with or without impaired function, made of all types of materials. Stage III includes destructive methods for and material-specific protocols for detailed failure, microstructural, and chemical analysis as well as determination of physical and mechanical properties.

5. Significance and Use

5.1 The investigation of retrieved implantable medical devices and adjacent tissues can be of value in the assessment of clinical complications associated with the use of a specific prosthetic device design; can expand the knowledge of clinical implant performance and interactions between implants and the body; provide information on implant performance and safety; and thus further the development of biocompatible implant materials and devices with improved performance.

5.2 A significant portion of the information associated with a retrieved implant is obtained with detailed studies of the device-tissue interface. Appropriate methods are provided to facilitate a study of the particles in the tissues, and chemical analysis for the byproducts of degradation of the implant, and histologic evaluation of the cellular response to the implant.

5.3 For the analysis to be accurate, it is essential that the

[15] *Annual Book of ASTM Standards*, Vol 14.02.

[16] *Annual Book of ASTM Standards*, Vol 13.01.

[17] Available from American National Standards Institute, 1430 Broadway, New York, NY 10018.

device and associated tissues be removed without alteration of their form and structure. It is also essential that the tissues be handled in such a way as to avoid microbial contamination of the work place or the investigator. Standard protocols for the examination and collection of data are provided for retrieval and handling of implantable medical devices, as well as for specific types of materials in relation to their typical applications. For particular investigational programs, additional, more specific, protocols may be required. If special analytical techniques are employed, the appropriate procedures must be specified.

5.4 In order to interpret the analysis of materials and tissues, it is also essential to capture a minimum data set regarding the clinical findings and laboratory studies documenting device performance and reasons for removal.

5.5 Any destructive analysis of implants must be done so as to not destroy any features that may become the subject of litigation, as per Practice E 860. This standard recommendation should be applied in accordance with state or national regulations or legal requirements regarding the handling and analysis of retrieved implants and tissues.

6. Interferences

6.1 Some critical features of the retrieved implant, tissue and the interface can only be accurately described by observation at the time of removal, and prior to sterilization or disinfection. Such observation must be made using appropriate aseptic precautions.

6.2 Due to the destructive nature of some of the analysis protocols provided in this practice, their use precludes any other type of analysis. It is therefore essential that handling of the device and tissues be done in concert with the requirements of all of the analyses to be performed, including analyses that may be done in the future.

7. Hazards

7.1 The handling of retrieved implants and tissues may involve handling of infectious material.

7.2 It is suggested that individuals handling the devices be vaccinated against Hepatitis B. As a precautionary measure, removed implants should be sterilized by an appropriate means that does not adversely affect the implant.

7.3 There are situations where tissues or implants can not be sterilized or disinfected prior to analysis, for example, requirements of specialized protocols in which sterilization will adversely effect tissue or material properties. In such cases, extreme care should be taken to use aseptic technique and disinfection. Where institutional guidelines for the handling of septic material do not exist, details for handling and sterilizing retrievals, and laboratory practice recommendations can be found in ISO 12891-1.

8. Clinical Information Gathered at the Time of Implant Explantation

8.1 The extent of clinical information to be obtained will depend in part on the type of implant and reasons for removal. Similarly, the amount of information provided about the implant site will depend on the circumstances regarding the removal. A detailed listing and format for documentation of the clinical information associated with removal are provided in Appendix X1.

8.2 As a minimum, the clinical information for device tracking should include the following information:

8.2.1 Date of implantation, and date of explantation.

8.2.2 Identification of hospitals, or physicians' offices, where device implantation and removal was performed.

8.2.3 Confidential, unique, patient ID Code to link to hospitals implantation and removal records.

8.2.4 Device identification (manufacturer's name and device catalogue number).

8.2.5 Device lot and serial number.

8.2.6 Indication for use and reason for explantation (clinical diagnosis).

8.3 For purposes of implant retrieval studies, the following information is considered essential:

8.3.1 Patient or animal age and sex.

8.3.2 A generic statement as to level of patient activity relative to the device.

8.3.3 A statement as to any gross evidence of inflammation, implant site infection, or tissue damage such as osteolysis.

8.3.4 Orientation of the implant relative to the patient. It is suggested that the proximal end of the device be identified with a nondestructive marking scheme.

8.4 More detailed clinical information should be gathered, where feasible, as indicated in Appendix X1. Obtaining an in situ, intraoperative photograph of the implant is highly desirable.

8.5 To facilitate subsequent analysis, it is recommended that the device be removed with the tissue interface intact.

8.5.1 In cases of animal studies of tissue responses to implants, the implant should be removed with at least a 4 mm thick layer of adjacent tissue, as per F 981.

9. Analysis of the Tissues and the Tissue-Implant Interface

9.1 *Macroscopic Examination of Tissue*:

9.1.1 Record a gross pathologic description of the tissue immediately adjacent to the implant, as to consistency and color, as seen by the naked eye, or with a hand lens or dissecting microscope. Record any differences between the implant-tissue interface and the tissues not in direct contact with the implant. Describe the specimen size either by dimensions or weight.

9.1.2 Since the color of tissue is altered by sterilization and fixation methods, it is recommended that gross observations be made prior to sterilization. Such observations should be made utilizing aseptic techniques.

9.1.3 Where appropriate and feasible, obtain photographic documentation of the explant and adjacent tissue, as well as a photographic record of subsequent dissections.

9.2 *Histopathological Analysis of Tissue*:

9.2.1 Process the excised tissue using standard laboratory procedures for the histological dehydration, embedding and sectioning. These procedures may be for paraffin embedding, methacrylate embedding or other special procedures. Routine staining with hematoxylin and eosin (H & E), or toluidine blue are recommended for light microscopy of soft tissues and bone.

Special stains, for example, von Kassa, Masson, Movat pentachrome, may be utilized as indicated and should be fully described.

9.2.2 Provide a detailed histopathologic description of the tissue-implant interface as well as all adjacent tissue specimens, for example, extracellular matrix, necrotic changes, thickness of fibrous capsule, cell types, particulates, hyperplasia, dysplasia, type of inflammatory reaction.

9.2.3 If the implant material is porous, then tissue analysis must include evaluation of the reaction within the pores as well as in the adjacent tissues. This should include the degree and nature of tissue ingrowth, and biological fixation.

9.2.4 For detailed studies of tissue reactions, the use of a quantitative scoring scheme, such as that in Practice F 981 is recommended.

9.2.5 Since some polymeric materials, for example, PMMA bone cement, are altered or dissolved by the solutions used for routine histology, special techniques may be indicated, or special note made of voids formerly occupied by the material.

9.3 *Immunohistochemical and Other Special Histopathology Protocols*:

9.3.1 These procedures can be used for identifying specific cell types and extracellular matrix tissue responses to implantable materials and prosthetic devices. This field is constantly changing, and therefore only one such approach is provided as an example.

9.3.1.1 Typical markers chosen are for the presence of immunoglobulins on lymphocytes to indicate B cells or on monocytes/macrophages to indicate activation, the presence of CD2 markers to indicate immature T cells, the presence of CD3 markers to indicate mature T cells, and markers to indicate activated macrophages.

9.3.1.2 The protocols consist of a series of steps or reactions which have been developed to amplify the reactions, and to be cost effective. First, an antibody specific for the CD marker is used (typically mouse anti-human). Then, a biotinilated antibody to the first antibody is applied (typically goat anti-mouse); biotin serves as a marker in this amplification phase of the reactions. Strept-avidine peroxidase is then added to bind to the biotin and immobilize the peroxidase. Finally, a substrate is added which will react with the peroxidase, change color and precipitate. Diaminobenzidine (DAB) is often used, although several substrates are available for different kits or automatic systems. The end result is the peroxidase oxidation of DAB to give a yellow-brown precipitate at the site of the reaction. The sections can be stained with hematoxylin to enhance the visibility of cells.

9.3.1.3 An example of a method to be used is briefly summarized below and is based on standard techniques. Although it was originally described for use on frozen tissues, the use of embedded tissues allows for examination of the same tissue blocks used for routine pathology. This is only one of many approaches.

9.3.2 *Reagents*:

9.3.2.1 The reagents used come from a variety of companies including DAKO, Becton Dickinson, Kirkegaard & Perry, and Oncogene.

9.3.2.2 Antibody for specific markers, for example, CD2, CD3.

9.3.2.3 Biotinilated goat anti-mouse or anti-rabbit IgG.

9.3.2.4 Strept-avidine peroxidase.

9.3.2.5 Diaminobenzidine (DAB), or other suitable substrate.

9.3.3 Sections are deparaffinated in xylene for 5 min twice, and then rehydrated with absolute ethanol for 3 min, 95 % ethanol for 3 min, and then in 70 % ethanol for 3 min.

9.3.4 The sections are then placed in a methanol-hydrogen peroxide solution for 30 min to diminish the background level of peroxidase in the tissue. The sections are rinsed in water, next placed in buffered saline, and then the slide around the section is dried.

9.3.5 The slide is then placed in a humidity chamber, covered with buffer, and the first antibody is added. This will be the antibody specific for the marker (for example, CD2) and will be either of mouse or rabbit origin. This is incubated overnight, then rinsed with buffer, drained, and the slide around the tissue dried.

9.3.6 The second antibody, which is biotinolated, is added. This is usually goat anti-mouse or anti-rabbit IgG. This is incubated for 30 min, rinsed, the slide dried, and then strept-avidin peroxidase is added.

9.3.7 The strept-avidin peroxidase is incubated for 30 min, rinsed, and then a substrate such as DAB is added. The development of the color is watched under the microscope, the action stopped with water, then the slides are dipped into osmium tetroxide for final fixation. The slides may be counterstained with hematoxylin for visualization of all cells. The slides are processed for mounting with eukitt and can be evaluated for presence of label.

9.3.8 This method can be used to detect the production of cytokines in the cells in the tissues. However, caution should be used in the interpretation of findings, since these are soluble mediators and rapidly leave the site of origin.

9.4 *Chemical Analysis of Tissues By Flame Atomic Absorption Spectroscopy (AAS), Graphite Furnace Atomic Absorption Spectroscopy (GFAAS), by Inductively Coupled Plasma Optical Emission Spectroscopy (ICP-OES) or Mass Spectroscopy (ICPMS)*:

9.4.1 *Reagents and Materials*:

9.4.1.1 Standard AAS grade solutions (MCB reagents, Fisher, and VWR) are used to make calibration curves. Calibration solutions should be prepared according to Practices E 1452 and D 3919, using the same matrix solution as the test specimen. Solutions of low concentration should be made fresh daily. The sensitivity and possible interferences depend on the particular element.

9.4.1.2 Any fixing agents, chemicals and solvents must be of analytic purity. The use of 70 % ethanol is recommended as a transport and storage solution. The use of double distilled, deionized water is necessary.

9.4.1.3 Handling of tissues for subsequent chemical analysis requires special precautions to be taken to insure that the specimens are not contaminated with the elements to be analyzed. Surgical knives or instruments used for tissue excision shall be free of any contamination or loose particulates.

The use of ceramic or glass knives is recommended for preparation of specimens associated with metallic implants. Glass knives are not recommended for subsequent silicone analysis.

9.4.1.4 Tissues should be transferred to plastic or glass containers of high quality which have been thoroughly acid cleaned or unused from a lot tested to be free of contamination. Acid cleaning which may etch the glass surfaces is not recommended for subsequent silicone analysis. Tissue transfer should be done in a dust free environment.

9.4.2 Test solutions should be analyzed in triplicate, either as is or after dilution with 1 % nitric acid to a concentration which falls within the standards, and the results averaged. Concentrations are determined in μ/l (ppb), or μ/g of tissue (ppm). Results from solutions of known volumes from *in vitro* studies can be converted to total micrograms in solution.

9.4.2.1 The concentration of metallic species in tissue may vary according to the location of the specimen relative to the implant. It is therefore important to carefully record the location of the specimen.

9.4.3 These methods of analysis require chemical digestion of the tissue samples prior to analysis, and therefore the samples can not be used for any other analysis. The ability to digest tissue is influenced by the method of tissue fixation. It is recommended that tissues be fixed in analytical grade 70 % ethanol in analytical grade water. The methods of digestion depend on the type of tissue to be analyzed.

9.4.3.1 *Blood* samples drawn from patients or animals should be done using polypropylene syringes. The blood can be allowed to clot at room temperature and centrifuged at 1850 g for 30 min to separate serum and clot fractions. Blood may also be drawn in heparinized vacutainer tubes. The blood may be allowed to settle so as to isolate red and white cells, or be centrifuged at 400 g and the plasma supernatant drawn off. Plasma is diluted at least 2× in 1 % nitric acid.

9.4.3.2 *Cells*, either red blood cells or cells from cell culture experiments may receive special treatment, such as separation of cell contents and cell membranes. The cells are washed and centrifuged 3 times with physiologic saline to remove trapped serum or growth media. The cell pellet is then lysed with 1 % Triton X100 to release intracellular contents, centrifuged and the supernatant harvested. This solution is pipetted off, diluted 2× in 1 % nitric acid, and referred to as "cell contents." The pellet of cell membranes is then washed and centrifuged 3 times in saline to remove the Triton and remaining contents. The membranes are then digested in 50 % nitric acid, diluted in 0.5 % nitric acid for analysis as "cell membranes."

9.4.3.3 *Tissue* from implant sites or joint capsules should be weighed and placed in plastic bags for the mechanical tissue digestion machine. These are then frozen until use. For preparation, 5 ml of 50 % nitric acid will be added to each bag. The tissue is then homogenized in a mechanical blender. The samples are then pipetted into the GFAAS for analysis. Dilution as necessary is done with nitric acid.

9.4.3.4 *Bone* specimens can be subjected to a two-stage digestion procedure to separate them into two phases, mineralized and demineralized (or organic). The bones are placed in 0.5 N HCl for 48 hrs at 4°C to demineralize them. The rubbery demineralized samples are then placed in 50 % nitric acid to digest the organic portion. Both the HCl and HNO_3 samples are diluted as necessary and analyzed by GFAAS.

9.4.4 Chemical analysis by flame AAS should be done according to manufacturer's instructions, in accordance with E 663 and E 135.

9.4.5 Analysis with graphite furnace (GFAAS) should be done according to D 3919 using the manufacturer's specifications for analyte wavelength and slit width. Calibration standards, as per E 1452, should be made up in the same matrix as the test specimens.

9.4.5.1 A multi-cycle protocol is recommended to insure complete drying of the specimen prior to charring and atomization; additional steps may be required for post analysis clearing of the tubes.

9.4.5.2 The use of ultra pure argon for clearing is essential.

9.4.5.3 There are two types of graphite tubes used in the furnace: pyrolytic carbon coated graphite tubes, and tubes with L'vov platforms. The analysis for Ni, Mo, Pt, Ti, and V are done from the wall of the tubes while Co, Cr and Al are done on platforms.

9.4.6 Chemical analysis by ICP should be done in accordance with Practice E 1479.

9.5 *Analysis of Tissues for Particulate Debris*:

9.5.1 Analysis for particulates can be done histopathologically as in 9.2, or by tissue or fluid digestion and particle separation. Tissues subjected to digestion become dedicated to this type of analysis.

9.5.1.1 Preparation of tissue for drying and digestion will depend on the state of the tissue. If the tissue is embedded in paraffin, the tissue block should be deparaffinized with xylene overnight at room temperature, and then washed with 100 % ethanol. If tissue is fixed in formalin, it should be dehydrated through a series of alcohols using standard histological protocol, and infiltrated with 100 % ethanol. If tissue is fresh, it should be frozen and free of embedding media.

9.5.1.2 The tissue will be weighed, or the fluid volume determined before digestion. If a wet weight is desired (only applicable for the fresh tissue), 0.3–0.5 g are typically weighed out. For a dry tissue weight, the tissue should be freeze dried, sliced with a ceramic knife, and 0.02–0.03 g weighed out with a microbalance. Weighed tissue should then be placed in acid washed polystyrene vials. Once weighed, the tissue is suitable for digestion.

9.5.1.3 Several digestion protocols are described in the literature. The choice of protocol depends in part on the type of particle of interest, for example, metal versus polymer, and on the type of tissue. Four methods of digestion are described in this recommended practice.

9.5.2 *Reagents for Digestion*:

9.5.2.1 *Ultrapure water*—Distilled H_2O filtered with 0.2 μm filter.

9.5.2.2 *Phosphate Buffer*—3.55 g Na_2HPO_4, 3.45 g NaH_2PO_4, 0.744 g EDTA, in 100 ml ultrapure water.

9.5.2.3 *Papain solution*—1 ml phosphate buffer, 100 μL pure papain, 3.26 mg N-acetylcysteine, 9 ml ultrapure water.

9.5.2.4 *Strong bases*—Tissues have been digested in solutions of sodium hydroxide ranging from 1–10 N NaOH (5–50 ml/g of tissue), or in potassium hydroxide 2 N KOH (10 ml/g of tissue), or 4 M KOH (2 ml/gram of tissue).

9.5.2.5 *Pronase*—2000 U/ml, 50 mM Tris, 75 mM NaCl.

9.5.2.5.1 Concentrated nitric acid (HNO_3) has been used when tissues are difficult to digest, especially after fixation and embedding.

9.5.3 *Procedure for Digestion in Papain*:

9.5.3.1 Place 1 gram of tissue sample in a clean 50 ml conical tube.

9.5.3.2 Add 5 ml of papain solution and vortex.

9.5.3.3 Incubate sample at 65°C for 24 h. If sample does not dissolve add an additional 100 μl papain and vortex.

9.5.3.4 Centrifuge in an ultracentrifuge for 1 h at 100 000 g. A variable gradient may be used comprising of 2.0 ml each of 5, 10, 20, and 50 % sucrose.

9.5.3.5 Wash particles in 10 cc of hot filtered water.

9.5.4 *Procedure for Digestion in Strong Base and Pronase*

9.5.4.1 Rinse tissue samples in phosphate buffered saline, and place 1 g in a 15 ml glass tube.

9.5.4.2 Add 2 ml of 4 M KOH.

9.5.4.3 Incubate sample at 56°C for 48 h. Mix samples occasionally.

9.5.4.4 Centrifuge at 1000 g for 1 h. To facilitate sedimentation of debris, add 6 ml of 95 % ethanol to the 2 ml aliquots. Discard clear supernatant, and repeat digestion and centrifugation steps.

9.5.4.5 Wash debris in distilled water, mix and place in 37°C for 8 h. Mix with excess amounts of ethanol, and centrifuge at 1000 g, 1 h. Repeat washing procedure 3 times.

9.5.4.6 Digest the organic material with debris in pronase at 37°C for 24 h. During the first 5 min in pronase, ultrasonicate the debris to disaggregate the particles.

9.5.4.7 Wash the debris 3 times in distilled water.

9.5.4.8 Resuspend debris (0.5 ml debris/3 ml of ethanol) and add an equal volume of hexane and vortex.

9.5.4.9 Transfer the cream colored fraction containing the polymeric particles, which stabilized at the hexane-ethanol interface into a clean, sterile tube. Metal debris and bone particles will be in the sediment at the bottom.

9.5.4.10 Repeatedly add hexane or ethanol to the original tube and vortex. Harvest and pool the polyethylene particles.

9.5.4.11 To the pooled particles, add 2 ml of ethanol and evaporate any remaining hexane.

9.5.4.12 Add excess ethanol to the tube and centrifuge at 1000 g for 30 min.

9.5.4.13 Discard the supernatant and resuspend debris in KOH at 56°C for 8 h.

9.5.4.14 Add excess ethanol to the tube and centrifuge at 1000 g for 30 min.

9.5.4.15 Discard the clear supernatant and resuspend particles in 1 ml of distilled water, incubate for 8 h followed by centrifugation in ethanol. Repeat wash procedure three times.

9.5.4.16 Resuspend approximately 0.5 ml of debris in 2 ml of ethanol. Ultrasonicate for 5 min before transfer to a stub for SEM and particle analysis.

9.5.5 *Procedure for Digestion in Nitric Acid*

9.5.5.1 With this protocol, the digest solution is never filtered, therefore, the submicron particles are not lost and can be evaluated (with SEM and Coulter), without complications that could arise from hemosiderin particles which remain with non-acid digestion protocols.

9.5.5.2 If paraffin embedded sections are deparaffinated in xylene or toluene, replace the solution with 2 changes of absolute ethanol.

9.5.5.3 Critical point dry the tissue specimen, slice it and place 0.02 to 0.03 g pieces in plastic tubes.

9.5.5.4 Add 1.0 ml of concentrated nitric acid.

9.5.5.5 Digest the tissue for 24 h at room temperature. Shake the tube and sonicate for 2 min. Continue digestion for an additional 24 h.

9.5.5.6 Centrifuge digestion solution at 9500 g for 5 min. Depending on the amount of debris, there will be a floating band of polymeric debris and a sedimented pellet of metallic debris. These can either be isolated separately, or together.

9.5.5.7 Separate the fluid from debris by aspirating the clear liquid between the floating band and the pellet.

9.5.5.8 Add 1 ml of concentrated nitric acid to the debris, sonicate for 2 min and centrifuge at 11 600 rpm for 5 min.

9.5.5.9 Aspirate the clear liquid and add 1 ml of acetone, sonicate 2 min, and centrifuge at 11 600 rpm for 20 min. Both metallic and polymeric debris will sediment in the acetone.

9.5.5.10 Aspirate the supernatant and resuspend the debris in 10 μl of dispersant (Coulter I B) and slowly add 1 ml of ultrapure water, with intermittent sonication.

9.5.6 *Procedure for Tissue or Dried Lubricant or Synovial Fluid Digestion in Sodium Hydroxide*:

9.5.6.1 For tissue only: mince 2.0–5.0 g of tissue and place in a glass container. To extract lipid, add 2:1 chloroform-:methanol solution and place on an orbital shaker overnight, or until the tissues sink to the bottom of the container. Rinse tissues with 3× filtered (0.2 μm) deionized H_2O.

9.5.6.2 For extracted tissues and dried (lyophilized) fluid, add 12 ml 5*N* NaOH and incubate at 65°C for 1 to 3 hours on a water bath-shaker.

9.5.6.3 Allow the digested solution to cool to room temperature, then ultrasonicate for 10 minutes.

9.5.6.4 Into two clean, particle-free polyallomer centrifuge tubes, place 7 ml each of the digested solution and top off with 5 ml of 5 % sucrose. Ultracentrifuge for 3 hours at 40 000 rpm, 5–15°C.

9.5.6.5 UHMWPE will rise to the top of each tube to form an opaque layer. Carefully pipette this band into another clean, particle-free vial. Other bands that sometimes appear can be collected separately or pooled with the UHMWPE.

9.5.6.6 To wash off the sucrose, add 3× filtered deionized H_2O to the collected band until the total volume is 21 ml. Ultrasonicate for 5 min, then heat sample for 1 h at 80°C.

9.5.6.7 Into three clean, particle-free polyallomer centrifuge tubes, place 7 ml each of the solution and top off with an isopropanol gradient consisting of 3 ml of 0.96 g/cm^3 isopropanol/deionized H_2O and 2 ml of 0.90 g/cm^3 solution. Ultracentrifuge for 1 h at 40 000 rpm, 20–25°C.

9.5.6.8 Collect the UHMWPE band at the 0.90 and 0.96 g/cm^3 interface into a clean, particle-free vial. Other bands that may appear can be collected separately.

9.5.7 *Isolation of Debris*:

9.5.7.1 The debris obtained by the above procedures may contain particles of a wide range of sizes and morphology. There may also be clumping or agglomeration of particles. As a result, several stages of filtration may be necessary to effectively isolate the different particles of interest.

9.5.7.2 The final common pathway for the above procedures is filtration with submicron filters. These are then subjected to optical or scanning electron microscopy, or particle counting. Particle morphology may be characterized.

9.5.7.3 To characterize retrieved particles with light microscopy, the particle solution should be sonicated for 10 min. Some particles may melt and agglomerate further by sonication for 10 min. For these, short bursts with time to cool are recommended. From this, 10 µl of the solution can be removed and filtered using a 0.1 µm filter (nitrocellulose, Millipore, Nucleopore). The filter should then be mounted and coverslipped on a glass slide. Since the filters become optically transparent when in contact with standard mounting media, the particles can be analyzed with a transmitted light microscope.

9.5.7.4 To characterize the morphology of retrieved particles with Scanning Electron Microscopy, 10–200 µl of particle solution should be filtered using a 0.2 µm polycarbonate filter, or 10 and 0.4 µm filters (nitrocellulose, Millipore, Nucleopore). The filtering vacuum should be stopped before all the liquid is removed, and the remaining liquid allowed to evaporate. The filter should then be fixed with double sided tape and copper conductive strip, on an SEM mount. Specimens may be coated with palladium or gold to make the polymeric particles conductive. Coating is not necessary when operating the SEM in the low vacuum Nature mode.

9.5.7.5 The large pore filters can be cut in half, dried at 50°C and coverslipped for viewing with transmitted polarized light microscopy.

9.5.7.6 Chemical analysis methods such as EDXA and FTIR may also be employed to determine the chemical nature of the particles.

10. Stage I Analysis of the Implant Components

10.1 Stage I examination and documentation should be conducted routinely on all retrieved devices. The procedures are intended to take the investigator a minimal amount of time and expense to complete, while providing sufficient information to permit device tracking.

10.1.1 Perform a separate analysis for each component of a device, if possible and necessary, as outlined below. A coating shall be considered as a separate component. A sample form is provided as Appendix X2.

10.1.2 Document chain of device custody as per Practice E 1188.

10.2 *Device Description*:

10.2.1 Identify the device type and describe all of the components retrieved.

10.2.2 Record the manufacturer and catalogue and serial numbers where possible.

10.2.3 Record any other information which describes the device.

10.3 *Macroscopic Examination*:

10.3.1 Perform this examination with the unaided eye or with the aid of a stereo-microscope.

10.3.2 Examine all surfaces of the components for evidence of in service or iatrogenic damage.

10.3.3 Record an estimate as to the degree of findings as per Appendix X2.

10.4 *Visual Examination for Evidence of Mechanical Failure*:

10.4.1 Observe the implant surface by suitable techniques to ascertain any mode of failure, as applicable. In no event should any surface of a failed implant be destructively evaluated at this time.

10.4.2 Sketch any significant features. These may also be recorded photographically, although this adds significant cost to routine, Stage I analysis.

11. Stage II Analysis

11.1 Stage II analysis should be carried out after Stage I, if deemed necessary, to further evaluate the characteristics, or failure mode, of the implant. This level of testing primarily relates to an assessment of the modes of failure and deterioration of an implant in the most non-destructive manner possible. Record the results on form Appendix X3.

11.1.1 Perform Stage II analysis for severely damaged components, or where optical fractography is sufficient to determine mechanisms involved in mechanical failure of the device.

11.1.2 Fabrication of surface replications may be indicated in some Stage II investigations. These could then be used for examination without damaging the specimen.

11.2 *Photography*:

11.2.1 A photographic documentation of findings should be made.

11.3 *Optical Fractographic Examination*:

11.3.1 If the implant is fractured, analyze the fracture surface by suitable techniques to ascertain the mode of fracture.

11.3.2 In no event should the fracture surface be destructively evaluated. If the device has mechanically failed, it is important to remember that it may be classified as legal evidence.

12. Stage III Analysis, Metallic Components

12.1 If further testing is necessary to assess the properties of the implant, the tests listed under Stage III Analysis, Metallic Components, in Appendix X4 shall be carried out as deemed necessary to further characterize the implant and its history.

12.1.1 Stage III examinations involve destructive methods for microscopy and chemical analysis. These should only be conducted when complete material characterization and failure analysis is indicated. Care should be taken to insure that potential legal evidence is not destroyed, as per Practice E 860.

12.2 *Microscopic Examination*:

12.2.1 Prepare appropriate metallographic sections in accordance with Methods E 3 and Terminology E 7.

12.2.2 Specimens should be etched as per Practice E 407, and examined microscopically using light microscopy as per Guide E 883.

12.2.3 Determine the inclusion content using Test Methods E 45 as a guide. Compare the observed content with that of the applicable material standard, if appropriate.

12.2.4 Determine the grain size as per Test Methods E 112 and compare results with the applicable material standard.

12.2.5 Characterize the grain boundaries in terms of inclusion content. Microscopic evidence of corrosion should be noted and recorded. Evidence of sensitization of stainless steels can be determined according to Practices A 262.

12.2.6 Any evidence of microporosity can be documented using Test Methods E 45 as a guideline.

12.2.7 The use of scanning electron microscopy as per Practice E 986 may be utilized for fractographic analysis.

12.3 *Material Characterization*:

12.3.1 Determine the physical and chemical composition and identity of the metallic alloy as per Test Methods A 751, E 353, E 354, and E 120. In the event that the composition does not meet a recognized material standard, the appropriate referee analysis procedure shall be used.

12.3.2 Chemical analysis can also be conducted with electron microprobe analysis.

12.4 *Mechanical Properties*:

12.4.1 The type of measurements to be carried out at this Stage of characterization will be dependent upon the implant and its use. Suggested property tests are shown in Appendix X4 under Mechanical Properties.

12.4.2 Determine the hardness as per Test Methods E 10, E 18, or E 92.

12.4.3 Determine the tensile, flexural, compressive, and the like properties in accordance with applicable material specification if indicated, and such other tests as are appropriate to the specimen which may be fabricated from the implant. Deviation from the specimen dimensions as described in the standard methods may be necessary to accommodate the shape and size of the device under investigation.

12.5 *Coated Samples*:

12.5.1 Examine coated samples microscopically for missing sections of coating. Estimate the fraction of coating missing.

12.5.2 Where possible determine the shear strength of the adherent coating as per Test Method F 1044.

12.5.3 Where possible determine the tensile strength of the adherent coating as per Test Method F 1147.

13. Stage III Analysis: Polymeric Components

13.1 If further testing is necessary to assess the properties of the implant, the tests listed under "Stage III Analysis, Polymeric Components," in Appendix X5 shall be carried out as deemed necessary to further characterize the implant and its history.

13.1.1 Stage III examinations involve destructive methods for microscopy and chemical analysis. These should only be conducted when complete material characterization and failure analysis is indicated. Care should be taken to insure that potential legal evidence is not destroyed, as per E 860.

13.1.2 A wide variety of polymeric materials are used in implantable devices. Actual identification of the material type may not be possible without Stage III chemical analysis. Where possible, classify the material according to Classification D 4000.

13.1.3 Each type or class of materials has an associated battery of tests designed for that specific type. As a result, the investigator is directed to the specific material standards to identify the specific tests which are appropriate. The methods and properties described in this section are intended to serve as a guide to the selection of test methods.

13.2 *Microscopic Examination*:

13.2.1 Examine the specimen for evidence of surface damage or degradation.

13.2.2 The use of thin sections (5–10 μm) and optical microscopy using reflected and transmitted, polarized and nonpolarized light has been found useful in identifying evidence of inclusions or porosity and for identification of changes in crystallinity or density.

13.2.3 In the case of mechanical failure, scanning electron microscopy (SEM) may provide insight into the mode of failure.

13.3 *Material Characterization*

13.3.1 Determine the molecular weight or weight distribution of the specimen. Possible methods and ASTM standards to be utilized are gel permeation chromatography (GPC) (Practice D 3016, Test Method D 5296), osmometry, light scattering (Test Method D 4001), viscometry (Test Methods D 3835, D 2857), or melt index (Test Method D 1238).

13.3.2 Determine the density by an appropriate method. Suggested methods are by displacement (Test Methods D 792), the gradient method (Test Method D 1505), or, for rigid cellular plastics, Test Method D 1622 is suggested.

13.3.3 Determine the thermal properties of the material. The glass transition (Tg), and melt temperature (Tm) can be determined by differential scanning calorimetry (DSC) as per Test Method D 3417. Phase identification by differential thermal analysis (DTA) as per Test Method D 3418. Softening point, thermomechanical properties, coefficient of expansion can be determined by thermomechanical analysis (TMA). The thermal stability can be determined by thermogravimetric analysis (TGA).

13.3.4 Determine the chemical composition and determine whether there has been any oxidation or degradation of the material. Analysis by infrared analysis and FTIR is suggested, as per Practices E 168 and E 204. Chemical composition and structure can be determined by nuclear magnetic resonance spectroscopy (NMR) as per Practice E 386. Free radicals can be identified with electronic spin resonance (ESR).

13.3.5 Of particular interest are the presence of any low molecular weight extractables. These may be from degradation of the polymer or from absorption of moieties such as lipids from the *in vivo* environment. There are a number of extraction protocols that could be utilized, for example, Test Methods D 1239, D 2842, D 4754, Practice D 5152, Test Method D 5227, Practice F 619. Appropriate chemical analysis assays can then be applied to identify the composition of the etractables. The results will depend on the method chosen.

13.4 *Mechanical Properties*:

13.4.1 The type of measurements to be carried out at this Stage of characterization will be dependent upon the implant and its use. In making such measurements, it is important to note and record the sample location and orientation.

13.4.2 Determine the hardness according to the applicable material standard. Testing by Rockwell, as per Test Method

D 785, or Durometer according to Test Method D 2240 are suggested.

13.4.3 Determine the tensile, flexural, compressive, etc. properties in accordance with applicable material specification if possible, and such other tests as are appropriate to the specimen which may be fabricated from the implant. Suggested test methods are: tensile (Test Methods D 412, D 638, D 1623, D 1708), flexural (Test Methods D 621, D 671, D 747, D 790), compression (Test Methods D 695, D 1621), shear (Test Method D 732), impact resistance (Test Methods D 256), tear resistance (Test Methods D 624, D 1004), abrasion resistance (Test Method D 1242), and tensile creep (Test Method D 2990). Deviation from the specimen dimensions as described in the standard methods may be necessary to accommodate the shape and size of the device under investigation.

13.4.4 Dynamic mechanical properties may also be of interest. These could be measured by means of a torsional pendulum as per Test Method D 4065 or in flexural fatigue as per Test Method D 671.

13.5 *Coated or Porous Specimens*:

13.5.1 Coatings should be microscopically and chemically characterized utilizing the methods as described in this section.

13.5.2 The porosity of porous materials or porous coatings should be determined according to Test Method D 2873, Practice E 562 or Test Method F 316.

13.6 *Polymer Matrix Composites*:

13.6.1 Analysis and characterization of polymer matrix should be as described in this section.

13.6.2 Analysis of the reinforcing material should be in accordance with the material type.

13.6.3 Of special interest with composites is the analysis of the interfacial relationships between matrix and the second phase. Microscopic methods should be utilized to establish degrees and nature of interfacial bonding, or degradation thereof.

14. Stage III Analysis: Ceramic and Glass Materials

14.1 If further testing is necessary to assess the properties of the implant, the tests listed under "Stage III Analysis: Ceramic and Glass Materials" In Appendix X6 shall be carried out as deemed necessary to further characterize the implant and its history.

14.1.1 Stage III examinations involve destructive methods for microscopy and chemical analysis. These should only be conducted when complete material characterization and failure analysis is indicated. Care should be taken to insure that potential legal evidence is not destroyed, as per Practice E 860.

14.1.2 There is a wide variety of materials and devices that fit this category. Therefore, these protocols shall serve as a guide to ascertaining the important features of retrieved devices.

14.2 *Microscopic Examination*:

14.2.1 Use standard light optical or electron optical microscopic preparation techniques suitable for the material under investigation.

14.2.2 Determine the inclusion content in accordance with the applicable material standard, if appropriate.

14.2.3 Determine the grain size in accordance with the applicable material standard and method.

14.2.4 Evidence of degradation should be noted and recorded as per Appendix X6. Surfaces should be examined for evidence of surface etching or grain excavation.

14.2.5 Fracture surfaces may be examined by scanning electron microscopy (SEM).

14.3 *Material Characterization*:

14.3.1 Determine the chemical composition and identity of the component. Chemical composition of glasses may be conducted according to Test Methods C 169. Composition of ceramics may be conducted according to Test Methods C 573.

14.3.2 Determine the density and apparent porosity, as per Test Methods C 20.

14.3.3 Appropriate x-ray diffraction (XRD) methods should be utilized to determine degree of crystallinity and phase composition. Phase composition may also be determined by FTIR.

14.3.4 Thermal properties may be determined by differential scanning calorimetry (DSC), or thermogravimetric analysis (TGA) as appropriate, and by differential thermal analysis (DTA).

14.4 *Mechanical Properties*:

14.4.1 The type of measurements to be carried out at this Stage of characterization will be dependent upon the implant and its use. Suggested property tests are shown in Appendix X6 under Mechanical Properties.

14.4.2 Determine the hardness as per Test Method C 730 for glasses or Test Method C 849 for ceramics.

14.4.3 Determine the tensile, flexural, compressive, etc. properties in accordance with applicable material specification, if possible. Modulus and Poisson's ratio may be determined as per Test Method C 623 for glasses, or Test Method C 1198 for ceramics. Flexural properties may be determined as per Test Methods C 158 for glasses, and Test Methods C 674 or C 1161 for ceramics.

14.5 *Porous and Coated Samples*:

14.5.1 Examine coated samples microscopically for missing sections of coating. Estimate the fraction of coating missing.

14.5.2 Determine the shear strength of the coating using the appropriate method, such as Test Method F 1658.

14.5.3 Determine the tensile strength of the coating using the appropriate method, such as Test Method F 1501.

14.5.4 Determine adhesion or cohesive strength of flame-sprayed coatings as per Test Method C 633.

14.5.5 Surface area of porous materials may be determined by Test Method C 1069. Porosity may be determined as per Practice E 562, or Test Method F 316.

14.6 *Ceramic Matrix Composites*:

14.6.1 Analysis and characterization of ceramic matrix should be as described in this section.

14.6.2 Analysis of the reinforcing material should be in accordance with the material type.

14.6.3 Of special interest with composites is the analysis of the interfacial relationships between matrix and the second phase. Microscopic methods should be utilized to establish degrees and nature of interfacial bonding, or degradation thereof.

15. Materials of Biological Origin or Tissue Engineering

15.1 If further testing is necessary to assess the properties of biologically derived implants, the tests shall be carried out as deemed necessary to further characterize the implant and its history.

15.1.1 Stage III examinations involve destructive methods for microscopy and chemical analysis. These should only be conducted when complete material characterization and failure analysis is indicated. Care should be taken to insure that potential legal evidence is not destroyed, as per Practice E 860.

15.2 The protocols in this document provide for analysis of biological tissues and of synthetic materials. The application of the appropriate methodologies should be utilized in the study of various biologic and synthetic components of retrieved biological or tissue engineered devices.

16. Keywords

16.1 ceramics; chemical analysis; composites; histology; implant retrieval; metals; particles; polymers

APPENDIXES

(Nonmandatory Information)

X1. CLINICAL INFORMATION SUGGESTED TO BE RECORDED DURING RETRIEVAL OF MEDICAL DEVICES

Minimum data set
Date of implantation, and date of removal
Hospital, or physician's office of implantation and of removal
Confidential patient ID Code to link to hospitals of implantation and removal records
Implant anatomical site
Device identification (manufacturer's name and device catalogue number), Device lot and serial number
Indication for use and Reason for explantation
Additional Clinical Information (confidential)
Surgeon (name & address)
Patient (name & address and/or ID number)
female [ ] male [ ] date of birth ____ occupation; weight height
History of substance abuse (smoking, etc.)
Reason for Investigation: routine series [ ], research [ ] documentation [ ], complaint [ ], liability claims [ ], clinical investigation [ ], other ______
Diagnosis at Insertion (or Reason for Insertion)
Additional Diagnoses and Complications
Antibiotics: pre op. [ ] peri op. [ ] post op. [ ] prophylactic [ ]
Relevant pharmaceuticals duration:

Post Operative Treatment:
Complications between insertion and removal: e.g. infection [ ]
Observations prior to removal (functional)
Clinical Reason for Removal:
routine [ ] pain [ ] revision [ ] failure [ ] infection [ ] allergy [ ] other _____
Patient level of activity at removal
Observations at Removal (indicate yes, no, not applicable,
doubt, etc.)

normal tissue [ ]	bursal fluid [ ]	scar tissue [ ]
granulation tissue [ ]	bone reaction [ ]	infection [ ]
loose implant [ ]	discoloration, implant debris [ ]	other _____

Additional Material Provided for Analysis

radiographs	no [ ]	yes [ ]	how many
tissue	no [ ]	yes [ ]	type origin
bacteriol. specimen	no [ ]	yes [ ]	type origin
immunol. specimen	no [ ]	yes [ ]	type origin
fluid	no [ ]	yes [ ]	type

photographs; pathology reports
surgical reports; additional documentation
Type of disinfection used

X2. STANDARD FORM FOR GUIDING THE STAGE I ANALYSIS OF RETRIEVED IMPLANTABLE MEDICAL DEVICES

Reason for Investigation:
routine clinical series [ ] animal study [ ] research [ ]
complaint [ ] liability claims [ ] other ____
Patient or animal ID code ____
Date Retrieved ____ Implant duration ____
Date of analysis ____
Record for all Components retrieved:
device type & component names ____________
manufacturer(s) ____________
catalog number(s) ____ Serial number(s) ____
identification marks, e.g. size: __________
material(s) ____________
Macroscopic examination (YES, NO, DOUBT, or NOT APPLICABLE)

		Location	Size/Area	Severity/ Degree
____ a)	wear or burnishing	____	____	____
____ b)	galling	____	____	____
____ c)	scratching	____	____	____
____ d)	change of shape	____	____	____
____ e)	mechanical damage	____	____	____
____ f)	macro porosity	____	____	____
____ g)	pitting or crevice corrosion	____	____	____
____ h)	fretting	____	____	____
____ i)	embedded particles	____	____	____
____ j)	discoloration or staining	____	____	____
____ k)	calcification	____	____	____
____ l)	thrombosis	____	____	____
____ m)	degradation	____	____	____
____ n)	stress cracking or crazing	____	____	____
____ o)	loss of coating	____	____	____
____ p)	mechanical failure	____	____	____
____ q)	cold flow			

Sketch(s):

X3. STANDARD FORM FOR GUIDING THE STAGE II ANALYSIS OF RETRIEVED IMPLANTABLE MEDICAL DEVICES

Photograph orientation and descriptions.
Mechanical failure (if YES, identify mode, indicate location of failure and method of identification)
a) static-overstress, causing plastic deformation
b) shear
c) fatigue
d) torsion
e) impact
f) stress corrosion or environmental cracking
g) fatigue, or corrosion-fatigue
h) combination of above (identify)
i) other (specify)____________
j) unable to identify

X4. STAGE III ANALYSIS: METALLIC MATERIALS

Standard form for guiding the Stage III analysis of retrieved metallic implantable medical devices

1. **Microscopic examination** (indicate location and orientation of sample)
a) Inclusion content
b) Grain size
c) Grain boundary constituents
d) Microporosity
e) Other distinguishing features
2. **Failure analysis** (if appropriate)
a) Presence of fatigue striations
b) Fraction of surface with ductile overload
c) Evidence of significant ductile overload
d) Defects associated with crack initiation
3. **Type of material** (indicate method of determination)
a) Chemical composition
4. **Mechanical properties** (indicate N/A if not available). Samples should be taken from areas representative of the original material.
a) Sample size and orientation
b) Hardness (indicate type and method)
c) Other ASTM tests as applicable (for example, tensile, or transverse bend tests)
5. **Metallic Coating**
a) Coating material
b) Estimated fraction of coating missing
c) Shear strength
d) Tensile strength

X5. STAGE III ANALYSIS: POLYMERIC MATERIALS

Standard form for guiding the Stage III analysis of retrieved polymeric components

Samples should be taken from areas representative of the original material, (D 1898).

1. **Microscopic examination** (indicate location and orientation of sample)
 a) Grain size
 b) Grain boundary constituents
 c) Microporosity
 d) Evidence of damage or degradation, or other distinguishing features.
2. **Failure analysis:**
 Mode of failure, delamination, oxidation, optical microscopy with polarized light.
3. **Material Characterization**
 a) Molecular weight (use most applicable technique)
  1) Gel permeation chromatography (GPC)
  2) Osmometry
  3) Light scattering
  4) Viscometry
  5) Melt index
 b) Density
 c) Thermal characterization (most appropriate techniques)
  1) Glass transition (Tg), melt temperature (Tm), by differential scanning calorimetry (DSC). Phase identification by differential thermal analysis (DTA).
  2) Softening point, thermomechanical properties, coefficient of expansion by thermomechanical analysis (TMA)
  3) Thermal stability by thermogravimetric analysis (TGA)
 d) Chemical analysis
  1) Infrared spectroscopy (IR, FTIR)
  2) Chemical composition and structure (NMR)
  3) Other chemical composition determinations
 e) Low molecular extractables, e.g. absorbed lipid content of implant.
4. **Mechanical properties** (indicate N/A if not available).
 a) Record sample size and orientation
 b) Hardness
 c) Other tests as appropriate, e.g. tensile, flexural, compression, shear, impact resistance, tear resistance, abrasion resistance, tensile creep.
 d) Dynamic mechanical measurements, fatigue.
5. **Porous or Coating materials**
 a) Coating material
 b) Any damage of loss of coating
 c) Porosity
6. **Composites**
 a) Type of composite materials
 b) Matrix phase relationships.

X6. STAGE III ANALYSIS: CERAMIC AND GLASS MATERIALS

STANDARD FORM FOR GUIDING THE STAGE III ANALYSIS OF RETRIEVED CERAMIC AND GLASS IMPLANTABLE MEDICAL DEVICES

1. **Microscopic examination** (indicate location and orientation of sample)
 a) Inclusion content
 b) Grain size
 c) Grain boundary constituents
 d) Microporosity
 e) Grain excavation, grain orientation, (texturing) of surface vs bulk
 f) Surface morphology (SEM)
 g) Other distinguishing features
2. **Failure Analysis** (if appropriate)
 a) Defects associated with crack initiation
 b) Fracture morphology indicative of failure stresses
3. **Material Characterization**
 a) Type of material (indicate method of determination)
 b) Chemical composition
 c) Surface chemistry, etching, new crystals
 d) Chemical glass transition (DSC or DTA)
 e) Crystallinity (XRD)
 f) Phase composition (FTIR)
4. **Mechanical properties** (indicate N/A if not available). Samples should be taken from areas representative of the original material.
 a) Sample size and orientation
 b) Hardness (indicate type and method)
 c) Other ASTM tests as applicable (for example, flexural properties)
5. **Porous or Ceramic Coatings**
 a) Coating material
 b) Estimated fraction of coating missing
 c) Shear strength
 d) Tensile strength
 e) Adhesive and cohesive strength
6. **Composite Materials**
 a) Material types
 b) Composite phase relationships

X7. RATIONALE

X7.1 The ultimate test for an implant or device and the materials out of which is fabricated, is its performance as an implant. In many situations, critical information can only be ascertained by examination of retrieved implants and the surrounding tissues. Such analysis could be part of experimental studies in animals, clinical studies, where devices are routinely removed or removed for revision, or in post-mortem autopsy studies. The information suggested for collection could also be of value in device tracking.

X7.2 This standard practice was first published in 1978 for analysis of retrieved metallic orthopaedic implants. Rather than develop a separate standard for each material type or class, the document was revised to cover all material types and analysis of the associated tissues.

X7.3 The intent of this document is to provide standard protocols for analysis of retrieved devices. It specifies standard methods of analysis and data collection for comparing similar sets of data between research centers. For information and data on retrieved devices to be useful on a national and international basis, standard methods of analysis and reporting are necessary. Therefore, collected data should conform to this standard practice.

X7.4 Because of the complexity of analysis of implant devices, and because of the large number of potential tests suggested in this standard, it has appeared desirable to divide the investigation into stages. The analyses of the implant are separated into three groups with the degree of characterization increasing from Stage I through Stage III. The implant characterizations may include macroscopic and microscopic examinations, chemical composition, as well as physical and mechanical property determinations to ascertain mechanisms and degree of degradation.

X7.5 The tests performed may depend upon the reason for removal of the implant. Furthermore, analysis can be an expensive and time consuming process. To facilitate capturing information on a large number of implants, a minimum dataset obtained by inexpensive means is proposed in the first two stages. Perform a Stage I analysis for all removals. Perform a Stage II analysis for severely damaged components, or where optical fractography is sufficient to determine mechanisms involved in mechanical failure of the device. Stage III examinations involve destructive methods for microscopy and chemical analysis. These should only be conducted when complete material characterization and failure analysis is indicated.

X7.6 The American Society for Metals, International, has published Metals Handbook, Failure Analysis and Prevention, which may be used as a reference to supplement the practices in this document. As part of an Implant retrieval meeting held at the National Bureau of Standards in 1980, an extensive collection of retrieval forms was assembled as an appendix **(9)**, which may also be used as a guide for documenting the analyses.

X7.7 This standard practice is intended for clinical and other research purposes. Users interested in product liability litigation may refer to E 860. In any event, care should be taken to insure that potential legal evidence is not destroyed.

REFERENCES

(1) L'Vov, B. V., "Electrothermal atomization—The Way Towards Absolute Methods of Atomic Absorption Analysis," *Spectrochimica Acta*, 33B, 153–193, 1978.

(2) Long, G. L., and Winefordner, J. D. "Limit of Detection. A closer look at the IUPAC definition. *Analyt. Chem.*, 55, 712A–724A, 1983.

(3) Jacobs, J. J., Skipor, A. K., Black, J., Urban, R. M., and Galante, J. O., "Release and Excretion of Metal in Patients Who Have a Total Hip-Replacement Component Made of Titanium-Base Alloy," *J Bone and Joint Surgery*, 73A (10), 1475–1486, 1991.

(4) Gill, R. J., "AAS or ICP-OES: Are They Competing Techniques?," *American Laboratory*, November, 24F–24K, 1993.

(5) Campbell, P., Ma, S., Schmalzried, T., and Amstutz, H. C., "Tissue Digestion for Wear Debris Particle Isolation," *J Biomedical Materials Research*, 28, 523–526, 1994.

(6) Shanbhag, A. S., Jacobs, J. J., Glant, T. T., Gilbert, J. L., Black, J., and Galante, J. O., "Composition and Morphology of Wear Debris in Failed Uncemented Total Hip Replacement," *J. Bone and Joint Surgery*, 76B, 60–67, 1994.

(7) Margevicius, K. J., Bauer, T. W., McMahon, J. T., Brown, S. A., and Merritt, K., "Isolation and Characterization of Debris in Membranes around Total Joint Prostheses," *J Bone Joint Surgery*, 76A, 1664–1675, 1994.

(8) Favero, M. S., and Bond, W. W., "Sterilization, Disinfection, and Antisepsis in the Hospital," Ch 24 in: *Manual of Clinical Microbiology*, Balows & Hausler, Herrman, Isenberg, Shadomy, ASM Washington, 1991.

(9) Weinstein, A., Gibbons, D., Brown, S., and Ruff, W., *Implant Retrieval: Material and Biological Analysis*, National Bureau of Standards Special Publication 601, 1981.

(10) Metals Handbook Vol 11, "Failure Analysis and Prevention," American Society of Metals, Metals Park, OH 1986.

Standard Specification for Wrought Cobalt-35 Nickel-20 Chromium-10 Molybdenum Alloy for Surgical Implant Applications UNS R 30035[1]

This standard is issued under the fixed designation F 562; the number immediately following the designation indicates the year of original adoption or, in the case of revision, the year of last revision. A number in parentheses indicates the year of last reapproval. A superscript epsilon (ε) indicates an editorial change since the last revision or reapproval.

1. Scope

1.1 This specification covers requirements of wrought cobalt-35 nickel-20 chromium-10 molybdenum alloy in the form of bars and wires, used for the manufacture of surgical implants. This alloy depends on combinations of work-strengthening, and work-strengthening and aging to attain a variety of combinations of strength and ductility.

1.2 The values stated in inch-pound units are to be regarded as the standard. The metric equivalents of the inch-pound units may be approximate.

2. Referenced Documents

2.1 *ASTM Standards:*

E 8 Test Methods for Tension Testing of Metallic Materials[2]

E 112 Test Methods for Determining the Average Grain Size[2]

E 354 Test Methods for Chemical Analysis of High-Temperature, Electrical, Magnetic, and Other Similar Iron, Nickel, and Cobalt Alloys[3]

F 981 Practice for Assessment of Compatibility of Biomaterials for Surgical Implants with Respect to Effect of Materials on Muscle and Bone[4]

2.2 *Federal Standard:*

Federal Test Method No. 151 Metals; Test Methods[5]

2.3 *Aerospace Material Specifications:*

AMS 2269 Chemical Check Analysis Limits—Wrought Nickel Alloys and Cobalt Alloys[6]

2.4 *American Society for Quality Standard:*

ASQC1 Specification of General Requirements for a Quality Program[7]

2.5 *Society of Automotive Engineers:*

SAE J1086 Practice for Numbering Metals and Alloys (UNS)[6]

3. Terminology

3.1 *Description of Term Specific to This Standard:*

3.1.1 *capability*—the word capability is used to indicate the ability of cold worked material to attain specific mechanical properties after thermal aging treatment.

4. Ordering Information

4.1 Inquiries and orders for material under this specification shall include the following information:

4.1.1 Quantity (weight or number of pieces),

4.1.2 ASTM designation and date of issue,

4.1.3 Form (1.1),

4.1.4 Condition (5.1),

4.1.5 Mechanical properties (if applicable),

4.1.6 Finish (9.2),

4.1.7 Applicable dimensions, including size, thickness, width, and length (exact, random, multiples), or print number,

4.1.8 Special tests, and

4.1.9 Special requirements.

5. Materials and Manufacture

5.1 *Condition*—Bar and wire shall be furnished , as specified, in the solution-annealed, cold-worked, or cold-worked and aged condition.

6. Chemical Requirements

6.1 The cobalt-35 nickel-20 chromium-10 molybdenum alloy shall conform to the chemical requirements prescribed in Table 1. The supplier shall not ship material that is outside the limits specified in Table 1.

6.1.1 Requirements for the major and minor elemental constituents are listed in Table 1. Also listed are important residual elements. Analysis for elements not listed in Table 1 is not required to verify compliance with this specification.

6.2 *Product Analysis*—The product analysis is either for the purpose of verifying the composition of a heat or lot or to determine variations in the composition within the heat.

6.2.1 Acceptance or rejection of a heat or lot of material

---

[1] This specification is under the jurisdiction of ASTM Committee F04 on Medical and Surgical Materials and Devicesand is the direct responsibility of Subcommittee F04.12on Metallurgical Materials.

Current edition approved May 10, 2000. Published August 2000. Originally published as F 562 – 78. Last previous edition F 562 – 95.

[2] *Annual Book of ASTM Standards*, Vol 03.01.

[3] *Annual Book of ASTM Standards*, Vol 03.05.

[4] *Annual Book of ASTM Standards*, Vol 13.01.

[5] Available from Standardization Documents Order Desk, Bldg. 4 Section D, 700 Robbins Ave., Philadelphia, PA 19111-5094, Attn: NPODS.

[6] Available from Society of Automotive Engineers, Inc., 400 Commonwealth Drive, Warrendale, PA 15096–0001.

[7] Available from American Society for Quality, 161 West Wisconsin Ave., Milwaukee, WI 53203.

TABLE 1 Chemical Requirements

Element	Composition,% (mass/mass)	
	min	max
Carbon	...	0.025
Manganese	...	0.15
Silicon	...	0.15
Phosphorus	...	0.015
Sulfur	...	0.010
Chromium	19.0	21.0
Nickel	33.0	37.0
Molybdenum	9.0	10.5
Iron	...	1.0
Titanium	...	1.0
Boron	...	0.015
Cobalt[A]	balance	balance

[A] Approximately equal to the difference between 100 % and the sum percentage of the other specified elements. The percentage cobalt content by difference is not required to be reported.

may be made by the purchaser on the basis of this product analysis.

6.2.2 Product analysis tolerances do not broaden the specified heat analysis requirements but cover variations between laboratories in the measurement of chemical content. Product analysis limits shall be as specified in Table 2.

7. Mechanical Requirements

7.1 Solution-annealed bar and wire product shall conform to the mechanical properties specified in Table 3. Test Methods E 8 shall apply.

7.2 Mechanical properties for the cold-worked and aged condition shall conform to the mechanical property requirements specified in Table 3.

7.3 Should it be necessary to illustrate the work strengthening capability of this alloy, the referee procedure will be the use of a straight draw bench at room temperature. A round bar shall be cold drawn 53 % to a smaller round bar.

7.4 The level of mechanical properties for material in other than the solution-annealed or 53 % cold-worked and aged condition shall be specified in the purchase order.

TABLE 2 Product Analysis Tolerances (% (mass/mass))[A]

Element	Tolerances over the max (upper limit) or under the min (lower limit), %[B]
Carbon	0.01
Manganese	0.03
Silicon	0.02
Phosphorus	0.005
Sulfur	0.005
Chromium	0.25
Nickel	0.30
Molybdenum	0.15
Iron	0.05
Titanium	0.04
Boron	0.005

[A] Refer to AMS 2269.
[B] Under minimum limit not applicable for elements where only a maximum percentage is indicated.

8. Special Tests

8.1 The grain size of bar product shall be predominantly No. 4 or finer with occasional grains as large as No. 2 permissible when tested in accordance with Test Methods E 112.

8.1.1 It is preferred that samples for grain size determination be selected after the last annealing operation and prior to the final cold-working operation.

8.1.2 If samples are selected after final cold-working operations, transverse specimens shall be prepared.

8.2 For other than bar product, the grain size shall be agreed upon between the purchaser and the manufacturer.

9. Workmanship, Finish, and Appearance

9.1 All products shall be free from external and internal imperfections detrimental to the intended purpose.

9.2 *Finish*—Types of finish available in bar and wire products are cold-drawn, pickled, ground, ground and polished, or as specified in the implant manufacturer's purchase order.

10. Test Methods

10.1 Chemical analysis shall be in accordance with Test Methods E 354, Federal Test Method No. 151, or as agreed upon between the purchaser and the manufacturer. The product after consumable electrode vacuum remelting may be used for reporting the chemical composition.

11. Certification

11.1 Upon request of the purchaser in the contract or order, a certification shall be provided by the manufacturer that the material was manufactured and tested in accordance with this specification. A report of the test results shall be furnished at the time of shipment.

12. Quality Program Requirements

12.1 The producer shall maintain a quality program, such as that defined in Specification ASQ 1.

12.2 The manufacturer of surgical implants or medical appliances shall be assured of the producer's quality program conformance to the intent of Specification ASQ 1, or any other recognized program.

13. Keywords

13.1 cobalt alloys (for surgical implants) cobalt-nickel alloy; metals (for surgical implants)-cobalt alloys

TABLE 3 Mechanical Properties (Bar Products)

Condition	Tensile Strength,[A] psi (MPa)	Yield Strength,[A] 0.2 % Offset, psi (MPa)	Elongation in 4D or 4W, min, %	Reduction of Area, min, %
Solution annealed[B]	115 000 to 145 000 (793 to 1000)	35 000 to 65 000 (241 to 448)	50.0	65.0
Cold-worked and aged[C]	260 000 (1793) min	230 000 (1586) min	8.0	35.0

[A] Tension and yield requirements apply to tests taken longitudinally to the direction of rolling.
[B] 1925 ± 25°F (1050° + 15°C), 1 to 2 h at temperature, air cool or water quench to room temperature.
[C] Cold worked 53 % and aged within the range 1000 to 1200°F ± 25°F (540 to 645°C± 15°C) for 4 h and air cool.

APPENDIXES

(Nonmandatory Information)

X1. RATIONALE

X1.1 The primary reason for this specification is to characterize the composition and properties to assure consistency in the starting material used in the manufacture of medical devices.

X1.2 The acceptable metal conditions include solution annealed, cold worked or cold worked and capability aged, the choice dependent upon the medical device design and its intended application.

X1.3 A boron limit has been added to the chemical requirements to coincide with industry melting practice for this alloy.

X2. BIOCOMPATIBILITY

X2.1 The alloy composition covered by this specification has been successfully employed in human implants **(1-5)**[8] for over a decade. This material has been found to produce a well characterized level of local biological response when tested in accordance with Practice F 981 or equivalent.

X2.2 No known surgical implant material has ever been shown to be completely free of adverse reactions in the human body; however, long-term clinical experience has shown an acceptable level of biological response can be expected, if this material is used in appropriate applications.

[8] The boldface numbers in parentheses refer to the list of references at the end of this standard.

REFERENCES

(1) Gaechter, A., Galante, G., "MP35N, A Corrosion Resistant High-Strength Alloy for Orthopaedic or Surgical Implants: Two Year Bioassay", *Journal of Biomedical Materials Research*, Vol 10, 1976, pp. 829–831.

(2) Escales, F., Galante, J., Rostoker, W., Coogan, P. S., "MP35N, A Corrosion Resistant High-Strength Alloy for Orthopaedic Surgical Implants: Bioassay Results", *Journal of Biomedical Materials Research*, Vol 9, No. 3, 1976, pp. 303–313.

(3) Kuehne, D., Willert, H. G., *The Tissue Compatibility of the Forging Alloy (Protasul 10) With the Hitherto Used Implant Alloys (Co-Cr- Mo Casting Alloy) and (AISI 316L) After an Implantation Period of One Year*, Doctoral Thesis, Osteological Research Laboratory of Orthopaedic University, Frankfurt am Main/Frg, 1975.

(4) Bauman, R., Semlitsch, M., *Biological and Mechanical Behavior or Newly Developed Implant Materials in Animal Studies,* Sulzer reprint, Re/28.09.00, 1974, pp 1–9.

(5) ISO/TC-150/SC-1/WG-1, Swiss Standard Association, Group 129-Surgical Implants, Draft Report of WG-1, Swiss Proposal 056509, Part 2, *Comments on Biocompatibility*, Davos Meeting, June 1974.

Designation: F 563 – 00

Standard Specification for Wrought Cobalt-20Nickel-20Chromium-3.5Molybdenum-3.5Tungsten-5Iron Alloy for Surgical Implant Applications (UNS R30563)[1]

This standard is issued under the fixed designation F 563; the number immediately following the designation indicates the year of original adoption or, in the case of revision, the year of last revision. A number in parentheses indicates the year of last reapproval. A superscript epsilon (ε) indicates an editorial change since the last revision or reapproval.

1. Scope

1.1 This specification covers the requirements for a wrought cobalt-20nickel-20chromium-3.5molybdenum-3.5tungsten-5 iron alloy in the form of bars, wires, and forgings used for the manufacture of surgical implants.

1.2 The values stated in inch-pound units are to be regarded as the standard. The SI units given in parentheses are for information only.

2. Referenced Documents

2.1 *ASTM Standards:*

A 751 Test Methods, Practices, and Terminology for Chemical Analysis of Steel Products[2]

E 8 Test Methods for Tension Testing of Metallic Materials[3]

E 18 Test Methods for Rockwell Hardness and Rockwell Superficial Hardness of Metallic Materials[3]

E 92 Test Method for Vickers Hardness of Metallic Materials[3]

E 112 Test Methods for Determining Average Grain Size[3]

E 140 Hardness Conversion Tables for Metals (Relationship Among Brinell Hardness, Vickers Hardness, Rockwell Hardness, Rockwell Superficial Hardness, Knoop Hardness, and Scleroscope Hardness)[3]

E 354 Test Methods for Chemical Analysis of High-Temperature, Electrical, Magnetic, and Other Similar Iron, Nickel, and Cobalt Alloys[4]

2.2 *Aerospace Material Specification:*

AMS 2269 Chemical Check Analysis Limits Wrought Nickel Alloys and Cobalt Alloys[5]

2.3 *ISO Standard:*

ISO 5832-8 Implant for Surgery—Metallic Materials—Part 8: Wrought Cobalt-Nickel-Chromium-Tungsten-Iron Alloy[6]

2.4 *ASQ Stamdard:*

Cl Specification of General Requirements for a Quality Program[7]

3. Ordering Information

3.1 Inquiries and orders for material under this specification shall include the following information:

3.1.1 Quantity (weight or number of pieces),

3.1.2 Condition (4.1),

3.1.3 Finish (4.2),

3.1.4 Mechanical properties (if applicable, for special conditions) (7.1),

3.1.5 Applicable dimensions, including size, thickness, width, and length (exact, random, multiples), or print number,

3.1.6 Special tests, and

3.1.7 Supplementary requirements (if applicable),

3.1.8 Product uniformity, and

3.1.9 Additional tests or inspections, supplementary composition limits, if any, as required by the manufacturing process and intended application, and other supplementary requirements.

4. Materials and Manufacture

4.1 *Condition*:

4.1.1 Bar and wire shall be furnished to the implant manufacturer as specified, in the annealed, medium hard, hard, or, for special applications, extra hard condition, depending on the degree of cold work and aging treatment, if any.

4.1.2 Forging shall be furnished to the implant manufacturer as specified, in the forged or forged and solution heattreated and aged condition.

4.2 *Finish*—Surface finish shall be as specified and required by the subsequent manufacturing process and the intended application, if pertinent.

5. Chemical Composition

5.1 The heat analysis shall conform to the requirements as

---

[1] This specification is under the jurisdiction of ASTM Committee F04 on Medical and Surgical Materials and Devices, and is the direct responsibility of Subcommittee F04.12 on Metallurgical Materials.

Current edition approved November 10, 2000. Published January 2001. Originally published as F 563 – 78. Last previous edition F 563 – 95.

[2] *Annual Book of ASTM Standards*, Vol 01.01.

[3] *Annual Book of ASTM Standards*, Vol 03.01.

[4] *Annual Book of ASTM Standards*, Vol 03.05.

[5] Available from Society of Automotive Engineers, 400 Commonwealth Drive, Warrendale, PA 15096.

[6] Available from American National Standards Institute, 11 W. 42nd St., 13th Floor, New York, NY 10036.

[7] Available from American Society for Quality, 161 West Wisconsin Ave., Milwaukee, WI 53203.

to chemical composition specified in Table 1. The product analysis tolerances shall conform to the requirements prescribed in Table 2.

5.1.1 Requirements for the major and minor elemental constituents are listed in Table 1. Also listed are important residual elements. Analysis for elements not listed in Table 1 is not required to verify compliance with this specification.

5.2 For referee purposes, Test Methods E 354 shall be used.

5.3 Methods and practices relating to chemical analysis required by this specification shall be in accordance with Test Methods A 751.

5.4 *Product Analysis*—Product analysis tolerances do not broaden the specified heat analysis requirements, but cover variations between laboratories in the measurement of chemical content. The manufacturer shall not ship material that is outside the limits specified in Table 1. Product analysis limits shall be as specified in Table 2.

5.4.1 The product analysis is either for the purpose of verifying the composition of a heat or lot or to determine variations in the composition within the heat.

5.4.2 Acceptance or rejection of a heat or lot of material may be made by the purchaser on the basis of this check analysis.

6. Metallurgical Requirements

6.1 The microstructure of the material shall be single phased as observed at 100× magnification.

6.2 The grain size shall be No. 5 or finer, based on the appropriate chart of Test Methods E 112.

TABLE 1 Chemical Requirements, Ladle Analysis

Element	Composition, (%), Mass/Mass	
	min	max
Carbon	...	0.05
Manganese	...	1.00
Sulfur	...	0.010
Silicon	...	0.50
Chromium	18.00	22.00
Molybdenum	3.00	4.00
Tungsten	3.00	4.00
Nickel	15.00	25.00
Titanium	0.50	3.50
Iron	4.00	6.00
Cobalt	balance	balance

TABLE 2 Product Analysis Tolerances[A]

Element	Tolerances over the max (upper limit) or under the min (lower limit), %, Mass/Mass	
Carbon	0.01	
Manganese	0.03	
Sulfur	0.003	
Silicon	0.03	
Chromium	0.25	
Molybdenum	0.10	
Tungsten	0.15	
	under min	over max
Nickel	0.20	0.25
Titanium	0.03	0.07
Iron	0.07	0.10

[A] Refer to AMS 2269.

7. Mechanical Requirements

7.1 The material shall conform to the appropriate minimum mechanical properties specified in Table 3. Test Methods E 8 shall apply.

7.2 When desired, hardness limits may be specified. Test Methods E 18 or E 92 and Standard Tables E140 shall be used. Hardness determination of cold-worked material shall be made on a product cross section, midway between the center and the surface, if the cross section size is adequate.

7.3 If any manufacturing operations of the implant manufacturer alter the properties of the material, the specimens shall be subjected to the same operations prior to testing.

8. Certification

8.1 The manufacturer's certification that the material was manufactured and tested in accordance with this specification together with a report of the test results requested shall be furnished at the time of shipment.

9. Quality Program Requirements

9.1 The producer shall maintain a quality program, such as that defined in ASQ Cl.

9.2 The manufacturer of surgical implants or medical appliances shall be assured of the producer's quality program for conformance to the intent of ASQ Cl, or any other recognized program.

10. Keywords

10.1 cobalt alloys; cobalt alloys (for surgical implants); cobalt-nickel alloy; metals (for surgical implants)

TABLE 3 Mechanical Properties

Conditions	Ultimate Tensile Strength, min, psi (MPa)	Yield Strength, (0.2 % Offset) min, psi (MPa)	Elongation[A] in 4*D* or 4*W*, min, %	Reduction of Area, min, %
Fully annealed	87 000 (600)	40 000 (276)	50	65
Cold worked or cold worked and aged[B]:				
medium hard	145 000 (1000)	120 000 (827)	18	50
hard	190 000 (1310)	170 000 (1172)	12	45
Cold worked and aged (for special purposes), extra hard	230 000 (1586)	190 000 (1310)	...	...

[A] 4 $D = 4 \times$ diameter: 4 $W = 4 \times$ width.
[B] Aging in the temperature range from 400 to 550°C.

APPENDIXES

(Nonmandatory Information)

X1. RATIONALE

X1.1 The primary purpose of this specification is to characterize composition and properties to assure consistency in the starting material used in the manufacture of medical devices.

X1.2 Acceptable metal conditions supplied to the medical device manufacturer include annealed, cold worked, and cold worked and aged depending upon the medical device design and its intended application.

X1.3 The title has been changed to include the nominal composition of the major elements; UNS designation has been added; the scope was changed to include the nominal analysis; ISO 5832-8 specification has been included under 2 on Referenced Documents; product analysis information was added in 5.4 and Section 8 on Certification; and Section 9 on Quality Program Requirements were updated; as well as Appendix X2 Biocompatibility added.

X2. BIOCOMPATIBILITY

X2.1 The material composition covered by this standard has been employed successfully in contact with soft tissue and bone for over a decade (**1-7**).[8]

X2.2 No known surgical implant material has ever been shown to be completely free of adverse reactions in the human body; however, long term clinical experience has shown an acceptable level of biological response can be expected, if the material is used in appropriate applications.

[8] The boldface numbers in parentheses refer to the list of references appended to this specification.

REFERENCES

(1) Hulliger, L., Pohler, O., and Straumann, F., "Effect of Pure Metals and Alloys on the Growth of Fibroblast Cultures," *Zeitschrift Fuer Die Gesamte Experimentelle Medizin,* Vol 114, 1967, p. 145.

(2) Straumann, F., Steinemann, S., Pohler, O., Willenegger, H., and Schenk, R., "Recent Experimental and Clinical Results on Metallosis," *Langenbecks Archiv Fuer Klinische,* Vol 305, 1963, p. 21.

(3) Contzen, H., Straumann, F., and Paschke, E., *Basics of the Alloplastic with Metals and Plastic Materials,* published by Georg Thieme, Stuttgart, 1967.

(4) Hagmann, R., "Investigations on New Bone Formation After Intrafemoral Implantation of Different Metal Screws in Rats," *Acta Anatomica,* Vol 64, 1966, p. 311.

(5) Hutzschenreuter, P., Perren, S. M., Steinemann, S., Geret, V., and Klebl, M., "Some Effects of Rigidity of Internal Fixation on the Healing Pattern of Osteotomies," *Injury 1,* 1969, p. 77.

(6) Wirz, J. "Die Transfixation von Stegpfeilern," *Zahnärztliche Rundschau,* Vol 79, 1970, p. 721.

(7) Wirz, J., *Die Transfixation von Stegpfeilern,* published by Alfred Huethig, Heidelberg, 1973.

Standard Specification and Test Methods for Metallic Bone Staples[1]

This standard is issued under the fixed designation F 564; the number immediately following the designation indicates the year of original adoption or, in the case of revision, the year of last revision. A number in parentheses indicates the year of last reapproval. A superscript epsilon (ε) indicates an editorial change since the last revision or reapproval.

1. Scope

1.1 This specification covers characterization of the design and mechanical function of metallic staples used in the internal fixation of the muscular skeletal system. It is not the intention of this specification to describe or specify specific designs for metallic bone staples.

1.2 This specification includes the following four test methods for measuring mechanical properties of metallic bone staples:

1.2.1 Test Method for Constant Amplitude Bending Fatigue Tests of Metallic Bone Staples—Annex A1.

1.2.2 Test Method for Pull-Out Fixation Strength of Metallic Bone Staples—Annex A2.

1.2.3 Test Method for Soft Tissue Fixation Strength of Metallic Bone Staples—Annex A3.

1.2.4 Test Method for Elastic Static Bending of Metallic Bone Staples—Annex A4.

1.3 Unless otherwise indicated, the values stated in SI units are to be regarded as standard. The values given in parentheses are given for information only.

1.4 *This standard does not purport to address all of the safety concerns, if any, associated with its use. It is the responsibility of the user of this standard to establish appropriate safety and health practices and determine the applicability of regulatory limitations prior to use.*

2. Referenced Documents

2.1 *ASTM Standards:*

E 4 Practices for Force Verification of Testing Machines[2]

E 122 Practice for Choice of Sample Size to Estimate a Measure of Quality for a Lot or Process[3]

E 467 Practice for Verification of Constant Amplitude Dynamic Loads in an Axial Load Fatigue Testing Machine[2]

F 75 Specification for Cast Cobalt-Chromium-Molybdenum Alloy for Surgical Implant Applications[4]

F 86 Practice for Surface Preparation and Marking of Metallic Surgical Implants[4]

F 382 Test Method for Static Bending Properties of Metallic Bone Plates[4]

F 565 Standard Practice for Care and Handling of Orthopedic Implants and Instruments[4]

F 601 Practice for Fluorescent Penetrant Inspection of Metallic Surgical Implants[4]

F 629 Practice for Radiography of Cast Metallic Surgical Implants[4]

3. Finish

3.1 Staples conforming to this specification shall be finished and identified in accordance with Practice F 86, as appropriate.

4. Inspection Practices

4.1 Staples made in accordance with Specification F 75 should be inspected in accordance with Practice F 601 or X-rayed in accordance with Practice F 629.

5. Care and Handling

5.1 Staples should be cared for and handled in accordance with F 565, as appropriate.

6. Keywords

6.1 bending test; bone fixation; fatigue test; fixation devices; metallic bone staples; orthopaedic medical devices; pullout test; soft tissue fixation; surgical implants

[1] This specification is under the jurisdiction of ASTM Committee F-04 on Medical and Surgical Materials and Devices and is the direct responsibility of Subcommittee F04.21 on Osteosynthesis.

Current edition approved May 10, 2000. Published August 2000. Originally published as F 564 – 85. Last previous edition F 564 – 85 (1997)$^{\epsilon 1}$.

[2] *Annual Book of ASTM Standards*, Vol 03.01.

[3] *Annual Book of ASTM Standards*, Vol 14.02.

[4] *Annual Book of ASTM Standards*, Vol 13.01.

ANNEXES

(Mandatory Information)

A1. TEST METHOD FOR CONSTANT AMPLITUDE BENDING FATIGUE TESTS OF METALLIC BONE STAPLES

A1.1 Scope

A1.1.1 This test method covers procedures for the performance of constant amplitude fatigue testing of metallic staples used in internal fixation of the musculoskeletal system. This test method may be used when testing in air at ambient temperature or in an aqueous or physiological solution.

A1.1.2 The values stated in SI units are to be regarded as the standard.

A1.1.3 *This standard does not purport to address all of the safety concerns, if any, associated with its use. It is the responsibility of the user of this standard to establish appropriate safety and health practices and determine the applicability of regulatory limitations prior to use.*

A1.2 Summary of Test Method

A1.2.1 Metallic bone staples are tested under bending loads until the specimen fails or a predetermined number of cycles has been applied to it. Bending tests may be performed in one of two modes: either pure, in-plane bending; or tension (or compression) combined with in-plane bending. Tests using either of these methods may be conducted at ambient conditions or in aqueous or physiological solutions (at either room temperature or 37°C).

A1.3 Significance and Use

A1.3.1 This test method is used to determine the fatigue resistance of metallic bone staples when subjected to repetitive loading for large numbers of cycles. This information may also be useful for comparing the effect of variations in staple material, geometry, surface condition, or placement under certain circumstances.

A1.3.2 It is essential that uniform fatigue practices be established in order that such basic fatigue data be comparable and reproducible and can be correlated among laboratories.

A1.3.3 The results of fatigue tests are suitable for direct application to design only when the service conditions parallel the test conditions exactly. This test method may not be appropriate for all types of bone staple applications. The user is cautioned to consider the appropriateness of the test method in view of the materials being tested and their potential application.

A1.4 Apparatus

A1.4.1 *Testing Machines*, conforming to the requirements of Practices E 4 and E 467. The loads used for determining strengths shall be within the loading range of the testing machine as defined in Practices E 4 and E 467.

A1.4.2 *Gripping Devices*:

A1.4.2.1 *Staple Extensions*—Pairs of specially designed metal blocks that permit the holding of individual staples for the application of bending fatigue loads. The legs of each staple are fitted into fixation holes in each block with minimal clearance to restrict bending of the staple within the hole. The staple is fixed securely in the block using a moldable filling or grouting agent. The extension design should minimize the weight to reduce the influence on the staple while maintaining sufficient stiffness to transfer the load to the staple without undesirable deflection. Holes for pin and clevis fixation are optional (see Figs. A1.1-A1.3).

NOTE A1.1—Variations in fixation hole configuration may be required for staple legs with noncircular cross sections. Also, it is necessary to provide a gap between the underside of the staple bridge and edge of the staple extender in most cases. This is necessary to eliminate contact between the staple bridge (or other bridge features such as tissue spikes) and the staple extender. However, this gap should be standardized within any test group as required.

A1.4.2.2 *4-Point Bend Fixture*—A standard or modified bending fixture that produces pure bending in the staple without appreciable shear or torsion when used to apply load to the staple through the staple extensions.

A1.4.2.3 *Pin and Clevice Fixture*—A standard or modified fixture used to apply a distractive or compressive load to the staple through the staple extensions to produce bending in the staple similar to that seen in vivo.

A1.4.3 *Filling or Grouting Agent*—A stiff, moldable filler, such as epoxy, acrylic cement, or a low-melting point alloy (for example, Wood's metal) used to secure the staple leg within the staple extension.

A1.4.4 *Aqueous Solution*—Tap water, distilled water, physiological saline, or similar aqueous solutions, used to immerse the test specimens fully during the test.

A1.4.5 *Constant Temperature Bath*—An aqueous bath capable of maintaining the samples and containers at physiologic

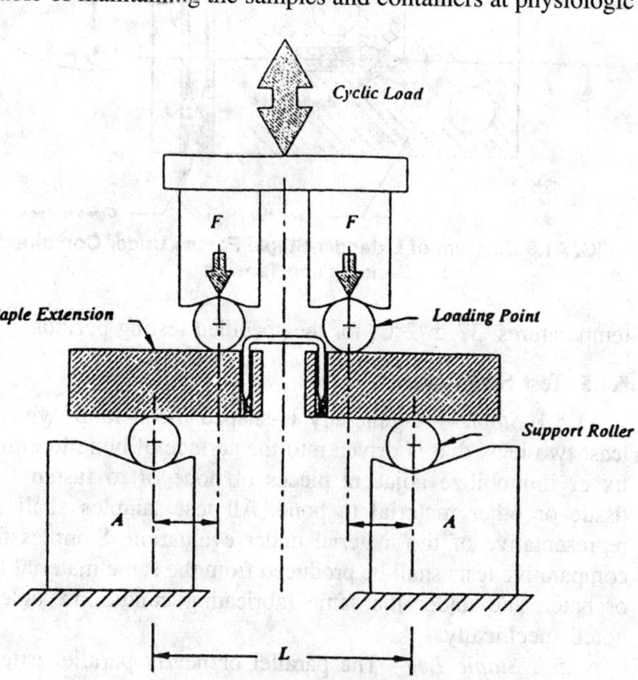

FIG. A1.1 4-Point Bending of Staples in Extension

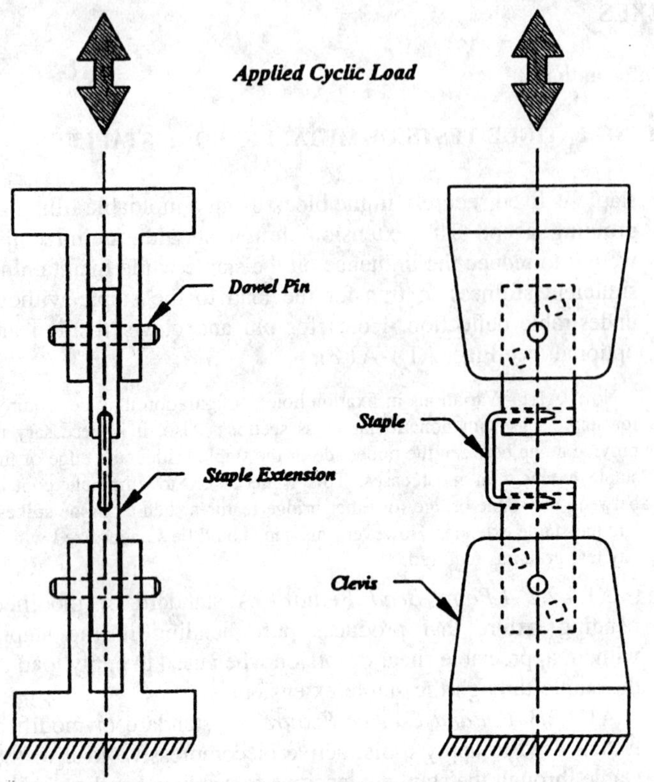

FIG. A1.2 Combined Tension (or Compression) and Bending of Staples

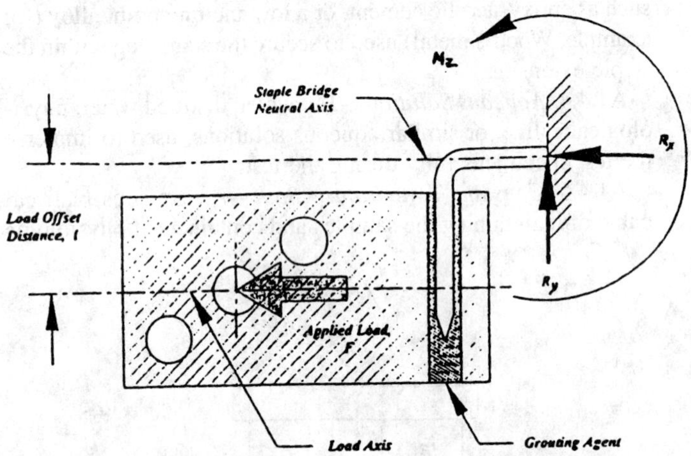

FIG. A1.3 Diagram of Extender-Staple Forces Under Combined Bending and Tension

temperatures, 37 ± 2°C, for the specified testing periods.

A1.5 Test Specimen

A1.5.1 *Staple*—A generally U-shaped metal loop, with at least two legs, that is driven into the surface of bone to either fix or immobilize adjacent pieces of bone or to fasten soft tissue or other material to bone. All test samples shall be representative of the material under evaluation. Samples for comparative tests shall be produced from the same material lot or batch and under the same fabricating conditions, unless noted specifically.

A1.5.2 *Staple Leg*—The parallel or nearly parallel extensions that are intended to penetrate the bone tissue; these may be round, square, or polygonal in cross section, and they may possess serrations or barbs to increase the fixation or purchase strength in the bone.

A1.5.3 *Staple Bridge*—The cross member of the staple connecting the legs; the bridge may be smooth or possess spikes or projections on the underside for the retention of soft tissue or other material.

A1.6 Procedure

A1.6.1 *Mounting the Specimen*—Fix the staple leg in an extension block using the filling agent. A fixture should be used to ensure proper in-plane alignment of the two extensions and the staple during this process. Also, each staple should be fixed such that the bridge is the same distance from the top of each extension.

NOTE A1.2—This distance is at the discretion of the operator, but it determines the portion of the staple subjected to the bending loads.

A1.6.2 *4-Point Bend Testing*:

A1.6.2.1 Place the staple and attached staple extensions in the 4-point bending fixture such that the loading point and support rollers contact the staple extensions on either side of the staple; direct contact of the rollers with the staple shall not be permitted during the test. Alignment of the loading point rollers shall be symmetric on the centerline between the support rollers (see Fig. A1.1).

A1.6.2.2 Apply cyclic loads (sinusoidal, sawtooth, etc.), generating bending moments in the staple without permanent deformation. Appropriate starting loads should be 50 to 75 % of the static bending strength, unless indicated otherwise.

NOTE A1.3—It may be necessary to provide a low-friction means of maintaining the position of the staple and attached extensions. Also, the fixtures should be designed so that loads are applied equally at the loading points during each deflection throughout the test.

A1.6.2.3 Compute the bending moment, M, by the following formula, where F = force applied at each loading point and A = distance between the loading point and support roller, $M_{bending} = FA$.

A1.6.2.4 Continue the test until failure of the staple or the fixation or a predetermined number of load cycles has been applied.

A1.6.3 *Combined Tension or (Compression) and Bending*:

A1.6.3.1 Place the staple and attached staple extensions in the axial bending fixture. The pins and clevices should permit free rotation of the staple extensions, with minimal friction, while maintaining alignment of the staple legs (and extensions) in the same plane (see Fig. A1.2).

A1.6.3.2 Apply cyclic loads (sinusoidal, sawtooth, etc.), generating bending moments in the staple without permanent deformation. Appropriate starting loads should be 50 to 75 % of the static yield strength, unless indicated otherwise.

NOTE A1.4—It may be necessary to maintain a minimum tensile or compressive load on the specimen throughout the test, since operating at or near zero load may result in either loss of machine control due to discontinuity in the load feedback loop or undesirable transient loading of the staple.

A1.6.3.3 Compute the bending moment in the staple bridge, M, by the following formula, where F = force applied at each center of each pin and L = distance between the load application axis, that is, the pin center, and the neutral axis of the staple bridge, $M_{bending} = FL$ (see Fig. A1.3).

NOTE A1.5—The application of this test method produces bending, tensile (or compressive), and shear stresses in the staple. The direction and magnitudes of these stresses should be analyzed using superposition theory or other suitable methods.

A1.6.3.4 Continue the test until failure of the staple or the fixation or a predetermined number of load cycles has been applied.

A1.6.4 *Stress Verification*—It is recommended that strain gages (or extensometry) be used to measure the bending strains induced in the specimen. This is accomplished most easily on the staple bridge, but it may be possible to perform on a portion of the staple leg or at the leg-bridge junction under certain circumstances and with certain staple designs. The recommended technique is to strain gage the actual fatigue test specimens, if possible, provided that the installation of strain gage will not influence the test results.

A1.7 Test Termination

A1.7.1 Continue the tests until the specimen fails or a predetermined number of cycles has been applied to the specimen. Failure should be defined as complete separation, a crack visible at a specified magnification, a crack of certain dimensions, or by some other criterion. State the criterion selected for defining failure when reporting the results.

A1.7.2 A test shall be considered invalid if a loosening of the staple occurs in the embedding medium or if noticeable yielding or permanent deformation occurs in the specimen.

A1.8 Report

A1.8.1 Report the following information:

A1.8.1.1 *Staple Description*—Type, size, special features (barbs, spikes, and so forth), manufacturer, material, batch or lot number, and dimensions (including leg length, bridge width, and length), as appropriate.

A1.8.1.2 *Test Type*—4-point or combined tension (or compression) and bending.

A1.8.1.3 *Fixation Geometry*—Load point separation distances (4-point bending), load offset distance (combined tension and bending), staple bridge-extension distance, and so forth.

A1.8.1.4 Minimum and maximum cycle loads, test frequency (for example, cycles/s), and forcing function type (sine, ramp, saw tooth, and so forth).

A1.8.1.5 Bending moment, M (N-m).

A1.8.1.6 Load ratio, R, where R = minimum load/maximum load.

A1.8.1.7 *Test Environment*—Ambient air or physiological solution.

A1.8.1.8 Number of cycles at failure or test termination (runout).

A1.8.1.9 Location of fatigue fracture (if applicable).

A1.8.1.10 Reason for test termination, that is, staple failure, fixation failure, runout to specified cycle limit, etc.

A1.9 Precision

A1.9.1 Intralaboratory and interlaboratory reproducibility have not been determined systematically.

A1.10 Rationale (Nonmandatory Information)

A1.10.1 This test method is intended to aid in characterizing the fatigue behavior of metallic bone staples used for the fixation of bone to bone or soft tissue to bone. The data obtained using this test method may be used to compare staple materials, designs, or placements under certain circumstances.

A1.10.2 This test method is intended to simulate potential in vivo staple loading conditions. However, in vitro testing of these devices may not duplicate their in vivo behavior adequately.

A2. TEST METHOD FOR PULL-OUT FIXATION STRENGTH OF METALLIC BONE STAPLES

A2.1 Scope

A2.1.1 This test method covers testing of the hard tissue pull-out fixation strength of metallic staples used in the internal fixation of the musculoskeletal system. This test method may be used with physiologic bone or a synthetic substitute. It may also be used when testing in an aqueous or physiological solution.

A2.1.2 The values stated in SI units are to be regarded as the standard.

A2.1.3 *This standard does not purport to address all of the safety concerns, if any, associated with its use. It is the responsibility of the user of this standard to establish appropriate safety and health practices and determine the applicability of regulatory limitations prior to use.*

A2.2 Summary of Test Method

A2.2.1 A thin, flat, flexible metal or fabric strap is fixed to bone (or a substitute) using a single staple. Tension is applied equally to both ends of the strap in a direction parallel to the staple legs until loss of staple fixation occurs. Tests using this test method may be conducted at ambient conditions or in aqueous or physiological solutions at either room temperature or 37°C.

A2.3 Significance and Use

A2.3.1 This test method is intended to help assess the axial holding strength of various metallic bone staples used to fix either soft or hard tissue to bone. This information may be useful for comparisons of staple materials, designs, or placement under certain circumstances.

A2.3.2 This test method may not be appropriate for all types of bone staple applications. The user is cautioned to consider the appropriateness of the test method in view of the materials being tested and their potential application.

A2.4 Apparatus

A2.4.1 *Testing Machines*, conforming to the requirements of Practices E 4. The loads used for determining strengths shall be within the loading range of the testing machine as defined in Practices E 4.

A2.4.2 *Gripping Devices*:

A2.4.2.1 *Hard Tissue Grips*—Grips designed specifically for secure grasping of bones, bone segments, or bone substitutes with minimal material effects at the staple fixation site during the application of tension to the metal or fabric strap. These grips must allow for variation in bone geometry and permit proper orientation and alignment of the bone (or substitute) during the test.

A2.4.2.2 *Metal or Fabric Strap Grips*—Grips designed for secure grasping of the metal or fabric strap with minimal damage during the application of tension. Typical grips may be actuated mechanically, pneumatically, or hydraulically to compress the strap between two flat grip faces parallel to the line of load application. The grip faces may be smooth or serrated.

A2.4.2.3 *Constant Temperature Bath*—An aqueous bath capable of maintaining the samples and containers at physiologic temperatures, 37 ± 2°C, for the specified testing periods.

A2.5 Test Specimen

A2.5.1 *Staple*—A generally U-shaped metal loop, with at least two legs, that is driven into the surface of bone to either fix or immobilize adjacent pieces of bone or to fasten soft tissue or other material to bone. All test samples shall be representative of the material under evaluation. Samples for comparative tests shall be produced from the same material lot or batch and under the same fabricating conditions, unless noted specifically.

A2.5.2 *Staple Leg*—The parallel or nearly parallel extensions that are intended to penetrate the bone tissue; these may be round, square, or polygonal in cross section, and they may possess serrations or barbs to increase the fixation or purchase strength in the bone.

A2.5.3 *Staple Bridge*—The cross member of the staple connecting the legs; the bridge may be smooth or possess spikes or projections on the underside for the retention of soft tissue or other material.

A2.5.4 *Bone*—Fresh, fresh frozen, or preserved bone with material properties representative of the staple placement site; either cadaveric or animal bone may be suitable.

A2.5.5 *Bone Substitute*—A material with known, consistent properties, similar in strength, density, or rigidity to fresh, fresh frozen, or preserved bone. Substitutes such as natural wood, solid plastics, composites, or rigid foams may be suitable, depending on type, material properties, and configuration.

A2.5.6 *Metal or Fabric Tension Strap*—A thin, flat, flexible, highly conformable metal strip or fabric (woven or braided) that is used to apply a balanced lifting or pull-out force under the staple bridge. The strap should have a width sufficient to support 90 % of the staple bridge and have sufficient tensile properties so that it does not deform plastically or rupture under the applied loads.

A2.5.7 *Aqueous Solution*—Tap water, distilled water, physiological saline, or similar aqueous solutions, used to either maintain hydration of the soft tissue and bone used in the test or bathe or immerse the test specimens fully during the test.

A2.6 Procedure

A2.6.1 Prepare the staple fixation site(s) on the bone (or substitute); this may require predrilling to accommodate the staple legs without damage or fracture of the bone (or substitute).

A2.6.2 Insert and seat the staple in the bone (or substitute) in a standardized, repeatable manner using all appropriate surgical instrumentation specified by the manufacturer. The staple should be positioned over the tension strap, interposing the metal or fabric between the staple bridge and bone surface, leaving equal lengths of the strap on either side of the staple bridge. The strap should also be centered under the staple bridge, and the strap bulk should permit the staple to be seated against the bone fully. The staple bridge should be perpendicular to the long axis of the strap.

NOTE A2.1—In order to either reduce the inherent variability of manual staple insertion techniques or investigate the effects of deliberate variation of insertion parameters, it is permissible to devise special instrumentation in addition to that provided by the manufacturer. These additional instruments may be used to limit staple angulation, control insertion depth, or standardize insertion forces. However, any use of nonstandard surgical instrumentation for staple insertion must be described and reported fully.

A2.6.3 Record the insertion method (manual or mechanical), staple orientation, and position from known landmarks (if applicable).

A2.6.4 Fix the bone (or substitute) in the machine grips and align so that tension can be applied to the strap ends parallel to the staple legs. The bone should be gripped at a sufficient distance from the staple fixation site so that the fixation site is left undamaged and undisturbed (see the schematic of staple pull-out testing in Fig. A2.1).

A2.6.5 Grasp the ends of the strap, place them together, and secure them between the flat grip faces under equal tension (see Fig. A2.1).

NOTE A2.2—It is recommended that self-alignment devices such as universal joints, pin pivots, and so forth be placed in the load train in order to minimize the eccentric loading of either the tension strap or the staple.

A2.6.6 Apply load to the strap at a constant displacement, load, or strain rate.

A2.6.7 Monitor the load-displacement continuously until one of the test termination criteria is reached.

NOTE A2.3—Elastic deformation in the strap may require a separate method of monitoring staple movement during the test.

A2.7 Test Termination

A2.7.1 Testing of the samples shall be terminated when one or more of the following has occurred:

A2.7.1.1 A significant drop in tensile load after peak,

A2.7.1.2 Visible tearing or rupture of the strap (or substitute),

A2.7.1.3 Fracture of the bone (or bone substitute), or

A2.7.1.4 Loosening of the staple(s) or disruption of the staple-bone interface.

A2.8 Report

A2.8.1 Report the following information:

A2.8.1.1 *Staple Description*—Type, size, special features (barbs, spikes, etc.), manufacturer, material, batch or lot

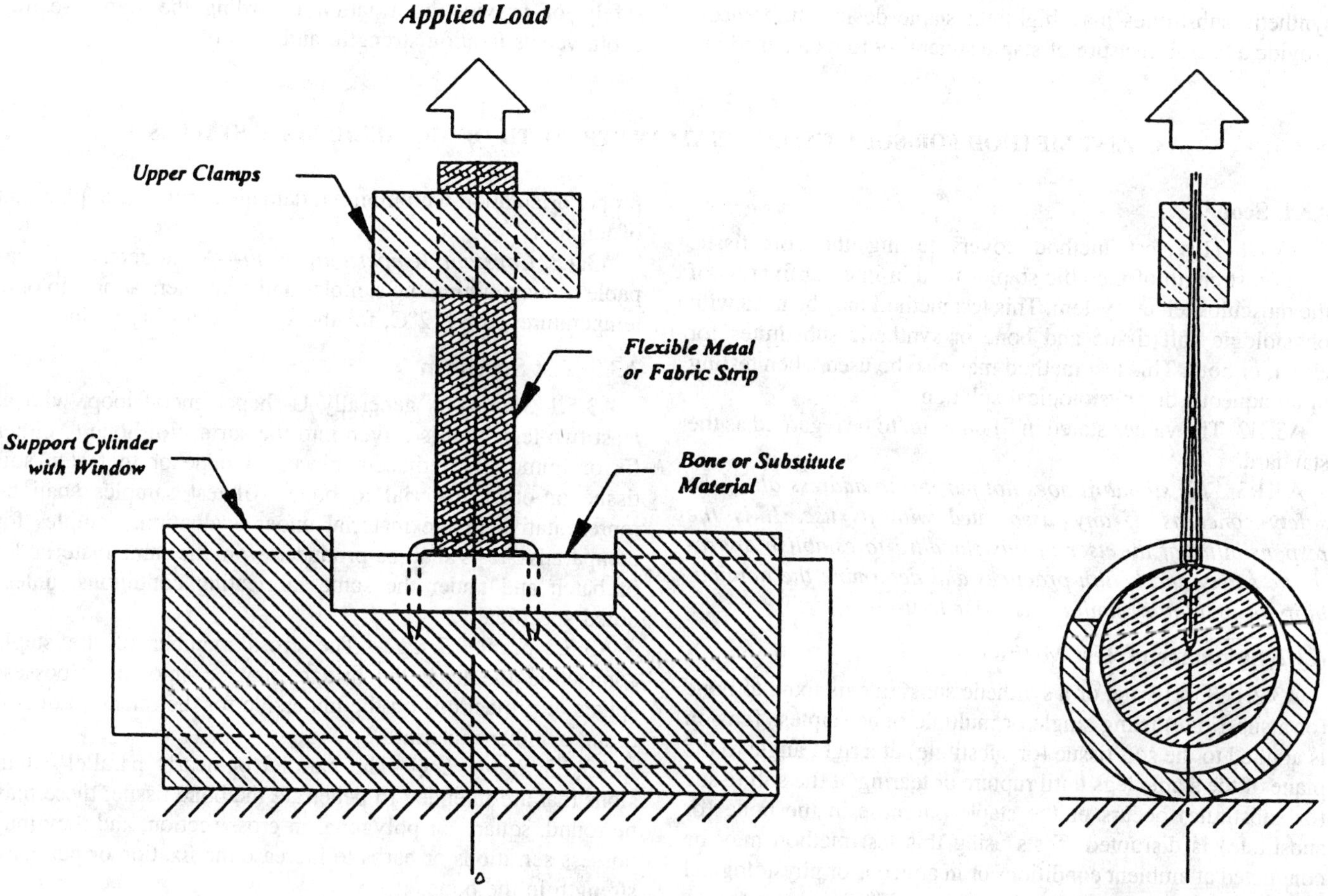

FIG. A2.1 Schematic of Staple Pull-Out Testing

number, and dimensions (including leg length, bridge width, and length), as appropriate.

A2.8.1.2 Fixation site and orientation (if applicable).

A2.8.1.3 Staple placement method, that is, manual or mechanical. Provide detail on the method used to insert the staples in a repeatable way.

A2.8.1.4 Speed of testing, that is, crosshead separation rate, load application rate, etc.

A2.8.2 *Test Materials*:

A2.8.2.1 *Bone*—Species, location, type (cancellous or cortical), cortical thickness, and method of preservation (if applicable).

A2.8.2.2 *Bone Substitute*—Material, thickness, density, tensile or compressive mechanical properties (strength, stiffness, and so forth.), grain direction, and so forth.

A2.8.2.3 *Strap*—Material, construction, tensile strength, and dimensions (width, thickness, and length).

A2.8.2.4 *Aqueous Solution (if used)*—Composition, temperature, and method of application.

A2.8.2.5 *Gage Length*—The minimum distance between the top of the staple bridge and lower end of the grip faces.

A2.8.2.6 Peak pull-out strength (average and standard deviation) or other fixation criteria (for example, load at the onset of defined staple movement), as deemed appropriate.

A2.8.2.7 Failure mode (pull-out of staple, rupture of strap, bone fracture, and so forth).

A2.9 Precision

A2.9.1 Intralaboratory and interlaboratory reproducibility have not been determined systematically.

A2.10 Rationale (Nonmandatory Information)

A2.10.1 This test method is intended to aid in determining the pull-out fixation strength of metallic bone staples used for the fixation of soft tissue to bone. Data obtained using this test method may be used to compare staple materials, design, or placement under certain circumstances.

A2.10.2 It is recognized that the use of substitute materials for bone may be necessary due to the practical limitations of obtaining sufficient suitable biological materials for comparing fixation strengths. Also, the inherent variability in biological materials makes the use of substitute materials preferable in some applications. However, in vitro testing, particularly with substitute materials, may not duplicate the in vivo behavior of implant devices adequately.

A2.10.3 The use of various tissue sources or synthetic substitutes is encouraged since this test method is intended to permit comparisons. Thus, the fixation of thinner, weaker tissue (for example, gracilis tendon) with a particular staple design may result in failure due to tearing or tissue rupture, while the use of the same staple to fix a thicker, stronger tissue (for example, patellar tendon) may produce a loss of fixation at higher loads due to staple movement. Similarly, the use of synthetic substitutes may highlight staple design differences, provide a useful measure of staple suitability to fix a substitute safely, or provide information regarding the staple seating depth versus fixation strength, and so forth.

A3. TEST METHOD FOR SOFT TISSUE FIXATION STRENGTH OF METALLIC BONE STAPLES

A3.1 Scope

A3.1.1 This test method covers testing the soft tissue fixation strength of metallic staples used in internal fixation of the musculoskeletal system. This test method may be used with physiologic soft tissue and bone or synthetic substitutes for either, or both. This test method may also be used when testing in an aqueous or physiological solution.

A3.1.2 The values stated in SI units are to be regarded as the standard.

A3.1.3 *This standard does not purport to address all of the safety concerns, if any, associated with its use. It is the responsibility of the user of this standard to establish appropriate safety and health practices and determine the applicability of regulatory limitations prior to use.*

A3.2 Summary of Test Method

A3.2.1 Soft tissue, or a synthetic substitute, is fixed to bone (or a substitute) using single or multiple bone staples. Tension is applied to the soft tissue (or substitute) at a right angle to the plane of the staple legs until rupture or tearing of the soft tissue (or substitute) occurs or the staple purchase in the bone (or substitute) is disrupted. Tests using this test method may be conducted at ambient conditions or in aqueous or physiological solutions (either at room temperature or 37°C).

A3.3 Significance and Use

A3.3.1 This test method is intended to help assess the tissue holding characteristics of various metallic bone staples used to fix soft tissue (tendons, ligaments, other grafts, etc.) to bone. This information may be useful for comparisons of staple materials, design, or placement under certain circumstances.

A3.3.2 This test method may not be appropriate for all types of bone staple applications. The user is cautioned to consider the appropriateness of the test method in view of the materials being tested and their potential application.

A3.3.3 *Measurement System*—Dimensions, loads, etc. shall be stated in SI units.

A3.4 Apparatus

A3.4.1 *Testing Machines*, conforming to the requirements of Practices E 4. The loads used in determining strengths shall be within the loading range of the testing machine as defined in Practices E 4.

A3.4.2 *Gripping Devices*:

A3.4.2.1 *Hard Tissue Grips*—Grips designed specifically for secure grasping of bones, bone segments, or bone substitutes with minimal material effects at the staple fixation site during the application of tension to the soft tissue (or substitute). These grips must allow for variation in bone geometry and permit proper orientation and alignment of the bone (or substitute) during the test.

A3.4.2.2 *Soft Tissue Grips*—Grips designed specifically for secure grasping of soft tissue or a synthetic substitute in the proper orientation with minimal damage during the application of tension.

A3.4.3 *Constant Temperature Bath*—An aqueous bath capable of maintaining the samples and containers at physiologic temperatures, 37 ± 2°C, for the specified testing periods.

A3.5 Test Specimen

A3.5.1 *Staple*—A generally U-shaped metal loop, with at least two legs, that is driven into the surface of bone to either fix or immobilize adjacent pieces of bone or to fasten soft tissue or other material to bone. All test samples shall be representative of the material under evaluation. Samples for comparative tests shall be produced from the same material lot or batch and under the same fabricating conditions, unless noted specifically.

A3.5.2 *Staple Bridge*—The cross member of the staple connecting the legs; the bridge may be smooth or possess spikes or projections on the underside for the retention of soft tissue or other material.

A3.5.3 *Staple Leg*—The parallel or nearly parallel extensions that are intended to penetrate the bone tissue; these may be round, square, or polygonal in cross section, and they may possess serrations or barbs to increase the fixation or purchase strength in the bone.

A3.5.4 *Bone*—Fresh, fresh frozen, or preserved bone with material properties representative of the staple placement site; either cadaveric or animal bone may be suitable.

A3.5.5 *Bone Substitute*—A material with known, consistent properties, similar in strength, density, or rigidity to fresh, fresh frozen, or preserved bone. Substitutes such as natural wood, solid plastics, composites, or rigid foams may be suitable, depending on type, material properties, and configuration.

A3.5.6 *Soft Tissue*—Fresh, fresh frozen, or preserved soft tissue (ligament, tendon, etc.) representative of tissue affixed with staples; either cadaveric or animal tissue may be suitable.

A3.5.7 *Soft Tissue Substitute*—A material with known, consistent properties, similar in strength, stiffness, or behavior to fresh, fresh frozen, or preserved soft tissue. Suitable substitutes may be flat or round in cross section, consisting of either woven, twisted, or braided natural or synthetic fibers.

A3.5.8 *Aqueous Solution*—Tap water, distilled water, physiological saline, or similar aqueous solutions, used either to maintain hydration of the soft tissue and bone used in the test or to bathe or immerse the test specimens fully during the test.

A3.6 Procedure

A3.6.1 Prepare the staple fixation site(s) on the bone (or substitute); predrilling in accordance with the manufacturer's recommendation may be required to accommodate the staple legs without damage or fracture to the bone.

A3.6.2 Insert and seat the staples in the bone (or substitute) in a standardized, repeatable manner using all appropriate surgical instrumentation specified by the manufacturer. The staples should be centered over the soft tissue or substitute, interposing them between the staple bridge and bone surface. Record the insertion method (manual or mechanical), distance between the staples (if applicable), staple orientation, and position from known landmarks (if applicable).

NOTE A3.1—In order to either reduce the inherent variability of manual staple insertion techniques or investigate the effects of deliberate variation of insertion parameters, it is permissible to devise special instrumentation in addition to that provided by the manufacturer. These additional instruments may be used to limit or fix staple angulation, control insertion depth, or standardize insertion forces, provided that they do not alter the normal insertion mechanics substantially. Any use of nonstandard surgical instrumentation for staple insertion must be described and reported fully.

A3.6.3 Fix the bone (or substitute) in the machine grips and align so that tension can be applied to the soft tissue (or substitute) parallel to its long axis. Grip the bone or soft tissue a sufficient distance from the staple fixation site(s) so they are not damaged or disturbed (see Fig. A3.1).

NOTE A3.2—Failure of the bone or soft tissue (or their substitutes) at the interface with the grips shall not be considered a fixation failure.

A3.6.4 Apply load to the soft tissue (or substitute) at a constant displacement, load, or strain rate.

NOTE A3.3—It is recommended that self-alignment devices such as universal joints, pin pivots, etc. be placed in the load train in order to minimize eccentric loading of either the soft tissue or the staple.

A3.6.5 Monitor the load-displacement continuously until one of the test termination criteria is reached.

A3.7 Test Termination

A3.7.1 Testing of samples shall be terminated when one or more of the following has occurred:

A3.7.1.1 A significant drop in tensile load after peak,

A3.7.1.2 Visible tearing or rupture of the soft tissue (or substitute),

A3.7.1.3 Slippage of the soft tissue from under the staple(s),

A3.7.1.4 Fracture of the bone (or bone substitute), or

A3.7.1.5 Loosening of the staple(s) or disruption of the staple-bone interface.

A3.8 Report

A3.8.1 Report the following information:

A3.8.1.1 Staple type, size, special features (barbs, spikes, and so forth.), manufacturer, material, batch or lot number, and dimensions (including leg length, bridge width, and length), as appropriate,

A3.8.1.2 Staple placement configuration (that is, single, double, belt-buckle, and so forth) and orientation (along length, across width, and so forth),

A3.8.1.3 Staple placement method, that is, manual or mechanical. Provide details on the method used to insert the staples in a repeatable way, and

A3.8.1.4 Speed of testing, that is, crosshead separation rate, load application rate, and so forth.

A3.8.2 *Test Materials*:

A3.8.2.1 *Bone*—Species, location, type (cancellous or cortical), cortical thickness, and method of preservation (if applicable).

A3.8.2.2 *Bone Substitute*—Material, thickness, density, tensile or compressive mechanical properties (strength, stiffness, and so forth), grain direction, and so forth.

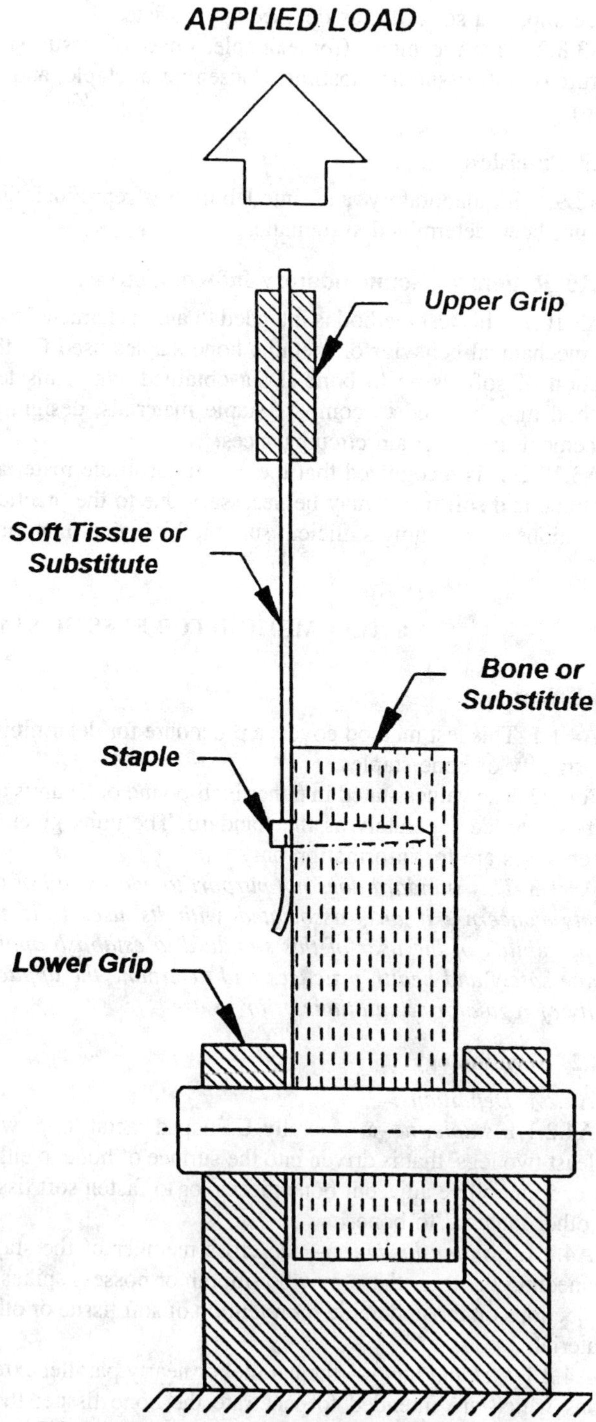

FIG. A3.1 Schematic of Tissue Fixation Strength Test

A3.8.2.3 *Soft Tissue*—Species, tissue type (ligament, tendon, and so forth), dimensions (thickness, width, and so forth), and method of preservation (if applicable).

A3.8.2.4 *Soft Tissue Substitute*—Material, geometry (width, thickness, diameter, and so forth), tensile strength and stiffness, and construction (braided, woven, and so forth).

A3.8.2.5 *Aqueous Solution*—Composition, temperature, and method of application.

A3.8.2.6 Peak fixation strengths (average and standard deviation) or other fixation criteria (peak load at the onset of tissue slip, and so forth), as deemed appropriate.

A3.8.2.7 Failure mode (for example, onset of tissue slip, rupture of soft tissue or substitute, loosening of staple, and so forth).

A3.9 Precision

A3.9.1 Intralaboratory and interlaboratory reproducibility has not been determined systematically.

A3.10 Rationale (Nonmandatory Information)

A3.10.1 This test method is intended to aid in characterizing the mechanical behavior of metallic bone staples used for the fixation of soft tissue to bone. Data obtained using this test method may be used to compare staple materials, design, or placement under certain circumstances.

A3.10.2 It is recognized that the use of substitute materials for bone and soft tissue may be necessary due to the practical limitations of obtaining sufficient suitable biological materials for comparing fixation strengths. Also, the inherent variability in biological materials makes the use of substitute materials preferable in some applications. However, in vitro testing, particularly with substitute materials, may not duplicate the in vivo behavior of implant devices adequately.

A3.10.3 The use of various tissue sources or synthetic substitutes is encouraged since this test method is intended to permit comparisons. Thus, the fixation of thinner, weaker tissue (for example, gracilis tendon) with a particular staple design may result in failure due to tearing or tissue rupture, while the use of the same staple to fix a thicker, stronger tissue (for example, patellar tendon) may produce a loss of fixation at higher loads due to staple movement. Similarly, the use of synthetic substitutes may highlight staple design differences, provide a useful measure of staple suitability to fix a substitute safely, or provide information regarding the staple seating depth versus fixation strength, etc.

A4. TEST METHOD FOR ELASTIC STATIC BENDING OF METALLIC BONE STAPLES[5]

A4.1 Scope

A4.1.1 This test method covers a procedure for determining the rigidity of bone staples.

A4.1.2 The values stated in either inch-pound or SI units are to be regarded separately as the standard. The units given in parentheses are for information only.

A4.1.3 *This standard does not purport to address all of the safety concerns, if any, associated with its use. It is the responsibility of the user of this standard to establish appropriate safety and health practices and determine the applicability of regulatory limitations prior to use.*

A4.2. Terminology

A4.2.1 *Definitions:*

A4.2.1.1 *staple, n*—a generally U-shaped metal loop, with at least two legs, that is driven into the surface of bone to either fix or immobilize adjacent bone pieces, or to fasten soft tissue or other material to bone.

A4.2.1.2 *staple bridge, n*—the cross member of the staple connecting the legs; these may be smooth or possess spikes or projections on the underside for retention of soft tissue or other material.

A4.2.1.3 *staple leg, n*—the parallel or nearly parallel extensions which are intended to penetrate the bone tissue; these may be round, square or polygonal in cross section, and may possess serrations or barbs to increase the fixation or purchase strength in the bone.

A4.3 Summary of Test Method

A4.3.1 This test method is based on a paper[5] that examined the bending rigidity of bone staples. The authors identified the initial slope of the bending curve as a parameter which could distinguish the staple stiffness from one staple to another. This parameter may be determined by placing each staple leg in a beam-like holder (see Fig. A4.1) and then bending the system in a four-point bending load apparatus (see Fig. A4.2). The applied force and displacement in the direction of the applied load will produce a bending curve from which the initial slope may be determined.

A4.4 Significance and Use

A4.4.1 This test method is intended to help assess the structural stiffness or rigidity of metallic bone staples for use in fixating or immobilizing bone or in fastening soft tissue or other material to bone. Under some circumstances, the test method may be of use in maintaining the batch uniformity of a test lot.

A4.5 Apparatus

A4.5.1 *Testing Apparatus*—Figs. A4.1 and A4.2 show the test apparatus. Fig. A4.1 is a holder designed to hold one of the

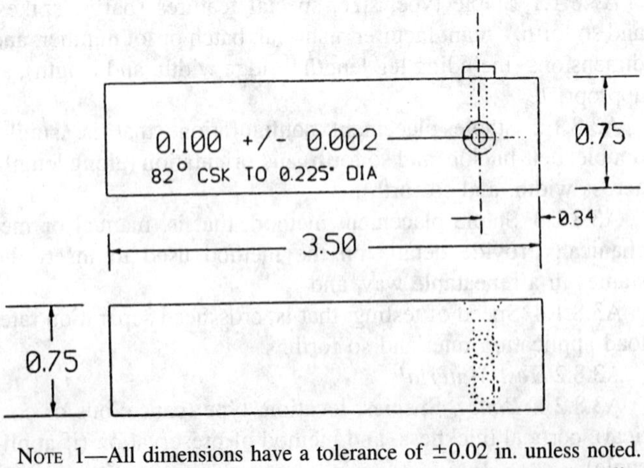

NOTE 1—All dimensions have a tolerance of ±0.02 in. unless noted.

NOTE 2—Extension block as shown is for a 3/32 in. staple only; adjust dimensions accordingly.

FIG. A4.1 Staple Extension Block

[5] Liberace, R., and Zvi L., "Mechanical Testing of Stainless Steel Bone Staples", *Journal of Testing and Evaluation*, Vol 20, No. 3, May 1992, pp. 217-224.

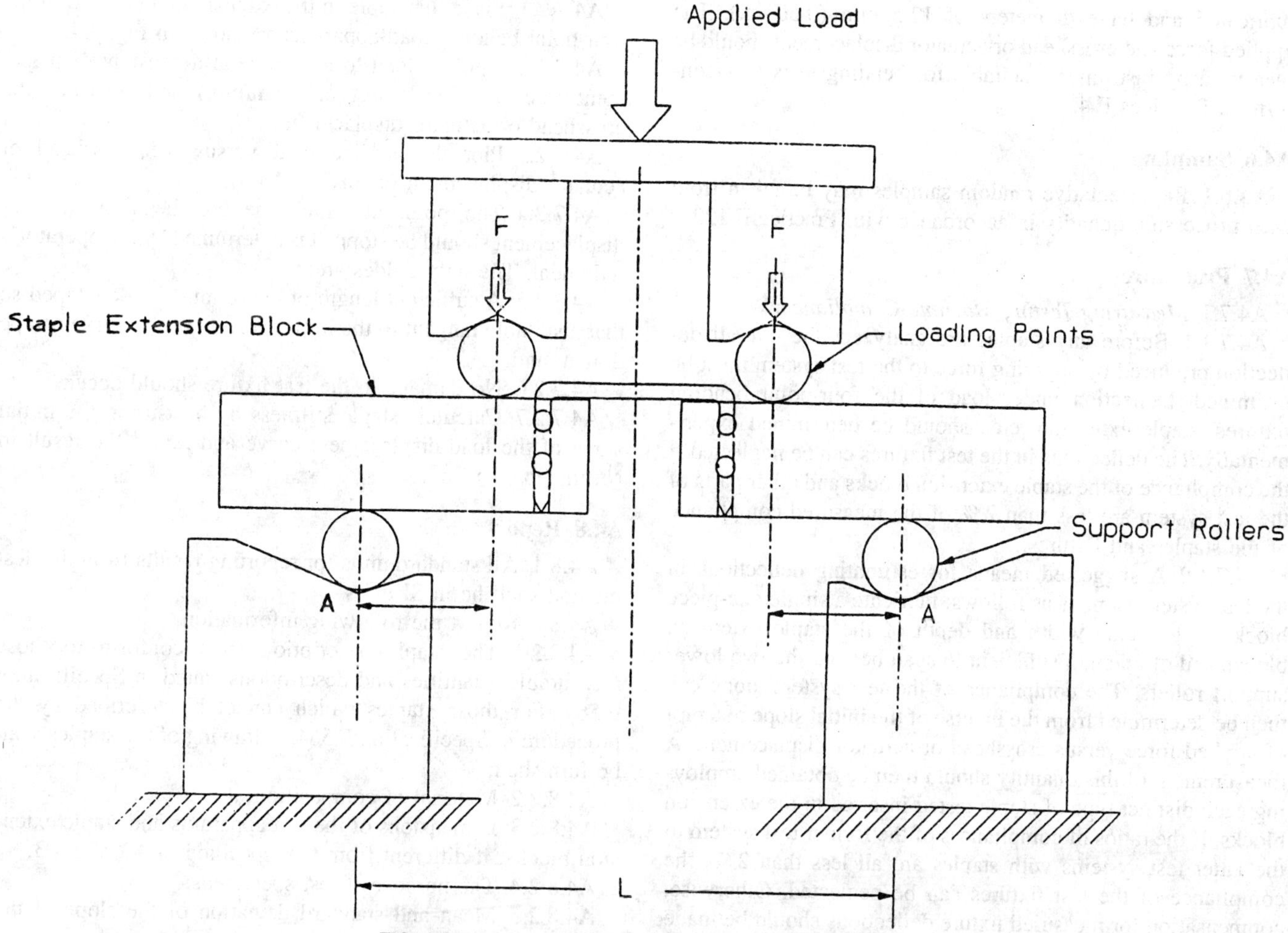

FIG. A4.2 Staple in Four-Point Bending Load Apparatus

staple legs as the entire assembly is placed in a four-point bending load apparatus (see Fig. A4.2). The design in this figure is only a suggested type for a cylindrical wire type staple.

A4.5.2 *Staple Extension Blocks*:

A4.5.2.1 The staple extension blocks shown in Fig. A4.1 can be constructed of aluminum, steel, iron or any other metallic material. Each must be long enough to fit over the support roller bearings and be much stiffer than the staple. The dimensions shown in Fig. A4.1 are suitable, but not mandatory. Fig. A4.1 shows a system which can accommodate a 3⁄32 in. staple. When the staples are placed in the holders, each leg is held in place by two set screws on the side of the holder. When the staple is fully inserted into the holder, the underside of the staple bridge should contact the top surface of the staple extension block. For those staples that have stiffening webs, additional countersinking of the holding holes or the cutting of notches in the staple extension block may be necessary so that the bridge of the staple will fit in the extension blocks as shown in Fig. A4.2.

A4.5.2.2 Other holding systems may be used. However, each system should firmly fasten the legs of the staple so that bending occurs only at the bends in the staple and not in the staple legs. The system shown uses two set screws for this purpose. For other shaped staples, triangular, square, etc., special holding blocks should be developed to custom fit the legs of the staples so that forces holding the staple legs are uniformly spread along the legs. For these staples an alternative holding procedure is to drill cylindrical holes large enough to accommodate the staple legs and then firmly cement the staple in place by using epoxy or some other agent. This procedure will eliminate the use of set screws that might produce uneven stresses upon the staple legs.

A4.5.3 *Four-Point Bending Fixture*:

A4.5.3.1 Fig. A4.2 shows the holders and a test staple placed in a four-point bending load apparatus. This apparatus is similar to that used in testing bone plates (see Test Method F 382):

L = the horizontal length between the two lower rollers' centers, and

A = the horizontal distance between upper and lower rollers' centers.

A4.5.3.2 The lower supports consist of two rollers, L = 120 mm (4.7 in.) apart and the upper loading apparatus has rollers placed 40 mm (1.57 in.) apart, which are one-third the distance from the lower support, so that all loads shall be equally supported by the rollers. Thus, the horizontal distance, A, between the centers of the upper and lower rollers will also be 40 mm (1.57 in.). The direction of the applied load shall be restricted to that shown in Fig. A4.2. All rollers should be well lubricated and have diameters of 12.5 mm (0.50 in.). The applied force and crosshead or actuator displacement should be measured by instruments suitable for bending tests that conform to Practices E 4.

A4.6 Sampling

A4.6.1 Representative random samples may be taken from each processing quantity in accordance with Practice E 122.

A4.7 Procedure

A4.7.1 *Measuring Testing Machine Compliance*:

A4.7.1.1 Before any staples are analyzed, the overall deflection produced by applying force to the test system must be examined. Deflection under load of the four-point bending fixtures, staple extension, etc., should be determined experimentally. The deflections in the test fixtures can be neglected if the compliance of the staple extension blocks and other parts of the test system are less than 2 % of the measured compliance of the staples and fixtures.

A4.7.1.2 A suggested means for estimating deflections in the test system alone is as follows: fabricate a single one-piece block of the same width and depth of the staple extension blocks and of a length sufficient to span beyond the two lower support rollers. The compliance of the test system alone can then be determined from the inverse of the initial slope of a plot of applied force versus crosshead or actuator displacement. A measurement of this quantity should then be obtained employing each distinct type of staple tested inserted in the extension blocks. If the ratios of compliances of the former test system to the latter test systems with staples are all less than 2 %, the compliance of the test fixtures can be neglected. Otherwise, compensation for measured fixture deflections should be made in the staple bending curves, or the staple extension blocks should be refabricated from a stiffer grade or type of metal.

A4.7.2 *Testing Procedures*:

A4.7.2.1 Place the staple in the extension blocks and in the four-point bending load apparatus as shown in Fig. A4.2.

A4.7.2.2 Apply a load to the staple at a constant displacement rate of 1 in./min (25.4 mm/min) and measure the crosshead or actuator displacement.

A4.7.2.3 Plot the applied load versus the crosshead or actuator displacement (as in Fig. A4.3).

A4.7.2.4 The point at which the crosshead or actuator displacement should be stopped is determined by the operator's judgment. The only guides are:

A4.7.2.5 A sufficient length of curve must be developed so that a suitable tangent to the initial portion of the curve can be drawn; and

A4.7.2.6 No damage to the test fixture should occur.

A4.7.2.7 Calculate staple stiffness by measuring the initial slope of the load-displacement curve and report the result in N/mm (lb_f/in.).

A4.8 Report

A4.8.1 All standard units for reporting results from this test method shall be in SI units.

A4.8.2 Report the following information:

A4.8.2.1 The staple description shall conform to those measurable quantities and descriptions stated in Specification F 564. For those staples which cannot be described by the procedure in Specification F 564, a drawing of the staples shall be furnished;

A4.8.2.2 Material of composition;

A4.8.2.3 Dimensions of the test apparatus and staple extension blocks, if different from that specified in 4.2 and 4.3;

A4.8.2.4 The number of test specimens;

A4.8.2.5 Mean and standard deviation of the slope of the bending curve; and

A4.8.2.6 Manufacturer, part number, and lot number if available.

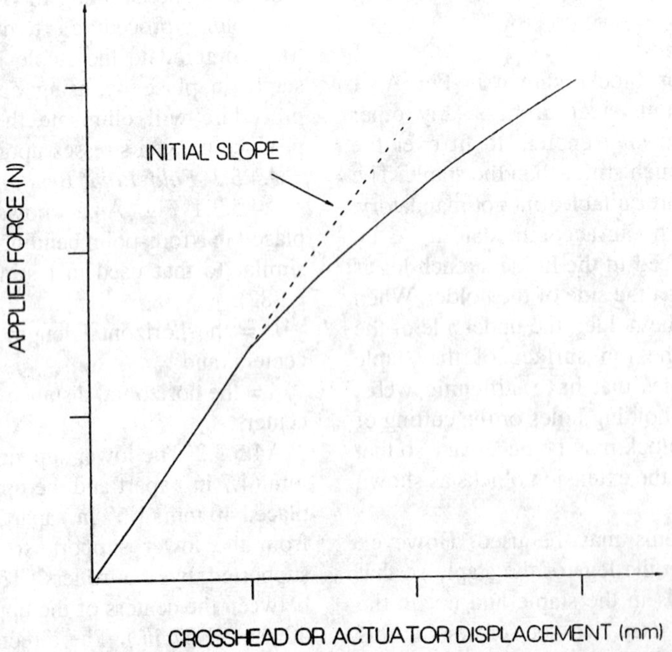

FIG. A4.3 Typical Load-Deflection Curve for Bone Staple in Four-Point Bending

A4.9 Precision and Bias

A4.9.1 Data establishing the precision and bias to be expected from this test method have not yet been obtained.

A4.10 Rationale (Nonmandatory Information)

A4.10.1 This test method provides a procedure that can measure the structural stiffness or rigidity of the staple. This property is an indication to the user of the relative stiffness of the staple from which the user can compare one staple with another.

Designation: F 565 – 00

Standard Practice for Care and Handling of Orthopedic Implants and Instruments[1]

This standard is issued under the fixed designation F 565; the number immediately following the designation indicates the year of original adoption or, in the case of revision, the year of last revision. A number in parentheses indicates the year of last reapproval. A superscript epsilon (ε) indicates an editorial change since the last revision or reapproval.

1. Scope

1.1 This practice covers recommended procedures for the handling of orthopedic implants and instruments.

1.2 Hospital receiving personnel, central supply personnel, operating room personnel, surgeons, and occasionally other individuals will handle orthopedic implants and instruments. All personnel should be informed of recommended care and handling procedures to prevent damage of orthopedic implants and instruments.

1.3 This practice does not cover producer level handling and packaging procedures.

1.4 *This standard does not purport to address all of the safety concerns, if any, associated with its use. It is the responsibility of the user of this standard to establish appropriate safety and health practices and determine the applicability of regulatory limitations prior to use.*

2. Terminology

2.1 *Definitions of Terms Specific to This Standard:*

2.1.1 *orthopedic implant*—a device introduced by surgically penetrating the skin or mucosa of the body with the intention that it remain within or attached to the skeleton within the body following the surgery. This device is referred to in this practice as an "implant."

2.1.2 *orthopedic instrument*—any cooperative device used during surgical procedures involving the implantation of orthopedic implants. This device is referred to in this practice as an "instrument."

3. Receiving Implants and Instruments

3.1 *Receipt*:

3.1.1 Many implants are wrapped in special sterilizable or pre-sterilized packages, envelopes, or other containers. These wrappings should not be removed by the receiving personnel.

3.1.2 Carefully unwrap and handle non-sterilized implants and instruments upon receipt to avoid scratching, marking, or abrasion by other implants, instruments, unpacking tools, or by dropping or otherwise endangering the surface finish or configuration.

3.2 *Transport*— Perform transport in a manner to preclude any damage or alteration to the received condition of the implant or instrument.

3.3 *Storage*:

3.3.1 Store implants or instruments prior to use in such a manner as to maintain the device's surface finish or configuration, or both.

3.3.2 Many implants are identified by a serial or lot number, or both, on the package label, package insert, or surface of the device. Record these control numbers and retain for transfer to patient records, to facilitate inventory, stock rotation, medical device reporting, and possible traceability to the manufacturer.

3.3.3 *Stock Rotation*— The principle of first in, first out, is recommended.

3.3.4 Store implants in the operating room in such a manner as to isolate and protect the implant's surface, sterility, and configuration. Keep implants made of different metals separated.

3.3.5 Store the implants and instruments in the operating room in such a manner as to isolate the instruments from the implants.

4. Handling

4.1 *Mixing Metals*— Maintain orthopedic implants and instruments of different metals separately to avoid the possibility of mixing during surgery.

4.2 *Cleaning and Sterilization*:

4.2.1 Prior to initial sterilization and promptly following each surgical procedure, thoroughly and carefully clean all instruments and implants. Ultrasonic cleaners, mechanized washers, or hand scrubbing are suitable methods, if carefully done. The method employed should be utilized to prevent impact, scratching, bending, or surface contact with any materials that might affect the implant or instrument surface or configuration.

4.2.2 Closely follow the manufacturer's recommendations on cleaning. In hand scrubbing, use soft brushes and avoid harsh chemicals or harsh cleaning solutions.

4.2.3 After cleaning, rinse the orthopedic implants and instruments completely free of all residuals, soap, detergent, or cleaning solutions. Following rinsing, dry them thoroughly. Devote special attention to hinges, pivots, box locks, and other recesses since these are points that entrap both chemicals and rinse water.

---

[1] This practice is under the jurisdiction of ASTM Committee F04 on Medical and Surgical Materials and Devices, and is the direct responsibility of Subcommittee F04.21 on Osteosynthesis.

Current edition approved Nov. 10, 2000. Published January 2001. Originally published as F 565 – 78. Last previous edition F 565 – 85 (1996).

4.2.4 Lubricate instruments that require lubrication immediately after drying. Follow the recommendations of the manufacturers of such instruments explicitly as to method, type, and amount of lubricant. Insufficient or excessive lubrication can be nearly as disastrous as no lubrication.

4.2.5 Carry out sterilization by steam autoclaving or other methods in a manner that protects the integrity of the implants and instruments.

4.2.6 Sterilize implants and instruments of polymeric materials in accordance with methods recommended by the manufacturer.

4.2.7 Do not sterilize implants in contact with instruments or implants of other materials. Metallic oxide could transfer to the implant, initiating an unacceptable conditioning.

4.2.8 Do not expose instrumental cutting edges and teeth to the hazard of dulling.

4.3 *Appearance*— Dispose of orthopedic implants that exhibit surface or configuration damage.

4.4 *Contouring and Modifying Implants and Instruments*:

4.4.1 Contouring or clamping of orthopedic implants, when necessary, shall be performed by the surgeon in a manner that will least damage the implant.

4.4.2 It is recommended that metallic orthopedic implants should not be sharply bent, re-bent, angulated at a screw hole, notched, or scratched.

4.4.3 Reshaping or contouring may cause complete loss of performance for instruments. It is recommended that orthopedic instruments be handled with care to prevent costly reworking or destruction. If modifications are necessary, the instrument should not be sharply bent, re-bent, or angulated.

4.4.4 Orthopedic instruments in general have a long service life, but mishandling or inadequate protection can quickly diminish the instrument's life expectancy.

4.4.5 Dispose of instruments whose performance capabilities have been jeopardized by mishandling or improper care.

5. Reuse

5.1 Avoid the reimplantation of previously implanted orthopedic implants.

5.2 Trial fitting of an orthopedic implant in a patient, followed by proper cleaning and sterilization if not immediately implanted in the same patient, shall not be considered as reimplantation.

6. Keywords

6.1 handling of implants; instruments; material handling

Designation: F 601 – 98

Standard Practice for Fluorescent Penetrant Inspection of Metallic Surgical Implants[1]

This standard is issued under the fixed designation F 601; the number immediately following the designation indicates the year of original adoption or, in the case of revision, the year of last revision. A number in parentheses indicates the year of last reapproval. A superscript epsilon (ε) indicates an editorial change since the last revision or reapproval.

1. Scope

1.1 This practice is intended as a guide for fluorescent penetrant inspection of metallic surgical implants.

1.2 *This standard does not purport to address all of the safety concerns, if any, associated with its use. It is the responsibility of the user of this standard to establish appropriate safety and health practices and determine the applicability of regulatory limitations prior to use.*

2. Referenced Documents

2.1 *ASTM Standards:*

D 95 Test Method for Water in Petroleum Products and Bituminous Materials by Distillation[2]

E 165 Test Method for Liquid Penetrant Examination[3]

E 433 Reference Photographs for Liquid Penetrant Inspection[3]

2.2 *ASNT Recommended Practice:*[4]

Recommended Practice No. SNT-TC-1A

2.3 *Military Standard:*[5]

MIL-I-25135 Inspection Material, Penetrant

3. Significance and Use

3.1 This practice is intended to confirm the method of obtaining and evaluating the fluorescent penetrant indications on metallic surgical implants.

3.2 The product acceptance and rejection criteria will be as agreed upon between the purchaser and the supplier.

4. Fluorescent Penetrant Method

4.1 Perform fluorescent penetrant inspection of metallic surgical implants in accordance with Practice E 165, Method A.

4.2 The penetrant system used shall conform to a minimum of Sensitivity Level 3, in accordance with the latest revision of MIL-I-25135.

4.3 All penetrant materials shall be compatible with each other.

5. Penetrant Method Materials Control

5.1 The penetrant method materials deteriorate in usefulness through contamination and age. The following controls should be used to evaluate the materials' usefulness unless the supplier's requirements are more stringent:

5.1.1 *Penetrants*:

5.1.1.1 *Water Content*—Where there is a possibility of water contamination to penetrant materials, the water content should be determined by Test Method D 95. The water content shall not exceed 10 %. The frequency of testing shall be at least once every 30 days for open containers.

5.1.1.2 *Fluorescent Brightness*—Fluorescent brightness should be determined at least once every 30 days or before use by comparison of samples of the working penetrant to a sample of new penetrant under black light. No visible difference shall be allowed.

5.1.2 *Developer*:

5.1.2.1 *Dry*—The developer should be dry and fluffy. Developers showing evidence of fluorescence when compared to new developer shall not be used.

5.1.2.2 *Wet*—A method should be employed to assure adequate suspension of the wet developer prior to use. The specific gravity of the developer should be from 1.018 to 1.034. This method does not apply to nonaqueous solvent developer due to the volatile nature of the product.

5.1.3 *Black Lights*—Black lights used for fluorescent penetrant inspection should be checked for black light output (with a filter) for a minimum of 800 μW/cm^2 at a distance of 381 mm (15 in.) from the lamp face. This measurement could be determined by using a calibrated black light meter. The

---

[1] This practice is under the jurisdiction of ASTM Committee F-4 on Medical and Surgical Materials and Devices and is the direct responsibility of Subcommittee F04.12 on Metallurgical Materials.

Current edition approved October 10, 1998. Published March 1999. Originally published as F 601 – 78. Last previous edition F 601 – 92.

[2] *Annual Book of ASTM Standards*, Vol 05.01.

[3] *Annual Book of ASTM Standards*, Vol 03.03.

[4] Available from American Society for Non-Destructive Testing, 3200 Riverside Dr., Columbus, OH 43221.

[5] Available form Standardization Documents Order Desk, Bldg. 4 Section D, 700 Robbins Ave., Philadelphia, PA 19111–5094, Attn: NPODS.

frequency of testing shall be at least once every 7 days or before use.

6. Evaluation

6.1 A general method of evaluating fluorescent penetrant indications is encompassed in reference photographs E 433.

7. Personnel Certification

7.1 The personnel performing fluorescent penetrant inspection under this practice shall be certified in accordance with ASNT Recommended Practice No. SNT-TC-1A or recognized national equivalent.

8. Keywords

8.1 fluorescent; penetrant inspection; testing methods; surgical implants

APPENDIX

(Nonmandatory Information)

X1. RATIONALE

X1.1 A method of nondestructive inspection, known as fluorescent penetrant inspection, is employed as a quality control tool for surgical devices. This method of inspection is not only used by the manufacturers, but by their suppliers and also independent testing laboratories. This method has been used for over twenty years for the nondestructive examination of surgical implants and devices. Fluorescent penetrant inspection provides a sensitive method of detecting surface imperfections such as scratches, cracks, surface porosity, and welding joint imperfections.

X1.2 Fluorescent penetrant inspection uses a specially formulated penetrating oil, manufactured by many sources, which also has a fluorescent dye as part of its formula. The method of inspection allows for the fluorescent penetrating oil to enter surface discontinuities; a subsequent process removes all other surface remnants of the penetrating oil, thus leaving the fluorescent material only in surface discontinuities. A final "developer" is applied to bring out the penetrating oil from the discontinuities. Then an ultra violet light (black light) is used to inspect the part for the presence of the fluorescent material. This method allows for highly sensitive examination of small discontinuities that normally would not be visible by unaided visual inspection.

X1.3 Due to a variety of specifications being applied to the inspection of surgical implants and devices, a task force was formed under Committee F-4 to standardize methods for fluorescent penetrant inspection of metallic surgical implants; the result was Practice F 601. The task force, comprised of a large cross section of manufacturers, testing experts, government representatives, and other interested parties, developed a universally accepted practice for surgical implants and devices.

X1.4 This is a *standard practice* and is only intended to confirm the standardized method of obtaining and evaluating the fluorescent penetrant indications, as well as the evaluation of the materials used in the testing method. This practice is not intended to set acceptance standards; this type of specification would be extremely difficult due to such variables as surface finish (that is, mechanically polished, vapor blasted, electro polished, etc.); manufacturing method (that is, wrought, forged, cast, etc.); as well as other variables in surface texture.

Designation: F 602 – 98a

Standard Criteria for Implantable Thermoset Epoxy Plastics[1]

This standard is issued under the fixed designation F 602; the number immediately following the designation indicates the year of original adoption or, in the case of revision, the year of last revision. A number in parentheses indicates the year of last reapproval. A superscript epsilon (ε) indicates an editorial change since the last revision or reapproval.

1. Scope

1.1 These criteria cover thermoset plastics based on diglycidyl ethers of bisphenol A (DGEBPA) and appropriate curing agents or catalysts as opposed to thermoplastics based on epoxy structures.

1.2 These criteria are generic and are intended to provide definitions and a standard description of epoxy plastics used in implantable devices. It is also intended to serve as a standard guide for the preparation of more specific documents with values and limits covering specific end uses.

1.3 Compliance with these criteria shall not be construed as an endorsement of implantability. The biocompatibility of epoxy plastics as a class has not been established. Epoxy plastic is a generic term relating to the class of polymers formed from epoxy resins, certain curing agents or catalysts, and various additives. Since many compositions and formulations fall under this class, it is essential that the formulator or fabricator ensure biocompatibility of the specific composition or formulation in its intended end use. Since these criteria provide guidance for the preparation of more specific documents covering specific end uses, these documents will provide bases for standardized evaluation of biocompatibility appropriate for a specific end use.

1.4 Each of the properties listed shall be considered in selecting materials for specific end uses. A list of selected properties with limiting values assigned is suggested for separate product specifications.

1.5 All of the properties and test methods listed may not be pertinent in any specific situation, nor may all of the tests outlined be required.

1.6 These criteria are limited to functionally or fully cured epoxy plastics. Uncured or incompletely cured formulations are specifically excluded.

1.7 The epoxy plastics covered by this standard are those to be evaluated for use in implantable biomedical devices. The term implantable is herein considered to include devices used in vivo for time periods in excess of 30 days.

1.8 *This standard does not purport to address all of the safety concerns, if any, associated with its use. It is the responsibility of the user of this standard to establish appropriate safety and health practices and determine the applicability of regulatory limitations prior to use.*

2. Referenced Documents

2.1 *ASTM Standards:*

D 149 Test Method for Dielectric Breakdown Voltage and Dielectric Strength of Solid Electrical Insulating Materials at Commercial Power Frequencies[2]

D 150 Test Methods for A-C Loss Characteristics and Permittivity (Dielectric Constant) of Solid Electrical Insulating Materials[2]

D 257 Test Methods for D-C Resistance or Conductance of Insulating Materials[2]

D 570 Test Method for Water Absorption of Plastics[3]

D 621 Test Methods for Deformation of Plastics Under Load[3]

D 638 Test Method for Tensile Properties of Plastics[3]

D 785 Test Method for Rockwell Hardness of Plastics and Electrical Insulating Materials[3]

D 792 Test Methods for Specific Gravity (Relative Density) and Density of Plastics by Displacement[3]

D 883 Terminology Relating to Plastics[3]

D 952 Test Method for Bond or Cohesive Strength of Sheet Plastics and Electrical Insulating Materials[3]

D 1042 Test Method for Linear Dimensional Changes of Plastics[3]

D 1434 Test Method for Determining Gas Permeability Characteristics of Plastic Film and Sheeting[4]

D 1763 Specification for Epoxy Resins[3]

D 2393 Test Method for Viscosity of Epoxy Resins and Related Components[5]

D 2471 Test Method for Gel Time and Peak Exothermic Temperature of Reacting Thermosetting Resins[5]

D 2562 Practice for Classifying Visual Defects in Parts Molded from Reinforced Thermosetting Plastics[5]

D 2566 Test Method for Linear Shrinkage of Cured Thermosetting Casting Resins During Cure[5]

D 2734 Test Method for Void Content of Reinforced Plastics[5]

D 2990 Test Method for Tensile, Compressive, and Flexural Creep and Creep Rupture of Plastics[5]

---

[1] These criteria are under the jurisdiction of ASTM Committee F-4 on Medical and Surgical Materials and Devices and are the direct responsibility of Subcommittee F04.11 on Polymeric Materials.

Current edition approved October 10, 1998. Published December 1998. Originally published as F 602 – 78. Last previous edition F 602 – 98.

[2] *Annual Book of ASTM Standards*, Vol 10.01.

[3] *Annual Book of ASTM Standards*, Vol 08.01.

[4] *Annual Book of ASTM Standards*, Vol 15.09.

[5] *Annual Book of ASTM Standards*, Vol 08.02.

D 3013 Specification for Epoxy Molding Compounds[5]

D 3137 Test Method for Rubber Property—Hydrolytic Stability[6]

E 96 Test Methods for Water Vapor Transmission of Materials[7]

F 74 Practice for Determining Hydrolytic Stability of Plastic Encapsulants for Electronic Devices[8]

F 619 Practice for Extraction of Medical Plastics[9]

F 748 Practice for Selecting Generic Biological Test Methods for Materials and Devices[9]

2.2 *AAMI Standard:*

EOS-D 10/75 Standard for Ethylene Oxide Sterilization[10]

3. Terminology

3.1 *Definitions:*

3.1.1 *accelerator*—an additive used to increase the rate of cure. An accelerator may also be a catalyst, or it may actually change composition and, therefore, not qualify as a catalyst.

3.1.2 *additive*—a chemical added to epoxy resins or hardeners to modify the handling characteristics or cured properties, or both, of the epoxy-hardener combination.

3.1.2.1 *diluent*—a chemical used in admixture to modify or enhance the properties of either or both the uncured or cured formulations. A primary use is to reduce the viscosity of the mixed system although other properties such as exotherm rate, stiffness, moisture absorption, etc., may be modified or enhanced also.

3.1.2.1.1 *nonreactive diluent*—a diluent not containing chemically reactive functional groups.

3.1.2.1.2 *reactive diluent*—a diluent that reacts chemically with the epoxy resin or hardener, or both, during cure.

3.1.2.2 *filler*—a relatively inert solid particulate material added to an epoxy formulation to modify its strength, permanence, working properties, or other qualities, or to lower costs.

3.1.3 *curing agent or hardener*—a compound normally used in a predetermined concentration to react chemically (copolymerize) by means of several different mechanisms (for example, condensation or addition polymerization) with or without heat or pressure in order to change its form from a liquid or fusible, friable, soluble solid to an infusible, insoluble solid having useful and desirable application or end-use properties.

3.1.3.1 *initiator*—an additive used to cause a thermosetting resin to react with itself (polymerize). Usually, these additives—used in relatively very small amounts—initiate homo-polymerization of the epoxy resin resulting in ether linkages.

NOTE 1—The term "catalyst" is frequently misused to denote any material added to a resin to cause a reaction to occur. This usage should be discouraged. The Society of Plastics Industries defines a catalyst as "a compound which alters the speed of a reaction without changing its original composition."

3.1.4 *epoxy*—oxirane ring structures.

O
R—CH—CH_2

3.1.4.1 *epoxy plastic*—thermoplastic or thermosetting plastics containing ether or hydroxyalkyl repeating units or both, resulting from the ring-opening reactions of lower molecular weight polyfunctional oxirane resins or compounds, with catalysts or with various polyfunctional acidic or basic coreactants.

3.1.4.2 *epoxy resin*—generally, any resin (liquid or solid) with a chemical structure at least difunctional in oxirane. Specifically for this standard, the diglycidyl ethers of bisphenol A or the equivalent. These compounds are defined as Grade 1 in Specification D 1763.

3.1.5 *Terms Relating to Cure:*

3.1.5.1 *cure, v*—to change the properties of a polymeric system into a final, more stable, usable condition by the use of heat, radiation, or reaction with chemical additives.

3.1.5.2 *cure cycle*—the schedule of time periods at specified conditions to which a reacting thermosetting material is subjected to reach a specified property level.

3.1.5.3 *cure time*—the interval of time from the start of reaction to the time at which specified properties of the reacting thermosetting composition are reached. For materials that react under the conditions of mixing, the start of reaction is the time of initial exposure to the conditions necessary for reaction to occur.

3.1.5.4 *functionally cured*—the term used to denote an epoxy plastic that has attained sufficient cure to achieve stable properties.

3.1.5.5 *fully cured*—the term used to denote total disappearance of epoxy groups as detected by infrared spectroscopy, or other equally sensitive physicochemical methods.

3.1.5.6 *one-component system*—a formulation based on an epoxy resin preblended with a heat, moisture, or otherwise activated curing agent or catalyst. The mixture is storable but cures under the appropriate activation conditions.

3.1.5.7 *postcure*—the additional and separate curing operations to which a "hardened" thermosetting plastic composition is subjected in order to enhance one or more properties. Also used to ensure stabilization of physical properties under use conditions.

3.1.5.8 *two-component system*—a formulation based on an epoxy resin to which a curing agent or catalyst is added just prior to use.

4. Chemical Composition

4.1 *Epoxy Resins*—Oxirane-terminated reaction products of epichlorohydrin and bisphenol A (DGEBPA) or the equivalent.

4.2 *Reactive Diluents*—The following are examples of compounds that may be included as reactive diluents:

4.2.1 Butyl glycidyl ether (BGE).

4.2.2 Phenyl glycidyl ether (PGE).

4.3 *Nonreactive Diluents*—The following are examples of compounds that may be included as nonreactive diluents:

4.3.1 Phthalate esters.

4.3.2 Nonyl phenols.

4.3.3 Miscible polymers.

4.3.4 Flexibilizers.

[6] *Annual Book of ASTM Standards,* Vol 09.01.

[7] *Annual Book of ASTM Standards,* Vol 04.06.

[8] *Annual Book of ASTM Standards,* Vol 10.04.

[9] *Annual Book of ASTM Standards,* Vol 13.01.

[10] Available from the Association for the Advancement of Medical Instrumentation, 1901 N. Ft. Myer Dr., Suite 602, Arlington, VA 22209.

4.4 *Fillers*—The following are examples of fillers that may be incorporated in the formulations:

4.4.1 Silicas:

4.4.1.1 Fumed silica.

4.4.1.2 Precipitated hydrated silica.

4.4.1.3 Diatomaceous earth.

4.4.2 Carbons.

4.4.3 Certain radiopaque materials:

4.4.3.1 Certain inorganic nonmetallic particles.

4.4.3.2 Certain metallic particles.

4.4.4 Certain pigments.

4.4.5 Glass fibers.

4.4.6 Glass ceramic particles.

4.4.7 Glass or plastic microballoons.

4.5 *Other Additives*—The following are examples of additives that may be used in the formulation:

4.5.1 Slip agents.

4.5.2 Optical brighteners.

4.5.3 Surfactants.

4.6 *Curing Agents*—The following are examples of curing agents for epoxy resins:

4.6.1 Amines (primary, secondary, and tertiary) such as triethylenetetramine (TETA).

4.6.2 Anhydrides, such as phthalic anhydride.

4.6.3 Acids such as phthalic acid.

4.6.4 Amine-terminated polyamides.

4.6.5 Acid or amine-terminated telomers.

4.6.6 Schiff's bases.

4.7 *Catalysts*:

4.7.1 Lewis bases such as tertiary amines.

4.7.2 Lewis acids such as BF_3.

4.8 *Accelerators*:

4.8.1 Tertiary amines.

4.8.2 Phenols.

NOTE 2—Since some curing agents and catalysts may be toxic by themselves, it may be necessary in specific end-use standards to require tests to limit their presence in the final product.

5. Physical Requirements

5.1 *Uncured Properties*—The following test methods may be conducted on the uncured mixed formulation or appropriate components:

5.1.1 *Peak Exotherm Temperature*—Test Method D 2471.

5.1.2 *Gel Time*—Test Method D 2471.

5.1.3 *Mix Ratio*—The mix ratio shall be calculated and maintained at the ratio recommended by the manufacturer of the formulation.

5.1.4 *Viscosity*—Test Method D 2393.

5.2 *Cured Properties* (Required)—The following test methods shall be conducted on the fully cured and properly conditioned material.

5.2.1 *Extraction*—Practice F 619.

5.2.2 *Foreign Particles*—Upon careful visual examination, the epoxy plastic shall be free of any extraneous debris that may adversely affect its safety, efficacy, or reliability.

5.2.3 *Hydrolytic Stability*—Practice F 74 or Test Method D 3137.

5.2.4 *USP Biological Tests*[11] —The material shall pass the biological tests for plastic containers, as is appropriate for the intended end use:

5.2.4.1 Short-term implantation test.

5.2.4.2 Saline extract test.

5.2.4.3 Cottonseed oil extract test.

5.2.4.4 Alcohol extract test.

5.2.5 *Sterilant Residues*—Testing regarding applicable methods of sterilization should be documented. In addition to degassing time necessary for EtO sterilization, the stability of the epoxy under steam and radiation sterilization should be specified if these types of sterilization are called for.

5.2.5.1 Sterilant residues shall be tested according to appropriate methods, such as AAMI EOS-D. The concentration of ethylene oxide, ethylene chlorohydrin, ethylene glycol, and dichlorodifluoromethane (or the equivalents) at the time of implant shall be shown to be within safe limits prescribed by the device manufacturer. Cell culture tests can be used to show absence of sterilant residues. When materials are sterilized by radiation, materials subjected to maximum radiation dose shall be qualified by performance tests.

5.2.6 *Water Absorption*—Test Method D 570.

5.3 *Cured Properties* (Optional)—The following test methods shall be conducted on the fully cured and properly conditioned material as is appropriate for the end use:

5.3.1 *Adhesion*—Test Method D 952.

5.3.2 *Bacteriostasis and Fungistasis*—Sterility Tests.[12]

5.3.3 *Compression Set*—Test Methods D 621.

5.3.4 *Dielectric Constant*—Test Methods D 150.

5.3.5 *Dielectric Strength*—Test Method D 149.

5.3.6 *Dissipation Factor*—Test Methods D 150.

5.3.7 *Elongation*—Test Method D 638.

5.3.8 *Flexural Strength*—Test Method D 1434.

5.3.9 *Gas Permeation*—Test Method D 1434.

5.3.10 *Hardness*—Test Method D 785.

5.3.11 *Hemolysis*—The material shall be tested for hemolytic properties by appropriate methods.

5.3.12 *Implantability*—The encapsulant shall be shown to be safe and effective for long-term implant by appropriate state-of-the-art tests.

5.3.12.1 Biological test procedures appropriate to determine biological safety and tissue reactions are described in Practice F 748 which recommends generic biological test methods for materials and devices according to end use applications.

5.3.13 *Moisture Vapor Transmission*—Test Methods E 96.

5.3.14 *Prothrombin Time*—The effect of the material on Prothrombin time shall be tested by appropriate methods.[13]

5.3.15 *Specific Gravity*—Test Methods D 792.

5.3.16 *Stability* (dimensional)—Test Method D 1042.

5.3.17 *Stypven Time*—The effect of the material on Stypven time shall be tested by appropriate methods.[12]

5.3.18 *Surface Resistivity*—Test Methods D 257.

5.3.19 *Tangent Modulus*—Test Method D 638.

5.3.20 *Tensile Strength*—Test Method D 638.

[11] *United States Pharmacopeia*, XXIII, 1995, pp. 1783–1786.

[12] Ibid, XXIII, 1995, pp. 1686–1690.

[13] *Human Blood Coagulation, Haemostasis, and Thrombosis*, Rosemary Biggs, ed., Blackwell Scientific Publications, 1972.

5.3.21 *Visual Defects*—Practice D 2562.
5.3.22 *Voids*—Test Method D 2734.
5.3.23 *Volume Resistivity*—Test Method D 257.

6. Identification

6.1 The following analytical methods may be used to characterize the materials:
6.1.1 Infrared spectroscopy.
6.1.2 Spectrographic analysis.
6.1.3 X-ray emission or diffraction.

7. Marking

7.1 The labels shall bear appropriate statements as to safety and handling precautions for each component and shall bear appropriate lot numbers.

8. Packaging

8.1 Packaging shall provide appropriate protection for the compound(s).

9. Keywords

9.1 epoxy (EP) plastics-surgical implants; plastics (thermosetting); plastic surgical devices/applications; polymers-surgical applications; resins-epoxy

APPENDIXES

(Nonmandatory Information)

X1. RATIONALE

X1.1 This document provides definitions and a standard description for thermoset epoxy plastics based on diglycidyl ethers of bisphenol A and appropriate curing agents and catalysts, compositions which are used in the manufacture of implantable devices. The guide enumerates relevant test methods and describes generic criteria which should assist in developing more specific specifications for implantable devices containing epoxy resins with values and limits covering end-use applications. This document should also help the fabricator to select ingredients for the medical device that ensure its biocompatibility.

X2. BIOCOMPATIBILITY

X2.1 The suitability of these materials from a human implant perspective is dependent on the specific application. The biologic tests appropriate for the specific site, such as recommended in Practice F 748 should be used as a guideline.

X2.2 No known surgical implant material has ever been shown to be completely free of adverse reactions in the human body. However, long-term clinical experience of use of specific compositions and formulations of this material class referred to in this standard has shown that an acceptable level of biological response can be expected, if the material is used in appropriate applications.

Designation: F 603 – 00

Standard Specification for High-Purity Dense Aluminum Oxide for Medical Application[1]

This standard is issued under the fixed designation F 603; the number immediately following the designation indicates the year of original adoption or, in the case of revision, the year of last revision. A number in parentheses indicates the year of last reapproval. A superscript epsilon (ε) indicates an editorial change since the last revision or reapproval.

1. Scope

1.1 This specification covers the material requirements for high-purity, dense aluminum oxide for load bearing surgical implant applications.

1.2 This specification does not cover finished parts (for example, femoral heads, acetabular inserts, dental implants and the like). It is intended as a qualification of the material as delivered to the parts manufacturer.

1.3 The values stated in SI units are to be regarded as standard.

2. Referenced Documents

2.1 *ASTM Standards:*

C 373 Test Method for Water Absorption, Bulk Density, Apparent Porosity, and Apparent Specific Gravity of Fired Whiteware Products[2]

C 1161 Test Method for Flexural Strength of Advanced Ceramics at Ambient Temperature[3]

C 1198 Test Method for Dynamic Young's Modulus, Shear Modulus, and Poisson's Ratio for Advanced Ceramics by Sonic Resonance[3]

C 1239 Standard Practice for Reporting Uniaxial Strength Data and Estimating Weibull Distribution Parameters for Advanced Ceramics[3]

C 1259 Test Method for Dynamic Young's Modulus, Shear Modulus and Poisson's Ratio for Advanced Ceramics by Impulse Excitation of Vibration[3]

C 1327 Standard Test Method for Vickers Indentation Hardness of Advanced Ceramics[3]

E 112 Methods for Determining Average Grain Size[4]

F 981 Practice for Assessment of Compatibility of Biomaterials for Surgical Implants with Respect to Effect of Materials on Muscle and Bone[5]

2.2 *American Society for Quality Control:*

C 1 Specification of General Requirements for a Quality Program[6]

2.3 *ISO:*

ISO 6474:1994 Implants for Surgery - Ceramic Materials Based on Alumina[7]

3. Chemical Requirements

3.1 The Chemical composition shall be as follows in Table 1, (measured by ICP-AES, XRF or mass spectrocopy):

4. Physical Requirements

4.1 The minimum bulk density shall be (3.94 ± .01) g/cm^3 as determined by Test Method C 373 as applied with the following modifications.

4.1.1 Weight determination, 3.1 and 5.1 of C 373 shall be made to the nearest 0.001 g.

4.1.2 The calculation of bulk density in 12.1 of C 373 shall be calculated as follows:

$$B = (D \cdot d)/(M - S) \quad (1)$$

where:

B = Bulk density (g/cm^3)
D = Dry weight (g)
M = Saturated weight (g)
S = Suspended weight (g)
d = Density of water at the temperature when measurement is taken.

4.2 The median grain size shall be 4.5 µm or less, in accordance with Section 10 of Methods E 112.

5. Mechanical Requirements (Table 2)

5.1 The average room temperature flexural strength for 10 samples shall be no less than 400 MPa (58,000 psi) by four point bend in accordance with Test Method C 1161 test configuration B. The specimen shall be prepared in accordance with Test Method C 1161 7.2.4 to a 500 grit finish.

5.2 The room temperature elastic modulus shall be measured in accordance with C 1259 or C 1198.

5.3 The minimum Vickers Hardness values for a 1 Kg load shall be 18 GPa (2.56 × 10^6 psi) in accordance with Test Method C 1327.

---

[1] This specification is under the jurisdiction of ASTM Committee F-4 on Medical and Surgical Materials and Devices, and is the direct responsibility of Subcommittee F04.13 on Ceramic Materials.

Current edition approved Jan 10, 2000. Published April 2000. Originally published as F 603 – 83. Last previous edition F 603 – 93 (95).

[2] *Annual Book of ASTM Standards*, Vol 15.02.

[3] *Annual Book of ASTM Standards*, Vol 15.01.

[4] *Annual Book of ASTM Standards*, Vol 03.01.

[5] *Annual Book of ASTM Standards*, Vol 13.01.

[6] Available from American Society for Quality Control, 161 West Wisconsin Ave., Milwaukee, WI 52303.

[7] Available from the American National Standards Institute 11 West 42nd St. 13th Floor, New York, NY 10036.

TABLE 1 Chemical Properties

Oxide	Weight Percent
Al_2O_3	≥ 99.5
MgO	≤ 0.5
Other Oxides	≤ 0.1

TABLE 2 Mechanical Properties

Compressive Strength GPa (ksi) Expected Minimum	4 (580)
Average Flexural Strength MPa (psi) Required Minimum	400 (58,000)
Elastic Modulus GPa (ksi) Required Minimum	380 (55,100)
Vickers Hardness GPa (ksi) Required Minimum	18 (2.56×10^6)
Weibull Modulus Required Minimum	8

5.4 The minimum Weibull modulus for 30 samples as calculated using C 1239 shall be no less than 8 by four point bend in accordance with Test Method C 1161, test configuration B. The specimens shall be prepared in accordance with Test Method C 1161 7.2.4 to a 500 grit finish.

6. Test Specimen Fabrication

6.1 Specific test specimens shall be prepared from the same batch of material and by the same processes as those employed in fabricating the ceramic implant device.

7. Quality Program Requirements

7.1 The producer shall maintain a quality program, such as the program defined in ASQC C 1.

7.2 The manufacturer of surgical implants shall be assured of the producer's quality program for conformance to the intent of ASQC C 1 or any other recognized program.

8. Keywords

8.1 advanced ceramics; alumina; aluminum oxide; ceramic; surgical implant

APPENDIXES

(Nonmandatory Information)

X1. RATIONALE

X1.1 This standard is needed to ensure a high quality material for use in biological applications. The chemical, physical and mechanical requirements serve as criteria for a high-purity, consistent product that can be implanted in the body. These requirements provide specifications for biocompatible grades of aluminum oxide for use in the physiological environments.

X2. BIOCOMPATIBILITY

X2.1 No known surgical implant has ever been shown to be completely free of adverse reactions in the human body. However, long term clinical experience has shown an acceptable level of biological response can be expected, if the material is used in appropriate applications.

X2.2 Aluminum oxide in accordance with Section 3 has been demonstrated to exhibit a well characterized biological response which is less than that exhibited by the reference materials cited and tested in Practice F 981 or equivalent (Refs **1-6**).

REFERENCES

(1) Hentrich, R.L., Graves, G.A., Stein, H.G. and Bajpai, P.K., "An Evaluation of Inert and Resorbable Ceramics for Future Clinical Orthopaedic Applications," Journal of Biomedical Materials Research, Vol. 5, 1971, p.25.

(2) Griss, P., et al.," Experimentelle Untersuchung zur Gewebsverträglichkeit oxidkeramischer (Al_2O_3) Abriebteilchen," Archiv für Orthopaedische und Unfallchirurgie, Vol. 76, 1973, pp. 270-279.

(3) Griss, P., et al., "Biological Activity and Histocompatibility of Dense Al_2O_3/MgO Ceramic Implants in Rats," Journal of Biomedical Materials Research Symposium No. 4, 1973, pp. 453-462.

(4) Griss, P., et al., "Experimental Analysis of Ceramic-Tissue Interactions: A Morphologic, Fluorescence-Optic and Radiographic Study on Dense Aluminum Oxide in Various Animals," Journal of Biomedical Materials Research, Symposium No. 5, Part 1, 1974, pp. 39-48.

(5) Richardson, W.C., et al., "Soft Tissue Response to a Series of Dense Ceramic Materials and Two Clinically Used Biomaterials," Publications 415, National Bureau of Standards, 1974, pp. 37-44.

(6) Wolfson, S.H., et al., "Load-Bearing Capacity of Functioning Alumina Dental Endosseous Implants," Journal of Dental Research, Vol. 44, No. 1, 1976, pp. 22-29.

(7) Dörre, E and Hübner, H., *Alumina: Processing, Properties and Applications*, Springer-Verlag, New York (1984) Chapter 3, pp. 74-187.

(8) Miyayama, M., et al., *Engineering Properties of Single Oxides*, Engineering Materials Handbook, Chapter 4: Ceramics and Glasses ASM, Int'l (1991) pp 748-757.

Last ASTM Designation: F 604 – 94

Standard Specification for
Silicone Elastomers Used in Medical Applications

This specification covers silicone elastomers intended for use as materials of construction for fabrication of medical devices.

Formerly under the jurisdiction of Committee F04 on Medical and Surgical Materials and Devices, this specification was withdrawn in January 2001 in accordance with Section 10.6.3.1 of the *Regulations Governing ASTM Technical Committees*, which requires that standards shall be updated by the end of the eighth year since the last approval date.

Standard Practice for Extraction of Medical Plastics[1]

This standard is issued under the fixed designation F 619; the number immediately following the designation indicates the year of original adoption or, in the case of revision, the year of last revision. A number in parentheses indicates the year of last reapproval. A superscript epsilon (ε) indicates an editorial change since the last revision or reapproval.

ε1 Note—Keywords were added editorially in May 1998.

1. Scope

1.1 This practice covers methods for extraction of medical plastics in liquids that simulate body fluids in their action on the plastics. This practice identifies two methods of extraction: one used for obtaining" extract liquid" to be analyzed by chemical and physical tests; and the other obtaining "extract liquid" for use in determining the biological response of animals. Further testing of the "extract liquid" is specified in other ASTM standards. The plastic after extraction may also be examined.

1.2 This practice may be used for, but is not limited to the following areas: partial evaluation of raw materials, auditing materials within the manufacturing process, and testing final products. This practice may also be used as a referee method for the measurement of extractables in plastics used in medical devices.

1.3 The values stated in SI units are to be regarded as the standard.

1.4 *This standard does not purport to address all of the safety concerns, if any, associated with its use. It is the responsibility of the user of this standard to establish appropriate safety and health practices and determine the applicability of regulatory limitations prior to use.*

2. Referenced Documents

2.1 *ASTM Standards:*

D 543 Test Method for Resistance of Plastics to Chemical Reagents[2]

D 570 Test Method for Water Absorption of Plastics[2]

D 618 Practice for Conditioning Plastics and Electrical Insulating Materials for Testing[2]

D 1193 Specification for Reagent Water[3]

D 1239 Test Method for Resistance of Plastic Films to Extraction by Chemicals[2]

D 1898 Practice for Sampling of Plastics[4]

E 171 Specification for Standard Atmospheres for Conditioning and Testing Materials[5]

3. Terminology Definitions

3.1 *extraction vehicle*—a liquid specified for use in testing the plastic. Specific extraction vehicles are to be designated by the ASTM standard that references this practice (see Section 7 for a list of standard extraction vehicles).

3.2 *extract liquid*— that liquid which is tested for biological and chemical/physical response; the end result of this practice.

3.3 *specimen portion*— the unit or units of plastic placed into the extraction vehicle.

3.4 *blank*—the extraction vehicle not containing the specimen under test which is used for comparison with the extract liquid.

4. Summary of Practice

4.1 Standard-size specimens of the plastic, which may closely simulate the intended device depending upon the use, are immersed in definite volumes of selected liquids (extraction vehicles) for the time and temperature specified.

4.2 A choice is made, based on the end use, of the extraction vehicles (see Section 7) and one of the combinations of time and temperature for the test (see Section 12).

4.3 The resultant test liquids (extract liquids) are kept in glass containers until used for testing. Test liquids for biological testing are kept in sterile glass containers. The test liquids for biological testing should be used within 24 h.

5. Significance and Use

5.1 These extraction procedures are the initial part of several test procedures used in the biocompatibility screening of plastics used in medical devices.

5.2 The limitations of the results obtained from this practice should be recognized. The choice of extraction vehicle, duration of immersion, and temperature of the test is necessarily arbitrary. The specification of these conditions provides a basis for standardization and serves as a guide to investigators wishing to compare the relative resistance of various plastics to extraction vehicles.

5.3 Correlation of test results with the actual performance or serviceability of plastics is necessarily dependent upon the

[1] This practice is under the jurisdiction of ASTM Committee F-4 on Medical and Surgical Materials and Devicesand is the direct responsibility of Subcommittee F04.16 on Biocompatibility.

Current edition approved May 31, 1979. Published August 1979. Originally published as F 619 – 79.

[2] *Annual Book of ASTM Standards,* Vol 08.01.

[3] *Annual Book of ASTM Standards,* Vol 11.01.

[4] *Annual Book of ASTM Standards,* Vol 08.02.

[5] *Annual Book of ASTM Standards,* Vol 15.09.

similarity between the testing and end-use conditions (see 12.1.2 and Note 7).

5.4 Caution should be exercised in the understanding and intent of this practice as follows:

5.4.1 No allowance or distinction is made for variables such as end-use application, for example, short-term versus long-term application or implantation.

5.4.2 No allowance is made to distinguish between a non-porous versus a porous plastic. Although no definitions are given in this practice for the following terms, such items as extraction vehicle surface tension at the specified extraction condition and plastic specimen physical structure should be taken into account.

5.5 Test Methods D 543, D 570, and D 1239 may be useful in providing supplemental information.

6. Apparatus

6.1 *Autoclave*, capable of maintaining a temperature of 121 ± 2.0°C (249.8 ± 3.8°F), and equipped with a thermometer, pressure gage, vent cock, and a rack to hold the extraction containers above the water level.

6.1.1 The autoclave preferably should have a water cooling system that will allow for the cooling of the extraction containers to about, but not less than, 22°C (71.6°F) immediately following the heating cycle.

6.1.2 Autoclaves not equipped with a water cooling system may be used. However, sealed, unvented, extraction vessels should not be removed from such an autoclave until internal temperature and pressure have reached ambient conditions. Such vessels, when hot, represent an extreme explosion hazard capable of causing serious injury or even death.

6.2 *Balance*, accurate to ±0.1 mg.

6.2.1 Caution should be exercised when performing weighings in glassware. Depending upon the required accuracy, the relative humidity should be the same for weighings at different times.

6.3 *Extraction Containers*—Suitable glass containers that protect the extract liquid from biological and chemical contamination or evaporation. One suggested container is the screw-cap culture test tube of borosilicate glass, unless a larger container is required for the size and shape for the material to be extracted. Screw caps, if used, shall have a rubber liner, whose exposed surface shall be completely covered with polytetrafluorethylene film 0.05 to 0.075 mm (0.002 to 0.003 in.) in thickness.

6.4 *Heating Equipment*:

6.4.1 *Oven*, forced air-circulation type that will maintain temperatures of 50 to 70 ± 2°C (122 to 158 ± 3.6°F).

6.4.2 *Water Bath*, capable of maintaining temperatures of 50 to 70 ± 2°C (122 to 158 ± 3.6°F).

6.5 *Micrometers*, capable of measuring dimensions of test specimens to 0.025 mm (0.001 in.).

6.6 *Room*, or enclosed space capable of being maintained at the Standard Laboratory Atmosphere, as prescribed in Practice D 618 (see 11.3).

7. Reagents and Materials

7.1 *Purity of Reagents*—Reagent grade chemicals shall be used in all tests. Unless otherwise indicated, it is intended that all reagents shall conform to the specifications of the Committee on Analytical Reagents of the American Chemical Society, where such specifications are available.[6] Other grades may be used, provided it is first ascertained that the reagent is of sufficiently high purity to permit its use without lessening the accuracy of the determination.

7.2 *Purity of Water*— Unless otherwise indicated, references to water shall be understood to mean reagent water conforming to Specification D 1193, Type II.

7.3 *Extraction Vehicles*—The following list of standard extraction vehicles is intended to simulate the main constituents of human body fluids. Aqueous solutions shall be made with distilled water. The extraction vehicles shall be:

7.3.1 *Sodium Chloride Injection*, USP, containing by weight not less than 0.85 % and not more than 0.95 % sodium chloride.

7.3.2 *Vegetable Oil*:

7.3.2.1 *Sesame Oil*, USP.

7.3.2.2 *Cottonseed Oil*, USP.

NOTE 1—To preclude the use of vegetable oil of poor or deteriorated quality, the following additional negative reactivity test, beyond the respective description in the USP, may be performed.

Select three healthy, thin-skinned albino rabbits, not previously used for any test, whose fur can be clipped closely and whose skin is free of mechanical irritation or trauma. On the day of the test, clip the fur from the dorsal surface. Divide the test area into a grid of suitably identified individual injection sites. Inject 0.2 ml intracutaneously at each of ten sites on each animal. In handling the animals, avoid touching the injection sites during observation periods. Examine the injected sites 24, 48, and 72 h after the injection. No site should show an edema or erythema over an area greater than 5 mm (0.197 in.) in diameter. Qualify a vegetable oil batch and store under adequate conditions until use. Ideal storage conditions may be under a nitrogen blanket in complete darkness. The primary objective is to prevent oxidative type reactions.

7.3.3 *Water for Injection*, USP.

7.3.4 Other extraction vehicles, as required.

NOTE 2—Depending upon the medical plastic under test and the user's needs, extraction vehicles other than those in 7.3 may be used. An example is pseudoextracellular fluid (PECF).[7]

8. Sampling

8.1 The application of this practice may be in various areas. Therefore, although some well-known quality sampling methods may be used, a statistician should be consulted to ensure a statistically valid sampling plan.

8.2 Practice D 1898 may also be consulted.

9. Test Specimen

9.1 This practice is designed primarily for application to plastics in the condition in which they are used. The plastic should be exposed to all conditions and substances as during a production run, such as washing, packaging, and sterilization.

[6] "Reagent Chemicals, American Chemical Society Specifications," Am. Chemical Soc., Washington, D.C. For suggestions on the testing of reagents not listed by the American Chemical Society, see "Reagent Chemicals and Standards," by Joseph Rosin, D. Van Nostrand Co., Inc., New York, N. Y., and the "United States Pharmacopeia."

[7] Homsy, C. A., "Bio-Compatibility in Selection of Materials for Implantation," *Journal of Biomedical Materials Research*, Vol. 4, 1970, pp. 341–356.

The extraction is to be done on the end-use item, specimen portions thereof, or representative molded or extruded test specimens of the formulated compound that are preconditioned by the same processing.

NOTE 3—Changes to a plastic formulation, specifically additives, such as plasticizers, stabilizers, antioxidants, pigments, and lubricants are perhaps more prone to produce differences in the extract liquid than the polymer itself.

9.2 *Specimen Size*— Use a surface-to-volume ratio that closely approximates or is greater than that of the final product. Suitable-size containers will allow a 20-mL extraction vehicle volume for each of the following specimen sizes:

9.2.1 The total surface area of a specimen (both sides) is equivalent to 120 cm^2(18.6 $in.^2$) when the specimen thickness is 0.50 mm (0.020 in.) or less, or equivalent to 60 cm^2 (9.3 $in.^2$) when the thickness is greater than 0.50 mm (0.020 in.).

9.2.2 An alternative for specimens of intricate geometry or those specimens with a thickness greater than 1.0 mm (0.039 in.) is a specimen whose weight is 4.0 g (0.14 oz).

9.2.3 Specimens shall be of such dimensions as to conveniently fit within the extraction container and their total surface area shall be completely covered by the extraction vehicle.

9.2.4 It may be necessary to subdivide the specimen, utilize inerts and noncontaminating spacers or weights or both, or initially agitate the extraction vehicle to ensure the entire specimen surface is contacted.

9.3 *Number of Specimen Portions*—In both procedures set forth in Section 12, test at least three specimen portions with each extraction vehicle to account for variability.

10. Preparation of Apparatus

10.1 Clean all reusable glassware thoroughly with a chromic acid cleansing mixture, or if necessary, with hot nitric acid, followed by prolonged rinsing with tap water and then at least two rinses with distilled water.

10.2 Clean cutting devices by an appropriate method, for example, successive cleaning with suitable solvents prior to use in subdividing the sample.

10.3 Clean all other equipment by thorough scrubbing with a suitable detergent and prolonged rinsing with tap water and then at least two rinses with distilled water.

10.4 Render containers and devices used for extraction and in transfer and administration of the extract liquids, sterile and dry by a suitable process.

NOTE 4—If ethylene oxide is used as the sterilizing agent, allow adequate conditioning for complete degassing. Ethylene oxide residuals may vary among different material formulations.

11. Specimen Portion and Conditioning

11.1 *Biological Response Extraction*—Select and cut to size, as in 9.2 and 9.3, at least three specimen portions for each extraction vehicle to be used.

11.2 *Extraction for Chemical/Physical Testing*:

11.2.1 Select and cut to size, as in 9.2 and 9.3, three specimen portions for each extraction vehicle to be used.

11.2.2 Unless otherwise indicated, there is no requirement to adhere to sterile procedure for this testing.

11.3 *Conditioning*— Although desirable, no conditioning is required. If a conditioning environment is required, the following shall be observed:

11.3.1 Unless otherwise specified, condition specimen portions in accordance with Procedure A of Practice D 618 in the Standard Laboratory Atmosphere which is 23 ± 2°C (73.4 ± 3.6°F) and 50 ± 5 % relative humidity, as described in Specification E 171. If closer tolerances are required, ±1°C (1.8°F) and ±2 % relative humidity may be specified.

11.3.1.1 *Specimen Portions 7 mm (0.28 in.) in Thickness and Under*—Condition in Standard Laboratory Atmosphere for 40 h.

11.3.1.2 *Specimen Portions Greater than 7 mm (0.28 in.) in Thickness*—Condition in the Standard Laboratory Atmosphere for 88 h.

NOTE 5—Care should be taken not to compromise sterility for biological response specimen portions.

12. Procedure

12.1 *Biological Response Extraction*:

12.1.1 Prepare a set of four 20-mL portions of each extraction vehicle. Place one specimen portion in each of three containers; the extraction vehicle in the fourth container will serve as a blank. Secure the cap on each container.

12.1.2 *Extraction Conditions*—Employ one of the following conditions in accordance with the specified requirements. Sufficient time, in addition to that specified, should be allowed for the liquid to reach the extraction temperature. Do not agitate the extraction vehicle or extraction container during the extraction.

12.1.2.1 37 ± 1°C (95 ± 1.8°F) for 120 h.

12.1.2.2 50 ± 2°C (122 ± 3.6°F) for 72 h.

12.1.2.3 70 ± 2°C (158 ± 3.6°F) for 24 h.

12.1.2.4 121 ± 2°C (250 ± 3.6°F) for 2 h.

NOTE 6—There may be the assumption that these conditions are equivalent to one another. The same combination of plastic and extraction vehicle, when subjected to different extraction conditions, is generally known to have significantly different responses when tested. The ideal evaluation of a material should employ times and temperatures that simulate the intended use of a plastic. Exaggerated conditions of extraction attempt to provide a margin of safety with a reasonable increase in temperature. The prescribed temperature and duration should be not so severe as to affect the character of the plastic, that is, no gross physical change. In general, most plastics can withstand 50°C (122°F) for 72 h with no thermal degradation.

12.1.3 Upon removal from the heat source, cool the containers to, but not below, 22°C (71.6°F). When cool, shake the containers vigorously for 30 s and decant the extract liquid into a dry sterile container.

NOTE 7—Sealed, unvented containers used at a temperature of 121 ± 2°C, should not be handled until the internal temperature and pressure have reached ambient conditions.

12.1.4 Store the extract liquids at 22 to 30°C (71.6 to 86°F). Use the extract liquids within 24 h.

12.1.5 To minimize the number of test animals required to determine a biological response, it is permissible to pool extract liquids from three specimen portions.

12.2 *Extraction for Chemical/Physical Testing*:

12.2.1 Prepare a set of four 20-mL portions of each extraction vehicle. Unless otherwise specified, the extraction vehicles are water for injection (7.3.3) or distilled water (7.2). In addition the use of a vegetable oil (7.3.2) is optional. Place one specimen portion in each of three containers; the extraction vehicle in the fourth container serves as a blank. Secure the cap on each container.

12.2.2 *Extraction Conditions*—Use the same conditions specified in 12.1.2.

12.2.3 Proceed in accordance with 12.1.3 and 12.1.4. In general, extract liquids do not have to be analyzed within 24 h. However, some analytical tests require that the extract liquid be analyzed within 24 h. There may be some absorption of certain species onto the borosilicate glass container. Vigorously agitate the extract liquid before removing it for testing.

13. Report

13.1 The report of any test referencing this practice shall include the following:

13.1.1 Designation of the standard referencing this practice.

13.1.2 Complete identification of plastic tested, including:

13.1.2.1 Type of device or plastic part,

13.1.2.2 Dimensions, sample and specimen portion weight,

13.1.2.3 Manufacturer's code, catalog, or formulation number, batch number or date of manufacture, trade name, and

13.1.2.4 Previous history in accordance with 9.1.

13.1.3 Extraction vehicle volume to specimen portion surface ratio (for example, 20 mL/120 cm^2 or 60 cm^2, not including edges) or weight of specimen portion to extraction vehicle volume (9.2.2).

13.1.4 Conditioning procedure used, including actual range of temperature if the standard tolerances are not used (see Practice D 618).

13.1.5 Extraction conditions; time and temperature.

13.1.6 Extraction vehicle.

13.1.6.1 If an extraction vehicle is used as allowed in 7.3.4, adequate description should be provided such that its formulation can be duplicated.

13.1.7 Results from biological and chemical/physical extract liquid tests.

13.1.8 Any observations on gross physical changes of the specimen portions or extract liquid. Such observations may include, but are not restricted to, specimen portion color change, exact liquid color change, light transmittance, and potential multiphase separation.

14. Precision

14.1 Under the accepted definitions of precisions, values cannot be given because of the variable nature of the plastics and procedures to be used. Some typical results will be reported, when available.

15. Keywords

15.1 biocompatibility; extraction; liquids; plastics; specimen size

Standard Specification for Alpha Plus Beta Titanium Alloy Forgings for Surgical Implants[1]

This standard is issued under the fixed designation F 620; the number immediately following the designation indicates the year of original adoption or, in the case of revision, the year of last revision. A number in parentheses indicates the year of last reapproval. A superscript epsilon (ε) indicates an editorial change since the last revision or reapproval.

1. Scope

1.1 This specification covers the requirements for alpha plus beta titanium alloy forgings for surgical implants when the material forged conforms to Specifications F136 (UNS R56401), F1295 (UNS R56700), or F1472 (UNS R56400).

1.2 The values stated in inch-pound units are to be regarded as the standard.

2. Referenced Documents

2.1 *ASTM Standards:*

E 8 Test Methods for Tension Testing of Metallic Materials[2]

E 10 Test Method for Brinell Hardness of Metallic Materials[2]

E 18 Test Methods for Rockwell Hardness and Rockwell Superficial Hardness of Metallic Materials[2]

E 92 Test Method for Vickers Hardness of Metallic Materials[2]

E 120 Test Methods for Chemical Analysis of Titanium and Titanium Alloys[3]

E 165 Test Method for Liquid Penetrant Examination[4]

E 1409 Test Method for Determination of Oxygen in Titanium and Titanium Alloys by the Inert Gas Fusion Technique[3]

E 1447 Test Method for Determination of Hydrogen in Titanium and Titanium Alloys by the Inert Gas Fusion Thermal Conductivity Method[5]

F 136 Specification for Wrought Titanium-6 Aluminum-4 Vanadium ELI (Extra Low Interstitial) Alloy (R56401) for Surgical Implant Applications[6]

F 601 Practice for Fluorescent Penetrant Inspection of Metallic Surgical Implants[6]

F 981 Practice for Assessment of Compatibility of Biomaterials for Surgical Implants with Respect to Effect of Materials on Muscle and Bone[7]

F 1295 Specification for Wrought Titanium-6 Aluminum-7 Niobium Alloy for Surgical Implant Applications [UNS R56700][6]

F 1472 Specification for Wrought Ti-6 Al-4V Alloy for Surgical Implant Applications[6]

2.2 *ASQC Standard:*

Cl Specifications of General Requirements for a Quality Program[7]

3. Ordering Information

3.1 Inquiries and orders for forgings under this specification shall include the following information:

3.1.1 Quantity, number of pieces,

3.1.2 ASTM designation, material grade,

3.1.3 Condition,

3.1.4 Mechanical properties (other than those specified herein),

3.1.5 Finish,

3.1.6 Applicable dimensions or print number,

3.1.7 Special tests, if any, and

3.1.8 Special requirements, if any.

4. Materials and Manufacture

4.1 Material for forgings shall be bars or wire fabricated in accordance with Specification F 136, F 1295, or F 1472.

4.2 The material shall be forged by hammering, pressing, extruding, or upsetting and shall be processed, if practicable, so as to cause metal flow during the hot-working operation in the direction most favorable for resisting stresses encountered in service, as may be indicated to the fabricator by the purchaser.

4.3 Forgings shall be free of splits, scale, cracks, flaws, and other imperfections not consistent with good commercial practice (see Note 1). Offset or mismatch allowance, dependent upon part size and configuration, shall be within standard forging tolerances.

NOTE 1—Compliance to these requirements may be verified by Test Method E 165 or Practice F 601 or other suitable methods.

4.4 After all hot-working operations, the forgings shall receive an annealing treatment, consisting of heating the parts to an appropriate elevated temperature for a specified dwell

---

[1] This specification is under the jurisdiction of ASTM Committee F-4 on Medical and Surgical Materials and Devicesand is the direct responsibility of Subcommittee F04.12 on Metallurgical Materials.

Current edition approved May 10, 2000. Published August 2000. Originally published as F 620 – 79. Last previous edition F 620 – 97.

[2] *Annual Book of ASTM Standards*, Vol 03.01.

[3] *Annual Book of ASTM Standards*, Vol 03.05.

[4] *Annual Book of ASTM Standards*, Vol 03.03.

[5] *Annual Book of ASTM Standards*, Vol 03.06.

[6] *Annual Book of ASTM Standards*, Vol 13.01.

[7] Available from American Society for Quality Control, 161 W. Wisconsin Ave., Milwaukee, WI 53203.

time followed by appropriate cooling to meet the applicable metallurgical requirements specified herein.

4.5 Optional identification marks, including the manufacturer's logo, material designation, heat code number, and impression number, may be placed upon each forging, the method and location of which shall be specified by the purchaser.

5. Chemical Composition

5.1 When specified by the purchaser, the chemical composition of either the forging bars or the completed forgings shall be determined and confirmed by the forger, and shall meet the product analysis limits of the appropriate material specification.

5.1.1 Hydrogen content must be determined for the annealed forgings. Samples for hydrogen analysis shall be taken after descaling, pickling, or chem milling, if these operations are performed.

5.2 For referee purposes, Test Methods E 120, E 1409, and E 1447 shall be used.

6. Mechanical Requirements

6.1 The mechanical properties of forgings shall be tested by the forger and shall comply with the minimum mechanical properties as specified in Specifications F 136, F 1295, or F 1472.

6.1.1 Test specimens shall be taken from a representative forging if possible, or from a representative forged test bar, only if the configuration does not lend itself to yielding the required specimen. Any specially forged test bar must be annealed with the forgings it represents.

6.1.2 Testing shall be in accordance with Test Methods E 8 using a strain rate of 0.003 to 0.007 in./in.·min (mm/mm·min) through the specified yield range, and then the crosshead speed shall be increased so as to produce fracture in approximately one additional minute.

6.2 When desired, hardness may be specified on the purchase order or drawing and shall be determined in accordance with Test Methods E 10, E 18,or E 92.

7. Special Requirements

7.1 The microstructure shall be a fine dispersion of the alpha and beta phases resulting from processing in the temperature range of the alpha plus beta phase field. There shall be no continuous alpha network at prior beta grain boundaries. There shall be no coarse, elongated alpha platelets. The alpha case, if present, shall be less than 0.020 in. (0.5 mm) in thickness.

8. Certification Requirements

8.1 The forger's certification that the material was manufactured and tested in accordance with this specification, together with a report of the test results, shall be furnished to the purchaser with each shipment.

9. Quality Program Requirements

9.1 The producer of material in accordance with this specification shall maintain a quality program as defined in ASQ Cl, or equivalent.

10. Keywords

10.1 forgings—surgical implants; metals (for surgical implants)—titanium alloys; orthopaedic medical devices—titanium/titanium alloy; titanium/titanium alloys (for surgical implants)

APPENDIXES

(Nonmandatory Information)

X1. RATIONALE

X1.1 The purpose of this specification is to characterize the chemical, mechanical, and metallurgical properties of wrought annealed alpha plus beta titanium alloy forgings for surgical implants.

X1.2 The microstructural requirements contained in this specification represent the current general consensus with respect to optimization of mechanical properties for implant applications.

X1.3 The title of the specification was changed to cover the alpha plus beta titanium alloy forgings and the Scope defines three specific compositions that have a similar microstructures and mechanical properties. The hydrogen content is now required to be determined in the final condition that the forgings will be shipped to the purchaser and mechanical properties are now required to be reported.

X2. BIOCOMPATIBILITY

X2.1 The material composition covered by this specification has been employed successfully in human implant applications in contact with soft tissue and bone for over a decade.

X2.2 No known surgical implant material has ever been shown to be completely free of adverse reactions in the human body. However, long term clinical experience has shown an acceptable level of biological response can be expected, if the material is used in appropriate applications.

The American Society for Testing and Materials takes no position respecting the validity of any patent rights asserted in connection with any item mentioned in this standard. Users of this standard are expressly advised that determination of the validity of any such patent rights, and the risk of infringement of such rights, are entirely their own responsibility.

This standard is subject to revision at any time by the responsible technical committee and must be reviewed every five years and if not revised, either reapproved or withdrawn. Your comments are invited either for revision of this standard or for additional standards and should be addressed to ASTM Headquarters. Your comments will receive careful consideration at a meeting of the responsible technical committee, which you may attend. If you feel that your comments have not received a fair hearing you should make your views known to the ASTM Committee on Standards, at the address shown below.

Designation: F 621 – 97

Standard Specification for Stainless Steel Forgings for Surgical Implants[1]

This standard is issued under the fixed designation F 621; the number immediately following the designation indicates the year of original adoption or, in the case of revision, the year of last revision. A number in parentheses indicates the year of last reapproval. A superscript epsilon (ε) indicates an editorial change since the last revision or reapproval.

1. Scope

1.1 This specification covers the requirements of forged stainless steel for surgical implants when the material forged conforms to F 138 (R31673), F 1314 (S21910), or F 1586.

1.2 The values stated in inch-pound units are to be regarded as the standard.

2. Referenced Documents

2.1 *ASTM Standards:*

A 262 Practices for Detecting Susceptibility to Intergranular Attack in Austenitic Stainless Steels[2]

A 370 Test Methods and Definitions for Mechanical Testing of Steel Products[2]

A 473 Specification for Stainless and Heat-Resisting Steel Forgings[3]

E 18 Test Methods for Rockwell Hardness and Rockwell Superficial Hardness of Metallic Materials[4]

E 112 Test Methods for Determining Average Grain Size[4]

E 165 Practice for Liquid Penetrant Inspection Method[5]

E 353 Test Methods for Chemical Analysis of Stainless, Heat-Resisting, Maraging, and Other Similar Chromium-Nickel-Iron Alloys[6]

F 138 Specification for Stainless Steel Bars and Wire for Surgical Implants (Special Quality)[7]

F 601 Practice for Fluorescent Penetrant Inspection of Metallic Surgical Implants[7]

F 1314 Specification for Wrought Nitrogen Strengthened-22 Chromium-12.5 Nickel-5 Manganese-2.5 Molybdenum Stainless Steel Bar and Wire for Surgical Implants[7]

F 1586 Specification for Wrought Nitrogen Strengthened–21 Chromium-10 Nickel-3 Manganese-2.5 Molybdenum Stainless Steel Bar for Surgical Implants[7]

2.2 *ASQC Standard:*

Cl Specifications of General Requirements for a Quality Control Program[8]

3. Ordering Information

3.1 Inquiries and orders for forgings under this specification shall include the following information:

3.1.1 Quality; number of pieces,

3.1.2 ASTM designation; material grade,

3.1.3 Condition,

3.1.4 Mechanical properties (other than those specified herein),

3.1.5 Finish,

3.1.6 Applicable dimensions or print number,

3.1.7 Special tests, and

3.1.8 Special requirements.

4. General Requirements for Delivery

4.1 Material furnished to this specification shall conform to the applicable requirements in the current edition of Specification A 473.

4.2 In the case where a conflict exists between this specification and that listed in 4.1, this specification shall take precedence.

5. Materials and Manufacture

5.1 Material for forgings shall be bars or wire fabricated in accordance with Specification F 138, F 1314, or F 1586, generally in the unannealed condition with a finish suitable for forging.

5.2 The material shall be forged by hammering, pressing, rolling, extruding, or upsetting, and shall be processed, if practicable, so as to cause metal flow during the hot-working operation in the direction most favorable for resisting stresses encountered in service, as may be indicated to the fabricator by the implant manufacturer.

5.3 Forgings shall be free of splits, scale, cracks, inequalities, flaws, and other imperfections not consistent with good commercial practice (see Note 1). Offset or mismatch allowance, dependent upon part size and configuration, shall be within standard forging tolerances.

NOTE 1—Compliance to these requirements may be verified by Practices E 165 or F 601 or other suitable methods.

---

[1] This specification is under the jurisdiction of ASTM Committee F-4 on Medical and Surgical Materials and Devicesand is the direct responsibility of Subcommittee F04.12 on Metallurgical Materials.

Current edition approved April 10, 1997. Published March 1998. Originally published as F 621 – 79. Last previous edition F 621 – 92.

[2] *Annual Book of ASTM Standards*, Vol 01.03.

[3] *Annual Book of ASTM Standards*, Vol 01.05.

[4] *Annual Book of ASTM Standards*, Vol 03.01.

[5] *Annual Book of ASTM Standards*, Vol 03.03.

[6] *Annual Book of ASTM Standards*, Vol 03.05.

[7] *Annual Book of ASTM Standards*, Vol 13.01.

[8] Available from American Society for Quality Control, 161 W. Wisconsin Ave., Milwaukee, WI 53203.

5.4 After all hot working-operations, the forgings shall receive an annealing treatment, when necessary, by heating the parts to an appropriate elevated temperature for a specified dwell time followed by rapid cooling to meet the applicable metallurgical requirements specified herein.

5.5 Optional identification marks, including the manufacturer's logo, material designation, heat code number, and impression number, may be placed upon each forging, the method and location of which shall be as specified by the purchaser.

6. Chemical Composition

6.1 When specified by the implant manufacturer, the chemical compositions of either the raw forging bars or the completed forgings shall be determined and confirmed by the forger, and shall meet the product analysis limits of Specification F 138, F 1314, or F 1586.

6.2 For referee purposes, Test Methods E 353 shall be used.

7. Mechanical Properties

7.1 The mechanical properties of stainless steel forgings produced from the three alloys of concern in this specification depend on a number of factors, including the specific alloy from which the forgings are produced and the fabrication practice. Different combinations of specific alloy and fabrication practice will provide substantially different mechanical properties.

7.2 When specified by the implant manufacturer, the mechanical properties of forgings shall be tested by the forger and shall comply with the minimum mechanical properties as specified by the implant manufacturer.

7.3 If tension testing is required, test specimens should be taken from a representative forging, if possible, or from a specially forged test bar only if the configuration does not lend itself to yielding the required specimen.

7.4 When desired, Rockwell hardness may be specified on the implant manufacturer's purchase order or print and shall be determined in accordance with Test Methods E 18.

7.5 The mechanical properties shall be determined in accordance with Test Methods A 370.

8. Special Requirements

8.1 *Corrosion Tests*— Forgings furnished to this specification shall be capable of passing the test for intergranular corrosion susceptibility in accordance with the current edition of Practices A 262, Practice E.

8.2 *Grain Size*—On the cross section examined, the grain size shall be predominately ASTM No. 4 or finer. No regions exhibiting grain size larger than ASTM No. 3 shall be allowed. Test procedures shall be in accordance with Test Methods E 112.

8.3 Other special requirements shall be as specified on the purchase order or print.

9. Certification

9.1 The fabricator's certification that the material was manufactured and tested in accordance with this specification, together with a report of the test results, shall be furnished to the implant manufacturer with each shipment.

10. Quality Program Requirements

10.1 The producer of material in accordance with this specification shall maintain a quality program as defined in ASQC C1 or equivalent.

10.2 The manufacturer of surgical implants or medical appliances shall be assured of or may audit the material producer's quality program for conformance to the intent of ASQC C1 or equivalent.

11. Keywords

11.1 forgings—surgical implants; metals (for surgical implants)—stainless steel; stainless steel—surgical applications

APPENDIXES

(Nonmandatory Information)

X1. RATIONALE

X1.1 The purpose of this specification is to characterize the chemical, mechanical, and metallurgical properties of wrought stainless steel forgings for surgical implants.

X1.2 The microstructural requirements contained in this specification represent the current general consensus with respect to optimization of mechanical properties for implant applications.

X1.3 This specification has been expanded to cover forgings of three specific alloys; each UNS designation has been included for clarification. A Biocompatibility section has been added as an appendix.

X2. BIOCOMPATIBILITY

X2.1 The material compositions covered by this standard have been employed successfully in human implant applications in contact with soft tissue and bone for over a decade.

X2.2 No known surgical implant material has ever been shown to be completely free of adverse reactions in the human body. However, long-term clinical experience has shown an acceptable level of biological response can be expected, if these materials are used in appropriate applications.

Designation: F 622 – 79 (Reapproved 1998)

Standard Specification for Preformed Cranioplasty Plates that can be Altered[1]

This standard is issued under the fixed designation F 622; the number immediately following the designation indicates the year of original adoption or, in the case of revision, the year of last revision. A number in parentheses indicates the year of last reapproval. A superscript epsilon (ϵ) indicates an editorial change since the last revision or reapproval.

1. Scope

1.1 This specification covers preformed cranioplasty plates that allow alteration for covering skull defects.

2. Referenced Documents

2.1 *ASTM Standards:*

F 67 Specification for Unalloyed Titanium for Surgical Implant Applications[2]

F 86 Practice for Surface Preparation and Marking of Metallic Surgical Implants[2]

F 90 Specification for Wrought Cobalt-Chromium-Tungsten-Nickel Alloy for Surgical Implant Applications[2]

F 136 Specification for Wrought Titanium 6A1-4V ELI Alloy for Surgical Implant Applications[2]

2.2 *ASQC Standard:*

C1-1968 Specifications of General Requirements for a Quality Program[3]

3. Terminology

3.1 *Definition*:

3.1.1 *cranioplasty plate*—an implanted prosthetic device used to repair or cover a skull defect or hole.

4. Materials

4.1 Cranioplasty plates conforming to this specification shall be fabricated from one of the materials covered by the following ASTM specifications or other such materials found acceptable for neurosurgical procedures only: F 67, F 90, and F 136.

5. Dimensions and Tolerances

5.1 Cranioplasty plates conforming to this specification shall be fabricated in a variety of dimensions to accommodate various sized skull defects. These plates may be altered in the operating room by the neurosurgeon in order to fit a particular skull defect.

5.2 The shape of the plate shall be contoured so as to reestablish the normal configuration and symmetry of the skull at various anticipated sites of defect, such as the parietal bosses, the inion, the brow, the linea temporalis, etc.

5.3 Plates shall contain multiple perforations.

5.4 Thickness and individual shapes shall vary with need. Thickness tolerances shall be as follows:

Specified Thickness, in. (mm)	Tolerances, in. (mm)
0.020 (0.51) to 0.035 (0.89), incl	±0.002 (0.05)
0.035 (0.89) to 0.050 (1.27), incl	±0.0025 (0.06)
0.050 (1.27) to 0.100 (2.54), incl	±0.003 (0.08)

5.5 For plates that are cast or hand-wrought, the establishment of tolerances is not practical and is the responsibility of the implant manufacturer.

6. Finish and Identification

6.1 Cranioplasty plates conforming to this specification shall be finished in accordance with Practice F 86.

6.2 Cranioplasty plates conforming to this specification shall be identified as to the material used for fabrication, in a manner in accordance with Practice F 86.

6.3 Tantalum cranioplasty plates shall be cleaned using a tantalum etching solution.

6.3.1 Prepare the tantalum etching solution as follows:

Hydrofluoric acid (H_2F_2)	48 vol %	4 parts
Sulfuric acid (H_2SO_4)	98 vol %	6 parts
Nitric acid (HNO_3)	70 vol %	3 parts
Water		13 parts

6.3.2 Use the tantalum etching solution at room temperature for a period of 15 min (Note 1). Wash with water immediately.

NOTE 1—The 15-min dip followed by a water bath is necessary to clean the tantalum cranioplasty plates.

6.3.3 **Warning**—The use of this solution should be under a hood as the fumes are toxic.

7. Precautions

7.1 When metallic sutures or screws are used to fasten the cranioplasty plates covered by this specification, they shall be of the same metallic composition as the specific plate being installed.

8. Packaging and Labeling

8.1 Cranioplasty plates conforming to this specification

[1] This specification is under the jurisdiction of ASTM Committee F04 on Medical and Surgical Materials and Devices and is the direct responsibility of Subcommittee F04.31 on Neurosurgical Standards.

Current edition approved March 30, 1979. Published May 1979.

[2] *Annual Book of ASTM Standards*, Vol 13.01.

[3] Available from American Society for Quality Control, 161 W. Wisconsin Ave., Milwaukee, WI 53203.

shall be packaged in accordance with federal regulations appropriate for such devices.

8.1.1 An insert shall be included in the package for the plate identifying the material from which it was fabricated. A recommendation against the use of fasteners other than the same material to secure the plate shall also be included.

8.1.2 Labeling shall include the nominal thickness of the plate.

9. Quality Program Requirements

9.1 The manufacturer of cranioplasty plates covered by this specification shall maintain a quality program such as defined in ASQC C1-1968.

10. Keywords

10.1 cranioplasty plates; neurosurgical medical devices/ applications

Designation: F 623 – 99

Standard Performance Specification for Foley Catheter[1]

This standard is issued under the fixed designation F 623; the number immediately following the designation indicates the year of original adoption or, in the case of revision, the year of last revision. A number in parentheses indicates the year of last reapproval. A superscript epsilon (ϵ) indicates an editorial change since the last revision or reapproval.

This standard has been approved for use by agencies of the Department of Defense.

INTRODUCTION

The objective of this specification is to describe those product requirements and associated test methods that will assure the safety and effectiveness of a disposable, 5-cm^3 (mL) balloon, retention-type catheter used in urinary bladder drainage.

This specification includes *referee test* methods that can be used to determine compliance with the stated performance requirements. Note that the test methods are not to be construed as production methods, quality control techniques, or manufacturer's lot release criteria. The product parameters addressed by the standard include those determined by the FDA Panel on Review of Gastroenterological-Urological Devices to be pertinent to the proposed classification of the Foley catheter to FDA Class II standards, plus other parameters determined by the ASTM task force to be pertinent to the product.

This specification represents the state-of-the-art at this time and is a minimum performance specification. It is recognized that the document must remain dynamic; suggestions for revision are encouraged, and should be directed to Committee F04 Staff Manager, ASTM, 100 Barr Harbor Dr., PO Box C700, West Conshohocken, PA 19428–2959.

1. Scope

1.1 This specification establishes performance requirements for the short-term utilization of a single-use, balloon-retention catheter, French sizes 12 through 26 inclusive, used by the medical professions for providing a means of bladder drainage by means of the urethra. The product is manufactured in various sizes and materials such as latex, silicone, rubber, and various polymers (as well as combinations of these) and is provided nonsterile for sterilization and sterile for single-use only. Catheters whose surface has been chemically treated to effect biocompatibility or microbial properties may be tested to this specification.

1.2 *Exclusions*—Long-term indwelling usage (over 30 days) is encountered with this product, but not commonly, and is therefore considered an exception to this specification. Similarly, the use of such catheters for nonurethral catheterization (such as for nephrostomy, suprapubic cystostomy, ureterostomy, gastrostomy, enemas, etc.) is excluded from the scope of this specification. Likewise, three lumen catheters, 30-cm^3 balloon and pediatric catheters, and catheters whose surface has been chemically treated to enhance their lubricity have not been tested to this specification and excluded from the scope of this specification and will require separate standard development.

1.3 *This standard may involve hazardous materials, operations, and equipment. This standard does not purport to address all of the safety concerns associated with its use. It is the responsibility of the user of this standard to establish appropriate safety and health practices and determine the applicability of regulatory limitations prior to use.*

2. Referenced Documents

2.1 *ASTM Standards:*

F 748 Practice for Selecting Generic Biological Test Methods for Materials and Devices[2]

2.2 *Other Documents:*

ISO/AAMI/ANSI 10993–1 Biological Testing of Medical and Dental Material and Devices — Part 1: Guidance on Selection of Tests[3]

U.S. Pharmacopeia[4]

3. Terminology

3.1 *Definitions of Terms:*

---

[1] This performance specification is under the jurisdiction of ASTM Committee F04 on Medical and Surgical Materials and Devices and is the direct responsibility of Subcommittee F04.34 on Urological Materials and Devices.

Current edition approved October 10, 1999. Published December 1999. Originally published as F 623 – 81. Last previous edition F 623 – 89.

[2] *Annual Book of ASTM Standards*, Vol 13.01.

[3] Available from American National Standards Institute, 25 W. 43rd St., 4th Floor, New York, NY 10036.

[4] Available from U.S. Pharmacopeia, 12601 Twinbrook Pkwy., Rockville, MD 20852.

3.1.1 *balloon (Foley) catheter*—an indwelling catheter retained in the bladder by a balloon that is inflated with liquid.

3.1.1.1 *Discussion*—A two-way balloon catheter has a drainage lumen and inflation lumen (see Fig. 1). Common balloon inflation sizes are 5 cm^3 with the 5-cm^3 balloon being used to hold the catheter in place for normal usage, and 30 cm^3 where so designated when a larger balloon is used. A three-way balloon catheter is used for continuous bladder irrigation, and features both a drainage lumen and an irrigation lumen (but as noted above is excluded from consideration in this specification).

3.1.2 *FDA*—the abbreviation for the Food and Drug Administration, the Federal agency under Health, Education, and Welfare responsible for the regulation of medical device products.

3.1.3 *French size*—a scale used for denoting the size of other tubular instruments and devices, each unit being roughly equivalent to 0.33 mm in diameter. Label French sizes are as follows:

French Size	Outside Diameter, in. (mm)
12	0.157 (4.0)
13	0.171 (4.3)
14	0.184 (4.7)
15	0.197 (5.0)
16	0.210 (5.3)
17	0.223 (5.7)
18	0.236 (6.0)
19	0.249 (6.3)
20	0.262 (6.7)
21	0.276 (7.0)
22	0.289 (7.3)
23	0.302 (7.7)
24	0.315 (8.0)
25	0.328 (8.3)
26	0.341 (8.7)

3.1.4 *lumen*—the channel within a tube.

3.1.5 *proximal*—refers to the balloon end of the catheter, since when in position for clinical use, the balloon end is proximal or closest to the patient.

3.1.6 *referee test method*—the method cited in the published specification for the device. This method and the corresponding requirements will be invoked when the performance of the medical device will be questioned. The manufacturer need not use this referee test method in his usual inspection and quality control.

3.1.7 *sterility*—generally, the state of being free of microorganisms. For purposes of this specification, sterility is defined as freedom from microorganisms when tested according to the methodology defined by the USP for nonparenteral devices.

3.1.8 *tolerances*—the allowable deviation from a standard size. In usual engineering practice, the maximum permitted size is denoted by a plus sign followed by the tolerance and the minimum permitted size denoted by a minus sign followed by the tolerance. In this standard the label French size has tolerances given for several dimensions. For example, +3, −1 means that a nominal 14 label French size can be permitted to go as high as 17, but not below 13. Another way of writing tolerance, when both tolerances are equal, is: ±2, meaning the 14 label French size must be between 12 French and 16 French.

3.1.9 *USP*—U.S. Phaarmacopeia

4. Requirements[5]

4.1 *Flow Rate through Drainage Lumen*—Label French size catheters 14 through 24 inclusive shall have a minimum average flow rate of 100 cm^3/min, and a label French size 12 catheter shall have a flow rate of 70 cm^3/min. Tests shall be conducted in accordance with 6.1.

4.2 *Balloon Integrity* (Resistance to Rupture)—The inflation balloon must be inflated easily with distilled or deionized water to labeled volume without showing any evidence of breakage throughout the test period. Leakage and failure to deflate are dealt with in 4.4 and 4.6. Tests shall be conducted in accordance with 6.2.

4.3 *Inflated Balloon Response to Traction*—The entire balloon of catheters label French size 14 through 26 shall not pass into or through the funnel barrel (Fig. 2). Tests shall be conducted in accordance with 6.3.

[5] Supporting data for this specification, which provides a rationale of the performance requirements and test methods, is available on loan from ASTM Headquarters, 100 Barr Harbor Dr., PO Box C700, West Conshohocken, PA 19428–2959. Request Research Report F04-1003.

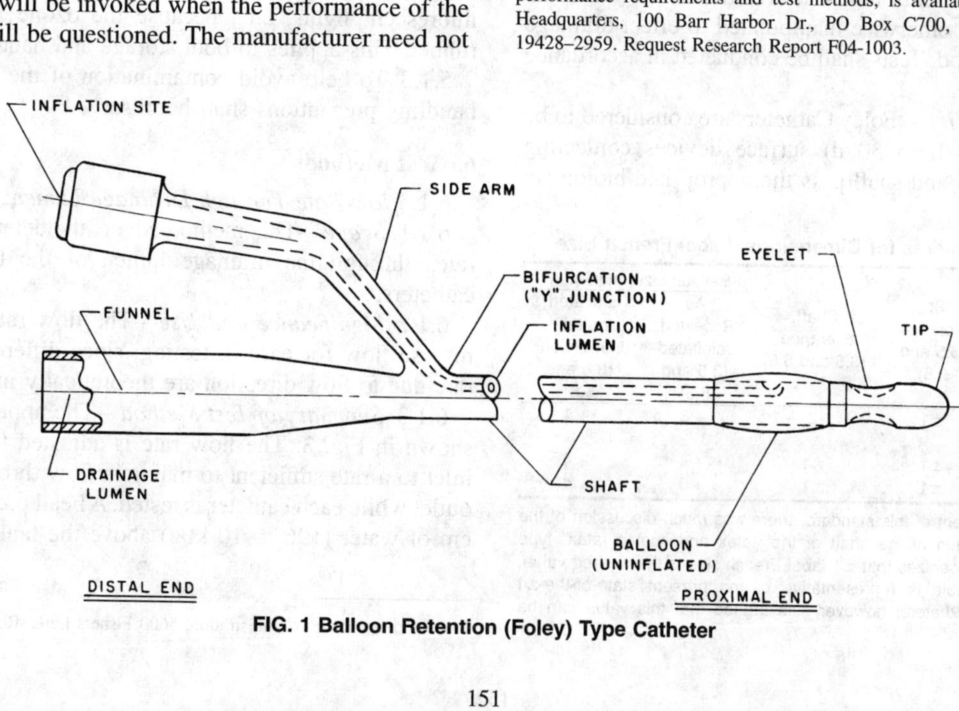

FIG. 1 Balloon Retention (Foley) Type Catheter

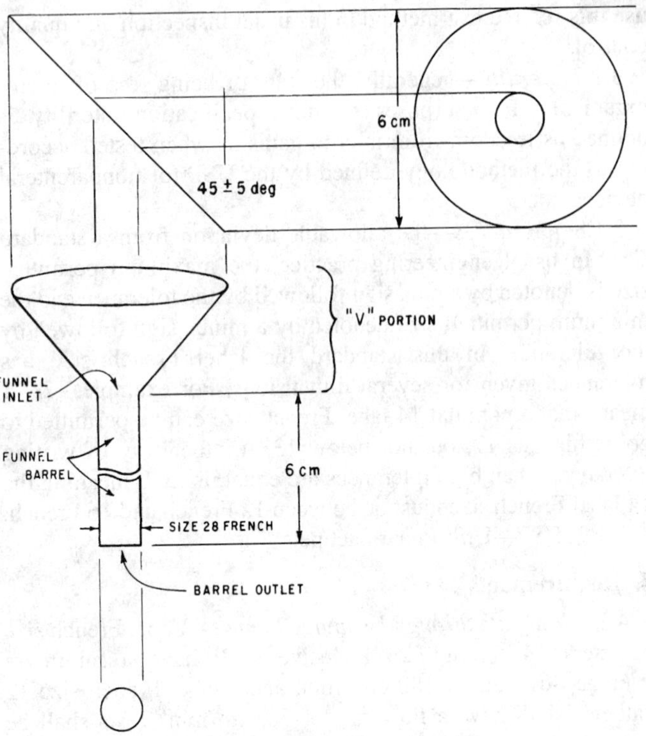

FIG. 2 Test Funnel

4.4 *Balloon Volume Maintenance*—The catheter shall maintain its volume throughout the test. Tests shall be conducted in accordance with 6.4.

4.5 *Balloon Size and Shaft Size*—The base dimension for the requirement on sizes and tolerances on the diameter of the catheter tip, the size of the balloon, and the diameter of the shaft is the "label French size." The proximal catheter tip, the balloon, and the shaft, for 10 in. distal to the balloon, shall meet the requirements on size and tolerances on diameter shown in Table 1. Tests shall be conducted in accordance with 6.5.

4.6 *Deflation Reliability* (Failure to Deflate)—The balloon shall deflate to within four French sizes of the label French size within 15 min or be otherwise manipulated to effect drainage within this time period. Tests shall be conducted in accordance with 6.6.

4.7 *Biocompatibility*— Foley Catheters are considered to be prolonged term (24 h to 30 d) surface devices contacting mucosal membranes and shall pass the appropriate biological tests conducted using the specification in ASTM Practice F 748 or similar guidance established by the U.S. Food and Drug Administration[6] or the International Organization for Standardization (ISO).[3]

4.7.1 The grading of any positive reaction that might be observed should reflect the degree of erythema or edema, or both, on the test sites. The pass or fail conclusion is based on the mild or severe nature of the reactions, respectively.

4.7.2 Criteria as to the microscopical evaluation of tissue reaction to the methods are included in this document. The question of pass or fail should be dealt with by reliable, competent scientists or pathologists and should be based on the degree of histological findings as compared with the response to the recommended USP polyethylene as "negative controls."

4.7.3 *Packaging and Labeling*—Packaged and individual items shall be properly labeled and conform to *(1)* legal requirements, *(2)* the needs of medical usage (such as size identification), *(3)* requirements for traceability and identification in event of failure, and *(4)* requirements for precautions in usage. In the majority of situations current GMP (good manufacturing practice) will provide guidelines for proper labeling.

TABLE 1 Requirements for Dimensions, Label French Size

Material Type	Tip, tolerance (3.5 and 5.5)	Shaft, tolerance (3.5 and 5.5)	Balloon size, maximum: As Received, Uninflated (3.5 and 5.5)	Balloon size, maximum: Deflated, after Immersion (3.6 and 5.6)
Latex and coated latex	±1	+ 2, − 1[A]	+ 3	+ 4
All-silicone	±1	±1	+ 4	+ 4
Others	±1	±1	+ 3	+ 4

[A] During the development of this standard, there was much discussion of the tolerance on the dimension of the shaft of the" latex and coated latex" type catheter. The industry recognizes that ±1 label French size is the desired value. The tolerance in this table is representative of the present state-of-the-art inmanufacturing Foley catheters; however it is argued that this value can be improved.

5. Special Precautions

5.1 The following cautionary comments recognize the sensitivity of the materials of construction to potential environmental conditions. These are outlined here to point out potential situations that could adversely affect the performance of the catheter during referee testing.

5.1.1 Care shall be taken during testing and use to prevent damage to the catheters. Such damage can be caused by abrasion and contact with sharp objects or chemical products. Contact shall be avoided with any of the following substances: vegetable oils, mineral oils or petrolatum, cleaning solvents, phenol, ether, cresols, oxidizing agents, copper, and manganese.

5.1.2 In addition, catheters should be kept away from the vicinity of generators, electric motors, diathermy machines, fluorescent lights, etc., because the ozone produced attacks rubber. This applies to both storage and handling.

5.1.3 To help avoid contamination of the catheters, proper handling precautions shall be observed.

6. Test Methods[5]

6.1 *Flow Rate Through Drainage Lumen*:

6.1.1 *Scope*—This method covers the determination of flow rates through the drainage lumen of the balloon retention catheters.

6.1.2 *Significance and Use*—The flow rate is measured in reverse flow for ease in testing, since differences in the flow rate due to flow direction are theoretically insignificant.

6.1.3 *Summary of Test Method*—The apparatus is set up as shown in Fig. 3. The flow rate is adjusted through the water inlet to a rate sufficient to maintain flow through the overflow outlet while each catheter is tested. A head pressure of 20 ± 1.0 cm of water (196 ± 10 kPa) above the tank bottom shall be

[6] Food and Drug Administration, 5600 Fishers Lane, Rockville, MD 20857.

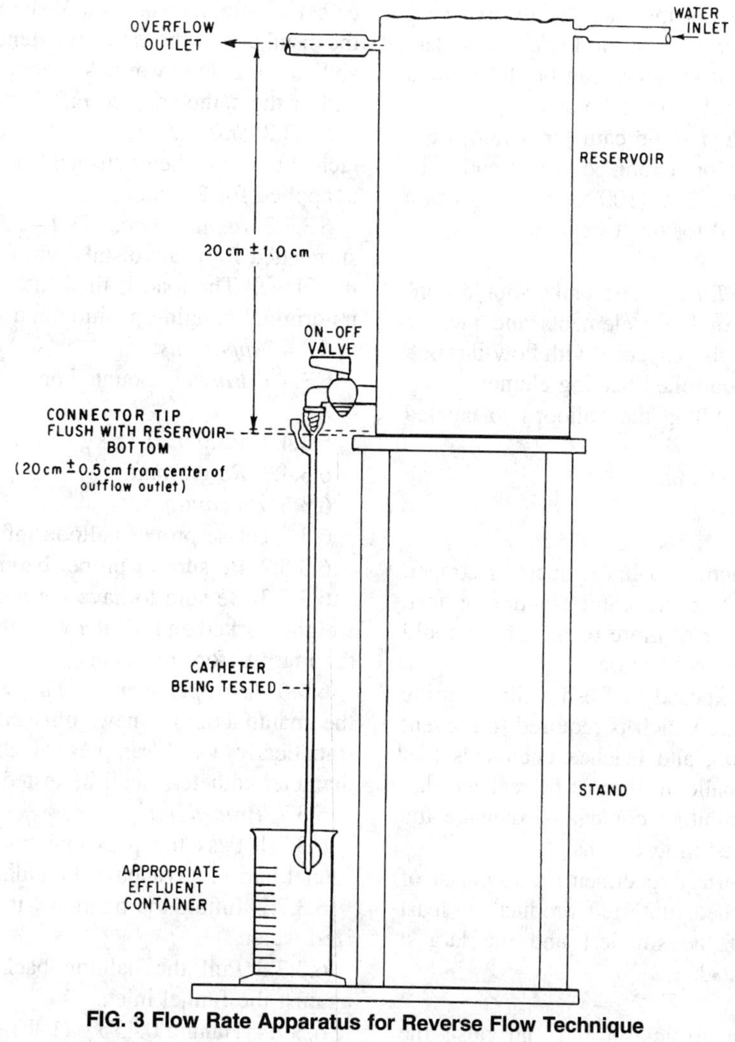

FIG. 3 Flow Rate Apparatus for Reverse Flow Technique

maintained throughout the test to approximate actual physiologic conditions. The overflow outlet should not be covered by water.

6.1.4 *Apparatus*:

6.1.4.1 *Water Reservoir*, capable of maintaining 20 ± 1.0 cm (7.9 ± 0.4 in.) of water (196 ± 10 kPa) above the tip of the catheter connection throughout the test as shown in Fig. 3.

6.1.4.2 *Graduated Cylinder*, calibrated for suitable measurement of the effluent.

6.1.4.3 *Syringe*, with appropriate tip for inflation of catheter balloon.

6.1.5 *Precautions*:

6.1.5.1 Overflow should not be covered. Head pressure must be kept constant; water should always be exiting through the overflow outlet.

6.1.5.2 Establish equilibrium prior to testing.

6.1.5.3 Flow rates through all fittings must exceed that of the catheter being tested.

6.1.6 *Test Specimen*— The test specimen shall consist of the manufacturer's new, finished, untested product; at least statistically valid samples of the smallest and the largest diameter catheters shall be tested.

6.1.7 *Procedure*:

6.1.7.1 Test at 23 ± 4°C (73.4 ± 7°F).

6.1.7.2 Inflate the retention balloon of the test specimen with distilled or deionized water to labeled volume. For example, a 5-cm^3 balloon should be inflated with 5 + 2, − 0 cm^3 of distilled or deionized water (or as recommended by the individual manufacturer on the label).

6.1.7.3 Connect the catheter to catheter connector and open the stopcock. The tip of the catheter connection at the junction of catheter on-off valve should be level with the bottom of the tank ±1 cm and it should deliver fluid at 20 ± 1 cm (196 ± 10 kPa) head pressure at that junction.

6.1.7.4 Establish the inflow and outflow equilibrium prior to test measurements.

6.1.7.5 Record the amount of water flowing through the catheter drainage lumen in 1 min. Express results in cubic centimetres per minute as flow rate. Test each catheter three times and calculate the average flow rate for each catheter.

6.1.8 *Interpretation of Results*—Flow rates for catheters tested must meet or exceed those established in the criteria section.

6.2 *Balloon Integrity* (Resistance to Rupture):

6.2.1 *Scope*—This method covers the determination of balloon integrity of Foley-type, balloon-retention, urinary drainage catheters.

6.2.2 *Significance and Use*—This method is designed to

simulate the actual intended use of the catheter, by exposing the balloon to body temperature for a period of 7 days. The balloon survival under effects of moisture can be determined during the usual life expectancy of the catheter.

6.2.3 *Summary of Test Method*—The catheter balloons are inflated with distilled distilled or deionized water and submerged in artifical urine at 37.8 ± 3° C (100 ± 5°F) for 7 days. The catheters are then examined for burst balloons.

6.2.4 *Apparatus*:

6.2.4.1 *Corrosion-Resistant Tanks*—The tanks should contain no exposed iron, copper or brass elements and include mixing and heating units of suitable capacity with flow-through water and a thermostatically controlled heating element.

6.2.4.2 *Device*, suitable for filling the balloons to labeled volume.

6.2.4.3 *Distilled or Deionized Water.*

6.2.4.4 *Artificial Urine.*

6.2.5 *Precautions*:

6.2.5.1 No materials destructive to latex, such as copper, manganese, or iron may contact the catheters during test. Copper content in the bath water of more than 50 ppm could seriously damage the balloons (see Section 5).

6.2.5.2 Catheters must be exposed to fresh artificila urine for each test period, a procedure which is required to prevent accumulation of bacteria, scum, and leached chemicals that could damage the catheter or balloon. It must be realized that bacteria or bacteriological inhibitors could also damage the balloons and should not be used in test baths.

6.2.6 *Test Specimens*— The test specimen shall consist of the manufacturer's new, finished, untested product; at least statistically valid samples of the smallest and the largest diameter catheters shall be tested.

6.2.7 *Procedure*:

6.2.7.1 Fill the tanks with artificial urine and raise the temperature to (37.8 ± 3°C).

6.2.7.2 Fill the balloons with distilled or deionized water to the labeled volume.

6.2.7.3 Fully submerge at least the entire balloon of the catheter in the tank.

6.2.7.4 After 7 days, inspect the catheters for ruptured balloons.

6.2.8 *Interpretation of Results*:

6.2.8.1 Any catheter whose balloon has burst during or after filling, up to the time of examination of the balloon shall have failed the test.

6.2.8.2 Any catheter whose balloon does not burst but which deflates during the test due to some form of leakage shall be an invalid test item.

6.3 *Inflated Balloon Response to Pullout*:

6.3.1 Scope—This method assesses the catheter's response to forces occurring during clinical use. Label French size 12 catheters shall be excluded from conforming to this test.

6.3.2 *Significance and Use*—The catheter, when subjected to reasonable traction forces, shall not be distorted and pulled through the bladder outlet of static and impact forces.

6.3.3 *Summary of Test Method*:

6.3.3.1 A funnel-like apparatus, with a size 28 French lumen, represents the bladder outlet and urethra. An inflated catheter balloon rests in the V-shaped portion of the funnel with the distal end of the catheter extended through the funnel barrel and hanging downward. A specified load hangs from the distal end of the catheter. (See Fig. 2 and Fig. 4.)

6.3.3.2 *Static Load Test*— A 0.45-kg (1-lb) weight is attached to the catheter suspended through the funnel. The load is applied for 2 min.

6.3.3.3 *Impact Load Test*— A 0.45-kg (1-lb) weight is suspended from the distal end of the catheter passing through the funnel. The load is then lifted vertically 0.6 m (2 ft) from its original hanging position and released.

6.3.4 *Apparatus*:

6.3.4.1 *Funnel*, mounted on a ring stand (see Fig. 2 and Fig. 4).

6.3.4.2 *Weight*, 0.45-kg (1-lb).

6.3.4.3 *Ring Stand.*

6.3.5 *Precautions*:

6.3.5.1 Use proper balloon inflation volume.

6.3.5.2 Be sure of proper balloon position before testing.

6.3.5.3 Be sure to have the natural suspension point of the weight marked and lift the weight vertically 0.6 m (2 ft) above the mark before releasing.

6.3.6 *Test Specimens*— The test specimen shall consist of the manufacturer's new, finished, untested product; at least statistically valid samples of the smallest and the largest diameter catheters shall be tested.

6.3.7 *Procedure*:

6.3.7.1 Pass the proximal tip of the catheter through the funnel barrel, advancing the balloon past the funnel inlet.

6.3.7.2 Inflate the balloon with 5 cm^3 of distilled or deionized water.

6.3.7.3 Pull the balloon back slowly until it fits snugly against the funnel inlet.

6.3.7.4 Hang a 0.45-kg (1-lb) weight from the distal end of the catheter.

(a) (a) Static Load Test—Observe the catheter balloon for 2 min.

(b) (b) Impact Load Test—There should be no obstruction to the free fall of the weight from a height of 305 mm (1 ft) above the base of the ring stand during its natural suspension.

6.3.7.5 Lift the weight 0.6 m (2 ft) from the point of its natural suspension and then release.

6.3.7.6 Observe the balloon position in the funnel inlet after the drop.

6.3.8 *Interpretation of Results*:

6.3.8.1 Passage of the entire balloon into or through the funnel barrel shall constitute a test failure.

6.3.8.2 Rupture (or other deflation) of the balloon shall constitute a test failure, regardless of catheter slippage.

6.4 *Balloon Volume Maintenance*:

6.4.1 Scope—This method may be applied to balloon-retention-type catheters to test their ability to retain injected balloon volume.

6.4.2 *Significance and Use*:

6.4.2.1 This method establishes a standard test method for determining the functional integrity of the inflation system of the balloon-retention catheter.

6.4.2.2 Since it is the function of the inflation balloon to

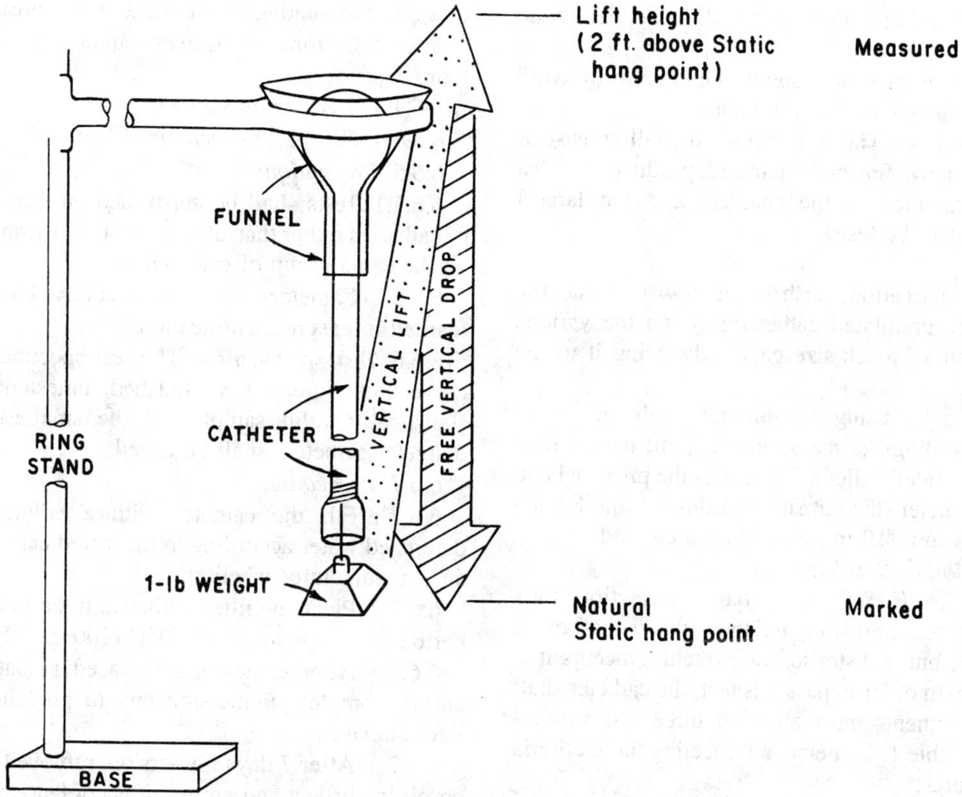

FIG. 4 Inflated Balloon Response to Pullout Test

keep the urinary catheter tip within the bladder and to permit drainage, it is imperative that the balloon inflate, retain inflation volume, and release that volume only when called upon to do so. The catheter balloon, therefore, is expected to maintain its volume throughout the test.

6.4.3 *Summary of Test Method*—The method is performed in order to identify inflation failure, and immediate retention failure irrespective of cause. A balloon is inflated to a labeled volume using colored solution from a device such as a syringe. The filled balloon catheter is then placed on a surface suitable for detecting color and leakage from the inflation system (such as a paper towel). The balloon remains filled for a 24-h period. After this time, the balloon is examined for leakage.

6.4.4 *Apparatus*:

6.4.4.1 *Syringe*, or other suitable inflation device.

6.4.4.2 *Distilled or Deionized Water*, for use as the inflation solution.

6.4.4.3 *Methylene Blue Crystal Solution or Equivalent*—Prepare 1 g of methylene crystals and dilute in 2000 cm^3 of water, to be detectable in the described retention test.

6.4.4.4 *Background Material*, suitable for detection of any leakage.

6.4.5 *Precautions*:

6.4.5.1 Assure that the syringe is properly seated in the valve.

6.4.6 *Test Specimens*— The test specimen shall consist of the manufacturer's new, finished, untested product; at least statistically valid samples of the smallest and the largest diameter catheters shall be tested.

6.4.7 *Procedure*:

6.4.7.1 Inflate the balloon with the methylene blue solution to the labeled volume.

6.4.7.2 Place on a surface suitable for detection of color leakage for a 24-h period. Cover or otherwise protect the catheters from light or ozone for the duration of the test.

6.4.7.3 After the test time has elapsed, observe the surfaces for any discoloration caused by content leakage from the catheter balloon-inflation system.

6.4.8 *Interpretation of Results*:

6.4.8.1 Failure to inflate is a failure of the liquid from the filling device (syringe) to enter the retention balloon.

6.4.8.2 Failure of retention is a discoloration of or leakage on the clean surface beneath the catheter.

6.5 *Balloon Size and Shaft Size*:

6.5.1 *Scope*—This method covers the determination of the Foley catheter balloon and shaft size.

6.5.2 *Significance and Use*—The overall outside diameter of the catheter during passage should conform to the expected urethral size.

6.5.3 *Summary of Test Method*—Using a French size gage, the proximal catheter tip is measured in holes close to the label French size. The balloon size is measured in larger holes. The catheter is then cut distal to the balloon and the shaft size is measured. The requirements are in Table 1.

6.5.4 *Apparatus*:

6.5.4.1 *French Size Calibration Gage*, having a tolerance of ±0.13 mm (±0.005 in.).

6.5.4.2 *Metric Scale Rule*.

6.5.5 *Precautions*:

6.5.5.1 No lubrication or undue force shall be applied to the catheter.

6.5.5.2 The edges of each hole should be smooth to avoid interference to the passage of the test catheter.

6.5.6 *Test Specimens*— The test specimen shall consist of the manufacturer's new, finished, untested product; at least statistically valid samples of the smallest and the largest diameter catheters shall be tested.

6.5.7 *Procedure*:

6.5.7.1 Without lubrication, push or otherwise thread the proximal end of the uninflated catheter through the various holes of the calibrated French-size gage, advancing it to the uninflated balloon.

6.5.7.2 Repeat 6.5.7.1, using the uninflated balloon.

6.5.7.3 After recording the measurements, cut the catheter just distal to the uninflated balloon. Then pass the proximal end of the remaining catheter (the cut surface) through the French scale to a point 254 mm (10 in.) distal to the cut end.

6.5.8 *Interpretation of Results*:

6.5.8.1 *Label French Size*—The balloon section may wrinkle but shall not tear or distort, and the catheter shaft or tip may offer resistance but if distortion or stretching occurs it is considered a failure. In order to pass this test, the catheter shaft and balloon measurements must meet all three test requirements as shown in Table 1. Catheters not meeting these criteria will be judged failures.

6.6 *Deflation Reliability (Failure to Deflate)*:

6.6.1 *Scope*—This method covers the determination of deflation failure risk of the balloon and deflation channel of the catheters.

6.6.2 *Significance and Use*—This test is designed to detect, in a wet medium, failures of the balloon and shaft lumen to deflate properly at the time of withdrawal. Proper deflation is critical to removal of the catheter from the patient following its use. Conditions of use are simulated.

6.6.3 *Summary of Test Method*—Inflated catheters that have been submerged for 7 days are deflated using a syringe (and "cut-off" method, if necessary).

6.6.4 *Apparatus*:

6.6.4.1 *Holding Bath*— A vessel of any suitable material (stainless steel, glass, fiberglass, or polyethylene) that will not deteriorate or discolor the material that the catheter is made of (see 6.2.4.1 and Section 5). The capacity of the vessel should be based on a minimum of 10 gal of liquid to 150 catheters. The liquid shall be kept at 37.8 ± 3°C (100± 5°F) by means of a suitable heating apparatus and thermostat.

6.6.4.2 *Calibrated Devices*, suitable for inflating the balloons.

6.6.4.3 *Scissors or Scalpel.*

6.6.4.4 *Distilled or Deionized Water.*

6.6.5 *Precautions*:

6.6.5.1 Tests shall be performed on separate sampling lots of catheters rather than attempting to perform three or four tests on the same group of catheters.

6.6.5.2 Catheters must be securely bundled and clearly marked to ensure identification.

6.6.6 *Test Specimens*— The test specimen shall consist of the manufacturer's new, finished, untested product; at least statistically valid samples of the smallest and the largest diameter catheters shall be tested.

6.6.7 *Procedure*:

6.6.7.1 Fill the catheter with a volume of distilled or deionized water according to the stated capacity of the balloon and manufacturer labeling.

6.6.7.2 Place the filled catheters in an immersion bath for a period of 7 days at 37.8 ± 3°C (100 ± 5°F).

6.6.7.3 After catheters are placed in bath, cover them to ensure complete immersion and to prevent evaporation and light damage.

6.6.7.4 After 7 days immersion, remove the catheters, place on clean surface and empty in accordance with the manufacturer's recommended technique or by use of the appropriate syringe or by the "cut-off" technique. Post-deflation shape of the balloon portion of the catheter shall pass through a calibrated French-size hole (or ring) no greater than four French sizes larger than the label French size. A force of no greater than 4.5 N (1-lbf) may be used to pull the catheter through.

6.6.7.5 Any catheter that fails to deflate using the syringe shall be cut off approximately 12.7 mm (½in.) proximal to the bifurcation of the inflation lumen and drainage lumen.

6.6.8 *Interpretation of Results*—Any cut-off catheter balloon that does not drain within 15 min shall be reported as a failure if it cannot be withdrawn through the appropriate French-size scale (not greater than four sizes larger than the label French size).

7. Keywords

7.1 balloon catheter; bladder drainage; urology

APPENDIXES

(Nonmandatory Information)

X1. RATIONALE

X1.1 Foley Catheters exhibit a range of physical properties that affect their clinical performance. These properties are affected by materials, manufacturing processes, and catheter geometry. This specification is intended to describe standard test methods to be used to measure the important functional characteristics of Foley catheters such as flow rate and balloon integrity, resistance to traction, volume maintenance, and deflation reliability.

X1.2 The objective of this specification is to describe the laboratory tests methods used to evaluate the safety and efficacy of disposable, 5mL balloon, retention–type catheters used for urinary bladder drainage. The minimum performance requirements presented include those determined by the FDS Panel of Review of Gastroenterologiacal-Urological Devices to be appropriate for a Class II medical device, as well as those determined by the ASTM Subcommittee to be relevant to Foley catheters.

X1.3 This specification includes referee test methods which are not to be construed as production methods, quality control techniques, or manufacturers' lot release criteria.

X2. CHEMICAL COMPOSITION OF ARTIFICIAL URINE

X2.1 This formulation artificial urine is based on the formulation propose by B. Finlayson **(4)** modified to include certain salts known to be present in human urine. The pH is adjusted to 5.5–7.0 range by adding a 1 normal (N) solution of NH4OH of NH4Cl to a 1,000 mL volumetric flask.

Salt	Mass (g)
NaCl	6.17
NaH2PO4	4.59
Na3Citrate	0.944
MgSO4	0.463
Na2SO4	2.41
KCl	4.75
CaCl2	0.64
Na2Oxalate	0.043
Distilled water	1000.

REFERENCES

(1) Autian, J., "The New Field of Plastics Toxicology-Methods and Results," *C.R.C. Critical Reviews In Toxicology*, Vol. 2, No. 1, 1973.

(2) Salthouse, T. N., and Matlaga, B. F., "An Approach to Numerical Quantitation of Acute Tissue Responses to Biomaterials," *Biomaterials Medical Device and Artificial Organs*, Vol. 3, No. 1, 1975.

(3) Wood, N. K., Kaminski, E. J., and Oglesby, R. J.," The Significance of Implant Shape in Experimental Testing of Biological Materials: Disc vs. Rod," *Journal of Biomedical Materials Research*, Vol. 4, No. 1, 1970.

(4) Burns, John R. and Finlayson, Birwell "A Proposal for a Standard Reference artificial Urine in In vitro Urolithiasis Experiments" *Investigational Urology*, Vol. 18, No. 2, pg. 167-169.

Designation: F 624 – 98a$^{\epsilon 1}$

Standard Guide for Evaluation of Thermoplastic Polyurethane Solids and Solutions for Biomedical Applications[1]

This standard is issued under the fixed designation F 624; the number immediately following the designation indicates the year of original adoption or, in the case of revision, the year of last revision. A number in parentheses indicates the year of last reapproval. A superscript epsilon (ε) indicates an editorial change since the last revision or reapproval.

ϵ^1 NOTE—10.1 was editorially corrected in May 2001.

1. Scope

1.1 This guide covers the evaluation of thermoplastic polyurethanes in both solid and solution form for biomedical applications. The polymers have been reacted to completion and require no further chemical processing.

1.2 The tests and methods listed in this guide may be referenced in specification containing minimum required values and tolerances for specific end use products.

1.3 Test values shall be stated in SI units with inch-pound units in parentheses.

1.4 Standard tests for biocompatibility are included to aid in the assessment of safe utilization in biomedical applications. Compliance with these criteria shall not be constructed as an endorsement of implantability. Since many compositions, formulations, and forms of thermoplastic polyurethanes in solid and solution forms are within this material class, the formulator or fabricator must evaluate the biocompatibility of the specific composition or form in the intended use and after completion of all manufacturing processes including sterilization.

1.5 Purchase specifications may be prepared by agreement between the buyer and seller by selection of appropriate tests and methods from those listed applicable to the specific biomedical end use.

1.6 *This standard does not purport to address all of the safety concerns, if any, associated with its use. It is the responsibility of the user of this standard to establish appropriate safety and health practices and determine the applicability of regulatory limitations prior to use.*

2. Referenced Documents

2.1 *ASTM Standards:*

D 149 Test Method for Dielectric Breakdown Voltage and Dielectric Strength of Solid Electrical Insulating Materials at Commercial Power Frequencies[2]

D 150 Test Methods for A-C Loss Characteristics and Permittivity (Dielectric Constant) of Solid Electrical Insulating Materials[2]

D 257 Test Methods for D-C Resistance or Conductance of Insulating Materials[2]

D 395 Test Methods for Rubber Property—Compression Set[3]

D 412 Test Methods for Vulcanized Rubber and Thermoplastic Rubbers and Thermoplastic Elastomers-Tension[3]

D 570 Test Method for Water Absorption of Plastics[4]

D 575 Test Methods for Rubber Properties in Compression[3]

D 671 Test Method for Flexural Fatigue of Plastics by Constant-Amplitude-of-Force[4]

D 790 Test Methods for Flexural Properties of Unreinforced and Reinforced Plastics and Electrical Insulating Materials[4]

D 792 Test Methods for Density and Specific Gravity (Relative Density) of Plastics by Displacement[4]

D 1238 Test Method for Flow Rates of Thermoplastics by Extrusion Plastometer[4]

D 1242 Test Methods for Resistance of Plastic Materials to Abrasion[4]

D 1434 Test Method for Determining Gas Permeability Characteristics of Plastic Film and Sheeting[5]

D 1544 Test Method for Color of Transparent Liquids (Gardner Color Scale)[6]

D 1638 Methods of Testing Urethane Foam Isocyanate Raw Materials[7]

D 2124 Test Method for Analysis of Components in Poly-(Vinyl Chloride) Compounds Using an Infrared Spectrophotometric Technique[8]

D 2240 Test Method for Rubber Property—Durometer Hardness[3]

D 2857 Test Method for Dilute Solution Viscosity of Polymers[9]

D 2990 Test Methods for Tensile, Compressive, and Flexural Creep and Creep Rupture of Plastics[9]

---

[1] This guide is under the jurisdiction of ASTM Committee F04 on Medical and Surgical Materials and Devices and is the direct responsibility of Subcommittee F04.11 on Polymeric Materials.

Current edition approved October 10, 1998. Published March 1999. Originally published as F 624 – 81. Last previous edition F 624 – 93.

[2] *Annual Book of ASTM Standards*, Vol 10.02.

[3] *Annual Book of ASTM Standards*, Vol 09.01.

[4] *Annual Book of ASTM Standards*, Vol 08.01.

[5] *Annual Book of ASTM Standards*, Vol 15.09.

[6] *Annual Book of ASTM Standards*, Vol 06.01.

[7] *Annual Book of ASTM Standards*, Vol 06.03.

[8] *Annual Book of ASTM Standards*, Vol 08.01.

[9] *Annual Book of ASTM Standards*, Vol 08.02.

D 3137 Test Method for Rubber Property—Hydrolytic Stability[3]

D 3418 Test Method for Transition Temperatures of Polymers by Thermal Analysis[10]

E 96 Test Methods for Water Vapor Transmission of Materials[11]

F 619 Practice for Extraction of Medical Plastics[12]

F 748 Practice for Selecting Generic Biological Test Methods for Materials and Devices[12]

3. Terminology

3.1 *Definitions:*

3.1.1 *chain extender*—(*1*) an active hydrogen containing compound such as a diol or diamine used to increase the molecular weight of an isocyanate-terminated prepolymer by chemical reaction; (*2*) a diisocyanate used to extend a polyol-terminated polyurethane by chemical reaction.

3.1.2 *chain terminating agent*—an active hydrogen containing a compound such as a monofunctional alcohol, amine, or acid that reacts with the isocyanate group of a prepolymer to prevent further chain growth.

3.1.3 *linear polyurethane*—a polymer whose backbone consists of urethane groups joined by hydrocarbon chains with little or no cross linking.

3.1.4 *segmented polyurethane*—A family of polymers in which ester or ether groups, connected by hydrocarbon chains, occur as blocks that are coupled by urethane and urea groups.

3.1.5 *thermoplastic polyurethane*—linear or segmented polyurethanes that can be melted for processing without significant crosslinking or degradation. They are most frequently synthesized by reacting diols with diisocyanates.

4. Significance and Use

4.1 This guide is intended to aid device fabricators in the selection of proper commercially available polyurethane solids and solutions for their application.

4.2 The polyurethanes covered by this guide may be thermoformed or solution cast into biomedical devices for use as surgical aids or for implantation as determined to be appropriate, based on supporting biocompatibility and physical test data.

5. Descriptive Chemical Information

5.1 *Diols*—Diols that can be used for biomedical applications are as follows:

5.1.1 Poly(oxypropylene).

5.1.2 Poly(oxytetramethylene).

5.1.3 Poly(caprolactone).

5.1.4 Poly(ethylene adipate).

5.1.5 1,4-dihydroxybutane.

5.1.6 Mixture of the above diols.

5.2 *Difunctional Diisocyanates*—Difunctional diisocyanates that can be used are:

5.2.1 Diphenylmethane 4,4-diisocyanate (MDI).

5.2.2 2,4-tolylene diisocyanate (TDI).

5.2.3 1,5-naphthalene diisocyanate.

5.2.4 1,6-hexamethylene diisocyanate (HMDI).

5.3 *Chain Extenders*—Chain extenders that can be used are:

5.3.1 Water.

5.3.2 Glycols.

5.3.3 Aliphatic and aromatic diamines.

5.4 *Chain-Terminating Agents*—Chain-terminating agents suitable for use are:

5.4.1 Monofunctional alcohols, such as methanol or ethanol.

5.4.2 Monofunctional amines, such as dibutylamine or diethylamine.

5.5 *Catalysts*—Stannous octoate is suitable for prepolymer preparation.

5.6 *Optional Additives*:

5.6.1 Pigments and dyes, such as titanium dioxide and copper phthalocyanine blue.

5.6.2 Radiopaque materials, such as barium sulfate.

5.6.3 Antiblocking agents and lubricants, such as natural and synthetic waxes.

5.6.4 Optical brighteners, antioxidants, and light and heat stabilizers.

5.6.5 The basic polymer bought may contain, as agreed upon between the purchaser and supplier, optional adjunct substances required in the production of the polymer or intended end use product, provided these substances are in minor amounts and are biocompatible in the recommended concentrations.

5.7 *Descriptive Information on Polyurethane Solutions*:

5.7.1 Solvent or solvents.

5.7.2 Percent solids.[13]

5.7.3 Solution viscosity—Test Method D 2857.

5.7.4 Infrared identity test—Test Method D 2124.

5.7.5 Recommended diluents.

5.7.6 Gardner color test—Test Method D 1544.

6. Processing Recommendations for Fabrication (by Supplier)

6.1 Drying conditions before fabrication.

6.2 Suggested optimum time, temperature, and pressure for injection molding, extrusion, or thermoforming to desired shapes.

6.3 Polymer stability at elevated temperatures of dry polymer in air or under an inert atmosphere.

6.4 Recommended storage conditions.

7. Suggested Physical Tests on a Solid Specimen or Film

7.1 *Tensile Strength*—Test Methods D 412.

7.2 *Ultimate Elongation*—Test Methods D 412.

7.3 *Compression Deflection Characteristics*—Test Methods D 575.

7.4 *Tensile Stress at 100, 200, and 300 % Strain*—Test Methods D 412.

7.5 *Flexural Strength*—Test Methods D 790.

[10] *Annual Book of ASTM Standards*, Vol 08.03.

[11] *Annual Book of ASTM Standards*, Vol 04.06.

[12] *Annual Book of ASTM Standards*, Vol 13.01.

[13] David and Staley, *Analytical Chemistry of the Polyurethanes*, Wiley Interscience Publishers, 1969, p. 359.

7.6 *Indentation Hardness (Durometer)*—Test Method D 2240.

7.7 *Flow Rate by Extrusion Plastometer*—Test Method D 1238.

7.8 *Compression Set*—Test Methods D 395.

7.9 *Abrasion Resistance (Taber)*—Test Methods D 1242.

7.10 *Specific Gravity*—Test Methods D 792.

7.11 *Hydrolytic Stability of Elastomers*—Test Method D 3137.

7.12 *Tensile Creep and Creep Rupture Test*—Test Methods D 2990.

7.13 *Gas Transmission Rate of Plastic Film*—Test Method D 1434.

7.14 *Water Vapor Transmission of Plastic Film*—Test Methods E 96.

7.15 *Water Absorption of Plastics*—Test Method D 570.

7.16 *Flexural Fatigue of Plastics*—Test Method D 671.

7.17 *Thermal Analyses*—Test Method D 3418.

8. Suggested Chemical Tests

8.1 *Isocyanate Group Content*—Methods D 1638.

8.2 *Amine Equivalent Weight.* [14]

8.3 *Ash.* [15]

9. Suggested Electrical Tests

9.1 *Volume Resistivity*—Test Methods D 257.

9.2 *Surface Resistivity*—Test Methods D 257.

9.3 *Dielectric Strength*—Test Method D 149.

9.4 *Dielectric Constant*—Test Methods D 150.

10. Suggested Biological Tests

10.1 The following tests are suggested for each product line offered for sale as a raw material for fabricating biomedical devices. Additional tests may be advised for certain devices as described by Practices F 619 and F 748 and USP Class VI testing guidelines.

10.1.1 Toxicological tests on individual batches of product may be made upon agreement between the purchaser and supplier.

11. Packaging, Labeling, and Preservation

11.1 The solid polymer should be packaged in a suitable container to avoid contamination and deterioration. An airtight container, capable of excluding moisture, should be used when necessary.

11.2 The polyurethane solutions should be packaged in nonreactive, noncontaminating containers to ensure product integrity.

11.3 The product should be properly identified including product and lot numbers, and, if necessary, a storage expiration date and conditions.

12. Keywords

12.1 plastic surgical devices/applications; polymers-surgical applications; polyurethane-medical applications

[14] *Ibid.*, pp. 87–89.

[15] *U.S. Pharmacopeia*, Vol 23, 1995.

APPENDIXES

(Nonmandatory Information)

X1. RATIONALE

X1.1 This document provides definitions and a standard description for thermoplastic polyurethanes in both solid and solution forms for biomedical applications. The guide enumerates relevant test methods and describes generic criteria which should assist in developing more specific specifications for implantable devices containing thermoplastic polyurethanes with values and limits covering end-use applications.

X2. BIOCOMPATIBILITY

X2.1 The suitability of these materials from a human implant perspective is dependent on the specific application. The biologic tests appropriate for the specific site, such as recommended in Practice 748 should be used as a guideline.

X2.2 No known surgical implant material has ever been shown to be completely free of adverse reactions in the human body. However, long-term clinical experience of use of specific compositions and formulations of this material class referred to in this standard has shown that an acceptable level of biological response can be expected, if the material is used in appropriate applications.

Designation: F 629 – 97

Standard Practice for Radiography of Cast Metallic Surgical Implants[1]

This standard is issued under the fixed designation F 629; the number immediately following the designation indicates the year of original adoption or, in the case of revision, the year of last revision. A number in parentheses indicates the year of last reapproval. A superscript epsilon (ϵ) indicates an editorial change since the last revision or reapproval.

1. Scope

1.1 This practice covers the procedure for radiographic testing of cast metallic surgical implants and related weldments.

1.2 *This standard does not purport to address all of the safety concerns, if any, associated with its use. It is the responsibility of the user of this standard to establish appropriate safety and health practices and determine the applicability of regulatory limitations prior to use.*

2. Referenced Documents

2.1 *ASTM Standards:*

E 94 Guide for Radiographic Testing[2]

E 142 Method for Controlling Quality of Radiographic Testing[2]

E 192 Reference Radiographs of Investment Steel Castings for Aerospace Applications[2]

2.2 *ASNT Standard:*

SNT-TC-1A Personnel Qualification and Certification in Nondestructive Testing[3]

3. Terminology

3.1 For definitions used in this practice, refer to the terms in Guide E 94, Method E 142, and Reference Radiographs E 192.

4. Significance and Use

4.1 The requirements expressed in this practice are intended to control the quality of the radiographic image of cast metallic surgical implants and related weldments.

5. Radiographic Methods

5.1 The radiographic method shall be agreed upon between the purchaser and supplier but should be in accordance with Guide E 94 and Method E 142.

5.1.1 Acceptance criteria should be derived from the reference radiographs presented in Reference Radiographs E 192.

5.2 Radiography of cobalt- or iron-base surgical implant castings may create film images resulting from grain diffraction. Radiographic techniques shall be utilized to ensure differentiation between these images and actual indications.

5.2.1 Generally, cobalt- or iron-base surgical implant castings require radiation intensities higher than normal, facilitating reduced exposure times.

5.2.1.1 Energies between 250 and 400 kV may be required to radiograph surgical implants with a ½-in. (12.7-mm) material thickness.

5.2.2 In some instances, filters, at the tube head, and relatively thick lead intensifying screens may reduce grain diffraction while sustaining adequate radiographic sensitivity.

5.2.3 Multiple radiographic exposures in which the implant is rotated between 5 and 180°, relative to the film, may help reduce grain diffraction. Additionally, multiple radiographic exposures in which the radiographic film is moved relative to the central ray of radiation also helps to change the diffraction pattern.

5.3 Radiography of titanium-base surgical implant castings may create a general mottled image, however standard low-energy radiation should produce acceptable sensitivity.

6. Sensitivity Requirements

6.1 Sensitivity of surgical implant castings shall be 2-2T, with the 2T hole clearly discernible, in the area of interest.

7. Metallurgical Requirements

7.1 In the absence of cast metallic implant standards at this time, the following requirements are suggested:

7.1.1 The product acceptance and rejection criteria shall be as agreed upon between the purchaser and supplier; however, indications which are linear in nature, generally, are unacceptable.

7.1.2 The mutually agreed upon acceptance or rejection limits shall employ ASTM reference radiographs or other radiographs, and where feasible, shall identify discontinuity of size and type levels.

8. Personnel Certification

8.1 The personnel performing radiography under this practice shall be certified in accordance with SNT-TC-1A, or recognized national equivalent.

8.1.1 The personnel performing radiographic interpretation shall be certified Level II or Level III individuals, or equivalent, in accordance with SNT-TC-1A or equivalent.

---

[1] This practice is under the jurisdiction of ASTM Committee F-4 on Medical and Surgical Materials and Devices and is the direct responsibility of Subcommittee F04.12 on Metallurgical Materials.

Current edition approved April 10, 1997. Published March 1998. Originally published as F 629 – 79. Last previous edition F 629 – 86 (1992).

[2] *Annual Book of ASTM Standards*, Vol 03.03.

[3] Available from American Society for Non-Destructive Testing, 3200 Riverside Drive, Columbus, OH 43221.

9. Report

9.1 A certified report shall be maintained showing radiographic test results including any rejected pieces.

9.1.1 Reports and radiographs, or an equivalent image of a radiograph shall be maintained by the purchaser for the life of the device.

APPENDIX

(Nonmandatory Information)

X1. RATIONALE

X1.1 The acceptance criteria for the radiographic examination of cast metallic surgical implants is based on reference radiographs presented in Reference Radiographs E 192.

X1.2 Specific radiographic techniques have been included to aid film image interpretation and ensure that adequate sensitivity has been maintained.

X1.3 Cobalt-, iron-, and titanium-base surgical implant castings may be radiographically examined according to the procedures referenced in this practice.

Standard Specification for Polyethylene Plastics for Medical Applications[1]

This standard is issued under the fixed designation F 639; the number immediately following the designation indicates the year of original adoption or, in the case of revision, the year of last revision. A number in parentheses indicates the year of last reapproval. A superscript epsilon (ε) indicates an editorial change since the last revision or reapproval.

1. Scope

1.1 This specification covers polyethylene plastics (as defined in Terminology D 883) intended for use in medical device applications involving human tissue contact devices, short term indwellings of 30 days or less, and fluid transfer devices. The biocompatibility of these materials as a class has not been established. Biocompatibility tests must be conducted on the final product.

1.2 This specification is not applicable to ultra-high molecular weight polyethylenes (UHMWPE) plastics, such as those used in joint implants, etc.

1.3 *This standard does not purport to address all of the safety concerns, if any, associated with its use. It is the responsibility of the user of this standard to establish appropriate safety and health practices and determine the applicability of regulatory limitations prior to use.*

2. Referenced Documents

2.1 *ASTM Standards:*

D 638 Test Method for Tensile Properties of Plastics[2]

D 671 Test Method for Flexural Fatigue of Plastics by Constant-Amplitude-of-Force[2]

D 695 Test Method for Compressive Properties of Rigid Plastics[2]

D 747 Test Method for Apparent Bending Modulus of Plastics by Means of a Cantilever Beam[2]

D 790 Test Methods for Flexural Properties of Unreinforced and Reinforced Plastics and Electrical Insulating Materials[2]

D 883 Terminology Relating to Plastics[2]

D 1238 Test Method for Flow Rates of Thermoplastics by Extrusion Plastometer[2]

D 1248 Specification for Polyethylene Plastics Molding and Extrusion Materials[2]

D 1505 Test Method for Density of Plastics by the Density-Gradient Technique[2]

D 1898 Practice for Sampling of Plastics[2]

D 1928 Practice for Preparation of Compression-Molded Polyethylene Test Sheets and Test Specimens[2]

D 2238 Test Methods for Absorbance of Polyethylene Due to Methyl Groups at 1378 cm^{-1} [2]

D 2576 Test Method for Metals in Water and Waste Water by Atomic Absorption Spectrophotometry[3]

F 619 Practice for Extraction of Medical Plastics[4]

F 748 Practice for Selecting Generic Biological Test Methods for Materials and Devices[4]

3. Significance

3.1 This specification describes polyethylene plastics used in the manufacture of medical devices or components of medical devices. The properties listed should be considered in selecting material according to the specific end-use requirements.

4. Classification

4.1 Types of polyethylene plastics molding and extrusion material are described in Specification D 1248.

5. General Requirements

5.1 Polyethylene plastics consist of basic polymers made with ethylene as essentially the sole monomer (as defined in Terminology D 883).

5.2 Polyethylene for use in medical applications shall have a maximum extractable fraction, expressed as weight percent in polymer, in *n*-hexane of 5.5 % at 50°C (**1**).[5]

5.3 The formulated compound may contain optional adjuvant substances required in the production of the polymer or in the fabrication or intended use of the end product. The biocompatibility of these adjuvant substances shall be established on the finished compound (see Section 9).

5.4 The formulated compound shall yield a consistent infrared absorption spectrum characteristic of the established formulation.

5.5 Maximum levels and type of extractable metals shall be established in accordance with the intended use of the formulated resin (**2**) (see Appendix X1).

NOTE 1—Appendix X1 is a suggested method for determining extractable metals utilizing the current state-of-the-art methodology. Alternative methods with equal reliability may be used.

5.6 The physical properties of polyethylene plastics may be

---

[1] This specification is under the jurisdiction of ASTM Committee F-4 on Medical and Surgical Materials and Devices and is the direct responsibility of Subcommittee F04.11 on Polymeric Materials.

Current edition approved October 10, 1998. Published March 1999. Originally published as F 639 – 79. Last previous edition F 639 – 98.

[2] *Annual Book of ASTM Standards*, Vol 08.01.

[3] Discontinued—See *1980 Annual Book of ASTM Standards*, Part 31.

[4] *Annual Book of ASTM Standards*, Vol 13.01.

[5] The boldface numbers in parentheses refer to the list of references at the end of this standard.

determined by the methods given in Section 7.

6. Sampling

6.1 The material should be sampled in accordance with standard sampling procedures such as those described in Practice D 1898.

7. Physical Methods

7.1 The following physical test procedures are suggested where applicable to the intended application:

7.1.1 *Density*—Test Method D 1505.

7.1.2 *Melt Flow*—Test Method D 1238.

7.1.3 *Tensile Properties*—Test Method D 638.

7.1.4 *Compressive Properties*—Test Method D 695.

7.1.5 *Stiffness*—Test Method D 747.

7.1.6 *Flexural Fatigue*—Test Method D 671.

7.1.7 *Flexural Properties*—Test Method D 790.

8. Packaging and Labeling

8.1 The product shall be packaged in a suitable container to prevent contamination of contents.

8.2 The material shall be identified including lot or batch numbers and recommended method of storage.

9. Biocompatibility

9.1 The biological safety of each polyethylene plastic formulation shall be established. Specific biological tests shall be determined in accordance with the intended use. Formulated compounds used in these tests should include all colorants and other additives present in the final product.

9.2 Biological tests are appropriate to determine biological safety and tissue reaction depending on the end use application. These tests should be conducted when indicated for specific applications. Additional tests may be necessary for certain cases; Practice F 748 and USP Class I–VI Biological Tests **(3)** may be used as guidelines.

10. Keywords

10.1 plastic surgical devices/applications; polyethylene (PE) plastics—surgical implant applications; polymers—surgical applications

APPENDIXES

(Nonmandatory Information)

X1. SUGGESTED PRACTICE FOR EXTRACTABLE METALS ANALYSIS OF PLASTIC BY ATOMIC ABSORPTION SPECTROSCOPY

X1.1 Scope

X1.1.1 This practice covers the analysis of extractable metals from plastics intended for use in medical device application.

X1.1.2 Formulated raw materials or finished products may be used.

X1.2 Referenced Documents

X1.2.1 *ASTM Standards*:

D 2576 Test Method for Metals in Water and Waste Water by Atomic Absorption Spectrophotometry[6]

E 117 Method for Spectrographic Analysis of Pig Lead by the Point-to-Plane Technique[7]

X1.3 Significance

X1.3.1 Concentrations of trace metals are measured as extracts in simulated body fluids. The metals concentration in extracts is based on the surface area of the plastic extracted from which the total amount of metal deliverable to the patient may be estimated.

X1.4 Preparation of Specimens

X1.4.1 Use suitable molded test strips of the formulated compound. The total surface area of the specimen to be exposed should be equivalent to 120 cm^2 when the specimen thickness is 0.5 mm or less or 60 cm^2 when the thickness is greater than 0.5 mm. Specimens may be separated from each other by suitable inert spacers to ensure contact with the extraction solvent.

X1.4.2 After the plastic sample has been prepared, extract the specimens using 20 ml of the desired solvent for 72 h at 50°C or 24 h at 70°C, as appropriate for the particular plastic. Then remove the plastic strips and analyze the extract for metals as described in Section X1.5.

X1.5 Preparation of Extract Solution

X1.5.1 Pipet 5.0 ml of the cottonseed oil (CSO) extract into a 10-ml volumetric flask and dilute to volume with hexane. Dilute the CSO atomic absorption standards and controls in the same manner.

X1.5.2 Run the saline eluate directly without dilution.

X1.6 Preparation of Atomic Absorption Standards

X1.6.1 Prepare certified aqueous standard solutions by diluting 1000 ppm of aqueous stock solutions with the 0.9 % saline solution used for extractions. Use the saline solution alone as the blank.

X1.6.2 Prepare the CSO standards by dissolving the appropriate organometallic compound in CSO to give intermediate solutions which are then diluted by volume 1 + 1 with hexane, giving final standard solutions of metal in the same matrix as the samples. Use a 1 + 1 dilution of CSO with hexane as the blank. Obtain the concentration analysis on organometallic standards from the manufacturer.

[6] *Annual Book of ASTM Standards*, Vol 11.01.

[7] *Annual Book of ASTM Standards*, Vol 03.06.

X1.7 Procedure

X1.7.1 Place the hollow cathode lamp for the element being tested in the instrument and set the instrument conditions for that element in accordance with the manufacturer's recommended procedure.

X1.7.2 When the lamp has warmed up, light the flame, adjust to the proper mixture, and allow to burn for 1 min to equilibrate the instrument. For the CSO-hexane mixtures, adjust the flame while aspirating the blank solution.

X1.7.3 Zero the instrument while aspirating the blank solution corresponding to the matrix to be analyzed.

X1.7.4 Aspirate a high standard and adjust the burner position and flame for the optimum signal and optimum signal-to-noise ratio.

X1.7.5 Rezero the instrument while aspirating blank solutions.

X1.7.6 Starting with the lowest, aspirate the standard solutions and record the absorbance corresponding to each. Between standards, aspirate the blank solution and check the zero.

X1.7.7 Aspirate the sample solutions and record the corresponding absorbance readings. Aspirate the blank solution and check the zero between samples.

X1.7.8 If there are many samples to be run, recheck the standards periodically during the analysis. In any case, reanalyze the standards after all the samples have been run.

X1.8 Calculation

X1.8.1 Prepare a calibration chart by plotting absorbance versus concentration.

X1.8.2 Calculate the concentrations of metal in the sample extracts by reference to the standard curve.

X1.8.3 Calculate the total amount of metal extracted as follows:

$$\frac{\mu\text{g metal}}{\text{ml extract}} \times \text{ml of extracts} = \text{total metal extracted, } \mu\text{g} \quad \text{(X1.1)}$$

X1.8.4 Calculate the amount of metal extracted per square centimetre of sample, μg/cm^2:

$$\frac{\text{total metal extracted, } \mu\text{g}}{\text{surface area of film, cm}^2} \quad \text{(X1.2)}$$

X1.9 Precision and Accuracy

X1.9.1 The precision and accuracy of this practice has not yet been determined. It is dependent upon several factors, such as, sample matrix, ionization interferences, sophistication of instrumentation, etc.

X1.9.2 Determine the precision for each test system in accordance with Method E 117.

NOTE X1.1—Pertinent data and other information regarding this specification may be reported to Committee F-4 Staff Manager, ASTM Headquarters, 1916 Race St., Philadelphia, PA 19103. Comments and suggestions will be considered in future standards development activities.

X2. BIOCOMPATIBILITY

X2.1 The suitability of these materials from a human implant perspective is dependent on the specific application. The biologic tests appropriate for the specific site, such as recommended in Practice F 748 should be used as a guideline.

X2.2 No known implant material has ever been shown to be completely free of adverse reactions in the human body. However, long-term clinical experience of use of specific formulations of this material class referred to in this standard has shown that an acceptable level of biological response can be expected, if the material is used in appropriate applications.

REFERENCES

(1) *Federal Register*, Vol 21, Part 177.1520.

(2) *Accuracy in Trace Analysis*, NBS Special Publication No. 422, U.S. Government Printing Office, Washington, DC, Catalog No. C-13.10:422.

(3) *U.S. Pharmacopeia*, Vol XXIII, 1995, pp. 1699–1703.

Standard Test Methods for Radiopacity of Plastics for Medical Use[1]

This standard is issued under the fixed designation F 640; the number immediately following the designation indicates the year of original adoption or, in the case of revision, the year of last revision. A number in parentheses indicates the year of last reapproval. A superscript epsilon (ε) indicates an editorial change since the last revision or reapproval.

This standard has been approved for use by agencies of the Department of Defense.

1. Scope

1.1 These test methods cover the determination, by radiography, of the radiopacity of plastic in the form of film, sheet, rod, tube, and moldings. The results of these measurements are an indication of the likelihood of locating the plastic part within the human body.

1.2 *Types of Tests*— There are three methods of tests described, differing in the method of calculating radiopacity.

1.2.1 *Method A*—Radiopacity is determined as a specific difference in optical density between the image of the plastic and the background on the X-ray film or equivalent.

1.2.2 *Method B*—Radiopacity is determined by comparing the images of the test piece and of a standard piece simulating the medical device.

1.2.3 *Method C*—The intrinsic radiopacity of a plastic is determined by measurements made on the image of a slab of a specific thickness of the formulation.

1.3 The values stated in SI units are to be regarded as the standard.

1.4 *This standard does not purport to address all of the safety concerns, if any, associated with its use. It is the responsibility of the user of this standard to establish appropriate safety and health practices and determine the applicability of regulatory limitations prior to use.*

2. Referenced Documents

2.1 *ASTM Standards:*

B 209 Specification for Aluminum and Aluminum-Alloy Sheet and Plate[2]

D 1898 Practice for Sampling of Plastics[3]

D 3182 Practice for Rubber—Materials, Equipment, and Procedures for Mixing Standard Compounds and Preparing Standard Vulcanized Sheets[4]

E 7 Terminology Relating to Metallography[5]

E 94 Guide for Radiographic Testing[6]

E 135 Terminology Relating to Analytical Chemistry for Metals, Ores, and Related Materials[7]

E 142 Test Method for Controlling Quality of Radiographic Testing[8]

F 647 Practice for Evaluating and Specifying Implantable Shunt Assemblies for Neurosurgical Application[9]

3. Terminology

3.1 *Definitions*—For definitions of terms relating to X-ray procedures, refer to Guide E 94 and Test Method E 142.

3.2 *Descriptions of Terms:*

3.2.1 *optical density*—in photographic photometry, the logarithm to the base 10 of the ratio of the incident light to the transmitted light (see Terminology E 135). The range of values of optical density expected in this test method is 0.5 to 1.5.

3.2.2 *contrast*—in this test method, contrast is the difference between optical density measurements made on the background (nominally 1.0 optical density) and on the test specimen.

3.2.3 *penetrameter*—a device employed to obtain evidence on a radiograph that the technique used is satisfactory. It is not intended for use in judging the size of discontinuities nor for establishing acceptance limits for materials or products.

3.2.4 *intrinsic radiopacity*—for this application, where the plastic is part of a medical device, the X-ray linear absorption coefficient is important. The following definition is excerpted from Terminology E 7:

absorption coefficient—specific factor characteristic of a substance on which its absorption radiation depends. The rate of decrease of the natural logarithm of the intensity of a parallel beam per unit distance traversed in a substance. For X rays, the linear absorption coefficient is the natural logarithm of the ratio of the incident intensity of an X-ray beam incident intensity of a beam of X rays, I_t the transmitted intensity, and X the thickness of the absorbing material, then:

$$I_t = I_e \exp(-\mu X).$$

Here μ is the linear absorption coefficient. The mass absorption is given by μ/ρ where ρ is the density.

3.2.5 *attenuation*—loss of energy per unit distance.

---

[1] These test methods are under the jurisdiction of ASTM Committee F04 on Medical and Surgical Materials and Devices and are the direct responsibility of Subcommittee F04.15 on Material Test Methods.

Current edition approved Oct. 26, 1979. Published January 1980.

[2] *Annual Book of ASTM Standards*, Vol 02.02.

[3] *Annual Book of ASTM Standards*, Vol 08.01.

[4] *Annual Book of ASTM Standards*, Vol 09.01.

[5] *Annual Book of ASTM Standards*, Vol 03.01.

[6] *Annual Book of ASTM Standards*, Vol 03.03.

[7] *Annual Book of ASTM Standards*, Vol 03.05.

[8] *Annual Book of ASTM Standards*, Vol 03.03.

[9] *Annual Book of ASTM Standards*, Vol 13.01.

4. Summary of Test Methods

4.1 The plastic specimen is laid on the cassette in the Xray apparatus and a 10-mm thick sheet of aluminum is placed on top of the specimen (or 15-mm thick, if so specified). The apparatus is equivalent to that used in a hospital. Radiographs are made at specified voltages, times, and currents that are typical of those used in the X-ray diagnosis of humans. The radiopacity of the material or medical device is evaluated in terms of the criteria described for the test method selected. Calibration is achieved by using both a standard specimen and an X-ray optical density standard.

5. Significance and Use

5.1 Plastics, being composed principally of chemical elements of low atomic weight, have little opacity to X rays. Compounds of elements of higher atomic weight are deliberately mixed into plastics to obtain radiopacity.

5.2 These methods are intended to determine whether the plastic part has the degree of radiopacity specified for its application as a medical device in the human body.

5.3 *Degree of Contrast*:

5.3.1 Using Method A, it is recommended that a specific difference in optical density between the background of 0.8 to 1.2 optical density (3.2.1) and the image of the test specimen be required in any specification for a radiopaque medical device.

5.3.2 Method B requires that the image of the medical device, or the image of the section of the medical device that is radiopaque, give as much contrast (same background optical density as above) as the image of a comparison standard simulating the medical device.

NOTE 1—It is expected that the dimensions and composition of the comparison standard will be specified in the standard for the medical device (see Appendix X1).

5.3.3 In Method C, the intrinsic radiopacity of a plastic is determined by comparison with an equal thickness of aluminum, and by the calculation of the relative linear X-ray attenuation (3.2.5) of the plastic based on measurements of optical density of the image of the sample, and of the image of the comparison aluminum piece.

6. Apparatus

6.1 *X-Ray Machine*, a medical-type (minimally full wave rectified).

6.2 *Inherent X-Ray Beam Filtration*, 2.5-mm aluminum equivalent minimum.

6.3 *X-Ray Film*, par-speed grade, used with par-speed intensifying screens. A grid may be used.

6.4 *Penetrameters*:

6.4.1 *Material*—The aluminum sheet on top of the test specimen and the step wedge (if used) shall be 99^+ % aluminum in accordance with Specification B 209 (typically, 1100 alloy). The comparison standard of Method B (7.1) shall be of the same metal, unless otherwise specified.

6.4.2 *Aluminum Sheet*— A 10.0 ± 0.15-mm thick aluminum sheet shall be used on top of the test specimen for all tests. If so specified in the standard for the medical device, a 15.0 ± 0.15-mm thick sheet shall be placed on top of the test specimen.

6.4.3 *Step Wedge*—A step wedge may be used instead of the aluminum sheet specified in 6.4.2, if it has the requisite thickness steps.

6.5 *Rubber Blankets*— Blankets incorporating X-ray absorbers may be used to mask areas outside that covered by the penetrameter (this prevents undercutting). Lead sheets may also be used for masking.

6.6 *Back-Scatter Protection*, as described in Guide E 94.

6.7 *Densitometer*— The densitometer shall be capable of measuring the optical density over the range from 0.0 to 3.0 optical density units, minimum. It shall have a measuring accuracy of ± 0.02 optical density units or better. The densitometer shall have been calibrated within 6 months previously by a method and calibration standard traceable to the U.S. National Bureau of Standards.

6.8 *Step Tablet*, [10] for calibrating densitometers.

7. Comparison Standards

7.1 *Method B*—The comparison standard shall be of similar dimensions to the medical device. Its exact dimensions and composition (see 6.4.1) shall be specified in the standard for the medical device.

7.2 *Method C*—The material of the comparison standard shall be Type 1100 aluminum (6.4.1), 2.0 mm thick, 25 mm wide, and 150 mm long.

8. Sampling

8.1 Sample fabricated stock shapes or molded items in accordance with Practice D 1898.

9. Test Specimens

9.1 *Film or Sheet*— The specimen shall be at least 150 mm long and 25 ± 1 mm wide. (For this specimen and the following it is assumed that the penetrameter covers an area of approximately 150 by 50 mm.)

9.2 *Rod or Tubing*— The specimen shall be at least 150 mm long.

9.3 *Molded Parts*— If the molded part has dimensions small with respect to the area covered by the penetrameter, then several moldings shall be placed under the penetrameter.

9.4 *Slab for Method C*—The dimensions of the specimen of the plastic shall be 2.0 by 25 by 150 mm.

NOTE 2—A 2.0-mm thick sheet is often molded especially for testing: for example, the description of sample in Practice D 3182.

10. Conditioning

10.1 The test shall be performed at Class 1 conditions (11.2.1), unless otherwise specified.

10.2 If other combinations of kilovolt peaks and milliampere·seconds are used, these exact conditions shall be described in the test report.

11. Procedure—Method A

11.1 Place the plastic test specimens on a cassette containing the X-ray film and the intensifying screens. Cover the test

[10] SRM 1001 has been found suitable for this purpose and is available from National Bureau of Standards, Office of Standard Reference Materials, Washington, DC 20234.

specimen with the penetrameter.

11.2 *X-Ray Exposure*— The recommended focus-film distance for all classes of exposure is 1000 ± 20 mm.

11.2.1 *Class 1*—The conditions for Class 1 exposure shall be:

80 to 85 kVp (full−wave rectified)

3.0 mA·s (must be varied)

11.2.2 The exposure shall be of such duration that an optical density of 1.0 ± 0.2 is obtained through a 10-mm thickness of aluminum (or 15.0 mm, if specified in the standard for the medical device).

11.3 *Film Development*— Develop the X-ray film in accordance with the manufacturer's instructions.

11.4 *Measurement of Optical Density*:

11.4.1 *Background*—Measure the background optical density to determine whether it is in the specified range, 0.8 to 1.2.

11.4.2 *Medical Device Image*—Measure the optical density of the image of the medical device.

12. Procedure—Method B

12.1 Expose the test specimen, with the comparison standard alongside it, to the X ray, in accordance with the procedure described in 11.1-11.3, inclusive.

12.2 *Measurement*— Compare the images of the medical device with the comparison standard on the developed film as to optical density.

13. Procedure—Method C

13.1 Expose the test specimen (9.4), with the comparison standard (7.2) alongside it, to the X ray, in accordance with the procedure described in 11.1-11.3 inclusive.

13.2 *Measurement*— Measure the optical density of the images of the test specimen (plastic slab) and the comparison standard, as well as the optical density of the background under the 10-mm thickness of aluminum.

14. Calculation

14.1 *Method A*—From the value of the optical density of the background (11.4.1), subtract the optical density value of the test specimen (11.4.2). Compare this difference, contrast (3.2.2), to the required contrast specified in the standard for the medical device.

14.2 *Method B*—Given that the background optical density is in the correct range (0.8 to 1.2), note whether the optical density of the image of the test specimen is less than, equal to, or greater than the optical density of the image of the comparison standard, as measured in 12.2. The radiopacity of the medical device meets the requirements if the optical density of its image on the developed film is less or equal to that of the comparison standard.

14.3 *Method C*—Calculate the percent relative linear attenuation coefficient, α, as follows:

$$\alpha = \frac{(B - S)}{(B - A)} \times 100$$

where:

B = background optical density, in the range 0.80 to 1.20,
A = optical density under the 2.0-mm thickness of aluminum, and
S = optical density of the image of the sample.

15. Report

15.1 The report shall include the following:

15.1.1 Test conditions, including the class, as described in 10, or the specific values of kVp and mA·s shall be listed. The focus-film distance shall also be listed.

15.1.2 Specification requirements, including the thickness of aluminum on top of the test specimen, the required contrast (Method A), the size of the comparison standard (Method B), or the percent relative linear attenuation coefficient (Method C), as listed in the requirements of the standard specification for the medical device. The number and title of the medical device specification shall also be listed.

15.1.3 Sample description, including name of manufacturer, type of device or plastic part, Catalog number or formulation number, dimensions of the test specimen, diameter, wall thickness, etc., and type of radiopaque additive and how it occurs in the part, such as a uniform dispersion, line of specific cross section, etc.,

15.1.4 Optical density readings for all optical density measurements as described in 11.4, 12.2, and 13, and

15.1.5 Calculations, reporting the contrast as calculated in 14.1, or whether the medical device is equivalent in contrast (optical density) to the comparison standard (14.2), or the percent relative linear attenuation coefficient (14.3).

16. Precision and Bias

16.1 The precision and bias of these test methods have not yet been established.

16.2 It is intended to develop data for the overall method and the measurement of density from a round-robin test.

17. Keywords

17.1 implants; plastic surgical devices; polymers; surgical applications; radiopacity; test methods; surgical implants

APPENDIXES

(Nonmandatory Information)

X1. VARIABLES IN RADIOPACITY OF PLASTICS IN MEDICAL DEVICES

X1.1 *General*—The initial development of this standard was based on the need to determine the location in the body of plastic parts of small diameter. This led to a proposed requirement for an optical density contrast measured on the medical device. However, radiopacity is a property of many types of medical devices and its required numerical level is influenced by many variables, some of the principal being: type of plastic; size, thickness, and configuration; part of body or circulatory system; and X-ray energy applied in the procedure.

X1.2 *Specification Values*—This standard does not have any requirements for minimum levels of radiopacity, nor that there be a preferred test method (of the three described). It is expected that a standard specification for the medical device will specify the required level of radiopacity, as determined by a particular test method (A, B, or C). The standard specification for the medical devices may also specify values for some parameters of the test method, such as: thickness of aluminum on top of the test specimen, whether 10 mm, 15 mm, or other; X-ray test voltage; and dimensions and composition of the comparison standard (Method B).

X2. COMPARISON OF THE THREE TEST METHODS

X2.1 *Method A*—It has been proposed that, for many applications, an optical density contrast of 0.10 is satisfactory. For larger pieces and thin sections of the human body, a contrast of 0.05 optical density units may be adequate.

X2.2 *Method B*—This test method has been considered to assure the radiopacity of a medical device. The dimension of the comparison standard, especially thickness in the direction of the X-ray path, does not have to correspond to the dimensions of the medical device.

X2.3 *Method C:*

X2.3.1 This test method is now being specified in Practice F 647.

X2.3.2 This test method may be necessary where it is difficult to characterize the radiopacity of the medical device, because of either its size or configuration. The remedy is to require a minimum radiopacity in the plastics formulation.

X2.3.3 From available reports on the development of medical devices, such as interuterine devices (IUDs) and from comments made by Committee F-4 members, it is obvious that radiopaque formulations are often measured by Method C. It has usually been done by comparing materials. Due to the variations in background optical density, it appears that a more reliable comparison and more reproducible test data can result if No. 1100 aluminum or other material with well-known X-ray absorption is used as a standard of radiopacity.

Designation: F 641 – 98a

Standard Specification for Implantable Epoxy Electronic Encapsulants[1]

This standard is issued under the fixed designation F 641; the number immediately following the designation indicates the year of original adoption or, in the case of revision, the year of last revision. A number in parentheses indicates the year of last reapproval. A superscript epsilon (ε) indicates an editorial change since the last revision or reapproval.

1. Scope

1.1 This specification covers thermoset plastics based on diglycidyl ethers of bisphenol A and amino functional curing agents or amine catalysts.

1.2 The epoxy encapsulants covered by this specification are intended to provide a tissue-compatible protective covering for implantable medical devices such as pulse generators, telemetry devices and RF receivers. The biocompatibility of epoxy plastics has not been established. Epoxy plastic is a generic term relating to the class of polymers formed from epoxy resins, certain curing agents or catalysts and various additives. Since many compositions and formulations fall under this category, it is essential that the fabricator assure safety of implantability of the specific composition or formulation for the intended use by current state-of-the-art test methods. This specification can be used as a basis for standardized evaluation of biocompatibility for such implantable encapsulants.

1.3 The encapsulants covered by this specification are for use in devices intended as long-term implants.

1.4 *Limitations*—This specification covers only the initial qualification of epoxy encapsulants for implantable electronic circuitry. Some of the requirements are not applicable to routine lot to lot quality control.

1.5 *This standard does not purport to address all of the safety concerns, if any, associated with its use. It is the responsibility of the user of this standard to establish appropriate safety and health practices and determine the applicability of regulatory limitations prior to use.*

2. Referenced Documents

2.1 *ASTM Standards:*

D 149 Test Method for Dielectric Breakdown Voltage and Dielectric Strength of Solid Electrical Insulating Materials at Commercial Power Frequencies[2]

D 150 Test Methods for A-C Loss Characteristics and Permittivity (Dielectric Constant) of Solid Electrical Insulating Materials[2]

D 257 Test Methods for D-C Resistance or Conductance of Insulating Materials[2]

D 570 Test Method for Water Absorption of Plastics[3]

D 638 Test Method for Tensile Properties of Plastics[3]

D 790 Test Methods for Flexural Properties of Unreinforced and Reinforced Plastics and Electrical Insulating Materials[3]

D 883 Terminology Relating to Plastics[3]

D 1042 Test Method for Linear Dimensional Changes of Plastics Under Accelerated Service Conditions[3]

D 1239 Test Method for Resistance of Plastic Films to Extraction by Chemicals[3]

D 1434 Test Method for Determining Gas Permeability Characteristics of Plastic Film and Sheeting[4]

D 1763 Specification for Epoxy Resins[3]

D 1898 Practice for Sampling of Plastics[3]

D 2240 Test Method for Rubber Property—Durometer Hardness[5]

D 2471 Test Method for Gel Time and Peak Exothermic Temperature of Reacting Thermosetting Resins[6]

D 2562 Practice for Classifying Visual Defects in Parts Molded from Reinforced Thermosetting Plastics[6]

D 2566 Test Method for Linear Shrinkage of Cured Thermosetting Casting Resins During Cure[6]

D 2734 Test Method for Void Content of Reinforced Plastics[6]

D 3137 Test Method for Rubber Property—Hydrolytic Stability[5]

F 74 Practice for Determining Hydrolytic Stability of Plastic Encapsulants for Electronic Devices[7]

F 135 Test Method for Embedment Stress Caused by Casting Compounds on Glass-Encased Electronic Components[7]

F 602 Criteria for Implantable Thermoset Epoxy Plastics[8]

F 748 Practice For Selecting Generic Biological Test Methods for Materials and Devices[8]

F 895 Test Method for Agar Diffusion Cell Culture Screening for Cytotoxicity[8]

F 981 Practice for Assessment of Compatibility of Biomaterials for Surgical Implants with Respect to Effect of Materials on Muscle and Bone[8]

---

[1] This specification is under the jurisdiction of ASTM Committee F-4 on Medical and Surgical Materials and Devices and is the direct responsibility of Subcommittee F04.11 on Polymeric Materials.

Current edition approved October 10, 1998. Published March 1999. Originally published as F 641 – 79. Last previous edition F 641 – 98.

[2] *Annual Book of ASTM Standards*, Vol 10.01.

[3] *Annual Book of ASTM Standards*, Vol 08.01.

[4] *Annual Book of ASTM Standards*, Vol 15.09.

[5] *Annual Book of ASTM Standards*, Vol 09.01.

[6] *Annual Book of ASTM Standards*, Vol 08.02.

[7] *Annual Book of ASTM Standards*, Vol 10.04.

[8] *Annual Book of ASTM Standards*, Vol 13.01.

2.2 *AAMI Standard:*
EOS-D E-O Sterilization Standard[9]

3. Classification

3.1 Encapsulants shall be classified as follows:

3.1.1 *Type I*—Those encapsulants which contact the tissue directly or indirectly.

3.1.2 *Type II*—Those encapsulants used only within hermetically sealed containers. The epoxy encapsulant has no contact with tissues or physiological fluids.

4. Chemical Composition

4.1 *Additives* (Type I Encapsulants Only):

4.1.1 *Reactive Diluents*—The following compounds when used as reactive diluents shall not be used in concentrations greater than 12 parts per hundred resin (phr).

4.1.1.1 Butyl glycidyl ether (BGE).

4.1.1.2 Phenyl glycidyl ether (PGE).

4.1.2 *Other Additives* (see Note 1)—Other additives shall be shown to be nonextractable in 37°C physiological saline for the device design life in concentrations sufficient to significantly affect the properties of the encapsulant or to produce a significant biological reaction.

NOTE 1—Other additives, as indicated in Criteria F 602, include compounds such as nonreactive diluents, fillers, release agents, and the like.

4.1.3 *Phthalate Esters*—Phthalate esters such as dibutyl phthalate shall not be used in concentrations ≥10 phr.

4.2 *Mix Ratios* (Type I and Type II Encapsulants):

4.2.1 *Amines*—The mix ratio shall be maintained at ±5 equivalent % of stoichiometry.

4.2.2 *Catalysts*—The mix ratio shall be maintained within the ranges recommended by the formulator.

4.3 *Carbonates* (Type I and Type II Encapsulants)—The encapsulant shall be poured under conditions such that the formation of amine carbonates is minimized. The device manufacturer may specify maximum limits of carbon dioxide or water vapor, or both, in the atmosphere in which the encapsulant is being mixed or poured.

5. Physical Properties

5.1 *Type I Encapsulants*:

5.1.1 *Peak Exotherm Temperature* (Test Method D 2471)—The peak exotherm temperature during cure shall be kept below the maximum acceptable value for the lowest temperature rated component of the device.

5.1.2 *Fully Cured Specimens*—The required properties measured on fully cured specimens conditioned as in 6.1 are as follows:

5.1.2.1 *Transparency*—In cases where no fillers or reinforcements are used, the encapsulant shall have sufficient transparency so that the circuitry may be visually inspected after encapsulation.

5.1.2.2 *Foreign Particles*—No foreign particles, particulate matter and gross contamination shall be observed when checked under 2× wide field magnification.

5.1.2.3 *USP Biological Tests Plastic Containers, Class IV*[10]—Pass.

5.1.2.4 USP Pyrogen Test[11] or other Pyrogen methods which have been demonstrated to be of equal or greater sensitivity—Pass.

5.1.2.5 *Sterilant Residues* (AAMI EOS-D)—Where applicable, the concentration of ethylene oxide, ethylene chlorohydrin, ethylene glycol, and dichlorodifluoromethane (or the equivalents) at the time of implant shall be shown to be within safe limits prescribed by the device manufacturer.

5.1.2.6 The cure shrinkage (Test Method D 2566) or embedment stress (Test Method F 135) shall be ≤2%. The stress shall not exceed the limits of the most pressure-sensitive components.

5.1.2.7 Tissue Culture Test (Agar Overlay)[12] or Test Method F 895—Pass.

5.1.2.8 While cell culture methods as described in Test Method F 895 may be appropriated for the batch-to-batch screening of fully cured specimens, the basic recipe used should have been qualified for its overall tissue response by methods such as those suggested in Practice F 748 for "Implanted Devices Principally Contacting Tissue and Tissue Fluid" including testing according to Practice F 981.

5.1.3 *Required Cured Properties Measured in Long-Term Immersion Tests for Type I Encapsulants*—The property values prescribed in Table 1 shall be obtained at 22 ± 3°C and 50 ± 10 % relative humidity on specimens conditioned as in 6.3. Samples shall be wiped dry prior to test with a lint-free tissue, as appropriate.

5.1.4 Optional cured properties measured after accelerated immersion for Type I encapsulants may be determined for screening purposes after conditioning as in 6.2.

5.2 *Type II Encapsulants*:

5.2.1 *Peak Exotherm Temperature* (Test Method D 2471)—The peak exotherm temperature during cure shall be kept below the maximum acceptable value for the lowest temperature rated component of the device.

5.2.2 The property values prescribed in Table 2 shall be determined at 22 ± 3°C (71.6 ± 5.7°F) and 50± 10 % relative humidity on fully cured samples conditioned as in 6.1.

6. Specimen Preparation

6.1 *Preparation*—Prepare specimens used for evaluation of properties of the cured material in the same manner as the intended product. Such conditioning shall include all specified relevant variables for the product prior to implant including specimen size or shape, cure time, cure temperature, post-cure, cleaning, packaging, sterilization, and aeration.

6.2 *Accelerated Immersion*:

6.2.1 For screening purposes, immerse specimens prepared as in 6.1 in refluxing physiological saline of pH 7.4 ± 0.2 for 7 days.

6.2.2 Prior to evaluation, allow the specimens to equilibrate to the test temperature of 22 ± 3°C (71 ± 5°F) in physiological

[9] Available from Association for Advancement of Medical Instrumentation, 1500 Wilson Blvd., Suite 417, Arlington, VA 22209.

[10] *U.S. Pharmacopeia*, XXIII, 1995, pp. 1783-1787.

[11] *Ibid.*, pp. 1696-1697.

[12] Guess, W. L., et al., *Journal of Pharmaceutical Sciences*, Vol 54, 1965, pp. 1545–1547.

TABLE 1 Cure Requirements for Long-Term Immersion Tests for Type I Encapsulants

Property	Requirement	ASTM Method
Extraction	<1 % in water	D 1239
Water absorption	≤4 %	D 570
Dielectric strength	>11.8 kV/mm	D 149
Dielectric constant	>2.0	D 150
Dissipation factor	<0.05	D 150
Elongation	>1.5 %	D 638
Flexural strength	≥1380 MPa	D 790
Gas permeation	[A]	D 1434
Hardness	≥60 Shore D	D 2240
Dimensional stability	<0.5 % change	D 1042
Tangent modulus	≥1380 MPa	D 638
Tensile strength (with outgassing power sources)	≥55 MPa	D 638
Tensile strength (without outgassing power sources)	≥7 MPa	D 638
Visual defects	none that adversely affect the safety, efficacy, or reliability of the device	D 2562
Voids	none that adversely affect the safety, efficacy, or reliability of the device	D 2734
Volume resistivity	$10^{10}\Omega\cdot$ cm	D 257

[A]For those devices containing gas-evolving power sources, the hydrogen permeation coefficient shall be 1.18×10^{-3}[(STP)(cm^3)(mm)/(atm)(day)(cm^2)]; or the encapsulant shall allow the escape of 0.06 cm^3 of hydrogen per cell day; or provision shall be made to ensure that gaseous material evolving from the power sources will be adequately disposed of in such a manner that the encapsulant is not comprised.

TABLE 2 Cure Requirements for Long-Term Immersion Tests for Type II Encapsulants

Property	Requirement	ASTM Method
Foreign particles	none visible	...
Cure shrinkage or embedment stress	≤2 %	D 2566 or F135, respectively
Dielectric constant	>2.0	D 150
Dielectric strength	>11.8 kV/mm	D 149
Dissipation factor	<0.05	D 150
Dimensional stability	<0.5 % change	D 1042
Visual defects	none that adversely affect the safety, efficacy, or reliability of the device	D 2562
Voids	none that adversely affect the safety, efficacy, or reliability of the device	D 2734
Volume resistivity	$10^{10}\Omega\cdot$cm	D 257

saline of pH 7.4 ± 0.2.

6.2.3 Condition one set of controls at 100 ± 3°C (212 ± 5°F) and another set at 22 ± 3°C (71.6 ± 5°F) for 7 days at 50 ± 10 % relative humidity.

6.2.4 Since two variables, heat and moisture, are inherent in this test, data from specimens refluxed 7 days in saline may be compared to controls conditioned dry at 100°C and at 22°C. Thus, one may estimate the long-term effects of moisture as opposed to the effects of moisture and heat or heat alone.

6.3 *Long-Term Immersion* (Test Method D 3137 or Practice F 74):

6.3.1 Prepare the specimens in accordance with 6.1.

6.3.2 During initial qualification of the formulation, immerse specimens in 37 ± 3°C (73 ± 5°F) aerated physiological saline of pH 7.4 ± 0.2 with periodic sampling for evaluation as is appropriate for a period of time consistent with projected service life. It is required that immersion continue for the projected service life of the device. For devices intended for long-term implant, however, it may not be practical to complete tank tests over the device's projected service life before one can claim compliance with the specification. One shall be considered in compliance with this section of the specification, therefore, if specimens meet the requirements of 5.4 after 1 year's immersion.

6.3.3 Store controls at 22 ± 3°C (71 ± 5°F) and 50 ± 10 % relative humidity.

7. Inspection

7.1 As a minimum, the following methods shall be used to characterize the formulation prior to mixing:

7.1.1 Infrared spectroscopy on each component.

7.1.2 Amine number on curing agent.

7.1.3 Epoxide equivalent weight on resin.

7.2 As a minimum, the following methods shall be used to characterize the "mixed" or "hardened" polymer:

7.2.1 Infrared spectroscopy.

7.2.2 Spectrographic analysis.

7.2.3 Total nitrogen.

8. Packaging and Package Marking

8.1 Packaging shall bear appropriate lot numbers that directly relate to the identification of the homogeneous batches which are the source of the encapsulant.

8.2 Packaging shall provide appropriate protection for the epoxy components of the device.

9. Keywords

9.1 encapsulants; evaluation of biocompatibility; implantable medical devices

APPENDIXES

(Nonmandatory Information)

X1. RATIONALE

X1.1 Epoxies as a general class of thermoset polymers may exhibit a wide range of properties depending upon the formulation. This specification is intended to describe minimum requirements for materials for use as encapsulants in implantable electronic components. It remains the responsibility of the device manufacturer to determine whether the particular formulation utilizes meets other specific requirements of the particular end use application.

X1.2 Epoxy encapsulants have been used in the manufacture of implantable electronic components for many years and have been found to exhibit acceptable tissue response. Whenever changes are made in the formulation of an encapsulant, the possibility exists that there may be changes in the tissue response. This specification therefore calls for requalification of different formulations to assure no adverse effects on the tissue response while allowing for cell culture screening batch-to-batch. This specification does not attempt to address the amount of change in formulation which would necessitate re-testing. The material and device manufactures will need to make that determination based upon their own experience, published data, and consultations with experts experienced in this area.

X2. BIOCOMPATIBILITY

X2.1 The suitability of these materials from a human implant perspective is dependent on the specific application. The biologic tests appropriate for the specific site, such as recommended in Practice F 748 should be used as a guideline.

X2.2 No known surgical implant material has ever been shown to be completely free of adverse reactions in the human body. However, long-term clinical experience of use of specific compositions and formulations of this material class referred to in this standard has shown that an acceptable level of biological response can be expected, if the material is used in appropriate applications.

Designation: F 647 – 94 (Reapproved 2000)

Standard Practice for Evaluating and Specifying Implantable Shunt Assemblies for Neurosurgical Application[1]

This standard is issued under the fixed designation F 647; the number immediately following the designation indicates the year of original adoption or, in the case of revision, the year of last revision. A number in parentheses indicates the year of last reapproval. A superscript epsilon (ε) indicates an editorial change since the last revision or reapproval.

INTRODUCTION

A hydrocephalus shunt assembly is a one-way pressure-activated or flow-controlling device or combination of devices intended to be surgically implanted in the body of a patient with hydrocephalus and designed to divert cerebrospinal fluid (CSF) from fluid compartments in the central nervous system (CNS) (the cerebral ventricles or other site within the cerebrospinal fluid system) to an internal delivery site (internal shunt) in another part of the body or an external collection site (external shunt), for the purpose of relieving elevated intracranial pressure or CSF volume.

A hydrocephalus shunt system typically consists of three basic elements: (1) an inflow (proximal) catheter, which drains CSF from the ventricular system, lumbar subarachnoid space or extraventricular structure and transmits it to (2) an arrangement of one or more valves which regulate(s) the differential pressure or controls flow through the system, and (3) an outflow (distal) catheter which drains CSF into the cardiovascular system via the peritoneal cavity, heart or other suitable drainage site. In addition, specialized accessory devices such as reservoirs, antisiphon devices and on-off valves and filters are added at the discretion of the physician to modify performance or adapt the basic system to the specialized needs of the patient.

Because of the considerable length of time over which a shunt or component may be required to function after implantation, it is felt that it should be type-tested to ensure its durability. It has not yet been found feasible to specify a test method of durability testing, but a test method is proposed in Appendix X1.

1. Scope

1.1 This practice covers requirements for the evaluation and specification of implantable shunts as related to resistance to flow, direction of flow, materials, radiopacity, mechanical properties, finish, sterility, and labeling of shunt assemblies.

1.2 Devices to which this practice is applicable include, but are not limited to, those that are temporarily implanted to effect external drainage; or permanently implanted to effect shunting of fluid from a cerebral ventricle, a cyst, the subarachnoid space to the peritoneal cavity, the venous circulation, or some other suitable internal delivery site, and intracranial bypass.

1.3 *Limitations*—Although this practice includes a standard test method for the evaluation of pressure/flow characteristics of shunts or shunt components, it does not include specific pressure/flow requirements.

1.4 The following components, that individually or in combination comprise shunt assemblies, are considered to be within the scope of this practice: catheters (such as atrial, peritoneal, ventricular), connectors, implantable accessory devices (such as antisiphon devices and reservoirs), valved catheters and valves.

1.5 *This standard does not purport to address all of the safety concerns, if any, associated with its use. It is the responsibility of the user of this standard to establish appropriate safety and health practices and determine the applicability of regulatory limitations prior to use.*

NOTE 1—The following standards contain provisions that, through reference in this text, constitute provisions of this practice. At the time of publication, the editions indicated are valid. All standards are subject to revision, and parties to agreements based on this practice are encouraged to investigate the possibility of applying the most recent editions of the standards indicated below. Devices or components, or both, whose structures are comparable to that outlined in these standards are acceptable.

---

[1] This practice is under the jurisdiction of ASTM Committee F04 on Surgical Materials and Devices and is the direct responsibility of Subcommittee F4.31 on Neurosurgical Standards.

Current edition approved June 15, 1994. Published August 1994. Originally published as F 647 – 79. Last previous edition F 647 – 85 (1993)$^{\epsilon 1}$.

2. Referenced Documents

2.1 *ASTM Standards:*

F 55 Specification for Stainless Steel Bar and Wire for Surgical Implants[2]

F 56 Specification for Stainless Steel Sheet and Strip for Surgical Implants[2]

F 67 Specification for Unalloyed Titanium for Surgical Implant Applications[3]

F 75 Specification for Cast Cobalt-ChromiumMolybdenum Alloy for Surgical Implant Applications[3]

F 90 Specification for Wrought Cobalt-Chromium-Tungsten-Nickel Alloy for Surgical Implant Applications[3]

F 138 Specification for Stainless Steel Bar and Wire for Surgical Implants (Special Quality)[3]

F 469 Practice for Assessment of Compatibility of Nonporous Polymeric Materials for Surgical Implants with Regard to Effect of Materials on Tissue[4]

F 604 Classification for Silicone Elastomers Used in Medical Use[3]

F 640 Test Methods for Radiopacity of Plastics for Medical Use[3]

F 897 Practice for Measuring Fretting Corrosion of Osteosynthesis Plates and Screws[3]

2.2 *ISO Standard:*[5]

NOTE 2—A suggested method of durability testing is given in Appendix X2.

3. Terminology

3.1 *Definitions of Terms Specific to This Standard:*

3.1.1 *antisiphon device*—a device implanted to counteract the affects of the hydrostatic column of the outflow catheter. This is to minimize the gravity (also termed "siphoning") effect of a hydrostatic pressure that may be created by the elevation of the proximal (inflow) catheter in relation to the distal (outflow) catheter thus preventing the excessive drainage of CSF caused by gravity.

3.1.1.1 *Discussion*—The Committee adopted the terms *siphon effect* and *antisiphon device* for this practice because they are used in the medical literature. However, such devices are designed to counteract the effects of gravity on the fluid in the distal catheter when the patient is standing.

3.1.2 *batch*—a quantity of material that consists of a homogeneous mixture of common ingredients or a quantity of devices processed and controlled as an integral production run.

3.1.3 *calibration*—the act of fixing, checking, or correcting on a schedule, the accuracy and precision of a measuring instrument and maintaining records of these activities.

3.1.4 *chambered valve*—an element of a hydrocephalus shunt containing one or more valve mechanisms that is to facilitate selective flushing in the proximal or distal direction.

3.1.5 *connector*—a device intended for the joining and fixation of implantable shunt components at operation.

3.1.6 *distal (outflow) catheter*—that part of a hydrocephalus shunt assembly that provides a passive outflow pathway for the diversion of fluid from a compartment of the central nervous system to the peritoneal cavity, venous circulation, or other internal delivery site. The outflow catheter may or may not contain a pressure/flow regulating device.

3.1.7 *flow-impedance device*—those components of a shunt assembly which, by virtue of their resistance properties, provide the principal means of controlling intracranial pressure or flow of cerebrospinal fluid, or both. Flow-impedance devices include valved catheters and valves and the relevant constituent parts thereof.

3.1.8 *fluid compartment*—the portion of the central nervous system (CNS) including the ventricles and subdural space, and extraventricular structures such as cysts and hygromas.

3.1.9 *functional range*—the representative pressure/flow characteristics of a shunt or shunt element usually expressed in graphical form.

3.1.10 *hydrocephalus*—the state of excessive accumulation of cerebrospinal fluid (CSF) within the ventricular system of the head due to a disturbance of secretion, flow or absorption, usually resulting in a pathological increase in intracranial pressure (ICP).

3.1.11 *hydrocephalus shunt*—a one-way pressure-activated or flow-controlling device or combination of devices intended to be surgically implanted in the body of a patient with hydrocephalus and designed to divert cerebrospinal fluid from a fluid compartment in the central nervous system or CNS (the cerebral ventricles or other site within the cerebrospinal fluid system) to an internal delivery site in another part of the body (internal shunt) or an external collection site (external shunt), for the purpose of relieving elevated intracranial pressure (ICP) or CSF volume.

3.1.12 *hydrocephalus shunt assembly*—a complete hydrocephalus shunt comprising all the components necessary for clinical use.

3.1.13 *implantable accessory device*—component intended to facilitate the treatment of hydrocephalus by: providing access to the shunt (such as reservoirs, antechambers, flushing devices) or; modifying the performance characteristics of the shunt (such as on/off and antisiphon devices) or; reducing hazards attendant to the presence of the shunt assembly (such as in-line filters).

3.1.14 *implantable external drainage catheter*—that element of an external drainage device which provides access to a fluid compartment of the central nervous system.

3.1.15 *kit*—a number of components in a common package to be used for a single purpose on the same occasion.

3.1.16 *magnetizable*—a metal that has the capacity to acquire magnetic properties of sufficient force to become dangerous due to movement or thermal effects, or both, or to degrade the MRI image to the point of making it diagnostically or therapeutically useless. A shunt system that is magnetizable is not MRI-compatible.

3.1.17 *modifiable connection*—a portion of the shunt assembly in which components are intended to be modified by the surgeon during a surgical procedure (for example, the

[2] Discontinued; see *1991 Annual Book of ASTM Standards*, Vol 13.01.

[3] *Annual Book of ASTM Standards*, Vol 13.01.

[4] Discontinued; see *1987 Annual Book of ASTM Standards*, Vol 13.01.

[5] Available from American National Standards Institute, 11 W. 42nd St., 13th Floor, New York, NY 10036.

length of a tube can be adjusted to accommodate the height of the patient).

3.1.18 *multipiece hydrocephalus shunt assembly*—a complete sterile, single-use hydrocephalus shunt, supplied either assembled by the manufacturer or in kit form for assembly by the physician typically consisting of an inflow catheter, pressure-activated or flow-controlling device or combination of devices and an outflow catheter with requisite connectors required for assembly.

3.1.19 *nominal category*—the generic performance category of the pressure/flow characteristics of the shunt assembly typically defined as "low,"" medium," "high," etc., the limits of which are defined by the manufacturer.

3.1.20 *nonmodifiable connection*—see *preassembled connection.*

3.1.21 *one-piece hydrocephalus shunt assembly*—complete sterile, single-use hydrocephalus shunt consisting of an inflow catheter integral with a pressure-activated or flow-controlling device or combination of devices and an integral outflow catheter.

3.1.22 *on-off device*—an accessory component specifically designed to permit alternate opening and closing of the shunt system upon external activation.

3.1.23 *packaging*—the protective wrapping of shunt systems or components:

3.1.23.1 *inner container*—the packaging that is in direct contact with the implant.

3.1.23.2 *multiple pack*—a pack containing a number of unit packs.

3.1.23.3 *outer container or shelf container*—a package, carton, or other container that may contain one or more unit containers. The packaging that envelopes the inner container such that sterility and the integrity of that container is maintained.

3.1.23.4 *sterile pack*—a pack intended to maintain the sterility of the contents and comprising an inner and outer container.

3.1.23.5 *transit container*—a package, carton, or other container that may contain one or more unit containers used to protect the contents during shipping of the product from the manufacturer to the end user.

3.1.23.6 *unit container*—a package containing a single item or a combination of procedure-related components or products.

3.1.23.7 *unit pack*—a pack containing a single unit or kit.

3.1.24 *preassembled connection*—a portion of the shunt assembly the components of which are preassembled at the time of manufacture and are intended to be permanently fixed and not modified during a surgical procedure (for example, the site where the valve is chemically bonded or mechanically joined to tubing).

3.1.25 *preimplantation test*—a test that is performed on the shunt assembly in the operating room prior to implantation.

3.1.26 *pressure/flow graph*—a graphic representation of the composite performance characteristics of a population of flow impedance devices.

3.1.27 *production line bench flow test*—a test method used by the manufacturer to verify that the pressure/flow characteristics of each individual flow impedance device conforms to its functional range.

3.1.28 *proximal (inflow) catheter*—that part of a hydrocephalus shunt assembly that is inserted into the cerebral ventricles or any other site in the craniospinal axis to provide access to a fluid compartment of the central nervous system (for example, into a lateral ventricle) and therefore constitutes the inflow pathway for the diversion of fluid through a shunt system.

3.1.29 *radiopacity*—the X-ray absorption properties that allow a shunt component to have clear and permanent visualization fluoroscopically or on X-ray film after implantation. (See Annex Annex A1).

3.1.30 *referee test method*—the methods in the published standard for the device. The method and the corresponding requirements will be invoked when the performance of the medical device will be questioned. The manufacturer need not use this referee test method in the usual inspection and quality control.

3.1.31 *reflux*—a flow of fluid within a hydrocephalus shunt towards the cerebral ventricles or cerebrospinal fluid system.

3.1.32 *shunt, v*—to drain CSF from the CNS.

3.1.33 *shunt assembly*—any device or combination of devices that functions to divert CSF from a fluid compartment of the central nervous system to an internal delivery site (internal shunt) or an external collection site (external shunt).

3.1.34 *shunt element*—any component of a hydrocephalus shunt.

3.1.35 *shunt filter*—a device intended to remove particulate matter from the CSF before it passes through the shunt.

3.1.36 *sterile*—in microbiology, free from all living organisms; in practice, the condition of a product that has been subjected to a validated sterilization process and maintained in this state by suitable protection.

3.1.37 *sterilized*—term used to denote an object that has been subjected to a validated sterilization process.

3.1.38 *test specimen*—a device or sample of devices representative of the population of devices.

3.1.39 *tip valve*—an element of a hydrocephalus shunt located at the distal catheter tip that controls pressure or establishes flow of cerebrospinal fluid and resists reflux of blood or other fluids into the shunt.

3.1.40 *traceability reference*—the number or other means of identification by which components can be traced to a specific manufacturing lot or batch.

3.1.41 *unit*—individual device(s) or object(s) defined in the relevant product standard or regulation.

3.1.42 *use by date*—a date that may be established by the manufacturer after which the device is not to be implanted.

3.1.43 *valve*—an element of a hydrocephalus shunt assembly that functions as a major resistance to the CSF flow thus controlling the relationship between pressure and flow of cerebrospinal fluid and resists reflux of blood or other fluids into the shunt assembly. In contrast to a valved catheter, it does not provide a significant portion of tubing for the fluid pathway.

3.1.44 *valved catheter*—an assembly or element of a shunt which provides a pathway for diversion of CSF to an internal delivery site and contains one or more valves, typically, a tip valve, and a significant portion of tubing for the fluid pathway.

4. Significance and Use

4.1 This practice provides minimum requirements for the ensurance of safety and efficacy. It provides a common language whereby the function of these surgical implants is described.

5. Materials

5.1 Metals used in the fabrication of implantable shunt components shall conform to specifications as referenced in 2.1.

5.2 All polymeric materials shall have total levels of extractable antimony, arsenic, bismuth, copper, lead, cadmium, mercury, and tin not exceeding 10 ppm (each), when tested by conventional methods of extraction and microanalysis conforming to the *United States Pharmacopeia* (*USP*), spectrographic analysis, or other machine methods that are proven reliable. The shunt manufacturer shall use Classification F 604 to provide guidance in the selection of silicone elastomeric materials appropriate for shunt application.

5.3 *Biocompatibility (Polymeric Materials)*:

5.3.1 Each polymeric formulation shall be shown to produce an acceptable level of tissue reaction by cell culture,[6] hemolysis (*USP*), pyrogenicity (*USP*), extraction and intracutaneous injection in rabbits (*USP*) and by Practice F 469 or any comparable procedures.

5.3.2 Each batch of polymeric material shall be biocompatible when tested by cell culture or seven-day rabbit implant (*USP*).

5.4 Interfacing surfaces of mated shunt components must be of the same material composition or recognized compatible materials (for example, connector-catheter interfacing materials).

5.5 Guidance for selection of materials is contained in Appendix X2.

6. General Requirements for Complete Shunts and Components

6.1 *Physical Requirements*:

6.1.1 *Surface Finish*—When examined with normal or corrected vision at a distance of 300 to 450 mm and at an illuminance of 2150 ± 215 lx, the surface of all implantable shunts and components of a shunt assembly that have passed through all stages of manufacture, including sterilization, shall be clean, smooth and free from surface irregularities, flash, molding and extrusion defects and extraneous particles that would be expected to compromise the function of the device.

6.1.2 *Radiopacity*—When tested by the method described in Annex Annex A1, all integral components and connectors of the shunt or component shall be radiopaque or shall carry radiopaque markers, so as to allow their visualization by X-rays. Composite structures or assemblies may contain radiolucent portions if surrounding or overlay material clearly identifies the location of nonradiopaque elements and enables any discontinuities to be readily apparent.

6.1.3 *Magnetic Resonance Imaging (MRI) Compatibility*—Imaging and investigative techniques such as nuclear magnetic resonance (NMR) (magnetic resonance imaging (MRI)) involve placing the patient in a strong magnetic field. This may result in severe stresses on magnetizable materials (that is, a metal that has the capacity to acquire magnetic properties of sufficient force to become dangerous due to movement or thermal effects, or both, or to degrade an MRI image to the point of making it diagnostically or therapeutically useless), even moving them through tissues. Magnetizable materials should be avoided if possible in hydrocephalus shunts but, if used, a suitable warning shall be included in the product labelling (see 6.4.2.6).

6.1.4 *Biological Properties*—In the absence of a test method for freedom from biological hazard, it is not possible to lay down requirements for toxicity or biocompatibility in this Standard. It is essential that such tests are carried out on the initial formulation of materials and whenever there is a major change in the formulation or processing, or both.

6.1.5 Specific guidance on the biological properties of materials is given in Appendix X2.

6.2 *Mechanical Properties*:

6.2.1 Where applicable, shunt assemblies, valved catheters, valves and catheters with integral valves shall be evaluated for security of assembly and absence of assembly leakage and for tensile strength. They shall be sufficiently strong and flexible as to permit manipulation and be resistant to stresses ordinarily associated with placement and use.

6.2.2 For any given shunt component and, where appropriate, the manufacturer shall subject device(s) (test specimens) to testing of those mechanical properties that are pertinent to *in vivo* performance.

6.2.3 Testing shall be performed on a finished product(s) selected in accordance with the manufacturer's usual quality assurance program.

6.2.3.1 The manufacturer shall specifically ensure the security of assembly of nonmodifiable junction sites, by subjecting a test specimen of the assembly to an applied load. Nonmodifiable junctions shall be as strong as modifiable junctions (assembled according to the manufacturer's instructions for use) when tested in a similar manner.

6.2.3.2 The manufacturer shall specifically ensure absence of assembly leakage (defined as the formation of two drops or 0.1 mL) at nonmodifiable junction sites, by subjecting a test sample of the assembly to an applied pressure of 300 mm H_2O for 1 min. Nonmodifiable junctions shall have the same properties to resist leakage as modifiable junctions (assembled according to the manufacturer's instructions for use) when tested in a similar manner.

6.2.3.3 The manufacturer shall specifically ensure that test specimens shall be tested by the method used or recommended after sterilization if the shunt is packaged and sold after sterilization.

6.2.3.4 Particulars of the test methodology used by each manufacturer, including test apparatus, etc., shall be documented and retained for a minimum of 25 years for permanently implanted products and in no case less than two years

[6] *Journal of Pharmacological Science*, Vol 54, No. 156, 1965.

from the date of release for commercial distribution by the manufacturer.

6.3 *Packaging*:

6.3.1 *Unit Container*:

6.3.1.1 Each shunt or component shall be individually packaged and sealed in a unit container, the materials of which shall be non-fibrous and lint-free.

6.3.1.2 The construction of the unit container shall be such that once it has been opened, this fact shall be evident.

NOTE 3—The packaging material should have no deleterious effects on the contents of the unit container. The unit container should provide adequate physical protection to the contents under normal conditions of handling, transit and storage, and be constructed so that, once opened, it cannot be easily resealed.

6.3.1.3 The unit container should maintain the sterility of the contents and be constructed so as to facilitate the aseptic presentation of the device for use.

6.3.1.4 If shunts or catheters are not packaged in the straight configuration, they should be packaged in such a manner that no permanent deformation is produced.

6.3.2 *Shelf Containers*—One or a number of unit containers, each containing the same model of shunt or component, shall be packaged in a shelf container.

NOTE 4—The shelf container should provide protection of the contents under normal conditions of handling, transit and storage. One or a number of shelf containers may additionally be packaged in an outer or transit container.

6.4 *Labeling, Packaging, and Sterility*:

6.4.1 *Shunts and Components*:

NOTE 5—It is recommended that shunts and components through which the fluid flow is uni-directional shall be marked to indicate the intended direction of flow (for example, by means of an arrow) using a method that is visible and obvious to the implanting surgeon.

6.4.2 *Unit Container*—The following information shall be marked on the unit container or given in a leaflet or insert:

6.4.2.1 The particular information specified in 6.1.2 and 6.1.3, as appropriate;

6.4.2.2 The words "STERILE" and "NONPYROGENIC";

6.4.2.3 The name or registered trademark, or both, of the manufacturer or supplier;

6.4.2.4 The batch number and date of manufacture (year and month) or a batch number from which the date of manufacture can be determined.

6.4.2.5 If appropriate, the word "RADIOPAQUE" or equivalent;

6.4.2.6 If appropriate, a warning that the contents contain magnetizable materials (including notation on patient ID card);

6.4.2.7 If the contents may be resterilized, full instructions for resterilization, indicating the recommended maximum number of sterilization cycles;

6.4.2.8 A warning against use of the contents if the unit container is open or damaged;

6.4.2.9 Directions for opening the container and aseptic presentation of the contents;

6.4.2.10 In the case of contents having a determined shelf-life, the Use Before Date (year) beyond which the contents should not be implanted;

6.4.2.11 The words "SINGLE USE" or equivalent phrase;

6.4.2.12 Any special instructions for storage of the unit container.

6.4.3 *Shelf Container*—The shelf container shall be either wholly or partially transparent so that the unit container markings are visible; or labelled or marked with the following information:

6.4.3.1 A description of the contents, as specified in clauses 6.1.2 or 6.1.3 (as appropriate), and number of contents,

6.4.3.2 The words "STERILE" and "NONPYROGENIC,"

6.4.3.3 The name and address of the manufacturer or supplier,

6.4.3.4 The batch number and date of manufacture (year and month) or a batch number from which the date of manufacture can be determined,

6.4.3.5 Any special instructions for storage, and

6.4.3.6 In the case of contents having a determined shelf-life, the expiry date (year) beyond which the contents should not be implanted.

6.5 *Additional Requirements for Complete Shunts, Valves and Catheters With Integral Valves and Components*:

6.5.1 *Type and Size Designation*—The type and size of the shunt shall be designated by means of the following information:

6.5.1.1 The function of the valve/catheter (for example, inflow, outflow, etc.);

6.5.1.2 The nominal operating characteristics of valve; (for example, high, medium, low)

6.5.1.3 The overall nominal length of component expressed in millimetres or centimetres, stating the unit used;

6.5.1.4 The nominal inside and outside diameters of the tubular portions of the component at connection point, expressed in millimetres.

6.5.2 *Connectors*—If additional connectors are supplied for use in conjunction with valves and catheters with integral valves, the dimensions of the connectors shall be such that the pressure and flow characteristics of the shunt with the connections in place shall not, when tested in accordance with Annex A2, differ by more than 10 % from the values determined for the shunt without the additional connectors in place.

6.5.3 *Resistance Properties*—The results for a preassembled shunt or a shunt sold as a kit, a valve or a catheter with valves, when tested in accordance with Annex A2, shall lie within a specified confidence interval of the functional range of the type of component stated by the manufacturer in accordance with published instructions for use.

6.5.3.1 The manufacturer shall be given the choice between providing pressure/flow characteristics of the assembled shunt and providing pressure/flow characteristics of each component in the kit, provided the manufacturer has obtained adequate data demonstrating the additive resistive effects of various shunt components, and the manufacturer properly explains these additive properties in the accompanying documentation.

6.5.3.2 Complete shunts, valved shunt assembly or integral valves shall be tested in accordance with Annex A2.

6.5.3.3 The pressure/flow properties of a complete shunt, valve, catheter with integral valve shall be such to provide resistance to flow of cerebrospinal fluid through the shunt, and to provide unidirectional flow in accordance with Annex A2.

6.5.3.4 Pressure/flow curves shall be plotted with flow rate on the horizontal axis and pressure on the vertical axis.

6.5.3.5 Evaluation of resistance properties shall be performed on a test specimen(s) prior to marketing and on a production-line basis thereafter.

6.5.4 *Freedom from Reflux*—When tested in accordance with Annex A3, the complete shunt, valve catheter with integral valve or component shall comply with the following requirements:

6.5.4.1 *Chambered Valves*—The meniscus shall remain static for at least 1 min at both test pressures (see A3.5.1). The meniscus shall remain static for at least 1 min (see A3.5.2). In the case of compressible valves, reflux shall not occur in the event that the chamber is compressed.

6.5.4.2 *Tip Valves*—Tip valves shall not show the continued formation of drops (less than one drop per minute) of liquid at the inlet end of the tubing at either test pressure (see A3.5.2).

6.6 *Security of Assembly/Assembly Leakage*—When assembled according to the manufacturer's instructions, all components supplied as a kit shall fit together securely without leakage.

6.6.1 Complete shunts, valves, and catheters with integral valves shall be evaluated for security of assembly and assembly leakage.

6.6.2 These components shall be evaluated to determine tensile force required to cause fracture, the test methodology and results being documented and retained by the manufacturer for a minimum of 25 years for permanently implanted products and, in no case, less than two years from the date of release for commercial distribution by the manufacturer.

6.6.3 Materials used in complete shunts, valves and catheters with integral valves shall be tested in accordance with Appendix X2.

6.7 *Marking and Labelling and Accompanying Documentation*:

6.7.1 Labelling and product identification of shunts sold as a kit, valves, catheters with integral valves and components shall include the following information:

6.7.1.1 A labelled and dimensioned diagram of the complete shunt, valve, catheter with integral valve or component showing the direction of fluid flow; where the design is such that the intended direction of flow is ambiguous, the device shall be marked accordingly;

6.7.1.2 A statement whether the shunt has been tested by the manufacturer and the suitable tests, if any, the manufacturer recommends to the surgeon to determine whether or not the shunt falls in a specific band range;

6.7.1.3 A statement of or a code for the nominal flow resistance of the valve in accordance with Annex A2 or other manufacturer's criteria.

6.7.2 *Accompanying Documentation*—Each complete shunt, valve, catheter with integral valve and components supplied as separate items shall be accompanied by documentation that includes the following information:

6.7.2.1 A description of the contents, including the type and size in accordance with 6.4;

6.7.2.2 Instructions for assembly of the shunt or use of the valve, catheter with integral valve and component(s) in the assembly of a shunt system;

6.7.2.3 A statement as to whether the preassembled shunt or shunt sold as a kit, a valve, or a catheter with integral valve should be tested prior to implantation using tests deemed by the manufacturer to be appropriate for use in the operating room and intended to assess the following: patency; freedom from reflux; and, whenever possible and practical, a simple test designed to assess operating (pressure or flow) characteristics and to verify that these are within the nominal range specified by the manufacturer.

6.7.2.4 The instructions shall emphasize the need for the use of sterile, lint-free apparatus and reagents and aseptic technique in carrying out the test.

6.7.2.5 A statement that non-proprietary details of the methods used to test materials and the results obtained are available on request, giving the address to which such requests should be sent;

6.7.2.6 A labelled diagram showing the dimensions of those connection points the user will use for assembly of the component into the system and its method of incorporation into the final shunt system, showing the direction of fluid flow through the component;

6.7.2.7 Details of the pressure and flow characteristics of the type of shunt, valve, or catheter with integral valve in accordance with A2.9.1.3 and A2.9.1.4 and the interval level that the product will perform within the specified ranges.

7. Additional Requirements for Implantable Accessory Devices Supplied Separately

7.1 *Other Components*:

7.1.1 *Implantable Accessory Devices*—Implantable accessory components of shunts such as reservoirs, antisiphon devices, and filters should not compromise the overall function of the shunt. Their contribution to the pressure/flow characteristics of the shunt should be tested and documented.

7.2 *External Drainage Catheters*:

7.2.1 *Mechanical Properties*—External drainage catheters shall be sufficiently strong and flexible as to permit manipulation and at the same time be resistant to stresses ordinarily associated with placement and use.

7.2.2 External drainage catheters shall be evaluated to determine tensile force required to cause failure, with test methodology and results documented and maintained.

7.3 *Antisiphon System*—The contribution to pressure/flow characteristics of an antisiphon device shall be specified at zero hydrostatic pressure (no siphon effect) and at a negative hydrostatic pressure (siphon effect) specified by the manufacturer.

8. Keywords

8.1 anti-sipon device; bio-compatibility; compatibility; hydrocephalus; magnetic resonance imaging (MRI); shunt; shunt assembly

ANNEXES

(Mandatory Information)

A1. TEST METHOD FOR DETERMINING RADIOPACITY OF SHUNT COMPONENTS

A1.1 Scope

A1.1.1 This test method provides the procedure and acceptance criteria upon which a judgment of acceptable radiopacity can be based and labeling claims substantiated.

A1.2 Significance and Use

A1.2.1 Radiopacity of shunt components is often desirable, in order to facilitate placement of the shunt at the time of surgery and to evaluate the continuity of the assembly and the position of individual shunt components after implantation.

A1.3 Apparatus and Materials

A1.3.1 *X-Ray Machine and Film*, of a type conventionally used (such as par-speed or hi-plus films) for clinical radiology. An industrial X-ray system may be used,[6] provided that clinical X-ray parameters are obtainable.

A1.3.2 *Sheet of Aluminum Alloy No. 1100*, having a thickness as specified by the manufacturer of a minimum 2.2 mm, interposed between the test samples and X-ray generator to identify discontinuities in the system.

A1.3.3 A standard number of specimens shall be tested to ensure that the observed radiographic properties are typical of the population.

A1.4 Test Specimens

A1.4.1 Test specimens shall consist of a finished product.

A1.4.2 A sufficient number of test specimens shall be tested as to assure that the observed radiographic properties are typical of the population.

A1.5 Control Specimens

A1.5.1 The control for each exposure shall consist of a strip of aluminum alloy No. 1100, having a width that is equivalent (to the nearest 0.1 mm) to the outer diameter of the test specimen. If the maximum thickness of the intended radiopaque region of the product is less than 1.3 mm, then the control specimen must have the same thickness. Otherwise, the control shall be at least 0.7 mm thick.

A1.6 Apparatus/Procedure

A1.6.1 Place the test and control specimen on a cassette containing the X-ray film and intensifying screens. Then cover all specimens with aluminum sheet described in A1.3.2. Position the lead blocker around the aluminum sheet to prevent undercutting.

A1.6.2 Expose the film using the following parameters: a peak kilovoltage (kVp) in the range from 65 to 80: a focal spot to film distance of at least 24 in. (610 mm) and a milliampere-second (mA-s) exposure time selected so as to achieve a background density of 0.8 to 1.2 optical density units.

A1.6.3 Develop the exposed film in accordance with the film manufacturer's instructions.

A1.6.4 Determine the radiographic opacity of test and control specimens by carefully centering the aperture of the densitometer over each image and recording the density. (The aperture size of the densitometer should be chosen so as to be slightly smaller than the size of the image in order to avoid confounding the density measurement with the background density of the film. In this application, an aperture size of 2 mm will typically be required.) The density of the background should be recorded and observed to be in the range of A1.6.2.

A1.7 Acceptance Criterion

A1.7.1 If the optical density of the test specimen image where the test sample thickness is 1.3 mm or greater (counting both walls) is observed to be as low as or lower than that of the control specimen (within the limits of precision of the densitometer), the test specimen may be termed radiopaque. If the thickness of the device is less than 1.3 mm (counting both walls), its linear attenuation shall be at least 56 % of the aluminum standard, when measured in Method C of Test Methods F 640.

A1.8 Report of Results

A1.8.1 Test results shall be documented and retained by the manufacturer in substantiation of radiopacity claims. The report shall include a description of the product tested (including physical dimensions, geometry, opacifier concentration, etc.) and of the procedure employed (with exposure parameters), and identification of test apparatus and materials.

A1.9 Precision and Bias

A1.9.1 The precision and bias of this test method have not yet been determined.

A2. REFERENCE METHOD FOR DETERMINING PRESSURE AND FLOW CHARACTERISTICS

A2.1 Scope

A2.1.1 This test method defines a means whereby shunts or shunt elements of differing design or manufacture can be related in terms of pressure/flow characteristics by pumping of liquid at a number of constant rates through the shunt or component and measuring the pressure required to maintain each flow rate to the reference standard defined herein.

A2.2 Summary of Test Method

A2.2.1 The resultant flow/pressure in a shunt or shunt element is a function of the restriction of the device to the rate of flow and the sum of the resistances of the device, if all other factors are held constant.

A2.2.2 The test is intended:

A2.2.2.1 As a type test to prepare a curve showing mean values and the functional range for a particular design of shunt or component (see 6.5.3); and

A2.2.2.2 To establish that the performance of an individual shunt or component falls within the predetermined functional range (see 6.5.3.1). Other methods of equal or better precision may be used, but, in cases of dispute, the method given in this annex shall be the reference method. All equipment utilized is to be subject to a documented calibration program.

A2.3 Significance and Use

A2.3.1 Results of this test method can be used to define a curve representing the pressure/flow characteristics of a shunt or shunt element over a physiologic range of flow rates.

A2.3.2 From the individual pressure/flow curves obtained, a composite graph can be plotted that describes these characteristics for a given functional range of flow rates.

A2.4 Test Medium

A2.4.1 *Test Fluid*—The fluid medium used for testing the shunt or shunt elements shall be deaerated and deionized or distilled water at 37 ± 2°C.

A2.5 Apparatus

A2.5.1 *Test Rig*:

A2.5.1.1 The test apparatus shall consist of a source reservoir, constant-temperature water bath, a variable-speed pump having a flow rate, in millilitres per hour, accurate to ±5 %, a water manometer or equivalent calibrated in millimetres H_2O, tee or y-connector, connecting tubing, an apparatus to maintain constant water level in the bath, the appropriate adaptor for the shunt or shunt element to be tested.

A2.5.1.2 The tee or y-connector shall be joined directly to the shunt or shunt element to be tested.

NOTE A2.1—For testing of valves with or without integral catheters, the outlet of the shunt system shall be submerged in the water bath.

A2.5.1.3 The test fluid temperature must be equal to the water-bath temperature prior to flow through the tee connector so as to be at 37 ± 2°C at the site of shunt or shunt element test.

A2.5.2 The test apparatus comprises the following elements:

A2.5.2.1 *Variable-Speed Pump*, capable of maintaining, within ±5 %, any pumping rate up to 65 mL/h in the test rig, and any necessary silicone elastomer pump tubing;

A2.5.2.2 *Water Bath*, capable of being controlled at 37 ± 2°C with means to maintain the water level constant within ±2 mm;

A2.5.2.3 *Means of Connecting the Shunt*, or component to the test rig without occluding inflow aperture(s);

A2.5.2.4 *Connecting Tubing*,

NOTE A2.2—This should contain a coiled portion of sufficient length that, when immersed in the water bath, allows the test fluid (see A2.4.1) to come to a temperature of 37 ± 2°C during its passage through it.

A2.5.2.5 *Manometer*, graduated in conventional millimetres of water (mm H_2O)[7,8] or suitably calibrated transducer.

A2.5.2.6 *Borosilicate Laboratory Glassware*.

A2.6 Test Specimens

A2.6.1 The test shall be carried out on shunts or components that have passed through all stages of manufacture, including sterilization but not previously implanted and within the manufacturer's use before date, and, in the case of multipiece complete shunts, have been assembled in accordance with the manufacturer's instructions.

A2.7 Procedure

A2.7.1 Prepare the test specimen by performing all pre-use steps included in the documentation.

A2.7.2 Prefill and soak the test specimen in deaerated water that is deionized or distilled at 37 ± 2°C for a sufficient period of time to reach an equilibrium state, maintaining the temperature by means of the water bath (see A2.5.2.2) to ensure a stable pressure/flow characteristic.

A2.7.3 Top up the water bath with the test fluid (see A2.4.1) and bring the contents to 37 ± 2°C. Connect the test specimen to the adaptor (as shown in Fig. A2.1) in such a manner as not to introduce air into the liquid pathway of the test system.

A2.7.4 Purge all air from the liquid pathway of the test element and the testing apparatus by irrigating at a gage pressure not to exceed 500 mm H_2O (0.71 psi; 4.9 kPa).

A2.7.5 Zero the pressure level of measuring device (manometer or equivalent) by having the zero level of the manometer by adjusting its position so that the zero graduation mark is level with the surface of the test fluid in the water bath (see Fig. A2.1). The level of the water bath shall remain constant within ±2 mm.

A2.7.6 Adjust the pump speed (see A2.5.2.1) to provide a flow rate of between 55 and 65 mL/h. Allow the flow rate to stabilize.

A2.7.7 Readjust the pump speed and read the manometer or pressure transducer pressure level after stabilization, in order

[7] The Hewlett-Packard Faxitron, or equivalent, has been found suitable for this purpose.

[8] 1 mm H_2O = 1 kgf/m^2 = 9807 Pa; the use of the unit "mm H_2O" is deprecated in ISO 31-3 (the unit "kPa" is preferred for fluid pressure), however, values are given in conventional millimetres of water since this unit is widely used in practice.

of diminishing flow rates and including one determination at 50 and 5 mL/h for a minimum of three flow rates at 30, 20, and 10 mL/h with a tolerance of ±5 mL/hr at each point or with a tolerance as stated in A2.5.2.1. An alternate method is to readjust the pump speed in increasing flow rates from 5 to 50 mL/h.

A2.7.8 Repeat A2.7 for each test specimen using the same flow rates.

A2.8 Interpretation of Results

A2.8.1 *Type Testing of Shunts or Components*—Calculate the mean pressure for all replicate test shunts or components at a flow rate of 50 mL/h. Note the lowest and the highest individual pressures. Repeat this calculation for each of the four remaining flow rates.

A2.8.1.1 Construct a graph of flow rate (expressed in millilitres per hour and plotted as the abscissa) against pressure (expressed in conventional millimetres of water and plotted as the ordinate) showing the average, lowest and highest pressures at each of the chosen flow rates.

A2.8.1.2 A composite graph shall be derived that is representative of the device population tested. The composite graph is used for labeling requirements (see 6.4.2, and 6.4.3) of this practice.

A2.8.1.3 Representation of this composite graph shall show the typical minimum and maximum data points for each flow rate. Flow rates shall be plotted on the horizontal axis and pressure on the vertical axis.

A2.8.1.4 A population of valves needs to be tested a sufficient number of times to establish the statistical confidence level for reproducibility of the pressure/flow characteristics. This information should be used in the labeling to report the statistical confidence that the device will perform between labeled minimum and maximum.

A2.8.2 *Shunts or Components with Intended Linear Pressure/Flow Response Curves*:

A2.8.2.1 For each design (nominal classification) of shunt or shunt component, note the lowest individual pressure, P_{min}, in millimetres of water, recorded at a flow rate of 5 mL/h and the highest individual pressure, P_{max}, in millimeters of water, recorded at a flow rate of 50 mL/h; express the final results in the following form:

$$\frac{P_{min}}{5\ \text{mL/h}} \quad to \quad \frac{P_{max}}{50\ \text{mL/h}} \tag{A2.1}$$

Example:

$$\frac{10\ \text{mm H}_2\text{O}}{5\ \text{mL/h}} \quad \text{to} \quad \frac{80\ \text{mm H}_2\text{O}}{50\ \text{mL/h}} \tag{A2.2}$$

A2.8.2.2 For each nominal classification of shunts or valved shunt components, the manufacturer shall make available a graph representative of the pressure/flow characteristics used to define the above nominal resistance range for that device population. The statistical confidence level for reproducibility of the pressure/flow characteristics shall be used in the labeling to report the statistical confidence that the device will perform between labeled minimum and maximum.

A2.8.2.3 This arrangement shall be referred to as the" functional range" of the shunt or component.

A2.9 Report

A2.9.1 Report the following information:

A2.9.1.1 Type testing of shunts or components;

A2.9.1.2 The identity of the type of shunt or component;

A2.9.1.3 The functional range of the type of shunt or component (see A2.8.2.2); and,

A2.9.1.4 A graph of pressure plotted against flow rate of the type of shunt or component (see A2.8).

A2.9.2 *Other Testing of Shunts or Components*:

A2.9.2.1 The identity of the test shunt or component;

A2.9.2.2 The pressures, as given in A2.8.2;

A2.9.2.3 A statement as to whether the performance of the individual shunt or component lies within the functional range for the design (that is, whether the values of [P_{min} (5 mL/h)] and [P_{max} (50 mL/h)] are higher and lower, respectively, than the corresponding values determined by type testing and stated by the manufacturer).

A3. REFERENCE TEST METHOD FOR REFLUX

A3.1 Principle

A3.1.1 Filling of the valve with liquid and application of hydrostatic pressure in an attempt to induce reflux.

A3.1.2 Other methods of equal or better precision may be used, but, in cases of dispute, the method given in this annex shall be the reference method.

A3.2 Reagent

A3.2.1 *Deaerated Water*, that is distilled or deionized.

A3.3 Apparatus

A3.3.1 *Connecting Tubing and Connectors.*

A3.3.2 *Borosilicate Laboratory Glassware.*

A3.3.3 *Tubing Clamps.*

A3.3.4 *Clock or Stop Watch.*

A3.4 Test Specimens

A3.4.1 Carry out the test on shunts or components that have passed through all stages of manufacture, including sterilization.

A3.5 Procedure

A3.5.1 *Testing of Chambered Valves*—If necessary, detach the chambered valve(s) from the shunt or component. Connect lengths of tubing to both ends of the valve under test. Fill the assembly with test fluid (deaerated water that is distilled or deionized), removing all air. Position the valve so that the outlet end is uppermost and press the valve chamber repeatedly until a meniscus forms in the tubing at a distance of 10 and 50 mm above the valve or fill the valve using a syringe. The inlet tubing shall be at the level of the valve unit. Stop pressing and observe the meniscus for 1 min to determine if it remains static. No more than two drops (0.1 cc) will form in 1 min.

A3.5.2 *Testing of Tip Valves*—If necessary, detach the tip valve from the shunt or component. Hold the valve and associated tubing vertically and fill it with test fluid, keeping the outlet and under the liquid surface. Dry the outer surface of the tubing. Lower the inlet end of the tubing to a distance of 10 mm and below the level of the liquid in the vessel. Observe the inlet end of the tubing for 1 min for signs of leakage and record the findings. Repeat the test with the inlet end of the tubing at distances of 50 and 140 mm (±2 mm at each point) below the level of the liquid.

APPENDIXES

(Nonmandatory Information)

X1. SUGGESTED TEST METHOD FOR DURABILITY

X1.1 General

X1.1.1 It is felt that shunts and at least certain components should be subjected to some form of accelerated durability test in order to demonstrate that they are able to meet the demands imposed upon them during the period (possibly several years) for which they may remain implanted. The main properties of interest are that:

X1.1.1.1 The pressure and flow characteristics remain within design limits;

X1.1.1.2 The valves continue to function correctly (particularly with regard to their resistance to reflux); and

X1.1.1.3 Connections and unions between components remain sound.

X1.1.1.4 Given that these properties relate chiefly to the design and materials of the shunt or component, a durability test is envisaged as being applied as a type test to preproduction devices, but not to routine production (although the test could be used in this way). Consequently it is suggested that the test be applied whenever, in view of the manufacturer, the design materials are significantly modified.

X1.1.1.5 Although it is feasible for all components to be tested for durability, practical considerations of time and cost may constrain the amount of testing that can be carried out. In this case, priority should be given to testing complete shunts (both one-piece and multipiece), valves, catheters with integral valves and other components having moving parts or containing permanent unions within their structure.

X1.1.1.6 It is recommended that the test method described in X1.2 to X1.7 be applied as outlined below in order to provide experience and data on which to base test conditions and pass/fail criteria for inclusion in a future edition of this practice.

X1.2 Principle

X1.2.1 Immersion of the shunt or component in water at elevated temperature; pumping of water in a pulsed fashion through the shunt or component so as to open and close the valve(s) repeatedly. Examination of the shunt or component for signs of mechanical damage; then test in accordance with Annex A2 and Annex A3 to establish if the functional range or the reflux properties have been impaired.

X1.3 Reagent—Test Fluid

X1.3.1 Deaerated water that is distilled or deionized.

X1.4 Apparatus

X1.4.1 *Test Rig*—The test rig shall comprise the following elements:

X1.4.1.1 *Variable Speed Pump*, capable of maintaining, within ±5 %, the selected pumping rate;

X1.4.1.2 *Water Bath*, capable of being controlled at 37 ± 2°C;

X1.4.1.3 *Means of Connecting the Shunt or Component to the Test Rig*, without occluding inflow aperture(s);

X1.4.1.4 *Silicone Elastomer Pump Tubing*, of dimensions to produce selected flow rate;

X1.4.1.5 *Silicone Elastomer Connecting Tubing;*

NOTE X1.1—This should contain a coiled portion of sufficient length that, when immersed in the water bath (see X1.4.1.3), allows the test fluid (see X1.3) to come to a temperature of 37 ± 2°C during its passage through it.

X1.4.1.6 *Manometer*, graduated in conventional millimetres of water (mm H_2O), or a suitable calibrated transducer.

NOTE X1.2—An example of the test rig is shown in Fig. A2.1 .

X1.5 Test Specimens

X1.5.1 Carry out the test shunts or components that have passed through all stages of manufacture, including sterilization, and, in the case of multipiece shunts, have been assembled in accordance with the manufacturer's instructions.

X1.6 Procedure

X1.6.1 Soak the test specimen in the test fluid (see X1.3) at 37 ± 2°C for at least 24 h, maintaining the temperature by means of the water bath (see Appendix X2.4.1.2).

X1.6.2 Top up the water bath with the test fluid and bring the contents to 37 ± 2°C.

X1.6.3 Purge all air from the liquid pathway of the test system by irrigating with test fluid at a pressure not exceeding 500 mm H_2O.

X1.6.4 Connect the test specimen as shown in Fig. A2.1 , taking care not to introduce air into the liquid pathway of the test system.

X1.6.5 Zero the manometer (see X1.4.1.6) by adjusting its position so that the zero graduation mark is level with the surface of the test fluid in the water bath.

X1.6.6 Start the pump (see X1.4.1.1) and adjust to a flow rate of between 5 and 15 mL/h greater than the flow rate selected for the test (see X1.6.7). Allow the flow rate to stabilize:

$$\frac{\text{Pulse frequency should be 0.5 Hz} \pm 0.25\text{ Hz.}}{\text{Pulse frequency should be 0.5 Hz} \pm 0.25\text{ Hz.}} \quad (X1.1)$$

X1.6.7 Adjust the pump to give a flow rate, either of a valve selected from the upper quartile of the range of flow rates for the shunt or component stated by the manufacturer, or (if no data are available) of 50 mL/h. When the flow rate has stabilized, record the manometer reading (see X1.4.1.6).

X1.6.8 Operate the pump at the rate described in X2.6.7 continuously for 28 days. Check the flow regularly and adjust if necessary. Check the manometer reading regularly. A change in pressure indicates the pressure of air bubbles, which should be purged from the system. If necessary, top up the water bath regularly.

X1.6.9 Remove the test specimen and rinse it twice with deaerated water. Examine the test specimen for breaks, loosening of unions and other evidence of mechanical damage.

X1.6.10 Determine the pressure and flow characteristics of the test specimen in accordance with Annex A2.

X1.6.11 Determine the reflux characteristics of the valves, if any, in accordance with Annex A3.

X1.7 Report

X1.7.1 Report the following information:

X1.7.1.1 The identity of the test specimen;

X1.7.1.2 The functional range of the test specimen (see Appendix X2.6.10) and a statement as to whether this falls within the range in any, stated by the manufacturer.

X1.7.1.3 The reflux properties (see Appendix X2.6.11) of the valves, if any, and a statement as to whether these comply with 6.5.4 and Annex A3; and

X1.7.1.4 A description of all defects and failures occurring during the 28-day test period, and during subsequent testing (see X1.6.9, X1.6.10, and X1.6.11).

X2. GUIDANCE ON MATERIALS

X2.1 The types of materials from which the shunt or component is made should be tested by appropriate published test methods to determine the following:

X2.1.1 The physical and chemical effects on the materials of body fluids and tissues with which the finished shunt or component is intended to come into contact; and

X2.1.2 The physical, chemical and biological effects of the materials on the body fluids and tissues with which the finished shunt or component is intended to come into contact.

X2.2 These records should be updated whenever the types or sources of materials are changed.

X2.3 Each polymeric formulation shall be shown to produce an acceptable level of tissue reaction by cell culture (or equivalent), hemolysis (*USP*), pyrogenicity (*USP* or equivalent), extraction and intracutaneous injection in rabbits (*USP* or equivalent), extraction and intracutaneous injection in rabbits (*USP*), and by Practice F 469 or equivalent.

X2.4 Each batch of polymeric material shall be biocompatible when tested by cell culture or seven-day rabbit implant (*USP*).

X2.4.1 Metals used in the fabrication of implantable shunt components shall conform with Specifications F 55, F 67, F 75, F 90, and F 138. The use of magnetizable materials should be avoided because of the possibility of movement of shunts or components through the body tissues when the patient is exposed to diagnostic investigations using high-strength magnetic fields, for example, nuclear magnetic resonance scanning (magnetic resonance imaging).

X2.5 All polymeric materials shall have total levels of extractable antimony, arsenic, bismuth, copper, lead, cadmium, mercury, and tin not exceeding 10 ppm (each), when tested by conventional methods of extraction and microanalysis conforming to the *United States Pharmacopeia* (*USP*), spectrographic analysis, or other machine methods that are proven reliable. The shunt manufacturer shall use Classification F 604 to provide guidance in the selection of silicone elastomeric materials appropriate for shunt application.

X2.6 The materials should be sufficiently flexible for the shunt or component to be manipulated without fracture, but should maintain resistance to kinking and applied pressure.

X2.7 Interfacing surfaces of mated shunt components must be of the same material composition or recognized compatible materials (for example, connector-catheter interfacing materials).

Designation: F 648 – 00

Standard Specification for Ultra-High-Molecular-Weight Polyethylene Powder and Fabricated Form for Surgical Implants[1]

This standard is issued under the fixed designation F 648; the number immediately following the designation indicates the year of original adoption or, in the case of revision, the year of last revision. A number in parentheses indicates the year of last reapproval. A superscript epsilon (ϵ) indicates an editorial change since the last revision or reapproval.

1. Scope

1.1 This specification covers Ultra-High Molecular Weight Polyethylene powder (UHMWPE) and fabricated forms intended for use in surgical implants.

1.2 The requirements of this specification apply to UHMWPE in two forms. One is virgin polymer powder (Section 4). The second is any form fabricated from this powder from which a finished product is subsequently produced (Section 5). This specification addresses material characteristics and does not apply to the packaged and sterilized finished implant.

1.3 The provisions of Specification D 4020 apply. Special requirements detailed in this specification are added to describe material which will be used in surgical implants.

1.4 The biological response to polyethylene in soft tissue and bone has been well characterized by a history of clinical use **(1, 2, 3)**[2] and by laboratory studies **(4, 5, 6)**.

1.5 The following precautionary caveat pertains only to the test method portion, Section 7, of this specification: *This standard does not purport to address all of the safety concerns, if any, associated with its use. It is the responsibility of the user of this standard to establish appropriate safety and health practices and determine the applicability of regulatory limitations prior to use.*

2. Referenced Documents

2.1 *ASTM Standards:*

D 256 Test for Impact Resistance of Plastics and Electrical Insulating Materials[3]

D 638 Test Method for Tensile Properties of Plastics[3]

D 648 Test Method for Deflection Temperature of Plastics Under Flexural Load[3]

D 790 Test Methods for Flexural Properties of Plastics and Electrical Insulating Materials[3]

D 792 Test Methods for Specific Gravity (Relative Density) and Density by Displacement[3]

D 1505 Test Method for Density of Plastics by the Density-Gradient Technique[3]

D 1898 Practice for Sampling of Plastics[3]

D 4020 Specification for Ultra-High Molecular Weight Polyethylene Molding and Extrusion Materials[4]

F 619 Practice for Extraction of Medical Plastics[5]

F 748 Practice for Selecting Generic Biological Test Methods for Materials and Devices[5]

F 749 Practice for Evaluating Material Extracts by Intracutaneous Injection in the Rabbit[5]

F 756 Practice for Assessment of Hemolytic Properties of Materials[5]

F 763 Practice for Short-Term Screening of Implant Materials[5]

F 813 Practice for Direct Contact Cell Culture Evaluation of Materials for Medical Devices[5]

F 895 Test Method for Agar Diffusion Cell Culture Screening for Cytotoxicity[5]

F 981 Practice for Assessment of Compatibility of Biomaterials (Nonporous) for Surgical Implants with Respect to Effect of Materials on Muscle and Bone[5]

2.2 *ISO Standards*

ISO 527 Plastics: Determination of Tensile Properties[6]

ISO 3451-1 Plastics—Determination of Ash, Part 1: General Methods[6]

ISO 11542/2, Plastics—Ultra-High Molecular Weight Polyethylene (UHMWPE) Moulding and Extrusion Materials—Part 2: Preparation of Test Specimens and Determination[6]

3. Terminology

3.1 *Definitions of Terms Specific to This Standard:*

3.1.1 *fabricated form*—any bulk shape of UHMWPE, fabricated from the virgin polymer powder, used during the process of fabricating surgical implants prior to packaging and sterilization.

3.1.1.1 *Discussion*—This form results from the application of heat and pressure to the virgin polymer powder, and the material characteristics of this form are subject to the applicable requirements of this specification. In present practice, this includes ram-extruded bars or molded blocks from which

[1] This specification is under the jurisdiction of ASTM Committee F04 on Medical and Surgical Materials and Devices and is the direct responsibility of Subcommittee F04.11 on Polymeric material.

Current edition approved May 10, 2000. Published August 2000. Originally published as F 648 – 96. Last previous edition F 648 – 98.

[2] The boldface numbers in parentheses refer to the list of references at the end of this specification.

[3] *Annual Book of ASTM Standards*, Vol 08.01.

[4] *Annual Book of ASTM Standards*, Vol 08.02.

[5] *Annual Book of ASTM Standards*, Vol 13.01.

[6] Available from American National Standards Institute, 11 W. 42nd St., 13th Floor, New York, NY 10036.

the final product form is machined, or a molded shape which is subsequently trimmed.

3.1.2 *generic property*—that property which is determined solely by the chemical composition and structure of the virgin polymer.

3.1.3 *morphology index (MI)*—material morphology quality shall be described by a morphology index (MI) defined as the ratio of the total number of Type A and Type B indications (See Annex A2) to the total surface area examined in cm^2.

3.1.4 *Type A non-fused flake*—a Type A non-fused flake (A2.4.1 and Fig. A2.1) is an indication visible under conditions described in A2.5.1 that has an essentially complete circumferential black boundary and a white center.

3.1.5 *Type B non-fused flake*—a Type B non-fused flake (A2.4.2 and Fig. A2.2) is an indication visible under conditions described in A2.5.1 that has a partially circumferential black boundary that appears to trace out 50 % to 99 % of a flake's perimeter.

3.1.6 *virgin polymer powder*—the form of UHMWPE as obtained from the powder manufacturer and prior to fabrication into a bulk shape.

4. Virgin UHMWPE Powder Requirements

4.1 *Generic Properties*:

4.1.1 The virgin polymer shall be a homopolymer of ethylene in accordance with Specification D 4020.

4.1.2 The resin type and solution viscosity number requirements are listed in Table 1.

4.2 *Nongeneric Properties*:

4.2.1 When a 300 g sample is prepared and viewed in accordance with 7.1.2, there shall be no more particles of extraneous matter than that specified in Table 1.

4.2.2 To promote uniformity between different lots of polymer powder, concentration limits for trace elements have been established and are listed in Table 1.

4.2.3 When determined as described in ISO 3451-1, the mean ash of duplicate samples shall not exceed the limits established in Table 1.

5. UHMWPE Fabricated Form Requirements

5.1 *Compositional Requirements*:

5.1.1 No stabilizers or processing aids are to be added to the virgin polymer powder during manufacture of a fabricated form.

5.2 *Physical Requirements*:

5.2.1 *Foreign Matter Requirements*:

5.2.1.1 When 3200 cm^2 is evaluated according to 7.2.2, there shall be no more than ten particles of extraneous matter visible on the surface when visually inspected by normal or corrected vision.

5.2.2 *Morphology Requirements*:

5.2.2.1 When evaluated according to Annex A2 the calculated morphology index (MI) and total surface area examined shall be reported.

5.3 *Mechanical Requirements*:

5.3.1 UHMWPE in fabricated form from which implants shall be made shall meet the requirements listed in Table 2.

5.3.2 The following mechanical tests may be conducted based on agreement between the vendor and purchaser:

5.3.2.1 Deflection temperature; Test Method D 648 (1.8 MPa), and Flexural modulus; Test Methods D 790 (secant, 2 % offset).

6. Sampling

6.1 Where applicable, the requirements of this specification shall be determined for each lot of powder and fabricated form by sampling sizes and procedures according to Practice D 1898, or as agreed upon between the purchaser and seller.

7. Test Methods

7.1 *UHMWPE Powder*:

7.1.1 Determine the solution viscosity number in accordance with the method given in Specification D 4020 at a concentration of 0.02 %.

7.1.2 Determine the amount of extraneous matter by the following procedure as agreed upon by the purchaser and seller.

7.1.2.1 A 300 g sample is divided into four 75 g samples. Place a 75 g sample in each of four 1000 mL Erlenmeyer flasks, add 400 mL isopropyl alcohol, shake 5 min, and let settle for 5 min. Count the total number of particles of extraneous matter in the four flasks.

7.1.2.2 Visually examine (20/20 corrected vision if necessary) the four flasks and count the total number of particles of extraneous matter.

7.1.3 Determine the following trace element concentrations

TABLE 1 Requirements for UHMWPE Powders

Property	Test Method	Requirement		
Resin Type		Type 1	Type 2	Type 3
Viscosity Number, mL/g,	ASTM D 4020 (0.02 %)	2000-3200	>3200	>3200
Ash, mg/kg, (Maximum)	ISO 3451-1	150	150	300
Extraneous Matter, No. Particles, (Maximum)	4.2.1	5	5	25
Titanium, mg/kg, (Maximum)	7.1.3.1	40	40	150
Aluminum, mg/kg, (Maximum)	7.1.3.1	40	40	100
Calcium, mg/kg, (Maximum)	7.1.3.1	50	50	50
Chlorine, mg/kg, (Maximum)	7.1.3.2	20	75	90

TABLE 2 Requirements for UHMWPE Fabricated Forms

Property	Test Method	Requirement		
Resin Type		Type 1	Type 2	Type 3
Density, kg/m^3	ASTM D 792 or D 1505	927-944	927-944	927-944
Ash, mg/kg, (Maximum)	ISO 3451-1	150	150	300
Tensile Strength, 23°C, MPa, (Minimum)[A]	ASTM D 638, Type IV, 5.08 cm/min			
Ultimate		35	27	27
Yield	ISO 527, 100 mm/min.	21	19	19
Elongation, %, (Minimum)[A]	ASTM D 638, Type IV, 5.08 cm/min ISO 527, 100 mm/min.	300	300	250
Izod Impact Strength, kJ/m^2, (Minimum)[B]	Annex A1	126	73	25
Charpy Impact Strength, kJ/m^2, (Minimum)[B]	ISO/CD 11542/2.3, Annex A2	180	90	30

[A]Either Test Method D 638 or ISO 527 may be used to determine tensile strength and elongation, however the ISO 527 method will be considered the referee method.

[B]Either Charpy or Izod impact strength may be determined, however, the Charpy test will be considered the referee method.

by the following methods, or by methods agreed upon by the purchaser and seller.

7.1.3.1 The elements Ti, Al, and Ca may be determined by atomic absorption (AA) or emission spectroscopy (ES); inductively coupled plasma mass spectroscopy (ICP/MS); or inductively coupled plasma spectroscopy (ICP).

7.1.3.2 The element chlorine (Cl) may be determined potentiometrically, titrametrically, by neutron activation analysis, by inductively coupled plasma mass spectroscopy (ICP/MS), or by the oxygen bomb combustion/UV-Vis spectroscopy method.

7.2 *UHMWPE Fabricated Form*:

7.2.1 The requirement that there will be no addition of any stabilizer or processing aid during fabrication of the fabricated form shall be met by certification of the fabricator.

7.2.2 Determine the amount of extraneous matter by the following procedure.

7.2.2.1 Prepare a number of test specimens from the fabricated form as agreed upon by the purchaser and seller.

7.2.2.2 Visually examine (20/20 corrected vision if necessary) a total area of 3200 cm^2 taken from locations within the fabricated form agreed upon by the purchaser and seller.

7.2.3 Determine the density in accordance with Test Methods D 792 or D 1505.

7.2.4 Determine specific mechanical properties in accordance with the methods listed in Table 2. Mechanical test specimens shall be produced by methods that represent those used to produce the fabricated form.

7.2.5 Unless otherwise specified, the testing described in Table 2 (except for ash) shall be conducted under standard conditions of 23 ± 2°C after storage of the test specimens for at least 16 h.

8. Biocompatibility

8.1 This material has been shown to produce a well characterized level of biological response following long term clinical use in laboratory animals. The results of these studies and the clinical history indicate an acceptable level of biological response in the applications in which the material has been utilized. When new applications of the material, or modification to the material or physical forms of the materials are being contemplated, the recommendations of Practice F 748 should be considered and testing considered as described in Practices F 619, F 749, F 756, F 763, F 813, and F 981 as well as Test Method F 895.

9. Keywords

9.1 fabricated forms; powdered form; ultra-high molecular weight polyethylene

ANNEXES

(Mandatory Information)

A1. IMPACT STRENGTH

A1.1 General Description

A1.1.1 This test method covers the determination of the impact resistance of Ultra-High Molecular Weight Polyethylene (UHMWPE) which is extremely impact resistant. When tested according to Test Method D 256, Method A, UHMWPE generally gives the NBF type for failure, rendering the test result invalid. This test method specifies the same type of pendulum impact test machine as given in Test Method D 256 but introduces a much higher degree of stress concentration into the specimen by double notching with a razor blade. It is advised that the user be familiar with Test Method D 256 before attempting to use this test method.

A1.2 Apparatus

A1.2.1 The Izod type impact machine which conforms to the requirements of Test Method D 256, including the calibration and checking methods, shall be used.

A1.3 Test Specimen

A1.3.1 The geometry and dimensions of the specimen are given in Fig. A1.1.

A1.3.2 The specimens shall be made from the fabricated form.

A1.3.3 Each specimen shall be free of twist and shall be bounded by mutually perpendicular pairs of plane parallel surfaces, free from scratches, pits, and sink marks.

A1.4 Notching of Specimens

A1.4.1 Notching shall be done on the sides parallel to the direction of application of molding pressure; if applicable.

A1.4.2 A 4.57± 0.076 mm (0.180 ± 0.003 in.) deep notch shall be made with a suitable machine by pressing in a 0.25 mm (0.010 in.) thick single edge razor blade with a 15° included angle at the cutting edge. The notching speed shall be less than 508 mm/min. (20 in./min.). A new blade shall be used after notching 40 specimens.

A1.4.3 The calibration of the notching machine shall be checked by direct measurement of the notch depth, perpendicularity, and offset of the two notches. One of the possible measurement methods is given in A1.8.

A1.5 Conditioning

A1.5.1 *Conditioning*—Condition the notched specimens at 23 ± 2 °C (73 ± 4 °F) for not less than 16 h prior to test.

A1.5.2 *Test Conditions*—Conduct the test in the standard laboratory atmosphere of 23 ± 2 °C (73 ± 4 °F).

A1.6 Procedure

A1.6.1 At least five and preferably ten individual determinations of impact value must be made on each sample to be tested under the conditions prescribed.

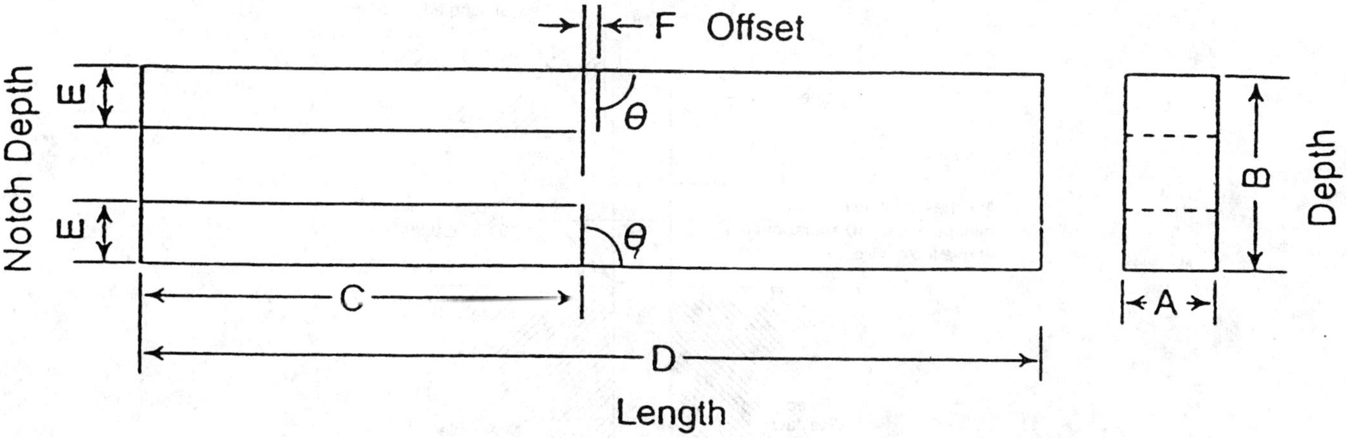

mm		in.	
A	6.35 ± 0.38	A	0.250 ± 0.015
B	12.70 ± 0.10	B	0.500 ± 0.004
C	31.75 ± 0.25	C	1.250 ± 0.010
D	63.50 ± 0.38	D	2.500 ± 0.015
E	4.57 ± 0.08	E	0.180 ± 0.003
F	0.00 ± 0.13	F	0.000 ± 0.005
O	90° ± 2°	O	90° ± 2°

FIG. A1.1 Dimensions of Double Notched Izod Test Specimen

A1.6.2 Measure the width of each specimen in the area between notches twice with a micrometer to the nearest 0.025 mm (0.001 in.) and record its average width. Carefully measure the distance between the notch roots on the two sides of the specimen. Use of an optical microscope may improve the accuracy of this measurement. Record the average value and multiply this number by the width of the specimen to get the remaining unnotched cross section area, AR. Also record the identifying markings of the specimen.

A1.6.3 Estimate the breaking energy for the specimen and select a pendulum of suitable energy. Start the test with a pendulum of 11 J (8 ft.-lb), if no prior test data is available. Use the lightest standard pendulum that is expected to break each specimen in the group with a loss of not more than 85 % of its energy.

A1.6.4 Before testing the specimens, perform the operations on the machine.

A1.6.4.1 With the excess energy indicating pointer in its normal starting position but without a specimen in the vise, release the pendulum from its normal starting position and note the position the pointer attains after the swing as one reading of Factor A.

A1.6.4.2 Without resetting the pointer, raise the pendulum and release again. The pointer should move up the scale an additional amount. Repeat this procedure until a swing causes no additional movement of the pointer and note the final reading as one reading of Factor B.

A1.6.4.3 Repeat the above two operations several times and calculate and record the average A and B readings.

A1.6.5 Position the specimen precisely and rigidly but not too tightly clamped in the vise. The relationship of the vise, specimen, and striking edge of the pendulum to each other is given in Fig. A1.2. Note that the top plane of the vise shall be 0.13 ± 0.13 mm (0.005± 0.005 in.) below the notches.

A1.6.6 Release the pendulum and note and record the excess energy remaining in the pendulum after breaking the specimen.

A1.6.7 From the breaking strength of the specimen and Factors A and B, determine the energy loss of the pendulum due to windage and friction using the correction charts from the commercial testing machine supplier. If these charts are not available, then use the method given in Appendix X2 or X3 of Test Method D 256. Subtract the correction so calculated from the indicated breaking strength of the specimen. If a pendulum of improper energy was used, discard the result and make additional tests on new specimens with the proper pendulum. If the proper pendulum was used, divide the net value so found by the unnotched area AR of the specimen as measured in A1.6.2 to obtain its double notched Izod impact resistance in kJ/m^2($ft.-lb/in.^2$).

A1.6.8 Record the type of failure for each specimen as one of the three coded categories defined as follows:

A1.6.8.1 *C (Complete Break)*—A break in which the specimen separates into two pieces and the fracture plane contains

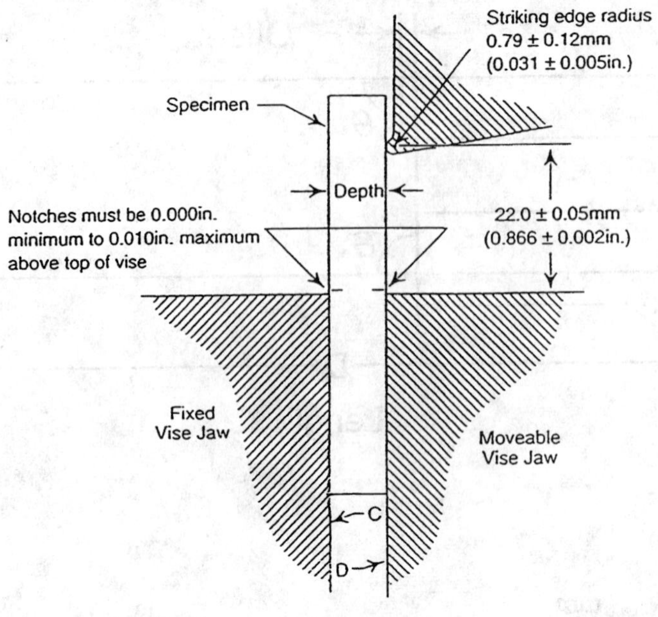

Planes C and D must be parallel to within 0.025mm (0.001in.)

FIG. A1.2 Relationship of Vise, Specimen, and Striking Edge to Each Other

both lines of the notch roots.

A1.6.8.2 *IB (Irregular Break)*—The specimen separates into two pieces but the fracture plane contains only one of the notch roots.

A1.6.8.3 *NB (Nonbreak)*—A break in which the specimen does not separate into two pieces.

A1.6.9 Calculate the average impact resistance and standard deviation of the group of specimens.

A1.7 Report

A1.7.1 Report the following information:

A1.7.1.1 Complete identification of the material tested, including type, source, and manufacturer's lot number,

A1.7.1.2 Capacity of the pendulum in joules (foot-pounds-force),

A1.7.1.3 Total number of specimens tested,

A1.7.1.4 Average double notched Izod impact resistance in kJ/m^2 (ft-lb/in^2),

A1.7.1.5 Standard deviation, and

A1.7.1.6 Percent of specimens failing in each category suffixed by the corresponding letter code from A1.6.8.

A1.8 Measurement Method of Imperfections in Specimen Notching

A1.8.1 The following is one of the possible test methods to directly measure the imperfections in specimen notching, which can be classified into three kinds: deviation from perpendicularity; incorrect notch depth, and; offset of notches (Fig. A1.3).

A1.8.2 *Apparatus*:

A1.8.2.1 An *Ocular*, 40 to 60×, reflective optical microscope with an X-Y stage accurate to 0.0025 mm (0.0001 in.);

A1.8.2.2 An *Eyepiece*, with a crosshair;

A1.8.2.3 *Fiber Optic Illumination*.

A1.8.3 *Procedure*:

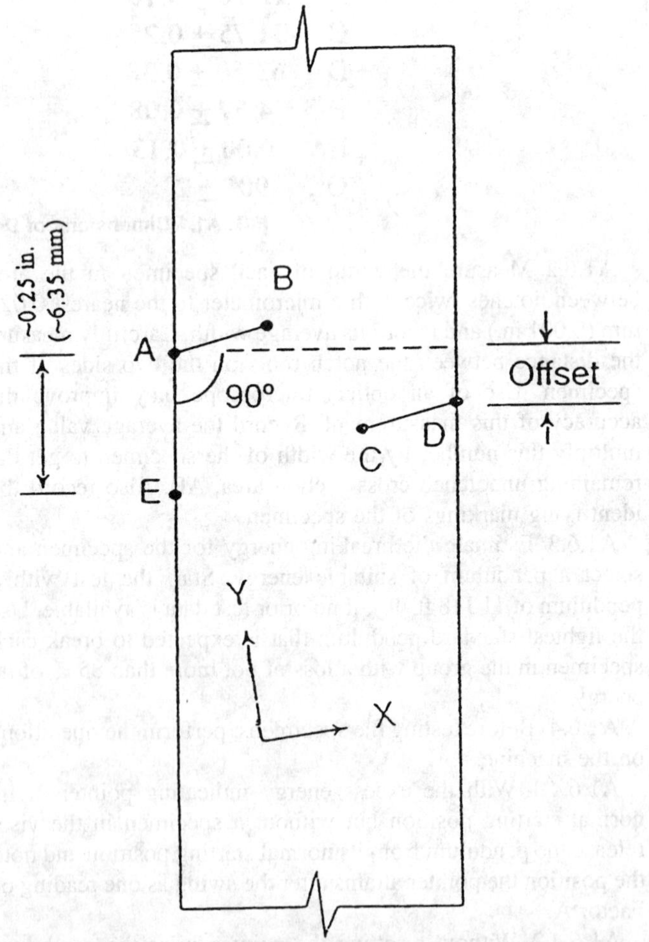

FIG. A1.3 Notch Geometry of Double Notched Izod Specimen

A1.8.3.1 Lay the specimen on one of its sides and mount it securely on the X-Y stage.

A1.8.3.2 The beginning and ending points of the notches are labeled from A to D in Fig. A1.3. Select one of the edges of the specimen as the datum line from which the perpendicularity of the notches to the edges is measured (in this case line *AE*). Note that point *E* is approximately 6.35 mm (0.25 in.) from point *A*.

A1.8.3.3 Both the microscope and the base of the X-Y stage should be stationary. Measure the coordinates of points *A* to *E* with respect to an arbitrarily selected coordinate system by moving the X-Y stage and by targeting the points by the crosshair of the eyepiece.

A1.8.4 *Calculation*

A1.8.4.1 The following equation is used to calculate perpendicularity of the notches:

$$\angle EAB = \tan^{-1}[(m_2 - m_1)/(1 + m_1 m_2)] \quad (A1.1)$$

where:

m_1 and m_2 are the slopes of line *AE* and *AB* with respect to the coordinate system. m_1 and m_2 are calculated from:

$$m = (y_2 - y_1)/(x_2 - x_1) \quad (A1.2)$$

where:

m is the slope, and $(x_1 y_1)$ and $(x_2 y_2)$ are the coordinates of the end points of the line. The distance between two points, I, is obtained from:

$$I = [(x_2 - x_1)^2 + (y_2 - y_1)^2]^{0.5} \quad (A1.3)$$

A2. MORPHOLOGY EVALUATION

A2.1 General Description

A2.1.1 This test method covers the determination of the morphology quality of fabricated forms of Ultra-High Molecular Weight Polyethylene (UHMWPE). Well consolidated UHMWPE will have none or few regions of incompletely fused UHMWPE flake particles. This procedure is designed to evaluate the relative consolidation quality (morphology) of fabricated forms of UHMWPE by measuring the number of incompletely fused UHMWPE particles.

A2.2 Test Specimens

A2.2.1 Test specimens are approximately 100 μm thick slices of the material.

A2.2.2 Test specimens shall be collected from locations known to be most prone to consolidation difficulties; otherwise, at the approximate center of the sample or as agreement between purchaser and seller.

A2.2.3 The number of test specimens collected shall be as agreed upon between the purchaser and seller.

A2.2.4 If multiple film specimens are taken from the same piece, they shall be spaced at least 0.5 mm apart.

A2.2.5 Approximately 2 cm^2 from the center region of each test specimen shall be examined according to A2.5.

A2.3 Preparing Thin Film Specimens

A2.3.1 Thin translucent film specimens approximately 100 μm thick shall be prepared. Films should be relatively uniform in thickness and essentially free of skives, tears, etc. commonly resulting from the use of dull cutting equipment.

A2.3.2 The thin films may be placed flat between two clean glass microscope slides for convenient microscopic examination.

A2.4 Definitions

A2.4.1 *Type A Non-Fused Flake*—A Type A non-fused flake is an indication visible under the conditions described in A2.5.1 that has an essentially complete circumferential black boundary and a white center. See Fig. A2.1.

A2.4.2 *Type B Non-Fused Flake*—A Type B non-fused flake is an indication visible under the conditions described in A2.5.1 that has a partially circumferential black boundary that appears to trace out 50 to 99 % of a flake's perimeter. See Fig. A2.2.

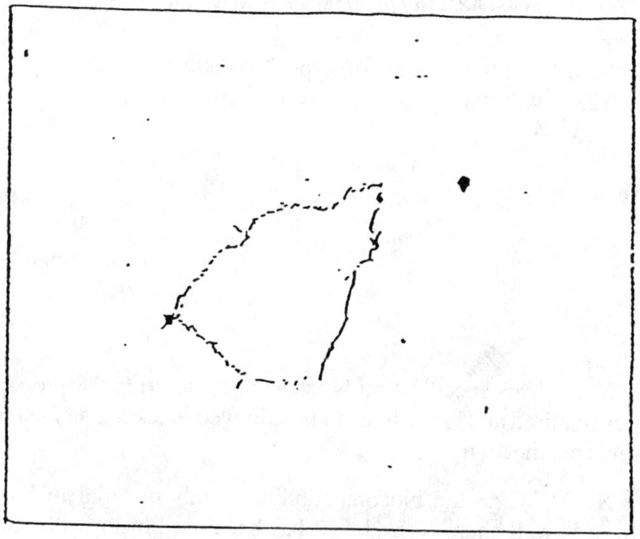

FIG. A2.1 Representative Type A Indication

A2.4.3 *Morphology Index (MI)*—Material morphology quality shall be described by a morphology index (MI) defined as the ratio of the total number of Type A and Type B indications to the total surface area examined in cm^2.

A2.5 Procedure

A2.5.1 Test specimens are evaluated by optical microscopy at no lower than 40x using thin films of the material illuminated by transmitted light. Dark field, reflection, or other such means may be used to visualize regions of incompletely fused flakes if they are demonstrated to give essentially equivalent results.

A2.6 Report

A2.6.1 Report the following for each material tested:

A2.6.1.1 Complete identification of the material tested, including virgin resin type consolidation method, and converter.

A2.6.1.2 Total number of Type A indications observed,

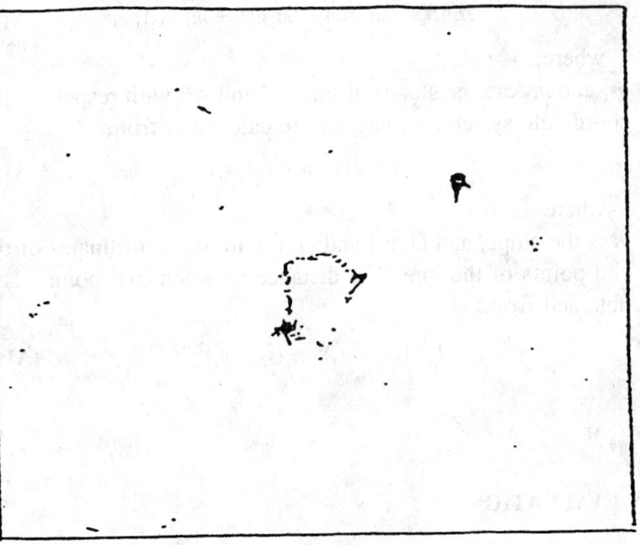

FIG. A2.2 Representative Type B Indication

A2.6.1.3 Total number of Type B indications observed,

A2.6.1.4 Total surface area examined in cm^2, and

A2.6.1.5 Calculated Morphology Index (MI) in accordance with A2.4.3.

APPENDIX

(Nonmandatory Information)

X1. RATIONALE

X1.1 This specification is intended to describe the properties required and procedures to be followed in testing and using this specification.

X1.2 While the biocompatibility of this material in bulk form is well characterized as it has been used historically, the data cannot necessarily be assumed to be applicable to modified forms or applications of the material. The material user should carefully analyze the published biocompatibility data and then decide whether additional testing may be necessary as a result of the changes which may have been made.

X1.3 Information on the degree of branching, methyl group concentration, and vinylidene content would be useful. Presently, there is not a suitable method to determine these parameters.

X1.4 While the precise relationship between the bulk properties and wear resistance of implants and the molecular weight of the polyethylene used to fabricate them has not been established quantitatively, it has been demonstrated that UHMWPE is more suitable for such applications than are polyethylenes of lower molecular weight.

X1.5 The viscosity number of dilute solutions of UHMWPE powder may be used as an adequate indicator that some minimum value of molecular weight is attained. At present, there is some uncertainty regarding the extension of the solution viscosity/molecular weight relationship to the UHMWPE range.

X1.6 Information on the molecular weight distribution may permit control of the weight fraction of low-molecular weight material. Presently, there is no adequate method for determining this distribution.

X1.7 There is no evidence at this time that the concentration of trace elements has any effect on the physical properties or the biological response of UHMWPE fabricated forms.

X1.8 The relationship between these mechanical properties and the in-vivo performance of a fabricated form has not been determined. While trends are apparent, specific property-polymer structure relationships are not well understood. These mechanical tests are frequently used to evaluate the reproducibility of a fabrication procedure and are applicable as quality control tests to determine lot to lot repeatability for a process of converting virgin polymer powder to a fabricated form. The mechanical properties are subject to variation as the fabrication process variables (such as temperature, pressure, and time) are changed.

X1.9 At the present time there are no clear correlations between a sample's morphology index and its functional characteristics. For this reason this document does not specify a maximum allowed index.

REFERENCE

(1) Charnley, J., Cupiz, A., "The Nine and Ten Year Results of the Low Friction Arthroplasty of the Hip," *Clinical Orthopaedics*, Vol 95, No. 9, 1973.

(2) Cimbrelo, E.G., Munera, L., "Early and Late Loosening of the Acetabular Cup After Low-Friction Arthroplasty", *The Journal of Bone and Joint Surgery*, Vol 74-A, No. 8, 1992.

(3) Mirra, J., Amstutz, H., Matos, M., Gold, R., "The Pathology of the Joint Tissues and Its Clinical Relevance in Prosthesis Failure," *Clinical Orthopaedics*, No. 117, 1976.

(4) Turner, J., Lawrence, W., Autian, J., "Subacute Toxicity Testing of Biomaterials Using Histopathologic Evaluation of Rabbit Muscle Tissue," *Journal of Biomedical Materials Research*, Vol 7, 1973.

(5) Laing, P., "Compatibility of Biomaterials," *Orthopedic Clinics of North America*, Vol 4, No. 2, 1973.

(6) Escalas, F., Galante, J., Rostoker, W., "Biocompatibility of Materials for Total Joint Replacement," *Journal of Biomedical Materials Research*, Vol 10, No. 2, 1976.

Designation: F 665 – 98

Standard Classification for Vinyl Chloride Plastics Used in Biomedical Application[1]

This standard is issued under the fixed designation F 665; the number immediately following the designation indicates the year of original adoption or, in the case of revision, the year of last revision. A number in parentheses indicates the year of last reapproval. A superscript epsilon (ε) indicates an editorial change since the last revision or reapproval.

1. Scope

1.1 This classification provides guidance to engineers and users in the selection of practical vinyl chloride plastics for medical applications and further provides a method for specifying these materials by use of a simple line call-out designation. This standard excludes vinyl chloride plastics used in long-term implants.

1.2 Use is made of a classification scheme based on the premise that the composition of vinyl chloride plastics, copolymers, fillers, plasticizers, stabilizers, and other additives in these systems can be arranged into characteristic material designations.

1.3 In all cases where the provisions of this classification system would conflict with those of the detailed specification for a particular device, the latter shall take precedence.

NOTE 1—For cases in which the vinyl chloride plastic may be used for purposes where the requirements are too specific to be completely described by this classification system, it is advisable for the purchaser to consult the supplier to secure adjustment of the properties to suit the actual conditions to which the device is to be subjected.

1.4 The biocompatibility of vinyl chloride plastics as a class of materials has not been established. Since many compositions and formulations fall under this class, it is essential that the fabricators/device manufacturers assure the safety and efficacy of the specific composition or formulation, in its intended application, using state-of-the-art test methods.

1.5 This classification is to assist the interface between the material supplier and the device manufacturer (fabricator) who purchases a formulated vinyl chloride plastic for a component. For those device manufacturers (fabricators) who do their own formulating, compounding, extrusion, molding, etc., this classification does not apply.

1.6 *This standard does not purport to address all of the safety concerns, if any, associated with its use. It is the responsibility of the user of this standard to establish appropriate safety and health practices and determine the applicability of regulatory limitations prior to use.*

2. Referenced Documents

2.1 *ASTM Standards:*

D 149 Test Method for Dielectric Breakdown Voltage and Dielectric Strength of Solid Electrical Insulating Materials at Commercial Power Frequencies[2]

D 150 Test Methods for A-C Loss Characteristics and Permittivity (Dielectric Constant) of Solid Electrical Insulating Materials[2]

D 257 Test Methods for D-C Resistance or Conductance of Insulating Materials[2]

D 543 Test Method for Resistance of Plastics to Chemical Reagents[3]

D 570 Test Method for Water Absorption of Plastics[3]

D 792 Test Methods for Specific Gravity (Relative Density) and Density of Plastics by Displacement[3]

D 882 Test Methods for Tensile Properties of Thin Plastic Sheeting[3]

D 955 Test Method of Measuring Shrinkage from Mold Dimensions of Molded Plastics[3]

D 1898 Practice for Sampling of Plastics[3]

D 2124 Method for Analysis of Components in Poly(Vinyl Chloride) Compounds Using an Infrared Spectrophotometric Technique[3]

D 2240 Test Method for Rubber Property—Durometer Hardness[4]

F 748 Practoce for Selecting Generic Biological Test Methods for Materials and Devices

2.2 *Other Standards:*

Title 21 Code of Federal Regulations[5]

3. Terminology

3.1 *Definitions:*

3.1.1 *filler*—a relatively inert material added to a plastic to modify its strength, permanence, working properties, or other qualities, or to lower costs.

3.1.2 *plasticizer*—a substance incorporated in a material to increase its workability, flexibility, or distensibility.

3.1.3 *stabilizer*—a substance added to a plastic that will retard the deterioration of the plastic due to the effects of heat, light, or oxidation.

3.1.4 *vinyl chloride plastics*—plastics based on polymers of vinyl chloride or copolymers of vinyl chloride with other

---

[1] This classification is under the jurisdiction of ASTM Committee F-4 on Medical and Surgical Materials and Devicesand is the direct responsibility of Subcommittee F04.11on Polymeric Materials.

Current edition approved October 10, 1998. Published March 1999. Originally published as F 665 – 80. Last previous edition F 665 – 80 (1993)$^{\epsilon 1}$.

[2] *Annual Book of ASTM Standards*, Vol 10.01.

[3] *Annual Book of ASTM Standards*, Vol 08.01.

[4] *Annual Book of ASTM Standards*, Vol 09.01.

[5] Available from Superintendent of Documents, U.S. Government Printing Office, Washington, DC 20402.

monomers, the vinyl chloride being the comonomer of the highest concentration by mass.

4. Significance and Use

4.1 This classification was developed to permit the addition of descriptive symbols and values for further new formulations with improved properties without complete reorganization of the standard and to facilitate the incorporation of future new test methods to keep pace with changing industry requirements.

5. Formulation Designation

NOTE 2—No judgment is made by ASTM as to the suitability of possible compounds classified by the following system to any specific biomedical use. Knowledge of formulation composition will only *aid* in evaluation of a composition for suitability.

5.1 A letter/number system shall be used that will give guidance to the engineer/user as to the nature of the formulation. A general knowledge of the types of additives employed will aid in the evaluation of a particular formulation's utility in a medical application.

5.2 *Homopolymer*—By definition, only one homopolymer is covered by this standard: poly(vinyl chloride).

5.3 *Copolymer*—The following is a representative list of major copolymers of poly(vinyl chloride). To specify the copolymer, use the prefix (A) followed by the number designation for the copolymer. In the event that more than one copolymer is present, separate the individual number designations by a comma.

Number Designation	Copolymer
1	none
2	vinyl acetate
3	vinylidene chloride
4	maleic ester
5	vinyl ether
6	propylene
7	ethylene
999	other

5.4 *Plasticizer*—The following is a representative list of primary monomeric and polymeric plasticizers with corresponding number designation and a list of secondary plasticizers with their corresponding letter designation. To specify the plasticizer system, use the prefix letter (B) followed by the secondary plasticizer number. In the event that there is more than one primary or secondary plasticizer, or both, separate the individual letter or number designations, or both, by a comma.

Letter Designation	Secondary Plasticizer
A	none
B	alkyl epoxy stearates
C	epoxidized tall oil
D	epoxidized soybean oil
E	epoxidized linseed oil
F	epoxidized sunflower oil
Z	other

Number	Primary Plasticizer
1	none
2	adipic acid derivatives
3	azelaic acid derivatives
4	benzoic acid derivatives
5	citric acid derivatives
6	isophthalic acid derivatives
7	myristic acid derivatives
8	phosphoric acid derivatives
9	phthalic acid derivatives
10	sebacic acid derivatives
11	terephthalic acid derivatives
12	polyethers
13	polyethylene glycols
14	polyesters
999	other

5.5 *Stabilizers*—Stabilization systems are usually composed of metal soap acceptors and auxiliary organic stabilizers. The metal soap acceptors are characterized by the metal(s) present. The following is a representative list of stabilizers. The designation is obtained by using the prefix (C) followed by the letter for the metal, followed by the number for the chelator used. In the event that more than one in each category is present, separate multiple letter or number designations, or both, by a comma.

Letter	Metal in Soap Acceptor
A	none
B	barium
C	calcium
D	cadmium
E	magnesium
F	lead
G	strontium
H	tin
I	zinc
Z	other

Number	Auxiliary Organic Stabilizer
1	none
2	organophospite
999	other

5.6 *Fillers*—The following is a representative list of fillers. The designation is obtained by using the prefix (D) followed by the number of the filler used. In the event that more than one is used, separate each number by a comma.

Number	Filler
1	none
2	clay
3	mica
4	talc
5	diatomaceous earth
6	titanium dioxide
7	calcium carbonate
8	carbon black
9	conductive carbon black
10	barium sulfate
11	Bi_2O_3
999	other

5.7 *Colorants*—The following is a representative list of colorants. The designation is obtained by using the prefix (E) followed by the number. In the event that more than one is used, separate each number by a comma.

Number	Colorant
1	none
2	titanium dioxide
3	ultramarine blue
4	phthalocyanines
5	benzidines
6	quinacridones
7	oxynaphthoic reds
8	FD & C colorants

999	other

5.8 *Lubricants*—The following is a representative list of lubricants. The designation is obtained by using the prefix (F) followed by the number. In the event that more than one is used, separate each number by a comma.

Number	Lubricant
1	none
2	stearic acid and derivatives
3	metal stearates
4	waxes
5	low molecular weight polyethylene
6	silicones
7	stearamides
999	other

5.9 *Example*—As an example of how this materials designation would be used, suppose there was a vinyl chloride plastic formulation with the following ingredients: PVC, 2 ethyl hexyl phthlate, expoxidized soybean oil, lead stearate, ultramarine blue, and stearic acid. This entire system would be characterized by the following designation: BD9CF1D1E3F2.

5.10 Many ingredients are cited by the FDA in the Food Additive Regulations (21 CFR). Since there is a very long list of possible additives to vinyl chloride plastics, it would serve as a starting point to know if all components to the formula are suitable for food contact applications. This can be designated as (Y) or (N) for yes or no at the end of the above example.

6. Main Number Designation

6.1 The main number shall define the basic physical properties of the plastic compound and will include hardness (Shore A), tensile strength, and elongation (%). Other properties and requirements shall be covered by a suffix code.

6.1.1 *Hardness*—The first number shall define the hardness of the plastic compound by the first number of the nominal ±5 point range:

Designation	Hardness (Shore A, Test Method D 2240)
0	below 5
1	10 ± 5
2	20 ± 5
3	30 ± 5
4	40 ± 5
5	50 ± 5
6	60 ± 5
7	70 ± 5
8	80 ± 5
9	See special note for special range requirement.

6.1.2 *Elongation*—The second set will be a two-digit code which shall define the minimum elongation in percent as follows:

Code	Elongation, min, % (Test Methods D 882)
10	100
29	290
99	990
00	See special note for special range requirement.

6.1.3 *Tensile Strength*—The second group shall be a threedigit code which shall designate the minimum allowable tensile strength in megapascals as follows:

Code	Tensile Strength, min, MPa (psi) (Test Methods D 882)
007	0.7 (100)
035	3.5 (500)
070	7.0(1000)
105	10.5(1500)
000	See special note for special range requirement.

7. Chemical, Mechanical, and Biological Properties

7.1 The specific chemical, mechanical, and biological properties will be determined by a purchaser-seller agreement based on end use.

7.2 The following is a representative list of referee tests that may be employed to determine those properties:

Specific gravity	D 792
Durometer	D 2240
Tensile strength	D 882
Percent elongation	D 882
Modulus at specified elongation	D 882
Dielectric strength	D 149
Dielectric constant	D 150
Volume resistivity	D 257
Surface resistivity	D 257
IR analysis of components	D 2124

8. Biocompatibility

8.1 The biocompatibility of vinyl chloride plastics, as a class of materials, has not been established. Since many compositions and formulations fall under this class, it is essential that the fabricator assure the safety and efficacy of the specific composition or formulation, in its intended application, using state-of-the-art test methods.

8.2 Biological tests are appropriate to determine biological and tissue reaction depending on the end-use application. These tests should be conducted when indicated for specific applications using F 748 and the United States Pharmacopeia[6] as a guide.**(1)**

9. Keywords

9.1 plastic surgical devices/application; vinyl chloride plastics

[6] The boldface numbers in parentheses refer to the list of references at the end of this standard.

APPENDIXES

(Nonmandatory Information)

X1. RATIONALE

X1.1 This document provides definitions and a standard description for vinyl chloride plastics for biomedical applications. The guide enumerates relevant test methods and describes generic criteria which should assist in developing more specific specifications for implantable devices containing vinyl chloride plastics with values and limits covering end-use applications.

X2. BIOCOMPATIBILITY

X2.1 The suitability of these materials from a human implant perspective is dependent on the specific application. The biologic tests appropriate for the specific site, such as recommended in Practice F 748 should be used as a guideline.

X2.2 No known surgical implant material has ever been shown to be completely free of adverse reactions in the human body. However, long-term clinical experience of use of specific compositions and formulations of this material class referred to in this standard has shown that an acceptable level of biological response can be expected, if the material is used in appropriate applications.

REFERENCES

(**1**) The United States Pharmacopeia, XXIII, 1995.

Designation: F 688 – 00

Standard Specification for Wrought Cobalt-35 Nickel-20 Chromium-10 Molybdenum Alloy Plate, Sheet, and Foil for Surgical Implants (UNS R30035)[1]

This standard is issued under the fixed designation F 688; the number immediately following the designation indicates the year of original adoption or, in the case of revision, the year of last revision. A number in parentheses indicates the year of last reapproval. A superscript epsilon (ε) indicates an editorial change since the last revision or reapproval.

1. Scope *

1.1 This specification covers the requirements for a wrought cobalt-35 nickel-20 chromium-10 molybdenum alloy plate, sheet, and foil used for the manufacture of surgical implants.

1.2 The values stated in inch-pound units are to be regarded as the standard. The SI units given in parentheses are for information only.

2. Referenced Documents

2.1 *ASTM Standards:*

A 480 Specification for General Requirements for Flat-Rolled Stainless and Heat-Resisting Steel Plate, Sheet, and Strip[2]

E 8 Methods for Tension Testing of Metallic Materials[3]

E 10 Test Method for Brinell Hardness of Metallic Materials[3]

E 18 Test Methods for Rockwell Hardness and Rockwell Superficial Hardness of Metallic Materials[3]

E 92 Test Method for Vickers Hardness of Metallic Materials[3]

E 112 Test Methods for Determining Average Grain Size[3]

E 140 Hardness Conversion Tables for Metals (Relationship Between Brinell Hardness, Vickers Hardness, Rockwell Hardness, Rockwell Superficial Hardness, and Knoop Hardness)[3]

E 345 Methods for Tension Testing of Metallic Foil[3]

E 384 Test Method for Microhardness of Materials[3]

F 562 Specification for Wrought Cobalt-Nickel-Chromium-Molybdenum Alloy for Surgical Implant Applications[4]

F 981 Practice for Assessment of Compatibility of Biomaterials for Surgical Implants with Respect to Effect of Materials on Muscle and Bone[4]

2.2 *Aerospace Materials Specification:*

AMS 2269 Chemical Check Analysis Limits—Wrought Nickel Alloys and Cobalt Alloys[5]

2.3 *American Society for Quality Standard:*

C 1 Specification of General Requirements for a Quality Program[6]

3. Terminology

3.1 *Descriptions of Terms Specific to This Standard:*

3.1.1 *foil*—material under 0.005 in. (0.127 mm) in thickness.

3.1.2 *plate*—as used in this specification, material 0.1875 in. (4.76 mm) and over in thickness.

3.1.3 *sheet*—as used in this specification, material 0.005 in. (0.127 mm) to under 0.1875 in. (4.76 mm) in thickness.

4. Ordering Information

4.1 Inquiries and orders for material under this specification shall include the following information:

4.1.1 Quantity (weight or number of pieces),

4.1.2 ASTM Designation,

4.1.3 Form (plate, sheet, foil),

4.1.4 Condition (see 5.1),

4.1.5 Mechanical properties (if applicable for special conditions),

4.1.6 Finish (see 5.2-5.4),

4.1.7 Applicable dimensions, including size, thickness, width, and length (exact, random, or multiples) or print number, and

4.1.8 Special requirements.

5. Manufacture

5.1 *Condition*—Plate, sheet, and foil shall be furnished to the implant manufacturer as specified in the annealed or cold-worked condition.

5.2 *Finishes Available for Plate*:

5.2.1 Ground finish produced by surface grinding or continuous belt sanding.

5.2.2 Dull finish produced by chemical descaling.

5.3 *Finishes Available for Sheet*:

---

[1] This specification is under the jurisdiction of ASTM Committee F04 on Medical and Surgical Materials and Devicesand is the direct responsibility of Subcommittee F04.12 on Metallurgical Materials.

Current edition approved Nov. 10, 2000. Published February 2001. Originally published as F 688 – 80. Last previous editioin F 688 – 95.

[2] *Annual Book of ASTM Standards*, Vol 01.03.

[3] *Annual Book of ASTM Standards*, Vol 03.01.

[4] *Annual Book of ASTM Standards*, Vol 13.01.

[5] Available from Society of Automotive Engineers, 400 Commonwealth Drive, Warrendale, PA 15096.

[6] Available from the American Society for Quality, 161 West Wisconsin Ave., Milwaukee, WI 53203.

***A Summary of Changes section appears at the end of this standard.**

5.3.1 Ground finish produced by continuous belt sanding for sizes 0.060 in. (1.524 mm) to under 0.1875 in. (4.76 mm).

5.3.2 Bright rolled finish for sizes under 0.060 in. (1.524 mm).

5.3.3 Dull finish on annealed or aged material.

5.4 *Finishes Available for Foil*:

5.4.1 Bright rolled finish.

5.4.2 Dull finish on annealed or aged material.

5.4.3 Mirror finish on rolled material.

5.5 *Edges Available for Plate*:

5.5.1 Rolled edge.

5.5.2 Approximate square edge produced by abrasive sawing.

5.6 *Edges Available for Sheet*:

5.6.1 For sizes greater than 0.060 in. (1.524 mm) in thickness, an approximate square edge produced by abrasive sawing.

5.6.2 For sizes under 0.060 in. (1.524 mm) an edge produced by slitting or shearing.

5.7 *Edge Available for Foil*—An edge produced by slitting or shearing.

6. Chemical Composition

6.1 The heat analysis and product analysis tolerance shall conform to the requirements as to chemical composition as specified in Specification F 562.

7. Mechanical Requirements

7.1 Material ordered in the annealed condition shall conform to the requirements as to mechanical properties as agreed upon between the implant manufacturer and the vendor. Minimum mechanical property requirements for annealed products are listed in Table 1.

7.2 The current edition of Specification A 480 shall be used as a reference in the selection of tension test specimens.

7.2.1 The tension test specimens shall conform to the appropriate sections of Methods E 8 and E 345.

7.3 Material ordered in the cold-worked condition shall conform to the requirements as to mechanical properties as agreed upon between the implant manufacturer and the vendor.

TABLE 1 Sheet Mechanical Properties

Condition	Ultimate Tensile Strength, min, psi (MPa)[A]	Yield Strength (0.2 % offset), min, psi (MPa)[A]	Elongation, min, % in 2 in. or 50 mm	Rockwell Hardness, min
Annealed[B]	115 000 (792)	45 000 (310)	45	87 HRB
48 % cold worked	197 000 (1357)	195 000 (1343)	3	43 HRC

[A] Tensile and yield requirements apply to tests taken longitudinally to the rolling direction.

[B] 0.0197 in. (0.5 mm) sheet, vacuum annealed at 1875°F (1022°C), 2 h at temperature.

Mechanical property requirements for a 48 % cold-worked sheet product, etc. listed in Table 1.

7.4 When desired, Rockwell hardness B scale (HRB), Rockwell hardness C scale (HRC) or Vickers hardness (HV) limits may be specified, as agreed upon between the implant manufacturer and the supplier. Test Methods E 10, E 18, E 92, E 384 and Standard Tables E 140 shall be used.

8. Special Tests

8.1 If supplied in the annealed condition, the average grain size shall be predominantly four or finer when tested in accordance with Methods E 112.

8.1.1 Samples for grain size determination shall be selected after the final annealing operation.

8.1.2 Any other special requirements shall be agreed upon between the implant manufacturer and the supplier.

9. Certification

9.1 The manufacturer's certification that the material was manufactured and tested in accordance with this specification, together with a report of the test results shall be furnished at the time of shipment.

10. Quality Program Requirements

10.1 The producer shall maintain a quality program, such as that defined in ASQ Specification C1 or any other recognized program.

11. Keywords

11.1 cobalt alloys (for surgical implants); cobalt-nickel alloy; metals (for surgical implants)-cobalt alloys

APPENDIXES

(Nonmandatory Information)

X1. RATIONALE

X1.1 The primary reason for this specification is to characterize the composition and properties to assure consistency in the starting material used in the manufacture of medical devices.

X1.2 The acceptable metal conditions include annealed, or cold worked. The choice is dependent upon the medical device design and its intended application.

X2. BIOCOMPATIBILITY

X2.1 The alloy composition covered by this specification has been successfully employed in human implants **(1-5)**[7] for over a decade. Due to the well characterized level of biological response exhibited by this alloy, it has been used as a control material in Practice F 981.

X2.2 No Known surgical implant material has ever been shown to be completely free of adverse reactions in the human body. However, long term clinical experience has shown an acceptable level of biological response can be expected, if the material is used in appropriate applications

[7] The boldface numerals in parentheses refer to the list of references at the end of this specification.

REFERENCES

(**1**) Gaechter, A., and Galante, G., "MP35N, A Corrosion Resistant High-Strength Alloy for Orthopaedic or Surgical Implants: Two Year Bioassay," *Journal of Biomedical Materials Research*, Vol 10, 1976, pp. 829–831.

(**2**) Escales, F., Galante, J., Rostoker, W., and Coogan, P. S., "MP35N, A Corrosion Resistant High Strength Alloy for Orthopaedic Surgical Implants: Bioassay Results," *Journal of Biomedical Materials Research*, Vol 9, No. 3, 1976, pp. 303–313.

(**3**) Kuehne, D., and Willert H. G., "The Tissue Compatibility of the Forging Alloy (Protasul 10) with the Hitherto Used Implant Alloys (Co-Cr-Mo Casting Alloy) and (AISI 316L) After an Implantation Period of One Year," Doctoral Thesis, Osteological Research Laboratory of Orthopaedic University, Frankfurt on Main/Frg, 1975.

(**4**) Bauman, R., and Semlitsch, M., "Biological and Mechanical Behavior of Newly Developed Implant Materials in Animal Studies," *Sulzer Reprint*, Re/28.09.00, 1974, pp 1–9.

(**5**) ISO/TC-150/SC-1/WG-1, Swiss Standard Association, Group 129-Surgical Implants, Draft Report of WG-1, Swiss Proposal 9056509, Part 2, Comments on Biocompatibility, Davos Meeting, June 1974.

SUMMARY OF CHANGES

Committee F04 has identified the location of selected changes to this standard since the last issue (F688–95) that may impact the use of this standard.

(1) The UNS designation has been added.
(2) Product analysis tolerance information was referred to F562.
(3) Test Specimens paragraph was deleted and requirements were included in the appropriate sub-paragraphs.
(4) F981, AMS 2269 and ASQ C1 specifications were updated.
(5) X2. Biocompatibility section was added to the Appendix.

Designation: F 700 – 93 (Reapproved 1998)

Standard Practice for Care and Handling of Intracranial Aneurysm Clips and Instruments[1]

This standard is issued under the fixed designation F 700; the number immediately following the designation indicates the year of original adoption or, in the case of revision, the year of last revision. A number in parentheses indicates the year of last reapproval. A superscript epsilon (ε) indicates an editorial change since the last revision or reapproval.

1. Scope

1.1 This practice covers recommended procedures for handling of neurosurgical intracranial aneurysm clips and the clip appliers (instruments).

1.2 This practice is intended to inform hospital receiving personnel, central supply personnel, operating room personnel, and other individuals who will handle intracranial aneurysm clips and the instruments related thereto of recommended care and handling procedures to prevent damage of intracranial aneurysm clips and instruments.

1.3 Handling and packaging procedures for the product are not a part of this practice and are covered in other practices.

2. Terminology

2.1 *Definitions:*

2.1.1 *clip applier*—any clip holder designed specifically for a particular type clip used during surgical procedures involving the implantation of intracranial aneurysm clips. This device is referred to in this practice as a clip applier.

2.1.2 *intracranial aneurysm clip*—a device introduced surgically to occlude the blood inlet into an intracranial aneurysm with the intention that it remain within the body following the surgery. This device is referred to in this practice as an "implant," specifically as an intracranial aneurysm clip.

3. Receiving Implants and Instruments

3.1 *Receipt*:

3.1.1 Many implants are wrapped in special packages, envelopes, or other containers. These wrappings should not be removed by the receiving personnel.

3.1.2 Carefully handle nonsterilized implants and instruments upon receipt to avoid scratching, marking, or abrasion by other implants, instruments, unpacking tools, or by dropping or otherwise endangering the surface finish or configuration.

3.2 *Transport*—Transport in a manner to preclude any damage or alteration to the received condition of the implant or instrument (clip applier).

3.3 *Storage*:

3.3.1 Store the aneurysm clips and appliers prior to use in such a manner to maintain the device's surface finish or configuration, or both.

3.3.2 Implants will be identified by a unique code on the surface of the device. When implanted, it is necessary that the type of aneurysm clip and its code be noted in the operative report.

3.3.3 *Stock Rotation*—The principle of first in, first out, is recommended.

3.3.4 Store implants in the operating room in such a manner as to isolate and protect the implant's surface, sterility, and configuration. Keep implants made of different metals separated.

4. Cleaning and Sterilization

4.1 Prior to resterilization and promptly following each surgical procedure, thoroughly and carefully clean all instruments and implants with approved cleaning techniques. Ultrasonic cleaners or hand scrubbing are suitable methods if carefully done. The method employed should be utilized to prevent impact, scratching, bending, or surface contact with any materials that might affect the implant or instrument configuration. Aneurysm clips must not be opened except by their specific applier.

4.2 Any clip that has been implanted or in direct contact with blood or body fluids and is not used in the procedure should not be reused in any subsequent procedure. The clips should be discarded; in accordance with tracing requirements, the manufacturer must be informed of each clip that is discarded.

4.3 After cleaning, rinse the neurosurgical intracranial aneurysm clips and instruments completely free of all residuals including soap, detergent, or cleaning solutions; and dry thoroughly. Devote special attention to hinges on the instruments and recesses on the clips since these are points that entrap both chemicals and rinse water. In so doing, the clip must not be opened except by its designated applier.

4.4 Lubricate clip appliers that require lubrication immediately after drying. Follow the recommendations of the manufacturers of such instruments explicitly as to the method, type, and amount of lubricant. Do not lubricate the clips.

4.5 Carry out sterilization by steam autoclaving or other methods in a manner that protects the integrity of the aneurysm clips and appliers.

---

[1] This practice is under the jurisdiction of ASTM Committee F-4 on Medical and Surgical Materials and Devicesand is the direct responsibility of Subcommittee F04.31 on Neurosurgical Standards.

Current edition approved March 15, 1993. Published May 1993. Originally published as F 700 – 81. Last previous edition F 700 – 81 (1986).

4.6 Do not sterilize implants in contact with instruments or implants of other materials. Metallic oxide could transfer to the implant, initiating an unacceptable condition.

5. Use of Neurosurgical Intracranial Aneurysm Clips and Appliers

5.1 Open and close an aneurysm clip with the clip applier specifically manufactured to handle that particular aneurysm clip. At no time should an aneurysm clip be opened with the fingertips.

5.1.1 Any aneurysm clip that has been opened with the fingertips should be discarded and never used in a patient.

5.2 No attempt should be made to alter the configuration of preformed aneurysm clip legs or springs.

5.2.1 Dispose of intracranial aneurysm clips that exhibit surface or configuration damage.

5.2.2 Dispose of intracranial aneurysm clips whose performance capabilities have been jeopardized by mishandling or improper care.

6. Keywords

6.1 handling of implants; instruments; material handling; neurosurgical medical/devices applications

The American Society for Testing and Materials takes no position respecting the validity of any patent rights asserted in connection with any item mentioned in this standard. Users of this standard are expressly advised that determination of the validity of any such patent rights, and the risk of infringement of such rights, are entirely their own responsibility.

This standard is subject to revision at any time by the responsible technical committee and must be reviewed every five years and if not revised, either reapproved or withdrawn. Your comments are invited either for revision of this standard or for additional standards and should be addressed to ASTM Headquarters. Your comments will receive careful consideration at a meeting of the responsible technical committee, which you may attend. If you feel that your comments have not received a fair hearing you should make your views known to the ASTM Committee on Standards, at the address shown below.

Standard Practice for Care and Handling of Neurosurgical Implants and Instruments[1]

This standard is issued under the fixed designation F 701; the number immediately following the designation indicates the year of original adoption or, in the case of revision, the year of last revision. A number in parentheses indicates the year of last reapproval. A superscript epsilon (ε) indicates an editorial change since the last revision or reapproval.

1. Scope

1.1 This practice covers recommended procedures for handling neurosurgical implants and instruments.

1.2 This practice is intended to inform hospital receiving personnel, central supply personnel, operating room personnel, and other individuals who will handle neurosurgical implants and instruments of recommended care and handling procedures to prevent damage of neurosurgical implants and instruments.

2. Terminlogy

2.1 *Definitions*:

2.1.1 *neurosurgical implant*—for the purpose of this practice, a device introduced by surgically penetrating the skin or mucosa of the body with the intention that it remain indefinitely within the body following surgery. This device is referred to in this practice as an "implant."

2.1.2 *neurosurgical instrument*—any cooperative device used during surgical procedures involving the implantation of neurosurgical implants. This device is referred to in this practice as an "instrument."

3. Receiving Implants and Instruments

3.1 *Receipt*:

3.1.1 Many implants are wrapped in special sterilizable or presterilized packages, envelopes, or other containers. These wrappings should not be removed by the personnel who receive the packages.

3.1.2 Carefully unwrap and handle nonsterilized implants and instruments upon receipt in such a manner to avoid scratching, marking, or abrasion by other implants, instruments, unpackaging tools, or by such mishaps as dropping or otherwise endangering the surface finish or configuration.

3.2 *Transport*—Transport in a manner to preclude any damage or alteration to the received condition of the implant or instrument when received.

3.3 *Storage*:

3.3.1 Store implants or instruments prior to use in such a manner as to maintain the device's surface finish or configuration, or both.

3.3.2 Many implants are identified by a serial or lot number, or both, on the package label, package insert, or surface of the device. Record these control numbers and retain for transfer to patient records to facilitate inventory, stock rotation, and possible traceability to the manufacturer.

3.3.3 *Stock Rotation*— The principle of first in, first out is recommended.

3.3.4 Store implants in the operating room in such a manner as to isolate and protect the implant's surface, sterility, and configuration. Keep implants made of different metals separated.

3.3.5 Store the implants and instruments in the operating room in such a manner as to isolate the instruments from the implants.

3.3.6 *Mixing Metals*— Maintain neurosurgical implants and instruments of different metals separately to avoid the possibility of mixing during surgery.

4. Cleaning and Sterilization

4.1 Prior to initial sterilization and promptly following each surgical procedure, thoroughly and carefully clean all instruments and implants. Ultrasonic cleaners, mechanized washers, or hand scrubbing are suitable methods if carefully done. The method employed should be utilized to prevent impact, scratching, bending, or surface contact with any materials that might affect the implant or instrument surface or configuration.

4.2 Closely follow the manufacturer's recommendations on cleaning. In hand scrubbing, use soft brushes and avoid harsh chemicals or harsh cleaning solutions.

4.3 After cleaning, rinse the neurosurgical implants and instruments completely free of all residuals, soap, detergent, or cleaning solutions. Dry thoroughly after rinsing. Devote special attention to hinges, pivots, chemicals, and water.

4.4 Lubricate instruments that require lubrication immediately after drying. Follow the recommendations of the manufacturers of such instruments explicitly as to method, type, and amount of lubricant. Insufficient or excessive lubrication can be nearly as disastrous as no lubrication.

4.5 Carry out sterilization by steam autoclaving or other methods in a manner that protects the integrity of the implants and instruments.

---

[1] This practice is under the jurisdiction of ASTM Committee F-4 on Medical and Surgical Materials and Devicesand is the direct responsibility of Subcommittee F04.31 on Neurosurgical Standards.

Current edition approved Jan. 30, 1981. Published March 1981.

4.6 Sterilize implants and instruments of polymeric materials in accordance with methods recommended by the manufacturer.

4.7 Do not sterilize implants in contact with instruments or implants of other materials. Metallic oxide could transfer to the implant initiating an unacceptable condition.

4.8 Do not expose instrument cutting edges and teeth to the hazard of dulling.

5. Contouring and Modifying Implants and Instruments

5.1 Attempts to contour an implant may alter its performance characteristics.

5.2 Neurosurgical instruments, in general, have a long service life, but mishandling or inadequate protection can quickly diminish the instrument's life expectancy.

5.3 Dispose of instruments whose performance capabilities have been jeopardized by mishandling or improper care. Dispose of neurosurgical implants that exhibit surface or configuration damage.

6. Reuse

6.1 Do not use neurosurgical implants that previously have been implanted and subsequently removed at surgery or autopsy.

7. Keywords

7.1 handling of implants; instruments; material handling; neurosurgical medical devices/applications

Designation: F 702 – 98a$^{\epsilon 1}$

Standard Specification for Polysulfone Resin for Medical Applications[1]

This standard is issued under the fixed designation F 702; the number immediately following the designation indicates the year of original adoption or, in the case of revision, the year of last revision. A number in parentheses indicates the year of last reapproval. A superscript epsilon (ε) indicates an editorial change since the last revision or reapproval.

ϵ^1 NOTE—Editorial corrections were made in Sections 1 and 2, 3.2, 8.2, and the References in May 2001.

1. Scope

1.1 This specification covers polysulfone resin (poly(oxy-*p*-phenylenesulfonyl-*p*-phenyleneoxy-*p*-phenyleneisopropylidene-*p*-phenylene)) for medical applications (as defined in Terminology D 883). This specification provides requirements and associated test methods for a form of this thermoplastic which is intended for use in manufacturing medical devices or components of medical devices.

1.2 As with any material, some characteristics may be altered by the processing techniques (such as molding, extrusion, machining, sterilization, and so forth) required for a specific application. Therefore, properties of fabricated forms of this resin should be evaluated using appropriate test methods to assure safety and efficacy.

1.3 The use of this resin in medical devices should be restricted to nonimplant applications until biocompatibility evaluations appropriate for the intended applications are successfully completed.

1.4 The biocompatibility of plastic compounds made up of polysulfone resin containing colorants, fillers, processing aids, or other additives as well as polymer blends which contain polysulfone should not be assumed on the basis of resin compatibility alone. Their biocompatibility must be established by testing the final (end-use) compositions using evaluation methods appropriate for the intended applications. Note that the types, levels, and biological effects of extractives yielded by the additives contained in a compound or blend may also have to be evaluated for some end-use applications.

1.5 All values in this standard are in SI units with the equivalent values in inch-pound units given in parentheses where applicable.

1.6 *This standard does not purport to address all of the concerns, if any, associated with its use. It is the responsibility of the user of this standard to establish appropriate safety and health practices and determine the applicability of regulatory limitations prior to use.*

2. Referenced Documents

2.1 *ASTM Standards:*

D 149 Test Method for Dielectric Breakdown Voltage and Dielectric Strength of Solid Electrical Insulating Materials at Commercial Power Frequencies[2]

D 256 Test Methods for Impact Resistance of Plastics and Electrical Insulating Materials[3]

D 570 Test Method for Water Absorption of Plastics[3]

D 638 Test Method for Tensile Properties of Plastics[3]

D 648 Test Method for Deflection Temperature of Plastics Under Flexural Load[3]

D 696 Test Method for Coefficient of Linear Thermal Expansion of Plastics Between – 30°C and 30°C[3]

D 883 Terminology Relating to Plastics[3]

D 955 Test Method of Measuring Shrinkage from Mold Dimensions of Molded Plastics[3]

D 1238 Test Method for Flow Rates of Thermoplastics by Extrusion Plastometer[3]

D 1505 Test Method for Density of Plastics by the Density-Gradient Technique[3]

D 1898 Practice for Sampling of Plastics[3]

D 3750 Practice for Determination of Number-Average Molecular Weight of Polymers by Membrane Osmometry[4]

F 619 Practice for Extraction of Medical Plastics[5]

F 748 Practice for Selecting Generic Biological Test Methods for Materials and Devices[5]

2.2 *Code of Federal Regulations:*

Title 21 CFR Subpart 177.1655[6]

3. Chemical Requirements

3.1 The polysulfone resin consists solely of the alternating copolymer which may be produced when the disodium salt of 4,4′-isopropylidenediphenol is made to react stoichiometrically with 4,4′-dichlorodiphenyl sulfone such that the finished resins have a minimum number average molecular weight of 24 000. The molecular weight shall be determined by osmotic pressure in monochlorobenzene using the method described in

[1] This specification is under the jurisdiction of ASTM Committee F04 on Medical and Surgical Materials and Devices and is the direct responsibility of Subcommittee F04.11 on Polymeric Materials.

Current edition approved October 10, 1998. Published March 1999. Originally published as F 702 – 81. Last previous edition F 702 – 98.

[2] *Annual Book of ASTM Standards,* Vol 10.01.

[3] *Annual Book of ASTM Standards,* Vol 08.01.

[4] *Annual Book of ASTM Standards,* Vol 08.03.

[5] *Annual Book of ASTM Standards,* Vol 13.01.

[6] Available from Standardization Documents Order Desk, Bldg. 4 Section D, 700 Robbins Ave., Philadelphia, PA 19111-5094, Attn: NPODS.

Practice D 3750 or an equivalent method. The weight average molecular weight shall be equal to or greater than two times the number average molecular weight.

3.2 Polysulfone resins shall conform to the requirements of 21 CFR 177.1655. In addition to the total extractables evaluation described in the CFR, maximum levels and types of extractable metals shall be established in accordance with the requirements of the intended use of the resin **(1, 2)**.[7]

3.3 The polysulfone resin shall yield an infrared transmittance spectrum which exhibits major transmittance bands only at the same wavelengths as appear on the attached reference spectrum (see Fig. 1).

4. Physical Requirements

4.1 Polysulfone resin may be processed by most techniques available for thermoplastic polymers. Medical devices and components of medical devices made of polysulfone may be repeatedly sterilized. Methods used successfully include steam, ethylene oxide, irradiation, and dry heat sterilization.

4.2 Except for nonvolatile content and melt flow, the properties listed in Table 1 are determined from specimens injection molded in accordance with the resin supplier's process recommendations. Additional or different treatments and processing steps (such as extrusion, molding, machining, sterilization, and so forth) may alter the material properties.

5. Sampling

5.1 The material shall be sampled in accordance with the procedure described in Practice D 1898 or equivalent.

6. Inspection, Marking, and Packaging

6.1 The resin shall be inspected for particulate foreign matter contamination using the following or equivalent procedure. Specimen plaques 2.67 ± 0.25 mm (0.105 ± 0.010 in.) thick shall be injection molded in accordance with the resin supplier's process recommendation. A sufficient number of plaques shall be made to provide 390 cm^2(60 in.^{2}) of viewing surface, based on one side of the transparent plaques. The plaques shall be examined visually under fluorescent light using a 2 to 3× magnifier to determine the number and size of any contaminant specks present, rating them in accordance with Table 2. The total level of contamination is then calculated by multiplying the number of specks in each size range by the appropriate numerical rating and summing. A total rating greater than 12 shall be cause for rejection of the material.

6.2 As determined by agreement between the purchaser and the supplier, polysulfone resin may be inspected for pyrogenic contamination using either of the following tests:

6.2.1 USP Pyrogen Test **(3)**.

6.2.2 Limulus Amebocyte Lysate (LAL) Test for Pyrogens **(3)**.

6.3 The material shall be properly identified including lot or batch numbers, date of manufacture, and recommended method of storage.

6.4 The material, before processing, as well as the end-use component, shall be packaged in a suitable container to prevent contamination of contents.

7. Certification

7.1 The manufacturer shall certify that each batch of the polysulfone resin passes Class VI Biological Tests **(5)**, Biological Reactivity Tests **(4)**, and Practice F 748 when indicated for specific applications.

8. Biocompatibility

8.1 Evaluation of the local and systemic tissue response to implant devices, made wholly or in part from polysulfone resin, must be carried out using biological tests appropriate to the intended functions and implantation site of the device.

8.2 Satisfactory tissue response must be established separately for any plastic compounds made up of polysulfone resin which contains colorants, fillers, processing aids, or other additives as well as for polymer blends which contain polysulfone. Note that the types, levels, and biological effects of extractives yielded by the additives contained in a compound or polymer blend may also have to be evaluated for some end-use applications as described in Practice F 619.

8.3 In choosing appropriate test protocols for the material, based upon end use, the recommendations found in Practice F 748 should be considered.

9. Keywords

9.1 plastic surgical devices/applications; polymers—surgical applications; polysulfone resins

[7] The boldface numerals in parentheses refer to the list of references at the end of this specification.

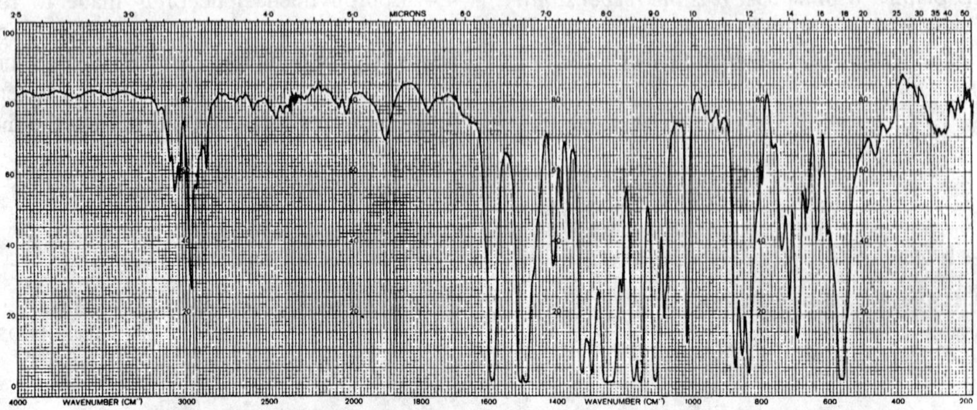

FIG. 1 Polysulfone Infrared Spectrum—Percent Transmittance for 0.0005 in. Film

TABLE 1 Physical Properties

Property	ASTM Test Method	Property Value
Electrical		
Dielectric strength of 3-mm (⅛-in.) specimen, kV/mm (kV/in.)	D 149	13 (350) min; 16 (425) avg
Mechanical/Physical:		
Density, kg/m^3	D 1505	1230 to 1250
Izod impact at 22°C (72°F) of 3 mm (⅛ in.) specimen, J/m (ft·lb/in.) of notch	D 256	50 (1.0) min; 69 (1.3) avg
Mold shrinkage, m/m	D 955	0.006 to 0.008
Tensile elongation at break, %	D 638	20 minimum; 50 to 100 average
Tensile modulus of elasticity, MPa (psi)	D 638	2300 (3.4 × 10^6) min; 2480 (3.6 × 10^6) avg
Tensile strength at yield, MPa (psi)	D 638	65 (9500) min; 70 (10 200) avg
Water absorption, gain in weight in 24 h, %	D 570	0.35 max; 0.30 avg
Nonvolatile content—burned, then heated to 585°C for 2 h, % by weight		0.010 max; 0.001 to 0.008 avg
Thermal:		
Coefficient of linear thermal expansion, m/m·°C (in./in.°F)	D 696	5.6 × 10^{-5}(3.1 × 10^{-5}) avg
Heat deflection temperature at 1820 kPa (264 psi), unannealed, °C (°F)	D 648	168 (335) min; 174 (345) avg
Melt flow at 343°C (650°F), 298.2 kPa (43.25 psi), g/10 min	D 1238 (modified)	9.0 max; 6.5 avg

TABLE 2 Rating Specimen Plaques

Speck Size [A]	Rating	
	Descriptive	Numerical
0.005 to 0.009	small	1
0.010 to 0.024	medium	2
0.025 and over	large	3

[A] The speck size is measured as the diameter, in inches, of the equivalent circular area.

APPENDIXES

(Nonmandatory Information)

X1. RATIONALE

X1.1 This specification was established to provide guidance in the testing of polysulfone resin intended for use in medical device applications. It recommends test methods for the measurement of chemical, physical, and mechanical properties of unfilled resin. Tests should be selected according to end-use applications. It is intended that biocompatibility be established on the finished product by the appropriate procedures, after it has gone through all processing steps and after all adjuvant substances have been incorporated.

X2. BIOCOMPATIBILITY

X2.1 No known surgical implant material has ever been shown to be completely free of adverse reactions in the human body. However, long-term clinical experience of use of specific compositions and formulations of this material referred to in this standard has shown that an acceptable level of biological response can be expected, if the material is used in appropriate applications.

REFERENCES

(**1**) *United States Pharmacopeia,* "Physico-Chemical Tests—Plastics," Vol 23, 1995, p. 1783.

(**2**) NBS Special Publication No. 422; "Accuracy in Trace Analysis," U.S. Government Printing Office, Washington, DC.

(**3**) *U.S. Pharmacopeia*, Vol 23, 1995, pp. 1696 and 1718.

(**4**) *U.S. Pharmacopeia*, Vol 23, 1995, pp. 1697–1699.

(**5**) *U.S. Pharmacopeia*, Vol 23, 1995, pp. 1699–1703.

Designation: F 703 – 96

Standard Specification for Implantable Breast Prostheses[1]

This standard is issued under the fixed designation F 703; the number immediately following the designation indicates the year of original adoption or, in the case of revision, the year of last revision. A number in parentheses indicates the year of last reapproval. A superscript epsilon (ε) indicates an editorial change since the last revision or reapproval.

1. Scope

1.1 This specification covers the requirements for silicone gel filled, saline inflatable silicone gel filled, and saline inflatable, smooth-shell implantable breast prostheses intended for use in surgical reconstruction, augmentation, or replacement of the breast.

1.2 *Limitations*— This specification does not cover custom fabricated implantable breast prostheses.

1.3 The values stated in SI units are to be regarded as the standard. The inch-pound units given in parentheses are for information only.

1.4 *This standard does not purport to address all of the safety concerns, if any, associated with its use. It is the responsibility of the user of this standard to establish appropriate safety and health practices and determine the applicability of regulatory limitations prior to use.*

2. Referenced Documents

2.1 *ASTM Standards:*

D 412 Test Methods for Vulcanized Rubber and Thermoplastic Rubbers and Thermoplastic Elastomers— Tension[2]

D 1349 Practice for Rubber—Standard Temperatures for Testing[2]

F 604 Specification for Silicone Elastomers Used in Medical Applications[3]

F 748 Practice for Selecting Generic Biological Test Methods for Materials and Devices[3]

F 1251 Terminology Relating to Polymeric Biomaterials in Medical and Surgical Devices[3]

3. Terminology

3.1 *Definitions:*

3.1.1 *barrier coat*—a silicone elastomer layer as a part of the shell of a silicone gel implantable breast prostheses that retards silicone bleed.

3.1.2 *fixation site*—an area of the shell of an implantable breast prosthesis containing material that allows tissue ingrowth.

3.1.3 *fused or adhered joints (seams)*—sites in the shell or other parts of an implantable breast prosthesis where materials have been joined (fused or bonded) together, with or without an adhesive, as part of the manufacturing process.

3.1.4 *gel bleed*—diffusion of liquid silicone components of silicone gel through the shell of an implantable breast prosthesis.

3.1.5 *gel filled breast prosthesis*—implantable breast prosthesis designed and provided with a pre-filled, fixed volume of silicone gel.

3.1.5.1 *Type I*—a fixed volume gel filled breast prosthesis—implantable breast prosthesis comprised of a single lumen containing a fixed amount of silicone gel. The lumen of Type I breast prostheses is not accessible for volume adjustments of any kind.

3.1.5.2 *Type II*—double lumen inflatable gel filled breast prosthesis—an implantable breast prosthesis comprised of two complete lumens, one inside the other. The inner lumen contains a fixed amount of silicone gel and is not accessible for volume adjustments of any kind. The outer lumen is provided with a valve to facilitate filling the void between the inner and outer lumens with saline to adjust the total volume of the prosthesis, only at the time of use.

3.1.5.3 *Type III*—reverse double lumen inflatable gel filled breast prosthesis—an implantable breast prosthesis comprised of two complete lumens, one inside the other. The volume between the inner and outer lumens contains a fixed amount of silicone gel and is not accessible for volume adjustments of any kind. The inner lumen is contained within the silicone gel contained in the outer lumen and has a valve system to facilitate filling the inner lumen with saline to increase the volume of the prosthesis at the time of use. The valve system is also designed to facilitate post-operative volume adjustment by following the instructions provided in product literature.

3.1.6 *inflatable breast prosthesis*—implantable breast prostheses not containing silicone gel—implantable breast prostheses designed and provided empty and to be filled, all or in part, with saline at the time of use to adjust the volume of the prosthesis.

3.1.6.1 *Type 1—fixed volume inflatable breast prosthesis*, an implantable breast prosthesis comprised of a single lumen, empty when supplied and having a valve to facilitate filling the lumen with the entire volume of saline at the time of use.

3.1.6.2 *Type II—adjustable inflatable breast prosthesis*, an implantable breast prosthesis comprised of a single lumen,

[1] This specification is under the jurisdiction of ASTM Committee F-4 on Medical and Surgical Materials and Devices and is the direct responsibility of Subcommittee F04.32 on Plastic and Reconstructive Surgery.

Current edition approved June 10, 1996. Published May 1997. Originally published as F 703 – 81. Last previous edition F 703 – 81 (1986).

[2] *Annual Book of ASTM Standards*, Vol 09.01.

[3] *Annual Book of ASTM Standards*, Vol 13.01.

empty when supplied and having a valve to facilitate filling the lumen with a system is designed to facilitate further post-operative adjustment with saline as instructed in product literature.

3.1.7 *low bleed*—silicone gel implantable breast prostheses designed to have minimal silicone bleed when tested by the method in 9.1.1.

3.1.8 *lumen*—a cavity within a shell of an implantable breast prosthesis. A lumen may contain either a fixed, non-adjustable volume of silicone gel, or it may be entirely or partly empty and intended to be inflated (filled) with saline. Inflatable lumens are accessible by valve to facilitate the addition of saline to adjust the volume of the prosthesis at the time of use. More than one lumen may be formed within a shell by silicone elastomer membrane partitions.

3.1.9 *orientation means*—any mark or palpable portion of an implantable breast prosthesis to assist the surgeon in positioning the implant.

3.1.10 *saline*—only sodium chloride injection USP is recommended for filling lumens of implantable breast prosthesis.

3.1.11 *shell*—a silicone elastomer continuous layer or membrane container (sac) that encloses a lumen or multiple lumens of an implantable breast prosthesis.

3.1.12 *silicone elastomer*—an elastomer containing cross-linked silicone polymer and fumed amorphous (non-crystalline) silica as a reinforcing filler.

3.1.13 *silicone gel*—a semisolid material consisting of a crosslinked silicone polymer network in which liquid silicone polymer is held (see definition of *gel* in Terminology F 1251).

3.1.14 *valve*—user sealable or self sealing opening in an inflatable or gel saline prosthesis, extending from the exterior surface of the shell into a lumen, designed to facilitate addition of saline at the time of use to fill the prosthesis and increase prosthesis volume.

4. Materials and Manufacture

4.1 *Silicone Elastomer*—Select and specify elastomers for use in implantable breast prostheses in keeping with Specification F 604.

4.1.1 *Shell*—The following describes suitable silicone elastomer compositions for use as the primary material of construction of the shell including the exterior (tissue contact) surface:

Polymer types	MQ or VMQ
Fillers	A, B or C
Additive	J (for radiopacity)
Catalysts	B, G, J, or K

4.1.2 *Barrier Coatings*— The following are suitable compositions of for use in barrier coat elastomers:

Polymer composition	FVMQ or VMP_2 M_2 Q
Fillers	B or C
Catalyst/cure	J or K

NOTE 1—The compositions listed in this section are not intended to limit the composition that may be used providing all other requirements of this specification are satisfied.

4.1.3 *Fabrication*— Fabrication techniques must necessarily be varied depending on the type of elastomer, the portion of an implantable breast prosthesis fabricated, its shape and its location and function on the prosthesis.

4.1.4 *Vulcanization and Postcure*—Time and temperature of vulcanization and postcure must be adjusted with consideration of the elastomer type and the multi-step fabrication requirements of specific prostheses. Final postcure is typically done only after the shell or shells and all other portions have been completely assembled. Time and temperature of final postcure shall be adequate to drive the chemistry of vulcanization of all elastomers to completion and remove by-products of the cure in keeping with the chemical stoichiometry of the specific cure systems (for example, after postcure no additional vulcanization should occur when heated additionally at recommended cure temperature).

4.1.5 *Physical Property Testing and Requirements*—Silicone elastomer shells shall demonstrate an acceptable response in physical property tests. Prostheses for testing should be selected from standard production batches which have gone through all manufacturing processes, including sterilization. With silicone gel prostheses, remove gel and clean shell with appropriate polar (for example, 2-propanol) or non-polar (aliphatic, aromatic, or chlorinated hydrocarbon) solvent, or both. If solvent cleaned, condition shell afterwards for 3 h 150°F (65.6°C) in an air circulation oven to remove solvent.

4.1.5.1 *Specimen Preparation*—Cut required tensile test specimens from shells with Test Methods D 412 dies. Specimens shall be conditioned before testing for at least 3 h at 23 ± 2°C (73.4 ± 3.6°F).

4.1.6 *Test Procedure*— Unless otherwise specified, the standard temperature for testing shall be 23 ± 2°C (73.4 ± 3.6°F). When testing at any other temperature is required, use one of the temperatures specified in Practice D 1349. Requirements are as follows:

4.1.6.1 *Percent Elongation*—Percent elongation shall be 350 % minimum when tested in accordance with Test Methods D 412.

4.1.6.2 *Breaking Strength*—Ultimate breaking force in tension shall be no less than 11.12 N (2.5 lbs) when tested in accordance with Test Methods D 412.

4.1.6.3 *Tensile Set*— Determine tensile set at 300 % elongation, stress the specimen for 3 min then allow 3 min for relaxation. The tensile set shall be <10 %, determined in accordance with Test Methods D 412.

4.1.6.4 *Critical Fused or Adhered Joints*—Joints or seams that are critical to the integrity of the prosthesis envelope shall not fail when the shell adjacent to the joint is stressed to 200 % elongation for 10 s (see Fig. 1).

4.1.6.5 *Non-Critical Fused or Adhered Joints*—Fused joints or seams that are bonded to the prosthesis envelope but are not critical to the envelope integrity (fixation sites, orientation means, valve covers etc.) shall not fail when the shell adjacent to the joint is stressed to 100 % elongation for 10 s (see Fig. 1).

4.1.7 *Shell Rupture/Failure Testing*—No standard test for assessing shell rupture/failure has yet been developed. When such test method has been developed it will be added to this standard.

4.1.8 *Shell Leakage Testing*—Fill a 5 to 8 qt stainless steel bowl with 70 % isopropyl alcohol. Submerge patched shell in bowl and gently apply pressure to the shell assembly. Visually

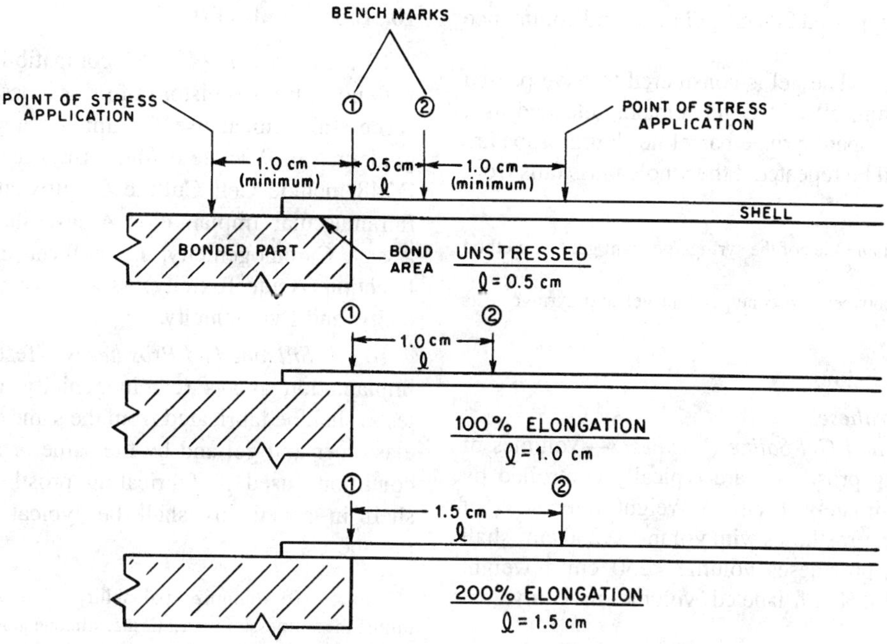

FIG. 1 Testing Fused or Adhered Joints

inspect for any bubbles. Reposition shell in hand until entire surface of shell has been tested while exposed. Reject shells whenever any bubbles are seen.

4.2 *Silicone Gel*— Select and specify ingredients in keeping with Specification F 604.

4.2.1 *Polymers and Catalysts*—The following are suitable for use in silicone gel:

Polymers	MQ and VMQ blend
Filler	A (no filler or additive)
Catalyst/cure	J or K

4.2.2 *Fabrication, Vulcanization and Postcure*:

4.2.2.1 *Fabrication and Curing*—Unvulcanized liquid gel is typically placed in the lumen of a shell and cured and postcured in situ while the shell is maintained in its desired final shape. Fabrication techniques must necessarily be varied to satisfy the requirements of the specific implant type and shape.

4.2.2.2 *Vulcanization and Postcure*—The time and temperature of vulcanization and postcure shall be adequate to drive the vulcanization chemistry of the gel to completion in keeping with the chemical stoichiometry of specific silicone gels. When postcure is adequate silicone gel does not undergo further vulcanization with additional heating at cure temperature.

4.2.3 *Testing and Requirements*:

4.2.3.1 *Specimens*—Remove test samples of gel from finished production batches of silicone gel—containing implantable breast prostheses after all manufacturing, including sterilization has been completed.

4.2.3.2 *Weight Loss From Heating*—When a 2 to 3 g sample is spread in an aluminum weighing cup and heated in an air circulating oven for 4 h at approximately 150°C the weight loss shall not exceed 1 %.

4.2.4 *Gel Cohesion*:

4.2.4.1 *Cone/Pendant Gel Test Method Described in Appendix* Appendix X1—This test is particularly useful to manufacturers for use in silicone gel development and quality control and quality control of unused silicone gel breast implants in that it provides quantitative results. The cohesive properties of silicone gel shall be considered suitable for use in silicone gel breast prostheses in the length of the pendant gel remains <4.5 cm when tested in accordance of the method in Appendix X1.

NOTE 2—The test results from cone/pendant gel testing are highly dependent on strict adherence to the specifications for the test apparatus and the procedures described in Appendix X1. A similar method contained in the 1986 edition and earlier editions of this specification was reported by most who used it to give highly variable and erratic results resulting in modifications of the test method as contained in Appendix X1. Precision and bias data for this method has not been established.

4.2.4.2 *Hypodermic Syringe/Pendant Gel Test Method*—A pass/fail test methods that can be used as an alternative to the cone/pendant gel test of 4.2.4.1. This test method may be applied by surgeon users, manufacturers, and others for evaluating the cohesive properties of silicone gel in breast prostheses including the gel from used, explanted devices.

4.2.5 *Test Fixture*— 60 cm^3 plastic hypodermic syringe with barrel having inside diameter of 26 to 28 mm. Prepare for use by sharply cutting off the tapered end circumferentially flush with the 0 cm^3 line leaving an unobstructed open barrel.

4.2.6 *Test Sample*— Cut the shell of the prosthesis to be tested diametrally across the apex from edge to edge. Push the plunger of the syringe forward until it is flush with the cut end of the barrel. Insert the plunger end of the syringe well into the gel on one side of the prosthesis and slowly draw the gel into syringe until the plunger is flush with the 60 cm^3 line. Care must be exercised to avoid drawing in either air or the shell. After one minute cut the gel sharply across the cut end of the syringe with scissors and remove syringe with test sample. Discard any samples where air was drawn in or if the shell interrupted obtaining the sample. With care, two gel samples may be obtained from most prosthesis.

4.2.7 *Testing*—Suspend the syringe in a vertical position with the open end down and at least 25 cm above a flat surface. Slowly move the plunger from the 60 cm^3 line to the 40 cm^3

line to extrude an unsupported 20 cm^3 gel mass and commence timing.

4.2.8 *Requirements*— The gel is considered to have passed this test if, after 30 min, all of the gel remains attached as a mass at the end of the open syringe barrel no liquid drops are visible. The test should be repeated if the whole mass falls from the syringe.

NOTE 3—The precision and bias of the syringe/pendant gel test method has not been established.

NOTE 4—Correlation between the cone/pendant gel and syringe tests has not been established.

5. Volume and Dimensions

5.1 *Volumes of Prostheses*:

5.1.1 *Silicone Gel and Gel-Saline Prostheses*—Volumes of silicone gel-containing prostheses are typically controlled by weight, 1 g = approximately 1 cm^3. Weight tolerances of silicone gel-containing prostheses with volume ≥250 cm^3 shall be ±5 g, and when prostheses volume <250 cm^3 weight tolerance shall be ±2 % of labeled volume in equivalent grams.

5.1.2 *Saline Inflatable and Gel-Saline Prostheses*—The design or maximum recommended volume of saline fill shall be listed in instructions for use.

5.2 *Dimensions*—The ranges of shapes, volumes, base sizes, and anterior projections are determined by the manufacturer. Pertinent information shall be contained in the package insert.

6. Significance and Use

6.1 This specification contains requirements based on state-of-the-art science and technology as applicable to various considerations that have been identified as important to ensure reasonable safety and efficacy in implantable breast prostheses.

6.1.1 This specification is not intended to limit the science and technology which may be considered and applied to ensure performance characteristics of subject breast prostheses in intended applications. When new information becomes available or changes in state-of-the-art science and technology occur and relevance to subject prostheses has been established by valid science, it is intended that this specification will be revised in keeping with this new information or advances in state-of-the-art science.

7. Fixation Sites

7.1 The presence of fixation sites on any type of implantable breast prosthesis is optional. When used, the size and locations of fixation sites shall be clearly stated in instructions for use.

8. Orientation Means

8.1 Orientation means are optional features of subject prostheses. When orientation means are claimed, the location and recommended techniques for use shall be clearly described in instructions for use.

9. Gel Bleed

9.1 *Test Method*— See Annex A2.

9.1.1 *Requirements*— The allowable quantities of gel bleed in this testing have not been established.

10. Biocompatibility

10.1 *Practice F 748*—Biocompatibility assays of materials with no or limited history of prior biocompatibility testing and successful clinical use for implant applications shall follow guidelines of Practice F 748. Assays recommended by Practice F 748 include Cell Culture Cytotoxicity Assays, Short-Term Intramuscular Implantation Assay, Short-Term Subcutaneous Assay, Carcinogenicity, Long-Term Implant Test, Systemic Injection (Acute Toxicity) Assay, Sensitization Assay, Mutagenicity, and Pyrogenicity.

10.1.1 *Silicone Gel Prostheses*—Test specimens for chronic implantation assays (carcinogenicity and long term implant tests) shall be fabricated from the same combination of silicone elastomer and gel and by the same or similar procedures and conditions used in fabricating prostheses. The thickness of shell in specimens shall be typical of thickness used in prostheses.

NOTE 5—To minimize palpability of prostheses and to effectively mimic the softness of breast tissue, silicone gels used in implantable breast prostheses must be soft (have low modulus). State-of-the-art silicone gels with required low modulus are also low strength. When implanted long term without an enclosing silicone elastomer shell, silicone gel may not retain its physical shape and integrity. Clinical implantation of free silicone gel sans shell is neither intended nor recommended. If shell rupture occurs in an implanted silicone gel breast prostheses resulting in direct contact between silicone gel and tissue, revision surgery for removal of ruptured prostheses and any free gel is recommended, with or without prosthetic replacement. To help assure relevancy of long term biocompatibility assays in animals to recommended clinical use of silicone gel implantable breast prostheses, the specimens used in chronic biocompatibility assays shall have silicone gel contained in an enclosing silicone elastomer shell, similar to silicone gel prostheses. Specimens of free silicone gel may be used in all other biocompatibility assays as specified in Practice F 748 for implants used in tissue and tissue fluid contact applications, including short term intramuscular implantation assay.

10.1.2 *Prior Biocompatibility Assays*—When prior biocompatibility data are available for silicone elastomers and gels that may also have histories of use in clinical use in breast implants, even if not done by the exact protocols described in more recently developed biocompatibility test method standards, such data may satisfy all or part of the specific biocompatibility requirements of Practice F 748.

11. Valve Competence

11.1 *Test Method*— Prior to testing manipulate valve to duplicate its use for filling an inflatable prosthesis with saline as described in instructions for use. Test such manipulated valve at both high and low retrograde pressures. Use air, distilled water or isotonic saline as test media. Pressures, in the order to be tested, are 30 cm and 30 cm H_2O pressure resp. Maintain each test pressure for 5 min. When air is test media immerse valve opening in water to check for leakage (bubbles). With water or isotonic saline check for droplets at the valve opening.

11.2 *Test Requirements*—No observable or detectable leakage.

12. Sterilization

12.1 Implantable breast prostheses may be supplied presterilized in accordance with current AMI AND PDA procedures and good manufacturing practices (GMP) established by FDA[4].

12.2 If user sterilization or re-sterilization of prostheses are intended, validated instructions for cleaning and sterilization shall be supplied with the package insert.

13. Packaging, Labelling, and Package Inserts

13.1 *Packaging*—Prostheses shall be packaged to protect against damage and maintain cleanliness and sterility during the customary conditions of processing, storage, handling and distribution.

13.2 *Labelling*—Each package shall be labelled in a manner that ensures the labelling arrives at the point of use with the prostheses. The package labelling shall include the following information:

13.2.1 Manufacturer's name and address,

13.2.2 Product name, shape, type and lot number,

13.2.3 Volume and dimension information,

13.2.4 Date (month and year) of sterilization or packaging,

13.2.5 Special storage requirements, if any,

13.2.6 Self-adhering label suitable for application to the patient's medical records containing following information:

13.2.6.1 Prosthesis name and manufacturer;

13.2.6.2 Lot number; and

13.2.6.3 Type and volume.

13.3 *Implant Marking*— Each individual implant unit shall be clearly and permanently marked with a manufacturer's unique identifying mark and the nominal volume of the device in millilitres (mL). The marking method shall not compromise the strength nor integrity of the device.

13.4 *Package Insert*— Shall contain information: to identify the manufacturer; to describe the prosthesis; on storage, handling, cleaning and sterilization; to provide directions for use to the surgeon, and warnings and precautions concerning known and potential patient adverse reactions and risks.

14. Keywords

14.1 breast prosthesis; gel-saline prosthesis; implant; saline inflatable prosthesis; silicone elastomer; silicone gel prosthesis; soft tissue implant

[4] Federal Register, Vol. 43, No. 141, Friday, July 21, 1978 Part II.

APPENDIXES

(Nonmandatory Information)

X1. RATIONALE

X1.1 Implantable breast prostheses are soft tissue implants used to simulate breast tissue in surgical procedures for breast augmentation, reconstruction, or replacement.

X1.2 Implantable breast prostheses are constructed with continuous, closed outer shells of silicone elastomer in various shapes, sizes and combinations. Lumens are spaces enclosed by shells. Prostheses may be have a single lumen or multiple lumens. Silicone gel prostheses contain fixed volume of silicone gel in the lumen or lumens and are implanted without alteration. The lumen or lumens of saline inflatable prostheses are empty as supplied and are filled through a valve at the time of use with isotonic, injection grade saline in fixed or variable volume. Gel saline prostheses contain a fixed volume of silicone gel with provisions for size adjustment at the time of use with either fixed or variable volumes of isotonic, injection grade saline.

X1.3 The only materials currently acceptable as materials of construction for implantable breast prostheses are silicone elastomer and silicone gel. This specification addresses the composition and vulcanization/cure of both silicone elastomer and gel and the physical properties of both materials as determined from specimens obtained from final prostheses. These requirements include bonded (fused, adhered or joined) areas of the shells. Provisions for softness and cohesiveness of silicone gel are included.

X1.3.1 There are a variety of other tests and considerations that have been proposed for incorporation into this specification including total energy to rupture, abrasion resistance, cyclic compression testing specific chemical characterization of all silicone species and others as such contained FDA's *Draft Guidance for Preparation of FDA Submissions of Silicone Gel-Filled Breast Prostheses.*[5] These proposals merit consideration, and the current content of this standard is not intended to limit its revision and updating to appropriately reflect changes and advancements in the state-of-the-art and the availability of relevant consensus test methods. The current content of this standard is believed to accurately represent currently available technology where there has been consensus on test methods and requirements.

X1.4 To ensure integrity of subject prostheses this specification contains provisions for testing shells and any associated inflation valves for leakage.

X1.5 Diffusion of liquid silicone component of silicone gel through the shell is commonly known as silicone bleed. This specification contains provisions for measuring silicone bleed in finished silicone gel—containing prostheses.

X1.6 *Biocompatibility Assays*—Because the prostheses

[5] Available from Food and Drug Administration, Rockville, MD 20850.

covered in this specification are soft tissue implants this specification contains provisions for state-of-the-art biocompatibility assays in accordance test methods as described in Practice F 748. Other biocompatibility assays were considered in the revisions to this standard as follows:

X1.6.1 *Tripartite Biocompatibility Guidance for Medical Devices*[6]—This guideline essentially duplicates Practice F 748, and in addition, references pharmacokinetics and reproductive and developmental toxicity, biological testing procedures typically associated with substances that are absorbed systemically and have biochemical reactivity.

X1.6.1.1 *Pharmacokinetics*—Young **(1)**[7] reported that in animal studies where data were available for analyses, including a study done at his own institution (National Center For Toxicological Research, FDA) little, if any, of injected silicone moved from the site of origin. He reported "Because of the extremely slow and limited movement of silicone from the initial site of administration, pharmacokinetics as a tool is really of limited usefulness." Further, "Based on these reports, it would appear that silicone implants would have very little or no movement and therefore any potential toxicity would be minimal." Young concluded "Regardless of the final placement of the PDMS and experimental design, any pharmacokinetics analysis of the data will be of limited usefulness due to the slow and limited movement of the material." In comparing injections of liquid silicone, as done in the studies analyzed, to the silicone gel of breast prostheses, Young noted that the enclosures (shells) would increase containment of the silicone. He also noted that pharmacokinetics is not the tool to use with silicone elastomers because some measurable movement is needed in order to use pharmacokinetics. Young's data demonstrate that techniques for conducting meaningful pharmacokinetics studies of polydimethylsiloxane elastomers and gels as used in the implantable breast prostheses covered by this specification have not been developed. When improved and validated techniques for conducting pharmacokinetics assays of polydimethylsiloxane have been developed evaluation of the elastomers and gels used in the implantable breast prostheses covered by this specification may be considered. Continued research on pharmacokinetics study techniques is encouraged.

X1.6.1.2 *Reproductive and Developmental Toxicology*—Bates reported **(2)** that Sprague-Dawley rats injected with up to 20 g/kg PDMS liquid, 350 cs, five days prior to insemination did not result in maternal toxicity or adversely affect fetal viability, fetal growth, or fetal development. Reporting on the findings from multiple studies, LeVier concluded that with regard to teratology no present evidence exists to lead to any serious concern about risk **(3)**. The reproductive and developmental toxicology of polydimethylsiloxane, the materials of concern in the implantable breast prostheses covered by this specification appear to have been well characterized.

X1.6.1.3 *Systemic Toxicological Considerations*—Anecdotal reports of systemic illness in patients with implantable breast prostheses have included immune disorders, human adjuvant disease, arthritis, connective tissue disease, scleroderma and others. These same health conditions are known to occur in persons who have not had implantable breast prostheses. There is no scientific evidence at present that persons with breast implants have an increased risk of adverse health effects **(4)**. Theories speculating a possible cause-and-effect relationship between silicone implants and immune phenomena were published more than a decade ago **(5, 6)**. With time these theories have changed and have become increasingly elaborate, but remain only hypothetical and unproven **(7, 8, 9)**. ASTM standards must be based on stable, proven and state-of-the-art technology. It was thus considered inappropriate and impossible to attempt development of new biological test methods for assay of biological or other considerations that are merely hypothetical, particularly since the hypotheses have not stabilized but are constantly changing. If cause-and-effect relationships between silicone implantable breast prostheses and systemic health conditions become established by valid science, rather than hypotheses, the need for testing in addition to Practice F 748 can then be considered and when validated standardized procedures are developed such procedures should be included in this specification and in Practice F 748.

X1.7 Implantable breast prostheses covered by this specification may vary widely in shape, size, design, intended use and other features. This specification contains provisions for labeling and package inserts to help ensure subject prostheses are appropriately identified and that adequate directions for use are available to users.

X1.8 Sterility of implantable breast prostheses is essential to prevention of infection. This specification addresses sterility by manufacturers and cleaning/sterilization/resterilization by users.

X1.9 Packaging is also addressed in this specification because prostheses must be protected against damage and all types of contamination (including microorganisms) during expected conditions of exposure in the course of distribution and handling.

X1.10 Identified limitations in technology and test methods have been noted in this specification.

---

[6] Prepared by Toxicology Sub-Group of the Tripartite Subcommittee on Medical Devices, representatives of governmental regulatory agencies of Canada, United Kingdom, and United States, September, 1986.

[7] The boldface numbers given in parentheses refer to a list of references at the end of the text.

X2. FEASABILITY PROTOCOL FOR GEL BLEED IN–VITRO TESTING BY MEANS OF A SILICONE DISK

X2.1 Scope

X2.1.1 The following test protocol details a method to evaluate the diffusion of silicone gel through the silicone elastomeric membrane or shell of silicone gel-filled mammary implants. This diffusion is commonly referred to as "gel-bleed."

X2.1.2 The results of this bleed test method can not be correlated with the actual physiological performance of an implant since the chemical gradient is not replicated. Attempts to devise a test method representative of the aqueous in vivo environment by ASTM to date, have been unsuccessful.

X2.1.3 This test method, which utilizes a silicon disk substrate in direct contact with a gel-filled mammary prosthesis can be used however for comparison of gel bleed diffusion rate's of various product configuration in a laboratory setting.

X2.1.4 Since the silicone disk, implant shell and implant gel are similar in chemical composition and structure (primarily polydimethylsiloxane), the diffusion of gel bleed through the implant shell into the silicone disk is accelerated in comparison to other collection media due to the lower surface transport gradient.

X2.1.5 The intent of this test method is for the comparison of smooth, non-textured, impants only.

X2.2 Summary of Test Method

X2.2.1 This test is performed at 110°F, a temperature exceeding an extremely high fever condition in humans. This serves to expose the breast prosthesis to a worst case temperature condition that can occur after implantation. Test results, however, are not intended to be indicative of the actual in vivo situation.

X2.2.2 A cleaned gel-filled breast prosthesis test specimen is placed on top of a pre-weighed silicone disk.

X2.2.3 Gravimetric analysis will be employed to determine weight gained by the disk after contact with the prosthesis. The weight gained on the disk is equated with the amount of gel that diffuses from the breast prosthesis at the localized contact surface area. Environmental control disks which do not come in contact with breast prostheses are gravimetrically analyzed to measure weight gain and loss as a result of factors such as humidity in the test facility. The test shall be run for a total of 8 weeks.

X2.3 Apparatus

X2.3.1 *Test containers*, standard outer polycarbonate thermoforms, or glass dishes of suitable size,

X2.3.2 *Silicone disks*, with 19.635 cm^2 surface area. Silicone disks are cut from platinum cured 70 durometer slabs having a thickness of 0.125 in. ± .010 in. A50 mm cutter is used to cut the disks,

X2.3.2.1 It is recommended when possible, that the disks used for any particular study be within ± .002 in thickness of each other.

X2.3.3 *Analytical balance* (Mettler AE 260 Precision Instrument with accuracy ± .0001 gm),

X2.3.4 *Incubator*, or oven capable of maintaining 110°F ± 3°F,

X2.3.5 *Isopropyl alcohol*, electronic or ACS reagent grade,

X2.3.6 *Non-Talc gloves,*

X2.3.7 *Kimwipes,*

X2.3.8 *Metal tray*, and

X2.3.9 *Forceps.*

X2.4 Test Specimen Configuration

X2.4.1 Test specimens shall be in the same form as breast prostheses intended for implantation. Alterations will not be necessary prior to testing. Unless otherwise specified test specimens should be sterilized in the same manner as actual end use implants.

X2.5 Number of Test Specimens

X2.5.1 For each product type, at least 3 test specimens and corresponding sets of silicone disks shall be used to measure the amount and rate of gel diffusion. Three additional silicone disks shall be used as environmental controls to measure unalterable factors which cause the silicone disks to gain or lose weight (for example, humidity).

X2.6 Test Specimen Preparation

X2.6.1 Test specimens shall be wiped clean (not soaked or submerged), using lint-free tissue and isopropyl alcohol, then left to dry patch side down at room temperature for at least two hours. Silicone disks shall be immersed in isopropyl alcohol and scrubbed to remove possible mold release agents or skin oil from handling. The cleaned disks shall be handled with gloved hands at all times to prevent contamination. They shall be placed on Kimwipes on a clean tray and allowed to equilibrate in the preheated incubator held at 110°F ± 3°F for at minimum of 12 hours.

X2.7 Procedure for Cleaning Test Containers

X2.7.1 Test containers shall be cleaned with an appropriate cleaning agent. They shall then be further wiped with Kimwipes soaked with isopropyl alcohol anbd allowed to dry for at least 10 minutes. They shall be labeled with an appropriate numbering system representing test specimens as well as the environmental controls.

X2.8 Procedure for Testing

X2.8.1 Non-talc gloves shall be worn when handling the test specimens and all manipulations shall be at the periphery of the specimen only. Forceps shall be used for handling the silicone disks.

X2.8.2 Remove silicone disk from incubator and allow to equilibrate for one hour at room temperature. Weigh each disk with analytical insrument to ± .0001 g. Place each test specimen, patch side up, on top of the silicone disk. It is necessary to ensure good contact between the surfaces of the test specimen and disk. Environmental control specimens are placed alone in their own test containers. Place uncovered containers with specimens in incubator.

X2.8.3 At weekly intervals, test containers will be removed from the incubator. The test specimens will be removed from the containers and placed patch side down on top of clean Kimwipes. An equilibration period of one hour at room temperature and room humidity shall be allowed. Each silicone disk shall then be weighed individually to ±.0001 g. It is necessary to ensure that the side of the silicone disk in contact with the test specimens shall be facing upward at all times. After each weighing, each silicone disk shall be returned to the bottom of its test container. The test specimen corresponding to the test container shall be placed, patch side up, on top of the silicone disk. Again, it is necessary to ensure good contact between the surfaces of the test specimen and disk. Environmental control specimens will also be weighed and returned to their containers. Return containers with specimens to incubator until the next measurement.

X2.8.4 The test shall be run for 8 weeks with measurements at one week intervals.

X2.9 Recording of Data

X2.9.1 Record all information on data sheet provided in Appendix Appendix X1 of this test protocol.

X2.10 Calculation

X2.10.1 Express the results of the gel diffusion test as the amount of silicone gel per surface area and rate of gel diffusion, calculated as follows:

$$W_g = [(T_t - T_i) - (C_t - C_i)]/A_s \quad (X2.1)$$

$$R_g = W_g/t$$

where:

W_g = average weight of gel diffusion per surface area (g/cm^2),
R_g = average weight of gel diffusion per surface area per time interval (g/cm ^{2}/t),
T_t = average weight of test disks at each time interval (g),
T_i = average weight of test disks at beginning of test (g),
C_t = average weight of environmental control disks at each time interval (g),
C_i = average weight of environmetal control disks at beginning of test (g),
A_s = surface area of silicone disk (cm^2), and
t = cumulative time from beginning of test to each interval (weeks).

X2.11 Test Limitations

X2.11.1 The conditions of this test method do not replicate physiological conditions. This test method is designed to accelerate the bleed diffusion process in order to evaluate various implant designs comparatively, in a reasonable time frame.

X2.11.2 Validation of the repeatability and accuracy of this test method has not been demonstrated. Typically a round robin test battery at different laboratories at different locations around the country is done for this validation.

X2.11.3 The variation in climate, particularly (humidity) in different locations may to some degree affect results.

X2.11.4 Although control specimens are always used to compensate for humidity changes, the exposed area of the conrols differs from that of the test disks since the test disks are covered by a prosthesis. This again may alter the accuracy of the test method.

X2.11.5 The intent of this test method is for the comparison of smooth, non-textured, implants only.

X2.12 Report

X2.12.1 The report shall include the following:

X2.12.1.1 Records of all measurements of silicone disk weight for each time interval,

X2.12.1.2 Records of temperature and humidity of laboratory at each time period,

X2.12.1.3 Calculated average amount of gel per surface area diffusing out of test specimens,

X2.12.1.4 Calculated average rate of gel diffusing out of test specimens,

X2.12.1.5 Records of any non-anticipated events that may affect measurements of gel diffusion during the test period, and

X2.12.1.6 Records of test specimens information and traceability (when available).

X2.12.1.6.1 Lot No.,

X2.12.1.6.2 Part No.,

X2.12.1.6.3 Volumes(s) of devices,

X2.12.1.6.4 Type of product,

X2.12.1.6.5 Sterilization Method, and

X2.12.1.6.6 Sterilization Lot Nos.

REFERENCES

(1) Young, J. F., "Disposition, Storage, Degradation, Removal, and Excretion of the Different Silicones," *Proceedings from the Conference on Silicones in Medical Devices*, CDRH/FDA, Baltimore, 1991.

(2) Bates, H. K., Cunny, H. C., and LaBorde, J. B., "Developmental Toxicity Evaluation of Polydimethylsiloxane in the Sprague-Dawley Rat," *Proceedings from the Conference on Silicone in Medical Devices*, CDRH/FDA, Baltimore, 1991.

(3) LeVier, R. R., "Toxicology of Silicone Mammary Implant Materials," *Proceedings from the Conference on Silicone in Medical Devices*, CDRH/FDA, HHS Publication FDA 92-4249, U.S. Government Printing Office, Baltimore, 1991.

(4) Department of Health and Human Services, Public Health Service, Food and Drug Administration (HFZ-30), *Medical Devices Bulletin*, Vol XI, No. 2, Center for Devices and Radiological Health, February 1993.

(5) Parsons, R. W., et al., *Observations of Cellular Immune Phenomena Provoked by Silicone*, Transactions of the VIII International Congress of Plastic Surgery, Montreal, Canada, 1983.

(6) Kossovsky, N., et al., *Ventricular Shunt Failure: Evidence of Immunologic Sensitization*, American College of Surgeons Surgical Forum Vol XXXIV, 1983.

(7) Kossovsky, N., *Bioreactivity and the Growing Controversy of Silicone Breast Prosthesis*, Guest Editorial Biomaterials Forum, 1991, Society for Biomaterials.

(8) Goldblum, R. M., et al., "Antibodies to Silicone Elastomers and Reactions to Ventriculorperitoneal Shunts," *The Lancet*, Vol 340, August 29, 1992.

(9) Kossowsky, N., et al., "Surface Dependent Antigens Identified by High Binding of Serum Antibodies in a Subpopulation of Patients with Breast Prostheses," *Jo. Applied Biomaterials*, Vol 4, No. 4, 1993, John Wiley& Sons, New York, NY.

Designation: F 719 – 81 (Reapproved 1996)$^{\epsilon 1}$

Standard Practice for Testing Biomaterials in Rabbits for Primary Skin Irritation[1]

This standard is issued under the fixed designation F 719; the number immediately following the designation indicates the year of original adoption or, in the case of revision, the year of last revision. A number in parentheses indicates the year of last reapproval. A superscript epsilon (ε) indicates an editorial change since the last revision or reapproval.

ϵ^1 NOTE—Keywords were added editorially in December 1996.

1. Scope

1.1 This practice covers a procedure by which the irritancy of a biomaterial may be assessed through contact with abraded and intact skin of rabbits.

1.2 The results of this practice depend upon the effectiveness with which contact between skin and the test material is established and maintained. Because of the operator technique included in performing this test, it is important that the test be performed by personnel with appropriate training.

1.3 *This standard does not purport to address all of the safety concerns, if any, associated with its use. It is the responsibility of the user of this standard to establish appropriate safety and health practices and determine the applicability of regulatory limitations prior to use.*

2. Referenced Documents

2.1 *ASTM Standards:*

F 619 Practice for Extraction of Medical Plastics[2]

3. Summary of Practice

3.1 Exposure of skin to the test material is accomplished by means of a patch test technique employing two intact and two abraded sites on the back of each of six albino rabbits. The skin is clipped free of hair one day prior to testing. The test substance is applied using 0.5 mL for liquids, 0.5 g for solids or semisolids, and a 2.5 by 2.5-cm square patch for films. After application, each test site is covered with a 2.5 by 2.5-cm gauze flat, and the entire trunk is occluded with a polyethylene sleeve. After 24 h, the sleeve, flat, and test material are removed, and test sites are evaluated for erythema and edema.

4. Significance and Use

4.1 Materials that are to be in contact with the skin should not cause irritation to the skin. Since it is probably the substances leached from a material that cause the irritation, this practice provides for direct material-skin contact testing or for skin exposure to the liquid extract of the test material. The rationale for this rabbit test is that it is a comparatively quick and inexpensive method which, through use over the years, has become a generally accepted method.

5. Materials and Manufacture

5.1 *Young New Zealand Albino Rabbits*,

5.2 *Gauze Flats*, 2.5 by 2.5-cm^2,

5.3 *Polyethylene Sleeves*, extra clear, and

5.4 *Adhesive Tape*, ½-in.

6. Test Specimen

6.1 The test specimen may be one of three forms:

6.1.1 Test 0.5 mL of liquids or saline extract liquids obtained in accordance with Practice F 619.

6.1.2 Test 0.5 mL of solids or semisolids.

6.1.3 Test films 2.5 by 2.5 cm.

NOTE 1—A vehicle control for liquids is required because of the potential for false positive due to skin temperature changes when handling rabbits. Positive controls may be used to validate the test method. The use of 5 % procaine HCl as a positive control is suggested.[3]

6.2 The pH of the solutions should be measured and reported.

7. Procedure

7.1 *Preparation of Test Animals*:

7.1.1 Twenty-four hours before the test, clip the hair from the backs of the animals so as to expose two test areas on each side of the spine, which are 10 cm apart.

7.1.2 To obtain more effective contact between the skin and the test substance it may be necessary to use a nonirritating depilatory agent. This test method may be used to ensure that the depilatory agent is nonirritating.

7.1.3 Test sites may be designated as two on each side of the spine. Alternatively, the area may be divided into quadrants with test and control substances applied to each quadrant.

7.2 *Test Procedure*:

7.2.1 Wipe the exposed area of the back with alcohol.

7.2.2 Using a sterile blade, abrade two of the four sites by moving the blade at right angles to the cutting surface in a scraping motion to create a denuded area of skin. Alternatively,

[1] This practice is under the jurisdiction of ASTM Committee F-4 on Medical and Surgical Materials and Devices and is the direct responsibility of Subcommittee F04.16 on Biocompatibility Test Methods.

Current edition approved April 24, 1981. Published July 1981. Originally published as F 791 – 81.

[2] *Annual Book of ASTM Standards*, Vol 13.01.

[3] H. H. Draize, *Appraisal of the Safety of Chemicals in Foods, Drugs, and Cosmetics*, 1965, p. 46.

make four epidermal incisions (which penetrate the stratum corneum but not the dermis), with two perpendicular to the other two.

7.2.3 Place the appropriate amount of the test material, as described in 6.1, on one intact and one abraded or incised site. Place the control material on the other abraded and intact sites.

7.2.4 Immediately occlude the sites by placing gauze flats on the test and control sites. Secure the patches with adhesive tape.

7.2.5 Tightly wrap the animal's trunk with a clear polyethylene sleeve.

7.3 *Test Site Examination and Scoring*:

7.3.1 Remove the polyethylene sleeve, gauze flats, test and control materials, and any excess test or control liquids 24 h after applying the test and control substances. Use alcohol solutions for removing excess liquids.

7.3.2 Using the criteria of Table 1, score test sites for erythema and edema 1 h after removal.

7.3.3 Rescore test sites for erythema and edema at 24 and 48 h after removal in accordance with Table 1. Take care to distinguish test site erythema from minor skin temperature changes.

NOTE 2—There is a possibility of infection associated with skin abrasion. Since infection would cause the same symptoms (erythema and edema) as would primary irritation, it is essential to ensure that the reaction is not due to infection. Any reaction at the control sites would be an indication of infection. If infection is suspected, the test should be repeated with a new animal, and the test substance cultured.

8. Interpretation and Calculation of Results

8.1 Score abraded and intact test sites for erythema and edema in accordance with Table 1.

8.2 The primary irritation index (PII) for each test animal and substance is the total of the abraded (incised) and intact skin scores for erythema and edema at 1, 24, and 48 h after removal, divided by six. The average primary irritation index is equal to the sum of the PIIs for each substance for all test animals divided by the number of test animals.

TABLE 1 Scoring Criteria for Test Reactions

Reaction	Description	Score
Erythema (ER)	Erythema and Eschar	
	No erythema	0
	Very slight erythema (barely perceptible)	1
	Well-defined erythema (pale red in color)	2
	Moderate to severe erythema (red and area well defined)	3
	Severe erythema (beet redness to slight eschar formation)	4
Edema (ED)	Edema Formation	
	No edema	0
	Very slight (barely perceptible)	1
	Slight edema (edges of area well defined by definite raising)	2
	Moderate edema (edges raised approximately 1 mm)	3
	Severe edema (raised more than 1 mm and extending beyond area of exposure)	4

9. Report

9.1 The report should contain a description of the test material, batch or lot number, vehicles, and extraction procedure used.

9.2 Report the pH value of test solution and vehicle solution if appropriate.

9.3 Report test data for erythema and edema in accordance with Fig. 1.

10. Keywords

10.1 acute toxicity tests; biocompatibility; rabbits; skin irritation; test animals

Primary Skin Irritation Test for Albino Rabbits

Test Material ____________________

Control Material ____________________

Results

Animal Number	Irritation Scores for Abraded Skin Sites after Removal						Irritation Scores for Intact Skin Sites after Removal						PII
	1 h		24 h		48 h		1 h		24 h		48 h		
	ER	ED	ER	ED	ER	ED	ER	ED	ER	ED	ER	ED	
1													
2													
3													
4													
5													
6													

Subtotal (PII sum) ____________________

Average Primary Irritation Index (sum/6) ____________________

FIG. 1 Sample Report Form

Designation: F 720 – 81 (Reapproved 1996)[ε1]

Standard Practice for Testing Guinea Pigs for Contact Allergens: Guinea Pig Maximization Test[1]

This standard is issued under the fixed designation F 720; the number immediately following the designation indicates the year of original adoption or, in the case of revision, the year of last revision. A number in parentheses indicates the year of last reapproval. A superscript epsilon (ε) indicates an editorial change since the last revision or reapproval.

ε[1] NOTE—Keywords were added editorially in December 1996.

1. Scope

1.1 This practice is intended to determine the potential for a substance, or material extract, to elicit contact dermal allergenicity.

1.2 *This standard does not purport to address all of the safety concerns, if any, associated with its use. It is the responsibility of the user of this standard to establish appropriate safety and health practices and determine the applicability of regulatory limitations prior to use.*

2. Referenced Documents

2.1 *ASTM Standards:*

F 619 Practice for Extraction of Medical Plastics[2]

3. Summary of Practice

3.1 After a two-stage induction employing Freund's complete adjuvant and sodium lauryl sulfate, the substance or extract is placed on patches and then placed on the skin of guinea pigs. After 24 h, the patches are removed and the skin examined for allergic reaction, and the intensity of the reaction scored at the time of removal and 24 and 48 h subsequent to removal.

4. Significance and Use

4.1 In selecting a new material for human contact in medical applications, it is important to ensure that the material will not stimulate the immune system to produce an allergic reaction. The reaction would be due to substances which could leach out of a material. Therefore, this practice provides for using material extracts. The rationale for this practice is based on the fact that the guinea pig has been shown to be the best animal model for human allergic contact dermatitis. The use of Freund's complete adjuvant and sodium lauryl sulfate tends to enhance the potential of a material to cause an allergy. Therefore, this test, while not guaranteeing that a material is nonallergenic, is the most severe animal test in common use today.

5. Materials and Manufacturer

5.1 *Hartley Strain Guinea Pigs*, male, 300 to 500 g.

5.1.1 Ten animals are used for each test material.

5.2 *Freund's Complete Adjuvant.*

5.3 *Occlusive Surgical Tape*, 3.75 cm in width.

5.4 *Elastic Bandage.*

5.5 *Sodium Lauryl Sulfate* (10 weight %) in USP petroleum jelly.

5.6 *Positive Control Substance.*

5.6.1 5 % formaldehyde for water-soluble test substances.

6. Preparation of Test Samples

6.1 *Samples for Intradermal Injection*:

6.1.1 *Water-Soluble Constituents or Water Extract Liquids*:

6.1.1.1 Dissolve the water soluble constituent up to its maximum solubility, not to exceed a concentration of 10 weight %, or obtain a water extraction liquid as described in Practice F 619.

6.1.1.2 Combine equal volumes of the liquid described in 6.1.1.1 and Freund's complete adjuvant. Homogenize by continuous and vigorous vortex mixing for a minimum of 5 min. Emulsification is complete when a drop placed on the surface of a water-ice bath remains intact.

6.1.1.3 Also prepare the constituent or extract to the same concentration in water without Freund's complete adjuvant.

6.1.2 *Oil Soluble Constituents*:

6.1.2.1 Dissolve oil-soluble constituents in Freund's complete adjuvant to concentration of 10 weight %.

6.1.2.2 Combine equal volumes of the 10 % Freund's adjuvant solution with an equal volume of water by slowly adding the water to the adjuvant while homogenizing with a rotating stirrer. Homogenize by continuous and vigorous mixing for a minimum of 5 min. Emulsification is complete when a drop placed on the surface of a water-ice bath remains intact.

6.1.2.3 Also prepare the constituent to an equal concentration without Freund's complete adjuvant.

6.1.3 *Vegetable Oil Extract Liquids*:

6.1.3.1 Mix equal volumes of oil extract liquid obtained in

[1] This practice is under the jurisdiction of ASTM Committee F-4 on Medical and Surgical Materials and Devicesand is the direct responsibility of Subcommittee F04.16 on Biocompatibility Test Methods.

Current edition approved April 24, 1981. Published July 1981. Originally published as F 720 – 81.

[2] *Annual Book of ASTM Standards,* Vol 13.01.

accordance with Practice F 619 with an equal volume of Freund's complete adjuvant.

6.1.3.2 Also prepare extract to an equal concentration in water without Freund's complete adjuvant.

6.1.4 Prepare control substances consistent with 6.1.1-6.1.3.2.

NOTE 1—If the final concentration of the suspected allergen results in deleterious effects such as ulceration, necrosis, or systemic toxicity, use the maximum tolerable concentration.

6.2 *Samples for Topical Application*:

6.2.1 *Liquids*—For all liquids, use highest concentration not causing excessive irritation or deleterious to general health of test animals.

6.2.1.1 For oil-miscible liquids, dilute with petroleum jelly if necessary.

6.2.1.2 For water-miscible liquids, dilute with water if necessary.

7. Procedure for Test and Control Substances

7.1 *Induction*:

7.1.1 *Intradermal Injection*:

7.1.1.1 Clip the shoulder region of each guinea pig free of hair exposing a 4 by 6-cm area.

7.1.1.2 Three injection sites on each side of the spine should be identified with at least 1.5 cm between sites. Intradermal injections are then made as indicated below, with Site 1 being closest to the animal's head.

(1) Site 1—0.1 mL of adjuvant without test sample

(2) Site 2—0.1 mL of test sample without adjuvant

(3) Site 3–0.1 mL of test sample emulsified in complete adjuvant

7.1.2 *Topical Application*:

7.1.2.1 One week after the intradermal injections, clip test area of guinea pigs.

7.1.2.2 If test sample is nonirritating, treat each test area with 10 % sodium lauryl sulfate (SLS) in petroleum jelly, 24 h before applying test patches. Massage SLS into skin with a glass rod.

7.1.2.3 Apply test sample to a 2 by 4-cm patch of qualitative filter paper. Apply test agent in petroleum jelly to filter in a thick, even layer. Apply test liquid to test paper until saturated.

7.1.2.4 Apply filter paper to injection site of guinea pigs. Occlude with 3.75-cm occlusive surgical tape, and wrap an elastic bandage around the torso to secure tape.

7.1.2.5 Leave in place for 48 h.

7.2 *Challenge*:

7.2.1 Perform two weeks following induction described in 7.1.

7.2.2 Shave a 5 by 5-cm area on animal's flank.

7.2.3 *Delivery of Test Sample*:

7.2.3.1 Test solids as a 25 % concentration (providing this concentration is not irritating) in petroleum jelly by weight. Apply on a 2 by 2-cm piece of filter paper as outlined in 7.1.2.3.

7.2.3.2 Test liquids in undiluted form consistent with 6.1.5. Apply on a 2 by 2-cm piece of filter paper as outlined in 7.1.2.3.

7.2.4 Occlude filter paper, and sample with occlusive surgical tape and elastic bandage as described in 7.1.2.4.

7.2.5 Leave samples in place for 24 h.

8. Interpretation of Results

8.1 Read the challenge sites within 1 h after removing the patches and at 24 and 48 h after removing the patches. Grade each site for erythema and edema in accordance with Table 1.

8.2 Prepare a tabular listing of the reactions at 1, 24, and 48 h. Any animal showing a reaction at 24 or 48 h of two or greater for erythema and edema shall be considered sensitized.

8.3 Rate the allergenicity of the test material in accordance with Table 2.

8.3.1 If a significant number (more than 50 %) of animals show a reaction score of one, repeat the test with an additional ten animals.

8.3.2 If 60 % of the animals in the positive control group do not show a reaction of two or greater, repeat the test.

9. Report

9.1 The report shall include the following:

9.1.1 Test material description, generic name, product name, and lot number.

9.1.2 Method of preparation, that is, extraction liquid used, and form of exposure.

9.1.3 Any necessary dilutions due to severe reactions.

9.1.4 General conditions of animal health.

9.1.5 Scoring of erythema and edema for each animal.

9.1.6 Rating of sensitization response.

10. Keywords

10.1 acute toxicity tests; allergenicity; biocompatibility; guinea pigs; sensitization; test animals

TABLE 1 Scoring Criteria for Test Reactions

Reaction	Description	Score
Erythema	erythema and eschar	
	no erythema	0
	very slight erythema (barely perceptible)	1
	well-defined erythema (pale red in color)	2
	moderate to severe erythema (red and area well defined)	3
	severe erythema (beet redness to slight eschar formation)	4
Edema	edema formation	
	no edema	0
	very slight edema (barely perceptible)	1
	slight edema (edges of area well-defined by definite raising)	2
	moderate edema (edges raised approximately 1 mm)	3
	severe edema (raised more than 1 mm and extending beyond area of exposure)	4

TABLE 2 Rating of Sensitization Response

% Sensitized	Grades	Classification
0 to 8	I	no different than control
9 to 28	II	mild
29 to 64	III	moderate
65 to 80	IV	strong
81 to 100	V	extreme

Designation: F 732 – 00

Standard Test Method for Wear Testing of Polymeric Materials Used in Total Joint Prostheses[1]

This standard is issued under the fixed designation F 732; the number immediately following the designation indicates the year of original adoption or, in the case of revision, the year of last revision. A number in parentheses indicates the year of last reapproval. A superscript epsilon (ε) indicates an editorial change since the last revision or reapproval.

1. Scope

1.1 This test method describes a laboratory method for evaluating the wear properties of combinations of materials that are being considered for use as bearing surfaces of human total joint prostheses. The body of this standard contains general methods which apply to all types of prosthesis wear applications while individual annexes describe specific wear test methods and clinical validation criteria tailored to each distinct wear application (for example, linear reciprocating motion, ball-cup ("hip-type") wear, delamination wear, etc.). It is the intent of this test method to rank materials, within each wear application, for polymer wear rates under simulated physiological conditions. It must be recognized, however, that contact geometries and wear motions are simplified using such methods. This test method, therefore, represents only an initial stage in the full wear characterization of a candidate material.

1.2 All candidate materials should be tested in an appropriate joint simulator apparatus using prototype prostheses before being used in clinical trials in patients. The tests described in this test method are used to quickly and reliably screen material combinations for wear performance in different orthopaedic wear applications prior to committing them to more expensive and time-consuming joint simulator testing. In addition, these simplified tests can be used to relate material, surface finish, or other parameters to wear behavior on a more practical basis than is possible in joint simulator tests.

2. Referenced Documents

2.1 *ASTM Standards:*

D 883 Definitions of Terms Relating to Plastics[2]

F 75 Specification for Cast Cobalt-Chromium-Molybdenum Alloy for Surgical Implant Applications[3]

F 86 Practice for Surface Preparation and Marking of Metallic Surgical Implants[3]

F 648 Specification for Ultra-High-Molecular-Weight Polyethylene Powder and Fabricated Form for Surgical Implants[3]

F 799 Specification for Thermomechanically Processed Cobalt-Chrome-Molybdenum Alloy for Surgical Implants[3]

F 1537 Specification for Wrought Cobalt-28-Chromium-6 Molybdenum Alloy for Surgical Implants[3]

F 2025 Practice for Gravimetric Measurement of Polymeric Components for Wear Assessment

G 40 Terminology Relating to Erosion and Wear[4]

3. Terminology

3.1 *Definitions of Terms Specific to This Standard:*

3.1.1 *wear*—for the purpose of this test method, the progressive loss of material from the polymer specimen as a result of the oscillating motion against the counterface under load. Wear may be generated by several mechanisms including adhesion, two or three body abrasion, surface fatigue, or other processes.

3.1.2 *wear rate*—the volume of material lost due to wear per unit of sliding distance (or per million wear cycles if complex motion patterns result in a non-uniform sliding distance across the specimen; see 4.3).

4. Significance and Use

4.1 This test method is intended to be performed in conjunction with pin-on-flat wear machines or similar machines that are designed to evaluate simplified specimen geometries.

4.2 This test method is designed to evaluate combinations of materials with respect to the amount of polymer wear, where quantifiable wear occurs primarily on the polymeric component. With some combinations of materials, significant wear of the counterface may occur, with subsequent embedding of counterface debris particles in the polymer. Such an occurrence will render the weight loss of the polymer specimen unreliable as an indicator of the polymer wear.

4.3 Wear is reported as volume loss of the polymeric specimen as a function of sliding distance; however, if the sliding distance is not constant across the polymeric specimen surface due to complex motion patterns, wear may be reported as volume loss of the polymeric specimen as a function of wear cycles (in which case a "wear cycle" shall be defined). Volume loss of the polymer specimen is determined by dividing the experimental weight loss by the density of the polymer. For ease of interpretation, wear should be reported as a function of

---

[1] This test method is under the jurisdiction of ASTM Committee F-4 on Medical and Surgical Materials and Devices and is the direct responsibility of Subcommittee F04.15 on Materials Test Methods.

Current edition approved May 10, 2000. Published August 2000. Originally published as F 732–82. Last previous edition F 732–98.

[2] *Annual Book of ASTM Standards*, Vol 08.01.

[3] *Annual Book of ASTM Standards*, Vol 13.01.

[4] *Annual Book of ASTM Standards*, Vol 03.02.

both the number of wear cycles and the sliding distance, when possible.

4.4 The reference for the comparative evaluation of candidate materials shall be the wear rate of ultra-high-molecular-weight polyethylene (UHMWPE) conforming to Specification F 648 bearing against counterfaces of cobalt-chromium-molybdenum alloy (in accordance with Specifications F 75, F 799, or F 1537), having prosthetic-quality surface finish and lubricated with bovine blood serum (see 5.2).

5. Apparatus and Materials

5.1 *Orthopaedic Wear Application*:

5.1.1 For linear reciprocating wear motion applications, refer to Annex A1.

5.1.2 For fixed-bearing ball-cup ("hip-type") wear motion applications, refer to Annex A2.

5.1.3 For nominally linear motion delamination wear applications, refer to Annex A3.

NOTE 1—Other types of applications may be addressed in later revisions.

5.2 *Lubricant (see also* Annex A4*)*:

5.2.1 The specimen shall be lubricated with bovine blood serum unless an alternative medium can be justified as described in section 5.2.8. Since different sera differ in composition (protein concentration, etc.), dilution with deionized water of up to 75 % (volume fraction) may be appropriate. The appropriate dilution shall be based on satisfaction of the clinical validation criteria in the appropriate annex.

5.2.2 A filter-sterilized serum rather than pooled serum should be used since the former is less likely to contain hemolyzed blood material, which has been shown to adversely affect the lubricating properties of the serum **(1)**[5]. Serum must be filtered to remove hard, abrasive, particulate contaminants that might otherwise affect the wear properties of the specimens being tested.

5.2.3 Maintain the volume, concentration, and temperature of the lubricant nearly constant throughout the test. This may be accomplished by sealing the chambers so that water does not evaporate, by periodically or continuously replacing evaporated water with deionized water, or by recirculating the lubricant in a sealed environment.

5.2.4 To retard bacterial degradation, freeze and store the serum until needed for testing. In addition, it is recommended that the serum contains a mass fraction of 0.2 to 0.3 % sodium azide (or other suitable antibacterial agent) to minimize bacterial degradation.

NOTE 2—Sodium azide is a poison and must be handled very carefully.

5.2.5 It is recommended that ethylene-diaminetetraacetic acid (EDTA) be added to the serum at a concentration of 20 mM (7.45 g/L) to bind calcium in solution and minimize precipitation of calcium phosphate onto the bearing surfaces. The latter event has been shown to strongly affect the friction and wear properties, particularly of polyethylene/ceramic combinations **(2)**.

5.2.6 Additives such as sodium azide and EDTA shall be dissolved in deionized water and passed through a 0.2-μm filter before adding to bovine serum.

5.2.7 The appropriate interval for replacing used serum depends on how long the serum maintains its composition (for example, lubricating properties) under the specific test conditions/materials being used and the additives present in the serum. There is no minimum replacement interval. The maximum replacement interval is two weeks. The selected interval must meet the validation requirements in the appropriate annex.

5.2.8 A lubricant other than bovine serum shall be used only when it can be shown that the lubricant reproduces clinical wear mechanisms as well or better than bovine serum. In such case the lubricant shall be specified in the test report.

6. Preparation of Specimens

6.1 The governing rule for specimen preparation is that the fabrication process parallels that used or intended for use in the production of actual prostheses, in order to produce a specimen with comparable bulk material properties and surface characteristics (see Practice F 86).

6.2 *Polymers and Composites*:

6.2.1 Obtain a fabrication history for each polymeric or composite specimen, including information such as grade, batch number, and processing variables, including method of forming (extruding, molding, etc.), temperature, pressure, and forming time used, articulation surface preparation methods (see Annex A5) and any post-forming treatments, including sterilization.

6.2.2 Pre-test characterization may include measurement of bulk material properties, such as molecular-weight range and distribution, percent crystallinity, density, or others. The surface finish of specimens may be characterized by profilometry, photomicrography, replication by various plastics, or other techniques.

6.2.3 *Sterilization*—Sterilize the specimens in a manner typical of that in clinical use for such devices unless it can be proven that this has no effect on wear properties of the materials. Report sterilization processing parameters with the aging time prior to each test, if known. Sterilization of all test and control specimens within a specific test group should be done simultaneously (in a single container), when possible, to minimize variation among the specimens.

6.2.4 *Cleaning of Polymer Specimens*— Prior to wear testing, careful cleaning of the polymer specimens is important to remove any contaminants that would not normally be present on an actual prosthesis. During the wear test, the specimens must be re-cleaned and dried before each wear measurement to remove any extraneous material that might affect the accuracy of the measurement. The required procedure for cleaning and drying of polymeric specimens, as defined in Practice F 2025, is given in Annex A6.

6.3 *Soaking of Polymeric and Composite Specimens*:

6.3.1 Polymeric and composite specimens should be presoaked in the wear test lubricant to minimize fluid-sorption during the wear test. Without presoaking, specimens made from very low-wear polymers such as UHMWPE could show a net increase in weight or volume during the initial wear

[5] The boldface numbers in parentheses refer to a list of references at the end of this test method.

intervals due to fluid sorption (**1, 3**). The error due to fluid sorption can be reduced through presoaking and use of control soak specimens. The length of presoaking depends on the variability and magnitude of fluid sorption encountered (**3**). A minimum of one control soak specimen per material condition is required.

6.4 *Counterfaces of Metal Alloys, Ceramic, or Other Materials*:

6.4.1 *Characterization*—Pretest characterization of the counterface material shall include recording of fabrication variables, such as composition, forming method (forging, casting, molding, etc.) and any postforming processing, such as annealing. Obtain data on material properties relevant to wear (for example, grain structure, hardness, and percentage of contaminants).

6.4.2 *Surface Finish*—In tests that are intended to evaluate an alternate counterface material bearing against the standard UHMWPE, ensure that the counterface finish is appropriate for components intended for clinical use. In test of alternate materials where a reference metal or ceramic is used, polish the counterface to the prosthesis quality.

6.4.3 Ensure that cleaning of specimens produces a surface free of any particles, oils, greases, or other contaminants that might influence the wear process.

7. Procedure

7.1 Make any initial measurements required to determine the subsequent amount of wear of the polymeric specimen (see Practice F 2025 for the gravimetric measurement method).

7.2 Place the control soak specimen(s) in a soak chamber of test lubricant, such that the total surface area exposed to the lubricant is equal to that of the wear specimens when mounted in the test chambers. Maintain the soak chamber lubricant temperature at the same nominal temperature as the test chambers. This temperature shall be 37 ± 3°C unless justification can be provided that use of a different temperature will not affect the results.

7.3 Place the wear test specimens in their test chambers, add the lubricant, and activate load(s) and motion(s).

7.4 As testing is commenced, monitor the specimens for signs of erratic behavior that might require early termination of the test.

7.5 Remove the wear and soak specimens at desired intervals, wash, rinse, concurrently in accordance with the procedure in Annex A6 (also defined in Practice F 2025). It is important that both the wear and soak components be treated identically to ensure that they have the same exposure to the wash, rinse, and drying fluids. This will provide the most accurate correction for fluid sorption by the wear specimens, and correction for any other factors which could affect wear measurements.

7.6 After rinsing and drying, conduct wear measurements.

7.7 Thoroughly rinse all test assembly surfaces which have contacted bovine serum using deionized water.

7.8 Inspect the bearing surfaces of the test specimens and note the characteristics of the wear process. Visual, microscopic, profilometric, replication, or other inspection techniques can be used. Care must be taken, however, that the surfaces do not become contaminated or damaged by any substance or technique that might affect the subsequent wear properties. If contamination occurs, thoroughly reclean the specimens prior to restarting the wear test.

7.9 Replace the wear specimens, maintaining original couples and orientation, and soak control(s) in fresh lubricant and continue wear cycling.

7.10 The appropriate wear test duration depends on the objective of the specific test, the duration of run-in effects, the linearity of wear rates, and the potential for wear mechanism transitions. The minimum duration shall be two million wear cycles. The minimum number of wear measurements, subsequent to the initial measurement shall be four.

8. Report

8.1 *Materials*:

8.1.1 Provide material traceability information from a raw material and fabrication or manufacturing standpoint for each material counterface. Examples of such information include material grade, batch number, and processing variables.

8.1.2 Pretest characterization for a plastic counterface may include measurement of bulk material properties, such as molecular-weight average, range, and distribution, percent crystallinity, density, degree of oxidation, or others. The surface finish of both counterfaces may be characterized by profilometry, photomicrography, replication, or other applicable techniques. Surface finish of the harder counterface shall be reported.

8.1.3 Report the method of sterilization, the sterilization and test dates, if known, and the means of storage post-sterilization and pretest.

8.2 *Test Apparatus*—Report the number of stations on the machine and the number of stations used for this test. Report if replicate tests were conducted during more than one test series. Describe the mechanisms used to generate motions and forces, the systems used to measure motions and forces, the arrangement for mounting specimens, a detailed description of the lubricant used, the arrangement for lubricating the articulating surfaces, arrangement for lubricant temperature control, the measured lubricant temperatures, total lubricant volume per station, lubricant replacement interval, and arrangement for the exclusion of contaminant particles. Report the nature and frequency of all calibrations conducted on the test apparatus. Define what constitutes one wear cycle. Confirm and explain how this test method satisfies all eleven test parameter requirements set forth in the corresponding annex.

8.3 *Wear Rates*:

8.3.1 Graphically plot the wear of each specimen as a function of sliding distance and/or wear cycles. Wear shall be reported as the volumetric loss of the bearing component(s) as a function of sliding distance and/or the number of wear cycles. If weight measurements were made, this will require knowing the density of the wear specimen(s).

8.3.2 In tests where the wear rate is nearly constant over the test run, calculate the volumetric wear rate by the method of least squares linear regression.

8.3.3 If the wear rate changes during the test, as with a decrease due to wearing-in of the specimens or an increase due to the onset of fatigue wear, linear regression may be applied to separate intervals of the test to indicate the change in wear rate.

8.3.4 At the discretion of the investigator, more complex, nonlinear models may be fit to the wear-test data.

8.3.5 Report the test duration in cycles. Explain why the selected test duration was used.

8.3.6 Report the method of calculating polymer sliding distance per wear cycle. Report the test duration in polymer sliding distance in addition to cycles.

8.3.7 An explanation of how the wear rates meet the designated criteria (in the appropriate annex) shall be reported.

8.4 *Wear Mechanisms*:

8.4.1 Provide a description of the articulating surfaces of both components.

8.4.2 An explanation of how the wear mechanisms meet the designated criteria (in the appropriate annex) shall be reported.

8.5 *Accuracy and Repeatability*:

8.5.1 In multiple tests where the wear rate is determined from the slope of the graph comparing wear versus test duration (cycles) for each specimen, report the individual rates, mean wear rate, and the 95 % confidence intervals for each rate.

8.5.2 In cases where the mean wear rate for two materials is different, evaluate and report the level of statistical significance of this difference.

8.6 Since the accumulation of wear debris in the lubricant may influence the wear rate, report any filtering of the lubricant during operation (continuously or periodically) and the lubricant replacement intervals.

8.7 Report the loading conditions, if any, on the soak control specimen(s). Load soaking, which is defined as a pulsing load profile equivalent to the wear profile without the tangential movement, may increase the fluid sorption rate.

8.8 Include a reference to this test method and to the method used for wear measurement.

9. Precision and Bias

9.1 In order that the screening test wear data be reproducible and comparable among laboratories, it is essential that uniform procedures be established. Sufficient data has not yet been produced using identical materials in different laboratories to permit determining the precision and bias of this procedure. The publication of this test method is intended, in part, to facilitate uniform testing and reporting of data from screening test wear studies. Validation of this methodology, may be achieved through round-robin testing.

10. Keywords

10.1 joint prosthesis materials; pin-on-disk; wear testing

ANNEXES

(Mandatory Information)

A1. TEST METHOD FOR LINEAR RECIPROCATING WEAR MOTION APPLICATIONS

A1.1 Scope

A1.1.1 The "linear reciprocating wear motion" test method describes a laboratory method for evaluating the friction and wear properties of combinations of materials that are being considered for use as the bearing surfaces of human total joint replacement prostheses which experience only linear reciprocating (straight or rotatory) wear motion. Such applications include hinged knees, other hinged joints, trunnion bearings, axle bearings, some mobile bearing knee applications in which the insert/tibial tray attachment mechanisms allow for linear motion only, and any other application in which the wear path at any given contact point reciprocates along a fixed line. Applications which are not relevant to this test method include head/socket articulation in hips and shoulders, fossa/condyle articulation in temporomandibular joints, liner/shell relative motion in hips, all patellofemoral and femorotibial articulation in knees where internal-external rotation may occur, and tibial insert/tibial tray relative motion in knees where rotation may occur. It is the intent of this test method to rank the materials with regard to friction levels and polymer wear rates under simulated physiological conditions. However, it must be recognized that, since any one design of joint replacement, even within this restricted scope, performs under unique conditions of load, motion, and contact geometry, there can be no single universally applicable wear screening test. This test method therefore represents only the first stage in the full characterization of a candidate material.

A1.1.2 All candidate materials should be tested in a joint simulator apparatus using prototype prostheses before being used in clinical trials in patients. The pin-on-disk test described in this test method is used to quickly and reliably identify those low-friction, low-wear materials for which the more expensive and time-consuming joint simulator testing is justified. In addition, the pin-on-disk test can be used to relate wear to material parameters such as polymer molecular weight or counterface surface finish, on a more practical basis than is possible in joint simulator tests.

A1.2 Criteria for Appropriate Test Results

A1.2.1 *Rationale*—Because there are subtle test method variables which will exist, even for a highly detailed test method such as this, it is necessary to identify characteristics of test results which must be met to ensure that they are representative of clinical results. Baseline testing should be conducted utilizing material combinations with significant clinical history such as cast CoCr and gamma-sterilized UHMWPE.

A1.2.2 *Reproduction of* in vivo *wear quantities*—The baseline test wear quantities should be compared to clinical results. Clinical data for linear reciprocating wear motion applications are quite sparse. At this time, a suitable guideline for relevant wear quantities is not clear.

A1.2.3 *Reproduction of* in vivo *wear mechanisms*—The baseline test wear mechanisms should be representative of those seen clinically. For linear reciprocating wear motion applications, a baseline CoCr/UHMWPE test should exhibit mild microadhesive/micro-abrasive wear mechanisms, resulting in a mild burnished or smeared UHMWPE wear surface and no significant loss of material. The wear motion direction should be apparent on this wear surface. A very thin transfer film may be visible on the CoCr surface.

A1.2.4 *Repeatability and reproducibility of results*—A minimum of three replicate tests per condition should be conducted; more if the repeatability relative to mean wear or aggregate wear rate is poor. If the same specimen condition were tested in separate series, there should be no significant difference in results.

A1.3 Apparatus and Materials

A1.3.1 *Description of Specimens and Test Parameters*:

A1.3.1.1 *Polymer Specimen*—The standard polymer specimen is a flat-ended circular cylinder 13 mm (0.50 in.) long and 9.00 mm (0.354 in.) in diameter, providing a cross-sectional area of 63.6 mm^2(0.0986 in^2). In the wear machine, the polymer specimen is loaded end-wise against the counterface in a flat-on-flat configuration. This specimen geometry provides a known contact area that remains constant as the test progresses and wear occurs. Care should be taken to ensure alignment of the specimen end face with the counter face.

A1.3.1.2 *Counterface*— The wear counterface may be fabricated in any convenient shape, provided that the contact surface is flat in the plane of motion of the polymer specimen and extends beyond the extremes of travel of the polymer specimen.

A1.3.1.3 *Wear Machine*:

*(1) Specimen Chambers*In the case of a multiple specimen machine, the specimens shall be contained in individual isolated chambers to prevent contamination of one set of specimens with debris from another test specimen. The chamber shall be made entirely of corrosion-resistant materials such as acrylic plastic and shall be easily removable from the machine for thorough cleaning between tests. The wear chambers shall be designed such that the specimen surfaces are immersed in the lubricant for the duration of the test.

*(2) Load*The test load of 225 N (50.6 lbf) shall be applied along the longitudinal axis of the polymer specimen, such that the average contact stress is 3.54 MPa (513 psi). The loading apparatus must be free to follow the specimen as wear occurs, such that the applied load is constant to within ± 3 % for the duration of the test

*(3) Motion*Relative motion between the specimen and the counterface shall be oscillatory. The orientation between sliding direction and the lay of the surface roughness in each test should be noted. It is recommended that the relative orientation of the pin and disk be maintained by suitable specimen-holder keying.

*(4) Sliding Speed*Specimens shall be run through a 25 mm stroke at a rate of 1 cycle/s, producing an average sliding speed of 50 mm/s.

*(5) Cycle Counter*The machine shall include a cycle counter to record the total number of wear cycles.

*(6) Friction*It is recommended that the machine include strain gage instrumentation or other transducers capable of providing a continuous readout of the tangential (friction) force transmitted across the specimen interface during the test.

A1.3.2 *Summary of Test Parameter Requirements*:

A1.3.2.1 Motion track: linear reciprocating sliding

A1.3.2.2 Polymer concave/flat/convex: flat-ended cylindrical pin

A1.3.2.3 Metal concave/flat/convex: flat

A1.3.2.4 Contact stress: 3.54 MPa

A1.3.2.5 Lubricant exclusion/exposure: metal re-exposed, polymer not

A1.3.2.6 Contact "coverage": polymer surface 100% coverage

A1.3.2.7 Contact area interaction ratio: metal wear surface area at least 100% greater than polymer wear surface area

A1.3.2.8 Cross-shear of polymer (change in angle of motion relative to metal surface) during a wear cycle: none (0°)

A1.3.2.9 Wear cycle frequency: 1 Hz

A1.3.2.10 Mean polymer sliding distance per wear cycle: 50 mm

A1.3.2.11 Mean polymer sliding speed: 50 mm/s

A2. TEST METHOD FOR FIXED-BEARING BALL-CUP ("HIP-TYPE") WEAR APPLICATIONS

A2.1 Scope

A2.1.1 The "hip-type" wear test method describes a laboratory method for evaluating the friction and wear properties of combinations of materials that are being considered for use as the bearing surfaces of fixed-bearing ball/cup devices for total hip replacement. It is the intent of this test method to rank the materials with regard to friction levels and wear rates under simulated physiological conditions. However, it must be recognized that, since any one design of fixed-beating ball-cup joint replacement, even within this restricted scope, performs under slightly different conditions of load, motion, and contact geometry, there may be no single universally applicable wear screening test for this application. This test method therefore represents only the first stage in the full characterization of a candidate material.

A2.1.2 All candidate materials should be tested in a joint simulator apparatus using prototype prostheses before being used in clinical trials in patients. The pin-on-disk test described in this test method is used to quickly and reliably identify those low-friction, low-wear materials for which the more expensive and time-consuming joint simulator testing is justified. In addition, the pin-on-disk test can be used to relate wear to material parameters such as polymer molecular weight or counterface surface finish, on a more practical basis than is possible in joint simulator tests.

A2.2 Criteria for Appropriate Test Results

A2.2.1 *Rationale*—Because there are test method variables which will exist, even for a highly detailed method such as this, it is necessary to identify characteristics of test results which must be met to ensure that they are representative of clinical results. Clinical history of ball-cup wear predominantly involves the CoCr ball/gamma-sterilized UHMWPE cup material combination. This combination should be used in a baseline test series to meet the requirements below.

A2.2.2 *Reproduction of* in vivo *wear quantities*—The baseline test wear quantities should be compared to clinical results: 69 ± 33 mm^3/yr for 22 mm balls, 85 ± 33 mm^3/yr for 28 mm balls, and 90 ± 44 mm^3/yr for 32 mm balls **(4)**. The wear area of the UHMWPE pin for this test method is roughly ten times smaller than that of a 22 mm cup, so the UHMWPE wear rate for this baseline test should be on the order of 7 mm^3/million cycles (under the assumption that the average patient generates one million activity cycles per leg per year). This is considered a rough guideline; the baseline test should not generate more than three times more or less wear. Another approach is to consider that typical linear penetration rates of cups have historically been in the 0.07 to 0.2 mm/yr range. A baseline pin-on-disk test generating this rate of linear wear (per million cycles) would satisfy this requirement. An additional approach to wear rate validation would be to test different polymers with known clinical history and demonstrate the proper wear rate ranking; for example, PTFE >> polyester > polyacetal ≥ UHMWPE **(4)**.

A2.2.3 *Reproduction of in vivo wear mechanisms*—Wear surfaces and particulate debris from retrieved UHMWPE cups have been characterized **(5, 6, 7, 8)**. Typical "clean conditions" macroscopic wear appears as a glossy "wear-polishing" of the UHMWPE surface **(6, 7)**. This pin-on-disk test method should reproduce this appearance. There should not be noticeable pitting or smearing of the UHMWPE or the development of a chemically bonded transfer film on the CoCr counterface. If UHMWPE debris particles are evaluated, they should have characteristics similar to those reported in **(5)** and **(8)**; size distributions should be similar to that reported in **(9)**.

A2.2.4 *Repeatability and reproducibility of results*—A minimum of three replicate tests per condition should be conducted; more if the repeatability relative to mean wear or aggregate wear rate is poor. If the same specimen condition were tested in separate series, there should be no significant difference in results.

A2.3 Apparatus and Materials

A2.3.1 *Description of Specimens and Test Parameters*:

A2.3.1.1 *Polymer Specimen*—The standard polymer specimen is a flat-ended circular cylinder. As in the linear reciprocating wear motion method (Annex A1), this specimen may be 13 mm (0.50 in.) long and 9.00 mm (0.354 in.) in diameter, providing a cross-sectional area of 63.6 mm^2(0.0986 in^2), but minor modifications to this geometry are acceptable if the other requirements are met. In the wear machine, the polymer specimen is loaded end-wise against the counterface in a flat-on-flat configuration. This specimen geometry provides a known contact area that remains constant as the test progresses and wear occurs. Care should be taken to ensure alignment of the specimen end face with the counterface.

A2.3.1.2 *Counterface*— The wear counterface may be fabricated in any convenient shape, provided that the contact surface is flat in the plane of motion of the polymer specimen and extends beyond the extremes of travel of the polymer specimen.

A2.3.1.3 *Wear Machine*:

*(1)Specimen Chambers*In the case of a multiple specimen machine, the specimens shall be contained in individual isolated chambers to prevent contamination of one set of specimens with debris from another test specimen. The chamber shall be made entirely of corrosion-resistant materials such as acrylic plastic and shall be easily removable from the machine for thorough cleaning between tests. The wear chambers shall be designed such that the specimen surfaces are immersed in the lubricant for the duration of the test.

*(2) Load*Because different loads (contact stresses) may be required to achieve the same wear characteristics for different motion patterns, one specific load or contact stress is not required. Load may even be varied using, for example, a physiological load profile if desired. The peak load within each wear cycle should correlate to a peak UHMWPE contact stress in the range of 2 to 10 MPa. The loading apparatus must be free to follow the specimen as wear occurs, such that the applied load (or load profile) stays constant to within ± 3% for the duration of the test.

*(3) Motion*Relative motion between the specimen and the counterface must be multidirectional to achieve wear rates and wear mechanisms representative of those in a fixed-bearing ball-cup application **(6, 7)**. More specifically, a certain degree of UHMWPE cross-shear must be achieved. The general requirement for relative motion for this test method is that the UHMWPE wear surface must change direction relative to the counterface at an angle of 60° to 90° at some point during the wear cycle. If there is a primary sliding direction, the orientation between sliding direction and the lay of the counterface surface roughness in each test shall be noted. It is recommended that the relative orientation of the pin and flat specimens be maintained by suitable specimen-holder keying.

*(4) Sliding Speed*Complex motions may complicate the determination of sliding speeds. The polymer sliding speed should be between 12.5 and 75 mm/s. Wear cycle frequency may be varied from 0.5 to 2.0 Hz as necessary to achieve this sliding speed.

*(5) Cycle Counter*The machine shall include a cycle counter to record the total number of wear cycles.

*(6) Friction*It is recommended that the machine include strain gage instrumentation or other transducers capable of providing a continuous readout of the tangential (friction) force transmitted across the specimen interface during the test.

A2.3.2 *Summary of Test Parameter Requirements*:

A2.3.2.1 Motion track: sliding with non-linear polymer specimen motion

A2.3.2.2 Polymer concave/flat/convex: flat-ended cylindrical pin

A2.3.2.3 Metal concave/flat/convex: flat

A2.3.2.4 Contact stress: peak during wear cycle anywhere from 2 to 10 MPa

A2.3.2.5 Lubricant exclusion/exposure: metal re-exposed, polymer not

A2.3.2.6 Contact "coverage": polymer surface 100% coverage

A2.3.2.7 Contact area interaction ratio: metal wear surface area at least 100% greater than polymer wear surface area

A2.3.2.8 Cross-shear of polymer (change in angle of motion relative to metal surface) during a wear cycle: 60° to 90°

A2.3.2.9 Wear cycle frequency: 0.5 to 2.0 Hz

A2.3.2.10 Mean polymer sliding distance per wear cycle: 25 to 150 mm

A2.3.2.11 Mean polymer sliding speed: 12.5 to 75 mm/s

A3. TEST METHOD FOR NOMINALLY LINEAR MOTION DELAMINATION WEAR APPLICATIONS

A3.1 Scope

A3.1.1 The delamination wear test method describes a laboratory method for evaluating the potential of a polymer material condition to exhibit delamination wear, a wear mechanism in which surface and sub-surface crack propagation eventually leads to the removal of relatively large pieces of surface material in the form of sheets or chunks. This wear mechanism has been observed clinically in polymer tibial components and patellar components, especially where the following conditions apply:

- oxidized (aged) polymer
- incongruent metal/polymer contact
- predominantly linear reciprocating sliding motion

It is the intent of this test method to determine a threshold for acceptable resistance to delamination wear and evaluate various polymer material conditions for their performance relative to this threshold under simulated physiological conditions. It must be recognized, however, that there may be multiple clinical applications where delamination is possible; thus, there may be no universally applicable wear screening test for this application. This test method therefore represents only an initial stage in the full characterization of a candidate material.

A3.1.2 All candidate materials should be tested in a joint simulator apparatus using prototype prostheses before being used in clinical trials in patients. The pin-on-disk test described in this test method is used to identify potential limitations in alternative materials or material conditions which are not targeted in other types of wear tests such as biaxial sliding or abrasive wear.

A3.1.3 Because the delamination test method focuses more on the onset and progression of delamination-related wear features, quantitative wear measurements are not required. Thus, all references to mid-test cleaning and wear measurement procedures in the body of this standard may be ignored. Details on measurement procedures for this test are given in A3.4.

A3.2 Criteria for Appropriate Test Results

A3.2.1 *Rationale*—Because there are test method variables which will exist, even for a highly detailed method such as this, it is necessary to identify characteristics of test results which must be met to ensure that they are representative of clinical results. Baseline testing for this method should be based on clinical history of materials known to delaminate. The most common material condition in this category is gamma-air-sterilized/shelf-aged UHMWPE. Based on published reports **(10, 11, 12, 13)**, this material condition should exhibit rapid and severe delamination wear with ten years of shelf aging; it should exhibit slower and more moderate delamination wear with five years of shelf-aging. This performance, however, will vary with the precise radiation dose, the resin grade, the device geometry, and other factors.

A3.2.2 *Reproduction of* in vivo *wear quantities*—Assessment of the delamination test does not require quantitative wear measurements. The onset and progression of delamination-related wear features are the relevant indicators, but these are more qualitative than quantitative (A3.2.3). The investigator may follow the procedures for wear measurement specified in the body of this standard, but it is not a requirement for conducting or assessing this test method.

A3.2.3 *Reproduction of in vivo wear mechanisms*—The investigator shall demonstrate that, using this test method, a severely aged gamma-air-sterilized UHMWPE specimen exhibits similar delamination-related features to those reported on retrieved devices of similar material condition. To evaluate candidate material conditions, the investigator should select and justify a baseline material condition which is believed to be representative of the minimum acceptable (or better) clinical performance (resistance to delamination) and show that the candidate material exhibits similar or better resistance to delamination. To satisfy this requirement, the candidate material must demonstrate a similar or longer period until the onset of visible signs of cracking or delamination, and a similar or milder progression of delamination-related wear features such as surface or subsurface cracking and removal of large sheets or chunks of material from the wear surface than the baseline material, under the same test conditions. The test shall be conducted for a minimum of 2 million cycles.

A3.2.4 *Repeatability and reproducibility of results*—A minimum of three replicate tests per condition should be conducted, more if the repeatability is poor. If the same specimen condition were tested in separate series, there should be no significant differences in results.

A3.3 Apparatus and Materials

A3.3.1 *Description of Specimens and Test Parameters*:

A3.3.1.1 *Polymer Specimen*—The standard polymer specimen is a flat rectangular or disk-shaped coupon with nominal dimensions of 51 mm (2 in.) x 25 mm (1 in.) x 6 mm (0.25 in.) thickness; minor modifications in this geometry are acceptable if the requirements in A3.3.2 are met. Specimen thickness, however, may be a critical dimension for a delamination wear test. It is recommended that, for purposes of conducting a "worst-case" test, the minimum thickness for a comparable device for this application, be used. In addition, test coupons of the same nominal dimensions cut from actual devices may be used provided there is not excessive curvature of the surface within the wear region and that all comparative tests are prepared similarly. This may be necessary for evaluating shelf-aged materials as the baseline conditions. In this case, the original articular surface of the device must be maintained and not machined down.

A3.3.1.2 *Counterface*— The wear counterface shall be fabricated from CoCr alloy (F 75, F 799, or F 1537) and shall have a hemispherical contact surface which creates a ball-on-flat contact geometry with the polymer specimen. The radius of this hemispherical tip shall be within a range necessary to meet the requirements specified in A3.3.2. The wear surface of this counterface shall be polished to a surface roughness (Ra) of 0.05 um (2 uinch) or smoother to avoid any influence of an abrasive wear mechanism.

A3.3.1.3 *Wear Machine*:

*(1) Specimen Chambers*In the case of a multiple specimen machine, the specimens shall be contained in individual isolated chambers to prevent contamination of one set of specimens with debris from another test specimen. The chamber shall be made entirely of corrosion-resistant materials such as acrylic plastic and shall be easily removable from the machine for thorough cleaning between tests. The wear chambers shall be designed such that the specimen surfaces are immersed in the lubricant for the duration of the test.

*(2) Load*In a metal ball on polymer flat configuration, contact stresses will vary within the contact region (Hertzian stress distribution) and they will also vary during the course of the test (due to wear and plastic deformation). The investigator shall determine the appropriate load (and corresponding contact stress) through development of the baseline test. If possible, calculations of the initial peak Hertzian contact stress (see X1.7) and initial average contact stress (load divided by initial contact area) shall be determined. They should fall within the ranges specified in A3.3.2.

*(3) Motion*Incidences of delamination observed in clinical applications are typically associated with nominally linear sliding motions such that cross-shear from multiaxial motions would not have a chance to dominate the wear mechanism. Thus, relative motion in this test method shall be linear (unidirectional or reciprocating). If the polymer specimen is removed during this test, there must be provisions to ensure that it is replaced in exactly the same orientation.

*(4) Sliding Speed*The polymer sliding speed should be between 12.5 and 75 mm/s. Wear cycle frequency may be varied from 0.5 to 2.0 Hz as necessary to achieve this sliding speed.

*(5) Cycle Counter*The machine shall include a cycle counter to record the total number of wear cycles.

*(6) Friction*It is recommended that the machine include strain gage instrumentation or other transducers capable of providing a continuous readout of the tangential (friction) force transmitted across the specimen interface during the test.

A3.3.2 *Summary of Test Parameter Requirements*:

A3.3.2.1 Motion track: linear (unidirectional or reciprocating) sliding

A3.3.2.2 Polymer concave/flat/convex: flat (or slightly dished) plate or disk

A3.3.2.3 Metal concave/flat/convex: convex (hemispherical wear surface)

A3.3.2.4 Contact stress (or peak contact stress if a cyclic load waveform is used) specific to the baseline [CoCr-on-UHMWPE] condition:

- Initial average contact stress: 19 to 24 MPa (2800 to 3450 psi)
- Initial peak Hertzian contact stress (optional; see X1.7): 29 to 36 MPa (4200 to 5200 psi)

A3.3.2.5 Lubricant exclusion/exposure: polymer re-exposed, metal not

A3.3.2.6 Contact "coverage": polymer surface less than 50% coverage

A3.3.2.7 Contact area interaction ratio: polymer wear surface area at least 100% greater than metal wear surface area

A3.3.2.8 Cross-shear of polymer (change in angle of motion relative to metal surface) during a wear cycle: none (0°)

A3.3.2.9 Wear cycle frequency: 0.5 to 2.0 Hz

A3.3.2.10 Mean polymer sliding distance per wear cycle: 25 to 150 mm

A3.3.2.11 Mean polymer sliding speed: 12.5 to 75 mm/s

A3.4 Measurement Methods

A3.4.1 As for other pin-on-disk test methods, the delamination test shall be conducted for at least 2 million cycles and at least four wear "measurements" shall be made. Quantitative wear measurements, however, are not required for this test. All references to mid-test cleaning and wear measurement procedures in the body of this standard may be ignored. Measurements will consist of periodic observations of the polymer wear surface including notation of the onset of delamination-related features such as cracking and qualitative assessments of the progressing severity of these features relative to the baseline condition. Photographs of the wear surfaces should be taken at the end of the test, and, if feasible, during observation periods. Observation intervals should be weighted towards the beginning of the test with recommended intervals of 50,000, 200,000, 500,000, 1,000,000, and 2,000,000 cycles. Prior to observations and/or photographs, minimum preparation of the wear surfaces shall include scrubbing with a nonabrasive material or device and thorough rinsing with deionized water.

A4. CHOICE OF WEAR TEST LUBRICANT

Comparative experiments have shown that distilled or deionized water or saline solutions do not duplicate the lubricating properties of fluids such as serum or synovial fluid that contain physiological concentrations of proteins (**1**). In particular, the heavy transfer of polyethylene to the surface of metal or ceramic implant that is typically observed with water or saline lubrication is not typical of serum-lubricated specimens and is not typical of retrieved components after extended use *in vivo*. Care must be taken in the choice and dilution of bovine serum to ensure that when used in simulated wear tests, it approximates the wear found clinically (see clinical validation criteria in the appropriate annex). Report the choice of lubricant along with the proof of validation for its use.

A5. PRECAUTIONS IN PREPARING SPECIMEN SURFACES

Do not polish or otherwise attempt to improve the polymer surfaces with abrasives, for example, aluminum oxide. Particles of the polishing compound may remain embedded in the polymeric material and could strongly affect the wear performance of the bearing materials. The exception to this is if the intent of the wear test is to investigate the effects of different surface finishing methods in which case a detailed description of all surface finishing methods shall be reported.

A6. METHOD FOR CLEANING OF POLYMER SPECIMENS (SEE ALSO PRACTICE F 2025)

A6.1 Rinse with tap water to remove bulk contaminants.

A6.2 Wash in an ultrasonic cleaner in a solution of 1 % detergent for 15 min.

A6.3 Rinse in a stream of distilled water.

A6.4 Rinse in an ultrasonic cleaner in distilled water for 5 min.

A6.5 Rinse in a stream of distilled water.

A6.6 Dry with lint-free tissue.

A6.7 Immerse in methyl alcohol (Note A6.1) for 3 min.

NOTE A6.1—This is a suggested cleaning procedure suitable for UHMW polyethylene. Methyl alcohol should be used only for polymers that are essentially insoluble in this solvent. For polymers that are dissolved or degraded in methyl alcohol a more appropriate volatile solvent should be substituted. The purpose of this step is to remove the water from the surface layer of the specimen that otherwise tends to evaporate during the weighing process. Other aspects of this procedure might require modification for the particular polymer being tested.

A6.8 Dry with lint-free tissue.

A6.9 Air-dry in a dust-free environment at room temperature for 30 min.

APPENDIX

(Nonmandatory Information)

X1. RATIONALE

X1.1 There is not one single screening wear test which can generate the relevant wear mechanisms for the many different types of orthopaedic wear applications. At the Fall 1997 ASTM F.04.15.09 meeting, Dr. Harry McKellop, originator of F 732 (later revised to F 2025), explained that there are at least four factors in addition to those addressed in the existing standard which should be considered, even for a screening test. These include: 1) motion track, 2) contact geometry (convex/concave/flat), 3) surface area ratio (size of specimens relative to each other, and 4) lubricant exclusion at wear surfaces. The present standard attempts to correlate such factors with the specific clinical wear application to generate the appropriate wear mechanism and prevent misleading results.

X1.2 The screening test wear studies of materials may involve three types of evaluation:

X1.2.1 Comparing the wear rate of a candidate polymeric material to that of polyethylene, both bearing against one of the reference metal or ceramic counterfaces.

X1.2.2 Comparing the polyethylene wear on the candidate counterface material to that of polyethylene wear on the reference metal or ceramic component.

X1.2.3 Comparing the wear rate of a new combination of candidate materials to the reference combinations.

X1.3 For the purpose of this test method, wear is defined as the progressive loss of material from a test specimen as a result of tangential motion against its mating component under load. For this test method, the polymeric specimen bearing against metal, ceramic, composite, or carbon specimens will be the sacrificial member, that is, the polymer will be the predominant source of wear debris. The metallic or other non-polymeric specimens, however, also may contribute either ionic or particulate debris. Depending on circumstances, therefore, wear may be generated by adhesion, two or three body abrasion, surface or subsurface fatigue, or some other process. Depending on the candidate materials selected, it may be desirable in some instances to add additional techniques to identify the nature and magnitude of the wear process.

X1.4 While wear results in a change in the physical dimensions of the specimen, it is distinct from dimensional changes due to creep or plastic deformation in that wear results in the removal of material in the form of debris particles, causing loss in weight of the specimen **(1, 14)**.

X1.5 Wear rate is the gravimetric or volumetric wear per million wear cycles of test.

X1.6 During wear testing in serum, calcium phosphate may precipitate on the surface of the test specimens, particularly those of ceramic, and strongly affect the friction and wear properties. The addition of 20 mM EDTA in the lubricant may reduce such precipitation.

X1.7 Hertzian contact stress distributions occur when a rigid ball is pressed into a deformable flat surface. The peak Hertzian contact stress occurs at the center of the contact region, assuming normal loading. Hertzian stress calculations assume elastic deformation of the deforming material. The test conditions described in A3.3.2.4 involve stresses which begin to exceed the yield stress of the deforming material (UHMWPE, approximately 21 MPa). Thus, there is an increasing degree of error involved in this calculation as loads are increased. The initial average contact stress (load divided by contact area) is the primary requirement for this method; calculations of Hertzian stresses are optional and are to be used as relative values only.

REFERENCES

(1) McKellop, H.A., Clarke, I.C., Markolf, K., and Amstutz, H.C., "Wear Characteristics of UHMW Polyethylene: A Method for Accurately Measuring Extremely Low Wear Rates." *J. Biomed. Mat. Res.*, 12: 895, 1978.

(2) McKellop, H., Lu, G., and Benya, P., "Friction, Lubrication, and Wear of Cobalt-Chromium, Alumina, and Zirconia Hip Prostheses Compared on a Joint Simulator," Ceramors. 92.

(3) Clarke, J.C., Starkebaum, W., Hosseinian, A., McGuire, P., Okuda, R., Salovey, R., and Young, R., "Fluid-Sorption Phenomena in Sterilized Polyethylene Acetabular Prostheses," *J. Biomat.*, 6: 184, 1985.

(4) Saner, W.L. and Anthony, M.E., "Predicting the Clinical Wear Performance of Orthopaedic Bearing Surfaces," *Alternative Bearing Surfaces in Total Joint Replacement*, ASTM STP 1346, J.J. Jacobs and T.L. Craig, Eds., American Society for Testing and Materials, 1998.

(5) McKellop, H.A., Campbell, P.C., Park, S.H., Schmalzfied, T.P., Grigoris, P., Amstutz, H.C., and Sarmiento, A., "The Origin of Submicron Polyethylene Wear Debris in Total Hip Arthroplasty," *Clin. Orthop.*, 311 (1995): 3-20.

(6) Bragdon, C.R., O'Connor, D.O., Lowenstein, J.D., Jasty, M., and Syniuta, W.D., "The Importance of Multidirectional Motion on the Wear of Polyethylene," *I Mech E-Proc. Instn. Mech. Engrs.* (Part H: Journal of Engineering in Medicine) 210 (1996): 157-165.

(7) Wang, A., Stark, C., and Dumbleton, J.H., "Mechanistic and Morphological Origina of Ultra High Molecular Weight Polyethylene Debris in Total Joint Replacement Prostheses," *I Mech EProc. Instn. Mech. Engrs.* (Part H: Journal of Engineering in Medicine) 210 (1996): 141-155.

(8) Campbell, P., Doom, P., Dorey, F., and Amstutz, H.C., "Wear and Morphology of Ultra-High Molecular Weight Polyethylene Wear Particles from Total Hip Replacements." *I Mech E-Proc. Instn. Mech. Engrs.* Part H: Journal of Engineering in Medicine) 210 (1996): 167-174.

(9) Schmalzried, T.P., Campbell, P., Brown, I.C., Schmidt, A.K., and Amstutz, H.C., "Polyethylene Wear Particles Generated *In Vivo* by Total Knee Replacements Compared to Total Hip Replacements," Trans. 21st SFB, San Francisco, March 1995: 210.

(10) Fisher, J., Chan, K.L., Hailey, J.L., Shaw, D., and Stone, M., "The Effect of Ageing Following Irradiation on the Wear of Ultra High Molecular Weight Polyethylene in Acetabular Cups," *J. Bone and Joint Surg.*, 77-B: Supp I (1995): 88.

(11) Sperling, D.K., Currier, J.H., Collier, J.P., Wooding, R.E., and Williams, I.R., "Role of Gamma Sterilization in the Damage of Tibial Knee Components," *63rd AAOS*, (1996): 225.

(12) Currier, B.H., Currier, J.H., Collier, J.P., Mayor, M.B., and Scott, R.D., "Shelf Life and In Vivo Duration," *Clin. Orth. Rel. Res.*, (342) (1997): 111-122.

(13) Bohl, J.R., Rohl, W.R., Postak, P.D., and Greenwald, A.S., "The Effects of Shelf Life on Clinical Outcome for Gamma Sterilized UHMWPE Tibial Components," *Scientific Exhibit SE020, 66th AAOS*, 1999.

(14) McKellop, H.A., and Clarke, I.C., "Degradation and Wear of Ultra-High-Molecular-Weight Polyethylene," *ASTM Special Technical Publication 859*, ASTM 1985.

Designation: F 745 – 00

Standard Specification for 18Chromium-12.5Nickel-2.5Molybdenum Stainless Steel for Cast and Solution-Annealed Surgical Implant Applications[1]

This standard is issued under the fixed designation F 745; the number immediately following the designation indicates the year of original adoption or, in the case of revision, the year of last revision. A number in parentheses indicates the year of last reapproval. A superscript epsilon (ϵ) indicates an editorial change since the last revision or reapproval.

1. Scope

1.1 This specification covers the requirements for 18chromium-12.5nickel-2.5molybdenum stainless steel alloy shot, bar, or ingot used for the manufacture of cast and solution-annealed surgical implants.

1.2 The values stated in inch-pound units are to be regarded as the standard.

1.3 *This standard does not purport to address all of the safety concerns, if any, associated with its use. It is the responsibility of the user of this standard to establish appropriate safety and health practices and determine the applicability of regulatory limitations prior to use.*

2. Referenced Documents

2.1 *ASTM Standards:*

A 744/A 774M Specification for Castings, Iron-Chromium-Nickel, Corrosion Resistant, for Severe Service[2]

E 8 Test Methods for Tension Testing of Metallic Materials[3]

E 353 Test Methods for Chemical Analysis of Stainless, Heat-Resisting, Maraging, and Other Similar Chromium-Nickel-Iron Alloys[4]

2.2 *American Society for Quality (ASQ) Standard:*[5]

ASQC 1 Specification of General Requirements for a Quality Program

3. Ordering Information

3.1 Inquiries and orders for material under this specification shall include the following information:

3.1.1 Quantity (weight or number of pieces),

3.1.2 ASTM Designation,

3.1.3 Form (Section 4.1),

3.1.4 Special tests, and

3.1.5 Special requirements.

4. Materials and Manufacture

4.1 The base material furnished to the implant manufacturer for purposes of casting surgical implants shall be supplied in the form of bar, shot, or ingot.

5. Chemical Composition

5.1 The heat analysis shall conform to the chemical composition listed in Table 1. The manufacturer shall not ship material that is outside the limits specified in Table 1.

5.1.1 Requirements for the major and minor elemental constituents are listed in Table 1. Also listed are important residual elements. Analysis for elements not listed in Table 1 is not required to verify compliance with this specification.

5.2 *Product Analysis*—The product analysis is either for the purpose of verifying the composition of a heat or lot or to determine variations in the composition within the heat.

5.2.1 Acceptance or rejection of a heat or lot of material may be made by the purchaser on the basis of this product analysis.

5.2.2 Product analysis tolerances do not broaden the specified heat analysis requirements but cover variation between laboratories in the measurement of chemical content. Product analysis limits shall be as specified in Table 2.

5.3 For referee purposes, Test Methods E 353 shall be used.

6. Mechanical Properties

6.1 The material shall conform to the mechanical property requirements prescribed in Table 3.

6.2 Specimens for tension tests shall be cast from remelted material from each master heat by the same general procedures used in casting surgical implants.

6.2.1 Specimens may be cast, ground, or machined to final dimensions in accordance with the 0.25 in. (6.35 mm) diameter specimen in Fig. 8 of Test Methods E 8.

6.2.2 Specimens shall be solution annealed using the same procedures used to solution anneal surgical implants.

6.3 A minimum of two tension specimens shall be tested. If one specimen fails below the specified mechanical requirements, two additional specimens shall be tested and both must pass.

6.3.1 Test results for any specimen which fractures outside of the gage length shall be considered invalid and void; and a

[1] This specification is under the jurisdiction of ASTM Committee F04 on Medical and Surgical Materials and Devicesand is the direct responsibility of Subcommittee F04.12 on Metallurgical Materials.

Current edition approved Nov. 10, 2000. Published February 2001. Originally published as F 745 – 81. Last previous edition F 745 – 95.

[2] *Annual Book of ASTM Standards,* Vol 01.02.

[3] *Annual Book of ASTM Standards,* Vol 03.01.

[4] *Annual Book of ASTM Standards,* Vol 03.05.

[5] Available from American Society for Quality Control, 161 West Wisconsin Ave., Milwaukee, WI 53203.

TABLE 1 Chemical Requirements (Heat Analysis)

Element	Composition, %	
	min	max
Carbon	...	0.06
Manganese	...	2.0
Phosphorus	...	0.045
Sulfur	...	0.030
Silicon	...	1.0
Chromium	17.00	19.00
Nickel	11.00	14.00
Molybdenum	2.00	3.00
Iron	balance	balance

TABLE 2 Product Analysis Tolerances

NOTE 1—Tolerances are over the maximum limit or under the minimum limit.

Element	Tolerance, %
Carbon	0.01
Manganese	0.04
Phosphorus	0.010
Sulfur	0.005
Silicon	0.05
Chromium	0.20
Nickel	0.15
Molybdenum	0.10

replacement specimen shall be tested.

7. Special Tests

7.1 Other tests may be required by agreement, between the purchaser and the supplier.

8. Special Requirements

8.1 Special requirements shall be specified on the purchase order by the purchaser.

TABLE 3 Mechanical Property Requirements (As-Cast and Solution-Annealed)

Property	Requirement
Tensile strength, min, psi (MPa)	70000 (483)
Yield strength (0.2 % offset), min, psi (MPa)	30000 (207)
Elongation (in 4× diameter), min, %	30
Reduction of area, min,%	50

9. Certification

9.1 Upon request of the purchaser in the contract or order a manufacturer's certification that the material was manufactured and tested in accordance with this specification together with a report of the test results requested shall be furnished at the time of shipment.

10. Quality Program Requirements

10.1 The producer shall maintain a quality program as defined in ASQC 1.

10.2 The purchaser shall be assured of the producer's quality program conformance to the intent of ASQC 1, or other recognized programs.

11. Keywords

11.1 castings; metals (for surgical implants); stainless steel; surgical applications

APPENDIXES

(Nonmandatory Information)

X1. STATEMENT OF RATIONALE FOR SPECIFICATION F745

X1.1 The intent of this document is to provide a standard material specification by specifying the chemical and mechanical properties of the material used to manufacture cast stainless steel surgical implants.

X1.2 This specification states that requirements are included for the stainless steel alloy from which cast surgical implants will be produced. The specification document does not cover the requirements for the implants themselves.

X1.3 Implants made from this material are solution-annealed to redissolve any carbides that have precipitated on the grain boundaries during casting. This treatment greatly improves the intergranular corrosion resistance of the casting.

X2. Biocompatibility

X2.1 The material composition covered by this standard has been employed successfully in contact with soft tissue and bone for over a decade.[6]

[6] Bechtol, C.O.; Failure of Femoral Implant Components in Total Hip Replacement Operations; Orphopedic Revue; Vol. IV, Number XI, p. 23-29, November 1975.

X2.2 No known surgical implant has ever been shown to be completely free of adverse reactions in the human body. However, long term clinical experience has shown an acceptable level of biological response can be expected, if the material is used in appropriate applications.

Designation: F 746 – 87 (Reapproved 1999)

Standard Test Method for Pitting or Crevice Corrosion of Metallic Surgical Implant Materials[1]

This standard is issued under the fixed designation F 746; the number immediately following the designation indicates the year of original adoption or, in the case of revision, the year of last revision. A number in parentheses indicates the year of last reapproval. A superscript epsilon (ε) indicates an editorial change since the last revision or reapproval.

1. Scope

1.1 This test method covers the determination of resistance to either pitting or crevice corrosion of metals and alloys from which surgical implants will be produced. It is a modified version of an established test[2] and is used as a screening test to rank surgical implant alloys in order of their resistance to localized corrosion.

1.2 This test method applies only to passive metals and alloys. Nonpassive alloys (other than noble alloys) are susceptible to general corrosion and are not normally suitable for implant use.

1.3 The test method is intended for use as a laboratory screening test of metals and alloys which undergo pitting or crevice corrosion, or both.

1.4 The values stated in SI units are to be regarded as the standard.

1.5 *This standard does not purport to address all of the safety concerns, if any, associated with its use. It is the responsibility of the user of this standard to establish appropriate safety and health practices and determine the applicability of regulatory limitations prior to use.*

2. Referenced Documents

2.1 *ASTM Standards:*

G 3 Practice for Conventions Applicable to Electrochemical Measurements in Corrosion Testing[3]

G 5 Standard Reference Test Method for Making Potentiostatic and Potentiodynamic Anodic Polarization Measurements[3]

G 15 Terminology Relating to Corrosion and Corrosion Testing[3]

3. Summary of Test Method

3.1 A cylindrical specimen fitted with an inert tapered collar is immersed in a saline electrolyte at 37°C for 1 h to establish a corrosion potential. Pitting (or crevice corrosion) is then stimulated by potentiostatically polarizing the specimen to a potential much more noble than the corrosion potential. Stimulation of pitting (or crevice corrosion) will be marked by a large and generally increasing polarizing current.

3.2 Immediately after the stimulation step, the potential is decreased as rapidly as possible to one of several preselected potentials at, or more noble than, the corrosion potential. If the alloy is susceptible to pitting (or crevice corrosion) at the preselected potential, the polarizing current will remain at relatively high values and will fluctuate or increase with time. A post-test examination of the metal specimen establishes whether localized corrosion has occurred by pitting of the exposed surface or by preferential attack at the crevice formed by the tapered collar, or both.

3.3 If the pit (or crevice) surface repassivates at the preelected potential and localized corrosion is halted, the polarizing current will drop to values typical for passive surfaces and the current will decrease continuously. The parameter of interest, the critical potential for pitting (or crevice corrosion), is defined as the highest (most noble) preselected potential at which pit (or crevice) surfaces repassivate after the stimulation step.

4. Significance and Use

4.1 This method is designed solely for determining comparative laboratory indices of performance. The results may be used for ranking alloys in order of increasing resistance to pitting and crevice corrosion under the specific conditions of this method. It should be noted that the method is intentionally designed to reach conditions that are sufficiently severe to cause breakdown of at least one alloy (Type 316 L stainless steel) currently considered acceptable for surgical implant use, and that those alloys which suffer pitting or crevice corrosion during the more severe portions of the test do not necessarily suffer localized corrosion when placed within the human body as a surgical implant.

5. Apparatus

5.1 The following required equipment is described in Practice G 5:

5.1.1 *Standard Polarization Cell*, of 1000 cm^3.

5.1.2 *Electrode Holders*, for auxiliary and working electrodes.

5.1.3 *Potentiostat*, calibrated in accordance with Practice G 5.

---

[1] This test method is under the jurisdiction of ASTM Committee F-4 on Medical and Surgical Materials and Devices and is the direct responsibility of Subcommittee F04.15 on Material Test Methods.

Current edition approved March 27, 1987. Published May 1987. Originally published as F 746 – 81. Last previous edition F 746 – 81.

[2] Syrett, B. C., *Corrosion*, Vol 33, 1977, p. 221.

[3] *Annual Book of ASTM Standards*, Vol 03.02.

5.1.4 *Potential-Measuring Instrument.*
5.1.5 *Current-Measuring Instrument.*
5.1.6 *Anodic Polarization Circuit.*
5.1.7 *Platinum Auxiliary Electrodes.*
5.1.8 *Saturated Calomel Electrode* (SCE).
5.1.9 *Salt Bridge Probe.*

5.2 A cylindrical working electrode is fabricated from the test material by machining, grinding, and suggested final polishing with 600-grit metallographic paper. It is suggested that the part of the cylindrical specimen that is exposed to the test solution have a length of 20.00 ± 1.00 mm (0.787 ± 0.039 in.) and a diameter of 6.35 ± 0.03 mm (0.250 ± 0.001 in.) (see Fig. 1).

5.3 A crevice is created by fitting the cylindrical specimen with a tapered collar, machined from commercial purity polytetrafluoroethylene (PTFE). The collar should have an outer diameter of 12.70 ± 0.05 mm (0.500 ± 0.002 in.) and a thickness of 3.18 ± 0.20 mm (0.125± 0.008 in.). The inside diameter of the tapered collar should range from 0.38 mm (0.015 in.) smaller than the diameter of the specimen to 0.38 mm (0.015 in.) larger. To be consistent with the dimensions suggested in 5.2, the inside diameter should taper from 5.97 ± 0.05 mm (0.235 ± 0.002 in.) to 6.73 ± 0.05 mm (0.265 ± 0.002 in.). See Fig. 1 for drawing of the tapered collar. The relatively fine tolerances are needed to ensure a reproducible fit and crevice.

5.4 In Practice G 5, the method of specimen attachment is to drill and tap the specimen to receive a threaded stainless steel connection rod. A 4-40 thread is used, typically. However, because many surgical implant alloys are not easily drilled, external threads may also be machined, ground, or cast, as illustrated in Fig. 1. A small stainless steel adapter is fitted on to these threads and the adapter then accepts the connection rod.

5.5 Determine the total exposed surface area of the specimen before placement of the PTFE collar, A_T; determine the area on the internal surface of the collar (the creviced area), A_C; and determine the exposed surface area of the specimen after placement of the collar, A_S (where: $A_S = A_T - A_C$). Dimensions should be measured to the nearest 0.1 mm.

5.5.1 *Example*—Using the dimensions suggested previously for the specimen diameter (d = 6.35 mm), the specimen length (l = 20.00 mm), and the collar thickness (t = 3.18 mm),

$$A_T = \pi dl + \frac{\pi d^2}{4} = 431 \text{ mm}^2 \quad (1)$$

$$A_C = \pi dt = 63 \text{ mm}^2 \quad (2)$$

$$A_S = A_T - A_C = 386 \text{ mm}^2 \quad (3)$$

6. Reagents

6.1 *Electrolyte*—Dissolve 9 g of reagent grade sodium chloride (NaCl) in distilled water to make 1000 cm^3 of solution.

6.1.1 After transferring the appropriate amount of electrolyte to the test cell (7.5), the pH is to be measured both before and after the test (see rationale in X1.6).

7. Preparation of Specimens and Conditioning

7.1 Prepare the test specimen surface within 1 h of the start of the experiment by the method described in Practice G 5.

7.2 Using a suitable mechanical jig, force-fit the PTFE collar onto the cylindrical specimen so that the base of the collar is up 10 ± 2 mm (0.393 ± 0.079 in.) from the bottom of the specimen (see Fig. 2). Care should be taken to avoid scratching the metal surface.

NOTE 1—Once the collar is removed from the specimen, it should not be reused.

7.3 Mount the specimen on the holder and on the electrode rod as described in Practice G 5.

7.4 Ultrasonically degrease the electrode assembly in either acetone, toluene, or boiling benzene (with caution, under hood), rinse in distilled water, and dry.

7.5 Transfer 500 mL of electrolyte solution to a clean polarization cell. Bring the temperature of the solution to 37 ± 1°C by immersing the test cell in a controlled temperature water bath or by other suitable means.

7.6 Place the platinum auxiliary electrodes, salt bridge probe and other components in the test cell and temporarily

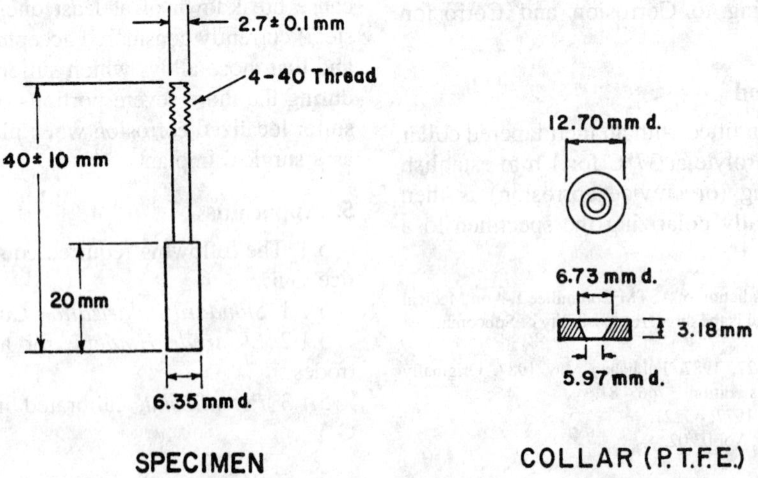

NOTE 1—Unless shown, dimensional tolerances are given in text.
FIG. 1 Dimensions of Specimen and Collar

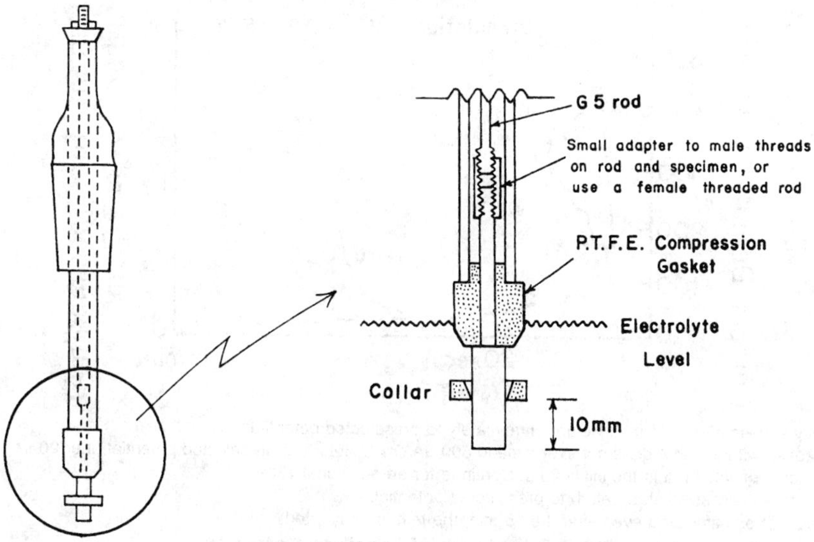

FIG. 2 Assembly into G5 Electrode Holder

close the center opening with a stopper. Fill the salt-bridge with the electrolyte.

NOTE 2—The levels of the solution in the reference and the polarization cells should be the same to avoid siphoning. If this is not possible, a solution-wet (not greased) stopcock can be used in the salt-bridge to eliminate siphoning.

7.7 Transfer the specimen electrode assembly to the test cell and adjust the submerged salt bridge probe tip so it is about 2 mm (0.08 in.) from the center of the bottom portion of the specimen (below the collar).

8. Procedure

8.1 Continuously record the corrosion potential of the working electrode (specimen) with respect to the saturated calomel electrode for 1 h, starting immediately after immersing the specimen. The potential observed upon immersion in the electrolyte shall be called the initial corrosion potential. The potential at the end of the 1 h shall be known as the final corrosion potential, E_1.

8.2 After the 1-h period, the potential should be potentiostatically shifted to + 0.8 V (SCE) to stimulate pitting (or crevice corrosion).

NOTE 3—In the stimulation step, the change in potential either from E_1 or from one of the preselected potentials to + 0.8 V (SCE) should be essentially instantaneous. Such instantaneous changes are facilitated by use of a two-channel potentiostat in which the new control voltage can be selected on the channel not in use. However, if a single channel potentiostat is used, it should be switched temporarily to the standby mode (no impressed current) while the set-potential control is being adjusted to a setting of + 0.8 V (SCE); after so adjusting, the potentiostat should be switched from the standby mode to the operate mode to allow stimulation of localized corrosion. After stimulation, the single-channel potentiostat must remain in the operate mode during the shift to the preselected potential, and the latter shift should be performed manually as rapidly as possible. Manual shifting of the potential may also be necessary after the stimulation step when using a two-channel potentiostat if the switch from + 0.8 V (SCE) to the preselected potential would result in a potential transient to values more active than the preselected potential. Such transients could lead to repassivation and to the incorrect assumption that the repassivation occurred at the preselected potential.

8.3 Record the current using a strip chart recorder with a minimum chart speed of 60 mm/min and a maximum current scale of 0 to 3 mA. The current will be recorded at + 0.8 V (SCE) for a period that depends upon the reaction (see Fig. 3).

8.3.1 If localized corrosion is not stimulated in the initial 20 s, the polarizing currents will remain very small or decrease rapidly with time. Proceed to 8.4.

8.3.2 Stimulation of localized corrosion will be marked either by polarization currents that generally increase with time or by current densities that exceed 500 μA/cm^2 (for the suggested specimen size this would be equivalent to a current of approximately 2 mA).

8.3.2.1 If the current generally increases with time, after 20 s proceed to 8.5.

8.3.2.2 If at any time a current density of 500 μA/cm ^{2} is exceeded, proceed immediately to 8.5. In some instances, upon shifting to + 0.8 V (SCE), the current density will almost instantaneously exceed 500 μA/cm^2. In such cases, proceed directly to 8.5 without pause.

8.4 If localized corrosion is not stimulated within the initial 20 s, continue at + 0.8 V (SCE) for an additional 15 min; the chart speed may be reduced to a minimum of 5 mm/min after the initial 20 s. If localized corrosion is eventually stimulated, proceed to 8.5. If localized corrosion cannot be stimulated even in 15 min, the test is terminated, and the material is considered to have a very high resistance to localized corrosion in the test environment. Report the critical potential as > + 0.8 V (SCE).

8.5 If localized corrosion is stimulated at + 0.8 V (SCE), the potential is then returned as rapidly as possible (see Note 3) to E_1 (which is the first preselected potential) to determine if the specimen will repassivate or if localized corrosion will continue to propagate at the preselected potential.

8.6 If the pitted or creviced local regions repassivate at the preselected potential, the polarizing current will drop quickly to zero or to low values consistent with a passive surface condition (see Fig. 4(*a*) for examples). Monitor this current for 15 min.

8.6.1 During this 15 min, the chart speed may be reduced to

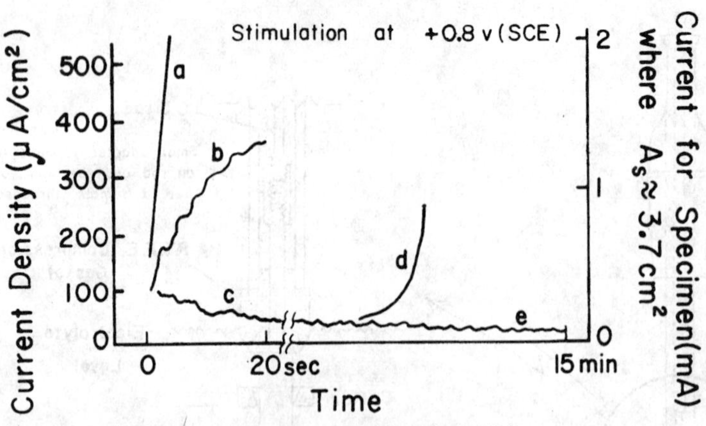

Note a—Current density instantly exceeds 500 μA/cm [2]. Return immediately to preselected potential.
Note b—Current generally increases with time but does not ever exceed 500 μA/cm [2]. Return to preselected potential after 20 s.
Note c—Localized corrosion is not stimulated within the initial 20 s. Continue for an additional 15 min.
Note d—If localized corrosion is eventually stimulated, return to preselected potential.
Note e—If localized corrosion cannot be stimulated even after the 15 min, the test is terminated.

FIG. 3 Stimulation of Localized Corrosion

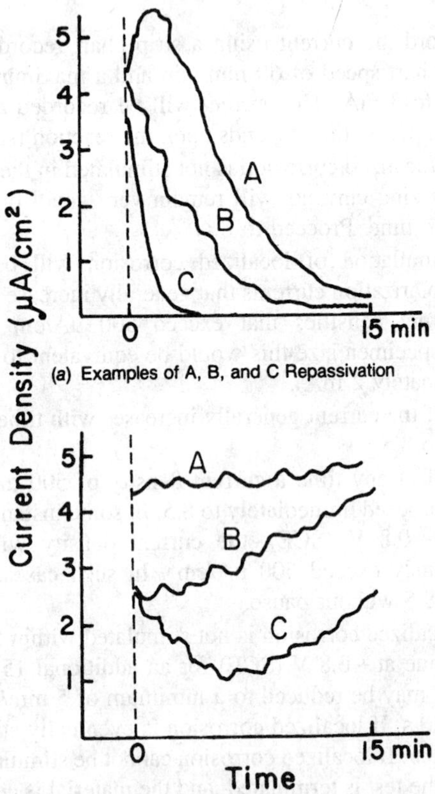

(a) Examples of A, B, and C Repassivation

(*b*) Examples of A, B, and C Continued Localized Corrosion

FIG. 4 Examples of Typical Current – Time Curves at a Preselected Potential

a minimum of 5 mm/min.

8.6.2 Adjust the current scale to obtain satisfactory accuracy. The range used for monitoring the relatively large current during stimulation is almost certainly unsuitable for accurately monitoring the much smaller repassivation currents.

8.6.3 If the pitted or local regions do not repassivate at E_1, then the critical voltage shall be reported as E_1, with the notation that the specimen never repassivated following the initial stimulation. The test shall be terminated.

8.7 After ensuring repassivation at E_1 by observing low, decreasing (or constant) polarization currents for 15 min, repeat the stimulation step (8.2 and 8.3) at + 0.8 V (SCE) and then change the potential as rapidly as possible (see Note 3) to the second preselected potential which should be the nearest 0.05-V increment more noble than E_1 (on the SCE scale). Repeat 8.6.

8.7.1 *Example*—If E_1 is any value in the range – 0.100 to – 0.051 V (SCE), then the second preselected potential would be – 0.050 V (SCE).

8.8 The test consists of alternating between stimulation at + 0.8 V (SCE) and returning to a preselected potential to see if repassivation occurs. After the second preselected potential, increase subsequent preselected potentials (that is, to more noble values) in increments of 0.05 V.

8.8.1 *Examples*—If E_1 were – 0.090 V (SCE), the second preselected potential would be – 0.050 V (SCE), the third preselected potential would be 0.000 V (SCE), the fourth + 0.050 V (SCE), followed by + 0.100 V (SCE), + 0.150 V (SCE), etc.

8.9 At some preselected potential, the localized corrosion may continue to propagate rather than repassivate, heralded by continuous increases or large fluctuations in current during the 15-min observation period (see Fig. 4(*b*) for example). At this point, terminate the test.

8.10 At whatever stage the test is terminated (8.4 or 8.9), remove the collar and holder and examine the specimen at 20× for evidence of pitting, crevice corrosion or discoloration.

9. Report

9.1 The report shall include the following:

9.1.1 Alloy composition, product name, trademark, or similar markings that identify the specimen.

9.1.2 Any special treatments such as heat treatments, amount of hot or cold working, surface finish other than the standard 600-grit metallographic polish, passivation treatments (chemicals, temperatures, times).

9.1.3 Total exposed surface area of the specimen before placement of the collar, A_T; the surface area under the collar,

A_C; and the exposed surface area of the specimen after placement of the collar, A_S.

9.1.4 Initial corrosion potential.

9.1.5 Final corrosion potential, E_1, at the end of the first hour.

9.1.6 Critical potential for pitting (or crevice corrosion): that is, the most noble preselected potential at which pit (or crevice) surfaces still repassivate after the stimulation step.

9.1.7 Plot of polarizing current density (that is, polarizing current divided by A_S) versus time for the 15-min period at the preselected potentials both at and immediately above the critical potential (see Fig. 4 and Fig. 5). By convention, the current densities are reported in μA/cm ^{2}.

9.1.8 Observations made during the microscopic examination including the type of localized corrosion that occurred (pitting in the exposed area, or crevice corrosion in the area under the collar), approximate size and spatial distribution of any pits, and appearance and approximate extent of any crevice corrosion or discoloration.

9.1.9 The pH both before and after the test.

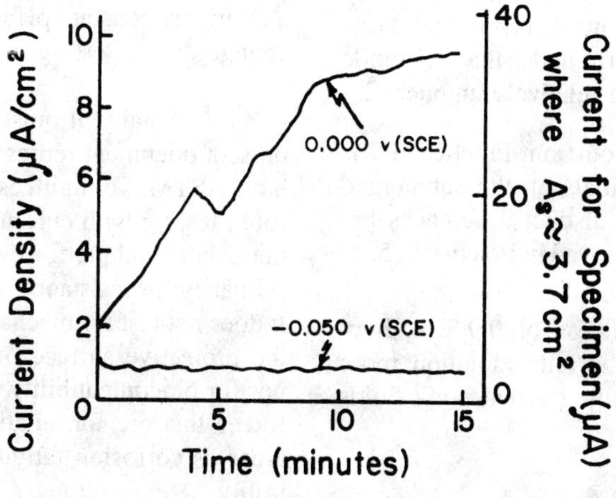

NOTE 1—Typical polarizing current densities during 15-min at (*a*) critical potential, – 0.050 V (SCE), and (*b*) the next more noble step, 0.000 V (SCE), where repassivation no longer occurs. This data is from a specimen of 316 LVM stainless steel in an "as-received" (not yet passivated in accordance with Practice F 86) condition.

FIG. 5 Typical Polarizing Current Densities

APPENDIX

(Nonmandatory Information)

X1. RATIONALE FOR CORROSION SPECIFICATION[4]

X1.1 Corrosion of any metallic implant or device is undesirable for two reasons. First, the corrosion or degradation of the metal may make it structurally weaker or less able to function properly. Second, the resulting corrosion products may react unfavorably with the tissue immediately adjacent to the metal implant or even at distant sites in the body.

X1.2 Most candidate materials for modern implants cannot be differentiated or screened for corrosion by simple conventional immersion testing. For instance, if a candidate alloy is placed in a relevant solution such as blood, salt water, saliva, or mild acid for 10 years, less than 0.1 % weight change would occur during that entire period. Therefore, to screen candidate materials in a reasonable period, corrosion processes must be

[4] Committee F-4 requires a rationale to accompany all standards. This rationale should be readable to lay consumers as well as technical experts.

promoted or accelerated in some way. In this method, electrochemical stimulation is used to accelerate the corrosion processes.

X1.3 In Practice G 5, the electrochemical potential impressed upon a metallic specimen immersed in an acid solution is steadily increased until the protective oxide film on the metal surface (the "passive film") breaks down and localized corrosion ensues. This breakdown is monitored by a rather sudden increase in the current flowing in the solution. With this method, the alloys are ranked in terms of the potential at which breakdown first occurs: the higher this potential, the more resistant the alloy is to passive film breakdown and to localized corrosion.

X1.4 It has been demonstrated[5] that slipping a polymeric ring over a small portion of a submerged cylindrical specimen can cause a concentrated attack in the creviced area between the metal and the ring. The environment within the crevice may become depleted in oxygen and concentrated in aggressive species, leading to a more aggravated attack than would have occurred without the creviced region. Some materials are very susceptible to this particular attack mechanism, and large amounts of corrosion products may form under the ring while the remainder of the specimen may be relatively untouched.

X1.5 In this method, instrumentation from Practice G 5 is employed to obtain the desired potentials on the submerged specimen; however, there are several distinct differences between this method and the method employed in Practice G 5, as follows:

X1.5.1 Instead of mild acid, a solution of 0.9 % sodium chloride in distilled water is used; the latter solution more closely simulates fluids within the body. (Actual body fluids cannot presently be employed because their organic components tend to foul the immersed corrosion detection instruments).

X1.5.2 A polymeric ring is placed on the specimen to create a crevice condition.

X1.5.3 This method requires less ancillary equipment than Practice G 5, so reducing capital costs; and potential inaccuracies in the interpretation of the results are avoided by eliminating the effects of incubation time for localized corrosion. A modified version of the method[2] is utilized in which the potential is first set at + 0.800 V measured with reference to a saturated calomel electrode (SCE). At this very high overvoltage, localized breakdown and corrosion occurs immediately in many alloys. After this corrosion stimulation step, the overvoltage is dropped immediately to lower values to determine if the alloy can repair itself (repassivate) under these less severe conditions.

X1.6 Committee efforts are underway to evaluate the importance of pH control to the outcome of the test. Conditions being examined include phosphate buffering the electrolyte to a relatively constant pH of 7.2 ± 0.2 versus allowing the pH to change during testing.

X1.7 Finally, it must be emphasized that even though this present document represents the results of combined efforts of both ASTM Committees F-4 and G-1, plus extensive round-robin testing with current implant metals, it is not intended as the sole technique for evaluation of implant materials. It tests primarily for resistance to certain forms of localized corrosion. It does not test for mechanical stability (ability of the metal and the protective surface oxide to withstand mechanical forces) nor for biocompatibility per se. There are currently active task forces that are formulating additional corrosion tests in such areas as corrosion fatigue, fretting corrosion, and biocompatibility.

[5] *Journal of Material Science*, Vol 7, 1972, p. 126.

Standard Practice for Selecting Generic Biological Test Methods for Materials and Devices[1]

This standard is issued under the fixed designation F 748; the number immediately following the designation indicates the year of original adoption or, in the case of revision, the year of last revision. A number in parentheses indicates the year of last reapproval. A superscript epsilon (ε) indicates an editorial change since the last revision or reapproval.

1. Scope

1.1 This practice recommends generic biological test methods for materials and devices according to end-use applications. While chemical testing for extractable additives and residual monomers or residues from processing aids is necessary for most implant materials, such testing is not included as part of this standard practice. The reader is cautioned that the area of materials biocompatibility testing is a rapidly evolving field, and improved methods are evolving rapidly, so this standard is by necessity only a guideline. A thorough knowledge of current techniques and research is critical to a complete evaluation of new materials.

1.2 These test protocols are intended to apply to materials and medical devices for human application. Biological evaluation of materials and devices, and related subjects such as pyrogen testing, batch testing of production lots, and so on, are also discussed. Tests include those performed on materials, end products, and extracts. Rationale and comments on current state of the art are included for all test procedures described.

1.3 The biocompatibility of materials used in single or multicomponent medical devices for human use depends to a large degree on the particular nature of the end-use application. Biological reactions that are detrimental to the success of a material in one device application may have little or no bearing on the successful use of the material for a different application. It is, therefore, not possible to specify a set of biocompatibility test methods which will be necessary and sufficient to establish biocompatibility for all materials and applications.

1.4 The ethical use of research animals places the obligation on the individual investigator to determine the most efficient methods for performing the necessary testing without undue use of animals. Where adequate prior data exists to substantiate certain types of safety information, these guidelines should not be interpreted to mean that testing should be unnecessarily repeated.

1.5 *This standard does not purport to address all of the safety concerns, if any, associated with its use. It is the responsibility of the user of this standard to establish appropriate safety and health practices and determine the applicability of regulatory limitations prior to use.*

2. Referenced Documents

2.1 *ASTM Standards:*

E 1262 Guide for Performance of the Chinese Hamster Ovary Cell/Hypoxanthine Guanine Phosphoribosyl Transferase Gene Mutation Assay[2]

E 1280 Guide for Performance of the Mouse Lymphoma Assay for Mammalian Cell Mutagenicity[2]

F 719 Practice for Testing Biomaterials in Rabbits for Primary Skin Irritation[3]

F 720 Practice for Testing Guinea Pigs for Contact Allergens: Guinea Pig Maximization Test[3]

F 749 Practice for Evaluating Material Extracts by Intracutaneous Injection in the Rabbit[2]

F 750 Practic for Evaluating Material Extracts by Systemic Injection in the Mouse[3]

F 756 Practice for Assessment of the Hemolytic Properties of Materials[3]

F 763 Practice for Short-Term Screening of Implant Materials[3]

F 813 Practice for Direct Contact Cell Culture Evaluation of Materials for Medical Devices[3]

F 895 Test Method for Agar Diffusion Cell Culture Screening for Cytotoxicity[3]

F 619 Standard Practice for Extraction of Medical Plastics[3]

F 981 Practice for Assessment of Compatibility of Biomaterials for Surgical Implants with Respect to Effect of Materials on Muscle and Bone[3]

F 1027 Practice for Tissue and Cell Compatibility of Orofacial Prosthetic Materials and Devices[3]

F 1408 Practice for Subcutaneous Screening Test for Implant Materials[3]

F 1439 Guide for Performance of Lifetime Bioassay for the Tumorigenic Potential of Implant Materials[3]

2.2 *Other Referenced Documents:*

ISO/AAMI/ANSI 10993-1 Biological Testing of Medical and Dental Materials and Devices - Part 1: Guidance on Selection of Tests[4]

---

[1] This practice is under the jurisdiction of ASTM Committee F-4 on Medical and Surgical Devices and is direct responsibility of Subcommittee F04.16 on Biocompatibility Test Methods.

Current edition approved August 10, 1998. Published October 1998. Originally published as F 748 – 82. Last previous edition F 748 – 95.

[2] *Annual Book of ASTM Standards*, Vol 11.04.

[3] *Annual Book of ASTM Standards*, Vol 13.01.

[4] Available from American National Standards Institute, 11 West 42nd St., 13th Floor, New York, NY 10036.

EN 30993–1 Biological Testing of Medical and Dental Materials and Devices - Part 1: Guidance on Selection of Tests[4]
General Program Memorandum #G95-1 FDA[5]
Immunotoxicity Testing Guidance-FDA[5]

3. Summary of Practice

3.1 A matrix listing biological test methods versus materials (devices) and their applications is included in Table 1. The expected duration of use of the device is also considered. Intra-operative is less than 24 h, short-term is up to and including 30 days, chronic is greater than 30 days. The position of row and column intersection is marked to indicate whether the test is recommended for a material or device for the specific application indicated. The terms relating to device or material type and application are addressed in Section 5. Discussion of applicability, current state of the art, and rationale for individual test methods also appears in that section.

4. Significance and Use

4.1 The objective of this practice is to recommend sufficient biological testing to establish a reasonable level of confidence concerning the biological response to a material or device, while at the same time avoiding unnecessary testing.

4.2 This document is intended to provide guidance to the materials investigator in selecting the proper procedures to be carried out for the screening of new or modified materials. Because each material and each implant situation involves its own unique circumstances, these recommendations should be modified as necessary and do not constitute the only testing that will be required for a material nor should these guidelines be interpreted as minimum requirements for any particular situation. While an attempt has been made to provide recommendation for different implant circumstances, some of the recommended testing may not be necessary or reasonable for a specific material or application.

5. Classification of Materials and Devices by End-Use Applications

5.1 *General*:

5.1.1 When new materials are sought for a medical application for use on humans, the material(s) may comprise the whole final device product, or may be one of many component materials in the device. The first step is a thorough literature search for previous use of the material or biocompatibility testing studies to assure that it has not been known to produce an adverse biological response that exceeds the expected benefit in the use of the device. Note that the final fabricated product may differ chemically, physically, or biologically from the raw materials used to fabricate the product due to processing and this has to be considered when designing test protocols. For some devices it may be necessary or desirable to take material test samples directly from the final device product. Samples should be fully representative of the finished product in terms of processing, cleaning, packaging, sterilization, and any other procedures that are performed on the materials before the device is used.

[5] Available from CDRH, Rockville, MD.

5.1.2 At this point preliminary material screening may be employed, depending on the expertise of the organizations evaluating the materials. Since preliminary screening is normally an option to minimize the economic impact of a candidate material failing final biological tests after extensive time and effort, it is not a required procedure. The investigator should be aware that, should an adverse tissue response be observed with a final product, it may be impossible to determine which component or process is responsible without these initial screening tests.

5.1.3 This practice addresses two dimensions of tissue-material interactions: duration and tissue type. A third dimension, which should be considered is the relative size difference between the host and the material, that is, to how much material surface area is the host exposed. The material surface area to body weight ratio may become a significant factor for porous materials, and devices of repeated short-term applications (for example, dialysis products). While this practice does not address the issue of "intensity factor" of increased surface area, the biocompatibility testing facility personnel should consider it in their material screening and testing protocol design.

5.1.4 For the purposes of this document, devices, and the materials that comprise them, are classified as to end-use human application as outlined in 5.2-5.4.

5.2 *External Devices*:

5.2.1 *Devices That Contact Intact Body Surfaces Only*—examples include electrodes, splints, external prostheses, certain dressings, monitors of various types, or ostomy appliances.

5.2.2 *Devices That Contact Breached Body Surfaces*—examples include ulcer, burn, and granulation tissue dressings, or healing devices.

5.3 *Externally Communicating Devices*:

5.3.1 *Devices Communicating with Intact Natural Channels*:

5.3.1.1 *Intraoperative (<24 hours)*—examples include intraintestinal devices (such as sigmoidoscopes, colonoscopes, stomach tubes, or gastroscopes), tracheal tubes, bronchoscopes and any parts of ancillary equipment that are in contact with materials entering the body, and irrigation sets.

5.3.1.2 *Short-term (up to and including 30 days)*—examples include contact lenses, urinary catheters, and intravaginal devices.

5.3.1.3 *Chronic (>30 days)*—examples include urinary catheters for chronic use and intrauterine devices.

5.3.2 *Devices Communicating with Body Tissues and Fluids*:

5.3.2.1 *Intraoperative (<24 hours)*—examples include hypodermic needles, penetrating electrodes, biopsy instruments, arthroscopes, laparoscopes, irrigation equipment, surgical instruments, trochars, and any parts of ancillary equipment that are in contact with materials entering the body.

5.3.2.2 *Short-term (up to and including 30 days)*—examples include cranial calipers, perfusion apparatus, drainage apparatus, stabilizing orthopedic devices, and any parts of ancillary equipment that are in contact with material entering the body.

5.3.2.3 *Chronic (>30 days)*—examples include percutaneous electrodes, active penetrating electrodes, stapedectomy

TABLE 1 Applicable Tests

Classification of Material or Device and Application	Cell Culture Cytotoxicity	Sensi-tization	Skin Irritation or Intra-cutaneous	Mucous Membrane Irritation	Systemic Toxicity, Acute or Subchronic	Blood Compatibility	Hemolysis	Pyrogen Test	Short-term Implantation	Long-term Implantation	Immune Response	Genotoxicity	Carcinogenicity
External devices													
Intact surfaces (all time periods)	x	x	x										
Breached surfaces													
Intraoperative	x	x	x										
Short-Term	x	x	x		x								
Chronic	x	x	x		x							x	
External Devices Communicating with:													
Intact Natural Channels													
Intraoperative	x	x	x	x									
Short-term	x	x	x	x	x				x				
Chronic	x	x	x	x	x				x		x	x	x
Body Tissues and Fluids													
Intraoperative	x	x	x		x			i[A]					
Short-term	x	x	x		x			i[A]	x		x		
Chronic	x	x	x		x			i[A]	x		x	x	x
Blood Path, indirect													
Intraoperative	x	x	x		x	x	x	x					
Short-term	x	x	x		x	x	x	x					
Chronic	x	x	x		x	x	x	x			x	x	
Blood Path, direct													
Intraoperative	x	x	x		x	x	x	x					
Short-term	x	x	x		x	x	x	x	x		x		
Chronic	x	x	x		x	x	x	x	x		x	x	x
Implanted Devices principally contacting Bone/Tissue/tissue fluid													
Intraoperative	x	x	x		x								
Short-term	x	x	x		x			x	x				
Chronic	x	x	x		x			x	x	x	x	x	x
Blood													
Intraoperative	x	x	x		x	x	x	x					
Short-term	x	x	x		x	x	x	x	x			x	x
Chronic	x	x	x		x	x	x	x	x	x	x	x	x

[A](i) Pyrogenicity testing may be considered for all devices contacting the central nervous system.

prostheses, partial and total ossicular replacement prostheses, or tympanoplasty ventilation tubes.

5.3.3 *Blood Path, Indirect*—Products contacting blood path at one point for usually less than 24 hours, and serves as a conduit for fluid entry into the vascular system. Examples include solution administration sets, extension sets, transfer sets, or blood administration sets.

5.3.3.1 Products that are used for >24 hours or that are used repeatedly in the same patient will be considered as chronic usage and should undergo extended testing.

5.3.4 *Blood, Path, Direct*—Single recirculating blood exposure or product is in blood path generally less than 24 hours. Examples include intravenous catheters, oxygenators, extracorporeal oxygenator tubing and accessories.

5.3.5 *Blood Path, Direct, Short Term, or Chronic, or repeated exposure*—Examples include dialyzers or dialysis tubing and accessories, shunts.

5.4 *Implanted Long-Term Devices*:

5.4.1 *Devices Principally Contacting Bones*—examples includd orthopedic pins, screws, replacement joints, bone prostheses, cements, or dental implants.

5.4.2 *Devices Principally Residing in the Subcutaneous Space*—examples include pacemakers, neuromuscular stimulators, facial augmentation devices, tissue expander devices, and breast prostheses.

5.4.3 *Devices Principally Contacting Soft Tissue and Tissue Fluids*—examples include drug supply devices, neuromuscular sensors, replacement tendons, penile, and other implants, cerebrospinal fluid drains, artificial larynx, vas deferens valves, or ligation clips.

5.4.4 *Devices Principally Contacting Blood*—examples include pacemaker leads, artificial arteriovenous fistulae, heart valves, vascular grafts, blood monitors, internal drug delivery catheters, or ventricular assist pumps.

6. Selection of Test Procedures

6.1 *General*—Biocompatibility testing involves tests of either the material itself, or an extract from it, or both, depending on the nature of the end-use application. While this practice does not address specific chemical methods for evaluating the extractable substances or residuals from implant materials, several of the recommended tests (see 6.2, 6.7, 6.6, and 6.3) utilize extracts rather than the original material for testing. If sensitive chemical assay techniques (such as GC, HPLC, and AA) should revel no detectable substances being extracted into the medium, consideration may be given to deletion of these tests from the test battery. The investigator is cautioned, however, that the detection limit of the analytical chemistry procedures may not be adequate to detect trace extractables that may generate a tissue response. Before analysis of extracts is substituted for actual biocompatibility testing of the extracts, validation procedures may be necessary to show the relative tissue response to levels of extractable which are slightly above the detection limit. It is particularly appropriate that animal testing involving extracts be considered for deletion if there are no detectable substances being extracted.

6.2 *Cell Culture Cytotoxicity Assays*—This test evaluates *in vitro* toxicity of substrate materials to cultured cells.

6.2.1 Generally materials that do not pass the cytotoxicity assays are not considered for further biocompatibility testing and are not used in devices for human application. Thus the direct relation between results of cytotoxicity testing and biocompatibility of materials has not been documented and there is some controversy as to the value of the testing since some good materials may be excluded and some others that are not biocompatible may pass this test. Cytotoxicity testing is recommended as an early screening test and also to provide information that will aid in the development of cytotoxicity tests predictive of in vivo performance.

6.2.2 Several different tests are included under this heading, such as Agar Diffusion, Fluid Medium, Agar Overlay, Flask Dilution, etc. All of these tests emphasize *in vitro* toxicity of either substrate materials or extract solutions to cultured cells. Cellular damage is observed and graded. Two available versions are included in Practice F 813 and Test Method F 895. An application-specific method is included in Practice F 1027. An HIMA/PMA guideline is available from the FDA for a discussion and references on other versions of this test.

6.2.3 Since the biological reaction to particles generated during function may differ from the reaction to soluble products, *in vitro* testing of macrophage/monocyte interaction with representative particles may be considered.

6.3 *Sensitization Test*—The guinea pig maximization test (Practice F 720) is a procedure whereby the material (or extracts thereof) is mixed with Freund's complete adjuvant and administered to the test animals during a 2-week induction period. After 2 weeks rest, the guinea pigs are challenged with the test substance and the skin graded for allergic reaction after 24 hours. Other test methods such as the repeated dermal patch may also be used. The mouse local lymph node assay should be considered as an alternative to the guinea pig maximization test. Controls are necessary for all tests.

6.3.1 These tests are for sensitization of the cell mediated type (Type IV). Since there are concerns about materials causing sensitization of the atopic type (Type I), measurement of IgE antibodies in test animals should also be considered. Similarly, measurement of IgE antibodies in humans in clinical trials may be considered.

6.4 *Skin Irritation Assay*—This is a patch test on the skin of rabbits, and after 24 hours the patches are removed and skin graded for erythema and edema. One available version is included in Practice F 719.

6.5 *Mucous Membrane Irritation*—The end use of the device product must be considered when deciding what tests to undertake. In some circumstances the mucous membrane should be considered for the testing site. Numerous tests utilizing different mucous membranes and different animals have been reported. There remains some controversy about the applicability of the results of these tests to human clinical use. The material investigator should consider the appropriateness of a particular test site and published discussion of these methods when planning testing. The intracutaneous irritation test (see section 6.6) may be the more suitable test.

6.6 *Intracutaneous Injection (Irritation) Assay*—This assay is designed to determine biological response of rabbits to the single-dose intracutaneous injection of appropriate extracts prepared from test samples. All rabbits are observed for signs of erythema (tissue redness) and edema (tissue swelling) at the injection site for periods up to 72 h. Significant reactions are recorded and the test extract is graded. A USP test has been in use for many years, and Practice F 749 may be consulted for additional information.

6.7 *Systemic Injection (Acute Toxicity) Assay*—This assay is designed to determine the biological response of animals (mice) to the single-dose intravenous or intraperitoneal injection of extracts prepared from test samples. The preferred extracts are saline, vegetable oil, or other liquids simulating body fluids or the vehicles of pharmaceutical products that may contact and potentially extract the material before reaching the patient. All mice are observed for signs of toxicity immediately after injection and again at specified intervals. Significant responses are recorded, and the test extract is graded. A USP procedure has been in use for many years, and many variations exist, including Practice F 750.

6.8 *Blood Compatibility*—Hemolysis and thrombosis are the most obvious examples of blood materials incompatibility, although adverse effects on plasma proteins, enzymes, and formed blood elements can also occur. Thrombogenicity can be studied through specifically designed *in vitro*, or *ex vivo* procedures specific to the type of product being tested. Normally these tests are dynamic, simulated in-use procedures, with each being developed specifically by the organization interested in evaluating the device in question. Hemolysis is covered in 6.9.

6.9 *Hemolysis*—While hemolysis testing is frequently performed in combination with other tests for blood compatibility as specified in 6.8, several methods are in use whereby both materials and extracts are utilized for determining hemolysis. Test rods and extracts of the materials are incubated with human or rabbit blood in dynamic and static test tubes. The amount of plasma hemoglobin is measured and compared to reference materials and controls. Practice F 756 describes one method for the performance of hemolysis testing. In addition, hemolysis may be evaluated in finished devices by means of dynamic *in vitro, in vivo,* or *ex vivo* procedures designed to emphasize the hemolytic effect of the entire device. These tests tend to be proprietary to the various organizations who employ them.

6.10 *Complement Activation*—The interaction of blood with some materials, especially large surfaces (such as in dialysis membranes), may lead to the activation of the complement cascade leading to patient morbidity. Testing for activation of the various complement components using *in vitro* systems is available and recommended for blood contacting materials and devices.

6.11 *Pyrogenicity*—Pyrogenic (fever producing) substances are either components of gram negative bacterial cell membranes (called endotoxin or lipopolysaccharide (LPS), or are chemical in origin, called chemical pyrogens. Sterile devices designed to contact the human vascular system are commonly labeled "nonpyrogenic," and each batch of product is tested for pyrogenicity by either the USP Rabbit Test or the Limulus Amebocyte Lysate Test (LAL) (USP bacterial endotoxin test). While endotoxin contamination is detectable by either the USP rabbit test or the LAL test, use of the LAL test for endotoxin detection is the preferred method whenever possible. Substances that are LAL positive should not be tested by the rabbit test. Chemical pyrogens can only be detected by the USP rabbit test and this may be done on LAL negative substances.

6.11.1 Since depyrogenating endotoxin-contaminated devices is difficult, costly, and often impractical, pyrogen testing is sometimes performed on incoming raw materials or components as a screening method. The LAL test should be used for these screening purposes for LPS before any rabbit test for chemical pyrogens. If the identity of possible chemical pyrogens is known, every effort should be made to detect chemical pyrogens by analytical or other means not involving the USP rabbit test.

6.12 *Implantation Tests*—The end use application should be considered when choosing the most suitable site for testing.

6.12.1 *Short-Term Subcutaneous Implantation Test*—Since many implants are intended specifically for subcutaneous use it is important to consider the reaction of this tissue space to implants and materials. The potential for mobility of implants and tissue of the subcutaneous plane makes this site significantly different from other tissue implantation sites. Inflammatory responses may be increased with motion. Practice F 1408 provides one method for short-term implant testing in a subcutaneous site.

6.12.2 *Short-Term Intramuscular Implantation Test*—This type of test is designed to evaluate the reaction of living tissue to a sample material that is surgically implanted into animal tissue (preferably the rabbit, but larger animals (such as the dog) may be considered where necessary). At the conclusion of the assay period, the sites of implantation are examined for significant reaction, and the test material is graded. A USP test has been in use for many years and 7- and 30-day evaluation is available in Practice F 763.

6.12.3 *Long-Term Implant Test*—Practice F 981 is a long-term implantation test in muscle and bone for metals, plastics, and ceramics. Other long-term implant tests may be appropriate for long-term implant applications.

6.13 *Genotoxicity*—A number of tests are available to assess genotoxic potential. The Ames test may be used as a preliminary screening study with materials. Two methods that have been developed for genotoxicity testing in mammalian cells are included in Guide E 1262 and Guide E 1280. Additionally, other tests may be suggested by regulatory agencies for certain implant applications and sites. No single test yet developed can detect all types of mutagens.

6.14 *Carcinogenicity*—Carcinogenicity testing is usually quite specific for the test substance, with no standard procedures available at this time. Guide F 1439 provides guidelines for the performance of these types of tests on implant materials. The National Toxicology Program has published a very comprehensive document[6] relating to the conduct of carcinogenicity testing of chemicals. While much of this document may not be applicable to implant materials, many of the recommendations for animal care, selection of model, and methods for ensuring the integrity of data may be applicable.

[6] General Statement of Work for the Conduct of Toxicology and Carcinogenicity Studies in Laboratory Animals, *National Toxicology Program,* April 1987.

The user of this document should be aware that very little is known about the latency periods for the development of tumors due to implant materials in the human or the relationship between the results of animal testing and the long-term clinical response. The primary measure of the carcinogenic potential of implant materials will be the results of long term clinical use.

6.15 *Immunotoxicity*—Materials may influence the immune system of the host in various ways. There may be toxicity to the cells in the immune system resulting in decreased responsiveness to antigens. There may be stimulation of the immune system resulting in increased immune responses to antigens. There may be stimulation of an immune response to components or extracts of the materials, which may or may not result in patient morbidity or unsatisfactory performance of the device. Testing for immunotoxicity and specific immune responses may be considered, especially for materials of natural origin or materials that are oil, wax, or gel in nature.

6.16 *Batch Testing of Materials and Devices for Biocompatibility*—Biocompatibility testing of materials may, in some circumstances, be done on samples from a batch of material to be used and the methods used for testing depend on the type of industry, product, and manufacturing and quality control operations in use. Periodic biocompatibility audits may be performed, depending on the manufacturer's degree of assurance that the supplier will not change his product or process, intentionally or otherwise. Additional biocompatibility testing must be performed when changes are made in the composition or processing of the materials.

7. Keywords

7.1 animal testing; biocompatibility; in vivo testing; laboratory testing; toxicity

APPENDIX

(Nonmandatory Information)

X1. RATONALE

X1.1 Application of any biocompatibility test to a material requires judgment about its appropriateness. No counsel can be given which will be correct under all circumstances. Regulatory agencies may be extremely helpful when available but such guidelines do not exist for all materials or products. It is for such circumstances that a biocompatibility guideline is needed.

X1.2 With time, greater emphasis has been placed on speed and reduced expense in the performance of biocompatibility screening procedures. It is incumbent on the researcher to reduce the numbers of animals used in experimental testing whenever possible. For primary screening, tissue culture testing may satisfy these requirements but no test is universally applicable.

X1.3 Test selection is based upon a stable manufacturing process and for materials that have been characterized chemically. Intended use and duration of use should affect the direction of more extensive testing. Since the results of biological testing may be affected by the cleaning and sterilization processes used, cleaning and sterilization methods, which are representative of final processing should be used for test specimens.

X1.4 The rationale for both the standard and the various sections is integrated into the text, since the nature of this document is such that understanding of the reasoning behind the statement, requirements, and discussion is required as one reads the standard.

X1.5 Biocompatibility has traditionally been associated with materials and devices that do not stimulate an adverse biological response. However, there is a growing number of devices that are designed to be bioactive or biointeractive. With these materials and devices, the presence of, or enhancement of a biological reaction is desirable. Therefore, interpretation of results of biological testing should be done in light of the intended end use of the material and device.

X1.6 Since this Practice was originally written, the International Standards Organization has prepared a document with similar intent and content. (See ISO 10993-1) This ISO standard has been adopted as a European standard, EN 30993-1, and as an American National Standard. The FDA has enacted a document, General Program Memorandum #G95-1, with guidelines and a table of tests for consideration for evaluation of biocompatibility. Manufacturers and other investigators may want to consult these document to assure that any differences are addressed in the planning of tests.

X1.7 The user of this guideline and the methods that are recommended should be aware that these methods reflect the best available knowledge concerning the assessment of possible physiological effects of materials and their components. No test can guarantee the biocompatibility of a material.

X1.7.1 *In vitro* testing and animal testing are only models of the human clinical environment. The actual clinical experience with a material will only be determined after a period of clinical use. It has been suggested that a clinical use period of several years in a carefully controlled trial with adequate follow-up will be necessary for reasonable assurance of biocompatibility.

X1.7.2 The latency period for the appearance of malignant tumors in response to carcinogenic agents may be 20 years or more in the human. It is unknown what the relationship between the latency period in animals and in the human will be for undiscovered tumor-causing materials.

Standard Practice for Evaluating Material Extracts by Intracutaneous Injection in the Rabbit[1]

This standard is issued under the fixed designation F 749; the number immediately following the designation indicates the year of original adoption or, in the case of revision, the year of last revision. A number in parentheses indicates the year of last reapproval. A superscript epsilon (ϵ) indicates an editorial change since the last revision or reapproval.

1. Scope

1.1 This practice is a nonspecific, acute toxicity test used to help determine the biocompatibility of materials used in medical devices.

1.2 The liquids injected in the rabbits are those obtained by Practice F 619 where the extraction vehicles are saline, vegetable oil, or other liquids simulating human body fluids.

1.3 This practice is one of several developed for the assessment of the biocompatibility of materials. Practice F 748 may provide guidance for the selection of appropriate methods for testing materials for a specific application.

2. Referenced Documents

2.1 *ASTM Standards:*

F 619 Practice for Extraction of Medical Plastics[2]

F 748 Practice for Selecting Generic Biological Test Methods for Materials and Devices[2]

3. Summary of Practice

3.1 The extract liquid is prepared in accordance with Practice F 619. The extraction vehicles are saline and vegetable oil, or other extraction vehicles can be used, as described in Practice F 619. The extract liquid is injected into rabbits and the animals are observed at regular intervals for 72 h for erythema, edema, and necrosis.

4. Significance and Use

4.1 This practice is to be used to help assess the biocompatibility of materials used in medical devices. It is an acute toxicological test designed to detect the presence of injurious leachable substances.

4.2 This practice may not be appropriate for all types of implant applications. The user is cautioned to consider the appropriateness of the method in view of the materials being tested, their potential applications, and the recommendations contained in Practice F 748.

4.3 The only limitation applicable is the extract preparation. Refer to Sections 4.3 and 4.4 of Practice F 619 for a description of this limitation.

5. Apparatus

5.1 *Cages*—There shall be one cage for each rabbit exposed to one extract liquid. Each rabbit will be uniquely identified with this identity recorded.

5.2 *Syringes*—Sterile syringes, not greater than 2 mL in volume, with a precision of no less than ± 0.10 mL shall be used. Sterile needles of 21 to 26 gage shall be used.

6. Test Animals

6.1 *Rabbits*—The rabbits shall be thin-skinned albino type, healthy, and not previously used for any test. Animal care shall be in accordance with Guide for Care and Use of Laboratory Animals.[3] Rabbits with significant scars or wounds are not suitable for this test. For each extraction vehicle a minimum of two rabbits are used in the test. If the results of the first test are inconclusive, three more rabbits are needed to complete the test with that extraction vehicle for one material.

6.1.1 During the test the rabbits shall be fed normally, with commercially available feed and tap water.

7. Sampling

7.1 Sample in accordance with Practice F 619.

8. Sample and Test Specimen

8.1 The sample is the extract of the test article (that is, plastic or other material) exposed to the extraction procedure. As a result of the extraction in Practice F 619, for each extraction vehicle there are available: (*1*) sample extract liquid, and (*2*) a blank extract liquid. These extract liquids are to be injected into the test animals within 24 h of the end of the extraction procedure. Record storage conditions if not used immediately after preparation.

8.1.1 There are usually four extract liquids prepared from two extraction vehicles available for test, those based on saline and vegetable oil. Samples based on other extraction vehicles may be available, as described in Practice F 619, or as required by the standard for the medical device.

8.2 The test specimen is the combination of the test site and

[1] This practice is under the jurisdiction of ASTM Committee F-4 on Medical and Surgical Materials and Devices and is the direct responsibility of Subcommittee F04.16 on Biocompatibility Test Methods.

Current edition approved February 10, 1998. Published June 1998. Originally published as F 749 – 82. Last previous edition F 749 – 87 (1996)$^{\epsilon 1}$.

[2] *Annual Book of ASTM Standards*, Vol 13.01.

[3] U.S. Department of Health, Education, and Welfare, *Guide for the Care and Use of Laboratory Animals*, Publication No. NIH 78-23, Bethesda, MD.

0.2 mL of the injected extract liquid. A total of 10 sites are to be injected with the sample extract liquid and 10 sites with the blank extract liquid.

9. Procedure

9.1 *Preparation of Rabbits*—On the day (no more than 24 h) before the test, closely clip the fur on the animal's back on both sides of the spinal column over a sufficiently large test area. Avoid mechanical irritation and trauma. Remove loose hair by means of a vacuum. The use of a depilatory agent that does not cause skin irritation in place of or in addition to clipping may be desirable. Swab the skin slightly with diluted alcohol, and dry the skin prior to injection.

9.2 Agitate each extract liquid vigorously prior to withdrawal of each injection dose, to ensure even distribution of the extracted matter. If the extract liquid appears to contain particulates, record and consider in reporting results.

9.3 Inject intracutaneously 0.2 mL of the sample extract liquid at five sites on one side of each of two rabbits. Similarly, at five other sites on the other side of each rabbit, inject 0.2 mL of the corresponding blank extract liquid.

9.4 Examine the injected sites 24, 48, and 72 h after the injection for gross evidence of tissue reaction, such as erythema, edema, and necrosis. To facilitate the examination, swab the skin lightly with diluted alcohol, and clip the fur, if necessary. Rate the tissue reaction for all ten sites of the sample and for the five sites of the blank extract at each observation period for each type of tissue reaction. The rating scales for erythema and edema are given in Tables 1 and 2.

10. Interpretation of Results

10.1 A sample extract passes the test if each type of tissue reaction of the test and blank extracts are similar for all observation periods.

10.2 *Retest*—If either rabbit has a sample extract tissue reaction of moderate or severe but the other does not, repeat the test using fresh extracts in three more rabbits. The sample extract passes if in this retest the tissue responses for the sample extracts are not biologically different from those for the blank extract liquid.[4]

10.3 A retest (see 10.2) requires that the extraction procedure be done a second time, since the extraction fluids must be used within 24 h of the end of the extraction.

TABLE 1 Severity Rating for Erythema

Severity of Erythema	Numerical Rating
No erythema	0
Very slight erythema (barely perceptible)	1
Well-defined erythema	2
Moderate to severe	3
Severe erythema (beet redness) to slight eschar formation (injuries in depth)	4

TABLE 2 Severity Rating for Edema

Severity of Edema[A]	Numerical Rating
No edema	0
Very slight edema (barely perceptible)	1
Slight edema (edges of area defined by definite raising)	2
Moderate edema (area raised approximately 1 mm)	3
Severe edema (area raised more than 1 mm and extending beyond area of injection)	4

[A] Edema is tissue swelling. Apparent swelling attributable to the injection vehicle is not considered edema.

11. Report

11.1 Describe the sample that was extracted, including generic name, trade name, manufacturer's code, catalog number, date of manufacture, formulation, fabrication procedures or processes, etc., as appropriate. Describe the extraction vehicle and the conditions of the extraction (temperature and time).

11.2 Report the scores for each type of tissue reaction at each observation period as described in 10.1 for the test and control extracts.

11.3 If a retest was made, report the data for that test, as in 11.2.

12. Precision and Bias

12.1 Intralaboratory and interlaboratory reproducibility have not been systematically determined. Reproducibility may be inferred from previous round robin studies.[5,6]

13. Keywords

13.1 acute toxicity tests; biocompatibility; intracutaneous injection; rabbits; test animals

[4] *U. S. Pharmacopeia*, Vol 23, Rand McNally, Taunton, MA, 1994, pp. 1699–1703.

[5] Brewer, John H., "Toxicity Standards for Plastics," Bulletin of Parenteral Drug Association, Vol 19, 1965, pp. 22–28.

[6] Materials Science Toxicology Laboratories, University of Tennessee Center for the Health Sciences, Memphis, Tenn., "Determination of Levels of Chemical Purity for Biomaterials Used as Surgical Implants," *Round Robin Evaluation of Primary Acute Toxicity Screening Protocols*, Quarterly Report No. 15–16, Part II, Contract No. FDA 223-73-5231, 1978.

Standard Practice for Evaluating Material Extracts by Systemic Injection in the Mouse[1]

This standard is issued under the fixed designation F 750; the number immediately following the designation indicates the year of original adoption or, in the case of revision, the year of last revision. A number in parentheses indicates the year of last reapproval. A superscript epsilon (ε) indicates an editorial change since the last revision or reapproval.

1. Scope

1.1 This practice covers a nonspecific, acute toxicity test used for detecting leachables from materials used in medical devices.

1.2 The liquids injected in the mouse are those obtained by Practice F 619 where the extraction vehicles are saline, vegetable oil, or other liquids simulating human body fluids.

1.3 Two procedures are outlined: Method A for intravenous injection and Method B for intraperitoneal injection.

1.4 This practice is one of several developed for the assessment of the biocompatibility of materials. Practice F 748 may provide guidance for the selection of appropriate methods for testing materials for a specific application.

2. Referenced Documents

2.1 *ASTM Standards:*

F 619 Practice for Extraction of Medical Plastics[2]

F 748 Practice for Selecting Generic Biological Test Methods for Materials and Devices[2]

3. Summary of Practice

3.1 The extract liquid is prepared in accordance with Practice F 619. The extraction vehicles are saline and vegetable oil, or other extraction vehicles, as described in Practice F 619. The extract liquid is injected into mice, and the animals are observed at regular intervals for 72 h for reactions, survival, etc.

4. Significance and Use

4.1 This practice is intended to help assess the biocompatibility of materials used in medical devices. It is an acute toxicological test designed to detect the presence of injurious leachable substances.

4.2 This practice may not be appropriate for all types of implant applications. The user is cautioned to consider the appropriateness of the method in view of the materials being tested, their potential applications, and the recommendations contained in Practice F 748.

4.3 The only limitation applicable is the extract preparation. Refer to Sections 4.3 and 4.4 of Practice F 619 for a description of this limitation.

5. Apparatus

5.1 *Mice*—The mice shall be albino-type, healthy and not previously used, and shall weigh between 17 and 23 g. Animal care shall be in accordance with the "Guide for Care and Use of Laboratory Animals."[3] Age, sex, and weight shall be recorded and reported. All the mice for each extraction vehicle shall be from the same source. For each extraction vehicle, a minimum of ten mice are used in the test. If the results of this first test group are inconclusive, then 20 more mice are needed to complete the test of one extraction vehicle for one plastic.

5.1.1 During the test the mice shall be fed normally with commercially available feed and tap water.

5.2 *Cages*—There shall be one cage for the five mice exposed to one extract liquid. Each mouse in a cage shall be uniquely identified, and this identification shall be recorded. Male and female mice are housed separately, and their cages are positioned in a manner which prevents the accidental transfer of feces or bedding from cage to cage.

5.3 *Syringe*—Sterile syringes, not greater than 3 mL in volume, with a precision of ± 0.10 mL shall be used.

5.3.1 *Method A*—Sterile needles of 25 to 27½ gage shall be used.

5.3.2 *Method B*—Sterile needles of 21 to 26 gage shall be used.

6. Sampling

6.1 Sample in accordance with Practice F 619.

7. Sample and Test Specimen

7.1 *General*—The sample is the plastic or other material exposed to the extraction procedure. As a result of the extraction in Practice F 619, for each extraction vehicle there are available: (*1*) a sample extract liquid, and (*2*) a blank extract liquid. These extract liquids are to be injected into the test animals within 24 h of the end of the extraction procedure. Record storage conditions if not used immediately after preparation.

---

[1] This practice is under the jurisdiction of ASTM Committee F-4 on Medical and Surgical Materials and Devices and is the direct responsibility of Subcommittee F04.16 on Biocompatibility Test Methods.

Current edition approved Sept. 25, 1987. Published November 1987. Originally published as F 750 – 82. Last previous edition F 750 – 82.

[2] *Annual Book of ASTM Standards*, Vol 13.01.

[3] U.S. Department of Health, Education, and Welfare, *Guide for Care and Use of Laboratory Animals*, Publication No. NIH 78-23, Bethesda, MD, 1978.

7.1.1 There are usually two extract liquids prepared from an extraction vehicle available for test. Samples based on other extraction vehicles may be available, as described in Practice F 619, or as required by the standard for the medical device.

7.2 *Method A, Intravenous*:

7.2.1 The extract liquid is prepared from a saline extraction vehicle. The dose of the extract liquid is 50 mL/kg of body weight for each mouse, injected at a steady rate of not more than 0.1 mL/s. If a hypotonic or hypertonic extract liquid is used, then the injection rate is adjusted proportionally.

7.2.2 Aqueous extract liquids shall be nominally isosmotic before injection. For example, sodium chloride may be added to distilled water extracts.

7.3 *Method B, Intraperitoneal*—The extract liquid is prepared from a vegetable oil extraction vehicle. The dose of the extract liquid is 50 mL/kg of body weight for each mouse.

8. Procedure

8.1 *Method A, Intravenous*:

8.1.1 Use saline, and similar extraction vehicles designated for intravenous injection.

8.1.2 Agitate each extract liquid vigorously prior to withdrawal of each injection dose to ensure even distribution of the extracted matter. If particulates are clearly present, then the extract liquids are injected by the intraperitoneal method. Optional: measure and record pH.

8.1.3 For each extraction vehicle, use ten mice, five for the sample extract liquid and five for the blank extract liquid. Weigh all mice, and record their weights. Use a system of marking to identify each individual mouse within each group of five.

8.1.4 Inject the predetermined amount (see 7.2.1) of the sample extract liquid into the tail vein of each of the five mice. Inject the blank extract liquid in the same way into five other mice. The use of warm water or a heat lamp may help dilate the tail veins for ease of injection.

8.1.5 Observe all animals immediately after injection, again 4 h after injection, and then not earlier than 24, 48, and 72 h, respectively, after injection for symptoms of slight, moderate, or marked toxicity or death (Table 1). Record the observations. Measure and record the body weights of all animals at 24, 48, and 72 h postinjection.

8.2 *Method B, Intraperitoneal*:

8.2.1 Method B is to be used with vegetable oil and similar extraction vehicles designated for intraperitoneal injection.

8.2.2 Agitate each extract liquid vigorously prior to withdrawal of each injection dose, to ensure even distribution of extracted matter. If the extract liquid contains particulates, record and report observations.

8.2.3 For each extraction vehicle use ten mice, five for the sample extract liquid and five for the blank extract liquid. Weigh all mice, and record their weight. Use a system of marking to identify each individual mouse within each group of five.

8.2.4 Inject the predetermined amount (see 7.3) of the sample extract liquid intraperitoneally into each of the five mice. Inject the blank extract liquid in the same way into five other mice.

8.2.5 Observe all animals immediately after injection, again 4 h after injection, and then not earlier than 24, 48, and 72 h, respectively, after injection for symptoms of slight, moderate, or marked toxicity or death (Table 1). Record the observations. Measure and record the body weights of all animals at 24, 48, and 72 h postinjection.

9. Interpretation of Results

9.1 If during the 72-h observation period none of the animals treated with the sample extract liquid shows a substantially greater biological reaction than the animals treated with the blank extract liquid, the sample meets the requirements of the test.

9.2 *Reaction*—If two or more animals show either marked symptoms of toxicity or die, then the sample does not meet the requirements of the test.

9.3 *Retest*—If any animals injected with the sample show slight signs of toxicity, and not more than one animal shows marked symptoms of toxicity or dies, repeat the test using groups of ten mice each. A substantial decrease in body weight for all animals in the group, even without other symptoms of toxicity, requires a retest using groups of ten mice each. In this

TABLE 1 Response to Systemic Injection Assay

Response	Description
Normal, no symptoms	Mouse exhibits no adverse physical symptoms after injection.
Slight	Mouse exhibits slight but noticeable symptoms of hypokinesia, dyspnea, or abdominal irritation after injection.
Moderate	Mouse exhibits definite evidence of abdominal irritation, dyspnea, hypokinesia, ptosis, or diarrhea after injection. (Weight usually drops to between 15 and 17 g.)
Marked	Mouse exhibits prostration, cyanosis, tremors, or severe symptoms of abdominal irritation, diarrhea, ptosis, or dyspnea after injection. (Extreme weight loss; weight usually less than 15 g.)
Dead, expired	Mouse dies after injection.

repeated test, the requirements of the test are met if none of the animals injected with the sample shows a substantially greater reaction than that observed in the animals injected with the blank.

9.4 A retest (see 9.3) requires that the extraction procedure be done a second time, since the extraction fluids must be used within 24 h of the end of the extraction.

10. Report

10.1 Describe the sample that was extracted, including, generic name, trade name, manufacturer's code, catalog number, date of manufacture, formulation, fabrication procedures or processes, etc., as appropriate. Describe the extraction vehicle and the conditions of the extraction (temperature and time).

10.2 Report the number of mice used, each mouse's weight, sex and age, and whether the mouse was exposed to the sample or blank extract.

10.3 Report whether a retest was necessary and if so, the reasons for the retest.

10.4 For each mouse used, including those used in a retest, report the clinical signs and the extract response: whether the reaction was none, slight, moderate, marked, or death. This applies to all mice, whether injected with the sample extract liquid or with the blank extract liquid.

11. Precision

11.1 *Precision*—Intralaboratory and interlaboratory reproducibility has not been systematically determined. Reproducibility may be inferred from previous round robin studies.[4,5]

12. Keywords

12.1 acute toxicity tests; biocompatibility; intravenous injection; mouse/mice; test animals

[4] Brewer, John H., "Toxicity Standards for Plastics," Bulletin Parenteral Drug Assn. Vol 19, 1965, pp. 22–28.

[5] Materials Science Toxicology Laboratories, University of Tennessee Center for the Health Sciences, Memphis, Tenn., "Determination of Levels of Chemical Purity for Biomaterials Used as Surgical Implants," Round Robin Evaluation of Primary Acute Toxicity Screening Protocols, Quarterly Report No. 15–16, Part II, Contract No. FDA 223-73-5231, 1978.

Designation: F 754 – 00

Standard Specification for Implantable Polytetrafluoroethylene (PTFE) Polymer Fabricated in Sheet, Tube, and Rod Shapes[1]

This standard is issued under the fixed designation F 754; the number immediately following the designation indicates the year of original adoption or, in the case of revision, the year of last revision. A number in parentheses indicates the year of last reapproval. A superscript epsilon (ε) indicates an editorial change since the last revision or reapproval.

1. Scope

1.1 This specification describes the performance of polytetrafluoroethylene (PTFE) fabricated in sheet, tube, and rod shapes which may be used for surgical implants. PTFE is a member of the generic class of perfluorocarbon (containing only the elements fluorine and carbon) polymers.

1.2 Perfluorocarbon high polymers are solids exhibiting extraordinary thermal and chemical stability. They do not require stabilizing additives of any kind.

1.3 The biological response to PTFE in soft tissue and bone has been well characterized by a history of clinical use and animal studies **(1-9)**.[2]

1.4 This specification does not apply to specific surgical implants. Such implants would be subject to appropriate end-use performance standards.

1.5 *This standard does not purport to address all of the safety concerns, if any, associated with its use. It is the responsibility of the user of this standard to establish appropriate safety and health practices and determine the applicability of regulatory limitations prior to use.*

2. Referenced Documents

2.1 *ASTM Standards:*

D 1457 Specification for PTFE Molding and Extrusion Materials[3]

D 1710 Specification for Polytetrafluoroethylene (PTFE) Basic Shapes, Rod, and Heavy–Walled Tubing[4]

D 1898 Practice for Sampling of Plastics[4]

D 3293 Specification for PTFE Resin Molded Sheet[5]

F 748 Practice for Selecting Generic Biological Test Methods for Materials and Devices[6]

F 749 Practice for Evaluating Material Extracts by Intracutaneous Injection in the Rabbit[6]

F 750 Practice for Evaluating Material Extracts by Systemic Injection in the Mouse[6]

F 813 Practice for Direct Contact Cell Culture Evaluation of Materials for Medical Devices[6]

F 895 Test Method for Agar Diffusion Cell Culture Screening for Cytotoxity[6]

F 981 Practice for Assessment of Compatibility of Biomaterials (Non-porous) for Surgical Implants with Respect to Effect of Materials on Muscle and Bone[6]

3. Significance and Use

3.1 Fabricated PTFE meeting the requirements of this specification will exhibit consistent and reproducible chemical, physical, and biological properties.

3.1.1 This specification ensures the absence of adulterants, additives, or processing aids.

3.1.2 This specification ensures the absence of extractable organic contaminants from fabricated configurations.

3.1.3 Fabricated configurations satisfying this specification should be compatible with tissue.

3.1.4 This specification addresses the characteristics of virgin raw molding powders obtained from resin manufacturers and used for producing implant configurations and of configurations packaged in either nonsterile or sterile states.

3.2 PTFE configurations were first used for implantation in the early 1950's and have served as compatible implants in large numbers of patients since that time with some implant durations beyond 20 years **(1)**. Reports of reaction to particulate debris of PTFE in load bearing applications outside of the pressure-velocity (PV) limits for the polymer **(10, 11)** have not been correlated with other biocompatibility assays for this polymer and clinical experience with molding powders or intact implants of this polymer **(1, 12)**. The shape and size of wear particles of this polymer and other implanted high polymers have been suggested as factors in elicited tissue reaction **(1, 11, 13)**. Therefore, care should be exercised not to construe this specification for applications where particulate debris may be anticipated.

4. Physical Property Requirements

4.1 *Molding and Extrusion Powders*:

4.1.1 *PTFE Polymer*— Molding and extrusion powders used for fabrication of implant configurations shall be virgin product which conform to Specification D 1457.

4.2 *PTFE Standard Shapes*:

---

[1] This specification is under the jurisdiction of ASTM Committee F-4 on Medical and Surgical Materials and Devicesand is the direct responsibility of Subcommittee F04.16 on Biocompatibility.

Current edition approved May 10, 2000. Published August 2000. Originally published as F 754 – 83. Last previous edition F 754 – 88 (95).

[2] The boldface numbers in parentheses refer to the list of references at the end of this specification.

[3] *Annual Book of ASTM Standards*, Vol 08.01.

[4] *Annual Book of ASTM Standards*, Vol 08.02.

[5] *Annual Book of ASTM Standards*, Vol 08.03.

[6] *Annual Book of ASTM Standards*, Vol 13.01.

4.2.1 Standard shapes such as molded sheet, rod, or tube shall have been prepared from virgin molding or extrusion materials which meet Specification D 1457.

4.2.2 PTFE molded sheet shall comply with Type I, Grade I, Class A requirements in Specification D 3293.

4.2.3 PTFE rod and tube shall comply with Type I, Grade I, Class D specifications in Specification D 1710. Material purchased for conversion into final implant shapes may meet Classes A, B, C, or D by vendor and vendee agreement.

4.3 *Surface Contamination*—The surface of a fabricated shape shall not contain particles of residue of diameter greater than 300 μm. The concentration of visible particles under 8× magnification shall not be greater than 10 particles per 400 cm^2.

4.4 Physical properties for other than standard shapes are not encompassed by this specification and must be addressed by appropriate performance standards for given configurations.

5. Chemical Property Requirements

5.1 *Carbon Tetrachloride Extraction*—PTFE sampled in accordance with Practice D 1898, from packaged-for-sale stock shall be extracted with carbon tetrachloride by the method described in Annex A1.

5.1.1 *Extractable Hydrocarbons*—The absence of extractable hydrocarbons shall be demonstrated by infrared analysis of the carbon tetrachloride extract using the methodology and acceptance criteria described in Annex A1.

5.1.2 *Appearance*—A sample should be obtained from packaged-for-sale stock and examined under daylight conditions with the naked eye immediately following carbon tetrachloride extraction as described in Annex A1. This sample while still wet with carbon tetrachloride shall not be apparently changed in size or consistency. When dried for 4 h in a 100°C air-circulating oven, the appearance of the extracted polymer sample shall be unchanged as compared to an unextracted specimen.

5.2 *Extraction with Distilled Water*—PTFE sampled from packaged-for-sale stock shall be extracted with distilled water by the methodology described in Annex A2.

5.2.1 *Extractable Electrolytes*—The resistivity of the water as measured by a resistivity conductivity meter shall be greater than 0.05 MΩ·cm.

5.2.2 *Appearance*—When examined by unaided vision in daylight, the appearance of PTFE sampled from stock immediately following water extraction shall be unchanged except for being obviously wet with water. When dried for 4 h at 100°C in an air-circulating oven the appearance shall be unchanged from pre-extraction appearance.

6. Biocompatibility

6.1 *Extractables Under Simulated and Accelerated In Vivo Exposure*—The polymer sampled from packaged-for-sale stock shall be tested under the general methodology and Practices F 749 and F 750 with specific conditions and criteria described in Annex A3.

6.2 *Acute Biocompatibility Requirements*—The polymer sampled from packaged-for-sale stock shall show no cytopathic effect when evaluated by a tissue culture test using direct contact of specimen with cell layer technique **(13, 14)** or ASTM Practice F 813 and Test Method F 895.

6.3 *Chronic Biocompatibility Requirements*—Vendor and vendee agreement may utilize the large, long-term and benign animal and clinical history of this generic class of polymer as equivalent to Practice F 748 and Practice F 981 certification.

7. Sterility

7.1 Fabricated configurations of PTFE are thermally stable to indefinite exposure at 200°C. The fabricated polymer shall, after sterilization, pass the USP Sterility Test **(15)**. Therefore, primary or repetitive sterilization by reliable steam autoclave technique is suggested. An alternative sterilization technique of using ethylene oxide may be adopted with due consideration for degassing rates for the particular specimen configuration. Sterilization by irradiation may cause molecular degradation of the polymer above certain radiation levels. Depending on the intended use of the implant, this molecular degradation could affect its mechanical and biocompatible properties.

8. Keywords

8.1 high polymer; polymer; polytetrafluoroethylene; PTFE; surgical implant

ANNEXES

(Mandatory Information)

A1. INFRARED ANALYSIS OF HYDROCARBONS EXTRACTABLE IN CARBON TETRACHLORIDE

A1.1 Stir at least 1 g of chopped sample, all of which passes a No. 40 mesh screen, for 30 min with 7-mL of reagent-grade carbon tetrachloride. When decanted, the carbon tetrachloride shall be clear and colorless.

A1.2 Perform infrared analysis with a Beckman Infrared Spectrophotometer IR-8, with Beckman Cell Part No. 580012, or equivalent.

A1.2.1 The requirements of this analysis shall be satisfied when transmission between 3 and 4 μm is essentially 100 % for the reagent grade control and at least 95% of that of the control scan for carbon tetrachloride in which the chopped sample was stored.

A2. EXTRACTION WITH WATER FOR ELECTROLYTES

A2.1 The specimens shall be cubes or rectangles with no edge dimension greater than 1 cm. The total specimen weight shall be 10 ± 1 g.

A2.2 Place the specimens in a suitable container, such as a100-cm^3 suction flask, along with 50 mL of distilled water. Store the flask 48 h at ambient temperature.

A2.3 After 48 h, decant the water. The water shall remain clear and colorless. The extractable electrolyte requirements shall be satisfied when the resistivity of the water is greater than 0.05 MΩ·cm.

A3. INFRARED ANALYSIS FOR ORGANIC SUBSTANCES EXTRACTABLE UNDER ACCELERATED, SIMULATED IN VIVO CONDITIONS (4)

A3.1 Use a total sample size of 150 squares each measuring 1 by 5 by 5 mm or a sample size having equivalent volume and surface area.

A3.2 *Extracting Media*—Prepare pseudo-extracellular fluid by dissolving 6.68 g of NaCl, 2.50 g of $NaHCO_3$, 0.174 g of K_2HPO_4, and 0.220 g of KCL in 1000 mL of distilled water.

A3.3 *Extraction Technique*—Place the sample in a monel metal screen cage and submerge in 250 mL of the extracting media. Conditions of extraction shall be 66 h at 96°C.

A3.4 *Infrared Analysis*—After extraction is complete, decant the pseudo-extracellular fluid. Its color shall be unchanged from pre-extraction. Extract the decanted liquid with 14 mL of reagent-grade carbon tetrachloride in a separatory funnel. Separate the carbon tetrachloride and dry with anhydrous $MgSO_4$. Compare a sample of the dried extractant sample with fresh reagent-grade carbon tetrachloride using an infrared spectrophotometer (Beckman IR-8 spectrophotometer or equivalent, Beckman Part No. 580012 cell, or equivalent). If hydrocarbons are present infrared absorption will occur between 3 and 4 μm.

A3.4.1 The requirements of this test shall be satisfied when transmission between 3 and 4 μm is essentially 100% for reagent-grade carbon tetrachloride and at least 95% of that for that of the control scan for the carbon tetrachloride extract.

APPENDIXES

(Nonmandatory Information)

X1. STATEMENT OF RATIONALE

X1.1 This specification was established to provide guidance in the testing of polytetrafluorethylene intended for use in medical device applications. It recommends test methods for the measurement of chemical, physical and mechanical properties of unfabricated and fabricated forms. Tests should be selected according to end-use applications. It is intended that biocompatibility be established on the finished product by the appropriate procedures, after it has gone through all processing steps.

X1.2 The scope section of this document defines the term "PTFE" and limits the specific scope of the document to fabricated sheet, tube, and rod shapes. It further makes clear that the specification does not apply to specific surgical implants that would be subject to appropriate specific end-use performance standards. This section emphasizes the extraordinary chemical and thermal stability and inherent absence of additives in PTFE; these factors are no doubt responsible for the large bibliography of successful implant use for this polymer in the absence of any previous implant grade specification guidance.

X1.3 The significance section sets out the capability of this standard by ensuring consistent and reproducible behavior. Section 3.2 explains the caution against construing this specification for applications where particulate debris may be anticipated.

X1.4 In 4.1 the specific raw polymer properties consistent with the scope and intent of this specification are defined in terms of existing ASTM specifications so that the raw polymers will be virgin products providing the highest purity available under current manufacturing technology. Similarly, 4.2 relates the finished shape physical properties consistent with the scope and objectives of this standard specification to existing ASTM specifications for such standard shapes. These requirements would provide the superior properties for such shapes available with current fabrication technology.

X1.5 Section 5 provides appearance and extractable criteria for PTFE-fabricated shapes sampled from packaged-for-sale stock to establish the absence of extractable organic or electrolytic contaminants that may have contaminated the product during its preparation and packaging. These tests would then signal the need for review of manufacturing protocol to determine where a breach may have occurred of the Good Manufacturing Practices regulations detailed in the U.S. Code of Federal Regulations.

X1.6 Section 6 prescribes specific biocompatibility assays that may be readily conducted on samples from packaged-for-sale stock to ensure biocompatibility. Although ASTM Practices F 749 and F 750 are the primary references for the evaluation of extractables under accelerated simulated in vivo exposure, more stringent test conditions are recommended in Annex A3 which the unique chemical and thermal stability and absence of additives of PTFE make feasible. These more stringent test conditions have provided assurance of safe and effective long-term in vivo implant performance for fabricated PTFE (**1, 12**).

X1.7 Finally, in Section 7 factors relating to mode of sterilization and reference to the USP sterility test protocols are described.

X2. Biocompatibility

X2.1 No known surgical implant material has ever been shown to be completely free of adverse reactions in the human body. However, long term clinical experience of use of specific compositions and formations of this material referred to in this standard has shown that an acceptable level of biological response can be expected, if the material is used in appropriate applications.

REFERENCES

(1) Homsy, C. A., "Biocompatibility of Perfluorinated Polymers and Composites of These Polymers," *Biocompatibility of Clinical Implant Materials*, O.F. Williams, ed., Chap. 3, Vol II, Boca Raton, FL, C.R.C. Press, Inc., 1982, pp 59–77.

(2) Calnan, J., "The Use of Inert Plastic Material in Reconstructive Surgery," *British Journal of Plastic Surgery*, Vol 16, 1963, p. 1.

(3) Homsy, C. A., and Anderson, M. S., "Functional Stabilization of Soft Tissue and Bone Prostheses with a Porous Low Modulus Materials System," *Biocompatibility of Implant Materials*, Williams, D. F., Ed., Sector Publishing, Ltd., Tunbridge Wells, 1976, Chapt. 10.

(4) Sullivan, B., Homsy, C. A., Woods, G. W., and Tullos, H. S., "Stabilization of Thompson Femoral Head Prosthesis with a Porous Stem Coating: A Case Report," *Clinical Orthopedics*, Vol 132, 1978, p. 136.

(5) Rice, R. M., Hegyeli, A. F., Gourlay, S. J., Wade, C. W. R., Dillon, J. G., Jaffe, H., and Kulkarni, R. K., "Biocompatibility Testing of Polymers: In Vitro Studies with In Vivo Correlation," *Journal of Biomedical Material Research*, Vol 12, 1978, p. 43.

(6) Gourlay, S. J., Rice, R. M., Hegyeli, A. F., Wade, C. W. R., Dillon, J. G., Jaffe, H., and Kulkarni, R. K., "Biocompatibility Testing of Polymers: In Vivo Implantation Studies," *Journal of Biomedical Materials Research*, Vol 12, 1978, p. 219.

(7) Harrison, J. H.," The Use of Teflon as a Blood Vessel Replacement in Experimental Animals," *Surgery, Gynecology, and Obstetrics*, Vol 104, 1975, p. 81.

(8) Friedenberg, Z. B., "Bone Growth into Teflon Sponge," *Surgery, Gynecology, and Obstetrics*, Vol 116, 1963, p. 588.

(9) U.S. Food and Drug Administration, Minutes of Panel Hearings, General and Plastic Surgery Devices Classification Panel, Washington, D.C., March 24, 1978.

(10) Charnley, J., "Factors in the Design of an Artificial Hip Joint, Lubrication and Wear in Living and Artificial Human Joints," *Proceedings of the Institute of Mechanical Engineers* , Vol 181, 1966–1967, pp. 104–111.

(11) Swanson, S. A. V., and Freeman, M. A. R., *The Scientific Basis of Joint Replacement*, John Wiley and Sons, New York, N.Y. 1977, pp. 46–85.

(12) Homsy, C. A., et al, "Rapid In-Vitro Screening of Polymers for Biocompatibility," *Journal of Macromolecular Science, Chemistry*, Vol , No. 3, 1970, pp. 615–634.

(13) Wilsnack, R. E., Meyer, F. J., and Smith, M. S., "Human Cell Culture Testing of Medical Devices and Correlation to Animal Tests," *Bio-materials, Medical and Artificial Organs* , Vol 1, 1973, pp. 543–562.

(14) Wilsnack, R. E., "Quantitative Cell Culture Biocompatibility Testing of Medical Devices and Correlation to Animal Tests," *Biomaterials, Medical Devices and Artificial Organs* , Vol 4, 1976, pp. 235–261.

(15) *U.S. Pharmacopeia,* Vol 21, 1985, pp. 1156–1160.

(16) Anderson, B. C., Barton, L. R., and Collette, J. W., Trends in Polymer Development, *Science*, 208,826, 1980.

Designation: F 755 – 99$^{\epsilon 1}$

Standard Specification for Selection of Porous Polyethylene for Use in Surgical Implants[1]

This standard is issued under the fixed designation F 755; the number immediately following the designation indicates the year of original adoption or, in the case of revision, the year of last revision. A number in parentheses indicates the year of last reapproval. A superscript epsilon (ϵ) indicates an editorial change since the last revision or reapproval.

ϵ[1] NOTE—Editorial corrections were made in 2.2 and 5.1 in May 2001.

1. Scope

1.1 This specification covers the properties and test methods for porous high density and ultra high molecular weight polyethylenes intended for use in surgical implants. The porous polyethylene may be used as a free standing product or as a coating on a substrate in nonloaded applications..

1.2 Evaluation of tissue response to a porous polyethylene must be completed. Guidance in establishing biocompatibility may be found in the list of references.

1.3 Clinical experience and animal studies have shown that tissue will grow into the open pores of porous polyethylene. The tissue ingrowth into the pores may allow for the establishment of implant fixation.

1.4 *This section does not purport to address all of the safety concerns, if any, associated with its use. It is the responsibility of the user of this standard to establish appropriate safety and health practices and determine the applicability of regulatory limitations prior to use.*

2. Referenced Documents

2.1 *ASTM Standards:*

D 638 Test Method for Tensile Properties of Plastics[2]

D 732 Test Method for Shear Strength of Plastics by Punch Tool[2]

D 790 Test Methods for Flexural Properties of Unreinforced and Reinforced Plastics and Electrical Insulating Materials[2]

D 883 Definitions of Terms Relating to Plastics[2]

D 1238 Test Method for Flow Rates of Thermoplastics by Extrusion Plastometer[2]

D 1505 Test Method for Density of Plastics by the Density-Gradient Technique[2]

D 1621 Test Method for Compressive Properties of Rigid Cellular Plastics[2]

D 1623 Test Method for Tensile and Tensile Adhesion Properties of Rigid Cellular Plastics[2]

D 1898 Practice for Sampling of Plastics[2]

D 2238 Test Methods for Absorbance of Polyethylene Due to Methyl Groups at 1378 cm^{-1} [2]

D 2873 Test Method for Interior Porosity of Poly(Vinyl Chloride) (PVC) Resins by Mercury Intrusion Porosimetry[3]

E 562 Practice for Determining Volume Fraction by Systematic Manual Point Count[4]

F 316 Test Method for Pore Size Characteristics of Membrane Filters for Use with Aerospace Fluids[5]

F 469 Practice for Assessment of Compatibility of Nonporous Polymeric Materials for Surgical Implants With Regard to Effect of Materials on Tissue[6]

F 648 Specification for Ultra-High-Molecular-Weight Polyethylene Powder and Fabricated Form for Surgical Implants[6]

F 748 Practice for Selecting Generic Biological Test Methods for Materials and Devices[6]

F 763 Practice for Short-Term Screening of Implant Materials[6]

F 981 Practice for Assessment of Compatibility of Biomaterials (Non-porous) for Surgical Implants with Respect to Effect of Materials on Muscle and Bone[6]

2.2 *Other Documents:*

Code of Federal Regulations Title 21, Paragraph 177.1520

U.S. Pharmacopeia, Vol 23, 1995

3. Significance and Use

3.1 Porous polyethylene is a matrix of substantially open cells, interconnected to form multidirectional paths. Performance of these structures, including tissue ingrowth, depends upon the biocompatibility of the polymer, average pore and interstitial opening diameters (ordinarily referred to as average pore size) in conjunction with void volume (referred to as pore volume or percent porosity).

3.2 This specification is applicable to all device standards in which a porous polyethylene is used. A complete list of end uses has not been established. In those cases where the use of

[1] This specification is under the jurisdiction of ASTM Committee F04 on Medical and Surgical Materials and Devices and is the direct responsibility of Subcommittee F04.11 on Polymeric Materials.

Current edition approved August 10, 1999. Published September 1999. Originally published as F 755 – 82. Last previous edition F 755 – 98.

[2] *Annual Book of ASTM Standards*, Vol 08.01.

[3] *Annual Book of ASTM Standards*, Vol 08.02.

[4] *Annual Book of ASTM Standards*, Vol 03.01.

[5] Discontinued—See *1995 Annual Book of Standards*, Vol 11.02.

[6] *Annual Book of ASTM Standards*, Vol 13.01.

a porous polyethylene has not been established, the mechanical and physical characteristics required shall be determined by proper testing. The pore size, pore volume, and the mechanical properties will be specified in the particular device standard.

4. Raw Material Requirements

4.1 The polyethylene plastic shall consist of basic polymers made with ethylene as essentially the sole monomer as defined in Terminology D 883.

4.2 High-density polyethylene shall exhibit a density of not less than 0.941 g/cm^3 when tested in accordance with Test Method D 1505.

4.3 Ultra-high-molecular-weight polyethylene shall conform to those sections of Specification F 648 that apply to base resin.

4.4 Particular raw materials shall contain no dirt or other foreign matter which will cause the end product to fail to meet the product requirement specified in 5.2.

4.5 The polyethylene resin shall conform to all parts of Paragraph 177.1520 of Title 21 which apply to polyethylene.

4.6 The polymer shall be characterized by determining the infrared absorption spectrum. An acceptable procedure may be found in Test Methods D 2238.

4.7 The polymer shall be characterized by one or more of the following test methods:

4.7.1 The polymer shall be characterized by determining the melt point range and rate of melt by thermal analysis.

4.7.2 The compositional characteristics of the polymer shall be analyzed by thermogravimetric analysis.

4.7.3 The flow rate of high density polyethylene shall be determined in accordance with Test Method D 1238.

5. Product Requirements

5.1 Until a porous polymer biocompatibility standard is available, porous polyethylene shall be screened by biocompatibility and toxicology tests applicable to its end use. Biological test procedures appropriate to determine biological safety and tissue reactions are described in Practices F 748 and F 981 and the United States Pharmacopeia which recommends generic biological test methods according to end use applications. Short term screening for implant materials are described in Practice F 763.

5.2 The surface of the porous polyethylene shall not contain particles of residue or loose particles of plastic of a diameter greater than 300 μm. The concentration of particles visible at 8× magnification shall not be greater than 10 particles/400 cm^2.

5.3 The level of extractables found in the porous product when tested in accordance with 4.5 shall not increase from that found in the raw material.

5.4 The porous product shall be inspected under 8× magnification to assure that the surface porosity is open.

5.5 The average pore size shall be specified by vendor-user agreement and shall be held to within 20% of the nominal value unless the end-use application requires less deviation.

5.6 Porous product quality and uniformity shall be assured by the appropriate test methods as specified by vendor-user agreement and listed in Section 6.

6. Test Methods

NOTE 1—The shape and end use of the porous product dictates which tests are appropriate. For example, it is impossible to perform a bubble point analysis on a total ossicular replacement, while mercury intrusion porosimetry is quite acceptable. A flexural test may be an acceptable nondestructive test where tensile strength tests are destructive.

6.1 All mechanical and physical tests shall be sampled as required in Practice D 1898.

6.2 Average pore size shall be established by appropriate test methods such as is found in Method F 316 or by mercury intrusion porosimetry. Test Method D 2873 is an acceptable method.

6.3 Average pore volume shall be established using one of the following methods:

6.3.1 Pore volume can be measured by mercury intrusion porosimetry. Test Method D 2873 is an acceptable method.

6.3.2 Pore volume can be approximated by measurement of weight of a nonsolvent saturant of known gravity and relating its volume to the matrix volume.

6.3.3 Pore volume can be estimated by optical microscopy as described in Practice E 562.

6.4 The tensile properties shall be determined in accordance with Test Method D 638. Test Method D 1623 may be used as an alternative method.

6.5 The compressive properties shall be determined in accordance with Test Method D 1621.

6.6 The flexural properties shall be determined in accordance with Test Methods D 790.

6.7 The shear properties shall be determined in accordance with Test Method D 732.

7. Certification

7.1 *Vendor of Porous Materials*:

7.1.1 Vendor shall certify that the raw material conforms to Section 4 of this specification.

7.1.2 Vendor shall certify that the porous polyethylene conforms to Section 5 of this specification and is made of the same raw material as has been characterized by Section 4.

7.1.3 Vendor shall certify that the mechanical properties as determined by 6.4-6.7 conform to the vendor-user agreement.

7.1.4 Porosity requirements as determined by 6.2 and 6.3 shall be certified by the vendor to conform to the vendor-user agreement.

7.1.5 Vendor shall specify in the certification report all test methods used.

NOTE 2—Certification is employed since verification would alter or destroy functionality.

8. Keywords

8.1 plastic surgical devices/applications; polyethylene (PE) plastics/surgical implant applications; polymers-surgical applicant

APPENDIXES

(Nonmandatory Information)

X1. RATIONALE

X1.1 The use of some solid polyethylenes in vivo has been well established. Because of their mechanical and physical properties, some porous polyethylenes have also shown considerable promise for many in vivo applications. The list of applications currently being investigated is quite lengthy but, even so, does not exhaust the possibilities. It is to be expected that as applications are developed the properties of the porous polyethylene which are acceptable for a given application will be uniquely specified. This will necessitate the writing of a standard for each end-use product.

X1.2 It is not the purpose of this generic standard to eliminate *a priori* any candidate porous polyethylene. For this reason, it is seen that in some respects the requirements for this are rather broad. The pore size and pore volumes are not specified since they will be a function of the end use and the type of tissue ingrowth desired. The same is true of the mechanical properties. The function of this specificiation is to specify those characteristics and tests to which a material is expected to conform to be used as a surgical implant and to be called porous polyethylene. To this end, the following five areas are addressed: (*1*) raw material requirements; (*2*) limits of impurities and extractables; (*3*) end product property test methods; (*4*) tissue response test methods; and (*5*) responsibilities of vendor certification.

X1.3 Porous polyethylenes which conform to this specification will be safe for selected applications and of a uniform high quality. Those properties which are critical to its being efficacious are the responsibility of an end-use product standard.

X2. BIOCOMPATIBILITY

X2.1 The material covered by this standard has been employed successfully in human implant applications in contact with soft tissue and bone for over a decade. Due to the well characterized level of biological response exhibited by this material, the ultra high molecular weight form (Practice F 648) has been used as a control material in Practice F 981

X2.2 No known surgical implant material has ever been shown to be completely free of adverse reactions in the human body. However, long-term clinical experience of use of this material referred to in this standard has shown that an acceptable level of biological response can be expected, if the material is used in appropriate applications.

Designation: F 756 – 00

Standard Practice for Assessment of Hemolytic Properties of Materials[1]

This standard is issued under the fixed designation F 756; the number immediately following the designation indicates the year of original adoption or, in the case of revision, the year of last revision. A number in parentheses indicates the year of last reapproval. A superscript epsilon (ε) indicates an editorial change since the last revision or reapproval.

1. Scope

1.1 This practice provides a protocol for the assessment of hemolytic properties of materials used in the fabrication of medical devices that will contact blood.

1.2 This practice is intended to evaluate the acute *in vitro* hemolytic properties of materials intended for use in contact with blood.

1.3 This practice consists of a protocol for a hemolysis test under static conditions with either an extract of the material or direct contact of the material with blood.

1.4 This practice is one of several developed for the assessment of the biocompatibility of materials. Practice F 748 may provide guidance for the selection of appropriate methods for testing materials for a specific application.

1.5 *This standard does not purport to address all of the safety concerns, if any, associated with its use. It is the responsibility of the user of this standard to establish appropriate safety and health practices and determine the applicability of regulatory limitations prior to use.*

1.6 *Identification of a supplier of materials or reagents is for the convenience of the user and does not imply single source. Appropriate materials and reagents may be obtained from many commercial supply houses.*

2. Referenced Documents

2.1 *ASTM Standards:*

F 619 Practice for Extraction of Medical Plastics[2]

F 748 Practice for Selecting Generic Biological Test Methods for Materials and Devices[2]

3. Terminology

3.1 *Definitions:*

3.1.1 *plasma hemoglobin*—the amount of hemoglobin in the plasma.

3.1.2 *% hemolysis*—the quotient of the free plasma hemoglobin (mg/ml) released as a result of contact with test material or extract divided by the total hemoglobin (mg/ml) present in the blood solution multiplied by 100. (This is synonymous with hemolytic index).

3.1.3 *comparative hemolysis*—comparison of the hemolytic index produced by a test material compared with that produced by a standard reference material such as polyethylene at the same test conditions.

3.1.4 *direct contact test*—a test for the hemolytic property performed with the test material in direct contact with the blood.

3.1.5 *extract test*—a test for the hemolytic property performed with an isotonic extract of the test material, as described in F 619, in contact with the blood.

3.1.6 *hemolysis*—destruction of erythrocytes resulting in the liberation of hemoglobin into the plasma or suspension medium.

3.1.7 *negative control*—a material, such as a polyethylene, that produces little or no hemolysis (<2 % after subtraction of the blank) in the test procedure. It is desirable that the control specimens have the same configuration as the test samples.

3.1.8 *positive control*—a material capable of consistently producing a hemolysis of at least 8 % after subtraction of the results of the blank. Suggested materials include, but are not limited to, BUNA N (Aero Rubber and other suppliers), and plastisol (Plasti-Coat, Watertown CT.).

3.1.9 *cyanmethemoglobin reagent*—a reagent to which whole blood, plasma, or test supernatant is added that quickly converts most of the forms of hemoglobin to the single cyanmethemoglobin form for quantification at its 540 nm spectrophotometric peak. The reagent (based on that by van Kampen and Zijlstra (**1**), pH 7.0-7.4), is made with 0.14 g potassium phosphate, 0.05 g potassium cyanide, 0.2 g potassium ferricyanide, and 0.5-1 ml of nonionic detergent diluted to 1 L with distilled water. The conversion time of this reagent is 3-5 minutes. This reagent is recommended by the National Commission for Clinical Laboratory Studies (NCCLS) and may be made from the chemicals or purchased from supply houses.

The first cyanmethemoglobin reagent used to measure total blood hemoglobin concentration was Drabkin's Reagent (1 g of sodium bicarbonate, 0.05g of potassium cyanide, 0.2 g of potassium ferricyanide and diluted with distilled water to 1 L). The disadvantages of using the Drabkin's reagent versus the NCCLS cyanmethemoglobin reagent are that it has a conversion time of 15 minutes, and pH of 8.6 which may cause

---

[1] This practice is under the jurisdiction of ASTM Committee F-4 on Medical and Surgical Materials and Devices and is the direct responsibility of Subcommittee F04.16 on Biocompatibility.

Current edition approved July 10, 2000. Published October 2000. Originally published as F 756 – 82. Last previous edition F 756 – 93.

[2] *Annual Book of ASTM Standards*, Vol 13.01.

turbidity. However, it is still available as individual chemicals or kits such as Sigma 525-A.

The Drabkin's and cyanmethemoglobin reagents were developed to quantify the high hemoglobin concentration normally found in whole blood (e.g. 15,000 mg/dl). By modifying the sample dilution volumes and accounting for background interference, these reagents can also be used to measure much lower plasma or supenatant hemoglobin concentrations as well (Moore et al, Malinauskas **(2)**, **(3)**).

3.1.10 *PBS*—phosphate buffered saline (Ca and Mg free). The use of phosphate buffered saline is preferable to the use of saline in order to maintain the pH. The use of magnesium and calcium free PBS is necessary to maintain the anticoagulant properties of the chelating agents used in collecting the blood. It is used as the background or "blank" for a hemolysis test.

3.1.11 *A*—absorbance value of cyanmethemoglobin reaction product measured at 540 nm.

3.1.12 *F*—slope of the hemoglobin curve. The units are [(mg/ml)/A] such that multiplication by an absorbance value yields a hemoglobin concentration. Implicit assumption: The y-intercept of the hemoglobin calibration curve is approximately zero and its effect on converting absorbance values to concentration values is negligible.

3.1.13 *PFH*—plasma free hemoglobin concentration.

3.1.14 *C*—total blood hemoglobin concentration.

3.1.15 *T*—diluted blood hemoglobin concentration.

3.1.16 *B*—blank (i.e. no material added to this tube, only the isotonic medium).

3.1.17 *S*—sample (i.e. test material sample, or negative and positive control sample).

4. Summary of Practice

4.1 Test and control material specimens or extracts are exposed to contact with rabbit blood under defined static conditions and the increase in released hemoglobin is measured. Comparisons are made with the control and test specimens tested under identical conditions.

5. Significance and Use

5.1 The presence of hemolytic material in contact with the blood may cause loss of, or damage to, red blood cells and may produce increased levels of free plasma hemoglobin capable of inducing toxic effects or other effects which may stress the kidneys or other organs.

5.2 This practice may not be predictive of events occurring during all types of implant applications. The user is cautioned to consider the appropriateness of the method in view of the materials being tested, their potential applications, and the recommendations contained in Practice F 748.

6. Preparation of Test and Control Specimens

6.1 Specimens with a determinable surface area will be used at a ratio of 3 cm^2 surface area to 1 ml of test blood solution. For irregular materials or powders, a weight of 0.2 to 0.5 g per ml of liquid will be used. A minimum of 6 of each positive and negative control and each test sample should be prepared to be used in the direct contact test and the test with the extract.

6.2 The final sample should be prepared with a surface finish consistent with end-use application.

6.3 The sample shall be sterilized by the method to be employed for the final product.

6.4 Care should be taken that the specimens do not become contaminated during preparation but aseptic technique is not required.

7. Hemoglobin Determination (Direct Method)

7.1 Prepare a hemoglobin calibration curve consistent with the specifications of the International Committee for Standardization in Hematology (ICSH). For hemoglobin standardization use reference standards such as the Sigma Hemoglobin Reference Standard No 525 or equivalent and the suggested reagent diluent. The spectrophotometer used should be high resolution and provide at least 3 decimal places.

7.2 Prepare a standard curve from stock hemoglobin in 8 dilutions to accommodate the range of 1.4 to 0.03 mg/ml (140-3 mg/dl). The cyanmethemoglobin reagent diluent serves as a zero blank in the spectrophotometer. Measure the absorbance at 540 nm. Plot a calibration curve from these values using mg/ml Hb on the y axis and A_{540} on the x-axis. The calibration coefficient (F) is the slope of this plot. The y-intercept should be approximately zero.

NOTE 1—If local restrictions or other problems contraindicate use of these cyanmethemoglobin reagents, then another method for measuring total blood hemoglobin concentration, plasma free hemoglobin concentration, and supernatant hemoglobin concentration may be substituted provided that it is validated and shown to be substantially equivalent to the cyanmethemoglobin method. Methods which quantify oxyhemoglobin alone may not be appropriate since some materials can convert oxyhemoglobin to other forms or alter the absorbance spectrum. Investigators should be aware that their results of determining supernatant hemoglobin concentration may be compromised by absorption of hemoglobin by the test materials, precipitation of hemoglobin out of solution, or alteration of the spectrophotometric absorbance spectrum by material leachables.

8. Collection and Preparation of Blood Substrates

8.1 Obtain anti-coagulated rabbit blood from at least 3 donors for each test day. The preferred anticoagulant is citrate (0.13 M). Approximately 5 ml should be drawn from each rabbit. Store the blood at 4 ± 2° C and preferably use within 48 h. Blood may be used up to 96 h after collection if the plasma free hemoglobin is not excessive. Equal quantities of blood from each rabbit should be pooled.

8.2 Do not wash cells; use them suspended in the original plasma.

8.3 *Determination of Plasma Free Hemoglobin (PFH)*:

8.3.1 Centrifuge a 3-ml sample of the pooled blood at 700-800 G in a standard clinical centrifuge for 15 min.

8.3.2 Add 0.5 ml of plasma to 0.5 ml of cyanmethemoglobin solution or validated diluent.

8.3.3 Read the absorbance of the resulting solution at 540 nm. Obtain the concentration from the standard curve. Multiply by 2 to obtain, and record, the total plasma free hemoglobin concentration (PFH), although it has not been corrected for the plasma background interference. Plasma free hemoglobin (mg/ml):

$$PFH = A^{PFH} * F * 2 \quad (1)$$

8.3.4 Proceed with the testing if the value of the PFH is less than 2 mg/ml. If the PFH is 2mg/ml or greater this sample should be discarded and another blood sample should be obtained.

8.4 *Determination of Total Blood Hemoglobin Concentration*:

8.4.1 Add 20 μL of well-mixed pooled whole blood specimen to 5.0 ml of cyanmethemoglobin solution or validated diluent.

8.4.2 Allow the resulting solution to stand 15 minutes for Drabkins or 5 min for cyanmethemoglobin reagent and then read the absorbance of the solution with a spectrophotometer at a wavelength of 540 nm.

8.4.3 Determine blood hemoglobin concentration from the standard curve and multiply by 251 to account for dilution. This should be performed in duplicate. Total blood hemoglobin concentration:

$$C = A^{C} * F * 251 \quad (2)$$

8.4.4 Adjust the total hemoglobin content of the blood sample to 10 mg/ml ± 1 mg/ml by diluting with an appropriate amount of calcium and magnesium free PBS. Verify the hemoglobin concentration by repeating 8.4.1-8.4.3 in triplicate but using 400 μl of the diluted blood to 5 ml of reagent to remain on the standard curve. This is a dilution factor of 13.5.

$$T = A^{T} * F * 13.5 \quad (3)$$

9. Procedure for the Test

9.1 *Extract*:

9.1.1 Prepare an extract of each of 3 replicate samples of each test, positive control, negative control material, and PBS blank according to Practice F 619 using the appropriate ratio of material to extractant. (The extractant is Mg Ca free PBS). A sample of 30 cm^2 surface area or 2-5 gram is recommended for use in 10 ml of extractant.

9.1.2 Use the highest temperature conditions of Practice F 619 that the material will withstand.

NOTE 2—If the extraction is done at 121° C, borosilicate tubes must be used and any volume lost should be noted. At lower temperatures either polystyrene or glass tubes may be used.

9.1.3 Transfer 7 ml of the resultant extract of each sample into individual screw capped test tubes of borosilicate glass or polystyrene approximately 16 x 125 or 16 x 150 mm.

9.1.4 Using an appropriate blank to zero the spectrophotometer, the absorbance of the extracts should be checked for background interference which could affect the supernatant hemoglobin concentration calculation.

9.2 *Direct Contact*:

9.2.1 Samples are cut into appropriate pieces. Transfer each of 3 nonextracted samples of test and control specimens into individual tubes as described in 9.1.3. For samples with a determinable surface area, the surface area should be 21 cm^2 or 1.4 to 3.5 g if the specimen is irregular or a powder. The recommended tube size is 16 x 125 mm. However the tube size may be any such that the specimen is covered by 7 ml of PBS liquid. Place 7 ml of PBS into each tube containing the nonextracted sample. Place 7 ml of PBS into each of 3 tubes to serve as the blank.

9.3 *Test*—Add 1 ml of blood prepared in 8.4.4 to each tube containing extract, each tube containing a specimen, and the blanks. Cap all tubes.

NOTE 3—This procedure calls for preparing the sample, adding the diluent to the sample and then adding the blood which minimizes the time difference for contact of sample with blood. Alternatively, the blood may be added to the diluent and then the sample added to the prepared solution. Whichever method is chosen must be used for the controls as well as the test specimens.

9.4 Maintain tubes in a suitable test tube rack for at least 3 h at 37° ± 2 C in a water bath. Gently invert each tube twice approximately every 30 min to maintain contact of the blood and material. In some cases of samples with complicated configurations, it may be necessary to do more inversions to adequately mix the sample.

9.5 At the end of the specified incubation time, transfer the fluid to a suitable tube and centrifuge at 700-800 G for 15 min in a standard clinical centrifuge.

9.6 Remove the supernatant carefully to avoid disturbing any button of erythrocytes which may be present. Place the supernatant into a second screw cap tube. Record the presence of any color to the supernatant and any precipitate.

9.7 Analyze the samples from 9.6 for supernatant hemoglobin concentration using the method in 9.8.

9.8 *Supernatant Hemoglobin Determination*:

9.8.1 Add 1.0 ml of supernatant to 1.0 ml of cyanmethemoglobin reagent, or validated diluent.

9.8.2 Allow the sample to stand for 15 min for Drabkin's or 3-5 min for cyanmethemoglobin reagent. Read the absorbance of the solution with a spectrophotometer at a wavelength of 540 nm.

9.8.3 In the unlikely event that A_{540} exceeds 2, dilute the 1 ml of the supernatant with 3 ml of diluent and repeat 9.8.

9.8.3.1 Determine the hemoglobin concentration in each supernatant from 9.8 using the calibration curve.

9.8.3.2 Multiply the results from 9.8.2 by 2 (or the results from 9.8.3 by 4) to correct for the dilution. Hemoglobin concentration of supernatant from test sample or control tubes:

$$S = A^{S} * F * 2 \quad (4)$$

Hemoglobin concentration of the blank tube:

$$B = A^{B} * F * 2 \quad (5)$$

9.8.3.3 Calculate the % hemolysis or hemolytic index as:

$$\%\ hemolysis = \frac{Concentration\ of\ hemoglobin\ released\ in\ supernatant * 100\%}{Total\ hemoglobin\ concentration\ in\ Tube} \quad (6)$$

(To account for the dilution factor introduced by putting 1 ml of diluted blood into each tube that contains 7 ml of isotonic solution, the total hemoglobin concentration in each tube (W) is defined as W = T/8). Then,

$$\%\ hemolysis = \frac{S}{W} * 100\% \quad (7)$$

In the above equation, the "total Hemoglobin in Tube" is calculated by dividing the total blood hemoglobin concentration obtained in 8.4.4 by 8 to account for the blood dilution in PBS in the test tubes. Use of this equation assumes that background interference from endogenous plasma and free hemoglobin, and from the extracts, is negligible. This assumption can be verified by measuring the supernatant absorbance of the extract solutions and of blood diluted in a test tube containing 7 ml of PBS and 1 ml of diluted blood (10 mg/ml) which has been incubated along with the test sample tubes.

9.8.3.4 % hemolysis corrected for the blank:

$$\textit{Blank corrected \% hemolysis} = \frac{(A^S*F*2)-(A^B*F*2)}{(A^T*F*13.5/8)-(A^B*F*2)}*100\% \quad (8)$$

The final equation can then be simplified:

$$\textit{Blank corrected \% hemolysis} = \frac{A^S—A^B}{(0.844)A^T—A^B}*100\% \quad (9)$$

10. Report

10.1 Express results in the form of the corrected % hemolysis index as described in 9.8.3.4.

10.2 The final report, as a minimum shall include the following:

10.2.1 Detailed sample and control preparations including generic or chemical names, catalog number, lot or batch number, and other pertinent available designations or descriptions.

10.2.2 Detailed sample and control preparations, including sample size, thickness, configuration of test specimens, and method of sterilization.

10.2.3 Age of blood and type and concentration of anticoagulant used.

10.2.4 Method of hemoglobin determination.

10.2.5 Tabulation of total supernatant hemoglobin levels.

10.2.6 % Hemolysis for the test samples, the negative controls, the positive controls, and the blanks. Include mean and standard deviation for each of the replicate samples, blanks, and positive and negative controls.

10.2.7 Other pertinent observations of the experiment.

10.3 *Conversion of % Hemolysis for reporting purposes*—This practice provides a method for determining the propensity of a material to cause hemolysis. Pass/fail criteria for the material are subject to consideration of the nature of the tissue contact, duration of contact, and surface area to body ratios, and the nature of the device. Historically a hemolytic grade had been assigned. However, the hemolytic grade is an arbitrarily derived scale, has not been validated, and is based on previous results using a slightly different procedure. If the assignment of a hemolytic grade is required, the following are suggested: The mean hemolytic index of the blank should be subtracted from the mean hemolytic index of the controls and the test samples. The results of the test sample should be compared to the results of the negative control.

Hemolytic Index above the negative control	Hemolytic Grade
0–2	nonhemolytic
2–5	slightly hemolytic
>5	hemolytic

In addition, if the mean from the replicate test samples is less than 5 but one or more samples gave a hemolytic index of greater than 5, then the test should be repeated with double the number of test articles.

11. Precision and Bias

11.1 *Precision*—The precision of this test method is being established. Although this method has been shown to have intralaboratory repeatability, especially with regards to classification of hemolytic response, interlaboratory variation is still significant.

11.2 *Bias*—The bias of this test method includes the quantitative estimates of the uncertainties of the calibration of the test equipment and the skill of the operators. At this time, statements of bias should be limited to the documented performance of particular laboratories.

12. Keywords

12.1 biocompatibility; blood compatibility; direct contact; extract; hemoglobin; hemolysis testing

APPENDIX

(Nonmandatory Information)

X1. RATIONALE

X1.1 The presence of hemolytic material in contact with blood may produce increased levels of blood cell lysis and increased levels of plasma hemoglobin. This may induce toxic effects or other effects which may stress the kidneys or other organs.

X1.2 This practice is presented as a screening procedure for comparing the hemolytic potential of a material with that of a negative control material which is generally acknowledged to be appropriate for blood contact applications. Materials with a hemolytic potential above that of the specified negative control material, which is known to have excellent performance in blood contacting situations, should be carefully considered for use since they may or may not be a potential cause of *in vivo* hemolysis.

X1.3 The procedure as presented is intended as a routine reproducible screening procedure. It is not to be represented as being the most sensitive nor the most specific procedure for assessing the hemolytic potential of all materials in all use applications. The results obtained with this procedure are intended to be used in conjunction with the results of other tests in assessing the blood compatibility of the test material.

REFERENCES

(1) International Committee for Standardization in Haematology. J Clin. Pathol, 1978, 31: 139-143, 1978.

(2) Moore GL, Ledford ME, Merydith A., A micromodification of the Drabkin hemoglobin assay for measuring plasma hemoglobin in the range of 5 to 2000 mg/dl. Biochem. Med. 1981; 26:167-173.

(3) Malinauskas, RA., Plasma hemoglobin measurement techniques for the in vitro evaluation of blood damage caused by medical devices. Artificial Organs 1997; 21:1255-1267.

Standard Practice for Short-Term Screening of Implant Materials[1]

This standard is issued under the fixed designation F 763; the number immediately following the designation indicates the year of original adoption or, in the case of revision, the year of last revision. A number in parentheses indicates the year of last reapproval. A superscript epsilon (ϵ) indicates an editorial change since the last revision or reapproval.

1. Scope

1.1 This practice provides guidelines for short-term testing or screening of candidate materials, both porous and dense, as to the effects of the material on animal tissue in which it is implanted. This is a rapid screening prodedure for determining acceptability of candidate materials.

1.2 This practice, along with other appropriate biological tests (including other appropriate ASTM tests) may be used in the biocompatibility assessment of the candidate materials for use in the fabrication of devices for clinical application.

1.3 This experimental protocol is not designed to provide a comprehensive assessment of the systemic toxicity, carcinogenicity, teratogenicity, or mutagenicity of the material since other standards deal with these issues.

1.4 This practice is one of several developed for the assessment of the biocompatibility of materials. Practice F 748 provides guidance for the selection of appropriate methods for testing materials for a specific application.

2. Referenced Documents

2.1 *ASTM Standards:*

F 75 Specification for Cast Cobalt-Chromium Molybdenum Alloy for Surgical Implant Applications[2]

F 86 Practice for Surface Preparation and Marking of Metallic Surgical Implants[2]

F 90 Specification for Wrought Cobalt-Chromium-Tungsten-Nickel Alloy for Surgical Implant Applications[2]

F 136 Specification for Wrought Titanium- 6 Aluminum–4 Vanadium 4V ELI (Extra Low Interstiitial) Alloy (UNS R56401) for Surgical Implant Applications[2]

F 138 Specification for Wrought 18 Chromium–14 Nickel–2.5 Molybdenum Stainless Steel Bar and Wire for Surgical Implants (UNS S31673)[2]

F 562 Specification for Wrought Cobalt-35 Nickel-20 Chromium-10 Molybdenum Alloy for Surgical Implant Applications[2]

F 563 Specification for Wrought Cobalt-Nickel-Chromium-Molybdenum-Tungsten-Iron Alloy for Surgical Implant Applications[2]

F 603 Specification for High-Purity Dense Aluminum Oxide for Surgical Implant Application[2]

F 648 Specification for Ultra-High-Molecular-Weight Polyethlene Powder and Fabricated Form for Surgical Implants[2]

F 748 Practice for Selecting Generic Biological Test Methods for Materials and Devices[2]

F 981 Practice for Assessment of Compatibility of Biomaterials for Surgical Implants with Respect to Effect of Materials on Muscle and Bone[2]

3. Terminology

3.1 *Description of a Term Specific to this Standard:*

3.1.1 *biocompatibility assay*—a comparison of the tissue response produced through the close association of the implanted candidate material to its implant site within the host animal to that tissue response recognized and established as suitable with control materials.

4. Summary of Practice

4.1 Under aseptic conditions, test specimens of the candidate material and of controls are inserted into a muscle or group of muscles of the animal host. After a period of time the animals are euthanized. The tissue reactions to implants of the candidate material during the acute to subchronic time period of healing are compared with tissue reactions to control materials which have a well characterized response. The implants are not subject to major stress while *in situ.*

5. Significance and Use

5.1 The use of *in vivo* implantation techniques for characterizing the biocompatibility of materials to be utilized in various medical applications provides a unique assessment of such materials not achieved by other procedures. Physical characteristics (that is, form, density, hardness, surface finish) can influence the character of the tissue response to the test materials.

5.2 This practice is intended as a rapid screening procedure for determining the acceptability of candidate materials. It would be invoked prior to using the long-term tests described in Practice F 981. It is understood that for some applications additional tests, including long-term implantation studies, may be required to assess the final suitability of the candidate materials.

5.3 This practice may not be appropriate for all types of

[1] This practice is under the jurisdiction of ASTM Committee F-4 on Medical and Surgical Materials and Devicesand is the direct responsibility of Subcommittee F04.16 on Biocompatibility.

Current edition approved May 10, 1999. Published August 1999. Originally published as F 763 – 82. Last previous edition F 763 – 87(1993)ϵ1.

[2] *Annual Book of ASTM Standards,* Vol 13.01.

implant applications. The user is cautioned to consider the appropriateness of the method in view of the materials being tested, their potential applications, and the recommendations contained in Practice F 748.

6. Test Preparation

6.1 Rabbits, rats, or other animals may be used as test hosts. The following procedure is written for New Zealand white rabbits, a commonly used test host but the procedure can be adapted with few alterations to other test hosts.

6.2 *Test Hosts and Sites*:

6.2.1 Choose healthy adult rabbits that weigh more than 2.5 kg and whose paravertebral muscles are sufficiently large to allow for implantation of the test specimens.

6.2.2 The paravertebral muscle shall serve as the test site for implants. (The gluteal muscles of rats have been used as test sites by some investigators.)

6.2.3 *Preparation of Rabbits*—On the day of the implantation or up to 20 h before implantation, clip the fur of the animals on both sides of the spinal column. Remove loose hair.

6.3 *Selection of Control Materials*:

6.3.1 Selection of control material(s) should be based on their prior acceptable use in medical applications similar to those proposed for the candidate test material and is not restricted to those listed in 6.3.2.

6.3.2 Metallic control materials, which have been demonstrated to elicit minimal tissue reactions, are the metal alloys, such as in Specifications F 75, F 90, F 136, F 138, F 562, or F 563, or a ceramic, such as, alumina F 603. A suitable polymeric control material is found in polyethylene Specification F 648.

NOTE 1—There are times when use of a positive control can help to clarify the character of the tissue response to the candidate test sample.

6.3.3 If the most appropriate control material is expected to elicit a tissue response greater than that normally observed with Negative Control Plastic or the alloys cited above, samples of these latter materials may be implanted as controls on the surgical technique.

7. Test Specimens

7.1 *Fabrication*—Each implant shall be fabricated, finished, and its surface cleaned in a manner appropriate for its projected application in humans. Dense metal implants should be finished in accordance with Practice F 86. The size, shape, and surface of test and control implants shall be as similar as is practically possible.

7.2 Implant sizes are left to the discretion of the investigator. Implants in the size range 1 by 10 mm (0.04 by 0.4 in.) to 3.2 by 12 mm (0.125 by 0.5 in.) have often been used. They may be of circular or square cross section. The edges of the specimens should be as smooth as possible to avoid additional mechanical trauma upon implantation.

7.3 *Implantation Period*:

7.3.1 The insertion of all implants into any one animal shall be done at the same surgical session.

7.3.2 Implant evaluation should be performed at 7 and 30 d so that an accurate characterization of both the test and control materials can be made during the acute and subchronic stages of the healing tissue response. Three animals will be used for each sample period, that is, 3 at 7 d, and 3 at 30 d.

NOTE 2—Some investigators have found that extending the test to include a third group of animals maintained for 90 d can provide additional data on the host response to the implant material.[3]

8. Procedure

8.1 *Implantation*:

8.1.1 The recommended method of implantation is by hypodermic needle or tube and trochar. For larger diameter samples, an incision of appropriate size will be required to permit passage of the larger diameter tube. If this technique is not convenient, however, other equivalent implantation techniques judged appropriate may be used. These should be reported as in 9.1. The implantation must be done using aseptic procedures.

8.1.2 *Preparation of Test Specimens*—The specimens should be fabricated as described in 7.1 and prepared for implantation following the procedure in either 8.1.2.1 or 8.1.2.2.

8.1.2.1 Sterilize each specimen as appropriate for final application and, using aseptic technique, insert it into a sterile needle or tube; or,

8.1.2.2 Insert the specimen into a needle or tube, protect the ends with an appropriate cover, and sterilize the assemblies in an appropriate manner.

NOTE 3—Allow for proper degassing if sterilizing agents such as ethylene oxide are used.

NOTE 4—If the materials to be tested are harder than the materials from which the handling instruments are made, there is the danger of surface contamination of the test specimens by wear from the instruments which can disturb the results (for example, ceramic test specimens implanted with metal instruments). If such test specimens must be handled, soft textile or plastic should be used between the implants and the instruments. Of course, care must be taken that none of these auxiliary protecting materials remain in the implantation wound.

8.1.3 The animals should be anesthetized with a commonly used anesthetic agent to a degree deep enough to prevent muscular movement, such as twitching. Properly scrub the clipped skin surface of the animal.

8.1.4 Implant four specimens of the sample into the paravertebral muscle on one side of the spine of each rabbit, about 2.5 cm from the mid-line and parallel to the spinal columns, and about 2.5 cm apart from each other. In a similar fashion, implant four specimens of the control material in the corresponding muscle on the opposite side of the spine of each animal.

8.1.5 In cases where the negative control is other than specified in 6.3.2 and may be expected to elicit more than a minimal response, use only two test specimens of this negative control. Implant these two control specimens in a location that will not interfere with the test samples.

8.1.6 When using a sterile needle for insertion, insert a sterile stylet into the needle to hold the test specimen in the tissue while withdrawing the needle. With trocar implantation,

[3] Turner, E., Lawrence, W. H., and Autian, J., "Subacute Toxicity Testing of Biomaterials Using Histopathological Evaluation of Rabbit Muscle Tissue," Journal of Biomedical Materials Research, Vol 7, 1973, pp. 39–58.

insert the test specimen after withdrawing the central point and use a stylet to hold the sample while withdrawing the cannula.

8.1.7 If excessive bleeding is observed after implantation of a test specimen, place a duplicate test specimen at another site. Close the incision after implantation is complete, if applicable. If a test host other than the rabbit is chosen, use as many animals as are necessary to permit the implantation of 12 test specimens and 12 controls for each sacrifice interval.

8.2 *Postoperative Care*:

8.2.1 All animal studies must be done, in a facility approved by a nationally-recognized organization and in accordance with all appropriate regulations.

8.2.2 Carefully observe each animal during the period of assay and report any abnormal findings.

8.2.3 If an animal dies prior to the expected date of sacrifice, perform a necropsy to determine the cause of death. Include the animal in the assay of data if the cause of death is related to the procedure or test material.

8.2.4 A successful test is one in which eight test specimens and eight controls for each test period are available for histologic evaluation.

8.2.5 Should infection or injury of the test implant site invalidate the results, replace the animal with another if necessary as described in 8.2.4.

8.3 *Sacrifice and Implant Retrieval*:

8.3.1 Sacrifice animals at the intervals suggested in 7.3.2.

8.3.2 At sacrifice, record any gross abnormalities of color or consistency observed in the tissue surrounding the implant. Documentation of findings using photography for a permanent record is highly recommended.

8.4 *Gross Observations, Acute Test (7-d)*:

8.4.1 Macroscopically examine the area of the tissue surrounding the center portion of each implanted test specimen. Use a magnifying glass, if necessary.

8.4.2 The requirements of the test are met if, in each rabbit, the reaction to three of four sample test specimens is not significantly greater than that of the reaction to the corresponding negative control. In situations in which two types of negative controls are included, these criteria apply to the tissue surrounding specimens of the minimally reactive material.

8.5 *Histopathological Observation, Acute Test (7–d) and Subchronic Test (30 d)*:

8.5.1 *Tissue Sample Preparation*—

8.5.1.1 Remove each implant with an intact envelope of surrounding tissue. The tissue sample should include a 4-mm thick layer of tissue surrounding the implants. If less than 4 mm of tissue is removed, report in accordance with 9.1. Process the excised tissue block containing either a test implant or control implant for histopathological and such other studies as are appropriate. Cut the tissue sample into appropriate specimens for each study. Record the gross appearance of the implant and the tissue immediately adjacent to the implant as to consistency and color, as seen by the naked eye, and with a hand lens or stereomicroscope (see 9.2).

8.5.1.2 If possible, process the specimen with the implant in place. This allows easy identification of the implant site and minimizes distortion during fixation. After fixation, the implant material can be removed if necessary, and the tissue specimens processed for sectioning using standard laboratory practice for embedding and staining. If an implant is removed from its tissue bed, report the amount of tissue removed with the implant as required in 9.1.

8.5.1.3 Histological sections can be prepared using conventional microtomy section, or grinding of plastic embedded specimens as appropriate.

8.5.1.4 For porous implant materials, the quality and quantity of tissue ingrowth may also be examined using the appropriate prepared sections.

8.5.2 *Histopathological Schedule*:

8.5.2.1 Process at least two tissue microscope slides from each sample of control and test implant, including the tissue envelope surrounding the implant so as to obtain adequate histopathological assessment of tissue reaction.

8.5.2.2 If special stains are deemed necessary, prepare additional sections, and make appropriate observations.

8.5.3 *Histopathological Observations*—Compare the amount of tissue reaction adjacent to the test implant to that adjacent to a similar location on the control implant as regards thickness of scar, presence of inflammatory or other cell types not normally present at the site, presence of particles, and any other indications of an interaction between tissue and material. The use of a scoring system similar to that in Practice F 981 is highly recommended. Report in accordance with 9.3.

9. Report

9.1 A report shall be made to include all details of implant characterization and size, fabrication, conditioning, (including cleaning, handling, and sterilization techniques employed), and procedures for implantation and implant retrieval. The control material characteristics of chemical composition, mechanical and thermal condition, and finish should be reported. Also details of any special procedure (such as unusual or unique diet fed to test animals) shall be included in the report.

9.2 A report shall be made to include the observations of each control and test implant at each time interval, as well as the gross appearance of the surrounding tissue in which the implants were implanted.

9.3 A report shall be made on the observation of each histopathological examination.

10. Keywords

10.1 biocompatibility; biomaterials; New Zealand white rabbits; orthopaedic medical devices; short-term implantation; tissue compatibility

APPENDIX

(Nonmandatory Information)

X1. RATIONALE

X1.1 Within ASTM, there is a standard which addresses the question of material biocompatibility through *in vivo* testing: Practice F 981. This standard is intended as a long-term test with experiments running as long as 2 years, therefore manufacturers, implant developers, and researchers cannot use it on a routine basis to rapidly test or screen candidate materials.

X1.2 This testing protocol, patterned after the USP-Implantation Test which calls for tests of very short duration (3 d), is intended as a short-term screening test for candidate materials. It would be invoked prior to using the long-term test of Practice F 981.

X1.3 Both porous and dense candidate materials are included within the scope of this practice and their effects on tissue are compared to dense control materials. There are, of course, very large differences between porous and dense materials; however, porous negative controls are not yet available. Hence, provision is made for comparing the tissue effects of the porous candidate material to both other suitable controls of a like material and to dense negative controls. This same problem also applies to certain polymers that have proven to have application as medical implants but which elicit a greater tissue response than the dense negative control. Such candidate materials can also be compared to other similar, already medically accepted materials as well as dense negative controls.

X1.4 This practice excludes, as beyond its scope, biodegradable implants or other biological implants such as gels, liquids, allografts or xenografts and immune responses to implanted materials.

Designation: F 799 – 99

Standard Specification for Cobalt-28Chromium-6Molybdenum Alloy Forgings for Surgical Implants (UNS R31537, R31538, R31539)[1]

This standard is issued under the fixed designation F 799; the number immediately following the designation indicates the year of original adoption or, in the case of revision, the year of last revision. A number in parentheses indicates the year of last reapproval. A superscript epsilon (ε) indicates an editorial change since the last revision or reapproval.

1. Scope

1.1 This specification covers requirements of cobalt-28chromium-6molybdenum alloy (UNS R31537, R31538, R31539) high-strength forgings for the manufacture of surgical implants. Material conforming to this specification has been evaluated for biocompatibility and corrosion resistance[2] and has been found to be comparable to material conforming to Specification F 75. The properties specified in this document specifically apply to finished or semifinished parts that receive no subsequent metallurgical processing.

1.2 The values stated in inch-pound units are to be regarded as the standard. The metric equivalents of the inch-pound units may be approximate.

1.3 Wrought material to be used as forging stock in the manufacture of forgings conforming to this specification, typically hot worked and unannealed with a surface finish suitable for forging, shall be fabricated and supplied in accordance with F 1537.

2. Referenced Documents

2.1 *ASTM Standards:*

E 8 Test Methods for Tension Testing of Metallic Materials[3]

E 18 Test Methods for Rockwell Hardness and Rockwell Superficial Hardness of Metallic Materials[3]

E 112 Test Methods for Determining the Average Grain Size[3]

E 165 Test Method for Liquid Penetrant Examination[4]

E 930 Test Methods for Estimating the Largest Grain Observed in a Metallographic Section (ALA Grain Size)[3]

F 75 Specification for Cast Cobalt-Chromium-Molybdenum Alloy for Surgical Implant Applications[5]

F 601 Practice for Fluorescent Penetrant Inspection of Metallic Surgical Implants[5]

F 981 Practice for Assessment of Compatibility of Biomaterials (Non-porous) for Surgical Implants with Respect to Effect of Materials on Muscle and Bone[5]

F 1537 Specification for Wrought Cobalt-28 Chromium-6 Molybdenum Alloy for Surgical Implants[5]

2.2 *American Society for Quality Standard:*[6]

ASQ C1 Specification of General Requirements for a Quality Program

3. Significance and Use

3.1 The purpose of this specification is to characterize the properties of currently available cobalt-28chromium-6molybdenum forgings.

4. Ordering Information

4.1 Inquiries and orders for material under this specification shall include the following information:

4.1.1 Quantity,

4.1.2 ASTM designation and date of issue,

4.1.3 Mechanical properties,

4.1.4 Form (semifinished parts, part No.),

4.1.5 Applicable dimensions or print number,

4.1.6 Condition (forged, heat treated, annealed),

4.1.7 Special tests, and

4.1.8 Other requirements.

5. Condition

5.1 The material shall be forged by hammering, pressing, rolling, extruding, or upsetting, and shall be processed, if practicable, so as to cause metal flow during the hot-working operation in the direction most favorable for resisting stresses encountered in service, as may be indicated by the implant manufacturer.

5.2 Forgings shall be free of splits, scale, cracks, flaws, and other imperfections not consistent with good commercial practice.

5.3 Optional indentification marks, including the manufacturer's logo, material designation, heat code number, and impression number, may be placed upon each forging, the

---

[1] This specification is under the jurisdiction of ASTM Committee F-4 on Medical and Surgical Materials and Devicesand is the direct responsibility of Subcommittee F04.12 on Metallurgical Materials.

Current edition approved June 10, 1999. Published September 1999. Originally published as F 799 – 82. Last previous edition F 799 – 96.

[2] Supporting data are available from ASTM Headquarters, 100 Barr Harbor Dr., West Conshohocken, PA 19428.

[3] *Annual Book of ASTM Standards*, Vol 03.01.

[4] *Annual Book of ASTM Standards*, Vol 03.03.

[5] *Annual Book of ASTM Standards*, Vol 13.01.

[6] Available from American Society for Quality, 161 W. Wisconsin Ave., Milwaukee, WI 53203.

method and location of which shall be as specified by the purchaser.

6. Chemical Compostion

6.1 The chemical composition of forgings shall meet the chemical requirements of F 1537

7. Mechanical Requirements

7.1 *Tensile Properties*:

7.1.1 Tensile properties shall be determined in accordance with Test Methods E 8.

7.1.2 The mechanical properties of test specimens prepared from finished or semifinished parts shall conform to the requirements in Table 1.

7.1.3 Tension specimens shall be produced from finished or semifinished parts or from material having the same process history as that which exists in the final forging. Tension specimens may have a ground finish on the reduced section and may be taken in a direction parallel to the long axis of the finished or semifinished part.

7.1.4 A minimum of two test specimens shall be tested. If one specimen falls below the specified tensile requirements, two additional specimens shall be tested and both must pass. If a specimen breaks outside the gage, the test is null in accordance with Methods E 8, and a retest should be performed.

7.1.5 In some instances mechanical test pieces may not be obtainable directly from forged parts due to their configuration or small size. In lieu of mechanical testing, these parts shall exhibit hardness of HRC 35 to 45 when tested in accordance with Test Methods E 18.

7.2 *Hardness*—Finished or semifinished parts conforming to this specification shall have a minimum Rockwell C hardness of 35 HRC. The hardness determination shall be performed in accordance with Test Methods E 18.

TABLE 1 Mechanical Requirements

Ultimate Tensile Strength, min, psi, (MPa)	Yield Strength (0.2 % offset), min, psi (MPa)	Elongation,[A] min, %	Reduction in Area, min, %	Hardness, R_C, min
170 000 (1172)	120 000 (827)	12	12	35

[A] Gage length = 4 × diameter.

8. Special Tests

8.1 The grain size of forgings shall be five or finer when tested in accordance with Test Methods E 112. In forgings it may not be possible to fully recrystallize the entire microstructure to a fine grain size. Duplex microstructures exhibiting areas of unrecrystallized grains as large as ASTM No. 2 (or ALA No. 2, as applicable, see E 930) shall be acceptable provided a minimum of 50 % of the area of each section examined displays an average grain size of ASTM No. 5 or finer; and the average microhardness of the larger grained regions is the equivalent of HRC 38 or greater. In quantities of 10 % (by area of the metallographic section in question) or less, unrecrystallized grains as large as ASTM No. 0 (or ALA No. 0, as applicable) shall be acceptable provided the average microhardness of the larger grained regions is the equivalent of HRC 40 or greater.

8.2 When specified by the implant manufacturer, liquid penetrant inspection or fluorescent penetrant inspection shall be performed on forgings. These penetrant inspections shall be performed in accordance with Practices E 165 and F 601.

9. Certification

9.1 The fabricator's certification that the material was manufactured and tested in accordance with this specification, together with a report of the test results, shall be furnished to the implant manufacturer with each shipment.

10. Quality Program Requirements

10.1 The alloy producer and any processors shall maintain a quality program such as, for example, is defined in ASQ C1.

10.2 The manufacturer of surgical implants or medical devices shall be assured of the producer's quality program for conformance to the intent of ASQ C1 or other recognized programs.

11. Keywords

11.1 cobalt alloys; cobalt alloys (for surgical implants); cobalt-chromium-molybdenum; forgings; metals (for surgical implants)

APPENDIXES

(Nonmandatory Information)

X1. RATIONALE

X1.1 The purpose for this standard is to characterize composition and properties to assure consistency in thermo-mechanically processed cobalt-28 chromium-6 molybdenum finished or semifinished parts used in the manufacturing of medical devices that receive no subsequent metallurgical processing.

X1.2 Published data[7,8] indicate that material with a fine-grained homogeneous metallurgical structure resulting from forging will be superior with respect to tensile strength and fatigue resistance compared to material conforming to Specification F 75. Based upon this, requirements include fine-grained microstructure and high tensile strength.

X1.3 The maximum iron content has been lowered to coincide with compositions that are commercially available.

X1.4 Some complex metallic phases, such as carbides, oxides, or carbonitrides, or combinations thereof, may be present in the microstructure of this alloy.

X1.5 The chemical requirements section has been made to reference Specification F 1537. A section concerning penetrant inspection and Appendix X2 on biocompatibility have been added.

[7] Bardos, D. I., "High Strength Co-Cr-Mo Alloy for Prostheses," *Current Concepts of Internal Fixation of Fractures*, edited by H. Uhthoff, Springer Verlag, New York, NY, 1980, p 111.

[8] Weisman, S., "Vitallium FHS Forged High-Strength Alloy," *Current Concepts of Internal Fixation of Fractures*, p 118.

X2. BIOCOMPATIBILITY

X2.1 The material composition covered by this specification has been employed successfully in human implant applications in contact with soft tissue and bone for over a decade.

X2.2 No known surgical implant material has ever been shown to be completely free of adverse reactions in the human body; however, long-term clinical experience has shown an acceptable level of biological response can be expected, if this material is used in appropriate applications.

Designation: F 813 – 83 (Reapproved 1996)[ε1]

Standard Practice for Direct Contact Cell Culture Evaluation of Materials for Medical Devices[1]

This standard is issued under the fixed designation F 813; the number immediately following the designation indicates the year of original adoption or, in the case of revision, the year of last revision. A number in parentheses indicates the year of last reapproval. A superscript epsilon (ε) indicates an editorial change since the last revision or reapproval.

ε[1] NOTE—Footnote 4 was corrected editorially December 1996.

1. Scope

1.1 This practice covers a reference method of direct contact cell culture testing which may be used in evaluating the cytotoxic potential of materials for use in the construction of medical materials and devices.

1.2 This method may be used either directly to evaluate materials or as a reference against which other cytotoxicity test methods may be compared.

1.3 This is one of a series of reference test methods for the assessment of cytotoxic potential, employing different techniques.

1.4 Assessment of cytotoxicity is one of several tests employed in determining the biological response to a material, as recommended in Practice F 748.

1.5 The L-929 cell line was chosen because it has a significant history of use in assays of this type. This is not intended to imply that its use is preferred; only that the L-929 is an established cell line, well-characterized and readily available, that has demonstrated reproducible results in several laboratories.

1.6 *This standard does not purport to address all of the safety concerns, if any, associated with its use. It is the responsibility of the user of this standard to establish appropriate safety and health practices and determine the applicability of regulatory limitations prior to use.*

2. Referenced Documents

2.1 *ASTM Standards:*

F 748 Practice for Selecting Generic Biological Test Methods for Materials and Devices[2]

2.2 *Other Documents:*

The American Type Culture Collection (ATCC), Catalogue of Strains II[3]

USP Negative Control Plastic Reference Standard[4]

3. Summary of Practice

3.1 Cell cultures are grown to a confluent monolayer in Petri dishes. The growth medium is aspirated and replenished to provide a resting, confluent cell layer. Test and control specimens are placed in direct contact with the cell layer to provide an accelerated assessment of the presence or absence of a cytotoxic effect from a given material or device.

4. Significance and Use

4.1 This practice is useful for assessing cytotoxic potential both when evaluating new materials or formulations for possible use in medical applications, and as part of a quality control program for established medical materials and medical devices.

4.2 This practice assumes that assessment of cytotoxicity potential provides one method for predicting the potential for cytotoxic or necrotic reactions to medical materials and devices during clinical applications to humans. In general, cell culture testing methods have shown good correlation with animal assays and are frequently more sensitive to toxic moieties.

4.3 This cell culture test method is suitable for adoption in specifications and standards for materials for use in the construction of medical devices that are intended to be implanted in the human body or placed in contact with tissue, tissue fluids, or blood on a long-term basis.

5. Apparatus

5.1 The following apparatus shall be used:

5.2 *Incubator*, to maintain 37 ± 2°C and 4 to 6 % CO_2 with greater than 90 % relative humidity.

5.3 *Tissue Culture Grade Petri Dishes*, that are sterile and 35 mm in diameter by 10 mm deep.

NOTE 1—Plastic dishes are recommended because they provide a flat surface that contributes to the formation of a uniform cell monolayer.

5.4 *Disposable, Sterile, Centrifuge Tubes.*

5.5 *Inverted Optical Microscope*, with magnifications of 40×, 100×, and 200×.

---

[1] This practice is under the jurisdiction of ASTM Committee F-4 on Medical and Surgical Materials and Devices and is the direct responsibility of Subcommittee F04.16 on Biocompatibility Test Methods.

Current edition approved April 29, 1983. Published June 1983.

[2] *Annual Book of ASTM Standards,* Vol 13.01.

[3] American Type Culture Collection, 12031 Parklawn Drive, Rockville, MD 10852.

[4] *U.S. Pharmacopeia*, Vol 23, Rand McNally, Taunton, MA, 1994, pp. 1652–1653. Use latest supplement to ensure current cumulative revisions are used.

5.6 *Clinical Centrifuge.*

5.7 *Filter Disks*—10 mm in diameter (for evaluation of liquids).

NOTE 2—Millipore AP2501000 filter disks have been found satisfactory for use in cytotoxicity evaluations because they elicit no cytopathic effect. Other filter disks that do not elicit a cytopathic effect may also be used.

5.8 *Water Bath*, capable of maintaining a temperature of 37 ± 2°C.

NOTE 3—A laminar flow work area capable of filtering out 99.99 % of all particles greater than 0.5 μm in diameter, or a class 100 clean room may be necessary to prevent contamination of cultures.

6. Reagents

6.1 The following reagents shall be used:

6.1.1 *Minimum Essential Medium* (MEM), prepared without L-glutamine and augmented by the addition of Earle's salts and 10 % fetal bovine serum.

NOTE 4—Glutamine is omitted from this formulation in order to maximize the shelf life of the medium. Immediately before use, 5 mL of L-glutamine solution (see 6.1.2) are added to each 500 mL of MEM.

NOTE 5—Opened containers of MEM may be stored at a temperature of 2 to 8°C for periods of not more than one week.

NOTE 6—Antibiotics, such as penicillin G and streptomycin, may be added to the medium to reduce the incidence of bacterial contamination. This may, however, have an adverse effect on the viability of the cell cultures.

6.1.2 *L-glutamine Solution*, 29.2 mg/mL of sterile water.

6.1.3 *Hanks' Solution*, calcium-and magnesium-free (store at room temperature).

6.1.4 *Trypsin*, 0.1 % solution in Hanks' solution or calcium- and magnesium-free, phosphate-buffered saline (store frozen).

6.1.5 *Water*, distilled, deionized, and sterile, with a minimum resistivity of 1 MΩ·cm.

6.2 All reagents shall be tissue-culture grade or equivalent.

6.3 Reagents shall be reconstituted in accordance with the manufacturer's directions, using aseptic technique.

6.4 Reagents shall be stored in accordance with the manufacturer's directions unless otherwise indicated in 6.1.

7. Cell Cultures

7.1 Cell cultures used in this assay shall be the ATCC, CCL 1 NCTC clone 929 strain (clone of Strain L, mouse connective tissue) designated L-929.

8. Control Materials

8.1 Prepare negative control specimens in accordance with Section 10 from a material that consistently ellicits negligible cellular response in this assay (for example, USP Negative Control Plastic Reference Standard).

8.2 Prepare positive control specimens in accordance with Section 10 from a material that consistently ellicits a predictable, moderate degree of cytotoxicity.

8.2.1 Use aqueous phenol (0.45 ± 0.05 % by volume) as a positive control for a diffuse reaction of cellular degeneration and sloughing. Take care to ensure that the preparation is homogenous.

8.2.2 Latex rubber (for example, cut from a Foley catheter) has been used as a positive polymeric control for a zone of inhibition.

9. General Technique

9.1 Use the aseptic technique throughout this assay to minimize microbial contamination.

NOTE 7—Mouth pipetting should not be employed to transfer cells, medium, or reagents.

9.2 Warm all solutions and materials to a temperature of 37 ± 2°C before placing in contact with cells.

10. Preparation of Specimens

10.1 Sterilize all specimens by a method appropriate to the end use of the device.

10.2 Where a device is sufficiently small (see 10.3 and 10.4) to fit into the Petri dish leaving an adequate margin of cells for evaluation, use the entire device as a specimen.

10.3 Cut large solid materials and devices in cross-section to obtain a flat surface having an area of 100 to 250 mm^2 to be placed in direct contact with the cell monolayer.

10.4 Prepare specimens of rod or tubing or of rod- or tube-shaped devices as follows:

10.4.1 Where the diameter is less than 6.4 mm, cut 5 to 15 mm in length.

10.4.2 Where the diameter is 6.4 to 15 mm, cut 2 to 8 mm in length.

10.4.3 Where the diameter exceeds 15 mm, prepare cross-sections as described in 10.3.

10.5 Obtain specimens from larger medical items from locations with relatively large cross-sections in order to expose interior material.

10.6 If a device is constructed of two or more materials, cut either the test specimen from the materials' interface or test separate specimens from each material.

10.7 Prepare specimens for evaluating the cytotoxicity of liquids or extracts by saturating a sterile filter disk and allowing the excess liquid to drain off while maintaining asepsis. Use the saturated filter disk as a test specimen.

NOTE 8—When ethylene oxide or other chemical sterilants are used, adequate aeration time should be allowed, to permit dissipation of residues which may adversely affect the results recorded in this assay.

NOTE 9—In general, specimens should be cleaned to remove any residues from specimen preparation, and sterilized after they have been cut to size. If the large solid materials are very hard, like ceramics, which require cutting with metal or diamond saws, care should be taken to remove any contamination from the metal blade or from the metal bonding the diamonds to the blade. When evaluating the cytotoxicity potential of medical materials or devices that are contained in the final sterile package, resterilization, further processing, or delay between the time of opening the package and starting the test must be avoided. With small items the entire content of the sterile package may be used as the test specimen. When the size of the sterile packaged item is too large, an appropriate, representative, small-sized specimen must be obtained. The application of this assay to items in the final sterile package is limited to items that are small or can be cut and reshaped with aseptic technique.

NOTE 10—The size and shape of test specimens may vary considerably, providing they physically fit into the Petri dish. This test is intended only to provide a qualitative assessment of cytotoxicity potential with no quantitative measurement of cytotoxicity magnitude, and thus specimen size is not considered important.

11. Preparation of Cell Layer

Prepare confluent cell monolayers as follows:

11.1 Aspirate the medium from a 150 cm^2-cell culture flask containing a near-confluent cell monolayer.

11.2 Rinse the cells with 5 ± 0.5 mL of Hanks' solution.

11.3 Aspirate the rinse solution.

11.4 Add 5 ± 0.5 mL of trypsin solution (0.1 %) to the flask.

11.5 Incubate for 5 to 10 min to suspend the cells.

11.6 Transfer the cell suspension to a centrifuge tube.

11.7 Centrifuge at 1300 g for 6 min.

11.8 Discard the supernatant.

11.9 Resuspend the cells in 10 ± 0.1 mL of fresh medium, and mix the suspension thoroughly.

11.10 Add 2.0 ± 0.1 mL of medium to each Petri dish.

11.11 Using a sterile 10 mL serological pipette, add 5 to 7 drops of cell suspension to each dish.

11.12 Incubate until a near-confluent monolayer has formed, as observed by microscopic examination.

NOTE 11—The formation of a near-confluent monolayer usually requires 3 to 5 days. By counting cells with a hemacytometer (to ensure the concentration of the inoculum) the time required for monolayer formation may be regulated. A cell concentration of 1.3×10^5 cells/mL will give a consistent time of 24 h. It should be recognized, however, that this procedure may increase the risk of bacterial contamination.

11.13 If cell suspension remains unused after step 11.11, a subculture may be prepared by adding 9 mL of fresh medium to each millilitre of each suspension in a cell culture flask with a surface area of approximately 3 cm^2 for each millilitre of diluted cells and incubating it until a near-confluent monolayer has formed, as determined by microscopic examination.

12. Test Procedure

12.1 Perform the direct-contact cytotoxicity assay as follows:

12.2 Microscopically examine the cell cultures and reject any in which the cell monolayer is not of correct confluency or the cells show signs of granulation or sloughing.

12.3 Aspirate the medium from all the acceptable cultures and replace it with 1.5 to 2 mL of fresh medium.

12.4 Place a single test or control specimen in each dish in direct contact with the cell monolayer. Prepare duplicate cultures for each test material and both positive and negative controls.

NOTE 12—Low-density materials that tend to float in the medium may be held in contact with the cell monolayers by placing a piece of negative control on top to weigh them down.

12.5 Incubate all cultures for 24 ± 1 h.

12.6 Examine each culture microscopically.

NOTE 13—The use of an histologic stain such as 2 % crystal violet in 20 % ethanol is helpful in assessing the cell cultures.

13. Evaluation of Results

13.1 A cell culture shall be deemed to show a cytotoxic effect if microscopic examination (see 12.6) reveals the following:

13.1.1 Malformation, degeneration, sloughing, or lysis of cells extending beyond the perimeter of the specimen of material; or

13.1.2 Moderate to severe reduction of cell layer density.

NOTE 14—A slight reduction of cell layer density is acceptable, provided that there is no evidence of the conditions specified in 13.1.1.

13.2 If, for a given set of specimens, a cytotoxic effect is observed for the negative controls or no cytotoxic effect is elicited by the positive controls, the results for that set of specimens shall be considered invalid.

13.3 If neither specimen of a test material elicits a cytotoxic effect as described in 13.1, the material shall be considered to pass this assay.

13.4 If both specimens of a test material elicit a cytotoxic effect, the material shall be considered to fail this assay.

13.5 If only one specimen of a test material elicits a cytotoxic effect, the assay shall be repeated on an additional four specimens. The material shall be considered to pass this assay only if none of the retest specimens elicits a cytotoxic effect, otherwise, it shall be considered to fail.

14. Report

14.1 The report of the assay results shall include at least the following:

14.1.1 Test date.

14.1.2 Cell strain used.

14.1.3 Culture history of cells.

14.1.4 Medium used (noting whether antibiotics were used).

14.1.5 Description of all test and control specimens, including:

14.1.5.1 Material or device name (including ASTM designation number, where appropriate).

14.1.5.2 Lot or batch number.

14.1.5.3 Source of supply.

14.1.5.4 Size and method of preparation.

14.1.5.5 Method of sterilization.

14.1.6 Statement of whether each test material passed or failed the assay.

14.1.7 Any other pertinent observations, including any deviations from the exact method described herein.

15. Precision and Bias

15.1 Quantitative precision and bias have not been determined.

16. Keywords

16.1 biocompatibility; cell culture; cytotoxicity testing; direct contact cytotoxicity

APPENDIX

(Nonmandatory Information)

X1. RATIONALE FOR EVALUATING DIRECT CONTACT CELL CULTURE OF MATERIALS FOR MEDICAL DEVICES[5]

X1.1 Medical devices such as implants and certain other devices intended for intimate contact with organs should not produce adverse biological reactions.

X1.2 Laboratory cell culture methods provide a rapid method[6,7,8] for assessment of cytotoxicity potential of both finished medical devices and materials used in their construction. The direct contact method is but one of several such techniques that are in common use. The cell culture method described in this standard is a modification of methods that have been routinely used for more than 10 years. A positive control which produces a cytopathic effect and a negative control which produces no cytopathic effect are assayed with each test to assure that the cell cultures have expected cytotoxicity responses. Test results are considered valid only when the expected responses for both controls are obtained.

[5] Committee F-4 requires a rationale to accompany all standards. This rationale should be readable to lay consumers as well as technical experts.

[6] Guess, W. L., Autian, J., "Toxicity Evaluation of Lexan, Kyonar, Rilsan Short-Term Studies," *Journal of Oral Therapeutics and Pharmacology*, Vol 3, No. 2, 1966, pp. 116–123.

[7] Wilsnack, R. E., Meyer, F. S., Smith, J. G., "Human Cell Culture Toxicity Testing of Medical Devices and Correlation to Animal Tests," *Biomaterials, Medical Devices, and Artificial Organs* Vol 1, 1973, pp. 543–562.

[8] Wilsnack, R. E., "Quantitative Cell Culture Biocompatibility Testing of Medical Devices and Correlation to Animal Tests," *Biomaterials Medical Devices and Artificial Organs*, Vol 4, 1976, pp. 235–261.

Designation: F 881 – 94 (Reapproved 2000)

Standard Specification for Silicone Elastomer Facial Implants[1]

This standard is issued under the fixed designation F 881; the number immediately following the designation indicates the year of original adoption or, in the case of revision, the year of last revision. A number in parentheses indicates the year of last reapproval. A superscript epsilon (ϵ) indicates an editorial change since the last revision or reapproval.

1. Scope

1.1 This specification covers the requirements for silicone elastomer implants used in facial surgery (that is, chin, nasal, malar, and ear implants).

1.2 *Limitations*—This specification does not cover implants containing silicone gels or other gels or liquids. It does not necessarily cover any custom-fabricated prosthesis manufactured to any other specification.

1.3 The following safety hazards caveat pertains only to the mechanical testing and test methods portion, Section 7, of this specification: *This standard does not purport to address all of the safety problems, if any, associated with its use. It is the responsibility of the user of this standard to establish appropriate safety and health practices and determine the applicability of regulatory limitations prior to use.*

2. Referenced Documents

2.1 *ASTM Standards:*

D 412 Test Methods for Rubber Properties in Tension[2]

D 624 Test Method for Rubber Property—Tear Resistance[2]

D 2240 Test Method for Rubber Property—Durometer Hardness[2]

F 604 Classification for Silicone Elastomers Used in Medical Applications[3]

F 748 Practice for Selecting Generic Biological Test Methods for Materials and Devices[3]

F 981 Practice for Assessment of Compatibility of Biomaterials for Surgical Implants with Respect to Effect of Materials on Muscle and Bone[3]

F 1251 Terminology Relating to Polymeric Biomaterials in Medical and Surgical Devices[3]

2.2 *Other Documents:*

United States Pharmacopeia, Volume XX[4]

Federal Register, Title 21,Part 820[5]

Dow Corning Corporate Test Method— CTM 0930—Adhesion—OneHundred Eighty Degree Shear—Thin Elastometric Substrates[6]

3. Terminology

3.1 *Definitions:*

3.1.1 *fixation site*—an area on the surface of the implant which has material on it that allows tissue ingrowth.

3.1.2 *fused or adhered joints*—all junctures of dissimilar materials; and all junctures of fully or partly formed or preformed materials bonded or fused together to form a single implant unit.

3.1.3 *Discussion*—Implants made from one material by a single charge of unvulcanized elastomer by one-step compression, transfer, or reactive injection molding are not considered to have fused or adhered joints.

3.1.4 *orientation means*—any locus on the surface of the implant that is modified to assist the surgeon to position the implant.

4. Significance and Use

4.1 The prostheses described in this specification are intended for implant use in the facial area.

5. Materials

5.1 The primary material of construction shall be fully vulcanized silicone elastomer.

5.1.1 Implants may have orientation means or sites of attached fixation materials, or both.

5.2 *Biocompatibility*:

5.2.1 Biological testing to ensure the safety of facial implant devices shall be selected and conducted in accordance with Practices F 748 and F 981.

5.2.2 In addition to biological testing as recommended by Practices F 748 and F 981, other biological testing may be appropriate.

6. Dimensions

6.1 The individual shape, range of sizes, and measurements are determined by the manufacturer.

6.1.1 Define sizing codes by typical dimensions and volumes, where applicable.

7. Mechanical Testing and Test Methods

7.1 *Typical Physical Properties of Elastomers*:

---

[1] This specification is under the jurisdiction of ASTM Committee F04 on Medical and Surgical Materials and Devices and is the direct responsibility of Subcommittee F04.32 on Plastic and Reconstructive Surgery.

Current edition approved May 15, 1994. Published July 1994. Originally published as F 881 – 84. Last previous edition F 881 – 84.

[2] *Annual Book of ASTM Standards*, Vol 09.01.

[3] *Annual Book of ASTM Standards*, Vol 13.01.

[4] Available from Mack Publishing Co., 1991 N Hampton St. Easton, PA. 18042.

[5] Available from Standardization Documents Order Desk, Bldg. 4 Section D, 700 Robbins Ave., Philadelphia, PA 19111-5094, Attn: NPODS.

[6] Available from Dow Corning Corp., Midland, MI 48686-0994 Phone: (517) 496-5461

7.1.1 *Elongation at Failure*—The elongation at failure shall be 200 %, minimum, when tested in accordance with Test Methods D 412.

7.1.2 *Durometer*—The durometer shall have a maximum of shore A80, depending on application, when tested in accordance with Test Method D 2240.

7.1.3 *Tensile Strength*—The minimum tensile strength of all silicone elastomers and adhesives used to fabricate facial implants shall be 200 psi when tested in accordance with Test Methods D 412.

7.1.4 *Modulus*—Test in accordance with Test Methods D 412.

7.1.5 *Tear*—Test in accordance with Test Method D 624.

7.1.6 *Durometer*—Test in accordance with Test Method D 2240.

7.2 *Fused or Adhered Joints*:

7.2.1 Techniques and materials used for adhered or fused joints or seams that are critical to the integrity of the implant shall demonstrate a strength greater than 20 ppi when test specimens made of the same materials and fabricated by similar techniques are tested in accordance with Dow Corning Corporate Test Method-CTM 0930.

8. Sterilization

8.1 The units may be supplied presterilized in accordance with the United States Pharmacopeia and good manufacturing practices released by the Food and Drug Administration (FDA).

8.2 Instructions for cleaning and sterilization shall be supplied with the package insert.

9. Packaging, Labeling, and Package Inserts

9.1 *Packaging (Primary)*:

9.1.1 Packages shall be sealed to prevent contamination and to maintain sterility.

9.1.2 Units shall be packaged with suitable containers that will prevent damage in transit.

9.2 *Labeling*:

9.2.1 Each implant shall be labeled in a manner that ensures the labeling arrives at the point of use with the device. Labeling shall include the following information:

9.2.1.1 Product name and manufacturer.

9.2.1.2 Configuration or type.

9.2.1.3 Size, dimensions, and durometer.

9.2.1.4 Special storage requirements, if any.

9.2.2 With each unit, a self-adhering tab shall be provided that is suitable for attaching to the patient's chart. The tab shall include the following information:

9.2.2.1 Product name and manufacturer.

9.2.2.2 Product lot number.

9.2.2.3 Product size and dimensions.

9.3 *Package Insert*—The package insert shall provide specific instructions for use, cleaning, sterilization, and storage.

APPENDIX

(Nonmandatory Information)

X1. STATEMENT OF RATIONALE FOR SPECIFICATION F 881

X1.1 Silicone elastomer facial implants described in this specification have generally been available to hospitals and physicians for surgical procedures requiring tissue augmentation in both aesthetic and reconstructive surgery. The uses of silicone elastomer implants for chin, nasal, malar, and ear augmentation have been reviewed by the plastic and reconstructive surgery sections of the Medical Device Classification Panels in keeping with the provisions of the Medical Device Amendments of 1976 to the Federal Food, Drugs, and Cosmetic Act. This panel recommended a Class II (standards) classification. This specification is thus needed both to satisfy regulatory considerations, and to provide enduser physicians and other health-care professionals with an adequate description of the properties and characteristics of silicone materials used for implant construction.

X1.2 The potential risk and hazards to health identified at the time of review by FDA classification panels included the possible presence of adulterants, adverse tissue reaction, extrusion, rejection, and infection. The test methods and requirements suggested in this specification have been selected specifically to provide reasonable assurance that none of the identified risks and hazards to health occur as a result of defective or adulterated materials. Label copy requirements include directions for handling and use, sterilization, and storage to minimize the occurrence of risks and hazards to health due to technique-of-use considerations.

X1.3 This specification includes suggested test methods and requirements for physical, chemical, and biological properties for silicone elastomer used in facial implant surgery. Criteria for dimensions, volume, physical characteristics, sterilization, packaging, and labeling are discussed thoroughly. Pertinent ASTM methods for biological testing of implant materials are cited. This specification assumes the following: (*1*) all formulations of various ingredients have been qualified by biological testing; (*2*) formulation ingredients and processing procedures are not changed from those used with biological test specimens; (*3*) all manufacturing starts with characterizable, well-characterized materials and is performed in plants that fully comply with regulatory GMPS; and (*4*) when the conditions stated in X1.1, X1.2 and X1.3 are satisfied and all the requirements as described in this specification for ingredients, and for physical and chemical properties, have been satisfied, silicone elastomers are duplicated adequately on a batch-to-batch basis to provide reasonable assurance of suitability for implant use.

Designation: F 882 – 84 (Reapproved 1996)

Standard Performance and Safety Specification for Cryosurgical Medical Instruments[1]

This standard is issued under the fixed designation F 882; the number immediately following the designation indicates the year of original adoption or, in the case of revision, the year of last revision. A number in parentheses indicates the year of last reapproval. A superscript epsilon (ε) indicates an editorial change since the last revision or reapproval.

This standard has been approved for use by agencies of the Department of Defense.

INTRODUCTION

This performance and safety specification was developed by Task Force F04.08 on Cryosurgical Medical Instruments.

This specification is intended to provide the user of Cryosurgical Medical Instruments with the assurance that the equipment will meet or exceed all safety and performance levels established by this document as claimed by the manufacturer. This is predicated on the requirements that the equipment is operated according to the manufacturer's recommendations.

Since, in the pursuit of improved health care and reduced medical costs, the medical industry is required to be innovative and dynamic, this standard must be capable of being upgraded in a swift and efficient manner. All inquiries regarding this standard should be addressed to: Committee F-4 Staff Manager, ASTM, 100 Barr Harbor Drive, West Conshohocken, PA 19428.

1. Scope

1.1 This specification covers standards a manufacturer shall meet in the designing, manufacturing, testing, labeling, and documenting of cryosurgical medical instruments, but it is not to be construed as production methods, quality control techniques, or manufacturer's lot release criteria, or clinical recommendations.

1.2 This specification represents the best currently available test procedures at this time and is a minimum safety and performance standard.

1.3 This specification covers only those cryosurgical devices intended for use on humans or animals for therapeutic purposes. This specification assumes the user is well-trained in the procedures of cryosurgery and has the ability to determine if an abnormality is treatable by cryosurgery, particularly by the type of equipment to be used.

1.4 Cryosurgical medical instruments produce low temperatures either inside a cryoprobe or directly on the target tissue by the principle of Latent Heat of Vaporization or the Joule-Thompson Effect, or both. The cryogen may be transported from the source as a liquid or a gas. These systems may be closed or open depending on the application and cryogen. In the open cryotip system, the cryogen is applied directly to the target tissue, while in the closed cryotip system, the cryogen is applied indirectly and is exhausted away from the target area.

1.5 Cryosurgical medical instruments are used to produce cryonecrosis, inflammatory response, or cryoadhesion.

1.6 Monitoring the progress of treatment during application is sometimes very important. Such monitoring is done by accessories that indicate the temperature of the cryotip or the target area being frozen. The temperature of the tissue may be measured directly (for example, by a thermocouple). These accessories are also covered by this specification.

1.7 The following precautionary caveat pertains only to the Test Method portion, Sections 8 through 13, of this specification: *This standard may involve hazardous materials, operations, and equipment. This standard does not purport to address all of the safety concerns, if any, associated with its use. It is the responsibility of the user of this standard to establish appropriate safety and health practices and determine the applicability of regulatory limitations prior to use.*

2. Referenced Documents

2.1 *ANSI Standard:*
ANSI B40.1-1974 Use and Installation of Pressure Gauges[2]

2.2 *ANSI/AAMI Document:*
ANSI/AAMI SCL 12/78[3]

2.3 *Canadian Standards Association (C.S.A.) Standard:*
C22.2-125 Electromedical Equipment 1973[4]

2.4 *International ElectroTechnical Commission (IEC) Document:*

[1] This specification is under the jurisdiction of ASTM Committee F-4 on Medical and Surgical Materials and Devices and is the direct responsibility of Subcommittee F04.33 on Medical/Surgical Instruments.

Current edition approved Sept. 11, 1984. Published February 1985.

[2] Available from the American National Standards Institute, 1430 Broadway, New York, NY 10018.

[3] Available from the Association for the Advancement of Medical Instrumentation (AAMI). 1901 North Fort Myer Drive, Suite 602, Arlington, VA 22209.

[4] Available from the Canadian Standards Association (C.S.A), 173 Rexdale Blvd., Rexdale, Ontario M9W 1R3, Canada.

IEC 601-1 1977[5]

2.5 *Compressed Gas Association Document:*

CGA V-1 1977[6]

2.6 *FDA Document:*

21CFR801: Labeling Specifications[7]

2.7 *NBS Document:*

Table IPTS-68 NBS Monograph 125[8]

3. Terminology

3.1 *Definitions:*

3.1.1 *closed cryotip*—a hollow, closed end usually shaped to fit a particular anatomical site where the cryogen cools the external surface which is applied to the target tissue.

3.1.2 *closed cryotip reference temperature*—the average of the minimum/maximum cycle temperature variation at the end of the freeze cycle.

3.1.3 *compressed gas cylinder*—a container that is specifically designed to store a gas or liquid under elevated pressure conditions.

3.1.4 *compressed gas cylinder connector*—a device specifically designed to attach to a cylinder for proper and safe removal of its contents.

3.1.5 *cryoadhesion*—cryotip attachment to target tissue.

3.1.6 *cryogen*—a substance used to obtain reduced temperatures. Cryogens are usually classed by their boiling points. The most common cryogens and their respective boiling points are as follows:

Cryogen	Boiling Point at S.T.P., °C
Freon 12	−29.8
Freon 22	−49.8
Carbon Dioxide (CO_2)	−78.6
Nitrous Oxide (N_2O)	−88.5
Liquid Nitrogen (LN_2)	−195.8

3.1.7 *cryometer*—a device for measuring low temperature(s) when used with a temperature sensor such as a thermocouple.

3.1.8 *cryonecrosis*—destruction of tissue cells using a cryosystem.

3.1.9 *cryoprobe*—the instrument used to deliver the cryogen to the cryotip or open tip. For a cryotip, a cryoprobe also directs the cryogen away from the target tissue.

3.1.10 *cryosystem*—all parts of a system excluding the cryogen and its container, unless supplied by the manufacturer, that is designed to apply or use a cryogen.

3.1.11 *defrost*—the ability to return the cryotip to ambient temperature.

3.1.12 *Dewar*—a vacuum insulated container that is specifically designed to store a liquid cryogen.

3.1.13 *Dewar withdrawal device*—a device specifically designed to attach to a dewar for proper and safe removal of its contents.

3.1.14 *disposable*—any device which is designated to be discarded after use.

3.1.15 *inflammatory response*—irritation of tissue cells as a result of using a cryosystem.

3.1.16 *mechanical integrity*—the ability of all components of a cryosystem to withstand the pressures and temperatures that may be encountered during use as recommended by the manufacturer.

3.1.17 *open cryotip*—a device specifically designed to apply the cryogen directly to the target tissue.

3.1.18 *target tissue*—the specific anatomical area intended to be treated.

3.1.19 *thermal insulation*—a material or technique, or both, used to prevent unintended cryonecrosis, inflammatory responses, or cryoadhesion to nontarget tissue.

3.1.20 *thermocouple*—a junction of two dissimilar metals that produce an output voltage proportional to the temperature of the junction. When used in conjunction with a cryometer(s), the output is directly correlated to the temperature to which the sensing junction is exposed.

3.1.21 *tractive forge*—the cryoadhesive attraction between the cryotip and the target tissue.

3.1.22 *worst case conditions*—the maximum pressures or temperatures, or both, a cryosystem may encounter when used according to the manufacturer's instructions.

4. Conformance

4.1 Presently, this specification is voluntary and not mandated by law. A manufacturer may label his product as conforming to these standards only if the product indeed meets the requirements of this specification.

5. Cryosystem Performance and Reproducibility Requirements

5.1 The purpose of these requirements is to ensure that a cryosystem of the same design or accessories, or both, shall meet the minimum performance and reproducibility requirements as originally designed. The cryosystem and accessory requirements shall not vary from procedure to procedure provided they are used and maintained according to the manufacturer's recommendations.

5.2 *Closed Cryotip Temperature Reproducibility*:

5.2.1 Cryosystem requirements are divided into three primary categories in accordance with their clinical application: cryonecrosis, inflammatory response, and cryoadhesion. The manufacturer's test procedures must be categorized into these groups and tested accordingly.

5.2.2 All cryosystems manufactured with closed cryotips of the same model, temperature sensing or nontemperature sensing, shall meet the requirements of Table 1.

5.2.3 *Test Method*—See Section 11.

5.3 *Closed Cryotip Tractive Force*:

5.3.1 All cryosystems specifically designed for cryoadhesion shall be capable of attaching to, lifting, and holding a minimum weight of 60 g for a minimum of 45 s.

5.3.2 *Test Method*—See Section 12.

5.4 *Monitoring Devices*:

5.4.1 *Cryogen Monitors, Regulators, and Gages*—Cryogen monitors include any instrument, device, or accessory intended

[5] Available from the International Electro-Technical Commission (IEC), Committee 62D, Rue de Varembe, CH-1211, NIOSH, Geneva 20, Switzerland.

[6] Available from the Compressed Gas Association, 500 Fifth Ave., New York, NY 10036.

[7] Available from the Food and Drug Administration (FDA), Bureau of Medical Devices, 8757 Georgia Ave., Silver Spring, MD 20910.

[8] Available from the National Bureau of Standards-Monograph 125, Gaithersburg, MD 10877.

TABLE 1 Time and Temperature Requirements

Manufacturers Specified Intended Use	Freeze Mode Duration	Cryotip Temperature Reproducibility (°C)	
	Time per Cycle (s)	Range 0 to − 100°C	Range − 100.1 to − 200°C
Cryonecrosis	180	±5	±10
Inflammatory Response	30	±5	±10
Cryoadhesion	30	±10	±10

to display or control any cryogen parameter. The cryogen monitors include, but are not limited to, pressure gages, pressure regulators, flow gages, and flow regulators.

5.4.1.1 Pressure gages on all cryosystems shall meet or exceed the ANSI Specification B 40.1.

5.4.1.2 Cryogen monitors shall be compatible with the type of cryogen employed and be of such design and construction to display or control the cryogen safely.

5.4.1.3 The manufacturer shall assure the user that the safety, performance, and reproducibility of a cryosystem will be maintained at the maximum error points of the cryogen monitor(s). See disclosure requirement in 6.2.10.

5.4.2 *Temperature Monitors, Cryotip*—Temperature monitors include, but are not limited to: analog cryometers, digital cryometers, chart recorders. A thermocouple is most commonly used as the temperature sensor.

All cryotip temperature monitor(s) shall be representative of the temperature of the cryotip when tested using the simulated tissue model. The following requirements shall be applied to cryosystems containing cryotip temperature monitors:

Temperature	Range °C
0 to − 100	−100.1 to − 200
±5°	±10°C

5.4.3 *Temperature Monitors, Tissue Temperature*—All cryosystems of accessories with tissue temperature monitors that use an invasive on noninvasive technique to monitor actual tissue temperature shall adhere to the requirements listed in 5.4.2.

6. Disclosure, Labeling, and Documentation Requirements

6.1 These requirements are intended to ensure a manufacturers' written dissemination of all necessary information that allow a user to determine properly a cryosystem's (and its accessories) operation, application, and limitation. These disclosure, labeling, and documentation requirements also ensure clear identification of the product and make available all pertinent data a user may require. A manufacturer may label his product as conforming to this standard only if the product fulfills the requirements of this specification.

6.2 *Disclosures*—A manufacturer shall disclose each specification listed, where applicable.

6.2.1 *Warning Statement*—A manufacturer of a cryosystem shall provide a warning statement to inform the user where contact with the cryosystem may cause user/patient harm. This statement shall appear in the instrument's instruction manual and, if possible, on sections of the instrument that become 0°C or colder.

6.2.2 A cryosystem designed to spray a cryogen onto a target tissue must have a disclosure statement warning the user to provide adequate protection to himself and the patient due to excess or residual cryogen droplets or mist.

6.2.3 A disclosure statement shall be required that states the normal operating pressure at +20°C, the boiling point, and the type of cryogen for which the instrument is designed.

6.2.4 *Sterilization*—A disclosure statement that states exactly what items of the cryosystem and its accessories can be sterilized and the recommended sterilization procedures shall be included with each cryosystem.

6.2.5 *Presterilized Cryosystem*—A disclosure statement shall be included with each presterilized cryosystem. This statement shall include the following information: (*1*) the device is sterile, (*2*) the expiration date of sterilization, and (*3*) notes of caution concerning means of shipping, storage, and use of the instrument.

6.2.6 All a-c powered cryosystems and accessories shall be prominently labeled "Danger-Explosion Hazard. Do Not Use in Presence of Flammable Anesthetics".

6.2.7 *Tissue Temperature Monitors*—The following description and specifications shall be included in the disclosure statement for tissue temperature monitors.

6.2.7.1 Type of cryometer (analog, digital, recorder),

6.2.7.2 Temperature range: minimum to maximum,

6.2.7.3 Type of thermocouple (for example, Type "T"),

6.2.7.4 Temperature limits for storage, shipping, and operation, and

6.2.7.5 Power requirements.

6.2.8 *Cryogen Use, Handling, and Storage*—The manufacturer shall disclose all safety requirements for use, handling, and storage of cryogens as recommended by the cryogen supplier.

6.2.9 *Optimum Operating Pressure*—The optimum operating pressure for each open cryotip shall be disclosed to maximize control and where appropriate minimize liquid run off.

6.2.10 *Cryogen Containers*—The manufacturer shall recommend or supply containers designed for the specific cryogen employed.

6.2.11 *Cryogen Monitors, Regulators and Gages*—A disclosure statement is required stating the recommended operating pressures, the minimum and maximum pressure limits, the optimum cryogen flows, the pressure or flow gage accuracy, and the accuracy and reproducibility of all regulators used in a cryosystem or accessory, where applicable.

6.3 *Labeling*:

6.3.1 All labeling shall be of a size that is legible, in size and color dictated by FDA guidelines, durable to last the life of the cryosystem, and permanently attached so as not to be lost.

6.3.2 All cryosystems shall be labeled so as to contain the following information:

6.3.2.1 Model of cryosystem,

6.3.2.2 Manufacturer's or distributor's name and address,

6.3.2.3 Type(s) of cryogen(s) used,

6.3.2.4 Power requirements,

6.3.2.5 Additional items needed such as water, air, venting, etc.,

6.3.2.6 Serial number or lot and batch number, and

6.3.2.7 Operational instructions.

6.3.3 If labeling is not conducive to direct attachment to the cryosystem, then all information should be provided in the manufacturer's instruction manual or, for disposable cryosystems, the final packaging itself.

6.4 *Documentation*:

6.4.1 All cryosystems shall include instruction manuals.

6.4.2 All instruction manuals for cryosystems shall include the following information, where applicable.

A Brief Theory of Operation
Operating Instructions
Set up
Use
Dismantle
Calibrations
Intended Applications

6.4.2.1 *Specifications—Cryosystem and Cryogen*:

Size
Weight
Type(s) of Cryogen(s) Used
Minimum and Maximum Operation Pressure
Power Requirements
Temperature Control Description
Cryosystem and Cryoprobe Performance Check
Defrost Features
Temperature Sensor
Serviceable Parts
Manufacturer's Recommended Cryogen Containers
Thermal Insulation
Specifications - Cryogen Container

6.4.2.2 *Recommended Withdrawal Devices*:

Type(s) of Cryogen Employed
Size
Weight
Capacity
Static Hold Time: Container Only
Static Hold Time: Container and Withdrawal Device
Optimum and Maximum Operating Pressure
Rating on Pressure Limiting Device
Filling Directions
Serviceable Parts

6.4.3 *Servicing Instructions*:

Trouble-Shooting Chart
Cryogen Flow Chart
Electrical Schematics
User Serviceable Part Numbers
Preventive Maintenance Recommendations
Warranty Information

6.4.4 *Electrical and Cryogen Safety Instructions*:

User Related
Patient Related

6.4.5 *Available Accessories.*

7. Cryosystem Safety Requirements

7.1 These cryosystem safety requirements are intended to protect the user and patient from harm during the use and storage of the cryosystem.

7.2 *Mechanical Integrity*:

7.2.1 The purpose of this requirement is to ensure the user that the cryosystem is capable of withstanding the pressure and temperatures normally encountered during operation.

7.2.2 All related assemblies of new or repaired cryosystems must be able to withstand static overpressure of at least two times the normal operating pressure that the assembly shall encounter. The pressure normally encountered shall be calculated based on the following conditions:

7.2.2.1 A cryosystem that uses a cryogen regulated by the Compressed Gas Association (CGA) shall withstand two times the CGA designated pressure at standard temperature and pressure for that or those specific cryogens.

7.2.2.2 A cryosystem with a pressure limiting device shall withstand two times the pressure of the maximum rating of the device's set operating pressure.

7.2.2.3 A cryosystem without a pressure limiting device shall withstand two times the maximum pressure it can normally encounter under the worst case conditions, (for example, storage and shipping temperature) as specified by the manufacturer.

7.2.3 *Test Method*—See Section 9.

7.3 *Cryogen Exposure*:

7.3.1 The purpose of this requirement is to minimize direct user or patient contact or exposure to the cryogen or to excessive gas concentrations.

7.3.2 *Cryogen Exhaust*—All cryosystems are required to vent the exhausted cryogen in such a manner that the user or patient cannot come into contact with cryogen droplets or mist, or both, under normal operating conditions.

Exception—This requirement does not apply to those cryosystems that spray the cryogen directly onto the target tissue.

7.3.3 *Ambient Concentrations of Nitrous Oxide*—Ambient concentrations of nitrous oxide shall not exceed 25 ppm in accordance with the test procedure. (25 ppm is a recommended level as suggested by NIOSH 77-140. All nitrous oxide cryosystems shall be equipped with a gas collection system that can be conveniently routed for safe disposal. To minimize nitrous oxide exposure, the disposition of the gas collected and exhausted from the system is the responsibility of the user.)

7.3.4 *Test Method*—See Section 10.

7.4 *Thermal Insulation*:

7.4.1 The purpose of this requirement is to prevent accidental injury to both the user and the patient due to contact with the cold sections of a cryosystem.

7.4.2 Where feasible, the manufacturer is responsible for adequate insulation designed into the cryosystem to prevent accidental injury. See disclosure requirement in 6.2.1.

7.5 *Device Sterilization*:

7.5.1 The purpose of this requirement is to inform the user of sterilizing methods suitable for the cryosystem(s).

7.5.2 See disclosure requirement in 6.2.4.

7.6 *Safe Current Limits for Cryosystems*:

7.6.1 The purpose of this requirement is to protect the user or patient from electrical hazard.

7.6.2 All alternating-current (a-c) powered cryosystems shall meet at a minimum, the requirement in Table 2.

7.6.3 Refer to the IEC 601-1 for test procedures.

7.7 *Use in the Presence of Flammable Anesthetics*:

7.7.1 The purpose of this requirement is to eliminate the possibility of explosion due to the ignition of flammable

TABLE 2 Maximum Leakage Current

Direction	Normal	Patient Connections Micro Amps (A/C)	Chassis/Enclosure Micro Amps (A/C)
		Heart	(Ground/Open)
Source	50	10	100
Sink	50	10	N/A

anesthetics by cryosystems.

7.7.2 All ac powered cryosystems and accessories shall be prominently labeled as described in 6.2.5.

7.8 *Cryogen Cylinder Connector(s)*—All cryosystems that use a cryogen regulated by the CGA, shall meet all the requirements of CGA V-1 1977.

TEST METHODS

8. Significance and Use

8.1 Sections 9-13 specify test methods for selecting, using, calibrating, controlling, and maintaining measurement standards and measuring devices used to determine conformance with this specification.

8.2 All measuring devices or systems shall be used in a manner which ensure that measurement uncertainty is known and is consistent with the required measurement capability. Measurement errors shall be recorded or, where possible, eliminated by calibration of the measuring device.

9. Test Method for Mechanical Integrity

9.1 *Apparatus*:

9.1.1 *Timing Device* (for example, clock).

9.1.2 *Hydraulic or Pneumatic Pressure Testing System.*

9.1.3 *Other Components*, to make the cryosystem functional in accordance with the manufacturer's operational instructions.

9.2 *Sampling*—For cryosystems of the same model, test and record five individual systems. For limited production, or for a unique cryosystem, test and record one unit.

9.3 *Procedure*:

9.3.1 Connect and operate the cryosystem as described in the manufacturer's operating instructions.

9.3.2 Thermally cycle the cryosystem in air under no load through five stimulated freezing modes of 3 min duration, followed by five defrost modes of 5 min each. For disposable cryosystems, one freeze defrost mode expending the total cryogen shall be sufficient prior to pressure test.

9.3.3 Begin timing once the cryosystem has stabilized at the coldest operating temperature in the freeze mode and at ambient temperature in the defrost mode.

9.3.4 Pressure test the item under investigation immediately following the thermal cycling. (See 7.2).

9.4 *Conformance*—Conformance with the requirements (7.2) shall be checked by inspection of the cryosystem or any of its components for absence of adverse effects such as bursting, rupturing, leaking, or other indications which compromise the integrity of the cryosystem.

10. Test Method for Determining Ambient Concentration of Nitrous Oxide

10.1 *Apparatus*:

10.1.1 *Standard Test Room*, as described in Fig. 1.

10.1.1.1 *Room Volume*, 1000 cubic feet maximum, nominally 10 by 10 by 10 ft.

10.1.1.2 *Ceiling Height*, 7 ft minimum.

10.1.1.3 *Fan Flowrate*, 500–600 cu. ft/min, fixed position household fan style to circulate air is required.

10.1.1.4 *Infrared Spectrophotometer.* [9]

10.2 *Sampling*—For a cryosystem of a similar design, test one cryosystem in accordance with 10.4. This cryosystem shall be a representative sample of a currently marketed production system.

10.3 *Preparation of Apparatus*:

10.3.1 Locate fan one foot from two walls and floor to the center of the fan. Make sure the flow is parallel to the wall and floor.

10.3.2 The room is to be leaktight with essentially zero room air changes.

10.3.3 Place the entire cryosystem including nitrous oxide cylinders in geometric center of room and confine about center

[9] A Wilks Miran 1A Infrared Spectrophotometer has been found satisfactory for this purpose.

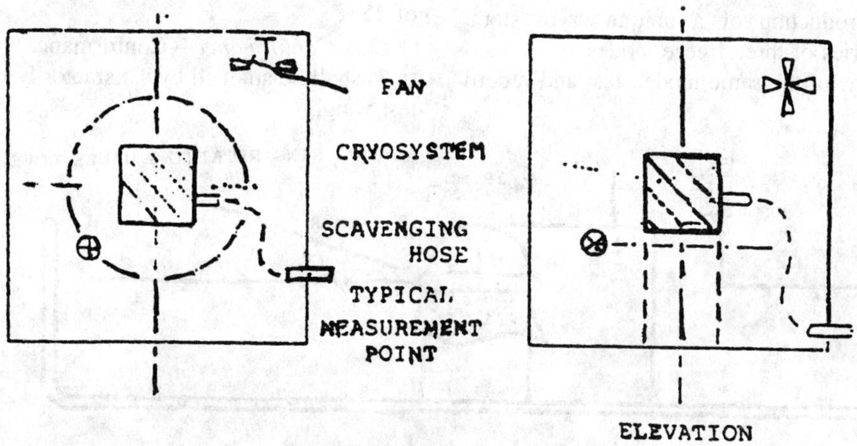

FIG. 1 Standard Test Room

1000 mL of distilled water at 30 ± 2°C. Brass weight: 60 g minimum.

as close as is practical.

10.3.4 Rout the scavenging hose out of the test room. Locate the sampling point at any point on a 3-ft radius from geometric center, 3 ft above floor level.

10.4 *Procedure*:

10.4.1 Position the cryosystem in the test room as specified in Fig. 1.

10.4.2 Turn on the circulating fan.

10.4.3 Zero and calibrate the spectrophotometer in accordance with the manufacturer's specification.

10.4.4 Monitor 12 data points at 1-min intervals. The total test for each cryosystem shall last 12 min.

10.4.5 Perform each test in accordance with the recommended operating procedure as specified in the cryosystem operational instructions.

10.4.6 Perform the test for two freeze modes of 3 min each, followed by two wait modes of 3 min each. The "wait" period shall consist of defrost, standby, or shut off modes in accordance with the manufacturer's recommended operating procedure.

10.4.7 To calculate the resultant ambient nitrous oxide concentration, average the readings from the 12 data points.

10.4.8 Vent the room of residual nitrous oxide gas prior to subsequent tests.

10.5 *Conformance*—Conformance with the requirements shall be checked by comparison of the calculated average nitrous oxide concentration with the maximum NIOSH recommended level of 25 ppm.

11. Test Method for Determining Closed Cryotip Temperature Reproducibility

11.1 *Apparatus*:

11.1.1 *Simulated Tissue Model*—The tissue model shall be 1000 mL of distilled water in a standard 1000-mL beaker. The water shall be maintained at 30 ± 2°C by a constant temperature bath. The water in the beaker shall not be circulated artificially during the actual test.

11.1.2 *Low Thermal Mass Thermocouple Sensor*.

11.1.3 *Temperature Indicator or Chart Recorder*.

11.1.4 *Other Components*, to make the cryosystem functional in accordance with the manufacturer's operational instructions.

11.2 *Sampling*:

11.2.1 For limited production of a unique cryosystem, perform and record a series of three freeze modes.

11.2.2 For cryosystems of the same model, test and record three individual systems.

11.2.3 Test in accordance with the requirements of Table 1.

11.3 *Procedure*:

11.3.1 Attach the thermocouple sensor to the therapeutic surface of the cryotip as determined by the manufacturer.

11.3.2 Immerse the closed cryotip into the simulated tissue model in a way which simulates the intended application as determined by the manufacturer.

11.3.3 Follow all parameters as described in the manufacturer's operational instructions to make the cryosystem functional.

11.3.4 Allow the cryotip to defrost between cycles.

11.3.5 Include disposable devices.

11.3.6 A precycle for the cryosystem to normalize operating conditions is permitted.

11.3.7 Calculate the reference temperature and limits of deviation from the recorded data.

11.4 *Conformance*—Conformance with the requirements (6.2.1) shall be checked by comparison of the deviation between the closed cryotip reference temperature and Table 1.

12. Tractive Force Test Method

12.1 *Apparatus*:

12.1.1 *Tractive Force Model*, as described in Fig. 2.

12.1.2 *Other Components*, to make the cryosystem functional in accordance with the manufacturer's operational instructions.

12.2 *Sampling*:

12.2.1 Test closed cryotips used for cryoadesion for tractive force. For limited production, or a unique cryosystem, perform and record a series of three cryoadhesion tests.

12.2.2 For cryosystems of the same model, test and record three individual cryosystems.

12.3 *Procedure*:

12.3.1 Place ambient temperature closed cryotip onto the top of the gauze covered weight.

12.3.2 Follow all normal operational procedures as described in the manufacturer's operational instructions.

12.3.3 Activate the cryosystem freeze mode.

12.3.4 When the cryotip has adhered sufficiently to the gauze, lift the weight out of the water, and hold for a minimum of 45 s.

12.4 *Conformance*—Conformance with the requirements (6.3) shall be attained by satisfactorily lifting and retaining the test weight.

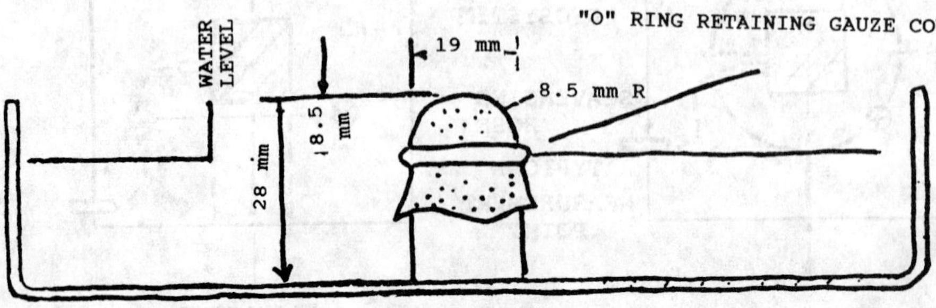

NOTE 1—All dimensions given are minimum values.

FIG. 2 Tractive Force Model

13. Test Method for Determining the Accuracy of Temperature Monitors (Cryotip and Tissue)

13.1 *Thermocouple Type*.

13.2 *Apparatus*:

13.2.1 *Direct-Current (d-c) Millivolt Generator*, with an output source resistance equivalent to the thermocouple resistance as specified by the manufacturer and a suitable test lead.

13.2.2 A method of measuring ambient or reference junction temperature.

13.2.3 *Thermocouple Reference Tables*, based on IPTS-68, refer to NBS Monograph 125.

13.2.4 *Direct-Current (d-c) Millivoltmeter*, and a suitable test lead.

13.2.5 *Calibration Medium*, such as ice/ice water, liquid nitrous oxide, dry ice, or liquid nitrogen.

13.3 *Sampling*—Test any cryosystem or accessory containing a cryometer for accuracy of temperature indication. For cryosystems of the same model, test and record three individual monitoring systems. For limited production, or a unique cryosystem, test and record each monitoring system. Accuracy may be checked as a complete monitoring system or by summing the cumulative errors of the cryometer and thermocouple tested individually. Testing shall be in accordance with the requirements of 5.4.2 for any temperature within the noted range.

13.4 *Procedure*:

13.4.1 *Determination of Cryometer Accuracy*:

13.4.1.1 Connect the test apparatus to the cryometer. Ensure that there is temperature uniformity. The reference ambient temperature shall be displayed on the measuring device located adjacent to, and preferably in thermal contact with, the reference junction.

13.4.1.2 With zero dc millivolts inserted via the test lead, the cryometer shall display the actual ambient temperature ±5°C.

NOTE 1—The cryometer may be calibrated to precisely display at 0°C, the cryogen boiling point, or any other specific operating temperature relevant to the intended use.

13.4.1.3 From the thermocouple tables, calculate the d-c millivolts signal equivalent to the calibration temperature relative to the reference ambient temperature, for the thermocouple type specified by the manufacturer. With the calculated d-c input voltage applied, the cryometer shall display the calibration temperature. Record the temperature deviation between the calibration temperature and the displayed value.

13.4.2 *Determination of Thermocouple Accuracy*:

13.4.2.1 Connect the d-c millivoltmeter to measure the thermocouple emf. The reference ambient temperature shall be displayed on the measuring device located adjacent to, and preferably in contact with, the reference junction. Ensure that there is temperature uniformity.

13.4.2.2 Insert the thermocouple measuring junction into the calibration medium and allow the temperature to stabilize. Measure the thermocouple electromotive force (emf).

13.4.2.3 From the thermocouple reference tables, calculate the emf value of the reference ambient temperature for the thermocouple type specified by the manufacturer. Subtract the reference ambient temperature emf from the value measured with the thermocouple in the test medium.

13.4.2.4 Determine the measuring junction temperature from the resultant emf according to the thermocouple reference tables.

13.4.2.5 Record the temperature deviation between the calibration medium temperature and the determined value.

13.5 *Conformance*—Conformance with the requirements (6.4) shall be checked by test.

Designation: F 895 – 84 (Reapproved 2001)$^{\epsilon 1}$

Standard Test Method for Agar Diffusion Cell Culture Screening for Cytotoxicity[1]

This standard is issued under the fixed designation F 895; the number immediately following the designation indicates the year of original adoption or, in the case of revision, the year of last revision. A number in parentheses indicates the year of last reapproval. A superscript epsilon (ε) indicates an editorial change since the last revision or reapproval.

This standard has been approved for use by agencies of the Department of Defense.

ϵ^1 NOTE—Editorial corrections were made throughout and keywords were added in June 2001.

1. Scope

1.1 This test method is appropriate for materials in a variety of shapes and for materials that are not necessarily sterile. This test method would be appropriate in situations in which the amount of material is limited. For example, small devices or powders could be placed on the agar and the presence of a zone of inhibition of cell growth could be examined.

1.1.1 This test method is not appropriate for leachables that do not diffuse through agar or agarose.

1.1.2 While the agar layer can act as a cushion to protect the cells from the specimen, there may be materials that are sufficiently heavy to compress the agar and prevent diffusion or to cause mechanical damage to the cells. This test method would not be appropriate for these materials.

1.2 The L-929 cell line was chosen because it has a significant history of use in assays of this type. This is not intended to imply that its use is preferred, only that the L-929 is an established cell line, well characterized and readily available, that has demonstrated reproducible results in several laboratories.

1.3 *This standard does not purport to address all of the safety concerns, if any, associated with its use. It is the responsibility of the user of this standard to establish appropriate safety and health practices and determine the applicability of regulatory limitations prior to use.*

2. Referenced Documents

2.1 *ASTM Standards:*

F 748 Practice for Selecting Generic Biological Test Methods for Materials and Devices[2]

2.2 *ATCC Document:*

American Type Culture Collection, (ATCC) Catalogue of Strains II[3]

USP Negative Control Plastic Reference Standard[4]

3. Summary of Test Method

3.1 Cell cultures are grown to a monolayer in culture dishes. The medium is aspirated and replaced with an agar-containing medium that is allowed to solidify. Test control articles are placed on the agar surface to evaluate the cytotoxic properties of a given material or device. Toxic components in the test article can diffuse into the culture medium forming a concentration gradient and adversely affecting cells at varying distances from the test article. This method is well suited for low-density materials (film, paper, and so forth), powders, liquids, and high-density materials that could physically damage the cells if placed in direct contact with the cell monolayer.

4. Significance and Use

4.1 This test method is useful for assessing the cytotoxic potential of new materials and formulations and as part of a quality control program for established medical devices and components.

4.2 This test method assumes that assessment of cytotoxicity provides useful information to aid in predicting the potential clinical applications in humans. Cell culture methods have shown good correlation with animal assays and are frequently more sensitive to cytotoxic agents.

4.3 This cell culture test method is suitable for incorporation into specifications and standards for materials to be used in the construction of medical devices that are to be implanted into the human body or placed in contact with tissue fluids or blood on a long-term basis.

4.4 Some biomaterials with a history of safe clinical use in medical devices are cytotoxic. This test method does not imply that all biomaterials must pass this assay to be considered safe for clinical use (Practice F 748).

5. Apparatus

5.1 The following apparatus shall be used:

5.2 *Incubator*, which maintains the cultures at 37 ± 2°C, 5 ± 1 % CO_2, and greater than 90 % relative humidity.

5.3 *Water Bath*, capable of maintaining a temperature of 37 ± 2°C and 45 ± 2°C.

5.4 *Microscope*, with inverted phase contrast optics and magnifications of 40, 100, and 200X.

5.5 *Clinical Centrifuge*, capable of attaining 1000 xg.

---

[1] This test method is under the jurisdiction of ASTM Committee F04 on Medical and Surgical Materials and Devices and is the direct responsibility of Subcommittee F04.16 on Biocompatibility Test Methods.

Current edition approved Sept. 28, 1984. Published February 1985.

[2] *Annual Book of ASTM Standards*, Vol 13.01.

[3] Fourth edition, 1983, is available from American Type Culture Collection, 12031 Parklawn Dr., Rockville, MD 10892. Library of Congress No. 76-640122.

[4] *U.S. Pharmacopeia*, current edition, Rockville, MD.

5.6 *Sterile, Disposable 150-cm² Tissue Culture Flasks.*

5.7 *Sterile, Tissue Culture Dishes*, 35 mm in diameter and 10 mm deep.

NOTE 1—Plastic dishes are recommended because they provide a flat surface that promotes the formation of a uniform monolayer of cells.

5.8 *Sterile, Disposable, Centrifuge Tubes.*

5.9 *Sterile Pipettes*, 1, 5, and 10 mL.

5.10 *Filter Disks*, 10 mm in diameter for evaluation of liquids.

NOTE 2—Millipore AP2501000 filter disks have been found satisfactory for use in cytotoxicity evaluations because they elicit no cytopathic effect. Other filter disks that do not elicit a cytopathic effect may also be used.

NOTE 3—A laminar flow work area capable of filtering out 99.99 % of all particles greater than 0.3 μm in diameter, or a Class 100 clean room may be necessary to prevent contamination of cultures.

6. Reagents

6.1 The following reagents shall be used:

6.1.1 *For Cell Culture Maintenance*, 1X Media. Minimum Essential Medium (MEM) is prepared by mixing 90-mL Eagle's MEM (with Earle's salts, without L-glutamine), adjust solution to pH 7.15, add 5- to 10-mL fetal bovine serum, and 1-mL 100X nonessential amino acids (L-glutamine).

6.1.1.1 Opened containers of prepared MEM may be stored at a temperature of 2 to 8°C for periods of not more than two weeks. Glutamine is omitted from this formulation to maximize the shelf life. Immediately before use, 1 mL of L-glutamine solution (see 6.1.3) is added to each 100 mL of MEM.

6.1.1.2 Antibiotics, such as penicillin G10 000 I.U./mL, and streptomycin 10 000 I.U./mL, may be added to the medium to reduce thc incidence of bacterial contamination. Use 1 mL of antibiotic per 100-mL media. Care shall be taken to ensure that the antibiotics do not have an adverse effect on the viability of the cell cultures.

6.1.2 *For Agar Media Overlay*, to prepare 2X Media (100-mL final volume). Twice concentrated (2X) MEM is prepared by mixing 20 mL of 10X Eagle's MEM (with Earle's Salts without L-glutamine), 0.22-g sodium bicarbonate (buffer) and sterile distilled water to bring to 70 % volume (70 mL). Adjust pH to 7.15. Add 20-mL fetal bovine serum and 2-mL 100X nonessential amino acid (L-glutamine). Bring to final volume (100 mL) with sterile distilled water. Filter sterilize the 2X media. Mix with equal amounts of sterilized 3 % agar nobel to give the final concentration of the media as 1X.

6.1.3 *L-Glutamine Solution (Lyophilized)*, 29.2 mg/mL. Rehydrate with sterile distilled water. (Store frozen.)

6.1.4 *Hanks' Balanced Salt Solution*, calcium- and magnesium-free (store at room temperature).

6.1.5 *Trypsin*, 0.1 % solution in Hanks' balanced salt solution or calcium- and magnesium-free, phosphate-buffered saline (store frozen).

6.1.6 *Water*, sterile, deionized, or distilled water should be used.

6.1.7 *Noble Agar*, 3 %.

6.1.8 *Neutral Red Stain*, 0.01 % by weight in phosphate-buffered saline.

6.2 All reagents shall be tissue-culture grade or equivalent.

6.3 Reagents shall be reconstituted in accordance with the manufacturer's directions, using aseptic technique.

7. Cell Culture

7.1 Cell cultures used in this assay shall be the ATCC, CCL I NCTC clone 929 strain (clone of Strain L, mouse connective tissue) designated L-929. Other suitable validated cell lines may be considered.

8. Control Materials

8.1 Prepare negative control specimens in accordance with Section 10 from a material that consistently elicits negligible cellular response in this assay (for example, USP Negative Control Plastic Reference Standard).

8.2 Prepare positive control specimens in accordance with Section 10 from a material that consistently elicits a moderate and reproducible degree of cytotoxicity (for example, an aqueous solution of phenol (0.45 ± 0.05 % by volume), or other material producing a known cytotoxic response, for example, latex rubber).

8.2.1 Use an aqueous solution of phenol to give a diffuse reaction of cellular degeneration and sloughing; a latex rubber will give a zone of toxicity.

8.2.2 Take care when preparing aqueous solutions of phenol to ensure the homogeneity of the solution since phase separations may occur.

8.2.3 Latex rubber is a widely used control material that has demonstrated reproducible results in several laboratories.

9. General Technique

9.1 Use aseptic technique throughout this assay to minimize microbial contamination.

NOTE 4—Mouth pipetting should not be used to transfer cells, medium, or reagents.

9.2 Warm all solutions and material to a temperature of 37 ± 2°C before being placed in contact with cells.

9.3 Wash all glass vessels thoroughly with a cleaning solution and rinse thoroughly with copious amounts of deionized water.

9.4 Clean all work surfaces with a disinfectant solution before use.

9.5 Record the culture history of the cells.

9.6 Stock cultures should be periodically screened for mycoplasma contamination.

10. Specimen Preparation

10.1 Sterilize all specimens by a method appropriate to the end use of the device.

10.2 Where a device is sufficiently small (see 10.3 and 10.4) to fit into the culture dish leaving an adequate margin of cells for evaluation, use the entire device as a specimen.

10.3 Cut large solid materials and devices in cross section to obtain a flat surface having an area of 100 to 250 mm² to be placed in direct contact with the agar surface.

10.4 Prepare specimens of rod or tubing or of rod- or tube-shaped devices as follows:

10.4.1 Where the diameter is less than 6.4 mm, cut 5 to 15 mm in length.

10.4.2 Where the diameter is 6.4 to 15 mm, cut 2 to 8 mm in length.

10.4.3 Where the diameter exceeds 15 mm, prepare cross sections as described in 10.3.

10.5 Obtain specimens from larger medical items from locations with relatively large cross sections to expose interior material.

10.6 If a device is constructed of two or more materials that are intended to contact body fluids or tissues, either cut the test specimen from the materials' interface or test separate specimens of each material or both.

10.7 Prepare specimens for evaluating the cytotoxicity of liquids or extracts by saturating a sterile filter disk and allowing the excess liquid to drain off while maintaining asepsis. Use the saturated filter disk as a test specimen.

NOTE 5—When ethylene oxide or other chemical sterilants are used, adequate aeration time should be determined to permit dissipation of residues which may adversely affect the results recorded in this assay.

NOTE 6—In general, specimens should be cleaned to remove any residues from specimen preparation and sterilized after they have been cut to size. If the specimen is very hard (for example, ceramics), care should be taken to remove the residues that may be left on the freshly cut surface by the cutting tool. When evaluating the cytotoxic potential of medical materials or devices that are contained in the final sterile package, resterilization, further processing, or delay between the time of opening the package and starting the test must be avoided. With small items, the entire content of the sterile package may be used as the test specimen. When the size of the sterile packaged item is too large, an appropriate, representative, small-sized specimen must be obtained. The application of this assay to items in the final sterile package is limited to items that are small or can be cut and reshaped using aseptic technique.

10.8 Absorbant materials tested in this method must be prewetted with culture medium to prevent loss of water from the agar and subsequent cellular damage.

11. Cell Culture Maintenance

11.1 Use the following procedures to maintain the cells by serial subculture:

11.2 Aspirate the medium from a 150-cm^2 cell culture flask containing a near-confluent monolayer.

11.3 Rinse the cells with a sufficient volume of Hanks' balanced salt solution to remove residual serum (for example, 5 to 10 mL).

11.4 Aspirate the rinse solution.

11.5 Add a sufficient volume of trypsin solution (0.1 %) to the flask to cover the cell monolayer (approximately 5 mL).

11.6 Incubate for 5 to 10 min to suspend the cells.

11.7 Transfer the cell suspension to a centrifuge tube.

11.8 Centrifuge at 1300 xg for 6 min.

11.9 Discard the supernatant.

11.10 Resuspend the cells in 10 ± 0.1 mL of fresh medium and mix the suspension thoroughly.

11.11 Distribute the cell suspension equally among each of two to eight 150-cm^2 tissue culture flasks.

11.12 Add a sufficient volume of fresh medium so that each flask will contain approximately 50 mL.

11.13 Change the medium every two to three days until the monolayer is nearly confluent, then repeat Steps 11.2-11.12.

12. Cell Layer Preparation

12.1 Prepare confluent cell monolayers as follows:

12.2 Follow Steps 11.1-11.9 to prepare a cell suspension.

12.3 Add 2.0 ± 0.1 mL of medium to each culture dish.

12.4 Using a sterile 10-mL serological pipette, add five to seven drops of cell suspension to each dish. Rotate the dishes to ensure even distribution of cells.

12.5 Incubate until a near-confluent monolayer has formed, as observed by microscopic examination.

NOTE 7—The formation of a near-confluent monolayer usually requires three to five days. By counting cells with a hemacytometer (to ensure the concentration of the inoculum), the time required for monolayer formulation may be regulated. A cell concentration of 1.3×10^5 cells/mL will give a consistent time of 24 h.

12.6 If cell suspension remains unused after Step 12.3, a subculture may be prepared by adding 9 mL of fresh medium to each millilitre of cell suspension in a cell culture flask with a surface area of approximately 3 cm^2 for each millilitre of diluted cells and incubating it until a near-confluent monolayer has formed, as determined by microscopic examination.

13. Test Procedure

13.1 Perform the agar diffusion cytotoxicity assay as follows:

13.2 Microscopically examine the cell cultures and reject any in which the cell monolayer is not of correct confluency or the cells show signs of granulation or sloughing.

13.3 Autoclave 3 % Nobel Agar for 15 min at 121°C.

13.4 Place the autoclaved agar into a 45°C waterbath and allow it to cool to 45°C.

13.5 Place 2X MEM into a 45°C waterbath and allow it to warm to 45°C. Do not allow the medium to remain at 45°C longer than 1 h.

13.6 Mix equal volumes of the 2X MEM and 3 % Nobel Agar thoroughly. Allow the mixture to cool to approximately 39°C.

13.7 Aspirate the medium from all acceptable cultures, and replace it with 2.0 mL of agar medium.

13.8 Place the cultures on a flat surface to solidify at room temperature.

13.9 Place a single test or control specimen in each dish in contact with the agar surface. Prepare duplicate cultures for each test material and both positive and negative controls.

NOTE 8—This method may be modified by using larger culture dishes to accommodate the positive and negative control specimens in the same dish as the test specimen. Quantities of cells and reagents must be increased appropriately if larger dishes are used.

13.10 Incubate all cultures for 24 ± 1 h.

13.11 Mark the outline of the specimen on the bottom of the culture dish with a permanent marker, and then remove the specimen.

13.12 Add 2 mL of Neutral Red solution to each dish and incubate for 1 h.

13.13 Pour off the Neutral Red solution and examine each culture microscopically under and around each control and test specimen.

14. Evaluation of Results

14.1 A cell culture shall be deemed to show a cytotoxic effect if microscopic examination reveals malformation, degeneration, sloughing, or lysis of the cells within the zone or a moderate to severe reduction in cell layer density.

14.2 The Zone Index (Table 1) measures the clear zone in which cells do not stain with neutral red.

14.3 The Lysis Index (Table 2) measures the number of cells affected within the zone of toxicity.

NOTE 9—A slight reduction of cell layer density is acceptable, provided there is no other evidence of cytotoxicity as specified in 14.1.

14.4 A Response Index may be determined by assigning a fraction with the Zone Index in the numerator and the Lysis Index in the denominator to each specimen (RI = ZI/LI).

$$\text{Response Index} = \frac{\text{Zone Index (0–5)}}{\text{Lysis Index (0–5)}} \quad (1)$$

The response index should be reported as a fraction, for example, 3/2.

14.5 If, for a given set of specimens, a cytotoxic effect is observed for the negative controls or no cytotoxic effect is elicited by the positive controls, the results for that set of specimens shall be considered invalid.

15. Report

15.1 The report of the assay results shall include, but not be limited to the following information:

TABLE 1 Zone Description

Zone Index	Description of Zone
0	No detectable zone around or under specimen
1	Zone limited to area under specimen
2	Zone extends less than 0.5 cm beyond specimen
3	Zone extends 0.5 to 1.0 cm beyond specimen
4	Zone extends greater than 1.0 cm beyond specimen but does not involve entire dish
5	Zone involves entire dish

TABLE 2 Lysis Description

Lysis Index	Description of Zone
0	No observable cytotoxicity
1	Less than 20 % of zone affected
2	20 to 39 % of zone affected
3	40 to 59 % of zone affected
4	60 to 80 % of zone affected
5	Greater than 80 % of zone affected

15.2 Test date.

15.3 Cell strain used.

15.4 Medium used (noting whether antibiotics were used).

15.5 A description of all test and control specimens, including:

15.5.1 Material or device name (including ASTM specification number, where appropriate).

15.5.2 Lot or batch number.

15.5.3 Source of supply.

15.5.4 Size and method of preparation.

15.5.5 Method of sterilization.

15.6 Numerical values for Zone Index, Lysis Index, and Response Index.

15.7 Any other pertinent observations, including any deviations from the exact method described herein.

16. Precision and Bias

16.1 Quantitative precision and bias have not yet been determined for this standard.

17. Keywords

17.1 agar diffusion; biocompatibility; cell culture; cytotoxicity testing

APPENDIX

(Nonmandatory Information)

X1. Rationale

X1.1 Laboratory cell culture methods provide a rapid method for assessment of cytotoxic potential of both finished medical devices and materials used in their construction. The agar diffusion method is but one of several such techniques that are in common use. The cell culture method described in this standard is a modification of methods that have been routinely used for decades. A positive control that produces a cytopathic effect and a negative control that produces no cytopathic effect are assayed with each test to assure that the cell cultures have expected cytotoxicity responses. Test results are considered valid only when the expected responses for both controls are obtained.

REFERENCES

(1) Guess, W. L., Rosenbluth, S. A., Schmidt, B., and Autian, J., "Agar Diffusion Method for Toxicity Screening of Plastics on Cultured Cell Monolayers," *Journal of Pharmaceutical Science*, Vol 54, 1965, pp. 1545–1547.

(2) Wilsnack, R. E., Meyer, F. S., and Smith, J. G., "Human Cell Culture Toxicity Testing of Medical Devices and Correlation to Animal Tests," *Biomaterials Medical Devices and Artificial Organs*, Vol 1, 1973, pp. 543–562.

(3) Autian, J., "New Fields of Plastic Toxicology—Methods and Results," *Critical Reviews in Toxicology*, Vol 2, CRC Press, Inc.

Designation: F 896 – 90 (Reapproved 1999)

Standard Specification for Flexible Fiberoptic Bronchoscopes[1]

This standard is issued under the fixed designation F 896; the number immediately following the designation indicates the year of original adoption or, in the case of revision, the year of last revision. A number in parentheses indicates the year of last reapproval. A superscript epsilon (ε) indicates an editorial change since the last revision or reapproval.

1. Scope

1.1 This specification covers definitions, requirements, and methods of test for flexible fiberoptic bronchoscope and certain endoscopic accessories used in the practice of medicine.

1.2 *Field of Application*—The standard applies to medical flexible fiberoptic bronchoscopes, those endoscopes accessories through which these bronchoscopes are used and those endoscopic accessories which are passed through these bronchoscopes in use.

2. Terminology

2.1 *Definitions:*

2.1.1 *bronchoscope*—a medical instrument having viewing means with or without optics introduced into the lung for examination, diagnosis, and/or therapy.

2.1.2 *endoscopic accessory*—a medical instrument inserted into a natural or surgically created body opening through which an endoscope is inserted; or a medical instrument inserted through or with an endoscope for examination, diagnosis or therapy.

2.1.3 *rigid endoscope or endoscopic accessory*— an endoscope or endoscopic accessory whose insertion portion is intended to be unyielding to natural or surgically created body cavities, or instrument lumens.

2.1.4 *flexible endoscope or endoscopic accessory*— an endoscope or endoscopic accessory whose insertion portion is intended to conform to natural or surgically created body cavities, or instrument lumens.

2.1.5 *distal*—refers to the location of that portion of an endoscope or endoscopic accessory which is farther from the user than some referenced point.[2]

2.1.6 *proximal*—refers to the location of that portion of an endoscope or endoscopic accessory which is closer to the user than some referenced point.

2.1.7 *insertion portion*—that portion of an endoscope or endoscopic accessory which is intended to be inserted into a natural or surgically created body opening; or which is intended to be inserted into the lumen of an endoscope or endoscopic accessory.[3]

2.1.8 *maximum insertion portion width*—the maximum external width of endoscopes or endoscopic accessories throughout the length of the insertion portion.

2.1.9 *minimum lumen width*—the minimum internal width at any endoscope or endoscopic accessory lumen through which an endoscope or endoscopic accessory is intended to pass.[4]

2.1.10 *working length*—the maximum length of the insertion portion.

2.1.11 *field of view*—the size of the object field viewed through a bronchoscope and is stated by the vertex angle (in degrees) of the cone whose vertex is at the distal window surface of the endoscope. (See Fig. 1.) The endoscope is not intended to be in contact with the object.

2.1.12 *Discussion*—These two definitions, (2.1.11 and 2.1.13) as illustrated, describe characteristics of endoscopes paramount for effective use, with the endoscopist selecting instruments of specific values for particular medical purposes. The field of view is not appropriate when the endoscope is intended to be in contact with the object.

2.1.13 *direction of view*—the location of the center of the object field relative to the normal axis of the bronchoscope and stated as the angle in degrees between the normal axis of the endoscope (0) and the center of the field of view. (See Fig. 2 and 2.1.11.)

2.1.14 *controllable portion*—that part of insertion portion of an endoscope or endoscopic accessory whose motion is intended to be remotely controlled by the user.

2.1.15 *Discussion*—Many endoscopes, both rigid and flexible, incorporate provisions for user remote control of the motion of the distal tip. The mechanisms for these controls vary widely; and are obviously of interest to the user. These include, for example, distal tips of flexible endoscopes and elevators of rigid and flexible endoscopes. In order to avoid constraining future designs, control characteristics are defined in the most general terms.

3. Characteristic Requirements

3.1 The maximum insertion portion width shall not be larger

---

[1] This specification is under the jurisdiction of ASTM Committee F-29 on Anesthetic and Respiratory Equipmentand is the direct responsibility of Subcommittee F29.13on Laryngoscopes and Bronchoscopes .

Current edition approved Dec. 28, 1990. Published March 1991.

[2] These terms, commonly used in endoscopy are defined in their most general form to avoid the need for such definitions as: "distal tip"," distal end", "area proximal to ...", "X cm, distal the ...".

[3] Although the terms defined seem self-explanatory, different expressions for the same portion of the instrument are used by different manufacturers; hence, the appropriateness of a definition.

[4] By defining external sizes as maximums and lumen sizes as minimums, sufficient instrument selection information will be provided to practitioners.

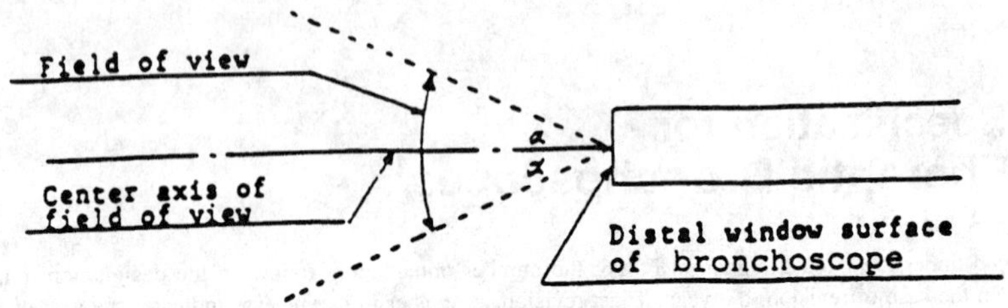

FIG. 1 Field of View

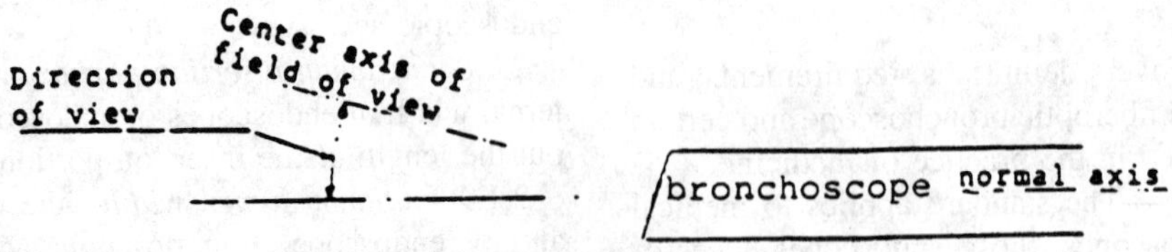

FIG. 2 Direction of View

than that stated by the manufacturer (see Note 1).

3.2 The minimum lumen width shall not be smaller than that stated by the manufacturer (see Note 1).

3.3 Insertion portion width and lumen width units shall be millimeters. Working length units shall be metric.

NOTE 1—These sizes are given to help the user to select the procedures which may be carried out with the instrument. Compatibility of instruments combination requires, however a certain clearance between the insertion portion width and the lumen width; the clearance required depending on the form, length and property of the instruments. There is no guarantee that the instruments combination selected solely by this criteria will be compatible.

3.4 Endoscopes and endoscopic accessories shall conform to relevant electrical safety standards.

NOTE 2—Users have reported that shocks and/or burns are a potential hazard when endoscopes and endoscopic accessories are connected to electromedical accessories such as electrosurgical units, pumps and light sources. Although electromedical accessories are beyond the scope of this standard, it is recognized that endoscopes, endoscopic accessories or portions thereof are conductors of or insulators from electrical energy; and, as such, can contribute to the reported hazard. As the need for explicit requirements becomes apparent, such requirements will be proposed for inclusion in subsequent revisions of this standard.

3.5 When tested in accordance with Section 4.2, a solid steel ball bearing, having a diameter equal to the minimum lumen width specified by the bronchoscope manufacturer, shall pass through the entire length of the operating lumen, while the bronchoscope is flexed to the minimum radius or maximum deflection angle specified by the manufacturer, with no applied force other than due to gravity. If any other lumen preconditioning is specified by the manufacturer such preconditioning shall also apply to this test (see Note 3).

NOTE 3—This requirement is intended to assure forceps passage during maximum deflection of the bronchoscope. According to a study performed by the Emergency Care Research Institute, difficulty in passing the forceps is a common problem which can degrade the procedure. (See above reference.) A ball bearing is used, in preference to forceps, because it isolates the effects due to collapse or deformation of the lumen from the effects due to stiffness of the forceps.

4. Test Methods

4.1 *Dimensional characteristics*:

4.1.1 The dimensional characteristics in 4 shall be verified by measuring instruments whose calibration is traceable to international standards.

NOTE 4—Specific test methods can impose real design constraints; however, test methods must be developed which can evolve over time into viable standard test methods. There must be some traceability of calibration of test instruments to standards in order to resolve issues of dimensional anomalies.

4.2 Forceps passage shall be tested as follows:

4.2.1 Attach the bronchoscope to the test fixture shown in Fig. 3. The bronchoscope should be positioned such that it's controllable portion is flexed to the minimum radius or maximum deflection angle specified by the manufacturer.

4.2.2 If any other lumen preconditioning is specified by the manufacturer such preconditioning shall also apply to this test.

4.2.3 Rotate the fixture to the position which directs the proximal portion of the bronchoscope upward.

4.2.4 Place a solid steel ball bearing, having a diameter equal to the minimum lumen width specified by the bronchoscope manufacturer, within the proximal end of the lumen.

4.2.5 Rotate the fixture in the direction which would cause the bearing to pass through the bronchoscope, motivated only

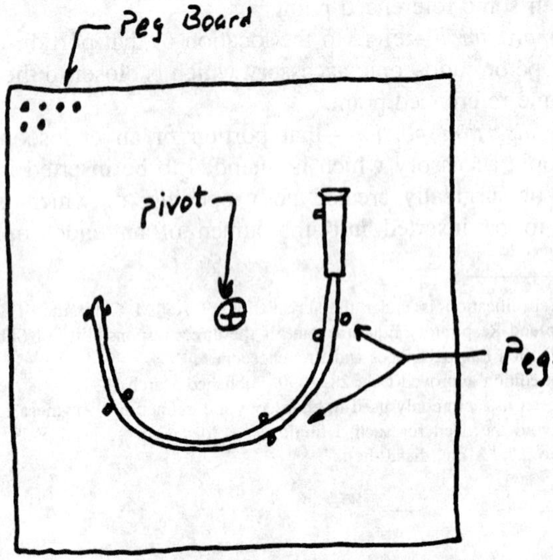

FIG. 3 Text for Forceps Passage

by the effect of gravity, until the bearing emerges from the distal end of the lumen.

4.2.6 Repeat 4.2.1-4.2.5 for each direction of tip deflection specified by manufacturer.

5. Marking, Labeling and Packaging

5.1 *Marking*:

5.1.1 *Instrument marking*—Each individual endoscope and endoscopic accessory shall have the following minimum marking: (see Note 5).

5.1.1.1 Catalog number and/or other mark sufficient to identify the instrument and its manufacturer.

5.1.1.2 Maximum insertion portion width, minimum lumen width, working length, field of view and/or direction of view where such identification is necessary for the intended use of the endoscope or endoscopic accessory.

NOTE 5—The identification of the instrument and insertion portion or lumen widths are sufficient to permit the user to select the appropriate instrument when necessary. All other instrument marking should be determined by the manufacturer providing that such marking, where appropriate for the user's information, is identified in the instrument labeling.

5.1.2 *Marking legibility*—The marking required in 5.1.1 shall remain legible throughout the expected life of the instrument when it is used, cleaned, disinfected, sterilized and stored in accordance with the manufacturer's labeling (see Note 6).

NOTE 6—The primary requirement of instrument marking is that it be legible. Any more detailed requirements on marking methods, materials, sizes and other characteristics are design solutions which could inhibit design and process innovation.

5.1.3 *Marking exceptions*—When the marking required in 5.1.1 and 5.1.2 is impossible to achieve due to instrument size or configuration, the required marking shall accompany the instrument.

NOTE 7—Design innovation in the trend toward smaller endoscopes and endoscopic accessories would be seriously inhibited without such a marking exception. The substitute requirement in such cases assures the objectives of the marking requirements.

5.2 *Labeling* (see Note 8)—The manufacturer of endoscopes or endoscopic accessories shall provide the user with labeling containing the following minimum information.

5.2.1 A statement of intended uses of the instrument.

5.2.2 Instructions on the functions and proper use of the instrument.

5.2.3 An annotated illustration of the instrument as appropriate to permit the user to identify pertinent parts and characteristics of the instrument which are referenced in the labeling and are consistent with Section 2 of this document.

5.2.4 The identification and specifications of the instrument including the following:

5.2.4.1 Manufacturer or distributor name and address.

5.2.4.2 Instrument catalog number and catalog name.

5.2.4.3 Maximum insertion portion width and working length.

5.2.4.4 The field of view, excluding any reference indicators and the direction of view; and the medium (if other than air) for which the claims are made.

5.2.4.5 The remote controls and the associated controllable portion positions available to the user.

NOTE 8—A significant number of hazards and performance problems of endoscopes and endoscopic accessories are best addressed by user education. The objective of the labeling section requirements are to provide a part of the user education process without engaging in the practice of medicine.

5.2.4.6 Identification of any user replaceable parts and instructions for their replacement.

5.2.4.7 Identification of where the user can obtain authorized service on the instrument.

5.2.4.8 Minimum lumen width of each instrument.

5.2.5 Instructions as required for assembling the instrument for its intended uses and for the disassembling of the instrument and reassembling after cleaning, disinfection and/or sterilization processes.

5.2.6 Cautions and instructions applicable in the intended uses of the instrument, including those related to electrical, electronic, electro-optical, or electromedical apparatus intended to be used with the instrument.

5.2.7 Inspection instructions to provide reasonable assurance that the instrument is in working order.

5.2.8 Instructions for the cleaning of reusable instruments including cleaning agents which can be used and identification of any specific cleaning tools or equipment.

5.2.9 The specific disinfection and sterilization environments which the equipment can survive.

5.2.10 Recommended procedures for the storage of the instrument prior to use and for reusable instruments, between uses.

5.3 *Packaging* (see Note 9)—The manufacturer shall package the instrument in a manner to protect the instrument from the adverse effects of shipping environments.

NOTE 9—Problems due to improper packaging have been reported. Rather than impose innovation limiting design requirements on the manufacturer, we believe that the disclosure approach cited above is more appropriate.

Designation: F 897 – 84 (Reapproved 1997)

Standard Test Method for Measuring Fretting Corrosion of Osteosynthesis Plates and Screws[1]

This standard is issued under the fixed designation F 897; the number immediately following the designation indicates the year of original adoption or, in the case of revision, the year of last revision. A number in parentheses indicates the year of last reapproval. A superscript epsilon (ε) indicates an editorial change since the last revision or reapproval.

1. Scope

1.1 This test method provides a screening test for determining the amount of metal loss from plates and screws used for osteosynthesis (internal fixation of broken bones) due to fretting corrosion in the contact area between the screw head and the plate hole countersink area. The implants are used in the form they would be used clinically. The machine described generates a relative motion between plates and screws which simulates one type of motion pattern that can occur when these devices are used clinically.

1.2 Since the environmental and stress conditions used in this test may not be identical to those experienced by bone plates in the human body, this test may produce fretting corrosion rates that are lower or higher than those experienced in practice. The recommended axial load of 400 N was selected as being in a range where the amount of fretting corrosion is not sensitive to small changes in axial load **(1)**.[2] The combination of the recommended load and angular displacement are such that a measurable amount of fretting corrosion of surgical alloys occurs in a comparatively short period of time (7 to 14 days). **(1-3)**

1.3 The device is designed so as to facilitate sterilization of the test specimens and test chambers to permit testing with proteinaceous solutions that would become contaminated with microbial growth in nonsterile conditions.

1.4 The specimens used can be standard osteosynthesis implants or can be materials fabricated into the appropriate shapes.

1.5 This test method may be used for testing the fretting corrosion of metal plates and screws of similar or different alloy compositions, or it may be used for testing the fretting corrosion of metal-nonmetal combinations. This test method may also be used for wear or degradation studies of nonmetallic materials. This test may be used as a screening test to rank the corrosivities of saline or proteinaceous solutions, or to rank metal-to-metal couples for resistance to fretting corrosion, or to study other material combinations.

1.6 *This standard may involve hazardous materials, operations, and equipment. This standard does not purport to address all of the safety concerns associated with its use. It is the responsibility of whoever uses this standard to consult and establish appropriate safety and health practices and determine the applicability of regulatory limitations prior to use.*

2. Referenced Documents

2.1 *ASTM Standards:*

D 1886 Test Methods for Nickel in Water[3]

F 86 Practice for Surface Preparation and Marking of Metallic Surgical Implants[4]

F 367 Specification for Holes and Slots for Inch Cortical Bone Screws[4]

F 543 Specification for Cortical Bone Screws[4]

G 1 Practice for Preparing, Cleaning, and Evaluating Corrosion Test Specimens[5]

3. Summary of Test Method

3.1 A two-hole plate is attached to two plastic rods with bone screws, with flexible spacers between the plate and the rods, placed in a glass beaker, and the beaker sealed with a flexible rubber cover. This assembly is steam sterilized, and then a sterile solution is injected through the rubber cover into the beaker. This assembly is then mounted in the fretting apparatus which, when set in motion, produces a rocking motion and, therefore, a small cyclic displacement between the mating surfaces of the plate and screws. The amount of fretting corrosion is determined at the end of the test by measurement of the weight loss of the plates and screws and by chemical analysis of the solutions.

4. Significance and Use

4.1 It is well known from examination of implants after use that plates and screws used for osteosynthesis are subjected to metal loss due to corrosion at the plate-screw interfaces. One of the mechanisms of this corrosive attack is fretting corrosion due to relative motion (micromotion) between the screw heads and plate-hole countersinks.

4.2 It is also known that release of corrosion products into the tissues surrounding an implant may have adverse effects on

---

[1] This test method is under the jurisdiction of ASTM Committee F-4 on Medical and Surgical Materials and Devicesand is the direct responsibility of Subcommittee F04.15 on Material Test Methods.

Current edition approved Sept. 28, 1984. Published February 1985.

[2] The **boldface** numbers in parentheses refer to the list of references at the end of this standard.

[3] *Annual Book of ASTM Standards,* Vol 11.01.

[4] *Annual Book of ASTM Standards,* Vol 13.01.

[5] *Annual Book of ASTM Standards,* Vol 03.02.

local tissue or have systemic effects. Thus, it is important to minimize the amount of tissue exposure to corrosion products.

4.3 Screws and plates are available in different configurations in accordance with Specifications F 543 and F 367. This test method may be used to evaluate the effects of different combinations of screw and plate designs. As new materials and device designs are developed for use in the treatment of fractured bones, it is important to determine the effects these developments have on the amount of metal loss due to fretting corrosion.

4.4 This test method provides a standardized screening test for ranking metal plates and screws in terms of resistance to fretting corrosion and for determining the influence of different solutions on fretting corrosion rates.

4.5 This test method may also be used to generate corrosion products either for chemical analysis of the products or for testing for biological reactions to corrosion products using animal or cell culture methods.

4.6 It is well known that fretting corrosion rates depend on normal load or pressure, frequency, sliding amplitude, materials, surface treatments, and environmental factors. **(4)** Therefore, when determining the effect of changing one of these parameters (for example, material or environment), all others must be kept constant to facilitate interpretation of the results.

5. Apparatus

5.1 *Steam Autoclave*, capable of maintaining 121 ± 2°C (250 ± 4°F), and equipped with a thermometer, pressure gage, vent cock, and a rack to hold the test assemblies above the water level.

5.2 *Microbalance*, with a 0.01-mg scale.

5.3 *Fretting Apparatus*, as described in 5.3.1-5.3.4 and illustrated in Fig. 1.

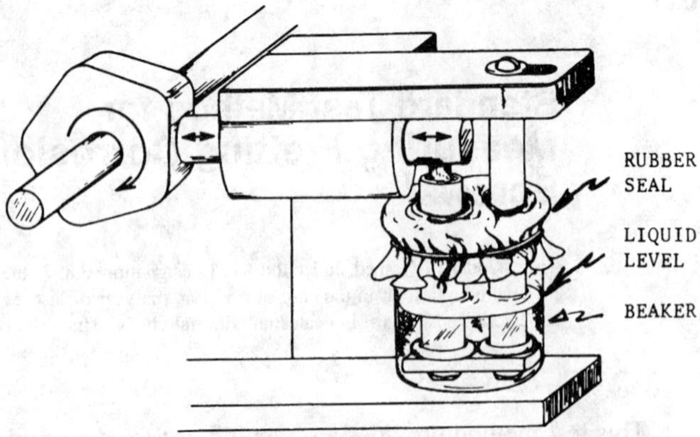

FIG. 2 Assembled Test Chamber with Rubber Seal

5.3.1 The fretting apparatus is driven by a slow speed gear motor connected to a horizontal rotating shaft. Round disks with machined flats (cams) are mounted on the shaft as shown in Fig. 1. For multiple specimen testing, there may be more than one cam on the drive shaft.

5.3.2 The flats on the cams are machined so as to produce 2° of relative motion between the posts of the test assemblies.

NOTE 1—A suggested combination of short post length and plunger displacement is a 5-cm post with a 1.9-mm displacement.

5.3.3 The shaft rotation rate and the number of machined flats shall be such that the flats produce one oscillation of the plunger per second.

5.3.4 Test assembly holding and driving frames are mounted symmetrically on each side of the rotating cams. The oscillating plunger is springloaded and held in the guide sleeve. The hole in the top plate is slotted to permit adjustment of the position of the test assemblies.

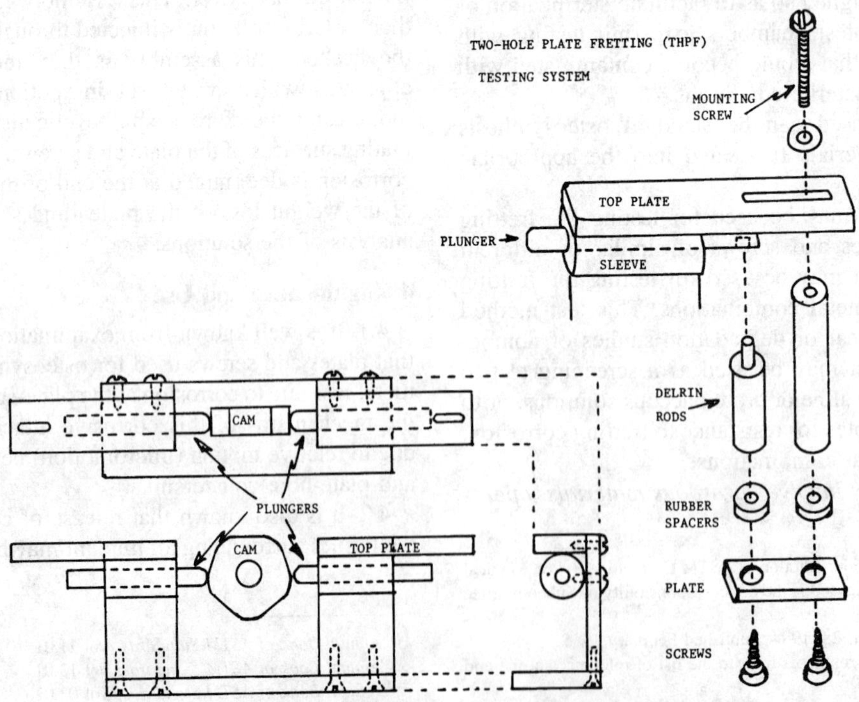

NOTE 1—Figure shows assembly drawings of one pair of test positions on each side of a cam, and of the relationships between the screws, plate, spacers, and polyacetal rods.

FIG. 1 Two-Hole Plate Fretting (THPF) Testing System

5.4 *Test Assemblies*, consisting of two plastic rods, and two flexible spacers, the two-hole plate, two bone screws, one beaker, and the rubber cover.

5.4.1 The longer rod is threaded at one end to mate with a mounting screw, while the other end is threaded to mate with the bone screw.

5.4.2 The shorter rod has a reduced diameter at one end to mate with the oscillating horizontal plunger, while the other end is threaded to mate with a bone screw.

5.4.3 The flexible spacers made of, for example, polydimethylsiloxane or buna-n, are used to maintain axial loads on the screws and to permit the necessary axial displacements associated with the rocking motion of the screws, while at the same time preventing fatigue failure of the screws. The screws are tightened such that there is a 400 ± 50 N load on the screws; a different load may be used, but in such cases the load must be reported (see 10.1). In actual operation, it may be easier to measure the screw torque rather than the axial load; a method for determining the relationships between torque and load is given in Appendix X2.

5.4.4 *Test Specimen Plates and Screws*, as described in Section 7.

5.4.5 *Beakers*, autoclavable borosilicate glass.

5.4.6 *Rubber Cover*, made from a thin piece of flexible rubber with two holes punched out to make a tight fit around the plastic rods. Heavy gage (0.3 mm thick) latex dental dam has been used effectively for this purpose. The cover is secured to the beaker with wire, rubber bands, or by some other appropriate device.

6. Reagents and Materials

6.1 The basic test solution shall be 0.9 % NaCl in distilled water. Measure the pH of the solutions before conducting the test. If necessary, buffer them to ensure they are in the range of 6.5 to 7.5.

6.2 Other solutions may include other "physiologic" saline and electrolyte solutions for injection (USP) or saline and protein solutions. If proteins are used, the solutions shall be sterile in accordance with 8.1.5. Protein solutions may either be purchased sterile, or sterilized by filtration. These shall be reported in accordance with 10.1.

7. Test Specimens

7.1 *Plates*:

7.1.1 The plates used for these tests may be cut from commercially available plates for osteosynthesis.

7.1.2 Plates may be fabricated from 4-mm or thicker metal sheet or strip. Holes may be prepared in accordance with Specification F 367. Holes may be round, or slotted, or "self-compressing" type.

7.2 *Screws*:

7.2.1 Screws used for this test may be commercially available bone screws. Heads should be spherical, although other shapes may be used.

7.2.2 Screws may be fabricated from rod stock in accordance with Specification F 543.

7.3 Test specimens may be used in the condition as received from the implant manufacturer; custom fabricated specimens should be prepared in accordance with Practice F 86.

8. Procedure

8.1 *Test Assembly Preparation* (see Fig. 1*b*):

8.1.1 Clean the plates and screws ultrasonically with detergent or other degreasing agent to ensure that they are free from grease and dirt. Rinse them with distilled water, and immediately dry them in warm air.

8.1.2 Weigh the plate and each screw separately. Then weigh the three together on a microbalance to an accuracy of 0.01 mg.

8.1.3 Attach the plates to the posts with the rubber spacers and bone screws. Tighten the screws so as to create a 400 ± 50 N axial load on the screws. After a correlation has been developed for relating torque and axial load for the particular metal(s), screw head, and plate hole configuration used, determine the load indirectly by measurement of the screw torque.

8.1.4 Place the assembled test specimens in a borosilicate beaker, add the test solution, and seal the top with the rubber cover with the tops of the posts projecting through the gasket.

8.1.5 If the test solution contains proteins that might support microbial growth, then the test assembly and solution must be sterile. Steam sterilize the test assembly for 20 min at 121°C prior to adding the liquid. Inject the sterile test liquid into the beaker using a sterile syringe and needle by carefully opening a small space between the post and the gasket.

8.2 *Test Assembly Mounting*:

8.2.1 Mate the short plastic rod to the horizontal plunger, and attach the longer rod to the top plate of the assembly holder with the mounting screw.

8.2.2 Start the motor and check that there is full motion of the horizontal plunger. It may be found that the elastic recoil of the elastomeric spacers is such that the plunger springs do not maintain plunger-cam contact during the complete oscillation cycle. Adjust the position of the mounting screw to ensure that contact is maintained. Run the test continuously for one million cycles. If the test is not run continuously, report details of all interuptions.

8.3 *Test Completion*:

8.3.1 At the completion of the designated number of days of fretting corrosion, stop the motor and remove the test assembly.

8.3.2 Remove the gasket seal, and remove the screws and plates from the spacers and plastic rods.

8.3.3 Ultrasonically clean the test specimens in their test liquids to remove all excess corrosion products.

8.3.4 Pour the test liquid and residue into a screw cap container, measure the pH of the solution, and store the liquid for chemical analysis. If the solutions contain organic materials, the container should be sterile. Determine the concentration of the appropriate metals by atomic absorption spectrophotometry. The concentration of nickel may be determined in accordance with Test Methods D 1886.

8.3.5 Ultrasonically clean the plates and screws in detergent and rinse with distilled water. Dry with warm air prior to reweighing. Additional cleaning with a stronger solution may be necessary, for example, with 10 % oxalic acid or other solutions in accordance with Practice G 1.

8.3.6 Weigh the plates and screws separately. Then weigh them together on a microbalance to an accuracy of 0.01 mg.

9. Calculation or Interpretation of Results

9.1 Calculate the change in weight of the plate and each screw separately, and as a total weight loss when the three are weighed together.

10. Report

10.1 The report shall contain a detailed description of the materials used for manufacture of the plate and screws, for example, chemical composition, grain size, hardness, and inclusion content, the design and dimensions of the plate and screws, the surface condition of the metal(s), the axial load on the screws if other than 400 ± 50 N, the pH before and after the test and the composition of the test solution, and the details of the fretting cycle and type of cleaning solution used.

10.2 Report the amount of fretting corrosion as follows:

10.2.1 the weight loss of the individual components,

10.2.2 the total weight loss, and

10.2.3 the amount of corrosion products in the solution.

10.3 Describe the appearance and damage associated with the region that underwent fretting corrosion.

11. Precision and Bias

11.1 The precision and bias of this test method have not been determined.

12. Keywords

12.1 corrosion-surgical implants; cracking-stress-corrosion; loading tests-surgical materials/applications; orthopaedic medical devices-bone plates; orthopaedic medical devices-bone screws; osteosynthesis; seals; stress-metallic materials; testing methods-surgical implants

APPENDIXES

(Nonmandatory Information)

X1. STATEMENT OF RATIONALE FOR TEST METHOD F 897

X1.1 This test method was developed as an ASTM standard based on the published results of Brown and Merritt **(1-3)**. They have shown that this type of device can be used to generate a measurable amount of weight loss and metal release due to fretting corrosion in a comparatively short time of 7 to 14 days. The results were sufficiently reproducible to permit comparison between metals or test solutions with comparatively small sample groups. Their results also have demonstrated that the method can be used to generate sufficient amounts of corrosion products for studies of the biological effects of corrosion products. The device presented is an example of how to get the relative motion pattern desired; other drive mechanisms may be employed.

X1.2 The load of 400 N was not selected to simulate load that would be incurred in vivo, but rather to permit the system to function with small return springs. It has also been reported **(1)** that the amount of fretting corrosion is not sensitive to small load variation in this range. The cycle rate was selected to simulate an *in vivo* condition, and to minimize effects due to heating and fluid agitation. The rubber gasket seals are used to minimize fluid concentration changes due to evaporation, as well as to permit the use of proteinaceous solutions with minimal risk of microbial contamination. Sterilization of the components and solutions is necessary when proteinaceous solutions are used, but is not necessary for electrolytes without proteins. Operation of the test at room temperature, rather than 37°C body temperature was selected to minimize the problems of evaporation, equipment breakdown, and microbial growth associated with the higher temperature.

X1.3 This test method may be used to compare the fretting corrosion rates of different metals and the effects of different solutions. It is not intended to be a quality control type of test, nor a required test for new material development.

X2. METHOD TO DETERMINE THE RELATIONSHIPS BETWEEN SCREW TORQUE AND AXIAL LOAD

X2.1 This method uses an electromechanical load cell from a testing machine that is capable of measuring tensile loads.

X2.2 Attach a polyacetal rod to the load measuring end of the load cell. Mate one end of the rod to the cell, and thread the other end of the rod to match the thread of the screws used in the fretting corrosion test.

X2.3 Construct a metal platform perpendicular to the load measuring axis. Support the platform with metal rods attached to the mounting frame of the load cell. The support rods should be long enough to leave 3 mm clearance between the platform and the end of the polyacetal rod. Drill a hole in the platform to permit insertion of the test screw through the platform and into the polyacetal rod.

X2.4 Insert the test screw through a test plate hole, through the elastomeric spacer, through the hole in the platform and into the threaded polyacetal rod. Tighten the screw with a torque measuring instrument capable of reading torque to ± 0.1 Nm. Record the torque required to produce axial loads of 300, 350, 400, 450, and 500 N.

REFERENCES

(1) Brown, S. A., and Merritt, K., "Fretting Corrosion of Plates and Screws: An In Vitro Test Method," ASTM Symposium, May 1983.

(2) Brown, S. A., and Merritt, K., "Fretting Corrosion in saline and serum," *Journal of Biomedical Materials Research*, Vol 15 (1981), pp. 479–488.

(3) Brown, S. A., and Merritt, K., "The Effects of Serum Proteins on Corrosion Rates In Vitro, *Clinical Applications of Biomaterials*, Lee, Albrektsson, and Branemark, eds., John Wiley, Chichester, 1982, pp. 195–202.

(4) Sherwin, M. P., Taylor, D. E., and Waterhouse, R. B. "An Electrochemical Investigation of Fretting Corrosion of Stainless Steel," *Corrosion Science*, Vol 11 (1971), pp. 419–429.

Designation: F 899 – 95

Standard Specification for Stainless Steel Billet, Bar, and Wire for Surgical Instruments[1]

This standard is issued under the fixed designation F 899; the number immediately following the designation indicates the year of original adoption or, in the case of revision, the year of last revision. A number in parentheses indicates the year of last reapproval. A superscript epsilon (ϵ) indicates an editorial change since the last revision or reapproval.

This standard has been approved for use by agencies of the Department of Defense.

1. Scope

1.1 This specification covers the requirements for stainless steel billet, bar, and wire used for the manufacture of surgical instruments. Billet or bar intended for forging into special shapes may also be purchased in accordance with this specification.

2. Referenced Documents

2.1 *ASTM Standards:*

A 276 Specification for Stainless and Heat-Resisting Steel Bars and Shapes[2]

A 314 Specification for Stainless and Heat-Resisting Steel Billets and Bars for Forging[2]

A 484/A484M Specification for General Requirements for Stainless and Heat-Resisting Bars, Billets, and Forgings[2]

A 555/A555M Specification for General Requirements for Stainless and Heat-Resisting Steel Wire and Wire Rods[3]

A 564 Specification for Hot-Rolled and Cold-Finished Age-Hardening Stainless and Heat-Resisting Steel Bars and Shapes[2]

A 582 Specification for Free-Machining Stainless and Heat-Resisting Steel Bars, Hot-Rolled or Cold-Finished[2]

A 751 Test Methods, Practices, and Terminology for Chemical Analysis of Steel Products[3]

2.2 *ISO Draft International Standard:*

ISO/DIS 7153/1 Instruments For Surgery—Metallic Materials—Part 1: Stainless Steel[4]

2.3 *American Society for Quality Control (ASQC) Standard:*

C1-1985 Specification of General Requirements for a Quality Program[5]

3. Classification and Type

3.1 *Classes*—Stainless steel material requirements for surgical instruments shall conform to one of the following classes, as specified:

3.1.1 *Class 3*—Austenitic Stainless Steel.

3.1.2 *Class 4*—Martensitic Stainless Steel.

3.1.3 *Class 5*—Precipitation Hardening Stainless Steel.

3.1.4 *Class 6*—Ferritic Stainless Steel.

3.2 *Type*—Where applicable, the commercially recognized type of stainless steel is included in Tables 1 and 2.

4. Ordering Information

4.1 Inquiries and orders for material under this specification shall include the following information:

4.1.1 Quantity (weight or number of pieces),

4.1.2 Classification, optional (see 3.1),

4.1.3 Type (see 3.2),

4.1.4 Form (billet, bar, wire),

4.1.5 Condition (see 5.1),

4.1.6 Finish (see 5.3),

4.1.7 Mechanical properties or hardness (see Section 8), and

4.1.8 Applicable dimensions including size, thickness, width, and length (exact, random, or multiples) or print number.

5. Manufacture

5.1 *Condition*—Billet, bar, and wire shall be furnished to the instrument manufacturer, as specified, in the hot finished, cold finished, annealed, solution treated, solution treated and aged, quench hardened, quench hardened and tempered, or as specified in the instrument manufacturer's purchase order.

Cautionary Note—Highly hardenable martensitic stainless billets and bars such as Types 420A, 420B, 420C, 420F, 420F Mod., 440A, 440B, and 440C intended for forging are commonly annealed prior to shipment and so specified in order to avoid the possibility of thermal cracking. Other hardenable martensitic grades such as Types 403, 410, 416, 416 Mod., and 431, which also may require annealing, depending on their composition and size, are furnished suitable for cold cutting when so specified on the purchase order.

5.2 *Conditioning*—Billet and bar intended for forging may be conditioned by chipping, grinding, or other suitable means

---

[1] This specification is under the jurisdiction of ASTM Committee F-4 on Medical and Surgical Materials and Devices and is the direct responsibility of Subcommittee F04.33 on Medical and Surgical Instruments.

Current edition approved Oct. 10, 1995. Published November 1995. Originally published as F 899 – 84. Last previous edition F 899 – 94.

[2] *Annual Book of ASTM Standards*, Vol 01.05.

[3] *Annual Book of ASTM Standards*, Vol 01.03.

[4] Available from American National Standards Institute, 1430 Broadway, New York, NY 10018.

[5] Available from American Society for Quality Control, 161 West Wisconsin Avenue, Milwaukee, WI 53203.

TABLE 1 Composition of Class 3, Austenitic Stainless Steels, %

Type	Carbon, max	Manganese	Phosphorus, max	Sulfur	Silicon, max	Chromium	Nickel	Other Elements
301	0.15	2.00 max	0.045	0.030 max	1.00	16.00–18.00	6.00–8.00	—
302	0.15	2.00 max	0.045	0.030 max	1.00	17.00–19.00	8.00–10.00	N 0.10 max
303	0.12	2.00 max	0.060	0.15–0.35	1.00	17.00–19.00	8.00–10.00	Mo 0.70 max^A
304	0.07	2.00 max	0.045	0.030 max	1.00	17.00–19.00	8.00–11.00	N 0.10 max
316	0.07	2.00 max	0.045	0.030 max	1.00	16.50–18.50	10.50–13.50	Mo 2.00–2.50 N 0.10 max
317	0.08	2.00 max	0.045	0.030 max	1.00	18.00–20.00	11.00–15.00	Mo 3.00–4.00 N 0.10 max
XM-7	0.10	2.00 max	0.045	0.030 max	1.00	17.00–19.00	8.00–10.00	Cu 3.00–4.00
—	0.15	17.00–19.00	0.040	0.040 max	1.00	17.00–19.00	—	Mo 0.75–1.25 Cu 0.75–1.25 N 0.40–0.60

^{A}Optional.

TABLE 2 Composition of Class 6, Ferritic Stainless Steels, %

Type	Carbon, max	Manganese, max	Phosphorus, max	Sulfur	Silicon, Max	Chromium	Other Elements
430 F	0.08	1.50	0.060	0.15–0.35	1.00	16.00–18.00	Mo 0.60 max
XM-34	0.08	2.50	0.040	0.28–0.41	1.00	17.50–19.50	Ni 1.00 max Mo 1.50–2.50

to remove injurious surface defects.

5.3 *Finish*—Types of finish available for bar and wire products are cold drawn, pickled, ground, ground and polished, or as specified in the instrument manufacturer's purchase order.

6. General Requirements for Delivery

6.1 In addition to the requirements of this specification, all requirements of the current editions of Specification A 484/A 484M and A555/A 555M shall apply as applicable.

6.2 This ASTM specification compliments the ISO applicable document covering stainless steel for surgical instruments and, by reference, includes all of the stainless grades in ISO/DIS 7153/1.

7. Chemical Requirements

7.1 The heat analysis shall conform to the requirements as to chemical composition specified in Tables 1-2.

7.2 Restricted carbon and sulfur limits for certain Class 4 martensitic stainless steels are specified to ensure consistency in the materials used for the manufacture of surgical instruments.

7.3 The chemical composition requirements for Types 301, 303, 304, 316, 410, 420A, 420B, 420C, and 430F will meet the composition requirements in ISO/DIS 7153/1.

7.4 Methods and practices relating to chemical analysis required by this specification shall be in accordance with Test Methods, Practices, and Definitions A 751.

8. Mechanical Requirements

8.1 Material shall conform to the mechanical property requirements cited in the appropriate ASTM standards (see 2.1) or shall meet the mechanical property requirements specified in the instrument manufacturer's purchase order.

8.2 When desired, Brinell hardness number (HB), Rockwell hardness, B scale (HRB) or Rockwell hardness, C scale (HRC), limits may be specified. Hardness guidelines for selected Class 4 martensitic stainless steels in the annealed condition are listed in Table 5.

TABLE 3 Composition of Class 4, Martensitic Stainless Steels, %

Type	Carbon	Mn Max	P Max	Sulfur S	Silicon Max	Chromium	Other Elements
410	0.09–0.15	1.00	0.040	0.030 max	1.00	11.50–13.50	Ni 1.00 max
410X	0.16–0.21	1.00	0.040	0.030 max	1.00	11.50–13.50	Ni 1.00 max
416	0.09–0.15	1.25	0.060	0.15–0.27	1.00	12.00–14.00	—
416 Mod	0.09–0.15	1.25	0.060	0.28–0.41	1.00	12.00–14.00	—
420A	0.16–0.25	1.00	0.040	0.030 max	1.00	12.00–14.00	Ni 1.00 max
420B	0.26–0.35	1.00	0.040	0.030 max	1.00	12.00–14.00	Ni 1.00 max
420X	0.36–0.41	1.00	0.040	0.030 max	1.00	12.00–14.50	Ni 1.00 max
420C	0.42–0.50	1.00	0.040	0.030 max	1.00	12.50–14.50	Ni 1.00 max
420F	0.30–0.40	1.25	0.060	0.20–0.34	1.00	12.50–14.00	Cu 0.60 max^A Ni 0.50 max^A
420F Mod	0.20–0.26	2.00	0.040	0.15–0.27	1.00	12.50–14.00	Mo 1.10–1.50 Ni 0.75–1.50
431	0.20 max	1.00	0.040	0.030 max	1.00	15.00–17.00	Ni 1.25–2.50
440A	0.60–0.75	1.00	0.040	0.030 max	1.00	16.00–18.00	Mo 0.75 max
440B	0.75–0.95	1.00	0.040	0.030 max	1.00	16.00–18.00	Mo 0.75 max
440C	0.95–1.20	1.00	0.040	0.030 max	1.00	16.00–18.00	Mo 0.75 max
440F	0.95–1.20	1.25	0.060	0.15–0.27	1.00	16.00–18.00	Cu 0.60 max^A Ni 0.50 max^A

^{A}Optional.

TABLE 4 Composition of Class 5, Precipitation Hardening Stainless Steels, %

Type	Carbon, max	Manganese, max	Phosphorus, max	Sulfur, max	Silicon, max	Chromium	Nickel	Copper	Columbiun + Tantalum	Other Elements
630	0.07	1.00	0.040	0.030	1.00	15.00–17.50	3.00–5.00	3.00–5.00	0.15–0.45	—
631	0.09	1.00	0.040	0.030	1.00	16.00–18.00	6.50–7.75	—	—	A1 0.75–1.50
XM-25	0.05	1.00	0.030	0.030	1.00	14.00–16.00	5.00–7.00	1.25–1.75	—	Mo 0.50–1.00 Cb 8 x C min
XM-16	0.03	0.50	0.015	0.015	0.50	11.00–12.50	7.50–9.50	1.50–2.50	0.10–0.50	Ti 0.90–1.40 Mo 0.50 max

TABLE 5 Hardness Guidelines[A] for Selected Class 4 Martensitic Stainless Steels in The Annealed Condition

Type	Brinell Hardness,[B] max (HB)
410	210
410X	220
416	262
416 Mod	262
420A	220
420B	235
420X	262
420C	262
420F	262
420F Mod	262
431	285
440A	285
440B	285
440C	285
440F	285

[A]Excludes billets and bars for forging.
[B]Or equivalent Rockwell hardness.

9. Heat Treatment

9.1 Material shall be heat treated as applicable for the stainless composition involved.

9.2 Heat treating guidelines and typical hardness values for selected Class 4 martensitic stainless steels are listed in Table 6.

9.3 Heat treating guidelines for Class 5 precipitation hardening stainless steels are included in Specification A 564.

10. Special Information

10.1 Some examples of selected stainless steels that have been used for various surgical instrument applications are listed in Table 7 and Table 8 for information purposes.

11. Quality Program Requirements

11.1 The producer shall maintain a quality program, such as defined in ASQC C1-1985.

11.2 The manufacturer of surgical instruments may audit the producer's quality program for conformance to the intent of ASQC C-1985, or other recognized program.

12. Keywords

12.1 instruments; stainless steel—bar; billets; wire

TABLE 6 Heat Treating Guidelines and Typical Hardness Values for Selected Class 4 Martensitic Stainless Steels

Type	Typical Hardening[A] Heat Treatment	Typical Hardness at Indicated Tempering Temperature[B] °F	°C	Hardness (HRC)
410	1850°F (1010°C) + Oil quench or air cool	500	260	43
		700	371	43
		900[C]	482	42
		1000[C]	538	30
		1100	593	24
410X	1875°F (1024°C) + Oil quench or air cool	500	260	46
		700	371	46/47
		900[C]	482	48
		1000[C]	538	44
		1100	593	31
416 Mod	1800°F (982°C) + Oil quench	300	149	38
		500	260	37
		700	371	37
		900[C]	482	35
		1000[C]	538	30
		1100	593	22
416	1800°F (982°C) + Oil quench	300	149	41
		500	260	39
		700	371	41
		900[C]	482	36
		1000[C]	538	31
		1100	593	26
420A	1850°F (1010°C) + Warm oil quench	300	149	53
		400	204	50
		500	260	48
		600	315	48
		700	371	48
		800[D]	427	48
420B	1900°F (1038°C) + Warm oil quench	300	149	52
		400	204	52
		500	260	50
		600	315	50
		700	371	49
		800[D]	427	49
420X	1900°F (1038°C) + Warm oil quench	300	149	52
		400	204	52
		500	260	50
		600	315	50
		700	371	49
		800[D]	427	49
420C	1900°F (1038°C) + Warm oil quench	300	149	58
		400	204	55/56
		500	260	53/54
		600	315	53/54
		700	371	54/55
		800[D]	427	55
420F	1900°F (1038°C) + Warm oil quench	300	149	52
		400	204	52
		500	260	50
		600	315	50
		700	371	49
		800[D]	427	49
420F Mod	1900°F (1038°C) + Warm oil quench	300	149	53
		400	204	50
		500	260	48
		600	315	48
		700	371	48
		800[D]	427	48
431	1900°F (1038°C) + Oil quench	500	260	42
		700	371	42
		900[C]	482	45
		1100[C]	593	34
440A Mod	1900°F (1038°C) + Warm oil quench	300	149	56/57
		400	204	23
		500	260	54
		600	315	51/52
		700	371	51
		800[D]	427	50
440B	1900°F (1038°C) + Warm oil quench	300	149	58/59
		400	204	56/57
		500	260	53/54
		600	315	53
		700	371	54
		800[D]	427	54
440C	1900°F (1038°C) + Warm oil quench	300	149	60
		400	204	59
		500	260	57
		600	315	56
		700	371	56
		800[D]	427	56
440F	1900°F (1038°C) + Warm oil quench	300	149	60
		400	204	59
		500	260	57
		600	315	56
		700	371	56
		800[D]	427	56

[A] Time at temperature depends on section size. Controlled heat treating atmosphere or alternate quench media may be used in accordance with good commercial practice.
[B] Temper at least one hour at indicated temperature and air cool. Large section sizes require longer time at temperature.
[C] Tempering in the range of 750/1050°F (399/566°C) results in decreased impact strength and reduced corrosion resistance.
[D] Tempering over 800°F (427°C) results in reduced corrosion resistance.

TABLE 7 Examples of Selected Stainless Steels That Have Been Used for Surgical Instruments in Accordance with ISO/DIS 7153/1

Type	Cutting Instruments	Non-Cutting Instruments
303	Chisels and gouges, bone curettes	probes
304		retractors
410		tissue, forceps, dressing forceps, retractors, probes
420A	Bone rongeurs, conchotomes, bone cutting forceps, chisels and gouges, bone curettes, scissors with carbide inserts	forceps, retractors, probes, forceps with bow handles, branch forceps
420B	bone rongeurs, scissors	
420C	scissors, bone rongeurs, bone cutting forceps, conchotomes, scalpels, knives, bone curettes, chisels and gouges	

TABLE 8 Examples of Selected Stainless Steels That Have Been Used For Surgical Instruments in the United States

Type	Cutting Instruments	Non-Cutting Instruments
302	knives, chisels, gouges, curettes	cannula, forceps, guides, needle vents, retractors, specula, spreaders, tendor passers, springs
303[A]	chisels, curettes, knives	cannula, clamps, drills, forceps, handles, hammers, mallets, needle vents, punches, retractors, rulers, screws, skin hooks, specula, spreaders, suction tubes, tendon strips, tongs, tunnelers, probes
304		cannula, clamps, forceps, holders, handles, needle vents, retractors, specula, spreaders, suction tubes, tendon passers
316		specula
410	chisels, curettes, dissectors, osteotomes, reamers, scissors with inserts	clamps, clip applicators, elevators, forceps, hemostats, holders, needle holders, punches, retractors, skin hooks, sounds, spreaders, probes, dilators
410X	curettes, dissectors, rongeurs	clamps, forceps, hemostats, holders, punches, retractors
416[A]	chisels, curettes, dissectors	clamps, punches, retractors, skin hooks, spreaders
420[B]	chisels, curettes, cutters, bone cutting forceps, knives, scissors, rongeurs, scalpels, skin punches, conchotomes	clamps, elevators, punches, rounds, dissectors, retractors, skin hooks, needles
420F[A]	cutters	burrs
431		cheak retractors, insertion wrenches, orthopeadic instruments
440[C]	chisels, knives, osteotomes, scalpels	drills, retractors, spreaders, tongs
630	reamers	
XM-16	scissors	drills, needles

[A]It is not recommended that free-machining grades be used for critical portions of surgical instruments.
[B]Types 420A, 420B, or 420C may be used depending on instrument design and application.
[C]Types 440A, 440B, or 440C may be used depending on instrument design and application.

APPENDIX

(Nonmandatory Information)

X1. STATEMENT OF RATIONALE FOR SPECIFICATION F 899

X1.1 The primary reason for this standard is to characterize composition and mechanical requirements to assure consistency in wrought materials used, directly or modified by forging in the manufacture of stainless steel surgical instruments.

X1.2 The chemical compositions of certain grades covered by this specification have been modified in order to meet the composition requirements in the most recent ISO Draft International Standard for stainless steels used in the manufacture of surgical instruments.

X1.3 Carbon and sulfur limits have been modified to provide an extra measure of uniformity for certain Class 4 stainless steel compositions used in the manufacture of surgical instruments.

X1.4 Acceptable metal conditions supplied to the instrument manufacturer include hot finished, cold finished, annealed, solution treated, solution treated and aged, quench hardened, or quench hardened and tempered, the choice dependent upon the alloy type, instrument design, and application.

X1.5 Mechanical requirements for Classes 3, 5, and 6 stainless steels covered in this specification are included in the appropriate ASTM standards listed in Section 2.

X1.6 Hardness and heat-treating guidelines for selected Class 4 stainless steels are included in this specification since the martensitic grades are the predominant class of stainless steel used for surgical instruments.

X1.7 Examples of selected stainless steels that have been used for surgical instrument applications are included in this standard for information purposes.

Standard Specification for Minimum Performance and Safety Requirements for Resuscitators Intended for Use With Humans[1]

This standard is issued under the fixed designation F 920; the number immediately following the designation indicates the year of original adoption or, in the case of revision, the year of last revision. A number in parentheses indicates the year of last reapproval. A superscript epsilon (ϵ) indicates an editorial change since the last revision or reapproval.

INTRODUCTION

In January of 1989, ASTM Subcommittee F29.03.03 met in Boston with representatives of the American Heart Association and the U.S. Department of Defense to discuss the revision of this specification. It was unanimously determined that until a revised version of this specification that would be consistent with the American Heart Association's revised Standards and Guidelines for Cardiopulmonary Resuscitation and Emergency Cardiac Care was available, ISO 8382-1988, should be used as the specific reference for manually-triggered gas-powered resuscitators. Shortly thereafter, the Subcommittee Chairman published a letter to this effect in the *Journal of the American Medical Association.*[2] The Subcommittee reaffirmed this stance at a subsequent meeting in March of 1990. This specification is therefore similar in content to ISO 8382.

1. Scope

1.1 This specification covers ventilatory resuscitators, that is, small portable ventilators intended to be used in emergencies both outside and inside hospitals. These devices are intended for use by medical personnel and for emergency use by personnel with varying degrees of training. They are intended to be used at the site of an emergency and during patient transport. Resuscitators intended for use on all age groups are included within the scope of this specification.

1.1.1 This specification does not intend to discourage or impede future innovation or development of resuscitators.

1.2 The effective and safe use of a resuscitator is determined not only by the performance of the resuscitator, but also by the skill of the operator. This specification does not describe the content of the training programs to develop such skill and does not state who should or should not use a resuscitator. This will be determined by the organizations involved in teaching resuscitation.

1.2.1 In certain countries, resuscitators are intended for use by nontrained personnel and lower pressure limits are set. Some countries also reserve the use of automatic gas-powered resuscitators to trained individuals under medical supervision. This specification is not intended to conflict with these established practices.

1.3 Annex A1 details test methods, while Annex A2 provides tables of resistances and compliances required to set up the test lung. Annex A3 gives a rationale for various clauses in this specification and is included to provide additional insight into the reasoning that led to the requirements and recommendations that have been given. Annex A4 and Annex A5 provide advice concerning materials to be used in resuscitators and face masks.

1.4 The values stated in SI units are to be regarded as the standard.

1.5 *This standard does not purport to address all of the safety problems, if any, associated with its use. It is the responsibility of the user of this standard to establish appropriate safety and health practices and determine the applicability of regulatory limitations prior to use.*

2. Referenced Documents

2.1 The following standards contain provisions that, through reference in this text, constitute provisions of this specification. At the time of publication, the editions indicated were valid. All standards are subject to revision, and parties to agreements based on this specification are encouraged to investigate the possibility of applying the most recent editions of the standards listed below.

2.2 *ASTM Standards:*

F 1054 Specification for Conical Fittings of 15 mm and 22 mm Sizes[3]

F 1243 Specification for Tracheal Tube Connectors[3]

2.3 *ANSI Standard:*

[1] This specification is under the jurisdiction of ASTM Committee F29 on Anesthetic and Respiratory Equipment and is the direct responsibility of Subcommittee F29.14 on Ventilators.

Current edition approved March 15, 1993. Published May 1993. Originally published as F 920 – 85. Last previous edition F 920 – 85.

[2] American Heart Association, "Standards and Guidelines for Cardiopulmonary Resuscitation (CPR) and Emergency Cardia Care (ECC)," *Journal of the American Medical Association*, Vol 255, No. 21, June 6, 1986, pp. 2905-2984.

[3] *Annual Book of ASTM Standards*, Vol 13.01.

ANSI/CAA V-1 Compressed Gas Cylinder Valve Outlet and Inlet Connections[4]

2.4 *ISO Standards:*

ISO 407 Small Medical Gas Cylinders—Yoke-Type Valve Connections[4]

ISO 4135 Anaesthesiology—Vocabulary[4]

ISO 5356-1 Anaesthetic and Respiratory Equipment—Conical Connectors—Part 1: Cones and Sockets[4]

ISO 5359 Low-Pressure Flexible Connecting Assemblies (Hose Assemblies) for Use with Medical Gas Systems[4]

ISO 7228 Tracheal Tube Connectors[4]

ISO 8382 Resuscitators Intended for Use with Humans[4]

3. Terminology

3.1 *Definitions*—Some of these definitions have been taken from ISO 4135, but are included in this specification for convenience. Other definitions, that are given in ISO 4135, for apparatus in general, have been modified slightly for the purposes of this specification as they apply specifically to resuscitators:

3.1.1 *airway*—the passageway for gas into and out of the lungs.

3.1.2 *apparatus deadspace* $V_{D,app}$— that volume of previously exhaled gas that is delivered from the resuscitator in the succeeding inspiratory phase.

3.1.3 *automatic resuscitator*—a resuscitator in which the cyclic flow of gas for inflation of the lungs is independent of any inspiratory effect of the patient or repetitive action of the operator.

3.1.3.1 *Discussion*—The expiratory phase may also be automatically cycled.

3.1.4 *back leak*—the volume of expired gas which does not pass through the expiratory port but returns to the resuscitator.

3.1.5 *bag inlet valve*—a valve activated by the subatmospheric pressure in the compressible unit of the resuscitator to refill the compressible unit from a compressed gas source.

3.1.6 *bag refill valve*—a valve, with no manual trigger, activated by the subatmospheric pressure in the compressible unit of the resuscitator to refill the compressible unit from a compressed gas source.

3.1.7 *compliance, C*—volume change of the gases in the compartment produced by a unit pressure change, expressed in litres per kilopascal (L/kPa).

3.1.8 *compressible unit*—that part of an operator-powered resuscitator that, when compressed by the operator, delivers a volume of gas, for example, a bag or bellows.

3.1.9 *delivered oxygen concentration*—the average concentration of oxygen in the gas delivered from the resuscitator.

3.1.10 *demand (intermittent flow) apparatus*—a device delivering a flow of gas, patient-triggered, during inspiration only at ambient pressure (or at respiratory pressure).

3.1.11 *expiratory port*—an opening through which gases or vapors, or both, pass from the patient during expiration.

3.1.12 *forward leak*—the volume of gas produced by the resuscitator during the inspiratory phase that does not pass through the patient port to the patient but passes to the atmosphere.

3.1.13 *gas-powered resuscitator*—a resuscitator powered by the energy of compressed gas.

3.1.14 *infant*—an individual weighing up to 10 kg, or being approximately one year of age.

3.1.15 *manually cycled, gas-powered resuscitator*— an operator-activated resuscitator whereby the work of resuscitation is accomplished by the energy of compressed gas and not the operator.

3.1.16 *maximum delivery pressure*—the highest gage pressure that can be attained at the patient connection port when the apparatus is functioning normally.

3.1.17 *minute volume,* $\mathring{V}$—the volume of gas, expressed in litres per minute, entering or leaving the patient or the lung model.

3.1.18 *Discussion*—The physical conditions under which measurements are made should be given.

3.1.19 *operator-powered resuscitator*—a resuscitation device in which ventilation of the lungs is produced by the operator compressing the compressible unit of the device.

3.1.20 *patient connection port*—that opening at the patient end of an expiratory value unit; a Y-piece fitting or a unidirectional valve to which may be connected either a tracheal tube or a face mask angle piece.

3.1.21 *patient connector*—that part of the resuscitator that connects directly to a face mask or an appropriate mating airway device.

3.1.22 *patient valve*—a valve in the breathing system that directs gas into the lungs for the inspiratory phase and into the atmosphere during the expiratory phase.

3.1.23 *pressure limiting system*—a mechanism for limiting the maximum delivery pressure.

3.1.24 *resistance, R*—pressure drop per unit of flow at a specified flow, expressed in kilopascals per litre per second [kPa/(L/s)].

3.1.24.1 *Discussion*—According to conventional practice, this has generally been expressed in centimetres of water per litre per second [cmH_2O/(L/s)].

3.1.25 *resuscitator*—a portable device used in emergency situations to provide lung ventilation to individuals whose breathing is inadequate.

3.1.26 *stroke volume*—the volume of gas deliverable from the resuscitator to the end of the patient connector during an inspiratory phase of the ventilatory cycle.

3.1.27 *tidal volume,* V_T—the volume of gas, expressed in millilitres, entering or leaving the patient or the lung model during the inspiratory or expiratory phase time.

3.1.27.1 *Discussion*—The physical conditions under which gas volumes are measured should be given.

3.1.28 *ventilatory cycle*—the cycle comprising the inspiratory phase plus the expiratory phase.

3.1.29 *ventilatory frequency, f*—the number of ventilatory cycles per minute.

3.1.29.1 *Discussion*—This definition differs from the one given in ISO 4135 because it refers to the number of ventilatory cycles of the resuscitator, not the patient breaths.

3.2 *Symbols:* In addition to the symbols given in clause 3,

[4] Available from American National Standards Institute, 25 W. 43rd St., 4th Floor, New York, NY 10036.

the following symbols are used in this specification:

3.2.1 $V_{D,system}$—system deadspace.

3.2.2 $F_{O_2,bag}$— oxygen concentration in bag.

4. Connectors

4.1 *Patient Connection Port (See also* Annex A3*)*—The patient connection port of the resuscitator shall have 15 mm female and 22 mm male coaxial connectors with dimensions in accordance with ISO 5356-1 and Specification F 1054.

4.2 *Expiratory Port for Breathing Gases (See also* Annex A3*)*—If a tapered connector is provided at the expiratory port, it shall be a 30 mm male conical connector or a 19 mm male conical connector in accordance with ISO 5356-1 and Specification F 1054.

4.2.1 The connector shall incorporate a baulk, for example, ridges in the internal lumen of the connector, so that it cannot accept a 22 mm male conical connector as specified in ISO 5356-1 and Specification F 1054.

NOTE 1—Such a baulk should not significantly increase the resistance to gas flow through the connector.

4.3 *Face Mask Connectors (See also* Annex A3*)*—If provided with the resuscitator, face masks shall have either a 22 mm female connector or a 15 mm male connector that will mate with the corresponding connectors specified in ISO 5356-1 and Specification F 1054.

4.4 *Bag Refill Valve Connectors (See also* Annex A3*)*—If a conical connector is provided at the inlet port for the attachment of a bag refill valve, it shall be a 32 mm female conical connector providing a secure fit with the gages shown in Fig. A1.1.

4.5 *Bag Inlet Valve Connectors*—Bag inlet valve connectors shall not be compatible with connectors dimensioned in accordance with ISO 5356-1 and Specification F 1054.

NOTE 2—For resuscitators intended for use in hazardous environments, attention is drawn to CEN 148, a draft standard on threaded gas filter connections.

5. Operational Requirements

5.1 *General*—Ideally, patient respiration through the resuscitator, that is, through connectors, the bag for hand-powered resuscitators, and any filtration apparatus, should be obtained within the inspiratory and expiratory resistance requirements given in this specification. All performance requirements in this specification should be satisfied when the resuscitator is operated by one person, since frequently only one person will be available to operate the resuscitator. This should be attainable when the resuscitator is used with either a face mask or an artificial airway device.

5.2 *Dismantling and Reassembly (See also* Annex A3*)*—The manufacturer shall recommend a functional test of operation to be carried out after reassembly (see 10.3.2.3(*d*)).

NOTE 3—A resuscitator intended to be dismantled by the user, for example, for cleaning, etc., should be designed so as to suppress the risk of incorrect reassembly when all parts are mated.

5.3 *Patient Valve Function After Contamination with Vomitus (See also* Annex A3*)*— After the resuscitator has been tested in accordance with the test described in A1.5.3, it shall meet the requirements specified in 7.3, 7.5, 7.8.1, 7.8.2, 7.9, 7.10.1, 7.10.2, and 7.10.3, as appropriate.

NOTE 4—It is preferable that the valve housing be constructed so that operation of the mechanism may be observed by the operator, for example, through a transparent housing. Observation of the functioning mechanism of the patient valve may assist the operator in detecting abnormal operation.

5.4 *Mechanical Shock*:

5.4.1 *Drop Test (See also* Annex A3*)*—If the resuscitator is intended to be operated outside of its carrying case, plastic bag, mounting bracket, etc., it shall meet the requirements specified in 7.3, 7.5, 7.8.1, 7.9, 7.10.1, 7.10.2, and 7.10.3 as appropriate, following the drop test described in A1.5.4. If the resuscitator is intended for operation only inside its carrying case, it may be so tested, but the case shall be open and in its "ready-for-use" condition.

5.4.2 *Mechanical Shock Test for Resuscitator Fixtures that are Mounted on Castors or on Wheels (See also* Annex A3*)*—The resuscitator shall meet the requirements specified in 7.3, 7.5, 7.8.1, 7.8.2, 7.9, 7.10.1, 7.10.2, and 7.10.3, as appropriate, after being tipped over from its normal operating position onto a concrete floor as described in A1.5.5.

5.5 *Immersion in Water (See also* Annex A3*)*—After immersion in water by the method described in A1.5.6, the resuscitator shall comply with the requirements specified in 7.3, 7.5, 7.8.1, 7.8.2, 7.9, 7.10.1, 7.10.2, and 7.10.3, as appropriate.

5.6 *Bag Refill Valves (See also* Annex A3*)*—Bag refill valves for use with operator-powered resuscitators shall not have provisions for manual operation.

6. Physical Properties

6.1 *Size (See also* Annex A3*)*—The resuscitator, with a container, if provided, shall pass through a rectangular opening 300 by 600 mm in size, in at least one position.

6.2 *Resuscitator Mass*—Except for gas-powered resuscitators designed to be an integral part of a neonatal critical care system, the mass of the resuscitator container and contents (including any full gas cylinders) shall not exceed 18 kg.

7. Performance Requirements

7.1 *Supplementary Oxygen and Delivered Oxygen Concentration*:

7.1.1 *Operator-Powered Resuscitators (See also* Annex A3*)*—When tested by the method described in A1.5.7 in accordance with the requirements of this classification (see 7.8.1), an operator-powered resuscitator shall deliver a minimum oxygen concentration of at least 40 % (V/V) when connected to an oxygen source supplying not more than 15 L/min, and shall be capable of delivering at least 85 % (V/V) (see Note 5). The manufacturer shall state the range of concentrations at representative flows, for example, 2 L/min, 4 L/min, 6 L/min, 8 L/min, etc. If the resuscitator is intended to be hand-operated, only one hand shall be used to compress the compressible unit, and the hand of the person carrying out the test shall not exceed the dimensions given in Fig. A1.2.

NOTE 5—The 85 % (V/V) requirement may be accomplished with the use of an attachment.

7.1.2 *Gas-Powered Resuscitators (See also* Annex A3*)*—When tested by the method described in A1.5.8, a gas-powered resuscitator shall deliver an oxygen concentration of at least 85 % (V/V). If the resuscitator is capable of delivering other oxygen concentrations, the manufacturer shall state the conditions under which the various concentrations may be delivered.

7.2 *Resistance to Inspiration and Expiration*—See the requirement for information to be provided by the manufacturer under 10.3.2.3(*c*).

7.3 *Expiratory Resistance (See also* Annex A3*)*—In the absence of positive end-expiratory devices, and when tested by the method described in A1.5.9, the pressure generated at the patient connection port shall not exceed 0,5 kPa (≈5 cmH_2O). (See also 10.3.2.3(*c*).)

7.4 *Inspiratory Resistance (See also* Annex A3*)*—When tested by the method described in A1.5.10, the pressure at the patient connection port shall not exceed 0,5 kPa (≈5 cmH_2O) below atmospheric pressure. (See also 10.3.2.3(*c*).)

7.5 *Patient Valve Malfunction (See also* Annex A2*)*—When tested by the method described in A1.5.11, the patient valve of the resuscitator shall not jam in the inspiratory position at an added input flow of up to 30 L/min when this flow is added in accordance with the manufacturer's instructions.

7.6 *Patient Valve Leakage—Forward Leakage (See also* Annex A3*)*—Where forward leakage is a design feature, it shall be so stated in the instruction manual.

7.7 *Apparatus Deadspace (See also* Annex A3*)*—When tested by the method described in A1.5.12, the apparatus deadspace shall not exceed 5.0 to 5.5 % of the tidal volume specified for the classification of the resuscitator (see 7.8.1).

7.8 *Ventilation Performance*:

7.8.1 *Tidal Volume (See also* Annex A3*)*—Resuscitators intended for use with infants and children up to 40 kg body mass shall be classified according to the body mass range for which they are suitable. This body mass range shall be derived from a requirement for a tidal volume of 15 mL/kg body mass.

7.8.1.1 Resuscitators delivering a tidal volume of 600 mL and over shall be classified as adult resuscitators. The tidal volumes specified shall be delivered under the test conditions listed in Table 1 using the methods described in A1.5.13, without the use of the override mechanism on any pressure-limiting system.

NOTE 6—Resuscitators designed to deliver a tidal volume of 20 to 50 mL are usually suitable for use with neonates.

7.8.2 *Pressure Limitation (Operator-Powered Resuscitators) (See also* Annex A3*)*:

7.8.2.1 For resuscitators classified for use with neonates and infants, a pressure-limiting system shall be provided so that the airway pressure does not exceed 4.5 kPa (≈45 cmH_2O) under the test conditions described in A1.5.15.

NOTE 7—An override mechanism may be provided.

7.8.2.2 If a pressure-limiting system is provided for a resuscitator classified for use with patients of over 10 kg body mass, the pressure at which it operates shall be stated in the instruction manual (see 10.3.2.3(*c*)). Any pressure limiting device provided that it limits pressure to below 6 kPa (≈60 cmH_2O), shall be equipped with an override mechanism. If provided with a locking mechanism, pressure override mechanisms shall be so designed that the operating mode, that is, on or off, is readily apparent to the user by obvious control position, flag, etc.

NOTE 8—If the resuscitator is equipped with a pressure-limiting system, there should be an audible or visible warning to the operator when the pressure-limiting system is operating.

7.9 *Gas-Powered Resuscitators*:

7.9.1 *Pressure-Limiting System (See also* Annex A3*)*—A pressure-limiting system shall be incorporated in gas-powered resuscitators. When the resuscitator is supplied with gas at the range of pressures specified in 10.5, the airway pressure shall not exceed 6 kPa (≈60 cmH_2O). An override mechanism shall be provided to enable the operator to select a higher pressure. However, automatic, pressure-cycled, gas-powered resuscitators shall not be equipped with any type of override mechanism. If provided with a locking mechanism, pressure override mechanisms shall be so designed that the operating mode, that is, on or off, is readily apparent to the user by obvious control position, flag, etc.

NOTE 9—A setting for the pressure-limiting system higher than 6 kPa (≈60 cmH_2O) may be made available for certain patients, although the selection of such a setting requires medical advice.

NOTE 10—There should be an audible or visible warning to the operator when the pressure-limiting system is operating.

7.9.2 *Inspiratory Flow*—All gas-powered resuscitators shall be capable of delivering 40 L/min ± 10 % inspiratory flow against a back pressure of 2 kPa (≈20 cmH_2O) when tested by the method described in A1.5.14.

NOTE 11—Devices with fixed flows should be set to this value. Devices with operator-adjustable flows should include this value in their range of adjustment.

7.9.3 *Manually Cycled, Gas-Powered Resuscitators*—Manually cycled gas-powered resuscitators shall meet the requirements specified in 7.1.2, 7.9.1, and 7.9.2 when tested by the methods described A1.5.8, A1.5.13, A1.5.14, and A1.5.16.

7.9.4 *Automatic Pressure-Cycled, Gas-Powered Resuscitators*—Automatic pressure-cycled resuscitators shall have positive cycling pressures in the range of 2 to 3 kPa (≈20 to ≈30 cmH_2O) when tested by the method described in A1.5.17 (see also 10.1.1).

NOTE 12—A negative-pressure phase may cause a decrease in arterial oxygen partial pressure (pO_2) or functional residual capacity (FRC).

TABLE 1 Test Conditions

Classification, kg	Compliance, L/kPa	Resistance, kPa/(L/s)	Inspiration: Expiration Ratio ± 20 %	Frequency f ± 10 %	Tidal Volume (V_T), mL
≤5	0,01	40	1:1	60	20
>5 ≤10	0,1	2	1:2	25	150
>10≤ 40	0,2	2	1:2	20	15 × B[A]
>40	0,2	2	1:2	20	>600

[A]Body mass, in kilograms, stated by the manufacturer in the manual.

7.9.5 *Automatic Time-Cycled, Gas-Powered Resuscitators*—Automatic time-cycled, gas-powered resuscitators shall meet the requirements specified in 7.1.2, 7.8.1, 7.9.1, and 7.9.2, when tested by the methods described in A1.5.8, A1.5.13, A1.5.14, and A1.5.16.

7.9.6 *Volume-Cycled, Gas-Powered Resuscitators*—Volume-cycled, gas-powered resuscitators shall meet the requirements specified in 7.1.2, 7.8.1, 7.9.1, and 7.9.2, when tested by the methods described in A1.5.8, A1.5.13, A1.5.14, and A1.5.16.

7.10 *Demand Valves*:

NOTE 13—These devices are subject to the requirements of this specification only when included as an integral part of a resuscitator.

7.10.1 *Pressure for Initiation (See also* Annex A3*)*—When tested by the method described in A1.5.18, the pressure drop needed to initiate gas flow shall be no more than a negative 0.2 kPa (≃2 cmH_2O).

7.10.2 *Peak Inspiratory Flow (See also* Annex A3*)*—When tested by the method described in A1.5.18.2, the minimum peak inspiratory flow shall be 100 L/min for at least 10 s, at an outlet pressure of no more than 0.8 kPa (≃8 cmH_2O).

7.10.3 *Termination Pressure (See also* Annex A3*)*—Demand flow shall terminate either when the negative input pressure equals atmospheric pressure or at a pressure stated by the manufacturer, when tested by the method described in A1.5.18.3.

8. Resistance to Environment

8.1 *Storage*—The resuscitator and the resuscitator kit (if provided) shall after storage at temperatures of – 40 and + 60°C and at any relative humidity between 40 and 95 %, meet the general requirements and the specific requirements for the category of resuscitator being tested, that is operator-powered or gas-powered, etc., specified in Section 7.

8.2 *Operating Conditions (See also* Annex A3*)*—When tested by the method described in A1.5.19, the resuscitator shall meet the general requirements and the specific requirements for the category of resuscitator being tested, specified in Section 7, throughout the temperature range from –18 to + 50°C and a humidity range from 40 to 95 % relative humidity.

NOTE 14—Problems due to ice formation will occur during use at temperatures below – 4°C and may render the unit inoperable.

9. Gas Supply

9.1 *Gas Cylinders, Cylinder Valves and Yoke Connections*—If provided, gas cylinders, cylinder valves and yoke connections of the pin index type shall meet the requirements given in ISO 407.

NOTE 15—Small cylinders with special fittings are frequently used in special situations.

9.2 *Indication of Contents*—Each gas supplied at cylinder pressure shall be monitored by a cylinder pressure gage or contents indicator.

9.3 *Captive Valve Key*—If detachable, the hand wheel, key or other device shall be made captive by means of a retaining chain or similar attachment capable of withstanding a static load of not less than 200 *N* (20 kg) without breaking.

9.4 *Connections for Compressed Gas (See also* Annex A3*)*—Gas connections between different gas services shall be noninterchangeable and shall not allow parts of the resuscitator to be incorrectly connected. If the device has a threaded connection, it shall meet the requirements given in ISO 5359.

NOTE 16—If provided, a press-fit connection should give an easy and reliable connection with 6 mm inside diameter elastomeric tubing.

9.5 *Supply Pressures (See also* Annex A3*)*—When supplied with gas at a pressure between 270 and 550 kPa (see 10.3.2.3(*n*)), the resuscitator shall meet the general requirements and any specific requirements for the type of resuscitator being tested, that is, automatically or manually cycled, specified in Section . Testing shall be as described in A1.5.20.

10. Information to be Supplied by Manufacturer

10.1 *Marking*:

10.1.1 *Manufacturer's Warning (See also* Annex A3*)*—For automatic pressure-cycled, gas-powered resuscitators, the manufacturer shall provide a warning on the resuscitator and the resuscitator case, and in the instructions for use shall be a warning that the unit is not designed to be used with closed-chest cardiac compression.

NOTE 17—Where possible, simple operating instructions should be provided on the resuscitator or the container.

10.1.2 *Range of Supply Pressures*—The range of supply pressures through which the resuscitator will operate shall be marked on the resuscitator.

10.1.3 *Gas Source for Spontaneously Breathing Patients*—If supplied, the gas source supplying a spontaneously breathing patient, if it is other than the reservoir, shall be indicated on the resuscitator.

10.1.4 *Indication of Pressure-Limiting System Setting*—If the resuscitator is supplied with a pressure-limiting system set at one fixed pressure, the nominal pressure setting at which the system is activated shall be marked on the resuscitator.

10.2 *Training*—The instructions provided shall include a warning that the unit must only be used by persons who have received training in resuscitation techniques.

10.3 *Information to be Provided by Manufacturer in Operating and Maintenance Instructions*:

10.3.1 *General*—The manufacturer shall provide instructions for use and maintenance instructions. The size and shape of this (these) manual(s) shall be such that it (they) may be enclosed within or attached to the resuscitator container. The instructions for use shall state that additional copies are available on request from the manufacturer.

10.3.2 *Contents*—The manual shall be divided into sections to facilitate understanding of the instructions and shall include the following information:

10.3.2.1 A warning that the resuscitator must be used only by persons who have received adequate training.

10.3.2.2 Instructions on how to make the resuscitator operational in all intended modes of operation.

10.3.2.3 A specification detailing the following information:

(a) *(a)* The body mass range for which the resuscitator is suitable for use,

(b) *(b)* Range of ventilatory frequency,

(c) *(c)* Attainable delivery pressures,

(d) (d) Operating environmental limits,

(e) (e) Storage environmental limits,

(f) (f) Delivered oxygen concentrations under various test conditions,

(g) (g) Characteristics or dimensions, or both, of the gas inlet connection,

(h) (h) Stroke-volume range for operator-powered resuscitators,

(i) (i) Apparatus deadspace (backward leakage and forward leakage, where appropriate),

(j) (j) Expiratory resistance and inspiratory resistance, and any special fittings that impose such resistance,

(k) (k) The value of end-expiratory pressure generated by the resuscitator in normal use, if greater than 0,2 kPa (≃2 cmH 2O),

(l) (l) Details of the pressure-limiting system and override mechanism operation, if any,

(m) (m) External dimensions of the resuscitator and, if provided, the resuscitator case, and

(n) (n) Mass of the resuscitator and, if provided, the resuscitator case.

10.3.2.4 Instructions for the dismantling and reassembly of components for cleaning and sterilization (if applicable). This shall include an illustration of the parts in their correct relationship. The manufacturer shall recommend a functional test of operation to be carried out after reassembly,

10.3.2.5 Recommendations for the preferred methods of cleaning and disinfection or sterilization of the resuscitator and its components,

10.3.2.6 A recommended functional test for operation to be carried out immediately prior to use,

10.3.2.7 A list of operator-replaceable parts,

10.3.2.8 Recommendations for frequency of approved or factory service,

NOTE 18—If no service is required, this should also be stated in the manual.

10.3.2.9 Resuscitator flow capabilities (if gas-powered) at 2 and at 4 kPa (≃20 and at ≃40 cmH_2O) airway pressure,

10.3.2.10 Recommendations for use in hazardous or explosive atmospheres, including a warning that if the resuscitator will entrain or permit the patient to inhale gas from the atmosphere, its use in contaminated environments may be hazardous unless entrainment is prevented. If applicable, the manufacturer shall describe how to prevent such entrainment or inhalation, for example, by the use of a filter,

10.3.2.11 Warnings that in the presence of high oxygen concentrations there is danger from smoking or open flames and that oil should not be used with the resuscitator,

10.3.2.12 Date of publication or revision of the manual, or both,

10.3.2.13 The approximate duration of the gas supply, expressed as time per litre cylinder volume when charged to the maximum nationally approved filling pressure and when the resuscitator is delivering a minute volume of 10 L/min (or the nearest setting to this) of at least 85 % (V/V) oxygen, and the manufacturer's elected value less than 85 % (V/V) oxygen, if the resuscitator is so capable; and

10.3.2.14 The range of supply pressures with which the resuscitator meets the applicable requirements specified in Section 7 and details of any necessary adjustments for particular supply pressures.

11. Keywords

11.1 artificial breathing apparatus; intensive care equipment; medical equipment; resuscitators; specifications; tests

ANNEXES

(Mandatory Information)

A1. TEST METHODS

A1.1 General Test Conditions

A1.1.1 The ambient temperature for the duration of the tests shall be between 20 and 25°C, except where otherwise stated. The relative humidity shall be within the range from 45 to 75 %, except where otherwise stated.

A1.2 (A2) Apparatus

A1.2.1 Typical test apparatus is shown in Figs. A1.1-A1.6; alternative test apparatus of equivalent or greater accuracy may be used (see A1.3).

A1.2.2 (A2.1) *Test Lung* (see Figs. A1.4 and A1.5 for examples), with appropriate compliance and resistance characteristics (see Table 1).

A1.2.3 (A2.2) *Resistors*, if not provided with the test lung.

A1.2.4 (A2.3) *Pressure, Flow, and Volume-Measuring and Recording Apparatus*, including a pneumotachograph.

A1.2.5 (A2.4) *Temperature-Measurement Apparatus.*

A1.2.6 (A2.5) *Deadspace-Measurement Apparatus*, (see Fig. A1.3 for typical example).

A1.2.7 (A.2.6) *Negative Pressure Generator*, (see Fig. A1.6 for typical example).

A1.2.8 (A.2.7) *Graduated Cylinder*, of at least 200 mL capacity.

A1.2.9 (A.2.8) *Oxygen Analyzer.*

A1.2.10 (A.2.9) *Water Reservoir*, minimum 1 by 1 by 1 m.

A1.2.11 (A.2.10) *Template*, 300 by 400 mm.

A1.2.12 (A.2.11) *Compressed Air Source*, capable of varying over the range from 270 to 550 kPa, and of producing a flow rate from 5 min to 60 L/min.

NOTE A1.1—This apparatus is only required if the resuscitator uses compressed air within the stated pressure ranges during normal operation.

NOTE A1.2—Flow rates exceeding 60 L/min may be required if the

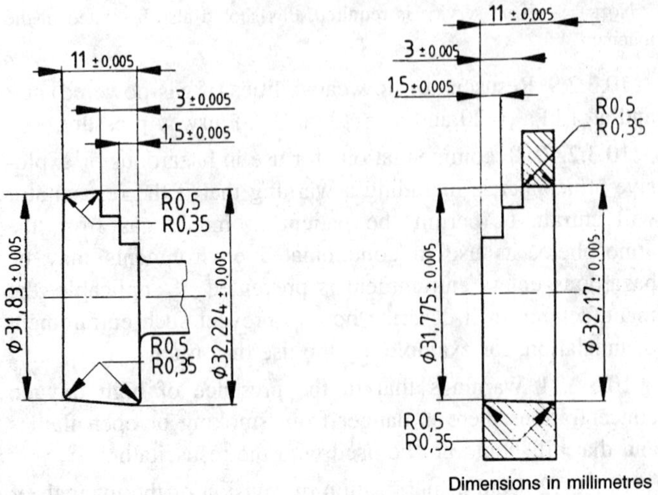

NOTE 1—Basic taper is 1:28 on diameter.

NOTE 2—Engagement is 9.5 nom.

FIG. A1.1 32-mm Ring and Plug Gages

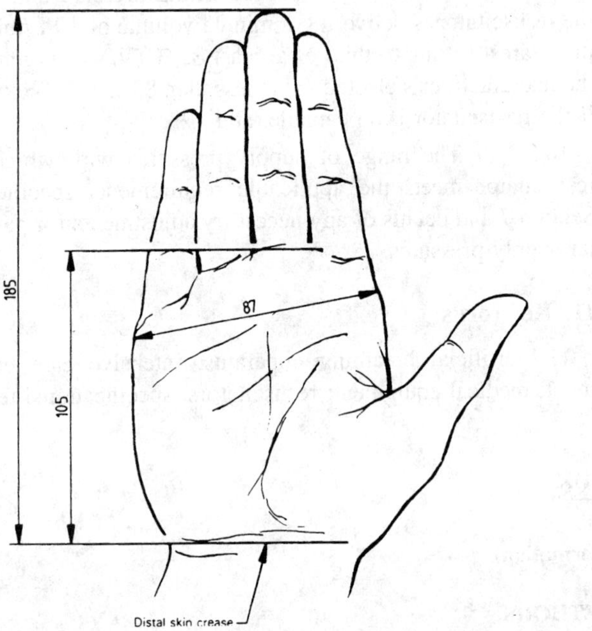

FIG. A1.2 Maximum Hand Dimensions

resuscitator is capable of flow rates exceeding 60 L/min (see A1.5.16).

A1.2.13 (A.2.12) *Environmental Chamber*, capable of maintaining temperatures from −40 ± 1°C to +60 ± 1°C and relative humidity from 40 to 95 % for periods of up to seven days.

A1.2.14 (A.2.13) *Oxygen Supply*, capable of varying over the range from 270 to 550 kPa and of producing a flow rate of at least 30 L/min.

A1.2.15 (A.2.14) *Vacuum Source*, capable of producing flow rates from 5 to 50 L/min.

A1.2.16 (A.2.15) *Gas Source*, capable of varying through the range of pressures from 270 to 550 kPa.

A1.3 (A.3) Test Apparatus Tolerances

A1.3.1 Test apparatus shall have the following minimum tolerances:

A1.3.1.1 (A.3.1) *Oxygen Analyzer*—±1 % (V/V) of the concentration being measured with a response time of greater than 90 % in 10 s.

A1.3.1.2 (A.3.2) *Compliances*—±5 % of the required compliance value throughout a range of inspiratory phase times from 0.5 to 6 s (see Annex A3).

A1.3.1.3 (A.3.3) *Pressure, Flow, and Volume*—±2.5 % of the reading plus ±2.5 % of the full scale reading. The reading accuracy of the associated recording device shall be maintained at a frequency of up to 10 Hz.

A1.3.1.4 (A.3.4) *Resistances*—±20 % for linear resistances and ±10 % for parabolic resistances within the designated flow range (see Annex A2).

A1.3.1.5 (A.3.5) *Temperature Measurement*—±0.5°C.

A1.4 (A.4) Conditioning and Reference Conditions

A1.4.1 (A.4.1) *Conditioning of Resuscitator and Test Apparatus*—Unless otherwise specified in particular tests, place the resuscitator and test apparatus in the test location and allow sufficient time for the resuscitator and apparatus to reach equilibrium with ambient conditions.

A1.4.2 (A.4.2) *Reference Conditions*—Correct all test readings to the reference conditions of ATPD (20°C, 1 atm, 0 % relative humidity).

A1.5 (A.5) Procedures

A1.5.1 (A.5.1) *Bag Refill Valve Connectors*—Using a 32 mm gage (see Fig. A1.1), measure the internal and external diameters of the connector.

A1.5.2 (A.5.2) *Dismantling and Reassembly*—Verify by inspection of the resuscitator and accompanying documents that a functional test has been provided to test operation after reassembly.

A1.5.3 (A.5.3) *Valve Function After Contamination with Vomitus:*

A1.5.3.1 (A.5.3.1) *Test Material*—Simulated vomitus, prepared by mixing two parts of baby meal beef with vegetable meal and one part water.

A1.5.3.2 (A.5.3.2) *Procedure*—Warm the simulated vomitus to 37 ± 3°C and pour 175 mL into the patient connection port while cycling the resuscitator at a rate of 30 breaths per minute for resuscitators suitable for use with patients of a body mass up to 10 kg, and at a rate of 12 breaths per minute for all other models. Perform this test with the resuscitator connected to the test lung (see A1.2.2). Continue to cycle the resuscitator for 30 s. Clear the resuscitator of the mixture according to the manufacturer's instructions and verify the resuscitator's performance.

NOTE A1.3—Some of the test solution may spill over when poured into the patient connection port.

A1.5.4 (A.5.4) *Drop Test*—Drop the resuscitator from a height of at least 1 m onto a concrete floor in the worst case orientation. For the purposes of this test, the resuscitator shall be a complete unit, including the face mask, valve, hose, regulator and cylinder, as appropriate. If the resuscitator kit

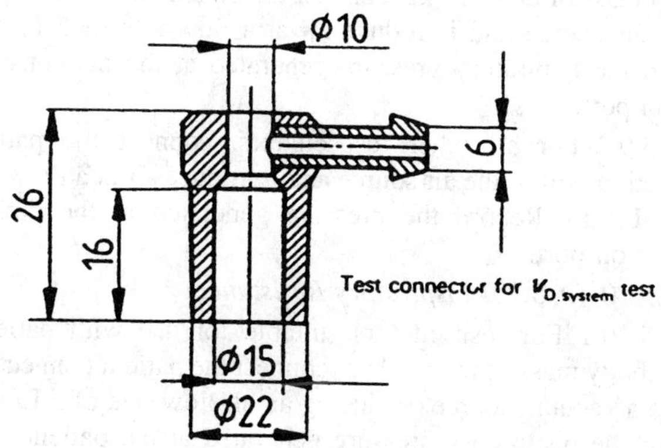

Dimensions in millimetres

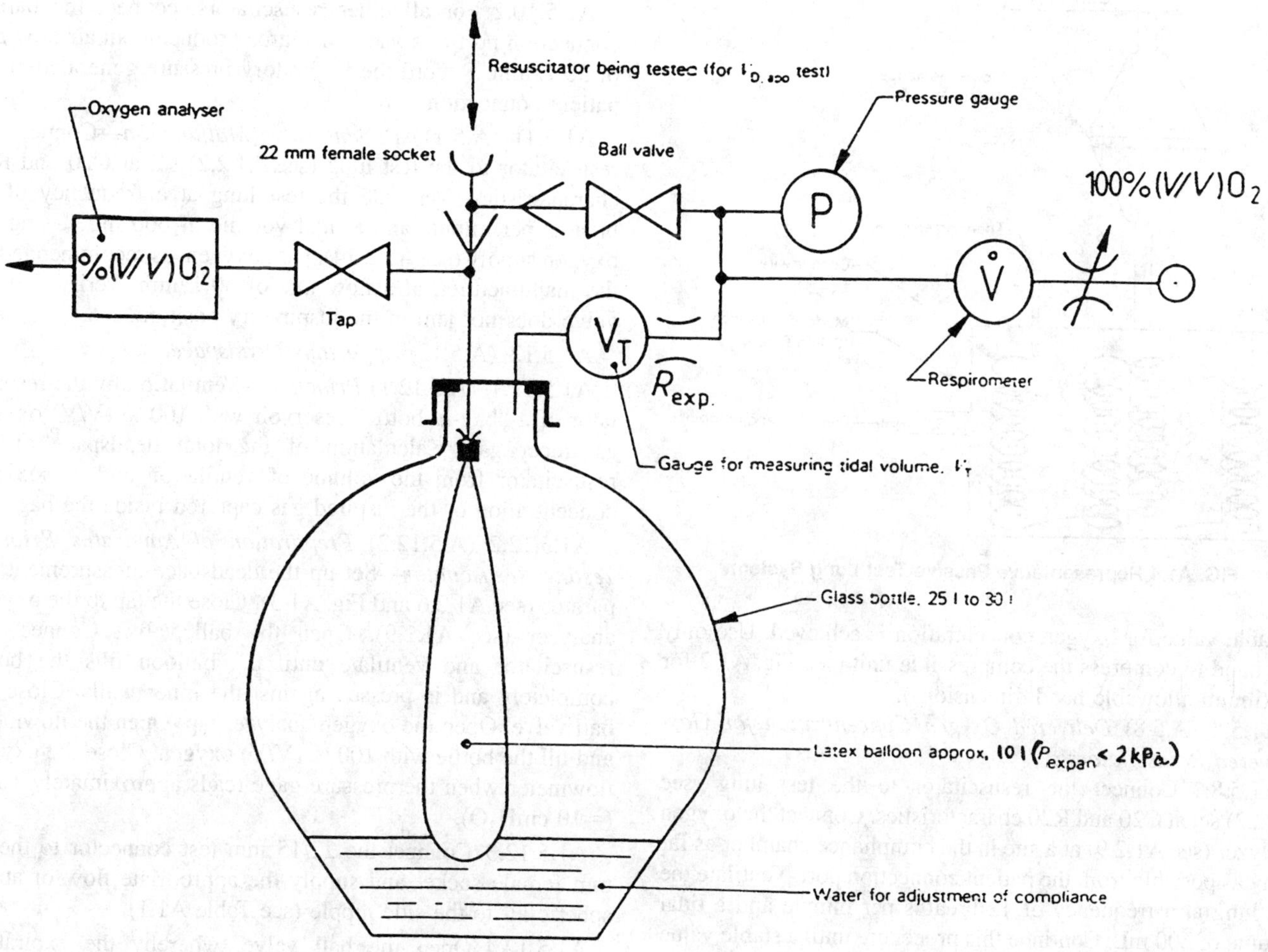

Dimensions in millimetres

FIG. A1.3 Test Setup for Measuring Total Apparatus Deadspace

includes a cylinder, perform the test with the cylinder empty.

A1.5.5 (A.5.5) *Mechanical Shock Test for Resuscitator Fixtures that are Mounted on Castors or on Wheels*—Place the resuscitator in its recommended operating position. Tip the resuscitator over in its worst case orientation. This test shall only be performed once.

A1.5.6 (A.5.6) *Immersion in Water*—Arrange the resuscitator in its ready-for-use condition, that is, gas on, gas off, etc. and drop it from a height of 1 m into the water reservoir (see A1.2.10). Take the resuscitator out after 10 s and shake out the water for not more than 20 s. Begin ventilating the test lung (see A1.2.2) immediately.

A1.5.7 (A.5.7) *Supplementary Oxygen and Delivered Oxygen Concentration*—Connect the resuscitator to the test lung (see A1.2.2) set at C20 and R20 characteristics. Connect an oxygen analyzer (see A1.2.9) at a site in the compliance chamber as far away as possible from the patient connection port. Ventilate the test lung at a frequency of 12 breaths per minute and a tidal volume of 600 mL. Introduce input oxygen flows of no more than 15 L/min. Continue this procedure until

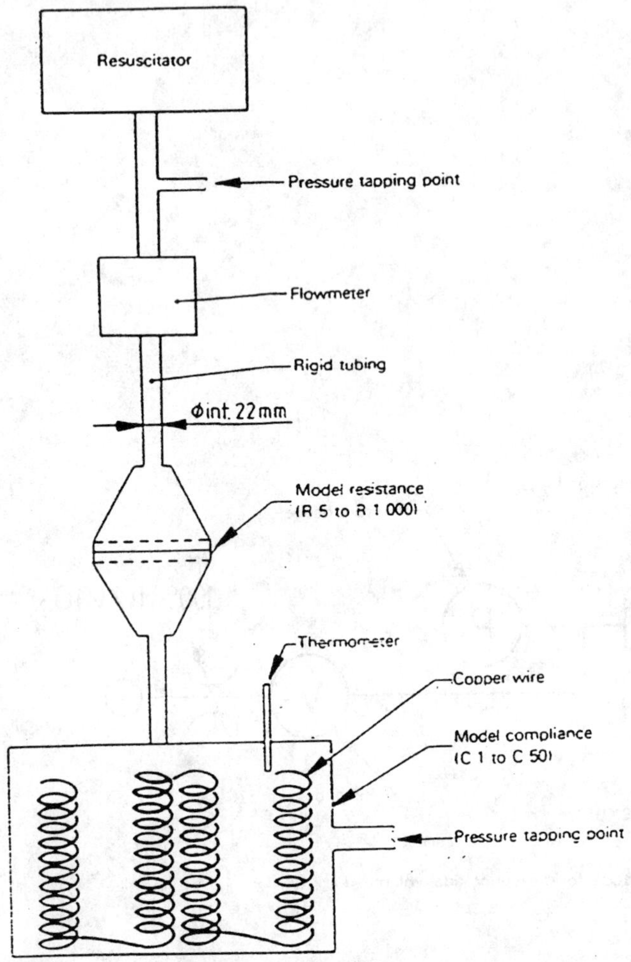

FIG. A1.4 Representative Passive Test Lung System

a stable value for oxygen concentration is achieved. Use only one hand to compress the compressible unit (see Fig. A1.2 for maximum allowable hand dimensions).

A1.5.8 (A.5.8) *Delivered Oxygen Concentration for Gas-Powered Resuscitators:*

A1.5.8.1 Connect the resuscitator to the test lung (see A1.2.2) set at C20 and R20 characteristics. Connect the oxygen analyzer (see A1.2.9) at a site in the compliance chamber as far away as possible from the patient connection port. Ventilate the test lung at a frequency of 12 breaths per minute and a tidal volume of 600 mL. Continue this procedure until a stable value for oxygen concentration is reached. Confirm that the resuscitator delivers an oxygen concentration of at least 85 % (V/V). If the resuscitator is capable of delivering other oxygen concentrations, arrange the resuscitator as recommended by the manufacturer and confirm that the oxygen concentration delivered to the test lung is within the range given by the manufacturer.

A1.5.8.2 Repeat the whole procedure using the test lung set at C50 and R5 characteristics.

A1.5.8.3 Perform both tests at the maximum and minimum flow settings recommended for the resuscitator.

A1.5.9 (A.5.9) *Expiratory Resistance:*

A1.5.9.1 For resuscitators suitable for use with patients with a body mass of up to 10 kg, connect the patient connection port to the air source and introduce air at a flow rate of 5 L/min. Record the expiratory pressure generated at the patient connection port.

A1.5.9.2 For all other resuscitators, connect the patient connection port to the air source and introduce air at a flow rate of 50 L/min. Record the pressure generated at the patient connection port.

A1.5.10 (A.5.10) *Inspiratory Resistance:*

A1.5.10.1 For resuscitators suitable for use with patients with a body mass of up to 10 kg, connect the patient connection port to a vacuum source producing an air flow rate of 5 L/min. Record the inspiratory pressure generated at the patient connection port.

A1.5.10.2 For all other resuscitators, connect the patient connection port to a vacuum source producing an air flow rate of 50 L/min. Record the inspiratory pressure generated at the patient connection port.

A1.5.11 (A.5.11) *Patient Valve Malfunction*—Connect the resuscitator to the test lung (see A1.2.2) set at C20 and R20 characteristics. Ventilate the test lung at a frequency of 12 breaths per minute and a tidal volume of 600 mL. Using the oxygen supply (see A1.2.14), pass oxygen, as recommended by the manufacturer, at a flow rate of 30 L/min. Verify that the valve does not jam in the inspiratory position.

A1.5.12 (A.5.12) *Apparatus Deadspace:*

A1.5.12.1 (A.5.12.1) *Principle*—Ventilation by the resuscitator of a "bag-in-bottle" reservoir with 100 % (V/V) oxygen as tracer gas. Calculation of the total deadspace of the resuscitator from the volume of ventilation and the oxygen concentration of the inspired gas captured inside the bag.

A1.5.12.2 (A.5.12.2) *Preparation of Apparatus Prior to Testing Resuscitator*—Set up the deadspace-measurement apparatus (see A1.2.6 and Fig. A1.3). Close the tap to the oxygen analyzer (see A1.2.9). Open the ball valve. Connect the resuscitator and ventilate until the balloon fills the bottle completely and is pressed against the inner walls. Close the ball valve. Open the oxygen analyzer tap. Open the flowmeter and fill the bottle with 100 % (V/V) oxygen. Close the oxygen flowmeter when the pressure gage reads approximately 1 kPa (≃10 cmH_2O).

A1.5.12.3 Connect the 22/15 mm test connector to the 22 mm female socket and supply the appropriate flow of atmospheric air to the side nipple (see Table A1.1).

A1.5.12.4 Open the ball valve, whereby the expiratory flowpath is flushed with 100 % (V/V) oxygen.

A1.5.12.5 Ventilate the lung by covering and opening the 10 mm diameter hole with a finger. Hold the tidal volume constant by means of the respirometer and pressure gage. The number of ventilating cycles is given in Table A1.1.

A1.5.12.6 Close the ball valve and open the analyzer tap. Adjust the 100 % (V/V) oxygen flow to approximately 5 L/min. Record the reading for the oxygen concentration in the bag, $F_{O2,bag}$, of the oxygen analyzer. Close off the oxygen flow when the pressure gage reads 1 kPa (≃10 cmH_2O) again.

A1.5.12.7 Determine the internal deadspace of the test apparatus for every combination of test parameters used.

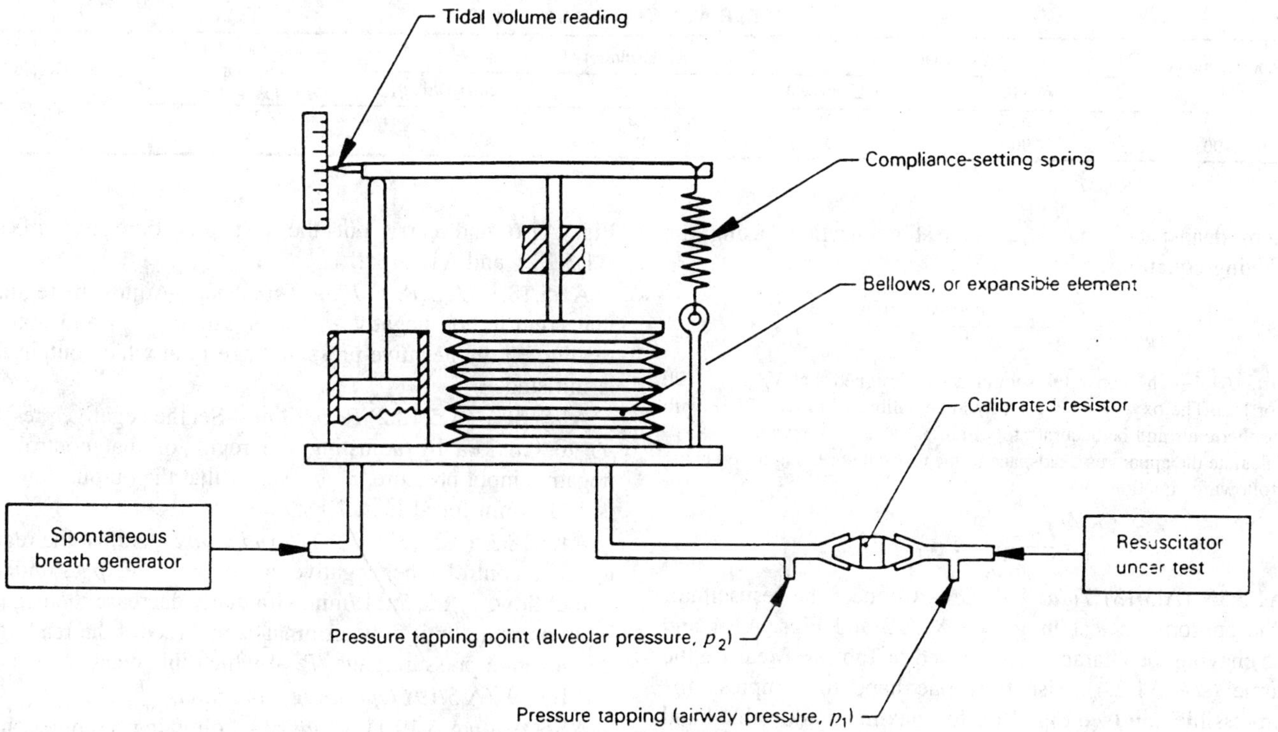

FIG. A1.5 Example of Active Test Lung System

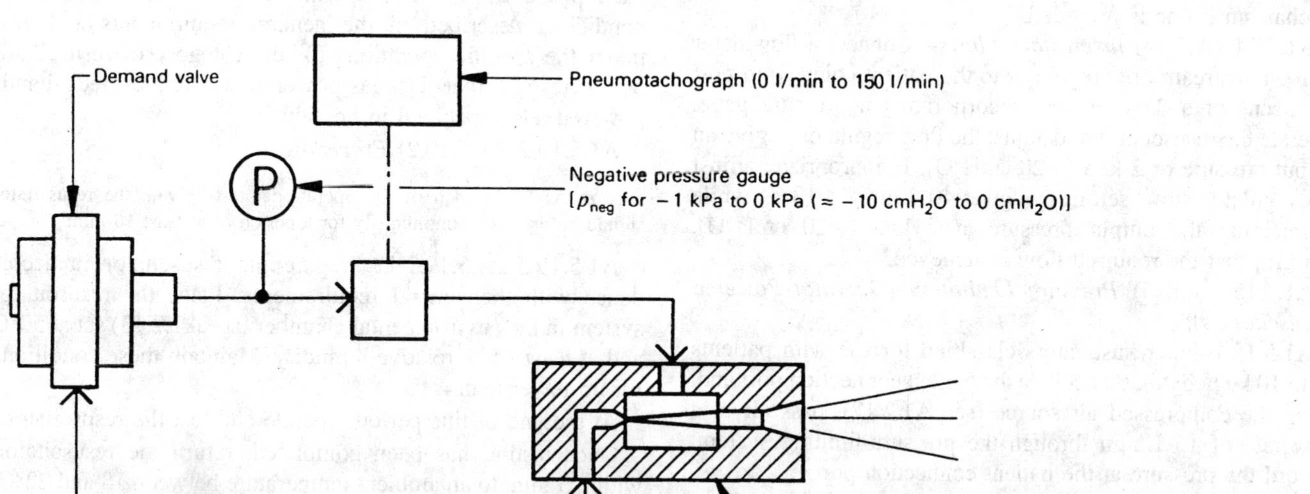

FIG. A1.6 Example of Test Apparatus for Testing Demand Valves (Threshold and Peak Flows)

A1.5.12.8 The apparatus is now ready for testing the resuscitator.

A1.5.12.9 (A.5.12.3) *Procedure*—Test the resuscitator using the same procedure as described for the test connector (see A1.5.12.2).

A1.5.12.10 (A.5.12.4) *Expression of Results*—Calculate the

TABLE A1.1 Test Parameters

Tidal Volume (V_T), mL	Compliance, C		Expiratory Resistance, R_{exp}		Test Flow for Internal Deadspace, L/min	Test Cycles
	mL/kPa	(mL/cmH_2O)	kPa/(L/s)	(cmH_2O/(L/s))		
600	200	(20)	0,5	(5)	30	>15
100	100	(10)	2	(20)	5	>50

system deadspace (that is, with test connection) using the following equation:

$$V_{D,system} = \frac{F_{O2,bag}(test\ connection)^{-21}}{79} \times V_T$$

NOTE A1.4—The apparatus should be so designed that $V_{D,system} = 20$ mL or less. The oxygen analyzer should be calibrated to read 21 % with atmospheric air and be accurate to within± 1 % (V/V) oxygen.

Calculate the apparatus deadspace of the resuscitator being tested using the following equation:

$$V_{D,system} = \frac{F_{O2,bag}^{-21}}{79} \times V_T - V_{D,system}$$

A1.5.13 (A.5.13) *Tidal Volumes*—Connect the resuscitator to the appropriate test lung (see A1.2.2 and Figs. A1.4 and A1.5) having the characteristics stated in Table 1. Measure the volume (see A1.2.4). Use only one hand to compress the compressible unit (see Fig. A1.2 for maximum allowable hand dimensions). Perform these tests without the use of an override mechanism if one is provided.

A1.5.14 (A.5.14) *Inspiratory Flows*—Connect a flowmeter with an upstream flow regulator to the patient connection port by means of a 22 mm hose incorporating a pressure gage. Operate the resuscitator and adjust the flow regulator to give an output pressure of 2 kPa (≃20 cmH_2O). If appropriate, adjust the regulator flow setting to give 40 L/min ±10 % while maintaining the output pressure at 2 kPa (≃20 cmH_2O). Confirm that the required flow is achieved.

A1.5.15 (A.5.15) *Pressure Limitation (Operator-Powered Resuscitators):*

A1.5.15.1 For resuscitators classified for use with patients up to 10 kg body mass, occlude the patient connection port and, using the compressed air source (see A1.2.12), pass air at a flow rate of 15 L/min through the pressure-limiting system. Record the pressure at the patient connection port.

A1.5.15.2 For resuscitators classified for use with patients of over 10 kg body mass and equipped with pressure-limiting systems, occlude the patient connection port and, using the compressed air source (see A1.2.12), pass air at a flow rate of 60 L/min through the pressure-limiting system. Record the pressure at the patient connection port.

A1.5.16 (A.5.16) *Pressure-Limiting System (Gas-Powered Resuscitators)*—Follow the method described in A1.5.14, substituting flows of 60 L/min or the maximum flow delivered by the resuscitator, whichever is greater.

A1.5.17 (A.5.17) *Pressure-Cycling System (Automatic, Pressure-Cycled, Gas-Powered Resuscitators)*—Connect the resuscitator to the appropriate test lung (see A1.2.2 and Figs. A1.4 and A1.5) having the characteristics stated in Table 1. Operate the resuscitator and record the pressure at which the resuscitator cycles from inspiration to expiration.

A1.5.18 (A.5.18) *Peak Inspiratory Flow and Flow Threshold*—Connect the demand valve to be tested as shown in Fig. A1.6 and carry out the test procedure described in A1.5.18.1 and A1.5.18.2.

A1.5.18.1 (A.5.18.1) *Flow Threshold*—Adjust the regulator that controls the negative input pressure, $p_{neg,1}$ and note the reading on the negative pressure gage *P*, at which output flow is initiated.

A1.5.18.2 (A.5.18.2) *Peak Flow*—Set the negative pressure, $p_{neg}$to 0.8 kPa by adjusting the regulator that controls the negative input pressure, $p_{neg,i}$. Verify that the output flow, $q_{v,o}$, is 100 L/min for at least 10 s.

A1.5.18.3 (A.5.18.3) *Flow Termination*—Adjust the regulator that controls the negative input pressure, $p_{neg,i}$until the output flow, $q_{v,o}$, is 5.0 L/min. Gradually decrease the negative input pressure until flow terminates, and record the reading on the negative pressure gage, *P*, at which this occurs.

A1.5.19 (A.5.19) *Operating Conditions:*

A1.5.19.1 (A.5.19.1) *General*—Following completion of each phase of the test, operate the resuscitator under the conditions described in the general requirements and also under the specific conditions for the category of resuscitator being tested, that is, gas-powered volume-cycled, hand-powered, etc., specified in Section 7.

A1.5.19.2 (A.5.19.2) *Procedure:*

NOTE A1.5—In each of the operational tests given, the resuscitator should be operated continuously for a period of at least 10 min.

A1.5.19.3 (A.5.19.2.1) Prepare the resuscitator in accordance with the general requirements. Place the resuscitator system in the environmental chamber (see A1.2.13) set at 50°C and at least 95 % relative humidity. Maintain these conditions for no fewer than 4 h.

At the end of this period, operate and test the resuscitator.

Once testing has been completed, return the resuscitator, within 5 min, to an ambient temperature between 18 and 22°C. Allow the resuscitator to stabilize for at least 4 h.

At the end of this period, operate and test the resuscitator.

A1.5.19.4 (A.5.19.2.2) Place the resuscitator in the environmental chamber set at – 40°C for a period of at least seven days, or until the resuscitator stabilizes.

At the end of this period, return the resuscitator, within 5 min, to an ambient temperature between 18 and 22°C. Alloy the resuscitator to stabilize for at least seven days.

At the end of this period, operate and test the resuscitator.

(A.5.19.2.3) Place the resuscitator in the environmental chamber at + 60°C and at 40 to 70 % relative humidity for a period of not less than seven days.

At the end of this period, return the resuscitator, within 5 min, to ambient conditions of 18 to 22°C and 40 to 70 % relative humidity. Allow the resuscitator to stabilize for at least seven days.

At the end of this period, operate and test the resuscitator.

Place the resuscitator in the environmental chamber set at − 18°C for 4 h.

At the end of this period, operate and test the resuscitator.

Once testing has been completed, return the resuscitator to ambient conditions of 18 to 22°C.

Within 5 min, operate and test the resuscitator.

A1.5.20 (A5.20) *Supply Pressures*—Connect the resuscitator to the gas source (see A1.2.16) and test its performance at source pressures of 270 and 550 kPa using the test methods described for the general requirements and any specific requirements for the type of resuscitator being tested, that is, automatically or manually cycled, specified in Section 7.

A2. COMPLIANCES AND RESISTANCES REQUIRED TO SET UP TEST LUNG

TABLE A2.1 Required Compliances

Classification[A]	Compliance, *C*	
	mL/kPa	mL/cmH_2O
C 50[B]	500	(50)
C 20	200	(20)
C 10	100	(10)
C 1	10	(1)

[A] The classification was originally based on conventional centimetres of water.
[B] Not used in test procedure.

TABLE A2.2 Required Resistances

Classification[A]	Resistance				Range of Air Flow[B] (for linear or parabolic resistances) is
	Linear, *R*		Parabolic[C], *R*•		
	kPa/(L/s)	[cmH_2O/(L/s)]	kPa/(L/s)	[cmH_2O/(L/s)]	
R 5	0.5	[5]	0.77	[7.7]	0 to 2
R 20	2	[20]	0.56	[5.6]	0.5 to 1
R 50[D]	5	[50]	0.39	[3.9]	0.25 to 0.5
R 100	40	[400]	0.14	[1.4]	0.05 to 0.075

[A]The classification was originally based on conventional centimetres of water.

[B]The tolerances for the flow range values are ±20 % for linear resistances and = 0•• for parabolic resistances.

[C]The values for parabolic resistances refer to the nominal inside diameter in millimetres sharp-cornered orifices needed to achieve these resistance values. Other geometric shapes may be used, for example, thicker orifices with rounded corners, but nominal diameters would be different.

[D]Not used in test procedure.

A3. RATIONALE STATEMENT

A3.1 This annex provides a concise rationale for the important requirements of this specification and is intended for those who are familiar with the subject of the specification but who have not participated in its development. An understanding of the reasons for the main requirements is considered to be essential for its proper application. Furthermore, as clinical practice and technology change it is believed that a rationale for the present requirements will facilitate any revision of the specification necessitated by those developments. The clauses in this annex have been so numbered to correspond to the clauses in the specification to which they refer. The numbering is, therefore, not consecutive.

A3.1.1 (5.1) *Patient Connection Port*—The patient connector dimensions permit connection to standard 15 mm tracheal tube connectors (see ISO 7228) and face masks having a 22 mm female connector or a 15 mm male connector.

A3.1.2 (5.2) *Expiratory Port for Breathing Gases*—The exhaust connection described is that used for connection to the transfer tubes of anesthetic gas scavenging systems. It is essential that breathing system conical connectors are not compatible with this port. It is also important that the exhaust port be designed such that it cannot be confused with the inspiratory port during use of the resuscitator.

A3.1.3 (5.3) *Face Mask Connectors*—It is important that resuscitator face masks should be generally interchangeable.

A3.1.4 (5.4) *Bag Refill Valve Connectors*—The size of this connector is chosen to prevent the accidental fitting of demand valves with manual controls.

A3.1.5 (6.2) *Dismantling and Reassembly*—Wrongly assembling a resuscitator so that it causes incorrect operation or complete malfunction is a serious hazard that may result in inadequate ventilation of the patient.

A3.1.6 (6.3) *Patient Valve Function After Contamination with Vomitus*—It is important that vomitus can be quickly and effectively cleared from a resuscitator so that resuscitation can be continued with a minimum of interruption.

A3.1.7 (6.4.1) *Drop Test*—It is important that resuscitators can withstand severe shock caused by falls from ambulances, hospital beds, etc.

A3.1.8 (6.4.2) *Mechanical Shock Test for Resuscitator Fixtures That are Mounted on Castors or on Wheels*—Castor-mounted or wheeled resuscitators may be tipped over either on the way to or during a resuscitation. This should not render the unit inoperative.

A3.1.9 (6.5) *Immersion in Water*—Resuscitators are often used in areas where the device may be inadvertently dropped into water during the resuscitation. If the unit is recovered quickly from the water, it should still function.

A3.1.10 (6.6) *Bag Refill Valves*—It is imperative that demand valves with manual controls are not accidentally substituted for bag refill valves. Demand valves are capable of high gas flows that may cause resuscitator patient valves to jam.

A3.1.11 (7.1) *Size* —Resuscitators may be required where access to patients is difficult, such as in crawl spaces and through manholes.

A3.1.12 (8.1.1) *Operator-Powered Resuscitators*—Although 40 % (V/V) oxygen concentration is adequate under some circumstances, 85 % (V/V) or higher oxygen concentrations are preferable for the treatment of severely hypoxemic patients during resuscitation. This concentration should be achievable at supplementary oxygen flows of 15 L/min or less because to specify greater than 15 L/min would exceed the normal calibration of standard, clinically used flowmeters for adult use and could potentially lead to inaccurate control of oxygen flows and jamming of the patient valve in the inspiratory position.

A3.1.13 (8.1.2) *Gas-Powered Resuscitators*—High oxygen concentrations are important in resuscitating patients who are extremely hypoxemic. Lower percentages of oxygen will lengthen the duration of oxygen supply. The performance of air-entrainment" mixing" devices is influenced by the flow settings of the resuscitator and the compliance and resistance of the patient.

A3.1.14 (8.3) *Expiratory Resistance*—To facilitate exhalation, expiratory resistance should be minimized unless there are special clinical indications to impose such resistance.

A3.1.15 (8.4) *Inspiratory Resistance*—The design of a resuscitator should be such that it is possible for the patient to breathe spontaneously without excessive subatmospheric pressure when the resuscitator is applied to the patient's airway but is not activated by the operator.

A3.1.16 (8.5) *Patient Valve Malfunction*—Valve malfunction or jamming in the inspiratory position at high supplementary oxygen flows may lead to failure of the resuscitator and transmission of excessive pressures to the patient. Resuscitators are commonly used at oxygen input flows of 15 L/min, but flowmeter valves are often capable of permitting flows of over 30 L/min. It is essential to follow the manufacturer's instructions and to use only attachments recommended for use with the resuscitator.

A3.1.17 (8.6) *Patient Valve Leakage*—Forward leakage If forward leakage is a design feature of a resuscitator, it should be disclosed so that the user does not confuse this leakage with a malfunction.

A3.1.18 (8.7) *Apparatus Deadspace*—It is essential to minimize apparatus deadspace in order to limit rebreathing of expired gases.

A3.1.19 (8.8.1) *Tidal Volume*—For adult ventilation a typical tidal volume is approximately 600 mL. The compliances and resistances listed in Table 1 are representative of the possible compliances and resistances found in adults and children needing resuscitation. The tidal volume requirements of 15 mL/kg are higher than normal and are commonly used during resuscitation to allow for mask leakage. The ventilatory frequencies are typical values used in pediatric and adult resuscitation.

A3.1.20 (8.8.2) *Pressure Limitation (Operator-Powered Resuscitators)*—Experience with infant resuscitation suggests that a maximum inspiratory pressure of 4.5 kPa (≈45 cmH_2O) will not produce lung damage and will permit adequate tidal volumes in most patients weighing under 10 kg.

A3.1.21 Pressure-limiting systems are not specified for operator-powered resuscitators designated for use with patients weighing over 10 kg. However, it is essential that resuscitators with such systems satisfy the tidal volume requirements specified in this specification (see Table 1) without the use of any override mechanism. When airway pressure is limited to below 6 kPa (≈60 cmH_2O), it was felt that an override mechanism is essential in order to ventilate those patients with low lung compliance or high airway resistance, or both.

A3.1.22 (8.9.1) *Pressure-Limiting System*—It is essential that maximum delivery pressure is limited on all gas-powered resuscitators. Airway pressure at 4.5 kPa (≈45 cmH_2O) was considered adequate for ventilation of the lungs, but unlikely to produce barotrauma. The selection of higher settings for difficult clinical problems necessitates risk of barotrauma.

A3.1.23 (8.9.2) *Inspiratory Flow*—To minimize the risk of gastric distension, 40 L/min is considered to be the maximum flow that should be used when resuscitating with a mask. This is in accordance with the recommendations of the American Heart Association,[5] and these recommendations are generally accepted worldwide. Higher flows may be used with intubated patients because of the decreased risk of gastric distension.

A3.1.24 (8.9.4) *Automatic Pressure-Cycled, Gas-Powered Resuscitators*—It is required that pressure-cycled resuscitators meet the performance requirements of this specification, but they are of limited use on patients with poor lung compliance or high airway resistance, or both, because the cycling pressure is achieved without adequate ventilation. A "negative" pressure phase should not be used as it is associated with a fall in functional residual capacity (FRC) and arterial oxygen partial pressure (pO_2).

A3.1.25 (8.10.1) *Pressure for Initiation*—It is important that the patient should not have to generate large amounts of negative pressure to initiate gas flow from the demand valve in order to minimize respiratory work. A negative pressure of – 0,2 kPa (≈–2 cmH_2O) is physiologically acceptable.

A3.1.26 (8.10.2) *Peak Inspiratory Flow*—Peak flows as outlined in A3.1.26 are necessary in order to satisfy the inspiratory needs of the typical patient; large amounts of negative pressure should not be required to generate these flows as it would cause fatigue in a spontaneously breathing patient.

A3.1.27 (8.10.3) *Termination Pressure*—Positive pressure indicates that adequate tidal volume has been delivered. When the pressure becomes slightly positive it indicates that the patient should be allowed to exhale and hence flow should stop.

A3.1.28 (9.2) *Operating Conditions*—Resuscitators can be expected to be exposed to the temperature extremes outlined in 8.2 since such temperatures frequently occur throughout the world in environments where resuscitators are used.

A3.1.29 (10.4) *Connections for Compressed Gas*—It is essential to be easily able to connect resuscitator oxygen tubing, for example, while the resuscitator is in use.

A3.1.30 (10.5) *Supply Pressures*—The range of supply pressures reflects the variety of pressures used internationally and the tolerances of pressure-regulating systems.

A3.1.31 (11.1.1) *Manufacturer's Warning*—These resuscitators are unacceptable for use during closed chest cardiopulmonary resuscitation because the increased intrathoracic pressure caused during chest compression causes the resuscitator to cycle from the inspiratory mode to the expiratory mode prior to adequate ventilation of the lungs.

A3.1.32 (11.3.2) *Duration of Gas Supply (See 10.3.2.3(m))*—Small, easily portable cylinders are commonly used with resuscitators. It is important that the operator have some idea of the duration of this size of oxygen supply under simulated conditions of use.

[5] "American Heart Association Standards for CPR and ECC," *Journal of American Medical Association*, Vol 25, No. 1, June 6, 1986.

A4. MATERIALS

A4.1 *Cleaning and Disinfection or Sterilization (See also A4.5)* —Components that are subject to contamination should either withstand the methods of cleaning and disinfection or sterilization recommended by the manufacturer, or be labelled "for single use only" (disposable).

A4.2 *Oxygen Compatibility (See also A4.5)* —All resuscitator components should be compatible with and resistant to ignition with oxygen concentrations and pressures to which the component is exposed.

A4.3 *Resistance to Corrosion and Deterioration (See also A4.5)* —Resuscitator performance should not be degraded because of corrosion during a period of twelve months after being stored in accordance with the manufacturer's instructions.

A4.4 *Patient Valve Housing*—The valve housing should be constructed of materials such that the functioning mechanism is readily visible to the operator.

A4.5 *Rationale:*

A4.5.1 Cleaning and disinfection or sterilization Resuscitators are likely to become contaminated by bacteria and foreign matter during use. It is therefore essential that manufacturers recommend suitable methods of cleaning and disinfection or sterilization.

A4.5.2 For many applications, cleaning and disinfection alone is adequate. However, in certain situations, the user may require resuscitators that can withstand steam or ethylene oxide gas sterilization of the contaminated components. The user should appreciate that some methods of disinfection and sterilization may shorter the usable life of the resuscitator.

A4.6 *Oxygen Compatibility*—Selection of materials for use in high oxygen concentrations, especially at elevated supply pressures, involves consideration of both compatibility and ease of ignition. Materials that burn in air will burn violently in high concentrations of oxygen at atmospheric pressure and may explode at higher pressures. Many materials, including metals, will not burn in air but may do so in pure oxygen, particularly under pressure. Materials may be ignited by the friction of a valve seat or stem packing or by the adiabatic compression produced when oxygen at high pressure is suddenly introduced into a system at low pressure. Therefore, easily ignitable materials, such as some rubber and plastics, should be avoided in valves and fittings, especially in high-pressure oxygen systems, unless tested or experience-rated for such services. These conditions and requirement also apply to the use of nitrous oxide.

A4.7 *Resistance to Corrosion and Deterioration*—Since resuscitators are often stored and used in the proximity of sea water, it is important that resuscitators are capable of meeting the performance requirements of this specification after being used and stored in such an environment.

A5. FACE MASKS

A5.1 A face mask provided with or recommended for use with a resuscitator should comprise a body, a face seal, and a port to receive the patient connector of the resuscitator.

A5.2 If the face mask is constructed of more than one part, then the parts should be easily assembled and securely held together in use.

A5.3 The face seal should be capable of providing a fit that minimizes leaks at the operating pressures and temperatures specified in this specification.

A5.4 The body of the mask should be transparent to allow the operator to observe the patient's nose and mouth for breath condensation as evidence of breathing and also for the possible appearance of vomitus. It is not intended that this specification should prohibit the use of nontransparent or translucent masks. Under certain circumstances, their use may be preferable.

Standard Definitions of Terms Relating to Hemostatic Forceps[1]

This standard is issued under the fixed designation F 921; the number immediately following the designation indicates the year of original adoption or, in the case of revision, the year of last revision. A number in parentheses indicates the year of last reapproval. A superscript epsilon (ε) indicates an editorial change since the last revision or reapproval.

1. Scope

1.1 These definitions cover basic terms and considerations for the components of hemostatic forceps. Instruments in these definitions are limited to those fabricated from stainless steel and for general surgical procedures. See Figs. 1 and 2 .

2. Referenced Documents

2.1 *ASTM Standards:*

F 899 Specification for Stainless Steel Billet, Bar, and Wire for Surgical Instruments[2]

2.2 *ISO Document:*

ISO/DIS 7151/1 Instruments for Surgery—Hemostatic Forceps—General Requirements[3]

Definitions of Hemostatic Forceps

3. Terminology

box lock—the junction where the female member and the male member are secured forming the pivoting feature.

distal end—the working end, comprised of two jaws, that is furthest from the surgeon when in use.

female member—the component that accommodates and encloses the male member at the box lock junction.

finger rings—the feature of both the female and the male members that forms the gripping surface for the surgeon (commonly classified as the ring-handled feature in ISO/DIS 7151/1).

hemostatic forceps—an instrument, available in various sizes and configurations, used in surgical procedures for the compression of blood vessels and the grasping of tissue.

jaws—parts that contain serrations to interrupt the flow of blood through any vessel.

male member—the component that is inserted through the female member and secured to the female member at the box lock junction.

proximal end—that portion of the instrument that is closest to the surgeon when in use.

ratchets—the portion of both the female and the male members possessing inclined teeth that forms the locking mechanism.

serrations or teeth—the gripping or clamping surfaces of the jaws.

shank—the part of either the female or the male member that yields configuration, length, and leverage.

Definitions of Physical Properties of Hemostatic Forceps

chamfer—the broken edge of the jaw serrations and the external edges of the box lock surfaces.

corrosion—the formation of rust.

elasticity—the capacity of the instrument to undergo induced stress without permanent distortion or breakage of any component.

finish—the final surface visual appearance of the instrument classified as follows:

(1) bright or mirror finish—highly reflective surfaces.

(2) satin, matte, or black finish—reduced reflected surfaces (as compared to bright or mirror finish).

hardness—a measurement of the resistance to indentation.

interdigitation—the interlocking or meshing of the female and male jaw serrations.

jaw alignment—the positioning of the female and male jaws with respect to interdigitation (related to box lock function and ratchet performance).

passivation—the changing of the chemically active surface of stainless steel to a much less reactive state.

stainless steel—the raw material on the instrument that is in accordance with Specification F 899.

---

[1] These definitions are under the jurisdiction of ASTM Committee F-4 on Medical and Surgical Materials and Devices and is the direct responsibility of Subcommittee F04.33 on Medical/Surgical Instruments.

Current edition approved June 5, 1985. Published August 1985.

[2] *Annual Book of ASTM Standards*, Vol 13.01.

[3] Available from American National Standards Institute, 1430 Broadway, New York, NY 10018.

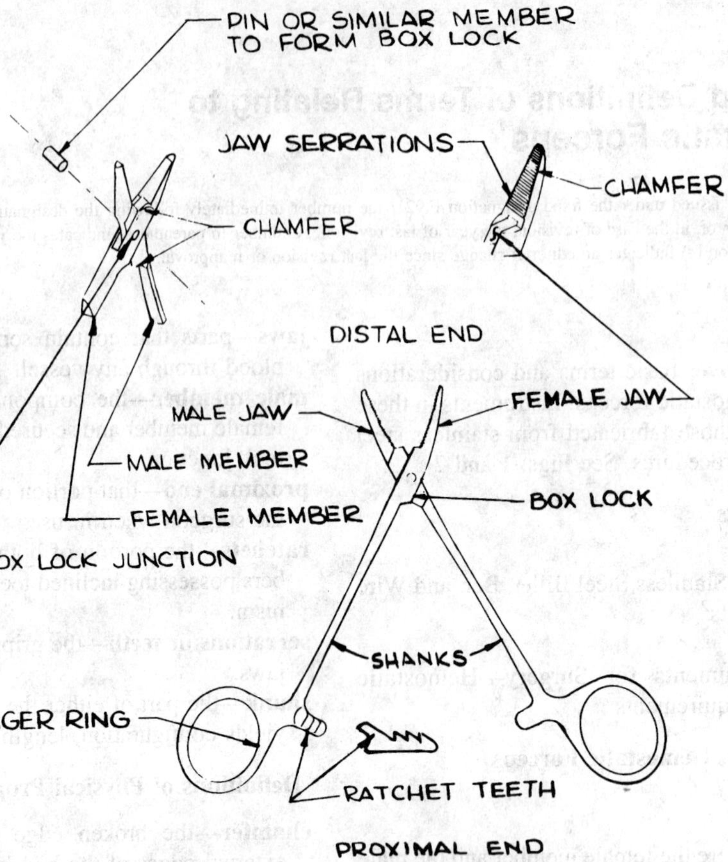

FIG. 1 Components of a Hemostatic Forceps

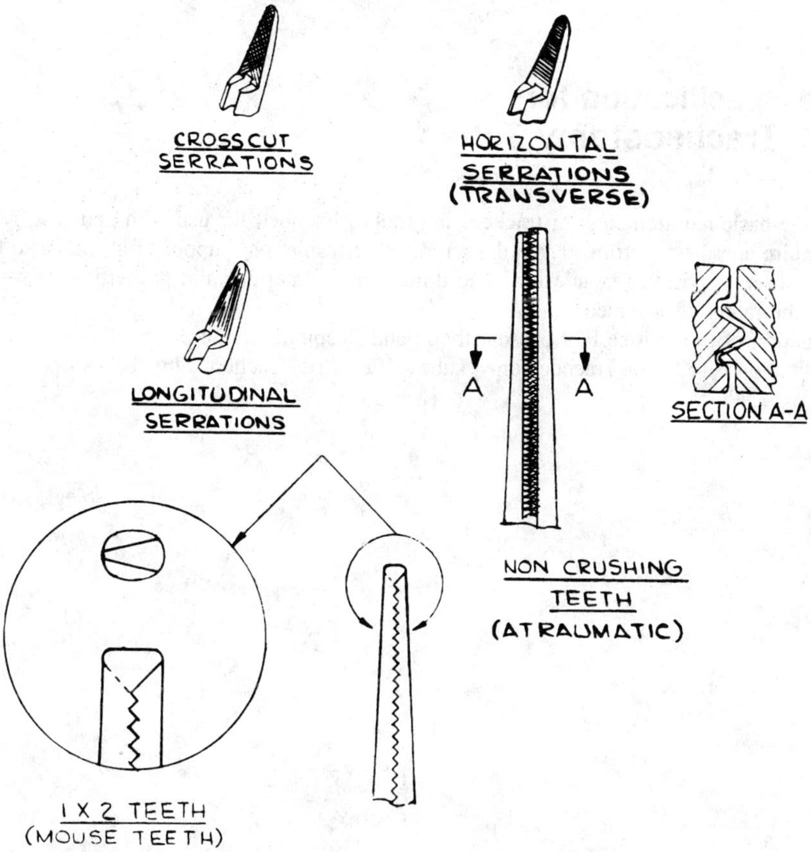

FIG. 2 Typical Types of Serrations and Teeth for Hemostatic Forceps

APPENDIX

(Nonmandatory Information)

X1. RATIONALE

X1.1 Because there is a clinical need for a variety of instruments for general and surgical procedures, they are manufactured in various configurations and from various types of stainless steel. For practical purposes and patient safety, these devices supplied by different manufacturers necessitate a defined system of categorization, materials, and performance requirements.

X1.2 This is the first standard of a multiple part standard that defines the components of a hemostatic forceps designed for repeated use, including various terminology that describes performance considerations.

X1.3 *Box Lock*—The box lock construction defined in these definitions is the most commonly produced junction for hemostatic forceps. However, the intent is not to prohibit technological innovation or to exclude instruments manufactured with other types of pivoting features such as lap joints.

X1.4 Disposable instruments are not included in these definitions, nor are the instruments designed for specific surgery. However, a part or all of the terminology defined herein may be applicable to specific and disposable surgical instruments.

Last ASTM Designation: F 927 – 86 (Reapproved 1994)

Standard Specification for Pediatric Tracheostomy Tubes

This specification covers the basic requirements for tracheostomy tubes intended for use with pediatric patients. Such tubes may be selected for patients who require anesthesia, artificial ventilation, or other respiratory support, but may also be used for others who do not require mechanical ventilation. Provision is made for basic dimensions, materials, and properties, as well as for related items, for example, inner cannula and obturators, if provided.

Formerly under the jurisdiction of Committee F29 on Anesthetic and Respiratory Equipment, this specification was discontinued in 1999 and replaced by Specification F 1627 for Tracheostomy Tubes—Pediatric Tracheostomy Tubes[1].

---

[1] *Annual Book of ASTM Standards*, Vol 13.01.

Standard Specification for Medical and Surgical Suction and Drainage Systems[1]

This standard is issued under the fixed designation F 960; the number immediately following the designation indicates the year of original adoption or, in the case of revision, the year of last revision. A number in parentheses indicates the year of last reapproval. A superscript epsilon (ε) indicates an editorial change since the last revision or reapproval.

This standard has been approved for use by agencies of the Department of Defense.

1. Scope

1.1 This specification describes minimum safety and performance requirements for medical and surgical suction and drainage apparatus.

1.2 This specification covers apparatus to be used for:

1.2.1 Oral, nasal, tracheal (ONT) suction,

1.2.2 Gastrointestinal drainage,

1.2.3 Pleural space and mediastinal drainage,

1.2.4 Closed wound drainage, and

1.2.5 Surgical suction (including uterine aspiration).

1.2.6 This specification also covers devices powered by centrally piped vacuum systems, compressed gases, electricity, and manual operation.

1.3 This specification does not cover the following:

1.3.1 Central vacuum pumps and piping systems of vehicles and buildings,

1.3.2 Catheters, tubes, drains, curettes, and suction tips inserted into the patient,

1.3.3 Syringes,

1.3.4 Breast pumps,

1.3.5 General dentistry suction equipment,

1.3.6 Waste gas scavenging systems,

1.3.7 Laboratory suction,

1.3.8 Fetal vacuum extractor or vacuum forceps with self-contained suction,

1.3.9 Autotransfusion,

1.3.10 Cardiopulmonary bypass pumps, and

1.3.11 Urinary drainage.

1.4 The following precautionary caveat pertains only to the test method portion, Section 5, of this specification: *This standard does not purport to address all of the safety problems, if any, associated with its use. It is the responsibility of the user of this standard to consult and establish appropriate safety and health practices and determine the applicability of regulatory limitations prior to use.* See 5.3.3.

2. Terminology

2.1 *Definitions of Terms Specific to This Standard:*

2.1.1 *aspiration*—the withdrawal, by means of suction, of fluids or friable tissue.

2.1.2 *collection vessel assembly*—a container whose primary function is to collect liquids.

2.1.3 *disclosure*—information on performance and test methods to be made available by manufacturers.

2.1.4 *drainage*—the removal of fluids from a body cavity or wound by a process utilizing gravity; drainage may be assisted by the application of vacuum.

2.1.5 *filter*—a device for reducing airborne particulate matter.

2.1.6 *flow-direction sensitivity*—performance is dependent on the direction of fluid flow.

2.1.7 *free air flow*—the flow of air into a vacuum source when its inlet is open to atmosphere.

2.1.8 *gastrointestinal drainage*—the removal of gastrointestinal contents, consisting of fluids and solid particles, by means of an indwelling tube which may be supplemented by gravity syphon or by vacuum.

2.1.9 *graduation indicators*—visible means of displaying measurement increments.

2.1.10 *inlet*—the port of a component into which fluid enters under use conditions.

2.1.11 *mediastinal drainage*—the removal of fluids from the mediastinum which may be supplemented by vacuum.

2.1.12 *outlet*—the port of a component from which fluid exits in normal use.

2.1.13 *patient connection*—the point at which the suction catheter, curette, or drainage tube inserted into the patient is attached to the suction system.

2.1.14 *pleural drainage*—the removal of fluids from the pleural space, maintaining a relatively constant partial vacuum within that space.

2.1.15 *regulator*—a device, which may be adjustable, that limits vacuum to a predetermined level.

2.1.16 *reprocessing*—preparation for reuse.

2.1.17 *shutoff mechanism*—a device designed to avoid overflow of suctioned material.

2.1.18 *stand-alone component*—a device which is not an integral part of any other component of the suction system.

2.1.19 *static vacuum*—the vacuum level without fluid movement.

2.1.20 *suction*—the removal of fluids or solids by the application of vacuum.

2.1.21 *suction system*—a series of components, devices, or assemblies which may include tubing, connectors, filters,

[1] This specification is under the jurisdiction of ASTM Committee F-29 on Anesthetic and Respiratory Equipmentand is the direct responsibility of Subcommittee F29.17 on Medical Surgical Suction and Drainage.

Current edition approved Jan. 8, 1986. Published March 1986.

collection vessels, shutoff mechanisms, regulators, portable pumps, safety overflow traps, and gages, beginning at the point of connection with the patient.

2.1.22 *vacuum*—a pressure less than atmospheric pressure.

2.1.23 *wound drainage*—the removal of fluids from a wound; removal may be supplemented by vacuum.

3. General Requirements

3.1 *Shutoff Mechanisms*—A suction or vacuum-assisted drainage system shall incorporate a shutoff mechanism which may stand alone or may be an integral part of a component of the system, unless the system is intended to continue operating after invasion or overflow of aspirated liquids and solids.

3.2 *Tubing Considerations*—Tubing used in suction and drainage systems should be kept as short as practical and should be arranged to minimize loops and drapes which can accumulate liquid and increase the potential for occlusion from pinching and kinks. Tubing diameter influences the total system resistance (see Appendix X1).

3.3 *Liquid Connections*—The connections which conduct liquids should be designed to minimize occlusion.

3.4 *Stand Alone Suction Tubing Connectors*:

3.4.1 *Lumen Size and Characteristics*—The size of stand alone suction tubing connector lumen chosen should not be less than 80 % of the nominal inside diameter of the suction tubing or 5 mm, whichever is greater. Internal passageways should be smooth. This requirement does not apply to wound and gastrointestinal drainage systems.

4. Performance Requirements

4.1 *Shutoff Mechanism Performance*—The shutoff mechanism shall not pass more than 5 mL of water distal to the shutoff mechanism. If the shutoff mechanism is integral to a collection vessel, it shall not activate before 90 % of the stated useable collection capacity of the system is reached.

4.2 *Electric Conductivity*—All components labeled conductive shall have a resistance not greater than 1 MΩ.

4.3 *System Performance*—When assembling the components of a suction or drainage system, the user should consider the flow resistance characteristics of the components in series and ensure that the system has the necessary performance characteristics for the suction procedure (see Appendix X2). The user should consider whether the system performance will be compromised by the use of a Y-piece or other multiport connector.

4.3.1 *Maximum Pleural Drainage System Pressure*—Pleural drainage systems shall not develop a pressure in excess of +10 cm H_2O at the patient inlet, at a flow of 10 L/min. If the pleural drainage system requires periodic adjustment to prevent intrapleural pressures above 10 cm H_2O, this shall be stated in the labeling.

4.3.2 *Leakage*—The leakage of a suction or drainage system is affected by the leaks of its components. Therefore, individual components shall not exceed their respective allowable leakage rates. Pumps and regulators are excluded (see 4.4 and 4.6.1.2).

4.3.3 *Resistance to Implosion*—If the collection vessel assembly will not resist loss of integrity and implosion at an applied vacuum of 690 mm Hg (27 in. Hg) for suction vessels, and at 200 cm H_2O (147 mm Hg) applied vacuum for pleural and mediastinal drainage vessels, labeling shall state the maximum vacuum the collection vessel assembly will withstand. This requirement does not apply to wound drainage.

4.4 *Vessel Air Leak Capacity*:

4.4.1 *Suction Collection Vessels*—The maximum leak rate of suction collection vessels shall be less than 10 bubbles in 10 s (approximately 13 mL/min) when exposed to a vacuum level of 300 mm Hg.

4.4.2 *Closed-Wound Drainage Vessels*—Closed-wound drainage vessels shall not lose more than 20 % of their maximum capacity after 2 h.

4.4.3 *Pleural Drainage Collection Vessels*—Pleural drainage collection vessels should not leak between the patient and the underwater seal (or one-way valve, if used).

4.5 *Indicator Performance*:

4.5.1 *Accuracy of Indicators*—Indicators shall be accurate to within ±10 % of full-scale calibration. The graduation increments of the indicator should not be less than the accuracy of the indicating device.

4.5.2 *Stability*—The regulator reading shall return to its original setting within ±10 % of full scale when the flow is cycled off and on.

4.6 *Tubing Performance*:

4.6.1 *If Connectors are Permanently Attached to Suction, Pleural, and Mediastinal Drainage Tubing*:

4.6.1.1 *Inside Diameter (ID)*—The smallest inside diameter of the connector shall not be less than 80 % of the nominal ID of the tubing, or 5 mm, whichever is greater.

4.6.1.2 *Integrity of Connector Attachment*—For connectors which are formed (molded) separately and subsequently attached to the tube, the bond shall be sufficiently strong to withstand a pull of 24.5 N (5.5 lbf) for 10 min and not exceed the leakage requirement of less than 10 bubbles in 10 s (approximately 13 mL/min) when exposed to a vacuum of 300 mm Hg. Tubing intended for use with drainage systems should not leak.

4.6.1.3 *Resistance to Collapse*—Tubing shall retain at least 50 % of its outside diameter throughout its length for at least 5 min when subjected to the disclosed vacuum (6.6.2).

4.6.1.4 *Connector Strength*—Connectors should resist collapse under normal use conditions.

4.6.2 *Flexibility*— Tubing should be flexible to permit bending and positioning and to reduce strain on connections.

4.6.3 *Translucency*— Tubing should be sufficiently translucent to permit observation of the contents.

4.7 *Filtering Device Performance (If used in a suction system)*:

4.7.1 *Filtering Device Integrity*—The filtering device shall maintain integrity of housing, if present, and filter medium when subjected to the flow and vacuum tests in 5.7.1.

5. Test Methods

5.1 *Shutoff Mechanism*—Connect the shutoff mechanism in the system in accordance with the manufacturer's instructions. Suction (draw) room temperature water into the system until the shutoff mechanism is activated. Measure the volume of water which passed the shutoff. Measure the volume collected in the vessel if the shut-off mechanism is an integral part of a vessel.

5.2 *Electric Conductivity*—Measure the electrical resistance of the component between inlet and outlet with an ohm meter. Resistance shall not be greater than 1 MΩ.

5.3 *System Performance*:

5.3.1 *Maximum Pleural Drainage System Pressure*—Attach the patient end of the pleural drainage system set up for normal operation in accordance with manufacturer's recommendations, to a pressure source adjusted to produce a flow of 10 L/min and measure the pressure at that point (Fig. 1).

5.3.1.1 *Reprocessing of Reuseable Components*—Reprocess the component as recommended and assure that the manufacturer's stated performance is not impaired. Check the labeling for conformance.

5.3.2 *Leakage*—The leakage of the system is affected by the leaks of its components. See 5.4 and 5.6.1.2.

5.3.3 *Resistance to Implosion*—Place the collection vessel in a protective enclosure, that is, a box, bag, etc. Attach a vacuum source to the collection vessel outlet and occlude all other collection vessel openings. Evacuate suction collection vessels to not less than 690 mm Hg (27 in. Hg) vacuum; pleural or mediastinal drainage collection vessels to 200 cm H_2O (147 mm Hg), or to the manufacturer's labeled maximum vacuum. Hold vacuum for 5 min. Release vacuum. Repeat cycle once (see Fig. 2). **Warning**—This test can be hazardous and proper care should be taken to protect personnel from possible flying debris.

5.3.3.1 *Graduation Indicator Accuracy*—The accuracy of the collection vessel graduation indicators shall be tested by filling the vessel with a premeasured amount of liquid and checking the volume indication to be within the disclosed accuracy.

5.4 *Vessel Air Leak Capacity Tests*:

5.4.1 *Suction Collection Vessels*—Set the regulator to 300 mm Hg. Open the valve and allow test component to reach the set vacuum. Close valve. Observe water bottle for bubbles. The test is passed if no more than 9 bubbles are observed in 10 s.

5.4.2 *Closed-Wound Drainage Vessels*:

5.4.2.1 Activate the vacuum in accordance with manufacturer's instructions.

5.4.2.2 Cap or plug all ports tightly.

5.4.2.3 Allow 2 h to elapse. Avoid excessive temperature fluctuations.

5.4.2.4 Place the unit in a water bath so that the patient port is immersed approximately 2 cm deep.

5.4.2.5 Open the cap of the patient port and allow water to enter the vessel until the vacuum is spent.

5.4.2.6 Remove from bath and expel all the aspirated water into a graduated cylinder to measure the residual capacity.

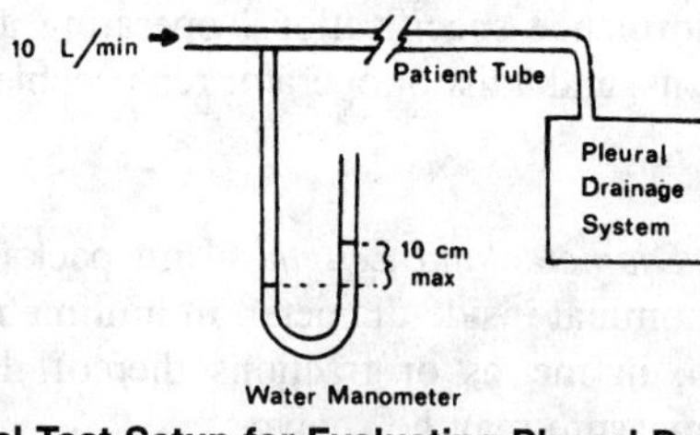

FIG. 1 Typical Test Setup for Evaluating Pleural Drainage System Performance

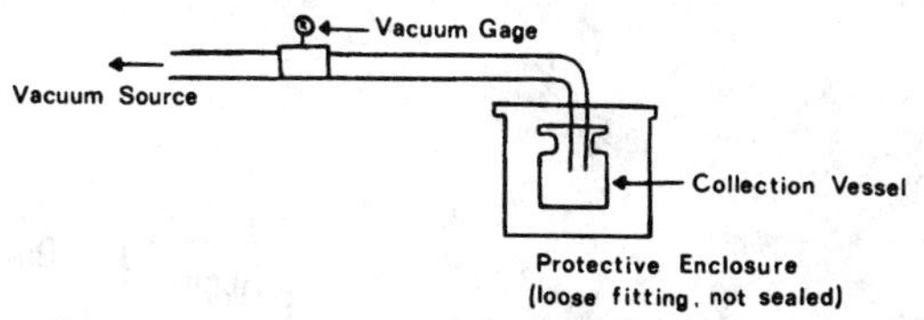

FIG. 2 Suction and Drainage Collection Vessel Assembly

5.4.2.7 Reactivate the vessel and seal all ports.

5.4.2.8 Repeat the residual capacity determination of the vessel immediately after activation. This is the maximum capacity.

5.4.2.9 The capacity remaining after 2 h (5.4.2.6) shall be at least 80 % of the maximum capacity (5.4.2.8).

5.5 *Indicators and Suction Regulators*:

5.5.1 *Accuracy of Indicators*—Check accuracy of the indicator against a mercury or water column as appropriate for the device.

5.5.2 *Stability*—Set regulator at 50 % of the maximum setting at any vacuum level with the inlet occluded. Open and close the inlet several times and observe that the vacuum indicator returns to the set value with ±10 % of full-scale calibration.

5.5.3 *Vacuum Indicator (gage)*—Check the markings for conformance.

5.5.4 *Vacuum Control Mechanism*—Attach the vacuum source, occlude inlet, and observe that adjusting the vacuum control mechanism in the indicated direction will change the level of vacuum in that direction.

5.5.5 *Operation and Repair Manual for Regulators*—Check the manual for conformance.

5.6 *Tubing*:

5.6.1 *Connectors Permanently Attached to Suction, Pleural, and Mediastinal Drainage Tubing*:

5.6.1.1 *Inside Diameter*— Direct measurement.

5.6.1.2 *Integrity of Connector Attachment*—Securely plug one end of the tube and attach the other connector to the set up of Fig. 3. Apply a 2.5-kg weight to the vertically suspended tube. After 10 min, with the weight attached, test for air leaks in accordance with the test in 5.4.

5.6.1.3 *Resistance to Collapse Under Vacuum*—At 20 to 25°C, uncoil the test specimen to its full length and plug one end to prevent any air flow through the tube. Attach a vacuum source to the other end of the tube and adjust the level of vacuum to the disclosed maximum (see Fig. 4). The specimen passes the test if the tube retains at least 50 % of the nominal diameter throughout its length for at least 5 min. The calculation of the degree of collapse may be determined by measurements performed on the outside diameter, as illustrated in Fig. 5.

5.7 *Filtering Devices (If used in a suction system)*:

5.7.1 *Filtering Device Integrity*—Attach by tubing, the filtering device to a regulated vacuum source and occlude the inlet of the filtering device. Apply 300 mm Hg vacuum for 15 s. Release the vacuum. Visually inspect housing for damage and then subject the test component to a leak test (5.4, Fig. 3).

5.7.2 *Suggested Method for Exposing the Filtering Device to Electrocautery Smoke*—Connect the vacuum port of the

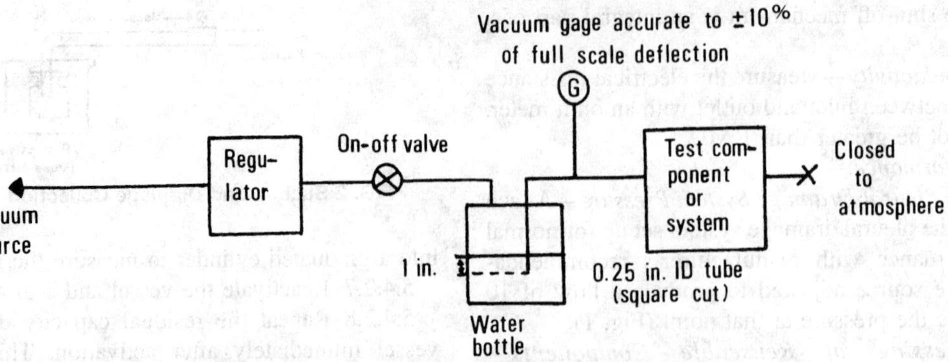

FIG. 3 Typical Test Setup for Evaluating Leakage

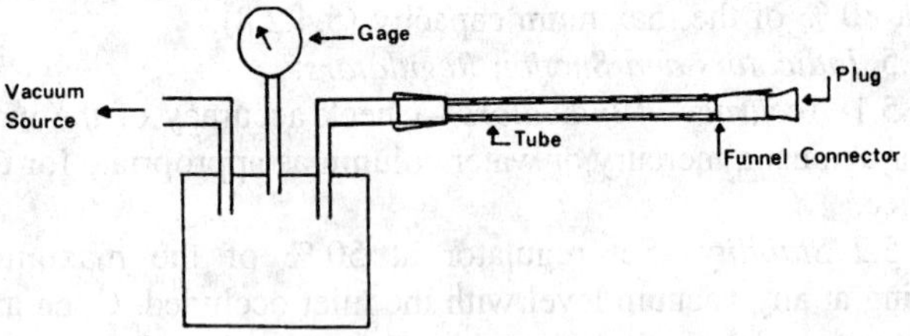

FIG. 4 Vacuum Assembly

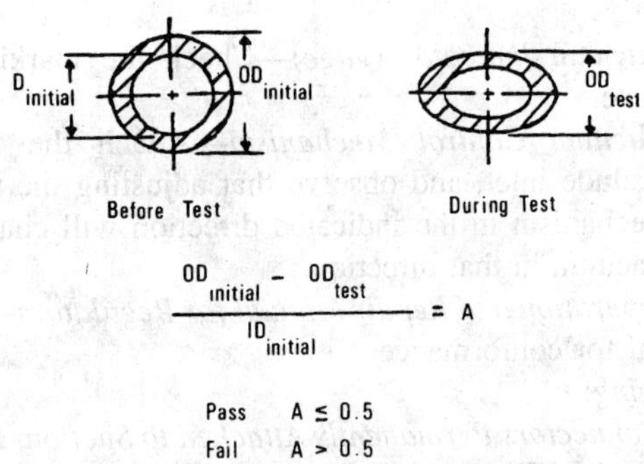

FIG. 5 Measurements for Calculation of Degree of Collapse

filtering device to the vacuum source with a 6-ft length of tubing. Connect the outlet of the filtering device to a regulated vacuum source with a 6-ft length of tubing. Establish a flow rate of 20 L/min. Place the suction tip 4 in. above a 1½-lb flank steak. Make a cut in the steak 2 cm deep and 5 cm long in 5 s, using the active electrode of an electrosurgical unit (Bovie setting at "60," Cut 2 mode). Perform this for 5 s each minute for 10 min. Measure the filtering device's performance.

5.8 *Portable and Mobile Suction Pumps*:

5.8.1 *Available Static Vacuum*—With the suction equipment in its operating mode, connect a vacuum measuring indicator to the suction inlet. Observe the indicated static vacuum. Check the manual for conformance.

5.8.2 *Available Free Airflow*—With the suction equipment in its operating mode, connect a flow meter indicator to the suction inlet. Check the manual for conformance.

5.8.3 *Equipment Noise Level*—With the suction equipment operating under conditions disclosed, and a sound level meter (dampened mode) positioned at one meter from the equipment, read the meter. Check the manual for conformance.

6. Labeling and Operating Manual Requirements

6.1 *General Requirements*:

6.1.1 *Legibility*—All markings pertaining to the operation of the device (for example, controls, gages, graduation indicators) must be legible to a person with 20/20 vision (corrected) at a distance of 1 m at a light level of 215 lux.

6.1.2 *Connection Labeling*—Means, preferably marking, shall be provided to identify correct connections when misconnection is possible.

6.1.3 *Single Use*—Components that are not intended for reuse shall be marked, in substance, "for single use."

6.2 *Electric Conductivity*—All components labeled conductive shall have a resistance not greater than 1 MΩ.

6.3 *System Performance*:

6.3.1 *Reprocessing*— If the component is intended for reuse, recommended methods for reprocessing shall be stated in the labeling. The component shall withstand the methods of reprocessing stated in the labeling.

6.4 *Suction and Drainage Collection Vessels*:

6.4.1 *Capacity*—Product labeling shall indicate the useable capacity, in millilitres, of the collection vessel.

6.4.2 *Positioning*— Labeling shall include instructions for positioning of the collection vessel assembly for proper function.

6.5 *Indicators*:

6.5.1 *Graduation Indicator Accuracy*—Graduation indicator accuracy shall be stated in the labeling or identified as being for approximation only.

6.5.2 *Vacuum Indicator (gage)*—The indicator shall be marked, in substance, "vacuum" to indicate the gas service and shall be appropriately graduated in any of the following units: kilopascals, mm Hg, cm H_2O, or in. Hg.

6.5.3 *Vacuum Control Mechanism*—If a vacuum level control mechanism is present, it shall show clearly the direction for increase or decrease in vacuum level.

6.5.4 *Operation and Repair Manual for Regulators*—A manual containing warnings and limitations, reprocessing instructions, performance specifications, operating and maintenance instructions, and a list of operator replaceable parts shall be included.

6.6 *Tubing*:

6.6.1 *Inside Diameter and Length*—Unit package labeling shall state the nominal inside diameter, in millimetres, and the nominal length, in metres or fractions thereof. In addition, other units of measure may be shown.

6.6.2 *Resistance to Collapse Under Vacuum*—Unit labeling

shall include a statement of the maximum vacuum for which the tubing is intended to be used.

6.6.3 *Sterility*—The labeling shall state whether the tubing is sterile.

6.7 *Filtering Devices (If used in a suction system)*:

6.7.1 *Flow Resistance*— The manufacturer shall disclose the filter flow resistance under dry, "wet," and electrocautery smoke conditions.

6.7.2 *Flow Direction*— If the filtering device is" stand-alone" and flow-direction sensitive, the flow direction shall be marked on the device.

6.7.3 *Accompanying Information*—Instructions for use shall accompany the filtering device.

6.7.4 *Reduction of Airborne Particulate Matter*—The manufacturer shall disclose the test method and filtration efficiency in reduction of airborne particulate matter.

6.8 *Portable and Mobile Suction Sources*:

6.8.1 *Operating Manual*— The manual shall contain appropriate operating environment warnings and limitations, specifications, operating and maintenance instructions, warranty statement, list of user replaceable parts, and, where intended to be user repairable, detailed repair instructions. For non-user repairable items, information on how to obtain service shall be provided where applicable.

6.8.2 *Power Requirement Label*—Labeling shall include operational power requirements for the device, except operator-powered vacuum sources.

6.8.3 *Operating Environment Information*—Environmental limitations shall be marked on the suction source.

6.8.3.1 If the source is electrically powered and is not an "explosion-proof" design, it shall be marked, in substance, that the device is *NOT FOR USE IN THE PRESENCE OF FLAMMABLE GASES.*

6.8.3.2 If the source is gas powered and oxygen may be used, it shall be marked, *USE NO OIL.*

6.8.4 *Source Connection Marking*—Where misconnection is possible, the suction inlet port shall be clearly marked, in substance, *SUCTION.*

6.8.5 *Available Static Vacuum*—The manufacturer shall disclose in the manual the maximum static vacuum capability of the source and the time required to achieve maximum static vacuum. This does not apply to drainage systems.

6.8.6 *Available Free Air Flow*—The manufacturer shall disclose in the manual the free air flow capability of the source. This requirement does not apply to closed wound, mediastinal, and gastrointestinal drainage systems.

6.8.7 *Equipment Noise Level*—The manufacturer shall disclose in the manual the maximum sound pressure level (dBA) at a distance of 1 m, during normal operation. This does not apply to operator-powered vacuum sources.

7. Keywords

7.1 drainage; suction

APPENDIXES

(Nonmandatory Information)

X1. LUMEN (PASSAGEWAY) SIZE AND ITS EFFECTS ON FLOW

X1.1 The laminar flow of fluid (gas or liquid) is approximately proportional to the fourth power of the inside diameter (ID) of the lumen, and inversely proportional to the length.

X1.2 For each system setup it is suggested that the largest diameter and shortest tube practical should be used.

X1.3 Table X1.1 shows the relative flow rates of various sizes of straight tubing under similar conditions. The flow through a 6.35-mm (¼-in.) ID tube is designated as 100 %.

TABLE X1.1 Relative Flow Rates of Straight Tubing

Diameter, in. (mm)	Flow, %	Estimated Pressure Drop for 2-m (6-ft) Length, mm Hg[A]	Approximate Water Flow (mL/min) through 2-m (6-ft) Length[B]
3/16 (4.76)	30	47	2.7
(5)	40	39	3.2
7/32 (5.56)	60	25	4.0
(6)	80	19	4.7
1/4[C] (6.35)	100	15	5.5
(7)	150	10	6.2
9/32 (7.14)	160	8	6.5
5/16 (7.14)	240	5	7.7
(8)	250	4.8	7.8

[A] Estimated vacuum loss per 2-m (6-ft) length of straight tubing flowing 20 L/min air at a source vacuum of 300 mm Hg. Specific brands of tubing may give slightly different results depending on smoothness of lumen and properties of material.

[B] These flow rates are for horizontally positioned tubing at ambient temperature and an applied vacuum of 300 mm Hg.

[C] Suggested minimum diameter.

X2. MINIMUM AND MAXIMUM FREE AIR FLOW RATES AND VACUUM LEVELS FOR SUCTION AND DRAINAGE

X2.1 The committee felt the flow rates and vacuum levels for the types of procedures given in Table X2.1 may be experienced in clinical practice. Systems and their components should be selected to provide appropriate performance capability. Performance disclosure should help in making this selection.

TABLE X2.1 Air Flow Rates and Vacuum Levels[A]

Type of Procedure	Static Vacuum Level	Flow Rate, L/min
Infant Oral-Nasal Tracheal Suction	0–100 mm Hg	0–40
Adult Oral-Nasal Tracheal Suction	0–160 mm Hg	0–40
Surgical Suction	0–500 mm Hg	0–40
Gastrointestinal Abdominal Drainage	0–120 mm Hg	0–8
Wangensteen Drainage	0–60 mm Hg	0–3
Wound Drainage	0–95 mm Hg	0–2
Pleural or Mediastinal Drainage	0–50 cm H_2O	0–10
Pleural or Mediastinal Drainage (Pediatric)	0–10 cm H_2O	0–8
Nasal-Gastric Drainage	0–120 mm Hg	0–3
Sump Drainage	0–50 mm Hg	0–3

[A] This table should not be used as a specification for equipment performance, nor is it a recommendation to users in selecting airflow rates and vacuum levels; airflow rates and vacuum levels should be based on clinical considerations.

X3. RATIONALE

X3.1 The rationales for the requirements of this standard are set forth in this Appendix X3. The following is a sequence of annotations to specific sections of this standard:

X3.1.1 *Shutoff Mechanism*:

Section 3.1—A shutoff mechanism is necessary to prevent aspirated liquids and solids from adversely affecting the internal components of the suction system. The committee realizes that this requirement addresses the entire system rather than individual components, and that a user may choose a suction system consisting of components from several different manufacturers. It is the committee's intent to convey the importance of using a shutoff mechanism and encourage the user to ensure that one is incorporated into each system.

Section 4.1—The function of the shutoff mechanism is to interrupt suction flow when a collection vessel is full. This feature needs to be self-actuating to protect suction systems during suctioning procedures as the user is unable to continuously monitor the liquid flow.

NOTE X3.1—The committee realizes that variables of turbulence, foam, and special hookup are encountered in clinical practice and recognizes that users may choose to devise alternate tests to evaluate products best suited to their needs.

X3.1.2 *Electric Conductivity*:

Section 4.2—Users need assurance that components labeled conductive will dissipate static charges.

X3.1.3 *System Performance*:

Section 3.2—Occlusion of passageways result in reduction of flow and inadequate suction.

Section 4.3.1—If a patient has air in the pleural space and coughs there may be relatively high flows from the patient through the drainage system. It is important to keep the positive pressure below 10 cm H_2O since intrapleural pressure levels above this may cause an acute physiological disturbance. In single bottle drainage systems, adjustment of the underwater seal or emptying of the drainage bottle may be required to reduce the positive pressure during exhalation.

Section 4.3.2—When developing this standard, the committee was unaware of any suction system that would be compromised by small leaks. This requirement recognizes that multiple components are used in a system, and if each leaked at a rate of 10 bubbles in 10 s (approximately 13 mL/min) the total leak of the system would not compromise its function.

Section 4.3.3—Safety to personnel from implosion of the suction collection vessel, as well as the integrity of the collection vessel, are deemed necessary. This requirement does recognize the use of collection vessels with a vacuum of less than 690 mm Hg (27 in. Hg). Collection vessels used in pleural and mediastinal drainage are typically exposed to vacuum levels up to −20 cm H_2O, but may occasionally be used at up to − 60 cm H_2O. Nasogastric and gastrointestinal drainage typically utilizes vacuum levels up to −120 mm Hg. If continuity of operation is important to patient safety, it is important that there be no loss of integrity of the system when subjected to these vacuum levels. The use of −200 cm H_2O adds a factor of safety for testing pleural and mediastinal drainage collection vessels.

Section 6.3.1—The proper method of reprocessing the device is necessary to ensure that the performance is not compromised. Products sold with the intent of reuse need to be able to withstand the suggested reprocessing.

X3.1.4 *Vessel Air Leak Capacity*:

Section 4.4—Excessive air leakage can impair the proper function of a suction collection vessel to the point where adequate suction is no longer available; this could pose a hazard to the patient.

Section 4.4.2—Closed-wound drainage systems must provide continuous drainage for proper function; therefore, leaks should be minimal.

Section 4.4.3—In the event of a leak in that portion of the system defined by the underwater seal (or one-way valve, if employed) at one end and the patient at the opposite end, fluids drained from the pleural cavity may be returned.

Section 6.4—Required capacity and translucency of suction collection vessels have not been addressed in this standard because these may vary according to the needs and preferences of the user.

Section 6.4.1—The capacity is important for user selection and proper use of the collection vessel.

Section 6.4.2—The collection vessel may be sensitive to positioning and may fail to function correctly if not positioned correctly. Accuracy of the graduation markings may be adversely affected if the collection vessel is tilted from upright. Additionally, the shutoff mechanism may activate prematurely if the vessel is tilted. The user needs to be provided this information for proper function.

X3.1.5 *Indicators*:

Section 4.5.1—The user relies on the indicating device to determine the level of vacuum applied. Inaccuracy of the indicating device can result in inadequate or excessive suction, which can be hazardous to the patient.

Section 4.5.2—If the vacuum level varies, inadequate or excessive suction can result. Repeatability ensures a return to a previously set vacuum level.

Section 6.5.1—Monitoring of the aspirated liquid volume may be necessary.

Section 6.5.2—The user needs to be able to readily determine that the gas service being supplied is vacuum.

Section 6.5.3—Adjusting the regulator the wrong way could cause excessive or insufficient suction.

Section 6.5.4—This information is for users to select, operate, and when indicated, to maintain the regulator.

X3.1.6 *Tubing*:

Section 3.2—This is for educational purposes. The committee felt this an important point to convey and recognizes that current hospital practice may include the use of loops and drapes which may give rise to changes in diameter and kinking and adversely affect flow. See Appendix X1 for the effects of tubing diameter on flow.

Section 3.4.1—Connectors chosen with less than 7-mm ID (minimum ¼-in. ID) tubing create further significant reduction in flow. Smooth passageways reduce turbulence and the collection of particulate matter, which can cause a reduction in flow.

Section 4.6.1.1—To ensure proper fit with connectors and minimize restrictions, consideration was given to establishing a single requirement that the smallest ID of the connector shall not be less than the ID of the tubing. However, it was concluded that this could impose problems because of the variety of connectors presently used by hospitals.

Section 4.6.1.2—This requirement is intended to safeguard the integrity of the connector and tube. In some situations, a leak might be mistaken for a slow flow. Accordingly, a requirement was adopted to aid in assuring that any slow flow observed would not actually be a leak.

Section 4.6.1.3—See 6.6.2.

Section 4.6.1.4—Weak connectors compromise system function.

Section 4.6.2—Flexibility is desirable for ease of handling and use.

Section 4.6.3—Translucency may be necessary to identify the location of obstructions.

Section 6.6.1—Inside diameter is the commonly accepted identifier for tubing size. Metric measurements are used for standardization.

Section 6.6.2—Depending on the application, medical tubing may be subjected to a vacuum level that might cause the tube to collapse and thus limits its ability to transmit fluids. A statement in the labeling, disclosing the level of vacuum for which the product is suitable, will aid users in selecting appropriate units. In order for such selections to be valid, however, a standard test method is necessary (see 4.6.1.3).

Section 6.6.3—The user needs to know this information for proper selection.

X3.1.7 *Filtering Devices*:

Section 4.7.1—Filtering devices may be used in surgical suction systems. There are two major areas of concern that have been voiced with respect to contaminants generated in surgical suction:

(1) Airborne particulates reaching the regulator or pump, or both, causing increased maintenance and its associated costs.

(2) Microbial contaminants from the patient's suctionate reaching the environment as airborne particulate, or through touch contamination.

The majority of the subcommittee thought that item (*1*) was a nearly universal concern, but that the clinical consequences of item (*2*) had not been sufficiently documented so as to merit inclusion in the standard. Therefore, the standard for filtering devices addresses only the function of reducing airborne contaminants to protect the regulator or pump, or both.

Concerning test procedures for performance, the subcommittee decided that disclosure was the best method of meeting this requirement because there exists in the filtration industry a wide variety of techniques and conditions for evaluating filter performance.

An imploded filtering device may produce increased flow resistance. A leak in the filtering device housing will reduce air flow rate at the catheter tip. A damaged filtering device may produce a reduction in efficiency and may compromise the filtering characteristics of the device.

Section 6.7.1—The user should know the resistance of a suction filter to ensure that the minimum suction required is available. The user needs to know the flow resistance of a filtering device under "wet" conditions, since the flow may be reduced. Electrocautery smoke may obstruct certain filtering devices and impede system performance.

Section 6.7.2—The user may need an indication of how to attach a filter to the suction circuit for proper performance.

Section 6.7.3—The user may need to have instructions for proper use of the filtering device readily available.

Section 6.7.4—The user needs assurance of the ability of the filtering device to reduce airborne particulates.

X3.1.8 *Portable and Mobile Suction Sources*:

Section 6.8.1—This information is necessary for users to

select, operate, and, when indicated, maintain the suction source.

Section 6.8.4—Labeling is necessary to assure correct connection.

Sections 6.8.5, 6.8.6, and 6.8.7—This information is necessary for users to determine which equipment is appropriate for the intended purpose and if it is functioning properly.

X3.1.9 *General Marking Requirements*:

Section 6.1.1—Without clearly legible instructions, the user may not be sufficiently familiar with the control movements or procedures to make necessary manipulations.

Section 6.1.2—If the component is flow direction sensitive, the function of the system will be jeopardized if the correct connections are not used.

Section 6.1.3—It is important for the user to know when a vessel should not be reused; reuse of a vessel intended for single use may compromise the vessel's integrity.

Standard Specification for Cobalt-35 Nickel-20 Chromium-10 Molybdenum Alloy Forgings for Surgical Implants (UNS R30035)[1]

This standard is issued under the fixed designation F 961; the number immediately following the designation indicates the year of original adoption or, in the case of revision, the year of last revision. A number in parentheses indicates the year of last reapproval. A superscript epsilon (ε) indicates an editorial change since the last revision or reapproval.

1. Scope

1.1 This specification covers the requirements for cobalt-35 nickel-20 chromium-10 molybdenum alloy forgings for surgical implants.

1.2 The values stated in inch-pound units are to be regarded as the standard.

2. Referenced Documents

2.1 *ASTM Standards:*

A 751 Test Methods, Practices, and Terminology for Chemical Analysis of Steel Products[2]

E 8 Test Methods for Tension Testing of Metallic Materials[3]

E 10 Test Method for Brinell Hardness of Metallic Materials[3]

E 18 Test Methods for Rockwell Hardness and Rockwell Superficial Hardness of Metallic Materials[3]

E 112 Test Methods for Determining the Average Grain Size[3]

E 140 Hardness Conversion Tables for Metals[3]

E 165 Practice for Liquid Penetrant Examination[4]

F 562 Specification for Wrought Cobalt-35 Nickel-20 Chromium-10 Molybdenum Alloy for Surgical Implant Applications[5]

F 601 Practice for Fluorescent Penetrant Inspection of Metallic Surgical Implants[5]

F 688 Specification for Wrought Cobalt-35 Nickel-20 Chromium-10 Molybdenum Alloy Plate, Sheet, and Foil for Surgical Implants[5]

F 981 Practice for Assessment of Compatibility of Biomaterials for Surgical Implants with Respect to Effect of Materials in Muscle and Bone[5]

2.2 *Federal Standard:*

Federal Test Method No. 151 Metals; Test Methods[6]

2.3 *American Society for Quality Control Standard:*

Cl Specification of General Requirements for a Quality Program[7]

3. Terminology

3.1 *Definition of a Term Specific to This Standard:*

3.1.1 *capability*—the word "capability" is used to indicate the ability of cold-worked material to attain specific mechanical properties after thermal aging treatment.

4. Ordering Information

4.1 Inquiries and orders for material under this specification shall include the following information:

4.1.1 Quantity (weight or number of pieces),

4.1.2 ASTM designation and date of issue,

4.1.3 Form,

4.1.4 Condition,

4.1.5 Mechanical properties (if applicable),

4.1.6 Finish,

4.1.7 Applicable dimensions, including size, thickness width, and length (exact, random, multiples), or print number,

4.1.8 Special tests, and

4.1.9 Special requirements.

5. Materials and Manufacture

5.1 Material for forgings shall be bars, plate, sheet, or wire fabricated in accordance with Specification F 562 or Specification F 688. The material shall be generally in the solution-annealed condition with a finish suitable for forging.

5.2 The material shall be forged by hammering, pressing, rolling, extruding, or upsetting and shall be processed, if practicable, so as to cause metal flow to be in the most favorable direction for resisting stresses encountered in service, as may be indicated to the fabricator by the implant manufacturer.

5.3 Forgings shall be free of splits, scale, cracks, inequalities, flaws, and other imperfections not consistent with good commercial practice.

NOTE 1—Compliance to these requirements may be verified by Practice E 165 or Practice F 601 or other suitable methods.

5.4 When specified by the implant manufacturer, a thermal treatment shall be performed, as specified, after all forging

[1] This specification is under the jurisdiction of ASTM Committee F04 on Medical and Surgical Materials and Devices and is the direct responsibility of Subcommittee F04.12 on Metallurgical Materials

Current edition approved Oct. 10, 1996. Published January 1997. Originally published as F 961 – 85. Last previous edition F 961 – 92.

[2] *Annual Book of ASTM Standards*, Vol 01.03.

[3] *Annual Book of ASTM Standards*, Vol 03.01.

[4] *Annual Book of ASTM Standards*, Vol 03.03.

[5] *Annual Book of ASTM Standards*, Vol 13.01.

[6] Available from Standardization Documents Order Desk, Bldg. 4 Section D, 700 Robbins Ave., Philadelphia, PA 19111-5094, Attn: NPODS.

[7] Available from American Society for Quality Control, 161 West Wisconsin Ave., Milwaukee, WI 53203.

operations are performed.

5.5 Optional identification marks, including the manufacturer's logo, material designation, heat code number, and impression number, may be placed upon each forging. The method and location of identification shall be as specified by the purchaser.

5.6 Forgings shall be supplied in the as-forged or forged-and-capability-aged condition, as specified by the implant manufacturer.

6. Chemical Composition

6.1 The heat analysis shall conform to the chemical composition requirements prescribed in Specification F 562, Table 1.

6.2 The chemical composition of samples taken for product analysis shall conform to the check tolerances prescribed in Specification F 562, Table 2.

6.3 Methods and practices relating to chemical analysis required by this specification shall be in accordance with Test Methods A 751.

7. Mechanical Requirements

7.1 When specified by the implant manufacturer, the mechanical properties of forgings shall be tested by the forger and shall comply with the minimum mechanical properties as specified by the implant manufacturer. Specification F 562, Section 7, shall be used as a guideline.

7.2 If tension testing is required, test specimens should be taken from a representative forging, if possible, or from a specially forged test bar only if the configuration does not lend itself to yielding the required specimen.

7.3 When desired, Rockwell hardness may be specified on the implant manufacturer's purchase order or print. Rockwell hardness shall be determined in accordance with Test Methods E 18.

NOTE 2—When desired, Brinell hardness may be taken as described in Test Method E 10 and converted to Rockwell hardness in accordance with Hardness Conversion Tables E140.

7.4 The mechanical properties shall be determined in accordance with Test Methods E 8 using a strain rate of 0.003 to 0.007 in./in. min. (mm/mm min.) through the specified yield range, and then the crosshead speed shall be increased so as to produce fracture in approximately one additional minute.

8. Special Tests

8.1 The grain size shall be agreed upon between the purchaser and the manufacturer and shall be tested in accordance with Test Methods E 112.

8.2 Other special requirements shall be as specified on the purchase order or print.

9. Certification

9.1 The fabricator's certification that the material was manufactured and tested in accordance with this specification, together with a report of the test results, shall be furnished to the implant manufacturer with each shipment.

10. Quality Program Requirements

10.1 The producer shall maintain a quality program, such as that defined in Specification ASQC C1.

10.2 The manufacturer of surgical implants or medical appliances shall be assured of the producer's quality program for conformance to the intent of Specification ASQC C1, or any other recognized program.

11. Keywords

11.1 cobalt alloys (for surgical implants); cobalt-nickels alloy; forgings; surgical implant; metals (for surgical implants)

APPENDIXES

(Nonmandatory Information)

X1. RATIONALE

X1.1 The primary reason for this specification is to characterize the composition and properties to assure consistency in the starting material used in the manufacture of medical devices.

X1.2 The acceptable metal conditions include as-forged or as-forged-and-capability aged, the choice dependent upon the medical device design and its intended application.

X1.3 The UNS designation has been added for clarification, and a Biocompatibility section has been added as an appendix.

X2. BIOCOMPATIBILITY

X2.1 The material composition covered by this specification has been employed successfully in human implant applications in contact with soft tissue and bone for over decade. Due to the well characterized level of local biological response established by this material, it has been used as a control material in Practice F 981.

X2.2 No known surgical implant material has ever been shown to be completely free of adverse reactions in the human body. However, long term clinical experience has shown an acceptable level of biological response can be expected, if the material is used in appropriate applications.

REFERENCES

(1) Willert, H. G., Buchhorn, U., Zichner, L., "Clinical Experience with Mueller Total Hip Endoprostheses of Different Design and Material," *Archives of Orthopaedic and Traumatic Surgery*, 97, 1980, pp. 197–205.

Standard Specification for Rigid Laryngoscopes for Tracheal Intubation—Hook-On Fittings for Laryngoscope Handles and Blades with Lamps[1]

This standard is issued under the fixed designation F 965; the number immediately following the designation indicates the year of original adoption or, in the case of revision, the year of last revision. A number in parentheses indicates the year of last reapproval. A superscript epsilon (ε) indicates an editorial change since the last revision or reapproval.

This standard has been approved for use by agencies of the Department of Defense.

1. Scope

1.1 This specification covers critical dimensions and considerations for the junction of any blade and any handle of a hook-on type laryngoscope to allow engagement, lamp illumination, and disengagement through multiple cycles. An electrical lamp is fixed to the blade and supplied with energy through the handle.

1.2 This standard does not cover: (*1*) the blade form or handle design beyond the interchangeability aspects of the connection between the blade and the handle; (*2*) the measurement and specificiation of the lamp illumination intensity; and (*3*) disposable, flexible, or fiber-illuminated laryngoscopes designed for surgery.

1.3 The state-of-the-art of laryngoscope performance does not permit sufficient reproducibility to allow inclusion of mandatory force values in this standard; therefore, only recommended values have been provided.

1.4 The values stated in SI units are to be regarded as the standard.

2. Referenced Documents

2.1 *ANSI Standard:*

ANSI Y14.5 Dimensions and Tolerances[2]

3. Terminology

3.1 *Definitions of Terms Specific to This Standard:*

3.1.1 *blade*—a separate rigid device to provide direct vision of the larynx, incorporating a hook-on base and a socket connection for a laryngoscope lamp and an electrical connection to the hook-on end.

3.1.2 *contacts*—conductive components of the hook-on fittings, both handle and blade, which come together to make an electrical circuit when the handle and blade are in the locked, operating position.

3.1.3 *engagement*—the blade and handle are engaged when the hinge pin is positioned against the closed end of the hinge slot, and remains coupled in all positions.

3.1.4 *folded position*—the position of the engaged blade when the tip of the blade is as close as possible to the handle.

3.1.5 *handle*—a separate, rigid device which is held in the hand during use, containing the hook-on connection that retains the blade and supplies electrical energy for the lamp.

3.1.6 *hinge*—the mechanical feature of the handle and blade that allows them to be engaged and disengaged. The hinge also allows the blade to be placed into the operating, folded, and all intermediate positions while engaged.

3.1.7 *hinge pin*—the component of the handle that inserts into the blade hinge slot.

3.1.8 *hinge slot*—the surfaces of the blade hook-on fitting that engage the hinge pin.

3.1.9 *locking mechanism*—the feature that retains the blade hook-on fitting in the operating position.

3.1.10 *locking slots*—the surfaces of the handle hook-on fitting that accept the locking surfaces of the blade hook-on fitting.

3.1.11 *locking surfaces*—the components of the blade locking mechanism that fit into the locking slots to resist the blade displacement from the normal operating position.

3.1.12 *operating position*—the position of the engaged blade and handle when the lamp is lit and the instrument is ready for use.

3.1.13 *retainer*—the surface, component, or feature of the blade hinge slot that retains the blade hook-on fitting to the handle hinge pin. The retainer maintains the engagement of the blade in the operating, folded, and all intermediate positions.

3.1.14 *seating surfaces*—the surface or surfaces of the blade hook-on fitting that contact the handle hook-on fitting to support the blade in the locked operating position.

4. Significance and Use

4.1 The primary objective of this specification is to ensure interchangeability concerning mechanical fit and electrical contact between the hook-on type handle and laryngoscope blade by specifying only the critical dimensions of the handle hook-on fitting that affect interchangeability, and by designating the minimum performance requirements.

4.2 The secondary objective is to provide test procedures and values for performance.

---

[1] This specification is under the jurisdiction of ASTM Committee F-29 on Anesthetic and Respiratory Equipmentand is the direct responsibility of Subcommittee F29.13on Laryngoscopes and Bronchoscopes.

Current edition approved July 10, 1999. Published September 1999. Originally published as F 965 – 85. Last previous edition F 965 – 85 (1993)$^{\epsilon 1}$.

[2] Available from American National Standards Institute, 1430 Broadway, New York, NY 10017.

5. Performance Requirements

5.1 *Hook-on Blade and Handle Fittings*—Detachable hook-on blade and handle combinations that engage shall lock and the lamp will light when in the operating position.

NOTE 1—For rationale statements for the performance requirements, see Appendix X1.

5.2 *Handle Fittings (Hook-On)*:

5.2.1 *Critical Dimensions*—Measurements shall be made with the accuracy and precision necessary to determine conformance with the dimensions specified in Fig. 1. The measurements shall be taken from datum plane A, datum B, and the hinge pin centerline. The total clearance between the width of the handle slot and the width of the blade hook-on fitting shall not exceed 0.011 in. (0.28 mm). Dimensions and configurations not shown shall be at the discretion of the manufacturer to ensure strength and safe operation. The method of dimensioning is in accordance with ANSI Y14.5.

5.2.2 *Electrical Contact*—The insulated central contact shall press against the central contact on the blade to maintain conductivity and ensure lamp illumination while in the operating position (see 5.9).

5.3 *Blade Fittings (Hook-On)*—Blade hook-on fittings shall engage the handle hook-on fitting as specified in Fig. 1 and 5.9. Typical blade hook-on fittings are shown in Fig. 2.

5.4 *Engagement, Hinge Slot*—The slot and hinge pin should engage when a force between 10 N and 45 N is applied. This force should be applied along the axis shown in Fig. 3 (Note 2).

5.5 *Blade Retention*—The retainer shall secure the hinge pin to the closed end of the blade hinge slot in all positions when the blade is in the engaged, folded position (see 5.10).

5.6 *Operating Position*:

5.6.1 *Locking*—Locking of the folded blade into the operating position should occur when a torque between 0.35 N · m and 1.35 N · m is applied to the blade.

5.6.2 *Unlocking*—Unlocking of the blade from the operating position to the folded position should occur when a torque between 0.25 N · m and 1.35 N · m is applied to the blade.

5.7 *Disengagement, Hinge Slot*—Disengagement of the folded blade from the handle and hinge pin should occur when a force between 10 N and 45 N is applied.

NOTE 2—The laboratory of the Defense Logistics Agency, Defense Personnel Support Center, Philadelphia, PA, constitutes the source for the data specified. Testing included components from various manufacturers, totalling 25 blades of three types and two handles of different manufacture. Measurements were obtained by the use of a 60 g load cell with 10 lb adapter and universal transducer readout. The laboratory results were verified with a calibrated spring gage. Results showed that the slot and hinge pin should engage when a force of less than 44.5 N is applied, locking of the blade into operating position should occur when a force of

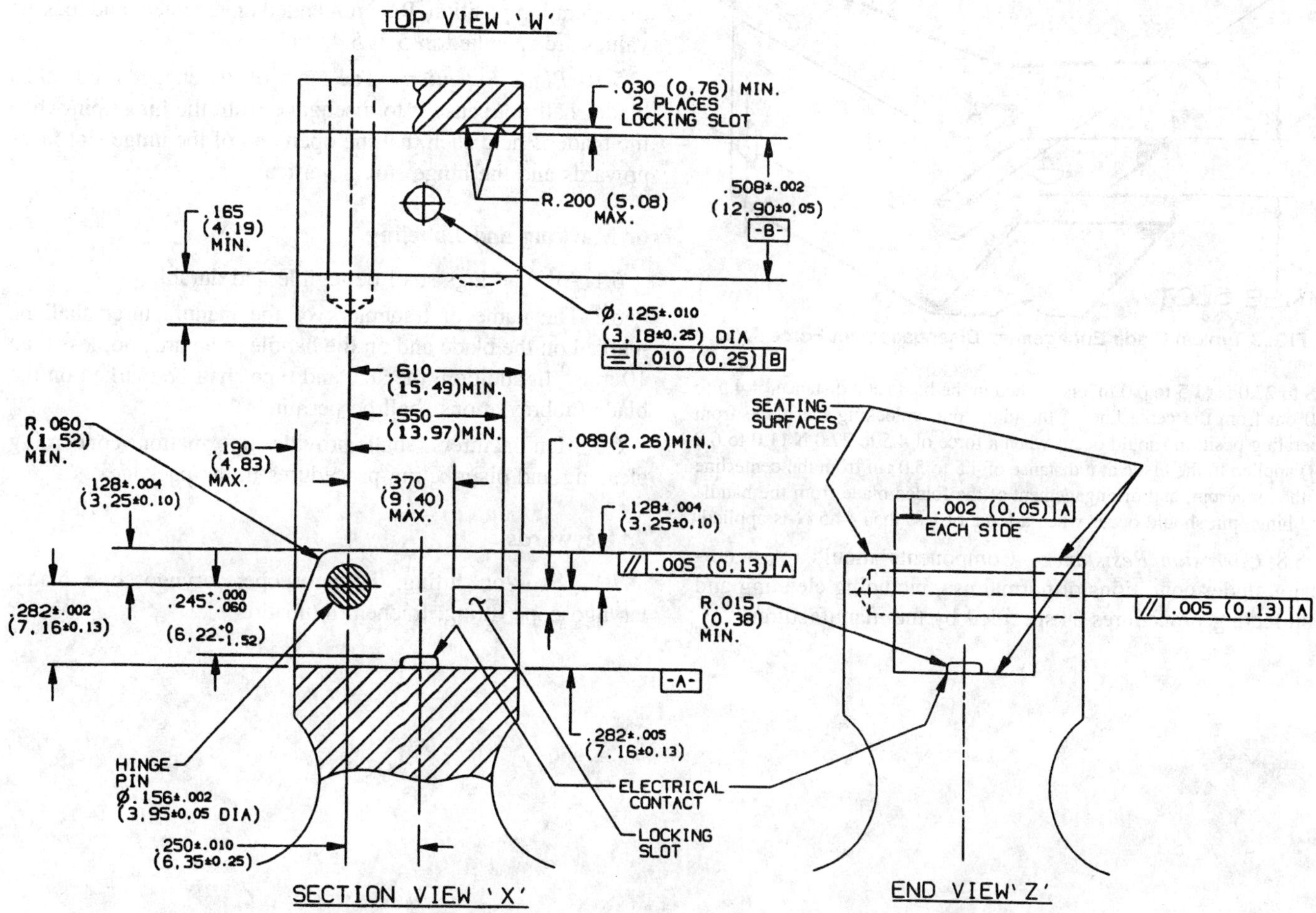

NOTE 1—(*1*) Dimensions are in inches. Dimensions in parenthesis [( )] are in millimetres, (*2*) Datum A is the plane of the handle slot seating surfaces, and (*3*) Datum B is the width of the handle slot.

FIG. 1 Handle Hook-On Fitting

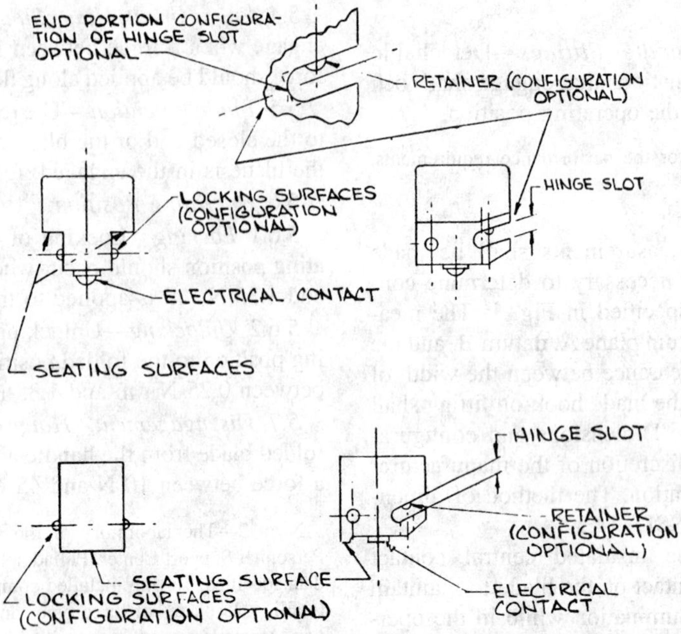

FIG. 2 Typical Blade Hook-On Fitting Configurations

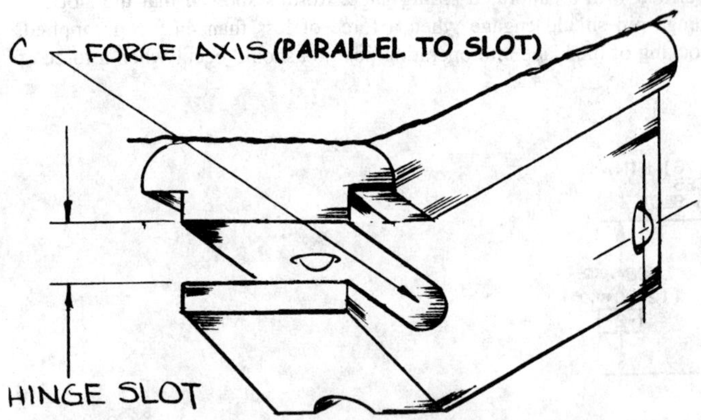

FIG. 3 Typical Blade Engagement/Disengagement Force Axis

6.8 to 27.0 N (1.5 to 6.0 lbf) is applied to the blade at a distance of 4.5 to 5.0 cm from the centerline of the hinge pin, unlocking the blade from operating position should occur when a force of 4.5 to 27.0 N (1.0 to 6.0 lbf) applied to the blade at a distance of 4.5 to 5.0 cm from the centerline of the hinge pin, and disengagement of the folded blade from the handle and hinge pin should occur when a force of less than 44.5 N is applied.

5.8 *Corrosion Resistance*—Components should resist corrosion under conditions of normal use, including cleaning and disinfecting procedures as specified by the manufacturer.

5.9 *Hook-On Blade and Handle Fittings and Electrical Contacts*—The lamp shall light when the blade is placed into the operating position. Recommended engagement and locking values are specified in 5.3, 5.4, and 5.6.

5.10 *Blade Retention*—The mass of the engaged, unlocked blade shall not cause it to disengage from the hinge pin when the blade is held such that the open end of the hinge slot faces upwards and the hinge slot is vertical.

6. Marking and Labeling

6.1 All markings shall be legible and durable.

6.2 The name or trademark of the manufacturer shall be marked on the blade and on the handle in an area not less than 10 mm.^{2} In addition, the size and type shall be marked on the blade (abbreviations shall be permitted).

6.3 Manufacturers shall provide information concerning cleaning and disinfecting procedures in the package.

7. Keywords

7.1 hook-on fitting; laryngoscope; laryngoscope blade; laryngoscope fitting; tracheal intubation

APPENDIXES

(Nonmandatory Information)

X1. RATIONALE FOR PERFORMANCE REQUIREMENTS

X1.1 *Hook-On Blade and Handle Fittings (Section 5.1)*—This is required for patient safety at the time of laryngoscopy.

X1.2 *Critical Dimensions (Section 5.2.1)*—Critical dimensions of the handle hook-on fittings require precise description to allow interchangeability of different manufacturers' blades and handles, and to ensure rigidity and illumination during use.

X1.3 *Electrical Contact (Section 5.2.2)*—To ensure illumination during use, electrical contacts must be maintained.

X1.4 *Blade Fittings (Hook-On) (Section 5.3)*—Engagement is required to allow use of laryngoscope blades. Because a variety of blades and handles made by different manufacturers are used in clinical practice, all blades should engage all handles.

X1.5 *Engagement, Hinge Slot (Section 5.4)*—Repeated engagement and disengagement are required during clinical use.

X1.6 *Blade Retention (Section 5.5)*—In non-operating positions, retention of the slot on the hinge pin must be sufficient to prevent inadvertent disengagement.

X1.7 *Locking, Operating Position (Section 5.6.1)*—The engaged blade and handle should lock in a stable fashion to provide exposure and illumination of the larynx.

X2. RATIONALE FOR TYPICAL BLADE HOOK-ON FITTING CONFIGURATIONS

X2.1 *Fig. 2*—This figure illustrates two types of laryngoscope blade hook-on fittings. The figure is not for manufacturing or design purposes, but illustrates some typical configurations that permit engagement of the blade and handle hook-on fittings.

Designation: F 981 – 99

Standard Practice for Assessment of Compatibility of Biomaterials for Surgical Implants with Respect to Effect of Materials on Muscle and Bone[1]

This standard is issued under the fixed designation F 981; the number immediately following the designation indicates the year of original adoption or, in the case of revision, the year of last revision. A number in parentheses indicates the year of last reapproval. A superscript epsilon (ϵ) indicates an editorial change since the last revision or reapproval.

1. Scope

1.1 This practice provides a series of experimental protocols for biological assays of tissue reaction to nonabsorbable biomaterials for surgical implants. It assesses the effects of the material on animal tissue in which it is implanted. The experimental protocol is not designed to provide a comprehensive assessment of the systemic toxicity, immune response, carcinogenicity, teratogenicity, or mutagenicity of the material since other standards deal with these issues. It applies only to materials with projected applications in humans where the materials will reside in bone or soft tissue in excess of 30 days and will remain unabsorbed. It is recommended that short-term assays, according to Practice F 763, first be performed. Applications in other organ systems or tissues may be inappropriate and are therefore excluded. Control materials will consist of any one of the metal alloys in Specifications F 67, F 75, F 90, F 136, F 138, or F 562, high purity dense aluminum oxide as described in Specification F 603, ultra high molecular weight polyethylene as stated in Specification F 648 or USP polyethylene negative control.

1.2 This document is a combination of Practice F 361 – 80 and Practice F 469 – 78. The purpose, basic procedure, and method of evaluation of each type of material are similar; therefore, they have been combined.

1.3 *This standard does not purport to address all of the safety concerns, if any, associated with its use. It is the responsibility of the user of this standard to establish appropriate safety and health practices and determine the applicability of regulatory limitations prior to use.*

2. Referenced Documents

2.1 *ASTM Standards:*

F 67 Specification for Unalloyed Titanium for Surgical Implant Applications[2]

F 75 Specification for Cast Cobalt-Chromium-Molybdenum Alloy for Surgical Implant Applications[2]

F 86 Practice for Surface Preparation and Marking of Metallic Surgical Implants[2]

F 90 Specification for Wrought Cobalt-Chromium-Tungsten-Nickel Alloy for Surgical Implant Applications[2]

F 136 Specification for Wrought Titanium-6 Aluminum-4 Vanadium ELI (Extra Low Interstitial) Alloy (UNS R56401) for Surgical Implant Applications[2]

F 138 Specification for Wrought-18 Chromium–14 NIckel–2.5 Molybdenum Stainless Steel Bar and Wire for Surgical Implants (UNS S31673)[2]

F 361 Practice for Assessment of Compatibility of Metallic Materials for Surgical Implants with Respect to Effect of Materials on Tissue[3]

F 469 Practice for Assessment of Compatibility of Nonporous Polymeric Materials for Surgical Implants with Regard to Effect of Materials on Tissue[4]

F 562 Specification for Wrought Cobalt-35 Nickel–20 Chromium-10 Molybdenum Alloy for Surgical Implant Applications[2]

F 603 Specification for High-Purity Dense Aluminum Oxide for Surgical Implant Application[2]

F 648 Specification for Ultra-High-Molecular-Weight Polyethylene Powder and Fabricated Form for Surgical Implants[2]

F 763 Practice for Short-Term Screening of Implant Materials[2]

3. Summary of Practice

3.1 This practice describes the preparation of implants, the number of implants and test hosts, test sites, exposure schedule, implant sterilization techniques, and methods of implant retrieval and tissue examination of each test site. Histological criteria for evaluating tissue reaction are provided.

4. Significance and Use

4.1 This practice covers a test protocol for comparing the local tissue response evoked by biomaterials, from which medical implantable devices might ultimately be fabricated, with the local tissue response elicited by control materials currently accepted for the fabrication of surgical devices. The

---

[1] This practice is under the jurisdiction of ASTM Committee F-4 on Medical and Surgical Materials and Devicesand is the direct responsibility of Subcommittee F04.16 on Biocompatibility.

Current edition approved May 10, 1999. Published August 1999. Originally published as F 981 – 86. Last previous edition F 981 – 93.

[2] *Annual Book of ASTM Standards*, Vol 13.01.

[3] Discontinued—See *1986 Annual Book of ASTM STandards*, Vol 13.01.

[4] Discontinued—See *1987 Annual Book of ASTM STandards*, Vol 13.01.

materials may include metals (and metal alloys), dense aluminum oxide, and polyethylene that are standardized on the basis of acceptable long-term well-characterized long-term response. The controls consistently produce cellular reaction and wound healing to a degree that has been found to be acceptable to the host.

5. Test Hosts and Sites

5.1 Rats (acceptable strains such as Fischer 344), New Zealand White rabbits, and other small laboratory animals may be used as test hosts for soft tissue implant response. It is suggested that the rats be age and sex matched. Rabbits or larger animals may be used as test hosts for bone implants. When larger animals such as dogs, goats, or sheep are used, the decision should be based upon special considerations of the particular implant material or study.

5.2 The sacro-spinalis, paralumbar, gluteal muscles, and the femur or tibia can serve as the test site for implants. However, the same site must be used for test and material implants in all the animal species.

5.3 There shall be a minimum of four animals at each sacrifice interval for a total of twelve animals per study. If larger animals are used, in which a greater number of implants can be placed, there shall be at least two animals sacrificed at each time period.

6. Implant Specimens

6.1 *Fabrication*— Each implant shall be made in a cylindrical shape with hemispherical ends (see 6.3 and 6.4 for sizes). If the ends are not hemispherical, this shall be reported. Each implant shall be fabricated, finished, and its surface cleaned in a manner appropriate for its projected application in human subjects in accordance with Practice F 86. If the specimens are porous, the method of preparation of the porous specimens shall be representative of the contemplated human implant application and shall yield a specimen with characteristic pore size, pore volume, and pore interconnection diameter. The choice between using solid core specimens with porous coatings and specimens that are porous throughout shall be a decision of the investigator and shall be reported.

6.2 Reference metallic specimens shall be fabricated in accordance with 6.1 from materials such as the metal alloys in Specifications F 67, F 75, F 90, F 138, or F 562, ceramic in Specification F 603, or polymers such as in Specification F 648 polyethylene or USP Negative Control Plastic. If the test materials are porous, consideration should be given to using porous specimens for reference specimens. Alternatively, nonporous reference specimens may be used.

6.3 *Suggested Sizes and Shapes of Implants for Insertion in Muscle*:

6.3.1 The implants shall be cylindrical in shape and may range from 1 mm to 6 mm in diameter and from 10 mm to 20 mm in length depending upon the relative size of the species under study.

6.3.2 The dimensions used shall be reported in accordance with 8.1.

6.3.3 Depending upon the particular device application, other sample shapes may be used. For instance, an investigator might wish to test the biocompatibility of a new material for screws in the form of a screw. If an alternative specimen shape is used, this should be reported in accordance with 8.1.

6.4 *Sizes and Shapes of Implants for Insertion in Bone*:

6.4.1 Implant diameters for use in bone shall be approximately equal to the cortex thickness. Implant lengths shall allow them to reside in one cortex and the medulla without excessive protrusion beyond the periosteum.

6.4.2 The dimensions used shall be reported in accordance with 8.1.

6.5 *Number of Test and Control Implants*:

6.5.1 In each rat, due to size, there may be two implants; one each test and control material implant.

6.5.2 In each rabbit, due to size, there may be six implants; four test materials and two control material implants.

6.5.3 In larger animals, there may be twelve implants; eight test materials and four control material implants.

6.5.4 In rabbits or larger animals, there shall be tested at least sixteen test material implants and eight control material implants at each time period.

6.6 *Conditioning*:

6.6.1 Remove all surface contaminants with appropriate solvents and rinse all test and control implants in distilled water prior to sterilization. It is recommended that the implant materials be processed and cleaned in the same way the final product will be.

6.6.2 Clean, package, and sterilize all implants in the same way as used for human implantation.

6.6.3 After final preparation and sterilization, handle the test and control implants with great care to ensure that they are not scratched, damaged, or contaminated in any way prior to insertion.

6.6.4 Report all details of conditioning in accordance with 8.1.

6.7 *Implantation Period*—Insert all implants into each animal at the same surgical session for implantation periods of 12, 26, and 52 weeks.

7. Procedure

7.1 *Implantation (Muscle)*:

7.1.1 Place material implants in the paravertebral muscles in such a manner that they are directly in contact with muscle tissue.

7.1.2 Introduce material implants in larger animals by the technique of making an implantation site in the muscle by using a hemostat to separate the muscle fibers. Then insert the implant using plastic-tipped forceps or any tool that is non-abrasive to avoid damage to the implant.

7.1.3 Introduce material implants using sterile technique. Sterile disposable needles or hypodermic tubing and trochar may be used to implant the material implants into the paravertebral muscles along the spine. In rats insert a negative control implant on one side of the spine and a test material implant on the other side. In rabbits implant one negative control material on each side of the spine and implant two test materials on each side of the spine. If larger diameter specimens are used, an alternative implantation technique is that described in 7.1.2.

7.2 *Implantation (Femur)*—Expose the lateral cortex of each rabbit femur and drill undersized pilot holes through the lateral cortex using the technique and instrument appropriate for the procedure. Final reaming of the holes should be performed by hand to yield holes which are smaller than the implant specimens by 0.1 mm or less. Into each one of these holes, insert one of the implants by finger pressure. Then close the wound.

NOTE 1—Caution should be taken to minimize the motion of the implant in the tissue to prevent the effects of motion on the desired result.

7.3 *Postoperative Care*:

7.3.1 All animal studies must be done in a facility approved by a nationally recognized organization and in accordance with all appropriate regulations.

7.3.2 Carefully observe each animal during the period of assay and report any abnormal findings.

7.3.3 Infection or injury of the test implant site may invalidate the results. The decision to replace the animal so that the total number of retrieved implants will be as represented in the schedule shall be dependent upon the design of the study.

7.3.4 If an animal dies prior to the expected date of sacrifice, perform a necropsy in accordance with the procedure in 7.4 to determine the cause of death. Replacement of the animal to the study shall be dependent upon the design of the study. Include the animal in the assay of data if the cause of death is related to the procedure or test material.

7.4 *Sacrifice and Implant Retrieval*:

7.4.1 Euthanize animals by a humane method at the intervals specified in 6.7.

NOTE 2—The necropsy periods start at 12 weeks because it is assumed that acceptable implant data has been received for earlier periods from short term implant testing according to Practice F 763. If the 90–day sacrifice period has been utilized under Practice F 763, that group need not be repeated under this protocol, and thus, the 12-week group may be eliminated.

7.4.2 At necropsy, record any gross abnormalities of color or consistency observed in the tissue surrounding the implant. Remove each implant with an intact envelope of surrounding tissue. Include in the tissue sample a minimum of a 4-mm thick layer of tissue surrounding the implant. If less than a 4-mm thick layer of tissue is removed, report in accordance with 8.1.

7.5 *Postmortem Observations*—In accordance with standard laboratory practice, perform a necropsy on all animals that are sacrificed for the purposes of the assay or die during the assay period. Establish the status of the health of the experimental animal during the period of the assay. Report as described in Section 8.

7.6 *Histological Procedure*:

7.6.1 *Tissue Sample Preparation*—Prepare appropriate blocks from each implantation site and indicate the orientation of the axis of the femur relative to the axis of the implant (for bone implants). Also indicate the orientation of the implant relative to the axis of rotation of the femoral condyles.

7.6.1.1 Process the excised tissue block containing either a test implant or control implant for histopathological examination and such other studies as are appropriate. Cut the sample midway from end to end into appropriate size and in the appropriate orientation for each study. Transfer, or record, or both, the orientational details noted in 7.6.1 to each part of the sample. Record the gross appearance of the implant and the tissue. If the sample is porous, it is imperative that sectioning procedures be used that maintain the implant within its tissue envelope to allow the evaluation of tissue within the pores. Such procedures may include ground section preparation.

7.6.1.2 If special stains are deemed necessary, prepare additional sections and make appropriate observations.

7.7 *Histopathological Observations*—Compare the amount of tissue reaction adjacent to the test implant to that adjacent to a similar location and orientation on the control implant with respect to thickness of scar, presence of inflammatory or other cell types, presence of particles, and such other indications of interaction of tissue and material as might occur with the actual material under test. A suggested method for the evaluation of tissue response after implantation is Turner, et al. **(1)**[5]. If a porous sample is being tested, the evaluation of the tissue reaction must include areas within the pores of the test and control samples at similar locations.

7.7.1 *Suggested Method for Tissue Response Evaluation*:

7.7.1.1 A suggested format with tissue response and cell accumulation to be evaluated and a scoring range of 0 to 3 is shown in Table 1.

7.7.1.2 The scoring system of 0 to 3 is based upon the observation of high power fields (400–500X) and an average of five fields.

Tissue Response/Cell Accumulation	Score
0	0
1–5	0.5
6–15	1
16–25	2
26 or more	3

[5] The **boldface** numbers in parentheses refer to the list of references at the end of this standard.

TABLE 1 Suggested Evaluation Format and Scoring Range

Animal Number						
Duration of Implant (weeks)						
Sample Description						
Gross Response						
Histopath-Number						
Score		0	0.5	1	2	3
Necrosis						
Degeneration						
Inflammation						
	Polymorphonuclear Leukocytes					
	Lymphocytes					
	Eosinophils					
	Plasma Cells					
	Macrophages					
Fibrosis						
Giant Cells						
Foreign Body Debris						
Fatty Infiltration						
Relative Size of Involved Area in mm						
Histopathologic Toxicity Rating						

7.7.1.3 The necrosis and/or degeneration score is determined using the same range of 0 to 3, as follows:

Degree	Score
No reaction	0
Very slight reaction	0.5
Mild reaction	1
Moderate reaction	2
Marked reaction	3

7.7.1.4 An overall rating of test samples may be given using a rating range of 0 to 4, as follows:

Rating	Score
No reaction	0
Very slight reaction	1
Mild reaction	2
Moderate reaction	3
Marked reaction	4

7.7.1.4.1 Pathologists may choose to use the scoring system of comparing the negative control to the test material as an aid in their evaluation. The overall reaction to the test material as compared to the negative control is to be evaluated independently for all time periods.

8. Report

8.1 Report the following information:

8.1.1 All details of implant characterization, fabrication, conditioning (including cleaning, handling, and sterilization techniques employed). For porous implants, a measure of the porosity and pore interconnection diameters shall have been measured and reported.

8.1.2 Procedures for implantation and implant retrieval.

8.1.3 Details of any special procedure (such as unusual or unique diet fed to test animals).

8.1.4 The observations of each control and test implant as well as the gross appearance of the surrounding tissue in which the implants were implanted.

8.1.5 The observation of each histopathological examination including a descriptive pathology narration and the pathologist's evaluation as to the reaction to the test material provided.

9. Keywords

9.1 biocompatibility; bone implant materials; cellular reaction; histology/histopathology; implants muscle; New Zealand rabbits; orthopaedic medical devices—bone; plastic surgical devices/applications; polyethylene (PE)—surgical implant applications; rabbits; rats; scar; test animals; tissue compatibility; tissue response evaluation

APPENDIX

(Nonmandatory Information)

X1. RATIONALE FOR PRACTICE F981

X1.1 This practice is based on the research techniques utilized by Cohen **(2)**, and by Laing, Ferguson, and Hodge **(3, 4)** in the early 1960's. These studies involved the implantation of metal cylinders in paravertebral muscle of rabbits. The biological reaction to the cylinders was described as the thickness of the fibrous membrane or capsule formed adjacent to the implant. The thickness of the capsule and the presence of inflammatory cells was used as a measure of the degree of adverse reaction to the test material.

X1.2 As first published in 1972, Practice F 361 was a test for the biological response to metallic materials. The scope had been expanded beyond that of the published reports to include bone as well as muscle as an implant test site. To avoid species specific reactions, the method called for the use of rats and dogs as well as rabbits. Cylindrical test specimens with rounded ends were used to avoid biological reactions associated with sharp corners or other variations in specimen shape.

X1.3 In 1978, Practice F 469 was published as a parallel document for the test of polymeric materials. In that the methods were essentially the same, the scope of Practice F 361 has been expanded to include the testing of specimens made of metallic, polymeric or ceramic materials, thereby including and superseding Practice F 469.

X1.4 Stainless steel, cobalt chromium, and titanium alloys are used as reference materials since the biological response to these materials has been well characterized by their extensive use in research. The response to these materials is not defined as compatible, but rather the response is used as a reference against which reactions to other materials are compared.

X1.5 This practice is a modification of the original Practice F 361 in that it only involves long term test periods. The short term response to materials is to be evaluated using Practice F 763.

X1.6 This practice was revised in 1987 to allow for alternative specimen dimensions for rats and rabbits for muscle implantation. The original specimen dimensions were intended to be implanted through a needle, which was a change from Practice F 361 and Practice F 469. The alternate dimensions restore those specified since 1972, which some members felt were more appropriate for some material types.

X1.7 This practice was revised in 1990 to add a ceramic material (Specification F 603) as a reference material when testing ceramics.

X1.8 In 1991, this practice was revised to add the testing of porous materials to the scope of the practice. Previously, the committee had been unable to achieve consensus on the appropriate modifications to the technique to allow the testing of porous materials.

X1.9 This method is based upon over 30 years of published

experience in the use of these techniques for the evaluation of the response of tissue to implant materials. In revision, there was discussion of the appropriate length of a long term study. Comments received suggested that one or two year studies were excessive. It was the decision of the task force that the one year sacrifice interval would be maintained but that the two year interval for larger animals could be removed.

X1.10 The revision of this document in 1992 removed all reference to the use of the canine for these studies to encourage the use of rats and rabbits when practical. Larger animals such as dogs, goats, and sheep may be utilized when found to be appropriate by the investigator.

REFERENCES

(1) Turner, J. E., Lawrence, W. H., and Autian, J., "Subacute Toxicity Testing of Biomaterials using Histopathologic Evaluation of Rabbit Muscle Tissue," *Journal Biomedical Material Research*, Vol. 7, No. 39, 1973.

(2) Cohen, J., "Assay of Foreign-Body Reaction," *Journal of Bone and Joint Surgery*, No. 41A, 1959, pp. 152–166.

(3) Ferguson, A. B., Jr., Laing, P. G., and Hodge, E. S.," The Ionization of Metal Implants in Living Tissues," *Journal of Bone and Joint Surgery*, No. 42A, 1960, pp. 77–90.

(4) Laing, P. G., Ferguson, A. B., Jr., and Hodge, E. S.," Tissue Reaction in Rabbit Muscle Exposed to Metallic Implants," *Journal Biomedical Materials Research*, No. 1, 1967, pp. 135–149.

Designation: F 982 – 86 (Reapproved 1998)

Standard Specification for Disclosure of Characteristics of Surgically Implanted Clamps for Carotid Occlusion[1]

This standard is issued under the fixed designation F 982; the number immediately following the designation indicates the year of original adoption or, in the case of revision, the year of last revision. A number in parentheses indicates the year of last reapproval. A superscript epsilon (ε) indicates an editorial change since the last revision or reapproval.

1. Scope

1.1 This specification covers requirements for the disclosure of specific characteristics of screw-type adjustable clamps that are designed for the gradual permanent occlusion of carotid arteries. These devices consist of an implantable portion and an externally projecting removable screwdriver (see Fig. 1).

1.2 The following precautionary caveat pertains only to the test method portion, Section 5, of this specification: *This standard does not purport to address all of the safety problems, if any, associated with its use. It is the responsibility of the user of this standard to establish appropriate safety and health practices and determine the applicability of regulatory limitations prior to use.*

2. Referenced Documents

2.1 The designations and titles of the applicable documents for this specification are listed in Annex A1 in the following groups:

2.1.1 Materials,

2.1.2 Finishing,

2.1.3 Biocompatibility,

2.1.4 Handling, and

2.1.5 Analysis.

3. Terminology

3.1 *Descriptions of Terms Specific to This Standard (see Fig. 1):*

3.1.1 *access plate*—portion of the device that closes the frame.

3.1.2 *cap*—covering device to seal the lumen of the stem when the screwdriver is not in place.

3.1.3 *collar*—threaded portion of the frame that acts as a guide and counter torque surface for the pressure plate screw.

3.1.4 *frame*—encircling portion of the device, usually U-shaped.

3.1.5 *guide*—cylinder within the stem to provide counter torque and guidance for the screwdriver.

3.1.6 *hinge*—means of attaching the access plate to the frame.

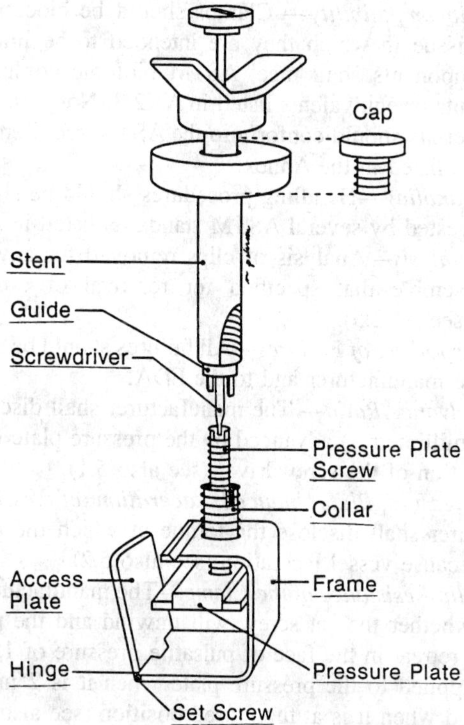

FIG. 1 Screw-Type Adjustable Clamp Components

3.1.7 *pressure plate*—movable compressing plate.

3.1.8 *pressure plate screw*—threaded shaft that advances the pressure plate.

3.1.9 *screwdriver*—device used to provide torque to the pressure plate screw. The screwdriver should have permanently marked scale indicating advance ratio by millimetres.

3.1.10 *set screw*—screw that secures the access plate to the frame.

3.1.11 *stem*—cylinder that is used to hold the frame and to provide counter torque for the screwdriver.

4. General Requirements

4.1 This section contains requirements for disclosure of information on screw-type adjustable clamps.

4.2 *Performance Disclosure*:

4.2.1 *Materials*:

4.2.1.1 The manufacturer shall disclose the generic names of the materials used in the manufacture of the clamp.

[1] This specification is under the jurisdiction of ASTM Committee F-4 on Medical and Surgical Materials and Devices and is the direct responsibility of Subcommittee F04.50 on Neurosurgical Standards.

Current edition approved March 27, 1986. Published May 1986.

Whenever available, ASTM material specification nomenclature shall be used (Annex A1). If multiple components are used, the names of each component shall be disclosed.

4.2.1.2 The metals and alloys or other materials used in clamps that conform to this specification should be fabricated of approved materials in accordance with the ASTM specifications listed in A1.2.1.

4.2.2 *Finishing*—Surface cleanliness and characteristics should meet the requirements of the ASTM specifications listed in A1.2.2. There should be no debris visible at 20X and no imperfections visible to the naked eye.

4.2.3 *Biocompatibility*— Clamps should be biocompatible with the tissue in which they are intended to be implanted. Metal components shall meet ASTM biologic compatibility requirements or equivalents listed in A1.2.3. Nonporous polymeric materials should conform to the ASTM requirements or equivalents listed in the Annex.

4.2.4 *Handling*—Handling procedures should be similar to those suggested by several ASTM standards listed in A1.2.4.

4.2.5 *Analysis*—Analysis of clips removed for any reason should resemble that specified for removal of orthopedic implants (see A1.2.5).

4.2.6 *Reporting of Failures*—All failures should be reported both to the manufacturer and to the FDA.

4.2.7 *Advance Ratio*— The manufacturer shall disclose the distance (millimetres) advanced by the pressure plate for each full revolution of the screwdriver (see also 5.1).

4.2.8 *Pressure Plate Induced Laceration of Vessel*—The manufacturer shall disclose the torque at which the pressure plate will cause vessel laceration (see also 5.2).

4.2.9 *Slip Resistance of the Clamp*—The manufacturer shall disclose whether the set screw will unwind and the pressure plate will retreat in the face of pulsatile pressure of 150/80 at 80 cpm applied to the pressure plate when it is 2 mm from closure and when it is at the closed position (see also 5.3).

5. Test Methods

5.1 *Advance Ratio*— This measurement must be accurate to ± 0.35 mm.

5.2 *Vessel Damage*— Implant the clamp aseptically around a dog carotid artery and close using a torque wrench. Implant several animals, each having their clamp tightened to a different torque. Sacrifice the animals two weeks later and examine microscopically as well as histologically to determine if there is laceration. Clamps can be tightened to a torque just below that which will cause laceration.

5.3 *Slip Resistance*— Perform the study "in vitro" using dog carotid arteries (average diameter 5 mm) or tubes of similar distensibility and a pulse duplicator system. Set the pulse duplicator to create a pulsatile cycle of pressure similar to the physiologic systolic - diastolic pattern (150/80 at 80 cpm). During the experiment, keep the artery in a normal saline bath and connect it to the pulse duplicator system. Close the clamp to a gap of 2 mm. Turn on the pulse duplicator and measure the position of the pressure plate relative to the basis of the frame every 24 h for 72 h to determine if there has been any retreat of the pressure plate. Perform a second test keeping the pulse duplicator functioning at the same setting but with the clamp closed down to occlude the artery using the torque determined safe as detailed in 5.2. Again, measure the position of the pressure plate every 24 h for 72 h. A backoff of 0.2 mm (90° turn) will be the maximum permitted. Measurement must be accurate to ±0.35 mm.

6. Labeling Requirements

6.1 All labeling must be consistent with applicable Federal Regulations. In addition, the labeling for carotid occlusive clamps within the scope of this specification should comply with the following requirements:

6.1.1 *Package Label*— The following information shall be available with the unit package:

6.1.1.1 Manufacturer's name,

6.1.1.2 Trade name,

6.1.1.3 Catalog number,

6.1.1.4 Manufacturer's identification or lot number,

6.1.1.5 Material(s),

6.1.1.6 Magnetic properties,

6.1.1.7 Advance ratio,

6.1.1.8 Torque which causes vessel laceration, and

6.1.1.9 Slip resistance.

6.1.2 *Product Insert*— The product insert should include the following information:

6.1.2.1 Manufacturer's name,

6.1.2.2 Trade name,

6.1.2.3 Catalog number,

6.1.2.4 Manufacturer's identification or lot number,

6.1.2.5 Size,

6.1.2.6 Length of compression plate,

6.1.2.7 Width of compression plate,

6.1.2.8 Compression surface,

6.1.2.9 Advance ratio,

6.1.2.10 Internal dimensions of clamp when fully opened,

6.1.2.11 Material(s),

6.1.2.12 Magnetic properties,

6.1.2.13 Torque which causes vessel laceration, and

6.1.2.14 Slip resistance.

6.1.3 *Catalog Information*—Recommendation that only the screwdriver specifically designed for the particular clamp be used (specify catalog number).

7. Keywords

7.1 cardiovascular surgical devices; carotid occlusion; clamps; disclosure; occlusions; resistance-slip; screw-type clamps

ANNEX

(Mandatory Information)

A1. APPLICABLE DOCUMENTS AND RATIONALE

A1.1 Background

A1.1.1 It is believed that the major sources for device-specific complications will result from suboptimal control of the following:

A1.1.1.1 Functional failure,

A1.1.1.2 Vessel trauma, and

A1.1.1.3 Biocompatibility.

A1.1.2 The ASTM standards listed in A1.2 were designed to prevent such possibilities.

A1.2 Referenced Documents

A1.2.1 *ASTM Standards for Materials:*[2]

F 55-82 Specification for Stainless Steel Bar and Wire for Surgical Implants

F 56-82 Specification for Stainless Steel Sheet and Strip for Surgical Implants

F 67-83 Specification for Unalloyed Titanium for Surgical Implant Applications

F 75-82 Specification for Cast Cobalt-Chromium-Molybdenum Alloy for Surgical Implant Applications

F 90-82 Specification for Wrought Cobalt-ChromiumTungsten-Nickel Alloy for Surgical Implant Applications

F 136-79 Specification for Wrought Titanium 6A1-4V ELI Alloy for Surgical Implant Applications

F 138-82 Specification for Stainless Steel Bars and Wire for Surgical Implants (Special Quality)

F 139-82 Specification for Stainless Steel Sheet and Strip for Surgical Implants (Special Quality)

F 560-78 Specification for Unalloyed Tantalum for Surgical Implant Applications

F 562-84 Specification for Wrought Cobalt-Nickel-Chromium-Molybdenum Alloy for Surgical Implant Applications

F 563-83 Specification for Wrought Cobalt-Nickel-Chromium-Molybdenum-Tungsten-Iron Alloy for Surgical Implant Applications

F 602-78 Criteria for Implantable Thermoset Epoxy Plastics

F 603-83 Specification for High-Purity Dense Aluminum Oxide for Surgical Implant Application

F 604-78 Classification for Silicone Elastomers Used in Medical Applications

F 620-79 Specification for Titanium 6A1-4V Alloy Forgings for Surgical Implants

F 621-79 Specification for Stainless Steel Forgings for Surgical Implants

F 624-81 Guide for Evaluation of Thermoplastic Polyurethane Solids and Solutions for Biomedical Applications

F 639-79 Specification for Polyethylene Plastics for Medical Applicatons

F 648-83 Specification for Ultra-High-Molecular-Weight Polyethylene Powder and Fabricated Form for Surgical Implants

F 665-80 Classification for Vinyl Chloride Plastics Used in Biomedical Application

F 688-80 Specification for Wrought Cobalt-Nickel-Chromium-Molybdenum Alloy Plate, Sheet, and Foil for Surgical Implants

F 702-81 Specification for Polysulfone Resin for Medical Applications

F 745-81 Specification for Stainless Steel for Cast and Solution Annealed Surgical Implant Applications

F 754-83 Specification for Implantable Polytetrafluoroethylene (PTFE) Polymer Fabricated in Sheet, Tube, and Rod Shapes

F 755-82 Specification for Selection of Porous Polyethylene for Use in Surgical Implants

F 799-82 Specification for Thermomechanically Processed Cobalt-Chromium-Molybdenum Alloy for Surgical Implants

A1.2.2 *ASTM Standards for Finishing:*[2]

F 86-76 Practice for Surface Preparation and Marking of Metallic Surgical Implants

F 601-78 Practice for Fluorescent Penetrant Inspection of Metallic Surgical Implants

F 746-81 Test Method for Pitting or Crevice Corrosion of Metallic Surgical Implant Materials

A1.2.3 *ASTM Standards for Biocompatibility:*[2]

F 361-80 Practice for Assessment of Compatibility of Metallic Materials for Surgical Implants with Respect to Effect of Materials on Tissue[3]

F 469-78 Practice for Assessment of Compatibility of Nonporous Polymeric Materials for Surgical Implants with Regard to Effect of Materials on Tissue[3]

F 619-79 Practice for Extraction of Medical Plastics

F 719-81 Practice for Testing Biomaterials in Rabbits for Primary Skin Irritation

F 720-81 Practice for Testing Guinea Pigs for Contact Allergens: Guinea Pig Maximization Test

F 748-82 Practice for Selecting Generic Biological Test Methods for Materials and Devices

F 749-82 Practice for Evaluating Material Extracts by Intracutaneous Injection in the Rabbit

F 750-82 Practice for Evaluating Material Extracts by Systemic Injection in the Mouse

F 763-82 Practice for Short-Term Screening of Implant Materials

F 813-83 Practice for Direct Contact Cell Culture Evaluation of Materials for Medical Devices

A1.2.4 *ASTM Standards for Handling:*[2]

F 565-78 Practice for Care and Handling of Orthopedic

[2] *Annual Book of ASTM Standards,* Vol 13.01.

[3] Discontinued—See *1986 Annual Book of ASTM Standards,* Vol 13.01.

Implants and Instruments

F 700-81 Practice for Care and Handling of Intracranial Aneurysm Clips and Instruments

F 701-81 Practice for Care and Handling of Neurosurgical Implants and Instruments

A1.2.5 *ASTM Standards for Analysis:*[2]

F 561-78 Practice for Retrieval and Analysis of Metallic Orthopedic Implants

Designation: F 983 – 86 (Reapproved 2000)

Standard Practice for Permanent Marking of Orthopaedic Implant Components[1]

This standard is issued under the fixed designation F 983; the number immediately following the designation indicates the year of original adoption or, in the case of revision, the year of last revision. A number in parentheses indicates the year of last reapproval. A superscript epsilon (ε) indicates an editorial change since the last revision or reapproval.

1. Scope

1.1 It is common practice for orthopaedic implant manufacturers to apply permanent identification to implant components. In this regard, Practice F 86 describes recommended locations and methods of marking for metallic implants.

1.2 The purpose of this practice is to (*1*) recommend that orthopaedic implants be permanently marked, and (*2*) recommend practical amounts of information that should be included in the marking. It is recognized, however, that marking is not practical in some cases (see 4.1).

1.3 *This standard does not purport to address all of the safety concerns, if any, associated with its use. It is the responsibility of the user of this standard to establish appropriate safety and health practices and determine the applicability of regulatory limitations prior to use.*

2. Referenced Documents

2.1 *ASTM Standards:*

F 86 Practice for Surface Preparation and Marking of Metallic Surgical Implants[2]

3. Methods of Marking

3.1 For metallic implants, the procedures described in Practice F 86 should be followed.

3.2 For nonmetallic implants, other methods should be devised and utilized.

3.3 In any case, however, the marking method should (*a*) not compromise implant performance significantly, and (*b*) provide legibility over the anticipated service life of the implant.

4. Information Included in Permanent Marking

4.1 Orthopaedic implants vary widely in size (for example, from wire to total joint prostheses), and the amount of information that practically can be included in marking varies accordingly. Some implants, such as threaded pins and cerclage wire and very small bone screws, do not provide any surfaces which can be marked practically.

4.2 *Standard Information*—Where implant size and shape allow, it is recommended that the following information be included in permanent marking:

4.2.1 *Manufacturer*:

4.2.2 *Material*—The use of generic names or ASTM standards, or both, in addition to or in place of trade names is recommended, where applicable.

4.2.3 Implant component catalog number or model number.

4.2.4 Implant component serial number or lot number.

4.3 *Minimum Information*—Where implant size and shape allow, it is recommended that the manufacturer mark smaller implants with symbols or letters selected by the manufacturer which identify (*a*) the manufacturer and (*b*) the material from which the component is made. The system of symbols or letters should be described in the manufacturer's product literature.

4.4 *Optional Information*—Manufacturers may wish to include additional information in the permanent marking, indicating, for example, implant size and whether an implant is intended for right limb or left limb reconstruction.

---

[1] This practice is under the jurisdiction of ASTM Committee F04 on Medical and Surgical Materials and Devices and is the direct responsibility of Subcommittee F04.21 on Osteosynthesis.

Current edition approved March 27, 1986. Published May 1986.

[2] *Annual Book of ASTM Standards*, Vol 13.01.

APPENDIX

(Nonmandatory Information)

X1. RATIONALE

X1.1 The intent of this practice is to provide needed information to users of orthopaedic implants under two different circumstances. First, many implants are removed from their packages outside the operating room long before surgery takes place, so that they may be sterilized or otherwise prepared for use. Permanent, readily understood marking will provide for positive identification of the implants under such circumstances. Second, when an implant is surgically removed, positive identification is desirable information for deciding the course of subsequent patient care and for purposes of research in implant utilization and performance.

Last ASTM Designation: F 984 – 86 (Reapproved 1992)

Standard Specification for Cutaneous Gas Monitoring Devices for Oxygen and Carbon Dioxide

This specification covers all devices intended for use as non-invasive monitoring systems of the partial pressure of oxygen or carbon dioxide at the skin's surface. This specification covers cutaneous monitors used with adults, children, and neonates, and may include the use of these devices in fetal monitoring prior to birth.

Formerly under the jurisdiction of Committee F-29 on Anesthetic and Respiratory Equipment, this specification was discontinued in 1999.

Designation: F 997 – 98a$^{\epsilon 1}$

Standard Specification for Polycarbonate Resin for Medical Applications[1]

This standard is issued under the fixed designation F 997; the number immediately following the designation indicates the year of original adoption or, in the case of revision, the year of last revision. A number in parentheses indicates the year of last reapproval. A superscript epsilon (ε) indicates an editorial change since the last revision or reapproval.

ϵ^1 NOTE—Editorial corrections were made to 2.3 and 6.1 in May 2001.

1. Scope

1.1 This specification covers polycarbonate resin and provides requirements and associated test methods for this thermoplastic when it is to be used in the manufacture of medical devices or components of medical devices.

1.2 As with any material, some characteristics may be altered by the processing techniques (such as molding, extrusion, machining, assembly, sterilization, and so forth) required for the production of a specific part or device. Therefore, properties of fabricated forms of this resin should be evaluated using those test methods that are appropriate to assure safety and efficacy.

1.3 The properties included in this specification are those applicable for polycarbonate only. The biocompatibility of plastic compounds made up of polycarbonate resin containing colorants, fillers, processing aids, or other additives, as well as polymer blends which contain polycarbonate, should not be assumed. The biocompatibility of these modified polycarbonates must be established by testing the final (end-use) compositions using the appropriate methods of evaluation. In addition, the biocompatibility of the material depends to a large degree on the nature of the end-use application. It is, therefore, necessary to specify a set of biocompatibility test methods for each new and distinct application.

1.4 *This standard does not purport to address all of the safety concerns, if any, associated with its use. It is the responsibility of the user of this standard to establish appropriate safety and health practices and determine the applicability of regulatory limitations prior to use.*

2. Referenced Documents

2.1 *ASTM Standards:*

D 256 Test Methods for Impact Resistance of Plastics and Electrical Insulating Materials[2]

D 570 Test Method for Water Absorption of Plastics[2]

D 638 Test Method for Tensile Properties of Plastics[2]

D 648 Test Method for Deflection Temperature of Plastics Under Flexural Load[2]

D 790 Test Methods for Flexural Properties of Unreinforced and Reinforced Plastics and Electrical Insulating Materials[2]

D 792 Test Methods for Specific Gravity (Relative Density) and Density of Plastics by Displacement[2]

D 883 Terminology Relating to Plastics[2]

D 955 Test Method of Measuring Shrinkage From Mold Dimensions of Molded Plastics[2]

D 1003 Test Method for Haze and Luminous Transmittance of Transparent Plastics[2]

D 1238 Test Method for Flow Rates of Thermoplastics by Extrusion Plastometer[2]

D 1600 Terminology for Abbreviated Terms Relating to Plastics[2]

D 1898 Practice for Sampling of Plastics[2]

D 3892 Practice for Packaging/Packing of Plastics[3]

D 3935 Specification for Polycarbonate (PC) Unfilled and Reinforced Materials[3]

F 748 Practice for Selecting Generic Biological Test Methods for Materials and Devices[4]

2.2 *Underwriter's Laboratories Document:*

UL Standard 94 Tests and Flammability of Plastic Materials for Parts in Devices and Appliances[5]

2.3 *Code of Federal Regulations:*

Title 21 CFR Subpart 177.1580[6]

3. Significance and Use

3.1 This specification is designed to recommend physical, chemical, and biological test methods to establish a reasonable level of confidence concerning the performance of unfilled polycarbonate resins for use in medical devices. The properties listed should be considered in selecting material according to the specific end-use requirements.

4. Classification

4.1 Types of polycarbonate plastics, molding, and extrusion grades are described in Specification D 3935.

[1] This specification is under the jurisdiction of ASTM Committee F04 on Medical and Surgical Materials and Devices and is the direct responsibility of Subcommittee F04.11 on Polymeric Materials.

Current edition approved October 10, 1998. Published March 1999. Originally published as F 997 – 86. Last previous edition F 997 – 98 .

[2] *Annual Book of ASTM Standards,* Vol 08.01.

[3] *Annual Book of ASTM Standards,* Vol 08.02.

[4] *Annual Book of ASTM Standards,* Vol 13.01.

[5] Available from Underwriter's Laboratories, Publication Stock, 333 Pfingsten Rd., Northbrook, IL 60062.

[6] Available from Standardization Documents Order Desk, Bldg. 4 Section D, 700 Robbins Ave., Philadelphia, PA 19111–5094, Attn: NPODS.

5. General Requirements

5.1 Polycarbonate resin may be processed by most techniques available for thermoplastic polymers. Medical devices and components of medical devices made of polycarbonate may be sterilized. Methods used successfully include steam, ethylene oxide, and irradiation. Repeated sterilization may weaken parts molded of any plastic material. The number of times a given part may be sterilized safely without fear of subsequent breakage depends on a number of factors, for example, the design of the part, the method of manufacture, the method of sterilization, the application or use of the part. Therefore, it is imperative that the manufacturer test the part to determine the maximum number of sterilization cycles to which it can be safely subjected. The function of the part should be very carefully evaluated if repeated sterilization is desired.

5.2 Polycarbonate resin is the thermoplastic carbonic-acid polyester of bisphenol-A (BPA), or 4,4′-isopropylidenediphenol, or as defined in Terminology D 883.

5.3 Polycarbonate resins used in medical applications may comply with the Food and Drug Administration (FDA) Regulation 21 CFR 177.1580 which covers both wet and dry food contact applications.

5.4 The formulated compound may contain optional adjuvant substances required in the production of the polymer or in the fabrication or intended use of the end product. The biocompatibility of these adjuvant substances shall be established on the finished product in accordance with Practice F 748.

6. Physical Properties

6.1 The physical properties of polycarbonate may be determined by the following: Test Methods D 256, Test Method D 570, Test Method D 638, Test Method D 648, Test Methods D 790, Test Methods D 792, Terminology D 883, Test Method D 955, Test Method D 1003, Test Method D 1238, Terminology D 1600, and UL Standard 94.

7. Biocompatibility

7.1 Biocompatibility shall be determined in accordance with Practice F 748, unless otherwise agreed upon by packager and consumer.

8. Sampling

8.1 The material should be sampled in accordance with standard sampling procedures, such as those described in Practice D 1898, or other sampling techniques unless otherwise agreed upon between consumer and supplier.

9. Packaging and Labeling

9.1 Packaging material shall meet the standards set forth in Practice D 3892, unless otherwise agreed upon by packager and consumer.

10. Keywords

10.1 plastics (thermoplastic); plastic surgical devices/applications; polycarbonate (PC) plastics; polymers-surgical applications; resins-polycarbonate; seals

APPENDIXES

(Nonmandatory Information)

X1. RATIONALE

X1.1 This specification was established to provide guidance in the testing of polycarbonate resins intended for use in medical device applications. It recommends test methods for the measurement of chemical, physical, and mechanical properties of unfilled resins. Tests should be selected according to end-use applications. It is intended that biocompatibility be established on the finished product by the appropriate procedures, after it has gone through all processing steps and after all adjuvant substances have been incorporated.

X2. BIOCOMPATIBILITY

X2.1 No known surgical implant material has ever been shown to be completely free of adverse reactions in the human body. However, long-term clinical experience of use of specific formulations and grades of this material referred to in this standard has shown that an acceptable level of biological response can be expected, if the material is used in appropriate applications.

Standard Specification for General Workmanship and Performance Measurements of Hemostatic Forceps[1]

This standard is issued under the fixed designation F 1026; the number immediately following the designation indicates the year of original adoption or, in the case of revision, the year of last revision. A number in parentheses indicates the year of last reapproval. A superscript epsilon (ε) indicates an editorial change since the last revision or reapproval.

This standard has been approved for use by agencies of the Department of Defense.

1. Scope

1.1 This specification covers general workmanship aspects of hemostatic forceps fabricated from stainless steel and intended for reuse in surgery.

2. Referenced Documents

2.1 *ASTM Standards:*

E 18 Test Methods for Rockwell Hardness and Rockwell Superficial Hardness of Metallic Materials[2]

E 92 Test Method for Vickers Hardness of Metallic Materials[2]

E 140 Hardness Conversion Tables for Metals[2]

F 899 Specification for Stainless Steel Billet, Bar, and Wire for Surgical Instruments[3]

F 921 Definitions of Terms Relating to Hemostatic Forceps[3]

3. Terminology

3.1 Definitions applicable to hemostatic forceps shall be in accordance with Definitions F 921.

4. Material

4.1 All of the component parts of the instruments shall be made of martensitic stainless steel of Type 410, 410X, 416, 416MOD, 420A, or 420B of Specification F 899.

5. Physical Requirements

5.1 *Heat Treatment and Hardness for Component Parts*:

5.1.1 The component parts of the instruments shall be heat treated under conditions recommended for the material used. Typical heat treating guidelines and hardness values are shown in Specification F 899.

5.1.2 The hardness of all opposing parts of the same instrument shall not vary in hardness by more than 4 units on the Rockwell Hardness C scale (HRC) or equivalent.

5.2 *Passivation*—Instruments and instrument components shall be passivated after completion of all fabricating and finishing operations.

6. Performance Requirements

6.1 *Finger Rings*—Inside surfaces shall be well rounded and polished and shall comply with the requirements in 7.1.

6.2 *Jaw Serrations and Teeth*—Jaw serrations and teeth shall be of the types specified in Definitions F 921. The serrations and teeth shall be of uniform depth and height and well defined to provide effective gripping. The serrations and teeth shall interdigitate. The edges of the serrations shall be chamfered.

6.3 *Box Lock*—The hemostatic forceps shall be of box lock construction, as defined in Definitions F 921. The pin, or other fastening component, shall be permanently secured. The joint performance of the box lock shall be smooth, of equal resistance, and non-binding when opening or closing the forceps to an included angle of 90 ± 5° (the lock may be lubricated).

6.4 *Clearance*—The maximum clearance between the male and female members of the forceps in the lock area shall be 0.4 mm (0.015 in.). The clearance is the visible gap that exists when the instrument is viewed from both the front and side profile or end view of the instrument (excluding bevel) (See Fig. 1).

6.5 *Ratchets*—Ratchet and ratchet catch shall securely engage at each ratchet position in a smooth and progressive manner.

6.6 *Jaw and Ratchet Setting*—The jaw tips shall close and interdigitate when the first ratchet position is engaged, and there shall be no visible misalignment of the jaws. The jaws shall progressively tighten with each succeeding ratchet engagement. Each ratchet position shall hold firmly and release easily. The jaws shall be fully closed and the serrations interdigitated when the last ratchet is engaged. The jaws shall not open as the result of engaging any ratchet position.

6.7 *Elasticity*—The instrument by design shall be capable of passing the test for elasticity as specified in 8.2. After completion of the test, no visible distortion, cracks, or other visible damage to the instrument shall be evident.

7. Workmanship, Finish, and Appearance

7.1 *Surfaces*—The surfaces of the instrument shall be uniformly finished and free of burrs, sharp edges, cracks, coarse marks, and manufacturing materials.

7.2 *Type*—The finish shall be one of the types defined in

---

[1] This specification is under the jurisdiction of ASTM Committee F-4 on Medical and Surgical Materials and Devices and is the direct responsibility of Subcommittee F04.33 on Medical/Surgical Instruments.

Current edition approved Sept. 26, 1986. Published November 1986.

[2] *Annual Book of ASTM Standards*, Vol 03.01.

[3] *Annual Book of ASTM Standards*, Vol 13.01.

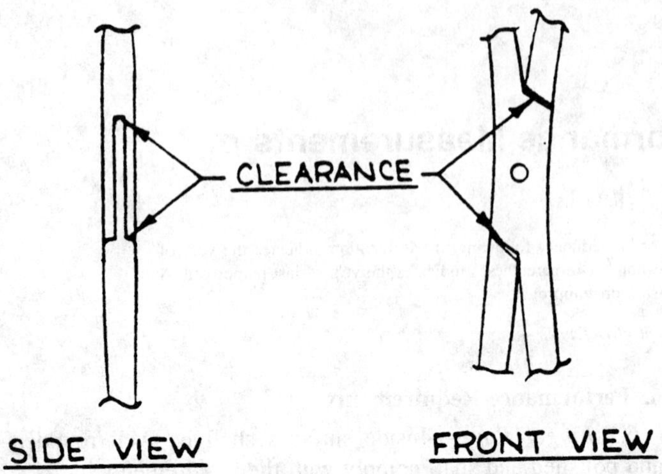

FIG. 1 Clearance of Forceps

Definitions F 921, or as required by the purchaser.

8. Test Methods

8.1 *Hardness*—Hardness shall be determined in accordance with Test Methods E 18 or Test Method E 92. Conversion of Vickers hardness values to Rockwell values shall be in accordance with Conversion Tables E140.

8.2 *Elasticity*—The instrument shall have a segment of basswood, leather strap, or stainless steel wire test material placed between the jaws at the tip. The instrument shall be engaged in the last (tightest) ratchet position for 24 h at room temperature. The thickness of the test material shall be as listed in Table 1.

8.3 *Corrosion Resistance*—Instruments or instrument components shall be subject to the corrosion tests.

9. Marking and Labeling

9.1 All markings shall be legible.

9.2 The instrument shall bear: the manufacturer's or contractor's name or registered trademark; the country of origin, when the instrument is not manufactured in the United States; and other markings as required by the purchaser, manufacturer, or contractor.

9.3 The location of markings shall be on a suitable surface of the instrument.

TABLE 1 Test Material Thickness and Instrument Length

Thickness or Diameter of Test Material, mm (in.)	Nominal Overall Length of Instrument, mm (in.)
1.98–2.00 (0.0781–0.0787)	Up to and including 127 (5)
3.00–3.18 (0.1181–0.1250)	Over 127 to 150 (5 to 5.906)
3.97–4.00 (0.1563–0.1575)	Over 150 to 177.8 (5.906 to 7.000)
4.76–5.00 (0.1875–0.1969)	Over 177.8 (7.000)

The American Society for Testing and Materials takes no position respecting the validity of any patent rights asserted in connection with any item mentioned in this standard. Users of this standard are expressly advised that determination of the validity of any such patent rights, and the risk of infringement of such rights, are entirely their own responsibility.

This standard is subject to revision at any time by the responsible technical committee and must be reviewed every five years and if not revised, either reapproved or withdrawn. Your comments are invited either for revision of this standard or for additional standards and should be addressed to ASTM Headquarters. Your comments will receive careful consideration at a meeting of the responsible technical committee, which you may attend. If you feel that your comments have not received a fair hearing you should make your views known to the ASTM Committee on Standards, at the address shown below.

Standard Practice for
Assessment of Tissue and Cell Compatibility of Orofacial Prosthetic Materials and Devices[1]

This standard is issued under the fixed designation F 1027; the number immediately following the designation indicates the year of original adoption or, in the case of revision, the year of last revision. A number in parentheses indicates the year of last reapproval. A superscript epsilon (ε) indicates an editorial change since the last revision or reapproval.

ϵ^1 NOTE—Editorial changes were made throughout November 1995.

1. Scope

1.1 This practice describes a procedure to assess the cytotoxic potential of materials for use in the construction of medical materials and devices using human excised donor (HED) tissues and their derived primary cells taken from the orofacial region.

1.2 This practice may be used either directly to evaluate materials or as a reference against which other cytotoxicity methods may be compared.

1.3 This practice is one of a series of reference methods for assessment of cytotoxic potential, employing different techniques.

1.4 Assessment of cytotoxicity is one of several procedures employed in determining the biological response to a material, as recommended in Practice F 748.

1.5 *This standard does not purport to address all of the safety concerns, if any, associated with its use. It is the responsibility of the user of this standard to establish appropriate safety and health practices and determine the applicability of regulatory limitations prior to use.*

2. Referenced Documents

2.1 *ASTM Standards:*

D 883 Terminology Relating to Plastics[2]

F 604 Specification for Silicone Elastomers Used in Medical Applications[3]

F 703 Specification for Implantable Breast Prostheses[3]

F 748 Practice for Selecting Generic Biological Test Methods for Materials and Devices[3]

F 813 Practice for Direct Contact Cell Culture Evaluation of Materials for Medical Devices[3]

3. Terminology

3.1 Nomenclature relating to the physical, mechanical, and chemical characteristics of plastics shall conform to Definitions D 883.

3.2 The nomenclature and glossary of terms related to tissue culturing shall conform to that of the Tissue Culture Association **(1)**.[4]

3.3 For other definitions used in this practice, see Annex A1.

4. Summary of Practice

4.1 Primary human orofacial tissue or cells and established human cell lines are cultured in Medium A3 or any medium supporting primary cell growth with homologous processed human serum or serum components in cell culture flasks or appropriate containers. The following series of cultures is set up:

4.1.1 Test material placed in contact with the cell layer.

NOTE 1—One or more replicates of 4.1.1 may be necessary.

4.1.2 Primary control wherein no material contacts the cell layer.

4.1.3 Positive control wherein the cell layer is contacted by a material eliciting a known cytotoxic response, such as a toxic chemical published in the Toxic Substances List **(2)**.

4.1.4 Negative control wherein the cell layer is contacted by polystyrene used in tissue culture labware.

4.2 The test culture shall be observed daily for growth and signs of toxicity. The test shall be terminated upon the attainment of confluency.

NOTE 2—For an established cell line cultured with Holmes alpha growth factor (AGF), confluency is usually achieved in slightly more than 5 days.

NOTE 3—For first passage cells from HED cultures, confluency is usually achieved between 10 to 20 days with an upper limit of 30 days.

5. Significance and Use

5.1 This practice is useful for assessing the cytotoxic potential both when evaluating new materials or formulations for possible use in medical applications, and as part of a quality control program for established medical devices.

5.2 This practice is used for assessing the cytotoxic potential of materials intended for the fabrication of inserts or implants in the orofacial region.

5.3 This practice is restricted to normal nontransformed,

[1] This practice is under the jurisdiction of ASTM Committee F-4 on Medical and Surgical Materials and Devicesand is the direct responsibility of Subcommittee F04.16 on Biocompatibility.

Current edition approved Sept. 26, 1986. Published November 1986.

[2] *Annual Book of ASTM Standards*, Vol 08.01.

[3] *Annual Book of ASTM Standards*, Vol 13.01.

[4] The **boldface** numbers in parentheses refer to the list of references at the end of this practice.

human orofacial tissues using cells cultured in human serum factors and does not depend upon cells and serum from nonhuman sources.

5.4 This practice incorporates procedures to monitor the quality of ingredient materials and the uniformity of the production process for formulating stock compositions.

5.5 This practice may be useful to determine the effects of age and radiation, and the state of carcinogenicity on the sensitivity of HED tissues to materials and devices used for orofacial prosthesis.

6. Apparatus

6.1 *Incubator*, capable of maintaining a temperature of 37 ± 1°C and an atmosphere of 95 % air and 5 % CO_2 with at least 90 % relative humidity.

6.2 *Plastic and Glassware*, that is specified by chemical type and is traceable to source of supply by catalog number or trade designation of the manufacturer or vendor.

6.3 *Laminar Flow Cabinet*, that meets the Class 100 clean room requirements of the U. S. Federal Standard 209B or the National Standard Foundation Standard NSF 49.

6.4 *Fluid Filters*, capable of removing 95 % of particles 0.22 µm or greater.

6.5 *Water Purification System*, with filtration capability for organic contaminants, capable of producing water with resistivity of 18 MΩ-cm or greater.

6.6 *Inverted Stage Microscope*, with phase contrast optics.

6.7 *Bright Field Microscope*, or a photomicroscope with magnification to 200×.

7. Reagents

7.1 *Medium A3*—Chemically defined medium A3 described by Holmes **(3)**.[5]

NOTE 4—Other chemically defined media shall be acceptable provided the test human cell adapts within 1 to 3 days to a steady growth rate from low cell density for a period of 7 to 30 days.

7.2 *Trypsin 0.25 % Solution*, stored in lyophilized form at 3 to 5°C. A solution may be prepared as needed and used at 37°C.

7.3 *Insulin*, 6.6 U/100 mL, used as supplement for primary cell and cell line cultures.

7.4 *Miscellaneous Fixatives*, dehydrating solutions, stains, etc. for making permanent record microscopic slides.

8. Human Serum

8.1 The human serum shall be processed in accordance with the method described in Annex A2.

NOTE 5—The dialysis treatment serves to remove suspect toxicants, ingested medication, unneeded adventitiae, and unidentified growth inhibitants with exclusion up to molecular weight of 3500 Daltons.

9. Cell Growth Factors

9.1 *Alpha Growth Factor (AGF)*—AGF, separated from the dialyzed human serum as described in Annex A3, shall be used as needed to enhance cell growth.

NOTE 6—Initially designated alpha-1-protein **(4)**, AGF can be used in place of whole serum to maintain the reference established cell line (ECL) cultures for the 7 to 30 test period when added to a chemically defined medium (7.1).

10. Reference ECL Cells

10.1 Human non-transformed established cell line (ECL) cell obtainable from a repository source, such as the American Type Culture Association (ATCC), shall be used as a reference to monitor the procedural details for uniformity of the testing system and for indication of quality and reliability of culture medium, human serum preparation, and quality of selected growth factors.

NOTE 7—For interlaboratory comparison of these procedural details, the clinically accessible gingival orofacial tissue cell, as well as the mucosal (nasal, maxillo, etc.), shall be selected and appropriately designated.

11. (HED) Cells

11.1 Human tissues of the orofacial region, obtained from patient donors, shall be cultured as explants until sufficient cell density is attained for succeeding passages into a valid primary cell line.

12. Preparation of Specimens

12.1 Aseptic techniques shall be used throughout the procedure.

12.2 Warm all solutions and materials to a temperature of 37 ± 2°C before placing in contact with cells.

12.3 *Specimens*:

12.3.1 Test materials shall range from 0.1 to 1 mm in thickness, cut into square or triangular geometries, 10 to 15 mm on a side.

12.3.2 Test specimens shall be sterilized by the method used in the preparation of the finished device.

12.3.3 The test arrangement must provide total immersion and immobilization of specimens (see Fig. 1). A pair of slots is cut in the specimen and a suitably cleaned cover glass (9 by 50 mm, No. 1) is threaded through the slots. One or more round holes (3 mm in diameter) are pre-cut in the center of the specimen. This provides an area of high leaching concentration as well as a focus for a photomicrographic record.

NOTE 8—If contamination of the assembled test material-microslip is suspected, it may be autoclaved before insertion into a sterile culture flask.

12.4 Conventional practices of maintaining contaminant free working conditions shall be applied in handling tissues, cells, and glassware with well-established techniques as already prescribed in numerous texts and handbooks. In this connection, see the work by John Paul **(5)** as one of several texts dealing with prevention of aerial and fluid contamination in cell culture practices.

13. Preparation of (ECL) Cultures

13.1 The reference cell line (see 10.1) shall be routinely maintained as stock cultures, either in completely chemically defined A3 medium or in Annex A3 medium containing the alpha growth factor (AGF), or in A3 medium supplemented with 10 % processed human serum.

13.2 Medium changes are made every 48 to 72 h or on a

[5] Commercially available as Holmes A3 medium from Grand Island Biologicals (GIBCO) Laboratories, 3175 Staley Rd., Grand Island, NY, 14072.

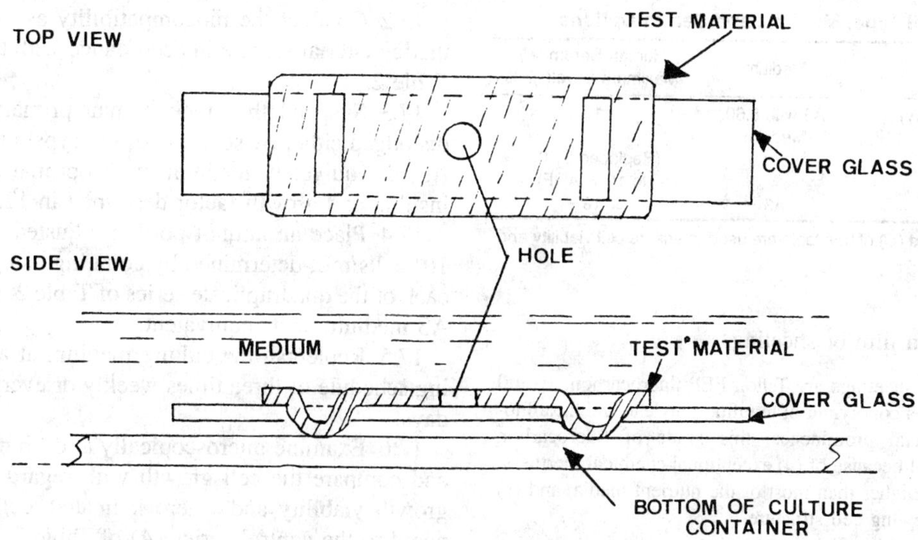

NOTE 1—Test specimens less than 1 mm in thickness tend to float. The figure depicts one means of maintaining submerged contact between specimens and cell cultures.

NOTE 2—Dimensions and configuration of the hole, serving for initial cell seeding, may be optionally modified and appropriately specified.

FIG. 1 Arrangement for Submersing and Immobilizing Specimens

triweekly schedule, such as Mondays, Wednesdays, and Fridays. Cultures are checked microscopically at the time and observed for any morphological changes or contamination, delayed or incidental.

13.3 Cell stock cultures of established cell line are maintained not only as source of cells for the biocompatibility assessment but also as a means to ascertain and verify the quality and titer of the production lots of processed human serum and preparation lots of separated AGF.

14. Preparation and Maintenance of Primary Human Cells

14.1 Place the human excised donor tissue (explant) asceptically onto a sterile petri dish holding gauze covered with A3 medium containing 10 % of processed human serum.

14.2 Dissect explant immediately into small pieces, cut into 1 to 2 mm thin slices of approximately 2 to 4 mm^2 dimension.

14.3 Incubate at 37 ± 1°C in a 5 % CO_2 and 95 % air atmosphere in quadruplicate series of culturing containers until a monolayer is formed and confirmed microscopically.

14.4 Trypsinize with fresh, ready prepared 0.25 % trypsin solution.

NOTE 9—Other methods of enzyme treatment may be utilized provided the outcome of the assay has been substantially equivalent.

14.5 Place the trypsinized cells in sterile culture flasks to prepare a stock of first passage cells for the biocompatibility test (see Section 17).

14.6 Check the first passage cultured cells for native contamination by virus, bacteria, and pleuropneumonia-like organisms (PPLO). Discard if present and identified and replace with new donor explants.

NOTE 10—Such microorganisms are often entrapped in oral mucosal tissues as contaminants which could compromise the validity of the test result by imposing foreign, nonspecific cytotoxicity in the procedure in Section 17.

14.7 Harvest the cultured propagated cells for use in amounts needed in 17.3. Store any unused portion in glycerol or dimethyl sulphoxide (DMSO) at –70°C for new sets of tests, using the procedure described in Chapter XIX of Ref. 5.

15. Ascertaining Minimum Effective Titer of Growth Factor

15.1 The selected reference human ECL cell shall be adapted to grow in the Holmes A3 medium or in a culturing medium of equivalent effectiveness using:

15.1.1 Initial low density cell level of 10^3 to 10^4 cells/mL,

15.1.2 One percent processed (Annex A2) human serum,

15.1.3 A series of alpha growth factor comprising 0, 0.1, 1.0, and 10 µg (dry basis) per millilitre of media.

15.1.4 Grown to confluent monolayer with a schedule of three fresh media maintenance replenishments per week as indicated in 13.2.

NOTE 11—It is essential to recognize the various phases of cell growth, which includes adaptation (I), usually with decreasing cell population for one or more days, followed by log growth (II), usually referred to in population doubling time, leading to monolayer confluency (III), and ultimately to decline (IV) in cell population by reason of senescence or toxicity. In this connection, appropriate, periodic cell counts to confluency (IV) can be applied as described by Lontz (**6**).

15.2 Following the attained confluency in the above AGF 0 to 10 µg/mL range, the minimal supplementation by AGF is noted for use in the ensuing procedure for biocompatibility of prosthetic material samples (Section 17).

16. Reference Control and Materials

16.1 The *negative* control shall be a material that consistently does not inhibit cell growth as observed visibly or by an appropriate increase in cell count during growth to confluency. The following material may be used:

16.1.1 USP Negative Control Plastic Reference Standard (**7**).

TABLE 1 Test Cell Type, Medium, and Serum Options

Cell Type	Medium	Human Serum (*P*) Maximum Level(*), %
(*A*) Human Orofacial (primary)	A3 with 6.60 Medium	10
(*B*) Established Cell Line[A]	A3	(Replaced by 0.1 to 10 % AGF)
(*C*) Established Cell Line	A3	10

[A] The combinations (*B*) and (*C*) of this table are used to ensure cell viability and procedural consistency.

16.1.2 Fluorocarbon film or sheeting.

NOTE 12—Satisfactory sheetings are Teflon FEP fluorocarbon, 10 mil (0.010 in.) thickness[6] and a copolymer of tetrafluorethylene and hexafluoropropylene of commercial prominence; this grade of fluorocarbon polymer is uniquely useful because of (*a*) exceptional chemical inertness, (*b*) high specific gravity, higher than most of the nutrient media, and (*c*) exceptional clarity for viewing cell structure.

16.1.3 Polystyrene culturing flask used in the test procedure.

16.2 The *positive* control shall be a material as required in other cell culture test methods, such as Practice F 813, section 8.2.2, or specially compounded at a level of 1 %, mixed in RTV grade of commercial silicone with known toxic agent, such as listed in Registry of Toxic Substance **(2)**.

NOTE 13—Although phenol is a common reference toxicant (Practice F 813, Section 8.7.1), its aqueous solubility and hence leachability is too rapid. For suitable, less soluble alternatives, use any of its aryl substituted chloro or nitro derivatives listed in the Registry.

16.3 Prosthetic material used in the device shall be in the chemically converted form, appropriately polymerized or otherwise consolidated to the final fabricated stage of the prosthetic device.

16.4 All prosthetic test materials, including the positive and negative controls, shall be in the substantially similar or equivalent form of thin film or sheeting in the range of 0.1 to 1.0 mm thickness, within a range of surface area of 2 to 4 cm^2 with mensurations of each of the test material specimens in terms of:

16.4.1 Shape description, that is, square, rectangle, etc.

16.4.2 Density or specific gravity.

16.4.3 Thickness (mm).

16.4.4 Weight (mg).

16.4.5 Surface area (m^2).

16.4.6 Volume (mL).

16.4.7 Surface/volume ratio.

16.5 In case of low density test material specimens that tend to float on the culture medium and away from the developing, culturing monolayer, submerge the test specimen with an appropriate weighting, such as depicted in Fig. 1.

17. Assessment of Biocompatibility of Prosthetic Material

17.1 Conduct concurrently the biocompatibility assessment of the prosthetic material samples by using the three combinations (a, b, and c) of cell type, medium and serum options shown in Table 1.

[6] Available from E. I. du Pont de Nemours and Co., Inc., Plastic Products and Resins Department, Wilmington, DE, 19898.

17.2 Conduct the biocompatibility assessment of the prosthetic material sample in accordance with the format shown in Table 2.

17.3 Suspend the stock human primary cells, (see 14.7), dislodged either by scraping or by trypsin treatment, into fresh A3, or equivalent medium, with optimal additives of serum, insulin, and growth factor described in 17.1, Table 1.

17.4 Place an aliquot portion adjusted to a level of 10^3 to 10^4 cells/mL, determined by counting using a hemocytometer, each of the quadruplicate series of Table 2, with the appropriate A3 medium or its equivalent.

17.5 Replenish the culture medium at a maintenance feeding schedule of three times weekly or every 48 h for at least 7 days.

17.6 Examine microscopically at each maintenance feeding and compare the cell growth with regard to evidence of cell growth viability and where indicated, cell abnormality compared to the control series (*A*) of Table 2.

NOTE 14—These abnormalities shall include visual evidence of (a) malformation or degeneration in structure, (b) cell lysis, or (c) reduced cell population or actual cell count.

17.7 Prepare photomicrographs at 100 to 200 magnification of each Table 2 series at culture days of 1, 3, 5, and 7 days for qualitative rating of cell, applying an appropriate system rating of toxicity.

NOTE 15—The appropriate system of rating shall be any of the following conventional, precedental methods of grading or scoring described by Johnson and Northrop **(8)** and Horres et al **(9)**. Both references apply a grade or rating of 0 for nontoxicity to 1 + to 4 + for degree of cell degeneration or inhibiton.

17.8 Where required for continued monolayer confluency beyond the 7-day maintenance period, continue the maintenance of the culture series with cytotoxic grading and microphotographs at approximately weekly intervals to 30 days, or until sooner terminated due to total of severe (more than 75 %) cell demise.

17.9 At the end of the 7-day or extended 30-day test period, the cells grown on the coverslip depicted in Fig. 1 shall be,

TABLE 2 Biocompatibility Format[A] for Primary Human Cells (for 12.4.7) for 7 or 30 Days (optional)[B]

Test Material in Culturing Series	Number of Culture Flasks	
	Morphological Assessment	Optional[C] Biochemical Assessment
(*A*) None—Procedural Control[D]	4	4
(*B*) Prosthetic Material Test Specimen	4	4
(*C*) Positive Control (cytotoxic reference)	4	4
(*D*) Negative Control (nontoxic reference)	4	4

[A] The cell stocks in this test matrix shall be drawn from a pool of stock cultures maintained in the same A3 or equivalent medium as supplemented and selected for this format.

[B] The optional 30-day test period, or longer, shall be acceptable with cells or from media modifications where diverse human cell growth adaptation may require extended periods.

[C] For use as collateral, adjunctive assessment for cell viability or cell transformations, or both.

[D] When using sterile polystyrene plastic containers of established non-cytoxicity, series (*A*) may be used as the negative control in lieu of series (*D*).

according to the conventional matter, fixed with formalin, dehydrated, and stained with hematoxylin and eosin.

17.10 An optional, corollary biochemical and biophysical assessment, as indicated in Table 2, shall be applied for evidence of cell transformations during the course of the 7 to 30 days maintenance, and as a check on potential or possible cytogenetic changes of stock primary and stock reference cells.

NOTE 16—Such biochemical assessments shall include key enzyme activities, for instance, lactose dehydrogenase and chromosomal aberrations such as described by Lontz et al **(10)**.

17.11 The cultured cells for optional biochemical assessment and or cell count shall be rinsed at least twice with 4 mL of fresh A3 medium or its selected equivalent, containing no additives.

17.12 The rinsed cells, on the completion or termination of a test phase, shall be collected from the culture flask in 1 mL of A3 medium, or its selected equivalent, for the selected biochemical assessment with the further option of freezing for storage at −70°F until used for the biochemical assessment or cell counts, or both.

18. Validity and Standardization

18.1 The rating of biocompatibility in accordance with 17.7 shall be deemed valid only when the morphological responses are evident with the negative and positive controls.

18.2 Wherever cell counting is applied during the 7-day or the extended 30-day culturing periods, conventional statistical assessment shall be by appropriate P^* (null hypothesis) values for paired comparisons with nontoxic and toxic reference controls.

18.3 Cytotoxicity shall be based on any one of the following criteria:

18.3.1 Visible cell lysis or cell demise, or both, in the vicinity of the test material.

18.3.2 Marked reduction in cell count by direct counting or equivalent means, such as DNA analysis.

18.3.3 Marked changes in enzyme levels when compared to controls, as determined by analyses of selected target enzymes.

18.4 Nontoxicity shall be so stated based on non-evident toxic assessments in 17.6 or 17.7, or both.

19. Report

19.1 Report the following information:

19.1.1 Test cells utilized.

19.1.1.1 Designate established cell line utilized (Table 1 (*a*) and (*b*)).

19.1.1.2 Designate human cell utilized; anatomical classification, viz, facial skin, lip, gingiva, palate, nasal pharyngeal, etc.

19.1.1.3 Prior history from primary culturing, media adaptation, passages, etc.

19.1.1.4 Results in accordance with Table 2.

19.1.2 Media.

19.1.3 Growth Factor(s), that is AGF or substitutes, or both.

19.1.3.1 General preparative method, whether human plasma or from serum, and the concentration or assay employed.

19.1.3.2 Commercially available source of media, cell growth factors, etc., with designated concentration used in test.

19.1.4 Prosthetic device test sample.

19.1.4.1 General chemical designation of principal polymer or elastomer component according to nomenclature established by American Chemical Society Chemical Abstracts.

19.1.4.2 Commercial designation of principal component, if provided as article of commerce, by classification, type or grade, with lot or batch identity.

19.1.4.3 Molecular characterization of principal component, in terms of molecular weight, infrared (IR) group frequency spectra, and differential thermal analyses (DTA) or differential scanning calorimetry (DSC).

19.1.4.4 Component additives, such as catalyst, stabilizers, fillers, and pigments or colorants with conventional chemical designation.

19.1.5 General method of processing or conversion of ingredient materials into fabricated prosthetic device.

19.1.6 Principal end-use tensile properties and tear resistance on: (*a*) fabricated unexposed test specimen, and (*b*) test specimens appropriately exposed to selected metabolite replicating reagents, namely, at least (*1*) glyceride selected from an edible vegetable oil, and (*2*) lactic acid.

19.1.7 Test specimen quantification and mensuration.

19.1.7.1 Density of specimen (g/cm^3 at stated temperature).

19.1.7.2 Weight, g.

19.1.7.3 Thickness (cm), width (cm), length (cm).

19.1.7.4 Volume (cm^3) from 19.1.7.3.

19.1.7.5 Volume (cm^3) of test medium per maintenance.

19.1.7.6 Total volumes (cm^3) of 19.1.7.5 to rated cytotoxicity.

19.1.7.7 Calculated ratios (quotients) for:

19.1.7.7.1 Surface area/sample weight from 19.1.7.3/19.1.7.2.

19.1.7.7.2 Sample weight/volume of test medium from 19.1.7.2/19.1.7.6.

19.1.7.8 Provide summarizing statement with a graded rating, as per 17.6, from 0 for nontoxicity to + 4 for extreme toxicity.

19.1.7.9 Permanent mounted slide stained and containing the test material, or photographs of the slide mentioned above and any other photographs taken during the test duration which may serve as a permanent record of the results.

19.1.7.10 All quantitative data derived from cell counts, DNA analyses, enzyme analyses, etc.

ANNEXES

(Mandatory Information)

A1. STANDARD DEFINITIONS OF TERMS RELATING TO TISSUE CULTURE TESTING FOR CYTOTOXICITY

A1.1 *Introduction*—The following is a list of specific terms taken with modifications from Appendix 4 of Ref. 11, based on recommendations of the Committee on Nomenclature of the Tissue Culture Association, **(1),** and supplemented by definitions taken from the text of the *Medical Dictionary* **(12).**

A1.2 *List of Terms*:

cell—a general non-specific term describing a small microscopic mass protoplasm bounded externally by a semipermeable membrane; should be used with descriptive and specific modifier as listed sequentially herein.

cell alteration—a change in the character of a cell line (seq.) usually associated with the emergence of an established cell line with alteration of morphology, contact inhibition, karyotype, viral susceptibility, and ability to grow in suspension.

cell culture—the growing of cells *in vitro* in which the cells are no longer organized into tissues.

cell line—a "cell line" arises from a primary culture at the time of the first subculture and implies that cultures from it consist of numerous lineages of the cells with further characterizations as to form and chromosome constitutions.

cell senescence—a marked change in any significant growth and/or morphology indicative of a pronounced lack of cell vitality.

cell strain—a type of cell derived from either a primary culture or from a cell line (vide supra) having specific characteristics, notably biochemical and/or biophysical markers that persist during subsequent culturing. In describing a cell strain, its specific features should be defined, as for instance, a cell strain with certain marker chromosome, or a cell strain which has acquired resistance to a certain virus, or a cell strain having a specific antigen, and so on.

chemically defined medium (media)—a medium (media) composed entirely of known chemical components in which cells may be cultured without any undefined additives.

cytotoxicity—an effect or range of effects, microscopic and/or visual, linked to the presence of test materials. These range from impairment in growth to complete cell lysis or dissolution when test cultures are compared to the reference blank.

cytotoxic effect—effects on cell culture may include decreased plating efficiency, cell lysis, inhibition of macromolecular synthesis and cell growth and detachment of cells from the substrate.

cytotoxic substance—any substance that inhibits or prevents the function of cells, or causes destruction of cells or both.

dialysis—the process of separating crystalloids and colloids in solution by the difference in their rates of diffusion through a semipermeable membrane.

established cell line—a cell line having and demonstrating the potential to be subcultured indefinitely *in vitro.*

explant—an excised fragment of a tissue or organ used to initiate a culture.

granulation—the visual microscopic formation of minute discrete masses within a cell.

growth—an increase in the mass of living substance and/or the number of cells.

lysis—the breaking up or disintegration of cells.

media renewal or maintenance—all or part of the used medium is removed and replaced with fresh medium.

medium—a mixture of substances which are essential, beneficial, or harmless to cells in culture.

mitotic figure—microscopic appearance of the achromatic spindle with chromosomes attached; it is an indication of cell division.

monolayer—a single layer of cells growing on a surface.

passage—this term is synonymous with subculture, and can denote the passage of cells from one culture vessel to another.

PPLO—initials standing for pleuropneumonia-like organisms, which are a group of filterable microorganisms, belonging to the genus *Mycoplasma.* This term may be used loosely to include *L*-forms of a variety of bacterial species.

primary culture—a culture started from cells, tissues, or organs taken directly from an organism; a primary culture may be regarded as such until it is subcultured for the first time, it then becomes a cell line.

rounding—the auto-conversion of a cell culture from a monolayer into loosely attached or floating spherically shaped cells.

serum—the fluid portion of the blood obtained after dialysis and coagulation.

subculture—the transfer of cells from one culture vessel to another.

tissue culture—the maintenance of tissue fragments *in vitro*; culture conditions may or may not be designed to preserve primordal tissue morphology.

A2. PREPARATION OF HUMAN SERUM FOR USE IN CULTURE MEDIUM FOR THE SEPARATION AND PREPARATION OF CELL GROWTH FACTOR

A2.1 The best serum is obtained from freshly clotted human blood containing no additives. However, this type of serum is difficult to obtain and satisfactory results may be obtained from plasma furnished by a Blood Bank, even though this plasma contains an anticoagulant ACD.

A2.2 Whole bank blood shall be utilized when obtained not later than within 48 h of its expired shelf life. The plasma is obtained by allowing whole blood to settle at 2 to 4°C (35 to 39°F) in the original blood pack for at least 48 h.

A2.3 The plasma is decanted and centrifuged at 17 210 g (Sorval RC-2) for 20 min at 20°C (68°F) to remove any residual blood cells.

A2.4 The plasma is dialyzed against a balanced salt solution consisting of 84 g NaCl, 4.8 g KCl, 2.4 g $MgSO_4 \cdot 7H_2O$, 1.68 g $CaCl_2 \cdot 2H_2O$, 1.37 g $Na_2HPO_4 \cdot 7H_2O$, and 0.72 g KH_2PO_4 in 12 L of deionized or distilled water in the cold. The dialysis is carried out in Spectrapor membrane tubing of 3500 molecular weight exclusion. The total dialysis time is 48 h. The balanced salt solution is changed after the first 24 h period.

A2.5 At the termination of the dialysis, the plasma is clotted within the tubing as the result of removing anticoagulant and the introduction of calcium into A2.4. The resulting serum is squeezed from the tubing and stored cold (2 to 4°C) for either direct use in culture or fractionation on a glass bead column.

NOTE A2.1—Other human plasma or serum derived cell growth factors shall be appropriate for use as a substitute, particularly as available commercially with appropriate specifications and analysis. As an example, alternate growth factors derived from blood components, such as the heat-stable human platelet derived growth factor **(29)**, may be considered.

A3. PRODUCTION OF ALPHA GROWTH FACTOR (AGF)

A3.1 *Preparation of the Glass Microbead*[7]*:*

A3.1.1 Place the dry beads in a 2-L glass beaker to a volume of 500 mL.

A3.1.2 Add 50 g of Haemosol enzyme active (EA) grade followed by 1 L of hot (65 to 70°C) distilled or deionized water while stirring for 1 min.

A3.1.3 Allow the slurry to stand at room temperature over night or approximately 16 h.

A3.1.4 Remove water the next day by decantation or suction from the setted microbeads.

A3.1.5 Wash the microbeads four times with 1 L of distilled or deionized water to remove the surfactant Haemosol.

A3.1.6 Add 250 mL of concentrated hydrochloric acid and adjust the volume and microbeads to 1 L with added distilled or deionized water.

A3.1.7 Stir the resulting suspension of microbeads for 2 min and let stand overnight, appropriately covered to contain the acid (HCl) vapor.

A3.1.8 Decant the acid liquid with at least 5 rinses of 1 L of distilled or deionized water.

NOTE A3.1—The washed microbeads are stored at this stage for ensuing or future use for an extended period of time.

A3.2 *Preparation of Microbead Column:*

A3.2.1 Glass Column Description (See Fig. A1.1):

A3.2.1.1 *Length*—40 cm.

A3.2.1.2 *Diameter*—5 cm.

A3.2.1.3 *Effluent Drain.*

A3.2.1.4 *Pressure Head.*

A3.2.2 Wash the column with 50 mL Haemosol and rinse with 500 mL distilled or deionized water, regulating the effluent flow at 2 to 5 mL/minute.

A3.2.3 Prior to packing into the column, wash the prepared, stored microbeads with 2 L of 0.6 *M* sodium bicarbonate ($NaHCO_3$) solution.

NOTE A3.2—This pretreatment neutralizes the chance acidity in the acid washed stock of microbeads, thus preventing formation of entrapped bubbles in the column.

A3.2.4 Pour the microbead slurry conditioned with 0.6 *M* sodium bicarbonate ($NaHCO_3$) into the column to the depth of 25 cm.

A3.2.5 Place a 5 cm disk of high grade chromatography paper (Whatman 3 mm thickness, basic weight 185 g/m^2), on top of the microbead as settled.

NOTE A3.3—The paper must be floated onto the column so that no air bubbles are trapped between it and the microbead layer.

A3.2.6 Drain off the superfluent above the settled microbeads bicarbonate solution to the boundary of the filter paper–microbead interface, shutting off the flow by the bottom Teflon adaptor.

A3.2.7 Place a preconditioning solution of 200 mL of 0.6 *M* sodium bicarbonate ($NaHCO_3$), pH 8.0, on top of the column and allow it to run through by gravity at the rate of 30 to 40 drops/min.

NOTE A3.4—Make sure that the column is never allowed to dry. To assist the flow rate, the column is pressured by compressed air with no more than 18 in. of water head (Fig. A3.1, C).

A3.2.8 When the superfluent bicarbonate layer reaches the paper–head interface, stop the flow by closing off the Teflon adaptor drain; the column is now ready for fractionation of the dialyzed human serum (Annex A2).

[7] Glass microbeads available from Ferro Cataphote Corporation, Microbeads Division, Jackson, MS have been found satisfactory for this purpose. The beads are Class IV A and range from 20 to 25 μm in diameter.

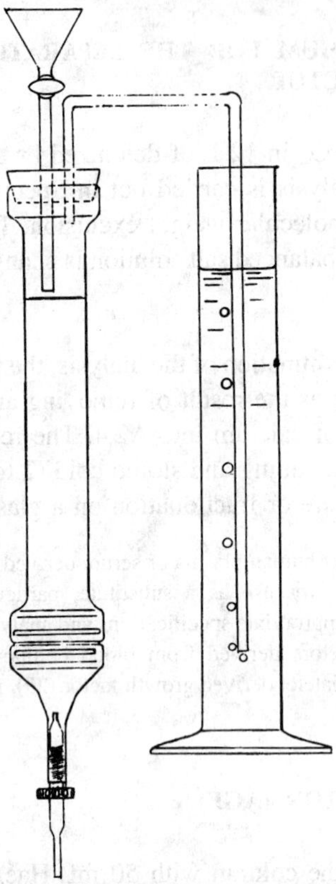

FIG. A3.1 Schematic Diagram for Chromatographic Separation of Holmes Alpha-1-Protein Growth Factor (AGF) from Dialyzed Human Serum

A3.3 *Preparation of Solutions of Column Elution*—Prepare the series of stock solutions listed in Table A3.1 and Table A3.2, stored in stoppered bottles and useable for a maximum of 12 weeks.

A3.4 *Column Separation Procedure:*

A3.4.1 Prepare beforehand the series listed in Table A3.3 of progressive additions added to microbead column.

A3.4.2 Add gently 20 mL of dialyzed human serum (A2.4) in two 10-mL pipette portions following the preliminary column conditioning with 0.8 *M* sodium bicarbonate (A3.2.3).

A3.4.3 Once the 20 mL of serum has settled in the column, add 200 of 0.6 *M* sodium bicarbonate ($NaHCO_3$), pH 8.0, solution with an initial 10-mL pipette portion directed to the internal wall of the column to rinse off the absorbed serum.

A3.4.4 Once the initial 10 mL bicarbonate has settled down into the column, the remaining 190 mL is carefully poured into

TABLE A3.1 Stock Solutions for Elution Buffers

Solution	Stock Quantity	pH
0.6 *M* $NaHCO_3$	100.0 g/2 L	8.0
0.2 *M* Na_2CO_3	42.4 g/2 L	Unadjusted
0.4 K_2CO_3	130.6 g/2 L	Unadjusted
1.2 $KHCO_3$	340.2 g/2 L	Unadjusted
0.2 *M* Na_2CO_3	42.4 g/2 L	Unadjusted
0.4 K_2CO_3	130.6 g/2 L	Unadjusted
1.2 $KHCO_3$	340.2 g/2 L	Unadjusted

TABLE A3.2 Elution Buffer Preparation

Solution	Volume	Final pH	Volume per/rim
0.6 *M* $NaHCO_3$	200 mL	...	...
0.2 *M* Na_2CO_3	390 mL	9.5 ± 0.02	100 mL
0.4 *M* K_2CO_3	429 mL	...	...
1.2 *M* $KHCO_3$	572 mL	9.6 ± 0.1	200 mL

TABLE A3.3 Additions to Column

Solution	Procedure Section	Volume
Human Serum	A3.4.2	20 mL
$NaHCO_3$	A3.4.3	200 mL
$NaHCO_3$ – Na_2CO_3	A3.4.3	100 mL
Distilled Water	A3.4.7	150 mL
$KHCO_3$ – K_2CO_3	A3.4.8	200 mL
Distilled Water	A3.4.9	250 mL

the column making sure not to disturb the lay of the filter paper and the underlying microbeads.

A3.4.5 Adjust the flow rate to 30 to 40 drops per minute by means of the Teflon stop cock in a series of 10 to 12 mL test tube fraction collection system.

NOTE A3.5—Any conventional type fraction collector shall be used with a variable wavelength detector to locate peak collection for the alpha growth factor at 280 mm.

A3.4.6 With the depletion of the sodium bicarbonate elution, proceed next with the 100 mL of $NaHCO_3$-Na_2CO_3 solution with continued fraction collection and absorbance monitoring at 280 mm.

A3.4.7 Following uninterruptedly the depletion of the $NaHCO_3$-Na_2CO_3 solution, proceed next with 150 mL distilled water elution.

A3.4.8 Following uninterruptedly the depletion of the distilled water elution, proceed next with the 200 mL $KHCO_3$-K_2CO_3 elution.

A3.4.9 Following uninterruptedly the depletion of the $KHCO_3$-K_2CO_3 elution, proceed next with the last, distilled water elution.

NOTE A3.6—It is necessary to elute a total of 670 mL from the column in order to assure that all fractions of the active growth factor have been eluted in the $KHCO_3$-K_2CO_3 buffer eluant.

A3.5 *Identification and Collection of AGF Fractions*:

A3.5.1 Using the 280 mm detection of the AGF fraction from A3.4.8 following the potassium ion (pH 9.6) buffer, collect and consolidate the 280 nm absorptive fractions, usually in the range of 6 to 10 test tubes.

A3.5.2 Place the consolidated fractions in a dialysis membrane (Spectra/Por 2. Membrane, 12 000 to 14 000 MWCO).

A3.5.3 Suspend the dialysis membrane contents in 8 to 10 L of distilled or deionized water at 4°C with constant stirring.

A3.5.4 After a minimum of 6 h, change the water and continue dialysis for 16 h.

A3.5.5 Sterilize the dialyzed AGF factor by filtering through a 0.2 mm filter.

A3.5.6 Store the AGF factor in a sterile container.

APPENDIX

(Nonmandatory Information)

X1. RATIONALE FOR ASSESSMENT OF CELL GROWTH COMPATIBILITY OF PROSTHETIC MATERIALS AND DEVICES

X1.1 This practice utilizes normal, nontransformed human excised donor (HED) tissue cells in a homologous human cell – human serum culturing system as a means for assessing biocompatibility of prosthetic materials directly relevant to specific orofacial reconstructive prosthetic devices. This HED tissue cell culturing system, with alternatives and options on use of separated human serum growth factors and corollary use of established cell lines, takes cognizance of the extensive variability of human source tissues and human serum and its separated components.

X1.2 This practice utilizes human serum processed to remove native and adventitious molecular entities by specified dialysis and further separations of the processed serum by buffered ionic elutions through glass microbead chromatography for specified cell growth factors. Thus, the human serum processing and separation provide a ready means for monitoring, with an established cell line for quality and uniformity of the serum preparations, serving as a reference standard for the ensuing cultures with specific HED orofacial tissue cell culturing for biocompatibility. The corollary use of established cell line reference, with defined growth factors, provides a means of comparison of relative sensitivity of the HED tissue cell culture test system.

X1.3 Accordingly, this practice using homologous human cell – human serum appropriately processed provides significant relevance on which to assess the biocompatibility and safety of the prosthetic material for the specific orofacial device.

X1.4 *Precedental Use of Adult Human Cell Culture Methods*—The procedure relates to the precedental usage disclosed in the published literature, listed in Refs. **(13)** thru **(28)** using adult human tissues, and heeds the suggestion of employing actual cell types at the anatomical sites at which the specific biomaterial is to be used **(17).** The published literature provides numerous studies of *in vitro* cell culture methods and procedures of normal, nontransformed human cells, exclusive of cells derived from neoplastic tumor or cancer cells, derived from various anatomical regions in a variety of culture systems media supplemented with heterologous (bovine) and homologous (human) serum derivations, as well as culturing in chemically-defined media with specific cell growth factors. This method provides for the procedural details that are in consonance with this precedental trend toward assessing biocompatibility in relation to anatomical site prosthetic application.

X1.5 Table X1.1 provides a summary of the continued development and modifications of cell culture methods, some salient features of which are: the employment of adult cells that are attributed with more clinical cogency than embryo cells; the involvement of not just the stabilized confluent stage of the test, but rather at the cell division stage with low cell density that must be taken into account as being more sensitive than that at matured confluency; and the extension of the short term, one-day test exposure to long term involvement of adaptation to media, log growth, and possible senescence or toxicity, or both, **(25)** and **(26).**

TABLE X1.1 Development and Modifications of Human Cell Culture Methods

Designation Authorship	Species Source	Cell Type	Prime Nutrient	Serum Type	Cell Growth Test Stage	Test Days	Toxicity Criteria	Clinical Implication
A. Heterologous Cell-Serum Culturing Methods								
ASTM F813 – 83 (Autian) (1968)	Mouse	Connective tissue	MEM	Bovine	Confluency	1	Morphologic inhibition, lysis, etc.	General safety screening
Wilsnack (1976)	Human fetal	Lung Foreskin	MEM MEM	Bovine Bovine	Confluency Confluency	1	Morphologic inhibition, lysis, etc.	General safety screening
Hensten-Pettersen (1977)	Human adult	Gingival cell lines	MEM	Bovine	Proliferation	3	Morphologic, inhibition, 51-Cr rel.	Dental resins safety to human tissues
VA (Lontz, et al) (1977)	Human adult	Orofacial	MEM	Bovine	Proliferation	30	Morphologic, inhibition, lysis, etc.	Maxillofacial and oral (at site safety)
B. Homologous Human Cell-Human Serum Culturing Methods								
Davison, et al (1980)	Human newborn	Endothelial, foreskin	MEM	Human	Proliferation	10	Morphologic, growth rate, patterns,	(Potential)
Davison, et al (1983)	Human adult	Endothelial, (melo-plasty, mammo-plasty)	MEM	Human + (growth factors)	Proliferation	16	Morphologic, growth rate, age variable.	(Proposed assay)
VA (Lontz, et al (1978)	Human adult	Orofacial	MEM and A-3 med.	Human + (growth factors)	Proliferation	30	Morphologic, inhibition, lysis, etc.	Maxillofacial and oral (at site safety)

REFERENCES

(1) Federeoff, S., *Experimental Cell Research,* Tissue Culture Association, 46, 1967, p. 642.

(2) *Registry of Toxic Substances,* National Institute for Occupational Safety and Health, Vol II, 1977.

(3) Holmes, R., *Journal of Biophysical and Biochemical Cytology,* Vol. 6, 1959, pp. 535–536.

(4) Holmes, R., *Journal of Cell Biology,* Vol 32, No. 2, 1967, pp. 297–308.

(5) Paul, John, *Cell and Tissue Culture,* 5th Ed., Chapter IX, Churchill Livingstone, New York, 1975.

(6) Lontz, J. F., et al, *Determining Cell Dynamic Constants for Assessing and Comparing Efficacy of Nutrient Media Modification,* Abstract, 35th Annual Meeting, Tissue Culture Association, Texas, 1984.

(7) *USP Negative Control Plastic Reference Standard,* U.S. Pharmacopeia, Vol XXIII, Mack Publishing, Easton, PA, 1995, p. 1652–1653. Use latest supplement to ensure current cumulative revisions are used.

(8) Johnson and Northrop, *Tissue-Culture Biocompatibility* Testing Program, pp. 25–34.

(9) Horres, et al, "Evaluation of Materials Used for the Fabricating of Medical Devices: Cytotoxicity Testing," *Cell Culture Test Methods, ASTM STP 810,* ASTM, 1983, pp. 35–50.

(10) Lontz, et al, "Use of Human Excised Donor Tissue Culture Systems to Evaluate Safety of Polydimethyl-Siloxane for Orofacial Prosthesis," *Biomaterials,* John Wiley and Sons, London, 1980, pp. 805–810.

(11) Paul, John, *Cell and Tissue Culture,* 5th Ed., Churchill Livingstone, New York, 1975, Appendix 4, pp. 466–470.

(12) *Medical Dictionary,* Stedman, Williams, and Wilkens Co., Baltimore, 1961.

(13) Wilsnack, R. E., Meyer, F. S., and Smith, J. G., "Human Cell Culture Toxicity Testing of Medical Devices and Correlation to Animal Tests," *Biomaterials, Medical Devices, and Artificial Organs,* Vol. 1, 1973, pp. 543–562.

(14) Wilsnack, R. E., "Quantitative Cell Culture Biocompatibility Testing of Medical Devices and Correlation to Animal Tests," *Biomaterials, Medical Devices, and Artificial Organs,* Vol. 4, 1976, pp. 235–261, quoted from the Abstract, "Positivity (toxicity) in animal tests (USP XIX up to 7 days) did not correlate quantitatively to cytotoxic titers in cell culture (1 day). Discrepancies between cell culture tests and animal tests, specifically rubber compounds, were attributable, in some instances, to differentials in elution efficiency between saline, cottonseed, and complete MEM culture medium."

(15) Rheinwald, J. G., and Green, H., "Serial Cultivation of Strains of Human Epidermal Keratinocytes: The Formation of Keratinizing Colonies," *Cell,* Vol. 6, 1975, pp. 331–344.

(16) Hensten-Pettersen, Arne, and Helgelan, Kristen, "Evaluation of Biologic Effects of Dental Materials Using Four Different Cell Culture Techniques" *Scand. J. Dent. Res.,* 1977: 85, pp. 291–296, quoted from the Abstract, "It is concluded that the effects obtained by the (four) cell culture techniques did not mimic the reactions obtained when the (dental) materials are tested under conditions which reflect their clinical use."

(17) Oser, Z., Abodeely, R. A., and McGunnigle, R. G., "Evaluation of Elastomers for Biomedical Applications Utilizing *in vivo* and *in vitro* Model Systems—State of the Art and Future Trends," *Intern. J. Polymeric Mater.,* Gordon Breach Science Publishers, Ltd. 1977, Vol. 5, pp. 177–187.

(18) Lontz, J. F., and Schweiger, J. W., "Maxillofacial Restorative Biomaterials and Techniques," *Bull. Prosth. Res.,* Fall 1977, pp. 183–184.

(19) Lechner, J. F., Shankar-Narayyan, K., Ohnuki, T., Babcock, M. S., Jones, L. W., and Kaighn, M. E., "Replicative Epithelial Cell Cultures from Normal Human Prostate Gland," *Journal National Cancer Institute,* Vol. 60, 1978, pp. 797–802.

(20) Autrup, H., Barrett, L. A., Jackson, F. E., Jesudason, M. L., Stoner, G., Phelps, P., Trump, B. F., and Harris, C. C. "Explant Culture of Human Colon," *Gastroenterology,* Vol. 74, 1978, pp. 1248–1257.

(21) Trump, B. F., and Harris, C. C., "Human Tissues in Biomedical Research," *Human Pathology,* Vol. 10, No. 3, 1979, pp. 245–248.

(22) Davison, P. M., Bensch, K., and Karasek, M. A., "Isolation and Growth of Endothelial Cells from Microvessels of the Newborn Human Foreskin in Cell Culture," *J. Invest. Dermat.,* 75, 1980, pp. 316–321.

(23) Lontz, J. F., and Schweiger, J. W., "Maxillofacial Restorative Biomaterials and Techniques," *Bull. Prosth. Res.,* Fall 1978, pp. 230–40; also Spring 1981, pp. 165–71.

(24) Davison, P. M., Beensch, K., and Karasek, M. A., "Isolation and Long-term Serial Cultivation of Endothelial Cells from the Microvessels of the Adult Human Dermis," *In Vitro,* Vol. 19, 1983, pp. 937–435.

(25) Lontz, J. F., Nadijcka, M. D., Gugel, E. A., Mohamed, N., and Hanson, V. A.," Determining Cell Dynamic Constants for Assessing Efficacy of Nutrient Media Modifications," Abstract No. 169, *In Vitro,* Vol. 20, No. 3, Part II, March 1984, pp. 409–415. Based on long term, 11 days culturing.

(26) Trewyn, R. W., and Gatz, H. B., "Altered Growth Properties of Normal Human Cells Induced by Phorbol 12, 13 Didecanoate," *In Vitro,* Vol. 20, No. 5, May 1984, pp. 409–415. Depicts long term cell growth curver up to 8 days from low cell count to confluency.

(27) Spiegel, J., Carey, T. E., Shimura, S., and Krause, C. J., "In Vitro Sensitivity and Resistance of Human Squamous Carcinoma Cells to cis-Platinum and Methotrexate," *Otolaryngology—Head and Neck Surgery,* Vol. 92, No. 5, October 1984, pp. 524–531. Depicts long term cell growth up to 12 days from moderate cell count to confluency and, in toxic modifications, to severe toxic loss of cell count.

(28) Antoniades, H. N., "Platelet-Derived Growth Factor and Malignant Transformation," *Biochemical Pharmacology,* Vol. 33, No. 18, 1984, pp. 2823–2828.

(29) Nardone, R. M., "Toxicity Testing in Vitro," *Growth, Nutrition and Metabolism of Cells in Culture,* Academic Press, 1977, Chapter 11, pp. 471–495.

(30) Merchant, D. J., Kahn, R. H., and Murphy, W. H., *Handbook of Cell and Organ Culture,* 2nd Ed., Burgess Publishing Co., Minneapolis, MN, 1964.

(31) *Manual of Cell, Tissue and Organ Culture Procedures,* Tissue Culture Association, Vol 7 and antecedents, ISSN 0271–8057, see Procedure No. 27072.

(32) The American Type Culture Collection, ATCC, *Catalog of Strains II,* 12031 Parklawn Drive, Rockville, MD, 10852.

Designation: F 1031 – 00

Standard Practice for Training the Emergency Medical Technician (Basic)[1]

This standard is issued under the fixed designation F 1031; the number immediately following the designation indicates the year of original adoption or, in the case of revision, the year of last revision. A number in parentheses indicates the year of last reapproval. A superscript epsilon (ε) indicates an editorial change since the last revision or reapproval.

1. Scope

1.1 This practice covers a standard course for the training of the emergency medical technician (basic) which will prepare a person to perform those skills commonly required to render lifesaving aid at the scene of an emergency and during transportation to a definitive care facility.

1.2 It is not the intent of this practice to require that the curriculum be used exactly as presented, but only that the knowledge and skill objectives that are part of the curriculum be included in any course purporting to train the emergency medical technician (basic). It is not the intent of this practice to limit the addition of knowledge and skill objectives as required by local conditions.

2. Referenced Documents

2.1 *U.S. Department of Transportation/National Highway Traffic Safety Administration*:

DOT Emergency Medical Technician-Ambulance: National Standard Curriculum, Course Guide , latest version[2]

DOT HS Emergency Medical Technician-Ambulance: National Standard Curriculum, Instructor's Lesson Plans, latest version.[2]

3. Description of Term Specific to This Standard

3.1 *emergency medical technician (basic)—as outlined in this practice,* a person who has successfully completed the course of training, may provide emergency medical care, and may transport the sick and injured. Legal functioning as an EMT (basic) will be based upon licensure/certification requirements, as established by the authority or authorities having jurisdiction.

4. Significance and Use

4.1 The purpose of this practice is to provide a standard means of providing Emergency Medical Technician (Basic) training. The practice should be used by all individuals and agencies that train such persons.

4.2 Successful completion of this course of training neither constitutes nor implies certification or licensure.

4.3 This practice adopts the knowledge and skill objectives contained in the DOT curriculum (latest version) as the standard practice for training those persons who provide emergency medical care at the basic life support level and are known as emergency medical technicians (basic). The actual lesson plans contained in the referenced document are recommended for use; however, each instructor may modify the order of presentation according to local needs.

4.4 This practice outlines a comprehensive course that covers most common emergencies encountered by the emergency medical technician. EMT-basic courses that do not include all of the knowledge and skill objectives of this practice may not be referred to as meeting this standard.

5. Contents of Course

5.1 The practice for training the emergency medical technician (basic) is a course consisting of, at a minimum, the knowledge and skill objectives contained in DOT curriculum (latest version). The knowledge and skill objectives are delineated as Objectives and are listed at the beginning of each of the designated lessons contained in the document. The course shall also include the objectives listed in the In-hospital Clinical Guidelines, Appendix C, of DOT curriculum (lastest version).

6. Course Implementation

6.1 The course shall be conducted in accordance with the regulations of the governmental authority having jurisdiction.

6.2 It is highly recommended that all courses adhere to the procedure for presentation outlined in DOT curriculum (latest version).

7. Keywords

7.1 EMS; EMT; curriculum

---

[1] This practice is under the jurisdiction of ASTM Committee F-30 on Emergency Medical Services and is the direct responsibility of Subcommittee F30.02 on Personnel Training and Education.

Current edition approved Oct. 10, 2000. Published January 2001.

Originally published as F1031-86. Discontinued February 1999 and reinstated F1031-00.

[2] Available from Superintendent of Documents, US Government Printing Office, Washington, DC 20402.

Designation: F 1044 – 99

Standard Test Method for
Shear Testing of Calcium Phosphate Coatings and Metallic Coatings[1]

This standard is issued under the fixed designation F 1044; the number immediately following the designation indicates the year of original adoption or, in the case of revision, the year of last revision. A number in parentheses indicates the year of last reapproval. A superscript epsilon (ε) indicates an editorial change since the last revision or reapproval.

1. Scope

1.1 This test method covers shear testing of continuous calcium phosphate coatings and metallic coatings adhering to dense metal substrates at ambient temperatures. It assesses the degree of adhesion of coatings to substrates, or the internal cohesion of a coating in shear, parallel to the surface plane.

1.2 The values stated in SI units are to be regarded as the standard. The values given in parentheses are for information only.

1.3 *This standard may involve hazardous materials, operations, and equipment. This standard does not purport to address all of the safety concerns, if any, associated with its use. It is the responsibility of the user of this standard to establish appropriate safety and health practices and determine the applicability of regulatory limitations prior to use.*

2. Referenced Documents

2.1 *ASTM Standards:*

C 633 Test Method for Adhesion or Cohesive Strength of Flame-Sprayed Coatings[2]

E 4 Practices for Force Verification of Testing Machines[3]

E 6 Terminology Relating to Methods of Mechanical Testing[3]

E 8 Test Methods for Tension Testing of Metallic Materials[3]

3. Terminology

3.1 *Definitions*—Terminology E 6 shall be considered as applying to the terms used in this test method.

4. Summary of Test Method

4.1 *Shear Method for Calcium Phosphate or Metallic Coatings*—

4.1.1 This test method consists of subjecting a specimen assembly composed of one coated and one uncoated component to a shear load. The components to be tested may be bonded together directly by thermomechanical means (for example, sintering or diffusion bonding) or may be bonded together by use of a polymeric adhesive. The adhesive may be in film form or bulk form, but it must have a minimum bulk shear strength of 34.5 MPa (5000 Psi).

4.1.2 The shear load must be applied parallel to the plane of the coating utilizing a tensile machine, which is capable of determining the maximum strength of the coating or coating attachment to the substrate interface.

4.2 *Shear Method for Metallic Coatings Only*—The lap shear method consists of subjecting a porous coated area to single shear loading, generally utilizing suitable polymeric adhesive or bone cement adhesive and test jig in a tension machine, and determining the maximum shear stress required to obtain separation (that is, the shear strength of the coating/substrate bond or shear strength of the coating).

5. Significance and Use

5.1 The shear test method is recommended for shear testing of calcium phosphate and metallic/substrate combinations and can provide information on the adhesive or cohesive strength of coatings under a uniaxial shear stress.

5.2 The test method may be useful for comparative evaluation of adhesive or cohesive strengths of a variety of types of coatings. Information developed using this test method may be useful for certain quality control and design purposes.

5.3 The test method should not be considered to provide an intrinsic values for utilization directly in making calculations such as determining the ability of a coating to withstand specified environmental stresses.

5.4 Processing variables, such as substrate preparation prior to coating, surface texture, coating technique variables or post-coating heat treatment, or heat may introduce a significant effect on the results of the shear test. The specimen being evaluated must be representative of the actual end-use coating.

6. Apparatus

6.1 *Testing Machines*—Machines used for testing shall conform to the requirements of Practices E 4. The loads used in determining shear strength and yield strength shall be within the loading range of the testing machine as defined in Practices E 4.

6.2 *Gripping Devices*:

6.2.1 *General*—Various types of grips may be used to transmit the load applied to the specimens by the testing machine. To ensure axial shear stress, it is important that the specimen axis coincide with the centerline of the heads of the

---

[1] This test method is under the jurisdiction of ASTM Committee F-4 on Medical and Surgical Materials and Devices and is the direct responsibility of Subcommittee F04.15 on Material Test Methods.

Current edition approved October 10, 1999. Published January 2000.

[2] *Annual Book of ASTM Standards*, Vol 02.05.

[3] *Annual Book of ASTM Standards*, Vol 03.01.

testing machine and that the coating test plane be parallel to the axial load. Any departure from this requirement (that is, any eccentric loading) will introduce bending stresses that are not included in the usual stress calculation (force/cross-sectional area).

6.2.2 *Aligned Interface Method for Calcium Phosphate or Metallic Coatings*:

6.2.2.1 A drawing of a typical gripping device for the test assembly is shown in Fig. 1.

6.2.2.2 A drawing of the adapter to mate the shear fixture to the tensile machine is shown in Fig. 2.

6.2.2.3 A schematic of the test assembly is shown in Fig. 3.

6.2.3 *Lap Shear Method for Metallic Coatings Only*:

6.2.3.1 *Lap Shear Testing Bonding Fixture*—A bonding fixture of the type shown in Fig. 4 or equivalent shall be designed and machined with sufficient precision to minimize movement of the specimen during curing of the adhesive. Some coatings, such as porous fiber metal coatings, may be bonded by sintering without the use of this fixture.

6.2.3.2 *Lap Shear Test Loading Grips*—A loading jig of the type shown in Fig. 5 or equivalent shall be used. It shall be made of hardened steel having a hardness of not less than Rockwell C60. To minimize the possible effect of distortion of the device under load, fitted and machined steel bolts may be used to hold the components together. The interfaces between the tongue and clevises shall be smooth.

7. Adhesive Bonding Materials

7.1 *Adhesive Bonding Agent*—A polymeric adhesive bonding agent in film form, or filled viscous adhesive cement, when used, shall be identified and shall meet the following requirements:

7.1.1 The bonding agent shall be capable of bonding the coating on the test specimen components with an adhesive shear strength that is at least 34.5 MPa (5000 Psi) or as great as the minimum required adhesion or cohesion strength of the coating, whichever is greater.

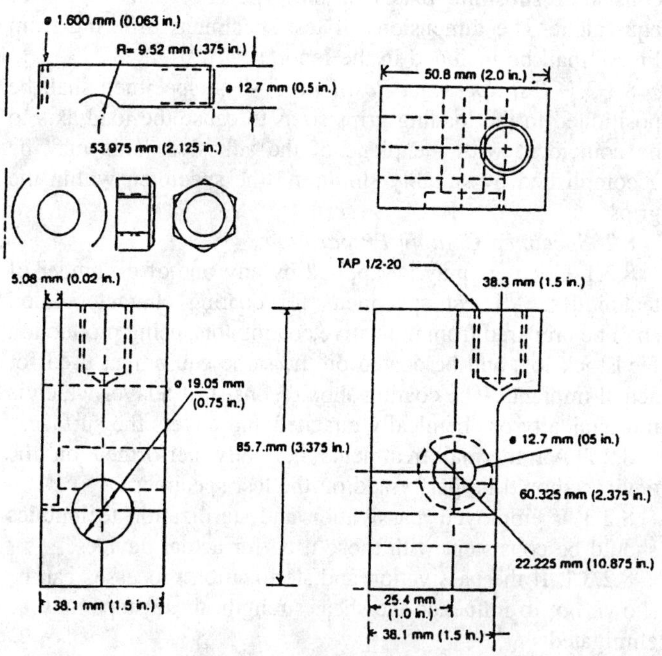

FIG. 1 Gripping Device for Shear Testing

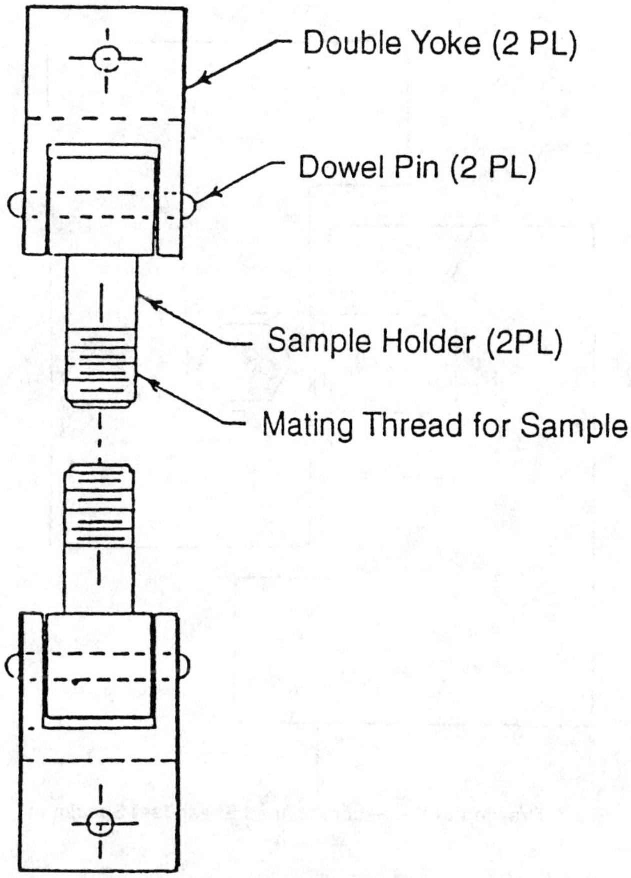

FIG. 2 Adapter to Mate the Gripping Device to the Tensile Machine

7.1.2 In instances where porosity extends to the coating/substrate interface, the bonding agent shall be sufficiently viscous and application to the coating sufficiently careful to assure that it will not penetrate through the coating to the substrate. The FM 1000 Adhesive Film[4] with a thickness of 0.25 mm (0.01 in.) has proven satisfactory for this test.

7.1.3 If a material other than FM 1000 is used, or the condition of the FM 1000 is unknown, it must be tested to establish its equivalence to fresh FM 1000. Testing should be performed without the presence of the calcium phosphate coating to establish the performance of the adhesive.

8. Test Specimen

8.1 *General*:

8.1.1 In order to assure precision and accuracy in test results, it is important that care be exercised in the preparation of specimens, both in machining and in the case of multi-part specimens, in the assembly. Specimen components must be properly aligned in order that generated stresses be purely axial, that is, parallel to the coated surface.

8.1.2 *Aligned Interface Method Specimen*—This shear test specimen is illustrated in Fig. 6. A complete, assembled test

[4] Available from Cytec, Harve de Grace, Maryland.

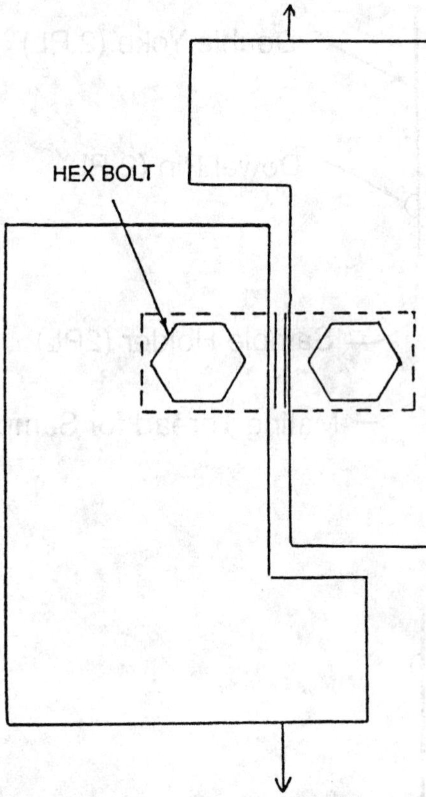

FIG. 3 Drawing of the Recommended Shear Test Specimen Assembly

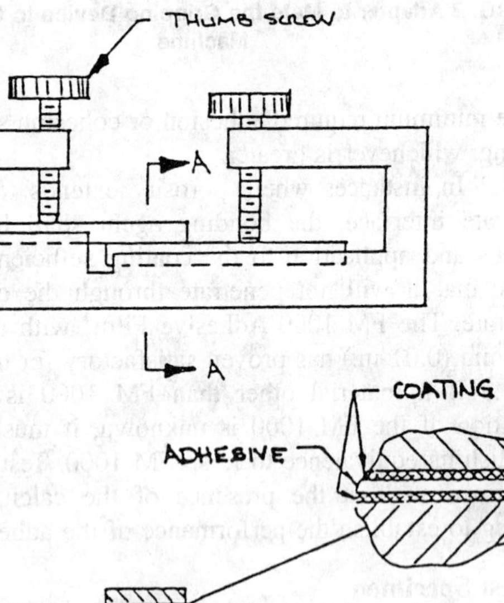

FIG. 4 Lap Shear Bonding Fixture

assembly consists of two solid pieces; one with a coated surface and the other with an uncoated surface. The uncoated surface may be roughened to aid in the bonding of the adhesive.

8.1.2.1 The cross-sectional area of the substrate upon which the coating is applied shall be nominal 2.84 cm^2 (0.44 $in.^2$). When specimens of another cross-sectional area are used, the data must be demonstrated to be equivalent to 2.84 cm^2

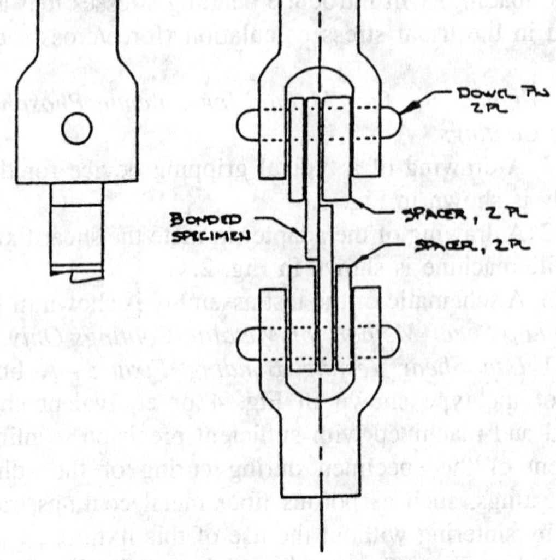

FIG. 5 Lap Shear Loading Grips

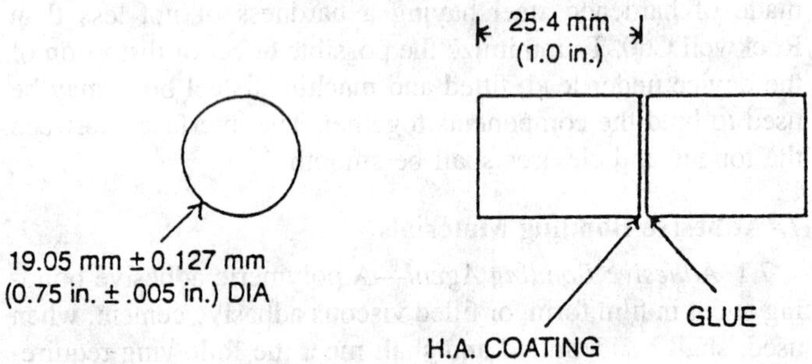

FIG. 6 Aligned Interface Specimen

standard cross-sectional area and the specimen size should be reported.

8.1.3 *Lap Shear Specimen*—Lap shear specimens shall consist of substrate plates of the type shown in Fig. 7 or equivalent. The dimensions of test specimens differing from Fig. 7 shall be included in the report.

8.1.3.1 *Test Specimen Positioning*—The specimen shall be positioned in the loading grips so as to cause the load axis to be coincident with the plane of the adhesive. This may be accomplished by suitably shimming the specimen within the grips.

8.2 *Specimen Coating Preparation*:

8.2.1 Coatings may be applied by any one of a number of techniques. All test specimens for coating characterization shall be prepared from indicative coating lots, using production feedstock lots and be coated on the same equipment used for actual implants. The coating should consist of a layer which is mechanically or chemically attached and covers the surface.

8.2.2 All thermal treatments normally performed on the devices should be performed on the test specimens.

8.2.3 If employed, passivation and sterilization techniques should be consistent with those used for actual devices.

8.2.3.1 If the passivation and sterilization processes can be shown not to influence the shear strength, these steps may be eliminated.

8.2.4 *Inspection*—Before testing, visual inspections should

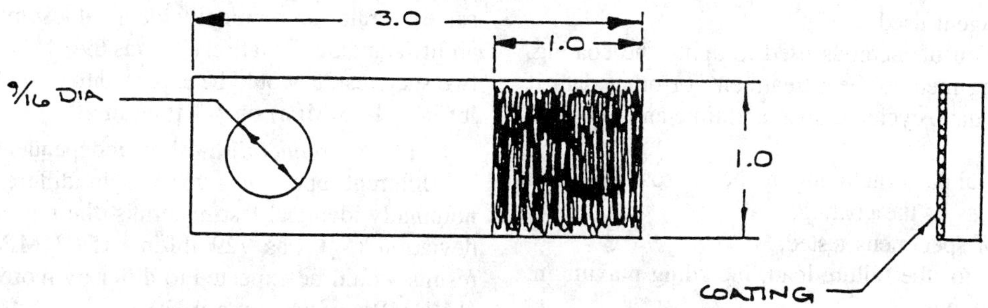

FIG. 7 Lap Shear Specimen (Metal Coatings Only)

be performed on 100 % of the test specimens. Lack of coating in highly stressed regions, as well as nonuniform coating appearance, shall be cause for specimen rejection.

8.2.4.1 *Coating Thickness Measurement*—The dimensions of the coating planar surface shall be measured to the nearest 0.80 mm (1⁄32 in.). For lap shear specimens, the thickness should be measured at the center and all four corners of the coated area to 0.03 mm (0.001 in.). Coating thickness may not vary by more than ± 15 % of the thickness at the center.

9. Procedure

9.1 Prepare a minimum of five test specimens and apply the coating of interest to the face of each in the same manner as for actual production devices.

9.2 *FM–1000 Glue Curing*—The test results achieved are greatly dependent upon the adhesive used and the way in which it is cured. One suggested adhesive commonly used with calcium phosphate coatings is FM 1000 having a thickness of 0.25 mm (0.01 in.). This material has successfully been cured using the following cycle:

9.2.1 Align the adhesive with the surface of the coating, taking precautions to align the adhesive in the center of the coating.

9.2.2 Apply a constant force using a calibrated high temperature spring, resulting in a stress of 0.138 MPa (20 psi) between the coating and the opposing device that will test the coating.

9.2.2.1 Maintain alignment of the coating and the matching counterface during the curing of the adhesive.

9.2.3 Place the assembly in an oven and heat at 176°C (350°F) for 2 to 3 h.

9.2.3.1 The exact amount of time necessary to cure the adhesive will need to be determined by each user, as oven temperature may vary with load size and oven type. It is suggested that initially the curing cycle be optimized without the coating present.

9.2.4 Remove the cured assembly from the oven and allow it to cool to room temperature.

9.2.5 Remove all excess glue which has protruded from the coated surface without compromising the integrity of the sample.

9.3 *3M Scotch - Weld 2214 - NMF Structural Adhesive Gluing Procedure*:

9.3.1 Ensure that surface to be bonded is clean, degreased, and free of any loose particles and beads.

9.3.2 Apply a thin layer of the adhesive evenly to the coated surface of the test coupons. A spatula or tongue depressor may be used as an application device.

9.3.3 Squeeze excess adhesive out of the assembly using hand pressure while coated faces of the test coupons are butted together.

9.3.4 Place the specimen thus prepared in the fixture shown in Fig. 5. During curing, ensure that the fixture maintains a mild pressure at the joint, and force bonding faces to remain parallel and maintain the axial alignment.

9.4 *Direct Thermomechanical Fabrication*—Metallic coating specimens may be tested in either the aligned interface or single lap configuration. For sintered or diffusion bonded coating systems, the test specimen configurations indicated in Figs. 4-7 may be constructed in a single process with the coating application without the use of adhesive. The details of the specimen fabrication process will necessarily be unique to each coating system. Perform appropriate inspections to assure that the microstructure and morphology of the coating in the test specimen configuration are representative of finish production parts (see 8.2).

9.5 *Aligned Interface Test*:

9.5.1 Place the specimen assembly in the grips so that the long axis of the specimen is perpendicular to the direction of applied shear load through the centerline of the grip assembly.

9.5.2 Apply a shear load to each test specimen at a constant rate of cross-head speed of 0.25 cm/min (0.1 in./min). Continue the test until complete separation of the components has been achieved. Record the maximum load applied.

9.6 *Lap Shear Test*:

9.6.1 Following curing, place the specimen in the test assembly shown in Fig. 6.

9.6.2 Load the specimens at a constant rate of cross-head speed of 0.25 cm/min (0.1 in./min). Continue the test until complete separation of the components has been achieved. Record the maximum load applied.

9.7 Discard specimens for which the adhesive has penetrated to the substrate and do not include the results in the analysis and report.

10. Stress Calculation

10.1 Calculate the substrate area upon which the coating is applied to the nearest 0.06 cm^2 (0.01 $in.^2$). Record peak (failure) load and calculate failing stress in MPa (psi) of adhesive bond area, as follows:

$$\text{adhesion or cohesion strength} = \text{maximum load/cross-section area} \quad (1)$$

11. Report

11.1 Report the following information:

11.1.1 Identification of the materials used in the specimen, including bonding agent used,

11.1.2 Identification of methods used to apply the coating, including the coating method, heat-treatment, or other data if available, including date, cycle number, and time and temperature of run,

11.1.3 Dimensional data, including the bond cross-sectional area and the thickness of the coating,

11.1.4 Number of specimens tested,

11.1.5 All values for the failure load, including maximum, minimum, and mean, and

11.1.6 The mode of failure (for example, cohesive versus adhesive) for each test specimen.

12. Precision and Bias

12.1 *Precision*—The precision of this test method was established by an interlaboratory comparison among six laboratories. The specimens tested were of the lap shear design and were plasma-spray coatings of Titanium – 6 Aluminum – 4 vanadium on a Titanium – 6 Aluminum – 4 vanadium substrate. The population mean shear strength was 4292 lbf/in.^{2}(29.6 MPa) for all samples tested by all laboratories.

12.1.1 *Repeatability*—For replicate results obtained by the same operator on nominally identical test materials, the repeatability standard deviation (S_r) was 698 lbf/in.^{2} (4.81 MPa). Any two such results would be expected to differ by more than 1954 lbf/in.^{2} (13.5 MPa) only 1 time in 20.

12.1.2 *Reproducibility*—For independent results obtained by different operators working in different laboratories on nominally identical test materials, the reproducibility standard deviation (S_R) was 729 lbf/in.^{2} (5.03 MPa). Any two such results would be expected to differ by more than 2041 lbf/in.^{2} (14.1 MPa) only 1 time in 20.

12.1.3 *Bias*—Since the measurement of coating shear strength by this test method is a destructive test measurement unique to each individual test sample, no independent determination of a correct or reference value is possible. Thus, no statements regarding the deviation of values measured in accordance with these procedures, from accepted values, is possible.

13. Keywords

13.1 ceramic materials; hydroxylapatite; shear testing; tribasic calcium phosphate

APPENDIX

(Nonmandatory Information)

X1. RATIONALE

X1.1 This standard is needed to aid in the development of a high quality material for use in load-bearing implant applications. The influence of coatings on the resulting shear behavior of the system must be viewed as a combination of the surface roughening treatments required to apply the coating, the thermal effects of the coating process, and any other secondary treatments employed. The purpose of this standard is to provide the following information: 1) the influence of the above processing steps, and 2) the integrity of the coating and the coating/substrate interface.

Designation: F 1054 – 01

Standard Specification for Conical Fittings[1]

This standard is issued under the fixed designation F 1054; the number immediately following the designation indicates the year of original adoption or, in the case of revision, the year of last revision. A number in parentheses indicates the year of last reapproval. A superscript epsilon (ϵ) indicates an editorial change since the last revision or reapproval.

1. Scope

1.1 This specification specifies dimensions and gaging requirements for cones and sockets intended for connecting anesthetic and respiratory care equipment including, but not limited to, breathing systems (resuscitators, ventilators, and anesthesia gas machines), anesthetic gas scavenging systems, and vaporizers. This specification gives requirements for the following cones and sockets:

1.1.1 15- and 22-mm sizes intended for general use in breathing systems;

1.1.2 22-mm size latching connectors (including performance requirements) intended for general use in breathing systems;

1.1.3 23-mm size intended for use with vaporizers intended for use outside the breathing system; and

1.1.4 30-mm size intended for the connection of a breathing system to an anesthetic gas scavenging system.

1.2 It is expected that standards for particular medical devices will provide details on the application and implementation of these conical connectors.

2. Referenced Documents

2.1 *ASTM Standards:*

F 1205 Specification for Anesthesia Breathing Tubes[2]

2.2 *ISO Standards:*[3]

ISO R129 Engineering Drawings—Dimensioning

ISO 1302 Technical Drawings—Methods of Indicating Surface Texture on Drawings

ISO 3040: 1990, Technical Drawings—Dimensioning and Tolerancing—Cones

ISO 4135: 1995, Vocabulary

3. Terminology

3.1 *Definitions:*

3.1.1 *22-mm latching connector*—female connector for engagement with a male connector of 22-mm size complying with this specification, and that has a feature to reduce the possibility of accidental disconnection.

3.1.2 Additional terms used in this specification are defined in accordance with ISO 4135.

4. Conical Connectors Made of Metal

4.1 *General Requirements*—The dimensions of conical connectors made of metal including those made of composite materials in which the mating surfaces are metal, shall be as shown in Figs. 1-3 and Table 1.

NOTE 1—See Annex A5 for dimensions of plug and ring gages for the connectors.

4.2 *Additional Requirements for Conical Connectors of 22-mm Size*:

4.2.1 If a 22-mm male conical connector incorporates a circumferential groove or grooves, the total width of the groove or grooves at the surface shall not exceed 8 mm.

4.2.2 If a 22-mm male conical connector incorporates a recess, the recess shall be as shown in Fig. 2.

4.2.3 If a 22-mm male conical connector incorporates a shoulder, the shoulder or equivalent construction shall be as shown in Fig. 3.

5. Conical Connectors Made of Materials Other Than Metal

5.1 *General Requirements*—Conical connectors made of materials other than metal shall meet the following requirements when they are type tested with gages having dimensions as shown in Fig. A1.1 and Table A1.1.

5.1.1 Conical connectors made of materials other than metal shall meet the dimensional requirements in Fig. 1 and Table 1, with the exception that the Dimensions A and B and Ratio F may vary from those shown.

5.1.2 When the connector is engaged in the appropriate plug or ring test gage shown in Fig. A1.1 and Table A1.1, its leading edge shall lie between the minimum and maximum diameter steps of the gage when an axial force of 35 ± 3.5 N for 15-mm connectors, and 50 ± 5 N for 22- and 30-mm connectors, is applied and while maintaining the same axial force the connector is rotated up to 20°. The connectors and gages shall be maintained at a temperature of 20 ± 3°C during the test.

NOTE 2—Because connectors made from plastic materials, for example, polyamide, polyacetal, polycarbonate, polysulfone, and so forth, may vary greatly in their physical characteristics, it is not considered practicable to specify their dimensions; for this reason, gaging requirements have been included. It is also considered impracticable to generalize on matters, such

[1] This specification is under the jurisdiction of ASTM Committee F29 on Anesthetic and Respiratory Equipmentand is the direct responsibility of Subcommittee F29.10on Anesthesia Workstations.

Current edition approved March 10, 2001. Published May 2001.

[2] *Annual Book of ASTM Standards*, Vol 13.01.

[3] Available from American National Standards Institute, 11 W. 42nd St., 13th Floor, New York, NY 10036.

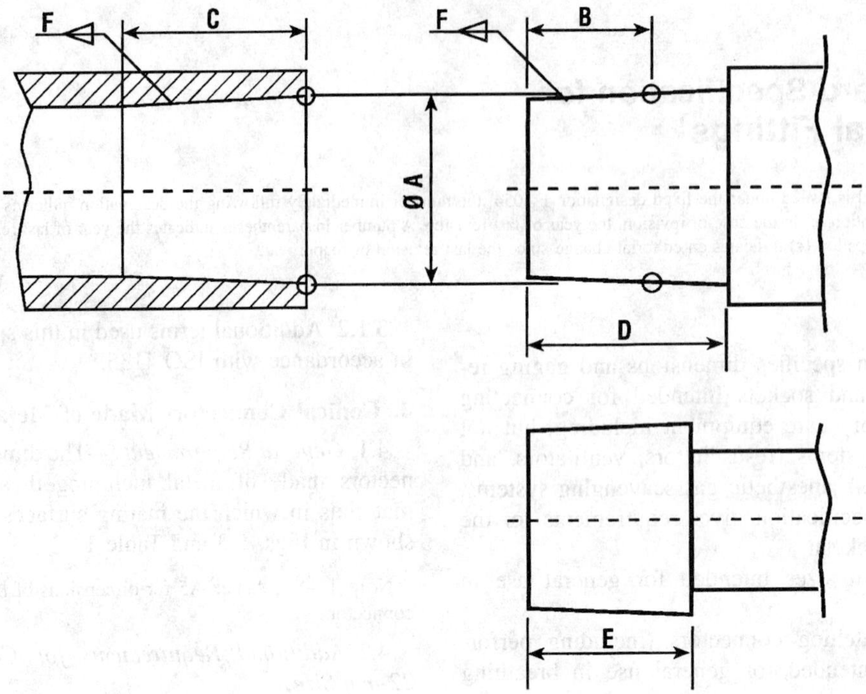

Ø = Diameter (per ISO R129).
∇ = Taper [per unit of length on diameter (ISO 3040)]. Note: Symbol is turned 90° to the left in diagram above.
Note: Maximum radius on the entrance to the female connector and on the leading edge of the male cone should be not less than 0.5 mm and not more than 0.8 mm.

FIG. 1 Conical Connectors Made of Metal (All dimensions in millimetres)

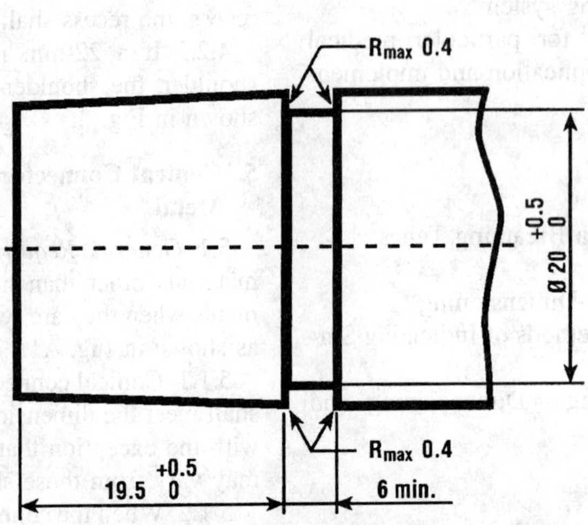

Note: Circumferential grooves may be incorporated on the surface of the male cone if required (see 4.2.1).

FIG. 2 Conical Connector of 22-mm Size Made of Metal—Supplementary Dimensions (All dimensions in millimetres)

as cold flow and thermal instability, as well as possible changes in physical characteristics with solvents, and so forth.

5.1.3 It is the responsibility of the manufacturer to make certain that adequate tests have been carried out to ensure that a suitable material is chosen for the connectors.

5.2 *Additional Requirements for Conical Connectors of 22-mm Size*—The requirements given in 4.2 apply.

6. 22-mm Latching Connectors

6.1 22-mm latching connectors shall not become disconnected when tested in accordance with Annex A2.

6.2 22-mm latching connectors shall have a leakage rate of less than 5 mL/min (corrected to 20°C and 101.3 kPa) when tested in accordance with Annex A3.

6.3 22-mm latching connectors shall meet the requirements specified in 6.1 and 6.2 after being subjected to the drop procedure described in Annex A4.

6.4 22-mm latching connectors which are intended for reuse shall meet the requirements specified in 6.1-6.3 after being subjected to the cleaning, disinfection, or sterilization procedures recommended by the manufacturer.

7. Keywords

7.1 anesthetic equipment; cones; sockets

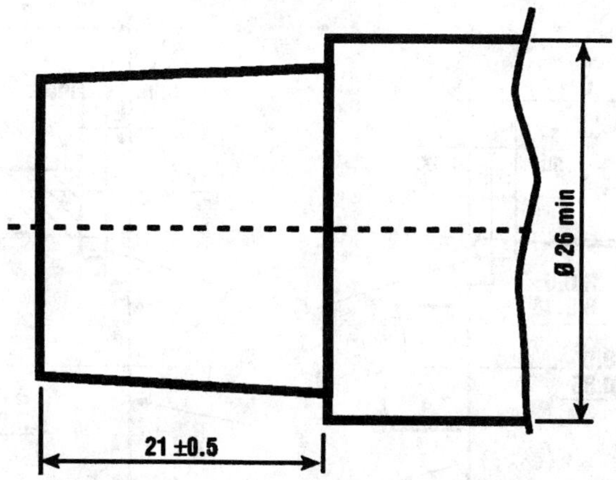

Note: Circumferential grooves may be incorporated on the surface of the male cone, if required (see 4.2.1).

FIG. 3 Connector Intended for Face Mask (with Shoulder) (All dimensions in millimetres)

TABLE 1 Conical Connectors Made of Metal—Dimensions (see Fig. 1)

Connector Size, mm	A Diameter, mm	B Gage Point, mm	C Length of Taper, mm	D Clearance to Shoulder (if Present), mm	E Length to Taper, mm	F Taper per Unit of Length on Diameter
15	15.47 ± 0.04	10	≥16	≥16	≥14.5	1:40
22	22.37 ± 0.04	15	≥21	see Fig. 2	see Fig. 2	1:40
23	23.175 ± 0.02	13	≥18	≥18	≥15	1:36
30	30.9 ± 0.05	14	≥18	≥18	≥14	1:20

ANNEXES

(Mandatory Information)

A1. PLUG AND RING TEST GAGES FOR CONICAL CONNECTORS MADE OF MATERIALS OTHER THAN METAL

A1.1 *General*—Fig. A1.1 and Table A1.1 give details of plug and ring gages for use in checking conical connectors made of materials other than metals.

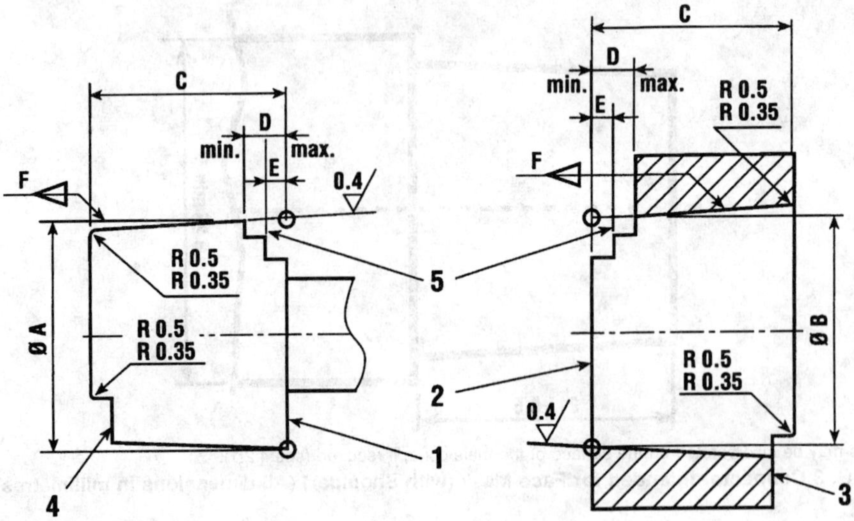

0.4 with symbol = surface roughness (per ISO 1302)—values in micrometres.
1. Face A.
2. Face B.
3. Step to check mating gages ground flush to Face A.
4. Step to check mating gages ground flush to Face B.
5. Basic steps.
Note: Basic and mating gage steps are optional.

FIG. A1.1 Plug and Ring Test Gages for Conical Connectors Made of Materials Other than Metal

TABLE A1.1 Plug and Ring Test Gages for Conical Connectors Made of Materials Other Than Metal—Dimensions (see Fig. 1)

Connector Size, mm	A, mm	B, mm	C, mm	D, mm	E, mm	F	Tolerance on Taper per Unit of Length on Diameter, mm
15	15.525 ± 0.005	15.165 ± 0.005	14.5 ± 0.005	4.3 ± 0.005	2.2 ± 0.005	1:40	0.025 ± 0.0002
22	22.425 ± 0.005	21.94 ± 0.005	19.5 ± 0.005	5.2 ± 0.005	2.2 ± 0.005	1:40	0.025 ± 0.0002
30	30.98 ± 0.005	30.12 ± 0.005	17.25 ± 0.005	3.1 ± 0.005	1.6 ± 0.005	1:20	0.050 ± 0.0002

A2. TEST FOR SECURITY OF ENGAGEMENT OF 22-MM LATCHING CONNECTOR TO MALE CONICAL CONNECTOR

A2.1 Condition a male 22-mm conical connector complying with Fig. 2 and the 22-mm latching connector for 1 h at a temperature of 35 ± 3°C and relative humidity of at least 80 %, and carry out the tests under the same conditions.

A2.2 Engage the 22-mm latching connector with the male connector in accordance with the manufacturer's instructions.

A2.3 After 1 min of engagement without activation of any disengagement mechanism, apply an axial separation force of 50 ± 5 N for 10 s. Unless the 22-min latching connector permits free radial rotation, also apply a torque of 25 ± 5 N cm at a rate not exceeding 20 N/s.

A2.4 Observe whether the assembled connectors become disengaged.

NOTE A2.1—Examples of suitable apparatus that can be used to test security of engagement, together with a more detailed test procedure are given in Annex A6.

A3. TEST FOR LEAKAGE FROM 22-MM LATCHING CONNECTORS

A3.1 Take the engaged male connector and 22-mm latching connector that have been tested as described in Annex A2 and condition them at 35 ± 3°C.

A3.2 Using air, apply an internal static pressure of 8 ± 0.5 kPa above ambient to the assembly and determine the leakage rate from the assembly, for example, by pressure drop or volumetric methods.

A4. DROP PROCEDURE FOR 22-MM LATCHING CONNECTORS

A4.1 Condition a male conical connector complying with Fig. 2 and the 22-mm latching connector for 1 h at a temperature of 20 ± 3°C and relative humidity of at least 80 % and carry out the tests under the same conditions.

A4.2 Engage the 22-mm latching connector with the male conical connector in accordance with the manufacturer's instructions. Attach the male conical connector to a breathing tube complying with Specification F 1205 and having a length of 2 m.

A4.3 Attach the opposite end of the breathing tube to a point 1-m above a 50-mm thick hardwood board, for example, hardwood having a density greater than 700 kg/m^3, standing on a rigid base, for example, a concrete block.

A4.4 Raise the engaged connectors to a point 1 m above the board and 2 m distant from the other end of the breathing tube and release them so that they fall onto the hardwood board. Repeat this five times.

A4.5 Proceed with the desired test.

A5. PLUG AND RING GAGES FOR CONICAL CONNECTORS MADE OF METAL

A5.1 *General*—Fig. A5.1 and Table A5.1 give details of plug and ring test gages that may be used to check metal conical connectors.

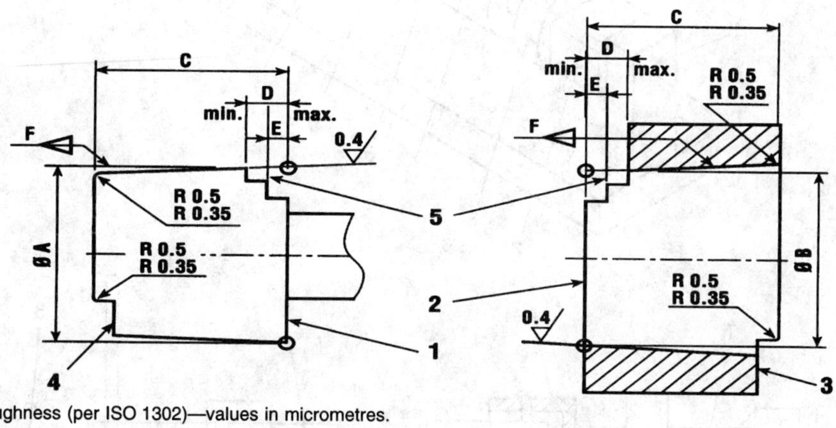

0.4 with symbol = surface roughness (per ISO 1302)—values in micrometres.
1. Face A.
2. Face B.
3. Step to check mating gages ground flush to Face A.
4. Step to check mating gages ground flush to Face B.
5. Basic steps.

Note: Basic and mating gage steps are optional.

FIG. A5.1 Plug and Ring Test Gages for Conical Connectors Made of Metal (All dimensions in millimetres)

TABLE A5.1 Plug and Ring Test Gages for Conical Connectors Made of Metal—Dimensions (see Fig. 1)

Connector Size, mm	A, mm	B, mm	C, mm	D, mm	E, mm	F	Tolerance on Taper per Unit of Length on Diameter, mm
15	15.51 ± 0.005	15.18 ± 0.005	14.5 ± 0.005	3 ± 0.005	1.6 ± 0.005	1:40	0.025 ± 0.0002
22	22.41 ± 0.005	21.955 ± 0.005	19.5 ± 0.005	3 ± 0.005	1.6 ± 0.005	1:40	0.025 ± 0.0002
23	23.195 ± 0.003	22.794 ± 0.003	16 ± 0.005	1.33 ± 0.005	0.72 ± 0.005	1:36	0.0278 ± 0.0002
30	30.95 ± 0.005	30.15 ± 0.005	17 ± 0.005	1.9 ± 0.005	1 ± 0.005	1:20	0.050 ± 0.0002

A6. EXAMPLES OF APPARATUS AND METHODS FOR TESTING THE SECURITY OF ENGAGEMENT OF 22-MM LATCHING CONNECTORS

A6.1 *Method 1—Bench-Mounted Test Equipment*:

A6.1.1 *Apparatus*:

A6.1.1.1 A typical bench-mounted apparatus for testing the security of engagement of 22-mm latching connectors is shown in Fig. A6.1. The male test piece should be a 22-mm male conical connector dimensioned as shown in Fig. 2 but with all of the tolerances reduced to ±0.0005 mm and a surface finish of 0.4 μm.

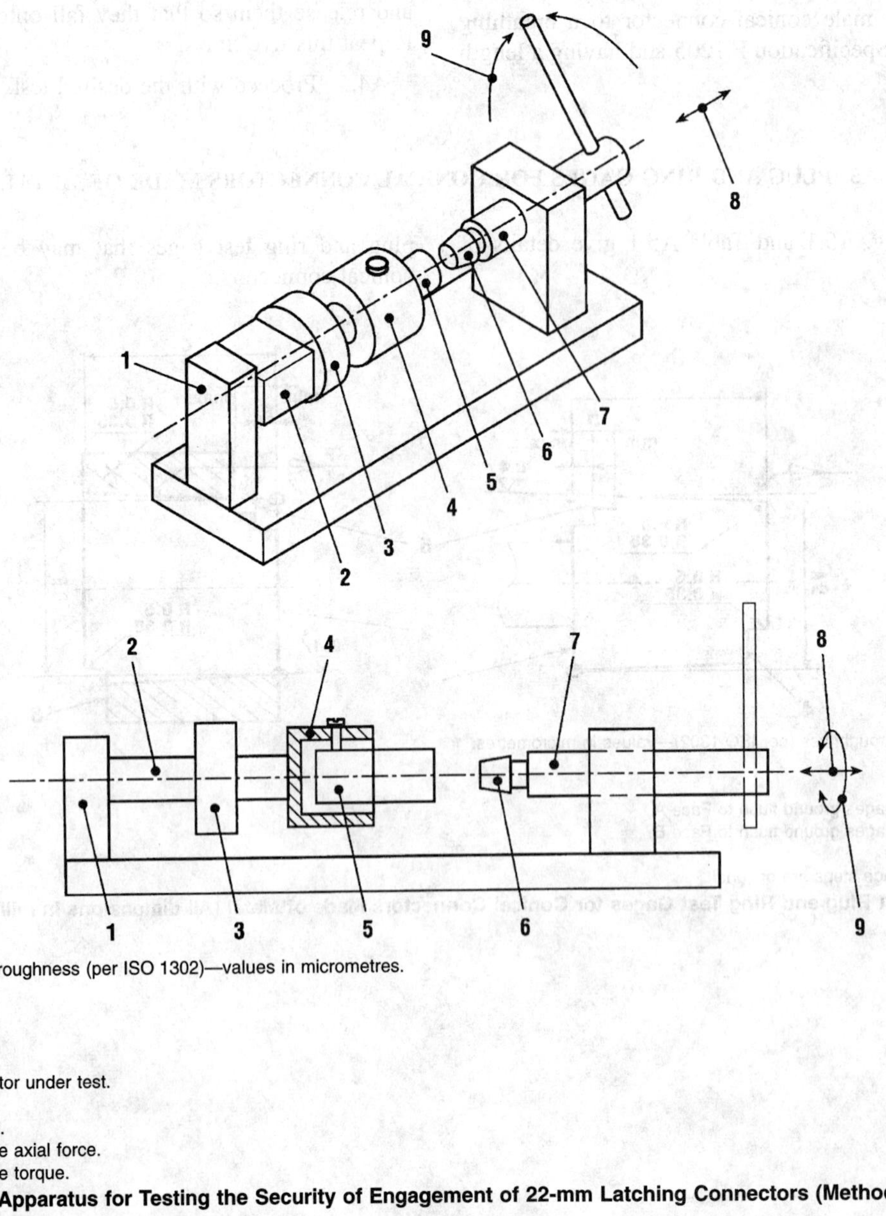

0.4 with symbol = surface roughness (per ISO 1302)—values in micrometres.
1. Rigid support.
2. Axial load meter.
3. Torque meter.
4. Holder.
5. 22-mm latching connector under test.
6. 22-mm male test piece.
7. Free to slide and rotate.
8. Application of adjustable axial force.
9. Application of adjustable torque.

FIG. A6.1 Example of Apparatus for Testing the Security of Engagement of 22-mm Latching Connectors (Method 1—Bench-Mounted)

NOTE A6.1—There are a number of methods for applying the test forces, and Fig. A6.1 is illustrative of only one approach. Other methods include the use of gravity loading by weights and liquid containers.

A6.1.1.2 The apparatus should ensure that the tensile force can be applied in a truly axial direction and that the torque can be applied without changing the tensile force. To minimize the effects of friction, the tensile force should be measured directly between the 22-mm latching connector and the male test piece.

A6.1.2 *Procedure*:

A6.1.2.1 Secure the 22-mm latching connector to be tested in the self-centering holder of apparatus (see A6.1.1) ensuring that the method of securing the 22-mm latching connector does not deform the section(s) that are intended to engage with the male test piece.

A6.1.2.2 Condition the 22-mm latching connector and the apparatus at a temperature of 35 ± 3°C and a relative humidity of at least 80 % for 1 h.

NOTE A6.2—If a number of 22-mm latching connectors are to be tested, some may be conditioned at the required temperature and relative humidity without being secured to the apparatus, provided that they are conditioned again for at least 5 min after being secured to the apparatus.

A6.1.2.3 Engage the 22-mm latching connector with the male test piece in accordance with the manufacturer's instructions.

A6.1.2.4 After 1 min, attach the force measuring device and apply an axial separation force at a rate not exceeding 20 N/s, until a force of 50 ± 5 N is reached. Maintain this force for 10 s without activating any disengagement mechanism, and observe whether the engaged 22-mm latching connector and male test piece become disconnected.

A6.1.2.5 Without reducing the tensile load and without activation of any disengagement mechanism, apply a torque of 25 ± 5 N cm or rotate the male test piece through an angle of 20°, whichever occurs first. Maintain this torque or position for 10 s and observe whether the engaged 22-mm latching connector and male test piece become disconnected.

A6.2 *Method 2—Hand-Held Test Equipment*:

A6.2.1 *Apparatus*—A typical hand-held apparatus for testing the security of engagement of 22-mm latching connectors is shown in Fig. A6.2.

A6.2.2 *Procedure*:

A6.2.2.1 Condition the 22-mm latching connector and the apparatus at a temperature of 35 ± 3°C and a relative humidity of at least 80 % for 1 h.

A6.2.2.2 Engage the 22-mm latching connector with the male test piece on the apparatus in accordance with the manufacturer's instructions.

A6.2.2.3 After 1 min, manually apply an axial separation force at a rate not exceeding 20 N/s, until a force of 50 ± 5 N is reached. Maintain this force for 10 s without activation of any disengagement mechanism, and observe whether the engaged 22-mm latching connector and male test piece become disconnected.

A6.2.2.4 Without reducing the tensile load and without activation of any disengagement mechanism, apply a torque of 25 ± 5 N cm or rotate the male test piece through an angle of 20°, whichever occurs first. Maintain this torque or position for 10 s and observe whether the engaged 22-mm latching connector and male test piece become disconnected.

A6.2.2.5 Repeat the procedure described in A6.2.2.4 with the torque applied in the opposite direction.

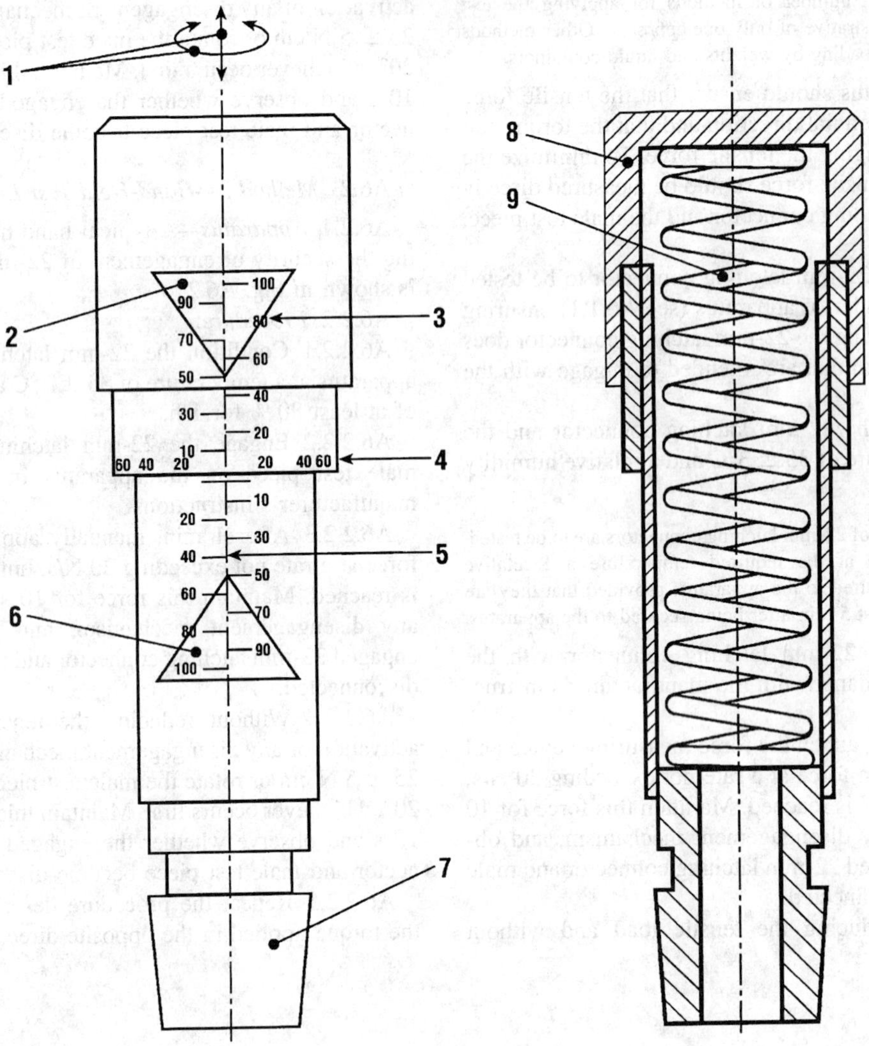

1. Application of torque or push or pull by hand.
2. Area of scale indicating acceptable pull and twist forces.
3. Pull-force scale.
4. Torque scale.
5. Push-force scale.
6. Area of scale indicating acceptable push and twist forces.
7. 22-mm male test piece.
8. Knob.
9. Coil spring fixed at both ends.

FIG. A6.2 Example of Apparatus for Testing the Security of Engagement of 22-mm Latching Connectors (Method 2—Hand-Held)

Designation: F 1058 – 97

Standard Specification for Wrought Cobalt-Chromium-Nickel-Molybdenum-Iron Alloy for Surgical Implant Applications[1]

This standard is issued under the fixed designation F 1058; the number immediately following the designation indicates the year of original adoption or, in the case of revision, the year of last revision. A number in parentheses indicates the year of last reapproval. A superscript epsilon (ε) indicates an editorial change since the last revision or reapproval.

1. Scope

1.1 This specification covers the requirements for two grades of wrought cobalt-chromium-nickel-molybdenum-iron alloy in the form of wire and strip used for the manufacture of surgical implants.

1.2 The values stated in inch-pound units are to be regarded as the standard.

2. Referenced Documents

2.1 *ASTM Standards:*

A 751 Methods, Practices, and Definitions for Chemical Analysis of Steel Products[2]

E 8 Methods of Tension Testing of Metallic Materials[3]

E 18 Test Methods for Rockwell Hardness and Rockwell Superficial Hardness of Metallic Materials[3]

E 45 Practice for Determining the Inclusion Content of Steel[4]

E 92 Test Method for Vickers Hardness of Metallic Materials[3]

E 112 Methods for Determining the Average Grain Size[4]

E 140 Hardness Conversion Tables for Metals (Relationship Between Brinell Hardness, Rockwell Hardness, Rockwell Superficial Hardness, and Knoop Hardness)[3]

2.2 *Aerospace Material Specifications:*

AMS 2269 Chemical Check Analysis Limits Wrought Nickel and Alloys and Cobalt Alloys[5]

AMS 5833 Alloy Wire, Corrosion and Heat Resistant 20Cr-15Ni-40Co-7.0Mo-16Fe Solution Treated and Cold Drawn[5]

AMS 5834 Alloy Wire, Corrosion and Heat Resistant 20Cr-15Ni-40Co-7.0Mo-16Fe Solution Heat Treated, Cold Drawn, and Aged[5]

AMS 5875 Alloy Strip, Corrosion and Heat Resistant 20Cr-15Ni-40Co-7.0Mo-16Fe Solution Heat Treated, Cold Rolled, and Aged[5]

AMS 5876 Alloy Strip, Corrosion and Heat Resistant 20Cr-15Ni-40Co-7.0Mo-16Fe Solution Heat Treated and Cold Rolled[5]

2.3 *American Society for Quality Control:*

C1 Specification of General Requirements for a Quality Program[6]

2.4 *ISO Standard:*

ISO 5832-7 Implants for Surgery—Metal Based Products—Part 7 Forgeable and Cold Formed Co-Cr-Ni-Mo-Fe Alloy[7]

3. Ordering Information

3.1 Inquiries and orders for material under this specification shall include the following information:

3.1.1 Quantity (weight or number of pieces),

3.1.2 Condition (4.11),

3.1.3 Finish (4.2),

3.1.4 Mechanical properties (if applicable, for special conditions) (7.1),

3.1.5 Applicable dimensions, including size, thickness, width, and length (exact, random, multiples), or print number,

3.1.6 Special tests, and

3.1.7 Supplementary requirements (if applicable):

3.1.7.1 Product uniformity, and

3.1.7.2 Additional tests or inspections, supplementary composition limits, if any as required by the manufacturing process and intended application, and other supplementary requirements.

4. Materials and Manufacture

4.1 *Condition*—Wire and strip shall be furnished to the implant manufacturer in the cold worked or cold worked and aged condition, as specified.

4.2 *Finish*—Surface finish shall be as specified and required by the subsequent manufacturing process and the intended application.

5. Chemical Requirements

5.1 The heat analysis shall conform to the requirements as to chemical composition specified in Table 1.

---

[1] This specification is under the jurisdiction of ASTM Committee F-4 on Medical and Surgical Materials and Devices, and is the direct responsibility of Subcommittee F4.12 on Metallurgical Materials.

Current edition approved July 10, 1997. Published March 1998. Originally approved as F 1058 - 91. Last previous edition F 1058 - 91.

[2] *Annual Book of ASTM Standards*, Vol 01.03.

[3] *Annual Book of ASTM Standards*, Vol 03.01.

[4] *Annual Book of ASTM Standards*, Vol 03.03.

[5] Available from Society of Automotive Engineers, 400 Commonwealth Drive, Warrendale, PA 15096.

[6] Available from American Society for Quality Control, 161 West Wisconsin Ave., Milwaukee, WI 53203.

[7] Available from American National Standards Institute, 1430 Broadway, New York, NY 10018.

TABLE 1 Chemical Requirements, Heat Analysis

Element	Composition, (%)			
	Grade 1		Grade 2	
	min	max	min	max
Carbon	...	0.15	...	0.15
Manganese	1.5	2.5	1.0	2.0
Silicon	...	1.20	...	1.20
Phosphorus	...	0.015	...	0.015
Sulfur	...	0.015	...	0.015
Cobalt	39.0	41.0	39.0	42.0
Chromium	19.0	21.0	18.5	21.5
Nickel	14.0	16.0	15.0	18.0
Molybdenum	6.0	8.0	6.5	7.5
Beryllium	...	0.10	...	0.001
Iron[A]	balance	balance	balance	balance

[A] Approximately equal to the difference between 100 % and the sum percentage of the other specified elements. The percentage iron content by difference is not required to be reported.

5.1.1 Requirements for the major and minor elemental constituents for this alloy are listed in Table 1. Also listed are important residual elements. Analysis for elements not listed in Table 1 is not required to verify compliance with this specification.

5.2 Product analysis tolerances do not broaden the specified heat analysis requirements, but cover variations between laboratories in the measurement of chemical content. The manufacturer shall not ship material that is outside the limits specified in Table 1. Product analysis limits shall be specified in Table 2 and in accordance with AMS 2269.

5.3 Methods and practices relating to chemical analysis required by this specification shall be in accordance with Methods A 751.

6. Metallurgical Requirements

6.1 The material shall have a homogeneous cold worked microstructure as observed at 100× magnification.

6.2 The grain size shall be ASTM 5 or finer, based on the appropriate chart of Methods E 112.

6.3 The microcleanliness of the alloy as determined by Practice E 45, Method A, except using Plate III for counts ½ through 2½ and Plate I for counts 3 through 5, on representative billet, bar, or hot band samples from the heat shall not exceed the following:

Inclusion Type	A (Sulfide)	B (Alumina)	C (Silicate)	D (Globular Oxide)
Thin	1	3	1	3
Heavy	0	0	0	0

TABLE 2 Product Analysis Tolerances[A]

Element		Tolerances over the max (upper limit) or under the min (lower limit), %
Carbon		0.01
Manganese		0.04
Silicon		0.10
Phosphorous		0.005
Sulfur		0.003
Cobalt		0.50
Chromium		0.25
Nickel		0.20
Molybdenum		0.15
Beryllium,[B]	max 0.10	0.01
	max 0.001	0.0001

[A] Refer to AMS 2269.

[B] Based on beryllium analysis by flame atomic absorbtion with a detection limit of 0.0000001 % (1 ppb).

TABLE 3 Mechanical Requirements, Cold Worked Wire

Diameter inch (mm)	Ultimate Tensile Strength, min, psi (MPa)
0.001 to 0.005, incl (0.02 to 0.12)	260 000 (1795)
Over 0.005 to 0.040, incl (0.12 to 1.00)	240 000 (1655)
Over 0.040 to 0.060, incl (1.00 to 1.50)	235 000 (1620)
Over 0.060 to 0.100, incl (1.50 to 2.50)	225 000 (1550)
Over 0.100 to 0.140, incl (2.50 to 3.50)	220 000 (1515)

TABLE 4 Mechanical Requirements, Cold Worked and Aged[A] Wire

Diameter inch (mm)	Ultimate Tensile Strength, min, psi (MPa)	Yield Strength (0.2 % offset), min, psi (MPa)
0.001 to 0.005, incl (0.02 to 0.12)	330 000 (2275)	...
Over 0.005 to 0.040, incl (0.12 to 1.00)	290 000 (2000)	210 000 (1450)
Over 0.040 to 0.060, incl (1.00 to 1.50)	285 000 (1965)	200 000 (1380)
Over 0.060 to 0.080, incl (1.50 to 2.00)	275 000 (1895)	200 000 (1380)
Over 0.080 to 0.100, incl (2.00 to 2.50)	275 000 (1895)	195 000 (1345)
Over 0.100 to 0.120, incl (2.50 to 3.00)	270 000 (1860)	185 000 (1275)
Over 0.120 to 0.140, incl (3.00 to 3.50)	270 000 (1860)	180 000 (1240)

[A] Thermally aged by heating to a temperature within the range 900° to 1000°F (480° to 540°C), holding at the selected temperature within ±25°F (±15°C) for 5 to 5½ h, and cooling in air to room temperature.

TABLE 5 Mechanical Requirements, Cold Worked Strip

Thickness, inch (mm)	Ultimate Tensile Strength, min, psi (MPa)
Up to 0.0043, incl (0.110)	260 000 (1795)
Over 0.0043 to 0.01875, incl (0.110 to 0.4688)	250 000 (1725)
Over 0.01875 to 0.025, incl (0.4688 to 0.62)	240 000 (1655)
Over 0.025 to 0.047, incl (0.62 to 1.18)	220 000 (1515)
Over 0.047 to 0.075, incl (1.18 to 1.88)	180 000 (1240)
Over 0.075 to 0.100, incl (1.88 to 2.50)	130 000 (895)

7. Mechanical Requirements

7.1 The material shall conform to the appropriate minimum mechanical properties specified in Table 3, Table 4, Table 5, or Table 6. Methods E 8 shall apply.

7.2 When desired, hardness limits may be specified. Test Methods E 18 or E 92 and Tables E 140 shall be used. Hardness determination of cold worked or cold worked and aged material shall be made on a product cross section,

TABLE 6 Mechanical Requirements, Cold Worked and Aged[A] Strip

Thickness, inch (mm)	Ultimate Tensile Strength, min, psi (MPa)	Yield Strength (0.2 % offset) min, psi (MPa)	Elongation in 2 in. or 50 mm, min, %
Up to 0.0043, incl (0.110)	325 000 (2240)	250 000 (1725)	...
>0.0043 to 0.01875, incl (0.110 to 0.4688)	315 000 (2170)	225 000 (1550)	...
>0.01875 to 0.025, incl (0.4688 to 0.62)	300 000 (2070)	225 000 (1550)	1
>0.025 to 0.047, incl (0.62 to 1.18)	275 000 (1895)	225 000 (1550)	1
>0.047 to 0.075, incl (1.18 to 1.88)	225 000 (1550)	160 000 (1105)	3
>0.075 to 0.100, incl (1.88 to 2.50)	170 000 (1170)	100 000 (690)	17

[A] Thermally aged by heating to a temperature within the range 850° to 950°F (455° to 510°C), holding at the selected temperature within ± 25°F (±15°C) for 5 to 5½ h, and cooling in air to room temperature.

midway between the center and surface, if the cross section size is adequate.

7.3 If any manufacturing operations of the implant manufacturer alter the properties of the material, the specimens shall be subjected to the same operations prior to testing.

8. Special Tests

8.1 Unless otherwise permitted, samples for grain size determination shall be selected after the last annealing operation prior to the final cold working or cold working and aging operation.

8.1.1 If samples are selected after a final cold working or cold working and aging operation, transverse specimens shall be prepared.

8.2 Any other special requirements shall be specified on the purchase order.

9. Certification

9.1 The manufacturer's certification that the material was manufactured and tested in accordance with this specification together with a report of the test results shall be furnished at the time of shipment.

10. Quality Program Requirements

10.1 The producer shall maintain a quality program, such as defined in ASQC C1.

10.2 The manufacturer of surgical implants may audit the producer's quality program for conformance to the intent of ASQC C1, or other recognized program.

11. Keywords

11.1 cobalt alloys (for surgical implants); cobalt-chromium

APPENDIXES

(Nonmandatory Information)

X1. RATIONALE

X1.1 The primary purpose of this specification is to characterize composition and properties to assure consistency in the starting material used in the manufacture of medical devices.

X1.2 The chemical composition and mechanical properties of Grade 1 and the mechanical properties of Grade 2 are in accordance with AMS 5833, 5834, 5875, and 5876. The chemical composition of Grade 2 is in agreement with the composition limits specified in ISO 5832-7.

X1.3 There is a general consensus that a homogeneous metallurgical structure will be superior with respect to corrosion and fatigue resistance, based upon this, metallurgical requirements include fine grained single phase microstructure with low micro-inclusion content.

X1.4 Acceptable alloy conditions supplied to the implant manufacturer include cold worked or cold worked and thermally aged, the choice dependent upon the implant design and application.

X1.5 Grade 1 is commonly referred to as Elgiloy alloy while Grade 2 is commonly referred to as Phynox alloy.

X2. BIOCOMPATIBILITY

X2.1 The alloy composition covered by this standard has been employed successfully in human implant applications in contact with soft tissue and bone for overa decade.**(1-6)**

X2.2 No known surgical implant material has ever been shown to be completely free of adverse reactions in the human body. However, long-term clinical experience of the use of the material referred to in this standard has shown that an acceptable level of biological response can be expected, if the material is used in appropriate applications.

REFERENCES

(1) Yokoo, A., Sugita, K., and Kobayashi, S., "Tissue Reaction Caused by Implanted Aneurysm Clips", *Shinsu Medical Journal*, Volume 28, 1980. pp. 555–557.

(2) Greatbach, W., "Electrochemical Polarization of Physiological Electrodes" *Medical Research Engineering*, Volume 6, No. 2, 1967, pp. 13–18.

(3) Braunwald, N., "Accelerated Fatigue Testing of Available Pacemaker Electrodes and Elgiloy Wire Coils", *Surgery*, 1965, p. 846.

(4) Wible, J., "Spring Valve Mitral Prosthesis", *Journal of the Michigan State Medical Society*, June 1957, p. 731.

(5) Dujovny, M., Kossovsky, N., Kossowsky, R., Segal, R., Diaz, F., Kaufman, H., Perlin, A., Cook, E., "Mechanical and Metallurgical Properties of Carotid Artery Clamps", *Neurosurgery*, 1985, pp. 760–767.

(6) Winkler, W., Ungethum, M., "Metallic Materials in Neurosurgery and Vascular Surgery", *Aesculap Scientific Information*, March 1987, 1st Edition.

Standard Terminology for Surgical Scissors—Inserted and Non-Inserted Blades[1]

This standard is issued under the fixed designation F 1078; the number immediately following the designation indicates the year of original adoption or, in the case of revision, the year of last revision. A number in parentheses indicates the year of last reapproval. A superscript epsilon (ϵ) indicates an editorial change since the last revision or reapproval.

This standard has been approved for use by agencies of the Department of Defense.

1. Scope

1.1 This terminology defines basic terms and considerations for the components of scissors with either inserted or non-inserted blades (see Fig. 1). Instruments in this terminology are limited to those fabricated having scissor blades made from stainless steel and used for surgical procedures.

2. Referenced Documents

2.1 *ASTM Standards:*

F 899 Specification for Stainless Steel Billet, Bar, and Wire for Surgical Instruments[2]

F 1079 Specification for Inserted and Noninserted Surgical Scissors[2]

2.2 *ISO Draft International Standard:*

ISO/DIS 7741— Instruments for Surgery—Scissors and Shears General Requirements, Testing[3]

3. Terminology

DEFINITIONS OF THE INSTRUMENTS

blade—the segment that contains the cutting edge which may be with or without serrations.

bottom scissor half—the component which contains the threaded end of the screw.

distal end—the working end, comprised of two blades, that is furthest from the surgeon when in use.

finger rings—the feature of the scissors that forms the gripping surface for the surgeon (commonly classified as the ring-handled feature).

joint—the junction where the scissor blades are secured by a screw allowing the instrument to pivot.

proximal end—that portion of the instrument that is closest to the surgeon when in use.

ride—the edge which acts as a cam.

ride relief—the contoured area between the shank and ride

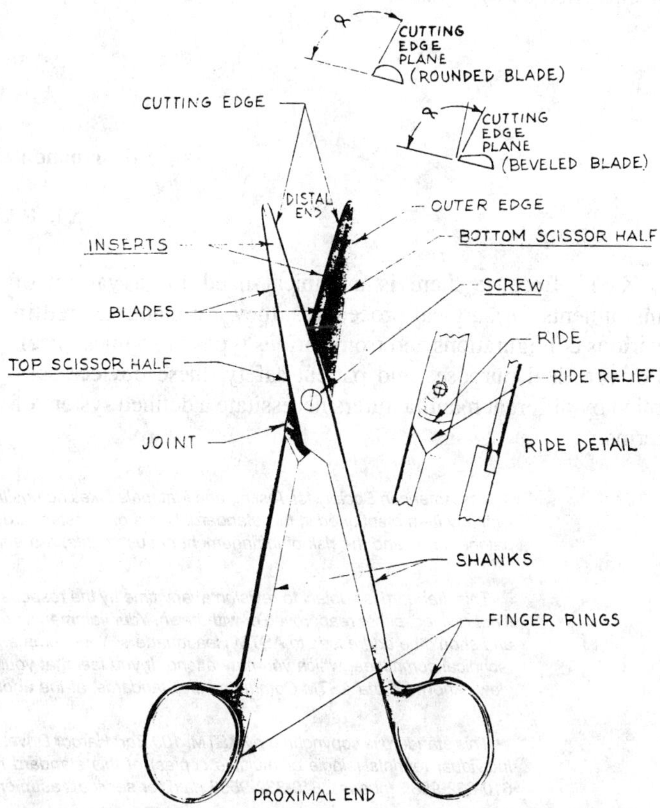

FIG. 1 Components of a Scissors (Inserted and Non-Inserted)

rounded blade—a blade having a radius on its outer surface which forms a transition between the outer edge and the cutting edges.

screw—the fastener which joins the scissor halves

serrations—corrugations in the cutting edge of the blades.

shank—(*1*) the part of either scissor half that yields configuration, length, and leverage (*2*) the part of the scissor between the finger ring and joint.

surgical scissors with inserts—a stainless steel instrument, available in various sizes and configurations, used in surgical procedures for cutting body tissue, gauze, and suture. An instrument of this type has tungsten carbide, stellite, or other inserts.

---

[1] This terminology is under the jurisdiction of ASTM Committee F04 on Medical and Surgical Materials and Devices and is the direct responsibility of Subcommittee F04.33 on Medical/Surgical Instruments. Current edition approved Sept. 25, 1987. Published November 1987.

[2] *Annual Book of ASTM Standards*, Vol 13.01.

[3] Available from American National Standards Institute, 25 W. 43rd St., 4th Floor, New York, NY 10036.

top scissor half—the component which contains the screw head at assembly.

DEFINITIONS OF PHYSICAL PROPERTIES OF THE INSTRUMENT

blade alignment—the positioning of the blades with respect to tip match-up and blade setting.

chamfer—the broken external edges of the instrument.

corrosion—the formation of rust.

finish—the final surface visual appearance of the instrument classified as follows:

(1) **bright or mirror finish**—highly reflective surfaces.

(2) **satin, matte, or black finish**—reduced reflected surfaces (as compared to bright or mirror finish).

hardness—a measurement of the resistance to indentation.

passivation—a process to render the surface condition of stainless steel chemically inactive.

set—the positioning of the blade for proper cutting action.

stainless steel—the raw material of the instrument that is in accordance with Specification F 899.

APPENDIX

(Nonmandatory Information)

X1. RATIONALE

X1.1 Because there is a clinical need for a variety of instruments for surgical procedures, they are manufactured in various configurations and from various types of stainless steel. For practical purposes and patient safety, these devices supplied by different manufacturers necessitate a defined system of terms.

X1.2 The terms defined in this standard are the most commonly used for scissors. However, the intent is not to prohibit technological innovation or to exclude instruments manufactured with other types of features.

Standard Specification for Inserted and Noninserted Surgical Scissors[1]

This standard is issued under the fixed designation F 1079; the number immediately following the designation indicates the year of original adoption or, in the case of revision, the year of last revision. A number in parentheses indicates the year of last reapproval. A superscript epsilon (ε) indicates an editorial change since the last revision or reapproval.

1. Scope

1.1 This specification covers general workmanship aspects of inserted and noninserted stainless steel scissors fabricated from stainless steel and intended for reuse in surgery.

1.2 The following safety hazards caveat pertains only to the test method described in this specification: *This standard does not purport to address all of the safety problems, if any, associated with its use. It is the responsibility of the user of this standard to establish appropriate safety and health practices and determine the applicability of regulatory limitations prior to use.*

2. Referenced Documents

2.1 *ASTM Standards:*

A 380 Practice for Cleaning and Descaling Stainless Steel Parts, Equipment, and Systems[2]

E 18 Test Methods for Rockwell Hardness and Rockwell Superficial Hardness of Metallic Materials[3]

E 92 Test Method for Vickers Hardness of Metallic Materials[3]

E 140 Hardness Conversion Tables for Metals (Relationship Between Brinell Hardness, Vickers Hardness, Rockwell Hardness, Rockwell Superficial Hardness, and Knopp Hardness)[3]

F 899 Specification for Stainless Steel Billet, Bar, and Wire for Surgical Instruments[4]

F 1078 Terminology for Surgical Scissors—Inserted Blades[4]

F 1089 Test Method for Corrosion of Surgical Instruments[4]

3. Terminology

3.1 Definitions applicable to surgical scissors shall be in accordance with Terminology F 1078.

4. Material

4.1 All the component parts of the instrument shall be made of martensitic stainless steel type 410, 410K, 416, 420, 420A, and 420B of Specification F 899. Inserts shall be made of stellite or tungsten carbide or other suitable material.

5. Physical Properties

5.1 *Rockwell Hardness*—The Rockwell hardness of the scissor halves and inserts shall be within the range of 40 HRC and 58 HRC (approximately equivalent to Vickers hardness 530 HV and 670 HV). Opposite halves and inserts shall not vary in hardness by more than 4 points on the Rockwell hardness scale (HRC) or equivalent.

5.2 *Passivation*—Instruments and instrument components shall be passivated after completion of all fabricating and finishing operations as specified in Practice A 380.

5.3 *Heat Treatment*—The component parts of the instruments shall be heat treated under conditions recommended for the material used. Typical heat treating guidelines and hardness values are shown in Specification F 899.

6. Performance Requirements

6.1 *Corrosion Resistance*—Instruments or instrument components shall be subject to corrosion tests specified in Test Method F 1089.

6.2 *Cutting Ability*—The test material shall comply with the material specified in Table 1, Table 2, or Table 3. Clean scissors to be tested prior to test. Perform three separate, consecutive tests with each scissor. Each test shall consist of a nonstop cut along the distal two-thirds of the blade length using the test material at right angles to the threads (if present) of the material. Each cut shall be made using the scissors in the normal manner, that is, with the examiner's fingers in the finger rings of the instrument, except that no lateral pressure shall be exerted. Any bending or snagging of the test material anywhere along the cut including the distal tips shall be cause for rejection.

7. Workmanship, Finish, and Appearance

7.1 *Finger Rings*—Inside surfaces shall be well rounded and polished and comply with the requirements in 7.5.1.

7.2 *Joint*—The instrument shall have a smooth moving joint (ride) and shall close and open easily.

7.3 *Cutting Edges*—Inside surfaces of blades and cutting edges shall be ground uniformly to provide a smooth nongrating action.

7.4 *Pivot Screw*—The pivot screw shall be permanently set, peened, and ground flush or peened over.

7.5 *Finish*:

7.5.1 *Surfaces*—The surfaces of the instrument shall be uniformly finished and free from burrs, sharp edges (except

[1] This specification is under the jurisdiction of ASTM Committee F-4 on Medical and Surgical Materials and Devices and is the direct responsibility of Subcommittee F 04.33 on Medical and Surgical Instruments.

Current edition approved Sept. 25, 1987. Published November 1987.

[2] *Annual Book of ASTM Standards*, Vol 01.03.

[3] *Annual Book of ASTM Standards*, Vol 03.01.

[4] *Annual Book of ASTM Standards*, Vol 13.01.

TABLE 1 Testing Materials for Lightweight and Micro, Neuro, and Ophthalmologic Scissors

Example of Acceptable Testing Materials	Thickness, in.	Examples
Synthetic (50 % polyester, 50 % cotton)	0.007 (1 layer)	Iris Scissors Strabismus Scissors Stevens Scissors Dissecting Scissors (Kilner)
Synthetic (65 % polyester, 35 % cotton)	0.006/0.007	Potts-DeMartell Joseph
Latex rubber sheet	0.009/0.0115	
Latex rubber sheet	0.004/0.008	
Wet facial tissue paper[A] (2 layers)	N/A	
Silicone tubing[A]	0.030 ID, 0.065 OD	
Suture—twist polyester fiber[A]	0.025 (G-207)	

[A] This material may also be used with the aforementioned materials to test extra fine micro, neuro, and ophthalmologic scissors.

TABLE 2 Testing Materials for Medium Weight Scissors

Example of Acceptable Testing Materials	Thickness, in.	Examples
Coarse flannel cotton	0.025/0.035 (1 layer)	Mayo Scissors Metzenbaum Scissors Nail Scissors
Stockinette (JJ-S-746 Type I)	1 layer	Sims Uterine Scissors Dressing Scissors DAPHINE
Latex rubber sheet	0.009/0.0115	Tonsil Scissors
Latex rubber sheet	0.006/0.010	

TABLE 3 Testing Materials for Heavyweight Scissors

Example of Acceptable Testing Materials	Thickness, in.	Examples
Coarse cotton flannel	0.050/0.070 (2 layers of 0.025/0.035)	Lister Bandage Scissors Smith Bandage Scissors Bowel Scissors Doyen Flesh Scissors
Stockinette (JJ-S-746 Type I)	2 layers	
Latex rubber sheet	0.006/0.010	

cutting edges), cracks, coarse marks, and processing materials.

7.5.2 *Type*—The finish shall be one of the types specified in Terminology F 1078 or as specified by the purchaser.

8. Keywords

8.1 instruments; stainless steel—surgical applications

Standard Guide for Structures and Responsibilities of Emergency Medical Services Systems Organizations[1]

This standard is issued under the fixed designation F 1086; the number immediately following the designation indicates the year of original adoption or, in the case of revision, the year of last revision. A number in parentheses indicates the year of last reapproval. A superscript epsilon (ϵ) indicates an editorial change since the last revision or reapproval.

1. Scope

1.1 This guide establishes optimum guidelines for the structures and responsibilities that will facilitate development, delivery, and assessment of Emergency Medical Services (EMS) on state, regional, and local levels.

1.1.1 *State Level*—At the state level, this guide sets forth a basic structure for the organization and management of a state emergency medical services program and outlines the responsibilities of the state in the planning, development, coordination, and regulation of emergency medical services throughout the state.

1.1.2 *Regional Level*—At the regional level, this guide addresses the planning, development, and coordination of a functional and comprehensive EMS system which consists of all personnel, equipment, and facilities necessary for the response to the emergently ill or injured patient, according to national and state lead agency standards.

1.1.3 *Local Level*—At the local level, this guide sets forth a basic structure for the organization and management of a local EMS system and outlines the responsibilities that a local EMS should assume in the planning, development, implementation, and evaluating of its EMS system.

2. Significance and Use

2.1 This guide is not meant to mandate a specific structure or responsibility at the various levels but rather to suggest a means or method that will allow for the creation or further development of a state, regional, or local EMS system.

2.2 This guide will assist state, regional, or local organizations in establishing EMS systems or refining existing EMS systems.

3. Descriptions of EMS Systems

3.1 *State EMS System*—A state EMS system includes all of the components of all EMS systems within the state, however, particular emphasis is placed upon the following:

3.1.1 Legislation establishing authority and responsibility for EMS systems.

3.1.2 Development and enforcement of minimum regulations and standards.

3.1.3 Development and dissemination of a statewide plan and goals for EMS systems.

3.1.4 Provision of technical assistance.

3.1.5 Funds for the development, maintenance, and enhancement of EMS systems.

3.1.6 Supportive components, including training, communications systems, record keeping and evaluation, public education, and acute care center designation.

3.1.7 Overall coordination of EMS programs within the state and in concert with other states or federal authorities as needed.

3.2 *Regional EMS System*—A recommended method of structuring substate EMS systems to provide for EMS planning, development, and coordination is to delineate specific geographic areas within which one organization is designated as responsible for the arrangement of personnel, facilities, and equipment for the effective, coordinated, and expeditious delivery of health care services in a region (3.2.1) under emergency conditions occurring as a result of the patient's condition or because of accidents, natural disasters, or similar situations.

3.2.1 *Region*—To implement a regional EMS system, the state lead agency will identify the geographic or demographic area that is a natural catchment area for EMS provision for most, if not all, patients in the designated area. Since this cannot be a perfect definition from an EMS delivery point of view, administrative and coordinating efficiency considerations will have to be made in establishing boundaries. The state lead agency should determine and define the substate structure for planning, coordination, and provision of emergency medical services. When a regional EMS system lies near a state border such that appropriate and efficient care of patients will require cooperation of prehospital system in another state and medical centers in another state, the state lead agency will develop a plan with the adjoining state lead agency. This plan must provide for the triage and transfer of patients across the state border under supervision of the REMSO.

3.2.2 *Regional EMS Organization (REMSO)*—A REMSO is a staffed organization responsible and accountable to the state EMS lead agency for coordinating the system in a region

[1] This guide is under the jurisdiction of ASTM Committee F-30 on Emergency Medical Services and is the direct responsibility of Subcommittee F30.03 on Organization/Management.

Current edition approved Oct. 15, 1994. Published December 1994. Originally published as F 1086 – 87. Last previous edition F 1086 – 87.

including system operations, and organization and coordination of resources. A REMSO should have a medical director and other technical expertise in order to provide the necessary assistance to its EMS system. A REMSO should work on a regional or subregional basis in liaison with professional societies, public safety, other governmental agencies, local EMS systems, and legislative bodies to establish standards and program policies for continued system improvement.

3.2.2.1 The REMSO should be a substate unit of government or a private entity that may be single or multi-jurisdictional. The REMSO should have the capacity and authority to receive and disburse public and private funds and must be designated by the state EMS lead agency.

3.3 *Local EMS System*—The local EMS system may be organized as a community EMS council and should include all provider groups, private and public, involved in EMS delivery including ambulance or rescue services, hospitals or hospital councils, psychosocial services, local boards of health, police and fire departments, other related governmental and quasi-governmental or political subdivisional bodies, and consumers.

3.3.1 The local EMS system must have linkages to substate and state EMS systems.

3.3.2 The local EMS system should be in compliance with local ordinances and state and federal laws that govern EMS delivery.

4. Standardization

4.1 Standard setting is a major component of the state EMS system operation. This includes, but is not limited to:

4.1.1 Legislation.

4.1.2 Regulations.

4.1.3 Guidelines.

4.1.4 Licensure.

4.1.5 Training.

4.1.6 Certification.

4.1.7 Data collection and evaluation.

5. System Coordination

5.1 System coordination is a function of the state EMS system but may be delegated to a regional EMS organization (REMSO). System coordination includes, but is not limited to:

5.1.1 Regional system planning.

5.1.2 Operational coordination at a regional level.

5.1.3 Regional data collection and processing.

5.1.4 Evaluation.

5.1.5 Continuing education.

5.1.6 Coordination of mass casualty incident response.

NOTE 1—If there are no regional organizations within the state, the state EMS will need to accomplish these tasks.

6. Service Delivery

6.1 Service delivery is the major component of local EMS systems. Realizing that patient care is the ultimate goal of EMS systems, service delivery includes, but is not limited to:

6.1.1 Public information and education.

6.1.2 Notification.

6.1.3 Dispatch.

6.1.4 First response.

6.1.5 BLS/ALS ambulance.

6.1.6 Air transport.

6.1.7 Medical facilities.

6.1.8 Psycho-social services.

6.1.9 Evaluation and quality assurance.

7. State EMS System Structure

7.1 *Agency Organization*—Each state should have a single agency with overall responsibility for the state's role in emergency medical services.

7.1.1 Organizationally, this agency should be located in the state government structure such that it reflects the program's health orientation.

7.1.2 The agency should have a representative advisory council, commission, or board to provide advice to the executive and legislative branches on policies, procedures, programs and funding for emergency medical services statewide. Alternatively, the agency may have a board with the authority to adopt or approve rules and regulations. Such a body should also serve as a mechanism for obtaining public support and participation in the program.

7.2 *Personnel*—The agency should have adequate managerial, technical, and clerical staff to carry out its responsibilities.

7.2.1 There should be a designated director who is a full-time employee of the state.

7.2.2 If the director is not a physician, there should be a medical director who serves at least on a part-time basis, depending on the needs of the program.

7.3 *Legislation*:

7.3.1 There should be comprehensive legislation that establishes the EMS program, outlines its basic responsibilities, and provides the authority necessary to effectively carry out these responsibilities.

7.3.2 There should be legislation authorizing the establishment of minimum standards for emergency medical services in the state.

7.3.3 There should be legislation specifying penalties for noncompliance with the established minimum standards.

7.3.4 There should be legislation to provide funding for the EMS program.

7.4 *Substate Structure*:

7.4.1 The state EMS agency should determine and define the substate framework for the planning, coordination, and provision of emergency medical services. This guide suggests that certain responsibilities, authority, and accountability may be delegated to regional and local EMS systems. Although specific suggestions are offered in this guide, the intent is to allow flexibility in configuring state and substate structures to meet the functional needs of the system.

7.4.2 The state should designate the regional boundaries, the regional EMS organization within each region, and the regional organization's responsibilities, authority, accountability, and provisions for servicing the EMS needs of its constituent state political subdivisions. When a REMSO falls near the border of another state it is essential that the state lead agency develop a plan with the bordering state's lead agency so that the regional EMS system can triage and transfer patients across the border as required by the patient's condition.

7.4.3 If local EMS systems have a "council" or similar organizational structure, the state should have appropriate communication channels to apprise them and the regional EMS systems of relevant information.

8. State EMS System Responsibilities

8.1 *Regulatory*:

8.1.1 The state should have the authority and responsibility for establishing minimum standards for the essential elements of the EMS system.

8.1.2 The state EMS agency should ensure that ambulance services are licensed and certified, that vehicles and equipment are inspected, and that ambulance personnel are licensed and certified.

8.1.3 The state EMS agency should have the responsibility to enforce the regulations, including the authority to take appropriate action to revoke or suspend the license or certification of those not in compliance. Revocation and suspension procedures should afford all litigants due process and provide for appeal.

8.2 *Planning and Standard Development*:

8.2.1 The state EMS agency should develop and disseminate a state EMS plan that does the following:

8.2.1.1 Describes the structure and framework for the development of EMS on a statewide basis.

8.2.1.2 Describes the current status of EMS and identifies statewide needs and priorities.

8.2.1.3 Outlines statewide goals for emergency medical services.

8.2.1.4 Is reviewed in accordance with the review cycle of the state health plan and with appropriate revisions made.

8.2.1.5 Is coordinated with the health planning agency and is integrated into the overall state health plan.

8.2.1.6 Is coordinated with the state emergency management agency and integrated where appropriate into the state emergency operations plan.

8.2.2 The state EMS agency should establish standards and guidelines for the development of EMS systems which:

8.2.2.1 Address all components of an EMS system. These components include but are not limited to: transportation, planning, critical care system development, evaluation, public information and education, training, certification, medical control, communications, mass casualty care, and others referred to within this guide.

8.2.2.2 Address the needs of patients in the following clinical target groups: behavior, burns, cardiac emergencies, obstetrical/perinatal emergencies, neonatal/pediatric emergencies, poisoning, head and spinal cord injuries, trauma, and other medical emergencies.

8.2.2.3 Identify the responsibilities of the various entities and levels of government involved in the system.

8.3 *Technical Assistance*—The state EMS agency should provide technical assistance to local units of government, EMS providers, and to the REMSOs. This should include, but not be limited to, the following:

8.3.1 Developing guidelines, model procedures, manuals, etc.

8.3.2 Serving as a clearinghouse and referral center for information.

8.3.3 Consulting with public officials, hospital administrators, ambulance service directors, EMS medical directors, etc.

8.3.4 Centralize EMS statistical data processing and provide activity reports to EMS providers and organizations involved in the provision and coordination of EMS.

8.4 *Funding*—The state government should provide funds to support the development, maintenance, and enhancement of emergency medical services systems including, but not limited to, the following:

8.4.1 Administrative and programmatic support of the state EMS agency.

8.4.2 Administrative and programmatic support of regional EMS organizations (REMSOs) in the form of direct funding or facilitation of other funding.

8.4.3 Grants to local EMS systems (or community EMS councils), ambulance providers, local governments, hospitals, and other appropriate agencies for improvement of the EMS system if such funds are available.

8.5 *Programs*—The state EMS agency should establish and/or operate supportive statewide programs for the development of emergency medical services to include, but not necessarily be limited to, the following:

8.5.1 Programs for the training and certification of prehospital EMS personnel.

8.5.2 Programs for planning, developing, and coordinating EMS communication systems. This should include citizen access, coordination, dispatch, and medical command/control.

8.5.3 Programs for the evaluation of the system including the establishment of an EMS patient record keeping system with, at a minimum, a standard run form or data set; the collection and tabulation of general statistics; and the development of programs to monitor, evaluate and outline definitive action steps to ensure optimal systems integrity of substate (regional) and local EMS systems.

8.5.4 Programs of statewide public education (PE) including the development of PE materials of importance to the citizens and EMS providers of the state.

8.5.5 Programs for application for designation as specialized acute care (trauma, burns, poison, pediatrics, etc.) centers, as necessary, to include evaluation of designated specialized acute care centers and systems.

8.5.6 Programs for preparedness, response, and evaluation of mass casualty incidents.

8.6 *Coordination*:

8.6.1 The state agency should have the primary responsibility for coordinating EMS activities with other state and federal agencies and with other states.

8.6.2 The state EMS agency should establish and maintain a liaison with other state and national EMS and EMS related organizations.

8.6.3 The state EMS agency should have a role in coordinating the EMS aspects of the state's disaster response. The state EMS agency should coordinate disaster programs affecting hospitals through state health planning agencies, professional associations and other appropriate organizations to maximize cooperation and obtain implementation assistance.

8.6.4 The state EMS agency should have a defined role in the state's highway safety program as established by statute or executive order.

9. Regional EMS System Structure

9.1 Regional EMS organizations (REMSO) can be established either as units of government or as private entities. The basic structures of a regional EMS system should consist of the following:

9.1.1 *When Structured as a Unit of Government*:

9.1.1.1 The REMSO should have a specific individual assigned as the lead person or coordinator responsible for the region's EMS system. This person is responsible to the designating state agency and to the governmental organization by which employed or from which a portion of his or her earnings are derived, and responsive to a REMSO advisory council.

9.1.1.2 A REMSO advisory council should consist of representatives designated by constituent state political subdivisions to provide guidance to the organization through the coordinator. All local EMS systems must be represented on the advisory council.

9.1.2 *When Structured as a Private Entity Organization*:

9.1.2.1 The REMSO board should consist of individuals willing to accept fiduciary responsibility for the governance of the organization designated as the REMSO, for the supervision of the REMSO director and actions of the REMSO staff.

9.1.2.2 The REMSO director, directly and through delegation to any REMSO staff, should be an individual who has the responsibility for the direction of the REMSO.

9.1.2.3 The REMSO advisory council should consist of individuals designated by constituent state political subdivisions to represent their constituencies on EMS matters. All local EMS systems must be represented on the advisory council. The council should be separate from the REMSO board, although individuals may serve as members of both. This separability is to ensure continued representation of key constituencies in the guidance of the REMSO operation regardless of the organization (board, director, staff) designated as the REMSO for that region by the state lead agency and any future changes in that designation.

9.1.2.4 A contract (or written agreement) between the state lead agency, the REMSO and constituent state political subdivisions should be executed defining the responsibilities and objectives of both parties.

9.1.2.5 The contract should identify any funding arrangement utilizing state funds and contain provisions for monitoring and auditing of expenditures.

9.1.2.6 The REMSO board should be the policy making body for the designated REMSO.

9.1.2.7 The REMSO advisory council (or sub-regional councils if practical) should also include provider and consumer participants of the EMS system in the region. The council(s) advise(s) the REMSO on EMS matters.

9.1.3 REMSO should be represented individually or collectively on the state lead agency advisory council.

10. Regional EMS System Responsibilities

10.1 The state lead agency should designate and contract with the REMSOs in the state. The state lead agency should provide state funding or facilitate other funding sufficient for the operation of REMSOs.

10.2 The REMSO board sets organizational policy for the REMSO and contracts with the state lead agency and state constituent political subdivisions. It must be responsive to the demands of the state lead agency and of the REMSO advisory council in order to hold the REMSO designation for the region.

10.3 The REMSO advisory council(s) should provide guidance to the REMSO in planning its activities.

10.4 The REMSO should maintain adequate staff and facilities to conduct ongoing planning, implementation, technical assistance, and evaluation of at least the following EMS system components (described as follows unless future ASTM standards substitute) in its region utilizing national standards adopted as state minimum standards for each (the REMSO itself need not be the implementing agency in each case; the local EMS agency may be the implementing agency as long as the REMSO can demonstrate that the component is being addressed adequately):

10.4.1 *Staffing and Training*—An adequate number of hospital and prehospital health professionals should exist to provide EMS on a 24-h basis. Provision should be made for the initial and ongoing training of these personnel utilizing curricula consistent with state and national criteria for each.

10.4.2 *Transportation*—There should exist an adequate system of ground, air, and water transport with vehicles that meet appropriate standards regarding location, design, performance, equipment, personnel, and safety. Basic life support (BLS) and advanced life support (ALS) prehospital and interhospital transport of critical patients should be addressed.

10.4.3 *Communications*—There should be provision for two-way communication between personnel and facilities within the coordinated communication system(s). Elements within the system(s) include public access to the EMS system, resource allocation, and medical control on both the BLS and ALS levels.

10.4.4 *Patient Transfer*—A system of identifying the most appropriate facility to manage a patient's clinical problem should be developed. This will be under medical control and will utilize pre-existing transfer policies. A mechanism to provide a continuum of care for each patient in the EMS system should be identified including protocols for selection of the primary receiving facility and subsequent transfer to an appropriate facility meeting the overall needs of the patient.

10.4.5 *Medical Control*—Medical control implies involvement of the medical community and ensures medical accountability in all phases of the EMS system and consists of the following elements that must be implemented:

10.4.5.1 Designation of a medical director for the region's EMS program, who is responsible for overall supervision and implementation of all medical requirements.

10.4.5.2 Effective emergency medical planning and designation of on-line medical control resources.

10.4.5.3 Design and utilization of treatment protocols that establish the standards for levels of care at both the BLS and ALS level from the scene to the appropriate level of hospital care in case of failure or interruption of provisions for on-line medical control.

10.4.5.4 New EMS technology that supports the training and operations of the program.

10.4.5.5 An effective process for accountability (records, case review, audits of day-to-day incidents and mass casualty incidents, etc.).

10.4.6 *Public Access and Education*—Provisions should be made to provide programs of public education and information to establish an awareness of the EMS system, how to access the system, and how to use the system properly. All patients should have access to the entire EMS system regardless of their ability to pay for such services. The public should have access to the governing boards and advisory councils regarding EMS in their area. Public CPR/First Aid training should be established.

10.4.7 *System Evaluation*—A regional prehospital patient record should be established in combination with a system, for central collection and processing of such records. The record should cover the patient's initial entry into the prehospital system through to the patient's transfer to the hospital emergency unit. A mechanism for tie-in to hospital patient visit and discharge information should exist. Analysis should be done on a routine basis, using this data (returned to the regions by the state if a statewide system exists) and appropriate process or outcome indicators, to determine the effectiveness of the EMS system.

10.4.8 *Emergency Responder Coordination*—The system should include provisions for appropriate system response to incidents beyond the day-to-day resource capacities of individual EMS provider organizations. Written mutual aid arrangements should be established with neighboring REMSO/local EMS systems to ensure integration of care and should consider the role of non-EMS public safety agencies, their roles, relationships, and responsibilities in standard operation.

10.4.9 *Disaster/Mass Casualty Incident Coordination*—Provisions should be made for expanding standard operations to meet the needs created by mass casualty and disaster incidents. This will include plans for integrating state, regional, and local communications systems.

10.5 The REMSO should develop a written plan addressing all of the components in 10.4 and any additional components as may be prescribed in an EMS state plan. The plan should be assessed for progress made in each of the component areas and revised as necessary to be consistent with state standards. These assessments are to be reported to the state EMS lead agency and should be made available within the EMS region.

10.6 The REMSO should recommend appropriate minimum levels of EMS for each unit of local government within the EMS region, and include this in the plan and annual report described in 10.5. Designated minimum levels should be consistent with state minimum standards and should be influenced by such characteristics as population, geography, health status demographics, and local economy.

10.7 The REMSO should develop regional policies, protocols, and standards that meet state minimum standards.

10.8 The REMSO should coordinate with the state lead agency to ensure that state and regional minimum standards are actively enforced.

10.9 The REMSO should coordinate with local government, EMS provider organizations, consumer groups, local EMS systems, and other entities to promote fair representation and active participation on the REMSO provider/consumer council.

11. Local EMS System Structure

11.1 The local EMS system may have a coordinating body (or community EMS council) composed of representatives from public and private provider groups involved in the delivery of EMS including ambulance and rescue services, medical society, emergency nurses, hospitals or hospital councils, psychosocial services, local boards of health, police and fire departments, other related governmental and quasi-governmental or political subdivisional bodies and representatives of the public or consumers of emergency medical sciences.

11.2 *Access to the System*—Public access should be through a centralized access such as a 911.

11.3 *Dispatch*:

11.3.1 There should be coordinated dispatch of resources.

11.3.2 It is desirable to have prearrival assistance or specific instructions to aid caller before help arrives on the scene. The instructions provided to the dispatcher should have medical control approval prior to implementation.

11.4 *Personnel*:

11.4.1 *Basic Life Support (BLS)*:

11.4.1.1 *First Responder*—Non-ambulance responders (police, etc.) should have minimum of DOT First Responder capability.

11.4.1.2 *EMT-Ambulance Attendants*—Attendants should have a minimum of DOT EMT-Basic capability. (Defibrillation and starting IVs are optional capabilities in accordance with state standards.)

11.4.2 *Advanced Life Support (ALS)*—Advanced life support should also include such techniques as endotracheal intubation and the use of intravenous medications and certain lifesaving procedures as defined in the state certification process.

11.5 *Medical Direction*—There should be physician control on all treatment protocols including on-line procedures and off-line standing orders.

11.6 *Psycho-Social Services*—There should be prior arrangements for availability, appropriate training, and utilization of trained mental health providers.

11.7 *Communications*—There should be provisions made for dispatch and communication between the field personnel and the receiving hospital or resource hospital.

11.8 *Transportation*—A transportation network (land, air, and water) should be established to ensure an adequate response time to the site as well as a minimal transit time from the site to the receiving facility. Provisions should include transportation to acute care centers.

11.9 *Receiving Facility*—A receiving facility should be in operation 24 hours a day, seven days a week with emergency care capability. Each facility should be identified as to its level of capability. Provisions should be made to identify special capabilities based on specific standards (trauma care, mental health units, poison control, cardiac care, pediatrics, etc.).

12. Local EMS System Responsibilities

12.1 *Planning and Development*—To implement the level(s) of service local EMS system wants or is capable of providing, consideration must be given to the following:

12.1.1 *First Responder*—Firefighters, police officers, and others who may respond to emergencies and provide emergency care but do not transport.

12.1.2 *Emergency Medical Technician*—Basic life support (BLS) ambulance attendant responders who provide initial stabilization at the scene of the emergency and transportation to the medical facility.

12.1.3 If a local EMS system has elected to have advanced life support (ALS) capability they will have advanced life support responders who, because of training and medical control, are permitted to utilize more advanced procedures prior to transporting victims to specialized acute care centers.

12.2 *Standards*—The local EMS agency should develop standards that meet state regulations. Those standards should include, but not be limited to:

12.2.1 *Level of Continuing Education*—The amount of annual continuing education will meet that required by the state.

12.2.2 *Staff*—The minimum number of qualified ambulance attendants consistent with state requirements.

12.2.3 *Training*—The hours of initial training must meet the minimum specified by the state. The local EMS agency should establish local quality control standards and provide for auditing competency.

12.3 *Coordination*:

12.3.1 The local EMS agency should assist in maintaining coordination between EMS providers and their medical direction. This may be best accomplished through regularly scheduled meetings between providers and medical administrators.

12.3.2 Other primary roles of coordination include oversight and assistance with communication problems, assisting the local training agency in preparation and conduct of courses, assuring that all EMS providers have mutual aid agreements as necessary, and participation in the preparation and development of emergency and disaster plans.

12.3.3 The local EMS system is directly responsible to the REMSO for all of its activities and the local EMS system activities must conform to REMSO policies. If there is no REMSO, the local EMS system is directly responsible to the state lead agency.

12.4 *Quality Assurance*—The primary responsibility is at local level and is achieved by high-quality initial training, continuing medical education, medical direction, monthly run reviews by medical control group, and periodic medical audits of patient care.

12.5 *Funding*—Financial support of service is a primary responsibility of local EMS and would include appropriate fee structuring, grants, donations, and government budget processes.

12.6 *Safety*—EMS system should ensure that standards for safety of rescuers, providers, patients, and bystanders are developed and enforced.

Designation: F 1088 – 87 (Reapproved 1992)$^{\epsilon 1}$

Standard Specification for Beta-Tricalcium Phosphate for Surgical Implantation[1]

This standard is issued under the fixed designation F 1088; the number immediately following the designation indicates the year of original adoption or, in the case of revision, the year of last revision. A number in parentheses indicates the year of last reapproval. A superscript epsilon (ϵ) indicates an editorial change since the last revision or reapproval.

ϵ^1 NOTE—Section 7 was added editorially in December 1992.

1. Scope

1.1 The specification defines the chemical and crystallographic properties of beta-tricalcium phosphate intended for surgical implantation. It also informs the user that manufacturers and distributors are obligated to meet certain federal requirements.

1.2 It has been found that material meeting this specification engenders an acceptable biocompatible response as defined in Practice F 981 **(1)**.[2] Other properties of calcium phosphates such as grain size, density, strength, and resorption rates are dependent upon certain process parameters **(2-9)**.

1.3 This specification excludes tribasic calcium phosphate, whitlockite, alpha-tricalcium phosphate, and hydroxyapatite.

2. Referenced Documents

2.1 *ASTM Standards:*

C 674 Test Methods for Flexural Properties of Ceramic Whiteware Materials[3]

F 981 Practice for Assessment of Compatibility of Biomaterials (Non-porous) for Surgical Implants with Respect to Effect of Materials on Muscle and Bone[4]

NOTE 1—Test Methods C 674 is referenced only to guide the future writers or users of performance standards that may yet be deemed necessary to promulgate. Test Methods C 674 does not contain any material specifications for beta-tricalcium phosphate.

2.2 *United States Code of Federal Regulations:*

Title 21 Part 820 Good Manufacturing Practices for Medical Devices[5]

3. Chemical Composition

3.1 Elemental analyses of calcium and phosphorus will be consistent with the expected stoichiometry of tricalcium phosphate.

NOTE 2—The precision of wet chemical methods for calcium and phosphorus are not sufficient to easily establish a 95 % purity of tricalcium phosphate. The theoretical calcium and phosphorus content of tricalcium phosphate is 38.76 and 19.97 %, respectively. The addition of 5 weight % hydroxyapatite results in calcium and phosphorous values of 38.82 and 19.90, respectively. To identify 5 weight % hydroxyapatite in tricalcium phosphate a maximum standard deviation for the calcium method must be 0.03; for phosphorus, 0.04 ($n = 10$, alpha = 0.05, power (1-beta) = 0.90). Precision of this order of magnitude is not expected.

3.2 *Trace Metals*:

3.2.1 The maximum allowable limits of individual heavy metals are as shown:

Metal	ppm, max
Lead	30
Mercury	5
Arsenic	3
Cadmium	5

For referee purposes, Limit Tests 251, 261, 211, **(10)** and Ref **(11)** will be used.

NOTE 3—These maximum values are based upon historical levels found in commercial calcium phosphates manufactured in the United States intended for surgical implantation.

3.2.2 The maximum allowable limit of all heavy metals determined as lead will be 50 ppm as described in Heavy Metals (231) Method 1 **(10)** or equivalent. Sample preparation will be identical to that for tribasic calcium phosphate as specified in the National Formulary Official Monograph on Tribasic Calcium Phosphate **(12)** except that approximately 1 g of material will be dissolved in approximately 30 mL of 5 % hydrochloric acid and boiled.

3.2.3 It is recommended that all metals or oxides not detected as lead present in concentrations equal to or greater than 0.10 % be listed on the package insert.

4. Crystal Structure

4.1 X-ray diffraction will confirm the beta phase of tricalcium phosphate and establish a minimum phase purity of 95 % according to a method equivalent to those cited in Refs **(13 and 14)**.

5. Test Specimens

5.1 Test specimens from each production run will be inspected according to Title 21 CFR 820.160 and will be shown to meet the standards of this ASTM specification by an acceptable statistical rationale.

---

[1] This specification is under the jurisdiction of ASTM Committee F-4 on Medical and Surgical Materials and Devices and is the direct responsibility of Subcommittee F04.13 on Ceramic Materials.

Current edition approved Oct. 30, 1987. Published December 1987.

[2] The boldface numbers in parentheses refer to the list of references at the end of this specification.

[3] *Annual Book of ASTM Standards*, Vol 15.02.

[4] *Annual Book of ASTM Standards*, Vol 13.01.

[5] Available from U.S. Government Printing Office, North Capital and H Streets NW, Washington, DC 20401.

6. Government Regulations

6.1 Material intended for commercial distribution will meet all applicable requirements imposed by the country of origin. If the material is manufactured for sale or imported within the United States or its territories the manufacturer and its authorized distributors will conform to the good manufacturing practices as described in Title 21 CFR 820.

7. Keywords

7.1 bioceramic; bone graft; hydroxy-apatite; tricalcium phosphate; whitlockite

APPENDIX

(Nonmandatory Information)

X1. RATIONALE

X1.1 Due to similar nomenclatures and chemical formulas other calcium phosphates have been confused with beta-tricalcium phosphate (beta-$Ca_3(PO_4)_2$). This specification excludes three such materials: tribasic calcium phosphate, whitlockite, and alpha-tricalcium phosphate. Tribasic calcium phosphate is a non-stoichiometric mixture: it is not a hydrated form of tricalcium phosphate. Tribasic calcium phosphate is assigned the same chemical formula as hydroxyapatite, $Ca_{10}(PO_4)_6(OH)_2$, by suppliers. Whitlockite and beta-tricalcium phosphate have been considered equivalent because of the similarity of their X-ray powder diffraction patterns. Whitlockite is a naturally occurring mineral containing magnesium and iron in octahedral coordination sites **(15)**; beta-tricalcium phosphate is prepared synthetically.

REFERENCES

(1) Metsger, D. S., et al., "Tricalcium Phosphate Ceramic—A Resorbable Bone Implant: Review and Current Status," *Journal of the American Dental Association*, 1982, Vol 105, No. 6, pp. 1035–1038.

(2) Klein, C., et al., "Relation Between Physical/Chemical Properties of Biodegradeable Calcium Phosphate Ceramics and Their Biodegradation Behavior," *Transactions of the Ninth Annual Meeting of the Society for Biomaterials*, Vol VI, Abstract 88, Birmingham, AL, April 1983.

(3) Klein, C., et al., "Biodegradation Behavior of Various Calcium Phosphate Materials in Bone Tissue," *Journal of Biomedical Material Research*, 1983, Vol 17, pp. 769–784.

(4) Krajewski, A., and Ravaglioli, A., "A Physico-Chemical Study of Crystal Growth of Hydroxyapatite Bioceramic," *Biomaterials*, 1981, Vol 2, No. 2, pp. 105–111.

(5) Niwa, S., "Synthetic Hydroxyapatite For Bone Graft," *Transactions of the Eighth Annual Meeting of the Society for Biomaterials*, Vol V, Abstract 76, April 1982, Birmingham, AL.

(6) Niwa, S., et al., "Preparation of Porous and Granular Hydroxyapatite and Possibility of Application as a Bone Graft," *Transactions of Ninth Annual Meeting of the Society for Biomaterials*, Vol VI, Abstract 24, April 1983, Birmingham, AL.

(7) Takayanagi, F., et al., "The Effect on Blood Coagulation System of Synthetic Hydroxyapatite," *Transactions of the Eleventh Annual Meeting of the Society for Biomaterials*, Vol VIII, Abstract 172, April 1985, Birmingham, AL.

(8) Winter, M., et al., "Comparative Histocompatibility Testing of Seven Calcium Phosphate Ceramics," *Biomaterials*, 1981, Vol 2, No. 3, pp. 159–160.

(9) Young, R. A., and Holcomb, D. W., "Variability of Hydroxyapatite Preparations," *Calcified Tissue International*, 1982, Vol 34, Supplement 2, pp. S17–S32.

(10) *United States Pharmacopeia*, Vol XXI, Identification Tests for: Calcium and Phosphate (191), Lead (251), Mercury (261), Arsenic (211), and Heavy Metals (231) Method I.

(11) Crock, J. G., Lichte, F. E., and Briggs, P. H., "Determination of Elements in National Bureau of Standards, Geological Reference Materials SRM 278 Obsidian and SRM 688 Basalt by Inductively Coupled Argon Plasma-Atomic Emission Spectroscopy," *Geostandards Newsletter*, Vol 7, No. 2, 1983, pp. 335–340.

(12) *National Formulary* XVI, Official Monograph on Tribasic Calcium Phosphate.

(13) Balmain, N., et al, "X-Ray Diffraction of Calcined Bone Tissue: A Reliable Method for the Determination of Bone Ca/P Molar Ratio," *Calcified Tissue International*, 1982, Vol 34, Supplement 2, pp. S93–S98.

(14) Foreman, D. W., and Metsger, D. S., "The Determination of Phase Composition of Calcium Phosphate Ceramics by X-Ray Diffraction," *Transactions of the Seventh Annual Meeting of the American Society for Bone and Mineral Research*, Kelseyville, CA, 1985, p. 391.

(15) Gopal, R., and Calvo, C.," Structural Relationship of Whitlockite and Beta-Tricalcium Phosphate," *Nature Physical Science*, 1972, Vol 237, pp. 30–32.

Designation: F 1089 – 87 (Reapproved 1994)$^{\epsilon 1}$

Standard Test Method for Corrosion of Surgical Instruments[1]

This standard is issued under the fixed designation F 1089; the number immediately following the designation indicates the year of original adoption or, in the case of revision, the year of last revision. A number in parentheses indicates the year of last reapproval. A superscript epsilon (ϵ) indicates an editorial change since the last revision or reapproval.

ϵ^1 NOTE—Section 8 was added editorially in April 1994.

1. Scope

1.1 This test method covers general test procedures and evaluation criteria for the corrosion resistance of surgical instruments fabricated from stainless steel and intended for reuse in surgery.

1.2 Austenitic (Class 3), martensitic (Class 4), and precipitation hardening (Class 5) materials are to use the boil test and the copper sulfate test.

1.3 Ferritic (Class 6) materials are to use the copper sulfate tests.

1.4 The copper sulfate test is used in austenitic materials to detect chromium depletion at the grain boundaries caused by improper heat treatment or improper cold working.

1.5 For martensitic steels, the copper sulfate test is used to detect improper heat treatment.

1.6 The boil test is applicable to martensitic, austenitic, and precipitation hardened materials to detect surface imperfections.

1.7 *This standard does not purport to address all of the safety concerns, if any, associated with its use. It is the responsibility of the user of this standard to establish appropriate safety and health practices and determine the applicability of regulatory limitations prior to use.*

2. Referenced Documents

2.1 *ASTM Standards:*

A 380 Practice for Cleaning and Descaling Stainless Steel Parts, Equipment, and Systems[2]

F 899 Specification for Stainless Steel Billet, Bar, and Wire for Surgical Instruments[3]

F 921 Definitions of Terms Relating to Hemostatic Forceps[3]

3. Significance and Use

3.1 This test method provides a test methodology and means of evaluation consistent to both producers and users alike. The corrosion tests serve as an indicator of proper material processing selection by the manufacturers and proper care by the user.

4. Reagents and Materials

4.1 *Cupric Sulfate*—Cupric sulfate crystals ($CuSO_4 \cdot 5H_2O$), 1 g.

4.2 *Sulfuric Acid*—Sulfuric acid AR (H_2SO_4), sp gr 1.84, 2.5 g.

4.3 *Distilled Water.*

4.4 *Isopropyl Alcohol or 95 % Ethyl Alcohol.*

4.5 *Nonreactive Vessel*, such as a glass or ceramic container.

5. Specimen Preparation

5.1 *Boil Test*:

5.1.1 Wash the instrument(s) with mild soap using a nonmetallic hard bristle brush and warm tap water (80 to 125 °F).

5.1.2 Rinse the instruments thoroughly at room temperature in distilled water, 95 % ethyl alcohol, or isopropyl alcohol.

5.1.3 Dry using paper towel or soft cloth.

5.2 *Copper Sulfate Corrosion Test*:

5.2.1 Wash the instrument(s) with mild soap using a nonmetallic hard bristle brush and warm (80 to 125 °F) tap water.

5.2.2 Rinse the instruments thoroughly at room temperature in distilled water followed by rinsing in 95 % ethyl alcohol or isopropyl alcohol.

5.2.3 Air dry (ambient air).

6. Procedure

6.1 *Boil Test*:

6.1.1 Immerse the instrument(s) into a nonreactive container of distilled water.

6.1.2 Bring the water to a boil.

6.1.3 Maintain boiling temperature for 30 ± 1 min.

6.1.4 Ensure that the instrument(s) remains immersed.

6.1.5 Remove the heat source and let the instrument(s) stand for 3 h± 15 min.

6.1.6 Remove the instrument(s) from the water and set on a towel to air dry (ambient air) for 2 h ± 10 min.

6.1.7 It is recommended that the pH level of test water is recorded before discarding. If the pH is outside the 6.5 to 7.0 range, the instrument was not cleaned thoroughly and should be retested accordingly.

[1] This test method is under the jurisdiction of ASTM Committee F-4 on Medical and Surgical Materials and Devices and is the direct responsibility of Subcommittee F04.33 on Medical/Surgical Instruments.

Current edition approved Oct. 30, 1987. Published December 1987.

[2] *Annual Book of ASTM Standards*, Vol 01.03.

[3] *Annual Book of ASTM Standards*, Vol 13.01.

6.2 *Copper Sulfate Corrosion Test*:

6.2.1 *Copper Sulfate Solution Preparation*:

6.2.1.1 Fill a nonreactive container with 22.5 mL of warm distilled water (80 to 125 °F).

6.2.1.2 Add 1 g of cupric sulfate crystals and stir until the crystals are completely dissolved.

6.2.1.3 Add 2.5 g of sulfuric acid and mix thoroughly.

6.2.2 *Test Procedure*:

6.2.2.1 Submerge the instrument(s) into a nonreactive container of copper sulfate solution of 63 to 67 °F.

6.2.2.2 Instruments too large for complete immersion shall have partial immersion or test by drops of the solution.

6.2.2.3 Copper sulfate solution shall be allowed to remain in contact with the instrument for 5½08to 6½ min.

6.2.2.4 Rinse the instrument(s) thoroughly with tap water and vigorously clean with cloth or nonmetallic soft bristle brush to remove any nonadherent copper plating.

7. Interpretation of Results

7.1 *Boil Test*:

7.1.1 All surfaces are to show no signs of corrosion (without magnification).

7.1.2 A slight evidence of rust (ferrous oxide) in serrations, teeth, locks, ratchets, inserts (brazed or soldered junctions), etc., shall not be cause for rejection.

7.2 *Copper Sulfate Corrosion Test*:

7.2.1 All surfaces are to show no visual signs of copper plating (without magnification) with the exceptions noted in 7.2.1.1 and 7.2.1.2.

7.2.1.1 Copper plating in serrations, teeth, locks, ratchets, braze junctions, solder junctions or dulling of polished surfaces shall not be cause for rejection.

7.2.1.2 Copper plating at the periphery of the copper sulfate solution drops shall not be cause for rejection.

8. Keywords

8.1 boil test; copper sulfate corrosion test; corrosion-surgical implants; immersion

APPENDIX

(Nonmandatory Information)

X1. RATIONALE

X1.1 The function of this test method is to provide a test methodology and means of evaluation consistent to both producers and users alike.

X1.2 The corrosion tests serve as indicator of proper material processing selection by the manufacturers and proper care by the user.

X1.3 Both the boil test and copper sulfate test serve as an indicator that the surface has achieved a passive state as well as remove chemical and free iron contaminants. Heat treatment has an important effect on corrosion resistance in martensitic stainless steel. Carbide formation does reduce corrosion resistance. Proper heat treatment dissolves free carbon. The copper sulfate detects carbide formation from free carbon. The copper sulfate test is used in austenitic materials to detect chromium depletion at the grain boundaries caused by improper heat treatment or improper cold working. The boil test is applicable to martensitic, austenitic, and precipitation hardened materials to detect surface imperfections.

NOTE X1.1—Practice 4380 states that a specialized copper sulfate test is used extensively on surgical and dental instruments made of hardenable martensitic stainless steel.

X1.4 Specific instrument design/manufacturing processes will influence corrosion test results. Accumulated testing experience is an important factor in determining the significance of corrosion results obtained for stainless steel.

X1.5 The copper sulfate test was developed to detect chromium depletion at the grain boundaries of austenitic material due to improper heat treatment (in the 900 to 1100 °F range) or improper cold working. The boil test would not readily show these defects, but would show cracks and pitting. The austenitic materials should be subjected to both tests. Improper heat treatment can result in carbide formation in the martensitic materials. Proper heat treatment results in the dissolution of free carbon into the martensitic structure. It is recognized in 7.2.1.1 that plating of unpolished surfaces may occur, and trouble areas are specifically excluded. This exclusion would negate the phenomena of plating in these areas with Type 410. The boil test is important for these materials for surface imperfections. The copper sulfate test is important to detect improper heat treatment. The precipitation hardening steels are included for the same rationale as the austenitics.

Designation: F 1091 – 91 (Reapproved 2000)

Standard Specification for Wrought Cobalt-20 Chromium-15 Tungsten-10 Nickel Alloy Surgical Fixation Wire [UNS R30605][1]

This standard is issued under the fixed designation F 1091; the number immediately following the designation indicates the year of original adoption or, in the case of revision, the year of last revision. A number in parentheses indicates the year of last reapproval. A superscript epsilon (ε) indicates an editorial change since the last revision or reapproval.

1. Scope

1.1 This specification covers the requirements for the manufacture of wrought cobalt-20 chromium-15 tungsten-10 nickel surgical fixation wire.

1.2 The values stated in metric units are to be regarded as standard. The inch-pound equivalents may be approximate.

2. Referenced Documents

2.1 *ASTM Standards:*

E 8 Methods of Tensile Testing of Metallic Materials[2]

F 90 Specification for Wrought Cobalt-Chromium-Tungsten-Nickel Alloy for Surgical Implant Applications[3]

F 86 Practice for Surface Preparation and Marking of Metallic Surgical Implants[3]

2.2 *USP Standards:*[4]

Nonabsorbable Surgical Suture, U.S. Pharmacopoeia

3. Material Requirements

3.1 Surgical fixation wire shall conform to the specified chemical composition of Specification F 90. Conformance with this standard shall be so identified by suitable packaging or labeling, or both.

3.2 Surgical fixation wire shall be furnished in the bright annealed condition and finish.

4. Mechanical Requirements

4.1 Surgical fixation wire shall conform to the appropriate mechanical properties specified in Table 1.

4.2 Mechanical testing shall be performed in accordance with Methods E 8 using a 254 mm (10 in.) gage length and cross-head speed of 254 mm/min (10 in./min).

4.3 The wire shall meet the requirements of USP for Nonabsorbable Surgical Sutures, (latest version) when tested in accordance with 4.2.

5. Dimensional Requirements

5.1 Surgical fixation wire shall be fabricated in accordance with the dimensions and tolerances specified in Table 1.

6. Surface Condition and Handling

6.1 The surface of surgical fixation wire conforming to this specification shall be free of imperfections such as toolmarks, nicks, scratches, cracks, cavities, spurs, and other defects that would impair the serviceability of the wire. The surface shall be free of embedded or deposited finishing materials and other undesirable contaminants.

6.2 The wire may be subjected to a passivation process if requested by the customer. Such passivation process shall be performed in accordance with F 86.

6.3 Surgical fixation wire shall be handled with care and packaged adequately to prevent damage and contamination of the surface.

7. General Requirements

7.1 In addition to the requirements of this specification, all requirements of the current edition of Specification F 90 shall apply.

7.2 In cases of conflict between this standard and those listed in 2.1, this standard shall take precedence.

8. Keywords

8.1 fixation; mechanical properties; surgical implant; suture; tolerances; wire; wrought cobalt-chromium alloy

---

[1] This specification is under the jurisdiction of ASTM Committee F04 on Medical and Surgical Materials and Devicesand is the direct responsibility of Subcommittee F04.21 on Osteosynthesis.

Current edition approved Feb. 22, 1991. Published June 1991.

[2] *Annual Book of ASTM Standards*, Vol 03.01.

[3] *Annual Book of ASTM Standards*, Vol 13.01.

[4] Available from U.S. Pharmacopeia, Mack Publishing Co., Easton, PA.

TABLE 1 Mechanical and Dimensional Requirements for Wrought Cobalt-Chromium Alloy Surgical Fixation Wire

Range of Sizes Diameter, mm (in.)	USP Size[A]	Diameter Tolerance[B,C]	Tensile Strength max, MPa (ksi)[D]	Elong. min, %[E]
0.010 to under 0.020 (0.0004 to 0.0008)	...	0.0015 (0.00006)	1730 (250)	20
0.020 to under 0.030 (0.0008 to 0.0012)	10-0	0.0015 (0.00006)	1660 (240)	20
0.030 to under 0.040 (0.0012 to 0.0016)	9-0	0.0025 (0.0001)	1590 (230)	25
0.040 to under 0.050 (0.0016 to 0.0020)	8-0	0.0025 (0.0001)	1555 (225)	30
0.050 to under 0.070 (0.0020 to 0.0028)	7-0	0.0025 (0.0001)	1520 (220)	30
0.070 to under 0.100 (0.0028 to 0.0039)	6-0	0.0025 (0.0001)	1385 (215)	35
0.100 to under 0.150 (0.0039 to 0.0059)	5-0	0.0050 (0.0002)	1450 (210)	35
0.150 to under 0.200 (0.0059 to 0.0079)	4-0	0.0050 (0.0002)	1415 (205)	35
0.200 to under 0.250 (0.0079 to 0.0098)	3-0	0.0075 (0.0003)	1380 (200)	40
0.250 to under 0.300 (0.0098 to 0.0118)	...	0.0075 (0.0003)	1380 (200)	40
0.300 to under 0.340 (0.0118 to 0.0134)	2-0	0.0100 (0.0004)	1310 (190)	40
0.340 to under 0.350 (0.0134 to 0.0138)	...	0.0100 (0.0004)	1310 (190)	40
0.350 to under 0.400 (0.0138 to 0.0158)	1-0	0.0100 (0.0004)	1275 (185)	40
0.400 to under 0.500 (0.0158 to 0.0197)	1	0.0100 (0.0004)	1275 (185)	40
0.500 to under 0.600 (0.0197 to 0.0236)	2	0.0100 (0.0004)	1275 (185)	45
0.600 to under 0.700 (0.0236 to 0.0276)	3 and 4	0.0130 (0.0005)	1240 (180)	45
0.700 to under 0.800 (0.0276 to 0.0315)	5	0.0130 (0.0005)	1240 (180)	45
0.800 to under 0.900 (0.0315 to 0.0354)	6	0.0200 (0.0008)	1240 (180)	45
0.900 to under 1.000 (0.0354 to 0.0394)	7	0.0200 (0.0008)	1170 (170)	45
1.000 to under 1.100 (0.0394 to 0.0433)	...	0.0200 (0.0008)	1170 (170)	45
1.100 to under 1.600 (0.0433 to 0.0630)	...	0.0250 (0.0010)	1140 (165)	45

[A] For reference purposes only. (U.S. Pharmacopoeia.)
[B] Diameter tolerances are over and under as given in this table. Also, round wire can be produced to tolerances all over and nothing under, or all under and nothing over, or any combination over and under, if the total spread in diameter tolerance for a specified diameter is not less than the total spread given in this table.
[C] The maximum out-of-round tolerance for round wire is one half of the total size tolerance given in this table.
[D] Maximum tensile strength is specified to assure proper wire-handling characteristics.
[E] Minimum elongation for spooled wire is 6 percentage points lower than table value.

APPENDIX

(Nonmandatory Information)

X1. RATIONALE

X1.1 The primary reason for this standard is to characterize the mechanical properties of annealed wrought cobalt-chrome monofilament wire for implant applications.

X1.2 This standard combines and replaces F 643 and F 644; Standard Specification for Wrought Cobalt-Chromium Alloy Flexible Wire for Surgical Fixations for Soft Tissue and Standard Specification for Wrought Cobalt Chromium Alloy Flexible Wire for Surgical Fixations for Bone.

X1.3 The title has been changed and the UNS designation has been added to more readily identify the material.

Standard Specification for Ventilators Intended for Use in Critical Care[1]

This standard is issued under the fixed designation F 1100; the number immediately following the designation indicates the year of original adoption or, in the case of revision, the year of last revision. A number in parentheses indicates the year of last reapproval. A superscript epsilon (ε) indicates an editorial change since the last revision or reapproval.

1. Scope

1.1 *General*—This specification establishes minimum performance and safety requirements for all ventilators and ventilator circuits intended for use with adult, child, or infant patients in critical care within the hospital and introduced for sale after the acceptance date of this specification, except as noted below. Definitions, performance requirements, test methods, and rationale are included. Several definitions have been included in Section 3.1 and Appendix X1 that are not used in the text of this specification. This material has been included for the sake of completeness, and for any possible educational benefit that may be served.

1.2 *Exclusions*—This specification does not apply to body ventilators such as the tank ventilator or the chest cuirass nor does it apply to ventilators utilizing the Sanders technique or "jet" ventilation, (venturi effect type) high frequency ventilators (greater than 2.5 Hz), or anesthesia ventilators. This specification does not apply to ventilators intended for use in transport applications or home care, nor does it apply to those ventilators developed for veterinary applications. The application of critical care ventilators in the home environment is not covered by this specification nor is the hospital use of transport or home care ventilators. (See also X2.1.)

1.3 The following precautionary caveat pertains to the test methods portion only, Section 6, of this specification: *This standard does not purport to address all of the safety concerns associated with its use. It is the responsibility of the user of this standard to establish appropriate safety and health practices and determine the applicability of regulatory limitations prior to use.*

2. Referenced Documents

2.1 *ASTM Standards:*

F 1054 Specification for Conical Fittings of 15-mm and 22-mm Sizes[2]

2.2 *ANSI Standards:*

ANSI Z-79.9, 1978, Humidifiers and Nebulizers for Medical Use[3]

ANSI Z-79.10, 1979, Requirements for Oxygen Analyzers for Monitoring Patient Breathing Mixtures[3]

2.3 *ISO Standards:*

ISO 4135 Anesthesiology Vocabulary[4]

ISO 5356 Anesthetic and Respiratory Equipment Conical Connectors[4]

2.4 *Other Standards:*

CGA V-5 Specifications for DISS Connections[5]

MDS 201 Electromagnetic Compatibility Standard for Medical Devices[6]

3. Terminology

3.1 *Descriptions of Terms*—For the purposes of this specification the definitions in 3.1.1-3.1.49 shall apply.

3.1.1 *airway pressure* (P_{aw})—pressure at a specified point in the patient's airway. The site and conditions under which measurements are made should be given.

3.1.2 *alarm*—a means of alerting the operator that a particular condition exists.

3.1.3 *alveolar pressure* (P_A)—pressure in the alveoli. In the case of the lung model, this is represented by the pressure in the compliance chamber.

3.1.4 *apparatus internal compliance*—volume/pressure relationship, expressed in millilitres per kilopascal (or millilitres per centimetre H_2O) of those portions of the patient system that are pressurized during the inspiratory phase time (see also 8.1).

3.1.5 *continuous positive airway pressure* (CPAP)—P_{aw} maintained above ambient.

3.1.5.1 *Discussion*—Common usage of this term references spontaneous ventilation.

3.1.6 *control*—a means available to the operator of directly adjusting a ventilator function.

3.1.7 *cycling pressure*—that pressure which, when reached in the patient system, causes the ventilator to cycle from inspiratory to expiratory phase or from expiratory to inspiratory phase.

3.1.8 *differential inspiratory triggering pressure* (ΔP_{tr})—changes in airway pressure at the patient connection port which must be generated by the patient to initiate the ventilator inspiratory phase.

[1] This specification is under the jurisdiction of ASTM Committee F29 on Anesthetic and Respiratory Equipment and is the direct responsibility of Subcommittee F29.14 on Ventilators.

Current edition approved May 18, 1990. Published June 1990.

[2] *Annual Book of ASTM Standards*, Vol 13.01.

[3] Available from the American National Standards Institute, 25 W. 43rd St., 4th Floor, New York, NY 10036.

[4] Available from the International Standards Organization, 1, Rue de Varembe, Case postale 56, CH-1211 Geneve 20, Switzerland.

[5] Available from the Compressed Gas Association, 1725 Jefferson Davis Highway, Suite 1004, Arlington, VA 22202–4102.

[6] Available from the National Technical Information Service (NTIS), Accession #PB271635, 5285 Port Royal Rd., Springfield, VA 22161.

3.1.8.1 *Discussion*—Pressure shall be expressed in terms of gage pressure in units of kilopascals (or centimetres H_2O) to follow the kilopascal units.

3.1.9 *expiratory pause time* (T_{EP})—interval from the end of expiratory flow to the start of inspiratory flow.

3.1.10 *expiratory phase time* (T_E)—interval from the start of expiratory flow to the start of inspiratory flow.

3.1.11 *expiratory positive airway pressure* (EPAP)—P_{aw} above ambient during the expiratory phase, generally approximated by P_{ps}.

3.1.12 *expiratory (sub-atmospheric) sub-ambient pressure*—pressure lower than ambient, during the expiratory phase time.

3.1.12.1 *Discussion*—Sub-ambient pressure may be constant throughout the expiratory phase time or it may vary through the phase time, depending upon the method by which such pressure is generated.

3.1.13 *frequency (ventilatory) (f)*—number of breathing cycles per minute.

3.1.14 *heat and moisture exchanger* (HME)—a passive device which is designed to conserve some of the patient's exhaled moisture and heat, and to release heat and moisture to the patient's airway during inspiration.

3.1.15 *inspiratory-expiratory phase time ratio (I:E ratio)*—ratio of the inspiratory phase time to the expiratory phase time.

3.1.16 *inspiratory minute volume* ($\dot{V}_I$)—volume of gas inspired per minute by the patient, measured by litres (L).

3.1.17 *inspiratory pause time* (T_{IP})—interval from the end of inspiratory flow to the start of expiratory flow.

3.1.18 *inspiratory phase time* (T_I)—interval from the start of inspiratory flow to the start of expiratory flow.

3.1.19 *inspiratory positive airway pressure* (IPAP)—P_{aw} above ambient during the inspiratory phase of CPAP, generally approximated by P_{ps}.

3.1.20 *inspiratory relief valve*—unidirectional valve designed to admit air to the patient system when the patient inspires spontaneously and the supply of inspiratory gases from the ventilator is inadequate.

3.1.21 *inspiratory relief valve resistance*—pressure difference across the inspiratory relief valve at a constant flow of 30 L/min.

3.1.22 *inspiratory triggering flow* ($\dot{V}_{Tr}$)—flow which must be generated by the patient at the patient connection port to initiate the ventilator inspiratory phase.

3.1.23 *inspiratory triggering pressure* (P_{tr})—airway pressure at the patient connection port which must be generated by the patient to initiate the ventilator inspiratory phase.

3.1.24 *inspiratory triggering response time* (T_{tr})—time delay between the satisfaction of the inspiratory triggering pressure or flow, or both, volume requirements, and the start of inspiratory flow.

3.1.25 *inspiratory triggering volume* (V_{tr})—volume, measured at the patient connection port, which must be moved by the patient to initiate the ventilator inspiratory phase.

3.1.25.1 *Discussion*—In some devices there exists a complex relationship between the multiple parameters as defined in 3.1.22-3.1.25.

3.1.26 *intermittent mandatory ventilation* (IMV)—a mode of operation of the ventilator that permits spontaneous breathing of a controlled inspiratory gas mixture between the predetermined ventilator-derived breaths, using the same inspiratory gas mixture.

3.1.27 *maximum limited pressure* ($P_{L\,max}$)—the highest gage pressure which can be attained in the patient system during malfunction of the ventilator but with functioning safety mechanisms.

3.1.27.1 *Discussion*—The title of this definition is different from the title given in ISO 4135. However, the text is identical to that in ISO 4135. The title of the ISO definition is *maximum safety pressure.*

3.1.28 *maximum working pressure* ($P_{w\,max}$)—the highest gage pressure which can be attained in the patient system during the inspiratory phase when the ventilator is functioning normally.

3.1.28.1 *Discussion*—This may be limited by a controllable ventilator mechanism to less than $P_{L\,max}$.

3.1.29 *minimum limited pressure* ($P_{L\,min}$)—the highest numerical value of sub-atmospheric gage pressure which can be attained in the patient system during malfunction of the ventilator but with functioning safety mechanisms.

3.1.29.1 *Discussion*—The title of this definition is different from the title given in ISO 4135. However, the text is identical to that in ISO 4135. The title of the definition in ISO 4135 is *minimum safety pressure.*

3.1.30 *minimum working pressure* ($P_{w\,min}$)—highest numerical value of sub-atmospheric gage pressure which can be attained in the patient system during the expiratory phase when the ventilator is functioning normally.

3.1.30.1 *Discussion*—This may be limited by a controllable ventilator mechanism to a sub-atmospheric pressure that is numerically smaller than $P_{L\,min}$.

3.1.31 *minute volume* ($\dot{V}$)—volume of gas, expressed in litres per minute entering or leaving the patient or lung model. The physical conditions under which measuring was made should be given.

3.1.32 *monitor (indicator display)*—a means of informing the operator of the status or numerical value of ventilation or a ventilator.

3.1.33 *nebulizing humidifier*—device designed to add water to the inspired gas in the form of droplets.

3.1.34 *negative end expiratory pressure* (NEEP)—the P_{ps} at the end of expiration, below ambient.

3.1.35 *patient system*—that part of the gas system of a ventilator through which respired gas travels at appropriate respiratory pressures.

3.1.36 *patient system compliance*—volume/pressure relationship, expressed in mL/kPa (or mL/cm H_2O), of those portions of the patient system that are pressurized during the inspiratory phase time.

3.1.37 *positive end-expiratory pressure* (PEEP)—P_{ps} at the end of expiration, above ambient.

3.1.38 *pressure, patient system* (P_{ps})—pressure at a specified point in the patient system.

3.1.38.1 *Discussion*—Conditions under which measurements are made shall be given.

3.1.39 *pressure support*—a ventilator mode designed to

augment the patient's ventilation synchronously with his inspiratory effort until a preset pressure is met.

3.1.40 *sigh (ventilator)*—deliberate increase in tidal volume for one or more breaths at intervals.

3.1.41 *spirometer*—device designed to measure a volume of gas.

3.1.42 *synchronous intermittent mandatory ventilation (SIMV) or assisted ventilation*—a ventilator mode which provides a mechanism for synchronizing the ventilator-delivered breaths with a patient's inspiration, as detected by the ventilator.

3.1.43 *tidal volume* (V_T)—volume of gas, expressed in millilitres (mL), entering or leaving the patient or the lung model during the inspiratory or expiratory phase time. The physical conditions under which gas volumes are measured should be given.

3.1.44 *time constant*—time in which an exponential process is 63 % complete.

3.1.45 *vaporizing humidifier*—device designed to add water to the inspired gas in the form of vapor.

3.1.46 *ventilator expiratory resistance*—for ventilators in which expiration is not assisted, the total resistance to gas flow from the patient connection port through the expiratory port of the patient system to atmosphere. This is expressed in kPa (or cm H_2O) referred to a flow of 0.5 L/s.

3.1.47 *ventilator pressure* (P_{vent})—pressure at a specified point in the ventilator. The site and conditions under which measurements are made should be given.

3.1.48 *ventilators intended for use with anesthesia*—ventilator designed to be used with or integral to an anesthesia breathing system.

3.1.49 *volumetric displacement*—that volume, under specific conditions and expressed in millilitres, passed per cycle during the inspiratory phase through the patient connection port when the pressure at the intake to the ventilator and the outlet from the patient's connection port is equal to the atmospheric pressure.

3.2 *Symbols:*

3.2.1 *C*—compliance in units of mL/kPa (or mL/cm H_2O), for example, *C*20 = 2.0 mL/kPa (20 mL/cm H_2O).

3.2.2 *R*—resistance to flow in units of kPa/L/s (or cm H_2O/L/s), for example, *R*5 = 0.5 kPa/L/s (5 cm H_2O/L/s).

3.2.2.1 *Discussion*—In the interest of brevity and clarity, all other abbreviations have been provided in parentheses following the related term in Section 3.

4. Materials and Manufacture

4.1 Components of a spirometer that come in direct contact with the patient's exhaled gas shall be capable of being sterilized or disinfected or shall be labelled for single use only, or isolated in some manner from the respired gas in the patient breathing circuit. (See also X2.2.)

5. Performance Requirements

5.1 *Determination of Ventilator Endurance, Wave-form, and Volume Characteristics—General*—Compliance with the requirements given in 5.2-5.4 shall be determined with one or more samples of production ventilators with the assurance that the results, which shall be made available to customers, are representative of all production ventilators of that type.

NOTE 1—The requirements given in 5.2-5.4 and the tests described in 6.3 delineate first article or design qualification tests and are not intended to be lot sampling tests. The disclosure of information referred to in 6.3 is intended to include periodic maintenance necessary during the endurance test and the results of work performed.

5.2 *Ventilator Endurance*—Each ventilator (as described in 5.1) shall be tested for endurance as described in 6.3.1 with respect to each group of patients for which its use is recommended, that is, for adults, for children, and for infants. The ventilator shall run for 2000 h against the appropriate conditions as shown in Table 1. A separate machine may be used for each group or the period of tests may be divided equally between groups. If the ventilator is provided with an assist mechanism, the mechanism shall be part of the test. If IMV or SIMV is provided, that mechanism shall be a part of the test. Data resulting from these tests shall be available on request from the manufacturer.

5.3 *Wave-form Performance*—The ventilator shall be tested as described in 6.3.2 with each of the compliance and resistance combinations appropriate to its intended use (that is, for adults, for children, or for infants), in the order shown in Table 2.

5.4 *Volume Performance*—The ventilator shall be tested against the combinations of compliance (*C*) and resistance (*R*) appropriate to its sphere of use, as shown in Table 3. The manufacturer shall determine the range of tidal volumes that the ventilator is capable of delivering to the lung at the specified frequencies with an inspiratory/expiratory phase time ratio as close to 1:2 as possible. Further measurements at different frequencies and with different compliance and resistance combinations may be included if desired. All results shall be expressed in the form of a table or a diagram similar to Fig. 1. The conditions under which the tests are carried out shall be stated (see 6.3.2 and 6.3.2.1).

5.5 *Power Sources*:

5.5.1 *Electrical*—The ventilator shall continue to function within the manufacturer's specifications at any control setting throughout a range of ±10 % fluctuation of the stated nominal voltage and ±1 % fluctuation of the stated frequency for electrical power sources.

5.5.2 *Pneumatic*—When tested according to the methods outlined in 6.5, the ventilator shall continue to function within the manufacturer's specifications at any control setting throughout a range of supply pressures of 379 kPa (55 psig) +20 %, −25 %. (See also Appendix X3.3.2.)

5.5.2.1 The ventilator's gas connection(s) shall be non-interchangeable. If the device has a threaded connection, it shall conform to the appropriate CGA V-5 1978 specification for DISS connections. If the ventilator is capable of being

TABLE 1 Endurance Test

Group	Minute Volume V_E, L	Ventilatory Frequency, f, breaths/min[A]	Compliance	Resistance
Adult	10	20	*C*50	*R*20 or R_p20
Child	4.5	30	*C*20	*R*50 or R_p50
Infant	0.8	60	*C*3	*R*200 or R_p200

[A] Or nearest possible.

TABLE 2 Procedure for Performance Test—Waveform[A]

Test Number[B]	Compliance	Resistance		Tidal Volume V_t± 5 %, mL	Ventilation Frequency *f*: ± 5 % (breaths/min)	Sample Time Constant, s	Ventilation Pressure Limit, cm H_2O[C]
		Linear	Parabolic				
Adult							
[1]	*C*50	*R*5	R_p5	500	20	0.25	12.5
2	*C*50	*R*20	R_p20	500	20	1.0	20.0
3	*C*20	*R*5	R_p5	500	20	0.1	27.5
4	*C*20	*R*20	R_p20	500	20	0.4	35.0
Children							
[1]	*C*20	*R*20	R_p20	300	20	0.4	21.0
2	*C*20	*R*50	R_p50	300	20	1.0	30.0
3	*C*10	*R*20	R_p20	300	20	0.2	36.0
4	*C*10	*R*50	R_p50	300	20	0.5	45.0
[5]	*C*3	*R*20	R_p20	50	30	0.06	18.5
6	*C*3	*R*50	R_p50	50	30	0.15	20.8
7	*C*3	*R*200	R_p200	50	30	0.6	32.0
Infant							
[1]	*C*3	*R*50	R_p50	30	30	0.15	12.3
2	*C*3	*R*200	R_p200	30	30	0.6	19.0
3	*C*1	*R*50	R_p50	30	30	0.05	32.3
4	*C*1	*R*200	R_p200	30	30	0.2	39.0
[5]	*C*1	*R*200	R_p200	15	60	0.2	24.0

[A] Inspiratory/expiratory phase time ratio as close to 1:2 as possible; see 6.3.2.

[B] The ventilator controls shall be reset to suit the chosen standard conditions (bracketed) before undertaking each subsequent test. Thus, the order of recordings obtained on adults would be Test [1]; Test 2 (controls unchanged); Test 2 (controls adjusted if necessary); controls reset to satisfy Test [1] conditions; Test 3 (controls unchanged); Test [3] (controls readjusted if necessary), etc.

[C] Ventilation Pressure Limit = Calculated pressure applied by constant-flow generators at the machine side of the airway resistance to achieve the required tidal volume during the set inspiratory time. These pressures will be in excess of the corresponding lung pressure that will be developed by the end of the inspiratory phase.

TABLE 3 Volume Performance Test

Type of Ventilator	Compliance	Resistance		Ventilatory Frequencies
		Linear	Parabolic	
Adult	*C*20	*R*20	R_p20	10, 15, 20, 30
Child	*C*10	*R*50	R_p50	15, 20, 30, 40
	*C*3	*R*200	R_p200	15, 20, 30, 40
Infant	*C*1	*R*200	R_p200	20, 30, 40, 60

Tidal Volume, V_T (ml)	Ventilatory Frequency, *f* (bpm)			
	10	15	20	30
Max	—	—	—	—
Min	—	—	—	—

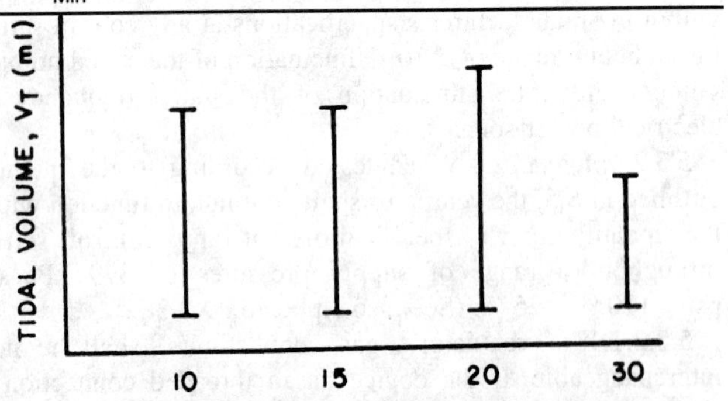

FIG. 1 Suggested Format for Volume Performance Test Report Form

independently connected to the gas piping system it shall have permanently attached a Nut and Gland Fitting No. 1240 (oxygen), if intended to be powered by oxygen, or a Nut and Gland Fitting No. 1160 (air), if intended to be powered by air, or both fittings if both gases are used. (See also Appendix X3.3.2.1.)

5.6 *Accuracy of Calibrated Controls, Indicators, and Pressure Relief Devices*:

5.6.1 *Calibrated Controls*—When tested according to the methods outlined in 6.6.1, controls for $P_{w\,max}$ on infant ventilators shall be accurate to within ±0.196 kPa (±2 cm H_2O) over the entire range. Controls for $P_{w\,max}$ in all other ventilators shall be accurate to within ±0.49 kPa (±5 cm H_2O) up to 2.94 kPa (30 cm H_2O) and± 0.98 kPa (±10 cm H_2O) for settings above 30 cm H_2O. All other calibrated controls, when working at nominal power inputs, should be accurate to within ±10 % of the setting. (See also X2.3.3.1.)

5.6.1.1 *Maximum Working Pressure*—If provided in the patient breathing circuit, positive pressure control devices shall restrict the airway pressure to within ±0.49 kPa (±5 cm H_2O) up to a point of 2.94 kPa (30 cm H_2O) and to within ±0.98 kPa (±10 cm H_2O) for settings above 30 cm H_2O, when tested by the methods described in 6.6.2. (See also X2.3.3.2.)

5.6.2 *Indicators*—All other indicators should be accurate to within ±10 % of the reading.

5.6.3 *Limited Pressure Relief Controls*— If the pressure in the breathing circuit reaches a level greater than the usual operator adjusted peak pressure, the device (ventilator) shall activate a pressure reduction mechanism within 3 s when tested as outlined in 6.6.3. This pressure reduction mechanism shall bring the breathing circuit to a predetermined baseline pressure equal to or less than the end-expiratory pressure. The limited pressure relief mechanism may also be activated without delay when the preset maximum limiting pressure is reached. A coupled visual/audible alarm shall be activated in this event. The visual signal shall be retained when the pressure is reduced and shall require a manual reset. (See also X2.3.3.3.)

5.6.4 When tested by the methods described in 6.6.4, devices indicating ventilatory frequency shall be accurate to one breath per minute or 10 % of the setting, whichever is greater.

5.6.4.1 When tested by the methods described in 6.6.4, devices controlling ventilator frequency shall be accurate to within one breath per minute or 10 % of the setting, whichever is greater. (See also X2.3.3.4.)

5.7 *Spirometers and Other Devices for Indication of Ventilator Function Integral to the Ventilator*:

NOTE 2—Continuous flow ventilators are exempt from the requirements of 5.7.

5.7.1 Provision shall be made for connection of a spirometer or other device for the measurement of expired volume if not provided as an integral part of the ventilator. The fitting for the attachment of this spirometer shall be a standard 30-mm conical male connector.

5.7.2 When tested as described in 6.7, any spirometer integral with the ventilator shall be accurate to within ±10 % of the reading over the flow ranges specified by the manufacturer. The pressure drop with a steady gas flow of 50 L/min shall not exceed 0.196 kPa (2.0 cm H_2O). Conditions of calibration shall be disclosed. (See also X2.3.4.1.)

5.7.3 When tested as described in 6.7.2, the spirometer shall continue to function within the limits of accuracy delineated in 5.7.2 whatever the humidity and within the temperature range of 20 to 37°C (due allowance being made for the difference between gas temperature and humidity in the spirometer and the temperature and humidity at which the spirometer was calibrated). Spirometers should be designed in such a manner that they cannot become obstructed by secretions from the patient. (See also X2.3.4.2.)

5.8 *Accuracy of Gas Mixture Controls*:

5.8.1 When tested as described in 6.8, ventilators that incorporate as a primary control an inspiratory gas mixture control shall provide a mean delivered oxygen concentration within ±10 % of the set oxygen concentration or 3 % oxygen, whichever is greater, throughout the range of pressures, frequencies, and tidal volumes for which the ventilator is capable. At a given setting of the ventilator, the mean delivered oxygen concentration shall be within ±3 % oxygen for at least one hour. (See also X2.3.5.)

5.9 *Expiratory Resistance*:

5.9.1 *Adult and Child Ventilators*—When tested in accordance with the methods described in 6.9, and in the absence of expiratory resistors or positive end expiratory pressure devices, the pressure at the patient connection port for adult and child ventilators shall not exceed 0.49 kPa (5 cm H_2O) at a flow of 50 LPM when spirometer or breathing attachments, or both, as specified by the manufacturer are used. (See also X2.3.6.)

5.9.2 *Constant Flow Infant Ventilators*— When tested according to the methods described in 6.9, positive end-expiratory pressure inherent in the design of constant flow infant ventilators shall not exceed 0.29 kPa (3 cm H_2O) at a constant machine flow of 20 L/min, 60 breaths per minute, 1:1 I:E ratio, R = 4.9 kPa/L/s (50 cm H_2O/L/s), and C = 3 mL/0.29 kPa (3 mL/cm H_2O). If expiratory assistance is necessary to comply with this requirement, it shall be so stated. (See also Appendix X2.6.)

5.10 *Fittings Connecting Adult Ventilator, Patient, and Spirometer*—The patient connection port shall be a 15⁄22 mm conical coaxial fitting in accordance with Specification F 1054.

5.10.1 For flow direction-sensitive devices, the direction of flow shall be permanently marked on the connector, and the connector should be designed so that it cannot be installed in the reverse direction. (See also X2.3.7.1.)

5.10.2 If a connector for a bag for manual ventilation is provided on the ventilator, it shall face downward and shall be situated away from the connectors for the patient breathing tubes. The bag mount should provide a secure connection. The term *bag* shall be marked on the connector. (See also X2.3.7.2.)

5.10.3 If there is a separate outlet for the spirometer on the breathing tubes or the machine, the gas outlet leading to the spirometer should be a 30-mm male cone in accordance with ISO 5356. In any case, it shall not be compatible with a 15, 19, or 22-mm fitting. (See also 6.10.3 and X2.3.7.3.)

5.10.4 If an ambient air inlet is fitted to the ventilator, it shall not be a 19, 22, 15, or 30-mm male cone and shall be clearly marked as *air inlet*. (See also 6.10.4 and X2.3.7.4.)

5.10.5 If an expired gas outlet (other than an outlet for spirometer) is fitted to the machine, it shall be designed in such a way that when tested as outlined in 6.10.5 it cannot easily be connected to either 22, 15, or 30-mm cones or sockets, or to 22-mm internal diameter tubing. (See also X2.3.7.5.)

5.11 *Alarm Systems*:

5.11.1 *General*—The alarm system shall provide a warning signal(s) if the function of the ventilator deviates from the control settings by more than preset levels as specified in the appropriate sections of this draft standard or in the instructions for use. Signal(s) shall be appropriate to the nature of the response expected from the operator. In general, if an immediate response is required of the operator, an audible and a visual signal shall be provided. If a less than immediate response is required, a lower priority visible signal may be used. This may be coupled with an audible signal so long as it is distinctly different from any audible signal requiring immediate operator response. Monitoring functions (for example, *ventilator on*) should not have coupled audible and visual alarms. Alarm signal outputs shall be provided.

5.11.2 *Testing of Alarm Function*—A means shall be provided to test the audible and visual annunciation of all alarms.

5.11.3 *Required Alarms*—The following alarms shall be provided on all critical care ventilators:

5.11.3.1 *Loss of Main Power Supply*—A loss of main power alarm shall be provided, and when tested as described in 6.11, shall have a duration of at least two min at a constant sound pressure level. A means shall be provided for silencing this alarm following disconnection from the main power supply. This means of silencing the alarm shall not be remote from the ventilator, and the alarm silencing mechanism shall automatically reset when the main power is restored. (See also X2.3.8.1.)

5.11.3.2 *Breathing Circuit Integrity*—When tested in accordance with the manufacturer's instructions, the breathing circuit integrity alarm(s) shall respond within 15 s or one complex cycle of the ventilator if the breathing circuit is compromised by disconnection or leakage. This alarm shall be activated within ±20 % of the control setting. The manufacturer shall disclose a method for complying with this requirement. A means shall be provided to silence the audible portion of this alarm. This period of audible alarm silencing shall not exceed 2 min. (During this period of time the visible alarm shall still be activated.) Means should be provided to remote the audible disconnect alarm's silencing mechanism a minimum of 4 ft and a maximum of 8 ft from the ventilator control panel. Monitoring of breathing circuit integrity may be accomplished utilizing any of several different technologies. The manufacturer shall disclose how breathing circuit integrity is monitored. (See also X2.3.8.2.)

5.11.3.3 *High Airway Pressure*—Alarms for high airway pressure shall be provided. This alarm may either sound immediately when the high alarm pressure limit set point is reached, or at the end of 3 s (see 5.6.3). The audible portion of this alarm may either automatically reset, or may require manual resetting. However, the visual portion of this alarm shall only be provided with a manual resetting mechanism. (See also X2.3.8.3.)

5.11.4 *Alarm Battery Power Supplies*—If any alarm incorporates a battery power supply, the battery should be of a type readily obtainable and the system shall include a means whereby the use may, with a simple operation, determine that the battery needs to be replaced or recharged.

5.11.5 *Alarm Operating Instructions* (see 7.2 and 8.3).

5.12 *Humidification (where applicable)*— Humidifiers that are integral to or recommended for use with critical care ventilators shall comply with the requirements of ANSI Z-79.9, 1978.

5.13 *Electromagnetic Interference*—MDS-201 may be used as a guide during the design and development of mechanical ventilators. This material was developed following a study of specific hospital environments in several areas of the United States (see section 2.4).

5.14 *Kinking and Occlusion of Breathing Tubing*:

5.14.1 *Kinking*—When preconditioned as described in 6.12.1, and tested as outlined in 6.12.2, tubing shall be sufficiently rigid (for example, wire guarded or wound) or so constructed (for example, corrugated) as to minimize the possibility of kinking. (See also X2.3.9.1.)

5.14.2 *Occlusion*—When preconditioned as described in 6.12.1, and tested as outlined in 6.12.3, the tubing shall be designed so as to prevent occlusion when a 2.5-kg weight bears on a 5-cm segment in the middle of a 1 m length of tubing. (See also X2.3.9.2.)

5.15 *Measurement of Oxygen Concentration*—The manufacturer shall either provide an oxygen monitor with the ventilator or shall recommend a monitor for use with the ventilator. If no oxygen monitor is provided with the ventilator, the manufacturer shall make provisions to facilitate the mounting of an oxygen analyzer on the ventilator and for the connection of an oxygen analyzer in the ventilator circuit.

5.15.1 If provided with the ventilator or recommended for use with a ventilator, the oxygen analyzer shall comply with the requirements of ANSI Z-79.10, 1979.

6. Test Methods

6.1 *General*—Measurements of pressure, flow, and volume shall be made as shown in Figs. 1 and 2, and shall be accurate to within ±2.5 % of the reading plus ±2.5 % of the full scale reading. The reading accuracy of the recording device shall be maintained at frequencies up to 10 Hz. Ambient conditions shall be recorded and converted to NTPD (20°C, 760 mm Hg, 0 % relative humidity). Dry air shall be used as the test gas unless specified otherwise in the individual test method.

6.2 *Test Equipment*:

6.2.1 *Lung Models*—Lung models are designed to provide impedances to the ventilator output that simulate both normal and diseased lung states. The impedances to ventilator output are lung elastance and airflow resistance, which can be simulated in the lung models by a compliance and a resistance connected in series (see Figs. 1 and 2). The various combinations of compliances and resistances used in the test procedures are given in Table 2. The passive lung model in Fig. 2 is intended for the testing of the controlled ventilation mode (see Appendix X1) only. Fig. 3 illustrates an active test system for the testing of IMV modes and other ventilator functions. These lung models do not preclude the development of different or more sophisticated lung models with the same ranges of compliance and linear or nonlinear resistances. If nonlinear resistances are used, their characteristics must be specified.

6.2.2 *Compliances*—The required compliances are given in Table 4. These compliances shall include the compliances of all components of the lung model system. The volume-pressure characteristics of the model compliances including connections shall be determined as in 6.1 and shall be within ±5 % of the required compliance values shown in Table 4 throughout a range of inspiratory gage pressures from − 1.96 to + 9.80 kPa (−20 to + 100 cm H_2O) and throughout a range of inspiratory phase times as specified by the manufacturer.

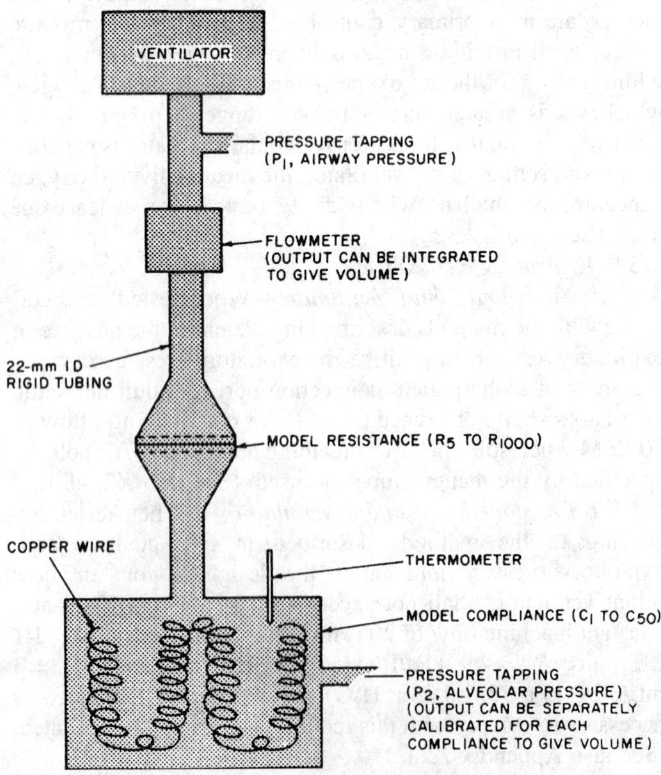

FIG. 2 Representative Passive Lung Model

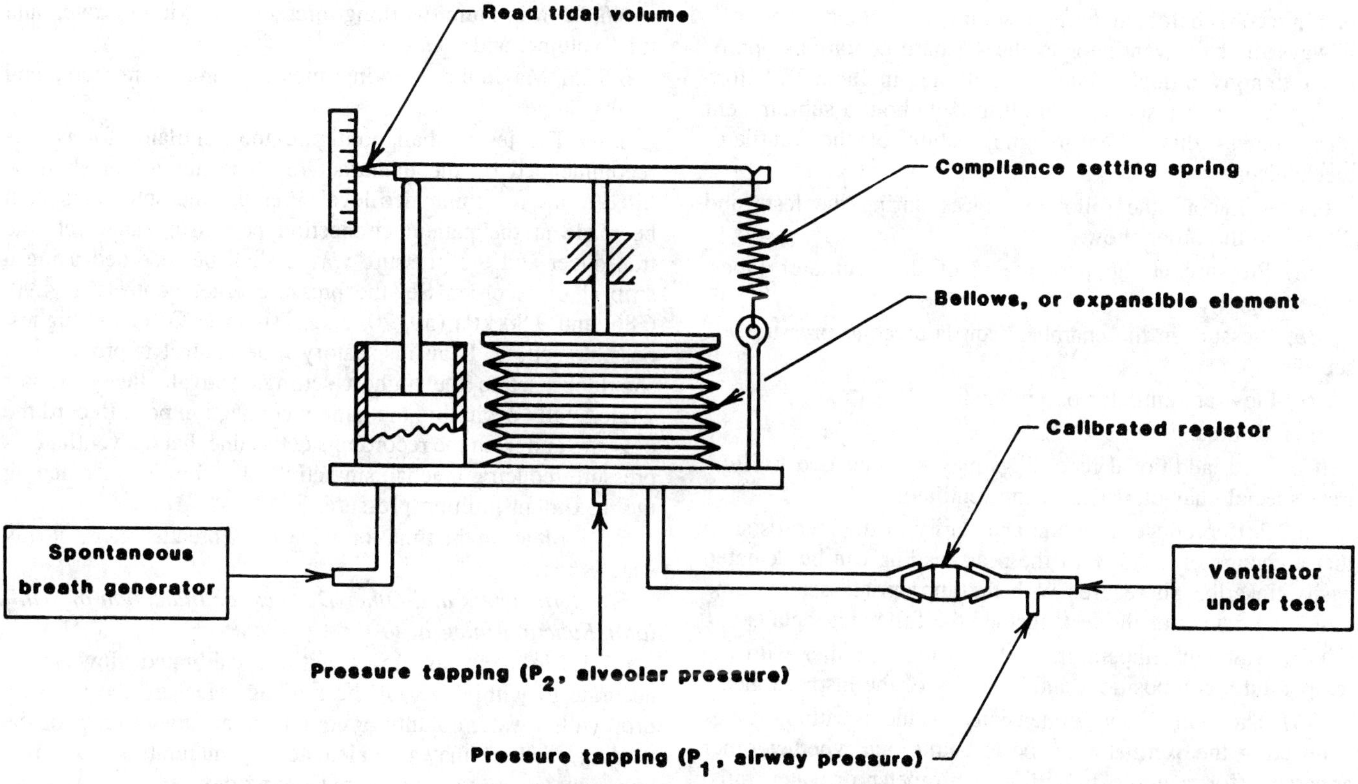

FIG. 3 Representative Active Lung Model

TABLE 4 Required Compliances

Compliance	Value	
	mL/kPa	(mL/cm H_2O)
*C*50	510	(50)
*C*20	204	(20)
*C*10	102	(10)
*C*3	30.6	(3)
*C*1	10.2	(1)

6.2.3 *Resistances*—The required resistances are given in Tables 5 and 6. These values relate to dry air at ambient pressure and at 20C. They include the resistance of the flow measuring device.

6.3 *Test Procedures—General*— This section includes one test for endurance and two tests for performance. Perform the endurance test first and the performance tests immediately thereafter. Routine maintenance as specified by the manufacturer may be carried out during these tests, but include details of all such maintenance in the test report.

6.3.1 *Endurance Test*—Make the inspiratory/expiratory phase time ratio as close to 1:2 as possible, and run the ventilator for 2000 h against the appropriate condition shown in Table 1. If provided, run IMV or SIMV functions at ten breaths per minute, with an additional ten breaths being provided by the machine. Otherwise the frequency of ventilation shall be as listed in Table 1.

6.3.2 *Wave-form Performance Test*—At the beginning of the test, adjust the ventilator controls to obtain the desired frequency and tidal volume at an inspiratory/expiratory ratio that is as close to 1:2 as possible. Record the ventilator control positions required to obtain these settings. If it is necessary to reset the ventilator controls to match the ventilator to the new set of conditions, note this in the results. In such an event,

TABLE 5 Required Resistances (Linear)

Resistance	Value in Flow Range		Range of Airflow (L/s)
	±20 % kPa/L/s	(cm H_2O/L/s)	
*R*5	0.49	(5)	0 to 2.0
*R*20	1.96	(20)	0 to 1.0
*R*50	4.90	(50)	0 to 0.5
*R*200	19.6	(200)	0 to 0.1
*R*500	49.0	(500)	0 to 0.075
*R*1000	98.1	(1000)	0 to 0.05

TABLE 6 Required Resistances (Parabolic)[A]

Parabolic Resistor	K ± 10 %	Pressure Drop		@	Flow (L/s)
		$\Delta P = K \dot{V}^2$ cm H_2O ($\dot{V}$ = L/s)			
		kPa	(cm H_2O)		
R_p5	2.70	0.26	(2.70)	@	1.0
		1.06	(10.80)	@	2.0
R_p20	17.61	0.43	(4.40)	@	0.5
		1.73	(17.60)	@	1.0
R_p50	108.70	0.67	(6.79)	@	0.25
		2.67	(27.20)	@	0.5
R_p200	2440.00	0.60	(6.10)	@	0.05
		2.39	(24.40)	@	0.1

[A] Linear and parabolic resistances may be used interchangeably. Representative test lungs and the appropriate parabolic resistances available from Michigan Instruments, Inc., 6300 28th Street, SE, Grand Rapids, MI 49506; BioTek Instruments, Highland Park, Winooski, VT 05404; or Hyco-Anlas Ganthier, S.A., Bureau a Paris, 13, rue Guyton-de-Morveau, 75013 Paris, France, or their equivalents have been found satisfactory for this purpose. Resistances will have different performance values, depending on the manufacturer and the individual resistor configuration. The ventilator manufacturer shall supply data on the resistors used during testing upon request.

obtain records before and after resetting the ventilator controls. Always reset the ventilator to the standard conditions appropriate to a given tidal volume (as indicated in Table 2), before each subsequent test. Perform all tests without a sub-ambient phase unless this is an integral feature of the ventilator mechanism.

6.3.2.1 Record the following traces during the tests and display in the order shown:

(a) Pressure at the patient end of the ventilator tubes, P_1(see Fig. 1),

(b) Pressure in the chamber (equals alveolar pressure P_2, see Fig. 1),

(c) Flow at ventilator output, and

(d) Volume.

If desired, additional recordings may be appended to illustrate special characteristics of the ventilator.

6.3.2.2 Reproduce the scale and clarity of the records such that a change of ±2.5 % of the peak reading can be detected easily. Inscribe all records with the appropriate scales, time base, and details of the test. Include the following details:

(a) Ambient temperature and pressure, together with the temperature, composition, and humidity of the inspired gas.

(b) The nature and dimensions of the breathing tubes connecting the ventilator to the test lung and whether other apparatus (for example, humidifier, spirometer, or water traps) were included in the part of the circuit which is pressurized during inspiration. If such apparatus is included, the type and position shall be specified. If a humidifier is included it shall be filled to the "full" water level with a relatively noncompressible substance. If this is not practicable, the humidifier shall be replaced with an equivalent compliance and resistance.

(c) A listing of all settings of controls, as applicable.

(d) Any other relevant information (for example, source and pressure of driving gas, use of special ventilator circuits, or type of humidifier).

6.4 Inspect the sterilization or disinfection instructions as supplied by the manufacturer.

6.5 Vary the gas supply pressure and electrical supply voltage independently and perform the tests in 6.3.2 under the worst possible conditions. That is, Test No. 4 for adults, children, and infants, respectively. These tests are to be conducted at both the upper and lower extremes as indicated in 5.5.1 and 5.5.2.

6.6 *Accuracy of Calibrated Controls, Indicators, and Pressure Relief Devices*:

6.6.1 Connect the device to a calibrated test apparatus (generally with an accuracy five times greater than the required accuracy), and test the accuracy of the controls over the entire range.

6.6.2 Either set the maximum limited pressure ($P_{L\ max}$) control above the test point for the $P_{w\ max}$ control or temporarily inactivate the $P_{L\ max}$ control. Occlude the ventilator output to the patient system, and verify that the $P_{w\ max}$ control functions within the limits specified in 5.6.1.1 when the ventilator is configured in each of the test modes listed below:

6.6.2.1 Minimum working pressure, minimum rate, and tidal volume,

6.6.2.2 Minimum working pressure, maximum rate, and tidal volume, and

6.6.2.3 Maximum working pressure, maximum rate, and tidal volume.

6.6.3 The tester shall configure the ventilator for use as recommended by the manufacturer. The humidifier shall be filled to the recommended level. Pressure measurements shall be made at the patient connection port using an electronic transducer and the pressure waves shall be recorded using a strip chart recorder. Set the pressure relief controls at 4.90, 6.86, and 9.80 kPa (50, 70, and 100 cm H_2O) or the highest possible setting. If an inspiratory time control is provided, it should be set to the highest setting. Activate the ventilator while totally occluding the patient connection port. Record the pressure and from the recordings determine that the ventilator's pressure reducing mechanism activated within 3 s of reaching the maximum limiting pressure.

6.6.4 Measure the time for at least 100 breaths after a steady state is reached.

6.7 *Spirometers and Other Devices for Indication of Ventilator Function Integral to the Ventilator*:

6.7.1 Measure gas flows with a calibrated flow meter accurate to within 5 % of the reading. Measure the pressure drop with a water column or equivalent accurate to 5 % of the reading. Volume may be calculated by integrating flow over one cycle, or by volumetric measuring device.

6.7.2 Test the spirometer in an ambient environment with the temperature of 20 to 24°C. Set ventilator humidifiers on the maximum output and run the ventilator in a steady state for 8 h with a reservoir bag of at least 1.5 L volume attached to the ventilator outlet. Determine that accuracy requirements of 5.7.2 have been met at the end of the 8-h test.

6.8 *Characteristics of Delivered Gas*— Measure delivered oxygen concentrations at the allowable extremes of pipeline pressures, that is, at 41.2 psig and 66 psig. Also measure concentrations at the extremes of resistance and compliance and before and after all ventilator changes during the *Endurance and Wave Form Performance Tests.* Collect gases from ten breaths and record the reading when the analyzer has reached a steady state.

6.9 *Expiratory Resistance*:

6.9.1 *Adult*:

6.9.1.1 Generate 50 L/min of gas flow through the patient breathing system with no PEEP.

6.9.1.2 Measure the pressure drop from the patient connection port to ambient. Pressure shall not exceed 0.49 kPa (5 cm H_2O).

6.9.2 *Infant*:

6.9.2.1 Generate 20 L/min of gas flow through the patient breathing system with no PEEP.

6.9.2.2 Connect a simulated patient with a resistance of 4.9 kPa/L/s (50 cm H_2O/L/s) and a compliance of 30 mL/kPa (3 mL/cm H_2O) to the circuit.

6.9.2.3 Cycle the ventilator at 60 breaths per minute, 1:1 I:E ratio.

6.9.2.4 Measure the pressure drop from the patient connection to ambient. Pressure shall not exceed 0.29 kPa (3 cm H_2O).

6.10 *Fittings Connecting Adult Ventilator, Patient, and Spirometer*:

6.10.1 Visually inspect the connector and attempt to change connector direction.

6.10.2 Inspect the ventilator in its normal configuration as supplied by the manufacturer.

6.10.3 Attempt to fit a 15, 19, or 22-mm fitting into the spirometer outlet.

6.10.4 Attempt to connect the fittings listed in 5.10.4 to the air inlet. Check the marking to assure that, if provided, the inlet is marked as required in 5.10.4.

6.10.5 Attempt to connect the fittings listed in 5.10.5 to the expired gas outlet. The test is passed if none of the connectors will provide a secure fit.

6.11 *Alarm Systems*—Connect the power supply to the ventilator and run according to the manufacturer's instructions. Then disconnect the ventilator from the main power supply, and determine that the alarm sounds, and maintains a constant sound pressure level ± 3 dBa, for at least 2 min. Repeat the test as outlined above, and silence the loss of main power supply alarm. Reconnect the ventilator main power immediately after silencing the alarm, and then disconnect the ventilator from the main power supply again and determine that the alarm silencing mechanism has reset.

6.12 *Kinking and Occlusion of Breathing Tubing*:

6.12.1 *Preconditioning of Tubing*—Condition all tubing at 42°C and 100 % relative humidity for 1 h prior to testing as outlined below.

6.12.2 *Kinking*—Suspend a length of tubing at least 1 m long over a metal cylinder with a 2.5-cm diameter, all at room temperature. Hang a 0.5-Kg weight on each end, and establish a steady 75 L/min flow (25 L/min for tubing smaller than 22 mm inside diameter which is intended for use with infants and neonates) through the tubing and measure the pressure above atmospheric pressure (Δ P) necessary to drive the flow through the tubing. The test is passed if Δ P is less than 0.98 kPa (10 cm H_2O).

6.12.3 Place a 2.5-Kg weight on a 5-cm segment in the middle of a 1-m length of tubing. Establish a steady 75 L/min flow (25 L/min for tubing smaller than 22 mm inside diameter which is intended for use with infants and neonates) through the tubing and measure the pressure above atmospheric pressure (Δ P) necessary to drive the flow through the tubing. The test is passed if Δ P is less than 0.98 kPa (10 cm H_2O).

7. Warnings and Markings

7.1 If an ambient air inlet is provided, it shall be clearly marked as *air inlet*.

7.2 *Alarm Operating Instructions*—The manufacturer shall provide instructions for testing and setting of the alarms. These instructions (abbreviated if necessary) shall be either permanently marked on or attached to the ventilator or ventilator alarm. (See also X2.3.10.)

8. Operation and Maintenance Manual

8.1 *Apparatus Internal Compliance*— The manufacturer shall disclose the internal compliance of the ventilator and shall provide, upon request, the test methods used to determine the derived values. Manufacturers of ventilator tubing that recommend the use of their tubing with several ventilators, or who do not manufacture ventilators, shall provide the data on tubing compliance on the labeling of their product. (See also X2.3.11.1.)

8.2 *Measurement of Oxygen Concentration*—The manufacturer shall either provide an oxygen monitor with the ventilator or shall recommend a monitor for use with the ventilator.

8.3 *Alarm Operating Instructions*—The manufacturer shall provide instructions for testing and setting of the alarms. These instructions (abbreviated if necessary) shall be either permanently marked on or attached to the ventilator or ventilator alarm. (See also X2.3.11.2.)

8.4 *Assisted Ventilation, or Synchronous Intermittent Mandatory Ventilation*—If the ventilator incorporates a mode of operation where the patient effort initiates a mechanical (for example, assisted, SIMV) breath, then the manufacturer shall disclose the following parameters as applicable: inspiratory triggering pressure, differential inspiratory triggering pressure, inspiratory triggering flow, inspiratory triggering volume, and inspiratory triggering response time.

8.4.1 The manufacturer shall disclose the conditions under which this information was obtained. The manufacturer shall also disclose the recommended patient breathing system (and its characteristics) used in these tests. (See also X2.3.11.3.)

APPENDIXES

(Nonmandatory Information)

X1. CLASSIFICATION AND TYPES OF BREATHING MACHINES

X1.1 *Lung Ventilator*—An automatic device that is connected to the patient's airway and is designed to augment or provide for the patient's ventilation.

X1.1.1 There are four types of lung ventilators:

X1.1.1.1 *Controller*— A device, or mode of operation of a device, that inflates the patient's lungs independently of the patient's inspiratory effort.

X1.1.1.2 *Assister*—A device designed to augment the patient's breathing synchronously with his inspiratory effort.

X1.1.1.3 *Assister-Controller*—An apparatus that is designed to function either as an assister or a controller, and that may, in default of the patient's inspiratory effort, automatically function as a controller.

X1.1.1.4 *Assister-Controller—Spontaneous Breathing*— Those devices that incorporate various modes of operation which allow the patient to breath spontaneously (1) at or above ambient pressure levels or, (2) with or without supplemental mandatory positive pressure breaths.

X1.2 *Resuscitator*—A portable device used in emergency situations to provide lung ventilation to individuals whose breathing is inadequate. Resuscitators are classified according to their prime movers as follows: (1) operator-powdered, (2) gas-powered, or (3) electrically powered. Auxiliary apparatus and methods for use in emergency situations are classified as follows: (1) manual resuscitation, or (2) exhaled air (mouth-to-mouth or mouth-to-nose) resuscitation.

X1.3 *Respiratory Therapy Ventilator*—A device that is connected to the patient's airway and is primarily designed to deliver an aerosol along with augmented ventilation.

X1.4 *External Body Ventilator*—A machine designed to augment or replace the patient's ventilation by means of the application of intermittent or alternating pressures to the trunk.

X1.4.1 External body ventilators are classified as follows:

X1.4.1.1 *Tank or cabinet*— An external body ventilator in which the patient is enclosed to his neck in a rigid airtight chamber.

X1.4.1.2 *Cuirass*—An external body ventilator in which all or part of the patient's trunk is in an airtight enclosure, forming or incorporating a rigid frame.

X1.4.1.3 *Belt*—An external pneumatic body ventilator consisting of a flexible wrapper which contains an airtight bag wrapped around the patient's abdomen. When inflated, the bag produces forced expiration, followed by inspiration upon deflation.

X1.5 *Rocking Apparatus*—A device used to produce or aid ventilation by rocking the patient and using the weight of the abdominal contents to move the diaphgram.

X1.6 *Electrostimulator*—Apparatus in which activity of the respiratory muscles is induced by electric impulses acting on the corresponding nerves or muscles.

X1.7 *High Frequency Ventilators*—Those ventilators that employ a frequency of greater than 2.5 Hz.

X1.8 *Characteristics of Lung Ventilators*—An outline of the modes of operation of lung ventilators is given in 2.1.1 through 2.1.9.[7]

X1.8.1 *Modes of Operation During the Inspiratory or Expiratory Phase*:

X1.8.1.1 Flow Generator
X1.8.1.2 Pressure Generator
X1.8.1.3 Combined Flow and Pressure Generator
X1.8.2 *Volume Control*:
X1.8.2.1 Pressure Preset
X1.8.2.2 Volume Preset
(*a*) Tidal
(*b*) Minute
X1.8.2.3 Combined
X1.8.3 *Cycling Control*:
X1.8.3.1 *Inspiration to Expiration*
(*a*) Volume
(*b*) Pressure
(*c*) Time
(*d*) Flow
(*e*) Combined
(*f*) Manual Override
(*g*) Other
X1.8.3.2 *Expiration to Inspiration*:
(*a*) Pressure
(*b*) Time
(*c*) Flow
(*d*) Combined
(*e*) Patient
(*f*) Manual Override
(*g*) Other
X1.8.3.3 *Types of Safety Limits*:
(*a*) Volume
(*b*) Pressure
(*c*) Time
(*d*) Other
X1.8.3.4 *Types of Pressure Patterns*:
(*a*) Positive-ambient
(*b*) Positive-subambient
(*c*) Positive-positive
X1.8.3.5 *Source of Power*:
(*a*) Pneumatic
(*b*) Electric
(*c*) Other
X1.8.3.6 *Power Transmission*:
(*a*) Direct
(*b*) Indirect
X1.8.3.7 *Source of Inspired Gas*:
(*a*) Driving gas
(*b*) Fresh gas
(*c*) Mixed
X1.8.3.8 *Type of Control*:
(*a*) Pneumatic
(*b*) Electronic
(*c*) Mechanical
(*d*) Combined

[7] See also Mushin, W., Rendell-Baker, L., Thompson, P. W., and Mapleson, W. W., *Automatic Ventilation of the Lungs*, Oxford, England. Blackwell, 1980. (Distributed in the U.S.A. by C.V. Mosby, St. Louis, MO.)

X2. RATIONALE

X2.1 Scope

X2.1.1 The scope of this specification is limited to critical care ventilators intended for use in hospitals because the operating environment outside the hospital is considerably different from that found in most hospitals. It was the opinion of the subcommittee that applications such as transport ventilation and ventilation in the home should be addressed in a separate standard. As well, ventilators intended for use during anesthesia have been addressed in another standard because the conditions of operation and the level of supervision present differ greatly from that found in the critical care environment. It was the opinion of the subcommittee that high frequency or jet ventilation had not as yet reached a point where a standard should be developed for devices used to provide this type of patient support.

X2.2 Although ideally all components in the breathing circuit should be sterilizable, certain types of pressure measuring devices cannot be sterilized with currently available methods without causing damage to the device. The same holds true for certain types of oxygen analyzer sensors. These devices should be capable of being disinfected with a high-level disinfectant[8] or should be isolated from other portions of the patient breathing circuit.

X2.3 *Performance Requirements:*

X2.3.1 *Volume Performance Test*—This test is designed to demonstrate that the ventilator can provide adequate ventilation under relatively severe circumstances, that is, low compliance and high resistance. However, the values given in Table 6 are not considered the worst case. These values are instead considered to be median values.

X2.3.2 *Power Sources*— Fluctuations within the ranges specified in 5.1 are known to occur in both electrical and pneumatic power supply systems in hospitals. The causes for such variation may be outside the control of the ventilator user. For example, a decrease in the power supplied by the local electric utility, or the variation that may result from demand for power caused by equipment such as elevator motors and air-handling apparatus within the hospital will cause these types of fluctuations. The periodic testing of emergency generators may also create this type of variation. Pneumatic power sources may show transient variations as well. The filling of liquid oxygen bulk reservoirs and changes in pressure switch settings on compressed air reservoirs are examples of functional variations that could cause the supply pressure to change. The ranges specified will also accommodate the fluctuations that would be anticipated in adapting equipment to European gas piping systems.

X2.3.2.1 The fittings specified in 5.5.2.1 vary from those presently supplied with critical care ventilators. Nut and gland fittings have been specified for the ventilator so that hoses supplying gas to the ventilator may be checked for the correct fittings by threading the connectors on both ends of the hose together. The subcommittee is aware of problems caused by the fitting of the wrong connector to one end of a hose during repair, and by specifying the nut and gland fitting on the ventilator it has provided a means for testing hoses for the appropriate fitting.

X2.3.3 *Accuracy of Calibrated Controls, Indicators, and Pressure Relief Devices*

X2.3.3.1 These control limits were the minimum that the subcommittee felt were acceptable for maintaining the safety of the ventilator and for maintaining operator confidence in ventilator settings.

X2.3.3.2 Maximum working pressure required for adequate patient ventilation will vary with changes in resistance and compliance. If provided, $P_{w\ max}$ controls provide an additional means for assuring that an injurious overpressure incident does not occur.

X2.3.3.3 The subcommittee felt that the requirement as written would reduce the possibility of barotrauma and would also reduce complications resulting from decreased cardiac output secondary to increased intrathoracic pressure, caused when ventilator pressure relief mechanisms *plateaued* in pressure rather than *dumping* the tidal volume to ambient. The subcommittee also felt for this requirement to be truly effective that a combined test should be performed to measure the performance of the limited pressure relief device during the tubing crush and kink tests.

X2.3.3.4 Limits specified in the requirements in 5.6.4 and 5.6.4.1 encompass the range of accuracy that the members of the subcommittee felt were necessary and appropriate for clinical performance and that were achievable within currently available technology.

X2.3.4 *Spirometers and Other Devices for Indication of Ventilator Function Integral to the Ventilator*

X2.3.4.1 The accuracy specified in this requirement will allow the clinician to adjust the ventilator tidal volume according to the physiologic dead space and carbon dioxide production of the patient or for other causes.

X2.3.4.2 Visual indication that the patient is being adequately ventilated is essential feedback provided to the operator by the spirometer. Partial reduction of flow to the spirometer may cause erroneous indication of ventilator malfunction, and complete occlusion of flow to the spirometer will have the same effect. The latter may render the unit inoperative for some period of time. Condensate formation due to temperature variations in the patient system and occlusion of the tubing by patient secretions are known to be potential causes for this type of malfunction. These potential problems should be compensated for in the design of the spirometer and the spirometer/ventilator interface.

X2.3.5 *Characteristics of Delivered Gas*—Maintaining the accuracy of delivered oxygen concentrations throughout the range of ventilator performance is important in order to allow

[8] See Garner, J. S., "CDC Guidelines for the Prevention and Control of Nosocomial Infections-Guideline for Handwashing and Hospital Environmental Control," *American Journal of Infection Control*, 1986, Section 2, pp. 116–129.

for the rapid and often frequent adjustment of the ventilator without significant variation in the oxygen concentration. The range of accuracy for oxygen analyzers in ANSI Z-79.10[3] is specified as ±3 % oxygen. Limiting the fluctuation to this level at any given ventilator setting is technologically possible, and will minimize the time spent making control adjustments. This should enhance operator confidence in the accuracy of control settings provided on the gas mixing device.

X2.3.6 *Expiratory Resistance:*

X2.3.6.1 *Adult*—Although expiratory resistances of less than 5 cm H_2O at 50 L/min are desirable, the subcommittee realizes that such values may not be uniformly achievable. Patient system configurations, tubing length, connector sizes, and gas flow through the system are all factors that may combine to raise end-expiratory pressure to the 0.49 kPa (5 cm H_2O) maximum under certain ventilator settings. End-expiratory resistance above the 0.49 kPa (5 cm H_2O) level are not acceptable because of the adverse effect they may have on the patient's respiratory pattern or cardiovascular flow.

X2.3.6.2 *Infant*—Positive end-expiratory pressure is inherent in the design of constant flow infant ventilators, and is caused by a combination of three factors: ventilator setting, patient circuit components, and the patient's condition. Ventilator inherent PEEP will increase because of an increase in either the machine flow, the resistance of the patient circuit, or patient expiratory flow. The level of positive end-expiratory pressure will also increase because of a decrease in the expiratory phase time. The increase in positive end-expiratory pressure may be nonlinear with respect to a linear increase in machine flow.

X2.3.7 *Fittings Connecting Adult Ventilator, Patient, and Spirometer*

X2.3.7.1 Flow-direction-sensitive devices such as one-way valves or humidifiers may be caused to malfunction by inadvertent connection in the reverse manner, and it is also possible for injury to the patient to occur if flows of gas are misdirected or humidifier contents are emptied into the breathing circuit as a result of such a misconnection.

X2.3.7.2 The positioning of the connector for a bag mount, if provided, is important so that it is not mistaken for a connector to a patient breathing tube. The marking of the connector is important for the same reason.

X2.3.7.3 This requirement is intended to minimize the possibility of inappropriate connection of the ventilator breathing circuit tubing to the spirometer outlet.

X2.3.7.4 The sizes of fittings outlined in 5.10.4 are commonly used for other types of apparatus on ventilators and should be prevented from being connected to the air inlet. Marking the inlet will also minimize the possibility of this occurring.

X2.3.7.5 The sizes of fittings listed in 5.10.5 are commonly used for other purposes on mechanical ventilators and connection of these tubings of the expired gas port could result in ventilator malfunction.

X2.3.8 *Alarm Systems*

X2.3.8.1 The subcommittee felt that a loss of main power supply alarm with a duration of 2 min was adequate to allow personnel to reach the ventilator and determine the cause of the alarm. The subcommittee also felt that a means for silencing this alarm when main power was disconnected was important in order to minimize the number of spurious alarm signals in the critical care environment. If such a means for silencing an alarm was not provided, every time the ventilator was disconnected to be moved from the patient area, the loss of main power alarm would sound for 2 min, distracting personnel. However, the subcommittee also felt that the means of silencing the loss of main power alarm should not be remote from the ventilator proper, and that when the alarm sounded the operator should be forced to walk to the ventilator to determine the cause of the alarm and correct the situation.

X2.3.8.2 Because breathing circuit disconnection can result in serious injury or death, the alarm used to indicate this event should be of the highest priority. Alarm response within 15 s or one ventilator cycle will allow for appropriate alarm setting when using IMV modes with slow ventilatory rates. The audible alarm should not be capable of being silenced for longer than 2 min because disconnection for longer than this period without an alarm could result in serious patient injury. Activation of the visual alarm during this 2 min audible delay will provide indication that the alarm is still functioning. In many clinical environments it is not possible to position the mechanical ventilator so that the alarm can be silenced from the operator's work position. As well, it may be necessary to silence the alarm for longer than 2 min (repeated activation of the delay) while wearing sterile gloves. Both of these problems have led to disconnect alarms being shut off. The failure to turn the alarm back on and a subsequent disconnection has been reported to have caused injuries and deaths. If an optional means for remoting the alarm silencing mechanism is provided, the user can then determine when this may be necessary, given the clinical environment where the ventilator is to be applied. Because of the various technologies available to provide this type of alarm function, no specification of a particular type of alarm has been made in this draft. The manufacturer should provide the user with a detailed explanation of how this alarm function is accomplished.

X2.3.8.3 Alarms for high airway pressure are necessary to indicate potentially injurious conditions that may be the result of either ventilator malfunction or change in patient pathophysiology. Often these alarms occur intermittently and the condition creating the alarm will have been cleared by the time the operator reaches the bedside. For this reason, the visual signal indicating that an overpressure condition has occurred should remain for operator information. The 3-s delay is permitted in order to minimize the possibility that transient conditions of short duration will cause spurious alarm signals.

X2.3.9 *Kinking and Occlusion of Tubing*:

X2.3.9.1 It is often necessary for ventilator tubing to be placed over the top of bedrails, or through the top or doors of incubators where the tubing may be subject to kinking. The tests outlined for this requirement are intended to simulate these conditions.

X2.3.9.2 It is often necessary for ventilator tubing to be placed in areas around the patient where it may be occluded (for example, movement of the patient's head onto the tubing, etc.). Tests for requirement 5.14.2 are intended to simulate this type of occlusion.

X2.3.10 *Warnings and Markings*—The permanent marking or attachment of the instructions to the ventilator or ventilator alarm is necessary because often these devices are used where the general instruction manual is not readily available.

X2.3.11 *Operation and Maintenance Manual*:

X2.3.11.1 *Apparatus Internal Compliance*—Increasing internal compliance will (1) decrease the actual volume delivered to the patient from a *set* volume, (2) increase measured volume above the patient's actual minute volume, and (3) decrease the pressure at the patient (both proximal and lung pressures) if not compensated for by the ventilator.

X2.3.11.2 *Alarm Operating Instructions*—The permanent marking or attachment of the instructions to the ventilator or ventilator alarm is necessary because often these devices are used where the general instruction manual is not readily available.

X2.3.11.3 *Assisted Ventilation, or Synchronous Intermittent Mandatory Ventilation*—The information required in 8.4 will allow the clinician to decide whether the ventilator is appropriate for application with a particular patient population, and whether one type of ventilator may be used for several different patient groups, that is, infants and adults.

Designation: F 1101 – 90 (Reapproved 1996)

Standard Specification for Ventilators Intended for Use During Anesthesia[1]

This standard is issued under the fixed designation F 1101; the number immediately following the designation indicates the year of original adoption or, in the case of revision, the year of last revision. A number in parentheses indicates the year of last reapproval. A superscript epsilon (ε) indicates an editorial change since the last revision or reapproval.

1. Scope

1.1 This specification applies to all ventilators specifically introduced for sale following acceptance of this specification and intended for use during the administration of anesthesia. Definitions, performance requirements, test methods, and a rationale for all mandatory requirements are included.

1.2 The anesthesia ventilator cannot protect against malfunctions within the anesthesia machine, nor can it protect against inappropriate or inadvertent use of the oxygen flush valve, and therefore, no attempt has been made to address problems that may arise from malfunctions with these devices in this specification. (See also X3.1.)

1.3 Several definitions have been included in Section 2 and Appendix X1 that are not used in the text of this specification. This material has been included for the sake of completeness, and for any possible educational benefit that may be served. Appendix X1 also outlines various characteristics of ventilators intended for use during anesthesia and defines the main classes of breathing machines that may be used in medical practice and indicates how these may be subdivided according to their mode of action.

1.4 The following precautionary caveat pertains to the test methods portion, Section 6 of this specification. *This standard may involve hazardous materials, operations, and equipment. This standard does not purport to address all of the safety concerns associated with its use. It is the responsibility of the user of this standard to establish appropriate safety and health practices and determine the applicability of regulatory limitations prior to use.* For an additional safety precaution, see Note 6.

2. Referenced Documents

2.1 *ASTM Standards:*

F 1054 Specification for Conical Fittings of 15-mm and 22-mm Sizes[2]

F 1161 Specification for Minimum Performance and Safety Requirements for Components and Systems of Anesthesia Gas Machines[2]

2.2 *ANSI Standards:*

Z-79.10 Standard for Oxygen Analyzers[3]

Z-79.11 Standard for Scavenging Systems for Excess for Anesthetic Gases[3]

2.3 *ISO Standard:*

ISO 4135 Anesthesiology Vocabulary[4]

2.4 *Other Standards:*

IEC 601-1 Safety of Medical Electrical Equipment[5]

CGA V-5, 1978 Specifications for DISS Connections[6]

3. Terminology

3.1 *Definitions*—For the purposes of this specification, the definitions in 3.1.1-3.1.51 shall apply.

3.1.1 *airway pressure* (P_{aw})—pressure at a specified point in the patient's airway. The site and conditions under which measurements are made should be given.

3.1.2 *alarm*—a means of alerting the operator that a particular condition exists.

3.1.3 *alveolar pressure* (P_A)—pressure in the alveoli. In the case of the lung model, this is represented by the pressure in the compliance chamber.

3.1.4 *apparatus internal compliance*—volume/pressure relationship, expressed in millilitres per kilopascal (or millilitres per centimetre H_2O) of those portions of the patient system that are pressurized during the inspiratory phase time (see also 5.8 and 3.1.36).

3.1.5 *continuous positive airway pressure (CPAP)*—P_{aw} maintained by the ventilator above ambient.

3.1.5.1 *Discussion*—Common usage of the term references spontaneous ventilation.

3.1.6 *control*—a means available to the operator of directly adjusting a ventilator function.

3.1.7 *cycling pressure*—that pressure which, when reached in the patient system, causes the ventilator to cycle from inspiratory to expiratory phase or from expiratory to inspiratory phase.

3.1.8 *differential inspiratory triggering pressure* (ΔP_{tr})—change in airway pressure at the patient connection port which

[1] This specification is under the jurisdiction of ASTM Committee F-29 on Anesthetic and Respiratory Equipmentand is the direct responsibility of Subcommittee F29.10on Anesthesia Workstations.

Current edition approved April 4, 1990. Published May 1990.

[2] *Annual Book of ASTM Standards*, Vol 13.01.

[3] Available from the American National Standards Institute, 1430 Broadway, New York, NY 10018.

[4] Available from International Standards Organization, 1, Rue de Varembe, Case postale 56, CH-1211.

[5] Available from International Electrotechnical Commission, 3 rue de Varembé, 1211 Geneva 20, Switzerland.

[6] Available from Compressed Gas Association, 1235 Jefferson Davis Highway, Arlington, VA 22202.

must be generated by the patient to initiate the ventilator inspiratory phase.

3.1.8.1 *Discussion*—Pressure shall be expressed in terms of gage pressure in units of kilopascals (or centimetres H_2O) to follow the kPa units.

3.1.9 *expiratory pause time* (T_{EP})— interval from the end of expiratory flow to the start of inspiratory flow.

3.1.10 *expiratory phase time* (T_E)— interval from the start of expiratory flow to the start of inspiratory flow.

3.1.11 *expiratory positive airway pressure (EPAP)*—P_{aw} above ambient during the expiratory phase, generally approximated by P_{ps}.

3.1.12 *expiratory (sub-atmospheric) subambient pressure*—pressure lower than ambient, during the expiratory phase time.

3.1.12.1 *Discussion*—Subambient pressure may be constant throughout the expiratory phase time or it may vary through the phase time, depending upon the method by which such pressure is generated.

3.1.13 *frequency (ventilatory) (f)*—number of breathing cycles per minute.

3.1.14 *heat and moisture exchanger (HME)*—a passive device which is designed to converse some of the patient's exhaled moisture and heat, and to release heat and moisture to the patient's airway during inspiration.

3.1.15 *high priority alarm*—signal which indicates a condition requiring immediate action.

3.1.16 *inspiratory-expiratory phase time ratio (I:E ratio)*—ratio of the inspiratory phase time to the expiratory phase time.

3.1.17 *inspiratory minute volume* ($\dot{V}_I$)—volume of gas inspired per minute by the patient, measured in litres (L).

3.1.18 *inspiratory pause time* (T_{IP})— interval from the end of inspiratory flow to the start of expiratory flow.

3.1.19 *inspiratory phase time* (T_I)— interval from the start of inspiratory flow to the start of expiratory flow.

3.1.20 *inspiratory positive airway pressure (IPAP)*—P_{aw} above ambient during the inspiratory phase of CPAP, generally approximated by P_{ps}.

3.1.21 *inspiratory triggering flow* ($\dot{V}_{Tr}$)—flow which must be generated by the patient at the patient connection port to initiate the ventilator inspiratory phase.

3.1.22 *inspiratory triggering pressure* (P_{tr})—airway pressure at the patient connection port which must be generated by the patient to initiate the ventilator inspiratory phase.

3.1.23 *inspiratory triggering response time* (T_{tr})—time delay between the satisfaction of the inspiratory triggering pressure or flow, or both, volume requirements, and the start of inspiratory flow.

3.1.24 *inspiratory triggering volume* (V_{tr})—volume, measured at the patient connection port, which must be moved by the patient to initiate the ventilator inspiratory phase.

3.1.25 *intermittent mandatory ventilation (IMV)*— a mode of operation of the ventilator that permits spontaneous breathing of a controlled inspiratory gas mixture between predetermined ventilator-delivered breaths using the same inspiratory gas mixture.

3.1.26 *low priority alarm*—signal which indicates a condition which requires operator awareness, but not necessarily action.

3.1.27 *maximum limited pressure* ($P_{L\,max}$)—highest gage pressure which can be attained in the patient system during malfunction of the ventilator but with functioning safety mechanisms.

3.1.27.1 *Discussion*—The title of this definition is different from the title given in ISO 4135. However, the text is identical to ISO 4135. The title of the ISO definition is *maximum safety pressure*.

3.1.28 *maximum working pressure* ($P_{w\,max}$)—highest gage pressure which can be attained in the patient system during the inspiratory phase when the ventilator is functioning normally.

3.1.28.1 *Discussion*—This may be limited by a controllable ventilator mechanism to less than $P_{L\,max}$.

3.1.29 *medium priority alarm*—signal which indicates a condition requiring prompt action.

3.1.30 *minimum limited pressure* ($P_{L\,min}$)—highest numerical value of sub-atmospheric gage pressure which can be attained in the patient system during malfunction of the ventilator but with functioning safety mechanisms.

3.1.30.1 *Discussion*—The title of this definition is different from the title given in ISO 4135. However, the text is identical to ISO 4135. The title of the ISO definition is *minimum safety pressure*.

3.1.31 *minimum working pressure* ($P_{w\,min}$)—highest numerical value of sub-atmospheric gage pressure which can be attained in the patient system during the expiratory phase when the ventilator is functioning normally.

3.1.31.1 *Discussion*—This may be limited by a controllable ventilator mechanism to a sub-atmospheric pressure that is numerically smaller than $P_{L\,min}$.

3.1.32 *minute volume* ($\dot{V}$)—volume of gas, expressed in litres per minute, entering or leaving the patient or lung model. The physical conditions under which measuring was made should be given.

3.1.33 *monitor (indicator display)*—a means of informing the operator of the status or numerical value of ventilation or a ventilator.

3.1.34 *nebulizing humidifier*—device designed to add water to the inspired gas in the form of droplets.

3.1.35 *negative end expiratory pressure (NEEP)*— the P_{ps} at the end of expiration, below ambient.

3.1.36 *patient system*—that part of the gas system of a ventilator through which respired gas travels at appropriate respiratory pressures.

3.1.37 *patient system compliance*—volume/pressure relationship, expressed in millilitres per kilopascals (or millilitres per centimetre H_2O) of those portions of the patient system that are pressurized during the inspiratory phase time.

3.1.38 *positive end-expiratory pressure (PEEP)*—P_{ps} at the end of expiration, above ambient.

3.1.39 *pressure, patient system* (P_{ps})— pressure at a specified point in the patient system. Conditions under which measurements are made shall be given.

3.1.40 *pressure support*—a ventilator mode designed to augment the patient's ventilation synchronously with his inspiratory effort until a preset pressure is met.

3.1.41 *selector valve*—a valve that routes the breathing

mixture to the breathing bag of the anesthesia circuit or to a ventilator.

3.1.42 *sigh (ventilator)*—deliberate increase in tidal volume for one or more breaths at intervals.

3.1.43 *spirometer*—device designed to measure a volume of gas.

3.1.44 *synchronous intermittent mandatory ventilation (SIMV)*—an IMV mode which provides a mechanism for synchronizing the ventilator-delivered breaths with a patient's inspiration, as detected by the ventilator.

3.1.45 *tidal volume* (V_T)—volume of gas, expressed in millilitres (mL), entering or leaving the patient or the lung model during the inspiratory or expiratory phase time. The physical conditions under which gas volumes are measured should be given.

3.1.46 *time constant*—time in which an exponential process is 63 % complete.

3.1.47 *vaporizing humidifier*—device designed to add water to the inspired gas in the form of vapor.

3.1.48 *ventilator expiratory resistance*—for ventilators in which expiration is not assisted, the total resistance to gas flow from the patient connection port through the expiratory port of the patient system to atmosphere. This is expressed in kilopascals (or centimetres H_2O) referred to a flow of 0.5 L/s.

3.1.48.1 *Discussion*—This definition is applicable in those types of ventilators in which expiration is not assisted.

3.1.49 *ventilator-patient system*—that part of the ventilator gas system through which inspired gas travels at respiratory pressures.

3.1.50 *ventilators intended for use with anesthesia*—ventilator designed to be used with or integral to an anesthesia breathing system.

3.1.51 *ventilator pressure* (P_{vent})— pressure at a specified point in the ventilator. The site and conditions under which measurements are made should be given.

3.2 *Symbols:Symbols:*

3.2.1 *C*—indicates compliance in units of mL/kPa (or mL/cm H_2O), for example, C20 = 20 mL/kPa (20 mL/cm H_2O).

3.2.2 *R*—indicates resistance to flow in units of kPa (or cm H_2O)/L/s; for example, *R*5 = 0.5 kPa/L/s (5 cm H_2O/L/s).

3.2.2.1 *Discussion*—For the purposes of clarity, all other abbreviations have been listed in parentheses following the related term or phrase in Section 2.

4. Materials and Manufacture

4.1 *Sterilization or Decontamination or Both*:

4.1.1 All components of the ventilator that come in contact with the patient's respired gases shall be capable of being sterilized, or shall be for single use only. (See also 6.2.)

4.1.2 All external surfaces of the ventilator shall be capable of being disinfected. (See also 6.2 and X3.2.)

5. Performance Requirements

5.1 *Volume and Wave-Form*—The tests in 6.1.3 and 6.1.4 shall be carried out on one or more samples of production ventilators with the assurance that the results, which shall be made available to customers, are representative of all production ventilators of that type. These tests include one test for endurance and two tests for performance. The endurance test shall be performed first and the performance tests immediately thereafter.

5.2 *Ventilator Endurance*—Each tested ventilator (as described in 5.1) shall be tested for endurance with respect to each group of patients for which its use is recommended, that is, for adults, for children, and for infants. A separate machine may be used for each group or the period of tests may be divided equally between groups. Inspiratory/expiratory phase time ratio shall be as close to 1:2 as possible and the ventilator run for 72 h against the appropriate condition shown in Table 1. (See also X3.3.1.)

5.3 *Power Sources*:

5.3.1 *Electrical*—When tested as outlined in 6.3.1, the ventilator shall continue to function within the manufacturer's specifications at any control setting throughout a range of ± 10 % fluctuation of the stated nominal voltage and ±1 % fluctuation of the stated frequency for electrical power sources. For all other aspects, ventilators intended for use during anesthesia shall comply with the electrical requirements of IEC 601-1. (See also X3.3.3.)

NOTE 1—The IEC is presently developing electrical safety standards specifically addressing ventilators. When approved, these will take precedence over the requirements in IEC 601-1.

5.3.2 *Pneumatic*—When tested as outlined in 6.3.1, the ventilator shall continue to function within the manufacturer's specifications at any control setting throughout a range of supply pressures of 55 psig + 20 % and − 25 %. The device's gas connection shall be non-interchangeable. If the device has a threaded connection, it shall conform to the appropriate CGA V-5 1978 specification for DISS connections. If the ventilator is capable of being independently connected to the gas piping system, it shall have permanently attached a Body Fitting number 1240 (oxygen) if intended to be powered by oxygen, or a Body Fitting number 1160 (compressed air) if intended to be powered by air. (See also X3.3.3.)

5.4 *Accuracy of Calibrated Controls, Indicators, and Pressure Relief Devices*:

5.4.1 *Calibrated Working Pressure Control*—If provided, calibrated controls for $P_{w\,max}$ shall be accurate to 0.245 kPa (± 2.5 cm H_2O) up to 2.94 kPa (30 cm H_2O) and to 0.49 kPa (± 5 cm H_2O) above 2.94 kPa (30 cm H_2O) when tested as described in 6.4.1. (See also X3.3.4.1.)

5.4.2 *Indicators*—The manufacturer shall disclose the accuracy of all indicators when tested as outlined in 6.4.1 unless accuracy is otherwise addressed in this draft standard. (See also X3.3.4.2.)

5.4.3 *Maximum Working Pressure Control*— A maximum working pressure control may be provided in the anesthesia

TABLE 1 Ventilator and Test Lung Settings for Endurance Test

	Compliance[A]	Resistance	Frequency	Tidal Volume, mL
Adult	*C* 20	*R*20 (R_p 20)	10/min	600
Pediatric	*C* 10	*R*50 (R_p 50)	20/min	200
Infant	*C* 3	*R*200 (R_p 200)	40/min	50

[A] *C* 20 refers to a compliance of 20 mL/0.098 kPa (1 cm H_2O), and *C* 10 to a compliance of 10 mL/0.098 kPa (1 cm H_2O), and *C* 3 refers to a compliance of 3 mL/0.098 kPa.

ventilator. If provided, these devices shall limit $P_{w\ max}$ and shall be accurate to within ±10 % of the set value (if calibrated) when tested as outlined in 6.4.2. If the ventilator derives its patient breathing mixture from a continuous flow anesthesia machine, then the manufacturer shall disclose the pressure at the breathing system connection port when a flow of 75 L/min is passed through the ventilator system with the $P_{w\ max}$ control activated. (See also X3.3.4.3.)

5.4.4 *Maximum Limited Pressure Mechanism ($P_{L\ max}$)*—A maximum limited pressure mechanism may be provided in the ventilator. If provided, these devices shall control $P_{L\ max}$) during ventilator malfunction, and may be operator adjustable. These devices shall be accurate to within 0.98 kPa (± 10 cm H_2O) of the set value at the opening pressure when tested as described in 6.4.3. (See also X3.3.4.3.)

NOTE 2—The maximum limited pressure control may not protect against malfunction in the anesthesia machine.

5.4.5 If provided, integral devices indicating ventilatory frequency shall be accurate to one breath per min or 10 % of actual (whichever is smaller) when tested as described in 6.4.4. (See also X3.3.4.3.)

5.4.5.1 Calibrated devices controlling ventilator frequency shall be accurate to within one breath per min or 10 % of actual (whichever is smaller) when tested as described in 6.4.4.

NOTE 3—This accuracy specification is not considered as an additive error in combination with the requirement of 5.4.5.

5.5 *Delivered Volume*—Delivered volume of the ventilator shall be indicated to the operator by some means and shall be accurate to ±15 % and shall be repeatable to ±5 % over a 1 h period. Test conditions shall be stated.

5.6 *Accuracy of Gas Mixture Controls*— When ventilators have incorporated as a primary control an inspiratory gas mixture control, the accuracy of the mean delivered oxygen concentration shall be within± 10 % of the set oxygen concentration or 3 % oxygen, whichever is greater, throughout the range of pressures, frequencies, and tidal volumes of which the ventilator is capable when tested as described in 6.6. At a given setting of the ventilator, the delivered oxygen concentration shall be ±3 % oxygen for at least 1 h. (See also X3.3.6.)

5.7 *Expiratory Resistance*:

5.7.1 *Adult and Child Ventilators*—When tested as described in 6.7, and in the absence of expiratory resistors or positive end expiratory pressure devices, the pressure at the breathing system connection for adult and child ventilators shall not exceed 0.49 kPa (5 cm H_2O) at a flow of 50 LPM when spirometer or breathing attachments, or both, as specified by the manufacturer, are used. If the ventilator is integral to the anesthesia machine, the manufacturer shall disclose the expiratory resistance when the flush valve is activated. The manufacturer should specify the maximum negative pressure created by the anesthesia ventilator with no fresh gas flow when the bellows does not reach the limiting stop. (See also X3.3.7.1.)

5.7.2 If the ventilator incorporates a weighted descending bellows, the manufacturer shall specify the maximum negative pressure created when tested as outlined in 6.7.2. (See also X3.3.7.2.)

5.8 *System Internal Compliance*—The manufacturer shall disclose the internal compliance of the ventilator and shall provide, upon request, the test methods used to determine the derived values. Manufacturers of ventilator tubing that recommend the use of their tubing with several ventilators, or who do not manufacture ventilators, shall provide the data on the compliance of their tubing in the labeling of their product. (See also 6.8 and X3.3.8.)

5.9 *Fittings Connecting Ventilator, Ventilator Circuit and Spirometer*:

5.9.1 The fitting for the tubing connecting the ventilator to the breathing circuit shall be a standard 22-mm male conical fitting, according to the dimensions specified in Specification F 1054. For flow direction-sensitive devices, the direction of flow shall be permanently marked on the connector, and the connector should be designed so that it cannot be installed in the reverse direction. (See also 6.9.1 and X3.3.9.1.)

5.9.2 If a 22-mm connector for a bag for manual ventilation is provided on the ventilator, it shall be marked *bag* with either the symbol or the word, and should face downward and shall be situated away from the connectors for the patient breathing tubes. No valve shall be permitted on the ventilator which will channel the patient's exhaled gas into the manual bag. The bag mount should provide a secure connection. (See also 6.9.2 and X3.3.9.2.)

5.9.3 If there is a separate outlet for the spirometer on the breathing tubes or the machine, the gas outlet leading to the spirometer should be a 30-mm male conical fitting.

5.9.4 If an ambient air inlet is fitted to the ventilator, it shall not be a 22, 15, 19, or 30-mm male cone and shall be clearly marked as *air inlet*. (See also 6.9.3 and X3.3.9.3.)

5.9.5 Outlets for anesthetic gas pollution control devices shall conform with ANSI Z-79.13. If an expired gas outlet (other than an outlet for spirometer) is fitted to the machine, it shall be designed in such a way that it cannot easily be connected to either 22 or 15-mm cones or sockets, or to 22-mm internal diameter tubing. (See also 6.9.4 and X3.3.9.3.)

5.10 *Mechanical Stability and Transportability*—Ventilators intended for use during anesthesia that are not an integral part of an anesthesia machine shall comply with Clause 24 of IEC 601-1.

5.11 *Ventilatory Monitoring and Alarms*— If provided as an integral part of the ventilator, ventilatory monitoring and alarms shall comply with the relevant sections set forth in Specification F 1161 and with the requirements of this section.

5.11.1 The alarm characteristics of monitors specified in this specification shall be grouped in three categories: (I) High Priority, (II) Medium Priority, and (III) Low Priority (see Table 2).

5.11.1.1 The audible components of these alarms should be designed to allow silencing until the anesthesia ventilator is placed in use (in other words, connected to the patient) in order

TABLE 2 Alarms

Category	Priority	Auditory	Visual	Operator Response
I	High	Not II or III	Not II or III	Immediate
II	Medium	Not I or III	Not I or III	Prompt
III	Low	Not I or II	Not I or II	Awareness

to reduce nuisance alarms.

5.11.1.2 The visual indicators for these alarms shall conform to the requirements given in the first two sentences of 5.13.

5.11.1.3 The audible component of these alarms at minimum volume should be discernible, to a person with normal hearing, above a background white noise level of 55 dB(A) at a distance of 3m from the front of the anesthesia gas machine.

5.11.1.4 There should be a visual indication that an audible alarm has been silenced.

5.11.1.5 The set points of adjustable alarms shall be indicated continuously or on user demand.

5.11.1.6 *Testing of Alarm Function*—A means shall be provided to test the function of the audible and visual annunciation of all alarms.

5.11.2 *High Priority Alarms*:

5.11.2.1 There shall be a visual indication of the high priority alarm. It shall be different and distinguishable from the visual signals specified in 5.11.3 and 5.11.4.

5.11.2.2 There shall be a simultaneous audible indication of the high priority alarm. This audible indication shall be different and distinguishable from the audible signals specified in 5.11.3 and 5.11.4.

5.11.2.3 The audible indicators shall reset automatically when the condition causing the alarm has cleared. The maximum time an audible high priority alarm can be silenced shall be 120 s.

5.11.3 *Medium Priority Alarms*:

5.11.3.1 There shall be a visual indication of the medium priority alarm. It shall be different and distinguishable from the visual signals specified in 5.11.2 and 5.11.4.

5.11.3.2 There shall be a simultaneous audible indication of the medium priority alarm. This audible indication shall be different and distinguishable from the audible signals in 5.11.2 and 5.11.4.

5.11.3.3 The audible indicator shall reset automatically when the condition causing the alarm has cleared. The audible indicator may be silenced for not more than 120 s, or until a different medium priority alarm condition occurs.

5.11.4 *Low Priority Alarms*:

5.11.4.1 There shall be a visual indication of the low priority alarm. It shall be different and distinguishable from the visual signals in 5.11.2 and 5.11.3.

5.11.4.2 There shall be a simultaneous audible indication of the low priority alarm. This audible indication shall be different and distinguishable from the audible signals specified in 5.11.2 and 5.11.3.

5.11.4.3 The audible indicator shall reset automatically when the condition causing the alarm has cleared. The audible indicator may be silenced until a different low priority alarm condition occurs.

5.11.5 *Required Alarms*—The following alarms shall be provided in association with all ventilators or ventilator/patient systems intended for use during anesthesia:

5.11.5.1 *Loss of Main Power Supply—Alarm Category: High Priority*—A loss of main power alarm shall be provided, and shall have a duration of at least 2 min at a constant sound pressure level when tested as outlined in 6.10. A means shall be provided for silencing this alarm following disconnection from the main power supply. This means of silencing the alarm shall not be remote from the ventilator, and the alarm silencing mechanism shall automatically reset when the main power is restored (see 6.10). If alternatively an alarm is provided to indicate loss of main power with backup power functioning, it shall be assigned to the *Low Priority* category. (See also X3.3.10.)

5.11.6 *Battery Power Supplies*—If any alarm incorporates a battery power supply: (*1*) the system shall include a means whereby the user may determine that the battery needs to be replaced for disposable batteries or recharged, and (*2*) the battery should be of a type readily obtainable.

5.12 *Anesthetic Gas Pollution Controls*— If provided as a part of the ventilator, pollution control devices shall comply with the requirements of ANSI Z-79.11.

5.13 *Controls and Indicators*—The faces of all scales and gages shall be legible and all controls and indicators shall be visible at a distance of 1 m (3.3 ft) and at a light level of 215 lux (20 footcandles) to an operator with 6.5 (20-20) vision (corrected), seated or standing in front of the anesthesia machine. The markings and calibrations should be readily identified with the controls, gages, meters, or indicators with which they are associated. Flowmeters, gages, controls, and other displays that need to be read most frequently should be grouped together and should be placed as close as possible to the operator's field of vision when in the normal position of operating the anesthesia machine and observing the patient. (See Appendix X4.)

6. Test Methods

6.1 *Lung Models and Method of Testing Performance of Lung Ventilators*:

6.1.1 *Test Equipment*—The lung models illustrated in Figs. 1 and 2 do not preclude the development of different or more sophisticated lung models with the same ranges of compliance and linear or alinear resistances. If nonlinear resistances are used, their characteristics must be specified.

6.1.1.1 *Lung Models*—Lung models are designed to provide impedances to the ventilator output that simulate both normal and diseased lung states. The impedances to ventilator output are lung elastance and airflow resistance, which can be simulated in the lung models by a compliance and a resistance connected in series (see Figs. 1 and 2). The various combinations of compliances and resistances used in the test procedures are given in Table 1.

6.1.1.2 *Compliances*—The required compliances are given in Table 2. These compliances shall include the compliances of all components of the lung model system. The volume-pressure characteristics of the model compliances including connections shall be determined at ambient pressure and temperature and shall be determined as in 6.1.2 and shall be within ±5 % of the required compliance values shown in Table 1.

6.1.1.3 *Resistors*—The required resistors are given in Table 1. Values for these resistors are given in Tables 3 and 4. These values relate to measurements at NTPD (20°C, 760 mm Hg, and 0 % RH).

6.1.2 *Test Methods—General*—Make measurements of pressure, flow, and volume as shown in Fig. 1 accurate to

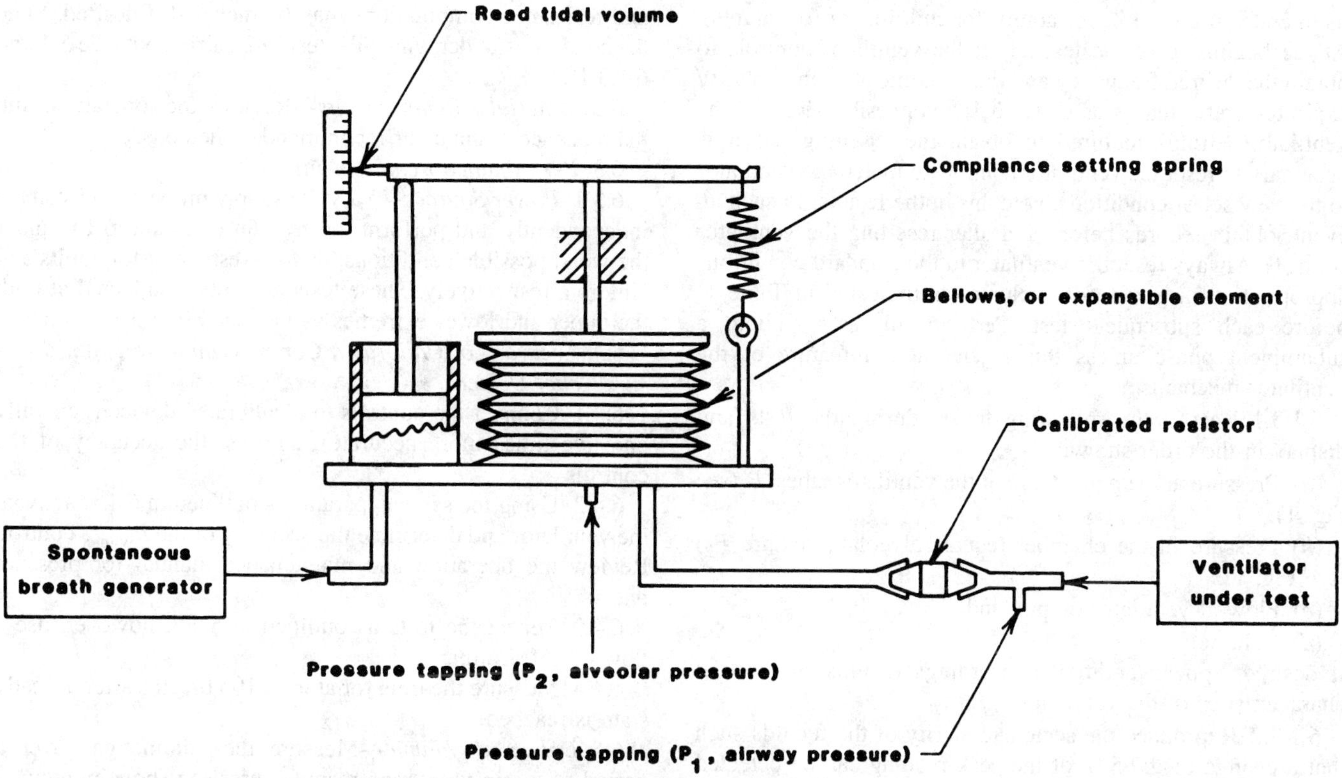

FIG. 1 Representative Active Lung Model

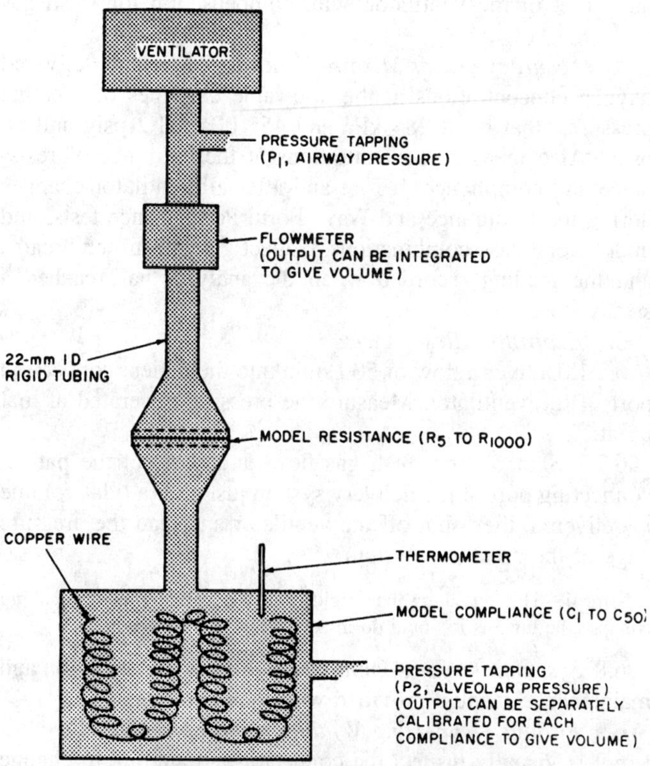

FIG. 2 Representative Passive Lung Model

TABLE 3 Linear Resistances

Resistance	Value in Flow Range ±20 % kPa/L/s	(cm/H_2O/L/s)	Range of Airflow (L/s)
*R*20	1.96	(20)	0 to 1.0
*R*50	4.90	(50)	0 to 0.5
*R*200	19.60	(200)	0 to 0.1

TABLE 4 Parabolic Resistances[A]

$\Delta P = K\,V^2$ cm H_2O (where V = L/s)

Resistances	$K \pm 10$ %	$P \pm 10$ % kPa	(cm H_2O)	@	V, L/s
R_p20	17.60	0.43	(4.40)	@	0.5
		1.73	(17.60)	@	1.0
R_p50	108.70	0.67	(6.79)	@	0.25
		2.67	(27.20)	@	0.5
R_p200	2440.00	0.60	(6.10)	@	0.05
		2.39	(24.40)	@	0.1

[A] Linear and parabolic resistances may be used interchangeably. Representative test lungs and the appropriate parabolic resistances are available from Michigan Instruments, Inc., 6300 28th Street, SE, Grand Rapids, MI 49506; BioTek Instruments, Highland Park, Winooski, VT 05404, or Hyco-Aulas Gauthier S.A., Bureau a Paris, 13, rue Guyton-de-Morveau, 75013 Paris, France or their equivalents have been found satisfactory for this purpose. Resistances will have different performance values, depending on the manufacturer and individual resistor configuration. The ventilator manufacturer shall supply data on the resistors used during testing upon request.

within ±2.5 % of the reading. Allow an additional tolerance of ±2.5 % of the full scale reading. Make measurements of power and work accurate to within ±5 % of the reading. Allow an additional tolerance of ±5 % of the peak reading. Maintain the reading accuracy of the recording device at frequencies up to 10 Hz. Record ambient conditions, and report all results at NTPD even though other conditions might exist during actual testing. Dry air, unless otherwise specified in an individual requirement, is the test gas.

6.1.3 *Wave-form Performance Test*—Connect the ventilator to the compliance and resistance combinations appropriate to its intended use (that is, for adults, for children, or for infants). At the beginning of the test adjust the ventilator controls to obtain the desired frequency and tidal volume at an inspiratory/expiratory ratio that is as close to 1:2 as possible. Record the ventilator settings required to obtain these settings. If it is necessary to reset the ventilator controls to match the ventilator to the new set of conditions, note this in the results. In such an event, obtain records before and after resetting the ventilator controls. Always reset the ventilator to the standard conditions appropriate to a given tidal volume (as indicated in Table 1) before each subsequent test. Perform all tests without a subambient phase unless this is an integral feature of the ventilator mechanism.

6.1.3.1 Record the following traces during the tests and display in the order shown:

(*a*) Pressure at the patient end of the ventilator tubes, P_1(see Fig. 1),

(*b*) Pressure in the chamber (equals alveolar pressure P_2) (see Fig. 1),

(*c*) Flow at ventilator output, and

(*d*) Volume.

If desired, append additional recordings to illustrate special characteristics of the ventilator.

6.1.3.2 Reproduce the scale and clarity of the records such that a change of ±2.5 % of the peak reading can be detected easily. Inscribe all records with the appropriate scales, time base, and details of the test. Include the following:

(*a*) Ambient temperature and pressure, together with the temperature, composition, and humidity of the inspired gas.

(*b*) The nature and dimensions of the breathing tubes connecting the ventilator to the test lung and whether other apparatus (for example, humidifier, spirometer, or water traps) were included in the part of the circuit which is pressurized during inspiration. If such apparatus is included, specify the type and position. If a humidifier is included, fill it to the *full* water level with a relatively non-compressible substance. If this is not practicable, replace the humidifier with an equivalent compliance and resistance.

(*c*) A listing of all settings of controls, if possible.

(*d*) Any other relevant information (for example, source and pressure of driving gas, use of special ventilator circuits, or type of humidifier).

6.1.4 *Volume Performance Test*—Test the adult ventilator against a compliance of *C* 20, and a resistance of *R* 20 (R_p20), at tidal volumes ranging from 300 to 1200 mL, and a range of frequencies from 6 to 20 breaths per min. Test pediatric ventilators at three representative volumes, that is, min, mean, and max, within the range of 50 to 300 mL tidal volume against a compliance of *C* 10 and a resistance of *R* 50 (R_p50) at a frequency of 20 breaths/min. Test the infant ventilator against a compliance of *C* 3, and a resistance of *R* 200 (R_p200), at a tidal volume range of 30 to 200 mL and a ventilatory frequency of 40 breaths per min.

6.1.5 The manufacturer shall determine the range of tidal volumes that the ventilator is capable of delivering to the lung at the specified frequencies with an inspiratory/expiratory phase time ratio as close to 1:2 as possible. Further measurements at different frequencies and with different compliance and resistance combinations may be included if desired. State the conditions under which the tests are carried out (see 5.1 and 6.1.3.1).

6.2 *Materials Requirements*—Review the operation and maintenance manual for recommended methods.

6.3 *Performance Requirements*:

6.3.1 *Power Sources*—Vary the supply pressure and voltage independently and perform the tests in 6.1.3 and 6.1.4 under the worst possible conditions, that is, Test No. 4 for adults and children, respectively. These tests are to be conducted at both the upper and lower extremes as indicated in 5.3.1 and 5.3.2.

6.4 *Accuracy of Calibrated Controls, Indicators, and Pressure Relief Devices*:

6.4.1 Connect the controls to a calibrated device (generally one five times more accurate), and test the accuracy of the controls.

6.4.2 Using the same apparatus as outlined in 6.4.1, activate the ventilator and determine the accuracy of the $P_{w\ max}$ control. Review the operation and maintenance manual for pressure data.

6.4.3 Repeat the tests as outlined in 6.4.2, however, use a flow of 150 L/min.

6.4.4 Measure the time for at least 100 breaths after a steady state is reached.

6.5 *Delivered Volume*—Measure the volume gas over a period of 5 min unless the manufacturer can show an equivalent accuracy with a lesser collection time, when measured at the outlet of the ventilator, with compensation for fresh gas flow.

6.6 *Accuracy of Gas Mixture Controls*— Measure delivered oxygen concentrations at the allowable extremes of pipeline pressures, that is, at 284 kPa and 455 kPa (41.2 psig and 66 psig). Also measure concentrations at the extremes of resistance and compliance, before and after all ventilator changes during the Endurance and Wave Form Performance tests, and under worst case combinations. Collect gases from ten breaths and the reading recorded when the analyzer has reached a steady state.

6.7 *Expiratory Resistance*:

6.7.1 Deliver a flow of 50 L/min into the patient connection port of the ventilator. Measure the pressure generated at that point.

6.7.2 Shut off the fresh gas flow, and obstruct the patient connecting port of the delivery system just after a tidal volume is delivered, then shut off the ventilator and read the pressure gage of the breathing system.

NOTE 4—The test lung has rigid walls; negative pressure *cannot* collapse the lung as it would do in actual patient application.

6.8 *System Internal Compliance*—Review the operation and maintenance manual provided with the ventilator.

6.9 *Fittings Connecting Ventilator and Spirometer*:

6.9.1 Visually inspect the connector and attempt to change connector direction.

6.9.2 Inspect the ventilator for appropriate marking and connector position, and review the ventilator circuit diagram.

6.9.3 Attempt to fit a 15, 19, or 22-mm or 30-mm fitting.

6.9.4 Repeat the test as outlined in 6.9.3 for 15 and 22-mm connectors.

6.10 *Alarms*—Connect the power supply to the ventilator, run according to the manufacturer's instructions, then disconnect the ventilator from the main power supply and determine that the alarm sounds, and maintains a constant sound pressure level ±3 dB for at least 2 min. Repeat the test as outlined above, and silence the loss of main power supply alarm. Reconnect the ventilator main power immediately after silencing the alarm, and then disconnect the ventilator from the main power supply again and determine that the alarm silencing mechanism has reset.

7. Warnings and Markings

7.1 *Marking*:

7.1.1 All breathing circuit components in which the direction of gas flow is critical shall be permanently marked in such a way that the intended direction of gas flow is immediately apparent to the operator.

7.1.2 For the purposes of this specification, all ventilator system components that contain a valve or valves, the purpose of which is to establish the direction of gas flow, are considered to be flow critical and shall be so marked. Examples include inhalation check valves, exhalation check valves, and non-rebreathing valves.

7.1.3 Where markings are applied to breathing system components in order to indicate the direction of gas flow, the minimum acceptable marking shall consist of at least one headed arrow permanently affixed to the component. Where a component contains more than one check valve, the minimum acceptable marking shall consist of at least one headed arrow indicating the direction of flow through each check valve.

7.1.4 All markings applied to breathing system components for the purpose of indicating direction of gas flow should be located, if possible, so that they will fall in the operator's normal field of view when equipment is in use.

7.1.5 Breathing system components in which the direction of gas flow is not critical need not be marked to indicate specific flow direction.

7.1.6 If possible, ventilators should be clearly marked with the following:

7.1.6.1 Adequate instructions for lubrication and routine maintenance,

7.1.6.2 Operating instructions, if a means of hand operation is provided,

7.1.6.3 Required operating gas pressure for equipment operated by gas,

7.1.6.4 Relief pressure of non-adjustable safety valves and maximum relief pressure of adjustable safety valves,

7.1.6.5 The maximum volumetric displacement, if less than 1400 mL,

7.1.6.6 The manufacturer's name or trademark and the country of manufacture,

7.1.6.7 Inlets and outlets of the machine, and

7.1.6.8 Voltage and current requirements.

NOTE 5—If it is not possible to mark this information on the ventilator, an instruction to refer to the instruction manual shall be marked on the ventilator.

7.1.7 All connectors for electrical and gas supply shall be marked with identification labels.

NOTE 6—**Precaution:** In addition to other precautions, if electrical components are included in the ventilator, the device should be marked with the phrase **Not For Use in the Presence of Flammable Anesthetic Agents**.

7.1.8 If multiple connection ports are provided, their intended use shall be marked.

7.1.9 *Alarm Operating Instructions*—The manufacturer shall provide instructions for testing and setting of the alarm. These instructions shall be either permanently marked on or attached to the ventilator or ventilator alarm.

8. Supplementary Requirements

8.1 *Information to be Included by the Manufacturer*—The following information shall be included in the information provided by the manufacturer:

8.1.1 Recommended means of sterilization or decontamination, or both, of the ventilator, and

8.1.2 Recommended power supply.

APPENDIXES

(Nonmandatory Information)

X1. CHARACTERISTICS OF VENTILATORS INTENDED FOR USE DURING ANESTHESIA

X1.1 *Volume Control:*

X1.1.1 Pressure Preset
X1.1.2 Volume Preset
X1.1.2.1 Tidal
X1.1.2.2 Minute
X1.1.3 Combined

X1.2 *Cycling Control:*

X1.2.1 Inspiration to Expiration
X1.2.1.1 Volume
X1.2.1.2 Pressure
X1.2.1.3 Time
X1.2.1.4 Flow
X1.2.1.5 Combined
X1.2.1.6 Manual override
X1.2.1.7 Other
X1.2.2 *Expiration to Inspiration*:
X1.2.2.1 Pressure
X1.2.2.2 Time
X1.2.2.3 Flow
X1.2.2.4 Combined
X1.2.2.5 Patient

X1.2.2.6 Manual override
X1.2.2.7 Other

X1.3 *Types of Safety Limits:*

X1.3.1 Volume
X1.3.2 Pressure
X1.3.3 Time
X1.3.4 Other

X1.4 *Types of Pressure Patterns:*

X1.4.1 Positive-ambient
X1.4.2 Positive-subambient
X1.4.3 Positive-positive

X1.5 *Source of Power:*

X1.5.1 Pneumatic
X1.5.2 Electric
X1.5.3 Other

X1.6 *Power Transmission:*

X1.6.1 Direct
X1.6.2 Indirect

X1.7 *Source of Inspired Gas:*

X1.7.1 Driving gas
X1.7.2 Fresh gas
X1.7.3 Mixed

X1.8 *Type of Control:*

X1.8.1 Pneumatic
X1.8.2 Electronic
X1.8.3 Mechanical
X1.8.4 Combined

X1.9 *Classification and Definitions of Types of Breathing Machines:*

X1.9.1 *Lung Ventilator*— An automatic device that is connected to the patient's airway and is designed to augment or provide for the patient's ventilation.

X1.9.2 *There are four types of lung ventilators*:

X1.9.2.1 *Controller*— A device, or mode of operation of a device, that inflates the patient's lungs independently of the patient's inspiratory effort.

X1.9.2.2 *Assister*—A device or mode of operation designed to augment the patient's breathing synchronously with his inspiratory effort.

X1.9.2.3 *Assister/Controller*—An apparatus or mode of operation that is designed to function either as an assister or a controller, and that may, in default of the patient's inspiratory effort, automatically function as a controller.

X1.9.2.4 *Assister/Controller—Spontaneous Breathing*—Those devices that incorporate various modes of operation which allow the patient to breath spontaneously (1) at or above ambient pressure levels, or (2) with or without supplemental mandatory positive pressure breaths.

X1.9.3 *High Frequency Ventilation*—Those ventilators that employ a frequency of greater than 2.5 Hz.

X2. DEFINITIONS OF ALARM CATEGORIES AND ASSOCIATED VISUAL INDICATORS

X2.1 *Category I*—A sound or indication of potential danger meaning that urgent action is required. Visual indicator—flashing indicator, colored red if indicator lights are used.

X2.2 *Category II*—A sound meaning that increased vigilance or prompt action is required. Visual indicator—flashing indicator, colored yellow if indicator lights are used.

X2.3 *Category III*—A sound meaning that alertness to a particular condition is required. Visual indicator—continuous indicator, colored yellow if indicator lights are used.

X3. RATIONALE

X3.1 *Scope:*

X3.1.1 This specification defines minimum performance and safety requirements for all types of anesthesia ventilators. The Subcommittee preparing this draft was of the opinion that the major problems with these devices would be addressed by the requirements that have been included, but was well aware that not all types of failures (double-fault, triple-fault, etc.) can be allowed for, and that it is not possible to design a totally safe or a totally effective ventilator.

X3.2 *Materials Requirements:*

X3.2.1 Although ideally all components of the ventilator should be sterilizable, certain components may not be able to be sterilized with currently available methods without causing damage to the device. These components should be capable of being disinfected with a high level disinfectant[7] or should be isolated from other portions of the patient breathing circuit.

X3.3 *Performance Requirements:*

X3.3.1 *Volume Performance*—The tests used to demonstrate compliance with these requirements were designed to demonstrate that the ventilator can provide adequate ventilation under relatively severe circumstances, that is, low compliance and high resistance. However, the values given in 6.1.4 are not considered the worst case. These values are instead considered to be median values.

[7] Garner, J. S. et al, "CDC Guidelines for the Prevention and Control of Nosocomial Infections–Guideline for Handwashing and Hospital Environmental Control, 1985" *American Journal of Infection Control*, 14:110–129, 1986, Section 2, pp. 116–129.

X3.3.2 *Wave-Form and Endurance*—The Subcommittee felt that 72 h was a reasonable length of time for an anesthesia ventilator to be able to meet the requirements of the standard without requiring readjustment or recalibration. The clinicians on the Subcommittee felt that it was quite possible that an anesthesia ventilator would be required to be used for this length of time without any possibility for recalibration.

X3.3.3 *Power Sources*— Fluctuations within the ranges specified in 5.3 are known to occur in both electrical and pneumatic power supply systems in hospitals. The causes for such variation may be outside the control of the ventilator user. For example, a decrease in the power supplied by the local electric utility, or the variation that may result from demand for power caused by such equipment as elevator motors and air-handling apparatus within the hospital will cause these types of fluctuations. The periodic testing of emergency generators may also create this type of variation. Pneumatic power sources may show transient variations as well. The filling of liquid oxygen bulk reservoirs, changes in pressure switch settings on compressed air reservoirs, and the temperature effects on regulator components in nitrous oxide systems are examples of functional variations that could cause the supply pressure to change.

X3.3.4 *Accuracy of Calibration Controls, Indicators, and Pressure Relief Devices*:

X3.3.4.1 The Subcommittee felt that this was the level of accuracy that was available with current technology.

X3.3.4.2 Accurate limiting of $P_{w\,max}$ may be desirable in certain conditions, for example, ventilation of small premature infants. The disclosure of the $P_{w\,max}$ at 75 L/min provides clinically useful information as it describes the maximum potential pressure generated in the patient system if the flush valve on the continuous flow anesthesia machine is activated during the inspiratory phase of anesthetic ventilation.

X3.3.4.3 Limits specified in requirements in 5.4.5 and 5.4.5.1 encompass the range of accuracy that the members of the Subcommittee felt were necessary and appropriate for clinical performance and that were achievable within current technology.

X3.3.5 *Delivered Volume*—The removal of carbon dioxide depends upon ventilation and the accurate measurement of the minute or tidal volumes is helpful to facilitate the control of carbon dioxide levels.

X3.3.6 *Accuracy of Gas Mixture Controls*—Maintaining the accuracy of delivered oxygen concentrations throughout the range of ventilator performance is important in order to allow for the rapid and often frequent adjustment of the ventilator without significant variation in the oxygen concentration. ANSI Z-79.10 specifies $\pm$ 3 % oxygen as the range of accuracy for oxygen analyzers. Limiting the fluctuation to this level at any given ventilator setting is technologically possible, and will minimize the time spent making control adjustments. This should enhance operator confidence in the accuracy of control settings provided on the gas mixing device. With the exception of some critical care ventilators intended for use during anesthesia, the gas mixing device is often the anesthesia machine itself and not the anesthesia ventilator.

X3.3.7 *Expiratory Resistance*:

X3.3.7.1 The Subcommittee felt that it was important to test ventilators by the methods described in 6.7 to assure that *ventilator inherent PEEP* greater than 0.49 kPa (5 cm H_2O) was not generated during exhalation in the breathing system of the ventilator.

X3.3.7.2 Anesthesia ventilators utilizing weighted descending bellows generate negative pressure when the bellows are not seating on the stop. This condition may occur during anesthesia if the fresh gas flow is low and there is a slight leak in the breathing circuit, or during closed-circuit anesthesia.

X3.3.8 *System Internal Compliance*—Increasing internal compliance will (*1*) decrease the actual volume delivered to the patient from a *set* volume, and (*2*) increase measured volume above the patient's actual minute volume.

X3.3.9 *Fittings Connecting Ventilator and Spirometer*:

X3.3.9.1 Flow-direction-sensitive devices such as one-way valves or humidifiers may be caused to malfunction by inadvertent connection in the reverse manner, and it is also possible for injury to the patient to occur if flows of gas are misdirected or humidifier contents are emptied into the breathing circuit as a result of such a misconnection.

X3.3.9.2 The positioning of the connector for a bag mount, if provided, is important so that it is not mistaken for a connector to a patient breathing tube. The marking of the connector is important for the same reason. If selector valves that provide for channeling of the patient's exhaled volume into the manual bag are allowed on anesthesia ventilators, it is possible to then have two selector valves, one on the anesthesia machine and one on the anesthesia ventilator, creating a potentially serious device complication if both selector valves are set so that no flow goes into the patient.

X3.3.9.3 These requirements are intended to minimize the possibility of inappropriate connection of the ventilator breathing circuit components to the spirometer outlet, ambient air inlets or anesthetic gas scavenging connections.

X3.3.10 *Alarms*:

X3.3.10.1 The Subcommittee felt that a loss of main power supply alarm with a duration of 2 min was adequate to allow personnel to reach the ventilator and determine the cause of the alarm. The Subcommittee also felt that a means for silencing this alarm when main power was disconnected was important in order to minimize the number of spurious alarm signals in the operating room environment. If such a means for silencing an alarm was not provided, every time the ventilator was disconnected to be moved from the patient area the loss of main power alarm would sound for 2 min, distracting personnel. However, the Subcommittee also felt that the means of silencing the loss of main power alarm should not be remote from the ventilator proper, and that when the alarm sounded the operator should be forced to walk to the ventilator to determine the cause of the alarm and correct the situation.

X4. HUMAN FACTORS CONSIDERATIONS

TABLE X4.1 Applications of Various Types of Mechanical Displays

USE	SCALES: Moving Pointer	SCALES: Fixed Pointer	COUNTERS	PRINTERS	FLAGS
QUANTITATIVE INFORMATION	FAIR May be difficult to read while pointer is in motion.	FAIR May be difficult to read while scale is in motion.	GOOD Minimum time and error for exact numerical value.	GOOD Minimum time and error for exact numerical value. Provides reference records.	N/A
QUALITATIVE INFORMATION	GOOD Location of pointer easy. Numbers and scale need not be read. Position change easily detected.	POOR Difficult to judge direction and magnitude of deviation without reading numbers and scale.	POOR Numbers must be read. Position changes not easily detected.	POOR Numbers must be read. Position changes not easily detected.	GOOD Easily detected. Economical of space.
SETTING	GOOD Simple and direct relation of motion of pointer to motion of setting knob. Position change aids monitoring.	FAIR Relation to motion of setting knob may be ambiguous. No pointer position change to aid monitoring. Not readable during rapid setting.	GOOD Most accurate monitoring of numerical setting. Relation to motion of setting knob less direct than for moving pointer. Not readable during rapid setting.	N/A	N/A
TRACKING	GOOD Pointer position readily controlled and monitored. Simplest relation to manual control motion.	FAIR No position changes to aid monitoring. Relation to control motion somewhat ambiguous.	POOR No gross position changes to aid monitoring.	N/A	N/A
GENERAL	Requires largest exposed and illuminated area on panel. Scale length limited unless multiple pointers used.	Saves panel space. Only small section of scale need be exposed and illuminated. Use of tape allows long scale.	Most economical of space and illumination. Scale length limited only by number of counter drums.	Limited application.	Limited application.

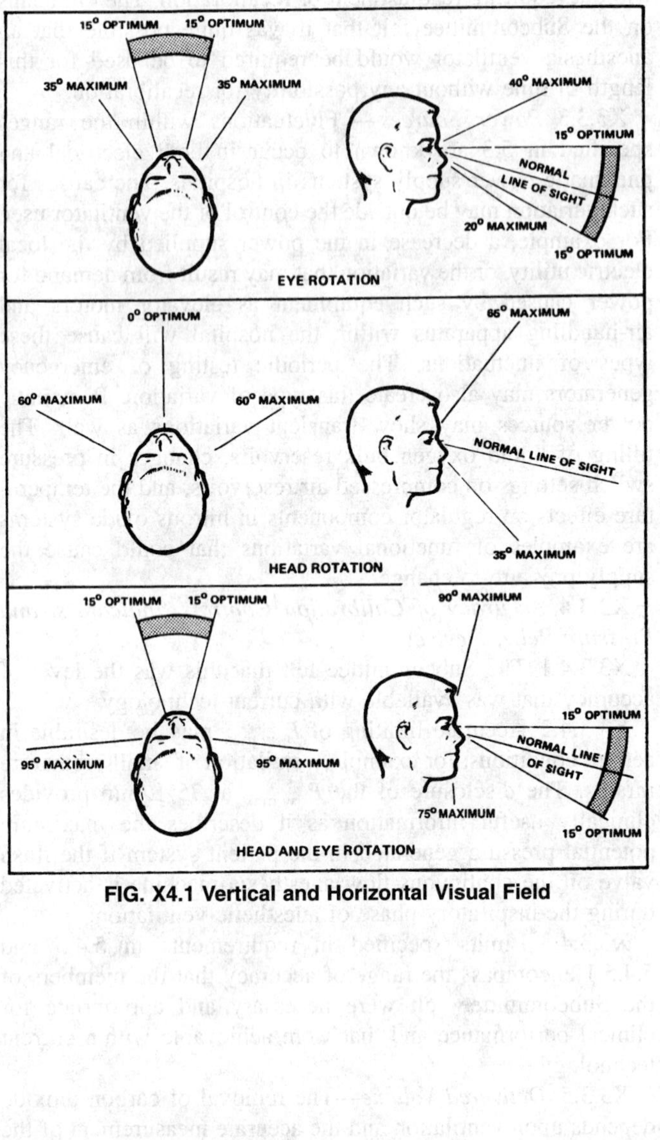

FIG. X4.1 Vertical and Horizontal Visual Field

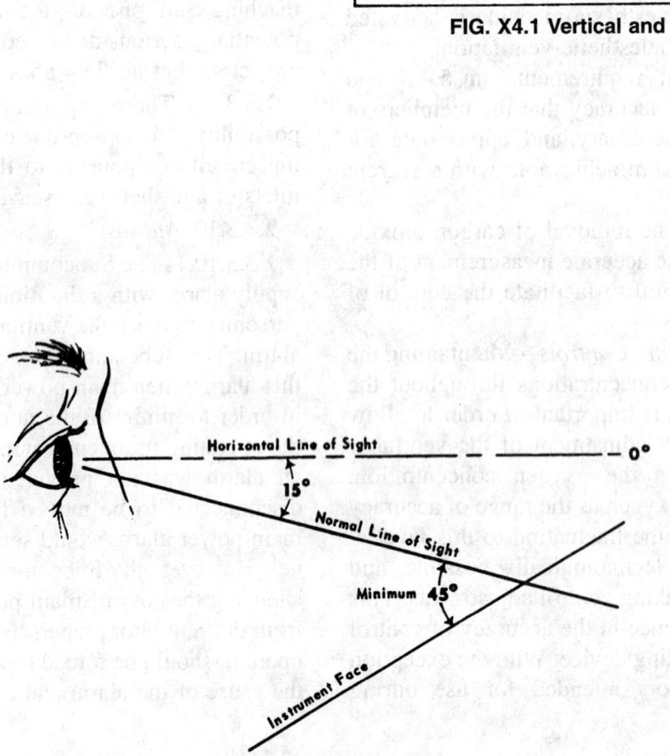

FIG. X4.2 Lines of Sight

Standard Specification for Titanium-6 Aluminum-4 Vanadium Alloy Castings for Surgical Implants (UNS R56406)[1]

This standard is issued under the fixed designation F 1108; the number immediately following the designation indicates the year of original adoption or, in the case of revision, the year of last revision. A number in parentheses indicates the year of last reapproval. A superscript epsilon (ϵ) indicates an editorial change since the last revision or reapproval.

1. Scope

1.1 This specification provides material requirements for titanium-6 aluminum-4 vanadium alloy castings to be used in the manufacture of surgical implants.

1.2 The values stated in inch-pound units are to be regarded as the standard. The metric equivalents of inch-pound units may be approximate.

2. Referenced Documents

2.1 *ASTM Standards:*

B 367 Specification for Titanium and Titanium Alloy Castings[2]

B 381 Specification for Titanium and Titanium Alloy Forgings[2]

B 600 Practice for Descaling and Cleaning Titanium and Titanium Alloy Surfaces[2]

E 8 Test Methods of Tension Testing of Metallic Materials[3]

E 120 Test Methods for Chemical Analysis of Titanium and Titanium Alloys[4]

E 1409 Test Method for Determination of Oxygen in Titanium and Titanium Alloys by the Inert Gas Fusion Technique[4]

E 1447 Test Method for Determination Hydrogen in Titanium and Titanium Alloys by the Inert Gas Fusion Thermal Conductivity Method[5]

F 136 Specification for Wrought Titanium 6A1-4V ELI Alloy for Surgical Implant Applications[6]

F 601 Practice for Fluorescent Penetrant Inspection of Metallic Surgical Implants[6]

F 629 Practice for Radiography of Cast Metallic Surgical Implants[6]

2.2 *ASQC Standard:*

C1 Specification of General Requirements for a Quality Control Program[7]

3. Materials and Manufacture

3.1 Parts conforming to this specification shall be produced by vacuum investment casting.

3.2 Parts covered by this specification shall be an annealed condition in the hot isostatically pressed condition.

NOTE 1—While hot isostatic processing (HIP) may enhance mechanical properties of Ti6A14V castings, it has also been shown to reduce the scatter in mechanical properties and therefore increases the confidence in reliability of castings.

3.3 Surface defects may be repaired by welding.

3.3.1 Weld repair shall be carefully executed as per written procedures by individuals qualified to perform those procedures.

3.3.2 ELI weld rod conforming to Specification F 136 shall be used where filler metal is needed.

3.3.3 Weld repairs shall be performed prior to final thermal processing.

NOTE 2—Under certain circumstances, a weld repair will act as a stress riser. Therefore, care should be exercised in the location and extent of weld repair as it relates to regions of the implant where significant stresses might be incurred.

NOTE 3—While not covered by this specification, there are other thermal processes which meet specific needs of the implant manufacturer. These thermal treatments may be mutually agreed upon by the casting vendor and the implant manufacturer.

3.4 All alpha case shall be removed by suitable means such as chemical milling or machining prior to HIP processing.

3.5 Parts shall be furnished in the descaled and cleaned condition in accordance with B 600.

4. Chemical Composition

4.1 The analysis for chemical composition of the castings shall conform to the requirements prescribed in Table 1. Chemical analysis shall be performed on a representative specimen cast from each heat using the same general procedures used in casting implants.

4.1.1 Requirements for the major and minor elemental constituents are listed in Table 1. Also listed are important

---

[1] This specification is under the jurisdiction of ASTM Committee F04 on Medical and Surgical Materials and Devices and is the direct responsibility of Subcommittee F04.12 on Metallurgical Materials.

Current edition approved April 10, 1997. Published March 1998. Originally published as F 1108 - 88. Last previous edition F 1108 - 97.

[2] *Annual Book of ASTM Standards*, Vol 02.04.

[3] *Annual Book of ASTM Standards*, Vol 03.01.

[4] *Annual Book of ASTM Standards*, Vol 03.05.

[5] *Annual Book of ASTM Standards*, Vol 03.06.

[6] *Annual Book of ASTM Standards*, Vol 13.01.

[7] Available from American Society for Quality Control, 161 W. Wisconsin Ave., Milwaukee, WI 53203.

TABLE 1 Chemical Composition

Element	Composition, Weight %
Nitrogen	0.05 max
Carbon	0.10 max
Hydrogen	0.015 max
Iron	0.30 max
Oxygen	0.20 max
Aluminum	5.5 to 6.75
Vanadium	3.5 to 4.5
Titanium	Balance[A]

[A] The remainder of the percent of titanium is determined by the difference. Residual metallic element tolerance levels will be agreed upon between producer and manufacturer.

residual elements. Analysis for elements not listed in Table 1 is not required to verify compliance with this specification.

4.2 Check analysis chemical requirements for samples taken from castings shall conform to the tolerances prescribed in Table 2.

4.2.1 *Product Analysis*—Product analysis tolerances do not broaden the specified heat analysis requirements, but cover variations between laboratories in the measurement of chemical content. The manufacturer shall not ship material that is outside the limits specified in Table 1.

4.3 For referee purposes, Test Methods E 120, E 1409, and E 1447 shall be used.

NOTE 4—Use care in sampling titanium for chemical analysis because of its affinity for elements such as oxygen, nitrogen, and hydrogen. Therefore, in cutting samples for analysis, carry out the operation, insofar as possible, in a dust free atmosphere. Collect the sample from clean metal and use clean and sharp tools. Store samples for analysis in suitable containers.

5. Mechanical Requirements

5.1 Material supplied under this specification shall conform to the mechanical property requirements prescribed in Table 3.

5.2 Specimens for tension tests shall conform to the mechanical property requirements prescribed in Table 3.

5.3 Specimens for tension tests shall be machined and tested in accordance with the methods in Test Methods E 8 using a strain rate of 0.003 to 0.007 in./in. min. (mm/mm min.) through the specified yield range and then the crosshead speed shall be increased so as to produce fracture in approximately one additional minute.

TABLE 2 Product Analysis Tolerances

Nitrogen	0.02
Carbon	0.02
Hydrogen	0.0030
Iron	0.08
Oxygen	0.04
Aluminum	0.40
Vanadium	0.15

TABLE 3 Mechanical Requirements[A]

Ultimate Tensile Strength	125 000 psi (860 MPa) min
Yield Strength (0.2 % offset)	110 000 psi (758 MPa) min
Elongation[B]	8 % min
Reduction of Area	14 % min

[A] In the cast, HIP, and annealed condition.
[B] Gage length = 4 × diameter.

5.4 Mechanical test specimens shall be produced by the same general procedures used in casting surgical implants and shall be tested in accordance with Test Methods E 8 which may have a ground finish on the reduced section. Alternatively, test specimens may be machined from surgical implant castings.

5.5 A minimum of two test specimens per heat shall be tested. If one specimen fails below the specified mechanical requirements or breaks outside the gage limits, two additional specimens shall be tested and both must pass.

6. Quality Program Requirements

6.1 The producer shall maintain a quality program such as, for example, is defined in ASQC C1, or equivalent.

6.2 The manufacturer of surgical implants or medical appliances shall be assured of and may audit the producer's quality program for conformance to the intent of ASQC C1 or other recognized program.

7. Nondestructive Examination

7.1 *Liquid Penetrant Examination*—Each individual part shall be subject to liquid penetrant examination in accordance with Practice F 601.

7.2 *Radiographic Examination*—Each individual part shall be subject to radiographic examination in accordance with Specification B 367, Section S1.

7.3 Other additional methods of nondestructive inspection may be used as mutually agreed upon by vendor and implant manufacturer.

8. Certification and Rejection

8.1 Certification and rejection shall be as specified in Specification B 367 and Specification B 381.

9. Packaging and Package Marking

9.1 Marking and packaging shall be as specified in Specification B 367 and Specification B 381.

10. Keywords

10.1 castings-surgical; orthopaedic medical devices-titanium/titanium alloy; titanium/titanium alloys (for surgical implants)

APPENDIXES

(Nonmandatory Information)

X1. RATIONALE

X1.1 This specification is intended to provide general guidelines for material requirements for Ti6A14V castings for use in surgical implants. It is in no way intended to usurp the role of the design engineer in the development and manufacture of a functionally sound implant. For example, this specification does not preclude the use of ELI grade titanium; and the weld repair of defects. The engineer needs to be aware of the ramifications of such processing, though, on the safety and efficacy of the implant for its intended use.

X1.2 The UNS designation has been added for clarification, and a biocompatibility section has been added as an appendix.

X2. BIOCOMPATIBILITY

X2.1 The material compositions covered by this specification have been employed successfully in human implant application in contact with soft tissue and bone for over a decade.

X2.2 No known surgical implant material has ever been shown to be completely free of adverse reactions in the human body. However, long term clinical experience has shown an acceptable level of biological response can be expected, if these materials are used in appropriate applications (**1,2,3,4**).[8]

[8] The boldface numbers in parentheses refer to the list of references at the end of this standard.

REFERENCES

(1) Laing, P. G., Ferguson, A. B., Jr., and Hodge, E. S., "Tissue Reaction in Rabbit Muscle Exposed to Metallic Implants," *Journal of Biomedical Materials Research*, Vol 1, 1967, pp 135–149.

(2) Laing, P. G., "Compatibility of Biomaterials," *Orthopedic Clinics of North America*, Vol 4, No. 2, April 1973, pp 249–273.

(3) Street, D. M., and Stevens, P. S., "A Humeral Replacement of Prosthesis for the Elbow," *Journal of Bone and Joint Surgery*, Vol 56A, No. 6, September 1974.

(4) Lynch, J. A., "Replacement Arthroplasty of the Elbow with Coonrad Total Elbow Prosthesis," *Orthopaedic Digest*, January 1976.

Standard Specification for National Air Medical Transport Units Resources Catalog[1]

This standard is issued under the fixed designation F 1118; the number immediately following the designation indicates the year of original adoption or, in the case of revision, the year of last revision. A number in parentheses indicates the year of last reapproval. A superscript epsilon (ε) indicates an editorial change since the last revision or reapproval.

INTRODUCTION

Committee F30 was established on a voluntary basis to edit, update, and create where necessary, voluntary standards for all facets of emergency medical services (EMS).

Task Group F30.01.02 is responsible for water and air vehicles and has prepared standards that cover the medical transport units for the three levels of general patient care, namely basic, advanced, and specialized.

This specification complements these standards in that it presents a unique method of cataloging EMS resources. It consists of a format that, when completed and submitted by the air ambulance providers, will give a complete catalog of medical air transport capabilities. The catalog will be known as the "National Air Medical Transport Units Resources Catalog." The short title "Resources Catalog" may be used when the meaning is clear.

The "Resources Catalog" is designed for use by planners, particularly in the time of a major national emergency. The format contained in this specification provides a standard method of presenting the key data so that communications during a stressful time will be quicker and easier.

Special attention has been taken to identify that information that is needed for immediate reference. For example, the concern during an emergency will be for the numbers of patients that can be carried, and at what level of care, rather than the commercial details about a particular name brand.

1. Scope

1.1 This specification provides the format and guidelines for producing a catalog of current resources of air medical transport units, showing the patient care capability of each, in standard form.

1.2 This specification applies to all the air transports involved in patient care that meet one or more applicable ASTM medical transport unit specifications.

1.3 This specification incorporates only the information that is considered essential for use by the planners during an emergency. The intent is to provide information on what is available, what level of care it can provide, where it is, and the earliest it can respond, so that the most efficient use can be made of each unit, in accordance with the emergency plans.

1.4 Information contained in the unit's operations manual,[2] such as the weight and balance calculations for the "Specialized Medical Resources" listed in Appendix X1, is not included in the catalog but it will be available to the planners, on request.

2. Significance and Use

2.1 The intent of the "Resources Catalog" is to tabulate the national capability for medical air transportation and to enumerate the level of patient care that each unit can provide. The level of care is based on the ASTM Specifications related to each type of medical air transport.

2.2 The "Resources Catalog" will provide a resource with which the emergency planners can identify the capability, availability, and response times for those units outside their local areas. With such up-to-date information, they can request the air medical transport unit that most closely meets the mission profile within the time frame required.

2.3 This catalog will increase public awareness of the availability and the high standard of emergency medical transportation.

3. Format

3.1 Appendix X1 is the format to be completed for each individual unit that meets one or more of the ASTM rotary wing or fixed wing medical transport standards. The format will be completed by the air ambulance provider and the unit's

[1] This specification is under the jurisdiction of ASTM Committee F30 on Emergency Medical Services and is the direct responsibility of Subcommittee F30.01 on EMS Equipment.

Current edition approved April 1, 1991. Published June 1991.

[2] See FAA Advisory Circular 135-14 for recommended content and layout of the unit operation manual. Available from Superintendent of Documents, U.S. Government Printing Office, Washington, DC 20402.

medical director and submitted to the state EMS director (or equivalent official).

3.2 Using this same procedure, the format will be updated by the air ambulance provider[3] annually and each time significant changes occur that affect operational or patient care capability. (This does not include temporary changes such as maintenance down-time.)

3.3 The completed formats will be reviewed by the state EMS director (or equivalent official) and, with state (or equivalent) approval, will be submitted to the F30.01.02 Task Group Chairman for consolidation into this specification. Annual up-dates will be forwarded to the Task Group Chairman prior to the Committee F30's regular year-end meeting.

3.4 The task group will assemble the formats, as submitted, provide a comprehensive index and a map showing the locations and declared areas.

3.5 The catalog will be updated by the task group at the regular year-end meeting and will be published annually by ASTM.

4. Keywords

4.1 air-medical; national resource catalog

[3] *Air Ambulance Provider*—The individual or entity that holds the air ambulance provider certificate and is responsible for and manages the operation of the fixed wing medical transport unit.

APPENDIX

(Nonmandatory Information)

X1. RESOURCES CATALOG FORMAT
EMERGENCY MEDICAL SERVICES
NATIONAL AIR MEDICAL TRANSPORT UNITS RESOURCES CATALOG

Date ______________

1. State ______________
2. City ______________
3. Unit N Number ______________
4. Role
   (a) EMS Level (Check each that apply)
      (i) Unit Category
      Basic ______ Advanced ______ Specialized ______
      (As per ASTM Standard Specifications)
      (ii) Dedicated EMS ______, or
      Multi-mission
      Police ______ Fire ______ Rescue ______
      Other ______________
   (b) EMS Capability
      (i) Number of stretcher patients that can be carried at one time:
      Normal ______________ Maximum ______________
      (ii) Number of seated patients that can be carried at one time:
      ____
      (iii) Comments on the adaptability of the configuration for patient transport in a multi incident situation.
      ____
      ____
      ____
      (iv) Number and titles of Transport Personnel normally on board:
      Flight crewmembers,
      ____
      Air-medical crewmembers,
      ____
      ____
   (c) Specialized Medical Resources (If applicable)
      (i) Neonatal Capability
      (Including number and type of isolettes ______________
      ____
      ____
      (ii) Special Cardiac Capability
      (Including number and type of intra-aortic balloon pumps)
      ____
      (iii) Hyperbaric Capability
      (Including number and type of chambers)
      ____
      (iv) Other ______________
   (d) Specialized Air-Medical Personnel (If applicable)
      ____
      ____
   (e) Rescue Equipment
      (i) None ______________
      (ii) Hoist ______ Capacity ______________
      (iii) Rescue nets (number and size) ______________
      (iv) Sling load capability ______________
      (v) Other ______________
5. Dispatch Information
   (a) Emergency Notification Phone Numbers
   (   ) ______-______, (   ) ______-______

(b) Radio Contact Frequencies for the Unit
_______________, _______________, _______________

(c) Specialized Communications Equipment on Board, Such as Frequency Agile Radios, Cellular Telephones, etc.
____

(d) Time Normally Required Between Mission Acceptance and Liftoff of the Unit
____

(e) Cruise Speed _______________

(f) N Number ___________ Call Sign ___________

(g) Logo (Identifiable Markings) _______________

6. Operational Capabilities

(a) IFR Day Yes _____ No _____
Night Yes _____ No _____

(b) Night Yes _____ No _____

(c) Over Water Yes _____ No _____

(d) Mountain Experience Yes _____ No _____

(e) Normal Days/Hours of Operation ___________

(f) Declared Effective Service Range
_______________ (attach map when applicable)

(g) Aircraft Gross Weight When On:
Skids _______ Wheels _______ Floats _______
(Weight and balance calculations for the practical combinations of specialized equipment and personnel, contained in the unit's operations manual, will be available on request)

(h) Rotary Wing Minimum Landing Area Diameter
____

(i) Fixed Wing Runway Landing/Takeoff Minimums at Gross Weight
____

(j) Transient Deviations (if applicable)
____

7. Contacts

(a) Program Director
Name _______________
Phone _______________
Address _______________

(b) Medical Director
Name _______________
Phone _______________
Address _______________

(c) Air Ambulance Provider[3]
Name _______________
Phone _______________
Address _______________

The American Society for Testing and Materials takes no position respecting the validity of any patent rights asserted in connection with any item mentioned in this standard. Users of this standard are expressly advised that determination of the validity of any such patent rights, and the risk of infringement of such rights, are entirely their own responsibility.

This standard is subject to revision at any time by the responsible technical committee and must be reviewed every five years and if not revised, either reapproved or withdrawn. Your comments are invited either for revision of this standard or for additional standards and should be addressed to ASTM Headquarters. Your comments will receive careful consideration at a meeting of the responsible technical committee, which you may attend. If you feel that your comments have not received a fair hearing you should make your views known to the ASTM Committee on Standards, at the address shown below.

Last ASTM Designation: F 1119 – 91

Standard Specification for
Rotary Wing Basic Life Support Transport Units

This specification pertains to rotary wing transport units involved in patient transportation and care at the basic life support level.

Formerly under the jurisdiction of Committee F-30 on Emergency Medical Services, this specification was withdrawn in January 2000.[1]

[1] Annual Book of ASTM Standards, Volume 13.01.

Last ASTM Designation: F 1124 – 91

Standard Specification for Rotary Wing Advanced Life Support Transport Units

This specification pertains to rotary wing transport units involved in patient transportation and care at the advanced life support level. Formerly under the jurisdiction of Committee F30 on Emergency Medical Services, this practice was withdrawn in February 2000.

Last ASTM Designation: F 1146 – 91

Standard Specification for
Rotary Wing Specialized Medical Transport Units

This specification pertains to rotary wing transport units involved in patient transportation and care at the specialized medical transport level.

Formerly under the jurisdiction of Committee F-30 on Emergency Medical Services, this specification was withdrawn in January 2000.[1]

---

[1] Annual Book of ASTM Standards, Volume 13.01.

Standard Test Method for Tension Testing of Calcium Phosphate and Metallic Coatings[1]

This standard is issued under the fixed designation F 1147; the number immediately following the designation indicates the year of original adoption or, in the case of revision, the year of last revision. A number in parentheses indicates the year of last reapproval. A superscript epsilon (ε) indicates an editorial change since the last revision or reapproval.

1. Scope

1.1 This test method covers tension testing of calcium phosphate and porous metallic coatings adhering to dense metal substrates at ambient temperatures. It assesses the degree of adhesion of coatings to substrates, or the internal cohesion of a coating in tension normal to the surface plane.

1.2 The values stated in inch-pound units are to be regarded as the standard.

1.3 *This standard does not purport to address all of the safety concerns, if any, associated with its use. It is the responsibility of the user of this standard to establish appropriate safety and health practices and determine the applicability of regulatory limitations prior to use.*

2. Referenced Documents

2.1 *ASTM Standards:*

C 633 Test Method for Adhesion or Cohesive Strength of Flame-Sprayed Coatings[2]

E 4 Practices for Force Verification of Testing Machines[3]

E 6 Terminology Relating to Methods of Mechanical Testing[3]

E 8 Test Methods for Tension Testing of Metallic Materials[3]

3. Terminology

3.1 The definitions of terms relating to tension testing appearing in Terminology E 6 shall be considered as applying to the terms used in this test method.

4. Summary of Test Method

4.1 The tensile test method consists of subjecting a specimen assembly composed of one coated and one uncoated component to a tensile load. In the case of the calcium phosphate coatings, the components to be tested must be bonded together by use of a polymeric adhesive. In the case of the metallic coatings, the components may either be bonded with the adhesive, or sintered together. The adhesive may be in film form or bulk form, but it must have a minimum bulk tensile strength of 34.5 MPa (5000 psi).

4.2 The tensile load must be applied normal to the plane of the coating utilizing a tension machine which is capable of determining the maximum strength of the coating or coating attachment to the substrate interface.

5. Significance and Use

5.1 The tensile test method is recommended for tension testing of calcium phosphate/substrate or porous metal coating/substrate combinations and can provide information on the adhesive or cohesive strength of coatings under (uniaxial) tensile stress.

5.2 The test method may be useful for comparative evaluation of adhesive or cohesive strengths of a variety of types of coatings. Coatings may be applied using a variety of methods, including but not limited to plasma-spraying and sintering. Information developed using this method may be useful for certain quality control and design purposes.

5.3 The test should not be considered to provide an intrinsic value for utilization directly in making calculations such as determining the ability of a coating to withstand specified environmental stresses.

5.4 Processing variables such as substrate preparation prior to coating, surface texture, coating technique variables or postcoating heat treatment variables may introduce a significant effect on the results of the tension test. The specimen being evaluated must be representative of the actual end use coating.

6. Apparatus

6.1 *Testing Machines*—Machines used for testing shall conform to the requirements of Practices E 4. The loads used in determining tensile strength and yield strength shall be within the loading range of the testing machine as defined in Practices E 4.

6.2 *Gripping Devices*:

6.2.1 *General*—Various types of grips may be used to transmit the load applied to the specimens by the testing machine. To ensure axial tensile stress, it is important that the specimen axis coincide with the centerline of the heads of the testing machine and that the coating test plane be perpendicular to the axial load. Any departure from this requirement (that is,

---

[1] This test method is under the jurisdiction of ASTM Committee F-4 on Medical and Surgical Materials and Devices and is the direct responsibility of Subcommittee F04.15 on Materials Test Methods.

Current edition approved March 10, 1999. Published June 1999. Originally published as F 1147 – 88. Last previous edition F 1147 – 95.

[2] *Annual Book of ASTM Standards*, Vol 02.05.

[3] *Annual Book of ASTM Standards*, Vol 03.01.

any eccentric loading) will introduce bending stresses that are not included in the usual stress calculation (force/cross-sectional area).

6.2.2 *Yoke and Dowel Pin Grips*—A schematic diagram of a typical gripping device for specimens with holes drilled for pin loading is illustrated in Fig. 1. There should be two perpendicular pins in order to maximize off axis loading.

7. Materials

7.1 *Adhesive Bonding Agent*—A polymeric adhesive bonding agent in film form, or filled viscous adhesive cement, when used, shall be identified and shall meet the following requirements.

7.1.1 The bonding agent shall be capable of bonding the coating on the test specimen components with a tensile strength that is at least 34.5 MPa (5000 psi) or as great as the minimum required adhesion or cohesion strength of the coating.

7.1.2 In instances where porosity extends to the coating substrate interface, the bonding agent shall be sufficiently viscous and application to the coating sufficiently careful to assure that it will not penetrate through the coating to the substrate. The FM 1000 Adhesive Film[4] with a thickness of 0.25 mm (0.01 inc.) has proven satisfactory for this test. If a material other than FM 1000 is used, or the condition of the FM 1000 is unknown, it must be tested to establish its equivalence fresh FM 1000. Testing should be performed without the presence of the coating to establish the performance of the adhesive.

8. Test Specimens

8.1 *General*:

8.1.1 In order to ensure precision and accuracy in test results, it is important that care be exercised in the preparation of specimens, both in machining and in the case of multi-part specimens, in the assembly. Specimen components must be properly aligned in order that generated stresses be purely axial, that is, normal to the coated surface.

8.1.2 *Tensile-Type Specimens*—Three general types of test specimens are illustrated in Figs. 2 and 3. A complete, assembled test assembly consists either of two solid pieces; one with a coated surface and the other with an uncoated surface or three solid pieces; two with uncoated surfaces and one with a coating applied on one side. The uncoated surface may be roughened to aid in the bonding of the adhesive.

8.1.3 The cross-sectional area of the substrate upon which the coating is applied shall be nominal 5.07 cm^2 (0.78 in^2).

[4] Available from Cytec, Harve Grace, Maryland.

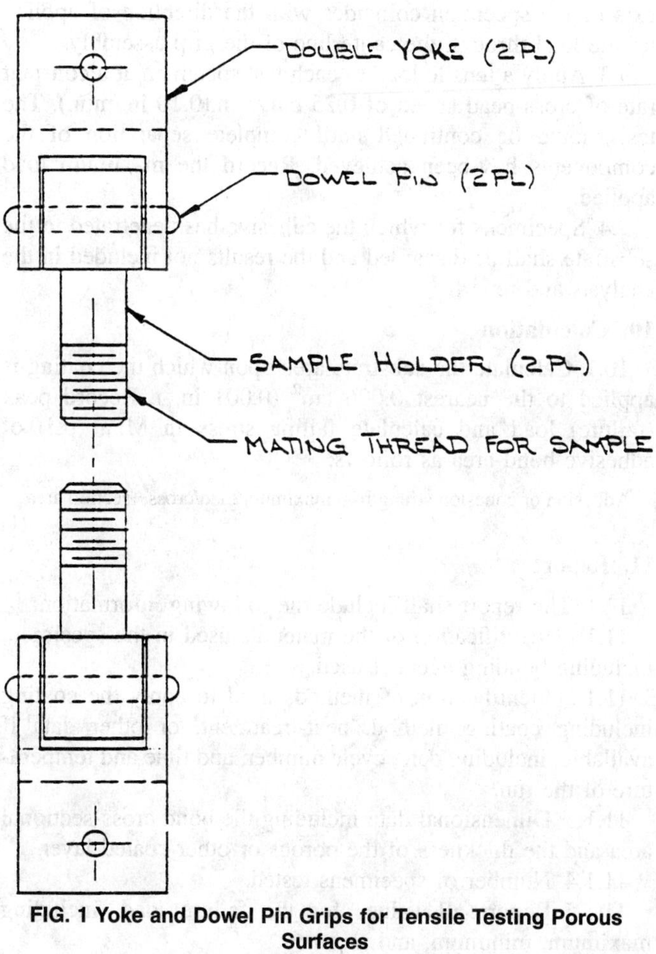

FIG. 1 Yoke and Dowel Pin Grips for Tensile Testing Porous Surfaces

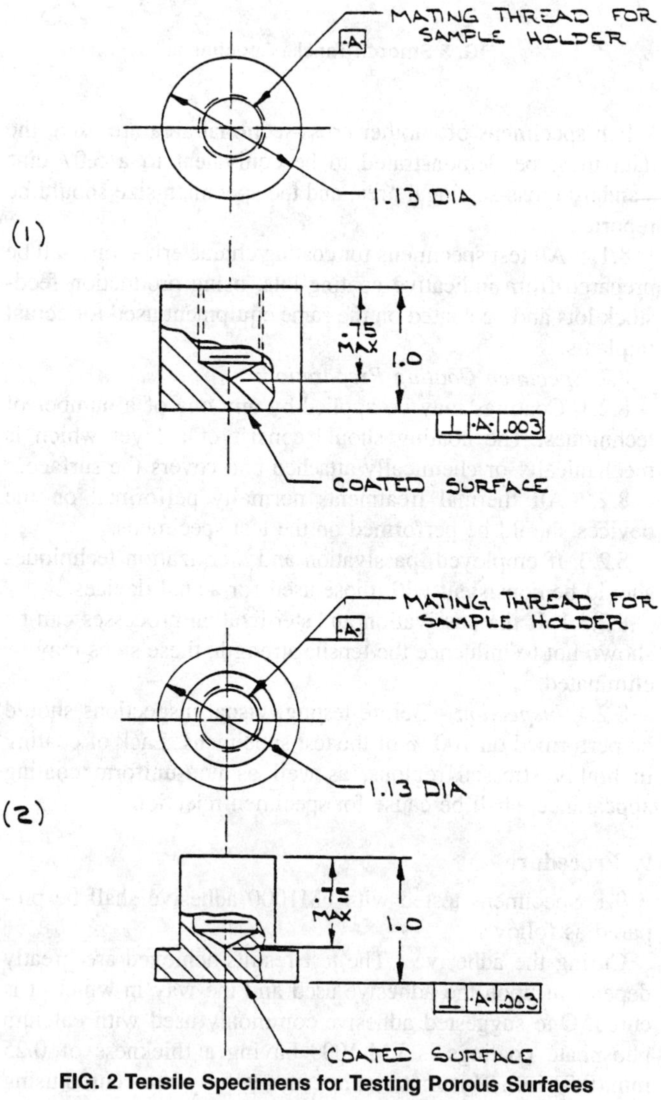

FIG. 2 Tensile Specimens for Testing Porous Surfaces

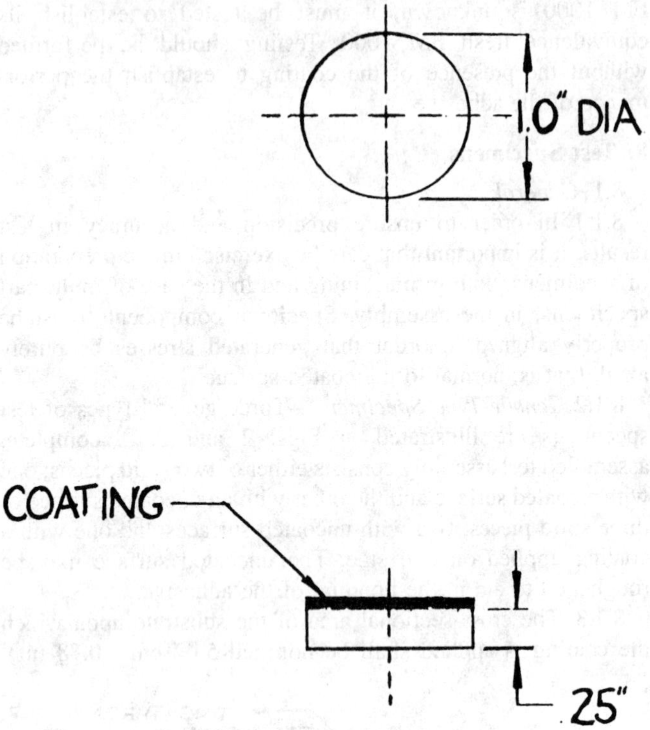

FIG. 3 Smooth Tensile Specimens

When specimens of another cross-sectional area are used, the data must be demonstrated to be equivalent to a 5.07 cm^2 standard cross-sectional area, and the specimen size should be reported.

8.1.4 All test specimens for coating characterization shall be prepared from indicative coating lots, using production feedstock lots and be coated on the same equipment used for actual implants.

8.2 *Specimen Coating Preparation*:

8.2.1 Coatings may be applied by any one of a number of techniques. The coating should consist of a layer which is mechanically or chemically attached and covers the surface.

8.2.2 All thermal treatments normally performed on the devices should be performed on the test specimens.

8.2.3 If employed, passivation and sterilization techniques should be consistent with those used for actual devices.

8.2.3.1 If the passivation and sterilization processes can be shown not to influence the tensile strength, these steps may be eliminated.

8.2.4 *Inspection* - Before testing, visual inspections should be performed on 100 % of the test specimens. Lack of coating in highly stressed regions, as well as non-uniform coating appearance, shall be cause for specimen rejection.

9. Procedure

9.1 Specimens tested with FM1000 adhesive shall be prepared as follows:

Curing the adhesive - The test results achieved are greatly dependent upon the adhesive used and the way in which it is cured. One suggested adhesive commonly used with calcium phosphate coatings is FM-1000 having a thickness of 0.25 mm.(0.01 in.). This material has successfully been cured using the following cycle: Where testing porous coatings, more than one layer of glue may need to be employed.

NOTE 1—In the case of porous coatings, care must be taken to guarantee that the adhesive does not bond to the substrate.

9.1.1 Align the adhesive with the surface of the coating, taking precautions to align the adhesive in the center of the coating.

9.1.2 Apply a constant force using a calibrated high temperature spring, resulting in a stress of 0.138 MPa.(20 Psi.) between the coating and the opposing device that will test the coating.

9.1.2.1 Care must be taken to maintain alignment of the coating and the matching counterface during the curing of the adhesive.

9.1.3 Place the assembly in an oven and heat at 176°C (350°F) for 2–3 h.

9.1.3.1 The exact amount of time necessary to cure the adhesive will need to be determined by each user, as oven temperature may vary with load size and oven type. It is suggested that the curing cycle be optimized without the coating present, first.

9.1.4 Remove the cured assembly from the oven and allow it to cool to room temperature.

9.1.5 Remove all excess glue which has protruded from the coated surface. This process must not compromise the integrity of the sample.

9.2 Place the specimen assembly in the grips so that the long axis of the specimen coincides with the direction of applied tensile load through the centerline of the grip assembly.

9.3 Apply a tensile load to each test specimen at a constant rate of cross-head speed of 0.25 cm./min.(0.10 in./min.). The test should be continued until complete separation of the components has been achieved. Record the maximum load applied.

9.4 Specimens for which the adhesive has penetrated to the substrate shall be discarded and the results not included in the analysis and report.

10. Calculation

10.1 Calculate the substrate area upon which the coating is applied to the nearest 0.006 cm^2 (0.001 $in.^2$). Record peak (failure) load and calculate failing stress in MPa (psi) of adhesive bond area as follows:

$$\text{Adhesion or cohesion strength} = \text{maximum load/cross-section area} \quad (1)$$

11. Report

11.1 The report shall include the following information:

11.1.1 Identification of the materials used in the specimen, including bonding agent if used.

11.1.2 Identification of methods used to apply the coating including coating method, heat-treatment, or other data if available, including date, cycle number, and time and temperature of the run.

11.1.3 Dimensional data including the bond cross-sectional area and the thickness of the porous or other coated layer.

11.1.4 Number of specimens tested.

11.1.5 Report all values for the failure load, including maximum, minimum, and mean.

11.1.6 The mode of failure (for example, cohesive versus adhesive) for each test specimen.

12. Precision and Bias

12.1 *Precision (beaded F75)*—The precision of this method was established by an interlaboratory comparison among six (6) laboratories. The specimens tested were sintered-bead coatings of F75 (Co-Cr-Mo) alloy on F75 substrates. The population mean tensile strength was 4325 lbf/in^2 (29.8 MPa) for all samples tested by all laboratories.

12.1.1 *Repeatability*—For replicate results obtained by the same operator on nominally-identical test materials, the repeatability standard deviation (S_r) was 613 lbf/in^2 (4.23 MPa). Any two such results (would be expected to differ by more than) 1715 lbf/in^2 (11.8 MPa) only 1 time in 20.

12.1.2 *Reproducibility*—For independent results obtained by different operators working in different laboratories on nominally-identical test materials, the reproducibility standard deviation (S_R) was 772 lbf/in^2 (5.32 MPa). Any two such results (would be expected to differ by more than) 2160 lbf/in^2 (14.8 MPa) only 1 time in 20.

NOTE 2—The precision study under Section 12.1 was conducted using coupons which had a one square inch area (1.13 in. diameter). The bead tensile strength was intentionally lowered for this round robin comparison to produce coating fractures rather than glue failures in the coupons.

12.2 *Precision (HA Coating)*—The precision of this method was established by an interlaboratory comparison among seven (7) laboratories. The substrate of the specimens tested was Titanium -6 Aluminum -4 vanadium, which was hydroxylapatite coated. The mean tensile strength was 8405 lbf/in^2 (58.0) MPa for all samples tested by all laboratories.

12.2.1 *Repeatability*—For replicate results obtained by the same operator on nominally-identical test materials, the repeatability standard deviation S_r was 1016 lbf/in^2 (7.0 MPa). Any two such results (would be expected to differ by more than) 2845 lbf/in^2 (19.6 MPa) only one time in 20.

12.2.2 *Reproducibility*—For independent results obtained by different operators working in different laboratories on nominally-identical test materials, the reproducibility standard deviation (S_R) was 1758 lbf/in^2 (12.1 MPa). Any two such results (would be expected to differ by more than) 4922 lbf/in^2 (33.9 MPa) only one time in 20.

NOTE 3—The precision study under Section 12.2 was run using a cross-head speed of 0.05 in/min (0.12 cm/min).

12.3 *Bias*—Since the measurement of porous-coating tensile strength by this method is a destructive test measurement unique to each individual test sample, no independent determination of a "correct" or "reference" value is possible. Thus, no statements regarding the deviation of values, measured in accordance with these procedures, from accepted values is possible.

13. Keywords

13.1 ceramic materials; hydroxylapatite; tribasic calcium phosphate; tension testing; adherence; interface; porous coating

ANNEXES

(Mandatory Information)

A1. PROCEDURE FOR BONDING POROUS COATED TEST SPECIMENS USING 3M SCOTCH-WELD 2214-NMF STRUCTURAL ADHESIVE

A1.1 Surface to be bonded must be clean, degreased, and free of any loose particles/beads.

A1.2 A thin layer of the adhesive shall be applied evenly to the coated surface of the test coupons. A spatula or tongue depressor may be used as application device.

A1.3 Excess adhesive shall be squeezed out of the assembly using hand pressure while coated faces of the test coupons are buffed together.

A1.4 The specimen thus prepared will be placed in a suitable fixture. During curing, the fixture shall be able to maintain a mild pressure at the joint. At the same time, it shall also force bonding faces to remain parallel and maintain the axial alignment.

A1.5 The specimen joint shall be cured at 250 ± 10°F (121 ± 5.7°C) in air for 1.25 h (a sharp pointed pin must not be able to penetrate the adhesive joint after optimum curing).

A1.6 Air cool to room temperature prior to testing.

A2. PROCEDURE FOR BONDING POROUS COATED TEST SPECIMENS USING FM 1000 FILM ADHESIVE

A2.1 Clean the specimen holders. If the holders have test coupons on them from a previous test, place the holders in the oven at 270°C for 1 h.

A2.1.1 After 1 h, put oven gloves on and take the holders out of the oven.

A2.1.2 Break the coupons off of the holders with gloved hands or with a pair of pliers.

A2.1.3 Cool the holders in water or air cool.

A2.1.4 The adhesive will stay on the holder; this will have to be removed. The adhesive is removed by polishing it off on a fiber wheel. If necessary, face off the holders in a lathe, as the faces must be parallel. The holders are then grit blasted.

A2.1.5 Test coupons to be run should not have any proud beads, nor should the beads extend past the side of the specimen.

A2.1.6 The holders and test coupons are placed in a set of pliers and dipped in trichlorotrifluoroethane, or equivalent, which is to clean and degrease the parts.

A2.1.7 The holders and test coupons are placed on tissues to evaporate the trichlorotrifluoroethane.

NOTE A2.1—Handle all of the test material with gloved hands because the test can vary with the amount of oil absorbed from the skin.

NOTE A2.2—Follow all manufacturer's instructions concerning the storage procedure and shelf life of the adhesive.

NOTE A2.3—**Precaution:** Handle the trichlorotrifluoroethane with care and use under a vent-hood.

NOTE A2.4—**Precaution:** Avoid inhalation of fumes during heating cycles.

A2.2 The adhesive that is used is FM 1000 film, 0.06 or 0.05 lb/sq ft produced by the American Cyanamid Company. Cut disks out of the adhesive to match the shape and dimensions of the test coupon.

A2.3 Typical assembly of components will include placing one adhesive disk between the back of the sample coupon and the specimen holder and two disks between the porous coated surface of the coupon and the other specimen holders. The amount of glue (the thickness of the sheets, as well as the number of sheets) is selected by a balance between having enough glue to fully bond the specimen holder with the test coupon, but not so much as to force the glue to the coupon's substrate which would render the test invalid. The fixturing of the assembly should maintain alignment during the glue curing cycle. A small compressive pressure placed on the components helps to prevent sliding and misalignment. This is best accomplished with a spring in the fixturing. An excessive pressure or amount of glue must not be used as the glue will be squeezed out and distort test values.

A2.4 Turn the oven on and preheat to 177°C (350°F). When the oven reaches the temperature, place the assembled curing fixtures in the oven on a level surface.

A2.5 Maintain this temperature for 2.5 h.

A2.6 Allow curing holders to air cool to room temperature before removing specimens.

A2.7 Samples cured at elevated temperatures should be allowed to remain at room temperature for 24 h before testing. This time period will allow for the adhesive to full cure, eliminating variations that may result if the adhesive has not reached an equilibrium temperature.

NOTE A2.5—A fan can be used to speed up the cooling process.

APPENDIXES

(Nonmandatory Information)

X1. RATIONALE

X1.1 This standard is needed to aid in the development of a high quality material for use in load-bearing implant applications. The influence of coatings on the resulting tensile behavior of the system must be viewed as a combination of the surface roughening treatments required to apply the coating, the thermal effects of the coating process, and any other secondary treatments employed. The purpose of this specification is to provide the following information: 1) the influence of the above processing steps, and 2) the integrity of the coating and the coating/substrate interface.

X2. PRECISION AND BIAS (EXAMPLE)

X2.1 Precision and Bias

X2.1.1 Review of the Round Robin - Seven laboratories were involved in round-robin testing. Each laboratory was provided with six (6) specimens coated with hydroxylapataite and an appropriate amount of FM 1000.

X2.1.2 Table 1 shows the raw data generated from each laboratory.

X2.1.3 *h Graph*:

X2.1.3.1 The h value evaluates the consistency of the test results from laboratory to laboratory.

X2.1.3.2 There are three patterns in these plots. In one pattern, all values are either positive or negative. In the second pattern, there are roughly the same number of laboratories which exhibit positive values as those which exhibit negative values. In the third type, one laboratory exhibits a value which is opposite of the other laboratories. The first two types are considered normal.

X2.1.3.3 Fig. X2.1 shows the h values for each laboratory.

X2.1.4 *k Graph*:

X2.1.4.1 The k value evaluates the consistency of the test results within each laboratory.

X2.1.4.2 The pattern to look for in the k graph is one laboratory having a very large or a very small k value. High k values indicate imprecision. Very small k values indicate a very insensitive measurement scale or other measurement problems. A k value greater than 1 indicates greater variability than other laboratories.

X2.1.4.3 Fig. X2.2 shows the k values for each laboratory.

X2.1.5 *Precision Statistics*—The precision statistics are shown in Table 2. These statistics are also reported in Section 12.2.

X2.1.6 ASTM would like to acknowledge the following companies for their help in the round-robin testing: Bio-Coat, Bio-vac, EML, FDA, Howmedica, Osteonics, and Steri-OSS.

TABLE 1 ASTM F 1147 Round Robin, Tensile Strength (psi)[A]

Company #1	Company #2	Company #3	Company #4	Company #5	Company #6	Company #7
9790	8945	10770	8612	5206[B]	9786	7222
7430	8150	10986	7949	9495	9469	4897
5510	6680	11712	6841	8832	11383	8402
8390	7144	11330	7261	8965	9048	8459
6750	5230	10922	7911	8743	9208	5919
7330	4815	10680	8230	8515	10614	7735
7533 ± 1455	6502 ± 1241	11067 ± 387	7801 ± 646	8910 ± 366	9918 ± 907	7106 ± 1429

[A] Data previously published in ASTM F 1501.
[B] Value excluded due to improper alignment.

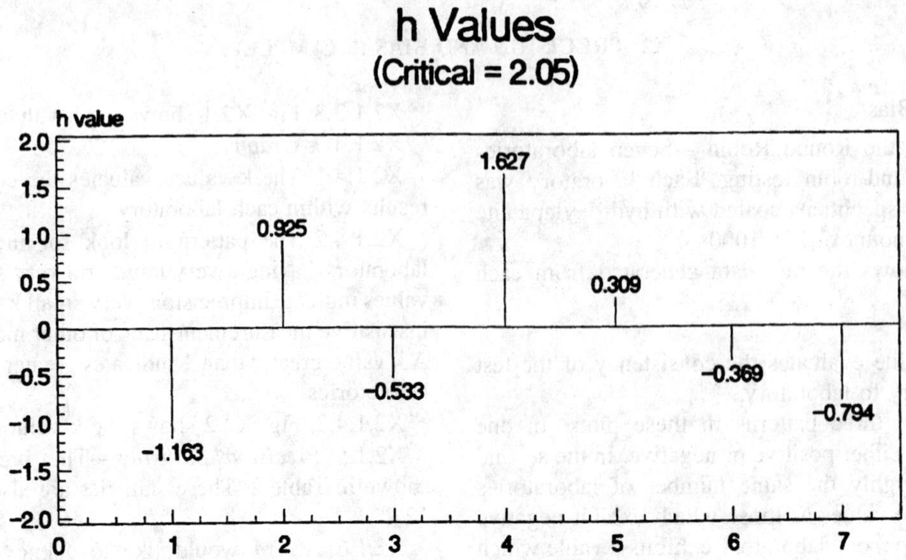

FIG. X2.1 h Values (Critical = 2.05)

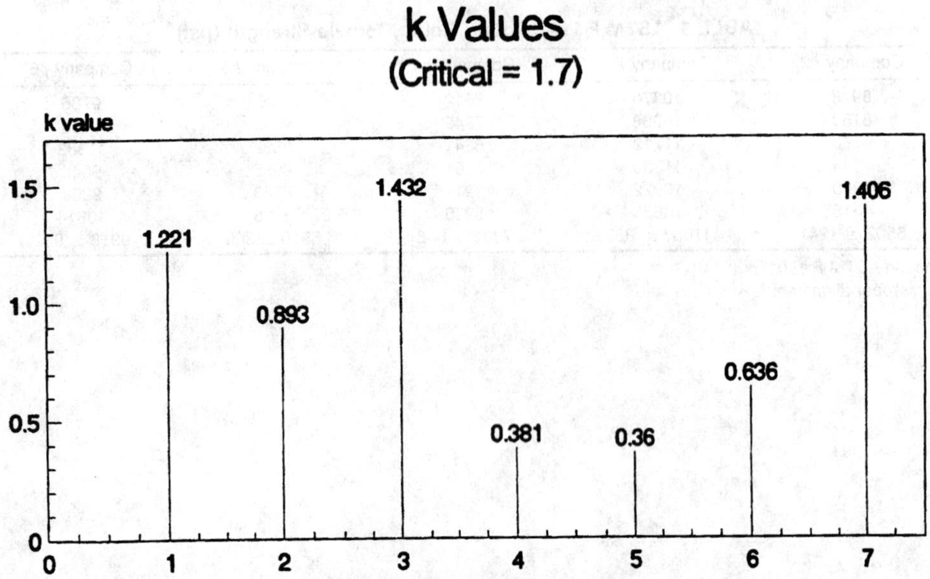

FIG. X2.2 k Values (Critical = 1.7)

TABLE 2 PRECISION STATISTICS

X	S_x	S_r	S_R	r	R
8405	1636	1016	1758	2845	4922

X = average of the cell averages
S_x = standard deviation of the cell averages
S_r = repeatability standard deviation
S_R = reproducibility standard deviation
r = 95 % repeatability limit, and
R = 95 % reproducibility limit

Designation: F 1149 – 93 (Reapproved 1998)

Standard Practice for Qualifications, Responsibilities, and Authority of Individuals and Institutions Providing Medical Direction of Emergency Medical Services[1]

This standard is issued under the fixed designation F 1149; the number immediately following the designation indicates the year of original adoption or, in the case of revision, the year of last revision. A number in parentheses indicates the year of last reapproval. A superscript epsilon (ε) indicates an editorial change since the last revision or reapproval.

1. Scope

1.1 This practice covers the qualifications, responsibilities, and authority of individuals and institutions providing medical direction of emergency medical services.

1.2 This practice addresses the qualifications, authority, and responsibility of a Medical Director (off-line) and the relationship of the EMS (Emergency Medical Services) provider to this individual.

1.3 This practice also addresses components of on-line medical direction (direct medical control) including the qualifications and responsibilities of on-line medical physicians and the relationship of the prehospital provider to on-line medical direction.

1.4 This practice addresses the relationship of the on-line medical physician to the off-line Medical Director.

1.5 The authority for control of medical services at the scene of a medical emergency is addressed in this practice.

1.6 The requirements for a Communication Resource are also addressed within this practice.

2. Referenced Documents

2.1 *ASTM Standards:*

F 1031 Practice for Training the Emergency Medical Technician (Basic)[2]

F 1086 Guide for Structures and Responsibilities of Emergency Medical Services Systems Organizations[2]

3. Terminology

3.1 *Description of Terms Specific to This Practice*

3.2 *communication resource*—an entity responsible for implementation of direct medical control. (Also known as medical control resource.)

3.3 *delegated practice*—only physicians are licensed to practice medicine; prehospital providers must act only under the medical direction of a physician.

3.4 *direct medical control*—when a physician or authorized communication resource personnel, under the direction of a physician, provides immediate medical direction to prehospital providers in remote locations. (Also known as on-line medical direction.)

3.5 *emergency medical services system (EMSS)*—all components needed to provide comprehensive prehospital and hospital emergency care including, but not limited to; Medical Director, transport vehicles, trained personnel, access and dispatch, communications, and receiving medical facilities.

3.6 *intervener physicians*—a licensed M.D. or D.O., having not previously established a doctor/patient relationship with the emergency patient and willing to accept responsibility for a medical emergency scene, and can provide proof of a current Medical License.

3.7 *medical direction*—when a physician is identified to develop, implement, and evaluate all medical aspects of an EMS system. (*syn.* medical accountability.)

3.8 *medical director off-line*—a physician responsible for all aspects of an EMS system dealing with provision of medical care. (Also known as System Medical Director.)

3.9 *on-line medical physician*—a physician immediately available, when medically appropriate, for communication of medical direction to non-physician prehospital providers in remote locations.

3.10 *prehospital provider*—all personnel providing emergency medical care in a location remote from facilities capable of providing definitive medical care.

3.11 *protocols*—standards for EMS practice in a variety of situations within the EMS system.

3.12 *standing orders*—strictly defined written orders for actions, techniques, or drug administration when communication has not been established with an on-line physician.

4. Significance and Use

4.1 Implementation of this practice will ensure that the EMS system has the authority, commensurate with the responsibility, to ensure adequate medical direction of all prehospital providers, as well as personnel and facilities that meet minimum criteria to implement medical direction of prehospital services.

4.1.1 The state will develop, recommend, and encourage use of a plan that would assure the standards outlined in this document can be implemented as appropriate at the local, regional, or state level (see Guide F 1086).

---

[1] This practice is under the jurisdiction of ASTM Committee F-30 on Emergency Medical Services and is the direct responsibility of Subcommittee F30.03 on Organization/Management.

Current edition approved August 15, 1993. Published October 1993. Originally published as F 1149 – 88. Last previous edition F 1149 – 88.

[2] *Annual Book of ASTM Standards*, Vol 13.01.

4.1.2 This practice is intended to describe and define responsibility for medical directions during transfers. It is not intended to determine the medical or legal, or both, appropriateness of transfers under the Consolidated Omnibus Budget Reconciliation Act and other similar federal and/or state laws.

5. Medical Director

5.1 *Position*—System Medical Director (Off-line Medical Director).

5.1.1 Each EMS system shall have an identifiable Medical Director who, after consultation with others involved and interested in the system, is responsible for the development, implementation, and evaluation of standards for provision of medical care within the system.

5.1.1.1 All prehospital providers (including EMT (Emergency Medical Technician) basics) shall be medically accountable for their actions and are responsible to the Medical Director of the EMS agency (local, regional, or state) that approves their continued participation.

5.1.1.2 All prehospital providers, with levels of certification above EMT basic, shall be responsible to an identifiable physician who directs their medical care activity.

5.1.2 The Medical Director shall be appointed by, and accountable to, the appropriate EMS agency in accordance with Guide F 1086.

5.2 *Requirements of a Medical Director*:

5.2.1 The medical aspects (see 5.3) of an emergency medical service system shall be managed by physicians who meet the following requirements:

5.2.1.1 Licensed physician, M.D. or D.O.

5.2.1.2 Experience in, and current knowledge of, emergency care of patients who are acutely ill or traumatized.

5.2.1.3 Knowledge of, and access to, local mass casualty plans.

5.2.1.4 Familiarity with Communication Resource operations where applicable, including communication with, and direction of, prehospital emergency units.

5.2.1.5 Active involvement in the training of prehospital personnel.

5.2.1.6 Active involvement in the medical audit, review, and critique of medical care provided by prehospital personnel.

5.2.1.7 Knowledge of the administrative and legislative process affecting the local, regional, and/or state prehospital EMS system.

5.2.1.8 Knowledge of laws and regulations affecting local, regional, and state EMS.

5.3 *Authority of a Medical Director Includes but is not Limited to*:

5.3.1 Establishing system-wide medical protocols (including standing orders) in consultation with appropriate specialists.

5.3.2 Recommending certification or decertification of non-physician prehospital personnel to the appropriate certifying agencies.

5.3.2.1 Every system shall have an appropriate review and appeals mechanism, when decertification is recommended, to assure due process in accordance with law and established local policies. The Director shall promptly refer the case to the appeals mechanism for review, if requested.

5.3.3 Requiring education to the level of approved proficiency for personnel within the EMS system. This includes all prehospital personnel, EMTs at all levels, prehospital emergency care nurses, dispatchers, educational coordinators, and physician providers of on-line direction (see Practice F 1031).

5.3.4 Suspending a provider from medical care duties for due cause pending review and evaluation.

5.3.4.1 Because the prehospital provider operates under the license (delegated practice) or direction of the Medical Director, the director shall have ultimate authority to allow the prehospital provider to provide medical care within the prehospital phase of the EMS system.

5.3.4.2 Whenever a Medical Director makes a decision to suspend a provider from medical care duties, the process shall be prescribed by previously established criteria.

5.3.5 Establishing medical standards for dispatch procedures to assure that the appropriate EMS response unit(s) are dispatched to the medical emergency scene when requested, and the duty to evaluate the patient is fulfilled.

5.3.6 Establishing under what circumstances non-transport might occur.

5.3.6.1 All decisions by prehospital providers regarding non-transport shall be based on defined protocol or on-line communications.

5.3.6.2 Develop a procedure for record keeping when the reason for non-transport was the result of a patient's refusal, including the appropriate forms and review process.

5.3.7 Establishing under which circumstances a patient may be transported against his or her will; in accordance with state law including, procedure, appropriate forms, and review process.

5.3.8 Establishing criteria for level of care and type of transportation to be used in prehospital emergency care (that is, advanced life support versus basic life support, ground, air, or specialty unit transportation).

5.3.9 Establishing criteria for selection of patient destination.

5.3.10 Establishing educational and performance standards for Communication Resource personnel.

5.3.11 Establishing operational standards for Communication Resource.

5.3.12 Conducting effective system audit and quality assurance.

5.3.12.1 The Medical Director shall have access to all relevant EMS records needed to accomplish this task. These documents shall be considered quality assurance documents and shall be privileged and confidential information.

5.3.13 Insuring the availability of educational programs within the system and that they are consistent with accepted local medical practice.

5.3.14 May delegate portions of his or her duties to other qualified individuals.

6. Direct Medical Control (On-Line Medical Direction)

6.1 *The Practice of Direct Medical Control*:

6.1.1 On-line medical direction capabilities shall exist and be available within the EMS system, unless impossible due to distance or geographic considerations.

6.1.1.1 All prehospital providers, above the certification of

EMT basic, shall be assigned to a specific on-line communication resource by a predetermined policy.

6.1.2 Specific local protocols shall exist which define those circumstances under which on-line medical direction is required.

6.1.3 On-line medical direction is the practice of medicine and all orders to the prehospital provider shall originate from or be under the direct supervision and responsibility of a physician.

6.1.4 The receiving hospital shall be notified prior to the arrival of each patient transported by the EMS system unless directed otherwise by local protocol.

6.2 *The On-Line Medical Physician*:

6.2.1 This physician shall be approved to serve in this capacity by the system Medical Director (off-line).

6.2.1.1 This physician shall have received education to the level of proficiency approved by the off-line Medical Director for proper provision of on-line medical direction, including communications equipment, operation, and techniques.

6.2.1.2 This physician shall be appropriately trained in prehospital protocols, familiar with the capabilities of the prehospital providers, as well as local EMS operational policies and regional critical care referral protocols.

6.2.2 This physician shall have demonstrated knowledge and expertise in the prehospital care of critically ill and injured patients.

6.2.3 This physician assumes responsibility for appropriate actions of the prehospital provided to the extent that the on-line physician is involved in patient care direction.

6.2.4 The on-line physician is responsible to the system Medical Director (off-line) regarding proper implementation of medical and system protocols.

7. Authority for Control of Medical Services at the Scene of Medical Emergency

7.1 *General*:

7.1.1 Control of a medical emergency scene shall be the responsibility of the individual in attendance who is most appropriately trained and knowledgeable in providing prehospital emergency stabilization and transport.

7.1.2 When an advanced life support (ALS) squad, under medical direction, is requested and dispatched to the scene of an emergency, a doctor/patient relationship has been established between the patient and the physician providing medical direction.

7.1.3 The prehospital provider is responsible for the management of the patient and acts as the agent of medical direction.

7.2 *Patient's Private Physician Present*:

7.2.1 When the patient's private physician is present and assumes responsibility for the patient's care, the prehospital provider should defer to the orders of the private physician if they do not conflict with established system protocols and the private physician documents the orders in a manner acceptable to the EMS system.

7.2.2 The Communication Resource shall be contacted for recordkeeping purposes to notify the on-line medical physician.

7.2.3 When the medical orders of the private physician differ from system protocol, Communication Resource shall be contacted and the private physician placed in communication with the on-line physician. If the private physician and the on-line physician are unable to agree on treatment, the private physician must either continue to provide direct patient care and accompany the patient to the hospital, or defer all remaining care to the on-line physician.

7.2.4 The prehospital provider's responsibility reverts to the systems Medical Director or on-line medical direction any time the private physician is no longer in attendance.

7.3 *Intervener Physician Present and Non-Existent On-Line Medical Direction*:

7.3.1 When an intervener physician has been satisfactorily identified as a licensed physician and has expressed his or her willingness to assume responsibility and document his or her intervention in a manner acceptable to the local emergency medical services system (EMSS), the prehospital provider should defer to the orders of the physician on the scene if they do not conflict with system protocols.

7.3.2 If treatment by the intervener physician at the emergency scene differs from that outlined in a local protocol, the physician shall agree in advance to assume responsibility for care, including accompanying the patient to the hospital.

7.3.3 In the event of a mass casualty incident or disaster, patient care needs may require the intervener physician to remain at the scene.

7.4 *Intervener Physician Present and Existent On-Line Medical Direction*:

7.4.1 If an intervener physician is present and on-line medical direction does exist, the on-line physician should be contacted and the on-line physician is ultimately responsible.

7.4.2 The on-line physician has the option of managing the case entirely, working with the intervener physician, or allowing him or her to assume responsibility.

7.4.2.1 If there is any disagreement between the intervener physician and the on-line physician, the prehospital provider should take orders from the on-line physician and place the intervener physician in contact with the on-line physician.

7.4.3 In the event the intervener physician assumes responsibility, all orders to the prehospital provider shall be repeated to the Communication Resource for purposes of recordkeeping.

7.4.4 The intervener physician should document his or her intervention in a manner acceptable to the local EMS.

7.4.5 The decision of the intervener physician to accompany the patient to the hospital should be made in consultation with the on-line physician.

7.5 Nothing in this section implies that the prehospital provider can be required to deviate from system protocols.

7.6 Air Medical Emergency Medical Service (EMS) Assistance at the Scene of a Medical Emergency (non-mass casualty):

7.6.1 Dispatch of air medical EMS assistance should be according to a pre-established state/regional/local EMS plan. Dispatch according to this pre-established EMS plan should take into account, for example, the patient's condition, response time, proximity of the receiving facility, geographical ease of access by ground, flight safety, and mechanism of injury.

7.6.1.1 The decision to request air medical EMS assistance at the scene of a medical emergency shall be the responsibility of a qualified individual, identified to assume such authority by the pre-established state/regional/local EMS plan.

7.6.2 When the air medical EMS assistance has arrived on the scene, the following shall apply:

7.6.2.1 There will be an orderly transfer of responsibility from the local EMS unit to the air medical EMS unit and its medical control authority, according to local protocols. These protocols should include a method of determining when air transport is appropriate.

7.6.2.2 Medical direction (on-line/off-line) of the local EMS unit retains responsibility until formally relinquished to the medical direction (on-line/off-line) of the receiving air medical EMS unit.

7.6.2.3 If there is a physician on-board the air medical EMS unit, this physician shall be considered an intervenor physician, unless on-line medical direction transfers responsibility to the physician. (See 7.3 and 7.4.)

7.6.2.4 After responsibility has been transferred to the air medical EMS unit, the local EMS unit should cooperate with the air medical EMS unit, and/or assist the air medical EMS unit crew as long as they are not required to exceed the levels of intervention permitted by their certification.

7.6.3 Air medical EMS should offer assistance only when invited or requested, or both, unless no ground unit is available.

7.6.4 The transport destination for the patient should be based upon a pre-established EMS plan that considers time and distance as well as the patient's medical condition and the capability of the receiving facility.

7.6.4.1 If no pre-established EMS plan for patient transport exists, the transport should follow the usual transport pattern of the requesting local EMS unit, unless otherwise indicated by medical considerations.

8. Requirements for Communication Resource (Medical Control Resource)

8.1 Communication Resource shall be designated to participate in the EMS system according to a plan developed by a state or regional authority.

8.2 The Communication Resource shall meet the following requirements:

8.2.1 The Communication Resource shall assure adequate staffing for the communication equipment at all times by health care personnel who have achieved a minimal level of competence and skill and are approved by the system Medical Director.

8.2.2 The Communication Resource shall assure that all requests for medical guidance, assistance, or advice by prehospital personnel will be promptly accommodated with an attitude of utmost participation, responsibility, and cooperation.

8.2.3 The Communication Resource shall provide assurance that they will cooperate with the EMS system in collecting and analyzing data necessary to evaluate the prehospital care program as long as patient confidentiality is not violated.

8.2.4 The Communication Resource will consider the prehospital provider to be the agent of the on-line physician when they are in communication, regardless of any other employee/employer relationship.

8.2.5 The Communication Resource shall assure that the on-line physician will issue transportation instructions and hospital assignments based on system protocols and objective analysis of patient's needs and facility capability and proximity.

8.2.5.1 No effort will be made to obtain institutional or commercial advantages through the use of such transportation instructions and hospital assignments.

8.2.6 When the Communication Resource is acting as an agent for another hospital, the information regarding patient treatment and expected time of arrival will be relayed to the receiving hospital in an accurate and timely fashion.

8.2.7 Communication Resource shall conduct regular case conferences involving the on-line physicians and prehospital personnel for purposes of problem identification and provide continuing education to correct any identified problems.

8.3 If the Communication Resource is located within a hospital facility, the hospital shall meet the requirements listed in 8.1 and 8.2 and the equipment used for on-line medical direction shall be located within the Emergency Department.

9. Medical Direction During Interfacility Transfers (Non-Mass Casualty):

9.1 *General Principles*:

9.1.1 When an emergency patient arrives for initial evaluation at a medical facility, that patient becomes the responsibility of that facility and its medical staff. This responsibility continues until the patient is appropriately discharged, or until the patient is transferred and the responsibility is assumed by the personnel of a facility with equal or greater capability.

9.1.2 All transferring personnel should have standing orders or protocols available for use as appropriate, in the event of inability to communicate with on-line medical direction.

9.1.3 Patient medical records for any interfacility transfer shall be the responsibility of the transferring facility.

9.1.4 A patient not receiving treatment, and expected to remain stable during interfacility transport may, with physician approval, be transferred by an appropriate medical transportation provider with personnel certified at the level of Emergency Medical Technician-Basic, or greater.

9.1.5 When the patient has a probability of experiencing complications which cannot be managed within the scope of practice of non-physician personnel, the transfer shall be managed by an appropriately trained physician, either on-line or off-line.

9.2 *Interfacility Transfers Conducted by the Transferring Facility*:

9.2.1 When a patient is transferred to another facility, is receiving treatment, medically unstable, or potentially medically unstable, it is the responsibility of the transferring facility to assure that the medical transport agency has qualified personnel and transportation equipment to complete the transfer.

9.2.2 The transferring personnel shall act as the agents of the transferring facility and the physician approving the transfer, regardless of any other employer/employee relationship.

Communication between the transferring physician, the pre-hospital on-line medical direction, and the transferring personnel is required, with agreement between physicians regarding medical care. (See 7.2.1 and 7.2.3.)

9.2.3 When a patient experiences complications beyond situations addressed in physician written orders, or beyond off-line protocols, the medical transport provider should, if possible, contact the transferring facility or the receiving facility for additional orders. Or, if deemed necessary, the EMS on-line medical direction should be contacted for consultation.

9.3 Interfacility transfers conducted by a receiving facility when the transferring personnel are agents of the receiving facility:

9.3.1 When the transferring personnel includes a physician, the patient becomes the responsibility of the receiving facility as soon as the patient leaves the transferring facility.

9.3.2 When the transferring team does not include a physician, the physician from the receiving facility who authorizes the transfer is responsible for the patient. The receiving facility must assure that the medical transport team has qualified personnel and transportation equipment to complete the transport.

10. Keywords

10.1 aeromedical; interfacility; medical control; medical direction; on-line/off-line

Designation: F 1160 – 00$^{\epsilon 1}$

Standard Test Method for Shear and Bending Fatigue Testing of Calcium Phosphate and Metallic Medical and Composite Calcium Phosphate/ Metallic Coatings[1]

This standard is issued under the fixed designation F 1160; the number immediately following the designation indicates the year of original adoption or, in the case of revision, the year of last revision. A number in parentheses indicates the year of last reapproval. A superscript epsilon (ϵ) indicates an editorial change since the last revision or reapproval.

ϵ^1 NOTE—Editorial corrections were made to 1.1, 8.1, 8.2, and 9.5.1.2 in June 2001.

1. Scope

1.1 This test method covers the procedure for determining the shear and bending fatigue performance of calcium phosphate coatings and of porous and nonporous metallic coatings and for determining the bending fatigue performance of metallic coatings oversprayed with calcium phosphate. This test method has been established based on plasma-sprayed titanium and plasma-sprayed hydroxylapatite coatings. The efficacy of this test method for other coatings has not been established. In the shear fatigue mode this test method evaluates the adhesive and cohesive properties of the coating on a metallic substrate. In the bending fatigue mode this test method evaluates both the adhesion of the coating as well as the effects that the coating may have on the substrate material. These methods are limited to testing in air at ambient temperature. These test methods are not intended for application in fatigue tests of components or devices; however, the test method which most closely replicates the actual loading configuration is preferred.

1.2 The values stated in SI units are to be regarded as the standard.

1.3 *This standard does not purport to address all of the safety concerns, if any, associated with its use. It is the responsibility of the user of this standard to establish appropriate safety and health practices and determine the applicability of regulatory limitations prior to use.*

2. Referenced Documents

2.1 *ASTM Standards:*

E 6 Terminology Relating to Methods of Mechanical Testing[2]

E 206 Definitions of Terms Relating to Fatigue Testing and the Statistical Analysis of Fatigue Data[3]

E 466 Practice for Conducting Force Controlled Constant Amplitude Axial Fatigue Tests of Metallic Materials[2]

E 467 Practice for Verification of Constant Amplitude Dynamic Loads on Displacements in an Axial Load Fatigue Testing Machine[2]

E 468 Practice for Presentation of Constant Amplitude Fatigue Test Results for Metallic Materials[2]

E 1012 Practice for Verification of Specimen Alignment Under Tensile Loading[2]

3. Definitions

3.1 The definitions of terms relating to shear and fatigue testing appearing in Terminology E 6 shall be considered as applying to the terms used in this test method.

4. Summary of Test Method

4.1 *Shear Fatigue Testing*:

4.1.1 The intent of the shear fatigue test is to determine the adhesive or cohesive strength, or both, of the coating.

4.1.2 This test method is designed to allow the coating to fail at either the coating/substrate interface, within the coating, or at the glue/coating interface between the coating and the adhesive bonding agent used to transmit the load to the coating.

4.2 *Bending Fatigue Testing*:

4.2.1 The primary intent of the bending fatigue test is to quantify the effect that the coating has on the substrate it is applied to. Secondarily, it may be used to provide a subjective evaluation of coating adhesion, (that is, spalling resistance, cracking resistance, and so forth).

4.2.2 This test is designed to first provide a substrate fatigue strength to serve as a baseline to assess the effects of the coating on the resulting fatigue strength of the system.

5. Significance and Use

5.1 The shear and bending fatigue tests are used to determine the effect of variations in material, geometry, surface condition, stress, and so forth, on the fatigue resistance of coated metallic materials subjected to direct stress for up to 10^7 cycles. These tests may be used as a relative guide to the selection of coated materials for service under condition of repeated stress.

[1] This test method is under the jurisdiction of ASTM Committee F04 on Medical and Surgical Materials and Devices and is the direct responsibility of Subcommittee F04.15 on Materials Test Methods.

Current edition approved Nov. 10, 2000. Published January 2001. Originally published as F 1160 – 91. Last previous edition F 1160 – 98.

[2] *Annual Book of ASTM Standards*, Vol 03.01.

[3] Discontinued 1988, see *Annual Book of ASTM Standards*, Vol 03.01; replaced by Terminology E 1823.

5.2 In order that such basic fatigue data be comparable, reproducible, and can be correlated among laboratories, it is essential that uniform fatigue practices be established.

5.3 The results of the fatigue test may be used for basic material property design. Actual components should not be tested using these test methods.

6. Equipment Characteristics

6.1 Equipment characteristics shall be in accordance with Practice E 466, Section 7.

6.2 *Shear Fatigue Test Grips*:

6.2.1 *General*—Various types of grips may be used to transmit the load to the specimens by the testing machine. To ensure axial shear stress, it is important that the specimen axis coincide with the centerline of the heads of the testing machine and that the coating test plane be parallel to the axial load. Any departure from this requirement (that is, any eccentric loading) will introduce bending stresses that are not included in the usual stress calculation (force/cross-sectional area).

6.2.2 A drawing of a typical gripping device for the test assembly is shown in Fig. 1.

6.2.3 Fig. 2 shows a drawing of the adaptor to mate the shear fixture to the tensile machine

6.2.4 Figs. 3 and 4 show a schematics of the test setup.

6.3 *Bending Fatigue Test Grips*—There are a variety of testing machines that may be employed for this test (that is, rotating beam fatigue machines and axial fatigue machines). The gripping method for each type of equipment shall be determined by either the manufacturer of that equipment (rotating beam machines) or the user.

7. Adhesive Bonding Materials

7.1 *Adhesive Bonding Agent*—A polymeric adhesive bonding agent in film form, or filled viscous adhesive cement, shall be identified and shall meet the following requirements.

7.1.1 The bonding agent shall be capable of bonding the coating on the test specimen components with an adhesive shear strength that is at least 34.5 MPa (5000 psi) or as great as the minimum required adhesion or cohesion strength of the coating, whichever is greater.

7.1.2 In instances where coating porosity extends to the coating/substrate interface, the bonding agent shall be sufficiently viscous and application to the coating sufficiently detailed, to ensure that it will not penetrate through the coating to the substrate. The FM 1000 Adhesive Film[4] with a thickness of 0.25 mm (0.01 in.) has proven satisfactory for this test.

7.1.3 If a material other than FM 1000 is used, or the condition of the FM 1000 is unknown, it must be tested to establish its equivalence to fresh FM 1000. Testing should be performed without the presence of the coating to establish the performance of the adhesive.

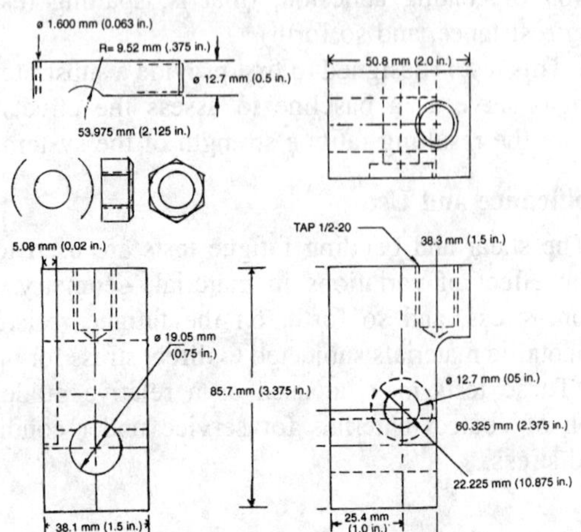

FIG. 1 Gripping Device for Shear Testing

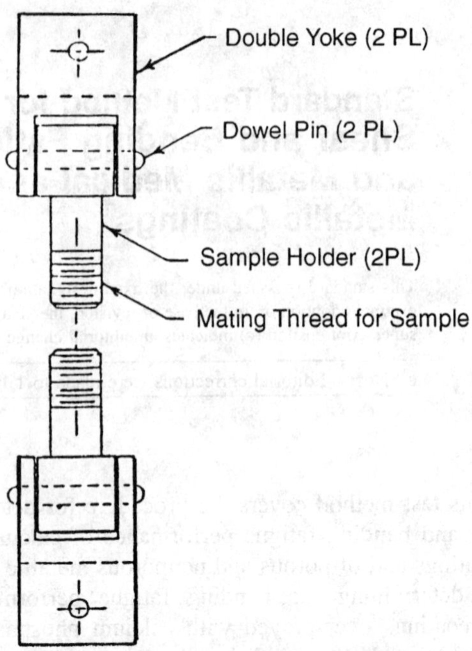

FIG. 2 Adaptor to Mate the Gripping Device to the Tensile Machine

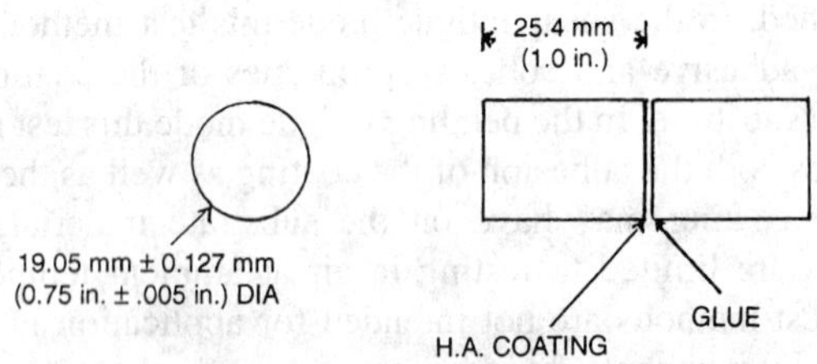

FIG. 3 Schematic of the Shear Test Setup

8. Test Specimen

8.1 *Shear Fatigue Specimen for Calcium Phosphate and Metallic Coatings Only*:

8.1.1 The recommended shear test specimen and setup is illustrated in Figs. 3 and 4, respectively. A complete assembled test assembly consists of two solid pieces, one with a coated surface and the other with an uncoated surface. The uncoated surface may be roughened to aid in the adhesion of the adhesive bonding agent.

8.1.2 The cross-sectional area of the substrate upon which the coating is applied shall be a nominal 2.85 cm^2 (0.44 in.^{2}). When specimens of another cross-sectional area are used, the

[4] Available from Cytec, Harve de Grace, MD.

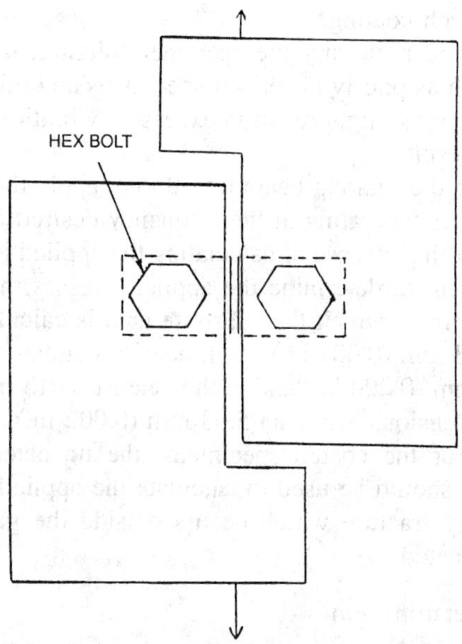

FIG. 4 Drawing of the Recommended Shear Test Specimen Assembly

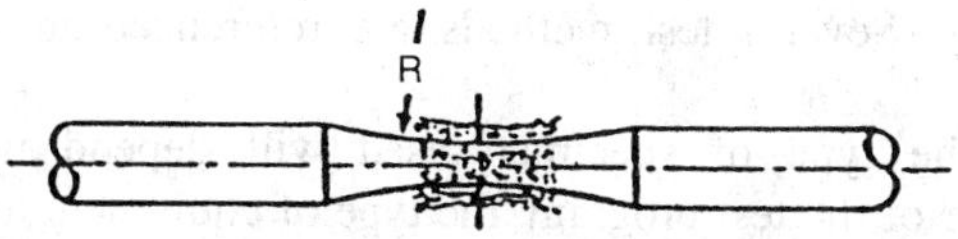

FIG. 6 Specimens With a Continuous Radius Between the Ends for Rotating Beam or Axial loading

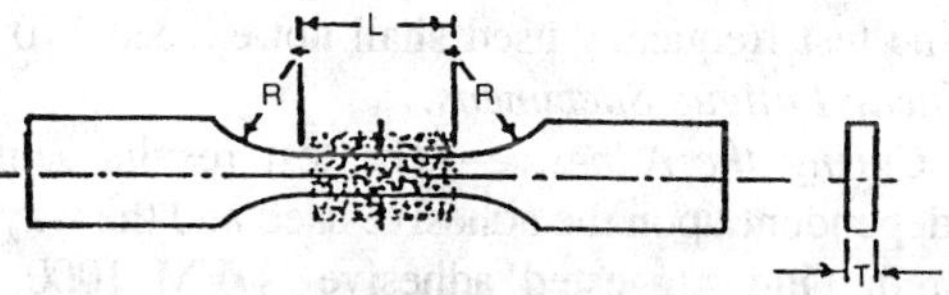

FIG. 7 Specimens With Tangentially Blending Fillets Between the Uniform Test Section and the Ends for Axial Loading

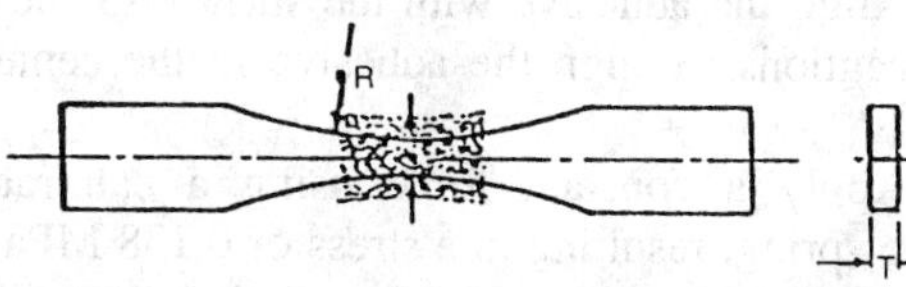

FIG. 8 Specimens With a Continuous Radius Between the Ends for Axial Loading

data must be demonstrated to be equivalent to the results produced using the 2.85-cm^2 standard cross-sectional area and the specimen size should be reported.

8.2 *Bending Fatigue Specimen for Calcium Phosphate, Metallic, and Calcium Phosphate-Metallic Composite Coatings*:

8.2.1 The type of specimen used will depend upon the objective of the test program, the type of equipment, the equipment capacity, and the form in which the material is available. However, the design must meet certain general criteria as follows:

8.2.1.1 The design of the specimen should be such that if specimen failure should occur, it should occur in the test section (reduced area as shown in Figs. 5-8).

8.2.1.2 Specimens using a flat tapered beam configuration should be designed such that a constant surface stress exists in the test section when the specimen is constrained at one end and point loaded perpendicular to the beam axis at the other end (that is, cantilever loading).

8.2.1.3 Rotating beam specimens may have unique dimensions, depending upon the type of machine used. Appropriate manufacturers' specifications for these specimens should be used.

8.3 *Specimen Coating Preparation*:

8.3.1 Coatings may be applied by any one of a number of techniques. All test specimens for coating characterization shall be prepared from indicative coating lots, using production feedstock lots and be coated on the same equipment used for

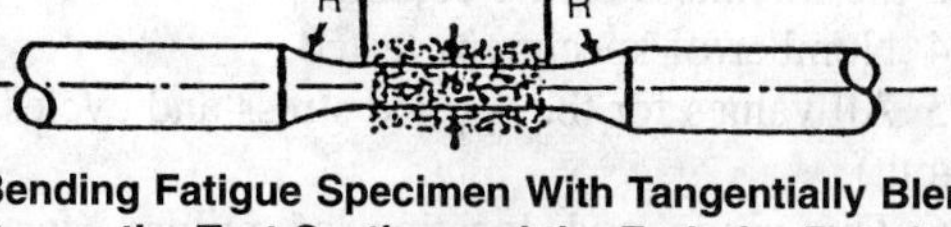

FIG. 5 Bending Fatigue Specimen With Tangentially Blending Fillets Between the Test Section and the Ends for Rotating Beam or Axial Loading

actual implants. The coating should consist of a layer which is mechanically or chemically attached and covers the surface.

8.3.2 Coatings should be applied as follows:

8.3.2.1 For the shear fatigue specimens, the coating should be applied to the 19.05-mm (0.75-in.) diameter face only (see Fig. 3).

8.3.2.2 For the bending fatigue specimens, the coating should be applied to the reduced section only, with the exception of the constant stress specimen which should have coating in the entire region of constant stress (see Figs. 5-9).

8.3.3 All thermal treatments normally performed on the devices should be performed on the test specimens.

8.3.4 If used, passivation and sterilization techniques should be consistent with those used for actual devices.

8.3.5 *Inspection*—Before testing, visual inspections should be performed on 100 % of the test specimens. Nonuniform coating density shall be cause for specimen rejection. For the shear fatigue specimen, lack of coating on the coated face shall be cause for specimen rejection. For the bending fatigue specimen, lack of coating in highly stressed regions shall be cause for specimen rejection.

9. Procedure

9.1 The number of specimens required for testing, as well as the test methods in which the fatigue data may be interpreted,

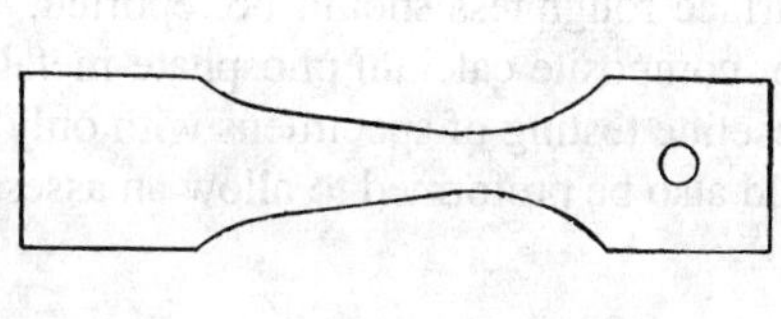

FIG. 9 Tapered Beam Configuration for Bend Testing

can vary. Several test methods are referenced in this test method.[5,6,7]

9.2 The type of specimen used will depend upon the objective of the test program, the type of equipment available, the equipment capacity, and the form in which the material is available. The specimen chosen should come as close to matching the intended application as possible.

9.3 The test frequency used shall not exceed 170 Hz.

9.4 *Shear Fatigue Specimens*:

9.4.1 *Curing the Adhesive*—The test results achieved are greatly dependent upon the adhesive used and the way in which it is cured. One suggested adhesive is FM 1000 having a thickness of 0.25 mm (0.01 in.). This material has successfully been cured using the following cycle:

9.4.1.1 Align the adhesive with the surface of the coating, taking precautions to align the adhesive in the center of the coating.

9.4.1.2 Apply a constant force using a calibrated high temperature spring, resulting in a stress of 0.138 MPa (20 psi) between the coating and the opposing device that will test the coating.

9.4.1.2.1 Care must be taken to maintain alignment of the coating and the matching counterface during the test.

9.4.1.3 Place the assembly in an oven and heat at 176°C for 2 to 3 h.

9.4.1.3.1 The exact amount of time necessary to cure the adhesive will need to be determined by each user, as oven temperature may vary with load size and oven type. It is suggested that the curing cycle be optimized first without the coating present.

9.4.1.4 Remove the cured assembly from the oven and allow it to cool to room temperature.

9.4.1.5 Remove all excess adhesive which has protruded from the coated surface. This process must not compromise the integrity of the sample.

9.4.2 Place the specimen assembly in the grips so that the long axis of the specimen is perpendicular to the direction of the applied shear load through the centerline of the grip assembly (see Fig. 3).

9.4.3 Specimens for which the adhesive has penetrated to the substrate shall be discarded and the results not included in the analysis and report.

9.5 *Bending Fatigue Specimens*:

9.5.1 Appropriate testing of the uncoated substrate material, upon which the coating will be applied, should be performed to establish a baseline from which to assess the effect of the coating.

9.5.1.1 The baseline test specimens may or may not be grit-blasted depending upon the objective of the test. In either event, the surface roughness should be reported.

9.5.1.2 For composite calcium phosphate-metallic coatings, additional baseline testing of specimens with only the metallic coating should also be preformed to allow an assessment of the effects of each coating.

9.5.2 When mounting the specimen, alignment is crucial. Factors such as poorly machined specimens and misalignment of machine parts might result in excessive vibration leading to erroneous results.

9.5.3 For the rotating beam test, do not apply the load until the machine is operating at the frequency desired for testing.

9.5.4 For the purpose of calculating the applied loads on the test specimen, to determine the applied stresses, measure the dimensions from which the substrate area is calculated to the nearest 0.03 mm (0.001 in.) for dimensions equal to or greater than 5.08 mm (0.200 in.) and to the nearest 0.013 mm (0.0005 in.) for dimensions less than 5.08 mm (0.002 in.).

9.5.4.1 For the coated specimens, the uncoated substrate dimensions should be used to calculate the applied stress.

9.5.5 Any fracture which occurs outside the gage section shall be rejected.

10. Test Termination

10.1 Continue the testing until the specimen fails or until a predetermined number of cycles has been reached (typically 10^7 cycles). Failure may be defined as: (*1*) complete separation of the coating, (*2*) visible cracking at a specified magnification, (*3*) a crack of certain dimensions, (*4*) or by some other criterion.

11. Stress Calculation

11.1 *Shear Fatigue Specimens*—Calculate the substrate area upon which the coating is applied to the nearest 0.06 cm^2 (0.01 $in.^2$). Record peak (failure) load and calculate failing stress in megapascals (pound-force per square inch) of adhesive area as follows:

Adhesion or cohesion strength = maximum load/cross-sectional area

11.2 *Bending Fatigue Specimens*—For the purpose of calculating the applied loads on the test specimen to determine the applied stresses, measure the dimensions from which the substrate adhesive area is calculated to the nearest 0.03 mm (0.001 in.) for dimensions equal to or greater than 5.08 mm (0.200 in.) and to the nearest 0.013 mm (0.0005 in.) for dimensions less than 5.08 mm (0.002 in.).

12. Report

12.1 The test report procedure and results shall be in accordance with Practice E 468 and include the following information:

12.1.1 Identification of the materials used in the specimen, including bonding agent used,

12.1.2 Identification of methods used to apply the coating including the coating method, heat treatment, or other data if available including date, cycle number, and time and temperature of run,

12.1.3 Dimensional data including the bond cross-sectional area and the thickness of the coating,

12.1.4 Number of specimens tested,

12.1.5 All values for the applied stress and cycles to failure (or run-out),

12.1.6 The mode and location of failure (for example, cohesive versus adhesive) for each test specimen. (This may

---

[5] Collins, J.A., *Failure of Materials in Mechanical Design*, John Wiley & Sons, New York, 1981.

[6] *Handbook of Fatigue Testing, ASTM STP 566*, ASTM, 1974.

[7] Frost, N. C., Marsh, K. J., and Pook, C. P., *Metal Fatigue*, Oxford University Press, London, 1974.

also be performed at various intervals during the test.),

12.1.7 The criteria selected for failure, including the number of cycles chosen for run-out,

12.1.8 Report the *R* ratio (minimum stress/maximum stress),

12.1.9 The test frequency,

12.1.10 The specimen size for the shear fatigue test if different than the standard size,

12.1.11 The substrate surface roughness for the baseline bending fatigue test, and

12.1.12 Location of the fracture.

13. Precision and Bias

13.1 *Review of the Round Robin*—Six laboratories were involved in round-robin testing. Each laboratory was provided with 12 Ti-6Al-4V rotating beam specimens coated with plasma-sprayed titanium. Specimens were tested at 90 000 psi.

13.2 Table 1 shows the cycles to failure raw data generated from each laboratory.

13.3 *h Graph*:

13.3.1 The *h* value evaluates the consistency of the test results from laboratory to laboratory.

13.3.2 There are three patterns in these plots. In one pattern, all values are either positive or negative. In the second pattern, there are roughly the same number of laboratories that exhibit positive values as those that exhibit negative values. In the third type, one laboratory exhibits a value that is opposite of the other laboratories. The first two types are considered normal. The third type warrants further evaluation.

13.3.3 Fig. 10 shows the *h* values for each laboratory.

13.4 The *k* value evaluates the consistency of the test results within each laboratory.

13.4.1 *k Graph*:

13.4.1.1 The *k* value evaluates the consistency of the test results within each laboratory.

13.4.1.2 The pattern to look for in the *k* graph is a laboratory having a very large or a very small *k* value. High values indicate imprecision. Very small values indicate a very insensitive measurement scale or other measurement problems. A *k* value greater than 1 indicates greater variability than other laboratories.

13.4.1.3 Fig. 11 shows the *k* values for each laboratory.

13.5 *Precision Statistics*—The precision statistics are shown in Table 2.

14. Keywords

14.1 ceramic coatings; composite coatings; fatigue testing; hydroxylapatite; metallic coatings; plasma-sprayed coatings; porous coatings; tribasic calcium phosphate

TABLE 1 ASTM F 1160 Round Robin, Cycles to Failure

Source[A]	1	2	3	4	5	6
	83 300	78 000	run out	64 700	64 200	71 900
	53 500	62 300	26 800	78 800	136 300	51 000
	80 400	92 200	16 900	137 200	57 000	88 100
	67 900	36 300	28 700	175 100	48 700	51 200
	64 900	73 400	17 900	116 400	32 100	58 200
	89 400	98 200	70 700	211 100	61 300	42 400
	51 000	49 100	52 900	183 100	45 100	58 400
	72 500	63 600	22 500	200 500	77 900	84 200
	46 600	118 200	23 300	161 200	40 000	64 600
	54 800	40 700	38 000	111 100	55 400	44 800
	48 100	82 800	36 800	277 500	38 100	73 300
	97 700	72 700	. . .	183 100	56 800	66 400
Average	67 517 ± 17 277	72 292 ± 22 009	33 450 ± 11 622	158 317 ± 60 157	59 408 ± 27 312	62 875 ± 14 653

[A]1 = Biomet.
2 = Osteonics.
3 = Wright Medical.
4 = EML.
5 = Zimmer.
6 = Howmedica.

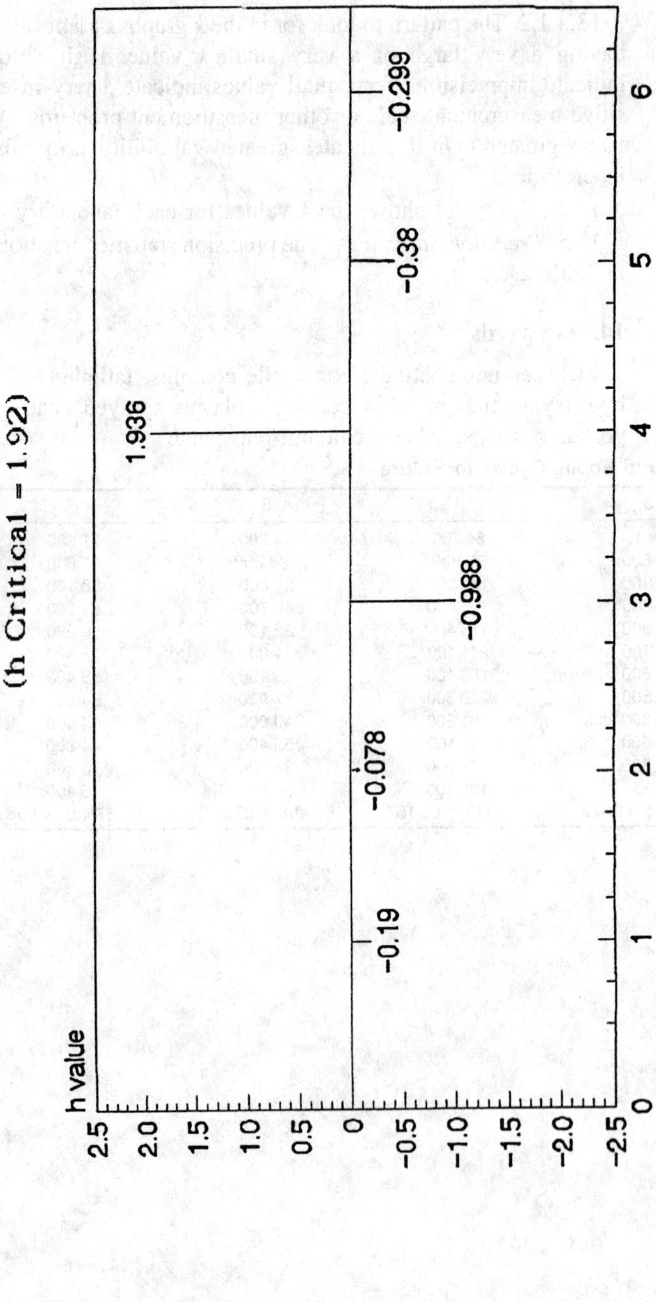

FIG. 10 *h* Values

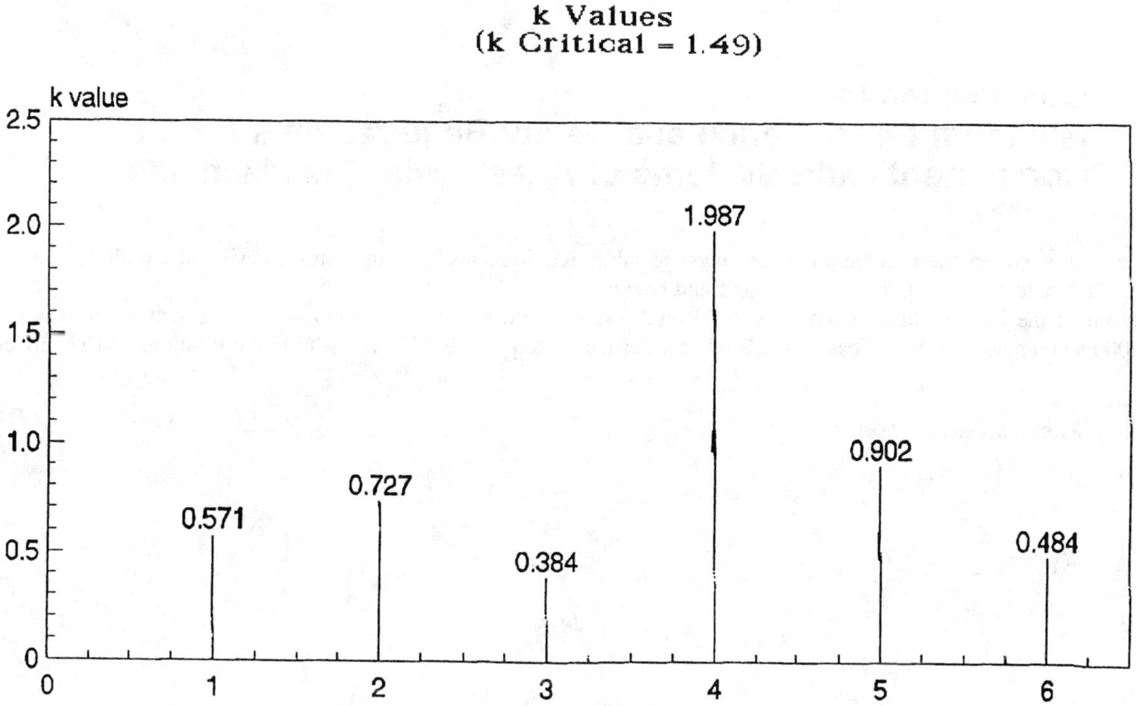

FIG. 11 *k* Values

TABLE 2 Precision Statistics

X^A	S_x^B	S_r^C	S_R^D	r^E	R^F
75 643	42 706	30 269	51 611	84 753	144 511

[A] X = average of the cell averages.
[B] S_x = standard deviation of cell averages.
[C] S_R = reproducibility standard deviation.
[D] S_r = repeatability standard deviation.
[E] r = 95 % repeatability limit.
[F] R = 95 % reproducibility limit.

APPENDIX

(Nonmandatory Information)

X1. RATIONALE

X1.1 These test methods are needed to aid in the development of a high-quality material for use in load-bearing implant applications. The influence of coatings on the resulting fatigue behavior of the system must be viewed as a combination of the surface-roughening treatments required to apply the coating, the thermal effects of the coating process, and any other secondary treatments used. The purpose of this specification is to provide the following information: (*1*) the influence of the preceding processing steps and (*2*) the integrity of the coating and the coating/substrate interface.

Last ASTM Designation: F 1161 – 88 (Reapproved 1994)

Specification for Minimum Performance and Safety Requirements for Components and Systems of Anesthesia Gas Machines

This specification covers the minimum performance and safety requirements to be used in the design of anesthesia gas machines for human use in order to enhance safety of the patient and operator.

Formerly under the jurisdiction of Committee F-29 on Anesthetic and Respiratory Equipment, this specification was withdrawn in February 2000 and replaced by Specification F1850–00 for Particular Requirements for Anesthesia Workstations and Their Components.[1]

[1] Annual Book of ASTM Standards, Volume 13.01.

Designation: F 1177 – 96a

Standard Terminology Relating to Emergency Medical Services[1]

This standard is issued under the fixed designation F 1177; the number immediately following the designation indicates the year of original adoption or, in the case of revision, the year of last revision. A number in parentheses indicates the year of last reapproval. A superscript epsilon (ε) indicates an editorial change since the last revision or reapproval.

1. Scope

1.1 This terminology covers standard definitions of terms which apply to all F-30 standards but which are more precise than common usage.

2. Terminology

2.1 Appropriate definitions for interpretation of terms used in ASTM Emergency Medical Services standards shall be determined in the following order:

2.1.1 Specific definitions of terminology or description of terms provided in the standard. These will apply to use of the term in that standard only.

2.1.2 ASTM Standard Terminology Relating to Emergency Medical Services (Standard F-1177).

2.1.3 Taber's Cyclopedic Medical Dictionary, 16th Edition (Philadelphia: F. A. Davis Company, 1989).

2.1.4 Mosby's Emergency Dictionary (St. Louis: C.V. Mosby Company, 1989).

2.2 *Definitions:*

adjunct instructor—an individual with specialized subject matter expertise, who, on occasion, instructs a specific topic of a curriculum under the direction of the course instructor/coordinator. **F 1256, F 1257**

advanced life support—medically accepted life sustaining, invasive or non-invasive procedures; provided at the detection of a physician or other authorized health care provider.

ambulance—a vehicle for transportation of the sick and injured, equipped and staffed to provide emergency medical care during transit.

ambulance service—a qualified provider of medical transportation for patients requiring treatment and/or monitoring due to illness or injury.

ambulance service provider—a person or organization, either public or private, responsible for operation, maintenance, and administation of an ambulance service.

associate instructor—an individual who possesses the qualifications and education/training of a course instructor/coordinator, but, in a specific course, assumes a supportive or assisting role to the course instructor/coordinator. This individual may substitute for the course instructor/coordinator in case of necessity or, in other courses, serves as a course instructor/coordinator. **F 1256, F 1257**

basic life support—medically accepted non-invasive procedures used to sustain life.

basic life support/cardiopulmonary resuscitation (BLS/CPR)—a set of skills that includes airway management, chest compressions, and others as defined by the American Heart Association. **F 1254, F 1255, F 1287**

call rotation—a system in which emergency medical responses are allocated sequentially to multiple providers.

clinical certification—a standardized process for evaluation and recognition of an acceptable level of competence in a specific aspect of patient care. **F 1256, F 1257**

clinical experience—exposure to and practice in an area of patient care. **F 1256, F 1257**

clinical/field preceptor—an individual who supervises and evaluates the students during clinical or field experiences under the direction of the course instructor/coordinator. **F 1256, F 1257**

clinical medical practice—patient diagnosis and treatment, including treatment protocols, which are the purview of qualified professionals (as determined by the state or other appropriate authority).

communication resource—an entity responsible for implementation of direct medical direction and/or entities responsible for response and scene two-way communication (a. k. a. medical control resource).

course administrator—an individual responsible for managing administrative details of a course, separate from actual instruction of the course. **F 1256, F 1257**

course instructor/coordinator (I/C)—an individual who is authorized by the appropriate entity to present and assess competence in all of the subject matter contained in a curriculum. This person also oversees all instruction in the course and makes final evaluations concerning student competence. **F 1256, F 1257**

definitive care—a level of therapeutic intervention capable of providing comprehensive health care services for a specific condition.

delegated practice—the medical activities of providers performed under the authority and direction of a licensed physician.

[1] This terminology is under the jurisdiction of ASTM Committee F-30 on Emergency Medical Services and is the direct responsibility of Subcommittee F30.06 on Terminology.

Current edition approved June 10 and Dec. 10, 1996. Published May 1997. Originally published as F 1177 – 88. Last previous edition F 1177 – 94a.

direct medical control—the process of providing immediate physician orders to EMS personnel through direct communication (a.k.a. on-line medical control, indirect medical direction).

dispatch life support—the knowledge, procedures, and skills used by trained emergency medical dispatchers in guiding care by means of post-dispatch (pre-arrival) instruction to callers.

EMS region—a defined geographic area used for EMS planning, development, and coordination.

emergency medical dispatcher (EMD)—a trained public safety telecommunicator with additional training and specific emergency medical knowledge essential for the efficient management of emergency communications.

emergency medical facility—a physical structure, excluding mobile vehicles, which has been approved by the appropriate regulatory authority to receive emergency patients and which is equipped and staffed to evaluate and treat patients with life threatening conditions.

emergency medical services (EMS) system—a coordinated arrangement of resources (including personnel, equipment, and facilities) organized to respond to medical emergencies, regardless of the cause.

emergency medical services—the provision of services to patients requiring immediate assistance due to illness or injury, including access, response, rescue, prehospital and hospital treatment, and transportation.

health care provider—an organization, institution, or individual authorized to provide direct patient care.

indirect medical direction—the physician management of all clinical aspects of an EMS system, including but not limited to planning, training, implementation, and evaluation (a.k.a. off-line medical control direct medical direction).

intervenor physician—a licensed M.D. or D.O., having not previously established a doctor/patient relationship with the emergency patient, who is willing to accept responsibility for patient care, and who can provide proof of a current medical license.

medical direction—physician responsibility for the development, implementation, and evaluation of the clinical aspects of an EMS system (a.k.a. medical direction).

medical director—off-line—a physician responsible for all aspects of an EMS system dealing with the provision of medical care (also known as System Medical Director).

medical protocol—pre-established physician authorized procedures or guidelines for medical care of a specified clinical situation, based on patient presentation (a.k.a. standing orders).

medical transportation services—the moving of patients from one location to another. Specific services include any or all of the following: emergency and non-emergency medical response and transportation; scheduled and non-scheduled interfacility transfers, medical standbys, long-distance medical transfers, air medical response and transport (helicopter and fixed wing aircraft); and stretcher and wheelchair transport services.

medical transportation system—a sub-system of the emergency medical services system consisting of an organization or collection of medical transport services which provide transportation, treatment, and observation of patients for a specific geographic area.

mutual aid—the furnishing of resources, from one individual or agency to another individual or agency, including but not limited to facilities, personnel, equipment, and services, pursuant to an agreement with the individual or agency, for use within the jurisdiction of the individual or agency requesting assistance.

on-line medical physician—a physician immediately available, when medically appropriate for communication of medical direction to non-physician prehospital care providers in remote location.

pertinent patient information—information obtained from all available resources that relates to the patient's condition and problems. This information must be continuously updated. All information must be recorded and reported. **F 1219, F 1253**

practical skills instructor—an individual who assists with practical skills instruction under the direction of the course instructor/coordinator. **F 1256, F 1257**

prehospital emergency medical services—a sub-system of the emergency medical services system which provides medical services to patients requiring immediate assistance due to illness or injury, prior to the patients' arrival at an emergency medical facility.

prehospital provider—all personnel providing emergency medical care in a location which is remote from facilities which are capable of providing definitive medical care.

sequential response—The assignment, according to local protocols, of emergency medical resources with varying levels of care capability to the scene of an illness or injury based on information received from previously arrived, medically trained, on-scene responders. A sequential response differs from a simultaneous response.

simultaneous response—The assignment of multiple emergency medical resources to the scene of an illness or injury based on initially available information and local operational policies. These may have varying levels of care capability (for example ALS and BLS, ground and air). Subsequent care and/or transportation of the patient is provided by the unit which most closely meets the patient's needs. A simultaneous response differs from a sequential response.

standing orders—a type of medical protocol which provides specific-written orders for actions, techniques, or drug administration when communication has not been established for direct medical direction.

tiered response—a predetermined, protocol driven, level of medical care and vehicle operation mode based on multiple levels of resource response. The two types of tiered response are sequential responsee (q.v.) and simultaneous response (q.v.).

trauma care system—a subsystem within the EMS system designed to manage the treatment of the trauma patient.

vehicle operation mode—the manner of operation of an emergency medical vehicle, involving the use of warning devices and the exercise of driving privileges legally allowed for emergency vehicles.

wilderness setting—situations in which the delivery of patient care by EMS providers is complicated by the remoteness with respect to logistics and access; a significant delay in the delivery of care to the patient; an environment that is physically stressful to both patients and rescuers; or the lack of equipment, supplies, and transporation. **F 30.02.05**

Designation: F 1185 – 88 (Reapproved 1993)$^{\epsilon 1}$

Standard Specification for Composition of Ceramic Hydroxylapatite for Surgical Implants[1]

This standard is issued under the fixed designation F 1185; the number immediately following the designation indicates the year of original adoption or, in the case of revision, the year of last revision. A number in parentheses indicates the year of last reapproval. A superscript epsilon (ϵ) indicates an editorial change since the last revision or reapproval.

ϵ^1 NOTE—Keywords were added and Section 3 editorially corrected in March 1993.

1. Scope

1.1 This specification covers material requirements for ceramic hydroxylapatite intended for surgical implants. For a material to be called ceramic hydroxylapatite, it must conform to this specification. (See Appendix X1.)

1.2 The biological response to ceramic hydroxylapatite in soft tissue and bone has been characterized by a history of clinical use **(1-3)**[2] and by laboratory studies **(4-6)**.

1.3 This specification specifically excludes hydroxylapatite coatings, non-ceramic hydroxylapatite, ceramic-glasses, tribasic calcium phosphate, whitlockite, and alpha- and beta-tricalcium phosphate. (See Specification F 1088.)

2. Referenced Documents

2.1 *ASTM Standards:*

F 1088 Specification for Beta-Tricalcium Phosphate for Surgical Implantation[3]

2.2 *Code of Federal Regulations:*[4]

Title 21, Part 820.

2.3 *National Formulary:*[5]

Tribasic Calcium Phosphate

2.4 *United States Pharmacopeia:*[6]

Identification Tests for Calcium and Phosphate <191>

Lead <251>

Mercury <261>

Arsenic <211>

Heavy Metals <231> Method 1

2.5 *U. S. Geological Survey Method:*[7]

Cadmium

3. Terminology

3.1 *Descriptions of Terms Specific to This Standard:*

3.1.1 *calcining*—the heat treatment of a ceramic precursor for the purpose of eliminating volatile constituents. Calcining is also accompanied by some surface area and bulk volume reductions. Increases in mechanical properties are not usually significant.

3.1.2 *ceramic hydroxylapatite*—hydroxylapatite which has been fired at sintering temperatures. Firing time is mass dependent, and should be sufficiently long to cause significant densification and formation of a biologically stable form.

3.1.3 *hydroxylapatite*—the chemical substance having the empirical formula $Ca_5(PO_4)_3OH$.[8]

3.1.4 *sintering*—an integration of time and temperature of a ceramic precursor which develops a coherent body with useful properties. Sintering is a non-melting process accompanied by significant surface area and bulk volume reductions (densification), grain growth, and increases in mechanical properties.

4. Chemical Requirements

4.1 Elemental analysis for calcium and phosphorus will be consistent with the expected stoichiometry of hydroxylapatite.

4.2 A quantitative X-ray diffraction analysis shall indicate a minimum hydroxylapatite content of 95 % **(7)**. Analysis of relative peak intensities shall be consistent with published data.[9]

4.3 The concentration of trace elements in the hydroxylapatite shall be limited as follows:

Element	ppm, max
As	3
Cd	5
Hg	5
Pb	30

[1] This specification is under the jurisdiction of ASTM Committee F-4 on Medical and Surgical Materials and Devices and is the direct responsibility of Subcommittee F04.13 on Ceramic Materials.

Current edition approved Oct. 31, 1988. Published December 1988.

[2] The boldface numbers in parentheses refer to the list of references at the end of this specification.

[3] *Annual Book of ASTM Standards*, Vol 13.01.

[4] Available from U.S. Government Printing Office, Washington, DC 20402.

[5] National Formulary XVI. Available from U.S. Pharmacopeia Convention, Inc., 12601 Twinbrook Parkway, Rockville, MD 20852.

[6] United States Pharmacopeia XXI. Available from U.S. Pharmacopeia Convention, Inc., 12601 Twinbrook Parkway, Rockville, MD 20852.

[7] Crock, J. G., Felichte, F. E., and Briggs, P. H., "Determination of Elements in National Bureau of Standards Geological Reference Materials SRM 278 Obsidian and SRM 688 Basalt by Inductively Coupled Argon Plasma—Atomic Emission Spectrometry," *Geostandards Newsletter*, Vol 7, 1983, pp. 335-340.

[8] Chemical Abstracts Service Registry Number [1306-06-5].

[9] The Joint Committee on Powdered Diffraction Standards has established a Powder Diffraction File. The Committee operates on an international basis and cooperates closely with the Data Commission of the International Union of Crystallography and ASTM (American Society for Testing and Materials). Hydroxylapatite data can be found on file card number 9-432 and is available from the Joint Committee on Powder Diffraction Standards, 1600 Park Lane, Swarthmore, PA 19081.

total heavy metals (as lead)	50

For referee purposes, methods in 2.4 and 2.5 shall be used.

4.4 The maximum allowable limit of all heavy metals determined as lead will be 50 ppm as described in 2.4 or equivalent. Sample preparation will be identical to that for tribasic calcium phosphate as specified in the National Formulary (2.2) except that approximately 1 g of material will be dissolved in approximately 30 mL of 5 % HCl and boiled.

4.5 It is recommended that all metals or oxides not detected as lead present in concentrations equal to or greater than 0.1 % be listed on the package insert.

5. Test Specimen Fabrication

5.1 Prepare test specimens from the same batch of material and by the same processes as those employed in fabricating the ceramic implant device.

6. Quality Program Requirements

6.1 The manufacturer shall conform to Good Manufacturing Practices (2.2) or its equivalent.

7. Keywords

7.1 bioceramic; bone graft; hydroxylapatite (HAP); tricalcium phosphate (TCP); whitlockite

APPENDIX

(Nonmandatory Information)

X1. RATIONALE

X1.1 Ceramic hydroxylapatite is commercially available as a synthetic bone-grafting material. As with any implant material, the bioresponse is critically dependent upon the material properties. To achieve reliable biocompatibility these must be known and consistent. This material standard provides specifications for a biocompatible grade of hydroxylapatite. Trace element content and leachability, physical form, and size must be within established biocompatibility standards.

X1.2 X-ray powder diffraction analysis provides better differentiation between hydroxylapatite and several commonly occurring second phases than traditional wet chemical methods.

X1.3 It is recognized that a separate performance standard may be necessary for each end-use product. For this reason, physical and mechanical properties were not specified. A source of general test methods for ceramics may be found in Ref **(8)**.

REFERENCES

(1) Cranin, A. N., Tobin, G., Gelbman, J., Varjan, R., "A Seven Year Follow-up of Patients with (H/A) Ridge Augmentation," *Transactions of the Society for Biomaterials*, 1986, p. 155.

(2) Kent, J. N., Quinn, J. H., Zide, M. F., Guerra, L. R., Boyne, P., "Augmentation of Deficient Alveolar Ridges with Nonresorbable Hydroxylapatite or with Autogenous Cancellous Bone," *Journal of Oral and Maxillofacial Surgery*, Vol 41 (10), 1983, pp. 629-642.

(3) Yukna, R. A., Mayer, E. T., Brite, D. V., "Longitudinal Evaluation of Durapatite Ceramic as an Alloplastic Implant in Periodontal Osseous Defects After Three Years," *Journal of Periodontology*, Vol 55 (11), 1984, pp. 633-637.

(4) Jarcho, M., Kay, J. F., Gumaer, K. I., Doremus, R. H., and Drobeck, H. P., "Tissue, Cellular and Subcellular Events at a Bone-Ceramic Hydroxylapatite Interface," *Journal of Bioengineering*, Vol 1, 1977, pp. 79-92.

(5) Drobeck, H. P., Rothstein, S. S., Gumaer, K. I., Sherer, A. D., and Slighter, R. G., "Histologic Observation of Soft Tissue Responses to Implanted, Multifaceted Particles and Discs of Hydroxylapatite," *Journal of Oral and Maxillofacial Surgery*, Vol 42, 1984, pp. 143-149.

(6) Tracy, B. M. and Doremus, R. H., "Direct Electron Microscopy Studies of the Bone-Hydroxylapatite Interface," *Journal of Biomedical Materials Research*, Vol 18, 1984, pp. 719-726.

(7) Balmain, N., Legros, R., and Bonel, G., "X-Ray Diffraction of Calcified Bone Tissue: A Reliable Method for the Determination of Bone Ca/P Molar Ratio," *Calcified Tissue International*, Vol 34, 1982, pp. S93-S98.

(8) *Annual Book of ASTM Standards*, Vol 15.02.

Last ASTM Designation: F 1187 – 91

Specification for
Fixed Wing Basic Life Support Transport Units

This specification pertains to fixed wing transport units involved in patient transportation and care, at the basic life support level. Formerly under the jurisdiction of Committee F30 on Emergency Medical Services, this specification was withdrawn in February 2000.

Designation: F 1195 – 99

Standard Specification for Rigid Laryngoscopes for Tracheal Intubation—Hook on Fittings for Fiberilluminated Blades and Handles[1]

This standard is issued under the fixed designation F 1195; the number immediately following the designation indicates the year of original adoption or, in the case of revision, the year of last revision. A number in parentheses indicates the year of last reapproval. A superscript epsilon (ε) indicates an editorial change since the last revision or reapproval.

INTRODUCTION

In clinical anesthesia and resuscitation a variety of laryngoscopes are used. Because there is a clinical need for a variety of blade forms, they are manufactured as detachable blade and handle units. In the interest of patient safety, defined dimensions and performance standards are necessary. The aim of this specification is to ensure compatibility of rigid, folding, fiber-illuminated blades and handles within a given system without restricting innovation or design.

1. Scope

1.1 The purpose of this specification is to ensure that reusable, detachable fiber-illuminated hook-on blade and handle combinations that engage shall lock and illuminate when in the operating position.

1.2 Dimensions and tolerances of fiber-illuminated systems shall be provided.

1.3 This specification provides methods of identifying by color the various fiber-illuminated systems and compatible blades and handles within the system.

1.4 This specification covers reusable handles and blades. It does not cover disposable components or systems.

1.5 Nonfiber-illuminated blades and handles with the lamp in the blade shall conform to Specification F 965.

2. Referenced Documents

2.1 *ASTM Standards:*

F 965 Specification for Rigid Laryngoscopes for Tracheal Intubation—Hook-On Fittings for Laryngoscope Handles and Blades with Lamps[2]

2.2 *Federal Standard:*

FED-STD-595A Colors[3]

3. Terminology

3.1 *Descriptions of Terms*—In addition to the terms defined in Specification F 965, the following terms are defined:

3.1.1 *fiber-illuminated laryngoscope blade*, *n*—a blade which utilizes optical fibers to transmit light from a source in the handle.

3.1.2 *fiber-illumination handle*, *n*—a hand-held rigid device which provides a power source for illumination of a fiber-illuminated blade. It shall include the light source.

3.1.3 *contact/switch*, *n*—components of the hook-on fittings, both handle and blade, which come in contact to energize the light source when the blade and handle are in the locked, operating position.

3.1.4 *engagement*, *n*—the blade and handle are engaged when mechanically attached and the blade remains coupled to the handle in all positions.

3.1.5 *operating position*, *n*—the position of the engaged blade and handle when illumination is produced and the instrument is ready for use.

4. Performance Requirements

4.1 *Blade and Handle Fittings*—Detachable fiber-illuminated blade and handle combinations that engage shall lock and illuminate when in the operating position, and shall have the same color identification (see Section 7).

4.2 *Mechanical Restrictions*—Fiber-illuminated blades shall be mechanically incompatible with nonfiber-illuminated handles to prevent engagement (see Specification F 965).

4.3 *Blade Retention*—The blade shall be retained on the handle in all attitudes when engaged.

4.4 *Corrosion Resistance*—Components should resist corrosion under conditions of normal use, including cleaning and disinfecting procedures as specified by the manufacturer.

4.5 *Critical Dimensions*—All handle hook-on fittings shall conform to the dimensions of one of the systems described by Fig. 1 and Fig. 2. The hook-on blade fitting must engage, lock, and operate at any tolerance specified within any one of the Fig. 1 and Fig. 2. The total clearance between the width of the handle slot and the blade hook-on fitting shall not exceed 0.011 in. (0.28 mm).

4.6 *Component Compatibility*—A handle and blade hook-on fitting which engage shall lock and illuminate. This feature

[1] This specification is under the jurisdiction of ASTM Committee F-29 on Anesthetic and Respiratory Equipmentand is the direct responsibility of Subcommittee F29.13 on Laryngoscopes and Bronchoscopes.

Current edition approved July 10, 1999. Published October 1999. Originally published as F 1195 - 88(1993)$^{\epsilon 1}$. Last previous edition F 1195 - 88(1993)$^{\epsilon 1}$.

[2] *Annual Book of ASTM Standards*, Vol 13.01.

[3] Available from the Naval Publications and Forms Center, 5801 Tabor Ave., Philadelphia, PA 19120.

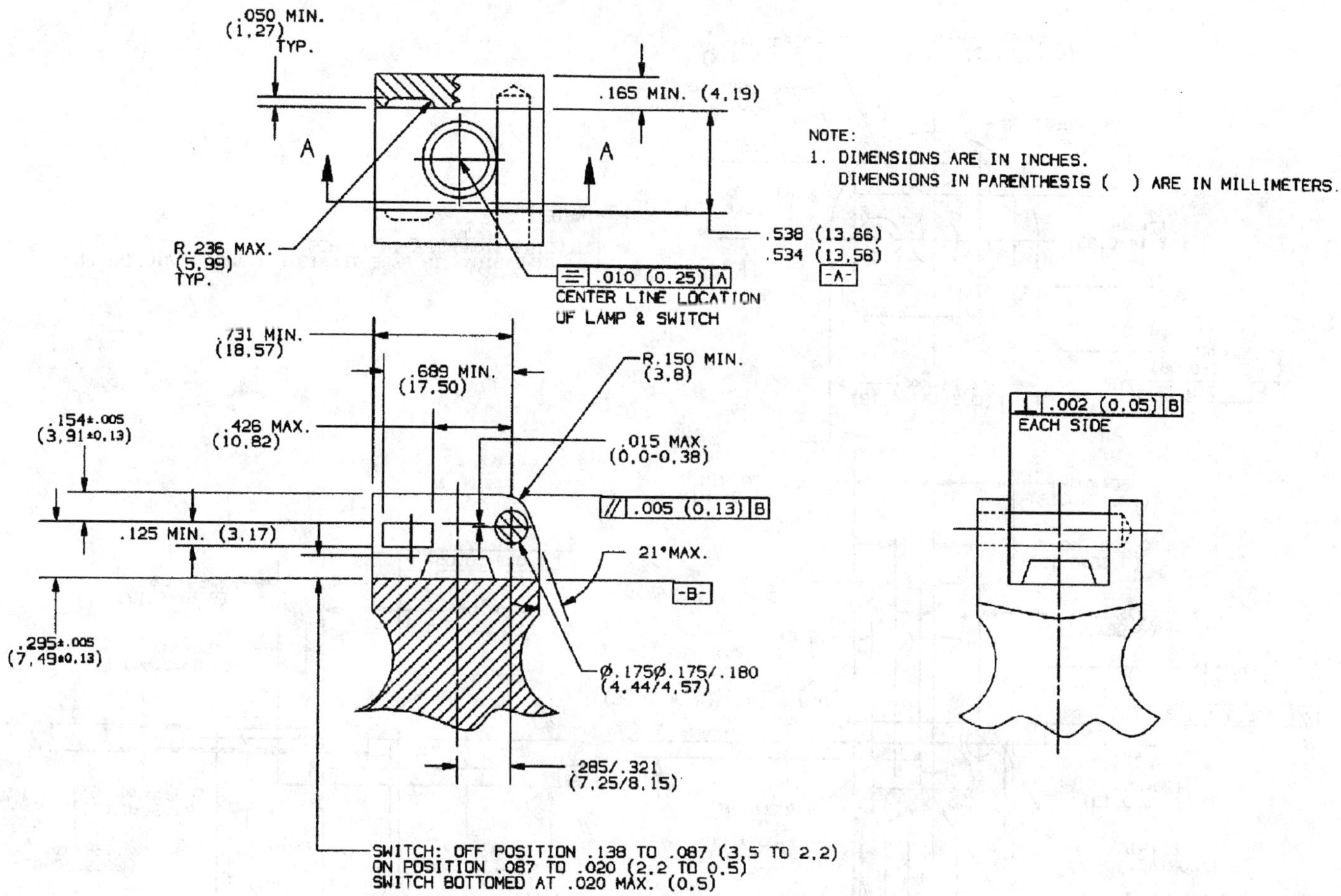

FIG. 1 Handle Hook-on Configuration for Green System

shall also apply to handles which engage either nonfiber-illuminated or fiber-illuminated blades.

5. Marking and Labeling

5.1 All markings shall be legible and durable.

5.2 The name or trademark of the manufacturer shall be marked on the blade fitting and on the handle in an area not less than 10 mm^2. In addition, the blade shall be marked with its size, type, country of origin, and either s/s, or stainless, if made of stainless steel.

5.3 Manufacturers shall provide information concerning cleaning and disinfecting procedures in the package.

5.4 Any removable fiber-optic components should be marked to indicate type and size.

6. Test Methods and Values

6.1 *Illumination*—The blade shall illuminate whenever placed in the operating position.

6.2 *Engagement and Locking*—Engagement and locking values are specified in Appendix X2.

6.3 *Blade Retention*—The engaged blade shall not disengage from the handle in any position because of its mass.

6.4 *Locking-Operating Position*—Locking of the blade into the operating position should occur when a reasonable force is applied (see Test Methods, Appendix X2.1).

6.5 *Unlocking—Operating Position*— Unlocking of the blade from the operating position should occur when a reasonable force is applied (see Test Methods, Appendix X2.2).

7. Identification of Compatible Systems

7.1 Compatible system components shall be identified by identical colors (see Appendix X3).

7.2 *Handle Identification*—Handles for fiber-illuminated systems shall be identified by a circumferential band of a color distinct from the handle. The band shall be located between the hook-on fitting and the midpoint of the handle. The width shall be 0.197 ± 0.079 (5 mm ± 2 mm).

7.3 *Blade Identification*—Blades shall be color coded by means of a mark on the heel of the blade or on light guide as specified in Appendix X3 (see Fig. 3). The mark shall be clearly visible when the rigid laryngoscope is in the operating position. The size of the mark shall not be less than 10 mm^2. In addition to the marking on the blade, if the fiber-illuminated component is detachable, it shall also be color marked, and such color marking should be visible when the laryngoscope is in the operating position.

NOTE 1—These marks should be resistant to friction, cleaning, handling, and sterilization.

8. Addition of New Systems

8.1 Any system of hook-on fitting which is incompatible with fittings included in this specification, but otherwise complies with this specification, shall be assigned a color for markings distinct from those previously assigned (see Appendix X3).

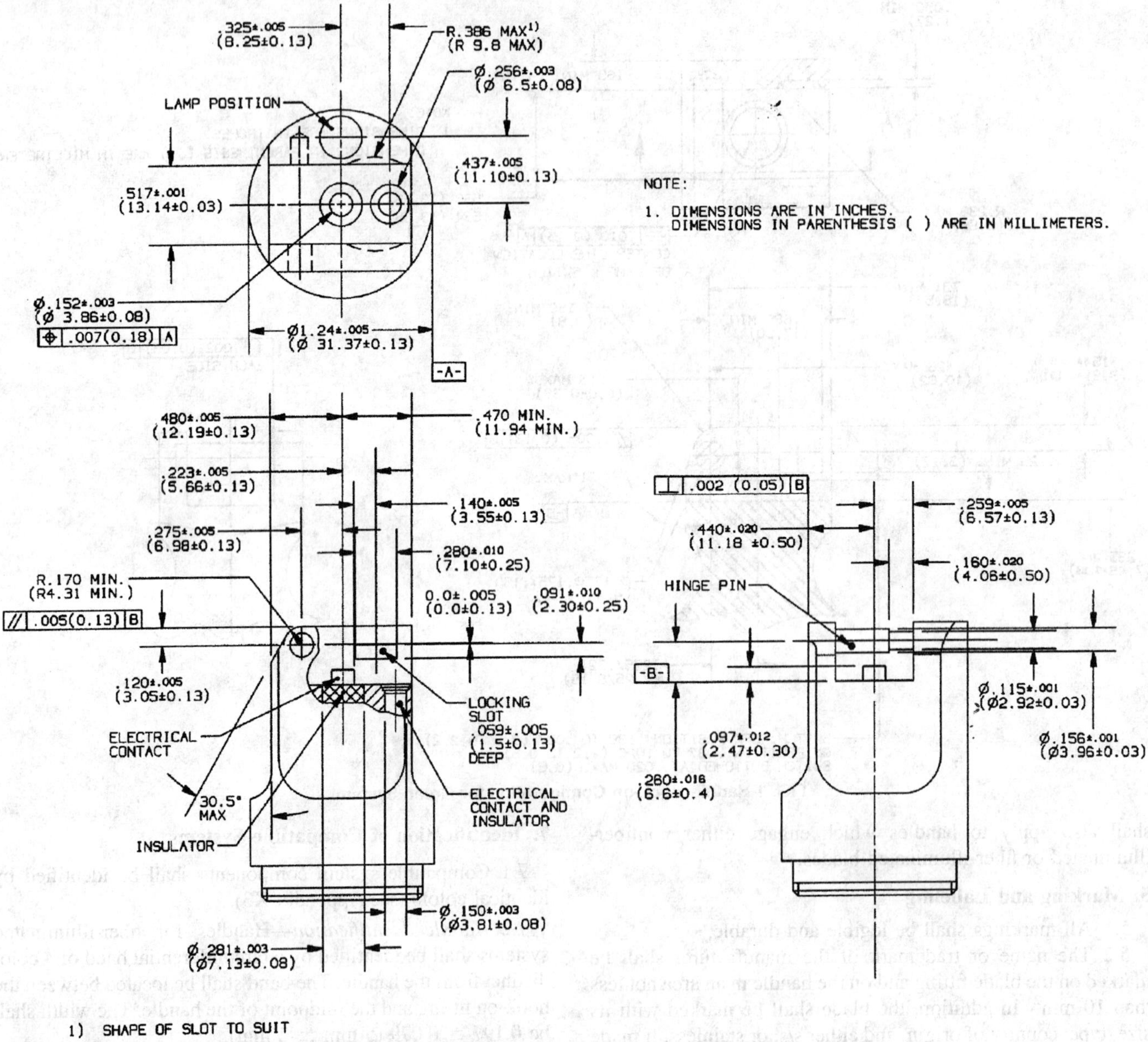

FIG. 2 Handle Hook-on Configuration for Blue System

9. Keywords

9.1 intubation; laryngoscope; trachael intubation

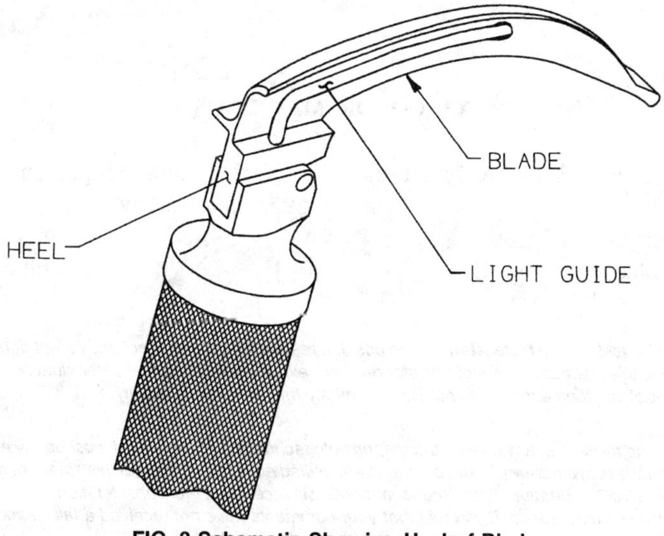

FIG. 3 Schematic Showing Heel of Blade

APPENDIXES

(Nonmandatory Information)

X1. RATIONALE

X1.1 *Blade and Handle Fittings* (4.1)—This is required for patient safety at the time of laryngoscopy.

X1.2 *Mechanical Restrictions* (4.2)—This is required for patient safety at the time of laryngoscopy.

X1.3 *Blade Retention* (4.3)—In nonoperating positions retention of the slot on the hinge pin must be sufficient to prevent inadvertent disengagement.

X1.4 *Corrosion Resistance* (4.4)—Corrosion may cause inadequate electrical and mechanical performance.

X1.5 *Critical Dimensions* (4.5)—The handle hook-on fittings require precise description to ensure compatibility of blades and handles within a given system.

X1.6 *Component Compatibility* (4.6)—In the interest of patient safety, handles and blades which engage should lock and illuminate.

X1.7 *Marking and Labeling* (Section 5)—Legible and durable markings of the manufacturer's trademark, the size, and the type of the blade are necessary to ensure easy identification of the blade by the user. Also, see Section 7. Removable components should be marked to facilitate proper reassembly.

X1.8 *Test Methods and Values* (Section 6)—A major goal of this specification is to ensure that fiber-illuminated components which engage shall lock and illuminate. Further, the components shall engage and disengage with reasonable force in the interest of patient safety at the time of laryngoscopy.

X1.9 *Identification of Compatible Systems* (Section 7)—Identification is necessary to facilitate rapid and accurate recognition of compatible handle and blade components.

X1.10 *Addition of New Systems* (Section 8)—Development of new systems necessitates a mechanism for inclusion in this specification.

X2. TEST METHODS AND VALUES

X2.1 *Locking—Operating Position*—Locking of the blade into the operating position should occur when a torque between 0.35 N•m and 1.35 N•m is applied to the blade.

X2.2 *Unlocking—Operating Position*—Unlocking of the blade from the operating position should occur when a torque between 0.25 N•m and 1.35 N•m is applied to the blade.

X2.3 *Engagement and Disengagement*—Engagement or disengagement of the blade from the handle should occur when a force between 10 N and 45 N is applied (see Fig. X2.1 and

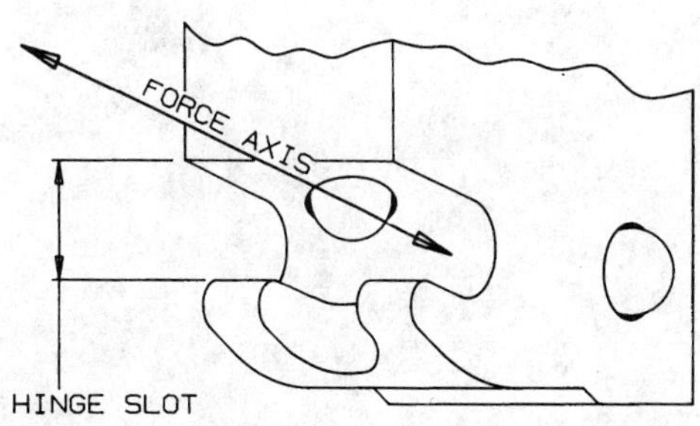

FIG. X2.1 Schematic of Force Axis During Locking and Unlocking

Specification F 965).

X3. COLOR MARKINGS

X3.1 The systems designated in 7.3 are assigned the following colors:

Fig. 1—green
Fig. 2—blue

X3.2 Color assignment in accordance with FED-STD-595A is as follows:

green—38901
blue—15180

Standard Specification for Anesthesia Reservoir Bags[1]

This standard is issued under the fixed designation F 1204; the number immediately following the designation indicates the year of original adoption or, in the case of revision, the year of last revision. A number in parentheses indicates the year of last reapproval. A superscript epsilon (ϵ) indicates an editorial change since the last revision or reapproval.

1. Scope

1.1 This specification covers reservoir bags for use with anesthesia breathing systems. For purposes of this specification, the reservoir bag includes the neck, body, and neck bushing, if provided. Special-purpose bags, for example, bellows, evacuation, and self-expanding bags are excluded from the scope of this specification.

1.2 The following subjects are covered: material, construction, neck, size, compliance (pressure-volume relationship), electrical conductivity, marking and labeling, and test methods to substantiate compliance with the requirements. Alternative test methods may be employed provided they can be shown to be equivalent or better. (A rationale is given in Appendix X1.)

NOTE 1—This specification supersedes ANSI Standard Z 79.4–1974.

1.3 *This standard does not purport to address all of the safety concerns, if any, associated with its use. It is the responsibility of the user of this standard to establish appropriate safety and health practices and determine the applicability of regulatory limitations prior to use.*

2. Referenced Documents

2.1 *ANSI Standard:*
ANSI/NFPA 99 Healthcare Facilities[2]

3. Terminology

3.1 *Definitions of Terms*—For the purpose of this specification, the following descriptions of terms shall apply:

3.1.1 *ambient temperature and pressure*—room temperature and pressure, dry gas (rtpd); indicates conditions of 20°C and 101.3 kPa (760 mm Hg) and dry gas.

3.1.2 *anesthesia reservoir bag*—collapsible container from which the patient may draw his tidal volume.

3.1.3 *compliance (pressure-volume relationship)*— a change of volume per change in pressure. Units of compliance are expressed as millilitres per kilopascals (millilitres per centimetre H_2O).

3.1.4 *conductive*—a property of an anesthesia reservoir bag and any integrally attached components with electrical conductivity acceptable in accordance with the applicable test (see 9.1.1).

3.1.5 *disposable*—an item intended to be used once and discarded.

3.1.6 *hanging loop*—a loop for hanging which may be provided near the tail of the bag (used to facilitate drying).

3.1.7 *labeling*—information and literature accompanying the device, such as brochures, package inserts, and manuals.

3.1.8 *marking*—information directly on the device.

3.1.9 *neck*—the end of the anesthesia reservoir bag that connects with the anesthesia breathing system.

3.1.10 *nonconductive*—a property of an anesthesia reservoir bag and any integrally attached components with insufficient electrical conductivity to meet the requirements of the applicable test (see 9.1.1).

3.1.11 *reusable*—an item intended for repeated use on one or more patients.

3.1.12 *size*—the size of the anesthesia reservoir bag is defined as the nominal or labeled capacity expressed in litres (L).

3.1.13 *tail*—the end of the bag opposite of the neck.

4. Material

4.1 *Requirements*:

4.1.1 The bag should be made of elastomeric material suitable for the intended use and should function satisfactorily in the presence of anesthetic agents and gases commonly used and not elute toxic substances.

4.1.2 Unless designated as disposable (for single use), the bag should be resistant to deterioration by methods of cleaning, disinfection, and sterilization as recommended by the manufacturer or the supplier. It is desirable that such products should withstand accepted methods of steam sterilization.

4.1.3 The material forming the body of the bag should be pliable to the extent that it remain elastic when the bag is inflated to its nominal size.

5. Construction

5.1 *Requirements*:

5.1.1 The bag shall not leak within a 10-s period when tested in accordance with 5.2.1.

5.1.2 The bag shall not be constructed in a manner such that the body or neck can cause a valve-like action (occlusion)

---

[1] This specification is under the jurisdiction of ASTM Committee F-29 on Anesthetic and Respiratory Equipmentand is the direct responsibility of Subcommittee F29.12 on Airways.

Current edition approved Dec. 30, 1988. Published February 1989.

[2] Available from American National Standards Institute, 1430 Broadway, New York, NY 10018.

under conditions of use.

5.1.3 The bag shall be free of visible defects or imperfections.

5.2 *Test Procedure*:

5.2.1 Inflate the bag with air to a pressure of 3.0 kPa (30 cm H_2O). Immerse the bag in a tank of water and observe for leakage as indicated by air bubbles. There shall not be air bubbles visible within a 10-s period.

5.2.2 Inflate the bag to its nominal size. Allow the bag to passively deflate (without assistance). Any indication of obstruction to flow as evidenced by failure of the bag to fully deflate is cause for failure.

5.2.3 Verify by visual inspection.

6. Neck

6.1 *Requirements*:

6.1.1 An integral neck bushing, if provided, shall be considered as part of the neck for purposes of this section.

6.1.2 The neck shall provide a secure fit on the nominal 22-mm plug gage shown in Fig. 1 such that it shall not disengage when tested in accordance with 6.2.2.

6.1.3 The axial length of the neck shall not be less than 25 mm.

6.2 *Test Procedure*:

6.2.1 Determine by inspection.

6.2.2 *Disconnection Test*—Lubricate the neck with distilled water and engage with the plug gage (see Fig. 1). The connection of the neck and gage shall be capable of withstanding a minimum tensile load of 15 N (3.4 lbf) applied on the body in any direction for a period of 1 min. The neck shall not become detached from the plug gage nor shall the bag detach from the bushing.

6.2.3 Verify by inspection.

7. Size

7.1 *Requirements*:

7.1.1 The size shall be determined in accordance with 7.2.1.

7.1.2 The accuracy of the labeled size shall be within± 15 % of the nominal size.

NOTE 2—The common nominal sizes are 0.5, 1.0, 2.0, 3.0, and 5.0 L.

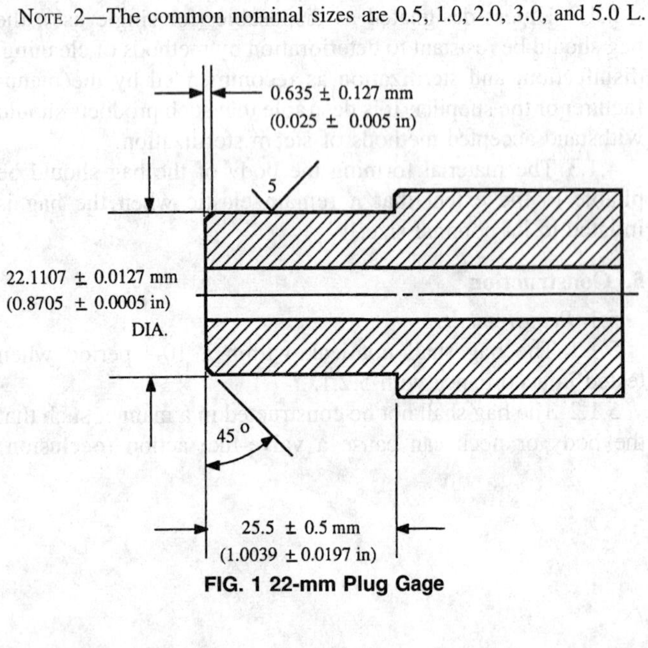

FIG. 1 22-mm Plug Gage

7.2 *Test Procedure*:

7.2.1 *Size Test*—Place the bag in a tank of water with the top rim of the neck held 25 mm above the water level. Seal lower opening of the bag (tail), if present. Fill the bag, held vertically, with water to the top rim of the neck. The water shall be at a temperature of 20 ± 3°C. Then remove the bag and measure the water volume. The measured volume is the size expressed in litres.

7.2.2 Verify by inspection.

8. Compliance

8.1 *Requirements*:

8.1.1 When tested in accordance with either 8.2.1 or 8.2.2, the bag shall expand uniformly. For bag sizes 1.5 L and smaller, the pressure shall not be less than 3.0 kPa (30 cm H_2O) nor shall it exceed 5.0 kPa (50 cm H_2O) when the bag is expanded to four times its size. For bag sizes greater than 1.5 L, the pressure shall not be less than 3.5 kPa (35 cm H_2O) nor shall it exceed 6.0 kPa (60 cm H_2O) when the bag is expanded to four times its size. After this test, the bag should revert to its original measured size within a tolerance of + 10 %, − 0 %. See Note 3.

8.2 *Test Procedure*:

8.2.1 *Water Test*—Seal the lower opening of the bag, if present. Place the bag in a tank of water with the neck held 25 mm above the water level. Fill the bag with water to the top rim of the neck. Insert an appropriately sized stopper into the neck of the bag. Insert a tube through the stopper to the water level in the tank. The bore of the tube shall not be less than 10 mm and it shall be of sufficient length to provide a pressure head of 6.0 kPa (60 cm H_2O). Add water through the tube until a total of four times the size of the bag is reached. Measure the pressure head when the water in the tube has reached a maximum height and has stabilized. The duration of the test shall not exceed 5 min with a water temperature of 20 ± 3°C. Measure the pressure to an accuracy of± 0.1 kPa (±1.0 cm H_2O).

8.2.2 *Air Test* (Optional)—Connect the bag to a pressure source with in-line flowmeter (compensated for pressure) and water manometer. Introduce air into the bag at a constant rate of two times nominal size per minute for a period of 2 min. Allow the system to stabilize. Record the pressure indicated on the manometer. The flow rate shall be accurate to within ±5.0 % with air temperature at 20± 3°C. Measure the pressure to an accuracy of ±0.1 kPa (±1.0 cm H_2O).

NOTE 3—The electrical conductivity of a conductive reservoir bag which has undergone either of these tests may be reduced. The bag may not meet electrical resistance requirements appropriate to new products.

9. Electrical Conductivity

9.1 *Requirements*:

9.1.1 The electrical characteristics of bags and integral neck bushings made of conductive material shall be as specified and tested in accordance with the requirements of ANSI/NFPA 99.

9.1.2 Bags and integral neck bushings made of conductive materials shall be marked "CONDUCTIVE."

9.1.3 Black bags and black integral neck bushings made of nonconductive materials shall be marked "NONCONDUCTIVE."

9.2 *Test Procedure*:

9.2.1 Test in accordance with ANSI/NFPA 99.

9.2.2 Verify by visual inspection.

9.2.3 Verify by visual inspection.

10. Marking

10.1 *Requirements*:

10.1.1 *Reusable Reservoir Bags*:

10.1.1.1 The name, trademark, or unique identifying mark of the manufacturer shall be marked on or affixed to the bag.

10.1.1.2 The size expressed in litres shall be marked on or affixed to the bag.

10.1.1.3 Conductive bags shall be marked "CONDUCTIVE."

10.1.1.4 The month and year of manufacture or equivalent code should be marked on or affixed to the bag.

10.1.2 *Disposable Reservoir Bags*:

10.1.2.1 The information required in 10.1.1.1-10.1.1.4 through may be marked on the bag but is not required.

10.1.2.2 Conductive bags included with nonconductive circuits need not be marked "CONDUCTIVE."

10.2 *Test Procedure*:

10.2.1 *Reusable Reservoir Bags*:

10.2.1.1 Verify by visual inspection.

10.2.1.2 Verify by visual inspection.

10.2.1.3 Verify by visual inspection.

10.2.1.4 Verify by visual inspection.

11. Labeling

11.1 *Requirements*:

11.1.1 *Reusable Reservoir Bags*:

11.1.1.1 When bags are supplied with the intention that they can be reused, this shall be indicated. Information shall be provided to recommend acceptable methods for cleaning, disinfection, and sterilization.

11.1.1.2 The size of the bag expressed in litres shall be stated.

11.1.1.3 The name or trademark of the manufacturer shall be stated.

11.1.1.4 If the bag is conductive as determined in Section 9, this shall be stated.

11.1.1.5 The month and year of manufacture or equivalent code shall be stated unless it is marked on or affixed to the bag.

11.1.2 *Disposable Reservoir Bags*:

11.1.2.1 With disposable bags, the unit package shall be labeled as such, for example, "Disposable."

11.1.2.2 The size of the bag expressed in litres shall be stated.

11.1.2.3 The name or trademark of the manufacturer shall be stated.

11.1.2.4 If the bag is conductive as determined in Section 9, this shall be stated.

11.1.2.5 The month and year of manufacture or equivalent code shall be stated.

11.2 *Test Procedure*:

11.2.1 *Reusable Reservoir Bags*:

11.2.1.1 Verify by visual inspection.

11.2.1.2 Verify by visual inspection.

11.2.1.3 Verify by visual inspection.

11.2.1.4 Verify by visual inspection.

11.2.1.5 Verify by visual inspection.

11.2.2 *Disposable Reservoir Bags*:

11.2.2.1 Verify by visual inspection.

11.2.2.2 Verify by visual inspection.

11.2.2.3 Verify by visual inspection.

11.2.2.4 Verify by visual inspection.

11.2.2.5 Verify by visual inspection.

12. Keywords

12.1 anesthesia; compliance; pressure testing—medical equipment; pressure volume relationship (compliance); water test

APPENDIX

(Nonmandatory Information)

X1. RATIONALE

NOTE X1.1—Paragraph numbers in parentheses correspond with sections in this specification.

X1.1 (5.1.2) The purpose of this requirement is to minimize the risk of gas flow interruption during ventilation. A valve-like action (occlusion) may result from reinforcement of the body or neck or use of an integral neck bushing, or both.

X1.2 (5.2) Pressurization to 3.0 kPa (30 cm H_2O) allows adequate distension of the elastomeric material for accurate leakage detection while maintaining the bag at a reasonable volume for testing. Due to the elastomeric characteristics of the material, a test method equating leakage with pressure loss may be inappropriate.

X1.3 (6.1.2) Since the physical characteristics of the materials used for neck construction may vary widely, specifying actual dimensions is not practical. The intent of this section is that necks must fit properly and securely, regardless of actual dimensions or materials used for their construction.

X1.4 (7.1.2) A clinical necessity was expressed for this accuracy.

X1.5 (7.2) The bag is immersed in water to provide uniform distribution of pressure.

X1.6 (8.1.1) The 3.0 to 5.0-kPa (30 to 50-cm H_2O) pressure limits are considered to be appropriate for safety and for effective use of the smaller size bags. For bags larger than 1.5 L, the lower pressure limit is 3.5 kPa (35 cm H_2O) to provide for effective use in ventilating patients with high airway resistance or low pulmonary compliance. The upper limit was set at 6.0 kPa (60 cm H_2O) because that is typical of reusable bags that have been used and considered safe for many years. Reusable bags generally are reinforced and are thus stiffer than disposable bags because the reusables must remain safe and effective for a much longer time.

X1.7 (8.2.1) The water test enables the user to perform a pressure test with simple equipment available. The air test enables the user to perform a pressure test on an anesthesia machine and is more analogous to clinical use.

Standard Specification for Anesthesia Breathing Tubes[1]

This standard is issued under the fixed designation F 1205; the number immediately following the designation indicates the year of original adoption or, in the case of revision, the year of last revision. A number in parentheses indicates the year of last reapproval. A superscript epsilon (ε) indicates an editorial change since the last revision or reapproval.

1. Scope

1.1 This specification covers anesthesia breathing tubes, integrally attached end fittings, and integrally attached components for use with anesthesia breathing systems. Excluded are similar tubes for specific other purposes, such as those used with some breathing machines, pediatric anesthesia circuits, and gas scavenging tubes.

1.2 The following subjects are covered: terminology, dimensions, labeling and marking, selected performance requirements, and test methods to substantiate compliance with the requirements. Alternative test methods may be employed provided that they can be shown to be equivalent or better.

NOTE 1—This specification supersedes ANSI Standard Z 79.6-1975.

1.3 *This standard does not purport to address all of the safety problems, if any, associated with its use. It is the responsibility of the user of this standard to establish appropriate safety and health practices and determine the applicability of regulatory limitations prior to use.*

2. Referenced Documents

2.1 *ASTM Standards:*

F 1054 Specification For Conical Fittings Of 15 mm and 22 mm Sizes[2]

2.2 *ANSI Standard:*

ANSI/NFPA 99 Healthcare Facilities[3]

3. Terminology

3.1 *Descriptions of Terms*—For the purpose of this specification, the following descriptions of terms shall apply:

3.1.1 *ambient temperature and pressure*—room temperature and pressure, dry gas (rtpd); indicates conditions of 20°C and 101.3 kPa (760 mm Hg) and dry gas.

3.1.2 *assembled end*—a fitting integrally attached by the manufacturer to the end of the tube.

3.1.3 *breathing tube*—a large-bore (greater than or equal to 15 mm) nonrigid tube, usually corrugated, used to convey gases or vapors, or both, to and from the patient.

3.1.4 *compliance* (pressure-volume relationship)—a change of volume per change in pressure. Units of compliance are expressed as millilitres per kilopascal (millilitres per centimetre H_2O) per metre length of tube.

3.1.5 *conductive*—a property of a breathing tube and any integrally attached components with electrical conductivity acceptable in accordance with the applicable test (see 10.1.1).

3.1.6 *disposable*—an item intended to be used once and discarded.

3.1.7 *flow resistance*—the pressure difference from inlet to outlet of a device caused by flow. Units of resistance are kilopascal per litre per second (centimetre of H_2O per litre per second) per meter length of tube.

3.1.8 *labeling*—information and literature accompanying the device, such as brochures, package inserts, and manuals.

3.1.9 *machine end*—that end of the breathing tube which is toward the machine.

3.1.10 *marking*—information directly on the device.

3.1.11 *nonconductive*—a property of a breathing tube and any integrally attached components with insufficient electrical conductivity to meet the requirements of applicable test (see 10.1.1).

3.1.12 *patient end*—that end of the breathing tube which is toward the patient.

3.1.13 *reusable*—an item intended for repeated use on one or more patients.

4. Material

4.1 *Requirements*:

4.1.1 Tubes should be made of materials suitable for the intended use and should function satisfactorily in the presence of anesthetic agents and gases commonly used and not elute toxic substances.

4.1.2 Reusable tubing should be able to withstand ordinary methods of cleaning, disinfection, and sterilization (see 12.1.1.1). It is desirable that such products should withstand accepted methods of steam sterilization.

5. Dimensions and Tolerances

5.1 *Requirements*:

5.1.1 *Measure System*—SI units shall be used.

5.1.2 *End Connectors*:

5.1.2.1 *Single Breathing Tube(s)*—Both ends of the tube shall mate with 22-mm male fittings which comply with Specification F 1054. The ends may be assembled, plain,

[1] This specification is under the jurisdiction of ASTM Committee F-29 on Anesthetic and Respiratory Equipmentand is the direct responsibility of Subcommittee F29.12 on Airways.

Current edition approved Dec. 30, 1988. Published February 1989.

[2] *Annual Book of ASTM Standards*, Vol 13.01.

[3] Available from American National Standards Institute, 1430 Broadway, New York, NY 10018.

cylindrical, or tapered.

5.1.2.2 *Assembled Sets* (integrally attached Y-piece and tubing, not intended to be disassembled):

(*a*) *Patient End*—The patient end of the Y-piece shall be a 22-mm/15-mm male/female coaxial fitting complying with Specification F 1054.

(*b*) *Machine End*—The machine end of both breathing tubes shall mate with 22-mm male fittings which comply with Specification F 1054. The ends may be assembled, plain, cylindrical, or tapered.

5.1.3 *Length*—The length of the breathing tube shall be designated as the nominal overall length when measured in the relaxed condition and shall be stated with a tolerance of ± 5 %.

5.2 *Test Procedure*:

5.2.1 Verify by inspection.

5.2.2 Test in accordance with 6.2.1.

5.2.2.1 (4.1.2.2(*a*)) Verify by inspection that the patient end fittings comply with Specification F 1054.

5.2.3 Verify by measuring.

6. Connections

6.1 *Requirements*:

6.1.1 All connections shall withstand a minimum tensile load of 15 N for 1 min in all directions, except the axial direction, which shall withstand a tensile load of 40 N for 1 min.

6.1.2 For breathing tubes with assembled ends, the joint between the tubing and assembled end fitting shall withstand an axial tensile load of 45 N for 1 min applied 250 mm from the end of the fitting. The breathing tube shall not become detached from the assembled end fitting.

6.2 *Test Procedure*:

6.2.1 Lubricate the mating surfaces of the end of the breathing tube with distilled water and engage with the appropriate plug gate (see Specification F 1054, Fig. 5 or Fig. 6). Apply a tensile load of 15 N at 45° to the axis for a period of 1 min. For the axial direction, apply a load of 40 N. Test each end separately. The breathing tube shall not become detached from the plug gage.

6.2.2 To test the integral joint between the assembled end fitting and the tube, affix the assembled end fitting and apply a 45-N axial tensile load to the tubing 250 mm from the joint for 1 min.

7. Leakage

7.1 *Requirements*:

7.1.1 When tested as specified in 7.2, leakage of one tube shall not exceed 25 mL/min at a pressure of 3.0 kPa (30 cm H_2O).

7.1.2 When tested as specified in 7.2, leakage of an assembled set as supplied by the manufacturer (two tubes plus integral Y-piece) shall not exceed 75 mL/min at a pressure of 3.0 kPa (30 cm H_2O).

7.2 *Test Procedure*:

7.2.1 The system shown in Fig. 1 is used to test for leakage of a single tube at ambient temperature and pressure (rtpd). Seal the end of the breathing tube and connect to the system as shown. Apply an airflow through the flowmeter (compensated for pressure) until the system pressure has stabilized at 3 kPa (30 cm H_2O). Record the flowmeter reading in millilitres per minute.

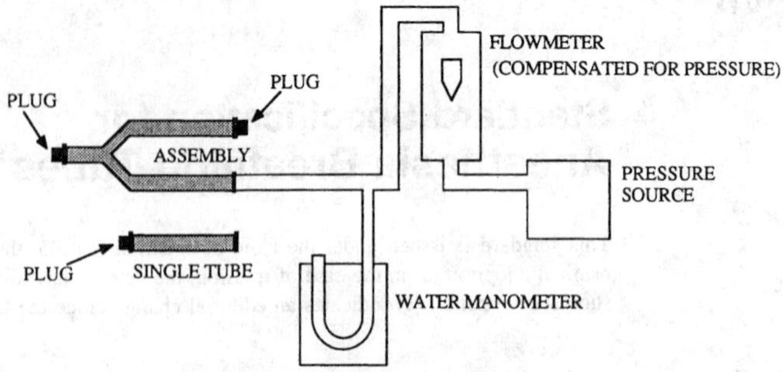

FIG. 1 Leakage Test Set-Up

7.2.2 The system shown in Fig. 1 is used to test for leakage of an assembled set (two tubes plus Y-piece) as supplied by the manufacturer at ambient temperature and pressure (rtpd). Seal the end of the Y-piece and one end of one of the tubes of the assembled set and connect to the system as shown. Apply an airflow through the flowmeter (compensated for pressure) until the system pressure has stabilized at 3 kPa (30 cm H_2O). Record the flowmeter reading in millilitres per minute.

8. Flow Resistance

8.1 *Requirements*:

8.1.1 Resistance of a single tube shall not exceed 0.1 kPa (1.0 cm H_2O)/m of length at 1.0 L/s.

8.1.2 Resistance of the inspiratory pathway of an assembled set (two tubes plus Y-piece) as supplied by the manufacturer shall not exceed 0.1 kPa (1.0 cm H_2O)/m of length at 1.0 L/s.

8.1.3 Resistance of the expiratory pathway of an assembled set (two tubes plus Y-piece) as supplied by the manufacturer shall not exceed 0.1 kPa (1.0 cm H_2O)/m of length at 1.0 L/s.

8.2 *Test Procedure*:

8.2.1 The system shown in Fig. 2 or Fig. 3 is used to determine the pressure drop (resistance) across a single tube. A buffer chamber may be placed between the source and the flowmeter to minimize pressure fluctuation. Connect the single tube as shown and set the airflow to 1.0 L/s. Record the pressure drop (resistance) from the water manometer as kilopascals per litre per second per meter length (centimetre H_2O per liter per second per meter length).

8.2.2 The system shown in Fig. 2 is used to determine the inspiratory pathway pressure drop (resistance). A buffer chamber may be placed between the source and the flowmeter to minimize pressure fluctuation. Connect the assembled set (two

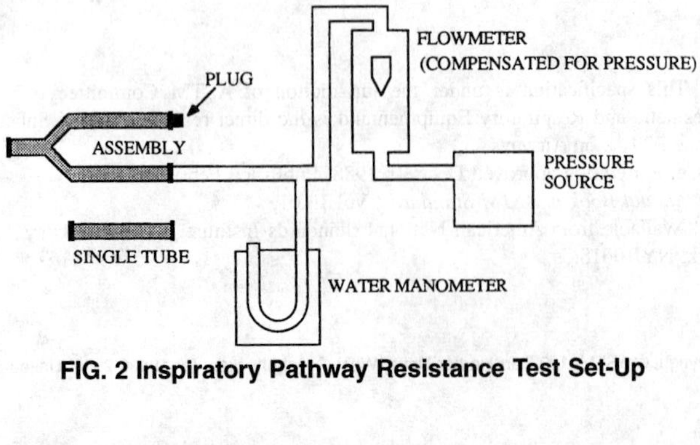

FIG. 2 Inspiratory Pathway Resistance Test Set-Up

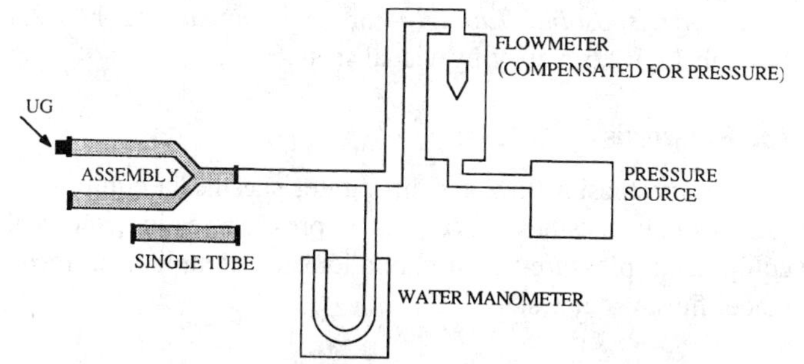

FIG. 3 Expiratory Pathway Resistance Test Set-Up

tubes plus Y-piece) to the test set-up at the end of the tube on the inspiratory side and seal the expiratory end as shown and set the airflow to 1.0 L/s. Record the pressure drop (resistance) from the water manometer as kilopascals per litre per second per meter length (centimetre H_2O per litre per second per meter length).

8.2.3 The system shown in Fig. 3 is used to determine the expiratory pathway pressure drop (resistance). A buffer chamber may be placed between the source and the flowmeter to minimize pressure fluctuation. Connect the assembled set (two tubes plus Y-piece) to the test set-up at the end of the Y-piece and seal the inspiratory end as shown and set the airflow to 1.0 L/s. Record the pressure drop (resistance) from the water manometer as kilopascals per litre per second per meter length (centimetre H_2O per litre per second per meter length).

9. Internal Compliance

9.1 *Requirements*—The typical compliance shall be measured at 2.0 kPa (20 cm H_2O) and 4.0 kPa (40 cm H_2O) and shall be expressed in the labeling at 2.0 kPa (20 cm H_2O) and 4.0 kPa (40 cm H_2O) as millilitres per kilopascal (millilitres per centimetre H_2O) per meter of length of tube(s). For assembled sets, the total compliance at 2.0 kPa (20 cm H_2O) and 4.0 kPa (40 cm H_2O) should be expressed in the labeling.

9.2 *Test Procedure*:

9.2.1 The system shown in Fig. 4 is used to determine the internal compliance (pressure-volume relationship) of a single tube or an assembled set as supplied by the manufacturer. The tubing volume connecting the manometer should not be more than 1/100 of the volume of the test sample. Connect the single tube or assembled set as shown and seal all ends. Inject and record the volume of air necessary to create 2.0 kPa (20 cm H_2O) of pressure. Inject an additional volume of air until the pressure reaches 4.0 kPa (40 cm H_2O) and record the total volume necessary to reach 4.0 kPa (40 cm H_2O).

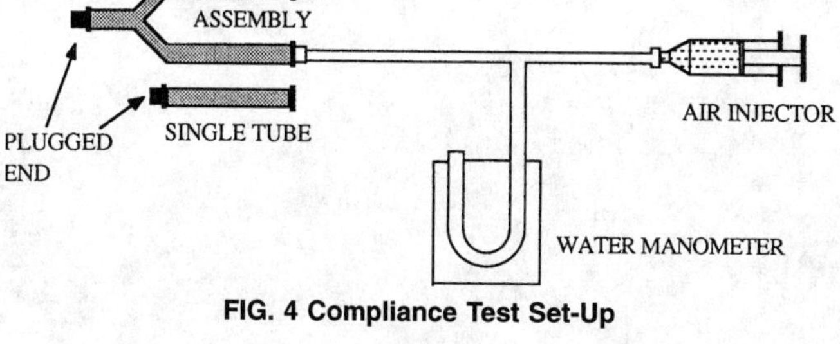

FIG. 4 Compliance Test Set-Up

10. Electrical Conductivity

10.1 *Requirements*:

10.1.1 The electrical characteristics of tubes and any integrally attached components made of conductive material shall be as specified and tested in accordance with the requirements of ANSI/NFPA 99.

10.1.2 Breathing tubes and integrally attached nonmetal components made of conductive materials shall be marked "CONDUCTIVE."

10.1.3 Black breathing tubes and black components made of nonconductive materials shall be marked "NONCONDUCTIVE."

10.2 *Test Procedure*:

10.2.1 Test in accordance with ANSI/NFPA 99.

10.2.2 Verify by visual inspection.

10.2.3 Verify by visual inspection.

11. Marking

11.1 *Requirements*:

11.1.1 *Reusable Tubing*:

11.1.1.1 The name, trademark, or unique identifying mark of the manufacturer shall be marked on or affixed to the tubing.

NOTE 2—The manufacture of reusable tubing without the name, trademark, or unique identifying mark of the manufacturer is permitted for 2 years after the initial publication of this specification.

11.1.1.2 Conductive tubes shall be marked "CONDUCTIVE."

11.1.1.3 The month and year of manufacture or equivalent code should be marked on or affixed to the tubing.

11.2 *Test Procedure—Reusable Tubing*:

11.2.1 Verify by visual inspection.

11.2.2 Verify by visual inspection.

12. Labeling

12.1 *Requirements*:

12.1.1 *Reusable Tubing*:

12.1.1.1 When tubes are supplied with the intention that they can be reused, this shall be indicated. Information shall be provided to recommend acceptable methods for cleaning, disinfection, and sterilization.

12.1.1.2 The typical compliance as determined in Section 9 shall be stated.

12.1.1.3 Tubing length as determined in 5.1.3 shall be stated.

12.1.1.4 The name or trademark of the manufacturer shall be stated.

12.1.1.5 If the tubing is conductive as determined in Section 10, this shall be stated.

12.1.1.6 The month and year of manufacture or equivalent code shall be stated unless it is marked on or affixed to the tubing.

12.1.2 *Disposable Tubing*:

12.1.2.1 The unit package shall be labeled as such, for example, "Disposable."

12.1.2.2 The typical compliance as determined in Section 9 shall be stated.

12.1.2.3 Tubing length as determined in 5.1.3 shall be stated.

12.1.2.4 The name or trademark of the manufacturer shall be stated.

12.1.2.5 If the tubing is conductive as determined in Section 10, this shall be stated.

12.1.2.6 The month and year of manufacture or equivalent code shall be stated unless it is marked on or affixed to the tubing.

12.2 *Test Procedure:*

12.2.1 *Reusable Tubing*—For requirements in 12.1.1.1 through 12.1.1.6, verify by visual inspection.

12.2.2 *Disposable Tubing*—For requirements in 12.1.2.1 through 12.1.2.6, verify by visual inspection.

13. Keywords

13.1 anesthesia; flow and flow rate; anesthesia equipment; leak testing; anesthesia equipment; pressure testing; medical equipment; pressure-volume relationship compliance; resistance; flow water test

Designation: F 1208 – 89 (Reapproved 2000)

Standard Specification for Minimum Performance and Safety Requirements for Anesthesia Breathing Systems[1]

This standard is issued under the fixed designation F 1208; the number immediately following the designation indicates the year of original adoption or, in the case of revision, the year of last revision. A number in parentheses indicates the year of last reapproval. A superscript epsilon (ε) indicates an editorial change since the last revision or reapproval.

1. Scope

1.1 This specification covers breathing systems and components employed with anesthesia gas machines for humans. This specification considers the circle system as a whole and some of its components individually. A particular emphasis is placed upon component arrangement in the circle absorber-type system, and submits a system of standard description and notation. Excluded are ventilators for use during anesthesia, Mapelson nonrebreathing type systems, as well as breathing systems and related components of dental *analgesia* machines. (For rationale, see Appendix X1.)

1.2 *This standard does not purport to address all of the safety concerns, if any, associated with its use. It is the responsibility of the user of this standard to establish appropriate safety and health practices and determine the applicability of regulatory limitations prior to use.*

1.3 This specification is arranged as follows:

2. Referenced Documents

2.1 *ASTM Standards:*

F 1054 Specification for Conical Fittings[2]

F 1204 Specification for Anesthesia Reservoir Bags[2]

F 1205 Specification for Anesthesia Breathing Tubes[2]

2.2 *ANSI/ASME Standard:*

ANSI/ASME B40.1M-1985 Standard for Pressure Gauge[3]

3. Terminology

3.1 *Definitions:*

3.1.1 *absorber assembly*—a container(s) for CO_2 absorbent, and may include, but need not be limited to, the inspiratory and expiratory unidirectional valves, APL valve, and bag mount.

3.1.2 *adjustable pressure limiting valve* (APL valve)—a user-adjustable valve which releases gas and is intended to provide control of the breathing system pressure.

3.1.3 *breathing system*—a gas pathway in direct connection with the patient through which gas flows occur at respiratory pressures, in which directional valves may be present, and into which a mixture of controlled composition may be dispensed.

3.1.4 *circle breathing system*—a breathing system in which circular gas flow (through separate inspiratory and expiratory pathways) is determined by unidirectional valves.

3.1.5 *common gas outlet*—that port through which the mixture dispensed from the anesthesia gas machine is delivered to the breathing system.

3.1.6 *compliance*—the change of volume per unit change in pressure within a closed system. Units of compliance are: L/kPa or L/cm H_2O (litres per kilopascal or litres per centimetre of water).

3.1.7 *expiratory pathway*—that portion of the gas pathway through which expired gases flow at respiratory pressures.

3.1.8 *fresh gas inlet*—that port on breathing systems to which the fresh gas supply is attached.

3.1.9 *fresh gas supply tube (or hose)*—that conduit conveying gases from the common gas outlet, or other gas source, to the fresh gas inlet of the breathing system.

[1] This specification is under the jurisdiction of ASTM Committee F29 on Anesthetic and Respiratory Equipment and is the direct responsibility of Subcommittee F29.01.02 on Anesthesia Breathing Systems/Performance.

Current edition approved Jan. 27, 1989. Published March 1989.

[2] *Annual Book of ASTM Standards*, Vol 13.01.

[3] Available from the American National Standards Institute, 25 W. 43rd St., 4th Floor, New York, NY 10036.

3.1.10 *inspiratory pathway*—that portion of the gas pathway through which inspiratory gases flow at respiratory pressures.

3.1.11 *kilopascal (kPa)—SI unit of pressure*, 1 kPa approximates 10 cm of H_2O.

3.1.12 *labeling*—information and literature accompanying the device (for example, brochure, package insert, manual, etc.).

3.1.13 *marking*—information directly on a device.

3.1.14 *may*—denotes an optional feature or consideration.

3.1.15 *resistance*—the pressure difference from inlet to outlet of the device per unit of flow, expressed in kPa/L/s (kilopascals per litre per second). For the purposes of this specification, pressure drops are noted at flows of 0.5 L/s and 1.0 L/s.

3.1.16 *room temperature and pressure, dry gas* (rtpd)—*forthe purposes of this specification*, 20 ± 3°C, at ambient barometric pressure.

3.1.17 *shall*—denotes a mandatory feature or consideration.

3.1.18 *should*—denotes a desirable but not mandatory feature or consideration.

4. System Classification

4.1 Symbols were devised, diagramatic rules established, and a standard method of notation utilized. In addition, these symbols, diagramatic rules, and method of notation may be used in labeling and marking.

4.1.1 *Notation*—The method of notation consists of two parts: that of graphic notation (see Fig. 1), and that of numeric designation of functional segments of the circle system (see

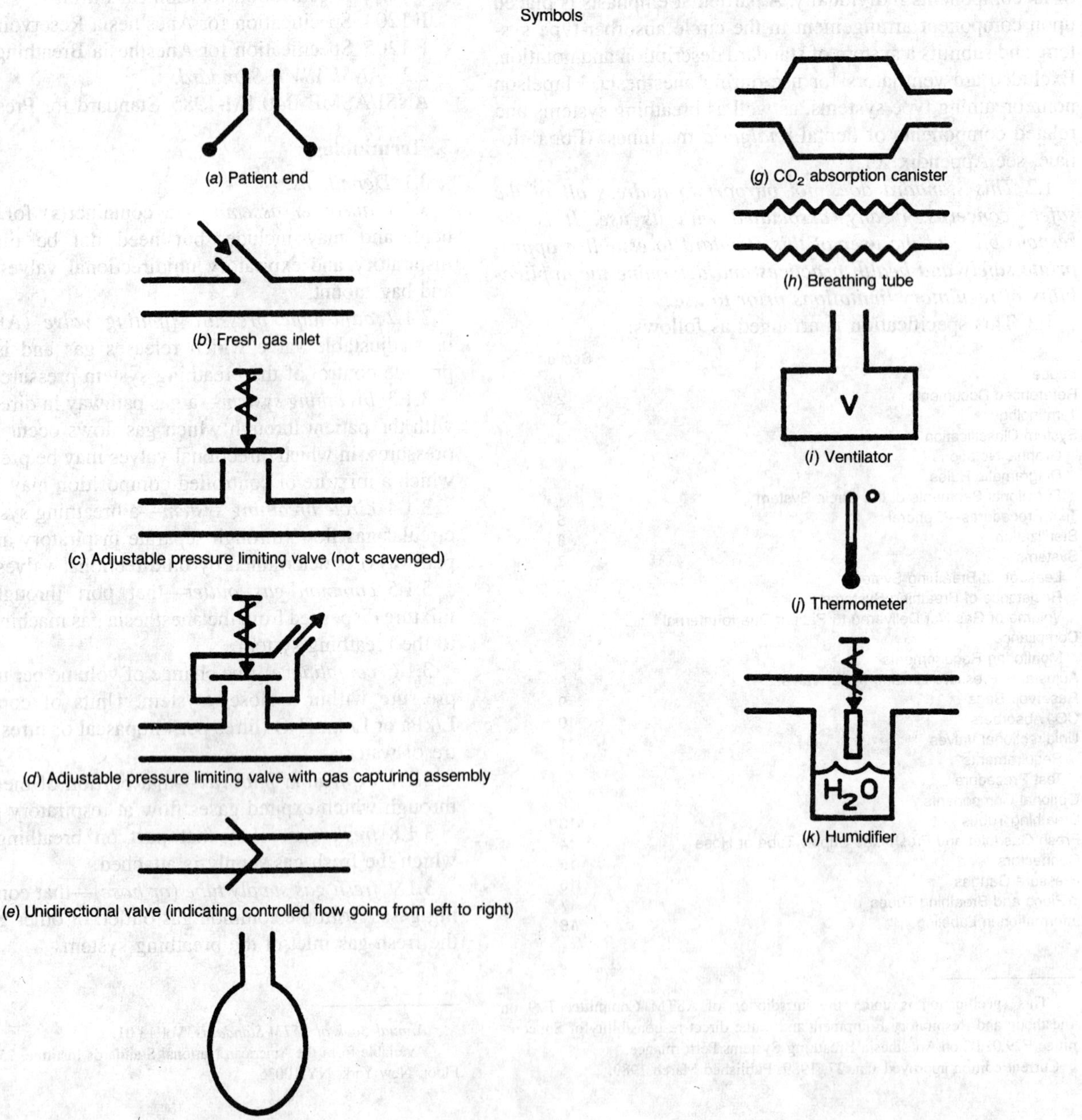

FIG. 1 Symbols

section 3.2 and Fig. 2).

4.1.1.1 *Diagramatic Rules*:

(a) Gas flow in circuit proceeds in counter-clockwise direction.

(b) Patient end symbol is on the right side of circle.

(c) Reservoir bag symbol is on the left side of circle opposite the patient symbol.

4.1.2 *Functional Divisions of the Circle System—Segmentation*—The circle system is divided into four segments (see Fig. 2) to illustrate specific functional characteristics. These segments include the following areas where components may be located, or in some cases, shall be located.

Segment 1—From patient to expiratory valve.
Segment 2—From expiratory valve to reservoir bag.
Segment 3—From reservoir bag to inspiratory valve.
Segment 4—From inspiratory valve to patient.

An example of the use of these symbols in a circle system is shown in Fig. 3 and is presented *for illustrative purposes only.*

5. Test Procedures

5.1 *General*—The test methods are included after each requirement (and each requirement will be referenced by section number in parentheses) to provide a means to substantiate compliance with the requirement. Other test methods may be employed if they can be shown to be equivalent.

5.1.1 *Accuracy*—Unless otherwise specified, accuracy shall be ±5 % of reading for each variable to be measured, and flow meters shall be compensated for pressure.

5.1.2 *Environmental Conditions*—Run all tests at rtpd except where otherwise stated.

5.1.3 *Test Gases*—All tests shall be performed with dry oxygen, or dry medical air, or dry nitrogen, unless otherwise specified in a particular test method.

6. Sterilization

6.1 *Disassembly*—The reuseable components of the breathing system, including the absorber and valves, shall be capable of being disassembled as required for cleaning and sterilization.

6.1.1 *Methods*—The manufacturer shall state suitable means of sterilization. The reuseable components of the breathing system should be sterilizable by autoclaving.

6.2 *Test Procedure*:

6.2.1 Disassemble according to instructions in the labeling.

6.2.2 Verify by reading the appropriate instructions in the labeling.

7. Systems

7.1 *Requirements*—The requirements of this section refer to breathing system assemblies as supplied complete by the manufacturer, that is, absorber, inspiratory and expiratory valves, APL valve, breathing tubes, Y-piece, and right angle

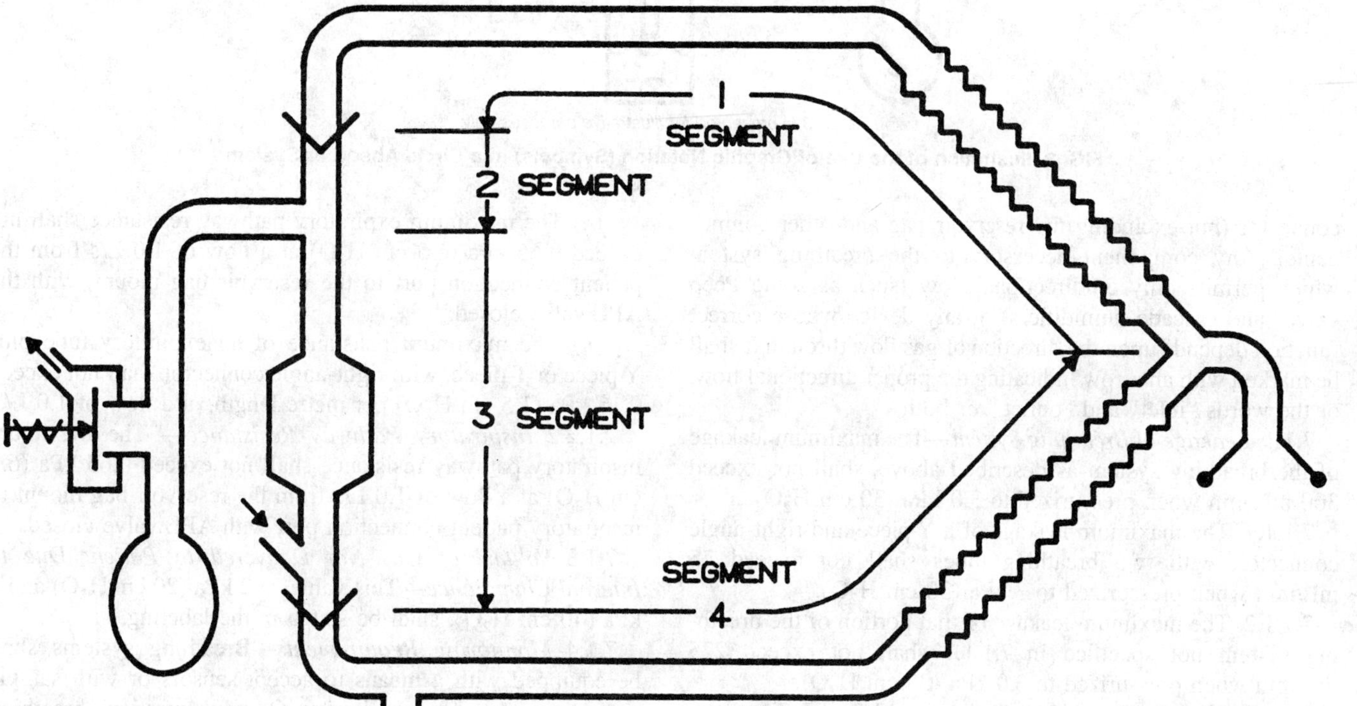

Segment 1—From patient to expiratory valve.
Segment 2—From expiratory valve to reservoir bag.
Segment 3—From reservoir bag to inspiratory valve.
Segment 4—From inspiratory valve to patient.

FIG. 2 Functional Segments of a Circle System

This example of the Use of these symbols in a circle system is *for illustrative purposes only.*

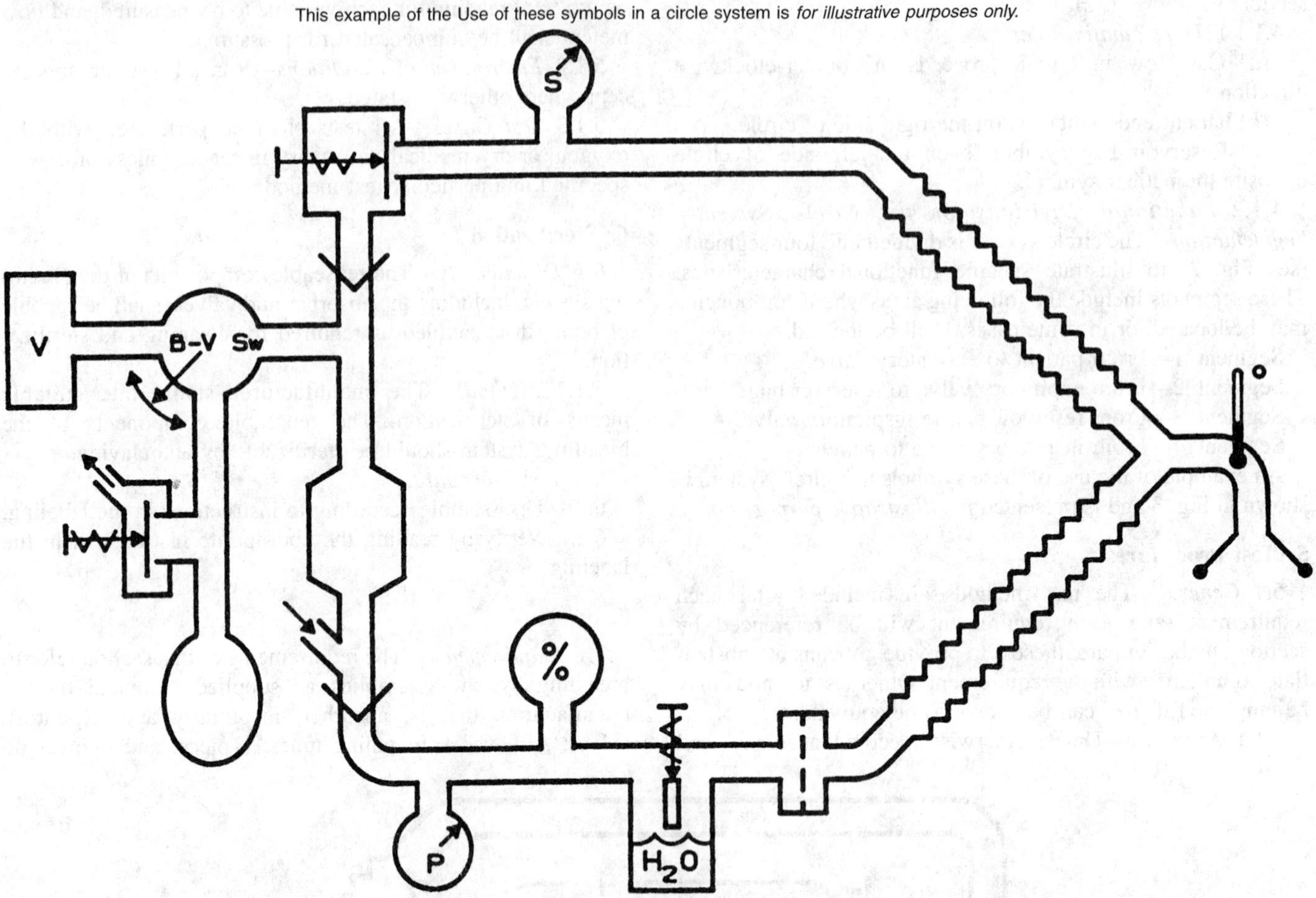

Figure 3 is presented for illustrative purposes only.

FIG. 3 Illustration of the Use of Graphic Notation (Symbols) in a Circle Absorber System

connector (but excluding the reservoir bag and other components). Any component accessory to the breathing system which permits only unidirectional flow (such as some Peep valves and cascade humidifiers) or any device whose correct function depends upon the direction of gas flow through it shall be marked with an arrow indicating the proper directional flow, or the words "inlet" and "outlet," or both.

7.1.1 *Leakage of Breathing System*—The maximum leakage of the breathing system as described above, shall not exceed 300 mL/min when pressurized to 3.0 kPa (30 cm H_2O).

7.1.1.1 The maximum leakage of a Y-piece and right-angle connector, with two breathing tubes shall not exceed 75 mL/min when pressurized to 3 kPa (30 cm H_2O).

7.1.1.2 The maximum leakage of that portion of the breathing system not specified in 7.1.1.1 shall not exceed 225 mL/min when pressurized to 3.0 kPa (30 cm H_2O).

7.1.1.3 Manufacturers shall disclose in their labeling conformance with 7.1.1.

7.1.2 *Resistance of Breathing Systems* (see 7.2.2)—Manufacturers shall disclose in their labeling the typical pressure drops due to inspiratory and expiratory gas flow in their breathing system at reference flows of 0.5 and 1.0 L/s. For pediatric systems resistance at appropriately lower flow rates should be disclosed.

7.1.2.1 *Expiratory Pathway Resistance*:

(a) The maximum expiratory pathway resistance shall not exceed 0.65 kPa (6.5 cm H_2O) at a flow of 1.0 L/s from the patient connection port to the reservoir bag mount, with the APL valve closed.

(b) The maximum resistance of an expiratory tube plus Y-piece or T-piece, with right-angle connector shall not exceed 0.15 kPa (1.5 cm H_2O) per metre length, at a flow of 1.0 L/s.

7.1.2.2 *Inspiratory Pathway Resistance*— The maximum inspiratory pathway resistance shall not exceed 0.65 kPa (6.5 cm H_2O) at a flow of 1.0 L/s from the reservoir bag mount to inspiratory patient connection port with APL valve closed.

7.1.3 *Volume of Gas Not Delivered to Patient Due to Internal Compliance*—This value, at 2 kPa (20 cm H_2O) and 4 kPa (40 cm H_2O), shall be stated in the labeling.

7.1.4 *Monitoring Requirements*—Breathing systems shall be equipped with a means to accept sensors or with sample extraction ports for monitoring O_2 concentration, breathing pressure, and either exhaled volume or ventilatory CO_2.

7.2 *Test Procedures*:

7.2.1 *Leakage of Breathing System*:

7.2.1.1 *Apparatus Required*—Pressure measuring device and flowmeter(s).

7.2.1.2 *Procedure*—Remove the reservoir bag and seal the bag port and patient connection. The pressure tap should be at the patient connection port. Introduce gas into the system or the component(s) until pressure is stabilized at 3.0 kPa (30 cm H_2O). Then record the flowmeter reading as the leak. If the system or component(s) incorporate(s) values designed to allow gas to leak at pressures below 3.0 kPa (30 cm H_2O), seal them for the test.

7.2.2 *Resistance of Breathing System*:

7.2.2.1 *Resistance Measurement of the Inspiratory Pathway*—Seal the expiratory pathway and close the APL valve. Inject air at both 0.5 L/s and 1.0 L/s and measure pressure at the bag port with the patient port open.

7.2.2.2 *Resistance Measurement of the Expiratory Pathway*—The inspiratory limb is sealed and the APL valve is closed. Inject air at both 0.5 L/s and 1.0 L/s and measure pressure at the patient port with bag port open.

7.2.3 *Measurement of Internal Compliance*:

7.2.3.1 The absorber shall be filled with fresh absorbent for this test. Seal the bag and patient ports as well as instrumentation ports and check that the system is gas tight. Add measured volumes of gas through the fresh gas inlet until 2.0 kPa (20 cm H_2O) and then 4.0 kPa (40 cm H_2O) pressures are achieved.

7.2.3.2 Internal compliance is the added volume (divided by 20) needed to achieve 20 cm H_2O pressure and the total of the two added volumes needed to achieve 40 cm H_2O pressure (divided by 40).

8. Adjustable Pressure-Limiting (APL) Valves

8.1 *Requirements*—These requirements apply to APL valves as separate components and as part of a gas collection assembly.

8.1.1 *Placement*—In a circle system an APL valve shall not be placed between the inspiratory valve and the patient (segment 4) though it may be placed at the Y-piece. The APL valve should be located in segment 2 or immediately adjacent to the bag mount.

8.1.2 *Marking*—An arrow or other marking shall be provided to indicate the direction of movement required to close the valve.

8.1.3 *Pressure-Flow Characteristics*— The influence of flow and control setting on the resistance of the APL valve shall be illustrated in the manual by charting the pressure-flow data curve between 0.5 and 1.0 L/s. For pediatric systems the data should be given for appropriately lower flows with the valve fully open.

8.1.4 *Direction of Motion*—Valves with rotating controls shall be so designed that a clockwise motion increases the limiting pressure and closes the valve. The full range of relief pressures should be adjusted by less than one full turn of the control.

8.1.5 *Resistance at Low Flow*—Fully open valves should have a pressure drop of between 0.1 and 0.3 kPa (1.0 and 3.0 cm H_2O) at an air flow of 3.0 L/min.

8.1.6 *Resistance at High Flow*—Valves, when adjusted to the fully open position, should have a pressure drop at 30 L/min of not less than 0.1 kPa (1.0 cm H_2O) and not greater than 0.5 kPa (5.0 cm H_2O).

8.2 *Test Procedures*:

8.2.1 *Apparatus Required*—Flowmeters and a water manometer.

8.2.2 *Procedure*—This system, shown in Fig. 4, is used to determine the pressure drop across the valve. The valve is isolated and connected as shown. A buffer chamber may be

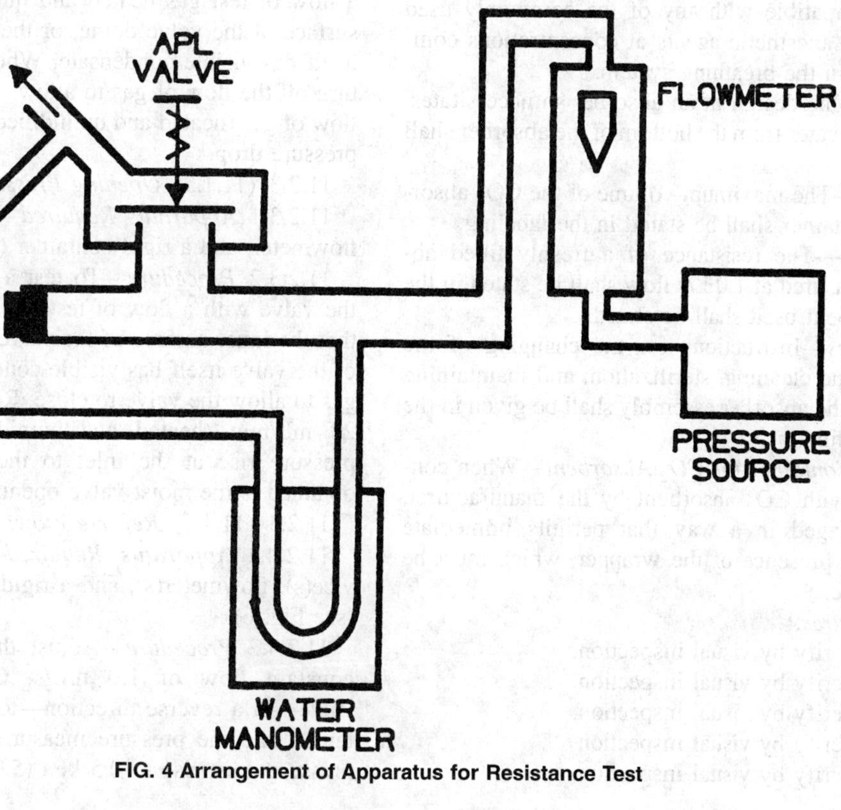

FIG. 4 Arrangement of Apparatus for Resistance Test

necessary to minimize pressure fluctuation. The proper flowmeter must be selected for each test. Valves must be in fully open position or adjusted as necessary.

8.2.3 *Resistance at Low Flow*—Increase the flow through the valve gradually until 3.0 L/min is reached. At that constant flow, measure the pressure drop across the valve. The valve passes the test if the pressure drop is not less than 0.1 kPa (1.0 cm H_2O) and not more than 0.3 kPa (3.0 cm H_2O).

8.2.4 *Resistance at High Flow*—Increase the flow to 30 L/min and measure the pressure drop across the valve. The valve passes the test if the pressure drop is not less than 0.1 kPa (1.0 cm H_2O) and not greater than 0.5 kPa (5.0 cm H_2O).

9. Reservoir Bag Connectors and Reservoir Bags

9.1 *Requirements*—See Specification F 1204.

9.1.1 *Placement*—Reservoir bag connectors shall not be placed on the patient side of the inspiratory or the expiratory valves in a circle system (segments 1 and 4).

9.1.2 The reservoir bag connector shall be male nominal 22 mm outside diameter. The outside configuration may be cylindrical, tapered, or manufacturer-specific in design.

9.2 *Test Procedure*:

9.2.1 Verify by visual inspection.

9.2.2 Verify by visual inspection and measurement.

10. CO_2 Absorbers

10.1 *Requirements*:

10.1.1 *Placement*—The absorber in the circle system should not be placed in segment 1 (from patient to expiratory valve) or at the patient end of segment 4 (from inspiratory valve to patient).

10.1.2 *CO Absorbent Container*—The walls of the container of CO_2 absorbent should be constructed of a transparent material that is compatible with any of the commonly used absorbents and with anesthetic agents at concentrations commonly encountered in the breathing system.

10.1.3 *Drain*—If the design of an absorber so necessitates, a means of draining water from the bottom of the absorber shall be provided.

10.1.4 *Capacity*—The maximum volume of the CO_2 absorbent held in the container shall be stated in the labeling.

10.1.5 *Resistance*—The resistance of a freshly filled absorber assembly measured at 1.0 L/s flow shall be stated in the labeling. The absorbent used shall be stated.

10.1.6 *Instructions*—Instructions for the changing of the absorbent, and for the cleaning, sterilization, and maintaining the gas tightness of the absorber assembly shall be given in the marking or the labeling.

10.1.7 *Prefilled Container for CO_2 Absorbent*—When container(s) are filled with CO_2 absorbent by the manufacturer, they shall be packaged in a way that permits immediate identification of the presence of the wrapper, which must be removed prior to use.

10.2 *Test Procedures*:

10.2.1 (10.1.3) Verify by visual inspection.

10.2.2 (10.1.4) Verify by visual inspection.

10.2.3 (10.1.5) Verify by visual inspection.

10.2.4 (10.1.6) Verify by visual inspection.

10.2.5 (10.1.7) Verify by visual inspection.

11. Unidirectional Valves

11.1 *Requirements*:

11.1.1 *Placement*—Inspiratory and expiratory unidirectional valves shall not be placed in a Y-piece.

11.1.2 *Flow Direction*—The direction of the intended gas flow shall be permanently marked on the valve housing or near its associated hose terminal, with either a directional arrow or with the marking "inspiration," or "expiration," so that it is visible to the user when the equipment is being assembled for use.

11.1.3 *Visibility*—The functioning of valves should be visible.

11.1.4 *Resistance*—The resistance of dry and moist inspiratory or expiratory valve assemblies shall not exceed a pressure drop of 0.15 kPa (1.5 cm H_2O) at 1.0 L/s flow.

11.1.5 *Opening Pressure*—The pressure to open moist inspiratory and expiratory valves should not exceed 0.15 kPa (1.5 cm H_2O).

11.1.6 *Reverse Flow and Valve Dislocation*— Reverse flow shall not exceed 60 mL/min at any differential pressure to 0.5 kPa (5 cm H_2O). The valve shall not become dislocated with a reversed differential pressure of 5.0 kPa (50 cm H_2O).

11.1.7 *Sterilization*—Reusable unidirectional valves should be capable of withstanding sterilization by autoclaving, or the manufacturer shall state another means of sterilization that may be used.

11.2 *Test Procedures*:

11.2.1 Verify by visual inspection that no directional valves are present in the Y-piece.

11.2.2 (11.1.4) *Resistance*—Introduce a 1.0-L/s flow of gas through the valve and measure the pressure drop.

11.2.2.1 To test a moist valve, first condition the valve with a flow of test gas heated and humidified such that the inner surface of the valve dome, or the visible surface of the valve itself has visible condensate. When all surfaces are saturated, turn off the flow of gas to allow the valve to close. Adjust the flow of gas (heated and humidified) to 1.0 L/s and measure the pressure drop.

11.2.3 (11.1.5) *Opening Pressure:*

11.2.3.1 *Apparatus Required*—Pressure measuring device, flowmeter, and a rigid container (see Fig. 5).

11.2.3.2 *Procedure*—To test a moist valve, first condition the valve with a flow of test gas heated and humidified such that the inner surface of the valve dome or the visible surface of the valve itself has visible condensate. Turn off the flow of gas to allow the valve to close. Reintroduce the flow of gas at 20 mL/min (heated and humidified) while recording the pressure rise at the inlet to the valve. The peak pressure obtained is the moist valve opening pressure.

11.2.4 (11.1.7) *Reverse Flow:*

11.2.4.1 *Apparatus Required*—(Pressure measuring device(s), flowmeter(s), and a rigid container of 5.0-L capacity (see Fig. 6).

11.2.4.2 *Procedure*—Adjust the flowmeter to maintain a constant flow of 1.0 mL/s. Connect the unidirectional valve—in a reverse direction—to the flowmeter, a rigid container, and the pressure measuring device (see Fig. 6). The pressure must rise to 0.5 kPa (5.0 cm H_2O) in 5 min or less.

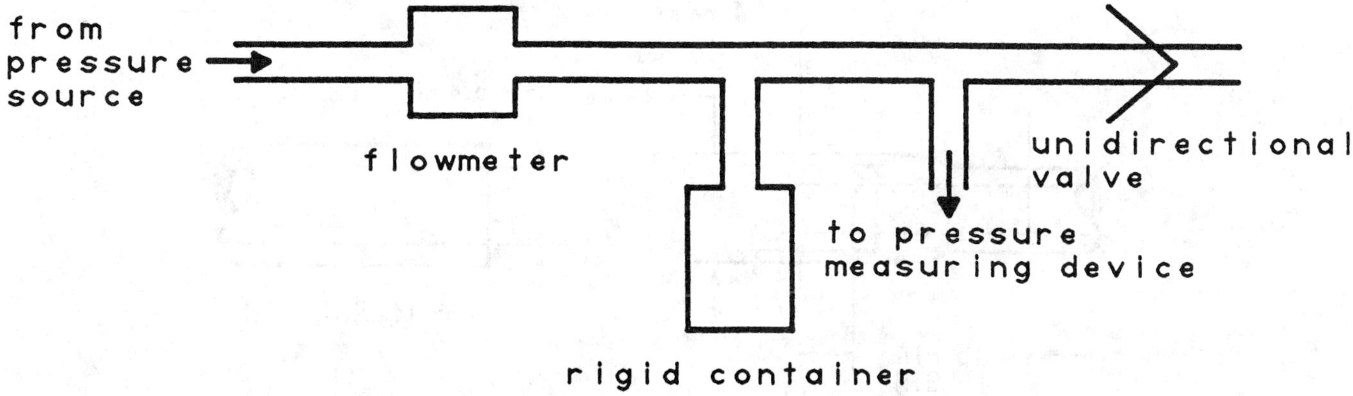

FIG. 5 Arrangement of Apparatus to Test for Opening Pressure

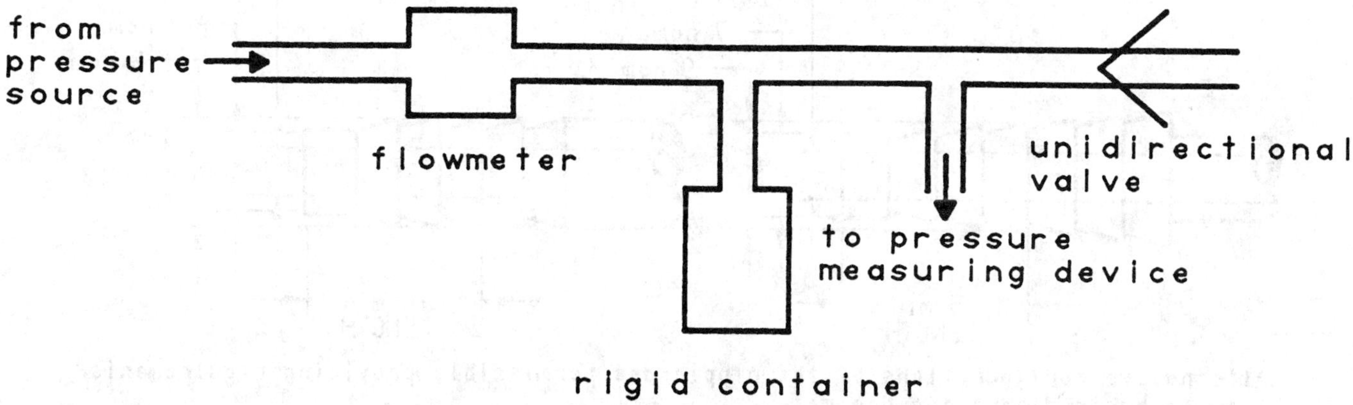

FIG. 6 Arrangement of Apparatus to Test for Reverse Flow

Adjust the flowmeter as necessary to pressurize the valve assembly to 5.0 kPa (50 cm H_2O), inspect the valve for dislocation, and repeat reverse flow test.

12. Optional Components

12.1 *Requirements*:

12.1.1 Components such as humidifiers, bacterial filters, and respirometers also may be used in the anesthesia breathing system. If these optional components are supplied by the manufacturer of the breathing system, they shall not cause the system to exceed the maximum permitted leakage of the total breathing system. Any manufacturer who sells these devices separately shall disclose in the component labeling the maximum leakage of the device at 3 kPa (30 cm H_2O), its resistance at 0.5 and 1.0 L/s flow, and its compliance at 2.0 and 4.0 kPa (20 and 40 cm H_2O) in a similar manner to those requirements and tests listed in Section 7.

12.1.2 *Flow Direction—Sensitive Components*—Any component or accessory to the breathing system which permits only unidirectional flow (such as PEEP valves and cascade humidifiers) or any device whose correct function depends on the direction of gas flow through it shall be so labeled by the manufacturer, and shall be marked with an arrow indicating the proper direction of flow or the words "inlet" and "outlet," or both.

12.1.3 *Bag/Ventilator Selector Switch*—The bag/ventilator selector switch shall be designed such that selection of the ventilator mode automatically excludes the APL valve from the breathing system or closes the valve.

12.2 *Test Procedures*:

12.2.1 *Leakage, Resistance, and Compliance*—Read the manual or verify by visual inspection, or both.

12.2.2 *Flow Direction-Sensitive Components*—Read the manual, then verify by visual inspection.

12.2.3 *Bag/Ventilator Selector Switch*—Open the APL valve, move the switch to the ventilator mode, and pressurize the breathing system. If the system cannot be pressurized, or if the system loses pressure through the APL valve, the requirement in 12.1.3 is not met.

13. Breathing Tubes

13.1 *Requirements*—Breathing tubes shall comply with the requirements of Specification F 1205.

14. Fresh Gas Inlet and Fresh Gas Supply Tube or Hose

14.1 *Requirements*:

14.1.1 *Placement*—The fresh gas inlet shall not be placed in segment 1 (from patient to expiratory valve) and should be in segment 3 (from reservoir bag to inspiratory valve) of a circle system.

14.1.2 *Fresh Gas Inlet*—The fresh gas inlet port, or nipple, if provided, should be of a manufacturer-specific design with a nominal inside diameter of at least 4.0 mm (see Fig. 7 for possible designs).

14.1.3 *Fresh Gas Delivery Tube or Hose*—If provided, the fresh gas delivery tubing shall have a nominal inside diameter of at least 6.4 mm and shall have an anesthesia machine end connector that mates to the common gas outlet and a breathing

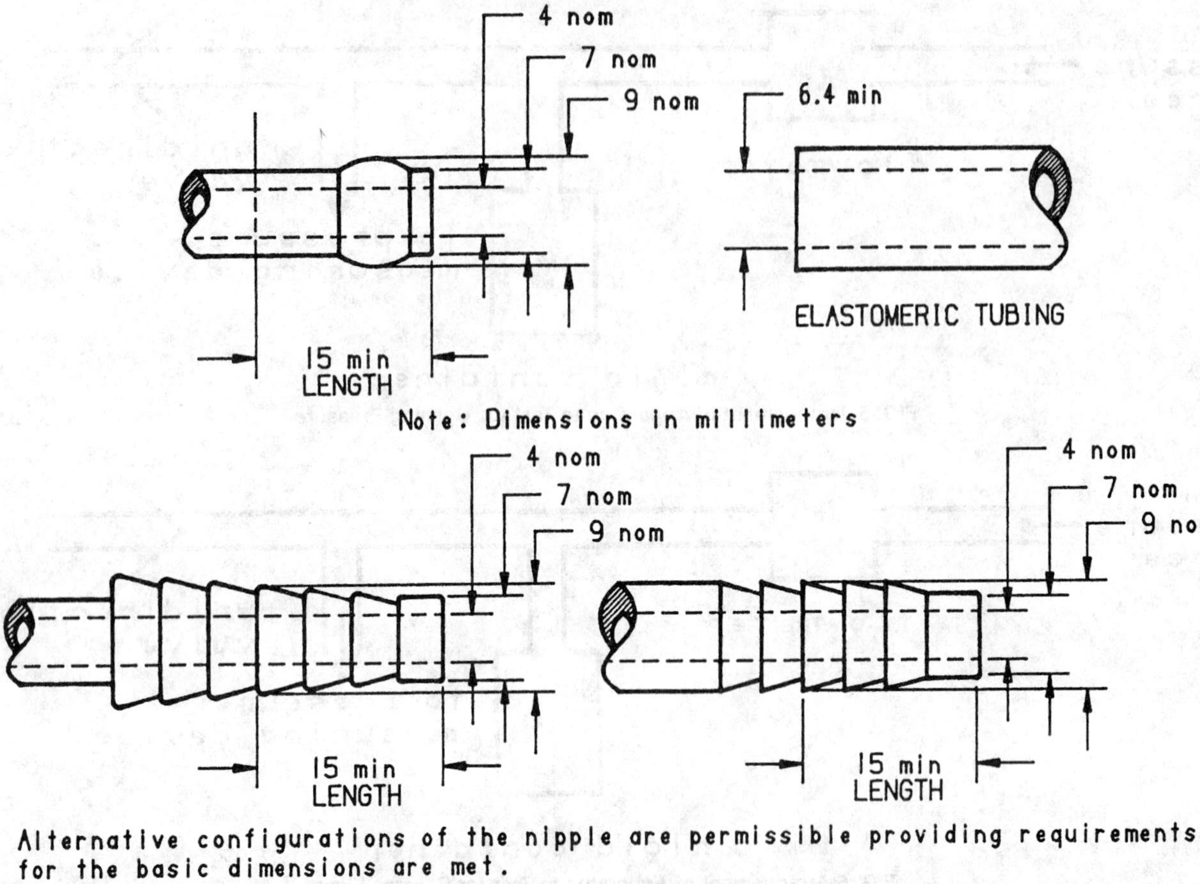

FIG. 7 Examples of Fresh Gas Inlet Nipples

system end connector that mates with the fresh gas inlet.

14.2 *Test Procedures*:

14.2.1 (14.1.1) Verify by visual inspection.

14.2.2 (14.1.3) Verify by measurement that the fresh gas delivery tube or hose has a nominal inside diameter of at least 6.4 mm. Verify by connection and engagement that the anesthesia machine end connector mates with the common gas outlet and the breathing system and connectors mate with the fresh gas inlet.

15. Connectors

15.1 Except for the reservoir bag connectors, the 15-mm and 22-mm fittings mentioned in this specification shall comply with Specification F 1054 – 87$^{\epsilon 1}$. More specifically, the inspiratory port and the expiratory port (traditionally mounted on the absorber) shall be 22-mm conical male fittings.

16. Pressure Gauges (Pressure Indicators)

16.1 Pressure gauges, if provided, shall be marked in units of kilopascals or centimetres H_2O, or both. Bourdon tube type pressure gauges shall conform to the appropriate requirements of ANSI/ASME B40.1M-1985. Units of calibration shall be marked on the gauge or indicator. The gauges should be easily detachable to permit sterilization of other components of the breathing system.

17. Y-Pieces and Breathing Tubes

17.1 The Y-piece and breathing tubes shall comply with the requirements given in Section 7. The patient connection port on the Y-piece shall have a 22-mm male fitting coaxial with the 15-mm female. The Y-piece may be designed so that the 15/22-mm coaxial patient port swivels.

18. Information in Labeling

18.1 The following information shall be provided by the manufacturer in the labeling for complete systems—or for components addressed by this specification, if sold separately as original equipment:

18.1.1 Illustration or schematic of total system showing recommended placement of components.

18.1.2 Expiratory resistance of breathing system (as per 7.1.2).

18.1.3 Inspiratory resistance of breathing system (as per 7.1.2).

18.1.4 A statement that the pressure to open moist inspiratory and expiratory valves meets the requirements of 11.1.5.

18.1.5 Volume of gas lost due to internal compliance of the breathing system, or of components (as per 7.1.3).

18.1.6 Leakage of breathing system (as per 7.1.1).

18.1.7 Information required by Specification F 1204.

18.1.8 Information required by Specification F 1205.

18.1.9 Pressure-flow data for APL valves (as per 8.1.3).

18.1.10 Absorber capacity of CO_2 absorbent in volume (as per 10.1.4).

18.1.11 Resistance of the absorber assembly (as per 10.1.5).

18.1.12 Instructions for changing absorbent (as per 10.1.6).

18.1.13 Instructions for draining absorber assembly.

18.1.14 Recommended sterilization method(s) for reusable equipment (as per Section 6). The manufacturer shall provide the user a method for determining whether a sterilized device retains characteristics for clinical re-use.

18.1.15 Devices that meet the requirements of this specification should be so marked or labeled by the manufacturer, for example, "Meets ASTM Standard Specification for Anesthesia Breathing Systems F1208."

18.2 Verify any, or all of the above by visual inspection.

19. Keywords

19.1 anesthesia absorber assembly; anesthesia breathing systems; anesthesia breathing system components; (symbols for); anesthesia breathing system pressure gauge; anesthesia circle system

APPENDIX

(Nonmandatory Information)

X1. RATIONALE

X1.1 This appendix gives the rationale on which the requirements of this specification and, where necessary, test methods are based. To the extent possible, it summarizes the discussions of the participants in the meetings of the writing group. What follows is not a continuous text but rather a sequence of annotation to specific sections of the specification. Each rationale statement references the corresponding requirement in parentheses, by requirement number.

X1.1.1 *General*—In many cases the methods of testing and limitations in performance of the components given in this specification are those developed under an FDA-sponsored contract (**1**),[4] later modified during committee discussion.

X1.2 *System Classification* (Section 4)—The circle absorption anesthesia breathing system is designed to:

X1.2.1 Convey the mixture of gases and vapor dispensed by the anesthesia apparatus to the patient.

X1.2.2 Eliminate some or all of the expired CO_2 from the system.

X1.2.3 Minimize atmospheric exposure to waste gases and vapors in anesthetizing locations.

X1.2.4 Minimize resistance to the patients' spontaneous ventilatory efforts.

X1.2.5 Permit assisted or artificial ventilation.

X1.3 *Sterilization* (Section 6)—The manufacturer cannot control the number of times a device will be sterilized, nor may he be able to quantitatively predict the effects of sterilization on performance. Therefore the user should at least be provided an operational test to verify that the device is suitable for reuse (even though the device may no longer meet original performance specifications).

X1.4 *Systems* (Section 7):

X1.4.1 *Leakage of Breathing Systems* (7.1.1)—The limit of 300 mL/min for the entire system was established for two reasons (1) to restrict the loss of gas volume intended to be delivered to the patient, and (2) to limit anesthesia gas pollution in the anesthetizing locations. This limit was considered minimally acceptable in view of all the other potential sources of gas leaks. The committee allocated for leaks between the various components of the anesthesia breathing system. The maximum limit of leak (300 mL/min) was based on realistic data, such as found in Ref (**1**). Individual component limits were established to allow flexibility in design; for example, a design can include a swivel adapter on the Y-piece, a potential source of increased leak, provided the rest of the components or connections, or both, leak minimally. In this case, the tubes plus Y-piece could perform at the maximum permitted leak of 75 mL/min, if the absorber leak is held to less than 225 mL/min and all other components are manufactured to close tolerances.

X1.4.2 *Resistance of the Breathing System* (7.1.2)—Total expiratory and total inspiratory resistance were established at a maximum of 0.65 kPa (6.5 cm H_2O) each in order to reduce the work of breathing for the spontaneously breathing patient and to restrict positive end-expiratory pressure. In setting the maximum, the committee considered the resistances of commercially available devices and selected a value between those considered and the ideal of zero resistance. A resistance of 0.65 kPa (6.5 cm H_2O) was considered to be a generally acceptable physiological maximum by clinicians.

X1.4.2.1 Since there are cases where one would require a system with resistance much less than the maximum or require the use of components that would increase the resistance above the maximum, the requirement for disclosure of the actual system's resistances was included to provide information for informed use.

X1.4.3 *Volume of Gas Lost Due to Internal Compressible Volume* (7.1.3)—It is important when providing a patient with artificial ventilation to know the volume of gas *actually* delivered to the patient's lungs. Gas will be compressed within both the rigid and distensible components as the pressure rises. To provide the user with a guide to the additional volume of ventilation required, compliance data is required to be stated at the commonly achieved pressures of 2.0 kPa and 4.0 kPa (20 cm H_2O and 40 cm H_2O).

X1.4.4 *Monitoring Requirements* (7.1.4)—It is important when administering anesthesia to be able to monitor the

[4] The boldface numbers in parentheses refer to the references at the end of this standard.

oxygen concentration, breathing pressure, and either exhaled volume or expiratory CO_2. Knowledge of oxygen concentration whenever the machine is in use is required for the safe administration of anesthesia and cannot be obtained without appropriate ports for gas sampling within the breathing circuit. It is equally essential for safe anesthesia to have sampling sites available to monitor "continuing pressure" and "high pressure" as mentioned in the anesthesia gas machine standard as well as sampling for monitoring either exhaled volume or ventilatory carbon dioxide. The reasons for this are as follows: excessive high airway pressure, or prolonged airway pressure may impede venous return, drop cardiac output, interfere with ventilation or cause barotrauma (for example, pneumothorax). The varying physical condition of patients or different disease processes will affect the susceptibility of a given patient to high airway pressure or continuing airway pressure. Monitoring ventilation by the use of exhaled volume or ventilatory CO_2 will aid in detecting inadvertent changes in ventilation caused by malfunction or disconnections within the breathing system. In addition measurement of exhaled CO_2 will provide evidence of alveolar hypoventilation, metabolic changes such as malignant hyperthermia, esophageal intubation, and pulmonary embolic phenomena.

X1.5 *APL Valves* (Section 8):

X1.5.1 *Placement* (8.1.1)—An open APL valve in segment 4 permits free return of exhaled gas into the inspiratory pathway with subsequent rebreathing.

X1.5.1.1 An APL valve in segment 2 or opposite the reservoir bag, with the fresh gas inflow and absorber in segment 3, will facilitate the removal of the maximum amount of CO_2—containing expired gas by permitting the retrograde flow of fresh gas during expiration. This will minimize exhaustion of the absorbent use and conserve fresh gas for delivery to the patient.

X1.5.2 *Pressure-Flow Characteristics* (8.1.3)—The authors of the breathing system study **(1)** stated that the APL valve was a component that has a significant effect on CO_2 elimination, work of breathing, and inadvertent positive end-expiratory pressure. Information on its function is paramount for patient safety. It was thus required that the resistance of the valve at different flows and valve settings be stated in the labeling.

X1.5.3 *Direction of Motion* (8.1.4)—Since rotary flow control valves are typically closed by clockwise rotation, the committee felt it necessary to standardize this to prevent inappropriate valve adjustment.

X1.5.4 *Resistance at Low Flow* (8.1.5)—The valve must offer some resistance at low flow in order to create a small positive pressure to keep the anesthesia reservoir bag from collapsing.

X1.5.5 *Resistance at High Flow* (8.1.6)—Valve resistance, although it must be present to keep the reservoir bag from collapsing, it must not be so high as to impede emptying of the lung.

X1.6 *Reservoir Bags* (Section 9):

X1.6.1 *Placement* (9.1.1)—A reservoir bag on the patient side of either unidirectional valve will fill with exhaled gas, which will be rebreathed on subsequent inhalation.

X1.6.2 (9.1.2) Previous experience has shown that the reservoir bag connection using a standard 22-mm male conical fitting did not always provide for a secure attachment of the reservoir bag to the reservoir bag connector. For this reason, it was decided to allow variations in designs centered around a nominal 22-mm outside diameter dimension.

X1.7 *CO_2* Absorbers (Section 10):

X1.7.1 *Placement* (10.1.1)—An absorber in segment 1 will be exposed to CO_2-laden, exhaled, gas which normally would be partially expelled from the system before reaching the absorber, thereby wasting absorbent. An absorber at the patient end of segment 4 offers the likeliest possibility of absorbent dust being delivered to the patient.

X1.7.2 *CO_2 Absorbent Container* (10.1.2)—It is desirable to see the actual absorbent material to determine color change in order to know when to replace spent absorbent.

X1.7.3 *Drain* (10.1.3)—Water is produced during the process of CO_2 absorption.

X1.7.4 *Absorbent Capacity* (10.1.4)—After taking into account other factors (such as gas flows, minute volume, and breathing system arrangement), the user can utilize these pieces of information to make an intelligent estimate of how long the absorbent charge will last.

X1.7.5 *Resistance*— See X1.4.2.

X1.7.6 *Instruction* (10.1.6)—Instructions for proper use, such as changing the absorbent, sterilization of the assembly, and obtaining a gas-tight seal, are necessary to ensure correct functioning.

X1.7.7 *Prefilled Container* (10.1.7)—Failure to remove the wrapper from prefilled containers has resulted in lack of CO_2 absorption or total obstruction of the breathing system, or both.

X1.8 *Unidirectional Valves* (Section 11):

X1.8.1 *Placement* (11.1.1)—A Y-piece with valves could be placed in reverse orientation to another set of unidirectional valves on an absorber, making ventilation impossible.

X1.8.2 *Flow Direction* (11.1.3)—Direction of flow markings reduce the possibility of incorrect placement of the value and harm to the patient.

X1.8.3 *Resistance* (11.1.4)—Maximum resistance was set in order to limit the work of breathing for the spontaneously breathing patient. In setting the maximum, the committee considered the resistances of commercially available devices and selected a value between those considered and the ideal of zero resistance. (Also read the rationale in X1.4.2.) Testing of a dry valve is not necessary since valve resistance is always greater when a valve is moist.

X1.8.4 *Opening Pressure* (11.1.5)—The pressure to open moist unidirectional valves may be higher than that to open dry valves. The value is chosen to limit the work of breathing (also see X1.8.3).

X1.8.5 *Reverse Flow and Dislocation* (11.1.6)—Reverse flow, dislocation, or incompetence of inspiratory or expiratory valves could result in rebreathing of end-expiratory gases and a reduction of CO_2 elimination. The most significant leak with disk-type valves may be at low pressures, whereas with flapper valves, the most significant leak may be closer to a pressure of

0.5 kPa (5.0 cm H_2O). A60-mL/min reverse flow was considered clinically acceptable, and obtainable using current manufacturing techniques. This flow is detectable by currently available volume monitors.

X1.8.6 *Sterilization* (11.1.7)—For reusable valves, this information is necessary in order not to damage the valves.

X1.9 *Optional Components* (Section 12)—This requirement is an attempt to deal with breathing systems that may include various components supplied by the system manufacturer, or other manufacturers, or both. The basic system leakage and resistance requirements (7.1.1 and 7.1.2) are for a defined set of components. If other components are included in the breathing system, or are sold for use in breathing systems, it is recommended that their leakage be considered in regard to the overall system leakage and that resistance values be disclosed to the user.

X1.9.1 *Flow Direction-Sensitive Components* (12.1.2)—Reverse connection of a flow direction-sensitive component may result in no flow to or from the patient. An example would be the reverse connection of a cascade humidifier. The same situation could arise if a circulator were connected backwards in a breathing system so that flow from the circulator was directed toward the patient exhalation port. Also when the sensor of a pressure alarm is located downstream from the expiratory valve (segments 2 and 3), a low pressure alarm may not be activated despite zero pressure at the Y-piece, since substantial pressure is generated at the sensor with each positive pressure breath. See Refs **(2-5)**.

X1.9.2 *Bag/Ventilator Selector Switch* (12.1.3)—Failure of the operator to manually close the APL valve (in the ventilator mode) has resulted in inadequate ventilation. Pressure alarms with relatively low thresholds (such as 8 cm of water) may be satisfied despite a substantial leak out the APL valve with each positive pressure breath. See Ref **(6)**.

X1.10 *Fresh Gas Inlet and Fresh Gas Supply Tube* (Section 14):

X1.10.1 *Placement* (14.1.1)—If the fresh gas inlet is placed in segment 1, loss of between fresh gas through the APL valve will occur. If the fresh gas inlet is placed between the expiratory valve and the absorber, the humidification of the fresh gas mixture will be enhanced; however, with this arrangement loss of fresh gas through the APL valve may occur if the latter is not placed at a sufficient distance from the fresh gas inlet. Placement in segment 4 vents that fresh gas flow which passes by the Y-piece during exhalation. This prevents the use of a spirometer in the exhalatory limb of the breathing system. Placement in segment 3 provides greater overall economy of the anesthetic agent and CO_2 absorbent.

X1.10.2 *Fresh Gas Inlet* (14.1.2)—The use of a manufacturer-specific fresh gas inlet would minimize the potential hazard of mismatching breathing systems and gas machines, and also prevents potentially dangerous increases in pressure behind (proximal to) the fresh gas inlet.

X1.10.3 *Fresh Gas Delivery Tube or Hose* (14.1.3)—Same as X1.10.2.

X1.11 *Connectors* (Section 15)—See X1.6.2.

X1.12 *Pressure Gauges or Indicators* (Section 16)—Consistent scale marking will reduce reading errors. Gauges are easily damaged by current methods of sterilization.

X1.13 *Y-Pieces* (Section 17) (see X1.5.1.1)—A 15/22-mm coaxial patient fitting on the Y-piece is mandatory to permit connection of the breathing system to either a mask or a tracheal tube.

X1.14 *Information in Manual* (Section 18)—The initial statement is written to require that manufacturers of complete breathing systems, and manufacturers of components sold separately, provide the information with the original sales of equipment and components but *not* with replacement parts. This information permits the user to reasonably predict the performance of a total breathing system even though the component parts may have been obtained from different manufacturers.

REFERENCES

(1) Saklad, M., et al, Final Report FDA Contract No. 223-76-5021, "Testing and Evaluating the Characteristics and Arrangements of Components in the Gas Conduction System of Continuous-Flow Anesthesia Machines," 1978.

(2) Schreiber, P., *Safety Guidelines for Anesthesia Systems*, Telford, PA: North American Drager, 1985, p. 34.

(3) Rendell-Baker, L., "Problems With Anesthetic and Respiratory Therapy Equipment," International Anesthesiology Clinic, fall 1982; 20: 3, p. 60.

(4) Dorsch, J. A., Dorsch, S. E., *Understanding Anesthesia Equipment*, Second Edition, Williams and Wilkins, Baltimore, 1984, p. 157.

(5) Andrews, J. J., "Anesthesia Systems," Barash, P. G., Cullen, B. F., Stoelting, R. K., eds. *Clinical Anesthesia* , Philadelphia, J. B. Lippincott, in press.

(6) Dorsch, J. A., Dorsch, S. E., *Understanding Anesthesia Equipment*, Second Edition, Williams and Wilkins, Baltimore, 1984, pp. 303 and 306.

Standard Specification for Bronchoscopes (Rigid)[1]

This standard is issued under the fixed designation F 1218; the number immediately following the designation indicates the year of original adoption or, in the case of revision, the year of last revision. A number in parentheses indicates the year of last reapproval. A superscript epsilon (ε) indicates an editorial change since the last revision or reapproval.

1. Scope

1.1 This specification covers definitions and requirements for rigid bronchoscopes and certain bronchoscopic accessories used in the practice of medicine.

2. Referenced Documents

2.1 *ASTM Standards:*

F 1054 Specification for Conical Fittings of 15 mm and 22 mm Sizes[2]

3. Terminology

3.1 *Definitions:*

3.1.1 *bronchoscopes (rigid)*—a medical instrument having viewing means, with or without optics, introduced into the larynx or tracheobronchial airway, or both, through a natural or surgically created body opening for examination, diagnosis, or therapy, and intended to be unyielding to natural or surgically created body cavities.

3.1.2 *optical endoscope*—a medical instrument with optics, having viewing means, which may be introduced into a body cavity through a bronchoscope, or through a naturally or surgically created body opening for examination, diagnosis, or therapy. An optical endoscope may be of rigid or flexible design.

3.1.3 *endoscopic accessory*—a medical instrument inserted through a bronchoscope for diagnosis or therapy.

3.1.3.1 *rigid accessory*—an accessory whose insertion portion is intended to be unyielding to natural or surgically created body cavities or instrument lumens.

3.1.3.2 *flexible accessory*—an accessory whose insertion portion is intended to conform to natural or surgically created body cavities or instrument lumens.

3.1.3.3 *Discussion*—The intent is to include forceps, snares, electrodes, and other such instruments which can be passed through a bronchoscope or with a bronchoscope through another accessory. The intent is also to exclude certain instruments, such as electrosurgical units, light sources, other such instruments, and ventilation systems external to the bronchoscope.

3.1.4 *distal*—the location of that portion of a bronchoscope or endoscopic accessory which is farther from the user than some reference point.

3.1.4.1 *Discussion*—The terms given in 3.1.4 and 3.1.5, commonly used in endoscopy, are defined in their most general form to avoid the need for such definitions as "distal tip," "distal end,"" area proximal to ...," "X cm distal to the ... ."

3.1.5 *proximal*—the location of that portion of a bronchoscope or endoscopic accessory which is closer to the user than some reference point.

3.1.5.1 See 3.1.4.

3.1.6 *insertion portion*—that portion of a bronchoscope or endoscopic accessory which is intended to be inserted into a natural or surgically created body opening; or which is intended to be inserted into the lumen of a bronchoscope or endoscopic accessory.

3.1.6.1 *Discussion*—Although the term defined seems self-explanatory, different expressions for the same portion of the instrument are used by different manufacturers.

3.1.7 *maximum insertion portion width*—the maximum external width of a bronchoscope or endoscopic accessory throughout the length of the insertion portion.

3.1.7.1 *Discussion*—By defining external sizes as maxima and internal sizes as minima, sufficient instrument information for selection of an instrument will be provided to users.

3.1.8 *minimum lumen width*—the minimum internal width of a bronchoscope or endoscopic accessory through which a bronchoscope or endoscopic accessory is intended to pass.

3.1.8.1 See 3.1.7.

3.1.9 *working length*—the maximum length of the insertion portion.

3.1.10 *overall length*—the distance between the proximal and distal ends of a rigid bronchoscope or bronchoscopic accessory, expressed in metric units.

3.1.11 *field of view*—the size of the object field viewed through an optical endoscope and stated by the vertex angle (in degrees) of the cone whose vertex is at the distal window surface of the instrument.

3.1.11.1 *Discussion*—The endoscope is not intended to be in contact with the object. (See Fig. 1.)

3.1.11.2 *Discussion*—The definitions given in 3.1.11 and 3.1.12, as illustrated, describe characteristics of optical endoscopes paramount for effective use, thereby allowing the user to select instruments of specific values for particular medical purposes.

3.1.12 *direction of view*—the location of the center of the

[1] This specification is under the jurisdiction of ASTM Committee F-29 on Anesthetic and Respiratory Equipmentand is the direct responsibility of Subcommittee F29.13 on Laryngoscopes and Bronchoscopes .

Current edition approved March 31, 1989. Published July 1989.

[2] *Annual Book of ASTM Standards*, Vol 13.01.

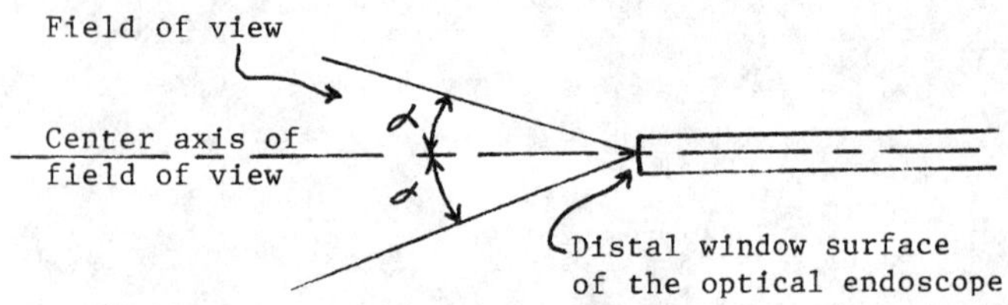

FIG. 1 Field of View

object field relative to the normal axis of the optical endoscope, and stated as the angle (in degrees) between the normal axis of the optical endoscope and the center of the field of view. (See Fig. 2.)

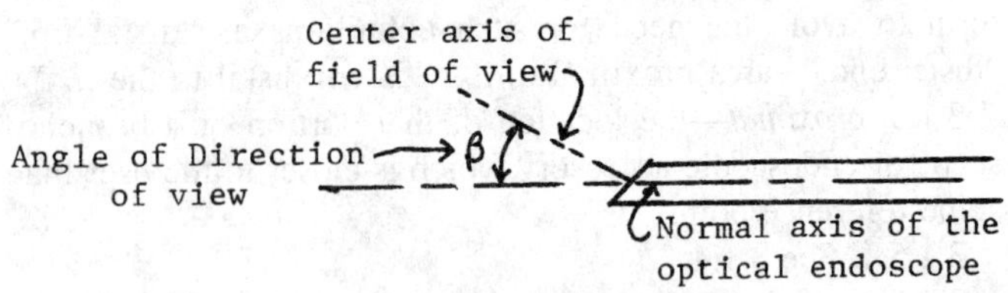

FIG. 2 Direction of View

3.1.12.1 See 3.1.11.

3.1.13 *controllable portion*—that part of the insertion portion of an optical endoscope whose motion is intended to be remotely controlled by the user.

3.1.13.1 Many optical endoscopes incorporate provisions for remote control of the motion of the distal tip by the user. The mechanisms for these controls vary widely, and are obviously of interest to the user. In order to avoid constraint of future designs, control characteristics are defined in the most general terms.

3.1.14 *French (Charriere) size (Fr)*—a measure of the size of certain endoscopic accessories of circular and noncircular cross-section. The measure has several definitions:

$$Fr = 3 \times u/3.1416 \text{ (pi) for noncircular cross-section}$$

where u is the perimeter of the cross-section, mm.

$$Fr = 3.1416(pi) \times d \text{ for circular cross-section}$$

where d is the diameter of the cross-section, mm.

$$Fr = 3.0 \times d \text{ for circular cross-section}^3$$

where d is the diameter of the cross-section, mm.

3.1.14.1 *Discussion*—This measure of size enjoys worldwide favor in many branches of medicine. In usage, the measurement is imprecise, as shown in 3.1.14. The user should be provided with the manufacturer's definition if the term is to be of any value. Metric measures appear to be more precise.

4. Significance and Use

4.1 This specification applies to rigid bronchoscopes, those endoscopic accessories through which rigid bronchoscopes are used, those accessories which are passed through rigid bronchoscopes in use, and those associated accessories which are inserted into the body.

[3] Commonly used by many manufacturers of endoscopic accessories.

5. Required Characteristics

5.1 *Critical Dimensions*:

5.1.1 The maximum insertion portion width shall not exceed that stated by the manufacturer. (See Note 1.)

NOTE 1—These sizes are given to help the user to select the instruments for a given procedure. Compatibility of instruments in combination requires certain clearances between the insertion portion width and the lumen width; the clearance required depends upon the configuration and dimensions of the instruments. There is no guarantee that the instruments selected solely by these criteria will be compatible in combination.

5.1.2 The minimum lumen width shall not be less than that marked on the bronchoscope. (See Note 1.)

5.1.3 The overall length shall not exceed that marked on the bronchoscope.

5.1.4 The working length shall not be less than that marked on the bronchoscope.

5.2 *Ventilation Connectors*—Ventilation connectors shall meet the requirements of Specification F 1054 or shall be provided with an adaptor to connect with the 15/22-mm connector.

6. Marking, Labeling, and Packaging

6.1 *Marking*:

6.1.1 *Instrument Marking* (see Note 2)—Dimensions shall be given in metric units. Each individual bronchoscope and endoscopic accessory shall have, as a minimum, the following markings:

NOTE 2—The identification of the instrument and markings listed in 6.1.1 are sufficient to permit the user to select the appropriate instrument when necessary.

6.1.1.1 A catalog number and other mark sufficient to identify the instrument and its manufacturer,

6.1.1.2 Maximum insertion portion width, minimum lumen width, overall length, and working length for rigid bronchoscope, and

6.1.1.3 Maximum insertion portion width, working length, field of view, and direction of view of the optical endoscope.

6.1.2 *Marking Legibility* (see Note 3)—The marking required in 6.1.1 shall remain legible throughout the expected life of the instrument when it is used, cleaned, disinfected, sterilized, and stored in accordance with the manufacturer's instructions.

NOTE 3—The primary requirement of instrument marking is that it be legible. Any more detailed requirements on marking methods, materials, sizes, and other characteristics could inhibit design and process innovation.

6.1.3 *Marking Exceptions* (see Note 4)—When the marking required in 6.1.1 and 6.1.2 is impossible to achieve due to instrument size or configuration, the required markings shall accompany the instrument.

NOTE 4—Design innovation in the trend towards smaller endoscopes and endoscopic accessories would be seriously inhibited without this marking exception.

6.2 *Information to Be Supplied by the Manufacturer* (see Note 5)—The manufacturer of rigid bronchoscopes or endoscopic accessories shall provide the user with at least the following information:

NOTE 5—A significant number of hazards and performance problems of endoscopes and endoscopic accessories are best addressed by education of the user. The objective of 6.2 is to provide a part of the educational process without engaging in the practice of medicine.

6.2.1 A statement of intended uses of the instrument and directions for proper assembly for each use,

6.2.2 Instructions for proper maintenance of the instrument,

6.2.3 An annotated illustration of the instrument, if necessary, to identify pertinent parts and characteristics of the instrument which are referenced in the information supplied, and

6.2.4 The specifications of the instrument, including the following:

6.2.4.1 The name and address of the manufacturer, or supplier, or both,

6.2.4.2 The catalog number and name of the instrument,

6.2.4.3 The dimensional characteristics specified in 6.1.1,

6.2.4.4 If applicable, the field of view and the direction of view,

6.2.4.5 If applicable, the remote controls and associated controllable portion positions available to the user,

6.2.4.6 An identification of any parts replacable by the user and instructions for their replacement, and

6.2.4.7 A listing of the names and addresses of authorized service agents.

6.2.5 Instructions for assembling the instrument for its intended uses and for the dismantling and reassembly of the instrument after cleaning, disinfection or sterilization, or combination thereof,

6.2.6 Precautions and other instructions applicable to the intended uses of the instrument, including those related to electrical, electronic, electro-optical, electrosurgical, or ventilatory apparatus intended to be used with the instrument,

6.2.7 Inspection instructions to provide assurance that the instrument is in working order,

6.2.8 Instructions for the cleaning of reusable instruments, including recommended cleaning agents and equipment,

6.2.9 Details of disinfection and sterilization environments which the instrument can withstand without damage, and

6.2.10 Recommended procedures for the storage of the instrument prior to use, and, for reusable instruments, between uses.

6.3 *Packaging.*

NOTE 6—Problems due to improper packaging have been reported. Rather than impose innovation-limiting design requirements on the manufacturer, we believe that the disclosure approach cited above is more appropriate.

NOTE 7—The manufacturer should package the instrument in a manner to protect the instrument from the adverse effects of shipping environments.

7. Keywords

7.1 bronchoscope; bronchoscopy; endoscope; endoscopy; optical endoscope

Designation: F 1219 – 00

Standard Guide for Training the Emergency Medical Technician (Basic) to Perform Patient Initial and Detailed Assessment[1]

This standard is issued under the fixed designation F 1219; the number immediately following the designation indicates the year of original adoption or, in the case of revision, the year of last revision. A number in parentheses indicates the year of last reapproval. A superscript epsilon (ϵ) indicates an editorial change since the last revision or reapproval.

1. Scope

1.1 This guide establishes the minimum training standard for the performance of the initial assessment of ill or injured patients of all ages.

1.1.1 Frequently repeated inital surveys are an essential and integral part of the complete care of the acutely ill or injured patient.

1.2 This guide establishes the minimum training standard for the detailed assesment of ill or injured patients of all ages.

1.3 This guide identifys the components of the focused detailed assessment.

1.4 This guide is one of a series which together describe the minimum training standard for the emergency medical technician (basic).

1.5

1.6 *This standard may involve hazardous materials, operations, and equipment. This standard does not purport to address all of the safety concerns associated with its use. It is the responsibility of the user of this standard to establish appropriate safety and health practices and determine the applicability of regulatory limitations prior to use.*

2. Referenced Documents

2.1 *ASTM Standards:*

F 1031 Practice for Training the Emergency Medical Technician (Basic)[2]

3. Terminology

3.1 *Definitions of Terms Specific to This Standard:*

3.1.1 *focused detailed assessment*—identification of the patient's real or perceived problem(s) by means of documentation and evaluation of additional data from the detailed survey and pertinent patient information.

3.1.2 *focused detailed survey*—the methodical physical examination of the patient to evaluate conditions discovered during the primary survey and to find conditions not previously identified.

3.1.3 *initial assessment*—the identification of a patient's real or perceived problem(s) by means of the accumulation and evaluation of data from a scene evaluation, an initial and pertinent patient information.

3.1.4 *initial survey*—the rapid assessment and management of the patient's immediately life-threatening conditions.

3.1.5 *pertinent patient information*—information obtained from all available resources that relates to the patient's condition and problems. This information must be continuously updated. All information must be recorded and reported.

3.1.6 *scene evaluation*—a rapid evaluation of the environment, conditions, and necessary resources.

4. Significance and Use

4.1 This guide establishes the minimum national training standard for the performance of the initial assessment of the ill and injured patient of any age by the emergency medical technician (basic).

4.2 This guide shall be used by those who wish to identify the minimum training standard of the emergency medical technician (basic) as it relates to patient initial assessment.

4.3 This guide establishes a minimum national standard for training the emergency medical technician (basic) in the preformance of the detailed assessment of ill and injured patients of all ages.

4.4 This guide shall be used by those who wish to identify the minimum training standard of the emergency medicial technician (basic) as it relates to a focused patient detailed assessment.

4.5 This guide shall be used as the basis to revise Practice F 1031.

4.6 Every person who is identified as an emergency medical technician (basic) shall be trained in accordance with this guide.

5. Scene Evaluation

5.1 While approaching the scene and the patient the emergency medical technician (basic) will assess the scene for hazards, number of patients, need for additional resources, and then take appropriate action.

5.2 While approaching the patient the emergency medical

[1] This guide is under the jurisdiction of ASTM Committee F-30 on Emergency Medical Services and is the direct responsibility of Subcommittee F30.02 on Personnel, Training, and Education.

Current edition approved Oct. 10, 2000. Published January 2001.

Originally published as F1219-89. Discontinued August 1998 and Reienstated as F 1219-00.

[2] *Annual Book of ASTM Standards*, Vol 13.01.

technician (basic) will assess the patient and the environment for clues relating to the mechanism of injury or illness.

6. Initial Survey

6.1 Frequently repeated initial surveys are an essential and integral part of the complete care of the acutely ill or injured patient. This guide identifies the preferred sequence for patient Primary Initial assessment; however, it must be emphasized that much of the initial assessment is done simultaneously and not necessarily sequentially. The Initial survey addresses:

6.1.1 The ability of the patient to communicate,

6.1.2 Cervical spine stability,

6.1.3 Airway patency,

6.1.4 Adequacy of ventilations,

6.1.5 Adequacy of circulation,

6.1.6 Life-threatening external bleeding

6.1.7 Level of consciousness, and

6.1.8 Clothing will be removed or loosened as needed to evaluate life threatening conditions.

6.2 The Initial survey shall be interrupted to manage immediately life threatening problems.

6.3 Patients with life-threatening problems that cannot be adequately corrected, as identified in the initial survey, shall be transported immediately as an emergency transport.

7. Pertinent Patient Information

7.1 Obtaining pertinent patient information shall be an ongoing process of collecting information from all available resources throughout the entire contact with the patient.

7.2 Identify the chief complaint.

7.3 Obtain pertinent information about present illness or injury, including current medication.

7.4 Suggested acronym: SAMPLE.

7.5 Obtain a pertinent past medical history, including allergies.

7.6 Locate any medical identification information.

8. Secondary Assessment

8.1 A detailed assessment is conducted only after the field treatment of all life threatening conditions has been initiated.

8.2 the detailed assessment may be focued on medical, trumatic or both entites.

8.3 The components of the detailed survey should be preformed following the completion of the initial survey. The selection and sequence of the components are dictated by the patient's condition and exisiting circumstances. The components of the primary survey will be monitored during the detailed. The components of the detailed survey are:

8.3.1 Stabilize the cervical spine as indicated until in-line immobilization can be preformed.

8.3.2 Assess for altered mental status.

8.3.3 Determine vital signs:

8.3.3.1 Determine rate, rhythm and quality of respirations.

8.3.3.2 Determine rate, regularity and quality of the pulse.

8.3.3.3 Measure blood pressure.

8.3.3.4 Asses caapillary refill time in pediatric patients.

8.3.4 Examine the head:

8.3.4.1 Inspect and palpate head for any signs of injury or other abnormalities.

8.3.4.2 Inspect for blood, fluid or freign objects in ears, nose and mouth.

8.3.4.3 Extamine the eyes for signs of injury or other abnormalities.

8.3.5 Examine the skin-mucous membranes for any signs of injury or edema for color, temperature, and moistness.

8.3.6 Inspect and palpate the neck for any signs of injury or other abnormalities.

8.3.7 Examine the chest:

8.3.7.1 Inspect and palpate the chest for any sins of injury or other abnormalities.

8.3.7.2 Asses breath sounds, including auscultation of the chest.

8.3.8 Inspect and palpate the abdomen for any signs of injury of other abnormalities.

8.3.9 Assess the integrity of the pelvis.

8.3.10 Examine the perineal area:

8.3.10.1 Inspect the perneal for any signs of injury or other abnormalities.

8.3.10.2 In the event of an assault, evidence protection techniques must be practiced.

8.3.10.3 Assess for any signs of impending birth in women of childbearing age.

8.3.11 Examine each extremity:

8.3.11.1 Inspect and palpate for any signs of injury or other abnormalities.

8.3.11.2 Assess peripheral circulation, movement and sensation.

8.3.11.3 Suggested acronym "PMS" (pulses-motor-sensory).

8.3.12 Inspect and palpate the back and buttocks for any signs of injury or other abnormalities.

9. Emergency Transport

9.1 Patients with life-threatening problems idenified in the focused detailed survey shall be transported as an emergency transport.

9.2 ALS intercept should be considered for critical or deterorating patients.

10. Keywords

10.1 assesment; detailed assessment; EMS; EMT; focused medical; focused truama; initial assessment

Designation: F 1220 – 95 (Reapproved 2001)

Standard Guide for Emergency Medical Services System (EMSS) Telecommunications[1]

This standard is issued under the fixed designation F 1220; the number immediately following the designation indicates the year of original adoption or, in the case of revision, the year of last revision. A number in parentheses indicates the year of last reapproval. A superscript epsilon (ε) indicates an editorial change since the last revision or reapproval.

1. Scope

1.1 This guide covers telecommunications practices and performance standards required to support all of the functions of community EMSS on a statewide basis. It defines state planning goals and objectives for EMSS communications.

1.2 This guide is for planning, coordinating, integrating, and evaluating telecommunications resources statewide to satisfy the functional needs of comprehensive community EMSS systems.

1.3 To facilitate a two-tiered planning approach recommended for EMSS communications, this guide identifies those communications system features that should be coordinated on a statewide basis and defined in statewide (first tier) EMSS communications planning guidelines. Local (second tier) EMSS communications plans prepared in accordance with the statewide guidelines should then be tailored to satisfy local EMSS needs while providing compatibility and interoperability of communications with other EMSS.

1.4 The sections in this guide appear in the following sequence:

1.5 *This standard does not purport to address all of the safety concerns, if any, associated with its use. It is the responsibility of the user of this standard to establish appropriate safety and health practices and determine the applicability of regulatory limitations prior to use.*

2. Referenced Documents

2.1 *ASTM Standards:*

F 1031 Practice for Training the Emergency Medical Technician (Basic)[2]

F 1149 Practice for Qualifications, Responsibilities, and Authority of Individuals and Institutions Providing Medical Direction of Emergency Medical Services[2]

F 1221 Guide for Interagency Information Exchange[2]

F 1229 Guide for Establishing the Qualifications, Education, and Training of EMS, Air-Medical Patient Care Providers[2]

F 1254 Practice for Performance of Prehospital Manual Defibrillation[2]

F 1258 Practice for Emergency Medical Dispatch[2]

F 1287 Guide for Scope of Performance of First Responders Who Provide Emergency Medical Care[2]

F 1381 Guide for Planning and Developing 9-1-1 Enhanced Telephone Systems[2]

F 1418 Guide for Training the Emergency Medical Technician (Basic) in Roles and Responsibilities.[2]

F 1453 Guide for Training and Evaluation of First Responders Who Provide Emergency Medical Care[2]

[1] This guide is under the jurisdiction of ASTM Committee F30 on Emergency Medical Services and is the direct responsibility of Subcommittee F30.04 on Communications.

Current edition approved Oct. 10, 1995. Published February 1996. Originally published as F 1220 – 89. Last previous edition F 1220 – 89.

[2] *Annual Book of ASTM Standards*, Vol 13.01.

F 1517 Guide for Scope of Performance of Emergency Medical Services Ambulance Operations[2]

F 1552 Practice for Training, Instructor Qualification, and Certification Eligibility of Emergency Medical Dispatchers[2]

F 1560 Practice for Emergency Medical Dispatch Management[2]

2.2 *Federal Standards:*

Communications Act of 1934 (47 U.S.C. 405) (as amended)[3]

Title 47, United States Code of Federal Regulations (47 CFR) on Telecommunications[3]

3. Terminology

3.1 *Definitions of Terms Specific to This Standard:*

3.1.1 *goal*—a statement of broad direction, general purpose, or intent. A goal is general and timeless and is not concerned with a specific achievement within a given time period.

3.1.2 *objective*—a statement of desired accomplishment that can be measured within a specified time frame and under determinable conditions. The attainment of an objective moves the system toward a directly related goal.

3.1.3 Communications terminology used in this guide and references are defined in Appendix X1, Acronyms and Glossary for EMSS Communications.

4. Summary of Guide

4.1 This guide identifies the functions and requirements of EMSS telecommunications. Observance of the state EMSS communications planning goals and objectives contained in this guide permits planning and implementation of compatible, interoperable, and reliable local EMSS communications which meet local needs while not interfering with the needs of adjoining EMSS.

4.2 EMSS communications should satisfy all of the performance goals and objectives specified by those who use it and those who are served by it. However, many constraints such as costs, political, demographic and social preferences, existing legislation and time, limit what can be achieved.

5. Significance and Use

5.1 In situations in which the coordination of EMSS communications among political subdivisions affects the health and safety of the state's population, it is appropriate for state government to take a coordinating role. Statewide planning for coordinated use of radio frequencies for EMSS communications is specifically needed.

5.2 The state is the logical unit to formulate the statutory and regulatory framework for EMSS planning. State planning for area-wide EMSS communications provides authority to accomplish coordination in the use of available radio frequencies, thus promoting multiagency cooperation to best serve the public needs.

5.3 With statewide planning, communities, counties, and multicounty EMSS regions are provided with guidance to achieve the performance goals and objectives of their EMSS communications systems.

5.4 The statewide EMSS communications performance goals and objectives in Sections 10-15 address specific roles of state governments in EMSS communications systems planning. These performance goals and objectives should be considered by states for evaluating, planning, and implementing of acceptable EMSS communications statewide.

6. Functions and Categories of EMSS Communications

6.1 *Telecommunications Functions*—The report "Communications in Support of Emergency Medical Services," given in Ref **(1)**,[4] defines the following EMSS functions that require telecommunications:

6.1.1 Medical emergencies requiring EMSS response should be reported immediately to appropriate community agencies that manage and control EMSS resources and services.

6.1.2 Appropriate EMSS resources should respond to human health emergencies at any time and place.

6.1.3 Recognition of the need for and immediate response by EMSS resources to life threatening and serious injuries and illness should be provided within a time period that will ensure the greatest saving of lives and reduction of morbidity.

6.1.4 EMSS and other health agencies and professionals should marshal their individual and collective resources (staff, equipment, supplies, and facilities) and coordinate their responses in the shortest effective time to meet individual and mass medical emergency needs.

6.1.5 Emergency medical dispatchers should have special training to provide guidance and direction to persons at the scene of a medical emergency pending arrival of trained prehospital EMSS personnel.

6.1.6 EMSS must be coordinated with other community public safety emergency response services.

6.1.7 The use of EMSS facilities (emergency departments, intensive care, and coronary care units, burn and trauma facilities, and so forth) should be coordinated so as to avoid preventable delays in access to definitive emergency medical care.

6.1.8 For life threatening and serious medical emergencies and in other instances requiring invasive prehospital emergency medical care, appropriate physiological data and patient assessment information should be collected and transmitted from the site of the emergency to the EMSS facility providing on-line medical direction.

6.1.9 Telecommunications relating to EMSS should be recorded, documented, saved, and used by EMSS managers to review, evaluate, revise, and reorganize EMSS as necessary to meet changing conditions and needs.

6.1.10 Telecommunications should exist between EMSS facilities and transport vehicles for safe interhospital transfer of patients with life threatening and serious medical emergencies.

6.1.11 Telecommunications should be used as needed, to improve utilization of all EMSS resources and to prevent or mitigate adverse effects of medical emergencies.

---

[3] Available from Superintendent of Documents, U. S. Government Printing Office, Washington, DC 20402.

[4] The boldface numbers in parentheses refer to the references at the end of this guide.

6.2 *Telecommunications Categories*—Based on the above EMSS needs, the following categories of information exchange requiring telecommunications are defined in Ref **(1)** as being necessary to support of EMS operations.

6.2.1 *EMSS Access*—Exchanges of information related to public access for reporting emergency medical situations to appropriate EMSS response organizations.

6.2.2 *EMSS Dispatch and Control*—Exchanges of information related to reducing response time, such as alerting, dispatching, and controlling the movement of EMS vehicles.

6.2.3 *Medical Coordination/Direction*—Exchanges of information related to the emergency patient and his care, such as transmission of physiological information and exchange of patient assessment information and treatment information between EMS personnel at the scene and physicians providing on-line medical direction.

6.2.4 *EMSS Resource Coordination*—Exchanges of information necessary for the effective coordination of all EMS resources.

6.2.5 *Interservice Coordination*—Exchanges of information for coordination of EMS activities with police, fire, government agencies, and other resources, such as public utilities and private contractors.

6.2.6 *Disaster Coordination*—Exchanges of information related to the coordination of EMS activities with those of local, state, and national disaster response authorities.

7. EMSS Functional Communications Requirements

7.1 An EMSS communications system should provide the means by which emergency resources can be accessed, mobilized, managed, and coordinated. To accomplish this, a communications system must incorporate operational provisions to use sufficient wire-line and radio linkages and channels among all EMSS participants over the service area of the EMSS (and for disaster response, between EMSS service areas) to facilitate the EMSS functional needs described in 7.2 through 7.5 for communications.

7.2 *Citizen Access*:

7.2.1 The EMSS communications system should have the ability to receive and process any incoming calls that report emergencies and request emergency medical assistance. Persons should be able to summon help rapidly in an emergency situation. They should be able to call for police, fire, rescue, and other emergency aid promptly, without confusion, and without familiarity with a particular community. Local, statewide, and nationwide uniformity is needed to accomplish this objective.

7.2.2 For several years, numerous governmental commissions, legislative bodies, private organizations, and citizen groups have recommended the establishment of a single, universal "Nationwide 9-1-1 Emergency Telephone Number" to meet this need for improved emergency communications. The achievement of this recommendation was stated as a matter of national policy in Bulletin No. 73-1 "National Policy for Emergency Telephone Number '911'" issued by the Executive Office of the President on March 21, 1973. The "nine-one-one" concept provides a single number that is easy to use and remember. Moreover, implementation of the three-digit emergency telephone number 9-1-1, encourages coordinated efforts between those providing communications services and emergency responses. The 9-1-1 concept should be included in EMSS communication planning with other methods of citizen access, primarily for its impact on response time and enhanced coordination among participants. Citizen access communications, primarily uses telephones, both public and private, to call 9-1-1 Public Safety Answering Points (PSAP).

7.2.3 On the nation's highways, citizen access to EMSS is facilitated by use of mobile communications services that enable drivers to rapidly report observed motor vehicle accidents and other emergency conditions to public safety service providers. In areas having cellular telephone coverage, motor vehicle occupants with cellular telephone may make direct calls to the local 9-1-1 PSAP. This use of cellular telephone for accessing public safety services is being facilitated through rule changes initiated in 1994 by provisions of the Federal Communications Commission Rules under RM-8143 Docket No. 94-102; to ensure compatibility of cellular 9-1-1 calls with enhanced 911 emergency calling systems. Also, Citizen Band (CB) mobile radio operators can report observed emergencies to volunteer CB base station radio monitors who in turn relay the information to appropriate public safety response agencies via the 9-1-1 emergency telephone number or some other prearranged telephone number. Similarly, mobile equipped amateur radio operators can report observed emergencies to appropriate public safety authorities via the 9-1-1 emergency telephone number using amateur radio/telephone interconnect services. Finally, motorists not equipped with mobile radio communications, can report emergencies by stopping at the nearest roadside site having a public telephone and dialing 9-1-1. In some locations, a statewide toll-free 800 telephone access number is available for calling state police. The availability of such 800 service should be indicated by road signs. Such 800 calls may also be made via cellular radio. Calls received by the state police may be transferred to the appropriate 9-1-1 answering point or directly to the designated response agency. The use of these numbers should include provisions for assuring caller identification and location and special screening by trained PSAP communicators.

7.2.4 In areas in which the 9-1-1 system has not been implemented, citizens may have to search through telephone directories for one of several listed police, fire, ambulance, and hospital emergency room numbers when a medical emergency arises. Continuation of this practice delays the availability of emergency medical assistance and, in life threatening and serious medical emergencies, can cost lives and limbs. There is no technical reason why a basic or enhanced 9-1-1 emergency telephone number cannot be planned and implemented by any telephone company in the United States. The universal "National 9-1-1 Emergency Telephone Number" should be implemented without further delay as a matter of national public safety.

7.2.5 Telephone calls for emergency services made by unattended automatic telephone calling devices should be received and screened by a private answering service and shall not be dialed in directly to the primary 9-1-1 or other general public access number.

7.3 *EMSS Vehicle Dispatch and Coordination*—When notified of the need for an emergency medical response, the communications system is used by trained emergency medical dispatchers:

7.3.1 To interrogate emergency callers to determine the nature and severity of the medical emergency,

7.3.2 To provide on-site callers with pre-arrival instructions,

7.3.3 To dispatch the most appropriate EMS vehicles to the site of the emergency promptly,

7.3.4 To guide them directly to the site with minimum delays,

7.3.5 To direct them to an appropriate emergency medical facility, and

7.3.6 To ensure that they become available for further assignment as soon as possible.

7.3.7 While EMS vehicles are enroute to a patient, the communications system is used to keep them informed regarding access to the patient and patient condition.

7.4 *Medical Coordination/Direction*—The EMSS communications system should provide EMS field personnel with a channel of communications that permits the exchange of treatment information with an EMSS hospital, while at the scene of the medical emergency, in an EMS ambulance and while enroute to an EMS hospital. Such communications also serves to alert the receiving medical facility before the patient's arrival and to provide for coordination between medical facilities. In areas in which the need frequently arises, consideration should be given to equipping EMS ambulances with high-power portable radios or vehicular relay equipment and hand-held portables to permit the exchange of patient treatment information while away from an EMS ambulance. Guidelines for medical coordination/direction are contained in Practice F 1149.

7.5 *Interservice Communications*—Medical emergencies often involve the response of other public safety and emergency services. Interservice communications are needed to support daily EMSS operations and mutual aid agreements and for mobilization, command, and control of all emergency response units during a disaster situation. Although the various services generally operate on different radio frequencies, interservice radio communications can be provided by use of mobile relays, cross-band operations, cross-frequency patching at the radio consoles, interservice use of common radio frequencies, trunked radio services, or other measures. Telephone lines between communications control centers for various emergency response agencies can also be used for interservice coordination. Provisions for such interservice radio communications should be included in the system design.

8. Radio Frequency Spectrum and Service Requirements

8.1 *Radio Frequencies*—All nonfederal telecommunications systems in the United States are subject to the regulations of the Federal Communications Commission (FCC). There are radio frequencies nationally allocated primarily for dispatch of ground emergency medical vehicles, transport of patients, and other EMS-related communications. Such radio communications are allowed under FCC Rules and Regulations (47 CFR, Part 90) Private Land Mobile Radio Services, Subpart B, Public Safety Radio Services. These current FCC Rules clearly distinguish between emergency medical service communications, other types of medical communications, and other types of emergency communications. Section 90.27 of the FCC Rules, defines the Emergency Medical Radio Services (EMRS), and allocates radio frequencies exclusively for licensing eligible applicants to use for EMS communications. FCC Rules and Regulations also permit EMS use of radio frequencies allocated to other land mobile services such as the Special Emergency Radio Service, Local Government Radio Service; Law Enforcement Radio Service; Fire Radio Service; and Business Radio Service.

8.1.1 *Radio Frequencies for EMSS Communications*—Section 90.27 of the FCC Rules identifies users eligible for licensing on frequencies allocated for EMRS.

8.1.2 *Eligibility Criteria*—As stated in the FCC Rules, the following are eligible for licensing to use the radio frequency spectrum allocated by the FCC for the Emergency Medical Radio Service:" Persons or entities engaged in the provision of basic or advanced life support services on an ongoing basis are eligible ... to operate stations for transmission of communications essential for the delivery or rendition of emergency medical services for the provision of basic or advanced life support." EMRS applicants are also eligible for licensing to use frequencies in the Special Emergency Radio Service (SERS): "in order to interface with other entities using SERS channels and to conduct necessary non-emergency communications."[5]

8.2 *EMSS Radio Service Coverage*—This guide addresses radio frequencies and radio service coverage currently authorized and available under FCC Rules for use for land mobile communications for EMSS. In the Emergency Medical Radio Service, there are seven high-band VHF frequencies, five 220 MHz frequency pairs, and 35 UHF band frequency pairs. Many of these frequencies are restricted for specific uses, such as paging, intersystem use, medical coordination, vehicle coordination, or shared with other Public Safety Radio Services. Appendix X1 lists the frequencies and usage limitations. While there are no 800-MHz band frequencies specifically allocated to EMS, all EMRS eligible may license 800-MHz frequencies allocated for Public Safety Radio Services. In addition, there are other land mobile communications services such as cellular systems, citizen band radio, and prospective satellite relayed land mobile radio communications systems that are available for public use. It is not intended that this guide exclude EMSS usage of such communications systems. In 1987, The FCC Report on Docket No. 87-112 points out, however, that such public communications systems that are merely extensions of the public telephone net are not amenable to planned usage for public safety services. The usage of any available radio spectrum for EMSS communications should be based on the capability of such systems of communications to provide the necessary linkage to satisfy criteria with respect to reliability of coverage of the EMSS operating area, grade of service (probability of blockage and delay), and accountability, that apply to EMSS communications as well as to other public safety communications such as fire and law enforcement communications.

[5] Summary of FCC Report and Order, PR Docket No. 91-72, *Federal Register*, March 3, 1993.

8.2.1 Radio frequencies listed in Appendix X1, and currently available for EMSS communications are in the VHF "low band" (33 to 48 MHz), the VHF "high band" (150 to 173 MHz), the UHF band (453 to 468 MHz) and in the 800-MHz frequency range. The VHF high band and the UHF frequency bands, which are most commonly used for EMS communications, and the 800-MHz frequencies are line of sight, with communications range primarily a function of transmitter power output, antenna gain, antenna height, and terrain. For planning purposes, estimates of the geographic area over which intelligible voice radio reception can be achieved between a specific radio base station site and a vehicle equipped with mobile radio can be made using computerized communications model services such as those described in Ref (**2**).

8.2.2 Preinstallation estimates of radio geographic coverage should be verified by postinstallation field tests using operational communications equipment. It is important to ensure that the transmitted signal strength from EMSS communications base stations is adequate to provide good radio reception in EMSS ambulances and other response vehicles over the entire area services by an EMSS.

8.2.3 A single radio base station operating on a specific radio frequency channel or channel pair permits separate two-way communications with a single radio-equipped EMSS ambulance operating on the same radio frequency channel or channel pair. If the need exists to communicate separately with multiple EMSS mobile units simultaneously, then base station sites must be equipped with multiple radio transmitter/receivers each equipped to operate on a separate radio frequency. To communicate by radio in an area provided with multiple transmitter/receivers, and EMSS mobile unit must use a radio transmitter/receiver that can be adjusted to operate on any base station frequency that may be available at a given time.

8.2.3.1 Specific estimates of radio frequency requirements to support EMSS communications demands for large populations are contained in Ref (**3**). Guidelines for determining the number of base station radio transmitter/receivers and radio frequencies needed to assure reliable EMSS communications in support of the EMS demands of various populations will be set forth in a future ASTM standard guide.

8.2.3.2 In instances of mass casualty response, when the need exists for an EMSS base station to communicate the same information to several ambulances, the ambulances involved should all be directed to adjust their radio equipment for operation on the selected base station frequency and to respond in sequence as required. Usage of radio frequencies can thereby be expanded to satisfy mass casualty and disaster EMS communications needs.

8.2.4 Geographic coverage and control for EMSS radio communications can be provided by various communication subsystem arrangements as illustrated in Figs. 1-4.

8.3 *Operational Considerations*:

8.3.1 Statewide communications planning, including interstate, regional, and local planning, is essential to successful EMSS operation. EMSS operational control should be carefully established and supported with communications operational procedures.

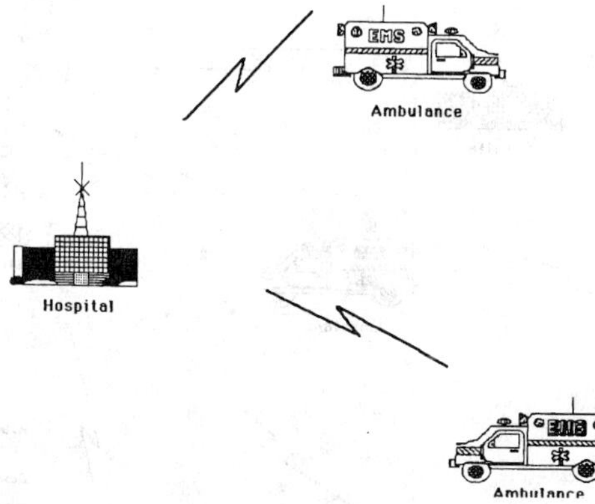

NOTE 1—*FCC Definitions (47 C.F.R. Sec. 90.7):*

mobile station—a station in the mobile service intended to be used while in motion or during halts at unspecified points. This includes hand carried transmitters.

base station—a station at a specified site authorized to communicate with mobile stations.

mobile service—a service of radiocommunication between mobile and base stations or between mobile stations.

NOTE 2—EMTs in ambulances equipped as "mobile stations" conduct two-way radio communications directly with medical control personnel at EMSS resource hospitals equipped as "base stations."

FIG. 1 An EMS Base/Mobile Communications System

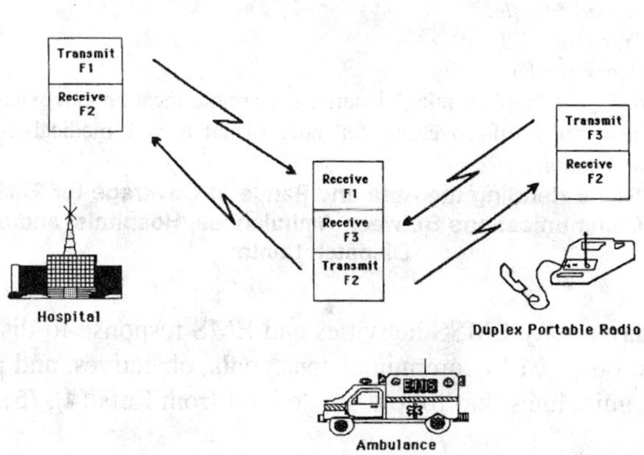

NOTE 1—*FCC Definitions (47 C.F.R. Sec. 90.7):*

mobile repeater station—a mobile station authorized to retransmit automatically on a mobile service frequency, communications to or from hand-carried transmitters.

hand carried transmitters—See definition of *mobile station* under Fig. 1.

mobile service–See definition under Fig. 1.

portable radio—Syn. for *hand-carried transmitter.*

NOTE 2—An EMT equipped with a "hand-carried" (portable) duplex radio, while located outside of an ambulance equipped as a duplex "mobile repeater station" can conduct two-way radio communications via the ambulance, with medical control personnel at EMSS resource hospitals equipped as "base stations." This extends the range of on-line medical control communications for patients outside of, but within portable radio communications range of, an ambulance.

FIG. 2 Extending the Range of Communications for EMTs While Outside of an Ambulance—Typical Both-Way Vehicular Repeater

8.3.2 EMSS communications systems should be planned and operated so as to be compatible and not interfere with the communications of adjacent EMSS. Compatibility means that EMS vehicles from one community can communicate with EMS vehicles and EMSS facilities in surrounding communities. Communications compatibility of EMS vehicles is needed

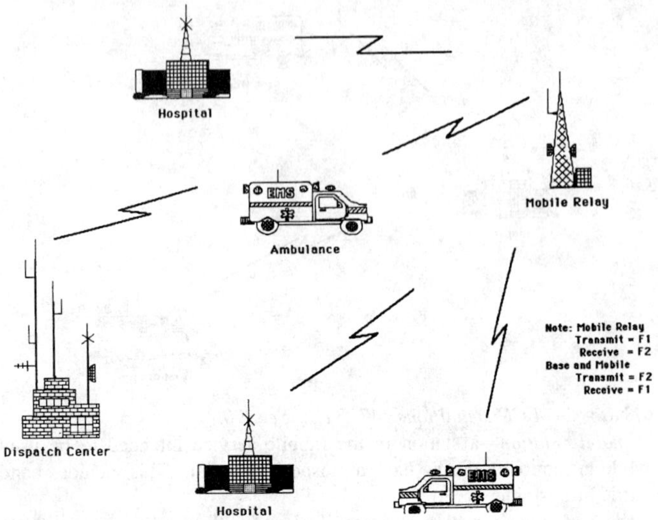

NOTE 1—*FCC Definition (47 C.F.R. Sec. 90.7):*

mobile relay station—a base station in the mobile service authorized to retransmit automatically on a mobile service frequency communications which originate on the transmitting frequency of the mobile station.

NOTE 2—*Mobile Relay:*

Transmit = F1.

Receive = F2.

Base and Mobile:

Transmit = F2.

Receive = F1.

NOTE 3—A "mobile relay" located at a remote location can extend the area and range of coverage for both dispatch and medical control communications.

FIG. 3 Extending the Area and Range of Coverage for EMSS Communications Between Ambulances, Hospitals, and a Dispatch Center

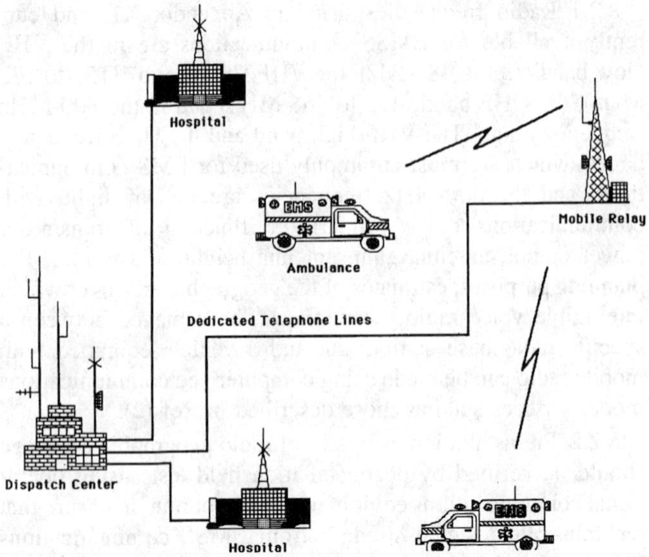

NOTE 1—*FCC Definitions (47 C.F.R. Sec. 90.7):*

land mobile radio system—a regularly interacting group of base, mobile, and associated control and fixed relay stations intended to provide land mobile communications service over a single area of operation.

land mobile radio service—mobile service between base stations and land mobile stations, or between land mobile stations.

NOTE 2—Real-time centralized coordination/control of base station and mobile relay frequencies and operations in an EMSS "land mobile radio" can be accomplished by use of dedicated telephone lines, microwave links, or combinations of both. In this illustration, the Dispatch Center also serves as the EMSS communications control center.

FIG. 4 Centralized Control of Radio Communications in an EMSS Land Mobile Radio System

for day-to-day EMSS activities and EMS response-to-disaster situations. EMSS communications goals, objectives, and planning guidelines that follow are derived from Refs **(4)**, **(5)**, and **(6)**.

9. Goals and Objectives for EMSS Communications

9.1 Determination of state goals and objectives require a definition of the specific role of state government in EMSS communications in its jurisdiction and in boundary areas with adjacent states. In general, state governments do not own or operate EMSS communications systems and do not exercise control over local systems. Instead, state governments act more in the role of planners, coordinators, regulators, and facilitators.

9.2 A state can be thought of as divided into a number of local EMS communications systems. The state's primary concern is with the external interfaces and interactions of these local EMS communications systems with each other and with their environments. The state government is not so much concerned with the other details of the design and operation of the individual local systems. Following is a description and comments on some of the important interfaces and relationships.

9.3 The most important interface is the one between a local EMS communications system and the population it serves. Here, the concern of the state government should be that the system serves its intended functions. The focus is on the end results: the character, quantity, and quality of service provided to the population, rather than the mechanics of how the service is provided. Items of interest include the degree to which the communications system supports the medical requirements for basic life support or advanced life support, communications parameters such as probability of place and time of coverage, communications practices, and operator training standards.

9.4 The second level of interface is between a local EMS communications system and other EMSS communications systems in neighboring areas. There are two main concerns. First, as a minimum, the various communications systems should not interfere with each other. This requires consideration of coverage boundaries, fixed allocation of unique frequencies, and real-time coordination and sharing of common frequencies. Second, systems should be able to cooperate constructively with each other in such matters as point-to-point communications and communications within an area to mobile units passing through from other regions. Items such as voice brevity codes and language must be standardized between regions.

9.5 A third level of interface is between a local EMS communications system and other types of emergency communications systems, such as law enforcement and emergency management and fire services, within the same area and with neighboring areas. The concerns are again the avoidance of interference (such as at shared radio sites) and assurance of compatibility for multiagency operations. With the creation of the Emergency Medical Radio Service, EMS agencies maintain their eligibility in the Special Emergency Radio Service (SERS). For EMS communications using frequencies in the SERS, there is a concern for interference from school bus radio communications and from hospital, veterinary and physician business communications that are permitted by the FCC. A "frequency coordination" process must be carried out as part of the statewide EMS communications system planning process to lessen instances of this interference potential.

9.6 A fourth interface is from the local communications system to the state government. The primary concern of the state is in ensuring that its population receives timely and appropriate emergency medical care in accordance with state statutes and regulations and health care standards. Additional concerns are efficient and effective use by the local systems of resources provided by the state or otherwise shared in common with multiple users. These might include radio sites, statewide microwave and telephone systems, and various services such as maintenance and purchasing. Complaints from adjoining states concerning radio communications interference in boundary areas should also be the concern of state government.

9.7 A fifth interface is from the state to the federal government. The state acts as a representative of local EMSS in dealing with federal agencies and other national organizations.

9.8 Finally, the state must be concerned with management of the state-level program. The management functions include ongoing planning; state and upper-level regional organizations; personnel qualifications, standards, and training; direction of the program by laws, rules, funding incentives, other means; and control of the program by means of information feedback, analysis, evaluation, and corrective action.

9.9 In summary, therefore, the areas of concern for definition of statewide goals and objectives are as follows:

9.9.1 Functional performance standards,

9.9.2 Interface with other EMS systems,

9.9.3 Interface with other types of systems,

9.9.4 Utilization of state and common resources,

9.9.5 National representation, and

9.9.6 State level management.

9.10 Each of these areas is addressed as a separate goal in the remaining sections of this guide. Each goal is followed by a listing of specific related objectives and a discussion of the implications of each objective. Note that progress can be made in many of these areas without substantial costs. In other cases, the achievement of certain objectives will involve substantial costs, and therefore, given the national and state economies, those objectives must be considered long term.

10. Goal 1—State EMSS Communication Systems Should Meet Recognized Standards for Functional Performance

10.1 State government should work to ensure that recognized standards for functional performance (end result delivery of service to the public) are met. Specifically, EMS communications systems should conform at least to minimum performance standards for public safety communications system contained in "Report on Police" (Ref **(7)**) and "Report on the Criminal Justice System" (Ref **(8)**), which have been broadly accepted by state and local public safety services and APCO as the basis for public safety communications systems planning and design. To the extent possible in view of local needs, resources, and capabilities, the standards should be applied uniformly throughout the state so that residents in rural areas do not necessarily receive lower levels of service than do urban residents.

10.2 *Objective*—EMSS requirement should be explicitly considered in plans for improvement of citizen-access communications.

10.2.1 Citizen-access communication systems (such as 9-1-1) handle all types of emergencies and are thus inherently broader in scope than EMSS. State EMSS authorities generally do not have the lead role in the development of citizen-access systems. The statewide development of 9-1-1 in many states, for example, has been assigned to the state emergency management or law enforcement authorities. State EMSS authorities should however participate in the statewide planning for expanding the coverage and enhancing existing 9-1-1 systems to ensure that EMSS requirements are taken into account. Guidelines for planning and developing 9-1-1 enhanced telephone systems are contained in Guide F 1381. Additional information regarding Emergency Medical Dispatch (EMD) is contained in Practice F 1258, Practice F 1552, and Practice F 1560. Following is a summary of the requirements for 9-1-1 enhanced telephone systems as set forth in Guide F 1381:

10.2.1.1 In any given area, there should be only one telephone number to call for requesting emergency assistance. It is a national goal that this number should be "9-1-1." A variety of supplemental and alternative arrangements exist in various areas of the United States and new alternative provisions for citizens access are being introduced and evaluated in areas in which 9-1-1 implementation is not operationally or economically feasible. These alternatives include roadway telephone call boxes, cellular radio emergency telephone numbers, and area code 800 toll free emergency numbers. Such alternatives should include a single telephone number other than 9-1-1 for all types of emergencies or barring that, at least a single telephone number or other means of access for reporting the existence of all medical emergencies. The single telephone number or means of access should be published on the inside cover of telephone directories, displayed in public telephone booths and otherwise prominently displayed to the public. Citizens should not have to look up EMSS ambulance companies in the telephone directories to request emergency medical assistance. They should not have to know their location in relation to jurisdictional boundaries to determine the proper number to call. Whatever means are provided, citizen public telephone access to emergency services should incorporate the following features:

10.2.1.2 There should be no financial barrier to requesting emergency medical assistance. Coins should not be required for EMS calls from public phones. (This "dial tone first" feature is usually provided in 9-1-1 systems.) Long distance EMS calls should be toll-free.

10.2.1.3 Sufficient lines should be provided to ensure that no more than one call for emergency medical assistance in 100 attempts receive a busy signal during the average busy hour

(P.01 grade of service).

10.2.1.4 Sufficient answering positions and operators should be provided to ensure that at least 90 % of the calls for emergency medical assistance are answered within 10 s during the average busy hour.

10.2.1.5 Call answerers should be provided with written protocols for distinguishing calls for emergency medical assistance from other types of emergencies and should have adequate training to use the protocols effectively.

10.2.1.6 Call transfer or information relay, if used, should be fast and reliable. Call referral (telling the caller to hang up and call a different number) should never be used for calls for emergency medical assistance.

10.2.1.7 If call transfer is used, the caller should never have to talk to more than two people (for example, the 9-1-1 call answerer and the EMSS dispatcher).

10.2.1.8 Where feasible and appropriate, the development of alternative and backup systems for citizen access to emergency medical care should be encouraged. Such systems might include the use of citizen band radio and monitoring networks, cellular telephone, and radio call boxes. Also, police stations, fire stations, and government buildings equipped with two-way public safety radio service should be posted and made available for walk-in access to emergency medical care.

10.2.1.9 There should be a plan of action to maintain public access to emergency medical care when the primary telephone service of the 9-1-1 system becomes inoperative. The plan might include provisions for stationing radio equipped personnel at central locations such as malls, major intersections, schools, and so forth. The plan should include provisions for public safety announcements and alerts on local radio and television advising the public of the situation and what should be done to report emergencies.

10.3 *Objective*—EMSS resources should be coordinated:

10.3.1 EMSS communications in a local area should be organized so as to guarantee for each caller that the nearest or most appropriate EMSS response unit(s) will be assigned to the call. This objective may be met by the use of "staging or move-up" plans to handle periods of peak EMS demand; by dynamic positioning of ambulances to enhance area-wide response readiness; by use of resource allocation protocols to assure that the most appropriate response unit is used; and by the development of an EMSS dispatch center usually in conjunction with a combined public safety dispatch center. The following requirements apply to an effective EMSS dispatch center:

10.3.1.1 The EMSS dispatch center should at all times monitor and be aware of the current location, status, and capability of all EMS response units in the area including private and public aeromedical units, ground ambulances, fire department EMS units, first responders, and so forth.

10.3.1.2 The EMSS dispatch center should be authorized and able to optimize the allocation of resources by preassigning specific units to particular locations in anticipation of need and relocating units as conditions change.

10.3.1.3 The EMSS dispatch center should have written policies and procedures for the assignment of specific combinations of units to particular types of EMS incidents.

10.3.2 Computer-aided dispatching, which includes provisions for dispatching EMSS and other public safety services, can facilitate coordination of emergency medical responses.

10.4 *Objective*—EMSS dispatch should be as direct as possible:

10.4.1 In the ideal case, the person who answers the call for emergency medical assistance is the radio dispatcher who can make direct contact with the units to be assigned to the incident. More commonly, however, one or more call transfers or information relays are necessary before the emergency information gets out to the response units who can actually act upon it. In any case, the chain of communications should be as short, simple, and direct as possible. The EMS caller should never have to talk to more than two people, for example, the 9-1-1 call answerer and the EMS dispatcher. Where the EMSS dispatcher must communicate with multiple units and locations for a given incident, the communications to all should occur simultaneously (or as nearly so as possible) using common or similar means of communications. There should also be some arrangement for positive feedback or an acknowledgment from each unit that the dispatch message has been received and understood.

10.4.2 EMSS dispatch should be prompt. The delay between the time of first notification of a medical emergency and the receipt of the dispatch message by the responding EMSS unit (ambulance or first responder) should never exceed 2 min. Using the standard practice described in Practice F 1258, 2 min is sufficient for an emergency medical dispatcher, trained in accordance with Practice F 1552, to interrogate a caller to determine the nature, severity, and most appropriate resource to dispatch.

10.5 *Objective*—EMSS communications systems should support statewide EMSS program requirements and local EMSS standard operating procedures by providing the following land mobile radio communications capabilities:

10.5.1 Provisions should exist for dispatch and coordination communications as described in 7.3. Statewide EMSS program requirements and local standard operating procedures should provide for prompt, reliable interagency coordination and direct access to communications for EMSS ambulance dispatch and coordination as described in 10.3 and 10.4.

10.5.2 Provisions for medical coordination/direction communications are described in 7.4. These provisions should conform with statewide EMSS program requirements and communication guidelines and should be incorporated in local EMSS communication plans so as to support local protocols for on-line medical direction to prehospital EMS response personnel.

10.5.2.1 A local (regional) EMSS communications plan should be prepared in accordance with state guidelines and should be kept updated. The plan should define the purposes and scope of the system and communication system features selected to support normal EMSS medical coordination procedures.

10.5.2.2 In areas where EMS ambulances frequently encounter medical emergencies in which patients are remote from ambulance access, consideration should be given to providing for two-way radio voice communications from EMS ambulance personnel at the immediate site of a medical emergency to an EMSS hospital. This communication capability permits on-line medical direction preparatory to moving a patient from a remote site to an EMS ambulance.

10.5.2.3 Provisions should exist for two-way voice communications between EMS ambulances and designated EMSS hospitals for consultation on patient status, treatment, and transport destination.

10.5.2.4 Provisions should exist for two-way voice communications between EMS ambulances and non-EMSS hospitals destined to receive EMS patients, for consultation regarding patient arrivals, patient condition, and need for transfer to EMSS hospitals.

10.5.2.5 The decision to require that an EMSS have provisions for biomedical telemetry from EMS ambulances and from the immediate site of medical emergencies, is an "off-line" EMSS medical control decision. If a decision is made to provide for biomedical telemetry, it should be incorporated into the system design.

10.5.2.6 Delay in EMSS hospital access to the channel being used for medical direction should be minimized. This can be accomplished by prescribing communications procedures restricting the duration of ambulance to hospital transmissions or by including design features to permit hospital preemption of the ambulance to hospital communications channel. The decision to provide communications system design features to permit EMSS hospitals to preempt a channel in use by an EMS ambulance (doctor interrupt) should be a matter for "off-line" medical control.

10.5.2.7 Provisions should exist for EMSS hospitals to arrange for direct two-way voice communications, as the need arises, with any other hospital within the EMSS area of responsibility that is destined to receive patients by EMSS ambulance. This may be accomplished by a variety of means such as direct radio link, if such exist, by radio-telephone interconnect, or by telephone.

10.6 *Objective*—EMSS communications systems should meet recognized standards while conforming to statewide EMSS program requirements and local EMSS communications plans. Some of these statewide requirements are listed below:

10.6.1 Statewide and local EMSS communications plans should contain provisions for reliable communications between EMSS ambulances for dispatch and routing from designated EMSS dispatch centers and for medical direction from designated EMSS hospitals over the entire territory defined by statewide EMSS program requirements.

10.6.1.1 Each EMSS hospital should be able to communicate with any EMS ambulance within its area of responsibility, or to ambulances at any location which the hospital is the nearest or most appropriate emergency medical facility for issuing medical direction, or for exchange of patient pre-arrival information, or both.

10.6.1.2 Each EMS ambulance should be able to communicate with any radio-equipped EMSS hospital in the state, when within range for mobile radio communications.

10.6.1.3 Each EMSS ambulance should be able to communicate by radio with any EMSS dispatch facility in the state when within range for mobile radio communications.

10.6.2 State and local (regional) EMSS communications plans should provide for statewide compatibility and interoperability of communications by defining statewide radio frequency requirements and compatibility factors for EMSS dispatch centers and for EMSS hospitals.

10.6.3 EMSS communications plans should specify a sufficient number of dispatch and medical coordination frequencies to reliably support the peak demand for EMSS communications with the same reliability as other public safety services.

10.6.3.1 For instances of peak EMS demand such as multiple casualty accidents, each EMSS hospital should be provided with sufficient radio frequencies and base stations to support reliably a simultaneous EMS communications demand equal to its capacity for simultaneous treatment of life threatening and serious medical emergencies for the duration of prehospital emergency medical care and transport to an EMSS hospital.

10.6.3.2 EMSS base stations should be equipped to avoid interference from reception of radio communications intended for other radio stations.

10.6.3.3 Consideration should be given to providing for selective calling of EMSS hospitals by EMSS ambulances.

10.6.4 In developing the statewide EMSS communication plan, consideration should be given to FCC licensing provisions, the number of frequencies available, their transmission characteristics, other authorized users of the various radio frequencies available for EMSS, and the impact of these features on the range of communication, and their adequacy for providing reliable communication for EMSS communication demands. Implementation of the FCC Rules on EMRS should result in a gradual reduction in the probability of interference and blockage of EMSS communications on these exclusive EMS radio frequencies. However, there may be increased probability of interference and blockage of EMSS communication by other authorized users on frequencies that are shared with non-EMS communications services.

10.7 *Objective*—The EMSS communications system design should ensure continued communications during disasters:

10.7.1 EMSS communications are particularly important during disasters. To ensure that an EMS communications system can satisfy the special needs for emergency medical response during a disaster, and not itself become disabled by the disaster, the system design should include the following considerations:

10.7.1.1 The public-switched telephone network is susceptible to traffic overload and physical disruption during disasters. Leased private lines are protected from traffic overload but not physical outage. The system design should therefore provide alternative and backup communication links, such as radio and microwave. Telephone lines coming into communication centers should be protected from damage, and where possible, alternate routing from multiple telephone company central offices should be used.

10.7.1.2 Means should be provided to allow police, fire, rescue, and ambulance units from different agencies to communicate with each other directly during disaster operations. Available techniques include use of common disaster channels, multiagency multichannel radios, or cross-patch of channels at public safety communications base stations.

10.7.1.3 Fixed communications facilities should be provided with independent standby power sources to avoid dependency on commercial power.

10.7.1.4 Important locations in an area should be covered by more than one radio site so that communication is not totally lost in the event of failure of one radio site.

10.7.1.5 Sufficient telephone lines, radio channel capacity, and operating positions (or rapid expansion capability) should be designed into the system to handle heavy traffic loads generated by disasters.

10.7.1.6 Disaster communications procedures should be well defined with emphasis on interagency coordination. Disaster procedures should be straight forward expansions of day-to-day procedures rather than radical changes.

10.7.1.7 Disaster systems and procedures should be periodically exercised.

10.8 *Objective*—Communication operators should be trained in both emergency medical services and in communications:

10.8.1 Problems can be caused by physicians, nurses, and EMTs inexperienced in the use of communications equipment and also by public safety communications center personnel not familiar with EMSS concepts and terminology. Sufficient cross-training should therefore be provided on both sides to ensure that EMSS protocols and technical communications procedures are clearly understood and uniformly applied throughout the system. Physicians, nurses, and EMTs should be cross-trained in EMD communications practices and procedures as described in Practice F 1258 on the EMD practice, and Practice F 1552 on EMS training.

10.9 *Objective*—EMSS communications systems should meet technical standards applicable to all public safety communications systems:

10.9.1 The system must meet all applicable FCC rules and regulations.

10.9.2 All EMS communications should be recorded. The recording should include date and time signals. As a minimum, communication recordings should be retained at least as long as other local public safety communication recordings and beyond that for the period determined appropriate by applicable state EMS communications guidelines.

10.9.3 The reliability of radio coverage for two-way voice communications between an EMSS hospital and an EMS ambulance should be 0.95 or 95 %. This means that the medial signal level to and from an EMSS ambulance should exceed that necessary to provide 20 dB of quieting in the presence of ambient noise in 95 % of the randomly selected locations within the service area. Proof-of-performance tests should be made with the EMSS ambulance in motion.

10.9.4 The equipment must be durable and easy to operate. This is particularly true for equipment to be used by EMTs, physicians, and nurses.

11. Goal 2—Local EMSS Communications Should be Compatible with, and Should Not Interfere with, EMSS Communications in Neighboring Areas

11.1 *Objective*—EMSS communications coverage boundaries should be defined and respected:

11.1.1 Normal radio communication coverage boundaries between neighboring EMSS should be mapped out and mutually agreed upon. Measures should be taken to respect the boundaries and minimize interference outside the boundaries by prudent base station transmitter site designs, including use of directional antennas, limiting antenna elevations and radiated power, and other technical design features.

11.1.1.1 Interference can also be avoided by adoption of appropriate standard operating procedures, for example, for VHF communications, adopt "listen-before-talk" channel monitoring policies.

11.1.1.2 In UHF communications, centralized monitoring of all MED channel traffic and real-time centralized assignment of operating frequencies is one strategy for limiting interference with other EMSS communications as well as with non-EMSS users of the same spectrum. Digitally Addressed Trunked Communications Systems (DATCS) technology defined in APCO Project 16A, includes provisions for minimizing such interference. This technological approach to minimizing interference was recommended in Ref **(3)**.

11.2 *Objective*—Frequency allocations and usage should be coordinated statewide and nationally when appropriate. State EMSS radio frequency usage plans are subject to changing provisions of the FCC Rules and Regulations. The State Office of Emergency Medical Services should assist with frequency coordination to establish a statewide frequency sharing pattern. The following advisory sections describe some of the implications of current FCC Rules and Regulations on statewide planning for coordinating the usage of radio frequencies available for communications so as to satisfy state EMSS program goals and objectives.

11.2.1 EMS dispatching is done on both VHF and UHF frequencies and on frequencies in the 800 MHz band. In some areas, where EMS is provided by local government or fire services, local government or fire service frequencies are being used for EMS dispatching. In EMS systems in which dispatching is to be performed on frequencies in different bands or radio services, state EMS authorities should use frequency coordination services in planning and selecting frequencies and in planning base station radio coverage for EMS radio-dispatching systems.

11.2.2 The UHF frequencies of MED-1 through MED-10 are subject to statewide use and must be coordinated by a state frequency coordinator. The state EMS communications plan is used as the framework for coordination of these frequencies and all mobile and portable radio equipment on these frequencies must incorporate all of the MED-1 through MED-10 channels. The state EMS communications plan should require that a minimum of four channels be operational within each station, unless a specifically identified need is demonstrated to and approved by the Office of Emergency Medical Services.

11.2.3 In some regions, such as large cities with populations greater than 4 000 000, it may be desirable to implement all eight MED channels to prevent unsatisfactory communications because of overloading during the average daily busy hour. Real-time frequency coordination, where channels are assigned on an "as needed real-time basis," in these instances should be used to reduce interference. The communications design should be coordinated within the region. In the largest cities, even this communication capacity is insufficient to prevent unsatisfactory communication blockage because of overloading during the average daily busy hour. In such instances, consideration should be given to various alternatives for reducing communication blockage such as changing communication protocols to reduce channel loading; using communication technology to facilitate real-time communication channel sharing (digitally addressed trunking technology) or; based on FCC Rules on FCC Docket No. 87-112, planning for the use of additional spectrum in the 821- to 824-/866-to 869-MHz bands. Whatever means is used, both dispatching and medical coordination communication for EMSS should have a grade of service such that blockage occurs no more than five times in a hundred attempts to access a channel (grade of service P.05).

11.2.4 In smaller cities and in rural areas, frequency coordination services can be used to establish area-wide frequency sharing pattern to provide a suitable grade of service for EMSS. Spare communication capacity should be provided for multicasualty incidents and for disaster situations. Frequency coordination services must be used and may be helpful in assisting small communities to develop EMS communication plans that include provision for coordinated sharing of base station usage among EMSS users.

11.2.5 In smaller cities and in rural areas, frequency coordination services can be used to establish area-wide frequency sharing pattern to provide a suitable grade of service for EMSS. Spare communication capacity should be provided for multicasualty incidents and for disaster situations. Communication capacity can be used to advantage for medical administrative communication and to permit rural physicians to stay in contact with their hospitals while they are on the road and otherwise away from their offices. Frequency coordination services must be used and may be helpful in assisting small communities to develop EMS communication plans that include provision for coordinated sharing of base station usage among EMSS users and other non-EMSS eligible medical use of the MED channels.

11.3 *Objective*—The provisions for continuous tone-coded squelch system (CTCSS) tones and other control tones and codes should be coordinated statewide, including along interstate boundaries. This coordination function is not provided by FCC-esignated frequency coordinators and should be done by state EMS authorities. All agencies should advise the state EMS authority of the tones used. Records and database should be established and maintained.

11.4 *Objective*—Regional and local systems should be interconnected with fixed radio links:

11.4.1 At least one frequency should be designated within a state as the standard frequency for interhospital communications for coordinating resources or response. This frequency should be implemented in all emergency hospitals and should extend to EMS dispatch and communications control centers to permit hospital resources to be effectively coordinated with other public safety resources. Operating procedures should be established on a uniform basis regionally and statewide. The VHF frequencies 155.400 and 155.340 MHz have been used in many states for this purpose.

11.5 *Objective*—Mobile unit parameters should be standardized statewide for intersystem compatibility (interoperability):

11.5.1 The objective of interoperability is to enable every EMS mobile unit to travel anywhere in the state (for example, on a mutual aid assignment, or on a patient transport to a distant specialty care facility, or for disaster response) and to remain in communications with an EMSS at all times. Achievement of this objective would require the following:

11.5.1.1 All EMSS in a state should adhere to a common mobile frequency plan. The plan should provide for a statewide set of common calling frequencies by which an EMS ambulance operating out of its home region can call EMSS hospitals for selection of a locally available radio frequency for medical coordination communications.

11.5.1.2 EMSS ambulances should be equipped for and informed of selective calling codes, and related equipment, and selective calling procedures to enable them to communicate with EMSS hospitals statewide.

11.5.1.3 EMSS ambulances should be equipped with and informed of tone-coded squelch, equipment, and procedures to enable them to communicate with EMSS hospitals statewide.

11.5.1.4 Equipment and procedures should be provided for maintenance of radio contact with an EMSS ambulance traveling from one EMSS region to another.

11.5.1.5 There should be statewide uniform training of communications operators. For the EMS communications system to function, the people, including the field teams, dispatchers, hospital personnel, and the system users, must know how to operate the telephone and radio equipment required for their communications. For example, the system users who use public telephones to call for emergency assistance must know what number to call. The field teams, dispatchers, telecommunicators, and hospital and medical personnel must know how to operate their radio equipment and the procedures to use to establish and maintain radio contact. Although this may sound elementary, if the people who must operate the EMS communications equipment do not understand how the equipment or the system functions, they will not use it. This leads to misunderstandings, confusion and frustration at a minimum and could result in interference or a more serious consequence, including loss of life at ALS levels. Provisions for such training should be explicitly included in ASTM standards for training of EMS personnel. See Practice F 1031*, Practice F 1149, Guide F 1229, Guide F 1287*, Guide F 1418, and F 1453*.

NOTE 1—ASTM standard numbers marked with an "*" do not include explicit provisions for communications training. Liaison should be conducted between Subcommittees F30.02 on Training and F30.04 on Communications to recommend changes to these standards. New standards being developed for the paramedic and the ambulance operator should be reviewed to ensure that appropriate communications training is included.

12. Goal 3—Local EMSS Communications Should Be Compatible With, and Should Not Interfere With, Other Types of Communications Systems

12.1 EMSS communications should be coordinated with the law enforcement, fire, emergency management services and other public safety radio systems in their areas in terms of frequency usage, site engineering, and intersystem communications.

12.2 *Objective*—EMSS frequencies should be coordinated with other public safety frequencies.

12.2.1 Radio systems have the potential for mutually interfering with collocated and nearby systems in the other public safety services, even if the systems operate on other frequencies. For this reason EMS frequency assignments, site selection, elevation, and radiated power should be coordinated and examined each time systems are modified or expanded. Such problems can usually be resolved by local communications technicians. State EMS offices should provide technical communications assistance to resolve such problems that may arise if needed technical assistance is not available locally.

12.3 *Objective*—EMSS should be "good neighbors" at shared radio sites:

12.3.1 EMS radio equipment cannot be arbitrarily installed at a site without consideration of the effect on systems already using the site. Factors to be considered include the following:

12.3.1.1 Intermodulation analysis should be performed to predict likely levels of interference.

12.3.1.2 All of the radio equipment, including EMSS, should use isolators and bandpass cavity filters.

12.3.1.3 The minimum number of antennae should be used with adequate spacing to avoid interference.

12.3.1.4 Directional antennae should be used where appropriate.

12.3.1.5 Minimum radiated power should be used.

12.4 *Objective*—EMS radio systems should be compatible with other public safety systems for multiagency operations:

12.4.1 Compatibility can be achieved in the following ways:

12.4.1.1 EMSS and other public safety radios can be equipped with one or more special common mutual operating frequencies.

12.4.1.2 EMSS radios can be equipped with some of the working frequencies of the other public safety agencies and vice versa.

12.4.1.3 Cross-channel radio patch equipment can be used to establish a temporary functional interconnection of multiple agency channels.

12.4.1.4 Verbal relay of messages by a dispatcher is possible if the dispatch communications center has base stations or control equipment, or both, on all of the multiple agency frequencies.

13. Goal 4—EMSS Communications Should Make Maximum Use of State and Common Resources Where Appropriate, Cost Effective, and Authorized

13.1 Cost savings can be achieved by sharing such resources as radio sites, microwave and telephone systems, and system services such as centralized purchasing and training. This type of sharing also promotes interchange of ideas, standardization of equipment and procedures, and effective system interfaces.

13.2 *Objective*—EMSS communication planners should be encouraged to share radio sites:

13.2.1 In many states, the advantageous mountain top radio sites have already been developed. Some of these sites are operated by state agencies such as the Department of Transportation, state police, and state educational organizations. Some sites developed for specific EMSS communications may also be usable by neighboring EMSS. The state should encourage sharing of sites by the following practices:

13.2.1.1 Identifying advantageous sites that could be shared.

13.2.1.2 Cataloging site characteristics such as location, elevation, frequencies in use, shelter, rack and tower space available, and availability of commercial and standby power and telephone service.

13.2.1.3 Developing uniform policies for cost allocation, maintenance, interference avoidance by means of appropriate use of cavities, filters, and so forth.

13.3 *Objective*—EMSS communication planners should be encouraged to share state and common system components such as microwave and telephone:

13.3.1 There are many extensive state-operated microwave systems for statewide interconnection of communication control centers and mountain-top radio sites and for support of state-owned government telephone services. These and similar resources could be advantageously used in EMSS communications for such purposes as control of remote base stations and repeaters, a backup alternative to commercial telephone facilities, and replacement of expensive leased telephone lines. To encourage sharing of these resources, states should inventory them, make their characteristics and capabilities known to EMSS planners, and develop policies for shared use.

13.4 *Objective*—EMSS communication planners should be encouraged to make effective use of state-provided services.

13.4.1 State government should act on behalf of local EMSS to take advantage of economies of scale and efficiencies not otherwise available to the local systems. Examples of opportunities in this area include the following:

13.4.1.1 Provide centralized purchasing through state contracts. This can be particularly advantageous for the purchase of EMSS radio equipment using federal grants, and it probably could be extended to cover "pooled" purchases with private funds.

13.4.1.2 Develop arrangements for statewide maintenance services.

13.4.1.3 Offer engineering design services to local EMSS communications planners.

13.4.1.4 Develop and provide standardized equipment specifications and request for proposal and contract boilerplate materials.

13.4.1.5 Offer or sponsor EMSS communications operator training programs.

14. Goal 5—The State Should Act as the Representative of Local EMSS in Dealing with Federal Agencies and National Organizations

14.1 In most states, a state EMSS director, in the state department of health acts as a fiscal agent in application and distribution of grants for EMSS from a number of federal programs. There is a need for broadening the scope of activity to encompass functions that affect EMSS statewide, may be beyond the capability of small local EMSS, and are legitimate functions for state government. Following are some examples of such functions:

14.1.1 Monitoring activity at the federal and national level including federal and private foundation grant programs, laws, and rule changes affecting EMSS communications.

14.1.2 Seeking out and securing new sources of funding.

14.1.3 Participating in the regulatory decision-making process at the federal level, particularly by commenting on FCC dockets that may impact on EMSS communications.

14.2 *Objective*—The state government should monitor federal and national level activity affecting EMSS communications:

14.2.1 The state should have a systematic mechanism for maintaining awareness of EMSS activity at the federal and national level, assessing the effects of that activity on EMSS communications, and communicating the findings to local EMSS planners. Activities of interest include:

14.2.1.1 Announcements of new federal or private foundation grant programs, changes in existing programs, and grant awards.

14.2.1.2 Significant new advances in EMSS communications technology or system management.

14.2.1.3 New or changed laws affecting EMSS.

14.2.1.4 Changes in FCC Rules and Regulations and in federal agency EMSS grant criteria.

14.3 *Objective*—The state should assist local EMSS planners in identifying and securing outside sources of funds:

14.3.1 State EMSS directors play a critical role in this area by administering grant funds for EMSS from various federal programs. The federal grant programs are generally limited to "seed funding" and at best are limited and unreliable as long range funding sources. Local funding sources are also severely limited. The need remains for specific improvements in EMSS communications. States should become active in locating and using new sources of funding such as private foundation grant programs. In some states, statutes have been enacted to raise funds for EMSS by requiring a mandatory additional financial penalty for each traffic violation. Other states have imposed a surcharge for EMSS for each renewal of a passenger motor vehicle registration.

14.4 *Objective*—The state should take an active role to influence federal communication law and rule-making decisions.

14.4.1 Local EMSS communications planners have little power and few opportunities to affect or influence the development of federal laws and regulations that have impact on them. The state government has the power to affect events at the national level and has many opportunities to do so. What is needed is an organized program to channel states efforts in this area. Such a program might include the following:

14.4.1.1 Review and comment, where appropriate, on FCC notices of inquiry and rule-making proposals affecting EMSS communications.

14.4.1.2 Review and comment on proposed regulatory changes in other federal agencies, such as NHTSA, DHHS, and FEMA.

14.4.1.3 Use of state lobbyists in matters affecting EMSS communications.

14.4.1.4 Informing state-elected representatives of the significance of issues affecting EMSS communications.

15. Goal 6—The State Should Have a Program for Positive Management of Its EMSS Communications Activities

15.1 State EMSS directors should have an EMSS communication management program to identify and resolve interstate as well as intrastate communication coordination problems.

15.2 *Objective*—EMSS communication planning should be established as an ongoing process. In developing a state plan, the planner should be cognizant of the requirements of the FCC rules and address differences between the rules and the plan. For example, the state plan may require more frequencies for specific uses above and beyond the requirements of the federal rules.

15.2.1 Current detailed guidance and information for statewide EMSS communications planning is contained in **(4)**.

15.2.2 Statewide EMSS communications planning is needed to resolve issues arising from shortages of spectrum and other uncertainties. For example, in some situations, the FCC rules permit EMSS to use radio frequencies allocated to other land mobile services such as the Special Emergency Radio Service, local Government Radio Service, Law Enforcement Radio Service, Fire Radio Service, Business Radio Service, and others. Such use, however, must meet eligibility requirements or be covered by cooperative use agreements with an existing licensee. These requirements should be considered in the planning process. Even with the creation of the Emergency Medical Radio Service, there are still insufficient radio frequencies available to meet the demands of all eligible users. Additionally, there are no specific provisions within the FCC Rules and Regulations for EMS aeromedical or helicopter communications. These unique communications, including flight following and wide range radio coverage must be addressed in future FCC rules and communications guidelines.

15.2.3 The completion of a statewide EMSS communication master plan and regional planning guidelines should be a primary planning objective. As a next step, the state should encourage and support development of subsidiary regional level plans. After that, all of the plans at all levels should be reviewed at frequent intervals (at least every two years) and adjusted to adapt to changing conditions. While these plans are important, the planning process, and continuing contacts among state and local EMSS communication planners are paramount. Only through such an ongoing planning process is it possible to get consensus on the many communication system features that must be standardized statewide if EMSS functional performance objectives are to be achieved.

15.3 *Objective*—Statewide aeromedical communications radio frequency plans should be developed and implemented to enable emergency aeromedical services to communicate with all necessary elements of other emergency medical and public safety services. These plans should include:

15.3.1 Radio frequencies for air/ground vehicle communications to ensure that any aeromedical rotor-wing aircraft can communicate with any ground EMS vehicle.

15.3.2 Radio frequencies for air/hospital communications to

ensure that any aeromedical rotor-wing aircraft can communicate with hospital emergency departments.

15.3.3 Provisions for an aeromedical communications center to ensure that any aeromedical rotor-wing aircraft can communicate with their communications center.

15.3.4 As a precondition for such planning, state EMS authorities should support for authorization of such frequencies from the Federal Communications Commission, The Federal Aviation Administration, and certified frequency coordinators.

15.4 There is a need for some type of statewide organizational structure to carry out planning, implementation, and management of regional and local EMSS communications. This structure should be made responsive to current needs by shifting the focus of its work from the pursuit of specific grant funding objectives to the more substantive concerns of system functional performance such as interregional cooperation, noninterference, utilization of shared and common resources, and overall system management. In addition, the organization must be provided with state-level technical staff support.

15.5 *Objective*—States should strengthen their own EMSS communications personnel resources and assist with local and regional personnel standards and training.

15.5.1 The agency of state government having overall responsibility for EMSS should be concerned and involved in technical communication matters. There should be a communication specialist on the state EMSS staff. This person should assume responsibility for much of the total state involvement outlined in its EMSS communication master plan including observance of functional performance standards, arbitration of intersystem interference problems, development of compatibility standards, promotion of sharing of state and common resources, interface with federal and national organizations, and overall communication program management.

15.5.2 In addition, the state should help regional and local systems in certain personnel areas. For example, the state should establish qualifications and standards for EMSS communication operators along the lines of existing EMT standards. The state should also provide or sponsor communication training programs for communication center operators (professional telecommunicators), hospital communication equipment operators (doctors and nurses), and mobile communication equipment operators (EMTs).

15.5.3 The State EMS authority should participate in the frequency coordination process required under Section 90.27 of FCC Rules to assist eligible nongovernmental applicants to obtain licenses from the FCC to operate on the EMRS frequencies. This requires coordination with the International Municipal Signal Association (IMSA) and the International Association of Fire Chiefs (IAFC), which are the Federal Communication Commission recognized frequency coordinators for the Emergency Medical Radio Service and the Special Emergency Radio Service.

15.5.3.1 For radio license applications by entities in the EMRS, FCC Rules Section 90.27 requires that an application be accompanied by a statement prepared by the governmental body having jurisdiction over the state's emergency medical service plans indicating that the applicant is included in the state's emergency plan or otherwise supporting the application. The essential components of this statement attest that: the applicant provides basic or advanced life support services on a ongoing basis, the application is in conformance with (or not in conflict with) the state's EMC communications plan, and the statement is supported by an authorized signature.

15.5.3.2 The state office of emergency medical service should establish a method by which the statement (letter or authorization) is provided. This authorization procedure should be documented and filed with the IMSA/IAFC frequency coordinator. There should be a method established to determine the applicant's eligibility under the FCC's Rules. The state EMS Director, or his designee, is normally the signatory for establishing this eligibility. The designated person must be knowledgeable of the technical aspects of the EMS communications systems within the state.

15.6 *Objective*—The state should provide positive direction by means of laws, rules, and funding policies.

15.6.1 Generally, state laws and regulations regarding communications are nonexistent or weak because of preeminence of FCC Rules and Regulations relative to communications. Ways should be sought by states to regulate communications in matters affecting the safety of life, as with EMSS communications. One obvious need is regional and local adherence to the statewide EMS communication master plan, when approved, should be mandatory. There should be legal minimum qualifications and requirements for EMSS communication operators since these people are just as important to patient safety and well-being as EMTs, and the state should ensure that they are well-qualified. State-level management responsibilities and organizational structures for EMSS communications should be clearly defined in state law.

15.7 *Objective*—Mechanisms should be developed to provide for feedback of information on EMSS communications, evaluation of the information, and corrective action.

15.7.1 These mechanisms could include methods such as the use of periodic questionnaires, meetings, and problem referrals. They could also extend to more direct and forceful methods such as an inspection program. In general, the state should assist local communications managers in early identification of problems and prompt and effective solutions.

16. Keywords

16.1 emergency medical services; telecommunications

APPENDIXES

(Nonmandatory Information)

X1. EMERGENCY MEDICAL RADIO SERVICE (EMRS) FREQUENCIES (MHz)

X1.1 VHF High Band

X1.1.1 *Base or Mobile*:

155.325 ... Biomedical telemetry allowed in some areas.[6]
155.340 ... Biomedical telemetry allowed in some areas.

X1.1.1.1 May be designated by common consent as an intersystem mutual assistance frequency under an area-wide medical communications plan.

155.355 ... Biomedical telemetry allowed in some areas.[6]
155.385 ... Biomedical telemetry allowed in some areas.[6]
155.400 ... Biomedical telemetry allowed in some areas.[6]

X1.1.2 *Mobile-only*:

150.775
150.790

X1.1.3 *Base/Mobile:*

220.9025/221.9025[7]
220.9075/221.9075[7]
220.9125/221.9125[7]
220.9175/221.9175[7]
200.9225/221.9225[7]
220.8025/221.8025.Public Safety/Mutual Aid (except PS)[7]
220.8075/221.8075.Public Safety/Mutual Aid (except PS)[7]
220.8125/221.8125.Public Safety/Mutual Aid (except PS)[7]
220.8175/221.8175.Public Safety/Mutual Aid (except PS)[7]
220.8225/221.8225.Public Safety/Mutual Aid (except PS)[7]
220.8275/221.8275.Public Safety/Mutual Aid (except PS)[7]
220.8325/221.8325.Public Safety/Mutual Aid (except PS)[7]
220.8375/221.8375.Public Safety/Mutual Aid (except PS)[7]
220.8425/221.8425.Public Safety/Mutual Aid (except PS)[7]
220.8475/221.8475.Public Safety/Mutual Aid (except PS)[7]

X1.2 *UHF Band:*

X1.2.1 *Base/Mobile*:

453.025/458.025 . . Biomedical telemetry permitted.[8,9]
453.075/458.075 . . Biomedical telemetry permitted.[8,9]
453.125/458.125 . . Biomedical telemetry permitted.[8,9]
453.175/458.175 . . Biomedical telemetry permitted.[8,9]
460.525/465.525 . . Shared with Police and Fire services[10]
460.550/465.550 . . Shared with Police and Fire services[10]
462.950/467.950 . . MED 9—Vehicle Coordination[11,12]
462.975/467.975 . . MED 10—Vehicle Coordination[11,12]
463.000/468.000 . . MED 1—Medical Coordination[13]
463.025/468.025 . . MED 2—Medical Coordination[12]
463.050/468.050 . . MED 3—Medical Coordination[13]
463.075/468.075 . . MED 4—Medical Coordination[13]
463.100/468.100 . . MED 5—Medical Coordination[14]
463.125/468.125 . . MED 6—Medical Coordination[14]
463.150/468.150 . . MED 7—Medical Coordination[14]
463.175/468.175 . . MED 8—Medical Coordination[14]

X1.2.2 *Shared With All Other Public Safety Radio Services:*

453.050/458.050	453.400/458.400	453.750/458.750
453.100/458.100	453.450/458.450	453.800/458.800
453.150/458.150	453.500/458.500	453.850/458.850
453.200/458.200	453.550/458.550	453.900/458.900
453.250/458.250	453.600/458.600	453.950/458.950
453.300/458.300	453.650/458.650	
453.350/458.350	453.700/458.700	

X1.3 *90.53 Frequencies Available:*

X1.3.1 Table X1.1 indicates frequencies available for assignment to stations in the Special Emergency Radio Service, together with the class of station(s) to which they are normally assigned and the specific assignment limitations that are explained in X1.3.2. (Frequencies below 450 MHz indicated for base or mobile stations may be authorized to fixed stations on a secondary basis to stations in the mobile service):

X1.3.2 Explanation of assignment limitations appearing in Table X1.1:

(1) Appropriate frequencies in the band 2000 to 3000 kHz which are designated in Part 80 of this chapter as available to Public Ship Stations for telephone communications with Public Coast Stations may be assigned on a secondary basis to Special Emergency fixed stations for communication with Public Coast Stations only, provided such stations are located in the United States and the following conditions are met:

(i) That such fixed station is established pursuant to the eligibility provisions of §90.47 and that the isolated area involved in an island or other location not more than 480 km (300 statute miles) removed from the desired point of communication and isolated from that point by water.

(ii) That evidence is submitted showing that an arrangement has been made with the coast station licensee for the

[6] Licensees may transmit one-way alert paging to ambulance and rescue squad personnel on a secondary basis on these frequencies.

[7] See FCC Rules 47 CFR, Subpart T for "Regulations Governing Licensing and Use of Frequencies in the 220-222 MHz Band".

[8] Paging licenses as of March 20, 1991 may continue to operate on a primary basis until January 14, 1998.

[9] Highway radio call box operations first licensed before March 31, 1980 permitted in accordance with FCC Rules §90.17(c) **(11)**.

[10] Intra- and inter-system mutual assistance allowed.

[11] Licensees may transmit one-way alert paging to ambulance and rescue squad personnel on a secondary basis on these frequencies.

[12] This frequency is primarily authorized for use in the dispatch of medical care vehicles and personnel for the rendition of medical services. This frequency may also be assigned for intra- and inter-system mutual assistance. The frequency pairs 462.950/467.950 and 462.975/467.975 may be referred to as MED-9 and MED-10, respectively.

[13] This frequency is authorized for use for operations in biomedical telemetry stations. Entities eligible in this Radio Service may use this frequency on a secondary basis for any other permissible communications consistent with FCC Rules 90.27(a).

[14] This frequency is authorized for communications between medical facilities and personnel related to medical supervision and instruction for the treatment and transport of patients in the rendition or delivery of medical services. Entities eligible in this Radio Service may use this frequency on a secondary basis for any other permissible communications consistent with FCC Rules 90.27(a).

TABLE X1.1 Special Emergency Radio Service Frequency Table

Frequency or Band	Class of Station(s)	Limitations
Kilohertz:		
2000 to 3000	Fixed	1
2726	Base or mobile	2
3201	do	...
Megahertz:		
33.02	do	3, 25
33.04	do	25
33.06	do	3, 25
33.08	do	25
33.10	do	3, 25
35.02	Mobile	27
35.64	Base	4
35.68	do	4
37.90	Base or mobile	3, 25
37.94	do	3, 25
37.98	do	3, 25
43.64	Base	4, 28
43.68	do	4
45.92	Base or mobile	25
45.96	do	25
46.00	do	25
46.04	do	25
47.42	do	5, 25
47.46	do	25
47.50	do	25
47.54	do	25
47.58	do	25
47.62	do	25
47.66	do	25
72.00 to 76.00	Operational-fixed	6
150 to 170	Base or mobile	30
Megahertz:		
152.0075	Base	4, 31
155.160	Base or mobile	25
155.175	do	25
155.205	do	25
155.220	do	25
155.235	do	25
155.265	do	25
155.280	do	25
155.295	do	25
157.450	Base	4, 11
163.250	do	4
169–172	Mobile	33
450–470	Fixed	12
453.025	Base	26
453.075	do	26
453.125	do	26
453.175	do	26
Megahertz:		
806 to 824	Mobile	21
851 to 869	Base or mobile	21
928 and above	Operational-fixed	22
929 to 930	Base only	7
1427 to 1435	Operational-fixed, base or mobile	23
2450 to 2500	Base or mobile	24
10 550 to 10 680	do	9

handling of emergency communications permitted by §80.453 and §90.47(d) of this chapter.

(iii) That operation of the special emergency fixed station shall at no time conflict with any provision of Part 80 of this chapter and further, that such operation in general shall conform to the practices employed by Public Ship Stations for radiotelephone communication with the same Public Coast Station.

(2) This frequency is shared with the Local Government Radio Service where it is available for state guard operations.

(3) This frequency is shared with the Highway Maintenance Radio Service.

(4) This frequency will be assigned only for one-way paging communications to mobile receivers. Transmissions for the purpose of activating or controlling remote objects on this frequency are not authorized.

(5) This frequency is reserved for assignment only to national organizations eligible for disaster relief operation under§ 90.41.

(6) The frequencies available for use at operational fixed stations in the band 72 to 76 MHz are listed in §90.257(a) (1). These frequencies are shared with other services and are available only in accordance with the provisions of §90.257.

(7) Frequencies in this band are available only for one-way paging operations in accordance with §90.494 of this part.

(8) (Reserved).

(9) The frequencies in the band 10.55 to 10.68 GHz are available for digital termination systems and for associated internodal links in the Point-to-Point Microwave Radio Service. No new licenses will be issued under this subpart but current licenses will be renewed.

(10) (Reserved).

(11) Operations on this frequency are limited to 30-W transmitter output power.

(12) The requirements for secondary fixed use of frequencies in this band are set forth in §90.261.

(13) (Reserved).

(14) (Reserved).

(15) (Reserved).

(16) (Reserved).

(17) (Reserved).

(18) (Reserved).

(19) (Reserved).

(20) (Reserved).

(21) Subpart S contains rules for assignment of frequencies in the 806- to 824-MHz and 851- to 869-MHz bands.

(22) Assignment of frequencies above 928 MHz for operational-fixed stations is governed by Part 94 of this chapter.

(23) This frequency band is available in this service subject to the provisions of §90.259.

(24) Available only on a shared basis with stations in other services, and subject to no protection from interference as a result of the operation of industrial, scientific, or medical (ISM) devices. In the 2483.5- to 2500-MHz band, no applications for new or modification to existing stations to increase the number of transmitters will be accepted. Existing licensees as of July 25, 1985, or on a subsequent date following as a result of submitting an application for license on or before July 25, 1985, are grandfathered and their operation is coprimary with the Radio Determination Satellite Service.

(25) A licensee regularly conducting two-way communication operations on this frequency may, on a secondary basis, also transmit one-way alert-paging signals to ambulance and rescue squad personnel.

(26) Paging licensees as of March 20, 1991 may continue to operate on a primary basis until January 14, 1998.

(27) This frequency is available in this service only to persons eligible under the provisions of §90.38(a) for operation of transmitters having a maximum power output of 3 W using

A1A, A1D, A2B, A2D, F1B, F1D, F2B, F2D, G1B, G1D, G2B, or G2D emission. This frequency is also available in the Business Radio Service on a coequal basis with the Special Emergency Radio Service users.

(28) No new licenses will be granted for one-way paging under§ 90.487 for use on this frequency after August 1, 1980. This frequency is available to persons eligible for station licenses under the provisions of §90.38(a) on a coequal basis with one-way paging users under §90.487 before August 1, 1985 and on a primary basis after August 1, 1985. Only A1A, A1D, A2B, A2D, F1B, F1D, F2B, F2D, G1B, G1D, G2B, G2D emissions and power not exceeding 10 W will be authorized. Antennas having gain greater than 0 dBd will not be authorized. Transmissions shall not exceed a 2-s duration.

(29) (Reserved).

(30) Rules concerning the use of this band for narrowband operations are set forth in §90.271.

(31) This frequency is removed by 22.5 kHz from frequencies assigned to other radio services. Utilization of this frequency may result in, as well as be subject to, interference under certain operating conditions. In considering the use of this frequency, adjacent channel operations should be taken into consideration. If interference occurs, the licensee may be required to take the necessary steps to resolve the problem. See §90.173(b).

(32) (Reserved).

(33) Frequencies in this band will be assigned for low power wireless microphones in accordance with the provisions of§ 90.265.

(34) (Reserved).

(c) Additional frequencies available. In addition to the frequencies shown in the frequency table of this section, the following frequencies are available in this service. (See also §90.253.)

(1) Substitution of frequencies available below 25 MHz may be made in accordance with the provisions of§ 90.263.

(2) (Reserved).

(3) Frequencies in the band 73.0 to 74.6 MHz may be assigned to stations authorizing their use on or before December 1, 1961, but no new stations will be authorized in this band, nor will expansion of existing systems be permitted. (See also §90.257.)

(4) The frequency bands 31.99 to 32.00 MHz, 33.00 to 33.01 MHz, 33.99 to 34.00 MHz, 37.93 to 38.00 MHz, 39.00 to 39.01 MHz, 39.99 to 40.00 MHz, and 42.00 to 42.01 MHz are available for assignment for developmental operation subject to the provisions of Subpart Q.

(5) Frequencies in the 421- to 430-MHz band are available in the Detroit, Cleveland, and Buffalo areas in accordance with the rules in §§90.273 through 90.281.

(d) Limitation on number of frequencies assignable. Normally only one frequency below 450 MHz will be assigned for mobile service operations by a single applicant in a given area. The assignment of an additional frequency will be made only upon a satisfactory showing of need, except that:

(1) Additional frequencies above 25 MHz may be assigned in connection with the operation of mobile repeaters in accordance with §90.247, notwithstanding this limitation.

(2) An additional frequency may be assigned for paging operations from those frequencies available under §90.53(b)(4).

(3) The frequency 155.340 MHz may be assigned as an additional frequency when it is designated as a mutual assistance frequency as provided in §90.53(b)(10).

(4) Additional frequencies may be assigned for fixed station operations.

(5) Frequencies in the 25 to 50 MHz, 150 to 170 MHz, and 450 to 512 MHz bands, and the frequency bands 903 to 904 MHz, 904 to 912 MHz, 918 to 926 MHz, and 926 to 927 MHz may be assigned for the operation of automatic vehicle monitoring (AVM) systems in accordance with §90.239, notwithstanding this limitation.

X2. ACRONYMS AND GLOSSARY FOR EMS COMMUNICATIONS

X2.1 Acronyms

A

AAT—above average terrain.
AC—alternating current.
ACD—automatic call distributor.
ACLS—advanced cardiac life support.
ACSB—amplitude compandored single-sideband.
ADP—automatic data processing.
AGL—above ground level.
ALS—advanced life support.
ALERT—automatic law enforcement response team.
ALI—automatic location identification.
AM—amplitude modulation.
AMSL—above mean sea level.
ANI—automatic number identification.
APB—all points bulletin.
APCO—Associated Public-Safety Communications Officers.
ASCII—American standard code for information interchange.
ASTM—American Society for Testing and Materials.
ASTRA—Automated Statewide Telecommunications and Records Access.
ATLS—Advanced Trauma Life Support.
AT&T—American Telephone and Telegraph Company.
AVC—automatic volume control.
AVI—automatic vehicle identification.

B

balun—balanced-to-unbalanced line transformer.
BCD—binary coded decimal.
BFO—beat frequency oscillator.
BIT—binary digit.
BLS—basic life support.
BPS—bits per second.
BSC—binary synchronous communications.

C

C—Celsius.
CAD—computer-aided dispatch.
CB—citizens band.
CCH—computerized criminal history.
CCITT—International Telegraph and Telephone Consultative Committee.
CCSA—common control switching arrangement.
CCTV—closed circuit television.
CCU—Coronary Care Unit or Critical Care Unit.
CDC—Cooperative Dispatch Center.
CG—Channel Guard (R) Trademark of General Electric.
CMED—Central Medical Emergency Dispatch.
CMR—Common Mode Rejection.
CMRR—Common Mode Rejection Ratio.
CNIL—Calling Number Identification and Location.
CO—Central Office.
COG—Council of Governments.
COR—Coronary Observation Radio.
CPR—cardiopulmonary resuscitation.
CJIS—Criminal Justice Information System.
CTCSS—continuous tone controlled squelch system.

D

dB—decibel.
dBm—decibel referenced to 1 mW.
dBu—decibel referenced to 1 μV/m.
dBv—decibel referenced to 1 V.
dBW—decibel referenced to 1 W.
DC—direct current.
DCS—Division of Computer Services.
DDD—direct distance dialing.
DID—direct inward dialing.
dod—direct outward dialing.
DOD—U.S. Department of Defense.
DOT—U.S. Department of Transportation.
DRG—diagnosis related grouping.
DP—double pole.
DPDT—double pole double throw.
DTMF—dual-tone multifrequency.
DPST—double pole single throw.

E

EACOM—emergency and administrative communications system.
EAS—extended area service.
E & M—the receive and transmit leads of a signaling system.
EAX—electronic automatic exchange.
ECC—emergency communications center.
ECG—electrocardiogram.
EDP—electronic data processing.
EIA—Electronic Industries Association.
EMD—emergency medical dispatcher.
EMF—electromotive force.
EKG—electrocardiogram.
EMDPRS—emergency medical dispatch priority reference system.
EMS—emergency medical service.
EMSS—emergency medical service system.
EMT—emergency medical technician.
EMT-B—emergency medical technician-basic.
EMT-AI—emergency medical technician-advanced intermediate.
—emergency medical technician-defibrillator.
EMT-I—emergency medical technician-intermediate.
EMT-IV—emergency medical technician-intraveneous certified.
EMT-P—emergency medical technician-paramedic.
EOC—emergency operations center.
EOM—end of message.
ERCC—emergency resource coordination center.
ERP—effective radiated power.
ESS—electronic switching system.
EST—Eastern Standard Time.
ETA—Estimated Time of Arrival.
ETV—Educational Television.

F

F—Fahrenheit.
FCC—U.S. Federal Communications Commission.
FCCA—Forestry Conservation Communications Association.

FEMA—Federal Emergency Management Agency.
FET—field-effect transistor.
FM—frequency modulation.
freq.—frequency.
FORTRAN—formula translation (computer language).
FSK—frequency-shift keying.
FX—foreign exchange.

G

GE—General Electric.
GESS—General Electric Service Station.
GFW—ground fault warning.
GHz—gigahertz (1000 MHz).
GIGO—garbage in, garbage out.
GMT—Greenwich mean time (Zulu).
GSA—General Services Administration.
GT&E—General Telephone and Electronics.

H

HEAR—hospital emergency administrative radio.
HF—high frequency.
HYSIS—highway safety information system.
HV—high voltage.
Hz—hertz.

I

I—current in amperes.
IAFC—International Association of Fire Chiefs.
IACP—International Association of Chiefs of Police.
IC—integrated circuit.
ICO—individual channel oscillator.
ICOM—integrated circuit oscillator module.
ICU—intensive care unit.
ICX—intercity exchange link.
IEEE—Institute of Electrical and Electronic Engineers.
IF—intermediate frequency.
IMSA—International Municipal Signal Association.
IMTS—improved mobile telephone service.
IRAC—interdepartmental radio advisory committee.
ISPERN—Illinois State Police Emergency Radio Network.
IT&T—International Telephone and Telegraph Corporation.
ITU—International Telecommunication Union.

J

JAN—Joint Army-Navy Specifications.
JETEC—joint electron tube engineering council.
JFET—junction field-effect transistor.
JEMS—Journal of Emergency Medical Services.

K

kbps—kilobits per second.
kHz—kilohertz (1000 hertz).

L

LATA—local access transport area.
LMR—land mobile radio.
LEAA—law enforcement assistance administration.
LETS—Law Enforcement Teletypewriter Service.
LORAN—long-range navigation.
LSI—large-scale integration.
LOS—line of sight.
LRO—lead regional organization.
LSU—life support unit.

M

MAST—Military Assistance to Safety and Traffic.
MCCU—mobile coronary care unit.
MF—medium frequency.
MHz—megahertz.
MICT—Mobile Intensive Care Technician.
MICU—Mobile Intensive Care Unit.
MRCC—Medical Resource Coordination Center.

N

NABER—National Association of Business and Educational Radio, Inc.
NCIC—National Crime Information Center.
NCMCN—North Carolina Medical Communications Network.
NEAR—National Emergency Aid Radio.
NHTSA—National Highway Traffic Safety Administration.
NLETS—National Law Enforcement Telecommunications System.
—see definition in glossary section.
NPA—number plan area.

O

O-D—origin-destination.
ONI—operator number identification.
OTP—Office of Telecommunications Policy.

P

PABX—Private Automatic Branch Exchange.
PBX—Private Branch Exchange.
PL—Private Line (R) Trademark of Motorola.
PM—Pulse Modulation.
PSAP—public safety answering point.
PSCC—Public Safety Communications Council.
PTT—press to transmit or push to talk.

Q

QEI—quantifiable evaluation indicator.

R

RCU—remote control unit.
RF—radio frequency.
Rx—receive.

S

SERS—Special Emergency Radio Service.
SIRSA—Special Industrial Radio Service Association, Inc.
SMR—Specialized Mobile Radio.
SMSA—standard metropolitan statistical area.
SPA—State Planning Agency.
SWR—Standing Wave Radio.

T

TASI—time assignment speech interpolation.
TCAM—telecommunications access method.
Telco—telephone company.
TELPAK—see definition in glossary section.
TPL—terminal per line.
TPS—terminal per station.
TSPS—see definition in Glossary section.
Tx—transmit.

U

UHF—ultra-high frequency.
UL—Underwriters Laboratories, Inc.
UPS—uninterruptible power supply.
USITA—U.S. Independent Telephone Association.
USFS—U.S. Forest Service.

V

V—volts.
VAC—volts, alternating current.
VDC—volts, direct current.
VHF—very high frequency.
VOM—volt-ohm meter.
VOR—voice operated relay.
VOX—voice operated switch.
VSWR—voltage standing wave ratio.
VTVM—vacuum tube voltmeter.
VU—Volume Unit.

W

WATS—Wide Area Telephone Service.
WECO—Western Electric Company.
WPM—words per minute.

X

Xcvr.—transceiver.
Xfmr.—transformer.
Xmit.—transmit.
Xmtr.—transmitter.
Xtal—crystal.

Z

Z—impedance.
ZULU—time zone at Greenwich, England.

X2.2 FCC Codes and Names of Radio Services

Industrial:
IB—business
IF—forest products
IM—motion picture
IP—petroleum
IS—special industrial
IT—telephone maintenance
IW—power
IX—manufacturers
IY—relay press

Motor Carrier:
LI—interurban passenger
LJ—interurban property
LU—urban passenger
LV—urban property

Land Transportation:
LA—automobile emergency
LR—railroad
LX—taxicab

Public Safety:
PF —fire
PH —highway maintenance
PL—local government
PP —police
PO —forestry conservation
PS—special emergency
RS—radiolocation
ZA—general mobile

Classes of Radio Stations (FCC):
FB—base
FB2—mobile relay
FB4—community repeater
FX1—control
MO—mobile
MO3—mobile/vehicular repeater
FXO—operational fixed
FX2—fixed relay
FX—fixed
FLT—auxiliary test
FXY—interzone
FXZ—zone
LR—radio location
MR—radio location mobile

806- to 821-/851- to 866-MHz Bands:

Conventional	Category	Trunked
GB	business	YB
GO	industrial/land transportation	YO
GP	public safety/special emergency	YP
GX	commercial (SMRS)	YX

929 to 930-MHz Band:
GS—private carrier paging systems

X2.3 Glossary

X2.3.1

A

acoustic feedback—the transfer of sound waves from a loud speaker or end terminal to any previous component within an audio system, such as a microphone. Acoustic feedback may be audible, subaudible, or superaudible.

activity—the expenditure of time and resources.

adapter—a device used for changing the terminal connections of a circuit or part to connect to another circuit or part with unlike connections.

alphabet, phonetic—a method of passing alphabetic information over a poor communication path with word substitution for letters. One phonetic alphabet is: Alfa; Bravo; Charlie; Delta; Echo; Foxtrot; Golf; Hotel; India; Juliett; Kilo; Lima; Mike; November; Oscar; Papa; Quebec; Romeo; Sierra; Tango; Uniform; Victor; Whiskey; X-ray; Yankee; Zulu.

American Standard Code for Information Interchange (ASCII)—an eight-level code for data transfer adopted by the American Standards Association to achieve compatibility between data devices.

amplitude compandored single-sideband—a form of sideband modulation used for narrow channel transmission that incorporates a pilot tone.

amplitude modulation (AM)—modulation in which the amplitude of the carrier-frequency current is varied above and below its normal value in accordance with the audio, picture, or other intelligence signal to be transmitted.

analog—physical representation of information such that the representation bears an exact relationship to the original information. Pertaining to data in the form of continuously variable physical qualities.

analog communication—system of telecommunications

used to transmit information other than voice which is sometimes used in telemetry.

antenna—a system of wires or electrical conductors used for reception or transmission of radio waves. Specifically, a radiator that couples the transmission line or lead-in to space for transmission or reception of electromagnetic radio waves. It changes electrical currents into electromagnetic radio waves and vice versa.

antenna, isotropic—a theoretical antenna with identical radiation in every direction.

antenna, parabolic—a directional antenna with a radiating (or receiving) element and a paraboloid reflector that concentrates the power into a beam.

antenna polarization—the direction of the radiated electric field in relation to the surface of the earth. Generally vertical in mobile radio use.

arc—a discharge of electricity.

arrester, lightning—a device designed to protect electrical equipment or property from damage by lightning.

assigned frequency—the frequency appearing on a station authorization from which the carrier frequency may deviate by an amount not to exceed that permitted by the frequency tolerance.

Associated Public-Safety Communications Officers (APCO) —a nonprofit public safety radio users group composed of administrators and communications technical, operations, and command personnel.[15]

ASTM—a scientific and technical organization formed for the development of standards on characteristics and performance of materials, products, systems, and services.[16]

attack time—the interval required after a sudden increase in input signal to a transducer (transmitter, receiver, and so forth) to attain a percentage of final output level as a result of this increase.

attenuation—the decrease in amplitude of a signal during its transmission from one point to another. It may be expressed as a ratio or, by extension of the term, in decibels.

attenuator—a device for reducing the energy of a wave without introducing distortion. Also called a pad, gain control, level adjustor, volume control, and so forth.

audible signal—a buzzer, bell, or other audible sound device that indicates an incoming call.

audio—pertaining to frequencies corresponding to normally audible sound waves. These frequencies range from 15 to 20 000 Hz.

aural—pertaining to the ear or sound.

automatic gain control (AGC)—a receiver circuit that maintains the output constant with wide variations in the receiver input level.

automatic volume control (AVC)—a self-acting gain control that maintains the output of a receiver constant despite variations in received signal strength.

automatic number identification (ANI)—equipment for recording the calling party's number without operator intervention.

B

back bone—a point-to-point communications system using several stations.

back-to-back repeater—a repeater consisting of a receiver and transmitter with the output of the receiver connected directly to the input of the transmitter.

band (radio frequency)—a range of frequencies between two definite limits. By international agreement, the radio spectrum is divided into nine bands. For example, the very high-frequency (VHF) band extends from 30 to 300 MHz.

bandpass filter—passes frequencies within a specified band and attenuates all frequencies outside that band.

bandwidth—(1) the width of a band of frequencies used for a particular purpose and (2) the range of frequencies within which a performance characteristic of a device is above specified limits. For filters, attenuators, and amplifiers these limits are generally taken to be 3 dB (half-power) below the average level.

baseband—for microwave systems, the available frequency band that the RF equipment is capable of transmitting.

base station—an item of fixed radio hardware consisting of a transmitter and a receiver.

baud—used to define the operating speed of a printing telegraph or data system. It is the total number of discrete conditions or signal events per second.

baudot code—a five-unit code used for teletypewriter signals.

beacon—a radio transmitter or lights designed to indicate exact geographical location or direction.

beam—a configuration of radiated energy whose rays are sharply directional and parallel.

beat—a regularly recurring pulsation from the combination of two-tone or frequency waves of different frequencies.

beat frequency—the frequency produced when signals of two different frequencies are combined and refracted. The beat frequency is equal in value to the difference between the original frequencies.

bel—a unit of relative power, named after Alexander Graham Bell, and used to express differences in power.

beeper—a pocket-paging receiver that emits a beeping sound upon receiving a page specifically directed to it.

biomedical telemetry (biotelemetry)—the technique of monitoring or measuring vital biological parameters and transmitting data to a receiving point at a remote location.

Biophone—trade name of Biocom, Inc. for portable telemetry devices.

bit—a unit of digital information (abbreviation of "binary digit").

boom microphone—a microphone arranged on an arm-type mechanical support to permit better placement of the microphone.

braid—a group of fibrous or metal filaments or threads woven into a cylindrical shape to form a covering over one or more wires.

broadcast—radio or television transmission intended for general reception.

Business Radio Service—a subpart of the Industrial Radio

[15] Headquarters office is in New Smyrna Beach, FL 32070.

[16] ASTM Committee F30 is developing consensus standards for emergency medical services. ASTM Headquarters is in West Conshohocken, PA.

Services section of the FCC rules.

busy indicator—an indicator provided at a control point to indicate the in use condition of a circuit or channel.

C

cable—one or more insulated or noninsulated wires used to conduct electrical current or impulses. Grouped insulated wires are called a multiconductor cable.

calibrate—to determine error by comparison with a known standard.

call, all—the alerting of all decoder-equipped units in a system by the transmission of a single coded signal.

call, group—the alerting of subdivided selective call groups by function, type of vehicle, location, and so forth by sending a single coded signal.

call, individual—the alerting of a specific coded decoder unit by sending a single coded signal.

call answerer—the initial answerer of a call for assistance whether by 9-1-1 or other telephone method.

call sign—Federal Communications Commission assigned identifying letters and numbers used for identification of a radio station, transmitter, or transmission.

call referral method—the calling party is referred to a secondary number.

call relay method—the call is answered at the PSAP where the pertinent information is gathered and then the interrogator relays the information to the proper public safety agency for their action. This can be accomplished by radio, intercom, telephone, and so forth.

call transfer method—the PSAP interrogator determines the proper responding agency and connects the user to that agency which then performs the necessary dispatching in accordance with prearranged plans with cooperating agencies.

call party hold—enables the public safety answering point to control the connection for confirmation and tracing of a call.

capture effect—an effect occurring in FM reception when the stronger of two signals on the same frequency suppresses the weaker signal.

cardioid microphone—a microphone having a heart-shaped space response pattern of 180° in front and minimum response in the rear.

carrier—a radio signal generally without voice or other information.

carrier control timer (CCT)—a device that limits the length of time that the transmitter carrier is on.

carrier frequency—the frequency of an unmodulated electromagnetic wave produced by the transmitter.

cavity resonator—a space enclosed by a metal conductor in which oscillating electromagnetic energy is stored and whose resonant frequency is determined by the geometry of the enclosure.

cellular radio—a commercially available mobile or portable radio telephone service.

Celsius—the metric scale of temperature in which water freezes at 0° and boils at 100°C. To convert a Celsius temperature to Fahrenheit, multiple by 9/5 and add 32.

central medical emergency dispatch (CMED)—see **command and control center**.

central office—sometimes called a wire center; the smallest subdivision within the telephone system which has relatively permanent geographic boundaries.

change out—to replace.

channel element—a temperature-compensated crystal oscillator.

channel guard—General Electric's trademark for continuous tone-coded squelch system (CTCSS).

channel, point-to-point—a radio channel used for radio communications between two definite fixed stations.

channel, radio—an assigned band of radio frequencies of sufficient width to permit its use for radio communication. The necessary width of a channel depends on the type of transmission and the tolerance for the frequency of emission.

channel, television—a band of radio frequencies 6 MHz wide used for television broadcast.

channelization—the assignment of circuits to channels and the arrangement of those channels into groups.

charge—to replenish the electrical potential in a battery or capacitor.

charge, fast or quick—a method of quickly recharging batteries under controlled conditions.

charge, trickle—the continuous charge of a battery at a slow rate.

chart, 4/3 earth's radius—a radio profile chart whose horizontal lines are curved to correspond to an earth having a radius ⁴⁄₃ times larger than actual earth radius.

chassis—the framework on which parts of a radio or other electronic circuits are mounted.

circuit merit—a rating of overall circuit quality. Circuit merit '5' is clear circuit. Merit '3' is readable with noise. Any rating below '3' is not readable and generally unacceptable.

class of service—service order code designation of the combination of telephone service features (equipment, calling area units, dial types) to which business and residence customers subscribe. It is used for rating, identification, and assignment purposes.

coaxial cable—a transmission line in which one conductor completely surrounds the other, the two being coaxial and separated by a continuous solid dielectric or by dielectric spacers.

code dialing—a method of signaling or encoding and decoding address codes by the use of standard telephone dial.

command and control center (central communications center)—a system that is responsible for establishing communications channels and identifying the necessary equipment and facilities to permit immediate management and control of an EMS patient. This operation must provide access and availability to public safety resources essential to the effective and efficient EMS management of the immediate EMS problem.

common mode rejection (CMR)—the ability of a differential amplifier to reject unwanted signals.

communications subsystem—comprises those resources and arrangements for notifying the EMS system of an emergency, for mobilizing and dispatching resources, for exchanging information, for remote monitoring of vital indicators, and for the radio transmission of treatment procedures and directions.

communications system—a collection of individual communication networks, transmission system, relay stations, control and base stations, capable of interconnection and interoperations that are designed to form an integral whole. The individual components must serve a common purpose, be technically compatible, use common procedures, respond to control, and operate in unison.

comparator—a circuit that compares two or more signals and selects the strongest or best.

compression—in audio systems, reducing the volume range of the input signal so that the minimum output has less noise and the maximum output has less distortion.

compressor—a variable gain audio device used to provide a relatively constant output level for a wide range of varying input levels.

computer—an electrical device that can accept information, process it mathematically in accordance with previous instructions, and provide the results of this processing.

cone of silence—the area directly over or under a vertical transmitting antenna in which little or no signal is radiated.

console—a cabinet housing electronic circuitry normally used in controlling other equipment such as transmitters and receivers installed at a remote location.

continuous tone-controlled squelch system (CTCSS)—a system wherein radio receiver(s) are equipped with a tone responsive device which allows audio signals to appear at the receiver audio output only when a carrier modulated with a specific tone is received. The tone must be continuously present for continuous audio output. CTCSS functions are sometimes referred to by various trade names such as private line or PL (Motorola Communications & Electronics), Channel Guard or CG (General Electric Mobile Radio), or Quiet Channel (RCA).

control console—a desk-mounted, enclosed piece of equipment which contains a number of controls or circuits used to operate a radio station.

control head—a device with appropriate controls, microphone, volume, squelch, on/off, and so forth, generally mounted in a vehicle, from which control of the radio or mobile unit is performed.

control point—a position from which a radio system is controlled and supervised.

control, remote—a control scheme for a radio system in which all control functions are performed remotely via telephone lines.

consolette—(1) Motorola Communications name for a desk top radio station and (2) a device for mounting a mobile microphone, control head and speaker.

continuous duty—(1) an unending transmission, (2) operating 100 % of the time, (3) EIA—full-load output under the manufacturers normal loading conditions for the class of service for 24 h.

control, local—a control system packaged with the control unit mounted directly on the base station.

coordination, frequency—the cooperative selection and allocation of radio frequencies such that all systems can operate with minimum interference.

couple—to connect two circuits so that signals are transferred from one to the other.

coverage—in a radio communications system, the geographic area where reliable communications exist; usually expressed in terms of miles extending radially from a fixed radio station.

crosstalk—the unwanted transfer of energy from one communication circuit to another by means of a mutual coupling.

crystal—a piece of quartz or similar material that has been ground thin and to the proper size to produce vibrations at the desired frequency. Used in radio transmission to generate, with a high degree of accuracy, the assigned carrier frequency of a station.

cut over—to transfer from one system to another.

cycle—one complete reversal of an alternating current, including a rise to the maximum level in one direction and a return to zero. The number of cycles occurring in 1 s is the frequency of the current. The word cycle is commonly used to mean cycles per second (now called hertz).

D

dBm—decibels referenced to 1 mW. Used in communication work as a measure of absolute power. Zero dBm equals 1 mW.

dBV—decibels referenced to 1 V.

dBW—decibels relative to 1 W (1 dBw = 30 dBm).

decibel (dB)—a unit that expresses the level of power value relative to a reference power value. Specifically, the level of power, value P, relative to a reference value, PR, in decibels is defined as $dB = 10*\log_{10}(P/PR)$.

DC control—a remote base station control scheme that requires metallic conductors and currents of different values to control the station's various functions.

decoding—the conversion and recognition by the addressed (receiving) unit of numerical address codes that have been transmitted through a communications system.

dedicated telephone line—a telephone wire pair, originating at one point, and terminating at another point, operating in a closed circuit. Also called a private line.

defibrillator—an electrical device used to eliminate fibrillation of the heart muscle by the application of high voltage impulses.

demodulation—the process of recovering the modulating information from a modulated signal.

deviation ratio—the ratio of the maximum frequency deviation of the RF carrier to the highest frequency contained in the modulating band.

dial tone first—allowance of a 9-1-1 or '0' operator calls to be completed without the deposit of a coin in a telephone pay station.

digital—data represented in discrete, discontinuous form, as contrasted with analog data represented in continuous form.

digital dial code—a signaling technique generally used in VHF radio systems to bypass a receiver CTCSS system.

diplexer—a device that enables the use of two radio transmitters, operating on different frequencies, on the same antenna simultaneously.

direct—in terms of communications circuits, means a dedicated, instant method of communications. A dial telephone is not direct, a radio or a ring down line are direct.

direct dispatch method—a system in which all 9-1-1 call answering and radio dispatching is performed by the personnel at the public safety answering point.

direct distance dialing (DDD)—telephone service that permits subscribers to dial their own long distance calls.

direct leased land lines—dedicated or designated point-to-point wire circuits (telephone) used in transmitting voice or data communications. See: **dedicated telephone line**.

direct trunking—an arrangement in which a telephone line connection has no intermediate points before reaching the final destination (called) party.

directional antenna—an antenna that radiates radio waves more effectively in some directions than in others.

directivity—the value of the direction gain of an antenna in the direction of its maximum value.

dish—a type of antenna. A parabolic reflector used in microwave systems.

dispatch point—a position from which a radio system is used but not a supervision or control point. Dispatch points are not usually listed on a station radio license.

distortion—unfaithful reproduction of audio or video signals as a result of change occurring in the wave form of the original signal somewhere in the course of its transmission or reception. The lower the percentage of distortion, the more distortion free the system is and the more intelligible the message.

diversity—a method of radio transmission, or reception, or both, that counteracts the effects of fading by combining several signals all bearing the same information.

doctor-interrupt—the ability of a physician or hospital-based communicator to interrupt the voice or telemetry transmission from a radio in the field.

dual-tone-multifrequency (DTMF)—the simultaneous generation of two audio tones generally compatible to AT&T's standard "Touch-Tone" frequencies. Used for control or signaling purposes. A method of sending numerical information from an encoder by sending specific pairs of audio tones for each digit, up to a total of 16.

duplex—the operation of transmitting and receiving apparatus at one location in conjunction with associated transmitting and receiving apparatus at another location: the process of transmission and reception being simultaneous. The simultaneous transmission and reception of information. A duplexed piece of equipment is capable of transmitting and receiving simultaneously. Duplex systems generally use different transmitting and receiving frequencies.

duplexed operation—the operation of associated transmitting and receiving apparatus concurrently as in ordinary telephones without manual switching between talking and listening periods. For comparison, see **simplex operation**.

duplexed/multiplexed telemetry unit—a radio device capable of simultaneous transmission and reception and concurrent transmission of both voice and EKG information.

duplexer—a device that is used in radio equipment to provide simultaneous transmit and receive capabilities on a single antenna.

duplex, half—a system in which communication may be in either direction but only one way at a time. Transmission in one direction at a time over a single channel.

E

E & M signaling—an arrangement by which signaling between two points on a radio or carrier path is accomplished. An *M* lead is associated with the transmit (or mouth) while the *E* lead is associated with the receiver (or ear).

EACOM—Emergency and Administrative Communications for hospitals. Tradename for a VHF radio system operating on standard frequencies with a selective calling system between stations. The system is similar to Motorola Communications HEAR radio system.

effective height—the true electrical height of an antenna corresponding to a "perfect" antenna that will produce the same field strength. The height of its center of radiation above the effective ground level.

effective radiated power (ERP)—the calculated power output from an antenna system which incorporates all the gains and losses in the antenna system. ERP is calculated as follows (1) convert power output of transmitter to dB referenced to 1 W (dBw); (2) subtract all transmission line losses including losses in equipment between the transmitter and antenna (filter, diplexers, circulators, duplexers, and so forth) expressed in dB; (3) add the antenna's power gain (expressed in dB reference to a half-wave dimple; and (4) convert the results into watts.

effective signal radiated—the rating basis for licensing radio transmitters. Equal to the square root of the effective radiated power times the antenna height in feet above ground level.

EKG display console—a unit of electronic equipment located in a hospital emergency room, or cardiac care unit, or both, which displays EKG and records voice and data information received from an EMS scene by transmission via radio or telephone path. A demodulation display console.

electrocardiogram (ECG or EKG)—a visual or hard copy trace of a patient's electrical heartbeat information.

electrode—(1) either of the two terminals of an electric source, such as a battery; (2) a conducting element through which electric current enters or leaves an electrolyte, gas, or vacuum; (3) a conducting element, usually metallic (such as silver/silver chloride), with a conducting medium or electrolyte (such as sodium chloride and water) attached to a patient to obtain the electrical signals of the heart.

electromagnetic radiation—radiation associated with a periodical varying electric and magnetic field and is traveling at the speed of light, including radio waves, light waves, X-rays, and gamma radiation.

electromagnetic wave—a wave of electromagnetic radiation, characterized by variations of electric and magnetic fields.

emergency call—a call that requires immediate action.

emergency medical dispatcher (EMD)—a trained public safety telecommunicator with additional training and specific emergency medical knowledge essential for the efficient management of emergency medical communications.

emergency medical dispatching—the reception and management of requests for emergency medical assistance.

emergency medical dispatch priority reference system (EMDPRS)—a medically approved reference system used by a local dispatch agency to dispatch aid to medical emergencies, which includes: systematized caller interrogation questions, systematized prearrival instructions, and protocols matching the dispatcher's evaluation of injury or illness severity with vehicle response mode and configuration.

Emergency Medical Service (EMS)—the service used in responding to the perceived individual need for immediate medical care to prevent loss of life or aggravation of physiological or psychological illness or injury.

emergency operations center (EOC)—(1) a secure, protected facility designed and equipped for the use of community officials to manage response of a community in time of emergency and (2) a communications center designed and operated by a community or within a geographic area for a combination of emergency resources, such as police, fire, and EMS.

emergency resource coordination center (ERCC)—generally a facility that has the resources and ability to coordinate all emergency services (police, fire, EMS, and so forth) within a given geographic area. ERCC works in conjunction with a public safety answering point (PSAP) and may be in the same facility or location.

enclosure—a housing such as a case, cabinet, cabinet rack, or console that is designed to provide protection and support to equipment.

encoding—the conversion of numerical address codes, such as telephone number or message codes, into a format of tone or on-off pulses of audio tones for transmission over a communications system, usually for individual or group addressing, such as for paging or selective calling.

exchange—a defined area, served by one or more telephone central offices, within which the telephone company furnishes service.

exciter—the low-level stages of a transmitter which normally consist of an oscillator, modulator, and multiplier.

extender board—a printed circuit board that plugs into a module's circuit connector at one end and the module on the other to maintain a circuit so that the module may be conveniently tested out of an inaccessible position.

F

facility—a communications facility is anything used or available for use in the furnishing of communications service.

facsimile—the process by which pictures, images, and other fixed graphic materials are scanned and the information converted into electrical signals for local use or transmission remotely to produce a likeness of the subject copy.

fading—the variation of radio field strength caused by a gradual change in the transmission medium.

fade margin—the number of decibels of attenuation that can be added to a specified radio frequency propagation path before the signal-to-noise ratio of the channel falls below a specified minimum.

FCC Part 90—the section of the Federal Communications Commissions Rules and Regulations that affects most EMS communications.

Federal Communications Commission (FCC)—a board of commissioners appointed by the President under the Communications Act of 1934 to formulate Rules and Regulations and to authorize use of radio communications. The FCC regulates all communications in the United States by radio or wireline, including television, telephone, radio, facsimile, and cable systems.

feedback—the act of returning a portion of the output voltage of a circuit which includes amplification to the input of that circuit.

feedback, acoustic—the feeding back of sound waves from a loudspeaker to a microphone in the same audio system.

field strength—the strength of an electric, magnetic, or electromagnetic field. Electromagnetic (radio) field strength is expressed in microvolts per metre or millivolts per metre.

fixed service—a service or radio communication between specified fixed points. Fixed station—(1) a radio station that is not mobile, (2) a station that is permanently installed, and (3) a base station in a mobile radio system.

fixed relay station—an operational fixed station established from the automatic retransmission of radio communications received from either one or more fixed stations or from a combination of fixed and mobile stations and directed to a specified location.

F-Layers—the upper layers of ionization in the ionosphere. The f-1 layer is about 130 miles above the earth. The f-2 layer height varies from about 250 miles during the day to about 150 miles at night.

float—to operate a storage battery in parallel with a charger and a load at such voltage that the charger supplies the load current and the battery supplies only transient peaks above the normal load.

FM transmitter—a radio transmitter that emits or radiates a frequency modulated wave.

folded dipole—a receiving or transmitting antenna composed of two parallel dimples connected at the ends. The connection to the receiver or transmitter is made at the center of one of the poles.

forced disconnect—the capability of the 9-1-1 center to disconnect a 9-1-1 call to avoid caller jamming of the incoming phone lines.

four wire operation—telephone operation in which the inbound audio signal is carried on one pair of wires and the outbound signal on another pair.

free space loss—the theoretical radiation loss that would occur in transmission if all variable factors were disregarded. Free space loss depends only on the frequency and the distance between antennas.

frequency—the number of cycles, repetitions, or oscillations of a periodic process completed during a unit of time. The frequency of waves in the electromagnetic spectrum (radio waves) is designated in hertz (Hz), kilohertz (kHz = 1000 Hz). One hertz is equivalent to one cycle per second.

frequency band—a continuous range of frequencies extending between two limiting frequencies.

frequency coordination—see **coordination, frequency**.

frequency deviation—frequency deviation of an FM signal is the change in the carrier frequency produced by the modulating signal. The frequency deviation is proportional to the instantaneous amplitude of the modulating signal.

frequency modulation (FM)—a method of modulating a carrier-frequency signal by causing the frequency to vary above and below the unmodulated value in accordance with the intelligence signal to be transmitted. The amount of deviation in frequency above and below the resting frequency is at each instant proportional to the amplitude of the intelligence signal being transmitted. The number of complete deviations per second above and below the resting frequency corresponds at each instant to the frequency of the intelligence signal being transmitted.

frequency response—the transmission loss or gain of a system, measured over the useful bandwidths, compared to the loss or gain at some reference frequency (generally 1000 Hz).

fresnel zone—the circular zone about the direct path between a transmitter and a receiver at such a radius that the distance from a point on this circle to the receiving point has a path length that is some multiple of a half wave length longer than the direct path.

fringe area—an area or locality at such a distance from the transmitter that the signals received are weak.

full-duplex operation—a method of operation of a radio system that provides simultaneous two-way communications between two points. In EMS radio systems, provides for mutual interrupt capabilities between the field technician and the physician or medical direction at a hospital location.

G

gain, of an antenna—the effectiveness of a directional antenna in a particular direction, compared against a standard (usually an isotopic antenna). The radio of standard antenna power to the directional antenna power that will produce the same field strength in the desired direction.

generator, standby power—a device that develops electrical voltage from mechanical energy. An ac electrical power source held in reserve and used to supply the necessary ac power when commercial power fails.

generator, signal—a portable test oscillator that can be adjusted to provide a test signal at some desired frequency, voltage, modulation, or waveform.

geographical assignment—the assignment and use of communications channels on a dedicated used basis within a given geographic area.

GHz—gigahertz (billion hertz, 1000 MHz).

gin pole—a pole which is used together with ropes and pulleys as a derrick for lifting heavy loads and for erecting poles or towers.

ground—a reference point. Also a connection, intentional or accidental, between an electrical circuit and the earth or its equivalent.

ground plane antenna—a type of vertical transmitting or receiving antenna used primarily for short wavelength or high band communications. A ground plane antenna consists of a quarter-wave vertical element, and four radial elements spaced 90° apart, and mounted on the base of the vertical element. Antennas of this type are nondirectional and have a low angle of radiation.

ground wire—a conductor leading from the radio equipment to an electrical connection with the ground.

guard band—a narrow band of frequencies provided between adjacent channels in certain portions of the radio spectrum to prevent interference between stations.

guy anchor—the buried weight or mass to which the lower end of a guy wire is attached.

H

half-duplex channel—a communication channel providing duplex operation at one end of the channel, but not the other. Sometimes, the base station is operated in the duplex mode; however, in EMS, the portable or mobile radio is often operated in the duplex mode, and the base station at the hospital operated simplex, to permit the medical direction physician to interrupt transmissions from the field technician. See also **simplex.**

half-duplex operation—generally refers to the ability of directing medical personnel in EMS radio system to interrupt or 'break in' on radio transmissions from field personnel to give instructions or ask questions. Sometimes referred to as "physician interrupt." Requires duplexed communications equipment in the field.

half-wave dipole antenna—a straight, ungrounded antenna having an electrical length equal to half the wave length of the signal being transmitted or received. Mounted vertically, it has a donut-shaped pattern, circular in the horizontal plane.

ham—a term applied to an amateur radio operator, as opposed to business or commercial operators. A person that makes amateur radio operation a hobby.

harmful interference—any emission, radiation, or induction that endangers the functioning of a radio service or seriously degrades, obstructs, or repeatedly interrupts a radio communication service.

hand microphone—a microphone designed to be held in the hand. Sometimes called a "palm" microphone.

handset—a device similar to a telephone handset used in place of a hand microphone.

hardcopy—a tangible printed copy of a message such as that obtained from a teleprinter.

hardware—the screws, nuts, clamps, anchors, connectors, and so forth, used in the installation and maintenance of communications systems.

hardwire—to wire or cable directly between units of equipment without passing through other media.

harmonic—an integral multiple of a fundamental frequency. The third harmonic of 20 Hz is 60 Hz. The fifth harmonic of 40 Hz is 200 Hz.

hash—noise signal produced by an electrical or mechanical source.

headphone—a device that can be placed on the head to allow individual listening to messages.

HEAR—Hospital Emergency Administrative Radio—Motorola Communications and Electronics trade name for a VHF radio system operating on standard frequencies with a selective calling system between stations. The system is similar to General Electric Mobile Radio Departments EACOM radio system.

helix—a single-layer, spiral wound coil usually having air or foamed polyethylene core.

hetrodyne—(1) pertaining to the production of difference in frequencies (beat frequencies) by the combination of the two frequencies and (2) to shift an incoming radio signal to a different frequency, often to a lower intermediate frequency.

Hetordyne frequency—the beat frequency, which is the sum or difference between two frequency signals.

hertz (Hz)—international unit of frequency identical to and used instead of the old term cycles. One hertz is equal to one cycle per second.

high band—a portion of the VHF radio frequency spectrum from 150 to 174 MHz in which two-way radio operates.

hollerith code—a twelve-level code which defines the relation between an alphanumeric character and the punched holes in an 80-column data card.

hookswitch—the device on which a handset or microphone hangs when not in use. The handset operates a switch, or switches, that open the associated circuits.

hop—(1) the number of reflections from the ionosphere encountered by the radio wave in traveling from the transmitter to the receiver and (2) the number of radio links required to span a given path.

hot line—direct circuit between two or more points for immediate use without patching or switching. (See direct leased land lines.) The hot line can use various signalling configurations (that is, ringdown, audio amplifier, and so forth).

hot standby operation—a method of achieving reliable operation by energizing two identical equipments fed by and to a switchable input and output. A sensing device causes transfer of input and output circuits when a failure is indicated.

hum—audio frequency interference which is at the frequency of the power supply or its harmonics.

humidity, relative—the ratio of the amount of water vapor the air contains to the maximum amount it could hold at the same temperature and pressure expressed in percent.

hybrid—(1) made up of several different components or a mixture of technologies. (2) A circuit required to convert four-wire operation to two wire, while maintaining isolation of the four-wire circuit.

I

ignition noise—interference produced by sparks or other ignition discharged in a vehicle.

image—one of the two groups of sidebands generated in the process of modulation, so called because one is the reverse (mirror image) of the other with respect to operating frequency.

image frequency—in hetrodyne frequency converters, an undesired input frequency that can beat with the local oscillator to produce the intermediate frequency and thus appear in the receiver output.

image rejection—the action of a receiver in suppressing the image frequency.

impedance—the total resistance that a circuit offers to the flow of alternating current. Impedance is a combination of resistance and reactance. The ohm is used as a unit of impedance measurement.

impedance match—the condition in which the impedance of one component is the same as the component to which it is connected or attached.

impedance, characteristic—the importance of characteristic impedance lies in the fact that when a transmission line is terminated, as with an antenna, in an impedance matching its own, then all of the energy or power flowing along the line is radiated by the antenna. If the impedance of the termination (antenna) is not matched to the transmission line, a portion of the energy will be reflected at the mismatch resulting in a lower output from the antenna.

Improved Mobile Telephone Service (IMTS)—a mobile radio telephone offering of a telephone company.

impulse—a surge of electricity having a single polarity.

indicator—a device used to inform of a condition or change in condition.

induced—produced as a result of exposure to a changing electric or magnetic field.

Industrial Radio Service—an FCC-designated radio service.

in-band signaling—the transmission of signaling tones within the frequency band of the channel.

insertion loss—the loss introduced when a device or line section is interposed between two elements of a circuit.

insulation—any nonconductive material used to prevent the leakage of electricity from a conductor, such as rubber, glass, mica, and so forth.

integrated circuit—a complete circuit consisting of transistors, capacitors, resistors, diodes, and so forth that is formed on a single semiconductor substrate.

Integrated Circuit Oscillator Module (ICOM)—a frequency determining circuit used in General Electric radios containing a crystal oscillator circuit and other circuits used to generate the oscillator frequency.

interface—a concept involving the specification of the interconnection between two equipments or systems. The specification includes the type, quantity, and function of the interconnection circuits and the type and form of the signals to be interchanged via these circuits.

interference—interference in a signal transmission path is either extraneous power which tends to interfere with the reception of the desired signals or the distribution of signals which results in loss of signal or distortion of information.

intermittent—not continuously present; disappearing and reappearing.

intermittent duty cycle—a duty cycle of 1 min on, 4 min off, or 20 % per electronic industries association (EIA).

intermodulation—the combination of two signals beating together to form a third unusable signal that interferes with reception of the desired signal. In a radio receiver the method of expressing in dB below the desired signal, the receiver's rejection of the unwanted signal to its acceptance of correct signals.

intrinsically safe—a laboratory (UL) rating for equipment considered approved to operate in areas in which hazardous concentrations of flammable gases exist.

inverter—(1) any of several devices used to convert direct current to alternating current, (2) a single input, single output device that changes the polarity of (inverts) a signal when passing it from input to output. A negative signal at the input produces a positive signal at the output and vice versa. A differential EKG amplifier has a normal and an inverting input.

ionosphere—the upper portion of the earth's atmosphere beginning at about 50 miles above the surface of the earth; the cause of radio signals being bent, and returned to earth.

isolator—a passive RF device that permits transmission in only one direction, absorbing energy in the opposite direction.

J

jack—a connecting device ordinarily used to make electrical contact with mating contacts of a plug.

jacket—the outer covering on an insulated wire or cable.

jamming—the deliberate radiation, reradiation, or reflection of electromagnetic energy with the object of impairing the use of electronic devices, equipment, or systems.

jumper—a short length of conductor used to bridge electrical connections.

junction box—a metal or other container into which wires or cables are led and connected.

K

key—a push-to-operate switch used for operating a transmitting circuit in a radio system.

key telephone equipment—an instrument that has the capability of multiple line terminations. Each line is accessed by depressing an association button (key).

keypunch—a machine controlled by a typewriter-like keyboard that enables an operator to punch holes in predescribed places in a hollerith code.

kilo—a prefix meaning one thousand.

kbps—thousands of bits per second.

kilohertz (kHz)—equal to 1000 cycles per second. Replaces the term kilocycle.

klystron—an electron tube in which the electrons are periodically bunched by electric fields. Used as an RF oscillator for microwave equipment.

knockout—a metal disk punched in the side of a metal terminal junction box or cabinet which can be punched out to allow entry of a cable or conduit.

L

land line—a generic term which refers to the public-switched telephone system.

lag—the difference in phase angle expressed in electrical degrees between the voltage and current that produced it.

land-mobile—an abbreviation for land to mobile communications such as between base stations and mobile radios or from mobile radio to mobile radio.

Land Mobile Radio Service—a mobile radio service defined by the Federal Communications Commission—FCC Rules and Regulations Part 90.

LATA—local access and transport area boundaries for telephone companies. The geographic area within which the local telephone company provides local and long distance service.

Law Enforcement Assistance Administration (LEAA)—an administration under the United States Department of Justice established by the Omnibus Crime Control and Safe Streets Act of 1968, restructured by the Justice Improvement Act of 1979 and abolished two years later.

leased line—a pair of wires or a circuit, usually leased or rented from a telephone company, designed for exclusive use between two fixed points for various communication control functions.

life cycle—a test performed on a material device to determine the length of time before failure.

line—a transmission line or power line. A system of one or more wires.

linear—describing a device in which the signal output voltage is directly proportional to the signal input voltage. A straight line relationship.

line, balanced—a two-wire line that has identical impedance from each wire.

line equalizer—a connection in series with a telephone line that will alter the frequency response characteristics of the line.

line, four-wire—a two-way transmission circuit using separate paths for transmit and receive functions.

line, lossy—a transmission line, usually a coaxial cable, that is designed to have very high transmission loss per unit length. Used in tunnels, underground, or buildings for radio communications systems.

line of sight—an unobstructed path between two points. Radio waves at those frequencies where signals travel in a straight line and are not reflected by the ionosphere.

line-of-sight distance—the straight-line distance from a radio station antenna to horizon. This represents the normal transmitting range of FM transmitting stations.

link—the portion of a radio relay system between adjacent radio stations.

load—(1) a device that receives power from a transmission system and (2) the amount of electric power drawn by an electric or electronic device.

load, dummy—a device that can dissipate energy (into heat) without radiating it.

loading, antenna—insertion of reactance in an antenna circuit to improve its transmission characteristic in a given frequency band.

loading, ice—the stress imposed on an antenna or antenna structure caused by ice forming on its members.

loading, wind—the stress imposed on an antenna or antenna structure caused by wind.

lobe—one of the three-dimensional petals representing the radiation or reception efficiency of a directional antenna.

local government radio service—a service of radio communication defined by the FCC essential to official activities of states, possessions, and territories, including counties, towns, cities, and similar governmental subdivisions.

local service area—that area that can be called on the telephone without incurring multimessage units or a toll charge.

log—a list of radio stations showing frequency, location, power, and other data. Also a communication record for a station showing calls made, time, date, and other data. A detailed record.

loop—(1) a short transmission line that connects a subscriber to a switchboard and (2) a closed path in which a signal may circulate. This path may be within a piece of equipment, such as a repeater or carrier terminal, or may be a complete carrier circuit.

loop resistance—the resistance presented to the signaling portion of the terminating set by the wireline when the far end of the wireline is short circuited.

loss—a decrease in power suffered by a signal as it is transmitted from one point to another, usually expressed in decibels. Energy dissipated without accomplishing useful work.

loss, free space—the theoretical transmission loss between two radio antennas dependent only upon distance and frequency.

loss, path—the reduction or attenuation of signal strength that occurs between the transmitted strength and the received signal strength.

low band—a section of the VHF radio frequency spectrum from 25 to 50 MHz in which mobile radio equipment is licensed to operate.

low loss—describing circuits and transmission line in which little energy is lost from the input to the output.

lower sideband—the lower of two frequencies or of two groups of frequencies produced by a modulation process.

lug, spade—a connector which has an open end to slip under a terminating screw.

M

marginal—operating at the borderline of permissible limits.

matrix—an array of horizontal and vertical input or output leads with cross points at the intersections, used as a means of switching from any input to any output.

mean—the arithmetic middle point of a range of values, obtained by adding the highest and lowest values and dividing by two.

median—the point below which there are as many instances as there are above.

medical communications control console—an installation of communications control equipment, usually located at a hospital, which provides for control of the transmitting and receiving equipment necessary for the medical communications.

microwave—a term applied to radio waves in the frequency range of 1000 MHz and upward. Microwave radio generally performs the same functions as telephone cables and may be used for radio remote control purposes.

mobile—term used to describe equipment designed for vehicular installation.

mobile relay station—a fixed station established for the automatic retransmission of mobile service radio communications that originate on the transmitting frequency of the mobile stations and are retransmitted on the receiving frequency of the mobile stations.

mobile repeater station—a mobile station in the mobile service authorized to retransmit automatically on a mobile service frequency communications originated by hand-held or portable units or by other mobile or base stations directed to such hand-carried units.

mobile service—a service of radio communications between mobile and land stations, or between mobile stations.

mobile station—a two-way radio station in the mobile service intended to be used while in motion or during halts at unspecified points.

mobile telephone service (MTS)—telephone service between a fixed mobile radio base station and several vehicles equipped with mobile radios.

mobile transmitter—a radio transmitter designed for installation in a vehicle, vessel, or aircraft and normally operated while in motion.

mobile unit—a two-way radio equipped vehicle or person. Also, sometimes the two-way radio itself, when associated with a vehicle or person.

modem—contraction of modulator-demodulator.

modular—a construction technique incorporating the use of standard size units for interchangeability.

modulate—to vary the amplitude (AM), frequency (FM), or phase of a high-frequency wave or carrier in step with amplitude variations of another wave (the modulating wave). The carrier is usually a sine wave while the modulating wave is often a complex voice or EKG signal.

modulator—the electronic circuit that combines the modulating wave with the carrier wave. In radio transmitters, the final audio-frequency stage that mates the audio signal with the carrier signal. In EKG telemetry, the circuit that combines the amplified EKG signal with the subcarrier (audio) signal for transmission by radio or telephone.

multichannel system—a radio system that uses more than one radio channel. Also known as a multifrequency system.

multicoupler, receiver—a device that permits several radio receivers to use the same antenna. Usually a broadband amplifier with several output ports.

multifrequency operation—using radio equipment capable of operation on two or more frequencies.

multijurisdictional system—a system covering more than one political boundary or agency.

multipath—the propagation phenomenon that results in signals reaching a radio receiving antenna by two or more paths usually resulting in a degradation of the original signal.

multiplex—transmitting two or more signals over the same medium. In EKG telemetry equipment, the ability to transmit electrocardiograph (EKG) signals and voice signals concurrently over the same transmitter.

multiplex, frequency division—a multiplex system in which the total transmission bandwidth is divided into narrower bands each used for a single separate channel.

multiplex, time division—a method of multiplexing in which the total frequency spectrum available is used by each channel, but only for part of the time. A sharing of transmission ability, first by one parameter, then by another.

multitone—a method of signaling that involves two or more tone signals produced simultaneously or sequentially.

mute—to silence or reduce sound level.

N

netting—the process of adjusting a system's transmitters and receivers to the same operating frequencies.

net loss—the algebraic sum of the gains and losses between two terminals of a circuit.

network—an orderly arrangement of stations interconnected through communications channels to form a coordinated entity.

nine-one-one (9-1-1)—a three-digit emergency telephone number accepted and promulgated by the telephone industry as the nationwide emergency number.

Nxx—the first three digits of a local telephone number that uniquely identifies that central office switching location within its area code number for nationwide long distance call routing.

noise—interference characterized by undesirable random voltages caused by an internal circuit defect or from some external source. Any extraneous signal tending to interfere with the proper and easy perception of those signals which are intended to be received.

noise blanker—a device used in mobile radio applications that senses the presence of undesired noise on the desired channel and causes the desired signal to be interrupted for the time period that the undesired noise signal is present. The time period is controlled and measured in milliseconds so that the interruption of the desired signal is not audible.

noise level—volume of noise usually expressed in decibels.

noise limiter—a circuit that cuts off the noise peaks that are stronger than the highest peak of the desired signal being received.

nomograph—a chart having three or more scales across which a straightedge can be placed to provide a graphical solution for a particular problem. In mobile radio nomographs may be used to determine frequency spread, estimated radio range, antenna height, and so forth.

O

octave—the interval between two frequencies having a ratio of two to one.

ohm—an electrical unit of resistance.

ohm's law—the current in an electric circuit is directly proportional to the electromotive force in the circuit. In the form $E = I*R$, where E is the electromotive force (voltage), I is the current (amperage), and R is the resistance of the circuit (ohms).

omnidirectional—equally effective in all directions.

open—a break in circuit continuity.

outage—a disruption of communications from any cause, whether planned or accidental.

out-of-band signaling—transmission of signals by frequencies outside of the voice band.

overload—a load greater than a device is designed to handle.

P

paging—a one-way communications service from a base station to mobile or fixed receivers that provide signaling or information transfer by such means as tone, tone-voice, tactile, optical readout, and so forth.

pair—two wires of a signal circuit generally applied to telephone wherein one wire is designated "tip" and the second wire "ring."

passive—a device that does not contribute energy to the signal it passes.

passive repeater—a device intentionally interposed in a microwave transmission path to redirect or reflect energy.

patch—a means of connecting one system to another. A patch may be between radio systems, or radio to telephone, as in a radio/phone patch.

path, signal—the route by which intelligence is conveyed from transmitter to receiver or through a circuit.

personal radio—a small portable radio intended to be carried by hand or on the person of the user.

PERT—program evaluation and review technique. A management tool for comparing actual with scheduled program progress.

phase—the position at any instant which the periodic wave occupies in its cycle of 360°.

phone patch—an interconnection between radio and telephone communications circuits which permits direct voice interchange between telephone lines and radio system.

pigtail—a splice made by twisting together the bared ends of two conductors.

plug-in—describing any device having terminals so it can be connected by simply pushing it into a suitable socket or connector.

portable—an easily transportable radio.

primary power—a reliable source of electrical power normally serving as the principle source of energy to equipment, such as the commercial 120-V ac power main.

private automatic branch exchange (PBX)—a telephone switchboard with many stations not individually identifiable to the telephone company's switching network requiring an operator.

private line (PL)—Motorola's trademarked name for continuous tone-controlled squelch system, CTCSS.

propagation, electromagnetic—the travel of electromagnetic waves through a medium or the travel of a sudden electric disturbance along a transmission line. Also called wave propagation.

protect—to equip with devices for safeguarding from damage by excessive voltages, current, or physical abuse.

public safety agency—a functional division of a public agency that provides fire fighting, police, ambulance, emergency medical, or other emergency services.

public safety answering point (PSAP)—the initial answering location of a 9-1-1 call and other calls for assistance.

public safety telecommunicator—an individual trained to communicate by electronic means with persons seeking emergency assistance and with agencies and individuals providing such assistance.

pull box—a box with a removable cover installed in a conduit run to facilitate pulling wire or cable into the conduit.

pulse—a signal of short duration.

pulsed tone—a system of selective signaling using a keyed on-off tone signal.

push-to-talk or press-to-talk (PTT)—in radio or telephone systems, that method of communication over a speech circuit in which transmission occurs from only one station at a time, the talker being required to keep a switch operated while he is talking. The keying button used to operate a radiotelephone transmitter.

Q

quarter-wave antenna—an antenna electrically equal to one fourth of the wavelength of the signal to be transmitted or received.

quartz—an element consisting of pure silicon dioxide. The original piezoelectric material widely used to control the frequency of oscillators.

quartz crystal—a thin square or rectangular slice of quartz which will vibrate at a frequency determined by its thickness.

quiet channel—RCA Corporation's trademarked name for

continuous tone-controlled squelch system (CTCSS).

quieting—reduction of system noise.

quick-call—Motorola Communications Company trademarked name for a system of selective calling, normally using two pairs of two tones each in sequence. Quick Call II uses a pair of sequential tones similar to General Electric's Type 99 tone system.

R

rack mounting—a method of mounting equipment in which metal panels supporting the equipment are attached to predrilled steel channel rails or racks. The dimensions of the panels, the spacing of the rails, and the size of the mounting screws are standardized.

rack unit—in mobile radio, generally a rack mounting 19 in. between rails and a height of 1.75 in. per unit.

radio—the transmission and reception of signals by means of electromagnetic waves without a connecting wire.

radio-frequency power—the power associated with any signal consisting of electromagnetic radiation which is used for telecommunications.

radio interference—undesired disturbance of radio reception. Man-made interference is generated by electric devices, with the resulting interference signals either being radiated through space as electromagnetic waves or traveling over power lines or other conducting media. Radio interference is also due to natural sources such as atmospheric phenomena, such as lightning. Radio transmitters themselves may additionally interfere with each other.

radio network—a number of radio stations, fixed and mobile, in a given geographical area that are jointly administered or communicate with each other by sharing the same radio channel or channels.

radio common carrier (RCC)—an enterprise that is licensed by the FCC and Public Utilities Commission to provide radio communications service to the public.

radio receiver—an instrument that amplifies radio frequency signals, separates the intelligence signal from the rf carrier, amplifies the intelligence signal additionally, and converts the intelligence signal to its original form.

radio relay system (radio relay)—a point-to-point radio transmission system in which the signals are received and retransmitted by one or more intermediate radio stations.

radio transmitter—a radio-frequency power source that generates radio waves for transmission through space.

radome—a dome-shaped cover for a parabolic antenna that protects the antenna from the elements and their attenuating effects.

range—distance over which a radio signal can be transmitted for effective reception or the distance at which a usable signal can be received.

receiver—an electronic device used to detect and amplify transmitted radio signals.

receiver, paging—a small, light, pocket-sized receiver used for alerting individuals when they are away from their normal communication instruments.

referral method—the calling party to a public safety answering point is referred to a secondary telephone number.

refraction—the change of direction experienced by a wave of any form of radiated energy when passing from one medium to another having a different dielectric constant or index of refraction.

regional EMS system—an emergency medical service area (trade, catchment, market, patient flow, geographic, or governmental) that provides essentially all of the definitive emergency medical care for all emergencies and for the most critically ill and injured patients within the area.

relay—transmission forwarded through an intermediate station.

relay station—radio stations that rebroadcast signals the instant they are received, so that the signal can be passed on to another station outside the range of the originating transmitter.

reliability—the ability of an item to perform a required function under stated conditions for a stated period of time.

remote base station—a base station located away from the operating console to take advantage of improved coverage offered by a better geographical location.

remote control—the operation of a device from a distance either electrically or by radio waves.

remote control equipment—the apparatus used for performing monitoring, controlling, supervisory control, or a combination of these functions at a distance by electrical means.

repeater—a combination of apparatus for receiving either one-way or two-way communication signals and delivering corresponding signals which are either amplified or reshaped or both.

repeater station—an operational fixed station established for the automatic retransmission of radio communications received from any station in the mobile service.

repeater station, remodulating—a microwave repeater station in which the signal is demodulated to the original baseband frequencies and reinjected onto the modulator for transmission to the distant station.

resource management center—a center responsible for the allocation of those resources essential to the most effective and efficient resolution, or management or both, of the immediate problem. In most communities these resources include police, fire and emergency medical services. The resource management center is most effective when its responsibilities encompass the whole of public safety response.

ringback—in a public safety answering center, permits the answering point to ring the hung-up telephone on a held circuit. The feature is useful when a calling party has failed to provide all necessary information to the answering point before hanging up.

ringdown—a type of signaling used in manual operation telephone (as compared to dial) which uses a continuous or pulsing ac signal transmitted over the line.

S

schematic diagram—a diagram or drawing that shows electrical connections of a radio or other electrical device by means of symbols which are used to represent the components.

search lock monitor—a receiver channel scanning scheme that locks the receiver on the first channel received.

selective call—a system for alerting individual or groups of stations by means of coded signals.

selectivity—the ability to select one particular signal from other signals at nearby frequencies. This specification is important in urban areas where radio spectrum congestion exists. The more negative the dB rating, the better the specification.

selective routing—a routing of telephone call to terminate at a PSAP determined by the location of the calling telephone. This is accomplished by using a computer to process the calling telephone number.

sensitivity—the characteristic of a radio receiver which determines the minimum input signal strength required for a given signal output. In FM, sensitivity is the signal level required to produce a given ratio of signal to noise. The more sensitive a receiver is, the weaker the signal it can receive.

service channel—in a microwave system, a voice channel fused for maintenance and fault location. Also called an order wire.

service life—the life expectancy of equipment under normal conditions of use.

side tone—the signal that reaches a telephone receiver from the transmitter of the same set by way of a local path within the set.

signal—the form of a radio wave in relation to the frequency serving to convey intelligence in communication.

signal-to-noise ratio—the ratio of the intensity of the desired signal to that of the undesired noise signal, usually expressed in decibels.

signal strength—a measure of the field intensity caused by a radio transmitter at a particular location within its operating range. Usually expressed as microvolts or millivolts of signal.

simplex—(1) single frequency operation whereby all base stations and mobiles operate on one common frequency and (2) operation on two different frequencies in a system that can communicate in two directions, but not simultaneously, such as when a base station and a mobile radio operate on reversed pairs of frequencies without duplexing.

simplex channel—a communication channel providing transmission in one direction only at any given time. For comparison see duplex channel.

simplex operation—a method of radio operation in which communication between two stations takes place in only one direction at a time. This includes ordinary transmit-receive operation, press-to-talk operation, voice-operated transmit, and other forms of manual or automatic switching from transmit to receive. Also called simplex.

SINAD—the ratio of signal plus noise plus distortion to the noise plus distortion; expressed in decibels. An EIA standard method of measuring receiver sensitivity. Basically a measure of RF signal strength that will result in a readable signal.

siren—an acoustical or electromechanical device used as a warning signal on emergency vehicles.

software—the programs or instructions required to use a computer or data processing device.

solid state—denoting the use of semiconductors instead of vacuum tubes or relays.

Special Emergency Radio Service (SERS)—that portion of radio communications frequency resources authorized by the FCC for use in the alleviation of emergency situations endangering life or property. See FCC Part 90.

spectrum—a continuous range of frequencies arranged in order of wavelength or frequency within which waves have some common characteristics, such as audio spectrum, radio spectrum, and so forth. The entire range of electromagnetic radiation extending from the longest known radio waves to the shortest known cosmic rays.

spurious response—the response of a radio receiver to an undesired frequency.

squelch—a circuit function that acts to suppress the audio output of a receiver when noise power exceeding a predetermined level is present.

squelch, carrier—a squelch system that responds to the presence of an RF carrier signal.

squelch circuit—a circuit that reduces or lowers the noise that would otherwise be heard in a radio receiver between transmissions.

stability, frequency—the ability of a radio transmitter to maintain any predetermined frequency, such as its assigned frequency. Measured in percent of the carrier. The lower the percentage the better the stability.

standing wave ratio (SWR)—a measure of the amount of lost transmitting power as a result of impedance differences between the transmission line and the antenna. The ratio of reflected to incident waves that exists at some particular point on a transmission line.

statewide EMS system—a network of EMS systems, integrated and coordinated at the state level.

strip chart recorder—an electromechanical device used to make paperchart recordings of EKG information. Usually it uses a heat-sensitive paper and a heated stylus.

subcarrier—a frequency sensitive device used to generate a modulated wave which in turn is applied as a modulating wave to modulate another carrier. For EMS telemetry, the subcarrier frequency is 1400 Hz.

supergroup—in microwave systems, groups of 60 channels each, occupying a particular range of frequencies.

switched network—a complex of diversified channels and equipment that automatically routes communications between the calling and called person or data equipment. The public telephone system.

synthesizer, frequency—a highly precise crystal oscillator with frequency dividers used to provide the precise radio frequency. A typical synthesizer can be set to small frequency increments and have an accurate output at the desired output frequency.

synchronization—the process of making the carrier at the receiving end of a line or system match the frequency of the carrier at the transmitting end.

system—a combination of two or more stations in such a way as to provide communications.

T

tandem trunking—an arrangement in which a telephone-line connection has one or more intermediate points that are required or permitted usually on a controlled dial pulse basis before reaching the final destination (called) party.

tariff—a document filed by a communications company with the Public Utilities Commission which lists the services offered the public and a schedule of rates and charges.

tarnish—a discoloration or stain on the surface of metal caused by exposure to chemicals or the atmosphere. To dull or destroy the luster of metal.

tee—a three-way connection in the shape of the letter *t*.

telecommunicator—see public safety telecommunicator.

telecommunications—all forms of electrical transmission of intelligence including: telegraph, telephone, radio, and television. Pertaining to the art and science of communication by these methods.

telemetry—the sensing and measuring of information at some remote location and transmitting the data to a convenient location to be read and recorded.

telpak—an acronym for "telephone package" a schedule of bulk discount rates for multiple private line telephone services such as AT&T long-lines series 500 tariff offering.

telephone line—a telephone line from a telephone company central office that is connected to key or nonkey telephone equipment.

teletypewriter—an electromechanical device, similar to a typewriter, such that messages typed on the keyboard of the transmitter unit are converted into electrical signals, which when conveyed to the receiver unit, are printed on paper.

ten signals—a series of coded messages designed to reduce air transmission time and confusion in busy mobile radio systems.

thermal noise—very small noise voltages that are present in all conductors, caused by the thermal agitation of charged particles within the conductor.

third harmonic—a frequency wave having three times the fundamental frequency value.

threshold—in an FM receiver, the point at which the peaks of the incoming RF signal exactly equal the peaks of the internally generated thermal noise power or the point above which increasing the input signal strength provides only a dB for dB improvement in the output signal-to-noise ratio.

tip—the ball-shaped contact on the cord (tip) of a plug. One of a pair of telephone wires (the other of which is called the ring).

tone—an audio or carrier of controlled amplitude and frequency used in a selective signaling system, or for equipment control purposes.

tone code—a specified character of transmitted tone signals required to effect a particular selection or function.

tone-coded squelch—a system whereby a superimposed tone is transmitted with the radio carrier to protect against nuisance-type interference.

tone, Type 90—General Electric's name for a system of single-tone signaling. The tones are generally between 1000 and 2400 Hz in two bands.

tone, Type 99—General Electric's name for its two-tone sequential selective signaling system. Sometimes called Sel-Call. The tones are generally between 520 and 953 Hz.

topographic map—an accurately scaled map having contour lines which show the elevation above sea level. Used in preparing profiles of radio propagation paths.

touch pad—a method of signaling or encoding and decoding address codes by the use of a simple numerical push button keyboard.

Touchtone—a Bell System trademark used to describe their method of signaling and use of dual tone multifrequency (DTMF) tones.

tower, antenna—a tall antenna support structure used to support one or more antennas or when an antenna must be mounted high above the ground or other support formation such as a building.

traffic—used for messages handling by a radio communications system.

transceiver—the combination of radio transmitting and receiving equipment in a common housing, usually for portable or mobile use, and using common circuit components for both transmitting and receiving.

transformer—an electrical device for voltage current transformation, or impedance matching, or both.

transfer method—the PSAP interrogator determines the proper responding agency and connects the user to that agency. To perform the necessary dispatching in accordance with prearranged plans with cooperating agencies.

transient—a rapid, sometimes violent, fluctuation of voltage or current in a circuit usually of short duration caused by switching or changes in load.

transmitter—apparatus for the production and modulation of radio frequency energy for the purpose of radio communication.

transmission line—a waveguide, coaxial line, or other system of conductors used to transfer signal energy efficiently from one location to another. In communications systems, the coaxial line between the base station and the antenna.

trunk—a circuit used for connecting a subscriber in a central office to all other services in/out of the switching equipment.

trunk line—a telephone line that terminates at a switchboard rather than a telephone.

TSPS—an electronic operating position system whereby operator-handled traffic is routed to its final destination via a central switching machine.

turret—a section of a communications control console, containing switches, controls, meters, and so forth.

two-way radio—a radio that is able to transmit and to receive.

two-wire operation—uses a single pair (two wires) for both transmitting and receiving.

U

Ultra High Frequency (UHF)—frequencies between 300 and 3000 MHz.

ultrasonic—describing frequencies higher than those which are audible. Generally above 20 000 Hz.

unbalanced line—a transmission line in which the voltages on the two conductors are unequal.

Underwriters Laboratories, Inc—a laboratory sponsored by the National Board of Fire Underwriters that examines and tests devices, material, and equipment whose action may affect casualty, fire, and life hazards.

unmodulated—without modulation; the RF carrier signal alone as it exists during pauses in conversations.

upper sideband—the higher of two frequencies or groups of frequencies produced by a modulation process.

utility—a power, gas, or water service available to the public.

V

Van Allen belts—radiation belts that surround the earth, consisting of electrons and protons at high energy levels.

varactor—a semiconductor diode used as a variable capacitor. Used as a harmonic generator, frequency multiplier, and amplifier.

vehicular repeater station—a mobile station in the mobile services authorized to retransmit automatically on a mobile service frequency, communications originated by hand-carried portable units or by other mobile or base stations directed to such hand-carried units.

Versatone—General Electric company tradename for a solid state tuned tone determining element.

vertical antenna—a vertical steel tower, rod, or shaft used as an antenna.

Very High Frequency (VHF)—frequencies between 30 and 300 MHz.

Vibrasponder—Motorola Communications company tradename for a tone determining vibrating reed element.

voice grade—a communications circuit that is nominally 300 to 3000 Hz.

voltage standing wave ratio (VSWR)—the ratio of the maximum voltage to the minimum voltage along a transmission line. It is the measure of the mismatch between the load and the line.

volume control—a potentiometer voltage divider used to adjust the loudness of an audio circuit.

volume unit (VU)—a measure of the magnitude of sound from an electrical wave. Measured in decibels.

voting—automatic selection of remote radio receiver. All incoming signals are compared for signal strength and the first signal found that meets or exceeds a preset level is selected and sent to the audio amplifier.

W

watt—the unit of power.

wattmeter—a meter to indicate the rate at which electrical energy is being used or produced.

wave—a propagated periodic disturbance such as a radio, light, or sound wave.

waveguide—a transmission line comprising a hollow conducting tube within which electromagnetic waves may be propagated. Generally used in microwave communications systems.

wavelength—the distance measured along the direction of propagation between two points that are in phase on adjacent waves. A wavelength is the distance traveled by a wave in the time of one cycle. Electromagnetic waves include both light and radio waves and travel in space at approximately 300 000 000 m/s. To determine the exact length of a wave, divide 300 000 000 m by the frequency in hertz.

wave, radio—an electromagnetic wave that travels through space at the speed of light.

wave, refracted—a radio wave that is bent (refracted) as it travels into a second medium of propagation, such as from the atmosphere to the ionized layers of the stratosphere.

weatherproof—so constructed or protected that exposure to the weather elements will not prevent proper operation.

weathertight—so constructed that exposure to a driven rain will not result in the entrance of water.

wire—a single metallic conductor.

REFERENCES

(1) "Communications in Support of Emergency Medical Services," Executive Office of the President, Office of Telecommunications Policy, November 1973.

(2) "Telecommunications Analysis Services—Reference Guide," Institute of Telecommunications Sciences, January 1983.

(3) "Emergency Medical Communication System Requirements for the Emergency Medical Communications Research Study, Contract No. FCC-0058, Federal Communications Commission," Advanced Technology Systems, Inc., October 9, 1973.

(4) "Planning Emergency Medical Communications—Volume One State-Level Planning Guide," National Association of State EMS Directors, 1995.

(5) "Emergency Medical Services Communications System Technical Planning Guide," Report NTIA-SP-79-3, U.S. Department of Commerce, March 1979.

(6) "Master Plan for Emergency Medical Services Communications in Oregon, Vol I, State-Level Plan," Oregon State Health Division, Emergency Medical Services Division, June 1982.

(7) "National Advisory Commission on Criminal Justice Standards and Goals, Report on Police," GPO, Washington, DC, 1973.

(8) "National Advisory Commission on Criminal Justice Standards and Goals, Report on the Criminal Justice System," GPO, Washington, DC, 1973.

Designation: F 1221 – 89 (Reapproved 2001)

Standard Guide for Interagency Information Exchange[1]

This standard is issued under the fixed designation F 1221; the number immediately following the designation indicates the year of original adoption or, in the case of revision, the year of last revision. A number in parentheses indicates the year of last reapproval. A superscript epsilon (ε) indicates an editorial change since the last revision or reapproval.

INTRODUCTION

This guide has been developed to address the need to provide for effective information exchange between agencies involved in responding to emergency medical services (EMS) situations.

Communications in the context of this guide refers to the communications that need to occur (1) *prior* to the EMS event, (2) *during* the EMS event, and (3) *after* the EMS event. *Communications* in this guide includes face-to-face communications, telecommunications, and written communications.

Before EMS events, the agencies that need to work closely together in emergency medical situations need to hold face-to-face meetings to develop communication plans that include an interagency communications component. These communication plans need to include written protocols outlining how the emergency response agencies will interface with each other during EMS events.

During the actual event, the agencies need to communicate either directly between emergency units, or through dispatch centers, or face-to-face (for example, communications related to implementing protocols or communications regarding decision making between agencies' senior officials, or combination thereof). After an emergency, there is a need for the agencies to critique the response. This may include face-to-face meetings to review the events, written critique reports of the emergency events, and revisions to the written protocols as may be found necessary by review of the events. (See the Rationale in Appendix X1.)

1. Scope

1.1 This guide covers the planning, operations, and evaluation phases of interagency communications as part of a comprehensive EMS system.

1.2 This is a guide for interagency communications within an EMS system. Interagency communications involves the EMS responder and support agencies whose primary mission is *not* to deliver prehospital emergency medical care.

1.3 The primary focus of this guide is to address interagency communications necessary for ongoing EMS responses.

1.4 The guide also addresses interagency communications in any major EMS incident, including man-made or natural disasters.

1.5 The recommendations for drills/exercises for the evaluation of interagency communications during an EMS event are also incorporated into this guide.

1.6 Additional information can be found in Guide F 1220 and Refs **1-5**.[2]

1.7 The sections in this guide appear in the following sequence:

1.8 *This standard does not purport to address all of the safety concerns, if any, associated with its use. It is the responsibility of the user of this standard to establish appropriate safety and health practices and determine the applicability of regulatory limitations prior to use.*

2. Referenced Documents

2.1 *ASTM Standards:*

F 1220 Guide for Emergency Medical Services System (EMSS) Telecommunications[3]

3. Terminology

3.1 *Definitions of Terms:*

[1] This guide is under the jurisdiction of ASTM Committee F30 on Emergency Medical Services and is the direct responsibility of Subcommittee F30.04 on Communications.

Current edition approved March 31, 1989. Published May 1989.

[2] The boldface numbers in parentheses refer to the references at the end of this guide.

[3] *Annual Book of ASTM Standards*, Vol 13.01.

3.1.1 *citizen access*—act of requesting emergency assistance for a specific event.

3.1.2 *dispatch*—act of sending emergency resources in response to a specific event.

3.1.3 *interagency communication evaluation phase*—interagency communications following an EMS incident for evaluation purposes.

3.1.4 *interagency communication operations phase*—interagency communications during an EMS incident for operational purposes.

3.1.5 *interagency communication planning phase*—interagency communications before an EMS incident for planning purposes.

3.1.6 *interagency communications*—communications that take place between EMS responders and agencies, nonmedical in nature, that respond in conjunction with emergency medical services.

3.1.7 *intra-agency communications*—communications that take place between agencies, medical in nature, within an EMS system.

3.1.8 *ongoing EMS incident*—any EMS incident that is managed without multiple EMS response units.

3.1.9 *significant EMS incident*—any EMS incident requiring multiple EMS response units including: multiple-casualty incidents, man-made or natural disasters.

3.1.10 *support agency*—any agency providing nonmedical support to EMS responders.

3.1.11 *vehicles*—all modes of transportation, including air, ground, or water, or combination thereof.

4. Significance and Use

4.1 This guide has been developed to facilitate communications between agencies involved in the delivery of emergency medical services. This guide is intended to be applied by agencies providing emergency medical services to improve their communications with EMS support agencies. It recommends necessary communication before, during, and after an EMS event.

5. Procedure

5.1 *Interagency Communication Planning Phase*:

5.1.1 *Methods*—A plan is needed for the coordination of interagency communication activities during ongoing and significant EMS responses. This plan must include alternatives for events which exceed or overwhelm the systems' communication capability. Contingency plans for diminished system capabilities, due to equipment or other failures, should also be addressed. The following methods should be used to develop the plan:

Meeting notices
Meeting documentation
Interagency communication agreement documents
Interagency communication protocols
Public information documents

At a minimum one or more of the following communication processes shall be used annually to develop, review, or amend, or combination thereof, interagency communication documents and protocols: face-to-face, telephone, or teleconference.

5.1.2 *Drills*—Interagency communication drills shall be conducted at a minimum of once annually. This drill should be used to evaluate procedures, protocols, communication path availability, grade of service, and communication path activation time. The exercise plans shall include performance parameters that will permit evaluation of interagency communication, procedures, protocols, communication paths, and executive times.

5.2 *Interagency Communications Operation Phase*:

5.2.1 *Off-Line Communications*—Documents developed in the planning phase are used for training and on-line reference to implement operational procedures. Documents shall include information on agencies such as law enforcement, fire protection, public utilities, special response agencies, and public information. This material shall uniquely identify each agency and provide an interagency protocol for each agency. Each protocol shall clearly identify resources by: who, what, when, and where for each EMS response.

5.2.2 *On-Line Communications*—On-line methods that include face-to-face, telephone, teleconference, one-way, and two-way radio shall be identified for each of the following elements of an EMS response for interagency communications:

5.2.2.1 *EMS Access*—Any agency that receives requests for EMS assistance (for example, citizens, public safety personnel) shall have immediate direct access to the EMS dispatcher.

5.2.2.2 *EMS Dispatch/Coordination*—Any EMS dispatch/coordination agency shall have immediate direct access to all supporting agencies.

5.2.2.3 *Enroute to or from an EMS Incident*—Interagency coordination to or from vehicles enroute to or from the EMS incident shall use two-way radio communication to the dispatch/coordination center and its immediate direct access interagency links.

5.2.2.4 *Scene Coordination*—Interagency communications by the first arriving emergency agency at the scene of an EMS incident shall be by two-way radio communication to the dispatch/coordination center and its immediate direct access interagency links. Direct two-way radio communication for on-scene interagency coordination is recommended. Alternative methods for interagency coordination at the scene may include: relay through the dispatch/coordination center(s), face-to-face communication, messenger, or other radio facilities such as cellular radio telephone. When an on-scene command post is established, additional communication capabilities are required to provide on-scene interagency communication and communication between the command post and the dispatch/coordination center or EOC.

5.2.3 *Drills/Exercises*—During drills or exercises, additional qualified personnel must be available to monitor and measure the process without affecting operations.

5.3 *Interagency Communication Evaluation Phase*:

5.3.1 *Methods*—The following methods should be used to evaluate interagency communication activities during ongoing and significant EMS responses:

Meeting notices
Meeting documentation
Interagency evaluation reports
Interagency communication agreement document reviewed or revised
Interagency communication protocol reviewed or revised
Public information documents

At the earliest opportunity, not more than 60 days following a drill or a significant EMS incident, an evaluation of interagency communication agreements and protocols shall be conducted using one or more of the following communication processes: face-to-face, telephone, teleconference. This process shall be in addition to the recommended annual planning process.

5.3.2 *Drills/Exercises*—Within 60 days following a significant EMS incident, exercise, or drill, an evaluation report shall be completed and distributed to all involved agencies including recommended changes in procedures, protocols, and other system elements.

6. Keywords

6.1 communications; emergency medical services; interagency information exchange

APPENDIX

(Nonmandatory Information)

X1. RATIONALE

X1.1 Those agencies who use this guide should carefully document when, why, and how specific rules or regulations, or both, were developed. This will allow revisions to be made as changes occur in communication technology or emergency medical practices, or both.

REFERENCES

(1) *Communications Act of 1934* (47 U.S.C. 405) as amended and Title 47 United States Code of Federal Regulations (47 CFR) on Telecommunications.

(2) *Communication Manual*, U.S. Department of Transportation, National Highway Traffic Safety Administration, June 1978, DOT, HS-802976, Department of Transportation, National Highway Traffic Safety Administration, Washington, DC.

(3) *EMS Communications Compatibility Study*, November 1978, DOT, HS-803858, final report prepared for Department of Transportation, National Highway Traffic Safety Administration, Washington, DC 20590.

(4) *Emergency Medical Services Communication Systems Technical Planning Guide*, March 1979, NTIA, Reports Series NTIA SP793, U.S. Department of Commerce, National Telecommunications and Information Administration.

(5) *Guidelines for Developing an EMS Communications Plan*, March 1977, HSA-772036, U.S. Department of Health, Education and Welfare, Public Health Service Administration, Bureau of Medical Services, Box 911, Rockville, MD 20852.

Designation: F 1223 – 96

Standard Test Method for Determination of Total Knee Replacement Constraint[1]

This standard is issued under the fixed designation F 1223; the number immediately following the designation indicates the year of original adoption or, in the case of revision, the year of last revision. A number in parentheses indicates the year of last reapproval. A superscript epsilon (ε) indicates an editorial change since the last revision or reapproval.

1. Scope

1.1 The purpose of this test method is to establish a database of total knee replacement (TKR) motion characteristics with the intent of developing guidelines for the assignment of constraint criteria to TKR designs. (See the Rationale in Appendix X1.)

1.2 This test method covers the means by which a TKR constraint may be quantified according to motion delineated by the inherent articular design as determined while under specific loading conditions in an *in vitro* environment.

1.3 Tests deemed applicable to the constraint determination are antero-posterior draw, medio-lateral shear, rotary laxity, and distraction, as applicable. Also covered is the identification of geometrical parameters of the contacting surfaces which would influence this motion and the means of reporting the test results. (See Practices E 4.)

1.4 *This standard does not purport to address all of the safety concerns, if any, associated with its use. It is the responsibility of the user of this standard to establish appropriate safety and health practices and determine the applicability of regulatory limitations prior to use.*

2. Referenced Documents

2.1 *ASTM Standards:*

E 4 Practices for Force Verification of Testing Machines[2]

3. Terminology

3.1 *Definitions*—Items in this category refer to the geometrical and kinematic aspects of TKR designs as they relate to their human counterparts:

3.1.1 *anterior curvature*—a condylar design which is generally planar except for a concave—upward region anteriorly on the tibial component.

3.1.2 *anterior posterior* (AP)—any geometrical length aligned with the AP orientation.

3.1.3 *AP displacement*—the relative linear translation between components in the AP direction.

3.1.4 *AP draw load*—the force applied to the movable component with its vector aligned in the AP direction causing or intending to cause an AP displacement.

3.1.5 *biconcave*—a condylar design with pronounced AP and ML condylar radii seen as a "dish" in the tibial component or a "toroid" in the femoral component.

3.1.6 *bearing surface*—those regions of the component which are intended to contact its counterpart for load transmission.

3.1.7 *condyles*—entity designed to emulate the joint anatomy and used as a bearing surface primarily for transmission of the joint reaction force with geometrical properties which tend to govern the general kinematics of the TKR.

3.1.8 *distraction*—the separation of the femoral component(s) from the tibial component(s) in the *z*-direction.

3.1.9 *flexion angle*—the angulation of the femoral component (about an axis parallel to the *y*-axis) from the fully extended knee position to a position in which a "local" vertical axis on the component now points posteriorly.

3.1.9.1 *Discussion*—For many implants, 0° of flexion can be defined as when the undersurface of the tibial component is parallel to the femoral component surface that *in vivo* contacts the most distal surface of the femur. This technique may not be possible for some implants that are designed to have a posterior tilt of the tibial component. In these cases, the user shall specify how the 0° of flexion position was defined.

3.1.10 *hinge*—a mechanical physical coupling between femoral and tibial components which provides a singular axis about which flexion occurs.

3.1.11 *hyperextension stop*—a geometrical feature which arrests further progress of flexion angles of negative value.

3.1.12 *internal-external rotation*—the relative angulation of the moveable component about an axis parallel to the *z*-axis.

3.1.13 *joint reaction force*—the applied load whose vector is directed parallel to the *z*-axis, generally considered parallel to tibial longitudinal axis.

3.1.14 *medio-lateral* (ML)—the orientation that is aligned with the *y*-axis in the defined coordinate system.

3.1.15 *ML condylar radius*—the geometrical curvature of the component's condyle in the frontal plane.

3.1.16 *ML dimension*—any geometrical length aligned with the ML orientation.

3.1.17 *ML displacement*—the relative linear translation between components in the ML direction.

3.1.18 *ML shear load*—the force applied to the moveable component with its vector aligned in the ML direction causing or intending to cause an ML displacement.

---

[1] This test method is under the jurisdiction of ASTM Committee F-4 on Medical and Surgical Materials and Devices and is the direct responsibility of Subcommittee F04.15 on Material Test Methods.

Current edition approved April 10, 1996. Published June 1996. Originally published as F 1223 – 89. Last previous edition F 1223 – 95.

[2] *Annual Book of ASTM Standards*, Vol 03.01.

3.1.19 *post-in-well feature*—a TKR design which tends to influence kinematics through the coupling of a prominent eminence with a recess or housing in a mating component.

3.1.20 *rotary laxity* (RL)—degree of relative angular motion permitted of moveable component about the *z*-axis as governed by inherent geometry and load conditions.

3.1.21 *rotary torque*—the moment applied to the moveable component with its vector aligned to an axis parallel to the *z*-axis and causing or intending to cause an internal or external rotation.

3.1.22 *tibial eminence*—a raised geometrical feature separating the tibial condyles.

3.2 *Definitions of Terms Specific to This Standard:*

3.2.1 *constraint*—the relative inability of a TKR to be further displaced in a specific direction under a given set of loading conditions as dictated by the TKR's geometrical design. This motion is limited, as defined in this test, to the available articular or bearing surfaces found on the tibial component. The actual relative motion values will be provided as an indicator of this type of constraint.

3.2.2 *coordinate system* —(see Fig. 1) a set of arbitrary cartesian coordinates affixed to the stationary component and aligned such that the origin is located at the intersection of the *y* and *z* axes.

3.2.2.1 *Discussion*—The *y*-axis is parallel to the ML direction, directed medially, and is coincident with the mated components' contact points when the knee is in the neutral position (see 7.2). The *z*-axis is located midway between the mated components' contact points (or in the case of a singular contact point, located at that point) and aligned in the superior-inferior direction of the distal component. A third axis, *x*, mutually orthogonal to the two previous axes is directed posteriorly. For determination of contact points, see Annex A1 and Fig. 2. The contact point shall be located to a tolerance of ±1 mm. In the case of multiple contact points on a condyle, an average location of the contact points shall be used.

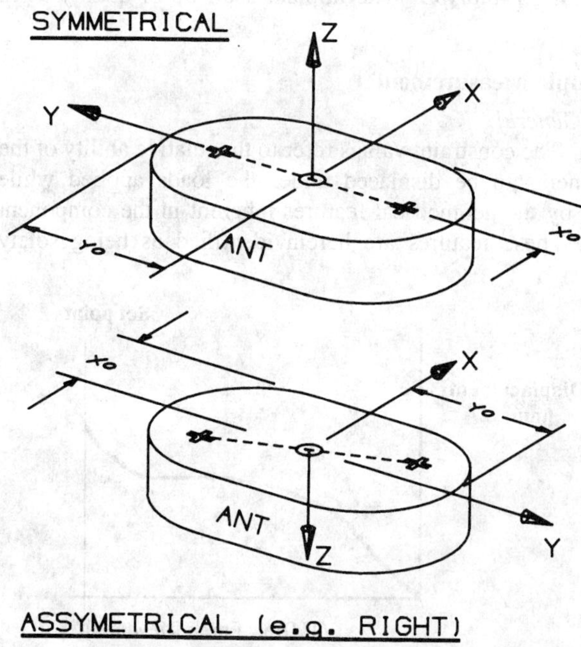

FIG. 1 Defined Coordinate System Examples

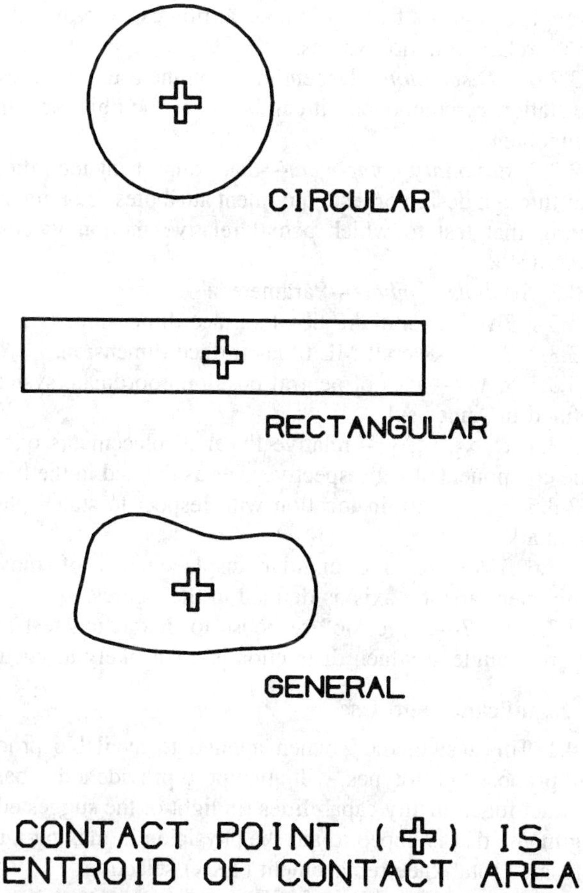

FIG. 2 Tibial Condyle Contact Point Location Examples

3.2.3 *degrees of freedom*—although the knee joint is noted to have 6 df, or directions in which relative motion is guided (three translations: AP, ML, vertical; three angulations: flexion, internal-external, varus-valgus), the coupling effects due to geometrical features reduce this number to the four which are the bases of this test method: AP draw, ML shear, internal-external rotation, and distraction.

3.2.4 *neutral position* (see 7.2)—that position in which the TKR is at rest with no relative linear or angular displacements between components.

3.2.4.1 *Discussion*—This is design-dependent and there may be a unique neutral position at each flexion angle. It may be indicated that the femoral component, when implanted, be positioned at some angle of hyperextension as seen when the patient's knee is fully extended; this, then becomes the neutral position for negative flexion angle tests. The neutral position may be determined by either applying a compressive force of 100 N and allowing the implant to settle or by measuring the vertical position of the movable component with respect to the stationary and using the low point of the component as the neutral point. In those implants with a flat zone and no unique low point, the midpoint of the flat zone can be used as the neutral point. For those implants having a tibial component with a posterior tilt, the user may use other means to define the neutral point, but will report on how it was found.

3.2.5 *set point*—that numeric quantity assigned to an input such as a load.

3.2.6 *movable component*—that component identified either

through design or test equipment attributes as providing the actual relative motion values.

3.2.6.1 *Discussion*—Depending upon the user's fixtures and the stationary component, it can be either the tibial or femoral component.

3.2.7 *stationary component*—that component identified either through design or test equipment attributes as being at rest during that test to which actual relative motion values are referenced.

3.3 *Symbols:Symbols*—Parameters:

3.3.1 *TAP*—overall AP tibial surface dimension.

3.3.2 *TML*—overall ML tibial surface dimension.

3.3.3 *x, y, z*—axes of neutral position coordinate system as defined in Annex A1.

3.3.4 x_1, x_2, y_1, y_2—relative linear displacements of movable component along respective axes as defined in the figures.

3.3.5 x_o, y_o—origin location with respect to stated plateau landmark.

3.3.6 *ANG*—relative angular displacements of movable component about *z*-axis as defined in the figures.

3.3.7 *DIST*—a "yes/no" response to distraction test at the reported angle at which distraction is most likely to occur.

4. Significance and Use

4.1 This test method, when applied to available products and proposed prototypes, will attempt to provide a database of product functionality capabilities (in light of the suggested test regimens) that is hoped to aid the physician in making a more informed total knee replacement (TKR) selection.

4.2 A proper matching of TKR functional restorative capabilities and recipient's (patient's) needs is more likely provided for by a rational testing protocol of the implant in an effort to reveal certain device characteristics pertinent to the selection process.

4.3 The TKR product designs are varied and offer a wide range of constraint (stability). The constraint of the TKR in the *in vitro* condition is dependent on several geometrical and kinematic interactions among the implant's components which can be identified and quantified. The degree of TKR's kinematic interactions should correspond to the recipient's needs as determined by the physician during clinical examination.

5. Apparatus

5.1 *General*:

5.1.1 The stationary component should be free to move only in directions parallel to the *z*-axis and not permitted to rotate about this axis in all but the distraction test. In the distraction test it is fully fixed.

5.1.2 The movable component shall be the displaced member when under loads specific to that test and shall be instrumented accordingly to obtain data pertinent to that test.

5.1.3 Load or torque actuators producing input vectors which tend to displace the movable component relative to the stationary component according to the guidelines of the specific tests shall be provided with a means of gradually applying the load or torque to the set point of that test.

5.1.4 Displacement sensing devices shall be arranged so as to measure relative motion between components in accordance with the prescribed coordinate system.

5.1.5 Output graphs depicting the relationship of load and displacement may provide the investigator with insight into the device's behavior or test setup, or both. It is therefore recommended that such capabilities of the apparatus be included in these tests. (See Fig. 3.)

5.2 *Antero-Posterior Draw Test*—The movable component shall be rigidly set in a fixture free to move in linear directions parallel to the *x*-axis only.

5.3 *Medio-Lateral Shear Test*—The movable component shall be rigidly set in a fixture free to move in linear directions parallel to the *y*-axis only.

5.4 *Rotary Laxity Test*—The movable component shall be rigidly set in a fixture free to move in angular displacements about an axis parallel to the *z*-axis only.

5.5 *Distraction Test*:

5.5.1 The movable component shall be rigidly set in a fixture free to move in only those directions tending to permit such distraction. Should distraction be possible at more than one angle of flexion the test should be conducted at that angle which would most likely permit the distraction.

5.5.2 The stationary component shall be rigidly set in a fixture and not permitted to move in those directions allowed to the movable component.

6. Test Specimens

6.1 *TKR Specimens*:

6.1.1 The TKR should be the manufacturer's designated" standard" or "medium" size as this is more suitable to the loading regimes encountered in the tests.

6.1.2 The implant shall be procured in its original packaging as supplied to the user by the manufacturer.

6.1.3 If the implant is not available in its package state, the condition of the device must meet all geometry and material specifications, but may contain slight surface irregularities (that is, "cosmetic rejects") not considered influential in those regions of the device deemed critical to the specific test.

6.2 *TKR Prototype*—The implant shall be of quality as in 6.1.3.

7. Sample Measurement

7.1 *General*:

7.1.1 The constraint values refer to the relative ability of the components to be displaced under the loads applied while guided by the geometrical features inherent in the component design. These features are herein identified as being solely

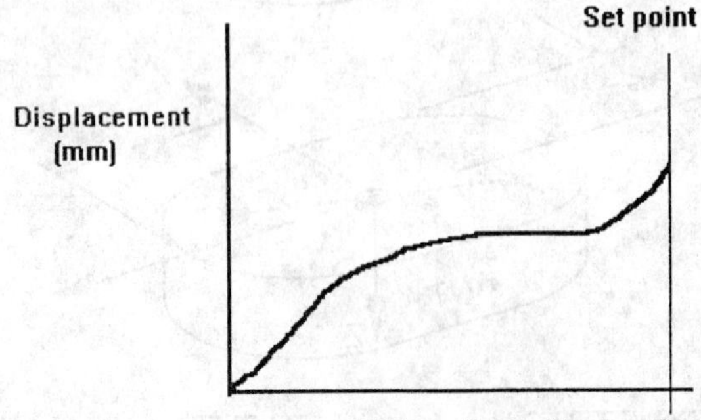

FIG. 3 Output Graph Example

based on bearing surfaces, although certain designs offer enhanced constraint (stability) due to other structures. The tibial bearing surfaces are used as a reference for relative displacement since the components should not move beyond the limits of these features, this being disarticulation.

7.2 *Neutral Position* (NP)—The neutral position is used as the initial at-rest condition prior to any test as defined in 3.2.4. It also corresponds to the measurement coordinate system which is affixed to the stationary component and aligned along anatomical planes. The location of the origin of the coordinate system is determined in Annex A1.

7.3 *Tibial Bearing Surface Dimensions*:

7.3.1 The TML and TAP reflect the medial-lateral width and antero-posterior length of the tibial tray. Typically TML shall be the maximum width of the implant. The TAP shall be the maximum antero-posterior dimension, typically at the medial-lateral center of the implant.

7.3.2 Overall tibial surface dimensions are measured from their projection onto the coronal or *xy*-plane. Refer to Figs. 1-6, and (TAP, TML, X_o, and Y_o).

8. Conditioning

8.1 Expose the test specimens to a clean atmosphere at a temperature of 25 ± 5°C for 24 h prior to testing.

8.2 At the time of the test, the tibial bearing surface will be lightly coated with a film of silicon to reduce frictional effects. The lubricant shall not have any viscoelastic properties and shall have a constant viscosity between 50 and 350 centistokes. An example of a lubricant used during the intralaboratory testing is poly(dimethysiloxone) 200 (Aldrich Chemical Co., viscosity 100 cSt). Either a liquid silicon oil can be used or a silicon mist. If a mist is used, the solvent shall be allowed to boil off. Before testing, the implant must be moved cyclically three times in the desired direction before data are acquired. These three repetitions can be performed by hand or using the method described in Section 9-Procedure.

9. Procedure

9.1 *General*:

9.1.1 Distraction test instructions are a special case, refer to 9.5

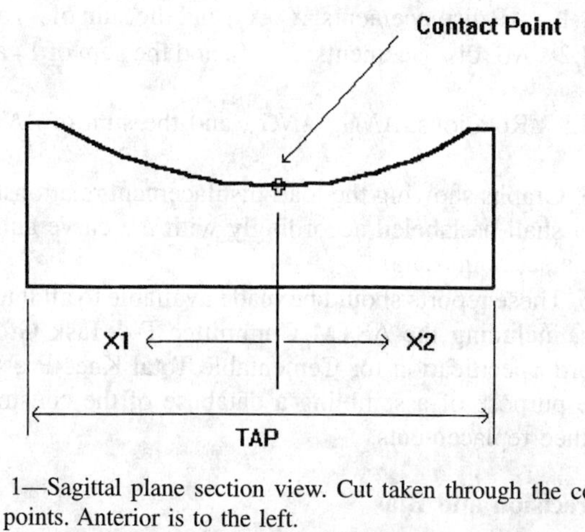

NOTE 1—Sagittal plane section view. Cut taken through the condylar contact points. Anterior is to the left.

FIG. 4 AP Dimensions and Displacement Examples

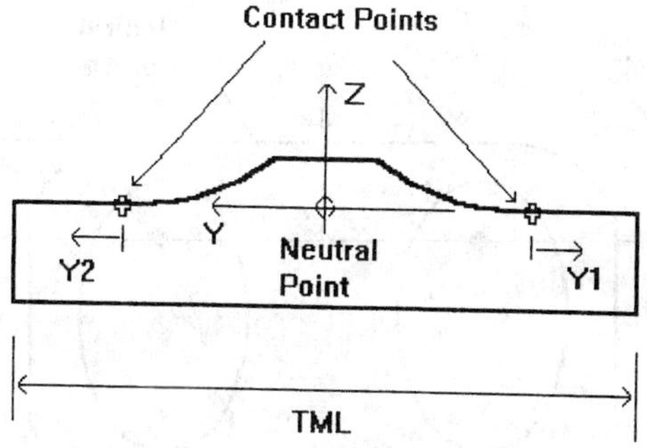

NOTE 1—Coronal plane section view. Cut taken though the condylar contact points. Medial is to the left.

FIG. 5 ML Dimensions and Displacements Example

9.1.2 Prior to installation of the tibial component, measure all relevant bearing surface dimensions as described in 7.3.

9.1.3 Install the stationary component in the apparatus such that the imaginary coordinate system attached to the stationary component is aligned with that of the fixturing, that is, loading devices are aligned with their respective axes.

9.1.4 The tests shall be performed at flexion angles specified by Specification for Cementable Total Knee Prostheses.[3]

9.1.5 Install the movable component such that when mated to the stationary component the condylar contact points seen are the same as those used to describe the neutral position and, hence, the coordinate system for that flexion angle.

9.1.6 Null all output instrumentation.

9.1.7 Apply the joint reaction force to a set point of 44.5 N.

9.1.8 If the AP draw, ML shear, or rotary laxity tests are stopped before reaching the set point load or torque, due to possible dislocation of the components, the maximum load or torque reached will be recorded and included in the report.

9.1.9 Each test must be completed within 2 min from initiation of the AP drawer force, the ML shear force, or the torque. If the time required to complete the test is greater than 2 min, it shall be reported.

9.1.10 If an *xy* slider is used to allow antero-posterior or medial motion, the slider friction will be measured and compensated for in the applied set point values.

9.1.11 If an implant has movable meniscal bearing inserts, they should not be constrained during each test.

9.2 *AP Draw Test*:

9.2.1 Apply the AP draw load gradually to a set point of 10 N, directed anteriorly, or until disarticulation of the components is imminent or a mechanical stop prevents further motion.

9.2.2 Record the AP displacement (in millimetres) and note as X_1.

9.2.3 Remove the loads and relocate the movable component to the neutral position.

9.2.4 Repeat 9.1.6 and 9.1.7 and 9.2.1, but direct the AP load posteriorly.

9.2.5 Record the AP displacement (in millimetres) and note as X_2.

[3] This document is currently under development in Subcommittee F04.02 and may be obtained by contacting the Committee F-4 staff manager.

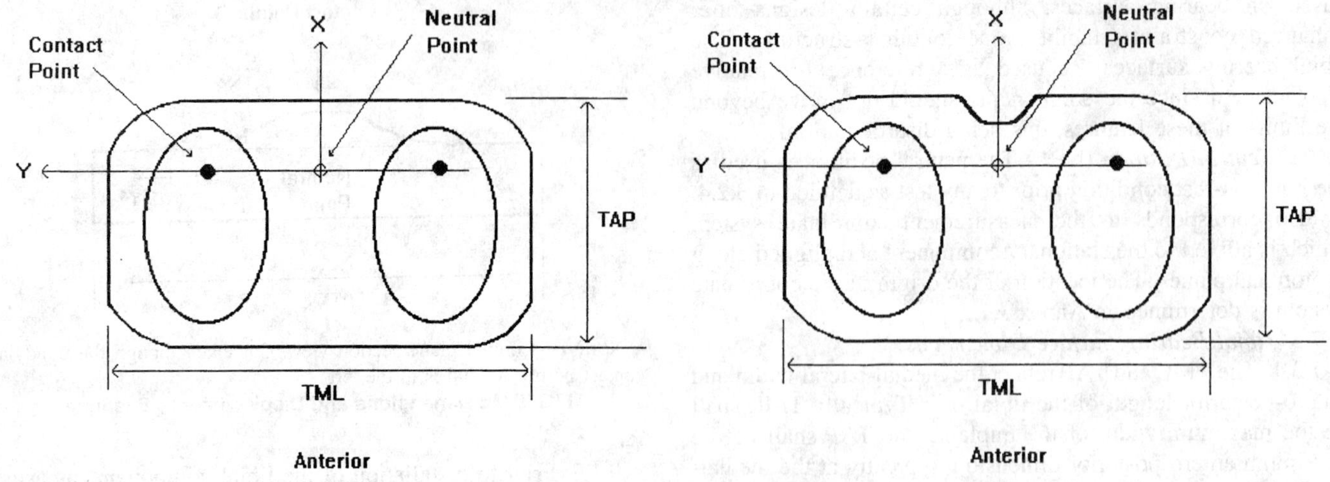

Note—Transverse plane section view. Center of rotation for rotary laxity test is about the neutral point.

Note—Transverse plane section view. Center of rotation for rotary laxity test is about the neutral point.

FIG. 6 A,B Neutral Point Determination Example

9.2.6 For additional flexion angles repeat 9.1.5-9.1.7 and 9.2.1-9.2.5.

9.3 *ML Shear Test*:

9.3.1 Apply the ML shear load gradually to a set point of 15 N, directed medially or until disarticulation of the component is imminent or a mechanical stop prevents further motion.

9.3.2 Record the ML displacement (in millimetres) and note as Y_1.

9.3.3 Remove the loads and relocate the movable component to the neutral position.

9.3.4 Repeat 9.1.6 and 9.1.7 and 9.3.1, but direct the ML shear load laterally.

9.3.5 Record the ML displacement (in millimetres) and note as Y_2.

9.3.6 For additional flexion angles repeat 9.1.5-9.1.7 and 9.3.1-9.3.5.

9.4 *Rotary Laxity Test*:

9.4.1 Apply the rotary torque gradually to a set point of 0.5 N·m directed internally, or until disarticulation of the components is imminent or a mechanical stop prevents further motion or a rotation of 90° is reached.

9.4.2 Record the internal rotation (in degrees) and note as ANG_i.

9.4.3 Remove the loads and relocate the movable component to the neutral position.

9.4.4 Repeat 9.1.5-9.1.7 and 9.4.1, but direct the rotary torque externally.

9.4.5 Record the external rotation (in degrees) and note as ANG_e.

9.4.6 For additional flexion angles repeat 9.1.5-9.1.7 and 9.4.1-9.4.5.

9.5 *Distraction Test*:

9.5.1 If distraction is deemed possible at more than one flexion angle, select that flexion angle at which distraction is most likely to occur.

9.5.2 Install the components in the apparatus such that the distraction force vector is in line with those design features normally providing the coupling for which distraction is being tested.

9.5.3 Apply the distraction force gradually to the movable component to a set point of 44.5 N.

9.5.4 If distraction occurred prior to or at the set point, report only that distraction occurred and the flexion angle for the occurrence.

10. Report

10.1 Product codes, lot and heat numbers, serial numbers, and special processes that might influence the test results should be noted.

10.2 Product sizing and specific dimensions relative to the performance of the tests that shall be recorded include *TAP* and *TML* (see Figs. 4-6).

10.3 Report the location (in millimetres) of origin of each neutral position with respect to prominent landmarks on the movable component (see Fig. 1).

10.4 Report the following test results to one decimal place using standard rounding convention.

10.4.1 AP displacements: X_1, X_2, and the sum of X_1 and X_2,

10.4.2 ML displacements: Y_1, Y_2, and the sum of Y_1 and Y_2, and

10.4.3 Rotations: ANG_i, ANG_e, and the sum of ANG_i and ANG_e.

10.5 Graphs showing the load-displacement relationship for the test shall be labeled accordingly with the curve annotated with the set point data.

10.6 These reports should be made available to all interested parties, including the ASTM Committee F-4 Task Group on Standard Specification for Cementable Total Knee Prostheses, for the purpose of assembling a database of the constraint of total knee replacements.

11. Precision and Bias

11.1 At the current time, a round-robin test is underway.

Although four participants have completed the testing, additional testing is required before a statement on the precision and bias of this test method can be made.

12. Keywords

12.1 arthroplasty; constraint; joint; laxity; prosthesis; total knee replacement

ANNEX

(Mandatory Information)

A1. NEUTRAL POSITION (NP) COORDINATE SYSTEM

A1.1 The origin is located on the stationary component at the intersection of three mutually orthogonal axes which are positioned with respect to the contact point(s) of the two components when at rest at a specific flexion angle (see Fig. 6).

A1.2 The contact point(s) on the components, which may be found using a variety of visual techniques (for example, removable dye, pressure-sensitive film, fingerprint dust, vacuum grease with carbon black, or a molding material), are the geometric centers of the contact area(s) (see Fig. 2).

A1.3 Should a line connecting the two contact points be parallel to the ML direction, and perhaps to the anterior border, then this is the *y*-axis. If the line is not aligned with the ML direction, then a point midway between the contact points is chosen through which the *y*-axis will pass being aligned in the ML direction. If only one contact point exists, then the *y*-axis passes through this point. The *y*-axis is directed medially.

A1.4 The *x*-axis is perpendicular to the *y*-axis at the midpoint between the line connecting the contact points. If only one contact point exists then the *x*-axis passes through this point. It is directed posteriorly.

A1.5 The *xy*-plane is thus at the level of the contact points and is aligned with the coronal plane. The location of the origin may now be noted referencing reported landmarks particular to the design.

A1.6 The *z*-axis is perpendicular to the *xy*-plane through the origin. It is directed using right-hand rule conventions: upward for left and symmetrical TKR, downward for right TKR (see Fig. 1).

A1.7 The geometry of the TKR may cause the contact points to shift at different flexion angles resulting in unique coordinate systems and hence neutral positions. These must be reported with reference to stated plateau landmarks.

APPENDIX

(Nonmandatory Information)

X1. RATIONALE

X1.1 In clinical practice there are significant differences among patients' requirements for total knee prostheses. These requirements will be determined by available bone stock and soft tissue capacities for stabilization. Because of these differences a method of classification of prosthetic total knee replacement (excluding patello-femoral interaction) is desirable to allow the surgeon to assess the applicability of the knee prosthesis to the particular patient problem under consideration.

X1.2 For instance, the patient with good soft tissue restraints will perhaps require a lesser constraint prosthesis, whereas the patient with major bone loss or destroyed ligamentous structures will more probably require a prosthesis with a higher degree of constraint.

X1.3 Biomechanical testing methods may take many directions depending upon the investigator or the facilities available, or both. Quite important to the standardization is the need for uniformity throughout the various testing programs. To provide comparable data from individual investigators, a standard test protocol is desired. These data, then, will provide some of the criteria for the selection of the prosthesis which will best fit the patient's needs. This test method provides quantitative data on the degree of constraint a prosthesis may provide and does not intend to contradict the three levels of constraint defined by the (Federal Drug Administration) FDA. The Specification for Cementable Total Knee Prostheses can use these results to classify prostheses into different categories by considering the end use of the devices and the data. Note that these tests are not intended to be nor are they related to the durability or reliability of the prosthetic device. The loads that were chosen are for relative comparison of devices and are not intended to be related to any physiological loads. They are intended to test geometrical design factors without introducing viscoelastic effects or causing deformation of the implants. It has been suggested that different results would be obtained at higher compressive pre-loads, but it has been shown that in one mode of testing, rotary, laxity, and the amount of compressive load does not alter the relative classification order of the knee implants tested. More data will need to be examined in the future to determine whether the magnitude of the compressive pre-load alters the classification of total knee replacements. The extremes in the TKR's range-of-motion or the manner in which such is arrested or not, as the case may be, are not covered in this test method. The speed of the test has not been specified to allow the test to be completed using deadweights. Sections 9.2.1, 9.3.1, and 9.4.1 simply indicate the load should be applied gradually to eliminate any displacement spikes. During the course of the round robin testing, users of this test method have completed the test in times ranging from five seconds to one minute.

X1.4 Test Method F 1223 has been revised from its original version approved in 1989 to clarify or simplify, or both, how certain measurements are made. As a result of the round-robin testing, it was decided to not continue to require the calculation of a constraint ratio.

X1.5 In 1995, In Test Method F 1223 was further revised to increase the contact point determination tolerance (3.2.2); to not require any humidity control (8.1); to allow the preliminary motions to be performed by hand or in accordance with Section 9 (8.2); to clarify the test time limits (9.1.9 and X1.3); add descriptive title in 104; and add reference to the Rationale (X1.3).

Standard Guide for Providing System Evaluation for Emergency Medical Services[1]

This standard is issued under the fixed designation F 1224; the number immediately following the designation indicates the year of original adoption or, in the case of revision, the year of last revision. A number in parentheses indicates the year of last reapproval. A superscript epsilon (ε) indicates an editorial change since the last revision or reapproval.

ϵ^1 NOTE—Section 12, Keywords, was added editorially in June 1996.

1. Scope

1.1 This guide covers providing system evaluation for emergency medical services **(1)**,[2] including authority, responsibility, objectives, approaches, data, applications, and implementation.

NOTE 1—This guide does not address evaluation for individual prehospital, hospital, or posthospital providers. (Related guides will be developed.)

2. Referenced Documents

2.1 *ASTM Standards:*

F 1149 Practice for the Qualifications, Responsibilities, and Authority of Individuals and Institutions Providing Medical Direction of Emergency Medical Services[3]

F 1177 Terminology Relating to Emergency Medical Services[3]

3. Terminology

3.1 *Definitions of Terms Specific to This Standard:*

3.1.1 *system evaluation*—a review of the performance of emergency medical services systems by qualified, experienced individuals.

3.1.2 *minimum data set*—the minimum number of data elements required for system evaluation.

3.2 *Definitions*—See Terminology F 1177.

4. Significance of Use

4.1 This guide establishes system evaluation as an essential component of emergency medical services systems.

4.2 This guide covers the methods and materials that are necessary to evaluate quality for emergency medical services systems at both the system operations and patient care levels.

5. Authority

5.1 The authority for providing system evaluation for emergency medical services rests with the entity that is utlimately legally responsible for system operation and evaluation.

6. Responsibility

6.1 The responsibility for providing system evaluation for emergency medical services systems rests with the directors of the entities specified in 5.1.

6.2 The responsibility for providing adequate financial resources and appropriate medical confidentiality for system evaluation for emergency medical services rests with the entities specified in 5.1.

6.3 Independent evaluation of individual parts of the emergency medical services system by prehospital, hospital, or posthospital providers must be integrated with and must not be substituted for system evaluation.

7. Objectives

7.1 System evaluation of quality for emergency medical services entails five objectives **(2)** including:

7.1.1 Setting priorities,

7.1.2 Assessing outcome,

7.1.3 Identifying problems,

7.1.4 Effecting changes, and

7.1.5 Reassessing outcome.

8. Approaches

8.1 System evaluation of quality entails approaches of structure, process, and outcome, singly or combined **(3)**.

8.2 The approaches specified in 8.1 should be applied at both the system operations and patient care levels.

8.2.1 Applied at the system operations level (Table 1) these approaches provide a means of identifying issues that require further attention, including:

8.2.1.1 System operation, and

8.2.1.2 Individual patients.

8.2.2 Applied at the patient care level these approaches provide a means of evaluating care for patients that are specified in 8.2.1.2.

8.3 Audits performed using the approaches specified in 8.1 should examine two aspects of care, including:

8.3.1 Compliance with system standards, and

8.3.2 Appropriateness of system standards.

[1] This guide is under the jurisdiction of ASTM Committee F-30 on Emergency Medical Services and is the direct responsibility of Subcommittee F30.03 on Organization/Management.

Current edition approved July 7, 1989. Published August 1989.

[2] The boldface numbers in parentheses refer to the references at the end of this guide.

[3] *Annual Book of ASTM Standards*, Vol 13.01.

TABLE 1 Approaches and Methods for System Evaluation for Emergency Medical Services

Evaluation Approaches	Evaluation Methods
Structure (standards)	ASTM guides (to be developed)
Process (care)	Medical direction (Guide F 1149) **(1)**
Outcome (results)	Intermediate: preventable morbidity **(4)**
	Final: preventable morbidity
	preventable mortality **(5)**
Combined	Preventable morbidity
	Preventable mortality
	Tracers **(6)**
	Registries **(7)**
	Generic Screens **(8)**

TABLE 2 Evaluation Criteria

High-Yield **(8)**	
Deaths	
High-Risk	
Critical care admissions	
Morbidity	
Instability—Symptoms:	severe pain, dyspnea, etc.
Signs:	severe injury, tachypnea, etc.
Procedures:	thoracostomy, air transport, etc.
Diagnoses:	shock, respiratory failure, etc.
Regionalized Care	
Prospective—prehospital or emergency department triage	
Transfers—interfacility	
Retrospective—discharges, deaths	
Administrative Review	
Complaint—patient, provider or third-party	
Prehospital Protocol Deviation—exceeding standard of care	
Patient Refusing Prehospital Care—against medical advice	
Outliers	
Medical—mortality, morbidity, timeliness, etc.	
Administrative—diagnostic related groups, cost, etc.	
Randomized	

9. Data

9.1 Systemwide uniform recordkeeping constitutes an essential element of medical evaluation of emergency medical services systems.

9.2 Emergency medical services system data sources subject to uniform recordkeeping include:

9.2.1 Prehospital care: dispatches, first responders, prehospital providers, base stations;

9.2.2 Facility care: nonhospital-based emergency facilities, hospitals;

9.2.3 Posthospital care: rehabilitation facilities, home care programs; and

9.2.4 Government agencies: medical examiners.

9.3 Each source specified in 9.2 must collect and report the data contained in the minimum data set as determined by the entity specified in 5.1.

9.3.1 Data comprise three types, including:

9.3.1.1 Patient demographic data such as patient origin, etiologic factors, condition severity, and resource utilization;

9.3.1.2 System operation data such as elapsed times, patient volumes, and protocol compliance; and

9.3.1.3 Patient care data such as procedures, diagnoses, and outcomes.

10. Applications

10.1 Patients who should be considered for evaluation by emergency medical services systems include, but are not limited to, those exhibiting the characteristics identified in Table 2.

10.2 Emergency medical services systems incorporating subsystems, such as those for burn, behavioral, cardiac, pediatric, perinatal, toxicologic, or traumatic emergencies, may require categories in addition to those specified in Table 2. When required, such categories should be identified in their respective subsystem standards.

11. Implementation

11.1 Implementation of system evaluation for emergency medical services entails eight steps, including:

11.1.1 Defining existing authority, responsibility, standards, and resources,

11.1.2 Establishing goals and objectives,

11.1.3 Selecting an approach and method,

11.1.4 Assembling data,

11.1.5 Analyzing results,

11.1.6 Modifying standards,

11.1.7 Periodically disseminating findings, and

11.1.8 Continually reevaluating the system.

12. Keywords

12.1 emergency medical service; emergency medical services system; system evaluation

REFERENCES

(1) Cayten, C. G., Evans, W. J.," EMS Systems Evaluation," Boyd, D. R., Edlich, R. F., Micik, S., eds, *Systems Approach to Emergency Medical Care*, Norwalk, CT, Appleton-Century-Crofts, 1983, Chapter 8.

(2) Williamson, J. W., Aronovitch, S., Simonson, L., et al, "Health Accounting: An Outcome-Based System of Quality Assurance: Illustrative Application to Hypertension," *Bulletin of the New York Academy of Medicine*, 1975, pp. 727–738.

(3) Donabedian, A., "Evaluating the Quality of Medical Care," *Milbank Memorial Fund Quarterly*, 1966, Vol 44, pp. 166–206.

(4) Pozen, M., et al, "Confirmation Parameters for Assessing Prehospital Care," final report for the National Center for Health Services Research, Hyattsville, MD, 1980.

(5) Rutstein, D. D., Berenberg, W., Chalmers, T. L., et al, "Measuring the Quality of Medical Care: A Clinical Method," *New England Journal of Medicine*, 1976, Vol 294, pp. 582–584.

(6) Kessner, D. M., Kalk, C. E., Singer, J., "Assessing Health Quality—The Case for Tracers," *New England Journal of Medicine*, 1973, Vol 288, pp. 189–194.

(7) Brooke, E. M., *The Current and Future Use of Registers in Health Information Systems*, Geneva, Switzerland, World Health Organization, 1974.

(8) Shortell, S. M., Richardson, W. C., *Health Program Evaluation*, St. Louis, MO, 1978.

Designation: F 1229 – 00

Standard Guide for Establishing the Qualifications, Education, and Training of EMS, Air-Medical Patient Care Providers[1]

This standard is issued under the fixed designation F 1229; the number immediately following the designation indicates the year of original adoption or, in the case of revision, the year of last revision. A number in parentheses indicates the year of last reapproval. A superscript epsilon (ϵ) indicates an editorial change since the last revision or reapproval.

INTRODUCTION

This guide describes the minimal qualifications, education, and training of five, definitive, air-medical providers. These guidelines are built on a foundation of recognized courses that are used to credential patient care providers; emergency medical technicians, nurses, and physicians. The members of the task group are experienced air-medical providers and users with broad and distinctive EMS backgrounds.

1. Scope

1.1 This guide applies only to personnel involved in the provision of *emergency* medical air transport, and does not necessarily address the qualifications, education, and training of specialty care responders or other allied health professionals.

1.2 This guide establishes air-medical nomenclature.

1.3 This guide establishes *minimal* qualifications, education, and training requirements for the air-medical crew member(s) and the air-medical director.

1.4 This guide identifies the general content of the curricula for air-medical education and training.

1.5 It is expected that a standard guide for education and training curricula, certification, and air-medical operations will be developed.

1.6 *This standard does not purport to address all of the safety concerns, if any, associated with its use. It is the responsibility of the user of this standard to establish appropriate safety and health practices and determine the applicability of regulatory limitations prior to use.*

2. Referenced Documents

2.1 *ASTM Standards:*

F 1031 Practice for Training the Emergency Medical Technician (Basic)[2]

3. Terminology

3.1 *Descriptions of Terms:*

3.1.1 *aeromedicine*—the branch of medicine that deals with the physiological, psychological, pathological, and epidemiological conditions, diseases, and disturbances that arise from flying.

3.1.2 *air-medical*—the practice of air-medicine.

3.1.3 *air-medical crew member(s)* (ACM)—patient care providers on-board medical flights. Identified by the prefix *flight* before their credentialed title (that is, *flight nurse*).

3.1.4 *air-medical director*—a physician who is licensed or otherwise legally authorized to practice and who functions within an air-medical operation as the individual ultimately responsible for the quality of patient care.

3.1.5 *air-medical operations*—that aspect of air-medicine involving policies, procedures, and protocols.

3.1.6 *air-medical patient care providers*—air-medical crew members and air-medical directors.

3.1.7 *air-medicine*—a discipline of medicine associated with the care and management of patients transported by aircraft.

3.1.8 *care*—patient care.

3.1.9 *educational experience*—the accumulation of knowledge and skills through education, training, and clinical practice.

3.1.10 *emergency medical air transport*—the transport of EMS patients by air.

3.1.11 *mission*—the specific patient care task and responsibility that an EMS provider has accepted.

3.1.12 *qualification*—possessing a recognized definable body of knowledge or specific credential (certificate, license, registration, or degree).

3.1.13 *specialty-care responder*—emergency air-medical responders whose mission is clearly defined and exclusively dedicated to the care of patients with specific illness or injuries.

3.1.14 *training*—supervised acquisition of specific skill or judgment, or both.

4. Significance and Use

4.1 This guide provides minimal criteria for development of

---

[1] This guide is under the jurisdiction of ASTM Committee F30 on Emergency Medical Services and is the direct responsibility of Subcommittee F30.02 on Personnel, Training and Education.

Current edition approved Oct. 10, 2000. Published December 2000. Originally published as F 1229 - 89. Last previous edition F 1229 - 89 (1998).

[2] *Annual Book of ASTM Standards*, Vol 13.01.

air-medical education and training programs.

4.2 This guide aids in the selection of education and training programs that will correspond to the level of the defined patient care mission.

4.3 It is recognized that the body of knowledge encompassed by an education and training program, not the degree, certificate, or license, is crucial, although documentation of such training may be difficult without said credentials.

4.4 This guide pertains to education, training, and curricula development and is not intended to be used operationally to select the level of patient care provider.

AIR-MEDICAL CREW MEMBERS

5. Flight EMT-Basic—Qualifications, Education, and Training

5.1 The education and training provided at this level is recognized as producing the minimally qualified ACM. The training shall include the knowledge and skills identified by both the required and optional objectives contained in Practice F 1031. Additional training in the following areas is required:

5.1.1 Air-medical patient handling considerations,

5.1.2 Aircraft safety,

5.1.3 Altitude physiology, and principles of atmospheric physics (gas laws),

5.1.4 Aviation communication,

5.1.5 Crash and survival procedures,

5.1.6 Familiarization with EMS systems in the service area,

5.1.7 Hazardous materials response procedures,

5.1.8 In-flight treatment modalities,

5.1.9 Infection control,

5.1.10 Mapping/aircraft orientation,

5.1.11 Oxygen therapy in relation to altitude,

5.1.12 Patient assessment in the airborne environment,

5.1.13 Quality assurance,

5.1.14 Roles and responsibilities,

5.1.15 Stress recognition and management,

5.1.16 Urinary catheter, nasogastric tube, feeding tubes, and ostomy devices: indications, complications, and monitoring of these devices in the airborne environment, and

5.1.17 Vital sign determination in the airborne environment.

5.2 Additional, desirable, education and training includes adult and pediatric cardiac, trauma, and burn life support.

6. Flight EMT-Intermediate—Qualifications, Education, and Training

6.1 The minimal entry level for a flight EMT-intermediate shall be the body of knowledge and skills identified by the required and optional objectives contained in EMT-I as defined in the DOT, National Standard Curriculum.[3] The flight EMT-intermediate shall possess all of the knowledge and skills required of a flight EMT-basic. Commensurate with the patient care mission, additional education and training is at the discretion of the air-medical director.

7. Flight EMT-P (Flight Paramedic)—Qualifications, Education, and Training

7.1 The minimum entry level for a flight EMT-paramedic shall be the body of knowledge and skills identified by both the required and optional objectives contained in the EMT-Paramedic DOT National Standard Curriculum.[4] The flight EMT-paramedic shall possess all of the knowledge and skills required of a flight EMT-intermediate. Commensurate with the patient care mission, additional education and training is at the discretion of the air-medical director and shall include:

7.1.1 Airborne endotracheal intubation/ventilation and needle cricothyroidotomy.

7.1.1.1 Rapid sequence induction as an adjunctive technique to intubation.

8. Flight Nurse—Qualifications, Education, and Training

8.1 The minimum entry level for a flight nurse shall be the body of knowledge and skills identified by the objectives contained in an accredited registered nursing program. Additional education and training in the areas 5.1.1-5.1.17. Commensurate with the patient care mission, the flight nurse shall possess all of the knowledge and skills required of a flight EMT-paramedic including those areas in 5.2, and may have additional education and training in the assessment and management of patients with special needs as prescribed by the air-medical director. Education and training shall include the airborne operation of monitoring and therapeutic devices and equipment.

9. Flight Physician—Qualifications, Education, and Training

9.1 The flight physician will be a doctor of medicine or osteopathy who is licensed or otherwise legally authorized to practice and who is educated and trained in areas 5.1.1-5.1.17 and, commensurate with the patient care mission, area 5.2.

10. Air-Medical Director, Flight Medical Director—Qualifications, Education, Training, and Educational Experience

10.1 The air-medical director shall be a physician who is licensed or otherwise legally authorized to practice and who has had educational experience in those areas of medicine and prehospital care that are commensurate with the patient care mission(s) including 5.2. Additional educational experience shall include areas listed in 5.1.1-5.1.17.

11. Keywords

11.1 aeromedicine; flight nurse; paramedic

[3] Training Program for the Emergency Medical Technician-Intermediate: National Standard Curriculum (see latest version).

[4] Training Program for the Emergency Medical Technician-Paramedic: National Standard Curriculum DOT (see latest version).

Designation: F 1242 – 96[ε1]

Standard Specification for Cuffed and Uncuffed Tracheal Tubes[1]

This standard is issued under the fixed designation F 1242; the number immediately following the designation indicates the year of original adoption or, in the case of revision, the year of last revision. A number in parentheses indicates the year of last reapproval. A superscript epsilon (ε) indicates an editorial change since the last revision or reapproval.

ε[1] NOTE—Editorial changes were made May 1997.

1. Scope

1.1 This specification covers the dimensions, rationale, labeling specifications, selected performance requirements, and test methods of cuffed and uncuffed Magill and Murphy-type tracheal tubes. These tubes are commonly used as airway catheters in human patients in the practice of anesthesiology and in respiratory care. This specification represents the state of the art at the time of publication and will be subject to periodic review.

1.2 This specification also provides test protocols to assess the performance and safety of cuffed oral and nasal tracheal tubes for prolonged use. Supporting rationale for the requirements is provided in Appendix X1, and references are included. Required safety and performance tests, together with availability of results, are relied upon in this specification, whenever possible, to allow a manufacturer the maximum use of technological alternatives in design and materials.

1.3 The values stated in SI units are to be regarded as standard.

1.4 The following precautionary caveat pertains to the test method portions, Annex A1 and Appendix X2, of this specification: *This standard does not purport to address all of the safety concerns, if any, associated with its use. It is the responsibility of the user of this standard to establish appropriate safety and health practices and determine the applicability of regulatory limitations prior to use.*

1.5 The following is a list of subject headings and subheadings included in this specification and the sections in which they appear:

[1] This specification is under the jurisdiction of ASTM Committee F-29 on Anesthetic and Respiratory Equipmentand is the direct responsibility of Subcommittee F29.12 on Airways.

Current edition approved Feb. 10, 1996. Published June 1996. Originally published as F 1242 – 89. Last previous edition F 1242 – 89.

This specification, which is a consolidation and revision of ANSI Z79.14-1983 and ANSI Z79.16-1983, supersedes these older standards. No attempt has been made to delineate all types of tracheal tubes. This specification is not intended to inhibit innovation, variation, and future development.

2. Referenced Documents

2.1 *ASTM Standards:*

NOTE 1—This specification is intended to be used in conjunction with the following standards. When the standards referred to in this specification are superseded by an approved revision, the revision shall apply.

F 640 Test Methods for Radiopacity of Plastics for Medical Use[2]

F 813 Practice for Direct Contact Cell Culture Evaluation of Materials for Medical Devices[2]

2.2 *ANSI Standards:*[3]

ANSI/HIMA MD70.1-1983 American National Standard for Medical Material—Luer Taper Fittings—Performance

ANSI Z79.14-1983 American National Standard For Anesthetic Equipment—Tracheal Tubes

ANSI Z79.16-1983 American National Standard for Anesthetic Equipment—Cuffed Oral Tracheal and Nasal Tracheal Tubes for Prolonged Use

3. Terminology

3.1 *Definitions:*

3.1.1 *bevel*—the slanted patient end of the tracheal tube (see Figs. 1 and 2).

3.1.2 *disposable*—an item intended for single use.

3.1.3 *inflation lumen*—the lumen within the wall of the tracheal tube for inflating the tracheal tube cuff.

3.1.4 *inflation tube*—the attached secondary tube for inflating the tracheal tube cuff (see Fig. 2).

3.1.5 *inflation valve*—a valve attached to the inflation system for inflating and deflating the cuff.

3.1.6 *machine end*—the end of the tracheal tube intended to project from the patient.

3.1.7 *Murphy eye*—a hole through the wall of a tracheal tube near the patient end and on the side opposite to the bevel. A Murphy type eye is illustrated in Fig. 3(*a*) to Fig. 3(*d*).

3.1.8 *patient end*—the end of the tracheal tube intended to be inserted into the patient's trachea.

3.1.9 *pilot balloon*—a small balloon attached to the inflation tube to indicate inflation or deflation of the tracheal cuff.

[2] *Annual Book of ASTM Standards*, Vol 13.01.

[3] Available from American National Standards Institute, 1430 Broadway, New York, NY 10018.

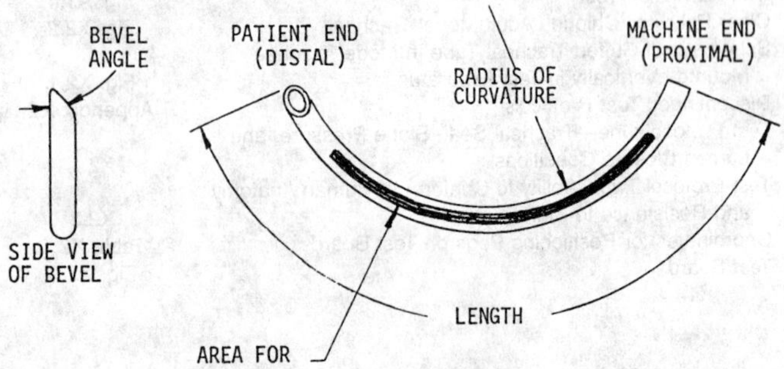

FIG. 1 Tracheal Tube

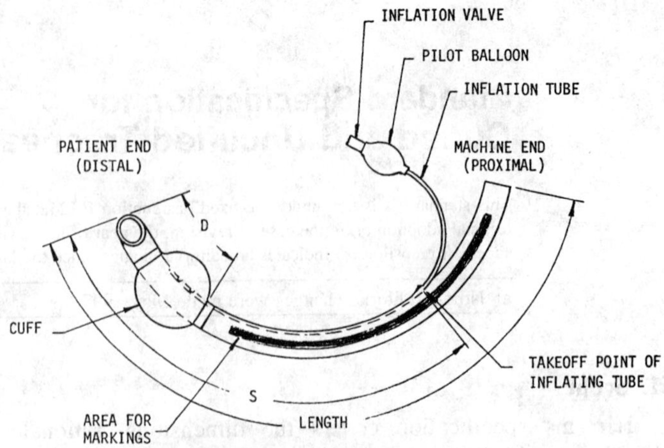

FIG. 2 Cuffed Tracheal Tube

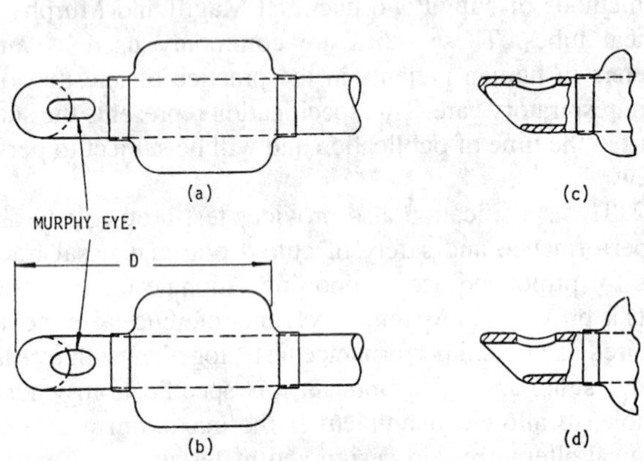

FIG. 3 Typical Murphy Tips

3.1.10 *tracheal tube*—a tube inserted either orally or nasally to convey gases or vapors to and from the trachea. This term shall be used rather than synonyms such as "endotracheal", "intratracheal", or "catheter". Typical tracheal tubes are illustrated in Figs. 1 and 2.

3.1.10.1 *Magill-type tracheal tube*—a Magill-type tracheal tube is illustrated in Fig. 1. Adult sizes of Magill tubes usually are provided with cuffs as illustrated in Fig. 2. A Magill tracheal tube does not have a Murphy eye.

3.1.10.2 *Murphy-type tracheal tube*—a tracheal tube that has a Murphy eye at the patient end as illustrated in Fig. 3(*a*) to Fig. 3(*d*). (See Refs **(1)**[4] and **(2)** for the original descriptions of Magill-type and Murphy-type tracheal tubes.)

3.1.11 *tracheal tube cuff*—an inflatable sleeve fastened to the patient end of the tracheal tube to provide an effective, leak-resistant fit between the tube and the trachea. A tracheal tube cuff is illustrated in Fig. 2.

3.1.12 *tracheal tube cuff resting diameter*—the diameter of the cuff when tested in accordance with A1.5.

4. Materials

4.1 *Inertness*:

4.1.1 Materials intended to be inserted into the patient shall be of a nontoxic substance compatible with human tissue, as

[4] The boldface numbers in parentheses refer to a list of references at the end of this specification.

determined by A1.1. Other tests may be used, including cell culture tests, provided they are shown to be equivalent. The biologic test procedure shall be applied to those portions of the finished product intended for insertion into the patient and in the form that they are supplied to the consumer. For tubes supplied sterile, the test shall be applied after sterilization. For tubes supplied nonsterile, the test shall be applied after the recommended method of sterilization. The test is designed to determine the suitability of formulations and is not intended to be used as a routine test for every lot.

4.1.2 Reusable tracheal tubes should be reasonably resistant both to deterioration by agents used in chemical cleansing and sterilizing and to deterioration from autoclaving, if steam sterilization is recommended.

4.1.3 Conditions of use require that all tracheal tubes be resistant to deterioration from anesthetic agents.

4.2 *Surface Characteristics*:

4.2.1 *Tubes*—The patient end of the tube shall be rounded without sharp points or rough edges. The tube surface should be smooth externally and internally. The external edge of the Murphy eye, if provided, and all bevel edges shall be smooth and well rounded. See Fig. 3.

4.2.2 *Cuffs*—The external surface should be smooth.

4.3 *Rigidity*—All sizes of tracheal tubes should be sufficiently flexible or should soften sufficiently at body temperature, to conform to the patient's airway anatomy without kinking.

4.4 *Integrity of Lumen*—The materials should be such as to allow construction of tracheal tubes with the thinnest possible walls, whose lumen will not be compromised by collapse under the inflated cuff at body temperature. Tubes shall be able to pass the tube collapse test (see A1.2).

5. Requirements for Tubes with Cuffs

5.1 *Cuffs*—The cuff shall be reliably attached to the tracheal tube. (See Ref **(3)** for information on cuff characteristics.) The maximum distance, *D*, from the tip of the tube to the machine end of the cuff shall be as illustrated in Figs. 2 and 3 and stated in Table 2. Upon visual inspection, the bonded edge of the cuff shall not encroach upon the Murphy eye, if present. The general requirement for tracheal tube materials shall also apply to cuff materials (see Section 4). The cuff position and size shall not cause the cuff to herniate over the tube tip under normal conditions of use (see Annex A1.4). The cuff shall inflate symmetrically (see Annex A1.3).

5.2 *Cuff Pressure, Volume, and Diameter Characteristics*—The manufacturer shall determine the resting diameter of the cuff. The diameter shall be stated in millimetres. (See Refs **(4)**, **(5)**, and **(6)** for background information on assessments of cuffs; see Refs **(7)** and **(8)** for reports on variations in sizes and shapes of human tracheas.) The cuff resting diameter shall be tested in accordance with A1.5 and be within ±15 % of the marked value referenced in Section 8.7.

5.3 *Inflation System*— The typical inflation system includes an inflation lumen in the wall of the tracheal tube, an external inflation tube, an optional pilot balloon, and an optional inflation valve (see Fig. 2). The inflation lumen within the wall of the tracheal tube shall not encroach upon the lumen of the tracheal tube and should not bulge outward. The external inflation tube shall not exceed 2.5 mm external diameter and should be attached to the tracheal tube at a small angle without undue projection. The external inflation tube shall be fitted, either with an inflation valve with an inlet that will mate with a male luer syringe tip or shall have a female end capable of accepting a standard luer syringe tip. (See ANSI/HIMA MD70.1.) The external inflation tube shall be attached to the tracheal tube at a distance *S* as described in Fig. 2 and stated in Table 2. The external inflation tube shall extend at least 3 cm beyond the machine end of the tracheal tube, in accordance with minimum tube length in Table 1, before any system is incorporated, for example, pilot balloon, valve, or connector. The pilot balloon, if provided, should give an indication of the degree of inflation or deflation of the cuff. The inflation system shall not leak when tested in accordance with X1.7. If the inflation tube is clamped, the lumen of the inflation tube should reopen after unclamping to enable the intentional deflation of the cuff.

TABLE 1 Tracheal Tube Dimensions

Inside Diameter, mm		Minimum Tube Length, mm	Precut Length, mm[A]
Size	Tolerance		
2.0	±0.15	140	110
2.5	±0.15	140	110
3.0	±0.15	160	120
3.5	±0.15	180	130
4.0	±0.15	200	140
4.5	±0.15	220	150
5.0	±0.15	240	160
5.5	±0.15	270	170
6.0	±0.15	280	190
6.5	±0.20	290	210
7.0	±0.20	300	230
7.5	±0.20	310	240
8.0	±0.20	320	250
8.5	±0.20	320	260
9.0	±0.20	320	270
9.5	±0.20	320	280
10.0	±0.20	320	280
11.0	±0.20	320	280

[A] Manufacturers desiring to market prepackaged sterilized oral tracheal precut tubes with connectors inserted may be guided by the lengths shown. However, the user is cautioned that anatomical variations, conditions of use, actual outside diameter of the tube, length of tube inserted, or other factors may well result in use of a tracheal tube either too long or too short for a given patient. Use of a tracheal tube precut to a standard length should not, under any circumstances, be substituted for expert clinical judgment in selecting tube size and length.

TABLE 2 Dimensions of Cuffed Tracheal Tubes

Size	Inflation Tube Take-Off Distance, (*S*), mm, ±10 mm[A]	Maximum Distance, (*D*), mm, from Tip to Machine End of Effective Cuff[B]
5.0	120	56
5.5	130	56
6.0	150	58
6.5	170	62
7.0	180	66
7.5	190	69
8.0	205	72
8.5	210	75
9.0	220	78
9.5	230	81
10.0	230	85
10.5	230	85
11.0	230	85

[A] See Fig. 2.
[B] See Figs. 2 and 3.

6. Dimensions and Permissible Variations of Tracheal Tubes

6.1 *Measurement System*—The SI (metric) system shall be the standard of measurement used.

6.2 *Size and Dimensions*—The size shall indicate the tube's inside diameter (ID) in millimetres, rather than be described by any other system, for example, French or Magill. The tube sizes with inside diameter tolerances, and the minimum tube lengths, shall be as listed in Tables 1 and 2.

6.3 *Radius of Curvature*—Both oral and nasal tracheal tubes shall have a radius of curvature of 140 ± 20 mm (see Fig. 1).

6.4 *Bevel*:

6.4.1 Tubes shall have a bevel angle of 38 ± 10° in relation to the long axis (see side view of bevel in Fig. 1).

6.4.2 The bevel opening of tubes shall be oriented as indicated in Figs. 1 and 2.

6.5 *Murphy Eye*—The area of a Murphy eye, if included, shall not be less than 80 % of the cross-sectional area of the tube lumen. The location of the eye shall be on the side of the tube opposite to the bevel (see Fig. 3(*a*) to Fig. 3(*d*). The size, shape, and location of the eye should not significantly weaken the patient end of the tube.

7. Product Marking

7.1 *Marking Materials*—Marking materials on the tracheal tube shall be nontoxic and tissue compatible (see A1.1). Marking materials on the tracheal tube should resist deterioration by anesthetic agents. The markings should not be easily rubbed off and should remain legible during use of the tube. If the tracheal tube is intended for reuse, the materials should also resist deterioration by recommended agents used in cleansing and sterilizing.

7.2 *Tracheal Tube Markings*—Markings should be of sufficient size and contrast to be clearly legible, shall be located on the bevel side of the tube within the shaded areas shown in Figs. 1 and 2, and shall read from left to right.

7.3 *Required Markings*:

7.3.1 Required markings shall include the word "Oral,"" Nasal," or "Oral/Nasal" as appropriate.

7.3.2 The size shall be marked in accordance with 6.2 and Table 1 and positioned between the cuff and take-off point, *S*, for cuffed tracheal tubes (see Fig. 2). For uncuffed tracheal tubes, size marking shall be towards the patient end and within the precut length (see Table 1).

7.3.3 For size 6.0 and smaller, the outside diameter (OD) shall be marked and that nominal marking shall be within 0.15 mm of the actual outside diameter. Marking of the outside diameter on larger tubes is optional.

7.3.4 The size markings shall be similar to one of the following specimens with the size marking inside diameter (ID) larger and bolder:

ID **6.0** Oral 8.4 OD
ID **6.0** Oral/Nasal 8.4 OD
ID **6.0** 8.4 OD Oral/Nasal
ID **6.0** Nasal 8.4 OD

ID **8.0** Oral
ID **8.0** Oral/Nasal
ID **8.0** Nasal

7.3.5 The name or trademark of the manufacturer or supplier shall be marked.

7.3.6 Tubes that comply with all requirements of this specification should be marked "F-29". Manufacturers shall state in their labeling the standard or standards for which the notation "F-29" indicates compliance.

7.3.7 Length (depth) markings in centrimetres, measured from the patient end, shall be provided.

7.3.8 Other markings not in conflict with required markings may be applied.

7.3.9 Individually packaged, sterile tubes being marketed as disposables shall be marked on the tube, "DO NOT REUSE," or" SINGLE USE ONLY," or equivalent.

7.3.10 *Radiopaque Marker*—A radiopaque marker shall be placed at the patient end or along the full length of the tube and the image of the tracheal tube marker shall have an optical density less than or equal to that of the aluminum comparison standard. The radiopaque marking shall be tested in accordance with A1.6.

8. Packaging and Labeling

8.1 *Gas Effects*— Cuff volume or pressure may either increase or decrease due to diffusion of nitrous oxide, oxygen, or air. This shall be stated in the product labeling and recommendations shall be included for minimizing this effect, if applicable. (The rapidity with which this diffusion occurs is shown in Refs **(9)** through **(14)**.)

8.2 *Sterile Tubes*— The markings shall be clearly legible through the intact package. The size should also be marked clearly on the right-hand end of the package in print at least 10 mm high.

8.3 *Nonsterile Tubes*— When tracheal tubes are not supplied sterile, the package information shall recommend a suitable method or methods of sterilization.

8.4 *Disposable Tubes*— Packages for disposable tubes shall be marked "DO NOT REUSE," or "FOR SINGLE USE ONLY," or equivalent.

8.5 *Reusable Tracheal Tubes*—When tracheal tubes are supplied with the intention that they can be reused, this shall be stated in the package information. The package information also shall recommend a method or methods for cleaning, sterilizing, and inspecting.

8.6 *Storage Conditions*—The manufacturer shall caution against known conditions of storage likely to result in rapid deterioration of the tubes and cuffs, for example, high temperature, ultraviolet light, or fluorescent lighting.

8.7 *Cuff Diameter*—For cuffed tubes the marking of packages or package inserts shall included the cuff resting diameter expressed in millimetres as determined in A1.5.

ANNEX

(Mandatory Information)

A1. TEST METHODS

A1.1 *Implantation Test*—See Ref **(18).** Other test methods, including cell cultures, may be used, provided that they are shown to yield equivalent results. One acceptable alternate is Practice F 813.

A1.2 *Tube Collapse:*

A1.2.1 *Apparatus*—Suitable apparatus is illustrated in Fig. A1.1 and includes the following:

A1.2.1.1 *Tube*, made of glass or transparent plastics material. The length of the tube shall be about twice the effective length of the cuff. The inside diameter of the transparent tube is to be within 5 % of two times the tracheal tube size, plus 4 mm. This is approximately two times the outside diameter of the tracheal tube.

A1.2.1.2 *Water Bath*, thermostatically controlled at 40 ± 1°C.

A1.2.1.3 *Air Supply.*

A1.2.1.4 *Air-Pressure Indicating Device.*

A1.2.1.5 *Rigid Ball*, of diameter not less than 75 % of the nominal size of the tracheal tube undergoing test. (Not shown in figure.)

A1.2.2 *Determination of the Test Inflation Pressure*—The test inflation pressure shall be determined as follows:

A1.2.2.1 Set up the apparatus as illustrated in Fig. A1.1.

NOTE A1.1—Fig. A1.1 includes a pressure gage, but this could be isolated by a stopcock for this test.

A1.2.2.2 Place the patient end of the tracheal tube into the test tube so that the cuff is centrally located.

A1.2.2.3 Attach the inflating tube to the air supply.

A1.2.2.4 Inflate the cuff with air until it makes circumferential contact with the test tube.

A1.2.2.5 Immerse the tracheal tube and the test tube in a water bath that is thermostatically controlled at 40 ± 1°C.

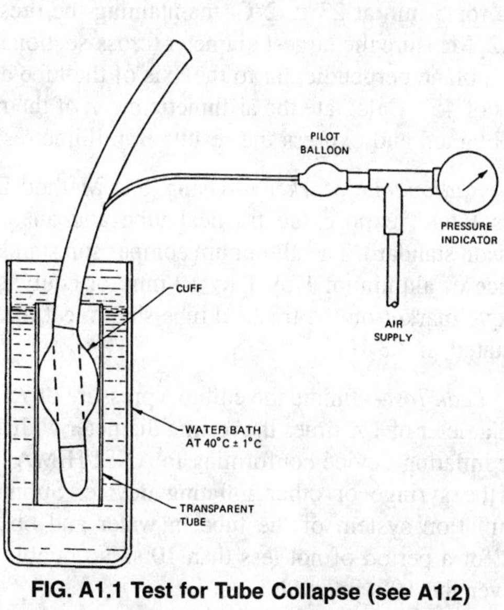

FIG. A1.1 Test for Tube Collapse (see A1.2)

A1.2.2.6 Periodically adjust the inflation volume of the air in the cuff so that circumferential contact is only just maintained.

A1.2.2.7 After 30 min in the water bath and with the inflation volume of air in the cuff adjusted so that minimum circumferential contact is maintained, record the inflation pressure of the cuff defined as the reference inflation pressure in Table A1.1. Select the test inflation pressure from Table A1.1.

A1.2.3 *Method of Test for Tube Collapse*—The following procedure shall be used to test for tube collapse:

A1.2.3.1 After determination of the test inflation pressure in accordance with A1.2.2, inflate the cuff with air at the test inflation pressure and leave for 24 h in the water bath at 40 ± 1°C. Regularly, check and maintain the test inflation pressure in the cuff during the test period.

A1.2.3.2 Check the patency of the lumen by means of a gravitational fall of a rigid ball having a diameter of not less than 75 % of the nominal size of the tracheal tube. This test is satisfied if the ball passes freely through the tube.

A1.3 *Cuff Symmetry*—The object of the test is to assess symmetrical expansion of the cuff in planes at right angles to the long axis of the tube. The following procedure shall be used to test cuff symmetry.

A1.3.1 Mount the tube on the test rig as illustrated in Fig. A1.2. The diameter of the mandrel shall be 1.0 mm less than the inside diameter of the tube. The mandrel may be designed to rotate on the base of the test rig.

A1.3.2 Inflate the cuff without external constraint until at least one diameter of the inflated cuff measures not less than 2.5 times the outside diameter of the tube. Note the inflation pressure and, if it is less than 4 kPa (30 mm Hg), continue the inflation until that pressure level is obtained.

A1.3.3 Visually inspect the inflated cuff for freedom from protuberances, obvious local areas of thinning or outpouching (bulging) (see Fig. A1.3). The presence of any of these defects shall constitute failure of this test.

A1.3.4 Adjust the height of the pointer to approximately midpoint of the cuff as in Fig. A1.2 and rotate the tube through 360° and measure the maximum distance, *B*.

A1.3.5 Without any further adjustment of the height of the pointer, rotate the tube relative to the pointer through 360° and

TABLE A1.1 Determination of the Test Inflation Pressure

Reference Inflation Pressure, kPa, (mm Hg)	Test Inflation Pressure, kPa (mm Hg)
Up to 16.6 (125)[A]	two times the reference inflation pressure or 2.7 (20), whichever is greater
Over 16.6 (125) to 33.3 (250)	33.3 (250)
Over 33.3 kPa (250)	the reference inflation pressure

[A] It is desirable that a cuff have a reference inflation pressure well below this figure, in the range of 10 to 20 mm Hg.

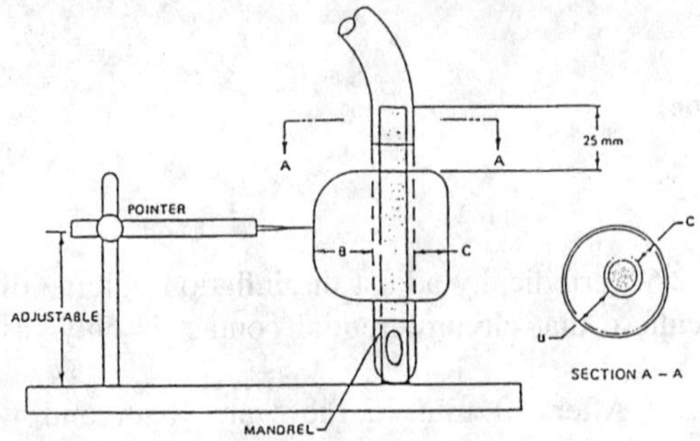

FIG. A1.2 Test Rig

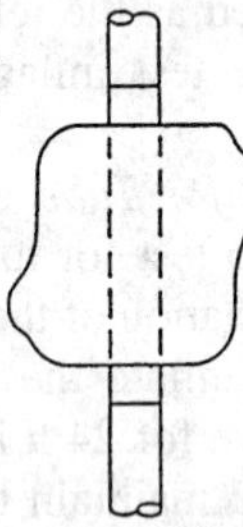

FIG. A1.3 Visual Inspection of Tube Cuff

measure the minimum distance, *C* , in Fig. A1.2.

A1.3.6 If the value calculated according to the formula, $((B-C)/C) \times 100$, is greater than 50, the tube failed the test.

A1.3.7 Readjust the height of the pointer away from the midpoint to the point between 25 and 75 % of the cuff length, where asymmetry appears greatest. Rotate the tube through 360° to measure distance *B* and repeat A1.3.5 and A1.3.6 (see Figs. A1.2 and A1.3).

A1.4 *Cuff Herniation:*

A1.4.1 *Apparatus*—Suitable apparatus is illustrated in Fig. A1.1 and Fig. A1.4 and includes the following:

A1.4.1.1 *Tube*, made of glass or rigid transparent plastics material. The length of the tube shall be about twice the effective length of the cuff. The inside diameter of the transparent tube is to be within 5 % of two times the tracheal tube size.

A1.4.1.2 *Water Bath*, thermostatically controlled at 40 ± 1°C.

A1.4.1.3 *Air Supply*.

A1.4.1.4 *Air-Pressure Indicating Device*.

A1.4.1.5 *100-g weight*.

A1.4.2 *Conditions*:

A1.4.2.1 Set up the apparatus as illustrated in Fig. A1.1, inflate the cuff with air at the Test Inflation Pressure determined in Table A1.1 and maintain that pressure in a water bath at 40 ± 1°C for 24 h.

A1.4.2.2 After 24 h, remove the inflated tracheal tube and transparent tube from the water bath. Invert and suspend the 100-g weight from the tracheal tube (see Fig. A1.4). Progressively deflate the cuff over a period of 10 s and continuously observe cuff conformation. No portion of the cuff shall encroach upon any part of the lumen at the patient end of the tube during the observation period up to the time when the tracheal tube falls freely from the transparent tube. Occlusion of a Murphy eye shall be ignored.

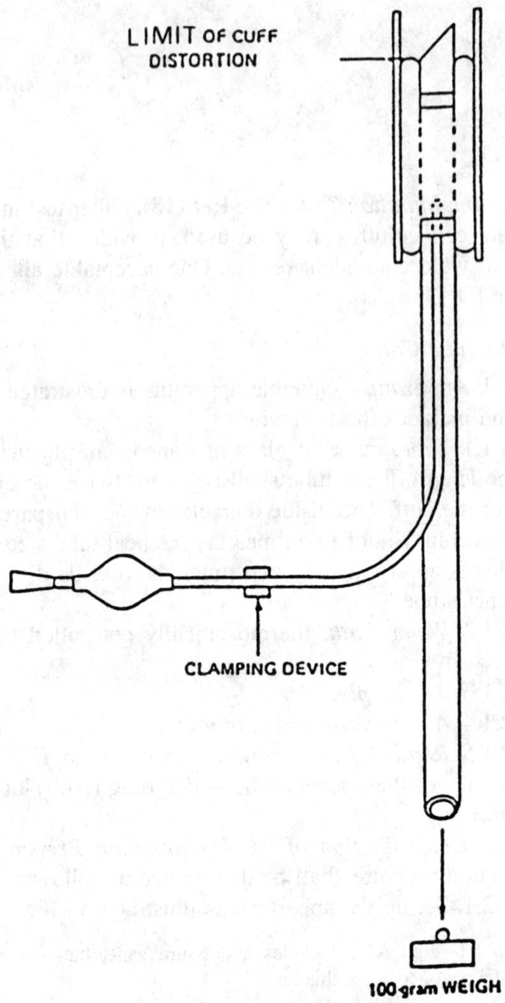

FIG. A1.4 Cuff Herniation Test

A1.5 *Cuff Diameter Assessment; and Tube Lumen Closure*—The following shall be completed to conduct this test protocol:

A1.5.1 Inflate the cuff with a 50-cm^3 syringe to an intracuff pressure of 2.0 kPa (20.4 cm H_2O) ±5 % and leave it to stabilize for 5 min at 23 ± 2°C, maintaining the pressure.

A1.5.2 Measure the largest diameter (cross-sectional dimension) in a plane perpendicular to the axis of the tube at rotated intervals of 45°. Calculate the arithmetic mean of the measurements obtained and express the results in millimetres.

A1.6 *Radiopaque Markers*—Using Test Method B in Test Methods F 640, expose the tracheal tube and an aluminum comparison standard. The aluminum comparison standard shall be a piece of aluminum 1 by 1 by 10 mm, or equivalent. The radiopaque marker on the tracheal tube shall meet the requirements stated in 7.3.10.

A1.7 *Leak Test*—Inflate the cuff to a pressure of 75 cm H_2O or to a diameter of 1½ times the resting diameter with a syringe or other inflating device conforming to ANSI/HIMA MD70.1. Detach the syringe or other inflating device. Submerge the entire inflation system of the tube in water and observe for bubbles for a period of not less than 10 s. No bubble shall be noted over the 10-s interval.

APPENDIXES

(Nonmandatory Information)

X1. RATIONALE FOR REQUIREMENTS

NOTE X1.1—This rationale is provided for the requirements in this specification. The section and subsection numbers given in parentheses at the end of each paragraph refer to the correspondingly numbered sections and subsections in the specification.

X1.1 *Tubes*—Sharp points or rough edges on the patient end of the tracheal tube, the bevel, and the eye may cause mucosal damage, particularly to the posterior nasopharynx during nasal intubations and to the cords. The internal edge of a Murphy eye is excluded because it is much less important compared with the external edges and much more difficult to round during the manufacturing process. (See 4.2.1.)

X1.2 *Rigidity*—Tracheal tube design is a trade-off of many factors; kinking and laryngeal loading are only two. (See 4.3.)

X1.3 *Integrity of Lumen*—Tube collapse due to cuff inflation is documented in Refs **(16)** and **(17)**. (See 4.4.)

X1.4 *Cuffs*—If the distance from the machine end of the cuff to the tip of the tube is too great, the tip of the tube may rest on the carina while the cuff impinges on the vocal cords. (See 5.1).

X1.4.1 Cuff and eye placement are important so that the cuff attachment sleeve does not encroach upon the eye, producing a knife-edge-like projection. (See 5.1.)

X1.4.2 The pressure versus volume and pressure versus diameter data are considered to be valuable in selecting a low-pressure cuff. Simply stated, a low-pressure, high-volume cuff must have a diameter greater than the diameter of the trachea into which the tube is to be placed. (See 5.2.)

X1.4.3 *Inflation System*—An unusually large inflation tube may project from the tracheal tube and may possibly exert pressure on airway structures. The 2.5-mm size limits this projection while allowing adequate size for the proper function of the cuff inflating system. (See 5.3.)

X1.5 *Size*—A standard system of size markings enables the user to readily select the desired tube. The tracheal tube lumen must be circular in shape to maximize cross-sectional area and reduce the potential of kinking. (See 6.2.)

X1.6 *Radius of Curvature*—A radius of curvature of about 14 cm seems to facilitate intubation. Clinical practice for more than 50 years with this curvature has proved satisfactory. Clinical data are not available to establish exact tolerance for the 14-cm requirement, but ASTM Committee F-29 consensus of ± 2 cm allows considerable variation. (See 6.3.)

X1.7 *Bevels:*

X1.7.1 Although a longer bevel (smaller angle) may facilitate passage through the nares, it increases the risk of occlusion. Tracheal tubes with shorter bevels (larger angles) may be more difficult to pass through the nares or larynx. This wide tolerance on bevel angle allows for a tube to have an angle of 30° for nasal intubation or 45° for oral intubation. (See 6.4.1.)

X1.7.2 The required placement of the bevel provides better visibility during intubation because the cords can be seen before passing the bevel through. (See 6.4.2.)

X1.8 *Murphy Eye*—Although the clinical benefit of a Murphy eye has not been proven, the eye, if included, should be safe, that is, it should be placed and sized so that it does not weaken the tip, and should be large enough so that it would not impose too much resistance to flow if required to pass respiratory gases. (See 6.5.)

X1.9 For tubes used in pediatrics, outside diameter is paramount in sizing the tube for tracheal seal and for passage with minimum trauma. (See 7.3.3.)

X1.10 It is required that the inside diameter marking be particularly prominent to distinguish it as *the* number that designates size. (See 7.3.4.)

X1.11 *Identification of Tubes*—It was the intention of the committee that tubes manufactured to meet all the requirements of this specification should be identified by "F-29." ASTM Committee F-29 felt that the confusing and sometimes misleading "F-29/IT" should not be used and particularly wanted to make it clear that the markings" F-29/IT" would not indicate compliance with this specification. (See 7.3.6.)

X1.12 *Sterile Tubes*—Bold type designating the inside diameter on the package is necessary so that tube size may be rapidly determined under emergency conditions where lighting may be less than ideal. (See 8.2.)

X2. DISCONTINUED TEST PROTOCOLS

NOTE X2.1—The following test protocols have been retained in this specification for informational purposes only. These tests came from predecessor documents ANSI Z79.14-1983 and Z79.16-1983. This appendix is numbered in accordance with ASTM form and style. This also applies to the numbering of figures. The numbers in parentheses at the end of each paragraph refer to the original numbering of sections used in ANSI Z79.14-1983 and Z79.16.-1983.

X2.1 *Test Protocol One—Tracheal Seal, Slope Pressure, and Lumen Closure Conditions*—The test apparatus (see Fig. X2.1) shall consist of a vertically mounted model trachea (Fig. X2.2), a test lung (or equivalent), mechanical ventilator, a pressure tap for measuring airway pressure, and a means for maintaining a specified temperature at 37 ± 1°C and relative humidity at 90± 10 %. Tracheal seal ventilation shall be defined as a condition in which a leak not to exceed 5 % of the tidal volume is evident in the flowmeter during mechanical ventilation. Conditions for mechanical ventilation shall consist of the ventilator and test lung settings necessary to produce a compliance of 150 to 350 mL/kPa (15.3 to 35.7 mL/cm H_2O), a resistance of 1 to 3 kPa/L/s (10.2 to 30.6 cm H_2O/L/s), a tidal volume of 500 mL, a frequency of 20/min, and a peak pressure of 3 to 4 kPa (30.6 to 40.8 cm H_2O). The inspiratory to expiratory ratio (I:E ratio) may be adjusted to meet these conditions, but shall not exceed 1:1 (8.1, 8.1.1).

X2.2 *Test Procedure*—The following steps shall be completed to conduct test protocol one (8.1.2):

X2.2.1 Assemble the test apparatus (see Fig. X2.1) in the following manner:

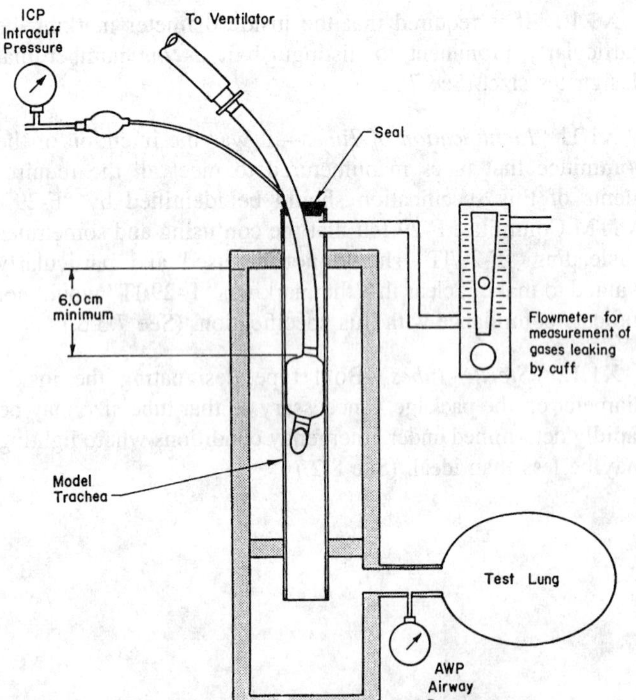

FIG. X2.1 Schematic of Cuffed Tracheal Tube in Model Trachea Mounted Vertically in Test Apparatus

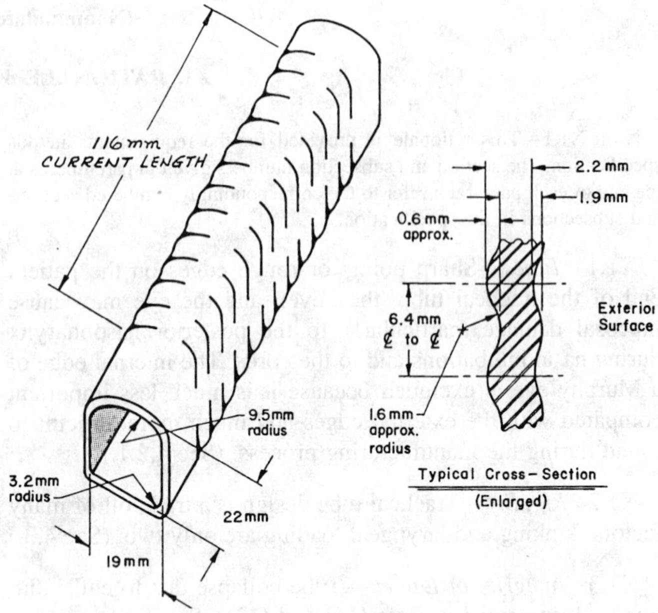

FIG. X2.2 Clear Polyvinyl Chloride (PVC) Adult Model Trachea

X2.2.1.1 Connect the pressure indicator to test apparatus at the junction with the test lung to determine airway pressure (AWP). (Record the accuracy and frequency response of the indicator.)

X2.2.1.2 Attach tubing and flowmeter for measurement of gases leaking past cuff.

X2.2.2 Place the size 8.0 cuffed tracheal tube in the model trachea for 4 h under specified conditions (see 8.1), prior to the test. Position the tube so that the upper margin of the cuff is at least 6 cm below the lower margin of the seal of the test apparatus. Seal the upper margin of the test apparatus.

X2.2.3 Connect the ventilator to the tracheal tube. Under specified conditions (see 8.1), ventilate the model trachea and test lung with heated, humidified air for 10 min with cuff deflated.

X2.2.4 Determine the intracuff volume and pressure necessary for tracheal seal ventilation in the following manner:

X2.2.4.1 Inflate cuff. Carefully adjust the cuff pressure until the desired leak is obtained. This pressure is defined as the intracuff pressure (ICP) for tracheal seal ventilation and the volume is defined as the intracuff volume (ICV) for tracheal seal ventilation. Record the ICP and the ICV, and the maximum and minimum AWP. Repeat this procedure on the same tube four additional times.

X2.2.4.2 Calculate the mean and standard deviation of at least these five determinations.

X2.2.5 Determine the overinflation slope-pressure curve and lumen patency as follows:

X2.2.5.1 Disconnect ventilator and test lung; remove the base of the test apparatus.

X2.2.5.2 Inflate the cuff to tracheal seal ventilation pressure, ±0.05 kPa (±0.5 cm H_2O), and record the volume in the cuff.

X2.2.5.3 Further inflate the cuff in 1.0-mL increments until a larger volume (either two times the tracheal seal ventilation volume or two times the testing volume) is reached. Check lumen patency by means of the free gravitational fall of a steel ball having a diameter of not less than 75 % of the nominal marked inside diameter of the tracheal tube.

X2.2.5.4 Record the ICV and ICP at each point.

X2.2.5.5 Perform this procedure four additional times on the same tube.

X2.2.5.6 Calculate the mean ±1 standard deviation of X2.2.5.4.

X2.3 *Ability to Conform to Human Anatomy and Resistance to Kinking*—Ten size 6.0-mm tubes and 10 size 8.0-mm tubes shall be used to determine the force (mean value ±1 standard deviation) required to achieve conformity. By placing the pegs on the test board so that the closest point to the tube is given by the coordinates in Table X2.1, the desired anatomical configuration is defined by both size 6.0 and 8.0 tubes. Other equivalent systems may be used (see Fig. X2.3) (8.2).

X2.3.1 *Storage Conditions*—With cuff removed or deflated, store each tube (unstressed) in a conditioning environment of 24 ± 1°C and 60 % relative humidity (RH)± 10 % RH for at least 60 ± 10 min (8.2.1).

X2.3.2 *Test Procedure*— Immediately after removing the tube from the conditioning environment, place the tube on the test board (see Fig. X2.3), with the cuff area placed under Peg F. Follow the tube's natural curvature for this placement. For reference in subsequent tube positioning, mark the most vertical uppermost surface at each end of the tube and mark the portion of the tube resting directly over Peg J (8.2.2).

X2.3.2.1 Loop a 1-cm-wide strap around the tube midway between Pegs J and K. Attach the strap to a force gage.

X2.3.2.2 Lift the tube 0.5 mm with the strap, pulling only in the direction of the *Y* axis. Record the force required to move the tube this distance.

X2.3.2.3 Immediately after the measurement, relax tension on the strap, and check the patency of the tube lumen by means

TABLE X2.1 Coordinates for Positioning Pegs on Test Board (Force Necessary to Conform to Human Anatomy)

Peg[A]	*X*-Coordinate, mm	*Y*-Coordinate, mm
A	−102	44
B	−92	44
C	−66	10
D	−53	5
E	−38	2
F	80	6
G	−96	−10
H	−82	−30
I	−50	−18
J	0	0
K	20	0

[A] Peg placements represent anatomical structures that establish limits on the positions a tracheal tube may occupy in human airways.

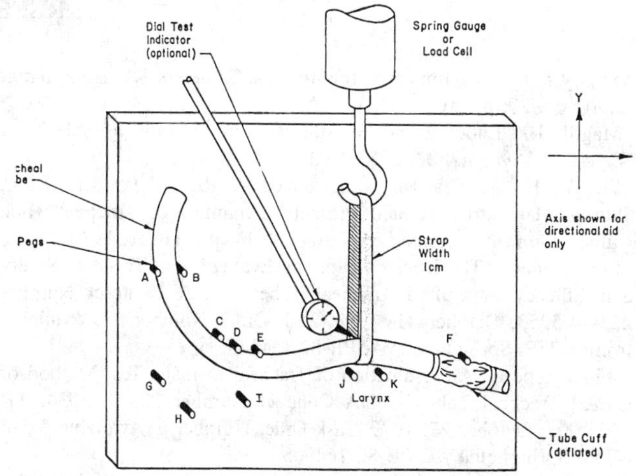

FIG. X2.3 Test Board

of the free gravitational falls of a steel ball having the diameter of not less than 75 % of the labeled internal diameter of the tracheal tube. This test is performed with the test board's *Y* axis parallel to the force of gravity.

X2.3.2.4 Store each tube to be tested on the test board or on a fixture with an equivalent positional restraint(s), in an environment of 37 ± 1°C and 90 ± 10 % RH for a period of 60 ± 10 min or until thermal equilibrium is reached. If the tube is transferred from the test board to another fixture, maintain the same orientation with respect to the tube's natural curvature, using the indexing marks specified in this procedure, and, with the same orientation, return the tube to the test board after environmental conditioning.

X2.3.2.5 Repeat X2.3.2.1-X2.3.2.3, inclusive. Again, be careful to maintain the same orientation with respect to the tube's natural curvature, using the indexing marks specified in this procedure.

X2.4 *Tracheal Seal:*

X2.4.1 For size 8.0 tubes, the manufacturer shall make available upon request the intracuff pressure and volume (mean values ± one standard deviation (SD) necessary to provide a seal in the model trachea. (See Refs **(2)**, **(3)**, and **(4)** for background information.)

X2.4.2 The tracheal seal shall be tested in accordance with the method in X2.1.

X2.5 *Cuff Slope Pressure Effects:*

X2.5.1 For size 8.0 tubes, the manufacturer shall make available upon request a plot of pressure versus volume as determined in the model trachea for volumes ranging from tracheal seal ventilation volume (see X2.2) to a larger volume (either two times the tracheal seal ventilation volume or two times the resting volume (see section 8.1.2) (A1.5).

X2.5.2 Slope pressure effects shall be tested in accordance with the method in X2.1.

REFERENCES

(1) Murphy, F. J., "Two Improved Intratracheal Catheters," *Anesthesia and Analgesia*, 20: pp. 102–103, 1941.

(2) Magill, I., "Endotracheal Anesthesia," *Proceedings of the Royal Society of Medicine*, 22: p. 83, 1928.

(3) Wu, W. H., Arteaga, M., Mlodezeniec, A. R., and Poppers, R. J., "Surface Ultrastructure and Pressure Dynamics of Tracheal Tube Cuffs," *Journal of Biomedical Research*, 14: pp. 11–21, 1980.

(4) Final Report: "The Development and Evaluation of Tests for Safety and Efficacy or Cuffed Tracheal Tubes," FDA Contract Number 223-74-5253, October 31, 1978, Task Order Number 21. Available from: NTIS, Springfield, VA, PB 82 154543.

(5) Final Report:" An Evaluation of Tracheal Damage Test Method of Cuffed Tracheal Tubes," FDA Contract Number 223-77-5034, TR 1705-003; October 27, 1979, Task Order Number 6. Available from: NTIS, Springfield, VA, PB 82 164906.

(6) Bernhard, W. N., Cottrell, J. E., Swakumaran, C., Patel, K., Yost, L., and Turndorf, H., "Adjustment of Intracuff Pressure to Prevent Aspiration," *Anesthesiology*, 50(4): pp. 363–366, April 1979.

(7) Mackenzie, C. F., Shin, B., Whitely, N., et al., "The Relationship of Human Tracheal Size to Body Habitus" *Anesthesiology*, 51(3, Supplement): p. 378, 1979.

(8) Bernhard, W. N., Yost, L., Turndorf, H., and Danziger, F., "Cuffed Tracheal Tubes—Physical and Behavioral Characteristics," *Anesthesia and Analgesia*, 61(1): pp. 36–41, January 1982.

(9) Stanley, T. H., "Effects of Anesthetic Gases on Endotracheal Tube Cuff Gas Volumes," *Anesthesia and Analgesia*, 53(3): pp. 480–482, May–June, 1974.

(10) Stanley, T. H., Kawamura, R., and Graves, C., "Effects of Nitrous Oxide on Volume and Pressure of Endotracheal Tube Cuffs," *Anesthesiology*, 41(3): pp. 256–262, September 1974.

(11) Stanley, T. H., and Liu, W. S., "Tracheostomy and Endotracheal Tube Cuff Volume and Pressure Changes During Thoracic Operations," *Annals of Thoracic Surgery*, 20(2): pp. 144–155, August 1975.

(12) Stanley, T. H., "Nitrous Oxide and Pressures and Volumes of High- and Low-Pressure Endotracheal-Tube Cuffs in Intubated Patients," *Anesthesiology*, 42(5): pp. 637–640, May 1975.

(13) Stanley, T. H., Foote, J. L., and Liu, W. S., "A Simple Pressure-Relief Valve to Prevent Increases in Endotracheal Tube Cuff Pressure and Volume in Intubated Patient," *Anesthesiology*, 43(4): pp. 478–481, October 1975.

(14) Bernhard, W. N., Yost, L. C., Turndorf, H., Cottrell, J. E., and Paegle, R. D., "Physical Characteristics of and Rates of Nitrous Oxide Diffusion into Tracheal Tube Cuffs," *Anesthesiology*, 48(6): pp. 413–417, June 1978.

(15) Steen, J. A., Lindholm, C. E., Brdlik, G. C., and Foster, C. A., "Tracheal Tube Forces on the Posterior Larynx: Index of Laryngeal Loading," *Critical Care Medicine*, 10(3): pp. 186–189, March 1982.

(16) Ketouer, A. D., et al., "Collapse of Disposable Endotracheal Tube by its High-Pressure Cuff," *Anesthesiology*, 13: pp. 108–110, 1975.

(17) Jacobson, J., "A Hazard of Armored Endotracheal Anesthesia," *Anesthesia and Analgesia* , 48: pp. 37–41, 1969.

(18) *United States Pharmacopia XXIII*, Mack Publishing Company, Easton, PA, 1995: p 1702.

Standard Specification for Tracheal Tube Connectors[1]

This standard is issued under the fixed designation F 1243; the number immediately following the designation indicates the year of original adoption or, in the case of revision, the year of last revision. A number in parentheses indicates the year of last reapproval. A superscript epsilon (ε) indicates an editorial change since the last revision or reapproval.

1. Scopc

1.1 This specification covers the general objectives, terminology, dimensions and tolerances, labeling, and materials for nominal 15-mm connectors utilized in joining tracheal tubes to breathing systems.

1.2 The purpose of this standard is to specify minimum and performance and safety requirements and to further promote interchangeability of components for tracheal tube connections.

1.3 The values stated in SI units are to be regarded as standard.

2. Referenced Documents

2.1 *ASTM Standards:*

F 1054 Specification for Conical Fittings of 15-mm and 22-mm Sizes[2]

3. Terminology

3.1 *Definitions:*

3.1.1 *machine end*—the end of the connector nearest the machine.

3.1.2 *patient end*—the end of the connector nearest the patient.

3.1.3 *tracheal tube connector*—a straight or curved connector that inserts directly into a tracheal tube.

4. Materials and Manufacture

4.1 The connector should be light in weight and be of sufficient strength to resist deformation under normal conditions of use.

4.2 Connectors should be made of materials suitable for the intended use and function satisfactorily in the presence of anesthetic agents and gases commonly used.

5. General Requirements

5.1 Connectors described in this specification should be designed primarily for patient safety and only secondarily for the convenience of the anesthesiologist and manufacturer.

5.2 Connectors described in this specification should be designed to have a minimum of dead space and cause a minimum of turbulence, consistent with other requirements in this specification.

5.3 Connections with components specified in this specification should not leak and should have sufficient stability to resist accidental disconnection during ordinary usage. Ordinarily the security of the connection may be increased by twisting (or turning) the mating components during engagement.

5.4 By visual inspection there shall be no shoulder within the lumen and transitions in the internal diameter shall be tapered to give an adequate lead-in for smooth passage of a suction catheter.

5.5 For connection and disconnection, tracheal tube fittings should provide a means to facilitate grasping.

5.6 The connectors may be provided with lugs, knobs, or other protrusions to which elastic bands or other devices may be attached to resist accidental separations.

5.7 The machine end shall conform with applicable requirements of Specification F 1054.

6. Dimensions and Tolerances of Tracheal Tube Connectors

6.1 *Measurement System*—Dimensions shall be stated in the International System of Units (SI).

TABLE 1 Size Designation, Tolerance, and Length of Patient End, mm

Inside Diameter (ID)		Length of L^A		
Size Designation	Tolerance	Suggested Length	min	max
2.0	±0.15	11	9.0	19.0
2.5	±0.15	11	9.0	19.0
3.0	±0.15	11	11.0	19.0
3.5	±0.15	13	11.0	19.5
4.0	±0.15	13	12.0	19.5
4.5	±0.15	14	12.0	20.0
5.0	±0.15	14	13.0	20.0
5.5	±0.15	15	13.0	20.5
6.0	±0.15	15	16.0	20.5
6.5	±0.15	18	16.0	21.0
7.0	±0.15	18	16.0	21.0
7.5	±0.15	18	16.0	21.5
8.0	±0.15	18	16.0	21.5
8.5	±0.15	18	16.0	22.0
9.0	±0.15	18	16.0	22.0
9.5	±0.15	18	16.0	22.5
10.0	±0.15	18	16.0	22.5
11.0	±0.15	18	16.0	23.0

^{A} See Figs. 1-3.

6.2 *Size*—The size of the tracheal tube connectors shall be

[1] This specification is under the jurisdiction of ASTM Committee F-29 on Anesthetic and Respiratory Equipmentand is the direct responsibility of Subcommittee F29.12 on Airways.

Current edition approved Sept. 29, 1989. Published March 1990.

[2] *Annual Book of ASTM Standards*, Vol 13.01.

defined by the size of the tracheal tube with which it is intended to mate and shall conform to the dimensions and tolerances indicated in Table 1.

6.3 *Wall Thickness*— The wall thickness of the patient end should be adequate to resist kinking and should be tapered or bevelled to facilitate insertion.

6.4 *Types of Tracheal Tube Connectors*—Connectors may be either straight or curved and shall conform to the specifications indicated in Table 1.

6.4.1 *Patient End of Tracheal Tube Straight Connectors*—The length of the patient end, *L* (see Fig. 1), shall be in accordance with Table 1. The cross-sectional area of the lumen throughout a straight connector shall not be less than that of the corresponding tracheal tube into which the connector is designed to fit.

6.4.2 *Tracheal Tube Curved Connectors*—Desirable included angles are 60 and 90° (see Fig. 2 and Fig. 3). The minimum inside diameter of a curved connector shall not be less than 80 % of the nominal diameter and the cross-sectional area of the lumen throughout a curved connector shall not be reduced by more than 10 % of the equivalent straight connector.

6.4.2.1 Curved connectors intended for nasal use may be shortened by one third of length *L* from the suggested length. (See Table 1.)

7. Product Marking

7.1 *Marking of Tracheal Tube Connectors*—The connector shall be marked as to size. This marking of size should be readily visible during use.

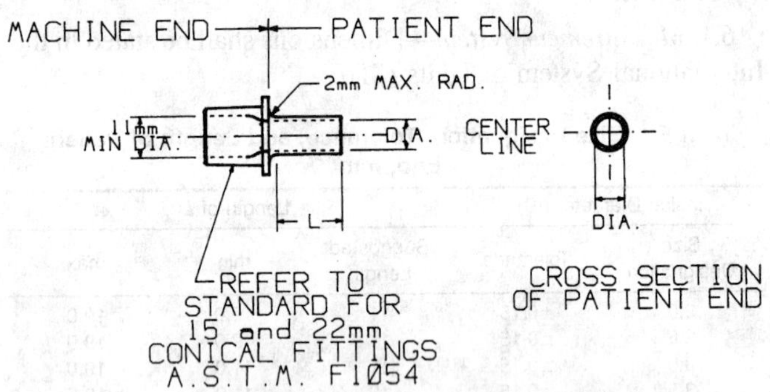

FIG. 1 15-mm Tracheal Tube Straight Connector

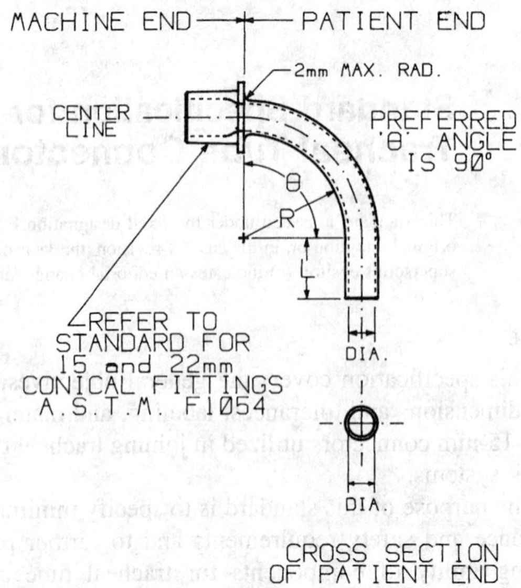

FIG. 2 Typical 15-mm Tracheal Tube Right Angle/Curved Connector

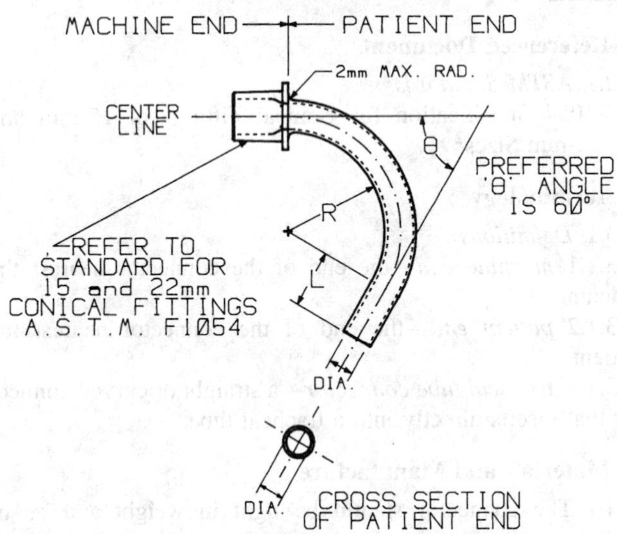

FIG. 3 Typical 15-mm Tracheal Tube Acute Angle/Curved Connector

Standard Specification for Electrically Powered Home Care Ventilators, Part 1—Positive-Pressure Ventilators and Ventilator Circuits[1]

This standard is issued under the fixed designation F 1246; the number immediately following the designation indicates the year of original adoption or, in the case of revision, the year of last revision. A number in parentheses indicates the year of last reapproval. A superscript epsilon (ε) indicates an editorial change since the last revision or reapproval.

1. Scope

1.1 This specification covers all electrically powered lung ventilators and ventilator circuits specifically intended for use in the home environment, and marketed after the final date of approval for this specification. Breathing circuits intended specifically for use with home care ventilators are also included within the scope of this specification. The application of critical care ventilators, anesthesia ventilators, emergency care transport ventilators, and resuscitators in the home environment is not covered by this specification. As well, this specification does not cover high frequency ventilators or external body ventilators. Part 1 of this specification addresses positive pressure ventilators, and Part 2 addresses negative pressure ventilators. (See also X1.1.1.)

1.2 The values stated in SI units are to be regarded as standard.

1.3 The following precautionary caveat pertains to the test method portion only, Section 6, of this specification. *This standard may involve hazardous materials, operations, and equipment. This standard does not purport to address all of the safety problems associated with its use. It is the responsibility of the user of this standard to establish appropriate safety and health practices and determine the applicability of regulatory limitations prior to use.*

2. Referenced Documents

2.1 *ASTM Standards:*

F 1054 Specification for Conical Fittings of 15 mm and 22 mm Sizes[2]

3. Terminology

3.1 *Definitions of Terms Specific to This Standard:*

3.1.1 *breathing system*—gas pathways in direct connection with the patient through which intermittent or reciprocating gas flow occurs and into which a mixture of controlled composition may be dispensed.

3.1.2 *end-expiratory pressure*—pressure in the breathing system at the end of the expiratory phase time, prior to the beginning of the inspiratory phase time.

3.1.3 *expiratory phase time, (T_E)*— interval from the start of expiratory flow to the start of inspiratory flow.

3.1.4 *home care ventilator*—ventilator intended for use in the home environment.

3.1.5 *home environment*—the patient's place of residence outside the hospital. This usually refers to the patient's home, but may include nursing homes, and personal or other means of transportation.

3.1.6 *inspiratory phase time, (T_I)*— interval from the start of inspiratory flow to the start of expiratory flow.

3.1.7 *maximum limited pressure, ($P_{L\ max}$)*—highest gage pressure that can be attained in the patient system during malfunction of the ventilator, but with functioning safety mechanisms.

3.1.7.1 *Discussion*—This term has not been changed in accordance with ISO 4135, however, the text is identical. The ISO term is "maximum safety pressure."

3.1.8 *maximum working pressure, ($P_{w\ max}$)*—highest gage pressure that can be attained in the patient system during the inspiratory phase when the ventilator is functioning normally.

3.1.8.1 *Discussion*—This may be limited by a controllable ventilator mechanism to less than $P_{L\ max}$.

3.1.9 *patient connection port*—that opening at the patient end of an expiratory valve unit; a *Y*-piece fitting or a unidirectional valve to which may be connected either a tracheal tube adaptor or a face mask angle piece.

3.1.10 *patient system*—that part of the gas system of a ventilator through which respired gas travels at appropriate respiratory pressures.

3.1.11 *peak pressure*—the maximum gage pressure achieved during the inspiratory phase time, with all pressure limiting mechanisms functioning.

3.1.12 *positive end-expiratory pressure (PEEP)*— pressure, patient system, (P_{ps}) at the end of expiration, above ambient.

3.1.13 *pressure, patient system (P_{ps})*— pressure at a specified point in the patient system.

3.1.14 *ventilator*—a device capable of automatically main taining or replacing a patient's entire pulmonary ventilation.

3.1.14.1 *Discussion*—Conditions under which measurements are made shall be given.

3.2 *Descriptions of Abbreviations Specific to This Standard:*

3.2.1 *C*—indicates compliance in units of mL/kPa (or mL/cm H_2O), for example, C 20 = 2.0 mL/kPa (20 mL/cm H_2O).

---

[1] This specification is under the jurisdiction of ASTM Committee F-29 on Anesthetic and Respiratory Equipmentand is the direct responsibility of Subcommittee F29.14 on Ventilators.

Current edition approved April 15, 1991. Published June 1991.

[2] *Annual Book of ASTM Standards*, Vol 13.01.

3.2.2 *R*—indicates resistance to flow in units of kPa/L/s (or cm H_2O/L/s), for example, R5 = 0.5 kPa/L/s (5 cm H_2O/L/s).

NOTE 1—In the interest of brevity and clarity, all other abbreviations have been provided in parentheses following the related term in 3.1.

4. Performance Requirements

4.1 *Power Sources*:

4.1.1 *Electrical*—The ventilator shall continue to function within the manufacturer's specifications at any control setting throughout a line voltage range of 90 to 130-V a-c, rms, and throughout a frequency range of 50 to 70 Hz. Testing shall be in accordance with 6.1.1 and 6.1.2.

4.1.2 An integral battery power source shall be provided that will activate automatically when line voltage conditions fall below the range specified by the manufacturer. This power source shall maintain the performance of the ventilator within the requirements of this specification for no less than 15 min. Testing shall be in accordance with 6.1.2. (See also X1.2.2.)

4.1.2.1 Battery use event alarm (see 4.12.3).

4.1.2.2 External battery connections (if supplied) shall be for a nominal 12-V d-c supply. (See also 5.1.7.)

4.2 *Accuracy of Controls, Indicators, and Pressure Relief Devices*:

4.2.1 *Calibrated Controls and Indicators*—All calibrated controls and indicators shall be accurate to within ±10 %.

4.2.2 *Pressure Controls, (calibrated, or uncalibrated with independent indicators)*—The actual pressure at the sensing site (see 5.1.8) shall agree with the control setting within ±5 cm H_2O up to 30 cm H_2O and± 10 cm H_2O over 30 cm H_2O. Testing shall be in accordance with 6.2.1. (See also X1.2.3.)

4.2.3 *Limited Pressure Relief Controls*—If the pressure in the breathing circuit reaches a level greater than the usual operator adjusted peak pressure, a pressure reduction mechanism shall activate within 3 s. This pressure reduction mechanism shall bring the breathing circuit to a predetermined baseline pressure equal to or less than the end-expiratory pressure, but in no case shall this pressure be subatmospheric. Alternately, the limited pressure relief mechanism may be activated without delay when the preset maximum limiting pressure is reached. A coupled visual/audible alarm shall be activated in this event. The visual signal shall be retained when the pressure is reduced and shall require a manual reset. Testing shall be in accordance with 6.2.2. (See also X1.2.4.)

4.3 *Volume Controls*— The actual minute or tidal volume delivered at the patient outlet of the ventilator shall be within± 10 % of the control setting for calibrated controls or indicated setting for uncalibrated controls. If both a calibrated control and indicator are used, both shall meet this requirement. Testing shall be in accordance with 6.2.3, Table 1, and Annex A1. (See also X1.2.5.)

TABLE 1 Lung Model and Ventilator Settings For Use in Testing

Compliance	Resistance	V^t Set, mL	Frequency Set	I:E Set
C 1	R 50	50	30	1:2
C 3	R 20	100	30	1:2
C 10	R 20	300	20	1:2
C 20	R 20	500	20	1:2
C 50	R 5	1000	15	1:2

4.3.1 *Volume Stability*— The volume delivered by the ventilator shall not vary by more than ±10 % of the set tidal volume or by more than ±10 % of the expired volume when tested as outlined in 6.2.3 and Annex A1 using all power sources as supplied by the manufacturer. (See also 5.1.10.)

4.3.2 *Exhaled Volume Measurement Devices, (if provided)*—See 5.1.11.

4.3.3 *Delivered Volume*— Interdependence of controls, see 5.1.12.

4.4 *Frequency*:

4.4.1 Devices controlling ventilator frequency shall be accurate to within one breath per minute or ±10 % of the setting, whichever is greater. Testing shall be in accordance with 6.2.3 and Annex A1. (See also 5.1.14 and X1.2.7.)

4.4.2 *Stability of Control Setting*—The ventilator controls shall not vary more than ±10 % of the set value. Testing shall be in accordance with 6.2.3 and Annex A1. (See also 5.1.15 and X1.2.7.)

4.4.3 *Frequency Controls*—Interdependence of control functions, see 5.1.16.

4.5 *Accuracy of Inspiratory Time Controls Calibrated or Uncalibrated with Associated Indicators* , (if provided)—Inspiratory time controls shall be accurate to within± 10 % of the set or indicated value. Testing shall be in accordance with 6.2.4.

4.5.1 *Stability of Inspiratory Time Controls*, (if provided)—The inspiratory time controls shall be stable to ±10 % of the set value. Testing shall be in accordance with 6.2.5 and Annex A1. (See also 5.1.17 and X1.2.9.)

4.6 *Inspiratory Flow Control*:

4.6.1 *Accuracy*—If provided, peak inspiratory flow shall be accurate to within ±10 % of the set value over the range as specified by the manufacturer. Testing shall be in accordance with 6.2.3 and Annex A1. (See also 5.1.18 and X1.2.10.)

4.6.2 *Stability*—If provided, inspiratory peak flow shall be stable to within ±10 % of the set value over the range as specified by the manufacturer. Testing shall be in accordance with 6.2.3 and Annex A1. (See also 5.1.18 and X1.2.10.)

4.7 *Intermittent Deep Breath (Sigh) Volume*—If provided, this feature shall be accurate to ±10 % of the set value. Testing shall be in accordance with 6.2.6. (See also 5.1.19.)

4.8 *Human Factors Requirements*:

4.8.1 The markings of all controls and indicators shall be legible from a distance of 1 m by an operator with 20/20 vision (corrected if necessary), in an illuminance level of 215 lx.

4.8.2 All controls shall be provided with some means to minimize the possibility of inadvertent control manipulation.

4.9 *Fittings*:

4.9.1 Fittings provided by the ventilator manufacturer, or the breathing system manufacturer (if different).

4.9.1.1 For flow direction sensitive devices, the direction of flow shall be permanently marked on the fitting. The fitting should be designed so that it cannot be installed in the reverse direction. Testing shall be in accordance with 6.3.1. (See also X1.3.1.)

4.9.2 If there is a separate outlet for the spirometer on the breathing tubes or the machine, the gas outlet leading to the spirometer should be designed such that it cannot be connected with the breathing tubes. (See also X1.3.2.)

4.9.3 If an ambient air inlet is fitted to the ventilator it shall not be a 15- or 22-mm male or female cone as defined in Specification F 1054, and it shall be clearly marked as "air inlet." Testing shall be in accordance with 6.3.2. (See also X1.3.3.)

4.9.4 If an expired gas outlet (other than an outlet for a spirometer) is fitted to the machine, it shall be designed in such a way that it cannot be easily connected to either 22-, 15-, or 30-mm cones or sockets, or 22-mm internal diameter tubing. Testing shall be in accordance with 6.3.3. (See also X1.3.4.)

4.9.5 *Gas Connections for Pressurized Gases*—If the device has a threaded connector on a pressurized gas connection, it shall be gas specific and non-interchangeable. If the ventilator is capable of being independently connected to a gas piping system or cylinder, it shall have a permanently attached CGA[3] nut and gland No. 1240 (oxygen) fitting, if intended to be supplied with oxygen, or a CGA[3] nut and gland No. 1160 (air) fitting, if intended to be supplied with compressed air, or both fittings if both gases are used. Testing shall be in accordance with 6.3.4.

4.9.5.1 Small tubing connections, for example, 3- to 6-mm (⅛- to 3⁄16-in.) inside diameter (ID) tubing for powering an exhalation valve and for proximal sampling of respired gases, if provided, shall be so designed as to be non-interchangeable and the connection point shall be clearly marked as to its intended purpose. Testing shall be in accordance with 6.3.5. (See also X1.3.5.)

4.10 *Breathing Circuits, General*—In addition to the relevant requirements set forth in 4.9 and 5.1.20, breathing circuits and breathing circuit components either supplied by the manufacturer or recommended for use with a home care ventilator shall comply with the following requirements:

4.10.1 *Expiratory Resistance*—In the absence of expiratory resistors or positive end-expiratory pressure devices, the pressure drop at the patient connection port shall not exceed 5 cm H_2O at a flow of 50 L/min when spirometer or breathing attachments specified by the manufacturer, or both, are used. Testing shall be in accordance with 6.4.1. (See also X1.4.1.)

4.10.2 *Kinking and Occlusion of Tubing*:

4.10.2.1 *Kinking*—Tubing shall be sufficiently rigid (for example, wire guarded or wound) or so constructed (for example, corrugated) as to minimize the possibility of kinking. Testing shall be in accordance with 6.4.2. (See also X1.4.2.)

4.10.2.2 *Occlusion*—The tubing shall be designed so as to prevent occlusion when a 2.5-kg weight bears on a 5-cm segment in the middle of a 1-m length of tubing. Testing shall be in accordance with 6.4.3. (See also X1.4.3.) The test is passed if ΔP is less than 10 cm H_2O.

4.10.3 All patient circuit components that are flow direction sensitive shall be permanently marked with the direction of flow and should be designed to minimize the risk of misassembly. Testing shall be in accordance with 6.4.4. (See also X1.4.4.)

4.10.4 All breathing circuits complying with the requirements as outlined in this specification should be either marked or labeled as complying with ASTM Specification F 1246.

4.11 *Provisions for Supplemental Oxygen*—The ventilator shall be capable of being provided with supplemental oxygen. (See also 5.1.21.)

4.12 *Alarms*—The following alarms shall be provided on all home care ventilators:

4.12.1 *Breathing Circuit Alarm*—The breathing circuit alarm(s) shall respond within 15 s or two complete breath cycles of the ventilator if the breathing circuit is compromised by disconnection. This alarm shall be activated within ± 20 % of the control setting. A means shall be provided to silence the audible portion of this alarm. This period of audible alarm silencing shall not exceed 60 s. (During this period of time the visual alarm shall remain activated.) (See also 5.1.21 and X1.5.1.)

4.12.2 *High Airway Pressure*—Alarms for high airway pressure shall be provided. This alarm may function in any of the following three ways:

4.12.2.1 Upon reaching a preset pressure the ventilator may plateau at that pressure or "dump" to ambient pressure, and then alarm on the next breath that meets or exceeds a preset value,

4.12.2.2 The ventilator may alarm on the second breath where the preset value has been met or exceeded, or

4.12.2.3 The ventilator may alarm on each breath where the preset value has been met or exceeded. (See Fig. 1 and X1.5.2.)

4.12.3 The audible portion of this alarm may automatically reset, or may require manual resetting. However, the visual portion of this alarm shall only be provided with a manual resetting mechanism.

4.12.4 *Battery Use Event Alarm*—A coupled, audible (cancellable), and visual event alarm shall be provided to indicate when the ventilator has switched to the integral battery power source. The visual alarm shall be automatically resetting only with restoration of external power. A non-cancellable audible advisory indicator other than the event alarm shall be periodically activated throughout the duration of integral battery power supply use. A low battery audible and visual indicator shall be enabled at all times. Testing shall be in accordance with 6.5.1. (See also X1.5.3.)

4.13 *Anti-Asphyxia Valves and Negative Pressure Relief Valves*—If an anti-asphyxia valve or a negative pressure relief valve is provided separate from the spontaneous breathing inlet valve, the ventilator or breathing circuit, or both, shall provide a means for the patient to inhale ambient air in the event of ventilator failure. The cracking pressure of this valve shall be no less than 3 cm of H_2O and no greater than 10 cm of H_2O. The resistance to flow shall not exceed 10 cm of H_2O per L/sec (measured at the patient connection port). The function of the anti-asphyxia or negative pressure relief valve shall not be compromised by the state of the power supply of the ventilator. Testing shall be in accordance with 6.6.1. (See also X1.6.1.)

4.14 *Electrical Safety*:

4.14.1 *Accessory Outlets, (if provided)*—Accessory outlets shall be separately fused in a circuit parallel to the circuit providing the ventilator power.

4.14.2 *Battery Charging Systems*—See 5.1.23.

4.14.3 *Electromagnetic Interference*—The ventilator should

[3] Available from Compressed Gas Association, 1235 Jefferson Davis Highway, Arlington, VA 22202.

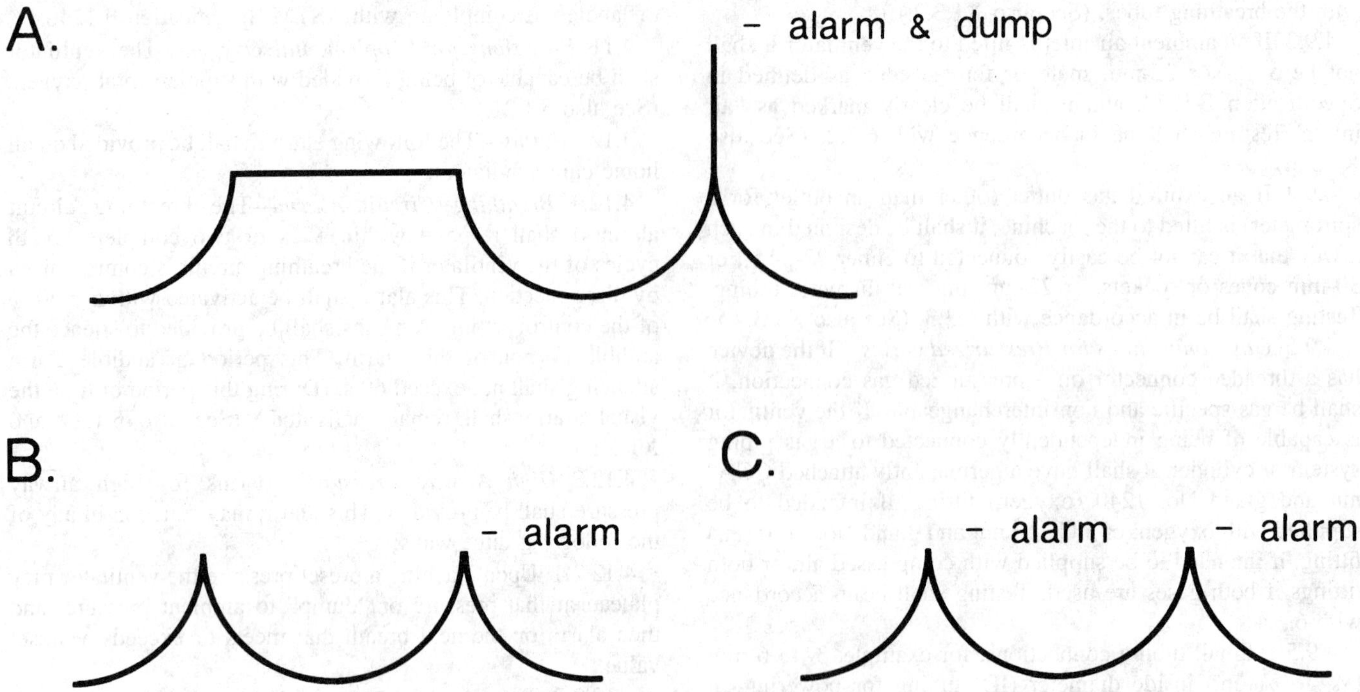

FIG. 1 Three Different Pressure Patterns That May Activate the Airway Overpressure Alarm

meet the requirements of MDS-201.[4] (See also X1.7.1.)

4.14.3.1 *Electrostatic Discharge*—The ventilator should continue to function within the manufacturer's specifications at any control setting following exposure to contact electrostatic discharges between 2 and 8 kV and air discharges between 2 and 15 kV applied using a probe that simulates electrostatic discharges from humans. The test discharges should be applied to the area of the ventilator most likely to conduct the discharge into the ventilator electric circuitry, for example, front panel controls or other conductive parts exposed to contact by the user. (See also X1.7.2.)

5. Labeling and Product Marking

5.1 The manufacturer shall provide the following information:

5.1.1 Intended environments for use (and recommended power supply or power supply limitations).

5.1.2 A recommended checklist for use in determining that the ventilator is functioning within the manufacturer's specifications following changes in ventilator settings or reassembly of the breathing circuit.

5.1.3 The recommendation that an alternative means of ventilation be available and the procedures to be followed if the ventilator ceases to function properly.

5.1.4 If the ventilator is intended for use during patient transport via ambulance, it shall be marked with instructions to use the 12-V d-c power supply rather than the 115-V a-c power supply.

5.1.5 The ventilator shall be marked with the following: **Warning**—Portable (external 115-V a-c) power supplies should not be used to power the ventilator unless it is known by the user that the voltage variations from such a power supply are within the operating limits recommended by the manufacturer.

5.1.6 The periodicity of the integral power source use indicator, (see 4.1.2.1).

5.1.7 The exact range of voltages over which the ventilator will operate.

5.1.8 Where in the ventilator breathing circuit the pressure for each pressure control is sensed, (for example, ventilator output, patient, etc.).

5.1.9 Volume performance of the ventilator when tested in accordance with 6.3.

5.1.10 The period of time during which the ventilator meets the volume control accuracy requirements of 4.3. The manufacturer shall disclose upon request the method of statistical analysis used to support the disclosed value.

5.1.11 The accuracy of any exhaled volume measurement devices, if provided with the ventilator, and the gas conditions during the accuracy testing shall be referenced.

5.1.12 The limits of frequency, inspiratory time, or I:E ratio, or combination thereof, beyond which the interdependence of control functions may cause the tidal volume specification not to be met. (See also X1.8.1.)

5.1.13 The tidal volume and minute volume range for which the ventilator is intended to function.

5.1.14 The period of time (utilizing both internal and external power supplies) during which the ventilator is capable of meeting the frequency control requirements of 4.4.1. The manufacturer shall disclose upon request the method of statistical analysis used to support the disclosed value.

5.1.15 The period of time during which the ventilator controls meet the requirements in 4.4.2. (See also X1.2.7.) The

[4] MDS-201 "Electromagnetic Compatibility Standard for Medical Devices," is available as Accession No. PB271635 from the National Technical Information Service, (NTIS), 5285 Port Royal Road, Springfield, VA 22161.

manufacturer shall disclose upon request the method of statistical analysis used to support the disclosed value.

5.1.16 The limits of inspiratory time, volume, and I:E ratio control interdependence that may cause the frequency requirements in 4.4.1 not to be met.

5.1.17 The period of time during which the inspiratory time controls, if provided, meet the requirements in 4.5.1. The manufacturer shall disclose upon request the method of statistical analysis used to support the disclosed value.

5.1.18 The period of time during which the ventilator will meet the requirements in 4.6.1 and 4.6.2. The manufacturer shall disclose upon request the method of statistical analysis used to support the disclosed value.

5.1.19 The range for sigh rate and sigh volume, if provided.

5.1.20 The tubing circuit manufacturer shall disclose the recommended continuous duration of use for "single patient use" or "disposable" circuits. (See also X1.8.2.)

5.1.21 The expected FiO_2 for various oxygen flows and ventilator settings. (See also X1.8.3.)

5.1.22 A test method for compliance with the requirements in 4.12.1.

5.1.23 Information concerning the input/output characteristics of the battery charging systems.

6. Test Methods

6.1 *Test Method for Power Source Requirements*:

6.1.1 While performing the tests for requirements 4.2-4.7 through , vary the supply voltage from 90 to 130-V a-c, and vary the frequency from 50 to 70 Hz.

6.1.2 Lower the line power to a point below the minimum specified by the manufacturer and verify that the ventilator switches to the integral battery power supply and continues to operate without degradation of performance. Next, configure the ventilator in such a manner as to create the maximum power consumption within the manufacturer's recommended operating range, and ensure that the integral battery powers the ventilator adequately to meet the requirements of this specification for no less than 15 min.

6.2 *Test Method for Accuracy of Controls, Indicators, and Pressure Relief Devices*:

6.2.1 Connect the ventilator to a calibrated test apparatus (generally with an accuracy five times greater than the required accuracy) and test the accuracy of controls over the entire range.

6.2.2 Configure the ventilator for use as recommended by the manufacturer. Fill the humidifier to the recommended level. Make pressure measurements at the patient connection port using an electronic transducer and record the pressure waves using a strip chart recorder. Set the pressure relief controls at 50, 70, and 100 cm H_2O, or the highest possible setting. If an inspiratory time control is provided, it should be set to the highest setting. Activate the ventilator while totally occluding the patient connection port. Record the pressure and from the recordings determine that the ventilator's pressure reducing mechanism activates within 3 s of reaching the maximum limiting pressure.

6.2.3 Test the ventilator against the parameters outlined in Table 1 using the general methods, etc. prescribed in Annex A1 as applicable, and record the volume control accuracy. The results of testing under this requirement, shall be made available by the manufacturer on request, and the values disclosed as the mean of the tests performed plus or minus the standard deviation.

NOTE 2—See Annex A1 for additional details.

6.2.4 Test the inspiratory time controls at the minimum, mid, and maximum inspiratory time against the conditions as outlined in 6.2.3 with the methods described in Annex A1.

6.2.5 Test the ventilator under the conditions as outlined in 6.2.3 and with the methods described in Annex A1 utilizing both the internal and external power sources and record the duration of time where the controls remain within the limits set in 4.5.1.

6.2.6 Activate the sigh mechanism as recommended by the manufacturer, repeat through five cycles, and determine the rate and volume. (See also 5.1.19.)

6.3 *Test Method for Human Factors Requirements*:

6.3.1 Visually inspect the connector for the appropriate markings under the conditions outlined in 4.8.1, and attempt to change the fitting direction.

6.3.2 Attempt to fit a 15- or 22-mm male or female cone into the ambient air inlet.

6.3.3 Attempt to connect 22-, 15-, and 30-mm cones and sockets, and 22-mm internal diameter tubing to the expired gas outlet.

6.3.4 Check the connectors to establish that the appropriate CGA[3] designated fitting has been supplied. Disconnect the hose(s) from the ventilator and connect the two ends of the hose together to verify that the connectors on both ends of the hose are for the same type of gas.

6.3.5 Inspect the connection point for markings under the conditions outlined in 4.8.1 and attempt to cross-connect or interchange the fittings or tubing.

6.4 *Tests for Breathing Circuit Requirements*:

6.4.1 Generate a 50 L/min gas flow through the patient breathing system with no PEEP. Measure the pressure drop from the patient connection port to ambient.

6.4.2 Condition all tubing at 42°C and 100 % relative humidity with gas flowing through the tubing for 1 h prior to testing as outlined as follows: suspend a length of tubing at least 1-m long over a metal cylinder with a 2.5-cm diameter, all at room temperature; hang a 0.5-kg weight on each end; and establish a steady 75 L/min flow (25 L/min for tubing smaller than 22-mm inside diameter (ID) that is intended for use with infants and neonates) through the tubing and measure the pressure above atmospheric pressure (ΔP) necessary to drive the flow through the tubing. The test is passed if ΔP is less than 10 cm H_2O.

6.4.3 Condition all tubing at 42°C and 100 % relative humidity with gas flowing through the tubing for 1 h prior to testing as outlined as follows: place a 2.5-kg weight on a 5-cm segment in the middle of a 1-m length of tubing; establish a 75 L/min flow (25 L/min for tubing smaller than 22-mm inside diameter (ID) that is intended for use with infants and neonates) through the breathing system, and use on an ambient air inlet could lead to misconnection of breathing circuit components to the ambient air inlet.

6.4.4 Visually inspect the circuit components under the

conditions outlined in 4.8.1, and attempt to change connector direction.

6.5 *Test Methods for Alarm Requirements*:

6.5.1 During performance of the tests for compliance with 4.4.1, check to ensure that the audible and visual event alarms sound as the transition from line power to battery power occurs, and that the periodic audible advisory indicator functions, annunciating at the interval outlined by the manufacturer in the accompanying documents.

6.6 *Test Method for Anti-Asphyxia Valve and Negative Pressure Relief Valves Requirements*—Configure the ventilator and breathing system as it is when connected to the patient. Measure pressure and flow at the patient connection port of the breathing system. Generate a breath at the minimum recommended tidal volume and record the opening pressure of the valve and the resistance to flow. Repeat the test at the maximum recommended tidal volume. Record the opening ("cracking") pressure and resistance to flow at both tidal volume settings.

ANNEX

(Mandatory Information)

A1. GENERAL TEST CONDITIONS, APPARATUS AND METHODS

A1.1 *General Test Conditions*—All tests shall be conducted at NTPD (20°C, 760 mm Hg, 0 % RH) or corrected to NTPD with the ventilator configured for use as recommended by the manufacturer.

A1.2 *Test Apparatus:*

A1.2.1 *Lung Models, Compliances and Resistances*—The lung models illustrated in Figs. A1.1 and A1.2 do not preclude the development of different or more sophisticated lung models with the same ranges of compliance and linear or nonlinear resistances. If nonlinear resistances are used, their characteristics must be specified.

A1.2.1.1 *Lung Models*— Lung models are designed to provide impedances to the ventilator output that simulate both normal and diseased lung states. The impedances to ventilator output are lung elastance and airflow resistance, that can be simulated in the lung models by compliance and a resistance connected in series (see Figs. A1.1 and A1.2). The various combinations of compliances and resistances used in the test procedures are given in Table 1.

A1.2.1.2 *Compliances*— The required compliances are given in Table 1. These compliances shall include the compliances of all components of the lung model system. The volume-pressure characteristics of the model compliances, including connections, shall be determined at ambient pressure and temperature, and shall be determined as in 6.1.2 and shall be within ±5 % of the required compliance values shown in Table 1.

A1.2.1.3 *Resistances*— The required resistances are given in Table 1. These values relate to measurements at NTPD. They include the resistance of the flow measuring device.

A1.3 *General Methods of Testing Performance of Lung Ventilators* —Measurements of pressure, flow, and volume shall be made as shown in Figs. A1.1 and A1.2 and shall be accurate to within± 2.5 % of the reading. An additional tolerance of ±2.5 % of the full scale reading shall be allowed. The reading accuracy of the recording device shall be maintained at frequencies up to 10 Hz. Ambient conditions shall be recorded, and all results are to be reported at NTPD (20°C, 760 mm Hg, and 0 % RH) even though other conditions may exist during actual testing. Dry air, unless otherwise specified in an individual requirement, is to be the test gas.

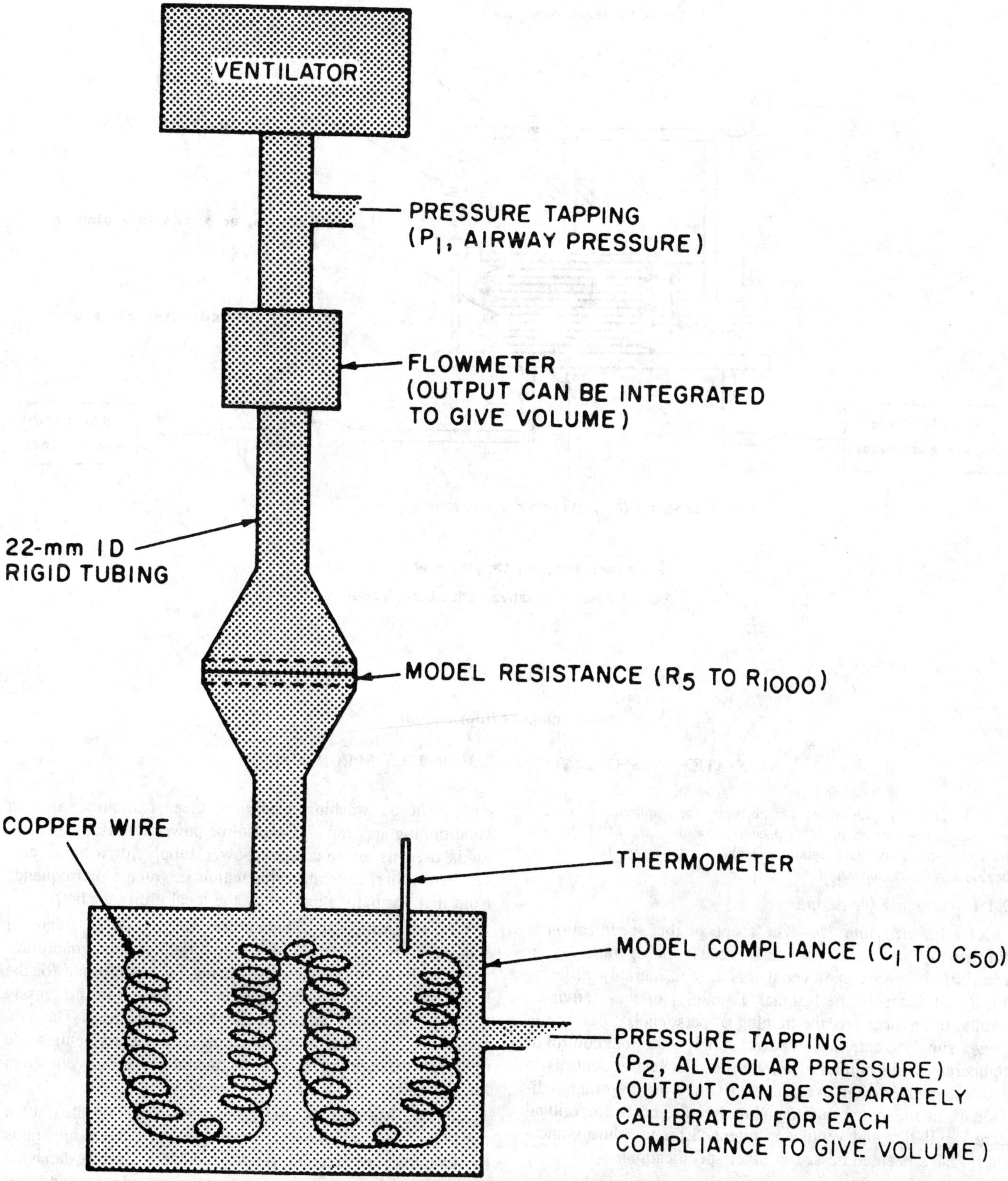

FIG. A1.1 Representative Passive Lung Model

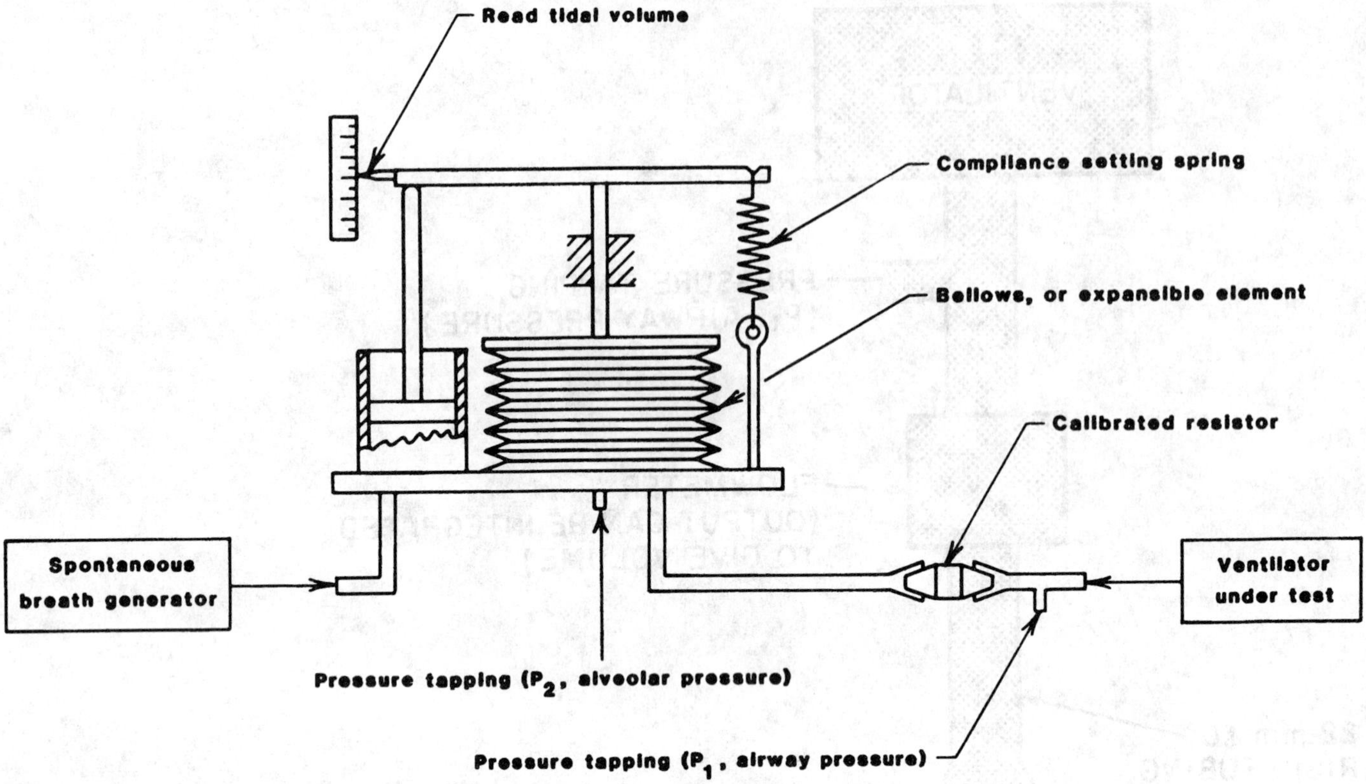

FIG. A1.2 Representative Active Lung Model

APPENDIX

(Nonmandatory Information)

X1. STATEMENTS OF RATIONALE FOR THIS SPECIFICATION

NOTE X1.1—The rationales for many of the requirements of this specification are given in this Appendix. For the sake of clarity, the paragraph to which each rationale applies is given in italics at the beginning of each subsection.

X1.1 Rationale for Scope

X1.1.1 *Paragraph 1.1*—The scope of this specification is limited to home care ventilators because the operating environment for home care ventilators is considerably different from that found in the hospital. Examples of these environmental differences are: the training of personnel, difference in power supplies, extremes in power supply variation, control of temperature and humidity, and the need to secure controls to prevent inadvertent movement and tampering by other individuals in the home environment. Requirements for critical care ventilators and ventilators intended for use during anesthesia have been addressed in other specifications.

X1.2 Rationale for Performance Requirements

X1.2.1 *Paragraph 4.1.1*—Fluctuation within the ranges specified in 4.1.1 is known to occur in electrical power supplies. The causes for such variations may be outside the control of the ventilator user. For example, a decrease in the voltage in the power supply by the local electric utility, or the variations that may result from demands for power by such equipment as washing machines, freezer motors, and air conditioning apparatus. If a gasoline powered portable generator is used as an emergency power supply for a home care ventilator, this may cause fluctuation in voltage or frequency from that normally supplied by the local utility, or both.

X1.2.1.1 Although Subcommittee F29.03.09 is aware of specific problems caused by extreme high voltage conditions, particularly in ambulances, it was not felt appropriate for the home care ventilator to be required to function in the grossly aberrant conditions described for some ambulances. The subcommittee is also aware that attempts are currently being made to correct these problems with the manufacturers of generators for ambulances.

X1.2.1.2 Members of Subcommittee F29.03.09 also noted that there were a number of other types of clinical apparatus (for example, apnea monitors, etc.) that were severely damaged or destroyed by the power variations in ambulances, and that this problem would be most appropriately addressed via standards for ambulances.

X1.2.2 *Paragraph 4.1.2*—Subcommittee F29.03.09 members present agreed that for safety purposes it was necessary to mandate that all ventilators intended for home care should have a power source integral to the ventilator to provide for patient needs in the event of an emergency such as an electrical storm or other such incidents that might interrupt the line power supply to the ventilator. "Integral" is intended to mean as a component part of the ventilator system. This power source may, or may not, be enclosed within the ventilator housing.

X1.2.2.1 Subcommittee F29.03.09 also agreed that the 15 min time period was intended to provide a safety factor so that the patient or the care giver could find an alternative source of power to operate the ventilator, or an alternative source of ventilation for the patient. The subcommittee agreed that it was not intended that the integral battery be used regularly as a power source for the ventilator during movement and transport of the patient.

X1.2.2.2 It was felt that to mandate switching to a battery power source under both low and high voltage conditions would significantly increase the cost of the ventilator while addressing a problem caused in a relatively small part of the ventilator use environment, and that the excessive voltage problem was better addressed by improving the specification for power supplies in ambulances. The subcommittee did note, however, that marking on the ventilator should be provided to the effect that the ventilator should be operated off the 12-V d-c power supply in the ambulance as opposed to the 115-V a-c generator supply.

X1.2.3 *Paragraph 4.2.2*—The limits set forth in 4.2.2 were the minimum acceptable to the subcommittee in order to maintain operator confidence and provide for patient safety.

X1.2.4 *Paragraph 4.2.3*—Subcommittee F29.03.09 felt that the requirement in 4.2.3 would reduce the possibility of barotrauma and would also reduce complications resulting from decreased cardiac output secondary to increased intrathoracic pressure, caused when ventilator pressure relief mech anisms "plateaued" in pressure rather than "dumping" the tidal volume until ambient pressure is reached. The subcommittee also felt for this requirement to be truly effective that a combined test would need to be developed ensuring that tubing met a given level of resistance to crushing and kinking.

X1.2.5 *Paragraph 4.3*—The requirement for disclosure of accuracy if both a calibrated control and indicator are used is intended to address the issue of a coarse gradation on the control and a fine gradation on the indicator that is associated with it. Under these circumstances it is important to clarify for the user which (the control or the indicator) meets the specified accuracy. The compliances and resistances given in the test method, the frequency, and I:E ratio are representative of conditions that would be found during the ventilation of an adult patient with normal pulmonary physiology. The members of the subcommittee felt that the accuracy specified would provide for adequate reproducibility of control movement to ensure effective modification of ventilator function.

X1.2.5.1 The parameters specified in Table 1 include a wide range of resistances, compliances, tidal volumes, and ventilatory rates reflective of the use environment and will provide the user with the necessary information to determine whether or not a particular ventilator is capable of providing for the needs of a specific patient.

X1.2.6 *Paragraph 4.3.1*—A variation of ±10 % of tidal volume or minute volume reflects a possible variation of 7 mm of mercury $PaCO_2$, and this is within acceptable limits for this type of ventilation.

X1.2.7 *Paragraph 4.4.1*—A variation of ±10 % of tidal volume or minute volume reflects a possible variation of 7 mm of mercury $PaCO_2$, and this is within acceptable limits for this type of ventilation.

X1.2.8 *Paragraph 4.5.1*——The required accuracy of inspiratory times will allow the clinician to control ventilation in situations where airway leaks prevent using set volume as the parameter to determine minute ventilation. Errors caused by inaccuracies in inspiratory time settings will also effect impedance of venous return.

X1.2.9 *Paragraph 4.5.1*—Variation in stability of inspiratory time controls will lead to variation in ventilation in cases where airway leak is the determinant of ventilation, and will affect venous return, and may therefore cause injury to the patient if variation outside of the limits stated in 4.5.1 occur.

X1.2.10 *Paragraph 4.6*—Peak flow in some types of ventilators may be the determinant of inspiratory time, and in other types of ventilators it may be the determinant of tidal volume. Therefore, the accuracy and stability need to fall within the specifications of 4.6.1 and 4.6.2 in order for the device to function safely in the clinical environment.

X1.3 Rationale for Human Factors Requirements

X1.3.1 *Paragraph 4.9.1.1*—Flow direction sensitive devices such as one-way valves or humidifiers may be caused to malfunction by inadvertent connection in the reverse manner, and it is also possible for injury to the patient to occur if flows of gas are misdirected or humidifier contents are emptied into the breathing circuit as a result of such a misconnection.

X1.3.2 *Paragraph 4.9.2*—This requirement is intended to minimize the possibility of inappropriate connection of the ventilator breathing circuit tubing to the spirometer outlet.

X1.3.3 *Paragraph 4.9.3*—In other standards for anesthetic and respiratory care equipment both 19- and 30-mm fittings have been prohibited from use as ambient air inlets. However, for ventilator use in the home environment, it was felt that both of these standard fittings should be allowed. The 19-mm fitting is conventionally used for scavenging anesthetic waste gases, and the 30-mm fitting is designated for use with spirometers. Subcommittee F29.03.09 felt that neither of these applications pertained to use of home care ventilators, and that it would be acceptable to allow the use of the 19- and 30-mm fitting on home care ventilators.

X1.3.4 *Paragraph 4.9.4*—The use of 15- or 22-mm fittings for a ventilator air inlet in these applications is unacceptable because 15- or 22-mm fittings are routinely a part of the requirements of 4.9.4. The requirements given in 4.9.4 will minimize the possibility of inadvertent connection of breathing system components to the expired gas outlet.

X1.3.5 *Paragraph 4.9.5*——These connections are manipulated every time the circuit is changed, and significant problems have been reported with misconnection of these tubings.

X1.4 Rationale for Breathing Circuit Requirements

X1.4.1 *Paragraph 4.10.1*—Although expiratory resistances of less than 5 cm H_2O at 50 L/min are desirable, the subcommittee realizes that such values may not be achievable.

Patient system configurations, tubing length, connector sizes, and gas flow through the system are factors that may combine to raise end-expiratory pressure to the 5 cm H_2O maximum under certain conditions of ventilation. Device-inherent resistance above the 5 cm H_2O level is not acceptable because of the adverse effect that these levels may have on the patient's respiratory pattern or cardiovascular flow.

X1.4.2 *Paragraph 4.10.2.1*—It is often necessary for ventilator tubing to be placed over the tops of bedrails, over the rails of wheelchairs, over crib railings, and in other places where it may be subject to kinking. The tests outlined for this requirement are intended to simulate these conditions.

X1.4.3 *Paragraph 4.10.2.2*—It is often necessary for ventilator tubing to be placed in areas around the patient where it may be occluded (for example, movement of the patient's head on the tubing, passing of the tubing over a wheelchair arm where it may be occluded by the patient's arm, etc.). Tests for this requirement are intended to simulate this type of occlusion.

X1.4.4 *Paragraph 4.10.3*—Flow direction sensitive devices such as one-way valves or humidifiers may be caused to malfunction by inadvertent connection in the reverse manner, and it is also possible for injury to the patient to occur if flows of gas are misdirected or humidifier contents are emptied into the breathing circuit as a result of such a misconnection.

X1.5 Rationale for Alarms Requirements

X1.5.1 *Paragraph 4.12.1*—A means of silencing the ventilator breathing circuit alarm is necessary in order to perform procedures such as measuring volumes, suctioning, etc., where the patient is briefly disconnected from the ventilator. The subcommittee felt that the time period of 60 s (rather than the requirement for 2 min that is included in other ventilator specifications) was more appropriate in this specification due to the lower level of supervision that most patients on home care ventilators are subject to.

X1.5.2 *Paragraph 4.12.2*:

X1.5.2.1 *Paragraph 4.12.2.1*—The type of alarm mechanism described in 4.12.2.1 is essential in certain types of ventilation where a variable leak is present, and in the first part of the illustration in Fig. 1 where the leak from the patient is equal to the flow of gas being sent to the patient, a plateau is reached. This type of ventilation is often used for pediatric patients. The portion of Fig. 1 illustrated in (A) defines a situation where a patient is being ventilated by a volume ventilator with a leak, and an obstruction occurs to decrease that leak.

X1.5.2.2 *Paragraph 4.12.2.2*—The type of alarm described in 4.12.2.2 is intended to reduce the number of spurious alarms in the home environment, in a situation where the upper pressure limit is frequently reached on an individual breath during routine ventilation, and may only indicate a malfunction or obstruction on repeated breaths.

X1.5.2.3 *Paragraph 4.12.2.3*—The type of alarm described in 4.12.2.3 is intended to provide the maximum indication of overpressure in applications where any overpressure condition may be injurious to the patient.

X1.5.3 *Paragraph 4.12.3*—Indicators for several different purposes have been addressed in this requirement. The coupled audible and visual event alarm to be activated when the ventilator begins operating on the battery power source was intended to provide notification to both the patient and the care-giver that line power was no longer being provided to the ventilator. The requirement states that the audible portion of this event alarm is manually cancelable, because once the care-giver has attended to the ventilator, the audible portion of the alarm has fulfilled its intended purpose. However, it was felt necessary to maintain the visual portion of the alarm as a reminder that the integral battery power source was still in use, and to provide an audible advisory indicator on a periodic basis (for example, every 4 or 5 min) to additionally remind both the patient and the care-giver that the integral battery power source was in use. The subcommittee felt that this approach to alarms and indicators on the power supply would provide the necessary safety while minimizing the nuisance factor that is inherent in continuously sounding alarms.

X1.6 Rationale for Anti-Asphyxia Valves and Negative Pressure Relief Valve Requirements

X1.6.1 *Paragraph 4.13*—The subcommittee included requirements for the valve to open at no less than 3 cm of H_2O and no greater than 10 cm of H_2O because it was felt that this was the range necessary in order to prevent the anti-asphyxia valve from opening during the initial negative pressure phase of assisted ventilation while still providing for function in the event of ventilator malfunction.

X1.7 Rationale for Electrical Safety Requirements

X1.7.1 *Paragraph 4.14.3*—Electromagnetic interference can cause improper operation of ventilators. There are numerous sources of such interference, including electrical appliances, telemetry transmitters, and nearby radio broadcasting stations. However, several manufacturers of medical devices have experienced field failures caused by conducted or radiated electromagnetic interference in devices that meet the requirements of MDS-201,[4] and further or additional requirements may be necessary in order to address application of home care ventilators in specific environments.

X1.7.2 *Paragraph 4.14.3.1*—Electrostatic discharge can cause improper operation of home care ventilators. Operators of medical devices in the home are likely to become electrostatically charged from contact with synthetic garments and carpets. Discharges to medical equipment from operators is likely, particularly in conditions of low humidity. Ventilators are life support devices, and must therefore continue to function within the manufacturer's specifications.

X1.7.2.1 Although test probes are necessary for effective testing, no accepted standards for electrostatic discharge testing exist at present. The specifications contained in a recent proposed revision of IEC Publication 801-2[5] describe a type of probe and waveforms that effectively model electrostatic discharges from humans.

X1.8 Rationale for Marking and Labeling Requirements

X1.8.1 *Paragraph 5.1.2*——Unpredictable degradation of performance due to interdependence of controls can seriously

---

[5] IEC Publication 801-2 is available from International Electrotechnical Commission, 3 rue de Varembé, 1211 Geneva 20, Switzerland.

affect the ability of the operator to accurately adjust the ventilator's function, and can thus result in jeopardy to the patient.

X1.8.2 *Paragraph 5.1.20*——Although "single patient use" tubing is often changed every 24 to 48 h in the hospital setting, the duration of use in the home care setting may considerably exceed this time period. It is necessary for the user/consumer to know the recommended duration of use so that the tubing can be changed prior to any physical degradation that might compromise performance of the ventilator.

X1.8.3 *Paragraph 5.1.21*——The expected FiO_2 for various flows and settings referenced in this requirement refer to operation during controlled ventilation only. Members of the subcommittee were well aware of the possibility of variation in FiO_2 during the assist mode, but it was agreed that it was not appropriate to mandate the use of such devices as gas blenders, etc. in order to maintain concentration during the assist mode because of the increased expense and complexity involved, and because of the decrease in portability that such equipment would cause.

Designation: F 1251 – 89 (Reapproved 1995)

Standard Terminology Relating to Polymeric Biomaterials in Medical and Surgical Devices[1]

This standard is issued under the fixed designation F 1251; the number immediately following the designation indicates the year of original adoption or, in the case of revision, the year of last revision. A number in parentheses indicates the year of last reapproval. A superscript epsilon (ε) indicates an editorial change since the last revision or reapproval.

1. Scope

1.1 This terminology covers polymeric biomaterials in medical and surgical devices. Terms are defined as they are used relative to medical and surgical materials and devices. Terms that are generally understood and in common usage or adequately defined in other readily available references are not included except where particular delineation to biomaterials may be more clearly stated.

1.2 This terminology is therefore intended to be selective of terms used generally in materials science and technology and published in a number of documents, such as those listed in the succeeding sections. The listing is also intended to define terms that appear prominently within other ASTM standards and do not appear elsewhere.

1.3 The definitions are substantially identical to those published in other ASTM standards on metals, ceramics and glass, rubbers and polymers, etc., or published by other standards writing organizations, such as International Standards Organization (ISO), American Institute of Mechanical Engineers (AIME), American Society of Plastic and Reconstructive Surgeons (ASPR), and Tissue Culture Association (TCA).

1.4 A need exists for this terminology to supplement current documents on terminology which concentrate on materials. This terminology covers each of the following disciplines: plastics (polymers), rubber (elastomers), and textiles (polymer derived).

1.5 An increasing number of product (polymeric, metallurgical, and ceramic types) designations and designations for chemical, physical, mechanical, and analytical tests and standards are coming into common usage in the literature and commerce of biomaterials in medical and surgical devices and clinical services. Section 2 lists those documents referenced in this terminology.

1.6 Table 1 lists abbreviated, anagramic designations. Annex A1 is a thesaurus of general usage terms relating to biomaterials.

2. Referenced Documents

2.1 *ASTM Standards:*

D 638 Test Method for Tensile Properties of Plastics[2]

D 747 Test Method for Apparent Bending Modulus of Plastics by Means of a Cantilever Beam[2]

D 790 Test Methods for Flexural Properties of Unreinforced and Reinforced Plastics and Electrical Insulating Materials[2]

D 882 Test Methods for Tensile Properties of Thin Plastic Sheeting[2]

D 1003 Test Method for Haze and Luminous Transmittance of Transparent Plastics[2]

E 380 Practice for Use of the International System of Units (SI) (the Modernized Metric System)[3]

3. Terminology

3.1 *Definitions:*

acetal plastic, *n*—a plastic based on polymers having a predominance of acetal linkages in the main chain. (See also polyoxymethylene.) **D-20**

acrylic plastic, *n*—a plastic based on polymers made with acrylic acid or a structural derivative of acrylic acid. **D-20**

addition polymerization, *n*—polymerization in which monomers are linked together without the splitting off of water or other simple molecules and involves the opening of a double bond. **D-20**

aging, *n*—the process of exposing materials to an environment for an interval of time. **D-20**

aging effect, *n*—a change in a material brought about by exposure of the material to an environment for an interval of time.

alkyd resin, *n*—a polyester convertible into a crosslinked form; requiring a reactant of functionality higher than two, or having double bonds. **D-20**

apparent density—see **density, apparent.**

artificial weathering, *n*—exposure of a material to laboratory conditions that simulate outdoor weathering.

DISCUSSION—Exposure conditions may be cyclic, involving changes in temperature, relative humidity, radiant energy, and many other elements found in the atmosphere in various geographical areas. The laboratory exposure conditions are usually intensified beyond those encountered in actual out-door exposure to accelerate the effect. **D-20**

blister, *n*—in sheet plastics, an imperfection, a rounded elevation of the surface, with boundaries that may be more or less

[1] This terminology is under the jurisdiction of ASTM Committee F-4 on Medical and Surgical Materials and Devices and is the direct responsibility of Subcommittee F04.11 on Polymeric Materials.

Current edition approved Nov. 24, 1989. Published January 1990.

[2] *Annual Book of ASTM Standards*, Vol 08.01.

[3] *Annual Book of ASTM Standards*, Vol 14.02. Excerpts in Related Material sections of all other volumes.

TABLE 1 Abbreviated, Anagramic Designations—Acronyms[A,B]

Term	Classification	Descriptive Term in Full
AAS	analytic, chemical	atomic absorption spectroscopy
ABC	plastic, polymer	acryline bone cement
ABS	plastic, polymer	acrylonitrile-butadiene-styrene polymer
AN	polymer, monomer	acrylonitrile
ATR-IR	analytic, chemical	attenuated total reflectance—infrared
CA	plastic, polymer	cellulose acetate (sheet X ray)
CAB	plastic, polymer	cellulose acetate-butyrate
CP	plastic, polymer	cellulose propionate or cellulose acetate-propionate
DSC	analytic, physical	differential scanning calorimetry
DTA	analytic, physical	differential thermal analysis
EDTA	analyses	ethylene dinitrilo tetraacetic acid
EPM/EPDM	elastomer	ethylene-propylene terpolymer
EPR	elastomer	see EPM/EDPM above
ESCA	analytic, chemical	used for X-ray photoelectron spectroscopy
ETFE	analytic, chemical	(ethylene-tetrafluoroethylene-fluoroplastics)
FEP	plastics, polymers	perfluoro(ethylene-propylene) copolymer
GC	analytic, chemical	gas chromatography
HEMA	plastic, polymer	hydroxyethyl methacrylate (polymer)
HPLC	analytic, chemical	high performance liquid chromatography
IR	analytic, physical	infrared spectroscopy (for example, IR scan)
kPA	mechanical, physical	kiloPascal (unit of pressure—see Practice E 380, Appendix)
MPa	mechanical, physical	megaPascal (unit of pressure—see Practice E 380, Appendix)
MW (mw)	physical, molecular	molecular weight
MWD (mwd)	physical, molecular	molecular weight distribution (see mw, above)
MRI	clinical	magnetic resonance imaging (diagnostic application of nmr)
MRS	analytic, chemical	magnetic resonance spectroscopy (diagnostic application of nmr)
NBR	elastomer, polymer	nitrile-butadiene rubber
NMR (nmr)	analytic, physical	nuclear magnetic resonance
PB	elastomer, polymer	polybutylene
PC	plastic, polymer	polycarbonate
PCTFE	plastic, polymer	polychlorotrifluoroethylene
PDMS	elastomer, polymer fluid	silicone, polydimethyl siloxane
PE	plastic, polymer	polyethylene
PET	plastic, polymer	poly(ethylene terephthalate)
PFA	plastic, polymer	perfluoroalkoxy fluorocarbon polymer
PMMA	plastic, polymer	poly(methyl methacrylate)
PTFE	plastic, polymer	polytetrafluoroethylene
PU	plastic or elastomer polymer	polyurethane
PVA	plastic, polymer	poly(vinyl alcohol) (often poly(vinyl acetate))
PVAc	plastic, polymer	poly(vinyl acetate)
PVC	plastic, polymer	poly(vinyl chloride)
PVDC	plastic, polymer	poly(vinylidene chloride)
PVP	polymer	poly(vinyl pyttolidone)
RTV	elastomer, plastic	room temperature vulcanization
SAN	elastomer, polymer	styrene-acrylonitrile polymer
SB	elastomer, polymer	styrene-butadiene polymer
SEM	analytic, microscopy	scanning electron microscopy (cf TEM)
SR	elastomer, polymer	styrene rubber (elastomer)
TEM	analytic, microscopy	transmission electron microscopy (cf SEM)
TAR	device or prosthesis	total ankle replacement
TER	device or prosthesis	total elbow replacement
THR	device or prosthesis	total hip replacement
TJR	device or prosthesis	total joint replacement
TKR	device or prosthesis	total knee replacement
TSR	device or prosthesis	total shoulder replacement
TWR	device or prosthesis	total wrist replacement
UHMW	plastic, polymer	ultrahigh molecular weight polyethylene (stated polymer)
UMHWPE	plastic, polymer	ultrahigh molecular weight polyethylene (see UHMW)
UV	analytic, physical	ultraviolet light spectroscopy
VCM	polymer, monomer	vinyl chloride monomer content
XPS	analytic, chemical	X-ray photoelectric spectroscopy (also called ESCA)
XRD	analytic, physical	X-ray diffraction

[A] If a method or name is used for the first time in a text (paper, etc.), it must be presented in full with the abbreviation in brackets.
[B] If the text is long or consists of several chapters, the full name must be repeated in reasonable sequences, at least when first mentioned in a new chapter.

sharply defined, somewhat resembling in shape a blister on the human skin. **D-20**

block copolymer, *n*—an essentially linear copolymer in which there are repeated sequences of polymeric segments of different chemical structure. **D-20**

bloom, *n*—a visible exudation or efflorescence of a performance additive on the surface of a material. **D-20**

bulk density—the weight per unit volume of a material including voids inherent in the material as tested.

DISCUSSION—This term is sometimes used synonymously with apparent density.

bulk factor, *n*—the ratio of the volume of a given mass of molding material to its volume in the molded form.

DISCUSSION—The bulk factor is also equal to the ratio of the density of the material to its apparent density in the unmolded form. **D-20** **ISO**

butylene plastic—plastic based on resins made by the polymerization of butene or copolymerization of butene with one or more unsaturated compounds, the butene being in greatest amount by weight. **D-20**

cast film, *n*—a film made by depositing a layer of plastic, either molten, in solution, or in a dispersion, onto a surface, solidifying the deposit and removing the film from the surface. **D-20**

cell, *n*—a small partially or completely enclosed cavity. **D-20**

cell, closed—see **closed cell.**

cell, open—see **open cell.**

chemically foamed polymeric material, *n*—a cellular material in which the cells are formed by gases generated by thermal decomposition or other chemical reaction. **D-20**

chlorofluorocarbon plastic, *n*—a plastic based on polymers made with monomers composed of chlorine, fluorine, and carbon only. **ISO**

chlorofluorohydrocarbon plastic, *n*—a plastic based on polymers made with monomers composed of chlorine, fluorine, hydrogen, and carbon only. **ISO**

closed cell, *n*—a cell totally enclosed by its walls and hence not interconnecting with other cells. (See also **cell** and **open cell.**) **ISO**

closed-cell foamed plastic, *n*—a plastic in which almost all the cells are noninterconnecting. **D-20**

cold flow—see preferred term **creep.**

compression molding, *n*—a process for molding a material in a confined cavity by applying pressure and usually heat. **D-20**

condensation polymer, *n*—polymerization in which during an acid/base reaction a small molecule is often split out.

copolymer, *n*—a polymer consisting of molecules characterized by the repetition (neglecting ends, branch junctions and other irregularities) of two or more different types of monomeric units. See **polymer.** **D-20**

copolymerization—see **polymerization** and **copolymer.**

crazing, *n*—apparent fine cracks at or under the surface of a plastic.

DISCUSSION—The crazed areas are composed of polymeric material of lower density than the surrounding matrix.

creep, *n*—the time-dependent part of strain resulting from stress.

cure, *v*—to change the properties of a polymeric system into a more stable, usable condition by the use of heat, radiation, or reaction with chemical additives.

DISCUSSION—Cure may be accomplished, for example, by removal of solvent or crosslinking. **ISO**

degradation, *n*—a deleterious change in the chemical structure, physical properties, or appearance of a plastic.

density, apparent, *n*—the weight in air of a unit of volume of a material.

DISCUSSION—This term is sometimes used synonymously with bulk density.

density, bulk, *n*—the weight in air of a unit of volume of a material.

DISCUSSION—This term is commonly used synonymously with apparent density (1973). **D-20**

elastomer, *n*—a macromolecular material that at room temperature returns rapidly to approximately its initial dimensions and shape after substantial deformation by a weak stress and release of the stress. **D-20**

epoxy plastic, *n*—a thermoplastic or thermosetting plastic containing ether or hydroxyalkyl repeating units, or both, resulting from the ring-opening reactions of lower-molecular weight polyfunctional oxirane resins, or compounds, with catalysts or with various polyfunctional acidic or basic coreactants.

DISCUSSION—Epoxy plastics often are modified by the incorporation of diluents, plasticizers, fillers, thixotropic agents, or other materials. **D-20**

ethylene plastic—a plastic based on polymers of ethylene or copolymers of ethylene with other monomers, the ethylene being in greatest amount by mass. **ISO**

filler, *n*—a relatively inert material added to a plastic to modify its strength, performance, working properties, or other qualities, or to lower costs. (See also **reinforced plastic.**)

film, *n*—in plastics, term for sheeting having a nominal thickness not greater than 0.25 mm (0.01 in.). (See also **sheeting.**)

fluorocarbon plastic, *n*—a plastic based on polymers made with monomers composed of fluorine and carbon only.

DISCUSSION—When the monomer is essentially tetrafluoro-ethylene, the prefix TFE may be used to designate these materials. When the resins are copolymers of tetrafluoro-ethylene and hexafluoropropylene, the resins may be designated with the prefix FEP. Other prefixes may be adopted to designate other fluorocarbon plastics. **ISO**

fluorohydrocarbon plastic, *n*—a plastic based on polymers made with monomers composed of fluorine, hydrogen, and carbon only. **ISO**

fluoroplastic, *n*—a plastic based on polymers with monomers containing one or more atoms of fluorine or copolymers of such monomers with other monomers, the fluorine-containing monomer(s) being in greatest amount by mass. (See also **fluorocarbon plastic, chlorofluorocarbon plastic, fluorohydrocarbon plastic,** and **chlorofluorohydrocarbon plastic.**)

gel, *n*—*in polymer*, a semisolid system consisting of a network of solid aggregates in which liquid is held.

DISCUSSION—Gels have very low strengths and do not flow like a liquid. They are soft, flexible, and may rupture under their own weight unless supported externally.

gel, *n*—*in polymerization*, the initial jelly-like solid phase that develops during the formation of a resin from a liquid.

gel, *n*—*with vinyl plastisols*, a state between liquid and solid that occurs in the initial stages of heating, or upon prolonged storage.

haze, *n*—*in plastics*, the cloudy or turbid aspect or appearance of an otherwise transparent material caused by light scattered from within the specimen or from its surfaces.

Discussion—For the purpose of Test Method D 1003, haze is the percentage of transmitted light which, in passing through the specimen, deviates from the incident beam through forward scatter more than 2.5° on the average.

isotactic, *adj*—pertaining to a type of polymeric molecular structure containing a sequence of regularly spaced asymmetric atoms arranged in like configuration in a polymer chain.

laminate, *n*—a product made by bonding together two or more layers of material or materials.

Discussion—A single resin-impregnated sheet of paper, fabric, or glass mat, for example, is not considered a laminate. Such a single-sheet construction may be called a "lamina." **ISO**

laminate, cross-plied, *n*—a nonparallel laminate.

laminate, parallel, *n*—a laminate in which all layers or plies are oriented with their principal direction (grain or strongest direction in tension) parallel with the principal direction of the laminate.

melamine plastic, *n*—plastic based on resins made by the condensation or melamine and aldehydes. **D-20**

monomer, *n*—a relatively simple compound which can react to form a polymer. (See also **polymer.**) **D-14, D-20**

nylon plastic, *n*—a plastic based on resins composed principally of a long-chain synthetic polymeric amide which has recurring amide groups as an integral part of the main polymer chain. **D-20**

olefin plastic, *n*—a plastic based on polymers made by the polymerization of olefins or copolymerization of olefins with other monomers, the olefins being at least 50 mass %. **D-11, D-20, F-17**

oligomer, *n*—a polymer consisting of only a few monomer units such as a dimer, trimer, tetramer, etc., or their mixtures.

open cell, *n*—a cell not totally enclosed by its walls, and hence interconnecting with other cells. (See **closed cell.**)

organosol, *n*—a suspension of a finely divided plastic in a plasticizer, together with a volatile organic liquid.

Discussion—The volatile liquid evaporates at elevated temperatures, and the resulting residue is a homogeneous plastic mass, provided the temperature is high enough to accomplish mutual solution of the plastic and plasticizer. **D-20**

phenolic plastic, *n*—a plastic based on resins made by the condensation of phenols, such as phenol and cresol, with aldehydes. **D-20**

pit, *n*—*in plastics*, an imperfection, a small crater in the surface, the depth and width of which are approximately the same order of magnitude.

plastic, *n*—any of numerous polymeric materials that are usually thermoplastic or thermosetting, of high molecular weight and that can be molded, cast extruded, drawn, laminated, or otherwise fabricated into objects, powders, beads, films, filaments, fibers, or other shapes (*Webster Modified*).

plasticizer, *n*—a substance incorporated into a material to increase its workability, flexibility, or distensibility of the material.

plastisol, *n*—a liquid suspension of a finely divided PVC polymer or copolymer in a plasticizer.

Discussion—The polymer does not dissolve appreciably in the plasticizer at room temperature but does dissolve at elevated temperatures to form a homogeneous plastic mass (plasticized polymer).

polybutylene, *n*—a polymer prepared by the polymerization of butene as the sole monomer. (See also **polybutylene plastic** and **butylene plastic.**)

polybutylene plastic, plastic based on polymers made with butene as essentially the sole monomer. **D-20**

polycarbonate, *n*—a polymer in which the repeating structural unit in the chain is a carbonic acid ester of Bisphenol A. **D-20**

polyester, *n*—a polymer in which the repeated structural unit in the chain is of the ester type.

Discussion—The polyester is linear and thermoplastic if derived, either actually or formally, from (*a*) mono-hydroxy-mono-carboxylic acids by selfesterification, or (*b*) the interaction of diols and dicarboxylic acids. **ISO**

polyether, *n*—a polymer in which the repeated structural unit in the chain is of the ether type. **D-20**

polyethylene, *n*—a polymer prepared by the polymerization of ethylene as the sole monomer. (See also **polyethylene plastic** and **ethylene plastic.**)

polyethylene plastic—a plastic based on polymers made with ethylene as essentially the sole monomer.

Discussion—In common usage for this plastic, essentially means no less than 85 % ethylene and no less than 95 % total olefins.

polyethylene terephthalate, *n*—a polymer derived from terephthalic acid and ethylene glycol by condensation polymerization.

polymer, *n*—a substance consisting of molecules characterized by the repetition (neglecting ends, branch junctions, and other minor irregularities) of one or more types of monomeric units. (See **copolymer.**) **IUPAC**

polymerization—a chemical reaction in which monomers are linked together to form polymers. (See also **polycondensation** and **polyaddition.**) **D-20**

polyolefin, *n*—a polymer prepared by the polymerization of an olefin(s) as the sole monomer(s). (See also **polyolefin plastic, olefin plastic.**) **D-20**

polyolefin plastic—a plastic based on polymers made with an olefin(s) as essentially the sole monomer(s).

polyoxymethylene, *n*—a polymer in which the repeated structural unit in the chain is oxymethylene.

Discussion—Polyoxymethylene is theoretically the simplest member of the generic class of polyacetals. **ISO**

polypropylene, *n*—a polymer prepared by the polymerization of propylene as the sole monomer. (See also **polypropylene**

plastic, propylene plastic.) **D-20**

polystyrene, *n*—a polymer prepared by the polymerization of styrene as the sole monomer. (See also **styrene plastic.**) **D-20**

polyterephthalate, *n*—a thermoplastic polyester in which the terephthalate group is a repeated structural unit in the polymer chain. **D-20**

poly(vinyl acetate), *n*—a polymer prepared by the polymerization of vinyl acetate as the sole monomer. **D-20, E-12**

poly(vinyl alcohol), *n*—a polymer prepared by the essentially complete hydrolysis of polyvinyl ester. **D-20**

poly(vinyl chloride), *n*—a polymer prepared by the polymerization of vinyl chloride as the sole monomer. **D-20**

prepolymer, *n*—a polymer of degree of polymerization between that of the monomer or monomers and the final polymer. **ISO**

propylene plastic, *n*—a plastic based on polymers of propylene or copolymers of propylene with other monomers, the propylene being in the greatest amount by mass. **ISO**

reinforced plastic, *n*—a plastic with high strength fillers imbedded in the composition, resulting in some mechanical properties superior to those of the base resin. (See also **filler.**)

DISCUSSION—The reinforcing fillers are usually fibers, fabrics, or mats made of fibers.

reins, *n*—a solid or pseudosolid organic material often of high molecular weight, which exhibits a tendency to flow when subjected to stress, usually has a softening or melting range, and usually fractures conchoidally.

DISCUSSION—In a broad sense, the term is used to designate any polymer that is basic material for plastics. **D-20**

rigid plastic—for purposes of general classification, a plastic that has a modulus of elasticity either in flexure or in tension greater than 700 MPa (100 000 psi) at 23°C and 50 % relative humidity when tested in accordance with Test Methods D 747, D 790, D 638, or D 882. **D-20**

rubber, *n*—an elastic substance derived from various tropical plants, such as the general Hevea and Ficus, essentially a polymer of isoprene; the term is frequently applied to both natural and synthetic elastic substances. (*Webster Modified*)

saran plastic—see **vinylidene chloride plastic.**

semirigid plastic—for purposes of general classification, a plastic that has a modulus of elasticity either in tension of between 70 and 700 MPa (10 000 and 100 000 psi) at 23°C and 50 % relative humidity when tested in accordance with Test Methods D 747, D 790, or D 882. **D-20**

sheeting, *n*—a form of plastic in which the thickness is very small in proportion to length and width and in which the plastic is present as a continuous phase throughout, with or without filler. (See also **film.**) **D-20**

silicone elastomer, *n*—an elastomer containing cross-linked silicone polymer and fillers, usually silica. **D-20**

silicone polymer, *n*—a polymer of alternating silicon-oxygen atoms consisting of repeating of diorganosiloxy groups. **D-20**

stress-crack, *n*—an external or internal crack in a plastic caused by tensile stresses less than its short-time mechanical strength.

DISCUSSION—The development of such cracks is frequently accelerated by the environment to which the plastic is exposed. The stresses which cause cracking may be present internally or externally or may be combinations of these stresses. **D-20**

styrene plastic, *n*—a plastic based on polymers of styrene or copolymers of styrene with other monomers, the styrene being greatest amount by mass. **ISO, D-20**

telomer, *n*—a polymer composed of molecules having terminal groups incapable of reacting with additional monomers, under the conditions of the synthesis, to form larger polymer molecules of the same chemical type. **D-20, F-17**

thermoplastic, *n*—a plastic that repeatedly can be softened by heating and hardened by cooling through a temperature range characteristic of the plastic, and that in the softened state can be shaped by flow into articles by molding or extrusion. **D-20**

thermoset plastic, *n*—a plastic that, after having been cured by heat or other means, is substantially infusible and insoluble. **D-20**

urethane plastic—a plastic based on polymers in which the repeated structural units in the chains are of the urethane type, or on copolymers in which urethane and other types of repeated structural units are present in the chains. **ISO, D-20**

viscosity, *n*—the property of resistance of flow exhibited with the body of a material.

DISCUSSION—In testing, the ratio of the shearing stress to the rate of shear of a fluid. Viscosity is usually taken to mean "Newtonian viscosity," in which case the ratio of shearing stress to rate of shearing strain is constant. In non-Newtonian behavior, which is the usual case with plastics materials, the ratio varies with the shearing rate. Such ratios are often called the" apparent viscosities" at the corresponding shear rates. (See **viscosity coefficient.**) **D-20**
ISO

void, *n*—(*1*) in a solid plastic, an unfilled space of such size that it scatters radiant energy such as light, (*2*) a cavity unintentionally formed in a cellular material and substantially larger than the characteristic individual cells. **ISO, D-20**

ANNEX

(Mandatory Information)

A1. THESAURUS OF GENERAL USAGE TERMS PERTINENT TO BIOMATERIALS

A1.1 *Designated Term:*

additive (in formulation)
additive, adventitious
amorphous
biocompatible
biomaterial
biomechanical
biomedical
catalyst (in polymerization)
carcinogen
chromatography
collagen
compliance
conversion (non-metric to metric units)
cosmetic
crystalline
dalton
delivery system
drug release
elastic (in elasticity)
encapsulated
explant
extractive
etched (surfaces)
filled (in composition)
formulation
primary culture
rounding
serum
subculture
tissue culture

Last ASTM Designation: F 1253 – 90

Standard Guide for Training the Emergency Medical Technician (Basic) to Perform Patient Secondary Assessment

This guide establishes the minimum training standard for the secondary assessment of ill or injured patients of all ages.

Formerly under the jurisdiction of Committee F30 on Emergency Medical Services, this guide was discontinued in February 1999 in accordance with Section 10.6.3.1 of the Regulations Governing ASTM Technical Committees, which requires that standards shall be updated by the end of the eighth year since the last approval date.

Standard Practice for Performance of Prehospital Manual Defibrillation[1]

This standard is issued under the fixed designation F 1254; the number immediately following the designation indicates the year of original adoption or, in the case of revision, the year of last revision. A number in parentheses indicates the year of last reapproval. A superscript epsilon (ε) indicates an editorial change since the last revision or reapproval.

1. Scope

1.1 This practice covers guidelines for prehospital providers performing manual defibrillation.

1.2 This practice is one in a set of performance guidelines for prehospital defibrillation.

1.3 This practice is specifically not meant to deal with equipment specifications, quality assurance, or training.

1.4 This practice is limited to external defibrillators used in the prehospital setting.

1.5 *This standard does not purport to address all of the safety concerns, if any, associated with its use. It is the responsibility of the user of this standard to establish appropriate safety and health practices and determine the applicability of regulatory limitations prior to use.*

2. Referenced Documents

2.1 *ASTM Standards:*

F 1031 Practice for Training the Emergency Medical Technician (Basic)[2]

F 1149 Practice for Qualifications, Responsibilities, and Authority of Individuals and Institutions Providing Medical Direction of Emergency Medical Services[2]

F 1177 Terminology Relating to Emergency Medical Services[2]

2.2 *American Heart Association Document:*

National Standards and Guidelines for Cardiopulmonary Resuscitation (CPR) and Emergency Cardiac Care (ECC), American Heart Association (Current Edition)[3]

3. Terminology

3.1 *Definitions of Terms Specific to This Standard:*

3.1.1 *basic life support/cardiopulmonary resuscitation (BLS/CPR)*—a set of skills that includes airway management, chest compressions, and others defined by the American Heart Association.

3.1.2 *defibrillation*—the discharge of an electrical current through the heart for the purpose of restoring a perfusing cardiac rhythm. For the purpose of this document, defibrillation may include cardioversion.

3.1.3 *manual defibrillator*—a monitor/defibrillator that has no capability for rhythm analysis and will charge and deliver a shock only at the command of the operator.

3.1.4 *operator*—as outlined in this practice, an Emergency Medical Technician (Practice F 1031) who has successfully completed a course of training and may treat prehospital cardiac arrest with a manual defibrillator. Legal functioning as an operator will be based upon licensure/certification requirements as established by the authority or authorities having jurisdiction.

3.1.5 *protocols*—see Terminology F 1177.

3.1.6 *service medical director*—the physician who is medicolegally responsible for the patient care provided by the operator (Practice F 1149).

3.1.7 *standing orders*—see Terminology F 1177.

4. Significance and Use

4.1 This practice establishes minimum guidelines for prehospital manual defibrillation.

4.2 Any person who is identified as prehospital manual defibrillation operator shall be an Emergency Medical Technician, as defined by the authority or authorities having jurisdiction, and shall meet the requirements of this practice.

4.3 Using this practice, emergency medical service institutions, organizations, and certification/licensing agencies should be able to develop standards for the certification/licensing and practice of the prehospital manual defibrillation operator.

5. Standards for Prehospital Manual Defibrillation

5.1 The operator shall be familiar with all operations of the defibrillator.

5.2 The operator shall be capable of performing prehospital defibrillation in accordance with standing orders or protocols, or both, developed or approved, or both, by the service medical director or other medical authority or authorities, or both, having jurisdiction.

5.3 The operator shall be capable of recognizing a patient who is unresponsive, apneic and pulseless.

5.4 The operator shall be capable of applying and activating the defibrillator according to manufacturer's recommendations and standing orders/protocols.

5.5 The operator shall be capable of assessing certain cardiac rhythms, including at least ventricular fibrillation, ventricular tachycardia, and asystole.

5.6 If the operator determines from 5.4 that the cardiac

[1] This practice is under the jurisdiction of ASTM Committee F30 on Emergency Medical Services and is the direct responsibility of Subcommittee F30.02 on Personnel, Training, and Education.

Current edition approved March 5, 1990. Published April 1990.

[2] *Annual Book of ASTM Standards*, Vol 13.01.

[3] Available from the American Heart Association, 7320 Greenville Ave., Dallas, TX 75231.

rhythm appears to be ventricular fibrillation, ventricular tachycardia, or asystole, then the operator must be capable of reassessing the rhythm by checking the cables, leads, battery, and switches for potential operational malfunctions.

5.7 The operator shall ensure that no one is in contact with the patient or the defibrillator, and that no one present in the vicinity of the patient is exposed to any danger of accidental shock during charging and defibrillation.

5.8 The operator shall be capable of accomplishing the tasks listed in 5.3-5.7 within 90 s following patient contact.

5.9 The operator shall be capable of recognizing that defibrillation energy was delivered.

5.10 The operator shall be capable of assessing the rhythm resulting from the defibrillation, and will be able to respond according to standing orders/protocol.

5.11 The operator shall be capable of determining whether an organized rhythm is perfusing and whether BLS/CPR is indicated.

5.12 The operator shall be capable of performing BLS/CPR as indicated.

5.13 The operator shall be capable of recognizing and responding, in accordance with the standing orders/protocols, to patients who return to or remain in an unresponsive, apneic, and pulseless condition.

5.14 The operator shall be capable of preparing the defibrillator for the next use.

5.15 The operator or the service, or both, utilizing the manual defibrillator shall be capable of providing, at a minimum, the following information for quality assurance purposes:

5.15.1 Patient data, including age; sex; whether arrest was witnessed or unwitnessed; and initial cardiac rhythm.

5.15.2 EMS system data, including time of:

5.15.2.1 Collapse/arrest,

5.15.2.2 Call for help,

5.15.2.3 Dispatch (include advanced life support, where available),

5.15.2.4 Initiation of BLS/CPR,

5.15.2.5 Arrival of the defibrillator at patient's side,

5.15.2.6 Initial defibrillation,

5.15.2.7 Departure to hospital, and

5.15.2.8 Arrival at hospital.

5.15.3 EMS system data in those systems that include these elements, including time of:

5.15.3.1 Activation of on-line medical control, and

5.15.3.2 Arrival of advanced life support.

5.15.4 Treatment, including documentation of treatment for each rhythm encountered.

5.15.5 Cardiac arrest patient outcome, including the rhythm after each defibrillation attempt; return of pulse or spontaneous respiration, or both; and level of consciousness. Also, the discharge disposition of the patient from the emergency department and the hospital.

5.16 The operator or the service, or both, using the defibrillator shall ensure that it is maintained in accordance with manufacturer's recommendations.

5.17 The operator shall be capable of recognizing any of the possible failure modes of the device and shall document any such failures to the service medical director.

6. Operator Proficiency Requirements

6.1 The operator shall demonstrate continued proficiency in rhythm recognition and manual defibrillation in accordance with standing orders/protocol.

6.2 Proficiency shall include performance skills demonstrating the ability to use the manual defibrillator correctly in a simulated environment.

6.3 There shall be documented evidence of initial and continuing education sufficient to establish and maintain proficiency in use of the manual defibrillator as approved by the service medical director.

7. Keywords

7.1 defibrillation; emergency medical services; manual defibrillation; prehospital manual defibrillation; prehospital defibrillation

Standard Practice for Performance of Prehospital Automated Defibrillation[1]

This standard is issued under the fixed designation F 1255; the number immediately following the designation indicates the year of original adoption or, in the case of revision, the year of last revision. A number in parentheses indicates the year of last reapproval. A superscript epsilon (ε) indicates an editorial change since the last revision or reapproval.

ε[1] NOTE—Section 7 on Keywords was added editorially November 1995.

1. Scope

1.1 This practice covers guidelines for the performance of automated defibrillation.

1.2 This practice is one in a set of performance guidelines for prehospital defibrillation.

1.3 This practice is specifically not meant to deal with equipment specifications, quality assurance, or training.

1.4 This practice is limited to external defibrillators used in the prehospital setting.

1.5 *This standard does not purport to address all of the safety concerns, if any, associated with its use. It is the responsibility of the user of this standard to establish appropriate safety and health practices and determine the applicability of regulatory limitations prior to use.*

2. Referenced Documents

2.1 *ASTM Standards:*

F 1149 Practice for the Qualifications, Responsibilities and Authority of Individuals and Institutions Providing Medical Direction of Emergency Medical Services[2]

F 1177 Terminology Relating to Emergency Medical Services[2]

2.2 *American Heart Association Document:*

National Standards and Guidelines for Cardiopulmonary Resuscitation (CPR) and Emergency Cardiac Care (ECC), American Heart Association (Current Edition)[3]

3. Terminology

3.1 *Definitions of Terms Specific to This Standard:*

3.1.1 *automated defibrillator*—an automatic or semi-automatic device, or both, capable of rhythm analysis and defibrillation after electronically detecting the presence of ventricular fibrillation and ventricular tachycardia.

3.1.2 *basic life support/cardiopulmonary resuscitation (BLS/CPR)*—a set of skills that includes airway management, chest compressions, and others defined by the American Heart Association.

3.1.3 *defibrillation*—the discharge of an electrical current through the heart for the purpose of restoring a perfusing cardiac rhythm. For the purpose of this practice, defibrillation may include cardioversion.

3.1.4 *operator*—as outlined in this practice, a person who has successfully completed a course of training and may treat prehospital cardiac arrest with an automatic or semi-automatic defibrillator. Legal functioning as an operator will be based upon licensure or certification requirements, or both, as established by the authority or authorities having jurisdiction.

3.1.5 *protocols*—See Definitions F 1177.

3.1.6 *service medical director*—the physician who is medico-legally responsible for the patient care provided by the operator (Practice F 1149).

3.1.7 *standing orders*—See Definitions F 1177.

4. Significance and Use

4.1 This practice establishes minimum guidelines for prehospital automated defibrillation.

4.2 This standard does not preclude the use of automated defibrillators as prescribed by a licensed physician.

4.3 All persons who are identified as prehospital automated defibrillation operators shall meet the requirements of this practice.

4.4 Using this practice, emergency medical service institutions, organizations, and certification/licensing agencies should be able to develop standards for the certification/licensing and practice of the prehospital automated defibrillation operator.

5. Guidelines for Prehospital Automated Defibrillation

5.1 The operator shall be familiar with all operations of the automated defibrillator.

5.2 The operator shall be capable of performing prehospital defibrillation in accordance with standing orders, protocols developed, approval by the service medical director or other medical authority or authorities having jurisdiction, or a combination thereof.

5.3 The operator shall be capable of recognizing a patient who is unresponsive, apneic and pulseless.

5.4 The operator shall be capable of preparing the automated defibrillator for operational use.

5.5 The operator shall be capable of applying and activating the automated defibrillator according to the manufacturer's recommendations and standing orders/protocols.

---

[1] This practice is under the jurisdiction of ASTM Committee F-30 on Emergency Medical Services and is the direct responsibility of Subcommittee F30.02 on Personnel, Training, and Education.

Current edition approved March 5, 1990. Published April 1990.

[2] *Annual Book of ASTM Standards*, Vol 13.01.

[3] Available from the American Heart Association, 7320 Greenville Ave., Dallas, TX 75231.

5.6 The operator shall ensure that no one is in contact with the patient or the automated defibrillator, and that no one present in the vicinity of the patient is exposed to any danger of accidental shock during charging and defibrillation.

5.7 The operator shall be capable of accomplishing the tasks listed in 5.3-5.5 and 5.6 within 90 s following patient contact.

5.8 The operator shall be capable of recognizing that defibrillation energy was delivered.

5.9 The operator shall be capable of recognizing the success or lack of success of defibrillation and treat the patient accordingly.

5.10 The operator shall be capable of performing BLS/CPR as indicated.

5.11 The operator shall be capable of recognizing and responding, in accordance with the standing orders or protocols, or both, to patients who return to or remain in an unresponsive, apneic and pulseless condition.

5.12 The operator shall be capable of preparing the automated defibrillator for the next use.

5.13 The operator or the service, or both, utilizing the automated defibrillator shall be capable of providing, at a minimum, the following information for quality assurance purposes:

5.13.1 *Patient data*, including age; sex; whether the arrest was witnessed or unwitnessed; pulselessness; and initial cardiac rhythm as identified by the automated defibrillator.

5.13.2 *EMS system data*, including time of:

5.13.2.1 Collapse/arrest,

5.13.2.2 Call for help,

5.13.2.3 Dispatch (include advanced life support, where available),

5.13.2.4 Initiation of BLS/CPR,

5.13.2.5 Arrival of automated defibrillator at patient's side,

5.13.2.6 Initial defibrillation,

5.13.2.7 Departure to hospital, and

5.13.2.8 Arrival at hospital.

5.13.3 *EMS System Data*, in those systems that include these elements, including time of:

5.13.3.1 Activation of on-line medical control, and

5.13.3.2 Arrival of advanced life support.

5.13.4 *Treatment*, including documentation of treatment for each rhythm encountered.

5.13.5 *Cardiac arrest patient outcome*, including the rhythm after each defibrillation attempt; the return of pulse or spontaneous respiration, or both; and the level of consciousness.

5.14 The operator or the service, or both, utilizing the automated defibrillator shall ensure it is maintained in accordance with manufacturer's recommendations.

5.15 The operator shall be capable of recognizing any of the possible failure modes of the device and shall document any such failures to the service medical director.

6. Operator Proficiency Requirements

6.1 The operator shall demonstrate continued proficiency in automated defibrillation in accordance with standing orders/protocol.

6.2 Proficiency shall include performance skills demonstrating the ability to use the automated defibrillator correctly in a simulated environment.

6.3 There shall be documented evidence of initial and continuing education sufficient to establish and maintain proficiency in use of the automated defibrillator as approved by the service medical director.

7. Keywords

7.1 automated defibrillation; defibrillation; emergency medical services; prehospital automated defibrillation; prehospital defibrillation

Designation: F 1256 – 90 (Reapproved 1996)ε1

Standard Guide for Selection and Practice of the Emergency Medical Services Instructor for Basic Life Support/Emergency Medical Technician (BLS/EMT) Training Programs[1]

This standard is issued under the fixed designation F 1256; the number immediately following the designation indicates the year of original adoption or, in the case of revision, the year of last revision. A number in parentheses indicates the year of last reapproval. A superscript epsilon (ε) indicates an editorial change since the last revision or reapproval.

ε1 NOTE—Keywords were added editorially in October 1996.

1. Scope

1.1 This guide is intended to assist emergency medical services (EMS) agencies and institutions in selecting and utilizing individuals who teach in EMT (emergency medical technician) training programs which include instruction in basic life support knowledge and skills.

1.2 This guide identifies six categories of instructor in a BLS/EMT (basic life support/emergency medical technician) training program: adjunct instructor, clinical/field preceptor, practical skills instructor, associate instructor, course instructor/coordinator (I/C), and course administrator. The guide recognizes that an individual may, depending on his/her level of practice and the training program involved, function in any or all of these categories.

1.3 This guide includes specific guidelines for qualifications, training, education, experience, scope of authority, responsibilities, continuing education, evaluation, and maintenance of competency when applicable.

1.4 This guide does not include specific guidelines for the course administrator or the adjunct instructor. While the guide recognizes, by offering a definition of each category, that these types of individuals function in many BLS/EMT training programs, the limited instructional roles played by these individuals precludes the need for specific selection and utilization guidelines.

1.5 This guide is intended to apply to any individual who teaches in BLS/EMT training programs regardless of the individual's present level of clinical practice.

1.6 This guide intentionally omits references to length of prehospital care experience, teaching experience, and continuing education requirements. This guide also omits reference to waiver or equivalency. These issues should be addressed by the appropriate agency.

1.7 This guide applies only to instructors who teach in basic life support training courses designed to prepare an individual for certification to practice as an EMT (basic) or first responder. It does not apply to instructors who teach in specialized courses that do not in themselves qualify the individual for a level of EMT certification.

1.8 This guide does not establish certification requirements. Such requirements should be established by the certifying agency in the jurisdiction in which the BLS/EMT instructor will function. This guide may be used to provide considerable guidance to the jurisdiction responsible for establishing certification standards.

1.9 *This standard does not purport to address all of the safety concerns, if any, associated with its use. It is the responsibility of the user of this standard to establish appropriate safety and health practices and determine the applicability of regulatory limitations prior to use.*

NOTE 1—Also see Practice F 1031.

2. Referenced Documents

2.1 *ASTM Standards:*

F 1031 Practice for Training the Emergency Medical Technician (Basic)[2]

3. Terminology

3.1 *Definitions of Terms Specific to This Standard:*

3.1.1 *adjunct instructor*—an individual with specialized subject matter expertise, who, on occasion, instructs a specific topic of a curriculum under the direction of the course instructor/coordinator.

3.1.2 *associate instructor*—an individual who possesses the qualifications and education/training of a course instructor/coordinator, but, in a specific course, assumes a supportive or assisting role to the course instructor/coordinator. This individual may substitute for the course instructor/coordinator in case of necessity or, in other courses, serve as a course instructor/coordinator.

3.1.3 *basic life support*—a level of pre-hospital emergency

[1] This guide is under the jurisdiction of ASTM Committee F-30 on Emergency Medical Services and is the direct responsibility of Subcommittee F30.02 on Personnel, Training and Education.

Current edition approved Jan. 10, 1990. Published February 1990.

[2] *Annual Book of ASTM Standards*, Vol 13.01.

medical care that includes any or all first responder and EMT-basic procedures as defined by the National Standard Curricula.[3,4]

3.1.4 *basic life support/emergency medical technician (BLS/EMT) training program*—a course of instruction that provides an individual with the knowledge and clinical skills of emergency medical care necessary to function at a level of first responder or EMT (basic) level of care. Such courses include, but are not limited to, first responder and EMT-basic training programs.

3.1.5 *BLS/EMT instructor*—an individual who provides instruction in a training or education program for prehospital BLS/EMT personnel. This term includes any individual who functions as an adjunct instructor, clinical/field preceptor, practical skills instructor, associate instructor or course instructor/coordinator.

3.1.6 *certification*—current, formal approval by the appropriate certifying agency to function at a specific level of practice. This may also be referred to as approval or licensure.

3.1.7 *clinical certification*—a standardized process for evaluation and recognition of an acceptable level of competence in a specific aspect of patient care.

3.1.8 *clinical experience*—exposure to and practice in an area of patient care.

3.1.9 *clinical/field preceptor*—an individual who supervises and evaluates the students during clinical or field experiences under the direction of the course instructor/coordinator.

3.1.10 *course administrator*—an individual responsible for managing administrative details of a course, separate from actual instruction of the course.

3.1.11 *course instructor/coordinator (I/C)*—an individual who is authorized by the appropriate entity to present and assess competence in all of the subject matter contained in a curriculum. This person also oversees all instruction in the course and makes final evaluations concerning student competence.

3.1.12 *course medical director*—the licensed physician who provides medical direction for all didactic and clinical instruction and clinical practice experience included in a BLS/EMT training program.

3.1.13 *evaluation*—the process of verifying clinical and educational skills and knowledge competencies of a BLS/EMT instructor.

3.1.14 *instructor training program*—an educational program that provides a foundation of essential educational principles to assist individuals to instruct in, or coordinate, BLS/EMT programs. It must, at a minimum, contain the elements of the DOT EMS Instructor National Standard Curriculum.[5]

3.1.15 *practical skills instructor*—an individual who assists with practical skills instruction under the direction of the course instructor/coordinator.

3.1.16 *qualification*—a requirement which shall be met by a BLS/EMT instructor candidate prior to selection and practice as a BLS/EMT instructor.

4. Significance and Use

4.1 Since the quality of prehospital BLS/EMT training depends, in large measure, on the instructional abilities and competencies of the BLS/EMT instructor, it is imperative that the individual selected and used in this capacity possess the qualifications and capabilities necessary to provide effective instruction.

4.2 A BLS/EMT instructor must possess clearly defined knowledge and skills competencies, have clearly defined responsibilities and scope of authority related to instructional programs and meet other specific requirements pertinent to the level of instruction.

4.3 Using this guide, EMS institutions and organizations should be able to develop requirements for selection and utilization of BLS/EMT instructors for BLS/EMT training and education programs.

BASIC LIFE SUPPORT INSTRUCTOR GUIDELINES

5. Course Instructor/Coordinator

5.1 An individual shall be considered eligible to serve as a BLS/EMT course I/C (instructor/coordinator) when requirements as outlined in 5.1.1 and 5.1.2 have been met by that individual.

5.1.1 *Qualifications*—Prior to entering the instructor training program, the course I/C candidate shall:

5.1.1.1 Be at least a high school graduate or have a General Equivalency Diploma (GED); preferably a higher education degree in a supportive discipline,

5.1.1.2 Have prehospital patient care experience at least at the level being taught,

5.1.1.3 Be certified at least at the level being taught,

5.1.1.4 Demonstrate, at the level being taught, current competence in and knowledge of emergency care of the acutely ill or traumatized patient to the satisfaction of the appropriate agency, and

5.1.1.5 Demonstrate to the instructor training agency, reading and language skills commensurate with resource materials to be utilized in the BLS/EMT training program.

5.1.2 *Education/Training/Experience*—The course I/C candidate shall:

5.1.2.1 Have served as a practical skills instructor, clinical or field preceptor, and successfully completed a supervised probationary teaching experience in a BLS/EMT training program at the level to be taught to the satisfaction of the appropriate agency,

5.1.2.2 Have advanced clinical certifications, provider or intructor, or both, as appropriate for the curriculum being taught,

5.1.2.3 Be certified as a CPR instructor according to the current standards as promulgated by the American Heart Association or the American Red Cross,

5.1.2.4 Become familiar with appropriate record keeping processes for students, sponsoring agency, or state EMS agency, or both, and

[3] Emergency Medical Services, First Responder Training Course—Instructor's Lesson Plans (U.S. DOT/NHTSA Report No. DOT HS 900–, 1984).

[4] Emergency Medical Technician—Ambulance: National Standard Curriculum—Instructor's Lesson Plans (U.S. DOT/NHTSA Report No. DOT HS 900–, 1984).

[5] Emergency Medical Services Instructor Training Program: A National Standard Curriculum—Instructor's Lesson Plans, First Edition, 1986 (U.S. DOT/NHTSA Report No. HS 900–086, February 1986).

5.1.2.5 Successfully complete an instructor training program that includes the knowledge and skills objectives contained in the DOT Instructor Curriculum.[5]

5.1.3 *Scope of Authority*—The course I/C shall have the authority to:

5.1.3.1 Conduct BLS/EMT training programs with approval of appropriate EMS agency,

5.1.3.2 Document to the appropriate agency those students successfully completing the BLS/EMT training program, and

5.1.3.3 Regulate student behavior within the scope of the training program under the institutional guidelines for due process.

5.1.4 *Responsibilities*—The course I/C:

5.1.4.1 Should provide a positive role model by:

(*a*) Maintaining personal mental and physical health,

(*b*) Maintaining appropriate personal hygiene and appearance,

(*c*) Actively pursuing personal and professional development,

(*d*) Recognizing personal limitations and seeking assistance when appropriate,

(*e*) Demonstrating competent, respectful, and caring interactions with students, coworkers, and patients at all times, and

(*f*) Demonstrating professional behavior in the classroom or in the presence of students.

5.1.4.2 Shall ensure a safe and effective learning environment,

5.1.4.3 Shall ensure competent training staff,

5.1.4.4 Shall maintain appropriate training records,

5.1.4.5 Shall teach the curriculum as adopted and defined by the appropriate certifying agency,

5.1.4.6 Shall inform students of the criteria for successful course completion,

5.1.4.7 Shall consistently monitor student progress toward terminal course objectives and provide appropriate feedback to the students within guidelines established by the appropriate certifying agency,

5.1.4.8 Shall uphold state and national clinical standards for practice at the appropriate BLS/EMT level,

5.1.4.9 Shall evaluate the students for safe and effective performance,

5.1.4.10 Shall orient, supervise and evaluate adjunct, practical skills, associate instructors, and clinical/field preceptors,

5.1.4.11 Shall coordinate student field or clinical activities with the clinical/field preceptors,

5.1.4.12 Shall ensure that practical skills training equipment is maintained in a safe and acceptable operating condition,

5.1.4.13 Shall protect the privacy of students and the confidentiality of training course records as required by applicable laws and standards,

5.1.4.14 Should have knowledge of the administrative and legislative processes affecting the local, regional, or state prehospital EMS system, or combination thereof, and

5.1.4.15 Should have knowledge of the laws and regulations affecting the local, regional, or state prehospital EMS system, or combination thereof.

5.1.5 *Evaluation*—The evaluation of a course I/C shall include:

5.1.5.1 Analysis of student outcomes,

5.1.5.2 Classroom observation of the I/C, and

5.1.5.3 Review of students' course evaluations.

5.1.6 *Maintenance of Competency*—In order to maintain competency, the course I/C shall:

5.1.6.1 Maintain certification at least at the level being taught,

5.1.6.2 Teach BLS/EMT related curriculum,

5.1.6.3 Participate in continuing education programs, which may include:

(*a*) Practice-related topics, for example, management or administration, vehicle maintenance, or communications,

(*b*) Clinical topics, and

(*c*) Educational methods and materials.

6. Associate Instructor

6.1 The associate instructor shall possess the same qualifications, training and education as the course I/C.

6.2 The associate instructor differs from the course I/C in that the associate instructor assumes a supportive and assisting role to the course I/C in a specific BLS/EMT training program.

7. Practical Skills Instructor

7.1 *Qualifications*—The practical skills instructor candidate:

7.1.1 Should be at least a high school graduate or have a General Equivalency Diploma (GED),

7.1.2 Shall have pre-hospital care experience or approval by course I/C and course medical director, or both, and

7.1.3 Shall demonstrate to the satisfaction of the course I/C and course medical director current competence in and knowledge of the skill(s) being taught.

7.2 *Education/Training/Experience*—The practical skills instructor candidate shall:

7.2.1 Demonstrate mastery of the knowledge and skills objectives contained in lessons 1, 8, and 9 of the DOT Instructor Curriculum,[5]

7.2.2 Successfully complete a supervised probationary teaching experience for the skill(s) to be taught to the satisfaction of the appropriate agency,

7.2.3 Be certified as a CPR instructor according to the current standards as promulgated by the American Heart Association or the American Red Cross, if CPR is among the skills to be taught, and

7.2.4 Become familiar with appropriate record keeping processes for students, sponsoring agency, or state EMS agency, or both.

7.3 *Scope of Authority*—The practical skills instructor shall have authority to:

7.3.1 Conduct practical skills sessions under the direction of the course I/C,

7.3.2 Verify successful achievement of course skill objectives, under the direction of the course I/C, and

7.3.3 Regulate student behavior within the scope of the practical skills training program under the institutional guidelines for due process.

7.4 *Responsibilities*—Under the direction of the course I/C, the practical skills instructor:

7.4.1 Should provide a positive role model by:

7.4.1.1 Maintaining personal mental and physical health,

7.4.1.2 Maintaining appropriate personal hygiene and appearance,

7.4.1.3 Actively pursuing personal and professional development,

7.4.1.4 Recognizing personal limitations and seeking assistance when appropriate,

7.4.1.5 Demonstrating competent, respectful, and caring interactions with students, co-workers, and patients at all times, and

7.4.1.6 Demonstrating professional behavior in the classroom or in the presence of students.

7.4.2 Shall ensure a safe and effective learning environment,

7.4.3 Shall provide consistent and competent training assistance to students,

7.4.4 Shall maintain appropriate student skills training records,

7.4.5 Shall teach the skills contained in the curriculum as adopted and defined by the appropriate certifying agency,

7.4.6 Shall consistently monitor students' progress toward established course skill objectives and provide appropriate feedback to the course I/C and the students within guidelines of the appropriate certifying agency,

7.4.7 Shall evaluate, according to the curriculum, and differentiate among students for safe and effective performance,

7.4.8 Shall uphold state and national clinical standards for practice at the level being taught,

7.4.9 Shall ensure that practical skills training equipment is maintained in a safe and acceptable operating condition, and

7.4.10 Shall protect the privacy of students and the confidentiality of training course records as required by applicable laws and standards.

7.5 *Evaluation*—The evaluation by the course I/C of a practical skills instructor shall include:

7.5.1 Analysis of student practical skills outcomes,

7.5.2 Classroom observation of the practical skills instructor, and

7.5.3 Review of students' course evaluations.

7.6 *Maintenance of Competency*—In order to maintain competency, the practical skills instructor shall:

7.6.1 Maintain, to the satisfaction of the course I/C and course medical director, current competence in and knowledge of the skill(s) being taught.

7.6.2 Teach the skills contained in a BLS/EMT related curriculum.

8. Clinical/Field Preceptor

8.1 *Qualifications*—The clinical/field preceptor candidate shall:

8.1.1 Be certified in his/her area of practice,

8.1.2 Have experience in his/her area of expertise, and

8.1.3 Demonstrate to the satisfaction of the course I/C a willingness and competence to work with students to assist them in meeting pertinent course objectives in the setting in which the clinical/field preceptor will function.

8.2 *Education/Training/Experience*—The clinical/field preceptor shall complete an orientation that includes:

8.2.1 Roles and responsibilities of the BLS/EMT,

8.2.2 Roles and responsibilities of the clinical/field preceptor, and

8.2.3 Guidelines for carrying out, meeting or accomplishing assigned responsibilities and duties.

8.3 *Scope of Authority*—The clinical/field preceptor shall have authority to:

8.3.1 Supervise student activities in the clinical/field setting as determined by stated course objectives,

8.3.2 Document student performance in the clinical/field setting, and

8.3.3 Regulate student behavior within the scope of the clinical/field setting under the institutional guidelines for due process.

8.4 *Responsibilities*—Under the direction of the course I/C, the clinical/field preceptor:

8.4.1 Should provide a positive role model,

8.4.2 Shall provide a safe and effective learning environment,

8.4.3 Shall provide consistent and competent supervision to students,

8.4.4 Shall maintain appropriate training records,

8.4.5 Shall assist the students in meeting the clinical/field skills objectives,

8.4.6 Shall consistently monitor students and provide appropriate feedback to the course I/C and the students,

8.4.7 Shall assess students for safe and effective performance, and

8.4.8 Shall protect the privacy of students and the confidentiality of training course records as required by applicable laws and standards.

8.5 *Evaluation*—The evaluation by the course I/C of a clinical/field preceptor in a BLS/EMT training program shall include:

8.5.1 Quality of training records,

8.5.2 Clinical/field observation of the preceptor, and

8.5.3 Review of students' clinical experience evaluations.

8.6 *Maintenance of Competency*—In order to maintain competency, the clinical/field preceptor shall:

8.6.1 Maintain certification in his/her area of practice, and

8.6.2 Maintain, to the satisfaction of the course I/C and course medical director, current competence in and knowledge of the areas precepted.

9. Keywords

9.1 basic life support; emergency medical services instructor; emergency medical technician; training programs

Designation: F 1257 – 90 (Reapproved 1996)$^{\epsilon 1}$

Standard Guide for Selection and Practice of the Emergency Medical Services Instructor for Advanced Life Support/Emergency Medical Technician (ALS/EMT) Training Programs[1]

This standard is issued under the fixed designation F 1257; the number immediately following the designation indicates the year of original adoption or, in the case of revision, the year of last revision. A number in parentheses indicates the year of last reapproval. A superscript epsilon (ε) indicates an editorial change since the last revision or reapproval.

ϵ^1 NOTE—Keywords were added editorially in October 1996.

1. Scope

1.1 This guide is intended to assist emergency medical services (EMS) agencies and institutions in selecting and utilizing individuals who teach in EMT (emergency medical technician) training programs which include instruction in advanced life support knowledge and skills.

1.2 This guide identifies six categories of instructor in an ALS/EMT (advanced life support/emergency medical technician) training program: adjunct instructor, clinical/field preceptor, practical skills instructor, associate instructor, course instructor/coordinator (I/C), and course administrator. The guide recognizes that an individual may, depending on his/her level of practice and the training program involved, function in any or all of these categories.

1.3 This guide includes specific guidelines for qualifications, training, education, experience, scope of authority, responsibilities, continuing education, evaluation, and maintenance of competency when applicable.

1.4 This guide does not include specific guidelines for the course administrator or the adjunct instructor. While the guide recognizes, by offering a definition of each category, that these types of individuals function in many ALS/EMT training programs, the limited instructional roles played by these individuals precludes the need for specific selection and utilization guidelines.

1.5 This guide is intended to apply to any individual who teaches in ALS/EMT training programs regardless of the individual's present level of clinical practice.

1.6 This guide intentionally omits references to length of prehospital care experience, teaching experience, and continuing education requirements. This guide also omits reference to waiver or equivalency. These issues should be addressed by the appropriate agency.

1.7 This guide applies only to instructors who teach in advanced life support training courses designed to prepare an individual for certification to practice as an EMT above the level of the EMT (basic). It does not apply to instructors who teach in specialized courses that do not in themselves qualify the individual for a level of EMT certification.

1.8 This guide does not establish certification requirements. Such requirements should be established by the certifying agency in the jurisdiction in which the ALS/EMT instructor will function. This guide may be used to provide considerable guidance to the jurisdiction responsible for establishing certification standards.

1.9 *This standard does not purport to address all of the safety problems associated with its use. It is the responsibility of the user of this standard to establish appropriate safety and health practices and determine the applicability of regulatory limitations prior to use.*

NOTE 1—Also see Practice F 1031.

2. Referenced Documents

2.1 *ASTM Standards:*

F 1031 Practice for Training the Emergency Medical Technician (Basic)[2]

3. Terminology

3.1 *Definitions of Terms Specific to This Standard:*

3.1.1 *adjunct instructor*—an individual with specialized subject matter expertise, who, on occasion, instructs a specific topic of a curriculum under the direction of the course instructor/coordinator.

3.1.2 *advanced life support*—a level of pre-hospital emergency medical care that includes all EMT-basic procedures and any or all additional procedures, interventions, or techniques defined by the National Standard Curricula.[3,4]

3.1.3 *advanced life support/emergency medical technician (ALS/EMT) training program*—a course of instruction that provides an individual with the knowledge and clinical skills of

[1] This guide is under the jurisdiction of ASTM Committee F30 on Emergency Medical Services and is the direct responsibility of Subcommittee F30.02 on Personnel, Training, and Education.

Current edition approved Jan. 10, 1990. Published February 1990.

[2] *Annual Book of ASTM Standards*, Vol 13.01.

[3] Emergency Medical Technician—Intermediate: National Standard Curriculum—Instructor's Lesson Plans (U.S. DOT/NHTSA Report No. DOT HS 900–091, August 1986).

[4] Emergency Medical Technician—Paramedic: National Standard Curriculum—Instructor's Lesson Plans, 1985 (U.S. DOT/NHTSA Report No. DOT HS 900–089, August 1986).

emergency medical care necessary to function at a level of EMT practice beyond the level of EMT (basic). Such courses include, but are not limited to, EMT–intermediate and EMT-paramedic training programs.

3.1.4 *ALS/EMT instructor*—an individual who provides instruction in a training or education program for prehospital ALS/EMT personnel. This term includes any individual who functions as an adjunct instructor, clinical/field preceptor, practical skills instructor, associate instructor, or course instructor/coordinator.

3.1.5 *associate instructor*—an individual who possesses the qualifications and education/training of a course instructor/coordinator, but, in a specific course, assumes a supportive or assisting role to the course instructor/coordinator. This individual may substitute for the course instructor/coordinator in case of necessity or, in other courses, serve as a course instructor/coordinator.

3.1.6 *certification*—current, formal approval by the appropriate certifying agency to function at a specific level of practice. This may also be referred to as approval or licensure.

3.1.7 *clinical certification*—a standardized process for evaluation and recognition of an acceptable level of competence in a specific aspect of patient care.

3.1.8 *clinical experience*—exposure to and practice in an area of patient care.

3.1.9 *clinical/field preceptor*—an individual who supervises and evaluates the students during clinical or field experiences under the direction of the course instructor/coordinator.

3.1.10 *course administrator*—an individual responsible for managing administrative details of a course, separate from actual instruction of the course.

3.1.11 *course instructor/coordinator (I/C)*—an individual who is authorized by the appropriate entity to present and assess competence in all of the subject matter contained in a curriculum. This person also oversees all instruction in the course and makes final evaluations concerning student competence.

3.1.12 *course medical director*—the licensed physician who provides medical direction for all didactic and clinical instruction and clinical practice experience included in an ALS/EMT training program.

3.1.13 *evaluation*—the process of verifying clinical and educational skills and knowledge competencies of an ALS/EMT instructor.

3.1.14 *instructor training program*—an educational program that provides a foundation of essential educational principles to assist individuals to instruct in, or coordinate, ALS/EMT programs. It must, at a minimum, contain the elements of the DOT EMS Instructor National Standard Curriculum.[5]

3.1.15 *practical skills instructor*—an individual who assists with practical skills instruction under the direction of the course instructor/coordinator.

3.1.16 *qualification*—a requirement which shall be met by an ALS/EMT instructor candidate prior to selection and practice as an ALS/EMT instructor.

4. Significance and Use

4.1 Since the quality of prehospital ALS/EMT training depends, in large measure, on the instructional abilities and competencies of the ALS/EMT instructor, it is imperative that the individual selected and used in this capacity possess the qualifications and capabilities necessary to provide effective instruction.

4.2 An ALS/EMT instructor must possess clearly defined knowledge and skills competencies, have clearly defined responsibilities and scope of authority related to instructional programs and meet other specific requirements pertinent to the level of instruction.

4.3 Using this guide, EMS institutions and organizations should be able to develop requirements for selection and utilization of ALS/EMT instructors for ALS/EMT training and education programs.

ADVANCED LIFE SUPPORT INSTRUCTOR GUIDELINES

5. Course Instructor/Coordinator

5.1 An individual shall be considered eligible to serve as an ALS/EMT course I/C when requirements as outlined in 5.1.1 and 5.1.2 have been met by that individual.

5.1.1 *Qualifications*— Prior to entering the instructor training program, the course I/C candidate shall:

5.1.1.1 Be at least a high school graduate or have a General Equivalency Diploma (GED); preferably a higher education degree in a supportive discipline,

5.1.1.2 Have prehospital patient care experience at least at the level being taught,

5.1.1.3 Be certified at least at the level being taught,

5.1.1.4 Demonstrate, at the level being taught, current competence in and knowledge of emergency care of the acutely ill or traumatized patient to the satisfaction of the appropriate agency, and

5.1.1.5 Demonstrate to the instructor training agency, reading and language skills commensurate with resource materials to be utilized in the ALS/EMT training program.

5.1.2 *Education/Training/Experience*—The course I/C candidate shall:

5.1.2.1 Have served as a practical skills instructor, clinical or field preceptor, and successfully completed a supervised probationary teaching experience in an ALS/EMT training program at the level to be taught to the satisfaction of the appropriate agency,

5.1.2.2 Have advanced clinical certifications, provider or instructor, or both, as appropriate for the curriculum being taught,

5.1.2.3 Be certified as a CPR instructor according to the current standards as promulgated by the American Heart Association or the American Red Cross,

5.1.2.4 Become familiar with appropriate record keeping processes for students, sponsoring agency or state EMS agency, or both,

5.1.2.5 Successfully complete an instructor training program that includes the knowledge and skills objectives contained in the DOT Instructor Curriculum.[5]

[5] Emergency Medical Services Instructor Training Program: A National Standard Curriculum—Instructor's Lesson Plans, First Edition, 1986 (U.S. DOT/NHTSA Report No. HS 900–086, February 1986).

5.1.3 *Scope of Authority*—The course I/C shall have the authority to:

5.1.3.1 Conduct ALS/EMT training programs with the approval of the appropriate EMS agency,

5.1.3.2 Document to the appropriate agency those students successfully completing the ALS/EMT training program, and

5.1.3.3 Regulate student behavior within the scope of the training program under the institutional guidelines for due process.

5.1.4 *Responsibilities*— The course I/C:

5.1.4.1 Should provide a positive role model by:

(a) Maintaining personal mental and physical health,

(b) Maintaining appropriate personal hygiene and appearance,

(c) Actively pursuing personal and professional development,

(d) Recognizing personal limitations and seeking assistance when appropriate,

(e) Demonstrating competent, respectful, and caring interactions with students, coworkers, and patients at all times, and

(f) Demonstrating professional behavior in the classroom or in the presence of students.

5.1.4.2 Shall ensure a safe and effective learning environment,

5.1.4.3 Shall ensure competent training staff,

5.1.4.4 Shall maintain appropriate training records,

5.1.4.5 Shall teach the curriculum as adopted and defined by the appropriate certifying agency,

5.1.4.6 Shall inform students of the criteria for successful course completion,

5.1.4.7 Shall consistently monitor student progress toward terminal course objectives and provide appropriate feedback to the students within guidelines established by the appropriate certifying agency,

5.1.4.8 Shall uphold state and national clinical standards for practice at the appropriate ALS/EMT level,

5.1.4.9 Shall evaluate the students for safe and effective performance,

5.1.4.10 Shall orient, supervise and evaluate adjunct, practical skills, associate instructors, and clinical/field preceptors,

5.1.4.11 Shall coordinate student field or clinical activities with the clinical/field preceptors,

5.1.4.12 Shall ensure that practical skills training equipment is maintained in a safe and acceptable operating condition,

5.1.4.13 Shall protect the privacy of students and the confidentiality of training course records as required by applicable laws and standards,

5.1.4.14 Should have knowledge of the administrative and legislative processes affecting the local, regional, or state prehospital EMS system, or combination thereof, and

5.1.4.15 Should have knowledge of the laws and regulations affecting the local, regional, or state prehospital EMS system, or combination thereof.

5.1.5 *Evaluation*—The evaluation of a course I/C shall include:

5.1.5.1 Analysis of student outcomes,

5.1.5.2 Classroom observation of the I/C, and

5.1.5.3 Review of students' course evaluations.

5.1.6 *Maintenance of competency*—In order to maintain competency, the course I/C shall:

5.1.6.1 Maintain certification at least at the level being taught,

5.1.6.2 Teach ALS/EMT related curriculum, and

5.1.6.3 Participate in continuing education programs, which may include:

(a) Practice-related topics, for example, management or administration, vehicle maintenance, communications,

(b) Clinical topics, and

(c) Educational methods and materials.

6. Associate Instructor

6.1 The associate instructor shall possess the same qualifications, training and education as the course I/C.

6.2 The associate instructor differs from the course I/C in that the associate instructor assumes a supportive and assisting role to the course I/C in a specific ALS/EMT training program.

7. Practical Skills Instructor

7.1 *Qualifications*— The practical skills instructor candidate:

7.1.1 Should be at least a high school graduate or have a General Equivalency Diploma (GED),

7.1.2 Shall have pre-hospital care experience or approval by the course I/C and course medical director, or both, and

7.1.3 Shall demonstrate to the satisfaction of the course I/C and course medical director current competence in and knowledge of the skill(s) being taught.

7.2 *Education/Training/Experience*—The practical skills instructor candidate shall:

7.2.1 Demonstrate mastery of the knowledge and skills objective contained in lessons 1, 8, and 9 of the DOT Instructor Curriculum,[5]

7.2.2 Successfully complete a supervised probationary teaching experience for the skill(s) to be taught to the satisfaction of the appropriate agency,

7.2.3 Be certified as a CPR instructor according to the current standards as promulgated by the American Heart Association or the American Red Cross, if CPR is among the skills to be taught, and

7.2.4 Become familiar with appropriate record keeping processes for students, sponsoring agency or state EMS agency, or both.

7.3 *Scope of Authority*—The practical skills instructor shall have authority to:

7.3.1 Conduct practical skills sessions under the direction of the course I/C,

7.3.2 Verify successful achievement of course skill objectives, under the direction of the course I/C, and

7.3.3 Regulate student behavior within the scope of the practical skills training program under the institutional guidelines for due process.

7.4 *Responsibilities*— Under the direction of the course I/C, the practical skills instructor:

7.4.1 Should provide a positive role model by:

7.4.1.1 Maintaining personal mental and physical health,

7.4.1.2 Maintaining appropriate personal hygiene and appearance,

7.4.1.3 Actively pursuing personal and professional development,

7.4.1.4 Recognizing personal limitations and seeking assistance when appropriate,

7.4.1.5 Demonstrating competent, respectful, and caring interactions with students, co-workers, and patients at all times, and

7.4.1.6 Demonstrating professional behavior in the classroom or in the presence of students.

7.4.2 Shall ensure a safe and effective learning environment,

7.4.3 Shall provide consistent and competent training assistance to students,

7.4.4 Shall maintain appropriate student skills training records,

7.4.5 Shall teach the skills contained in the curriculum as adopted and defined by the appropriate certifying agency,

7.4.6 Shall consistently monitor students' progress toward established course skill objectives and provide appropriate feedback to the course I/C and the students within guidelines of appropriate certifying agency,

7.4.7 Shall evaluate, according to the curriculum, and differentiate among students for safe and effective performance,

7.4.8 Shall uphold state and national clinical standards for practice at the level being taught,

7.4.9 Shall ensure that practical skills training equipment is maintained in a safe and acceptable operating condition, and

7.4.10 Shall protect the privacy of students and the confidentiality of training course records as required by applicable laws and standards.

7.5 *Evaluation*—The evaluation by the course I/C of a practical skills instructor shall include:

7.5.1 Analysis of student practical skills outcomes,

7.5.2 Classroom observation of the practical skills instructor, and

7.5.3 Review of students' course evaluations.

7.6 *Maintenance of Competency*—In order to maintain competency, the practical skills instructor shall:

7.6.1 Maintain, to the satisfaction of the course I/C and course medical director, current competence in and knowledge of the skill(s) being taught, and

7.6.2 Teach the skills contained in an ALS/EMT related curriculum.

8. Clinical/Field Preceptor

8.1 *Qualifications*— The clinical/field preceptor candidate shall:

8.1.1 Be certified in his/her area of practice,

8.1.2 Have experience in his/her area of expertise, and

8.1.3 Demonstrate to the satisfaction of the course I/C a willingness and competence to work with students to assist them in meeting pertinent course objectives in the setting in which the clinical/field preceptor will function.

8.2 *Education/Training/Experience*—The clinical/field preceptor shall complete an orientation which includes:

8.2.1 Roles and responsibilities of the ALS/EMT,

8.2.2 Roles and responsibilities of the clinical/field preceptor, and

8.2.3 Guidelines for carrying out, meeting or accomplishing assigned responsibilities and duties.

8.3 *Scope of Authority*—The clinical/field preceptor shall have authority to:

8.3.1 Supervise student activities in the clinical/field setting as determined by stated course objectives,

8.3.2 Document student performance in the clinical/field setting, and

8.3.3 Regulate student behavior within the scope of the clinical/field setting under the institutional guidelines for due process.

8.4 *Responsibilities*— Under the direction of the course I/C, the clinical/field preceptor:

8.4.1 Should provide a positive role model,

8.4.2 Shall provide a safe and effective learning environment,

8.4.3 Shall provide consistent and competent supervision to students,

8.4.4 Shall maintain appropriate training records,

8.4.5 Shall assist the students in meeting the clinical/field skills objectives,

8.4.6 Shall consistently monitor students and provide appropriate feedback to the course I/C and the students,

8.4.7 Shall assess students for safe and effective performance, and

8.4.8 Shall protect the privacy of students and the confidentiality of training course records as required by applicable laws and standards.

8.5 *Evaluation*—The evaluation by the course I/C of a clinical/field preceptor in an ALS/EMT Training Program shall include:

8.5.1 Quality of training records,

8.5.2 Clinical/field observation of the preceptor, and

8.5.3 Review of students' clinical experience evaluations.

8.6 *Maintenance of Competency*—In order to maintain competency, the clinical/field preceptor shall:

8.6.1 Maintain certification in his/her area of practice, and

8.6.2 Maintain, to the satisfaction of the course I/C and course medical director, current competence in and knowledge of the areas precepted.

9. Keywords

9.1 advanced life support; emergency medical services instructor; emergency medical technician; training programs

Standard Practice for Emergency Medical Dispatch[1]

This standard is issued under the fixed designation F 1258; the number immediately following the designation indicates the year of original adoption or, in the case of revision, the year of last revision. A number in parentheses indicates the year of last reapproval. A superscript epsilon (ε) indicates an editorial change since the last revision or reapproval.

1. Scope

1.1 This practice covers the definition of responsibilities, knowledge, practices, and organizational support required to implement, perform, and manage effectively the emergency medical dispatch function.

1.2 This practice is useful for planning and evaluating the training, implementation, and organizational support to satisfy the functional needs of emergency medical dispatching.

1.3 *This standard does not purport to address all of the safety concerns, if any, associated with its use. It is the responsibility of the user of this standard to establish appropriate safety and health practices and determine the applicability of regulatory limitations prior to use.*

2. Referenced Documents

2.1 *ASTM Standards:*

F 1031 Practice for Training the Emergency Medical Technician (Basic)[2]

F 1381 Guide for Planning and Developing 9-1-1 Enhanced Telephone Systems[2]

F 1552 Practice for Training Instructor Qualification and Certification Eligibility of Emergency Medical Dispatchers[2]

F 1560 Practice for Emergency Medical Dispatch Management[2]

3. Terminology

3.1 *Definitions of Terms Specific to This Standard:*

3.1.1 *emergency medical dispatcher (EMD)*—a trained public safety telecommunicator with additional training and specific emergency medical knowledge essential for the efficient management of emergency medical communications.

3.1.2 *emergency medical dispatching*—the reception and management of requests for emergency medical assistance.

3.1.3 *emergency medical dispatch priority reference system (EMDPRS)*—a medically approved system used by a dispatch agency to provide aid to medical emergencies that includes: systematized caller interrogation questions, systematized prearrival instructions, and protocols matching the dispatcher's evaluation of injury or illness severity with vehicle response mode and configuration.

3.1.4 *medical direction*—the management and accountability for the medical care aspects of an emergency medical dispatch (EMD) program including: the medical monitoring oversight of the training of the EMD personnel; approval and medical control of the operational emergency medical dispatch priority reference system (EMDPRS); evaluation of the medical care and prearrival instructions rendered by the EMD personnel; direct participation in the EMD system evaluation, quality, assurance, and quality improvement process and mechanisms; and, responsibility for the medical decisions and care rendered by the emergency medical dispatcher and emergency medical dispatch program.

3.1.5 *public safety telecommunicator*—an individual trained to communicate remotely with persons seeking emergency assistance and with agencies and individuals providing such assistance.

3.1.6 *telephone aid*—consists of "ad-libbed" telephone instructions provided by either trained or untrained dispatchers and differs from DLS-based prearrival instructions in that the instructions provided to the caller are based on the dispatcher's knowledge or previous training in a procedure or treatment without following a scripted prearrival instruction protocol. They cannot be medically preapproved since they do not exist in written form.

3.1.7 *telephone treatment sequence protocols*—specific treatment strategies designed in a conversational script format that direct the EMD step by step in giving critical prearrival instructions such as CPR, Heimlich maneuver, mouth-to-mouth breathing, and childbirth instruction.

3.1.8 *vehicle response configuration*—the specific vehicle(s) of varied types, capabilities, and numbers responding to render assistance.

3.1.9 *vehicle response mode*—the use of emergency driving techniques, such as warning lights and siren, versus a routine driving response.

4. Summary of Practice

4.1 An emergency medical dispatcher is a trained public safety telecommunicator with additional training and specific emergency medical knowledge essential for assessment of medical emergencies and limited remote treatment and apportionment of medical priorities. The EMD functions under the medical authority of an off-line medical director to receive and

[1] This practice is under the jurisdiction of ASTM Committee F30 on Emergency Medical Services and is the direct responsibility of Subcommittee F30.04 on Communications.

Current edition approved Oct. 10, 1995. Published December 1995. Originally published as F 1258 – 90. Last previous edition F 1258 – 90.

[2] *Annual Book of ASTM Standards*, Vol 13.01.

manage calls for emergency medical assistance through the systematic interrogation of callers, using procedures established by the off-line medical director who remains responsible for the medical quality assurance of the EMD program.

4.1.1 The EMD's role includes the ability to:

4.1.1.1 Remotely evaluate the patient or incident,

4.1.1.2 Interpret the requirement and need for emergency medical resources,

4.1.1.3 Allocate the appropriate resources,

4.1.1.4 Identify conditions requiring prearrival instructions and provide them to the caller when necessary, possible and appropriate,

4.1.1.5 Coordinate the response of emergency medical and other public safety resources,

4.1.1.6 Provide information to the responding units regarding the emergency scene and patient, and

4.1.1.7 Record and retrieve emergency medical response records.

4.1.2 There must be continuity in the delivery of EMD care. To provide correct medical care safely and effectively, the EMD that is medically directing, evaluating, and coding must maintain direct access to the calling party and must use a medically approved emergency medical dispatch priority reference system. The person giving the medical instruction to the caller must be the same person that asks the systematic interrogation questions.

4.1.3 To accomplish the above safely and effectively, the EMD must use a medically approved EMDPRS that includes:

4.1.3.1 Systematized caller interrogation questions,

4.1.3.2 Systematized prearrival instructions, and

4.1.3.3 Protocols that determine vehicle response mode and configuration based on the EMD's evaluation of injury or illness severity.

4.2 This practice is intended to be used by agencies as a baseline for establishing a certifying emergency medical dispatch training program that includes the implementation of the emergency medical dispatch priority reference system, under medical direction, and provides a means of evaluating the EMD program.

4.3 This practice will provide a common set of expectations for training, performance, and preplanned response based on understanding of the medical condition, thorough interrogation, caller intervention, safe responses, and prearrival instructions.

4.4 This practice establishes the EMD's role and responsibilities in receiving, managing, and dispatching calls for medical assistance and related agency coordination.

4.5 An organizational structure as defined in Practice F 1560 must be in place before implementing the EMD program; therefore, this practice establishes some general recommendations concerning the development of a supportive structure and program content.

4.6 Use of this practice is not intended to protect the EMD or dispatch organization from liability for negligent actions or failure to perform in accordance with established and approved medical practices and protocols.

4.7 The EMD must be certified through either state government processes or by professional medical dispatch standard-setting organizations.

4.7.1 When certification is achieved by recognition of a professional medical dispatch standard-setting organization, it shall clearly demonstrate compliance with all criteria enumerated in this practice and within Practice F 1560 and Practice F 1552.

5. Significance and Use

5.1 This practice is intended to promote the use of trained telecommunicators in the role of emergency medical dispatcher. It defines the basic skills and medical knowledge to permit understanding and resolution of the problems that constitute their daily routine. To use trained telecommunicators fully as functioning members of the emergency medical team, it is deemed necessary to upgrade the telecommunicators' training by the addition of the concept of emergency medical dispatch priorities.

5.2 All agencies or individuals who routinely accept calls for emergency medical assistance from the public and dispatch emergency medical personnel shall have in effect an emergency medical dispatcher program in accordance with this practice. The program shall include medical direction and oversight and an emergency medical dispatch priority reference system.

5.3 The successful use of the EMD concept depends on the medical community's awareness of the "prearrival" state of EMS affairs and their willingness to provide medical direction in dispatch.

5.4 This practice may assist in overcoming some of the misconceptions regarding emergency medical dispatching. These include the uncontrollable nature of the caller's hysteria, lack of time of the dispatcher, potential danger and liability to the EMD, lack of recognition of the benefits of dispatch prearrival instructions, and misconceptions that red lights, siren, and maximal response are always necessary.

5.5 The EMD is the member of the EMS response team with the broadest view of the entire emergency system's current status and capabilities. The EMD has immediate lifesaving capability in converting the caller into an effective first responder. This practice recognizes the EMD's role as including:

5.5.1 Interrogation techniques,

5.5.2 Triage decisions,

5.5.3 Information transmission,

5.5.4 Telephone medical intervention, and

5.5.5 Logistics and resource coordination during the event.

5.6 For the EMD, this practice supersedes any other EMSS standards under which an individual may be qualified, such as Practice F 1031. It is not the role of the EMD to generate a specific diagnosis but rather to elicit accurately a finite body of information, assign the appropriate response, and to communicate clearly among persons and units involved in the response. The protocols for inquiry, response, and resource coordination are essential and must not be modified based on an individual's possible experiences as a responder.

5.7 As an initial contact with the EMS system, the EMD is subject to questioning of actions as they relate to medical practice. This practice may be used by agencies as a recognized baseline for EMD training, practice, and organization and is intended to supplant de facto standards that exist in some areas. This practice will assist in developing sound EMD programs that will reduce the need and potential for legal action and provide a common set of expectations for performance.

5.8 It will bring more accurate information into the dispatch office by way of appropriate understanding of the medical condition and therefore better interrogation, caller intervention, and decision-making. It allows for preplanned responses, safer responses (fewer units responding with lights and siren), fuel and energy savings (smaller units and fewer units used when possible), and may save advanced lifesupport resources for true advanced life-support emergencies when a tiered-level response is available.

6. System Components

6.1 *Emergency Medical Dispatch Priority Reference System (EMDPRS)*:

6.1.1 This system is a written, reproducible document in a uniform format based on medical and administrative protocols. The emergency medical dispatch priority reference system directs the EMD to complete a full, programmed interrogation. The information from the caller is paired with preset problem groups to determine the appropriate response level. It shall include the following:

6.1.1.1 A set of systematized caller interrogation (key) questions. The key questions must obtain the minimum amount of information necessary to:

6.1.1.1.1 (*a*) Adequately establish the correct level of response,

6.1.1.1.2 (*b*) Establish the need for prearrival instructions, and

6.1.1.1.3 (*c*) Provide responders with adequate patient and incident information.

6.1.2 A set of systematized coding and response protocols that include:

6.1.2.1 Protocols that predetermine vehicle response mode and configuration based on the EMD's evaluation of injury and illness severity as determined through key question interrogation. These protocols must reflect a given EMS systems varied ability to respond, ranging from single-unit squads through multiple-level (tiered) response.

6.1.2.2 An established, medically approved, quantitative coding system for quality assurance/improvement and statistical analysis.

6.1.3 A set of systematic prearrival instructions that include:

6.1.3.1 Chief complaint specific caller and EMD advise, and

6.1.3.2 Scripted prearrival instructions.

6.1.4 In addition to the EMDPRS, an emergency medical dispatch system should include:

6.1.4.1 A mass casualty plan for notification and operation in a disaster situation,

6.1.4.2 A directory of emergency response resources and information resources,

6.1.4.3 A written description of the communications system configuration for the service area, and

6.1.4.4 A record-keeping system, including report forms or a computer data management system to permit evaluation of EMD compliance with the EMDPRS, evaluation of protocol effectiveness, and timeliness of interrogation and dispatch.

7. Functions of Emergency Medical Dispatch

7.1 *Receive and Process Calls for Assistance*—The EMD must receive and record calls for emergency medical assistance from various sources. This function includes the establishment of effective communication with the person requesting assistance, using the EMDPRS to evaluate the patient or situation, provide appropriate prearrival instructions, and select the most appropriate EMS system action in response to each call.

7.2 *Dispatch and Coordinate Appropriate, Available Response Resources*—The EMD must select and dispatch the necessary EMS vehicles and personnel to the scene of an emergency in an appropriate time frame. The EMD functions in coordinating the movements of EMS vehicles en route to the scene, en route to the medical facility, and back to the base of operations. This requires that the EMD have current knowledge of the status of all EMS resources in the dispatch area and the geographic constraints that will affect the EMS response. This also requires that the EMD have dispatch-specific medical training and understands the use of systematized interrogation and response assignment protocols.

7.3 *Provide Information and Prearrival Instructions*:

7.3.1 To the caller, the EMD is the contact with the emergency response agency and must be prepared to provide emergency care instructions to callers waiting for an EMS response. These instructions should enable the caller to prevent or reduce further injury to the victim and to do as much as possible under the circumstances to intervene in any life-threatening situation that exists. These instructions should also include appropriate warnings and safety messages regarding potential dangers that can be reasonably foreseen through correct use of the EMDPRS.

7.3.2 All dispatch life-support-based instructions and information should be given directly from the EMDPRS rather than ad lib. Federal Publication NIH No. 94-3287 on Emergency Medical Dispatching[3] categorizes ad-lib instructions as "telephone aid" which, further defined, "may only ensure that the dispatcher has attempted to provide some sort of care to the patient through the caller but does not ensure that such care is correct, standard, and medically effective or even necessary in the first place. Telephone aid, therefore, is usually considered as inappropriate and an unreliable form of dispatcher-provided medical care."

7.3.3 To the responding unit(s), the EMD must provide accurate information regarding the patient, conditions at the scene of response, other public safety unit responses, and other information regarding the situation. This information always includes the chief complaint, patient's age, status of consciousness, and status of breathing.

7.4 *Coordinate With Other Agencies and Emergency Services*—The EMD must ensure the existence and maintenance of an effective communication link between and among

[3] U.S. Department of Health and Human Services, Public Health Service, National Institutes of Health, National Heart, Lung, and Blood Institute. NIH Publication No. 94-3287, *Emergency Medical Dispatching: Rapid Identification and Treatment of Acute Myocardial Infarction*, July 1994.

all public safety services (that is, fire, police, rescue, aeromedical, hazardous materials, utility, and so forth) involved in the EMS response to facilitate mutual aid and to coordinate services including such items as traffic control, fire suppression, and extrication.

7.5 *Necessary Skills of the Emergency Medical Dispatcher*:

7.5.1 Ability to read and write English proficiently and other language or communications skills necessary to function in given area,

7.5.2 Ability to speak clearly and distinctly on radio and telephone,

7.5.3 Ability to remain calm, use reasoned judgment, and communicate effectively in stressful or crisis situations,

7.5.4 Ability to use established interrogation and response assignment protocols,

7.5.5 Ability to provide prearrival instructions appropriate for the emergency situation to both the caller and responders, and

7.5.6 Ability to retain a professional attitude with the caller specifically regarding courtesy and empathy for the situation encountered.

7.5.7 *Inappropriate EMD Activities*:

7.5.7.1 Display of hostility toward or arguing with the caller,

7.5.7.2 Judgment of a situation based on past experience with the caller,

7.5.7.3 Judgment of a situation severity based on previous personal experiences,

7.5.7.4 Unreasonably refusing to dispatch available units in accordance with the approved dispatch protocol,

7.5.7.5 Premature termination of call for assistance, and

7.5.7.6 Failure to act or to dispatch in accordance with protocol.

8. Medical Dispatch Practice

8.1 The role of the EMD is to obtain specific medical information to prioritize accurately each medical response as listed in the emergency medical dispatch priority reference system (EMDPRS). Using this system, the EMD asks key questions about patient condition and incident types, determines the necessity for and gives prearrival instructions, and selects predetermined response levels based on the medical significance of the information obtained. To accomplish this, the EMD must:

8.1.1 Understand the basic philosophy of medical interrogation. Medical dispatch experts have shown that through the use of proper techniques and interrogation protocols significantly more vital information can be obtained. While it may seem the emotional, and at times, hysterical caller's behavior is random and unpredictable, there are some very predictable, generic components present in most cases. Some of these are noted in Appendix X1.

8.1.2 Understand the difference between key questions asked in medical as opposed to trauma cases:

8.1.2.1 Medical case questions are generally based on symptoms such as chest pain, breathing, level of consciousness, and so forth. The caller usually is with the victim or is personally familiar with the patient or their problem.

8.1.2.2 Trauma case questions are generally based on the type of incident rather than specific symptoms, since the caller usually is a third-party observer not directly associated with the patient. The question" How far did the patient fall?," as opposed to, "What are the patient's injuries?," is more appropriate to successful, useful information gathering.

8.1.3 Understand the third-party caller limitation in regards to the difficulty of obtaining useful information when the caller is not with the patient and does not know the patient.

8.1.4 The EMD must be able to apply the following points:

8.1.4.1 The concept of the hysteria threshold and the method of attaining it, for example, repetitive persistence.

8.1.4.2 Until the hysteria threshold is broken, the EMD cannot be in control of a call.

8.1.4.3 The EMD must realize that this threshold exists and can be reached in most all cases so that they do not give up prematurely before obtaining control of the caller.

8.1.4.4 Increases in firmness or continued repetition in questioning or requests may not be successful initially until the threshold (that is different for each caller) is attained. At this point the EMD obtains control.

8.1.4.5 Handling an unpleasant, uncooperative, or hysterical caller by only obtaining the location of the incident and sending the response unit(s) is not acceptable.

8.2 *Prearrival Instructions*:

8.2.1 The objectives of giving prearrival instructions are:

8.2.1.1 To assist the caller in keeping the patient from further injury,

8.2.1.2 To enable the caller to do as much as possible to save a patient in a life-threatening situation, and

8.2.1.3 To transform a hysterical caller into a calmer rescuer who no longer feels helpless.

8.2.2 The following general instructions pertain to most callers:

8.2.2.1 Calm down,

8.2.2.2 Don't move the patient (except in situations that endanger the patient, such as fire, carbon monoxide, and so forth),

8.2.2.3 Observe the area for hazardous situations,

8.2.2.4 Observe what the patient is doing,

8.2.2.5 Identify the incident location by blinking the porch lights, opening garage door, describing house, identifying landmarks, and so forth,

8.2.2.6 Remove obstacles to the responders by locking up pets, sending children to neighbors, unlocking doors, obtaining elevators, opening gates, and so forth,

8.2.2.7 Preserve material or articles relating to the injury, and

8.2.2.8 Gather medications for responders.

8.2.3 General medical instructions commonly given to callers are as follows:

8.2.3.1 Airway management (head tilt/chin lift),

8.2.3.2 Heimlich maneuver,

8.2.3.3 Mouth-to-mouth ventilation,

8.2.3.4 Remove pillows from behind head,

8.2.3.5 CPR,

8.2.3.6 Direct-pressure hemorrhage control, and

8.2.3.7 Cool small burns in cold water.

8.2.4 The requisites of providing these instructions are as follows:

8.2.4.1 The EMD must be trained in basic life-support techniques before the provision of prearrival instructions,

8.2.4.2 Master the use of telephone treatment sequence cards, and

8.2.4.3 Understand the role of the trained versus untrained citizen at the scene of the emergency.

8.3 Roles of the EMD in emergency dispatch centers may differ such as assigned subroles:

8.3.1 *The Interrogator's Role*:

8.3.1.1 Obtain from the calling party the address or location of the emergency (first and most important),

8.3.1.2 Obtain from the calling party, or verify (in the case of E9-1-1 systems) the call-back telephone number at the calling location,

8.3.1.3 Obtain from the calling party the chief complaint,

8.3.1.4 Determine if the caller is with the patient,

8.3.1.5 Obtain the approximate age of the patient,

8.3.1.6 Determine if the patient is conscious (yes, no, or unknown),

8.3.1.7 Determine if the patient is breathing (yes, no, or unknown),

8.3.1.8 Use the EMD priority reference system to:

(1) Ask the systematized caller interrogation questions,

(2) Convey to the "dispatcher" the appropriate response assignment, and

(3) Give the calling party the listed telephone prearrival treatment instructions.

8.3.2 *The Dispatcher's Role*:

8.3.2.1 Alert the appropriate response unit(s) as determined by the interrogator's use of the EMD priority reference system,

8.3.2.2 Relay to responding unit(s):

(1) Location of incident,

(2) Age and sex of patient,

(3) Chief complaint,

(4) Status of conscious,

(5) Status of breathing,

(6) Other pertinent information, and

(7) Number of victims (if applicable).

8.3.3 *Other Functions*:

8.3.3.1 Assist the emergency response unit(s) in finding the address or patient location, or both,

8.3.3.2 Relay information between various units and responding agencies,

8.3.3.3 Monitor and relay information between units, especially those that do not have compatible radio frequencies,

8.3.3.4 Understand the immediate transport concept based on the nearness of the scene to advanced life support or the hospital with regard to the criticality of the patient,

8.3.3.5 Understand how to assist in coordinating a rendezvous, and

8.3.4 Solitary EMDs must perform all functions in an integrated fashion.

9. Organizational Support

9.1 The organizational support for the EMD function must consist minimally of the following:

9.1.1 Provision of EMS physician medical direction regardless of whether the EMD function is carried on in a freestanding EMS communications center or a consolidated public-safety answering point or communications center.

9.1.2 Provision of prospective, concurrent, and retrospective supervision of the EMD function. Such supervision shall consist of:

9.1.2.1 Reoccurring continuing education,

9.1.2.2 A real-time supervisor having medical dispatch experience and expertise,

9.1.2.3 A quality assurance program with random case audit including logging tape reviews on a regular scheduled basis, and

9.1.2.4 A risk management program including problem review.

9.1.3 Provision of written procedures and protocols including:

9.1.3.1 A clear formal chain of command for establishment of policies, procedures, and resolution of grievances related to emergency medical dispatch,

9.1.3.2 Administrative procedures for real-time resource allocation in alternative response assignments,

9.1.3.3 An emergency medical dispatch priority reference system, and

9.1.3.4 Other local resource materials covering specific situations affecting the EMD, such as, disaster plans, hospital resources, specialty facilities, and so forth.

9.1.4 Provision of complete written and recorded documentation of EMD activity and retention of these records.

9.2 Provision of initial EMD training and certification.

9.3 Probationary on-the-job training.

9.4 Provision of continuing professional education and recertification:

9.4.1 Ongoing medical education,

9.4.2 Basic life-support education and recertification,

9.4.3 Skills practicum,

9.4.4 Crisis management, and

9.4.5 Field experience and accompaniment during actual EMS field calls on a "ride-a-long" basis.

9.5 Provision for maintaining and upgrading equipment to meet EMSS needs.

NOTE 1—See Appendix X2.

10. Keywords

10.1 communications; dispatch; emergency medical dispatch

APPENDIXES

(Nonmandatory Information)

X1. MEDICAL INTERROGATION TECHNIQUES

X1.1 *Hysteria Threshold*—Many distraught callers have been shown to have a "threshold of hysteria" that can be overcome and controlled by the practice of "repetitive persistence." This practice will assist with uncooperative caller interrogation and facilitates giving prearrival instructions. The hysteria control threshold frequently may be easily attained, and once established, the caller is completely in control and repeats instructions word perfect.

X1.2 *Repetitive Persistence*—The most successful method of attaining the hysteria control threshold is repetitive persistence. Repetitive persistence is performed by the EMD repeating over and over again, in the exact same wording, a request to calm down or to perform any other act desired. It has been demonstrated that this approach works nearly universally after a limited number of repetitions. Altering the wording of a request, it is believed, appears to the caller's subconscious as indecision or lack of control on the EMD's part and is less effective.

X1.3 *Bring-the-Victim-to-the-Phone Problem*—The EMD must determine the location of the patient relative to the caller at the outset of the call. This will help avoid a possible later interruption of the telephone treatment sequence that may occur when the caller directs others by yelling, "Bring him in here to the phone." The EMD should always ask where the patient is at the beginning of the telephone treatment sequence.

X1.4 *"Nothing's Working" Phenomenon*—The exception to the control obtained once the hysteria threshold is reached occurs when the caller is reminded of the distressed state of the victim at three different stages. First, when the victim is brought to the phone, they are also brought back into the sight of the caller, who is unfortunately reminded of how bad the victim looks. Second, when the EMD asks for verification of absent vital signs (breathing or pulse), the caller is likewise reminded. Third, when the caller is finally dutifully performing CPR or the Heimlich, and the victim is not revived from their initial actions, the caller may state, "nothing's working" and in frustration and despair will sometimes stop trying.

X1.5 Some callers have the misconception that because they are performing the EMD's instructions, the victim should respond or be revived. Callers will sometimes become frustrated and may lose composure when the victim fails to respond to first-aid measures. This results in an event that can interrupt the treatment sequence. The EMD can overcome this problem with appropriate encouragement, repetitive persistence, and by mentioning that, "You are keeping the victim going until the paramedics get there."

X2. MEDICOLEGAL ISSUES OF EMERGENCY MEDICAL DISPATCH

X2.1 The agency and the EMD should understand the importance of EMD performance evaluation.

X2.1.1 Inappropriate performance or procedures, or both, can cause injury or death, or both, to field personnel or civilians.

X2.1.2 Poor work habits can lead to lawsuits against the EMD and the parent department or agency.

X2.1.3 It is important that the EMD remain informed on the correct procedures and protocols and follow them explicitly.

X2.1.4 If procedures appear faulty, the EMD should inform a supervisor for appropriate review.

X2.2 Civil liability for the EMD or his organization can result from the following:

X2.2.1 Caused action or omission by the EMD,

X2.2.2 Failure to supervise on the part of EMD supervisor,

X2.2.3 Failure to observe recognized agency standards by the EMD or the parent organization, and

X2.2.4 Failure to observe recognized community or national practice standards.

X3. TELECOMMUNICATION ISSUES OF EMERGENCY MEDICAL DISPATCH

X3.1 The telecommunicator should be thoroughly familiar with the applications of the following telecommunications equipment, procedures, and Federal Communications Commission (FCC) rules:

X3.1.1 Radio communications control console,

X3.1.2 Telephone equipment and recorders,

X3.1.3 Alert paging equipment and encoders,

X3.1.4 Telephone patch equipment,

X3.1.5 Biotelemetry equipment and MED radio systems,

X3.1.6 Computer equipment, CAD equipment, and record keeping,

X3.1.7 Logging recorder equipment and tape management, and

X3.1.8 Other specialized equipment, generators, tower lighting, and so forth.

X3.2 *Relevant FCC Rules* :

X3.2.1 Only trained and authorized personnel are permitted to operate radio equipment.

X3.2.2 Provisions for access to remote radio sites and base radio equipment shall be maintained.

X3.2.3 The station call sign shall be broadcast in accordance with FCC rules.

X3.2.4 The FCC personnel are authorized to inspect communication records and transmitter equipment at reasonable times with proper identification and notice.

X3.2.5 Transmission of false or deceptive information is prohibited.

X3.2.6 Disclosure of radio messages monitored or intercepted to any uninvolved third party is prohibited.

X3.2.7 Transmission of profane language is prohibited.

X3.2.8 The radio station license shall be displayed at the control points and transmitter location.

X3.2.9 Radio equipment shall be maintained to required technical standards.

X3.2.10 Users shall take reasonable precautions to avoid causing harmful interference, including monitoring before transmission where practical.

X3.3 *Public Safety Telecommunicator-Caller Communication*—The public safety telecommunicator is the contact an emergency caller has with the emergency response system. Prompt and efficient information gathering by the telecommunicator aids in the dispatch of appropriate resources, allows preparation time for responding units, and alerts the telecommunicator to significant events requiring prearrival instructions to the caller. As such, the public safety telecommunicator should:

X3.3.1 Answer telephone calls promptly (within 10 s of the first ring).

X3.3.2 Identify the service to the caller in accordance with the local protocol.

X3.3.3 Speak at a rate of no more than 80 to 100 words per minute.

X3.3.4 Speak directly into the microphone mouthpiece.

X3.3.5 Take control through an authoritative but courteous manner.

X3.3.6 Focus the caller's response to obtain key incident information.

X3.3.7 Elicit and record the following basic information from the person requesting assistance:

X3.3.8 *Location Information (Where)*:

X3.3.8.1 Location of the incident,

X3.3.8.2 Location to which the responding unit(s) should be sent (if different), and

X3.3.8.3 Directions to the incident (if not commonly recognized).

X3.3.9 *Incident Information (What)*:

X3.3.9.1 Primary nature of the event as described by the caller, and

X3.3.9.2 Nature of the response needed.

X3.3.10 *Caller Information (Who)*:

X3.3.10.1 Call back telephone number,

X3.3.10.2 Caller's name when appropriate, and

X3.3.10.3 Victim's name when appropriate.

X3.3.11 *Time/Duration Information (When)*:

X3.3.11.1 Time the incident occurred,

X3.3.11.2 How long incident has been underway (according to caller's perception), and

X3.3.11.3 When call was received.

X3.3.12 Maintain a professional demeanor even when dealing with hostile callers.

X3.3.13 Repeat questions to obtain additional necessary information or to clarify information.

X3.3.14 Record appropriate information in accordance with local protocol.

X3.3.15 Use plain language (not codes) and avoid jargon or slang.

X3.3.16 Allow the caller to hear the dispatch of units, or inform the caller that the dispatch has been or is being made.

X3.3.17 Explain any waiting period such as having to relay or transfer the caller to another agency or individual.

X3.3.18 Inform the caller not to hang up until they are told to do so.

X3.3.19 Show interest in the caller:

X3.3.19.1 Use the caller's name when possible (last name with appellation for adults; first name for children and teenagers).

X3.3.19.2 Calm and continually reassure the caller.

X3.3.20 Direct the caller to perform helpful activities before the arrival of responders.

X3.3.21 Accept responsibility for all emergency calls received (whenever possible the system should provide internal methods for transferring or relaying of information).

X3.3.22 Never leave an assigned work station (console) without relief personnel in place.

X3.4 *Dispatch Procedures:*

X3.4.1 Dispatch the appropriate units in a timely manner upon determination of needed location and incident information.

X3.4.2 Relay to appropriate responding units such items as:

X3.4.2.1 The location of the incident.

X3.4.2.2 Nature of incident/chief complaint.

X3.4.2.3 All important supplemental information including: age and sex of patient(s), status of consciousness, status of breathing, number of patients, and so forth.

X3.4.3 Avoid use of contractions or homonyms in directing responding units.

X3.4.4 Break long messages into short (10-s) segments.

X3.4.5 Confirm receipt of and understanding of information.

X3.4.6 Assist responding units by giving directions to the incident address, hazards and obstacles en route, and accessibility and conditions.

X3.4.7 Update responders on changes in the status of the incident.

X3.4.8 Relay information between other responding units.

X3.4.9 Record information upon receipt, using a standard report and recording format to document call reception, dispatch, scene arrival, scene departure, destination arrival, clear scene, and unit in service times.

X3.4.10 Provide supplemental or incident information as received from other sources.

X3.4.11 Use appropriate signalling methods and techniques

based on a thorough knowledge of the communications system.

X3.4.12 Use proper radio communications techniques.

X3.4.13 Perform all activities in compliance with FCC rules and local standard operating procedures and protocols.

The American Society for Testing and Materials takes no position respecting the validity of any patent rights asserted in connection with any item mentioned in this standard. Users of this standard are expressly advised that determination of the validity of any such patent rights, and the risk of infringement of such rights, are entirely their own responsibility.

This standard is subject to revision at any time by the responsible technical committee and must be reviewed every five years and if not revised, either reapproved or withdrawn. Your comments are invited either for revision of this standard or for additional standards and should be addressed to ASTM Headquarters. Your comments will receive careful consideration at a meeting of the responsible technical committee, which you may attend. If you feel that your comments have not received a fair hearing you should make your views known to the ASTM Committee on Standards, at the address shown below.

Standard Specification and Test Methods for Intramedullary Fixation Devices[1]

This standard is issued under the fixed designation F 1264; the number immediately following the designation indicates the year of original adoption or, in the case of revision, the year of last revision. A number in parentheses indicates the year of last reapproval. A superscript epsilon (ϵ) indicates an editorial change since the last revision or reapproval.

1. Scope

1.1 This specification is intended to provide a characterization of the design and mechanical function of intramedullary fixation devices (IMFDs) specify labeling and material requirements, provide test methods for characterization of IMFD mechanical properties and identify needs for further development of test methods and performance criteria. The ultimate goal is to develop a standard which defines performance criteria and methods for measurement of performance-related mechanical characteristics of IMFDs and their fixation to bone. It is not the intention of this specification to define levels of performance or case-specific clinical performance of these devices, as insufficient knowledge is available to predict the consequences of the use of any of these devices in individual patients for specific activities of daily living. It is not the intention of this specification to describe or specify specific designs for IMFDs.

1.2 This specification describes IMFDs for surgical fixation of the skeletal system. It provides basic IFMD geometrical definitions, dimensions, classification, and terminology; labeling and material specifications; performance definitions; test methods and characteristics determined to be important to in-vivo performance of the device.

1.3 This specification includes four standard test methods:

1.3.1 Static Four-Point Bend Test Method—Annex A1, and

1.3.2 Static Torsion Test Method—Annex A2.

1.3.3 Bending Fatigue Test Method—Annex A3.

1.3.4 Test Method for Bending Fatigue of IMFD Locking Screws—Annex A4.

1.4 A Rationale is given in Appendix X1.

1.5 The values stated in SI units are to be regarded as the standard.

2. Referenced Documents

2.1 *ASTM Standards:*

A 214/A 214M Specification for Electric-Resistance-Welded Carbon Steel Heat Exchanger and Condenser Tubes[2]

A 450/A 450M Specification for General Requirements for Carbon, Ferritic Alloy, and Austenitic Alloy Steel Tubes[2]

D 790 Test Methods for Flexural Properties of Unreinforced and Reinforced Plastics and Electrical Insulating Materials[2]

E 4 Practices for Force Verification of Testing Machines[3]

E 691 Practice for Conducting an Interlaboratory Study to Determine the Precision of a Test Method[4]

F 86 Practice for Surface Preparation and Marking of Metallic Surgical Implants[5]

F 138 Specification for Wrought-18 Chromium-14 Nickel-12.5 Molybdenum Stainless Steel Bar and Wire for Surgical Implants (UNS S31673)[5]

F 339 Specification for Cloverleaf Intramedullary Pins[6,7]

F 383 Practice for Static Bend and Torsion Testing of Intramedullary Rods[5]

F 565 Practice for Care and Handling of Orthopaedic Implants and Instruments[5]

F 1611 Terminology for Sizing of IMFDs for Application to Reamed Diaphyseal Bone and Associated Instrumentation[5]

2.2 *AMS Standard:*

AMS 5050[8] Steel Tubing, Seamless, 0.15 Carbon, Maximum Annealed

2.3 *SAE Standard:*

SAE J524[9] Seamless Low-Carbon Steel Tubing Annealed for Bending and Flaring

3. Terminology

3.1 *Definitions for Geometric:*

3.1.1 *closed section, n*—any cross section perpendicular to the longitudinal axis of a solid IMFD, or hollow IMFD where there is no discontinuity of the outer wall. In order to orient the IMFD for testing and for insertion, the desired relationship of any irregularities, asymetries, etc., to the sagittal and coronal planes should be described for the intended applications.

3.1.2 *IMFD curvature, n*—dimensions of size and locations of arcs of the curvature, or mathematical description of the curvature, or other quantitative descriptions to which the curvature is manufactured along with tolerances. In order to

[1] This specification is under the jurisdiction of ASTM Committee F-4 on Medical and Surgical Materials and Devices and is the direct responsibility of Subcommittee F04.21 on Osteosynthesis.

Current edition approved May 10, 2000. Published August 2000. Originally published as F 1264 – 89. Last previous edition F 1264 – 99a.

[2] *Annual Book of ASTM Standards*, Vol 08.01.

[3] *Annual Book of ASTM Standards*, Vol 03.01.

[4] *Annual Book of ASTM Standards*, Vol 14.02.

[5] *Annual Book of ASTM Standards*, Vol 13.01.

[6] Discontinued; see *1998 Annual Book of ASTM Standards*, Vol 13.01.

[7] Discontinued; see *1996 Annual Book of ASTM Standards*, Vol 13.01.

[8] Available from the Society of Automotive Engineers, 400 Commonwealth Dr., Warrendale, PA 15096.

[9]

orient the IMFD for testing and for insertion, the desired relationship of the curvature to the sagittal and coronal planes should be described for the intended applications.

3.1.3 *IMFD diameter, n*—The diameter of the circumscribed circle, which envelops the IMFDs' cross section when measured along the IMFDs' working length. If the diameter is not constant along the working length, then the site of measurement should be indicated.

3.1.4 *IMFD length, n*—the length of a straight line between the most proximal and distal ends of the IMFD.

3.1.5 *open section, n*—any cross section perpendicular to the longitudinal axis of a hollow IMFD where there is a discontinuity of the outer wall. In order to orient the IMFD for testing and insertion, the desired relationship of the discontinuity to the sagittal and coronal planes should be described for the intended applications.

3.1.6 *potential critical stress concentrator (CSC), n*—any change in section modulus, material property, discontinuity, or other feature of a design expected to cause a concentration of stress, which is located in a region of the IMFD expected to be highly stressed under the normal anticipated loading conditions.

3.1.7 *working length, n*—a length of uniform cross section of the IMFD intended to obtain some type of fit to the medullary canal in the area of the diaphysis.

3.1.8 *tolerance*—the acceptable deviations from the nominal size of any dimension describing the IMFD.

3.2 *Definitions—Mechanical/Structural:*

3.2.1 *bending compliance, n*—the reciprocal of the stiffness of the IMFD under a bending load in a specified plane as defined and determined in the static four-point bend test described in Annex A1.

3.2.2 *fatigue strength at N cycles, n*—the maximum cyclic force parameter (for example, load, moment, torque, stress, etc.,) for a given load ratio, which produces device structural damage or meets some other failure criterion in no less than N cycles as defined and measured according to the test conducted.

3.2.3 *failure strength, n*—the force parameter (for example, load, moment, torque, stress, etc.) required to meet the failure criteria defined and measured according to the test conducted.[10]

3.2.4 *yield strength, n*—the force parameter (for example, load, moment, torque, stress, etc.) which initiates permanent deformation as defined and measured according to the test conducted.

3.2.5 *no load motion*—some devices have a degree of free motion at fixation points which allows relative motion to occur between the device and the bone with no elastic strain in the device and no (or minimal) change in load. This is termed "no load motion."[10]

3.2.6 *structural stiffness, n*—the maximum slope of the elastic portion of the load-displacement curve as defined and measured according to the test conducted. For bending in a specified plane this term is defined and determined in the static four-point bend test described in Annex A1.

3.2.7 *ultimate strength, n*—the maximum force parameter (for example, load, moment, torque, stress, etc.) which the structure can support defined and measured according to the test conducted.

3.2.8 *N*—a variable representing a specified number of cycles.

4. Classification

4.1 The following IMFDs may be used singly, multiply, with or without attached supplemental fixation.

4.2 Types of IMFDs: solid cross section, hollow cross section (open, closed, combination).

4.3 Intended application or use for particular IMFD designs:

4.3.1 *Preferred Orientation*:

4.3.1.1 Right versus left,

4.3.1.2 Sagittal versus coronal plane,

4.3.1.3 Proximal versus distal, and

4.3.1.4 Universal or multiple options.

4.3.2 *Preferred Anatomic Location*:

4.3.2.1 Specific bone,

4.3.2.2 Proximal versus distal versus midshaft, and

4.3.2.3 Universal or multiple options.

4.3.3 *Preferred Use Limited to Specific Procedures*:

4.3.3.1 Acute care of fractures,

(*a*) Specific types,

(*b*) Specific locations,

4.3.3.2 Reconstructive procedures, and

4.3.3.3 Universal or multiple options.

5. Material

5.1 All IMFDs made of materials which have an ASTM standard shall meet those requirements given in the ASTM standards (2.1).

6. Performance Considerations and Test Methods

6.1 *Cross-Section Dimensional Tolerances* affect matching the bone preparation instruments (that is, reamers) to the IMFD diameter, and fit the fixation of IMFDs in the bone.

6.1.1 Terminology related to sizing of IMFD devices and instruments is provided in Terminology F 1611.

6.2 *Longitudinal Contour Tolerances* (along with bending compliance), affect the fit and fixation of IMFDs in the bone.[8]

6.3 *Fatigue Strength*, affects the choice of implant in cases where delayed healing is anticipated (that is, infected nonunions, allografts, segmental loss, multiple trauma, etc.).

6.3.1 The fatigue strength or fatigue lives, or both for IMFD's subjected to cycle bending forces shall be determined using the cyclic bending fatigue test method described in Annex A3.

6.3.2 The fatigue strength or fatigue lives, or both, for IMFD locking screws subjected to cyclic bending forces shall be determined using the cyclic bending fatigue test method for locking screws described in Annex A4.

6.4 *Bending Strength*, affects the choice of implant where load sharing is minimized or loading is severe, or both (that is, with distal or proximal locking, subtrochanteric fractures, comminuted fracture, segmental loss, non-compliant patient, etc.).

6.4.1 Yield, failure, and ultimate strength for IMFDs subjected to bending in a single plane shall be determined using

[10] No present testing standard exists related to this term for IMFDs.

the static four-point bend test method described in Annex A1.

6.5 *Bending and Torsional Stiffness*, may affect the type and rate of healing (primary or secondary healing) depending upon the fracture type (transverse, oblique, etc.).

6.5.1 Bending structural stiffness for IMFDs subjected to bending in a single plane shall be determined using the static four-point bend test method described in Annex A1.

6.5.2 Torsional stiffness for IMFDs subjected to pure torsion shall be determined using the static torsion test method described in Annex A2.

6.6 *No-Load Axial and Torsional Motion Allowed in Devices Using Secondary Attached Fixation*, affects degree of motion at the fracture site.[10]

6.7 *Extraction System*, Mechanical Failures Should Occur in the Extraction Device Before They Occur in the IMFD, prevents need to remove IMFD without proper tools.[10]

7. Marking, Packaging, Labeling, and Handling

7.1 Dimensions of IMFDs should be designated by the standard definitions given in 3.1.

7.2 Mark IMFDs using a method specified in accordance with Practice F 86.

7.3 Use the markings on the IMFD to identify the manufacturer or distributor and mark away from the most highly stressed areas, where possible.

7.4 Packaging shall be adequate to protect the IMFD during shipment.

7.5 Include the following on package labeling for IMFDs:

7.5.1 Manufacturer and product name,

7.5.2 Catalog number,

7.5.3 Lot or serial number,

7.5.4 IMFD diameter (3.1.3), and

7.5.5 IMFD length (3.1.4).

7.6 Care for and handle IMFDs in accordance with Practice F 565.

8. Means for Insertion and Extraction

8.1 For IMFDs which are to be extracted using a hook device, the following requirements apply:

8.1.1 The slot at the end of the IMFD shall have the dimensions shown in Fig. 1.

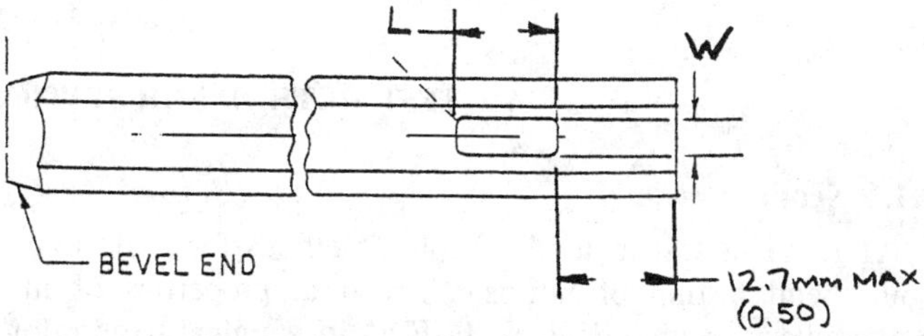

IMFD Diameter, mm	Hook Size	Slot Length, *L*, mm (in.)	Slot Width, *W*, mm (in.)
6, 7	2	9.50 (0.375)	1.91 (0.075)
8 and larger	1	9.50 (0.375)	3.23 (0.127)

FIG. 1 Dimensions of Extractor Hook Slot

8.1.2 The hook used for extraction shall have the dimensions shown in Fig. 2.

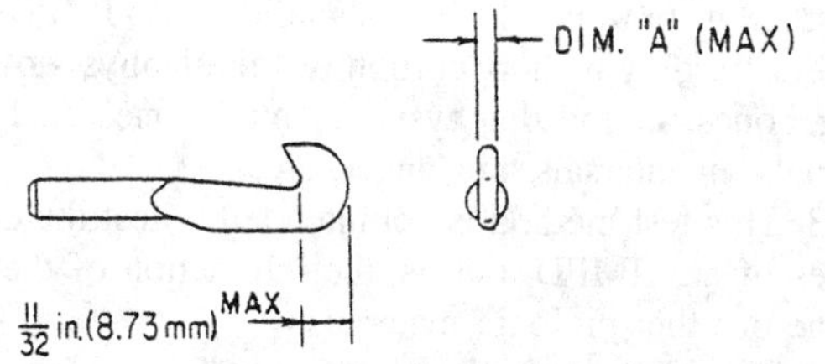

Hook Size	Hook Width, *A*, mm (in.)
1	3.18 (0.120)
2	1.78 (0.070)

FIG. 2 Dimensions of Extractor Hook

9. Keywords

9.1 bend testing; definitions; extraction; fatigue test; fracture fixation; implants; intramedullary fixation devices; orthopaedic medical device; performance; surgical devices; terminology; test methods; torsion test; trauma

ANNEXES

(Mandatory Information)

A1. TEST METHOD FOR STATIC FOUR-POINT BEND TEST METHOD

A1.1 Scope

A1.1.1 This test method describes methods for static four-point bend testing of intrinsic, structural properties of intramedullary fixation devices (IMFDs) for surgical fixation of the skeletal system. This test method includes bend testing in a variety of planes defined relative to the major anatomic planes. The purpose is to measure bending strength and bending stiffness intrinsic to the design and materials of IMFDs.

A1.1.2 This test method is designed specifically to test IMFD designs which have a well-defined working length (*WL*) of uniform open or closed cross section throughout the majority of its length ($WL \geq 10\times$ diameter), and is to be applied to the full length of the diaphysis of a femur, tibia, humerus, radius or ulna. This is not applicable to IMFDs which are used to fix only a short portion of the diaphysis of any of the long bones, or the diaphysis of small bones such as the metacarpals, metatarsals, phalanges, etc.

A1.1.3 This test method is not intended to test the extrinsic properties of any IMFD, that is, the interaction of the device with bone or other biologic materials.

A1.1.4 This test method is not intended to define case-specific clinical performance of these devices, as insufficient knowledge is available to predict the consequences of the use of any of these devices in individual patients.

A1.1.5 This test method is not intended to serve as a quality assurance document, and thus statistical sampling techniques for batches from production of IMFDs are not addressed.

A1.1.6 This test method may not be appropriate for all types of implant applications. The user is cautioned to consider the appropriateness of the method in view of the devices being tested, the material of their manufacture, and their potential applications.

A1.1.7 The values stated in SI units are to be regarded as the standard.

A1.1.8 *This standard does not purport to address all of the safety concerns, if any, associated with its use. It is the responsibility of the user of this standard to establish appropriate safety and health practices and determine the applicability of regulatory limitations prior to use.*

A1.2. Terminology

A1.2.1 *Definitions:*

A1.2.1.1 *bending compliance, n*—the reciprocal of the stiffness of the IMFD under a bending load in a specified plane ($1/EI_e$ for the IMFD, y/F for the system tested).

A1.2.1.2 *bending moment to failure, n*—the moment required to meet predetermined failure criteria measured in accordance with A1.5.1. (Failure may be defined by permanent deformation, breakages or buckling.)

A1.2.1.3 *bending moment to yield, n*—the moment which produces plastic deformation as defined by the 0.2 % strain off-set method from the load-displacement curve.

A1.2.1.4 *bending structural stiffness, n*—the resistance to bending of an IMFD tested in accordance with the procedures of A1.5.1, normalized to the cross-sectional properties of the working length without regard to the length of IMFD tested, by the calculations described in A1.5.1.8 (the effective EI_e for the region tested).

A1.2.1.5 *fixture/device compliance, n*—a measurement of the combined compliance of the IMFD on the test fixture with co-aligned load-support points (such as, A1.5.2). This value is dependent upon IMFD orientation, load direction and load and support spans.

A1.2.1.6 *ultimate bending moment, n*—the moment at the maximum or ultimate load as measured on the load-displacement curve for any test in accordance with A1.5.1.

A1.2.2 *Definitions of Terms Specific to This Standard:*

A1.2.2.1 The testing mode shall consist of an applied compression load cycle, at a constant displacement rate, to a defined failure.

A1.2.2.2 The testing mode shall be single cycle of load applied at least three diameters of the IMFD from the nearest critical stress concentration point (CSC) unless otherwise specified or unless the CSC is a characteristic of the normal cross section in the working length.

A1.3 Classification

A1.3.1 *Types of Test Covered by This Specification Are*:

A1.3.1.1 Measurement of structural mechanical behavior inherent to IMFDs—Intrinsic Properties.

A1.3.1.2 Measurement of single-cycle elastic stiffness and strength in four-point bending.

A1.3.1.3 Measurement of a single-cycle fixture/device elastic compliance.

A1.4 Procedure

A1.4.1 *Bending Test for Intrinsic Properties of the Working Length (WL)*:

A1.4.1.1 Determine the spans to be used as described in A1.4.1.2 and A1.4.1.3 and set the spans, *s, c* and *L* within 1 % of the determined values.

A1.4.1.2 Conduct four-point bending at room atmospheric conditions as shown in Fig. A1.1 using two rolling supports spaced from 10 to 50 cm apart, *L*, with the span between the loading points, *c*, no greater than *L*/3. Loading points should also be of the rolling type, and the diameter of both the loading and support rollers should be between 1.0 and 2.6 cm. Choice of spans should be made based upon the guidelines given in A1.7.1.

A1.4.1.3 A recommendation for load and support spans is provided below to minimize interlaboratory variability and provide consistency with the previous ASTM standard for four-point bend testing of IMFDs. The suggested long or short

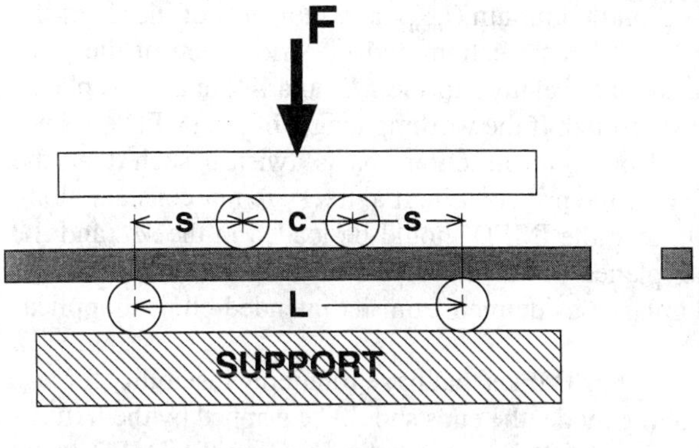

FIG. A1.1 4-Point Bend Test Setup

span should be used whenever possible, provided the general guidelines of A1.7.1 are achieved. The short span is identical to that used in the previous standard, Practice F 383, and the long span is based upon the experience of several laboratories testing a broad range of design and sizes of current (1995) IMFD designs.

Short span	$s = c = 3.8$ cm (1.5 in.)	$L = 11.4$ cm (4.5 in.)
Long span	$s = c = 7.6$ cm (3.0 in.)	$L = 22.8$ cm (9.0 in.)

A1.4.1.4 Apply equal loads at each of the loading points (a single load centered over the load points as shown in Figs. A1.1 and A1.2 is the usual method) at a constant rate of displacement no greater than 1 mm/s. Measure the relative deflections between the support and loading points (inner versus outer), y. For devices made of strain-rate-sensitive materials, the displacement rate for a given strain rate may be estimated by using the following approximations:

$$y_R = S_{t\,1\,\%}, \text{ and } c = L - 2s \tag{A1.1}$$

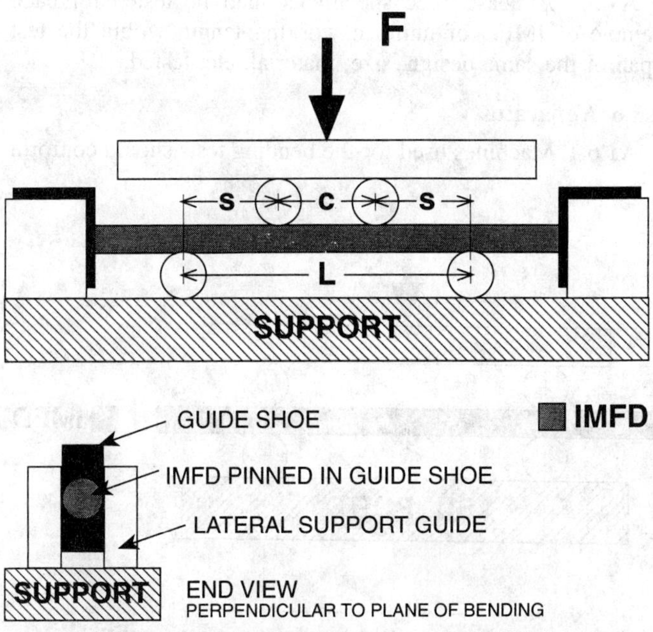

FIG. A1.2 4-Point Bend Test with Guide Shoes

$$y_{1\,\%} = s(L + 2c)/300\ D_{IMFD} = s(3L - 4s)/300\ D_{IMFD} \tag{A1.2}$$

or

$$= s(sc + 2s)/300\ D_{IMFD}$$

where:

S_t = the desired strain rate,
$y_{1\,\%}$ = the deflection at the loading point for an estimated 1 % maximum strain in the IMFD,
s = the span from a load point to the nearest support,
c = the center span,
L = the total span ($c + 2s$), and
D_{IMFD} = the diameter of the IMFD.

NOTE A1.1—The estimate of the deflection rate which corresponds to the desired strain rate is only a rough estimate based upon the assumptions of plane strain for closed-section tubes or solid rods so that the neutral axis of the cross section lies uniformly throughout the working length in the center of the circumscribed circle of the cross section and that there is material in the cross section touching the circumscribed circle where it intersects the plane of bending.

A1.4.1.5 Compute the bending moment, M, as used in A1.2.1:

$$M = Fs/2 \tag{A1.3}$$

where:

F = the force applied to the system (two times the force applied to each of the loading points),
s = the span from a load point to the nearest support.

A1.4.1.6 Compute an estimate for the maximum strain in the IMFD:

$$S_{MAX} = FS\ D_{IMFD}\ (4\ EI_e)^{-1} \tag{A1.4}$$

$$y = Fs^2\ (L + 2c)\ (12\ EI_e)^{-1} \tag{A1.5}$$

where:

S_{MAX} = estimate of maximum strain in the IMFD,
F = force on the system,
s = span from a load point to the nearest support point,
EI_e = effective structural stiffness of the IMFD portion tested,
D_{IMFD} = diameter of the IMFD,
L = the total span between supports ($2s + c$), and
c = the center span.

A1.4.1.7 Compute the bending moment to yield by estimating the load at 0.2 % maximum plastic strain. This can be approximated by calculating as follows:

$$y_{0.2\,\%} = s(L + 2c)/1500\ D_{IMFD} \tag{A1.6}$$

where:

$y_{0.2\,\%}$ = the permanent deflection at the loading point for 0.2 % maximum plastic strain (estimated by measuring the offset displacement from the linear region of the load-displacement curve),
s = the span from a load point to the nearest support,
c = the center span,
L = the total span ($c + 2s$), and
D_{IMFD} = the diameter of the IMFD.

At this point on the load-deflection curve read the yield

force, F_y. From F_y the bending moment to yield is computed from:

$$M_y = F_y s/2, \text{ (see Fig. A1.3)} \quad (A1.7)$$

Likewise, the ultimate bending moment, M_{MAX}, may be determined from the load-deflection curve:

$$M_{MAX} = F_{MAX} s/2, \text{ (see Fig. A1.3)} \quad (A1.8)$$

NOTE A1.2—The estimate of the deflection which corresponds to the 0.2 % desired strain is only a rough estimate based upon the assumptions of plane strain for closed section tubes or solid rods so that the neutral axis of the cross-section lies uniformly throughout the working length in the center of the circumscribed circle of the cross-section and that there is material in the cross-section touching the circumscribed circle where it intersects the plane of bending.

A1.4.1.8 Compute the bending structural stiffness:

$$EI_e = s^2(L + 2c)(F/y)/12 \quad (A1.9)$$

or

$$EI_e = s^2(3L - 4s)(F/y)/12 \quad (A1.10)$$

where:
- F/y = the slope of the elastic portion of the load-displacement curve,
- s = the span from a load point to the nearest support,
- c = the center span, and
- L = the total span ($c + 2s$).

NOTE A1.3—If no linear range can be easily approximated from the load-displacement curve, the ratio of the bending load to yield, as defined in A1.2.1.1, to the total deflection produced by that load at the loading point, when tested in accordance with the procedures of A1.5.1 can be used to estimate the average slope of the elastic range of bending.

A1.4.1.9 Bending should be applied in the planes of maximum (I_{max}) and minimum (I_{min}) area moments of inertia of the working length cross-section, and the orientation of the principal inertia axes relative to the *ML* and *AP* anatomic planes should be reported. If the working length of the IMFD does not have a uniform cross-section, or is twisted such that the orientation of the principal inertial axes are not constant along its length, then the IMFD should be loaded in the *ML* and *AP* anatomic planes, with the IMFD oriented relative to the anatomic planes as defined from its intended clinical application.

A1.4.1.10 For IMFDs that have rotational instability for any given bending mode, the ends should be gripped by the fixtures shown in Fig. A1.2. This fixture will allow the IMFD to be constrained outside the actively loaded region by plates that prevent rotation of the IMFD while allowing the in-plane bending with supported, free ends in such a manner that the ends are stable when the IMFD rests on the outer support rollers. The use of guide shoes will produce a mixed loading condition due to friction, in the portion of the system that resists rotation, that will contribute to the bending resistance. The magnitude of this effect is not easily measured or estimated but should be noted in the report.

A1.4.2 *Fixture/Device Compliance Test for the Intrinsic Properties of the Working Length*:

A1.4.2.1 Align both of the supports directly in line with the load points (see Fig. A1.4).

A1.4.2.2 Place the working length of the IMFD between the load point and support. Orient the IMFD so that load is applied in the desired plane (*AP, ML* or another specified direction).

A1.4.2.3 Load the IMFD in compression at a constant displacement rate of 0.1 mm/s. Record the slope of the load-displacement curve.

A1.4.2.4 Calculate the fixture/device compliance by calculating the reciprocal of the slope of the load-displacement curve in the elastic region and express in mm/N.

A1.5 Number of Specimens

A1.5.1 At least three specimens shall be tested for each sample of IMFD of uniform working length within the test span of the same design, size, material, etc. tested.

A1.6 Apparatus

A1.6.1 Machines used for the bending tests should conform

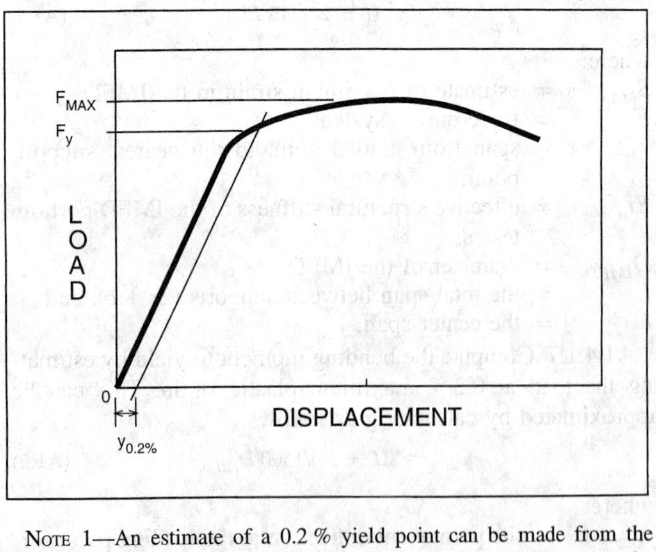

NOTE 1—An estimate of a 0.2 % yield point can be made from the "load cell versus ram displacement" measurements. Load represents the total load on the system (2× the load at each support) and the displacement represents the deflection at the load point(s) relative to the supports in the *y* (or vertical) direction. Setting S_{MAX} = 0.002 in the strain estimate equation (A1.5.1.6) and substituting into *y* gives:

$$y_{0.2\,\%} = 2\, s\, (L + 2c)\, (3D_{IMFD})^{-1} \times 10^{-3}$$

where: $y_{0.2\,\%}$ = an estimate of the deflection at the load point which corresponds to 0.2 % strain.

FIG. A1.3 Load Cell versus Ram Displacement Graph

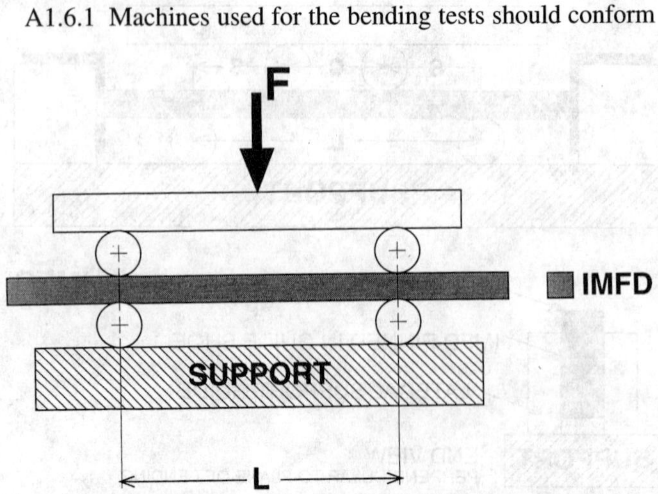

FIG. A1.4 Fixture/Device Compliance Test Setup

to the requirements of Practices E 4.

A1.6.2 The purpose of allowing a variety of spans and roller diameters for the bending tests is to allow one to accommodate the design differences of devices while maintaining standard techniques. For hollow and open-section IMFDs, long spans and large-diameter rollers will minimize local artifacts at the load and support points as much as possible. For long, small-diameter, solid section IMFDs, much smaller rollers and smaller spans are adequate to measure the bending of the IMFD (see A1.4.1.2).

A1.7 Precision and Bias

A1.7.1 *Minimizing and Correcting for Test Errors*:

A1.7.1.1 Because of differences in cross sectional shapes, areas, working lengths, etc., sensitivity to potential sources of measurement error will be different for each device. Typical sources of error include: *1*) span measurements, *2*) compliance of the IMFD at the support, *3*) fixture compliance and *4*) shear load produced at the load and support points in proportion to bending produced.

A1.7.1.2 *Span Measurement*—In general, longer spans minimize the effect of measurement error. However, the effect of particular measurement errors can be minimized by proper selection of the support and load spans. For example, calculated structural stiffness, EI_e, is more sensitive to errors in measurement of load-to-support point distance, s, than in the center span, c, because stiffness is dependent on s^2 and only linearly dependent on c. Therefore, maximizing s and minimizing c within the guidelines of A1.5.1 will reduce stiffness measurement errors.

A1.7.1.3 *Shear Load Errors*—Test Methods D 790 recommends a 16:1 support span-to-depth (such as, specimen thickness) ratio in order to minimize the effects of shear and compressive loads at the load and support points on the structural bending strength. This ratio should be used within the guidelines of A1.4.1.2, unless the device has insufficient working length to provide such spans.

A1.7.1.4 *Compensating for Fixture/Device Compliance*—Fixture/device compliance can be measured by setting the supports and load points coincident (so that $s = 0$, $c = L$ as described in A1.4.2). An elastic measure in this set up gives the combined device/fixture compliance, y/F_{F+D}. By subtracting this measurement from the system compliance measurements, y/F_{SYS}, during the bending tests, one is left with the bending compliance, y/F_{BEND}.

$$y/F_{BEND} = y/F_{SYS} - y/F_{F+D} \quad \text{(A1.11)}$$

The reciprocal of the bending compliance is the bending stiffness for the set up, which should be used in A1.4.1 to compute the structural bending stiffness of the IMFD, EI_e. By using this technique of compensating for the effect of local compliance, shear loading and fixture compliance, it is possible to keep these artifacts within reasonable limits for support span to IMFD diameter ratios of less than 20. This helps to ensure that the bending test, in fact, measures bending. Note that the fixture/device and fixture compliances may not be linear for all load ranges, thus these measurements should be carried out within the load ranges used for IMFD testing.

A1.7.1.5 *Toe Region Compensation*—Toe region compensation may be necessary to determine system, device, or fixture compliance/stiffness measurements. If a toe region exists, or if a true linear region cannot be identified, compliance/stiffness measures can be estimated by use of standard techniques such as in Test Methods D 790, Appendix X1, Toe Compensation.

A1.7.2 Tables A1.1-A1.4 provide the precision statistics for the following test parameters: load-displacement slope, bending structural stiffness, bending moment to yield, and ultimate bending moment, respectively. These results are based on a round robin interlaboratory study (ILS) conducted during the Fall of 1997 in accordance with Practice E 691. The precision statistics were determined using the Practice E 691 software (Version 2).

A1.7.3 The ILS utilized specimens from three types of cylindrical steel tubes, with the characteristics described in Table A1.5. The strength, stiffness, and geometry of the three specimen groups were intended to represent the range of likely values for IMFDs. For each specimen group, the samples were cut from a single length of bar stock.

A1.7.4 A total of eight laboratories participated in the testing. Three samples from specimen Group A were typically tested by each laboratory, and five samples from specimen Groups B and C were tested typically. In order to have a balanced statistical study and meet the requirements of the Practice E 691 software, four replicates were used for the statistical analysis. If only two or three specimen results were available from a particular laboratory, then the average from that laboratory was used to make up for the missing data points. Likewise if five specimen results were available from a particular lab, then the farthest outlying result was discarded. Labs were only included if they provided results for all three specimen groups. For the four parameters investigated, a minimum of 6 labs were included, satisfying the Practice E 691 requirements.

A1.7.5 *Repeatability, r*—In comparing two test results for the same material, obtained by the same operator using the same equipment on the same day, the two test results should be judged not equivalent if they differ by more than the *r* value for that material.

A1.7.6 *Reproducibility, R*—In comparing two test results for the same material, obtained by different operators using different equipment on different days, the two test results should be judged not equivalent if they differ by more than the *R* value for that material.

NOTE A1.4—The explanations for *r* and *R* (A1.7.5 and A1.7.6) only are intended to present a meaningful way of considering the approximate precision of this test method. The data in Tables A1.1-A1.4 should not be applied rigorously to acceptance or rejection of material, as those data are

TABLE A1.1 Precision Statistics for Load-Displacement Slope, F/y

Specimen Group	Mean (N/mm)	S_r[A]	S_R[B]	r[C]	R[D]	No. of Labs
A	905.23	9.03	28.15	25.28	78.81	8
B	1667.63	59.11	127.34	165.51	356.56	8
C	132.20	4.02	11.18	11.26	31.32	8

[A] S_r = within-laboratory standard deviation of the mean,
[B] S_R = between-laboratories standard deviation of the mean,
[C] $r = 2.83\ S_r$, and
[D] $R = 2.83\ S_R$.

TABLE A1.2 Precision Statistics for Bending Structural Stiffness, EI_e

Specimen Group	Mean (N/m^2)	S_r^A	S_R^B	r^C	R^D	No. of Labs
A	179.59	2.16	7.82	6.04	21.89	6
B	396.49	17.56	41.47	49.16	116.13	6
C	25.30	0.73	1.05	2.04	2.95	6

^AS_r = within-laboratory standard deviation of the mean,
^BS_R = between-laboratories standard deviation of the mean,
^Cr = 2.83 S_r, and
^DR = 2.83 S_R.

TABLE A1.3 Precision Statistics for Bending Moment to Yield, M_y

Specimen Group	Mean (N-m)	S_r^A	S_R^B	r^C	R^D	No. of Labs
A	183.47	3.26	12.78	9.12	35.77	8
B	79.13	1.44	6.85	4.02	19.19	8
C	11.03	0.30	0.58	0.83	1.62	8

^AS_r = within-laboratory standard deviation of the mean,
^BS_R = between-laboratories standard deviation of the mean,
^Cr = 2.83 S_r, and
^DR = 2.83 S_R.

TABLE A1.4 Precision Statistics for Ultimate Bending Moment, M_{MAX}

Specimen Group	Mean (N-m)	S_r^A	S_R^B	r^C	R^D	No. of Labs
A	237.22	1.75	2.77	4.90	7.76	7
B	107.15	1.44	4.15	4.04	11.61	7
C	12.75	0.18	0.27	0.49	0.75	7

^AS_r = within-laboratory standard deviation of the mean,
^BS_R = between-laboratories standard deviation of the mean,
^Cr = 2.83 S_r, and
^DR = 2.83 S_R.

specific to the round robin and may not be representative of other lots, materials, or laboratories. Users of this test method should apply the principles outlined in Practice E 691 to generate data specific to their laboratory and materials.

A1.7.7 Any judgment in accordance with A1.7.5 and A1.7.6 would have an approximate 95 % (0.95) probability of being correct.

A1.7.8 *Bias*—No statement may be made about bias of these test methods since there is no standard reference device or material that is applicable.

A1.8 Report

A1.8.1 *Purpose*—Reports of results should be aimed at providing as much relevant information as necessary for other investigators, designers or manufacturers to be able to duplicate the tests being reported. Thus the choices for all relevant parameters from the methods must be reported. Other relevant observations that influence the interpretation of results such as distortion of cross section, localized buckling at support points, cracks at stress concentration points, etc. should also be reported. Criteria for failure and observed modes of failure should also be reported.

A1.8.2 Report the following information:

A1.8.2.1 Complete identification of the device(s) tested including: type, manufacturer, catalogue number(s), lot number(s), material specifications, principal dimensions (and precision of measurements of those dimensions) and previous history (if applicable).

A1.8.2.2 Direction of loading of specimens and the location.

A1.8.2.3 Conditioning procedure, if any.

A1.8.2.4 Total support span, *L*; load to support span, *s*; and precision of each measurement made.

A1.8.2.5 Fixture/device compliance measured in mm/N.

A1.8.2.6 Support span to depth ratio and methods of compensation chosen for small ratios or radially compliant devices, or both.

A1.8.2.7 Use of outriggers or supports for control of rotation during testing.

A1.8.2.8 Methods to compensate for toe regions or compensation for any other phenomenon encountered (see Test Methods D 790).

A1.8.2.9 Radius of supports and loading roller and precision of those measurements.

A1.8.2.10 Rate of crosshead motion.

A1.8.2.11 Slope of the linear portion of the load-displacement curve, *F/y*, in N/mm; estimate of structural stiffness of the IMFD, EI_e, in N-m^2, from *F/y, s, c* and *L*; and, explanation of adjustments for fixture/device compliance.

A1.8.2.12 Load at yield, *F*, in N and the estimate of moment at yield, M_y, in *NM*; and any other failure criteria/measures made.

A1.8.3 *Statistical Report*:

A1.8.3.1 The mean value, number of specimens in the sample and the sample deviations should be reported for each measurement and calculation of values so that precision and accuracy of the test method as well as the behavior of the specific IMFD design and size can be established.

A1.8.3.2 The report shall include the results and methods of tests used to determine outliers and normality of the data.

A1.9 Rationale (Nonmandatory Information)

A1.9.1 IMFDs are bone fracture fixation devices intended for use as temporary, adjunctive stabilizing devices for skeletal parts with a limited mechanical service life only until the injured hard or soft tissue parts, or both, have healed. These devices are not designed to support the skeletal parts indefinitely if the injured parts do not heal. This is far different from prosthetic devices which are intended to permanently replace the mechanical function of a skeletal or soft tissue part and serve as the sole load-bearing member.

A1.9.2 The bending stiffness of IMFDs throughout the working length is known to have an effect upon the level of load transfer and level of stress in the surrounding bone and callus and to influence the rate and strength of healing of the bone as well as long term remodeling. The specific level of stress and load in the bone related to a specific bending stiffness is an unknown and dependent upon multiple factors such as level and type of activity of the patient, condition of the surrounding bone and soft tissue, stability of the fracture pattern and its fixation, size of the bone, weight of the patient, etc. Thus, measurements of structural bending stiffness using this standard testing technique are only of value for comparative purposes between devices of different sizes, designs, and materials.

A1.9.3 The single-cycle bending strength of IMFDs is known to be an important factor in cases where bone support

TABLE A1.5 Description of Specimen Groups in ILS

Specimen Group	Outer Diameter (in.)	Inner Diameter (in.)	Material	Material Yield Strength (ksi)	Material Tensile Strength (ksi)	Material Elongation (%)
A	0.472 ± 0.003	0.199 ± 0.002	316LVM Stainless steel (Specification F 138, Grade 2)	100 min	125 min	12 min
B	0.625 ± 0.004 (Specification A 450/A 450M)	0.495 (Specification A 450/A 450M)	Carbon steel (Specification A 214/A 214M)	39.5	51.6	51
C	0.313 (SAE J524)	0.243 (SAE J524)	Carbon steel (AMS 5050)	36.1	54.2	40

is minimal and a secondary trauma occurs. In such cases a plastic deformation (load beyond the yield moment) may occur necessitating a secondary surgical procedure for correction of any anatomic deformity which is clinically unacceptable. Since secondary trauma is uncontrollable and unpredictable, there is no acceptable limit which can be set for bending strength in any plane. Thus, measurements of structural bending strength using this standard testing technique are only of value for comparative purposes between devices of different sizes, designs, and materials. The separation between the bending moment to yield and the bending moment to ultimate reflects the ductility of a given design. This may be important in cases where a single event of secondary trauma has created plastic deformity in the IMFD which requires reverse bending beyond yield to straighten the IMFD sufficiently for removal. An IMFD with minimal ductility is at increased risk of breaking instead of bending in either the secondary trauma or an intraoperative correction maneuver which may result in greater risk to some patients.

A1.9.4 Recommended load and support spans are based upon consistency with the old Practice F 383 for short spans; laboratory experiences with larger hollow femoral devices for the long spans; and reflects common practice.

A2. TEST METHOD FOR STATIC TORSIONAL TESTING OF INTRAMEDULLARY FIXATION DEVICES

A2.1 Scope

A2.1.1 This test method covers the test procedure for determining the torsional stiffness of intramedullary fixation devices (IMFD). The central part of the IMFD, with a straight and uniform cross-section and away from screw holes or other interlocking features, is tested in a static test.

A2.1.2 IMFDs are indicated for surgical fixation of the skeletal system and are typically used in the femur, tibia, humerus, radius, or ulna. Devices that meet the IMFD specifications of Section 4, and other similar devices, are covered by this test method.

A2.1.3 This test method does not intend to test or provide information that will necessarily relate to the properties of fixation that an IMFD may obtain in a bone or any other connection with other devices.

A2.1.4 This test method is not intended to define case-specific clinical performance of these devices, as insufficient knowledge is available to predict the consequences of the use of any of these devices in individual patients.

A2.1.5 This test method is not intended to serve as a quality assurance document, and thus, statistical sampling techniques for batches from the production of IMFDs are not addressed.

A2.1.6 Unless otherwise indicated, the values stated in SI units are to be regarded as the standard. The values in parentheses are given for information only.

A2.1.7 *This standard does not purport to address all of the safety concerns, if any, associated with its use. It is the responsibility of the user of this standard to establish appropriate safety and health practices and determine the applicability of regulatory limitations prior to use.*

A2.2 Summary of Test Method

A2.2.1 An intramedullary fixation device is secured in a fixture so that a straight, uniform cross section of specified length is in the gage section. The IMFD is loaded under a pure torsional moment and the resulting angular deflection (rotation) is measured. The slope of the torque-rotation curve provides the elastic torsional stiffness of the IMFD.

A2.3 Terminology

A2.3.1 *Definition of Term Specific to This Standard:*

A2.3.1.1 *torsional stiffness (N-m/°),n*—the slope of the torque-rotation curve, as determined in A2.9.1.

A2.4 Significance and Use

A2.4.1 This test method describes a static torsional test to determine the torsional stiffness of the central and uniform portion of an intramedullary fixation device.

A2.4.2 This test method may not be appropriate for all types of implant applications. The user is cautioned to consider the appropriateness of the method in view of the devices being tested and their potential application.

A2.5 Apparatus

A2.5.1 *Torsional Load Frame*, a testing machine capable of applying torsional loads at a constant angular displacement rate and capable of either applying axial loads in load control or being free to move in axial displacement.

A2.5.2 *Axial Load Frame*, a testing machine capable of applying tensile or compressive loads at a constant displacement rate.

A2.5.3 *Test Fixture*, a fixture capable of gripping both ends of the IMFD and ensuring that only torsional moments are applied to the IMFD. If the fixture is used with an axial load frame, the fixture must be free to slide in the longitudinal direction of the test specimen. The test fixture should be sufficiently rigid so that its rotational deformation under the maximum torque is less than 1 % of the deformation of the test specimen.

A2.5.4 *Torque Transducer*, a calibrated device capable of measuring torsional moments with an accuracy of ±1 % of its rated full scale capacity and providing output readable by a suitable recording device.

A2.5.5 *Rotational Transducer*, a calibrated device capable of measuring angular displacement with an accuracy of ±1 % of its rated full scale capacity and providing output readable by a suitable recording device.

A2.5.6 *Recording Device*, a recording device capable of plotting the output of the torque transducer and rotation transducer to provide a torque-rotation curve.

A2.6 Test Specimen

A2.6.1 A straight section of IMFD with an approximate length of 28 cm (11.02 in.) is recommended. Approximately 2.5 cm (1 in.) at each end will be gripped by the test fixture. A straight section is required to prevent the simultaneous introduction of bending under the application of the torsional moment.

A2.6.2 The central portion of the test specimen must have a uniform cross section along the recommended gage length of 23 cm (9.06 in.). The ends of the gage length must be at least one IMFD diameter from any type of stress concentration or change in geometry. The gage length may be changed to accommodate IMFDs that cannot meet the requirement of a 23 cm length of straight and uniform section. In that case, report the gage length used.

A2.6.3 All test components shall be representative of implant quality products with regard to material, cross-section, surface finish, and manufacturing processes. IMFDs may differ from actual implant products if the difference is required to obtain a straight nail section. Report any differences.

A2.7 Procedure

A2.7.1 Prepare the ends of the test specimens for gripping. This may include machining three flats along the grip section for securing in Jacob's type chucks. For slotted (open section) IMFDs, the grip section at each end may be potted with a suitable potting agent such as PMMA or potting metal, provided the potting material does not extend into the gage section. Some members have used a clearance-fit pin inside of the grip ends of the open section IMFDs to support the cross-section while gripping with a Jacob's type chuck. Report the method used for gripping the specimen.

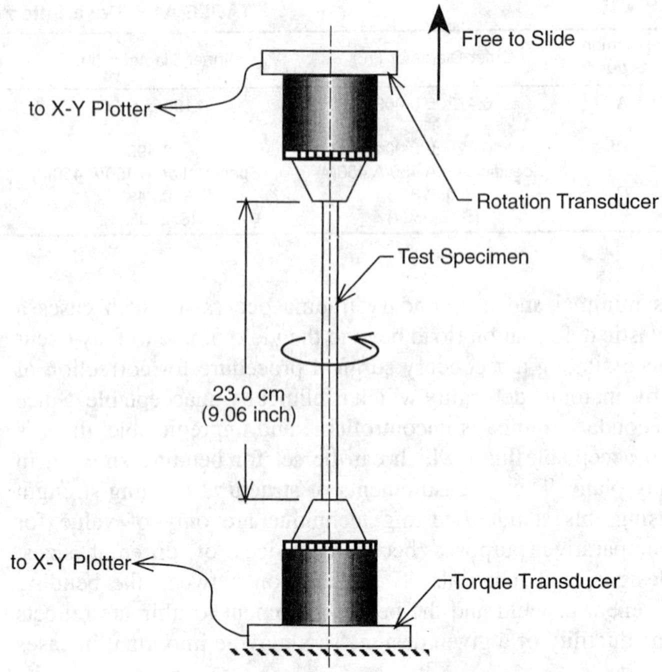

FIG. A2.1 Torsional Load Frame Set-Up

A2.7.2 Secure the ends of the test specimen into the test fixture to provide the gage length of 23 cm (9.06 in.). As indicated in A2.6.2, deviations from the specified gage length are permitted if necessary, provided the gage length is reported. The grips will directly grip the surface of the nail or the potting material, if applicable.

A2.7.2.1 When a torsional load frame is used, the fixture usually will consist simply of two gripping devices, such as Jacob's chucks, which will prevent rotation of the test specimen inside of the grips. This set-up is shown in Fig. A2.1. The axis of the test specimen must be coincident with the axis of the load frame. Place the axial load controller in load control to apply a small compressive axial load (5 to 10 N [1 to 2 lb]) during the course of the test. If the load frame is not capable of applying axial loads in load control, then one of the fixtures should be free to displace in the longitudinal direction of the test specimen.

A2.7.2.2 When an axial load frame is used, a more sophisticated test fixture is required. An example of such is shown in Fig. A2.2. It consists of two gripping devices that prevent rotation of the test specimen inside of the grips. The axis of the test specimen must be coincident with the axis of the two grips. One grip is secured to the torque transducer, which in turn is

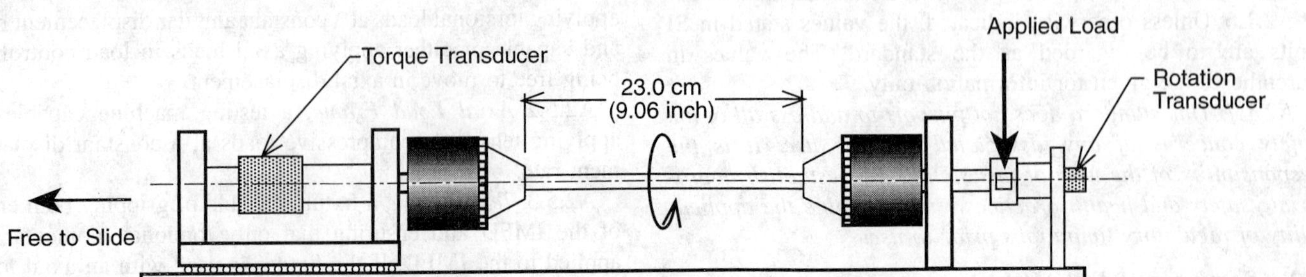

FIG. A2.2 (a) Axial Load Frame Set-Up Side View

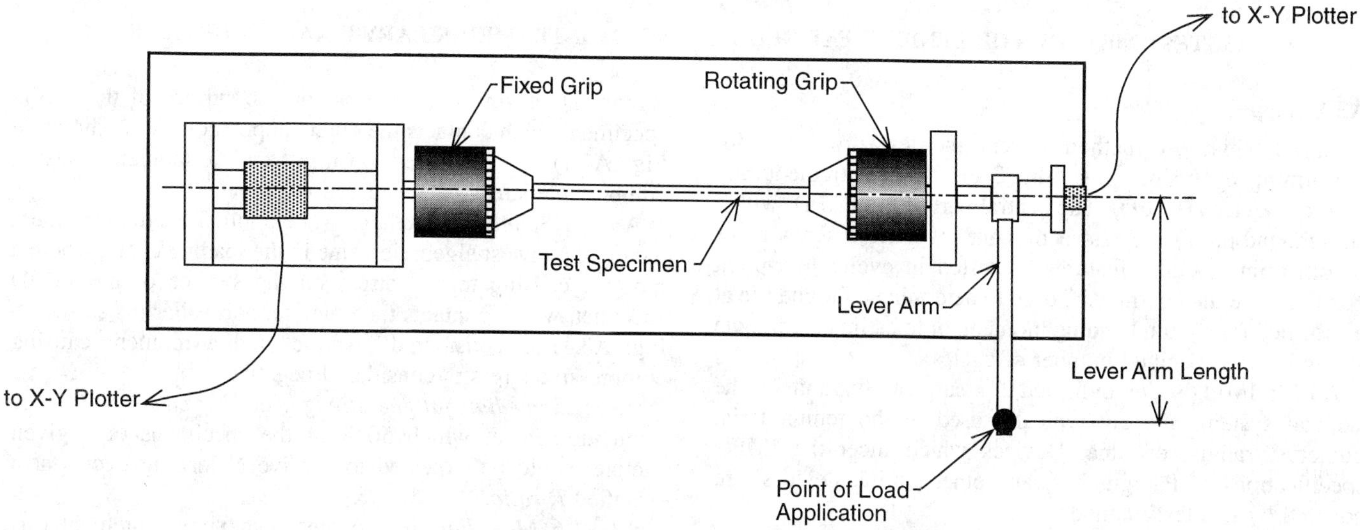

FIG. A2.2 (b) Axial Load Frame Set-Up Top View *(continued)*

secured to the test fixture. This grip should be free to displace in the longitudinal direction of the test specimen. The other grip is attached to the test fixture through a bearing that allows the grip to rotate freely. A lever arm is attached to the rotating grip and is used to apply a torsional moment to the test specimen through its contact with the axial load frame actuator. The load actuator will contact the level arm through a roller some distance from the axis of the test specimen. The roller diameter and lever arm distance may be chosen by the user but must be reported. The rotation transducer measures the angular displacement of the rotating grip.

A2.7.3 The recording device will be configured to record a torque-rotation curve. Choose the torque and rotation axes scales to provide sufficient data to determine the slope of the curve.

A2.7.4 The load frame will be configured to rotate at a constant rate of 5°/min when a torsional load frame is used. When an axial load frame is used, choose a constant displacement rate that will result in a rotation rate that is approximately 5°/min.

A2.7.5 The load frame will be activated and the torque applied until the test specimen rotates through approximately 5°, or until a straight-line portion of the torque-rotation curve is achieved.

A2.8 Calculation or Interpretation of Results

A2.8.1 The initial slope of the straight-line portion of the torque-rotation curve will provide the torsional stiffness of the test specimen.

A2.9 Report

A2.9.1 Include the following information in the test report:

A2.9.1.1 Manufacturer of IMFD specimen;

A2.9.1.2 IMFD size and catalog number (if applicable);

A2.9.1.3 Material of IMFD specimen;

A2.9.1.4 Deviations from normal implant product;

A2.9.1.5 Method of gripping, and potting agent and potting diameter used (if applicable);

A2.9.1.6 Gage or grip length used, or both, if different from that specified;

A2.9.1.7 Average torsional stiffness, standard deviation, and sample size; and

A2.9.1.8 Any deviations from the test method.

A2.10 Precision and Bias

A2.10.1 Data establishing the precision and bias to be expected from this test method have not yet been obtained.

A2.11 Rationale (Nonmandatory Information)

A2.11.1 This test method determines the torsional stiffness of an intramedullary fixation device (IMFD). These devices are intended for use as temporary, adjunctive stabilizing devices of skeletal parts. The torsional stiffness of IMFDs is known to have an affect upon the level of load transfer and level of stress in the surrounding bone and callus and to influence the rate and strength of healing of the bone, as well as long-term remodeling. The specific level of stress and load in the bone related to a specific torsional stiffness is unknown and dependent upon multiple factors such as level and type of activity of the patient, condition of the surrounding bone and soft tissue, stability of the fracture pattern, size of the bone, weight of the patient, etc. Measurements of torsional stiffness using this test method, therefore, are only of value for comparative purposes between devices of different sizes, designs, and materials, and the results are not intended to define case-specific clinical performance of the tested devices.

A3. TEST METHOD FOR BENDING FATIGUE TESTING OF INTRAMEDULLARY FIXATION DEVICES

A3.1 Scope

A3.1.1 This test method covers` the test procedure for performing cyclic bending fatigue testing of intramedullary fixation devices (IMFD). The central part of the IMFD, with a straight and uniform cross-section and away from screw holes or other interlocking features, is tested in cyclic four-point bending. The method may be used to determine a fatigue life at a specified maximum bending moment, or to estimate a fatigue strength for a specified number of cycles.

A3.1.2 IMFD's are indicated for surgical fixation of the skeletal system, and are typically used in the femur, tibia, humerus, radius, or ulna. Devices which meet the IMFD specifications of Paragraph 4, and other similar devices, are covered by this test method.

A3.1.3 This test method does not intend to test or provide information which will necessarily relate to the properties of fixation which an IMFD may obtain in a bone, or any other connection with other devices.

A3.1.4 This test method is not intended to define case-specific clinical performance of these devices, as insufficient knowledge is available to predict the consequences of the use of any of these devices in individual patients.

A3.1.5 This test method is not intended to serve as a quality assurance document and thus statistical sampling techniques for batches from the production of IMFD's are not addressed.

A3.1.6 Unless otherwise indicated, the values stated in SI units are to be regarded as the standard. The values in parentheses are given for information only.

A3.1.7 *This standard does not purport to address all of the safety concerns, if any, associated with its use. It is the responsibility of the user of this standard to establish appropriate safety and health practices and determine the applicability of regulatory limitations prior to use.*

A3.2 Referenced Documents

A3.2.1 *ASTM Standards:*

E 467 Practice for Verification of Constant Amplitude Dynamic Loads in an Axial Fatigue Testing Machine[3]

E 1150 Definitions of Terms Relating to Fatigue[11]

A3.3. Terminology

A3.3.1 *Definitions*—Unless otherwise given, the definitions for fatigue terminology given in ASTM E 1150 will be used.

A3.3.1.1 *R-ratio*—the algebraic ratio of the two loading parameters of a fatigue cycle. For the purposes of this test method the R-ratio is defined as:

R = Minimum moment/Maximum moment

A3.3.1.2 *Nominal stress*—The stress at a point calculated in the net cross-section by simple elastic theory without taking into account the increase in stress that may be caused by a local stress concentrator, such as a hole.

A3.3.1.3 *maximum moment*—The applied bending moment having the highest algebraic value in the loading cycle, where a moment causing tensile stress on the surface of the IMFD specimen which contacts the outer support rollers (as shown in Fig. A3.1) is considered positive, and a moment causing compressive stress is considered negative.

A3.3.1.4 *minimum moment*—The applied bending moment having the lowest algebraic value in the loading cycle, where a moment causing tensile stress on the surface of the IMFD specimen which contacts the outer support roller (as shown in Fig. A3.1) is considered positive, and a moment causing compressive stress is considered negative.

A3.3.1.5 *median fatigue strength at N cycles*—The maximum moment at which 50 % of the specimens of a given sample would be expected to survive N loading cycles at a specified *R-ratio.*

A3.3.1.6 *M-N diagram*—A plot of maximum moment versus the number of cycles to a specified failure point.

A3.3.1.7 *runout*—A predetermined number of cycles at which the testing on a particular specimen stopped, and no further testing on that specimen will be performed. When the intent of the fatigue test program is to determine the fatigue strength at N cycles, the runout is usually specified as N cycles.

A3.4 Summary of Test Method

A3.4.1 An intramedullary fixation device is placed on a four-point bending fixture so that a straight, uniform cross section of specified length is in the gage section. The IMFD is loaded under four-point bending, in a sinusoidal cyclic manner at a specified frequency. The fatigue loading is continued until the specimen fails, a limit is reached which terminates the test, or a predetermined number of cycles (runout limit) is reached.

A3.5 Significance and Use

A3.5.1 This test method describes a cyclic bending fatigue test to characterize the fatigue performance of an IMFD. The method may be used to determine a fatigue life at a specified maximum bending moment, or to estimate a fatigue strength for a specified number of cycles.

A3.5.2 This test method may not be appropriate for all types of implant applications. The user is cautioned to consider the appropriateness of the method in view of the devices being tested and their potential application.

A3.6 Apparatus

A3.6.1 *Axial Load Frame*—A testing machine capable of

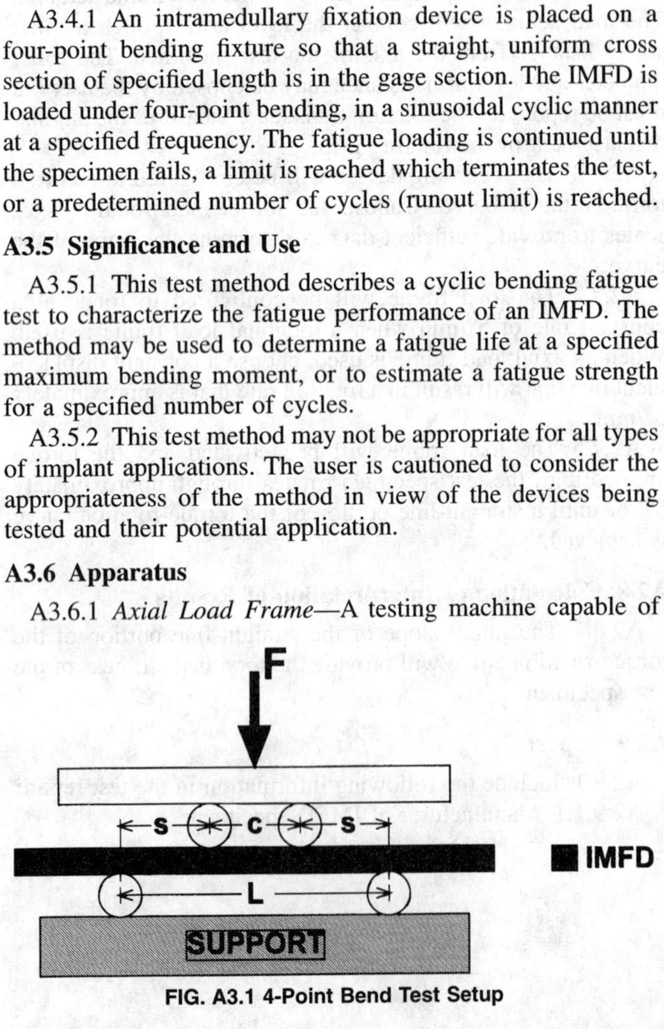

FIG. A3.1 4-Point Bend Test Setup

[11] Discontinued 1996; Replaced by E 1823.

applying cyclic sinusoidal tensile, or compressive loads.

A3.6.2 *Cycle Counter*—A device capable of counting the number of loading cycles applied to a specimen during the course of a fatigue test.

A3.6.3 *Four Point Bend Fixture*—A two part fixture (top and bottom) capable of applying a uniform bending moment to the central portion of an IMFD. The IMFD specimen is supported by two outer support rollers, and the moment is applied through two inner loading rollers. This is shown in Fig. A3.1 and is similar to that used for static testing, as described in Annex A1.

A3.6.4 *Load Cell*—A load cell capable of measuring dynamic tensile and/or compressive loads in accordance with Practice E 467.

A3.6.5 *Limit*—A device capable of detecting when a test parameter (e.g. load, actuator displacement, DC error, etc.) reaches a limiting value, at which time the test is stopped and the current cycle count recorded.

A3.7 Test Specimen

A3.7.1 A straight section of an IMFD or an IMFD with curvature in a single plane is recommended. It is recommended that the central portion of the test specimen have a uniform cross section along the gage length, unless any geometrical features are characteristic of the normal cross-section along the IMFD's working length. Deviations from this may be appropriate, as described in A3.7.2.

A3.7.2 The addition of a geometrical feature, such as a hole, may be located in the gage section. For the stated example, this may be useful for evaluating the bending fatigue performance of IMFD screw holes. Any type of feature should be placed in the center of the gage section to maintain a symmetric deflection profile.

A3.7.3 All test components should be representative of implant quality products, with regard to material, cross-section, surface finish, and manufacturing processes. Any differences must be reported.

A3.8 Procedure

A3.8.1 Prior to testing, the load level for testing must be determined. To evaluate the fatigue performance of an IMFD, the user has several alternatives or approaches.

A3.8.1.1 *M-N or S-N Diagram*—One may test at several load levels to characterize the general fatigue behavior of an IMFD over a range of loads or stresses. The applied moment and the cycles to failure are plotted on a M-N diagram. Alternatively, the nominal stress due to the applied moment may be determined using analytical, experimental, or computational stress analysis methods, and a S-N diagram generated. A curve fit may be applied to the data to develop a M-N or S-N curve.

A3.8.1.2 *Fatigue Strength Determination*—Another approach is to determine the fatigue strength of a particular IMFD device. For the purposes of standardization, the fatigue strength in this standard is determined at 1 million cycles of loading. A rationale for this criterion is given in A.X1. The up and down method for determining fatigue strength is a generally accepted manner for conducting fatigue testing to determine fatigue strength.**(1)**

For bending fatigue testing described in this test method, the load level is expressed as the maximum moment, M, applied to the IMFD specimen.

A3.8.2 The four point bend fixture should be adjusted so that the span of the outer support rollers, L, is between 10 and 50 cm (3.94 to 19.69 inches). The inner loading span, c, should be no greater than L/3. The two span dimensions are shown in Fig. A3.1. The diameter of the load and support rollers should be between 1.0 and 2.6 cm (0.39 to 1.0 inches). The spans should be set to within 1 % of their determined values. The choice of load and support spans should be based upon the guidelines given in A1.8.1 of Annex A1.

A3.8.3 *Suggested Load Spans*—A recommendation for load and support spans is provided below to minimize interlaboratory variation and provide consistency with the previous ASTM standard and with the static test method specified in Annex A1. The suggested long or short spans should be used whenever possible, provided the general guidelines of A1.8.1 are achieved.

Short Span	s = c = 3.8 cm (1.5 in.)	L = 11.4 cm (4.5 in.)
Long Span	s = c = 7.6 cm (3.0 in.)	L = 22.8 cm (9.0 in.)

A3.8.4 The IMFD specimen should be placed on the support rollers so that any CSC or geometrical feature in the gage section is at least 3 diameters of the IMFD from any load or support roller. If the IMFD is curved, the device should be placed so that the applied bending moment is in the same plane as the IMFD curvature. The orientation of the applied bending relative to the ML and AP anatomic planes should be reported.

A3.8.5 For IMFD's which have rotational instability, the fixtures described in A1.5.1.10 of Annex A1 may be used. During fatigue testing, specimens can have the tendency to "walk" during the application of cyclic loading, if they are not constrained against such behavior. This can be a problem during 4-point bending fatigue tests as the specimens are typically only resting on support rollers. This can be prevented by constructing appropriate guides in combination with the test fixture such to prevent the specimens from shifting their position during testing. The guides, of course, must not interfere with load application or specimen deformation.

A3.8.6 Apply equal loads at each of the loading points. The maximum applied load, *F*, is determined from:

$$F = 2M/s, \tag{A3.1}$$

where *M* is the maximum moment. The maximum nominal stress applied to the IMFD may be determined using analytical, experimental, or computational methods.

A3.8.7 The loads shall be applied in a sinusoidal cyclic manner at a frequency no greater than 5 Hz. For strain-rate sensitive materials, an appropriate cyclic rate may be determined using the equation for strain-rate given in A1.5.1.4 of Annex A1.

A3.8.8 The recommended *R-ratio* is 0.1. Any deviations from this should be reported.

A3.8.9 The cycle counter shall record a cumulative number of cycles applied to the test specimen, and the appropriate limits should be set to indicate specimen failure or deviations from the intended load system performance.

A3.8.10 Testing shall continue until the specimen breaks, a

limit is reached which terminates the test, or the runout criterion is reached.

A3.9 Calculation and Interpretation of Results

A3.9.1 The maximum moment (or stress) and cycles to failure should be recorded and plotted on a M-N (or S-N) diagram. Various techniques may be used to estimate mean or median fatigue lives, statistical differences between groups, curve fits to the fatigue data, probability of survival curves, and so on **(1-3)**[12].

A3.9.2 If determining fatigue strength *at N cycles*, it is recommended that the fatigue strength be determined as the median fatigue limit (50 % probability of survival), using a technique or criteria described in the literature. **(1)**

A3.10 Report

A3.10.1 The test report shall include the following:

A3.10.1.1 Manufacturer of IMFD specimen.

A3.10.1.2 IMFD *diameter* and catalog number (if applicable).

A3.10.1.3 Material of IMFD specimen, including applicable ASTM or ISO specifications.

A3.10.1.4 Description of deviations from a uniform cross-section in the gage length, if any.

A3.10.1.5 Deviations from normal implant product.

A3.10.1.6 Outer support span, L; Inner loading span, c; Span between inner and outer rollers, s; and roller diameters.

A3.10.1.7 *R-ratio* and the test frequency.

A3.10.1.8 Description of the testing environment.

A3.10.1.9 A summary of the maximum moment (and stress) and the resulting cycles to failure or runout for each specimen tested. The data should be plotted on a M-N or S-N diagram. A description of the analytical or statistical techniques used for interpretation of the fatigue data should be included.

A3.10.1.10 A description of the failure mode and failure location for each specimen which failed.

A3.10.1.11 If appropriate, an estimate of the fatigue strength should be reported. A description of the analytical or statistical techniques used for determining the fatigue strength should be included.

A3.11 Precision and Bias

A3.11.1 Data establishing the precision and accuracy to be expected from this test method have not yet been obtained.

A3.12 Rationale

A3.12.1 The low cycle bending fatigue strength of IMFD's is known to be an important factor in cases where bone support is minimal and when healing is delayed. In such cases, major stresses may occur in the unsupported region of the working length of the IMFD over several weeks, prior to development of adequate mechanical support from the healing bone to reduce the level of stresses in the IMFD. Since the rate and amount of healing are uncontrollable and unpredictable, as well as the levels of load which the IMFD must bear in any given case, there is no "acceptable" limit which can be set for the bending moment or number of cycles of load which the IMFD should withstand in any plane.

A3.12.2 One of the objectives of this test is to estimate a fatigue strength at 10^6 cycles for comparison of different devices. Since these are trauma fixation devices whose service life is limited and mechanical demands are finite in time, no definition of endurance limit is necessary. One million cycles has been arbitrarily chosen as the number of cycles for testing, recognizing that no IMFD in clinical service is expected to withstand 10^6 loading cycles *of high stresses* in clinical use. Fractures and skeletal reconstructions generally heal in 2–3 months normally (about 150 000 to 250 000 cycles). Therefore, the fatigue resistance at 10^6 cycles is beyond the expected clinical need for these devices.

A3.12.3 Finally, measurements of cyclic bending fatigue strength or fatigue life using this standard testing technique are only of value for comparative purposes between devices of different sizes, designs, materials, and materials.

[12] The boldface numbers in parentheses refer to the list of references at the end of this standard.

A4. TEST METHOD FOR BENDING FATIGUE TESTING OF IMFD LOCKING SCREWS

A4.1 Scope

A4.1.1 This test method covers the test procedure for performing cyclic bending fatigue testing of locking screws utilized for the fixation of intramedullary fixation devices (IMFD). The central part of the screw is tested in cyclic three-point or four-point bending. The method may be used to determine a fatigue life at a specified maximum bending moment or to estimate a fatigue strength for a specified number of cycles.

A4.1.2 This test method is specifically applicable to screws described by Specification F 543, which are used to provide fixation of IMFDs in bone by transversely crossing through the IMFD from one cortex to another. This test method may or may not be applicable to other types of orthopaedic bone screws.

A4.1.3 This test method does not address the connection between the IMFD and the screw.

A4.1.4 This test method is not intended to define case-specific clinical performance of these devices, as insufficient knowledge is available to predict the consequences of the use of any of these devices in individual patients.

A4.1.5 This test method is not intended to serve as a quality assurance document, and thus, statistical sampling techniques for batches from the production of screws are not addressed.

A4.1.6 Unless otherwise indicated, the values stated in SI units are to be regarded as the standard. The values given in parentheses are provided for information only.

A4.1.7 *This standard does not purport to address all of the safety concerns, if any, associated with its use. It is the responsibility of the user of this standard to establish appropriate safety and health practices and determine the applicability of regulatory limitations prior to use.*

A4.2 Referenced Documents

A4.2.1 *ASTM Standards:*

E 467 Practice for Verification of Constant Amplitude Dynamic Loads in an Axial Fatigue Testing Machine[3]

E 1150 Definitions of Terms Relating to Fatigue[12]

F 543 Specification for Cortical Bone Screws[5]

A4.3. Terminology

A4.3.1 *Definitions*—Unless otherwise given, the definitions for fatigue terminology given in Definitions E 1150 will be used.

A4.3.2 *Definitions of Terms Specific to This Standard:*

A4.3.2.1 *maximum moment, n*—the applied bending moment having the highest algebraic value in the loading cycle, where a moment causing tensile stress on the surface of the screw specimen, which contacts the outer support rollers (see Fig. A4.1) is considered positive, and a moment causing compressive stress is considered negative.

A4.3.2.2 *median fatigue strength at N cycles, n*—the maximum moment at which 50 % of the specimens of a given sample would be expected to survive *N* loading cycles at a specified R-ratio.

A4.3.2.3 *minimum moment, n*—the applied bending moment having the lowest algebraic value in the loading cycle, where a moment causing tensile stress on the surface of the screw specimen which contacts the outer support rollers (see Fig. A4.1) is considered positive, and a moment causing compressive stress is considered negative.

A4.3.2.4 *M-N diagram, n*—a plot of maximum moment versus the number of cycles to a specified failure point.

A4.3.2.5 *R-ratio, R, n*—the algebraic ratio of the two loading parameters of a fatigue cycle. For the purposes of this test method the *R*-ratio is defined as follows:

$$R = \text{Minimum moment/Maximum moment}$$

A4.3.2.6 *runout, n*—a predetermined number of cycles at which the testing on a particular specimen will be stopped, and no further testing on that specimen will be performed. When the intent of the fatigue test program is to determine the fatigue strength at *N* cycles, the runout usually is specified as *N* cycles.

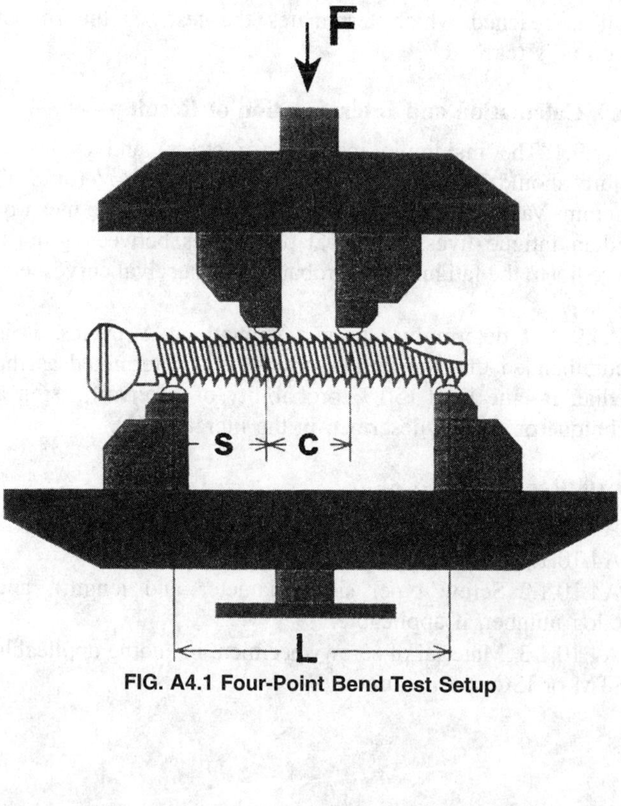

FIG. A4.1 Four-Point Bend Test Setup

A4.4 Summary of Test Method

A4.4.1 A screw is placed on a three-point or four-point bending fixture so that a straight and regular section of specified length is in the gage section. The screw is loaded under three-point or four-point bending, in a sinusoidal cyclic manner at a specified frequency. The fatigue loading is continued until the specimen fails, a limit is reached, which terminates the test, or a predetermined number of cycles (runout limit) is reached.

A4.5 Significance and Use

A4.5.1 This test method describes a cyclic bending fatigue test to characterize the fatigue performance of an IMFD locking screw. The method may be used to determine a fatigue life at a specified maximum bending moment or to estimate a fatigue strength for a specified number of cycles.

A4.5.2 This test method may not be appropriate for all types of implant applications. The user is cautioned to consider the appropriateness of the method in view of the devices being tested and their potential application.

A4.6 Apparatus

A4.6.1 *Axial Load Frame*—A testing machine capable of applying cyclic sinusoidal tensile or compressive loads.

A4.6.2 *Cycle Counter*—A device capable of counting the number of loading cycles applied to a specimen during the course of a fatigue test.

A4.6.3 *Four-Point Bend Fixture*—A two-part fixture (top and bottom) capable of applying a uniform bending moment to the central portion of a screw. The screw specimen is supported by two outer support rollers, and the moment is applied through two inner loading rollers (see Fig. A4.1).

A4.6.4 *Three-Point Bend Fixture*—A two-part fixture (top and bottom) capable of applying a three point bending moment to the central portion of a screw. The screw specimen is supported by two outer support rollers, and the moment is applied through a single roller which is centered between the two outer support rollers (see Fig. A4.2).

A4.6.5 *Load Cell*—A load cell capable of measuring dynamic tensile, or compressive loads, or both, in accordance with Practice E 467.

A4.6.6 *Limit*—A device capable of detecting when a test parameter, for example, load, actuator displacement, DC error, etc., reaches a limiting value, at which time the test is stopped and the current cycle count recorded.

A4.7 Test Specimen

A4.7.1 A straight and regular section of a screw thread, or the central portion of screw, shall be used for testing. The thread diameter and core diameter shall be consistent throughout the intended gage section with no steps or other geometric

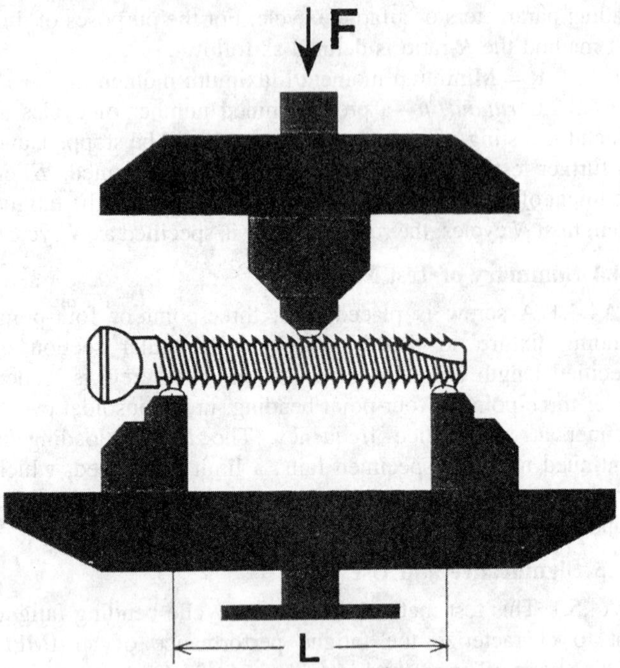

FIG. A4.2 Three-Point Bend Test Setup

discontinuities, other than from the threads themselves.

A4.7.2 All test components should be representative of implant quality products, with regard to material, cross-section, surface finish, and manufacturing processes. Any differences must be reported.

A4.8 Procedure

A4.8.1 Prior to testing, the load level for testing must be determined. To evaluate the fatigue performance of a screw, the user has several alternatives or approaches.

A4.8.1.1 *M-N or S-N Diagram*—One may test at several load levels to characterize the general fatigue behavior of a screw over a range of loads or stresses. The applied moment and the cycles to failure are plotted on a *M-N* diagram. Alternatively, the stress due to the applied moment may be determined using analytical, experimental, or computational stress analysis methods, and a *S-N* diagram generated. A curve fit may be applied to the data to develop a *M-N* or *S-N* curve.

A4.8.1.2 *Fatigue Strength Determination*—Another approach is to determine the fatigue strength of a particular screw. For the purposes of standardization, the fatigue strength in this test method is determined at one million cycles of loading. A rationale for this criterion is given in A3.X1. The "up and down" method for determining fatigue strength generally is an accepted manner for conducting fatigue testing to determine fatigue strength **(1)**.

For bending fatigue testing described in this test method, the load level is expressed as the maximum moment, *M*, applied to the screw.

A4.8.2 Depending on the length of the screw, either a three-point or four-point bending fixture shall be utilized. Generally, it is favorable to use four-point bending because the central portion of the specimen is subjected to a uniform bending moment; however, for short screws, it may not be practical to fit all four loading points along the screw length. The choice of three-point or four-point bending, and the span lengths to use in either case, is left to the discretion of the user. The choice of support spans should be based upon the guidelines given in A1.8.1.

A4.8.2.1 *Four-Point Bend*—The four-point bend fixture should be adjusted to the chosen span of the outer loading rollers, *L*. The inner loading span, *c*, should be no greater than *L*/3. The test setup is shown in Fig. A4.1.

A4.8.2.2 *Three-Point Bend*—The three-point bend fixture should be adjusted to the chosen span of the outer support rollers, *L*. The upper loading roller shall be centered between the outer support rollers. The test setup is shown in Fig. A4.2.

A4.8.3 The load and support rollers shall be made of hardened steel and have a diameter which is two to four times greater than the thread pitch of the screw being tested. The screw shall be placed on the loading fixture such that the support rollers sit between the crests of two adjacent threads. This may require some adjustment of the fixture spans to accommodate the particular screw being tested.

A4.8.4 Apply equal loads at each of the loading points. The maximum applied load, *F*, is determined from the following:

$$F = 2M/s \qquad \text{(A4.1)}$$

where:

M = the maximum moment. The maximum stress applied to the IMFD may be determined using analytical, experimental, or computational methods.

A4.8.5 The loads shall be applied in a sinusoidal cyclic manner at a frequency no greater than 5 Hz.

A4.8.6 The recommended *R*-ratio is 0.1. Any deviations from this should be reported.

A4.8.7 The cycle counter shall record a cumulative number of cycles applied to the test specimen, and the appropriate limits should be set to indicate specimen failure or deviations from the intended load system performance.

A4.8.8 Testing shall continue until the specimen breaks, a limit is reached which terminates the test, or the runout criterion is reached.

A4.9 Calculation and Interpretation of Results

A4.9.1 The maximum moment (or stress) and cycles to failure should be recorded and plotted on a *M-N* (or *S-N*) diagram. Various techniques may be used to estimate mean or median fatigue lives, statistical differences between groups, curve fits to the fatigue data, probability of survival curves, etc. **(1-3)**.

A4.9.2 If determining fatigue strength at *N* cycles, it is recommended that the fatigue strength be determined as the median fatigue limit (50 % probability of survival), using a technique or criteria described in the literature **(1)**.

A4.10 Report

A4.10.1 The test report shall include the following:

A4.10.1.1 Manufacturer of screw.

A4.10.1.2 Screw type, size (diameter and length), and catalog number, if applicable.

A4.10.1.3 Material of screw specimen, including applicable ASTM or ISO specifications.

A4.10.1.4 Description of deviations from a regular cross-section in the gage length, if any.

A4.10.1.5 Deviations from normal implant product.

A4.10.1.6 Type of bending applied, outer support span, *L*; Inner loading span, *c*, if applicable; Span between inner and outer rollers, *s*, if applicable; and, roller diameters.

A4.10.1.7 *R*-ratio and the test frequency.

A4.10.1.8 Description of the testing environment.

A4.10.1.9 A summary of the maximum moment, or stress, and the resulting cycles to failure or runout for each specimen tested. The data should be plotted on a *M-N* or *S-N* diagram. A description of the analytical or statistical techniques used for interpretation of the fatigue data should be included.

A4.10.1.10 A description of the failure mode and failure location for each specimen that failed.

A4.10.1.11 If appropriate, an estimate of the fatigue strength should be reported. A description of the analytical or statistical techniques used for determining the fatigue strength should be included.

A4.11 Precision and Bias

A4.11.1 Data establishing the precision and bias to be expected from this test method have not yet been obtained.

APPENDIX

(Nonmandatory Information)

X1. RATIONALE

X1.1 This standard is intended to provide useful and consistent information related to the terminology, performance, test methods, and application of intramedullary fixation devices. IMFD geometrical definitions, dimensions, classification and terminology; material specifications; and performance definitions are provides in Sections 1-5. A rationale for the importance of particular performance characteristics and a reference to applicable test methods are given in Section 6. Some of the applicable test methods are given in the Annexes. Currently, standard test methods for static four-point bending, static torsion and cyclic bending fatigue are provided in Annex A1-Annex A3, respectively.

X1.2 The orthopaedic surgeon should be able to chose the size, design, and orientation of an implant and the manner of preparation of the bone for the appropriate fit of the IMFD to each individual patient. In order to do this the surgeon must have confidence that the designation of size of the implant and its instrumentation has a specific, known meaning which is quantifiable and reliable regardless of the manufacturer or design. The mechanical behavior and material properties must also be described in a reliable, known manner which is irrespective of the manufacturer or design. In order to accomplish this uniformity of designations, the terminology, dimensions, tolerances, mechanical properties, material properties, and test methods for obtaining and reporting these parameters must be standardized.

X1.3 The original standard (F 1264 – 89) defined the performance characteristics important to the in-vivo clinical performance of the device. Previous revisions modified the standard to incorporate three test methods (static four-point bending static torsion, and cyclic fatigue bending) which define the criteria and methods to be used in determining some of the performance characteristics. The task group is currently working on additional test methods which can be used to determine the remaining performance characteristics defined in Section 6. Those test methods will be added to this standard as Annexes when they become available. It is the intent of the task group to provide specifications and test methods for all performance characteristics of Section 6 in one document for easy reference, and to eventually replace F 339 and all design-specific standards for IMFDs with this specification. The latest revision of this specification adds the dimension for the extractor hooks and accompanying slots used to extract some intramedullary pin designs (currently specified in F 339), and includes repeatability and reproducibility information for the test method described in Annex A1 as determined in an interlaboratory round-robin test program.

REFERENCES

(1) Little, R. E., and Jebe, E. H.: *Manual on Statistical Planning and Analysis for Fatigue Experiments*, STP 588, American Society of Testing and Materials, 100 Barr Harbor Drive, West Conshohocken, PA 19428, 1975.

(2) Conway J. B., and Sjodahl, L. H.: *Analysis and Representation of Fatigue Data*, ASM International, Materials Park, OH, 1991.

(3) Collins, J. A.: *Failure of Materials in Mechanical Design*, John Wiley and Sons, New York, NY, 1981.

Standard Performance Specification for Cerebral Stereotactic Instruments[1]

This standard is issued under the fixed designation F 1266; the number immediately following the designation indicates the year of original adoption or, in the case of revision, the year of last revision. A number in parentheses indicates the year of last reapproval. A superscript epsilon (ε) indicates an editorial change since the last revision or reapproval.

1. Scope

1.1 This specification covers stereotactic instruments used by neurosurgeons to assist in the placement of probes, such as cannulae, needles, forceps, or electrodes or to direct radiation into brain regions or anatomical targets that are not visible on the surface. The general location of these regions is determined by measurements from landmarks visualized by X ray or other means, such measurements being based on atlases derived from anatomical studies and autopsy. Because of the anatomical variability, more precise location in any single patient may be determined by physiological responses in that patient. The degree of success in stereotactic surgery depends upon the experience of the surgeon as well as the precision of the stereotactic instrument. Nevertheless, minimum standards of accuracy for stereotactic instruments that are within the range of variability of human anatomy must be maintained.

1.2 For the purpose of this specification, a stereotactic instrument is a guiding device used in human neurosurgery for the purpose of directing an instrument or treating modality to a specific point within the brain by radiographic or other visualization of landmarks.

1.3 Stereotactic instruments must be constructed to afford the surgeon reliably reproducible accuracy in placing instruments into target areas. Proper positioning of the probe is often verified by X rays to control errors in calculation and to correct deflection of the probe during insertion. Physiological parameters may be used to further define the optimal target.

1.4 At the present time, stereotactic instruments are used most frequently, but not exclusively in the following operations. The list is presented only to present examples and should not be construed to restrict advances or developments of new procedures. For some applications it is not required to hit a point in space, but to hit a volume or make a lesion within a mass. For that purpose, devices other than those covered by this specification may be employed, but should be restricted to such uses.

1.4.1 Thalamotomy for parkinsonism and other types of tremor,

1.4.2 Electrode implantation for epilepsy,

1.4.3 Needle or magnetic insertion, or both, for aneurysm thrombosis,

1.4.4 Thalamic or subthalamic operations for dystonia,

1.4.5 Thalamic or subthalamic operations for involuntary movements such as chorea or hemiballismus,

1.4.6 Ablation of deep cerebellar nuclei for spasticity,

1.4.7 Cingulotomy and thalamic or subthalamic surgery for pain,

1.4.8 Mesencephalotomy or tractotomy for pain,

1.4.9 Ablations of subcortical temporal lobe structures for treatment of epilepsy,

1.4.10 Psychosurgical procedures,

1.4.11 Implantation of depth stimulating electrodes for pain,

1.4.12 Insertion of forceps or needle for obtaining biopsy specimens,

1.4.13 Foreign body removal,

1.4.14 Implantation of radioactive material, and

1.4.15 Biopsy or treatment of tumors.

1.5 *This standard does not purport to address all of the safety concerns, if any, associated with its use. It is the responsibility of the user of this standard to establish appropriate safety and health practices and determine the applicability of regulatory limitations prior to use.*

2. Referenced Documents

2.1 *NFPA Standard:*

NFPA 99 Health Care Facilities Code (56A and 76B-T)[2]

2.2 *UL Standard:*

UL 544 Electrical, Medical, and Dental Equipment[3]

3. Terminology

3.1 *Descriptions of Terms*—The following descriptions of terms are for the purposes of this specification only. Other nomenclature may be used throughout the literature and by various manufacturers:

3.1.1 *anatomical accuracy*—the reliability or accuracy with which the tip of a probe can be introduced into a given anatomical target. Because of anatomical variability, a given anatomical structure or anatomical target may vary relative to the position of the reference atlas position of that structure. Consequently, it is not possible to relate the reliability of a stereotactic apparatus to anatomical accuracy, but only to mechanical accuracy.

[1] This specification is under the jurisdiction of ASTM Committee F-4 on Medical and Surgical Materials and Devices and is the direct responsibility of Subcommittee F04.31 on Neurosurgical Standards.

Current edition approved Nov. 24, 1989. Published January 1990.

[2] Available from National Fire Protection Association, Batterymarch Park, Quincy, MA 02269.

[3] Available from Underwriters Laboratories, 333 Pfingsten Rd., Northbrook, IL 60062.

3.1.2 *anatomical target*—that anatomical structure within the central nervous system into which it is intended to insert a probe.

3.1.3 *anatomic variability*—a variation in position, size or configuration of an anatomical structure from one human brain to another.

3.1.4 *angular accuracy*—the accuracy to which the probe holder can be adjusted to a given angle from reference planes.

3.1.5 *angular scale*—the scale on the stereotactic apparatus which indicates at which angle the electrode probe holder directs a probe in relation to one or more reference planes of the coordinate system of the apparatus.

3.1.6 *atlas*—a topographical map of the brain or spinal cord based on autopsy studies, used to define the relationship between anatomical structures and landmarks, sometimes including information about the anatomical variability.

3.1.7 *direct visualization*—the visualization of an anatomical target by direct visual observation or roentgenographically with or without the assistance of air or contrast material.

3.1.8 *disconnect system*—a system to afford adequate access to the patient.

3.1.9 *electrode*—a probe usually insulated except for a specific portion or portions, commonly the end, which is stereotactically inserted into a desired anatomical target for the purpose of recording electrical activity, stimulating nervous tissue, producing a lesion in nervous tissue by passage of a direct or rapidly alternating electrical current, or measuring impedance.

3.1.10 *frame*—that part of the stereotactic apparatus which is attached to the skull.

3.1.11 *guide tube*—a tube through which an electrode or probe can be directed to a target. The tube imparts additional strength and less likelihood of deviation from a true trajectory. The guide tube can be attached to the electrode probe holder or stereotactic apparatus or attached to the electrode or insertional probe in a sleeve-like fashion.

3.1.12 *landmark*—a structure than can be visualized radiographically, with or without contrast material or air, from which measurements are made to define the position of the stereotactic target.

3.1.13 *linear accuracy*—the positioning accuracy of a linear movement of the probe holder in the direction of one or more of the reference planes of the stereotactic apparatus.

3.1.14 *linear scale*—the scale on the stereotactic apparatus which indicates linear movement of the electrode probe holder in relation to one or more of the reference planes, or a point within the coordinate system.

3.1.15 *mechanical accuracy*—the accuracy with which a stereotactic apparatus can bring the tip of a straight probe to a given coordinate within the stereotactic coordinate system.

3.1.16 *probe*—any type of long, thin device stereotactically inserted into a desired anatomical target. The most common type of probe is an electrode, but probes can also be cryoprobes, leukotomes, needles, biopsy devices, devices to insert radioactive or other material, magnetic probes, needles or injection devices, cannulae, forceps, etc.

3.1.17 *probe holder*—that part of the stereotactic apparatus that holds the electrode or probe. It is ordinarily attached to the frame either directly or indirectly, depending on the type of apparatus.

3.1.18 *simulated skull*—any device to which a stereotactic apparatus might be attached to simulate the stresses imparted to the apparatus when it is attached to the patient's skull. Because of the differences in how various stereotactic apparatus are attached to the skull, no universal simulated skull can be described.

3.1.19 *stereotactic apparatus*—any guiding device used in human neurosurgery for the purpose of directing a probe into the brain, under guidance of radiographic visualization of landmarks, direct radiographic visualization, or other means.

3.1.20 *stereotactic target*—that point in space, defined by the coordinate system of some types of stereotactic apparatus, to which it is desired to insert a probe.

3.1.21 *undamaged—in regard to electrodes*—not damaged to an extent where the electrical properties would be affected as to make an electrode unacceptable for clinical use.

4. Classification of Stereotactic Apparatus

4.1 Four basic types of stereotactic instruments, or a combination thereof are presently used and will be referred to herein as the arc (polar coordinate), rectilinear type, (c) aiming type, and (d) interlocking arc type. Types with comparable or greater accuracy should be recognized as they are developed.

4.1.1 *Arc Type*—The arc type apparatus is constructed according to the spherical radius principle so that the target point lies at the center of an arc along which the probe holder moves so that when a probe inserted into the probe holder perpendicular to a tangent of the arc and for a distance equal to the radius of the arc, the tip of the probe arrives at a single point in space, the center of the circle defined by the arc, that is, the stereotactic target. This occurs regardless of the position of the probe holder along the arc or the angle the arc subtends with the base of the apparatus. Generally, the apparatus is adjusted so that the stereotactic target point corresponds to the anatomical target point, so the probe might be introduced at any angle yet accurately find the stereotactic target.

4.1.2 *Rectilinear Type*— The rectilinear type provides individually for the longitudinal, transverse and vertical movements of the probe and probe holder. Ordinarily, a rectilinear stereotactic apparatus also provides for sagittal and transverse angle adjustment as well. Calculations can be made so the probe can be adjusted to the scales to aim and advance the probe to the desired target point along a predetermined trajectory.

4.1.3 *Aiming Type*— The aiming type of stereotactic apparatus is attached to a burr hole in the skull. The angles of insertion can be adjusted and the depth of insertion of the electrode or probe controlled so the probe can be pointed to the desired target point and then advanced to it.

5. Significance and Use

5.1 The purpose of a stereotactic apparatus is to guide the advance of an electrode or other probe accurately and in a controlled fashion to a given point in space, relative to the apparatus, to the stereotactic target. Thus, when the apparatus is attached to the skull, the electrode or probe can be advanced to a given geographical point within the cranial cavity, near the base of the skull or in the spinal canal.

5.1.1 As generally employed, the ventricles or cavities within the brain or other neurosurgical landmarks are identified roentgenographically by other means and, by consulting an atlas or other table, the mean distance and direction between the visualized landmark and a given anatomical target are measured. The electrode or probe is then inserted to the stereotactic target, that is, the point in space which is calculated from the distance and direction between the visualized landmark and the desired target in relation to the coordinate system of the stereotactic apparatus.

5.1.2 It is recognized that there is considerable anatomical variability in the size and shape of the central nervous system so that the target point that is identified from the atlas or table is only approximate. Usually, where possible, physiological verification may also be obtained. One must distinguish between the anatomical accuracy, which is inexact because of the variability of brains, and the mechanical accuracy, which is a function of the precision of the stereotactic instrument.

5.1.3 The requirements set forth herein are concerned only with the mechanical accuracy of stereotactic instruments. It is also recognized that once minimum standards for mechanical accuracy have been obtained, increased mechanical precision will not necessarily lead to increased anatomical precision.

6. Application

6.1 *Attachment to the Skull*—It is necessary to fix the stereotactic apparatus to the skull firmly in order to maintain an accurate relationship between the stereotactic apparatus and the skull. Those stereotactic apparatus which are attached to a platform or operating table shall provide for the rigid fixation of the skull to the apparatus or to the supporting platform. There shall be no visible movement of the frame of the apparatus in relation to the skull with the application of forces of magnitude and direction as would ordinarily be encountered during stereotactic surgery. Furthermore, fixation shall be secured enough to maintain mechanical accuracy. Design and construction of the apparatus shall be such that forces incidental to screwing its attachment pins into the skull do not distort the system to the extent of compromising its mechanical accuracy.

6.2 *Access for Radiology or Other Visualization*—Since the central nervous system landmarks are identified roentgenographically or by other means, the apparatus or that part of the apparatus from which movements are made, when properly applied to the patient, shall be arranged in such a way that radiographs can be made in more than one plane or other visualization obtained. Means shall also be available to reposition the X-ray tubes accurately and conveniently. The stereotactic apparatus shall be constructed in such a way that no mechanical part interferes with X-ray, computerized tomography or other necessary visualization of landmarks during the part of the procedure when radiographs are being made.

6.3 *Accuracy of the Probe Placement*—The accuracy of placement in an anatomical target is dependent on anatomical variability which exceeds the mechanical inaccuracies of the stereotactic system. Nevertheless, specifications for mechanical precision, to a practical extent, are appropriate to obtain maximum target accuracy with an electrode or other probe. In general, the mechanical precision of a stereotactic apparatus should be sufficient to place a probe at a given point in space one half the diameter of the probe. Since most electrodes or probes are larger than 1.2 mm in diameter, a mechanical accuracy of 0.6 mm at the 99 % confidence level would ensure that a given point is generally included within the probe tract. Although probes less than 1.2 mm in diameter are sometimes employed, they are generally used for specialized purposes which require direct visualization of the target.

6.4 *Probe Holder*—The probe holder shall be designed so that it mechanically grasps the electrode or probe along sufficient length to prevent deviation, so the accuracy of the instrument is maintained, and so that its insulation is undamaged. A system to identify the appropriate target length of the electrode or probe, either on a depth scale or by a system preventing electrode overtravel shall be employed. If the procedure requires that the probe be advanced only to the target point, the system shall be designed so that the probe can be stopped accurately at the chosen target so that penetration beyond the target can be avoided. If the system is designed to advance the electrode along a calculated trajectory, a mechanical or other drive system shall be employed so that the millimetre-by-millimetre advance can be controlled.

6.5 *Adjustability of Probe Holder*—The apparatus shall be designed so that the probe holder may be locked at the proper angular scale or linear scale reading and can be moved in a controlled fashion along the appropriate scale, either by a continuous mechanical drive system, by a mechanical drive system in 1-mm steps or less, or manually. The system shall be free of binding. The system should be designed to allow clear and legible visibility by the operator performing the adjustments of the scale to which adjustments are being made.

6.6 *Linear Accuracy*— A mechanical linear accuracy one half the diameter of the probe or electrode is desired, but accuracy of greater than 0.6 mm at the 99 % confidence level is not required.

6.7 *Angular Accuracy*— A stereotactic device, such as the arc type, which requires only the advancement of the electrode probe tip to a specific target point regardless of the angle of insertion need not have an angular accuracy of greater than 1°.

6.7.1 A stereotactic device that uses a phantom target point shall have an angular accuracy that provides a mechanical accuracy of at least 0.6 mm for the whole system.

6.7.2 For repositioning without the use of the phantom, the angular accuracy of the apparatus shall be such that a probe of the length ordinarily used in stereotactic surgical procedures will fall within 0.6 mm of the intended stereotactic target coordinates at the 99 % confidence level. For example, if a stereotactic apparatus is designed for use with a probe 250 mm in length, an angular accuracy to introduce a given angle into a rectilinear system would be. 0.256° or better. Less angular accuracy would be required to consistently fall within 0.6 mm of a point for an arc type stereotactic apparatus used with a probe of identical length.

7. Insertional Devices/Brain Instrument Interface

7.1 *Desirability for Intracranial Guiding*—When it is necessary to introduce a fine gage probe into central nervous tissue and thermal tissue resistance may cause a flimsy probe to deviate excessively, means shall be provided to increase probe rigidity to prevent deviation. Probe deviation may be prevented by stepped diameters along the shaft to increase rigidity or by introducing the probe through a rigid guide tube extended subdurally along the probe trajectory to a point beyond deflective tissue.

7.1.1 *Materials Used in Intracranial Guides*—Whether such guides are insulated or uninsulated shall be a matter of calculated design, and if insulated, the same criteria for electrode insulation shall apply. If uninsulated, the guide tube extension shall be grounded separately or through the electrode holder so as to prevent potentials being induced on it by its inherent or by other means, whereby such intermediate potentials might have effects which are clinically detectable or undesirable for recording purposes.

NOTE 1—Standards for electrodes and other probes will be dealt with in a separate document under the jurisdiction of a separate working group.

8. Calibration of Apparatus

8.1 *Test Probes*— A probe used in the calibration and recalibration of the apparatus shall consist of a steel rod no less than 1.5 mm or greater than 2.5 mm in diameter which will be straight to better than ½mm. The dimensions of the test probe shall be similar to that of an electrode probe ordinarily used with the apparatus under test and shall be capable of being held securely by the electrode holder of that apparatus.

8.2 *Test Method*— The accuracy of an instrument shall be determined by the maximum error found in a significant number of tests performed by moving the probe time from any given starting position to any other predetermined position within the recommended working area for that instrument.

8.3 *Frame Distortion*— Frame accuracy of each type of apparatus shall be measured by the manufacturer on a suitable simulated skull or test phantom. The range of distortions which would be anticipated in normal use shall be included in the calibration measurement procedure unless a method is presented to eliminate such distortion effects.

8.4 *Recalibration*— A system shall be included, with appropriate instructions by the manufacturer, to make it possible for the operator to recalibrate the apparatus between cases or at any time there is likelihood that the apparatus may have become damaged or distorted. Such recalibration may involve either advancing a test probe to a simulated stereotactic target within the apparatus or the alignment of a test probe with specified reference lines defining reference planes or reference points.

9. Radiologic Safety Aspects

9.1 It is recognized that although roentgenographically is an indispensable part of many stereotactic procedures, the radiologic aspects concern separate equipment which is not part of the stereotactic frame. Refer to standards for intra-operative use of roentgenographic equipment for specific standards pertaining thereto.

9.2 *Safety*—Any stereotactic apparatus that requires the direct contact with a radiologic apparatus shall include provision for electrical safety, to ensure that the patient is protected from harmful current flow in the event of a short circuit or grounding failure of the radiologic equipment. The requirements and techniques of such provisions shall be clearly defined in the information supplied by the manufacturer.

9.2.1 *Radiologic Safety*—Standards for preventing overexposure of patient and personnel to harmful radiation during a stereotactic procedure are a function of safety procedures established for the use of radiologic equipment and consequently do not involve the manufacturer of stereotactic instruments. Nevertheless, it is recognized that those individuals qualified to use stereotactic equipment should likewise be knowledgeable about safe radiologic techniques with stereotactic procedures.

9.2.2 The stereotactic apparatus shall be constructed in a manner such that it does not interfere with alignment and use of radiologic equipment.

9.2.3 The stereotactic apparatus shall not include any component that would hinder X-ray visualization of anatomical structures of interest since this would necessitate the use of inordinately large doses of X rays to perform the studies necessary for precision and safety of the stereotactic operation.

10. Anesthesia and Operating Room Safety

10.1 *Scope*—This specification is concerned with the definitions and standards that are required in the manufacture of stereotactic instruments to ensure patient and operating room personnel safety during the administration of anesthesia for stereotactic surgery.

10.2 *Definition*—For the purpose of this specification, general anesthesia may be defined as a state of altered consciousness occurring as a result of drug administration by intravenous, intramuscular, inhalation or oral routes. However, most stereotactic surgery is performed with local anesthetic, the choice being the responsibility of the operating surgeon.

10.3 *General Requirements*—It is desirable to designate the operative area as a nonflammable anesthetizing location in accordance with NFPA Standard Nos. 56A and 76B-T both included in NFPA No. 99. To this end, appropriate signs shall be posted.

10.4 *Specific Requirements*:

10.4.1 *Disconnect System*—The mechanism to connect or rapidly disconnect the patient from that part of the stereotactic apparatus as may be necessary in an emergency must be easily accessible, quickly operative, and independent of electrical supply, as may be necessary to manage any untoward drug reactions from excess secretions to cardiopulmonary failure.

10.4.2 *Airway Maintenance*—The apparatus shall allot free access to the head and neck for maintenace of an airway either by endotracheal intubation or suctioning.

10.4.3 *Other Monitoring*— The apparatus shall also be constructed to allow monitoring of vital signs including blood pressure, electrocardiograms, etc.

10.4.4 *Avoidance of Facial Damage*—The apparatus shall be constructed to avoid undue pressure on the eyes, ears, or other susceptible areas of the skin.

10.4.5 *Electrical Safety*—The apparatus shall not interfere with the maintenance of electrical safety and electrical isolation as defined in governmental regulations.

11. Electrical Safety

11.1 *Scope*—This specification is concerned with the definitions and standards that are required to ensure operating room safety to prevent electrical shock to the patient or to the operating room personnel, and to prevent distressing secondary effects such as skin burns. It must be recognized that the stereotactic frame and the patient become part of an electrical circuit when an electrode is introduced into the body. When electrical devices other than those directly concerned with the conduct of the procedure are connected to the patient, it is mandatory that any electrical currents that can flow in the complex network, thereby created, be held to safe levels by adherence to the safety procedures used with those devices. Unless overall instrumentation standardization is set up, it must be assumed that a variety of grounded output or isolated output systems may be connected to the patient. It must be further assumed that attempts to apply a UL Standard 544 to the design of the stereotactic frame and its electrodes would make electrode systems so awkward and cumbersome as to preclude their use in the desired manner. Consequently, responsibility falls on the operator to use informed judgment in providing for all aspects of electrical safety since, by the very nature of the stereotactic apparatus, it is not possible to design sufficient safeguards for electrical safety into the apparatus.

11.2 *Reference Potential of the Frame*:

11.2.1 A common characteristic of almost all stereotactic frames is that they are fixed to the skull by pointed metallic screws or other metallic parts. Each screw may therefore be assumed to be in some degree of electrical contact with the patient, the contact impedance depending on several factors.

11.2.2 Ideally, the frame should be fabricated of materials and surface finishes which are conductors or which afford very low electrical resistance between the various parts, so that the frame can be considered as one piece electrically; accordingly, the frame also should be electrically bonded to the operating table or have a common ground, so that the patient could not contact metal parts which were not at the same potential as the stereotactic frame.

11.2.3 Although one might theoretically consider that frames made of surface treated aluminum might not have sufficient electrical contact between parts so that a small electrical potential might exist between the parts of the apparatus, current flow which might result from the discharge of these potentials are far from those parts of the body which would be adversely affected by brief flow of current at such levels. Indeed, historically the good safety record of surface coated aluminum stereotactic devices indicates that such construction is satisfactory from the standpoint of electrical safety.

11.3 *Electrode Systems*—The electrode should be electrically isolated from the stereotactic apparatus. Ordinarily, this is a function of the manufacture of the electrode. The electrical or grounding characteristics of the lesion generator are beyond the scope of this specification. Electrical hazards caused by spurious current pathways associated with electrical connections to auxiliary equipment can only be prevented by the precautions ordinarily employed in an operating room environment.

11.4 *Explosion Hazard*— To prevent explosion hazards, the usual precautions in the operating room must be taken. If possible, electrical ground connections between the stereotactic frame and auxiliary apparatus shall be made before the line cord is plugged into the explosion proof wall receptacle.

12. Sterilizability of Devices

12.1 *Scope*—This specification establishes requirements for sterilizability of stereotactic devices. Examples of devices included are the (*a*) arc type, (*b*) rectilinear type, and (*c*) the aiming type of stereotactic devices as described in 4.1. Excluded are insertional devices/brain instrument interface which will be included in a separate standard.

12.2 *Requirements*:

12.2.1 The patient-invasive components of the stereotactic apparatus must be sterilizable by an accepted procedure for sterilization of neurosurgical instruments.

12.2.2 If detached from the main apparatus during the sterilization procedure, it must be possible to reattach these patient invasive components to the apparatus with preservation of sterility.

12.2.3 The probe holder must satisfy the requirement of sterilizability by an accepted procedure for sterilization of surgical instruments.

12.2.4 If the design of the apparatus permits intraoperative adjustments of the probe holder, the apparatus design must reasonably permit the operator to make such adjustments while preserving the sterility of both the probe and the patient-invasive components.

13. Instructions and Warnings

13.1 *General*—Instructions to be included with every stereotactic apparatus sold by the manufacturer shall include the following information:

13.1.1 Description of the apparatus and nomenclature for the component parts.

13.1.2 Instructions or diagrams for a recommended method of positioning the patient's head or attachment of the apparatus to the patient's head.

13.1.3 Recommended procedure for positioning or changing position of the probe holder indicating a technique that is compatible with the design of the apparatus.

13.1.4 Instructions for a recommended technique for insertion of electrode or other probes into the probe holder to minimize risk to the straightness or insulation of the device.

13.1.5 Recommended procedure for repositioning the probe holder or the patient's head in order to properly adjust the instrument to aim the insertional device to the target.

13.1.6 Recommended procedure for aligning and taking X rays with safeguards to ensure the reproducibility of alignment and X ray safety, if appropriate.

13.1.7 Recommended procedure for rapidly disconnecting the patient from the apparatus for quick access to the head in the event of an emergency, if required by instrument design.

NOTE 2—It is recognized that there is no standard technique for the conduct of stereotactic surgery and that it is not appropriate for the manufacturer to dictate surgical procedures. Instructions should pertain only to matters regarding the design of the apparatus. It is recognized that the surgeon has the ultimate responsibility for the welfare of patients and that surgeons have a variety of surgical approaches. The manufacturer cannot include all possible acceptable techniques in any instructional manual, but should include a recommended technique and sufficient detail so that one familiar with stereotactic surgery might know how to use the specific stereotactic instrument, even if the operator has had not prior experience with it. It is recognized that the experience, training and innovation of the operator may lead him to use or develop a technique other than the single technique outlined in the instruction manual.

13.2 *Sterilizability*:

13.2.1 Instructions shall be included for the sterilization of necessary parts of the stereotactic apparatus using techniques ordinarily available in an operating suite. These instructions shall include any special requirements for cleaning, disassembling and reassembling, packaging requirements, or special handling of any parts of the apparatus if such a procedure does not conform to the usual techniques for sterilization of surgical instruments.

13.2.2 Any contraindications to sterilization of all or part of the stereotactic apparatus by the use of any standard sterilization technique shall be noted. For instance, it is not possible to sterilize some plastic parts by steam autoclave without distorting them.

13.3 *Hazards*:

13.3.1 Any reported hazards particular to a specific instrument shall be noted.

13.3.2 Hazards related to the attachment of the instrument to the skull shall be specifically noted.

13.4 *Calibration and Recalibration*:

13.4.1 Instructions for calibration, recalibration, or verification of the proper alignment of the stereotactic instrument shall be included. These should be sufficiently clear and concise so that a nurse or surgeon or one not familiar with engineering or mechanical testing can perform the testing procedure accurately.

13.4.2 A recommended schedule of recalibration shall be included to ensure that the apparatus maintains the mechanical accuracy defined above. This may involve testing of the procedure for alignment and configuration between or just prior to each stereotactic procedure and may be incorporated in the procedure for X ray alignment. Alternatively, it may be recommended at reasonable intervals depending upon the mechanical stability of each type of apparatus.

13.5 *Manufacturer's Warranty*:

13.5.1 The limits of the manufacturer's warranty shall be clearly specified in the information originally supplied with the stereotactic apparatus.

13.5.2 A source for service or repair of the apparatus shall be clearly indicated in the information supplied by the manufacturer.

13.5.3 Where appropriate, instructions for readjustments or repairs of the most common repairs that can be performed locally shall be included in the information originally supplied by the manufacturer.

13.6 *Serial Number*— Each apparatus shall be assigned a unique serial number by the manufacturer who will keep a record of the original owner. If information is received by the manufacturer of the transfer of the apparatus to new owner, it shall be incorporated in his records. If, at any time, the device is returned to the manufacturer for repairs, but proper repairs are not possible, the current owner shall be notified and this information shall be recorded by the manufacturer.

13.7 *Clinical Information*—It is not required that the manufacturer include information of a clinical nature with the apparatus, nor information concerning the physiologic recommendations for monitoring or anatomical variabilities.

Designation: F 1268 – 90 (Reapproved 1998)

Standard Guide for Establishing and Operating a Public Information, Education, and Relations Program for Emergency Medical Service Systems[1]

This standard is issued under the fixed designation F 1268; the number immediately following the designation indicates the year of original adoption or, in the case of revision, the year of last revision. A number in parentheses indicates the year of last reapproval. A superscript epsilon (ε) indicates an editorial change since the last revision or reapproval.

INTRODUCTION

The Emergency Medical Service (EMS) system exists for only one reason—to serve the public. If the system is to perform its functions, the public must be aware of it and must use it to the fullest extent. Because the public is an essential part of the EMS system, every EMS system must support a public information, education, and relations (PIER) component. However, because other elements such as categorization, critical care protocols, communications, and provider training require as much time and energy, plus the fact that most administrators lack orientation to public information principles, there is a tendency to approach the public information, education, and relations component in a less organized and scientific way. Consequently, PIER may suffer a lower priority and may become a random or fragmented activity.

The fact is that people do not readily change their attitudes and behavior unless it is specifically and immediately demonstrated to them that there is a need to do so. In this day of complex media message sending, it is often difficult to get the attention of the general public in the first place. To achieve a successful PIER program, it should be an organized and systematic effort, including:

(*1*) An assessment of the attitudes, awareness and knowledge about one's health and access to the health delivery system;

(*2*) A determination of the knowledge needs and identifiable components of the general public;

(*3*) A method for delivery of information that is relevant, accessible, understandable, acceptable, usable, timely, and cost-effective;

(*4*) Ensure that, as much as possible, the information is integrated into attitudes and behaviors of daily living; and

(*5*) Evaluate PIER objectives to assess whether or not behavioral changes have occurred, with beneficial effect upon the individual and ultimately society, and adjusting future PIER activities as indicated.

Education about health matters has to be interesting, enjoyable, uncomplicated, relevant, and have some evidence of immediate concrete benefit to the individual's activities. In EMS, some of the programs are intrinsically appealing: for example, people might readily participate in CPR training as it represents a dramatic and demonstrable learning process. However, citizens are less enthusiastic about access information, abuse and misuse messages, or other facts which are to them, less dramatic and apparently less relevant.

1. Scope

1.1 The purpose of this guide is to provide national voluntary standards and recommendations to effectively provide emergency medical service system information and education to the public.

2. Referenced Documents

2.1 *ASTM Standards:*

F 1086 Guide for Structures and Responsibilities of Emergency Medical Services Systems Organizations[2]

3. Terminology

3.1 *Descriptions of Terms:*

3.1.1 *demographics*—the study of the descriptive characteristics of the population. They have long been used to divide or

[1] This guide is under the jurisdiction of ASTM Committee F-30 on Emergency Medical Services and is the direct responsibility of Subcommittee F30.03 on Organization/Management.

Current edition approved Jan. 10, 1990. Published February 1990.

[2] *Annual Book of ASTM Standards*, Vol 13.01.

segment the population.

3.1.2 *external PIER attributes*—for the public or user of the EMS system.

3.1.3 *internal PIER attributes*—within the EMS system for its participants and providers.

3.1.4 *public education*—an activity that conveys knowledge or training, or both, in specific skills.

3.1.5 *public information*—an activity that factually teaches what the EMS system is and how to enter and use it.

3.1.6 *public information, education and relations (PIER) program*—the totality of efforts in all three areas. It is ideally well integrated, unified, focused, with planning and systematic execution.

3.1.7 *public information officer*—a person who disseminates appropriate and timely facts.

3.1.8 *public relations*—an activity used to foster positive public attitudes and enhance trust and credibility about the EMS system and its providers.

4. Significance and Use

4.1 It is essential to have the public's understanding and support for the EMS system to ensure its proper development and utilization.

4.2 This guide encompasses those procedures, considerations, and resources that are necessary for a successful EMS public information, education, and relations program. Complex EMS systems may integrate or augment, or both, this guide in its entirety. Less complex systems may need to collaborate with other EMS organizations and related agencies. Responsibility for this guide will vary by level of authority, that is, state, regional, and local. (See Guide F 1086.)

4.3 The PIER tasks involve research, planning, production, distribution, and evaluation. Production requires significant resources and expertise and may be done most appropriately at the higher level, such as regional, state, and national levels.

5. Statement of the Problem

5.1 Despite the development and rapid expansion of emergency medical services following the passage of the Highway Safety Act of 1966 and the Emergency Medical Services System Act of 1973, underutilization and improper utilization of services still exists in the system. The general public lacks information on how to access and use the EMS system appropriately.

5.2 The public needs to learn what EMS is and especially that it is a system, the importance of utilizing EMS, how to access it, and what to do and not to do until the ambulance and therefore the EMS system arrives. If the public knowledge concerning EMS can be improved, then it is likely that appropriate utilization of EMS will increase.

6. Elements of a PIER Program for EMS

6.1 The essential elements of an effective public information, education, and relations program include, but are not limited to:

6.1.1 An understanding of EMS system design and operation.

6.1.2 Proper access to the system (9-1-1, telephone, call box).

6.1.3 Self help, for example, CPR, First Aid, Vial of Life, Medic Alert, and other emergency data devices.

6.1.4 Provision for the appropriate and timely release of information on EMS related events, issues, and public relations (damage control).

6.1.5 Evaluation of EMS.

6.1.5.1 Importance of user and provider input.

6.1.5.2 How to effectively collect and assimilate input.

6.1.6 Current health and safety habits as they relate to prevention and reduction of health risks for the public and providers.

6.1.7 Provision for recruitment campaigns for career and volunteer personnel in EMS.

7. Organizational Commitment to and Authority for PIER

7.1 There must be an organizational commitment from the EMS system (See Fig. 1.)

7.2 To have an effective PIER program the chief executive officer (CEO) must be personally committed to PIER and be able to make definitive decisions concerning committment of organizational resources. This CEO must assign a PIER director who has access to the CEO. This person may in some small areas also be the CEO. The CEO must be continually apprised of the progress of the PIER program.

7.3 The organization must designate a responsible and committed public information and education person with demonstrated ability, who is accountable for the PIER program. This person will also provide the mechanism for establishing standard operating procedures for the occurrence of unplanned events, and appropriate training for PIO's or others assuming that role. The PIO's responsibility may include, but not be limited to the news media concerning the nature and extent of an incident and emergency medical care, for planned or unplanned events.

8. Identify Resources and Funding

8.1 A successful PIER program must have a source of funding exclusively dedicated to PIER. Funding sources exist at federal, state, and local levels.

8.2 Greater expenditures may be required in areas where hard costs such as media space and time, and morbidity and

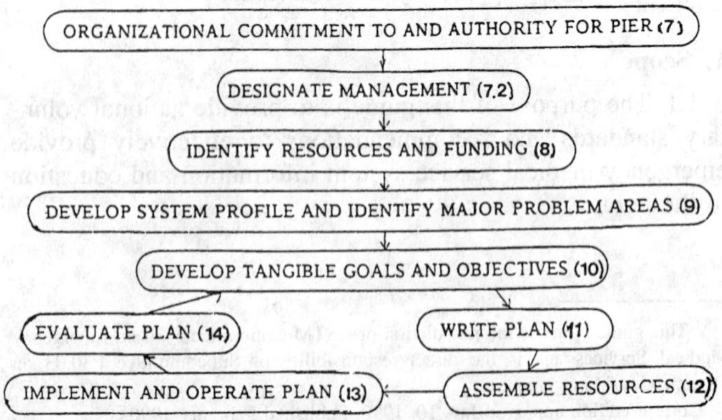

NOTE 1—In order to provide the elements of the PIER program, this planning model should be followed.

FIG. 1 PIER Planning Model

mortality from medical/trauma emergencies are higher than national norms.

9. Develop System Profile and Identify Major Problem Areas

9.1 In developing the system profile you should utilize existing data included in 9.2.1 to 9.3.1.10. If public perception data is not readily available it may be necessary to collect the data using a valid research methodology. Development of the profile will enable PIER personnel to identify broad problem areas or possible problem areas, and other factors that may affect the PIER program in a positive or negative manner.

9.2 A statistically valid comprehensive poll must be taken to establish a baseline of information on the EMS system operation. The required baseline components of the poll should include:

9.2.1 *Demographic Variables*—These include age, race, sex, population characteristics and trends, income levels, predominant languages, education levels, cultural factors, and other socioeconomic factors (religion, employment, and related).

9.2.2 *System Utilization Variables*—These include number and type of EMS personnel (volunteer and paid) and attrition rate, trends in EMS responses (coverage and response time), access type (9-1-1, tele, multi or single, number, radio, etc.), appropriate use or abuse problems, or both, and outcome costs and other utilization data.

9.2.3 *Medical Facilities*—These include number, location (and service area), beds, type, trauma center designation, teaching facility, and the interface/cooperation with the EMS system.

9.2.4 *Current Public Information and Education Programs*—These include type and scope of existing programs, effectiveness, program costs and funding sources, and related programs of other organizations and institutions (for example, AHA, ARC, etc.).

9.2.5 *Current Public Perceptions and Knowledge*—This includes knowledge of existing system structure, capabilities, and quality, access to the system, self help programs (CPR, first aid, and related programs), and current health habits, for example, diet, smoking, exercise, substance abuse, etc., as it is related to prevention and reduction of emergency health risks.

9.2.6 *Emergency Health Data*—This includes morbility/mortality from critical care, subgroups of cardiac, trauma, poison, drugs, burns, neonate, CNS, behavioral, and other emergency health data that may affect the EMS system. This includes prehospital, hospital, and rehabilitation data.

9.2.7 *Risk Variables (Possible Public Health Hazards and Possible Dangers in Particular Area or System)*—These include insufficient medical facilities, cultural, occupational, criminal, recreational, transportation, system maturity (ALS versus BLS capabilities), weather, sanitation, disease, and geographic considerations (rivers, mountains).

9.2.8 *Media Resources*—These include type (radio, TV, print, public, private), availability, cost, public relations and marketing firms, and contacts.

9.2.9 *Contributory Variables*—These include adjoining systems/resources, political and financial considerations, type and effectiveness of EMS management at all levels, and applicable regulatory factors.

9.3 *Methods to Accomplish System Profile and Baseline Study*:

9.3.1 Compile data already in existence from:

9.3.1.1 Census,

9.3.1.2 Vital statistics (health, government, and planning agencies, phone companies, realtors, etc.),

9.3.1.3 Commercial sources,

9.3.1.4 Voluntary organizations (AHA, ARC, ATS),

9.3.1.5 National and state agencies,

9.3.1.6 Current EMS system data,

9.3.1.7 College/universities,

9.3.1.8 Chambers of commerce,

9.3.1.9 Cultural/civic organizations, and

9.3.1.10 Medical facilities registries.

9.3.2 Collect data not currently in existence using valid research methodologies. Identify appropriate technical expertise who can assist with the research methodology.

10. Develop Goals and Objectives

10.1 This guide requires the development of tangible PIER goals and objectives. Goals must be realistic and should be consistent with program needs. PIER objectives whether long or short term, must be concise, consistent, attainable, measurable, written, flexible, revised periodically, reliable, and accountable. Since objectives are, by definition, measurable, their impact can be estimated.

10.1.1 Measurement criteria and evaluation mechanisms should be identified in advance and minimal standards for performance should be set. Baseline data will also help to determine priorities of the goals and objectives identified. Goals and broad objectives should be analyzed according to the public as a whole, and specific objectives may be addressed to a distinct public segment.

NOTE 1—By way of example, baseline data can be gathered from system analysis to determine the false alarm rate, and from survey to determine the percentage of adult population who know 9-1-1. One goal might then be to "increase the appropriate use of 9-1-1." Objectives might be (*1*) to ensure that 80 % of the adult population knows to dial 9-1-1 for medical emergencies, and (*2*) to decrease false alarms to less than 2 % of the total calls by ___ (date).

10.2 The final product of the goal setting process is a work plan that should include explicit goals and objectives.

11. Writing the PIER Plan

11.1 The work plan should include goals, objectives, implementation steps, required resources, and time lines. Management roles, functions, and activities should be identified. Identify specific problems anticipated in accomplishment of a goal: develop alternative solutions that are more realistic if necessary.

11.2 This guide requires the written preparation of a PIER plan and then the implementation of that plan, as well as the evaluation of the effectiveness of the PIER plan and proper modification to meet changing needs on an ongoing basis.

11.3 There must be a process for the identification of public information needs for the PIER plan and several methods and requirements are noted within this guide.

11.4 The development of a PIER plan must include the

following information to ensure the PIER plan is realistic and that it has tangible goals and measurable objective and is an improvement over past performance data (see 9.2).

12. Assemble Resources

12.1 There are four types of resources that can be assembled: human, information, financial, and materials/equipment. Select from these resources as necessary to implement the plan.

12.2 Large organizations and institutions (for example, universities, corporations, hospitals, trauma centers, etc.) are excellent resources to assist with marketing, survey development, and other PIER activities.

13. Implementation and Operation of PIER Plan

13.1 The PIER director must assign the work to his/her employees.

13.2 Each employee must be trained for his/her task.

13.3 The relationship of public information goals and objectives to the development of other system components should be analyzed to assess appropriate timing. Timing can be the most important element.

13.4 The director and employees must follow the schedule of events devised for each project.

13.5 The director and employees must confer quickly when problems arise in carrying out a project. They must promptly specify and phase in solutions, amending workplans in that process.

13.6 Employees must continually report project results to their supervisors.

14. Evaluate Plan

14.1 Evaluation is a process of assessing past or proposed actions and their results against the criteria, goals and objectives, and other normative elements of the plan and defined problem. Assessment and appraisal are usually used as more general terms than evaluation, connoting the drawing of conclusions from the examination of a situation and its elements. Additionally, evaluation and measurement are not synonymous, as measurement is basically a counting mechanism, which is part of evaluation. For instance, criteria are measurable components or test of a standard that permits determinations to be made of when or in what respect that standard has been met. Standards are explicit conditions to be fulfilled, either in operating a process or as a characteristic or an end state.

14.2 A basic evaluation process model includes information about procedures; a comparison with a norm (expression of what is desired); decision about program actions to be taken, compiling and reporting back their findings, and recycling as often as necessary to solve the original problem. Essential evaluation components include:

14.2.1 Resource allocation,

14.2.2 Media/communication used,

14.2.3 Quality of technical/production aspects,

14.2.4 Funding resource status (increasing, stable, decreasing),

14.2.5 Relationship between media and systems,

14.2.6 Number of people reached by media type and message disseminated,

14.2.7 Analysis of system utilization information as it relates to PIER,

14.2.8 Behavioral change/knowledge perception change, and

14.2.9 Timing of evaluation should also be considered (what is reasonable or necessary deadline for completion/evaluation).

14.3 And finally consider the needs as defined by goals and objectives, in relation to available time, money, and expertise. It may be that one or more lower priorities must be revised or totally dismissed until additional money becomes available. In other words, measure your goals and objectives against the reality of expectations to achieve them.

15. Performance Standards for Evaluation of EMS PIER Programs

15.1 A statistically valid survey or other scientific valid method of measuring the PIER will be completed annually. The public's knowledge and attitudes established in the baseline evaluation, will be updated every 3 years, as a minimum.

15.2 An ultimate goal is that 100 % of a community should know how to access the EMS system at all times.

15.3 There should be a 5 % improvement per year in the public's knowledge and attitude as established in the initial system survey. An accepted minimum national practice will be that 50 % of the population in every community have the knowledge. The areas addressed in this requirement include: prevention, knowing when to call, who to call, how to call, what to say, and what to do and not to do until the system arrives, including knowledge of resuscitation such as CPR and knowledge of what to expect from the EMS system, to facilitate the systems effective performance.

15.4 A minimum of 50 % of the distributed population should know the direct or most effective way of accessing the EMS system under usual circumstances. In extraordinary circumstances, such as vacationing in a rural area, the 50 % should have enough knowledge to choose an appropriate means for insuring EMS system activation and response.

Last ASTM Designation: F 1274 – 91

Specification for
Fixed Wing Advanced Life Support Transport Units

This specification pertains to fixed wing transport units involved in patient transportation and care, at the advanced life support level. Formerly under the jurisdiction of Committee F30 on Emergency Medical Services, this specification was withdrawn in February 2000.

Last ASTM Designation: F 1283 – 91

Standard Specification for
Fixed Wing Specialized Medical Transport Units

This specification pertains to fixed wing transport units involved in patient transportation and care at the specialized medical transport level.

Formerly under the jurisdiction of Committee F30 on Emergency Medical Services, this practice was withdrawn in February 2000.

Standard Guide for Training the Emergency Medical Technician (Basic) to Perform Patient Examination Techniques[1]

This standard is issued under the fixed designation F 1285; the number immediately following the designation indicates the year of original adoption or, in the case of revision, the year of last revision. A number in parentheses indicates the year of last reapproval. A superscript epsilon (ε) indicates an editorial change since the last revision or reapproval.

1. Scope

1.1 This guide covers the minimum patient examination techniques that the emergency medical technician (basic) shall be trained to use when assessing ill or injured patients of all ages.

1.2 This guide is one of a series which together describe the minimum training standard for the emergency medical technician (basic).

1.3 *This standard does not purport to address the safety problems associated with its use. It is the responsibility of the user of this standard to establish appropriate safety and health practices and determine the applicability of regulatory limitations prior to use.*

2. Referenced Documents

2.1 *ASTM Standards:*

F 1031 Practice for Training the Emergency Medical Technician (Basic)[2]

3. Terminology

3.1 *Definitions of Terms Specific to This Standard:*

3.1.1 *auscultation*—examination by listening with a stethoscope.

3.1.2 *inspection*—examination by careful visualization of the body or a part of the body.

3.1.3 *palpation*—examination by touching with the hand.

4. Significance and Use

4.1 This guide establishes the minimum national standard for training the emergency medical technician (basic) to perform patient examination techniques on patients of all ages.

4.2 This guide shall be used by those who wish to identify the minimum training standard for the emergency medical technician (basic) as it relates to the performance of patient examination techniques.

4.3 This guide shall be used as the basis to revise Practice F 1031.

4.4 Every person who is identified as an emergency medical technician (basic) shall have been trained in accordance with this guide.

4.5 This guide does not stand alone and must be used in conjunction with the applicable documents cited in Section 2.

5. Examination Techniques

5.1 The emergency medical technician (basic) shall be trained to perform the following examination techniques and to recognize the differences that exist because of age and sex:

5.1.1 Assess respirations for rate, rhythm, and quality,

5.1.2 Auscultate for breath sounds,

5.1.3 Assess rate and regularity of the following pulses: carotid, brachial, radial, femoral, and pedal,

5.1.4 Palpate blood pressure,

5.1.5 Auscultate blood pressure,

5.1.6 Assess mental status and level of consciousness,

5.1.7 Inspect the body,

5.1.8 Palpate the body,

5.1.9 Assess sensory perception,

5.1.10 Assess motor function, and

5.1.11 Assess airway patency.

[1] This guide is under the jurisdiction of ASTM Committee F-30 on Emergency Medical Services and is the direct responsibility of Subcommittee F30.02 on Personnel, Training and Education.

Current edition approved June 21, 1990. Published August 1990.

[2] *Annual Book of ASTM Standards*, Vol 13.01.

Designation: F 1286 – 90 (Reapproved 1996)$^{\epsilon 1}$

Standard Guide for Development and Operation of Level 1 Pediatric Trauma Facilities[1]

This standard is issued under the fixed designation F 1286; the number immediately following the designation indicates the year of original adoption or, in the case of revision, the year of last revision. A number in parentheses indicates the year of last reapproval. A superscript epsilon (ε) indicates an editorial change since the last revision or reapproval.

ϵ^1 NOTE—Keywords were added editorially in May 1996.

1. Scope

1.1 This guide establishes minimum guidelines for the development and operation of a pediatric trauma facility in a children's or general hospital. A pediatric trauma facility is an institution whose medical and administrative leadership has expressed the personal, institutional, and financial commitment to optimal care of the injured child 24 h a day, 365 days a year.

1.2 This guide defines the system, organizational structure, clinical personnel, and physical equipment necessary for a pediatric trauma facility, whether freestanding or a joint adult/pediatric facility in either a children's hospital or general hospital committed to the care of injured children.

1.3 The criteria outline in this guide incorporates levels of categorization and their essential or desired characteristics.

2. Referenced Documents

2.1 *ASTM Standards:*

F 1224 Guide for Providing System Evaluation for Emergency Medical Services[2]

3. Terminology

3.1 *Definitions:*

3.1.1 *trauma care system*—a coordinated network of emergency medical systems (EMS) comprised of one or more trauma centers linked by triage protocols, appropriate communications, transportation services, and prehospital care to manage effectively the injured child from initial injury to complete rehabilitation. The trauma care system is a subsystem within the EMS system.

3.1.2 *trauma center*—a hospital that has made the institutional commitment to fulfill all criteria outlined in Sections 1 through 4 and where available be designated by the appropriate authority.

3.2 *Definitions of Terms Specific to This Standard:*

3.2.1 *pediatric patient*—a patient whose morphologic growth potential has not been completed. In general, a patient less than 15 years old or consistent with local practice.

4. Significance and Use

4.1 The purpose of this guide is to provide guidelines for categorizing pediatric trauma centers to ensure consistency of pediatric trauma care throughout the nation. The guidelines will form the quantitative basis for audit and ongoing quality assurance.

4.2 This guide can be used in conjunction with objective quality assurance outcome measures as outlined in Guide F 1224.

4.3 This guide can be used by local, regional, and national authorities to establish pediatric trauma centers.

5. Implementation of Pediatric Trauma Facilities

5.1 The implementation of a pediatric trauma facility designation will be conducted consistent with the regulation of local, state, and federal government authorities having jurisdiction for this process.

5.2 The most significant ingredient necessary for optimal care of the pediatric trauma patient is commitment, both personal and institutional. For the institutions, optimal care means providing capable personnel who are immediately available, sophisticated equipment, services that are frequently expensive to purchase and maintain, and priority of access to laboratory, radiology, operating suites, and intensive care facilities and services. For the medical and nursing staff, optimal care means a commitment to the concept of adequate staffing, prompt availability, continuing education, and quality assurance.

5.3 It is recognized that a Level I pediatric trauma center should be located in a facility providing comprehensive care for children. The institutions must demonstrate a continuing commitment to a high level of pediatric trauma care. Methods of demonstrating the commitment to the trauma system shall include, but not be limited to, a broad resolution that the hospital governing body agrees to do the following:

5.3.1 Participate in the operations and integration of a regional or statewide system, to ensure pediatric patient care data for system management, quality assessment, and operations research,

5.3.2 Establish policy and procedures for the maintenance of services essential for a trauma center/system,

5.3.3 Ensure that all pediatric trauma patients will receive

---

[1] This guide is under the jurisdiction of ASTM Committee F30 on Emergency Medical Services and is the direct responsibility of Subcommittee F30.03 on Organization/Management.

Current edition approved July 9, 1990. Published August 1990.

[2] *Annual Book of ASTM Standards*, Vol 13.01.

medical care to the level of the institution's accreditation, and

5.3.4 Establish a priority admission for the pediatric trauma patient to the full services of the institution, including adequate resuscitation facilities and personnel, operating room availability, and intensive care unit availability. The Level I pediatric trauma center must assume the responsibility for ensuring prompt access for all patients requiring trauma care.

5.3.5 Written transfer agreements to receive and transfer the pediatric trauma patient must be in place.

5.3.6 The pediatric trauma center must have the capability to receive the pediatric trauma patient by ground or by air.

6. Criteria for Level I Pediatric Trauma Facilities

6.1 *Participation Requirements*:

6.1.1 Designation as a Level I trauma center confers upon a facility the recognition that it has the commitment, personnel, and resources to provide optimum medical and psychological care for the critically injured child.

6.1.2 The center shall have appropriate support services for the child and the family and commitment to the ongoing care and total rehabilitation of the patient. This shall include the following:

6.1.2.1 Evidence of appropriate social service intervention and follow-up,

6.1.2.2 Identification of members of the rehabilitation team,

6.1.2.3 Discharge summary of the trauma care to the patient's private physician, where appropriate, and

6.1.2.4 Documentation in the patient's medical record of the post-discharge plan.

6.1.3 A Level I pediatric trauma center shall demonstrate its capability to manage injured and their sequelae to major injuries or critical conditions such as:

6.1.3.1 Signs of shock or hypotension associated with one or more system injuries,

6.1.3.2 Fractures of the axial skeleton,

6.1.3.3 Two or more proximal long-bone fractures,

6.1.3.4 Amputation or traumatic avulsion of one or more extremities proximal to digits,

6.1.3.5 Suspected or actual spinal cord injuries,

6.1.3.6 Head injuries,

6.1.3.7 One or more system injuries requiring pediatric intensive care, intracranial pressure monitoring, or mechanical ventilation support, and

6.1.3.8 Thermal or chemical injury.

6.2 *Service Requirements*:

6.2.1 Criteria guidelines embrace administrative and physical attributes of individual trauma centers. By this means, autonomous functioning of the trauma service may be ensured, and its staffing and direction sharply defined. The definition of bed capacity, intensive care unit, operating room capability, and proximity to an availability of supporting services (radiology, laboratory, etc.) are important features of the concept. The intent is to ensure the optimal coordination of services for the trauma patient.

6.2.2 The hospital shall have an organized, defined trauma service within the institutional structure that shall consist of the following:

6.2.2.1 A pediatric surgeon as chief of the pediatric trauma service who shall have special interest and experience in major pediatric trauma care and the leadership skills to head a multidisciplinary team approach to the management of the patient. This surgeon shall have a significant time commitment to major trauma care.

6.2.2.2 The pediatric trauma service shall have designated pediatric specialists available 24 h per day for care of the major trauma patients.

6.2.2.3 Children with significant injuries shall undergo evaluation by the trauma service and disposition to the appropriate hospital service.

6.2.2.4 All pediatric trauma patients shall be treated by personnel who are organized as a team and available in-house from the major trauma service and the pediatric service 24 h per day with attending coverage as specified.

6.2.2.5 A designated pediatric surgeon is responsible for multidisciplinary and interdepartmental coordination of effort to trauma care.

6.3 *Trauma Service Director*:

6.3.1 Fundamental to the establishment and organization of a hospital's pediatric trauma service is the recognition that the individual identified and accountable for the operation of this service must be qualified to serve in this capacity. The following indicators shall be present:

6.3.1.1 Evidence of qualifications, including pediatric educational preparation in pediatric surgery and a certificate of special qualifications in pediatric surgery,

6.3.1.2 Selection process as defined by the hospital's medical staff bylaws,

6.3.1.3 Participation in local/state/national trauma-related activities,

6.3.1.4 Educational involvement such as the Advance Trauma Life Support (ATLS) course, teaching in the undergraduate, graduate, and postgraduate level training programs within the department of surgery. There shall be evidence of interface and collaboration between nursing management responsible for the trauma nursing service and the physician management responsible for the trauma service,

6.3.1.5 Participation in research and publication efforts of pediatric trauma,

6.3.1.6 Evidence of active participation by the trauma program director in the resuscitation or surgery, or both, of multisystem trauma patients,

6.3.1.7 A job description and organizational chart depicting the relationship between the trauma program director and other hospital clinical services, and

6.3.1.8 Evidence that a multidisciplinary method of providing, monitoring, and evaluating trauma patients throughout their hospital stay is in effect through the hospital organizational plan.

6.4 *Nursing Requirements*:

6.4.1 The hospital organization must define the roles of the nursing team members and their areas of responsibility, accountability, and authority.

6.4.2 It is suggested that the trauma plan for the nursing department include the ability to immediately mobilize qualified nursing resources.

6.4.3 Essential to the overall coordination and integration of the trauma center or system in the hospital is the designation of an individual as the pediatric trauma nurse coordinator. The trauma nurse coordinator should be responsibile for monitoring and promoting all trauma-related activities associated with patient care, and for providing documented evidence thereof.

6.4.3.1 Participation in trauma educational activities separate from the institution's in-house trauma education program as either program coordinator, consultant, or faculty member shall be required. There must be evidence of specific pediatric nursing practice application. There must be evidence of documentation of this participation.

6.4.4 The following indicators shall be present:

6.4.4.1 Evidence of qualification to include educational preparation, certification, and experience in pediatrics,

6.4.4.2 Participation in local, state, and national pediatric trauma-related nursing activities,

6.4.4.3 Evidence of participation in trauma research through promotion or coordination,

6.4.4.4 A job description and organizational chart depicting the relationship between the trauma nurse coordinator and other services, and

6.4.4.5 Evidence of participation in the establishment of systems to influence the nursing care of pediatric trauma patients.

6.5 *Department Requirements*—There shall be surgery departments, divisions, services, or sections with designated chiefs and staffed by qualified specialists with expertise in pediatrics in the following areas:

6.5.1 Pediatric general surgery,

6.5.2 Orthopedic surgery,

6.5.3 Cardiac surgery,

6.5.4 Vascular surgery,

6.5.5 Neurosurgery,

6.5.6 Urology,

6.5.7 Ear, nose, and throat,

6.5.8 Plastic and maxillofacial surgery,

6.5.9 Oral surgery,

6.5.10 Ophthalmic surgery,

6.5.11 Transplant or transfer agreement,

6.5.12 Reimplantation, or appropriate transfer agreement, and

6.5.13 Obstetrics and gynecologic surgery consultation.

6.6 *Physician Requirements*:

6.6.1 *Specialists*—Specialists shall be available in-hospital 24 h per day, as follows:

6.6.1.1 Pediatric surgical attendant or resident,

6.6.1.2 Pediatric attendant or resident,

6.6.1.3 Anesthesiologist or resident, and

6.6.1.4 Neurosurgical attendant or resident, or surgical designee of chief of neurosurgery.

6.6.2 *Attending Staff*—Attending (on-site) staff with expertise in pediatrics shall be on-call and promptly available in the following areas:

6.6.2.1 Orthopedic surgery,

6.6.2.2 Ophthalmic surgery,

6.6.2.3 Ear, nose and throat,

6.6.2.4 Plastic surgery,

6.6.2.5 Oral surgery,

6.6.2.6 Urologic surgery,

6.6.2.7 Hand surgery,

6.6.2.8 Burn,

6.6.2.9 Radiology,

6.6.2.10 Vascular radiology,

6.6.2.11 Neuroradiology,

6.6.2.12 Mental health services,

6.6.2.13 Pediatric medicine,

6.6.2.14 Pediatric critical care,

6.6.2.15 Neurosurgery, and

6.6.2.16 Anesthesia.

6.6.3 *Pediatric Consultation*—Specialists shall be on-staff and available on-site to respond for pediatric consultation in the following areas:

6.6.3.1 Cardiology,

6.6.3.2 Gastroenterology,

6.6.3.3 Hematology,

6.6.3.4 Infectious disease,

6.6.3.5 Psychiatry,

6.6.3.6 Neurology,

6.6.3.7 Pulmonary disease,

6.6.3.8 Clinical pathology,

6.6.3.9 Rehabilitation medicine, and

6.6.3.10 Nephrology.

6.6.4 *Subspecialists*—All subspecialists in a Level I specialty pediatric trauma center shall be board certified subspecialists where appropriate.

7. Hospital Resource Requirements

7.1 *General*—A Level I pediatric trauma facility shall have all of the hospital resources described in this section.

7.2 *Emergency Department*:

7.2.1 The hospital shall have an easily accessible and identifiable designated resuscitation area used for neonate, pediatric/adolescent major trauma patients.

7.2.2 The physical environment shall have areas for at least two simultaneous resuscitations.

7.2.3 The hospital should demonstrate a commitment to pediatric emergency care, and demonstrate compliance with the following requirements:

7.2.3.1 The designated trauma resuscitation area must be of adequate size to accommodate the full trauma resuscitation team.

7.2.3.2 Adequate facilities and personnel must be available within the emergency department to care simultaneously for more than one multisystem trauma patient. Back up areas to accomplish this need not be separately designated but should be immediately available.

7.2.3.3 Under normal conditions, the emergency department shall be open at all times.

7.2.3.4 All closures of the emergency department, for whatever reasons, shall be documented with notification of appropriate authorities and institutions.

7.2.3.5 The institution shall develop formal written protocols with neighboring trauma centers to accept trauma patients when bypass is mandatory.

7.2.4 *Receiving Personnel*—Emergency department or trauma receiving area personnel shall be comprised of at least the following:

7.2.4.1 There shall be a designated physician qualified in

emergency care and pediatrics, and a nursing director of the emergency department.

7.2.4.2 There shall be 24-h in-house immediate coverage and response to the emergency department with a team approach to the initial management of the pediatric major trauma patient.

7.2.4.3 A paging system shall function to immediately mobilize the team.

7.2.5 *Emergency Department Team*—The team shall be comprised of at least the following personnel who are immediately available and responsible for resuscitation and stabilization of the patient:

7.2.5.1 *Physician*, with special competence in the care of the critically injured pediatric patient who is a designated member of the trauma team and physically present in the emergency department 24 h a day with training in emergency medicine and pediatrics, or appropriate subspecialities.

7.2.5.2 *Pediatric Resident or Staff*, PGY-3 (postgraduate year 3).

7.2.5.3 *Surgical Resident(s) or Staff*, PGY-3/4.

7.2.5.4 *Anesthesiologist Physician*—Initial response may be an anesthesiology resident at PGY 3/4 level responsible to attending anesthesiologist who is immediately available. When a residency trained pediatric anesthesiologist is not available there must be the ability to demonstrate the experience or special education of the anesthesiologist in the pediatric age group.

7.2.5.5 *Respiratory Therapist*.

7.2.5.6 *Registered Nurses*—A minimum of two registered nurses per shift, functioning in trauma resuscitation, who have documented experience in the care of injured children.

(a) (*a*) All registered nurses shall be educated in trauma nursing.

(b) (*b*) All registered nurses assigned to the department must receive training in pediatrics.

(c) (*c*) The patient classification system utilized by the institution should define the severity of injury or illness, which indicates the number of nursing staff needed to adequately provide patient care.

(d) (*d*) Appropriate nursing documentation for the trauma patient must be present.

(e) (*e*) Evidence of annual continuing education in pediatric trauma care is required.

7.2.6 *Equipment and Drugs*—Equipment and drugs shall be available to the emergency department 24 h per day for the resuscitation and stabilization of the following conditions or injuries in the pediatric patient:

7.2.6.1 Unstable or potentially unstable airway,

7.2.6.2 Unstable or potentially unstable cardio-vascular system,

7.2.6.3 Open and closed head injuries,

7.2.6.4 Open and closed fractures,

7.2.6.5 Spinal cord or column injuries,

7.2.6.6 Facial injuries,

7.2.6.7 Thoraco-abdominal injuries,

7.2.6.8 Amputation,

7.2.6.9 Burns, and

7.2.6.10 Toxicology.

7.2.7 Equipment and drugs in the emergency department, all sized as appropriate for the pediatric patient, shall include, but not be limited to, at least one of each of the following items:

7.2.7.1 Resuscitation stretcher,

7.2.7.2 Airway control ventilator available, bag mask oxygen (O_2) suction, endotracheal tubes, laryngoscopes, tracheostomy set, and other appropriate respiratory equipment,

7.2.7.3 Electrocardiographic (ECG) monitor, oscilloscope, intracranial pressure monitor, and defibrillators with internal paddles,

7.2.7.4 Central venous pressure monitors,

7.2.7.5 Intravenous insertion sets for pediatric patients,

7.2.7.6 Drugs and intravenous fluids for all emergency situations with appropriate administrative devices,

7.2.7.7 Pediatric dose chart, immediately accessible and prominently displayed,

7.2.7.8 Mobile X-ray capability with 24-h in-house technician,

7.2.7.9 Communication between emergency transport system and emergency room personnel,

7.2.7.10 Thoracotomy trays,

7.2.7.11 Peritoneal lavage tray,

7.2.7.12 Appropriate lighting for emergency surgery,

7.2.7.13 Pediatric pneumatic antishock garments,

7.2.7.14 Pediatric suction equipment,

7.2.7.15 Pediatric skeletal tongs and splinting,

7.2.7.16 Neck immobilization device,

7.2.7.17 Thermal control equipment for patient, blood, and environment,

7.2.7.18 Patient weighing devices,

7.2.7.19 Intraosseous infusion set,

7.2.7.20 Needle cricothyroidotomy set, and

7.2.7.21 Cranial burr hole set.

7.3 *Operating Suite (Special Requirements)*—The operating suite shall be staffed and equipped to handle all children who are present in the emergency department and are in need of immediate surgical intervention, and, at a minimum, shall meet the following requirements:

7.3.1 The operating room shall be adequately staffed and immediately available 24 h per day for trauma patients.

7.3.2 A second staffed operating room shall be promptly available and staffed.

7.3.3 *Nursing Personnel*:

7.3.3.1 The operating room registered nursing staff shall have experience and shall be trained as both scrub and circulating nurses in the operating room.

7.3.3.2 At least one registered nurse must be physically present in the operating room.

7.3.4 *Equipment*—The operating room shall contain at least the following equipment:

7.3.4.1 Cardiopulmonary bypass pump-oxygenator,

7.3.4.2 Operating microscope available,

7.3.4.3 Thermal control equipment for patient, blood, and environment,

7.3.4.4 X-ray capability,

7.3.4.5 Pediatric endoscopes, all varieties, or promptly available,

7.3.4.6 Burr hole capability,

7.3.4.7 *Monitoring Equipment*—Electrocardiographic (ECG), continuous blood pressure, ICP, and appropriate respiratory monitors (such as transcutaneous pO_2, CO_2 monitors),

7.3.4.8 Pediatric drug dose chart,

7.3.4.9 Pediatric anesthesia ventilator,

7.3.4.10 Image intensifier available,

7.3.4.11 Fracture table available, and

7.3.4.12 Auto transfuser.

7.4 *Postanesthetic Recovery Room (PAR)*—The postanesthetic recovery room (pediatric intensive care unit is acceptable) shall consist of at least the following:

7.4.1 *Nursing Personnel*—Registered nurses and other essential personnel shall be on duty 24 h a day, and must be competent in postanesthesia care of the pediatric trauma patient.

7.4.2 *Anesthesiologist*—An anesthesiologist with pediatric experience or physician with demonstrated experience in airway management shall be available in-hospital 24 h per day.

7.4.3 *Equipment*—Equipment for resuscitation and to provide life support for the critically or seriously injured neonate, pediatric/adolescent shall include but not be limited to the following:

7.4.3.1 Airway control and ventilation equipment, including laryngoscopes, assorted blades, airways, endotracheal tubes, and bag-mask resuscitators of all sizes (this equipment must be readily available),

7.4.3.2 Oxygen, air, and suction devices,

7.4.3.3 Electrocardiograph, internal and external pediatric paddles, and defibrillator,

7.4.3.4 Apparatus to establish and maintain hemodynamic and ICP monitoring,

7.4.3.5 Appropriate standard intravenous fluids and administration devices, including intravenous catheters,

7.4.3.6 Sterile surgical set for emergency procedures such as thoracotomy and cut-down,

7.4.3.7 Drugs and supplies necessary for emergency care,

7.4.3.8 Temperature control devices for the patient (that is, radiant warmers), for parenteral fluids, and for blood,

7.4.3.9 Temporary cardiac pacemaker, and

7.4.3.10 Appropriate pressure monitoring.

7.5 *Intensive Care Unit*—The hospital shall have a pediatric intensive care unit (ICU) that has separate comprehensive pediatric intensive care capability and is capable of treating all pediatric major trauma patients requiring an ICU.

7.5.1 *ICU Personnel*—The unit shall be staffed at a level to ensure appropriate nurse-patient ratios, as determined by written nursing standards. Pediatric ICU personnel shall, at a minimum, be comprised of the following:

7.5.1.1 A designated medical director for pediatric intensive care, and.

7.5.1.2 Physician on duty in ICU 24 h a day or immediately available from inside the hospital. This physician should be credentialed by the institution in trauma care. The physician on duty in the ICU is not the emergency department physician. There shall be another physician in-house who has experience in pediatric trauma care.

7.5.1.3 *Nursing Staff*:

(a) (*a*) The patient classification system utilized by the institution should define the patient care workload of the nursing staff.

(b) (*b*) The pediatric patient shall have nursing care given by a registered nurse who has experience in pediatric nursing.

7.5.2 *Patient Care*—ICU equipment, drugs, and supplies shall be available for the optimal treatment of the following critical conditions or injuries:

7.5.2.1 Unstable airway or pulmonary system,

7.5.2.2 Unstable cardiac system,

7.5.2.3 Unstable cardiovascular system,

7.5.2.4 Head injuries with or without coma,

7.5.2.5 Axial skeletal injuries or fractures,

7.5.2.6 Spinal cord injuries,

7.5.2.7 Fractures, pre- or post-reduction, with or without traction devices,

7.5.2.8 Fluid electrolytes, or metabolic derangements,

7.5.2.9 Visceral injuries,

7.5.2.10 Eye injuries, and

7.5.2.11 Burns, or transfer agreement.

7.5.3 *Equipment*—Equipment of all sizes, as appropriate for pediatric patients, shall include, but not be limited to, the following:

7.5.3.1 *Airway Control Devices*, including endotracheal tubes, ventilating equipment, O_2 source and O_2 concentration devices, and suction,

7.5.3.2 *Electronic Monitors*—Electrocardiographic monitor, heart rate monitors, respiratory monitors, doppler and temperature,

7.5.3.3 *Other Equipment*—Pediatric venous, intraosseous, arterial access trays and catheters including catheterization venous pressure and Swanganz catheters, compartment pressure monitors, pediatric temperature control devices, pediatric dialysis machine, pediatric scales, skeletal traction attachments and instruments, and sterile thoracotomy kit, pulse, oximetry, pressure monitors and other equipment necessary for the care of children,

7.5.3.4 *Drugs*—All necessary drugs for optimal treatment,

7.5.3.5 *Sets*—Intravenous, crystalloid solutions, and pediatric administration sets,

7.5.3.6 *In-Unit and Intra-Hospital Communications*, and

7.5.3.7 *Standard Microtechnique*, required for electrolytes, blood count, arterial blood gases and platelets, urine/serum osmolality, coagulation studies, and capability to accept bacterial cultures, available 24 h in the laboratory.

7.6 *Pediatric Medical-Surgical Units*—These are general medical-surgical nursing unit beds.

7.6.1 *Nursing Staff*:

7.6.1.1 The patient classification system utilized by the institution should define the work load that indicates the number of nursing staff to adequately provide patient care.

7.6.1.2 Pediatric trauma patients will receive nursing care from a registered nurse trained in pediatric care.

7.6.2 *Equipment*—The equipment should support the current status of the patient and be readily available. Equipment for resuscitation and to provide support for the injured neonate, pediatric/adolescent patient shall include, but not be limited to, the following:

7.6.2.1 Airway control and ventilation equipment, including

laryngoscopes, assorted blades, airways, endotracheal tubes, bag-mask resuscitator of all sizes (this equipment must be immediately available),

7.6.2.2 Oxygen, air, and suction devices,

7.6.2.3 Electrocardiograph, monitor, and defibrillator to include internal and external paddles,

7.6.2.4 All standard intravenous fluids and administration devices, including intravenous catheters designed with the capacity for delivering IV fluids and medication at rates and in amounts appropriate for children ranging in age from neonate to adolescent,

7.6.2.5 Drugs and supplies necessary for emergency care, and

7.6.2.6 Thoracotomy tube sets and cut down trays.

7.7 *Rehabilitation Medicine*:

7.7.1 *Rehabilitation Plan*—There must be a clearly identifiable comprehensive trauma rehabilitation plan developed for every pediatric trauma patient. If the patient is transferred to another institution for rehabilitation, then records, outcome, and follow-up must be obtained. If a rehabilitation facility is not associated with the institution, a formal written transfer agreement with a rehabilitation center specifically equipped for the care of the children shall be in place.

7.7.1.1 The multidisciplinary pediatric trauma team shall define and implement a mechanism for discharge planning for the pediatric trauma patient.

7.7.1.2 The pediatric trauma rehabilitation plan developed for the pediatric trauma patient shall be under the direction of a psychiatrist or a physician with special competence in pediatric trauma rehabilitation.

7.7.1.3 Ancillary services, such as physical therapy, occupational therapy, speech therapy, play therapy, nutritional therapy, etc., shall have a defined role in the rehabilitative care of the pediatric patient.

7.7.2 *Nursing Staff*:

7.7.2.1 Nursing staff ratios for medical-surgical units caring for the rehabilitation of the post-acute trauma neonate, pediatric/adolescent patients shall be based upon a patient classification system.

7.7.2.2 When a separate rehabilitation unit exists, the nursing staff ratios shall be based on the institution's classification system.

7.7.2.3 The education of the rehabilitation unit nurse shall have emphasis on the pediatric trauma patient's rehabilitation.

7.8 *Burn Center*—A transfer agreement with a burn center shall be in effect if not in-house.

7.9 *Spinal Cord Care*—A team approach to the initial and continued management of the acute spinal cord injury shall exist, and shall include the active participation of members of the rehabilitation service or as stated in a transfer agreement.

7.10 *Hemodialysis*—Hemodialysis capabilities shall be available.

7.11 *Radiology*—Radiological special capabilities shall be available and shall consist of the following:

7.11.1 Angiography of all types,

7.11.2 Sonography,

7.11.3 Nuclear scanning,

7.11.4 Computerized tomography, available 24 h per day, and

7.11.5 General angiography and cerebrovascular aortography, cardiac catheterization, and coronary capability.

7.12 *Blood Laboratory*—Clinical laboratory services shall be available 24 h per day and shall consist of the following:

7.12.1 Standard microtechnique analysis of blood, urine, and other body fluids,

7.12.2 Blood typing and crossmatching,

7.12.3 Coagulation studies,

7.12.4 Comprehensive blood bank with at least ten units of blood (all types) in-house, and access to community central blood bank and adequate hospital storage facilities,

7.12.5 Blood gases determinations immediately available,

7.12.6 Serum and urine osmolality,

7.12.7 Microbiology,

7.12.8 Written protocol that trauma patient receives priority, and

7.12.9 Toxicology testing.

7.13 *Social Service Capabilities*:

7.13.1 Social service intervention shall be available from the time of entry into the facility to the time of discharge. Social workers shall provide psycho-social services as part of an interdisciplinary team. They should be graduates of masters level programs in social work.

7.13.2 Social workers shall be available to the patient, patient's family, significant others, the community, and members of the interdisciplinary team as indicated.

7.13.3 There shall be adequate documentation in the patient's record of the social work services provided.

7.13.4 The social work team should participate in the development and delivery of in-service training for the trauma center staff and the community.

7.14 *Pastoral Counseling*—The opportunity for spiritual counseling should be available. As the injury or illness of a child frequently stresses the bonds of a family unit, it is suggested that there be the opportunity for all spiritual denominations to receive clerical support. This can be accomplished by developing a listing of clergy promptly available to the facility.

8. Education

8.1 Formal programs in continuing medical education specifically concerning pediatric trauma care shall be given by the hospital for the following personnel:

8.1.1 Staff physicians,

8.1.2 Nurses,

8.1.3 Allied health professionals (emergency medical technicians/paramedics),

8.1.4 Community physicians, and

8.1.5 Community nurses (registered nurses or licensed practical nurses).

8.2 Public education shall be provided by trauma hospitals.

8.3 The hospital shall exhibit existing or planned pediatric trauma prevention programs. There needs to be evidence of active programs to increase the public awareness of trauma prevention. The trauma prevention program needs to be internal and external to the facility. These programs can be presented collectively with other hospitals and organizations.

8.4 The hospital must be able to document active involvement in its local and regional emergency medical services (EMS) systems. The hospital can demonstrate involvement in local and regional EMS programs by the following means:

8.4.1 When appropriate, participation in pediatric emergency medical technician training programs,

8.4.2 Joint educational programs to include equipment, supplies, and drugs specific to the neonate and pediatric patient,

8.4.3 Participation in EMS system quality assessment and quality assurance mechanism, and

8.4.4 Assistance in the development of regional policy and procedures.

9. Disaster Plan

9.1 Each hospital shall incorporate into its master disaster plan the utilization of its pediatric major trauma area for children.

9.2 Each hospital shall participate in a process to incorporate its resources and activities into local and regional disaster plans.

10. Research in Pediatric Trauma

10.1 Each hospital shall participate in a registry of all pediatric major trauma admissions with pertinent treatment and outcome data as determined by the regional emergency medical services. The registry must include at a minimum:

10.1.1 Severity of injury, including the probability of dying,

10.1.2 Anatomic site of injury,

10.1.3 Nature of injury,

10.1.4 Mechanism of injury,

10.1.5 Classification of patient injuries, including sub groups,

10.1.6 Demographic information as to age, sex, etc.,

10.1.7 Outcome, and

10.1.8 Active involvement in the research of pediatric trauma care.

11. Protocols and Policies

11.1 The hospital shall provide written protocols and policies to support a systematic and comprehensive approach to the care of the pediatric trauma patient (including child abuse), as follows:

11.1.1 Trauma patient triage protocols,

11.1.2 Trauma team response protocols,

11.1.3 Trauma patient resuscitation and stabilization,

11.1.4 Operating room support, laboratory, X-ray, respiratory therapy, and pharmacy protocols; explicit recognition of the priority given to trauma patients,

11.1.5 Trauma patient transport protocols—emergency room to operating room, hospital to hospital,

11.1.6 Special audit for pediatric trauma deaths at least every month, including autopsy data, and

11.1.7 Monthly morbidity and cost-of-care review.

11.2 *Agreements*—The trauma center or unit shall have the following agreements:

11.2.1 The hospital shall implement a process of peer review regarding the care of the pediatric major trauma patient.

11.2.2 There shall be a system to permit all patients access to services regardless of financial status.

11.2.3 The pediatric trauma center shall agree to an area-wide mortality audit.

11.2.4 The trauma center shall provide evidence of consultation and appropriate transfer agreements with referring hospitals (including organ procurement).

11.2.5 The trauma center shall provide telephone consultation 24 h per day.

11.2.6 There shall be a written by-pass policy.

11.3 *Trauma Conferences*:

11.3.1 Regular trauma conferences, such as the following, are critical to the self evaluation and timely identification of problems for prompt resolution:

11.3.1.1 Pediatric nursing audit,

11.3.1.2 Medical records review, and

11.3.1.3 Long term follow-up of trauma care.

11.3.2 Every trauma admission shall be reviewed at these conferences. Departmental morbidity and mortality conferences do not exempt review by these conferences.

11.3.2.1 Conferences are intended to be major problem identification and problem solving sessions. Therefore, attendance of designated personnel from hospital administration is essential. Attendance is also expected to include physician and nursing personnel, pediatric transport team members, trauma call surgeons, involved consultants, the physician director of the ICU, social services, the prehospital agency, and rehabilitation personnel. The conference should be chaired by the trauma service director.

11.4 Adult and pediatric trauma may be reviewed at the same conference.

11.5 The multidisciplinary pediatric trauma conference, shall be held at least every 3 months.

12. Keywords

12.1 hospital; pediatric trauma; pediatric trauma facility; trauma center

Standard Guide for Scope of Performance of First Responders Who Provide Emergency Medical Care[1]

1. Scope

1.1 This guide covers minimum requirements for the scope of performance of first responders who may be responsible for the initial care of sick and injured persons of all ages in the prehospital environment.

1.2 This guide includes objectives based on an individual's acquired knowledge, including signs and symptoms; patient assessment; basic life support/cardiopulmonary resuscitation (BLS/CPR); bleeding and shock; injuries to the skull, spine, chest, abdomen, and extremities; moving patients; medical and environmental emergencies; triage; gaining access; and hazardous situations that the first responder may encounter.

1.3 *This standard does not purport to address all of the safety concerns, if any, associated with its use. It is the responsibility of the user of this standard to establish appropriate safety and health practices and determine the applicability of regulatory limitations prior to use.*

2. Referenced Documents

2.1 *ASTM Standards:*

F 1031 Practice for Training the Emergency Medical Technician (Basic)[2]

2.2 *American Heart Association/American Red Cross (AHA/ARC) Standards:*

Standards and Guidelines for Cardiopulmonary Resuscitation and Emergency Cardiac Care[3]

3. Terminology

3.1 *Definitions of Terms Specific to This Standard:*

3.1.1 *basic life support/cardiopulmonary resuscitation* (BLS/CPR)—a set of skills that includes airway management, chest compressions, and others as defined by the American Heart Association.

3.1.2 *first responder* (FR)—an individual trained to provide initial care for sick or injured persons in accordance with this guide.

4. Significance and Use

4.1 The purpose of this guide is to improve the quality of initial emergency medical care provided to the sick and injured. As the first trained person at an emergency medical scene, it is critical that the first responder be proficient in providing patient care and minimizing further complications until more highly trained emergency medical service personnel intervene.

4.2 In identifying these minima the guide acknowledges many types of first responder emergency medical care courses of study. This guide allows and encourages the addition of optional knowledge, skill, and attitudinal objectives. Programs such as those for law enforcement, firefighters, and ski patrol are examples of this diversity meeting specific local community needs.

4.3 This guide is intended to assist those who are responsible for defining the scope of performance for first responders.

4.4 This guide is *not* intended to be used as a scope of performance for emergency ambulance personnel.

5. Objectives

5.1 *Required Objectives*—These objectives are not in an order suggesting a particular performance sequence. The first responder shall be able to:

5.1.1 Identify the roles and responsibilities of a first responder within the local emergency medical services (EMS) system,

5.1.2 Function within the medical-legal scope of care as a first responder in the local EMS system,

5.1.3 Determine vital signs and identify normal ranges,

5.1.4 Identify and report various forms of emergency medical identification found on the patient,

5.1.5 Conduct a primary assessment for life threatening conditions,

5.1.6 Provide BLS/CPR in accordance with American Heart Association/American Red Cross (AHA/ARC) standards,

5.1.7 Control bleeding,

5.1.8 Dress and bandage soft tissue injuries,

5.1.9 Care for a person in shock,

5.1.10 Supplement respirations with available mechanical aids to breathing, including oxygen,

5.1.11 Perform a secondary assessment,

5.1.12 Immobilize musculoskeletal injuries,

5.1.13 Immobilize the spine,

---

[1] This guide is under the jurisdiction of ASTM Committee F-30 on Emergency Medical Services and is the direct responsibility of Subcommittee F30.02 on Personnel, Training and Education.

Current edition approved May 25, 1990. Published July 1990.

[2] *Annual Book of ASTM Standards*, Vol 13.01.

[3] Reprinted from the *Journal of the American Medical Association* (JAMA). Copies are available from the American Heart Association, 7320 Greenville Ave., Dallas, TX 75231.

5.1.14 Move a sick or injured person from a hazardous environment in such a manner that the chance of aggravating injuries is minimized,

5.1.15 Move a person in conjunction with patient care activities in such a manner that the chance of aggravating injuries is minimized,

5.1.16 Care for a person who has non-traumatic chest pain,

5.1.17 Care for a person who is experiencing respiratory distress,

5.1.18 Care for a person who is experiencing a diabetic emergency,

5.1.19 Care for a person who is experiencing seizure activity,

5.1.20 Care for a person who has ingested, injected, inhaled, or absorbed a poison,

5.1.21 Care for a person who is experiencing an altered level of consciousness,

5.1.22 Care for a person who has thermal, chemical, or electrical burns,

5.1.23 Care for a person who is adversely affected by the environment,

5.1.24 Provide initial care for:

5.1.24.1 Persons with behavioral problems,

5.1.24.2 Physically and sensory impaired persons,

5.1.24.3 Abused persons, and

5.1.24.4 Dying persons,

5.1.25 Recognize a multiple casualty incident and initiate an appropriate response,

5.1.26 Triage injured persons found at a multiple casualty incident,

5.1.27 Recognize potential dangers at an emergency scene and take appropriate actions to protect first responders and other persons,

5.1.28 Use available equipment to gain access to trapped and injured persons in order to provide life saving care, and

5.1.29 Assist with the delivery of a baby.

5.2 *Optional Objectives*—The roles and responsibilities for the provision of initial emergency medical care vary among first responders. When the responsibilities for initial emergency medical care are limited, the ability of a first responder to perform the tasks in 5.1 may be sufficient to ensure satisfactory care. When a first responder must care for a greater variety of illnesses and injuries, the scope of performance must be expanded accordingly.

6. Keywords

6.1 basic life support/cardiopulmonary resuscitation (BLS/CPR); emergency medical services (EMS); first responder (FR)

Standard Guide for Planning for and Response to a Multiple Casualty Incident[1]

This standard is issued under the fixed designation F 1288; the number immediately following the designation indicates the year of original adoption or, in the case of revision, the year of last revision. A number in parentheses indicates the year of last reapproval. A superscript epsilon (ε) indicates an editorial change since the last revision or reapproval.

1. Scope

1.1 This guide covers the planning, needs assessment, training, integration, coordination, mutual aid, implementation, provision of resources, and evaluation of the response of a local emergency medical service (EMS) organization or agency to a multiple patient producing situation that may or may not involve property loss. This guide is limited to the pre-hospital response and mitigation of an incident up to and including the disposition of patients from the incident scene.

1.2 This guide addresses the background on planning, scope, structure, application, federal, state, local, voluntary, and nongovernmental resources and planning efforts involved in developing, implementing, and evaluating an EMS annex, or component, to the local jurisdiction's emergency operations plan (EOP) as defined in the Federal Emergency Management Agency (FEMA) publication, Civil Preparedness Guide (CPG) 1–8.[2]

1.3 *This standard does not purport to address the safety problems associated with its use. It is the responsibility of the user of this standard to establish appropriate safety and health practices and determine the applicability of regulatory limitations prior to use.*

2. Referenced Documents

2.1 *ASTM Standards:*

F 1149 Practice for Qualifications, Responsibilities, and Authority of Individuals and Institutions Providing Medical Direction of Emergency Medical Services[3]

3. Terminology

3.1 *Definitions of Terms Specific to This Standard:*

3.1.1 *command post*—the physical location from which incident command exercises direction over the entire incident.

3.1.2 *disaster*—a sudden calamity, with or without casualties, so defined by local, county, or state guidelines.

3.1.2.1 *medical disaster*—a type of significant medical incident which exceeds, or overwhelms, or both, the capability of local resources and of routinely available regional or multijurisdictional medical mutual aid, and for which extraordinary medical aid from state or federal resources is very likely required for further diagnosis and treatment.

3.1.3 *EMS control/medical group supervision*— the first emergency medical services response at the incident scene, or designated by the local response plan or incident command to be responsible for the overall management of the incident's EMS operation.

3.1.4 *extrication management*—the function of supervising personnel who remove entrapped victims.

3.1.5 *fatality management*—the function designated by existing plans, or the EMS control/medical group supervisor, to organize, coordinate, manage, and direct morgue services.

3.1.6 *incident commander*—the individual responsible for the overall on-site management and coordination of personnel and resources involved in the incident.

3.1.7 *logistics resources management*—the function responsible for acquiring personnel, equipment (including vehicles), facilities, supplies, and services as requested by the incident commander.

3.1.8 *medical communications management*—the function designated by the incident commander or EMS control/ medical group supervisor to establish, maintain, and coordinate effective communication between on-site and off-site medical personnel and facilities.

3.1.9 *medical supplies management*—the function designated by the incident commander to manage equipment and report to EMS control/medical group supervisor.

3.1.10 *mental health coordinator*—a qualified mental health professional responsible for coordinating the psychosocial assessments and interventions for responders, affected individuals, and groups.

3.1.11 *multiple casualty incident (MCI)*—a type of significant medical incident that may fall into the following categories:

3.1.11.1 *extended*—an incident for which local medical resources are available and adequate to provide for field medical triage and stabilization, and for which appropriate local facilities are available and adequate for further diagnosis and treatment.

3.1.11.2 *major*—an incident producing large numbers of casualties, for which routinely available regional or multijurisdictional medical mutual aid is necessary and adequate for further diagnosis and treatment.

3.1.12 *mutual aid*—the coordination of resources, including but not limited to facilities, personnel, vehicles, equipment, and

---

[1] This guide is under the jurisdiction of ASTM Committee F-30 on Emergency Medical Services and is the direct responsibility of Subcommittee F30.03 on Organization/Management.

Current edition approved July 6, 1990. Published August 1990.

[2] Available from FEMA, P.O. Box 70274, Washington, DC 20024.

[3] *Annual Book of ASTM Standards*, Vol 13.01.

services, pursuant to an agreement between jurisdictions providing for such interchange on a reciprocal basis in responding to a disaster or emergency.

3.1.13 *needs assessment*—a preliminary survey of real or potential hazards in a specific geographic area.

3.1.14 *operations officer*—individual who assists the incident commander on issues relating to the operations of the incident.

3.1.15 *public information*—a function designated by the incident commander for the dissemination of factual and timely reports to the news media.

3.1.16 *safety management*—the function that identifies real or potential hazards, unsafe environment or procedures at the incident scene, and recommends the appropriate corrective or preventive actions under the authority of the incident commander, to ensure the safety of all personnel at the incident scene.

3.1.17 *sector officers (group supervisors/leaders/managers)*—qualified personnel who control a specific area or task assignment.

3.1.18 *staging area*—the location where responding emergency services equipment and personnel assemble for assignment.

3.1.19 *staging management*—the function designated by the incident commander that is responsible for the orderly assembly and utilization of resources in a designated area.

3.1.20 *transportation management*—the function designated by the EMS control/medical group supervisor that is responsible for the transportation of the patients from the incident scene and for coordination with EMS control/ medical group supervisor, communications, and the incident commander.

3.1.21 *treatment area*—the site at or near the incident for emergency medical treatment prior to transport.

3.1.22 *treatment management*—the function that is responsible for the definitive on-scene medical treatment of patients.

3.1.23 *triage*—the process of sorting and prioritizing emergency medical care of the sick and injured on the basis of urgency and type of condition present, and the number of patients and resources available in order to properly treat and transport them to medical facilities appropriately situated and equipped for their care.

3.1.24 *triage area*—a location near the incident site to which injured persons should be brought, triaged, and taken directly to the treatment area.

3.1.25 *triage management*—the function that is responsible for triage and preliminary treatment of casualties.

4. Summary of Guide

4.1 This guide is based upon a body of knowledge on the planning, implementation, and evaluation of the emergency medical components of the local pre-hospital response to multiple casualty incidents.

4.2 The body of knowledge on which the guide is based was drawn from a wide variety of sources, including individual authors, academic institutions, and federal, state, regional, and local organizations.

4.3 This guide is organized in such a way as to provide those responsible for planning, implementing, and evaluating the emergency medical components of the local pre-hospital response to multiple casualty incidents with information they can readily use to ensure that their response is as expedient and appropriate as is reasonably possible.

4.4 The guide was created to organize, collate, and distribute related information in such a way as to be readily accessible to people in the fields of emergency medical services and emergency management.

4.5 This guide should not be perceived as an inflexible rule or standard but as a guide that should be adapted to the needs of the individual community, and should be refined and improved as the body of knowledge on which it is based increases.

5. Significance and Use

5.1 This guide is intended to assist the management of the local EMS agencies or organizations in the design, planning, and response of their jurisdiction's resources to multiple casualty incidents (MCIs).

5.2 This guide does not address all of the necessary planning and response of pre-hospital care agencies to an incident that involves the total destruction of community services and systems.

5.3 This guide does not address the necessary design, planning, and response to be undertaken by a medical care facility to an internal or external event that necessitates the activation of the facility's disaster plan.

5.4 This guide provides procedures to coordinate and provide a systematic and standardized response by responsible parties, including the local elected officials, emergency management officials, public safety officials, medical care officials (pre-hospital and hospital), local EMS agencies/organizations and others with objectives and tasks for the pre-hospital management of a significant incident.

5.5 This guide provides for the establishment of an incident command system with position descriptions that identify mission, functions, and responsibilities of the command structure to be used at a MCI. The incident command functions include but are not limited to staging, logistics, rescue/extrication, triage, treatment, transportation (air, land, and water), communications, and fatality management.

5.6 This guide provides examples and other management tools that can assist in providing training objectives and decision making models for dispatch, response, triage, treatment, and transportation for local jurisdictions experiencing multiple casualty incidents.

PLANNING

6. Planning

6.1 *Purpose*—Planning should be a cooperative effort between local EMS providers and the jurisdiction in which they deliver services. The plan should be written to establish the emergency organization, basic policies, responsibilities, and actions required for support of local operations of emergency medical/health plans. Plans should ensure rapid medical assistance to persons requiring aid due to an incident. Plans should describe a system for coordination of alerting, dispatching, and uses of medical personnel and resources whenever a local emergency medical health agency requires assistance from another EMS agency/jurisdiction. The plan should be designed to be an extension of day to day service, facilities, and resources.

6.2 *Goal*—The plan ensures adequate and coordinated efforts that will minimize loss of life, disabling injuries, and human suffering by providing effective medical assistance through efficient use of medical and other resources in the event of emergencies resulting in multiple casualty incidents.

6.3 *Objectives*—The primary objectives of a plan should include a process whereby:

6.3.1 Each EMS agency/jurisdiction should have a plan to meet its own needs within its capabilities.

6.3.2 Each EMS agency/jurisdiction should enter into mutual aid agreements with other local or regional jurisdictions which can be invoked when local capability to manage a situation has been exceeded. Each jurisdictional plan should facilitate the access and utilization of local and state resources.

6.3.3 The EMS agency/jurisdiction's plan should conform to appropriate regional and state plans.

6.3.4 Each EMS agency/jurisdiction should define training requirements, and develop and utilize a training program based on the needs assessment of the community.

6.3.5 The plan should be a coordinated interagency effort. Responsible agencies should have regular interaction in order to facilitate working relations during an incident.

6.3.6 Plans and procedures should be reviewed and revised regularly on the basis of tabletop exercises, simulated incidents, or actual events.

6.4 *Needs Assessment and Hazards Analysis*:

6.4.1 A needs assessment is a preliminary survey of real or potential hazards in a specific geographic area. Basic to the planning process is an understanding of the problems that should be anticipated in the specific area.

6.4.1.1 A needs assessment lets the EMS agency/jurisdiction know what to expect.

6.4.1.2 It prevents planning for unnecessary events.

6.4.1.3 It provides an incentive for the EMS agency/jurisdiction's plan.

6.4.1.4 It might indicate preventive measures.

6.4.1.5 It creates an awareness of new hazards.

6.4.2 When the needs assessment is complete, the jurisdiction should be able to make the following decisions:

6.4.2.1 The type of planning desired,

6.4.2.2 What types of response to emphasize,

6.4.2.3 What resources will be needed to fulfill that response, and

6.4.2.4 The type and quantity of mutual aid and support services that might be required outside the normal jurisdictional services.

6.4.3 *Components*—There are three basic parts to a needs assessment:

6.4.3.1 Consideration of the potential for specific incidents,

6.4.3.2 Evaluation of the potential harm resulting from the incident, and

6.4.3.3 Evaluation of the resources required to respond to the incident.

6.4.4 *Approach*—The following are suggested approaches to completing a needs assessment:

6.4.4.1 Form a team to identify the potential hazards, risks, and impact relating to potential MCIs.

6.4.4.2 Consult the local or state civil defense/emergency preparedness offices for assessment information.

6.4.4.3 After identifying potential MCIs, evaluate them for their potential hazards, risks, and impact.

6.4.4.4 Evaluate the area's resources.

6.4.5 *Resources Assessment*—Consider the personnel required for performing such tasks as emergency medical services, firefighting, and rescue. Inventory equipment for the job and evaluate its ability to perform the task. Prepare a written description of what potential incidents exist, and the ability to respond to these incidents.

6.4.6 Once complete, the needs assessment becomes part of the plan.

6.5 *Plan Components*— The plan should include provision for the following:

6.5.1 *Organizational Structure for Response*:

6.5.1.1 The plan should define an overall incident organization based on a strategy of efficient and effective utilization of resources.

6.5.1.2 The plan should address chain of command, including transfer of authority of any officer or position.

6.5.2 *Organization of Manpower and Resources for Response*:

6.5.2.1 The plan should provide for delineation of responsibilities and authority for all involved response personnel and agencies.

6.5.2.2 The plan should address necessary resources for each level of event and prepare for availability and updating of those resources.

6.5.3 *Response*:

6.5.3.1 The plan should provide for appropriate response to MCIs.

6.5.3.2 The plan should provide for organization and implementation of the following during MCIs:

(*a*) Incident command system,

(*b*) Patient triage, treatment, and transportation areas,

(*c*) Transportation dispatch and routing (ground, air, and water),

(*d*) Coordination with receiving hospitals (patient care capacity inventory (PCCI)),

(*e*) Medical teams,

(*f*) Communications plan,

(*g*) Psychosocial services,

(*h*) Medical records, and

(*i*) Resource inventory list of equipment, services, and personnel.

6.5.4 *Coordination*— Each EMS agency/jurisdiction should have plans and procedures that facilitate working with other response agencies during a MCI. Communications with these organizations should be established on a regular basis to ensure a more effective response. The EMS agency/jurisdiction should effectively interact with the following:

6.5.4.1 Hospitals, hospital consortia, skilled nursing facilities, poison control centers, and other specialty care centers,

6.5.4.2 Health department and mental health agencies,

6.5.4.3 Law enforcement agencies,

6.5.4.4 Fire services,

6.5.4.5 Other EMS agencies,

6.5.4.6 Local companies and businesses,

6.5.4.7 Local/regional EMS councils,

6.5.4.8 Media,

6.5.4.9 Emergency management offices of the local jurisdiction,

6.5.4.10 Local emergency planning committees (as defined by law for hazardous materials (HAZMAT) mitigation),

6.5.4.11 Specialty services such as CHEMTREC, HAZMAT teams (medical and mitigation), mine rescue teams, search teams, etc.,

6.5.4.12 Social service agencies such as the American Red Cross, Salvation Army, churches, and religious and community service groups,

6.5.4.13 City or county government,

6.5.4.14 Neighboring jurisdictions,

6.5.4.15 *State Government*— Procedures for obtaining assistance from state resources, including resources of the National Guard, and

6.5.4.16 *Federal Government*—Procedures for obtaining assistance from local installations of these agencies, including military resources, U.S. Weather Service, or National Park Service; and procedures for obtaining assistance through the state from federal agencies such as the Department of Health and Human Services or the Environmental Protection Agency.

6.6 *Legal Issues*— Ensure that the plan is in compliance with local, state, and federal laws and regulations.

6.7 *Psychosocial Services*—Arrangements for psychosocial services should be an integral part of the planning process. Efforts should be made to solicit involvement from professional clinicians who are experienced with medical systems. A coordinator should be assigned who participates as an active member of the area planning effort. This team should be organized, in place, and available as part of any community response effort. Further, this team should participate in all phases of the response, including planning and evaluation.

6.8 *Mutual Aid*

6.8.1 *Planning Stage*:

6.8.1.1 Define who will respond where and when, and what advanced life support procedures are authorized, etc.

6.8.1.2 Establish formal written agreements between jurisdictions to mitigate potential problems before they occur. Establish protocols for requesting aid and conditions for refusing to provide aid.

6.8.1.3 Update the equipment inventory and distribution of resources.

6.8.2 *Formal Agreement*— The written agreement should also include:

6.8.2.1 *Objectives*:

(*a*) Definition of mutual aid,

(*b*) Assignment of review date,

(*c*) Amendments, and

(*d*) Definitions used in plan.

6.8.2.2 *Participation*:

(*a*) Extent and limit of participation: emergency agencies, adjacent counties and cities, state agencies, and out of state jurisdictions,

(*b*) Point of contact,

(*c*) Request for mutual aid,

(*d*) Obligations of the plan,

(*e*) Conditions for refusing to provide aid, and

(*f*) Withdrawal from plan.

6.8.2.3 *Organization*:

(*a*) Local organization chart,

(*b*) Extent of authority of person initiating plan,

(*c*) Line of authority in absence,

(*d*) Status of EMS agency,

(*e*) Maintenance of individual authority of requesting incident command or EMS control,

(*f*) Local mutual aid plan operations exclusive of city or county plan,

(*g*) Assisting state or private institution,

(*h*) Assisting federal institution,

(*i*) Operation of city or county dispatch center,

(*j*) Preparation and use of participants' inventory and resources,

(*k*) Participation in the state EMS mobilization and mutual aid plan,

(*l*) Procedures to obtain activation,

(*m*) Authority and responsibility of EMS agencies and services, and

(*n*) Coordination with other EMS services.

6.8.2.4 *Equipment Loss Replacement Procedures*:

6.8.2.5 *Reimbursement*.

6.8.2.6 *Liability*.

6.8.2.7 *Operation Command Procedures*.

6.8.2.8 *Post Incident Evaluation*.

6.8.3 *Request*—When requesting mutual aid for an incident, specify the following:

6.8.3.1 Nature and location of the MCI,

6.8.3.2 Type of equipment and number of personnel requested, and whether specialized personnel are needed,

6.8.3.3 Location where assisting units shall report (staging area), and

6.8.3.4 Radio frequencies assigned to the incident.

NOTE 1—The agency receiving the request should consider availability of resources and provide the estimated response time to the staging area.

6.8.4 *Decision Plan*— Develop a decision plan for determining when to activate mutual aid agreements, request state aid, or recommend a state request for federal aid. Base the decision on resources, personnel, and number of patients.

6.9 *Evaluation*—The evaluation of an effective pre-hospital EMS system response to a MCI must encompass an objective, as well as a subjective assessment of the planning, needs assessment, training, communication, integration, coordination, mutual aid, implementation, and provision of resources by all organizations and agencies written into that area's plan. Because of the lack of reliable EMS system MCI analysis, all evaluators are urged to share their findings with the EMS and emergency management communities.

6.9.1 *Post Incident Analysis*—A subjective assessment of response to an actual incident should be held for all organizations and agencies that participated in the response. All comments and concerns should be researched for validity and impact in changing the plan.

6.9.1.1 An objective assessment should involve all agencies involved in the response and use a pre-established critique tool developed or accepted by the local planners.

6.9.2 Though the format of the objective critique will differ from area to area, the following principles of evaluation are important to the goal of that area's EMS system's response to MCIs:

6.9.2.1 The critique tool should include but not be limited to a minimum data set that should be collected as close to the conclusion of the emergency state as is safe for responders and is considerate of medical well-being of victims and responders.

6.9.2.2 The minimum data set should include but not be limited to a collection of reproducible data that can be verified and validated by subsequent investigators.

6.9.2.3 Whereas summaries for the data should be a matter of public record accessible to responsible requesters, the actual collected data should be a matter of EMS confidentiality and subject to release and disclosure only under subpoena.

6.9.2.4 This confidentiality for information involving victims and responders must be ensured by the area EMS agency and must not be confused with the purpose of the evaluations, which is to improve the future response.

6.9.2.5 The collected data on MCIs should be summarized and made available.

6.9.2.6 The data should be available for analysis by EMS research groups.

6.9.3 The implementation of the system evaluation after an incident may be accomplished by any qualified researcher (for example, conducted by a formally trained researcher) or participant evaluation group that has received the permission of that area's medical control to collect data.

6.9.3.1 Multi-disciplinary teams are suggested as systems evaluators for timely and efficient completion of the entire critique tool.

IMPLEMENTATION

7. Incident Command Structure

7.1 *Introduction*

7.1.1 The concept of the incident command system (ICS) was first developed by Fire Suppression Services in an effort to organize an effective response to forestfires, brush fires, and major urban conflagrations. The ICS includes some fundamental practices of management and control of personnel and resources. The general concept currently used by a majority of public safety agencies includes an incident commander or unified command post with staff support officers, and then distinct operational areas: (*1*) Operations Branch/Section, in charge of the actual tactical deployment of personnel and resources; (2) Financial Branch/Section, for financial and expense/payment accountability, typically found and used with state or federal government response; (*3*) a Planning Branch/Section, to prepare short/long term objectives and strategic decisions for incident command; and (*4*) Logistics Branch/Section, in charge of securing resources and supplies.

7.1.2 The general ICS training courses currently taught throughout the country do not specifically discuss the needs for immediate on-scene responsibilities for EMS.

7.1.3 The concept used in the planning guide for incident command assumes that any EMS agency/jurisdiction having authority to develop and implement an effective multiple casualty incident response plan will have the necessary training and understanding of the generic incident command system. The intent of this planning guide, and specifically this section, is to reinforce the acceptable job responsibilities and functions specifically required to mitigate a multiple casualty incident. This section does not address all of the components of an ICS that may be necessary in order for an EMS agency/jurisdiction to develop, implement, or mitigate an incident within their jurisdiction.

7.1.4 This section does not include specific information for the operations section officer, fire operations, police operations, public works, or hazardous materials teams. It does provide suggested job junctions for the key EMS positions. It does not imply that all positions must be staffed in every incident. The ICS section was prepared and written to provide detailed information for guidance for any EMS agency/jurisdiction needing such information. It is not intended to replace an EMS agency/jurisdiction's existing ICS plan as it relates to the EMS job functions/descriptions of the agency's established ICS plans.

7.1.5 Job descriptions and functions should be developed for all key ICS positions by mutual agreement between responding, responsible EMS agencies/jurisdictions as they relate to the overall incident command plan for a jurisdiction. For the purposes of this planning guide, some job functions were merged together. It should be the responsibility of the EMS agency/jurisdiction writing the multiple casualty incident plans to address any or all of the job functions and ensure that the job functions developed are reviewed by the EMS agencies and jurisdictions having authority for multiple casualty planning, response, and mitigation.

7.1.6 The job descriptions and functions listed in this section are models only and are designed to particularly highlight functions and tasks that must be fulfilled in the EMS operations section of an overall ICS. The model can be implemented by a rural EMS agency/jurisdiction, as well as a municipal EMS agency/jurisdiction. The system is devised around functional areas of management rather than staffing all listed command positions.

7.1.7 Although specific functional areas are emphasized, it does not mean that other areas may not be developed, or that these may not be further subdivided. In any incident, any EMS agency or jurisdiction could have several operating sectors depending upon the incident situations. It is important to remember that, at most, a person given functional responsibility within the ICS should not have more than four or five people under his direct supervision, or supervision should be moved to the next lower level of command within the incident command structure.

7.1.8 The functions of extrication, triage, treatment, and transportation are generally performed on all calls whether it be for two people or 200 people. The incident command model presented here for inclusion for a multiple casualty incident plan is one that is flexible and expandable in the particulars of any given incident.

7.1.9 It should be the responsibility of the EMS agency/jurisdiction having authority to ensure that the participants in the development of the multiple casualty incident planning guide for their jurisdictions have necessary knowledge and training on general incident command concepts and organization.

7.2 *Incident Command Duties*—The function of incident command is the overall management and coordination of all responding personnel and resources. The person assuming this command will be identified primarily by the type of incident, fire, medical, traffic, etc.

7.2.1 Upon arrival at the scene, an individual predetermined by the jurisdiction having authority shall assume the incident command function, and announce his name and title to the communications center for announcement to all other agencies and others involved.

7.2.2 The incident commander should request a face-to-face briefing with the emergency services personnel in charge at that time to obtain the following information:

7.2.2.1 Nature and scope of the incident,

7.2.2.2 Current situation,

7.2.2.3 Operational decisions made,

7.2.2.4 Current manpower committed,

7.2.2.5 Current resources committed,

7.2.2.6 Number of injuries and number of expected injuries,

7.2.2.7 Radio frequencies currently being used for the incident, and

7.2.2.8 Hazards that may hinder incident operation.

7.2.3 The incident commander should ensure that the following tasks are accomplished:

7.2.3.1 Establish a command post that should house together the police, fire, EMS, and search and rescue, to facilitate making and implementing face-to-face decisions,

7.2.3.2 Announce location of command post,

7.2.3.3 Coordinate interagency on-scene and off-scene communications,

7.2.3.4 Ensure that proper record-keeping is done, including such information as who held what positions at what times, notes, victim data, decision/command orders, log, communications, resources, and personnel present,

7.2.3.5 Designate appropriate ancillary functions: EMS, fire or rescue, logistics, staging, public information,

7.2.3.6 Request additional manpower and equipment, as appropriate,

7.2.3.7 Coordinate and control aircraft traffic in the airspace around the incident,

7.2.3.8 Receive situation reports from ancillary functions regarding the status of operations,

7.2.3.9 Demobilize incident, and

7.2.3.10 Prepare written after-action report.

7.2.4 The flow charts shown in Fig. 1 and Fig. 2 provide two examples of incident command structures utilized during a multiple casualty incident.

7.3 *EMS Control Sectors/Areas/EMS Management Functions*

7.3.1 The EMS control/medical group supervisor is responsible for the overall EMS operations at an incident, and for designating EMS functions, as appropriate, managing prehospital emergency care resources, and forwarding recommendations to the incident command.

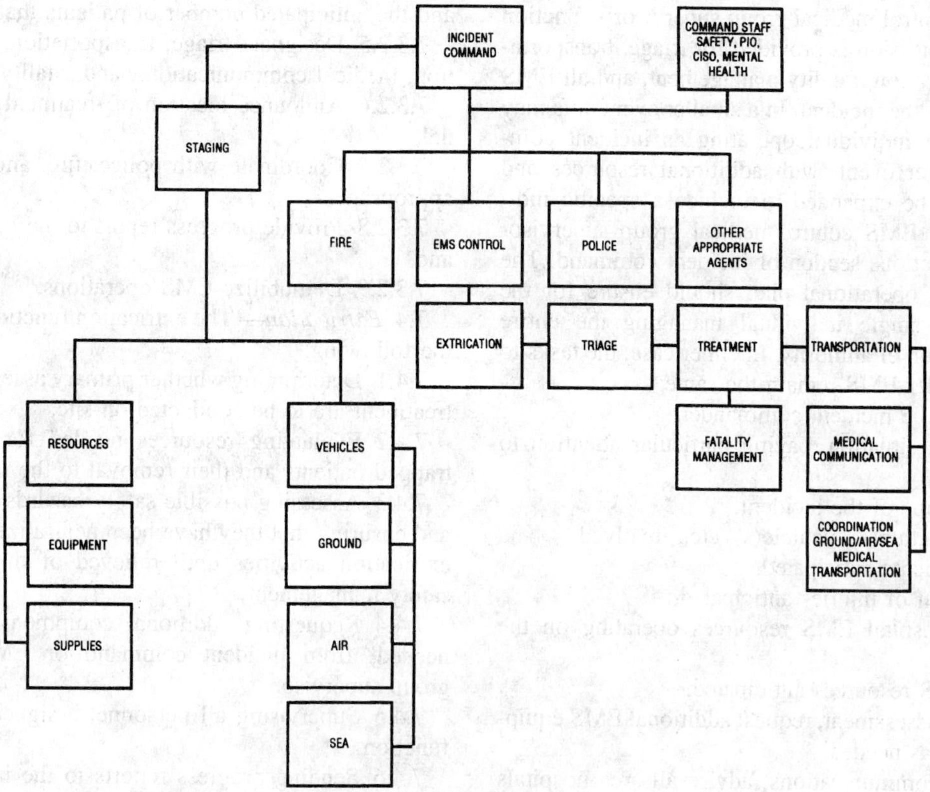

FIG. 1 Example 1—EMS Model for Management and Response

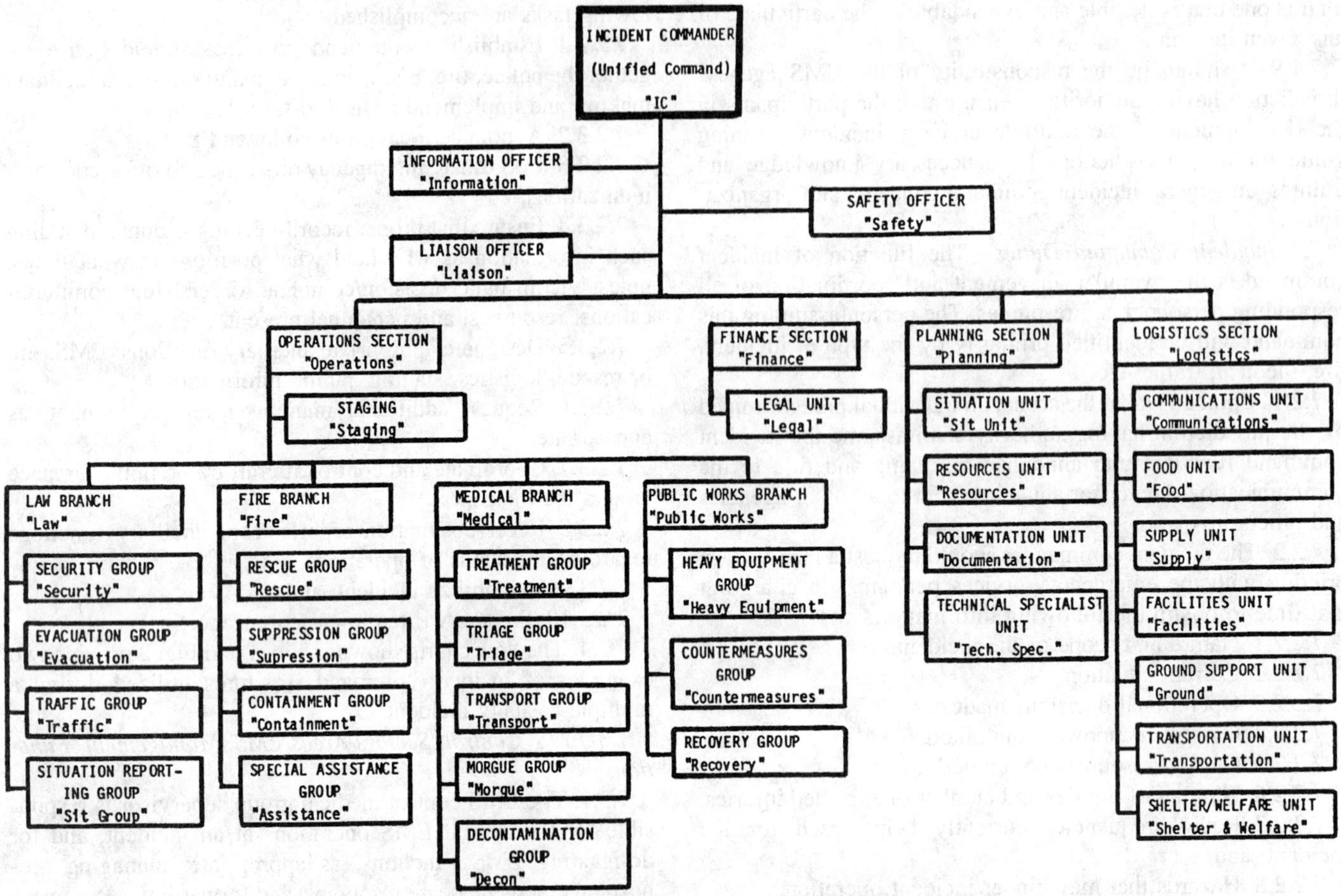

FIG. 2 Example 2—EMS Model for Management and Response

7.3.2 The EMS control/medical group supervisor's function is to ensure that supervision is provided for triage, transportation, treatment, extrication, fatality management, and all EMS personnel involved in the incident. In a smaller event, this may be done by a single individual operating as incident commander, or in a larger event, with additional resources and personnel, this may be expanded to include a specific individual designated as EMS control/medical group supervisor reporting to the operations section of incident command. The EMS agency's local operational plan should ensure for the changeover from a single individual managing the entire incident to a delegation of authority. In either case, the tasks to be accomplished under EMS remain the same:

7.3.2.1 Report to the incident commander,

7.3.2.2 Assess the situation, paying particular attention to the following:

(*a*) Nature and scope of the incident,

(*b*) Type(s) of structure(s), vehicle(s), etc., involved,

(*c*) Number of patients anticipated,

(*d*) Type and extent of injuries anticipated,

(*e*) Current pre-hospital EMS resources operating on the scene, and

(*f*) Additional EMS resources anticipated,

7.3.2.3 Based on assessment, request additional EMS equipment and personnel as needed,

7.3.2.4 Through communications, advise all area hospitals and specialty centers of the nature and scope of the incident, and the anticipated number of patients that are injured,

7.3.2.5 Designate triage, transportation, treatment, extrication, medical communications, and fatality management,

7.3.2.6 Announce location of treatment area to all personnel,

7.3.2.7 Coordinate with police, fire, and other agencies as appropriate,

7.3.2.8 Provide progress report to the incident commander, and

7.3.2.9 Demobilize EMS operations.

7.4 *Extrication*— The extrication function is responsible for the following:

7.4.1 Determining whether primary assessment and primary treatment are to be conducted on-site,

7.4.2 Evaluating resources needed for the extrication of trapped patients and their removal to the treatment area,

7.4.3 Assessing possible safety hazards in the environment and ensuring that they have been neutralized prior to initiating extrication activities until relieved of this responsibility by safety management,

7.4.4 Requesting additional equipment and personnel, as needed, from incident command or EMS control/medical group supervisor,

7.4.5 Supervising all personnel assigned to the extrication function,

7.4.6 Sending progress reports to the incident commander or EMS control/medical group supervisor,

7.4.7 Reporting to the incident command when all patients have been extricated and delivered to the treatment area, and

7.4.8 Coordinating activities with triage, treatment, and fatality management.

7.4.9 The extrication function reports to EMS control/medical group supervisor, and is designated by EMS control/medical group supervisor or the agency/jurisdiction having authority.

7.5 *Triage*—The triage function is responsible for the following (procedures for the triage process are contained in Section 9):

7.5.1 Sorting of patients to establish priorities for extrication, treatment, and transportation,

7.5.2 Ensuring that all patients are triaged,

7.5.3 Directing and controlling patient removal teams assigned to triage,

7.5.4 Ensuring that all patients are transferred to the appropriate treatment areas,

7.5.5 Transferring patient care to treatment area,

7.5.6 Maintaining communication and coordinating activities with treatment, extrication, and fatality management,

7.5.7 Requesting personnel and equipment, as needed,

7.5.8 Coordinating the activities of all pre-hospital personnel assigned to triage, and

7.5.9 Managing all triage activities at the site and providing update to EMS.

7.5.10 Triage reports to EMS control/medical group supervisor.

7.6 *Treatment*—The treatment function is responsible for the definitive on-scene treatment of patients, and for the following:

7.6.1 Determining the number and type of injured expected,

7.6.2 Establishing priority areas for treatment (primary, delayed, or minor),

7.6.3 Inventorying equipment and personnel necessary for the supervision of care in their area,

7.6.4 Providing for the proper deployment and utilization of personnel,

7.6.5 Receiving the transfer of patient care from triage as the patients are transferred from the triage area to the treatment area,

7.6.6 Ensuring that reassessment and re-triage of patients is done as needed,

7.6.7 Ensuring that appropriate treatment is rendered to patients within the treatment area,

7.6.8 Providing guidance and direction to treatment team personnel,

7.6.9 Maintaining constant communication with transportation to ensure coordinated patient loading area,

7.6.10 Coordinating activities with triage, transportation, extrication, and fatality management,

7.6.11 Managing all activities within the treatment area, and

7.6.12 Providing updates to EMS control/medical group supervisor.

7.6.13 Treatment reports to the EMS control/medical group supervisor and supervises all personnel assigned to the treatment area.

7.7 *Transportation*— The transportation function is responsible for the management of the transport of patients requiring medical treatment from the incident scene, and for the following:

7.7.1 Establishing a patient loading area,

7.7.2 Establishing or designating, or both, a medical communications function,

7.7.3 Arranging appropriate vehicles and methods of transport (ground or water vehicle or aircraft),

7.7.4 Maintaining a log of vehicle and patient destination,

7.7.5 Coordinating patient allocation and transportation with treatment and staging,

7.7.6 Determining hospital and specialty referral center capabilities, and, through communications, updating their status regularly,

7.7.7 Assigning patients to be transported to each facility, in accordance with pre-determined plans and policies or consultations with medical facilities, or both,

7.7.8 Communicating with receiving facility regarding patient condition and status,

7.7.9 Providing progress reports to EMS control/medical group supervisor, and

7.7.10 Reporting to EMS control/medical group supervisor when the last patient has been transported.

7.7.11 The transportation function reports to the EMS control/medical group supervisor and supervises ambulance, paramedic, and other transport crews, and all other personnel assigned to the transportation area.

7.8 *Medical Communications*—The medical communications function is responsible for establishing, maintaining, and coordinating medical communications at the incident scene between the hospital's medical control and the treatment and transportation functions as needed. These responsibilities include:

7.8.1 Establishing communications link with the designated hospital medical control system,

7.8.2 Acquiring hospital status information relating to patient handling capacity from hospital medical control and relaying it to transportation,

7.8.3 Obtaining patient-specific advanced life support orders as necessary,

7.8.4 Receiving basic patient information and injury status from triage/treatment and relaying it to hospital medical control,

7.8.5 Designating patient destination based on pre-determined bed availability assignment information to transportation,

7.8.6 Establishing additional medical communication as required, and

7.8.7 Providing ongoing progress reports to transportation.

7.8.8 Medical communications is a function designated by transportation. It reports to transportation or treatment, or both.

7.9 *Fatality Management*—The function of fatality management is to supervise all personnel assigned to the morgue area. Fatality management controls access to the area and organizes, coordinates, manages, and directs morgue functions, and is responsible for the following:

NOTE 2—The function of fatality management may be assigned to any emergency service responder until the arrival of the designated personnel (that is, medical examiner, coroner, funeral director). The function of fatality management should only be assigned to experienced emergency responders.

7.9.1 Establishing a morgue area remote from the treatment area and not readily available to other victims, but accessible to vehicles, such as, emergency vehicles, law enforcement, or coroner,

7.9.2 Assessing resources needed on the scene, such as equipment, supplies, personnel, and community health and social services,

7.9.3 Keeping area off-limits to all personnel, except those needed,

7.9.4 Coordinating with law enforcement and assisting the coroner's office as necessary,

7.9.5 Keeping identity of deceased victims confidential,

7.9.6 Maintaining records, including victims' identities (if available), personal effects, location found, etc., and

7.9.7 Providing appropriate security to the morgue area.

7.9.8 Fatality management is designated by and reports to EMS control/medical group supervisor or the agency/jurisdiction having authority.

7.10 *Support Functions*—Staging, logistics and resources, safety, public information, and critical incident stress teams are support functions to incident command.

7.10.1 *Staging*—The staging function is responsible for the orderly assembly (in a designated area) and on-scene dispatch of vehicles, equipment, and personnel, and for supervising air medical staging and all other personnel assigned to the staging area, and is responsible for:

7.10.1.1 Establishing a staging area,

7.10.1.2 Announcing the staging area location to incident command and communications center, so that all responding units will report to the staging area,

7.10.1.3 Establishing units for assignment as requested by incident command or transportation,

7.10.1.4 Requesting maintenance for vehicles, through logistics, at the staging area, as needed,

7.10.1.5 Updating incident command of the status of currently available units, and

7.10.1.6 Demobilizing staging area.

7.10.1.7 The staging function reports to an operations officer or the incident commander.

7.10.2 *Logistics and Resources*—The logistics and resources function is responsible for acquiring personnel, equipment (including vehicles), and supplies as requested by incident command, and for ensuring that the following tasks are accomplished:

7.10.2.1 Establishing an on-site equipment and supply resource area,

7.10.2.2 Inventorying equipment and supplies on the scene and determining requirements of additional equipment and supplies,

7.10.2.3 Receiving requests from the incident commander for equipment and resources that must be obtained from outside the incident area,

7.10.2.4 Requesting additional equipment and supplies as they arrive at the scene and notifying incident command, if appropriate, as to their assignment,

7.10.2.5 Maintaining inventory of arriving equipment and supplies,

7.10.2.6 Making provisions for service, repair, and fuel for all apparatus and equipment, and

7.10.2.7 Coordinating with other personnel, as appropriate.

7.10.2.8 The logistics and resources function reports to the incident commander.

7.10.3 *Safety*—The safety function monitors and assesses hazards and unsafe situations and develops measures to ensure personnel safety. Although emergency action may occur to stop unsafe actions, generally such actions should be corrected through the incident commander. Other tasks include:

7.10.3.1 Surveying incident areas and identifying hazards and potential hazards,

7.10.3.2 Advising incident command of special equipment, procedures, or teams needed to handle specific hazards,

7.10.3.3 Identifying and informing incident command of hazardous or potentially unsafe situations associated with the incident on an ongoing basis,

7.10.3.4 Exercising emergency authority to stop and prevent unsafe acts, and

7.10.3.5 Investigating and documenting accidents and injuries to emergency personnel and other events that have occurred within incident areas and recommending appropriate actions to eliminate or minimize risks.

7.10.3.6 The safety function reports to the incident commander.

7.10.4 *Public Information*—The public information function disseminates factual and timely reports to the news media. The individual performing this function should be the only person who deals with the media. The function is responsible for the following:

7.10.4.1 Contacting the incident commander for a briefing upon arrival,

7.10.4.2 Contacting the jurisdictional agency in charge to coordinate public information activities,

7.10.4.3 Establishing a media area located away from the command post,

7.10.4.4 Acting as liaison to the press to identify their needs and assist them in accessing special resources,

7.10.4.5 Deciding what information should be released,

7.10.4.6 Never releasing names of patients prior to notification of next of kin, and

7.10.4.7 Giving information such as patients' age, sex, a general description of injury (multi-trauma, burns, etc.), and hospital where patient was taken when describing injured patients.

7.10.4.8 The public information function reports to the incident commander.

7.10.5 *Critical Incident Stress Team*—The mental health coordinator leads the critical incident stress team. The critical incident stress team is a pre-organized unit that is responsible for the delivery of psychosocial support for victims and responders who experience acute stress reactions as the result of involvement in an incident. This function should include the following responsibilities:

7.10.5.1 Coordinating between incident command and providers in hospitals or other appropriate agencies, or both, which provide follow-up services,

7.10.5.2 Functioning as advisor to incident command on matters related to the psychosocial needs resulting from the incident,

7.10.5.3 Ensuring that training of psychosocial response personnel is established and is appropriate,

7.10.5.4 Verifying proper credentials of all psychosocial support staff,

7.10.5.5 Reporting the availability of the critical incident stress team at the scene to incident command,

7.10.5.6 Establishing an unobtrusive base of operations in the command post,

7.10.5.7 Assigning members of the team to cover the following:

(*a*) Assessing the psychological status of emergency personnel and victims of the incident,

(*b*) Providing the opportunity for emotional ventilation or participation in a defusing, which provides stress management education,

(*c*) Providing information and support to significant others who arrive at the scene,

(*d*) Referring for follow-up services, as needed, and

(*e*) Maintaining records as deemed appropriate.

7.10.5.8 The critical incident stress team function reports to the incident commander.

8. Communications

8.1 *Requirements*— EMS communications become particularly important during a MCI, in order to ensure that an EMS communications system can meet the special needs of an MCI, and not itself become disabled by the MCI. The system design should meet the following requirements:

8.1.1 *Interagency Communications*—Means should be provided to allow direct communications as needed among policy, fire, hospitals, and EMS units from different agencies. Available techniques include use of radios (common disaster channels, multiagency multichannel radios, or cross path of channels through dispatch center or mobile dispatch center), runner, and face-to-face communication. The fixed site facilities should be provided with independent standby power sources to avoid dependence on commercial power.

8.1.2 *Backup Systems*— All systems should strongly consider redundancy and backup communication systems.

8.2 *Support Functions*—An EMS communication system must provide the means by which emergency resources can be accessed, mobilized, managed, and coordinated. Telecommunications for support of EMS functions should include the following categories:

8.2.1 Dispatching and controlling movements of emergency vehicles,

8.2.2 Alerting and notifying receiving health care facilities,

8.2.3 Communicating the transportation priority and patient treatment care status,

8.2.4 Mobilizing medical response personnel,

8.2.5 Interfacing with law enforcement, fire, and local government agencies and other mutual providers, and

8.2.6 Communicating with field personnel to update incident response and response requirements.

9. Patient Care

NOTE 3—See Practice F 1149.

9.1 *Patient Care Capacity Inventory*—During an MCI the day-to-day hospital care system continues to provide care. In shifting to an MCI mode it is necessary for pre- and in-hospital planners to acknowledge that *people* take care of patients. Bed counts alone do not determine the ability to take care of patients. To provide the most effective care for the greatest number of victims of an MCI, hospitals must assess their capability to provide such MCI care. This assessment must be reported to the EMS control hospital, agency, or officer for assistance in the transportation of field ill or injured patients to appropriate hospitals. The communication of this patient care capacity inventory should be reported in two categories:

9.1.1 *Immediate*—The ability to devote one of each of the following to each patient for 1 hour:

9.1.1.1 Anesthesiologist,

9.1.1.2 Critical care or emergency care nurse,

9.1.1.3 Open surgical suite,

9.1.1.4 Physician (emergency medicine, critical care specialist, or general surgeon),

9.1.1.5 Respiratory therapist or certified nurse anesthetist,

9.1.1.6 Scribe, and

9.1.1.7 Surgical nurse.

9.1.2 *Delayed*—The ability to devote one of each of the following to each patient for ½hour:

9.1.2.1 Critical care nurse,

9.1.2.2 Physician, and

9.1.2.3 Scribe.

NOTE 4—These categories may be further broken down into more specific capacities or capabilities such as NDMS or Armed Services Medical Regulating Office (ASMRO) classifications.

9.2 *Triage: Field Triage During MCI*

9.2.1 The process of triage consists of three levels: primary, secondary, and tertiary, with the following objectives:

9.2.1.1 *Primary Triage*:

(*a*) Rapid patient assessment and tagging (documentation) into three groups (see Fig. 3), and

(*b*) Immediate (brief) life sustaining care, as necessary.

9.2.1.2 *Secondary Triage*:

(*a*) Document, tag, and sort patients, if not already performed, and

(*b*) Provide medical treatment as appropriate and available.

9.2.1.3 *Tertiary Triage*:

(*a*) Determine priority for disposition of the patient from the incident site, and

(*b*) Evaluate condition of patients relevant to resources, transportation, and available medical facilities. These factors will determine their priority for disposition from the scene.

9.2.2 *Triage Categories*—Victims are placed into the following categories in accordance with the local standard of medical care during an MCI. For example, see algorithm in Fig. 3.

9.2.2.1 *First Priority/Immediate*—Victims who have serious life threatening injuries but have a high probability of survival if they receive immediate care.

9.2.2.2 *Second Priority/Delayed*—Those victims who are

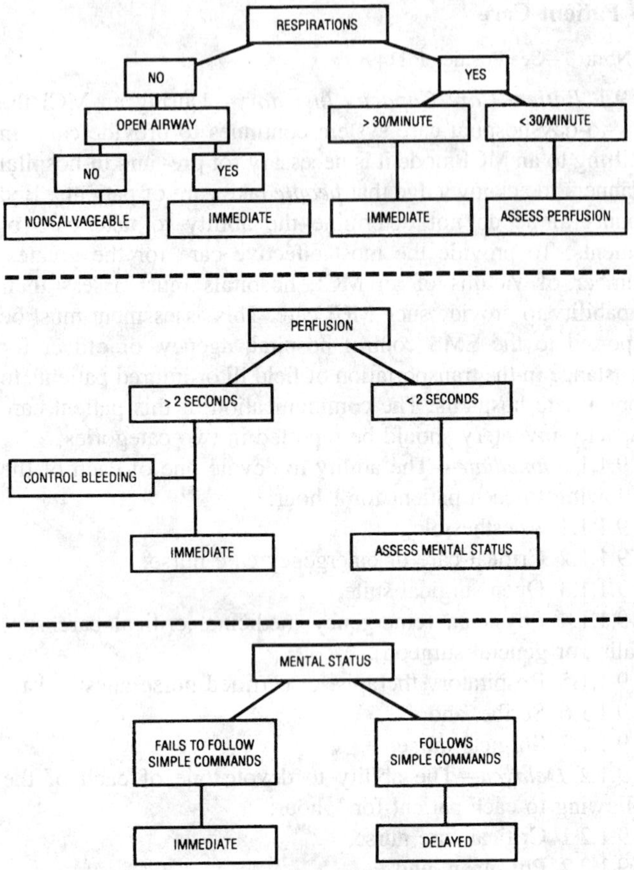

FIG. 3 Primary Triage

seriously injured and whose lives are not immediately threatened. Triage status of these patients may change to priority one patients based on medical resources at any time during the MCI, or upon consultation with on-line medical control, or both.

9.2.2.3 *Third Priority/Minor*—Those victims who are injured but do not require immediate medical attention, and those apparently not physically injured.

9.2.2.4 *Fourth Priority/Dead/Mortally Injured*—Those patients who are obviously dead as per local medical control or victims with severe injuries with low probability of survival, even with immediate care. Based on limited resources some patients who are expected to die may not receive immediate care. Those patients should be classified in the delayed or other category based on local policies. As this is a difficult field decision, actual practice may be to provide treatment and transportation.

9.3 *Standard Operations and Protocol Compatibility*—Cooperation of planning can minimize problems prior to occurrence of an MCI. Work within the local EMS region should be done to standardize basic life support (BLS) and advanced life support (ALS) procedures and protocols for all patients, including:

9.3.1 Airway management,

9.3.2 Shock,

9.3.3 Chest injuries,

9.3.4 Blunt trauma,

9.3.5 Head injuries,

9.3.6 Major orthopedic injuries, and

9.3.7 Medical emergencies.

9.4 *Field Medical Records*—Field medical records should be based on information as available, to include times of evaluation, treatment, and transport. The following information should be completed prior to the patient's arrival at the hospital:

9.4.1 Age, sex, name if known, and address,

9.4.2 Chief complaint, injuries found, and medical problem,

9.4.3 Treatment provided and vital signs,

9.4.4 Agency providing treatment or transportation, or both, and

9.4.5 Hospital to which patient is transported.

9.5 *Medical Response Teams*—Medical response teams can be activated from a number of sources, including the following:

9.5.1 *Local*:

9.5.1.1 *Hospital Based Response Teams*—Hospital based response teams may be able to respond to an incident in a short period of time. The team composition varies, but usually consists of a physician and nurse or EMT-P, or both, who are trained in triage, field medicine, and the incident command system. These teams will usually maintain an operational mode for a very short period of time until resupplied or until other personnel become available.

9.5.1.2 *HAZMAT Teams*— Hazardous materials teams are usually activated through the public health department or fire department. They are activated whenever the possibility of exposure to hazardous materials exists, or whenever decontamination due to hazardous materials is needed.

9.5.1.3 *Psychosocial Teams*—These teams are activated when calls are made to designated provider agencies and hospitals.

9.5.2 *State*—The State Office of Emergency Services should be contacted regarding state sponsored teams.

9.5.3 *National*—Disaster Medical Assistance Teams (DMATs) from the National Disaster Medical System (NDMS) can be activated by the federal government during a disaster. NDMS is a federally coordinated system that will supplement responses when the incident overwhelms local and state capacity to respond. DMATs can only be activated through a request from the state government. These are 29-member teams consisting of physicians, nurses, emergency medical technicians, and other personnel that can be mobilized to respond to a declared disaster. A unit of three DMATs can function independently. When teams are dispatched to the disaster site they will bring necessary supplies and equipment.

EVALUATION

10. Training

10.1 It is essential that EMS staff at all levels be trained to meet their responsibilities in the course of an MCI. This is critical for four reasons: (*1*) an MCI is unlikely to give advance warning, which means that response must be rapid and effective; (*2*) as neither the time nor place of an MCI can be predicted, all staff must be trained to respond; (*3*) an MCI response will differ significantly from single-patient response; and (*4*) the ability of the EMS organization to respond effectively can mean the difference between life and death, and health and disability, to MCI victims.

10.2 *Levels of Training*—Four levels of training are recommended for the training of emergency management personnel: basic, intermediate, mid-level, and senior management.

10.2.1 *Basic MCI Training* is recommended for all field responders who will need to recognize an MCI, report it properly, and respond as effectively as possible during the first crucial minutes and hours.

10.2.2 *Intermediate MCI Training* is recommended for field responders and managers who will need to initially assume incident command positions and responsibilities, mobilize additional EMS resources, and integrate the additional EMS resources into a well-coordinated response.

10.2.3 *Mid-Level MCI Training* is recommended for EMS managers who may need to assume senior incident command responsibility and interface the EMS response with other emergency response such as police, fire, search and rescue, and public works.

10.2.4 *Senior Management MCI Training* is recommended for senior EMS managers and directors who may need to interface with the news media, coordinate with local government officials, and request or mobilize resources from beyond their immediate jurisdiction.

10.3 *Curriculum*—An MCI training curriculum should address, at a minimum, the following:

10.3.1 Introduction/overview of National Interagency Management System response planning,

10.3.2 Developing the MCI response plan,

10.3.3 Roles, responsibilities, and resources of various responders, services, and levels of government,

10.3.4 Principles and practices for both pre-hospital and in-hospital MCI preparedness,

10.3.5 Field management of the MCI,

10.3.6 Triage,

10.3.7 Incident command system,

10.3.8 Drills and exercises,

10.3.9 Communications,

10.3.10 Coordination with other agencies and services,

10.3.11 Incident-specific guidelines, such as hazardous materials incidents, rural versus urban incidents, terrorist incidents, etc.,

10.3.12 Psychosocial impacts of MCIs on responders, victims, families, and the community, and

10.3.13 Evaluation and application of lessons learned from drills, exercises, and actual MCI response.

10.4 *Objectives*—At the end of a training session, trainees should be familiar with incident types, communication systems, pre-planning phase functions, scene command functions, scene triage, special resources, staging management, patient identification, procedures, medical control, transfer of command procedures, PCCI (patient care capacity inventory), and patient transport decision procedures.

10.5 *Training Drills and Exercises*

10.5.1 *Purpose*—The purpose of a drill is to test the plan, evaluate personnel performance, provide experience and training, meet licensure requirements, and draw attention to a problem.

10.5.2 *Defining Scope*:

10.5.2.1 Determine which agencies are involved and to what extent,

10.5.2.2 Determine a realistic scenario from community's problems, and

10.5.2.3 Define contingencies for bad weather, out of service equipment, etc.

10.5.3 *Planning the Drill*

10.5.3.1 Establish a committee with personnel from various sections or agencies. The committee should have defined responsibilities and appoint subcommittees as necessary.

10.5.3.2 Establish a timetable for the committee's work and for the drill date and times.

10.5.4 *Drill Management*— Safety is the primary concern. Identify a safety officer who has authority to stop any portion of the drill.

10.5.5 *Insurance*—The planning agency should consider a temporary insurance policy for participants.

10.5.6 *Evaluation*—Develop evaluation criteria to test the plan/drill exercise and provide timely review of evaluation data and outcome of the drill with participating agencies. A drill planning guidelines form is illustrated in Fig. 4.

Section I—To be completed during the first meetings of the committee.

1. Date and time of drill ______
2. Scenario ______
3. Total number of casualties and triage priority distribution
   Total ______
   Pr. I (RED) ______ Pr. II (YELLOW) ______
   Pr. III (GREEN) ______ Pr. IV (BLACK) ______
4. Committee Assignments and Service Liaisons
   a. Ambulance coordination ______
   b. Fire service ______
   c. Law enforcement ______
   d. Hospitals ______
   e. Staging ______
   f. Casualty coordination ______
   g. Moulage ______
   h. Press coordination ______
   i. Red Cross/blood bank ______
   j. Site selection and criteria ______
   k. Evaluation team ______
   l. Communications ______
   m. Chairman ______
   n. Military ______
   o. Mental health coordinator ______
   p. Medical examiner liaison ______
   q. Funeral directors liaison ______

Section II—To be completed during subsequent meetings by the committee chairman. There should be written reports from each member. This timetable and these reports can form the beginning of the written report of the exercise.

5. Ambulance Coordination Date of Report ______
   a. Participating squads or agencies No. of vehicles ______
   b. Will on-site treatment be simulated? ______
      If yes, by whom? ______
   c. Has a map showing the route from the scene to participating hospitals been prepared? ______
      When will it be distributed? ______
6. Fire Department Date of Report ______
   a. Extent of participation ______
   b. Name and phone numbers of contact persons ______
7. Law Enforcement Date of Report ______
   a. Extent of participation ______
   b. Name and phone numbers of contact persons ______
8. Hospitals Date of Report ______
   a. Extent of participation ______
   b. Name and phone numbers of contact persons ______
9. Staging Date of Report ______
   a. Location ______
   b. Permit obtained (if necessary) ______
   c. Conditions of use ______
   d. Name and phone number of contact person ______
10. Casualty Coordination Date of Report ______
    a. Names or organizations providing casualty volunteers
       Organizations Contact Person ______
    b. Who will provide training of the casualty volunteers? ______
    c. Who will provide food and transportation of casualties? ______
    d. Has a letter of instruction been prepared? ______
    e. Have injury assignments been made? ______
    f. Have arrangements been made for moulage removal? ______
    g. Have all volunteers signed the consent form? ______
11. Moulage Date of Report ______
    a. Names and organizations of moulagers ______
    b. Has the makeup been ordered? ______
    c. What time will the team arrive at staging to apply the moulage? ______
    d. Are there any injuries that might present a problem? ______
12. Press Coordination Date of Report ______
    a. Has a press release been prepared and by whom (attach a copy) ______
    b. Have members of the press been invited to observe the drill, and if so, who will attend? ______
    c. Have arrangements been made for photographs or videos? ______
    d. Who will be the spokesperson for the drill? ______
13. Red Cross/Blood Bank Date of Report ______
    a. Extent of participation ______
    b. Name and phone number of contact persons ______
14. Site Selection and Liaison Date of Report ______
    a. What site has been selected and who is the contact person? ______
    b. What special requests by this site owner must be adhered to? ______
    c. What forms of insurance need to be purchased? ______
    d. By whom, when, and at what cost? ______

FIG. 4 Drill Planning Guidelines

15. Evaluation Team Date of Report __________
    a. Names and assignments of team members
    ____
    ____
    ____
    ____
    b. Have critique sheets been prepared and shared with evaluators and participants? __________
    ____
    c. Where and when will the evaluation be conducted?
    ____
    ____
16. Communications Report Date of Report __________
    a. Who will need communications devices and what frequencies will they be using? __________
    ____
    ____
    b. What back-up systems are to be used in case of equipment failure? __________
    ____
    c. How will regular radio traffic be managed? __________
    ____
17. Chairman Date of Report __________
    a. Has a drill protocol, with injury list, been prepared? (attach a copy) __________
    b. Does the protocol describe the incident clearly? __________
    ____
    c. Does the protocol describe the exercise clearly and how and when each event is to take place? __________
    ____
    d. Does the protocol describe clearly who will start and terminate the exercise and at what times? Who stops drill in the event of a real disaster? __________
    ____
    e. What financial support is being given to this drill?
    ____

Section III—Attach a copy of your hospital-based community-wide disaster plan.

18. Medical Control
    a. Which facility will serve as medical control? __________
    ____
    b. Will the drill involve the need for victim decontamination, and if so, where will it be done (field or hospital)? __________
    ____
    c. Will med/surg teams be sent to the field, and if so, by whom? __________
    ____

Section IV—Other considerations:

19. Will aeromedical evacuation take place, and if so, by whom (name of service and contact person)? __________
    ____

Section V—Sample Consent Form

I, __________ give my permission for myself to participate in a disaster drill, sponsored jointly by __________ and the public agencies of __________, to be held on __________. I understand that the entire drill will be supervised. I permit photographs or videos to be taken of myself or my child while participating in the drill and agree that those photographs or videos may be used by any of the participating agencies. I understand that makeup may be applied to me to give the appearance of injury. I also agree not to hold any of the sponsoring agencies responsible for any injuries I may suffer in connection with the disaster drill.

____
Date

____
Signature of Participant

Witness

__________ Name	__________ Address
__________ Participant's name	__________ Participant's address
__________ Person to notify in emergency	__________ Phone number

FIG. 4 Drill Planning Guidelines *(continued)*

The American Society for Testing and Materials takes no position respecting the validity of any patent rights asserted in connection with any item mentioned in this standard. Users of this standard are expressly advised that determination of the validity of any such patent rights, and the risk of infringement of such rights, are entirely their own responsibility.

This standard is subject to revision at any time by the responsible technical committee and must be reviewed every five years and if not revised, either reapproved or withdrawn. Your comments are invited either for revision of this standard or for additional standards and should be addressed to ASTM Headquarters. Your comments will receive careful consideration at a meeting of the responsible technical committee, which you may attend. If you feel that your comments have not received a fair hearing you should make your views known to the ASTM Committee on Standards, 100 Barr Harbor Drive, West Conshohocken, PA 19428.

Standard Specification for Wrought Titanium-6 Aluminum-7 Niobium Alloy for Surgical Implant Applications [UNS R56700][1]

This standard is issued under the fixed designation F 1295; the number immediately following the designation indicates the year of original adoption or, in the case of revision, the year of last revision. A number in parentheses indicates the year of last reapproval. A superscript epsilon (ε) indicates an editorial change since the last revision or reapproval.

1. Scope

1.1 This specification covers the chemical, mechanical, and metallurgical requirements for wrought annealed titanium-6 aluminum-7 niobium alloy bar to be used in the manufacture of surgical implants **(1-4)**.[2]

1.2 The values stated in inch-pound units are to be regarded as the standard. The SI (metric) units given in parentheses are for information only.

2. Referenced Documents

2.1 *ASTM Standards:*

E 8 Test Methods for Tension Testing of Metallic Materials[3]

E 120 Test Methods for Chemical Analysis of Titanium and Titanium Alloys[4]

E 1409 Test Method for Determination of Oxygen in Titanium and Titanium Alloys by the Insert Gas Fusion Technique[4]

E 1447 Test Method for Determination of Hydrogen in Titanium and Titanium Alloys by the Insert Gas Fusion Thermal Conductivity Method[5]

F 981 Practice for Assessment of Compatibility of Biiomaterials for Surgical Implants with Respect to Effect of Materials in Muscle and Bone[6]

2.2 *Aerospace Material Specification:*

AMS 2249 Chemical Check Analysis Limits, Titanium and Titanium Alloys[7]

2.3 *ASQC Standard:*

C1 Specification of General Requirements for a Quality Program[8]

3. Ordering Information

3.1 Inquiries and orders for material under this specification shall include the following information:

3.1.1 Quantity (weight or number of pieces),

3.1.2 ASTM designation,

3.1.3 Dimensions,

3.1.4 Condition,

3.1.5 Finish, and

3.1.6 Special requirements.

4. Materials and Manufacture

4.1 The titanium alloy shall be manufactured from multiple vacuum melted material using conventional reactive metal processing methods. The bar product covered in this specification is normally formed with the conventional forging and rolling equipment found in ferrous and nonferrous plants.

4.2 *Finish*—Annealed bar may be furnished to the implant manufacturer as descaled or pickled, sandblasted, ground, or combinations of these operations.

5. Chemical Composition

5.1 The heat analysis shall conform to the chemical composition of Table 1. Ingot analysis may be used for reporting all chemical requirements, except hydrogen. Samples for hydrogen shall be taken from the finished mill product.

5.1.1 Requirements for the major and minor elemental constituents are listed in Table 1. Also listed are important residual elements. Analysis for elements not listed in Table 1 is not required to certify compliance with this specification.

5.2 *Product Analysis*:

5.2.1 Product analysis tolerances do not broaden the specified heat analysis requirements but cover variations between laboratories in the measurement of chemical content. The manufacturer shall not ship material that is outside the limits specified in Table 1. Product analysis limits shall be as specified in Table 2.

5.2.2 The product analysis is either for the purpose of verifying the composition of a heat or lot or to determine variations in the composition within the heat.

5.3 For referee purposes, Test Methods E 120, E 1409, and E 1447 shall be used or other analytical methods agreed upon between purchaser and supplier shall be used.

5.4 Samples for chemical analysis shall be representative of

---

[1] This specification is under the jurisdiction of ASTM Committee F-4 on Medical and Surgical Materials and Devicesand is the direct responsibility of Subcommittee F04.12 on Metallurgical Materials.

Current edition approved June 10, 1997. Published September 1997. Originally published as F 1295 – 92. Last previous edition F 1295 – 97.

[2] The boldface numbers in parentheses refer to a list of references at the end of the text.

[3] *Annual Book of ASTM Standards*, Vols 01.02, 02.01, 02.02, 02.03, and 03.01.

[4] *Annual Book of ASTM Standards*, Vol 03.05.

[5] *Annual Book of ASTM Standards*, Vol 03.06.

[6] *Annual Book of ASTM Standards*, Vol 13.01.

[7] Available from Society of Automotive Engineers, 400 Commonwealth Drive, Warrendale, PA 15096.

[8] Available from American Society for Quality Control, 161 West Wisconsin Ave., Milwaukee, WI 53203.

TABLE 1 Chemical Requirements

Element	Composition, %
Aluminum	5.50 to 6.50
Niobium	6.50 to 7.50
Tantalum	0.50 max
Iron	0.25 max
Oxygen	0.20 max
Carbon	0.08 max
Nitrogen	0.05 max
Hydrogen	0.009 max
Titanium[A]	Balance

[A] The percentage of titanium is determined by difference and need not be determined or certified.

TABLE 2 Product Analysis Tolerances[A]

	Tolerance Under the Minimum[B] or Over the Maximum Limit
Aluminum	0.10
Niobium	0.10
Tantalum	0.10
Iron	0.10
Oxygen	0.02
Carbon	0.02
Nitrogen	0.02
Hydrogen	0.002

[A] Refer to AMS 2249.
[B] Under minimum limit not applicable for elements where only a maximum percentage is indicated.

the material being tested. The utmost care must be used in sampling titanium for chemical analysis because of its affinity for elements such as oxygen, nitrogen, and hydrogen. Therefore, in cutting samples for analysis any contamination should be avoided. Chips should be clean and sharp cutting tools should be used. Samples for analysis should be stored in suitable containers.

6. Mechanical Properties

6.1 Material supplied under this specification shall conform to the mechanical properties given in Table 3.

6.2 Specimens for tension tests shall be machined and tested in accordance with Test Methods E 8. Tensile properties shall be determined using a strain rate of 0.003 to 0.007 in./in./min. through the specified yield strength and then the crosshead speed shall be increased so as to produce fracture in approximately one additional minute.

6.3 *Number of Tests*— A minimum of two tension tests shall be made from each lot. A lot is defined as the total number of a specific mill product produced under the same conditions at essentially the same time. Should either of the test specimens not meet the specific requirements or break outside the gage limits, two additional test pieces representative of the same lot shall be tested in the same manner. The lot shall be rejected if either of the additional test pieces fail to meet the specified requirements.

TABLE 3 Annealed Mechanical Properties for Bar[A]

Ultimate Tensile Strength, min, psi, (MPa)	Yield Strength (0.2 % offset), min, psi, (MPa)	Elongation, [B] min, %	Reduction of area, min, %
130 500 (900)	116 000 (800)	10	25

[A] Up to 3.94 in. (100 mm) diameter or thickness.
[B] Gage length = 5.65 $\sqrt{S_o}$ or 2 in. (50 mm), where S_o is the original cross-sectional area.

7. Microstructure

7.1 The microstructure shall be a fine dispersion of the alpha and beta phases resulting from processing in the alpha plus beta field. There shall be no continuous alpha network at prior beta grain boundaries. There shall be no coarse, elongated alpha platelets. There shall be no alpha case.

7.2 Products supplied with a machined or ground surface finish shall have no alpha case. For other products, there shall be no continuous layer of alpha case when examined at 100×.

7.3 A minimum of one sample per lot shall be examined.

8. Certification

8.1 A certificate of tests shall be provided with the following information:

8.1.1 Heat number,

8.1.2 Mill or purchase number, or both,

8.1.3 Chemical analysis including Al, Nb, Ta, Fe, O, C, N, and H,

8.1.4 Mechanical properties (tensile strength, yield strength, elongation, reduction of area),

8.1.5 Surface finish,

8.1.6 Quantity delivered,

8.1.7 Date of shipment,

8.1.8 Size and condition, and

8.1.9 Specification.

9. Product Marking

9.1 The name of the manufacturer, heat number, lot number, specification number, and year of issue shall be legibly and durably marked.

10. Quality Assurance

10.1 The producer shall maintain a quality assurance program, for example, such as defined in ASQC C1.

10.2 The manufacturer of surgical implants shall be assured of the producer's quality assurance program for conformance to the intent of ASQC C1 or other recognized program.

APPENDIXES

(Nonmandatory Information)

X1. RATIONALE

X1.1 The purpose of this specification is to characterize the composition and properties of wrought annealed Ti-6A1-7Nb titanium alloy bar to ensure consistency in the starting material used in the manufacture of medical devices, in particular of surgical implants.

X1.2 The microstructural requirements contained in this specification represent the current general consensus of opinion with respect to optimization of mechanical properties for implant applications.

X1.3 The minimum mechanical properties specified ensure a baseline of strength and ductility for the highly stressed devices that may be manufactured from this alloy.

X1.4 The stress corrosion cracking resistance of this alloy is similar to Ti-6A1-4V alloy.

X1.5 The UNS designation has been added, residual element language has been included, alpha case information has been clarified, the inclusion requirement has been deleted because no standard method exists for determining the inclusion content in titanium alloys, and Appendix X2 Biocompatibility section has been added to the Rationale.

X2. BIOCOMPATIBILITY

X2.1 The material composition covered by this standard has been employed successfully in contact with soft tissue and bone for over a decade.

X2.2 No known surgical implant has ever been shown to be completely free of adverse reactions in the human body. However, long term clinical experience has shown an acceptable level of biological response can be expected, if the material is used in appropriate applications.

X2.3 The material in this specification has been subjected to animal studies **(5)** and has been shown to produce a well characterized level of biological response that is equal to or less than that produced by the reference material titanium. This material has been used clinically since 1986 **(6 and 7)**.

REFERENCES

(1) Semlitsch, M., Straub, F., and Weber, H., "Titanium-Aluminium-Niobium Alloy, Development of Biocompatible, High Strength Surgical Implants," *Biomedizinische Technik 30*, 12, 1985, pp. 334–339.

(2) Maeusli, P. A., Block, P. R., Geret, V., and Steinemann, S. G., "Surface Characterization of Titanium and Titanium Alloys," *Biological and Biomechanical Performance of Biomaterials*, edited by Christel, Meunier, and Lee, Elsevier Science Publ., 1986, pp. 57–62.

(3) Simpson, J. P., "The Electrochemical Behaviour of Titanium and Titanium Alloys with Respect to their Use as Surgical Implant Materials," *Biological and Biomechanical Performance of Biomaterials*, 1986, pp. 63–68.

(4) Semlitsch, M., Staub, F., and Weber, H., "Development of a Vital, High-Strength Titanium-Aluminium-Niobium Alloy for Surgical Implant Materials," *Biological and Biomechanical Performance of Biomaterials*, 1986, pp. 69–74.

(5) Perren, S. M., Geret, V., Tepic, M., and Rahn, B. A., "Quantitative Evaluation of Biocompatibility of Vanadium-Free Titanium Alloys," *Biological and Biomechanical Performance of Biomaterials*, 1986, pp. 397–402.

(6) Semlitsch, M.," Titanium Alloys for Hip Joint Replacements," *Clinical Materials*, 2, 1987, pp. 1–13.

(7) Zweymüller, K. A., Lintner, F. K., and Semlitsch, M. F., "Biologic Fixation of a Press-Fit Titanium Hip Joint Endoprosthesis," *Clinical Orthopaedics and Related Research* 235, Oct. 1988, pp. 195–206.

Designation: F 1314 – 95

Standard Specification for Wrought Nitrogen Strengthened–22 Chromium–12.5 Nickel–5 Manganese–2.5 Molybdenum Stainless Steel Bar and Wire for Surgical Implants[1]

This standard is issued under the fixed designation F 1314; the number immediately following the designation indicates the year of original adoption or, in the case of revision, the year of last revision. A number in parentheses indicates the year of last reapproval. A superscript epsilon (ϵ) indicates an editorial change since the last revision or reapproval.

1. Scope

1.1 This specification covers the requirements for wrought nitrogen strengthened–22 chromium–12.5 nickel–5 manganese–2.5 molybdenum stainless steel bar and wire (except suture wire) used for the manufacture of surgical implants.

1.2 The values stated in inch-pound units are to be regarded as the standard. The values in parentheses are for information only.

2. Referenced Documents

2.1 *ASTM Standards:*

A 262 Practices for Detecting Susceptibility to Intergranular Attack in Austenitic Stainless Steels[2]

A 484/A 484M Specification for General Requirements for Stainless and Heat-Resisting Bars, Billets, and Forgings[3]

A 555/A 555M Specification for General Requirements for Stainless and Heat-Resisting Steel Wire and Wire Rods[2]

A 751 Test Methods, Practices, and Terminology for Chemical Analysis of Steel Products[2]

E 45 Practice for Determining the Inclusion Content of Steel[4]

E 112 Test Methods for Determining Average Grain Size[4]

F 746 Test Method for Pitting and Crevice Corrosion of Metallic Surgical Implant Materials[5]

F 981 Practice for Assessment of Compatibility of Biomaterials (Nonporous) for Surgical Implants with Respect to Effect of Materials on Muscle and Bone[5]

2.2 *American Society for Quality Control (ASQC) Standard:*

Cl Specification of General Requirements for a Quality Program[6]

3. Ordering Information

3.1 Inquiries and orders for material under this specification shall include the following information:

3.1.1 Quality (weight or number of pieces),

3.1.2 ASTM designation,

3.1.3 Form (bar or wire),

3.1.4 Condition (see 4.1),

3.1.5 Mechanical properties (if applicable, for special conditions),

3.1.6 Finish (see 4.2),

3.1.7 Applicable dimensions including size, thickness, width, and length (exact, random or multiples) or print number, and

3.1.8 Special requirements.

4. Materials and Manufacture

4.1 *Condition*—Bar and wire shall be furnished to the implant manufacturer, as specified, in the hot-worked, annealed, or cold-worked condition.

4.2 *Finish*—Types of finish available in bar and wire products are cold-drawn, pickled, ground, ground and polished, or as specified in the implant manufacturer's purchase order.

5. Chemical Composition

5.1 The heat analysis shall conform to the requirements as to chemical composition specified in Table 1.

5.2 Methods and practices relating to chemical analysis required by this specification shall be in accordance with Test Methods A 751.

5.3 Requirements for the major and minor elemental constituents are listed in Table 1. Also listed are important residual elements. Analysis for elements not listed in Table 1 is not required to verify compliance with this specification.

6. Metallurgical Requirements

6.1 The material shall exhibit no free ferrite phase when it is examined metallographically at 100× magnification.

6.2 The microcleanliness of the steel, as determined by Practice E 45, Method A, except using Plate III and Plate I, on representative billet or bar samples from the heat shall not exceed the following:

---

[1] This specification is under the jurisdiction of ASTM Committee F-4 on Medical and Surgical Materials and Devices and is the direct responsibility of Subcommittee F04.12 on Metallurgical Materials.

Current edition approved March 15, 1995. Published May 1995. Originally published as F 1314 – 90. Last previous edition F 1314 – 90.

[2] *Annual Book of ASTM Standards*, Vol 01.03.

[3] *Annual Book of ASTM Standards*, Vol 01.05.

[4] *Annual Book of ASTM Standards*, Vol 03.01.

[5] *Annual Book of ASTM Standards*, Vol 13.01.

[6] Available from American Society for Quality Control, 161 West Wisconsin Ave., Milwaukee, WI 53203.

TABLE 1 Chemical Requirements, Heat Analysis

Element	Composition, %
Carbon	0.030 max
Manganese	4.00 to 6.00
Phosphorus	0.025 max
Sulfur	0.010 max
Silicon	0.75 max
Chromium	20.50 to 23.50
Nickel	11.50 to 13.50
Molybdenum	2.00 to 3.00
Nitrogen	0.20 to 0.40
Niobium	0.10 to 0.30
Vanadium	0.10 to 0.30
Copper	0.50 max
Iron[A]	balance

[A] Approximately equal to the difference between 100 % and the sum percent of the other specified elements. The percent iron content by difference is not required to be reported.

Inclusion Type	A (Sulfide)	B (Alumina)	C (Silicate)	D (Globular oxide)
Thin	1.5	2.5	2.5	2.5
Heavy	1.5	1.5	1.5	1.5

NOTE 1—General practice is to use electroslag remelted steel to comply with these cleanliness requirements and to give other additional benefits.

7. Mechanical Requirements

7.1 Material shall conform to the appropriate requirements as to mechanical properties specified in Table 2. The level of mechanical properties for material in other than the annealed condition shall be specified in the implant manufacturer's purchase order.

7.2 Brinell hardness number (HB) is the preferred method of reporting the hardness of hot-worked material. Hardness determinations shall be made on a product cross section midway between the center and the surface, if the cross section size is adequate.

7.3 When desired, hardness limits may be specified. Hardness determination on cold-worked material shall be made on a product cross section, midway between the center and surface, if cross section size is adequate.

8. Special Tests

8.1 The steel shall be capable of passing the intergranular corrosion susceptibility test in accordance with Practices A 262, Practice E. The test shall be performed on a sample sensitized at 1250°F for 1 h.

8.2 The grain size shall be five or finer when tested in accordance with Test Methods E 112.

8.2.1 If grain size samples are selected after a final cold-working operation, transverse specimens shall be prepared.

8.3 Any other special requirements shall be specified on the purchase order.

9. General Requirements for Delivery

9.1 In addition to the requirements of this specification, all requirements of the current editions of Specifications A 484/A 484M and A 555/A 555M shall apply.

9.2 In cases where a conflict exists between this specification and the standards listed in 2.1 and 2.2, this specification shall take precedence.

10. Certification

10.1 The manufacturer's certification that the material was manufactured and tested in accordance with this specification together with a report of the test results shall be furnished at the time of shipment.

11. Quality Program Requirements

11.1 The producer shall maintain a quality program, such as defined in ASQC C1.

11.2 The manufacturer of surgical implants may audit the producer's quality program for conformance to the intent of ASQC Cl, or other recognized program.

12. Keywords

12.1 manganese; metals (for surgical implants); nitrogen strengthened; stainless steel; surgical applications

TABLE 2 Mechanical Requirements, Wire and Bar

Condition	Diameter or Thickness, in. (mm)	Ultimate Tensile Strength, min, psi (MPa)	Yield Strength (0.2 % Offset), min, psi (MPa)	Elongation[A] in 4*D*, min, %	Brinell[B] Hardness, max, HB
Hot-worked[C]	Up to 2 (50.8), incl	...	...	...	325
Annealed	all	100 000 (690)	55 000 (380)	35	
Cold-worked	1⁄16 to 3⁄4 (1.59 to 19.1)[D], incl	150 000 (1035)	125 000 (862)	12	

[A] 4D = 4 × diameter.
[B] 3000-kgf (20 400-N) load.
[C] Typically supplied as hot-rolled bar for forging applications.
[D] Other sizes may be furnished by agreement between the producer and the purchaser.

APPENDIX

(Nonmandatory Information)

X1. RATIONALE

X1.1 The primary purpose of this specification is to characterize composition and properties of a nitrogen strengthened austenitic stainless steel to ensure consistency in the starting material used, directly or as modified by forging, in the manufacturing of medical devices.

X1.2 The metallurgical requirements include fine-grained austenitic structure free of ferrite, with low micro-inclusion content and capability of passing an intergranular corrosion susceptibility test.

X1.3 Acceptable metal conditions supplied to the implant manufacturer include hot-worked, annealed, and all cold-worked conditions, the choice dependent upon the implant design and application.

X1.4 The material has been shown to produce an acceptable level of local biological response that is similar to F138, Grade 2 reference material.[7] The low-carbon composition has been selected to provide an extra measure of assurance that the material will be free from susceptibility to intergranular corrosion.

X1.5 This alloy is capable of being cold worked to ultimate tensile strengths exceeding 200 000 psi (1380 Mpa) for high-strength surgical implant applications.

X1.6 This alloy has been tested in accordance with Test Method F 746 and exhibits a pitting potential greater than F138, Grade 2 reference material.

X1.7 The nitrogen used for strengthening this steel can result in the formation of carbonitrides. Carbonitrides can be revealed by etching electrolytically in a solution of potassium hydroxide (56 g of K(OH) in 100 mL of water for 3 s at 2 V). These small dispersed second phase particles exert a strengthening effect but do not significantly alter the corrosion properties of the alloy. They may effect the finish of electropolished surfaces.

[7] FDA Submission No. K830196.

Designation: F 1325 – 91 (Reapproved 1996)

Standard Specification for Stainless Steel Suture Needle Holders-General Workmanship Requirements and Corresponding Test Methods[1]

This standard is issued under the fixed designation F 1325; the number immediately following the designation indicates the year of original adoption or, in the case of revision, the year of last revision. A number in parentheses indicates the year of last reapproval. A superscript epsilon (ϵ) indicates an editorial change since the last revision or reapproval.

1. Scope

1.1 This specification covers general workmanship aspects of stainless steel suture needle holders intended for reuse in surgery.

2. Referenced Documents

2.1 *ASTM Standards:*

E 18 Test Methods for Rockwell Hardness and Rockwell Superficial Hardness of Metallic Materials[2]

E 92 Test Method for Vickers Hardness of Metallic Materials[2]

E 140 Hardness Conversion Tables for Metals[2]

F 899 Specification for Stainless Steel Billet, Bar, and Wire for Surgical Instruments[3]

F 921 Definitions of Terms Relating to Hemostatic Forceps[3]

F 1089 Test Method for Corrosion of Surgical Instruments[3]

3. Terminology

3.1 *Definition:*

3.1.1 *modified working end*—working surfaces possessing superior hardness characteristics which are either the result of depositing various materials on the base metal or the result of permanently securing an insert (such as by brazing) to the base metal.

3.1.2 *Discussion*—The typical method of modifying the working end of the suture needle holder is to use jaw inserts or to plasma deposit (flame plate) materials with improved wear characteristics such as tungsten carbide or stellite. For the jaw insert method, the insert is brazed to the jaw face with a uniform deposit of silver solder which is free of crevices at all interfaces. For the flame plating method, a uniform layer of material is deposited which is 0.004 ± 0.001 in. thick.

3.2 Definitions applicable to stainless steel suture needle holders and the terms specified herein, shall be in accordance with Definitions of Terms F 921.

4. Materials

4.1 All component parts of the instrument other than the modified working end shall be fabricated from martensitic stainless steel type 410, 410X, 416, 420A, 420B, 420C, 420F, 420F Mod, and 440B per Specification F 899 (see Note 1). The modified working end may be made of stellite, tungsten carbide, or other suitable material.

NOTE 1—Free-machining grades of stainless steel are inappropriate for use due to their lower corrosion resistance and toughness.

5. Requirements

5.1 Heat treatment and hardness for component parts.

5.1.1 Stainless steel component parts of the instrument shall be heat treated under conditions recommended for the material used.

5.1.2 The Rockwell hardness of an instrument with the working end not modified shall be 42 HRC to 52 HRC. Instruments where the working end has been modified shall have a modified working surface whose Rockwell hardness is A77 minimum.

5.2 *Corrosion Resistance*—Holders with working ends not modified shall be subjected to corrosion tests as specified in Test Method F 1089. Holders with modified working ends shall be subject to corrosion tests as specified in Test Method F 1089 except for the modifying material.

6. Performance Requirements

6.1 *Needle retention test*—From Table 1, select a needle, sized for use with the holder being tested. The suture needle, with its axis held perpendicularly to the axis of the jaw shall, upon engagement of the second ratchet of the suture needle holder, show no lateral, rotational, or longitudinal motion when subjected to a one-half pound pull and a one-inch-pound torsion.

7. Workmanship, Finish, and Appearance

7.1 *Finish*:

7.1.1 *Surfaces*—Surfaces of the instrument shall be uniformly finished and free from burrs, sharp edges, cracks, coarse marks, and processing materials.

7.1.2 *Type*—The finish shall be one of the types specified in

[1] This specification is under the jurisdiction of ASTM Committee F-4 on Medical and Surgical Materials and Devices and is the direct responsibility of Subcommittee F04.33 on Medical/Surgical Instruments.

Current edition approved April 15, 1991. Published June 1991.

[2] *Annual Book of ASTM Standards*, Vol 03.01.

[3] *Annual Book of ASTM Standards*, Vol 13.01.

TABLE 1 Suture/Needle/Holder Relationship

Suture Needle Holder	Most Common Use	Recommended Teeth Per Square Inch	Compatible Suture Size Per USP[A]		Corresponding Wire Size (Diameter) of Needle
Debakey 7″ thru 12″	vascular and valve	2500	0	0.16 in.	.035 in.
			2-0	0.14	0.24
Hufnagel 8″ thru 10″	replacement	2500	3-0	.010	.024
			4-0	.008	.015
Webster	coronary	3500 or	5-0	.006	.015
Hegar-Mayo	bypass	smooth	6-0	.004	.009
Brown			7-0	.003	.009
Castrovieijo	microsurgery	smooth	8-0	.002	.006
			9-0	.0015	.006
Kalt		smooth	10-0	.0008	.006

[A]Mean average of USP absorbable and non-absorbable and Suture size averages.

Definitions of Terms F 921 or as specified by the purchaser.

7.2 *Workmanship*:

7.2.1 Finger rings-inside surfaces of the finger rings shall be well rounded and conform to the requirements of Section 7.1.1.

7.2.2 The pivot screw or pin shall be permanently set peened, and flush.

Standard Guide for Training Emergency Medical Technician (Basic) to Prepare Patients for Medical Transportation[1]

This standard is issued under the fixed designation F 1328; the number immediately following the designation indicates the year of original adoption or, in the case of revision, the year of last revision. A number in parentheses indicates the year of last reapproval. A superscript epsilon (ε) indicates an editorial change since the last revision or reapproval.

1. Scope

1.1 This guide establishes the minimum training standard for preparing ill or injured patients of all ages for medical transportation.

1.2 This guide is one of a series that together describe the minimum training standard for the emergency medical technician (basic).

2. Referenced Documents

2.1 *ASTM Standards:*

F 1031 Practice for Training the Emergency Medical Technician (Basic)[2]

F 1219 Guide for Training the Emergency Medical Technician (Basic) to Perform Patient Initial and Detailed Assessment[2]

2.2 *Other Documents:*[2]

Standards and Guidelines for Cardiopulmonary Resuscitation and Emergency Cardiac Care. Reprinted from Journal of the American Medical Association, lastest edition

3. Terminology

3.1 *Definitions of Terms Specific to This Standard:*

3.1.1 *management*—the step(s) that constitute action taken by the emergency medical technician (basic) for a patient in need of assistance due to a real or perceived traumatic or medical condition.

4. Significance and Use

4.1 This guide establishes the minimum national standard for training the emergency medical technician (basic) to prepare the ill and injured patient of all ages for medical transportation. This guide does not preclude additions to or modification of these as authorized by local medical direction.

4.2 This guide shall be used by those who wish to identify the minimum training standard for the emergency medical technician (basic) as it relates to moving, lifting, and transporting patients.

4.3 This guide shall be used as the basis to revise Practice F 1031.

4.4 Every person who is identified as an emergency medical technician (basic) shall have been trained to this standard.

4.5 This guide must be used in conjunction with Practice F 1031, Guides F 1219, and JAMA Standards and Guidelines.

5. General Guidelines

5.1 All emergency medical technicians (basic) shall be trained to accomplish the following:

5.1.1 All patients must be reassessed frequently and at least prior to and following every therapeutic intervention.

5.1.2 Patients may have more than one problem and these problems should be dealt with in the order of their severity.

5.1.3 Patients with life-threatening conditions which cannot be resolved in the field should be immediately transported in accordance with local protocol.

5.1.4 Patients shall be treated in a professional, caring, and reassuring manner.

5.1.5 The emergency medical technician (basic) is responsible for facilitating the delivery of definitive care by a higher level of care in both the field or hospital in the most expedient manner available.

5.1.6 Depending upon the patient's condition ALS intercept should be considered.

5.1.7 Transport should not be unnecessarily delayed. During transport the patient should be continuously reassessed. The patient's problem and status should be reported to the receiving hospital or medical control as soon as possible without compromising patient care. Patients should be transported in a safe manner.

5.1.8 The emergency medical technician (basic) shall provide all pertinent patient information to the receiving facility.

5.1.9 Upon completion of patient care responsibilities the emergency medical technician (basic) will prepare the ambulance and/or equipment and supplies to be ready to care for the next patient.

6. Position for Examination and Transport

6.1 The emergency medical technician (basic) shall be trained to place each patient in the position most comfortable to that patient. Exceptions are dictated by the following clinical situations:

---

[1] This guide is under the jurisdiction of Committee F-30 on Emergency Medical Services and is the direct responsibility of Subcommittee F30.02 on Personnel Training and Education.

Current edition approved Oct. 10, 2000. Published January 2001.

Originally published as F 1328-90. Discontinued

[2] *Annual Book of ASTM Standards*, Vol 13.01.

6.1.1 spinal and head injury,
6.1.2 rapid extrication, HAZMAT
6.1.3 shock,
6.1.4 musculoskeletal injuries,
6.1.5 obstetrical emergencies,
6.1.6 unconscious patient, and
6.1.7 dangerous or disruptive patient, or both.

7. Lifting and Moving

7.1 Utilizing proper body mechanics, the emergency medical technician (basic) must be able to safely lift and move patients with the following methods:
7.1.1 log roll,
7.1.2 straddle lift,
7.1.3 single and multiple rescuer lifts and carries, and
7.1.4 patient drags.

7.2 The emergency medical technician (basic) must be able to move patients utilizing the following mechanical devices:
7.2.1 stair chair,
7.2.2 scoop stretcher,
7.2.3 short/long board,
7.2.3.1 vehical extrication vests (KED, XP ect.)
7.2.4 simple stretcher,
7.2.5 standard ambulance cot,
7.2.6 improvised device, and
7.2.7 splinting devices.

8. Keywords

8.1 EMT; Emergency Medical Technician (basic); preparation for medicine transportation; training.

Designation: F 1329 – 00

Standard Guide for Training the Emergency Medical Technician (Basic) in Basic Anatomy and Physiology[1]

This standard is issued under the fixed designation F 1329; the number immediately following the designation indicates the year of original adoption or, in the case of revision, the year of last revision. A number in parentheses indicates the year of last reapproval. A superscript epsilon (ϵ) indicates an editorial change since the last revision or reapproval.

1. Scope

1.1 This guide establishes the minimum national standard for training the emergency medical technician (basic) in basic anatomy and physiology.

1.2 This guide is one of a series which together describe the minimum training standard for the emergency medical technician (basic).

2. Referenced Documents

2.1 *ASTM Standards:*

F 1031 Practice for Training the Emergency Medical Technician (Basic)[2]

F 1177 Terminology Relating to Emergency Medical Services[2]

F 1219 Guide for Training the Emergency Medical Technician (Basic) to Perform Patient Initial and Detailed Assessment[2]

3. Terminology

3.1 *Definitions of Terms Specific to This Standard:*

3.1.1 *anatomy*—the branch of science dealing with the structure of the human organism.

3.1.2 *physiology*—the science dealing with the functions of the human organism.

4. Significance and Use

4.1 This guide establishes the minimum national training standard in basic anatomy and physiology for the emergency medical technician (basic).

4.2 This guide shall be used by those who wish to identify the minimum training standard of the Emergency Medical Technician (basic) as it relates to basic anatomy and physiology.

4.3 This guide shall be used as a basis to revise Practice F 1031.

4.4 Every person who is identified as an Emergency Medical Technician (basic) shall be trained to this standard.

4.5 This guide must be used in conjunction with Practice F 1031, Guide F 1219 and Terminology F 1177.

5. Anatomy and Physiology

5.1 The Emergency Medical Technician (basic) shall describe the basic anatomy and physiology of the major body systems and the differences that exist because of age and gender, which include:

5.1.1 Respiratory,
5.1.2 Circulatory,
5.1.3 Muscular,
5.1.4 Skeletal,
5.1.5 Nervous,
5.1.6 Digestive,
5.1.7 Genitourinary,
5.1.8 Reproductive,
5.1.9 Integumentary, and
5.1.10 Endocrine.

6. Anatomic Terms

6.1 The Emergency Medical Technician (basic) shall define anatomic terms, which include:

6.1.1 Medial,
6.1.2 Lateral,
6.1.3 Proximal,
6.1.4 Distal,
6.1.5 Superior,
6.1.6 Inferior,
6.1.7 Anterior,
6.1.8 Posterior,
6.1.9 Midline,
6.1.10 Right,
6.1.11 Left,
6.1.12 Mid-clavicular, and
6.1.13 Mid-axillary.

7. Keywords

7.1 basic anatomy and physiology; emergency medical technician (basic); emt

---

[1] This guide is under the jurisdiction of ASTM Committee F30 on Emergency Medical Services and is the direct responsibility of Subcommittee F30.02 on Personnel, Training and Education.

Current edition approved Oct.10, 2000. Published December 2000. Originally published as F 1329 – 91. Last previous edition F 1329 – 91 (1998).

[2] *Annual Book of ASTM Standards*, Vol 13.01.

Standard Guide for Organization and Operation of Emergency Medical Services Systems[1]

This standard is issued under the fixed designation F 1339; the number immediately following the designation indicates the year of original adoption or, in the case of revision, the year of last revision. A number in parentheses indicates the year of last reapproval. A superscript epsilon (ε) indicates an editorial change since the last revision or reapproval.

1. Scope

1.1 This standard established guidelines for the organization and operation of Emergency Medical Services Systems (EMSS) at the state, regional and local levels. This guide will identify methods of developing state standards, coordinating/managing regional EMS Systems, and delivering emergency medical services through the local EMS System.

1.1.1 At the state level this guide identifies scope, methods, procedures and participants in the following state structure responsibilities: a) establishment of EMS legislation; b) development of minimum standards; c) enforcement of minimum standards; d) designation of substate structure; e) provision of technical assistance; f) identification of funding and other resources for the development, maintenance, and enhancement of EMS systems; g) development and implementation of training systems; h) development and implementation of communication systems; i) development and implementation of record-keeping and evaluation systems; j) development and implementation of public information, public education, and public relations programs; k) development and implementation of acute care center designation; 1) development and implementation of a disaster medical system; m) overall coordination of EMS and related programs within the state and in concert with other states or federal authorities.

1.2 At the regional level, this guide identifies methods of planning, implementing, coordinating/managing, and evaluating the emergency medical services system which exists within a natural catchment area and provides guidance on the use of these methods.

1.3 At the local level, this guide identifies a basic structure for the organization and management of a local EMS system and outlines the responsibilities that a local EMS should assume in the planning, development, implementation and evaluation of its EMS system.

2. Referenced Documents

2.1 *ASTM Standards:*

F 1086 Guide for Structures and Responsibilities of Emergency Medical Services Organizations[2]

F 1149 Practice for Qualifications, Responsibilities, and Authority for Individuals and Institutions Providing Medical Direction of Emergency Medical Services[2]

F 1220 Guide for Emergency Medical Services System (EMSS) Telecommunications[2]

F 1268 Guide for Establishing and Operating Public Information, Education and Relations Programs for Emergency Medical Services Systems[2]

F 1285 Guide for Training the Emergency Medical Technician (Basic) to Perform Patient Examination Techniques[2]

2.2 *American Ambulance Association*

Standards and Accreditation Document[3]

3. Significance and Use

3.1 This guide suggests methods for organizing and operating state, regional, and local EMS systems, in accordance with Guide F 1086. It will assist state, regional, or local organizations in assessing, planning, documenting, and implementing their specific operations. The guide is general in nature and able to be adapted for existing EMS Systems. For organizations that are establishing EMS System operations, the guide is specific enough to form the basis of the operational manual.

4. State Guide

4.1 *Establishment of EMS Legislation*:

4.1.1 *Methods and Procedures*—The legislative process varies from state to state. The EMS lead agency should seek a description of the process in its state from:

4.1.1.1 The legislature's staff or clerk offices.

4.1.1.2 The legislative liaison, or other appropriate staff of the governmental unit housing EMS (its "umbrella").

4.1.1.3 The legal counsel assigned to EMS.

4.1.2 Legislative proposals are commonly subject to the following processes:

4.1.2.1 *Drafting*—The standard-setting or other goal is put into general form by the agency, citing the sections of statute it believes are affected. The entities listed in 4.1.1-4.1.1.3 may be a resource, or may be required to be involved, in this proposal development.

4.1.2.2 *Sponsorship*— The proposal may be submitted through the agency's "umbrella" department to become an official part of the administration's legislative initiative.

---

[1] This guide is under the jurisdiction of ASTM Committee F-30 on Emergency Medical Services and is the direct responsibility of Subcommittee F30.03 on Organization/Management.

Current edition approved March 15, 1992. Published July 1992.

[2] *Annual Book of ASTM Standards*, Vol 13.01.

[3] Available from the American Ambulance Association.

TABLE 1

	State	Regional[A]	Local
Standard Setting	Legislation Regulations Guidelines/policies/procedures State protocols	Regional policies Regional protocols Assistance re: personnel	Employment standards Operating policies
System Coordination	Statewide coord. and planning Licensure/certification Facility licensure Service approval/licensure Training approval MIS/QA Inter-regional coord. Inter-state coord. Statewide SMI planning Design of sub-state structure	System planning Implementation Inter-organizational coordination Regional SMI Medical audit/QA Operational coordination System evaluation Personnel authorization accreditation	Daily operations
Service Delivery	Training Technical assistance Communications guidelines Funding PI&E	Training coordination Group purchasing Technical assistance PI&E	First response Ambulance (BLS, ALS; ground, helicopter, fixed wing) Hospital services PI&E

[A]If there are no regional organizations, within the state, the State EMS will need to accomplish, either directly or through delegation, regional tasks.

Whether this is true or not, the umbrella's legislative liaison will generally seek the sponsorship of appropriate legislators for the bill unless the bill is opposed by the administration. Sponsorship might be sought directly by the agency or by third parties on the agency's behalf under certain circumstances where practical.

4.1.2.3 *Final Drafting and Introduction*—The bill may be drafted in the form technically required for consideration by the legislature in the umbrella unit and/or legislative counsels offices. It is then read in the legislature and generally referred to a committee.

4.1.2.4 *Committee Consideration*—The committee usually holds a public hearing at which the agency and others may testify in favor of or against the bill, or neutrally. In subsequent, scheduled work sessions the bill is considered, changed as necessary, and some action usually voted. Agency and lobbyist attendance at work sessions is common and often influential.

4.1.2.5 *Adoption/Rejection*—Bills voted out to the legislature by committee, favorably or otherwise, are then read and voted on by that body.

4.1.2.6 *Governor*—Bills adopted by the legislature may be signed, not signed (but not vetoed), or vetoed by the governor. Bills that are vetoed may be returned to the legislature to attempt to override the veto. Bills that are not vetoed generally become law immediately if designated as emergency bills, or some time after the legislature adjourns as prescribed by law.

4.1.3 The timing of legislative proposal submissions, and the tracking of their progress to assure agency input are critical to their success. Hearing announcements and progress reports generated by the legislature or umbrella unit legislative liaison are useful. A legislative" hotline" is also commonly available and of use in tracking bills but personal contact with legislative aides and/or committee staff and legal counsels are even more useful.

4.1.4 *Participants in the EMS Legislative Process*:

4.1.4.1 Drafting/Sponsorship Resources may include:

A. Umbrella unit legislative liaison,

B. Assistant attorney general assigned to EMS,

C. Legislators/aides to legislators,

D. Staff/legal counsel to committee likely to consider bill, and

E. Agency staff, or staff of other agencies.

4.1.4.2 Formally Required Reviews/Approvals and/or Informal, Politically Expedient, Reviews/Approvals may be Sought From:

A. Umbrella unit commissioner/head (cabinet level),

B. Other agency heads with any potential interest,

C. State EMS and other advisory boards with potential interest,

D. REMSO staffs and advisory councils, and

E. EMS, fire, physician, nurse and other organized, active EMS-related professional associations.

4.1.4.3 *Resources for Monitoring Legislative Progress*:

A. Legislature staff/clerk offices and their publications (for example, hearing notices) and hotline,

B. Committee members and their aides,

C. Committee staffers and legal counsels, and

D. Sponsors of bill and their aides.

4.1.4.4 *Public Hearing Testimony Resources*:

A. Those listed in 4.1.4.1, *A* to *E*, (sponsoring), 4.1.4.2, *A* to *E*, (review/approval), and 4.1.4.3, *A* to *D*, (monitoring),

B. Hospital/prehospital personnel, and

C. Consumers.

4.1.4.5 *Governor's Office Resources*:

A. Umbrella unit commissioner/head (cabinet level),

B. Aides to Governor (if known and appropriate), and

C. Legislators and aides with links to Governor.

4.2 *Development of Minimum Standards*:

4.2.1 *Methods and Procedures*—A variety of standard-setting mechanisms exist, from that which is formal and explicitly housed in the state's laws to that which is the least formal, for instance, the non-binding opinion of EMS staff which is standard-setting to the extent of the dissemination and "rightness" of the opinion and the perceived expertise of the staff. The most commonly employed method and procedures are listed below.

4.2.1.1 *Origins of Standards*—State standards should be

derived from the ASTM process. When this process has not provided a standard in a needed area, standards set by the National Association of State EMS Directors and/or, secondarily, by other EMS-related professional associations should be used as a foundation.

4.2.1.2 When utilizing standards documents generated by other than the ASTM process, these should be critically reviewed by experts from a range of EMS-related clinical, administrative, training, planning, regulatory and other disciplines. In these cases, this process should assure that all interested parties have an opportunity to comment. Federal standards, in law and otherwise, may exist in certain areas of EMS which may affect a state's future receipt of federal funds; these should be reviewed for consistency with planned standards.

4.2.2 *Specific Methods and Procedures*:

4.2.2.1 *Legislation*— Used for setting broad, legally-binding standards. Sets the responsibilities of the state, regional, and local EMS structures; defines areas of rule or regulation-making authority, and sets general minimum standards for the system as a whole. See 4.1.

4.2.2.2 *Rules/Regulations*—Used to set more specific standards for system design and operation including, but not limited to, the interaction of state, regional, and local EMS structures in provider operation (for example, licensure, training course approval); requirements for and terms of operation (usually through licensure or certification) for EMS personnel, vehicles, equipment and services; organization of EMS training for certification or licensure; organization of certification or licensure testing; scope of practice; causes and procedures for disciplinary actions. This process is governed by the administrative procedures act ("APA") of the state and generally requires the EMS rule-making authority to publish notices and hold hearings on proposed changes. Consult the state's APA and discuss with the legal counsel assigned to EMS.

4.2.2.3 *Executive Order*— The Governor may be empowered to take actions which have a standard-setting impact. Consult the legal counsel assigned to EMS or the Governor's staff.

4.2.2.4 *Policies/Procedures*—Used by the state agency to govern the details of its operations and interactions with providers. Examples could include the personnel licensure/certification application form, procedures for in-state grant programs, or a policy for the administration of state licensure examinations. These are generally created outside of legislative or rule-making arenas. This makes them easier to create than laws or rules but also much less binding upon the EMS system and its providers. In fact, these are generally not considered to be legally binding. They are useful, though, in defining and clarifying required licensure/certification processes for providers and in providing immediate direction to providers where such direction is not provided in law, rules, or elsewhere.

4.2.2.5 *Protocols*—Virtually unique to EMS in their regional or statewide application, treatment protocols may be used to set clinical and operational standards and to define scope of practice. Protocols are most effective when they are given power of law by virtue of specific reference in statute (for example, "Treatment shall be in accord with protocols established by the medical director of the state (or regional) EMS agency"). Protocol-development may require a consensus-building process among the state's medical advisory committee, regional medical directors and others.

4.2.2.6 *Contracts and/or Letters of Agreement*—Generally in return for funding or other resources, regional and local structures and providers may agree to certain standards of performance. For example, state funding of training courses or ambulance equipment items may be afforded with agreement on standards for course content or equipment use. States generally have a standard process and forms for contracts and grants. Consult the purchasing and/or contracts office or legal counsel assigned to EMS.

4.2.3 *Participants in the Development of Minimum Standards*:

4.2.3.1 *By Legislation*— See 4.1.

4.2.3.2 *By Rules/Regulations*:

A. Agency staff (drafting),

B. Legal counsel assigned to EMS (review),

C. REMSO staffs/advisory councils/committees (review),

D. State advisory council/committees (review),

E. State EMS-related professional associations (review),

F. Impartial legal counsel (approval),

G. Secretary of state (records/announces proposals, certifies adopted rules),

H. Legislature (subject to review),

I. Umbrella unit staff and head (review/approval unless EMS agency has own rule-making authority), and

J. Providers/general public.

4.2.3.3 *By Executive Order*:

A. Agency staff (drafting),

B. Legal counsel assigned to EMS (review),

C. Umbrella unit head/commissioner (cabinet level),

D. Governor; governor's staff,

E. State advisory council/committees,

F. Consider those listed in 4.2.3.2 for review.

4.2.3.4 *By Policies/Procedures*:

A. Agency staff (drafting and review),

B. REMSO staff (review), and

C. Consider umbrella unit/advisory council review.

4.2.3.5 *By Protocols*:

A. Agency staff,

B. REMSO staff,

C. State/regional medical directors and medical advisory boards, and

D. Consider those listed in 4.2.2.2 for review.

4.2.3.6 *By Contracts/Letters of Agreement*:

A. Agency staff,

B. REMSO (contractor or reviewer),

C. Local system/provider (contractor),

D. Legal counsel assigned to EMS,

E. Consider umbrella unit/advisory council review,

F. Impartial legal counsel for contract approval,

G. Budget office if funding involved (approval/encumbrance), and

H. Purchasing/contract review if funding involved.

4.3 *Enforcement of Minimum Standards*:

4.3.1 *Methods and Procedures*—Enforcement may be accomplished in a variety of formal and informal ways. The more formal methods are discussed below, however, it is worth considering informal means (for example, peer pressure, training approaches, meetings with town and hospital officials and others with whom the non-complying individual or organization routinely interacts). If formal methods of enforcement are used, due process should be assured. The need to enforce may be discovered when a specific complaint is made, from incidental information derived from the media and other sources, from routine quality assurance processes, from service/vehicle inspections, and from the EMS management information system when it is used to link training, licensure, and run/patient reporting to monitor compliance with licensure requirements.

4.3.1.1 *Of Enforcing Laws, Rules or Regulations, Executive Orders*:

A. General information/education for those affected,

B. Specific verbal/written warnings of potential non-compliance and consequences,

C. Formal investigation by agency. Such investigations may lead to licensure action, fines, and/or imprisonment. Such penalties, conditions for penalties and avenues of appeal should be specified in law and rules/regulations. Refer to the Council of State Governments' certification curriculum for those who conduct administrative law investigations,

D. Criminal investigations as appropriate.

4.3.1.2 *Of Enforcing Policies/Procedures*:

A. General information/education for those affected,

B. Refusal to issue licenses/certifications for non-compliance (consult legal counsel assigned to EMS), and

C. Investigate and pursue policy non-compliance under a general "unprofessional conduct" or similar provision for licensure action under state EMS law.

4.3.1.3 *Of Enforcing Protocols*—Regional and/or state QA and EMS/MIS processes should exist to identify protocol non-compliance. If protocols are enforceable under state EMS law see 4.3.1.1. Other methods of enforcement include:

A. Withholding of medical control orders or privileges to practice at a regional or state level,

B, Withholding franchise to operate (dispatcher no longer calls the service), and

C. Withholding Medicaid, indigent fees, grants or other subsidies received by non-complying provider.

4.3.1.4 *Of Enforcing Contracts/Letters of Agreement*:

A. Withholding of grants, or the other resources or privileges identified in the particular document, and

B. Cancellation of contract.

4.3.2 *Participants*— Those involved in enforcement are usually state EMS agency officials or their agents. Agency staff, medical directors on the state and regional levels, REMSO staff, the legal counsel assigned to EMS, and others identified in 4.2.2 may be involved in enforcement on a formal or informal basis.

4.4 *Designation of Substate Structure*:

4.4.1 *Methods and Procedures*:

4.4.1.1 Determine purpose of substate structure (refer to Guide F 1086).

4.4.1.2 Determine maximum funding available to support structure established.

4.4.1.3 Given purpose and funding level, establish regional boundaries (ideally according to natural catchment areas).

4.4.1.4 Select REMSO for each Region, using RFP or other process, and establish a specific contract for services.

4.4.2 *Participants*— This is a decision with significant systems operation and political impact. Agency staff, state and local advisory councils, appropriate local governments, professional associations, provider services, hospitals and others should be involved.

4.5 *Provision of Technical Assistance*:

4.5.1 *Methods and Procedures*—States should have a mechanism for identifying needs for technical assistance.

4.5.1.1 Dissemination of current EMS information and description of technical assistance availability through statewide newsletter, computer bulletin board service, and special notices to providers or through REMSOs.

4.5.1.2 Participation of agency staff in statewide, regional, and local conferences and other educational programs.

4.5.1.3 Regular coordinating meetings with REMSO staffs, and agency staff attendance at regional council meetings.

4.5.1.4 State agency assistance in drafting EMS legislation and obtaining outside grant funding for local and regional projects.

4.5.1.5 State agency participation in ASTM and other national EMS technical and educational programs in order to represent interests of state and import new knowledge.

4.5.2 *Participants*— State agency and REMSO staffs and agents.

4.6 *Identification of Funding and Other Resources For The Development, Maintenance, and Enhancement of EMS Systems* :

4.6.1 See document of F30.03.05 ("Standard Guide for the Development of EMS Funding").

4.7 *Development and Implementation of Training Systems*:

4.7.1 *Methods and Procedures*—Development of standards (for example, specific objectives, curricula, instructor outlines) for training programs leading to certification/licensure. Determine purpose of substate structure (refer to F-1086-87).

4.8 *Development and Implementation of Communication Systems*:

(Refer to the work of, and standards developed by, Subcommittee F-30.04 on communications).

4.9 *Development and Implementation of Record-Keeping and Evaluation Systems*:

(Refer to the work of, and standards developed by, Task Group F-30.03.03 on Management Information Systems; 4.9.11 see the Centers for Disease Control's *Trauma Registry Patient Data Set*).

4.10 *Development and Implementation of Public Information, Public Education, and Public Relations Programs*:

(Refer to the work of, and standards developed by, Task Group F-30.03.06 on Public Information, Education, and Relations).

4.11 *Development and Implementation of Acute Care Center Designation*:

(Refer to work of, and standards developed by Subcommittee F-30.05 on Facilities;

4.11.1 See the American Medical Association Commission on EMS' *Guidelines for the Categorization of Hospital Emergency Capabilities* (most recent version).

4.12 *Development and Implementation of a Disaster Medical System*:

(Refer to the work of, and standards developed by Task Group F-30.03.07 on Disaster Management Response).

4.12.1 Resources for larger scale events involving out-of-state responses include the National Disaster Medical System (NDMS) and the Federal Emergency Management Agency (FEMA).

4.13 *Overall Coordination of EMS and Related Programs Within The State and In Concert With Other States Or Federal Authorities*:

4.13.1 This broad responsibility involves the establishment and on-going maintenance of efficient and effective communication with EMS and EMS impacting agencies and organizations in state government, federal government, and other state and national governments as issues of border necessitate.

4.13.2 With state government, public health, medical, nursing, emergency management, highway safety, public safety (state police and fire marshal), and state military agencies should be considered for on-going, general or special purpose, liaison.

4.13.3 Federal government agency contacts should include the U.S. Department of Transportation's National Highway Traffic Safety Administration which is involved in EMS funding through its Category 402/403 funding and standard setting (for example, 'KKK' standards for ambulance vehicles). Other EMS-impacting agencies include FEMA, the National Fire Academy, the National Disaster Medical System, the Federal Communications Commission, the Centers for Disease Control, and the Department of Defense.

4.13.4 Mutual aid agreements and compacts across border lines, and participation in the National Association of State EMS Directors, the National Council of State EMS Training Coordinators, ASTM, Multi-state EMS Associations, such as the New England and Mid-Atlantic EMS Councils, and other state and regional organizations and important activities in maintaining lines of communications.

5. Regional Guide

5.1 *General*:

5.1.1 EMS systems exist as a natural result of the interaction of ambulance services, first responder agencies, hospitals, and other providers. The role of EMS organizations, as defined by Guide F 1086, is to improve operation of this system.

5.1.2 Although they are usually independent organizations, providers within the EMS system have high degrees of interdependence. Their actions must be coordinated in order to ensure close cooperation, to limit conflict, and to ensure that the interests of the patients are primary in the system.

5.2 *Planning Functions*:

5.2.1 An EMS system plan should be developed for each system. The plan should:

5.2.1.1 Determine the optimal system design for the EMS system, based on appropriate ASTM standards, when not in conflict with state law, rules, or regulations, or with local ordinances. The system design should be based on predetermined, desired goals (for example, response time, clinical performance, fiscal performance, and the like) and should include:

A. The staffing level and level of training of hospital and pre-hospital personnel,

B. The number, location, and service level of pre-hospital providers,

C. Communications pathways and methods necessary to address citizen access, dispatch, coordination, and medical control,

D. The role of hospitals and speciality care centers, including initial patient triage, and interfacility transfer, and

E. Policies, procedures, personnel, and facilities, to provide medical control, as described in Practice F 1149,

F. A program for regular public information and education on system access, first aid, CPR, injury prevention, and system capabilities,

G. A program for system evaluation, as described in ASTM Standard Guide for Establishing and Operating EMS Management Information Systems (in progress),

H. Programs to ensure appropriate emergency response throughout the system,

I. Programs to ensure sufficient coordinated response to significant medical incidents, as described in Guide F 1285, and

J. The roles, responsibilities and relationships of agencies participating within the system.

5.2.1.2 Describe the area covered by the system

5.2.1.3 Determine what resources (including, but not limited to, personnel, vehicles, facilities, and services) are needed within the system, based on workload, geographic, demographic, and epidemiologic factors.

5.2.1.4 Determine system financial needs.

5.2.1.5 Inventory and assess the resources which are currently available within the EMS system.

5.2.1.6 Determine the needs of the system.

5.2.1.7 Provide a process for meeting the identified system needs, including identification of sources of funding.

5.2.2 The organization developing the EMS plan should ensure that consumers of emergency health services and existing EMS providers have an opportunity to participate in development of the plan.

5.3 *Implementation Functions:* (See Note 1)

NOTE 1—These functions, particularly those requiring regulatory powers may be performed by agencies at the state, regional, or local levels, depending on the division of responsibility and authority within the state.

5.3.1 The EMS system is generally implemented through the actions of participating provider agencies. The implementing organization is not required to perform any or all of the required functions, but instead should establish the framework to ensure that they are all done.

5.3.2 The implementing organization should promote the need for the system through education of the public, current providers, and public officials and should encourage and facilitate the voluntary participation of existing provider agencies.

5.3.3 Some components of the system may be implemented through regulatory processes. Regional organizations should evaluate the status of other regulatory programs, given regional standards. Such processes include:

5.3.3.1 Certification/licensure of personnel,

5.3.3.2 Accreditation/designation/certification of facilities,

5.3.3.3 Approval of pre-hospital provider services,

5.3.3.4 Licensing/permitting of emergency pre-hospital provider vehicles and equipment (not including non-emergency (for example, wheelchair) services),

5.3.3.5 Approval of training programs, and

5.3.3.6 Development of policies, procedures, and protocols.

5.3.4 Some components of the system may be implemented through use of competitive processes, including:

5.3.4.1 Ambulance franchising, and

5.3.4.2 Request for proposals for facility designation.

5.3.5 Some components of the system may be implemented through direct operation of a service by a state or regional EMS organization, including:

5.3.5.1 Training programs,

5.3.5.2 Recruitment of personnel,

5.3.5.3 Operation of a communications center,

5.3.5.4 Operation of a communications system,

5.3.5.5 Provisions of technical assistance to providers, and

5.3.5.6 Sponsorship of group purchasing programs.

5.4 *Coordination/Management Functions*:

5.4.1 Policies, regulations, guidelines, procedures, and protocols should be developed to determine appropriate actions where a decision by one agency impacts on another or where more than one agency must interact. These include, but are not limited to:

5.4.1.1 Triage and patient flow,

5.4.1.2 Pre-hospital treatment,

5.4.1.3 Inter-facility transfer,

5.4.1.4 Operations,

5.4.1.5 Communications,

5.4.1.6 Incident command system, compatible with NIIMS, including on-scene command,

5.4.1.7 Response to *multiple casualty* incidents *and medical disasters*, and

5.4.1.8 Medical control, in accordance with Practice F 1149.

5.4.2 Communications resources should be available to allow coordination of participating agencies, including:

5.4.2.1 A single access number for emergencies,

5.4.2.2 Common radio frequencies for:

A. Dispatch,

B. On-scene coordination

C. Hospital notification

D. Medical contro

E. Inter-facility coordination

5.4.2.3 Dispatch protocols,

5.4.2.4 Pre-determined response policies, and

5.4.2.5 Move-up and coverage plans.

5.4.3 Provision should exist for general coordination of public and private services, medical facilities, first responders and other appropriate public and private entities.

5.5 *Evaluation Functions*:

5.5.1 The evaluating organization must consider the overall effectiveness of the system and the day-to-day operation of the system.

5.5.2 Day-to-day operation of the system can be evaluated through:

5.5.2.1 Retrospective medical control, including chart and tape reviews, and audits,

5.5.2.2 Operational reviews,

5.5.2.3 Reviews of problems, and

5.5.2.4 Critique of significant medical incidents.

5.5.3 Overall operation and outcome of the system can be evaluated through:

5.5.3.1 Analysis of trends,

5.5.3.2 Outcome studies, and

5.5.3.3 Analysis of emergency medical care data bases.

5.5.4 Review and update of the EMS system plan.

6. Local Guide

6.1 *Structures*—The basic structures of a local EMS organization should consist of the following:

6.1.1 Local EMS Council or Committee composed of representatives from public and private provider groups involved in the delivery of EMS including but not limited to: ambulance services/rescue squads, medical society (all disciplines), emergency nurses, hospitals or hospital councils, local boards of health, police departments, fire departments, dispatch agency, and other related governmental or political subdivisional bodies.

6.1.2 *System Access*— It is desirable to have centralized access such as 9-1-1 or a single 7 digit number for all emergency services (for example, police, fire, EMS).

6.1.3 *Dispatch/Communications*—It is desirable to have coordinated dispatch of local resources and centralized communications with regional and state groups. If possible, dispatch personnel should have been trained consistent with the guidelines of the F30.02.04 committee on dispatch/communicator training.

6.1.4 *Personnel*:

6.1.4.1 *Basic Life Support (BLS)*—Should include all levels of training identified in the guidelines of the F30.02 committee on personnel training and education and state certification processes.

6.1.4.2 *Advanced Life Support (ALS)*—ALS capabilities should be consistent with state certification criteria and need should be determined by the local EMS council or committee.

6.1.5 *Medical Direction*—Should be provided by a physician(s), qualified in a manner consistent with the guidelines on medical control in Practice F 1149, who is involved with local EMS providers.

6.1.6 *Transportation*— Transportation guidelines for all aspects (land, air, and water) according to need should be developed by the local component council or committee. Establishment of minimum response times to the site as well as transit time to the receiving facility should be done by the local council or committee in accordance with state and regional guidelines. Provisions should also be included for interfacility transport in accordance with local and state laws.

6.1.7 *Receiving Facilities*—Each facility should be identified as to the hours of operation, level of care provided, and capacity for multiple casualties. Provisions should be made to identify special needs for the local area and facilities identified for provision of these needs. Input will have to be solicited from the local component medical control, REMSO groups, and appropriate state agencies.

6.2 *Responsibilities*:

6.2.1 *Planning/Development*—To implement the level(s) of services identified by the local committee or council consideration must be given to the following:

6.2.1.1 Determine local system design/needs with input from state, REMSOs, Federal, and Local Provider

A. Determine area of coverage, vehicle needs and staffing available,

B. Determine local resources available, and

C. Identify process to be used to meet system needs.

6.2.1.2 Personnel training levels as identified in section 3.1.4 and their availability. In addition to continuing education requirements that may be mandated by the state, the local council or committee should identify any other continuing education needed at the local level to maintain standards.

6.2.1.3 Medical Control as identified in 3.1.5 and in Practice F 1149.

6.2.1.4 Develop plan with participation from consumers of emergency health services and existing EMS providers.

6.3 *Implementation*:

6.3.1 Functions identified in this document may not necessarily be implemented by the local agency but by participatory provider agencies. The implementing organization is not required to perform any or all of the functions but to ensure that they are all done.

6.3.2 The implementing local council or committee should promote the need for the local system through public education and education of the local provider agencies.

6.3.3 Some processes utilized in the implementation of the local system include but are not limited to:

6.3.3.1 Regulatory processes (both Regional and State),

A. Certification/licensure of personnel,

B. Accreditation/designation/certification of facilities, and

C. Approval of training programs.

6.3.3.2 Competitive processes (both private and commercial),

A. Ambulance franchising, and

B. Proposals for complete local system development.

6.3.3.3 Direct provision of service by regional or state

A. Training programs,

B. Dispatch provision and operation,

C. Recruitment of personnel,

D. Technical assistance for participating agencies,

6.4 *Methods and Procedures for the Operation of a Local EMS System*:

6.4.1 The clear delineation of service ownership and organizational structure is necessary to assure accountability to consumers and governmental entities. Full disclosure of the agency ownership is required.

6.5 *Inter-Agency Relations*:

6.5.1 Inter-agency relations are necessary to provide high quality patient care services. A high quality EMS system depends on cooperation between various types of public-safety agencies as well as among all local EMS providers. These standards are to emphasize these relationship.

6.5.2 *Mutual Aid*—The ambulance service shall develop and maintain mutual aid relationships with other ambulance/EMS organizations in its immediate or neighboring service areas. (See Appendix X3)

6.5.3 *Disaster Coordination*—The service should play an active role in the regional disaster plan and response.

6.5.4 *Conflict Resolution*—The agency should develop and maintain a means to resolve conflicts among personnel of all organizations directly or indirectly involved in patient care (for example, other ambulance providers, police and fire departments, medical personnel, and the like). The conflict resolution policy should include appropriate follow-up activities.

6.6 *Coordination*:

6.6.1 The local council or committee should be the contact agency for coordination with REMSOs and state groups. The local council or committee should also assist in coordination with local providers, medical facilities, and medical control through utilization of guidelines developed by the local component in addition to guidelines developed by other group's (REMSOs, State, etc.) and hold regularly scheduled meetings of all involved agencies. (See Regional document F30.03.02).

6.6.2 The local council or committee should assist in the establishment of guidelines with the local provider(s) for communication, training, mutual aid, and participation in local mass casualty and emergency plans (See document from F30.03.04).

6.6.3 Responsibilities to REMSOs and state agencies should be guided by local identification of areas of need and implementing mechanisms for meeting those need requirements.

6.7 *Quality Assurance*—Local EMS agencies should provide mechanisms for medical review and quality assurance of runs with local medical control, local medical facilities, and local participating agencies. The local implementation of this should be consistent with regional guide 5.5.

6.8 *Funding*—Local responsibility should be developed within the local council or committee and should include provisions to identify funding mechanisms for financial support due to changes made in regulations from REMSO, State, or Federal agencies.

6.9 *Safety*—The local council or committee should emphasize usage of all applicable OSHA, FEMA, ASTM, and other available documents.

APPENDIXES

(Nonmandatory Information)

X1. THE EMS SYSTEM PLANNING PROCESS (see Fig. X1.1 and Fig. X1.2)

X1.1 EMS system planning begins with the question "what need will the system meet?" The answer to this question establishes the overall goals of the system. The goals identify the targets of the system, such as patients within various emergency clinical target groups. The system's boundaries are defined in this initial step.

X1.2 The second step of the planning process if to define the optimal system. The planner answers the question "If I could start this system totally from scratch, without any limitations or constraints caused by past practices or decisions, how would I design it?" This approach allows the planner to consider the ultimate system prior to determining legal constraints, financial limitations, political considerations, the inertia of the status quo, and other limiting factors. The optimal system is based on national, state, and local standards for emergency medical care and operations, legal minimums, and demands which are placed on the system through the public policy arena.

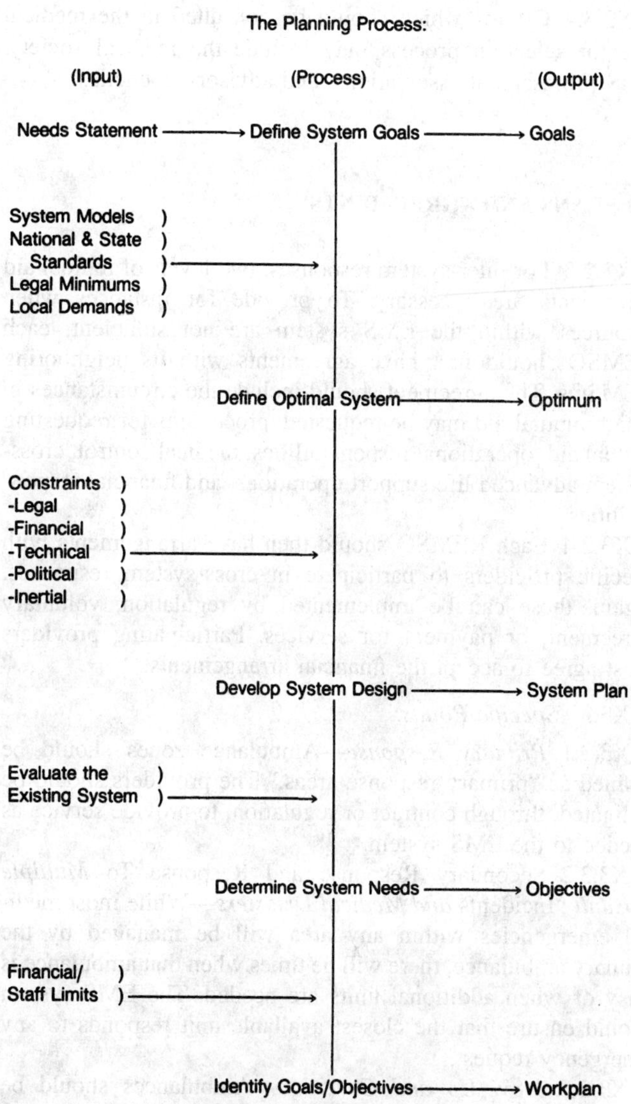

FIG. X1.1 The Planning Process

(Example of EMS Plan Objective)

STANDARD:

The REMSO should assess, and periodically reassess the EMS-related capabilities of acute care facilities in its service area.

CURRENT STATUS:

Hospitals in the region have not been categorized according to their capabilities in the critical care target categories.

NEED(S):

The REMSO has only limited information regarding the capabilities of hospitals and is unable to rationally develop a patient destination policy.

OBJECTIVE X.XX:

The REMSO should categorize hospitals according to state standards.

TIMEFRAME FOR OBJECTIVE:

[X] Annual Implementation Plan

[ ] Five Year Plan

FIG. X1.2 Example of EMS Plan Objectives

X1.3 After determining the optimal system, the planner can then look at the environment in which the system operates. At this stage, system constraints—legal, financial, political, technological—can be identified. The result is the system design—the ultimate system which is realistically possible, given the constraints which are present.

X1.4 The existing system is then examined and compared to the system design. Problem areas are identified and objectives are developed for overcoming these problems. With consideration of the resources which are available for system development, the objectives are prioritized into immediate and long-range. The result becomes part of the annual workplan for the agency.

X1.5 For each system need, an objective should be stated which explains what the need is and how it will be met. All areas in which the current system does not meet the system design should be identified.

X1.6 In planning, the process is often more important than the resulting document. The plan can be a tool to focus attention on system needs and to involve appropriate parties—both provider and consumer—in the system. The value of an open planning process should be self-evident.

X2. HOW TO RECRUIT AND SELECT AN EMS MEDICAL DIRECTOR

X2.1 Develop a position description, based on a job analysis of the tasks that the medical director will be expected to perform (refer to Practice E 1149 for further information on the roles and responsibilities for medical control). The analysis should include:

X2.1.1 A description of the tasks to be accomplished in both general and descriptive terms.

X2.1.2 Identification of key individuals and agencies with whom the medical director will need to work to accomplish these tasks.

X2.1.3 A description of the general political climate of the area (as it relates to the EMS community, medical community, and key agencies).

X2.1.4 A description of the time commitments involved.

X2.2 The position description based on this analysis should include the tasks to be accomplished, the specific skills (including interpersonal skills) needed to accomplish them, and other requirements of the agency (for example, ABEM board certification, and the like).

X2.3 Once the position description is established, the agency may select the most appropriate means for securing the services of a medical director, given local needs and the local climate. These may include:

X2.3.1 An informal recruitment process led by the advisory council/committee or agency staff, intended to bring on an individual physician known to meet the needs of the agency.

X2.3.2 A more formal recruitment process involving advertising, application, and interviewing several candidates. If this process is used and multiple candidates apply, the agency must establish a means of evaluating the candidates' credentials in light of structural interview panels using set questions and interview rating systems. More complex evaluation processes, such as assessment centers, may be used if the position involves a large time commitment, substantial remuneration, or a very sensitive political climate.

X2.3.3 Structural interview materials and recruiting aids are available from a wide variety of sources, including the American Personnel Association, etc.

X2.3.4 Groups which should be consulted in the medical director selection process may include the medical society, EMS professional associations, and advisory councils.

X3. DEVELOPMENT OF MUTUAL AID PLANS AND AGREEMENTS

X3.1 *Definition*—"Mutual aid" must be considered more broadly than as just an agreement between organizations for the provision of assistance. It includes:

X3.1.1 Policies and procedures to maintain coverage within the EMS system on a day-to-day basis and during significant medical incidents.

X3.1.2 Policies and procedures to provide for response when the primary ambulance is busy and for sufficient response to significant medical incidents.

X3.1.3 Agreements among counties for responses which cross EMS system lines.

X3.2 *General Framework for Mutual Aid:*

X3.2.1 All participants with the EMS system should function as part of that system, not as independent entities. The REMSO is responsible for coordinating the actions of all participating entities so as to ensure an optimal response to the entire EMS area. Policies and procedures can be implemented by regulation or by contract—with or without a subsidy payment.

X3.2.2 REMSOs should develop policies and procedures for day-to-day response and response to significant medical incidents. These should include response to day-to-day incidents within the ambulance's primary response area and other parts of the county, response to significant medical incidents, and a move-up and cover plan. The latter two responses should be considered part of an optimal system response, and not as mutual aid.

X3.2.3 For inter-system responses, two levels of mutual aid agreements are necessary. To provide for instances when resources within the EMS system are not sufficient, each REMSO should first have agreements with its neighboring REMSOs. The agreement should include the circumstances in which mutual aid may be requested, procedures for requesting mutual aid, operational responsibilities, medical control, cross-system advanced life support operations, and financial responsibilities.

X3.2.4 Each REMSO should then have arrangements with specific providers to participate in cross-system responses. Again, these can be implemented by regulation, voluntary agreement, or payment for services. Participating providers must agree to accept the financial arrangements.

X3.3 *Specific Points:*

X3.3.1 *Primary Response*—Ambulance zones should be defined as "primary response areas." The providers should be obligated, through contract or regulation, to provide service as needed to the EMS system.

X3.3.2 Secondary Response and Response To *Multiple Casualty* Incidents *and Medical Disasters*—While most medical emergencies within any area will be managed by the primary ambulance, there will be times when that ambulance is busy or when additional units are needed. The EMS system should ensure that the closest available unit responds to any emergency request.

X3.3.3 *Move-Up and Coverage*—Ambulances should be moved to pre-determined standby points as needed to ensure coverage throughout the EMS system. Move-ups may be appropriate when day-to-day demand has removed ambulance coverage within a portion of the area or when multiple ambulances are required to respond to a single incident. The policies and procedures which are required resemble a provider's "system status management plan" but encompass all providers within the system.

X3.3.4 *Mutual Aid Agreements*—Agreements, as described in the general framework above, are necessary to implement the cross-system portion of the above items.

Designation: F 1341 – 99

Standard Specification for Unalloyed Titanium Wire UNS R50250,[1] UNS R50400,[1] UNS R50550,[1] UNS R50700,[1] for Surgical Implant Applications[2]

This standard is issued under the fixed designation F 1341; the number immediately following the designation indicates the year of original adoption or, in the case of revision, the year of last revision. A number in parentheses indicates the year of last reapproval. A superscript epsilon (ε) indicates an editorial change since the last revision or reapproval.

1. Scope

1.1 This specification covers the chemical, mechanical, and metallurgical requirements for four grades of unalloyed titanium wire used for the manufacture of surgical implants.

1.2 The values stated in inch-pound units are to be regarded as the standard. The values given in parentheses are for information only.

2. Referenced Documents

2.1 *ASTM Standards:*

E 8 Test Methods for Tension Testing of Metallic Materials[3]

E 120 Test Methods for Chemical Analysis of Titanium and Titanium Alloys[4]

E 527 Practice for Numbering Metals and Alloys (UNS)[5]

E 1409 Test Method for Determinitation of Oxygen in Titanium Alloys by the Inert Gas Fusion Technique[4]

E 1447 Test Method for Determination of Hydrogen in Titanium and Titanium Alloys by the Inert Gas Fusion Thermal Conductivity Method[6]

F 67 Specification for Unalloyed Titanium for Surgical Implant Applications[7]

F 981 Practice for Assessment of Compatibility of Biomaterials for Surgical Implants with Respect to Effect of Materials on Muscle and Bone[7]

2.2 *Aerospace Material Specification:*

AMS 2249 Chemical Check Analysis Limits, Titanium and Titanium Alloys[8]

2.3 *American Society for Quality (ASQ) Standard:*

C1 Specifications of General Requirements for a Quality Program[9]

2.4 *Society of Automotive Engineers Standard:*

SAE J1086 Practice for Numbering Metals and Alloys (UNS)[8]

3. Product Classification

3.1 *Wire*—Round product with a diameter equal to or less than 0.3125 in. (7.94 mm). Flat and special shape wire with a major dimension equal to or less than 0.3125 in. (7.94 mm) may also be ordered as agreed upon between the supplier and the purchaser.

4. Ordering Information

4.1 Inquiries and orders for material under this specification shall include the following information:

4.1.1 Quantity (weight or number of pieces),

4.1.2 Grade (1, 2, 3, or 4),

4.1.3 ASTM designation,

4.1.4 Form (wire),

4.1.5 Condition (5.1),

4.1.6 Mechanical Properties (if applicable, for special conditions),

4.1.7 Finish (5.2),

4.1.8 Applicable dimensions including size, thickness, width, spool size, coil diameter, and length (exact, random, multiples) or print number, and

4.1.9 Special Tests, if any.

5. Manufacture

5.1 *Condition*—Material shall be furnished in the annealed or cold worked condition.

5.2 *Finish*—Types of finish available for wire products are bright annealed, pickled, cold drawn, cold rolled, ground, ground and polished, or as specified in the purchase order.

6. Chemical Composition

6.1 The heat analysis shall conform to the requirements as to chemical composition prescribed in Table 1. Ingot analysis may be used for reporting all chemical requirements except hydrogen, samples of which shall be taken from the finished product. The supplier shall not ship material that is outside the limits specified in Table 1 for the applicable grade.

6.1.1 Requirement for the major and minor elemental constituents are listed in Table 1. Also listed are important residual elements. Analysis for elements not listed in Table 1 is not required to verify compliance with this specification.

---

[1] New designation established in accordance with E 527 and SAE J1086.

[2] This specification is under the jurisdiction of ASTM Committee F-04 on Medical and Surgical Materials and Devices and is the direct responsibility of Subcommittee F04.12 on Resources.

Current edition approved May 10, 1999. Published August 1999. Originally published as F 1341 - 92. Last previous edition F 1341 - 92.

[3] *Annual Book of ASTM Standards*, Vol 03.01.

[4] *Annual Book of ASTM Standards*, Vol 03.05.

[5] *Annual Book of ASTM Standards*, Vol 01.01.

[6] *Annual Book of ASTM Standards*, Vol 03.06.

[7] *Annual Book of ASTM Standards*, Vol 13.01.

[8] Available from Society of Automotive Engineers, 400 Commonwealth Drive, Warrendale, PA 15096.

[9] Available from American Society for Quality, 1611 E. Wisconsin Ave., Milwaukee, WI 53203.

TABLE 1 Chemical Requirements

Element	Composition (wt %)			
	Grade 1 UNS R50250	Grade 2 UNS R50400	Grade 3 UNS R50550	Grade 4 UNS R50700
Nitrogen, max	0.03	0.03	0.05	0.05
Carbon, max	0.10	0.10	0.10	0.10
Hydrogen, max	0.0125	0.0125	0.0125	0.0125
Iron, max	0.20	0.30	0.30	0.50
Oxygen, max	0.18	0.25	0.35	0.40
Titanium	balance	balance	balance	balance

6.2 *Product Analysis*— Product analysis tolerances do not broaden the specified heat analysis requirements but cover variations between laboratories in the measurement of chemical content. Product analysis limits shall be as specified in Table 2.

6.2.1 The product analysis is either for the purpose of verifying the composition of a heat or lot or to determine variations in the composition within the heat.

6.2.2 Acceptance or rejection of a heat or lot of material may be made by the purchaser on the basis of this check analysis.

6.3 For referee purposes, Test Methods E 120, E 1409, and E 1447 shall apply.

6.3.1 Samples for chemical analysis shall be representative of the material being tested. **Precaution**—Extreme care must be taken in sampling titanium for chemical analysis because of its affinity for elements such as oxygen, nitrogen, and hydrogen. Therefore, when cutting samples for analysis, the operation should be carried out in a dust-free atmosphere, if possible. Chips should be collected from clean metal. Cutting tools should be clean and sharp. Samples for analysis should be stored in suitable containers.

7. Mechanical Requirements

7.1 Annealed round wire shall conform to the appropriate requirements as to mechanical properties prescribed in Table 3. Material may be ordered in the cold worked condition to higher ultimate tensile strengths and lower elongation levels as agreed upon between the supplier and the purchaser.

7.2 Tension testing shall be performed in accordance with Test Method E 8. Tensile properties shall be determined as listed in Table 3 using the appropriate gage length for the wire size being tested. For wire diameters 0.3125 to 0.062 in. (7.93 to 1.57 mm) (4D gage length) a strain rate of 0.003 to 0.007 in./in.(mm/mm)/min through the specified yield strength shall be used and then the crosshead speed shall be increased so as to produce fracture in approximately one additional minute. For wire diameters less than 0.062 in. a crosshead speed of 0.5 to 1.0 in./min (12.7 to 25.4 mm) shall be used. Once yielding has begun the crosshead speed may be increased to a maximum of 3.0 in./min. (76.2 mm).

7.3 Any other special tests shall be specified on the purchase order.

TABLE 2 Product Analysis Tolerances[A]

Element	Limit or Maximum of Specified Range, %	Tolerance Under the Minimum or Over the Maximum Limit[B]
Nitrogen	Up to 0.05	0.02
Carbon	Up to 0.10	0.02
Hydrogen	Up to 0.0125	0.0020
Iron	Up to 0.25	0.10
Iron	Over 0.25	0.15
Oxygen	Up to 0.20	0.02
Oxygen	Over 0.20	0.03

[A] Refer to AMS 2249C.
[B] Under minimum limit not applicable for elements where only a maximum percentage is indicated.

TABLE 3 Annealed Wire Mechanical Requirements

Diameter, in. (mm)	Grade	Ultimate Tensile Strength, min, ksi (MPa)	Yield Strength, (0.2 % offset), min, ksi (MPa)	Elongation[A,B,C] min, %	Red. in Area min, %
0.3125 to 0.125 (7.938 to 3.175)	1	35 (240)	25 (170)	24	30
	2	50 (345)	40 (275)	20	30
	3	65 (450)	55 (380)	18	30
	4	80 (550)	70 (483)	15	25
<0.125 to 0.062 (<3.175 to 1.575)	1	35 (240)	25 (170)	15	...
	2	50 (345)	40 (275)	12	...
	3	65 (450)	55 (380)	10	...
	4	80 (550)	70 (483)	8	...
<0.062 to 0.020 (<1.575 to 0.508)	1	35 (240)	...	12	...
	2	50 (345)	...	10	...
	3	65 (450)	...	8	...
	4	80 (550)	...	6	...
<0.020 to 0.005 (<0.508 to 0.127)	1	35 (240)	...	10	...
	2	50 (345)	...	8	...
	3	65 (450)	...	6	...
	4	80 (550)	...	4	...

[A] Report gage length on certification.
[B] 2 in. (50 mm) or 4D gage length for diameters 0.3125 to 0.062 in. (7.938 to 1.575 mm).
[C] 10 in. (250 mm) gage length for diameters <0.062 in. (<1.575 mm).

8. Special Requirements

8.1 Size variation and out-of-round tolerance for round wire shall meet the requirements specified in Table 4.

9. Certification

9.1 The supplier's certification that the material was manufactured and tested in accordance with this specification together with a report of the test results shall be furnished to the purchaser at the time of shipment.

10. Quality Program Requirements

10.1 The supplier shall maintain a quality program, such as defined in ASQ C1.

TABLE 4 Round Wire Size Tolerance

Diameter, in. (mm)	Size Variation, in., (mm)	Out-Of-Round,[A] in., (mm)
0.3125 to 0.250 (7.983 to 6.350)	±0.005 (0.127)	0.008 (0.203)
<0.250 to 0.125 (<6.350 to 3.175)	±0.003 (0.076)	0.005 (0.127)
<0.125 to 0.030 (<3.175 to 0.762)	±0.002 (0.051)	0.003 (0.076)
<0.030 to 0.020 (<0.762 to 0.508)	±0.001 (0.025)	0.0008 (0.020)
<0.020 to 0.010 (<0.508 to 0.254)	±0.001 (0.025)	0.0006 (0.015)
<0.010 to 0.005 (<0.254 to 0.127)	±0.0005 (0.013)	0.0005 (0.013)

[A] Out-of-round is the difference between the maximum and minimum diameters of the wire measured at the same cross section.

10.2 The purchaser shall be assured of the producer's quality program for conformance to the intent of ASQ C1-1985, or other recognized program.

11. Keywords

11.1 metals (for surgical implants); titanium alloys; orthopaedic medical devices; titanium/titanium alloy; titanium/titanium alloys (for surgical implants); wire

APPENDIXES

(Nonmandatory Information)

X1. RATIONALE

X1.1 The primary reason for this standard is to characterize composition and properties to assure consistency in the starting wire material used in the manufacture of medical devices.

X1.2 The choice of composition and mechanical properties is dependent upon the design and application of the medical device.

X1.3 Added UNS designations and biocompatibility statements.

X2. BIOCOMPATIBILITY

X2.1 The alloy compositions covered by this specification have been employed successfully in human implant applications in contact with soft tissue and bone for over a decade. Due to the well characterized level of biological response exhibited by these alloys, they have been used as control materials (Specification F 67) in Practice F 981.

X2.2 No known surgical implant material has ever been shown to be completely free of adverse reactions in the human body. Long-term clinical experience of the use of the materials referred to in this specification, however, has shown that an acceptable level of biological response can be expected, if the material is used in appropriate applications.

Last ASTM Designation: F 1343 – 91

Specification for Anestetic Equipment-Scavenging Systems for Anesthetic Gases

This specification covers the minimum performance and safety requirements to be used for systems for scavenging excess anesthetic gases from operating rooms.

Formerly under the jurisdiction of Committee F29 on Anesthetic and Respiratory Equipment, this specification was withdrawn in February 2000.

Designation: F 1350 – 01

Standard Specification for Wrought 18 Chromium-14 Nickel-2.5 Molybdenum Stainless Steel Surgical Fixation Wire (UNS S31673)[1]

This standard is issued under the fixed designation F 1350; the number immediately following the designation indicates the year of original adoption or, in the case of revision, the year of last revision. A number in parentheses indicates the year of last reapproval. A superscript epsilon (ε) indicates an editorial change since the last revision or reapproval.

1. Scope

1.1 This specification covers the requirements for the manufacture of stainless steel surgical fixation wire.

1.2 The values stated in metric units are to be regarded as standard. The inch-pound equivalents may be approximate.

2. Referenced Documents

2.1 *ASTM Standards:*

A 262 Practices for Detecting Susceptibility to Intergranular Attack in Austenitic Stainless Steels[2]

A 370 Test Methods and Definitions for Mechanical Testing of Steel Products[2]

A 555 Specification for General Requirements for Stainless Steel Wire and Wire Rods[2]

E 45 Test Methods for Determining the Inclusion Content of Steel[3]

F 86 Practice for Surface Preparation and Marking of Metallic Surgical Implants[4]

F 138 Specification for Wrought 18 Chromium-14 Nickel-2.5 Molybdenum Stainless Steel Bar and Wire for Surgical Implants (UNS S31673)[4]

2.2 *USP Standard:*

Nonabsorbable Surgical Suture, *U.S. Pharmacopeia*[5]

3. Materials and Manufacture

3.1 Surgical fixation wire shall conform to the specified chemical composition of Specification F 138 material. Conformance with this specification shall be so identified by suitable packaging or labeling, or both.

3.2 The microcleanliness of the steel as determined by Test Methods E 45, Method A shall conform to Specification F 138. Microcleanliness conformance shall be stated on the material certification.

3.3 The steel shall be capable of passing the intergranular corrosion susceptibility test in accordance with Practices A 262, Practice E as specified in Specification F 138. Conformance shall be stated on material certification.

3.4 Surgical fixation wire shall be furnished in the bright annealed condition and finish.

4. Mechanical Properties

4.1 Surgical fixation wire shall conform to the appropriate mechanical properties specified in Table 1.

4.2 Mechanical testing shall be performed in accordance with Test Methods A 370 using a 254-mm (10-in.) gage length and crosshead speed of 254 mm/min (10 in./min).

4.3 The wire shall meet the requirements of USP for Nonabsorbable Surgical Sutures, (latest revision) when tested in accordance with 4.2.

5. Dimensional Requirements

5.1 Surgical fixation wire shall be fabricated in accordance with the dimensions and tolerances specified in Table 1.

6. Surface Condition and Handling

6.1 The surface of surgical fixation wire conforming to this specification shall be free of imperfections such as toolmarks, nicks, scratches, cracks, cavities, spurs, and other defects that would impair the serviceability of the wire. The surface shall be free of embedded or deposited finishing materials and other undesirable contaminants.

6.2 The wire may be subjected to a passivation process if requested by the customer. Such passivation process shall be performed in accordance with Practice F 86.

6.3 Surgical fixation wire shall be handled with care and packaged adequately to prevent damage and contamination of the surface.

7. General Requirements

7.1 In addition to the requirements of this specification, all requirements of the current editions of Specifications A 555 and F 138 shall apply.

7.2 In cases of conflict between this specification and those listed in 2.1, this specification shall take precedence.

8. Keywords

8.1 fixation; mechanical properties; stainless steel; surgical implant; suture; tolerances; wire

[1] This specification is under the jurisdiction of ASTM Committee F04 on Medical and Surgical Materials and Devices and is the direct responsibility of Subcommittee F04.21 on Osteosynthesis.

Current edition approved May 10, 2001. Published May 2001. Originally published as F 1350 – 91. Last previous edition F 1350 – 96 (2000).

[2] *Annual Book of ASTM Standards*, Vol 01.03.

[3] *Annual Book of ASTM Standards*, Vol 03.01.

[4] *Annual Book of ASTM Standards*, Vol 13.01.

[5] Available from U.S. Pharmacopeia, 12601 Twinbrook Pkwy., Rockville, MD 20852.

TABLE 1 Mechanical and Dimensional Requirements for Stainless Steel Surgical Fixation Wire

Range of Sizes Diameter, mm (in.)	USP Size[A]	Diameter Tolerance[BC]	Tensile Strength max, MPa (ksi)[D]	Elong. min %[E]
0.010 to under 0.020 (0.0004 to 0.0008)	...	0.0015 (0.00006)	1380 (200)	15
0.020 to under 0.030 (0.0008 to 0.0012)	10–0	0.0015 (0.00006)	1240 (180)	15
0.030 to under 0.040 (0.0012 to 0.0016)	9–0	0.0025 (0.0001)	1100 (160)	20
0.040 to under 0.050 (0.0016 to 0.0020)	8–0	0.0025 (0.0001)	1100 (160)	20
0.050 to under 0.070 (0.0020 to 0.0028)	7–0	0.0025 (0.0001)	960 (140)	25
0.070 to under 0.100 (0.0028 to 0.0039)	6–0	0.0025 (0.0001)	965 (140)	25
0.100 to under 0.150 (0.0039 to 0.0059)	5–0	0.0050 (0.0002)	895 (130)	30
0.150 to under 0.200 (0.0059 to 0.0079)	4–0	0.0050 (0.0002)	895 (130)	30
0.200 to under 0.250 (0.0079 to 0.0098)	3–0	0.0075 (0.0003)	860 (125)	30
0.250 to under 0.300 (0.0098 to 0.0118)	...	0.0075 (0.0003)	860 (125)	30
0.300 to under 0.340 (0.0118 to 0.0134)	2–0	0.0100 (0.0004)	860 (125)	30
0.340 to under 0.350 (0.0134 to 0.0138)	...	0.0100 (0.0004)	860 (125)	30
0.350 to under 0.400 (0.0138 to 0.0158)	1–0	0.0100 (0.0004)	825 (120)	35
0.400 to under 0.500 (0.0158 to 0.0197)	1	0.0100 (0.0004)	825 (120)	35
0.500 to under 0.600 (0.0196 to 0.0236)	2	0.0100 (0.0004)	790 (115)	35
0.600 to under 0.700 (0.0236 to 0.0276)	3 and 4	0.0130 (0.0005)	790 (115)	35
0.700 to under 0.800 (0.0276 to 0.0315)	5	0.0130 (0.0005)	760 (110)	35
0.800 to under 0.900 (0.0315 to 0.0354)	6	0.0200 (0.0008)	760 (110)	35
0.900 to under 1.000 (0.0354 to 0.0394)	7	0.0200 (0.0008)	760 (110)	40
1.000 to under 1.100 (0.0394 to 0.0433)	...	0.0200 (0.0008)	690 (100)	40
1.100 to under 1.600 (0.0433 to 0.0630)	...	0.0250 (0.0010)	690 (100)	40

[A] For reference purposes only. (U.S. Pharmacopeia).
[B] Diameter tolerances are over and under as given in this table. Also, round wire can be produced to tolerances all over and nothing under, or all under and nothing over, or any combination over and under, if the total spread in diameter tolerance for a specified diameter is not less than the total spread given in this table.
[C] The maximum out-of-round tolerance for round wire is one half of the total size tolerance given in this table.
[D] Maximum tensile strength is specified to assure proper wire-handling characteristics.
[E] Minimum elongation for spooled wire is 6 percentage points lower than table value.

APPENDIX

(Nonmandatory Information)

X1. RATIONALE

X1.1 The primary reason for this specification is to characterize the mechanical properties of annealed stainless steel wire for implant applications.

X1.2 This specification combines and replaces Specifications F 642 and F 666.

X1.3 The title has been changed and the UNS designation has been added to more readily identify the material.

Designation: F 1357 – 99

Standard Specification for Articulating Total Wrist Implants[1]

This standard is issued under the fixed designation F 1357; the number immediately following the designation indicates the year of original adoption or, in the case of revision, the year of last revision. A number in parentheses indicates the year of last reapproval. A superscript epsilon (ε) indicates an editorial change since the last revision or reapproval.

1. Scope

1.1 This specification describes total wrist implants, including solid ceramic implants, used to provide functioning articulation by employing radial carpal components.

1.2 This specification excludes those implants with ceramic-coated or porous-coated surfaces, one piece elastomeric implants (with or without grommets), and those devices used for custom applications.

1.3 The values stated in SI units are standard. The English values in parentheses are for information only.

2. Referenced Documents

2.1 *ASTM Standards:*

F 67 Specification for an Unalloyed Titanium for Surgical Implant Application[2]

F 75 Specification for Cast Cobalt-Chromium-Molybdenum Alloy for Surgical Implant Applications[2]

F 86 Practice for Surface Preparation and Marking of Metallic Surgical Implants[2]

F 90 Specification for Wrought Cobalt-Chromium-Tungsten-Nickel Alloy for Surgical Implant Applications[2]

F 136 Specification for Wrought Titanium 6A1-4V ELI Alloy for Surgical Implant Applications[2]

F 562 Specification for Wrought Cobalt-Nickel-Chromium-Molybdenum Alloy for Surgical Implant Applications[2]

F 563 Specification for Wrought Cobalt-Nickel-Chromium-Molybdenum-Tungsten-Iron Alloy for Surgical Implant Applications[2]

F 601 Practice for Fluorescent Penetrant Inspection of Metallic Surgical Implants[2]

F 603 Specification for High-Purity Dense Aluminum Oxide for Surgical Implant Application[2]

F 629 Practice for Radiography of Cast Metallic Surgical Implants[2]

F 648 Specification for Ultra-High-Molecular-Weight Polyethylene Powder and Fabricated Form for Surgical Implants[2]

F 748 Practice for Selecting Generic Biological Test Methods for Materials and Devices[2]

F 799 Specification for Thermomechanically Processed Cobalt-Chromium-Molybdenum Alloy for Surgical Implants[2]

F 981 Practice for Assessment of Compatibility of Bio-Materials (Non-Porous) for Surgical Implants with Respect to Effect of Materials on Muscle and Bone[2]

F 983 Practice for Permanent Marking of Orthopaedic Implant Components[2]

F 1108 Specification for Ti6A14V Alloy Castings for Surgical Implants[2]

F 1537 Specification for Wrought Cobalt-28 Chromium-6 Molybdenum Alloy for Surgical Implants[2]

3. Terminology

3.1 *Definitions:*

3.1.1 *carpal component*—articulating member inserted into or through the carpal bones.

3.1.2 *radial component*—articulating member inserted into the radius for articulation with the carpal component.

3.1.3 *total wrist replacement*—prosthetic parts substituted for the native opposing radial and carpal articulating surfaces.

4. Classification

4.1 *Constrained*—A constrained joint prosthesis is used for joint replacement and prevents dislocation of the prosthesis in more than one anatomical plane and consists of either a single, flexible, across-the-joint component, or more than one component linked together or affined.

4.2 *Partially Constrained*—A semi-constrained joint prosthesis is used for partial or total joint replacement and limits translation and rotation of the prosthesis in one or more planes via the geometry of its articulating surfaces. It has no across-the-joint linkages.

4.3 *Unconstrained*—An unconstrained joint prosthesis is used for partial or total joint replacement and restricts minimally prosthesis movement in one or more planes. Its components have no across-the-joint linkages.

5. Materials and Manufacture

5.1 Proper material selection is necessary, but insufficient to ensure suitable function of a device.

5.2 All metal implant components shall conform to one of the following specifications for implant materials: Specification F 67, F 75, F 90, F 136, F 562, F 563 (nonbearing use only), F 799, F 1108, or F 1537.

---

[1] This specification is under the jurisdiction of ASTM Committee F-4 on Medical and Surgical Materials and Devicesand is the direct responsibility of Subcommittee F04.22 on Anthroplasty.

Current edition approved November 10, 1999. Published December 1999.Originally published as F 1357 - 91. Last previous edition F 1357 - 91 (1997).

[2] *Annual Book of ASTM Standards*, Vol 13.01.

5.3 All polymeric components shall conform to the following specification for implant materials: Specification F 648.

5.4 All solid ceramic components shall conform to Specification F 603 for implant materials.

5.5 *Biocompatibility*—Articulating implants shall be manufactured from the materials listed in 5.2-5.4. Before implants can be manufactured from other materials, their biocompatibility will be considered suitable only if they produce an acceptable response after testing in accordance with Practice F 981.

5.6 When required for metallic implants, fluorescent penetrant inspection shall be performed in accordance with Practice F 601.

5.7 When required for cast metallic implants, radiography shall be performed in accordance with Practice F 629.

6. Performance Requirements

6.1 *Polymeric Creep (Cold Flow)*—Ultra-high molecular weight polyethylene in implant form must conform to the requirements detailed in Specification F 648. When creep occurs, it must not impair the function or stability of the interface.

6.2 *Wear of Alternative Materials*—It is important to understand the wear performance for articulating surfaces. Any new or different material couple should not exceed the wear rates of the following material couple when tested under physiological conditions. The current wear couple is CoCrMo alloy (F75) against ultra high molecular weight polyethylene. This is an industry wide referenced wear couple and is considered by some to be the minimum. It has been proven to provide clinically acceptable results.

NOTE 1—In situations where the pin-on-flat test may not be considered appropriate, other test methods may be considered.

6.3 *Range of Motion of the Device Before Implantation*—The implant shall be evaluated to determine the maximum dorsiflexion, palmar flexion, radial deviation, and ulnar deviation possible before subluxation occurs or the motion is arrested by the implant. These results shall be reported in the product labeling.

6.4 *Guidelines for In-Vitro Laboratory Testing*—No ASTM standards for testing articulating wrist implants have not been developed. Laboratory testing that simulates the conditions of use is desirable to compare materials and designs and to provide an indication of clinical performance. Implant testing shall be done in keeping with the implants intended function, that is, implants intended to partially stabilize or stabilize a joint shall be subjected to the maximum destabilizing force anticipated in clinical application during flexural testing.

7. Dimensions

7.1 Dimensions of wrist joint replacement components shall be as designated in Figs. 1 and 2.

8. Finish and Marking

8.1 Items conforming to this specification shall be finished and marked in accordance with Practice F 86 where applicable.

8.2 *Metallic Bearing Surface*—Articulate surfaces shall be finished to an average roughness of 0.125 µm.

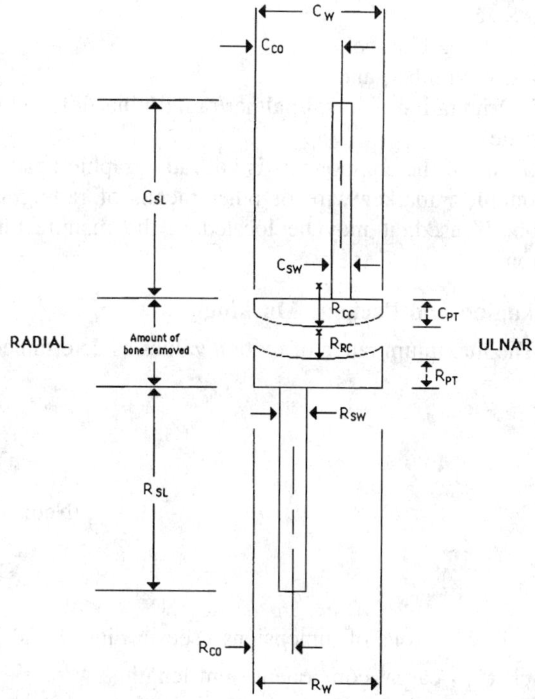

FIG. 1 Dimensions of Wrist Joint Replacements (Coronal Plane)

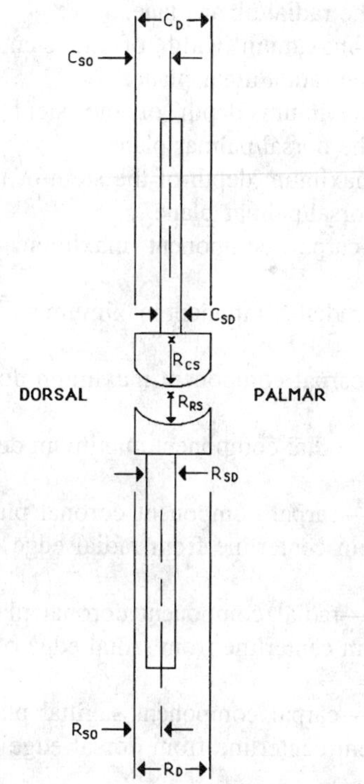

FIG. 2 Dimensions of Wrist Joint Replacements (Sagittal Plane)

8.3 *Polymeric Bearing Surface Finish*— shall conform to manufacturer's documented standards concerning concentricity, sphericity, and surface roughness, when applicable.

8.4 Items conforming to this specification shall be marked in accordance with Practices F 86, and F 983. Radial and carpal component marking shall include, as possible, the items below in the following order of importance:

8.4.1 Manufacturer,

8.4.2 Size,

8.4.3 Catalog Number,

8.4.4 Lot Number, and

8.4.5 Orientation (dorsal/palmar/radial/ulnar/left/right as appropriate).

8.5 If one of the components is not radiographic opaque, it shall contain a marker wire or other means of radiographic detection. If used, it may be located at the manufacturer's discretion.

9. Packaging and Package Marking

9.1 The maximum range of motion values as determined by 6.3 shall be included in the product labeling.

9.2 The dimensions shown in Figs. 1 and 2 and described in the glossary in Appendix X1 shall be included in the product labeling.

9.3 The material(s) used for the implant shall be specified on the package labels and inserts.

10. Keywords

10.1 arthroplasty; prosthesis; total wrist replacement

APPENDIXES

(Nonmandatory Information)

X1. GLOSSARY

X1.1 Descriptions of dimensions used in Figs. 1 and 2.

X1.1.1 C_{sl}—carpal component stem length.

X1.1.2 R_{sl}—radial component stem length.

X1.1.3 C_{sw}—maximum width of the stem of the carpal component in the radial/ulnar plane.

X1.1.4 R_{sw}—maximum width of the stem of the radial component in the radial/ulnar plane.

X1.1.5 *C*—maximum depth of the stem of the carpal component in the dorsal/palmar plane.

X1.1.6 *R*—maximum depth of the stem of the radial component in the dorsal/palmar plane.

X1.1.7 C_w—carpal component maximum width (radial/ulnar plane).

X1.1.8 R_w—radial component maximum width (radial/ulnar plane).

X1.1.9 C_d—carpal component maximum dorsal/palmar dimension.

X1.1.10 R_d—radial component maximum dorsal/palmar dimension.

X1.1.11 C_{co}—carpal component coronal plane stem offset (distance of stem centerline from radial edge of carpal component).

X1.1.12 R_{co}—radial component coronal plane stem offset (distance of stem centerline from radial edge of radial component).

X1.1.13 C_{so}—carpal component sagittal plane stem offset (distance of stem centerline from dorsal edge of carpal component).

X1.1.14 R_{so}—radial component sagittal plane stem offset (distance of stem centerline from dorsal edge of radial component).

X1.1.15 R_{pt}—radial plateau thickness; thickness of radial component from transverse resection plane to functional surface.

X1.1.16 C_{pt}—carpal plateau thickness; thickness of carpal component from transverse resection plane to functional surface.

X1.1.17 R_{cc}—radii of curvature at the low point of the carpal component in the radial/ulnar (coronal) plane.

X1.1.18 *R*—radii of curvature at the low point of the radial component in the radial/ulnar (coronal) plane.

X1.1.19 R_{cs}—radii of curvature at the low point of the carpal component in the dorsal/palmar (sagittal) plane.

X1.1.20 R_{rs}—radii of curvature at the low point of the radial component in the dorsal/palmar (sagittal) plane.

X1.1.21 *amount of bone resected*—amount of bone removed to allow insertion and use of implant ($R_{pt} + C_{pt}$).

X1.1.22 *palmarflexion (flexion)*—movement of the palm of the hand toward the palmar surface of the forearm.

X1.1.23 *dorsiflexion (extension)*—movement of the dorsum of the hand toward the dorsal surface of the forearm.

X1.1.24 *radial deviation*—movement of the hand toward the radius.

X1.1.25 *ulnar deviation*— movement of the hand toward the ulna.

X1.1.26 *neutral position*—a position of the hand that is parallel to the forearm.

RATIONALE

X2. RATIONALE

X2.1 The objective of this standard is the provision of guidelines for the physical characteristics of the components for total wrist replacement. Total wrist replacement parts are intended for use in a patient who is skeletally mature, under conditions of imposed dynamic loads, in a corrosive environment and virtually continuous motion at the bearing surfaces. Laboratory tests to accurately simulate imposed loads, aggressive electrolytes and complex constituents of body fluids have not been usefully accelerated at the present time for a complete joint evaluation. Long term projections of satisfactory performance over many decades can be suggested but not accurately predicted using available screening procedures. This document identifies those factors felt to be important to assure a satisfactory useful prosthetic life. It is here recognized that failure of an arthroplasty can occur, even while the components are intact. This is true owing to the composite nature of the arthroplasty procedure, which includes the implant, cement if any, and the physiological environment.

X2.2 Under applicable documents and materials, the list reflects the current state of the art. It is recognized that should materials not now included appear and be proved acceptable, they shall be inserted in the process of revision.

X2.3 Performance Considerations: Component performance can be predicted only indirectly at this stage, by referring to strength levels and other parameters. Reference to parameters applicable to materials may or may not adequately describe structures made from them. In a period of transition from device specification standards to device performance standards both methods of description may be appropriate.

X2.4 It is recognized that with wear between two materials can have both mechanical detrimental and biological adverse effects. However, section 6.2, *Wear of Alternative Materials*, applies only to the mechanical effect of minimizing wear and does not apply to the biological issues related to wear.

X2.5 Component performance shall be considered with regard to patient anatomy. It is well recognized that physical stresses resulting from events or activities out of the ordinary range, as in accidents or especially vigorous sports, predictably exceed allowable stress levels in any component design. It is also recognized here that other forms of arthroplasty failure are known to occur, related primarily to patient factors, such as osteoporosis, Paget's disease, misuse and disuse, and others.

X2.6 Specific criteria need to be established in assessing the biocompatibility of articulating wrist implants made of new materials. F 748, Practice for Selecting Generic Biological Test Methods for Materials and Devices, will need to be used to determine which additional biocompatibility tests are required.

X2.7 Range of motion data of devices before implantation will provide comparative information among implants.

X2.8 Dimensions: The methods of dimensional measurement must be sought to conform with the industry practice and, whenever possible, on an international basis.

X2.9 Finish and Markings: Dimensions and tolerances are as described by ANSI documents for sphericity, concentricity and surface finish. A maximum allowable roughness for the polymeric bearing surface is not specified at this time, but will be in the future. It is suggested if needed at the time of explanation that the material composition can be determined by referring to the manufacturers' information, instead of marking the material on each implant.

X2.10 If one of the components is not radiographic opaque, it should be appropriately marked for radiographic evaluation. If a marker wire is used, it is considered to be a non-critical element, as long as it is radiographically detectable.

X2.11 The manufacturers trademark must appear legibly on each of the components. It is desirable to have complete information, where space is available to do so, including size, orientation if any, and catalog number with date.

Designation: F 1377 – 98a

Standard Specification for Cobalt-28 Chromium-6 Molybdenum Powder for Coating of Orthopedic Implants (UNS-R30075)[1]

This standard is issued under the fixed designation F 1377; the number immediately following the designation indicates the year of original adoption or, in the case of revision, the year of last revision. A number in parentheses indicates the year of last reapproval. A superscript epsilon (ε) indicates an editorial change since the last revision or reapproval.

1. Scope

1.1 This specification covers the requirements for cobalt-28 chromium-6 molybdenum alloy powders for use in fabricating coatings on cobalt-28 chromium-6 molybdenum alloy orthopedic implants.

1.2 Powders covered under this specification may be used to form coatings by sintering or thermal spraying techniques.

1.3 This specification covers powder requirements only. It does not address properties of the coatings formed from them.

1.4 The values stated in inch-pound units are to be regarded as the standard. The SI units given in parentheses are for information only.

2. Referenced Documents

2.1 *ASTM Standards:*

B 214 Test Method for Sieve Analysis of Metal Powders[2]

B 215 Practices for Sampling Finished Lots of Metal Powders[2]

E 11 Specification for Wire-Cloth Sieves for Testing Purposes[3]

E 354 Test Methods for Chemical Analysis of High Temperature, Electrical, Magnetic, and Other Similar Iron, Nickel, and Cobalt Alloys[4]

F 75 Specification for Cobalt-28 Chromium-6 Molybdenum Casting Alloy and Cast Products for Surgical Implants (UNS-R30075)[5]

F 981 Practice for Assessment of Compatibility of Biomaterials for Surgical Implants with Respect to Effect of Materials on Muscle and Bone[5]

2.2 *ASQ Standards:*

C1 General Requirements for a Quality Program[6]

3. Significance and Use

3.1 Coatings formed from metallic powders have become widely used as a means of improving tissue attachment to uncemented orthopedic joint prosthesis. Such coatings have also been demonstrated to improve bonding of acrylic cement to prostheses. This specification addresses the special requirements of the metal powders used to form these coatings.

4. Materials and Manufacture

4.1 Powders may be manufactured by the rotating electrode process, inert gas atomization, or other methods capable of producing powder meeting the requirements of this specification.

5. Chemical Composition

5.1 The heat analysis of stock used to manufacture the powder shall conform to the chemical analysis set forth in Table 1 of Specification F 75.

5.2 The product analysis tolerance shall conform to the requirements set forth in Table 2 of Specification F 75.

5.3 For referee purposes, Test Methods E 354 shall be used.

6. Particle Size

6.1 Powder shall be sieved to the customer's requirements with screens conforming to Specification E 11. Analysis of the sieved powder for conformance to customer's particle size range requirements shall be according to Test Method B 214. Powder sampling shall be according to Test Method B 215.

7. Cleanliness

7.1 Powder shall be handled at all times so as to minimize possible contamination with nonmetallic materials or other metal alloy powders, or both.

7.2 Powder cleanliness shall be determined by examining a representative sample comprising at least 1 in.^{2} (645 mm^2) of a closely packed mono-layer of powder at 20× magnification. No foreign material shall be visible under these conditions.

8. Special Requirements

8.1 Various materials known as processing aids may be added to the powder to provide enhanced processability and, if applicable, the powder supplier shall include this information on the material certification.

---

[1] This specification is under the jurisdiction of ASTM Committee F-4 on Medical and Surgical Materials and Devicesand is the direct responsibility of Subcommittee F04.12on Metallurgical Materials.

Current edition approved April 10, 1998. Published March 1999. Originally published as F 1377–92. Last previous edition F 1377–98.

[2] *Annual Book of ASTM Standards*, Vol 02.05.

[3] *Annual Book of ASTM Standards*, Vol 14.02.

[4] *Annual Book of ASTM Standards*, Vol 03.05.

[5] *Annual Book of ASTM Standards*, Vol 13.01.

[6] Available from American Society for Quality, 611 East Wisconsin Ave., Milwaukee, WI 53203.

8.2 Processing aids shall have no detrimental effect on the corrosion resistance and biocompatibility of the final coating.

9. Certification

9.1 Powder shipped under this specification shall be accompanied by a certification that includes the following:

9.1.1 ASTM designation,

9.1.2 Quantity (weight),

9.1.3 Method of manufacture,

9.1.4 Chemical analysis in accordance with 5.1,

9.1.5 Sieve analysis in accordance with 6.1,

9.1.6 Powder cleanliness in accordance with 7.2,

9.1.7 Special requirements in accordance with 8.1, and

9.1.8 Other requirements.

10. Quality Program Requirements

10.1 The producer shall maintain a quality program, for example, such as defined in ASQ C1.

10.2 The manufacturer of surgical implants shall be assured of the producer's quality program for conformance to the intent of ASQ C1 or other recognized program.

11. Keywords

11.1 coatings, metallic; cobalt alloys (for surgical implants); metals (for surgical implants, cobalt alloys); orthopedic medical devices (cobalt alloys); porous coatings; powder

APPENDIXES

(Nonmandatory Information)

X1. RATIONALE

X1.1 Coatings formed from metallic powders have become widely used as a means of improving tissue attachment to uncemented orthopedic joint prosthesis. Such coatings have also been demonstrated to improve bonding of acrylic cement to prostheses.

X1.2 It should be recognized that the heat treatments used to form porous coatings can create microstructures which are substantially different from investment cast F 75 alloy. Porous coated implants also exhibit much greater surface area than monolithic implants. For these reasons, the biocompatibility and corrosion behavior must be characterized on finished coatings.

X1.3 Pore size and morphology are important factors influencing tissue ingrowth and acrylic penetration of porous coatings. Particle size and shape are critical to controlling the pore size and morphology in the final coating. Particle size is conventionally controlled by screening. The referenced ASTM and MPIF (Metal Powder Industries Federation) standards allow comparison of powder to a manufacturer's specifications for a given coating process.

X1.4 Other process parameters are also critical to determining final pore size and morphology in the final coating. Because these parameters are not directly related to the chemical and physical characteristics of the starting powder, they are not addressed in this standard.

X1.5 The requirements for powder cleanliness minimize contaminants which might adversely affect either the biocompatibility or the finished coatings or the ability to properly bond the coating during manufacturing. The test method in 7.2 is commonly used for relatively coarse spherical powders used to fabricate sintered porous coatings. Other types of powders may require different methods for cleanliness characterization. The development and implementation of such methods are the responsibility of the implant manufacturer.

X2. BIOCOMPATIBILITY

X2.1 The alloy composition, free of processing aids (see Section 8), covered by this standard has been employed successfully in human implant applications is contact with soft tissue and bone for over a decade. Due to the well characterized level of biological response exhibited by this alloy, it has been used as a control material in Practice F 981.

X2.2 No known surgical implant material has ever been shown to be completely free of adverse reactions in the human body. However, long-term clinical experience of the use of the material referred to in this standard has shown that an acceptable level of biological response can be expected, if the material is used in appropriate applications.

Designation: F 1378 – 00

Standard Specification for Shoulder Prostheses[1]

This standard is issued under the fixed designation F 1378; the number immediately following the designation indicates the year of original adoption or, in the case of revision, the year of last revision. A number in parentheses indicates the year of last reapproval. A superscript epsilon (ϵ) indicates an editorial change since the last revision or reapproval.

1. Scope

1.1 This specification covers shoulder prostheses for total or hemiarthroplasty used to provide functioning articulation by employing glenoid and humeral components.

1.2 Devices for custom applications are not covered by this specification. Modular prostheses are included in this specification.

1.3 The values stated in SI are to be regarded as the standard. The inch-pound units given in parentheses are for information only.

2. Referenced Documents

2.1 *ASTM Standards:*

F 75 Specification for Cast Cobalt-Chromium-Molybdenum Alloy for Surgical Implant Applications[2]

F 86 Practice for Surface Preparation and Marking of Metallic Surgical Implants[2]

F 90 Specification for Wrought Cobalt-Chromium-Tungsten-Nickel Alloy for Surgical Implant Application[2]

F 136 Specification for Wrought Titanium 6A1-4V ELI Alloy for Surgical Implant Applications[2]

F 138 Specification for Stainless Steel Bar and Wire for Surgical Implants (Special Quality)[2]

F 562 Specification for Wrought Cobalt-Nickel-Chromium-Molybdenum Alloy for Surgical Implant Applications[2]

F 563 Specification for Wrought Cobalt-Nickel-Chromium-Molybdenum-Tungsten-Iron Alloy for Surgical Implant Applications[2]

F 603 Specification for High-Purity Dense Aluminum Oxide for Surgical Implant Applications[2]

F 648 Specification for Ultra-High-Molecular-Weight Polyethylene Powder and Fabricated Form for Surgical Implants[2]

F 745 Specification for Stainless Steel for Cast and Solution-Annealed Surgical Implant Applications[2]

F 746 Test Method for Pitting or Crevice Corrosion of Metallic Surgical Implant Materials[2]

F 748 Practice for Selecting Generic Biological Test Methods for Materials and Devices[2]

F 799 Specification for Thermomechanically Processed Cobalt-Chromium-Molybdenum Alloy for Surgical Implants[2]

F 981 Practice for Assessment of Compatibility of Bio-Materials (Non-Porous) for Surgical Implants with Respect to Effect of Materials on Muscle and Bone[2]

F 983 Practice for Permanent Marking of Orthopaedic Implant Components[2]

F 1044 Test Method for Shear Testing of Porous Metal Coatings[2]

F 1108 Specification for Ti6A14V Alloy Castings for Surgical Implants[2]

F 1147 Test Method for Tension Testing of Porous Metal Coatings[2]

F 1537 Specification for Wrought Cobalt-Chromium-Molybdenum Alloy for Surgical Implants[2]

F 1829 Test Method for Static Evaluation of the Glenoid Locking Mechanism in Shear[2]

F 2028 Test Methods for the Dynamic Evaluation of Glenoid Loosening or Dissociation[2]

2.2 *ANSI Standard:*[3]

ASME B46.1–1995

3. Terminology

3.1 *Definitions of Terms Specific to This Standard:*

3.1.1 *collar*—flange at junction of neck and stem.

3.1.2 *glenoid component*—the prosthetic portion that replaces, in part or in total, the glenoid fossa of the scapula and articulates with the natural humeral head or a prosthetic replacement.

3.1.3 *head*—bearing member for articulation with the glenoid.

3.1.4 *humeral component*—the prosthetic portion that replaces, in part or in toto, the proximal humerus or humeral head and articulates with the natural glenoid fossa or a prosthetic replacement.

3.1.5 *keel, (or pegs)*—single or multiple projections that provide resistance to translation or rotation of the glenoid component, or both, by mating with cavities created in the glenoid fossa.

3.1.6 *neck*—segment connecting the head and the stem.

3.1.7 *stem*—segment intended for insertion within the humeral medullary canal.

[1] This specification is under the jurisdiction of ASTM Committee F04 on Medical and Surgical Materials and Devices and is the direct responsibility of Subcommittee F04.22 on Anthroplasty.

Current edition approved Nov. 10, 2000. Published January 2001. Originally published as F 1378–92. Last previous edition F 1378–99.

[2] *Annual Book of ASTM Standards*, Vol 13.01.

[3] Available from American National Standards Institute, 11 W. 42nd St., 13th Floor, New York, NY 10036.

4. Classification

4.1 *Constrained*— A constrained joint prosthesis is used for joint replacement and resists dislocation of the prosthesis in more than one anatomical plane and consists of either a single, flexible, across-the-joint component or more than one component linked together or affined.

4.2 *Partially Constrained*—A semi-constrained joint prosthesis is used for partial or total joint replacement and limits translation and rotation of the prosthesis in one or more planes via the geometry of its articulating surfaces. It has no across-the-joint linkages.

4.3 *Unconstrained*— An unconstrained joint prosthesis is used for partial or total joint replacement and restricts minimally prosthesis movement in one or more planes. Its components have no across-the-joint linkage.

5. Materials and Manufacture

5.1 The choice of materials is understood to be a necessary but not sufficient ensurance of function of the device made from them. All devices conforming to this specification shall be fabricated from materials, with adequate mechanical strength and durability, corrosion resistance, and biocompatibility.

5.1.1 *Mechanical Strength*—Various components of shoulder prostheses have been successfully fabricated from the following materials. However, not all of these materials may possess sufficient mechanical strength for critical highly-stressed components. See Specifications F 75, F 90, F 136, F 138, F 562, F 563 (nonbearing use only), F 603, F 648, F 745, F 799, F 1108, F 1537.

5.1.2 *Corrosion Resistance*—Materials with limited or no history of successful use for orthopedic implant application must be determined to exhibit corrosion resistance equal to or better than one of the materials listed in 5.1.1 when tested in accordance with Test Method F 746.

5.1.3 *Biocompatibility*— Materials with limited or no history of successful use for orthopedic implant application must be determined to exhibit acceptable biological response equal to or better than one of the materials listed in 5.1.1 when tested in accordance with Practices F 748 and F 981.

6. Performance Requirements

6.1 *Wear of Alternative Materials*—It is important to understand the wear performance for articulating surfaces. Any new or different material should not exceed the wear rates of the following material couple when tested under physiological conditions. The current standard wear couple is CoCrMo alloy (Specification F 75) against ultra high molecular weight polyethylene (Specification F 648), both having prosthetic quality surface finishes according to 8.2.

NOTE 1—In situations where the pin-on-flat test may not be considered appropriate, other test methods may be considered.

6.2 *Range of Motion of Shoulder Prosthesis Prior to Implantation*—Flexion shall be equal to or greater than 90°. Abduction shall be equal to or greater than 90°. Internal rotation shall be equal to or greater than 90°. External rotation shall be equal to or greater than 45°. Extension shall be equal to or greater than 45°.

6.3 Porous metal coatings shall be tested according to Test Method F 1044 (shear strength) and Test Method F 1147 (tensile strength).

6.4 *Guidelines for In-Vitro Laboratory Testing*:

6.4.1 Implant testing should reflect current clinical failures and potential failure modes particular to the implant. These tests may be directed towards subluxation, glenoid loosening, insert disassociation from a metal backing, and humeral head disassociation.

6.4.2 All modular implants should be tested in accordance with Test Method F 1829.

6.4.3 All prosthetic glenoid components should be tested in accordance with Test Method F2028.

7. Dimensions

7.1 Dimensions of shoulder joint replacement components shall be as designated in Figs. 1-3.

8. Finish and Product Marking

8.1 Items conforming to this specification shall be finished and marked in accordance with Practice F 86, where applicable.

8.2 *Articulating Surface Finishes*:

8.2.1 *Metallic Bearing Surface*— The main bearing surface shall have a surface finish no rougher than 0.10 μm (4 μin.) roughness average, R_a, with a cutoff length of 0.25 mm, when measured according to the principles given in ASME B46.1–1995.

8.2.2 *Polymeric Bearing Surface (if used)*—The main bearing surface shall have a surface finish no rougher than 2 μm roughness, R_a, with a cut-off length of 0.8 mm, when measured according to the priniciples given in ASME B46.1–1995.

8.3 In accordance with Practices F 86 and F 983, items conforming to this specification shall be marked as follows in order of priority where space permits: manufacturer, material, lot number, catalog number, and size. Additional information may include a designation for left or right and front.

8.3.1 Optional glenoid marking may specify orientation (top, if applicable; right or left, if applicable).

8.4 If one of the components is not radiographic opaque, it is strongly encouraged that it shall contain a marker wire or other means of radiographic detection. It may be located at the manufacturer's discretion.

9. Labeling

9.1 The dimensions shown in Figs. 1-3 shall be included in the product labeling.

9.2 The material(s) used for the implant shall be specified on the package labels and inserts.

10. Keywords

10.1 arthroplasty; glenoid; humeral; prostheses; hemi-shoulder replacement; total shoulder replacement

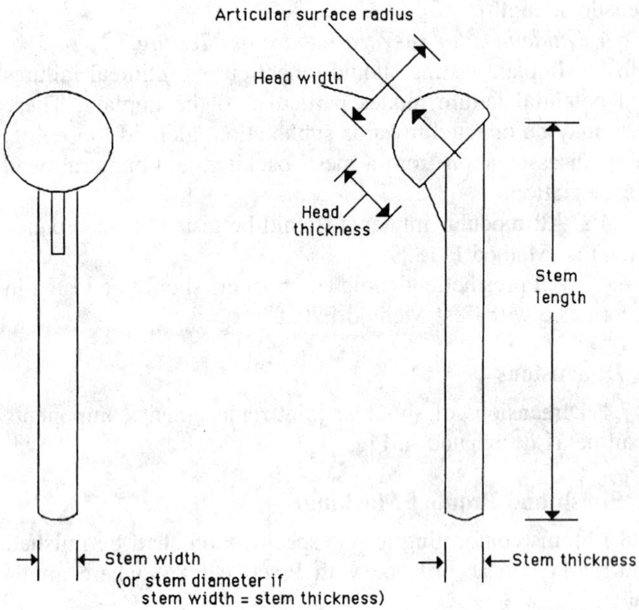

NOTE—A modular connection may be included in this device.

FIG. 1 Humeral Collarless Design

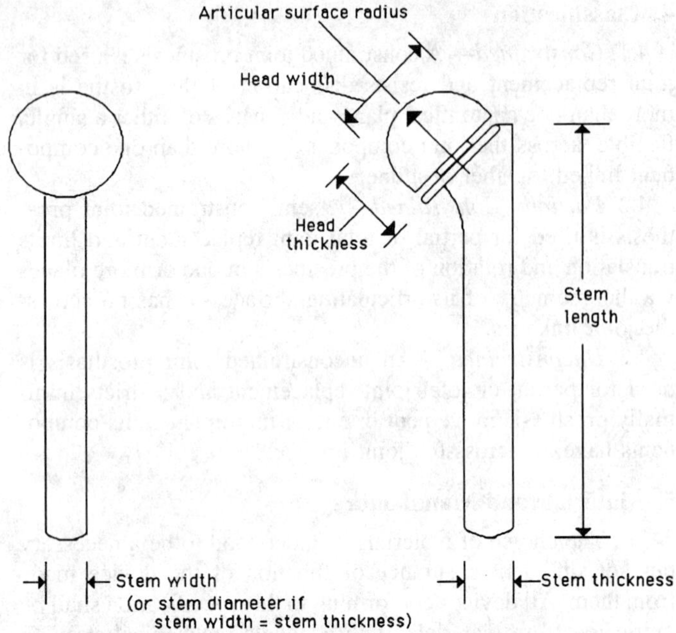

NOTE—A modular connection may be included in this device.

FIG. 2 Humeral Collared Design

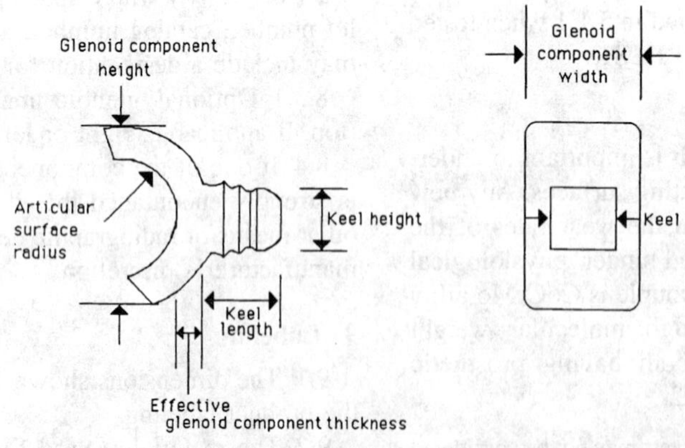

NOTE 1—If the glenoid component is not symmetric about the transverse plane, a minimum and maximum component width shall be specified.

NOTE 2—A modular connection may be included in this device.

FIG. 3 Glenoid Components

APPENDIX

(Nonmandatory Information)

X1. RATIONALE

X1.1 The objectives of this specification are the provision of guidelines for the manufacture and use of the components for total shoulder replacement. Total shoulder replacement parts are intended for use in a patient who is skeletally mature, under conditions of imposed dynamic loads, in a corrosive environment and virtually continuous motion at the bearing surfaces. Laboratory tests to accurately simulate imposed loads, aggressive electrolytes and complex constituents of body fluids have not been usefully accelerated at the present time for a complete joint evaluation. Long-term projections of satisfactory performance over many decades can be suggested but not accurately predicted using available screening procedures. This specification identifies those factors considered to be important to assure a satisfactory useful prosthetic life. It is here recognized that failure of an arthroplasty can occur, even while the components are intact. This is true owing to the composite nature of the arthroplasty procedure, which includes the implant, cement if any, and the physiological environment.

X1.2 Under applicable documents and materials, the list reflects the current state of the art. It is recognized that should materials not now included appear and be proved acceptable, they shall be inserted in the process of revision.

X1.2.1 *Performance Considerations*— Component performance should be considered with regard to patient anatomy. It is well recognized that physical stresses resulting from events or activities out of the ordinary range, as in accidents or especially vigorous sports, predictably exceed allowable stress levels in any component design. It is also recognized here that other forms of arthroplasty failure are known to occur, related primarily to patient factors, such as osteoporosis, Paget's disease, misuse and disuse, and others.

X1.2.1.1 No device specific wear test is specified in this specification. It is felt that at this time wear is not a major issue in existing or potential implant designs, that presently there are no techniques available to do device specific wear tests and that this consideration is already partly covered in 6.1.

X1.2.1.2 The range of motion parameters are specified as minimum values so that the implant itself does not restrict patient shoulder motion and thus allow potential dislocation or loosing of the implant. Initially the minimum range of motion parameters were larger but they were decreased to those given in 6.2.

X1.2.2 *Dimensions*—The method of dimensional measurement must be sought to conform with industry practice and, whenever possible, on an international basis.

X1.2.3 *Finish and Markings*—Dimensions and tolerances are as described by ANSI documents for sphericity, concentricity and surface finish.

X1.2.3.1 The manufacturer's trademark must appear legibly on each of the components. It is desirable to have complete information, where space is available to do so, including size, orientation if any, and catalog number with date.

Standard Guide for Planning and Developing 9-1-1 Enhanced Telephone Systems[1]

This standard is issued under the fixed designation F 1381; the number immediately following the designation indicates the year of original adoption or, in the case of revision, the year of last revision. A number in parentheses indicates the year of last reapproval. A superscript epsilon (ε) indicates an editorial change since the last revision or reapproval.

1. Scope

1.1 This guide recommends minimum performance requirements for enhanced access to public safety services using the North American standard emergency telephone number, 9-1-1.

1.2 This guide provides assistance to states, counties, and local jurisdictions in the development of 9-1-1 enhanced systems.

1.3 This guide makes recommendations for planning and organizational needs in the development of 9-1-1 enhanced systems.

1.4 This guide does not address access to public safety response services through means other than use of the 9-1-1 telephone number.

1.5 This guide applies only to the use of the number 9-1-1 to request a public safety response, from the point of initiation of the call through the point that the caller is connected to the responsible agency, or essential information needed for disposition of the call, or both, is received.

1.6 The sections in this guide are arranged in the following order:

1.7 *This standard does not purport to address all of the safety problems, if any, associated with its use. It is the responsibility of the user of this standard to establish appropriate safety and health practices and determine the applicability of regulatory limitations prior to use.*

2. Terminology

2.1 *Definitions:*

2.1.1 *9-1-1, n*—a three-digit telephone number to facilitate the reporting of an incident or situation requiring response by a public safety agency.

2.1.2 *Poisson Distribution, n*—a probability density function that is often used as a mathematical model of the number of outcomes obtained in a suitable interval of time and space. In 9-1-1 it is used to predict potential call blockage during normal busy periods.

2.2 *Definitions of Terms Specific to This Standard:*

2.2.1 *abandoned call, n*—a call placed to 9-1-1 in which the caller disconnects before the call can be answered by the public safety answering point (PSAP) attendant.

2.2.2 *action agency, n*—the public safety agency having a legal or consensual obligation to respond to a call for service.

2.2.3 *alternate routing, n*—the capability of automatically rerouting 9-1-1 calls to a designated alternate location(s) if all 9-1-1 trunks from a central office or to a primary PSAP are busy or out of service. May also be activated upon request, or automatically if detectable, when 9-1-1 equipment fails or the PSAP itself is disabled.

2.2.4 *answering position, n*—an appropriately equipped location within a PSAP that is used to receive incoming 9-1-1 calls.

2.2.5 *audible signal, n*—a sound that indicates an incoming 9-1-1 call.

2.2.6 *automatic call distributor (ACD), n*— equipment that distributes incoming calls to available PSAP attendants in the order the calls are received, or holds calls until an attendant becomes available.

2.2.7 *automatic location identification (ALI), n*—the automatic display at the PSAP of the caller's telephone number, the address for the telephone and supplementary information.

2.2.8 *automatic number identification (ANI), n*—the automatic display at the PSAP of the caller's telephone number.

2.2.9 *average busiest hour, n*—the 1-h period during the week statistically shown over time to be the hour in which the most emergency telephone calls are received.

2.2.10 *call detail logging, n*—a means of establishing chronological and operational accountability for each 9-1-1 call

[1] This guide is under the jurisdiction of ASTM Committee F-30 on Emergency Medical Services and is the direct responsibility of Subcommittee F30.04 on Communications.

Current edition approved Feb. 15, 1992. Published April 1992.

processed, consisting minimally of the caller's telephone number, the date and time the 9-1-1 telephone equipment established initial connection (trunk seizure), the time the call was answered, the time the call was transferred (if applicable), the time the call was disconnected, the trunk line used, and the identity of the PSAP attendant's position. Also known as *ANI printout*.

2.2.11 *called party hold, n*—the capability to maintain control of an incoming 9-1-1 call by a PSAP attendant for tracing or confirmation of an emergency even if the caller hangs up.

2.2.12 *call progress signals, n*—audible cues to advise 9-1-1 users of the status of their calls.

2.2.13 *call relay, n*—disposition of a 9-1-1 call by the notation of pertinent information by the PSAP attendant who forwards the information to the action agency.

2.2.14 *call referral, n*—disposition of a 9-1-1 call by advice to the caller of the appropriate numbers to call other than 9-1-1.

2.2.15 *call transfer, n*—the extending of a 9-1-1 call by a PSAP attendant to connect the caller with the action agency.

2.2.16 *central office (CO), n*—a telephone company facility that houses the switching and trunking equipment serving telephones in a defined area. Also known as *end office*.

2.2.17 *circuit routes, n*—a means of two-way communication between two terminal installations.

2.2.18 *class of service, n*—a service order code designation of the telephone service features to which business and residence customers subscribe.

2.2.19 *computer-aided dispatch (CAD), n*— a computer-based system intended to increase the efficiency and accuracy of public safety call handling and dispatching.

2.2.20 *computer-aided dispatch (CAD) interface, n*—the means of automatically introducing the ALI data into a computer-aided dispatch (CAD) system, as opposed to manually entering the information.

2.2.21 *conference transfer, n*—the capability of transferring a call to the action agency and allowing the PSAP attendant to monitor or participate in the call after it has been transferred to the action agency. Also known as *three-way calling*.

2.2.22 *contiguous agency, n*—a public safety agency whose jurisdiction is adjacent to the area served by a 9-1-1 system.

2.2.23 *cross tandem transfer, n*—the capability of transferring a call over the 9-1-1 network from a PSAP served by one tandem office to another PSAP served by a different tandem office.

2.2.24 *customer comments, n*—supplementary information useful in dispatching, provided in conjunction with ALI displays.

2.2.25 *customer premises equipment (CPE), n*— terminal equipment at a PSAP or secondary answering location.

2.2.26 *cutover, n*—the actuation of a new telephone call processing or switching system.

2.2.27 *data base, n*—a collection of information organized in a computer to facilitate rapid search and retrieval. In this guide, such data bases include MSAG, telephone number/ESN, and telephone customer records.

2.2.28 *data management system (DMS), n*—the combination of manual procedures and computer programs used to create, store, manipulate, and update data required to provide selective routing and ALI.

2.2.29 *dedicated trunk, n*—a telephone circuit used for one purpose only; that is, transmission of 9-1-1 calls.

2.2.30 *default routing, n*—the capability to route a 9-1-1 call to a designated (default) PSAP when the incoming 9-1-1 call cannot be selectively routed due to an ANI failure, garbled digits, or other cause.

2.2.31 *dial tone first, n*—the provision of dial tone to enable a caller to originate and complete 9-1-1 calls from public telephones without inserting a coin or any other device. Also known as *coin-free dialing*.

2.2.32 *direct dispatch, n*—the functions of 9-1-1 call answering and dispatching are both performed by personnel at the primary PSAP.

2.2.33 *diverse routing, n*—the practice of routing calls through different circuit paths in order to prevent total loss of the 9-1-1 system in the event an individual circuit is disabled.

2.2.34 *emergency service number (ESN), n*— a number used in the DMS to designate the public safety agencies responsible for service to the location of each telephone in a 9-1-1 service area, for the purpose of determining call routing. Also see *emergency service zone (ESZ)*.

2.2.35 *electronic switching system (ESS), n*— a central office with programmable switching logic. Can also be used as a tandem.

2.2.36 *emergency service zone (ESZ), n*—a defined geographical territory consisting of a specific combination of law enforcement, fire, and emergency medical coverage areas. Also see *emergency service number (ESN)*.

2.2.37 ***end office, n***—see *central office*.

2.2.38 *enhanced 9-1-1, n*—a telephone system which includes ANI, ALI, and (optionally) selective routing, to facilitate appropriate public safety response.

2.2.39 *exchange, n*—a defined area, served by one or more telephone central offices, within which a telephone company furnishes service.

2.2.40 *fixed transfer, n*—the capability of a PSAP attendant to transfer a 9-1-1 call to the agency associated with a single button.

2.2.41 *forced disconnect, n*—the capability of a PSAP attendant to disconnect a 9-1-1 call to prevent jamming of the incoming lines.

2.2.42 *foreign exchange (FX) service, n*— a telephone line switched in an exchange or central office other than the exchange or central office in which the telephone is located.

2.2.43 *interconnect, n*—the connection of the serving telephone company's equipment with the equipment of another vendor. Also a generic term used to refer to a non-telephone company vendor.

2.2.44 *interlocal services agreement, n*— an agreement among governmental jurisdictions or privately owned systems, or both, within a specified area to share 9-1-1 system costs, maintenance responsibilities, and other considerations.

2.2.45 *logging recorder, n*—a device that records date/time, voice communications, and other transactions involved in the processing of calls to a PSAP.

2.2.46 *main station, n*—a telephone that is connected directly to a central office and has a unique telephone number. It is not an extension.

2.2.47 *master street address guide (MSAG), n*— a data base of street names and address ranges within their associated communities defining emergency service zones for 9-1-1 purposes.

2.2.48 *network, n*—an arrangement of main stations interconnected by means of communications channels organized to perform or serve a common function.

2.2.49 *nonselective routing, n*—the capability of routing 9-1-1 calls by the use of the NXX or trunk group.

2.2.50 *NXX, n*—the first three digits of a local telephone number that identifies the central office switching location within its area code. Also erroneously referred to as NNX.

2.2.51 *P.01 grade of service, n*—a measure of emergency telephone service in which no more than one call in 100 attempts will be blocked during the average busiest hour.

2.2.52 *pilot number, n*—a telephone customer's main account number, lead number, listed number, or billing number.

2.2.53 *private branch exchange (PBX), n*— a private, internally switched telephone system, of significance to 9-1-1 systems because internal stations may not be individually contained in the DMS and, as a result, will not be displayed by ANI or ALI equipment.

2.2.54 *public safety agency, n*—an entity that provides firefighting, law enforcement, emergency medical, or other emergency service.

2.2.55 *public safety answering point (PSAP) attendant, n*—a person responsible for answering incoming 9-1-1 calls at a PSAP, determining the action to be taken, and executing the PSAP's procedures in the disposition of such calls.

2.2.56 *public safety answering point (PSAP), n*—a facility equipped and staffed to receive 9-1-1 calls. A primary PSAP receives the calls directly; if the call is relayed or transferred the next receiving PSAP is designated a secondary PSAP.

2.2.57 *public switched telephone network (PSTN), n*—the totality of equipment, lines, and controls assembled to establish communication paths between calling and called parties.

2.2.58 *ring back, n*—the capability permitting a PSAP attendant to cause the telephone on a held circuit to ring. Also known as *re-ring*.

2.2.59 *selective routing, n*—the capability of routing a 9-1-1 call to a designated PSAP based upon the location of the caller.

2.2.60 *selective transfer, n*—the capability of transferring a 9-1-1 call to the pre-programmed action agency by operation of one of several buttons typically designated as police, fire, or emergency medical; based on the origin of the incoming call and the nature of the response required.

2.2.61 *serving central office, n*—the central office (CO) from which a PSAP is served. Also see *central office*.

2.2.62 *splash ringing, n*—the capability to provide an audible signal simultaneously with trunk seizure on an incoming 9-1-1 call.

2.2.63 *tandem, n*—a switching system in the public switched telephone network or a privately owned system that establishes 9-1-1 call routing.

2.2.64 *tandem office, n*—the location of the routing table and equipment to direct 9-1-1 calls to the appropriate PSAP.

2.2.65 *TDD/TTY, n*—a telecommunication device for the hearing or speech impaired, or both.

2.2.66 *thousands number group, n*—the entire last four-digit group of numbers in an exchange, sometimes used to determine default routing locations.

2.2.67 *trunk, n*—a circuit connecting switching equipment at two sites (for example, between a PBX and central office, between two central offices).

2.2.68 *trunk group, n*—one or more trunks terminated at the same two points.

2.2.69 *trunk seizure, n*—the point at which a call is assigned to a trunk and acknowledgement is provided by the 9-1-1 call processing equipment.

2.2.70 *uninterruptible power system (UPS), n*— the capability of providing a continuous source of power without regard to the interruption or loss of commercial power. Also known as *uninterruptible power supply*.

2.3 *Abbreviations:*

2.3.1 *NHTSA*—National Highway Traffic Safety Administration, United States Department of Transportation.

2.3.2 *NTIA*—National Telecommunications and Information Administration, United States Department of Commerce.

2.4 *Acronyms:*

2.4.1 *ACD*—automatic call distributor.

2.4.2 *ALI*—automatic location identification.

2.4.3 *ANI*—automatic number identification.

2.4.4 *CO*—central office.

2.4.5 *CAD*—computer-aided dispatch.

2.4.6 *CPE*—customer premises equipment.

2.4.7 *DMS*—data management system.

2.4.8 *ESN*—emergency service number.

2.4.9 *ESS*—electronic switching system.

2.4.10 *ESZ*—emergency service zone.

2.4.11 *FX*—foreign exchange.

2.4.12 *MSAG*—master street address guide.

2.4.13 *PBX*—private branch exchange.

2.4.14 *PSAP*—public safety answering point.

2.4.15 *PSTN*—public switched telephone network.

2.4.16 *UPS*—uninterruptible power system.

3. Significance and Use

3.1 This guide recommends approaches for planning and developing access to public safety services through the telephone number 9-1-1.

3.2 This guide is of most value when a jurisdiction initiates planning for implementation of a 9-1-1 system or when expansion or consolidation of 9-1-1 systems is contemplated. It may be of particular value to state legislatures considering statewide 9-1-1 legislation.

3.3 This guide will help agencies provide effective response to requests for public safety services initiated through 9-1-1. It should be noted that the public perception of 9-1-1 often includes elements of response systems beyond the scope of this guide. This guide is significant because access to the response system through the public switched telephone network is a critical element of timely and appropriate service delivery.

3.4 This guide has significance for the radio telephone industries in that consideration should be given to provide compatibility with 9-1-1 enhanced features in both urban and rural areas.

3.5 This guide is not meant to address other response system elements such as public safety dispatching, prearrival instructions, or deployment of field forces.

4. Concept of Operation

4.1 The basic concept of 9-1-1 planning and operation embraces a simple principle: make the system easy to use. In an emergency situation, 9-1-1 allows a caller to contact the appropriate public safety agency and convey information rapidly and efficiently, without placing an unrealistic burden on the caller.

4.1.1 Inherent features of 9-1-1 increase communications efficiency. 9-1-1 is a simple telephone number, easy to remember, easy to dial, and consistently used throughout North America. The missing element is universality in that 9-1-1 is not available in some locations. Most metropolitan areas provide 9-1-1 service, and a handful of states have attained 100 % coverage. While 9-1-1 service is not universally available, the public often has the perception that it is. This may cause problems for persons attempting to use 9-1-1 in areas without 9-1-1 service.

4.1.2 Enhanced features further benefit 9-1-1 users by reducing average call handling time. Automatic number identification displays the caller's telephone number, ALI displays information about the location of that telephone, and selective routing sends the call to the appropriate PSAP for that location. Selective transfer allows rapid redirecting of calls, and alternate routing arrangements assure effective call handling during unusual conditions.

4.2 Performance requirements of 9-1-1 systems are intended to ensure an adequate number of trunks and answering positions available for the population served, the enhancements are accurate and reliable, and all associated equipment performs adequately.

4.2.1 The number of trunks required to provide adequate telephone service for a given population must be determined. To establish a reasonable number of trunks, agencies should provide at a minimum a level or grade of service at P.01. P.01 grade of service simply means that there is an expectation that no more than one call in 100 attempts will be blocked during the average busiest hour.

4.2.1.1 In determining a grade of service for any telecommunications system, the number of calls and the average call duration must be measured. There may be other local considerations that could have a substantial effect on such calculations. See appendix for a sample calculation using representative numbers.

4.2.1.2 A minimum of two trunks per exchange is recommended in all cases.

4.2.2 The method used to determine the number of positions is similar to calculations for the number of trunks, but also includes other call processing requirements.

4.2.3 Other design criteria are also important in planning 9-1-1 systems:

4.2.3.1 9-1-1 trunks should be diversely routed, using different circuit routes wherever feasible.

4.2.3.2 The network provider should ensure current 9-1-1 circuit routing profiles are maintained, circuits are individually tagged to prevent inadvertent disruption, and failure of any circuit element that involves 9-1-1 trunking is automatically detected. Affected PSAPs should be immediately notified of disruptions and corrective action taken in a timely way.

4.2.3.3 Standard call-progress signals should be used to inform the caller of the status of the call.

4.2.3.4 All public telephones, including coin and credit card telephones, shall be configured to allow a caller to dial and complete a 9-1-1 call without inserting a coin or any other device.

4.2.3.5 In order to prevent network disruption remote automatic alarms and automatic dialers should be prohibited by ordinance or law from being programmed to dial 9-1-1.

4.2.3.6 Rural and common carrier radio-telephone users should be able to access 9-1-1. A statewide plan for handling these calls should be developed.

4.2.3.7 Hearing impaired callers shall have equal access to 9-1-1. A statewide plan for handling calls from special population groups should be developed.

4.2.3.8 Non-English speaking callers should have equal access to 9-1-1. A statewide plan for handling calls from non-English speaking population groups should be developed.

4.2.3.9 Calls from all telephones with outgoing access to the public switched telephone network should not be blocked from access to 9-1-1. This includes FX and WATS lines.

4.2.3.10 Calls should enter the 9-1-1 system only after the caller dials all three digits to avoid false calls entering the system.

4.2.4 The ANI should be consistent and reliable from all classes of telephone service, including coin, centrex, PBX, two-party, multi-party, FX, and cellular.

4.2.4.1 The ANI should be transmitted to the PSAP during the call setup sequence so it is immediately available to the PSAP call attendant upon answering the 9-1-1 call.

4.2.5 The ALI should be consistent and reliable from all classes of telephone service, including coin, centrex, PBX, two-party, multi-party, FX, and cellular.

4.2.5.1 The ALI should include the subscriber name for all classes of service as well as the full street address (or functional equivalent in the case of mobile service), additional location information, and community.

4.2.5.2 The ALI display should indicate the correct PSAP and responsible law enforcement, fire, and EMS agencies.

4.2.5.3 Supplementary information regarding the caller location should include area code and number, pilot number, and class of service.

4.2.5.4 Call completion information should include time and date as well as ESN.

4.2.5.5 The ALI system should be maintained at a level sufficient to ensure that the ALI display will be retrieved in less than 5 s for 95 out of 100 attempts during the average busy hour.

4.2.6 Nonselective routing is accomplished through identifying the NXX of the calling party's telephone number or the trunk group associated with that central office.

4.2.6.1 Nonselective routing is appropriate where all the calls in a central office go to the same PSAP.

4.2.6.2 Nonselective routing can be accomplished either by reading the NXX (and sending the call to the appropriate PSAP by using a routing table), or by assigning each trunk group to a PSAP.

4.2.7 Selective routing should be based on the complete telephone number related to that location rather than just the NXX.

4.2.7.1 Selective routing tables should be updated within 24 h of DMS update.

4.2.8 Transfer capabilities should be consistent and reliable. Transfers between 9-1-1 enhanced PSAPs should include full ANI and ALI capabilities, even if a cross-tandem transfer is involved.

4.2.8.1 Fixed transfer should automatically transfer a 9-1-1 call to the agency associated with a single button as designated by the PSAP. Three-way calling among the 9-1-1 caller, the transferring agency, and the transferred-to agency should be initiated with a single keystroke.

4.2.8.2 Manual transfer should allow transfer of a received 9-1-1 call to a dialed seven-digit or abbreviated number. Three-way calling among the 9-1-1 caller, the transferring agency, and a transferred-to agency should be initiated with the operation of an add-on button (to obtain dial tone) and the dialing of that agency's number.

4.2.8.3 Selective transfer, with the operation of a single button, should automatically transfer a received 9-1-1 call to the action agency as designated by the ESN. Three-way calling among the 9-1-1 caller, the transferring agency, and the transferred-to agency should be enabled by a single keystroke of the button associated with the service required.

4.2.8.4 Release of the call should allow the transferring PSAP to leave the call without disrupting the connection between the 9-1-1 caller and the transferred-to-agency.

4.2.9 Alternate routing allows 9-1-1 calls to be routed to another PSAP or telephone number if conditions warrant.

4.2.9.1 Alternate routing should be automatically executed if all PSAP 9-1-1 trunks are busy.

4.2.9.2 Alternate routing to a predesignated number or another PSAP should be enabled automatically if detectable or, if not detectable by the provider, in less than 5 min of notification to the provider that the equipment at a PSAP is unable to accept 9-1-1 calls.

4.2.9.3 Alternate routing to a predesignated different PSAP should be enabled automatically if detectable or, if not detectable by the provider, in less than 5 min of notification to the provider that an entire PSAP is unable to accept 9-1-1 calls.

4.2.9.4 An automatic alternate routing mechanism should be developed in cases where an individual central office is isolated from the tandem office or both the tandem office and the public switched telephone network.

4.2.10 The PSAP answering equipment should be specially designed for 9-1-1 enhanced call answering.

4.2.10.1 Uninterruptible power systems or some alternate means should be employed to ensure power disruptions will not interrupt calls in progress or prevent new 9-1-1 calls from being received.

4.2.10.2 Splash ringing, or an instant audible signal in the case of automatic call distributors, should be provided to allow calls to be answered as quickly as possible.

4.2.10.3 To manage multiple calls the answering point should have the capability to place calls on hold.

4.2.10.4 Transfer and conference capability should be included in the equipment.

4.2.10.5 The ANI/ALI should be directed to each new position, to each position that picks up a call even if simultaneous pickup occurs, and on transfers to other 9-1-1 equipped PSAPs.

4.2.10.6 Call detail logging should be provided in a format readily adaptable to common commercially sold data base programs.

5. Coordinating 9-1-1 Systems

5.1 Congress has not enacted any legislation specifically funding or coordinating state and local 9-1-1 implementation. Congressional resolutions have been passed supporting the 9-1-1 concept, but it is clear that Congress regards the provision of 9-1-1 service as a state and local matter. What limited Federal funding is available is found in programs such as NHTSA grant funding, community development block grants, and certain other Federal agency programs. The NTIA has also supported the development and distribution of various 9-1-1 planning guides.

5.2 State 9-1-1 statutes are in effect in about three quarters of the states. They aid in resolution of political issues by providing a framework for inter-agency call-handling agreements. They aid in solving technical issues by establishing minimum standards for 9-1-1 implementation and operation. Financial issues are faced by providing a mechanism for funding 9-1-1 implementation and operation, that may involve spreading the costs over a broad population base to make 9-1-1 more affordable in sparsely populated areas.

5.3 Regional agencies, that coordinate planning beyond community, county, or state boundaries, or any combination thereof, have provided a framework for the implementation and administration of 9-1-1 systems in several areas of the country.

5.4 A county government is usually responsible for 9-1-1 system planning, because it is in the best position to secure the cooperation of different agencies and units of government within a reasonably sized area.

5.5 Community-based 9-1-1 systems often provide the starting point for county, regional, and statewide systems.

5.6 Privately operated 9-1-1 systems may be implemented by corporations, educational institutions, or federal facilities. In such circumstances, to ensure compatibility, the planning and development of these systems require that they should be coordinated with adjacent public 9-1-1 systems.

6. State 9-1-1 Statutory Provisions

6.1 Successful implementation of a 9-1-1 enhanced system rests on a clear understanding of the responsibilities of each participating jurisdiction.

6.1.1 While only one jurisdiction may be involved in a 9-1-1 enhanced system, the number of potential jurisdictions and agencies in a system is usually much larger. (In a few cases, the system may embrace the state and all of its subdivisions.)

6.1.2 If the state is contemplating or has enacted legislation supporting 9-1-1 enhanced system implementation, the responsibilities of the state, its subdivisions, and any privately owned 9-1-1 systems should be set forth explicitly.[2]

6.1.3 The greatest challenge in establishing a multi-user system is to ensure that jurisdictional autonomy in the handling of 9-1-1 calls is not adversely affected by virtue of the jurisdiction's participation in the system.

6.1.3.1 The advantages of the 9-1-1 enhanced system contribute substantially to ensuring that jurisdictional autonomy is preserved, but specific language addressing jurisdictional responsibilities and the responsibilities of privately owned 9-1-1 systems in memoranda of agreement or written protocols is still required.

6.1.3.2 If the state has not enacted legislation in regard to jurisdictional responsibility for 9-1-1 call handling, it is all the more important to ensure that system participants agree on the responsibilities to be assumed in a legally binding way. The responsibilities that should be described and assigned can be divided into management and operational concerns.

6.1.3.3 Among the management concerns are the creation and composition of the system's oversight board or committee; who appoints, who chairs, who may serve, when and where meetings are held; how expenses are met and audited; how a system manager is to be selected, compensated, and supervised; if the board is to be terminated upon system implementation, how termination is effected; and the board's legal authorities (in the employment of consultants, for example).

6.1.3.4 Among the operational concerns are the scope of the system; what specific services are to be included and what 9-1-1 enhanced system capabilities are to be supplied; the planning, design, and implementation of the system; who determines participants; who negotiates with representatives of the public switched telephone network; who evaluates proposals, who may contractually obligate the system and its participants; what legal obligations apply to the handling of calls (from call inception to call acknowledgment); who establishes and promulgates local standards, rules, and regulations, and how they are enforced (including supervision of that portion of the public switched telephone network used in forwarding calls to 9-1-1); who provides and who verifies the data upon which the 9-1-1 enhanced system depends; the financial support of the system (if not provided by state or other law); and the apportionment of expenses (where appropriate).

6.2 State legislation recommending, guiding, or mandating the provision of 9-1-1 service has taken a variety of forms, but all recognize that three system elements must be addressed: the community; the providers of public safety services (usually but not always governmental agencies); and the provider of the telephone network.

6.2.1 A situation of several communities served by different telephone companies and public safety agencies presents the 9-1-1 enhanced system designer with a substantial challenge. Successful implementation will be aided by specific delegation of authority among these groups.

6.2.2 The state legislature should delegate general planning oversight and the development of minimum performance standards to a state agency.

6.2.2.1 The state agency should develop administrative rules to establish standards for consistency in planning and operating 9-1-1 systems throughout the state.

6.2.2.2 A state agency is in a better position than a user group to coordinate and resolve the kinds of multijurisdictional problems that often arise, such as defining service areas or identifying primary response agencies.

6.2.2.3 An agency of the state government may also be more effective in dealing with its utility regulators, who must ensure that the interests of the public are properly balanced with the needs of the telephone network owners. Specific procedures for authorizing expenditures of state or local funds, or both, should be provided.

6.2.2.4 The active participation of a state regulatory commission may be appropriate in the event that telephone service suppliers seek state or local funding to pay for the costs of switching office modifications to accommodate 9-1-1 enhanced services.

6.2.2.5 The state agency should in turn delegate planning authority at the service level to its subdivisions, while retaining right of review and approval based on the state's administrative rules.

6.2.2.6 If a statewide funding mechanism is established to support the 9-1-1 enhanced system, delegation of authority to collect and distribute funds should be provided.

6.3 Implementation problems are best dealt with at the level of execution. Adequate delegation of authority to the overseer of the 9-1-1 enhanced system is critical in order to bring together the disparate system elements. Authority to undertake an area-wide education program, for example, upon the introduction of 9-1-1 enhanced service, should be vested in a system manager.

7. 9-1-1 Funding

7.1 The following are various options for funding a 9-1-1 emergency telephone system:

7.1.1 *General Funds*—Costs are met by line item or other provisions in the tax-supported general operating budgets of the state or participating jurisdictions.

7.1.2 *Service Fee*—Costs are met by a fee or surcharge applied against a specific type of service. In the case of 9-1-1 it is usually applied against local telephone service or long distance service and collected by the local exchange carrier or the inter-exchange carrier and remitted to the funding agency.

7.1.3 *Sales Tax*—Costs are met by a tax applied against goods at the time of sale. This tax may be applied at the local or state level and these funds may be dedicated to planning, implementing, and operating 9-1-1 telephone service.

7.1.4 *Base Telephone Rate*—The 9-1-1 funding requirements are taken into account in determining tariff rates for local telephone service.

7.2 The following are specific factors that must be considered in establishing funding for 9-1-1 telephone service:

7.2.1 *Personnel*—The number of personnel required to plan and administer a 9-1-1 system will vary with system design,

[2] "Suggested State Legislation," Vol 40, Council of State Governments, P.O. Box 11910, Lexington, KY 40578.

area of coverage, and responsibilities. The following are specific functions for which staffing is necessary:

7.2.1.1 Oversight/management of planning, implementation, and operation of the 9-1-1 telephone system,

7.2.1.2 Responsibility for the development, accuracy, and maintenance of the MSAG and 9-1-1 data base,

7.2.1.3 Development of regular and special public education campaigns and related materials, and

7.2.1.4 Development of a training program for PSAP call attendants and supervisors in the use and operation of the 9-1-1 telephone system.

7.2.2 *Telephone Service*—The major expense is for telephone service implementation. Some of the cost components are nonrecurring and funding responsibility may be negotiated in some cases. These components include the costs of modifying the telephone network to provide 9-1-1 service, such as costs of trunking, central office modifications, software upgrades, and other network considerations.

7.2.3 *Construction*—Costs of building, redesigning, or upgrading the PSAP facility so as to allow for the installation of the 9-1-1 customer premises equipment.

7.2.4 *Customer Premises Equipment (CPE)*— Costs of equipment needed at the PSAP to provide and operate the 9-1-1 telephone system. This includes ANI and ALI controllers, display terminals, telephone sets, recorders, printers, generators, UPS, and other equipment.

7.3 The following costs will recur over the life of the system:

7.3.1 Monthly billed costs for the operation and maintenance of the 9-1-1 system,

7.3.2 Charges for equipment maintenance and replacement or upgrade that will occur due to changes in technology, and

7.3.3 Costs that are incurred monthly for administration and operation, such as payroll, insurance, utilities, other telephone service, office equipment and supplies, and other operating expenses.

8. Geographical Data Bases

8.1 The development and maintenance of an accurate ALI data base is critical to enhanced 9-1-1 success, and may involve other community resources.

8.1.1 The ALI data base is located in the 9-1-1 computer, that contains the information to be displayed at the PSAP attendant position when a 9-1-1 call is received. This computer is typically located at the serving telephone company's facilities, but could be located at other nearby or remote sites.

8.1.2 The following ALI features are required:

8.1.2.1 The ALI file will be accessed from the PSAP when ANI data associated with the call is identified.

8.1.2.2 The ALI displays the name and address associated with the calling telephone number once the PSAP receives the 9-1-1 call.

8.1.2.3 The ALI identifies the time and date the ALI information is requested by or retrieved at the PSAP.

8.1.2.4 The ALI provides display of additional information related to the telephone number and address from which the 9-1-1 call originated.

8.1.2.5 The ALI identifies the type or class of telephone service, that is, coin phone, residence, business, business extension, FX, and TDD.

8.1.2.6 The ALI identifies the ESN (emergency service number) of the location, that in turn identifies law enforcement, fire, and EMS responders for the calling address.

8.1.3 The ALI data is retained and redisplayed when a call placed on hold is retrieved by a PSAP call attendant.

8.1.3.1 An address that does not have telephone service will not have a file in the ALI data base.

8.1.3.2 Updating of the telephone number specific records contained in the ALI data base should be done on a daily basis to maintain current information.

8.2 The 9-1-1 enhanced systems require a reliable addressing system throughout the areas covered. A state agency should take the lead in establishing an address program, or a county should establish an address program in conjunction with 9-1-1 enhanced implementation.

8.2.1 A statewide address program requires cooperative agreements among local government entities and political subdivisions to establish formal participation in an addressing project involving multiple governmental entities.

8.2.2 An address program at a level below a statewide program also requires many cooperative agreements and coordination requirements. Building a successful address program regardless of level involves the following considerations:

8.2.2.1 Developing organizational responsibilities and the staffing for assigning addresses.

8.2.2.2 Implementing an addressing project. This can range from six months to several years of planning and address mapping tasks.

8.2.2.3 The cost of a uniform address program will depend on number of properties to be addressed and the data base needs.

8.2.2.4 Critical system tools required include maps and specific procedures for locating parcels and structures.

8.2.2.5 Address ranges should be assigned to streets based on a predetermined addressing grid applied to the map.

8.2.3 Address assignment should include a system of record keeping and maintenance.

8.2.3.1 Notification to the affected specific residents or businesses is necessary for new addresses. Cooperation between the post office and the agency responsible for addressing is recommended.

8.2.3.2 Once new addresses are assigned, the responsibility for maintenance should be assigned to an appropriate body.

8.2.4 Posted street signs and house numbers are necessary for locating structures. Specifications should include size, material, longevity, and legibility. These requirements should be delineated in local or state addressing ordinances.

8.2.5 Telephone company standards and U.S. Postal Service guidelines should be considered when implementing a uniform addressing program.

8.2.5.1 The sequence of address elements should be as follows: street number, pre-directional, primary street name, designator, post directional, and secondary number if any. The sequence may vary depending on telephone company service order writing standards.

8.2.5.2 Specific addresses should be used and nonspecific

addresses, for example an intersection or PO Box, should be avoided.

8.2.5.3 Addressing continuity should be maintained throughout a community and, where possible, throughout a county.

8.2.5.4 Each street should have only one correct name. The use of directionals or designators to distinguish separate, noncontiguous streets should be avoided wherever possible (that is, Palm Court, Palm Avenue, Palm Street).

8.2.5.5 There should be no primary street names that are also used as designators or directionals (that is, Court Street or Southeast Blvd.).

8.2.5.6 There should be no sound alike street names (that is, Beach, Beech).

8.2.5.7 Street names should not be longer than fifteen (15) characters.

8.2.5.8 Special characters in street names (that is, hyphens, apostrophes, periods, decimals) should be avoided.

8.2.5.9 Official street numbers should proceed from a logical point of origin and should be in numerical sequence in relation to other lots with frontage on the same street.

8.2.5.10 Odd numbers should be assigned to properties on one street side and even numbers should be assigned to properties on the other side. Numbers should provide flexibility to accommodate additional development.

8.2.5.11 There should be no primary street numbers longer than six numerals.

8.2.5.12 There should be no fractions in the addresses.

8.2.5.13 Alphanumeric primary or secondary address numbers should be prohibited.

8.2.5.14 Multi-unit structures should be addressed with primary numbers and with apartment or suite numbers as secondary location indicators.

8.2.5.15 Streets within multi-structure complexes should be named and each structure individually addressed.

8.2.5.16 Streets within mobile home parks should be named and each lot should be individually addressed.

8.3 Selective routing is directed by selective routing tables that are defined by local jurisdictions.

8.3.1 The selective routing file resides in the 9-1-1 tandem.

8.3.2 Selective routing tables are developed by the telephone company. They consist of all telephone numbers and ESNs for telephone subscribers within boundaries of the 9-1-1 system and are programmed into the tandem for call routing. The tandem uses the ESN to identify and route the call.

8.3.3 The tandem uses the ANI from each call to retrieve the routing information and forward the 9-1-1 call to the appropriate PSAP.

8.3.4 If transfer to a secondary PSAP is required, the tandem, or a privately owned switch, also performs the transfer and selective transfer functions.

8.4 Service areas with specific combinations of responders for law enforcement, fire, and EMS are defined by local jurisdictions.

8.4.1 The ESN's in the 9-1-1 data base identify these combinations to the tandem for routing of the 9-1-1 call to the appropriate PSAP.

8.4.2 Each ESN corresponds to a set of law enforcement, fire, and EMS responders to be displayed on ALI at the PSAP.

9. Other Planning Concerns

9.1 Initial plans for public education should include an explanation of 9-1-1 service, noting the agencies and the area to be served.

9.1.1 All sectors of the public should be included, from preschool through senior citizens.

9.1.2 Prior to cutover a publicity plan should be formulated. This plan includes provisions for preparation, productions, and dissemination of materials involving various media such as brochures, audio visuals, billboards, public speaking engagements, press packets, novelty items, and children's items. The plan should also include an implementation schedule.

9.1.3 A plan for continuing public education should also be developed. This plan includes periodic release of performance statistics and other information regarding changes in the system, and means to gather and release information about significant actions resulting from 9-1-1 use.

9.2 The jurisdiction responsible for training should determine initial and ongoing training requirements and ensure that they are met.

9.2.1 Introductory training of 9-1-1 personnel in system operation should be provided.

9.2.2 Periodic refresher training is necessary to maintain an efficient system.

9.3 In order to maintain the system at an optimum operational level, a standard operating procedure should be developed by representatives of the agencies served in the system.

9.3.1 The system manager should be responsible for supervision of the system operation, equipment maintenance, data base accuracy, and continued refinement of thestandard operating procedures.

9.3.2 The system manager should be knowledgeable about developments and changes in 9-1-1 system technology and procedures, and should undertake to accomplish changes and enhancements that will benefit the 9-1-1 system. The manager should actively participate in public safety and communications conferences and seminars.

9.4 The CAD interface compatibility should be included in PSAPs which use or plan to install computer aided dispatch.

9.5 The many applications of technology to personal communications and other mobile telephone services are important to 9-1-1 planners. Such developments broaden the base of potential sources of 9-1-1 calls as well as the means used to access 9-1-1 service. The pace of technological development suggests that failure to recognize and accommodate such development may adversely affect the coordination and provision of effective 9-1-1 enhanced service.

9.5.1 For example, personal communications networks using mobile satellite technology are likely to proliferate if spectrum allocations can be gained. Political boundaries in consideration of network service areas are essentially meaningless. If a caller can access the PSTN and dial 9-1-1 special treatment is required. Similarly, "intelligent vehicle/highway systems" are being developed that transmit operational data that could include a sensory alarm of an accident. The translation of such signals into an acceptable format for 9-1-1 processing will require careful planning.

9.5.2 The use of "800" service may generate potential problems for 9-1-1 service providers. A crisis intervention center, for example, may advertise widely its "800" number through which its services may be obtained. The situation described by a caller may prompt crisis center personnel to place a call into the 9-1-1 system in the locality of the crisis center. Obviously, if the call is received on a 9-1-1 trunk, the ALI data displayed at the PSAP are meaningless. While 800 numbers may be programmed to generate 9-1-1 enhanced data, that information would be of little value in cases such as this. Such unusual conditions must be recognized by the 9-1-1 planner or system manager.

9.6 Some jurisdictions may opt to install a 9-1-1 enhanced system in which all features, except ANI, are locally provided and maintained. The requirements in this guide are equally applicable to these systems.

9.7 A man-made or natural disaster may produce various kinds of unanticipated malfunctions in a 9-1-1 system. Potential problems should be identified by continually testing the system under stress conditions, that could include simultaneous test calls by public safety personnel throughout the area served. Other disaster planning should be coordinated with state, local, and telephone company emergency preparedness planners to ensure that the needs of the 9-1-1 system are adequately addressed in such circumstances, including the provisioning and restoration of the PSTN.

10. Keywords

10.1 automatic location identification (ALI); automatic number identification (ANI); basic 9-1-1; emergency medical services (EMS); emergency service number (ESN); enhanced 9-1-1; fire; law enforcement; master street address guide (MSAG); 9-1-1; public safety; public safety answering point (PSAP); selective routing; tandem

APPENDIX

(Nonmandatory Information)

X1. GRADE OF SERVICE CALCULATIONS

X1.1 The best way to determine the number of lines needed in a communications system is to measure actual usage on existing lines over an extended period of time and at different hours of the day, adjusting the figures to account for such variables as the number of calls that will still be answered on the seven-digit numbered lines, the decrease in the length of the average call due to 9-1-1 feature-induced faster call handling, and the specimen in duplicate calls due to ease of dialing 9-1-1. This in-depth analysis requires special skills, is time consuming and expensive. Reasonable estimates are usually sufficient for the initial design of 9-1-1 systems. Estimates can be developed by using assumed or measured demographic and calling characteristics of the population to be served to calculate the amount of line loading, then referring to a distribution table, typically a Poisson table, to determine the number of lines that would handle that load at the desired grade of service. Poisson tables are based on call blockage on the first attempt. Other distribution tables, generally available through telephone traffic engineers, may be more accurate than Poisson tables since they account for unusual traffic patterns such as peakedness, fast retries of blocked calls, or all calls overflowing to another PSAP or another telephone number. Generally speaking, however, Poisson tables are sufficiently accurate to provide a good estimate of the number of lines needed.

X1.2 The following example contains assumptions based on the operational experience of 9-1-1 systems, but local jurisdictional requirements should be considered when using these calculations:

X1.2.1 There are 1.5 to 3.0 people per telephone main station.

X1.2.2 The length of the average 9-1-1 call is 90 s, measured from time of trunk seizure to the time of call termination. (Ninety seconds is allowed to provide for differences in technology, training, and operations. No special call handling techniques, such as pre-arrival instructions, hostage negotiations or other extenuating circumstances, have been considered in this calculation.)

X1.2.3 An estimated 10 % of the calls on the busiest day of the average week will be placed during a 1–h period.

X1.2.4 One 9-1-1 call per thousand people per day can be expected in a rural area.

X1.2.5 Two calls per thousand people per day can be expected in an area with over 25 000 population or within five miles of such an area.

X1.2.6 Three calls per thousand people per day can be expected in an area with over 100 000 population or within ten miles of such an area.

X1.3 The degree of loading on a network is generally measured in CCS (hundred call seconds). CCS can be determined by using the following calculation:

$$CCS = \frac{population \times 90 \times 0.1 \times CPT}{100 \times 1000}$$

or:

$$CCS = \frac{MS \times 2.8 \times 90 \times 0.1 \times CPT}{100 \times 1000}$$

where:

MS = telephone main stations,
2.8 = conversion to number of people,
90 = seconds of hold time,

0.1 = conversion to hours (10 % of daily calls), and
CPT = calls per thousand people per day.

X1.3.1 By that formula (and using a Poisson table for trunkage):

over 1600 lines (4400 people); two trunks (0.4 CCS)
over 10 700 lines (30 000 people); three trunks (5.4 CCS)
over 31 000 lines (87 000 people); four trunks (15.7 CCS)
over 39 000 lines (110 000 people); five trunks (29.6 CCS)
over 61 000 lines (171 000 people); six trunks (46.1 CCS)
over 85 000 lines (240 000 people); seven trunks (64.4 CCS)
over 111 000 lines (310 000 people); eight trunks (83.9 CCS)
over 139 000 lines (390 000 people); nine trunks (105 CCS)

REFERENCES[3]

(1) "Addressing Handbook for Local Governments," State of Texas Advisory Commission on State Emergency Communications, 1989.
(2) "The Addressing of Smith County, Texas," *APCO Bulletin*, November 1989, p. 29.
(3) "An Analysis of 911 Emergency Telephone Service and Tariffs," Transcomm, Inc. for U.S. Department of Commerce, NTIA, Washington, DC, February 1980.
(4) Yung, T. J. and Dayharsh, T. I., "The Design and Costing of 911 Systems—A Technical Manual," U.S. Bureau of Justice Statistics, Washington, DC, September 1980.
(5) Angel, Spence and Ehrlich, Roanne, "Enhanced 911 Implementation," Minneapolis, MN, June 1983.
(6) "9-1-1 MSAG Manual," Clackamas County Oregon, revised July 1989.
(7) Ivy, S. C., Dayharsh, T. I., and Bruce, P. H., "911 Public Education Assessment Guidelines," U.S. Bureau of Justice Statistics, Washington, DC, September 1980.
(8) "9-1-1 Service Planning Handbook," State of Texas Advisory Commission on State Emergency Communications, 1989.
(9) "State of Florida 9-1-1 Emergency Telephone System Plan," Division of Communications, Tallahassee, FL, revised 1990.
(10) Ehrlich, Roanne R., "A Study of Relationships During the Establishment of an Enhanced 911 System," Mankato State University, Mankato, MN, January 1984.
(11) "Suggested State Legislation," Volume 40, Council of State Governments, PO Box 11910, Lexington, KY 40578, 1981.

[3] These documents (and many others related to 9-1-1) are available through Associated Public Safety Communications Officers, Inc., APCO-IS, New Smyrna Beach, FL 32170.

Standard Specification for Search and Rescue Computer Software Information Exchange[1]

This standard is issued under the fixed designation F 1382; the number immediately following the designation indicates the year of original adoption or, in the case of revision, the year of last revision. A number in parentheses indicates the year of last reapproval. A superscript epsilon (ε) indicates an editorial change since the last revision or reapproval.

1. Scope

1.1 This specification covers the basic data formats to be used by search and rescue computer applications programs (software) for import from and export to other programs.

1.2 Additional data or word processing formats may be supported by search and rescue programs.

2. Referenced Documents

2.1 *ASTM Standards:*

E 1013 Terminology Relating to Computerized Systems[2]

2.2 *ANSI Standard:*

ANSI X3.4 Information Systems Codes[3]

3. Terminology

3.1 *Definitions:*

3.1.1 *applications program, n*—a generic term for a computer program written for a particular application, possibly unique to a particular installation (see Terminology E 1013).

3.1.2 *applications software, n*—the collection of applications programs used on a given computerized system (see Terminology E 1013).

3.1.3 *ASCII, n*—(pr. ass key′) American Standard Code for Information Interchange. A standard for representing characters and control codes for computers. The attached appendix contains an ASCII table of codes.

3.2 *Definitions of Terms Specific to This Standard:*

3.2.1 *data, n*—alphabetic, numeric, or logical information stored, transmitted, or otherwise processed by an applications program.

3.2.2 *export, v*—the process of writing data from an applications program for use by another program.

3.2.3 *field, n*—one specific attribute of a record, for example, a missing person's last name in a subject description record.

3.2.4 *file, n*—an aggregate of equivalent records, for example, a missing person physical description file with separate records for different subjects. Text files are functionally the same where lines of text may be considered records.

3.2.5 *import, v*—the process of reading data into an applications program from another program.

3.2.6 *record, n*—one complete item in a file, consisting of an aggregate of fields, for example, a missing person's physical description where individual fields contain first name, middle name, last name, hair color, and the like.

4. Classification

4.1 Two categories of search and rescue applications programs are covered by this specification: text processing and data processing.

4.1.1 Text processing applications programs are those which manipulate free-form text, as commonly found in notes, letters, and documents.

4.1.2 Data processing applications programs are those which manipulate formatted numeric, logical, or text fields of a data record, as commonly found in spreadsheets and database management systems.

4.2 Any given piece of applications software may combine elements of either type of program. Specifications for information interchange apply to the particular importing or exporting function.

4.3 Application programs designed to be self-contained and not interchange information with other programs are not covered by this standard.

5. General Requirements

5.1 *Text Processing Programs*—Search and rescue applications software capable of processing text shall be capable of importing and exporting data according to the following specifications:

5.1.1 consisting of only ASCII characters decimal 32 through 126 (printable characters), 10 (linefeed), 12 (formfeed), and 13 (carriage return) in accordance with ANSI X3.4;

5.1.2 a maximum line length of 78 characters, not counting the line termination codes; and

5.1.3 line termination using a carriage return/line feed combination (decimal 13 and 10, hexadecimal 0D and 0A, ASCII symbols CR and LF).

5.2 *Data Processing Programs—Export*—Search and rescue applications software capable of manipulating data other than purely text shall be capable of exporting data according to the following specifications:

[1] This specification is under the jurisdiction of ASTM Committee F32 on Search and Rescue and is the direct responsibility of Subcommittee F32.02 on Management and Operations.

Current edition approved Feb. 15, 1992. Published July 1992.

[2] *Annual Book of ASTM Standards*, Vol 14.01.

[3] Available from American National Standards Institute, 25 W. 43rd St., 4th Floor, New York, NY 10036.

5.2.1 consisting of only ASCII characters decimal 32 through 126 (printable characters), 10 (linefeed), and 13 (carriage return) in accordance with ANSI X3.4;

5.2.2 a maximum of 4000 data bytes per record;

5.2.3 a maximum of 128 fields per record;

5.2.4 a maximum of 254 data bytes for a character field;

5.2.5 a maximum of 1 data byte for a logical field, the character 'T' representing a true condition and 'F' representing a false condition;

5.2.6 a maximum of 19 bytes for a numeric field;

5.2.7 each field delimited by a comma (ASCII decimal 44), with an equal number of fields in each record;

5.2.8 each text field enclosed in double quotes (ASCII decimal 34); and

5.2.9 record termination using a carriage return/line feed combination (decimal 13 and 10, hexadecimal 0D and 0A, ASCII symbols CR and LF).

5.3 *Data Processing Programs—Import*—Search and rescue applications software capable of manipulating data other than purely text may require imported data files considerably smaller than the maximums specified above for exporting. They shall be capable of importing data following these specifications:

5.3.1 required record size, field size, and number of fields per record no greater than the maximums allowed for exporting;

5.3.2 each field delimited by a comma (ASCII decimal 44), with an equal number of fields in each record;

5.3.3 each text field enclosed in double quotes (ASCII decimal 34); and

5.3.4 record termination using a carriage return/line feed combination (decimal 13 and 10, hexadecimal 0D and 0A, ASCII symbols CR and LF).

APPENDIX

(Nonmandatory Information)

X1. ASCII CODE TABLE

X1.1 Printable Characters

Hex	Decimal	Symbol	Hex	Decimal	Symbol
20	32	SPACE	48	72	H
21	33	!	49	73	I
22	34	"	4A	74	J
23	35	#	4B	75	K
24	36	$	4C	76	L
25	37	%	4D	77	M
26	38	&	4E	78	N
27	39	'	4F	79	O
28	40	(	50	80	P
29	41	)	51	81	Q
2A	42	*	52	82	R
2B	43	+	53	83	S
2C	44	,	54	84	T
2D	45	–	55	85	U
2E	46	.	56	86	V
2F	47	/	57	87	W
30	48	0	58	88	X
31	49	1	59	89	Y
32	50	2	5A	90	Z
33	51	3	5B	91	[
34	52	4	5C	92	\
35	53	5	5D	93	]
36	54	6	5E	94	^
37	55	7	5F	95	_
38	56	8	60	96	`
39	57	9	61	97	a
3A	58	:	62	98	b
3B	59	;	63	99	c
3C	60	<	64	100	d
3D	61	=	65	101	e
3E	62	>	66	102	f
3F	63	?	67	103	g
40	64	@	68	104	h
41	65	A	69	105	i
42	66	B	6A	106	j
43	67	C	6B	107	k
44	68	D	6C	108	l
45	69	E	6D	109	m
46	70	F	6E	110	n
47	71	G	6F	111	o
			70	112	p

Hex	Decimal	Symbol
71	113	q
72	114	r
73	115	s
74	116	t
75	117	u
76	118	v
77	119	w
78	120	x
79	121	y
80	122	z
81	123	{
82	124	¦
83	125	}
84	126	~
85	127	DEL

Control characters

Hex	Decimal	Symbol	Code	Description
00	0	NUL	^@	Null
01	1	SOH	^A	Start of Heading
02	2	STX	^B	Start of Text
03	3	ETX	^C	End of Text
04	4	EOT	^D	End of Transmission
05	5	ENQ	^E	Enquiry
06	6	ACK	^F	Acknowledge
07	7	BEL	^G	Bell
08	8	BS	^H	Backspace
09	9	SH	^I	Horizontal Tab
0A	10	LF	^J	Line Feed
0B	11	VT	^K	Vertical Tab
0C	12	FF	^L	Form Feed
0D	13	CR	^M	Carriage Return
0E	14	SO	^N	Shift Out
0F	15	SI	^O	Shift In
10	16	DLE	^P	Data Link Escape
11	17	DC1	^Q	Device Control 1
12	18	DC2	^R	Device Control 2
13	19	DC3	^S	Device Control 3
14	20	DC4	^T	Device Control 4
15	21	NAK	^U	Negative Acknowledge
16	22	SYN	^V	Synchronous Idle
17	23	ETB	^W	End of Transmission Block
18	24	CAN	^X	Cancel
19	25	EM	^Y	End of Medium
1A	26	SUB	^Z	Substitute
1B	27	ESC	^[	Escape
1C	28	FS	^\	File Separator
1D	29	GS	^]	Group Separator
1E	30	RS	^^	Record Separator
1F	31	US	^_	Unit Separator
7F	127	DEL	DEL	Delete

^—Denotes control key combination

Designation: F 1408 – 97

Standard Practice for Subcutaneous Screening Test for Implant Materials[1]

This standard is issued under the fixed designation F 1408; the number immediately following the designation indicates the year of original adoption or, in the case of revision, the year of last revision. A number in parentheses indicates the year of last reapproval. A superscript epsilon (ε) indicates an editorial change since the last revision or reapproval.

1. Scope

1.1 This practice covers a short-term testing method to screen the subcutaneous tissue reaction to metallic or other implant candidate materials in small laboratory animals. The material may be dense or porous. The tissue reactions will be evaluated in comparison to those evoked by control materials that are accepted as clinical implant materials.

1.2 This practice, along with other appropriate biological tests (including other ASTM test methods), may be used to assess the biocompatibility of candidate materials for use in the fabrication of devices for clinical application. It may be also applied to evaluate the effect of special surface textures and preparations of known materials.

1.3 This experimental protocol is not designed to provide a comprehensive assessment of the systemic toxicity, carcinogenicity, teratogenicity, or mutagenicity of the material.

1.4 The values stated in SI units are to be regarded as the standard.

1.5 *This standard does not purport to address all of the safety concerns, if any, associated with its use. It is the responsibility of the user of this standard to establish appropriate safety and health practices and determine the applicability of regulatory limitations prior to use.*

2. Referenced Documents

2.1 *ASTM Standards:*

F 67 Specification for Unalloyed Titanium for Surgical Implant Applications[2]

F 75 Specification for Cast Cobalt-ChromiumMolybdenum Alloy for Surgical Implant Applications[2]

F 86 Practice for Surface Preparation and Marking of Metallic Surgical Implants[2]

F 136 Specification for Wrought Titanium 6Al-4V ELI Alloy for Surgical Implant Applications[2]

F 138 Specification for Stainless Steel Bar and Wire for Surgical Implants (Special Quality)[2]

F 648 Specification for Ultra-High-Molecular-Weight Polyethylene Powder and Fabricated Form for Surgical Implants[2]

F 763 Practice for Short-Term Screening of Implant Materials[2]

F 981 Practice for Assessment of Compatibility of Biomaterials for Surgical Implants With Respect to Effect of Materials on Muscle and Bone[2]

3. Summary of Practice

3.1 Under strict aseptic conditions, specimens of the candidate and control materials are implanted subcutaneously in the neck of mice (or other suitable animals). After one, three, and nine weeks the animals are anesthetized and the test samples are excised with an intact tissue envelope. On histologic sections the tissue reactions to the candidate materials are compared with the tissue response to clinically accepted control materials.

4. Significance and Use

4.1 This practice is a guideline for a short-term screening test for the evaluation of the tissue response to materials that may be selected for implantation in the human body. This test may be performed prior to longterm testing (for example, Practice F 981) to eliminate unsuitable candidate materials early and to save further animal testing.

4.2 This practice may be used to detect toxic effects of materials in general (see Appendix X1). However, it is particularly suitable for the testing of materials that are intended to have contact with subcutaneous tissues or soft tissues in general. For materials intended to be inserted specifically into muscle tissues, Practice F 763 should be considered as a short term test method.

4.3 The suggested implant specimens are cylindrical. A special grooved type of cylinder may be used (see Fig. X2.1 of Appendix X2) to allow tissue interlocking that could keep the implant in place and minimize tissue irritation through motion at the interface that otherwise could contribute to increased variance of the results. In case ungrooved cylinders are used (see Fig. X1.2 of Appendix X2), probable motion at the implant/tissue interface must be taken into account. Control cylinders should be shaped like the test cylinders.

4.4 The type of surface preparation of the specimens can affect the tissue reaction, therefore the preparation procedure should be noted in the report. The test may be used to compare the effect of different surface structures or conditions of the same material or to assess the effect of various treatments of modifications of a material.

---

[1] This practice is under the jurisdiction of ASTM Committee F-4 on Medical and Surgical Materials and Devices and is the direct responsibility of Subcommittee F04.16 on Biocompatibility Test Methods.

Current edition approved November 10, 1997. Published June 1998. Originally published as F 1408 - 92. Last previous edition F 1408 - 92 (1996).

[2] *Annual Book of ASTM Standards*, Vol 13.01.

5. Test Animals and Sites

5.1 Mice of an established strain, (preferably females), are used as test hosts. The test may be adapted to other suitable test animals (for example, rats).

5.2 The implant specimens of control and candidate materials are inserted subcutaneously in the neck of the host.

5.3 One implant is inserted per mouse. Therefore, the number of animals is identical with the number of test specimens. If rats or other larger suitable animals are used, more than one test specimen may be implanted, but the implants should never be allowed to come in contact with each other. If animals other than mice are large enough, cylinders of the candidate and control material may be implanted separately at the right and the left side of the neck in one animal.

6. Implant Specimens

6.1 *Specimen Design*— Cylinders of 7 mm length and 4 mm diameter are prepared for implantation in mice. Special specimens with two grooves are designed corresponding to the figures in Appendix X2. If larger animal hosts are used, the implant dimensions may be increased proportionally. If it is impossible to prepare specimens of this kind, the specimen configuration used must be described fully in the report. Implant specimens from the candidate and control material should always have the same dimensions.

6.2 *Selection of Control Materials*—Recommended metals for use as control materials include those given in Specifications F 67, F 75, F 136, and F 138. However, for specific applications any metal of known compatibility and standardized as implant material may be employed as control material for comparison. To study adverse tissue reactions, a non-compatible material like copper may be used as a positive control material. A suitable polymeric control material like the polyethylene USP negative control plastic, RS, or UHMWPE (see Specification F 648) may be used.

6.3 *Specimen Surface*— The surface of specimens from prospective implant materials should be treated in the same manner as the implant intended for clinical application in the human patient. Depending on the particular issue, the control specimens should have either a surface condition as it is normally used for clinical applications or a surface condition most similar to that of the tested candidate material. For preparation of metallic materials Practice F 86 should be considered.

6.4 *Numbers of Test and Control Implants*—Per each time period, at least six implant specimens of each candidate and control material should be evaluated in mice (one per mouse). If more than one specimen is implanted in larger test hosts, at least four animals should be used per material and time period.

6.5 *Conditioning*— The cleaning, sterilization, and packaging should be the same as used for implantation in the human patient. After surface preparation and sterilization the implant specimens should be protected from surface alterations and contamination and should be handled with non-metallic forceps when appropriate. When plastified forceps are used, be sure that no plastic material is transferred to the implant surface.

7. Procedure

7.1 *Implantation*:

7.1.1 Implant the specimens under sterile conditions in anesthetized animals. The incision site is remote from the implantation site to prevent infection around the implant. In mice, make a 1 cm long incision above the sacrum and prepare a subcutaneous tunnel toward the neck.

7.1.2 Push the implant through the tunnel and position at the neck. In some distance of the implant close the tunnel with three stitches with a thread of a non-metallic suture material to prevent moving of the implant. Then close the incision. (Do not place the implant directly underneath the incision to avoid infection.)

7.1.3 Keep the individually marked animals in standard cages that comply with current animal protection requirements. Keep mice up to three or four weeks in individual cages.

7.2 *Post-Operative Care*:

7.2.1 Care of the animals should be in accordance with accepted standards as outlined in the *Guide for the Care and Use of Laboratory Animals*.[3]

7.2.2 Carefully observe each animal during the period of assay, and report any abnormal clinical findings.

7.2.3 If infection or injury of the test implant site invalidates the results, replace the animal so that the number of retrieved implants will be at least that of the schedule.

7.2.4 If an animal dies prior to the expected date of sacrifice, autopsy it and determine the cause of death. Replace the animal if the cause of death is unrelated to the test procedure or the test material. Include the test animal in the assay of data if the cause of death is related to the procedure or test material.

7.3 *Sacrifice and Implant Retrieval*:

7.3.1 Sacrifice the animals after one, three, and nine weeks. If longer time intervals are of interest, mice may be kept up to 24 weeks. Examine and report the status of the health of the animals prior to euthanasia.

7.3.2 At sacrifice, record any gross abnormalities of color or consistency observed on the tissues surrounding the implant. Remove each implant with an intact tissue envelope. If the tissue envelope was damaged during the excision, such should be reported. Transfer the tissue specimen as soon as possible in a fixing agent that does not interfere with the implant material and its probable degradation products.

8. Histologic Evaluation

8.1 *Histological Preparation*:

8.1.1 In general, standard laboratory practices for histological preparation of the implant/tissue specimens and staining are used.

8.1.2 If the implant/tissue interface is to be studied, embedding of the intact tissue envelope with the implant in situ using hard plastics is preferred. Appropriate microtomes or cutting and grinding techniques must be employed for the preparation of histologic slides. Before sectioning, hard metals may be removed by an electrochemical technique. In this case, after

[3] *The Guide for Care and Use of Laboratory Animals*, Department of Health, Education, and Welfare, Publication No. 78-23, 1978. Available from the Superintendent of Documents, U.S. Government Printing Office, Washington, DC 20402.

embedding, one cuts the sample longitudinally through the implant and dissolves the implant parts electrochemically, providing that the electrochemical procedure does not markedly alter the contacting tissues embedded in the plastics. The empty space may be filled with plastic material to protect the original contacting surface during sectioning.

If the implant material is a ceramic or calcified material, other procedures may need to be considered. Where possible, the material may be dissolved after embedding, thus preserving the interface, and allowing standard histologic procedures. If the material cannot be dissolved after embedding, the use of thick sections and grinding to desired thickness may be preferable.

8.1.3 For quantitative evaluations the cutting geometry in relation to the cylinder must be considered. The implant orientation and cutting geometry shall be reported.

8.1.4 If techniques described under 8.1.2 are not available, conventional (for example, paraffin) embedding and standard microtomy may be employed. However, with this technique the tissue layers closest to the implant are usually destroyed.

8.1.5 If such conventional technique is used, the tissue envelope should be opened before or after exposure to a fixative and the condition of the implant surface and the tissue bed shall be reported.

8.1.6 The stained histologic sections of the surrounding tissues from the candidate- and control-material implants are compared, and their characteristics are reported. The comparison should be made between the same cylinder sections. With grooved implants the center portions between the grooves and the flat top surfaces of the implant are usually used for evaluation.

8.1.7 The counted cell populations at defined distances from the implant interface, and the thickness of the tissue capsula may be parameters for quantitative evaluation.

9. Report

9.1 Report the following information:

9.1.1 *Implants*—Describe implant material, material condition, fabrication, surface condition, and modifications of the recommended shape and size of implants.

9.1.2 *Conditioning*— Describe cleaning, handling, and sterilization techniques employed.

9.1.3 *Hosts and Implantation*—Report type of test host and number of implants inserted, if other animals than mice are used. Comment on age, sex, and strain of animals, insertion techniques, and special diet. Any pathologic signs shall be diagnosed and reported. If test animals are lost the cause of death should be noted.

9.2 Include a description of retrieval technique, observations made on control and test implants, as well as the gross appearance of the tissues surrounding the implants. The number of implants tested per time interval should be stated.

9.3 Report the observation of each histological examination. The techniques employed for the preparation of the histologic sections shall be described.

10. Keywords

10.1 biocompatibility; mice; orthopaedic medical devices; short-term tissue screening; subcutaneous tissue screening; tissue compatibility; toxicity/toxicology

APPENDIXES

(Nonmandatory Information)

X1. RATIONALE

X1.1 This practice complements existing ASTM standards on in vivo biocompatibility testing of prospective implant materials. The two particular related standards, Practices F 981 and F 763, provide only procedures for long term testing in muscle and bone and short term testing in muscles, respectively. Thus, a short term subcutaneous screening test is desirable for the assessment of the tissue response to materials intended to be used either for typical subcutaneous implants (for example, in plastic or tumor surgery) or for implants for fracture treatment that are usually in contact with subcutaneous tissues (for example, midface, hand, tibia), muscles, fasciae, tendons, etc. This practice is also of interest for the testing of materials for short term implants such as drains or leads.

X1.2 The test procedure in this practice is used during many years of in vivo implant material testing and is designed to give reproducible results.

X1.3 The use of mice as test hosts has the advantage that the tests are not expensive, and that the animals can be kept separate during the period of wound healing. However, the test method in this practice can be adapted when larger test animals are requested. Then, more than one implant of the same kind can be tested in one animal.

X1.4 The testing of a wide variety of metallic and plastic materials in mice has shown that the reaction to compatible and non-compatible materials is significantly different. The reaction scale ranges from the death of the animals after three weeks, over tissue necrosis, inflammation, indifferent material layers at the interface, and varying tissue capsulae. The thickness of the tissue capsula surrounding the implants, as well as the cell population, can vary significantly in response to different materials.

X1.5 For information the following literature references may be consulted:

Turner, E., Lawrence, W. H., and Autian, J. "Subacute Toxicity Testing of Biomaterials. Using Histopathological Evaluation of Rabbit Muscle Tissue," *Journal of Biomedical Materials Research, 7,* 39, 1973.

Geret, V., Rahn, B. A., Mathys, R., Straumann, F., and Perren, S. M., "In vivo Testing of Tissue Tolerance of Implant Materials: Improved Quantitative Evaluation through Reduction of Relative Motion at the Implant Tissue Interface," from *Current Concepts of Internal Fixation of Fracture*, Uhthoff, H. K., Springer Verlag, 1980.

Geret, V., Rahn, B. A., Mathys, R., Straumann, F., and Perren, S. M., "A Method for Testing Tissue Tolerance for Improved Quantitative Evaluation Through Reduction of Relative Motion at the Implant-Tissue Interface Evaluation of Biomaterials," Chapter 35, Edited by Winter, G. D., Leray, J. L., and de Groot, K., John Wiley and Sons Ltd., 1980.

Rahn, B. A., Geret, V., Capaul, C., Lardi, M., and Solothurmann, B., "Morphometric Evaluation of Tissue Reaction to Implants Using Low Cost Digitizing Techniques," *Clinical Applications of Biomaterials*, Edited by Lee, A. J. C., Albrektsson, T., and Branemark, P. I., John Wiley and Sons Ltd., 1982.

Rahn, B. A., Gerber, H. W., Simpson, J., Straumann, F., and Perren, S. M., *Cultured Cells Contacting Implant Material of Different Surface Treatment Biomaterials 1980*, Edited by Winter, G. D., Gibbson, D. F., and Plenk, Jr. H., John Wiley and Sons Ltd., 1982.

Rahn, B. A., Gerber, H. W., Geret, V., and Perren, S. M. *Assessment of Biocompatibility*, World Congress on Medical Physics and Biomedical Engineering, Hamburg, 1982.

Geret, V., Rahn, B. A., Mathys, R., and Perren, S. M., Quantitative Analyse der In vivo Gewebeverträglichkeit von Hydroxylapatit, Ceros 80, Hefte zur Unfallheilkunde, Heft 165, Hrsg: C. Burri/U. Heim/J. Poigenfürst, Springer-Verlag Berlin Heidelberg, 1983.

X2. SHAPE AND DIMENSIONS OF CYLINDERS FOR IMPLANTATION IN MICE (GIVEN IN MILLIMETRES)

X2.1 See Fig. X2.1 and Fig. X2.2

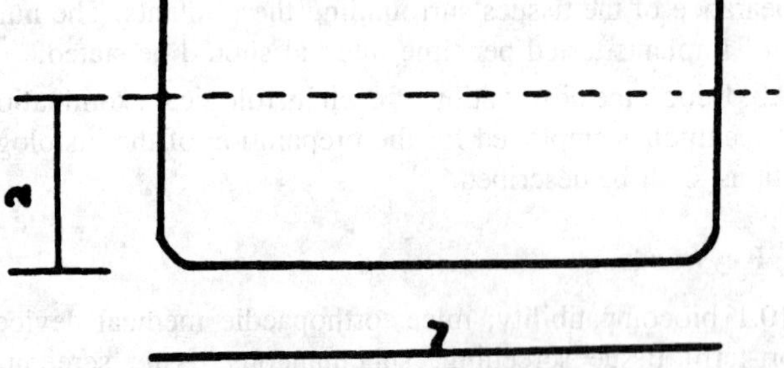

FIG. X2.1 Cylinders Without Grooves

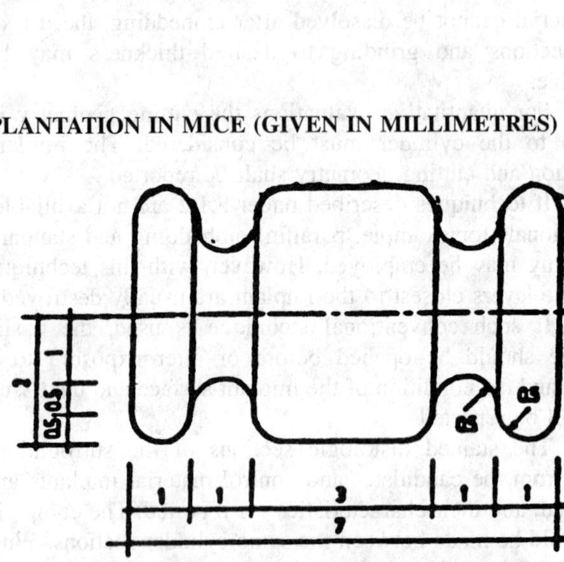

FIG. X2.2 Special Cylinders With Grooves

Standard Specification for Pulse Oximeters[1]

INTRODUCTION

The approximation of hemoglobin saturation through the use of pulse oximetry has become an increasingly common practice in many areas of clinical medicine. These areas include, but are not limited to anesthesia, respiratory therapy, pediatrics, and intensive care. A variety of devices are currently available that are intended for these applications. This specification covers minimum safety and performance requirements based on parameters that are believed to be achievable within the limits of existing technology.

Appendix X1 contains a rationale for the most important requirements. It is included to provide additional insight into the reasoning that led to the requirements and recommendations that have been incorporated in this specification.

This specification references IEC 601-1 for many of the general requirements for safety. Requirements specific to pulse oximeters not included in IEC 601-1.

1. Scope

1.1 The scope given in Clause 1 of IEC 601-1 applies except that 1.1 shall be replaced by the following:

1.1.1 This specification includes requirements for the safety and performance of pulse oximeters, as defined in 3.2.9 intended for use in approximating the saturation of arterial hemoglobin, non-invasively, from a light signal transmitted through the tissue, taking into account the pulsatile nature of volume changes with blood flow.

1.2 The field of application includes, but is not limited to: intraoperative and perioperative use; adult critical care application; pediatric and neonatal application; and general determination of saturation on hospitalized and non-hospitalized patients.

1.3 Pulse oximeters intended for use in laboratory research applications and "bench" type oximeters that require a blood sample from the patient are outside the scope of this specification.

2. Referenced Documents

2.1 The following standards contain provisions that, through reference in this text, constitute provisions of this specification. At the time of publication, the editions indicated were valid. All standards are subject to revision, and parties to agreements based on this specification are encouraged to investigate the possibility of applying the most recent editions of the standards listed below.

2.2 *ASTM Standards:*

F 1463 Specification for Alarm Signals in Medical Equipment Used in Anesthesia and Respiratory Care[2]

2.3 *ISO Standards:*

ISO 7249 Controls—Terms, Suitability, Design Requirements[3]

ISO 7250 Basic List of Anthropomorphic Measurements[3]

2.4 *IEC Standards:*

IEC 79-3:1972 Electrical Apparatus for Explosive Atmospheres Part III: Spark Test Apparatus for Intrinsically Safe Units[3]

IEC 79-4:1975 Electrical Apparatus for Explosive Atmosphere Part IV: Method of Test for Ignition Temperature[3]

IEC 601-1:1988 Safety of Medical Electrical Equipment—Part I: General Safety Requirements[3]

IEC 801-2 Electromagnetic Compatibility for Industrial Process Measurement and Control Equipment Part 2: Electrostatic Discharge Requirements (August, 1990—TC65 (Secreteriat) 136[3]

3. Terminology

3.1 *Definitions:*

3.1.1 For the purposes of this specification, the definitions given in Clause 2 of IEC 601-1 apply together with the following additional terms.

3.2 *Definitions of Terms Specific to This Standard:*

3.2.1 *alarm*—a warning signal.

3.2.2 *alarm set point*—the setting of the adjustment control,

[1] This specification is under the jurisdiction of ASTM F29 on Anesthetic and Respiratory Equipment and is the direct responsibility of Subcommittee F29.11 on Gas Monitors.

Current edition approved July 31, 1992. Published December 1992.

[2] *Annual Book of ASTM Standards*, Vol 13.01.

[3] Available from American National Standards Institute, 11 West 42 nd St., 13th Floor, NY, NY 10036.

or display value that indicates the SpO_2, at or beyond which the alarm is intended to be activated.

3.2.2.1 *Discussion*—Terms such as *alarm limits* or *alarm threshold* are frequently used to describe the same function.

3.2.3 *alarm system*—those parts of the pulse oximeter that establish the alarm set point(s); and activate an alarm when the SpO_2 is less than or equal to the low alarm set point, if provided, or is equal to or greater than the high alarm set point, if provided.

3.2.4 *calibration range*—the range of SpO_2 values over which the pulse oximeter has been tested and calibrated.

3.2.5 *display range*—the range of the SpO_2 values that may be displayed by the pulse oximeter.

3.2.6 *display update frequency*—the number of seconds or events, that is, pulses, between possible changes in the displayed value.

3.2.7 *probe*—the portion of the applied part of the pulse oximeter intended to come in direct contact with the patient. With some oximeters, the probe may be considered an accessory.

3.2.8 *probe fault*—a condition including, but not limited to, a probe component failure or disconnection of the probe from either the pulse oximeter or the patient.

3.2.9 *pulse oximeter*—a device for determination of saturation of hemoglobin non-invasively from a light signal transmitted through the tissue, taking into account the pulsatile nature of volume changes with blood flow.

3.2.10 *total Hb*—the sum of all hemoglobin species including, but not limited to, O_2Hb, Meth Hb, HHb, and COHb.

3.3 *Symbols:*

3.3.1 *O_2Hb/(total Hb)*—fractional saturation.

3.3.2 *$O_2Hb/(O_2 Hb + HHb)$*—functional saturation.

3.3.2.1 *Discussion*—HHb = deoxyHb.

3.3.3 *SaO_2*—hemoglobin saturation with oxygen in systemic arteries.

3.3.4 *SpO_2*—hemoglobin saturation with oxygen as measured by a pulse oximeter.

4. Classification

4.1 The requirements given in Clause 5 of IEC 601-1 apply except as follows:

4.1.1 In Clause 5.6 delete all but "continuous operation."

5. Relationship of This Specification to IEC 601-1

5.1 *Section One—General*:

	(A)	(N/A)	(AM/R)*
1. Scope and Object			X
2. Terminology and definitions			+X
3. General requirements	X		
4. General requirements for tests			X
5. Classification			X
6. Identification, marking and documents			X
7. Power input	X		

*A = Applies, NA = Not Applicable, AM/R - applies with an amendment, addition, or revision to the requirements in IEC 601-1.

5.2 *Section Two—Environmental Conditions*:

	(A)	(N/A)	(AM/R)*
8. (Not used)			
9. (Not used)			
10. Environmental conditions	X		
11. (Not used)			
12. (Not used)			

5.3 *Section Three—Protection Against Electric Shock Hazards*:

	(A)	(N/A)	(AM/R)*
13. General	X		
14. Requirements related to classification	X		
15. Limitation of voltage and/or energy	X		
16. Enclosures and PROTECTIVE COVERS	X		
17. Separation	X		
18. Protective earthing, functional earthing, and potential equalization	X		
19. PATIENT AUXILIARY CURRENTS			X
20. Dielectric strength			X

5.4 *Section Four—Protection Against Mechanical Hazards*:

	(A)	(N/A)	(AM/R)*
21. Mechanical strength			X
22. Moving parts	X		
23. Surfaces, corners, and edges	X		
24. Stability in NORMAL USE	X		
26. Vibration and Noise	X		
27. Pneumatic and hydraulic power		X	
28. Suspended masses		X	

5.5 *Section Five—Protection Against Hazards from Unwanted or Excessive Radiation*:

	(A)	(N/A)	(AM/R)*
29. X-radiation	X		

	(A)	(N/A)	(AM/R)*
30. Alpha, beta, gamma, neutron radiation and other particle radiation		X	
31. Microwave radiation	X		
32. Light radiation (including visual radiation and lasers)	X		
33. Infra-red radiation	X		
34. Ultra-violet radiation	X		
35. Acoustical energy (including ultrasonics)	X		
36. Electromagnetic compatibility			X

5.6 *Section Six—Protection Against Hazards of Ignition of Flammable Anaesthetic Mixtures*:

	(A)	(N/A)	(AM/R)*
37. Locations and basic requirements	X		
38. Marking and ACCOMPANYING DOCUMENTS	X		
39. Common requirements for Category AP and Category APG EQUIPMENT	X		
40. Requirements and tests for Category AP EQUIPMENT, parts or components thereof	X		
41. Requirements and tests for Category APG EQUIPMENT, parts or components thereof	X		

5.7 *Section Seven—Protection Against Excessive Temperatures and Other Safety Hazards*:

	(A)	(N/A)	(AM/R)*
42. Excessive temperatures	X		
43. Fire prevention	X		
44. Overflow, spillage, leakage, humidity, ingress of liquids, cleaning, sterilization, and disinfection	X		
45. Pressure vessels and parts subject to PRESSURE	X		
46. Human errors			X
47. Electrostatic charges	X		
48. Materials in APPLIED PARTS in contact with the body of the PATIENT	X		
49. Interruption of the power supply	X		

5.8 *Section Eight—Accuracy of Operating Data and Protection Against Hazardous Output*:

	(A)	(N/A)	(AM/R)*
50. Accuracy of operating data	X		
51. Protection against hazardous output			X

5.9 *Section Nine—Abnormal Operations and Fault Conditions: Environmental Tests*:

	(A)	(N/A)	(AM/R)*
52. Abnormal operation and fault conditions	X		
53. Environmental tests	X		

5.10 *Section Ten—Constructional Requirements*:

	(A)	(N/A)	(AM/R)*
54. General	X		
55. ENCLOSURES and covers	X		
56. Components and general assembly	X		
57. MAINS PARTS, components and layout	X		
58. Protective earthing—Terminals and connections	X		
59. Construction and layout	X		

5.11 *Section Eleven—Additional Clauses Specific to Pulse Oximeters*:

	(A)	(N/A)	(AM/R)*
60. Pulse amplitude or pulse strength display	X		

5.11.1 Clauses containing amendments, additions or replacements to the text in IEC 601-1.

NOTE 1—The clause numbers used reference the specific section in IEC 601-1.

6. General Requirements and General Requirements for Tests

6.1 Clauses 3 and 4 of IEC 601-1 apply together with the following addition:

6.1.1 Test methods other than those specified in this specification but of equal or greater accuracy may be used to verify compliance with the requirements of this specification. However, in the event of dispute, the methods specified in this specification shall be used as the reference methods.

7. Identification, Marking, and Documents

7.1 The requirements given in Clause 6 of IEC 601-1 apply with the following additions and modifications:

7.1.1 In 4.1, replace Item B by the following:

7.1.1.1 If the size of the pulse oximeter does not permit the complete marking as specified throughout this clause, at least the following shall be marked on the pulse oximeter: the name of the manufacturer, a serial number or lot or batch identifying number, Symbol Number 14 in Table D1 of IEC 601-1, and if the pulse oximeter is not provided with a low SpO_2 alarm, the words "NOT FOR MONITORING."

7.1.2 In 4.1, add the following item to Item F:

7.1.2.1 A serial number or other lot or batch identifying number.

7.1.3 In 4.1, add additional items as follows:

7.1.3.1 Displays of percent saturation shall be displayed in units of "% SpO_2." The units of measure shall be marked by (adjacent to) the display, or displayed on demand.

7.1.3.2 Marking shall be provided on the probe package or on the probe itself if the probe is for "single patient use."

7.1.3.3 If the pulse oximeter is not provided with a low SpO_2 alarm, the words "NOT FOR MONITORING."

7.2 Clause 6.7 of IEC 601-1 shall apply with the following modification:

7.2.1 Dot matrix, alphanumeric displays, and computer-generated graphics are not considered to be indicator lights.

7.2.2 Compliance shall be checked by functional tests and inspections.

7.3 In 6.8.2 delete Subclause b and add the following items:

7.3.1 The instructions for use shall additionally include the following information:

7.3.1.1 If the pulse oximeter is provided with adjustable alarm levels, the range of adjustment;

7.3.1.2 A method of disinfection or sterilization, or both, of both the probe and the body of the pulse oximeter, where applicable;

7.3.1.3 The display update interval of the pulse oximeter and the method by which the displayed value is determined;

7.3.1.4 The calibration range of the pulse oximeter;

7.3.1.5 The display range of the pulse oximeter;

7.3.1.6 Any types of interference known to influence the function of the pulse oximeter at the time that the instructions for use were prepared;

7.3.1.7 If the pulse oximeter requires in-service calibration, a suitable calibration procedure;

7.3.1.8 The mechanism and nature of alarm silencing, that is, during probe disconnection, probe off the finger, etc., and a method for manual self-testing of the alarm circuitry if an automatic self-test is not provided;

7.3.1.9 The default parameters for the alarm that occur upon pulse oximeter activation, if applicable;

7.3.1.10 If not provided with a low SpO_2 alarm, the statement "NOT FOR MONITORING"; and

7.3.1.11 The accompanying documents shall specify probes that may be used with the pulse oximeter.

7.3.2 In 6.8.2, add the following to Item D:

7.3.2.1 The manufacturer shall also state in the accompanying documents the maximum application time for each probe at a single site.

7.4 In 6.8.3 add the following:

7.4.1 *Accuracy*:

7.4.1.1 The accuracy and the range of hemoglobin saturation with oxygen over which the accuracy of the pulse oximeter is claimed shall be disclosed. The manufacturer shall also disclose whether the calibration was to functional or fractional saturation. Test methods shall be available from the manufacturer upon request.

7.4.1.2 If provided, the manufacturer shall disclose in the accompanying documents the accuracy and range for the pulse rate and the range over which this accuracy is claimed.

7.4.1.3 The test methods shall be available from the manufacturer upon request.

8. Continuous Leakage Currents and Patient Auxiliary Currents

8.1 The requirements given in Clause 19 of IEC 601-1 apply except for the following modification:

8.1.1 Replace the alternate saline test with the following:

8.1.1.1 Probes marked as watertight (using Symbol 13 in Table D1 of IEC 601-1) shall comply with the following test: immerse the probe for 1 min in a saline solution containing 0.9% sodium chloride that is maintained at a temperature between 20 and 25°C. While the probe is still immersed, perform the tests for patient leakage current as specified in Clause 19.4 g) 5) of IEC 601-1.

9. Dielectric Strength

9.1 The requirements given in Clause 20 of IEC 601-1 apply except for the following addition:

9.1.1 Probes marked as watertight (using Symbol 13 in Table D1 of IEC 601-1) shall comply with the following test: immerse the probe for 1 min in a saline solution containing 0.9 % sodium chloride that is maintained at a temperature between 20 and 25°C. While the probe is still immersed, perform the tests for dielectric strength as specified in Clause 20.4 a) of IEC 601-1.

10. Mechanical Strength

10.1 The requirements given in Clause 21 of IEC 601-1 apply except add the following to 21.5:

10.1.1 Patient probes that are hand held during normal use and cord-connected control switches shall not present a safety hazard as a result of a free fall from a height of 1 m onto a hard surface.

10.2 Compliance shall be checked by the following test:

10.2.1 Allow the sample to be tested to fall freely once from each of three different starting orientations from a height of 1 m onto a 50 mm thick hardwood board (that is, hardwood having a density of >700 kg/m ^{3}) that lies flat on a rigid base (concrete block). After this test no live parts shall become accessible. Cracks not visible to the naked eye and surface cracks in fiber-reinforced moldings and the like shall be ignored. If the sample appears operational after the fall, a dielectric strength test, according to Clause 20 of IEC 601-1 shall be carried out.

11. Electromagnetic Compatibility

11.1 The requirements in Clause 36 of IEC 601-1 apply with the following addition (the test method in 36.1 is derived from IEC 801-2):

11.1.1 *Protection from Electrostatic Discharge*—The pulse oximeter should continue to function and meet the requirements of this specification or should fail without causing a safety hazard. The discharges shall have a potential of 3 kV ± 5 % DC for a contact discharge and 8 kV ± 5 % DC for an air discharge from a network as described in IEC 801-2 (TC 65

Sec 136). If an anomaly occurs, such as, display interrupt, alarm activation, etc., it should be possible to restore normal operation within 30 s after the electrostatic discharge has been applied. (Silencing of an activated alarm should not be considered a failure.)

12. Human Errors

12.1 Twin-pole or multi-pole plugs and sockets for extra low voltage patient circuits shall not be interchangeable with plugs and sockets for mains connections and further shall minimize any electrical connection that may result in a safety hazard.

13. Protection Against Hazardous Output

13.1 The requirements given in Clause 51 of IEC 601-1 are replaced by the following:

13.1.1 *Control Function and Position*—If the intended test control function is not clearly distinguishable when displayed on the pulse oximeter, the corresponding control(s) shall automatically return from such control function position(s). The positions of measurement and test controls shall be clearly distinguishable. Calibration controls shall include a means to prevent inadvertent change from the intended position.

NOTE 2—User-operable function checks other than "power on" for test controls such as battery condition or signal operation should automatically return from the check, test, or override position.

NOTE 3—All other controls should also include means to prevent inadvertent changes from the intended position and should have clearly distinguishable positions.

13.1.2 *Movement of Controls*—For controls that consist of a movable part and a non-movable part, movement upwards, to the right, or in a clockwise direction shall increase the control function. Movement downwards, to the left, or in an anti-clockwise direction shall decrease the control function.

NOTE 4—The separation between control knobs, switches, toggles, pinwheels, or push buttons should conform to the recommendations given in ISO 7249 and ISO 7250.

NOTE 5—Controls and their associated markings should be visible or legible, or both, to a user having a visual acuity (corrected if necessary) of at least 1.0 when the user is located at least 1 m in front of the pulse oximeter and the illuminance level is 215 Lx. Markings should be clearly identified with their associated controls.

14. Alarms

14.1 *Alarm Prioritization*:

14.1.1 The alarm characteristics of monitors specified in this specification shall be grouped in three categories: high priority, medium priority, and low priority (see Table 1).

TABLE 1 Alarm Characteristics

Alarm Category	Operator Response	Audible Indicators*	Indicator Color***	Flashing Frequency (Hz)**
High priority	Immediate	Not medium or low priority I	Red	1.4 to 2.8 Hz (F_2)
Medium priority	Prompt	Not high or low priority	Yellow	0.4 to 0.8 Hz (F_1)
Low priority	Awareness	Nor high or medium priority	Yellow	Constant (On)

14.1.2 The audible components of these alarms should be designed to allow silencing until the PULSE OXIMETER is placed in use (that is, connected to the patient) in order to reduce nuisance alarms.

14.1.3 There shall be a visual indication that an audible alarm has been silenced.

14.1.4 The set points of adjustable alarms shall be indicated continuously or on user demand.

14.2 *High Priority Alarms*:

14.2.1 There shall be a visual indication of the high priority alarm. It shall be different and distinguishable from the visual signals specified in 14.3 and 14.4.

14.2.2 There shall be a simultaneous audible indication of the high priority alarm. This audible indication shall be different and distinguishable from the audible signals specified in 14.3 and 14.4.

14.2.3 The audible indicators shall reset automatically when the condition causing the alarm has cleared.

14.3 *Medium Priority Alarms*:

14.3.1 There shall be a visual indication of the medium priority alarm. It shall be different and distinguishable from the visual signals specified in 14.2 and 14.4.

14.3.2 There shall be a simultaneous audible indication of the medium priority alarm. This audible indication shall be different and distinguishable from the audible signals in 14.2 and 14.4.

14.3.3 The audible indicator shall reset automatically when the condition causing the alarm has cleared.

14.4 *Low Priority Alarms*:

14.4.1 There shall be a visual indication of the low priority alarm. It shall be different and distinguishable from the visual signals in 14.2 and 14.3.

14.4.2 There may be a simultaneous audible indication of the low priority alarm. This audible indication, if provided, shall be a low priority alarm. This audible indication shall be different and distinguishable from the audible signals specified in 14.2 and 14.3.

14.4.3 The audible indicator shall reset automatically when the condition causing the alarm has cleared.

NOTE 6—An ASTM standard (see Specification F 1463) is presently being developed for the general characteristics (audible and visual) of all alarms on anesthetic and respiratory care equipment.

14.5 *Alarm Characteristics*:

14.5.1 If intended for continuous monitoring, the pulse oximeter shall have a low SpO_2 alarm.

NOTE 7—In certain clinical applications a high saturation alarm may provide an additional safety feature.

14.5.2 The difference between the alarm set point and the SpO_2 when the alarm is activated shall not exceed 2 "% SpO_2."

14.5.2.1 Compliance shall be checked by the test given in 14.6.

14.6 *Method of Test for* SpO_2 *Alarm Set Point Accuracy*:

14.6.1 Generate at least four stable SpO_2 readings that span the range of the alarm system in approximately equal steps by varying the input to the pulse oximeter, or by adjusting the calibration control (if provided).

14.6.2 For each SpO_2 reading, adjust the alarm set point so that the alarm is deactivated. Incrementally adjust the alarm set point until the alarm is activated and record the SpO_2 reading at which the alarm is activated. The difference between the alarm set point and the corresponding SpO_2 reading shall not exceed 2 "% SpO_2."

NOTE 8—An alarm may be of a type that is activated at a SpO_2 reading above (high alarm) or below (low alarm) the alarm set point. A pulse oximeter may have either or both types of alarm.

14.6.3 If alarms are provided, alarm set points shall be operator adjustable. Operator adjustment of alarm set points or default parameters shall require a deliberate sequence of actions on the part of the operator.

14.6.4 Default limits on low SpO_2 alarms shall be 80 "% SpO_2" or greater.

14.6.5 Temporary silencing of audible alarms, if provided, shall not exceed 2 min. The visual signal shall remain until the condition is corrected. If permanent silencing of the audible alarm is provided, it shall require deliberate action on the part of the operator if the silencing is performed after the pulse oximeter is ready for use. The visual signal shall remain until the condition is corrected.

14.6.6 If intended for continuous monitoring, a probe fault alarm shall be provided, and its function shall be checked by the test given in 14.6.7.

14.6.7 Disconnect the probe from the pulse oximeter and replace it with a circuit with which each probe wire can be opened or shorted to any other probe wire. Verify that the alarm is activated.

15. Additional Clauses Specific to Pulse Oximeters

15.1 *Pulse Amplitude or Pulse Strength Display*—If a normalized pulse waveform display is provided, a visual display of pulse strength shall also be provided.

NOTE 9—Visual indication of the signal adequacy should be provided.

NOTE 10—If a variable pitch audible annunciation is provided for the pulse signal, a pitch or amplitude change in the sound indicator should be provided parallel to the reading, for example, as the SpO_2 reading lowers the sound pitch should also be lowered.

ANNEX

(Mandatory Information)

A1.

A1.1 Annexes A to M in IEC 601–1 together with Appendix X1 of this specification apply.

APPENDIX

(Nonmandatory Information)

X1. GENERAL

X1.1 Pulse oximetry facilitates patient care management by providing an approximation of arterial hemoglobin saturation with oxygen, and allows for the possibility of early detection of the catastrophic events associated with patient hypoxemia.

X1.2 The present technology requires an adequate concentration of hemoglobin, a volume change in blood flow, and light transmission through a tissue bed in order to provide effective in vivo approximation of human hemoglobin saturation with oxygen.

X1.3 Pulse oximeters may not function effectively during cardiopulmonary bypass or at extreme low-flow states, and are not at present intended as a means for the measurement of blood flow or blood volume.

X1.4 With the limitations of the present technology, pulse oximetry is not a precision measurement device. The presently marketed in vivo pulse oximeters are not a replacement for measurement of in vitro blood samples by bench-type oximeters.

X1.5 The values derived from pulse oximetry are not a measurement of blood or tissue oxygen tension.

Standard Guide for Training the Emergency Medical Technician (Basic) in Roles and Responsibilities[1]

This standard is issued under the fixed designation F 1418; the number immediately following the designation indicates the year of original adoption or, in the case of revision, the year of last revision. A number in parentheses indicates the year of last reapproval. A superscript epsilon (ϵ) indicates an editorial change since the last revision or reapproval.

1. Scope

1.1 This guide establishes the minimum training standard for emergency medical technicians (basic) as it relates to their roles and responsibilities.

1.2 This guide is one of a series which together describe the minimum training standard for the emergency medical technician (basic).

1.3 *This standard does not purport to address all of the safety concerns, if any, associated with its use. It is the responsibility of the user of this standard to establish appropriate safety and health practices and determine the applicability of regulatory limitations prior to use.*

2. Referenced Documents

2.1 *ASTM Standards:*

F 1031 Practice for Training the Emergency Medical Technician (Basic)[2]

F 1219 Guide for Training the Emergency Medical Technician (Basic) to Perform Patient Initial and Detailed Assessment[2]

F 1220 Guide for Emergency Medical Services Systems (EMSS) Telecommunications[2]

F 1285 Guide for Training the Emergency Medical Technician (Basic) to Perform Examination Techniques[2]

F 1288 Guide for Planning for and Response to a Multiple Casualty Incident[2]

F 1328 Guide for Training Emergency Medical Technician (Basic) to Prepare Patients for Medical Transportation[2]

F 1329 Guide for Training the Emergency Medical Technician (Basic) in Basic Anatomy and Physiology[2]

F 1419 Guide for Training the Emergency Medical Technician (Basic) to Manage Shock[2]

F 1420 Guide for Training the Emergency Medical Technician (Basic) to Perform Patient Management Techniques[2]

F 1421 Guide for Training the Emergency Medical Technician (Basic) to Manage Obstetrical Emergencies[2]

2.2 *Other Documents:*

Centers for Disease Control: Recommendations for Prevention of HIV Transmission in Health-Care Settings[3] MMWR (most current recommendation)

Centers for Disease Control: Update: Universal Precautions for Prevention of Transmission of Human Immunodeficiency Virus, Hepatitis B Virus, and Other Bloodborne Pathogens in Health-Care Settings[3] MMWR (most current recommendation)

3. Terminology

3.1 *Definitions:*

3.1.1 *EMSS communications subsystem, n*—comprises those resources and arrangements for notifying the EMS system of an emergency, for mobilizing and dispatching resources, for exchanging information, for remote monitoring of vital indicators, and for transmission of treatment procedures and directions (from F 1220).

3.1.2 *management, n*—refers to the step(s) that constitute action taken by the emergency medical technician (basic) for a patient in need of assistance because of a real or perceived traumatic or medical condition.

3.1.3 *stress, n*—nonspecific response of the body to any demand made upon it.

3.1.4 *triage, n*—the process of sorting and making priorities for emergency medical care of the sick and injured on the basis of urgency and type of condition present, number of patients and resources available to route them properly to medical facilities appropriately situated and equipped for their care.

4. Significance and Use

4.1 This guide establishes the minimum national standard for training the emergency medical technician (basic) as it relates to his/her roles and responsibilities.

4.2 This guide shall be used by those who wish to identify the minimum training standard for the emergency medical technician (basic) as it relates to his/her roles and responsibilities.

4.3 This guide shall be used as the basis to revise Practice F 1031.

4.4 Every person who is identified as an emergency medical technician (basic) shall have been trained to this standard.

---

[1] This guide is under the jurisdiction of ASTM Committee F30 on Emergency Medical Services and is the direct responsibility of Subcommittee F30.02 on Personnel, Training and Education.

Current edition approved Feb. 10, 2001. Published April 2001. Originally published as F 1418 - 92. Last previous edition F 1418 - 92.

[2] *Annual Book of ASTM Standards*, Vol 13.01.

[3] Available from Epidemiology Program Office, Centers for Disease Control, Public Health Service, U.S. Dept of Health and Human Services, Atlanta, GA 30333.

4.5 This guide does not stand alone and must be used in conjunction with all referenced documents cited in Section 2.

5. Roles and Responsibilities

5.1 The role and responsibilities of the emergency medical technician (basic) shall be patient care which includes:

5.1.1 Providing scene evaluation and control,

5.1.2 Carefully examining the patient for signs and symptoms of illness or injuries,

5.1.3 Communicating with and providing emergency management for victims of sudden illnesses or injuries,

5.1.4 Assuring that the patient receives the available resources appropriate to his condition, for example, advanced life support, heavy rescue, specialized rescue situations, and so forth, in accordance with local protocol,

5.1.5 Careful handling of the patient in moving to transport vehicle,

5.1.6 Safe and efficient transport of the patient while continuously reassessing the patient and providing any appropriate continuing care,

5.1.7 Orderly and expeditious transfer of the patient to the medical facility,

5.1.8 Communication with medical facility for medical direction or to notify of patient's condition, or both,

5.1.9 Documenting the care provided and maintaining accurate records,

5.1.10 Operating and maintaining the emergency vehicle and its equipment and supplies, and

5.1.11 Observing all safety precautions to protect self, patient, and others in all hazardous situations.

5.2 The emergency medical technician (basic) shall be trained to perform the following functions in the event other emergency services are not available at the accident scene:

5.2.1 Use of basic tools and procedures to gain access to and disentangle the patient, and

5.2.2 Control of the incident scene.

5.3 Special responsibilities shall be a component of minimum training standards for the emergency medical technician (basic), such as the following:

5.3.1 Professional manner,

5.3.2 Appearance, and

5.3.3 General conduct.

5.4 The emergency medical technician (basic) shall receive instruction in the organization of the emergency medical services system and the role of the emergency medical technician (basic) within the emergency medical services system.

5.4.1 The emergency medical technician (basic) shall be familiar with state and local EMS laws, codes, regulations, and policies.

5.4.2 The emergency medical technician (basic) shall be familiar with the role of medical direction in the delivery of prehospital emergency medical care.

6. Legal Issues

6.1 The emergency medical technician (basic) shall receive instruction in the following legal issues.

6.1.1 *Standard of Care*—Shall include the review of relevant federal, state, regional, and local customs, statutes, ordinances, case law, or administrative orders.

6.1.2 *Duty to Act*—Shall be reviewed in regard to the responsibilities relative to responding to the need for patient care according to the federal, state, regional, and local regulations, laws, or administrative orders.

6.1.3 The emergency medical technician (basic) shall have the responsibility to handle and report special situations according to the state, regional, or local laws or ordinances, as follows:

6.1.3.1 Child, adult, or elder abuse,

6.1.3.2 Injury as a result of criminal act,

6.1.3.3 Drug-related injuries,

6.1.3.4 Childbirth,

6.1.3.5 Animal bites,

6.1.3.6 Attempted suicides,

6.1.3.7 Assaults and rape,

6.1.3.8 Scene of a crime,

6.1.3.9 The deceased, and

6.1.3.10 Communicable disease.

6.1.4 *Patient Consent*—Shall be taught according to federal, state, regional, and local regulations, laws, or ordinances and shall include the following concepts:

6.1.4.1 Implied consent,

6.1.4.2 Informed consent,

6.1.4.3 Actual/express consent,

6.1.4.4 Minor's consent,

6.1.4.5 Consent of the mentally ill/diminished mental capacity,

6.1.4.6 Patient's right to refuse treatment,

6.1.4.7 Use of restraint,

6.1.4.8 Do not resuscitate orders and living wills, and

6.1.4.9 Voluntary/involuntary commitment.

6.1.5 Legal liability for the emergency medical technician (basic) shall be taught according to federal, state, regional, and local statutes, laws, and ordinances and shall include the following:

6.1.5.1 Malpractice insurance,

6.1.5.2 Torts,

6.1.5.3 Abandonment,

6.1.5.4 Negligence,

6.1.5.5 Good samaritan laws, and

6.1.6 Patient confidentiality.

7. Certification and Licensure

7.1 Licensure, certification and recertification shall be reviewed according to national, state, regional, and/or local requirements and shall include the following:

7.1.1 EMT statutes and

7.1.2 Exemption from Medical Practices Act.

8. Stress Management/Critical Incident Stress

8.1 The occupation of an emergency medical technician (basic) is highly stressful and the minimum training shall include the identification and management of stress.

8.2 The emergency medical technician (basic) shall be taught the concept of critical incident stress, its long-term consequences and how critical incident stress debriefing is used to mitigate its effects.

9. Patient Communication Problems

9.1 The emergency medical technician (basic) shall be

trained in the principles of effective communication techniques and be aware of the following types of patients/situations that may have specific communication needs that include, but are not limited to, the following:

9.1.1 Geriatric,
9.1.2 Speech/hearing-impaired,
9.1.3 Blind,
9.1.4 Non-english speaking,
9.1.5 Confused,
9.1.6 Mentally handicapped,
9.1.7 Sudden death crisis,
9.1.8 Terminal disease,
9.1.9 Abuse/assault,
9.1.10 Suicide, and
9.1.11 Pediatric patients.

10. Universal Blood and Body Fluid Precautions

10.1 The emergency medical technician (basic) shall be trained to implement current Center for Disease Control (CDC) recommendations when caring for all patients and when cleaning all equipment and supplies (see the latest MMWR recommendation.

11. Records and Reports

11.1 The emergency medical technician (basic) shall be trained to make and maintain run reports and records on each patient according to state, regional, or local protocol. The training shall include the use of reports for the following:

11.1.1 Providing for continuity of care,
11.1.2 Inclusion in the patient's permanent medical record,
11.1.3 Furnishing source of information for evaluating the quality of care,
11.1.4 Furnishing legal evidence,
11.1.5 Providing administrative information, and
11.1.6 Research purposes.

11.2 The emergency medical technician (basic) should assure that the following information is recorded:

11.2.1 Patient's name, sex, date of birth, and address,
11.2.2 Nature of illness or type and mechanism of injury,
11.2.3 Location of patient upon arrival to the scene,
11.2.4 Rescue and treatment measures provided by bystanders and first responders before the EMT's arrival,
11.2.5 Findings of initial and detailed survey,
11.2.6 Care given at the site and during transport,
11.2.7 Vital signs, patient condition, and any changes of either during transport,
11.2.8 Source of on-line medical direction and the receiving hospital,
11.2.9 Disposition of patient's valuables,
11.2.10 Signature of patient or legal guardian if patient care is refused, or notation and witnessed if patient refused to sign,
11.2.11 Circumstances involved in special situations identified in 6.1.3, and
11.2.12 Unusual circumstances that affected patient care.

11.3 The emergency medical technician (basic) shall consider all patient information confidential and shall release it only to the proper authorities as defined by state or local laws, regulations, or protocols.

12. Multiple Casualty Incidents

12.1 The emergency medical technician (basic) shall be able to perform triage in a multiple casualty incident in accordance with Section 9.3 of Guide F 1288.

12.2 The emergency medical technician (basic) shall be trained in the concept and application of the incident command system.

13. Hazardous Materials

13.1 The emergency medical technician (basic) shall be aware of national, state, and local standards or regulations regarding hazardous materials incidents.

13.2 The emergency medical technician (basic) shall be trained to provide emergency care to patients exposed to hazardous materials including radiation.

14. Quality Assurance

14.1 The emergency medical technician (basic) shall receive instruction in the purpose and importance of quality assurance programs.

14.2 The emergency medical technician (basic) shall receive instruction in how to participate in quality assurance activities.

15. Vehicle and Equipment Maintenance

15.1 The emergency medical technician (basic) will assure routine vehicle and equipment preventive maintenance, regular inspections, and inspections after each run.

16. Ground Emergency Vehicle Driving

16.1 The emergency medical technician (basic) shall be trained to identify the risks associated with ground emergency vehicle operations.

16.2 The minimum training standard for ground emergency vehicle driving shall include a review of state, regional, and local laws, regulations, or ordinances or protocols that specifically address the following:

16.2.1 Vehicle parking or standing regulations,
16.2.2 Intersections,
16.2.3 Speed limits,
16.2.4 Multilaned highways,
16.2.5 Standard emergency or disaster routes,
16.2.6 Traffic signals and control/warning signs and devices,
16.2.7 Use of audible warning devices,
16.2.8 Use of emergency lights,
16.2.9 Right-of-way,
16.2.10 Exemptions from direction-of-movement regulations or specified turns,
16.2.11 Safer following distances,
16.2.12 Interactions with other emergency vehicles, and
16.2.13 Common distractions.

16.3 The emergency medical technician (basic) shall receive instruction regarding the effects of vehicle operation on patient care, comfort, and safety.

16.4 The emergency medical technician (basic) shall receive didactic instruction in defensive driving, accident avoidance, and principles of vehicle control.

17. EMSS Communications Subsystem Use

17.1 The emergency medical technician (basic) shall be trained regarding the EMSS communications subsystem. Such training shall include:

17.1.1 Relevant FCC regulations,

17.1.2 Channel and frequency allocation,

17.1.3 The functions, procedures, and equipment used in the emergency medical dispatch process,

17.1.4 Notifying hospital emergency departments of incoming patients,

17.1.5 Typical communications equipment and protocol used for state, regions, or local areas,

17.1.5.1 Introduction to analog/digital/satellite communication.

17.1.6 Communicating pertinent patient information,

17.1.7 Receiving medical direction in accordance with local protocol,

17.1.8 Detection and reporting of motor vehicle crashes to the dispatcher,

17.1.9 Altering other emergency resources,

17.1.10 Maintaining contact between the vehicle, dispatcher, and hospital, and

17.1.11 Communicating with other emergency services.

18. Keywords

18.1 emergency medical technician (basic); EMT (basic); EMT; training; EMT; roles; EMT; responsibilities

Designation: F 1419 – 00

Standard Guide for Training the Emergency Medical Technician (Basic) To Manage Shock[1]

This standard is issued under the fixed designation F 1419; the number immediately following the designation indicates the year of original adoption or, in the case of revision, the year of last revision. A number in parentheses indicates the year of last reapproval. A superscript epsilon (ϵ) indicates an editorial change since the last revision or reapproval.

1. Scope

1.1 This guide establishes the minimum national standard for training in the management of shock in patients of all ages by the emergency medical technician (basic).

1.2 This guide is one of a series which together describe the minimum training standard for the emergency medical technician (basic).

1.3 *This standard does not purport to address all of the safety problems, if any, associated with its use. It is the responsibility of the user of this standard to establish appropriate safety and health practices and determine the applicability of regulatory limitations prior to use.*

2. Referenced Documents

2.1 *ASTM Standards:*

F 1031 Practice for Training the Emergency Medical Technician (Basic)[2]

F 1219 Guide for Training the Emergency Medical Technician (Basic) to Perform Patient Initial and Detailed Assessment[2]

F 1285 Guide for Training the Emergency Medical Technician (Basic) to Perform Patient Examination Techniques[2]

F 1328 Guide for Training the Emergency Medical Technician (Basic) to Prepare Patients for Medical Transportation[2]

F 1329 Guide for Training the Emergency Medical Technician (Basic) in Basic Anatomy and Physiology[2]

F 1418 Guide for Training the Emergency Medical Technician (Basic) in Roles and Responsibilities[2]

F 1420 Guide for Training the Emergency Medical Technician (Basic) to Perform Patient Management Techniques[2]

F 1421 Guide for Training the Emergency Medical Technician (Basic) to Manage Obstetrical Emergencies[2]

2.2 *Other Documents:*

Standards and Guidelines for Cardiopulmonary Resuscitation and Emergency Cardiac Care [3](see latest edition)

3. Terminology

3.1 *Definitions of Terms Specific to This Standard:*

3.1.1 *Management*—refers to the suggested step(s) that constitute action taken by the emergency medical technician (basic) for a patient in need of assistance due to a real or perceived traumatic or medical condition.

4. Significance and Use

4.1 This guide establishes the minimum national standard for training the emergency medical technician (basic) in the suggested management of shock in patients of all ages. This guide does not preclude additions to or modifications of the management of shock as authorized by local medical direction.

4.2 This guide shall be used by those who wish to identify the minimum training standard for the emergency medical technician (basic) as it relates to suggested management of shock.

4.3 This guide shall be used as the basis to revise Practice F 1031.

4.4 Every person who is identified as an emergency medical technician (basic) shall have been trained to this standard.

4.5 This guide does not stand alone and must be used in conjunction with all referenced documents cited in Section 2.

4.6 The management steps outlined in this document are not necessarily in sequential order and they will often vary with the patient's age, size, location and condition.

5. General Guidelines

5.1 All emergency medical technicians (basic) shall be trained to:

5.1.1 Reassess all patients frequently and at least prior to and following every therapeutic intervention.

5.1.2 Manage patient problems in the order of their severity.

5.1.3 Immediately transport patients with life-threatening conditions that cannot be resolved in the field in accordance with local protocol.

5.1.4 Treat all patients in a professional, caring and reassuring manner.

5.1.5 Transfer care of the patient to either ALS providers responding to the scene or an appropriate hospital or other medical facility in accordance with local protocols.

5.1.6 Report the patient's chief complaint and status to the receiving hospital or medical control as soon as possible without compromising patient care.

---

[1] This guide is under the jurisdiction of ASTM Committee F30 on Emergency Medical Services and is the direct responsibility of Subcommittee F30.02 on Personnel, Training and Education.

Current edition approved Oct. 10, 2000. Published December 2000. Originally published as F 1419 - 92. Last previous edition F 1419 - 92.

[2] *Annual Book of ASTM Standards*, Vol 13.01.

[3] Reprinted from Journal of the American Medical Association, June 6, 1986, Vol 255, pp. 2842–3044 (latest edition).

5.1.7 Transport patient expeditiously and safely.

5.1.8 The emergency medical technician (basic) shall provide all pertinent patient information to the receiving facility at the receiving facility.

5.1.9 Upon completion of patient care responsibilities, prepare the ambulance or equipment, or both, and supplies to be ready to care for the next patient.

6. Management of Patients in Shock

6.1 The emergency medical technician (basic) shall be trained to provide emergency care for the patient in shock as noted below. The selection and sequence of the components are dictated by the patient's condition and existing circumstances.

6.2 Administer high concentration oxygen.

6.3 Assist ventilations as necessary.

6.4 If necessary, control bleeding by any one or combination of the following:

6.4.1 direct pressure on site of bleeding,

6.4.2 elevation of the injured extremity, and

6.4.3 pneumatic anti-shock garment (PASG) inflation in accordance with local medical protocols.

6.5 Place the patient in the supine position with lower limbs elevated if not contraindicated.

6.6 Do not allow the patient to eat or drink.

6.7 Prevent loss of body heat.

7. Keywords

7.1 emergency medical technician (basic); EMT; shock; training

Designation: F 1420 – 01

Standard Guide for Training the Emergency Medical Technician (Basic) to Perform Patient Management Techniques[1]

This standard is issued under the fixed designation F 1420; the number immediately following the designation indicates the year of original adoption or, in the case of revision, the year of last revision. A number in parentheses indicates the year of last reapproval. A superscript epsilon (ε) indicates an editorial change since the last revision or reapproval.

1. Scope

1.1 This guide establishes the minimum national standard for training the emergency medical technician (basic) to perform patient management techniques for patients of all ages.

1.2 This guide is one of a series which together describe the minimum training standard for the emergency medical technician (basic).

1.3 *This standard does not purport to address all of the safety concerns, if any, associated with its use. It is the responsibility of the user of this standard to establish appropriate safety and health practices and determine the applicability of regulatory limitations prior to use.*

2. Referenced Documents

2.1 *ASTM Standards:*

F 1031 Practice for Training the Emergency Medical Technician (Basic)[2]

F 1219 Guide for Training the Emergency Medical Technician (Basic) to Perform Patient Initial and Detailed Assessment[2]

F 1255 Practice for Performance of Prehospital Automated Defibrillation[2]

F 1285 Guide for Training the Emergency Medical Technician (Basic) to Perform Patient Examination Techniques[2]

F 1328 Guide for Training Emergency Medical Technician (Basic) to Prepare Patients for Medical Transportation[2]

F 1329 Guide for Training the Emergency Medical Technician (Basic) in Basic Anatomy and Physiology[2]

F 1418 Guide for Training the Emergency Medical Technician (Basic) in Roles and Responsibilities[2]

F 1419 Guide for Training the Emergency Medical Technician (Basic) to Manage Shock[2]

F 1421 Guide for Training the Emergency Medical Technician (Basic) to Manage Obstetrical Emergencies[2]

2.2 *Other Documents:*

Standards and Guidelines for Cardiopulmonary Resuscitation and Emergency Cardiac Care[3]

Textbook of Pediatric Advanced Life Support[4]

3. Terminology

3.1 *Definition*

3.1.1 *management techniques, n*—refers to those skills that constitute actions or activities conducted by the emergency medical technician (basic) for a patient in need of assistance as a result of a real or perceived traumatic or medical condition.

4. Significance and Use

4.1 This guide establishes the minimum national standard for training the emergency medical technician (basic) to perform management techniques for patients of all ages. This guide does not preclude additions to or modifications of the management techniques used by the emergency medical technician (basic) as authorized by local medical protocol.

4.2 This guide shall be used by those who wish to identify the minimum training standard for the emergency medical technician (basic) as it relates to the performance of management techniques.

4.3 This guide shall be used as the basis to revise Practice F 1031.

4.4 Every person who is identified as an emergency medical technician (basic) shall have been trained to this standard.

4.5 This guide does not stand alone and must be used in conjunction with all referenced documents cited in Section 2.

4.6 The management techniques outlined in this guide are not necessarily in sequential order, and they will often vary with the patient's age, size, location and condition.

5. Management Techniques

5.1 Use of airway management techniques and devices.

5.2 Use of techniques for management of the compromised circulatory system.

5.2.1 Direct pressure to the source of bleeding.

5.2.2 Pressure dressings.

5.2.3 Patient positioning.

5.2.4 The pneumatic antishock garment in accordance with local medical control protocol.

---

[1] This guide is under the jurisdiction of ASTM Committee F30 on Emergency Medical Services and is the direct responsibility of Subcommittee F30.02 on Personnel, Training and Education.

Current edition approved Feb. 10, 2001. Published April 2001. Originally published as F 1420 - 92. Last previous edition F 1420 - 92.

[2] *Annual Book of ASTM Standards*, Vol 13.01.

[3] Reprinted from *Journal of American Medical Association*, June 6, 1986, Vol 255, pp 2842–3044.

[4] Chameides, et al., American Heart Association, Dallas, TX 1988.

5.3 Use of spinal immobilization techniques.
5.3.1 Manual spinal motion control.
5.3.2 Cervical spine immobilization devices.
5.3.3 Short spine boards.
5.3.4 Long spine boards.
5.3.5 Manual in-line spinal immobilization during rapid extrication.
5.4 Use of techniques for management of musculoskeletal injuries (nonspine).
5.4.1 Manual in-line stabilization.
5.4.2 External immobilization fixation devices:
5.4.2.1 Traction devices.
5.4.2.2 Rigid devices.
5.5 Use of techniques for management of soft tissue injuries.
5.5.1 Asceptic technique.
5.5.2 Management of amputations.
5.5.3 Bandaging techniques.
5.6 Use of medications and techniques in accordance with local medical control protocol.
5.6.1 Oxygen.
5.6.2 Activated charcoal.
5.6.3 Oral glucose.
5.6.4 Blind insertion airway device.
5.6.5 Patient-prescribed NTG.
5.6.6 Patient-prescribed bronchodilator (nebulizer/MDI).
5.6.7 Patient-prescribed epinephrine.
5.7 Use of basic life support as described in Standards and Guidelines for Cardiopulmonary Resuscitation and Emergency Cardiac Care and the Textbook of Pediatric Advanced Life Support.
5.8 Use of techniques for management of the normal spontaneous vertex vaginal delivery.
5.8.1 Uterine massage.
5.9 Use of techniques for management of the newborn.
5.10 Use of isolation techniques for communicable disease control.
5.11 Use of techniques for gaining entry/access to the patient.
5.12 Use of extrication techniques other than for spinal.
5.13 Use of techniques for restraining patients.
5.14 Use of patient positioning techniques for medical emergencies.
5.15 Use of techniques for managing penetrating injuries and blunt trauma which compromises the respiratory system.
5.16 Use of automated external defibrillation in accordance with Practice F 1255.
5.17 Endotracheal intubation in accordance with local medical control.
5.18 Insertion of nasogastric tube in accordance with local medical control.

6. Keywords

6.1 emergency medical technician (basic); EMT, training; EMT, management techniques; EMT, skills

Designation: F 1421 – 01

Standard Guide for Training the Emergency Medical Technician (Basic) To Manage Obstetrical Emergencies[1]

This standard is issued under the fixed designation F 1421; the number immediately following the designation indicates the year of original adoption or, in the case of revision, the year of last revision. A number in parentheses indicates the year of last reapproval. A superscript epsilon (ε) indicates an editorial change since the last revision or reapproval.

1. Scope

1.1 This guide establishes the minimum training standard for the management of obstetrical emergencies by the emergency medical technician (basic).

1.2 This guide is one of a series which together describe the minimum training standard for the emergency medical technician (basic).

1.3 *This standard does not purport to address all of the safety concerns, if any, associated with its use. It is the responsibility of the user of this standard to establish appropriate safety and health practices and determine the applicability of regulatory limitations prior to use.*

2. Referenced Documents

2.1 *ASTM Standards:*

F 1031 Practice for Training the Emergency Medical Technician (Basic)[2]

F 1219 Guide for Training the Emergency Medical Technician (Basic) to Perform Patient Primary Assessment[2]

F 1285 Guide for Training the Emergency Medical Technician (Basic) to Perform Patient Examination Techniques[2]

F 1328 Guide for Training the Emergency Medical Technician (Basic) to Prepare Patients for Medical Transportation[2]

F 1329 Guide for Training the Emergency Medical Technician (Basic) in Basic Anatomy and Physiology[2]

F 1419 Guide for Training the Emergency Medical Technician (Basic) to Manage Shock[2]

F 1420 Guide for Training the Emergency Medical Technician (Basic) to Perform Management Techniques[2]

2.2 *Other Documents:*

Standards and Guidelines for Cardiopulmonary Resuscitation and Emergency Cardiac Care[3]

Textbook of Pediatric Advanced Life Support[4]

3. Terminology

3.1 *Definitions:*

3.1.1 *management techniques, n*—refers to the step(s) that constitute action taken by the emergency medical technician (basic) for a patient in need of assistance as a result of a real or perceived traumatic or medical condition.

4. Significance and Use

4.1 This guide establishes the minimum national standard for training the emergency medical technician (basic) in the management of obstetrical emergencies in patients of all ages. This guide does not preclude additions to or modifications of the management of obstetrical emergencies by the emergency medical technician (basic) as authorized by local medical protocol.

4.2 This guide shall be used by those who wish to identify the minimum training standard for the emergency medical technician (basic) as it relates to management of obstetrical emergencies.

4.3 This guide shall be used as the basis to revise Practice F 1031.

4.4 Every person who is identified as an emergency medical technician (basic) shall have been trained to this guide.

4.5 This guide does not stand alone and must be used in conjunction with all referenced documents cited in Section 2.

4.6 The management steps outlined in this guide are not necessarily in sequential order, and they will often vary with the patient's age, size, location, and condition.

5. General Guidelines

5.1 All emergency medical technicians (basic) shall be trained to:

5.1.1 Reassess all patients frequently and at least before and following every therapeutic intervention.

5.1.2 Deal with patient problems in the order of their severity.

5.1.3 Immediately transport patients with life-threatening conditions that cannot be resolved in the field in accordance with local protocol.

5.1.4 Treat all patients in a professional, caring, and reassuring manner.

---

[1] This guide is under the jurisdiction of ASTM Committee F30 on Emergency Medical Services and is the direct responsibility of Subcommittee F30.02 on Personnel, Training and Education.

Current edition approved March 10, 2001. Published April 2001. Originally published as F 1421 - 92. Last previous edition approved F 1421 - 92.

[2] *Annual Book of ASTM Standards*, Vol 13.01.

[3] Reprinted from *JAMA*, 6 June 1986, Vol 255, pp 2842–3044.

[4] Chameides, et al., American Heart Association, Dallas, 1988.

5.1.5 Transfer care of the patient to either advanced life support (ALS) providers responding to the scene or an appropriate hospital or other medical facility in accordance with local protocols.

5.1.6 Report the patient's problem and status to the receiving hospital or medical control as soon as possible without compromising patient care.

5.1.7 Transport patient expeditiously and safely.

5.1.8 The emergency medical technician (basic) shall provide all pertinent patient information at the receiving facility.

5.1.9 Upon completion of patient care responsibilities, prepare the ambulance or equipment and supplies, or both, to be ready to care for the next patient.

6. Obstetrical Emergencies—Labor and Delivery

6.1 The emergency medical technician (basic) shall be trained to manage a patient in active labor as follows:

6.1.1 Place patient in position of comfort to the patient.

6.1.2 Administer oxygen as indicated.

6.1.3 Transport patient.

6.1.3.1 Recognize and allow appropriate interaction of "significant other" or labor coach.

6.1.4 Monitor the progress of labor.

6.2 The emergency medical technician (basic) shall be trained to manage a patient with an imminent delivery as follows:

6.2.1 Recognize the signs and symptoms of imminent delivery.

6.2.2 Position the patient in semireclining or position of comfort.

6.2.3 Identify abnormal presentations, administer oxygen, and immediately transport the patient in the knee-chest position or according to local protocols.

6.2.4 Don appropriate personal protective equipment.

6.2.5 Control but do not impede delivery of the head.

6.2.6 Suction the neonate when the head is delivered with either bulb-type or a filtered small-bore trap suction as appropriate.

6.2.7 Feel for umbilical cord around the neck, using index finger, and slip over shoulder or cut if necessary.

6.2.8 Identify meconium and suction it with a filtered small-bore trap suction (modified DeLee or similar device).

6.2.8.1 Recognize meconium staining as an emergent condition and request ALS assistance.

6.2.9 Support the head and shoulders during delivery.

6.2.10 Double clamp and cut the umbilical cord at least 5 in. from the infant and cut between the clamps.

6.2.11 Transport the patients.

6.2.12 If the placenta delivers, transport it to the hospital with the mother.

6.2.13 Following delivery of the placenta massage the mother's abdomen to cause the uterus to contract.

6.2.14 Allow the mother to nurse the infant if both are stable.

6.2.15 Document time and location of birth.

6.2.16 Request ALS intercept, as required.

7. Obstetrical Emergencies—Care of the Neonate

7.1 Suction the neonate when the head is delivered with either bulb-type or a filtered small-bore trap suction as appropriate.

7.2 Identify meconium and suction it with a filtered small-bore trap suction (modified DeLee or similar device).

7.2.1 Request ALS intercept, as required.

7.3 Stimulate breathing if necessary.

7.4 Administer oxygen as indicated.

7.5 Dry off infant and keep warm.

7.6 Allow the mother to nurse the infant if both are stable.

8. Obstetrical Emergencies—Uterine Atony

8.1 Identify uterine atony by excessive bleeding after delivery of the infant, or, soft noncontracted uterus, or both.

8.2 Perform uterine massage as in 6.2.13.

8.3 Have the mother stimulate her nipples.

8.4 Administer high concentration oxygen.

8.5 In accordance with local media direction, apply and inflate the pneumatic antishock garment.

9. Obstetrical Emergencies—Vaginal Bleeding in Late Pregnancy

9.1 Administer high concentration oxygen.

9.2 Transport with left side down.

9.3 Be prepared for delivery.

10. Obstetrical Emergencies—Miscarriage

10.1 Collect and transport all tissue passed from the vagina.

10.2 Transport the patient.

10.3 Manage excessive bleeding.

10.4 Administer high concentration oxygen.

11. Obstetrical Emergencies—Trauma in Pregnancy

11.1 Treat traumatic injuries.

11.2 Transport with left side down.

11.3 Be prepared for delivery.

11.4 Administer high concentration oxygen.

11.5 Request ALS intercept, as required.

12. Obstetrical Emergencies—Pre-eclampsia/Eclampsia

12.1 Minimize central nervous system stimulation.

12.2 Administer oxygen.

12.3 Manage seizures.

12.4 Request ALS intercept, as required.

13. Keywords

13.1 delivery; emergency medical technician (basic); EMT; labor; miscarriage; neonate; obstetric; pre-eclampsia/eclampsia; pregnancy; training; trauma; uterine atony; vaginal bleeding

Standard Guide for Using the Incident Command System Framework in Managing Civilian Search and Rescue Operations[1]

This standard is issued under the fixed designation F 1422; the number immediately following the designation indicates the year of original adoption or, in the case of revision, the year of last revision. A number in parentheses indicates the year of last reapproval. A superscript epsilon (ε) indicates an editorial change since the last revision or reapproval.

1. Scope

1.1 This guide covers the use of the Incident Command System (ICS), (as developed in ICS-120), as the management framework for civilian search and rescue (SAR) operations.

1.2 Except as otherwise specified herein, the methods and requirements of the 1983 version of ICS-120 form a part of this guide.

1.3 *This standard does not purport to address all of the safety problems, if any, associated with its use. It is the responsibility of the user of this standard to establish appropriate safety and health practices and determine the applicability of regulatory limitations prior to use.*

2. Referenced Documents

2.1 *Incident Command Systems Publications:*

ICS-120 Operational System Descriptions Manual[2]

ICS-420 Field Operations Guide[2,3]

3. Significance and Use

3.1 The ICS framework is designed to be used for all kinds of emergencies and is applicable to both small day-to-day situations as well as very large and complex incidents.[4]

3.2 ICS-120 describes the ICS framework, operating requirements, components, and procedures for organizing and operating an on-scene management structure only.

3.3 Users of this guide are expected to be familiar with the ICS.

3.4 Neither this guide nor ICS-120 provides a specific plan for managing a SAR operation, but rather outlines a process for developing a management framework.

3.5 Mission specific elements such as resource and strike team classifications and types, map symbols, T-card colors, position checklists, and staffing requirements do not form a part of this guide.

NOTE 1—These elements of the ICS are contained in ICS-420 and position checklists.[2] Information in these documents may be useful for managing a SAR operation but contains terminology specific to the fire services.

4. Procedure

4.1 SAR management personnel should develop the management structure in a top down manner similar to that outlined in ICS-120.

4.2 SAR management personnel should utilize the flexibility allowed by the ICS to modify the framework and fill only those functional positions necessary to conduct the operation.

4.3 Document the SAR operation for planning, analytical, legal, and historical purposes. Local forms, forms contained in Guide ICS-420, or similar forms may be used for documenting the operation.

---

[1] This guide is under the jurisdiction of ASTM Committee F-32 on Search and Rescue and is the direct responsibility of Subcommittee F32.02 on Search and Rescue Management.

Current edition approved Dec. 15, 1992. Published February 1993.

[2] Available from Fire Protection Publications, Oklahoma State University, Stillwater, OK 74078.

[3] The Field Operations Guide and Systems Description Manual are available combined in one volume from the same source. A Field Operations Guide, ICS-420-1, is also available.

[4] See ICS-120, p. 4.

Designation: F 1439 – 92 (Reapproved 1996)

Standard Guide for Performance of Lifetime Bioassay for the Tumorigenic Potential of Implant Materials[1]

This standard is issued under the fixed designation F 1439; the number immediately following the designation indicates the year of original adoption or, in the case of revision, the year of last revision. A number in parentheses indicates the year of last reapproval. A superscript epsilon (ε) indicates an editorial change since the last revision or reapproval.

1. Scope

1.1 This guide is intended to assist the biomaterials testing laboratory in the conduct and evaluation of tumorigenicity tests to evaluate the potential for new materials to evoke a neoplastic response. The procedure is generally reserved only for those materials which have not previously been used for human implantation for a significant period of time.

1.2 Assessment of tumorigenicity is one of several procedures employed in determining the biological response to a material as recommended in Practice F 748. It is assumed that the investigator has already determined that this type of testing is necessary for a particular material before consulting this guide. The recommendations of Practice F 748 should be considered before a study is commenced.

1.3 Whenever possible, it is recommended that a battery of genotoxicity procedures be initiated and proposed as an alternative to an in-vivo tumorigenicity bioassay. Genotoxicity assays may also be considered as initial screening procedures due to the sensitivity of the assays, the significant reduction in time to gain valuable data, and the desire to reduce the use of animals for testing. Genotoxicity assays that may be considered are outlined in Guides E 1262 and E 1280 and Practices E 1397 and E 1398. Additionally, other genotoxicity testing which might be considered (but which do not yet have ASTM test methods) include Salmonella/Mammalian-Microsomal Plate Incorporation Mutagenicity Assay, In Vivo Cytogenetics Bone Marrow Chromosomal Damage Assay, BALB/3T3 Morphological Transformation of Mouse Embryo Cells, and the Mouse Micronucleus Assay. The investigator is advised to consider carefully the appropriateness of a particular method for his application after a review of the published literature.

1.4 *This standard does not purport to address all of the safety concerns, if any, associated with its use. It is the responsibility of the user of this standard to establish appropriate safety and health practices and determine the applicability of regulatory limitations prior to use.*

2. Referenced Documents

2.1 *ASTM Standards:*

E 1262 Guide for the Performance of the Chinese Hamster Ovary Cell/Hypoxanthine Guanine Phosphoribosyl Transferase Gene Mutation Assay[2]

E 1280 Guide for Performing the Mouse Lymphoma Assay for Mammalian Cell Mutagenicity[2]

E 1397 Practices for the In-Vitro Rat Hepatocyte DNA Repair Assay[2]

E 1398 Practices for the In-Vivo Rat Hepatocyte DNA Repair Assay[2]

F 748 Practice for Selecting Generic Biological Test Methods for Materials and Devices[3]

2.2 *Other Documents:*

National Toxicology Program General Statement of Work for the Conduct of Toxicity and Carcinogenicity Studies in Laboratory Animals[4]

OECD Guidelines for Testing of Chemicals: Guideline 451, Carcinogenicity Studies[5]

OECD Guidelines for Testing of Chemicals: Guideline 453, Combined Chronic Toxicity/Carcinogenicity Studies[5]

Good Laboratory Practice for Nonclinical Laboratory Studies[6]

3. Terminology

3.1 *Definitions of Terms Specific to this Standard:*

3.1.1 *carcinogenic*—a substance is considered to be carcinogenic if it can be shown to be causally related to an increased incidence of malignant neoplastic formation.

3.1.2 *maximum implantable dose*—the maximum weight or volume of the test article which can be reasonably implanted into the test site taking into account the gross distention of tissue which can occur and its possible effects on test results.

3.1.3 *mutagenic*—a substance is said to be mutagenic if it induces alterations in the genetic code of the cell.

3.1.4 *tumorigenic*—a substance is said to be tumorigenic if it can be shown to be causally related to an increased incidence of neoplastic formation whether malignant or benign.

[1] This guide is under the jurisdiction of ASTM Committee F-4 on Medical and Surgical Materials and Devices and is the direct responsibility of Subcommittee F04.16 on Biocompatibility Test Methods.

Current edition approved Oct. 15, 1992. Published December 1992.

[2] *Annual Book of ASTM Standards*, Vol 11.05.

[3] *Annual Book of ASTM Standards*, Vol 13.01.

[4] Available from National Institute of Environmental Health Sciences, Research Triangle Park, NC, August 1988.

[5] Available from Organization for Economic Cooperation and Development, Washington, DC.

[6] Available from 21 CFR, Part 58, U.S. Government Printing Office, Washington, DC.

4. Significance and Use

4.1 This guide is not intended to specify the exact method of conducting a test for any particular material but only to present some of the criteria that should be considered in method design and possible problems that could lead to misleading results. In the development of the actual test protocol, it is recommended that recognized tumorigenesis bioassay procedures be consulted.

4.2 The recommendations given in this guide may not be appropriate for all applications or types of implant materials. These recommendations should be utilized by experienced testing personnel in conjunction with other pertinent information and the requirements of the specific material application.

5. Choice of Animal Model

5.1 These types of bioassays for chemical substances have traditionally been performed in mice or rats, or both, because of their small size, relative cost factors, and lifespan. For the testing of biomaterials, mice are not recommended because the small animal size is not conducive to the placement of solid implants. The investigator should seriously consider the use of one of the traditional models in order to draw upon the extensive information available about typical tumor formation rates and sites in control animals. The National Toxicology Program[4] recommends the use of Fischer 344 (F344/N) rats. However, other readily available species and strains may also be acceptable for the performance of these studies. Other rat species which have been recommended include Sprague-Dawley, Long-Evans, and Wistar. Some investigators have recommended the use of Long-Evans or Wistar Rats because of the difficulty of achieving a two-year lifespan for Fischer and Sprague-Dawley rats.

5.2 The currently accepted level of testing in a particular site of implantation or medical specialty should be carefully researched and regulatory requirements determined before a study design is finalized to assure acceptability of the final results.

5.3 The appropriate choice of male or female animals or a combination should be carefully considered in light of the particular material and application being investigated. If the device will ultimately be used only in the male or female, only one sex may need to be evaluated. Otherwise, both sexes should be used.

5.4 The decision to use other species for study should be carefully documented in terms of a clear need. The use of species which have not previously been used may reduce the amount of comparative data available on control animals. Typical tumor rates for hamsters, rats, and mice have been tabulated and are available in Refs. **(1, 2, 3)**.[7]

6. Selection of Size and Form of Implant

6.1 Tumorigenicity bioassays have traditionally been performed using chemical substances as the challenge. The evaluation of implant materials requires that solid material be implanted in some form. It is important to realize that the down-sized implants necessary for use in animals will have a greater surface area to volume ratio, and this difference must be considered in experimental design.

6.2 It may be important to determine the site of administration of the test material that is most appropriate to the end use before determining implant size. The site of implantation should be the paravertebral muscle unless the size of the implant causes this site to be unacceptable. Alternatively, the site of implantation should mimic the anticipated end use, if possible. Where a specific material may be utilized in more than one type of device, multiple sites of administration should be considered if different types of tissue will be contacted. (For instance, materials that may be in contact with bone or implanted into internal organ tissue might be tested in both tissues.)

6.3 It should be recognized that the response of the test animal to an extract of a material may not fully represent the response that might be seen if the material itself were to be implanted. In general, an extract should not be used as a substitute for the actual material of interest.

6.4 The physical form of the test material should be representative of that intended for use in human patients and should consider potential material debris, if appropriate. The investigator should be aware that tests have shown **(4)** that powdered polymeric materials may not elicit a tumorigenic response subcutaneously even when prepared from polymers that do induce tumors when implanted in the form of a film. The impact of physical form and surface properties on tumorigenesis must be carefully considered, in making decisions about the physical form of the implants **(5, 6, 7, 8, 9, 10)**.

6.5 Researchers have found that the aspect ratio (length/diameter) of fiber materials may play a role in the tumorigenesis of a particular material **(11, 12)**. When new fibrous materials are being tested, the actual fiber length to be anticipated in practice should be studied. If fragmentation can be anticipated or is a worse case possibility, an attempt should be made to document a clinically relevant fiber length.

6.6 The material to be tested should originate from sample(s) representative of all processing including surface finishing, passivation, and sterilization or other final processing that will occur to a finished device.

6.7 *Dosage*:

6.7.1 In most materials, the ratio between the surface area of the implant and the body weight of the animal or person will have an effect on the amount of extractable substances (if any) which leach out of the material. The total weight or volume of material used in each animal should be in excess of the anticipated dosages to be seen in clinical practice when calculated based upon the ratio of surface area of sample to body weight of the animal. Consideration should be given to using the maximum implantable dose as the dosage or as one of multiple dosage levels. For the special case of degradable materials, the sample size should be calculated based on the ratio of sample weight to animal body weight.

6.7.2 Whenever possible, more than one exposure level should be considered to evaluate a dose-response effect.

7. Choice of Control

7.1 Control groups for this type of study will usually consist

[7] The boldface numbers in parentheses refer to the list of references at the end of this guide.

of identical animals that have not received an implant of the test material but have been subjected to the remainder of the surgical procedures. Additional groups such as housing (animals which receive no treatment but are housed with the test animals) and reference control groups may be included in the study design.

7.2 The investigator should consider a negative control group in addition to the sham or untreated controls. These animals would receive an implant or treatment identical to the test animals but the implant would be manufactured from a selected negative reference material. This group would then serve to isolate any results due to the implant trauma or mechanically induced changes.

8. Size of Test Groups

8.1 The test group and the control group should each contain enough animals which will be scheduled to survive to the end of the study to allow statistically valid conclusions to be drawn from the study. If both male and female animals are being used, each group should contain an equal number of animals of each sex. The National Toxicology Program[4] requires 60 animals/sex/group for chemical studies with ten animals being sacrificed earlier than two years. Other international organizations recommend 50 animals/sex/group.[5] The investigator should ascertain that the number of animals in each group is adequate for statistical and regulatory purposes before proceeding. In order to ensure valid data analysis, the animals should be randomly assigned to control and experimental groups. Considerations specific to the particular implant application or medical specialty may mandate a greater number of animals in each group. Additional animals in interim sacrifice groups or satellite groups may be added.

8.2 The number of test animals in each group shall be determined based upon a sound statistical analysis of the scientific questions to be addressed by the study. This analysis should take into account predicted survival rates (if available) for the species being used as well as being consistent with responsible use of experimental animals. If a statistically valid experiment can be performed with fewer than the usual number of animals per group, that fact should be documented and the study design should proceed accordingly.

9. Duration of Study

9.1 Recommended durations for evaluation of tumorigenicity in rats is two years.

9.2 Depending upon the material being evaluated, the early results may suggest that the study can be terminated earlier than two years without compromising the validity of the study. Examples might include studies in which a significantly increased rate of tumor formation or toxicity is being seen in the test animals or in one or more dosage groups.

9.3 At the termination of the study, a majority of the animals in each group should have survived for euthanasia or been terminated early for study-related reasons such as increased tumor incidence, spontaneous tumors, or toxicity of the test article. It is expected that a minimum of 50 % of the animals per sex and per group should survive until final study termination barring the above reasons. Moreover, the number of survivors or study-related terminations should be sufficient for detection of effects at the $p < 0.05$ level of significance. If attrition is occurring due to reasons which cannot be attributed to the test articles or spontaneous tumor formation, other factors should be considered such as environmental and food and water problems. This type of attrition can adversely affect the validity of a study and the investigator should be cognizant of the importance of prompt investigation of attrition in animal numbers.

10. Housing and Postoperative Care

10.1 The animals shall be housed and care provided in accordance with the *Guide for the Care and Use of Laboratory Animals* **(13)** or other appropriate guidelines.

10.2 In addition to the requirements for humane treatment of animals in 10.1, the facilities and environment used, as well as any postoperative drug therapies or other treatments of the animals, must be carefully considered to prevent unexpected effects on the results of the study. The recommendation in 7.1 that a housing control be considered is related to the possibility that environmental factors could provide unexpected changes in study results if adequate care is not taken to eliminate the possibility.

11. Evaluation of Results

11.1 The test and control animals should be examined on a daily basis and any remarkable observations noted. This examination should include noticeable changes in eating habits, alertness, or obvious loss in body weight and palpation at least weekly for detectable masses. A complete record should be maintained of these examinations. When a mass is detected, the date of initial observation should be recorded and the record should document subsequent growth or change in each mass. If it is determined that humane considerations require that an animal be sacrificed early, or if an animal should die before its planned sacrifice date, a complete necropsy shall be performed in accordance with 11.2-11.6.

11.2 At termination or early death or sacrifice, a complete necropsy should be performed and gross observations recorded. Any abnormalities or lesions should be noted, photographed, and evaluated by histopathology. The implant site in particular should be identified and evaluated in detail, documenting all findings carefully. The list of tissues to be evaluated histologically is divided into a minimum list (see 11.4) to be evaluated for all studies and a list of additional tissues which may be appropriate (see 11.5) depending upon the type of material being tested, the route of administration, and the anticipated end use of the test material.

11.3 The investigator should consider performing appropriate hematology and blood chemistry assays on samples taken at the time of animal termination to identify possible effects on blood elements as well as to point to organs which may have been affected by the experiment.

11.4 The tissues to be evaluated shall include (at minimum):

11.4.1 Implant site,

11.4.2 Suspect lesions,

11.4.3 Lymph nodes in region of implant,

11.4.4 Heart,

11.4.5 Kidneys,

11.4.6 Liver,

11.4.7 Lungs,
11.4.8 Brain, and
11.4.9 Other tissues appropriate to the type of implant material being tested. The choice of additional sites should be carefully considered with the intent of not missing important information.

11.5 Depending upon the particular site of implantation and type of material being evaluated, it may be necessary to evaluate other tissues microscopically. Other tissues which should be considered in determining those appropriate to a particular material or application include:

11.5.1 Adrenal glands,
11.5.2 Esophagus,
11.5.3 Femur (effects on marrow cells, cartilage, and growth plates from substances which may enter the systemic circulation),
11.5.4 Gallbladder,
11.5.5 Intestines, large and small,
11.5.6 Mammary gland with adjacent skin,
11.5.7 Muscle adjacent to implant,
11.5.8 Sciatic nerve,
11.5.9 Nasal cavity,
11.5.10 Oral cavity, larynx, and pharynx,
11.5.11 Ovaries,
11.5.12 Pancreas,
11.5.13 Parathyroid gland,
11.5.14 Pituitary gland,
11.5.15 Prostate,
11.5.16 Salivary glands,
11.5.17 Seminal vesicles,
11.5.18 Skin,
11.5.19 Spinal cord,
11.5.20 Spleen,
11.5.21 Stomach,
11.5.22 Testes,
11.5.23 Thymus,
11.5.24 Thyroid gland,
11.5.25 Tongue,
11.5.26 Trachea,
11.5.27 Urinary bladder,
11.5.28 Uterus, and
11.5.29 Vagina.

11.6 In order to allow additional tissue to be evaluated if found necessary, all tissues in 11.4 and 11.5 shall be collected and should be preserved in neutral buffered formalin until the final report has been completed and approved. Retention beyond that time should be consistent with US FDA Good Laboratory Practice regulations or equivalent requirements of other countries.

12. Report

12.1 The study report should include a description of the study design in sufficient detail that it could be repeated if necessary.

12.2 A comparison of the types and incidence of tumors for the control and test series should be made and statistical techniques applied to measure the significance of any differences seen.

12.3 A complete record of the rationale for the study design decisions should be maintained as a part of the permanent record in accordance with FDA Good Laboratory Practice regulations.

12.4 The provisions of the FDA Good Laboratory Practice regulations must be followed in study design, conduct, and recordkeeping.

13. Keywords

13.1 biocompatibility; carcinogenicity testing; tumorigenicity testing

APPENDIX

(Nonmandatory Information)

X1. RATIONALE

X1.1 The medical industry in the United States is developing new materials and new applications of existing materials. Regulatory requirements have included the request for tumorigenesis bioassay for materials that have not previously seen clinical use and been recognized as safe. During the preparation of this guide, there was extensive discussion concerning the validity of this type of testing as any predictor of the tumorigenic potential of materials in humans. Among the issues raised were the Oppenheimer Effect and the effect of mechanical irritation on the production of tumors in rodents. While the occurrence of tumors due to these effects has been frequently reported in rodents, there is little evidence that similar phenomena exist in humans. The investigator is cautioned to carefully consider these possibilities in protocol development and the interpretation of results. The use of a negative control with exactly the same size and shape as the test article is strongly encouraged as an aid in the interpretation of results.

X1.2 The task force has attempted to identify the items that will need to be considered and some of the important steps to be taken in the performance of these types of studies. It is intended that this guide will be modified and made more specific as the industry and researchers gain more experience with the bioassay of solid materials.

X1.3 In the development of this guide, the possibility was raised that animals other than rats might be used for this testing. The large numbers of animals required and the current desire to reduce or eliminate the use of animals for testing would seem to suggest that canine and feline species would not be appropriate for this type of testing unless overpowering reasons can be developed for their use. The use of mice was eliminated because it was believed that mice were too small to allow the types and sizes of implants necessary for solid material testing to be implanted. The costs and logistics of such a study would seem to make it nearly impossible to use primates in these quantities. It is the feeling of the task force that rats should be used unless there is an overriding need for other species. The study should be designed to utilize the minimum number of animals consistent with adequate statistical treatment of the data.

X1.4 Typically, in the performance of tumorigenicity assays, a maximum tolerated dose is determined and that dosage level is utilized as one of the test groups. The physical effects of implanting gross amounts of solid materials into rats, such as tissue distension and its effects on the long-term results of the study, may make the definition of this maximum dosage and interpretation of the results difficult, at best. The task force determined, based upon comments received, that a maximum implantable dose should be recommended as one of the dosage levels despite the experimental problems which might result.

X1.5 There was extensive discussion about the appropriate way to address the Oppenheimer Effect relating to the tumorigenicity of plastics and the Stanton Hypothesis relating to the tumorigenicity of fibrous materials. Paragraphs 6.4 and 6.5 reflect this discussion. Much of the discussion centered around the extreme difficulty or impossibility of performing a valid study in light of these two phenomena. There was also discussion of the possibility of the development of neoplasia in rodents due to mechanical irritation.

X1.6 Data were presented during the development of this guide which reflected a possible decline in the average lifetime in the rats used for these studies. It was decided to address the issue in terms of the cause of early death. Since these strains are used because of their history of spontaneous tumor formation, it is to be expected that early deaths or termination may occur. The task force has attempted to present this concern in terms of the reasons for death rather than the absolute ratios of survivors.

REFERENCES

(**1**) Sher, S. P., "Tumors in Control Hamsters, Rats, and Mice: Literature Tabulation," *CRC Critical Reviews in Toxicology*, Vol 10, 1982, pp. 49–79.

(**2**) Sher, S. P., "Mammary Tumors in Control Rats: Literature Tabulation," *Toxicology and Applied Pharmacology*, Vol 22, 1972, pp. 562–588.

(**3**) Sher, S. P., "Review Article: Tumors in Control Mice: Literature Tabulation," *Toxicology and Applied Pharmacology*, Vol 30, 1974, pp. 337–359.

(**4**) Oppenheimer, E. T., Willhite, M., Danishefsky, I., and Stout, A. P., "Observations on the Effects of Powdered Polymer in the Carcinogenic Process," *Cancer Research*, Vol 21, 1961, pp. 132–134.

(**5**) Oppenheimer, B. S., Oppenheimer, E. T., Stout, A. P., Willhite, M., and Danishefsky, I., "The Latent Period in Carcinogenesis by Plastics in Rats and its Relation to the Presarcomatous Stage," *Cancer*, Vol 11, 1957, pp. 204–213.

(**6**) Brand, K. G., Johnson, K. H., and Buoen, L. C., "Foreign Body Tumorigenesis," *CRC Critical Reviews in Toxicology*, Vol 4, 1976, pp. 353–394.

(**7**) Moizhess, T. G., and Vasiliev, J. M., "Early and Late Stages of Foreign-Body Carcinogenesis Can Be Induced by Implants of Different Shapes," *International Journal of Cancer*, Vol 44, 1989, pp. 449–453.

(**8**) Brand, K. G., Buoen, L. C., Johnson, K. H., and Brand, I., "Etiological Factors, Stages, and the Role of the Foreign Body in Foreign Body Tumorigenesis: A Review," *Cancer Research*, Vol 35, 1971, pp. 279–286.

(**9**) Brand, K. G., "Diversity and Complexity of Carcinogenic Processes: Conceptual Inferences from Foreign-Body Tumorigenesis," *Journal of the National Cancer Institute*, Vol 57, 1976, pp. 973–976.

(**10**) Brand, K. G., Buoen, L. C., and Brand, I., "Foreign-Body Tumorigenesis Induced by Glass and Smooth and Rough Plastic: Comparative Study of Preneoplastic Events," *Journal of the National Cancer Institute*, Vol 55, 1975, pp. 319–322.

(**11**) Stanton, M. F., Layard, M., Tegeris, A., Miller, E., May, M., Morgan, E., and Smith, A., "Relation of Particle Dimension to Carcinogenicity in Amphibole Asbestoses and Other Fibrous Materials," *Journal of the National Cancer Institute*, Vol 67, 1981, pp. 965–975.

(**12**) Harington, J. S., "Fiber Carcinogenesis: Epidemiologic Observations and the Stanton Hypothesis," *Journal of the National Cancer Institute*, Vol 67, 1981, pp. 977–989.

(**13**) *Guide for the Care and Use of Laboratory Animals*, U.S. Department of Health and Human Services, National Institutes of Health, Publication No. 85-23, 1985.

Standard Practice for Cyclic Fatigue Testing of Metallic Stemmed Hip Arthroplasty Femoral Components Without Torsion[1]

This standard is issued under the fixed designation F 1440; the number immediately following the designation indicates the year of original adoption or, in the case of revision, the year of last revision. A number in parentheses indicates the year of last reapproval. A superscript epsilon (ϵ) indicates an editorial change since the last revision or reapproval.

1. Scope

1.1 This practice describes a method for the fatigue testing of metallic stemmed femoral components used in hip arthroplasty. The described method is intended to be used to evaluate the comparison of various designs and materials used for stemmed femoral components used in the arthroplasty. This practice covers procedures for the performance of fatigue tests using (as a forcing function) a periodic constant amplitude force.

1.2 This practice applies primarily to one-piece prostheses and modular components, with head in place such that prostheses should not have an anterior/posterior bow, and should have a nearly straight section on the distal 50 mm of the stem. This practice may require modifications to accommodate other femoral stem designs.

1.3 For additional information see Refs. **(1-5)** .

2. Referenced Documents

2.1 *ASTM Standards:*

E 4 Practices for Load Verification of Testing Machines[2]

E 466 Recommended Practice for Constant Amplitude Axial Fatigue Tests for Metallic Materials[2]

E 467 Practice for Verification of Constant Amplitude Dynamic Loads in an Axial Load Fatigue Testing Machine[2]

E 468 Recommended Practice for the Presentation of Constant Amplitude Fatigue Test Results for Metallic Materials[2]

3. Terminology

3.1 *Definitions and Symbols* (see Fig. 1(*a*) and 1(*b*)):

3.1.1 *cantilever plane*—a plane perpendicular to the line of load application at the level on the stem where the stem becomes unsupported.

3.1.2 *distal stem axis*—the centerline in the anterior/posterior projection of the most distal 50 mm of the stem.

3.1.3 *estimated maximum bending moment*—the maximum load times the unloaded moment arm.

3.1.4 *geometric centroid (cantilever plane)*— the point in a cross-sectional area of the cantilever plane whose coordinates are the mean values of the coordinates of all the points in the area.

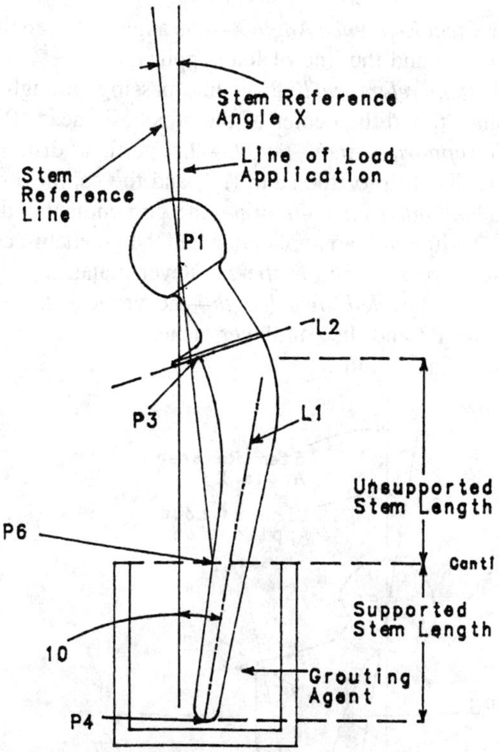

FIG. 1 Collared Device

3.1.5 *line of load application*—the loading axis of the test machine.

3.1.6 *Reference Line L1, distal stem axis*—the medial-lateral (M-L) centerline of the most distal 50 mm of stem in the A-P projection.

3.1.7 *Reference Line L2*:

3.1.7.1 *collared device*— the plane of the distal side of the collar in the A-P projection.

3.1.7.2 *collarless device*—the resection plane recommended for the device in the A-P projection.

3.1.8 *Reference Point P1*—the spherical center of the prosthesis head.

3.1.9 *Reference Point P3*:

3.1.9.1 *collared device*— the intersection of the principal axis of the collar (L2) with the medial surface of the stem in the A-P projection.

[1] This practice is under the jurisdiction of ASTM Committee F-4 on Medical and Surgical Materials and Devices and is the direct responsibility of Subcommittee F04.22 on Arthroplasty.

Current edition approved Sept. 15, 1992. Published November 1992.

[2] *Annual Book of ASTM Standards*, Vol 03.01.

3.1.9.2 *collarless device*—the intersection of the resection plane (L2) with the medial surface of the stem in the A-P projection.

3.1.10 *Reference Point P4*—the distal tip of the stem.

3.1.11 *Reference Point P6*[3]— the intersection of the cantilever plane with the medial surface of the stem in the A-P projection.

3.1.12 *R value*—the *R* value is the ratio of the minimum force to the maximum force.

$$R = \frac{\text{minimum force}}{\text{maximum force}}$$

3.1.13 *Stem Reference Angle X*—the angle between the stem reference line and the line of load application.

3.1.14 *stem reference line*—a line passing through Reference Point P6 and the center of the prosthesis head (P1).

3.1.15 *supported stem length*—the vertical distance between the distal tip of the stem (P4) and the cantilever plane.

3.1.16 *unloaded moment arm*—the perpendicular distance between the line of load application and the geometric centroid of the stem cross section at the cantilever plane.

3.1.17 *unsupported stem length*—the vertical distance between Point P3 and the cantilever plane.

3.2 See Figs. 1 and 2.

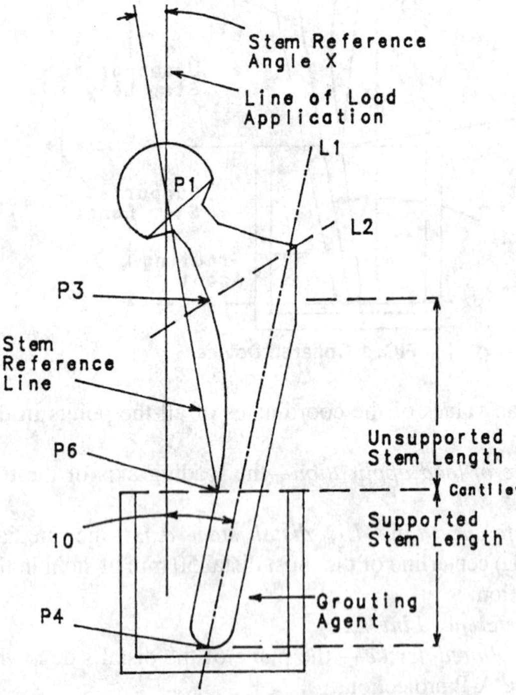

FIG. 2 Collarless Device

4. Significance and Use

4.1 This practice can be used to describe the effects of materials, manufacturing, and design variables on the fatigue resistance of metallic stemmed femoral components subjected to cyclic loading for relatively large numbers of cycles. The recommended test assumes a "worst case" situation where proximal support for the stem has been lost. It is also recognized that for some materials the environment may have an effect on the response to cyclic loading. The test environment used and the rationale for the choice of that environment should be described in the report.

4.2 It is recognized that actual *in vivo* loading conditions are not constant amplitude. However, there is not sufficient information available to crate standard load spectrums for metallic stemmed femoral components. Accordingly, a simple periodic constant amplitude force is recommended.

4.3 In order for fatigue data on femoral stems to be useful for comparison, it must be reproducible among different laboratories. Consequently, it is essential that uniform procedures be established.

5. Specimen Selection

5.1 The specimen selection should have the same geometry as the final finished product, and the stem should be in the final finished condition.

6. Apparatus

6.1 The specimen shall be constrained by a suitable grouting agent within a rigid cavity. A common grouting agent used is poly methyl methacrylate (PMMA—bone cement) that is polymerized in place. The minimum thickness of the grouting agent should be 1 cm. Although bone cement is the recommended grouting agent, other material may be used provided it does not chemically or mechanically interact with the test specimen.

6.2 The test fixtures shall be constructed so that the line of load application is in the implant anterior/posterior symmetry plane of the supported portion of the stem.

6.3 The test fixtures shall be constructed so that the line of load application passes through the ball center.

6.4 A ball- or roller-bearing low-friction mechanism shall be included in the loading apparatus to minimize loads not perpendicular to the cantilever plane. An example of such a mechanism is included in Appendix X1.

7. Equipment Characteristics

7.1 The action of the machine should be analyzed to ensure that the desired form and periodic force amplitude is maintained for the duration of the test. (See Practice E 467.)

7.2 The test machine should have a load monitoring system such as the transducer mounted in line with the specimen. The test loads should be monitored continuously in the early stages of the test and periodically thereafter to ensure the desired load cycle is maintained. The varying load as determined by suitable dynamic verification should be maintained at all times to within ±2 % of the maximum force being used.

8. Procedure

8.1 *Specimen Test Orientation*—The angle between the distal stem axis and the line of load application shall be 10 ± 1 deg %. An example of a method to accomplish mounting the stem at the desired angle is given in Appendix X2.

8.2 *Specimen Mounting*:

[3] The reference points and lines are consistent with the Proposed Standard Specification for Cementable Total Hip Prostheses with Femoral Stems. The reference points "P2" and "P5" in that proposed specification are not relevant to this practice. Consequently, they are not used in this practice.

8.2.1 Maintain the stem Reference Angle X within a range of ±1 deg over a test group.

8.2.2 Maintain the unsupported stem length at ±2 mm.

8.2.3 No relative motion between the prosthesis and the grouting agent is permitted during hardening of the grouting agent.

8.2.4 The surface of the grouting agent at the cantilever plane shall be approximately level and perpendicular to the line of load application.

8.2.5 An example of a technique for setting a specimen in the grouting agent in the correct orientation is given in Appendix X2.

8.3 *Test Frequency*— Run all tests at a test frequency of 30 Hz or less.

8.4 *R Value*—Run all tests with an R value of 10.0.[4]

8.5 Measure the unsupported stem length, stem reference angle, and moment arm for each test specimen prior to testing. A possible means would be to use a shadowgraph of the anterior posterior projection as shown in Fig. 1.

8.6 Estimate the amount of horizontal deflection of the head in response to the periodic forcing function one time after the beginning of each test. Possible methods included dial gages, optical micrometers, or linear scales viewed with a strobe light to slow the apparent motion of the deflection.

9. Test Termination

9.1 Continue the test until the specimen fails or until a predetermined number of cycles has been applied to the specimen. Failure should be defined as a complete separation, or exceeding of a deflection limit on a test machine. In reporting results, state the criteria selected for defining failure and the number of cycles shown as the predetermined runout of the test. Discard the data for a specific sample if the grouting agent fractured prior to test completion.

10. Report

10.1 Report the fatigue test specimens, procedures, and results in accordance with Recommended Practice E 468.

10.2 In addition, report the following parameters: Stem Reference Angle X, supported stem length, maximum force, R value, specimen material, cycles to failure, location of fractures in relation to the cantilever plane, average dimensions of the stem cross section in the cantilever plane, grouting agent, test environment, and test frequency.

11. Precision and Bias

11.1 The precision and bias of this practice is being established.[5]

12. Keywords

12.1 arthroplasty; femoral components; hip arthroplasty; metallic stemmed femoral components; orthopaedic medical devices

[4] In strict terms, since the force applied to the head is compressive, the maximum force is the smallest negative amplitude. Consequently the *R* value is 10 when the negative signs cancel each other. In terms of applied bending moment at the cantilever plane, the *R* value would be 0.1

[5] Test results that can be used to establish precision and bias are solicited.

APPENDIXES

(Nonmandatory Information)

X1. EXAMPLE OF A LOW-FRICTION MECHANISM

X1.1 See Fig. X1.1.

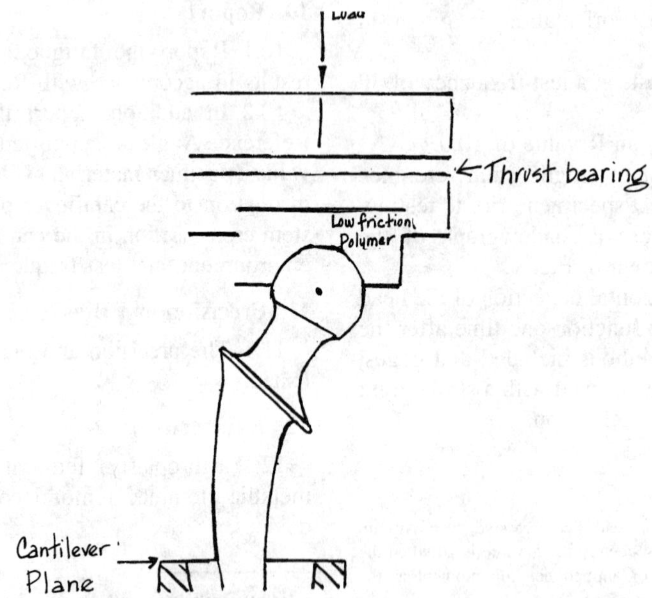

FIG. X1.1 Example of a Low Friction Mechanism

X2. EXAMPLE PROSTHESIS MOUNTING PROCEDURE

X2.1 A drawing or shadowgraph of the prosthesis should be available before mounting to establish the angular relationship between the distal stem axis and the stem reference angle.

X2.2 A gripping device as illustrated in Fig. X2.1 or a ringstand and test tube holder can be used to grip the head of the subject prosthesis.

X2.3 The prosthesis is held by the head permitting the distal tip to rest on a flat surface. The angle jig is positioned with the distal stem in the notch. The stem is adjusted so that it is centered in the notch of the angle jig. This will orient the distal stem at approximately 10 deg to the line of load application. The head is now firmly gripped to maintain the angular orientation of the stem.

X2.4 The angle jig can be removed and the prosthesis mounted at the appropriate depth in an appropriate specimen holder.

X2.5 Grouting material can be placed around the test prosthesis into the specimen holder and allowed to harden.

X2.6 After hardening of the grouting agent the grip on the head of the prosthesis is released and a shadowgraph may be prepared of the profile of the test specimen/specimen holder assembly.

X2.7 A second adjustable stop may be added below the grip and adjusted to rest against the medial surface of an appropriately oriented prosthesis to facilitate repeatable mounting of the test group.

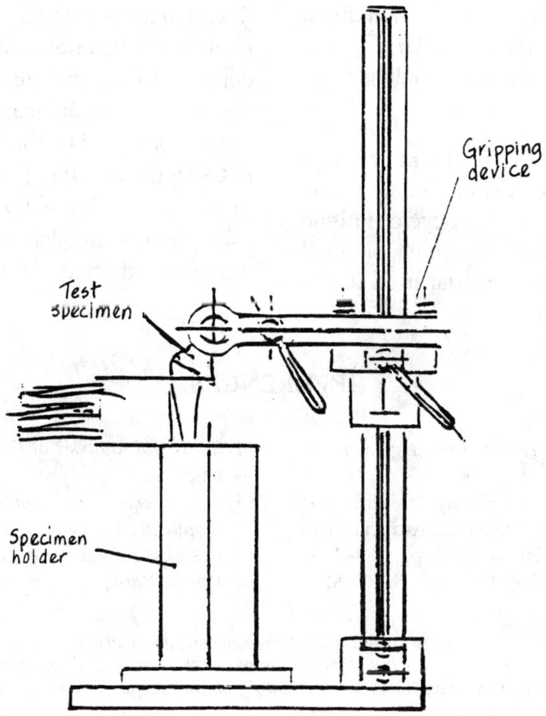

FIG. X2.1 Apparatus for Gripping the Test Specimen While Embedding it in the Correct Orientation

X3. RATIONALE

X3.1 Fracture of femoral stems in THA has been a problem in clinical application. The stem design, PMMA support, quality of bone, and other features contribute to stem fracture. One recognizable mode of failure is with the distal portion of the stem firmly anchored, while medial proximal support is lost. As the body loads are applied through the head of the prosthesis, significant stem stresses can result at the area where the cement is still firmly anchored. Because it is believed that this proximal cement breakdown model is the primary reason behind fracture of the femoral stems, this simplified model was chosen for the fatigue testing of actual stems. There are some problems with the proposed simplified model. The worst case assumes that proximal cement breakdown has already occurred. It does not address any features of a THA system that might help prevent cement breakdown or any features that aid in placing the femoral component in an optimal position with good cement support. While the latter approach is desirable, the test described can give information on the relative fatigue strengths.

X3.2 In 8.1 there is no specification of the number of cycles for test runout. The fundamental idea behind this type of test is that the number of cycles to runout represents a limiting point beyond which the material will not fracture no matter how many more cyclic loads are applied. This is referred to as a fatigue limit. However, in real life most materials do not possess a true fatigue limit. Consequently, a compromise must be made between the amount of testing, (the number of test cycles) and the relationship of the test to actual device performance and device life. Since most of these tests are plotted and evaluated on a semi-log or log-log plot, a typical runout point is often ten million cycles. Doubling or tripling the number of test cycles to twenty or thirty million contributes only a small amount to the trend analysis on the log scale, but it doubles or triples the length of the test. In Europe five million cycles has been used as a runout value for some stem tests.

X3.3 This test is a cantilever beam bend test. In a cantilever beam bend test the load point will tend to deflect in the direction of the applied load, the amount of deflection depending on the elasticity of the test sample With this test the head of the prosthesis is the cantilever load point. Since the direction of the load also applies a compressive force down the stem, only the vector portion of the force, perpendicular to the prosthesis long axis, will contribute to the beam deflection. That contribution of beam bending will deflect the head to the side. This motion effectively increases the bending moment arm. This motion must be permitted. If the head is not allowed to deflect in a near frictionless manner the portion of the test fixture that prevents the deflection is actually applying an unknown force against the head to keep it from deflecting. If the device is flexible enough, the magnitude of periodic motion of the head of the prosthesis (in the plane perpendicular to the line of load application) in response to the periodic forcing function; can significantly increase the applied maximum bending moment. It may be wise to estimate this deflection and include it in bending moment calculations.

X3.4 Any fatigue strength as predicted by tests following the method described herein must be considered on a relative basis, that is, these tests may yield valuable information about the relative merits of different devices for particular applications, but should not be used as a quantitative indicator of expected *in vivo* device lifetime.

X3.5 There is limited information in the literature as to whether the materials used in THA femoral components experience a significant degradation in high-cycle fatigue initiation properties due to the presence of a physiological environment. If there is concern that the material used in the device may degrade significantly in a physiological environment; such material characteristics would be more realistically determined fatigue testing a material test specimen in a simulated physiological environment at rates of one cycle per second or less. For these reasons, a particular environment is not specified in this practice. However, a simulated environment is not prohibited. However, if a simulated environment is used, the test frequency should be selected so as to not mask the expected effects of the environment.

REFERENCES

(**1**) *Manual on Statistical Planning and Analysis of Fatigue Experiments, ASTM STP 588,* Little and Jebe, eds.

(**2**) Semlitsch, M., and Panic, B., "Ten Years of Experience with Test Criteria for Fracture-Proof Anchorage of Stems of Artificial Hip Joints," *Engineering in Medicine*, Vol 12, No. 4, 1983, pp. 185–198.

(**3**) *Handbook of Fatigue Testing, ASTM STP 566,* Swanson, S. R., ed.

(**4**) *Statistical Analysis of Fatigue Data, ASTM STP 744,* Little and Evkal, eds.

(**5**) *Technolgische und biomechanische Aspekte der Hüft-und Kniealloar thoplastik*; Statisch-biomechanische spannungs—analysen und dynamische Prüfungen von Hüftprothesen, Ungethum pp. 90–110, Huns Huber, Bern.

Standard Specification for Soft-Tissue Expander Devices[1]

This standard is issued under the fixed designation F 1441; the number immediately following the designation indicates the year of original adoption or, in the case of revision, the year of last revision. A number in parentheses indicates the year of last reapproval. A superscript epsilon (ϵ) indicates an editorial change since the last revision or reapproval.

1. Scope

1.1 This specification covers the requirements for inflatable tissue expansion devices to be used intraoperatively or implanted for typically less than 6 months and then removed.

1.2 *Limitations*—This specification applies only to soft-tissue expander devices fabricated with elastomer shells. It does not necessarily cover any custom fabricated soft tissue expander device manufactured to any other specification.

1.3 The values stated in SI units are to be regarded as standard, values in parentheses are for information only.

1.4 The following statement pertains only to the test methods portion, Section 7, of this specification. *This standard does not purport to address all of the safety problems, if any, associated with its use. It is the responsibility of the user of this standard to establish appropriate safety and health practices and determine the applicability of regulatory limitations prior to use.*

2. Referenced Documents

2.1 *ASTM Standards:*

D 412 Test Methods for Rubber Properties in Tension[2]

D 624 Test Method for Rubber Property—Tear Resistance[2]

D 1349 Practice for Rubber—Standard Temperatures for Testing[2]

F 604 Classification for Silicon Elastomers Used in Medical Applications[3]

F 748 Practice for Selecting Generic Biological Test Methods for Materials and Devices[3]

F 1251 Terminology Relating to Polymeric Biomaterials in Medical and Surgical Devices[3]

2.2 *Federal Register:*

Title 21, Part 820[4]

3. Terminology

3.1 *Definitions:*

3.1.1 *injection port*—the port through which an injection to inflate or deflate the variable volume device is made.

3.1.1.1 *remote port*—a port that is remote from the shell and attached to the shell by means of tubing.

3.1.1.2 *self-contained (integrated) port*—a port that is integral to the device shell.

3.1.2 *injection surface*—the area of the injection port recommended by the manufacturer for needle insertion to inflate or deflate the device.

3.1.3 *needle stop*—the injection port component used to limit hypodermic needle penetration through the port.

3.1.4 *reinforced silicone elastomer*—a composite of silicone elastomer and an embedded textile made from polyethylene terephthalate (Dacron®) fibres.

3.1.5 *shell*—an outer sac of the device which is comprised of silicone elastomer (or other appropriate material).

3.1.6 *tubing length adapter*—the tissue expander component used to connect more than one piece of remote port tubing.

3.1.7 *tubing/shell junction*—the junction of the remote port tubing to the shell of the tissue expander.

3.2 For other terms used in this specification see Terminology F 1251.

4. Classification

4.1 *Type I: Chronic Tissue Expansion Device*—A soft tissue expander device intended to be inflated postoperatively.

4.2 *Type II: Immediate Tissue Expansion Device*—A soft tissue expander device only intended for intraoperative use.

5. Significance and Use

5.1 The devices described in this specification are intended for use in soft tissue expansion. This specification identifies those factors felt to be important to ensure safety as it relates to the device biocompatibility and the mechanical integrity of the device components.

6. Requirements

6.1 *Biocompatibility*:

6.1.1 Biological testing to ensure safety of soft tissue expander devices shall be selected and conducted in accordance with Practice F 748.

6.1.2 In addition to biological testing as recommended by Practice F 748, other biological testing may be appropriate.

6.2 *Physical Properties*:

6.2.1 *Tensile Set*—Maximum set shall be less than 10 % when tested in accordance with 7.2.1.

[1] This specification is under the jurisdiction of ASTM Committee F-4 on Medical and Surgical Materials and Devices and is the direct responsibility of Subcommittee F04.06 on Plastic and Reconstructive Surgery.

Current edition approved Dec. 15, 1992. Published February 1993.

[2] *Annual Book of ASTM Standards*, Vol 09.01.

[3] *Annual Book of ASTM Standards*, Vol 13.01.

[4] Available from U.S. Government Printing Office, Superintendent of Documents, Washington, DC 20402.

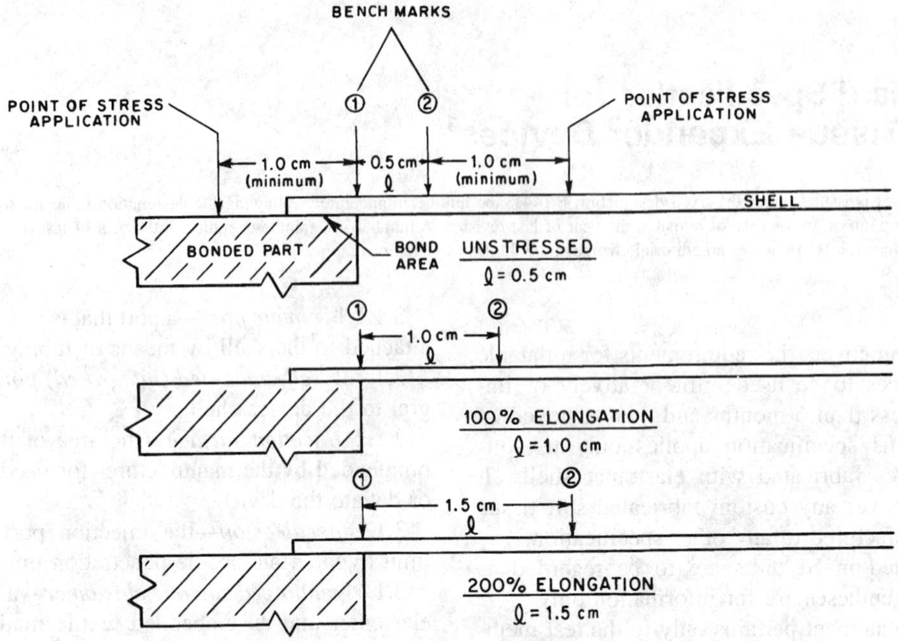

FIG. 1 Testing Fused or Adhered Joints

6.2.2 *Breaking Force*—Ultimate breaking force in tension shall be no less than 11.12 N (2.5 lb) when tested in accordance with 7.2.3.

6.2.3 *Tear Resistance*—Tear resistance shall be 3.5584 N (0.8 lb) minimum when tested in accordance with 7.2.3.

7. Test Methods

7.1 Tissue expander or component designs, or both, shall demonstrate an acceptable response to the following tests. Unless otherwise specified, the standard temperature for testing shall be 23 ± 2°C (73.4 ± 3.6°F). Condition the test specimens for at least 3 h when the test temperature is 23 ± 2°C. If the material is affected by moisture, maintain the relative humidity at 50 ± 5 % and condition the specimen for at least 24 h prior to testing. When testing at any other temperature is required, use one of the temperatures specified in Practice D 1349.

7.2 *Shell*—Cut the test specimens from units made by standard production processes including sterilization. Clean with appropriate (polar, for example, 2-propanol, or nonpolar, for example, 1,1,1-trichloroethane) solvent if necessary.

7.2.1 *Tensile Set*—At 300 % elongation, stress the test specimens for 3 min. Remove the load, then allow 3 min for relaxation. Test the set in accordance with Test Methods D 412 with the exception of sample thickness and cycle time.

7.2.2 *Breaking Force*—Test ultimate breaking force in tension in accordance with Test Methods D 412 Die C with the exception of sample thickness.

7.2.3 *Tear Resistance*—Test tear resistance in accordance with Test Method D 624 Die B or Die C with the exception of sample thickness. Include the indication of which die (B or C) is appropriate when citing tear resistance values.

7.3 *Tubing Shell Junction*—The tubing/shell junction of Type I tissue expanders shall not fail when tested under the following conditions:

7.3.1 *Tubing Greater Than 2.3 mm (0.090 in.) in Outer Diameter*—The tubing/shell junction shall not fail when stressed to 6.672-N (1.5-lb) tension.

7.3.2 *Tubing Less Than or Equal to 2.3 mm (0.090 in.) in Outer Diameter*—The tubing/shell junction shall not fail when stressed to 2.224-N (0.5-lb) tension.

7.4 *Injection Port Competence*—There shall be no Type I tissue expander port leakage observed when an injection port is tested under the following conditions. Apply 120-mm Hg intraluminal pressure to the port using water or test media with demonstrated equivalence. Using the prescribed gauge hypodermic needle, puncture the port 5 consecutive times within 1 mm^2 at a site near the center of the port. The port is considered leaking and fails the test if beads of fluid on the port surface are not static after 30 s.

7.4.1 *21 Gage Port*—An injection port may be labelled a 21G port only if it passes the injection port competence test when tested with a 21G hypodermic needle.

7.4.2 *23 Gage Port*—An injection port may be labelled a 23G port only if it passes the injection port competence test when tested with a 23G hypodermic needle.

7.4.3 *25 Gage Port*—An injection port may be labelled a 25G port only if it passes the injection port competence test when tested with a 25G hypodermic needle.

7.5 *Overexpansion*—There shall be no leakage or device rupture when the tissue expander is expanded (using water at ambient conditions) to 200 % of its maximum recommended inflation volume and kept at that volume for a minimum of 10 min.

7.6 *Tubing Length Adapter Strength*—Two pieces of remote port tubing attached by means of the tubing length adapter shall not separate when a 152.4-mm (6-in.) test specimen is stressed at 10 % elongation. Tubing length adapter shall not be ligated in this test method.

7.7 *Needle Stop Penetration*—Mount a 38.1-mm (1.5-in.)

21-gage hypodermic needle[5] to a syringe. Insert the needle into the injection port, perpendicular to the needle stop. Apply force along the axis of the needle, to push it into the needle stop. The needle must fail without penetrating the needle stop.

7.8 *Fused or Adhered Joints*—Requirements for adhered or fused materials shall be critical to their integrity.

7.8.1 Adhered or fused joints or seams that are critical to the integrity of the device envelope shall not fail when the shell adjacent to the joint is stressed to 200 % elongation for 10 s (see Fig. 1).

7.8.2 Adhered or fused joints or seams that are bonded to the device envelope, but are not critical to the envelope integrity (fixations, suture tabs, orientation bars, valve covers, etc.) shall not fail when the shell adjacent to the joint is stressed to 100 % elongation for 10 s (see Fig. 1).

8. Sterilization

8.1 The units may be supplied pre-sterilized in accordance with current USP[6] procedures and good manufacturing practices (GMP established by the FDA).

8.2 If re-sterilization of the device is intended, instruction for cleaning and sterilization shall be supplied with the package insert.

[5] Available from *U.S. Pharmacopeia*, Vol XX, Mack Publishing Co., Easton, PA.

[6] The Precision Glide hypodermic needle, available from Becton Dickinson, One Becton Drive, Franklin Lakes, NJ 07417, or its equivalent, has been found satisfactory for this purpose.

9. Packaging, Labelling, and Package Inserts

9.1 *Packaging*—The devices shall be packaged to protect them from damage, including maintenance of sterilization of pre-sterilized devices, during the customary conditions of processing, storage, handling, and distribution.

9.2 *Labelling*:

9.2.1 Each package shall be labelled in a manner that ensures the labelling arrives at the point of use with the device. The package labelling shall include the following information:

9.2.1.1 Product name,

9.2.1.2 Configuration or type,

9.2.1.3 Manufacturer's name and address,

9.2.1.4 Manufacturer lot number,

9.2.1.5 Volume or dimension,

9.2.1.6 Date of sterilization or packaging (year), and

9.2.1.7 Special storage requirements, if any.

9.2.2 With each unit, a self-adhering tab shall be provided which is suitable for attaching to the patient's chart. The tab shall include the following information:

9.2.2.1 Product name and manufacturer,

9.2.2.2 Product lot number, and

9.2.2.3 Product type and volume dimension.

9.3 *Package Insert*—The package insert shall provide recommended instructions for use.

10. Keywords

10.1 elastomer; implant; implant material; medicale device; plastic surgery; soft tissue

APPENDIX

(Nonmandatory Information)

X1. RATIONALE

X1.1 Tissue expanders are intended for use as temporary devices that are surgically placed under the muscle or in subcutaneous soft tissue. To assure biological safety of the materials and finished devices, this specification contains requirements for biocompatibility testing.

X1.2 Tissue expanders are intended to be inflated in situ, at intraimplant pressures sufficient to stretch soft tissue. Such stretching may also include the envelope or shell of the tissue expander, since it is reasonable to expect that expanders may be inflated beyond their normal volume in normal usage. To minimize the potential for leakage or deflation during use, this specification contains requirements for the physical properties of materials of construction, bonded or adhered areas and connectors.

X1.3 When expansion is accomplished by percutaneous hypodermic needle penetration of the tissue expander's injection port, multiple injections are typically required, spaced over a variable time period, in order to achieve adequate expansion. Thus, this specification contains requirements for resistance of the injection port to leakage after repeated needle punctures.

X1.4 The tissue expanders subject to this specification may reasonably be expected to vary widely in shape, size, and design. Tissue expander devices may vary significantly in design and the materials of construction to achieve their intended purpose. Thus, this specification contains requirements for labelling that includes defining the specific nature and function of the expander, and other appropriate use information.

X1.5 Because device sterility is an important consideration, this specification requires labelling to comply with GMP requirements set forth by the FDA regarding sterilization.

Standard Specification for Minimum Performance and Safety Requirements for Components and Systems of Anesthetic Gas Monitors[1]

This standard is issued under the fixed designation F 1452; the number immediately following the designation indicates the year of original adoption or, in the case of revision, the year of last revision. A number in parentheses indicates the year of last reapproval. A superscript epsilon (ϵ) indicates an editorial change since the last revision or reapproval.

INTRODUCTION

The measurement of the concentration of inhalation anesthetic gases is becoming common practice. This specification establishes minimum safety and performance requirements for anesthetic gas monitors that are achievable within the limits of existing technology.

The appendix that follows contains rationale for the most important requirements. It is included to provide additional insight for the reasoning that led to the requirements and recommendations that have been incorporated in this specification.

SECTION ONE—GENERAL

1. Scope

1.1 This specification applies to ANESTHETIC GAS MONITORS used with adults, children, and neonates. It does not apply to devices intended for use in laboratory research applications, non-human applications, or for calibration of anesthetic agent vaporizers.

2. Referenced Documents

2.1 The following standards contain provisions which, through reference in this specification, constitute provisions of this specification. At a time of publication of this document, the editions indicated were current. All standards are subject to revision, and parties using this specification are encouraged to investigate the possibility of applying the most recent editions of the standards listed below.

2.2 *ASTM Standards:*

F 1054 Specification for Conical Fittings of 15 mm and 22 mm Sizes[2]

F 1161 Specification for Minimum Performance and Safety Requirements for Components and Systems of Anesthesia Gas Machines[2]

F 1343 Specification for Anesthetic Equipment-Scavenging Systems for Anesthetic Gases[2]

2.3 *IEC Standards:*[3]

IEC 601-1:1988 Medical Electrical Equipment—Part 1: General Requirements for Safety. (This particular IEC standard is referred to as the General Standard throughout this document; the section and clause numbering as well as the titles used here follow those used in IEC 601-1.)

IEC 651:1979 Sound Level Meters

IEC 801-2:1993 Electromagnetic Compatibility for Industrial-Process Measurement and Control Equipment—Part 2: Electrostatic Discharge Requirements

2.4 *ISO Standards:*[3]

ISO 3744:1981 Acoustics—Determination of Sound Power Levels of Noise Sources: Engineering Methods for Free-Field Conditions over a Reflecting Plane

ISO 4135:1979 Anesthesiology—Vocabulary

ISO 5356-1:1986 Anesthetic and Respiratory Equipment—Conical Connectors—Part 1: Conical Connectors for the Breathing System

ISO 5356-2:1987 Anesthetic and Respiratory Equipment—Conical Connectors—Part 2: Screw-Threaded Weight-Bearing Connectors

ISO 7000-1984 Graphical Symbols For Use on Equipment—Index and Synopsis

ISO 7504:1984 Gas Analysis—Vocabulary

ISO 7767:1988 Oxygen Analyzers for Monitoring Patient Breathing Mixtures—Safety Requirements

2.5 *Other Documents:*[4]

CGA C-9-1982 Standard Color Markings of Compressed Gas Cylinders Intended for Medical Use in the United States

NFPA 70-1993 National Electric Code[5]

3. Terminology

3.1 *Definitions*—The definitions given in Clause 2 of the

[1] This specification is under the jurisdiction of ASTM Committee F-29 on Anesthetic and Respiratory Equipment and is the direct responsibility of Subcommittee F29.11 on Gas Monitors.

Current edition approved December 15, 1992. Published June 1993.

[2] *Annual Book of ASTM Standards*, Vol 13.01.

[3] Available from American National Standards Institute, 1430 Broadway, New York, NY 10018.

[4] Available from Compressed Gas Association, 1235 Jefferson Davis Highway, Arlington, Va 22202.

[5] Available from National Fire Protection Association (NFPA), 470 Atlantic Ave., Boston, MA 02210.

General Standard apply, with the following additions:

3.1.1 *accuracy*—the quality that characterizes the ability of a device to give indications approximating to the true value of the quantity measured.

3.1.2 *alarm*—an indication that some undesirable condition exists.

3.1.3 *alarm set point*—the setting of the adjustment control, or display value, that indicates the anesthetic gas reading, at or beyond which the alarm is intended to be activated.

3.1.3.1 *Discussion*—Terms such as "alarm limits" or "alarm threshold" are frequently used to describe the same function.

3.1.4 *alarm system*—those parts of the anesthetic gas monitor which: (*1*) establish the alarm set point(s); (*2*) activate an alarm when the anesthetic gas reading is less than or equal to the low alarm set point, if provided, or is equal to or greater than the high alarm set point.

3.1.5 *anesthetic gas level*—the volume percent of anesthetic gas in a gaseous mixture.

3.1.6 *anesthetic gas monitor*—a device for the measurement of the concentration or partial pressure of anesthetic gas(es) in ventilatory gases.

3.1.6.1 *Discussion*—The anesthetic gas monitor consists of all equipment, including accessories, sensor, and sampling tube (if a diverting type), specified by the manufacturer for the intended use of the anesthetic gas monitor.

3.1.7 *anesthetic gas reading*—the measured anesthetic gas level as indicated by the analyzer display.

3.1.8 *anesthetic gas scavenging systems*—systems that collect and remove the excess anesthetic gases and vapors released from equipment used in administering anesthetics under normal operating conditions, or exhaled by the patient. Scavenging is intended to reduce ambient concentrations of anesthetic agents in anesthetizing areas.

3.1.9 *anesthetic gas transducer*—a device for converting the partial pressure or volume percent of an anesthetic gas or vapor into a signal for monitoring or recording.

3.1.10 *common gas outlet*—that port through which the dispensed mixture from the anesthetic apparatus is delivered to the breathing system.

3.1.11 *default parameter (default setting)*—those operating parameters within the machine, which are pre-set at the factory, or by the operator, and which the machine itself sets, without further intervention, when it is turned on.

3.1.12 *delay time*—the time from a step function change in anesthetic gas concentration or partial pressure at the sampling site to the achievement of 10 % of the step change in anesthetic gas value in the analyzer (see Fig. 1).

3.1.13 *display*—the visual representation of output data.

3.1.14 *diverting anesthetic gas monitor*—a monitor that transports a portion of ventilatory gases from the sampling site through a sampling tube to the sensor, which is remote from the sampling site.

3.1.15 *drift*—(from ISO 7504:1984) change of the anesthetic gas level display of an analyzer for a given level of concentration over a stated period of time, under reference conditions that remain constant.

3.1.15.1 *Discussion*—It is necessary to distinguish the zero drift that concerns the operation of the instrument with samples of zero or low concentration from the drift considered at one or several levels of concentration.

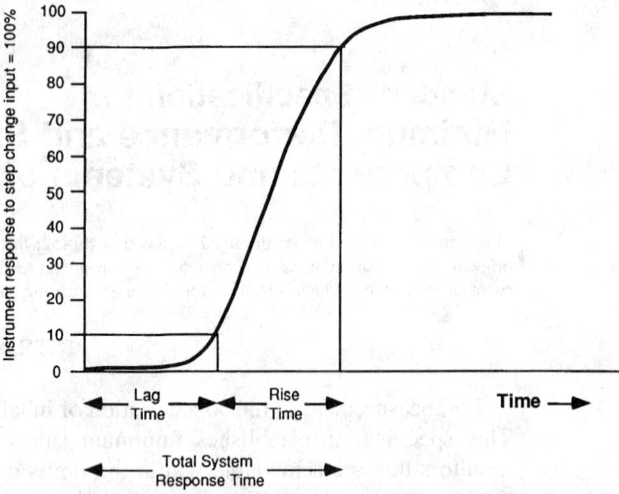

FIG. 1 Lag Time, Rise Time, and Total System Response (Delay Time is Synonymous with Lag Time and is the Preferred Term)

3.1.16 *high priority alarm*—a combination of audible and visual alarms indicating that immediate action on the part of the operator is required.

3.1.17 *interference with measurement accuracy*— the difference between the anesthetic gas readings in the presence and absence of an interfering gas(es).

3.1.18 *low priority alarm*—an indication of a condition that requires awareness, but not necessarily action, on the part of the operator.

3.1.19 *medium priority alarm*—a combination of audible and visual alarms indicating that prompt action on the part of the operator is required.

3.1.20 *non-diverting anesthetic gas monitor*—an anesthetic gas monitor that uses a sensor at the sampling site.

3.1.21 *partial pressure*—the pressure that each gas in a gas mixture would exert if it alone occupied the volume of the mixture at the same temperature.

3.1.22 *rise time*—the time required to display a rise from 10 to 90 % of the change in the anesthetic gas value by the anesthetic gas monitor when a step function change in anesthetic gas volume percent occurs at the sampling site (see Fig. 1).

3.1.23 *sampling site*—the location at which respiratory gases are diverted from measurement to a remote sensor in a diverting anesthetic gas monitor or the location of the sensor area in a non-diverting anesthetic gas monitor.

3.1.24 *sampling tube*—the conduit for transfer of respiratory gases from the sampling site to the sensor in a diverting anesthetic gas monitor.

3.1.25 *sensor*—the part of the anesthetic gas monitor that is sensitive to the presence of the anesthetic gas.

3.1.26 *total system response time*—the sum of the delay time and rise time (see Fig. 1).

3.1.27 *volume percent (V/V) of a gas or vapor*— the volume of an anesthetic gas (or other gas or vapor) in a mixture, expressed as a percent of the total volume.

4. Relationship of This Specification to the General Standard

	(A)	(NA)	(AM/R)[A]
Section One—General			
1. Scope and object			X
2. Terminology and definitions			X
3. General requirements			X
4. General requirements for tests			X
5. Classification			X
6. Identification, marking, and document			X
7. Power input	X		
Section Two—Environmental Conditions			
8. Not used[B]		X	
9. Not used		X	
10. Environmental conditions	X		
11. Not used		X	
12. Not used		X	
Section Three—Protection Against Electric Shock Hazards			
13. General	X		
14. Requirements related to classification	X		
15. Limitation of voltage or energy, or both	X		
16. Enclosures and protective covers	X		
17. Separation			X
18. Protective earthing, functional earthing, and potential equalization	X		
19. Patient auxiliary currents			X
20. Dielectric strength	X		
Section Four—Protection Against Mechanical Hazard			
21. Mechanical strength	X		
22. Moving parts	X		
23. Surfaces, corners, and edges	X		
24. Stability in normal use	X		
25. Expelled parts	X		
26. Vibration and noise			X
27. Pneumatic and hydraulic power	X		
28. Suspended masses	X		
Section Five—Protection Against Hazards from Unwanted or Excessive Radiation			
29. X-radiation	X		
30. Alpha, beta, gamma, neutron radiation and other particle radiation	X		
31. Microwave radiation	X		
32. Light radiation (including visual radiation and lasers)	X		
33. Infra-red radiation	X		
34. Ultra-violet radiation	X		
35. Acoustical energy (including ultrasonics)	X		
36. Electromagnetic compatibility			X
Section Six—Protection Against Hazards of Ignition of Flammable Anesthetic Mixtures			
37. Locations and basic requirements	X		
38. Marking and accompanying documents	X		
39. Common requirements for Category AP and Category APG equipment	X		
40. Requirements and tests for Category AP equipment, parts or components thereof	X		
41. Requirements and tests for Category APG equipment, parts or components thereof	X		
Section Seven—Protection Against Excessive Temperatures and Other Safety Hazards			
42. Excessive temperatures	X		
43. Fire prevention			X
44. Overflow, spillage, leakage, humidity, ingress of liquids, cleaning, sterilization, and disinfection			X
45. Pressure vessels and parts subject to pressure			X
46. Human errors			X
47. Electrostatic charges			X
48. Materials in applied parts in contact with the body of the patient	X		
49. Interruption of the power supply	X		
Section Eight—Accuracy of Operating Data and Protection Against Hazardous Output			
50. Accuracy of operating data			X
51. Protection against incorrect output			X
Section Nine—Abnormal Operation and Fault Conditions; Environmental Tests			
52. Abnormal operation and fault conditions	X		
53. Environmental tests	X		
Section Ten—Constructional Requirements			
54. General	X		
55. Enclosures and covers	X		
56. Components and general assembly			X
57. Main parts, components, and layout	X		
58. Protective earthing—terminals and connections	X		
59. Construction and layout	X		
Additional Clauses			
60. Interfering gas and vapor effects (other than water vapor)	X		
61. Pressure effects	X		
62. Sample gas exhaust port	X		
63. Breathing system connections	X		
64. Obstruction of sampling tube	X		
65. Contamination of breathing systems	X		

[A] A = applies, NA = not applicable, and AM/R = applies with an amendment, addition, or revision to the requirement in the General Standard.

[B] "Not used" means that material in this (these) section(s) of IEC 601-1:1977 has been deleted from the 1988 edition, but the section number is reserved for future use.

5. Clauses Containing Amendments, Additions, or Replacements to the Text in IEC 601-1:1988

NOTE 1—The clause numbers used refer to the specific section in the General Standard.

4. *General Requirements and General Requirements for Tests*—The requirements given in Clauses 3 and 4 of the General Standard apply, together with the following addition:

4.12 Test methods other than those specified in this draft specification, but of equal or greater accuracy, may be used to verify compliance with the requirements of this draft specification. However, in the event of dispute, the methods specified in this draft specification shall be used as the reference methods.

5. *Classification*—The requirements given in Clause 5 of the General Standard apply, with the following additions:

NOTE 2—An ANESTHETIC GAS MONITOR may have APPLIED PART(S) of different types (as classified in Clause 14.6 of the General Standard).

Clauses 5.4 and 5.6 are deleted and the following is added:

5.9 The method(s) of sterilization or disinfection recommended by the manufacturer shall be included in the labeling and may be included in the marking.

6. *Identification, Marking, and Documents*—The requirements given in Clause 6 of the General Standard apply, together with the following modifications:

Under" clearly legible," the first sentence shall be modified to read:

Warning statements, instructional messages, or drawings: affixed permanently and legible to an operator with a visual acuity of 1.0 (corrected if necessary) from a distance of 1 m at an illuminance level of 215 lx.

6.1 aa) All operator interchangeable components of an ANESTHETIC GAS MONITOR that are flow direction sensitive shall be marked clearly and durably with an arrow showing the direction of gas flow.

6.1 bb) If a sampled gas inlet and outlet are provided, their presence shall be marked clearly and durably.

6.1 cc) Packages for single use components shall be marked clearly with the following words:" SINGLE USE" or "SINGLE PATIENT USE."

NOTE 3—Additionally, Symbol No. 1051 given in ISO 7000 may be used.

6.5 Color of the insulation of conductors shall be according to NFPA 70.

6.6 a) Replace Clause 6.6 a) with the following:

Identification of the content of gas cylinders used in medical practice as a part of electrical equipment shall be in accordance with CGA C-9-1982. Colors of calibration gas cylinders not already specified in relevant national standards such as CGA C-9-1982 shall be color-coded differently from the colors specified for medical gases (see also Subclause 56.3a).

6.6 b) Replace Clause 6.6 b) with the following:

The point of connection of gas cylinders shall be so identified on equipment that errors are unlikely when a connection is made. If a sampled gas inlet and outlet are provided, the port shall be marked clearly..

6.6 c) If color coding of labels for halogenated anesthetic agents is used, they shall be in accordance with Table 1.

TABLE 1 Colors for Color Coding of Anesthetic Agents

Anesthetics	Color	Federal	Pantone	Munsell
Enflurane	orange	22510	144	2.5YR 6/16
Halothane	red	11105	200	5R4/14
Isoflurane	purple	none	252/253	7.5P 4/12

6.7 Clause 6.7 of the General Standard shall apply.

6.8 Clause 6.8 of the General Standard shall apply, with the following additions:

(*A*) The instructions for use shall additionally include the following information:

(*1*) A description of the purpose and intended use of the ANESTHETIC GAS MONITOR;

(*2*) A description of the principles of operation of the ANESTHETIC GAS MONITOR, including the relationship between gas concentration and its PARTIAL PRESSURE, and the effects of humidity.

A detailed specification including the following:

(*a*) The anesthetic gas measurement range and the accuracy and precision of measurement;
(*b*) If the ANESTHETIC GAS MONITOR is capable of identifying the halogenated anesthetic gas(es) without user intervention, the manufacturer shall make the test methods and results supporting the claim available upon request;
(*c*) The gas diversion flow, if gas diversion occurs;
(*d*) The stability of measurement accuracy;
(*e*) The RISE TIME;
(*f*) The anesthetic gas alarm range, its resolution, and delay time from detection to activation;
(*g*) The operating, nonoperating (standby), and storage temperature and humidity ranges, if applicable;
(*h*) Power requirements; and
(*i*) Time from switching on to obtaining specified operating performance.

(*4*) Details of any known adverse effects on stated function (for example, measurement accuracy and precision, integrity of electrical isolation, and the integrity of pneumatic components) due to the following;

(*a*) Humidity or condensate, including, for example, any adverse effects if an accessory is provided to improve the function of the sensor in the presence of condensation or particulate water;
(*b*) Interfering gases or vapors;
(*c*) Leaks or internal venting of sampled gas;
(*d*) Mechanical shock;
(*e*) Cyclic (ventilating) pressure in the breathing circuit;
(*f*) Barometric pressure;
(*g*) Fluctuation in ac mains or battery voltage;
(*h*) If automatic compensation for barometric pressure is not provided, then the accompanying documents shall contain an explanation that the readings in concentrations units are correct only under the pressure at which the anesthetic gas monitor is calibrated; and
(*i*) Other sources of interference, if any.

(*5*) An illustration of the features of the anesthetic gas monitor, indicating the function and location of all operating controls, adjustments, and system components necessary for correct operation.

(*6*) Instructions for operation of the anesthetic gas monitor, including the following:

(*a*) Checking and calibration before use;
(*b*) Routine inspection and testing;
(*c*) Recommended methods for cleaning and disinfection or sterilization;
(*d*) Recommended method for connecting an exhaust port of the ANESTHETIC GAS MONITOR to an ANESTHETIC GAS SCAVENGING SYSTEM, if applicable; and
(*e*) Recommended method of verifying alarm functions.

(*7*) A description of any recommended in-use calibration or verification, or both, procedure employing recommended test gas(es).

(*8*) A description of the correct installation of the ANESTHETIC GAS MONITOR and a detailed description of sampling arrangements and any connecting tubing.

(*9*) Upon request by the user, disclosure of the electromagnetic compatibility standard or test method to which the anesthetic gas monitor was tested.

(*10*) The instructions for use shall include information concerning any precautions to be taken if a specific unusual risk is associated with the disposal of a device, after its useful life.

7. *Power Input*—The requirements given in Clause 7 of the General Standard apply.

8. *Basic Safety Requirements*—Not used.

SECTION TWO—ENVIRONMENTAL CONDITIONS

9. *Removable Protective Means*—Not used. Replaced by Subclause 6.1.z.

10. *Environmental Conditions*—The requirements given in Clause 10 of the General Standard apply.

11. Not used.

12. Not used; transferred to Subclause 3.6.

SECTION THREE—PROTECTION AGAINST ELECTRIC SHOCK HAZARDS

13. *General Comments: Protection Against Electric Shock Hazards*—The requirements given in Clause 13 of the General Standard apply.

14. *Requirements Related to Classification*—The requirements given in Clause 14 of the General Standard apply.

15. *Limitation of Voltage and/or Energy*—The requirements given in Clause 15 of the General Standard apply.

16. *Enclosures and Protective Covers*—The requirements given in Clause 16 of the General Standard apply.

17. *Separation (Formerly Insulation and Protective Impedances)*—The requirements given in Clause 17 of the General Standard apply.

18. *Protective Earthing, Functional Earthing and Potential Equalization*—The requirements given in Clause 18 of the General Standard apply.

19. *Continuous Leakage Currents and Patient Auxiliary Currents*—The requirements given in Clause 19 of the General Standard apply with the following exception:

(*1*) When national standards mandate more restrictive limits, these more restrictive limits shall apply.

(*2*) In item 19.1 e), add the following:

(*a*) For non-diverting anesthetic gas monitors at the sensor;
(*b*) For diverting anesthetic gas monitors, at the junction of the sampling tubing and the body of the anesthetic gas monitor.

20. *Dielectric Strength*—The requirements given in Clause 20 of the General Standard apply.

SECTION FOUR—PROTECTION AGAINST MECHANICAL HAZARDS

21. *Mechanical Strength*—The requirements given in Clause 21 of the General Standard shall apply.

22. *Moving Parts*—The requirements given in Clause 22 of the General Standard shall apply.

23. *Surface, Corners and Edges*—The requirements given in Clause 23 of the General Standard shall apply.

24. *Stability in Normal Use*—The requirements given in Clause 24 of the General Standard shall apply.

25. *Expelled Parts*—The requirements given in Clause 25 of the General Standard shall apply.

26. *Vibration and Noise:*

26.1 If an ANESTHETIC GAS MONITOR is included as a part or integral to other equipment, the relevant specification for that equipment shall apply.

26.2 If, when tested, as described in 26.3, the A-weighted sound pressure level exceeds 60 dB, the circumstances under which it occurs shall be noted.

NOTE 4—If an accessory intended for a particular application reduces the A-weighted sound pressure level to 60 dB(A) or below, the manufacturer should state in which part or parts of the operating range this occurs.

26.3 The A-weighted sound pressure level shall be measured as follows:

26.3.1 *Measuring Instruments*—A precision sound level meter of Type 1, as specified in IEC 651, shall be used. Measurements shall be made with the A-weighted network in use and the "slow" meter characteristics selected. The sound level meter shall be calibrated in accordance with the manufacturer's instructions.

26.3.2 *Test Environment*—Measurement shall be made in a free field over a reflecting plane, such as that specified in ISO 3744.

NOTE 5—The necessary conditions may be achieved economically on a hard, flat surface outdoors, in a large room, or in a smaller room with sufficient sound absorptive materials on its walls and ceiling.

26.3.3 *Ambient Conditions*—At the microphone positions, the A-weighted sound pressure levels of the background noise shall be at least 10 dB below the sound pressure level to be measured.

NOTE 6—If barometric pressure, temperature, or relative humidity deviate from those of standard conditions, appropriate corrections may be used.

26.3.4 *Anesthetic Gas Monitor Installation*—The ANESTHETIC GAS MONITOR shall be mounted as recommended by the instructions for use and in a manner typical of its intended use. If it is intended to be table-mounted, the table top shall be a hard, acoustically reflecting surface, unless a resilient pad is recommended in the installation instructions. If it is wall-mounted, the wall shall be of hard, acoustically reflecting material.

26.3.5 *Procedure*—Operate the ANESTHETIC GAS MONITOR over its normal working range. Place the microphone at the position of maximum sound pressure level in the horizontal plane passing through the geometric center of the ANESTHETIC GAS MONITOR and at a radius of 1 m. At each setting, if the ANESTHETIC GAS MONITOR is intended for use with a sampling tube, make a second measurement using the recommended sampling tubing. Place the sampling tubing inlet so as to lie on the specified horizontal plane, with the axis of the sampling tubing vertical and 150 mm from the microphone on the axis between the ANESTHETIC GAS MONITOR and the microphone. If the length of the sampling tubing does not allow this disposition, move the microphone toward the ANESTHETIC GAS MONITOR until the distance between it and the sampling tubing is 150 mm. If the manufacturer recommends or supplies accessories for particular diagnostic applications and states that these reduce the A-weighted sound pressure level to 60 dB or less, repeat the measurements with the accessories fitted. If any such accessory incorporates a port intended for connection to a tracheal or tracheostomy tube, connect the tube of an internal diameter equal to or greater than that of the port and at a length such that its other end will be sufficiently distant from the sound level meter not to interfere with the noise measurements.

27. *Pneumatic and Hydraulic Power*—The requirements given in Clause 27 of the General Standard shall apply.

28. *Suspended Masses*—The requirements given in Clause 28 of the General Standard shall apply.

SECTION FIVE—PROTECTION AGAINST HAZARDS FROM UNWANTED OR EXCESSIVE RADIATION

(*1*) The requirements given in Clauses 29 through 35 of this section of the General Standard shall apply.

(*2*) The manufacturer shall mark the device with a warning to refer to the accompanying documents for the expected adverse effects on the performance of the anesthetic gas monitor when exposed to electrocautery, electrosurgery, defibrillation, X-ray (gamma radiation), infrared radiation, conducted transients, magnetic fields including magnetic resonance imaging (MRI), and radiofrequency interference that are known at the time of preparation of the accompanying documents.

36. *Electromagnetic Compatibility*—The requirements in Clause 36 of the General Standard apply, with the following addition (the test method in 36.1 is derived from IEC 801-2:1991:

36.1 *Protection from Electrostatic Discharge*—The ANESTHETIC GAS MONITOR shall continue to function and meet the requirements of this draft specification or shall fail without causing a safety hazard when tested in accordance with IEC 801-2. The discharges shall have a potential of 3 kV ± 5 % dc for a contact discharge and 8 kV± 5 % dc for an air discharge. Discharges shall be applied only to accessible parts and coupling planes (as defined in IEC 801-2). If an anomaly occurs, such as display interrupt, alarm activation, etc., it should be possible to restore normal operation within 30 s after the electrostatic discharge has been applied. (Silencing of an activated alarm shall not be considered a failure.)

SECTION SIX—PROTECTION AGAINST HAZARDS OF IGNITION OF FLAMMABLE ANESTHETIC MIXTURES

37. *Locations and Basic Requirements*—The requirements given in Clause 37 of the General Standard shall apply.

38. *Marking, Accompanying Documents*—The requirements given in Clause 38 of the General Standard shall apply.

39. *Common Requirements for CATEGORY AP and CATEGORY APG EQUIPMENT*—The requirements given in Clause 39 of the General Standard apply.

40. *Requirements and Tests for CATEGORY AP EQUIPMENT, Parts and Components Thereof* —The requirements given in Clause 40 of the General Standard shall apply.

41. *Requirements and Tests for CATEGORY APG EQUIPMENT, Parts and Components Thereof*—The requirements given in Clause 41 of the General Standard shall apply.

SECTION SEVEN—PROTECTION AGAINST EXCESSIVE TEMPERATURES AND OTHER SAFETY HAZARDS

42. *Excessive Temperatures*—The requirements given in Clause 42 of the General Standard shall apply.

43. *Fire Prevention*—The requirements given in Clause 43 of the General Standard apply, together with the following additional requirements:

43.1 In order to eliminate the risk of fires caused by electrical components which may be a source of ignition in oxygen or nitrous oxide enriched atmospheres (or mixtures of gases containing anesthetic gases referred to in Clause 37), at least one of the following requirements shall be met:

(a) Electrical components shall be separated from compartments in which accumulations of such gases can occur by a barrier complying with the requirements given in 43.2.

(b) Compartments containing electrical components shall be ventilated according to the requirements given in 43.3 of this draft specification.

(c) Electrical components, which in normal use and single fault condition can be a source of ignition, shall comply with the requirements given in Clause 43.5 of this draft specification.

43.2 Any barrier required under the provisions of 43.1(*a*) shall be sealed at all joints and at any holes for cables, shafts, or other purposes.

(*1*) Compliance shall be checked by the following methods, as appropriate:

(*a*) Inspection;
(*b*) By compliance test for enclosures with restricted breathing, given in 40.5 of the General Standard;
(*c*) If, under normal conditions, a pressure difference exists between the spaces separated by the barrier, the test method given in 43.4.

43.3 The ventilation required in 43.1(*b*) shall be such that, when tested by the method described in 43.5, the oxygen level in the enclosed compartment containing electrical components shall not exceed 4 % above the ambient oxygen level; if this requirement is met by forced ventilation, an alarm shall be provided to warn of failure of the ventilation.

43.4 Oxygen levels in enclosed compartments shall be tested as follows:

43.4.1 *Principle*—The oxygen level in the enclosed compartment is measured after the ANESTHETIC GAS MONITOR has been operated for 18 h under single fault conditions.

43.4.2 *Procedure*—Place the ANESTHETIC GAS MONITOR in a room in which the air exchange is between 3 and 10 room volumes per hour. Flow 100 % O_2 through the ANESTHETIC GAS MONITOR at the maximum diverting flow. Switch off the mains supply and measure the oxygen level in the enclosed compartment. Operate the ANESTHETIC GAS MONITOR under single fault conditions, with the least favorable control setting selected and with the mains voltage deviating by ±10 %, if applicable. After 18 h, switch off the supply mains and measure the oxygen level in the enclosed compartment.

43.4.3 *Expression of Results*—Record the oxygen levels measured at the beginning and end of the 18 h period.

43.5 Electrical circuits, which can produce sparks or generate increased surface temperatures and which can be a source of ignition, shall be so designed that no ignition occurs. The following requirement shall be satisfied in normal condition and single fault condition:

(*1*) The surface temperature of components shall not exceed 300°C, unless it can be shown that no ignition occurs when the component(s) is(are) exposed to 100 % O_2 at temperatures above 300°C.

(*2*) Short- and open-circuiting of resistors, capacitors, and inductances complying with the requirements given in Clause

14 of IEC 65:1985 are not considered to be single fault conditions.

43.6 Compliance shall be checked by measuring the surface temperatures of the components under normal and single fault conditions. If the surface temperature of the component(s) exceeds 300°C, inspect for ignition when the component(s) is(are) exposed to 100 % O_2 at the measured temperature.

44. *Overflow, Spillage, Leakage, Humidity, Ingress of Liquids, Cleaning, Sterilization and Disinfection*—The requirements given in Clause 44 of the General Standard apply, as well as those given in "Good Manufacturing Practices" issued by the Food and Drug Administration.[6]

45. *Pressure Vessels and Parts Subject to Pressure*—The requirements given in Clause 45 of the General Standard apply, except for 45.7(*b*), and with the following addition:

45.7(*c*) It shall be so installed that it is accessible for inspection, maintenance, and repair according to the accompanying documents.

46. *Human Errors*—The requirements given in Clause 46 of the General Standard apply, together with the following additional clauses:

46.1 Connections for calibration gases for which Diameter Index Safety System (DISS) or Pin Index Safety System (PISS) are not specified shall not be interchangeable with diameter or pin index systems.

46.2 Colors of calibration gas cylinders not already specified in relevant national standards, such as CGA C-9-1982, shall be color-coded differently from the colors specified for medical gases.

46.3 Compliance with the requirements in 46.1 and 46.2 shall be determined by inspection of the accompanying documents and the ANESTHETIC GAS MONITOR.

47. *Electrostatic Discharges*—The requirements given in Clause 47 shall apply.

48. *Materials in Applied Parts in Contact with the Body of the Patient*—The requirements given in Clause 48 of the General Standard apply.

49. *Interruption of the Power Supply*—The requirements given in Clause 49 of the General Standard apply.

SECTION EIGHT—ACCURACY OF OPERATING DATA AND PROTECTION AGAINST HAZARDOUS OUTPUT

50. *Accuracy of Operating Data*—The requirements given in Clause 50 of the General Standard apply, with the following additional clauses:

50.3 *Measurement Accuracy:*

(*1*) For halogenated anesthetic gases, the difference between the mean ANESTHETIC GAS READING and the ANESTHETIC GAS LEVEL shall be within ± (0.15 volume percent + 15 % of ANESTHETIC GAS LEVEL) over the full measurement range specified in the accompanying documents. In addition, six standard deviations of the ANESTHETIC GAS READINGS (for a given ANESTHETIC GAS LEVEL) shall be less than or equal to 0.6 volume percent.

(*2*) For nitrous oxide, the difference between the mean ANESTHETIC GAS READING and the ANESTHETIC GAS LEVEL shall be within ± (2.0 volume percent + 8 % of the ANESTHETIC GAS LEVEL) over the full measurement range specified in the accompanying documents. In addition, six standard deviations of the ANESTHETIC GAS READINGS (for a given nitrous oxide level) shall be less than or equal to 10.0 volume percent.

(*3*) Compliances shall be checked by the test given in 50.4.

50.4 *Test Method:*

50.4.1 *Principle*—ANESTHETIC GAS READINGS are determined at a number of anesthetic gas levels spanning the ANESTHETIC GAS MONITOR measurement range.

50.4.2 Test gases of an accuracy equal to or better than 0.03 % of the tolerance of the essential requirement stated in clause 50.3 as determined by gravimetric methods shall be used for these tests. Alternative methods of certifying gas composition accuracy may be substituted for the gravimetric method if the alternative method can be shown to be equivalent or better than the gravimetric method.

50.4.3 *Dry Gas Testing*—The anesthetic gas monitor shall be set up in accordance with the accompanying documents and tested using dry test gas mixtures, given in Table 1, at an ambient temperature of 23 ± 2°C. For each numerically displayed anesthetic gas, verify that the accuracy requirements of 50.3 are met.

50.4.4 *Water Saturated Gas Testing:*

(*1*) Connect the ANESTHETIC GAS MONITOR to a simulated breathing system containing air fully saturated with water at 37 ± 2°C, with the system being cycled at a frequency of 10 breaths/min between a pressure of ambient and 35 cm H_2O (3.5 kPa).

(*2*) Following the accompanying documents, with the sampling site connected to the breathing system, operate the monitor with condensate visible at the sampling site for a minimum of 1 h.

(*3*) At this point, perform an accuracy test using the gas mixtures given in Table 2 (with a dry gas accuracy of 0.03 volumes percent as in Clause 50.4.2) fully saturated at 37 ± 2°C.

TABLE 2 Dry Gas Test Mixtures

NOTE 1—5 % CO_2 is used for all gas mixtures containing halogenated gases except for the mixtures containing 0.5 % halothane, 1.0 % isoflurane, and 5.0 % enflurane, all of which contain no appreciable amounts of CO_2.

O_2, %	CO_2,%[A]	N_2O, %	Halothane, %	Isoflurane,%	Enflurane, %
100					
bal		65	0.5		
bal	5	65	1.0		
bal	5	65	4.0		
bal	5	65		0.5	
bal		65		1.0	
bal	5	65		5.0	
bal	5	65			0.5
bal	5	65			1.0
bal		65			5.0
bal	5	50			
		100			

[A] CO_2 may be excluded from the test gas mixture if the anesthetic gas monitor is not intended for use in gas mixtures containing CO_2.

[6] Available from Good Manufacturing Practices for Medical Devices, Food and Drug Administration, 5600 Fishers Lane (HF2-220), Rockville, MD 20857, or call 800-638-2041.

50.5 *Drift of Measurement Accuracy:*

(*1*) The anesthetic gas monitor shall meet the requirements specified in 50.3 for no less than 6 h when used in accordance with the accompanying documents.

(*2*) Compliance shall be checked by the test given in 50.6.

50.6 *Test Methods:*

50.6.1 *Test Method (Water Saturated):*

(*1*) This requirement does not apply to ANESTHETIC GAS MONITORS intended solely for use in dry fresh gas mixtures.

(*2*) Continue to operate the anesthetic gas monitor as specified in 50.4.4, sampling the gas test mixtures in Table 2 every 2 h for a minimum of 6 h.

50.6.2 *Test Method (Dry Gas):*

(*1*) If the ANESTHETIC GAS MONITOR is tested by the method in Clause 50.6.1, this clause does not apply.

(*2*) The ANESTHETIC GAS MONITOR shall be set up in accordance with the accompanying documents under the ambient conditions described in Clause 50.4.3. Connect the ANESTHETIC GAS MONITOR to a simulated common gas outlet supplying dry air at 23 ± 2°C into a simulated breathing system, with the system cycling at a frequency of 10 ± 1 breaths/min at an I:E ratio of 1:2 ± 20 %, between a pressure of ambient and 3.5 ± 0.5 kPa (35 ± 5 cm H_2O) above ambient.

(*3*) Operate the monitor for a minimum of 1 h, and after that time perform an accuracy test using the dry gas method as described in Subclause 50.4.3, with the test gas mixtures given in Table 2.

(*4*) Continue to operate the ANESTHETIC GAS MONITOR for a minimum of 6 h, repeating the accuracy test every 2 h.

50.7 *Displays:*

(*1*) ANESTHETIC GAS LEVEL displays shall be marked continuously or on operator demand with kPa or V/V % (volume percent) anesthetic gas.

(*2*) Displays should not be obscured by the hand normally adjusting the control(s) associated with the display.

(*3*) Compliance shall be determined by inspection of markings and instructions for use.

51. *Protection Against Hazardous Output*—The requirements given in Clause 51 of the General Standard are replaced by the following:

51.1 *Control Function and Position:*

(*1*) The measurement and test positions of controls shall be clearly distinguishable.

(*2*) When the display of a non-measurement mode is not obviously distinguishable from a normal monitoring display, the ANESTHETIC GAS MONITOR shall return automatically from such nonmeasurement mode to normal monitoring mode within a period not exceeding 1 min of no operator interaction.

(*3*) Calibration controls shall include a means to prevent inadvertent change from the intended position.

NOTE 7—User-operable function checks, other than "power on" for test controls such as battery condition or signal operation, should return automatically from the check, test, or override position within a period not exceeding 1 min of no operator interaction.

NOTE 8—All other controls should also include means to prevent inadvertent change from the intended position and should have clearly distinguishable positions.

51.2 *Movement of Controls:*

(*1*) For controls that consist of a movable part and a non-movable part, movement upwards, to the right, or in a clockwise direction shall increase the control function. Movement downwards, to the left, or in an anti-clockwise direction shall decrease the control function.

(*2*) Rotary gas flow controls are exempt from this requirement.

NOTE 9—Controls and their associated markings should be visible or legible, or both, to an operator having a visual acuity (corrected, if necessary) of at least 1.0 when the operator is located at least 1 m in front of the ANESTHETIC GAS MONITOR and the illuminance level is 215 lx. Controls should be identified clearly with their associated markings.

51.3 *ALARMS:*

51.3.1 *Alarm Prioritization*—The alarm characteristics of monitors specified in this specification shall be grouped in three categories: HIGH PRIORITY, MEDIUM PRIORITY, and LOW PRIORITY (see Tables 3-5).

51.3.1.1 The audible components of these alarms should be designed to allow silencing until the ANESTHETIC GAS MONITOR is placed in use (that is, connected to the patient) in order to reduce nuisance alarms.

51.3.1.2 There shall be a visual indication that an audible alarm has been silenced.

51.3.1.3 The set points of adjustable alarms shall be indicated continuously or on user demand.

51.3.2 HIGH PRIORITY ALARMS:

51.3.2.1 There shall be a visual indication of the HIGH PRIORITY ALARM. It shall be different and distinguishable from the visual signals specified in 51.3.3 and 51.3.4.

51.3.2.2 There shall be a simultaneous audible indication of the HIGH PRIORITY ALARM. This audible indication shall be different and distinguishable from the audible signals specified in 51.3.3 and 51.3.4.

51.3.2.3 The audible indicators shall reset automatically when the condition causing the alarm has cleared.

51.3.2.3.1 Alphanumeric or computer-generated graphic displays are exempt from color and flashing frequency requirements. However, if an alphanumeric or computer generated graphics display does not meet the visual requirements as given in Table 3, an alternative visual method that does meet those requirements shall be employed. The visual indicators of alarm categories in Table 3 shall conform to the requirements of ASTM F29.03.04, under consideration.

51.3.2.3.2 Compliance shall be checked by functional tests and inspections, to be furnished by the manufacturer in the operator's manual.

51.3.3 *MEDIUM PRIORITY ALARMS:*

TABLE 3 Alarms[A]

Priority	Operator Response	Audible Indicators	Indicator Color and Flashing Frequency
High	immediate	not medium or low priority	red/1.4 to 2.8 Hz
Medium	prompt	not high or low priority	yellow/0.4 to 0.8 Hz
Low	awareness	not high or medium priority	yellow/constant (on)

[A] A single color indicator per category is sufficient to satisfy the requirements in the table above.

TABLE 4 Test Concentrations of Interfering Gases or Vapors, %

Nitrogen	78 (use medical air)
Nitrous oxide	80
Helium	50
Halothane	5
Enflurane	5
Isoflurane	5
Ethanol	specified by manufacturer
Acetone	specified by manufacturer
(Chlorodifluoromethane)	5

TABLE 5 Test Gases for Pressure Effects

O_2, %fx	CO_2,%[A]	N_2O, %	Halothane, %	Isoflurane,%	Enflurane, %
bal	5	65	4.0		
bal	5	65		0.5	
bal	5	65			1.0

[A] CO_2 may be excluded from the test gas mixture if the anesthetic gas monitor is not intended for use in gas mixtures containing CO_2.

51.3.3.1 There shall be a visual indication of the MEDIUM PRIORITY ALARM. It shall be different and distinguishable from the visual signals specified in 51.3.2 and 51.3.4.

51.3.3.2 There shall be a simultaneous audible indication of the MEDIUM PRIORITY ALARM. This audible indication shall be different and distinguishable from the audible signals specified in 51.3.2 and 51.3.4.

51.3.3.3 The audible indicator shall reset automatically when the condition causing the alarm has cleared.

51.3.4 *LOW PRIORITY ALARMS:*

51.3.4.1 There shall be a visual indication of the LOW PRIORITY ALARM. It shall be different and distinguishable from the visual signals specified in 51.3.2 and 51.3.3.

51.3.4.2 The audible indicator, if provided, shall reset automatically when the condition causing the alarm has cleared.

51.4 *Alarm Characteristics:*

51.4.1 The ANESTHETIC GAS MONITOR shall have high anesthetic gas reading alarm(s) for halogenated ANESTHETIC GAS(ES).

51.4.2 The ANESTHETIC GAS MONITOR may have (a) low ANESTHETIC GAS READING.

51.4.3 Alarm set points for both high and, if provided, low ANESTHETIC GAS READING shall be operator-adjustable.

51.4.4 When the ANESTHETIC GAS MONITOR is switched on, the high ANESTHETIC GAS READING for halogenated anesthetic gas(es) shall be (a) medium priority signal(s).

51.4.5 If low ANESTHETIC GAS READING are provided, they shall be low priority signal(s).

51.4.6 If the ANESTHETIC GAS MONITOR has an operator-adjustable high ANESTHETIC GAS READING alarm priority control, it shall allow the operator to change the ALARM priority between MEDIUM and HIGH PRIORITY only after the ANESTHETIC GAS MONITOR is switched on.

51.4.7 If the ANESTHETIC GAS MONITOR has an automatic change in ALARM priority setting, it shall change only to a higher alarm priority, and only after activation of the MEDIUM PRIORITY ALARM.

(*1*) Compliance shall be checked by inspection.

51.4.8 The difference between the ALARM SET POINT and the ANESTHETIC GAS READING when the alarm is activated shall not exceed 0.2 volumes percent for halogenated anesthetic gas(es) and 2.0 volumes percent for nitrous oxide.

(*1*) Compliance shall be checked by the procedure given in 51.4.9.

51.4.9 Generate at least four stable ANESTHETIC GAS READINGS that span the range of the alarm system in approximately equal steps by varying the ANESTHETIC GAS LEVEL delivered to the SENSOR, or by electrically stimulating the SENSOR, or by adjusting the calibration control (if provided).

(*1*) For each ANESTHETIC GAS READING, adjust the ALARM SET POINT so that the alarm is deactivated. Incrementally adjust the ALARM SET POINT until the alarm is activated, and record the ANESTHETIC GAS READING at which the alarm is activated. The difference between the ALARM SET POINT and the corresponding ANESTHETIC GAS READING shall not exceed 0.2 volumes percent for halogenated gases and 2 volumes percent for nitrous oxide.

51.5 *Announcement of Alarm Condition:*

51.5.1 If ALARM SET POINTS are adjustable by the operator, operator adjustment of ALARM SET POINTS or DEFAULT PARAMETERS shall require a deliberate sequence of actions on the part of the operator. Temporary silencing of audible alarms, if provided, shall not exceed 2 min. The visual signals shall remain until the alarming condition no longer exists. If permanent silencing of the audible portion is provided, the control shall require deliberate action on the part of the operator and shall incorporate a design feature to impede accidental alarm silencing. The visual indication shall remain until the operator re-enables the audible alarm.

51.5.2 All alarms shall be provided with a DEFAULT SETTING, and that DEFAULT SETTING shall be disclosed in the accompanying documents.

SECTION NINE—ABNORMAL OPERATION AND FAULT CONDITIONS

(*1*) Clauses 52 and 53 of the General Standard apply.

SECTION TEN—CONSTRUCTIONAL REQUIREMENTS

(*1*) Clauses 54 and 55 of the General Standard apply.

56. *Components and General Assembly:*

(*1*) This clause of the General Standard applies, except as follows:

Components of the ANESTHETIC GAS MONITOR should be made of materials that are compatible with the gases and agents with which those components are designed to come into contact, thus minimizing health risks due to substance leached from the anesthetic agent monitor in use

(*2*) Clauses 57, 58, and 59 of the General Standard apply.

6. Additional Requirements Specifically Related to Anesthetic Gas Monitors

60. *Interfering Gas and Vapor Effects (Other Than Water Vapor):*

60.1 The manufacturer shall disclose, in the accompanying documents, known effect on ANESTHETIC GAS READINGS (if any) caused by the gases given at the nominal concentrations listed in Table 6. The manufacturer shall make available

TABLE 6 Test Gas Mixtures (Dry) for Water Saturated Testing

O_2, %	CO_2,%[A]	N_2O, %	Halothane, %	Isoflurane,%	Enflurane, %
100					
bal	5	65	4.0		
bal	5	65		0.5	
bal	5	65			1.0

[A] CO_2 may be excluded from the test gas mixture if the anesthetic gas monitor is not intended for use in gas mixtures containing CO_2.

upon request the test methods used to make such determination.

61. *Pressure Effects:*

61.1 ANESTHETIC GAS MONITORS shall either:

(a) Meet the requirements given in 50.3 following exposure of the sampling site to a nominal positive pressure of 10 kPa (100 cm H_2O) and a nominal negative pressure of 1.5 kPa (15 cm H_2O) for 5 s each for 20 cycles; or

(b) be marked with the warning "not for use in breathing systems," and a similar warning shall appear in the accompanying documents.

(*1*) Compliance with (*a*) shall be checked by the test given in 61.2.

61.2 Compliance shall be tested as follows:

61.2.1 *Principle*—The accuracy of the ANESTHETIC GAS READINGS is determined after exposure of the SENSOR to pressure changes.

61.2.2 *Procedure*—Cycle the pressure at the SAMPLING SITE between a positive pressure with respect to ambient of 10 $\pm$ 1 kPa (100 $\pm$ 10 cm H_2O) and a negative pressure with respect to ambient of 1.5 $\pm$ 0.2 kPa (15 $\pm$ 2 cm H_2O) for not less than 5 s each. Repeat this procedure 20 times, and then conduct the test for measurement accuracy using the dry gas method as described in Subclause 50.4.3, using the gases listed in Table 3.

62. *Sample Gas Exhaust Port:*

62.1 For DIVERTING ANESTHETIC GAS MONITORS, an exhaust port shall be provided to collect or route the diverting gas from the anesthetic gas monitor.

(*1*) Compliance shall be checked by inspection.

63. *Breathing System Connections*—If an ANESTHETIC GAS MONITOR is intended to be connected to the breathing system through a T-piece, the breathing system connection ports of the T-piece shall be a 15 or 22 mm, or both, conical connector in accordance with Specification F 1054 (or ISO 5356-1). The sampling gas and outlet ports of a DIVERTING ANESTHETIC GAS MONITOR shall not be interchangeable with the breathing system connection ports of a breathing system.

64. *Obstruction of the SAMPLING TUBE:*

64.1 The DIVERTING ANESTHETIC GAS MONITOR shall have a means to indicate obstruction of the SAMPLING TUBE.

(*1*) Compliance shall be checked by the test given in 64.2.

64.2 *Test Method*—With the ANESTHETIC GAS MONITOR operating according to the accompanying documents, obstruct the SAMPLING TUBE totally, and verify that the requirements of 64.1 are met.

65. *Contamination of Breathing Systems*—It shall not be possible to reverse the direction of flow through the SAMPLING TUBE in a DIVERTING ANESTHETIC GAS MONITOR.

APPENDIX

(Nonmandatory Information)

X1. RATIONALE

X1.1 *Rationale for Modification of Clause 6.7*—Dot matrix and alphanumeric displays, as well as computer generated graphics, are not considered, for purposes of this specification, to be indicator lights, so that they do not need to meet the IEC requirements of having specific colors according to whether they indicate a high priority or a medium priority alarm. It was thought that the displays and graphics were sufficiently "attention getting" so that they did not require associated alarm lights.

X1.2 *Rationale for Clause 6.7 Relating to Instructions for Use (Numbers 1 to 8)* —The need to know the basic workings of the anesthetic gas monitor, its principles of operation, and many of its detailed specifications should be self-evident. It is necessary that the user have any or all of this information available, and that he know well any possible adverse effect on the claimed function of the analyzer due to any of a number of different conditions, for example, condensation from excess humidity, interfering gases, sensitivity to mechanical shocks, fluctuations in barometric pressure or supply voltage, etc. It should be equally self-evident that the user must be provided with instructions for proper operation of the anesthetic gas monitor as listed in Numbers 6 and 7 of that clause.

X1.3 *Rationale for Clause 7: Power Input*—This is a typical statement which says that this particular requirement of the parent document, IEC 601-1 (1988), applies without any exemptions from, or additions to, the requirements as stated.

X1.4 *Rationale for Clause 8: Basic Safety Requirements* —The phase "not used" means that the original requirements in Clause 8 of the 1977 edition of IEC 601-1 are not used in the current (1988) edition of IEC 601-1.

X1.5 *Rationale for Clause 26.2*—It is important that the anesthetic gas monitor not generate so much noise in normal operation that it masks conversation or the sound of other alarms within the operating room.

X1.6 *Rationale for Clause 36.1*—Anesthetic Gas Monitors are not life-support devices, but a "vigilance adjunct." Therefore, it is acceptable if this device fails without creating a safety hazard (that is, without affecting patient safety directly) or presenting erroneous data. The test voltages of 8 kV for air discharges and 3 kV for contact discharges using the IEC 801-2 (1991) network and procedure are adequate to ensure good performance under the conditions in which anesthetic gas monitors are used. It is necessary to limit the application of discharges to accessible parts, since to allow the application of charges to the interior of the device would require the device to have internal barriers that would make service of the device more difficult and costly. It is reasonable to require any person opening a device for maintenance to exercise both common sense and accepted work practices, which include ESD precautions.

X1.7 *Rationale R43.5*—Historical perspective is that the 10 VA requirement was intended to provide a general criteria of good practice for the design of power dissipating elements which may be required to operate in an Oxygen-enriched atmosphere. The implication is that these specific design limitations prevent ignition-producing elements from being designed.

NOTE X1.1—Curiously enough, the criteria stated does little in a real sense to provide practical direction in design for a lower possibility of ignition, and that is why the requirement, "The product of the RMS value of the no-load voltage and the RMS value of the short circuit current shall not exceed 10 VA," was removed.(*1*) All electrical circuits dissipate power (there is no such thing as a 100 % efficient circuit). Dissipation of power naturally raises surface temperatures of components in the circuit. Therefore, the clause applies to *all* electrical circuits.

(*2*) The maximum surface temperature of the power-dissipating element is the primary parameter of interest with respect to ignition in an oxygen-rich environment. Every flammable compound has a unique and intrinsic surface temperature above which ignition occurs spontaneously if oxygen is present. Therefore, the specification should be written in such a manner that emphasis is placed on controlling surface temperatures below the intrinsic ignition point for all flammable elements.

(*3*) The requirement for 10 VA as the maximum product of RMS no-load voltage and RMS short-circuit current implies a maximum power dissipation and therefore implies "good practice" with respect to maintaining surface temperatures below the ignition temperature. In fact, it does not, as it does not limit power or temperature.

(*4*) The reason that it does not limit power is that it is not a measure of the power being dissipated under any" normal" circumstance. Under no load (zero current conditions), the power dissipated by the circuit element is zero. (Power = V × I, and RMS no-load voltage multiplied by zero current is zero.) Under short-circuit current, the power is undefined. This is because modern circuits, and especially power supplies, usually have provisions to actively reduce the drive voltage when abnormally low circuit resistance is detected ("foldback" under short-circuit conditions).

(*a*) Thus, the voltage and current used in the calculation specified occur under cases of either no power dissipation, or undefined (or abnormally low-by design) power dissipation, and do not indicate the maximum power dissipation of the circuit under worst-case load. Most high power circuits are designed to dissipate maximum power in some intervening condition of load between no load and short circuit.

(*5*) The maximum power dissipation of the circuit does not determine the surface temperature of the element. Circuit elements in common design are designed to dissipate 100 watts easily, ten times the implied power of the clause, without significant increase in surface temperatures. They simply have a large heat-sinking capability, designed to accommodate the high levels of power dissipated. Certainly, this is an example of "good practice" and should not be restricted by the specification.

(*a*) Because of these facts, it is very unlikely that any piece of equipment with significant electronics will meet the criteria stated in the clause for all elements of the design. Power supply designers, as a matter of practice, would not be able to meet the specification as presently stated; nor would they be likely to use the information to provide design direction, due to its simplistic view. Therefore, this clause is commonly disregarded, and other criteria are used to qualify the ignition-resistance of the equipment design.

(*b*) While this clause may have merit in providing guidance for relatively simple circuit designs, it is felt that it is not comprehensive enough to provide direction for the more complex modern designs and does not even speak to the issue of primary concern, assurance that ignition surface temperatures are not exceeded in normal or single fault conditions.

X1.8 *Rationale R50.3: Measurement Accuracy*—The required accuracies for halogenated anesthetic gases and nitrous oxide were probably the single most extensively discussed subject during committee deliberations. The committee furthermore had before it the results of extensive deliberations at the international level on the same subject. The final figures were arrived at after clinicians both nationally and internationally stated their "clinical requirements" for deviation from actual values at different concentrations of halogenated anesthetics and nitrous oxide (that is, clinically permissible inaccuracy of the readout). The resultant values, when the device is operating within these specifications, are compared in the table below with the statement of clinical requirements.

Actual Anesthetic Gas Concentration, %	Clinical Requirement for Accuracy	Resultant Performance Accuracy, %
	Halogenated Agents, %	
0.50	±0.20	±0.23
1.00	±0.30	±0.30
1.50	±0.30	±0.38
2.50	±0.50	±0.53
4.00	±1.00	±0.75
	Nitrous Oxide, %	
40	±5.0	±5.2
50	±5.0	±6.0
60	±6.0	±6.8
80	±8.0	±8.4

(*1*) There was concern among manufacturers that one random reading beyond the accuracy specified would be viewed as a failure to perform to the specification, and clinicians were concerned that the relatively simple accuracy specifications proposed would allow periodic cycling within the accuracy limits to be accepted.

To resolve both of these concerns, and provide a specification supported by classical statistical methods, two refinements were added. Specifically, the term "mean" was added to the accuracy specification, indicating that the monitor was to be tested in such a manner that deviation of the recorded value for the displayed gas reading from the true mean was to be statistically insignificant. The method by which this is to be accomplished is left to the discretion of the testing party, but methods are well known, and the confidence tests of methodology are well founded in the mathematics of statistics.

(*2*) The randomness of the data displayed (often referred to as "noise") is critical not only to the test methodology, but to the user as well. It is important not only to develop figures of merit for this parameter, but also to establish the method by which this parameter will be measured.

In general, randomness is found to occur in a Gaussian (normal) distribution. The mathematics of such distributions are well known and allow relatively simple calculations to be performed to establish the practical range of readings. As an example:

68.27 % of all the readings occur within ±1.0 sigma (standard deviation) from the mean.
95.45 % of all the readings occur within ±2.0 sigma from the mean.
99.73 % of all the readings occur within ±3.0 sigma from the mean.
99.9937 % of all the readings occur within ±4.0 sigma from the mean.

There is a general consensus that the limit of practical consideration for the values of a Gaussian set is bounded by ±3.0 sigma (99.73 %). While it is still possible for a reading to occur beyond this limit, it only occurs 0.27 % of the time. (Approximately 1 reading in 400 will be beyond this limit, versus 1 reading in 20 for± 2.0 sigma, or 1 reading in 15 000 for ±4.0 sigma.)

(*3*) The fact that the deviations of readings are easily quantifiable (by calculation of the standard deviation) then allows for simple methods to be used to establish limits of clinical acceptability.

(*4*) The randomness specification for halogenated agents states: "in addition, six standard deviations of the anesthetic gas readings (for a given anesthetic gas level) shall be less than or equal to 0.6 volumes percent."

Six standard deviations is equivalent to ±3.0 sigma (and shall not exceed 0.6 volumes percent).

This means that 68.27 % (just over 2/3) of all the readings occur within± 0.1 volumes percent from the mean reading; that 95.45 % (just over 19/20) of all the readings occur within ±0.2 volumes percent from the mean reading; and that 99.73 % (about 399/400) of all the readings occur within ±0.3 volumes percent from the mean reading.

(*5*) The randomness specification for nitrous oxide states: "in addition, six standard deviations of the anesthetic gas readings (for a given nitrous oxide level) shall be less than or equal to 10.0 volumes percent."

(*6*) Six standard deviations is equivalent to± 3.0 sigma (and shall not exceed 10.0 volumes percent). This means that 68.27 % (just over 2/3) of all the readings occur within ±1.7 volumes percent from the mean reading; that 95.45 % (just over 19/20) of all the readings occur within ±3.3 volumes percent from the mean reading; and that 99.73 % (about 399/400) of all the readings occur within ±5.0 volumes percent from the mean reading.

X1.9 *Rationale for Clause 50.4.2*—After review of many possibilities, the committee felt that it was reasonable, especially from the point of view of clinical requirements and economics, that test gases, in order to provide the required operating accuracies as stated in R50.3 just above, needed to be equal to or better than 1/5 of the required accuracies. That is to say, that test gases for halogenated anesthetic agents had to have a concentration known within± 0.04 volumes percent of the stated concentration; similarly, for nitrous oxide, the test gas would have to be certified to be within ±1 volume percent of the claimed concentration.

X1.10 *Rationale for Table 2, Which is Part of the Description of the Procedure to Confirm Accuracy of the Anesthetic*—The menu of test gases outlined in Table 1 was constructed in order to cover the complete spectrum of possible concentrations of background gases (that is, oxygen or carbon dioxide, or both) and halogenated anesthetics. It will be noted that the concentrations recommended may provide for testing of several gases at the same time. (For example, the third mixture listed in the table can be used to calibrate an anesthetic agent analyzer at 5 % carbon dioxide test point, a 65 % nitrous oxide test point, and a 1 % halothane concentration test point, with the background gas being oxygen.) Five percent carbon dioxide was chosen because it is the usual concentration of exhaled carbon dioxide. The values of 0.5, 1, and 4 % halogenated agent are used merely to span the usual range of concentrations of these anesthetics clinically available.

X1.11 *Rationale R50.4.4: Water Saturated Gas Testing*—This test is run after 1 h of simulated breathing system conditions so that the anesthetic agent analyzer is exposed to fully saturated gas and the varying pressures typically seen in an anesthetic breathing circuit. The test is designed to demonstrate that the anesthetic agent monitor will function well under these two potentially interfering conditions.

X1.12 *Rationale R50.5: Drift of Measurement Accuracy*—The test period of 6 h, during which the anesthetic gas monitor should have a limited drift in its measuring accuracy, was chosen because many anesthetic cases last that long and it is not unreasonable to use a gas monitor for that period of time without having to re-calibrate it.

X1.13 *Rationale R51.1: Control Function and Position, Note 7*—This note indicates a desirability to avoid a potential malfunction after the user tests some function, leaves the associated control in the test position, and then attempts to use the monitor clinically.

X1.14 *Rationale for Clause 51.3: Alarms*—This entire section has been constructed carefully to provide the following: a mandatory high concentration alarm, an optional low concentration alarm, and operator-adjustable alarm set points for both high and low concentration alarms. The committee also felt (Clause 51.3.4) that when the gas monitor was first turned on, the high concentration alarm should be a medium priority signal (that is, that operator response be prompt but need not be urgent). The committee was concerned with two factors when arriving at this conclusion: (*1*) they wanted to avoid a proliferation of high priority alarms on the anesthesia machine and in the operating room; and (*2*) a higher-than-expected-concentration of anesthetic agent required only a prompt operator response because, in most instances, this was not an immediate life threatening situation.

X1.15 *Rationale R51.4*—A great deal of effort has been expended in the discussion of alarm methodology for anesthetic gas monitors. A great deal of progress has been made to resolve the underlying conflict in existing equipment design philosophy between two "competing" alarm strategies.

(*1*) Most digital-based monitor alarm systems now allow the operator to set the high and low (if provided) alarming point by means of a digital display that reflects precisely the display value which will either:

(a) Cause the alarm to be activated when the anesthetic gas displayed concentration equals the *alarm* setting; or

(b) Causes the alarm to be activated when the anesthetic gas displayed concentration *exceeds* the alarm setting (further complicated by low alarms, as the alarm activation occurs when the display value is incrementally *less than* the alarm setting).

(*2*) It was decided to clarify (with terminology and a graphic representation) the full aspects of alarms. It was felt that clarifying all of the aspects of the alarm systems was required to bring resolution of this complex issue (see Fig. 2).

(*3*) Thus, a number of general terms were defined and assigned a name, and a corresponding graphic representation of these terms was generated. The ground rules were as follows:

(a) Define the alarm set point as the setting that relates to the intended displayed value at which alarm activation occurs. This definition speaks to the *intent* of the clinician, rather than the specific design strategy of the monitor.

(b) Alarm limit was removed as a defined term, and the specification (Clause 51.4.8) re-written to speak to alarm accuracy as simply the difference between the alarm set point and the displayed reading at which the alarm activation occurs. (Basically, this means that the alarm set point is now defined to be the *intended*alarm limit.)

(c) Accommodate the two alarm strategies within the tolerance of accuracy specified for the alarms. This, in effect, clarifies that the most important aspect to specify is the maximum acceptable difference between the displayed reading at alarm activation and the displayed reading at which the clinician intended the alarm to be activated (the new definition of alarm set point).

(*4*) This simplification could be reached when the monitor manufacturers realized that the practical implementation of digital monitoring systems caused very close correlation between the alarm set point display and the displayed reading, thereby allow alarm activation to Strategy B to occur one display digit past the alarm setting and still be well within the alarm accuracy tolerance under consideration. This, then, met the original intent of allowing both alarm strategies to occur within the same specification.

(*5*) To restate the present situation, Clause 51.4.8 specifies the maximum difference between the alarm set points and the displayed readings at which alarm activation occurs, with a maximum allowable difference that accommodates either alarm strategy.

Designation: F 1453 – 92 (Reapproved 1996)

Standard Guide for Training and Evaluation of First Responders Who Provide Emergency Medical Care[1]

This standard is issued under the fixed designation F 1453; the number immediately following the designation indicates the year of original adoption or, in the case of revision, the year of last revision. A number in parentheses indicates the year of last reapproval. A superscript epsilon (ε) indicates an editorial change since the last revision or reapproval.

1. Scope

1.1 This guide covers the minimum training standards for First Responders (FRs) who may be responsible for the initial care of sick and injured persons of all ages in the prehospital environment.

1.2 The scope of training will be in accordance with Guide F 1287.

1.3 Included in this guide is a standard for knowledge and skill evaluation.

1.4 This guide does not suggest a particular training sequence.

1.5 *Operating within the framework of this guide may expose emergency medical service personnel to hazardous materials, procedures and equipment. This standard does not purport to address all of the safety concerns, if any, associated with its use. It is the responsibility of the user of this standard to establish appropriate safety and health practices and determine the applicability of regulatory limitations prior to use.* For specific precautionary statements, see the documents cited in 2.2.

2. Referenced Documents

2.1 *ASTM Standards:*

F 1031 Practice for Training the Emergency Medical Technician (Basic)[2]

F 1177 Terminology Relating to Emergency Medical Services[2]

F 1287 Guide for Scope of Performance of First Responders Who Provide Emergency Medical Care[2]

2.2 *Code of Federal Regulations:*[3]

Part 1910.1030 of Title 29 of the Code of Federal Regulations Concerning Bloodborne Pathogens

Part 1910.120 of Title 29 of the Code of Federal Regulations Concerning Hazardous Materials Emergency Response & Training

Part 1910.132 of Title 29 of the Code of Federal Regulations Concerning Personal Protective Equipment

Part 331.000 of Title 21 of the Code of Federal Regulations Concerning Registration of Medical Devices

2.3 *Other Documents:*

Most recent Standards and Guidelines for Cardiopulmonary Resuscitation and Emergency Cardiac Care as reprinted from the Journal of the American Medical Association (JAMA)[4]

3. Terminology

3.1 *Definitions of Terms Specific to This Standard:*

3.1.1 *basic life support/cardiopulmonary resuscitation (BLS/CPR)*—a set of skills that includes airway management, chest compressions, and others as defined by the American Heart Association (AHA).

3.1.2 *first responder (FR)*—an individual trained to provide initial care for sick or injured persons in accordance with this guide.

4. Significance and Use

4.1 This guide is for those responsible for the development and implementation of training and evaluation programs for first responders (FRs).

4.2 At the beginning of the program, students shall be informed of the course objectives and requirements for successful completion.

4.3 This guide is not intended for use as a training guide for emergency ambulance personnel.

5. Required Performance Objectives

5.1 The FR shall be trained to perform the following skills. These skills are not necessarily listed in the order in which they are to be taught or that in which they may have to be performed during the prehospital care of a sick or injured person.

5.1.1 *Roles and Responsibilities*—Describe and demonstrate an understanding of the roles and responsibilities of the FR for the provision of prehospital emergency care within the local emergency medical services (EMS) system.

5.1.2 *Medicolegal Aspects*—Describe and demonstrate an understanding of the medicolegal aspects of a FR's provision of emergency medical care in the jurisdiction having authority, including, but not limited to, duty to act, standard of care,

[1] This guide is under the jurisdiction of ASTM Committee F-30 on Emergency Medical Services and is the direct responsibility of Subcommittee F30.02 on Personnel, Training and Education.

Current edition approved Dec. 15, 1992. Published March 1993.

[2] *Annual Book of ASTM Standards*, Vol 13.01.

[3] Available from Standardization Documents Order Desk, Bldg. 4 Section D, 700 Robbins Ave., Philadelphia, PA 19111-5094, Attn: NPODS.

[4] Available from American Heart Association, 7320 Greenville Ave., Dallas, TX 75231.

consent to care, forcible restraint, abandonment, documentation, and any applicable Good Samaritan Laws.

5.1.3 *Vital Signs and other Indicators of a Sick or Injured Person's Condition*—Determine and record vital signs exhibited by a sick or injured person, including pulse, respiration, skin color, temperature and moistness, level of consciousness, and an estimate of blood pressure.

5.1.4 *Emergency Medical Identification*—Identify the most commonly used medical identification devices and apply the information contained on or in the device to patient assessment and patient care procedures.

5.1.5 *Primary Assessment*—Conduct an assessment for problems that are a threat to life if not corrected immediately, including an inadequate airway, inadequate respirations, inadequate circulation, and profuse bleeding, using spinal precautions as appropriate.

5.1.6 *BLS/CPR*—Conduct basic life support procedures, including the establishment and maintenance of an open airway and the restoration of breathing and circulation by means of cardiopulmonary resuscitation.

5.1.7 *Bleeding*:

5.1.7.1 Control external bleeding by means of direct pressure and elevation.

5.1.7.2 Identify the likelihood of internal bleeding through the observation of signs, symptoms, and mechanisms of injury.

5.1.7.3 Care for a patient who exhibits the signs and symptoms of internal bleeding.

5.1.8 *Dressing and Bandaging*:

5.1.8.1 Identify items that can be used to control external bleeding and minimize the contamination of open wounds.

5.1.8.2 Apply pressure dressings that will control bleeding and minimize the contamination of open wounds.

5.1.9 *Shock*:

5.1.9.1 Recognize the likelihood that shock may occur or be present on the basis of patient assessment and observation of a mechanism of injury.

5.1.9.2 Provide anti-shock measures as a part of routine patient care.

5.1.10 *Mechanical Aids to Breathing*:

5.1.10.1 Use available mechanical devices to ensure the maintenance of an open airway.

5.1.10.2 Use available mechanical devices to assist ventilation.

5.1.10.3 Use available oxygen delivery equipment.

5.1.10.4 Use available suction equipment.

5.1.11 *Secondary Assessment*:

5.1.11.1 Conduct a methodical head-to-toe physical examination to discover conditions not found during the primary assessment.

5.1.11.2 Interview the sick or injured person to obtain facts relevant to the person's condition.

5.1.11.3 Interview co-workers, witnesses, family members, or other individuals to obtain facts relevant to the person's condition.

5.1.12 *Musculoskeletal Injuries*:

5.1.12.1 Identify the various types of musculoskeletal injuries.

5.1.12.2 Immobilize and otherwise care for suspected fractures, dislocations, sprains, and strains with available equipment.

5.1.13 *Spine Injuries*:

5.1.13.1 Determine the likelihood of a spinal injury on the basis of the patient assessment and an observation of a mechanism of injury.

5.1.13.2 Perform manual spinal stabilization.

5.1.13.3 Immobilize a person who has a suspected spinal injury with available equipment.

5.1.14 *Emergency Evacuation*—Alone or with a partner, use the most appropriate assist, drag, or carry to move a sick or injured person from a dangerous location to a safe place.

5.1.15 *Patient Transfer*—Use an available patient-carrying method or device to move a sick or injured person from the place of initial care to the location of transport.

5.1.16 *Non-Traumatic Chest Pain*:

5.1.16.1 Identify a patient who is experiencing non-traumatic chest pain on the basis of the patient assessment.

5.1.16.2 Care for a patient who is experiencing non-traumatic chest pain.

5.1.17 *Respiratory Distress*:

5.1.17.1 Identify a patient who is experiencing respiratory distress on the basis of the patient assessment.

5.1.17.2 Care for a patient who is experiencing respiratory distress.

5.1.18 *Diabetic Emergencies*:

5.1.18.1 Identify a diabetic emergency on the basis of the patient assessment.

5.1.18.2 Care for a patient who is experiencing a suspected diabetic emergency.

5.1.19 *Seizures*:

5.1.19.1 Identify a patient who is experiencing or has experienced a seizure on the basis of the patient assessment.

5.1.19.2 Care for a patient who is experiencing or has experienced a seizure.

5.1.20 *Poisoning*:

5.1.20.1 Identify poisoning as the possible cause of a patient's medical emergency on the basis of the patient assessment.

5.1.20.2 Care for a patient who has ingested a poisonous substance.

5.1.20.3 Care for a patient who has inhaled a poisonous substance.

5.1.20.4 Care for a patient who has absorbed a poisonous substance.

5.1.20.5 Care for a patient who has been injected with a poisonous substance.

5.1.21 *Altered Level of Consciousness*:

5.1.21.1 Identify a patient with an altered level of consciousness on the basis of the patient assessment and an observation of a mechanism of injury.

5.1.21.2 Care for a patient whose level of consciousness has been altered.

5.1.22 *Burns*:

5.1.22.1 Determine the severity of burns, including degree, body surface area, type, and location.

5.1.22.2 Care for a patient who has thermal burns.

5.1.22.3 Care for a patient who has chemical burns.

5.1.22.4 Care for a patient who has electrical burns.

5.1.23 *Environmental Emergencies*:

5.1.23.1 Determine that a medical emergency has resulted from exposure to heat or cold on the basis of the patient assessment.

5.1.23.2 Care for a patient who is experiencing heat cramps.

5.1.23.3 Care for a patient who is experiencing heat exhaustion.

5.1.23.4 Care for a patient who is experiencing heat stroke.

5.1.23.5 Care for a patient who is experiencing frostbite.

5.1.23.6 Care for a patient who is experiencing hypothermia.

5.1.24 *Special Patient Situations*—Care for patients who have special needs, such as children, the elderly, and the physically and developmentally challenged.

5.1.25 *Triage*:

5.1.25.1 Categorize the victims of multiple casualty incidents, according to the severity of injury or illness, on the basis of patient assessments.

5.1.25.2 Use triage tags or other identification devices available locally to indicate priorities for prehospital emergency care and transportation to medical facilities.

5.1.26 *Multiple Casualty Incidents*:

5.1.26.1 Work as a member of a team to perform triage at locations of multiple casualty incidents.

5.1.26.2 Work as a member of a team to perform patient assessments at locations of multiple casualty incidents.

5.1.26.3 Work as a member of a team to conduct patient care procedures at the locations of multiple casualty incidents.

5.1.27 *Potential Dangers*:

5.1.27.1 On the basis of an assessment of a scene, take steps to minimize the chance of injury or death to all involved when confronted with a potentially life-threatening situation.

5.1.27.2 Utilize appropriate precautions to minimize the risk of disease transmission.

5.1.28 *Entrapment Situations*:

5.1.28.1 Identify accident-related hazards and undertake hazard control measures consistent with the capabilities of the FR and available equipment.

5.1.28.2 Use available equipment safely to gain access to persons who are entrapped.

5.1.28.3 Use available equipment safely to disentangle persons from entrapment mechanisms.

5.1.29 *Childbirth*:

5.1.29.1 Evaluate a mother to determine whether delivery is imminent.

5.1.29.2 Assist with a normal delivery.

5.1.29.3 Care for the mother and baby.

5.1.29.4 Identify abnormal childbirth situations, and care for the mother and baby within the FR's capabilities.

5.1.30 *Critical Incident Stress*:

5.1.30.1 Identify stressors that may affect the performance of a FR.

5.1.30.2 Identify stressors that may affect the behavior of a sick or injured person.

5.1.30.3 Conduct procedures to minimize critical incident stress.

5.1.31 *Patient Information*—Communicate the observations and actions of the FR to whomever patient care is transferred.

6. Optional Objectives

6.1 The roles and responsibilities for the provision of initial emergency medical care vary among FRs. When the responsibilities for initial emergency medical care are limited, the ability of a FR to perform the tasks in Section 5 may be sufficient to ensure satisfactory care. When a FR must care for a greater variety of illnesses and injuries, additional training shall be necessary.

7. Evaluation

7.1 There shall be a final written and practical evaluation that measures the ability of the FR to meet the objectives listed in Section 5.

7.2 There shall be established pass/fail criteria or a method for grading, or both.

7.3 There shall be a method of remediation.

7.4 There shall be a method for retesting.

8. Keywords

8.1 basic life support; basic life support/cardiopulmonary resuscitation (BLS/CPR); emergency medical services (EMS); emergency medical technician (EMT); first responder (FR); prehospital; triage

Standard Specification for Capnometers[1]

This standard is issued under the fixed designation F 1456; the number immediately following the designation indicates the year of original adoption or, in the case of revision, the year of last revision. A number in parentheses indicates the year of last reapproval. A superscript epsilon (ϵ) indicates an editorial change since the last revision or reapproval.

INTRODUCTION

The measurement of carbon dioxide in a gaseous mixture has become a common practice in many areas of clinical medicine, such as anesthesia, respiratory therapy, pediatrics, and intensive care. This draft specification establishes minimum safety and performance requirements for capnometers based on parameters that are achievable within the limits of existing technology.

Appendix X1 contains a rationale for the most important requirements. It is included to provide additional insight for the reasoning that led to the requirements and recommendations that have been incorporated into this draft specification.

This draft specification references IEC 601-1:1988 (hereafter referred to as the General Standard) for many of the general requirements for safety. Requirements specific to capnometers begin at Clause 60.

1. Scope

1.1 The scope given in Clause 1 of the General Standard applies except that 1.1 shall be replaced by the following:

1.1.1 This specification specifies requirements for the safety and performance of capnometers as defined in Subclause 3.5. It applies to capnometers used with adults, children, and neonates.

1.1.2 It does not apply to devices solely intended for use as cutaneous monitors.

1.1.3 Capnometers intended for use in laboratory research applications are outside the scope of this specification.

2. Referenced Documents

2.1 The following standards contain provisions which, through reference in this text, constitute provisions of this specification. At the time of publication, the editions indicated were valid. All standards are subject to revision, and parties to agreements based on this specification are encouraged to investigate the possibility of applying the most recent editions of the standards listed below.

2.2 *ASTM Standards:*

F 1054 Specification for Conical Fittings of 15 mm and 22 mm sizes[2]

F 1463 Specification for Alarm Signals in Medical Equipment Used in Anethesia and Respiratory Care[3]

2.3 *ISO Standards:*[3]

ISO 32:1977 Gas Cylinders for Medical Use—Marking for Identification of Contents

ISO 5356/1:1987 Anaesthetic and Respiratory Equipment—Connectors, Part I: Cones and Sockets

ISO 5356/2:1987 Anaesthetic and Respiratory Equipment—Connectors, Part II: Screw-Threaded-Weight-Bearing Connectors

ISO 7249 Controls—Terms, Suitability, Design Requirements

ISO 7250 Basic List of Anthropomorphic Measurements

2.4 *IEC Standards:*[3]

IEC 65:1985 Safety Requirements for Mains Operated Electronic and Related Apparatus for Household and Similar Use

IEC 79-3:1972 Electrical Apparatus for Explosive Atmospheres—Part III: Spark Test Apparatus for Intrinsically Safe Units

IEC 79-4:1975 Electrical Apparatus for Explosive Gas Atmospheres—Part IV: Method of Test for Ignition Temperature

IEC 601-1:1988 Safety of Medical Electrical Equipment—Part I: General Safety Requirements

IEC 801-2:1991 Electromagnetic Compatibility for Industrial-Process Measurement and Control Equipment—Part 2: Electrostatic Discharge Requirements

3. Terminology

3.1 *Definitions*—For the purposes of this specification, the definitions given in Clause 2 of the General Standard apply, along with the following definitions:

3.1.1 *accuracy*—the quality that characterizes the ability of a device to give indications approximating to the true value of

[1] This specification is under the jurisdiction of ASTM Committee F-29 on Anesthetic and Respiratory Equipmentand is the direct responsibility of Subcommittee F29.11on Gas Monitors.

Current edition approved December 15, 1992. Published June 1993.

[2] *Annual Book of ASTM Standards*, Vol 13.01.

[3] Available from American National Standards Institute, 1430 Broadway, New York, NY 10018.

the quantity measured.

3.1.2 *alarm*—a warning signal.

3.1.3 *alarm set point*—the setting of the adjustment control, or display value, which indicates the carbon dioxide reading, at or beyond which the alarm is intended to be activated.

3.1.3.1 *Discussion*—Terms such as "alarm limits" or "alarm threshold" are frequently used to describe the same function.

3.1.4 *alarm system*—those parts of the capnometer which: (*1*) establish the alarm set point(s); and (*2*) activate an alarm when the carbon dioxide reading is less than or equal to the low-alarm set point, if provided, or is equal to or greater than the high-alarm set point.

3.1.5 *capnometer*—a device for the measurement of carbon dioxide concentration or partial pressure in ventilatory gases.

3.1.5.1 *Discussion*—The capnometer consists of all equipment including accessories, sensor, and sampling tubing (if a diverting capnometer) specified by the manufacturer for the intended use of the capnometer.

3.1.6 *carbon dioxide level*—the concentration of carbon dioxide in gaseous mixture.

3.1.6.1 *Discussion*—This may be expressed in any suitable unit such as percent by volume or partial pressure in kPa (or mm Hg).

3.1.7 *carbon dioxide reading*—the measured carbon dioxide level as indicated by the capnometer display.

3.1.8 *cutaneous oxygen and carbon dioxide partial pressure monitoring equipment*—equipment or associated transducers, or both, for the monitoring or recording, or both, of partial pressures of oxygen and carbon dioxide at the skin surface.

3.1.9 *delay time*—the time from a step function change in CO_2 concentration or partial pressure at the sampling site to the achievement of 10 % of final CO_2 value in the capnometer (see Fig. 1).

3.1.10 *display*—the visual representative of output data.

3.1.11 *diverting capnometer*—a capnometer that transports a portion of respired gases from the sampling site through a sampling tube to the sensor, which is remote from the patient.

3.1.12 *high-priority alarm*—an indication of danger and meaning that immediate action on the part of the operator is required.

3.1.13 *interference with measurement accuracy*— the difference between the carbon dioxide reading in the presence of an interfering gas mixture and the carbon dioxide reading in a corresponding mixture in which the interfering gas or vapor fraction has been replaced by nitrogen.

3.1.14 *low-priority alarm*—an indication of a condition that requires awareness on the part of the operator, but not necessarily action.

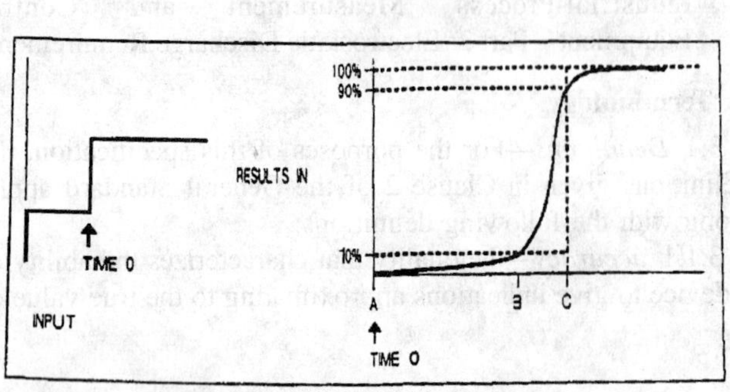

FIG. 1 Response Time (Total System Response)

3.1.15 *medium-priority alarm*—an indication meaning that prompt action on the part of the operator is required.

3.1.16 *non-diverting capnometer*—a capnometer that uses a sensor at the sampling site.

3.1.17 *oxygen level*—the concentration of oxygen in a gaseous mixture.

3.1.17.1 *Discussion*—This may be expressed in any suitable unit such as percent by volume or partial pressure in kPa (or mm Hg).

3.1.18 *partial pressure*—the pressure that each gas in a gas mixture would exert if it alone occupied the volume of the mixture at the same temperature.

3.1.19 *percent (%) v/v carbon dioxide (or other gases)*—the level of carbon dioxide (or other gas) in a mixture, expressed as a percent volume fraction.

3.1.20 *rise time*—the time required to achieve a rise from 10 to 90 % of the final CO_2 value in the capnometer when a step function change in CO_2 concentration or partial pressure occurs at the sampling site (see Fig. 1).

3.1.21 *sampling site*—the location at which respiratory gases are diverted for measurement to a remote sensor in a diverting capnometer or the location of the sensor area in a non-diverting capnometer.

3.1.22 *sampling tubing*—the conduit for transfer of respiratory gases from the sampling site to the sensor in a diverting capnometer.

3.1.23 *sensor*—the part of the capnometer that is sensitive to the presence of carbon dioxide.

3.1.24 *sensor area*—the part of the sensor at which carbon dioxide is detected.

3.1.25 *total system response time*—the sum of the delay time and the rise time (see Fig. 1).

3.1.26 *transducer*—a device for converting the partial pressure or concentration of a gas into a signal for monitoring or recording.

4. Relationship of This Specification to the General Standard

	(A)	(NA)	(AM/R)[A]
Section One—General			
1. Scope and object			X
2. Terminology and definitions			X
3. General requirements			X
4. General requirements for tests			X
5. Classification	X		
6. Identification, marking and documents			X
7. Power input	X		
Section Two—Environmental Conditions			
8. Basic safety requirements (not used)			
9. Removable protective means (not used)			
10. Environmental conditions	X		
11. Special measures with respect to safety (not used)			
12. SINGLE FAULT CONDITION (not used)			
Section Three—Protection Against Electric Shock Hazards			
13. General	X		
14. Requirements related to classification	X		
15. Limitation of voltage and/or energy	X		

16. Enclosures and PROTECTIVE COVERS	X		
17. Separation	X		
18. Protective earthing, functional earthing, and potential equalization	X		
19. Continuous LEAKAGE CURRENTS and PATIENT AUXILIARY CURRENTS			X
20. Dielectric strength	X		
Section Four—Protection Against Mechanical Hazard			
21. Mechanical strength			X
22. Moving parts	X		
23. Surfaces, corners, and edges	X		
24. Stability in NORMAL USE	X		
25. Expelled parts	X		
26. Vibration and noise (not used)			
27. Pneumatic and hydraulic power	X		
28. Suspended masses	X		
Section Five—Protection Against Hazards from Unwanted or Excessive Radiation			
29. X-radiation	X		
30. Alpha, beta, gamma, neutron radiation and other particle radiation	X		
31. Microwave radiation	X		
32. Light radiation (including lasers)	X		
33. Infra-red radiation	X		
34. Ultra-violet radiation	X		
35. Acoustical energy (including ultrasonics)	X		
36. Electromagnetic compatibility			X
Section Six—Protection Against Hazards of Ignition of Flammable Anaesthetic Mixtures			
37. General	X		
38. Marking, ACCOMPANYING DOCUMENTS	X		
39. Common requirements for Category AP and Category APG EQUIPMENT	X		
40. Requirements and tests for Category AP EQUIPMENT, parts or components thereof	X		
41. Requirements and tests for Category APG EQUIPMENT, parts or components thereof	X		
Section Seven—Protection Against Excessive Temperatures and Other Safety Hazards			
42. Excessive temperatures	X		
43. Fire prevention			X
44. Overflow, spillage, leakage, humidity, ingress of liquids, cleaning, sterilization, and disinfection			X
45. Pressure vessels and parts subject to pressure	X		
46. Human errors			X
47. Electrostatic charges	X		
48. Materials in APPLIED PARTS in contact with the body of the PATIENT	X		
49. Interruption of the power supply	X		
Section Eight—Accuracy of Operating Data and Protection Against Hazardous Output			
50. Accuracy of operating data (not used)			
51. Protection against hazardous output			X
Section Nine—Abnormal Operation and Fault Conditions; Environmental Tests			
52. Abnormal operation and fault conditions	X		
53. Environmental tests	X		
Section Ten—Constructional Requirements			
54. General	X		
55. ENCLOSURES and covers	X		
56. Components and general assembly	X		
57. MAIN PARTS, components and layout	X		
58. Protective earthing—terminals and connections	X		
59. Construction and layout	X		
Additional Clauses			
60. Interfering gas and vapor effects other than water vapor	X		
61. Sustained pressure	X		
62. Gas leakage and sampling loss	X		
63. Connectors	X		

[A] A = applies, NA = not applicable, and AM/R = applies with an amendment, addition, or revision to the requirement in the General Standard.

5. Clauses Containing Amendments, Additions, or Replacements to the Text in IEC 601-1:1988

NOTE 1—The clause numbers used reference the specific section in the General Standard.

4. *General Requirements and General Requirements for Tests*—Clauses 3 and 4 of the General Standard apply together with the following additions:

4.12 Test methods other than those specified in this draft specification, but of equal or greater accuracy, may be used to verify compliance with the requirements of this draft specification. However, in the event of dispute, the methods specified in this draft specification shall be used as the reference methods.

4.13 Components of the capnometer should be made of materials that are compatible with the gases and agents with which those components are designed to come into contact.

6. *Identification, Marking, and Documents*—The requirements given in Clause 6 of the General Standard apply together with the following additions and modifications:

(*1*) In the preamble to Clause 6, replace the first item under "clearly legible" by the following:

Warning statements, instructive statements, or drawings: affixed in a permanent location and legible to a user with a visual acuity of 1.0 (corrected if necessary) from a distance of 1 m at an illuminance level of 215 lx.

(*2*) In 6.1, replace item (*d*) by the following:

If the size of the capnometer does not permit the complete marking as specified throughout this clause, at least the following shall be marked on the capnometer: the name of the manufacturer, a serial or lot or batch identifying number, and Symbol 14 in Table D1 of the General Standard.

(*3*) In 6.1, add the following to item (*f*): a serial number or other lot or batch identifier.

(*4*) In 6.1, add the following to item (*q*): the words "not for use in breathing systems," if applicable.

(*5*) In 6.1, add additional items as follows:

(*zz*) Marking on the capnometer shall additionally include the following:

(*a*) For capnometers not for use with inhalational anesthetic agents, the phrase "not for use with inhalation anesthetic agents," if applicable.

(*b*) If moisture has an adverse effect on performance, either a statement that the operator or user shall see the accompanying documents for the effect of moisture on accuracy, or Symbol 14 in Table D1.

(*c*) Abridged operating instructions for those capnometers that are intended as "free standing" types of devices.

(*d*) *Other Sources of Interference*—The manufacturer shall mark the device with a warning to refer to the accompanying documents or Symbol 14 in Table D1 of the General Standard for the expected adverse effects on the performance of the capnometer when exposed to electrocautery, electrosurgery, defibrillation, X-ray (gamma radiation) infra-red radiation, conducted transients, magnetic fields (that is, magnetic resonance imaging (MRI)), and radiofrequency interference known at the time of preparation of the accompanying documents.

NOTE 2—It is recommended that illustrated service information be provided to include the following: instructions for preventive maintenance and service calibration, and those adjustments that are necessary to maintain the capnometer in the correct operating condition, as well as a description of those adjustments and replacements that can be performed by the user.

(*6*) Clause 6.7 of the General Standard shall apply with the following modifications:

(*a*) Dot matrix, alphanumeric displays, and computer-generated graphics are not considered to be indicator lights.

(*b*) Compliance shall be checked by functional tests and inspections.

(*7*) In 6.8.2, add the following to item (*a*): The instructions for use shall additionally include the following information:

(*a*) A description of the purpose and intended use of the capnometer.

(*b*) A description of the principles of operation of the capnometer, including the relationship between gas concentration and its partial pressure, and the quantitative effects of humidity.

(*c*) A detailed specification including the following:

The carbon dioxide measurement range and the accuracy of measurement;
If gas diversion occurs, the gas diversion flow;
The stability of measurement accuracy;
The rise time;
The carbon dioxide level alarm range and its accuracy;
The operating and non-operating (storage) temperature ranges;
For sampling type capnometers, the gas diversion rate;
Power requirements; and
Time from switching on to obtaining specified operating performance.

(*d*) Details of any adverse effect on stated function due to the following:

Humidity or condensate, including, for example, any adverse effects if an adaptor is provided to improve the function of the sensor in the presence of condensation or particulate water;
Interfering gases or vapors;
Mechanical shock;
Cyclic pressure;
Barometric pressure or pressure at the site of use of the capnometer;
Fluctuation in line or battery voltage; and
If automatic compensation for barometric pressure is not provided, then the accompanying documents shall contain an explanation that the readings in concentration units are correct only under the pressure at which the capnometer is calibrated.

(*e*) An illustration of the features of the capnometer, indicating the location of all operating controls, adjustments, and system components necessary for correct operation.

(*f*) Instructions for operation of the capnometer, including the following:

Checking and calibration before use;
Routine inspection and testing; and
Recommended methods for cleaning and disinfection or sterilization.

(*g*) A description of an in-service test using a recommended test gas as the calibration gas.

(*h*) A description of the correct installation of the capnometer and a detailed description of sampling arrangements and any connecting tubing.

NOTE 3—If the capnometer requires a sensor cable or sampling tubing for connection from the capnometer to the sensing area, the cable or tubing should be of sufficient length to reduce the likelihood of its being elongated beyond its elastic limit and being stressed at the point or connection.

19. *Continuous Leakage Currents and Patient Auxiliary Currents*—The requirements given in Clause 19 of the General Standard apply except as follows:

(*1*) In item 19.1(*e*), add the following:

(*a*) For non-diverting capnometers at the sensor; and

(*b*) For diverting capnometers, at the junction of the sampling tubing and the body of the capnometer.

NOTE 4—Sampling tubing usually non-conducting. Input port most likely to represent an electrical hazard.

(*2*) Where national standards mandate more restrictive limits, these more restrictive limits shall apply.

21. *Mechanical Strength:*

(*1*) The requirements given in Clause 21 of the General Standard are replaced by the following:

21.1 Free-standing capnometers (that is, those not intended for use as an integral inseparable component of a larger system) and all separable components, such as sensors, shall be able to withstand mechanical shock and vibration, such that electrically live parts shall not become accessible.

(*2*) Compliance shall be checked by the test given in 21.7.

21.7 *Method of Test:*

21.7.1 *Principle*—The accuracy of the carbon dioxide reading, the rise time, and, if applicable, the alarm accuracy are determined after the capnometer and all separable components have been subjected to a mechanical shock.

21.7.2 *Procedure:*

(*1*) Attach the unpackaged items to be tested rigidly to a shock table machine. Apply three shocks in both directions along three mutually perpendicular axes of each test item (a total of 18 shocks to each item), taking care to ensure the following:

(*a*) That the shape of the shock pulse is in accordance with Fig. 2;

(*b*) That the acceleration amplitude (A) of the ideal half-sine pulse is 300 m/s2 (30 × gravity) and its duration (D) is 11 ms.

(*c*) That the oscillogram of the shock pulse includes a time approximately 33 ms (3 × D) long;

(*d*) That the measured acceleration pulse is contained between the broken-line boundaries shown in Fig. 2;

(*e*) That the measured velocity change (which may be obtained by integration of the acceleration pulse) is within the limits Vi_ 0.1 Vi, where the velocity change associated with the ideal pulse is Vi 2 × A × D/3.1416 2 × 300 × 0.011/3.1416 2.1 m/s; and

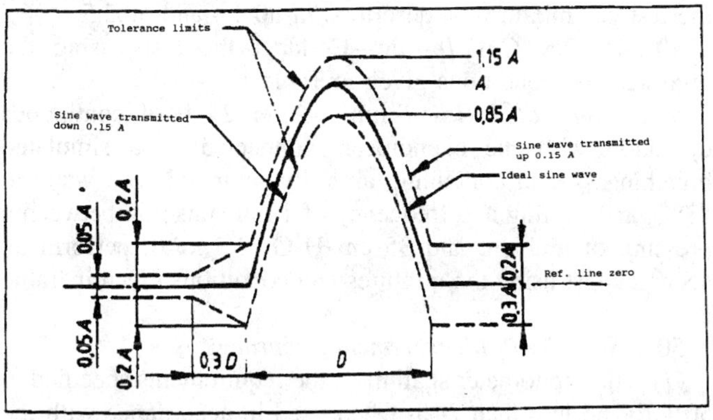

FIG. 2 Half Sine Shock Pulse Configuration and Its Tolerance Limits

(*f*) That the integration to determine velocity change extends from 4.4 ms (0.4 D) before the pulse to 1.1 ms (0.1 D) after the pulse.

(*2*) Inspect the capnometer to check that the appearance and condition of the capnometer, including the enclosure and warning or display indications or markings, have not been damaged or have not deteriorated in such a way as to prevent normal operation of the capnometer and that no electrically live parts have become accessible.

(*3*) Reattach any separable components to the capnometer and conduct the test for measurement accuracy as described in Clause 50.2 and the test for rise time as described in Clause 50.5 and, if the capnometer is fitted with a carbon dioxide level alarm, the test for carbon dioxide level alarm set point as described in Clause 51.4.9.

21.7.3 *Expression of Results*—Express the results as described in the relevant subclauses of Clause 51 and report any damage or the accessibility of live parts.

26. *Vibration and Noise:*

26.1 *Noise Output*—If a capnometer is included as a part or integral to other equipment, the relevant specification for that equipment shall apply.

26.2 If, when tested as described in 26.3, the A-weighted sound pressure level exceeds 60 dB, the circumstances under which it occurs shall be noted.

NOTE 5—If an attachment intended for a particular application reduces the A-weighted sound pressure level to 60 dB(A) or below, the manufacturer should state in which part or parts of the operating range this occurs.

26.3 The A-weighted sound pressure level shall be measured as follows:

26.3.1 *Measuring Instruments*—A precision sound level meter of Type 1, as specified in IEC Publication 651, shall be used. Measurements shall be made with the A-weighted network in use and the "slow" meter characteristics selected. The sound level meter shall be calibrated in accordance with the manufacturer's instructions.

26.3.2 *Test Environment*—Measurement shall be made in a free field over a reflecting plane such as that specified in ISO 3744.

NOTE 6—The necessary conditions may be achieved economically on a hard, flat surface outdoors, in a large room, or in a smaller room with sufficient sound absorptive materials on its walls and ceiling.

26.3.3 *Ambient Conditions*—At the microphone positions, the A-weighted sound pressure levels of the background noise shall be at least 10 dB below the sound pressure level to be measured.

NOTE 7—If barometric pressure, temperature, or relative humidity deviate from those of standard conditions, appropriate corrections may be used.

26.3.4 *Capnometer Installation*—The capnometer shall be mounted as recommended by the instructions for use and in a manner typical of its intended use. If it is intended to be table-mounted, the table top shall be a hard acoustically reflecting surface unless a resilient pad is recommended in the installation instructions. If it is wall-mounted, the wall shall be of hard acoustically reflecting material.

26.3.5 *Procedure*—Operate the capnometer over its normal working range. Place the microphone at the position of maximum sound pressure level in the horizontal plane passing through the geometric center of the capnometer and at a radius of 1 m. At each setting, if the capnometer is intended for use with a sampling tubing, make a second measurement using the recommended sampling tubing. Place the sampling tubing inlet so as to lie on the specified horizontal plane, with the axis of the sampling tubing vertical and 150 mm from the microphone. If the length of the sampling tubing does not allow this disposition, move the microphone toward the capnometer until the distance between it and the sampling tubing is 150 mm. If the manufacturer recommends or supplies attachments for particular diagnostic applications and states that these reduce the A-weighted sound pressure level to 60 dB or less, repeat the measurements with the attachments fitted. If any such attachment incorporates a port intended for connection to an endotracheal or tracheostomy tube, connect a tube of an internal diameter equal to our greater than that of the port and at a length such that its other end will be sufficiently distant from the sound level meter not to interfere with the noise measurements.

36. *Electromagnetic Compatibility*—The requirements in Clause 36 of the General Standard apply with the following addition (the test method in 36.1 is derived from IEC 801-2:1991):

36.1 Protection from electrostatic discharge.

43.4.1 *Principle*—The oxygen level in the enclosed compartment is measured after the capnometer had been operated for 18 h under single fault conditions.

43.4.2 *Procedure*—Place the capnometer in a room in which the air exchange is between 3 and 10 room volumes per hour. Set the oxygen flow through the capnometer so that it equals the maximum flows of oxygen and nitrous oxide under normal conditions. Switch off the mains supply, and measure the oxygen level in the enclosed compartment. Operate the capnometer under single fault conditions with the least favorable control setting selected and with the mains voltage deviating by ±10 %, if applicable. After 18 h, switch off the supply mains and measure the oxygen level in the enclosed compartment.

43.4.3 *Expression of Results*—Record the oxygen levels measured at the beginning and end of the 18 h period.

43.5 Electrical circuits which can produce sparks or generate increased surface temperatures, and which can be a source of ignition, shall be so designed that no ignition occurs. At least the following requirements shall be satisfied in normal and single fault condition:

(*1*) The surface temperature of components shall not exceed 300°C.

NOTE 8—If it can be shown that the component burns when subjected to overheating in 100 % oxygen but without propagating the fire, this component may have a surface temperature that exceeds 300°C.

(*2*) Short- and open-circuiting of resistors, capacitors, and inductances complying with the requirements given in Clause 14 of IEC 65:1985 are not considered to be single fault conditions.

(*3*) Compliance shall be checked by the test given in 43.6.

43.6 Measure or calculate the voltages and currents in stead state conditions and measure the surface temperatures in normal condition and single fault condition.

44. *Overflow, Spillage, Leakage, Humidity, Ingress of Liquids, Cleaning, Sterilization and Disinfection*—The requirements given in Clause 44 of the General Standard apply, with the following additions:

44.8 *Condensation Effects*—The manufacturer shall disclose in the accompanying documents the effects of the test listed in 66.2.5 on the performance of the capnometer other than accuracy.

44.9 *Obstruction of the Sensing Area or Sampling Tubing:*

(*1*) The capnometer shall have a means of indicating obstruction of the sensing area or sampling tubing.

(*2*) Compliance shall be checked by the test given in 44.10.

44.10 *Test Method*—Totally obstruct the sensing area or sampling tubing at the sampling site, and verify that the requirements of 44.11 are met.

44.11 *Contamination of Breathing Systems*—It shall not be possible to reverse the direction of flow through the sampling tube in order to purge the capnometer.

46. *Human Errors*—Clause 46 of the General Standard applies with the following addition:

46.1 Gas connections provided for calibration gases shall not be interchangeable with DISS or pin index systems, and cylinders shall be color-coded differently from the colors used for medical gases.

50. *Accuracy of Operating Data*—Replace Clause 50 of the General Standard with the following:

50.1 *Measurement Accuracy:*

(*1*) The carbon dioxide reading shall be within ± 12 % of the actual test gas value or ±4 mm Hg (0.53 kPa), whichever is greater, over the full range of the capnometer, corrected to one atmosphere (760 mm Hg).

(*2*) Compliance shall be checked by the test given in 50.2.

50.2 *Test Method:*

50.2.1 *Principle*—Carbon dioxide readings are determined at a number of carbon dioxide levels spanning the capnometer measurement range.

50.2.2 Test gases of an accuracy of 0.03 % as determined by gravimetric methods shall be used for these tests.

50.2.3 *Procedure*—The capnometer shall be set up in accordance with the accompanying documents and tested using the test gas mixtures as described in 50.2.4 and 50.2.5.

50.2.4 *Dry Gas Testing*—Conduct the tests using the mixtures and conditions given in Table 1.

50.2.5 *Saturated Gas Testing*—After 24 h of continuous operation with the capnometer connected to a simulated breathing system containing air fully saturated with water at 37°C, and cycling at a frequency of 10 breaths/min between a pressure of ambient and 35 cm H_2O (3.5 kPa), perform an accuracy test using the mixtures and conditions given in Table 2.

50.3 *Stability of Measurement Accuracy:*

(*1*) The capnometer shall meet the requirements specified in 50.1 for no less than 24 h when used in accordance with the accompanying documents.

(*2*) Compliance shall be checked by the test given in 50.4.

50.4 *Test Method*—Repeat the tests given in 50.2 at the end of 24 h.

50.5 *Rise Time*—The manufacturer shall disclose in the accompanying documents the rise time for a 10 to 90 % step change in concentration, when tested as described in 50.6 (both increase and decrease in concentration), and shall also disclose the flow required to meet the disclosed rise time.

50.6 *Test Method:*

(*1*) The capnometer shall be set up in accordance with the accompanying documents and arranged as in Fig. 3. Connect the carbon dioxide signal output of the capnometer to a suitable recording device with a resolution within 1 %, reproducibility within 1 %, and a time constant equal to or less than one-tenth of the expected rise time of the capnometer.

(*2*) Pass dry air at ambient temperature and at a flow of 10 L/min through the test apparatus and the capnometer with the capnometer switched to normal function. By means of the three-way tap, a dry calibrated gas at ambient temperature containing approximately 5 % (V/V) of carbon dioxide is passed through the apparatus and the rise time is calculated. Repeat the above procedure, switching from 5 % (V/V) carbon dioxide to air.

50.7 *Procedure*—Hold the ambient temperature of the capnometer constant to within ±2°C of a nominal value within the operating range specified in the accompanying documents. Generate at least four stable carbon dioxide readings that span the range of the alarm system in approximately equal steps by varying the carbon dioxide level delivered to the sensor, or by electrically stimulating the sensor, or by adjusting the calibration control.

50.8 *Displays*—Carbon dioxide (CO_2) level displays shall be marked with kPa, V/V %, or mm Hg. Units of measure shall be marked by (adjacent to) the display, or be displayed on demand.

NOTE 9—Displays should not be obscured by the hand normally

TABLE 1 Dry Gas Testing

Composition	Range in Percent	Temperature	Humidity
Mixture No. 1	Carbon Dioxide:[A] 0 %, 2.5, 5.0, and 10.0, balance nitrogen	23 ± 2°C	dry
Mixture No. 2	Carbon Dioxide: 0 %, 2.5, 5.0, and 10.0, balance air	23 ± 2°C	dry

[A] Carbon dioxide shall be expressed at one atmosphere, 23°C, as dry gas.

TABLE 2 Gas Testing Following Use in a Simulated Breathing System

Composition	Range in Percent	Temperature	Humidity
Mixture No. 1	Carbon Dioxide:[A] 0 %, 2.5, 5.0, and 10.0, balance nitrogen	37 ± 2°C	100 %
Mixture No. 2	Carbon Dioxide: 0 %, 2.5, 5.0, and 10.0, balance air	37 ± 2°C	100 %

[A] Carbon dioxide shall be expressed at ambient pressure, 37°C, saturated with water vapor.

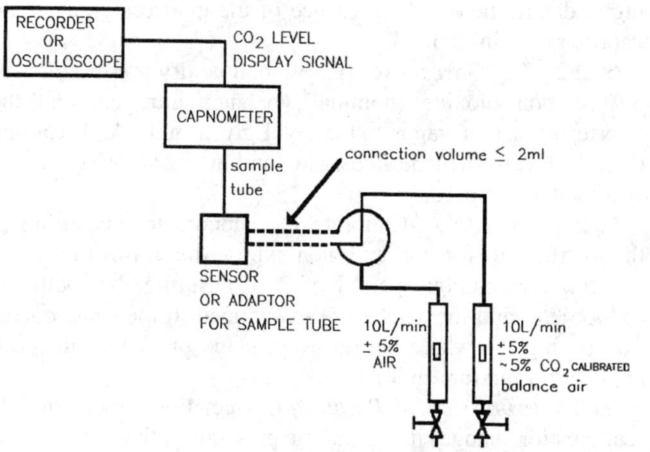

FIG. 3 Test Apparatus to Determine Response Time

adjusting the control(s) associated with the display.

51. *Protection Against Hazardous Output*—The requirements given in Clause 51 of the General Standard are replaced by the following:

51.1 *Control Function and Position:*

(*1*) If the intended test control function is not clearly distinguishable when displayed on the capnometer, the corresponding control(s) shall automatically return from such control function position(s). The positions of measurement and test controls shall be clearly distinguishable.

(*2*) Calibration controls shall include a means to prevent inadvertent change from the intended position.

NOTE 10—User-operable function checks other than "power on" for test controls, such as battery condition or signal operation, should automatically return from the check, test, or override position.

NOTE 11—All other controls should also include means to prevent inadvertent changes from the intended position and should have clearly distinguishable positions.

51.2 *Movement of Controls:*

(*1*) For controls that consist of a movable part and a non-movable part, movement upwards, to the right, or in a clockwise direction shall increase the control function. Movement downwards, to the left, or in an anti-clockwise direction shall decrease the control function.

(*2*) Rotary gas flow controls are exempt from this requirement.

NOTE 12—The separation between control knobs, switches, toggles, pinwheels, or push buttons should conform to the recommendations given in ISO 7249 and ISO 7250.

NOTE 13—Controls and their associated markings should be visible or legible, or both, to a user having a visual acuity (corrected, if necessary) of at least 1.0 when the user is located at least 1 m in front of the capnometer and the illuminance level is 215 lx. Markings should be identified clearly with their associated controls.

51.3 *Alarms:*

51.3.1 *Alarm Prioritization*—The alarm characteristics of monitors specified in this specification shall be grouped in three categories: high priority, medium priority, and low priority (see Table 3).

51.3.1.1 The audible components of these alarms should be designed to allow silencing until the capnometer is placed in use (that is, connected to the patient) in order to reduce nuisance alarms.

51.3.1.2 There shall be a visual indication that an audible alarm has been silenced.

51.3.1.3 The set points of adjustable alarms shall be indicated continuously or on user demand.

51.3.2 *High Priority Alarms:*

51.3.2.1 There shall be a visual indication of the high priority alarm. It shall be different and distinguishable from the visual signals specified in 51.3.3 and 51.3.4.

51.3.2.2 There shall be a simultaneous audible indication of the high priority alarm. This audible indication shall be different and distinguishable from the audible signals specified in 51.3.3 and 51.3.4.

51.3.2.3 The audible indicators shall reset automatically when the condition causing the alarm has cleared.

51.3.3 *Medium Priority: Alarms*

51.3.3.1 There shall be a visual indication of the medium priority alarm. It shall be different and distinguishable from the visual signals specified in 51.3.2 and 51.3.4.

51.3.3.2 There shall be a simultaneous audible indication of the medium priority alarm. This audible indication shall be different and distinguishable from the audible signals specified in 51.3.2 and 51.3.4.

51.3.3.3 The audible indicator shall reset automatically when the condition causing the alarm has cleared.

51.3.4 *Low Priority Alarms:*

51.3.4.1 There shall be a visual indication of the low priority alarm. It shall be different and distinguishable from the visual signals specified in 51.3.2 and 51.3.3.

51.3.4.2 There may be a simultaneous audible indication of the low priority alarm. This audible indication, if provided, shall be a low priority alarm. This audible indication shall be different and distinguishable from the audible signals specified in 51.3.2 and 51.3.3.

51.3.4.3 The audible indicator shall reset automatically when the condition causing the alarm has cleared.

51.4 *Alarm Characteristics:*

51.4.1 The capnometer shall have a high carbon dioxide

TABLE 3 Alarms

Alarm Category	Operator Response	Audible Indicators[A]	Indicator Color[B]	Flashing Frequency (Hz)[C]
High priority	immediate	not medium or low priority I	red	1.4 to 2.8 Hz (F_2)
Medium priority	prompt	not high or low priority	yellow	0.4 to 0.8 Hz (F_1)
Low priority	awareness	not high or medium priority	yellow	constant (on)

reading alarm for both inspired and exhaled carbon dioxide.

51.4.2 The capnometer should have a low carbon dioxide reading alarm for exhaled carbon dioxide.

51.4.3 Alarm set points for both high and (if provided) low carbon dioxide reading alarms shall be operator-adjustable.

51.4.4 When the capnometer is switched on, the high carbon dioxide reading alarms for carbon dioxide shall be a medium priority alarm.

51.4.5 If a low carbon dioxide reading alarm is provided, it shall be a medium priority alarm.

51.4.6 If the capnometer has an operator-adjustable high carbon dioxide reading alarm priority control, it shall allow the operator to change the alarm priority between medium and high priority only after the capnometer is switched on.

51.4.7 If the capnometer has an automatic change in alarm priority setting, it shall change only to a higher alarm priority, and only after activation of the alarm.

(*1*) Compliance shall be checked by inspection.

51.4.8 The difference between the alarm set point and the carbon dioxide reading when the alarm is activated shall not exceed 0.2 volumes percent (1.4 mm Hg at 760 mm Hg barometric pressure, BTPS) carbon dioxide.

(*1*) Compliance shall be checked by the procedure given in 51.4.9.

51.4.9 Generate at least four stable carbon dioxide readings that span the range of the alarm system in approximately equal steps by varying the carbon dioxide level delivered to the sensor, or by electrically stimulating the sensor, or by adjusting the calibration control (if provided).

(*1*) For each carbon dioxide reading, adjust the alarm set point so that the alarm is deactivated. Incrementally adjust the alarm set point until the alarm is activated, and record the carbon dioxide reading at which the alarm is activated. The difference between the alarm set point and the corresponding carbon dioxide reading shall not exceed 0.2 volumes percent.

51.5 *Announcement of Alarm Condition:*

51.5.1 If alarm set points are adjustable by the operator, operator adjustment of alarm set points or default parameters shall require a deliberate sequence of actions on the part of the operator.

(*1*) Temporary silencing of audible alarms, if provided, shall not exceed 2 min. The visual signals shall remain until the alarming condition no longer exists. If permanent silencing of the audible portion is provided, it shall require deliberate action on the part of the operator. The visual indication shall remain until the alarming condition no longer exists.

51.5.2 All alarms shall be provided with a default setting, and that default setting shall be disclosed in the accompanying documents.

6. Additional Requirements Specifically Related to Capnometers

60. *Interfering Gas and Vapor Effects (Other Than Water Vapor):*

60.1 The manufacturer shall disclose in the accompanying documents any adverse interference caused by the gases and vapors at the concentrations listed in Table 4.

60.2 Compliance shall be tested as follows:

60.2.1 *Principle*—The accuracy of the carbon dioxide reading is determined in the presence of the interfering gases and vapors given in Table 4.

TABLE 4 Test Concentrations of Interfering Gases or Vapor

Gas or Vapor	Concentration (vol %)
Oxygen	100
Nitrous oxide	80
Halothane	4
Enflurane	5
Isoflurane	5
Ethanol	specified by manufacturer
Acetone	specified by manufacturer
Chlorodifluromethane	5

60.2.2 *Test Gases*—Test gases shall be dry pre-mixtures of 5 % carbon dioxide (nominal), balance nitrogen, and the interfering gas or vapor at the level given in Table 4. Carbon dioxide levels shall be known to within ±2 % (V/V) of the specified value used.

60.2.3 *Procedure*—Calibrate the capnometer according to the instructions for use, and then expose the sensor to the test gas for a continuous period of 2 h, ensuring that both the capnometer and the sensor are maintained in the same condition during the whole period. Repeat the procedure for each application mixture in Table 4.

60.2.4 *Expression of Results*—Correct the carbon dioxide readings for changes in barometric pressure, if the errors due to this effect equal or exceed _0.1 % (V/V) carbon dioxide, and report the corrected readings.

61. *Sustained Pressure:*

61.1 Capnometers shall either:

(*1*) Meet the requirements given in 50.3 and 50.7 following exposure to a sustained positive pressure of 10 kPa (100 cm H_2O) and a negative pressure of 1.5 kPa (15 cm H_2O) for 30 s; or

(*2*) Be marked with the warning "not for use in breathing systems," and a similar warning shall appear in the accompanying documents.

(*3*) Compliance with (*1*) shall be checked by the test given in 61.2.

61.2 Compliance shall be tested as follows:

61.2.1 *Principle*—The accuracy of the carbon dioxide reading and the rise time are determined after exposure of the sensor to sustained pressure.

61.2.2 *Procedure*—Expose the sampling site to a sustained positive pressure with respect to ambient of 10 ± 1 kPa (100 ± 10 cm H_2O) and a sustained negative pressure with respect to ambient of 1.5 ± 0.2 kPa (15 ± 2 cm H_2O), in turn, for not less than 30 s each. Repeat this procedure four times, and then conduct the test for measurement accuracy as described in Clause 50.2 and the test for rise time as described in Clause 50.6.

62. *Gas Leakage and Sampling Loss:*

62.1 The rate of leakage for a non-diverting capnometer shall not be greater than 20 mL/min under the test conditions.

NOTE 14—The rate at which a sampling capnometer withdraws gas from a breathing system (the gas diversion rate) should not exceed 1.15 times the value stated in the accompanying documents.

NOTE 15—This requirement ensures that when fitted to a breathing system, the capnometer's rate of leakage at a continuous pressure of 3.0 kPa (30 cm H_2O) does not exceed more than 20 mL/min.

(*1*) Compliance shall be checked by the test given in 62.2.

62.2 Compliance shall be tested as follows:

62.2.1 *Apparatus*—A pressure gage having an accuracy to within ±0.3 kPa and a flow metering device having an accuracy within ± 2 mL/min shall be used.

62.2.2 *Procedure*—Tests shall be performed in both the ready for use and off configuration. Assemble the capnometer so that the sampling site is installed in a dimensionally suitable port of a test apparatus containing an inlet fitting to which a test gas and airflow metering device are attached. Connect the pressure gage to a third port of a test apparatus. Slowly adjust the flow to raise the pressure in the test apparatus to 3 kPa. Determine the flow necessary to maintain this pressure. This leakage flow shall be as specified in Clause 62.1.

62.3 The rate at which a sampling capnometer withdraws gas from a breathing system (the gas diversion rate) shall not exceed 1.15 times the value stated in the accompanying documents.

(*1*) Compliance shall be checked by the test given in 62.4.

62.4 *Method of Test:*

62.4.1 *Principle*—The rate at which a sampling capnometer withdraws gas from a simulated breathing system is measured.

62.4.2 *Test Gas*—Pressurized air at room temperature shall be used.

62.4.3 *Apparatus*—A pressure gage having an accuracy to within ±0.3 kPa, and a flow or volume measurement device having an accuracy to within ±2.5 % of the rate at which the capnometer withdraws gas from the breathing system as stated in the accompanying documents.

62.4.4 *Procedure*—Assemble the apparatus as described in 62.2.2 but using the flowmeter specified in 62.4.3. Adjust the pressurized air source to 3.0 kPa and monitor the flow reading for 1 min.

62.5 An exhaust port shall be provided to collect or route the diverting gas from the capnometer, and this exhaust port shall be incompatible with the inlet port of the capnometer.

(*1*) Compliance shall be checked by inspection.

63. *Breathing System Connections*—If a capnometer is intended to be connected to the breathing system through a T-piece, the breathing system connection ports of the T-piece shall be a 15 or 22 mm, or both, conical connector in accordance with Specification F 1054-88 (or ISO 5356/1:1987). The sampling gas and outlet ports of a diverting capnometer shall not be interchangeable with the breathing system connection port of a breathing system.

NOTE 16—Annexes A to M given in the General Standard, together with Appendix X1 in this draft specification, apply.

APPENDIX

(Nonmandatory Information)

X1. RATIONALE

X36.1 Capnometers are not life-support devices but are a "vigilance adjunct." Therefore, it is acceptable if this device fails without creating a safety hazard (that is, without affecting patient safety directly) or presenting erroneous data. The test voltages of 8 kV for air discharges and 3 kV for contact discharges using the IEC 801-2:1991 network and procedures are adequate to ensure good performance under the conditions in which capnometers are used. It is necessary to limit the application of discharges to accessible parts, since to allow the application of charges to the interior of the device would impose unnecessary design restrictions. It is reasonable to require any person opening a device for maintenance to exercise both common sense and accepted work practices, which include ESD precautions.

X50.1 Accurate knowledge of inspired and exhaled carbon dioxide concentration provides the clinician with information regarding the patient's cardiopulmonary status, function of the airway, and integrity of the breathing circuit. Adjustments to pulmonary ventilation, blood volume, and systemic circulation are often based on values of exhaled carbon dioxide. Recognition of unintended esophageal intubation, partial and complete airway obstruction, and rebreathing of exhaled carbon dioxide from the breathing system are often first recognized by changes in the respired carbon dioxide concentrations. For clinicians to use capnometers routinely for enhancement of patient safety and management, there must be confidence in the reliability and accuracy of the displayed data from the capnometer. The accuracy requirements detailed in Clause 50 are sufficient to meet these safety concerns.

Designation: F 1462 – 93

Specification for Oxygen Analyzers[1]

This standard is issued under the fixed designation F 1462; the number immediately following the designation indicates the year of original adoption or, in the case of revision, the year of last revision. A number in parentheses indicates the year of last reapproval. A superscript epsilon (ε) indicates an editorial change since the last revision or reapproval.

INTRODUCTION

Subcommittee F29.03.08 met in Boston in January of 1989 and August of 1990 and agreed to consider ISO 7767 as a possible replacement for the existing oxygen analyzer standard, ANSI Z-79.10. ISO 7767 is one of a series of standards developed for specific medical electrical equipment (a "particular standard") based on IEC 601-1 (the "general standard"). The text that follows has been taken from ISO 7767 and modified editorially. ISO 7767 references the first edition of IEC-601-1, published in 1977, and this specification references the second edition, published late in 1988.

Sections 1-3 of this specification are in keeping with the *Form and Style for ASTM Standards*-manual. Section 4 is a compilation of all the clauses in IEC 601-1:1988 with an indication as to whether the clause applies, does not apply, or applies with an amendment or addition.

Section 5 lists in numerical order all of the clauses in IEC 601-1:1988 that have amendments or additions in this specification. Additional requirements specific to oxygen analyzers begin with Clause 60.

Annex A1 provides a rationale for specific requirements.

1. Scope

1.1 The scope given in Clause 1 of IEC 601-1 1988 applies except that 1.1 shall be replaced by the following:

1.2 This specification covers safety requirements for oxygen analyzers, as defined in 3.11 (in this specification 3.1.11) intended for use in determining the oxygen level in breathing gas mixtures administered to patients. Both sampling and non-sampling oxygen analyzers are covered.

1.3 The field of application includes, but is not limited to:

1.3.1 Anesthetic machines and breathing systems,

1.3.2 Ventilators,

1.3.3 Baby incubators, and

1.3.4 Oxygen concentrators (domiciliary or clinical).

1.4 Oxygen analyzers intended for use in laboratory research applications are outside the scope of this specification.

1.5 The values stated in SI units are to be regarded as the standard.

1.6 *This standard does not purport to address all of the safety concerns, if any, associated with its use. It is the responsibility of the user of this standard to establish appropriate safety and health practices and determine the applicability of regulatory limitations prior to use.*

2. Referenced Documents

2.1 The following standards contain provisions that, through reference in the test, constitute provisions of this specification. At the time of publication, the editions indicated were valid. All standards are subject to revision, and parties to agreements based on this draft specification are encouraged to investigate the possibility of applying the most recent editions of the standards listed below:

2.2 *ASTM Standards:*

F 1463 Specifications for Alarm Signals in Medical Equipment Used in Anesthesia and Respiratory Care[2]

F 1054 Standard Specification for Conical Settings[2]

2.3 *IEC Standard:*

IEC 601-1:1988 Medical Electrical Equipment—Part 1—General Requirements for Safety[3]

2.4 *ANSI Standard:*

ANSI Z79.10 Requirements for Oxygen Analyzers for Monitoring Patient Breathing Mixtures[4]

2.5 *ISO Standards:*

ISO 7767 Oxygen Analyzers for Monitoring Patient Breathing Mixtures—Safety Requirements[4]

ISO 8158 Evaluation of the Performance Characteristics of Gas Analyzers

[1] This specification is under the jurisdiction of ASTM Committee F29 on Anesthetic and Respiratory Equipment and is the direct responsibility of Subcommittee F29.11 on Gas Monitors.

Current edition approved April 15, 1993. Published July 1993.

[2] *Annual Book of ASTM Standards*, Vol 13.01.

[3] Available from International Electrochemical Commission, 3 rue de Varembé, 1211 Geneva 20, Switzerland.

[4] Available from American National Standards Institute, 25 W. 43rd St., 4th Floor, NY, NY 10036.

2.6 *Military Standard:*

MIL-STD-810C Environmental Test Methods for Engineering Guidelines[5]

3. Terminology

3.1 *Definitions*—For the purposes of this specification, the definitions given in Clause 2 of IEC 601-1: 1988 apply together with the following additional definitions:

3.1.1 *alarm*—a warning signal that is activated when the oxygen reading reaches or exceeds the alarm limit.

3.1.2 *alarm set-point*—the setting of the adjustment control or display value that indicates the oxygen level at or beyond which the alarm is intended to be activated (the indicated alarm limit).

3.1.3 *alarm system*—those parts of the oxygen analyzer that establish the alarm set-point(s); activate an alarm when the oxygen level is less than or equal to the low alarm set-point, or is equal to or greater than the high alarm set-point.

3.1.4 *delay time*—the time from a step function change in oxygen concentration or partial pressure at the sampling site to the achievement of 10 % of final oxygen value in the oxygen analyzer.

3.1.5 *display*—a device that visually indicates quantitative or qualitative information.

3.1.6 *expected useful life*—the period during which the performance of an oxygen analyzer or any of its components is expected to meet the requirements of this specification, when used and maintained according to the accompanying documents.

3.1.7 *high priority alarm*—a combination of audible and visual signals indicating that immediate operator response is required.

3.1.8 *interference with measurement accuracy*— the difference between the oxygen reading in the presence of an interfering gas mixture and the oxygen reading in a corresponding mixture in which the interfering gas or vapor fraction has been replaced by nitrogen.

3.1.9 *low priority alarm*—a visual signal, or a combination of audible and visual signals indicating that operator awareness is required.

3.1.10 *medium priority alarm*—a combination of audible and visual signals indicating that prompt operator response is required.

3.1.11 *oxygen analyzer*—a device that measures and indicates the oxygen level in a gaseous mixture.

3.1.12 *oxygen level*—the concentration of oxygen in a gaseous mixture.

3.1.12.1 *Discussion*—This may be expressed in any suitable unit such as percent by volume or partial pressure in kPa (or mm Hg).

3.1.13 *oxygen reading*—the measured oxygen level as indicated by the oxygen analyzer.

3.1.14 *partial pressure*—the pressure that each gas in a gas mixture could exert if it alone occupied the volume of the mixture at the same temperature.

[5] Available from Standardization Documents Order Desk, Bldg. 4 Section D, 700 Robbins Ave., Philadelphia, PA 19111-5094. Attn: NPODS.

3.1.15 *percent (V/V) oxygen (or other gases)*— the level of oxygen (or other gas) in a mixture, expressed as a percentage volume fraction.

3.1.16 *response time*—the time required for the oxygen analyzer to achieve a 90 % response to a step change in oxygen level.

3.1.17 *sensing area*—the part of the oxygen analyzer that is in direct contact with the gas mixture of which the oxygen level is to be measured.

3.1.17.1 *Discussion*—An example of such a part is the membrane surface of an oxygen-sensing electrode.

3.1.18 *shelf life*—the period during which the oxygen analyzer or any of its components are stored in its original container according the the accompanying documents.

3.1.19 *useful life*—the period of time during which the performance of an oxygen analyzer or any of its components meets the requirements of this specification, when used and maintained according to the accompanying documents.

4. Relationship of This Specification to the General Standard

	(A)	(NA)	(AM/R)
Section One—General			
1. Scope and object			X
2. Terminology and definitions			X
3. General requirements			X
4. General requirements for tests			X
5. Classification			X
6. Identification, marking, and document			X
7. Power input			X
Section Two—Environmental Conditions			
8. Basic safety requirements	X		
9. Removable protective means	X		
10. Environmental conditions			X
11. Not used			
12. SINGLE FAULT CONDITION—Not used			
Section Three—Protection Against Electric Shock Hazards			
13. General	X		
14. Requirements related to classification	X		
15. Limitation of voltage and/or current	X		
16. Enclosures and PROTECTIVE COVERS	X		
17. Separation			X
18. Protective earthing, functional earthing, and potential equalization	X		
19. Continuous LEAKAGE CURRENTS and PATIENT AUXILIARY CURRENTS			X
20. Dielectric strength	X		
Section Four—Protection Against Mechanical Hazards			
21. Mechanical strength			X
22. Moving parts	X		
23. Surfaces, corners, and edges	X		
24. Stability and transportability	X		
25. Expelled parts	X		
26. Not used			
27. Pneumatic and hydraulic power	X		
28. Suspended masses	X		
29. X-radiation	X		
30. Alpha, beta, gamma, neutron radiation and other particle radiation	X		
31. Microwave radiation	X		
32. Light radiation (including visual radiation and lasers)	X		
33. Infra-red radiation	X		
34. Ultra-violet radiation	X		
35. Acoustical energy (including ultra-sonics)			X
36. Electromagnetic compatibility			X

	(A)	(NA)	(AM/R)
Section Six—Protection Against Hazards of Ignition of Flammable Anesthetic Mixtures			
37. Locations and basic requirements	X		
38. Marking ACCOMPANYING DOCUMENTS	X		
39. Common requirements for "AP" and "APG" EQUIPMENT	X		
40. Requirements and tests for Category AP equipment, and components thereof	X		
41. Requirements and tests for Category APG equipment, parts and components thereof	X		
42. Excessive temperatures			X
43. Fire prevention			X
44. Overflow, spillage, leakage, humidity, ingress of liquids, cleaning, sterilization, and disinfection			X
45. Pressure vessels and parts subject to PRESSURE	X		
46. Human errors—Not used			
47. Electrostatic charges—Not used			
NOTE: WG 13 of IEC 62A is currently preparing a draft standard for electrostatic discharges for medical equipment.			
48. Materials in APPLIED PARTS in contact with the body of the PATIENT—Not used			
49. Interruption of the power supply	X		
Section Eight—Accuracy of Operating Data and Protection Against Hazardous Output			
50. Accuracy of operating data—Not used			
51. Protection against incorrect output			X
Section Nine—Abnormal Operation and Fault Conditions; Environmental Tests			
52. Abnormal operation and fault conditions	X		
53. Environmental tests	X		
Section Ten—Constructional Requirements			
54. General	X		
55. Enclosures and covers—Not used			
56. Components and general assembly	X		
57. MAIN PARTS, components, and layout	X		
58. Protective earthing—terminals and connections	X		
59. Construction and layout	X		
Additional Clauses			
60. Interfering gas and vapor effects other than water vapor	X		
61. Cyclic pressure	X		
62. Gas leakage and sampling loss	X		
63. Replacement of oxygen sensor	X		
64. Alarms	X		
65. Connectors	X		
66. Measurement accuracy	X		

A = applies, NA = Not Applicable, AM/R = applies with an amendment, addition, or revision to the requirements in the General Standard.

"Not used" means that material in this (these) sections of IEC 601-1:1977 has been deleted from the 1988 edition, but the section number is reserved for future use.

5. Clauses Containing Amendments, Additions, or Replacements to the Text in IEC 601-1:1988, and Additional Clauses 60–67

NOTE 1—The clause numbers used reference the specific section in the general standard.

4. *General Requirements and General Requirements for Tests:*

Clauses 3 and 4 of the general standard apply together with the following additions:

Test methods other than those specified in this specification, but of equal or greater accuracy may be used to verify compliance with the requirements of this specification. However, in the event of a dispute, the methods specified in this specification shall be used as the reference methods.

In 3.6 (i) add the following: additional single fault conditions include short and open circuits of the sensor and associated circuitry that cause sparks to occur, or increase the energy of sparks, or increase temperatures.

In 4.5, add the following:

At 20°C if the tests are to be carried out at any nominal temperatures within the operating temperature range of the oxygen analyzer,

Unless otherwise specified in individual test methods, with dry test gas mixtures that have a relative humidity below 2 %, and

At ambient atmospheric pressure.

NOTE 2—Room air is considered to be 20.9 % oxygen.

NOTE 3—Care should be taken to ensure that room air used for testing is not contaminated, for example, from exhaust ducts, etc., and has a relative humidity below 95 %.

6. Classification

NOTE 4—Oxygen analyzers used in the home, for example, to monitor oxygen concentrators, should be designated as Class II equipment due to the fact that the protective earthing in many homes may be inadequate or nonexistent.

7. Identification, Marking, and Documents

The requirements given in Clause 6 of IEC 601-1 1988 apply except for the following additions and modifications:

a) In 6.1, replace Item (d) by the following:

If the size of the oxygen analyzer does not permit the complete marking as specified throughout this clause, at least the following shall be marked on the oxygen analyzer: the name of the manufacturer; a serial number or lot or batch identifying number; and symbol Number 14 in Table D.I. of IEC 601-1 1988.

b) In 6.1, add the following to Item (f):

Oxygen analyzers shall be marked with a serial number or other lot or batch-identifying number.

c) In 6.1, add the following to Item (q):

Oxygen analyzers shall be marked with the words "Not for use in breathing systems", if applicable (see Clause 62.1).

d) In 6.1, add additional items as follows:

(zz) The following shall either be marked on the body of the oxygen analyzer or be permanently attached to the oxygen analyzer:

Abridged operating instructions which shall include an indication of the period of time necessary, following a change in oxygen level, for the oxygen level to stabilize.

NOTE 5—Markings related to controls should be visible or legible, or both, to an operator having a visual acuity (corrected if necessary) of at least" one" when the operator is 1 m in front of the oxygen analyzer at an illuminance of 215 lx. Markings should be clearly identified with their associated displays or visual indicators.

a) Marking on the outside of the oxygen analyzer shall additionally include the following:

b) For oxygen analyzers not intended for use with inhalation anesthetic agents, the phrase "Note for use with inhalation anesthetic agents", if applicable (see Clause 60.1).

c) A statement that the operator should see the accompanying documents for the effect of moisture on accuracy, if applicable.

6.1.5.3 Symbol number 14 in Table D.I. of the general standard.

6.1.5.4 The words "Will not withstand mechanical shock", if applicable (see Clause 21.1), and symbol Number 14 in Table D.I.

6.1.5.5 The alarm set-point of the oxygen level, if the oxygen analyzer is provided with a non-adjustable oxygen level alarm.

6.1.6 In 6.3, add the following:

6.1.6.1 *Oxygen Level Displays*—Oxygen level displays shall be marked with the appropriate units of measurement.

NOTE 6—Displays should not be obscured by the hand normally adjusting the control(s) associated with the display.

6.1.7 In 6.7, replace Item (a) by the following:

If visual indicators are used on the oxygen analyzer, with the exception of alphanumeric displays, their coloring shall conform to the following requirements:

6.1.7.1 Red, with a flashing frequency of 1.4 to 2.8 Hz, shall be used as a high priority alarm.

6.1.7.2 Yellow, with a flashing frequency of 0.4 to 0.8 Hz, shall be used to indicate a medium priority alarm.

6.1.7.3 Yellow, with a constant signal, shall be used to indicate a low priority alarm.

6.1.7.4 Green shall be used to indicate that the oxygen analyzer is ready for use or in normal operation.

6.1.7.5 Blue shall be used only as an advisory indicator.

6.1.8 The function of all lights and displays shall be marked.

6.1.9 Compliance shall be checked by functional test and inspection.

NOTE 7—Visual indicators and their associated markings should be visible or legible, or both, to an operator having visual acuity (corrected if necessary) of at least "one" when the operator is located 1 m in front of the oxygen analyzer at an illuminance of 215 lux.

g) In 6.8.2, add the following to Item (a): The instructions for use shall additionally include the following information:

1) A description of the purpose and intended use of the oxygen analyzer.

2) A description of the principles of operation of the oxygen analyzer, including the relationship between gas concentration and its partial pressure and the effects of humidity.

3) A detailed specification, including the following:

a) The oxygen level measurement range and the accuracy of measurement (see Clauses 66.1, 66.2 and 66.3),

b) The stability of measurement accuracy (see Clauses 66.4 and 66.5),

c) The response time (see Clauses 66.6 and 66.7),

d) The oxygen level alarm range and its accuracy (see Clauses 64.3, 64.4 and 64.5),

e) The operating and non-operating temperature ranges (see Clause 10),

f) For sampling-type oxygen analyzers, the gas diversion rate (see Clause 62.3),

g) Power requirements, and

h) Time from switching on to obtaining specific operating performance.

4. Details of any effect on stated function due to the following:

a) Humidity or condensation including, for example, any adverse effects if an adaptor is provided to improve the function of the sensor in the presence of condensation or particulate water (see Clause 44.5),

b) Interfering gases or vapours (see Clause 60),

c) Mechanical shock (see Clauses 21.1 and 21.2),

d) Cyclic pressure (see Clause 61),

e) Barometric pressure or pressure at the site of use of the oxygen analyzer,

f) Fluctuations in line or battery voltages, and

g) Aging of the oxygen sensor or of the oxygen analyzer itself (see Clause 63).

NOTE 8—If the oxygen level is displayed in units of oxygen concentration, the accompanying documents should contain an explanation that readings in concentration units are correct only under the pressure at which the oxygen analyzer is calibrated.

5. The expected useful life of the oxygen sensors, if they are intended to be replaced during the useful lifetime of the oxygen analyzer. The useful life shall be stated as the number of hours, days, or months of continuous use in dry, 100 % (V/V) oxygen at 23°C during which the oxygen analyzer meets the requirements given in 60.3, 60.5, 60.6 and 60.8 of this specification (see Clause 63).

NOTE 9—Other operating conditions may also be used as a basis for useful life.

NOTE 10—The shelf life of oxygen sensors should be stated.

NOTE 11—The expected useful life of other expendable components of the oxygen analyzer, for example batteries, should be stated under specified conditions of use.

6. An illustration of the features of the oxygen analyzer indicating the location of all operating controls, adjustments and system components (for example, the battery compartment) necessary for correct operation and on site servicing by the user.

7. Instructions for operation of the oxygen analyzer, including the following:

a) Pre-use checking and calibration,

b) Routine inspection and testing, and

c) Recommended methods for cleaning and disinfection or sterilization.

8. A description of an in-service test using room air as the calibration gas.

9. Illustrated service information, including: instructions for preventive maintenance and service calibration, and those adjustments that are necessary to maintain the oxygen analyzer in correct operating conditions, as well as a description of those adjustments and replacements that can be performed by the operator.

10. A description of the correct installation of the oxygen analyzer and the connection of the oxygen sensor or sampling tubing. The maximum permissible distance of separation between the oxygen analyzer and the sensing area shall be stated.

NOTE 12—If the oxygen analyzer requires a sensor cable or sampling tubing for connection from the oxygen analyzer to the sensing area, the cable or tubing should be of sufficient length to reduce the likelihood of its being elongated beyond its elastic limit and being stressed at the connection points. In the event that the sensor cable becomes disconnected, this should be indicated by an alarm.

11. Unless it can be demonstrated that the oxygen analyzer is not susceptible to electromagnetic interference, a warning statement in the instructions for use to the effect that the function of the oxygen analyzer may be adversely affected by the operation of such equipment as high frequency apparatus, short-wave, microwave or magnetic resonance imaging equipment in the vicinity.

12. If the lowest temperature that the oxygen analyzer can withstand during transport is higher than − 40°C or if the highest temperature the oxygen analyzer can withstand during transport is lower than 70°C, or both, the recommended temperature shall be stated in the accompanying documents and the transport package shall be printed with a notice indicating the restrictions on temperature during transport.

SECTION TWO—ENVIRONMENTAL CONDITIONS

10. *Environmental Conditions*—Replace 10.1 and 10.2.1 with the following:

10.1 *Nonoperating Temperature Range:*

The oxygen analyzer shall meet the requirements given in 66.1 and 66.6, after it has been subjected to the extremes of the specified non-operating temperature range as detailed in the accompanying documents.

Compliance shall be checked by the test given in 10.1.1

10.1.1 *Test Method:*

10.1.1.1 *Principle*Determination of the accuracy of the oxygen reading and the response time at normal operating temperature after the oxygen analyzer, as packaged for transport, has been subjected to the extremes of the specified non-operating temperature range.

10.1.1.2 *Procedure*

Place the oxygen analyzer, as packaged for transport, in an atmosphere of room air having a relative humidity of less than 95 %, at the lower of the following temperatures until it has reached equilibrium: a) 70 ± 1°C; or, b) the highest temperature recommended during transport, as marked on the transport package.

NOTE 13—Equilibrium can be verified by a suitable means, such as placing a thermistor inside the oxygen analyzer.

Maintain the oxygen analyzer at this temperature for 4 h after equilibrium is attained.

Return the packaged oxygen analyzer to room temperature, unpack it and install it so that it is ready for use, as described in the accompanying documents.

Carry out the test for measurement accuracy as described in 66.2 and the test for response time as described in 66.7.

Repeat the procedure equilibrating the packaged oxygen analyzer at the higher of the following temperatures: a) − 40 ± 1°C; or b) the lowest temperature recommended during transport, as marked on the transport package.

10.1.1.3 *Expression of Results*—Express the results as described in 66.2 and 66.7 at both test temperatures.

10.2.1 *Operating Temperature Range:*

Oxygen analyzers shall meet the requirements given in 66.1 and 66.6 over a sample gas and ambient temperature range of 15 to 40°C.

Compliance shall be checked by the test given in 10.2.1.1.

10.2.1.1 *Test Method:*

10.2.1.1. *Principle*—Determination of the accuracy of the oxygen reading and the response time after equilibrating the oxygen analyzer at the extremes of the specified operating temperature range.

10.2.1.1.2. *Procedure:*

Place the oxygen analyzer in an atmosphere of room air at 40 ± 1°C having a relative humidity of less than 95 % until it has reached equilibrium.

NOTE 14—Equilibrium can be verified by a suitable means, such as placing a thermistor inside the oxygen analyzer.

Carry out the test for measurement accuracy as described in 66.2 and the test for response time as described in 66.7 except that both the oxygen analyzer and the test gases are to be maintained at 40 ± 2°C during both tests.

Repeat the procedure at the test temperature of 15 ± 1°C.

10.2.1.1.3 *Expression of Results*Express the results as described in 50.4 and 50.9 at both test temperatures.

17. *Separation*—The requirements given in Clause 17 of IEC 601-1:1988 apply together with the following additional item:

h) Deterioration of parts due to anesthetic agents and oxygen should be taken into account.

18. *Earthing and Potential Equalization*—See also Clauses 19 and 39.3.

19. *Continuous Leakage Currents and Patient Auxiliary Currents*—The requirements given in Clause 19 of IEC 601-1:1988 apply except in Item 19.1e), add the following: The patient leakage current shall be measured at the following positions:

For non-sampling (continuous monitoring) oxygen analyzers, at the oxygen sensor, and

For sampling (intermittent) oxygen analyzers, at the junction of the sampling tubing and the body of the oxygen analyzer.

SECTION FOUR—PROTECTION AGAINST MECHANICAL HAZARDS

21. *Mechanical Strength*—The requirements given in Clause 21 of IEC 601-1:1988 are replaced by the following:

21.1 *Free-Standing Oxygen Analyzers*—Such oxygen analyzers (that is, those not manufactured as an integral, inseparable component of a larger system) and all separable components, such as oxygen sensors shall either:

a) Meet the requirements given in 66.1 and 66.6 and, if applicable, 6.3, 60.12, and 64.3; electrically live parts shall not be accessible, compliance being checked by the test given in 21.2; or

b) Be marked with the warning to the effect that it does not meet this requirement (see section 6.1), with a similar warning appearing in the accompanying documents.

21.2 *Test Method:*

21.2.1 *Principle*—Determination of the accuracy of the oxygen reading, the response time and, if applicable, the alarm accuracy after the oxygen analyzer and all separable components have been subjected to a mechanical shock.

21.2.2 *Procedure*—Attach the unpackaged items to be tested rigidly to a shock machine table. Apply three shocks in both directions along three mutually perpendicular axes of each test item (a total of 18 shocks to each item), taking care to ensure the following:

8.2.2.1 That the shape of the shock pulse is in accordance with Fig. 1,

That the oscillogram of the shock pulse includes a time approximately 33 ms (3 D) long,

That the acceleration amplitude (A) of the ideal half-sine pulse is 300 m/s^2 (30 × gravity) and its duration (D) is 11 ms,

That the measured acceleration pulse is contained between the broken line boundaries shown in Fig. 1,

That the measured velocity change (that may be obtained by integration of the acceleration pulse) is within the limits $V^i \pm 0.1\ V_i$, where the velocity change associated with the ideal pulse is:

$$V_i = 2 \times \frac{A \times D}{\pi} = 2 \times \frac{300 \times 0.011}{3.1416} = 2.1 \text{ m/s} \quad (1)$$

That the integration to determine velocity change extends from 4.4 ms (0.4 D) before the pulse to 1.1 ms (0.1 D) after the pulse.

Inspect the oxygen analyzer to check that the appearance and condition of the oxygen analyzer, including the enclosure and warning or display indications or markings, have not been damaged or have not deteriorated in such a way as to prevent normal operation of the oxygen analyzer and that no electrically live parts have become accessible.

Reattach any separable components to the oxygen analyzer and carry out the test for measurement accuracy as described in Clause 66.2 and the test for response time as described in Clause 66.7 and, if the oxygen analyzer is fitted with an oxygen level alarm, a test for oxygen level alarm limit as described in Clause 64.4.

21.2.3 *Expression of Results*—Express the results as described in relevant subclauses of Clause 66 and report any damage or accessibility of electrically live parts.

35. *Acoustical Energy (Including Ultrasonics)*—The requirements given in Clause 35 of IEC 601-1:1988 apply, together with the following additional requirement:

Unless the analyzer is an integral inseparable component of a larger system, the relevant standards of the equipment shall apply.

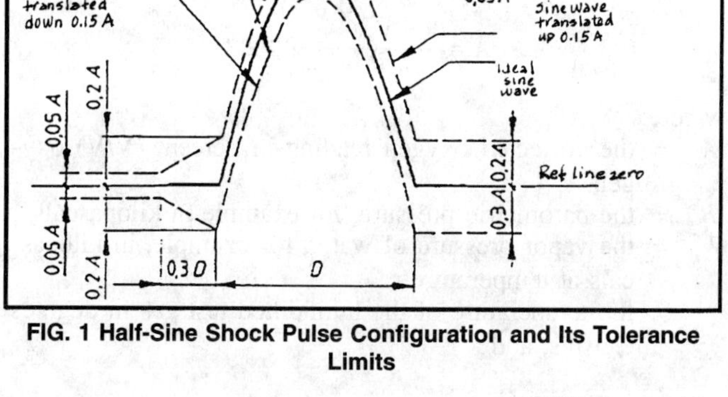

FIG. 1 Half-Sine Shock Pulse Configuration and Its Tolerance Limits

36. *Electromagnetic Compatibility*—The requirements given in Clause 36 of the general standard apply.

SECTION 6—PROTECTION AGAINST HAZARDS OF EXPLOSION IN MEDICALLY USED ROOMS

9.1 *Locations and Basic Requirements*—The requirements given in Clause 37 of IEC 601-1:1988 apply.

9.2 *Common Requirements for Category AP and Category APG Equipment*—The requirements given in Clause 39 of IEC 601-1:1988 apply.

SECTION 7—PROTECTION AGAINST EXCESSIVE TEMPERATURES, FIRE, AND OTHER HAZARDS, SUCH AS HUMAN ERRORS

42. *Excessive Temperatures*—The requirements given in Clause 42 of IEC 601-1:1988 apply except as follows: Replace 42.3 with the following:

42.3 Applied parts with intentionally come in contact with the patient and that are not intended to supply heat to the patient shall not have surface temperatures exceeding 41°C.

43. *Fire Prevention*—The requirements given in Clause 43 of IEC 601-1:1988 apply together with the following additional requirements:

43.1 In order to eliminate the risk of fires caused by electrical components that may be a source of ignition in oxygen or nitrous oxide enriched atmospheres (or mixtures of gases containing anesthetic agents referred to in Clause 37), at least one of the following requirements shall be met:

a) Electrical components shall be separated from compartments in which accumulations of such gases can occur by a barrier complying with the requirements given in 43.2.

b) Compartments containing electrical components shall be ventilated according to the requirements given in 43.5.

c) Electrical components that in normal use and single fault condition can be source of ignition shall comply with the requirements given in 43.7.

43.2 Any barrier required under the provisions of 43.1 (a) shall be sealed at all joints and at any holes for cables, shafts, or other purposes. Compliance shall be checked by the following methods, as appropriate:

Inspection,

By compliance test for enclosures with restricted breathing given in 40.5 of IEC 601-1:1988, and

If under normal use conditions a pressure difference exists between the spaces separated by the barrier, the test method given in 43.4.

43.3 The ventilation required in 43.1 (b) shall be such that when tested by the method described in 43.2, the oxygen level in the enclosed compartment containing electrical components shall not exceed 4 % above the ambient oxygen level; if this requirement is met by forced ventilation, an alarm shall be provided to warn of failure of the ventilation.

43.4 Oxygen levels in enclosed compartments shall be tested as follows:

43.4.1 *Principle*—Measurement of the oxygen level in the enclosed compartment is measured after the oxygen analyzer is operated for 18 h under single fault conditions.

43.4.2 *Procedure*—Place the oxygen analyzer in a room in which the air exchange is between three and ten room volumes per hour. Set the oxygen flow through the oxygen analyzer so that it equals the maximum flows of oxygen and nitrous oxide under normal conditions. Switch off the mains supply and measure the oxygen level in the enclosed compartment; operate the oxygen analyzer under single fault conditions with the least favorable control setting selected and with the mains voltage deviating by ±10 %, if applicable. After 18 h, switch off the supply mains and measure the oxygen level in the enclosed compartment.

43.4.3 *Expression of Results*—Record the oxygen levels measured at the beginning and the end of the 18 h period.

43.5 Electrical circuits that can produce sparks or generate increased surface temperatures and that can be a source of ignition shall be so designed that no ignition occurs. At least the following requirements shall be satisfied in normal condition and single fault condition:

The product of the R.M.S. value of the no load voltage and the R.M.S. value of the short circuit current shall not exceed 10 VA.

The surface temperature of components shall not exceed 300°C. Short- and open-circuiting of resistors, capacitors, and inductances complying with the requirements given in Clause 14 of IEC 65:1985 are not considered to be single fault conditions.

Compliance shall be checked by the test given in 43.6.

43.6 Measure or calculate the voltages and currents in steady state condition and measure the surface temperatures in normal condition and single fault condition.

43.5 Electrical circuits that can produce sparks or generate a high surface temperature and can be a source of ignition shall be so designed that in normal use and single fault condition, no ignition occurs; under these conditions, the product of the effective open circuit voltage and effective short circuit current shall not exceed 10 VA in each circuit.

43.6 The surface temperature of components that may constitute a source of ignition shall not exceed 300°C.

44. *Overflow, Spillage, Leakage, Humidity, Ingress of Liquids, Cleaning, Sterilization, and Disinfection:*

The requirements given in Clause 44 of IEC 601-1:1988 apply except (a) replace 44.3 by the following:

44.3 *Spillage*—Oxygen analyzers shall be so constructed that spillage does not wet parts which, if wetted, may cause a safety hazard.

44.3.1 Compliance shall be checked by the test given in 44.3.2.

44.3.2 Position the oxygen analyzer as in normal use. Pour 200 mL of water steadily on an arbitrarily chosen point on the top surface of the oxygen analyzer. After this the oxygen analyzer shall comply with the requirements of this specification; (b) replace 44.5 by the following:

44.5 *Humidity and Condensation Effects:*

44.5.1 *Humidity Effects*—When operated in accordance with the instructions for use, oxygen analyzers shall maintain ±5 % (V/V) measurement accuracy when used with air or comparable gas mixtures having any relative humidity between 0 % and 100 %.

NOTE 15—These requirements may be met with the addition of an adaptor if required.

Compliance shall be checked by the test given in 44.5.2.

44.5.2 *Test Method:*

44.5.2.1 *Principle*—Determination of the accuracy of the oxygen reading over a 2-h period of exposure of the oxygen sensor to a high relative humidity (non-condensing) after calibration in dry air.

44.5.2.2 *Test Gases*—Dry room or compressed air as the calibration gas mixture and humidified room or compressed air having a relative humidity between 95 and 100 % (non-condensing) shall be used as the test gas mixture.

44.5.2.3 *Procedure:*

Hold the ambient temperature of the oxygen analyzer constant to within ±1°C of a nominal value within the operating rate of the oxygen analyzer (see 10.2.1). Hold the temperature and calibration of the test gas mixtures delivered to the sensing area constant at ±2°C. Deliver the calibration and test gas mixtures to the sensing area at ambient barometric pressure. Set up the oxygen analyzer for the measurement of humidified gases as described in the accompanying documents (for example, by attachment of an adaptor or orientation of the oxygen sensor). Maintain the oxygen analyzer and oxygen sensor in the same position throughout the test.

Ensure that the oxygen sensor is at a temperature of 35 ± 2°C and that the oxygen analyzer is at ambient temperature. Calibrate the oxygen analyzer according to the accompanying documents using the calibration gas mixture. Do not recalibrate the oxygen analyzer during the test period. Expose the sensing area to the test gas mixture for a continuous period of 2 h. For continuous monitoring oxygen analyzers, record the oxygen reading at least once every 15 min. For intermittent sampling oxygen analyzers, sample the test gas mixture at least once every 15 min and record the oxygen reading. In either case, record the temperature to an accuracy of ±0.2°C and the barometric pressure to an accuracy of ±0.2 % of the reading every time an oxygen reading is recorded.

44.5.2.4 *Expression of Results:*

If the oxygen readings are not already in partial pressure use, convert each oxygen reading to partial pressure, P, for example in kilopascals using the equation:

$$P = (R/100) \times B \quad (2)$$

where:

R = the oxygen reading in percent (V/V) oxygen, and

B = the barometric pressure, for example, in kilopascals.

Correct each oxygen reading for the dilution effect of 100 % water vapor at the temperature and barometric pressure of each reading, using the following equation:

$$A = \frac{\frac{B}{B - V_t} \times P}{B} \times 100 \quad (3)$$

where:

A = the corrected oxygen reading in percent (V/V) oxygen,

B = the barometric pressure, for example in kilopascals,

V_t = the vapor pressure of water, for example, in kilopascals at temperature t,

t = the temperature of the humidified test gas in degrees Celsius, and

P = the oxygen partial pressure, for example in kilopascals.

Table 1 lists the vapor pressure of water at selected temperatures.

44.5.3 *Condensation Effects*—Oxygen analyzers intended for use in a breathing system shall meet the following requirements, either:

a) Oxygen analyzers shall maintain the oxygen measurement accuracy specified in 66.1 and 66.3 and the response time specified in 66.6. If the manufacturer recommends or supplics an attachment for use when measuring gases of high humidity, these requirements shall be met with the attachment in place.

b) Compliance shall be checked by the test given in 44.5.4, or

If the oxygen analyzer does not meet these requirements, a cautionary notice shall be included in the accompanying documents.

44.5.4 *Test Method:*

44.5.4.1 *Principle*—Determination of the accuracy of the oxygen reading and the response time over a 2-h period of exposure of the oxygen sensor to a relative humidity of 100 % (condensing) after calibration in dry air.

44.5.4.2 *Test Gases*—Dry room or compressed air as the calibration gas mixture and humidified room or compressed air having a relative humidity of 100 % (condensing) shall be used as the test gas mixture.

44.5.4.3 *Procedure*—Carry out the procedure described in 44.5.2 ensuring that the test gas is delivered to the sensing area in a fully saturated condensing state and that condensate forms at the sensing area. In addition, measure the response time by the method described in 50.9 after recording each oxygen reading.

44.5.4.4 *Expression of Results*—Express the results as described in 44.5.2.4.

47. *Electrostatic Charges*—This clause of the general standard applies.

SECTION 8—ACCURACY OF OPERATING DATA AND PROTECTION AGAINST INCORRECT OUTPUT

51. *Protection Against Hazardous Output*—The requirements given in Clause 51 of IEC 601-1:1988 apply together with the following additional requirements:

51.5 *Function and Position of Controls:*

Check or test controls for battery condition or signal operation and signal override shall automatically return from the check, test or override position, unless these functions are carried out automatically when switching to the operating mode.

The positions of measurement and test controls shall be clearly distinguishable.

Calibration controls shall include means to prevent an inadvertent change from the intended position (for example, by recessing the control or by providing a locking mechanism).

NOTE 16—All other controls should also include means to prevent inadvertent changes from the intended positions and should have clearly distinguishable positions.

SECTION 9—FAULT CONDITIONS CAUSING OVERHEATING OR MECHANICAL DAMAGE, OR BOTH; ENVIRONMENTAL TESTS

56. *Components and General Assembly*—The requirements given in Clause 56 of IEC 601-1:1988 apply except as follows:

In 56.8, add the following:

High priority signals provided with the oxygen analyzer for monitoring oxygen levels shall be both visual and auditory.

Medium priority signals provided with the oxygen analyzer shall be visual.

NOTE 17—Visual and auditory indicators may be accompanied by a display. Medium priority signals may be accompanied by an auditory signal.

In 56.10, add an additional item as follows:

d) *Movement of controls*—for controls that consist of a movable part and a non-movable part, movement upwards, to the right, or clockwise shall increase the control function.

Rotary gas flow controls are exempt from this requirement.

NOTE 18—The separation between control knobs, switches, toggles, pinwheels, or push buttons should conform to the recommendations given in DOD Handbook 743A.

NOTE 19—Controls and their associated markings should be visible or legible, or both, to an operator having visual acuity (corrected if necessary) of at least "one" when the operator is located at least 1 m in front of the oxygen analyzer at an illuminance of 215 lux. Markings should be clearly identified with their associated controls.

SECTION 11—ADDITIONAL REQUIREMENTS

60. *Interfering Gas and Vapor Effects:*

60.1 Oxygen analyzers shall either:

a) Have not more than 5 % (V/V) oxygen interference with measurement accuracy in the presence of any of the gases or vapors at the levels listed in Table 2; or

b) If the body of the oxygen analyzer is marked "Not for use with inhalation agents" or equivalent, the oxygen analyzer shall not have more than 5 % (V/V) oxygen interference with measurement accuracy in the presence of helium or carbon dioxide at the levels listed in Table 2. If the oxygen interference is greater than 1 % (V/V) this shall be stated in the accompanying documents.

Compliance shall be checked by the test given in 60.2.

60.2 Compliance shall be tested as follows:

TABLE 1 Vapor Pressure Over Water

Temperature, °C	Pressure, kPa	Pressure, mmHg
33	4.90	37.7
34	5.19	39.9
35	5.48	42.2
36	5.79	44.6
37	6.12	47.1

TABLE 2 Inhalation Anesthetics and Other Interfering Gases and Vapors

Gas or Vapor (In 30 % Oxygen, 70 % Nitrous Oxide)	Level Volume %
Nitrous Oxide[A]	80
Carbon Dioxide	5
Halothane[A]	4
Enflurane[A]	5
Isoflurane[A]	5

[A] Inhalation anesthetic agent.

60.2.1 *Principle*Determination of the accuracy of the oxygen reading in the presence of interfering gases and vapors given in Table 2.

60.2.2 *Test Gases*—Dry pre-mixtures of 30 % oxygen and 70 % nitrous oxide and the interfering gas or vapor at the level given in Table 2, the oxygen levels being known to within ± 5 % (V/V), shall be used.

60.2.3 *Procedure*—Carry out the test described in 66.2 with the following modification:

Expose the sensing area to the test gas for a continuous period of 2 h, ensuring that both the oxygen analyzer and the oxygen sensor are maintained in the same condition during the whole period. Repeat the procedure for each applicable mixture given in Table 2.

60.2.4 *Expression of Results*—Correct the oxygen readings for changes in barometric pressure, if the errors due to this effect equal or exceed ± 0.1 % (V/V) oxygen, and report the corrected readings.

61. *Cyclic Pressure:*

61.1 Oxygen analyzers shall either meet the requirements given in 66.1 and 66.6 following exposure to cyclic positive pressure of 10 kPa (100 cm H_2O) and negative pressure of 1.5 kPa (15 cm H_2O) in the breathing system, or be marked with the warning "Not for use in breathing systems" and a similar warning shall appear in accompanying documents.

Compliance shall be checked by the test given in 61.2.

61.2 Accuracy shall be tested as follows:

61.2.1 *Principle*—Determination of the accuracy of the oxygen reading and the response time after exposure of the sensing area to cyclic pressure.

61.2.2 *Procedure*—Expose the sensing area to a cyclic pressure waveform such that a positive pressure with respect to ambient of 10 ± 1 kPa (100 ± 10 cm H_2O) and a negative pressure with respect to ambient of 1.5 ± 0.2 kPa (15 ± 2 cm H_2O) are each maintained, in turn, for not less than 2 s each. Cycle the pressures at a rate of 0.167 ± 0.017 Hz (10 ± 1 cycle/minute) for 10 min.

Carry out the test for measurement accuracy as described in 50.4 and the test for response time as described in 50.9.

61.2.3 *Expression of Results*—Express the results as described in 66.2 and 66.7.

62. *Gas Leakage and Sampling Loss:*

62.1 The rate of leakage of a non-sampling oxygen analyzer shall not be greater than 20 mL/min.

NOTE 20—This requirement ensures that when fitted to a breathing system its rate of leakage at a continuous pressure of 3 kPa (30 cm H_2O) does not increase by more than 20 mL/min.

Compliance shall be checked by the test given in 62.2. The accuracy shall be tested as follows:

62.2.1 *Apparatus*—A pressure gage having an accuracy within ± 0.3 kPa and a flowmeter having an accuracy within ± 2 mL/min shall be used.

62.2.2 *Procedure*—Assemble the oxygen analyzer so that the oxygen sensor is installed in a dimensionally suitable port of a test apparatus containing an inlet fitting to which a test gas and air flow meter are attached. Connect the pressure gage to a third port of the test apparatus. Slowly open the flowmeter to raise the pressure in the test apparatus to 3 kPa. Determine the flow necessary to maintain this pressure. This leakage flow shall be as specified in Clause 62.1.

62.3 The rate at which a sampling oxygen analyzer withdraws gas from a breathing system (the gas diversion rate) shall not exceed 1.15 times the value stated in the accompanying documents.

Compliance shall be checked by the tests given in 62.4.

62.4 The rate of gas withdrawal shall be tested as follows:

62.4.1 *Principle*—Measurement of the rate at which a sampling (intermittent) oxygen analyzer withdraws gas from a simulated breathing system.

62.4.2 *Test Gas*—Pressurized air at room temperature shall be used.

62.4.3 *Apparatus*—A pressure gage having an accuracy within ±0.3 kPa, and a flowmeter having an accuracy to within ±10 % of the rate at which the oxygen analyzer withdraws gas from the breathing system as stated in the accompanying documents shall be used.

62.4.4 *Procedure*—Assemble the apparatus as described in 62.2.2 but using the flow meter specified in 62.4.3. Adjust the pressurized air source to 3 kPa and monitor the flowmeter reading for 1 min.

62.5 A means shall be provided to collect the gas from the oxygen analyzer.

63. *Replacement of Oxygen Sensor*

63.1 The accuracy of the oxygen reading and stability of measurement accuracy in response time shall meet the requirements given in 66.1, 66.3, 6.4, and 66.6, respectively, over a period of time, as described by the manufacturer in the accompanying documents.

Compliance shall be checked by the test given in 63.2.

63.2 The accuracy shall be tested as follows:

63.2.1 *Principle*—Determination of the accuracy of the oxygen reading, the stability of measurement accuracy and the response time over a period of time.

63.2.2 *Test gas*—A dry gas mixture containing oxygen at a level greater than 98 % (V/V) shall be used.

63.2.3 *Procedure:*

Hold the ambient temperature of the oxygen analyzer and the temperature of the test gas mixture delivered to the sensing area constant to within ± 1°C of a nominal value within the operating temperature range specified in the accompanying documents.

NOTE 21—The test gas mixture need not be at ambient temperature.

Deliver the test gas to the sensing area at ambient barometric pressure. Verify that the requirements given in 66.1, 66.3, 66.4, and 66.6 have been met.

13.5.3.3 Expose the sensing area to the test gas for at least 31 days.

NOTE 22—The ambient and test gas temperatures may vary over the full operating temperature range specified in accompanying documents during this period.

At the end of the period, carry out the test for measurement accuracy as described in 66.2, stability of measurement accuracy as described in 66.5, and response time as described in 66.7.

63.2.4 *Expression of Results*—Express the results as described in 66.2, 66.5, and 66.7, before and after the exposure period.

64. *Alarms:*

64.1 *Manual High Priority Signal Override*—If a manual control is provided to override the low oxygen level alarm, it shall only override the auditory high priority signal and shall automatically cancel after not more than 120 s following its most recent activation.

64.2.1 *Auditory Signal Frequency:*

Sound Quality—The fundamental frequency of auditory signals should lie between 150 and 1000 Hz, that shall be based on standard musical pitches, that is, the A440 system ±1 %. There shall be at least four frequency components ranging from 300 to 4000 Hz. These frequency components shall be related so that they form a distinct sound. These alarms should be non-startling. Rise times should exceed 15 mg.

64.2.2 *Sound Intensity*—Alarms that have an adjustable volume shall not be totally silenced by the adjustment, and shall have a minimum setting of 45 dB(A) or greater and a maximum setting of 85 dB(A) or less (peak output at 1 m) from the source in an anechoic chamber. Alarms with fixed intensity shall be between 70 and 85 dB(A) peak output at 1 m. If operator adjustment is provided, the control and its associated indicator shall be marked to indicate an increase or decrease in volume.

64.3 *Oxygen Level Alarms*—If an oxygen level alarm system is provided, is shall meet the following requirements:

a) The alarm shall be both visual and auditory.

b) The alarm limit shall lie within ±2 % (V/V) oxygen of the alarm set-point in the range of 15 % (V/V) to 60 % (V/V) oxygen and within ±5 % (V/V) oxygen of the alarm set-point elsewhere throughout the range.

Compliance shall be checked by the test given in 64.4.

64.4 *Test Method for Oxygen Level Alarm Limit*

64.4.1 *Principle*—Determination of the alarm limit values and the alarm set-point values at a number of oxygen readings across the range of the alarm system.

64.4.2 *Procedure:*

Hold the ambient temperature of the oxygen analyzer constant to within ±1°C of a nominal value within the operating temperature range specified in the accompanying documents. Generate at least four stable oxygen readings that span the range of the alarm system in approximately equal steps, by varying the oxygen level delivered to the sensor, or by electrically stimulating the oxygen sensor, or by adjusting the calibration control.

For each oxygen reading, adjust the alarm limit control so that the alarm is deactivated. Slowly adjust the alarm limit control until the alarm is activated. For each oxygen reading, record the alarm limit value, that is, the indicated oxygen reading, and the corresponding alarm set-point value, that is, the most precise set-point indication at the point of first activation of the alarm.

NOTE 23—An alarm may be of a type that is activated at an oxygen reading above (high alarm) or below (low alarm) the alarm limit. An oxygen analyzer may have either or both types of alarm.

64.5 *Low Alarm Limit Requirements*—If an adjustable low alarm limit is provided, it shall not be adjustable below an alarm set-point point value of 15 % (V/V) oxygen. If a non-adjustable low alarm limit is provided, the alarm set-point value shall not be below 15 % (V/V) oxygen. There shall be a visual indication to the user when a low alarm limit is adjusted to an alarm set-point value below 21 % (V/V) oxygen.

NOTE 24—This requirement may be met by methods such as red markings on the low alarm limit control in the range below 21 % (V/V) oxygen, or a caution signal that is activated when the low alarm limit control is set below 21 % (V/V) oxygen, or markings on the oxygen analyzer itself.

65. *Connections:*

If an oxygen sensor is intended to be connected to the breathing system through a T-piece, the breathing system connection ports of the T-piece shall be 15- or 22-mm conical connectors, or both, in accordance with ISO 5356-1:1987 or ISO 5356-2:1987.

If the oxygen sensor is mounted directly into the T-piece, the oxygen sensor connection port of the T-piece shall not be interchangeable with the breathing system connection ports of the T-piece.

The sampling gas and outlet ports of a sampling oxygen analyzer shall not be interchangeable with the breathing system connection port or with the oxygen sensor connection port.

66. *Measurement Accuracy:*

66.1 Oxygen readings shall be within ±3 % (V/V) oxygen of the actual oxygen level.

NOTE 25—This tolerance includes errors from all sources associated with the oxygen analyzer, such as its electrical circuits, calibration method, display resolution, and oxygen sensor, excluding the effects of interfering gases as listed in Table 2.

Compliance shall be checked by the method given in 66.2.

66.2 *Determination of Measurement Accuracy:*

66.2.1 *Principle*—Determination of the accuracy of the oxygen reading at a number of oxygen levels across the full range of the oxygen analyzer.

66.2.2 *Test gases*—At least the following four mixtures of oxygen and nitrogen shall be used: 15, 21, 40, and 60 % (V/V) oxygen. Ensure that the gas mixtures are dry, are pre-mixed, and that the oxygen level is known to within ±0.5 % (V/V) oxygen.

66.2.3 *Procedure:*

Operate the oxygen analyzer as described in the accompanying documents. Hold the ambient temperature of the oxygen analyzer and the temperature of the test gas mixture delivered to the oxygen sensor constant to within ±1°C of a nominal value within the operating range specified for the oxygen analyzer.

NOTE 26—The test gas mixtures need not be at ambient temperature.

Calibrate the oxygen analyzer as described in the accompanying documents. Deliver one of the test gas mixtures to the sensing area at ambient barometric pressure. Ensure that the oxygen analyzer is in equilibrium with the test gas mixture and that the oxygen analyzer is at ambient temperature. After a period of at least three times the response time in the accompanying documents, record the oxygen reading indicated by the oxygen analyzer. Repeat the procedure with the other gas mixtures.

66.2.4 *Expression of Results*—Correct the oxygen readings for changes in barometric pressure, if the errors due to this effect equal or exceed ±0.1 % (V/V) oxygen, and report the corrected readings.

66.3 *Digital Readings*—If an oxygen analyzer displays the oxygen reading digitally, there shall be: a) at least two digits, and b) a means for indicating that the oxygen reading is above the specified range of the display.

NOTE 27—This requirement may be met, for example, by a two-digit display that flashes or by a three-digit display that reads greater than 100 % (V/V) oxygen when the reading exceeds 100 % (V/V) oxygen, for instance, during calibration.

66.4 *Stability of Measurement Accuracy:*

Oxygen analyzers shall maintain the measurement accuracy specified in 66.1, 66.2, and 66.3 for a period of at least 8 h continuous use.

Compliance shall be checked by the test given in 66.5.

66.5 *Test Method:*

66.5.1 *Principle*—Determination of the accuracy of the oxygen reading in the central part of the oxygen measurement range of the oxygen analyzer during an eight-hour period after calibration.

66.5.2 *Test Gas*—A dry pre-mixture of oxygen and nitrogen containing oxygen at a level between 20 and 80 % of the full scale oxygen reading indicated on the oxygen analyzer shall be used, the oxygen level being known to within ±0.5 % (V/V) oxygen.

NOTE 28—If a reading of 21 % (V/V) oxygen lies within the required range, room air or compressed air may be used as the test gas mixture.

66.5.3 *Procedure:*

Operate the oxygen analyzer as described in the accompanying documents. Hold the ambient temperature of the oxygen analyzer and the temperature of the test gas mixture delivered to the sensing area constant to within ±1°C of a nominal value within the operating temperature range as specified in the accompanying documents.

NOTE 29—The test gas mixture need not be at ambient temperature.

Calibrate the oxygen analyzer as described in the accompanying documents. Deliver the test gas mixture to the sensing area at ambient barometric pressure. Ensure that the oxygen sensor is in equilibrium with the test gas mixture and that the oxygen analyzer is at ambient temperature. Expose the sensing area to the test gas for a continuous period of 8 h, ensuring that the oxygen analyzer is maintained in the same position during the whole period. For continuous monitoring oxygen analyzers, record the oxygen reading at least once every 15 min. For intermittent sampling oxygen analyzers, sample the test gas mixture at least once every 15 min and record the oxygen reading.

66.5.4 *Expression of Results*—Correct the oxygen readings for changes in barometric pressure, if the errors due to this effect equal or exceed ±0.1 % (V/V) oxygen, and report the corrected readings.

66.5 *Response Time*—The response time shall not be greater than 1.15 times the value stated in the accompanying documents.

Compliance shall be checked by the test given in 66.6.

66.6 *Test Method:*

66.6.1 *Principle*—Measurement of the time taken for the oxygen analyzer to respond to changes in oxygen level at the sensing area.

66.6.2 *Test Gases*—Two mixtures of oxygen and nitrogen that contain levels of oxygen equal to 95 to 100 % of the full scale oxygen reading and between 20 and 25 % of the full scale oxygen reading indicated on the oxygen analyzer shall be used.

NOTE 30—If a reading of 21 % (V/V) oxygen lies within the required range, room air or compressed air may be used as the test gas mixture.

66.6.3 *Procedure:*

Hold the ambient temperature of the oxygen analyzer and the temperature of the test gas mixtures delivered to the sensing area constant to within ±1°C of a nominal value within the operating temperature range specified in the accompanying documents.

NOTE 31—The test gas mixture need not be at ambient temperature.

Calibrate the oxygen analyzer at its full scale reading as described in the accompanying documents.

Deliver the test gas mixture to the sensing area at ambient barometric pressure. Ensure that the oxygen sensor is in equilibrium with the test gas mixture and that the oxygen analyzer is at ambient temperature.

Expose the sensing area to a test gas mixture with an oxygen level equivalent to 95 to 100 % of the full-scale oxygen reading. After a period of at least three times the response time as stated in the accompanying documents, record the oxygen reading indicated by the oxygen analyzer (R_1). Expose the sensing area to a test gas mixture with an oxygen level equivalent to 20 to 25 % of the full-scale oxygen reading. After a period of at least three times the response time as stated in the accompanying documents, record the oxygen reading indicated by the oxygen analyzer (R_2). With the oxygen analyzer measuring R_2, re-expose the sensing area to the 95 to 100 % full-scale oxygen reading test gas mixture. Measure the interval, to the nearest second, from the time at which the oxygen reading is at 10 % of the change above the initial reading (R_3) to the time at which the oxygen reading is 90 % of the change above the initial oxygen reading, that is, when the oxygen reading (R_4) is:

$$R_4 = R_2 + (0.9 \times [R_1 - R_2]) \quad (4)$$

$$R_3 = R_2 + (0.1 \times [R_1 - R_2]). \quad (5)$$

Finally, with the oxygen analyzer measuring R_1, re-expose the sensing area to the 20 to 25 % full-scale oxygen reading test gas mixture. Measure the interval, to the nearest second, from the time at which the oxygen reading is 10 % of the change above the initial reading, (R_6) to the time at which the oxygen reading is 90 % of the change below the initial oxygen reading, that is, when the oxygen reading (R_5) is:

$$R_5 = R_1 + (0.9 \times [R_1 - R_2]) \quad (6)$$

$$R_6 = R_1 + (0.1 \times [R_1 - R_2]). \quad (7)$$

66.6.4 *Expression of Results*—Report the times taken to reach the R_4 and R_6 readings.

NOTE 32—See also the requirements of Clauses 10.1, 21, 44.5.1, 61, and 63.1.

NOTE 33—The stated response time is the slowest that occurs when any one of the above referenced conditions is varied over its full range.

ANNEXES

(Mandatory Information)

A1. RATIONALE

INTRODUCTION

This annex provides a concise rationale for the important requirements of this specification and is intended for those who are familiar with the subject of this specification but who have not participated in its development. An understanding of the reasons for the main requirements is considered to be essential for its proper application. Furthermore, as clinical practice and technology change it is believed that a rationale for the present requirements will facilitate any revision of the specification necessitated by those developments. The clauses in this annex have been so numbered to correspond to the clauses in this specification to which they refer. The numbering is, therefore, not consecutive.

This annex presents the rationale on which the requirements, and, where necessary, the test methods are based. To the extent possible, it summarizes the discussions that were carried on by the participants in the meetings of the subcommittee that developed this specification.

NOTE A1.1—Annexes A to M given in IEC 601-1:1988 together with Annex A1 and Annex A2 in this specification apply.

A1.1 (X1.1) Scope

A1.1.1 There exists a great variety of devices for the measurement of oxygen level. The scope excludes devices used in laboratory research applications. Devices used in these applications are often experimental or intended primarily for non-medical uses. Imposition of the requirements of this draft standard on devices used for research might unduly limit development of beneficial new techniques or devices.

A1.1.2 It is expected that some devices that are not intended for clinical applications may eventually become used in the clinical environment. They would then be subject to the provisions of this draft standard if, for instance, the manufacturer suggested (for example, through advertising) applications that fall within the scope of this specification.

A1.2 (X1.3) Definitions

A1.2.1 (X1.3.1) *Alarm*—The distinction between the terms "alarm," "alarm system," and "alarm set-point" are important because they tend to be used imprecisely and somewhat interchangeably. Alarm is used in this specification only to refer to the high priority signal that occurs when the oxygen reading exceeds the alarm set-point. The alarm set-point value is the oxygen reading at which the alarm limit control or display indicates the alarm will activate. The alarm system comprises all of the preceding elements. The alarm set-point definition implies that the alarm set-point value need not be continuously displayed, but is capable of being readily displayed.

A1.2.2 (X1.3.6) *Display*—The term "display" is used to denote any device that visually conveys information to the operator. The term "visual indicator" is used to denote only those displays which present an indication of a condition, such as on (lamp illuminated) or off (lamp not illuminated).

A1.2.3 (X1.3.8) *Oxygen Analyzer*—Devices that do not "measure and indicate" are not intended to be covered by this specification. For instance, a device that has no function other than to signal an alarm at a specific oxygen level would not be considered to be an oxygen analyzer for use in direct patient monitoring applications.

A1.2.3.1 The term "in a gaseous mixture" implies that devices that measure or monitor oxygen in a liquid phase (for example, blood gas analyzers or indwelling catheters) are not covered by this draft specification.

A1.2.4 (X1.3.9) *Oxygen Level*—The term "oxygen level" was deliberately chosen and defined to allow oxygen readings in any accepted units, such as partial pressure or percent by volume. Oxygen level refers to the actual concentration of oxygen in a gas mixture.

NOTE A1.2—Most oxygen analyzers operate according to the partial pressure of oxygen present. Since, in medical applications, the gases measured are mixed by known volumes, it is normal practice to graduate analyzer scales in percent oxygen.

A1.2.5 (X1.3.10) *Oxygen Reading*—The term "oxygen reading" refers to the measured concentration of oxygen in the gas mixture. The oxygen reading will, in general, be different from the oxygen level. The magnitude of this difference will be the sum of the error (that is, the accuracy) of the analyzer and the error (again, the accuracy) of the reference method by which the gas mixture oxygen level was analyzed (for example, gas chromatography).

A1.2.6 (X1.3.14) *Sensing Area*—The term "sensing area" is not intended to be a synonym for "oxygen sensor". It is, rather, intended to define that location in the gaseous environment being measured at which oxygen molecules are considered to pass into the oxygen analyzer system. The actual oxygen sensor may be remote, as in the case of a sampling type analyzer.

A1.3 (X1.6.1) Identification, Marking, and Documents

A1.3.1 *Analyzer Markings*—(a) and (b) It is essential that users be able to identify the manufacturer, catalogue number and serial number of any medical device in order that problems, questions or complaints regarding the device can be communicated expeditiously. The absence of such information can, under some circumstances, render the instrument useless.

A1.3.2 (d) *Instructions*—Since it is common for oxygen analyzers to be operated in areas where the personnel using these change frequently, it is likely that full instructions will not be given in the use of an individual manufacturer's unit.

A1.3.2.1 Thus, it was generally agreed that some instructions and precautions needed to be placed on the analyzer itself, in addition to the detailed information contained in the accompanying documents. The requirement for instructions is intended to specify, in general, the minimal level of information that an unfamiliar user would need to operate the analyzer correctly and safely. It is recognized that there are limitations to the amount of information that can be placed on the analyzer without creating clutter or confusion. Thus, for this requirement, as well as throughout this entire clause, manufacturers are required to warn only of the more serious potential hazards on the analyzer itself, referring the user to the accompanying documents for details and cautions.

A1.3.3 (X1.6.3) *Marking of Controls and Instruments*—Since oxygen level may be stated in a number of different units of measure, such as % (V/V) oxygen, kPa or mmHg, it is necessary that the oxygen display be marked with the appropriate units of measure.

A1.3.4 (X1.6.7) If visual indicators are used on the oxygen analyzer, with the exception of alphanumeric displays, their color shall conform to the following requirements:

A1.3.4.1 (1) Red, with a flashing frequency of 1.4 to 2.8 Hz, shall be used as a high priority alarm.

A1.3.4.2 (2) Yellow, with a flashing frequency of 0.4 to 0.8 Hz, shall be used to indicate a medium priority alarm.

A1.3.4.3 (3) Yellow, with a constant signal, shall be used to indicate a low priority alarm.

A1.3.4.4 (4) Green shall be used to indicate that the oxygen analyzer is ready for use or in normal operation.

A1.3.4.5 (5) Blue shall be used only as an advisory indicator. Green indicators are reserved for indications of satisfactory function. Green is not intended to be used as a power-on indicator, unless the analyzer is ready for use and operating within tolerance without any warm-up delay. For example, it is not acceptable to have a green power-on indicator that illuminates simultaneously with a yellow warm-up delay indicator. In a case such as this, the green indicator illuminates only after the yellow indicator extinguishes.

A1.3.5 Blue indicators may not be used for any of the applications reserved for red, flashing red, yellow or green, in order to avoid confusion. Blue may only indicate information that has no connotation of good, marginal or poor performance of the analyzer or the monitored function(s).

A1.3.6 There are no color restrictions on displays, such as dot matrix displays or cathode ray tubes. Displays are generally monochromatic and are usually used to convey detailed information. The implication of the requirements of this draft specification is that if a monochromatic display is used, separate colored indicators are to be used to alert the operator to warning or caution conditions. A single indicator of each required color may be used, however, with the display providing the information on the nature of the problem.

A1.3.7 (X1.6.8.2) (f10) *Accompanying Documents*—It has been noted by some users that some oxygen analyzers have cables or sample tubing that are of insufficient length to be safely and conveniently mounted on apparatus, such as an anesthetic machine. It is difficult to specify universal lengths for all analyzers, since the required lengths may vary depending on the application. This requirement asks only that manufacturers recognize this problem and adequately inform users of the procedure for correct use.

A1.3.8 (f11) *Electromagnetic Interference*—Electromagnetic susceptibility is considered to be an important, but difficult to solve, medical device problem. Electrosurgery devices are the best-known primary offenders in terms of electromagnetic emissions. For these reasons, it was decided to compromise on a warning in the accompanying documents to educate the device user.

A1.3.8.1 There are no generally accepted specifications for minimum levels of electromagnetic interference to which medical devices should not be susceptible. When a recognized standard exists, this will be taken into account in the revision of this specification.

A1.3.8.2 (f) (12) An oxygen analyzer may be exposed to temperatures in the range of −40 to +70°C during transport. The extremes are those that might reasonably be expected to be met in transport by air, land, or sea. The objective of this requirement is to ensure that an analyzer will still be operable after exposure to these temperature extremes during transport.

A1.3.8.3 It is recognized that some types of oxygen sensor probably cannot withstand extremely low temperatures and that their response time or expected useful life, or both, are likely to be adversely affected. To account for this and to allow such oxygen sensors to be used because of their other desirable benefits, a narrower non-operating temperature range is permitted, provided that a notice to that effect is printed on the transport package and the actual range is disclosed in the accompanying documents. It is left to the manufacturer's discretion to determine the details of such precautionary instructions.

A1.4 (X1.10) Environmental Temperature Limitations

A1.4.1 Operating temperature range-temperatures as high as 40°C are often encountered in incubators. Temperatures as low as 15°C may be encountered during transport.

A1.5 (X1.19) Continuous Leakage Currents and Patient Auxiliary Currents

A1.5.1 It is essential that the leakage current is limited because the analyzer may come into contact with pacemaker leads or other conduction paths to the patient.

A1.6 (X1.21) Mechanical Strength

A1.6.1 Both line and battery powered oxygen analyzers, if easily portable or rack-mounted, will be subjected to frequent shock in the course of normal use. This requirement and test method is adapted from US MIL-STD-810C (Method 516.2). The intent of this requirement is not to require that severe shocks or drops (for example, from tabletops to floor) be withstood. Rather it is an attempt to set a baseline, minimum suggested standard for the moderate shocks or drops frequently encountered in portable or rack-mounted medical equipment. It appears that no data exist on average or extreme shock conditions in medical environments. However, it is generally agreed that medical equipment is typically subjected to abuse. A300 m/s_2, 11 ms, half-sine wave shock pulse has an energy content of 0.23 g/s, which is about equivalent to the 30 cm free fall of an object. A shock pulse time of 11 ms is reasonable for a fall to a typical hospital surface such as wood or tile. In summary, the test requires portable analyzers to have enough strength to withstand roughly the equivalent of a 30-cm free fall to a table.

A1.7 (X1.37.1) Protection Against Hazards of Explosion in Medically Used Rooms

A1.7.1 Since the worldwide use of flammable anesthetics is becoming rare, an analyzer that has a restricted use is considered acceptable.

A1.7.2 Two levels of safety for explosion hazards are set. The first, less stringent, level is for the analyzer body and oxygen sensor in a flammable environment not in direct communication with a patient (ambient atmosphere in an operating room). If there are no sparks possible, only thermal energy could ignite a flammable gas mixture and thus the temperature maximum has been specified. If there could be sparks, the maximum level of energy in the electrical circuit is additionally specified. This level is based on the ignition energy of the most flammable mixtures of diethyl ether and air.

A1.7.3 The second, more stringent, level is for oxygen sensors that are placed in a breathing system in direct communication with breathing gas mixtures and the patient airway. In this case, the supply voltage is restricted and, if sparks are possible, the maximum level of electrical circuit energy is specified, in addition.

A1.7.4 This level is based on the ignition energy level of the most flammable mixture of diethyl ether and oxygen.

A1.8 (X1.44.5) Humidity and Condensation Effects

A1.8.1 Analyzers are routinely used in humid environments or in environments where condensate could form on the oxygen sensor. It is essential that users are informed of any adverse effects of such conditions. There are four potential effects to be considered:

A1.8.1.1 (1) The addition of water vapor to a dry gas mixture under isothermal, isobaric conditions changes the partial pressure of gases in that mixture. This physical principle is not construed as an adverse effect of humidity and, therefore, needs no precautionary warning. Clause 6 requires that this physical principle be explained in the accompanying documents.

A1.8.1.2 (2) Water vapor may interfere with the measurement of oxygen, as may other gases or vapors listed in Table 1. For water vapor, this effect is covered by the test described.

A1.8.1.3 (3) The accuracy, stability, or response time of the analyzer may be affected under less than saturation conditions by mechanisms other than interference that would not be detected by the test described in 44.5.2. This effect is not examined separately in this draft specification; rather, it is assumed that such an effect would also be encountered under saturation conditions and is thus covered by the test described in 44.5.4.

A1.8.1.4 (4) The formation of condensate in breathing mixtures can have significant effects on oxygen measurement systems. It is probably the most serious humidity effect and is frequently encountered in clinical practice. This problem is checked by the test described in 44.5.4. This test requires, as does the test described in 44.5.2, that temperature equilibrium be attained to separate humidity effects from those of transient temperature effects.

A1.9 (X1.51.5) Function and Position of Controls

A1.9.1 An operator unaware that checking of test controls can cause a control to be permanently left in one position can lead to the mistaken assumption that oxygen levels are being measured when, in fact, they are not. An example would be a battery check that indicated good battery condition when the display indicates 20 to 22 % (V/V) oxygen. Distinguishable control positions are necessary to determine what is being displayed on multi-function displays.

A1.9.2 Inadvertent changes in the calibration control position will result in the display of erroneous measurements.

A1.9.3 Controls should operate according to stereotyped expectations to discourage inappropriate control settings.

A1.10 (X1.56.8) Indicators

A1.10.1 Operator attention is required when a condition occurs that results in the activation of a high, medium, or low priority signal. In the case of a high priority signal, immediate attention is required. The requirement for an auditory signal ensures that the operator will be made aware of a serious problem immediately, even if he or she is not looking at the analyzer. Since medium priority signals indicate conditions that do not require immediate action, an auditory component is not required. In either case, the visual indicator is intended primarily to identify which piece of equipment requires attention. The specific nature of the problem which resulted in the signal being activated can be identified by the use of multiple visual indicators or by a display such as a dot matrix display, a cathode ray tube, or a liquid crystal display.

A1.11 (X1.60) Interfering Gas and Vapor Effects

A1.11.1 One of the principal applications of oxygen analyzers is in anesthesia. It is essential that operators are informed of any additional errors in the oxygen reading that may be introduced as a result of cross-sensitivity of the oxygen sensor to any of the gases or vapors likely to be encountered during anesthesia. An interference greater than ± 2 % (V/V) oxygen is not permitted since, even though stated in the accompanying documents, it could produce an unsafe condition in the hands of the user unaware of this type of interference. An interference of less than ±1 % (V/V) oxygen is considered insignificant and, therefore, the value need not be stated.

A1.11.2 The use of oxygen for the balance of the mixture allows the test to identify interference errors that may only occur in the presence of oxygen.

A1.11.3 The operator should be aware that in some analyzers the combination of low battery and interfering gases or vapors can be especially misleading.

A1.12 Cyclic Pressure

This requirement does not deal with the "problem" of oxygen level changes due to breathing circuit pressure changes based on the fundamental physical principle of operation of oxygen analyzers—that is, that they measure the partial pressure of oxygen which is a function of ambient pressure. Instead, this requirement deals with permanent mechanical changes to oxygen sensors due to imposed cyclical pressure changes.

A1.12.1 The pressure extremes of +10 and −1.5 kPa are considered clinically relevant pressures that are occasionally attained.

A1.13 (X1.62) Gas Leakage and Sampling Loss

Sensors mounted in T-pieces have contributed to leakage in breathing systems due to both poor seals at the sensor and incorrect 22 mm connectors on the T-piece. As the breathing system normally contains a number of various components, it is essential that the maximum leakage rate from the oxygen analyzer be as low as possible. Otherwise, it will be impossible to achieve an acceptably low maximum leakage rate for the breathing system.

When sampling analyzers withdraw gas from the breathing system, it may have a significant effect on the gas volume delivered to the patient. The requirement to provide information on the sampling gas flow provides the use with the information necessary to assess its significance for various clinical situations. In closed circuit systems, high gas withdrawal flows are not acceptable with regard to patient safety and pollution effects.

Since oxygen analyzer manufacturers usually do not manufacture the fittings with which their T-pieces must mate, testing is performed with standard 22 mm fittings.

A1.14 (X1.63) Replacement of Oxygen Sensor

While it is recognized that the expected life may vary considerably as a function of test conditions, it is important that the operator is given some indication of the expected life of the analyzer's expendable components. Manufacturers are required to express expected life by the same conventions so that the user has a consistent set of information on which to base clinical and financial decisions.

The conditions for determining expected useful life were chosen somewhat arbitrarily to represent routine environments in which oxygen analyzers will be operated in anesthesia and respiratory therapy applications. The conditions will yield a conservative estimate of expected useful life, since they are a combination of that which tends to be a "worse case" environment for all sensing techniques employed at the time that this draft specification was developed.

In the test method, oxygen analyzer function is evaluated at 85 % of expected useful life rather than at 100 % of expected useful life. This allows the stated useful life to be at or closer to the nominal value rather than at the worst case value, allowing for variations between individual sensors. A tolerance of plus or minus one day is included to allow the test to begin and conclude when personnel are available.

A1.15 (X1.64) Alarms

Auditory signals with very low or very high fundamental frequencies may be difficult for some operators to hear. At such frequencies, it can be more difficult to locate the position in the room from which the signal is emanating. Also, more sound energy is required at low or high frequencies to achieve the same perceived sound intensity, since human hearing is less sensitive in those ranges.

Frequencies between 150 and 1000 Hz provide a reasonable combination of perceived loudness and directionality.

Warning signals are more effective in attracting the attention of the user when they are cyclic rather than continuous. A relatively slow cycle rate is recommended, in order to convey a sense of urgency without startling the people in the room.

A1.16 (X1.64.1) Manual High Priority Signal Override

Continuous signals may be used for the auditory component of high priority signals, yet they can be a significant distraction during the time that the operator is attempting to correct such a condition. Thus, a temporary silencing mechanism is desirable. In the case of a low oxygen level alarm, a prolonged deactivation of the auditory components of the high priority signal is allowed. It was considered that 120 s was the maximum time that would be required to correct any condition that results in the activation of a low oxygen level alarm.

This requirement implies that all high priority signals may have their auditory component overridden but only low oxygen level alarms are required to cancel automatically.

A1.17 (X1.64.3, X1.64.4, X1.64.5) Oxygen Level Alarms

Alarm systems, although a desirable feature, should be optional. Not all applications require alarms. The operator makes the final decision on whether an alarm system is required. An auditory warning signal is required, since the exceeding of an oxygen level alarm limit requires immediate attention by the user. A visual indicator is required, since there may be many instruments in the same room with similar sounding auditory warning signals. The visual indicator serves to identify which device is to be attended to. The requirements for alarm accuracy are based primarily on the minimum necessary for patient safety, although technical and financial constraints are also a consideration. An alarm accuracy of ±2 % (V/V) oxygen should be sufficient in the lower range of clinical applications where the concern is the accidental delivery of an hypoxic breathing mixture. The additive error of ±3 % (V/V) oxygen reading accuracy and ±2 % (V/V) oxygen alarm accuracy implies that a combined error of ±5 % (V/V) oxygen could occur in the worst case. It is believed that such an error could be tolerated for warning by the alarm of an unsafe condition. The individual and combined errors are believed to be achieved by reasonable means within the limitations of existing technology and the financial constraints of the marketplace. A lesser degree of accuracy can be tolerated over the balance of the alarm range, since the combined error of ±8 % (V/V) oxygen is within the range of any established, clinically significant effects on the patient (see 64.3).

A1.15.3 A low alarm limit that can be adjusted or is pre-set to a set-point value below 15 % (V/V) oxygen is considered unsafe. It is important to recognize that due to the cumulative nature of the permissible measurement and alarm accuracy errors, an analyzer with a low alarm limit that is adjusted to a set-point value of 15 % (V/V) oxygen may begin to alarm at an oxygen level as low as 10 % (V/V) oxygen (with a corresponding alarm limit of 13 % (V/V) oxygen) or at an oxygen level as high as 20 % (V/V) oxygen (with a corresponding alarm limit of 17 % (V/V) oxygen).

A1.16 (X1.66) Measurement Accuracy

X1.16.1 (X1.66.1, X1.66.2, X1.66.3) *Measurement Accuracy*—The accuracy of the oxygen reading is of major importance due to the critical applications of oxygen analyzers.

In this specification, accuracy takes into account all errors in the measurement system introduced between the sensing area and the displayed oxygen reading as perceived by the operator. This includes sampling system errors, oxygen sensor errors, electrical circuit errors, calibration errors and play errors, among others.

The maximum error allowance of ±3 % (V/V) oxygen satisfies the criteria of effective function for all three primary areas of medical use: anesthesia, pediatrics and respiratory therapy. For anesthesia, the requirement is particularly critical, because a patient being maintained on an indicated 21 % (V/V) oxygen reading would, in most cases, suffer no ill effects if the oxygen level were between 18 and 24 % (21 ± 3 %) (V/V) oxygen. Below an oxygen level of 18 % (V/V) oxygen, primary organ function could begin to be compromised. The maximum error allowance of ±3 % (V/V) oxygen is considered by pediatric anesthesiologists to be the maximum acceptable error in the normal range of their applications between 40 and 60 % (V/V) oxygen. The requirements of respiratory therapy are also satisfied. For diagnostic measurements where 90 to 100 % (V/V) oxygen is delivered (the most rigid need), an error of ±3 % (V/V) oxygen is the maximum permissible. Therefore, a maximum error allowance of ±3 % (V/V) oxygen has been chosen for the entire range of 0 to 100 % (V/V) oxygen.

(a) A simple, effective calibration method would be:

(b) Place the sensing area in 100 % (V/V) oxygen,

(c) Adjust the calibration control so that the oxygen reading is 100 % (V/V) oxygen,

Place the sensing area in room air and verify that the oxygen reading is 21 ± 3 % (V/V) oxygen.

The use of single point calibration methods (for example, only air) is discouraged, since anomalies such as non-linearities and zero offsets would not be detected.

The four points specified in the test method (66.2.2) have been chosen to allow a reasonably simple procedure for checking accuracy. For instance, an oxygen analyzer with a span of 0 to 100 % (V/V) oxygen might be tested at 0 and 100 % (V/V) oxygen. One of the two other points could be room air. The fourth point could then be a pre-mixed calibration standard of ±0.5 % (V/V) oxygen accuracy and containing between 40 and 80 % (V/V) oxygen. High purity mixtures of 0 and 100 % (V/V) oxygen are easily and inexpensively obtainable, as is dry room air. Pre-mixed gas standards of better than ±0.5 % (V/V) oxygen accuracy are not so readily available. Thus, this accuracy value was chosen.

NOTE A1.3—For further information, see Annex A2.

The requirement for digital displays was included to avoid unsafe situations such as display that indicates 99 % (V/V) oxygen when the actual electrical signal to the display is well over 100 % (V/V) oxygen. Such a display with a maximum reading of 99 would hide an otherwise clear device error or out-of-calibration state. Solutions to this problem include:

(a) A three-digit display and

(b) An indicator for oxygen levels above the specified range of the display.

A1.17 (A1.66.4, X1.66.5) Stability of Measurement Accuracy

It is reasonable that users should expect that an analyzer will not drift beyond its stated accuracy for a period of at least 8 h after it has been calibrated according to the accompanying documents. It is felt reasonable to require that the analyzer's calibration be confirmed at the change of each eight-hour working shift when in continuous use.

A1.17.2 This requirement implies that the stability will be within the specified limits at any constant temperature within the operating temperature range.

A1.18 (X1.66.6, X1.66.7) Response Time

Operators (especially those unfamiliar with the characteristics of a specific analyzer) should be given some indication of the period of time required for a reading to reach steady state after a change in oxygen level has been introduced. It is felt that the 90 % response time represents a reasonable approximation to steady state conditions and would thus indicate to the operator how long he or she should wait in order to ensure that a stable reading has been reached. With such information, calibration errors are less likely to occur. In the test method, the measured response time is allowed to be as much as 1.15 times slower than the value stated by the manufacturer. This allows the stated response time to be at or closer to the nominal value rather than at the worst case value, allowing for variations between individual sensors. The response time is measured with both increasing and decreasing oxygen levels, since response time can be a function of the direction of the change in oxygen level.[6]

[6] DOD Handbook 743 A: *Anthropometry of U.S. Military Personnel (Metric)*, February 13, 1991.

A2. INFORMATIVE

A2.1 For documents containing further information see ISO 8158, DOD Handbook 7434[6], and MIL-STD-810.

Designation: F 1463 – 93 (Reapproved 1999)

Standard Specification for Alarm Signals in Medical Equipment Used in Anesthesia and Respiratory Care[1]

This standard is issued under the fixed designation F 1463; the number immediately following the designation indicates the year of original adoption or, in the case of revision, the year of last revision. A number in parentheses indicates the year of last reapproval. A superscript epsilon (ε) indicates an editorial change since the last revision or reapproval.

INTRODUCTION

Medical practice in hospitals is increasingly dependent on equipment for observation and treatment of patients. Sounds and lights are frequently used to indicate the patient's physiological status and the functional state of the equipment. The sounds used are frequently too loud and not sufficiently distinctive, and it is often difficult to identify which item of equipment is signalling. The purpose of this specification is to specify signals, both audible and visual, to be used to draw attention to the fact that equipment has detected a disturbance and to indicate the degree of urgency.

The content of this specification was developed with contributions from clinicians, engineers, applied psychologists, and musicians. Some of the criteria considered during development of the sounds included optimal signal recognition in a relatively noise-filled environment, maximum transmission of information at the lowest practical sound pressure level, ease of learning and retention by operators who have to respond to the various signals, and perceived urgency of the sounds.

1. Scope

1.1 This specification covers defining the characteristics and requirements of electrically generated alarm signals for use with medical equipment intended for use in anesthesia and respiratory care. It does not specify the condition that activates the alarms, nor does it specify the devices used for the production of audible and visual signals. This specification does not address informational sounds produced by devices such as ECG monitors, surgical lasers, and electrocautery units.

1.2 The values stated in SI units are to be regarded as the standard.

2. Referenced Documents

2.1 *ISO Standard:*

ISO 3744: Acoustics—Determination of Sound Power Levels of Noise Sources—Engineering Methods for Free-Field Conditions Over a Reflecting Plane[2]

2.2 *IEC Standards:*[2]

IEC 651 Sound Level Meters

IEC 73 Colors of Indicator Lights and Push-Buttons[3]

IEC 601-1 Medical Electrical Equipment—Part 1: General Requirements for Safety[3]

3. Terminology

3.1 *Definitions:*

3.1.1 *burst*—a group of pulses with a distinctive rhythm.

3.1.2 *burst amplitude*—the A-weighted sound pressure level of the maximum pulse in the burst measured in decibels.

3.1.3 *burst spacing*—the period of time between the start of the first pulse in one burst and the start of the first pulse in the next burst.

3.1.4 *clearly legible*—the visual attribute of information displayed by the equipment that allows the operator to discern (or identify) quantitative values or functions under a specific set of environmental conditions.

3.1.5 *discriminate*—the ability of an operator to perceive a qualitative difference among visual signals under a specific set of environmental conditions.

3.1.6 *flashing frequency*—the number of light flashes per unit of time.

3.1.7 *high priority alarm*—a combination of audible and visual signals indicating that immediate operator response is required.

3.1.8 *low priority alarm*—a visual signal, or a combination of audible and visual signals indicating that operator awareness is required.

3.1.9 *medium priority alarm*—a combination of audible and visual signals indicating that prompt operator response is required.

3.1.10 *overall pulse duration*—the time over which the pulse amplitude exceeds 10 % of the maximum amplitude.

---

[1] This specification is under the jurisdiction of ASTM Committee F-29 on Anesthetic and Respiratory Equipment and is the direct responsibility of Subcommittee F29.15 on Harmonization of Alarms.

Current edition approved Feb. 15, 1993. Published June 1993.

[2] Available from American National Standards Institute, 11 W. 42nd Street, 13th Floor, New York, NY 10036.

[3] Patterson, R. D., *Guidelines for Auditory Warning Systems on Civil Aircraft*, Civil Aviation Authority (UK) Paper 82017, 1982.

3.1.11 *pulse*—a sound having a specific frequency spectrum and specific duration.

3.1.12 *pulse frequency*—the fundamental frequency of the pulse.

3.1.13 *pulse spacing (within a burst)*—the period of time between the start of one pulse and the start of the next pulse.

4. General Requirements

4.1 *High Priority Alarm Signal*—A high priority signal shall have the characteristics given in Table 1.

4.2 *Medium Priority Alarm Signal*—A medium priority signal shall have the characteristics given in Table 1.

4.3 *Low Priority Alarm Signal*—A low priority alarm signal shall have the characteristics given in Table 1.

4.4 When an alarm signal is generated, the cause of the alarm shall be indicated.

NOTE 1—This requirement is satisfied if the monitored variable or condition is identified.

5. Specific Requirements for Audible Signals

5.1 *Sound Quality*— Alarm sounds shall have a fundamental frequency of between 150 and 1000 Hz, based on standard musical pitches, that is, the A440 system ± 1 %. There shall be at least four frequency components ranging from 300 to 4000 Hz. These frequency components shall be related so that they form a distinct sound. These alarms should be nonstartling. Rise times should exceed 15 ms.

5.2 *Sound Intensity*— Alarms that have an adjustable volume shall not be totally silenced by the adjustment, and shall have a minimum setting of 45 dB(A) or greater and a maximum setting of 85 dB(A) or less (peak output at 1 m) from the source in an anechoic chamber. Alarms with fixed intensity shall be between 70 and 85 dB(A) peak output at 1 m. If operator adjustment is provided, the control and its associated indicator shall be marked to indicate an increase or decrease in volume.

5.3 There shall be a visual indication that a high or medium priority alarm audible signal has been disabled.

NOTE 2—The conditions for alarm silencing are specified in the relevant standards for particular devices.

5.4 *Duration of Alarm Sounds*—If the alarm sounds are limited in duration, for example, "power failure alarm," such limitations shall be disclosed by the manufacturer.

6. Visual Requirements

6.1 All visual signals for alarms shall be clearly legible at a distance of 1 m when tested in accordance with 6.1.1.

6.1.1 The test operator with a visual acuity of one (corrected if necessary), shall be able to read correctly from a distance of 1 m and at an angle of 30° from either side of a line perpendicular to the center of the display or control panel and under an ambient illuminance in the range of 100 to 1500 lx. The test is passed if the test operator can correctly perceive the quantitative value(s) or function(s) displayed by the visual alarm signal(s).

6.1.2 *Rationale*—The ability of an operator to perceive the quantitative information contained in any visual alarm display at a distance of 1 meter was considered by the committee to represent the minimum safety requirement in the operating room environment, or at an ICU bedside.

6.2 An operator shall be able to discriminate between high and medium priority alarm signals at a distance of 4 m when tested in accordance with 6.2.1.

6.2.1 The test operator with a visual acuity of one (corrected if necessary), shall be able to read correctly from a distance of 4 m and at an angle of 30° from either side of a line perpendicular to the center of the display or control panel and under an ambient illuminance in the range of 100 to 1500 lx. The test is passed if the test operator can perceive the high priority and medium priority visual signals, and discriminate between them.

6.2.2 *Rationale*—The ability to see the warning and caution indicators at a distance of 4 meters, and to discriminate between them, is important in large intensive care settings with multiple ventilators and the possibility of multiple simultaneous alarms. The operator can then make a decision as to which alarm to respond to first based on the alarm priority.

6.3 Alphanumeric or computer-generated graphics displays of alarm messages, including centralized alarm displays, are exempt from the color and flashing frequency requirements in Table 1 if the displays meet the requirements in 6.1 and 6.2. However, if an alphanumeric or graphics display of alarm messages does not meet the requirements in 6.1 and 6.2, then an alternate visual method that does meet the requirements in Table 1 shall be employed.

NOTE 3—A single color indicator per category is sufficient to satisfy the requirement in Table 1.

TABLE 1 Alarm Signal Requirements

Alarm Category	Operator Response	Audible Indicators[A]	Indicator Color[B]	Flashing Frequency (Hz)[C]
High priority	Immediate	Not medium or low priority I	Red	1.4–2.8 Hz (F_2)
Medium priority	Prompt	Not high or low priority	Yellow	0.4–0.8 Hz (F_1)
Low priority	Awareness	Not high or medium priority	Yellow	Constant (On)

[A] See 5.1, 5.2, and Annex A1.
[B] See 6.3.
[C] Reference to IEC 73.

ANNEX

(Mandatory Information)

A1. CONSTRUCTION OF PULSES AND BURSTS

A1.1 *Pulses*—A pulse is a small unit of sound lasting from 100 to 1000 ms. It is made from a set of harmonics of which the lowest if the fundamental, that usually gives the pulse its pitch. The harmonic content of a pulse would normally consist of a fundamental frequency and a set of higher component frequencies, known as harmonics. The relationship between the fundamental frequency and a set of higher component frequencies, known as components will produce the timbre, or sound quality, of the pulse. There should be at least four, and preferably more, of these harmonics in the pulse in order to avoid masking by other sounds and to aid localisation by the listener. In order to avoid startle responses, the pulses should have a shaped amplitude envelope, meaning that they do not come on at their loudest level. They should therefore be gated with cosine ramps at the onset and the offset. A200 ms pulse may, for example, possess a "standard" envelope consisting of a 25 ms onset and a 25 ms offset ramp. A "slow onset" ramp placed on a pulse of the same length might have a 175 ms onset ramp followed by a 25 ms offset, and a "slow offset" ramp would have the opposite construction. The pulse is the basic unit of sound from which the burst is constructed.

A1.2 *Bursts*—A burst is a unit of sound typically lasting several seconds, consisting of two or more pulses. These bursts will sound like melodies with a rhythm. Bursts are played at intervals to form a complete warning. The first one or two pulses should be played at a lower level in order to avoid startle reactions. Different bursts are more readily discriminated if their rhythms and pitch patterns differ from one another.

A1.3 *Perceived Urgency*—It is essential that the high priority warning is made to be more urgent than the medium priority warning, which in turn should be made to be more urgent than the low priority warning. This can be achieved by selecting spectral (pulse) characteristics that are known to produce high urgency ratings for high priority warnings, low-urgency pulse characteristics for low priority warnings, and the same principles applied to burst characteristics.

A1.3.1 In general, the pulse characteristics will carry less weight in determining the overall urgency of the warning than the burst characteristics. More emphasis should be placed on producing variation in the burst parameters to alter the urgency of the sounds to achieve their final urgency level.

A1.3.1.1 *Pulses*—The fundamental frequency of the pulse affects urgency; the higher the pitch of the pulse, the more urgent it is judged to be. However, the fundamental should not be so high as to produce annoyance, and the first four harmonics should be below 4 kHz. Thus the fundamental frequency should be below 1000 Hz. The harmonic components also affect the urgency of the pulse. Pulses where the harmonics do not bear an integer relationship to the fundamental are judged to be more urgent than completely harmonic, "musical" pulses. However, a very complex harmonic series will obscure the pitch of the pulse. Amplitude envelopes that are either "standard" or "slow onset" are sometimes judged to be more urgent than those with a "slow offset," although the effect is unclear and the changes in urgency produced are small.

A1.3.1.2 *Bursts*—Both temporal and melodic characteristics affect the perceived urgency of the burst. The temporal characteristics are determined by variations in pulse-to-pulse time, and the melodic characteristics are determined by variations in the fundamental frequency of the pulses.

A1.3.1.3 *Temporal Characteristics*—The primary determinant of the urgency of a burst is its speed, as measured by the pulse-to-pulse interval. Any interval below about 200 ms may be judged to be fairly urgent, although faster speeds may be necessary. Any interval greater than about 350 to 400 ms may be described as less urgent. The rhythm of the burst, determined by varying individual pulse-to-pulse intervals, also affects urgency. Regular rhythms are generally more urgent than irregular rhythms, although some sorts or irregularities, such as decreasing the pulse-to-pulse interval during the burst, can be effective. It is very important also to have different temporal patterns within a warning set in order to reduce confusions between warnings. Repeating a burst more often, or at shorter time intervals, may also increase the urgency of the overall warning.

A1.3.1.4 *Melodic Characteristics*—The pitch contour (pattern of ups and downs, produced by altering the fundamental frequency of individual pulses) can affect the urgency of a burst, but it is probably more useful as a discriminating factor between warnings. Larger pitch ranges (the frequency range from the highest to the lowest pulses in the burst) are more urgent than smaller ranges, and bursts which are musically resolved may sound less urgent than atonal or unresolved bursts. The amplitude envelope of a high priority burst should reach maximum output level after one or two pulses, and should stay at that level. A less urgent burst may be produced by reducing the level of the pulses again towards the end of the burst.

A2. Additional References[4,5]

[4] Patterson, R. D., "Guidelines for the Design of Auditory Warning Sounds," *Proc. Inst. Acoust. 11(5)*, pp. 17–24, 1989.

[5] Edworthy, J., Loxley, S., Geelhoed, E., and Dennis, I., "The Perceived Urgency of Auditory Warnings," *Proc. Inst. Acoust. 11(5)*, pp. 73–80, 1989.

Standard Specification for
Oxygen Concentrators for Domiciliary Use[1]

This standard is issued under the fixed designation F 1464; the number immediately following the designation indicates the year of original adoption or, in the case of revision, the year of last revision. A number in parentheses indicates the year of last reapproval. A superscript epsilon (ε) indicates an editorial change since the last revision or reapproval.

INTRODUCTION

Oxygen concentrators provide a safe source of oxygen-enriched air for patients in need. They are devices that raise the level of inspired oxygen by separating nitrogen or oxygen from ambient air.

Oxygen concentrators fall into two main classes according to the means whereby gas separation is effected, namely: oxygen concentrators in which oxygen selectively permeates or transports through a membrane or lattice, and pressure swing adsorbers (PSA) in which air is exposed at a certain pressure to molecular sieve material that selectively retains nitrogen and other components until they are subsequently released when the pressure is reduced.

The scope of this specification is not restricted to these two classes as alternative methods of concentrating oxygen may become available and it is not intended that this specification should restrict future developments.

This particular specification is one of a series of standards based on IEC 601-1 second edition and it amends and supplements IEC 601-1 second edition, hereinafter called the "general standard." As stated in 1.3 of the general standard, the requirements of this particular specification take precedence over those of the general standard.

As in the general standard the requirements are followed by compliance tests. The numbers of the sections and clauses in this specification refer to the related sections and clauses in the general standard. Clauses, sub-clauses or figures that are additional to those of the general standard are numbered starting after the last numbered clause in the general standard; additional annexes are lettered AA, BB, etc. and additional items (aa), (bb), etc. The changes from the text of the general standard are specified by the use of the following words:

"Replacement" means that the clause, sub-clause or specified paragraph of the general standard is replaced by the text of this specification.

"Amendment" means that the clause, sub-clause or specified paragraph of the general standard is amended as indicated by the text of this specification.

"Addition" means that the text of this specification is additional to the requirements of the general standard.

Details of the arrangement of test apparatus for carrying out a number of the tests to check compliance with certain requirements are given in Annex A1.

A rationale for the most important requirements is given in Annex A2. It is considered that a knowledge of the reasons for the requirements will not only facilitate the proper application of the standard, but will expedite any subsequent revision. This annex does not form part of the specification.

Test methods and apparatus other than those specified in this specification, but of equal or greater accuracy may be used to verify compliance with particular requirements. However, in the event of a dispute the methods and apparatus as specified in this specification shall be used to resolve the matter.

The format of this specification is similar to that of IEC "particular standards"; but differs in the following respects: Sections 1, 2, and 3 will appear in the format as recommended in *Form and Style for ASTM Standards Manual*. Section 4 includes a chart listing all of the clauses of IEC 601-1 and indicates whether that clause applies (A), does not apply (NA), or applies with an amendment or replacement (AM/R). For the text of clauses that either apply or do not apply, consult IEC 601-1 Second Edition, 1988. Section 5 includes, in numerical order, the text of all amendments, additions or replacements to the general standard, and includes tests for compliance.

1. Scope

1.1 This clause of the general standard applies except as follows (replacement): This particular specification specifies safety requirements for oxygen concentrators as defined in 3.1. This specification does not apply to oxygen concentrators intended to supply gas to several patients via a piped medical gas installation or to those intended for use in the presence of flammable anaesthetic or cleaning agents, or both.

1.2 The values stated in SI units are to be regarded as the standard.

2. Referenced Documents

2.1 *ISO Standards:*

ISO 3744 Acoustics—Determination of Sound Power Levels of Noise Sources—Engineering Method for Free-Field Conditions Over a Reflecting Plane[2]

ISO 8359 Oxygen Concentrators for Medical Use—Safety Requirements[2]

ISO 9703 Anaesthesia and Respiratory Care Alarm Signals—Part 1: Visual Alarm Signals[2]

2.2 *IEC Standards:*

IEC Publication 601-1 Medical Electrical Equipment Part I, General Requirements for Safety (Second Edition)

IEC Publication 651 Sound Level Meters[3]

3. Terminology

3.1 *Definitions:* For the purposes of this specification, the definitions given in Clause 2 of IEC 601-1:1988 apply, with the following replacements and additions.

3.1.1 *applied part*—the oxygen concentrator outlet.

3.1.2 *administration accessories*—all accessories for conducting the product gas from the oxygen concentrator outlet to the patient for example, tubing, humidifier, breathing system, mask or nasal cannulae, but excluding any fixed tubing extensions.

3.1.3 *flow adjuster*—a device that controls the flow of the product gas.

3.1.4 *flow indicator*—a device that shows the volume of gas passing through the oxygen concentrator in a unit of time.

3.1.5 *operator control*—a control to enable the user, without the need for tools, to cause the oxygen concentrator to perform its intended function.

3.1.6 *outlet pressure*—the gage pressure at the oxygen concentrator outlet under the test flow conditions.

3.1.7 *oxygen analyzer*—a device that measures and quantitatively indicates the concentration of oxygen present in a gaseous mixture.

3.1.8 *oxygen concentration status indicator*— a device that by measuring the proportion of oxygen in the product gas, indicates when that proportion is at an abnormal level.

3.1.9 *oxygen concentrator*—a device that, by separating out nitrogen or oxygen from ambient air, provides oxygen enriched air.

3.1.10 *oxygen concentrator outlet*—the port of the oxygen concentrator from which the product gas flows.

3.1.11 *product gas*—the output from the oxygen concentrator consisting of respirable oxygen-enriched air.

4. Relationship of This Specification to IEC 601-1, Second Edition:

Section One - General	(A)	(NA)	(AM/R)
1. Scope and object			X
2. Terminology and definitions			X
3. General requirements	X		
4. General requirements for tests	X		
5. Classification	X		
6. Identification, marking and documents			X
7. Power input	X		
Section Two - Environmental Conditions			
8. Basic safety categories		X	
9. (Not used in IEC-601-1 Second Edition)			
10. Environmental conditions	X		
11. (Not used in IEC-601-1 Second Edition)			
12. (Not used in IEC-601-1 Second Edition)			
Section Three - Protection Against Electric Shock Hazards			
13. General	X		
14. Requirements related to classification	X		
15. Limitation of voltage and/or energy	X		

[1] This specification is under the jurisdiction of ASTM Committee F-29 on Anesthetic and Respiratory Equipmentand is the direct responsibility of Subcommittee F29.14 on Ventilators.

Current edition approved Feb. 15, 1993. Published June 1993.

[2] Available from American National Standards Institute, 11 West 42nd St., New York, NY 10036.

	(A)	(NA)	(AM/R)
16. Enclosures and PROTECTIVE COVERS	X		
17. Separation	X		
18. Protective earthing, functional earthing and potential equalization	X		
19. Continuous LEAKAGE CURRENTS and PATIENT AUXILIARY CURRENTS	X		
20. Dielectric strength	X		
Section Four - Protection Against Mechanical Hazards			
21. Mechanical strength	X		
22. Moving parts	X		
23. Surfaces, corners and edges	X		
24. Stability in normal use	X		
25. Expelled parts	X		
26. (Not used in IEC-601-1 Second Edition)			
27. Pneumatic and hydraulic power (Under Consideration in IEC-601-1, 2nd Ed.)		X	
28. Suspended masses	X		
Section Five - Protection Against Hazards from Unwanted or Excessive Radiation			
29. X-radiation	X		
30. Alpha, beta, gamma, neutron radiation and other particle radiation (Under Consideration in IEC-601-1, 2nd Ed.)		X	
31. Microwave radiation (Under Consideration in IEC-601-1, 2nd Ed.)		X	
32. Light radiation (including lasers) (Under Consideration in IEC-601-1, 2nd Ed.)		X	
33. Infra-red radiation (Under Consideration in IEC-601-1, 2nd Ed.)		X	
34. Ultraviolet radiation (Under Consideration in IEC-601-1, 2nd Ed.)		X	

	(A)	(NA)	(AM/R)
35. Acoustical energy (Under Consideration in IEC-601-1, 2nd Ed.)		X	
36. Electromagnetic compatibility (Under Consideration in IEC-601-1, 2nd Ed.)			X
Section Six - Protection Against Hazards of Ignitions of Flammable Anaesthetic Mixtures			
37. Locations and basic requirements		X	
38. Marking, ACCOMPANYING DOCUMENTS		X	
39. Common requirements for CATEGORY AP and CATEGORY APG EQUIPMENT		X	
40. Requirements and tests for CATEGORY AP EQUIPMENT, parts and components thereof		X	
41. Requirements and tests for CATEGORY APG EQUIPMENT, parts and components thereof		X	
Section Seven - Protection Against Excessive Temperatures and Other Safety Hazards			
42. Excessive temperatures			X
43. Fire prevention			X
44. Overflow, spillage, leakage, humidity, ingress of liquids, cleaning, sterilization and disinfection	X		
45. Pressure vessels and parts subject to pressure	X		
46. (Not used in IEC-601-1 Second Edition)			
47. (Not used in IEC-601-1 Second Edition)			
48. (Not used in IEC-601-1 Second Edition)			
49. Interruption of the power supply	X		
Section Eight - Accuracy of Operating Data and Protection Against Hazardous Output			
50. Accuracy of operating data			X
51. Protection against hazardous output			X

	(A)	(NA)	(AM/R)
Section Nine - Abnormal Operation and Fault Conditions. Environmental Tests			
52. Abnormal operation and fault conditions	X		
53. Environmental tests	X		
Section Ten - Constructional Requirements			
54. General	X		
55. (Not used in IEC-601-1 Second Edition)			
56. Components and general assembly			X
57. MAINS PARTS, components and layout	X		
58. Protective earthing - TERMINALS AND CONNECTORS	X		
59. Construction and layout	X		
Additional Clauses			
60. Auditory indicators	X		
61. Malfunction indicator	X		
62. Noise	X		

5. CLAUSES CONTAINING AMENDMENTS, ADDITIONS, OR REPLACEMENTS TO TEXT IN IEC 601-1 SECOND EDITION

6. Identification, Markings and Documents

Additional Item—(aa) All markings pertaining to the operation of the oxygen concentrator shall be legible to an operator having visual acuity, corrected if necessary, of 1.0 when seated or standing 1 m from the oxygen concentrator, at an illuminance of 215 lx.

NOTE 1—All markings should have a luminance contrast of at least 50 %, when compared with the surrounding background material.

6.1 *Marking on the Outside of Equipment or Equipment Parts:*

5.2.1 *(Item e) Indication of Origin*—The oxygen concentrator shall be marked with its country of origin.

6.1 *Additional Item*—(aa) The marking on the outside shall additionally include the following:

1 A warning against removal of the covers by unauthorized persons
2 A warning stating "No Smoking or Open Flames."
3 The nominal concentration of oxygen in the product gas expressed in % oxygen v/v at a flow of 2 L/min, and at recommended maximum flow.
4 The statement "Use No Oil or Grease."
5 The flow indicator shall be marked so as to indicate output for example; output, gas flow, or the like.
6 If the operator adjustable controls are capable of setting the flow in excess of the maximum recommended rate or; if the flow indicator is marked above the maximum flow, or both, then markings in excess of the recommended maximum flow shall be uniquely marked on the flow indicator in red and a warning shall be marked on the device.

6.7 *Indicator Lights and Push Buttons:*

(a) *Colors of Indicator Lights*—Table 1, Recommended colors of indicator lights and their meaning for equipment (refer also to ISO 9703 for guidance) (replacement).

5.3.2 The function of all lights and displays shall be marked.

5.3.3 Compliance shall be checked by functional test and inspection.

6.8 *Accompanying Documents:*

6.8.2 *Instructions for Use*—(Item a) General information

TABLE 1 Recommended Colors of Indicator Lights and Their Meaning for Equipment

Color	Meaning
Red, non-flashing	Denotes oxygen concentrator has failed.
Red, flashing	Immediate response required to deal with a condition. High priority.
Yellow, non-flashing	Awareness of condition. Low priority.
Yellow, flashing	Prompt response to deal with a condition. Medium priority.
Green	Ready for action.
Any other color	None allowed.

The instructions for use shall additionally include the following information:

The intended use of the oxygen concentrator.

At least one type of humidifier which is suitable for use with the oxygen concentrator.

The statement "Use of certain humidifiers not specified for use with this oxygen concentrator may impair the performance."

The preferred location of any humidifier in the administration accessories.

A statement that in certain circumstances oxygen therapy can be hazardous and that seeking medical advice before using this machine is advisable.

A statement of the time taken from switching on the concentrator to reach a stated performance.

A statement that the air intake of the oxygen concentrator should be located in a well-ventilated space so as to avoid airborne pollutants or fumes.

Intervals at which cleaning procedures need to be performed and the items required for such cleaning.

A statement that no lubricants are to be used other than those recommended by the manufacturer.

A statement that advises operator to call for service when the oxygen concentration status indicator indicates an abnormal oxygen concentration level.

d Cleaning, disinfection and sterilization of parts in contact with the patient.

The instructions for use shall additionally include the following information:

1 A specification for at least one complete set of administration accessories that are suitable for use with the oxygen concentrator and, except for administration accessories intended for single-use, recommendations for their cleaning, sterilization, and disinfection.

2 The statement" Use of some administration accessories not specified for use with this oxygen concentrator may impair the performance."

6.8.3 *Technical Description:*

a *General*—The technical description shall additionally include the following information:

1 A table or graph showing values of oxygen concentration as a function of flow at specified operator settings at an outlet pressure of nominal zero.

2 The maximum recommended flow, expressed in L/min.

3 The flow values in liters per minute at a specified control setting for outlet pressures of nominal zero and 7 kPa.

4 The maximum outlet pressure when the oxygen concentrator is operated according to the method given to check compliance with Clause 50.8.

5 The maximum A-weighted sound pressure level in dB(A) when the oxygen concentrator is operated under the test conditions specified in Clause 62.

6 If a pressure relief mechanism is provided, the range of pressure in kPa at which the mechanism operates.

7 The nominal concentration of oxygen in the product gas expressed in percent oxygen v/v at a flow of 2 L/min.

8 A statement of the concentration of oxygen in the product gas expressed in % v/v at the maximum recommended flow.

9 d Restricted environmental condition for transport and storage.

1 The temperature range in which the concentrator is intended to be used must be specified (addition).

2 Any degradation of performance over the altitude range of from 0 to 4000 m above sea level must be specified (addition).

SECTION FIVE—PROTECTION AGAINST HAZARDS FROM UNWANTED OR EXCESSIVE RADIATION

36 *Electromagnetic Compatibility:*

36.1 *Protection from Electrostatic Discharge* (addition)—The oxygen concentrator shall continue to function and meet the requirements of this specification or shall fail without causing a safety hazard when tested in accordance with IEC-801-2. The discharge shall have a potential of 3 kv ± 5 % direct current for a contact discharge and 8 kilovolts ± 5 % direct current for an air discharge. A minimum of eight discharges shall be applied only to accessible parts and coupling planes (as defined in IEC 801-2). If an anomaly occurs, such as, display interrupt, alarm activation, etc., it should be possible to restore normal operation within 30 s after the electrostatic discharge has been applied. (Silencing of an activated alarm shall not be considered a failure.)

SECTION SEVEN—PROTECTION AGAINST EXCESSIVE TEMPERATURES, AND OTHER SAFETY HAZARDS

42 *Excessive Temperature*—

42.1 Amendment: Amend the last entry of Table Xa as follows:

Equipment parts that may in normal use have unintentional contact with a patient shall not attain temperatures exceeding 50°C, if made from metal, or 60°C, if made from non-metal.

42.3 Replace 42.3 with the following:

42.3.1 The gas temperature at the oxygen concentrator outlet shall not exceed 6°C above ambient temperature when the oxygen concentrator is operated in accordance with the manufacturer's instructions (replacement).

7.3 Compliance shall be checked by the following test:

7.3.1 Use the test apparatus described in Annex A1. With the variable restrictor fully open, set the flow adjuster to give approximately the maximum flow recommended by the manufacturer in the technical description. Operate the oxygen concentrator for 0.5 h and readjust the flow so that exactly the maximum flow recommended by the manufacturer is indicated on the flowmeter of the test apparatus. Operate the oxygen concentrator for a further 9 h and take readings of the product gas temperature at intervals not exceeding 0.5 h, the first reading being taken after 1 h.

The temperature of the product gas shall not exceed the specified value.

43.3.1 The gas temperature at the oxygen concentrator outlet shall not exceed 41°C when operated in accordance with the manufacturer's instructions over the range of ambient temperature recommended by the manufacturer.

Compliance shall be checked by repeating the test given in 42.3.1 with the oxygen concentrator in an atmosphere maintained at the maximum temperature at which the manufacturer recommends it should be used.

43 *Fire Prevention*—Additional subsections:

43.1 In order to minimize the risk of fire in normal use or in single fault conditions at least one of the following requirements shall be satisfied.

a) Electrical components shall be separated from compartments in which accumulations of oxygen can occur by a barrier complying with the requirements given in 43.2.

b) Compartments containing electrical components shall be ventilated according to the requirements of 43.3.

c) Electrical components which, in normal use or single fault conditions can be a source of ignition, shall comply with the requirements given in 43.4.

43.2 Any barrier separating electrical components from compartments where accumulations of oxygen can occur shall be sealed at all joints and holes for cables or for other purposes.

Compliance shall be checked by inspection and, if applicable, by the compliance test for sealed enclosures given in 40.5 of the General Standard (IEC 601-1 1988).

If, in normal use, a pressure difference of 0.4 kPa or greater exists between the spaces separated by the barrier, the compliance test described in 7.4.3 shall be used.

43.3 The ventilation required under the provision of 43.1(b) shall be such that the oxygen concentration in the compartment containing electrical components shall not exceed 25 % v/v.

Compliance shall be checked by the following test:

Measure the oxygen concentration under the following conditions and for such a period that the highest possible concentration of oxygen occurs and is maintained for 0.5 h.

a) Rupture or leakage of any component which carries oxygen-enriched air in close proximity to the test compartment.

b) Selection of the least favorable control settings for example, highest oxygen concentration or maximum flow.

c) Supply mains voltage variation of + 10 to – 15 %.

The oxygen concentration measured shall not exceed the specified value.

43.9 Electrical circuits that can produce sparks or generate increased surface temperatures and which can be a source of ignition shall be so designed that in normal use and single fault conditions no ignition occurs. The following requirements shall be satisfied:

a) The surface temperature of components shall not exceed 300°C, unless it can be shown that no ignition occurs when the component(s) is (are) exposed to 99.5 % oxygen at temperatures above 300°C.

7.5.2 Compliance shall be checked by measuring the surface temperatures of the components under normal and single fault conditions. If the surface temperature of the component(s) exceeds 300°C, inspect for ignition when the component(s) is (are) exposed to 99.5 % oxygen at the measured temperature.

SECTION EIGHT—ACCURACY OF OPERATING DATA AND PROTECTION AGAINST HAZARDOUS OUTPUT

50 *Accuracy of Operating Data*—A flow indicator shall be provided on the oxygen concentrator and shall indicate total product gas flow. It shall be graduated in L/min and be accurate to ± 10 % of the indicated flow or ± 0.5 L/min, whichever is the greater (addition).

Compliance shall be checked by the following test:

Use the test apparatus described in Annex AA. With the variable restrictor completely open set the flow adjuster on the oxygen concentrator so that the flow indicator shows 20 % of the maximum flow stated by the manufacturer. Operate the oxygen concentrator for 15 min and measure the flow of the product gas using the flowmeter of the test apparatus. Repeat the procedure at the 100 % flow indicated and at a 50 % flow. If a fixed orifice device is used to regulate flow, each orifice shall be tested.

The flow shown on the flow indicator shall be within the tolerance specified.

50.4 The concentration of oxygen in the product gas, at a flow of 2 L/min, shall be within ± 3 % v/v oxygen of the value stated by the manufacturer in the accompanying documents.

Compliance shall be checked by the following test:

Use the test apparatus described in Annex AA and set the mains voltage 10 % above the rated supply voltage. With the variable restrictor completely open, set the flow adjuster to give an output of approximately 2 L/min. Operate the oxygen concentrator for 0.5 h and then adjust the flow to exactly 2 L/min, as indicated on the flow meter of the test apparatus. Operate the oxygen concentrator for a further 1 h and take five consecutive readings of the concentration of oxygen in the product gas, as displayed on the oxygen analyzer, at intervals of 1 min. Repeat the test with the mains voltage set 15 % below the rated supply voltage.

The concentration of oxygen in the product gas shall be within the tolerance specified.

50.5 When the oxygen concentrator is operated at the maximum flow recommended by the manufacturer in the technical description, the mean concentration of oxygen in the product gas over an 8 h period shall be within ± 3 % v/v oxygen of the value stated by the manufacturer in the accompanying documents and no individual reading shall vary by more than ± 3 % v/v oxygen of the mean.

Compliance shall be checked by the following test:

Use the test apparatus described in Annex AA and set the mains voltage 10 % above the rated supply voltage. With the variable restrictor completely open, set the flow adjuster to give approximately the maximum flow recommended by the manufacturer in the technical description. Operate the oxygen concentrator for 0.5 h and re-adjust the flow so that exactly the maximum flow recommended by the manufacturer is indicated on the flow meter of the test apparatus. Operate the oxygen concentrator for a further 9 h and take readings of the concentration of oxygen in the product gas, as indicated on the oxygen analyzer, averaged over 1 min, at intervals of 0.5 h, the first reading being taken after 1 h. Calculate the arithmetic mean of the readings obtained. Repeat the test with the mains voltage set 15 % below the rated supply voltage.

The mean concentration of oxygen in the product gas and the individual readings shall be within the tolerances specified.

50.6 When the oxygen concentrator is set to the maximum flow recommended by the manufacturer in the technical description and operated for 8 h, the mean of the flows recorded at intervals of 0.5 h over the period shall be within ± 10 % of the stated value or ± 0.5 L/min, whichever is the greater, and no individual reading shall vary by more than ± 10 % of the mean value.

Compliance shall be checked by the following test:

During the test for compliance with 50.5, note the flow from the oxygen concentrator, as indicated on the flowmeter of the test apparatus, at the same time as taking readings of the concentration of oxygen in the product gas. Calculate the arithmetic mean of the flow readings obtained.

The mean of the flows recorded and the individual flows shall be within the tolerances specified.

50.7 The change in the maximum recommended flow when a back pressure of 7 kPa is applied shall be within ± 10 % of the figure stated by the manufacturer in the technical description.

Compliance shall be checked by the following test:

Use the test apparatus described in Annex A1. Set the flow from the oxygen concentrator so that its flow indicator shows the maximum flow recommended by the manufacturer in the technical description. Adjust the variable restrictor in the test apparatus to give a back pressure of 7 kPa. Operate the oxygen concentrator for 15 min and record the flow indicated on the flowmeter of the test apparatus. Subtract this figure from the manufacturer's recommended flow to give the change in flow when a back pressure of 7 kPa is applied.

The change in flow shall be within the tolerance specified.

50.8 The maximum outlet pressure shall be within ± 10 % of the value stated by the manufacturer in the technical description.

Compliance shall be checked by the following test:

Use the test apparatus described in Annex AA. Operate the oxygen concentrator at the maximum flow recommended by the manufacturer in the technical description and adjust the variable restrictor to stop the flow. Record the pressure indicated. The pressure indicated shall be within the tolerance specified.

51 *Protection Against Hazardous Output*—

51.1 Flow adjuster—Replace 51.1 with the following:

The oxygen concentrator shall be fitted with a flow adjuster. Compliance shall be checked by inspection.

The flow adjuster should be provided with a means to prevent adjustments by the user.

51.2 *Filter*: Replace 51.2 with the following:

A filter capable of retaining particles of 10 μm or greater shall be provided between the oxygen concentrating elements and the oxygen concentrator outlet.

Compliance shall be checked by inspection.

Oxygen Concentration Status Indicator—Replace 51.3 with the following:

An oxygen concentration status indicator shall be included to warn the operator of abnormality in the product gas.

Compliance shall be checked by operating the oxygen concentrator and inducing an oxygen concentration below the manufacturer's stated normal level.

SECTION TEN—CONSTRUCTIONAL REQUIREMENTS

56 Components and General Assembly—at 56.8 Indicators (addition):

An indicator(s) of continued mechanical and electrical function or of malfunction shall be provided on the oxygen concentrator.

Compliance shall be checked by operating the oxygen concentrator and inducing the following faults individually:

a) Compressor failure,
b) Pump failure,
c) Cycle failure,
d) Pressure failure,
e) Vacuum failure, and
f) Oxygen concentration failure.

A non-resetable elapsed time indicator showing the total operating time in hours shall be provided on the oxygen concentrator.

Compliance shall be checked by inspection.

56.9 *Pre-Set Controls*: (addition)

Pre-set controls shall either be inside the casing or shall require the use of a tool for adjustment.

Compliance shall be checked by inspection.

60 *Additional Clauses:*

Auditory Indicators—Any auditory indicator provided with the oxygen concentrator shall annunciate in a tone distinctly different from the sounds generated by the oxygen concentrator during normal operation in order to avoid masking. If an oxygen concentrator of the domiciliary type is to be used in a hospital, auditory indicators should meet ASTM guidelines or standards for such auditory indicators.

61 *Loss of Mains Power Indicator*—An auditory alarm shall be provided to indicate when mains power has been interrupted.

62 *Noise:*

62.1 In normal use the maximum A-weighted sound pressure level (steady or peak value) of the oxygen concentrator shall not exceed 60 dB(A).

Compliance shall be checked by the following test:

a) Place the microphone on a sound level meter complying with the requirements for Type 1 specified in IEC 651 at the position of maximum sound pressure level in the horizontal plane passing through the geometric center of the oxygen concentrator at a radius of 1 m. The measured sound pressure level shall not exceed the specified value.

b) For this test, operate the oxygen concentrator over its normal working range of flow including the maximum flow recommended by the manufacturer. Use the sound level meter with the "A" weighted network and the "fast" meter characteristics selected. Carry out the measurements in a free field over a reflecting plane as specified in ISO 3744.

c) The background level of extraneous noise shall be at least 10 dB(A) below that measured during the test.

ANNEXES

(Mandatory Information)

A1. (AA) TEST APPARATUS

A1.1 *Components:*

A1.1.1 (AA.1.1) *Flowmeter,* accurate to within ± 2 % of the flow to be measured.

A1.1.2 (AA.1.2) *Oxygen analyzer,* accurate to within ± 1 % of the oxygen concentration to be measured and which gives a reading equal to at least 90 % of the actual oxygen concentration within 10 s of the sensing element being exposed to the gas flow. If a pump is required to aspirate the gas sample, it shall neither reduce the pressure at the outlet of the flowmeter to below atmospheric pressure nor draw air back through the open end of the tube.

A1.1.3 (AA.1.3) *Pressure Indicator,* accurate to within ± 2 % of the pressure to be measured.

A1.1.4 (AA.1.4) *Thermometer,* accurate to within ± 0.5° of the temperature to be measured.

A1.2 (AA.21) *Component Assembly*—Assemble the components as shown in Fig. A1.1 (AA.1) using tubing of 6 ± 1 mm internal diameter to connect between the components.

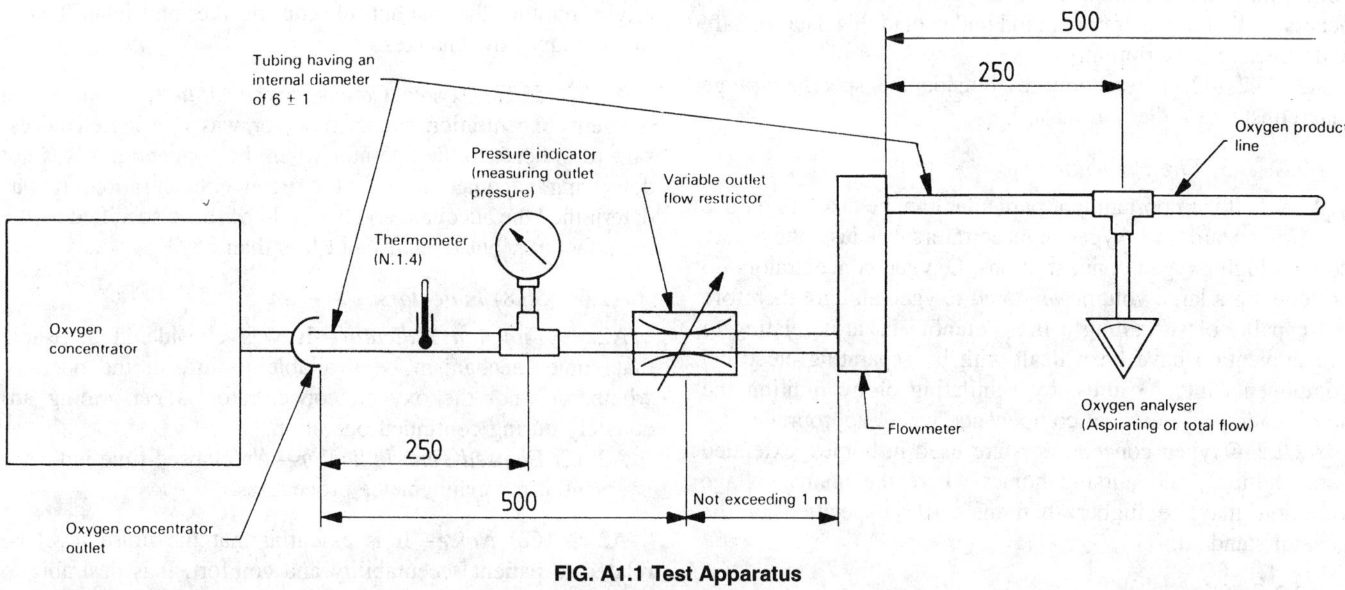

FIG. A1.1 Test Apparatus

A2. (BB) RATIONALE

This annex provides a concise rationale for the important requirements of this specification and is intended for those who are familiar with the subject of the standard but who have not participated in its development. An understanding of the reasons for the main requirements is considered to be essential for the proper application of the standard. Furthermore as clinical practice and technology change it is believed that a rationale for the present requirements will facilitate any revision of the standard necessitated by those developments.

A2.1 (BB) *Scope and Field of Application:*

A2.1.1 This international standard does not apply to institutional pressure swing adsorber devices (molecular sieve devices) which use the separation principle to deliver oxygen of a specified minimum concentration to a hospital or like distribution system at a minimum pressure of 400 kPa. The performance and safety requirements for this type of device vary considerably from the portable oxygen concentrators addressed in this specification.

A2.1.2 (6.1) *Marking on the Outside of Equipment or Equipment Parts*—(aa) To ensure the safety of the patients, it is important to visibly warn the operator whenever the manufacturers recommend maximum flow is exceeded. Flows in excess of those recommended can result in reduced oxygen concentration.

A2.1.3 (6.7a) *Colors of Indicator Lights*—(a), The use of the existing standardized color system for visible indicators decreases the likelihood of patient and operator error.

A2.1.4 (6.8.2) *Instructions for Use*—(Item a) General Information:

A2.1.4.1 (2) The need for humidification is a matter for clinical judgment and its assessment should take into consideration the method of delivery, the volume of entrained air and total flow.

A2.1.4.2 (3) It was recognized that the supplier cannot be required to test or approve all types of humidifiers that might be used with the oxygen concentrator. Such equipment which requires a high pressure might seriously degrade the performance of the oxygen concentrator.

A2.1.5 (d) *Parts in Contact with the Patient*—

(1) The supplier is required to recommend oxygen administration accessories that are suitable for use with the oxygen concentrator because administration accessories suitable for use with medical gas pipelines or cylinder regulators may not be satisfactory.

A2.1.6 (6.8.3) *Technical Description*:

A2.1.6.1 This performance data is important information concerning the functioning of oxygen concentrators. It is necessary that the operator should understand this data for safe and effective prescription.

A2.1.6.2 (42.1) Temperatures outside the specified range may constitute a thermal hazard.

A2.2 (43) *Fire Prevention:*

A2.2.1 It is important that particular care be taken to reduce the fire hazard of oxygen concentrators because they may contain high oxygen concentrations. Oxygen concentrators do not contain a large volume of stored oxygen and are therefore not capable of sustaining a fire. Potential hazards relating to fire prevention have been dealt with by separating electrical components into closures, by ventilating or by limiting the specification of electrical components, where appropriate.

A2.2.2 Oxygen concentrators are used in homes, extended care facilities, and nursing homes where the mains voltage variation may be higher than the + 10 % specified in the general standard.

A2.3 (50) *Accuracy of Operating Data:*

A2.3.1 (50.3) A medical need was expressed for these accuracies. The design of a molecular sieve oxygen concentrator is such that oxygen concentration decreases with increasing flow whilst the total volume of oxygen delivered generally increases with flow. Oxygen administration by flow adjustment should be accurate and related to the device used for administration, the patient minute ventilation and the desired arterial blood oxygen concentration.

A2.3.2 (50.4) There is a medical need for accurate oxygen concentrations. Deviations within ± 3 % v/v oxygen concentration were considered to be achievable by the manufacturer and were acceptable medically.

A2.3.3 (50.5) Measurement of stability of oxygen concentration over a long period is necessary to give a meaningful result.

A2.3.4 (50.6) A medical need was expressed for flow stability without attention on the part of the patient for this period of time. The maintenance of a stable flow with its resultant oxygen concentration is, therefore, important to the patient.

A2.4 (51.1) *Flow Adjuster*—A flow adjuster was considered necessary to match the output of the oxygen concentrator to variations in the needs of the patient. It was considered that in some clinical circumstances a deterrent to operator adjustment of flow was important. The presence of this deterrent might remind the patient to consult the physician before making any flow changes.

A2.5 (51.5) *Oxygen Concentration Status Indicator*—An oxygen concentration status indicator was considered necessary to indicate to the operator when the concentrator was not delivering adequate levels of oxygen concentration. It was determined the adequate levels should be those specified by the manufacturer, but typically not less than 85 %.

A2.6 (56.8) *Indicators:*

A2.6.1 *Function Indicator*—It was considered advisable that some mechanism be available to inform the operator whether or not the oxygen concentrator is performing adequately during continued operation.

A2.6.2 *Elapsed-Time Indicator*—An elapsed-time indicator is essential for maintenance procedures.

A2.7 (62) *Noise*—It is essential that the noise level be related to patient acceptability and comfort. It is desirable to reduce the noise level as far as possible for devices that might interfere with sleeping. It is recognized that oxygen concentrators (pressure swing adsorbers) may have both a steady sound level and a peak sound level. The peak sound pressure level was considered to be the more likely to be obtrusive to the patient during continuous machine performance.

Designation: F 1472 – 00

Standard Specification for Wrought Titanium-6Aluminum-4Vanadium Alloy (UNS R56400) for Surgical Implant Applications[1]

This standard is issued under the fixed designation F 1472; the number immediately following the designation indicates the year of original adoption or, in the case of revision, the year of last revision. A number in parentheses indicates the year of last reapproval. A superscript epsilon (ε) indicates an editorial change since the last revision or reapproval.

1. Scope

1.1 This specification covers the chemical, mechanical, and metallurgical requirements for wrought annealed titanium-6aluminum-4vanadium alloy (UNS R56400) to be used in the manufacture of surgical implants.

1.2 The values stated in inch-pound units are to be regarded as the standard. The values given in parentheses are provided for information only.

1.3 *This standard does not purport to address all of the safety concerns, if any, associated with its use. It is the responsibility of the user of this standard to establish appropriate safety and health practices and to determine the applicability of regulatory limitations prior to use.*

2. Referenced Documents

2.1 *ASTM Standards:*

B 265 Specification for Titanium and Titanium Alloy Strip, Sheet, and Plate[2]

B 348 Specification for Titanium and Titanium Alloy Bars and Billets[2]

B 381 Specification for Titanium and Titanium Alloy Forgings[2]

E 8 Test Methods for Tension Testing of Metallic Materials[3]

E 120 Test Methods for Chemical Analysis of Titanium and Titanium Alloys[4]

E 290 Test Method for Semi-Guided Bend Test for Ductility of Metallic Materials[3]

E 527 Practice for Numbering Metals and Alloys (UNS)[5]

E 1409 Test Method for Determination of Oxygen in Titanium and Titanium Alloys by the Inert Gas Fusion Technique[4]

E 1447 Test Method for Determination of Hydrogen in Titanium and Titanium Alloys by the Inert Gas Fusion Thermal Conductivity Method[6]

F 136 Specification for Wrought Titanium-6 Aluminum-4 Vanadium ELI (Extra Low Interstitial) Alloy (UNS R56401) for Surgical Implant Applications[7]

2.2 *Other Standard:*

ASQ C1 Specifications of General Requirements for a Quality Program[8]

2.3 *Aerospace Material Specifications:*

AMS 2249 Chemical Check Analysis Limits, Titanium and Titanium Alloys[9]

AMS 4928 Titanium Alloy Bars, Wire, Forgings and Rings 6Al-4V[9]

AMS 4965 Titanium Alloy, Bars, Wire, Forgings, and Rings 6.0Al-4.0V Solution Heat Treated and Aged[9]

3. Classification

3.1 *Strip*—Any product under 0.1875 in. (4.76 mm) in thickness and under 24 in. (610 mm) wide.

3.2 *Sheet*—Any product under 0.1875 in. (4.76 mm) in thickness and 24 in. (610 mm) or more in width.

3.3 *Plate*—Any product 0.1875 in. (4.76 mm) thick and over and 10 in. (254 mm) wide and over, with widths greater than five times the thickness. Plate up to 4.00 in. (101.60 mm) thick, inclusive, is covered by this specification.

3.4 *Bar*—Round bars and flats from 0.1875 in. (4.75 mm) to 4.00 in. (101.60 mm) in diameter or thickness (other sizes and shapes by special order).

3.5 *Forging Bar*—Bar as described in 3.4, used for production of forgings, may be furnished in the hot-rolled condition.

3.6 *Wire*—Rounds less than 0.1875 in. (4.76 mm) in diameter.

4. Ordering Information

4.1 Inquiries and orders for material under this specification shall include the following information:

4.1.1 Quantity (weight or number of pieces),

4.1.2 Applicable ASTM designation,

4.1.3 Form (sheet, strip, plate, wire, bar, or forging bar),

4.1.4 Condition (see 5.1),

4.1.5 Mechanical properties (if applicable, for special conditions),

[1] This specification is under the jurisdiction of ASTM Committee F04 on Medical and Surgical Materials and Devices and is the direct responsibility of Subcommittee F04.12 on Metallurgical Materials.

Current edition approved Nov. 10, 2000. Published March 2001. Originally published as F 1472 – 93. Last previous edition F 1472 – 99.

[2] *Annual Book of ASTM Standards*, Vol 02.04.

[3] *Annual Book of ASTM Standards*, Vol 03.01.

[4] *Annual Book of ASTM Standards*, Vol 03.05.

[5] *Annual Book of ASTM Standards*, Vol 01.01.

[6] *Annual Book of ASTM Standards*, Vol 03.06.

[7] *Annual Book of ASTM Standards*, Vol 13.01.

[8] Available from American Society for Quality, 611 E. Wisconsin Ave., PO Box 3005, Milwaukee, WI 53201–3005.

[9] Available from the SAE World Headquarters, 400 Commonwealth Dr., Warrendale, PA 15096–0001.

4.1.6 Finish (see 5.2),

4.1.7 Applicable dimensions including size, thickness, width, or drawing number,

4.1.8 Special tests, and

4.1.9 Special requirements.

5. Materials and Manufacture

5.1 *Finish*—Annealed material may be furnished to the implant manufacturer as descaled or pickled, sandblasted, ground, machined, vapor blasted, or combinations of these operations.

5.2 Alloy shall be multiple melted; at least one of the melting cycles shall be under vacuum. The first melt shall be made by consumable electrode, nonconsumable electrode, electron beam, or plasma arc melting practice. The subsequent melt or melts shall be made using consumable electrode practice with no alloy additions permitted in the last consumable electrode melt.

5.2.1 The atmosphere for nonconsumable electrode melting shall be inert gas at a pressure not higher than 250 mm of mercury.

5.2.2 The electrode tip for nonconsumable electrode melting shall be water-cooled copper.

5.2.3 The product, as received by the purchaser, shall be uniform in quality and condition, sound, and free from foreign materials and from internal and external imperfections detrimental to usage of the product.

6. Chemical Requirements

6.1 The heat analysis shall conform to the chemical composition of Table 1. Ingot analysis may be used for reporting all chemical requirements, except hydrogen. Samples for hydrogen shall be taken from the finished mill product. Supplier shall not ship material with chemistry outside the limits specified in Table 1.

6.1.1 Requirements for major and minor elemental constituents are listed in Table 1. Also listed are important residual elements. Analysis for elements not listed in Table 1 is not required to verify compliance with this specification.

6.2 The product analysis is either for the purpose of verifying the composition of a heat or lot or to determine variations in the composition within the heat.

6.2.1 Acceptance or rejection of a heat or lot of material may be made by the purchaser on the basis of this product analysis.

6.2.2 Product analysis tolerances do not broaden the specified heat analysis requirements but cover variation between laboratories in the measurement of chemical content. Product analysis limits shall be as specified in Table 2.

6.3 For referee purposes, Test Methods E 120, E 1409, and E 1447 shall be used.

6.4 Samples for chemical analysis shall be representative of the material being tested. The utmost care must be used in sampling titanium for chemical analysis because of its affinity for elements such as oxygen, nitrogen, and hydrogen. Therefore, in cutting samples for analysis, the operation should be carried out insofar as possible in a dust-free atmosphere. Cutting tools should be clean and sharp. Chips should be clean. Samples for analysis should be stored in suitable containers.

7. Mechanical Requirements

7.1 Material supplied under this specification shall conform to the mechanical property requirements given in Table 3.

7.2 Specimens for tension tests shall be machined and tested in accordance with Test Methods E 8. Tensile properties shall be determined using a strain rate of 0.003 to 0.007 in./in./min (mm/mm/min) through the specified yield strength, and then the crosshead speed shall be increased so as to produce fracture in approximately one additional minute.

7.3 For sheet and strip, the bend test specimen shall withstand being bent cold through an angle of 105° without fracture in the outside surface of the bent portion. The bend shall be made on a diameter equal to that shown in Table 3. Test condition shall conform to Test Method E 290.

8. Special Requirements

8.1 The microstructure shall be a fine dispersion of the alpha and beta phases resulting from processing in the alpha plus beta field. There shall be no continuous alpha network at prior beta grain boundaries. There shall be no course, elongated alpha platelets.

8.2 The beta transus temperature shall be determined by a suitable method and reported on the material's certification.

8.3 Products supplied with a machined or ground surface finish shall have no alpha case. For other products, there shall be no continuous layer of alpha case when examined at 100×.

9. Quality Program Requirements

9.1 The producer shall maintain a quality program such as that defined in Specifications ASQ C1.

TABLE 1 Chemical Requirements[A]

Element	Composition, %
Nitrogen, max	0.05
Carbon, max	0.08
Hydrogen, max[B]	0.015
Iron, max	0.30
Oxygen, max	0.20
Aluminum	5.5–6.75
Vanadium	3.5–4.5
Yttrium, max	0.005
Titanium[C]	balance

[A]Refer to AMS 4928.

[B]Billets shall have a maximum of 0.01 % hydrogen content.

[C]The percentage of titanium is determined by difference and need not be determined or certified.

TABLE 2 Permissible Variation in Product Analysis Tolerance[A]

Element	Tolerance Under the Minimum or Over the Maximum Limit (Composition %)[B]
Nitrogen	0.02
Carbon	0.02
Hydrogen	0.002
Iron	0.10
Oxygen	0.02
Aluminum	0.04
Vanadium	0.015
Yttrium	0.0006

[A]Refer to AMS 2249.

[B]Under minimum limit not applicable for elements in which only a maximum percentage is indicated.

TABLE 3 Annealed Mechanical Properties[A]

Nominal Diameter or Distance Between Parallel Sides, in. (mm)	Tensile Strength, psi, (MPa), min	Yield Strength at 0.2 % Offset, psi (MPa), min	Elongation[B] in 2 in. (50 mm), or 4D or 4T, %, min			Reduction of Area, %, min[C]		
			L	LT[D]	ST[D,E]	L	LT[D]	ST[D,E]
Bars and Forgings:								
Up to 2.0 (50), incl	135 000 (930)	125 000 (860)	10			25	20	
Over 2.0 to 4.0 (50 to 100), incl	130 000 (895)	120 000 (825)	10			25	20	15
Over 4.0 to 6.0 (100 to 150), incl	130 000 (895)	120 000 (825)	10		8	20	15	
Sheet, Strip, and Plate:								
Up to 0.008 (0.2), excl	134 000 (924)	126 000 (869)						
0.008 to 0.025 (0.2 to 0.6), excl	134 000 (924)	126 000 (869)	6					
0.025 to 0.063 (0.6 to 1.6), excl	134 000 (924)	126 000 (869)	8					
0.063 to 0.1875 (1.6 to 4.8), excl	134 000 (924)	126 000 (869)	10					
0.1875 to 4.00 (4.8 to 101.6), incl	130 000 (895)	120 000 (825)	10	10	10	20	20	15
Bending Parameters:								
Up to 0.07 (1.875), incl				bend factor[F] = 9T				
Over 0.07 to 0.1875 (4.8), excl				bend factor[F] = 10T				

[A]Mechanical properties for conditions other than those listed in this table may be established by agreement between the supplier and the purchaser.
[B]Elongation of material 0.062 in. (1.575 mm) or greater in diameter or thickness shall be measured using a gage length of 2 in. or 4D or 4T. Elongation of material under 0.062 in. in diameter or thickness may be obtained by negotiation.
[C]Applies to bar, plate, and forgings only. L = longitudinal; LT = long transverse; ST = short transverse.
[D]Transverse requirements in Table 3 apply only to product from which a tensile specimen not less than 2.50 in. (63.5 mm) in length can be obtained.
[E]Material tested in the short transverse direction need not be tested in the long transverse direction.
[F]Bend test applicable to sheet and strip products: T = thickness of bend specimen in reference to diameter of bend. (Bend factor is the mandrel diameter.)

9.2 The manufacturer shall be ensured of and may audit the producer's quality program for conformance to the intent of Specifications ASQ C1 or other recognized program.

10. Marking, Packing, Certification, and Rejection

10.1 Marking, packing, certification, and rejection shall be as specified in Specifications B 265, B 348, and B 381.

11. Keywords

11.1 metals (for surgical implants); orthopaedic medical devices; titanium alloys; titanium/titanium alloys; titanium/titanium alloys (for surgical implants)

APPENDIXES

(Nonmandatory Information)

X1. RATIONALE

X1.1 The purpose of this specification is to characterize the chemical, physical, mechanical, and metallurgical properties of wrought annealed Ti-6Al-4V alloy to be used in the manufacture of surgical implants.

X1.2 The alloy composition covered by this specification has been used successfully in human implants, exhibiting a well-characterized level of local biological response since 1983. **(1, 2)**.[10]

X1.3 The microstructural requirements contained in this specification represent the current general consensus of opinion with respect to optimization of mechanical properties for implant applications.

X1.4 This alloy exhibits similar mechanical properties to Specification F 136 required for the application of load-bearing orthopedic implants **(2-18)**.

X1.5 Melting requirements specified in AMS 4928 have been included to ensure that melting practice conforms to industry guidelines for titanium - 6aluminum - 4vanadium.

X1.6 This alloy can be solution treated and aged to achieve different properties according to, for example, AMS 4965 (titanium alloy bars, wire, forgings, and rings – titanium 6.0 aluminum 4.0 vanadium – solution heat treated and aged).

[10] The boldface numbers refer to references listed at the end of this standard.

X2. BIOCOMPATIBILITY

X2.1 The material composition covered by this specification has been used successfully in contact with soft tissue and bone since 1983 **(12)**.

X2.2 No known surgical implant has ever shown to be completely free of adverse reactions in the human body. However, long-term clinical experience has shown an acceptable level of biological response can be expected, if the material is used in appropriate applications.

X2.3 The material in this specification has been subjected to animal studies and has been shown to produce a well-characterized level of biological response that is equal to or less than that produced by the reference material titanium. This material has been used clinically since 1983 **(1, 2, 19)**.

REFERENCES

(1) Dobbs, H. S., and Scales, J. T., "Behavior of Commercially Pure Titanium and Ti-318 (Ti-6Al-4V) in Orthopedic Implants," Titanium Alloys in Surgical Implants, *ASTM STP 796*, H. A. Luckey and Fred Kubli, Jr., Eds., ASTM, 1983, pp. 173–186.

(2) Dobbs, H. S., and Robertson, J. L. M., "Tensile Strength, Fatigue Life and Corrosion Behavior of Ti-318 and Ti-550," Titanium Alloys in Surgical Implants, *ASTM STP 796*, H. A. Luckey and Fred Kubli, Jr., Eds., ASTM, 1983, pp. 227–237.

(3) Semlitsch, M. F., Panic, B., Weber, H., and Schoen, R., "Comparison of the Fatigue Strength of Femoral Prosthesis Stems Made of Forged Ti-Al-V and Cobalt Base Alloys," Titanium Alloys in Surgical Implants and Materials, 1983, pp. 120–135.

(4) Cook, S. D., Georgette, F. S., Skinner, H. B., and Haddad, R. J., Jr., "Fatigue Properties of Carbon- and Porous-Coated Ti-6Al-4V Alloys," *JBMR* Vol 18, 1984, pp. 497–512.

(5) Yue, S., Pilliar, R. M., and Weatherly, G. C., "The Fatigue Strength of Porous-Coated Ti-6Al-4V Implant Alloy," *JBMR* Vol 18, 1984, pp. 1043–1058.

(6) *Basic Design Facts About Titanium*, RMI Co., Niles, OH.

(7) *How To Use Titanium—Properties and Fabrication of Titanium Mill Products*, Timet, Pittsburgh, PA.

(8) Harrigan, M. J., Haplan, M. P., and Sommer, A. W., "Effect of Chemistry and Heat Treatment on the Fracture Properties of Ti-6Al-4V Alloy," *Titanium and Titanium Alloys Source Book*, 1982, pp. 50–79.

(9) Lewis, R. E., Bjelstich, J. G., Morton, T. M., and Crossley, F. A., "Effect of Cooling Rate on Fracture Behavior of Mill-Annealed Ti-6Al-4V," Cracks and Fracture, *ASTM STP 601*, ASTM, 1976, pp. 371–390.

(10) Chesnutt, J. C., Rhodes, C. G., and Williams, J. C., "Relationship Between Mechanical Properties, Microstructure and Fracture Topography in Alpha & Beta Titanium Alloys," Fractography Microscopic Cracking Process, *ASTM STP 600*, ASTM, 1976, pp. 99–138.

(11) Hieronymous, W. S., *Aviation Week and Space Technology*, July 1971, p. 42.

(12) Stubbington, C. A., and Bowen, A. W., "Improvements in the Fatigue Strength of Ti-6Al-4V through Microstructure Control," *J of Mat Sci* 9, 1974, pp. 941–947.

(13) Yoder, G. R., Cooley, L. A., and Crooker, T. W., "A Comparison of Microstructural Effects on Fatigue—Crack Initiation and Propagation in Ti-6Al-4V," *NRL Memorandum Report*, 4758, 1982.

(14) Bowen, A. W., and Stubbington, G. A., "The Effect of Heat Treatment on the Fatigue Strength of Ti-6Al-4V," *Titanium Science and Technology*, R. I. Joffee and H. M. Burte, Eds., Plenum Press, New York, 1973.

(15) Bartlo, L. J., "Effect of Microstructure on the Fatigue Properties of Ti-6Al-4V Bar," Fatigue at High Temperature, *ASTM STP 459*, ASTM, 1969, pp. 144–154.

(16) Seagle, S. R., Seeley, R. R., and Hall, G. S., "The Influence of Composition and Heat Treatment on the Aqueous-Stress Corrosion of Titanium," Applications Related Phenomena in Titanium Alloys, *ASTM STP 432*, ASTM, 1968, pp. 170–188.

(17) Stubbington, C. A., "Metallurgical Aspects of Fatigue and Fracture in Titanium Alloys," *AGARD Proceedings*, No. 185, 1976.

(18) *Titanium Alloys Handbook*, MCIC-HB-02 Battelle Columbus Laboratories and Wright Patterson Air Force Base, 1972, pp. 104:72–15.

(19) Semlitsch, M., "Titanium Alloys for Hip Joint Replacements," *Clinical Materials*, 2, 1987, pp. 1–13.

Standard Guide for Performance of Patient Assessment by the Emergency Medical Technician (Paramedic)[1]

This standard is issued under the fixed designation F 1489; the number immediately following the designation indicates the year of original adoption or, in the case of revision, the year of last revision. A number in parentheses indicates the year of last reapproval. A superscript epsilon (ε) indicates an editorial change since the last revision or reapproval.

1. Scope

1.1 This guide describes the patient assessment techniques to be used by the emergency medical technician (paramedic).

1.2 *This standard does not purport to address all of the safety problems, if any, associated with its use. It is the responsibility of the user of this standard to consult and establish appropriate safety and health practices and determine the applicability of regulatory limitations prior to use.*

2. Referenced Documents

2.1 *ASTM Standards:*

F 1149 Practice for Qualifications, Responsibilities, and Authority of Individuals and Institutions Providing Medical Direction of Emergency Medical Services[2]

3. Terminology

3.1 *Definitions of Terms Specific to This Standard:* Description of Terms Specific to This Guide:

3.1.1 *patient assessment*—the identification of a patient's real or perceived problem(s) by means of the accumulation and evaluation of data from a primary assessment and a secondary assessment.

3.1.2 *pertinent patient information*—information obtained from all available resources that relate to the patient's condition and problems: this information is continuously updated and all information is recorded and reported.

3.1.3 *primary assessment*—the identification of a patient's real or perceived problem(s) by means of the accumulation and evaluation of data from a scene evaluation, a primary survey, and pertinent patient information.

3.1.4 *primary survey*—the rapid assessment and management of the patient's immediately life-threatening conditions.

3.1.5 *scene evaluation*—a rapid evaluation of the environment, conditions, and necessary resources.

3.1.6 *secondary assessment*—Identification of the patient's real or perceived problem(s) by means of documentation and evaluation of additional data from the secondary survey and pertinent patient information.

3.1.7 *secondary survey*—the methodical physical examination of the patient to evaluate conditions discovered during the primary survey and to find conditions not previously identified.

3.1.8 *chief complaint*—a subjective statement made by a patient describing the patient's symptoms or signs of illness or dysfunction.

3.1.9 *field diagnosis*—a statement of a health problem or of a potential problem in the patient's health status based on the findings of the primary and secondary assessment.

4. Significance and Use

4.1 This guide establishes the national standard for the performance of patient assessment by the emergency medical technician (paramedic).

4.2 This guide shall be used by those who supervise and train the emergency medical technician (paramedic) as the recommended way to perform patient assessment.

4.3 Every person who is identified as an emergency medical technician (paramedic) shall have been trained to this standard.

4.4 It is understood that the scope of medical practice is constantly evolving. Where this guide contains recommendations for the management of illnesses and injuries those recommendations are not intended to supersede the protocols and standing orders of the system medical director or on-line medical physician (see Practice F 1149).

4.5 This guide does not standardize the scope of clinical practice of the emergency medical technician (paramedic).

4.6 The patient examination and management steps outlined in this document are not necessarily in sequential order and they will often vary with the patient's age, size, location and condition.

5. Initial Approach to the Patient

5.1 The emergency medical technician (paramedic) shall identify himself and his training level to the patient and appropriate bystanders, identify the patient and obtain consent to treat the patient. The point in the assessment where this is done varies with patient condition, age and the environment.

6. Primary Assessment

6.1 *Scene Evaluation*:

6.1.1 While approaching the scene and the patient the emergency medical technician (paramedic) will assess the scene for hazards, number of patients, need for additional resources and then take appropriate action.

[1] This guide is under the jurisdiction of ASTM Committee F-30 on Emergency Medical Services and is the direct responsibility of Subcommittee F30.02 on Personnel, Training and Education.

Current edition approved August 15, 1993. Published October 1993.

[2] *Annual Book of ASTM Standards*, Vol 13.01.

6.1.2 While approaching the patient the emergency medical technician (paramedic) will assess the patient and the environment for clues relating to the mechanism of injury or illness.

6.2 *Primary Survey*:

6.2.1 Frequently repeated primary surveys are an essential and integral part of the complete care of the acutely ill or injured patient. This guide identifies the preferred sequence for patient primary assessment; however, it must be emphasized that much of the primary assessment is done simultaneously and not necessarily sequentially. The primary survey addresses:

6.2.1.1 Cervical spine stability,

6.2.1.2 Airway patency,

6.2.1.3 Adequacy of ventilations,

6.2.1.4 Adequacy of circulation,

6.2.1.5 Life-threatening external bleeding, and

6.2.1.6 Level of consciousness.

6.2.2 The primary survey shall be interrupted to manage immediately life-threatening problems.

6.2.3 Patients with life-threatening problems that cannot be adequately corrected, as identified in the primary survey, shall be immediately transported.

6.3 *Pertinent Patient Information*—Obtaining pertinent patient information shall be an ongoing process of collecting information from all available resources throughout the entire contact with the patient.

7. Secondary Assessment

7.1 *Secondary Survey*—The secondary survey should be performed following the completion of the primary assessment. The selection and sequence of the components are dictated by the patient's condition and existing circumstances. The components of the primary survey shall be monitored during the secondary assessment. The components of the secondary survey are:

7.1.1 Stabilization of the cervical spine as indicated until in-line immobilization can be performed.

7.1.2 Assessment for altered mental status.

7.1.3 Determination of vital signs:

7.1.3.1 Determine rate, rhythm and quality of the respirations.

7.1.3.2 Determine rate, regularity and quality of the pulse.

7.1.3.3 Measure blood pressure.

7.1.3.4 Assess electrical activity of the heart.

7.1.4 Examination of the head:

7.1.4.1 Inspect and palpate head for any signs of injury or other abnormalities.

7.1.4.2 Inspect for blood, fluid or foreign objects in ears, nose and mouth.

7.1.4.3 Examine the eyes for signs of injury or other abnormalities.

7.1.5 Examination of the skin-mucous membranes for any signs of injury or edema and for color, temperature, and moistness.

7.1.6 Inspection and palpation of the neck for any signs of injury or other abnormalities.

7.1.7 Examination of the chest:

7.1.7.1 Inspect and palpate the chest for any signs of injury or other abnormalities.

7.1.7.2 Assess breath sounds.

7.1.8 Inspection and palpation of the abdomen for any signs of injury or other abnormalities.

7.1.9 Assessment of integrity of the pelvis.

7.1.10 Examination of the perineal area:

7.1.10.1 Inspect perineal area for any signs of injury or other abnormalities.

7.1.10.2 Assess for any signs of impending birth, if indicated.

7.1.11 Examination of each extremity:

7.1.11.1 Inspect and palpate for any signs of injury or other abnormalities.

7.1.11.2 Assess peripheral circulation, movement and sensation.

7.1.12 Inspection and palpation of the back and buttocks for any signs of injury or other abnormalities.

7.2 *Pertinent patient information*—The collection of pertinent patient information is part of the secondary survey and includes the following components:

7.2.1 Identification of the chief complaint.

7.2.2 Collection of pertinent information about present illness or injury including current medications.

7.2.3 Collection of a pertinent past medical history, including allergies.

7.2.4 Discovery of any medical indentification information.

7.2.5 Determination of the patient's age, sex and race.

7.3 *Emergency Transport*—Patients with life-threatening problems identified in the secondary survey shall be immediately transported.

8. Field Diagnosis and Management Plan

8.1 The emergency medical technician (paramedic) shall formulate a field diagnosis of the patient's problems and develop a plan to manage the patient's problems.

Designation: F 1490 – 96

Standard Terminology Relating to Search and Rescue[1]

This standard is issued under the fixed designation F 1490; the number immediately following the designation indicates the year of original adoption or, in the case of revision, the year of last revision. A number in parentheses indicates the year of last reapproval. A superscript epsilon (ϵ) indicates an editorial change since the last revision or reapproval.

1. Scope

1.1 This terminology standard is a compilation of definitions of terms, abbreviations and acronyms used in the search and rescue field collected in order to provide consistency in communication when used in actual operations, training and literature dealing with this field.

2. Terminology

access, *n*—the process of reaching the patients or subjects and establishing physical contact with them.

belayer, *n*—the one who performs the belay.

brake bar rack, *n*—a variable friction device consisting of a u-shaped metal bar to which are attached several metal bars that create friction on the rope. Also known as a rappel rack.

chest harness, *n*—a type of harness worn around the chest for upper body support.

evacuation, *n*—the process used to move the patient/subject between the completion of extraction and the beginning of transportation.

extraction, *n*—the process of removing the patient/subject from an immediately hazardous environment along with assessment, treatment, stabilization, and packaging.

---

[1] This terminology is under the jurisdiction of ASTM Committee F-32 on Search and Rescue and is the direct responsibility of Subcommittee F32.06 on Terminology.

Current edition approved March 10, 1996. Published June 1996. Originally published as F 1490 – 93. Last previous edition F 1490 – 93b.

Standard Specification for An Avalanche Beacon Frequency[1]

This standard is issued under the fixed designation F 1491; the number immediately following the designation indicates the year of original adoption or, in the case of revision, the year of last revision. A number in parentheses indicates the year of last reapproval. A superscript epsilon (ε) indicates an editorial change since the last revision or reapproval.

1. Scope

1.1 This specification establishes a National Avalanche Beacon Frequency.

2. Terminology

2.1 *Definitions of Terms Specific to This Standard:*

2.1.1 *avalanche beacon*—an electronic device for radio location of persons buried or trapped, usually by snow, and employing radio frequency electromagnetic induction.

3. Requirements

3.1 *Standard Frequency*—The avalanche beacon shall operate on a frequency of 457.0 kHz.

3.2 *Additional Interim Frequency*—The avalanche beacon may also operate on a frequency of 2.275 kHz.

3.3 *Frequency Priorities*—The standard frequency (457.0 kHz) is mandatory in all devices. Use of the interim frequency (2.275 kHz) shall not impair or disable effective operation with the standard frequency.

3.4 *Transition to Standard Frequency*—Both frequencies should be employed during the interim period. Incorporation of the interim frequency is intended to provide temporary backward interoperability with older beacons, until such devices can be replaced or retired. Beacons incorporating both frequencies should be employed until December 31, 1995. After this date, only single frequency (457.0 kHz) beacons should be employed and the use of 2.275 (kHz) should be discontinued.

4. Significance and Use

4.1 Avalanche beacons are used for the location of persons who are buried by avalanches. In operation, users wear the beacons, which are all set to transmit. After an incident, the rescuers switch their units to receive and search for the subject, whose units are still in transmit.

5. Keywords

5.1 avalanche; beacon; frequency; snow; transceiver

[1] This specification is under the jurisdiction of ASTM Committee F-32 on Search and Rescue and is the direct responsibility of Subcommittee F32.01 on Equipment, Testing, and Maintenance.

Current edition approved August 15, 1993. Published October 1993.

Standard Guide for Financing and Financial Accountability of Medical Transportation Systems[1]

This standard is issued under the fixed designation F 1493; the number immediately following the designation indicates the year of original adoption or, in the case of revision, the year of last revision. A number in parentheses indicates the year of last reapproval. A superscript epsilon (ε) indicates an editorial change since the last revision or reapproval.

1. Scope

1.1 This document establishes guidelines for understanding the financing of medical transportation systems. It identifies factors affecting financing, system design and performance requirements, revenue sources, financial accountability and management, and requirements for financially efficient systems.

2. Referenced Documents

2.1 *ASTM Standards:*

F 1177 Terminology Relating to Emergency Medical Services[2]

3. Terminology

3.1 *Definitions of Terms Specific to This Standard:* Description of Terms Specific to This Guide:

3.1.1 *patient transport price*—determined by summing all costs related to patient transports, to include all non allowed charges and contractual allowance and adjusted by any revenue generated by any subsidies, contributions and subscription fees. The resulting amount is divided by the total number of patient transports to determine the patient transport price.

3.1.2 *medical transportation system*—(see Terminology F 1177 for the definition of this term.)

3.1.3 *medical transportation services*—(see Terminology F 1177 for the definition of this term.)

4. Significance and Use

4.1 *Management*—Sound fiscal management is essential for all medical transportation systems. Without sufficient financial resources, a system will fail to consistently achieve its objectives. Therefore, finance is a primary responsibility in all systems; be they hospital owned/operated, private, public or volunteer organizations, or any combination thereof.

4.2 *Cost Determination*—This guide is designed to accurately determine actual and imputed costs of providing ambulance service. It provides methodology for understanding the value of services rendered and a basis for realistic industry-wide comparisons.

4.3 *Cost Accounting*—It is recognized that medical transportation services frequently are a part of a larger organization. However, the proper use of this guide mandates that all costs, real and imputed, directly or indirectly related to providing ambulance service, regardless of organizational structure, be totally and accurately accounted for through the use of generally accepted accounting principles.

4.4 *Application*—This guide, as part of the ASTM Standards and Practices, shall apply in its entirety whenever the entire document, or any part thereof, is used by any governmental authority to establish, operate, manage or regulate the delivery or payment for medical transportation services.

5. Environmental Factors

5.1 Several significant factors of a given service area affect its system's resources and related costs. They require careful examination and analysis. Understanding these factors will enhance the ability of those who direct, administer, manage and/or regulate medical transportation systems to more accurately determine anticipated needs and evaluate actual costs.

5.2 *Terrain*—Areas with mountains, valleys, waterways and bridges, etc., will usually be less accessible and require more resources resulting in reduced efficiency and a higher patient transport price.

5.3 *Roads and Highways*—Outdated and dangerous design of roads create hazards. These hazards create more demand for service and thus require a greater concentration of resources. The extra resources increase system costs.

5.4 *Weather*—Systems subject to extreme weather conditions (i.e., cold and snow, heavy rain and rock/mud slides, hurricanes, heat and dry conditions, wild/forest fires, and the like.) will need seasonal or periodic plans to meet area needs during such extremes. Maintenance of proper response plans and participation therein is a cost factor to the system. During such times maximum resources are required and system efficiency is reduced resulting in higher overall patient transport costs.

5.5 *Population Density*—Areas of high population density generate higher call volume and allow greater flexibility in utilization of resources resulting in lower overall patient transport costs.

5.5.1 *Demographics*—Areas with population characteristics with high concentrations of the elderly and economically disadvantaged, or both will result in higher call volume and a

---

[1] This guide is under the jurisdiction of ASTM Committee F-30 on Emergency Medical Services and is the direct responsibility of Subcommittee F30.03 on Organization/Management.

Current edition approved Sept. 15, 1993. Published November 1993.

[2] *Annual Book of ASTM Standards*, Vol 13.01.

greater demand on resources to meet the needs of these portions of the total service area.

5.6 *Natural/Man Made Disasters*—Systems subject to unpredictable events of extreme consequences (for example, earthquakes, airplane crashes, structural fires, hazardous material incidents, and the like.) will need emergency preparedness planning to meet area needs during disaster events. Maintenance of proper response plans and participation in exercise are cost factor to the system. During disasters maximum resources are required and system efficiency is reduced resulting in higher overall patient transport costs.

6. System Design Factors

6.1 *Service Area*—It is generally more economical for a medical transportation system to serve a larger population. Systems which provide a larger volume of transports within a given area will benefit from the inherent economies of scale and generate a lower average cost per transport.

6.2 *Medical Transport Providers*—The number of medical transport providers in a service area directly influences the cost per transport. Duplication of resources by multiple providers within a service area can negatively impact economies of scale.

6.3 *Health Care Facilities*—The number and location of hospitals, nursing homes, and the like, will influence costs. A significant number of transports to hospitals outside the service area can increase costs. A larger ratio of nursing home beds to a given general population can result in higher economies of scale than a smaller ratio and thereby lower costs.

6.4 *Start-Up Costs*—Sufficient funds must be available to ensure the success of initial start-up, or expansion of an existing service. To determine the required level of funding, consideration must be given to the following;

6.4.1 *Office/Service Facility*—Items to be included are building, office equipment, furniture and fixtures, computers, etc.

6.4.2 *Equipment*—Items to be included are ambulances, administrative vehicles, communication equipment, medical equipment and supplies, etc.

6.4.3 *Inventory*—Items to be included are sufficient levels of supplies for on-going operations of ambulance services and office functions for the period of time it is expected to take to establish cash flow to support on-going operation.

6.4.4 *Personnel*—Items to be included are expenses related to recruiting, hiring, training, salaries and benefits.

6.4.5 *Insurance*—Actual premium paid, or imputed costs for self-funding.

6.4.6 *Working Capital*—Funds adequate to support overall operations until such time as sufficient cash flow is established.

6.5 *Jurisdictional Responsibilities*—Jurisdictions exist at the federal, state, regional, and local level which have an impact on the operation of each EMS provider and the EMS system. They may include the following:

6.5.1 *EMS Regulations/Legislation*—EMS regulations and legislation are usually passed at the state or local units of government. They are usually influenced by EMS guidelines recommended at the federal level.

6.5.2 *Labor*—Federal labor laws cover issues related to Health & Safety, Collective Bargaining, and Wages & Hours.

6.5.3 *Taxes*—Federal, state, and local taxes apply to purchases, property, incorporation, and the like.

6.5.4 *Other Non-EMS Related Costs*—Other restrictions include building and zoning regulations.

7. System Factors Related to Expense

7.1 *Exclusionary Policies*—Systems that exclude providers from emergency or non-emergency calls, respectively, by design increase total system cost. Utilization of all resources within the service area is necessary to achieve maximum economy while maintaining performance requirements, thereby resulting in lower overall patient transport price.

7.2 *Performance Factors*—Jurisdictional authorities have a responsibility to establish performance requirements for the provider(s) of service and demand accountability and compliance thereof. In the design of such requirements, cost considerations, allowances for geography, population density, demographics, economies of scale, duplication and/or multiple responders and exclusionary policies, must be addressed. Precise accounting practices for the system must be initially established and routinely maintained so all cost factors within the system design can be identified and reviewed with relationship to the performance factors.

7.2.1 *Operations*—Factors include meeting standards for average response and total times, staffing patterns, etc. Systems that require shorter response and total time performance will demand greater resources and will cost more than those with less rigid requirements.

7.2.2 *Clinical Capability*—Factors include meeting standards for the license level of the service (Basic to Paramedic), the license level of the personnel, on-line medical control, quality assurance activities, and the like. Systems that require higher levels of clinical care, training and medical supervision will demand greater resources and will cost more than those with lesser requirements.

7.3 *Efficiency*—Efficiency is affected by policies, ordinances, and rules which limit the flexibility of the provider or which do not provide incentives to promote efficiency.

7.3.1 Efficient systems deploy ambulance, staffing, and equipment resources to eliminate duplication.

7.3.2 Efficient systems promote cooperation between the jurisdictional authorities and the providers to identify and eliminate waste, inefficiencies and restrictive regulations in order to reduce overall system cost while improving system efficiency.

8. System Factors Related to Revenue

8.1 *Revenue Sources*—Different types of revenue sources fund the providers within an EMS system. The different types of revenue, separately or in combination with each other, have different impacts on the operations of the system.

8.1.1 *Subsidies*—Revenue received from direct governmental funding. Subsidies range from total funding to supplemental compensation to affect shortfalls from other revenue sources.

8.1.2 *Subscription Fee*—Pre-paid fee for a family or individual who belong to a membership plan which agrees to provide ambulance service for reasons of medical necessity.

8.1.3 *Contributions/Donations*—Revenue received from individual or general solicitations, fund raising, grants, etc.

8.1.4 *Fee for Service*—Revenue received from charges for

specific services performed.

8.2 *Reductions in Revenue*—Revenue may be reduced because of management practices related to third party payor regulations, group purchases of service, or non-payment of fees.

8.2.1 *Non-Allowed Charges*—Third party payors such as Medicare and Medicaid reimburse specific service and supplies utilized at a lower rate than the normal billing rate. The unreimbursed amount is referred to as non-allowed charges. This is applicable only on transports where the provider accepts Medicare or Medicaid assignment.

NOTE 1—It is not mandatory that a provider must accept assignment on Medicare claims. Providers may submit claims as non-assigned and charge patients the full amount for services rendered, thereby avoiding the reduction in revenue for non-allowed charges.

8.2.2 *Contractual Allowances*—Specific group purchasers may be granted pre-determined discounts based upon negotiated agreements (for example, exclusive contract, accelerated payment, and the like).

8.2.3 *Bad Debt*—Although bad debt is a cost of doing business, it bears special mention with relationship to reduction in revenue.

8.2.3.1 An EMS provider will have a significant number of accounts (much higher than most other industries) which will not be paid. These accounts are bad debt, for which the responsible party is unwilling or unable (indigent) to pay.

8.2.3.2 Calculation of projected bad debt is determined by deducting a historical percentage from gross charges. This percentage will vary by provider, its ability to manage its collection policies and a given service area.

8.3 *Revenue Surplus/Profit*—A surplus in revenue occurs when revenue is greater than all expenses (operating, general & administrative, taxes). Profit making organizations define this surplus as profit. To survive, such organizations must generate a revenue surplus to provide for growth and improvements.

9. System Financial Accountability Requirements

9.1 Different types of reports exist to evaluate the financial status of the system.

9.2 *Balance Sheet*—A periodic look at a system's financial standing at a specific point in time shall include;

9.2.1 *Assets*—Tangible or non-tangible items of value to the system.

9.2.1.1 *Current Assets*—Assets whose value will be used or realized within a twelve month (fiscal year) period (for example, cash, accounts receivable, pre-paid expenses, and the like).

9.2.1.2 *Fixed Assets*—Assets which will have value to the system at the end of a twelve month (FY) period.

9.2.1.3 *Other Assets*—Assets whose length of value is indeterminable (for example, goodwill, tax credits, utility deposits, and the like).

9.2.2 *Liabilities*—Obligations owed by the system.

9.2.2.1 *Current Liabilities*—Obligations which will generally be paid within a twelve month (FY) period (for example, accounts payable, accrued payroll expenses, current portion of long-term debt, and the like).

9.2.2.2 *Long-Term Liabilities*—Obligations owed by the system whose payment term extends beyond a twelve month (FY) period (for example, bank notes, bond payments, advances from stockholders, and the like).

9.2.2.3 *Other Liabilities*—Obligations whose payment terms are indeterminable (for example, deferred taxes, and the like).

9.2.3 *Equity*—The value of the difference between total system assets and liabilities which reflect the net value of the system.

9.2.3.1 *Paid in Capital*—Initial or additional investment in the system.

9.2.3.2 *Retained Earnings/Reserves*—The total net income/loss which remains in the system at a specific point in time.

9.3 *Income Statement*—The measure of the financial performance of the system over a period of time.

9.3.1 *Revenue*—Total income from all revenue sources, less revenue reductions.

9.3.2 *Operating Expenses*—Total costs, real or imputed, which relate to producing the service (for example, service related salaries & associated costs, supplies, vehicle maintenance & depreciation, insurance, and the like).

9.3.3 *General and Administrative Expenses*—Total costs, real or imputed, which relate to administration and promotion of the service (for example, administrative/clerical salaries and associated costs, advertising, computer systems, professional fees, and the like).

9.3.4 *Income Taxes*—Federal, state and local income taxes required of providers who are not tax exempt.

9.4 *Reserve and Working Capital*—An annual capital and operating budget is an estimate of yearly expenses. As it is impossible to predict all expenses and occurrences, a reserve fund is an appropriate protective mechanism. This fund should be an amount which can cover most unexpected financial emergencies. Another important component is a planning budget allowance for sufficient funds to pay bills when due, recognizing that revenue income can be variable, inconsistent, and periodic. This is referred to as working capital and must be sufficient to pay bills until collections are received. Insurance companies and other parties often take several weeks to process reimbursements. Some services receive once-a-year subsidies. Careful planning is required to assure that these funds last until the next year's receipt of revenue. For subsidized services a subsidy advance may be necessary to provide working capital.

9.5 *Revenue Accounting*—Precise accounting practices must be established and routinely maintained with respect to specific categories of revenue and reductions thereof. This information is necessary for system directors, administrators and managers to assess income performance and make decisions when revenue must be increased, or decreased, and which revenue source, or reduction, or combination thereof, must be altered to achieve the desired result.

9.6 *Accounting Methodology*—The accrual method of accounting, as identified in the General Accepted Accounting Principals,[3] is the recommended way of determining costs and maintaining financial records.

[3] As promulgated by the Financial Accounting Standards Board.

10. Management Issues Related to Establishing the Patient Transport Price

10.1 *Total Patient Transport Cost*—This is comprised of all operating and administrative costs of the system (including bad debt), direct or indirect, real or imputed, including allowances for reserves/profit.

10.2 *Adjustment for Non-Allowed Charges*—Add to the patient transport cost the total amount of non-allowed charges by Medicare or Medicaid.

10.2.1 Non-allowed charges are amounts which, by law, cannot be billed, as a result of accepting assignment from Medicare or Medicaid. This occurs when a provider accepts assignment, and thereby agrees that what Medicare determines as the allowable payment, and Medicaid pays, is payment in full for services rendered.

10.2.2 A provider who accepts assignment on Medicare claims, will receive only a percentage of the charges billed. The provider's actual charge, minus Medicare's allowed charge, if lower, equals the non-allowed charge. The allowed charge is based upon the profile established by the Medicare carrier, within a given region, for a particular provider, and is reimbursed as 80 %. Medicaid reimbursement depends on the policies of various state programs.

10.2.3 Calculation of projected non-allowed charges is determined by deducting a historical percentage from gross Medicare and Medicaid billings. This percentage will vary by provider, its Medicare profile, its ability to manage billing policies, a given service area and state. This calculation must be made as a factor in determining the patient transport price.

10.3 *Adjustment for Contractual Allowances*—Add to the patient transport cost and non-allowed charges the total amount discounted to specific users.

10.3.1 Calculation of contractual allowances is determined by deducting the negotiated amount/percentage from gross charges to specific users with whom agreements exist. This amount will vary by provider, its ability to negotiate special agreements and the service area. This calculation is a factor in determining the patient transport price.

10.4 *Adjustment for Subsidy*—Subtract from the total patient transport cost, non-allowed charges and contractual allowances the amount of subsidy.

10.4.1 Many service areas need subsidies to achieve desired levels of availability and performance requirements. They may generate abnormally high patient transport costs, based on geographics, population density, demographics or a combination thereof, desired results. These areas must provide subsidy to offset these unique costs that are results of these factors. However, subsidy should not be used to arbitrarily reduce patient transport price beyond considerations for these factors.

10.4.2 Systems which subsidize patient charges by charging less than cost, by design, limit funds otherwise available from third party payers.

10.4.3 The level of subsidy should have no relationship to system efficiency, but does have a direct effect on the reduction of the unadjusted patient transport price. Reductions in the adjusted patient transport price will affect future reimbursement levels from third party payers.

10.4.4 Once the patient transport cost is established the effect of subsidy must be calculated. The provision of subsidy for ambulance service affects the patient transport price.

10.4.5 A variance in subsidy is not equivalent to a similar change in the patient transport price. Allowances for bad debt must be made (for example, at a collection rate of 50 %: for a $1.00 reduction in per patient transport subsidy, $2.00 must be added to fee for service billings; for a $1.00 increase in per patient transport subsidy, $2.00 may be eliminated from fee for service billings).

10.5 *Adjustment for Contributions/Donations*—Subtract from the patient transport cost, non-allowed charges and contractual allowances the amount of funding received from general or individual solicitations, divided by the total of all patients transported.

10.6 *Patient Transport Price*—The patient transport price is determined from all costs related to the transport of the patient, to which must be added non-allowed charges and contractual allowances, adjusted for revenue generated by subsidies, contributions/donations and/or subscription fees, as described herein. The resulting amount is divided by the total number of patient transports to determine the patient transport price.

11. Keywords

11.1 costs; finance; reimbursement; revenue

Standard Test Method for Determining Laser Resistance of the Shaft of Tracheal Tubes[1]

This standard is issued under the fixed designation F 1497; the number immediately following the designation indicates the year of original adoption or, in the case of revision, the year of last revision. A number in parentheses indicates the year of last reapproval. A superscript epsilon (ε) indicates an editorial change since the last revision or reapproval.

INTRODUCTION

Surgery in the airway in which a laser is used brings together an oxygen-enriched atmosphere, fuel, and high energy that can combine to create a fire. Various materials and devices have been used to minimize the chance of airway fire. This test method was developed to determine the laser resistance of a tracheal tube shaft for a defined set of conditions.

1. Scope

1.1 This test method covers a standard means of testing the laser resistance of the shaft of a tracheal tube.

1.2 This test method addresses the laser resistance of the shaft of the tracheal tube. Other components of the system, such as the inflation system and cuff, are outside the scope of this test method.

1.3 Caution should be observed since the direct applicability of the results of this test method to the clinical situation has not been fully established.

1.4 The values stated in SI units are to be regarded as the standard. The values given in parentheses are for information only.

1.5 *This test method should be used to measure and describe the properties of materials, products, or assemblies in response to heat and flame under controlled laboratory conditions and should not be used to describe or appraise the fire hazard or fire risk of materials, products, or assemblies under actual fire conditions. However, results of this test may be used as elements of a fire risk assessment that takes into account all of the factors that are pertinent to an assessment of the fire hazard of a particular end use.*

1.6 *This standard does not purport to address all of the safety concerns, if any, associated with its use. It is the responsibility of the user of this standard to establish appropriate safety and health practices and determine the applicability of regulatory limitations prior to use.* Specific precautionary statements are given in Notes 1-6.

2. Referenced Documents

2.1 *ASTM Standards:*

F 1242 Specification for Cuffed and Uncuffed Tracheal Tubes[2]

2.2 *ANSI Standards:*

ANSI Z136.1 American National Standard for the Safe Use of Lasers-1993[3]

ANSI Z136.3 American National Standard for the Safe Use of Lasers in Health Care Facilities-1996[3]

2.3 *CGA Standard:*

CGA G-4.3 Commodity Specification for Oxygen[4]

CGA G-10.1 Commodity Specification for Nitrogen[4]

3. Terminology

3.1 *Definitions:*

3.1.1 *blemish*—any apparent physical change to the shaft of the tracheal tube, other than damage or burning. Some examples of blemish are discoloration, surface pitting, and minor deformation.

3.1.2 *burning*—any continuing combustion process that occurs in or on the test specimen. Some signs of burning are flame, smoldering, and rapid evolution of smoke.

3.1.3 *damage*—any physical change (for example, local heating, melting, creation of holes, ashing without burning, pyrolysis), other than burning, that may affect the safety of the patient or efficacy of the shaft of the tracheal tube.

3.1.4 *laser resistance*—the relative ability of a material to withstand laser energy without burning or damage.

3.1.5 *power density*—the rate at which laser energy is delivered per unit area of irradiated surface, given in watts per square centimetre (W/cm^2).

3.1.6 *shaft*—the portion of the tracheal tube between the cuff and the machine end of the tube.

---

[1] This test method is under the jurisdiction of ASTM Committee F-29 on Anesthetic and Respiratory Equipmentand is the direct responsibility of Subcommittee F29.18 on Operating Room Fire Safety.

Current edition approved November 10, 1999. Published December 1999. Originally published as F 1497 - 94. Last previous edition F 1497 - 99.

[2] *Annual Book of ASTM Standards*, Vol 13.01.

[3] Available from American National Standards Institute, 11 W. 42nd St., 13th Floor, New York, NY 10036.

[4] Available from Compressed Gas Association, 1235 Jefferson Davis Highway, Arlington, VA 22202.

4. Summary of Test Method

4.1 The shaft of a tracheal tube will be exposed to laser energy of known characteristics while in an environment of 98 ± 2 % oxygen.

NOTE 1—This test method can result in a rocket-like fire involving the tracheal tube. This fire can produce high heat, intense light, and toxic gases.

5. Significance and Use

5.1 This test method determines a uniform and repeatable measurement of the laser resistance of the shaft of a tracheal tube. Most of the variables involved in laser ignition of a tracheal tube have been fixed in order to establish a basis for comparison. This measurement can be used to compare tracheal tubes having differing designs of laser protection.

5.2 There are a large number and range of variables involved in laser ignition of a tracheal tube. A change in one variable may affect the outcome of the test. Caution should be observed since the direct applicability of the results of this test method to the clinical situation has not been fully established.

5.3 Since it is conceivable that an oxygen enriched atmosphere may be encountered in the clinical situation, either intentionally or unintentionally, the test is performed in an environment of 98 (±2 %) oxygen.

5.4 A flow rate of 1 L/min in a 6.0-mm inner diameter tube was chosen as the best condition for tube ignition and establishment of a fire.

5.5 *Opportunities for Development*—Variations of this test method can be applied to study the effect of changing the test conditions but are outside the scope of this test method. For example, variation of the respiratory gas flow rate or different breathing gas mixtures may affect the laser resistance of the tracheal tube. Use of modes of laser energy delivery other than continuous, (for example, pulsed, superpulse, q-switched, and ultrapulsed), may alter the tracheal tube's ignition characteristics. Also, tubes of different diameter will have laser resistance different from that defined in this test method.

6. Apparatus

6.1 *Gas Supply System*:

6.1.1 The gas supply system shall provide oxygen to the containment box at a controllable flow rate. Also, the system shall be capable of rapidly flooding the containment box with nitrogen or other inert gas or stopping oxygen flow, or both, to extinguish any burning material. (See Fig. 1.) The nitrogen or inert gas supplied should be at a higher pressure and allow a flow at least an order of magnitude greater than the oxygen supplied to the containment box.

6.1.2 Other arrangements, such as an oxygen flood valve for rapidly purging the containment box or an inert gas flooding system for rapid extinguishment of burning material, may be made as long as the requirements of this test method are not affected.

6.2 *Containment Box*:

6.2.1 The containment box is a means to control the environment around the test specimen while allowing access of the laser delivery system to the test unit (see Fig. 2).

6.2.2 The typical containment box will have the following characteristics:

6.2.2.1 Allows direct access of the laser energy to the entire length of the tracheal tube shaft, and

6.2.2.2 Supports the shaft of the tracheal tube 7 to 10 cm (3 to 4 in.) below the opening for laser access as shown in Fig. 1.

6.2.2.3 Maintains an environment of at least 96 % oxygen

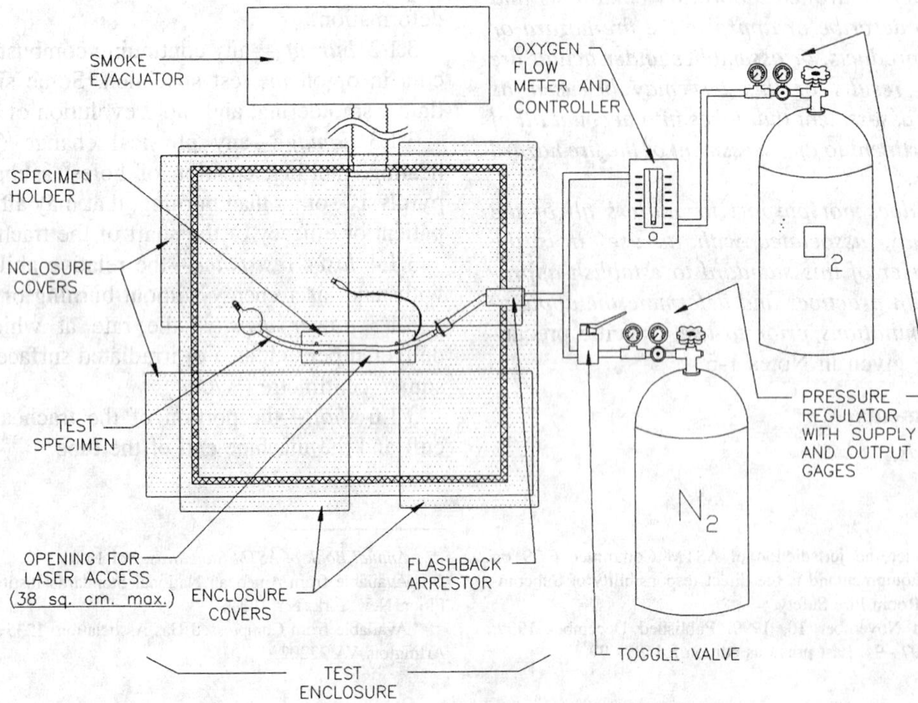

FIG. 1 Typical Testing Apparatus Schematic

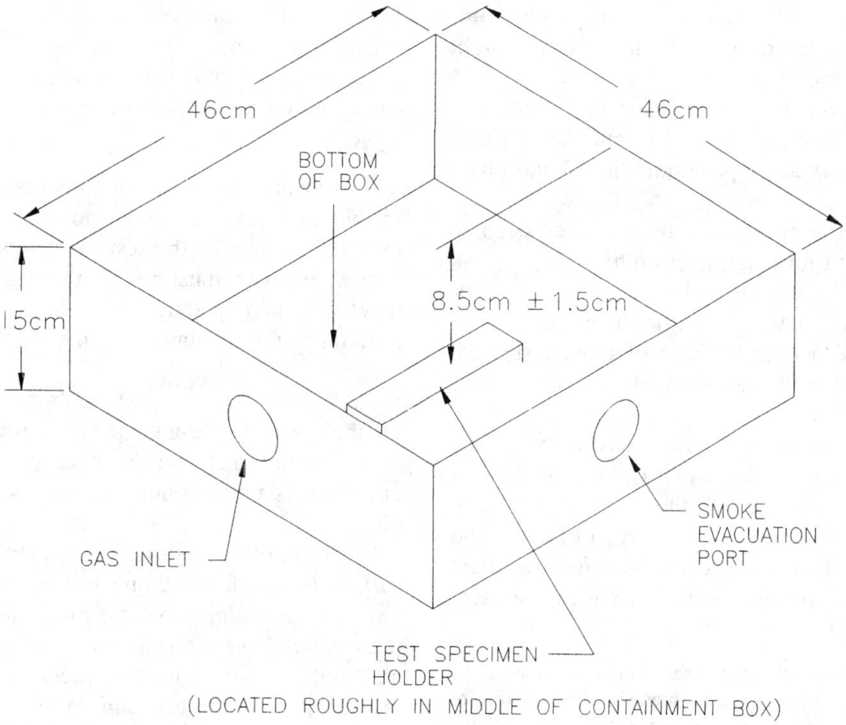

Construction Notes:
1) All tolerances are ±6 cm except as noted.
2) Gas inlet and smoke evacuation ports are to be sufficiently large to allow for appropriate plumbing access.
3) Commonly available electrical pull boxes with knockouts may be used.
4) A fume hood which encloses the containment box may be used in the place of a smoke evacuator.
5) The containment box should be covered with glass during testing. An opening large enough for laser access should be present. The area of this opening is not to exceed 6 in.^{2}

FIG. 2 Containment Box Drawings

around the tracheal tube,

6.2.2.4 Exhausts the gas flowing through the tube and any products of combustion to a safe area,

6.2.2.5 Is fireproof and easily cleaned of soot and residue from burned tracheal tubes,

6.2.2.6 Is a rectangular parallel pipe approximately 46 by 46 by 15 cm (18 by 18 by 6 in.),

6.2.2.7 Has transparent, nonflammable enclosure covers that are positioned on top of the box to allow visibility of and access to the test unit while maintaining the test environment. The covers must be able to define an opening of no longer than 38 cm^2 to allow laser access to the test unit. The covers shall be easily removable for access to the test unit, cleaning of the box, and cleaning of the covers themselves, and

6.2.2.8 Can be rapidly flooded with nitrogen or other inert gas to extinguish any fire inside the box.

6.2.3 Other configurations may be used as long as the requirements of this test method are not affected.

6.3 *Smoke Evacuation*:

NOTE 2—**Warning:** Combustion of most materials used in tracheal tubes produces toxic gases such as carbon monoxide, hydrogen chloride, and hydrogen cyanide. Also, the smoke produced in such fires contains hazardous particles of carbon, silica, unburned matter, and other materials.

6.3.1 A device to safely remove smoke resulting from any burning tube should be attached to the containment box so as to minimize the chance of drawing fire into the exhaust system. Alternately, the containment box can be placed in a fume hood that exhausts out-of-doors.

6.3.2 This device must not interfere with maintaining the oxygen environment within the containment box. For example, the flow of a fume hood should not create drafts that would enter or pull gas from the opening for laser access. A smoke evacuator, if used, should not be activated until after ignition of a fire.

6.4 *Lasers*:

NOTE 3—**Warning:** Surgical lasers emit concentrated, coherent light energy of sufficient power to damage living tissue or ignite fires directly or by reflected energy.

NOTE 4—**Precaution:** In addition to other precautions, test personnel should be schooled in the use of lasers and take proper safety measures based on the type of laser being used. These precautions should include laser safety eyewear, protective clothing, and controlled access to the test area. Refer to ANSI Z136.1-1993 and ANSI Z136.3-1996 for detailed guidelines for the safe use of lasers.

6.4.1 Lasers typically used during surgery shall be used. Some of these lasers are as follows:

6.4.1.1 *Carbon Dioxide Laser*, commonly known as CO^2 laser, that emits infrared light energy with a wavelength of 10 600 nm.

6.4.1.2 *Neodymium:Yttrium Aluminum Garnet Laser*, commonly known as Nd:YAG laser, that emits near-infrared light energy with a wavelength of 1064 nm.

6.4.1.3 *Frequency-Doubled Nd:YAG Laser*, that emits visible light energy with a wavelength of 532 nm. A particular design of this laser is known as the potassium titanyl phosphate laser or KTP laser.

6.4.1.4 Other types of lasers may be used as they become available, or become used for surgery, or both.

6.4.2 Other lasers, such as those used for aiming systems or industrial machining, that have capabilities (for example, 5 mW HeNe, 1000 W CO^2) outside those of typical surgical lasers, shall not be used for this test method.

6.4.3 *Laser Delivery Systems*:

6.4.3.1 The laser emission shall be by means of the typical systems used with the particular laser, that is, focusing lens or micromanipulator, in accordance with the manufacturer's instructions. These devices allow the laser energy of known and controllable size to be directed onto an area for treatment without physical contact. The system shall provide a spot size of 0.5-mm ± 10 % diameter.

NOTE 5—**Caution:** Cooling or clearing gases should be used at the minimum settings recommended by the laser manufacturer. Cooling or clearing gases are used by some lasers to maintain the quality of the delivery system. It is understood that the flow of these gases may alter the measured laser resistance, for example, by extinguishing nascent fire.

6.4.3.2 Bare fibers, contact tips, contact fibers, or other devices that convert some laser energy into heat energy and are used in physical contact with tissue are not covered by this test method. Heat energy affects materials differently than does laser energy and is inconsistent with this test method.

NOTE 6—**Caution:** The power transmitted by these systems should be verified as accurate. This can be accomplished by use of an external power meter or internal calibration systems. Fiber transmitted laser energy should be frequently checked, that is, at each new power level and after fiber cleaving, as the fiber ends are easily damaged by the testing performed in this procedure.

6.5 *Oxygen Analyzer*:

6.5.1 Any device that can measure the concentration of gaseous oxygen with a precision of at least 1 % of full scale and an accuracy of at least 1 % of full scale is satisfactory for use.

6.5.2 The oxygen sensor should be positioned to minimize the chance of its ignition by any resulting fire in the containment box.

7. Reagents and Materials

7.1 *Oxygen Produced by Air Liquefaction, U.S.P.*—Medical grade oxygen as defined by *United States Pharmacopoeia* and CGA G-4.3 typically at least 99 % pure oxygen.

7.2 *Nitrogen or Other Inert Gas (That Is, Non-Oxidizing, Nonflammable), such as Nitrogen Produced by Air Liquefaction, U.S.P.*—Medical grade nitrogen as defined by *United States Pharmacopoeia* and CGA G-10.1 typically at least 99 % pure nitrogen.

8. Test Units

8.1 The test units shall be any material, device, or system used as a tracheal tube, as generally defined in Specification F 1242, with whatever modifications used to protect the tracheal tube from laser energy.

8.2 Five test units shall be used for each time value tested each with 6.0-mm inside diameter.

9. Preparation of Apparatus

9.1 Ensure that the containment box is clean, that is, free of visible, gross contaminants and debris that may interfere with the performance of the test or evaluation of the results. The enclosure covers must be clean enough to allow test personnel to view laser interaction with the test unit. The containment box must not contaminate the test unit with any visible material.

9.2 Ensure that the gas supply system has sufficient gases for the test and extinguishment of any fire.

9.3 Ensure that the laser is in working order, that its operation is understood, and that personnel protection is in place.

9.4 Have other methods of fire extinguishment, for example, carbon dioxide fire extinguisher, at hand. Water is not advised as it will not extinguish some materials burning in oxygen and, if used, will cause considerable soiling of the containment box and will interfere with interpretation of the results of laser interaction with the test unit. Water is also not recommended and is hazardous for use on fire involving energized electrical equipment.

10. Conditioning

10.1 Prepare each test unit in accordance with the manufacturer's instructions for use. Some devices may require special preparation, for example, wetting of the tracheal tube, filling cuff with saline, or insufflation of inert gas, as part of the laser protection.

10.2 Test units shall be free from extraneous materials such as blood, mucous, lubricants, char, ash, or soot. Such materials can alter the laser resistance of the tracheal tube.

10.3 The test units, all apparatus, and all gases shall be at 20 ± 3°C, prior to the start of testing. This is done to standardize the test conditions rather than to simulate a clinical condition. The ignitability and flammability of most materials do not significantly change between room temperature and body temperature.

10.4 The test units shall not be preconditioned in an oxygen-enriched atmosphere. Some materials absorb oxygen and may have reduced laser resistance if exposed to oxygen for long periods.

11. Procedure

11.1 Perform the test at 20 ± 3°C.

11.2 Insert the test unit into the containment box. Connect the gas supply system to the test unit.

11.3 Place the enclosure covers on top of the containment box as shown in Fig. 1. Ensure that the opening for laser access is not larger than 38 cm^2 (6 $in.^2$) and allows laser access to the shaft of the test unit. Also, ensure that the test unit is visible through the enclosure covers.

11.4 Determine that the inert gas flush is working properly to extinguish any fire resulting from the test.

11.5 Determine that the smoke evacuation system is working properly and does not affect the gas environment of the containment box during the test.

11.6 Flow oxygen at a rate and time period sufficient to establish an environment of 98 (±2 %) oxygen in the containment box. Verify this environment of 98 (±2 %) oxygen by use of an oxygen analyzer measuring at the location of the test unit.

11.7 Establish a flow of oxygen at 1 L/min through the tracheal tube.

11.8 Position the laser so that the emitted energy will be perpendicular to the surface of the shaft of the test unit proximal to the cuff (see Fig. 3). Also, position the laser so that the spot size of the emitted beam on the surface of the test unit is 0.5 mm ± 10 % in diameter. Avoid pre-focus or post-focus of the beam as the spot size of the beam is a critical dimension and uniform absorption of the laser energy depends on focusing of the beam. Lateral motion of the laser spot must be minimized by some form of stabilization, for example, laser handpiece probe tip resting on the test unit.

11.9 Starting with a recommended 2 W, apply the laser energy to the test unit for a specified duration of 1 to 10 s and continuous laser emission mode. Stop laser emission upon evidence of tracheal tube burning or difficulty with the test apparatus.

NOTE 7—These test data shall be reported in addition to data collected at 10 s.

11.10 Increase the laser power by the minimum increment available with the type of laser being used, but not less than 2 W. Repeat the application of the laser energy at a cool, clean, undamaged area on the test unit for each new power. This can be accomplished by starting the test at one end of the shaft and proceeding toward the other end.

11.11 Continue testing by increasing the power density until burning occurs, or the maximum power of the laser is reached. If burning occurs, extinguish the fire with the nitrogen or inert gas system.

12. Interpretation of Results

12.1 Any test unit that experiences burning, as defined in 3.1.2 and 3.1.3 will be considered to have laser resistance up to the maximum power at which the burning did not occur under the specified test conditions.

12.2 Any damage or blemish occurring to the test unit other than burning (for example, melting, creation of holes) must be described in the test report, together with the laser settings which caused such change(s). These changes should be evaluated for their potential to harm the patient or operating-room personnel. For example, a tube that melts during the laser emission may become occluded and risk loss of the airway.

13. Report

13.1 Verify that the following standardized test parameters were correct during performance of the test:

13.1.1 Inside diameter of test unit = 6.0 mm,

13.1.2 Oxygen concentration = 98 (±2 %),

13.1.3 Oxygen flow rate = 1 L/min,

13.1.4 Laser spot size = 0.5 mm (±10 %), and

13.1.5 Mode of laser application = continuous.

13.2 Report the following information for each test unit:

13.2.1 Laser type and delivery system used,

13.2.2 Laser energy duration, in (seconds),

13.2.3 Maximum power of the laser, W,

13.2.4 Outside diameter of test unit, cm,

13.2.5 Length of the test unit, cm,

13.2.6 Power at which damage occurred, W,

13.2.7 Maximum power that did not cause damage, W,

13.2.8 Power at which burning occurred, W,

13.2.9 Maximum power that did not cause burning, W,

13.2.10 Physical description of the flame produced (for example, color, size),

13.2.11 Physical description of smoke evolved (for example, color, amount),

13.2.12 Physical description of ash produced (for example, color, texture),

13.2.13 Physical description of damage produced, and

13.2.14 Physical description of any blemish occurring at the

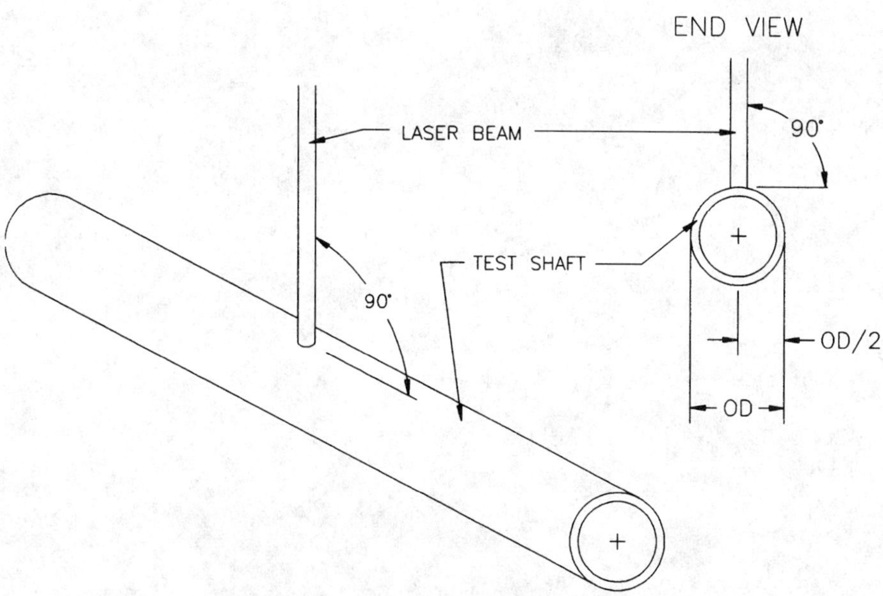

FIG. 3 Laser-Beam Firing-Angle Diagram

maximum power that did not cause burning or damage.

13.3 Report any other effect that could result in harm to the patient or operating-room personnel, for example, reflected laser energy.

14. Precision and Bias

14.1 *Precision*—The precision of the procedure in this test method for defining the laser resistance of the shaft of a tracheal tube is being evaluated. Preliminary intralaboratory results suggest that the laser resistance will be within ±4 W.

14.2 *Bias*—Since there is no accepted reference material suitable for defining the bias of the laser resistance of the shaft of a tracheal tube, bias has not been determined.

15. Keywords

15.1 burning; fire; laser; laser resistance; oxygen; power density; safety; tracheal tube

Last ASTM Designation: F 1501 – 95

Test Method for Tension Testing of Calcium Phosphate Coatings

This test method covers tension testing of continuous calcium phosphate coatings adhering to dense metal substrates at ambient temperatures.

Formerly under the jurisdiction of Committee F04 on Medical and Surgical Materials and Devices, this test method was withdrawn in November 2000 and replaced by Test Method F 1147 for Tension Testing of Calcium Phosphate and Metallic Coatings.[1]

---

[1] Annual Book of ASTM Standards, Volume 13.01.

Designation: F 1517 – 94

Standard Guide for Scope of Performance of Emergency Medical Services Ambulance Operations[1]

This standard is issued under the fixed designation F 1517; the number immediately following the designation indicates the year of original adoption or, in the case of revision, the year of last revision. A number in parentheses indicates the year of last reapproval. A superscript epsilon (ε) indicates an editorial change since the last revision or reapproval.

1. Scope

1.1 This guide covers minimum standards for the performance of emergency medical services (EMS) ambulance operators, including: operator qualifications, pre-run operation, and post-run aspects.

1.2 This guide shall promote the safe and efficient delivery of the ambulance, equipment, crew, passengers and patients, during all phases of the delivery of EMS involving the ambulance; at all times exercising the highest degree of care for the safety of the public. This guide may be applied to other EMS vehicles that do not necessarily provide patient transport.

1.3 This guide shall be used as the basis for training guides of the emergency medical services ambulance operator.

1.4 The values stated in SI units are to be regarded as the standard. The SI units given in parentheses are for information only.

1.5 *This standard does not purport to address all of the safety concerns, if any, associated with its use. It is the responsibility of the user of this standard to establish appropriate safety and health practices and determine the applicability of regulatory limitations prior to use.*

2. Referenced Documents

2.1 *ASTM Standards:*

F 1031 Practice for Training the Emergency Medical Technician (Basic)[2]

F 1177 Terminology Relating to Emergency Medical Services[2]

F 1230 Specification for Minimum Performance Requirements for Emergency Medical Service (EMS) Ground Vehicles[2]

F 1258 Practice for Emergency Medical Dispatch[2]

3. Terminology

3.1 *Definitions:*

3.1.1 The definitions given in Terminology F 1177 are applicable to this guide.

3.1.2 *ambulance*—See Terminology F 1177.

3.2 *Definitions of Terms Specific to This Standard:*

3.2.1 *ambulance operations*—the efficient delivery of the ambulance, equipment, crew, passengers and patients, during all phases of the delivery of EMS involving the ambulance at all times exercising the highest degree of care for the safety of the public.

3.2.2 *ambulance service provider*—as outlined in this guide, a person, company, corporation or political entity responsible for operation, maintenance, or policy making, or combination thereof, regarding emergency medical vehicle operations.

3.2.3 *bona fide occupational qualification (BFOQ)*—the skills and knowledge relevant to the performance of a specific task.

3.2.4 *departure check*—the visual check of the vehicle and surrounding area ensuring that equipment and supplies have been retrieved and properly stored and that all compartment doors are secured.

3.2.5 *egress check*—the visual check of the vehicle and surrounding area prior to operating the ambulance.

3.2.6 *emergency mode*—as defined by individual state statues that refer to emergency vehicles, equipment, and operations.

3.2.7 *full check*—a comprehensive and systematic evaluation of the ambulance at specified intervals, including documentation of the inspection, any deficiencies found and their corrective actions.

3.2.8 *operator*—a person who operates or assists with the operation of an ambulance.

3.2.9 *post-run*—the managed return of the ambulance and operators to optimal pre-run readiness.

3.2.10 *pre-run*—all aspects of assuring response readiness.

3.2.11 *quick check*—an abbreviated version of the full check, focusing on the major operational functions of the vehicle.

4. Significance and Use

4.1 This guide provides minimum guidelines for safe and efficient ambulance operation.

4.2 All ambulance operations and operators should follow this guide for the development of educational and training programs.

4.3 This guide is intended to promote safe and efficient ambulance operations and to reduce morbidity, mortality, and property loss associated with ambulance operations.

---

[1] This guide is under the jurisdiction of ASTM Committee F-30 on Emergency Medical Services and is the direct responsibility of Subcommittee F30.02 on Personnel, Training, and Education.

Current edition approved May 15, 1994. Published July 1994.

[2] *Annual Book of ASTM Standards*, Vol 13.01.

4.4 This guide is intended to assist those who are responsible for the development and implementation of policies and procedures for ambulance operations.

5. Medical Fitness to Drive

5.1 Because of the complex relationship of certain medical and mental impairments, a medical screening program shall be established by all EMS entities bestowing the privilege of ambulance driving.

5.2 The authorization of ambulance drivers must always be based on bona fide occupational qualifications (BFOQ) pursuant to the task of ambulance operation. The following considerations must be evaluated:

5.2.1 A medical exam of the applicant by a licensed M.D. or D.O. attesting that the history and physical reveals no evidence of any medical or physical condition which would prove detrimental to operating an ambulance.

5.2.2 Eye exam by a licensed ophthalmologist/optometrist to include:

5.2.2.1 Visual acuity,

5.2.2.2 Depth perception,

5.2.2.3 Peripheral vision,

5.2.2.4 Night blindness,

5.2.2.5 Color blindness, and

5.2.2.6 Amblyopia.

5.2.3 An examination of the medical history of the individual, designed to identify drivers who may be impaired by:

5.2.3.1 Loss of consciousness,

5.2.3.2 Cardiovascular disease,

5.2.3.3 Neurological/neurovascular disorder,

5.2.3.4 Mental illness,

5.2.3.5 Substance abuse/dependency,

5.2.3.6 Insulin-dependent diabetes, and

5.2.3.7 Rheumatic, arthritic, orthopedic, muscular, neuromuscular, or vascular disease that interferes with the ability to control and operate a motor vehicle safely.

5.2.4 The presence of a medical condition by itself may not constitute an impaired operator, but shall identify an area for consideration by the physician in making a determination of the medical fitness to operating an ambulance.

6. Qualifications to Drive

6.1 Authorization shall be based upon cognitive evaluation of the operator regarding laws, guidelines, and policies relating to ambulance operation during emergency and non-emergency modes.

6.1.1 The provider shall have a policy that addresses operator fatigue.

6.2 An ambulance driving evaluation by the provider covering warning device operation, passing, intersection approach precautions, turning, backing, and parking techniques during emergency and non-emergency modes.

6.3 A review of the state motor vehicle record for the previous three years with specific attention to traffic convictions concerning:

6.3.1 Speed,

6.3.2 Careless and imprudent driving,

6.3.3 Driving under the influence of alcohol or other mind-altering substances, and

6.3.4 Moving violations.

6.4 A review of motor vehicle accidents for the previous five years.

6.5 The operator shall possess a valid motor vehicle operators license, and any other certification required by state or local laws or regulations.

7. Pre-Run

7.1 The operator shall have knowledge of and shall comply with all applicable federal, state statues, local ordinances, and regulations.

7.2 The operator shall have knowledge of the provider's policies and procedures.

7.3 The operator shall have knowledge of roads, highways, and the locations of and accesses to major public facilities within the service area.

7.4 The provider shall have a process by which the operator is made aware of conditions that may affect traffic flow within the service area (street closures, construction, special events ...).

7.5 The provider shall have a process by which the operator is made aware of present or forecasted environmental conditions affecting traffic flow within the service area (ice, snow, rain ...).

7.6 Upon unit availability, the operator shall visually inspect the ambulance, and document the inspection in accordance with one of the methods as shown in Table 1. The vehicle shall be inspected for the following:

7.6.1 Apparent body or glass damage,

7.6.2 Proper function of emergency lights:

7.6.2.1 Beacons or strobe,

7.6.2.2 Light bar,

7.6.2.3 Tunnel lights/flashers, and

7.6.2.4 Other warning lights.

7.6.3 Vehicle operating lights:

7.6.3.1 Headlights (high/low),

7.6.3.2 Emergency flashers,

7.6.3.3 Parking/running lights,

7.6.3.4 Interior and exterior turn signal,

7.6.3.5 Brake lights,

7.6.3.6 Back up lights,

7.6.3.7 Flood or scene lights,

7.6.3.8 Dome lights: cab and patient compartment, and

7.6.3.9 Spotlights.

7.6.4 Damage, wear, and pressure in tires,

7.6.5 Damage, loose, or missing lugs on wheels,

7.6.6 Proper opening, closing, locking, and seals of entry and compartment doors,

7.6.7 Fluid levels:

7.6.7.1 Automatic transmission,

TABLE 1 Emergency Medical Services Ambulance Maintenance Guidelines for Checklist Completion

Runs per Week	Full Check, h	Quick Check, h
0 to 1	every 96	every 24
2 to 3	every 72	every 24
4 to 7	every 48	every 24
8 to 50	every 24	every 12
50 +	every 24	every 8

7.6.7.2 Battery,
7.6.7.3 Brakes,
7.6.7.4 Engine oil,
7.6.7.5 Engine coolant,
7.6.7.6 Power steering, and
7.6.7.7 Windshield washer.
7.6.8 Fluid leakage on, around, or under the vehicle,
7.6.9 Wear, abrasion, rigidity or sponginess of radiator, fuel, heater, and other hoses,
7.6.10 Wear, abraded, or cracked engine drive or accessory belts,
7.6.11 Cleanliness of exterior, crew cab, and patient compartments,
7.6.12 Wear, abrasion, and proper function of operator, passenger, and patient restraint,
7.6.13 Indications and function of gages:
7.6.13.1 Electrical charging system,
7.6.13.2 Emergency brake,
7.6.13.3 Fuel,
7.6.13.4 Oil pressure,
7.6.13.5 Tachometer, and
7.6.13.6 Temperature.
7.6.14 Wear, abrasion, and proper function of windshield wipers,
7.6.15 Proper function and aim of windshield washer,
7.6.16 Proper function and clarity of two-way radio and other communication devices,
7.6.17 Damage, stability, and adjustment of outside and inside mirrors,
7.6.18 Proper function and clarity of emergency siren, public address, and other warning devices,
7.6.19 Proper adjustment of all seats,
7.6.20 Proper adjustment and function of steering wheel,
7.6.21 Charged and properly stored fire extinguishers,
7.6.22 Proper function of heating and air conditioning systems,
7.6.23 Proper inventory and condition of medical equipment and supplies, and
7.6.24 Level and alignment of chassis.
7.7 The quick check shall be constituted by:
7.7.1 Visually checking for any fluid leakage on or around the ambulance,
7.7.2 Conducting vehicle warmup,
7.7.3 Checking fluid levels:
7.7.3.1 Fuel,
7.7.3.2 Engine oil,
7.7.3.3 Power steering,
7.7.3.4 Water/coolant level,
7.7.3.5 Brake fluid,
7.7.3.6 Transmission fluid,
7.7.3.7 Windshield washer fluid, and
7.7.3.8 Battery water level.
7.7.4 Wear and tension of belts,
7.7.5 Wear and pressure of tires,
7.7.6 Emergency lights,
7.7.7 Function of lighting systems:
7.7.7.1 Emergency lights,
7.7.7.2 Running lights,
7.7.7.3 Vehicle exterior, and
7.7.7.4 Vehicle interior.
7.7.8 Proper function of horn and each siren position,
7.7.9 Vehicle cleanliness, and
7.7.10 Proper function of two-way radio and other communications equipment.

8. Operations

8.1 *Response Mode Management*:
8.1.1 The response mode of the ambulance shall be determined by dispatch protocol based on dispatch determinants as approved by the medical director. These determinants shall be consistent with Practice F 1258.
8.2 The operator shall, on the basis of known information, determine the best route to the scene and end destination.
8.3 Before beginning the response, the operator shall conduct a brief egress check consisting of the following:
8.3.1 Vehicle doors are securely closed and latched,
8.3.2 Vehicle hood is closed and securely latched,
8.3.3 Vehicle shore line is disconnected,
8.3.4 All equipment is secured,
8.3.5 Egress door is open, and
8.3.6 Patient stretcher is in place and secured.
8.4 *Operational Check Sequence*:
8.4.1 Ensure crew is on board and properly restrained,
8.4.2 Adjust the operator's seat,
8.4.3 Adjust mirrors,
8.4.4 Turn on battery(s),
8.4.5 Start the engine,
8.4.6 Review all gages,
8.4.7 Adjust environmental controls consistent with applicable needs,
8.4.8 Turn radio on and contact dispatch,
8.4.9 Adjust the tilt wheel,
8.4.10 Turn the headlights on,
8.4.11 Activate the emergency warning lights (if applicable),
8.4.12 Turn on power to siren/public address control system (if applicable),
8.4.13 Partially open the driver side window,
8.4.14 Evaluate brake pedal resistance,
8.4.15 Place the vehicle in gear,
8.4.16 Activate the siren (if applicable), and
8.4.17 Activate the turn signal (if applicable).
8.5 *Crew Roles*—The operator/crew member is responsible for:
8.5.1 Operating the ambulance in a safe and efficient manner, exercising the highest degree of care,
8.5.2 Safely passing other vehicles,
8.5.3 Utilizing eye sweep,
8.5.4 Maintaining a 3 to 4-s following distance, and
8.5.5 Maintaining the vehicle at a speed that is safe for conditions.
8.5.5.1 Under emergency response conditions the speed shall not exceed that which is safe for road or environmental conditions; in no case shall the speed exceed ten miles per hour over the posted speed limit.
8.5.5.2 Under non-emergency operations the operator shall comply with all local and state traffic laws.

8.5.6 Controlling the operation of the appropriate audible warning device for the current traffic conditions.

8.5.7 Utilizing the vehicle communication system,

8.5.8 Applying policies and procedures in the driving of the ambulance,

8.5.9 Initiating a constant rate of acceleration,

8.5.10 Using engine compression in stopping of the ambulance,

8.5.11 Maintaining smooth braking and cornering of the ambulance,

8.5.12 Assuring adequate stopping distance in traffic,

8.5.12.1 The operator shall stop the ambulance in traffic so the operator can see the bumper, both rear tires of the vehicle in front of the ambulance, and a minimum of five feet of the road surface in front of the ambulance.

8.5.13 Utilizing the 10-s lane change procedure,

8.5.14 Maintaining a rear and side space cushion,

8.5.15 Backing with a ground guide,

8.5.15.1 The operator is responsible for the safe backing of the ambulance. The operator shall never begin to back the ambulance before it has come to a complete stop. A person serving as a ground guide should be in place, eight to ten feet directly behind the left rear of the ambulance. Audio and visual communications should be established between the operator and the ground guide.

8.5.16 Understanding special transport procedures,

8.5.17 Undertaking special safety precautions with multiple personnel in the patient compartment,

8.5.18 Safely using and loading patient handling equipment,

8.5.19 Utilizing other crew members in the operation of the ambulance,

8.5.20 Accepting constructive criticism from other crew members, and

8.5.21 Utilizing safe procedures for operating in oncoming traffic lanes.

8.6 Controlled intersection management during emergency response mode:

8.6.1 300 ft (91.44 m) prior to the intersection the siren should be in the wail mode.

8.6.2 150 ft (45.72 m) prior to the intersection the operator shall active the yelp mode of the siren.

8.6.3 The operator's foot should be removed from the accelerator to cover the brake pedal and allow compression to slow the vehicle enabling the operator to start to apply the brake to bring the ambulance to a complete stop at the crosswalk line.

8.6.4 If the ambulance has an air-driven audible airhorn, give two short blasts on the airhorn.

8.6.5 Look to the left, look to the immediate front, look to the right, and then again to the left. The operator may then proceed through the intersection under ten miles per hour if traffic is stopped in all lanes to the left, in front of, and to the right of the ambulance. After the operator has made eye contact with all stopped vehicle drivers, the ambulance may proceed through the intersection exercising the highest degree of care.

8.6.6 Continue the siren yelp mode activation and proceed through the intersection exercising the highest degree of care.

8.6.7 When there are vacant lanes to the left or right, the operator must complete the previous steps of clearing each lane of traffic prior to crossing that lane.

8.6.8 The operator should anticipate that any vacant lane to his left or right may become occupied by another vehicle which did not see or hear the ambulance's warning systems.

8.6.9 The operator should be aware that other emergency vehicles may be approaching the same intersection that the operator has taken control of and the ambulance should not enter the intersection until the other vehicles have stopped or proceeded through the intersection.

8.6.10 The operator should avoid passing stopped vehicles on the right.

8.6.11 The operator should turn right at the intersection only after all vehicles have stopped and drivers on the right are aware of the ambulance.

8.6.12 The operator should anticipate that any vehicles in front may make an unexpected left turn in front of the ambulance after it has started to enter the intersection.

8.6.13 The operator must be aware of other hazards at the intersection, for example, pedestrians, road hazards, defective traffic control systems.

8.7 *Opposing Lane Usage*—The operator shall not enter an opposing traffic lane until it is safe to do so and all other on coming vehicles are aware of the ambulance's presence.

8.8 *Moving Against Traffic*—The operator shall not enter a one-way street against traffic until all opposing traffic is aware of the ambulance's presence and has yielded the right of way.

8.9 *Passing*:

8.9.1 *Stopped Vehicles*—The operator should exercise extreme caution when passing a stopped vehicle on either the left or right.

8.9.2 *School Buses (or Other Like Vehicles)*—The operator shall not pass a school bus when its stop sign and warning lights are activated unless the operator of the school bus signals that it is safe to pass. The ambulance should then proceed using the highest degree of care.

8.9.3 *Moving Vehicles*:

8.9.3.1 The operator shall exercise extreme caution when passing another vehicle in order to assure ample space to overtake and reenter the lane of traffic.

8.9.3.2 Passing on the right is generally not permitted, except when traffic flow is obstructed on the left and the right on multiple-lane highways. The operator may pass between the two lanes of traffic exercising the highest degree of caution.

8.10 *U-Turns*—The operator shall not make U-turns in traffic until all traffic has stopped. When doing so, all warning devices must be activated prior to executing the U-turn.

8.11 *Defensive Driving Techniques*—The operator is responsible for practicing defensive driving techniques under all conditions using the highest degree of care.

8.12 *Parking*:

8.12.1 The operator shall not park the ambulance so as to create a traffic hazard unless warning or other traffic control devices, or both, are being utilized.

8.12.2 *Emergency Scene*:

8.12.2.1 The operator is responsible for safely parking the ambulance at the scene to protect the ambulance, it's crew members, possible patients, and the scene.

8.12.2.2 The operator is responsible for setting the parking brake when the transmission is in the park position.

8.12.2.3 When there is a significant electrical load on the ambulance that is parked, if available the automatic idle advance should be activated.

8.12.2.4 When appropriate, the vehicle should be positioned so that the ambulance will not be required to back into traffic when leaving the scene.

8.13 *Scene Approach and Size-Up*—The operator is responsible for scene evaluation and for safely approaching the scene and overall evaluation of the scene.

8.14 *Multiple-Responding Units*:

8.14.1 The operator is responsible for maintaining a 300-ft (91.44-m) buffer zone between the ambulance and other emergency vehicles in front of the ambulance.

8.14.2 The ambulance and other responding unit(s) should never enter an intersection in tandem.

8.14.3 The operator shall not utilize a law enforcement escort.

8.14.4 The operator shall strongly discourage private, non-emergency vehicles from following the ambulance during transport.

8.15 *Environmental Modifying Factors*—The operator is responsible for keeping the ambulance out of a potentially hazardous scene until such scene has been declared safe by an appropriate authority.

8.16 *Vehicle Operation at Scene*:

8.16.1 *Warning Device Operation*—The operator is responsible for utilization of appropriate warning devices to protect the scene and the vehicle.

8.16.2 *Mechanical/Electrical System*:

8.16.2.1 The operator is responsible for monitoring the mechanical and electrical systems of the vehicle when on scene for an extended period of time.

8.16.2.2 The operator is responsible for monitoring the environmental systems of the vehicle when on scene for an extended period of time.

8.16.3 *Doors/Compartments*—The operator is responsible for ensuring that all vehicle doors are closed at all times except when loading and unloading the patient or equipment.

8.16.4 *Lights*—Scene lights/floodlights/high beams should not be directed in such a way as to blind oncoming traffic.

8.17 *Departing the Scene*:

8.17.1 *Departure Check*:

8.17.1.1 The operator is responsible for performing a quick visual walk-around check of the vehicle, checking for any obvious fluid leakage, open compartments, equipment left on scene before departing the scene.

8.17.1.2 The operator shall be advised by the senior medical technician as to the mode of operation of the ambulance during transport based on the condition of the patient.

9. Post Run

9.1 *Decontamination*—Any contamination of the ambulance, operator, equipment, or crew shall be managed in accordance with applicable standards.

9.2 *Resupply*—The operator shall ensure that disposables and other equipment are replaced as necessary to return the ambulance to pre-run status.

9.3 *Fuel*:

9.3.1 The operator shall ensure that the vehicle is replenished and maintained with fuel and other fluids as necessary to return the ambulance to pre-run status.

9.3.2 The operator shall ensure that the proper quality and type of fuel is used in the ambulance pursuant to the manufacturer's specifications.

9.4 *Documentation*—The operator shall ensure that all applicable documentation is completed in accordance with company policy.

Designation: F 1518 – 00

Standard Practice for Cleaning and Disinfection of Flexible Fiberoptic and Video Endoscopes Used in the Examination of the Hollow Viscera[1]

This standard is issued under the fixed designation F 1518; the number immediately following the designation indicates the year of original adoption or, in the case of revision, the year of last revision. A number in parentheses indicates the year of last reapproval. A superscript epsilon (ε) indicates an editorial change since the last revision or reapproval.

1. Scope

1.1 This practice covers the flexible fiberoptic and video endoscopes that are fully immersible in liquid and are used in the examination of the hollow viscera (that is, colonoscopes, gastroscopes, duodenoscopes, sigmoidoscopes, and enteroscopes). These endoscopes will be referred to as flexible gastrointestinal (GI) endoscopes.

1.1.1 It is strongly recommended that only immersible endoscopes be used in order to assure that all parts of the endoscope will be high-level disinfected; however, it is recognized that, in some instances, portions of endoscopes that neither contact patients nor patient fluids may not be immersible. In these instances, care must be taken to disinfect the nonimmersible portions to the highest degree with which they are compatible, according to the manufacturer's directions.

1.2 This practice is intended to complement, not replace the instructions and labeling provided by product manufacturers. Endoscope manufacturers must provide instructions and labeling necessary for users to know the basic design, specifications, nomenclature, and components of specific flexible GI endoscopes and to properly inspect, prepare, use, clean, disinfect, rinse, dry, and store these instruments.

1.3 Endoscopic technique and the medical aspects of gastrointestinal endoscopy are not covered in this practice.

1.4 This practice details the steps necessary to properly reprocess flexible GI endoscopes and render them patient-ready.

1.5 This practice details manual reprocessing as well as automated reprocessing of flexible GI fiberoptic and video endoscopes.

1.6 The application of all practices relating to endoscopic reprocessing will ultimately fall into the purview of the individual assigned to that task in an endoscopic area.

1.6.1 To ensure the proper adherence to this practice, those personnel should themselves meet certain requirements as specified in 4.8.

1.7 This practice does not detail the steps necessary for the reprocessing of endoscopic accessories.

1.8 *This standard does not purport to address all of the safety concerns, if any, associated with its use. It is the responsibility of the user of this standard to establish appropriate safety and health practices and determine the applicability of regulatory limitations prior to use.* Specific precautionary statements are given in Note 1 and Note 2.

2. Terminology

2.1 *Definitions of Terms Specific to This Standard:*

2.1.1 *clean, adj*—visibly free from debris.

2.1.2 *endoscope, n—flexible GI endoscope*, flexible fiberoptic or video endoscopes used in the examination of the hollow viscera (that is, colonoscope, gastroscope, duodenoscope, sigmoidoscope, and enteroscopes).

2.1.3 *High-Level Disinfectant*—A liquid chemical sterilant used under the same contact conditions as for sterilization except for a shorter contact time. A sterilant is a liquid chemical germicide, which has passed the AOAC sporicidal test with no failures; therefore, to qualify for a high-level disinfection claim, a germicide must be a sterilant as defined by the AOAC sporicidal test. In addition, the claim should be supported by efficacy data from potency tests, simulated-use tests, and in-use tests.

2.1.3.1 *Discussion*—A high-level disinfectant is a liquid chemical germicide cleared by FDA for market with a claim for high-level disinfection.

2.1.4 *high-level disinfected, adj*—devoid of all vegetative bacteria, viruses, and fungal spores and some but not all bacterial endospores.

2.1.5 *patient-ready endoscope, n*—an endoscope rendered clean after being subjected to a validated cleaning procedure, subjected minimally to a high-level disinfection process, and rinsed so that it does not contain residual chemicals in amounts that can be harmful to humans.

2.1.5.1 *Discussion*—It is recognized that in limited circumstances, portions of an endoscope that neither contact patient fluids nor contact the patient directly, may not be immersible (for example, ultrasound endoscopes). In these instances, care must be taken to disinfect the non-immersible portions of the endoscope to the highest degree with which they are compatible according to the manufacturer's directions.

2.1.6 *reprocessing, n*—the cleaning and high-level disinfection necessary to render an endoscope patient-ready.

---

[1] This practice is under the jurisdiction of ASTM Committee F-4 on Medical and Surgical Materials and Devices and is the direct responsibility of Subcommittee F04.35 on GI Endoscopes.

Current edition approved April 10, 2000. Published July 2000. Originally published as F 1518 – 94. Last previous edition F 1518 – 94.

2.1.7 *reprocessing chemicals*, *n*—detergents and liquid chemical germicides used for reprocessing endoscopes.

2.1.8 *residual chemical*, *n*—freely extractable residual reprocessing chemicals in amounts that can be harmful to humans.

3. Summary of Practice

3.1 Each brand, type, and model of endoscope has unique specifications, nomenclature, interior design, function, and components.

3.2 Endoscopes used in gastrointestinal endoscopy are considered semi-critical medical devices because they normally only come into contact with mucous membranes.

3.3 To prevent the spread of microorganisms during endoscopy, semi-critical medical devices must receive scrupulous manual cleaning followed minimally by high-level disinfection.

3.4 Upon removal of the endoscope from the patient, the instrument should be manually cleaned followed by high-level disinfection, rinsing, and drying. If due to time constraints, it is not possible to complete the reprocessing immediately, the endoscope should be leak-tested, flushed, brushed, and allowed to soak in a detergent solution until it can be thoroughly reprocessed.

3.4.1 Follow the endoscope manufacturer's recommendations for the maximum liquid exposure time.

3.5 After cleaning and high-level disinfection, endoscopes must be stored in a manner that allows air to circulate around the endoscope.

3.6 Refer to the endoscope manufacturer's instructions for proper storage.

4. Significance and Use

4.1 Because endoscopes are used to diagnose disease in immunocompetent and immunocompromised individuals, care must be taken to ensure that only endoscopes that are patient-ready are used for each examination.

4.2 Endoscopy of patients with diagnosed or suspected infections such as hepatitis B or human immunodeficiency virus is not contraindicated. Further, endoscopes do not need to be dedicated for use in only these patients.

4.3 By nature of their design requirements, endoscopes are more difficult to reprocess than other medical instruments.

4.4 Endoscopes have long narrow internal channels making inspection for cleanliness difficult if not impossible.

4.5 Endoscopes made from elastomeric materials cannot be subjected to heat sterilization, thus requiring high-level disinfection or sterilization with compatible chemical agents. Contact the endoscope manufacturer for liquid chemical sterilant compatibility.

4.6 Each user needs to understand the specifications, nomenclature, function of component parts, and interior channel design of endoscopes in order to render them patient-ready.

4.7 Persons responsible for the reprocessing of endoscopes should follow this practice and associated labeling and instructions from manufacturers after each endoscopic procedure to ensure that the endoscope is patient-ready for the next patient.

4.8 Reprocessing of endoscopes should be the specific responsibility of appropriately trained personnel. Temporary employees without the requisite training should not be given these responsibilites.

4.8.1 The responsibility for this activity should not be delegated from person to person unless each has the appropriate credentials for the position.

4.8.2 Persons responsible for processing the endoscopes should have the ability to read, understand, and implement instructions from manufacturers and regulatory agencies as they relate to endoscopic disinfection.

4.8.3 Reprocessing personnel should have the opportunity to become completely familiar with the mechanical aspects of the endoscopic equipment. This should be done by study of the manufacturer's information, and demonstration by the manufacturer's representatives.

4.8.4 Reprocessing personnel should participate in an institutionally developed, competency-based training program dedicated to endoscope reprocessing.

4.8.4.1 The competency-based training program should incorporate currently published national standards, such as ASTM, SGNA, APIC, and ASGE.

4.8.5 Reprocessing personnel should be made fully aware of the potential chemical and infectious hazards for patients and health care personnel associated with the reprocessing of the endoscope.

4.8.5.1 Training should include a thorough background regarding the potential for negative patient outcomes resulting from lapses in compliance with written reprocessing guidelines.

4.8.5.2 Training should include a thorough background in infection control principles and concepts based on written in-house infection control procedures.

4.8.5.3 Training should include familiarization with Occupational Safety and Health Administration (OSHA) regulations and in-house policies regarding the appropriate and safe handling of liquid chemical reagents and equipment used during the reprocessing of the endoscopes. OSHA guidelines are directed only toward healthcare worker safety and health but also may benefit patient safety.

4.8.5.4 Training should include information on the safe handling of endoscopes contaminated with patient tissue and fluids. This should include familiarization with principles and practices of standard (Universal) precautions.

4.8.6 Each endoscopic unit should have appropriately motivated individuals with the proper educational background or experience, or both, to assume the responsibility for the reprocessing of endoscopes. Temporary employees without the requisite training should not be given this responsibility.

4.9 This practice is not intended to replace the cleaning and disinfection instructions provided by the manufacturers of the endoscope, endoscope disinfector, or chemicals used for cleaning and disinfection. Rather, it is to be used together with the manufacturer's instructions that provide specific instructions for specific products.

4.10 This practice is not intended to cover the endoscopic techniques, patient care, or other medical aspects of gastrointestinal endoscopy.

4.11 This practice does not include instructions for the use or reprocessing of endoscopic accessories.

5. Reagents

5.1 *Alcohol*—seventy percent isopropyl or seventy percent ethyl alcohol. Keep alcohol in a closed container. Alcohol stored in an open container is a fire hazard and may not remain effective because of evaporation. Do not reuse.

5.2 *Air*—Air flow provided by an air pump or compressor. Refer to the endoscope manufacturer's instructions and avoid using excessively high air pressure.

5.3 *Detergent*—Low-sudsing detergent formulations recommended by the manufacturer of the endoscopes.

5.4 *High-Level Disinfectant*—A liquid chemical germicide as defined in 2.1.3.

5.4.1 A high-level disinfectant is a liquid chemical sterilant used under the same contact conditions as for sterilization except for a shorter contact time. A sterilant is a liquid chemical germicide, which has passed the AOAC sporicidal test with no failures; therefore, to qualify for a high-level disinfection claim, a germicide must be a sterilant as defined by the AOAC sporicidal test. In addition, the claim should be supported by efficacy data from potency tests, simulated-use tests and in-use tests.

5.4.2 A high-level disinfectant is a liquid chemical germicide cleared by the FDA for market with a claim for high-level disinfection.

Subject valves and other removal parts to high-level disinfection by soaking in a basin of disinfectant, or if possible, place the valves and other removable parts in the designated accessory basket of the automated disinfector.

5.5 *Water*—Clean, potable water or potable water that has been filtered by passage through a 0.2-µm filter or otherwise treated by a method documented to improve the microbiological quality of the water.

6. Equipment and Supplies

6.1 *Reprocessing Adapters*—Adapters provided by the endoscope or disinfector manufacturer specifically for injecting fluids through the internal lumens of the endoscope, or for partially restricting or capping a lumen opening.

6.2 *Brushes*, must be high-level disinfected or disposed of after each use.

6.2.1 Cleaning brushes, of appropriate size and configuration, designed for use with specific endoscopes, and

6.2.2 Soft toothbrush or similar brush used for cleaning the exterior of the endoscope.

6.3 *Basin(s)*, must be large enough to totally immerse the endoscopes without coiling them too tightly. See the endoscope manufacturer's instructions for maximum coiling of specific endoscopes:

6.3.1 Cleaning basin, and

6.3.2 Disinfectant basin for soaking:

6.3.2.1 Nonmetal, and

6.3.2.2 Must include a tight-fitting lid to minimize escape of disinfectant vapors. This lid should be kept in place at all times except when transferring instruments into or out of the solution.

6.3.3 *Automated Disinfector*, must include a tight-fitting lid to minimize the escape of disinfectant vapors.

6.4 *Cloth*—Soft, lint-free cloth or sponge for wiping the exterior of the endoscope.

6.5 *Personal Protective Equipment*:

6.5.1 *Gloves*:

6.5.1.1 High-quality, impervious latex, butyl or nitrile rubber gloves should fit properly and be of adequate length to prevent skin exposure.

6.5.1.2 Gloves must be changed regularly as needed or as recommended by the manufacturer. They must be discarded if they are cracked, pealing, punctured, or when their ability to function as a barrier is compromised.

6.5.2 *Gowns*:

6.5.2.1 Impervious protective clothing must be worn when handling contaminated endoscopes and when working with liquid chemical germicides.

6.5.2.2 Gowns used during endoscope reprocessing must be removed prior to leaving the decontamination area.

6.5.3 Face masks or shields and protective eye gear should be worn to protect the face and eyes from contact with reprocessing chemicals and infectious material.

6.6 *Adequate Air Ventilation*—A large well-ventilated area with eight to ten air exchanges per hour is necessary to help protect personnel from chemical vapors.

7. Procedure

7.1 *Cleaning*:

7.1.1 Put on all necessary personal protective equipment.

7.1.2 Prepare detergent in accordance with the manufacturer's specifications.

7.1.3 Immediately after removing the endoscope from the patient:

7.1.3.1 Wipe all debris from the insertion tube using a soft lint free cloth and water to which you have added a lowsudsing detergent recommended by the endoscope manufacturer and diluted in accordance with the detergent manufacturer's instructions.

7.1.3.2 Place the distal end of the endoscope into the water and detergent solution and suction through the biopsy/suction channel until the exiting solution is visibly clean. Alternate suctioning detergent solution and air several times. Finish by suctioning air.

7.1.3.3 Flush or blow out air and water channels in accordance with the endoscope manufacturer's instructions.

7.1.4 Detach the endoscope from the light source and suction pump.

7.1.5 Take the endoscope to the reprocessing area. Put on all necessary personal protective equipment if this was not done in 7.1.1.

7.1.6 Attach any necessary water-tight caps to the electrical portion of the umbilicus.

7.1.7 Inspect and leak test the endoscope following the manufacturer's instructions.

7.1.7.1 Inspect the insertion tube and universal cord for damage and the bending section for deflection.

7.1.7.2 Leak test the endoscope to ensure the integrity of the water-tight design.

7.1.7.3 Follow the endoscope manufacturer's instructions if the instrument appears damaged.

7.1.8 Fill a sink or basin with a freshly made solution of water and a low-sudsing detergent recommended by the endoscope manufacturer and diluted in accordance with the detergent manufacturer's instructions.

7.1.9 Immerse the endoscope. Wash all debris from the exterior of the endoscope by brushing and wiping the instrument while submerged in the detergent solution. Whenever practical, leave the endoscope submerged in detergent solution when performing all subsequent cleaning steps.

7.1.10 Detach the distal end hood if present and brush the distal tip with a small soft brush.

7.1.11 Detach the suction and air/water valves, the biopsy channel cover, and all other removable parts.

7.1.11.1 Discard those parts that are labeled as single-use disposable.

7.1.11.2 Use a small soft brush to scrub all reusable, removable parts.

7.1.11.3 Use a brush to clean inside all reuseable vavles and valve housings including but not limited to suction, air/water, and biopsy port openings as per manufacturer's instructions.

7.1.12 Brush the entire channel system that includes the body, the insertion tube, and the umbilicus of the endoscope in accordance with the manufacturer's instructions.

7.1.12.1 After each passage, rinse the brush before retracting it and before reinserting it.

7.1.12.2 Continue brushing until there is no debris visible on the brush.

7.1.13 Attach channel adapters for suction/biopsy, air, and water channels.

7.1.13.1 Cover the biopsy port in accordance with the instructions from the manufacturer of the endoscope.

7.1.13.2 Attach any cleaning devices provided for special features of the endoscope.

7.1.14 Flush all channels with detergent to remove dislodged debris.

7.1.15 Fill all channels with detergent solution and soak in accordance with the detergent manufacturer's instructions.

7.2 *Rinse After Cleaning*:

7.2.1 Rinse the endoscope and all removable parts in clean water.

7.2.2 Rinse all channels well with water to remove debris and detergent.

7.2.3 Purge water from all channels and wipe dry the exterior of the endoscope with a soft clean cloth to prevent dilution of the disinfectant chemical used in subsequent steps.

7.3 *Manual Disinfection*:

7.3.1 Follow all steps in accordance with 7.1 and 7.2 for thorough manual cleaning and rinsing of the endoscope prior to disinfection.

7.3.2 Prepare disinfectant in accordance with the disinfectant label. If the disinfectant solution is reused, it should be tested regularly in accordance with the manufacturer's instructions or the individual institution's protocol to ensure the minimum effective concentration of active ingredients.

7.3.3 Attach reprocessing adapters for suction/biopsy, air, and water channels.

7.3.3.1 Cover the biopsy port in accordance with the instructions from the manufacturer of the endoscope.

7.3.3.2 Attach any reprocessing devices provided for special features of the endoscope.

7.3.4 Completely immerse the endoscope in a basin of disinfectant.

7.3.5 Inject disinfectant into all channels of the endoscope until it can be seen exiting the opposite end of each channel. Take care that all channels are filled with disinfectant and that no air pockets remain within the channels.

7.3.6 Subject all valves and other removable parts to highlevel disinfection by soaking in the basin of disinfectant.

NOTE 1—**Caution:** In order to prevent damage to the endoscope, DO NOT soak any other accessory equipment with the endoscope.

7.3.7 Cover the disinfectant soaking basin with a tightfitting lid to minimize chemical vapor exposure.

7.3.8 Immerse the endoscope in the disinfectant for the the recommended time and temperature as indicated on the label of the disinfectant. Use a timer to ensure adequate immersion time.

7.3.9 Before completely removing the endoscope from the disinfectant, flush all channels with air to remove disinfectant.

7.4 *Rinse After Manual Disinfection*:

NOTE 2—It is suggested that all rinsing after disnfection should be done with water that has been filtered by passage through a 0.2 micron filter or otherwise treated by a method documented to improve the microbiological quality of water.

7.4.1 Thoroughly rinse the exterior of the endoscope with large amounts of clean water.

7.4.2 Thoroughly rinse all of the channels by flushing with large amounts of clean water.

7.4.3 Purge all channels with air.

7.4.4 Flush all channels with alcohol until the alcohol can be seen exiting the opposite end of each channel.

7.4.5 Purge all channels with air.

7.4.6 Remove the cleaning/disinfection adapters and devices.

7.4.7 Dry the exterior of the endoscope with a soft clean towel.

7.4.8 Thoroughly rinse and dry all removable parts. Do not attach removable parts (valves, etc.) to the endoscope prior to storage.

7.5 *Automated Disinfection*:

7.5.1 Check with the automated disinfector manufacturer to confirm the ability of the disinfector to disinfect a particular endoscope model or channel, or both.

7.5.2 Follow all steps in accordance with 7.1 and 7.2 for thorough manual cleaning and rinsing of the endoscope prior to disinfection.

7.5.3 Carefully insert the endoscope into the disinfector in accordance with the directions of the manufacturer of the automated disinfector .

7.5.4 Subject valves and other removable parts to highlevel disinfection by soaking in a basin of disinfectant or if possible place the valves and other removable parts in designated accessory basket of the automated disinfector.

NOTE 3—**Caution:** If the disinfector does not have dedicated space for accessories, in order to prevent damage to the endoscope DO NOT disinfect any other accessory equipment along with the endoscope.

7.5.5 Attach all channel connectors from the disinfector to the endoscope including those for special features of the endoscope. Closely follow the directions provided by the manufacturer of the automatic disinfector.

7.5.6 If the machine has a wash or predisinfection cycle which uses detergent, use a formulation recommended by the manufacturer of the endoscope and disinfector. Dilute in accordance with the disinfector manufacturer's instructions.

7.5.7 Prepare disinfectant in accordance with the disinfectant label. If the disinfectant solution is reused, it should be tested regularly in accordance with the manufacturer's instructions or the individual institution's protocol to ensure the minimum effective concentration of active ingredients.

7.5.8 Set the machine for the time and temperature for the chosen disinfectant.

7.5.9 Start the machine and allow it to complete all cycles/phases.

7.6 *Drying*:

7.6.1 Flush all channels, with alcohol until the alcohol can be seen exiting the opposite end of each channel.

7.6.2 Dry all channels with air.

7.6.3 Remove the reprocessing adapters and devices.

7.6.4 Dry the exterior of the endoscope with a soft clean cloth.

7.6.5 Thoroughly rinse and dry all removable parts. Do not attach removable parts (valves, etc.) prior to storage.

7.7 *Storage*:

7.7.1 Do not attach the removable parts (valves, etc.) to the endoscope prior to storage.

7.7.2 Hang the endoscope vertically with the distal tip hanging freely in a well-ventilated, dust-free cabinet.

8. Keywords

8.1 cleaning; endoscope; flexible fiberoptic; high-level disinfection; reprocessing; video GI endoscopes

APPENDIX

(Nonmandatory Information)

X1. RATIONALE

X1.1 Manufacturers of endoscopic devices provide an operating manual for each type/model produced. These have not been standardized in the past. Professional organizations have produced guidelines for cleaning and disinfection which have also not been standardized. This has led to confusion among users of the devices as to how to properly care for the instrumentation.

X1.2 According to reports in the medical literature, many cases of patient infection or cross contamination are the result of "short cuts", breaks in proper reprocessing procedure, use of inappropriate chemicals, or a misunderstanding of the consequences of eliminating important steps of the reprocessing process.

X1.3 Avoid the use of excessively high air pressure. Highpressure air can damage the internal channels of flexible GI endoscopes. It is recommended that endoscope manufacturers publish the maximum allowable pressure for drying the internal channels of their instruments.

X1.4 *Low-Sudsing Detergents*—The presence of excessive suds can prevent good fluid contact with internal channels. Excessive suds will also inhibit the performance of some automated disinfectors.

X1.5 *High-Level Disinfectant*—The use of an improper disinfectant may result in unexpected disinfection outcome; for example, instrument is not high-level disinfected or is damaged.

X1.6 *Basin Size*—Coiling a flexible GI endoscope too tightly will damage the instrument. Refer to the endoscope manufacturer's instructions regarding the minimum radius of curvature.

X1.7 *Tight-Fitting Lid:*

X1.7.1 Disinfectant vapors can be irritating to personnel in the area.

X1.7.2 Exposure of patients and medical staff to disinfectant vapors should be minimized.

X1.8 *Soft, Lint-Free Cloth*—Abrasive materials will damage the endoscope. Lint may collect in or occlude the smaller internal channels of the endoscope.

X1.9 *Personal Protective Equipment:*

X1.9.1 Gloves and gowns help prevent the health-care worker from coming into contact with contaminated endoscopic equipment, patient secretions, blood, stool, and reprocessing chemicals, which may be irritating to the skin.

X1.9.2 Face masks and protective eye gear help prevent reprocessing chemicals from contacting the face or eyes.

X1.10 Immediate cleaning of flexible GI endoscopes prevents drying of organic material on the interior and exterior surfaces of the endoscope, removes large numbers of microorganisms from the endoscope, and is a necessary prerequisite to high-level disinfection.

X1.11 Alternate suctioning of fluid and air is more effective than suctioning fluid alone in removing debris.

X1.12 It is very important to either flush or blow out the small internal air and water channels of the endoscope immediately after the procedure. Debris that is allowed to dry in these channels both impedes the flow of air and prevents these channels from being adequately disinfected.

X1.13 Some types of electrical connectors are not water tight. These connectors must be capped prior to immersion in order to prevent invasion of fluid into the connector and into the interior portions of the endoscope.

X1.14 The leak test detects damage to the interior or exterior of the endoscope that allows fluids to pass into areas inside the endoscope that would be damaged by fluid exposure. The leak test is done before immersion of the endoscope in reprocessing chemicals in order to minimize further damage to the endoscope.

X1.15 All removable parts must be removed to be completely cleaned. In addition, the areas underneath these parts must be brushed to remove debris.

X1.16 Thorough manual brushing is required to remove all organic debris such as blood, mucus, and feces. High-level disinfection can not occur unless the organic debris is removed.

X1.17 It is important that all internal channels of the endoscope be adequately filled with detergent and disinfectant solution. Channel reprocessing adapters and reprocessing adapters for special features of endoscopes are the only means of filling these channels. Internal endoscope channels offer various resistances to fluid flow due to differences in diameter and length. In order to achieve adequate flow through all channels, various adapters or channel restrictors may be required. Refer to the manufacturer's instructions for specifics.

X1.18 Channels must be irrigated to remove dislodged organic debris before disinfection.

X1.19 The concentration of the disinfectant chemical must be routinely monitored since it may become ineffective through dilution, organic load, or expired life.

X1.20 It is critical that all internal channels be subjected to high-level disinfection. Only by direct injection of a liquid chemical sterilant into these channels can all air pockets be eliminated.

X1.21 All internal channels of the endoscope must be emptied of disinfectant chemical and flushed with water to avoid the possibility of retained disinfectant chemical which could be injected into a patient during the next examination.

X1.22 Alcohol evaporates rapidly and facilitates the drying of endoscope channels.

X1.23 Storage of endoscopes with the removable parts detached lowers the risk of trapping liquid inside the instrument and facilitates continued drying of the channels and channel openings. To prevent the growth of waterborne organisms, the endoscope and all detached parts should be thoroughly dried prior to storage.

X1.24 If the reprocessing procedure is performed correctly, all internal channels should be devoid of water droplets. However, hanging the endoscope in a ventilated environment versus coiling it in a closed environment (such as a carrying case) will further discourage growth of any potential residual organisms.

X1.25 This practice represents current standard practice and is generic in nature. The steps in this practice may be modified should an alternate reprocessing procedure be developed and appropriately validated.

Bibliography

(1) American Association of Medical Instrumentation (AAMI): Technical Report *Chemical Sterilants and High-Level Disinfectants-A Guide to Selection and Use.*

(2) American College of Gastroenterology (ACG), American Gastroenterology Association (AGA), and American Society of Gastrointestinal Endoscopy (ASGE) Position Statements, *Reprocessing of Flexible Gastrointestinal Endoscopes*

(3) Society of Gastroenterology Nurses and Associates (SGNA) Monograph Series 2000 *Standards of Infection Control in Reprocessing of Flexible Gastrointestinal Endoscopes*, 1999 *Guidelines for the Use of High-Level Disinfectants and Sterilants for Reprocessing Flexible Gastrointestinal Endoscopes*, 1996 *Safe and Effective Handling of Glutaraldehyde Solutions*

(4) Association of Practitioners in Infection Control and Epidemiology (APIC) 1997, 1998, and 1999 APIC Guidelines Commmittees, *APIC Guideline for Infection Prevention and Control in Flexible Endoscopy*

Standard Test Method for Determining Strength and Setting Time of Synthetic Water-Activated Polyurethane Fiberglass Orthopaedic Casting Tape[1]

This standard is issued under the fixed designation F 1536; the number immediately following the designation indicates the year of original adoption or, in the case of revision, the year of last revision. A number in parentheses indicates the year of last reapproval. A superscript epsilon (ε) indicates an editorial change since the last revision or reapproval.

1. Scope

1.1 This test method covers the functional diametral compression strength of cylindrical test specimens formed from synthetic fiberglass polyurethane casting materials. The test specimens employed in this test are similar in geometry and construction to casts used in orthopaedic applications. This test method is not intended to determine the strength of the base materials used for fabrication of the test specimen.

1.2 The values stated in inch-pound units are to be regarded as the standard. The SI units given in parentheses are for information only.

1.3 *This standard does not purport to address all of the safety concerns, if any, associated with its use. It is the responsibility of the user of this standard to establish appropriate safety and health practices and determine the applicability of regulatory limitations prior to use.* Specific precautionary statements are given in Note 1.

2. Referenced Documents

2.1 *ASTM Standards:*

E 4 Practices for Force Verification of Testing Machines[2]

E 691 Practice for Conducting an Interlaboratory Test Study to Determine the Precision of a Test Method[3]

3. Terminology

3.1 *Definitions of Terms Specific to This Standard:*

3.1.1 *diametral compression strength*—the load per unit width in lbs/in. (Newtons/mm), calculated by dividing either the peak failure load or the maximum deflection load by the nominal sample length (that is, manufacturer's stated tape width).

3.1.2 *maximum deflection load*—the test cylinder is compressed 0.4 in. (10 mm) from the initial load position without noticeable failure or a measurable decrease in load. The load at 0.4 in. (10 mm) deflection shall be called the maximum deflection load.

3.1.3 *peak failure load*—failure of the test cylinder with a concomitant decrease in load prior to 0.4 in. (10 mm) diametral compression. The highest load attained prior to the decrease shall be called the peak failure load.

4. Summary of Test Method

4.1 A test cylinder is prepared by immersing the casting tape in 75 ± 2°F (23.9 ± 1.1°C) water, squeezing per the manufacturer's instructions under the surface of the water, and then wrapping around either a 2.0 in. (50.8 mm) or 2.5 in. (63.5 mm) outside diameter cylindrical mandrel. The tape is wrapped layer upon layer producing a five layer cylinder. The test cylinder is removed from the mandrel after an initial setting period. After a specified time, the test specimen is positioned on its side between two flat platens in the testing machine and compressed to determine its strength. Ambient temperature and humidity are specified because of their pronounced effect on material properties during the curing period.

5. Significance and Use

5.1 Diametral compression strength is an important measure of the mechanical properties of casting materials. This test method simulates the loading pattern seen in lower extremity casting applications during ambulation. This method cannot be used to determine cast life or measure bending or other modes of cast failure.

5.2 This test method measures but does not prescribe values.

6. Apparatus

6.1 *Testing Machines*— Machines used for compression testing shall conform to the requirements of Practices E 4. For universal machines with a common test space, calibration shall be performed in compression.

6.1.1 The surfaces of the flat platens shall be perpendicular to the loading axis and parallel at all times within 0.005 in./in. (1.3 mm/mm). Platen surfaces should be clean and free of corrosion.

6.1.2 The testing machine shall be capable of producing a constant compression rate between 1 to 10 in./min (25.4 to 254 mm/min).

6.1.3 The testing machine shall be capable of measuring the compressive load within ±0.5 lbs (2.2 N).

[1] This test method is under the jurisdiction of ASTM Committee F-4 on Medical and Surgical Materials and Devicesand is the direct responsibility of Subcommittee F04.15 on Material Test Methods.

Current edition approved May 15, 1995. Published July 1995.

[2] *Annual Book of ASTM Standards*, Vol 03.01.

[3] *Annual Book of ASTM Standards*, Vol 14.02.

6.2 *Test Specimen Preparation Mandrel*—A solid, cylindrical aluminum mandrel of sufficient length to accommodate three test specimens without end contact shall be mounted in a horizontal position (see Fig. 1). Either of two mandrel diameters may be used: Type I—2.00 in. (50.8 mm) diameter, or Type II—2.50 in. (63.5 mm) diameter.

6.2.1 *Option*—Three individual mandrels, either Type I or Type II, each capable of holding one test specimen, may be substituted for a single, solid mandrel.

6.3 *Constant Tension Method*—Each layer of tape shall be wrapped on the mandrel at a constant tension of 0.25 lbs/in. (4.5 g/mm) width of tape. Suggested methods for accomplishing this include the use of a dead weight clamped to the free end of the tape while the horizontally mounted mandrel is manually rotated (see Fig. 1), or the use of an automated constant torque winding mechanism (see Fig. 2).

6.4 *Water Container*— A container capable of holding at least 1 gal (3.78 L) of water and of sufficient depth to allow complete immersion of the casting tape.

6.5 *Release Liner*— A sheet form liner of nominal thickness, such as waxed paper, shall be used to cover the mandrel and prevent adhesion of the resin to the mandrel. This liner must allow release of the cured specimen from the mandrel with minimal force, and must be easily removable from the specimen inner diameter prior to compression testing.

6.6 *Timer*—A timing device accurate to ±1 s.

6.7 *Gloves*—Gloves capable of protecting the hands from contact with the resin, for example, latex surgical gloves.

NOTE 1—**Precaution:** Contact with uncured or curing resins should be avoided. These resins may adhere to the skin and be difficult to remove. In addition, most polyurethane resins contain isocyanate to which some individuals are or may become sensitized. Gloves should be worn at all times when handling uncured or curing casting tape.

6.8 *Thermometer*— A device capable of measuring temperatures within ± 1°F (0.5°C) in the 70 to 80°F (21.1 to 26.7°C) range.

7. Reagents and Materials

7.1 At least three rolls of the casting tape shall be tested; one roll for each of the three specified time periods. Three test cylinders shall be prepared from each roll without the use of manual molding techniques.

NOTE 2—If testing of cylinders with the use of manual molding is desired, a secondary group of samples should be prepared using the desired molding technique.

7.2 Water for initiation of the curing process shall be maintained at 75 ± 2°F (23.9 ± 1.1°C).

7.2.1 The water shall be changed after three rolls have been prepared.

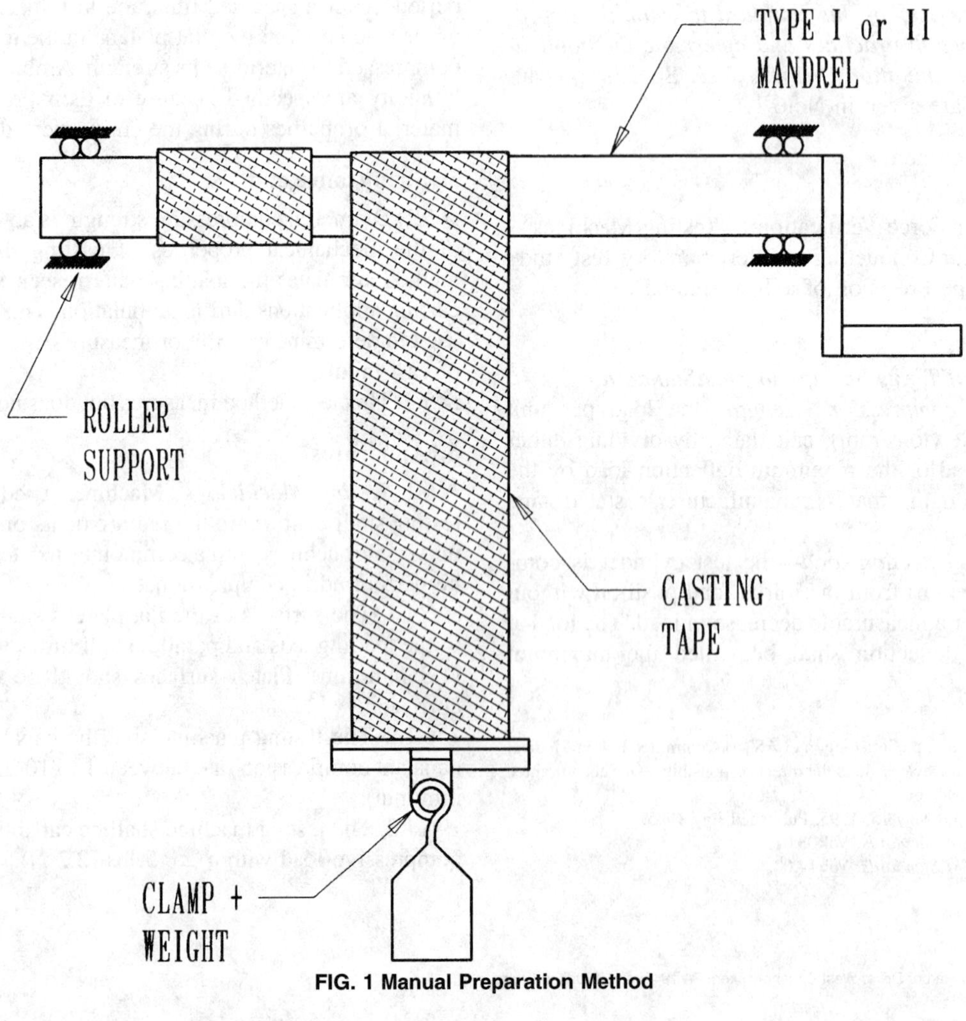

FIG. 1 Manual Preparation Method

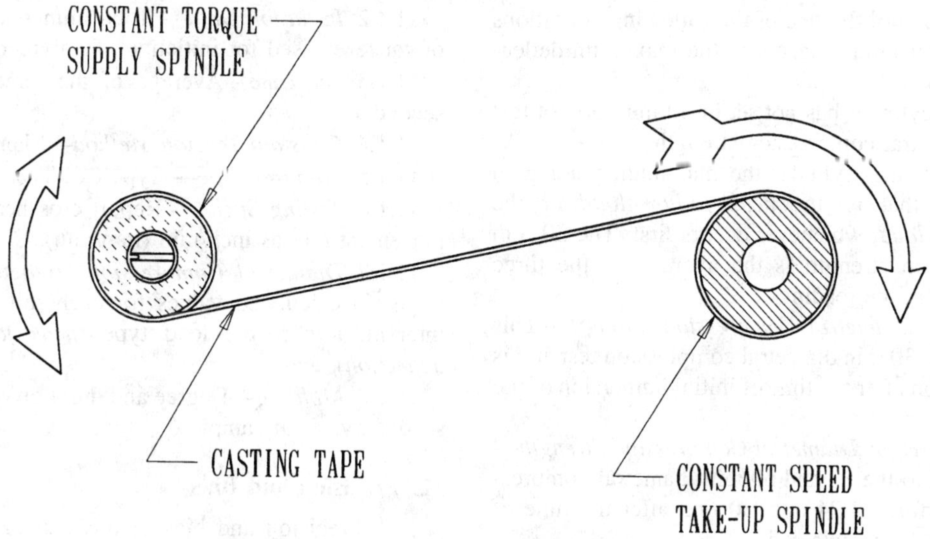

FIG. 2 Automated Constant Torque Preparation Method

8. Sample Conditioning

8.1 Store each package flat, with each roll on its side, at 70 ± 5°F (21.1 ± 2.8°C) for at least 24 h before use.

8.2 Open each package immediately prior to use.

9. Specimen Preparation

9.1 Before opening each package, record the manufacturer's name, product description, size (width and length), and lot number.

9.2 Wrap the release liner around test specimen preparation mandrel and secure with tape.

9.3 Open the package and loosely grasp roll with core perpendicular to fingers in palm of hand.

9.4 Start the timer, fully immerse roll in water and squeeze following manufacturer's instructions. Record immersion time and number of squeezes.

9.5 Remove roll from water and allow excess water to drain for not more than five seconds. DO NOT SQUEEZE to remove excess water.

9.6 Wrap a five-ply cylinder on mandrel as rapidly as possible using constant tension (see Fig. 1 or Fig. 2). Each succeeding layer shall be aligned directly over the preceding layer with complete overlap. Cut the tape at the end of the fifth ply within ± ¼ in. (6.4 mm) relative to the starting end of the first ply.

9.7 Immediately wrap a second five-ply cylinder as rapidly as possible by repeating 9.6.

9.8 Immediately wrap a third five-ply cylinder as rapidly as possible by repeating 9.6. Cut off excess tape.

9.9 *Molding*—Primary test samples should be prepared without the use of manual molding. If testing of samples with the use of manual molding is desired, a secondary group of samples should be prepared using the desired molding technique. Record the molding time and degree of manipulation used.

9.10 *Setting Time*— This is determined by a manual indentation test, that is, the time elapsed from the initial immersion until the test cylinder cannot be indented by moderate fingernail pressure. Begin indentation testing for material setting after all 3 samples from a single roll are wrapped. Repeat the test every 15 s until all samples are set. Record the three times and report the average as the *setting time*.

9.11 After the test cylinders have set, remove them from the mandrel taking care to avoid deforming them. Remove the release liner from the inside of the test cylinders.

9.12 Stand test specimens on end with enough space between samples to allow air to freely circulate between the cylinders.

10. Procedure

10.1 *Testing Speed*— The recommended constant crosshead (or actuator) speed shall be between 1 to 10 in./min (25.4 to 254 mm/min). Report the exact speed.

NOTE 3—Testing speeds outside the recommended range may be used provided that there are no demonstrable rate dependent effects on the material and that complete data capture is assured at higher rates.

10.2 *Load Range Selection*—Set the load range of the testing machine so that the maximum expected load is at least 20 % of the range selected.

10.3 *Thirty Minute Diametral Compression Strength*—This test is performed 30 ± 5 min after the time of initial immersion of the sample roll.

10.3.1 Place each specimen, one at a time, between the platens of the testing machine. Center the test cylinder on the lower platen, the platen being sufficiently large to support the specimen over its entire length. Orient the test cylinder so that the transition or overlap area, that is, where the first ply begins and the fifth ply ends, is in contact with either the upper or lower platen.

NOTE 4—The presence or absence of an overlap between the first and fifth ply affects the strength of the transition area, by either increasing or decreasing it from that of the surrounding area with a uniform number of plies. Since sample failure generally occurs in regions of high tensile stress on the free outer wall of the test cylinder, it is important that the overlap, or transition area, not be in the high tensile stress region.

10.3.2 Bring the platens together until they just touch the test cylinder, but no load has been applied.

10.3.3 Initiate the test at the prescribed rate. Continue the test at a uniform rate until the one of the following conditions occurs: either cylinder failure occurs or the maximum deflection is reached.

10.3.4 If the test cylinder has not set in 30 min, do not test for the 30 min diametral compression strength.

10.3.5 Record for each cylinder the maximum reading in pounds (Newtons), that is, the *peak failure load* or the *maximum deflection load*, whichever occurs first. The 30 min diametral compression strength is the average of the three values calculated from the readings.

10.4 *Sixty Minute Diametral Compression Strength*—This test is identical to the 30 min diametral compression test and is performed 60 ± 5 min after the time of initial immersion of the sample roll.

10.5 *Twenty-Four Hour Diametral Compression Strength*—This test is identical to the 30 and 60 min diametral compression tests and is performed 24 h ± 30 min after the time of initial immersion of the sample roll.

10.5.1 Maintain specimens for the 24 h diametral compression test at 75 ± 5°F (23.9 ± 2.8°C) and 50 ± 10 % relative humidity for the 24 h curing period.

11. Report

11.1 Report the following information:

11.1.1 *Product Identity*— Manufacturer, product description, product size (width and length) and manufacturing lot code,

11.1.2 *Initiation Data*— Total immersion time and number of squeezes used for initiation of polymerization,

11.1.3 *Set Time*—Average of the three measurements (in seconds),

11.1.4 *Constant Tension Method*—Manual or automated,

11.1.5 *Mandrel Type*— Type I or Type II,

11.1.6 *Testing Speed*— Report crosshead or (actuator) displacement rate as inch/min (mm/min),

11.1.7 *Diametral Compression Strengths*—Average of the three (3) calculated values for each roll tested at each time interval. Report the load type (*peak failure* or *maximum deflection*), and

11.1.8 *Molding*—Degree and duration of molding used on a secondary set of samples.

12. Precision and Bias

12.1 Precision and bias of this test method will be determined after interlaboratory tests are carried out and the results tabulated. The interlaboratory tests will be carried out following Practices E 691.

13. Keywords

13.1 orthopaedic casting tape—diametral compression strength; orthopaedic casting tape—mechanical testing; orthopaedic casting tape—setting time; polyurethane—biomedical applications; polyurethane/fiberglass orthopaedic casting tape

APPENDIX

(Nonmandatory Information)

X1. RATIONALE

X1.1 The primary purpose of this test method is to provide a standard method for determining the strength and setting time of synthetic water-activated polyurethane fiberglass orthopaedic casting tape. This includes sample preparation, testing procedure and data reporting.

X1.2 Specimen preparation in this test method is not intended to duplicate all actual casting tape use. It is intended to produce uniform samples upon which mechanical testing may be performed with minimal variability.

X1.3 Wrapping by hand may produce samples in which there are variations in adhesion between layers, or along the sample width because of variations in wrapping tension. Sample to sample variation may also be increased when using manual methods. Therefore, samples should be prepared using a method that employs constant tension during wrapping of the plies (see Fig. 1 and Fig. 2).

X1.4 Manual molding of the casting tape, while an integral part of the normal cast application process, is extremely subjective, making standardization of this process difficult. Variations in molding pressure and molding time can greatly influence test results. Therefore, this test method provides for testing to be performed on a primary set of specimens prepared *without* molding. Should it be desirable to quantify the effects of molding, a secondary set of samples should be prepared *with* a molding technique.

X1.5 The mandrel diameters (Type I and Type II) were selected based on the need to limit the number of possible diameters and still remain in a reasonable anatomic size range. Mandrel material has been limited to aluminum in order to maintain reasonable fixture mass, and to provide a material that was relatively corrosion resistant. Because ferrous metals, non-ferrous metals, and polymers have intrinsically different masses and heat conduction coefficients, changes in materials or design (that is, solid versus hollow) could alter heat conduction between the mandrel and the curing tape. If the peak exothermic temperature or the curing temperature profile were affected in this manner, unpredictable changes in setting time and measured compression strengths could result.

X1.6 The testing procedure in this method is not intended to replicate actual casting tape use, nor duplicate all failure modes. It is meant to provide a standard, repeatable test method for comparison of the relative strengths for various synthetic water-activated polyurethane fiberglass orthopaedic casting tapes. The prescription of tests at 30 min, 60 min and 24 h is intended to provide useful information regarding the curing profile for materials tested, and provide some objective measure of relative strengths for partially cured and fully cured casting tape samples.

X1.7 This test method is not intended to restrict the curing temperature regimes should alternate curing chemistries be developed.

Designation: F 1537 – 00

Standard Specification for Wrought Cobalt - 28Chromium - 6Molybdenum Alloys for Surgical Implants (UNS R31537, UNS R31538, and UNS R31539)[1]

This standard is issued under the fixed designation F 1537; the number immediately following the designation indicates the year of original adoption or, in the case of revision, the year of last revision. A number in parentheses indicates the year of last reapproval. A superscript epsilon (ϵ) indicates an editorial change since the last revision or reapproval.

1. Scope

1.1 This specification covers the requirements for three wrought cobalt - 28chromium - 6molybdenum alloys used for surgical implants. The properties specified apply specifically to wrought bar, rod, and wire.

1.2 The values stated in inch-pound units are to be regarded as the standard. The SI equivalents of the inch-pound units may be approximate.

2. Referenced Documents

2.1 *ASTM Standards:*

E 8 Test Methods for Tension Testing of Metallic Materials[2]

E 18 Test Methods for Rockwell Hardness and Rockwell Superficial Hardness of Metallic Materials[2]

E 112 Test Methods for Determining Average Grain Size[2]

E 354 Test Methods for Chemical Analysis of High Temperature, Electrical, Magnetic, and Other Similar Iron, Nickel, and Cobalt Alloys[3]

F 75 Specification for Cast Cobalt-Chromium Molybdenum Alloy for Surgical Implant Applications[4]

2.2 *Aerospace Material Specifications:*

AMS 2269 Chemical Check Analysis Limits, Nickel, Nickel Alloys and Cobalt Alloys[5]

AMS 2248 Chemical Check Analysis Limits, Corrosion and Heat Resistant Steels and Alloys, Maraging and Other Highly-Alloyed Steels, and Iron Alloys[5]

AMS 2630 Ultrasonic Inspection[5]

2.3 *American Society for Quality Standard:*

ASQ C1 Specification of General Requirements for a Quality Program[6]

3. Significance and Use

3.1 The purpose of this specification is to characterize the chemical, mechanical, and metallurgical requirements of wrought cobalt - 28chromium - 6 molybdenum bar, rod, and wire.

4. Ordering Information

4.1 Inquiries and orders for material under this specification shall include the following information:

4.1.1 Quantity,

4.1.2 ASTM designation and alloy number,

4.1.3 Mechanical properties (See Section 7),

4.1.4 Form (bar, rod or wire),

4.1.5 Applicable dimensions including size, thickness, width, and length (exact, random, or multiples) or drawing number,

4.1.6 Condition (See Section5,

4.1.7 Special tests (if any), and

4.1.8 Other requirements.

5. Condition

5.1 Product shall be furnished as specified below:

5.1.1 The annealed condition is typically supplied as a hot rolled and annealed product.

5.1.2 The hot worked condition is typically supplied as a hot rolled and unannealed product.

5.1.3 The warm worked condition is typically supplied as a thermomechanically processed product to achieve a strainhardened structure.

5.1.4 Other conditions may be provided as agreed upon between purchaser and supplier.

6. Chemical Requirements

6.1 The cobalt-28chromium-6molybdenum alloys shall conform to the chemical requirements prescribed in Table 1. The supplier shall not ship material that is outside the limits specified in Table 1 for the applicable alloy.

6.1.1 Requirements for the major and minor elemental constituents are listed in Table 1. Also listed are important residual elements. Analysis for elements not listed in Table 1 is not required to verify compliance with this specification.

---

[1] This specification is under the jurisdiction of ASTM Committee F04 on Medical and Surgical Materials and Devices and is the direct responsibility of Subcommittee F04.12 on Metallurgical Materials.

Current edition approved May 10, 2000. Published August 2000. Originally published as F 1537 – 94. Last previous edition F 1537 – 94.

[2] *Annual Book of ASTM Standards*, Vol 03.01.

[3] *Annual Book of ASTM Standards*, Vol 03.05.

[4] *Annual Book of ASTM Standards*, Vol 13.01.

[5] Available from Society of Automotive Engineers, Inc., 400 Commonwealth Drive, Warrendale, PA 15096-0001.

[6] Available from American Society for Quality, 611 East Wisconsin Avenue, Milwaukee, WI 53203.

TABLE 1 Chemical Composition

Element	Alloy 1 UNS R31537 (Low Carbon)		Alloy 2 UNS R31538 (High Carbon)		Alloy 3 UNS R31539 (Dispersion Strengthened)	
	Composition % (mass/mass)					
	min	max	min	max	min	max
Carbon	......	0.14	0.15	0.35	......	0.14
Aluminum	......	......	......	......	0.30	1.00
Lanthanum	......	......	......	......	0.03	0.20
Chromium	26.0	30.0	26.0	30.0	26.0	30.0
Molybdenum	5.0	7.0	5.0	7.0	5.0	7.0
Nickel	......	1.0	......	1.0	......	1.0
Iron	......	0.75	......	0.75	......	0.75
Silicon	......	1.0	......	1.0	......	1.0
Manganese	......	1.0	......	1.0	......	1.0
Nitrogen	......	0.25	......	0.25	......	0.25
Cobalt[A]	Balance		Balance		Balance	

[A]Approximately equal to the difference of 100 % and the sum percentage of the other specified elements. The percentage of cobalt difference is not required to be reported.

6.2 *Product Analysis*—The product analysis is either for the purpose of verifying the composition of a heat or lot or to determine variations in the composition within the heat.

6.2.1 Acceptance or rejection of a heat or lot of material may be made by the purchaser on the basis of this product analysis.

6.2.2 Product analysis tolerances do not broaden the specified heat analysis requirements but cover variations between laboratories in the measurement of chemical content. Product analysis limits shall be as specified in Table 2

TABLE 2 Product Analysis Tolerances[A,B]

Element	Permissible Variation Under the Minimum Limit or Over the Maximum Limit, % (mass/mass)[C]
Carbon	0.02
Aluminum ≤ 0.50	0.05
Aluminum > 0.50 up to 1.00	0.10
Lanthanum	0.01
Chromium	0.30
Molybdenum	0.15
Nickel	0.05
Iron	0.03
Silicon	0.05
Manganese	0.03
Nitrogen[D]	0.02

[A]See Test Methods E 354.
[B]Refer to AMS 2269 for chemical check analysis limits (except nitrogen).
[C]For elements in which only a maximum percentage is indicated, the "under minimum limit" is not applicable.
[D]Refer to AMS 2248.

7. Mechanical Requirements

7.1 *Tensile Properties*:

7.1.1 Tensile properties shall be determined in accordance with Test Methods E 8

7.1.2 The mechanical properties of test specimens shall conform to the requirements specified in Table 3.

7.2 *Hardness*:

7.2.1 Hardness values shall be determined in accordance with Test Methods E 18.

7.2.2 Hardness values are for information only and shall not be used as a basis for rejection.

8. Special Tests

8.1 Bar, rod, and wire conforming to this specification shall have a homogeneous microstructure with an average grain size of ASTM No. 5 or finer when measured in accordance with Test Methods E 112.

8.2 Ultrasonic inspection should be per AMS 2630, Class A1.

9. Certification

9.1 Certification shall be provided by the supplier that the material meets the requirements of this specification. A report of the test results shall be furnished at the time of shipment.

10. Quality Program Requirements

10.1 The alloy producer and any processors shall maintain a quality program such as that which is defined in ASQ C1.

11. Keywords

11.1 cobalt alloys (for surgical implants); cobalt-28chromium-6molybdenum; metals (for surgical implants)

TABLE 3 Mechanical Requirements

Condition	Ultimate Tensile Strength min, psi (MPa)	Yield Strength (0.2 % offset), min, psi (MPa)	Elongation[A] min, %	Reduction in Area min, %	Hardness HRC, Typical
Annealed	130 000 (897)	75 000 (517)	20	20	25
Hot Worked	145 000 (1000)	101 000 (700)	12	12	28
Warm Worked	170 000 (1192)	120 000 (827)	12	12	35

[A]Elongation of material 0.062 in. (1.575 mm) or greater in diameter or thickness shall be measured using a gage length of 2 in. or 4D or 4W. The gage length must be reported with the test results. The method for determining elongation of material under 0.062 in. (1.57mm) in diamter or thickness nay be negotiated.

APPENDIXES

(Nonmandatory Information)

X1. RATIONALE

X1.1 The purpose of this specification is to characterize composition and properties to ensure consistency in wrought cobalt-28chromium-6molybdenum bar, rod, and wire used in the manufacturing of medical devices.

X1.2 The carbon content of commercially available F 1537 barstock varies to meet specific customer needs. The chemical composition was expanded into low and high carbon alloys (Alloys 1 and 2 in Table 1). Alloy 2 contains a greater volume fraction of carbides compared to Alloy 1.

X1.3 Alloy 3 was added in Table 1 since bar, rod, and wire produced with this composition meet the current ASTM F 1537 requirements. Alloy 3 is a dispersion-strengthened alloy containing fine aluminum-lanthanum oxides/nitrides.[7,8]

X1.4 The minimum mechanical properties of wrought bar, rod, and wire conforming to this specification are superior to the minimum mechanical properties of Specification F 75 material in the as-cast condition.

X1.5 Some complex metallic phases, such as carbides, oxides, or carbonitrides, or combinations thereof, may be present in the microstructure of this alloy.

[7] Wang, Kathy K., Gustavson, Larry J., and Dumbleton, John H., U.S. Patent #4,668,290, "Dispersion Strengthened Cobalt-Chromium-Molybdenum Alloy Produced By Gas Atomization", Filed August 13, 1985, Issued May 26, 1987.

[8] Wang, Kathy K., Gustavson, Larry J., and Dumbleton, John H., "The Development of a New Dispersion Strengthened Vitallium Alloy for Medical Implants", *Modern Developments in Powder Metallurgy,* Volume 20, 1988, pp. 361-375, Metal Powder Industries Federation, 105 College Road East, Princeton, NJ 08540-6692

X2. BIOCOMPATIBILITY

X2.1 The alloy compositions covered by this specification have been employed successfully in human implant applications in contact with soft tissue and bone for over a decade (reference 510k #K852964 for Alloy 3, which has been used since 1985).

X2.2 No known surgical implant material has ever been shown to be completely free of adverse reactions in the human body. Long term clinical experience of the use of the material referred to in this specification, however, has shown that an acceptable level of biological response can be expected, if the material is used in appropriate applications.

Designation: F 1538 – 94

Standard Specification for Glass and Glass Ceramic Biomaterials for Implantation[1]

This standard is issued under the fixed designation F 1538; the number immediately following the designation indicates the year of original adoption or, in the case of revision, the year of last revision. A number in parentheses indicates the year of last reapproval. A superscript epsilon (ε) indicates an editorial change since the last revision or reapproval.

1. Scope

1.1 This specification covers the material requirements and characterization techniques for glass and glass-ceramic biomaterials intended for use as bulk porous or powdered surgical implants, or as coatings on surgical devices, but not including drug delivery systems.

1.2 The biological response to glass and glass-ceramic biomaterials in bone and soft tissue has been demonstrated in clinical use **1-9**[2] and laboratory studies **10-14**.

2. Referenced Documents

2.1 *ASTM Standards:*

C 158 Method for Flexural Testing of Glass (Determination of Modulus of Rupture)[3]

C 169 Method for Chemical Analysis of Soda-Lime and Borosilicate Glass[3]

C 623 Test Method for Young's Modulus, Shear Modulus, and Poisson's Ratio for Glass and Glass-Ceramics by Resonance[3]

C 633 Test Method for Adhesion or Cohesive Strength of Flame-Sprayed Coatings[4]

C 693 Test Method for Density of Glass by Buoyancy[3]

C 729 Test Method for Density of Glass by the Sink-Float Comparator[3]

C 730 Test Method for Knoop Indentation Hardness of Glass[3]

C 958 Method for Determination of Particle Size Distribution of Alumina or Quartz by X-Ray Monitoring of Gravity Sedimentation[3]

C 1069 Method for Specific Surface Area of Alumina or Quartz by Nitrogen Adsorption[3]

C 1070 Test Method for Determining Particle Size Distribution of Alumina or Quartz by Laser Light Scattering[3]

E 228 Test Method for Linear Thermal Expansion of Solid Materials with a Vitreous Silica Dilatometer[5]

F 748 Practice for Selecting Generic Biological Test Methods for Materials and Devices[6]

2.2 *Code of Federal Regulations:*[7]

Title 21, Part 820

2.3 *United States Pharmacopoeia:*[8]

Lead <252>

Mercury <261>

Arsenic <211>

Heavy Metals <231> Method found in Annual Book of ASTM Standards, vol 13.01.

2.4 *U.S. Geological Survey Method:*[7]

(7) Cadmium

3. Terminology

3.1 *Definitions of Terms Specific to This Standard:*

3.1.1 *bioactive glass*—an amorphous solid that is not intrinsically adhesive and that is capable of forming a cohesive bond with both hard and soft tissue when exposed to appropriate in vivo or in vitro environments, such as simulated body fluid or tris-hydroxymethylaminomethane buffer, by developing a surface layer of hydroxycarbonate apatite by release of ionic species from the bulk material.

3.1.2 *bioactive glass-ceramic*—an amorphous-derived crystalline solid that is not intrinsically adhesive and that is capable of forming a cohesive bond with bone and soft tissue when exposed to appropriate in vivo or in vitro environments, such as simulated body fluid or tris-hydroxymethylaminomethane buffer, by developing a surface layer of hydroxycarbonate apatite by release of ionic species from the bulk material.

3.1.3 *bulk material*—intended to describe a unit material used as a load bearing implant.

3.1.4 *coating*—intended to describe a surface layer that is relatively thin compared to the overall dimensions of the prosthetic part that has been coated.

3.1.5 *glass biomaterial*—any one of a number of compositions of amorphous inorganic solids that are used as implant materials for various medical or dental uses, or both.

3.1.6 *glass-ceramic biomaterials*—any one of a number of compositions of an amorphous-derived crystalline solid that is used as an implantable biomaterial for medical or dental use, or both.

---

[1] This specification is under the jurisdiction of ASTM Committee F-4 on Medical and Surgical Materials and Devices and is the direct responsibility of Subcommittee F04.13 on Ceramic Materials.

Current edition approved Dec. 15, 1994. Published February 1995.

[2] The boldface numbers in parentheses refer to the list of references at the end of this specification.

[3] *Annual Book of ASTM Standards*, Vol 15.02.

[4] *Annual Book of ASTM Standards*, Vol 02.05.

[5] *Annual Book of ASTM Standards*, Vols 03.01 and 14.02.

[6] *Annual Book of ASTM Standards*, Vol 13.01.

[7] Available from Standardization Documents Order Desk, Bldg. 4 Section D, 700 Robbins Ave., Philadelphia, PA 19111-5094, Attn: NPODS.

[8] Available from United Stated Pharmacopia, 12601 Twinbrook Parkway, Rockville, MD 20852.

3.1.7 *particulate material*—intended to describe several pieces (usually small size) used together within an implant construct.

4. Chemical Requirements

4.1 Bulk compositions shall be tested using Method C 169.

4.2 The concentration of heavy metals in the bioactive glass and glass-ceramics shall be limited as follows:

Element	ppm, max
As	3
Cd	5
Hg	5
Pb	30
total heavy metals (as lead)	50

For referee purposes, the methods listed in 2.2 and 2.3 shall be used.

5. Physical Characterization

5.1 The following physical and mechanical characterizations may be applicable to various bioactive glass and glass-ceramics products and should be used whenever possible to verify the material.

5.1.1 *Density*—The densities of glass and glass ceramic materials are related directly to the processing history and composition of the material. The density of the bulk material shall be measured using Test Method C 729 and shall be consistent for the specific materials.

NOTE 1—This test should use a non-aqueous liquid for bioactive glass and glass ceramic materials, which are known to react in an aqueous environment and could thereby affect the measurement.

5.1.2 *Flexural Strength*—When used as bulk materials in load bearing applications, the flexural strength of the bulk material shall be measured using Method C 158.

5.1.3 *Young's Modulus*—When used as a bulk material, Young's Modulus of glass and glass ceramic biomaterials shall be determined following Test Method C 623.

5.1.4 *Hardness*—Where applicable, for characterization of the material, the hardness of bulk samples shall be determined using Test Method C 730. The knoop indentation hardness is one of many properties that is used to characterize glasses. Attempts have been made to relate knoop hardness to tensile strength, but no generally accepted methods are available. Such conversion is limited in scope and should be used with caution, except for special cases in which a reliable basis for conversion has been obtained by conversion tests.

5.1.5 *Surface Area*—The surface area of a particulate may be important in determining the reliability of the bioactivity of the material. Whenever the specific surface area of the material relates to function, the surface area of particulate glass and glass ceramic biomaterials shall be measured using Method C 1069.

5.1.6 *Bond Strength of Glass or Glass Ceramic Coating*—When used as a coating on a metallic or ceramic substrate, the bond strength of the coating shall be measured following Test Method C 633.

5.1.7 *Crystallinity*—For glass-ceramic biomaterials, the percent crystallinity and crystal phases present in glass ceramic biomaterials shall be determined by means of X-ray diffraction analysis. While there is no single standard method for determining the crystallinity and crystal phases of glass ceramic materials, techniques such as those detailed in reference 10.16 and 10.17 should be followed to standardize methods as much as possible.

5.1.8 *Thermal Expansion*—Thermal expansion shall be measured using Test Method E 228, when materials are to be used for coatings (raw materials are to be measured), or on finished product as a quality control test.

6. Biocompatibility

6.1 Glass and glass-ceramic biomaterials should be evaluated thoroughly for biocompatibility before human use. Bioactive glass and glass-ceramic materials are unique in their mode of action when implanted in the body due to the released ionic species and the mechanisms by which these materials bond with bony tissue. These materials have been found to exhibit an excellent tissue response in laboratory studies **10-14** and clinical usage **1-7**. Before any new formulations are used clinically, the tissue response should be characterized by the methods recommended in Practice F 748.

7. Test Specimen Fabrication

7.1 Test specimens should be prepared concurrent with implant devices, as well as from the same batch of material and by the same processes as those used in fabricating the glass and glass-ceramic implant device.

8. Quality Program Requirement

8.1 The manufacturer shall conform to good manufacturing practices (2.1) or its equivalent.

9. Keywords

9.1 bioactive glass; bioactive glass-ceramics; glass biomaterials; glass-ceramic biomaterial; —surgical implants

APPENDIX

(Nonmandatory Information)

X1. RATIONALE

X1.1 A number of glass-ceramic materials are available commercially. Bioactive glass and glass-ceramic materials are available commercially as synthetic graft materials for maintenance of the alveolar ridge; as devices for spinal fushion; as implants for replacement of the vertebral body, iliac crest, and ossicular chain of the middle ear; as bone filler to substitute for bone defects remaining after the excision of bone tumors and extraction of loosened joint prostheses; and as coatings on dental and orthopedic implants. As with any implant material, the bioresponse is critically dependent on the material properties. To achieve reliable biocompatibility, these properties must be known and consistent. This specification provides specifications for biocompatible grades of bioactive glass and glass-ceramics.

X1.2 In order to be called bioactive, the materials must demonstrate that living tissue is bonding to a significantly higher level than non-bonding implant control, as well as demonstrate that ionic species are released from the material into solution in a controlled and reproducible manner.

X1.3 Bioactive glass and glass-ceramic materials are generally silicate-based materials, with additions of oxides of calcium, phosphorous, and various alkalis. They may be phosphate-based materials as well. These materials may also include fluoride and other alkali earth metals. Table X1.1 gives a few specific examples of the bioactive glass and glass-ceramic materials produced. Since the compositions of these materials may vary greatly from product to product, it is not possible to specify their exact compositions.

X1.4 It is recognized that separate performance standards may be necessary for each end-use product. Physical and mechanical properties were not specified for this reason. A source of general test methods for glass and ceramic materials may be found in Ref **(15)**.

TABLE X1.1 Typical Bioactive Glass and Glass-Ceramic Compositions (Compositions in Weight %)

	45S5 Bioglass®	45S5.4F Bioglass®	52S4.6 Bioglass®	KGC Ceravital	A-W-GC
SiO_2	45	45	52	46.2	34.2
P_2O_5	6	6	6		16.3
CaO	24.5	14.7	21	20.2	44.9
CaF_2		9.8			0.5
$Ca(PO_3)_2$				25.5	
MgO				2.9	4.6
Na_2O	24.5	24.5	21	4.8	
K_2O				0.4	

REFERENCES

(1) Reck, R., "Tissue Reactions to Glass Ceramics in the Middle Ear," *Clin. Otolaryngol*, Vol 6, 1981, pp. 59–63.

(2) Merwin, G. E., "Review of Bioactive Materials for Otological and Maxillofacial Applications," *Handbook of Bioactive Ceramics*, Vol 1, Ed. T. Yamamuro, L. L. Hench, and J. Wilson, CRC Press, Boca Raton, Florida, 1990, pp. 323–328.

(3) Douek, E., "Otological Applications of Bioglass® Implants," *Proceedings Fourth International Symposium on Bioceramics in Medicine*, Ed. W. Bonfield, London, United Kingdom, September 10 and 11, 1990.

(4) Stanley, H. R., et al., "Residual Alveolar Ridge Maintenance with a New Endosseous Implant Material," *J. Pros. Dent.*, Vol 58, No. 5, November 1987.

(5) Nakamura, T., et al., "A New Glass-Ceramic for Bone Replacement: Evaluation of its Bonding to Bond Tissue," *Journal of Biomedical Material Research*, Vol 19, 1985.

(6) Yamamuro, T., et al., "Novel Methods for Clinical Application of Bioactive Ceramics," *Bioceramics: Material Characteristics Versus in Vivo Behavior*, Ann. New York Acad. Sci., Vol 523, 1988, pp. 107–114.

(7) Yamamuro, T., "Reconstruction of the Iliac Crest with Bioactive Glass-Ceramic Prosthesis," *Handbook of Bioactive Ceramics Prosthesis*, Eds. T. Yamamuro, L. L. Hench, and J. Wilson, Vol 1, CRC Press, Boca Raton, FL, 1990, pp. 335–342.

(8) Yamamuro, T., "Replacement of the Spine with Bioactive Glass-Ceramic Prosthesis," pp. 343–352, idem.

(9) Taguchi, T., "A Bioactive Glass Powder-Ammonium Hydrogen Phosphate Composite for Repairing Bone Defects," *Journal of Appl. Biomater.*, Vol 1, pp. 217–223.

(10) Hench, L. L., and Paschall, H. A., "Histo-Chemical Responses at a Biomaterials Interface," *Journal of Biomedical Material Research*, Vol 5, 1974, p. 1.

(11) Kitsugi, T., et al., "Bonding Behavior of a Glass-Ceramic Containing Apatite and Wollastonite in Segmental Replacement of the Rat Tibia Under Load-Bearing Conditions," *Journal of Bone St. Surg.*, Vol 71A, 1989.

(12) Gross, U., et al., "The Response of Bone to Surface Active Glasses/Glass-Ceramics," *CRC Critical Reviews in Biocompatibility*, Vol 4, No. 2, 1988, pp. 155–179.

(13) Piotrowski, G., et al., "Mechanical Studies of the Bone Bioglass® Interfacial Bond," *Journal of Biomedical Material Research*, Vol 6, 1975, p. 47.

(14) Strunz, V., et al., "The Mechanical Strength of the Bond Between Bone and Implants of Glass-Ceramics with Apatite," *Dental Implants*, Ed. G. Heimke, Henser, Munich, 1980, pp. 27–34.

(**15**) Cullity, B. D., *Elements of X-ray Diffraction*, 2nd ed., Addison-Wesley Publishing Company, Reading, MA, 1978.
(**16**) Li, P., et al., "The Effect of Residual Glassy Phase in a Bioactive Glass-Ceramic on the Formation of its Surface Apatite Layer In-Vitro," *Journal Mater. Sci. in Med.*, Vol 3, 1992, pp. 452–456.

Last ASTM Designation: F 1539 – 95 (Reapproved 1999)

Test Method for
Consant Amplitude Bending Fatigue Tests of Metallic Bone Staples

This test method covers procedures for the preformance of constant amplitude fatigue testing of metallic staples used in internal fixation of the musculoskeletal system.

Formerly under the jurisdiction of Committee F04 on Medical and Surgical Materials and Devices, this test method was withdrawn in November 2000 and replaced by Specification F 564–00 for Metallic Bone Staples.[1]

[1] Annual Book of ASTM Standards, Volume 13.01.

Last ASTM Designation: F 1540 – 95 (Reapproved 1999)

Test Method for
Pull-Out Fixation Strength of Metallic Bone Staples

This test method covers testing of the hard tissue pull-out fixation strength of metallic staples used in the internal fixation of the musculoskeletal system.

Formerly under the jurisdiction of Committee F04 on Medical and Surgical Materials and Devices, this test method was withdrawn in November 2000 and replaced by Specification F 564–00 for Metallic Bone Staples.[1]

[1] Annual Book of ASTM Standards, Volume 13.01.

Standard Specification and Test Methods for External Skeletal Fixation Devices[1]

This standard is issued under the fixed designation F 1541; the number immediately following the designation indicates the year of original adoption or, in the case of revision, the year of last revision. A number in parentheses indicates the year of last reapproval. A superscript epsilon (ε) indicates an editorial change since the last revision or reapproval.

1. Scope

1.1 This specification provides a characterization of the design and mechanical function of external skeletal fixation devices (ESFDs), test methods for characterization of ESFD mechanical properties, and identifies needs for further development of test methods and performance criteria. The ultimate goal is to develop a specification, which defines performance criteria and methods for measurement of performance-related mechanical characteristics of ESFDs and their fixation to bone. It is not the intention of this specification to define levels of performance or case-specific clinical performance of the devices, as insufficient knowledge is available to predict the consequences of the use of any of these devices in individual patients for specific activities of daily living. Furthermore, it is not the intention of this specification to describe or specify specific designs for ESFDs.

1.2 This specification describes ESFDs for surgical fixation of the skeletal system. It provides basic ESFD geometrical definitions, dimensions, classification, and terminology; material specifications; performance definitions; test methods; and characteristics determined to be important to the in-vivo performance of the device.

1.3 This specification includes a terminology and classification annex and five standard test method annexes as follows:

1.3.1 *Classification of External Fixators*—Annex A1.

1.3.2 *Test Method for External Skeletal Fixator Connectors*—Annex A2.

1.3.3 *Test Method for Determining In-Plane Compressive Properties of Circular Ring or Ring Segment Bridge Elements*—Annex A3.

1.3.4 *Test Method for External Skeletal Fixator Joints*—Annex A4.

1.3.5 *Test Method for External Skeletal Fixator Pin Anchorage Elements*—Annex A5.

1.3.6 *Test Method for External Skeletal Fixator Subassemblies*—Annex A6.

1.3.7 *Test Method for External Skeletal Fixator/Constructs Subassemblies*—Annex A7.

1.4 A rationale is given in Appendix X1.

1.5 The values stated in SI units are to be regarded as the standard.

1.6 The following safety hazards caveat pertains only to the test method portions (Annex A2-Annex A6):

1.7 *This standard does not purport to address all of the safety concerns, if any, associated with its use. It is the responsibility of the user of this standard to establish appropriate safety and health practices and determine the applicability of regulatory limitations prior to use.*

2. Referenced Documents

2.1 *ASTM Standards:*

A 938 Test Method for Torsion Testing of Wire[2]

D 790 Test Methods for Flexural Properties of Unreinforced and Reinforced Plastics and Electrical Insulating Materials[3]

E 4 Practices for Force Verification of Testing Machines[4]

F 67 Specification for Unalloyed Titanium for Surgical Implant Applications[5]

F 90 Specification for Wrought Cobalt-20 Chromium-15 Tungsten-10 Nickel Alloy for Surgical Implant Applications (R30605)[5]

F 136 Specification for Wrought Titanium-6 Aluminum-4 Vanadium ELI (Extra Low Interstitial) Alloy (UNS R56401) for Surgical Implant Applications

F 138 Specification for Wrought 18 Chromium-14 Nickel-2.5 Molybdenum Stainless Steel Bar and Wire for Surgical Implants (UNS S31673)[5]

F 366 Specification for Fixation Pins and Wires[5]

F 543 Specification for Metallic Medical Bone Screws[5]

F 544 Reference Chart for Pictorial Cortical Bone Screw Classification[6]

F 1058 Specification for Wrought Cobalt-Chromium-Nickel Molybdenum-Iron Alloy for Surgical Implant Applications (UNS R30003 and UNS R30008)[5]

F 1264 Specification and Test Methods for Intramedullary Fixation Devices[5]

F 1472 Specification for Wrought Titanium-6 Aluminum-4 Vanadium Alloy for Surgical Implant Applications (UNS R56400)[5]

---

[1] This specification is under the jurisdiction of ASTM Committee F04 on Medical and Surgical Materials and Devices and is the direct responsibility of Subcommittee F04.21 on Osteosynthesis.

Current edition approved May 10, 2001. Published May 2001. Originally published as F 1541 – 94. Last previous edition F 1541 – 00.

[2] *Annual Book of ASTM Standards*, Vol 01.03.

[3] *Annual Book of ASTM Standards*, Vol 08.01.

[4] *Annual Book of ASTM Standards*, Vol 03.01.

[5] *Annual Book of ASTM Standards*, Vol 13.01.

[6] Discontinued; see 1998 *Annual Book of ASTM Standards*, Vol 13.01.

F 1713 Specification for Wrought Titanium-13 Niobium-13 Zirconium Alloy for Surgical Implant Applications[5]

3. Terminology

3.1 *Definitions*—The definitions of terms relating to external fixators are described in Annex A1.

4. Classification

4.1 External skeletal fixators are modular devices assembled from component elements.

4.2 Test methods can address individual elements, for example, anchorage elements, bridge elements; subassemblies of elements, for example, connectors, joints, ring elements; or the entire fixator.

4.3 Tests of an entire assembled fixator may include the fixator alone, or alternatively, the fixator as anchored to a representation of the bone(s) upon which it typically would be mounted in clinical usage.

5. Materials

5.1 All ESFDs made of materials, which have an ASTM standard, shall meet those requirements given in ASTM Standards listed in 2.1

6. Performance Considerations and Test Methods

6.1 *Individual Components*—The anchorage pins through which an ESFD is attached to a skeletal member or members typically experience high flexural, or torsional loads, or both. Often, the majority of the overall compliance of an ESFD is in its anchorage elements. A test method for evaluating the mechanical performance of an ESFD anchorage element in either of these loading modes is described in Annex A5.

6.2 *Subassemblies of Elements*:

6.2.1 The sites of junction between ESFD anchorage elements, for example, pins, and bridge elements, for example, rods, normally require specialized clamping or gripping members, known as connecting elements. Often, connecting elements are subjected to high loads, especially moments, so adequacy of their intrinsic mechanical stiffness, or strength, or both, is critical to overall fixator performance. A test method for evaluating the mechanical performance of ESFD connector elements is described in Annex A2.

6.2.2 ESFDs involving ring-type bridge elements are used widely both for fracture treatment and for distraction osteogenesis. The anchorage elements in such fixators usually are wires or thin pins, which pass transverse to the bone long axis and which are tensioned deliberately to control the longitudinal stiffness of the fixator. Tensioning these wires or pins causes appreciable compressive load in the plane of the ring element. A test method for evaluating the mechanical performance of ESFD ring elements in this loading mode is described in Annex A3.

6.2.3 The high loads often developed at ESFD junction sites are of concern both because of potentially excessive elastic deformation and because of potential irrecoverable deformation. In addition to the connecting element itself (Annex A2), overall performance of the junction also depends on the interface between the connecting element and the anchorage, or bridge elements, or both, which it grips. A test method for evaluating the overall strength, or stiffness, or both, at an external fixator joint, as defined in Annex A1 as the connecting element itself plus its interface with the anchorage, or bridge, or both, elements, which it grips, is described in Annex A4.

6.2.4 The modular nature of many ESFD systems affords the surgeon particularly great latitude as to configuration of the frame subassembly, as defined in Annex A1 as the bridge elements plus the connecting elements used to join bridge elements, but specifically excluding the anchorage elements. Since configuration of the frame subassembly is a major determinant of overall ESFD mechanical behavior, it is important to have procedures for unambiguously characterizing frame subassemblies, both geometrically and mechanically. Test methodology suitable for that purpose is described in Annex A6.

6.3 *Entire Assembled Fixator*—No test methods are yet approved for entire assembled fixators.

7. Keywords

7.1 anchorage element; bending; bridge element; connector; external skeletal fixation device; fracture fixation; joints; modularity; orthopedic medical device; osteosynthesis; ring element; subassembly (frame); terminology; torsion

ANNEXES

(Mandatory Information)

A1. CLASSIFICATION OF EXTERNAL SKELETAL FIXATORS

A1.1 Scope

A1.1.1 This classification covers the definitions of basic terms and considerations for external skeletal fixation devices (ESFDs) and the mechanical analyses thereof.

A1.1.2 It is not the intent of this classification to define levels of acceptable performance or to make recommendations concerning the appropriate or preferred clinical usage of these devices.

A1.1.3 *This standard does not purport to address all of the safety concerns, if any, associated with its use. It is the responsibility of the user of this standard to establish appropriate safety and health practices and determine the applicability of regulatory limitations prior to use.*

A1.2 Referenced Documents

A1.2.1 *ASTM Standards:*

F 366 Specification for Fixation Pins and Wires[5]
F 543 Specification for Cortical Bone Screws[5]
F 544 Reference Chart for Pictorial Cortical Bone Screw Classification[6]

A1.3 Background

A1.3.1 ESFDs are in widespread use in orthopedic surgery, primarily for applications involving fracture fixation or limb lengthening, or both. The mechanical demands placed on these devices often are severe. Clinical success usually depends on suitable mechanical integration of the ESFD with the host bone or limb.

A1.3.2 It is important, therefore, to have broadly accepted terminology and testing standards by which these devices can be described and their mechanical behaviors measured.

A1.3.3 Useful terminology and testing standards must take into account that the modular nature of most ESFDs deliberately affords a great deal of clinical latitude in configuring the assembled fixator.

A1.4 Significance and Use

A1.4.1 The purpose of this classification is to establish a consistent terminology system by means of which these ESFD configurations can be classified. It is anticipated that a companion testing standard using this classification system will subsequently be developed.

A1.5 Basis of Classification

A1.5.1 An assembled ESFD and the bone(s) or bone analog(s) to which it is affixed constitute a *fixator-bone construct.*

A1.5.1.1 The assembled ESFD itself, apart from the host bone, is termed the *fixator assembly.*

A1.5.1.2 The individual parts (or modules of individual parts) from which the end user assembles the fixator are termed its *elements.*

A1.5.2 An ESFD normally is configured to span a mechanical discontinuity in the host bone that otherwise would be unable to transmit one or more components of the applied functional load successfully. This bony discontinuity is termed the *mechanical defect.*

A1.5.3 Examples of mechanical defects are fracture surfaces, interfragmentary callus, segmental bone gaps, articular surfaces, neoplasms, and osteotomies.

A1.5.4 *Coordinate System(s)*—The relative positions of the bones or bone segments bordering the mechanical defect should be described in terms of an orthogonal axis *coordinate system* (Fig. A1.1).

A1.5.4.1 Where possible, coordinate axis directions should be aligned perpendicular to standard anatomical planes, for example, transverse (horizontal or axial), coronal (frontal), and sagittal (median).

A1.5.4.2 Where possible, translation directions should be consistent with standard clinical conventions, for example, ventral (anterior), dorsal (posterior), cranial (cephalad or superior), caudal (inferior), lateral, or medial.

A1.5.4.3 Rotation measurement conventions must follow the right-hand rule and, where possible, should be consistent with standard clinical terminology, for example, right or left lateral bending, flexion, extension, and torsion.

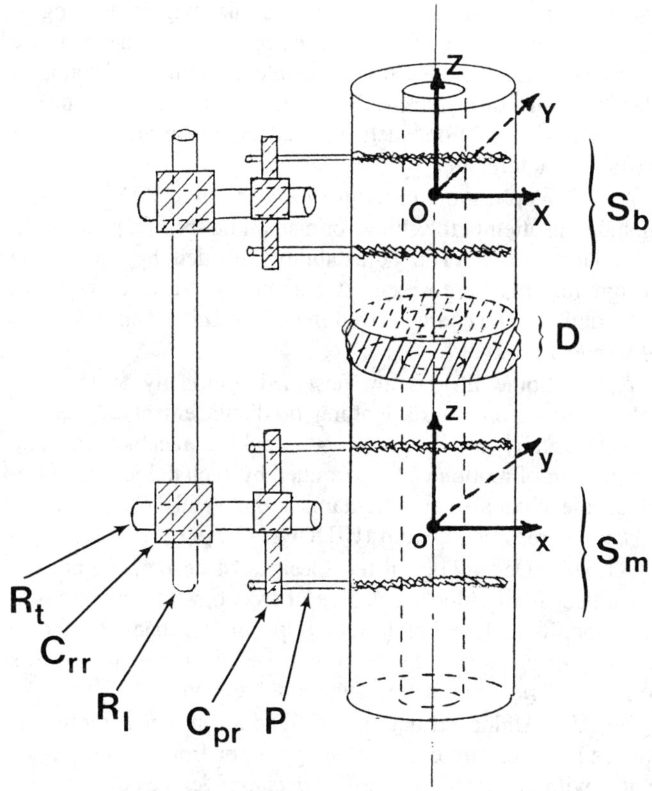

S_b	= base segment
S_m	= mobile segment
D	= mechanical defect
O	= origin of base reference frame
X, Y, and Z	= base reference frame axes
o	= origin of mobile reference frame
x, y, and z	= mobile reference frame axes
R_t	= transverse rod
R_L	= longitudinal rod
P	= pin
C_{rr}	= rod-rod connector
C_{pr}	= pin-rod connector

FIG. A1.1 External Fixator Definition Schematic

A1.5.5 A base coordinate system (X, Y, Z) should be affixed to one of the bones or major bone segments bordering the mechanical defect. This bone or bone segment is termed the *base segment,* S_b, and serves as a datum with respect to which pertinent motion(s) of bone segments or fixator elements, or both, can be referenced. Depending on context, S_b may be defined as being on either the proximal or the distal side of a mechanical defect.

A1.5.6 The other bone(s) or bone segment(s) bordering the mechanical defect, whose potential motion(s) with respect to S_b is of interest, is termed the *mobile segment(s),* S_m. If necessary, a local right-handed orthogonal coordinate system (x, y, z) may be embedded within the S_m(s).

A1.5.7 *Degrees of Freedom:*

Describing the position, or change in position, of S_m relative to S_b requires specifying one or more independent variables. These variables will be termed *positional degrees of freedom* (P-DOF).

A1.5.7.1 Depending on context, this may involve as many as six variables (three translation and three orientation).

A1.5.7.2 Also depending on context, P-DOFs may be used

to describe motions of interest in various magnitude ranges. For example, P-DOFs may be used to describe one or more components of visually imperceptible motion, for example, elastic flexure of a thick rod) or one or more components of grossly evident motion, such as, interfragmentary motion at an unstable fracture site.

A1.5.8 Application or adjustment of an ESFD normally includes an attempt to achieve or maintain a specific position of S_m relative to S_b. The adjustability afforded by the ESFD design for this purpose, most commonly, fracture fragment reduction, will be characterized in terms of *adjustment degrees of freedom* (A-DOF).

A1.5.9 Some ESFDs are designed optionally to transmit selected components of loading or displacement across the defect, usually by disengaging a locking mechanism. The component of motion of S_m permitted by such unlocking, often given the clinical name "dynamization," will be termed *unlocked* degrees of freedom (U-DOF).

A1.5.9.1 Depending on the specifics of design, the motion permitted in an unlocked degree of freedom may be opposed substantially and deliberately by a specific mechanism such as a spring or a cushion. Such an unlocked degree of freedom is termed a *resisted* unlocked degree of freedom.

A1.5.9.2 Unlocked degrees of freedom in which motion is induced actively by external energy input from devices associated with the fixator are termed *actuated* degrees of freedom.

A1.5.9.3 An unlocked degree of freedom in which motion is unopposed by a specific design mechanism is termed an *unresisted* unlocked degree of freedom. Incidental friction in a dynamizing element shall not be construed as representing deliberately resisted motion; however, conditions involving untoward resistance to motion, for example, substantial binding friction, in a supposedly unresisted degree of freedom should be identified.

A1.5.10 For adjustment or unlocked DOFs, the extrema of angular or translational displacement between which motion is permitted before encountering a fixed or adjustable constraint are termed that DOF's *range of motion* (ROM).

A1.5.11 A *fixator assembly* consists of a structurally purposeful arrangement of three basic types of *elements*: bone anchorage elements, usually transcutaneous, bridge elements, usually extracutaneous, and connection elements.

A1.5.12 *Anchorage elements* are those that attach directly to the bone. Examples are smooth pins, threaded pins, screws, wires, or cortex clamps.

A1.5.13 *Bridge elements* are structural members designed to transmit loads over relatively long distances, and they are joined to one another or to anchorage elements, or both, by connectors. Bridge elements can either be simple or complex and should be described in terms of their characteristic shape and, where appropriate, their orientation with respect to the bone or the mechanical defect.

A1.5.13.1 Examples of *simple bridge elements* are longitudinal rods, transverse rods, rings, or ring segments. Simple bridge elements need not be single-piece. If multipiece, however, the individual parts are joined rigidly rather than adjustable by the end user.

A1.5.13.2 *Complex bridge elements* are mechanisms that consist of two or more subelements designed to function together to achieve a specific kinematic objective. Examples of complex bridge elements are articulated or telescoping mechanisms.

A1.5.14 *Connectors* join bridge elements either to other bridge elements or to anchorage elements. Of the two elements comprising any joint or junction, the connector is that element to which the end user applies an active gripping force or torque to engage the attachment. Connectors should be described in terms of the types of elements that they connect and, where appropriate, in terms of their adjustment or unlocked degrees of freedom. Examples of connectors are pin(-rod) clamps, pin cluster(-rod) clamps, ring-rod clamps, and rod-rod clamps.

A1.5.15 That portion of the fixator assembly specifically excluding the bony anchorage elements and their associated connectors is termed the *frame*. Connectors that join only bridge elements, or that join bridge elements to bone anchors but are not user removable from bridge elements, are considered to be part of the frame.

A1.5.16 A joint or junction for which the relative positions between any two elements or subelements can be controlled by the end user is termed an *articulation*. The components of relative motion permitted between the fixator elements at an articulation should be described in terms of that articulation's degrees of freedom, either A-DOF or U-DOF, depending on context. Additionally, articulations should be described in terms of the types of elements that they connect.

A1.5.17 Joints at which the relative positions of the elements connected are fixed and cannot be controlled by the end user are termed *nonadjustable*. Nonadjustable joints should be described in terms of the types of elements that they connect.

A1.6 Attributes

A1.6.1 Coupling between the assembled frame and the host bone is achieved by anchorage elements such as wires, pins (threaded or unthreaded), screws, or cortex clamps (sometimes called claws or prongs). In long bone applications, anchorage elements normally transmit load transversely from the host bone segments to the frame structure.

A1.6.1.1 *Wires* are thin, smooth, constant cross-section (usually circular) anchorage elements that transmit load from the host bone to the frame primarily by axial tension as a result of transverse ("bow string") distention by the host bone; therefore, wires must transfix the bone and must be clamped to the frame at two sites. The stiffness of bone-frame coupling achieved using a wire depends sensitively on the tension in the wire, which normally is controlled by the end user. *Stoppers* ("olives") sometimes are used to oppose incidental slippage along the length of a transfixing wire.

A1.6.1.2 *Pins* are slender anchorage elements, again, usually of circular cross section or envelope, for which bone-to-frame load transmission occurs primarily by longitudinal bending stresses. Pins can penetrate one or (usually) both cortices of a long bone, and they can be clamped to the frame at one end ("half-pins") or both ends ("through-and-through pins" or "full-pins"). Pins can either be smooth or threaded. Threaded pins can be designed for achieving purchase in cortical bone, cancellous bone, or in a combination of the two. Pins can either be of constant cross section, shouldered, or tapered. They can be clamped to the frame either individually or in clusters. Depending on the flute or thread design, or both, pins can be classified as being one of the following:

(*1*) Self-drilling/self-tapping,

(*2*) Self-tapping/nonself-drilling, or

(*3*) Nonself-tapping/nonself-drilling.

A1.6.1.3 *Screws* are threaded anchorage elements, loaded primarily in axial tension or in transverse shear, or both. This term is sometimes (mis)used interchangeably as a descriptor for ESFD threaded pins, but it is reserved more properly for devices that have a head with a recess for wrenching (see Specification F 543 and Reference Chart F 544) and that are used to develop compression across a fracture site or across a bone/implant interface.

A1.6.1.4 *Cortex clamps* (claws/prongs) are anchors that grip the host bone externally at two or more sites, without penetrating through the full cortical thickness. Cortex clamps may or may not pierce the periosteum.

A1.6.2 Frame *bridge elements* are structural members configured in such a manner as to transmit functional load from the anchorage elements on one side of the mechanical defect to those on the other side of the defect. Bridge elements can be simple members such as smooth prismatic rods, threaded rods, bars, flat plates, curved plates, or arched plates. Alternatively, they can be complex assemblies of several members, designed to allow or induce specific motions such as fixed axis rotation, linear sliding, or active adjunct distraction. Most ESFD frames using simple bridge elements involve structural arrangements in which several simple bridge elements are linked to one another by connectors.

A1.6.3 *Fixator-Bone Construct Classifications*—Constructs may be classified in accordance with the anatomic skeletal structure to which the frame is applied. Common types are as follows:

A1.6.3.1 Long bone,

A1.6.3.2 Articular joint,

A1.6.3.3 Pelvis,

A1.6.3.4 Spinal, and

A1.6.3.5 Halo (skull).

A1.6.3.6 A *construct subunit* is one bony fragment plus its pins/wires and connectors and plus bridge elements not shared with other bony fragments.

A1.6.4 Long bone frames or frame subunits can be characterized in terms of limb access.

A1.6.4.1 Frames or frame subunits that encompass 90° or less of an extremity sector circumferentially are termed *unilateral*.

A1.6.4.2 Frames or frame subunits that encompass more than 90° of an extremity sector circumferentially are termed *multilateral*. Multilateral frames are often described in terms of their characteristic geometry: bilateral (two columns of longitudinal bridge elements), triangular (three longitudinal columns), quadrilateral (four columns), or circular (ring fixators).

A1.6.5 Long bone frames or frame subunits (unilateral or multilateral) can be classified according to pin configuration, as follows:

A1.6.5.1 As *one plane* if all of their pins lie approximately within a common plane,

A1.6.5.2 Or as *multiplane* if their pins lie in two or more distinct planes.

A1.6.6 Constructs may be classified in terms of the means by which the frame is coupled to the bone.

A1.6.6.1 A frame for which coupling to the bone is by a homogeneous group of primarily moment-transmitting anchors such as pins, screws, or cortex claws is termed a *pin-fixed* construct.

A1.6.6.2 If the coupling is by primarily tension-transmitting members instead, the construct is said to be *wire fixed.* The wire-fixed constructs involve ring-type bridge elements in almost all instances.

A1.6.6.3 If coupling involves a heterogeneous mixture of wires and pins (or screws or other anchorage elements, or both), the construct is said to incorporate *hybrid coupling*.

A1.6.7 Fixator constructs may be classified according to the degree of homology or similarity between the respective subunits.

A1.6.7.1 If the bone fragments on opposing sides of a mechanical defect are part of analogously assembled construct subunits, the overall fixator is said to be *symmetrically configured.* This does not imply strict geometric symmetry about the defect mid plane, but rather that each major element in each construct subunit possesses a similar counterpart in the other construct subunit.

A1.6.7.2 A construct whose subunits do not have such counterpart elements is said to have a *hybrid*, or *asymmetrically configured,* frame.

A1.6.8 Some pin-fixed constructs allow *independent control* of each pin's orientation and DOF of articulation with the frame. In other designs, *multipin clamps* are used to control the common orientation and DOF of frame articulation of a small group of pins termed a *pin cluster*. Pin cluster clamps most commonly enforce parallel alignment of the pins in the cluster. The specific A-DOF and U-DOF of pin/frame articulation in each instance, that is, either independent or clustered pins, depends on the design of the specific connecting element joining the pin(s) to the frame.

A1.6.9 *Ring fixators* have complex frames assembled from several transverse-plane ring or partial-ring bridge elements. The anchoring transfixation tensile wires are connected to the rings individually. Longitudinal rods normally are used to connect the transverse-plane rings.

A2. TEST METHOD FOR EXTERNAL SKELETAL FIXATOR CONNECTORS

A2.1 Scope

A2.1.1 This test method covers the procedures for determining the stiffness and strength of connecting elements (clamps) of external skeletal fixators under axial loads and bending moments. Depending on the design of the connector and its use in the overall construct, the connector needs to transmit one or more components of loading (tension, compression, torsion, or bending, or a combination thereof) between the elements it grips (anchorage elements or bridge elements), without itself undergoing either permanent deformation or excessive elastic deformation.

A2.1.2 *This standard does not purport to address all of the safety concerns, if any, associated with its use. It is the responsibility of the user of this standard to establish appropriate safety and health practices and determine the applicability of regulatory limitations prior to use.*

A2.2 Referenced Documents

A2.2.1 *ASTM Standards:*

E 4 Practices for Force Verification of Testing Machines[5]

A2.3. Terminology

A2.3.1 *Definitions of Terms Specific to This Standard:*

A2.3.1.1 *connectors, n*—external fixator elements used to join bridge elements either to other bridge elements, or to anchorage elements.

(1) Of the two elements comprising any joint or junction, the connector is that element to which the end user applies an active gripping force or torque to engage the attachment.

(2) Connectors should be described in terms of the types of elements, which they connect, and where appropriate, in terms of their adjustment or unlocked degrees of freedom.

(3) Examples of connectors are pin(-rod) clamps, pin cluster(-rod) clamps, ring-rod clamps, and rod-rod clamps.

A2.3.1.2 *input-loading axis, n*—the line of application in the case of a force input, or the axis about which a moment is applied in the case of a moment input.

A2.3.1.3 *input-loading platen, n*—a member, not normally part of the connector during clinical usage, through which the input force, or moment, is delivered from the testing machine actuator to the connector.

A2.3.1.4 *support platen, n*—a member, also not normally part of the connector during clinical usage, through which the connector is rigidly affixed to the testing machine base.

A2.4 Summary of Test Method

A2.4.1 Connecting elements (clamps) are obtained, and if applicable, assembled using the techniques and equipment recommended by the manufacturer. Platens substituting for the body, or anchorage elements, or both, are attached to the connector in such a manner that no slippage can occur relative to the connector. Axial loads or bending moments are applied to the connector, and a graphical plot of load (or moment) versus displacement is used to determine the intrinsic stiffness, and strength, if tested to failure, of the connector.

A2.5 Significance and Use

A2.5.1 These laboratory benchtop tests are used to determine values for the intrinsic stiffness, or strength, or both, of connectors, under force or moment loadings. Since different connectors have different materials and geometries, stresses within individual subcomponents or at subcomponent interfaces may differ substantially between designs. During testing, the connectors are loaded and supported in such a manner that all measured deformation occurs within the connector itself, rather than at the interface between the connector and the fixator element(s) gripped.

A2.5.2 The results obtained in this test method are not intended to predict the clinical efficacy or safety of the tested elements. This test method is intended only to measure the uniformity of the elements tested or to compare the mechanical performance of different connectors; however, the actual load that can be transmitted to the connector in clinical practice depends very much on the slippage resistance of the different subcomponent interfaces.

A2.5.3 This test method may not be appropriate for all types of external skeletal fixator applications. The user is cautioned to consider the appropriateness of the method in view of the materials and designs being tested and their potential application.

A2.6 Apparatus

A2.6.1 *Force or Moment or both Application Fixture:*

A2.6.1.1 The loading configuration is shown schematically in Fig. A2.1. The input loading axis must pass through one of the platens (the loading platen) rigidly affixed to the connector. The other platen (the support platen) is rigidly affixed to the base of the testing apparatus.

A2.6.2 *Load Frame*—Machines used for testing shall conform to the requirements of Practices E 4. The loads used for this test method shall be within the loading range of the test machine as defined in Practices E 4.

A2.6.3 *Data Acquisition Device*—A suitable recorder to plot a graph of load versus load frame displacement on prependicular axes. Optionally, this device may include the use of computer-based digital sampling and output of the load and displacement signals.

A2.7 Test Specimen

A2.7.1 All tested connectors should be representative of clinical quality products.

A2.7.2 If the connector(s) to be tested have been used previously, the nature of such prior usage should be described appropriately.

A2.7.3 The test specimens should be prepared in the manner in which they would normally be used clinically. For example, if a particular connector would normally be sterilized in a particular manner before clinical use, it should be similarly sterilized before mechanical testing.

A2.7.4 If the connector to be tested is a prototype, or under development, or both, the geometric and material information needed to characterize the component fully should either be

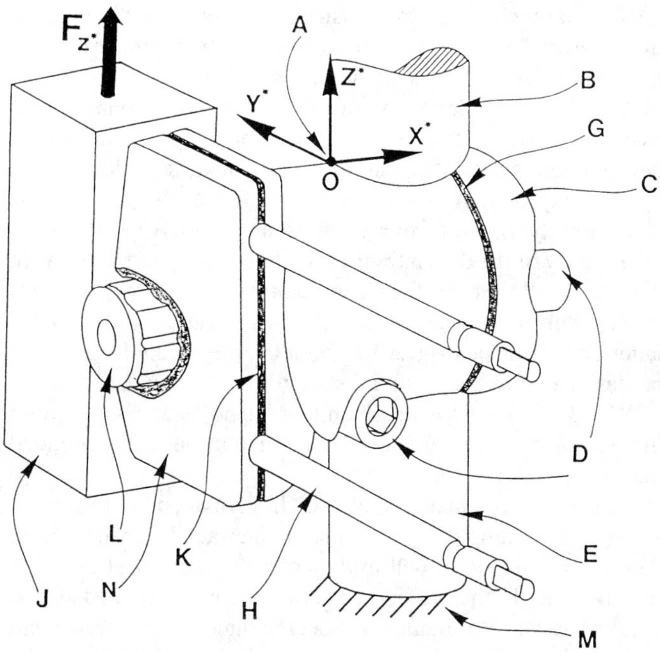

A = local coordinate system, defined with respect to landmark Point O
B = rod (as normally gripped by connector)
C = connector body
D = connector tightening mechanism(s)
E = rod grip platen (support platen)
G = rod grip interface
H = pins (as normally gripped by connector)
J = pin grip/clamp platen (loading input platen, rigidly bonded to pin grip)
K = pin clamping interface
L = pin grip/clamp tightening mechanism
M = testing machine base (fixed)
N = pin grip/clamp (in this illustration, the input loading is a force Fz^* in the z^* direction, delivered through a loading platen rigidly affixed to the pin grip/clamp. δ_z is the displacement of the loading platen in the z direction

FIG. A2.1 Schematic for Testing an External Fixator Connector (Example, Generic for a Pin-Rod Joint)

included in the report, or detailed descriptive information should be referenced.

A2.8 Procedure

A2.8.1 *Configuring the Connecting Element for Testing:*

A2.8.1.1 With the connecting element assembled in the configuration normally used, input and support platens are affixed in a manner that insures that all measured deformations are intrinsic to the connecting element itself and are not influenced by possible interfacial slippage between the connecting element and the fixator elements, for example, rods or anchorage pins, which it clamps.

(1) The input and support platens should made of steel or other metal and should have negligible compliance relative to that of the connecting element itself.

(2) The input and support platens should have recesses to accommodate those fixator elements geometrically, for example, anchorage pins or rods, normally clamped by the connecting element being tested.

(3) The input and support platens should be rigidly affixed to the connecting element, for example, by welding, epoxy, cyanoacrylate cement, or other appropriate means.

A2.8.1.2 The input and support platens serve as attachments for gripping by the testing apparatus. This test method is applicable only to those components of loading (force or moment, or both), which can be applied through such platens.

A2.8.1.3 A local right-handed coordinate system (X^*,Y^*,Z^*) should be defined with respect to a specific origin landmark point on (or in) the connecting element. The platen locations (position and orientation) should be identified relative to these local coordinate axes.

A2.8.2 *Mounting the Test Connector*:

A2.8.2.1 The platen through which the input force (or moment) is to be applied is gripped, appropriately aligned, in the testing machine. The support platen is rigidly affixed to the testing machine base.

A2.8.2.2 The grips and the testing machine itself should be sufficiently stiff that their deformation under load is negligible relative to that of the connecting element being tested. The tare compliance of the testing machine and grips, that is, without the connector mounted, should be measured and reported. Typically, the tare compliance of the testing machine plus grips should be less than 1 % of the compliance of the connector being tested. The gripping mechanism should be clearly described.

A2.8.3 Forces should be delivered through an input platen, which is rigidly bonded to the connector. Normally, the axis of loading will be referenced to that of a member, such as a rod or a pin, that would be clamped by the connector. The line of action of the input force should be recorded relative to the local coordinate system. Appropriate fixturing detail should be provided as to how that force is applied through the input platen.

A2.8.4 Moments may be delivered either by an eccentrically applied force, or alternatively, by a torsional actuator. In the former instance, the offset from the local coordinate system origin should be recorded. In either instance, the orientation of the moment axis should be recorded relative to the local coordinate system. Appropriate fixturing detail should be provided as to how that moment is applied through the input platen.

A2.8.5 For connectors made entirely of metal or other materials exhibiting elastic behavior, the load (or moment) may be applied quasistatically. An input rate sufficient to attain in 30-s force, or moment, magnitude in the range of typical clinical usage, or of connector failure, shall be deemed quasistatic. For connectors incorporating polymeric or other materials that exhibit viscoelastic behavior, load/stroke rates, which are in the range of those expected clinically, may instead be desirable. In either case, the rate(s) used and a rationale for its choice should be provided.

A2.8.6 Tests may be run under either load or displacement control. They may either be single- or multi-cycle, and can be either restricted to the elastic regime, or taken to failure of the connector. The specific conditions used should be described fully.

A2.8.7 If single-cycle testing is to be performed, the specimen must be subjected to several preconditioning load cycles to demonstrate that the reported load/deformation curve is repeatable from cycle to cycle.

A2.8.7.1 Preconditioning should be continued until the apparent stiffness of the connector changes less than 5 % between subsequent cycles.

A2.8.7.2 Normally, about five preconditioning load cycles are suitable for this purpose, with peak applied load within the elastic range, approximately 50 % of the expected physiologic service load or 50 % of the expected connector failure load, whichever is lower.

A2.8.7.3 Load/deformation curves for the preconditioning cycles should be recorded. Preconditioning cycle stiffnesses should be reported.

A2.8.8 *Data Recording*—The load (N) or torque (N-m) and linear (mm) or angular (°) displacement measured by the testing machine should be continuously recorded. The linear displacement should be measured at the point of load application. In some instances it may be appropriate also to record components of deformation in directions other than that of the applied loading. If so, the sensors used, for example, dial gages or LVDTs, and the points and directions of their measured deformations should be recorded.

A2.9 Calculation or Interpretation of Results

A2.9.1 Stiffness (units according to the chosen load and deflection configuration, for example, N/mm for force, N-mm/degree for moment) shall be calculated from the slope of the linear-most portion of the load/deflection curve, as apparent visually (Fig. A2.2, Point A). If an objective slope determination technique, for example, curve fitting of a digitized tracing, is used, this should be described. The load and deflection

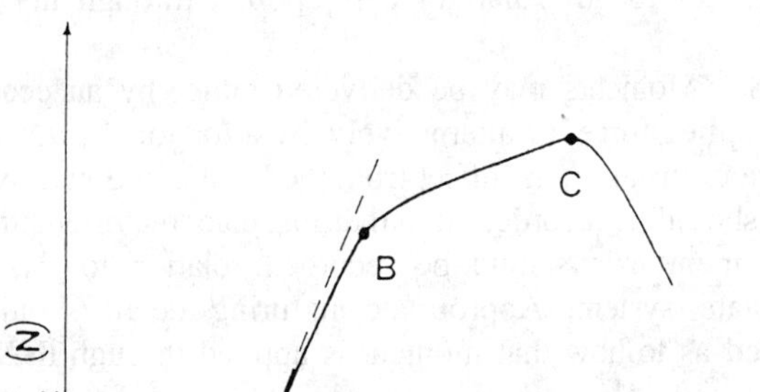

NOTE—Stiffness is defined as the slope of the linear-most portion of the curve, here evaluated by a tangent drawn at Point A. Point B illustrates a slope discontinuity (possibly indicative of interfacial slip or subcomponent failure within the connector), and Point C illustrates the maximal load acceptance (ultimate strength).

FIG. A2.2 Load/Deformation Curve (Generic, Here Illustrated for the z* Direction)

configuration (location of measuring element and direction of the measured vector) must be defined clearly with respect to the loading axis of the testing equipment (Fig. A2.1).

A2.9.2 Failure load (N or N-mm) of the connector is associated frequently with a discontinuity in the load/deformation curve. Depending on context, additional load uptake may or may not be possible after occurrence of this discontinuity. In the former circumstance (Fig. A2.2, Point B), the severity of the discontinuity should be measured in terms of change in slopes of the load/deformation curve for loads immediately below and above the discontinuity point. In the latter circumstance (Fig. A2.2, Point C), the failure load should be designated as the ultimate strength of the connector.

A2.9.3 In situations in which there is no clear discontinuity in the load displacement curve, other definitions of failure load may be used.

A2.9.3.1 For situations in which permanent deformation occurs, for example, as a result of interfacial slip or plastic deformation, or both, within the connector, an offset criterion may be used. In this instance, the failure load is defined as that load necessary to induce a specific amount of permanent deformation, either linear or angular, depending upon the degree of freedom being tested, upon release of the applied load.

A2.9.3.2 For situations in which excessive elastic deformation occurs within the connector, failure may be defined in terms of a specific fractional reduction of the connector's small-load stiffness. For example, failure might be defined in terms of the connector's tangent stiffness having fallen to 25 % of the tangent stiffness that was apparent at a load of 50 N.

A2.10 Report

A2.10.1 The test report shall include, but is not limited to, the following information:

A2.10.1.1 *Connecting Element Identification*, including manufacturer, part number, nomenclature, and quality control or lot number. If the part is a prototype, geometrical and material descriptions shall be included.

A2.10.1.2 Specimen preparation condition, for example, sterilization and description of prior usage history, if applicable.

A2.10.1.3 Connecting force or torque used to engage the connector's gripping mechanism.

A2.10.1.4 Configuration of the (bonded) platens and testing apparatus grips.

A2.10.1.5 Specific degrees of freedom tested, such as, tension or compression, torsion, or bending. In each case, the axis along which or about which loading is applied should be specified.

A2.10.1.6 Loading rate and number of cycles (fatigue tests).

A2.10.1.7 Stiffness, and, if loaded to failure, the failure criterion and strength, in the specific direction(s) tested.

A2.10.1.8 In cases in which the mode of failure is ascertainable, for example, visually apparent interfacial slippage of a specific subcomponent interface, the nature of such failure should be described.

A2.11 Precision and Bias

A2.11.1 Data establishing the precision and bias to be

expected from this test method have not yet been obtained.

12. Keywords

12.1 bending moments; connecting elements; connectors; external fixator; orthopedic device; stiffness; strength

A2.13 Rationale

A2.13.1 Connecting elements of various designs are used widely in external fixators. Both the elements connected and the pertinent directions of force, or moment, or both, transmission through them are design and site specific. This test method provides an outline by which the stiffness, or strength, or both, intrinsic to the connector itself, as opposed to the stiffness or strength by which it grips the elements it connects, can be measured. Since the joints of external fixators normally involve abrupt redirection of appreciable loads, substantial stresses often are developed within one or more of the subcomponents of the connector securing the joint.

A2.13.2 Even if there is no apparent interfacial slippage between the connector and the various bridge or anchorage elements it grips, the associated elastic deformations within the connector body itself may result in appreciable distension of the overall frame. Moreover, excessive forces, or more commonly, moments, applied to a connector may cause destructive failure of the connector body, even if gripped interfaces remain intact. This test method focuses on the intrinsic load/deformation behavior of the connector body, independent of whether or not there is interfacial slip between the connector and the bridge or anchorage elements, or both, which it grips. This goal is achieved by means of platens, which are bonded rigidly to the connector.

A3. TEST METHOD FOR DETERMINING IN-PLANE COMPRESSIVE PROPERTIES OF CIRCULAR RING OR RING SEGMENT BRIDGE ELEMENTS

A3.1 Scope

A3.1.1 This test method covers the test procedure for determining the in-plane compressive properties of circular or ring segment bridge elements of external skeletal fixators.

A3.1.2 *This standard does not purport to address all of the safety concerns, if any, associated with its use. It is the responsibility of the user of this standard to establish appropriate safety and health practices and determine the applicability of regulatory limitations prior to use.*

A3.2 Referenced Documents

A3.2.1 *ASTM Standards:*

E 4 Practices for Force Verification of Testing Machines[4]

A3.3. Terminology

A3.3.1 *Definitions of Terms Specific to This Standard:*

A3.3.1.1 *circular ring bridge element, n*—an external skeletal fixator component as described in Annex A1, which is circular, or may be assembled from several components to form a circular element, lies in a single plane, and has one center or curvature.

A3.3.1.2 *ring segment bridge element, n*—an external skeletal fixator component as described in Annex A1, which consists of a single ring segment, or is assembled from several components to form a ring segment, lies in a single plane, has one center of curvature, and whose arc spans 180° or more, but less than 360°.

A3.3.1.3 *test component, n*—a complete or assembled *circular ring bridge element* or *ring segment bridge element* prepared for testing according to A3.8.1 and A3.8.2.

A3.4 Summary of Test Method

A3.4.1 Complete circular ring elements (either a single component or an assembly of components to form a complete circular ring) or a ring segment (≥180° arc) are obtained for testing. In-plane compressive forces are applied quasistatically to the circular ring or ring segment, so that the load application points are 180° apart, measured along the arc of the ring. If appropriate, load is increased until part failure occurs. A graphical plot of load versus displacement is used to determine in-plane compressive strength and stiffness.

A3.5 Significance and Use

A3.5.1 This test method is used to measure the compressive strength and stiffness of circular ring or ring segment bridge elements of external skeletal fixators when loaded in the plane of the ring. The results obtained in this test are not intended to predict the clinical efficacy or safety of the tested products. This test method is intended only to measure the uniformity of the products tested or to compare the mechanical properties of different products.

A3.5.2 This test method may not be appropriate for all types of fixator applications. The user is cautioned to consider the appropriateness of the method in view of the materials being tested and their potential application.

A3.6 Apparatus

A3.6.1 *Pin and Clevis Fixture*—A U-shaped metal lug ("clevis") with a hole drilled across both legs of the "U" to accommodate a clearance fit steel pin. The opposite end of the Clevis is attached to the grip of the load frame. The pin diameter should be of the approximate size of the holes in the test components, if applicable; or, if a hole must be drilled for testing, the pin shall be no greater than half the width of the test component at the point of load application.

A3.6.2 *Shims*—Metallic flat washers of varying specified thickness, which will fit over the pin and between the sides of the clevis and the test component.

A3.6.3 *Torquemeter*—An electronic, or mechanical device, or both, which is capable of measuring torque applied to a screw or bolt.

A3.6.4 *Load Frame*—Machines used for testing shall conform to the requirements of Practices E 4. The loads used for the test shall be within the loading range of the test machine as defined in Practices E 4.

A3.6.5 *Recording Device*—A suitable recorder to plot a

graph of load versus load frame displacement on perpendicular axes.

A3.7 Test Specimen

A3.7.1 All test components, including connection components, shall be representative of clinical quality products.

A3.7.2 If one or more of the elements to be tested has been used previously, the nature of such prior usage should be appropriately described.

A3.7.3 The test component, when assembled (if applicable), shall form a full or partial ring in a single plane, with a single center of curvature.

A3.7.4 The test specimens should be prepared in the manner in which they normally would be used clinically. For example, if components, particularly polymeric rings or ring segments, normally would be sterilized in a particular manner before use, they should be sterilized similarly before mechanical testing.

A3.8 Procedure

A3.8.1 *Constructing the Test Component*—Some ring external fixation systems may fit into both the circular ring and ring segment descriptions in A3.8.1.1 and A3.8.1.2, depending on how many components are assembled. The two types are discussed separately here to be congruent with the separate descriptions given in Annex A1. The user must consider the appropriateness of the two test component options in view of the materials being tested, their potential application, and the manufacturer's recommendations.

A3.8.1.1 *Circular Ring Bridge Element*—For circular ring bridge elements, which are not a complete circle, the individual arcs or segments must be joined together to form a single circular ring. The arcs or segments shall be jointed using the equipment, for example, nut and bolts, recommended by the manufacturer. For screw or bolted connections, the tightening torque recommended by the manufacturer shall be applied using a torque wrench. If a recommended torque value is not available, a sufficient torque shall be chosen by the user, and then used for all components.

A3.8.1.2 *Ring Segment Bridge Elements*—For ring segments whose arc spans less than 180°, individual arcs or segments must be joined together to form a ring segment that spans more than 180° but less than 360°. The arcs or segments shall be joined using the equipment, for example, nut and bolts, recommended by the manufacturer. For screw or bolted connections, the tightening torque recommended by the manufacturer shall be applied using a torque wrench. If a recommended torque value is not available, a sufficient torque shall be chosen by the user, and then used for all components.

A3.8.2 *Preparing the Test Component*—The test component must have two holes that are positioned 180° from each other, as measured along the arc of the ring, for introduction of the load. For rings with holes provided by the manufacturer, two holes must be chosen that are 180° apart. For rings without two properly positioned holes, holes may be drilled through the test component. The diameter of the hole shall be less than one half of the width of the test component at the drilling location. If the test component is constructed from ring segments, the critical joint, as determined by the user, shall be 90° from the two loading holes.

A3.8.3 *Mounting the Test Component*—The two clevis fixtures shall be secured to the upper and lower grips of the load frame. The test component shall be inserted into the clevis fixture so that the loading holes are aligned with the clevis holes. A clearance-fit pin will be inserted through the clevis and through the test component, securing the test component to the upper and lower fixtures. As necessary, shims will be inserted between the sides of the clevis and the test components to insure that the test component is centered in the clevis and to reduce the lateral movement of the test component on the pin. The diameter of the shims must be less than the width of the test component at the loading hole location. The total lateral movement of the test component in the clevis shall be less than 0.5 mm. An example test setup of a circular ring bridge element, constructed from two 180° ring segments bolted together, is shown in Fig. A3.1. An example test setup of a single ring segment bridge element is shown in Fig. A3.2.

A3.8.4 *Data Recording*—The load (N) and displacement (mm) measured by the testing machine shall be recorded on the recording device. The displacement is measured at the point of load application.

A3.8.5 *Load Application*—An increasing compressive load shall be applied to the test component. Either load or stroke control may be used. It is recognized that no specific rate is applicable to all situations. For rings or ring segments comprised entirely of metal or other elastic materials, quasistatic loading may be applied. In this context, a quasistatic input loading rate should be interpreted as being sufficient to attain in approximately 30 s a load magnitude in the range of typical clinical usage or a load sufficient to cause ring or ring segment failure, whichever is lower. For rings or ring segments containing polymeric or other materials exhibiting viscoelastic behavior, load/stroke rates, which are in the range of those expected clinically, may be desirable. In either case, the rate(s) of loading and the rationale for its choice should be specified.

A3.8.6 If tested to failure, the load application shall continue until a peak load is observed on the load displacement

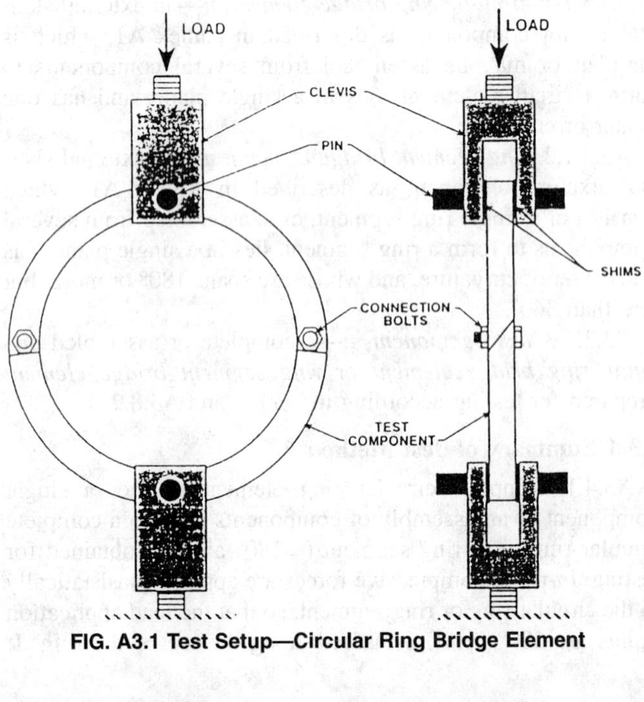

FIG. A3.1 Test Setup—Circular Ring Bridge Element

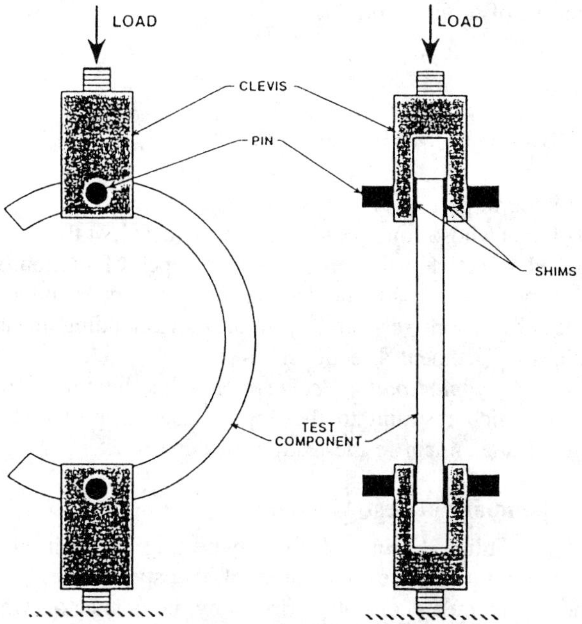

FIG. A3.2 Test Setup—Ring Segment Bridge Element

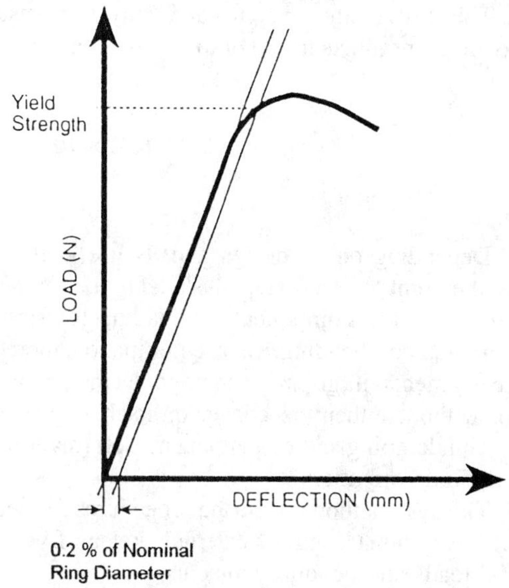

FIG. A3.3 Secant Offset Method

curve or until the load reaches a near constant value while significant irrecoverable deformation, typically 10 % of the nominal ring diameter, has occurred.

A3.8.7 *Test Component Examination*—After the test is complete, visual examination of the test component shall be made to determine the location and mode of failure of the test component.

A3.9 Calculation or Interpretation of Results

A3.9.1 *In-Plane Compressive Stiffness*—The in-plane compressive stiffness (N/mm) of the test component shall be determined from the maximum slope of the initial portion of the load-displacement curve.

A3.9.2 *In-Plane Compressive Yield Strength*—The in-plane compressive yield strength (N) of the component shall be determined from the load-displacement curve, using the secant-offset method shown in Fig. A3.3. A permanent deflection of 0.2 % of the nominal ring diameter is defined as yield.

A3.9.3 *In-Plane Maximum Compressive Strength*—The in-plane maximum compressive strength (N) of the test component shall be determined from the load-displacement curve, and is the maximum load (N) reached during the test, or the load level at which the component achieves a deflection of 10 % of the nominal ring diameter.

A3.10 Report

A3.10.1 The test report shall include the following information:

A3.10.1.1 *Ring Bridge Element Identification*, including manufacturer, part number(s), quality control or lot number(s), nominal size, element width and element thickness. For assembled components, a description of the connection method and components, and the final construct form and geometry is required.

A3.10.1.2 *Connection Torque*—Torque used on screws or bolts for connection, if applicable.

A3.10.1.3 Material composition and surface finish.

A3.10.1.4 *Load Pin Description*—Diameter of load pin used and explanation of whether holes were drilled in the test component for loading.

A3.10.1.5 In-plane compressive stiffness.

A3.10.1.6 In-plane compressive yield strength.

A3.10.1.7 *In-Plane Compressive Maximum Strength*—Identify whether the strength is determined from a maximum value or from when the load produced a deflection of 10 % of the nominal ring diameter.

A3.10.1.8 *Failure Mode and Location*—Identify the location of failure, for example, ring hole connection bolt, and the mode of failure, for example, yielding, localized buckling, interface slip, and so forth.

A3.11 Precision and Bias

A3.11.1 Data establishing the precision and bias to be expected from this test method have not yet been obtained.

12. Keywords

12.1 compression; external fixator; in-plane loading; ring element

A3.13 Rationale

A3.13.1 Circular ring and ring segment bridge elements commonly are found in commercial external skeletal fixators. They may consist of a single ring, two, or more ring segments connected to form a circular ring, or as individual ring segments. In clinical use, circular ring and ring segment bridge elements are subjected to a wide variety of loads, including in-plane compression. The in-plane compression loads are due primarily to tensioned wires connected from one side of the bridge element to the other.

A3.13.2 This test specification provides a relatively simple method to determine the in-plane compressive properties of single or joined-together circular ring or ring segment bridge elements. The results obtained in this test method are not intended to predict the clinical efficacy or safety of the tested products. This test method is intended only to measure the uniformity of the products tested or to compare the mechanical properties of different products.

A4. TEST PROCEDURE FOR EXTERNAL SKELETAL FIXATOR JOINTS

A4.1 Scope

A4.1.1 Depending on its design and its use in the overall construct, the joint of an external skeletal fixator needs to transmit one or more components of loading (tension, compression, torsion, or bending, or a combination thereof) between the elements it grips (anchorage elements or bridge elements), without either the connector itself or its gripping interface(s) undergoing either permanent deformation or excessive elastic deformation.

A4.1.2 This test method covers the procedures for determining the stiffness and strength of external skeletal fixator joints under axial loads and bending moments.

A4.1.3 This document also covers procedures for determining the range of adjustability in degrees of freedom for which the joint's configuration can be adjusted by the user and procedures for determining the joint's range of motion in degrees of freedom for which motion is permitted if the fixator is unlocked.

A4.1.4 *This standard does not purport to address all of the safety concerns, if any, associated with its use. It is the responsibility of the user of this standard to establish appropriate safety and health practices and determine the applicability of regulatory limitations prior to use.*

A4.2 Referenced Documents

A4.2.1 *ASTM Standards:*

E 4 Practices for Force Verification of Testing Machines[4]

A4.3. Terminology

A4.3.1 *Definitions of Terms Specific to This Standard:*

A4.3.1.1 *connector, n*—of the two (or more) elements comprising any joint or junction, the connector is that element to which the end user applies an active gripping force or torque to engage the attachment.

A4.3.1.2 *hysteresis, n—for cyclic loading,* the unity minus the ratio of energy recovered (during load release) to energy input (during load uptake).

A4.3.1.3 *input loading axis, n*—the line of application in the case of a force input or the axis about which a moment is applied in the case of a moment input.

A4.3.1.4 *input loading element, n*—that fixator element, for example, pins, rod, gripped by the joint, through which the applied force or moment loading is transmitted to the joint.

A4.3.1.5 *joint, n*—an external skeletal fixator subassembly consisting of a connecting element and one or more bridge or anchorage elements gripped by that connector. Bridge, anchorage, and connection elements are as defined in Annex A1.

(*1*) *Joints* should be described in terms of the types of elements that they connect, and where appropriate, in terms of their adjustment or unlocked degrees of freedom.

(*2*) Examples of joints are a pin/rod articulation, a pin-cluster/rod articulation, a ring/rod articulation, and a rod/rod articulation, in each case with the connector being considered as an integral part of the articulation.

(*3*) Joints whose configuration can be adjusted, or that can be unlocked selectively to permit specific types of motion, are said to possess adjustment degrees of freedom or unlocked degrees of freedom, respectively, in the corresponding linear or angular displacement directions.

A4.3.1.6 *output loading element, n*—that fixator element through which restraint to the applied load is provided, by means of attachment to the testing machine base.

A4.4 Summary of Test Method

A4.4.1 Unlike testing of the connecting element alone, testing a joint requires inclusion of the specific bridge or anchorage elements, or both, gripped by the connector, which in principle may slip with respect to the connector during load uptake.

A4.4.2 Connecting elements (clamps) are obtained, and if applicable, assembled using the techniques and equipment recommended by the manufacturer.

A4.4.3 Axial loads or bending moments are applied to the joint through one of the gripped elements, and a graphical plot of load (or moment) versus displacement is used to determine the effective stiffness (and strength, if tested to failure) of the joint.

A4.4.4 For range of adjustability/motion assessment, the joint is unlocked, and quasistatic linear or angular displacements are input until encountering a discontinuous increase in resisting force or moment, indicative of the limit of adjustability or motion of the joint in the particular degree of freedom considered.

A4.5 Significance and Use

A4.5.1 These laboratory tests are used to determine values for the effective stiffness, or strength, or both, of an external fixator joint, under force or moment loadings.

A4.5.1.1 The deformations accruing under loading consist of elastic deformation in the clamp body itself, plus any deformation, especially, slip, occurring at the interface between the clamp and the gripped element(s).

A4.5.1.2 Where appropriate, the joint's range of adjustability, or its range of motion when "dynamized," or both, also are measured.

A4.5.2 The results obtained in this test method are not intended to predict the clinical efficacy or safety of the tested elements. This test method is intended only to measure the uniformity of the elements tested or to compare the mechanical performance of different joints.

A4.5.3 This test method may not be appropriate for all types of external skeletal fixator applications. The user is cautioned to consider the appropriateness of the method in view of the materials and designs being tested and their potential application.

A4.6 Apparatus

A4.6.1 *Force, or Moment (or Both) Application Fixture*:

A4.6.1.1 The loading configuration is shown schematically in Fig. A4.1. The loading input axis must pass through the input loading element, that is, the bridge or anchorage element, gripped by the connector.

A4.6.1.2 Gripping of the input loading element by the testing apparatus should be at a site as close as possible to the body of the connector so as to minimize elastic flexure in the loading input element itself.

A4.6.1.3 Restraint is provided either by rigidly affixing the body of the connector to the testing machine base, in which case the only (potential slippage) interface included in the loading path is that between the loading input element and the connector body; or, by rigidly affixing another of the gripped elements, termed the loading output element, to the testing machine base, again, gripping as closely as possible to the connector. In this case, two potential slip interfaces are included in the loading path. An example of the input loading element and output loading element is shown in Fig. A4.1.

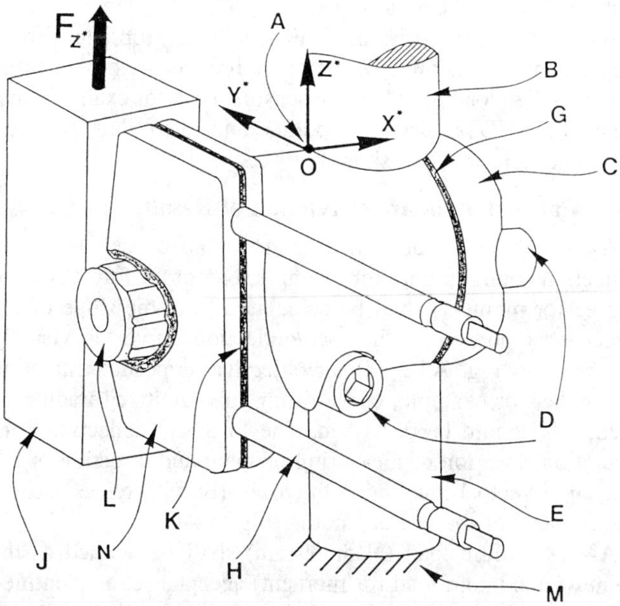

A = local coordinate system, defined with respect to landmark Point O
B = rod (as normally gripped by connector)
C = connector body
D = connector tightening mechanism(s)
E = output loading element (here, a rod gripped by the connector and rigidly affixed to the test machine base)
G = rod grip interface
H = pins (as normally gripped by connector)
J = loading platen, clamped to pins (the input loading element) as closely as possible to the site of connector gripping
K = pin clamping interface
L = pin grip/clamp tightening mechanism
M = testing machine base (fixed)
N = pin grip/clamp (in this illustration, the input loading is a force Fz^* in the z^* direction, delivered through an input platen clamped to the input loading element (the pins). δ_z is the corresponding displacement of the input platen in the *z* direction

FIG. A4.1 Schematic for Testing an External Fixator Joint (Example, Generic for a Pin-Rod Joint)

A4.6.2 *Load Frame*—Machines used for testing shall conform to the requirements of Practices E 4. The loads used for the test shall be within the loading range of the test machine as defined in Practices E 4.

A4.6.3 *Data Acquisition Device*—A suitable recorder to plot a graph of load versus load frame displacement on perpendicular axes.

A4.7 Test Specimen

A4.7.1 All tested elements should be representative of clinical quality products.

A4.7.2 If one or more of the elements to be tested has been used previously, the nature of such prior usage should be described appropriately.

A4.7.3 The test specimens should be prepared in the manner in which they normally would be used clinically. For example, if a particular joint normally would be sterilized in a particular manner before use, it should be sterilized similarly before mechanical testing.

A4.7.4 If the elements to be tested are prototypes, or are under development, or both, the geometric and material information needed to characterize fully all such elements should either be included in the report or detailed descriptive information should be referenced.

A4.8 Procedure

A4.8.1 *Assembling the Joint to Be Tested*:

A4.8.1.1 The input loading element, and, if appropriate, the output loading element, should be clamped by the connecting element according to the manufacturer's instructions. In situations in which this clamping force, or torque, is discretional, the magnitude of the applied tightening force, or torque, should be measured and recorded since this may affect interface slip.

A4.8.1.2 The input and output loading elements serve as attachments for gripping by the testing apparatus. This test method is applicable only to those components of loading (force or moment, or both), which can be applied through such elements.

A4.8.1.3 A local right-handed coordinate system (X^*, Y^*, Z^*) should be defined with respect to a specific origin landmark point on, or in, the connecting element. The input and output loading element locations (position and orientation) should be identified relative to these local coordinate axes.

A4.8.2 *Mounting the Joint to Be Tested*:

A4.8.2.1 The input loading element is gripped, appropriately aligned, in the testing machine. Restraint is applied by rigidly gripping and attaching to the testing machine base either the connecting element body or the output loading element (see A4.6.1.3).

A4.8.2.2 The test specimen should be mounted in such a manner that there is no discontinuity of the load/deformation curve as a result of shifting or settling of the specimen in the testing machine grip(s) during load uptake.

A4.8.2.3 The grips should be sufficiently stiff that their deformation under load is negligible relative to that of the joint being tested. Normally, the tare compliance (testing machine + grips) should be less than 1 % of the compliance of the joint being tested. The gripping mechanism should be described clearly, and its tare stiffness measured and reported.

A4.8.3 *Stiffness or Strength Testing*:

A4.8.3.1 Forces should be delivered through a platen rigidly affixed to the input loading element. Normally, the axis of joint loading will be referenced to that of an element, such as a rod or a pin, that would be clamped at the joint. The line of action of the input force should be recorded relative to the local coordinate system.

A4.8.3.2 Moments may be delivered either by an eccentrically applied force couple or, alternatively, by a torsional actuator. In the former instance, the offset from the local coordinate system origin should be recorded. In either instance, the orientation of the moment axis should be recorded relative to the local coordinate system.

A4.8.3.3 Appropriate fixturing detail should be provided as to how the input force or moment is applied to the input loading element by the testing machine actuator.

A4.8.3.4 It is recognized that no specific loading rate is applicable to all situations. For joints comprised entirely of metal or other materials exhibiting elastic behavior, the load (or moment) may be applied quasistatically. An input rate sufficient to attain in 30 s a force, or moment, magnitude in the range of typical clinical usage, or of joint failure, shall be deemed quasistatic. For joints incorporating polymeric or other materials that exhibit viscoelastic behavior, load/stroke rates, which are in the range of those expected clinically, may instead be desirable. In either case, the rate(s) used and the rationale for its choice should be provided.

A4.8.3.5 Stiffness or strength tests may be run under either load or displacement control. They may either be single- or multi-cycle and may be either restricted to the elastic regime, or taken to the point in which one of the interfaces slips, or the connector body destructively fails. The specific conditions used should be described fully.

A4.8.3.6 If single-cycle testing is to be performed, the specimen must be subjected to several preconditioning load cycles to demonstrate that the reported load/deformation curve is repeatable from cycle to cycle. Preconditioning should be continued until the apparent stiffness of the joint changes less than 5 % between subsequent cycles. Normally, about five preconditioning load cycles are suitable for this purpose, with peak applied load within the elastic range, approximately 50 % of the expected physiologic service load or 50 % of the expected joint failure load, whichever is lower. Load/deformation curves for the preloading cycles should be recorded. Preconditioning cycle stiffnesses should be reported.

A4.8.3.7 If multicycle testing is to be performed, load deformation curves also must be recorded for at least the first five cycles during test startup. As stated in A4.8.3.6, apparent stiffness values should be reported for each of these cycles. The number of cycles needed to reach the point at which apparent stiffness changes less than 1 % should be noted.

A4.8.3.8 The severity of hysteresis in each of these preconditioning cycles, and in the testing cycle(s), also should be reported. These energy values for hysteresis correspond to the areas under the respective load/deformation curves. The areas under the load/deformation curves may be determined by graphical integration, by numerical integration, or by other appropriate technique.

A4.8.4 *Range of Adjustability or Range of Motion Tests*:

A4.8.4.1 These tests should be run under displacement control since there may be negligible resisting force, or moment, over the permitted range of travel.

A4.8.4.2 These tests should be run quasistatically. In this context, quasistatic linear or angular displacement input should be interpreted as a displacement rate sufficient to cause the joint to reach the extrema of its permitted adjustment or motion range in approximately 30 s.

A4.8.4.3 The test should terminate when there is an abrupt increase in the force (or moment) developed to resist the input linear (or angular) displacement.

A4.8.5 *Data Recording*:

A4.8.5.1 The load (N) or torque (N-m) and linear (mm) or angular (°) displacement measured by the testing machine should be continuously recorded by a data acquisition device. Alternatively, a digital recording and display device can be used, operating at a sampling rate sufficiently fast to capture accurately any discontinuities in the load/deformation curve accompanying subcomponent failure or interface slippage.

A4.8.5.2 The linear displacement should be measured at the point of load application.

A4.8.5.3 In some instances, it may be appropriate also to record components of deformation in directions other than that of the applied loading. If so, the sensors used, for example, dial gages or LVDTs, and the points and directions of their measured deformations should be recorded.

A4.9 Calculation or Interpretation of Results

A4.9.1 Stiffness (units according to the chosen load and deflection configuration, for example, N/mm for force, N-mm/degree for moment) shall be calculated from the slope of the linear-most portion of the load/deflection curve, as visually apparent (in Fig. A4.2). If an objective slope determination technique, for example, curve-fitting of a digitized tracing, is used, this should be described. The load and deflection configuration (location of measuring element and direction of the measured vector) must be defined clearly with respect to the loading axis of the test apparatus (Fig. A4.1).

A4.9.2 Failure load (N or N-mm) shall be defined as the point of maximum load (or moment) acceptance, as identified by a discontinuity in the load/deformation curve.

A4.9.2.1 In situations in which there is no clear discontinuity in the load displacement curve, other definitions of failure load may be used. For situations in which interfacial slip, or plastic, deformation, or both, occurs within the joint, an offset criterion may be used. In this instance, the failure load is defined as that load necessary to induce a specific amount of permanent deformation (either linear or angular, depending upon the degree of freedom being tested), upon release of the applied load. For situations in which excessive elastic deformation occurs within the joint, failure may be defined in terms of a specific fractional reduction of the joint's small-load stiffness. For example, failure might be defined in terms of the joint's tangent stiffness having fallen to 25 % of the tangent stiffness that was apparent at a load to 50 N.

A4.9.3 The range of adjustability or motion in a specific degree of freedom shall be defined as that linear or angular displacement value at which the joint develops an abrupt

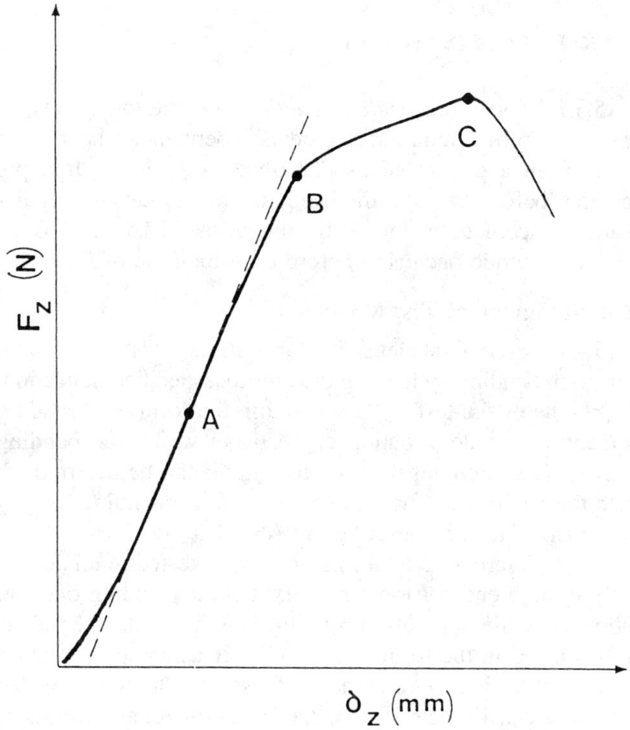

NOTE—Stiffness is defined as the slope of the linear-most portion of the curve, here evaluated by a tangent drawn at Point A. Point B illustrates a slope discontinuity (possibly indicative of interfacial slip or subcomponent failure within the connector), and Point C illustrates the maximal load acceptance (ultimate strength).

FIG. A4.2 Load/Deformation Curve (Generic, Here Illustrated for the z^* Direction)

increase in the force or moment resisting the input displacement.

A4.10 Report

A4.10.1 The test report shall include, but is not limited to, the following information:

A4.10.1.1 *Connecting Element and Bridge/Anchorage Element Identification*, including manufacturer, part number, nomenclature, and quality control or lot number. If the part is a prototype, geometrical and material descriptions shall be included.

A4.10.1.2 Assembly force or torque used to engage the connector's gripping mechanism.

A4.10.1.3 Configuration of the input loading element, and, for A4.6.1.3, the output loading element, and testing apparatus grips. Describe the method/apparatus used to grip the input and output loading elements.

A4.10.1.4 Specific degrees of freedom tested in tension, compression, torsion, or bending. In each case, the axis along which or about which loading is applied should be specified.

A4.10.1.5 Loading rate and number of cycles (fatigue tests).

A4.10.1.6 Stiffness in the specific direction(s) tested. The stiffness of the initial load cycle, the "stable" stiffness determined after the preconditioning cycles, and the number of cycles needed to attain a "stable" stiffness should be reported.

A4.10.1.7 If loaded to failure, the failure criterion, strength, and the specific mode of failure, for example, slip at the interface between the clamp and the loading input element.

A4.10.1.8 Where appropriate, the range of adjustability or the unlocked range of motion in specific degrees of freedom. For unlocked degrees of freedom, the joint may be further characterized as having resisted motion (for example, spring-loaded), in which case either the tangent resisting stiffness or, if resistance is nonuniform, the load/deformation curve in the permitted motion range, may be reported; actuated motion, in which case the available actuating force may be reported; or, unresisted motion, in which case any factors identified as causing appreciable increase in the normally incidentally small friction, that is causing binding, should be reported.

A4.11 Precision and Bias

A4.11.1 Data establishing the precision and bias to be expected from this test method have not yet been obtained.

12. Keywords

12.1 bending; connecting elements; external fixator; joints; orthopedic device; range of adjustability; range of motion; stiffness; strength; torsion

A4.13 Rationale

A4.13.1 Joints of various designs are used widely in external fixators. Both the types of elements connected and the pertinent directions of force, or moment, or both, transmission through joints are design and site specific. In many situations, elastic deformations at the joints between bridge elements, or between anchorage and bridge elements, account for a substantial fraction of the overall compliance of the fixator construct. Moreover, slippage between clamps and the bridge or anchorage elements they grip is often the major reason for overall structural failure of an external fixator.

A4.13.2 This test specification outlines a method by which the stiffness or strength, or both, of a joint can be measured, including both the connector body itself, and the one or more interfaces between the connector body and the bridge (or anchorage) elements so joined.

A4.13.3 The test specification also outlines a procedure by which the range of adjustability may be determined in specific degrees of freedom for which the joint's configuration can be adjusted by the end user. In the case of unlockable (dynamizable) joints, it outlines a method for determining the limits of motion permitted in the corresponding degrees of freedom.

A5. TEST METHOD FOR EXTERNAL SKELETAL FIXATOR PINS

A5.1 Scope

A5.1.1 This test method covers the procedure for determining the static bending strength and torsional strength of metallic pins used in external skeletal fixation systems. The described method is intended to provide a means of mechanically evaluating pins and not to define acceptable levels of performance. This test method is applicable only to pins made from materials exhibiting linearly elastic behavior. Pins are defined in Annex A1.

A5.1.2 *This standard does not purport to address all of the safety concerns, if any, associated with its use. It is the responsibility of the user of this standard to establish appropriate safety and health practices and determine the applicability of regulatory limitations prior to use.*

A5.2 Referenced Documents

A5.2.1 *ASTM Standards:*

A 938 Test Method for Torsion Testing of Wire[2]

E 4 Practices for Force Verification of Testing Machines[4]

F 1264 Specification and Test Methods for Intermedullary Fixation Devices[5]

A5.3. Terminology

A5.3.1 *Definitions of Terms Specific to This Standard:*

A5.3.1.1 *bending rigidity, n*—the resistance to bending of a pin tested in four-point bending, normalized to the cross-sectional properties of the working length, without regard for the length of the pin tested. This parameter is calculated as described in Guide F 1264 (EI_e). This theoretical equation is appropriate only for working lengths of constant cross section; it is not applicable to tapered pins.

A5.3.1.2 *bending stiffness, n*—the slope of Line *m-b* defined in A5.8.1.4.

A5.3.1.3 *bending yield strength, n*—the bending moment required to produce a 0.2 % permanent flexural strain in a pin tested as described in A5.8.1.4. If the pin fractures before the above-specified amount of permanent flexural strain is accrued, the maximum bending yield strength shall be defined as the bending moment occurring before or at the time of fracture.

A5.3.1.4 *maximum deformation, n*—in the four-point bending test of A5.8.1, the maximum vertical displacement measured at the point of load application while the load is applied.

A5.3.1.5 *permanent angular rotation, n*—in the torsion test of A5.8.2, the angle of rotation of the pin measured after the applied torque has been removed.

A5.3.1.6 *permanent deformation, n*—in the four-point bending test of A5.8.1, the vertical displacement of the point of load application after the applied loading has been removed.

A5.3.1.7 *thread runout, n*—the junction between the threaded and nonthreaded portions of the pin.

A5.3.1.8 *torsional rigidity, n*—a measure of the pin's normalized resistance to torsional shear when tested as described in A5.8.2. The value is calculated by dividing the torsional stiffness by the gage section length.

A5.3.1.9 *torsional stiffness, n*—the slope of line *m-b* defined in A5.8.2.4.

A5.3.1.10 *torsional yield strength, n*—in the torsion test of A5.8.2, the torque required to produce a permanent shear strain of 0.2 % in a pin tested as described in A5.8.2.4. If a pin fractures before the specified amount of permanent angular rotation is accrued, the torsional strength shall be defined as the maximum torque occurring before or at the time of fracture.

A5.4 Summary of Test Method

A5.4.1 External skeletal fixator pins are tested in static four-point bending by loading the pins to a specified deflection. The results of the test are displayed in the form of a bending moment versus deformation curve, from which the bending stiffness, and strength, if tested to failure, can be determined. Once the bending stiffness is determined, the bending rigidity can be calculated, as described in A5.3.1.1.

A5.4.2 External skeletal fixator pins are tested in torsion by gripping both ends of the pin in fixtures and holding one end stationary while applying torque to the other end. The results are displayed in the form of a torque versus angle of rotation curve, from which the torsional stiffness, and strength, if tested to failure, can be determined. Once the torsional stiffness is determined, the torsional rigidity can be calculated as described in A5.3.1.8.

A5.5 Significance and Use

A5.5.1 These benchtop tests are used to determine values for the mechanical response of external fixator pins under flexural loading conditions and under torsional loading conditions.

A5.5.2 The results obtained in these tests are not intended to predict the clinical efficacy or safety of the tested elements. The methods are intended only to measure the uniformity of the elements tested or to compare the mechanical performance of different pins.

A5.5.3 Since clinical failures often involve the threaded portions of the pin or the thread runout, it may be appropriate to perform bending tests (see A5.6.3.2), or torsional tests (see A5.6.4.2), or both, with working regions representing the corresponding portions of the pin.

A5.6 Test Apparatus

A5.6.1 Machines used for these tests shall conform to the requirements of Practices E 4.

A5.6.2 *Data Acquisition Device*—A suitable recorder to plot a graph of load versus load frame displacement, or torque versus load frame rotational displacement, on perpendicular axes. Optionally, this may include the use of computer-based digital sampling and output of the load and displacement signals.

A5.6.3 *Four-Point Bending Test*:

A5.6.3.1 The test configuration for the static four-point bending test is illustrated in Fig. A5.1.

A5.6.3.2 Since pins are available in a wide range of sizes, no single-testing geometry is appropriate in all circumstances; however, the following sizing criteria should be adopted. For testing the nonthreaded portion of the pin, the distance between

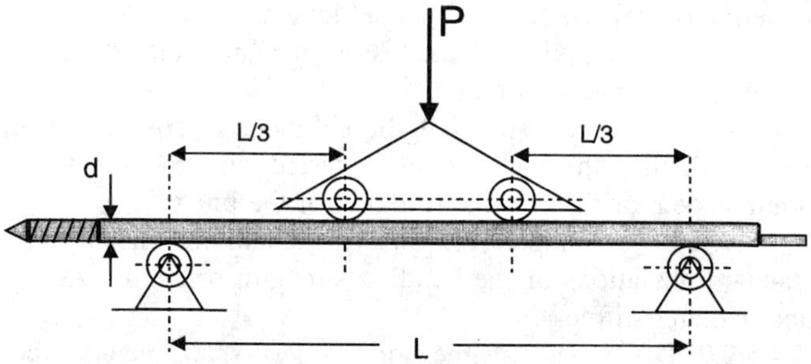

FIG. A5.1 Four-Point Bending Test for an External Skeletal Fixation Pin

the supports should be short enough that only a prismatic section of the pin is loaded; that is, the threaded portion of the pin plus at least a two-diameter length of the prismatic portion of the pin should overhang one outer (support) roller, and the keyed drive section and at least a two-diameter length of the prismatic portion of the pin should overhang the other outer (support) roller. For testing the threaded portion of the pin, the pin should be positioned such that its threaded portion completely spans the distance between the inner (loading) rollers. For testing to include the thread runout, the pin should be positioned such that the thread runout is positioned midway between the inner (loading) rollers. The diameter of the face of the rollers should be at least four times the diameter of the pin to insure negligible local deformation of the roller or the pin as a result of (Hertzian-like) contact stresses. The diameter of the roller face should be less than ⅒ the span length, so that roller/pin contact interface approximates point loading for purposes of beam flexure analysis.

A5.6.3.3 The load rollers will be placed at ⅓ points between the supports. The load shall be shared equally between both loading points.

A5.6.3.4 Deformation shall be measured as the displacement of the fixture applying the load.

A5.6.4 *Torsion Test*:

A5.6.4.1 A biaxial mechanical testing system is recommended for the torsion test.

A5.6.4.2 Two clamping heads, for example, collets, shall be used to clamp the pin. Care should be taken to not to damage the pin to the extent that failure initiates at the clamped surfaces during torsion. For testing the nonthreaded portion of the pin, the pin should be positioned in the clamps such that the free span of the pin between the clamps is prismatic and is at least two pin diameters from either the thread or the drive key. For testing the threaded portion of the pin, the pin should be positioned in the clamps such that the free span between the clamps is occupied only by the threaded portion of the pin. For testing the thread runout, the pin should be positioned in the clamps such that the junction between the threaded and nonthreaded portions of the pin lies mid way between the clamps.

A5.6.4.3 The clamping heads shall be affixed to the mechanical testing system, one to the test table and one to the torsional actuator.

A5.6.4.4 The pin and clamping heads should be aligned such that as the actuator rotates, negligible bending occurs.

A5.7 Test Specimen

A5.7.1 All tested pins should be representative of clinical quality products.

A5.7.2 If the pins to be tested have been used previously, the nature of such prior usage should be described appropriately.

A5.7.3 If the pin to be tested is a prototype, or under development, or both, the geometric and material information needed to characterize fully the pin should either be included in the report or detailed descriptive information should be referenced.

A5.8 Procedure

A5.8.1 *Four-Point Bending Test*:

A5.8.1.1 The pin should be placed into the test fixture (see Fig. A5.1). Quasistatic loads of progressively increasing magnitude should be applied, while recording the load P and corresponding deformation δ until either failure occurs or further deformation does not result in a corresponding increase in applied load.

A5.8.1.2 It is recognized that no specific rate is applicable to all situations; however, an input rate sufficient to attain in 30 s a pin flexural strain magnitude in the range of typical physiological usage, or of pin failure, shall be deemed quasistatic. The testing machine may be operated in either load or stroke control.

A5.8.1.3 The bending moment shall be computed as PL/6.

A5.8.1.4 On the bending moment versus deformation plot (see Fig. A5.2), lay off O-m on the abcissa from the origin of the curve to a point corresponding to a flexural strain of ϵ = 0.2 % the origin. Here, flexural strain is defined Mr/EI, where r is the pin radius. Draw a line parallel to the linear portion of the curve beginning as Point m and ending where the bending moment versus deformation curve is intersected, Point b. The location of this intersection corresponds to the bending moment, B, which is the bending yield strength.

A5.8.1.5 The bending stiffness is the slope of the Line *m-b*.

A5.8.1.6 The bending rigidity is defined as $(EI_e) = 0.0154\ L^3(F/y)$, where L is the distance between the support rollers and (F/y) is the slope of the Line O-m.

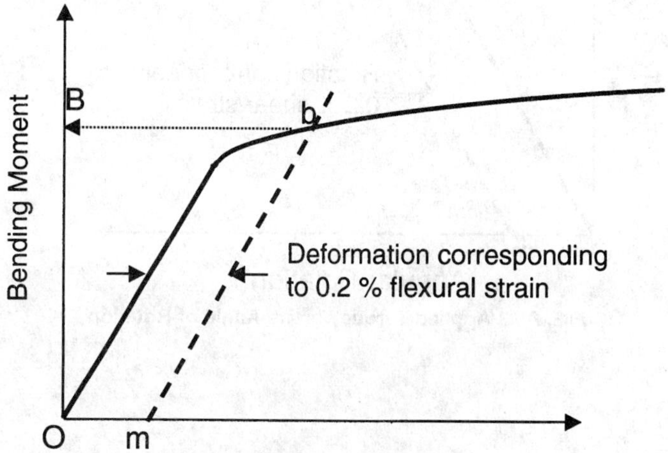

FIG. A5.2 Bending Moment Versus Flexural Deformation

A5.8.2 *Torsion Test*:

A5.8.2.1 Secure the pins in the clamping heads and affix the clamping heads to the mechanical test system table and torsional actuator such that the pin and clamping heads are aligned collinear with the axis of rotation of the actuator.

A5.8.2.2 Apply quasistatic torque via the torsional actuator and record the torque T and angle of rotation θ. The axial load on the pin should remain negligible at all times.

A5.8.2.3 It is recognized that no specific torsion rate is applicable to all situations; however, an input rate sufficient to attain in 30 s a pin shear strain magnitude in the range of typical physiological usage, or of pin failure, shall be deemed quasistatic. The testing machine may be operated in either torque or angular stroke control.

A5.8.2.4 Determine the torsional yield strength and stiffness as follows. On the torque versus angle of rotation plot (see Fig. A5.3), lay off O-m on the abcissa from the origin of the curve to a point corresponding to 0.2 % shear strain. Shear strain $\gamma = \theta\, r_{eff}/L_0$, where θ is the angle of rotation, r_{eff} is the effective radius, and L_0 is the free specimen length between the clamping heads. The effective pin radius may be taken as the root diameter of the threaded portion of the pin. For tests of nonthreaded pin portions, r_{eff} is the pin radius. Draw a line parallel to the linear portion of the curve beginning at Point m and ending where the torque versus angle of rotation curve is intersected, Point b. The location of this intersection corresponds to the Torque B, which is the torsional yield strength. The torsional stiffness is the slope of the Line M-B.

A5.8.2.5 The torsional rigidity is torsional stiffness divided by the free specimen length L_0.

A5.9 Report

A5.9.1 The report of the four-point bending test shall include the following information:

A5.9.1.1 Description of the pins, including manufacturer, part number, nomenclature, quality control or lot number, the material, overall length, unthreaded length.

A5.9.1.2 Description of the testing machine, including the make, model, and load range.

A5.9.1.3 Test rate, span length, and mode of control. Also, report whether the span segment tested was the threaded, nonthreaded, or thread-runout region of the pin.

A5.9.1.4 The number of pins tested and the means and standard deviations of the bending strength, bending rigidity, and bending stiffness.

A5.9.2 The report of the torsion test shall include the following information:

A5.9.2.1 Description of the pins, including manufacturer, part number, nomenclature, quality control or lot number, the material, overall length, unthreaded length.

A5.9.2.2 Description of the testing machine, including the make, model, and load range.

A5.9.2.3 Test rate, span length, and mode of control. Also, report whether the span segment tested was the threaded, nonthreaded, or thread-runout region of the pin.

A5.9.2.4 The number of pins tested and the means and standard deviations of the torsional strength, torsional rigidity, and torsional stiffness.

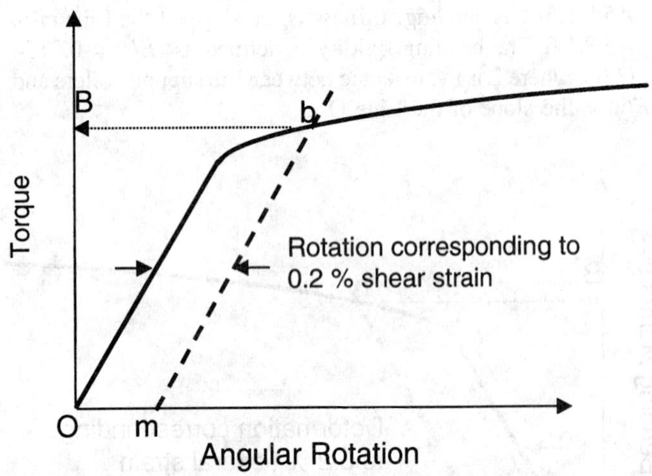

FIG. A5.3 Applied Torque Versus Angle of Rotation

A5.10 Precision and Bias

A5.10.1 Data establishing the precision and bias to be expected from this test method have not yet been obtained.

11. Keywords

11.1 external fixation; four-point bending; orthopedic device; pins; rigidity; stiffness; strength; torsion

A5.12 Rationale

A5.12.1 Partially threaded transcutaneous pins are the most commonly used anchorage elements for external fixation. Normally, the threaded portion of a fixation pin is self-tapping and engages both bony cortices. Once inserted, these pins are loaded primarily in flexure. In many external fixation constructs, flexural deformation of the pins is responsible for much or most of the total axial and bending deformations of the overall construct. Pins experience torsional loading during the threading/insertion process and in resisting construct bending about axes parallel to pins (in a cluster).

A5.12.2 Besides heavily influencing deformations at the fracture site, pin deformation during loading is a major determinant of interfacial motion at the pin/bone interface, frequently a problematic site in terms of bone remodeling, pin loosening, and sepsis. Also, in some situations, the loads borne by the pins are so high that the pins themselves are at risk of failure either by plastic deformation of by breakage. This test method outlines benchtop flexural and torsional testing protocols useful for determining the flexural and torsional stiffnesses and strengths of these key fixator elements.

A6. TEST METHOD FOR EXTERNAL SKELETAL FIXATOR SUBASSEMBLIES

A6.1 Scope

A6.1.1 This test method covers procedures for determining the stiffness and strength of external skeletal fixator subassemblies, under force loadings (axial, medial-lateral shear, anterior-posterior shear), or under moment loadings (torsion, medial-lateral bending, anterior-posterior bending), or a combination thereof.

A6.1.2 *This standard does not purport to address all of the safety concerns, if any, associated with its use. It is the responsibility of the user of this standard to establish appropriate safety and health practices and determine the applicability of regulatory limitations prior to use.*

A6.2 Referenced Documents

A6.2.1 *ASTM Standards:*

D 790 Test Methods for Flexural Properties of Unreinforced and Reinforced Plastics and Electrical Insulating Materials[3]

E 4 Practices for Force Verification of Testing Machines[5]

A6.3. Terminology

A6.3.1 *Definitions of Terms Specific to This Standard:*

A6.3.1.1 *subassembly, n*—that portion of an external fixator assembly specifically excluding the bony anchorage elements. Definitions of the terms used to describe various external skeletal fixator components are given in Annex A1.

A6.4 Summary of Test Method

A6.4.1 Subassemblies to be tested are assembled from individual bridge and connector elements. All geometric, material, and assembly parameters necessary to characterize the subassembly configuration unambiguously are recorded. The subassembly then is mounted within the testing machine, rigidly gripped at two sites: the input platen, at which load is input and deformation measured (or vice versa), and the support or restraint platen, which is rigidly coupled to the testing machine base. Loads, or displacements, are applied at the input platen, and the corresponding displacements, or loads, continuously recorded, allowing calculation of the subassembly's effective stiffness, or strength, or both, if loaded to failure, in one or more specific testing modes, for example, axial load, medial-lateral bending, and so forth.

A6.5 Significance and Use

A6.5.1 These laboratory tests are used to determine values for the effective stiffness, or strength, or both, of an external fixation subassembly, under force or moment loadings.

A6.5.2 The results obtained in this test are not intended to predict the clinical efficacy or safety of the tested subassemblies. This test method is intended only to measure the uniformity of the subassemblies tested or to compare the mechanical performance of different subassemblies.

A6.5.3 This test method may not be appropriate for all types of external skeletal fixator applications. The user is cautioned to consider the appropriateness of the method in view of the materials and designs being tested and their potential application.

A6.6 Apparatus

A6.6.1 *Force, or Moment (or Both), Application Fixture*:

A6.6.1.1 The loading configuration is shown schematically in Fig. A6.1. The line of application in the case of a force input, or the axis about which a moment is applied in the case of a moment input, is designated as the input loading axis.

A6.6.1.2 The subassembly undergoing testing is rigidly attached to two platens. One platen, termed the input platen, delivers the input load, or displacement, as a result of programmed motion of the actuator or crosshead of the testing machine. The other platen, termed the support or restraint platen, is affixed to the testing machine base, which in turn acts as a fixed support.

A6.6.1.3 Both the loading axis and the platen positions, orientations, and unrestrained degrees of freedom should be prescribed, or located, or both, with respect to a right-hand coordinate system defined with respect to the undeformed position of the subassembly being tested. Since positioning of the subassembly relative to anatomical orientations may vary from bone to bone, or with surgeon judgment, or both, the coordinate system should be defined relative to the major components of the subassembly. Normally, the axial direction will be associated with the longitudinal rod(s) or other longitudinal elements, and one of the transverse axes would be associated with the dominant direction of the anchorage elements.

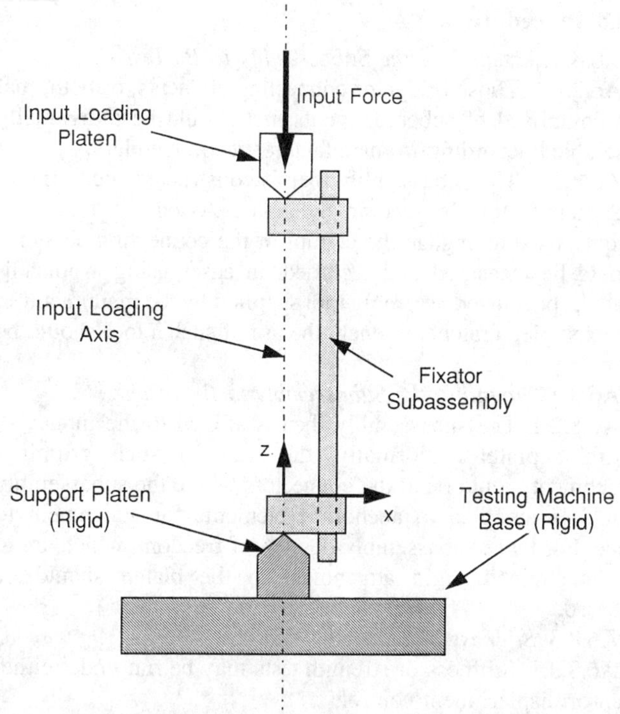

NOTE—Input force is delivered by the actuator (not shown) of the testing machine. Subassembly displacement is measured at the input loading platen.

FIG. A6.1 Schematic Test Configuration for Longitudinal (*z* Direction) Loading of an External Fixator Subassembly

A6.6.2 Machines used for testing shall conform to the requirements of Practice E 4. The loads used for the test shall be within the loading range of the test machine, as defined in Practices E 4.

A6.6.3 A suitable device should be used to record load versus input platen displacement. Such recordings may be either continuous, for example, magnetic tape, stripchart recorder, *x-y* flatbed plotter, storage oscilloscope, or discrete, that is, analog-to-digital samples written to computer disk, but must suffice to allow subsequent reconstruction of the load/deformation curve to determine stiffness and strength.

A6.7 Test Specimen

A6.7.1 All tested subassemblies should be assembled from elements representative of clinical quality products.

A6.7.2 If one or more of the elements in the frame to be tested has been previously used, the nature of such prior usage should be described appropriately.

A6.7.3 If any elements of the subassemblies to be tested are prototypes, or are under development, or both, the geometric and material information needed to characterize fully all such elements should either be included in the report, or a similarly detailed descriptive information should be referenced.

A6.7.4 The test specimens should be prepared in the manner in which they normally would be used clinically. For example, if a component normally would be sterilized in a particular manner before use, it should be sterilized similarly before mechanical testing. This is especially true for polymeric components and polymeric and metallic mechanisms used for connection or clamping.

A6.8 Procedure

A6.8.1 *Assembling the Subassembly to Be Tested*:

A6.8.1.1 Those bridge or connecting elements, or both, that are comprised of subcomponents first should be individually assembled according to manufacturer recommendations.

A6.8.1.2 The subassembly then is constructed according to the manufacturer's recommendations. Assembly forces or torques used to engage the clamps of the connecting elements should be measured and recorded. In cases using a noncalibrated, specialized assembly tool supplied by the manufacturer, for example, a ratchet wrench, the use of such a tool should be noted.

A6.8.2 *Mounting the Subassembly to Be Tested*:

A6.8.2.1 The subassembly then is affixed to the input and restraint platens. Normally, the sites of such gripping/attachment would be at the connectors where the subassembly would be coupled to anchorage elements for attachment to bone. For those subassembly degrees of freedom, which are to be constrained, rigid attachment to the platen should be ensured.

A6.8.3 *Stiffness or Strength Testing*:

A6.8.3.1 Stiffness or strength tests may be run under either load or displacement control.

A6.8.3.2 The tests may be either single- or multi-cycle and may either be restricted to the elastic regime or taken to the point of failure.

A6.8.3.3 If single-cycle testing is to be performed, the specimen must be subjected to several preconditioning load cycles to demonstrate that the reported load/deformation curve is repeatable from cycle to cycle. Preconditioning should be continued until the apparent stiffness of the joint changes less than 5 % between subsequent cycles. Normally, about five preconditioning cycles are suitable for this purpose, with peak applied load within the elastic range, approximately 50 % of the expected physiologic service load or 50 % of the expected subassembly failure load, whichever is lower. Load/deformation curves for the preconditioning cycles should be recorded. Preconditioning cycle stiffnesses should be reported.

A6.8.3.4 The input load (or displacement) should be applied quasistatically. The rate(s) used should be reported. It is recognized that no specific rate is applicable to all situations; however, in this context, a quasistatic input rate should be interpreted as being sufficient to attain, in approximately 30 s, a load, or moment, magnitude in the range of typical physiologic usage, or sufficient to cause frame failure as defined below. Input loading rates, which are in the range of those expected clinically may be desirable for testing components made of polymeric materials, that exhibit viscoelastic behavior, and for components that rely upon friction for fixation. A rationale should be provided for whatever input loading rate is used.

A6.8.3.5 For multicycle testing (fatigue or low cycle fatigue), the input loading frequency shall not exceed 5 Hz. Maximum and minimum values of the loading cycle, as well as the input waveform, should be included in the test report.

A6.8.3.6 A subassembly will be defined as having failed if it undergoes irrecoverable deformation, either from destructive failure of one or more of its elements, for example, plastic bending of a rod, or from slip at one or more of the interfaces between individual components.

A6.8.3.7 The threshold magnitude of irrecoverable deformation constituting failure is context specific, and often will depend on factors outside the scope of the immediate test, for example, clinically acceptable interfragmentary displacements at a fracture site. The specific threshold or irrecoverable deformation constituting failure must be reported, and the rationale for that specific value stated.

A6.8.3.8 Input forces, or linear displacements, should be delivered either along the subassembly longitudinal axis (axial load), or perpendicular to the subassembly longitudinal axis (shear load). The line of action of the input force should be recorded, with respect to the subassembly based right-hand orthogonal coordinate system.

A6.8.3.9 Input moments may be delivered either by an eccentrically applied force couple or by a torsional actuator. These moments should be either about the input loading axis or about an axis perpendicular to the input loading axis. If the moment is delivered by an eccentric force couple, the points and lines of application if the individual forces must be reported.

A6.8.4 *Data Recording*:

A6.8.4.1 The input load (N) or torque (N-mm) and the corresponding linear (mm) or angular (°) displacement of the input platen, or vice versa, should be recorded continuously. This may be done either as direct analog signals or using digital sampling at a rate sufficient to allow subsequent reconstruction of a visibly smooth load/deformation curve mimicking a continuous analog tracing.

A6.8.4.2 Linear or angular displacements should be measured at the site of the input load platen.

A6.8.4.3 In some situations, it may be appropriate to record displacement in a direction other than that of the loading input, or vice versa. If this involves releasing one or more degrees of restraint at the input platen, this should be noted. Any additional sensors used for recording such coupled motion, or force/torque, components should be described, and their sampling points and measurement directions noted.

A6.9 Calculation or Interpretation of Results

A6.9.1 Tangent stiffness, units according to the chosen load and deflection configuration, such as, N/mm for force, N-mm/degree for moment, shall be calculated from the slope of the linear-most portion of the load/deflection curve, as apparent visually (see Fig. A6.2). If an objective slope determination technique, such as, curve fitting of a digitized tracing is used, this should be described. The load and deflection configuration (location of measuring elements and direction of the measured vector) must be defined clearly with respect to the loading axis of the test apparatus (see Fig. A6.1).

A6.9.2 Chord stiffness (units according to the chosen load and deflection configuration, such as, N/mm for force, N-mm/degree for moment) shall be calculated as the change in load (force or moment), divided by the change in the corresponding displacement (linear or angular), between two specific points on the load/deformation curve. The load and deflection configuration (location of measuring elements and direction of the measured vector) must be defined clearly with respect to the loading axis of the test apparatus (see Fig. A6.1).

A6.9.3 Ultimate strength (N or N-mm) shall be defined as the point of maximum force, or moment, acceptance.

A6.9.4 Yield strength (N or N-mm) shall be defined using the chord offset method (see Fig. A6.2). Toe regions of the load (moment) versus displacement (angulation) curve, which may occur during the initial loading of the subassembly, may be compensated for using the techniques described in Test Methods D 790.

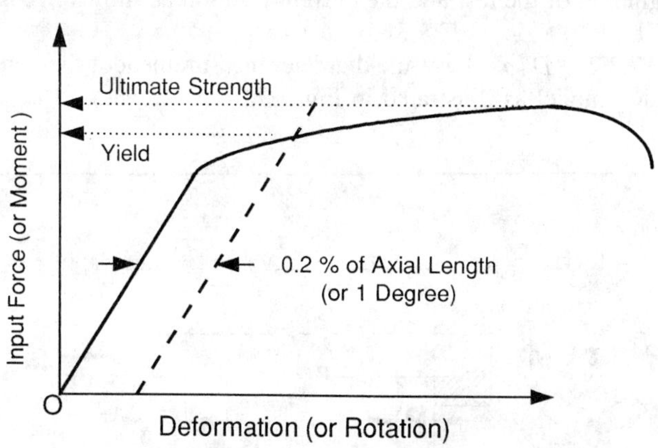

NOTE—Stiffness is defined as the slope of the linear portion of the force/deformation curve.

FIG. A6.2 Typical Force/Deformation Curve, Illustrating Definitions of Ultimate Strength and Offset Yield Strength

A6.9.4.1 Normally, yield should be based on an irrecoverable deformation of 0.2 % of the axial length of the subassembly for force inputs, or 1° for moment inputs.

A6.9.4.2 Other permanent deformation thresholds may be appropriate, depending on the subassembly configuration. If alternative yield definitions are used, they should be included in the report, with appropriate justification.

A6.10 Report

A6.10.1 The test report shall include, but is not limited to, the following information:

A6.10.1.1 Identification of the individual elements comprising the subassembly. This should include manufacturer, part number, nomenclature, and where possible, the quality control or lot number. If the part is a prototype, geometrical and material descriptions shall be included.

A6.10.1.2 Configuration of the subassembly. This should include a drawing, or photograph of the subassembly, or both, using multiple orthogonal views (antero-posterior view, medial-lateral view, superior-inferior view) as necessary to define unambiguously the relative positions and orientations of the individual elements comprising the subassembly. All physical dimensions, or element orientations within the subassembly, or both, that can be varied by the end user must be unambiguously specified, for example, clamp positions along rod elements, angle between rods connected by an adjustable clamp. For subassembly elements whose physical dimensions, or orientations, cannot be varied by the end user, or both, it is recognized that detailed dimensional, or material information, or both, may not be practical or appropriate to report when testing overall subassembly behavior. At a minimum, however, reference to public domain documentation reporting that specific information must be included. The assembly force or torque used to engage any connector grip mechanism(s) should be reported. If assembly is performed using noncalibrated specialty instruments often provided by manufacturers, such as ratchet drives, this should be reported and reference made to documentation reporting the actual force or torque delivered by such specialty instruments, if available.

A6.10.1.3 Test machine (manufacturer, model) and configuration of the subassembly relative to the test machine. A drawing, or photograph of the subassembly, or both, within the test machine setup should be provided. The positions of the load application platens must be identified. All physical dimensions, whether or not end user variable, which influence the load (or moment) delivered to the subassembly by the testing machine, must be specified. Constrained versus unconstrained degrees of freedom at the two platen/subassembly interfaces must be identified.

A6.10.1.4 Loading rate, and for fatigue tests, the number of cycles, maximum and minimum loads, and the waveform.

A6.10.1.5 Subassembly stiffness (tangent, or secant, or both) in the specific direction(s) tested.

A6.10.1.6 If the subassembly is loaded to failure, both the strength and the specific mode of failure, for example, slip at a particular clamped interface or yield of a specific bridge element, should be specified. If the specific mode of failure cannot be ascertained by gross observation, the technique(s) used to identify the mode or site of failure should be reported.

A6.11 Precision and Bias

A6.11.1 Data establishing the precision and bias to be expected from this test method have not yet been obtained.

A6.12 Rationale

A6.12.1 The modularity of most external fixation devices affords a great deal of variability in how subassemblies can be constructed. In many instances, it is desirable to compare the effective stiffness or strength of alternative subassembly configurations that can be assembled from a specific set of elements, such as perturbations of end-user-controlled variables, such as the distance between two connection clamps attached to a rod element. Also, there are many instances in which it is desirable to compare the effective stiffness or strength of similarly conceived subassemblies built up from different individual components, for example, choosing different rod diameters from within a given manufacturer's fixator set or assembling conceptually similar subassemblies using different manufacturers' fixator sets.

A6.12.2 Normally, the subassembly itself is the stiffest and strongest part of an overall external fixator assembly or construct. Also, the mechanical behavior of the subassembly, per se, is of interest because intrinsic subassembly properties do not depend upon the specifics how the subassembly is connected (via anchorage elements) to the skeletal elements being fixated, provided of course, that those anchorage elements connect to the subassembly at comparable locations. That is, many attributes of the mechanical behavior of an overall fixator assembly/construct can be influenced substantially by the structural characteristics of the subassembly itself without needing to confront anatomic or clinical constraints limiting the configuration(s) of anchorage elements.

A6.12.3 Because of the wide variety of fixator size ranges and anatomic sites, it is inappropriate to standardize the geometry or kinetics of subassembly loading tests. Rather, this test method emphasizes unambiguous specification of the subassembly being tested, clear identification of the site at which loading is applied and deformation is measured, and a formal definition of the subassembly's stiffness, or strength, or both, for each combination of load/deformation measured.

A7. TEST METHOD FOR EXTERNAL SKELETAL FIXATOR-BONE CONSTRUCTS

A7.1 Scope

A7.1.1 This test method covers procedures for determining the stiffness, strength, and repetitive loading performance characteristics of external skeletal fixator-bone constructs when subjected to force loading (axial, medial-lateral shear, anterior-posterior shear) and moment loading (torsion, medial-lateral bending, anterior-posterior bending).

A7.1.2 This test method establishes a universal fixator-bone construct's minimum configuration and set of laboratory tests for evaluating the external fixator device's (EFD) basic performance characteristics.

A7.1.3 *Units*—Unless otherwise stated, the values stated in SI units are to be regarded as standard.

A7.1.4 *This standard does not purport to address all of the safety concerns, if any, associated with its use. It is the responsibility of the user of this standard to establish appropriate safety and health practices and determine the applicability of regulatory limitations prior to use.*

A7.2 Referenced Documents

A7.2.1 *ASTM Standards:*

D 790 Test Methods for Flexural Properties of Unreinforced and Reinforced Plastics and Electrical Insulating Materials[3]

E 4 Practices for Force Verification of Testing Machines[4]

E 122 Practice for Choice of Sample Size to Estimate the Average Quality of a Lot or Process[7]

E 467 Practice for Verification of Constant Amplitude Dynamic Loads and Displacements in an Axial Fatigue Testing Machine[4]

E 1823 Terminology Relating to Fatigue and Fracture Testing[4]

E 1942 Guide for Evaluating Data Acquisition Systems Used in Cyclic Fatigue and Fracture Mechanics Testing[4]

A7.3. Terminology

A7.3.1 *Definitions*—Unless otherwise specified, the terms used to describe various external skeletal fixator components are defined in Annex A1. Unless otherwise defined in this method, the terminology to mechanical testing that is used in this method will be in accordance with the definitions of Terminology E 1823.

A7.3.2 *Definitions of Terms Specific to This Standard:*

A7.3.2.1 *angular displacement* (θ), (°), *n*—the relative change in the angle of the moment application point at the beginning of the test and the current position as shown in Fig. A7.1.

A7.3.2.2 *D (mm), n*—the diameter measurement of the bone analog model as illustrated in Fig. A7.2.

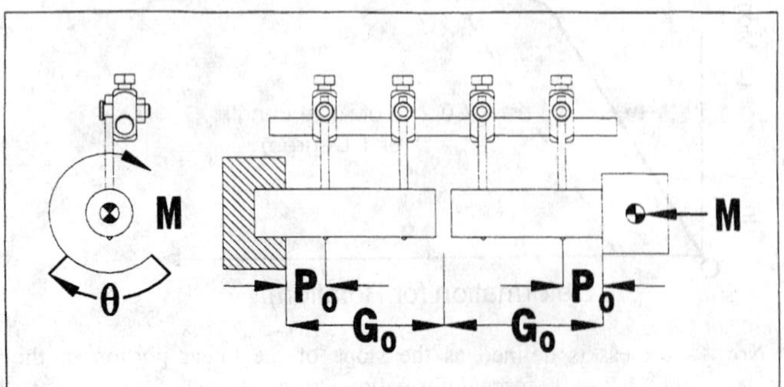

FIG. A7.1 Torsion Test Configuration

[7] *Annual Book of ASTM Standards*, Vol 14.02.

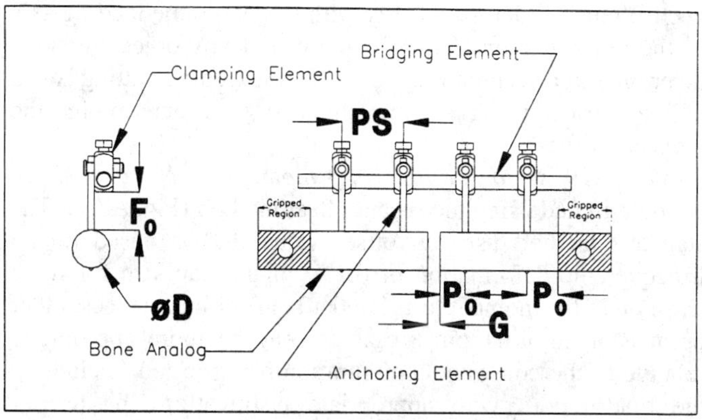

FIG. A7.2 Typical Fixator-Bone Construct

A7.3.2.3 *failure, n*—the point when the construct experiences either irrecoverable deformation or has reached a deformation limit. This can be a result of the destructive failure of an element, for example, plastic bending of a rod or pin or from slippage at an interconnection between individual components. The threshold magnitude of irrecoverable deformation constituting failure is context specific and often will depend on factors outside the scope of the immediate test, for example, clinically acceptable interfragmentary displacements at a fracture site.

A7.3.2.4 *fixator-bone construct, n*—the combination of an EFD and the bone analog to which it is anchored.

A7.3.2.5 *fracture gap offset (G_o), (mm), n*—the distance between the plane at the center of the fracture gap and the gripping (or loading) locations that are illustrated in Fig. A7.1 and Figs. A7.3-A7.5. If different fracture gap offset values are used in the same test construct, identify each offset with a unique subscript label.

A7.3.2.6 *frame offset (F_o), (mm), n*—the minimum clearance between the periosteal surface of the bone analog and any frame elements when measured normal to the bone analog surface (see Fig. A7.2).

A7.3.2.7 *gap size (G), (mm), n*—the minimum clearance between the distal end of the proximal bone analog segment and the proximal end of the distal bone analog segment (see Fig. A7.2).

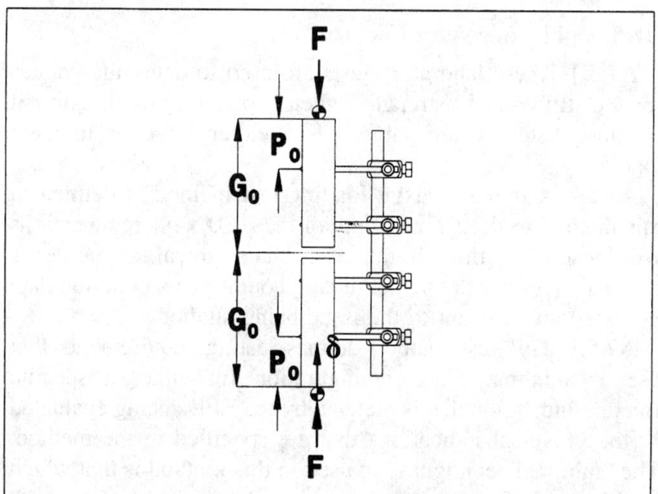

FIG. A7.3 Axial Load Test Configuration

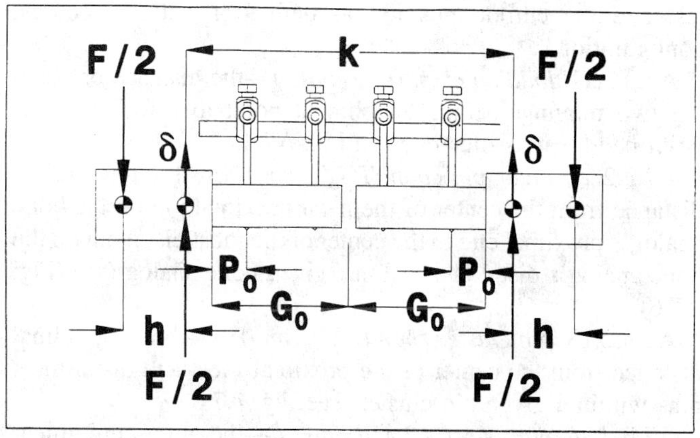

FIG. A7.4 Four-Point Bend Test Configuration

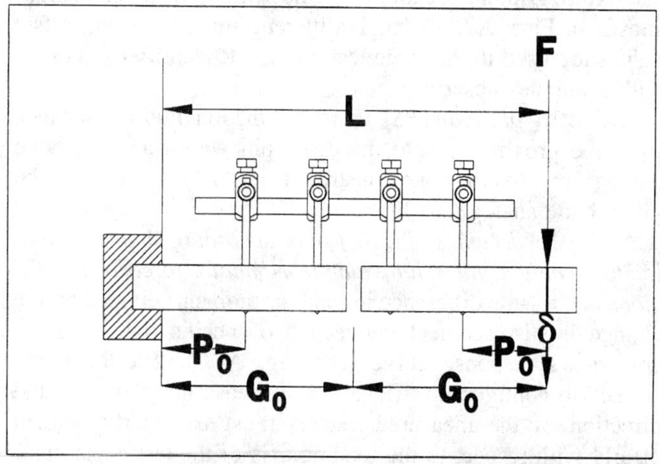

FIG. A7.5 Cantilever Bend Test Configuration

A7.3.2.8 *inner pin span (PS_I)*, (mm), *n*—the longitudinal distance from the center of the most distal pin on the bone analog's proximal end to the center of the most proximal pin on the bone analog's distal end within a given bone analog (see Fig. A7.6).

A7.3.2.9 *level arm (L), (mm), n*—the distance between either the test block anchor point or section of interest and the position of the load application point as illustrated in Fig. A7.5.

A7.3.2.10 *linear displacement* (δ), *(mm), n*—the relative change in the position of the load point at the beginning of the

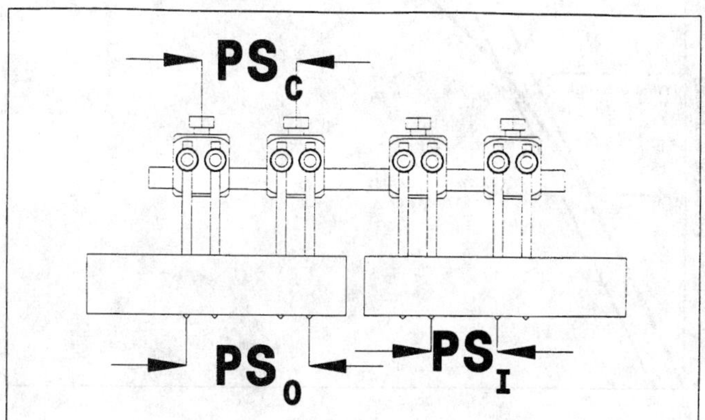

FIG. A7.6 Pin Cluster Illustration

test and the current position as defined for the given test configuration.

A7.3.2.11 *loading span (k), (mm), n*—the distance between the two moving loading attachment point axis for the four-point bend test as illustrated in Fig. A7.4.

A7.3.2.12 *outer pin span (PS_o), (mm), n*—the longitudinal distance from the center of the most proximal pin on the bone analog's proximal end to the center of the most distal pin on the bone analog's distal end within a given bone analog (see (Fig. A7.6).

A7.3.2.13 *pin cluster span (PS_c), (mm), n*—the longitudinal distance from the center of the proximal-most and distal-most pins within a given pin cluster (see Fig. A7.6).

A7.3.2.14 *pin offset (P_o), (mm), n*—the minimum linear distance between either the ends of the bone analog elements or test fixture gripping locations and the nearest anchor element as shown in Figs. A7.1-A7.5. If different anchor element offset values are used in the same test construct, identify each offset with a unique subscript label.

A7.3.2.15 *pin span (PS), (mm), n*—the longitudinal distance from the proximal pin to the distal pin within a given bone analog for a fixator-bone construct using only two pins in the given bone analog (see Fig. A7.2).

A7.3.2.16 *secant stiffness, (units according to the chosen loading configuration, for example, N/mm for force, N· m/° for moment), n*—the difference in load (or moment) divided by the change in displacement between two specific points on the construct's response curve (see Fig. A7.7). The load and deflection configuration (location of measuring elements and direction of the measured vector) must be clearly defined clearly with respect to the loading axis of the test apparatus.

A7.3.2.17 *support span (h), (mm), n*—the distance between the fixed support attachment point axis and the nearest loading attachment point axis for the four-point bend test as illustrated in Fig. A7.4.

A7.3.2.18 *tangent stiffness, (units according to the chosen loading configuration, for example, N/mm for force, N· m/° for moment), n*—calculated from the slope of the linear-most portion of the load versus deformation curve, as apparent visually (Fig. A7.6). The load and deflection configuration (location of measuring elements and direction of the measured vector) must be defined clearly with respect to the loading axis of the test apparatus. Describe the use of any objective slope determination techniques, for example, curve fitting of a digitized tracing) that are implemented when determining the tangent stiffness.

A7.3.2.19 *yield load (or moment), N or N·m), n*—determined using the secant offset method (Fig. A7.7). The standard method uses an offset value that is based on an irrecoverable deformation of 0.2 % of the gap size for force tests, or 1° for moment tests. Under some circumstances, other permanent deformation thresholds may be more appropriate relative to the construct configuration being tested. Include in the final report, with appropriate justification, the use of alternative yield definitions. Toe regions of the load (moment) versus displacement (angulation) curve, which may occur during the initial loading of the construct, may be compensated for using the techniques described in Test Methods D 790 Annex 1.

A7.3.2.20 *ultimate load (or moment), N or N·m), n*—the maximum reaction force (or torque) experienced by the construct during a static strength test. The load and deflection configuration (location of measuring elements and direction of the measured vector) must be defined clearly with respect to the loading axis of the test apparatus.

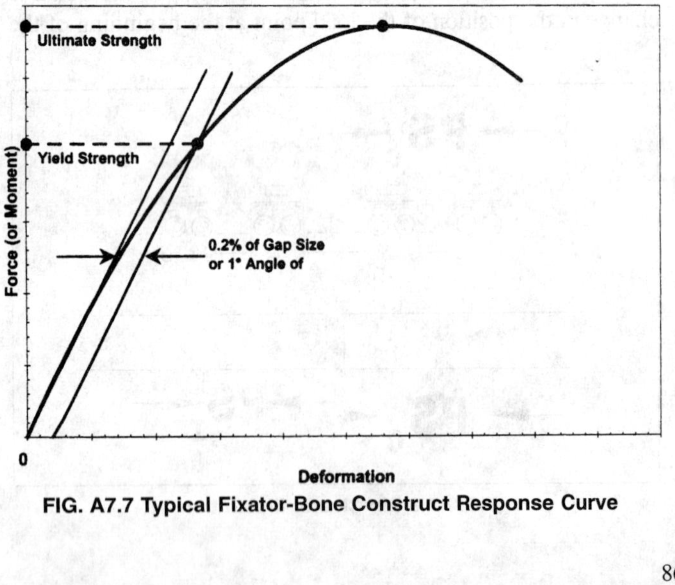

FIG. A7.7 Typical Fixator-Bone Construct Response Curve

A7.4 Summary of Test Method

A7.4.1 Fixator systems are assembled from individual bridge and connector elements. The assembled fixator system is anchored to upper and lower sections of a bone analog, producing a fixator-bone construct that simulates a segmental defect fracture. All geometric, material, and assembly parameters necessary to characterize the fixator configuration unambiguously are recorded. The fixator-bone construct is then mounted within the testing machine and subjected to a specific loading condition. For the static tests, the fixator-bone construct's reaction to the applied displacement (either linear or angular) is recorded which allows for the calculation of the fixator's stiffness and strength, when applicable, for the specific testing mode. For the dynamic test, the fixator-bone construct's ability to survive the application of repeated loading cycles is determined and reported.

A7.5 Significance and Use

A7.5.1 These laboratory tests are used to determine values for the stiffness and strength (when applicable) of an external fixation system when subjected to either force or moment loading.

A7.5.2 A dynamic axial loading test method is defined in this method to determine if any of the EFD's interconnections will loosen over time. In the event that a typical fatigue test is desired, carefully define the testing conditions so that the data provided are relevant to the issue being studied.

A7.5.3 This test method defines testing requirements that use a "minimal" EFD configuration for either a specific fracture indication that is dictated by the EFDs being evaluated or the universal indications that are specified in the method. The "minimal" configuration used in this method is that which is either specified by the manufacturer's surgical technique or by the requirements specified in this method. The user may elect to test other fixator system configurations using the methodology found in this specification.

A7.5.4 The results obtained in these tests are not intended to predict the clinical efficacy or safety of the tested fixator. The methods are intended only to measure the uniformity of the fixators tested or to compare the mechanical performance of different fixators.

A7.5.5 The test method may not be appropriate for all types of external skeletal fixator applications. Furthermore, the minimum recommended test series may not be adequate to evaluate performance characteristics fully that are unique to a given fixator system; therefore, the user is cautioned to consider the appropriateness of the method in view of the materials and designs being tested and their potential application.

A7.6 Apparatus

A7.6.1 *Test Fixture*:

A7.6.1.1 Use rigid test fixtures that are able to support the construct adequately for the test being performed and do not influence the final test results.

A7.6.1.2 This test specification concentrates on testing EFDs with the construct constrained as illustrated in Fig. A7.1 and Figs. A7.3-A7.5. Since no single universal set of constraints or boundary/loading conditions may be appropriate for all evaluations, the constraints or boundary/loading conditions may be modified depending upon the construct being tested. Document the rationale behind alternative loading constraint conditions that were adopted in the test report.

A7.6.1.3 The input loading axis is designated as either the line of application in the case of force input or the axis about which a moment is applied in the case of moment input.

A7.6.1.4 The construct undergoing testing is attached to two platens. One platen, termed the input platen, delivers the input displacement (or load) caused by the programmed motion of the actuator or crosshead of the testing machine. The other platen, termed the support or restraint platen, is affixed to the testing machine base, which in turn acts as a fixed support.

A7.6.2 *Test System*:

A7.6.2.1 Use a rigid mechanical test machine that is capable of a generating the forced displacement of the test sample's supporting (gripping) points at a constant displacement rate.

A7.6.2.2 Machines used for testing shall conform to the requirements of Practices E 4 and, when applicable, Practice E 467. The loads used for the test shall be within the loading range of the test machine, as defined in Practices E 4.

A7.6.2.3 Monitor the linear (angular) displacement of the input platen with a calibrated displacement (angle) transducer that has an accuracy of ±0.5 % of the selected full-scale range.

A7.6.2.4 In some situations, it may be appropriate to record displacements in a direction other than that of the loading input (or vice versa). Sensors used for recording such coupled motion components should be described, and their sample points and measurement directions noted. Monitor these secondary displacements with calibrated transducers that have an accuracy of ±0.5 % of the selected transducer's full-scale range.

A7.6.3 *Data Acquisition Systems*:

A7.6.3.1 Automatically record the test parameters with either an analog or a digital recorder.

A7.6.3.2 A suitable analog recorder would be capable of continuously monitoring the output from the test machine's load (moment) transducer and the displacement transducer to produce a load (moment) versus displacement curve.

A7.6.3.3 Alternatively, a multichannel analog-to-digital recording device with storage capabilities may be used to record the test's progress. The analog-to-digital hardware should meet the requirements of Guide E 1942 and be capable of collecting the necessary data at rates up to 1 kHz. Under any circumstance, the recorder must be able to reconstruct subsequently the load versus deformation curve to determine stiffness and strength parameters.

A7.7 Sampling

A7.7.1 The sample size used for static tests shall be determined according to the methods defined in Practice E 122 for any given loading condition. If insufficient information is available to determine a suitable sample size in accordance with Practice E 122, then test a minimum sample size of five for any given loading condition.

A7.7.2 For multicycle dynamic studies, test at least three constructs at any given load or moment level. If the study's goal is to generate a fatigue curve, then evaluate the fatigue properties for at least three different maximum load (or moment) levels for a specific loading condition. One of the three maximum load (or moment) levels selected for such studies should result in all three constructs reaching the fatigue runout cycle limit. Guidance and recommendations for selecting suitable sample sizes for fatigue studies used to develop a *P-N (M-N)* diagram can be found in the literature **(1, 2)**.[8]

A7.8 Test Specimen

A7.8.1 All tested fixators should be assembled from elements representative of clinical quality products.

A7.8.2 Select anchoring elements that have a sufficient threaded length so that they will at least pass through the test block.

A7.8.3 If one or more of the elements in the fixator to be tested has been used previously, the nature of such prior usage should be described appropriately.

A7.8.4 Record either the geometric and material information necessary to characterize fully any prototype elements that are contained in the tested fixator or provide references to similarly detailed descriptive information.

A7.8.5 Prepare all fixator system components for testing with the same methods that they would normally be prepared clinically. For example, if a component would normally be sterilized in a particular manner before use, it should be sterilized similarly before mechanical testing. This is true especially for polymeric components and polymeric and metallic mechanisms used for connections or clamping.

A7.8.6 The bone analog can be either a solid right circular cylinder or a thick-walled hollow cylinder of a size representative of the anatomic bone on which the fixator to be tested normally would be mounted (see Table A7.1).

[8] The boldface numbers in parentheses refers to the list of references at the end of this standard.

TABLE A7.1 Basic Fixator-Bone Construct Parameters

Test Construct Configuration Parameter	Fixator Size Classification		
	Large (that is, femur, tibia, and so forth)	Small (that is, forearm, wrist, and so forth)	Mini (that is, finger, and so forth)
Pin span, *PS* (mm)	90	45	18
Frame offset, F_o (mm)	50	25	10
Gap size, *G* (mm)	20	10	5
Bone analog diameter, *D* (mm)	30	15	6
Pin offset, P_o (mm)	20	10	5
Tightening torque (N·m)	10.0	5.0	2.5

A7.8.7 The material to be used for the bone analog will be such that elastic deformations within the two individual pieces of the bone analog can be considered negligible compared to elastic deformations in the fixator. Normally, this condition can be achieved if the stiffness of the bone analog in three-point bending (N/mm) is more than 100 times the axial compressive stiffness (N/mm) of the overall fixator-bone construct.

A7.8.8 Ensure that the bone analog material chosen is sufficiently tough so that the anchorage elements (usually pins) will remain tightly embedded throughout the test.

A7.8.9 Reuse of bone analogs should be avoided, unless it can be demonstrated that the test/retest variability generated is no greater than the variability of similarly conducted tests with fresh unused bone analogs.

A7.9 Construct Assembly

A7.9.1 The EFD construct being evaluated is attached to two bone analog test blocks. Prepare the typical "minimal" test construct (see Fig. A7.2) for testing in the following manner. The illustrated EFD configuration is considered the typical "minimal" test construct since it is a four-pin (two per bone analog) and clamp single-bar unilateral construct.

A7.9.2 Be sure to measure and record assembly forces or torque values that are used to engage the clamps of the connecting elements. Record the use of any noncalibrated specialized assembly tools supplied by the manufacturer, for example, a ratchet wrench.

A7.9.3 Install the anchoring elements into the test block using the insertion techniques, templates, and so forth, recommended by the manufacturer. If other procedures are used, this should be reported. Ensure that the anchoring elements are aligned, as they would be oriented for the clinical situation. Unless otherwise specified in the manufacturer's surgical technique, affix the anchoring elements along the centerline of the test block. Position the anchoring elements so that the anchor element offset is either in compliance with the manufacturer's surgical technique or is no less than four anchoring element diameters away from the ends of the test blocks.

A7.9.4 Loosely assemble multicomponent bridge, or connecting elements, or both, according to manufacturer's recommendations. Avoid tightening any interconnections any more than is necessary to ease the fixator-bone construct's assembly.

A7.9.5 Assemble the subassembly (frame) according to the manufacturer's recommendations leaving any interconnection loose that will affect the fixator-bone construct's alignment. Install the subassembly on the anchoring elements and position it so that the frame offset meets the requirement listed in Table A7.1. Tighten only those connecting element interconnections that are necessary to maintain the frame offset for the remainder of the fixator-bone construct's assembly process.

A7.9.6 Align the test blocks so that their longitudinal axes are coincident and positioned so that the gap size adheres to the requirements listed in Table A7.1.

A7.9.7 Tighten all EFD interconnections either to the manufacturer's recommendations or to the recommended tightening torque that is listed in Table A7.1.

A7.9.8 Check and record the fixator-bone construct's alignment before testing.

A7.10 Procedure

Construct Mounting

A7.10.1 Verify that the loading axis, input and restraint platen positions, orientations, and restrained and unrestrained degrees of freedom meet the requirements of the particular investigation. Record these parameters with respect to a right-hand coordinate system defined with respect to the undeformed position of the construct being tested.

A7.10.2 Input linear displacements (or forces) should be delivered either along the bone analog longitudinal axis (axial load) or perpendicular to the bone analog longitudinal axis (shear load). The line of action of the input displacement should be recorded, with respect to the fixator-based right-hand orthogonal coordinate system.

A7.10.3 Input angular displacements (or moments) should be delivered either by a torque actuator or by an applied force couple. These moments should be either about the symmetry axis of the bone analog or about an axis perpendicular to the input-loading axis. If the moment is delivered by a force couple system, the points and lines of application if the individual forces must be reported. Typical way to achieve this might be four-point bending or eccentric force (cantilever).

A7.10.4 Because of the inherent variability of available fixator systems, use the following hierarchy to determine the alignment and subsequent loading orientation designations for the tests.

A7.10.4.1 The fixator system is indicated for a specific anatomical indication with a fixed anatomical orientation. Align the test construct relative to the direction of the applied load for the given tests according to the fixator system's alignment relative to the anatomical axes for the indication being evaluated.

A7.10.4.2 One fixator system within the group being evaluated is indicated for a specific anatomical indication with a fixed anatomical orientation. Align all test constructs relative to the direction of the applied load for the given tests according to each fixator system manufacturer's recommended alignment relative to the anatomical axes for the indication being evaluated.

A7.10.4.3 All fixator systems being evaluated are universally indicated for multiple indications. The axes will be aligned according to the major axes of the major construct components as follows. The axial axis will be oriented with the longitudinal elements rods(s). The transverse axis will be oriented parallel to the longitudinal axis of the anchorage elements. The lateral axis will be oriented normal to both the transverse and axial axes.

A7.10.5 Position the test construct in the test apparatus so that the fracture gap offset and anchor element offset parameters are equivalent for the series of tests being performed.

A7.10.6 Affix the construct to the input and restraint platens.

A7.10.7 The sites used as construct gripping/attachment locations should be on the bone analog and located at least three pin diameters away from the outermost sites of anchorage element attachments.

Construct Conditioning

A7.10.8 Subject constructs destined for single-cycle static tests to several quasistatic preconditioning load cycles to demonstrate that the reported load versus deformation curve is repeatable from cycle to cycle.

A7.10.9 Preconditioning should be continued until the apparent stiffness of the construct changes less that 5 % between subsequent cycles.

A7.10.10 Normally, about five preconditioning cycles are suitable for this purpose, with peak applied load within the elastic range, approximately 50 % of the expected physiological service load or 50 % of the expected construct failure load, whichever is lower.

A7.10.11 Record the resulting load versus deformation curves for the preconditioning cycles and the preconditioning cycle stiffness for each preconditioning cycle.

Static Strength or Stiffness Tests

A7.10.12 Single-cycle static tests may either be restricted to the elastic regime or taken to a failure point.

A7.10.13 Run single-cycle static stiffness or strength tests in displacement control (either linear or angular). Tests may be run in load control as long as the construct's response is of a linear nature.

A7.10.14 The minimum series of static tests for any given fixator-bone construct should include the following types of tests.

A7.10.15 *Axial Load Test*:

A7.10.15.1 Axially load the test construct through spherical load points as illustrated in Fig. A7.3. This test configuration results in a minimally constrained condition during the axial load test.

A7.10.15.2 For this test configuration, displacement is defined as the relative change in the straight-line distance between the loading points (see Fig. A7.3). Monitor this distance directly with the displacement transducer. The reaction force is measured by the force transducer and shall be the force vector that is aligned with the direction of the displacement vector.

A7.10.16 *Bend Tests*—This test method tests the fixator-bone construct in bending with loading occurring in the two principle anatomical (or local relative) planes for a given fracture indication. For typical long bone indications (femur; tibia, and so forth), this would be bending on both the *M-L* and *A-P* planes. For a universal fixator system, this would be bending about both the transverse and longitudinal axes.

A7.10.16.1 *Four-Point Bend Test*:

A7.10.16.1.1 The four-point bend test is used primarily used to evaluate fixator systems that are symmetrical about the fracture gap plane. A constant bending moment is generated in the test construct because of the forced displacement of the load points as illustrated in Fig. A7.4; therefore, this test normally would not be used to evaluate a fixator system that does not normally experience a uniform bending moment when clinically applied, that is, a system that bridges a joint space.

A7.10.16.1.2 For this test configuration, displacement is defined as the relative change in the vertical distance between the loading points and the support points (see Fig. A7.4). Monitor this distance directly with the displacement transducer. The reaction force is measured by the force transducer and shall be the force vector that is aligned with the direction of the displacement vector.

A7.10.16.2 *Cantilever Bend Test*:

A7.10.16.2.1 This test is used primarily for fixator systems that are not symmetrical about the fracture gap plane. Additionally, this test normally would not be used for the evaluation of a fixator system that would normally experience a uniform bending moment when clinically applied.

A7.10.16.2.2 A variable bending moment is generated in the test construct as a result of a load applied at a distance L (mm) from the rigidly anchored end of the test construct (see Fig. A7.5). The test construct should be orientated so that the anatomical proximal end is rigidly anchored and the anatomical distal end is unconstrained.

A7.10.16.2.3 For this test configuration, displacement is defined as the relative change in the vertical position of the load application point (see Fig. A7.5). Monitor this distance directly with the displacement transducer. The reaction force is measured by the force transducer and shall be the force vector that is aligned with the direction of the displacement vector.

A7.10.17 *Torsion Test*:

A7.10.17.1 A moment is applied to the test construct about the axis of the bone analog segments as illustrated in Fig. A7.1. The test construct is orientated so that the anatomical proximal end is rigidly anchored and the anatomical distal end is unconstrained.

A7.10.17.2 For this test configuration, displacement is defined as the relative change in the angular position of the test system's grips about the test machine's drive axis (see Fig. A7.1). Monitor this position directly with the displacement transducer. The reaction moment is measured by the torque transducer and shall be the moment vector that is oriented in the direction of the displacement vector.

A7.10.17.3 Load the construct in a quasistatic manner at a constant rate. Use a rate that is sufficient to attain in approximately 30 s either a load (or moment) magnitude that is in the range of typical physiologic usage or that is sufficient to cause failure. Alternatively, rates that are in the range of those expected clinically may be desirable for testing components made of polymeric materials that exhibit viscoelastic behavior and for components which rely upon friction for fixation. A rationale should be provided for whatever input rate is used and the rate(s) should be reported.

A7.10.17.4 Continuously record the reaction load (or

torque) in response to the applied linear (or angular) displacement of the input platen.

A7.10.17.5 Continue the test until the construct has met the specified failure criteria.

Multicycle Dynamic Tests

A7.10.18 These types of tests should be run in either load or torque control.

A7.10.19 Restricted multicycle dynamic tests to loading conditions that are within the EFD's elastic regime.

A7.10.20 The input loading frequency should be limited to a frequency that does not result in dynamic heating of any test construct component. Typically, a limit of five cycles per second (5 Hz) is sufficient to prevent heating and still generate test results in a timely manner. Alternatively, rates that are in the range of those expected clinically (1 Hz) may be necessary for testing components made of polymeric materials, which exhibit viscoelastic behavior, and for components, which rely upon friction for fixation. A rationale should be provided in the final report for the test frequency used for these types of devices.

A7.10.21 The standard multicycle dynamic test is a dynamic axial loading test (see Fig. A7.3). The test construct is exercised with a fully reversed tension and compression ($R = -1.0$) true sinusoidal loading waveform. Set the runout cycle limit for the standard test at 50 000 cycles.

A7.10.22 Record the loading cycle's maximum and minimum values, the input waveform shape, and the test frequency for inclusion in the final report.

A7.10.23 Continue the test until the construct has met the specified failure criteria or until the runout cycle limit has been reached.

A7.10.24 Record the final cycle count and failure mode (if applicable) of the dynamic test for inclusion in the final report.

A7.11 Calculation or Interpretation of Results

Static Strength or Stiffness Tests

A7.11.1 Using the load (or moment) versus deformation curve, determine the tangent stiffness and secant stiffness, as applicable, according to the definitions found in A7.3.

A7.11.2 On the load (or moment) versus deformation curve, determine the yield load (or moment) and ultimate load (or moment), as applicable, according to the definitions found in A7.3.

A7.11.3 Perform the following additional analyses for bend-type tests.

A7.11.4 *Cantilever Bend Test*:

A7.11.4.1 Calculate the bending (tangent or secant) stiffness in the following manner:

$$\text{Bending Stiffness} = \text{Stiffness} \cdot L \quad \text{(A7.1)}$$

where:
L = lever arm length (as illustrated in Fig. A7.5).

A7.11.4.2 Calculate the yield bending moment in the following manner, when applicable:

$$\text{Yield Bending Moment} = \text{Yield Load} \cdot L \quad \text{(A7.2)}$$

A7.11.4.3 Calculate the ultimate bending moment in the following manner, when applicable:

$$\text{Ultimate Bending Moment} = \text{Ultimate Load} \cdot L \quad \text{(A7.3)}$$

A7.11.5 *Four-Point Bend Test*:

A7.11.5.1 Calculate the bending (tangent or secant) stiffness in the following manner:

$$\text{Bending Stiffness} = \frac{\text{Stiffness} \cdot h^2\,(2h + 3k)}{12} \quad \text{(A7.4)}$$

where:
h = loading span distance (as illustrated in Fig. A7.4) and
k = support span distance (as illustrated in Fig. A7.4).

A7.11.5.2 Calculate the yield bending moment in the following manner, when applicable:

$$\text{Yield Bending Moment} = \frac{\text{Yield Load} \cdot h}{2} \quad \text{(A7.5)}$$

A7.11.5.3 Calculate the ultimate bending moment in the following manner, when applicable:

$$\text{Ultimate Bending Moment} = \frac{\text{Ultimate Load} \cdot h}{2} \quad \text{(A7.6)}$$

A7.11.6 Calculate the mean and standard deviation of the tangent stiffness, secant stiffness, yield load (or moment), and ultimate load (or moment) for each group of fixator-bone constructs tested.

Multicycle Dynamic Tests

A7.11.7 Plot the maximum load (or moment) versus cycles to test termination data on a semi-log graph. Various techniques may be used to estimate the mean or median fatigue lives, statistical differences between groups, curve fits of the fatigue data, probability of survival curves, and so forth. **(3-7)**.

A7.11.8 If determining median fatigue load (or moment) at a specific cycle count, it is recommended that the fatigue load (or moment) be determined as the median fatigue load (or moment) (50 % probability of survival), using a technique or criteria described in the literature **(1-3, 6, 7)**.

A7.12 Report

A7.12.1 The test report shall include the following, at a minimum:

A7.12.2 Identification of the individual elements comprising the fixator, which should include the manufacturer, part number, nomenclature, and where possible, the quality control or lot number. If the part is a prototype, provide geometrical and material descriptions.

A7.12.3 A description of the fixator-bone construct's configuration.

A7.12.3.1 The geometry and material composition of the bone analog used.

A7.12.3.2 Include a drawing, or photograph, or both, of the construct, using multiple orthogonal views (anterior-posterior, medial-lateral, and superior-inferior views) as necessary to define unambiguously the relative positions and orientations of the individual elements comprising the fixator.

A7.12.3.3 The physical dimensions, or element orientations, or both, within the fixator that can be varied by the end-user must be unambiguously specified. Typically, this would include the following information: fracture gap offset, frame offset, gap size, inner pin span, outer pin span, pin cluster span, pin offset, pin span. Additional optional information would include the position of clamps along the rod elements or pins, the angle between rods connected by an adjustable clamp and unsupported pin length.

A7.12.3.4 For fixator elements whose physical dimensions, or orientations, or both, cannot be varied by the end user, it is recognized that detailed dimensional, or material information, or both, may not be practical or appropriate to report when testing overall construct behavior. At a minimum, however, reference to public domain documentation reporting that specific information must be included.

A7.12.3.5 Description of any prior usage for any fixator element that was tested.

A7.12.3.6 Alternative procedures that were used while installing the anchoring elements in the test blocks.

A7.12.3.7 The assembly force or torque used to engage any connector gripping mechanism(s). If assembly is performed using noncalibrated specialty instruments often provided by manufacturers, for example, ratchet drives, this should be reported, and reference made to documentation reporting the actual force or torque delivered by such specialty instruments, if available.

A7.12.3.8 The construct's alignment before testing.

A7.12.4 Number of constructs tested for each test configuration and the rationale for the sample size selected.

A7.12.5 A description of the test machine (manufacturer, model).

A7.12.5.1 Include the description of any secondary transducers that were used to record construct response data that is presented in the final report.

A7.12.6 A description of the testing configuration(s).

A7.12.6.1 Report the loading axis, input and restraint platen positions, and restrained and unrestrained degrees of freedom for each test configuration.

A7.12.6.2 Report the construct's orientation relative to the test machine's loading axis for each test configuration.

A7.12.6.3 A drawing, or photograph, or both, of the construct within the test machine setup should be provided.

A7.12.6.4 Rationale for the use of alternative or modifications to the defined test configurations.

A7.12.7 Description of the test environment if other than the recommended room temperature laboratory air environment.

Static Tests

A7.12.8 Pictures of the failure surfaces of any components that failed during the study.

A7.12.9 The loading rate used during static tests with a corresponding rationale.

A7.12.10 The load versus deformation curves for the preconditioning cycles and the preconditioning cycle stiffness for each preconditioning cycle.

A7.12.11 The load versus deformation curves for each test performed.

A7.12.12 Alternative methods that were used to determine the stiffness or yield point. Also, include any methods that were used to compensate for toe regions found in the construct's response curve.

A7.12.13 The tabulated construct stiffness (tangent, or scan, or both) in the specified directions tested including the mean and standard deviation for each data set.

A7.12.14 The tabulated yield load (or moment) data in the specified directions tested including the mean and standard deviation for each data set.

A7.12.15 *Failure-Type Tests*:

A7.12.15.1 The specific threshold of irrecoverable deformation constituting failure and the rationale for the specific value selected.

A7.12.15.2 The failure definition used and the rationale for the method selected.

A7.12.15.3 The tabulated ultimate load (or moment) data in the specified directions tested including the mean and standard deviation for each data set.

A7.12.15.4 Any failure modes observed during the tests, for example, slip at a particular clamped interface or yield of a specific bridge element. If the specific mode of failure cannot be ascertained by gross observation, the technique(s) used to identify the mode or site of failure should be reported.

Multicycle Dynamic Tests

A7.12.16 Test frequency, waveform shape, and runout cycle limit for multicycle dynamic tests. Include a rationale for the test frequency used while testing constructs that contain polymeric fixator components that exhibit viscoelastic behavior or components that rely upon friction for fixation.

A7.12.17 Tabular listing that summarizes the maximum and minimum load and the number of cycles until test termination for the specified directions tested.

A7.12.18 Description of the failure mode and failure location for each construct that failed.

A7.12.19 The semi-log diagram of the maximum load (or moment) versus number of cycles to test termination. Uniquely identify constructs that have not failed before reaching the runout cycle limit.

A7.12.20 Regression analysis results for the maximum load (or moment) versus number of cycles to failure data, when applicable.

A7.12.21 When applicable, include the results of any fatigue data analyses conducted on the final study results. Include descriptions of any analytical or statistical techniques used when interpreting the fatigue data.

A7.13 Precision and Bias

A7.13.1 *Precision*—Data establishing the precision of the test method have not yet been obtained.

A7.13.2 *Bias*—No statement of bias can be made, since no acceptable reference values are available, nor can they be obtained since this test is a destructive test.

14. Keywords

14.1 bend testing—orthopedic medical devices; fatigue testing—orthopedic medical devices; orthopedic medical devices—external fixation devices; test methods—surgical devices

APPENDIXES

(Nonmandatory Information)

X1. RATIONALE

X1.1 This specification is intended to provide useful and consistent information related to the terminology, performance, test methods, and application of external skeletal fixation devices. A rationale for the importance of particular performance characteristics and a reference to applicable test methods is given in Section 6. Some of the applicable test methods are given in the annexes. Currently, test methods for connectors, in-plane compression of ring elements, joints, anchorage pins, and subassemblies are provided in Annex A2, Annex A3, Annex A4, Annex A5, and Annex A6, respectively.

X1.2 The orthopedic surgeon should be able to choose the size, design, orientation, and configuration of an ESFD, and the manner of preparation of the bone, appropriate to the usage of a fixator for each individual patient. To do so, the surgeon must have confidence that the geometry of the individual components of the fixator and its subassemblies has a specific, known meaning, which is quantifiable and reliable regardless of the manufacturer or design. The mechanical behavior and material properties also must be described in a reliable, known manner, which is irrespective of the manufacturer or design. To accomplish this uniformity of designations, the terminology, dimensions, mechanical properties, material properties, and test methods for obtaining and reporting these parameters must be standardized.

X1.3 Because of the wide variety of ESFDs currently available, and the many assemblages that are possible as a result of the modularity of these devices, a wide variety of testing protocols is needed. This specification provides an overall framework within which several test methods for individual elements, subassemblies of elements, or entire ESFD assemblies are registered in the form of annexes. As additional test methods are developed, it is contemplated that they will be incorporated as new annexes.

X2. RATIONALE FOR ANNEX A7

X2.1 The modularity of most external fixation devices affords a great deal of variability of how fixators can be constructed; therefore, it is necessary to develop a standard test method that will evaluate any possible fixator configuration in a consistent and repeatable manner so that a surgeon will have useful information available for comparing various fixation devices.

X2.2 In many instances, it is desirable to compare the effective stiffness or strength of alternative fixator configurations (deviations from the manufacturer's recommended configuration) that can be assembled from a specific set of elements; therefore, this test method was developed with flexibility built into it.

X2.3 Normally, elastic flexure of anchorage elements is the greatest source of compliance in the overall fixator construct. Clinically, however, large apparent fixator compliance can also result from loose anchorage elements. This test procedure is not designed to document anchorage element loosening or to identify factors responsible for loosening; therefore, the choice of bone analog material and the method used to insert anchorage elements should ensure sound purchase of the anchorage elements throughout construct testing.

X2.4 Because of the variety of fixator size ranges and anatomic sites, it is inappropriate to standardize completely the geometry or kinetics of construct loading tests. This test method, therefore, emphasizes the unambiguous documentation of the construct being tested. This is accomplished by clearly identifying the site at which loading is applied and deformation is measured and a formal definition of the construct's stiffness, or strength, or both for each combination of load/deformation measured.

X2.5 A dynamic axial loading test method is defined in this test method instead of a typical fatigue test. The anticipated outcome for a typical fatigue test is the generation of a fatigue crack, which leads to the eventual failure of a component within the fixator system. Unfortunately, this type of failure is not a typical clinical failure of fixator systems. The typical cyclic loading clinical failure mode of fixator systems is a degradation of the interconnection strength at the bone/anchoring element interface. Since this type of failure cannot be consistently reproduced in the laboratory, this specification does not attempt to evaluate this failure mode. The only purpose then to perform cyclic loading tests would be to determine if any of the interconnections loosened over time; therefore, the standard dynamic test method stipulates a maximum runout cycle limit of only 50 000 cycles. In the event that a typical fatigue test is required, the testing conditions should be defined corresponding to the particular questions that need to be answered.

REFERENCES

(1) Little, R. E., *Statistical Planning and Analysis, ASTM STP 588*, American Society of Testing and Materials, West Conshohocken, PA.

(2) Little, R. E. and Ekvall, *Statistical Analysis of Fatigue Data, ASTM STP 744*, American Society of Testing and Materials, West Conshohocken, PA.

(3) Little, R. E. and Jebe, E. H., *Manual on Statistical Planning and Analysis of Fatigue Experiments, ASTM STP 588*, American Society of Testing Materials, West Conshohocken, PA, 1975.

(4) Conway, J. B. and Sjodahl, L. H., *Analysis and Representation of Fatigue Data*, ASTM International, Materials Park, OH, 1991.

(5) Collins, J. A., *Failure of Materials in Mechanical Design*, John Wiley and Sons, New York, 1981.

(6) Swanson, *Handbook of Fatigue Testing, ASTM STP 566*, American Society of Testing and Materials, West Conshohocken, PA.

(7) Little, R. E., "Optimal Stress Amplitude Selection in Estimating Median Fatigue Limits Using Small Samples," *Journal of Testing and Evaluation*, 1990, pp. 115–122.

Standard Specification for the Requirements and Disclosure of Self-Closing Aneurysm Clips[1]

This standard is issued under the fixed designation F 1542; the number immediately following the designation indicates the year of original adoption or, in the case of revision, the year of last revision. A number in parentheses indicates the year of last reapproval. A superscript epsilon (ε) indicates an editorial change since the last revision or reapproval.

1. Scope

1.1 This specification covers requirements for the specific characteristics of self-closing aneurysm clips that are intended for permanent implantation. Appropriate test requirements are also included.

1.2 Since all of the properties that contribute to aneurysm clip performance may not be known, this specification is intended to reflect the state of our knowledge to date.

1.3 Miniatures of "microclips" that are not intended for the obliteration of aneurysms are excluded from this specification.

2. Referenced Documents

2.1 *ASTM Standards:*

F 55 Specification for Stainless Steel Bar and Wire for Surgical Implants[2]

F 56 Specification for Stainless Steel Sheet and Strip for Surgical Implants[2]

F 67 Specification for Unalloyed Titanium for Surgical Implant Applications[3]

F 75 Specification for Cast Cobalt-Chromium-Molybdenum Alloy for Surgical Implant Applications[3]

F 90 Specification for Wrought Cobalt-Chromium-Tungsten-Nickel Alloy for Surgical Implant Applications[3]

F 136 Specification for Wrought Titanium 6A1-4V ELI Alloy for Surgical Implant Applications[3]

F 138 Specification for Stainless Steel Bar and Wire for Surgical Implants (Special Quality)[3]

F 139 Specification for Stainless Steel Sheet and Strip for Surgical Implants (Special Quality)[3]

F 361 Practice for Assessment of Compatibility of Metallic Materials for Surgical Implants with Respect to Effect of Materials on Tissues[4]

F 469 Practice for Assessment of Compatibility of Nonporous Polymeric Materials for Surgical Implants with Regard to Effect of Materials on Tissues[4]

F 560 Specification for Unalloyed Tantalum for Surgical Implant Applications[3]

F 562 Specification for Wrought Cobalt-Nickel-Chromium-Molybdenum Alloy for Surgical Implant Applications[3]

F 563 Specification for Wrought Cobalt-Nickel-Chromium-Molybdenum-Tungsten-Iron Alloy for Surgical Implant Applications[3]

F 688 Specification for Wrought Cobalt-Nickel-Chromium-Molybdenum Alloy Plate, Sheet, and Foil for Surgical Implants[3]

F 700 Practice for Care and Handling of Intracranial Aneurysm Clips and Instruments[3]

F 748 Practice for Selecting Generic Biological Test Methods for Materials and Devices[3]

F 981 Practice for Assessment of Compatibility of Biomaterials (Non-Porous) for Surgical Implants with Respect to Effect of Materials in Muscle and Bone[3]

2.2 *ISO Standard:*[5]

ISO TC 150

3. Requirements

3.1 *General*—This section contains requirements for the disclosure of information on aneurysm clip force measurements and requirements for labeling the materials and biocompatibility of the device.

3.2 *Performance Disclosure*:

3.2.1 *Force (See X1.2)*—The manufacturer shall disclose the closing force (measured in g) exerted by the blades when tested in accordance with 4.2.

3.2.2 *Force Range*—The manufacturer shall measure each clip as defined in 3.2.1 and report either the closing force of the individual clip, a minimum closing force for that specific clip, or a range within which the specific clip lies. If a range is reported, defined ranges shall be no greater than ±10 % of the median force.

3.2.3 *Materials*:

3.2.3.1 The manufacturer shall disclose the generic names of the materials used in the manufacture of the clip. ASTM material specification nomenclature shall be used whenever available. If the clips are made of multiple components, the name of the material for each component shall be disclosed.

3.2.3.2 Clips will be manufactured so as to be nonferromagnetic. The aneurysm clip must possess the following material

[1] This specification is under the jurisdiction of ASTM Committee F04 on Medical and Surgical Materials and Devices and is the direct responsibility of Subcommittee F04.31 on Neurosurgical Standards.

Current edition approved Aug. 15, 1994. Published October 1994.

[2] Discontinued 1991—See *Annual Book of ASTM Standards*, Vol 13.01.

[3] *Annual Book of ASTM Standards*, Vol 13.01.

[4] Discontinued—See *Annual Book of ASTM Standards*, Vol 13.01.

[5] Available from American National Standards Institute, 25 W. 43rd St., 4th Floor, New York, NY 10036.

property in order to be judged as nonferromagnetic. The force exerted on a finished aneurysm clip by a 1.5 tesla whole body MRI magnet must not exceed the gravitational force on the clip (that is, its own weight).

3.2.3.3 *(See X1.4)*—The materials and alloys used in aneurysm clips conforming to this specification should be fabricated in accordance with one of the following ASTM specifications: F 55, F 56, F 67, F 75, F 90, F 136, F 138, F 139, F 560, F 562, F 563, F 688, ISO TC 150, or subsequently approved ASTM Committee F04 standards. Clips manufactured with nonapproved materials must be labeled with a statement that they are made of a material for which there is no ISO or ASTM Committee F04 standard.

3.3 *Biocompatibility*—Aneurysm clips should be biocompatible with the tissue in which they are intended to be implanted. Components shall meet the biologic compatibility requirements of Practices F 361, F 469, F 748, and F 981, or other equivalent practices wherever applicable.

3.4 *Clip Nomenclature Disclosure*:

3.4.1 *General*—This section contains requirements for a standard nomenclature for self-closing aneurysm clips.

3.4.2 The manufacturer shall use the following type nomenclature to describe its clips and disclose this information where applicable:

3.4.2.1 *Blade Geometry*:

(1) Straight,
(2) Angled,
(3) Curved,
(4) Angled tip,
(5) Vessel encircling,
(6) Fenestrated,
(7) Bayonet, and
(8) Other (describe).

3.4.2.2 *Blade and Clip Dimensions*:

(1) Length of the blade (the blade being defined as the contact surfaces of the clip, when the clip is in the closed position; in straight blade clips, this being the measured contact surface and in curved blades, the measured arc cord length of the contact surface);
(2) Blade width (indicate mean width for tapered blade);
(3) Blade cross section (flat, rolled, round, or other (describe in detail));
(4) Clip length;
(5) Maximum opening at the tip; and
(6) Inside diameter of encircling clip.

3.4.2.3 *Spring Type*:

(1) Integral single bend,
(2) Integral coil,
(3) Inserted coil,
(4) Noncontinuous ring,
(5) Torsion bar, and
(6) Other (describe).

3.4.2.4 *Surface Finish*:

(1) Blade Gripping Surfaces:
(a) Smooth,
(b) Serrated, and
(c) Other (describe).

(2) *Clip Body:*
(a) Polished,
(b) Matte,
(c) Satin, and
(d) Other (describe).

(3) Material Treatment:
(a) Passivated,
(b) Electropolish, and
(c) Other (describe).

3.5 *Labeling Requirements (See X1.5)*—The labeling for aneurysm clips within the scope of this specification must comply with the following requirements as a minimum:

3.5.1 *Unit Labeling*—Each clip will have imprinted on it a unique code to allow traceability in accordance with FDA guidelines.

3.5.2 The following information shall be available with the unit package:

3.5.2.1 Manufacturer's identification or lot number;
3.5.2.2 Blade geometry (3.4.2.1);
3.5.2.3 Blade length (3.4.2.2);
3.5.2.4 Blade width (3.4.2.2);
3.5.2.5 Gripping surface (3.4.2.4);
3.5.2.6 Force (4.2);
3.5.2.7 Manufacturer's name;
3.5.2.8 Identification of catalog number;
3.5.2.9 Composition of material(s), including ASTM material specifications, if applicable, from which the clip is made; and
3.5.2.10 Specification of the ferromagnetic property(s) of the aneurysm clip or its component (see 4.3).

3.5.3 *Product Information*—As a minimum, the following data should be available in the manufacturer's and distributor's ordering information.

3.5.3.1 Blade geometry (3.4.2.1);
3.5.3.2 Blade length (3.4.2.2);
3.5.3.3 Blade width (3.4.2.2);
3.5.3.4 Spring type (3.4.2.3);
3.5.3.5 Surface finish (3.4.2.4);
3.5.3.6 Force (4.2);
3.5.3.7 Composition of materials, including ASTM material specifications, if applicable, from which the clip is made;
3.5.3.8 A statement suggesting that only applier(s) designed specifically for the particular clip(s) be used (specify catalog number);
3.5.3.9 A statement referencing Practice F 700;
3.5.3.10 Specification of the ferromagnetic property(s) of the aneurysm clip or its component (see 4.3); and
3.5.3.11 Identification or catalog number.

4. Tests

4.1 *Significance*—This force measurement test provides information on the closing force of the clip under circumstances approximating its neurosurgical application.

4.2 *Force Measurement*:

4.2.1 The closing force shall be measured at a point one-third the length of the blade measured from its tip at a blade separation distance of 1.0 mm. In the case of clips that are not designed for blade contact along the blade's entire working length, the closing force will be measured at the midpoint of the region of the blade contact.

4.2.2 The manufacturer will perform a test on each finished clip and report its performance as specified in 3.2.2.

4.3 *Non-Ferromagnetic Property*—The operational definition of a non-ferromagnetic aneurysm clip, stated in 3.2.3.2, is met if, and only if, the clip passes the following test:

4.3.1 The magnetic force on the clip is proportional to the product $\vec{B} \cdot \nabla\vec{B}$, where $\vec{B}$ = the magnetic field intensity and $\nabla\vec{B}$ = the gradient of magnetic field intensity.

4.3.1.1 In general, the $\vec{B} \cdot \nabla\vec{B}$ product is maximum in the vicinity (usually just inside) of the portal of the magnet. Note that the magnitudes of $\vec{B}$ and $\nabla\vec{B}$ are those at the local site at which the force measurement is made.

4.3.1.2 The clip is suspended at the end of a string and held stationary in the vertical direction (that is, perpendicular to the ground) while it is placed in position at the portal of the imaging magnet. Following release of the clip, the deflection of the string from the vertical is then observed. The magnetic force is less than the gravitational force (that is, the clip's weight) if the deflection of the string with respect to the vertical is less than 45°. The clip is then judged to be non-ferromagnetic and suitable for implantation.

4.3.2 There are four caveats. First, for a given magnet, it will be necessary to find the position at which the $\vec{B} \cdot \nabla\vec{B}$ product is maximum. Second, this position is likely to be different in magnets from different manufacturers. It may be necessary to collect data from these magnets using the test described in 4.3.1. Third, the specification described above deals only with the magnetic force on a finished, unimplanted clip. The possibility exists that nominally non-ferromagnetic clips may product image artifacts due to local distortion of the radiofrequency field or due to mild ferromagnetism induced by bending of the clips during placement. Fourth, a deflection of less than 45° at the portal of a 1.5 tesla magnet does not preclude a deflection exceeding 45° at a higher magnetic field strength.

APPENDIX

(Nonmandatory Information)

X1. RATIONALE FOR DEVELOPMENT OF THE SPECIFICATION

X1.1 *General Rationale*—This specification is intended to provide a common language for communication between producers, users, engineers, government agencies, and designers of self-closing aneurysm clips; to provide uniformity in reporting performance characteristics, test methodology, and nomenclature; and to be versatile enough to cover new products and test methods as they are introduced.

X1.2 The surgeon must have available quantitative data on the clip closing force to select an optimal clip for a particular aneurysm. Clips are marketed with a variety of closing forces and may be indistinguishable otherwise.

X1.3 Because of the increasing importance of magnetic resonance as an imaging modality at 1.5 tesla, the expectation that even higher strength magnets will be introduced in the future, and the fact that implanted aneurysm clips made of ferromagnetic alloys may move or even become dislodged in these magnetic fields, it is important that aneurysm clips be non-ferromagnetic. Inasmuch as non-ferromagnetic alloys may be converted to a ferromagnetic state by the working processes, it is essential that testing be conducted on the finished clip and that all clips be identified clearly as to the ferromagnetic (or non-ferromagnetic state).

X1.4 The materials designated are those shown to be reasonably corrosion resistant at the physiologic conditions of the biologic environment and are not susceptible to intergranular corrosion attack, are non-toxic, and are biocompatible. Other materials have been used successfully for aneurysm clips. Some clip designs made with these materials are considered by surgeons to be essential and potentially lifesaving but have not been able to be made of other materials. The use of these materials is therefore not proscribed, but appropriate labeling is required.

X1.5 Labeling requirements are to ensure that the medical community has available sufficient information to facilitate the proper selection of self-closing aneurysm clips for safe and effective use. Specific coding imprinted on each clip is necessary to allow traceability in accordance with FDA requirements.

Standard Terminology Relating to Underwater Search, Rescue, and Recovery Activities[1]

This standard is issued under the fixed designation F 1549; the number immediately following the designation indicates the year of original adoption or, in the case of revision, the year of last revision. A number in parentheses indicates the year of last reapproval. A superscript epsilon (ϵ) indicates an editorial change since the last revision or reapproval.

1. Scope

1.1 The purpose of this terminology is to establish uniformity in terminology used in the field of underwater search, rescue, and recovery.

1.2 The terminology is appropriate to those underwater search, rescue, or recovery activities that use self-contained or surface-supplied underwater breathing apparatuses to provide a breathing gas supply for the searcher(s).

1.3 *This standard does not purport to address all of the safety concerns, if any, associated with its use. It is the responsibility of the user of this standard to establish appropriate safety and health practices and determine the applicability of regulatory limitations prior to use.*

2. Significance and Use

2.1 This terminology is not intended to be used as a replacement for proper training and experience in the skills necessary to conduct an underwater search and rescue operation safely.

3. Terminology

3.1 *Definitions:*

ascent rate, *n*—the speed of vertical movement toward the water's surface.

bail-out bottle, *n*—A diver-carried supply of air or mixed gas (as appropriate) sufficient under standard operating conditions to allow the diver to reach the surface or another source of breathing gas, or to be reached by a safety diver.

bottom time, *n*—the total elapsed time measured in minutes from the time that the diver leaves the surface in descent to the time that the diver begins ascent.

console, *n*—an instrument package that contains one or more instruments used to monitor depth, bottom time, surface intervals, air pressure, compass direction, decompression status, or some combination thereof.

D.A.N., *n*—Divers Alert Network.[2]

DCS, *n*—decompression sickness, a medical condition with a variety of symptoms that may result from gas or bubbles in the tissues of divers after pressure reduction.

decompression, *n*—the technique used to allow the controlled removal of excess insert gas from the body during and after a dive to prevent decompression sickness (DCS).

dive computer, *n*—a microprocessor-based electronic instrument that provides data based on a specific decompression model.

dive profile, *n*—the depth/time history of a dive that typically consists of bottom time, maximum depth, and surface interval.

Doppler bubble detector, *n*—a device that uses the Doppler Effect to monitor specific areas of the circulatory system and detect the presence of bubbles as a measure of decompression stress.

hyperbaric chamber, *n*—a chamber in which the internal pressure can be elevated by the introduction of compressed air (or other gasses) that is used primarily for medical treatment (including decompression sickness and arterial gas embolism) and physiological studies.

J-valve, *n*—a manually operated, spring-loaded, SCUBA cylinder check valve that incorporates a low air warning/reserve air mechanism.

K-valve, *n*—a simple, manually operated on-off SCUBA cylinder valve.

line tender, *n*—the individual who controls the diver's search pattern.

nitrogen narcosis, *n*—a distinct anesthetic effect, characterized by loss of judgment and disorientation, caused from breathing nitrogen at increased partial pressures.

repetitive diving, *n*—any dive conducted while the decompression model being followed for the dives indicates that inert gases are still present in the tissues from a previous dive. This is within the context of a fixed time period, usually 12 to 24 h, depending on the model being followed.

repetitive group designation, *n*—an assigned letter on a decompression table that relates directly to the amount of residual inert gas in the diver's tissues following a dive. This group changes with time as the diver's body off-gases.

residual nitrogen, *n*—nitrogen gas that is still dissolved in a diver's tissues after he has surfaced from a dive using compressed air as a breathing gas.

RNT, *n*—residual nitrogen time.

safety diver, *n*—diver who is dressed completely in dive gear and who remains on the surface to go to the immediate aid

[1] This terminology is under the jurisdiction of ASTM Committee F-32 on Search and Rescue and is the direct responsibility of Subcommittee F32.06 on Terminology.

Current edition approved August 15, 1994. Published September 1994.

[2] D.A.N. is an organization that disseminates diving safety information, provides diving medical insurance, and offers telephone assistance for answering questions related to diving medicine and for locating hyperbaric treatment facilities that can provide medical care for barotrauma injuries. It can be contacted by telephone at 919-684-2948 for non-emergency questions and at 919-684-8111 for emergencies.

of a distressed diver underwater.

safety stop, *n*—additional time spent at shallow depths even though the dive computer or dive table indicates that a direct ascent to the surface is possible.

standby diver, *n*—a diver at the dive location available to assist a diver in the water.

treatment table, *n*—a recompression schedule used to treat decompression sickness or embolisms.

umbilical, *n*—in surface-supplied diving, diver's gas and a communication and safety line all in one bundle.

Designation: F 1552 – 94

Standard Practice for Training Instructor Qualification and Certification Eligibility of Emergency Medical Dispatchers[1]

This standard is issued under the fixed designation F 1552; the number immediately following the designation indicates the year of original adoption or, in the case of revision, the year of last revision. A number in parentheses indicates the year of last reapproval. A superscript epsilon (ε) indicates an editorial change since the last revision or reapproval.

INTRODUCTION

The emergency medical dispatcher (EMD) is the principal link between the public requesting emergency medical assistance and the emergency medical services (EMS) system. The EMD plays a key role in the ability of the EMS system to respond to a perceived medical emergency. The benefits of specifically trained emergency medical dispatchers are far reaching. Through medical dispatch, specific education, and compliance to medically sound policies and procedures, the EMD is able to accurately interrogate the caller, dispatch the appropriate responders, provide pertinent information to responders, and give instructions to aid patients via the caller.

This practice provides direction for the training and certification of emergency medical dispatchers to assist them in making appropriate decisions about EMS responses in a safe, consistent and non-arbitrary manner. EMS systems with emergency medical dispatchers trained to this practice provide pre-arrival instructions to the caller to assist the patient until pre-hospital care arrives. The EMD concept provides for safer vehicle response configurations and modes. It may reduce operating costs by preserving specialized EMS resources for those emergencies requiring them.

The EMD training curriculum is not intended to furnish all inclusive telecommunications education required for the emergency medical dispatcher or public safety telecommunicator. EMD training provides only the additional education affecting the practice of dispatching emergency medical resources such as ambulances, rescue units, first responder units and other types of responding units of an emergency medical nature; coordinating these response units with those of other public safety agencies; and providing instructions to the calling party to assist in preserving life prior to the arrival of responding units. The curriculum is intended to provide specific knowledge and medical information above that required of a previously trained and educated basic public safety telecommunicator. EMD training is only one module of education required of emergency medical services telecommunicators. It is a subspecialty of both public safety communications and emergency medical services systems that is required within a comprehensive public safety communications center where other disciplines of communications are practiced and should be present in all EMS systems. Additional disciplines include law enforcement, fire, and aeromedical telecommunications.

This practice is one of a set of applicable standards relating to the emergency medical dispatch function. The reader is directed to obtain related ASTM documents that encompass the administration of EMD programs and Practice F 1258.

1. Scope

1.1 This practice covers the training structure and primary function of emergency medical dispatchers. The primary function of the emergency medical dispatcher is the management of calls for emergency medical assistance as outlined in Practice F 1258 and NAEMSP Position Paper on emergency medical dispatch. Training as an emergency medical technician, paramedic, nurse, physician, or basic telecommunicator does not prepare a person to function as an EMD. The emergency medical dispatching functions have become so specialized that only an individual with dispatch specific medical training can perform the required tasks. This practice will delineate the training structure for the essential role of emergency medical dispatcher.

1.2 This practice is intended to outline the basic areas of knowledge required for an EMD, and to standardize the expectations and training between the various educational settings that are available to deliver the EMD training. This

[1] This practice is under the jurisdiction of ASTM Committee F-30 on Emergency Medical Services and is the direct responsibility of Subcommittee F30.02 on Personnel, Training and Education.

Current edition approved August 15, 1994. Published October 1994.

practice is not intended to serve as a curriculum for a training agency. All curricula developed or selected shall include the key components outlined in this practice.

1.3 It is understood that each agency may possess special and unique needs related to the training of EMDs. However, those specialty training areas that lie outside the scope of this standard shall not be included in selected 24 h minimum curriculum delineated by this practice. Additional training as desired may be annexed but may not supplant the learning goals required by this practice.

1.4 The scope of this standard includes:

1.4.1 EMD instructor qualifications,

1.4.2 Student selection criteria for emergency medical dispatcher candidates,

1.4.3 Emergency medical dispatcher training curriculum guideline,

1.4.4 Guidelines for EMD course goals and minimum time allocations,

1.4.5 Testing and evaluation of the student utilizing the stated course goals as basis for certification or certification eligibility as an emergency medical dispatcher,

1.4.6 Recommended equipment, materials, and facilities for training,

1.4.7 Guidelines for training course administration and record maintenance, and

1.4.8 Guidelines for an optional EMD preceptorship.

1.5 *This standard does not purport to address all of the safety concerns, if any, associated with its use. It is the responsibility of the user of this standard to establish appropriate safety and health practices and determine the applicability of regulatory limitations prior to use.*

2. Referenced Documents

2.1 *ASTM Standards:*

F 1177 Terminology Relating to Emergency Medical Services[2]

F 1258 Practice for Emergency Medical Dispatch[2]

3. Terminology

3.1 *Definitions of Terms Specific to This Standard:*

3.1.1 *coding*—the selection and assignment of an alphanumeric classification to a call by an EMD.

3.1.2 *emergency medical dispatcher (EMD)*—a trained public safety telecommunicator with additional training and specific emergency medical knowledge essential for the efficient management of emergency medical communications.

3.1.3 *emergency medical dispatch priority reference system (EMDPRS)*—a medically approved reference system used by a local dispatch agency to dispatch aid to medical emergencies, which includes: systematized caller interrogation questions, systematized pre-arrival instructions, and protocols matching the dispatcher's evaluation of injury or illness severity with vehicle response mode and configuration.

3.1.3.1 *Discussion*—An EMDPRS is not any particular proprietary set of cards or questions. It is a generic set of protocols meeting this description.

3.1.4 *EMD preceptorship*—a supervised dispatcher internship sponsored by the training agency.

3.1.5 *EMD selection*—the process that establishes criteria to identify a candidate for training as an emergency medical dispatcher (EMD).

3.1.6 *pre-arrival instructions*—telephone rendered, medically approved written instructions given by trained emergency medical dispatchers through callers that help to provide aid to the victim and control of the situation prior to patient access by pre-hospital care providers.

3.1.7 *public safety telecommunicator*—an individual trained to communicate by electronic means with persons seeking emergency assistance and with agencies and individuals providing such assistance.

4. Significance and Use

4.1 The emergency medical dispatcher should be a specially trained telecommunicator with specific emergency medical knowledge. These EMS personnel have traditionally performed this role without the benefits of dispatch specific medical training and medically sound protocols. Prompt, correct, and appropriate patient care can be enhanced with the use of a standardized approach to selection, training and performance assessment. This standard guide is intended for use by agencies, organizations and jurisdictions having the responsibility for providing the training, practice, and evaluation of emergency medical dispatchers.

5. Instructor Qualifications

5.1 All instructors shall be thoroughly knowledgeable about the emergency medical dispatching environment and with the working environment of public safety telecommunications.

5.2 It is essential that the emergency medical dispatch instructor be capable of understanding, adequately presenting, and defending ALS level-Dispatch Life Support information. This necessitates that the instructor responsible for teaching the medical portion of the training program have training, skill, and experience at the advanced EMT (EMT-I/EMT-P) level. Alternatively, this instructor may be a critical care trained physician, nurse or physician assistant. This level of instructor qualification is necessary to facilitate the student's understanding of medical classifications necessary to interrogate and evaluate the input of the caller, as well as their ability to systematically categorize the information obtained from the caller and assign appropriate and locally designed response configurations and modes.

5.3 The instructor shall have proven competence as an instructor in a related field.

5.4 EMD instructors shall be proficient in the specific skills and concepts taught in the EMD course.

5.5 Each instructor shall have successfully completed a recognized EMD training course.

6. Selection Criteria for Training

6.1 Each EMD training entity shall adopt a formal written policy delineating the selection procedures for individuals to be trained or employed as emergency medical dispatchers, or both. It must address the ability to:

6.1.1 Read and write at a high school graduate or GED level;

---

[2] *Annual Book of ASTM Standards*, Vol 13.01.

6.1.2 Perform those clerical skills as delineated by the employing agency;

6.1.3 Perform verbal skills in a clear and understandable manner, in the required language or languages established in the criteria as necessary to that dispatch provider agency;

6.1.4 Perform alpha-numeric transcription skills necessary to correctly record addresses, locations, and telephone numbers; and,

6.1.5 Demonstrate competency in basic telecommunications skills as defined by the training or hiring agency.

6.2 Selection criteria should also include the following traits:

6.2.1 A clear attribute of helpfulness and compassion toward the sick or injured patient and the caller advocate;

6.2.2 The attributes necessary to clearly guide callers in crisis through necessary interrogation procedures and the provision of telephone pre-arrival instructions;

6.2.3 The attributes of learning necessary to master the skills, philosophy, and knowledge required to successfully complete the training process;

6.2.4 The attributes necessary to efficiently and effectively organize multiple tasks and complicated situations and activities;

6.2.5 The ability to handle the known levels of emotional stress clearly present in caller/patient crisis intervention, death and dying situations, call prioritization and triage, and multiple tasking;

6.2.6 The abilities necessary to function within the team framework of public safety and EMS systems;

6.2.7 The abilities to elicit and assimilate caller information and then to prioritize but appropriately consolidate (summarize) this information in a format used to inform the public safety responders.

7. Emergency Medical Dispatcher Training Curriculum Guidelines

7.1 The EMD curriculum must be specific to this subspecialty of telecommunications and emergency medical systems.

7.2 The EMD curriculum used shall consist of lesson plans with defined educational goals and objectives. The lesson plans and their individual objectives shall coincide with the practice standards listed in reference documents and in the appendix. The EMD training curriculum shall address the concepts of design and the application of skills necessary for the appropriate use of the EMDPRS utilized within their dispatch agency.

7.3 The curriculum used shall include the learning goals contained in this practice.

7.4 The specific curriculum used must follow a logical and progressive sequence of presentation.

7.5 The medical portion of the emergency medical dispatch priority reference system (EMDPRS) shall not be modified or changed in any manner by the instructing agency or instructors.

8. Emergency Medical Dispatcher Course Goals and Minimum Time Allocations

8.1 This course provides instruction and skills practice sufficient to achieve EMD certification eligibility. The minimum time allocation of this course shall be 24 h.

8.2 The following EMD course goals are delineated with their associated minimum time allocations. Although 19 h are mandated, all 24 h of the EMD course must be utilized in teaching these required goals. The remaining 5 h are to be dispersed so the learning goals may be tailored to each training agencies requirements. It is imperative the "no less than" (NLT) hours be followed when developing an EMD course.

8.3 Develop a basic understanding of the rationale for emergency medical dispatching including (NLT 1 hour):

8.3.1 The history of EMD,

8.3.2 The evolution of EMD,

8.3.3 The philosophy of EMD,

8.3.4 Common misconceptions of EMD,

8.4 Develop a basic understanding of the roles and responsibilities of EMD: (NLT 1 h),

8.4.1 The sub-roles and segments of the duties,

8.4.2 Professional subspecialties,

8.4.2.1 Public safety community,

8.4.2.2 Law enforcement,

8.4.2.3 Fire communications,

8.4.2.4 EMS communications,

8.4.2.5 The medical community team,

8.4.2.6 A colleague of the medical profession,

8.5 Develop an understanding of the medical-legal aspects of EMD (NLT 1 h),

8.5.1 The legal concepts affecting the EMD,

8.5.1.1 Negligence,

8.5.1.2 Abandonment,

8.5.1.3 Foreseeability,

8.5.2 Misconceptions and inappropriate concerns, and

8.5.3 Appropriate concerns.

8.6 Gain the knowledge necessary to successfully interrogate callers to obtain relevant information (NLT 1 h):

8.6.1 Rationale for interrogation,

8.6.2 Understand the psychology of the caller,

8.6.3 Chief complaint determination,

8.6.4 The caller's hysteria threshold,

8.6.5 The concept of repetitive persistence, and

8.6.6 The types of callers (minority groups, third party, children, disabled and speech impaired, etc.).

8.7 Develop an understanding of the concepts of dispatch life support (DLS) and the psychological aspects of providing pre-arrival instructions (NLT 1 h):

8.7.1 Practical limitations confronting the EMD, and

8.7.2 Predictable events affecting DLS delivery.

8.8 Develop an understanding of the methodologies for delivering pre-arrival instructions and demonstrate the practical use of the pre-arrival instructions (NLT 1 h):

8.8.1 Understand the various categories of pre-arrival instructions contained in the employing agency's EMDPRS including written protocols and verbatim scripts,

8.8.2 Understand the requirements for formal pre-arrival instructions,

8.8.3 Understand the necessity for formal written treatment scripts,

8.8.4 Demonstrate the practical application of pre-arrival instruction, and

8.8.5 Demonstrate the verbatim delivery of formal treatment scripts.

8.9 Develop an understanding of those pre-hospital medical emergencies and emergency medical complaints as found in the employing agency's EMDPRS (NLT 8 h).

8.10 Develop a working knowledge of each EMDPRS chief complaint to include interrogation, coding, response, and related pre-arrival instructions (NLT 1 h):

8.10.1 Configuration of EMDPRS used by the employing agency,

8.10.2 Flow through the configuration, and

8.10.3 Interaction between EMDPRS elements.

8.11 Develop an understanding of how to handle all EMD functions in a prompt and accurate manner while being courteous and professional in dealing with all callers.

8.12 Demonstrate the ability to utilize all of the components of the employing agency's EMDPRS (NLT 2 h):

8.12.1 Interrogation,

8.12.2 Coding,

8.12.3 Response, and

8.12.4 Related pre-arrival instructions.

8.13 Gain an appreciation of the influence of the correct functioning of trained professional emergency medical dispatchers through their routine utilization the EMDPRS.

8.14 Understand the basic principles and components of quality assurance/improvement and their relationship to the application of correct dispatch processes (NLT 1 h).

8.15 Become certified or certification eligible emergency medical dispatcher via designated agency or government channels (NLT 1 h):

8.15.1 Required testing and evaluation.

9. Equipment, Materials, and Facilities

9.1 The need for the audio-video equipment will be determined by the types of audio-visual teaching materials utilized.

9.2 Suggested audio-visual equipment and materials needed for an EMD course may include:

9.2.1 Lectern/podium,

9.2.2 Chalk board or dry erase board,

9.2.3 Flip chart (if used),

9.2.4 Overhead slide or movie projector, or both,

9.2.5 Spare bulbs for projector,

9.2.6 Electrical extension cords as needed,

9.2.7 Projection screen,

9.2.8 Audio tape player,

9.2.9 Videotape player and monitor,

9.2.10 Pointer, and

9.2.11 Additional audio-video equipment and training aids as required.

9.3 Student and instructor textbooks and reference materials, including:

9.3.1 Instructor's lesson plan,

9.3.2 Lesson plans shall be based on the EMDPRS used by the employing dispatching agency,

9.3.3 Each lesson plan must contain a listing of the unit performance objectives, needed materials and equipment, textual content, practice exercises and review questions or evaluation mechanisms,

9.3.4 Student study guide (one for each student),

9.3.5 The study guide shall include the same performance objectives as the lesson plans and shall be used as a working document throughout the instructional course. The student study guide shall be retained by the student at the completion of the EMD course and may serve as a review tool after the student has completed the training program,

9.3.6 Course schedule (one for each student), and

9.3.7 Student performance objectives (one for each student).

9.4 Films, slides, overhead transparencies, audio and video tapes to accompany lessons, as required for instructional objectives.

9.5 Written final examination.

9.6 Written course evaluation.

9.7 Emergency medical dispatch priority reference system (EMDPRS) approved by the medical control physician (one for each student).

9.8 The classroom must be well lighted to permit students to take notes and refer to the study guide and handouts. The room must have adequate heating, ventilation, or air conditioning, or both, to ensure the comfort of the students and instructor.

9.9 Each student should have a chair and table or desk at which to take notes.

10. Training Course Administration

10.1 The collection, maintenance and dissemination of records required to document the conduct of the program and to assess how well the course achieves its objectives must occur. The following records shall be maintained:

10.1.1 Factual and accurate student attendance records,

10.1.2 Factual and accurate student performance records, including, comments regarding need for improvement in skills or knowledge,

10.1.3 Identity and qualifications of the instructor(s),

10.1.4 Records of the evaluation of instructor(s) performance, and

10.1.5 Records of course content evaluations.

11. Optional Preceptorship for Emergency Medical Dispatchers

11.1 Once an individual has successfully completed the initial EMD training course, an optional preceptorship program may allow the individual to experience the intense and demanding conditions that exist in an emergency communications center. It may include:

11.1.1 Orientation manual for new EMDs specific to the participating agency's operation,

11.1.2 Orientation through one-on-one preceptorship with a competent, experienced, trained, emergency medical dispatcher, and

11.1.3 Evaluation should be performed through the participating agency's quality assurance/quality improvement program.

12. Student Reference Texts

12.1 Textbooks and course material from established EMD programs may be utilized.

12.2 Students should have access to a selection of reference documents and training materials that deal with emergency medical dispatching.

13. Keywords

13.1 curriculum; dispatcher; dispatch life support (DLS);

emergency medical dispatch; emergency medical dispatcher (EMD); pre-arrival instructions; preceptorship; telecommunicator

APPENDIX

(Nonmandatory Information)

X1. RELATED PUBLICATIONS

X1.1 *Principles of EMS Systems: A Comprehensive Text for Physicians.* Roush, W. R. ed, American College of Emergency Physicians, Dallas, 1989.

X1.2 *EMS Medical Directors Handbook*, Kuehl, Alexander. C. V. Mosby Company, St. Louis, Second edition, 1993.

X1.3 *Principles of Emergency Medical Dispatch*, Clawson, Jeff J., M.D. and Dernocoeur, Kate B., Brady/Prentice Hall, Englewood Cliffs, NJ 1988.

X1.4 *APCO Basic Telecommunicator Student Manual*, APCO Inc., South Daytona Beach, FL.

X1.5 *Emergency Dispatching: A Medical Communicators Guide.* Steel, S., Brady/Prentice Hall, Englewood Cliffs, NJ, 1992.

Designation: F 1555 – 94

Standard Guide for Characteristics for Extremity Splints[1]

This standard is issued under the fixed designation F 1555; the number immediately following the designation indicates the year of original adoption or, in the case of revision, the year of last revision. A number in parentheses indicates the year of last reapproval. A superscript epsilon (ϵ) indicates an editorial change since the last revision or reapproval.

INTRODUCTION

The objective of this guide is to begin to address the recognized need to support and immobilize the injured extremity. Although this guide does not quantitatively address performance standards for this device, it does address the characteristics of the device(s) used to provide support and immobilization of the extremities in a patient suspected of receiving trauma to that portion of the body.

1. Scope

1.1 This guide covers minimum standards for devices, designated here as extremity splint(s) (ES), commonly known as splints. Extremity splints are designed to be used for the immobilization of an extremity by emergency medical service personnel.

1.2 This guide does not identify specific degrees of limitation of motion achieved by placement of a extrication device (ED) on a patient. Definitive requirements for immobilization of extremities in the out of hospital environment, and, in particular, the degree of limitation associated with the use of an ED in the out of hospital setting, has not been established in the medical literature.

1.3 *This standard does not purport to address all of the safety concerns, if any, associated with its use. It is the responsibility of the user of this standard to establish appropriate safety and health practices and determine the applicability of regulatory limitations prior to use.*

2. Referenced Documents

2.1 *ASTM Standards:*

F 1177 Terminology Relating to Emergency Medical Services[2]

2.2 *Centers for Disease Control Standard:*

Guidelines for Prevention of Transmission of HIV and HBV to Healthcare and Public Safety Workers[3]

2.3 *OSHA Standard:*

29 CFR 1910.1030 Occupational Exposure to Bloodborne Pathogens; Final Rule[4]

3. Terminology

3.1 *Definitions:*

3.1.1 *extremity(ies)*—limb; arm or leg.

3.1.2 *extremity immobilization*—immobilization of the injury site and its contiguous proximal and distal joints or bones.

3.1.3 *retention system*—a retention system is an adjunct to, or an integral part of a device that allows the device to be securely attached to the patient, used in whatever configuration and size necessary to accomplish the goal, while still allowing reasonable and necessary access to the patient.

3.2 *Definitions of Terms Specific to This Standard:*

3.2.1 *directions of movement*—movements include flexion, extension, rotation, distraction, lateral motion, and axial compression motion.

3.2.2 *extremity splint*—a device that can be secured to the extremity that will maintain the position and limit motion of the extremity.

3.2.3 *immobilization*—limitation of motion.

3.2.4 *pneumatic devices*—devices utilizing air pressure or vacuum to limit the motion of an extremity.

3.2.5 *traction device*—a device that aligns the extremity and limits its motion.

3.3 For definitions of other terms used in this guide, refer to Terminology F 1177.

4. Significance and Use

4.1 The intent of this guide is to identify characteristics that an ES should possess.

4.2 Varied clinical situations may require differing combinations of devices for adequate extremity immobilization, including traction or pneumatic devices, or both.

4.3 A device intended for use with adult patients shall accommodate the 95th percentile adult American male.

4.4 Devices that are labeled as intended for pediatric use shall not be required to accommodate adult patients.

---

[1] This guide is under the jurisdiction of ASTM Committee F-30 on Emergency Medical Services and is the direct responsibility of Subcommittee F30.01 on EMS Equipment.

Current edition approved Oct. 15, 1994. Published December 1994.

[2] *Annual Book of ASTM Standards*, Vol 13.01.

[3] Available from Centers for Desease Control, Atlanta, GA 30333.

[4] Available from Superintendent of Documents, U.S. Government Printing Office, Washington, DC 20402.

5. Capability

5.1 The ES shall allow for the use of adjunct devices as necessary such that immobilization is provided in the planes of motion as noted in 3.2.1.

5.2 Traction splints should facilitate full orthopedic and vascular assessment.

6. Durability

6.1 The ES shall maintain stated characteristics throughout its lifetime as indicated by manufacturer's recommendations.

7. Maintenance

7.1 The ES shall be disposable, or easily cleaned, consistent with CDC and OSHA decontamination procedures, without deterioration of the product or the retention of cleaning agents which may be harmful to the patient.

7.2 The cleaning/decontamination procedure shall be explained in the manufacturer's product information.

8. Capability

8.1 This guide does not presently quantify the limitation of motion expected to be imposed upon a patient as a result of the application of an ES. This capability has not been omitted due to a lack of need, but as a result of the fact that such quantitative requirements have not been identified in the medical literature. It is hoped that such requirements can be developed, and included in this guide at its next review.

9. Keywords

9.1 extremity splint; immobilization; splint

Designation: F 1556 – 94

Standard Guide for Spinal Immobilization and Extrication (Spined) Device Characteristics[1]

This standard is issued under the fixed designation F 1556; the number immediately following the designation indicates the year of original adoption or, in the case of revision, the year of last revision. A number in parentheses indicates the year of last reapproval. A superscript epsilon (ε) indicates an editorial change since the last revision or reapproval.

INTRODUCTION

The objective of this guide is to begin to address the recognized need to support and immobilize the components of the spine or spinal cord. Although this guide does not quantitatively address performance standards for this device, it does address the characteristics of the device(s) used to provide support and immobilization of the components of the central nervous system for the patient suspected of receiving trauma to that body system.

1. Scope

1.1 This guide covers minimum standards for devices, designated here as spinal immobilization and extrication device(s) (SPINED), commonly referred to as short spine board. The SPINED is designed to be used as the platform for immobilization and extrication of a patient with potential spine or spinal cord injury by emergency medical service personnel.

1.2 This guide does not identify specific degrees of limitation of motion achieved by placement of a SPINED on a patient. Definitive requirements for immobilization of the spine, and, in particular, the degree of limitation associated with the use of a SPINED, has not been established in the medical literature.

1.3 *This standard does not purport to address all of the safety concerns, if any, associated with its use. It is the responsibility of the user of this standard to establish appropriate safety and health practices and determine the applicability of regulatory limitations prior to use.*

2. Referenced Documents

2.1 *ASTM Standards:*

F 1177 Terminology Relating to Emergency Medical Services[2]

2.2 *Centers for Disease Control Standard:*

Guidelines for Prevention of Transmission of HIV and HBV to Healthcare and Public Safety Workers[3]

2.3 *OSHA Standard:*

29 CFR 1910.1030 Occupational Exposure to Bloodborne Pathogens; Final Rule[4]

3. Terminology

3.1 *Definitions:*

3.1.1 *retention system*—a retention system is an adjunct to or an integral part of the primary platform that allows the patient to be securely attached to that platform used in whatever configuration and size necessary to accomplish the goal, while still allowing reasonable and necessary access to the patient.

3.1.2 *spinal immobilization*—spinal immobilization shall refer to immobilization of the spine and its contiguous structures, the pelvis, and skull.

3.1.3 *spine*—the spine shall include the cervical, thoracic, lumbar, and sacral vertebrae.

3.2 *Definitions of Terms Specific to This Standard:*

3.2.1 *directions of movement*—directions include flexion, extension, rotation, distraction, lateral motion, and axial compression motion.

3.2.2 *immobilization*—limitation of motion.

3.2.3 *spinal immobilization and extrication device*—a platform to which the patient can be secured, which will support the patient's spine during immobilization and transportation.

3.3 For definition of other terms used in this guide, refer to Terminology F 1177.

4. Significance and Use

4.1 The intent of this guide is to identify characteristics that a SPINED shall possess.

4.2 As opposed to a full body spinal immobilization device, the SPINED incorporates additional features that assist in the extrication of a victim from a confined space.

4.3 It is not expected that the SPINED will be used alone to

[1] This guide is under the jurisdiction of ASTM Committee F-30 on Emergency Medical Services and is the direct responsibility of Subcommittee F30.01 on EMS Equipment.

Current edition approved Oct. 15, 1994. Published December 1994.

[2] *Annual Book of ASTM Standards*, Vol 13.01.

[3] Available from Center for Disease Control, Atlanta, GA 30333.

[4] Available from Superintendent of Documents, U.S. Government Printing Office, Washington, DC 20402.

provide the entire scope of required immobilization. Clinical situations may require differing combinations of devices for adequate total spinal immobilization. A SPINE device may be one of the devices.

4.4 A device intended for use with adult patients shall accommodate the 95th percentile adult, American male.

4.5 Devices that are labeled as intended for pediatric use shall not be required to accommodate adult patients.

4.6 The device shall be able to be used by the practitioner in an ergonomically sound manner.

5. Characteristics

5.1 The SPINED, when lifted in accordance with manufacturer's instructions, shall support the 95th percentile adult American male patient.

5.2 There shall be a retention system used in conjunction with the immobilization platform.

5.3 The SPINED shall incorporate a means to accommodate the ergonomically sound handling and lifting of the immobilized patient.

5.4 The SPINED shall allow X-ray to be taken through it, and be MRI compatible.

6. Durability

6.1 The SPINED shall maintain stated characteristics throughout its lifetime as indicated by manufacturer's recommendations.

7. Maintenance

7.1 The SPINED shall be disposable or easily cleaned consistent with CDC and OSHA decontaminated procedures, without deterioration of the product or the retention of cleaning agents that may be harmful to the patient.

7.2 The cleaning/decontamination procedure shall be explained in the manufacturer's product information.

8. Capability

8.1 This guide does not presently quantify the limitation of motion expected to be imposed upon a patient as a result of the application of a SPINED. This capability has not been omitted due to a lack of need, but as a result of the fact that such quantitative requirements have not been identified in the medical literature. It is hoped that such requirements can be developed, and included in this guide at its next review.

9. Keywords

9.1 extrication device; short spine board; spinal immobilization

Designation: F 1557 – 94

Standard Guide for Full Body Spinal Immobilization Devices (FBSID) Characteristics[1]

This standard is issued under the fixed designation F 1557; the number immediately following the designation indicates the year of original adoption or, in the case of revision, the year of last revision. A number in parentheses indicates the year of last reapproval. A superscript epsilon (ε) indicates an editorial change since the last revision or reapproval.

INTRODUCTION

The objective of this guide is to begin to address the recognized need to support and immobilize the components of the spine or spinal cord. Although this guide does not quantitatively address performance standards for this device, it does address the characteristics of the device(s) used to provide support and immobilization of the components of the central nervous system for the patient suspected of receiving trauma to that body system.

1. Scope

1.1 This guide establishes minimum standards for devices, designated here as full body spinal immobilization device(s) (FBSID), commonly known as long boards. The FBSID is designed to be used as the base structure for immobilization and transport of a patient with potential spine or spinal cord injury by emergency medical service personnel.

1.2 This guide does not identify specific degrees of limitation of motion achieved by placement of a FBSID on a patient. Definitive requirements for immobilization of the spine, and, in particular, the degree of limitation associated with the use of a FBSID, has not been established in the medical literature.

1.3 *This standard does not purport to address all of the safety concerns, if any, associated with its use. It is the responsibility of the user of this standard to establish appropriate safety and health practices and determine the applicability of regulatory limitations prior to use.*

2. Referenced Documents

2.1 *ASTM Standards:*

F 1177 Terminology Relating to Emergency Medical Services[2]

2.2 *Centers for Disease Control Standard:*

Guidelines for Prevention of Transmission of HIV and HBV to Healthcare and Public Safety Workers[3]

2.3 *OSHA Standard:*

29 CFR 1910.1030 Occupational Exposure to Bloodborne Pathogens; Final Rule[4]

3. Terminology

3.1 *Definitions:*

3.1.1 *retention system*—a retention system is an adjunct to or an integral part of the primary platform that allows the patient to be securely attached to that platform, used in whatever configuration and size necessary to accomplish the goal, while still allowing reasonable and necessary access to the patient.

3.1.2 *spinal immobilization*—spinal immobilization refers to immobilization of the entire spine and its contiguous structures, the pelvis and skull.

3.1.3 *spine*—the spine shall include the cervical, thoracic, lumbar, and sacral vertebrae.

3.2 *Description of Terms Specific to This Standard:*

3.2.1 *directions of movement*—include flexion, extension, rotation, distraction, lateral motion, and axial compression motion.

3.2.2 *full body spinal immobilization device*—a platform upon which a patient can be secured, that will support the entire length and weight of the patient during immobilization and transportation.

3.2.3 *immobilization*—limitation of motion.

3.3 For definitions of other terms used in this guide, refer to Terminology F 1177.

4. Significance and Use

4.1 The intent of this guide is to identify characteristics which a FBSID shall possess.

4.2 It is not expected that the FBSID will be used alone to provide the entire scope of required immobilization. Clinical situations may require differing combinations of devices for adequate total spinal immobilization. A FBSID may be one of the devices.

4.3 A device intended for use with adult patients shall accommodate the 95th percentile adult American male.

4.4 Devices that are labeled as intended for pediatric use

---

[1] This guide is under the jurisdiction of ASTM Committee F-30 on Emergency Medical Services and is the direct responsibility of Subcommittee F30.01 on EMS Equipment.

Current edition approved Oct. 15, 1994. Published December 1994.

[2] *Annual Book of ASTM Standards*, Vol 13.01.

[3] Available from Center for Disease Control, Atlanta, GA 30333.

[4] Available from Superintendent of Documents, U.S. Government Printing Office, Washington, DC, 20402.

shall not be required to accommodate an adult.

4.5 The device shall be able to be used by the practitioner in an ergonomically sound manner.

5. Characteristics

5.1 The FBSID, when lifted in accordance with manufacturer's instructions, shall support the 95th percentile adult American male patient, full length in the supine position.

5.2 The FBSID shall incorporate a means to accommodate the ergonomically sound handling and lifting of the device when fully loaded.

5.3 The FBSID shall allow X-ray to be taken through it, and be MRI compatible.

5.4 The FBSID shall allow for the use of adjunct devices as necessary such that immobilization is provided in the planes of motion as noted in 3.2.1.

5.5 The FBSID shall support lower extremities in such a manner that it prevents motion of the pelvis and spine.

5.6 There shall be a retention system used in conjunction with the immobilization platform.

6. Durability

6.1 The FBSID shall maintain stated characteristics throughout its lifetime as indicated by manufacturer's recommendations.

7. Maintenance

7.1 The FBSID shall be disposable, or easily cleaned, consistent with CDC and OSHA decontamination procedures, without deterioration of the product or the retention of cleaning agents that may be harmful to the patient.

7.2 The cleaning/decontamination procedure shall be explained in the manufacturer's product information.

8. Capability

8.1 This guide does not presently quantify the limitation of motion expected to be imposed upon a patient as a result of the application of a SPINE device. This capability has not been omitted due to a lack of need, but as a result of the fact that such quantitative requirements have not been identified in the medical literature. It is hoped that such requirements can be developed, and included in this guide at its next review.

9. Keywords

9.1 immobilization device; long board; spinal cord; spine

Standard Guide for Characteristics for Adjunct Cervical Spine Immobilization Devices (ACSID)[1]

This standard is issued under the fixed designation F 1558; the number immediately following the designation indicates the year of original adoption or, in the case of revision, the year of last revision. A number in parentheses indicates the year of last reapproval. A superscript epsilon (ϵ) indicates an editorial change since the last revision or reapproval.

INTRODUCTION

The objective of this guide is to begin to address the recognized need to support and immobilize the components of the spine or spinal cord. Although this guide does not quantitatively address performance standards for this device, it does address the characteristics of the device(s) used to provide support and immobilization of the components of the central nervous system for the patient suspected of receiving trauma to that body system.

1. Scope

1.1 This guide establishes minimum standards for devices designated here as adjunct cervical spine immobilization device (ACSID); a lateral stabilizer for the head is an example of this type of device. The ACSID is designed to be used to assist in the immobilization of the cervical spine, by emergency medical services personnel.

1.2 This guide does not identify specific degrees of limitation of motion achieved by placement of an ACSID on a patient. Definitive requirements for immobilization of the spine, and, in particular, the degree of limitation associated with the use of an ACSID, has not been established in the medical literature.

1.3 *This standard does not purport to address all of the safety concerns, if any, associated with its use. It is the responsibility of the user of this standard to establish appropriate safety and health practices and determine the applicability of regulatory limitations prior to use.*

2. Referenced Documents

2.1 *ASTM Standards:*

F 1177 Terminology Relating to Emergency Medical Services[2]

2.2 *OSHA Standard:*

20 CFR 1910.1030 Occupational Exposure to Bloodborne Pathogens; Final Rule[3]

2.3 *Centers for Disease Control Standard:*

Guidelines for Prevention of Transmission of HIV and HBV to Healthcare and Public Safety Workers[4]

3. Terminology

3.1 *Definitions:*

3.1.1 *retention system*—an adjunct to or an integral part of the primary platform that allows the patient to be securely attached to that platform used in whatever configuration and size necessary to accomplish the goal while still allowing reasonable and necessary access to the patient.

3.1.2 *spinal immobilization*—immobilization of the entire spine and its contiguous structures, the pelvis and skull.

3.1.3 *spine*—the spine shall include the cervical, thoracic, lumbar, and sacral vertebrae.

3.2 *Definitions of Terms Specific to This Standard:*

3.2.1 *directions of movement*—directions include flexion, extension, rotation, distraction, lateral motion, and axial compression motion.

3.2.2 *immobilization*—limitation of motion.

3.3 For definitions of other terms used in this guide, refer to Terminology F 1177.

4. Significance and Use

4.1 The intent of this guide is to identify characteristics that an ACSID shall possess.

4.2 It is not expected that the ACSID will be used alone to provide the entire scope of required immobilization. Clinical situations may require differing combinations of devices for adequate total spinal immobilization. An ACSID may be one of the devices.

---

[1] This guide is under the jurisdiction of ASTM Committee F-30 on Emergency Medical Services and is the direct responsibility of Subcommittee F30.01 on EMS Equipment.

Current edition approved Nov. 15, 1994. Published December 1994.

[2] *Annual Book of ASTM Standards*, Vol 13.01.

[3] Available from Superintendent of Documents, U.S. Government Printing Office, Washington, DC 20402.

[4] Available from Center for Disease Control, Atlanta, GA 30333.

4.3 An ACSID is intended to provide stabilization and/or support in addition to other immobilization devices in one or more of the planes of motion mentioned in 3.2.1 (see 4.2).

5. Characteristics

5.1 Placement or use of the ACSID shall not require or cause movement of the head or neck, or both, during treatment or transport of patient.

5.2 Once in place, the ACSID shall assist in the immobilization of the cervical spine.

5.3 It shall not cause vascular compression or airway compromise.

5.4 It shall provide access to see the ears once applied.

5.5 It shall provide for continued evaluation of cervical soft tissue or jugular vein distention, or tracheal deviation, or combination thereof.

5.6 It shall be capable of being applied without movement of the cervical spine.

5.7 It shall provide for the performance of normally accepted techniques of airway management/maintenance.

5.8 It shall allow X-ray to be taken through it, and be MRI compatible.

5.9 It shall be compatible with other devices used in the complete immobilization of the cervical spine.

6. Durability

6.1 The ACSID shall maintain stated characteristics throughout its lifetime as indicated by manufacturer's recommendations.

7. Maintenance

7.1 The ACSID shall be disposable or easily cleaned consistent with CDC and OSHA decontamination procedures, without deterioration of the product or the retention of cleaning agents that may be harmful to the patient.

7.2 The cleaning/decontamination procedure shall be explained in the manufacturer's product information.

8. Capability

8.1 This guide does not presently quantify the limitation of motion expected to be imposed upon a patient as a result of the application of a SPINE device. This capability has not been omitted due to a lack of need, but as a result of the fact that such quantitative requirements have not been identified in the medical literature. It is hoped that such requirements can be developed, and included in this guide at its next review.

9. Keywords

9.1 cervical spine immobilization device; spinal cord; spine

Designation: F 1559 – 94

Standard Guide for Characteristics for Cervical Spine Immobilization Collar(s) (CSIC)[1]

This standard is issued under the fixed designation F 1559; the number immediately following the designation indicates the year of original adoption or, in the case of revision, the year of last revision. A number in parentheses indicates the year of last reapproval. A superscript epsilon (ε) indicates an editorial change since the last revision or reapproval.

INTRODUCTION

The objective of this guide is to begin to address the recognized need to support and immobilize the components of the spine or spinal cord. Although this guide does not quantitatively address performance standards for this device, it does address the characteristics of the device(s) used to provide support and immobilization of the components of the central nervous system for the patient suspected of receiving trauma to that body system.

1. Scope

1.1 This guide establishes minimum standards for devices, designated here as cervical spine immobilization collar(s) (CSIC), commonly referred to as cervical collars. The CSIC is used as the initial device for immobilization of the cervical spine, of a patient by emergency medical service personnel.

1.2 This guide does not identify specific degrees of limitation of motion achieved by placement of a CSIC on a patient. Definitive requirements for immobilization of the spine, and, in particular, the degree of limitation associated with the use of a CSIC, has not been established in the medical literature.

1.3 *This standard does not purport to address all of the safety concerns, if any, associated with its use. It is the responsibility of the user of this standard to establish appropriate safety and health practices and determine the applicability of regulatory limitations prior to use.*

2. Referenced Documents

2.1 *ASTM Standards:*

F 1177 Terminology Relating to Emergency Medical Services[2]

2.2 *Centers for Disease Control Standard:*

Guidelines for Prevention of Transmission of HIV and HBV to Healthcare and Public Safety Workers[3]

2.3 *OSHA Standard:*

29 CFR 1910.1030 Occupational Exposure to Bloodborne Pathogens; Final Rule[4]

3. Terminology

3.1 *Definitions:*

3.1.1 *retention system*—a retention system is an adjunct to or an integral part of the primary platform that allows the patient to be securely attached to that platform used in whatever configuration and size necessary to accomplish the goal, while still allowing reasonable and necessary access to the patient.

3.1.2 *spinal immobilization*—spinal immobilization shall refer to immobilization of the spine and its contiguous structures, the pelvis, and skull.

3.1.3 *spine*—the spine shall include the cervical, thoracic, lumbar, and sacral vertebrae.

3.2 *Definitions of Terms Specific to This Standard:*

3.2.1 *cervical spine immobilization collar*—a device that can be applied and secured to a patient to support and immobilize the cervical spine during immobilization and transportation.

3.2.2 *directions of movement*—directions include flexion, extension, rotation, distraction, lateral motion, and axial compression motion.

3.2.3 *immobilization*—limitation of motion.

3.3 For definitions of other terms used in this guide, refer to Terminology F 1177.

4. Significance and Use

4.1 The intent of this guide is to identify characteristics that a CSIC shall possess.

4.2 It is not expected that the CSIC will be used alone to provide the entire scope of required immobilization. Clinical situations may require differing combinations of devices for adequate total spinal immobilization. A CSIC may be one of the devices.

4.3 Various configurations or sizes, or both, may be required to accommodate variation amongst individuals.

---

[1] This guide is under the jurisdiction of ASTM Committee F-30 on Emergency Medical Services and is the direct responsibility of Subcommittee F30.01 on EMS Equipment.

Current edition approved Oct. 15, 1994. Published December 1994.

[2] *Annual Book of ASTM Standards*, Vol 13.01.

[3] Available from Center for Disease Control, Atlanta, GA 30333.

[4] Available from Superintendent of Documents, U.S. Government Printing Office, Washington, DC 20402.

4.4 The CSIC shall be able to be used by the practitioner in an ergonomically sound manner.

4.5 The CSIC is intended to provide stabilization, not traction, and shall not be used to apply traction.

5. Characteristics

5.1 It shall allow X-ray to be taken through it, and be MRI compatible.

5.2 It shall have a rapid, accurate, and easily usable method for size selection.

5.3 Placement of the CSIC shall not require or cause movement of the head or neck, or both.

5.4 A CSIC shall provide support in all directions of motion mentioned in 3.2.1.

5.5 It shall be compatible with other devices used in the complete immobilization of the cervical spine.

5.6 It shall be capable of being applied with the patient in a prone, sitting, or supine position, without movement of the cervical spine.

5.7 Because during rapid extrication there may only be time to apply the CSIC, it shall provide a high degree of immobilization.

5.8 It shall not cause vascular compression or airway compromise.

5.9 It shall provide access to secure an airway established by a needle cricothyroidotomy.

5.10 It shall provide for continued evaluation of cervical soft tissue or jugular vein distention or tracheal deviation, or combination thereof.

5.11 It shall provide for the performance of normally accepted techniques of airway management/maintenance.

6. Durability

6.1 The CSIC shall maintain stated characteristics throughout its lifetime as indicated by manufacturer's recommendations.

7. Maintenance

7.1 The CSIC shall be disposable or easily cleaned consistent with CDC decontamination procedures, without deterioration of the product or the retention of cleaning agents that may be harmful to the patient.

7.2 The cleaning/decontamination procedure shall be explained in the manufacturer's product information.

8. Capability

8.1 This guide does not presently quantify the limitation of motion expected to be imposed upon a patient as a result of the application of a spine device. This capability has not been omitted due to a lack of need, but as a result of the fact that such quantitative requirements have not been identified in the medical literature. It is hoped that such requirements can be developed, and included in this guide at its next review.

9. Keywords

9.1 cervical spine immobilization collar; spinal cord; spine

Standard Practice for Emergency Medical Dispatch Management[1]

This standard is issued under the fixed designation F 1560; the number immediately following the designation indicates the year of original adoption or, in the case of revision, the year of last revision. A number in parentheses indicates the year of last reapproval. A superscript epsilon (ε) indicates an editorial change since the last revision or reapproval.

INTRODUCTION

The emergency medical dispatcher (EMD) is the principal link between the public caller requesting emergency medical assistance and the emergency medical service (EMS) resource delivery system. As such, the EMD plays a fundamental role in the ability of the EMS system to respond to a perceived medical emergency. With proper training, program administration, supervision, and medical direction, the EMD can accurately query the caller, select an appropriate method of response, provide pertinent information to responders and give appropriate aid and direction for patients through the caller. Through careful application and reference to a written, medically approved, emergency medical dispatch protocol, sound decisions concerning EMS responses can be made in a safe, reproducible, and non-arbitrary manner. These benefits are realized by EMS systems when appropriate implementation, sound medical management and quality assurance/quality improvement (QA/QI) at dispatch are provided within the EMD/EMS system. This practice assists in establishing these management and administrative standards.

1. Scope

1.1 This practice covers the function of the emergency medical dispatcher (EMD). This function is the prompt and accurate processing of calls for emergency medical assistance. The training and practice through the use of a written or automated medical dispatch protocol is not sufficient in itself to ensure continued medically correct functioning of the EMD. Their dispatch-specific medical training and focal role in EMS has developed to such a complexity that only through a correctly structured and appropriately managed quality assurance environment can the benefits of their practice be fully realized. The philosophies of emergency medical dispatch have established new duties to which the emergency medical dispatch agency must respond. It is important that their quality assurance/quality improvement (QA/QI) activities, including initial hiring, orientation, training and certification, continuing dispatch education, recertification, and performance evaluation be given appropriate managerial attention to help ensure the ongoing safety in the performance of the EMD. This practice establishes functional guidelines for these managerial, administrative and supervisory functions.

1.2 The scope of this practice includes:

1.2.1 The entry level selection criteria for hiring emergency medical dispatchers;

1.2.2 The orientation of new emergency medical dispatchers;

1.2.3 Development of QA/QI mechanisms, management strategies and organizational structures for use within a comprehensive emergency medical dispatch system;

1.2.4 Performance evaluation as a component of a comprehensive and ongoing quality assurance and risk management program for an emergency medical dispatch system;

1.2.5 Development and provision of continuing dispatch education activities for the emergency medical dispatcher;

1.2.6 Requirements for initial certification and recertification of the emergency medical dispatcher;

1.2.7 Provision for comparative analysis between different EMD program approaches available to the EMS community that conform to established EMD practice standards prior to implementation of an emergency medical dispatch program; and

1.2.8 Guidelines for implementation of an emergency medical dispatch program.

1.3 *This standard does not purport to address all of the safety concerns, if any, associated with its use. It is the responsibility of the user of this standard to establish appropriate safety and health practices and determine the applicability of regulatory limitations prior to use.*

2. Referenced Documents

2.1 *ASTM Standards:*

F 1258 Practice for Emergency Medical Dispatch[2]

---

[1] This practice is under the jurisdiction of ASTM Committee F30 on Emergency Medical Services and is the direct responsibility of Subcommittee F30.04 on Communications.

Current edition approved Oct. 10, 2000. Published January 2001. Originally published as F 1560 - 94. Last previous edition F 1560 - 94.

[2] *Annual Book of ASTM Standards*, Vol 13.01

F 1552 Practice for Training, Instructor Qualification, and Certification Eligibility of Emergency Medical Dispatchers[2]

3. Terminology

3.1 *Definitions of Terms Specific to This Standard:*

3.1.1 *case review template*—a structured performance evaluation document containing all necessary input and output actions required of dispatchers that parallels the EMDs' on-line protocols, policies, and procedures related to call-taking and processing. It contains check-off lists and compliance scoring mechanisms that objectively rate the EMDs' performance on a single call.

3.1.2 *dispatch life support*—the knowledge, procedures, and skills used by trained EMDs in providing care through pre-arrival instructions to callers. It consists of those BLS and ALS principles that are appropriate to application by medical dispatchers.

3.1.3 *emergency medical dispatch agency*—any organization or a combination of organizations working cooperatively, that routinely accepts calls for emergency medical assistance and facilitates the dispatch of prehospital emergency medical resources/personnel and provides medically oriented pre-arrival instructions pursuant to such requests.

3.1.4 *performance evaluation*—the documented, objective, quantitative measure of an individual emergency medical dispatcher's performance based upon compliance with departmental protocols, policies and procedures.

3.1.5 *pre-arrival instructions*—telephone-rendered, medically approved written instructions provided by trained EMDs through callers which help to provide aid to the victim and control of the situation prior to arrival of prehospital personnel.

3.1.6 *quality assurance/quality improvement (QA/QI)*—the comprehensive program of prospectively setting standards, concurrently monitoring the performance of clinical, operational and personnel components, and retrospectively improving these components in the emergency medical dispatch agency when compared with these standards.

3.1.7 *risk management*—a sub-component of the quality assurance/quality improvement program designed to: identify problematic situations and assist EMS medical directors, dispatch supervisors, and EMDs in modifying practice behaviors found to be deficient by quality assurance procedures; protect the public against incompetent practitioners; and modify structural, resource, and protocol deficiencies that may exist in the emergency medical dispatch system.

4. Summary of Practice

4.1 A comprehensive plan for managing the quality of care in an emergency medical dispatch system must include careful planning, EMD program selection, proper system implementation, employee selection, training, and certification, QA/QI, performance evaluation, continuing dispatch education, recertification, and risk management activities. These functions must be designed and implemented to assist the medical director, dispatch supervisor, and emergency medical dispatcher in monitoring and modifying EMD performance found deficient by QA/QI to protect the public against incompetent practitioners, as well as modify organizational structure, resource, or protocol deficiencies that exist in the emergency medical dispatch system.

4.1.1 *Entry Level Selection*—The selection and evaluation of new dispatchers must include clearly written objective standards to be adopted for qualifying candidates, interviewing applicants and pre-employment aptitude and skill testing pursuant to the hiring of dispatchers.

4.1.2 *Orientation*— A pre-planned process of events focusing on the development and acclimation of an employee who will function within the organization's standards, practices, policies, and procedures.

4.1.3 *Quality Assurance/Quality Improvement*—Within a physician medically directed emergency medical dispatch system, the development and implementation of employee performance thresholds, concurrent evaluation of compliance to these thresholds through on-line supervision, retrospective evaluation of non-edited logged recordings of requests for emergency service measuring compliance with policy, practice, and procedure to validate that the practices are appropriate, and to correct the employee and practice if they are found to be deficient.

4.1.4 *Performance Evaluation*—Each EMD in an emergency medical dispatch agency must regularly and routinely be evaluated with respect to his or her adherence to policy, protocol, and procedure through the QA/QI process. This determines conformance to these elements and measures how this performance affects the efficiency and effectiveness of the emergency medical dispatch agency. The evaluation must be quantitative and qualitative.

4.1.5 *Continuing Education*—Each emergency medical dispatch agency must provide for the development and implementation of a continuing dispatch education program for the benefit of that agency's EMD personnel. This program must provide the EMD with applicable educational topics designed to enhance their general knowledge and skill in the philosophy and application of the EMD program used within the emergency medical dispatch agency.

4.1.6 *Risk Management*— A written practice and procedure shall be established for each agency that provides guidelines for physician medical directors, EMS system administrators, agency supervisors, and/or QA/QI personnel to follow when an EMD is identified as failing to meet or follow established protocols. These may be acts of omission or commission identified through concurrent or retrospective review. This practice and procedure shall provide guidelines for proper investigative criteria relative to the medical or administrative nature of the perceived infraction, and the proper progressive disciplinary procedure to be followed in order to provide the EMD due process.

4.1.7 *Certification, Recertification*—All EMDs working in a medical dispatch agency shall be certified as competent in the use of the medically approved emergency medical dispatch priority reference system (EMDPRS) used within the medical dispatch center. Initial certification and recertification standards shall be established by each certifying entity associated with their EMDPRS protocols in accordance with ASTM-EMD standards that validate the individual EMD's knowledge and competency in their use.

4.1.8 *Reciprocal Certification*—Reciprocal certification shall be established between certifying agencies and organizations having programs that meet the standards contained in this practice.

4.1.9 *Registration and Maintenance of Certification Records*—All certifying entities, agencies, or organizations shall maintain records for all certified individuals and shall provide documents and reports regarding testing and certification status as required by using agencies, states, or governmental units. All records shall be maintained for a minimum period of ten years from initial certification, recertification or testing of the individual.

4.1.10 *Revocation of Certification*—This guide shall set forth guidelines for assessing grounds for a possible suspension or termination of certification when questionable situations arise in EMD conduct or performance.

4.1.11 *Program Selection and Implementation*—This is intended to assist the EMS administrator in the selection of the program that best suits the dispatch agency's needs from a medical, legal, and operational perspective and provide for comparative analysis between different EMD program approaches available to the EMS community that conform to established EMD practice standards.

4.1.12 *Physician Medical Director*—Each emergency medical dispatch agency shall have a physician medical director, who shall assist in evaluation and review of the EMD program under consideration. The physician medical director shall approve the selected EMD program written protocol. The physician shall be responsible for all medical aspects of the EMD program. Additional responsibilities include the medical oversight of the EMD training and certification program, continuing education requirements, recertification eligibility, QA/QI and risk management functions. These responsibilities include recommendations regarding the certification and employment eligibility of individuals found to be unsafe practitioners through employee evaluation and disciplinary due process.

5. Significance and Use

5.1 The emergency medical dispatcher should be a specially trained telecommunicator with specific emergency medical knowledge. Many of these personnel still perform in this role without the benefits of dispatch specific medical training and medically sound protocols. The majority perform their duties without appropriate medical management provided through a structured quality assurance/improvement environment. Training only prepares a new EMD for correct use of the EMDPRS. It cannot ensure that the EMDPRS is used as intended. Since the EMD is clearly defined as a pre-hospital medical professional, it is necessary to establish sound medical management processes through a multi-component QA/QI program administered by the EMD's agency in conjunction with the physician medical director. Prompt, correct, and appropriate patient care can be enhanced through the use of a standardized approach to quality assurance, especially the component of EMD performance assessment. This practice is intended for use by agencies, organizations, and jurisdictions having the responsibility for providing such services and assurances to the public through the correct management of the nation's emergency medical dispatchers.

6. EMD Entry Level Selection Criteria

6.1 Each emergency medical dispatch agency shall adopt a formal written policy delineating the selection procedures for individuals to be employed as emergency medical dispatchers. It must address the ability to:

6.1.1 Read and write at a high school graduate or GED level;

6.1.2 Perform those clerical skills as delineated by the employing agency;

6.1.3 Perform verbal skills in a clear and understandable manner, in the required language or languages established as necessary to that emergency medical dispatch agency;

6.1.4 Perform alphanumeric transcription skills necessary to correctly record addresses, locations, and telephone numbers; and

6.1.5 Demonstrate competency in basic telecommunications skills as required by the employing or training agency.

6.2 Selection criteria should also include the following:

6.2.1 A clear attribute of helpfulness and compassion toward the sick or injured patient and the caller advocate;

6.2.2 The ability to clearly guide callers in crisis through application of necessary interrogation procedures and the provision of telephone pre-arrival instructions;

6.2.3 The ability to learn and master the skills, philosophy and knowledge required to successfully complete the training process;

6.2.4 The ability to efficiently and effectively organize multiple tasks and complicated situations and activities;

6.2.5 The ability to handle the levels of emotional stress present in caller/patient crisis intervention, death and dying situations, call prioritization and triage, and multiple tasking;

6.2.6 The ability to function within the team framework of public safety and EMS systems; and

6.2.7 The ability to elicit and assimilate caller information and then to prioritize and appropriately consolidate and summarize this information in a format used to inform and direct public safety responders.

7. Orientation Guidelines for Emergency Medical Dispatchers

7.1 When an individual has successfully completed the initial EMD training and is employed by an emergency medical dispatch agency, a comprehensive orientation program must be in place to initiate this individual to the intense and demanding conditions that exist in dispatch centers. It must include:

7.1.1 An orientation manual for the new EMD;

7.1.2 A formal orientation for the new EMD in the communications and dispatch operation as well as the employing agency as a whole including all relevant policies, practices, and procedures.

7.1.3 Orientation with a one-on-one preceptor concurrent with the employee's probationary period;

7.1.4 Written evaluation of compliance through the agency's quality assessment practice as defined in this practice; and

7.1.5 Written evaluation of performance during orientation and frequent feedback and critique from those individuals responsible for training and evaluation of the new emergency medical dispatcher.

8. Performance Evaluation

8.1 The EMD must function using a medically approved EMDPRS to establish the template for performance and protocol compliance evaluation. The ongoing performance appraisal must evaluate the EMD's ability to follow and comply with the established agency policies and procedures.

8.2 Established performance criteria should be shared with new employees and measured on a regular basis. These should include evaluation of performance in:

8.2.1 Conformance to established policies of the employing agency, and

8.2.2 Compliance with the EMDPRS of the employing agency.

8.3 Performance appraisal of the EMD through case review should be accomplished by the following:

8.3.1 Multiple cases that an individual manages must be reviewed on a regular basis.

8.3.2 The selection of cases to be reviewed should provide a perspective of the individual's performance over the entire spectrum of call-types received. The review process should, as a minimum, review 7 to 10 % of calls received by the emergency medical dispatch agency.

8.3.3 Individuals performing dispatch case reviews must have an emergency medical background (preferably experienced at an ALS level) and be specially trained in the process of EMD case review.

8.3.4 These reviewers shall use a standardized *case review template* form that objectively outlines and quantifies all parameters of EMDPRS compliance by which the EMD will be evaluated.

8.3.5 Records must be kept showing at a minimum the following areas of compliance:

8.3.5.1 Compliance to asking the systematized interrogation questions. These should be subdivided to show different areas of interrogation in the EMDPRS.

8.3.5.2 Compliance to providing the systematized pre-arrival instructions (when possible and appropriate to do so); the record should show separate compliance for each type of pre-arrival instructions found within the EMDPRS.

8.3.5.3 Compliance to correctly selecting the dispatch response classification code.

8.3.6 Records should be kept showing cumulative compliance scores in the listed areas for the following groups:

8.3.6.1 Individual compliance averages;

8.3.6.2 Shift compliance averages, and

8.3.6.3 Emergency medical dispatch agency compliance averages.

8.3.7 Group compliance averages should be periodically purged of older records allowing the EMD to reasonably improve scores over time. All records should be maintained and archived.

8.3.8 The process of individual case review and the findings and recommendations should be managed by a specially trained diversified group of EMS and dispatch agency personnel. Participants in the management of the case review process should represent a cross-section of those individuals within the system affected by the emergency medical dispatch program. These should include, but not be limited to, line dispatchers, managers, administrators, medical control physicians or their representatives, or both, field personnel, and ancillary public safety groups such as 9-1-1, primary and secondary public safety answering points (PSAPs), that operate within the structure of an organized medical dispatch case review committee.

8.3.9 The specific policies and procedures to be utilized for performance appraisal activity must be carefully explained to the EMDs whose performance will be measured and must be objectively and impartially administered.

8.3.10 Regular feedback must be provided to the EMDs based on the findings of their performance appraisal.

8.3.11 The goal of the case review process is to enhance the performance of the EMD. This feedback should include both recognition of exemplary performance as well as behavior requiring remediation. This feedback must be provided in written form and maintained in the employee's records.

8.3.12 EMDs who consistently provide quality care should be recognized. Commendations, awards, advancements, media exposure, and other forms of positive reinforcement are important elements of performance appraisal.

8.3.13 The emphasis of any remedial activity should focus on re-training and modification of unacceptable practice patterns rather than on sanctions.

8.4 Field-to-dispatch feedback mechanisms should be established to monitor, inquire about and document issues relative to the application of medical dispatch practices witnessed in the total system.

8.4.1 Standardized forms should be used to collect, record, and report this information.

8.4.2 All reports generated should be carefully tracked through the system, investigated and evaluated, and written "feed back" provided to the initiator. These reports shall be maintained.

8.4.3 All reports should avoid any and all accusatory "non-colleagueal" tones.

9. EMD Certification

9.1 To become certified, an EMD shall successfully complete an EMD course that meets the requirements of this practice and the curriculum standard guidelines contained in Practice F 1552; and

9.2 Successfully pass a written or automated examination that evaluates the knowledge, comprehension and application of information required to function as an EMD as enumerated by Practice F 1258 and Practice F 1552.

9.3 The official sanctioning agency must evaluate the curriculum, testing, and EMDPRS of any emergency medical dispatch program to be approved through direct evaluation and approval by the physician medical director.

9.4 The initial certification period for a new emergency medical dispatcher shall be two years.

9.5 Certification of EMDs shall be documented and directly traceable to a nationally established organization with a recognized program sanctioned by the governmental body with jurisdiction for EMS systems in the state.

9.6 All certifying entities or organizations shall maintain

records for all certified individuals and shall provide documents and reports regarding testing and certification status as required by using agencies, states, or governmental units. All records shall be maintained for a minimum period of ten years from initial certification, recertification or testing of the individual.

10. Recertification

10.1 To become recertified as an EMD a candidate shall provide evidence of successful completion of a minimum of 12 h of approved continuing medical dispatch education per year during the required recertification period.

10.2 The content of the continuing medical dispatch education required shall be defined and approved by the certifying agency and be consistent with the requirements of this practice; and

10.3 The candidate shall also successfully pass a written or automated examination that evaluates the knowledge, comprehension and application of information required to function as an EMD as enumerated by Practice F 1258 and the minimum curriculum guideline of Practice F 1552.

10.4 After the initial two year certification, the subsequent recertification period of the emergency medical dispatcher shall be not less than two years and not more than four years.

10.5 If an EMD certification expires, the EMD shall have twelve months to recertify or the EMD shall be required to perform all requirements of initial certification.

11. Reciprocal Certification

11.1 Reciprocal certification shall be established between certifying agencies and organizations having programs that meet the requirements contained in this practice and Practice F 1552.

11.2 The diversified EMDPRS protocols require specific training and knowledge in their proper use; therefore, the emergency medical dispatcher wishing reciprocal certification must receive formal training on the specific EMDPRS that is used for the certification being sought and as used within the employing emergency medical dispatch agency.

12. Revocation of Certification

12.1 The goal of quality assurance is to correct deficiencies and encourage excellence, not just adhere to minimum standards. Demonstrated inabilities and failure to perform appropriate patient care through approved pre-arrival instructions and demonstrated inabilities and failure to perform according to the predetermined medically approved protocols are significant failures and cannot be tolerated within a comprehensive EMD program.

12.2 EMD certification or recertification may be suspended or revoked by the certifying entity for any of the following causes:

12.2.1 Habitual or excessive use of or addiction to narcotics or dangerous drugs, or conviction of any offense relating to the use, sale, possession, or transportation of narcotics, dangerous drugs, or controlled substances.

12.2.2 Habitual or excessive use of alcoholic beverages or being under the influence of alcoholic beverages, or controlled substances while on call or on duty as an EMD, or conviction of driving under the influence of alcohol or controlled substances.

12.2.3 Fraud or deceit in applying for or obtaining any certification, or fraud, deceit, incompetence, patient abuse, theft, or dishonesty in the performance of duties and practice as an EMD or other EMS professional.

12.2.4 Involvement in the unauthorized use or removal of narcotics, drugs, supplies or equipment from any emergency vehicle, agency, or health care facility.

12.2.5 Performing procedures or skills beyond the level of certification or not allowed by rules, or violation of laws pertaining to medical practice and drugs.

12.2.6 Conviction of a felony or a crime involving moral turpitude, or the entering of a plea of guilty or the finding of guilt by a jury or court, of commission of a felony, or a crime involving moral turpitude.

12.2.7 Mental incompetence as determined by a court of competent jurisdiction.

12.2.8 For good cause, including conduct that is unethical, immoral, or dishonorable.

12.2.9 Demonstrated inabilities and failure to perform appropriate patient care through approved pre-arrival instructions, and

12.2.10 Demonstrated inabilities and failure to perform according to the predetermined medically approved EMDPRS protocols.

13. Continuing Dispatcher Education (CDE)

13.1 A sound, ongoing program of continuing dispatcher education is essential. Without regular educational experiences specifically direct to their practice, the EMD will become less proficient in the understanding of and compliance to the EMDPRS. The agency's continuing dispatch education (CDE) program should be coordinated and organized for the EMDs through the emergency medical dispatch QA/QI personnel who, through the evaluation of on-line case review, identify the specific and individual needs of the EMD. Objectives of training should be for the EMD to:

13.1.1 Develop an understanding of telecommunications and the EMDs' roles and responsibilities;

13.1.2 Enhance the on-line skills in pre-arrival instructions and in all emergency telephone procedures within the practice of EMD;

13.1.3 Improve skills in the use and application of all component parts of the EMDPRS, including interrogation, prioritization, and appropriate provision of pre-arrival instructions;

13.1.4 Seek opportunities for discussion, skill practice, and critique of skill performance;

13.1.5 Maintain a current understanding of the evolving science of emergency medical dispatching methods, procedures, techniques, and standards.

13.2 *Elements of Continuing Dispatcher Education*—CDE at a minimum must include a review of the elements of the curriculum, with special emphasis on operational functions, protocol and policy compliance, new procedures, medical advancements, problematic situations, and greater in depth understanding of the medical conditions that are represented within the EMDPRS. CDE learning can be obtained through various educational methods and may include but is not limited to the following suggested CDE categories:

13.2.1 Scenario Drills/Role Playing—Workshops and seminars related to EMS, preferably related to the skills of an EMD; that is, airway management, review of essential telecommunication skills, telephone scenarios, medical legal issues, computer aided dispatch, stress management, refresher courses, etc. (maximum of eight instructional hours per year);

13.2.2 Local planning or management meetings, including general organization for disaster mass casualty, and HAZ-MAT related incidences (maximum of four instructional hours per year.),

13.2.3 Case Review Activities—Quality assurance/quality improvement case review, planning and analysis of issues or findings identified by dispatch QA/QI, theoretically or in practice (maximum of four instructional hours per year.),

13.2.4 Audio-visuals (films, video tapes, etc.), that illustrate and review proper emergency care and EMD procedures. Titles should be restricted to those specific to EMS, preferably EMD related (maximum of two instructional hours per year),

13.2.5 Didactic Lectures—Teaching the general public any topic within the scope of basic EMD/EMS relations. Synopsis of the subject taught should be included in the CDE documentation (maximum of two instructional hours per year),

13.2.6 EMS Field Experience—Miscellaneous categories may include on-duty work experience as an EMT (maximum of two instructional hours per year), and

13.2.7 Attendance at Remote Professional Conferences and Seminars—Workshops and seminars related to EMS, preferably related to the skills of an EMD.

14. Risk Management

14.1 The following attitudinal philosophy of risk management within a quality assurance program is derived from the *Guidelines for Quality Assurance*[3] from the Council on Medical Service of the American Medical Association and deals mainly with risk management-type issues. These ten guidelines should be utilized in any medical dispatch system, whether private or governmental operated and whether conducted by medical directors, administrators, supervisors, peers, or governmental authorizing agencies.

14.1.1 The specific policies and procedures to be utilized for performance evaluation activity must be carefully explained to the EMDs whose performance will be measured. All procedures must be objectively and impartially administered.

14.1.2 Any formal corrective activity related to an individual EMD should be triggered by concern for that individual's overall practice, rather than by deviation from specified criteria in single cases. Judgment as to the competence of specific dispatchers should be based on an assessment of their performance with a number of patients and not on the examination of single, isolated cases, except in extraordinary circumstances.

14.1.3 The institution of any corrective action or activity should be preceded by discussion with the EMD involved. There should be ample opportunity for the EMD to explain observed deviations from accepted practice patterns to supervisors, professional reviewers, or the medical director, or all three, before any remedial or corrective action is decided on.

14.1.4 Emphasis should be placed on retraining and modification of unacceptable practice patterns rather than on sanctions. The initial thrust of any remedial activity should be toward helping the EMD correct deficiencies in knowledge, skills, or technique, with practice restrictions or disciplinary action considered only for those not responsive to such remedial activities.

14.1.5 The employing agency must provide the appropriate educational resources needed to effect desired practice modifications whether they be peer consultation, continuing education, retraining or self-learning and self-assessment programs.

14.1.6 Feedback mechanisms should be established to monitor and document needed changes in practice patterns and allow for assessment of the effectiveness of any remedial activities instituted by or for an EMD.

14.1.7 Restrictions, sanctions or disciplinary actions should be imposed on those dispatchers not responsive to remedial activities, whenever the employing agency or medical director, or both, deem such action necessary to protect the public. Depending on the severity of the deficiency such restrictions may include loss of certification.

14.1.8 The imposition of restrictions, sanctions or disciplinary actions must be timely and consistent with due process. Before a restriction or disciplinary action is imposed, the EMD affected should be provided an explanation of the basis for such actions, ample opportunity to request reconsideration and to submit any documentation relevant to the request, and the right to meet with those considering its imposition. However, in cases where those considering the imposition of restrictions, sanctions or disciplinary action deem the dispatcher to pose an imminent hazard to the health of patients, personnel or the public at large, such restrictions or disciplinary actions may be imposed immediately.

14.1.9 Quality assurance systems for medical dispatch should be structured and operated so as to ensure immunity for those conducting or applying such systems who are acting in good faith. To ensure the active unfettered participation of all parties in the review process, all case reviews, and the documents and opinions generated by them, should be structured, if possible, for protection from subpoena and legal discovery. This incident review protection is common in most hospital and medical review environments. Reviewing state and federal legislation as well as pertinent court decisions as the basis for developing comprehensive guidelines on immunity in review activities is essential.

14.1.10 To the fullest degree possible, quality assurance systems should be structured to recognize care of high quality as well as correcting instances of deficient practice. The vast majority of practicing, professionally trained EMDs provide care of high quality. Quality assurance systems should explore methods to identify and recognize those treatment methodologies, procedures, and protocols that consistently contribute to improved patient outcomes, system efficiency, and safety. Information on such results should be communicated to the

[3] *Guidelines for Quality Assurance*, Council on Medical Service of the American Medical Association.

medical control community and dispatch agency administrations. EMDs providing high and consistent quality care should be rewarded. Commendations, awards, advancements and other forms of positive reinforcements are important facets of quality assurance.

15. Sequence of Implementation

15.1 This section is intended to serve as sequential steps guideline of activities that must be completed to implement an emergency medical dispatch program. All administrative and oversight functions must be established and in place prior to training the EMDs or any "on line" use of the EMDPRS.

15.1.1 Selection and orientation of:

15.1.1.1 The medical director (who also serves on the QA/QI and oversight committees noted below);

15.1.1.2 EMD project director;

15.1.1.3 Communications center manager;

15.1.1.4 Emergency medical service system(s) administrator(s);

15.1.1.5 EMD program QA/QI personnel;

15.1.1.6 Active on-line dispatcher(s);

15.1.1.7 Prehospital care provider representative (EMT or paramedic, or both);

15.1.1.8 EMD labor organization representative; and

15.1.1.9 Continuing dispatch education personnel;

15.1.2 Identification of the goals and objectives of the proposed EMD program by the oversight committee.

15.1.3 Selection of an EMDPRS by the oversight committee, with the written approval of the program medical director, conforming to the goals and objectives identified above.

15.1.4 Acquisition of the selected EMDPRS.

15.2 Orientation about the EMD program for all relevant governmental or municipal personnel, EMS personnel (field responders, supervisory, administrative) and communications managers, administrators, and oversight committee members.

15.3 Development of a QA/QI program for employee evaluation as indicated in the section on performance evaluation.

15.4 Ensuring that all oversight committee functions, QA/QI mechanisms, continuing education programs and other above outlined administrative functions are established prior to commencement of EMD training.

15.5 Arranging, scheduling and conducting all prerequisite or pre-EMD training programs such as CPR or emergency medical orientation (first responder) classes for communications personnel.

15.6 Arranging, scheduling and conducting the EMD training program for all communications personnel, all oversight committee members, and medical direction personnel.

15.7 Implemention of the EMDPRS in the communications center

15.8 Commencement performance evaluation of EMD cases according to the QA/QI program.

15.9 Initiation of the continuing dispatch education program (CDE).

15.10 Commencement of dispatch feedback mechanisms and performance remediation process.

15.11 Conduct orientation of ancillary public safety communications centers in the geographic area.

15.12 Provision for a public education component to orient the serviced population to the new EMD program.

15.13 Continuation of gathering and recording data relative to the effectiveness of the EMDPRS and evaluate the impact of the EMD program on the delivery of emergency medical services.

16. Keywords

16.1 case review; continuing dispatch education; dispatch life support; dispatch management; dispatch protocol; dispatcher; EMD; EMD administration; EMD certification; EMDPRS; emergency medical dispatcher; emergency medical dispatch management; emergency medical dispatch priority reference system; medical dispatch; medical director; performance evaluation; pre-arrival instructions; priority dispatch; PSAP; quality improvement; quality assurance; recertification; reciprocity; risk management; telecommunicator

Standard Specification for Anesthetic Equipment—Oropharyngeal and Nasopharyngeal Airways[1]

This standard is issued under the fixed designation F 1573; the number immediately following the designation indicates the year of original adoption or, in the case of revision, the year of last revision. A number in parentheses indicates the year of last reapproval. A superscript epsilon (ε) indicates an editorial change since the last revision or reapproval.

1. Scope

1.1 This specification covers minimum performance and safety requirements for oropharyngeal and nasopharyngeal airways for human use.

1.2 Size designations, dimensions, and tolerances; material compatibility; product marking and labeling; and packaging are considered.

1.3 Because of the wide variation in size and configuration of the human airway, various conditions of use, user preferences, and cost, this specification cannot cover all types of oropharyngeal and nasopharyngeal airways.

1.4 Standards for the types of airways not specifically addressed by this specification may be developed in the future.

1.5 This specification is not intended to limit the development of the other devices so long as the minimum safety and performance requirements stated herein are met.

2. Referenced Documents

2.1 *ASTM Standards:*

ANSI Z79.3-1983 Anesthetic Equipment—Oropharyngeal and Nasopharyngeal Airways[2]

3. Terminology

3.1 *Definitions of Terms Specific to This Standard:*

3.1.1 *buccal end (flanged end)*—the end of the airway that is flanged and is expected to fit between the teeth or gums or against the external nares.

3.1.2 *nasopharyngeal airway*—a device intended to maintain the patency of respiratory passages through the nasal cavity into the pharynx.

3.1.3 *oropharyngeal airway*—a device intended to maintain the patency of respiratory passages through the oral cavity into the pharynx.

3.1.4 *pharyngeal end*—the end of the airway that is intended to be inserted into the patient's pharynx.

3.1.5 *shall*—the word "shall," as used in this specification, is to be understood as denoting a mandatory requirement.

3.1.6 *should*—the word "should," as used in this specification, is to be understood as denoting a recommendation that is a sound safety practice: it does not denote a mandatory requirement.

4. Size Designation

4.1 *Measurement System*—The metric system shall be the standard of measurement used. Other units of measure may be provided as supplemental information.

4.2 *Size*:

4.2.1 *Oropharyngeal Airways*—The size of oropharyngeal airways shall be designated by a number giving the nominal length in centimetres in accordance with Table 1[3,4] and Fig. 1(*a*) and (*b*).

4.2.2 *Nasopharyngeal Airways*—The size of nasopharyngeal airways shall be designated by a number expressing the inside diameter in millimetres as the primary dimension, in accordance with tolerances given in Table 2[3,4,5] and Fig. 1(*c*).

5. Materials and Manufacture

5.1 Airways shall be fabricated from plastics, or elastomeric materials, or from combinations of these materials.

5.1.1 Airways shall be nontoxic and compatible with the human tissue with which they are intended to be used, as determined by the implantation test in the *United States Pharmacopeia*.[6]

NOTE 1—The designs shown in Fig. 1 and Fig. 2 are intended to illustrate typical common types of airways for the purpose of size designation and marking, but are not otherwise intended to form a part of this specification.

5.1.2 All material should be resistant to changes or deterioration from normal concentrations of substances encountered during routine use.

5.2 Reusable airways shall be made of material capable of being sterilized. The manufacturer shall supply recommended methods of sterilization.

---

[1] This specification is under the jurisdiction of ASTM Committee F29 on Anesthetic and Respiratory Equipmentand is the direct responsibility of Subcommittee F29.02 on Division Two on Endoscopes and Airways.

Current edition approved Jan. 15, 1995. Published April 1995.

[2] Available from American National Standards Institute, 11 W. 42nd St., 13th Floor, New York, NY 10036.

[3] Table 1 and Table 2 are intended to relate nominal size to the length (or diameter) of the airway. Clinical practice neither suggests nor requires the availability of all nominal sizes given in the tables.

[4] Sizes not shown may be added by interpolation.

[5] For nasopharyngeal airways, the actual outside diameter shall be designated on the product or the package label within ±0.5 mm (see X1.1.2).

[6] See *United States Pharmacopeia*, Easton, Pa: Mack Publishing Company.

TABLE 1 Dimensions and Tolerances of Oropharyngeal Airways

Nominal Size of Airway	Length (L), (mm)	Tolerance, Length (L), (mm)
3	30	±2.5
3.5	35	±2.5
4	40	±2.5
4.5	45	±2.5
5	50	±2.5
5.5	55	±2.5
6	60	±2.5
6.5	65	±2.5
7	70	+5.0
...	...	−2.5
8	80	±5.0
9	90	±5.0
10	100	±5.0
11	110	±5.0
12	120	±5.0

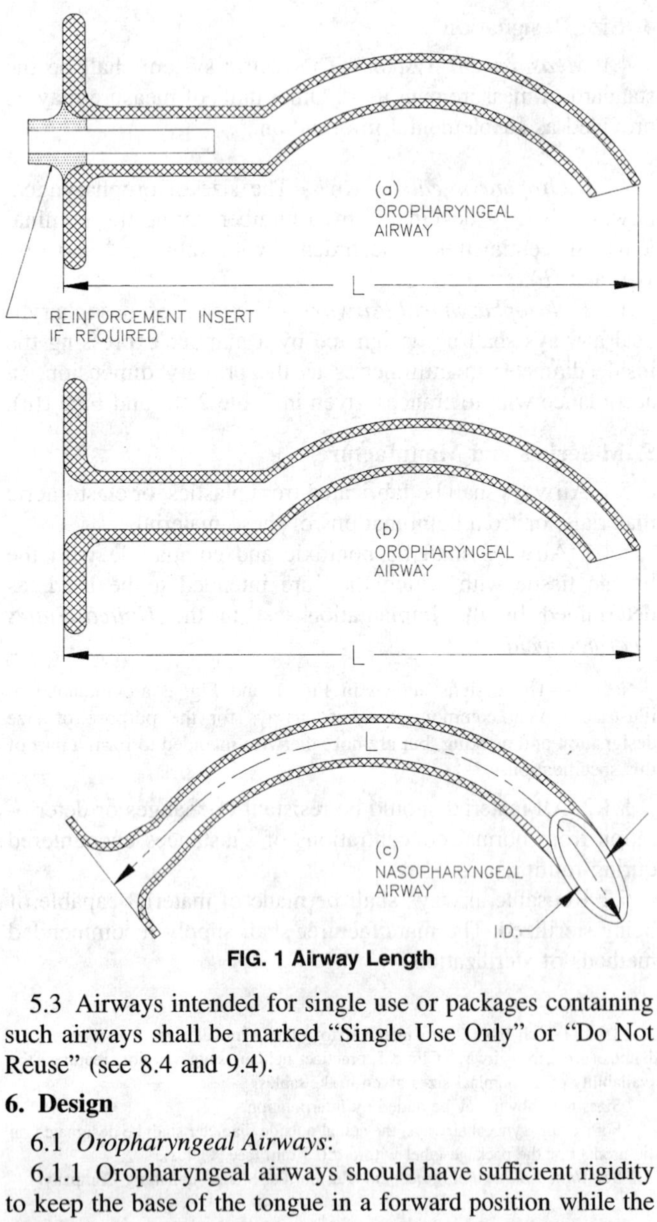

FIG. 1 Airway Length

5.3 Airways intended for single use or packages containing such airways shall be marked "Single Use Only" or "Do Not Reuse" (see 8.4 and 9.4).

6. Design

6.1 *Oropharyngeal Airways*:

6.1.1 Oropharyngeal airways should have sufficient rigidity to keep the base of the tongue in a forward position while the airway is in use.

6.1.2 Oropharyngeal airways shall have sufficient rigidity at the buccal (flanged) end (by use of an insert, if necessary) to prevent collapse when bitten by the patient. Collapse shall have occurred when the airway has narrowed to the point of interfering with the passage of a correctly sized suction catheter or to a 25 % reduction in available airflow under incisor bite of 225 *N*. (See X1.1.5.1 and X2.1.2).

6.1.3 Edges and corners that may come in contact with the patient's tissues should have a minimum radius of curvature of 0.5 mm.

6.1.4 The oropharyngeal airway (or its package or package insert) should be clearly marked with the designation, " *DO NOT USE AS A BITE BLOCK*" to prevent incisor luxation that is a common sequel to such use of oropharyngeal airways.

6.2 *Nasopharyngeal Airways*:

6.2.1 The nasopharyngeal airway shall be constructed to prevent kinking in use. Kinking shall have occurred when the airway, bent into the same curvature as the human nasopharynx, has flattened to the point of interfering with the passage of a steel ball that is 50 % of the diameter of the airway lumen. (See X1.1.5.1 and X2.1.2)

6.2.2 Nasopharyngeal airways that have been preformed into the correct anatomical curvature shall be straightened for testing and shall not kink or interfere with the passage of the steel ball described in 6.2.1.

6.2.3 The diameter of the flange shall be at least twice the outside diameter of the tube.

TABLE 2 Dimensions and Tolerances of Nasopharyngeal Airways

Nominal Size of Airway	Inside Diameter, (mm)	Suggested Length, (mm)
5.0	5.0 ± 0.2	90
5.5	5.5 ± 0.2	100
6.0	6.0 ± 0.2	110
6.5	6.5 ± 0.2	120
7.0	7.0 ± 0.2	130
7.5	7.5 ± 0.2	140
8.0	8.0 ± 0.2	150
8.5	8.5 ± 0.2	160
9.0	9.0 ± 0.2	170

7. Workmanship, Finish, and Appearance

7.1 Mismatch of surfaces produced by molds shall not cause a depression of one surface relative to another by more than 0.15 mm, if the surfaces were designed to produce a continuous surface. All surfaces shall be generally smooth and free of flash.

8. Product Marking

8.1 Each oropharyngeal airway shall be permanently and clearly marked with nominal size and name or trademark of the manufacturer as shown in Fig. 2(*a*) and 2(*b*). The nominal size should be further suffixed by the abbreviation," cm" (centimetres).

8.2 Each nasopharyngeal airway shall be permanently and clearly marked with the nominal size as shown in Fig. 2(*c*). The manufacturer's name or trademark shall also be marked on the airway as shown in Fig. 2(*c*). The actual outside diameter to within ±0.5 mm, shall be included in the package label or on the product itself.

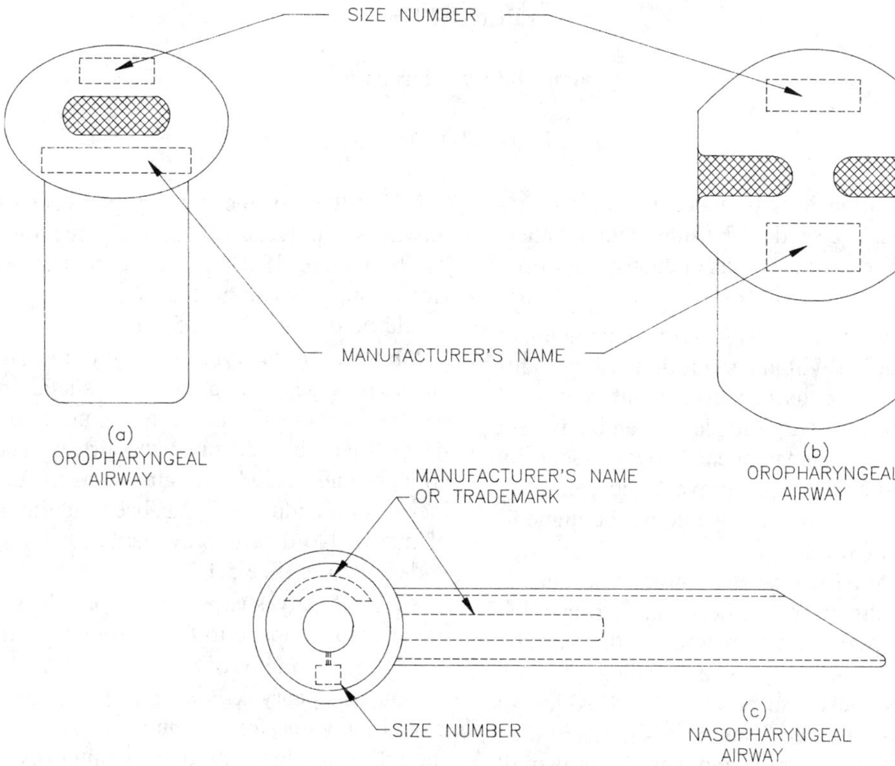

FIG. 2 Airway Marking

8.3 All required markings shall be clearly legible to the normal unaided eye.

8.4 All airways should be marked to differentiate those intended for single use from those that are intended to be reusable (see 5.3).

8.5 Airways shall be marked (or the package or package insert will record) either the date of manufacture, or a code that allows traceability to the date of manufacture.

9. Packaging and Package Marking

9.1 Airways may be marketed in a sterile or a nonsterile condition.

9.2 Airways marketed as sterile shall be in properly sealed packages capable of maintaining the sterile integrity of the airways under normal conditions of shipping and storage. The manufacturer shall disclose, upon request, the test method used to verify package integrity.

9.3 For airways supplied in sterile form, the word *"STERILE"* and the lot or batch number shall be readily apparent on examination of the package.

9.4 The packages containing airways intended for single use shall be clearly marked "Single Use Only" or "Do Not Reuse."

9.5 If individually packaged, the size of the airway shall be readily apparent on examination of the package. The size should be marked on the package label in bold print for ease of identification.

10. Precision and Bias

10.1 No statement is made about either the precision or bias of test methods of X2.1.2.1 or X2.1.3.2, since the results merely state whether there is conformance to the specification as described.

APPENDIXES

(Nonmandatory Information)

X1. RATIONALE

X1.1 The following rationale is provided for the requirements in this specification. The section and subsection numbers given in parentheses refer to the correspondingly numbered sections and subsections in the text.

X1.1.1 *Size of Oropharyngeal Airways*—A nominal number is assigned to airways falling within certain dimensions. This size designation provides the user with a rapid means of determination for the proper airway and also for an equivalent product. The marking of oropharyngeal airways only by millimetre length, for instance, might prove to be confusing because the actual measured dimension would not be immediately familiar to the user. (See 3.1.3.)

X1.1.2 *Nasopharyngeal Airways*—Both inside and outside diameter are important dimensions when considering what airways to use. The passage of the airway will be influenced by the outside diameter, and passage of a suction catheter through the lumen of the airway must also be considered. Although materials are specified in this specification, it is possible that, in the future, manufacturing processes and new materials will result in significant changes in the wall thickness of the airway. If only one dimension is provided, the user will have insufficient data for comparison. (See 3.1.2.)

X1.1.2.1 Tolerances must be specified so that in the worst case, the nearest possible size of suction catheter may be passed through the nasopharyngeal airway. For example, it should be possible to pass a 16 French (5.3 ± 0.15 mm) through a 6-mm airway. The tolerance of ±0.2 mm, that is possible under current manufacturing practice, would allow this passage to occur without reaching the point of an interference fit.

X1.1.2.2 The outside diameter is less critical than the inside diameter, and a tolerance of ±0.5 mm would be allowable if the airway conforms to the sizing given in Table 2.

X1.1.3 The nasal airway must flex and compress as it is passed through the nares. Metal is not sufficiently pliable for this purpose. (See 4.1.)

X1.1.3.1 Both oropharyngeal and nasopharyngeal airways will be in contact with the mucosa for prolonged periods and shall be compatible with these tissues. (See 4.1.1.)

X1.1.3.2 Anesthetic gases, water soluble lubricants, topical anesthetics, and other agents are commonly used with airways. To test all possible combinations of all possible substances would be prohibitively expensive. The committee has not been presented with sufficient data to justify such extensive testing. (See 4.1.2.)

X1.1.4 Manufacturers supply recommended methods of sterilization for reusable devices, as required by Food and Drug Administration regulations. (See 4.2.)

X1.1.4.1 Disposable airways are marked to differentiate them from reusable airways. These markings are important as a reprocessed disposable device may fail to perform adequately. (See 4.3.)

X1.1.5 One of the primary purposes of the oropharyngeal airway is to prevent soft tissue obstruction of the human airway by the tongue. If the oropharyngeal airway were to collapse (for example, when heated to body temperature), this purpose would be defeated. (See 5.1.1.)

X1.1.5.1 Oropharyngeal airways are often used to maintain an air passage or as a route for suctioning patients who are unconscious or suffering from seizure disorders. In these cases, patients may bite down on the airway. The airway should not collapse and occlude the air passage. The biting force of the incisor of an adult male has been determined to be an average of 225 *N*. No data was available for biting force of a patient under seizure. (See 5.1.2.)

X1.1.5.2 Any sharp corners or edges on the device may cause tissue damage to the surrounding mucosa. (See 5.1.3.)

X1.1.5.3 A radius of curvature has not been specified for the human nasopharynx due to wide anatomic variation. A suggested guideline for test purposes is 5 cm. The manufacturer should specify in the product labeling any limitations regarding radius of curvature. (See 5.2.1.)

X1.1.5.4 It is important that the flange diameter be twice the tube diameter, to minimize the possibility that the airway may slip into the patient's posterior pharynx. (See 5.2.3.)

X1.2 *Finish*—Flash and other rough surfaces may cause mucosal damage during airway use. (See Section 6.)

X1.2.1 Several reports have indicated that the semirigid Guedel-type oropharyngeal airway (among other types) does not adequately distribute the force of jaw closure, and that it prevents the upper and lower incisors from gliding past each other during biting. As a result, the forward luxation of the upper and lower incisors commonly results. An acceptable bite block is one which distributes force of biting to one or both sets of molars that are in direct opposition. (See 6.1.4.)

X1.2.2 These permanent markings provide the only means of size identification and product traceability. (See 7.1 and 7.2.)

X1.2.3 Unless the markings of "Do Not Reuse" or "Single Use Only" is on the device, the user cannot differentiate between reusable and disposable devices of similar appearance. Often, the individual who removes the airway is not the person who initially put the device in place and package information is of no value under these circumstances. (See 7.4.)

X1.2.4 No standardized test method for this requirement is possible, given the variety of packaging types and numerous test methods available. (See 8.2.)

X1.2.5 Materials used in the manufacture of oropharyngeal and nasopharyngeal airways may become less compliant and more susceptible to breakage with age. It has been noted, however, that only in rare circumstances will age affect the characteristics of airways, and a manufacturer's code will adequately identify airways.

X2. TEST METHODS

X2.1 The following test methods are provided for the requirements in this specification. The section and subsection numbers given in parentheses refer to the correspondingly numbered sections and subsections in the text.

X2.1.1 *Visual and Dimensional Inspection* (see 3.1.2):

X2.1.1.1 For reusable devices, read the instructions and sterilize or disinfect accordingly. Then perform the tests in accordance with X2.1.2 or X2.1.3, as applicable. (See 4.2.)

X2.1.1.2 For disposable devices, visually inspect the package or device for proper labeling. (See 4.3.)

X2.1.2 *Test Method for Collapse at Bit Block Area (Oropharyngeal Airways) (see* 5.1.2):

X2.1.2.1 *Apparatus*—A compression tester similar to that shown in Fig. X2.1 should be used. A tensile testing machine, with compression fixture, may be substituted.

X2.1.2.2 *Procedure*—Precondition test samples in accordance with applicable tests in *Plastics—General Test Methods, Nomenclature*, ASTM Part 35,[7] for the material being tested. Prior to insertion into the test fixture, bring the test unit to a temperature of ±1°C. Apply a force of 225 N to the bite block area of the airway for 3 min. The airflow through the airway, while holding constant pressure as measured on the flowmeter, shall be at least 75 % of the original value as measured before the force was applied. An initial flow of 10 L/min is suggested.

X2.1.2.3 Using radius gage, measure correct radius of curvature. (See 5.1.3.)

NOTE X2.1—The above procedure in X2.1.2.2 is feasible, though technically difficult, as a means of testing oropharyngeal airways of the Guedel, Connell, and Waters types. It is not feasible as a test for the Berman airway. It has been suggested that a steel ball test (see X2.1.3) be used as an alternative test for all oropharyngeal airways, including the Berman airway. (For descriptions of the various airway types, see Footnote 8.[8] (See 5.1.4.)

X2.1.3 *Test for Kinking (Nasopharyngeal Airways) (See 5.2.1)*:

X2.1.3.1 *Apparatus*—A test fixture similar to that shown in Fig. X2.2 should be used.

X2.1.3.2 *Procedure*—Precondition test samples in accordance with applicable tests in *Plastics—General Test Methods, Nomenclature*, ASTM, Part 35,[7] for the material being tested. Prior to insertion into the test fixture, bring the test specimen to a temperature of 37 ± 1°C. Position the test specimen in the fixture so its inside radius of curvature is placed on the 5-cm scribed line of the test fixture. Anchor the distal end of the test specimen between the pins provided on thescribed line. Drop a steel ball that is 50 % of the diameter of the airway lumen into the flanged end of the test specimen. The ball should pass through the lumen of the airway without interference. After the ball is removed, return the curved airway to the straight vertical position and anchor the distal end between the pin and right-angle retaining plate. Drop the steel ball into the flange of the test specimen. If the ball passes all the way through to the pinned areas at the distal end without interference, the airway passes the test.

X2.1.3.3 Using vernier calipers or optical comparator, measure the diameter of flange compared to the outside diameter of the airway tube. (See 5.2.3.)

[7] Available from ASTM, 1916 Race St., Phila., PA 19103.

[8] Dorsch, J. A., and Dorsch, S. E., *Understanding Anesthesia Equipment*, Second Edition, Wiliams and Wilkins, Baltimore, MD, 1984, pp. 332–333.

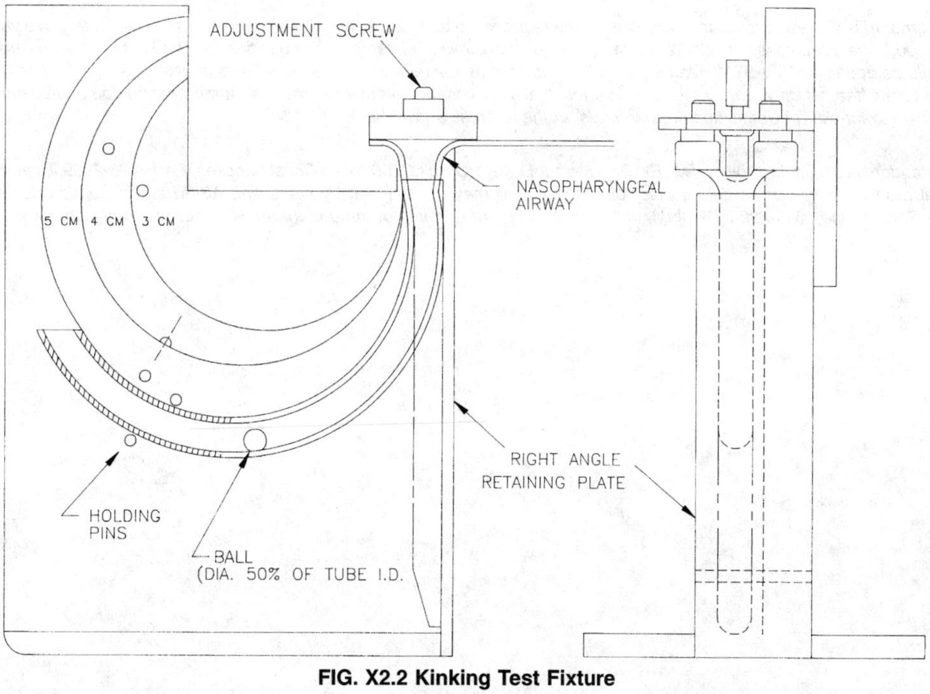

FIG. X2.2 Kinking Test Fixture

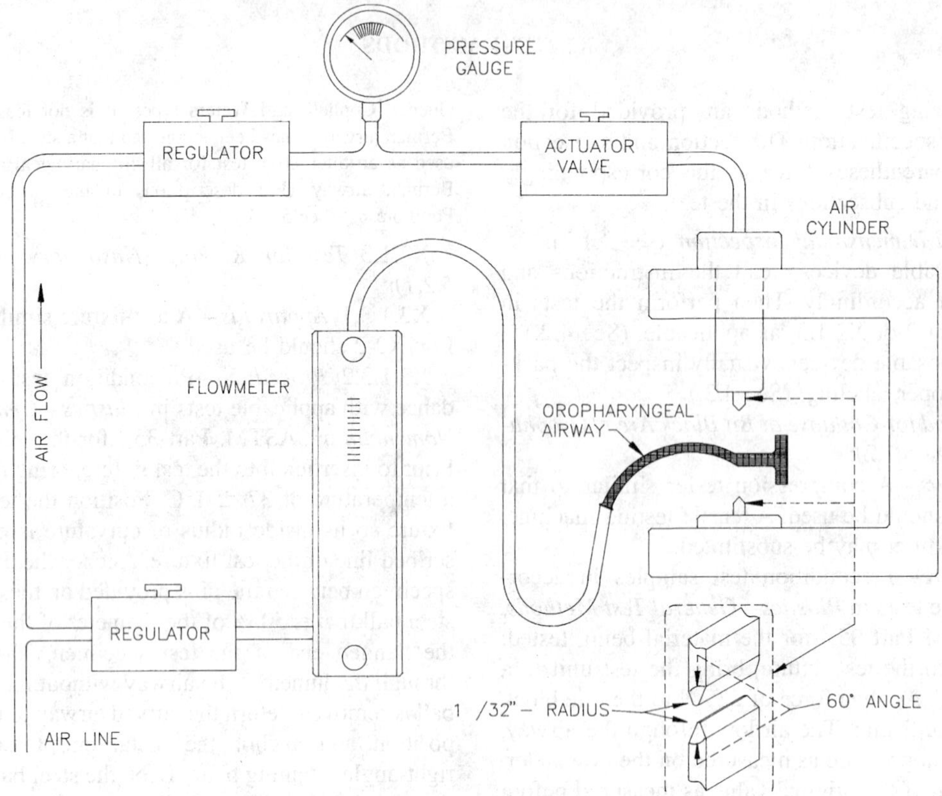

FIG. X2.1 Compression Tester

X2.2 *Finish*—Using calipers or micrometer, measure adjacent surfaces for mismatch resulting in sharp edges. (See Section 6.)

X2.2.1 For reusable devices, after processing in accordance with the manufacturer's instructions, visually inspect for deterioration of markings. (See 7.1 and 7.2.)

X2.2.2 Visual inspection. (See 8.3, 8.4, and 8.5.)

The American Society for Testing and Materials takes no position respecting the validity of any patent rights asserted in connection with any item mentioned in this standard. Users of this standard are expressly advised that determination of the validity of any such patent rights, and the risk of infringement of such rights, are entirely their own responsibility.

This standard is subject to revision at any time by the responsible technical committee and must be reviewed every five years and if not revised, either reapproved or withdrawn. Your comments are invited either for revision of this standard or for additional standards and should be addressed to ASTM Headquarters. Your comments will receive careful consideration at a meeting of the responsible technical committee, which you may attend. If you feel that your comments have not received a fair hearing you should make your views known to the ASTM Committee on Standards, at the address shown below.

Designation: F 1579 – 98

Standard Specification for Polyaryletherketone (PAEK) Resins for Surgical Implant Applications[1]

This standard is issued under the fixed designation F 1579; the number immediately following the designation indicates the year of original adoption or, in the case of revision, the year of last revision. A number in parentheses indicates the year of last reapproval. A superscript epsilon (ε) indicates an editorial change since the last revision or reapproval.

1. Scope

1.1 This specification covers polyaryletherketone (PAEK) resins in virgin forms as supplied by a vendor (flakes, pellets, blocks, etc.). It provides requirements and associated test methods for these thermoplastics when they are to be used in the manufacture of intracorporeal devices such as surgical implants or components of surgical or dental devices.

1.2 As with any material, some characteristics may be altered by the processing techniques (molding, extrusion, machining, assembly, sterilization, etc.) required for the production of a specific part or device. Therefore, properties of fabricated forms of these resins should be evaluated using test methods that are appropriate to ensure safety and efficacy as agreed upon by the vendor, purchaser, and regulating bodies.

1.3 The properties included in this specification are those applicable for PAEK resins only. Fabricated forms, material or forms containing colorants, fillers, processing aids, or other additives, as well as polymer blends that contain PAEK, are not covered by this specification.

1.4 This specification is designed to recommend physical, chemical, and biological test methods to establish a reasonable level of confidence concerning the performance of unfilled PAEK resins for use in medical devices. The properties listed should be considered in selecting material according to the specific end-use requirements.

1.5 When evaluating material to this specification hazardous materials, operations, and equipment may be involved. *This standard does not purport to address all of the safety concerns, if any, associated with its use. It is the responsibility of the user of this standard to establish appropriate safety and health practices and determine the applicability of regulatory limitations prior to use.*

2. Referenced Documents

2.1 *ASTM Standards:*

D 149 Test Methods for Dielectric Breakdown Voltage and Dielectric Strength of Solid Electrical Insulating Materials at Commercial Power Frequencies[2]

D 256 Test Methods for Impact Resistance of Plastics and Electrical Insulating Materials[2]

D 570 Test Method for Water Absorption of Plastics[2]

D 621 Test Methods for Deformation of Plastics Under Load[2]

D 638 Test Method for Tensile Properties of Plastics[2]

D 648 Test Method for Deflection Temperature of Plastics Under Flexural Load[2]

D 695 Test Method for Compressive Properties of Rigid Plastics[2]

D 696 Test Method for Coefficient of Linear Thermal Expansion of Plastics[2]

D 790 Test Methods for Flexural Properties of Unreinforced and Reinforced Plastics and Electrical Insulating Materials[2]

D 792 Test Methods for Specific Gravity (Relative Density) and Density of Plastics by Displacement[2]

D 955 Test Method for Measuring Shrinkage from Mold Dimensions of Molded Plastics[2]

D 1238 Test Method for Flow Rates of Thermoplastics by Extrusion Plastometer[2]

D 1505 Test Method for Density of Plastics by the Density-Gradient Technique[2]

D 1898 Practice for Sampling of Plastics[3]

D 3417 Test Method for Heats of Fusion and Crystallization of Polymers by Thermal Analysis[4]

D 3418 Test Methods for Transition Temperatures of Polymers by Thermal Analysis[4]

D 4000 Classification System for Specifying Plastic Materials[4]

F 748 Practice for Selecting Generic Biological Test Methods for Materials and Devices[5]

2.2 *ISO Documents:*

ISO 1133 Plastics—Determination of the Melt Mass-Flow Rate (MFR) and the Melt Volume-Flow Rate (MVR) of Thermoplastics[6]

ISO 1628/1 Plastics, Guidelines for the Standardization of Methods for Determination of Viscosity Number and Limiting Viscosity Number of Polymers in Dilute

[1] This specification is under the jurisdiction of ASTM Committee F-4 on Medical and Surgical Devices and is under the direct responsibility of Subcommittee F04.11 on Polymeric Materials.

Current edition approved April 10, 1998. Published September 1998. Originally published as F 1579 – 95. Last previous edition F 1579 – 95.

[2] *Annual Book of ASTM Standards,* Vol 08.01.

[3] *Annual Book of ASTM Standards,* Vol 08.02.

[4] *Annual Book of ASTM Standards,* Vol 08.03.

[5] *Annual Book of ASTM Standards,* Vol 13.01.

[6] Available from American National Standards Institute, 11 W. 42nd St., 13th Floor, New York, NY 10036.

TABLE 1 Required Properties of Some PAEK Virgin Resins

PAEK Type	T_B (°C)	T_m (°C)	Voscosity Number, (ml/g)	Melt Flow, (cm^3/10 min)	Heavy Netaksm (%)
	ASTM D 3418, 20°C/min	ASTM D 3418, 20°C/min	ISO 1628, Sulfuric Acid 0.5 %, 25°C	ISO 1133, 400°C, 10 kg	U.S. Pharmacopeia Test 231
PEKEKK	160–200	360–400	≥55	25–120	≤0.1
PEEK	125–165	320–360	≥77		≤0.1
PEKK	135–175	310–350		40–100	≤0.1
PEEKK	140–195	350–390			≤0.1
PEK	140–180	350–395			≤0.1

TABLE 2 Typical Mechanical Properties of Some PAEK Consolidated Forms

PAEK Type	Density, (kg/m^3) (Minimum)	Tensile Strength, (MPA) (Minimum)		Percent Elongation, (%) (Minimum)	Izod Impact Strength, (ft-lf/in) (Minimum)	Deformation Under Load, (%) (Maximum)
	ASTM D 1505	ASTM D 638, Type IV, 5.08 cm/min		ASTM D 638, Type IV, 5.08 cm/min	ASTM D 256, d = 0.254 cm, r = 0.025 cm	ASTM D 621 (A), 7 MPA, 24 hr, 23°C, 90 min Rec.
PEKEKK	1.2	90	70	10	0.7	2
PEEK	1.3	90	70	10	1.0	2
PEKK	1.3			10		2
PEEKK	1.3	90		10		2
PEK				10		2

Solution—Part 1: General Conditions[6]

ISO 10993 Biological Evaluation of Medical Devices, Parts 1–12[6]

2.3 *Other Documents:*

United States Pharmacopeia, Vol. XXI, or latest edition[7]

3. Terminology

3.1 *Definitions of Terms Specific to This Standard:*

3.1.1 *fabricated forms*—those items into which the virgin forms may be converted. These include shapes and forms produced by means of machining, extruding, and compression molding virgin forms into a subsequent entity (for example, rods, slabs, sheets, film, complex shaped parts and devices).

3.1.2 *formulated compound*—PAEK materials, parts, or devices fabricated from virgin forms in such a way as to contain intentional or unintentional adjuvant substances.

3.1.3 *virgin forms*—that form of the PAEK resin as obtained by the synthesizer after removal of residual monomers, solvents, catalysts, etc. It typically will be in the form of pellets, chips, or blocks. It is the material from which rods, slabs, sheets, films, or specific parts and devices are fabricated.

4. Classification

4.1 PAEK resins in the scope of this specification are pure semicrystalline homopolymers consisting of phenylene rings connected by ether and carbonyl groups. Their structures are commonly identified by the sequence of ether (E) and carbonyl (or ketone, K) groups along the polymer chain (for example, PEKEKK, PEEK, etc.) (see Appendix X2).

4.2 Types of PAEK plastics, molding, and extrusion grades are described in Classification D 4000.

5. General Properties

5.1 PAEK resins used in medical applications may comply with the Food and Drug Administration (FDA) regulation 21 CFR 177.1580[8] that covers both wet and dry food contact applications.

6. Chemical Properties

6.1 The required physical and chemical properties of some virgin PAEK resins are listed in Table 1.

6.2 The infrared spectrum[9] of these materials is characteristic of their molecular repeating units. Representative spectra are listed in Appendix X3. The PAEK resin shall yield an infrared transmittance spectrum which exhibits major bands only at the wavelengths listed for the standard reference spectrum for the material.

6.2.1 The infrared spectrum, as used herein, is to identify the specific type of PAEK present and does not necessarily indicate an acceptable degree of material purity.

6.2.2 The presence of additional bands in the sample's infrared spectrum compared to that of the reference material may indicate a different PAEK, impurities, or both.

7. Mechanical Properties

7.1 The mechanical properties of consolidated forms of these materials are dependent on the consolidation process. Additionally, the necessary mechanical properties of consolidated forms will vary from one application to another. Table 2 lists some typical mechanical properties expected for some of these resins.

7.2 The solution viscosity requirements listed in Table 1 may be supplemented, or replaced, by rheological or complex viscosity data as agreed upon by vendor and purchaser.

7.3 The mechanical properties of consolidated forms of PAEKs shall be determined on finished parts or test specimens processed similarly to finished parts.

[7] Available from U.S. Pharmacopeial Convention, Inc., Easton, PA.

[8] Available from the Food and Drug Administration, Pittsburgh, PA.

[9] Silverstein, R. M., Bassler, G. C., and Morrill, T. C., Spectroscopic Identification of Organic Compounds, 5th ed., John Wiley & Sons, Inc., New York, NY.

7.4 Tests and test procedures shall be such as to assure a high level of control and characterization of the virgin resin as received from the supplier. The following are some test methods that may be appropriate: Test Method D 149, Test Method D 256, Test Method D 570, Test Method D 638, Test Method D 648, Test Method D 695, Test Method D 696, Test Method D 790, Test Method D 792, Test Method D 955, Test Method D 1238, Test Method D 1505, Test Method D 3417, Test Method D 3418, and Test Method D 4000.

8. Sampling

8.1 The material should be sampled in accordance with standard sampling procedures, such as those described in Practice D 1898, or other sampling techniques unless otherwise agreed upon between consumer and supplier.

9. Biocompatibility

9.1 Biocompatibility of PAEK resins and implant devices made using these materials shall be determined in accordance with Practice F 748 or the ISO 10993 series, unless otherwise agreed upon by packager and consumer, and regulating bodies.[10]

10. Keywords

10.1 PAEK; PEEK; PEEKK; PEKEKK; PEKK; PEK; polyaryletherketone

[10] Other useful references for testing biocompatibility of materials include: Autian, J., "Toxicological Evaluation of Biomaterials: Primary Acute Toxicity Screening Program," *Journal of Artificial Organs,* Vol 1, No. 1, 1977, p. 53.

Autian, J., "The New Field of Plastic Toxicological Methods and Results," *CRC Critics Review in Toxicology,* 1973, p. 18.

Homsy, C. A., Ansevin, K. D., O'Brannon, W., Thompson, S. H., Hodge, R., and Estrella, M. E., "Rapid In Vitro Screening of Polymers for Biocompatibility," *Journal of Macromolecular Science, Chemistry,* Vol A4, No. 3, May 1970, pp. 615–634.

Rice, R. M., Hegyeli, A. F., Gourlay, S. J., Wade, C. W. R., Dillon, J. G., Jaffe, H., and Kulkarni, R. K., "Biocompatibility Testing for Polymers: In Vitro Studies With in Vivo Correlation," *Journal of Biomedical Materials Research,* Vol 12, 1978, p. 43.

APPENDIXES

(Nonmandatory Information)

X1. RATIONALE

X1.1 PAEK resins may be processed by most techniques available for thermoplastic polymers. Medical devices and components of medical devices made of PAEK resins may be sterilized. Sterilization methods successfully used include steam, ethylene oxide, and irradiation. Repeated sterilization may weaken parts fabricated of any plastic material. The number of times a given part may be sterilized safely without fear of subsequent failure depends on a number of factors including the molecular weight of resin and design, fabrication, intended function, and method of sterilization of the device. Therefore it is imperative that the manufacturer test the device in order to determine the maximum number of sterilization cycles to which it can be safely subjected.

X1.2 The potential to develop a significant level of crystallinity is an important characteristic of these materials. Performance characteristics are related to the percent crystallinity. Certain additives and processes (for example, excessive crosslinking) can limit these materials' ability to crystallize. Therefore, this feature of the resin and its fabricated form should be evaluated using appropriate test methods to ensure efficacy.

X1.3 A formulated compound or fabricated part or device may contain optional adjuvant substances required for the fabrication or intended use of the end product. The biocompatibility of these adjuvant substances and subsequent formulated compounds, parts, and devices shall be established in accordance with Practice F 748 or the ISO 10993 series.

X2. CHEMICAL STRUCTURES OF SOME PAEK MATERIALS

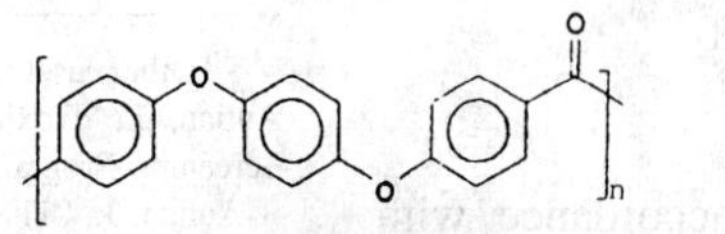

FIG. X2.1 PEEK

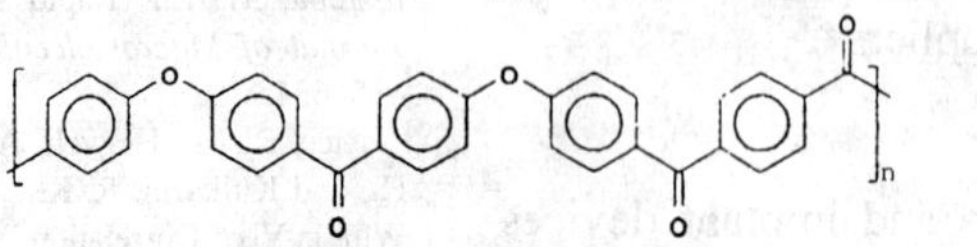

FIG. X2.2 PEKEKK

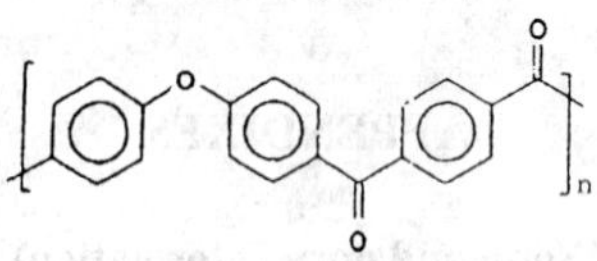

FIG. X2.3 PEKK

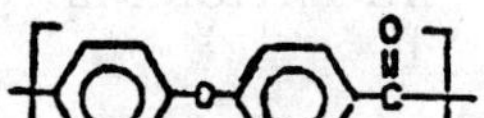

FIG. X2.4 PEK

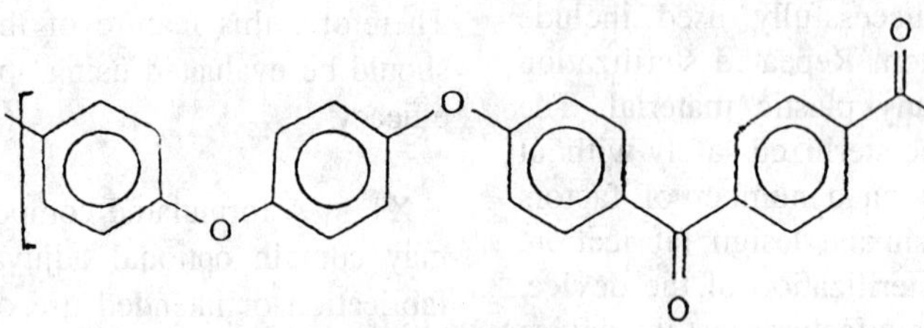

FIG. X2.5 PEEKK

X3. INFRARED SPECTRA OF SOME PAEK MATERIALS

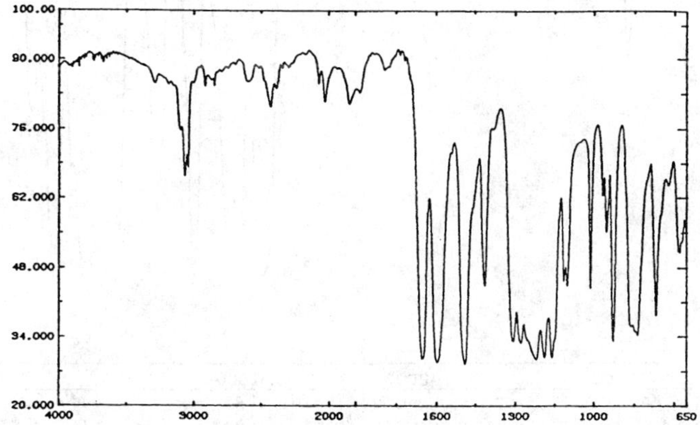

FIG. X3.1 Typical Infrared Spectrum for PEEK, 450G

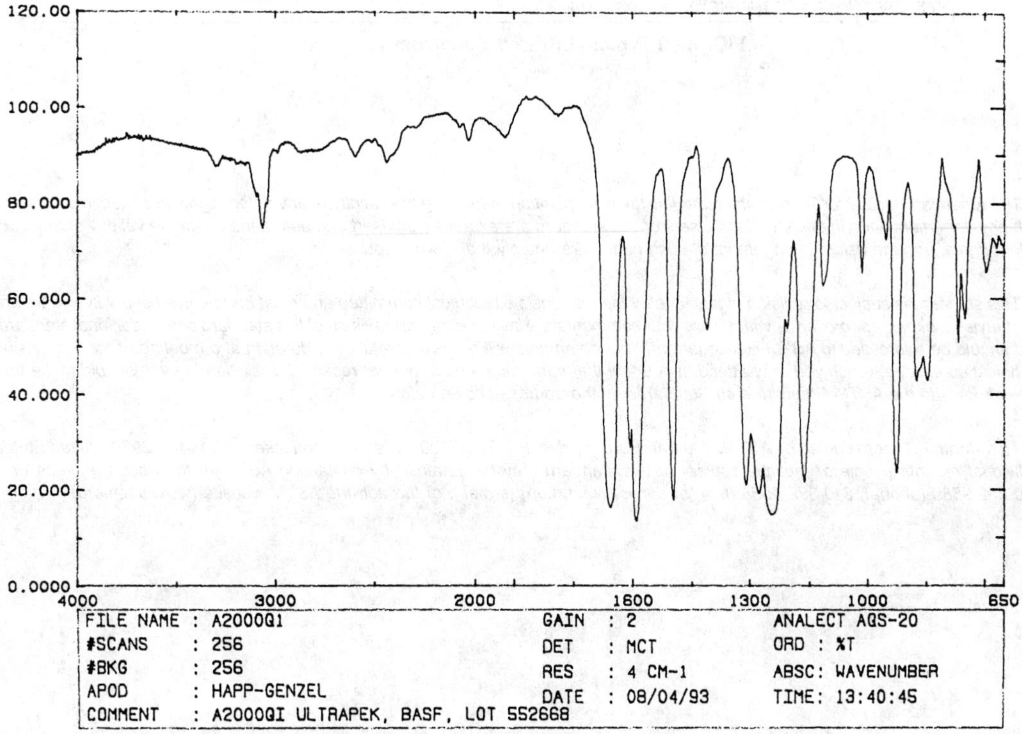

FIG. X3.2 Typical Infrared Spectrum for PEKEKK, A3000

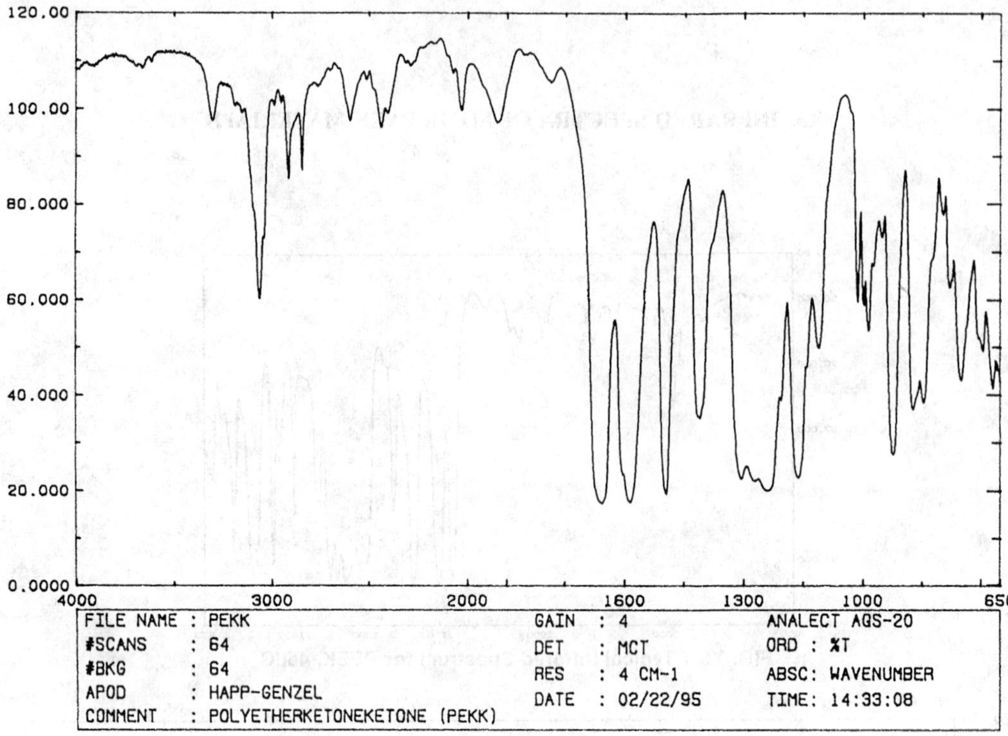

FIG. X3.3 Typical Infrared Spectrum for PEKK

Designation: F 1580 – 95$^{\epsilon 1}$

Standard Specification for Titanium and Titanium-6 % Aluminum-4 % Vanadium Alloy Powders for Coatings of Surgical Implants[1]

ϵ^1 NOTE—Table 1 was editorially corrected in May 2001.

1. Scope

1.1 This specification covers the requirements for unalloyed titanium and Ti-6Al-4V alloy powders for use in fabricating coatings on titanium alloy implants.

1.2 Powders covered under this specification may be used to form coatings by sintering or thermal spraying techniques.

1.3 This specification covers powder requirements only. It does not address properties of the coatings formed from them.

2. Referenced Documents

2.1 *ASTM Standards:*

B 214 Test Method Sieve Analysis of Granular Metal Powders[2]

B 215 Methods of Sampling Finished Lots of Metal Powders[2]

B 299 Specification for Titanium Sponge[3]

E 11 Specification for Wire-Cloth Sieves for Testing Purposes[4]

E 120 Test Methods for Chemical Analysis of Titanium and Titanium Alloys[5]

F 67 Specification for Unalloyed Titanium for Surgical Implant Applications[3]

F 1472 Specification for Wrought Ti-6Al-4V Alloy for Surgical Implant Applications[6]

2.2 *American Society for Quality Control (ASQC) Standards:*[7]

ASQC C1 General Requirements for a Quality Control Program

2.3 *Aerospace Material Specifications:*[8]

AMS 2249 Chemical Check Analysis Limits, Titanium and Titanium Alloys

AMS 4998A Powder, 6Al-4V, Premium Quality (noncurrent)

3. Significance and Use

3.1 Coatings formed from metallic powders have become widely used as a means of improving tissue attachment to implants. Such coatings have also been demonstrated to improve bonding of acrylic cement to prostheses. This specification addresses the special requirements of the metal powders used to form these coatings.

4. Methods of Manufacture

4.1 Powders may be manufactured by the plasma rotating electrode process, inert gas atomization, hydride-dehydride, or other method capable of producing powder meeting the requirements of this specification.

5. Chemical Requirements

5.1 The chemical analysis of the powder shall conform to the requirements set forth in Table 1. Analysis shall be performed before the addition of any processing aids.

5.1.1 Requirements for the major and minor elemental constituents for unalloyed titanium and Ti-6Al-4V alloy powders are listed in Table 1. Also listed are all important residual elements. Analysis for elements not listed in Table 1 is not required to verify compliance with this specification.

5.2 The product analysis tolerance shall conform to the requirements set forth in Table 2.

5.3 For referee purposes, Test Methods E 120 shall be used.

5.4 Intentional elemental additions other than those specified in Table 1 are not permitted.

5.5 For powder that includes particle size fractions finer than 200 mesh (74 μm), the oxygen content limits shall be agreed upon between buyer and seller.

6. Particle Size

6.1 Powder shall be sieved to the customer's requirements with stainless steel screens conforming to Specification E 11. Analysis of sieved powder for conformance to the customer's

[1] This specification is under the jurisdiction of ASTM Committee F04 on Medical and Surgical Devices and is under the direct responsibility of Subcommittee F04.12on Metallurgical Materials.

Current edition approved Feb. 15, 1995. Published July 1995.

[2] *Annual Book of ASTM Standards*, Vol 02.05.

[3] *Annual Book of ASTM Standards*, Vol 02.04.

[4] *Annual Book of ASTM Standards*, Vol 14.02.

[5] *Annual Book of ASTM Standards*, Vol 03.05.

[6] *Annual Book of ASTM Standards*, Vol 13.01.

[7] Available from the American Society for Quality Control, 161 W. Wisconsin Ave., Milwaukee, WI 53203.

[8] Available from Society of Automotive Engineers, 400 Commonwealth Dr., Warrendale, PA 15096.

TABLE 1 Chemical Requirements

Element	Unalloyed Ti Powder[A] % (Mass/Mass)		Ti Sponge Powder[B] % (Mass/Mass)		Ti-6Al-4V Powder[C] % (Mass/Mass)	
	min	max	min	max	min	max
Al				0.05	5.50	6.75
V					3.50	4.50
O		0.40		0.40[D]		0.20
Fe		0.50		0.15		0.30
C		0.10		0.03		0.08
H		0.05		0.03		0.015
N		0.05		0.02		0.05
Cu						0.10
Sn						0.10
Si				0.04		
Cl[E]				0.20[E]		
Na				F		
Ti	balance[G]		balance[G]		balance[G]	

[A]Chemistry per Specification F 67.
[B]Chemistry per Specification B 299, general purpose grade.
[C]Chemistry per Specification F 1472.
[D]Oxygen per Specification B 299 is 0.15 %. This level is reasonable for sponge product but not for powder because of the increased surface area of small particle powder product.
[E]Lower maximum chlorine content may be agreed upon between buyer and seller.
[F]Sodium or magnesium, 0.50 maximum.
[G]The percentage of titanium is determined by difference and need not be measured.

TABLE 2 Product Analysis Tolerances[A]

Element	Variation Under Min or Over Max
Aluminum	0.04
Vanadium	0.015
Oxygen	0.03[B]
Oxygen	0.02[C]
Iron	0.10
Hydrogen	0.002
Carbon	0.02
Nitrogen	0.02
Copper	0.05
Tin	0.15
Silicon	0.02

[A]Refer to AMS 2249.
[B]For unalloyed Ti powder.
[C]For Ti-6Al-4V alloy powder.

particle size range requirements shall be in accordance with Test Method B 214.

7. Cleanliness

7.1 Powder shall be handled at all times so as to ensure freedom from contamination with nonmetallic materials or other metal alloy powders, or both.

7.2 Powder cleanliness shall be determined by examining a representative sample, per Methods B 215 or as agreed upon between buyer and seller, comprising at least 1 in.^{2} (6.45 cm^2) of a closely packed mono-layer of powder per lot at 20× magnification. No foreign material shall be visible under these conditions. Powder cleanliness shall be determined before the addition of any processing aids.

8. Special Requirements

8.1 Various materials known as processing aids may be added to the powder to provide enhanced processibility. The powder supplier shall identify the chemical composition and weight percentage of any added processing aids on the material certification.

8.2 Processing aids shall have no detrimental effect on the corrosion resistance or biocomptability of the final coating.

NOTE 1—Finely divided titanium powder may be considered pyrophoric and should be handled in accordance with the appropriate guidelines in the Material Safety Data Sheet.

9. Certification

9.1 Powder shipped under this specification shall be accompanied by certification that includes:

9.1.1 ASTM designation.

9.1.2 Quantity (weight).

9.1.3 Method of manufacture.

9.1.4 Chemical analysis per 5.1.

9.1.5 Sieve analysis per 6.1.

9.1.6 Powder cleanliness per 7.2.

9.1.7 Special requirement per 8.2.

9.1.8 Other requirements.

10. Quality Program Requirements

10.1 The producer shall maintain a quality program, such as that defined in the ASQC C1, for example.

10.2 The manufacturer of surgical implants shall be ensured of the producer's quality program for conformance to the intent of ASQC C1 or other recognized programs.

11. Keywords

11.1 coatings; metallic; metals (for surgical implants titanium alloys); orthopaedic medical devices (titanium/titanium alloys); powder; porous coatings; titanium/titanium alloys (for surgical implants)

APPENDIX

(Nonmandatory Information)

X1. RATIONALE

X1.1 Coatings formed from metallic powders have become widely used as a means of improving tissue attachment to uncemented orthopedic joint prosthesis. Such coatings have also been demonstrated to improve bonding of acrylic cement to prostheses.

X1.2 The biocompatibility of metallic implants is a direct function of their composition. The compositions of titanium and titanium alloy powders allowed by this specification have been used in wrought form for surgical implants and are in widespread commercial use for fabrication of porous coatings.

X1.3 Chemical composition limits for O, Fe, C, and N in the unalloyed grade are taken from Specification F 67, Grade 4. Limits for Si, Cl, H, and Na are taken from Specification B 299, Grade SL.

X1.4 Chemical composition limits for Al, V, O, Fe, C, H, and N in the Ti-6Al-4V grade are taken from Specification F 1472. Limits for Cu and Sn are taken from AMS 4998.

X1.5 Product analysis tolerances are taken directly from AMS 2249. No recognized product analysis tolerances currently exist specifically for Cl or Na in titanium alloys.

X1.6 Processing aids are frequently used to facilitate powder processing and application of porous coatings to implant surfaces. It is beyond the scope of this specification to identify suitable processing aids or define their use. It is the responsibility of the implant manufacturer to ensure that any processing aid or residue of a processing aid has no detrimental effect on biocompatibility or coating properties.

X1.7 It should be recognized that the heat treatments used to form porous coatings can create microstructures that are substantially different from wrought titanium alloys. Porous coated implants also exhibit much greater surface area than monolithic implants. For these reasons, the biocompatibility and corrosion behavior must be characterized on finished coatings.

X1.8 Likewise, these heat treatments can create microstructures that give substantially different corrosion fatigue behavior from that of typical wrought titanium alloys. Corrosion fatigue behavior must be evaluated on finished coated substrates.

X1.9 Pore size and morphology are important factors influencing tissue ingrowth and acrylic penetration of porous coatings. Particle size, size distribution, and shape are critical to controlling the pore size and morphology in the final coating. Particle size and size distribution are conventionally controlled by screening. The referenced ASTM and MPIF (01, 05, 09) standards allow comparison of powder to a manufacturer's specifications for a given coating process. A number of methods to characterize particle shape exists. The coating manufacturer should select a means of particle shape characterization suitable for his process.

X1.10 This specification requires sampling for particle size and powder cleanliness on each powder lot. In some cases, sampling on each shipping container of powder may be appropriate.

X1.11 Other process parameters are also critical to determining final pore size and morphology in the final coating. Because these parameters are not directly related to the chemical and physical characteristics of the starting powder, they are not addressed in this specification.

X1.12 The requirements for powder cleanliness ensure freedom from contaminants that might adversely affect either the biocompatibility or the finished coatings or the ability to bond the coating properly during manufacturing. The method in 7.2 (Methods B 215) is commonly used for relatively coarse spherical powders used to fabricate sintered porous coatings. Other types of powders may require different methods for cleanliness characterization. The development and implementation of such methods are the responsibility of the implant manufacturer.

Designation: F 1581 – 99

Standard Specification for Composition of Anorganic Bone for Surgical Implants[1]

This standard is issued under the fixed designation F 1581; the number immediately following the designation indicates the year of original adoption or, in the case of revision, the year of last revision. A number in parentheses indicates the year of last reapproval. A superscript epsilon (ε) indicates an editorial change since the last revision or reapproval.

1. Scope

1.1 This specification covers material requirements for anorganic xenogeneic or allogeneic bone (apatite) intended for surgical implants. For a material to be called anorganic or deorganified bone, it must conform to this specification (see Appendix X1).

1.2 The biological response to apatite in soft tissue and bone has been characterized by a history of clinical use [2] and by laboratory studies **(1,2,3)**. Xenogeneic bone, with organic components present, has been shown to be antigenic in the human host **(4)** whereas the same material that has been completely deorganified has been shown to elicit no inflammatory or foreign body reactions in human clinical use **(5, 6, 7)**.

1.3 This specification specifically excludes synthetic hydroxylapatite, hydroxylapatite coatings, ceramic glasses, tribasic calcium phosphate, whitlockite, and alpha- and beta-tricalcium phosphate.

1.4 *This standard does not pruport to address all of the safety concerns, such as health concerns due to the presence of transmissible disease, associated with its use. It is the responsibility of the user of this standard to establish appropriate safety and health practices and determine the applicability of regulatory limitations prior to use.*(See Appendix X2).

2. Referenced Documents

2.1 *ASTM Standards:*

D 513 Test Methods for Total and Dissolved Carbon Dioxide in Water[3]

D 1688 Test Methods for Copper in Water[3]

D 2972 Test Methods for Arsenic in Water[3]

D 3557 Test Methods for Cadmium in Water[3]

D 3559 Test Methods for Lead in Water[3]

D 3919 Practice for Measuring Trace Elements in Water by Graphite Furnace Atomic Absorption Spectrophotometry[3]

D 4129 Test Method for Total and Organic Carbon in Water High Temperature Oxidation and Coulometric Detection[4]

E 1184 Practice for Electrothermal (Graphite Furnace) Atomic Absorption Analysis[5]

F 748 Practice For Selecting Generic Biological Test Methods for Materials and Devices[6]

F 1185 Specification for Composition of Ceramic Hydroxylapatite for Surgical Implants[6]

2.2 *Code of Federal Regulations:*[7]

Title 21, Part 820

2.3 *National Formulary:*[8]

Tribasic Calcium Phosphate

2.4 *United States Pharmocopeia:*[9]

Identification Tests for Calcium and Phosphate <191>

Lead <251>

Mercury <261>

Cadmium <461>

Arnsenic <211>

Heavy Metals <231> Method 1

Nitrogen Determination <4617>

2.5 *U.S. Geological Survey Method:*[10]

Cadmium

3. Terminology

3.1 *Definitions:*

3.1.1 *allogeneic, adj*—derived from different individuals of the same species.

3.1.2 *anorganic, adj*—denoting tissue (for example, bone) from which the organic material has been totally removed. Also referred to as *deorganified, deproteinized or deproteinated.*

3.1.3 *apatite, n*—the mineral substance having the molecular formula $Ca_{10}(X)_2(PO_4)_6$ where X=OH (hydroxyapatite or hydroxylapatite), CO_3(carbonated apatite), F or C1 **(8)**.

3.1.4 *xenogeneic, adj*—derived from individuals of a different, specified species. For example, bovine bone, when used as an implant material in humans, is xenogeneic.

---

[1] This specification is under the jurisdiction of ASTM Committee F-4 on Medical and Surgical Devices and is under the direct responsibility of Subcommittee F04.13 on Ceramic Materials.

Current edition approved Feb. 10, 1999. Published June 1999. Originally published as F 1581 – 95. Last previous edition F 1581 – 96.

[2] The boldface numbers in parentheses refer to the list of references at the end of this specification.

[3] *Annual Book of ASTM Standards*, Vol. 11.01.

[4] *Annual Book of ASTM Standards*, Vol. 11.02.

[5] *Annual Book of ASTM Standards*, Vol. 03.06.

[6] *Annual Book of ASTM Standards*, Vol. 13.01.

[7] Available from Standardization Documents Order Desk, Bldg. 4 Section D, 700 Robbins Ave., Philadelphia, PA 19111-5094, Attn: NPODS.

[8] National Formulary XVI. Available from U.S. Pharmacopeia Convention, Inc., 12601 Twinbrook Parkway, Rockville, MD 20852.

[9] United States Pharmacopeia XXI. Available from U.S. Pharmacopeia Convention, Inc., 12601 Twinbrook Parkway, Rockville, MD 20852.

[10] Crock, J. G., Felichte, F. E., and Briggs, P. H., "Determination of Elements in National Bureau of Standards Geological Reference Materials SRM 278 Obsidian and SRM 688 Basalt by Inductively Coupled Argon Plasma—Atomic Emission Spectrometry." *Geostandards Newsletter*, Vol 7, 1983, pp. 335–340.

4. Chemical Requirements

4.1 Elemental analysis for calcium and phosphorus will be consistent with the expected composition of the source of the biologically derived bone mineral **(9)**.

4.2 An X-ray diffraction analysis of the material shall be consistent with PDF card #9-432 for hydroxyapatite **(10)** or PDF card #35–180 for calcium phosphate carbonate (carbonated apatite). Analysis of relative peak intensities shall be consistent with published data.[11]

4.3 The concentration of trace elements in the anorganic bone shall be limited as follows:

Element	ppm, max
As	3
Cd	5
Hg	5
Pb	30
total heavy metals (as lead)	50

For referee purposes, use either inductively coupled plasma/mass spectroscopy (ICP/MS) **(11)** or the United States Pharmocopeia (USP) methods <191>, <251>, <261>, <211>, <231> Method 1, < 4617> and for cadmium either <461> or the U.S. Geological Survey Method on Cadmium. (See 2.4 and 2.5). Graphite furnace atomic absorption spectrophotometry may also be used for ananlysis of trace elements using (Test Methods D 2972), Cd (Test Method D 1688), Pb (Test Methods D 3559) with 1 g anorganic bone/100mL H_2O samples. G eneral guides for the application of the graphite furnace are given in Practices D 3919 and E 1184.

4.4 The maximum allowable limit of all heavy metals determined as lead will be 50 ppm as described in 2.4 or equivalent. Sample preparation will be identical to that for tribasic calcium phosphate as specified in the National Formulary (see 2.3), except that approximately 1 g of material will be dissolved in approximately 30 mL of 5 % HCl and boiled.

4.5 It is recommended that all minor constituents such as metals or oxides not detected as lead present in concentrations equal to or greater than 0.1 % be identified and quantified.

4.6 Organic content shall be measured either as total carbon or nitrogen (see Note 1) or total protein by amino acid analyses **(13)**. For all methods, a synthetic hydroxylapatite control that conforms to Specification F 1185 or an established NIST standard must be used. The maximum allowable limit of either nitrogen, carbon, or protein will be within two standard deviations of the mean value established for the control.

NOTE 1—The Kjeldahl process for nitrogen determination (USP <461>) is set forth by the Association of Official Analytical Chemists **(12)** as an appropriate measure of proteins. Alternatively, organic material (carbon) can be measured by the coulometric method (Test Method D 4129). Subtract from this value the carbonate content, which can be determined by Test Methods D 513.

4.7 Functional groups will be identified by infrared analysis. Typical functional groups of apatites have been described by Elliott **(8)**, LeGeros et al **(14)**, and Rey **(15,16,17)**.

4.8 Analysis of additional elements or ionic species associated with the source or with processing conditions should be specified for this material.

5. Test Specimen Fabrication

5.1 Prepare test specimens from the same batch of material and by the same processes as those employed in fabricating the implant device.

6. Quality Program Requirements

6.1 The manufacturer shall conform to Good Manufacturing Practices (see Title 21, Part 820, of the Code of Federal Regulations[7]) or its equivalent.

7. Biocompatibility

7.1 The biocompatibility of anorganic bone may depend upon processing conditions or source material history, or both, which may not be identified by the compositional requirements of this specification. The biocompatibility of these products should be ensured by a combination of preclinical testing and process controls. Material derived under the desired process conditions should be tested in accordance with the recommendations of Practice F 748 and manufacturing controls put in place to ensure that process variations outside of acceptable tolerances do not occur. Substantial changes in process conditions or source control parameters will necessitate additional biocompatibility testing to ensure maintenance of an acceptable tissue response.

8. Sterilization

8.1 Anorganic bone may be supplied presterilized in accordance with current procedures set forth by the Association for the Advancement of Medical Instrumentation (AAMI) and Good Manufacturing Practices (GMP) established by the Food and Drug Administration (FDA).[12]

8.2 If user sterilization or resterilization is intended, validated instructions for sterilization shall be supplied with the package insert.

9. Keywords

9.1 allogeneic; anorganic; apatite; bone; hydroxyapatite; hydroxylapatite; implant; xenogeneic

[11] The Joint Committee on Powdered Diffraction Standards has established a Powder Diffraction File. The Committee operates on an international basis and cooperates closely with the Data Commission of the International Union of Crystallography and ASTM. Hydroxylapatite data can be found on file card number 9-432 and is available from the Joint Committee on Powder Diffraction Standards, 1600 Park Lane, Swarthmore, PA 19801.

[12] Federal Register, Vol. 43, No. 141, Friday, July 21, 1978.

APPENDIXES

(Nonmandatory Information)

X1. RATIONALE

X1.1 Xenogeneic and allograft bone is commercially available as grafting material. To eliminate concerns about possible immunogenicity effects or partially purified bone, anorganic or deorganified bone has been developed. To achieve reliable biocompatibility as an implant material, this material must be characterized for its hydroxylapatite mineral component and trace element content as well as for the absence of organic material. At the current time, sufficient data do not exist to provide specific limits for carbon and nitrogen values. Individual laboratories must apply statistical analysis to show equivalence with the negative control. Test results that might provide data to assign specific limits for carbon and nitrogen are hereby solicited.

X2. BIOCOMPATIBILITY

X2.1 No known surgical implant material has ever been shown to be completely free of adverse reactions in the human body. However, long term clinical experience of the use of the material referred to in this standard has shown that an acceptable level of biological response can be expected, if the material is used in appropriate applications.

REFERENCES

(**1**) Hench, L.L., Wilson, J., *An Introduction to Bioceramics*, World Scientific, 1993, pp. 139–238.

(**2**) Damien, C. J., and Parsons, J. R., "Bone Graft and Bone Graft Substitutes: A Review of Current Technology and Applications," *Journal of Applied Biomaterials*, Vol 2, 1991, pp. 187–208.

(**3**) Jarcho, M., Kay, J. F., Gumaer, K. I., Doremus, R. H., and Drobeck, H. P., "Tissue, Cellular and Subcellular Events at a Bone-Ceramic Hydroxylapatite Interface," *Journal of Bioengineering*, Vol. 1, 1977, pp. 79–92.

(**4**) Salama, R., and Gazit, E., "The Antigenicity of Kiel Bone in the Human Host," *The Journal of Bone and Joint Surgery*, Vol. 60-B No. 2, 1978, pp. 262–265.

(**5**) Urist, M.R., O'Connor, B.T., Burwell, R.G., Bone Grafts, Derivatives and Substitutes, Butterworth-Heineman Ltd., 1994, pp 41–42.

(**6**) Begley, C.T., Doherty, M.J., Mollan, R.A., Wilson, D.J., "Comparative Study of the Osteoinductive Properties of Bioceramic, Coral and Processed Bone Graft Substitutes", Biomaterials, Vol 16. 1995, pp. 1181–1185.

(**7**) Callan, D.P., "Use of Bovine-Derived Hydroxyapatite in the Treatment of Endentulous Ridge Defects: A Human Clinical and Histologic Case Report", *Journal of Periodontology*, Vol. 64, 1993, pp. 575–582.

(**8**) Elliott, J.C., Structure and Chemistry of the Apatites and Other Calcium Orthophosphates, Elsevier Science B.V., 1994, p.4

(**9**) LeGeros, R.Z., LeGeros, J.P., Daculsi, G., Kijkowska, R., "Calcium Phosphate Biomaterials: Preparation, Properties, and Biodegradation", Encylopedic Handbook of Biomaterials and Bioengineering, Part A: Materials, Vol. 2, Marcel Dekker, 1995, pp. 1429–1463

(**10**) Balmain, N., Legeros, R., and Bonel, G., "X-Ray Diffraction of Calcified Bone Tissue: A Reliable Method for the Determination of Bone Ca/P Molar Ratio," *Calcified Tissue International*, Vol 34, 1982, pp. 593–594.

(**11**) Northington, D.J., "Inductively Couples Plasma-Mass Spectrometry for the Analysis of Metals on Membrane Filters", Am. Ind. Hyg. Assoc. J., Vol 48, 1987, pp. 977–979.

(**12**) Horwitz, W., Ed, *Official Methods of Analysis of the Association of Analytical Chemists*, Association of Official Analytical Chemists, Washington, DC, 1980, pp. 15,214.

(**13**) Ozols, J., "Amino Acid Analysis", in Guide to Protein Purification, Methods in Enzymology, Vol. 182, Editor M.P. Deutscher, 1990, pp. 587–601.

(**14**) LeGeros, R.Z., Calcium Phosphates in Oral Biology and Medicine, Karger, 1991

(**15**) Rey, C., Miquel, J.L., Facchini, L., Legrand, A.P., Glimcher, M.J., "Hydroxyl Groups in Bone Mineral", Bone, Vol 16, 1995, pp. 583–586.

(**16**) Rey, C., Collins, B., Goehl, T., Dickson, I.R., Glimcher, M.J., "The Carbonate Environment in Bone Mineral: A Resolution-Enhanced Fourier Transform Infrared Spectroscopy Study", Calcified Tissue International, Vol 45, 1989, pp. 157–164.

(**17**) Rey, C., Shimizu, M., Collins, B., Glimcher, M.J., "Resolution-Enhanced Fourier Transform Infrared Spectroscopy Study of the Environment of Phosphate Ions in the Early Deposits of a Solid Phase of Calcium-Phosphate in Bone and Enamel, and their Evolution with Age. I: Investigations in the υ_4 PO_4Domain" Calcified Tissue International, Vol 46, 1990, pp. 384–394

Designation: F 1582 – 98

Standard Terminology Relating to Spinal Implants[1]

This standard is issued under the fixed designation F 1582; the number immediately following the designation indicates the year of original adoption or, in the case of revision, the year of last revision. A number in parentheses indicates the year of last reapproval. A superscript epsilon (ϵ) indicates an editorial change since the last revision or reapproval.

1. Scope

1.1 This terminology covers basic terms and considerations for spinal implant devices and their mechanical analyses.

2. Referenced Documents

2.1 *ASTM Standards:*

E 6 Terminology Relating to Methods of Mechanical Testing[2]

E 1150 Definitions of Terms Relating to Fatigue[2]

3. Terminology

Definitions Related to Spinal Implant Devices

anchor, *n*—components that are directly attached to the bony elements of the spine (sacrum, lamina, pedicle, vertebral body, spinous process, transverse process, the pelvis, or ribs).

band, *n*—a flexible anchor component with a noncircular cross section that connects the bony elements of the spine, pelvis, or ribs to each other or to other implant components using a knot or similar tying mechanism, forming a locked, closed loop.

bolt, *n*—an anchor component that connects to the bony elements of the spine, pelvis, or ribs by means of threads with the lead threads accomodating a nut thus sandwiching the bony element or implant component between the nut or washer and bolt head or other fixed stop.

expansion anchor, *n*—a component that forms a connection to bony element by means of a mechanism which enlarges once the component is inserted into the bony elements.

hook, *n*—an anchoring component that fastens to the spine by means of a curved blade passed under or over lamina, transverse or spinous processes or into an anatomic or surgically created notch or opening.

hook blade, *n*— that portion of a spinal hook that is placed under, over, or into a bony structure to provide attachment.

hook body—that portion of a spinal hook that connects the hook blade to the longitudinal element.

post, *n*—a non-threaded anchor component that connects to the bony elements of the spine, pelvis, or ribs by means of a non-threaded hole in the bony element.

screw, *n*—an anchor component that connects to the bony elements of the spine, pelvis, or ribs by means of threads.

staple, *n*—an anchor component that connects the bony elements of the spine, pelvis, or ribs to each other or to other implant components by using at least two interconnected posts.

wire—a single strand flexible anchor component with a circular cross section that connects the bony elements of the spine, pelvis, or ribs to each other or to other implant components. A series of wire components can be bound together to form a cable (see **cable**).

assembly, *n*— a complete implant configuration (not including spine, pelvis, ribs, or substitute material) as intended for surgical use.

component, *n*— any single element used in an assembly.

construct, *n*— a complete implant configuration attached to and including the spine, pelvis, ribs or substitute material as intended for surgical use.

interbody spacer, *n*—a structure (biologic or synthetic) to replace (partially or totally) the vertebral body or intervertebral disk(s), or both.

intervertebral body fusion devices, *n*—a structure which is placed in the disc space between two adjacent vertebral bodies to provide support for eventual arthrodeses of the two adjacent vertebral bodies.

intervertebral body fusion cage, *n*—a hollow device which contains graft material.

partial replacement disc—a structure intended to restore a portion of the support and motion or a portion thereof, between adjacent vertebral bodies.

replacement disc, *n*—a structure intended to restore support and motion between adjacent vertebral bodies.

vertebral body replacement device, *n*—a structure which is designed to restore anatomic position and support to a section of spine lacking one or more vertebral bodies and intervening disc(s).

interconnection, *n*—the mechanical interface or connection mechanism between at least two components or between components and bony elements of the spine, pelvis, or ribs.

bolt interconnection, *n*—an interconnection having an implant component sandwiched between two nuts or between a nut and fixed stop.

clamp, *n*—an interconnection component whose mechanism

---

[1] This terminology is under the jurisdiction of ASTM Committee F-4 on Medical and Surgical Materials and Devices and is the direct responsibility of Subcommittee F04.31 on Spinal Terminology.

Current edition approved April 10, 1998. Published September 1998.

[2] *Annual Book of ASTM Standards*, Vol. 03.01.

to secure the longitudinal element is through a squeezing action.

DISCUSSION—For example, crimps, wedges, set screws.

screw interconnection, *n*—an interconnection having an implant component sandwiched between the screw head (or screw thread) and bony element or other implant components.

sleeve interconnection, *n*—an interconnection in which an implant component passes through any opening that limits motion in one or more planes.

interface, *n*— one of the two mating surfaces, lines or points of contact within an interconnection between two components, between any component and bone, or between two bony elements.

longitudinal element, *n*—a component whose long axis is parallel, or nearly so, to the long axis of the spine.

cable, *n*—a multi-strand, flexible longitudinal element designed primarily to resist axial tension loading.

hybrid longitudinal element, *n*—a longitudinal element consisting of two or more types of longitudinal elements of different size or cross-section manufactured into a single element.

plate, *n*—a longitudinal element asymmetrical in the transverse plane and designed to resist tension, compression, bending, and torsion.

rod, *n*—a longitudinal element symmetrical in the transverse plane designed to resist tension, compression, bending, and torsion.

motion segment, *n*—two adjacent vertebrae, the intervening disc, and the associated ligamentous structures.

subassembly, *n*— any portion of an implant assembly that is composed of two or more components.

subconstruct, *n*— any portion of an implant construct that is composed of two or more components including the spine, pelvis, ribs, or substitute structure.

transverse element, *n*—a component or subassembly that links longitudinal members together.

vertebral span, *n*—the number of vertebra that are spanned by the longitudinal element, including the vertebrae containing anchor components.

Definitions Related to Spinal Implant Testing Defined in Other Documents, or are Established Terminology

DISCUSSION—In certain instances, a value for moment or load can be substituted for *stress* when describing fatigue life. This is true in cases in which the actual stress values are unknown or not easily obtainable. The moment or load can be substituted when comparing devices assigned to perform the same mechanical function. The value for load or moment thus determined is subject to the same conditions as those that apply to *stress* in this terminology standard. However, whenever possible, *stress* should be the standard employed.

fatigue, *n*—the process of progressive localized permanent structural change occurring in a material subjected to conditions that produce fluctuating stresses and strains at some point or points and that may culminate in cracks or complete fracture after a sufficient number of fluctuations.

DISCUSSION—See Definitions E 1150.

fatigue life, *n*— the number of loading cycles, *N*, of a specified character that a given specimen sustains before failure of a specified nature occurs.

DISCUSSION—See Definitions E 1150

fatigue strength at N Cycles, $S_n[FL^{-2}]$, *n*—a value of stress for failure at exactly *N* cycles as determined from an *S-N* diagram. The value S_n thus determined is subject to the same conditions as those that apply to the *S-N* diagram.

DISCUSSION—The value of S_n which is commonly found in the literature is the value of S_{max} (*maximum stress*) or S_a (*stress amplitude*) at which 50 % of the specimens of a given sample could survive *N* stress cycles in which S_m (*mean stress*) = 0. This is also known as the median fatigue strength for *N* cycles (see Definitions E 1150).

fatigue test, *n*— a test designed to evaluate the cyclic load properties of a material, component, interconnection, subconstruct, construct, subassembly, or assembly.

load ratio, R, A, *n*—in fatigue loading, the algebraic ratio of the two loading parameters of a cycle.

DISCUSSION—The most widely used ratios are:

$$R = \frac{\text{Minimum Load}}{\text{Maximum Load}} = \frac{P_{\min}}{P_{\max}} \tag{1}$$

or

$$\frac{S_{\min}}{S_{\max}} \tag{2}$$

or

$$R = \frac{\text{Valley Load}}{\text{Peak Load}} \tag{3}$$

and

$$A = \frac{\text{Loading Amplitude}}{\text{Mean Load}} = \frac{Pa}{Pm} \tag{4}$$

or

$$\frac{Sa}{Sm} \tag{5}$$

or

$$A = \frac{(\text{Maximum Load} - \text{Minimum Load})}{(\text{Maxium Load} + \text{Minimum Load})} = \frac{(P_{\max} - P_{\min})}{(P_{\max} + P_{\min})} \tag{6}$$

S-N diagram, *n*— a plot of stress against the number of cycles to failure. The stress can be maximum stress S_{max}, minimum stress S_{min}, stress range *S* or S_r, or alternating stress S_a. The diagram indicates the *S-N* relationship for a specified value of S_m (*mean stress*) *A*, or *R* (*load or stress ratio*), and a specified probability of survival. For *N*, a log scale is almost always used. For *S*, a linear scale is used most often, but a log scale is sometimes used.

DISCUSSION—See Definitions E 1150.

static test, *n*— single cycle loading tests designed to evaluate the mechanical properties of materials, components, interconnections, subconstructs, constructs, subassemblies, or assemblies.

DISCUSSION—The mechanical properties can include stiffness, flexibility, failure loads and stresses, and yield and ultimate strengths defined in the associated test standard, that is, the properties associated with elastic and inelastic reactions when force is applied or those that involve a relationship between stress and strain.

stress, S, *n*— the intensity at a point in a body of the forces or components of force that act on a given plane through the point.

DISCUSSION—Stress is expressed in units of force per unit area (pounds-force per square inch, megapascals, etc.) (See Terminology E 6.)

4. Coordinate System Related to the Application of Spinal Implant Devices

4.1 The coordinate system used in the testing of spinal implant devices is a system of three orthogonal axes that are defined in terms of the standard anatomic planes that they are perpendicular to, for example, transverse (horizontal or axial), coronal (frontal), and sagittal (median). Translations are also defined in terms of standard clinical directions, for example, ventral (anterior), dorsal (posterior), cranial (cephalad or superior), caudal (inferior), lateral, or medial. All rotations follow the right hand rule and are defined using current clinical terminology, for example, right or left side bending, flexion, extension, or twist. In addition, translations and rotations should be broken down into their accordant anatomic components.

4.2 It is recommended that the origin of the axes be located in a rigid structure such as bone. In addition, the orientation of the coordinate system, the designation of the three axes and location of the origin should be reported.

APPENDIX

(Nonmandatory Information)

X1. RATIONALE

X1.1 Where available, the standard terms used in Definitions E 1150 or Terminology E 6 were used.

X1.2 The coordinate system proposed is based on standard engineering practices for defining an orthogonal coordinate system. For clinical relevancy, anatomic or clinical terms are recommended. The selection of this coordinate system was made to avoid the differences in the myriad coordinate systems used in the current published literature and by various institutions, for example, International Organization for Standardization (ISO), Department of Transportation, Armed Services, and so on.

Standard Practice for Communications Procedures—Phonetics[1]

This standard is issued under the fixed designation F 1583; the number immediately following the designation indicates the year of original adoption or, in the case of revision, the year of last revision. A number in parentheses indicates the year of last reapproval. A superscript epsilon (ϵ) indicates an editorial change since the last revision or reapproval.

1. Scope

1.1 *Establishment of Phonetics*—This practice covers the establishment of phonetics (including an alphabet, numerals, and punctuations), and the procedures for their use, in communications.

1.2 *Performance*— This practice is intended to facilitate the performance of communications personnel and systems under adverse communications conditions. This objective is achieved by employing easily recognized and used symbols and procedures that are highly resistant to errors. This system may be used with speech, print, or other media.

1.3 *Interoperability*— This practice is intended to facilitate the interoperability of communications personnel and systems among different organizations, especially if they use different internal practices. This system is also recommended for use within any organization for improved internal communications and uniformity of operations.

1.4 *English as Common Language*—This practice is intended for use with English. English has been designated by the International Civil Aviation Organization (ICAO) and others as a common interoperability language that is widely used in search and rescue, emergency, and international operations such as aviation, maritime, and military.

2. Terminology

2.1 The terminology used in this practice is derived from references **(1-10)**.[2,3]

2.2 *automatic repeat-request (ARQ)*—a system of error control for information transmission in which the receiving station is arranged to detect a transmission error and automatically transmit a repeat-request signal to the transmitting station. The transmitting station then retransmits the message until it is either correctly received or the error persists beyond a predetermined number of transmittals.

2.3 *error correcting code*—a code in which each symbol conforms to specific rules of construction so that departures from this construction in the received signals can generally be automatically detected and corrected. If the number of errors is not greater than the maximum correctable threshold of the code, all errors are corrected.

2.4 *error correcting system*—in information transmission, a system employing either forward error correction or automatic repeat-request techniques or both, such that most transmission errors are automatically removed from the data prior to delivery to the user.

2.5 *forward error correction (FEC)*—a system of error control for information transmission wherein the receiving station has the capability to detect and correct any character or message that contains fewer than a predetermined number of symbols in error.

2.6 *interoperability*—the condition achieved among communications stations or personnel when information can be exchanged directly and satisfactorily between them or their users or both. It is desirable that the exchanges are error free, rapid, and automatic.

2.7 *phonetics*—a system of symbols and procedures that is used to control errors in communications, validate selected parts of messages, and enhance the interoperability and performance of communications personnel and systems.

2.8 *phonetic alphabet*—a selected set of phonetic symbols that has a one-to-one correspondence to the set of individual letters in a language. Also, any of various systems of code words for identifying letters in voice communications.

2.9 *phonetic punctuation*—a selected set of phonetic symbols that has a one-to-one correspondence to the set of individual punctuation in a language.

2.10 *phonetic numerals*—a selected set of phonetic symbols that has a one-to-one correspondence to the set of individual numerals in a language.

2.11 *phonetic symbol*—a unique word or combination of letters that is used as a substitute for, or an addition to, a specific letter, numeral, or punctuation in a language. It has the characteristics of an error correcting code.

3. Summary of Practice

3.1 *Interoperability and Performance*—A set of easily recognized and used symbols and procedures are established. They are used to control the errors that may be encountered in messages, to validate selected parts of messages, and to enhance the interoperability and performance of communications personnel and systems. This phonetic system is intended

[1] This practice is under the jurisdiction of ASTM Committee F32 on Search and Rescue and is the direct responsibility of Subcommittee F32.07 on Communications and Electronics.

Current edition approved March 15, 1995. Published April 1995.

[2] The boldface numbers in parentheses refer to a list of references at the end of this practice.

[3] This practice is based on an extensive survey of multiple organizations. Their communications documents were consulted to determine or verify compliance and interoperability among their many known and accepted phonetic systems. These documents are hereby referenced.

to be directly interoperable with the majority of standard phonetic systems presently employed, both internationally and within the United States.

3.2 *Error Control*— Error control is accomplished by detection of the errors and either prompt correction (based on the available information) or a request for another copy (if the information is inadequate for error correction).

4. Significance and Use

4.1 *Communications Errors and Delays*—Communications systems, including their procedures and channels, are subject to errors due to noise, interference, weak signals, mistakes, and other causes. They are also subject to delays due to the necessity to detect and correct these errors. There may also be errors and delays due to the lack of trained and experienced operators.

4.2 *Error Control*— Phonetics enables the control of errors through error detection, and usually prompt correction, for words and characters in speech and printed text. It employs an error correcting system of symbols and procedures that are standardized and easily recognized under adverse or high error communications conditions.

4.3 *Symbol Characteristics*—The phonetic alphabet is an error detecting and correcting code composed of phonetic symbols that are carefully selected to have distinctive sounds or appearances (or other unique characteristics) that improve detection under adverse conditions (such as severe noise or high errors) and enhance differentiation from each other.

4.3.1 Phonetics are inherently language-dependent. For English text letters, there are 26 phonetic alphabet symbols, that correspond to the 26 letters (from A to Z) that may be used to compose the words in a message. Additional symbols are used for numerals and punctuations.

4.3.2 Phonetic symbols (including an alphabet, numerals, and punctuation) must have unique characteristics as mentioned above, and they should not be restricted to only one communications media.

4.4 *Procedures for Error Detection and Correction*:

4.4.1 Phonetic communications procedures are used to minimize or eliminate information errors and to facilitate the correct transmission of messages using trained operators.

4.4.2 The phonetic procedures are carefully structured to enable symbol differentiation and error detection based on simple examination of the received data. Using forward error correction (FEC), in most cases the symbols can be identified, and the errors can be corrected promptly with no additional information.

4.4.3 FEC is based on the error detection system, which is usually the more robust of the two. Essentially, in certain poor conditions, it is possible to detect errors even though they may not be correctable (at the moment).

4.5 *Procedures for Retransmission*—In most cases, prompt error detection and correction is achievable through FEC. If this is not possible or acceptable, manual or automatic repeat-request (ARQ) is employed. The process of error detection can be used to initiate the ARQ and therefore the retransmission of the information, such as an additional copy (or copies). The copy(ies) may be received error free or with correctable errors (especially when compared with previous copy(ies)).

4.6 *Use of Non-standard Systems*—This phonetic system is not intended to prohibit the use of non-standard brevity or error control systems that are used only internally within any single organization. It also does not preclude the use of additional methods for clarity.

4.7 *Use of Standard Systems*—This phonetic system is intended to be directly interoperable with the majority of standard phonetic systems presently employed, both internationally and within the United States, as noted in references **(1-9)**. These standard systems actually exhibit many variations among themselves. Some provide no procedures, and none include all of the symbols presented herein. Of all these known documents, this practice is the only one that presents an explanation of the phonetic system in terms of modern communications technology. To achieve interoperability and performance through bona fide standardization, system administrators should consider this comprehensive practice for superseding, or revising, these other standard systems.

5. Procedure

5.1 *Phonetic Alphabet*:

5.1.1 *Phonetic Alphabet and Pronunciations*—Table 1 presents the phonetic alphabet and the pronunciations used in this practice.

5.1.2 *Usage of Phonetic Alphabet*—Phonetic alphabet symbols are inserted in text that may be spoken, printed, or otherwise communicated.

NOTE 1—Examples of the usage of the phonetic alphabet in spoken and printed text are provided in the sections below. The word(s) to be validated are in bold for clarity. Phonetic pronunciations are included for speech, with a" *pause*" as indicated:

5.1.2.1 *Phonetic Alphabet in Speech*—For speech, the phonetic alphabet symbols are placed adjacent to the word(s) that are spelled, as follows:

TABLE 1 Phonetic Alphabet and Pronunciations

Letter	Symbol	Pronunciation[A]
A	ALFA	"AL-fah"
B	BRAVO	"BRAH-voh"
C	CHARLIE	"CHAR-lee"
D	DELTA	"DELL-tah"
E	ECHO	"ECK-oh"
F	FOXTROT	"FOKS-trot"
G	GOLF	"GOLF"
H	HOTEL	"hoh-TELL"
I	INDIA	"IN-dee-ah"
J	JULIET	"JEW-lee-ETT"
K	KILO	"KEY-loh"
L	LIMA	"LEE-mah"
M	MIKE	"MIKE"
N	NOVEMBER	"no-VEM-ber"
O	OSCAR	"OSS-cah"
P	PAPA	"pah-PAH"
Q	QUEBEC	"keh-BECK"
R	ROMEO	"ROW-me-oh"
S	SIERRA	"see-AIR-rah"
T	TANGO	"TANG-go"
U	UNIFORM	"YOU-nee-form"
V	VICTOR	"VIK-tah"
W	WHISKEY	"WISS-key"
X	XRAY	"ECKS-ray"
Y	YANKEE	"YANG-key"
Z	ZULU	"ZOO-loo"

[A] The pronunciations are in quotes and CAPITAL letters to indicate the verbal emphasis.

(1) Use the word(s) to be spelled;

(2) Add "I SPELL" (which indicates the start of phonetics);

(3) Spell the word(s) using the phonetic alphabet symbols (with a pause between spelled word(s));

(4) Again use the word(s) that were spelled (which indicates the end of phonetics);

(5) Return to normal words for the spoken text that follows.

5.1.2.2 For single letters in speech, such as initials in a name, the phonetic alphabet symbols replace the letter(s) that are spelled, as follows:

(1) Note and replace (but do not use) the letter(s);

(2) Add "INITIALS" (which indicates the start of phonetics);

(3) Spell the replaced letter(s) using the phonetic alphabet symbols (with a pause between spelled letter(s));

(4) Return to normal name or words (which indicates the end of phonetics) and continue with the spoken text that follows.

5.1.2.3 *Phonetic Alphabet in Speech, Examples*:

(1) As an example, the phrase

(... respond emergency to **Xylon** St. for a ...)

would be spoken as follows:

"... respond emergency to **Xylon** *pause* I SPELL *pause* ECKS-ray, YANG-key, LEE-mah, OSS-cah, no-VEM-ber *pause* **Xylon** *pause*

Street for a ..."

(2) As an additional example, the phrase

(... reported sight of D.B. Cooper near ...)

would be spoken as follows:

"... reported sight of *pause* INITIALS DELL-tah *pause* BRAH-voh *pause* Cooper near ..."

5.1.2.4 *Phonetic Alphabet in Print*—For print, the phonetic alphabet symbols are placed (as capital letters) within parentheses adjacent to the word(s) that are spelled, as follows:

(1) Use the word(s) to be spelled;

(2) Add the left parenthesis "(" (which indicates the start of phonetics);

(3) Spell the word(s) using the phonetic alphabet symbols (as capital letters if upper/lower case is available) (with a comma between the spelled words);

(4) Add the right parenthesis ")" (which indicates the end of phonetics);

(5) Return to normal words for the printed text that follow.

5.1.2.5 *Phonetic Alphabet in Print, Examples*:

(1) As an example, the phrase

(... land medevac at **Jim** and **Bob** Sts. for ...)

would be printed as follows:

" ... land medevac at Jim (JULIET INDIA MIKE) and Bob (BRAVO OSCAR BRAVO) Streets for ..."

In this example, the symbols enable validation or correction of the text, even if they are slightly garbled themselves. (Was it Jim or Gem or Jem? Was it Bob or Rob or Hob?)

(2) As a continued example, the phrase might have been received as follows (with errors " + "):

" ... 1 + nd med + v + c at + i + (JUL + E + + NDIA M + KE) a + d + ob (BR + VO + SCAR B + AVO) S + reets fo + ..."

Examination of the capitalized phonetic symbols that were received (even with errors) enable error correction of the essential words.

5.2 *Phonetic Numerals*:

5.2.1 *Phonetic Numerals and Pronunciations*—Table 2 presents the phonetic numerals and the pronunciations that shall be used in this practice.

5.2.2 *Modified Numbers and Sequences*—Certain specific numbers or combinations that are easily misunderstood, such as those ending with "teen" and "ty", shall not be used. They shall be modified for clarity and shall be "spelled out" as digits, as presented in Table 3.

5.2.3 *Usage of Phonetic Numerals*—Phonetic numeral symbols are inserted in text that may be spoken, printed, or otherwise, and they may be mixed with letters and punctuation. Examples of the usage of the phonetic numerals in spoken and printed text are provided in the sections below. The number(s) to be clarified or validated are in bold for clarity. Phonetic pronunciations are included for speech, with a "*pause*" as indicated:

5.2.3.1 *Phonetic Numerals in Speech*—For speech, the phonetic numeral symbols replace the number(s) that are clarified or validated, as follows:

(1) Note and replace (but do not use) the number(s);

(2) Add "FIGURES" (which indicates the start of phonetics);

(3) "Spell" the replaced number(s) using individual phonetic numeral symbols (with a pause between "spelled" number(s));

(4) Return to normal words (which indicates the end of phonetics) and continue with the spoken text that follows.

5.2.3.2 *Phonetic Numerals in Speech, Examples*:

(1) As an example, the phrase

(... subject license tag is Virginia **930FXZ** ...)

would be spoken as follows:

" ... subject license tag is Virginia *pause* FIGURES *pause* NIN-er, TREE, ZEE-roh, FOKS-trot, ECKS-ray, ZOO-loo *pause* ..."

(2) As an additional example, the phrase

(... meet medic unit 10-4 near ...)

would be spoken as follows:

"... meet medic unit *pause* FIGURES *pause* WUN, ZEE-roh, DASH, FO-wer *pause* near ..."

5.2.3.3 *Phonetic Numerals in Print*—For print, the phonetic numeral symbols are placed (as capital letters) within parentheses adjacent to the number(s) that are clarified or validated, as follows:

TABLE 2 Phonetic Numerals and Pronunciations

Letter	Symbol	Pronunciation[A]
0	ZERO	"ZEE-roh"
1	ONE	"WUN"
2	TWO	"TOO"
3	THREE	"TREE"
4	FOUR	"FO-wer"
5	FIVE	"fi-YEV"
6	SIX	"SIKS"
7	SEVEN	"SAY-ven"
8	EIGHT	"AIT"
9	NINE	"NIN-er"
'00	HUNDRED	"HUN-dred"
'000	THOUSAND	"THOU-zand"

[A] The pronunciations are in quotes, and CAPITAL letters indicate the verbal emphasis.

TABLE 3 Modified Numbers and Sequences

Number	Symbol	Pronunciation[A]	Comments
10	TEN	"WUN, ZEE-roh"	(NOT "ten")
11	ONE-ONE	"WUN, WUN"	(NOT "eleven")
12	ONE-TWO	"WUN, TOO"	(NOT "twelve")
13 to 19	ONE-THREE to ONE-NINE	"WUN, TREE" to "WUN, NIN-er"	(NOT "thirteen" to "nineteen")
20 to 90	TWO-ZERO to NINE-ZERO	"TOO, ZEE-roh" to "NIN-er, ZEE-roh"	(NOT "twenty" to "ninety")

[A] The pronunciations are in quotes, and CAPITAL letters indicate the verbal emphasis.

(1) Use the number(s) to be "spelled";

(2) Add the left parenthesis "(" (which indicates the start of phonetics);

(3) "Spell" using phonetic numeral symbols as letter words (as capital letters if upper/lower case is available) (with a comma between "spelled" number(s));

(4) Add the right parenthesis ")" (which indicates the end of phonetics);

(5) Return to normal words for the printed text that follows.

5.2.3.4 The use of phonetic numeral symbols (in parentheses) after the numbers in printed text is an essential technique to ensure the accuracy of any critical number(s) that may have been (or might be) garbled in transmission (due to errors from conditions, humans, or machines).

5.2.3.5 *Phonetic Numerals in Print, Examples*:

(1) As an example, the phrase

(... pickup Team ECHO at coordinates **A397258** for ...)

would be printed as follows:

"... pickup Team ECHO at coordinates A397258 (ALFA THREE NINE SEVEN TWO FIVE EIGHT) for ..."

(2) In this example, the symbols enable validation or correction of the text, even if they are slightly garbled themselves. The phrase might have been received as follows (with errors" + "):

" ... p + ckup T + am ECH + at + oord + nat + s + 3 + 7 + 58 (+ LFA + HR + E N + NE SEV + N TW + F + VE EI + HT) fo + ..."

(3) Examination of the capitalized phonetic symbols that were received (even with errors) enable error correction of the essential letters and numerals.

5.3 *Phonetic Punctuation and Pronunciations*—Table 4 presents phonetic punctuation and the pronunciations that shall be used in this practice. The pronunciations are in quotes, and capital letters indicate the verbal emphasis.

5.3.1 *Usage of Phonetic Punctuation*—Phonetic punctuation symbols are inserted in text that may be spoken, printed, or otherwise, and they may be mixed with letters and numerals.

5.3.1.1 *Phonetic Punctuation in Speech*—For speech, the phonetic punctuation symbols replace the punctuation(s) that are clarified or validated, as follows:

(1) Note and replace (but do not use) the punctuation(s);

TABLE 4 Phonetic Punctuation and Pronunciations

Punctuation	Symbol	Pronunciation[A]	Comments/ Alternates
.	PERIOD	"PEER-ee-odd"	or "FULL STOP", "DOT"[B]
?	QUESTIONMARK	"KWES-chin-MARK"	
!	EXCLAMATIONPOINT	"ECKS-kla-MAY-shin-POYNT"	
'	APOSTROPHE	"ah-PAH-stro-fee"	
,	COMMA	"KOM-mah"	
;	SEMICOLON	"SEM-my-KO-lon"	
:	COLON	"KO-lon"	
-	HYPHEN	"HY-fen"	or" DASH"
/	SLANT	"SLANT"	or "STROKE" or "SLASH"[B]
\	BACKSLANT	"BAKS-SLANT"	or "BAKS-STROKE" or "BAKS-SLASH"[B]
"	QUOTE	"QUOTE"	or "OPEN QUOTE"
"	UNQUOTE	"UNN-QUOTE"	or "CLOSE QUOTE"
(	PAREN	"PAIR-ren"	or "OPEN PAIR-ren"
)	UNPAREN	"UNN-PAIR-ren"	or "CLOSE PAIR-ren"
[	BRACKET	"BRA-ket"	or "OPEN BRA-ket"
]	UNBRACKET	"UNN-BRA-ket"	or "CLOSE BRA-ket"
.	DECIMAL	"DAY-see-mal"	or "DOT"[B]
=	EQUALS	"EE-quills"	
+	PLUS	"PLUSS"	or "PLUSS-sine"
–	MINUS	"MY-nuss"	or "MY-nuss-sine"
*	STAR	"STARR"	(NOT "asterick")
#	POUNDSIGN	"POWND-sine"	(NOT "tic-tac-toe")
$	DOLLARS	"DOLL-arrs"	
%	PERCENT	"purr-SENT"	

[A] The pronunciations are in quotes, and capital letters indicate the verbal emphasis.

[B] Several symbols have achieved widespread usage with personal computers, yet they are not recommended for phonetic use as they have not been demonstrated to provide the needed robust performance over poor channels: DOT, SLASH, and BACKSLASH.

(2) Use the individual phonetic punctuation symbols (which indicate the use of phonetics) with a pause before and after;

(3) Return to normal words for the spoken text that follows.

5.3.1.2 *Phonetic Punctuation in Print*—For print, the phonetic punctuation symbols (in capital letters) replace the punctuation(s) which are clarified or validated, as follows:

(1) Note and replace (but do not use) the punctuation(s);

(2) Use the individual phonetic punctuation symbols (which indicate the use of phonetics), using capital letters if upper/lower case is available;

(3) Return to normal words for the printed text that follows.

5.3.1.3 The use of phonetic punctuation symbols (in capital letters) in place of the punctuation in printed text is an essential technique to ensure the accuracy of any critical phrase(s) or structure(s) that may have been (or might be) garbled in transmission (due to errors from conditions, humans, or machines).

6. Keywords

6.1 alphabet; communications; English; error correction; error detection; interoperability; messages; numeral; performance; phonetic; procedures; punctuation; symbols

REFERENCES

(1) **ACP-125**
North Atlantic Treaty Organization (NATO), Allied Communications Procedures 125 (ACP-125), Radiotelephone Procedures.

(2) **American Heritage Dictionary**
American Heritage Dictionary, Second College Edition, Houghton Mifflin Company.

(3) **APCO**
Associated Public-Safety Communications Officers, Inc. (APCO), Public Safety Communications Standard Operating Procedures Manual.

(4) **ARRL**
American Radio Relay League (ARRL), Handbook for the Radio Amateur.

(5) **CAP**
Civil Air Patrol (CAP), Manual 100-1, Communications.

(6) **FED-STD 1037**
Federal Standard 1037 (FED-STD 1037), Telecommunications: Glossary of Telecommunications Terms.

(7) **ICAO**
International Civil Aviation Organization (ICAO), Volume II, Annex 10, Chapter 5.

(8) **ITU**
International Telecommunications Union (ITU) Radio Regulations, Appendix 24, "Phonetic Alphabet and Figure Code".

(9) **NAVY and MARS**
Naval Telecommunications Procedures, U.S. Navy-Marine Corps Military Affiliate Radio System (MARS), Naval Telecommunications Policy Eight (NTP-8).

(10) **SHARES**
National Communications System Manual NCSM 3-3, Telecommunications Operations, SHARES HF Radio Program User Manual.

Designation: F 1584 – 95

Standard Practice for Marking Buildings During Disaster Search Operations[1]

This standard is issued under the fixed designation F 1584; the number immediately following the designation indicates the year of original adoption or, in the case of revision, the year of last revision. A number in parentheses indicates the year of last reapproval. A superscript epsilon (ε) indicates an editorial change since the last revision or reapproval.

1. Scope

1.1 This practice covers the methodology for marking buildings that have been searched during disaster responses.

1.2 *This standard does not purport to address all of the safety concerns, if any, associated with its use. It is the responsibility of the user of this standard to establish appropriate safety and health practices and determine the applicability of regulatory limitations prior to use.*

2. Terminology

2.1 There are no terms in this standard that require new or other than dictionary definitions.

3. Significance and Use

3.1 Searching vacant or collapsed structures, or both, is an important part of emergency disaster response. A uniform marking system easily identifies, from the outside of structures, the number and status of any subjects found, hazards and the time of the search. The use of this methodology will reduce duplicate searches and wasted rescue efforts.

3.2 This methodology is also used at each interior space or room searched.

4. Procedure

4.1 Use contrasting color spray paint, crayon or other indelible, easily applied media on the exterior of the structure and each interior space to be searched. The size of the marking should be as large as is practical given the media used, the area available and the viewing distance. For example, the "X" on the interior would be 2′ × 2′ in size.

4.2 If the main access to the structure or interior space is not usable due to damage, this system shall be used as close as possible to the best available access. Directional markings shall be applied to the building as shown to indicate the best available access route.

Distinct markings will be made inside the four quadrants of the X to clearly denote the search status and findings at the time of this search. The following illustrations define the search marks:

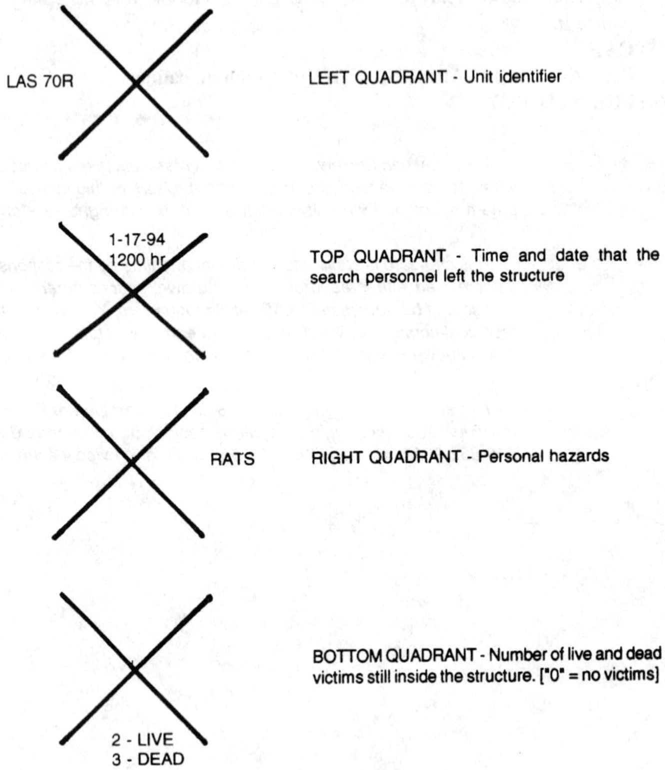

FIG. 1 Search Markings

4.3 Use symbols shown in Figs. 1 and 2.

4.4 Single slash drawn upon entry to a structure or area indicates search operations are currently in progress and by which unit. See following:

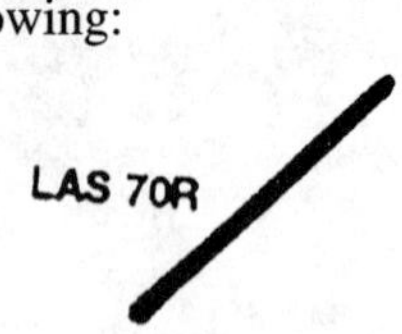

---

[1] This practice is under the jurisdiction of ASTM Committee F32 on Search and Rescue and is the direct responsibility of Subcommittee F32.02 on Management and Operations.

Current edition approved Feb. 15, 1995. Published April 1995.

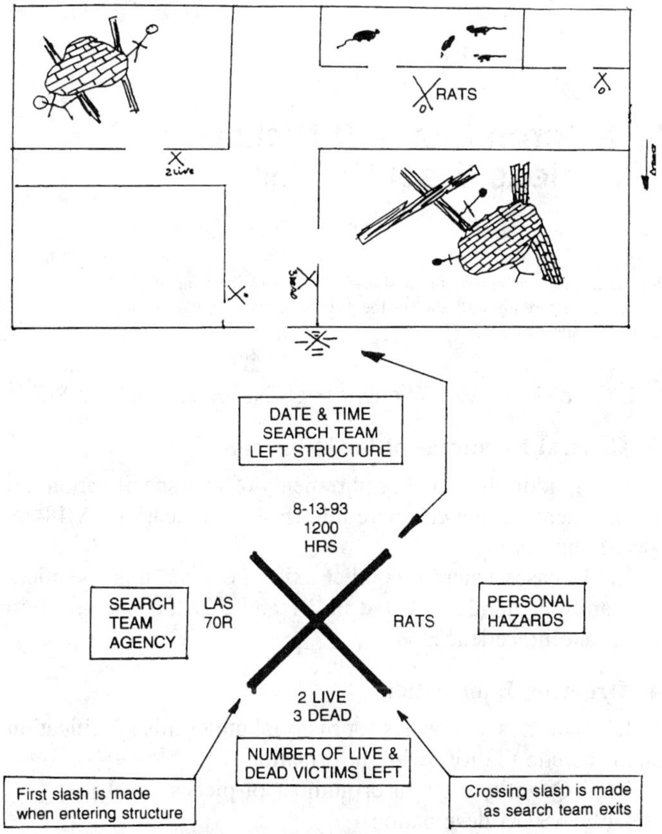

FIG. 2 Search Markings in Use

4.5 Crossing slash drawn upon exit of search personnel from the structure or area. After exiting the structure also add the appropriate subject, time and hazard information. See following:

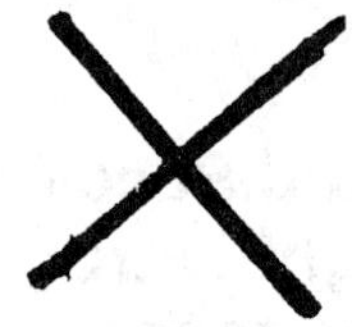

5. Keywords

5.1 collapsed structure; disaster; marking; search

Standard Specification for Wrought Nitrogen Strengthened-21 Chromium—10 Nickel—3 Manganese—2.5 Molybdenum Stainless Steel Bar for Surgical Implants[1]

This standard is issued under the fixed designation F 1586; the number immediately following the designation indicates the year of original adoption or, in the case of revision, the year of last revision. A number in parentheses indicates the year of last reapproval. A superscript epsilon (ϵ) indicates an editorial change since the last revision or reapproval.

1. Scope

1.1 This specification covers the requirements for wrought nitrogen strengthened-21 chromium—10 nickel—3 manganese—2.5 molybdenum stainless steel bar for the manufacture of surgical implants.

1.2 The values stated in inch-pound units are to be regarded as the standard. The SI units in parentheses are for information only.

2. Referenced Documents

2.1 *ASTM Standards:*

A 262 Practices for Detecting Susceptibility to Intergranular Attack in Austenitic Stainless Steels[2]

A 484/A 484M Specification for General Requirements for Stainless and Heat-Resisting Steel Bars, Billets, and Forgings[3]

A 751 Test Methods, Practices, and Terminology for Chemical Analysis of Steel Products[2]

E 10 Test for Brinell Hardness of Metallic Materials[4]

E 18 Tests for Rockwell Hardness and Rockwell Superficial Hardness of Metallic Materials[4]

E 45 Practice for Determining the Inclusion Content of Steel[4]

E 112 Test Methods for Determining Average Grain Size[4]

F 746 Test Method for Pitting or Crevice Corrosion of Metallic Surgical Implant Materials[5]

F 981 Practice for Assessment of Compatibility of Biomaterials (Nonporous) for Surgical Implants with Respect to Effect of Materials in Muscle and Bone[5]

2.2 *ASQC Standard:*

C1 Specification of General Requirements for a Quality Program[6]

2.3 *ISO Standard:*

ISO 5832-9/1992: Wrought High Nitrogen Stainless Steel[7]

3. General Requirement for Delivery

3.1 In addition to the requirements of this specification, all requirements of the current editions of Specifications A 484/A 484M shall apply.

3.2 In cases where a conflict exists between this specification and the standards listed in 2.1 and 2.2, this specification shall take precedence.

4. Ordering Information

4.1 Inquiries and orders for material under this specification shall include the following information:

4.1.1 Quantity (weight or number of pieces),

4.1.2 ASTM desgination,

4.1.3 Form,

4.1.4 Condition (see 5.1),

4.1.5 Mechanical properties (if applicable, for special conditions),

4.1.6 Finish (see 5.2),

4.1.7 Applicable dimensions including size, thickness, width, and length (exact, random, or multiples) or print number, and

4.1.8 Special requirements.

5. Materials and Manufacture

5.1 *Condition*—Bars shall be furnished to the implant manufacturer, as specified, in the annealed, medium hard, or hard condition.

5.2 *Finish*—Types of finish available in bar products are pickled, ground, ground and polished, or as specified in the implant manufacturer's purchase order.

6. Chemical Composition

6.1 The heat analysis shall conform to the requirements as to chemical composition specified in Table 1.

6.1.1 Requirements for the major and minor elemental constituents are listed in Table 1. Also listed are important residual elements. Analysis for elements not listed in Table 1 is not required to verify compliance with this specification.

[1] This specification is under the jurisdiction of ASTM Committee F-4 on Medical and Surgical Materials and Devices is under the direct responsibility of Subcommittee F04.12 on Metallurgical Materials.

Current edition approved March 15, 1995. Published June 1995.

[2] *Annual Book of ASTM Standards*, Vol 01.03.

[3] *Annual Book of ASTM Standards*, Vol 01.05.

[4] *Annual Book of ASTM Standards*, Vol 03.01.

[5] *Annual Book of ASTM Standards*, Vol 13.01.

[6] Available from American Society for Quality Control, 161 W. Wisconsin Ave., Milwaukee, WI 53203.

[7] Available from American National Standards Institute, 11 W. 42nd St., 13th Floor, New York, NY 10036.

TABLE 1 Chemical Requirements, Heat Analysis

Element	Composition, %
Carbon	0.08 max
Manganese	2.00 to 4.25
Phosphorus	0.025 max
Sulfur	0.01 max
Silicon	0.75 max
Chromium	19.5 to 22.0
Nickel	9.0 to 11.0
Molybdenum	2.0 to 3.0
Nitrogen	0.25 to 0.5
Niobium	0.25 to 0.8
Copper	0.25 max
Iron[A]	balance

[A] Approximately equal to the difference between 100 % and the sum percent of the other specified elements. The percent iron content by difference is not required to be reported.

6.2 Methods and practices relating to chemical analysis required by this specification shall be in accordance with Test Methods A 751.

7. Metallurgical Requirements

7.1 The material shall exhibit no free ferrite phase when it is examined metallographically at 100× magnification.

7.2 The microcleanliness of the steel, as determined by Method A in Practice E 45, except using Plate III and Plate I, on representative billet or bar samples from the heat shall not exceed the following:

Inclusion Type	A (Sulfide)	B (Alumina)	C (Silicate)	D (Globular oxide)
Thin	1.5	2.0	2.0	2.5
Heavy	1.5	1.5	1.5	1.5

NOTE 1—General practice is to use electroslag remelted steel to comply with these cleanliness requirements and to give other additional benefits.

8. Mechanical Requirements

8.1 Material shall conform to the appropriate requirements as to mechanical properties specified in Table 2. The level of mechanical properties for material in other than the annealed, medium hard, or hard condition shall be specified in the implant manufacturer's purchase order.

8.2 When desired, hardness limits may be specified. Hardness determination on cold-worked material shall be made in accordance with Test Method E 10 or Test Method E 18 on a product cross section, midway between the center and surface, if cross section size is adequate.

TABLE 2 Mechanical Requirements of Bars

Condition	Diameter or Thickness, in. (mm)	Ultimate Tensile Strength, min, psi (MPa)	Yield Strength (0.2 % Offset), min, psi (MPa)	Elongation[A] in 4D, min, %
Annealed[B]	all	107 000 (740)	62 400 (430)	35
Medium hard	1/16 to 3/4 (1.59 to 19.1)[C]	145 000 (1000)	102 000 (700)	20
Hard	1/16 to 3/4 (1.59 to 19.1)[C]	160 000 (1100)	145 000 (1000)	10

[A] $4D = 4 \times$ diameter.
[B] Corresponds to ISO 5832-9.
[C] Other sizes may be furnished by agreement between the producer and the purchaser.

9. Special Tests

9.1 The steel shall be capable for passing the intergranular corrosion susceptibility test in accordance with Practice E of Practices A 262. The test shall be performed on a sample sensitized at 1250°F for 1 h.

9.2 The grain size shall be five or finer when tested in accordance with Test Methods E 112.

9.2.1 If grain size samples are selected after a final cold-working operation, transverse specimens shall be prepared.

9.3 Any other special requirements shall be specified on the purchase order.

10. Certification

10.1 The manufacturer's certification that the material was manufactured and tested in accordance with this specification together with a report of the test results shall be furnished at the time of shipment.

11. Quality Program Requirements

11.1 The producer shall maintain a quality program, such as defined in ASQC C1.

11.2 The manufacturer of surgical implants may audit the producer's quality program for conformance to the intent of ASQC C1, or other recognized program.

12. Keywords

12.1 manganese; metals (for surgical implants); nitrogen strengthened; stainles steel; surgical applications

APPENDIX

(Nonmandatory Information)

X1. RATIONALE[8]

X1.1 The primary purpose of this specification is to characterize composition and properties of a nitrogenstrengthened austenitic stainless steel to ensure consistency in the starting material used, directly or as modified by forging, in the manufacturing of medical devices.

X1.2 The metallurgical requirements include fine-grained austenitic structure free of ferrite, with low micro-inclusion content and capability of passing an intergranular corrosion susceptibility test.

X1.3 Acceptable metal conditions supplied to the implant manufacturer include hot-worked, annealed, and all cold-worked conditions, the choice dependent upon the implant design and application.

X1.4 The material has been shown to produce an acceptable level of local biological response that is similar to F 138, Grade 2 reference material.

X1.5 This alloy has been tested in accordance with Test Method F 746 and exhibits a pitting potential greater than F 138, Grade 2 reference material.

X1.6 The nitrogen used for strengthening this steel can result in the formation of carbonitrides. Carbonitrides can be revealed by etching electrolytically in a solution of potassium hydroxide (56 g of K(OH) in 100 mL of water for 3 s at t 2 V). These small dispersed second-phase particles exert a strengthening effect but do not significantly alter the corrosion properties of the alloy.

[8] Supporting data available from ASTM Headquarters. Request RR: F04-1007.

Designation: F 1590 – 95

Standard Specification for Tracheostomy Tube Connectors[1]

This standard is issued under the fixed designation F 1590; the number immediately following the designation indicates the year of original adoption or, in the case of revision, the year of last revision. A number in parentheses indicates the year of last reapproval. A superscript epsilon (ϵ) indicates an editorial change since the last revision or reapproval.

INTRODUCTION

There are many advantages in harmonizing the requirements for connectors for tracheostomy tubes with those already widely used for tracheal tubes.

The patient connection port of the breathing system of an anaesthetic machine or ventilator is a coaxial 22-mm male/15-mm female conical connector, an important purpose of the smaller connector being to mate with the 15-mm male tracheal tube connector. It is, therefore, advantageous to use the same size of fitting for tracheostomy tubes used for patients during surgical operations and for those for whom artificial ventilation or other respiratory support may be required.

Inadvertent disconnection of the breathing system from the tracheostomy tube is a well-recognized hazard and it is therefore specified for the larger sizes of tube that the male 15-mm conical fitting shall be permanently attached to either the tracheostomy tube or inner cannula.

It is also recommended that the design should permit the fitting of a device to make a more secure attachment between the conical fittings if so desired. Such a device may, however, introduce other hazards such as that of accidental extubation. It should, therefore, be as light and compact as possible. Any protuberances should be designed so as to minimize the likelihood of their catching on attendants' hands, surgical dressings, or other equipment.

1. Scope

1.1 This specification covers basic requirements for connectors for tracheostomy tubes for use on patients undergoing surgical operations or those for whom artificial ventilation or other respiratory support may be required, or both. This specification does not apply to those tracheostomy tubes used when ventilatory support is not required.

2. Referenced Documents

2.1 *ASTM Standards:*

F 1054 Specification for Conical Fittings of 15 mm and 22 mm Sizes[2]

3. Terminology

3.1 *Definitions*—For the purpose of this specification, the following definitions apply:

3.1.1 *machine end*:

3.1.1.1 end of the tracheostomy tube that is intended to project from the neck of the patient; or

3.1.1.2 end of connector or the adaptor intended to mate with the breathing system of an anaesthetic machine or ventilator.

3.1.2 *tracheostomy (tracheotomy) tube*—tube designed for insertion into the trachea through a tracheostomy (tracheotomy).

4. Apparatus

4.1 *Connectors*:

4.1.1 Tracheostomy tubes shall have at the machine end an attached male 15-mm conical connector in accordance with Specification F 1054. This connector shall be permanently attached to either the outer tube or the inner cannula. If the connector is attached to the inner cannula, a mechanism must be provided to fasten the inner cannula to the outer tube. The inside diameter of the conical element shall be not less than the designated inside diameter of the outer tube or inner cannula with which it is intended to be used.

4.1.2 Any transition in inside diameter shall be tapered to give an adequate lead-in for passage of a suction catheter.

5. Keywords

5.1 connector; tracheostomy; tube

[1] This specification is under the jurisdiction of ASTM Committee F-29 on Anesthetic and Respiratory Equipment and is under the direct responsibility of Subcommittee F29.12 on Airways.

Current edition approved March 15, 1995. Published May 1995.

[2] *Annual Book of ASTM Standards*, Vol 13.01.

ANNEX

(Mandatory Information)

A1. GUIDANCE ON DESIGN

A1.1 *Retaining Devices:*

A1.1.1 A retaining or locking device may be incorporated in the design to provide added security of attachment of the conical fittings.

A1.1.2 Any projections (for example hooks, lugs, or studs) should be designed so as to minimize the risk of their catching on surgical dressings or other equipment.

Designation: F 1591 – 95 (Reapproved 2000)

Standard Practice for Visual Signals Between Persons on the Ground and in Aircraft During Ground Emergencies[1]

This standard is issued under the fixed designation F 1591; the number immediately following the designation indicates the year of original adoption or, in the case of revision, the year of last revision. A number in parentheses indicates the year of last reapproval. A superscript epsilon (ε) indicates an editorial change since the last revision or reapproval.

1. Scope

1.1 This practice covers the signals to be used between persons on the ground and in aircraft when two-way voice communications cannot be established during ground emergencies. Ground signals are limited to land-based ones that do not require special equipment. Flare, light, panel, and maritime signals are specifically excluded.

1.2 The signals are divided into two categories: those used by persons on the ground and those used by aircraft.

1.3 *This standard does not purport to address all of the safety concerns, if any, associated with its use. It is the responsibility of the user of this standard to establish appropriate safety and health practices and determine the applicability of regulatory limitations prior to use.*

2. Referenced Document

2.1 *International Civil Aviation Organization Standard:*
International Standards and Recommended Practices, Search and Rescue, Annex 12 to the Convention on International Civil Aviation[2]

3. Significance and Use

3.1 While many of the reasons for needing the signals contained in this practice have been overcome by technology development, situations still arise where voice communications cannot be established between aircraft and persons on the ground during emergencies. This is particularly true of persons in distress, who typically have no communications equipment. These signals continue to meet the need for communications.

3.2 Most of these signals have been adopted by international convention, the others by civilian and military agencies of the United States Government. The signals described in this practice are intended for use on land and can be made without special equipment such as flares or colored panels. Other signaling systems are described in the *National Search and Rescue (SAR) Manual.*[3]

3.3 The signals are also useful in situations where either complete or partial voice communications exist. Where only partial capabilities exist, for example, a ground unit with receive-only capability, the aircrew can transmit voice and the ground crew can respond with the appropriate signal.

3.3.1 The signals described in Section 4, by their nature, are not intended for real-time communications with aircraft. They can be left unattended as messages for aircrews. Persons on the ground (SAR or otherwise) can make a signal and continue on without contact with the aircraft. The SAR personnel should keep this in mind when encountering the signals of Fig. 1.

3.4 Search and rescue agencies utilizing this practice should disseminate these signals to the public as part of their preventative search and rescue (PSAR) efforts. The signals have changed over the years and a number of publications contain obsolete signals.

4. Ground-to-Air Signals

4.1 Signals for use by either SAR personnel or persons in distress on the ground are shown in Fig. 1.

4.1.1 The signals in Fig. 1 have been adopted by the Convention on International Civil Aviation. As defined in Annex 12 to the Convention (see 2.1), these signals are divided into those for use by SAR personnel and those for use by persons in distress. Several of the signals have only been adopted by certain countries.

4.1.2 Since the signals are useful regardless of the user's situation or location, this practice includes all of them without limitation. While there may be potential for this to cause confusion for aircrews seeing the signals, this would be a temporary condition and the aircrew's response should not be dependent on the user's status. The benefits of unlimited use of the signals outweighs any confusion caused by their use contrary to the Convention.

4.2 The signals in Fig. 1 shall have the meanings indicated. They shall be used only for the purpose indicated and no other signals likely to be confused with them shall be used.

4.3 All signals shall be as large as possible in the proportions shown in Fig. 2.

4.4 The signals shall be made in a manner that contrasts with the surface on which they are placed. Brush, vegetation, rocks, stones, or surface material can be piled up; trenches dug; soft material stomped down; brush or grass cut down; strips of material laid out; etc. Materials can be combined, such as

---

[1] This practice is under the jurisdiction of ASTM Committee F32 on Search and Rescue and is the direct responsibility of Subcommittee F32.02 on Management and Operations.

Current edition approved April 15, 1995. Published July 1995.

[2] Available from the International Civil Aviation Organization; Document Sales Unit; 1000 Sherbrooke St. West, Suite 400; Montreal, Quebec, Canada H3A 2R2.

[3] *National Search and Rescue (SAR) Manual*, Vol I, Joint Publication 3-50, Feb. 1, 1991. Available from United States Coast Guard; Washington, DC 20953-0001.

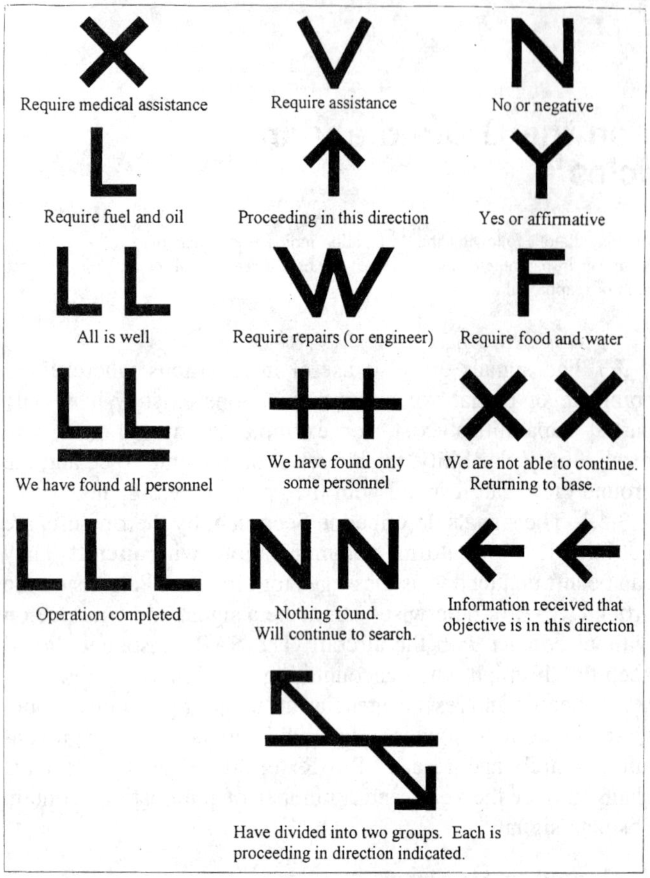

FIG. 1 Ground-to-Air Signals

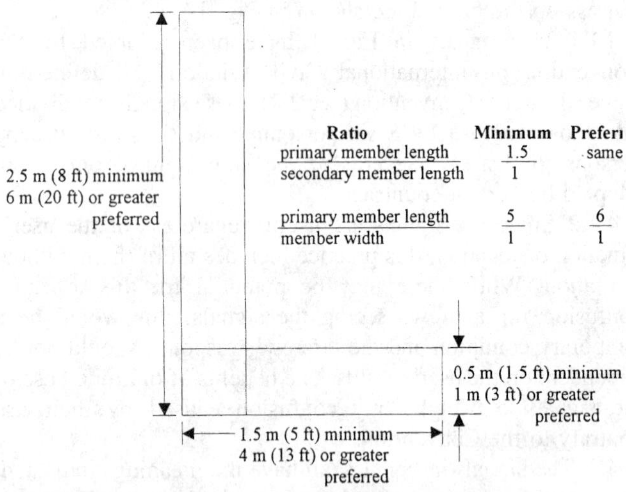

FIG. 2 Minimum Signal Dimensions and Proportions

stomping out the signal in snow, then filling it in with brush. The signals should have sufficient height or depth so that shadows will be cast in the shape of the signal to add contrast.

4.5 The signals shall be placed in the open away from the obstacles that could block the signals from the view of overflying aircraft or that could create shadows on the signals.

4.6 Fires, flares, smoke, mirror flashes, or lights may be used with the signals to attract attention. Attraction should be attempted only if aircraft are known to be in the area, however.

4.7 Once a signal has served its intended purpose, it shall be destroyed if at all possible, to prevent confusion and additional search effort later.

5. Ground-to-Air Body Signals

5.1 The signals of Fig. 1 are "messages," in that they take considerable time to prepare, and so are not suitable for direct communications when an aircraft is overhead. For real-time or spontaneous communications, the body signals of Fig. 3 shall be used.

5.1.1 The signals in Fig. 3 shall have the meanings indicated. They shall be used only for the purpose indicated and no other signals likely to be confused with them shall be used.

5.1.2 The person making the signal shall be in the open and as conspicuous as possible. Clothing worn should contrast with the background. Attraction techniques such as flares, signal mirrors, and smoke can be used to draw the aircrew's attention. These devices should not be used once contact has been made, to prevent the signal from being obscured or interfering with the aircrew's vision.

5.1.3 The signals in Fig. 3 are recognized by United States civil and military authorities but are not part of the International Convention. Therefore, their meanings may not be recognized outside the United States.

6. Air-to-Ground Signals for Responding to Specific Ground Signals

6.1 The following shall indicate that the aircrew has understood the ground signals of Fig. 1 or Fig. 3:

6.1.1 During daylight, by rocking the wings (rolling the aircraft) as shown in Fig. 4(*a*).

6.1.2 During darkness, by flashing the landing lights or the navigation lights, or both, on and off.

6.1.3 The U.S. military aircraft may flash a green light to acknowledge the ground signal. This is not internationally recognized or typically used by civilian aircrews so is presented here for coordination and reference only. This signal shall not be considered part of this practice.

6.2 Any of the following shall indicate the aircrew has not understood the ground signal:

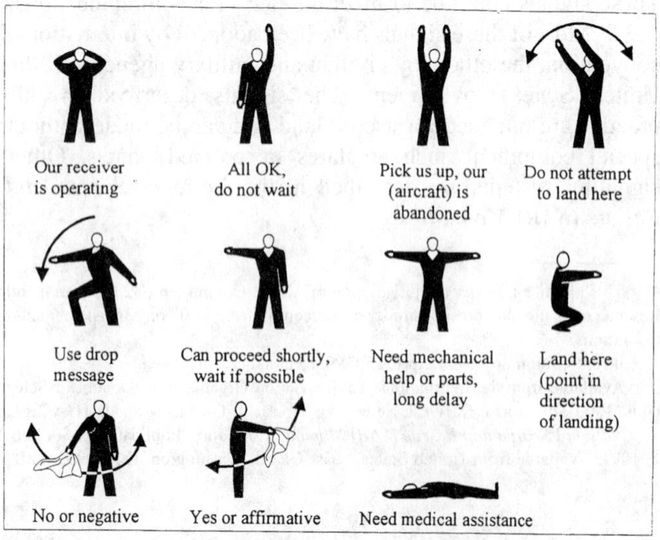

FIG. 3 Ground-to-Air Body Signals

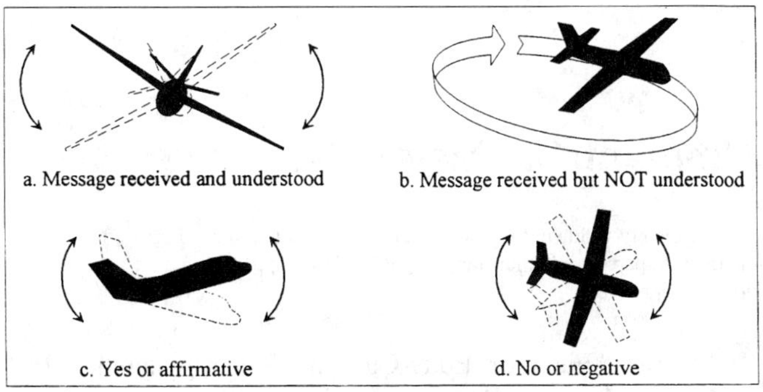

FIG. 4 Air-to-Ground Signals

6.2.1 No response in accordance with 6.1.1., 6.1.2, or 6.1.3.

6.2.2 A complete right-hand circle of the aircraft as shown in Fig. 4(*b*).

6.2.2.1 This positive response by the aircraft is an acknowledgment that the signal has at least been seen, and is recommended over not responding. A lack of aircraft response does not indicate to the persons on the ground whether the aircrew missed the signal or did not understand it. This signal is recognized by U.S. civil and military authorities but is not part of the International Convention. Therefore, its meaning may not be recognized outside the United States.

6.2.3 The U.S. military aircraft may flash a red light to indicate that the ground signal has not been understood. This is not internationally recognized or typically used by civilian aircrews so is presented here for coordination and reference only. This signal shall not be considered part of this practice.

6.3 An affirmative reply to a ground signal shall be indicated by raising and lowering the nose of the aircraft (pitching) as shown in Fig. 4(*c*).

6.4 A negative reply to a ground signal shall be indicated by moving the nose of the aircraft right and left (yawing) as shown in Fig. 4(*d*).

6.5 The signals of 6.3 and 6.4 are recognized by U.S. civilian and military authorities but are not part of the international convention. Therefore, their use may not be recognized outside of the United States.

7. Air-to-Ground Signals for Directing Persons on the Ground

7.1 The following signal, in the sequence listed, shall indicate the persons on the ground are to follow the aircraft or, if already moving, to proceed in a different direction:

7.1.1 Circling the ground personnel at least once, and

7.1.2 Flying off in the direction to be taken.

7.2 To stop a moving ground party, or to initially get its attention, the following signal shall be used:

7.2.1 Crossing ahead of the ground personnel at low altitude, and

7.2.2 While making this low pass, also rocking the wings (rolling the aircraft), or opening and closing the throttle, or changing the propeller pitch, or some combination thereof.

7.3 To indicate that the aircraft is no longer able to assist the persons on the ground, or to cancel the response of ground SAR personnel, the following signal shall be used:

7.3.1 Crossing behind the ground personnel at low altitude, and

7.3.2 While making this low pass, also rocking the wings (rolling the aircraft), or opening and closing the throttle, or changing the propeller pitch, or some combination thereof.

7.4 The signals of 7.1, 7.2, and 7.3 may be repeated until the ground parties comply.

8. Keywords

8.1 aircraft; communications; distress; emergencies; ground; search; signals; visual

Designation: F 1609 – 95

Standard Specification for Calcium Phosphate Coatings for Implantable Materials[1]

This standard is issued under the fixed designation F 1609; the number immediately following the designation indicates the year of original adoption or, in the case of revision, the year of last revision. A number in parentheses indicates the year of last reapproval. A superscript epsilon (ε) indicates an editorial change since the last revision or reapproval.

1. Scope

1.1 This specification covers the material requirements for calcium phosphate coatings for surgical implant applications.

1.2 In particulate and monolithic form, the calcium phosphate materials system has been well-characterized regarding biological response **(1, 2)**[2] and laboratory characterization **(2–4)**. Several publications **(5–10)** have documented the in vitro and in vivo properties of selected calcium phosphate coating systems.

1.3 This specification includes hydroxylapatite coatings, tricalcium phosphate coatings, or combinations thereof, with or without intentional minor additions (10 % or less, as opposed to trace elements) of other ceramic or metallics, and applied by methods including, but not limited to, the following: (*1*) mechanical capture, (*2*) plasma spray deposition, (*3*) dipping/sintering, (*4*) electrophoretic deposition, (*5*) porcelainizing, and (*6*) sputtering.

1.4 Substrates may include smooth, porous, textured, and other implantable topographical forms.

1.5 This specification excludes organic coatings that may contain calcium and phosphate ionic species.

2. Referenced Documents

2.1 *ASTM Standards:*

C 313 Test Method for Adherence of Porcelain Enamel and Ceramic Coatings to Sheet Metal[3]

C 501 Test Method for Relative Resistance to Wear of Unglazed Ceramic Tile by the Taber Abraser[4]

C 633 Test Method for Adhesion or Cohesive Strength of Flame-Sprayed Coatings[5]

C 674 Test Methods for Flexural Properties of Ceramic Whiteware Materials[4]

C 949 Test Method for Porosity in Vitreous Whitewares by Dye Penetration[4]

E 376 Practice for Measuring Coating Thickness by Magnetic-Field or Eddy-Current (Electromagnetic) Test Methods[6]

F 1044 Test Method for Shear Testing of Porous Metal Coatings[7]

F 1088 Specification for Beta-Tricalcium Phosphate for Surgical Implantation[7]

F 1147 Test Method for Tension Testing of Porous Metal Coatings[7]

F 1185 Specification for Composition of Ceramic Hydroxylapatite for Surgical Implants[7]

2.2 *Pharmacopeia Convention Documents:*[8]

National Formulary XVI, Tribasic Calcium Phosphate

United States Pharmacopeia:

U.S. Pharmacopeia XXI, Chemical Tests CaP (191), Lead <251>, Mercury <261>, Arsenic< 211>, and Heavy Metals <231> Method (1)

2.3 *Other Documents:*

U.S. Geological Survey Method, Cadmium[9]

21 CFR 820[10]

X-Ray Diffraction Analyses[11]

3. Terminology

3.1 *Definitions:*

3.1.1 *beta tricalcium phosphate*—a calcium phosphate substance of empirical chemical formula, $Ca_3(PO_4)_2$ (see Specification F 1088).

3.1.2 *calcium phosphate*—any one of a number of inorganic chemical compounds containing calcium and phosphate ions as its principal constituents.

3.1.3 *coating*—a layer of mechanically or chemically attached material covering a substrate material.

3.1.4 *hydroxylapatite*—A calcium phosphate crystalline

---

[1] This specification is under the jurisdiction of ASTM Committee F-4 on Medical and Surgical Materials and Devices and is the direct responsibility of Subcommittee F04.13 on Ceramic Materials.

Current edition approved Aug. 15, 1995. Published September 1995.

[2] The boldface numbers in parentheses refer to the list of references at the end of this specification.

[3] *Discontinued* 1991—See 1990 *Annual Book of ASTM Standards*, Vol 15.02.

[4] *Annual Book of ASTM Standards*, Vol 15.02.

[5] *Annual Book of ASTM Standards*, Vol 02.05.

[6] *Annual Book of ASTM Standards*, Vol 03.03.

[7] *Annual Book of ASTM Standards*, Vol 13.01.

[8] Available from U.S. Pharmacopeia Convention, Inc., 12601 Twinbrook Parkway, Rockville, MD 20852.

[9] Crock, J. G., Felichte, F. E., and Briggs, P. H., "Determination of Elements in National Bureau of Standards Geological Reference Materials SRM 278 Obsidian and SRM 688 Basalt by Inductively Coupled Argon Plasma—Atomic Emission Spectrometry," *Geostandards Newsletter*, Vol 7, 1983, pp. 335–340.

[10] Available from Standardization Documents Order Desk, Bldg. 4 Section D, 700 Robbins Ave., Philadelphia, PA 19111-5094, Attn: NPODS.

[11] The Joint Committee on Powdered Diffraction has established a Powder Diffraction File. The committee operates on an international basis and cooperates closely with the Data Commission of the International Union of Crystallinity and ASTM. Hydroxylapatite data can be found on file card No. 9-432; beta tricalcium phosphate data can be found on file card No. 9-169.

compound of empirical chemical formula, $Ca_5(PO_4)_3OH$ (see Specification F 1185).

4. Chemical or Crystallographic Requirements, or Both

4.1 *Chemical*:

4.1.1 Elemental analysis for calcium and phosphorous and intentional additions (other than trace elements) will be consistent with the expected stoichiometry of the specific calcium phosphate compound(s).

4.1.2 *Trace Element Analysis*—The concentration of trace elements in the coating shall be limited as follows:

Element	ppm, max
As	3
Cd	5
Hg	5
Pb	30
total heavy metals (as lead)	50

For reference purposes, the *U.S. Pharmacopeia XXI* and *U.S. Geological Survey Method, Cadmium*, shall be used.

4.1.3 The analysis of other trace elements may be required, based on the conditions, apparatus, or environments specific to the coating application technique used.

4.1.4 The analysis of intentional additional elements or compounds such as fluorine, manganese, magnesium, carbonate, etc. must be specified for calcium phosphate coatings.

4.2 *Crystallographic Characterization*:

4.2.1 This involves the degree of crystallinity, determined as a weight percent of the total substance.

4.2.2 This involves the identification of crystalline species and their weight percentages, expressed as a percent of the total substance.

4.2.3 This involves the identification of functional groups by infrared analysis.

4.3 *Environmental Stability*—The characterization of environmental stability shall be consistent with prior referenced methods using solutions best representing the potential in-service device environments.

5. Physical Characterization

5.1 *Coverage of Substrate*:

5.1.1 Microscopic examination of the surface will be made at 10× magnification; flaws, "bare" areas, "pinholes," and coating borders, etc. will be reported for those observed at 10× magnification.

5.1.2 Visible impurities shall be reported if observed at 10× magnification.

5.2 *Thickness*—The thickness will be measured from cross sections and will be reported as the mean and range of thickness. If distinct layers are noted, each layer should be so characterized.

5.3 *Porosity*—The microporosity and macroporosity characterization shall be determined.

5.4 *Color*—The color should be uniform and consistent in consideration of the specific process, substrate material and geometry, and coating thickness.

5.5 *Surface Topography*—the surface topography shall be measured using equipment designed to determine surface roughness dimensions as microinches or micrometres. Characterization of the surface topography of the underlying substrate may be required if applicable for the specific coating method. Scanning electron microscopy shall be used to establish the coating surface and cross-section morphology.

5.6 *Other Characterizations*—Other characterizations may be required or applicable, depending on the end-use application. Standard test methods should be used in all cases, where available, or acceptable alternatives developed. An additional ASTM test that may apply is Test Methods C 674.

6. Mechanical Characterization

6.1 The following mechanical characterizations may be applicable to a coating, depending on the substrate material or geometry, coating thickness or location, and coating methods(s), or some combination thereof. Characterization reports shall contain sufficient information regarding the test techniques, procedures, and standards used and details such as specimen orientation and proportional depth of thickness in order to represent the analysis accurately.

6.1.1 The tensile bond strength of the coating to the substrate shall be measured using a non-penetrating adhesive such as FM-1000 Adhesive Film. The measurement technique shall follow the general procedure of Test Methods C 633 and F 1147. The tensile test shall be considered invalid if any portion of the metal substrate is exposed to the surface before testing, allowing direct bonding of the adhesive to the metal.

6.1.2 Shear strength determinations shall be consistent with Test Method F 1044, or a demonstrated equivalent technique, as long as the adhesive is demonstrated to be non-penetrating and the test technique allows for the coating to be placed in a pure shear condition, minimizing "peeling stress" modes.

6.1.3 The fatigue strength shall be determined on an applicable full-scale device and as a materials system using appropriate testing methods applicable to the various service conditions.

6.1.4 Abrasion resistance shall be determined using a comparative model such as Test Method C 501, or a demonstrated equivalent, with two standards of comparison, one more abrasive and one less abrasive. A function-related installation abrasion test, specific to the device and its associated instrumentation, may additionally be required.

6.1.5 Other mechanical evaluations of calcium phosphate coatings shall be made, depending on service environments, installation techniques, or other load considerations.

7. Test Specimen Fabrication

7.1 All test specimens for coating characterizations shall be prepared from indicative coating lots and samples from the same production feedstock lots and prepared on the same equipment, representative of the coating as applied to the devices.

7.2 For device characterization, all test specimens should be subjected to the same processing and sterilization as the finished device, if applicable.

8. Quality Program Requirements

8.1 The manufacture of calcium phosphate coatings will conform to good manufacturing practices (21 CFR 820).

9. Keywords

9.1 bone implant; calcium phosphate; coating; dental implant materials; hydroxylapatite; mechanical tests; orthopedic medical devices; physical characterizations; tricalcium phosphate

APPENDIX

(Nonmandatory Information)

X1. RATIONALE

X1.1 Ceramic hydroxylapatite and beta-tricalcium phosphate are commercially available as synthetic bone grafting materials. Specifications F 1088 and F 1185 have been established for these substances as particulates. For most implant materials, the biological performance is critically dependent on the material's properties, including chemical and mechanical properties and physical form. These properties must be well-characterized and consistent in order to achieve reproducible clinical results and reliable biocompatibility. This specification provides biocompatible grades of calcium phosphate coatings.

X1.2 Powder X-ray diffraction analysis provides differentiation between crystalline forms of these various calcium phosphate crystalline species, one or more of which will be a major phase in coatings covered by this specification, while others may occur as second or minor phases. It is anticipated that a separate performance standard may be necessary for each separate coating as designated by the major crystalline phase. The physical and mechanical property assessments are not specific to any one type of coating for this reason, but rather they are listed generically as guidelines for analysis. Minor or significant modifications to these procedures may have to be made to result in useful characterization data for the maintenance of individual coating consistency. The sources of general test methods for these coatings are listed in Section 2.

REFERENCES

(**1**) Jarcho, M., Kay, J. F., Gumaer, K. I., Doremus, R. H., and Drobeck, H. P., "Tissue, Cellular and Subcellular Events at a Bone-Ceramic Hydroxylapatite Interface," *Journal of Bioengineering*, Vol 1, 1977, pp. 79–92.

(**2**) Jarcho, M., "Calcium Phosphate Ceramics as Hard Tissue Prosthetics," *Clin Orthop*, Vol 157, 1981, pp. 259.

(**3**) de Groot, K., "Ceramics of Calcium Phosphates: Preparation and Properties," *Bioceramics of Calcium Phosphate*, K. de Groot, ed., CRC Press, Inc., Boca Raton, FL, 1982.

(**4**) Jarcho, M., Bolen, C. H., Thomas, M. B., Bobick, J., Kay, J. F., and Doremus, R. H., "Hydroxylapatite Synthesis and Characterization in Dense Polycrystalline Form," *Journal of Materials Science*, Vol 11, 1976, pp. 2027–2035.

(**5**) "Bioceramics: Material Characteristics Versus In-Vivo Behavior," P. Ducheyne and J. Lemons, eds., *N.Y. Academy of Science*, Vol 523, 1988.

(**6**) Cook, S. D., Kay, J. F., Thomas, K. A., and Jarcho, M., "Interface Mechanics and Histology of Titanium and Hydroxylapatite-Coated Titanium for Dental Implant Applications," *International Journal of Oral Maxillofac Implants*, Vol 2, 1987, pp. 15–22.

(**7**) Cook, S. D., Kay, J. F., Thomas, K. A., and Jarcho, M., "Hydroxylapatite-Coated Porous Titanium for Use as an Orthopaedic Biological Attachment System," *Clin Orthop*, Vol 230, 1988, pp. 303–312.

(**8**) Kay, J. F., Golec, T. S., and Riley, R. L., "Hydroxylapatite-Coated Subperiosteal Dental Implants: Design Rationale and Clinical Experience," *Journal of Prosthet Dent*, Vol 58, 1987, pp. 339–343.

(**9**) Block, M. S., Kent, J. N., and Kay, J. F., "The Evaluation of Hydroxylapatite-Coated Dental Implants in Dogs," *Journal of Oral Maxillofac Surg*, Vol 45, 1987, pp. 601–607.

(**10**) Thomas, K. A., Kay, J. F., and Cook, S. D., "The Effect of Surface Macrostructure and Hydroxylapatite Coating on the Mechanical Strengths and Histologic Profiles of Titanium Implant Materials," *Journal of Biomed Mater Res*, Vol 21, 1987, pp. 1395–1414.

(**11**) Cullity, B. D., *Elements of X-Ray Diffraction*, Addison Wesley, Reading, MA, 1967.

(**12**) *Handbook of Bioactive Ceramics, II: Calcium Phosphate and Hydroxylapatite Ceramics*, Yamamuro, Hench, Wilson, eds., CRC Press, Boca Raton, FL, 1990.

(**13**) Balmain, N., Legros, R., and Bonel, G., "X-Ray Diffraction of Calcified Bone Tissue: A Reliable Method for the Determination of Bone Ca/P Molar Ratio," *Calc Tiss Res*, Vol 34, 1982, pp. 93–98.

(**14**) Toth, J., Hirthe, W., Hubbard, W., Brantley, W., and Lynch, K., "Determination of the Ratio of HA/TCP Mixtures by X-Ray Diffraction," *Journal of Applied Biomaterials*, Vol 2, 1991, pp. 37–40.

(**15**) Sendax, V., "Hydroxylapatite Coated Implants," *Dent Clin N Am*, Vol 36, 1992.

Last ASTM Designation: F 1610 – 95 (Reapproved 1999)

Test Method for Soft Tissue Fixation Strength of Metallic Bone Staples

This test method covers testing the soft tissue fixation strength of metallic staples used in internal fixation of the musculoskeletal system.

Formerly under the jurisdiction of Committee F04 on Medical and Surgical Materials and Devices, this test method was withdrawn in November 2000 and replaced by Specification F 564–00 for Metallic Bone Staples.[1]

---

[1] Annual Book of ASTM Standards, Volume 13.01.

Standard Specification for Intramedullary Reamers[1]

This standard is issued under the fixed designation F 1611; the number immediately following the designation indicates the year of original adoption or, in the case of revision, the year of last revision. A number in parentheses indicates the year of last reapproval. A superscript epsilon (ε) indicates an editorial change since the last revision or reapproval.

1. Scope

1.1 This specification provides requirements for material, dimensions and tolerances, finish and marking, and care and handling for reamers intended to cut a cylindrical path along the medullary canal of diaphyseal bone.

1.2 Intramedullary reamers are commonly used to prepare the medullary canal for the insertion of intramedullary fixation devices (IMFD). As such, the relationship between the intramedullary reamer diameter and the IMFD's diameter are considered.

1.3 The values stated in SI units are to be regarded as the standard.

2. Referenced Documents

2.1 *ASTM Standards:*

A 564/A 564M Specification for Hot-Rolled and Cold-Finished Age-Hardening Stainless Steel Bars and Shapes[2]

A 693 Specification for Precipitation-Hardening Stainless Steel and Heat-Resisting Steel Plate, Sheet, and Strip[2]

A 705/A 705M Specification for Age-Hardening Stainless and Heat Resisting Steel Forgings[2]

F 86 Practice for Surface Preparation and Marking of Metallic Surgical Implants[3]

F 565 Practice for Care and Handling of Orthopaedic Implants and Instruments[3]

F 899 Specification for Stainless Steel Billet, Bar, and Wire for Surgical Instruments[3]

F 983 Practice for Permanent Marking of Orthopaedic Implant Components[3]

F 1264 Specification and Test Methods for Intramedullary Fixation Devices[3]

3. Terminology

3.1 *Definitions of Terms Specific to This Standard:*

3.1.1 *cutting head, n*—the portion of the reamer, which consists of flutes, or edges, which cut the bone.

3.1.2 *reamer diameter, n*—the diameter of the circumscribed circle of the cutting head's cross-section (shown in Fig. 1).

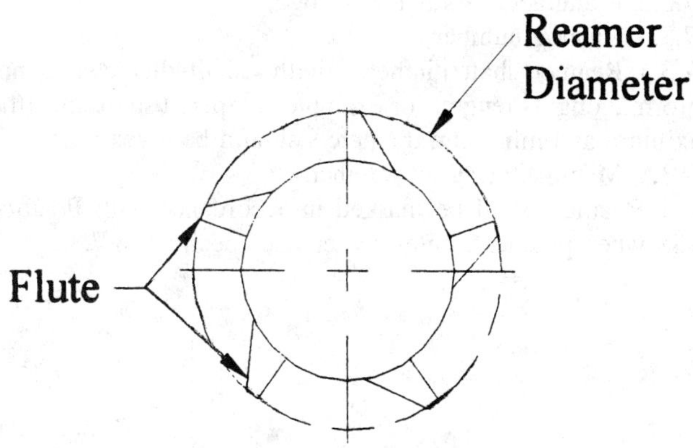

FIG. 1 Reamer Cutting Head

3.1.3 *reamer shaft diameter, n*—the diameter of the circumscribed circle of the long portion of the reamer, which connects the cutting portion of the reamer to the drill.

4. Classification

4.1 In general, intramedullary reamers consist of two types:

4.1.1 *One-piece reamer*—A design where the reamer shaft and cutting head are permanently attached to each other.

4.1.2 *Modular Reamer*—A design where the reamer shaft and cutting head are two separate components, fixed to each other temporarily at the time of use via a geometric connection, for example, dovetail joint.

5. Dimensions and Tolerances

5.1 The reamer diameter shall be measured at the largest portion of the cutting head's cross section and reported to the nearest 0.2 mm. The reamer diameter shall be measured using a micrometer or an appropriate ring gage. When using a micrometer to measure reamers with an odd number of flutes, a V-anvil micrometer (with the appropriate angle, based on the number of flutes) will be used to accurately determine the reamer diameter.

5.2 The tolerance of a reamer diameter shall be no more than ±0.075 mm.

6. Material Requirements

6.1 The reamer's shaft and cutting head shall be fabricated from materials with suitable strength, hardness, and corrosion resistance. The materials described in Specifications A 564, A 693, A 705, and F 899 have been found to be suitable for this use.

---

[1] This specification is under the jurisdiction of ASTM Committee F04 on Medical and Surgical Materials and Devices and is the direct responsibliltiy of Subcommittee F04.21 on Osteosynthesis.

Current edition approved Nov. 10, 2000. Published February 2001. Originally published as F 1611 – 95. Last previous edition F 1611 – 95.

[2] *Annual Book of ASTM Standards*, Vol 01.03.

[3] *Annual Book of ASTM Standards*, Vol 13.01.

7. Finish and Marking

7.1 The shaft and cutting head shall be free from burrs, nicks, dents, and scratches when examined in accordance with Practice F 86.

7.2 The flutes of the cutting head will be of the appropriate geometry to perform the intended use of reaming bone.

7.3 When space permits, the following information should be legibly marked on the reamer (in order of preference):

7.3.1 Reamer diameter,

7.3.2 Manufacturer's name or logo,

7.3.3 Catalog number,

7.3.4 Reamer shaft diameter, if the shaft diameter is not uniform along its length, for example, a tapered shaft, then the maximum and minimum diameters should be given.

7.3.5 Manufacturing lot number.

7.4 Reamers shall be marked in accordance with Practice F 983 when practical, unless otherwise specified in 7.3.

8. Care and Handling

8.1 The reamer should be cared for and handled in accordance with Practice F 565, as appropriate.

8.2 The flutes of the cutting head should be checked periodically for damage or wear. Reamers that are considered to be performing inadequately should be removed from service.

NOTE 1—No standards exist for the measurement of "sharpness." Reamer performance is the most reliable method for assessing reamer sharpness.

9. Keywords

9.1 intramedullary fixation device; orthopaedic medical device; reamer; surgical instruments

APPENDIX

(Nonmandatory Information)

X1. RATIONALE

X1.1 Intramedullary reamers commonly are used to prepare the medullary canal for the subsequent insertion of an IMFD. The relationship between the diameter of the hole prepared by the reamer and the IMFD's diameter are important in relation to the fit achieved by the implant in the bone and the avoidance of surgical complications. If the fit is too loose, the initial fixation may be inadequate to control the translation of the fragments. If the fit is too tight, it may be impossible to drive the IMFD into the bone, the bone fragments may burst, the IMFD may migrate out through the side of the bone, and so forth. It is important that the designation for the reamer size or diameter be related to the diameter of the reamer's cutting flutes so that instruments and IMFDs of different designs and manufacturers can be interchanged during use. Using the reamer diameter specified here and the IMFD diameter specified in Specification F 1264, the surgeon may have confidence in achieving the correct reamer/IMFD geometric relationship.

X1.2 The reamer shaft diameter may be an important dimension in the clinical use of the intramedullary reamer. Laboratory studies have suggested that larger reamer shaft diameters result in greater intramedullary pressure.[4,5,6]

[4] Muller, C.A., Schavan, R., Frigg, R., Perren, S.M., and Pfister, U., "Intramedullary Pressure Increase for Different Commercial and Experimental Reaming Systems: An Experimental Investigation," *Journal of Orthopaedic Trauma*, Vol 12, No. 8, pp. 540–46, 1998.

[5] Peter, R.E., Selz, T., and Koesti, A., "Influence of the Reamer Shape on Intraosseous Pessure During Closed Intramedullary Nailing of the Unbroken Femur: A Preliminary Report," *Injury*, Vol 24, Suppl. 3, pp. S48–55, 1993.

[6] Muller, C.A., Frigg, R., and Pfister, U., "Can Modifications to Reamer and Flexible Shaft Design Decrease Intramedullary Pressure During Reaming? An Experimental Investigation," *Techniques in Orthopaedics*, Vol 11, No. 1, pp. 18–27, 1996.

Standard Practice for Cyclic Fatigue Testing of Metallic Stemmed Hip Arthroplasty Femoral Components with Torsion[1]

This standard is issued under the fixed designation F 1612; the number immediately following the designation indicates the year of original adoption or, in the case of revision, the year of last revision. A number in parentheses indicates the year of last reapproval. A superscript epsilon (ε) indicates an editorial change since the last revision or reapproval.

1. Scope

1.1 This practice covers a method for the fatigue testing of metallic stemmed femoral components used in hip arthroplasty. The described method is intended to be used for evaluation in comparisons of various designs and materials used for stemmed femoral components used in the arthroplasty. This practice covers procedures for the performance of fatigue tests using (as a forcing function) a periodic constant amplitude force.

1.2 This practice applies primarily to one-piece prostheses and femoral stems with modular heads, with the head in place. Such prostheses should not have an anterior-posterior A-P bow or a medial-lateral M-L bow, and they should have a nearly straight section on the distal 50 mm of the stem. This practice may require modifications to accommodate other femoral stem designs.

1.3 The values stated in SI units are to be regarded as the standard.

1.4 *This standard does not purport to address all of the safety concerns, if any, associated with its use. It is the responsibility of the user of this standard to establish appropriate safety and health practices and determine the applicability of regulatory limitations prior to use.*

2. Referenced Documents

2.1 *ASTM Standards:*

E 4 Practices for Force Verification of Testing Machines[2]

E 466 Practice for Constant Amplitude Axial Fatigue Tests of Metallic Materials[2]

E 467 Practice for Verification of Constant Amplitude Dynamic Loads in an Axial Load Fatigue Testing Machine[2]

E 468 Practice for Presentation of Constant Amplitude Fatigue Test Results for Metallic Materials[2]

E 1150 Definitions of Terms Relating to Fatigue[2]

2.2 *ISO Document:*[3]

ISO 7206-3 (1988) Stem Test

3. Terminology (see Fig. 1 Fig. 2)

3.1 *Definitions of Terms Specific to This Standard:*

3.1.1 *cantilever plane*—a plane perpendicular to the line of load application at the level on the stem at which the stem becomes unsupported.

3.1.2 *distal stem axis*—the centerline in the A-P projection and the M-L projection of the most distal 50 mm of the stem.

3.1.3 *estimated maximum bending moment*—the maximum compressive load times the unloaded moment arm.

3.1.4 *geometric centroid (cantilever plane)*— the point in a cross-sectional area of the cantilever plane whose coordinates are the mean values of the coordinates of all of the points in the area.

3.1.5 *line of load application*—the loading axis of the test machine.

3.1.6 *R value*—the ratio of the minimum force to the maximum force,

$$R = \frac{minimum\ force}{maximum\ force}$$

3.1.7 *Reference Line L1:*

3.1.7.1 *distal stem axis*—the M-L centerline of the most distal 50 mm of stem in the A-P projection.

3.1.8 *Reference Line L2:*

3.1.8.1 *collared device*—the plane of the distal side of the collar in the A-P projection.

3.1.8.2 *collarless device*—the resection plane recommended for the device in the A-P projection.

3.1.9 *Reference Point P1*—the spherical center of the prosthesis head.

3.1.10 *Reference Point P3:*

3.1.10.1 *collared device*—the intersection of the principal axis of the collar (L2) with the medial surface of the stem in the A-P projection.

3.1.10.2 *collarless device*—the intersection of the resection

[1] This practice is under the jurisdiction of ASTM Committee F04 on Medical and Surgical Materials and Devicesand is the direct responsibility of Subcommittee F04.22on Arthroplasty.

Current edition approved Aug. 15, 1995. Published December 1995.

[2] *Annual Book of ASTM Standards*, Vol 03.01.

[3] Available from American National Standards Institute, 11 W. 42nd St., 13th Floor, New York, NY 10036.

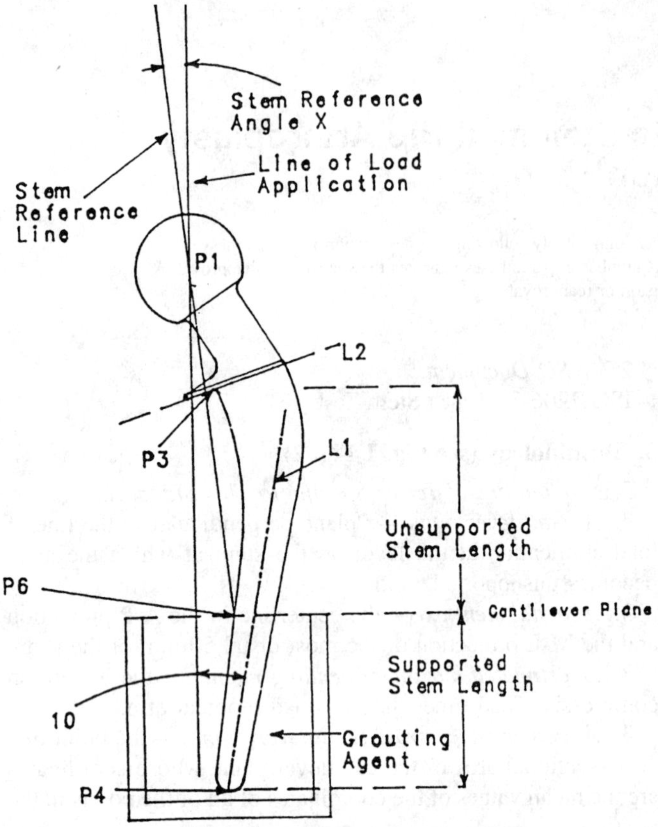

FIG. 1 1(a) Collared Device, M-L Projection

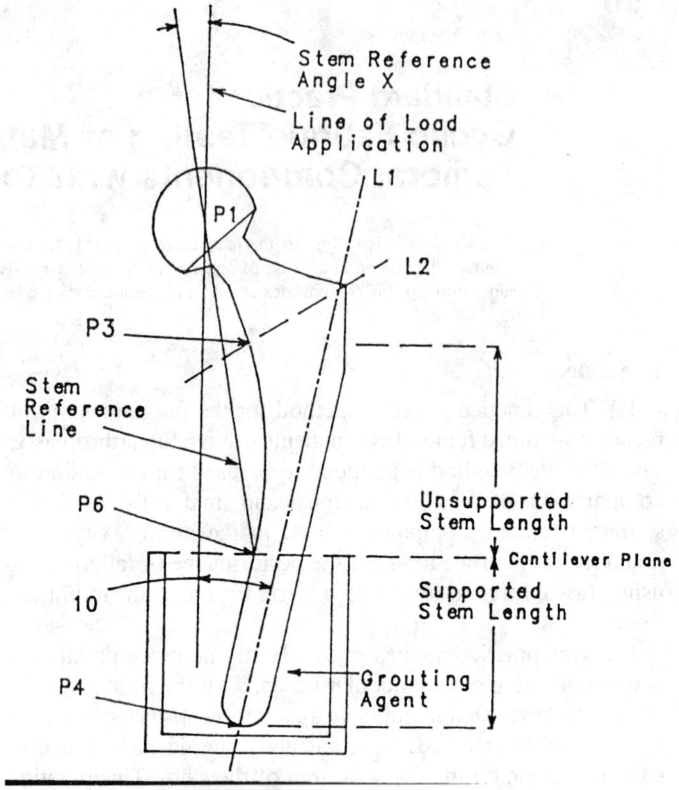

FIG. 2 1(b) Collarless Device, M-L Projection

plane (L2) with the medial surface of the stem in the A-P projection.

3.1.11 *Reference Point P4*—the distal tip of the stem.

3.1.12 *Reference Point P6*[4]— the intersection of the cantilever plane with the medial surface of the stem in the A-P projection.

3.1.13 *stem reference angles*—Since the distal stem axis is obscurred by the grouting agent after preparation of the test sample, the stem reference angles are to be used to measure the repeatability of the stem orientation. They may also be used to estimate the actual orientation of the distal stem to the line of load application if the stem geometry is well known.

3.1.13.1 *X (M-L)*—the angle between the stem reference line and line of load application in the M-L projection.

3.1.13.2 *X (A-P)*—the angle between the stem reference line and line of load application in the M-L and A-P projections.

3.1.14 *stem reference line*—a line passing through Reference Point P6 and the center of the prosthesis head (P1).

3.1.15 *supported stem length*—the vertical distance between the distal tip of the stem (P4) and cantilever plane.

3.1.16 *unloaded moment arm*—the vector sum of the perpendicular distance between the line of load application and geometric centroid of the stem cross section at the cantilever plane in the A-P and M-L projections.

3.1.17 *unsupported stem length*—the vertical distance between Point P3 and the cantilever plane.

4. Significance and Use

4.1 This practice can be used to describe the effects of materials, manufacturing, and design variables on the fatigue resistance of metallic stemmed femoral components subjected to cyclic loading for relatively large numbers of cycles. The recommended test assumes a worst case situation in which proximal support for the stem has been lost. It is also recognized that, for some materials, the environment has an effect on the response to cyclic loading (see section 12.7). The test environment used and rationale for the choice of that environment should be described in the test report.

4.2 It is recognized that actual in vivo loading conditions are not constant amplitude. However, sufficient information is not available to create standard load spectrums for metallic stemmed femoral components. A simple periodic constant amplitude force is accordingly recommended.

5. Purpose

5.1 In order for fatigue data on femoral stems to be useful for comparison, it must be reproducible among different laboratories. It is consequently essential that uniform procedures for testing and reporting test data be established.

6. Apparatus

6.1 The specimen shall be constrained by a suitable grouting agent within a rigid cavity. A common grouting agent used is polymethyl methacrylate (PMMA, bone cement). The minimum thickness of the grouting agent should be 1 cm. Although

[4] The reference points and lines are consistent with the proposed Specification for Cementable Total Hip Prostheses with Femoral Stems. The Reference Points P2 and P5 in that specification are not relevant to this practice. Consequently, they are not used in this practice.

bone cement is the recommended grouting agent, other material may be used, provided that it does not alter the test specimen chemically or mechanically.

6.2 The test fixtures shall be constructed so that the line of load application is in the implant A-P symmetry plane of the supported portion of the stem (Fig. 3).

6.3 The test fixtures shall be constructed so that the line of load application passes through the ball center.

6.4 A ball or roller bearing, low-friction mechanism shall be included in the loading apparatus to minimize loads not perpendicular to the cantilever plane. An example of such a mechanism is included in Appendix X2.

7. Specimen Selection

7.1 The specimen selected should have the same geometry as the final finished product, and the stem should be in the final finished condition.

7.2 The head of the prothesis should have the same geometry and surface finish as the final finished product, unless it can be demonstrated that differences in the condition of the head have no effect on the fatigue response of the stem in this test.

7.3 The length of the neck of the prosthesis contributes to the magnitude of the maximum bending moment. The length of neck (or head offset) should be the longest possible that will be used with the femoral stem being evaluated. This will inherently maximize the maximum bending moment.

8. Equipment Characteristics

8.1 The action of the machine should be analyzed to ensure that the desired form and periodic force amplitude is maintained for the duration of the test. (see Practice E 467).

8.2 The test machine should have a load monitoring system such as the transducer mounted in line with the specimen. The test loads should be monitored continuously in the early stages of the test and periodically thereafter to ensure that the desired load profile is maintained. The varying load as determined by suitable dynamic verification should be maintained at all times to within ±2 % of the largest compressive force being used.

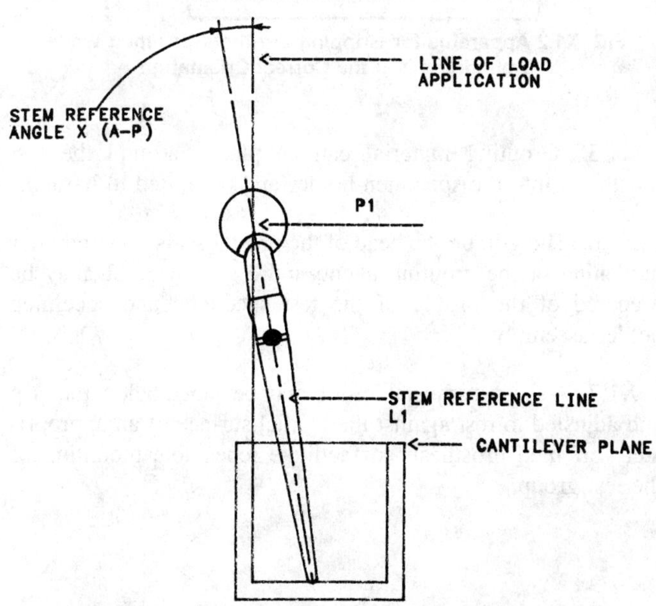

FIG. 3 Collared or Collarless Device, A-P Projection

9. Procedure

9.1 *Specimen Test Orientation*—The angle between the distal stem axis and the line of load application in the M-L projection shall be 10 ± 1° (Fig. 1 Fig. 2)), and the angle between the distal stem axis and the line of load application in the A-P projection shall be 9 ± 1° (Fig. 3). An example of a method of accomplishing mounting the stem at the desired angle is given in Appendix X1.

9.2 *Specimen Mounting*:

9.2.1 Maintain the stem reference angles X (M-L) and X (A-P) within a range of ±1° over a test group.

9.2.2 Maintain the unsupported stem length within ±2 mm.

9.2.3 Do not permit any relative motion between the prosthesis and grouting agent during hardening of the grouting agent.

9.2.4 Keep the surface of the grouting agent at the cantilever plane approximately level and perpendicular to the line of load application.

9.2.5 An example of a technique for setting a specimen in the grouting agent in the correct orientation is given in Appendix X1.

9.3 *Test Frequency*—Run all tests at a test frequency of 30 Hz or less (see section 12.8).

9.4 *R Value*—Run all tests with an *R* value of 10.0.[5]

9.5 Measure the unsupported stem length, stem reference angle, and moment arm for each specimen prior to testing. A possible means would be to use a shadowgraph of the A-P projection as shown in Fig. 1 Fig. 2 Fig. 3.

9.6 Measure the amount of horizontal deflection of the head in both the M-L and A-P projections in response to the periodic forcing function one time after the beginning of each test (see section 12.9).

10. Test Termination

10.1 Continue the test until the specimen fails or a predetermined number of cycles has been applied to the specimen. Specimen failure should be defined as a complete separation of the specimen, or exceeding of a deflection limit on a test machine. In reporting the results, state the criteria selected for defining specimen failure and the number of cycles shown as the predetermined runout of the test. Discard the data for a specific sample if the grouting agent fails prior to test completion.

11. Report

11.1 Report the fatigue test specimens, procedures, and results in accordance with Practice E 468.

11.2 In addition, report the following parameters: stem reference angles X (M-L) and X (A-P), unsupported stem

[5] In strict terms, since the force applied to the head is compressive, the maximum force is the largest algebraic value. The *R* value is consequently 10 when the negative signs cancel each other. As a numeric example, assume a test is conducted at a peak load of 3000 N (−3000). The least compressive load would be 10 % of that, or 300 N (−300). The *R* value would be – 3000/–300, or 10. The *R* value would be 0.1 in terms of applied bending moment at the cantilever plane.

length, supported stem length, largest compressive force, *R* value, specimen material, cycles to failure, estimated maximum bending moment, location of fractures in relation to the cantilever plane, average dimensions of the stem cross section in the cantilever plane, grouting agent, test environment, test frequency, head/neck offset of the stem (neck length), and deflection limit used to cut off testing (see 10.1).

12. Precision and Bias

12.1 The precision and bias of this practice is being established.[6]

[6] Test results that can be used to establish precision and bias are solicited.

APPENDIXES

(Nonmandatory Information)

X1. EXAMPLE PROSTHESIS MOUNTING PROCEDURE

X1.1 A drawing or shadowgraph of the prosthesis should be available before mounting to establish the angular relationship between the distal stem axis and stem reference angle.

X1.2 A gripping device, as illustrated in Fig. X1.1, or a ringstand and test tube holder can be used to grip the head of the subject prosthesis.

X1.3 The prosthesis is held by the head permitting the distal tip to rest on a flat surface. The angle jig illustrated in Fig. X1.2 is positioned with the distal stem in the notch. The stem is adjusted so that it is centered in the notch of the angle jig. This will orient the distal stem at approximately 10° to the line of load application. The head is now gripped firmly to maintain the angular orientation of the stem.

X1.4 The angle jig can be removed and the prosthesis mounted at the appropriate depth in an appropriate specimen holder.

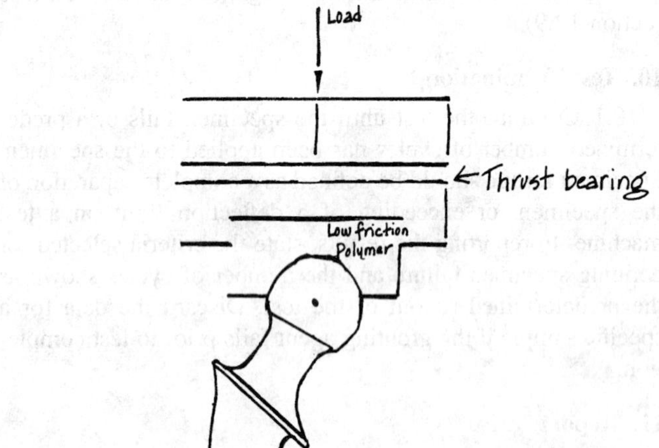

FIG. X1.1 Example of a Low-Friction Mechanism

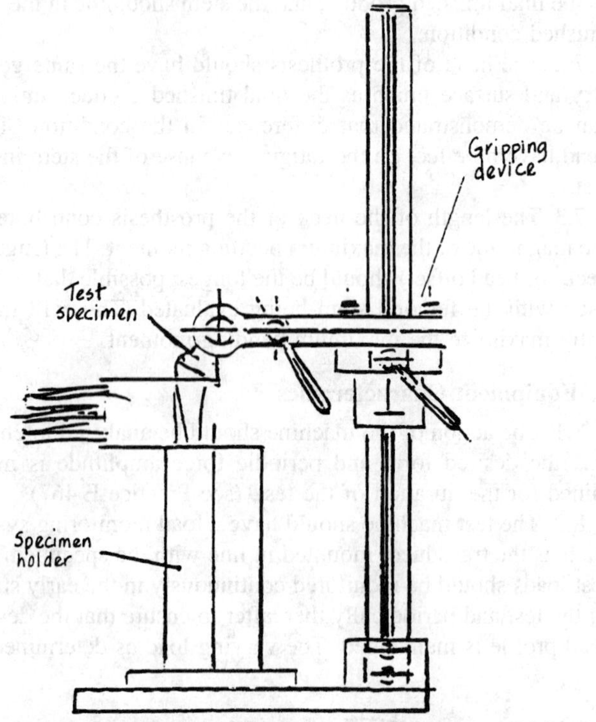

FIG. X1.2 Apparatus for Gripping the Test Specimen While Embedding it in the Correct Orientation

X1.5 Grouting material can be placed around the test prosthesis into the specimen holder and permitted to harden.

X1.6 The grip on the head of the prosthesis is released after hardening of the grouting agent, and a shadowgraph may be prepared of the profile of the test specimen and specimen holder assembly.

X1.7 A second adjustable stop may be added below the grip and adjusted to rest against the medial surface of an appropriately oriented prosthesis to facilitate repeatable mounting of the test group.

X2. RATIONALE

X2.1 The breakage of femoral stems in hip arthroplasty has occurred in clinical application. The stem design, PMMA support, quality of bone, and other features contribute to stem fracture. One recognizable mode of breakage is with the distal portion of the stem anchored firmly, while medial proximal support is lost. As the body loads are applied through the head of the prosthesis, significant stem stresses can result at the area where the cement is still firmly anchored. This simplified model was chosen for the fatigue testing of actual stems because it is believed that this proximal cement breakdown model is the primary reason behind breakage of the femoral stems. There are some problems with the proposed simplified model. The worst case assumes that proximal cement breakdown has already occurred. It does not address any features of a hip arthroplasty system that might help prevent cement breakdown or any features that aid in placing the femoral component in an optimal position with good cement support. While the latter approach is desirable, the test described can provide information on the relative fatigue strengths.

X2.2 This is a general purpose test method. It is not intended solely to be used on one specific test location on a stem but rather can estimate fatigue strengths at several different locations along the stem. There are various aspects of geometry or material features in the design of hip stems that could cause a local decrease in properties. The fatigue properties of these sections can be evaluated by changing the unsupported stem length to put the cantilever plane at or near the desired location.

X2.3 This practice attempts to model simply the orientation of the stemmed femoral component in relation to the peak loads that are applied in the human body. To accomplish this, the distal stem will have an anatomic orientation to the applied load in both the M-L and A-P plane of the prosthesis. Because of the A-P orientation, the applied load has a vector component that applies a rotation force to the main axis of the stem; this loading mode is designated "with torsion." The orientation of the applied load also causes a bending moment to be applied in two different planes. Local stresses in the prosthesis result from superposition of the stresses caused by the two bending moments and torsional component.

X2.4 It is also possible to use this practice for comparison of the relative fatigue strength of different stem designs. The unsupported stem length to select for this type of testing is difficult to select. Historically, earlier stem designs with clinical incidence of fracture fractured at several different locations along the stem. The selection of a single, unsupported stem length for all designs will have to be arbitrary. A stem performance document that references this practice will select a specific unsupported stem length. The ISO stem test document, ISO 7206-3 (1988), specifies an unsupported stem length of 80 mm. However, the ISO document defines the unsupported stem length using a simpler, but less consistent method. The ISO unsupported stem length is from the center of the head (Point P1) to the cantilever plane. The problem with this method is that the actual stem cross section in the cantilever plane can be different, depending on the neck length of the device. The definition of unsupported stem length in this practice will test the same approximate stem section on a stem, even if the neck length is different. The Reference Line L2 can be difficult to determine on some collarless prostheses. This line corresponds to the approximate osteotomy line in the bone. It may be necessary to review the documentation from the stem manufacturer if the location of Line L2 is not obvious on the prosthesis. The stem manufacturer's literature or X-ray templates will usually include the desired location of the prosthesis relative to the osteotomy line.

X2.5 In Section 10 of this practice, there is no specification of the number of cycles for test runout. The fundamental idea behind this type of test is that the number of cycles to runout represents a limiting point beyond which the material will not fracture, no matter how many more cyclic loads are applied. This is referred to as a fatigue limit. However, most materials do not possess a true fatigue limit in real life. A compromise must consequently be made between the amount of testing (the number of test cycles) and the relationship of the test to actual device performance and device life. A typical runout point is often 10 million cycles since most of these tests are plotted and evaluated on a semilog or log-log plot. Doubling or tripling the number of test cycles to 20 or 30 million contributes only a small amount to the trend analysis on the log scale, but it doubles or triples the length of the test. In Europe, 5 million cycles has been used as a runout value for some stem tests.

X2.6 This test is a cantilever beam bending test. The load point in a cantilever beam bend test will tend to deflect in the direction of the applied load, with the amount of deflection depending on the elasticity of the test sample. The head of the prosthesis is the cantilever load point with this test. Since the direction of the load also applies a compressive force down the stem, only the vector portion of the force, perpendicular to the prosthesis' long axis, will contribute to the beam deflection. That contribution of beam bending will deflect the head to the side. This motion increases the bending moment arm effectively. This motion must be permitted. If the head is not allowed to deflect in a near frictionless manner, the portion of the test fixture that prevents the deflection is actually applying an unknown force against the head to keep it from deflecting. If the device is flexible enough, the magnitude of periodic motion of the head of the prosthesis (in the plane perpendicular to the line of load application) in response to the periodic forcing function can increase the applied maximum bending moment significantly. It may be important to measure this deflection and include it in maximum bending moment calculations.

X2.7 Any fatigue strengths as predicted by tests following the method described herein must be considered on a relative basis, that is, these tests may yield valuable information concerning the relative merits of different devices for particular applications, but they should not be used as a quantitative indicator of the expected in vivo device lifetime.

X2.8 There is limited information in the literature regarding whether the materials used in hip arthroplasty femoral components experience a significant degradation in high-cycle fatigue initiation properties due to the presence of a physiological environment. If there is concern that the material used in the device may degrade significantly in a physiological environment, such material characteristics would be more realistically determined fatigue testing of a material test specimen in a simulated physiological environment at rates of 1 cycle/s or less. A particular environment is not specified in this practice for these reasons, but a simulated environment is not prohibited. However, if a simulated environment is used, the test frequency should be so as to not mask the expected effects of the environment.

X2.9 Possible methods include dial gages, optical micrometers, or linear scales viewed with a strobe light to slow the apparent motion of the deflection.

The American Society for Testing and Materials takes no position respecting the validity of any patent rights asserted in connection with any item mentioned in this standard. Users of this standard are expressly advised that determination of the validity of any such patent rights, and the risk of infringement of such rights, are entirely their own responsibility.

This standard is subject to revision at any time by the responsible technical committee and must be reviewed every five years and if not revised, either reapproved or withdrawn. Your comments are invited either for revision of this standard or for additional standards and should be addressed to ASTM Headquarters. Your comments will receive careful consideration at a meeting of the responsible technical committee, which you may attend. If you feel that your comments have not received a fair hearing you should make your views known to the ASTM Committee on Standards, at the address shown below.

Standard Specification for Surgical Tissue/Dressing/Pick-Up Forceps (Thumb Type)[1]

This standard is issued under the fixed designation F 1613; the number immediately following the designation indicates the year of original adoption or, in the case of revision, the year of last revision. A number in parentheses indicates the year of last reapproval. A superscript epsilon (ϵ) indicates an editorial change since the last revision or reapproval.

1. Scope

1.1 This specification covers general workmanship aspects of spring-action, tissue, dressing, or pick-up forceps (thumb-type) intended for the retraction, grasping, or dissection of tissue during surgical procedures.

1.2 The values stated in inch-pound units are to be regarded as the standard. The values given in parentheses are for information only.

2. Referenced Documents

2.1 *ASTM Standards:*

E 18 Test Methods for Rockwell Hardness and Rockwell Superficial Hardness of Metallic Materials[2]

E 92 Test Method for Vickers Hardness of Metallic Materials[2]

E 140 Hardness Conversion Tables for Metals (Relationship Between Brinell Hardness, Vickers Hardness, Rockwell Hardness, Rockwell Superficial Hardness, and Knoop Hardness)[2]

F 899 Specification for Stainless Steel Billet, Bar, and Wire for Surgical Instruments[3]

F 921 Definitions of Terms Relating to Hemostatic Forceps[3]

F 1026 Specification for General Workmanship and Performance Measurements of Hemostatic Forceps[3]

F 1089 Test Method for Corrosion of Surgical Instruments[3]

F 1638 Terminology for Surgical Tissue/Dressing/Pick-Up Forceps (Thumb-Type)

3. Terminology

3.1 *Definitions*—Definitions shall be in accordance with Terminology F 1638.

3.1.1 *modified working ends*—working surfaces possessing superior hardness characteristics that are the result of either depositing various materials on the base metal or securing an insert permanently (such as by brazing) to the base metal (see Note 3).

4. Material

4.1 All component parts of the instrument shall be fabricated from Class 4 martensitic stainless steel in accordance with Specification F 899. The modified working ends may be of stellite, tungsten carbide, or other suitable material.

5. Requirements

5.1 *Heat Treatment and Hardness for Component Parts*:

5.1.1 The stainless steel component parts shall be heat treated under conditions recommended for the material used.

5.1.2 The Rockwell hardness (HRC) of the instrument with the working end not modified shall be 40–49 HRC after appropriate processing. Instruments in which the working end has been modified shall have an HRC of A77.

5.2 *Corrosion Resistance*—Instruments shall be subjected to corrosion tests as specified in Test Method F 1089.

5.3 *Finish*:

5.3.1 *Surfaces*—Surfaces of the instruments shall be uniformly finished and free of burrs, sharp edges, cracks, coarse marks, and processing materials.

5.3.2 *Type*—The finish shall be one of the types specified in Definitions F 921 or as specified by the purchaser.

5.4 *Workmanship*:

5.4.1 *Symmetry*—Excluding functional differences, both forceps halves shall be symmetrical.

5.4.2 *Teeth*—Teeth shall be well formed, uniform in depth and spacing, and mesh without binding, unless designed otherwise.

5.4.3 *Handle Serrations*—Handle serrations shall be uniform in depth and spacing.

5.5 *Guide Pin and Guide Pin Hole*:

5.5.1 The guide pin shall pass through the guide pin hole without binding.

5.5.2 The guide pin length shall not protrude past the outside surface of the guide pin hole when the forceps' tips come in contact.

NOTE 1—Guide pin/guide pin holes are generally used on forceps 7½ in. (191 mm) or longer.

6. Performance

6.1 *Alignment*—Scissoring shall be 0.015 in. (0.38 mm) or less upon closure.

7. Marking and Labeling

7.1 All marking and labeling shall be legible.

7.2 The instruments shall bear the following: (*1*) the manufacturer's (or contractor's) name or registered trademark; (*2*)

[1] This specification is under the jurisdiction of ASTM Committee F-4 on Medical and Surgical Materials and Devices and is the direct responsibility of Subcommittee F04.65 on Medical/Surgical Instruments.

Current edition approved Aug. 15, 1995. Published September 1995.

[2] *Annual Book of ASTM Standards*, Vol 03.01.

[3] *Annual Book of ASTM Standards*, Vol 13.01.

the country of origin (when the instrument is not manufactured in the United States); and (*3*) other markings, as required, by the purchaser or the manufacturer (contractor).

7.3 The location of marking shall be on a suitable surface of the instrument.

NOTE 2—This specification is not intended to cover delicate tissue forceps such as those used in microsurgery or neurosurgery.

NOTE 3—Typical methods of modifying the working end of the forceps is to use jaw inserts or to plasma deposit (flame plate) materials with improved wear characteristics such as tungsten carbide or stellite. For the jaw insert methods, the insert is brazed to the jaw face with a uniform deposit of silver solder that is free of crevices at all interfaces. For the flame plating method, a uniform layer of material is deposited that is 0.004 ± 0.001 in. (0.1 ± 0.03 mm) thick.

Standard Guide for
Scope of Performance of First Responders Who Practice in the Wilderness or Delayed or Prolonged Transport Settings[1]

This standard is issued under the fixed designation F 1616; the number immediately following the designation indicates the year of original adoption or, in the case of revision, the year of last revision. A number in parentheses indicates the year of last reapproval. A superscript epsilon (ϵ) indicates an editorial change since the last revision or reapproval.

1. Scope

1.1 This guide covers minimum performance requirements for first responders who may initially provide care for sick or injured persons in the specialized pre-hospital situations of the wilderness or delayed or prolonged transport settings, including catastrophic disasters.

1.2 Individuals who will operate in the wilderness or delayed or prolonged transport settings need to be aware of the physical requirements necessary to be able to perform all identified objectives and necessary skills required for the setting.

1.3 This guide establishes supplemental or continuing education programs that will be taught to individuals trained to the first responder level by an appropriate authority.

1.4 This guide does not establish performance standards for use in the traditional emergency medical services (EMS) or ambulance transportation environment.

1.5 This guide does not establish medical protocols; nor does it authorize invasive procedures without specific authorization and medical control.

1.6 Successful completion of a course based on this guide does not constitute or imply certification or licensure.

1.7 *This standard does not purport to address all of the safety concerns, if any, associated with its use. It is the responsibility of the user of this standard to establish appropriate safety and health practices and determine the applicability of regulatory limitations prior to use.*

2. Referenced Documents

2.1 *ASTM Standards:*

F 1177 Terminology Relating to Emergency Medical Services[2]

F 1287 Guide for Scope of Performance of First Responders Who Provide Medical Care[2]

F 1453 Guide for the Training and Evaluation of First Responders Who Provide Emergency Medical Care[2]

F 1490 Terminology Relating to Search and Rescue[2]

2.2 *Code of Federal Regulations:*[3]

Title 29, Part 1910.1030, Bloodborne Pathogens

2.3 *Department of Transportation Document:*[3]

U.S. DOT HS 900-25, *Course Guide, Emergency Medical Services: First Responder Training Course*, 1979

3. Terminology

3.1 *Definitions:*

3.1.1 *access*—the process of reaching the patient/subject and establishing physical contact.

3.1.2 *basic life support/cardiopulmonary resuscitation (BLS/CPR)*—a set of skills that includes airway management, chest compressions, and others as defined by the American Heart Association (AHA).

3.1.3 *definitive care (see Terminology F 1177)*—a level of therapeutic intervention capable of providing comprehensive health care services for a specific condition.

3.1.4 *evacuation (see Terminology F 1490)*—the process used between the time of extraction and transportation.

3.1.5 *extraction (see Terminology F 1490)*—the process of initial assessment, treatment, stabilization, and packaging of the patient/subject as well as removal of the patient/subject from the immediately hazardous environment.

3.1.6 *first responder*—an individual trained to meet the requirements of Guide F 1287.

3.1.7 *transportation*—the use of a specially designed vehicle to move a patient to a medical facility or definitive care facility.

3.2 *Definitions of Terms Specific to This Standard:*

3.2.1 *delayed or prolonged transport setting*—when the time between patient injury and arrival at a definitive care facility is greater than 60 min.

3.2.2 *nontraditional EMS environment*—an environment that is not readily accessible to a ground ambulance.

3.2.3 *wilderness first responder (WFR)*—an individual trained to meet the requirements of this guide.

3.2.4 *wilderness setting*—situations in which the delivery of patient care by EMS providers is complicated by one or more of the following factors: (*1*) remoteness with respect to logistics and access; (*2*) a significant delay in the delivery of care to the patient; (*3*) an environment that is physically

[1] This guide is under the jurisdiction of ASTM Committee F-30 on Emergency Medical Services and is the direct responsibility of Subcommittee F30.02 on Education.

Current edition approved Aug. 15, 1995. Published October 1995.

[2] *Annual Book of ASTM Standards*, Vol 13.01.

[3] Available from Standardization Documents Order Desk, Bldg. 4 Section D, 700 Robbins Ave., Philadelphia, PA 19111-5094, Attn: NPODS.

stressful to both patients and rescuers; and (*4*) lack of equipment, supplies, and transportation.

4. Significance and Use

4.1 This guide is intended to expand the scope of the practice of first responders and improve the emergency medical care delivered to patients in the wilderness or delayed or prolonged transport settings.

4.2 This guide does not suggest a particular performance sequence.

4.3 Individuals will be trained initially or concurrently in accordance with the U.S. DOT HS 900-25, *Course Guide*, and Guide F 1453.

4.4 This guide may be used by individuals who develop training programs for nontraditional EMS environments.

4.5 This guide acknowledges the need for additional or specific training required for the wilderness or delayed or prolonged transport settings.

5. Required Objectives

5.1 The WFRs shall be able to accomplish the following:

5.1.1 Identify specific subjects included within the scope of Guide F 1287, where traditional patient care is not sufficient or appropriate, due to a patient being in the wilderness or delayed or prolonged transport settings; and manage such problems in an appropriate manner.

5.1.2 Demonstrate a knowledge of anatomy and physiology sufficient to apply emergency care principles to the unique problems found in the wilderness or prolonged or delayed transport settings.

5.1.3 Identify and manage the following medical problems in the wilderness or delayed or prolonged transport settings:

5.1.3.1 Abdominal pain,

5.1.3.2 Vomiting,

5.1.3.3 Diarrhea,

5.1.3.4 Diabetes,

5.1.3.5 Seizure disorders,

5.1.3.6 Respiratory distress (for example, asthma and altitude),

5.1.3.7 Allergies,

5.1.3.8 Hypertension,

5.1.3.9 Cardiac emergencies, and

5.1.3.10 Dental emergencies.

5.1.4 Identify and manage illness or injury related to or caused by the environment in the wilderness or delayed or prolonged transport settings, including the following:

5.1.4.1 Altitude illness (for example, acute mountain sickness, high-altitude pulmonary edema, and high-altitude cerebral edema);

5.1.4.2 Barotrauma;

5.1.4.3 Cold injury (for example, hypothermia and frostbite);

5.1.4.4 Heat illness (heat stroke and heat exhaustion);

5.1.4.5 Electrical and lightning injuries;

5.1.4.6 Exposure to plant or animal (for example, insect, reptile, arachnid, and marine) toxins;

5.1.4.7 Drowning, near-drowning, and cold water immersion; and

5.1.4.8 Dehydration.

5.1.5 Understand the proper disinfection of water, and identify and manage illnesses associated with improper water disinfection.

5.1.6 Identify and manage open wounds in the wilderness or delayed or prolonged transport settings.

5.1.7 Identify and manage orthopedic problems in the wilderness or delayed or prolonged transport settings, including dislocations, fractures, and open fractures.

5.1.8 Identify and manage spinal injuries and associated problems in the wilderness or delayed or prolonged transport settings.

5.1.9 Identify specific problems with managing cardiopulmonary arrest in the wilderness or delayed or prolonged transport settings.

5.1.10 Identify the uses, side effects, and administration concerns for nonprescription medications and prescription medications in the wilderness or delayed or prolonged transport settings.

5.1.11 Identify measures necessary to prevent illness or injury in the wilderness or delayed or prolonged transport settings, including the management of immediate stress reactions.

5.1.12 Identify unique problems related to rendering care in severe weather, in environmental extremes, when equipment is not readily available, access is limited, and there is little or no additional assistance.

5.1.13 Identify clothing, survival techniques, emergency communications, and bivouac considerations necessary to survive in environmental extremes.

5.1.14 Understand patient packaging in the wilderness or delayed or prolonged transport settings.

5.1.15 Understand the need to document all care provided to any patient.

5.1.16 Understand the EMS system and any unique legal aspects related to providing care in the wilderness or prolonged or delayed transport settings.

5.1.17 Understand the role of medical control as it relates to the WFR's practice, including patient care and quality improvement.

5.1.18 Understand and demonstrate familiarity with the principles of disease transmission, body fluid isolation, and the use of personal protective equipment.

5.1.19 The order of these objectives does not suggest a performance sequence.

6. Keywords

6.1 delayed; first responder; prolonged; nontraditional; prehospital; wilderness

REFERENCES

(1) Pre-Hospital Committee, Wilderness Medical Society, "Wilderness Pre-Hospital Emergency Care (WPHEC) Curriculum," *Journal of Wild Medicine*, Vol 2, No. 2, 1991, pp. 80–87.

(2) Rural Affairs Committee, National Association of EMS Physicians, "Clinical Guidelines for Delayed/Prolonged Transport: I, Cardiopulmonary Arrest," *Prehospital and Disaster Medicine*, Vol 6, No. 3, July–September 1991.

(3) Rural Affairs Committee, National Association of EMS Physicians, "Clinical Guidelines for Delayed/Prolonged Transport: II, Dislocations," *Prehospital and Disaster Medicine*, Vol 8, No. 1, January–March 1993.

(4) Rural Affairs Committee, National Association of EMS Physicians, "Clinical Guidelines for Delayed/Prolonged Transport: III, Spine Injury," *Prehospital and Disaster Medicine*, Vol 8, No. 2, April–June 1993.

(5) Rural Affairs Committee, National Association of EMS Physicians, "Clinical Guidelines for Delayed/Prolonged Transport: IV, Wounds," *Prehospital and Disaster Medicine*, Vol 8, No. 3, July–September 1993.

(6) *Emergency Medical Services: First Responder Training Course*, U.S. DOT HS 900-025, *Course Guide*, March 1979.

(7) "Guidelines for Cardiopulmonary Resuscitation and Emergency Cardiac Care—Recommendations of the 1992 National Conference," *Journal of the American Medical Association*, Vol 268, No. 16, Oct. 28, 1992, p. 2173.

Last ASTM Designation: F 1622 – 95 (Reapproval 2000)

Standard Test Method for Measuring the Torsional Properties of Metallic Bone Screws

This test method covers the testing of stainless steel, cobalt-based, and titanium-based bone screws for the determination of torsional yield strength, maximum torque, breaking angle, and torque versus angle of rotation. The described test method is intended to be used as a means of evaluating the mechanical properties of bone screws.

Formerly under the jurisdiction of Committee F04 on Medical and Surgical Materials and Devices, this test method was discontinued in 2001 and replaced by Specification and Test Methods F 543 for Metallic Medical Bone Screws[1] because the complete content of Test Method F 1622 is now contained in Specification and Test Methods F 543.

[1] *Annual Book of ASTM Standards*, Vol 13.01.

Standard Specification for Tracheostomy Tubes–Pediatric Tracheostomy Tubes[1]

This standard is issued under the fixed designation F 1627; the number immediately following the designation indicates the year of original adoption or, in the case of revision, the year of last revision. A number in parentheses indicates the year of last reapproval. A superscript epsilon (ε) indicates an editorial change since the last revision or reapproval.

INTRODUCTION

Pediatric tracheostomy tubes are primarily intended for use with infants and children who may require anesthesia, artificial ventilation, relief of upper airway obstruction, or other respiratory therapy.

An infant or child differs from an adult, not only in size but especially with regard to airway anatomy and respiratory physiology. Airway equipment for pediatric patients involves differences not only of size but also of basic design. The differences created a demand for a separate standard for tracheostomy tubes for pediatric use. It should be noted that, although this standard specifies some requirements for cuffs, cuffs are seldom provided on the smaller sizes of pediatric tubes.

This specification describes requirements for those characteristics of tracheostomy tubes that can be standardized and that are important for patient safety. It does not, however, limit the variety of tube designs necessary to conform to pediatric anatomy and the variety of lesions and space limitations encountered.

A tracheostomy tube may increase resistance to gas flow. For tubes with a given outside diameter, differences in wall thickness have a major influence on the resistance to gas flow, especially in the smaller sizes of pediatric tracheostomy tubes.

1. Scope

1.1 This specification describes basic requirements for tracheostomy tubes made of plastic materials or rubber, or both, having inside diameters less than 6.0 mm. Such tubes are primarily designed for pediatric patients who may require anesthesia, artificial ventilation or other respiratory support, but need not be restricted to these uses. Specialized tubes are excluded from the scope of this specification.

2. Referenced Documents

2.1 *ASTM Standards:*

F 640 Test Methods for Radiopacity of Plastics for Medical Use[2]

F 1054 Specification for Conical Fittings of 15 mm and 22 mm Sizes[2]

F 1242 Specification for Cuffed and Uncuffed Tracheal Tubes[2]

F 1666 Specification for Adult Tracheostomy Tubes

2.2 *ISO Standards:*[3]

ISO 7000 Graphical Symbols—Synopsis

ANSI/HEMA MD 70.1-Conical Fittings

3. Terminology

3.1 *Definitions*—For the purpose of this specification, the definitions given in Specification F 1666, together with the following definition, apply.

3.2 *pediatric tracheostomy tube*—tube designed for insertion into the trachea of an infant or child through a tracheostomy.

4. Size and Dimensions

4.1 *Designation of Tube Size*:

4.1.1 The size of a tracheostomy tube (outer tube) shall be designed by the nominal inside diameter (ID) of the tube expressed in millimetres, as measured at the minimum diameter, in accordance with Table 1, excluding any encroachment allowed by 6.6.1. When the ID of the tracheostomy (outer) tube does not fall within specified limits of the categories listed in Table 1, the actual ID may be used as the size designation with appropriate tolerances.

4.1.2 The size of a pediatric tracheostomy tube with inner cannula shall be designated in accordance with Specification F 1666.

4.2 *Outside Diameter*:

4.2.1 The outside diameter (OD) of sections A and B (see Fig. 1) of the tube, other than at the cuff if provided, shall be expressed in millimetres, subject to a tolerance of ±0.20 mm. Section C of the outer tube shall have a tolerance of ±0.50 mm.

NOTE 1—The marked outside diameter relates to that portion of the

[1] This specification is under the jurisdiction of ASTM Committee F-29 on Anesthetic and Respiratory Equipment and is under the direct responsibility of Subcommittee F29.12 on Airways.

Current edition approved Sept. 10, 1995. Published December 1995.

[2] *Annual Book of ASTM Standards*, Vol 13.01.

[3] Available from American National Standards Institute, 11 W. 42nd St., 13th Floor, New York, NY 10036.

TABLE 1 Size Range of Pediatric Tracheostomy Tubes

Dimensions and Tolerances, mm

Designated Size (nominal inside diameter, ID)	Inside Diameter and Tolerance
2.0	2.0 + 0.20 −0
2.5	2.5 + 0.20 −0
3.0	3.0 + 0.20 −0
3.5	3.5 + 0.20 −0
4.0	4.0 + 0.20 −0
4.5	4.5 + 0.20 −0.10
5.0	5.0 ± 0.20
5.5	5.5 ± 0.20
6.0	6.0 ± 0.20

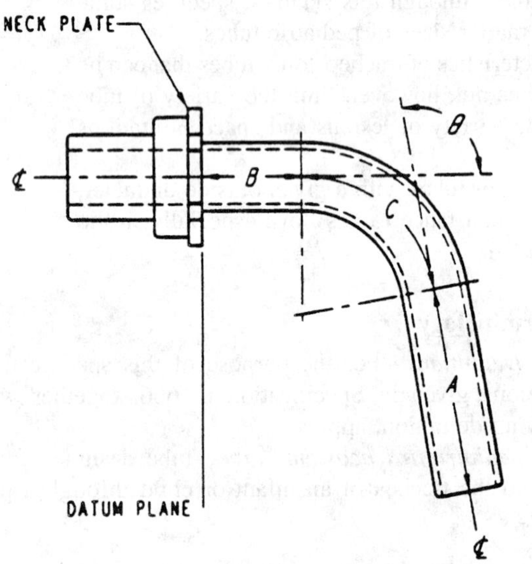

NOTE 1—The angle θ is an obtuse angle formed between the tangents to the longitudinal axes of the tube at the machine and patient ends. As dimensions A or B, or both, approach or equal zero, the angle θ shall be the obtuse angle formed between the tangents (planes perpendicular) to the longitudinal axes.

FIG. 1 Basic Dimensions of Pediatric Tracheostomy Tubes

tube intended to be within the wall and lumen of the trachea.

4.3 *Length*:

4.3.1 The center-line length (dimension A + B + C in Fig. 1) shall extend from the patient side of the neck-plate to the patient end of the outer tube including to the tip of the bevel, if present (see Fig. 2 Fig. insert) and expressed in millimetres.

4.3.2 The actual center-line length shall not vary by more than 1.5 mm from the marked length for tubes with a marked inside diameter of less than 4.5 mm, or by more than 2 mm for tubes with a marked inside diameter of 4.5 mm or greater.

4.3.3 Dimensions A, B and C shall be expressed in millimetres.

NOTE 2—Dimensions A or B, or both, may be, or approach, zero.

4.3.4 For tubes with an adjustable neck-plate, the range of measurements for center-line lengths shall be expressed in centimetres.

4.4 *Angle* θ:

4.4.1 The angle θ (see Fig. 1) shall be expressed in degrees. The angle θ shall be the obtuse angle formed between the tangents (planes perpendicular) to the longitudinal axes.

5. Materials

5.1 The materials of pediatric tracheostomy tubes shall comply with the requirements specified in Specification F 1666.

6. Design

6.1 *Inner Tube*:

6.1.1 The inner tube, if provided, shall extend to within 0.5 mm of the patient end of the tracheostomy (outer) tube and not more than 3.0 mm beyond the patient end.

6.1.2 The machine end of the inner tube shall be a 15-mm male connector conforming with the requirements of Specification F 1054. It shall not prevent the tracheostomy (outer) tube connector or adaptor, if provided, from mating with the breathing system of an anaesthetic machine or ventilator.

6.1.3 If the connector is attached to the inner cannula, a mechanism must be provided to fasten the inner cannula to the outer tube.

6.2 *Neck-plate*:

6.2.1 A tracheostomy tube shall have a neck-plate (see Fig. 1).

6.2.2 The neck-plate shall be provided with holes or other means to permit attachment to the patient.

6.2.3 If a tracheostomy tube has an adjustable neck-plate, it shall be securable to the tube, but not removable.

6.3 *Cuff*:

6.3.1 The cuff, if provided, shall be permanently attached to the tube.

6.3.2 Cuffs of tracheostomy tubes shall comply with the requirements specified in Specification F 1242.

6.3.3 The labeled cuff resting diameter shall be within ± 15 % of the normative value when determined in accordance with Annex A1-Annex A3.

6.4 *Inflating Tubes for Cuffs*:

6.4.1 *Inflating Tubes*:

6.4.1.1 The inflating tube, if fitted, shall have an outside diameter of not more than 2.5 mm. The secondary (inflation) lumen shall not encroach on the lumen of the tracheostomy tube by more than 10 % of the inside diameter of the tracheostomy tube.

NOTE 3—The wall around the secondary (inflation) lumen should not project substantially on the outside surface of the tracheostomy tube.

6.4.2 *Pilot Balloon*:

6.4.2.1 The inflating tube shall have a pilot balloon or other means, or both, to indicate inflation status of the cuff.

NOTE 4—This (these) device(s) may also serve as a pressure indicating or limiting device.

6.4.2.2 Neither the inflating tube nor any device shall act as a non-return valve to prevent the intentional evacuation of the cuff.

6.4.3 *Free End of Inflating Tubes for Cuffs*:

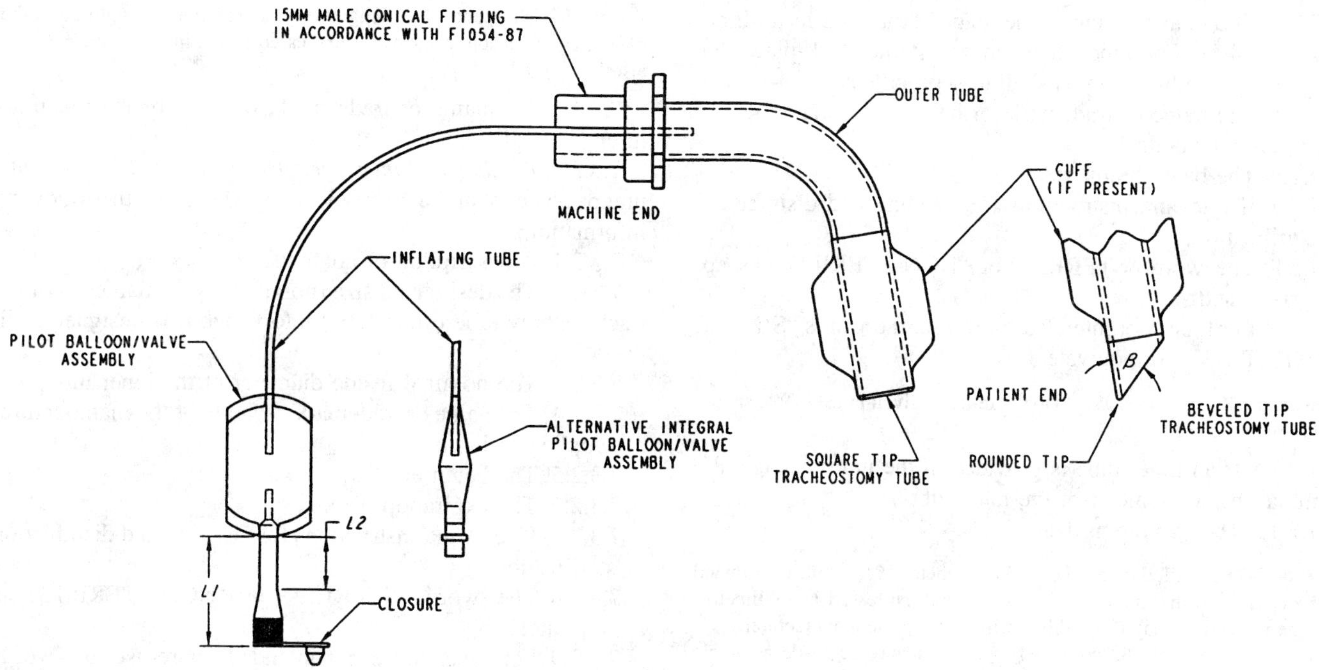

FIG. 2 Typical Tracheal Tube

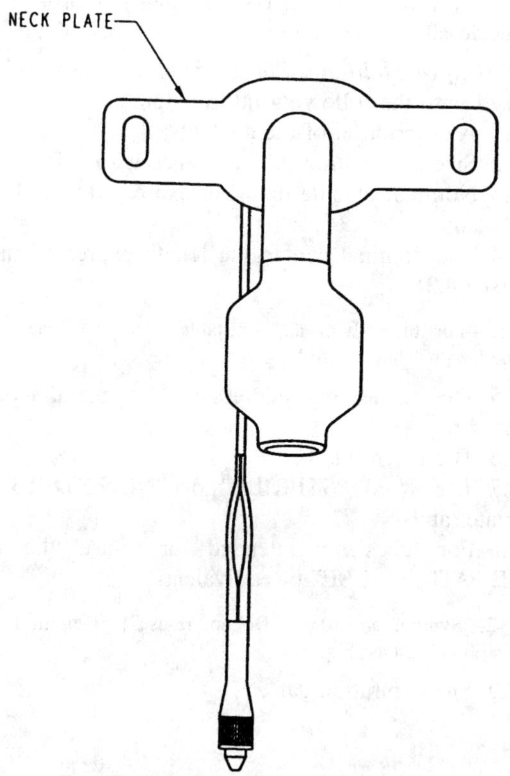

FIG. 2 *(continued)*

6.4.3.1 The end of the inflating tube may be open or sealed with a closure device or inflation valve, but in all instances it shall be capable of accepting a male conical fitting with a 6 % taper (Luer), complying with the requirements specified in ANSI/HEMA MD 70.1. The length, Fig. 2, Dimension L1 of the free end of the inflating tube shall not be less than 40 mm unless an inflation valve or closure device is provided.

6.4.3.2 If an inflation valve or closure device is provided, the length (Fig. 2, Dimension L2) between the pilot ballot (or other device) and the 6 % conical fitting shall not be less than 10 mm unless the pilot balloon and valve or closure device are integral.

6.5 *Patient End*:

6.5.1 The patient end may be square, beveled or of other configuration.

6.5.2 If a bevel is present, the angle of the bevel β shall be not less than 45° (see Fig. 2).

6.6 *Introducer (Obturator)*:

6.6.1 Provision of an introducer is optional.

6.6.2 The introducer shall be smooth and facilitate rapid intubation.

6.6.3 The introducer shall be easily inserted and removed.

6.6.4 When correctly seated the introducer should not fall out of the tracheostomy tube under its own weight when the tube is held by the neck-plate with the patient end uppermost.

7. Packaging and Labeling

7.1 *Unit Package*— The following information shall be apparent on visual examination of the intact unit package:

7.1.1 The size and shape of the tube;

7.1.2 Whether a cuff is provided; and

7.1.3 Whether a connector or adaptor is provided.

NOTE 5—The unit package may be transparent and the tube visible, or a drawing to scale, preferably full scale may be used. If a drawing is provided, product dimensions may be included.

7.2 The following information shall be provided either on the unit package or on an insert with the unit package:

7.2.1 A description of the contents;

7.2.2 The designated size expressed in millimetres in accordance with 4.1;

7.2.3 The nominal outside diameter expressed in millimetres (see 4.2);

7.2.4 The nominal center-line length expressed in millimetres (see 4.3). For tubes with an adjustable neck-plate, the range of center-line lengths shall also be given;

7.2.5 The name or trademark, or both, of the manufacturer or supplier, or both;

7.2.6 The batch number;

7.2.7 If relevant, instructions for cleaning and disinfection or sterilization;

7.2.8 The word "STERILE" or "NON-STERILE", as appropriate; and

7.2.9 For tubes not intended for re-use, the words "SINGLE PATIENT USE" or equivalent.

NOTE 6—Symbol no. 1051 ("Do not re-use") given in ISO 7000 should additionally be used (see Fig. 3).

7.2.10 If an inner tube is provided in the unit package, the nominal inside diameter of the inner tube.

7.2.11 The expiration date.

NOTE 7—For cuffed tubes, the resting diameter of the cuff, determined in accordance with Annex A1-Annex A3, and expressed in millimetres may be marked or may be readily available from the manufacturer.

NOTE 8—The angle θ, expressed in degrees may be made available upon request from the manufacturer.

7.3 *Marking*:

7.3.1 *Neck Plate*—The following information shall be marked on the neck-plate and shall be visible from the machine end of the tube:

7.3.1.1 The designated size (nominal inside diameter) expressed in millimetres in accordance with 4.1;

7.3.1.2 The nominal outside diameter expressed in millimetres (see 4.2);

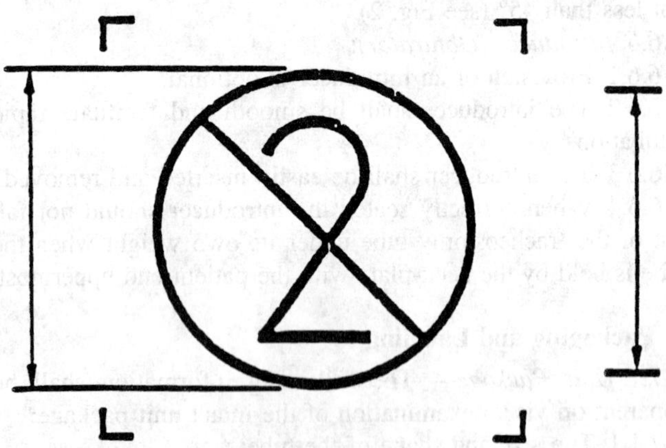

FIG. 3 ISO Symbol 7000/1051 "Do Not Re-Use"

NOTE 9—The center-line length (or the maximum length for tubes having an adjustable neck-plate) expressed in millimetres (see 4.3) may also be marked.

7.3.1.3 The name or trade mark, or both, of the manufacturer.

7.3.2 *Labelling of Inner Tube Unit Packages*—Inner tube unit packages shall be clearly labelled to indicate the following information:

7.3.2.1 A description of contents;

7.3.2.2 The designated size (nominal inside diameter) of the tracheostomy tube (outer tube) into which it is designed to fit (see 4.1);

7.3.2.3 The nominal inside diameter of the inner tube;

7.3.2.4 The name or trademark, or both, of the manufacturer or supplier, or both;

7.3.2.5 The batch number;

7.3.2.6 The expiration date.

7.3.2.7 If relevant, instructions for cleaning and disinfection or sterilization;

7.3.2.8 The word "STERILE" or "NON-STERILE", as appropriate;

7.3.2.9 For inner tubes not intended for re-use, the words "SINGLE PATIENT USE" or equivalent;

NOTE 10—Symbol no. 1051 ("Do not re-use") given in ISO 7000 should additionally be used (see Fig. 3).

7.3.3 *Shelf or Multi-unit Packs*—Shelf or multi-packs shall be marked with the following information:

7.3.3.1 A description of the contents;

7.3.3.2 Size designation in accordance with 4.1;

7.3.3.3 Nominal outside diameter expressed in millimetres (see 4.2); and

7.3.3.4 The nominal center-line length expressed in millimetres (see 4.3);

NOTE 11—For tubes with an adjustable neck-plate, the range of center-line lengths should also be given.

7.3.3.5 The name and address of the manufacturer or supplier;

7.3.3.6 The batch number;

7.3.3.7 The word "STERILE" or "NON-STERILE", as appropriate; and

7.3.3.8 For tubes not intended for re-use, the words" SINGLE PATIENT USE" or equivalent.

NOTE 12—Symbol no. 1051 ("Do not re-use") given in ISO 7000 should also be used (see Fig. 3).

7.3.3.9 The expiration date.

ANNEXES

(Mandatory Information)

A1. IMPLANTATION TEST

A1.1 See Specification F 1666.

A2. METHOD FOR DETERMINING THE RESTING DIAMETER OF THE CUFF

A2.1 *Principle*:

A2.1.1 The resting diameter of the cuff is measured when the cuff is inflated with a pressure which removes creases but minimizes stretching of its walls.

A2.2 *Apparatus*:

A2.2.1 Means to inflate the cuff with sufficient air to create an intracuff pressure of 2.0 kPa (20 cm H_2O) ±5 %.

A2.3 *Procedure*:

A2.3.1 Inflate the cuff with sufficient air to create an intracuff pressure of 2.0 kPa (20 cm H_2O) ±5 % and leave to stabilize for 5 min at (23 ± 2)°C, maintaining that pressure.

A2.3.2 Measure the maximum cuff diameter in a plane perpendicular to the axis of the tube at intervals of 45°.

A2.4 *Expression of Results*:

A2.4.1 Calculate the arithmetic mean of the measurements obtained in A2.3.2 and express the result in millimetres.

A3. GUIDANCE ON MATERIAL DESIGN AND FINISH

A3.1 See Specification F 1666.

Designation: F 1628 – 95 (Reapproved 2000)

Standard Specification for Labeling and Marking of Cuffed and Uncuffed Tracheal Tubes and Related Treatments Intended for Use During Laser Surgery[1]

This standard is issued under the fixed designation F 1628; the number immediately following the designation indicates the year of original adoption or, in the case of revision, the year of last revision. A number in parentheses indicates the year of last reapproval. A superscript epsilon (ε) indicates an editorial change since the last revision or reapproval.

1. Scope

1.1 This specification covers the labeling, marking, warnings, and precautions for cuffed and uncuffed tracheal tubes and related materials intended by the manufacturer for use during laser surgery of the airway.

1.2 Rationale for this specification is to provide a standard format for reporting results obtained from Test Method F 1497. Safety and performance tests, with availability of results, are described in this specification to allow a manufacturer the maximum use of technological alternatives in design and materials. This specification addresses the laser resistance of the shaft of the tracheal tubes. Other components of the system, such as the inflation system and cuff, are outside the scope of this specification.

1.3 The values stated in SI units are to be regarded as standard.

2. Referenced Documents

2.1 *ASTM Standards:*

F 1242 Specification for Cuffed and Uncuffed Tracheal Tubes[2]

F 1497 Test Method for Determining the Laser Resistance of the Shaft of Tracheal Tubes[2]

3. Terminology

3.1 *Definitions*—For definitions other than those listed below refer to Specification F 1242 and Test Method F 1497.

3.1.1 *device*—a tracheal tube or tracheal tube treatment material.

3.1.2 *marking*—information permanently affixed by the manufacturer to any surface of a tracheal tube or to any applied component of a laser resistant tracheal tube treatment that is affixed to or protects the component up to the point it is applied to the tracheal tube.

3.1.3 *product*—commercially available device in its packaged and labeled form.

3.1.4 *tracheal tube*—a tube to convey gases or vapors to and from the trachea. This term shall be used rather than synonyms such as "endotracheal," "intratracheal," or "catheter."

3.1.4.1 *laser resistant tracheal tube*—a tracheal tube that is intended by the manufacturer for use during laser surgery. This includes devices that are sold pre-assembled, or in kit form.

3.1.5 *laser resistant tracheal tube treatments*— coverings or surface treatment materials, or both, indicated by the manufacturer for use with standard tracheal tubes where this product is intended to adapt the standard tracheal tube for use in laser surgery.

3.1.5.1 *Discussion*—This definition does not include such materials when provided in kit form with the tracheal tube (see 3.1.4.1).

3.1.6 *tracheal tube cuff*—an inflatable sleeve fastened to the patient end of the tracheal tube to provide an effective, leak-resistant fit between the tube and the trachea.

3.1.7 *upper airway*—the segment of the anatomical airway above the laryngotracheal junction.

4. Product Marking and Labeling

4.1 All values shall be in SI units.

4.2 *Marking on the Device Shall Include*:

4.2.1 The name or trademark of the manufacturer or supplier.

4.2.2 Model or formulation code that is necessary to distinguish similar products from the same manufacturer, where this distinction is relevant to the laser resistance of the product.

4.2.3 A reference to any preparation steps designated by the manufacturer as essential to the laser resistance of the tracheal tube (that is, saturate covering with saline solution).

4.2.4 For cuffed tracheal tubes, a reference shall be included to any preparation steps designated by the manufacturer as essential for protection of the cuff from ignition (that is, inflate cuff with saline or water).

4.2.5 Depth markings are optional.

4.2.5.1 **Caution:** When markings on the device are applied to an area of the shaft considered to be laser resistant, the determination of laser resistance by the manufacturer must include testing of the shaft directly upon these markings.

4.3 *Labeling on the Unit of Use Package*:

---

[1] This specification is under the jurisdiction of ASTM Committee F29 on Anesthetic and Respiratory Equipment and is under the direct responsibility of Subcommittee F29.18 on Operating Room Fire Safety.

Current edition approved Sept. 10, 1995. Published November 1995.

[2] *Annual Book of ASTM Standards*, Vol 13.01.

4.3.1 The following information shall be included in product labeling on product container. This information is supplemental to other descriptive labeling regulated by applicable standards, and is not intended to replace said labeling.

4.3.1.1 A description of the package contents.

4.3.1.2 The name or trademark of the manufacturer or supplier.

4.3.1.3 The product code or catalog number.

4.3.1.4 A reference to the batch, lot, or control number.

4.3.1.5 The word "sterile," if appropriate.

4.3.1.6 For devices not intended for reuse, the words" single patient use."

4.3.1.7 For devices intended to be sterilized by the user, detailed information necessary to maintain laser resistance shall be included or referenced.

4.3.1.8 *Storage Conditions*—a caution statement of known conditions of storage likely to result in rapid deterioration of the materials, for example, high temperature, ultraviolet light, or fluorescent lighting.

4.3.1.9 Expiration date.

4.3.1.10 Prominent notice shall be listed to refer to information describing laser resistance required by 4.4.4.

4.4 The following information shall be included with each unit of sale package, such as in a package insert:

4.4.1 *Preparation and Use of the Device*—For protective treatments that require setup and routine maintenance to achieve the stated laser resistance, explicit information must include applicable precautionary statements.

4.4.2 Indications for use, including laser type, nominal wavelength, and contraindications.

4.4.3 Warnings and precautions relative to the use of the device including descriptions of damage and effects that are likely to occur from contact with lasers that could result in harm to the patient or operating room personnel. These sections shall include events other than ignition, which were reported during laser resistance testing conducted in accordance with Test Method F 1497.

4.4.4 The laser resistance test results for each laser type indicated including nominal laser wavelength. These test results shall be derived from testing conducted in accordance with Test Method F 1497. The presentation of the data shall be in graphical format depicting power from 0 to 100 W (unless warranted by higher power levels) versus laser energy duration from 1 to 30 s. No values less than 1 s or greater than 30 s shall be included. (See Fig. 1.)

4.4.4.1 Individual data points shall be connected by straight lines. Data shall be presented for laser energy durations of 1, 10, 20, and 30 s. Additional data points shall be included to limit the change from adjacent data points to no more than 20 % of the larger value, or 2 W, whichever is greater.

4.4.5 Graph axes shall be linear, with power (watts) as the vertical axis and laser energy duration (seconds) as the horizontal axis, as listed in Test Method F 1497. The power curves for each laser type and nominal wavelengths shall be clearly indicated. The graph shall be titled "Maximum Power Settings In Which Ignition Does Not Occur." The graph shall include a note stating that the data was derived from Test Method F 1497 (Fig. 1).

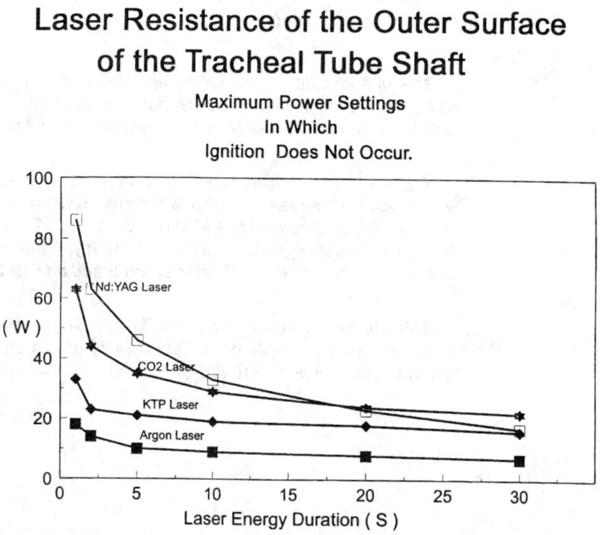

FIG. 1 Laser Resistance of the Outer Surface of the Tracheal Tube Shaft

4.4.5.1 The length of the horizontal axis at 30 s shall be 160 ± 10 % of the height of the vertical axis at 100 W.

4.4.6 The following statements must appear in reasonable proximity to the graphs, such that it is clear that the statements apply to the data presented in the graphs.

4.4.6.1 The test method used to obtain these data addresses the laser resistance of the shaft of the tracheal tube. Other components of the system, such as the inflation system and cuff, are outside the scope of this test method.

4.4.6.2 Caution should be observed since the direct applicability of the results of the test method to the clinical situation has not been fully established.

4.4.6.3 These data were derived with a 0.5 mm spot size laser beam continuously applied perpendicularly to the tracheal tube shaft in a 98 % oxygen atmosphere. Refer to Test Method F 1497 for further information.

4.4.6.4 The test method data measures and describes the properties of materials, products, or assemblies in response to heat and flame under controlled laboratory conditions and does not describe or appraise the fire hazard or fire risk of materials, products, or assemblies under actual fire conditions. However, results of this test may be used as elements of a fire risk assessment which takes into account all of the factors that are pertinent to an assessment of the fire hazard of a particular end use.

4.4.6.5 Storage conditions (see 4.3.1.8).

4.5 *Shelf or Multi-Unit Containers*—The following supplemental information shall be displayed in addition to the other regulated labeling requirements for the product:

4.5.1 The name or trademark of the manufacturer or supplier.

4.5.2 The product code or catalog number.

4.5.3 The descriptive name of the device (trademark, etc.).

4.5.4 A reference to the batch, lot, or control number.

4.5.5 The word "sterile" as appropriate.

4.5.6 For products not intended for reuse, the words" single patient use."

4.5.7 Expiration date.

4.5.8 Quantity of unit packages contained in the package.

4.5.9 Storage conditions (see 4.3.1.8).

Designation: F 1629 – 95

Standard Guide for Establishing Operating Emergency Medical Services and Management Information Systems, or Both[1]

This standard is issued under the fixed designation F 1629; the number immediately following the designation indicates the year of original adoption or, in the case of revision, the year of last revision. A number in parentheses indicates the year of last reapproval. A superscript epsilon (ε) indicates an editorial change since the last revision or reapproval.

1. Scope

1.1 The Emergency Medical Services Management Information System (EMS-MIS) serves as a framework for the management and linkage of data documenting the complete emergency episode from onset through the pre-hospital, emergency department, and hospital phases to final discharge. This document establishes a standard guideline for the planning, development, and maintenance of an EMS-MIS framework, including linkage among pre-hospital, hospital, and other public safety or government agencies. The resultant EMS-MIS should be capable of monitoring the compliance of an EMS system with its established system standards, and provide an objective basis upon which different EMS systems can be comparatively evaluated.

1.2 *EMS-MIS Goals*:

1.2.1 To manage data regarding response to a medical emergency.

1.2.2 To provide a process for obtaining and documenting objective, reliable data.

1.2.3 To provide information that can be used to affect operational changes in an EMS system leading to the delivery of better quality emergency medical care.

1.2.4 To provide information to guide the rational investment of local, state, and national resources to improve and maintain EMS.

1.3 This guide will standardize data needed for decision making at various levels of the EMS system, and offer suggestions as to the appropriate use of this information.

1.4 This guide comments on several possible configurations for information flow and data processing, recognizing that no one configuration is best suited to all circumstances.

1.5 This guide focuses on pre-hospital medical activities, including emergency responses, scheduled transports, and all interinstitutional transfers.

1.6 This guide addresses EMS-MIS techniques applicable to the internal operations of outpatient and inpatient facilities as well as pre-hospital care providers.

1.7 This guide will not address specialized data systems and applications such as trauma registries, but will allow for interfacing with such applications.

1.8 This guide will not address computer-aided dispatch (CAD) systems, nor system status management (SSM) applications, but will allow for interfacing with such applications.

2. Referenced Documents

2.1 *ASTM Standards:*

E 622 Guide for Developing Computerized Systems[2]

E 623 Guidelines for Developing Functional Requirements for Computerized Laboratory Systems[2]

E 624 Guide for Developing Implementation Designs for Computerized Systems[2]

E 625 Guide for Training Users of Computerized Systems[2]

E 627 Guide for Documenting Computerized Systems[2]

E 730 Guide for Developing Functional Designs for Computerized Systems[2]

E 1113 Guide for Project Definition for Computerized Systems[2]

E 1239 Guide for Description of Reservation/Registration-Admission, Discharge, Transfer (R-ADT) Systems for Automated Patient Care Information Systems[2]

E 1384 Guide for Description of Content and Structure of an Automated Primary Record of Care[2]

F 1177 Terminology Relating to Emergency Medical Services[3]

3. Terminology

3.1 Standard EMS terminology is referenced in Terminology F 1177. Definition of individual data elements is given in 5.3 and 5.4.

3.2 *Definitions of Terms Specific to This Standard:*

3.2.1 *Continuing Medical Education (CME)*—refers to data that identify all continuing medical education activity completed by an EMT in the system.

3.2.2 *Data Flow Diagram (DFD)*—Diagram that partitions system business functions into a series of events that enhances analysis and clarifies the purpose, events, and functions that take place for each process.

3.2.3 *Emergency Medical Services Management Information System (EMS-MIS)*—a framework for the management and linkage of data documenting the complete emergency

[1] This guide is under the jurisdiction of ASTM Committee F-30 on Emergency Medical Services and is the direct responsibility of Subcommittee F30.03 on Organization/Management.

Current edition approved Sept. 10, 1995. Published October 1995.

[2] *Annual Book of ASTM Standards*, Vol 14.01.

[3] *Annual Book of ASTM Standards*, Vol 13.01.

episode from onset through the pre-hospital, emergency department, and hospital phases to final discharge.

3.2.4 *Patient Care Record (PCR)*—refers to the data elements described in 5.3 which are to be completed by each PSO for every patient who is treated or transported, or both.

3.2.5 *Provider Service Organization (PSO)*—any public service or commercial organization that utilizes providers to deliver pre-hospital emergency medical care, and transports patients to healthcare facilities, on either an emergency or prescheduled, non-emergent basis.

3.2.6 *Public Safety Answering Point (PSAP)*—a dispatch center that receives incoming calls for help.

3.2.7 *Regional Emergency Medical Services Organization (REMSO)*—Political users of the EMS-MIS at the regional level. This could include an organizational entity such as a regional EMS council, a multi-county hospital consortium, and so forth, or a regional coordinating division within the prevailing EMS authority.

4. Summary of Guide

4.1 The ability to deliver high-quality, cost-effective pre-hospital care can be enhanced by analysis of information about the EMS system's structure, process, and outcomes. This guide defines a standardized terminology and recommends a conceptual design for a computerized EMS-MIS which can facilitate such analysis.

4.2 This guide is intended to serve as a blueprint for the initiation of such a system in geopolitical areas where computerized EMS-MIS is not available or is being updated and to provide a standard basis for data collection to allow for meaningful comparisons between EMS systems throughout the country. The EMS-MIS's already in operation should give serious consideration to restructuring their databases to be consistent with this guide.

4.3 Fig. 1 defines the major organizational entities involved in day-to-day EMS operations. This diagram is based upon the assumption that these organizations represent the potential sources of all data and policies needed for the EMS-MIS. It shows types of data and reports available from the various entities, and needed by them to optimize their operation.

4.4 Fig. 2 defines the political users of the EMS-MIS. It

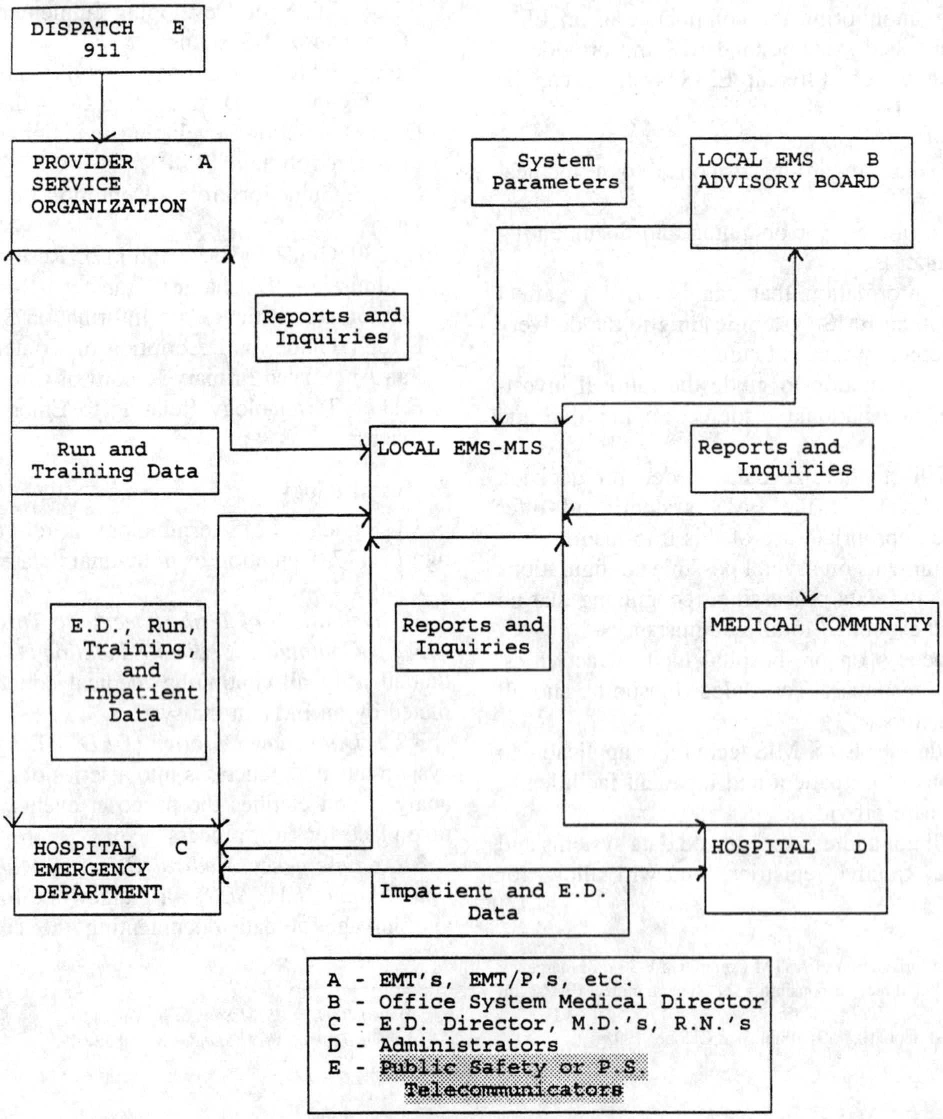

FIG. 1 EMS-MIS Context Diagram I

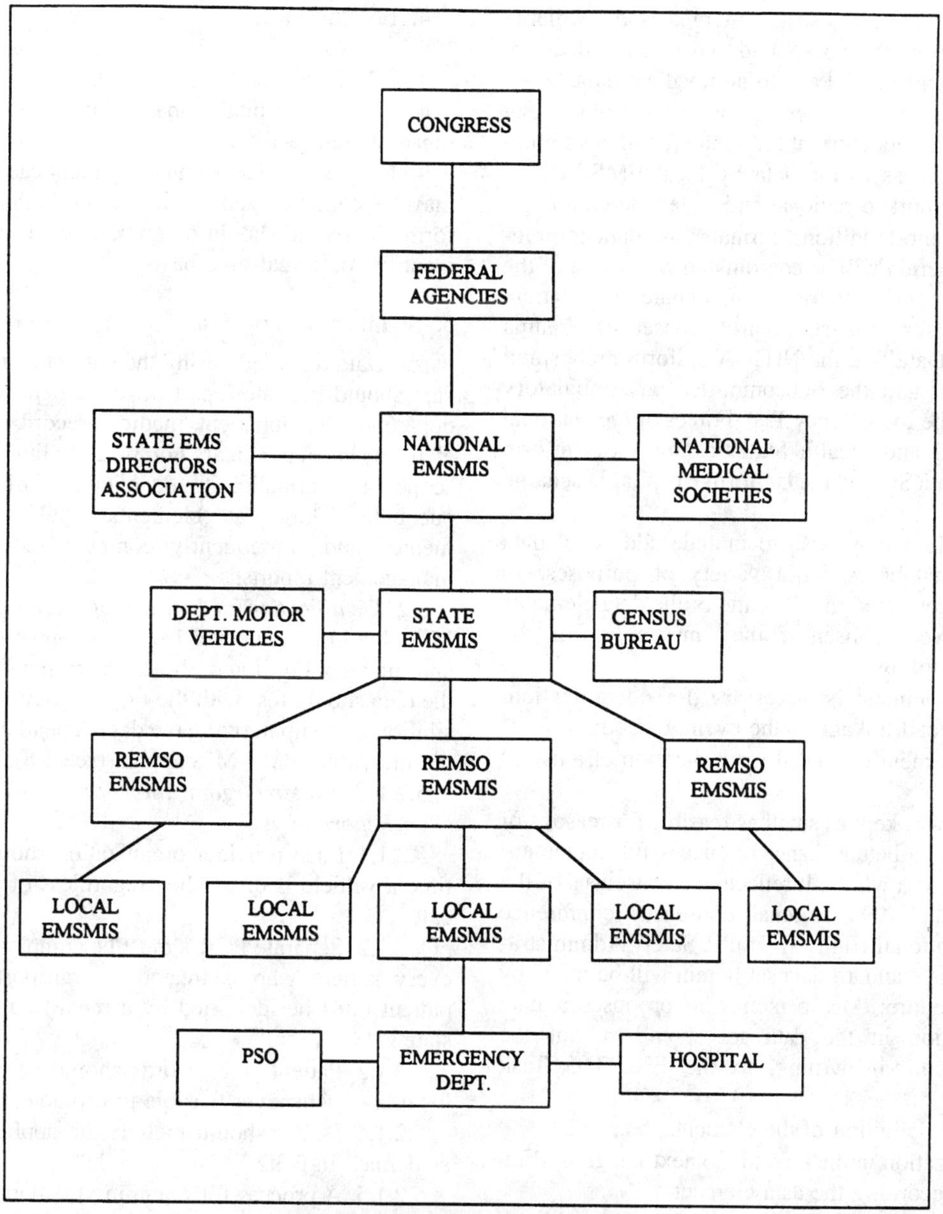

FIG. 2 EMS-MIS Context Diagram II

should be understood that such entities as LOCAL EMS-MIS, REMSO, EMS-MIS, and so forth, do not necessarily refer to distinct organizational entities, but may be coordinating divisions within the prevailing EMS authority.

4.5 The EMS-MIS defined herein recognizes a graduated process of data collection and analysis. This means that data elements collected at the provider and hospital levels may be useful only at the local levels. Emphasis has been given to the ability to capture information in an electromagnetic format as closely as possible to the time/source from which it was generated in order to enhance completeness, validity, reliability, and utilization of data. By observing the linkage parameters defined herein, it should be possible for higher levels of the pyramid to access detailed data through welldefined linkage mechanisms, when and if necessary, without resorting to costly duplication and centralization of all data elements.

4.6 The task group recommends that the data collected by the PSO be aggregated at the various levels that have responsibility for medical quality assurance, planning, and management activities. These levels include but are not limited to the emergency department, hospital(s), regional EMS, and statewide.

4.6.1 The emergency department is an important link between the pre-hospital and inpatient settings.

4.6.2 The medical direction for a PSO, on-line and frequently off-line as well, usually originates in an adjacent hospital emergency department. Analysis of pooled data at this level facilitates medical quality assurance activities and minimizes the necessity for uploading confidential and sensitive data to higher levels of the pyramid.

4.6.3 Access to hospital in-patient data may occur at the hospital or state level. More rapid feedback to medical care providers is possible when the in-patient data are accessed while the patient is hospitalized or shortly after discharge.

Statewide hospital data are usually merged and available within six months after the year's end. These state data are useful for planning and for linkage to nonmedical data.

4.6.4 Laptop/palmtop and other computer technology that permits computerized data entry at the scene facilitates immediate and efficient access to the data by local EMS-MIS in addition to timely export to regional and statewide entities.

4.7 All data element definitions, formats, and data communications protocols herein will be coordinated with those of the ASTM E31.12 Subcommittee on the Computerized Patient Record, the Center for Disease Control Consensus Trauma Registry Minimum Data Set, the NHTSA uniform prehospital EMS data elements, and the Subcommittee on Ambulatory Care Statistics and the Interagency Task Forces of the National Committee on Vital and Health Statistics for the Uniform Ambulatory Care Data Set and the Uniform Hospital Discharge Data Set.

4.8 The EMS-MIS's may wish to include additional data elements in their databases for a variety of purposes. In addition to the sources listed in 4.7, some of the data elements presented in 5.3 were chosen if they met either of the conditions listed as follows:

4.8.1 The data element is necessary for identification/documentation or recall/linkage of the event, or both.

4.8.2 The data element is needed for generation of a useful management report.

4.9 The data list was kept as small as feasible for reasons of practicality, cost, and a better chance of successful implementation of the system as a whole. It reflects the consensus of the Task Group and the 1994 national consensus conference sponsored by the National Highway Traffic Safety Administration. Additions to the standard data set herein will be made by the following procedure: Any person who proposes a data element for inclusion in the data set should submit the following information, in writing, to the F30.03.03 Task Group.

4.9.1 An explicit definition of the element.

4.9.2 The organization in the Level I Context Diagram (Fig. 1) responsible for recording the data element.

4.9.3 The logical database file the element should reside in. (See 5.8.6.7 for the list of database files.)

4.9.4 The organizations that should have possession of the element routinely and optionally.

4.9.5 Those who should have access to the element.

4.9.6 The purpose of the data element and its various uses.

4.10 After review of the information in 4.9.1 to 4.9.6, the task group will vote to include/exclude the element, and so advise Subcommittee F30.03.

4.11 Certain key identifiers must exist in a planned, coordinated manner in order for an EMS-MIS to function efficiently and without ambiguity. There should be a system in each state that allows for the assignment of unique identification or registration numbers to each of the following:

4.11.1 Individual providers.

4.11.2 Provider service organizations (PSO).

4.11.3 Individual vehicles owned or operated by PSO's, or both.

4.11.4 First responder organizations.

4.11.5 Physicians.

4.11.6 Nurses.

4.11.7 Hospitals.

4.11.8 Non-hospital in-patient institutions (nursing homes, rehabilitation facilities, etc.).

4.11.9 A statewide, standard, patient care record. The record may be computerized, or paper, or both. Regardless of the form, the record should be prenumbered or assigned a unique identifier on a real-time basis.

5. Significance and Use

5.1 Data recorded during the patient's pre-hospital phase of care should become a part of the patient's formal emergency department or inpatient medical record, or both. The data elements listed herein are not meant to limit or define the entire scope of information to be elicited during a given patient encounter. These data elements should, however, be documented and subsequently computerized for generation of management reports.

5.2 *Identification of Sources of Data*—Data for the EMS-MIS should be collected from the source organizations listed and shown in Fig. 1 and Fig. 2. The responsibility for collecting the data should rest with the organization as detailed. Responsibility for computerizing the data depend upon the specifics of the individual EMS-MIS design (see 5.8).

5.2.1 *Provider Organization Patient Care Records (PCR), (Run Reports)*:

5.2.1.1 Each provider organization should document every time a vehicle is dispatched regardless of the outcome of the call.

5.2.1.2 Separate PCR's must be completed by each PSO for every patient who is treated or transported, or both. Each patient must be identified by a record number that is unique statewide.

5.2.1.3 Patient care records should be computerized at the local level whenever feasible to promote efficient data access.

5.2.1.4 PCR's should include the applicable data elements as defined in 5.3.2.

5.2.1.5 A process for obtaining the data elements collected by the dispatcher should be established and followed by the provider.

5.2.1.6 The provider should maintain personnel records including the data elements listed in 5.3 and 5.4.

5.2.2 *Hospital Emergency Department Record*:

5.2.2.1 The hospital emergency department should document medical direction. The documentation should include all instances of radio or telephone contact with providers.

5.2.2.2 The hospital emergency department should generate a unique record for each emergency patient visit.

5.2.2.3 Emergency department data should be computerized and also merged at the regional or state level.

5.2.2.4 Data elements listed in 5.4.2 that are usually contained in the emergency department record are important for EMS-MIS evaluation.

5.2.3 *Hospital Discharge Record*:

5.2.3.1 A hospital discharge abstract should be completed for every emergency patient discharged from an inpatient facility.

5.2.3.2 Data elements listed in 5.4.3 that are usually contained in the hospital discharge abstract are important for EMS-MIS evaluation.

5.2.3.3 Hospital discharge data should be computerized and merged statewide.

5.2.3.4 Computerized hospital discharge data should be linked to pre-hospital EMS data in order to document all patients transported by EMS who were admitted and discharged from a hospital.

5.3 *Provider*:

5.3.1 The following data elements should be recorded about the patient by the provider and maintained in its respective "EMS RUN" database file (5.8.6.7(*1*). The following data elements are defined according to the NHTSA definitions for essential and desirable pre-hospital EMS data elements. Essential elements are marked with an asterisk and desirable elements are unmarked. Data elements marked with a bullet represent elements not included among the NHTSA elements but recommended during the ASTM consensus process.

5.3.2 All dates are coded numerically as YYYYMMDD. Time is coded numerically as HHMM. Multiple entries should be possible particularly for patient assessment criteria.

5.3.2.1 *Onset Date*—Date of onset of symptoms or injury date.

5.3.2.2 *Onset Time*—Time of onset of symptoms or injury time.

5.3.2.3 **Date Incident Reported*—Date the call is first received by a public safety answering point (PSAP) or other designated entity.

5.3.2.4 **Time Incident Reported*—Time the call is first received by a public safety answering point (PSAP) or other designated entity.

5.3.2.5 •*Public Safety Incident Number*—The incident number assigned by the PSAP when the call for help is received.

5.3.2.6 **Time EMS Dispatch Notified*—Time of first connection with EMS dispatch.

5.3.2.7 **Incident Number*—Unique number for each incident reported to EMS dispatch. This number is assigned by EMS. If there is a CAD system, this would be the CAD system incident number.

5.3.2.8 **Patient name*—The current name of the patient receiving emergency medical care services for whom the record is being created and about whom data are being collected. The name should be defined to include last name, first name, middle name, initial.

5.3.2.9 *Age*—The patients age:

{3 digits for age in years}
888 Not applicable
999 Unknown
000 For patients up to 1 year of age

5.3.2.10 **Date of birth*—Patient's date of birth.

5.3.2.11 **Gender*—The gender of the patient:

M Male
F Female
U Unknown

5.3.2.12 **Race/Ethnicity*—Patient's ethnic origin including:

1 White non-Hispanic
2 White Hispanic
3 Black non-Hispanic
4 Black Hispanic
5 American Indian/Alaskan Native
6 Asian or Pacific Islander
7 Other
8 Not applicable
9 Unknown

5.3.2.13 *Social Security Number*—Patient social security number:

{9 digit SSN}
888888888 Not applicable
999999999 Unknown

5.3.2.14 *Patient Street Address*—Patient's address of actual residence.

5.3.2.15 **City of Residence*—Patient's city or township of actual residence (if applicable):

{5 digit FIPS code}
88888 Not applicable
99999 Unknown

5.3.2.16 *County of Residence*—Patient's county actual residence (if applicable):

{3 digit FIPS code}
888 Not applicable
999 Unknown

5.3.2.17 *State of Residence*—State, territory, or province, or District of Columbia, where patient resides:

{2 digit FIPS code}
88 Not applicable
99 Unknown

5.3.2.18 **Zip Code of Residence*——Zip code of patient's residence:

{5 digit Zip Code}
88888 Not applicable
99999 Unknown

5.3.2.19 *Telephone Number*—Patient's primary telephone number:

{10 digit telephone number}
8888888888 Not applicable
9999999999 Unknown

5.3.2.20 **Agency/Unit Number*—Number that identifies the agency and unit responding to an incident (state specific).

5.3.2.21 **Patient Care Record Number*—Unique number for each patient care record (PCR) (state specific).

5.3.2.22 **Response Number*—Unique number for each individual response by a response team/vehicle to an incident (team/agency specific).

5.3.2.23 **Service Type*—Type of service requested:

1 Scene
2 Unscheduled interfacility transfer
3 Scheduled interfacility transfer
4 Standby
5 Rendezvous
8 Not applicable
9 Unknown

5.3.2.24 **Vehicle Type*—Type of vehicle that responded to the incident:

1 Ground (transport, non-transport)
2 Rotor craft
3 Fixed wing
4 Other
5 None

5.3.2.25 •*Mileage at Outset*—The mileage at the time the

vehicle is dispatched on a run.

5.3.2.26 •*Mileage at Scene*—The mileage on the vehicle when it arrives at the scene.

5.3.2.27 •*Mileage at Destination*—The mileage on the vehicle when the patient is transferred to the receiving health care facility.

5.3.2.28 •*Mileage at Return*—The mileage when the vehicle returns to its point of outset.

5.3.2.29 **Crew Member One Number*—Personnel certification/license number for crew member who is designated as responsible for the care of the patient. This person will be the signer of the patient care record. The personnel certification/license number should be a unique identifier statewide.

5.3.2.30 **Crew Member One Type*—Type of personnel certification/license for first crew member:

1 First responder
2 EMT basic
3 EMT intermediate
4 EMT paramedic
5 Nurse
6 Physician
7 Other health care professional
8 None of the above
9 Unknown

5.3.2.31 **Crew Member Two Number*—Personnel certification/license number for second crew member. This should be a unique identifier statewide.

5.3.2.32 **Crew Member Two Type*—Type of personnel certification/license for second crew member.

1 First responder
2 EMT basic
3 EMT intermediate
4 EMT paramedic
5 Nurse
6 Physician
7 Other health care professional
8 None of the above
9 Unknown

5.3.2.33 *Crew Member Three Number*—Personnel certification/license number for third crew member. This should be a unique identifier statewide.

5.3.2.34 *Crew Member Three Type*—Type of personnel certification/license for second crew member.

1 First responder
2 EMT basic
3 EMT intermediate
4 EMT paramedic
5 Nurse
6 Physician
7 Other health care professional
8 None of the above
9 Unknown

5.3.2.35 •*Highest Available Level of Care*—This should be determined by the ability to deliver care at the time of the patient encounter whether limited by certification status of the most senior individual or the type of equipment being carried at the time.

1 EMT—paramedic
2 EMT—advanced/intermediate
3 EMT—basic
4 EMT—other

5.3.2.36 •*Initiation of Service Request*:

1 Emergency, 911
2 Emergency, non-911
3 Scheduled transport
4 On-scene request (for example, squad happens to witness accident)
5 Other

5.3.2.37 *Date Unit Notified*—Date response unit is notified by EMS dispatch.

5.3.2.38 **Time Unit Notified*—Time response unit is notified by EMS dispatch.

5.3.2.39 •*Location/Status of Responding Unit*—Coded value to indicate the location/status (primary post, secondary post, enroute back, etc.) of the responding unit when notified by EMS dispatch. This element should be defined according to local dispatch configurations.

5.3.2.40 **Lights and Sirens to Scene*—The use of lights and sirens enroute to scene:

1 Non-emergent, no lights or sirens
2 Initial emergent, downgraded to no lights or sirens
3 Initial non-emergent, upgraded to lights or sirens
4 Emergent, with lights or sirens
8 Not applicable

5.3.2.41 **Time Unit Responding*—Time that the response unit begins physical motion.

5.3.2.42 **Time of Arrival at Scene*—Time EMS unit stops physical motion at scene (last place that the unit or vehicle stops prior to assessing the patient).

5.3.2.43 *Time of Arrival at Patient*—Time response personnel establish direct contact with patient.

5.3.2.44 **Time Unit Left Scene*—Time when the response unit began physical motion from scene.

5.3.2.45 **Time of Arrival at Destination*—Time when the patient arrives at destination or transfer point.

5.3.2.46 **Time Back in Service*—Time response unit back in service and available for response.

5.3.2.47 **Location Type/Scene Description*—Type of location of incident including:

849.0 Home/residence
849.1 Farm
849.2 Mine/quarry
849.3 Industrial place and premises
849.4 Place for recreation or sport
849.5 Street or highway
849.6 Public building
849.7 Residential institution
849.E Educational institution
849.8 Other specified location
849.9 Unspecified location
849.10 Unknown

5.3.2.48 **Incident Address*—Address (or best approximation) where patient was found, or, if no patient, address to which unit responded. Use route numbers and mileposts, or other landmarks, which can be coded in a consistent manner if a street address is not applicable. In maritime areas and in rural and wilderness areas, consideration should be given to use of geographic information system (GIS) coordinates or geographic positioning system (GPS) coordinates corresponding to the location of the incident site.

5.3.2.49 **Incident City*—City or township (if applicable) where patient was found, or to which unit responded (or best approximation):

{5 digit FIPS code}
88888 Not applicable

99999 Unknown

5.3.2.50 *Incident County*—County or parish (if applicable) where patient was found, or to which unit responded (or best approximation):

{3 digit FIPS code}
888 Not applicable
999 Unknown

5.3.2.51 *Incident State*—State, territory, or province, or District of Columbia, where patient was found or to which unit responded:

{2 digit FIPS code}
88 Not applicable
99 Unknown

5.3.2.52 *Factors Affecting EMS Delivery of Care*—Special circumstances affecting the EMS response or delivery of care:

01 Adverse weather
02 Adverse road conditions
03 Vehicle problems
04 Unsafe scene
05 Language barrier
06 Prolonged extrication (>20 min)
07 Hazardous material
08 Crowd control
09 Other
88 Not applicable

5.3.2.53 •*Complaint at Dispatch*—Patient's chief complaint as reported at the time of dispatch.

5.3.2.54 *Cause of Injury*—External cause of injury (E code):

81x.x Motor vehicle traffic crash
814.x Pedestrian traffic accident
82x.x Motor vehicle non-traffic crash
826.x Bicycle accident
83x.x Water transport accident
84x.x Aircraft related accident
85x.x Accidental drug poisoning
86x.x Accidental chemical poisoning
88x.x Accidental falls
890.x Fire and flames
890.2 Smoke inhalation
900.x Excessive heat
901.x Excessive cold
905.x Venomous stings (plants, animals)
906.x Animal Bites
907.x Lightning
907.x Lightning
910.x Drowning
913.x Mechanical suffocation
919.x Machinery accidents
925.x Electrocution (non-lightning)
925.x Electrocution (non-lightning)
926.x Radiation exposure
955.x Firearm self-inflicted (intentional)
960.1 Rape/sexual assault
965.x Firearm assault
966.x Stabbing assault
967.x Child assault/abuse

Other assault:

985.x Firearm injury (accidental)
000.8 Not applicable
000.9 Unknown
Other (Record as narrative)

5.3.2.55 *Safety Equipment*—Safety equipment in use by the patient at time of the injury.

00 None
01 Shoulder belt only used
02 Lap belt only used
03 Shoulder and lap belt device
04 Child safety seat
05 Helmet used
06 Airbag, not deployed
07 Airbag deployed, no belt used
08 Airbag deployed, shoulder belt used
09 Airbag deployed, lap belt used
10 Airbag deployed, lap and shoulder used
11 Airbag deployed, child safety seat used
12 Eye protection used
13 Protective clothing used
14 Personal flotation device used
15 Protective clothing/gear used
88 Not applicable
99 Unknown

5.3.2.56 *Suspected Alcohol/Drug Use*—Suspected alcohol or drug use by patient:

1 Alcohol, yes
2 Drugs, yes
3 Alcohol/Drugs, yes
8 Not applicable
9 Unknown

5.3.2.57 *Injury Intent*—Intent of individual inflicting injury:

1 Intentional, self
2 Intentional, other
3 Unintentional
8 Not applicable
9 Unknown

5.3.2.58 •*First Responder Organization Identification Number*—This should be a unique alphanumeric sequence assigned by the state which identifies each first responder organization in the state, and should be listed on the provider run PCR if a trained first responder was present at the scene.

5.3.2.59 •*Bystander Assistance*—This should indicate which type of first aid was administered by a non-first responder at the scene and be coded as:

1 Extrication
2 Airway assistance/Heimlich maneuver
3 Bleeding control
4 CPR
5 Multiple
6 Automatic external defibrillator
7 Other

5.3.2.60 *Chief Complaint*—Statement of problem by patient or other person to provider.

5.3.2.61 *Provider Impression*—Provider's clinical impression that led to the management given to the patient (treatments, medications, procedures):

789.00 Abdominal pain/problems
519.80 Airway obstruction
995.30 Allergic reaction
780.09 Altered level of consciousness
312.90 Behavioral
427.50 Cardiac arrest
427.90 Cardiac rhythm disturbance
786.50 Chest pain/discomfort
250.90 Diabetic symptoms (hypoglycemia)
994.80 Electrocution
780.60 Hyperthermia
785.59 Hypovolemia/shock
987.90 Inhalation injury (toxic gas)
798.99 Obvious death
977.90 Poisoning, drug ingestion
659.90 Pregnancy/OB delivery
799.10 Respiratory arrest
786.09 Respiratory distress
780.30 Seizure
959.90 Sexual assault/rape

987.90 Smoke inhalation
989.50 Stings/venomous bites
991.60 Hypothermia
436.00 Stroke/CVA
780.20 Syncope/fainting
959.90 Traumatic injury
623.80 Vaginal hemorrhage
623.80 Vaginal hemorrhage
000.77 Other
000.88 Not applicable
000.99 Unknown

5.3.2.62 •*Initial Assessment Acuity*—Coded value to indicate the initial assessment of patient acuity by provider at the scene before care is rendered. This data element should be defined according to local standards to facilitate quality assurance and managed care activities. The definition should be consistent with the definition for 5.3.2.99.

5.3.2.63 *Preexisting Condition Source of Data*—Source of information about the patient's preexisting condition recorded in 5.3.2.64:

01 Patient
02 Relative/Friend
03 Central monitoring agency (for example, private security organization storing health records)
04 Physician/patient provider
05 Other

5.3.2.64 **Preexisting Condition*, Preexisting medical conditions known to the provider:

493.90 Asthma
239.90 Cancer
585.00 Chronic renal failure
518.81 Chronic respiratory failure
250.00 Diabetes
492.80 Emphysema
401.90 Hypertension
312.90 Psychiatric problems
780.30 Seizure convulsions
V44.00 Tracheostomy
011.90 Tuberculosis

5.3.2.65 **Signs and Symptoms Present*—Signs and symptoms reported to or observed by provider:

789.00 Abdominal pain
724.50 Back pain
578.10 Bloody stools
786.09 Breathing difficulty
427.50 Cardiorespiratory arrest
786.50 Chest pain
933.10 Choking
558.90 Diarrhea
780.40 Dizziness
388.70 Ear pain
379.91 Eye pain
780.60 Fever/hyperthermia
784.00 Headache
401.90 Hypertension
787.00 Nausea
344.90 Paralysis
785.10 Palpitations
659.90 Pregnancy/childbirth/miscarriage
780.30 Seizures/convulsions
780.20 Syncope
780.09 Unresponsive/unconscious
Uncontrolled bleeding
623.80 Vaginal bleeding
787.00 Vomiting
780.70 Weakness (malaise)
991.60 Hypothermia

5.3.2.66 **Systolic Blood Pressure*—Patient's systolic blood pressure:

{Systolic BP}
888 Not obtained
999 Unknown

5.3.2.67 *Diastolic Blood Pressure*—Patient's diastolic blood pressure:

{Diastolic BP}
888 Not obtained
999 Unknown

5.3.2.68 **Pulse Rate*—Patient's palpated or auscultated pulse rate expressed in number per minute:

{Pulse rate}
888 Not obtained
999 Unknown

5.3.2.69 **Respiratory Rate*—Unassisted patient respiratory rate expressed as number per minute:

{Respiratory rate}
888 Not obtained
999 Unknown

5.3.2.70 *Respiratory Effort*—Patient's respiratory effort (this field is essential for children 18 years or less):

0 Normal
1 Increased, not labored
2 Increased and labored or decreased and fatigued
3 Absent
9 Not assessed

5.3.2.71 *Skin Perfusion*—Patient skin perfusion, expressed as normal or decreased (this field is essential for children 18 years or less):

1 Normal
2 Decreased
9 Not assessed

5.3.2.72 *Treatment Authorization*—Indicates the type, if any, of treatment authorization:

01 Protocol (standing orders)
02 On-line (radio telephone)
03 On-scene
04 Written orders (patient specific)
88 Not applicable
99 Unknown

5.3.2.73 •*Initiation of ALS*—Coded as:

Before contact with medical direction
After contact with medical direction
No ALS initiated

5.3.2.74 •*On Line Medical Direction Facility Number*—This should be the unique identification number of the radio resource facility, regardless of whether or not the radio resource/medical control facility ultimately received the patient.

5.3.2.75 •*Time on-line Medical Direction Established*—Best estimate of time medical director contacted or protocol implemented.

5.3.2.76 *Time of First CPR*—Best estimate of time of first CPR.

5.3.2.77 *Provider of First CPR*—Person who performed first CPR on patient:

1 Bystander
2 EMS responder
3 Not applicable
9 Unknown

5.3.2.78 *Time CPR Discontinued*—Time at which medical

control or responding EMS unit terminated resuscitation efforts (chest compressions and CPR) in the field.

5.3.2.79 •*Time of Witnessed Cardiac Arrest*—Time of witnessed cardiac arrest.

5.3.2.80 *Witness of Cardiac Arrest*—Person who witnessed the cardiac arrest:

1 Bystander
2 EMS responder
3 Not applicable
9 Unknown

5.3.2.81 *Time of First Defibrillatory Shock*—Time of first defibrillatory shock.

5.3.2.82 *Return of Spontaneous Circulation*—Whether a palpable pulse or blood pressure was restored following cardiac arrest and resuscitation in the field:

1 Yes
2 No
8 Not applicable

5.3.2.83 *Initial Cardiac Rhythm*—Initial monitored cardiac rhythm as interpreted by EMS personnel:

01 Sinus rhythm
02 Other rhythm from 60–100 (not otherwise listed)
03 Paced rhythm
04 Bradycardia
05 Extrasystole
06 Narrow complex tachycardia
07 Wide complex tachycardia
08 Ventricular fibrillation
09 Asystole
10 Pulseless electrical activity
88 Not applicable
99 Unknown

5.3.2.84 *Rhythm at Destination*—Monitored cardiac rhythm upon arrival at destination:

01 Sinus rhythm
02 Other rhythm from 60–100 (not otherwise listed)
03 Paced rhythm
04 Bradycardia
05 Extrasystole
06 Narrow complex tachycardia
08 Ventricular fibrillation
07 Wide complex tachycardia
09 Asystole
10 Pulseless electrical activity
88 Not applicable
99 Unknown

5.3.2.85 **Glasgow Coma Score, Eye*—A one-digit number denoting the eye component of the patient's Glasgow coma score at the time of the provider's arrival on scene.

1 None
2 Opens eyes in response to painful stimulation
3 Opens eyes in response to verbal stimulation
4 Opens eyes spontaneously
9 Unknown

5.3.2.86 **Glasgow Coma Score, Verbal*—A one-digit number denoting the verbal component of the patient's Glasgow coma score at the time of the provider's arrival on scene:

For patients >5 years:

1 None
2 Nonspecific sounds
3 Inappropriate words
4 Confused conversation or speech
5 Oriented and appropriate speech
9 Unknown

For patients 2–5 years:

1 None
2 Moans, whimpers, unintelligible sounds
3 Inappropriate words
4 Confused conversation or speech
5 Appropriate words or speech
9 Not assessed

For patients 0–23 months:

1 None
2 Moans, whimpers
3 Irritable cry words
4 Cries but inconsolable
5 Cries appropriately to stimulus, smiles, coos, fixes, and follows
9 Not assessed

5.3.2.87 **Glasgow Coma Score, Motor*—A one-digit number denoting the motor component of the patient's Glasgow coma score at the time of the provider's arrival on scene.

For patients >5 years:

1 None
2 Extensor posturing in response to painful stimulation
3 Flexor posturing in response to painful stimulation
4 General withdrawal in response to painful stimulation
5 Localization of painful stimulation
6 Obeys commands with appropriate motor response
9 Unknown

For patients up to 5 years:

1 None
2 Extensor posturing in response to painful stimulation
3 Flexor posturing in response to painful stimulation
4 General withdrawal in response to painful stimulation
5 Localization of painful stimulation
6 Spontaneous or purposeful movement
9 Not assessed

5.3.2.88 *Glasgow Coma Score Total*—A two-digit number denoting the patient's first GCS to be automatically calculated at the time of computerization.

5.3.2.89 *Revised Trauma Score*—Patient's revised trauma score.

Respiratory Rate Component:

4 10–29 min
3 >29 min
2 6–9 min
1 1–5 min
0 None spontaneous

Systolic Blood Pressure Component:

4 >89 mm Hg
3 76–89 mm Hg
2 50–75 mm Hg
1 1–49 mm Hg
0 No pulse

Neurologic Component:

4 Glasgow coma score 13–15
3 Glasgow coma score 9–12
2 Glasgow coma score 6–8
1 Glasgow coma score 4–5
0 Glasgow coma score 3

5.3.2.90 •*Other Severity Measures Implemented at the Scene*—Coded value to indicate severity determined from other measures, such as blood sugar, etc. This data element should be defined locally to support quality improvement activities.

5.3.2.91 **Injury Description*—Clinical description of injury type and body site to be organized as a matrix for data collection:

Body Sites:

A External (including burns)
B Head only (excluding neck, cervical, spine, and ear)
C Face (including ear)
D Neck
E Thorax (excluding thoracic spine)
F Abdomen (excluding lumbar spine)
G Spine
H Upper extremities
I Lower extremities or bony pelvis
J Body region unspecified

Injury types:

01 Amputation
02 Blunt injury
03 Burn
04 Crush
05 Dislocation/fracture
06 Gunshot
07 Laceration
08 Pain without swelling/bruising
09 Puncture/stab
10 Soft tissue swelling/bruising

5.3.2.92 **Medication Name*—Medication name, time, and identification of provider giving the medication. The medications include but are not limited to:

1.1 Diphenhydramine
2.1 Atropine
3.1 Albuterol
3.2 Terbutaline
3.3 Dopamine
3.4 Epinephrine
3.5 Isoproterenol
3.6 Metaproterenol
4.1 Succinylcholine
5.1 Heparin
6.1 Adenosine
6.2 Bretylium tosylate
6.3 Lidocaine
6.4 Procainamide
6.5 Verapamil
6.6 Nifedipine
7.1 Amyl nitrate
7.2 Nitroglycerin
8.1 Aspirin
9.1 Meperidine
9.2 Morphine
10.1 Naloxone
11.1 Acetaminophen
12.1 Diazepam
13.1 Magnesium sulfate
14.1 Lorazep
15.1 Sodium bicarbonate
16.1 Calcium chloride
16.2 Calcium gluconate
17.1 Dextrose and water (50 %)
18.1 Furosemide
18.2 Mannitol
18.3 Bumetanide
19.1 Charcoal, activated
20.1 Ipecac
21.1 Metoclopramide
22.1 Dexamethasone
22.2 Methylprednisolone
23.1 Glucagon
24.1 Thiamine

5.3.2.93 **Procedure or Treatment Name*—Procedure or treatment name, time, and identification of provider giving the medication. The procedures include but are not limited to:

96.70 Assisted ventilation (positive pressure)
93.59 Backboard
39.98 Bleeding controlled
93.57 Burn care
99.60 Cardiopulmonary resuscitation
93.52 Cervical immobilization
31.10 Cricothyrotomy
89.51 ECG monitoring
96.04 Endotracheal intubation
99.63 External cardiac massage
99.62 External defibrillation (includes auto)
38.93 Intravenous catheter
41.92 Intraosseous catheter
99.29 Intravenous fluids
93.58 MAST (military antishock trousers)
96.01 Nasopharyngeal airway insertion
96.05 Nasogastric tube insertion
73.59 Obstetrical care (delivery)
96.02 Oropharyngeal airway insertion
93.96 Oxygen by mask
93.96 Oxygen by cannula
93.54 Splint of extremity
93.54 Traction splint

5.3.2.94 *Procedure Attempts*—Total number of attempts for each procedure attempted, regardless of success.

5.3.2.95 **Destination Determination*—Reason a transport destination was selected:

01 Closest facility (none below)
02 Patient/family choice
03 Patient physician choice
04 Managed care
05 Law enforcement choice
06 Protocol
07 Specialty resource center
08 On-line medical direction
09 Diversion
10 Other
88 Not applicable
99 Unknown

5.3.2.96 **Lights or Sirens, or both, Used from Scene*—Use of lights or sirens, or both, from the scene:

1 Non-emergent, no lights or sirens
2 Initial emergent, downgraded to no lights or sirens
3 Initial non-emergent, upgraded to lights or sirens
4 Emergent, with lights or sirens
8 Not applicable

5.3.2.97 **Destination/Transferred to*—Health care facility or pre-hospital unit/home that received patient from EMS responder providing this record. Facilities will be recorded by unique identification numbers.

01 Home
02 Police/jail
03 Medical office/clinic
04 Other EMS responder (ground)
05 Other EMS responder (air)
06 Hospital
07 Morgue
08 Free-standing emergency center
09 Nursing Home
88 Not applicable

5.3.2.98 **Incident/Patient Disposition*—End result of EMS response.

01 Treated, transported by EMS
02 Treated, transferred care
03 Treated, transported by private vehicle
04 Treated and released
05 No treatment required
06 Patient refused care
07 Dead at scene
08 Canceled
88 Not applicable
99 Unknown
00 No patient found

5.3.2.99 •*Insurance Class*——This should reflect the patients payer classification as determined by the crew members.

01 Commercial insurance
02 Subscription to ambulance
03 Medicare
04 Champus
05 Workers compensation
06 State Medicaid
07 Public/county assistance
08 Self-pay or uninsured
09 No charge
10 Managed health care plan
11 Other

5.3.2.100 •*Change of Condition*—Coded value to indicate the level of change in the patient's condition upon arrival at the destination. This data element should be defined according to local standards to facilitate quality assurance and managed care activities.

5.3.3 The following data elements should be recorded for each EMS provider in the "EMS Training/Skill" Database File (5.8.6.7(2))

5.3.3.1 *Last Name*—The last name of the individual provider employed by the PSO observing the conventions.

5.3.3.2 *First Name*—The first name of the provider employed by the PSO.

5.3.3.3 *Address*—The mailing street address where the provider resides.

5.3.3.4 *City*—The city in which the provider resides.

5.3.3.5 *State*—The two letter state abbreviation as determined by the Postmaster General where the provider resides.

5.3.3.6 *Zip Code*—The five-digit code in which the provider resides.

5.3.3.7 *Phone Number*—The area code and phone number where the provider resides.

5.3.3.8 *State License or Certification Number*—This should be a unique identifier for each provider.

5.3.3.9 *Current Training Level*—This should describe the highest current certification for the crew member:

EMT—paramedic
EMT—advanced/intermediate
EMT—basic
EMT—defibrillation

5.3.3.10 *Most Recent Certification Date*—The certification date of the provider's current license.

5.3.3.11 *Most Recent Expiration Date*—The expiration date of the provider's current license.

5.3.3.12 *Most Recent ACLS Expiration Date*—The expiration date of the provider's ACLS certification.

5.3.3.13 *Most Recent BCLS Expiration Date*—The expiration date of the provider's BCLS certification.

5.3.3.14 *Other Certification One*—Other pertinent certification that the provider holds.

5.3.3.15 *Other Certificate Date One*—The expiration date of certification listed in 5.3.3.13.

5.3.3.16 *Other Certification Two*—Other pertinent certification that the provider holds.

5.3.3.17 *Other Certification Date Two*—The expiration date of certification listed in 5.3.3.15.

5.3.4 The following data elements should be recorded by the provider and maintained in a log recording continuing medical education (CME) (5.8.6.7.(*3*)).

5.3.4.1 *Last Name*—The last name of the provider who attended a CME course.

5.3.4.2 *First Name*—The first name of the provider who attended a CME course.

5.3.4.3 *State License Number*—The state license number of the provider who attended the CME course.

5.3.4.4 *Course Title*—The title of the CME course taken by the provider.

5.3.4.5 *Course Date*—The date of the CME course taken by the provider.

5.3.4.6 *Number of Hours*—The number of credit hours awarded for successful completion of the CME course.

5.3.4.7 *Type of Course*—A number describing the type of CME course completed:

1 Certification
2 Recertification
3 Continuing Education
4 Clinical Rotation
5 Other

5.3.4.8 *Sponsoring Agency*—The name of the agency or person sponsoring the CME course.

5.3.4.9 *Certifying Agency*—The name of the agency or person certifying the CME course.

5.4 *Hospital*:

5.4.1 *Medical Direction*—The following data elements should be logged at the emergency department and maintained, as appropriate, in a "Medical Direction" database file (5.8.6.7.(*4a*)).

5.4.1.1 *Medical Direction Document Number*—An internal control number that logs a request for on line medical direction or documents notification to the hospital of an impending patient arrival.

5.4.1.2 *Date Call Received*—The date that the request for on-line medical direction was received by the hospital.

5.4.1.3 *Time Call Received*—The time that a request for on-line medical direction was received by the hospital.

5.4.1.4 *PSO/Run Number*—The PSO identification number of the provider requesting on-line medical direction.

5.4.1.5 *Medical Direction Physician Number*—The state license number of the physician responsible for the episode of on-line medical direction.

5.4.1.6 *Medical Director Number*—The individual's state license number for anyone other than the responsible physician who gave on-line medical direction.

5.4.1.7 *Age*—The age of the patient being transported.

5.4.1.8 *Sex*—The sex of the patient being transported:

Male
Female
Unknown

5.4.1.9 *Chief Complaint*—The reason the patient accessed the EMS system.

5.4.1.10 *Type Injury/Illness*—As defined in 5.3.1.61.

5.4.1.11 *Allergies*—Known patient indication of allergies.

5.4.1.12 *Current Medications*—Known medications currently being taken by the patient.

5.4.1.13 *Initial Systolic Blood Pressure*—As defined in 5.3.2.65.

5.4.1.14 *Initial Diastolic Blood Pressure*—As defined in 5.3.2.66.

5.4.1.15 *Initial Pulse*—As defined in 5.3.2.67.

5.4.1.16 *Initial Respiratory Rate*—As defined in 5.3.2.68.

5.4.1.17 *Glasgow Coma Score*—As defined in 5.3.2.87.

5.4.1.18 *First Cardiac Rhythm*—As defined in 5.3.2.82.

5.4.1.19 *Last Cardiac Rhythm*—As defined in 5.3.2.83.

5.4.1.20 *Treatments*—As defined in 5.3.2.92.

5.4.1.21 *Medication*—As defined in 5.3.2.91.

5.4.1.22 *Call Disposition*—As defined in 5.3.2.96.

5.4.1.23 *Receiving Hospital Identification Number*—As defined in 5.3.2.96.

5.4.1.24 Flag to identify cases, such as major trauma, medication errors, unusual occurrence, and so forth, for quality assurance/improvement review.

5.4.2 *Emergency Outpatient Patient Record*:

5.4.2.1 Outcome information describing the status of patients after arrival at an emergency outpatient facility is needed to evaluate the structure, process, and outcome of emergency medical services delivered at the scene and enroute. For this type of evaluation to be successful, it is important to access information that describes the population receiving care and the population not receiving care prior to arrival.

5.4.2.2 The following data elements represent a subset of the information collected for the emergency patient receiving outpatient care. They have been chosen because of their usefulness for evaluating the effectiveness of the EMS system response and patient care at the scene and enroute and for linkage to other medical records. The data element specifications should be compatible with the variables listed in 5.3.2. These variables are referred to as "Emergency Department Patient Record" database file (5.8.6.7(*4b*)) in the logic model presented later and include the following:

Patient name
Address
City
State
Zip code
Telephone
Age
Gender
Medical record number
Arrival means
Arrival means
EMS agency number
Treating emergency physician
Date of visit
Time of arrival
Chief complaint
Severity
Vital signs
Procedures
Discharge diagnosis narrative
ICD-9-CM dx1-n
E code
V code
Date of discharge from ED
Time of discharge from ED
Disposition
Payer classification

5.4.3 Similar information is needed about emergency patients who receive treatment as an inpatient in order to evaluate the structure, process, and outcome of emergency medical services delivered at the scene and enroute.

5.4.3.1 The following data elements represent a subset of the information collected for the emergency inpatient receiving acute care. They have been chosen because of their usefulness for evaluating the effectiveness of the EMS system response and patient care at the scene and enroute and for linkage to other medical records. The following data elements are maintained in the "Hospital Discharge" file (5.8.6.7.(*4c*)):

Patient inpatient record number
Date of admission
Hour of admission
Attending physician
Principal surgeon
Discharge diagnosis codes (ICD-9-CM)
Procedure codes (ICD-9-CM)
Date of discharge
Disposition
Diagnosis related group
Major diagnosis category at discharge

5.5 *Procedure for Adoption of Statewide Minimum EMS Data Set*:

5.5.1 Establishment and utilization of a standard medical emergency data set should be encouraged to simplify EMS-MIS feedback at the state, regional, and local levels.

5.5.2 The standardized data to be collected should be relative to the goals and capabilities of the EMS-MIS system.

5.5.2.1 Some of the goals of standardization include:

(1) Enhancement of documentation of patient care.

(2) Enhancement of patient information reporting from the scene, enroute, and at the time of patient arrival at the receiving facility.

(3) Efficient and appropriate data capture.

(4) Enhancement of statistical analysis.

(5) Linkage of data elements for uploading to higher level data collection systems.

5.5.2.2 Some of the benefits of standardization include:

(1) Improved system resource allocation.

(2) Improved medical and legal documentation.

(3) Improved provider skill monitoring and feedback.

(4) Elimination of peripheral documentation.

(5) Improve EMS billing and collections.

5.5.3 Initial planning for standardization should allow the inclusion of the data elements in 5.3.2 to satisfy data requirements for local and higher level reporting needs.

5.5.4 The process for determining what information should be standardized should include consideration of the following:

5.5.4.1 Data collection should be efficient.

5.5.4.2 Data should be recorded in a logical sequence that parallels the process of dispatch, patient evaluation, treatment, and transport.

5.5.4.3 A narrative section should be included to record descriptive data deemed helpful by the provider. This section should be computerized if feasible.

5.5.4.4 Basic and advanced life support provider service organizations should be part of the same EMS-MIS system for both emergency or prescheduled calls.

5.5.4.5 Data elements should be congregated according to classification or usage.

5.5.4.6 The elements should include data collected at the scene, enroute, and at the hospital.

5.5.4.7 The data should be easily coded and computerized.

5.5.5 The development of the local EMS-MIS should be a collaborative process, involving a representative cross-sectional group of those individuals who own and use the information being collected including:

5.5.5.1 State or federal EMS representatives.

5.5.5.2 Regional EMS administrators.

5.5.5.3 Local EMS administrators.

5.5.5.4 Providers of emergency care (pre-hospital, hospital).

5.5.5.5 Injury control and other health organizations/agencies.

5.5.6 Drafts of the proposed EMS-MIS should be submitted for review to a broader representative sample of the group in 5.5.5 and appropriate suggestions and comments incorporated.

5.5.7 When a comprehensive draft of the proposed EMS-MIS has been developed, it should be submitted to representatives of other groups interested in EMS for additional scrutiny:

5.5.7.1 Medical records personnel.

5.5.7.2 Law enforcement officials.

5.5.7.3 Fire services.

5.5.7.4 Medical examiners.

5.5.8 The proposed EMS-MIS should be tested in a pilot study prior to statewide implementation.

5.5.9 After adoption, the EMS-MIS should be reviewed yearly by the group in 5.5.5 to measure its effectiveness and implement any needed changes.

5.5.10 Statewide legislation mandating compliance with the EMS-MIS by all PSOs has many benefits in areas of cost reduction and gaining 100 % participation.

5.6 *Confidentiality and Security of Data*:

5.6.1 The policies and procedures to protect confidentiality of individual patients and their families, hospitals, and ambulance services are extremely important and require special attention. Security requirements involve a number of issues, including:

5.6.1.1 Privacy rights of the patients.

5.6.1.2 Liability.

5.6.1.3 Potential inaccuracies.

5.6.1.4 Media coverage.

5.6.1.5 Ownership of data.

5.6.2 All formulated policies and procedures must be written taking into account any state laws pertaining to such matters. Efforts should be made to enact state legislation which deems EMS-MIS information non-discoverable.

5.6.3 A system should be based upon the supposition that users will have access to the data and information which they generated and to comparative local, regional, and state averages and totals for comparison.

5.6.4 Systems must provide an appropriate level of data security.

5.6.5 Security should be developed to protect aggregated data from unauthorized use.

5.6.5.1 The data collection center or its agent shall not make data available to any party other than the owner of the data without prior written consent by the owner.

5.6.5.2 The center, in collaboration with the data owner, shall disseminate summaries of the data that do not provide information identifying specific individuals or organizations, or both.

5.6.5.3 Written data release policies will include severe penalties for users who violate them.

5.6.6 A blanket confidentiality statement should preface all documents, procedures, and policies prepared or implemented by the EMS-MIS. An example blanket statement is as follows:

5.6.6.1 All information identifying an individual obtained by any central data collection center shall be held confidential and shall not be divulged without the individual's consent, except as may be required by law, or as may be necessary to provide service to the individual. Information may be disclosed in summary statistical or other form that does not identify particular individuals.

5.6.7 The following technical features should be incorporated in the system design as appropriate.

5.6.7.1 Individual user identification and password protection should be employed.

5.6.7.2 Confidentiality of patient data must be maintained during all phases of data collection, processing, and analysis.

5.6.7.3 Terminal identification should exist within a network, and terminal lock-out and time-out features should be incorporated.

5.6.7.4 File and record access should be uniquely identified and separately restricted.

5.6.7.5 Security violations should be reported at the central processing site and reported to the appropriate authority and involved organizations.

5.6.7.6 Software maintenance control should be enforced.

5.6.7.7 Report distribution procedures should be developed and followed.

5.7 Data Processing System Configurations:

5.7.1 Methodology for Data Collection:

5.7.1.1 Data capture must occur in a timely, efficient, complete manner if meaningful information about the system as a whole is to be generated.

5.7.1.2 Data capture involves the following sequences of events, as shown in Fig. 3.

5.7.2 *Data and Information Timeliness*:

5.7.2.1 Data capture will occur most reliably when the data are entered into the computer and validated as soon as possible after the event that generated the data. Ideally, this would be done by the observer who actually recorded the data, thereby eliminating delays due to report form illegibility, incompleteness, and lost forms.

5.7.2.2 Timely entering of data allows for faster generation of useful information and its return to managers who will utilize such information.

5.7.3 *Methods of Data Recording and Data Entry*:

5.7.3.1 In most circumstances, recording of data will involve the generation of handwritten records as diagrammed in Fig. 4, and subsequent computer entry of data from the records.

5.7.3.2 In some instances, portions of the records generated in Fig. 4 may be completed on a form that can be read by an optical scanning device. The optical scanner converts the coded information to electromagnetic format automatically. Advantages of this method are:

(1) That the forms are easy to enter into the computer thereby reducing transcription error.

(2) Data entry costs are minimal after the initial purchase of the scanner.

5.7.3.3 Disadvantages of this method are:

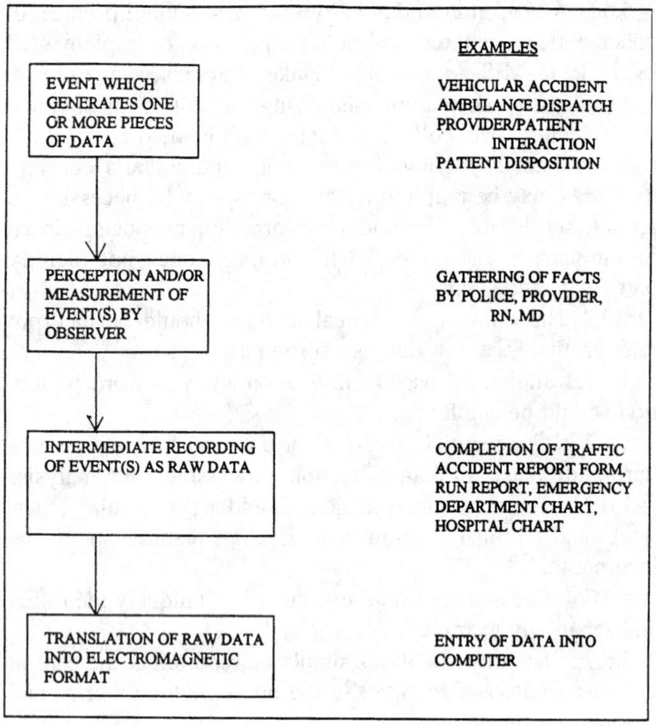

FIG. 3 Data Capture

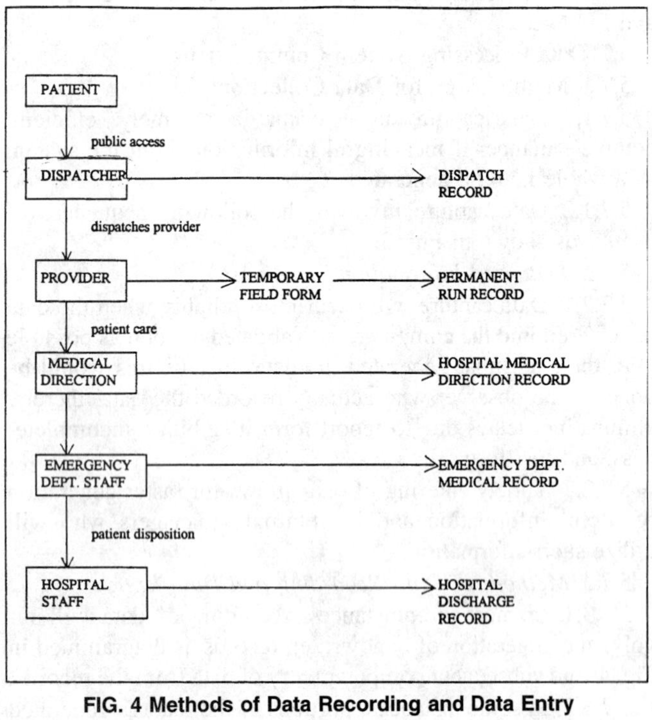

FIG. 4 Methods of Data Recording and Data Entry

(1) Cost of the forms is high because of the quality of paper needed.

(2) Alphanumeric data are difficult to enter.

(3) The form is cumbersome to fill out.

(4) The form is difficult to read.

(5) Forms must be collected and sent to a central input facility and are subject to loss.

(6) Staff are necessary to correct errors on records that have been rejected.

5.7.3.4 Keyboard entry of handwritten records has been a common and familiar data entry method.

5.7.3.5 Keyboard entry can be simplified by programmed menu-driven systems that allow the operator to choose from predefined options by a single keystroke.

5.7.3.6 Light pen/palm top/laptop computers provide a method to computerize data at the scene. Rapid developments in technology are making this option more costeffective.

5.7.3.7 Voice entry of data may be feasible in the future.

5.7.4 *Auditing the Accuracy of Data Entry*:

5.7.4.1 The EMS-MIS should include some means of measuring the accuracy of data entry. This is especially important in systems using keypunched or optically scanned data input.

5.7.4.2 Each organization that provides information to the EMS-MIS should routinely audit 5 % of its hard copy records on a quarterly basis for verification against the database. The transcription error rate should be compared with that of other similar organizations and a cause sought for any unusually high results. Well-functioning systems should have less than a 2 % transcription error rate.

5.7.5 Compliance with data collection and reporting is a major obstăcle to successful operation of any EMS-MIS. Compliance issues are most important with safety personnel, providers, and emergency department staff because the bulk of data must be obtained during their activities or it will be difficult to capture retrospectively. Methods to improve compliance include:

5.7.5.1 Routine monitoring of an individual's compliance rate as part of job performance appraisal.

5.7.5.2 Financial incentives/disincentives based on compliance for both the individual and the organizations.

5.7.5.3 Provision of timely and useful reports that illustrate the desirability of good compliance.

5.7.5.4 Utilization of feedback information into training programs.

5.7.5.5 Maintenance of satisfactory compliance rate as a requirement of certification or licensing, or both.

5.8 *Centralized Versus Decentralized Data Processing*:

5.8.1 Data recording must take place in all levels of the EMS-MIS. However, options exist as to where data entry, data processing, and report generation take place. To illustrate, we will take an example of an EMS-MIS dealing only with provider run sheets.

5.8.2 In a purely centralized data processing model, all completed handwritten run sheets would be sent to the State Data Processing Center, where an operator would enter the information into the computer. After all run sheets from across the state for a one-month period were entered, reports could be generated summarizing various types of activity for each provider organization, local EMS agency, REMSO, and the entire state. Reports would be sent back to the appropriate individuals.

5.8.3 In a purely decentralized data processing model, all data obtained by a provider would be initially handwritten or entered directly into a hand held computer at the time of observation and then input locally into the provider's own personal computer. Reports concerning the provider's internal operations would be generated on a daily basis or as frequently as desired. Periodically, the provider would upload certain designated data elements about each run to the local EMS agency computer, which would collect information from all local, and generate local aggregate summary reports. With the exception of the copy of the run sheet inserted into the patient's record, the actual run sheets would never leave the provider. Selected data from various local EMS agency computers would be uploaded to REMSO computers for generation of regional reports, and REMSO computers would upload a state computer for generation of statewide reports.

5.8.4 *Combination Centralized and Decentralized Models*:

5.8.4.1 In a combination model, flexibility would exist so that providers could utilize either the centralized or decentralized approach. Low-volume providers would probably opt to submit their records to a central facility (at either the local EMS agency or REMSO levels) for data entry, and would receive all their reports back from the central facility. Larger-volume providers, or any provider with the interest, would have the ability to locally enter their own data, run internal reports, upload selected data, and receive back aggregate summaries. Providers would be able to enter their own data on either an in-house personal computer and generate internal reports with it, or enter data on a remote access terminal to the central computer but have less ability to generate reports. This model allows providers to participate in the EMS-MIS initially by submitting handwritten records, and to develop computer capability at their own pace should they so desire.

5.8.5 *Logical Model*:

5.8.5.1 The following section describes a logical design prototype for an EMS-MIS. The data elements to be tracked are listed and defined in 5.3 and 5.4. The suggested output reports are detailed in 5.11. Implementation of this logical design may be accomplished with a variety of hardware/software combinations depending upon local preference and preexisting resources.

5.8.5.2 This design was developed through the use of structured analysis techniques. This approach uses a context diagram, data flow diagrams, procedure narratives, and a data dictionary to depict a conceptual design. This analytical process uses a top-down approach that begins by identifying major system functions during the conceptual design phase and decomposes the conceptual design to structure charts, process qualifications, and detail data definition in the detail design phase.

5.8.5.3 The Data Flow Diagrams (DFDs) are a way of partitioning system functions into a series of events that enhances analysis and clarifies what is being developed. Most important is that these models highlight business functions, as opposed to traditional flow charting of computer logic.

5.8.5.4 The logical model for the conceptual EMS-MIS includes the following:

(1) Context Diagram—Identifies the users of the system.

(2) Level 0 Diagram—Identifies the major system processes and data flows that are developed for the system under study. It also identifies the logical files and major system events for each process.

(3) Level 1 Diagram—Identifies the data flows of each type of process contained within the system. These business events are the initial indication of the physical components of the system in terms of computer programs, files, and reporting requirements.

(4) Brief Narratives—(DFD-Data Flow Diagrams)—Identifies the purpose, events, and functions that take place for each process.

5.8.5.5 The following graphic conventions have been used in the documentation:

(1) Process Event—Rectangle—These action-released boxes describe the procedures that act on data. Each process is numbered so they can be broken down from generalized functions into detailed ones. Each numbered event represents a process that must be developed. In the conceptual design phase, they are only decomposed to Level 1; however, during detail design, they will be converted to structure charts and programming specifications detailed in terms of specific events and data elements.

(2) Data Stores—Open-Ended Rectangle—These boxes represent the files necessary to store the information required by the system.

(3) Data Flow—Lines with Arrows—These lines depict the movement of data from one process to the next. If no definition is given, it is assumed to be an obvious one. As the level of data flows are broken down, (two and greater), the amount of information on these lines tends to be more explicit.

5.8.5.6 These structured techniques assist in developing streamlined efficient computer systems that meet user requirements. The use of these techniques reduces the amount of technical jargon and interference, allowing members to concentrate on business functionally and process control.

5.8.5.7 The key issue identified with the narratives are part of this methodology. The intention is to identify issues from early on in the project, which tend to be more user and policy related, and continue to raise issues throughout detail design. As the project progresses, these issues need to be resolved by project participants.

5.8.6 *Level 0 Diagram—System Overview*—This data flow diagram (Fig. 5) presents the major events which will occur within the system. It identifies major processes that must be developed to meet the system objectives.

5.8.6.1 *Enter Data*—This procedure will provide for the entering of, emergency department, patient, and EMT data into the EMS-MIS. It is designed to accommodate various types of input media, such as, source, on-line, electronic files, and computer. Unique procedures are defined for type of entry process and user group for data integrity and to provide consistent controls. Although not shown here, internal system files will be used to control and process the various types and formats of input that will be coming into the system.

5.8.6.2 *Record Skill Used*—The recognition of EMT skills performed will be an internal system process that is automatically maintained once entered with the run information. This data will be physically maintained on a separate file with restricted access.

5.8.6.3 *Generate Standard Reports*—This reporting process is designed as a series of events that will control to whom and

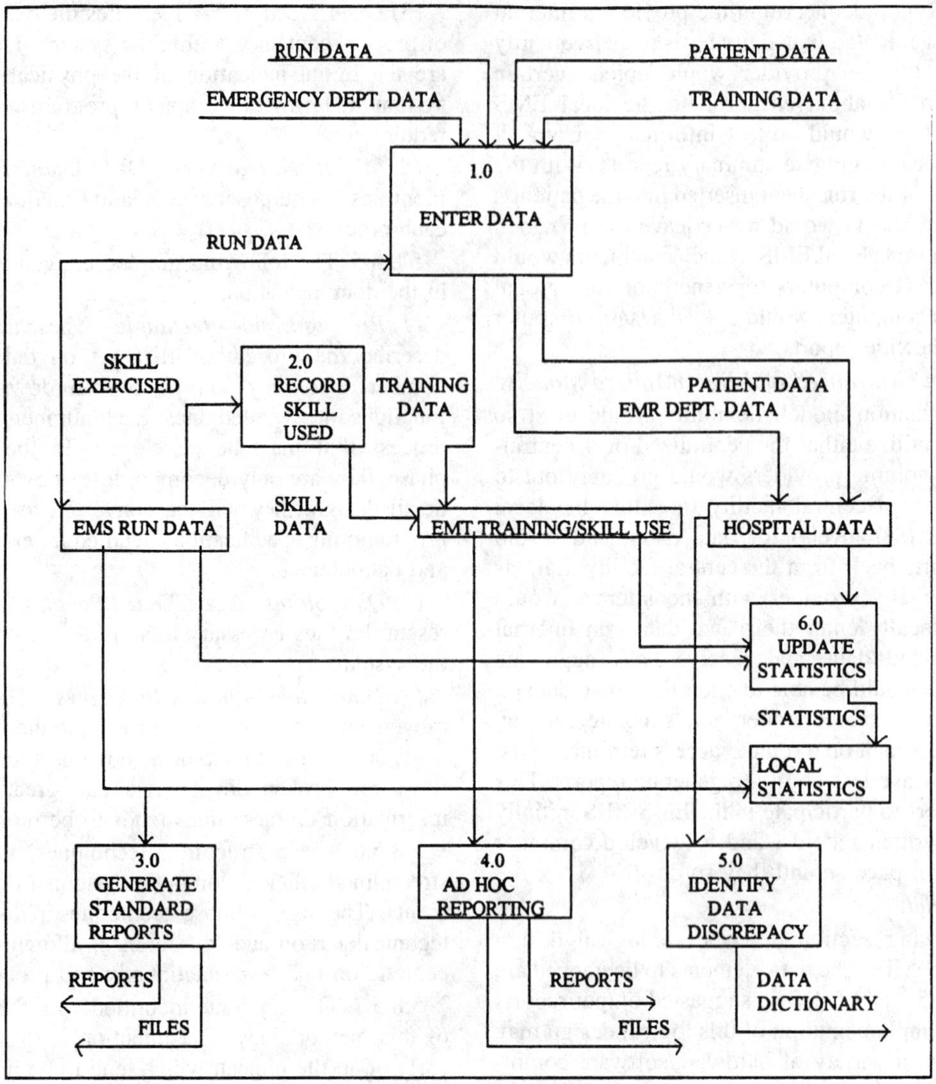

FIG. 5 EMS-MIS Level 0 Diagram

how information gets distributed. A report file will be created that is linked with pre-defined table information so authorization, distribution, copies, and hard copy or transmitted medium controls, can be placed on the reporting process. This process will produce all standard reports and special job requests. It will also include the creation of files to be used as input to other systems or personal computers.

5.8.6.4 *Ad Hoc Reporting*—This process is specifically designed so end users can obtain information as soon as possible. They can write their own customized reports or request predefined system reports. This interactive process allows a user to extract authorized data from the EMS-MIS database and create customized files. These files can be downloaded into a personal computer where conventional software or internal applications can process the data. Operation control requirements should be designed into the system to prevent abuse or the tying up of the system based on run time or file contention.

5.8.6.5 *Identify Data Discrepancy*—These procedures will be developed to enhance the integrity and completeness of the database. Processes can be built to compare data for reasonableness or discrepancies based on the different methods that data is compiled. It is not intended to provide a complex, analytical tool, but to list and report to end users for their subsequent follow up and individual correction. For example, if the run file indicates one treatment administered and the hospital indicates a different procedure, one could report this discrepancy in the information to both the hospital and the EMT provider, allowing them to resolve and correct the data. Queues containing data integrity issues will be held in suspense until resolved.

5.8.6.6 *Update Statistics*—Because of the complexity and potential for error, this function has been separated and made an internal system process. Statistics will be collected from each record in the system and maintained on a separate file. This file will not be maintainable through normal interactive file access, thereby the internal control procedures within the system will directly affect the accuracy of local statistical information.

5.8.6.7 *System Files*, The logical files that store the information in the EMS-MIS database, which are all related by keys, are summarized as follows:

(1) EMS RUN FILE—This is a unique file for each EMS provider which maintains the pre-hospital patient care record information (see 5.3.2).

(2) EMS TRAINING/SKILL USE FILE—This file identifies each EMT in the system, his qualifications, certifications, training, and skills utilized (see 5.3.3).

(3) EMS CONTINUING MEDICAL EDUCATION FILE—This file identifies all continuing medical education activity for each EMT in the system (see 5.3.4).

(4) HOSPITAL DATA FILES—These are unique files for each hospital that contain patient information, including emergency department and inpatient data.

(*a*) EMERGENCY DEPARTMENT MEDICAL DIRECTION FILE—This file contains data about on line medical direction given by E.D. personnel, regardless of whether or not the patient was transported to their institution (see 5.4.1).

(*b*) EMERGENCY DEPARTMENT PATIENT RECORD FILE—This file contains data about all E.D. patients, regardless of whether they used the EMS system or not (see 5.4.2).

(*c*) HOSPITAL DISCHARGE FILE—This file contains data about EMS system patients who were eventually admitted (see 5.4.3).

(5) STATISTICS FILE—This is a separate file where all raw data will be maintained for statistical reporting.

(6) TABLE FILES—During the detailed design phase, many user and system controlled tables will be created. The information in these tables will be used to control functions, provide unique user procedures, and be used as a means to easily change common routines instead of building them into computer program logic.

5.8.6.8 *Data Flow Name—1.0a Enter Run Data (*Fig. 6*)*—This process allows the EMS provider to select the method of inputing run data into the system. The EMS provider will be restricted to updating only run information related to his unit. These personnel will not be restricted from using any EMS-MIS terminal to which they have authorized access.

5.8.6.9 Enter run data on line in an interactive, userfriendly, menu-driven environment. Immediate validation and error reporting would be available to the person keying. Weekly log reports will be distributed which identify the activities of each run, which will then be verified by the EMT for accuracy.

5.8.6.10 Send run data to the central facility for key entry. These source documents will be tagged and logged for system control and verification purposes.

5.8.6.11 Special data entry procedures will be developed to accommodate multiple users and system control procedures at a centralized facility.

5.8.6.12 Transmit run data, using an existing non-EMS-MIS network or a direct computer-to-computer link.

5.8.6.13 Edit and validate electronic records submitted as input to the system. Ensure that only authorized, valid data in the proper format is accepted for processing.

5.8.6.14 Update the database in a controlled, organized process that does not interfere with other system processes or could destroy data.

5.8.6.15 Transfer run data on electronic media (tape, diskette, etc.).

5.8.6.16 *Key Issues*:

(1) Should an EMT be allowed to modify run data after it has been uploaded to the database?

(2) Does the EMT need to have access to the hospital patient information?

5.8.7 *Data Flow Name 1.0b—Enter Emergency Department Data (EDD)*—This process permits the emergency department to choose how it will submit patient or run information. Because of the unique environment and management approaches that exist within the hospitals and municipalities, a flexible approach is required for the computerization of EMS-MIS data. A hospital will have the ability to start to use the system using one method, while having the ability to select another at a later point, to better accommodate its needs.

5.8.7.1 Enter EDD data on-line in an interactive, userfriendly, menu-driven process. Validation and error reporting will be immediate to enhance the integrity of the system.

5.8.7.2 Collect, tag, log, and transfer EDD data to the central processing center.

5.8.7.3 Provide unique data entry procedures that accommodate the controls and special handling processes required at the central facility.

5.8.7.4 Provide temporary record storage for all data transmitted to the system prior to updating the EMS-MIS database.

5.8.7.5 Edit and validate electronic records submitted as input to the system. Ensure that only authorized, valid data in the proper format is accepted for processing.

5.8.7.6 Update the database in a controlled, organized process that does not interfere with other system processes or would destroy data.

5.8.7.7 Transfer EDD data on electronic media (tape, diskette, and so forth).

5.8.7.8 *Key Issues*:

(1) Should the emergency department be allowed to modify patient outcome data after the patient has been transferred to another department?

(2) Should the EDD department be allowed to modify run data whether or not the EMT provider uses the hospital to input its data?

5.8.8 *Data Flow Name 1.0c Enter Patient Data*—This process (Fig. 7) describes how hospital personnel can enter patient data into the system. These data entry procedures are uniquely defined for patient information entered by hospital employees as opposed to the emergency department staff or emergency medical technicians. This will facilitate linkage of pre-hospital, emergency department, and in-patient data, as well as uploading and downloading of aggregated data. This process allows the hospital flexibility in the manner it chooses to submit selected patient information to the EMS-MIS. The design of the information processing procedures was developed to ensure timeliness and accuracy of the data being recorded. These methods use a consistent approach to transferring data, as well as uploading and downloading of aggregated data.

5.8.8.1 Enter patient data using an on-line terminal. These interactive sessions limit access by hospital file and individual functions. The screens should be menu-driven and provide immediate feedback as to the results of the data entered. All activity is logged, summarized, and reported.

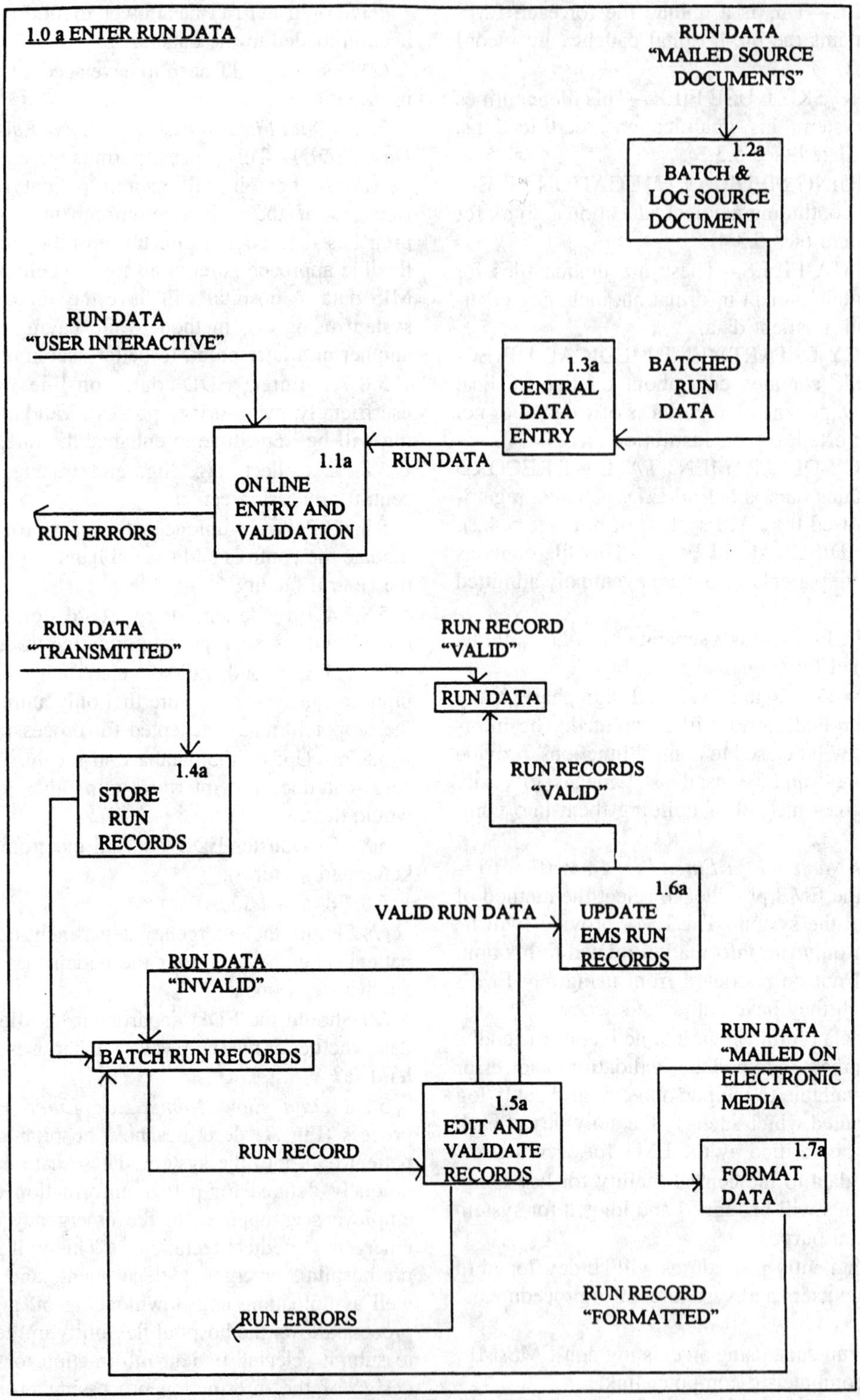

FIG. 6 EMS-MIS Level 1 Diagram

5.8.8.2 Transfer patient source document to the central facility to be tagged and logged by their staff.

5.8.8.3 Unique data entry procedures to accommodate processing controls at central processing site.

5.8.8.4 Transmit patient data, using an existing network or a computer-to-computer link, possibly through hospital emergency department.

5.8.8.5 Edit and validate electronic records submitted as input to another system. Ensure that only authorized, valid data in the proper format is accepted.

5.8.8.6 Update the database in a controlled, organized process that does not interfere with other system processors or destroy data.

5.8.8.7 Transfer patient data on electronic media (tape,

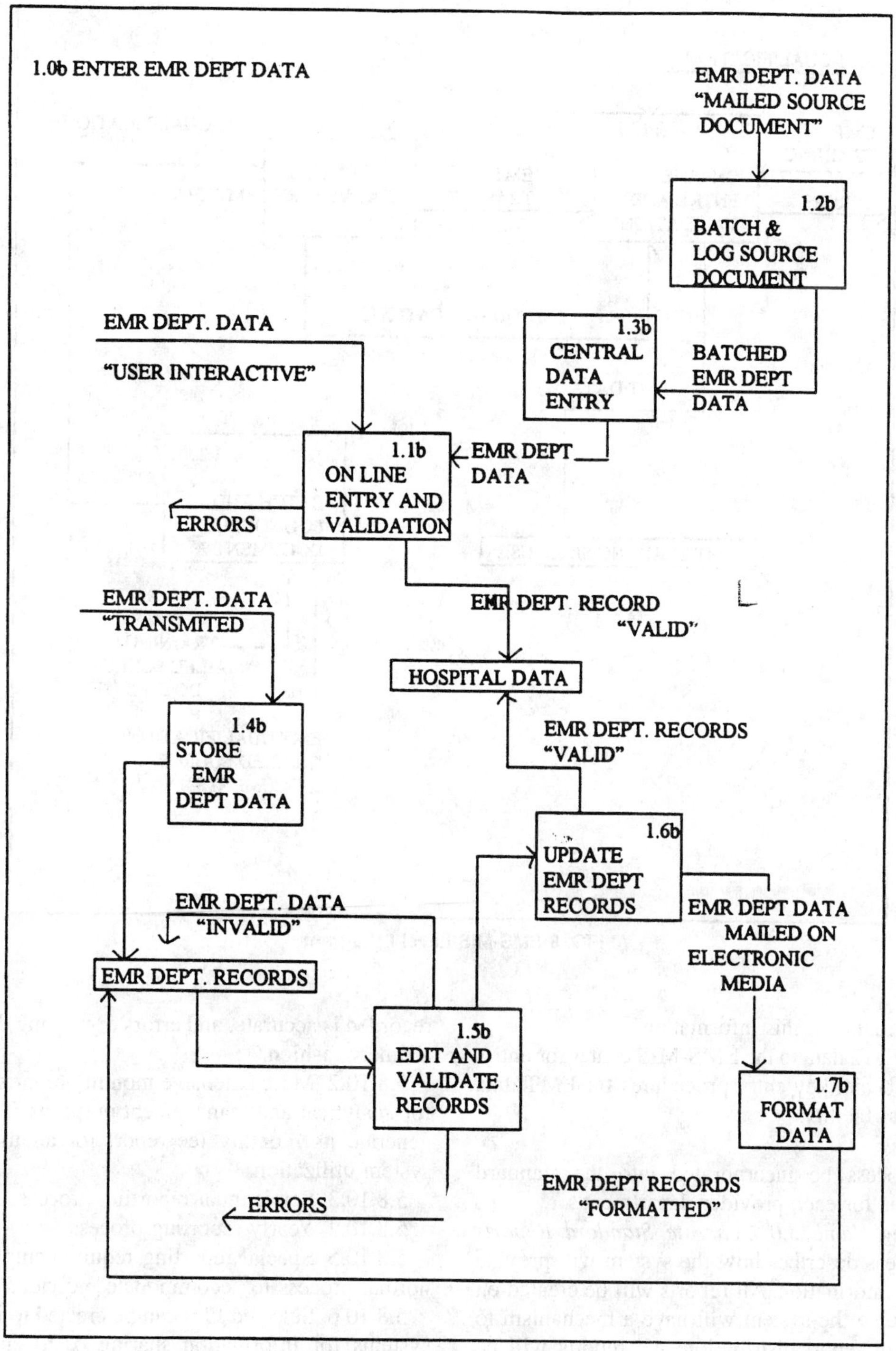

FIG. 7 EMS-MIS Level 1 Diagram

diskette, and so forth).

5.8.9 *Data Flow Name—Enter Training Data (*Fig. 8*)*—This process describes how the EMT profile information will be entered into the system. This is the process that identifies an EMT to the system, defines his background and qualifications, and reports his complete training. It is not the method of tracking EMT skill utilization defined in Process 2.0. This would contain his previous employment, qualifications, and possible practicing skills. Record training courses and the date completed, track recertification dates, and maintain continuing education credits. Since this process is temporary in nature, it is recommended that the inputing of information be limited to two methods: (*1*) on-line entry by an EMS provider unit, or (*2*) batch entry at the EMS-MIS center. The ability to maintain this information will be limited by department and individual. The qualification and training information is defined on a separate file to enhance the file security features and extend the individual protection of the EMT personnel.

5.8.9.1 Enter EMT information on-line from the service provider he is employed by. Access will be limited to only

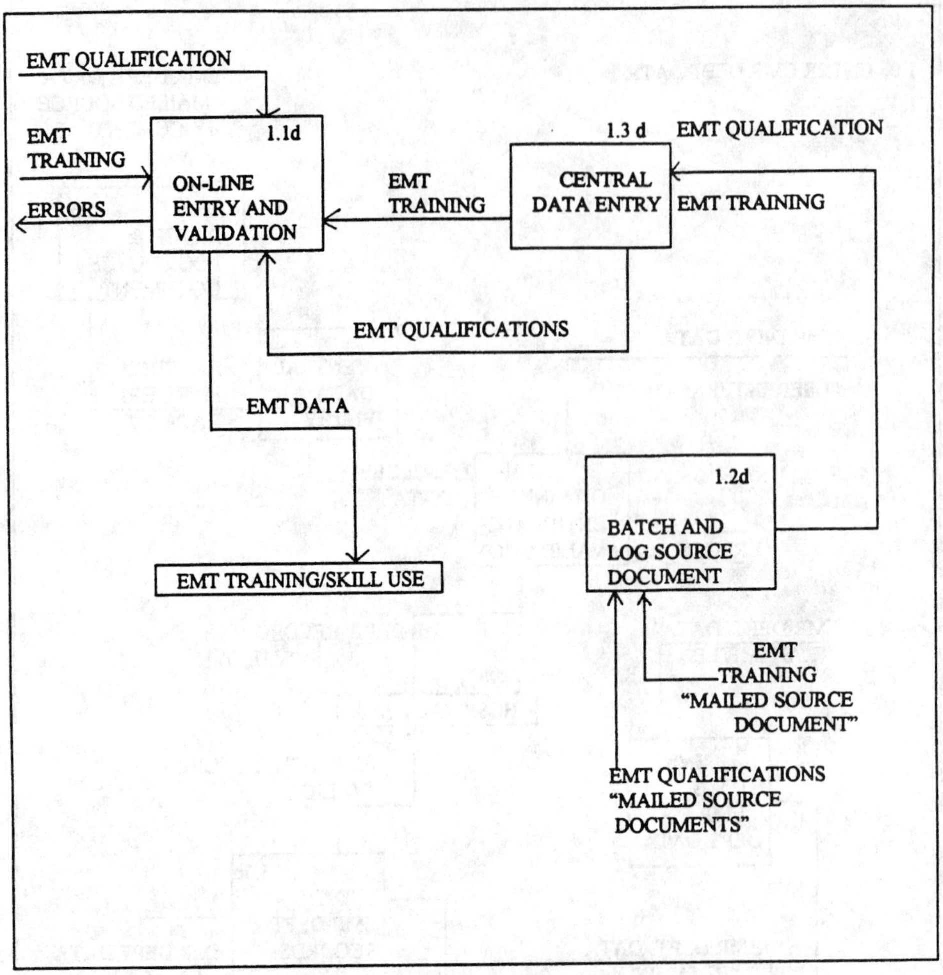

FIG. 8 EMS-MIS Level I Diagram

those authorized to maintain this information.

5.8.9.2 Transfer EMT data to the EMS-MIS center for entry.

5.8.9.3 Provide special key entry procedures for EMT data entered at the central facility.

5.8.9.4 *Key Issues*:

(1) Can this process be incorporated into the standard personnel procedures for each provider department?

5.8.10 *Data Flow Name 3.0 Generate Standard Reports* (Fig. 9)—This process describes how the system will provide users with standard information. All reports will be created on a special reports file so the system will have a mechanism to authorize and control report distribution. All reports will be defined in a table for each user. This allows each user to choose his reports, number of copies, define where they are to be sent, and determine the report distribution media. Minimum reporting will be a predefined requirement to ensure that all system controls and procedures are followed. This report file will contain associated distribution information to ensure reports are routed correctly and prevent unauthorized report distribution.

5.8.10.1 Produce weekly reports for system control purposes that reflect the activity recorded by all EMS-MIS system users. Weekly reports should be distributed to all departments that have activity as a means to ensure that the information recorded is accurate, and errors or missing data are corrected in a timely fashion.

5.8.10.2 More extensive monthly reports will be distributed for analytical and management purposes. The system will also generate its monthly fee report for all users based on their system utilization.

5.8.10.3 Semiannual reporting process.

5.8.10.4 Yearly reporting process.

5.8.10.5 Special reporting requirements can be set up as a normal process to accommodate individual reporting needs.

5.8.10.6 Selected files can be created to interface with other systems for information sharing or to enhance productivity where automated application already exists.

5.8.10.7 Print reports using the predefined distribution and authorization rules.

5.8.10.8 For users who request their reports to be transmitted, write the format and transmission protocols so the reports can be sent.

5.8.10.9 *Key Issues*:

(1) Should ad hoc (user report writer) reporting be processed through the report file procedure, or should interactive reporting based on individual access levels be allowed?

5.8.10.10 *Data Flow Name—Ad Hoc Reporting* (Fig. 10)—This process describes how end users can retrieve information

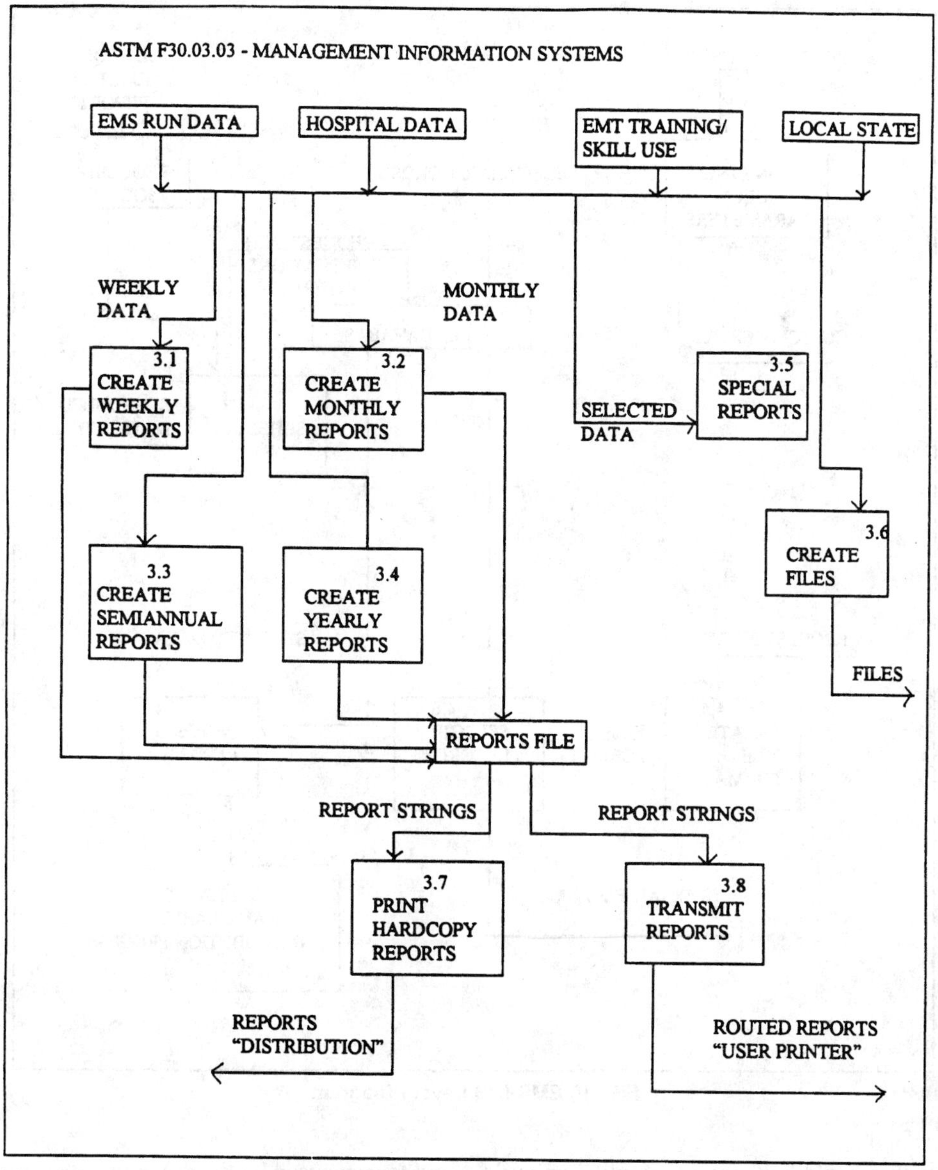

FIG. 9 EMS-MIS Level 1 Diagram

from the EMS-MIS databases. The process will be designed to allow flexible reporting from the user community, but at the same time, permit operation restrictions to ensure that information is extracted in a manner that does not degrade or significantly tie up the system. All access for ad hoc reporting and file creation will follow the predefined information security rules, in accordance with 5.6. Even though the process provides a means to easily extract information, the user will only be able to access data that is authorized.

5.8.10.11 The system should provide the ability to extract data by designing custom reports with an on-line query language. Another consideration is the ability to write generalized reports that could easily be modified for an individual's own use. A library process should be developed so custom, written reports can be stored and need not be rewritten for any future request.

5.8.10.12 The design has been developed to allow the user to request any job or predefined system report on an asneeded basis. In trying to put the information in the hands of the user community at his request, special control and scheduling processes must be designed to prevent unnecessary system abuse. Without an authorized job request and schedule performance criteria, users could tie up the network or incur extensive billing costs.

5.8.10.13 This process will allow individual users to request and schedule jobs as seen fit. The individual will also be able to receive the information based on the job run time and the fastest sport distribution available.

5.8.10.14 Provide a special report writing process for ad hoc reporting.

5.8.10.15 The system design incorporates the ability to create a file to be downloaded into the user's computer. Based on the user's information access level, the system can create files from the EMS-MIS database to be utilized by the user's computer and application software.

5.8.10.16 This feature permits specific information to be

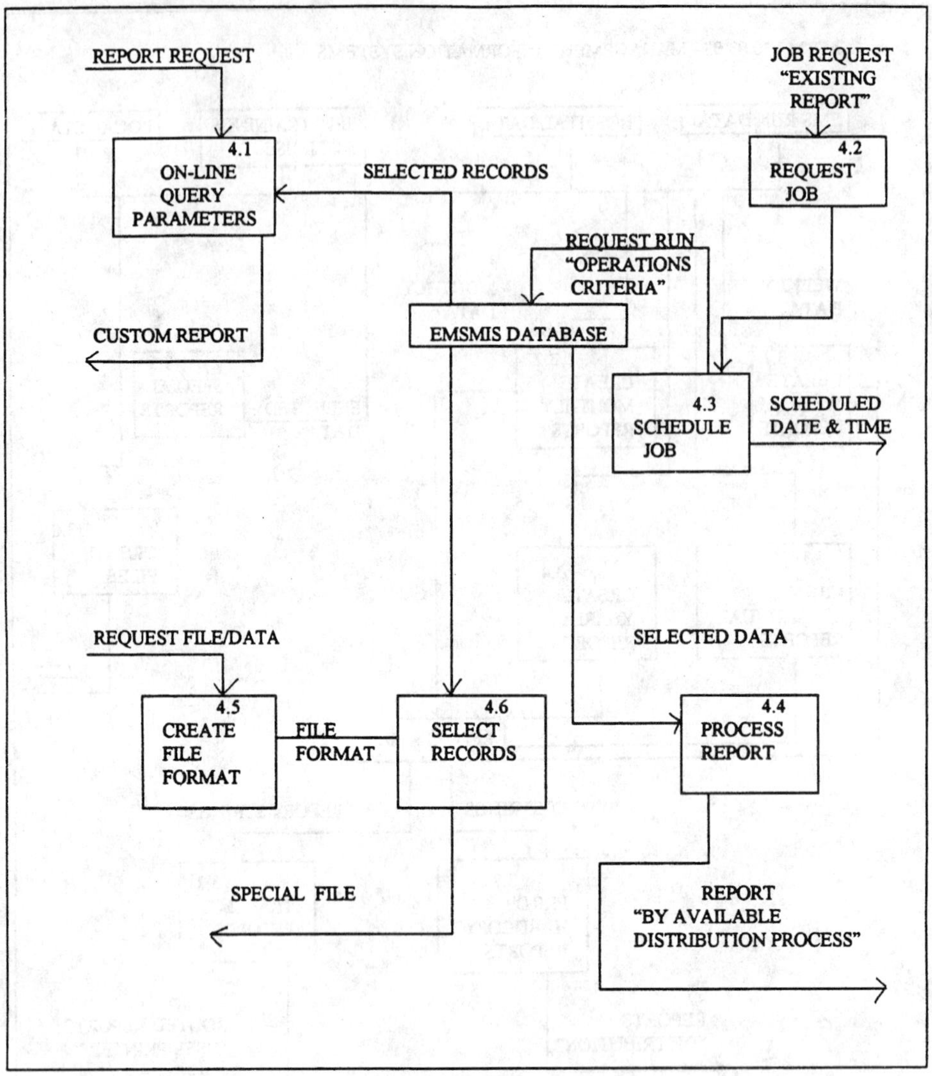

FIG. 10 EMS-MIS Level I Diagram

extracted in a format that could enhance or simplify unique reporting needs.

5.8.10.17 *Key Issues*:

(1) Should the system allow any type of report writer languages available to be used, or only one to be available to enhance controls?

(2) Who will determine the operations criteria for scheduling jobs?

(3) What role or level of commitment will be required by the technical staff to effectively support the ad hoc reporting?

(4) Should all reporting go through one reporting process, or should it be based on individual access as needed?

5.8.11 *Linkage Among Sources of Data*—Patient-based outcome evaluation requires linking multiple databases in order to trace the patient from the scene to final disposition. The EMS data are collected at different points of time and at different locations by the different providers responsible for the emergency victim. Some of the data, usually nonclinical, are routinely computerized and aggregated into statewide databases which can be linked. Many barriers to linkage exist. These include lack of standardization of definitions, measures, and formats used by the different data sources. Linkage of data sets is further impeded by incompatibilities in computer hardware and software systems. Data entry errors and omissions are common. Data may not be readily shared because of incompatible reporting periods and proprietary concerns. Additional administrative problems further limit linkage, specifically, cost and data management considerations. Sources of data may be linked directly or indirectly using single or multiple variables, respectively. The purpose of linking two EMS databases is to expand the usefulness of each database. Thus, for example, linkage of the accident report to the run report provides outcome data for highway safety analyses and mechanism of injury data to EMS analyses. The ultimate purpose is to trace an emergency patient from the scene, to discharge, and eventually through the rehabilitation phase in order to generate descriptive data describing what happens to the emergency victim, process data describing how well the system responded during the various phases of the emergency, and patient outcome data describing the effectiveness of EMS on mortality and morbidity. Data linkage makes it possible to perform tracer studies on large groups of patient (such as, motor vehicle injured), to use statewide data to describe how well the EMS system functions (such as, Sensitivity Index Project), and to create permanent patient registries for monitoring overtime (Trauma Registry).

5.8.11.1 Linkage is facilitated by the use of unique identifiers. Common unique identifiers include:

(1) Patient name.

(2) Social security number.

(3) Unique record number.

(4) Universal health identifier (not currently available).

(5) Ambulance run report number for each patient injured.

(6) Inpatient record number for each patient admitted.

(7) Insurance claim number.

(8) Coroner's report/death certificate number.

(9) Crash report number.

(10) Unique record number of any database.

(11) Provider License Number.

5.8.11.2 Unique identifiers identify a specific person.

5.8.11.3 Data collection forms must each be designed to collect the unique identifier and the data must be recorded accurately for linkage to be successful. Accurate recording of unique identifiers may be difficult if the identifier is not available at the time of primary data collection when the patient is being treated. For example, if the ambulance leaves the scene early, the policeman may have to obtain the run report number from the hospital to which the patient is transported. Also in most states, accident reports are not prenumbered but numbered later at the time of data entry.

5.8.11.4 Unique identifiers are useful for linking primary patient records or for linking databases, or both, consisting of abstracted (secondary) records (trauma registry, and so forth) when data quality is good.

5.8.12 Indirect linkage variables must be combined to identify a specific person. The data and the linkage process must be computerized except when volume is low enough to be managed manually.

5.8.12.1 Missing/inaccurate data (particularly age and time), multiple patients with the same age matched to the same record, and multiple records in the database for the same patient complicate linkage with a combination of indirect variables.

5.8.12.2 Unique identifiers reduce the need for manual verification but increase the probability of unmatched records when the linkage data are missing or are inaccurate, or both.

5.8.12.3 Systems with low volume have the option of developing manual verification procedures to increase the percentage of matches. Systems with high volume should consider using probability-based methods of recording linkage.

(1) Probabilistic linkage techniques do not require an exact match among the attributes of the linkage variables in order to identify valid matches. Values are assigned according to the frequency of occurrence among valid matched pairs and by chance agreement.

(2) The EMS researchers must be careful to evaluate the potential for false positives and false negatives before using the linked state for small area variation analyses. For example, a paramedic run report matched to a crash occurring in an area without paramedic service is more visible in small area analyses than in a statewide total.

(3) Linkage files should consist primarily of records which have the potential of linkage. Ineligible records should be eliminated whenever possible to increase the efficiency of the matching process without incurring systematic bias.

(4) Identifiers to be used for indirect matching should be chosen based on their capability to limit the need for verification of the match.

(5) The most common indirect identifiers are age/birth date, sex, date, location (injury, hospital destination).

(1a) Birthdate is more restrictive than age but is frequently computerized on only one file.

(2a) Race, when accurately recorded on both files, is also useful.

(3a) Times usually have a high rate of discrepancy, the inevitable result of multiple providers at different locations some of whom forget to use military time. Probabilistic linkage matches times within a predetermined range and prorates the weight accordingly.

(6) Sets of indirect identifiers found to be successful for linking crash to EMS patient care data:

(1a) Patient care record number.

(2b) Age/birth date.

(3b) Sex.

(4b) Date of crash/EMS run.

(5b) Crash location (FIPS geographical code)/EMS pickup location.

(7) Sets of indirect identifiers for linking the crash data directly to hospital discharge data:

(1c) Age/birth date.

(2c) Sex.

(3c) Date of crash/date of admission (may vary by one day if crash occurs after 9 a.m.).

(4c) Location of crash/hospital service area.

(5c) Time of crash/time of admission (use range from 1 to 4 h as match range).

(8) Sets of indirect identifiers for linking the EMS patient care data to the hospital discharge data

(1d) Age/birth date.

(2d) Sex.

(3d) Date of run/date of admission (may vary by one day if accident occurs after 9 p.m.).

(4d) The EMS destination/hospital identification.

(9) Sets of indirect identifiers for linking death certificate data and crash report:

(1e) Name.

(2e) Date of accident.

(10) Sets of indirect identifiers for linking death certificate data and EMS patient care data.

(1f) Age/birth date.

(2f) Sex.

(3f) Date of onset (usually not computerized)/date of run.

(4f) Hour of onset (usually not computerized)/time of run.

(11) Sets of indirect identifiers for linking death certificate data and hospital discharge data:

(1g) Age/birth date.

(2g) Sex.

(*3g*) Location of death/hospital identification.

(*12*) Sets of indirect identifiers for linking census data with crash or EMS data:

(*1h*) The FIPS geographical code.

5.9 *Generation of Management Information Reports*:

5.9.1 *Frequency*—Reports should be generated depending on:

5.9.1.1 The nature of the event or process being studied. Low-frequency events can only be assessed over relatively long periods of time in order to collect a large enough sample to study.

5.9.1.2 The frequency of the need for feedback to the users of the system. Large, complex PSOs, emergency department, and EMS systems may benefit from daily reporting to assist in day-to-day management. Smaller organizations may only require periodic review of operation for strategic planning or evaluation purposes, or both.

5.9.1.3 The nature of the report itself. Reports dealing with incomplete data or data discrepancies should be generated rapidly and frequently to maximize the changes of recovering accurate data.

5.9.1.4 The lag time necessary to obtain all needed data for the report. Reports describing hospital outcome will have a longer lag time than reports dealing with purely pre-hospital or emergency department phenomena.

5.9.1.5 Cost of production and distribution in terms of time, materials, and labor.

5.9.2 *Distribution of Routine Reports*—Once an EMS-MIS has decided which reports should be generated on a regular basis, distribution policies should be determined in accordance with the concern addressed in the confidentiality section (5.6).

5.9.2.1 Who is to receive the report on a regular basis.

5.9.2.2 The method by which the report will be sent (hard copy, electronic file, on-line availability).

5.9.2.3 Who may request a report on a nonroutine basis.

5.9.3 *Ad Hoc Reports*—The particulars of the software/hardware chosen to implement the conceptual design will affect the ease and practicality with which ad hoc reports can be generated.

5.9.3.1 Highly decentralized systems utilizing microcomputer offer end users the ability to analyze their own data in a timely and unlimited fashion. Opportunities for more extensive analysis exist at the local level since nonsensitive area-wide data can be downloaded as needed.

5.9.3.2 Centralized systems offer less flexibility due to potential cost issues (5.9.1.4) at the central processing center, and delays caused by insufficient personnel resources.

5.9.3.3 Generation of ad hoc reports must take into account data confidentiality concerns (5.6).

5.9.3.4 Policies must be established that define the process to be followed in requesting and distributing ad hoc reports, as well as the log to be completed recording all such activity.

5.10 *Utilization of Information*—The suggested management reports defined in 5.11 and 5.12 are designed to be used at the individual PSO, emergency department, and local EMS-MIS level. They can all be generated using the minimum recommended data set defined in 5.2 and 5.3. The information needs at higher levels in the EMS-MIS "pyramid" (REMSO, State, and National Context Diagram I) may be satisfied with a subset of the data elements necessary for local operations. In order to provide maximum benefit and to enhance compliance with data collection, the EMS-MIS must be geared to the day-to-day needs of those involved with patient care.

5.11 *Provider Reports*:

5.11.1 *Basic Run Information*—Transports, non transports, refusals, and so forth.

5.11.2 *Response Time Analysis*—By 3 to 15-min intervals, addressing nine basic time intervals (call received to dispatch, dispatch to enroute, enroute to on scene, on scene to destination, destination to back in service, total time call received to arrival at scene, total pre-hospital time, total out of service time).

5.11.3 Response time by geographical indicator.

5.11.4 Response time or cardiac arrests.

5.11.5 Runs by day and time.

5.11.6 Patient disposition by hospital.

5.11.7 Receiving hospital profile of transported patients by squad at 1.2.3—Average miles per call by squad.

5.11.8 On line medical direction by hospital per squad.

5.11.9 Illness/injury category by squad.

5.11.10 Mechanism of injury.

5.11.11 Pre-hospital procedures attempted/performed.

5.11.12 Drugs/IV's administered.

5.11.13 First cardiac rhythm.

5.11.14 Last cardiac rhythm.

5.11.15 Case severity—at dispatch versus scene.

5.11.16 Glasgow Coma Scale on arrival at scene.

5.11.17 Trauma score on scene.

5.11.18 Defibrillation success/failure in field.

5.11.19 CPR success/failure—none, first responder, bystander.

5.11.20 Disposition of patients from emergency department.

5.11.21 The CPR case disposition from emergency department.

5.11.22 Trauma score on scene by death versus discharge.

5.11.23 Trauma score by patient outcome and disposition.

5.11.24 Patient outcome by response time for major trauma.

5.11.25 Patient outcome by response time for cardiac arrest.

5.11.26 Individual paramedics by skills performed.

5.11.27 Drug administration by paramedics.

5.11.28 Individual paramedic practice profile.

5.11.29 Paramedics/EMT training profile.

5.11.30 Patient distribution by age and sex.

5.11.31 Call response by presenting problem.

5.11.32 Time on scene by presenting problem.

5.11.33 Medical communications summary.

5.11.34 Calls per 1000 population by FIPS area.

5.11.35 Simultaneous call analysis.

5.11.36 Response mode summary.

5.11.37 Arrivals by PSO.

5.11.38 On-line medical direction summary.

5.12 *System Funding Consideration*:

5.12.1 The most successful and cost-effective EMS-MIS will be flexible to respond to needs and be supported at the state, regional, and local levels.

5.12.2 System design should allow for as much decentralization as possible in order to reduce the costs of data entry.

5.12.3 Funds invested in an EMS-MIS will be justified by more efficient and effective resource allocation.

5.12.4 The cost of emergency patient care data collection is the responsibility of the physician outpatient, EMS, and hospital providers and is passed on to the patient as part of the cost of patient care.

5.12.5 The cost of computerizing, merging, linking, and analyzing emergency patient care data should be shared by the owners and users of these data.

5.12.6 Various funding strategies include:

5.12.6.1 Government subsidy at the federal, state, or local level.

5.12.6.2 Direct fees to system users.

5.12.6.3 Direct fees to third-party carriers.

5.12.6.4 Surcharges on license plates, moving violations, and so forth.

5.12.6.5 Subscription programs.

5.12.6.6 Donations.

5.12.7 Financial justification for EMS-MIS costs may be found in:

5.12.7.1 Documentation and evaluation of EMS activity for legislative bodies and state and federal funding agencies.

5.12.7.2 Availability of data to support state EMS regulatory functions such as training, licensing of personnel, and vehicles, etc.

5.12.7.3 On-going training and equipment needs based on run review information.

5.12.7.4 Licenses to local PSOs based on-call demand/needs assessment for the area to be served.

6. Keywords

6.1 data system; emergency medical services; EMS-MIS; Management Information Systems

Standard Guide for Techniques in Land Search[1]

This standard is issued under the fixed designation F 1633; the number immediately following the designation indicates the year of original adoption or, in the case of revision, the year of last revision. A number in parentheses indicates the year of last reapproval. A superscript epsilon (ϵ) indicates an editorial change since the last revision or reapproval.

1. Scope

1.1 This guide identifies and describes techniques that may be used by individuals or agencies when searching for persons, property or evidence, on land. The application of one or more of these techniques to any particular land search will depend upon the individual circumstances of the search and the judgment of the person responsible for conducting the search.

1.2 This guide assists individuals and agencies by providing a list of techniques for their consideration during a land search and by providing a brief description of the application of the technique to land search. Some advantages and disadvantages, as well as the most common uses of the techniques, are discussed in the guide. The guide does not, however, purport to discuss all aspects of conducting a land search.

1.3 *This standard does not purport to address all of the safety concerns, if any, associated with its use. It is the responsibility of the user of this standard to establish appropriate safety and health practices and determine the applicability of regulatory limitations prior to use.*

2. Referenced Documents

2.1 *ASTM Standard:*

F 1767 Guide for Forms Used in Search and Rescue[2]

3. Terminology

3.1 *Definitions:*

3.1.1 *attraction, n*—to get the attention of lost, missing or stranded subject(s) by sound or visual methods, or both, for example, whistle, light, smoke.

3.1.2 *clue awareness, n*—to be aware of evidence left by a subject(s) which may help to ascertain their location or direction of travel, or both.

3.1.3 *confinement, n*—the act of limiting the growth of the potential search area by minimizing the ability of the subject(s) leaving the search area undetected.

3.1.4 *electronic search, n*—technique(s) using electronic systems or devices to locate a subject(s) or evidence, or both.

3.1.5 *hasty search, v*—to send a fast moving, well-trained crew(s) of searchers to quickly check selected high probability area(s).

3.1.6 *investigation, n*—the systematic collection and analysis of information about the lost or missing subject(s) by interviewing (interrogation) or reviewing records or evidence, or both.

3.1.7 *line search, v*—to use searchers in a linear pattern(s) at specified intervals, to investigate a defined search segment.

3.1.8 *probability of area (POA), n*—the probability of a subject or clue being in the area or segment being searched.

3.1.9 *probability of detection (POD), n*— the probability that the subject or clue will be detected by the search action if the subject or clue is in the search area.

3.1.10 *search dog, n*—canine trained in techniques to locate a subject(s) or evidence or both.

3.1.11 *search dog crew(s), n*—canine and their handler(s) trained in search techniques to locate a subject(s) or evidence, or both.

3.1.12 *segment (search area), n*—a geographic unit within the search area established for the purpose of effective and efficient assignment of search resources.

3.1.13 *segmentation, n*—the process of partitioning the search area into segments.

3.1.14 *segmentation, binary, n*—to reduce the size of a search area through subdivision into increasingly smaller segments.

3.1.15 *tracking, v*—to follow a subject(s) footprint(s), track(s), or sign through varying types of terrain.

3.2 *Definitions of Terms Specific to This Standard:*

3.2.1 *breakage, n*—a physical rupture of material or the surface of material, such as frequently seen when vegetation is crushed or bent by external forces such as the passage of subjects.

3.2.2 *bruising, n*—changes in the subsurface of vegetation which generally leaves the surface intact but noticeably different and is the result of vegetation being crushed or squeezed by external forces such as the passage of a subject(s).

3.2.3 *color change, n*—changes in tone or contrast of a surface as a result of a disturbance which causes the disturbed area to appear different from the surroundings. An example of such a change would be the turning up of sub-soil with more moisture than the drier surface soil, thereby creating a darker pattern in the disturbed area. See also *shine*.

[1] This guide is under the jurisdiction of ASTM Committee F-32 on Search and Rescue and is the direct responsibility of Subcommittee F32.04 on Search Operations and Techniques.

Current edition approved July 10, 1997. Published March 1998. Originally published as F 1633 - 95. Last previous edition F 1633 - 95$^{\epsilon 1}$.

[2] *Annual Book of ASTM Standards*, Vol 13.01.

3.2.4 *disturbance, n*—evidence of recent change, displacement, or rearrangement such as dislodged rocks, pebbles, twigs, or bruised leaves. Other evidence could include breaks in branches, twigs, or bruised leaves at or above the ground.

3.2.5 *flattening, n*—when pebbles, twigs and other objects are pushed below their natural bed, indicating that something very hard such as a sole or hoof of an animal has stepped on them.

3.2.6 *scuff, n*—a disturbance caused by the dragging of a foot on a surface such as is evidenced by the displacement of a lichen on a rock.

3.2.7 *shine, n*—an apparent color change in the reflection of light from surfaces as a result of disturbance to the area. Frequently seen as dew laden grass that has had the moisture knocked from it as a subject walks through it or as flattened grass from foot pressure. This is most easily seen from distances between 5 and 10 m.

3.2.8 *sign, n*—any evidence of external forces acting upon the environment. Emphasis is placed on sign that indicates the passage of the subject(s) being sought. Examples include a sole pattern imbedded in the soil as a sign that a person or shoes have been there.

3.3 Terminology not defined in this guide but referenced in the text can be found in ICS 420,[3] *Managing the Search Function*,[4] and in *Search is an Emergency*.[5]

4. Summary of Guide

4.1 This guide presents the land search manager with a brief synopsis of various land search techniques that have been shown to be effective in locating missing subjects or evidence. Some known strengths and weaknesses are discussed to assist the land search manager in selecting the most appropriate set of techniques for the incident at hand.

4.2 Much of the information in the guide comes from classroom materials available through the National Association for Search and Rescue *Managing the Search Function*[4] Course and from the Emergency Response Institute's classroom text *Search is an Emergency*.[5]

5. Significance and Use

5.1 Lost persons are at risk of injury or death from extended periods of isolation, either mental, physical or both. Their inability to solve immediate problems requires that search and rescue (SAR) personnel use the most efficient and effective techniques to resolve the lost person's situation and to minimize the risks of injury or death.

5.2 Searching for immobile or unresponsive subjects, including those deceased, places further limitations upon the search options that are available to search managers. Where appropriate, the guide identifies these limitations.

5.3 The use of the listed techniques improves the probability of locating a lost or missing person when applied to land search incidents. These techniques may be employed at the discretion of and under the direction and control of a land search manager.

5.4 Terms used in this guide are not intended to be comprehensive, nor are they presumed to be inclusive of all terminology used in the search function.

6. General Considerations

6.1 Operational factors that are common to any search but not specific to any one phase or element of the operation are listed in Table 1. Each factor should be considered when initiating a search for a lost subject(s). Often these considerations can be summarized to a single form such as is given in the example in Appendix X1.

7. Land Search Techniques

7.1 *Attraction*—Method of searching, in which the searcher attempts to establish contact with the subject by audio or visual means, or both. When the technique is used it is important that the searcher remains stationary for a long enough period of time to be sure the subject will respond if able. This method is used when the subject is believed to be responsive. The subject(s) may or may not be mobile, although mobility improves the usefulness of the technique in many instances.

7.1.1 There are many ways of attracting a subject (see Table 2). Which method to use depends on a great variety of conditions that may exist during the search. Some of the conditions to be considered are local background noise, weather, natural and artificial lighting present, topography, time of day/year, and resources available.

7.1.2 Attraction can be used in conjunction with other search techniques. When searchers are moving it is important to stop at various intervals to look and listen for a response. Observation and listening posts may be established throughout a search area.

7.2 *Confinement*— A search technique that presumes the subject's ability to leave a search area can be prevented or at

TABLE 1 General Considerations for Land Search

Subject Considerations:	number of subjects
	age
	physical condition and abilities
	mental condition and attitude
	knowledge and training
	clothing
	equipment
	self-rescue likelihood
Terrain Considerations:	difficulty of travel
	difficulty of access
	remoteness
	exposure to object hazards
Weather Considerations:	recent past
	present
	future
Time Considerations:	last seen
	remaining light, if any
	sign age/longevity
Resource Considerations:	available personnel
	available equipment
	knowledge, training and experience
	available air-evac assets

[3] International Fire Service Training Association, *Incident Command System Field Operations Guide, ICS 420* available from the International Fire Service Training Association, Fire Protection Publications, Oklahoma State University, Stillwater, OK 74078.

[4] *Managing the Search Function*, Third Edition, 1987. Available from the National Association for Search and Rescue, P.O. Box 3709, Fairfax, VA 22038.

[5] LaValla, Rick and Stoffel, Skip. 1987. *Search is an Emergency*, Emergency Response Institute, 4537 Foxhall Drive, Olympia, Washington 98506.

TABLE 2 Examples of Attraction

Visual	Audio
lights	horns
flares	sirens
fires	voice
beacons	bells
strobes	firearms
smoke	PA systems
balloons	whistles

TABLE 3 Electronic Search Techniques

Subject Status/Technique	Examples
Not Specially Equipped, Not Responsive	
infrared thermal imaging	helicopter Forward Looking Infrared (FLIR)
infrared illumination	
light amplification	starlight or sniper scope
acoustic amplification	
magnetometer	
Not Specially Equipped, Responsive	
all of the above	
seismic sensing	
acoustic interrogation	loudspeaker, acoustic amplifier for listening
Specially Equipped, Not Responsive	
radio direction finding	automatically activated Emergency Locator Transmitter (ELT)
avalanche beacon	
transponder interrogation	RECCO™ personnel locator[5]
Specially Equipped, Responsive	
all of the above	
radio direction finding	manually activated transmitter
direct radio/telephone communication	

least detected. It is most useful when several items of pertinent information are known, thereby enabling the subject's rate of travel to be estimated. This information includes the point last seen (PLS), the time the person became lost, and the mobility of the subject keeping in mind that weather or darkness may further limit the subject's mobility.

7.2.1 Confinement is less effective when the search area is not well defined or is extremely large. If search tools such as string lines or other temporary boundaries must be built, it will require much time and manpower, thereby increasing the chances that the subject(s) may leave the search area undetected.

7.2.2 Terrain features may be conducive to the confinement technique if the borders of the search segment are well defined by natural or man-made boundaries.[3] Under these circumstances, boundaries tend to direct or restrict the subject's travel.

7.3 *Electronic Search*—The use of electronic systems or devices to locate a subject(s) or evidence, or both. Which electronic search techniques can be used depends upon what equipment is available, whether or not the subject or evidence is specially equipped (for example, RECCO™,[6] ELT), and whether or not the subject(s) are responsive. Table 3 summarizes the suitability of the various techniques to specific circumstances of a search.

7.3.1 All of these methods, except for infrared illumination and light amplification, which can be used only at night, can be used day or night. Most infrared thermal imaging systems work only at night, but systems that produce color images can be used during the day. All the methods can be used in any weather or terrain, but the acoustic and seismic techniques need a relatively quiet environment to function properly.

7.4 *Hasty Search*— A planned, rapid, non-thorough search, of high probability areas, by small, fast moving, clue conscious crews. This active method of searching is usually used in the early phases of a land search to search the areas where the subject is most likely to be located, or to find a clue to give direction of travel, or both. Some areas in which a hasty crew may be used include known or suspected routes (for example, trails), the area around the point last seen, areas which might be attractive to the subject (for example, ponds, rivers, meadows, vistas), drainages, and ridge tops.

7.5 *Investigation*— The act of gathering information, often referred to as intelligence, about the lost person(s). In the course of investigation, information is gathered regarding two elements of lost persons. The first involves subject behavior and survivability profiles within the boundaries of the search area. The second pertains to the potential whereabouts and plight of missing persons who are potentially outside the search area (staged incident[5] or "bastard" search[7]). This could be information needed by criminal investigators should the search become criminal in nature.

7.5.1 Intelligence is gathered from interviews with persons other than the subject(s), review of records, and examination of evidence found during the course of the search. Relatives, friends, associates, and persons in the search area are prime candidates for interviews. Record reviews might include use permits, rental agreements, Department of Motor Vehicles, criminal history, and personal records left by the missing subject(s). Evidence examination may include vehicles, campsites and other items found in the search area.

7.5.2 Many agencies have found it desirable to develop standardized missing subject forms similar to the examples given in F 1767. The forms help remind investigators of the types of information to be gathered as well as to document the investigator's findings. Forms are also a convenient way to communicate and review missing subject information during subsequent operational periods of a search.

NOTE 1—Missing subject forms come in a variety of lengths and complexities. Content and length vary to support the documentation requirements of the responsible agency and to supplement the abilities of the investigator. Many are designed to be specific to an agency's primary form of response (law enforcement, land search, marine rescue, etc).

7.6 *Line Search*— Includes many methods of searching, all of which use a number of searchers forming a line of some sort to sweep a selected segment of the search area. These methods vary in their manpower and time requirements according to the desired percent of detection. Some line search methods use

[6] RECCO is a registered trademark of RECCO Technologies, 2396 Caledonia Ave., North Vancouver, BC Canada V7G IT9.

[7] Stenicka, T. J., *Wilderness Search and Rescue*, 1985. Available from Appalachian Mountain Club, Boston, MA.

very tight spacing to find small clues or deceased subjects (for example, an avalanche probe line). Other methods use wide spacing while attempting to make sound contact with a responsive subject. In all cases the probability of detecting the missing subject is inversely related to the spacing between adjacent searchers.[4,5] The objective of line searching is to achieve the desired percent of detection for the complete segment, thoroughly, without duplication. Often this is done by marking the edge of the searched area with flagging or string, and using this as a guide for the next sweep. In some methods, searchers start and end on a common line, but work independently or in small groups using a compass bearing as a guide.

7.7 *Search Dog Crews*— The use of search dog crews in land search involves the fielding of a trained canine, trained handler and often at least one other trained searcher who handles navigation and radio communications for the crew. Search dog crews are typically used to identify and develop clues that will lead searchers to the location of a missing subject. Search dog crews, however, are also frequently used to establish the subject's direction of travel and to quickly decrease the probability of area (POA) of one or more search segments.

7.7.1 Search dog crews have one or more capabilities in trailing, tracking and air-scent detection of missing subjects. The appropriateness of utilizing a trailing, tracking or air-scenting dog crew will depend upon the specific circumstances of the search. These circumstances include but are not limited to:

7.7.1.1 The availability of a viable, uncontaminated scent article,

7.7.1.2 The prior identification of a point-last-seen,

7.7.1.3 The length of time the subject has been missing,

7.7.1.4 The current and previous days' weather, and

7.7.1.5 The population of search and non-search personnel in the search area.

7.7.2 Trailing and tracking dog crews can be utilized most effectively when the first three of the above listed circumstances are known. Trailing and tracking dog crews are especially useful to confirm the presence or absence of a missing subject along a specific route. Air-scenting dog crews, on the other hand, can be utilized without knowledge of the first three circumstances, but the effectiveness of these crews is influenced much more by the last two circumstances listed. Failure on the part of the search manager to control the number of searchers and other extraneous personnel in the search area, or to heed the limitations of weather, especially meteorological factors that affect air movement, will almost always diminish the usefulness of an air-scenting dog crew. All types of dog crews perform more effectively when all of the above circumstances are known.

7.8 *Segmentation*— A search strategy that involves dividing the area to be searched into smaller more manageable units called segments. Segments are constructed to assist search crews in achieving strategic objectives in a defined amount of time (usually a single operational period[4]). They may or may not be equal in size. Properly constructed segments will improve the coverage of the area being searched and will enhance a search manager's ability to set tactical priorities. Segmentation is also used as a basis for applying statistical probability theory to the prioritization of search resources and the estimation of and tracking of search success.

7.8.1 When distinct terrain features, and natural and man-made barriers exist (ridge lines, canyon bottoms, streams, fences, roads, etc.), segments may be created to limit search crews within these boundaries or to focus search coverage to these features. In the absence of such features, segments may be constructed to equally divide the area to be searched. Binary segmentation is often used in these situations to systematically reduce the search area (or segment) into smaller parts. The reduction is usually achieved by cutting for sign sequentially through the center of a search area and then eliminating from the search that portion of the area where no sign was found.

7.8.2 Segmentation is most often applied during preliminary steps to define and help record actions taken in the search area. The success of this strategy improves when the subject profile and knowledge of the terrain can be utilized to delineate the segments, and segment size can be limited to areas searched during a single operational period.

7.9 *Tracking*—The process of following a subject(s) over varying types of terrain based upon physical evidence of the subject's passage. This evidence may include footprints, bruised or broken vegetation, or far more subtle signs such as scuffs, flattening, color changes or shine. Highly skilled trackers can even suggest information about the subject's physical condition by studying their tracks and gait. For instance, long, even strides are often considered evidence of a subject in good physical condition while a deteriorating or otherwise uneven gait, foot dragging, aimless drifting from the trail, or frequent falls are often considered as an indication of a subject in poorer physical condition.

7.9.1 In concert with other search techniques, tracking can aid in verifying information and evidence provided by other land search techniques (for example, search dogs, eyewitness interviews, victim profiling). It can reduce the search area by establishing a known direction of travel of the missing subject(s). Finally, because it is basically a step-by-step technique, it can be especially helpful in locating hidden or otherwise unresponsive subjects.

7.9.2 Except for scent, footprints are usually the most numerous clues in a search area.[5] However, one of the most difficult parts of tracking is the proper identification of the subject's footprints. Very often, the subject's tracks are in areas where numerous other persons have walked, both before and after the subject's passage. In some areas (for example, the desert), track identification can be further complicated by the almost fresh appearance of tracks that are many days old. Accurate communication of a tracker's identifications must also be maintained to prevent search crews from following persons other than the subject. For these reasons trackers and search managers often use some type of standardized form, such as the examples given in Guide F 1767.

8. Keywords

8.1 investigation; lost persons; lost subjects; missing persons; search

APPENDIXES

(Nonmandatory Information)

X1. RELATIVE SEARCH URGENCY RATING FORM[8]

X1.1 On the following chart, the lower the numerical rating of the factor, the higher the relative urgency becomes. The chart is intended as a guide. It is a tool for the manager to use in evaluating individual incidents. All figures are relative and the total derived from the chart only indicates a possible relative urgency. All factors bearing on the incident must also be evaluated by the Incident Commander (search manager) in the process of finally establishing urgency.

Factor	Rating
Subject Profile	
Age	
Very Young	1
Very Old	1
Other	2–3
Medical Condition	
Known/suspected injured, ill or mental problem	1–2
Healthy	3
Known Fatality	2
Number of Subjects	
One alone	1
More than one (unless separation suspected)	2–3
Subject Experience Profile	
Not experienced, does not know area	1
Not experienced, knows area	1–2
Experienced, not familiar with area	2
Experienced, knows area	3
Weather Profile	
Past or existing hazardous weather, or both	1
Predicted hazardous weather (8 h or less)	1–2
Predicted hazardous weather (more than 8 h)	2
No hazardous weather predicted	3
Equipment Profile	
Inadequate for environment and weather	1
Questionable for environment and weather	1–2
Adequate for environment and weather	3
Terrain/Hazards Profile	
Known hazardous terrain or other hazards	1
Few or no hazards	2–3

[8] Derived from Figure 13.2 of *Managing the Search Function*, Third Edition, 1987. Available from the National Association for Search and Rescue, P.O. Box 3709, Fairfax, VA, 22038.

X2. MISSING SUBJECT FORM

X2.1 See Fig. X2.1 for example of a missing subject form.

LOS ANGELES COUNTY SHERIFF'S DEPARTMENT
SEARCH AND RESCUE CIRCUMSTANCE

DATE AND TIME OF CALL ______ FILE NO. ______
VICTIM ______ NICKNAME(S) ______
(MAKE OUT SEPARATE SHEET FOR EACH VICTIM)
ADDRESS ______ CITY ______ PHONE ______
SEX ___ RACE ___ AGE ___ HEIGHT ___ WEIGHT ___ BUILD ___ HAIR ___ EYES ___
MARKS/SCARS ______ PHOTO AVAIL ( ) SHOES ______
TYPE COLOR SIZE DIMENSION SOLE AGE
CLOTHING WORN ______
______ MONEY CARRIED $ ______

PERSONALITY: CALM ( ) NERVOUS ( ) CAUTIOUS ( ) CARELESS ( )
ATTITUDE WHEN LAST SEEN: WORRIED ( ) ANGRY ( ) FRIGHTENED ( ) HAPPY ( )
PHYSICAL COND: VERY GOOD ( ) GOOD ( ) SICK* ( ) TIRED ( ) WEAK ( ) *MEDICINE ______
SMOKER: YES ( ) NO ( ) TYPE FILTER ( ) CORK ( ) PLAIN ( ) BRAND ______
FAMILIARITY WITH AREA: NONE ( ) SLIGHT ( ) GOOD ( )
ABILITY IN MTS.: NONE ( ) AMATEUR ( ) GOOD ( ) EXPERT

ITEMS CARRIED: FOOD & CANDY ______
EQUIPMENT ______
NUMBER IN PARTY ___ NO. LOST ___ PERSONS W/VICTIM ______
LAST SEEN (PLACE/DATE) ______ TIME ______ AM PM
UATION: LOST ( ) FALL ( ) STRANDED ( ) INJURED ( ) SICK ( ) DEAD ( )
AREA: TRAIL ( ) STREAM ( ) RIDGE ( ) CANYON ( )
DESTINATION ______
ROUTE OF TRAVEL FROM ______ TIME ______ AM PM
TO ______ TO ARR. ______ AM PM
WAS THERE A CHANGE OF PLANS ___ WHAT ______
AREA/PLACES VICTIM FAMILIAR WITH ______
KNOWN FRIENDS ______
INFORMANT ______ WAS INFORMANT MEMBER OF PARTY ______
ADDRESS ______ CITY ______ PHONE ______
NEXT OF KIN ______ RELATIONSHIP ______
ADDRESS ______ CITY ______ PHONE ______
NOTE: IF VICTIM IS LOST, SECURE ARTICLE OF CLOTHING FOR TRACKING DOG. CLOTHING MUST HAVE BEEN WORN NEXT TO BODY AND MUST NOT HAVE BEEN LAUNDERED. DO NOT HANDLE, PICK UP WITH FORK OR STICK AND PLACE IN CLEAN PAPER BAG. USE REVERSE SIDE OF FORM FOR REMARKS.
DEPUTY ______ BADGE ______
MOUNTAINEER ______
SAR NUMBER ______ DESK ______ STATION ______

FIG. X2.1 Missing Subject Form

X3. STANDARDIZED FORM

X3.1 See Fig. X3.1 for example of standarized form trackers and search managers use to assist one another in describing footprints.

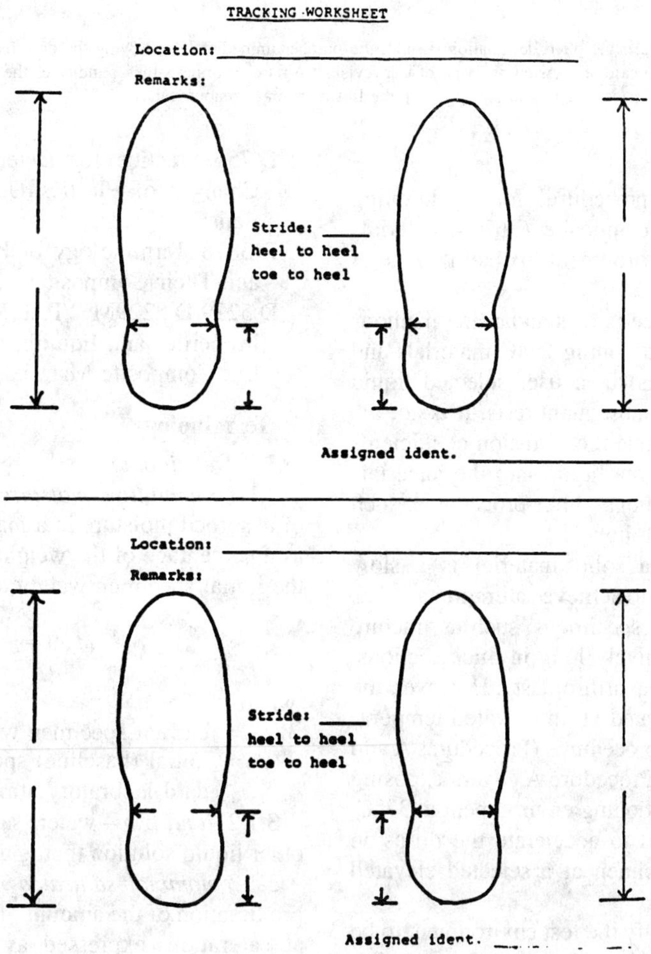

FIG. X3.1 Standardized Form

The American Society for Testing and Materials takes no position respecting the validity of any patent rights asserted in connection with any item mentioned in this standard. Users of this standard are expressly advised that determination of the validity of any such patent rights, and the risk of infringement of such rights, are entirely their own responsibility.

This standard is subject to revision at any time by the responsible technical committee and must be reviewed every five years and if not revised, either reapproved or withdrawn. Your comments are invited either for revision of this standard or for additional standards and should be addressed to ASTM Headquarters. Your comments will receive careful consideration at a meeting of the responsible technical committee, which you may attend. If you feel that your comments have not received a fair hearing you should make your views known to the ASTM Committee on Standards, at the address shown below.

Designation: F 1634 – 95 (Reapproved 2000)

Standard Practice for In-Vitro Environmental Conditioning of Polymer Matrix Composite Materials and Implant Devices[1]

This standard is issued under the fixed designation F 1634; the number immediately following the designation indicates the year of original adoption or, in the case of revision, the year of last revision. A number in parentheses indicates the year of last reapproval. A superscript epsilon (ϵ) indicates an editorial change since the last revision or reapproval.

1. Scope

1.1 This practice covers two procedures for conditioning non-absorbable polymer matrix composite (PMC) materials and implant devices in a liquid environment to obtain a state of saturation.

1.2 The purpose of this practice is to standardize methods and reporting procedures for conditioning PMC materials and implant devices (PMC specimens) in a user selected liquid environment prior to conducting subsequent tests. It is not the purpose of this practice to determine the diffusion coefficients or actual saturation levels of a given liquid into the materials and devices. For these determinations, other procedures, such as Test Method D 5229, may be followed.

1.3 Diffusion of liquid into a solid material is a slow process. While the time necessary to achieve saturation at 37°C may be sufficiently short for thin specimens, such as fracture fixation plates, it may be prohibitively long in thick sections, such as femoral components for hip arthroplasty. However, the diffusion process may be accelerated at an elevated temperature. Consequently, two separate procedures (Procedures A and B) are presented in this practice. Procedure A covers exposing the specimen to the desired conditioning environment at 37°C. Procedure B prescribes a method to accelerate the diffusion process by conditioning the specimen at a selected elevated temperature.

1.4 This practice does not specify the test environment to be used for conditioning. However, the pH value of immersion liquid shall be maintained at 7.4 ± 0.2 to simulate the in vivo environment.

1.5 *This standard does not purport to address all of the safety concerns, if any, associated with its use. It is the responsibility of the user of this standard to establish appropriate safety and health practices and determine the applicability of regulatory limitations prior to use.*

2. Referenced Documents

2.1 *ASTM Standards:*

D 618 Practice for Conditioning Plastics and Electrical Insulation Materials for Testing[2]

D 756 Practice for Determination of Weight and Shape Changes of Plastics Under Accelerated Service Conditions[2]

D 3878 Terminology of High-Modulus Reinforcing Fibers and Their Composites[3]

D 5229/D 5229M Test Method for Moisture Absorption Properties and Equilibrium Conditioning of Polymer Matrix Composite Materials[3]

3. Terminology

3.1 *Definitions:*

3.1.1 *cumulative moisture content, M_t (%), n*—the amount of absorbed moisture in a material at a given time *t*, expressed as a percentage of the weight of absorbed moisture divided by the initial specimen weight, as follows:

$$M_t, \% = \frac{W_i - W_b}{W_b} \times 100 \quad (1)$$

where:
W_t = current specimen weight, g, and
W_b = initial (baseline) specimen weight at $t = 0$ and standard laboratory atmosphere, g.

3.1.2 *liquid, n*—water, saline solution, calf serum, or any other liquid solution that is used to condition PMC specimens.

3.1.3 *nominal saturated moisture content, M_s(%)*—an approximation of the amount of moisture absorbed by a specimen at saturation, expressed as a percentage of the weight of absorbed moisture at approximate saturation divided by the initial specimen weight, as follows:

$$M_s, \% = \frac{W_s - W_b}{W_b} \times 100 \quad (2)$$

where:
W_s = specimen weight at approximate saturation, g, and
W_b = initial (baseline) specimen weight at $t = 0$ and standard laboratory atmosphere, g.

3.1.4 *standard laboratory atmosphere, n*— a laboratory atmosphere having a temperature of 23 ± 2°C and a relative humidity of 50 ± 10 %.

4. Summary of Test Method

4.1 In Procedure A, a specimen is immersed in a liquid bath at 37 ± 1°C with a pH value of 7.4 ± 0.2.

[1] This practice is under the jurisdiction of ASTM Committee F04 on Medical and Surgical Materials and Devices and is the direct responsibility of Subcommittee F04.14 on Composite Materials.

Current edition approved Nov. 10, 1995. Published January 1996.

[2] *Annual Book of ASTM Standards*, Vol 08.01.

[3] *Annual Book of ASTM Standards*, Vol 15.03.

4.2 In Procedure B, conditioning occurs in a liquid bath at a selected elevated temperature.

4.3 Weight change is monitored over time until specimens reach the nominal moisture saturation content.

4.4 Keep specimens in the conditioning bath for storage prior to subsequent tests.

5. Significance and Use

5.1 The conditioning procedures covered in this practice provide methods for saturating PMC specimens in a liquid environment prior to conducting other tests for property evaluation.

5.2 The conditioning may affect geometric and dimensional changes in specimens. In some severe cases, chemical changes may occur in the fiber, polymer and fiber-polymer interphase and interface.

5.3 Caution must be taken if Procedure B (10.2, Procedure B—Accelerated Moisture Saturation at Elevated Temperature) is followed to condition PMC specimens at an elevated temperature. Physical and chemical reactions in materials are normally temperature dependent. An increase in experimental temperature may accelerate a desirable moisture diffusion process. However, elevated temperatures above 37°C may also cause undesirable reactions that do not represent appropriate responses of materials at 37°C. Consequently, a pilot study is recommended in Procedure B to determine if a selected elevated temperature can be used for accelerated conditioning. If the properties of materials are determined to be irreversibly affected by this pilot study at the selected elevated temperature, then either an appropriate lower elevated temperature should be determined by repeating the pilot study, or Procedure B should not be used.

6. Apparatus

6.1 *Balance*—An analytical balance capable of measuring weight of specimens to within a resolution of at least 0.005 % of the total specimen weight.

6.2 *Conditioning Bath*—A temperature-controlled liquid bath shall be capable of maintaining the required temperature to within ±1°C. The bath shall be monitored either on an automated continuous basis or on a manual basis at regular intervals.

6.3 *Specimen Bag*— A sealable, flexible, moisture-proof bag made of material suitable for exposure to specimens that have been removed from the conditioning bath for cooling prior to weighing. Bags that meet the requirement of MIL-B-131 have been found to be satisfactory for use in such applications.

6.4 *Absorbent Cloth*— Clean, non-linting absorbent cloth for use in wiping excess liquid from surface of specimens.

6.5 *Gloves*—Clean, non-linting gloves for use when handling specimens.

6.6 *pH Measurement System*—An analytical system capable of measuring pH to within ±0.1.

6.7 *Differential Scanning Calorimeter*—An analytical system capable of heating a specimen at a controlled rate while measuring heat input and temperature.

7. Sampling and Test Specimens

7.1 *Preparation*— Precaution shall be taken to avoid the entrapment of moisture in uneven surfaces, or delamination due to inappropriate machining and manufacturing processes.

7.2 *Labeling*—Label the specimen so as to be distinct from each other in a manner that will both be unaffected by the test and not influence the test and, furthermore, will not be removed during conditioning.

8. Measurements of Test Specimens

8.1 The following measurements shall be made on specimens prior to immersion, after conditioning at the end of a test procedure, and at any intermediate stage as prescribed in the test procedures:

8.1.1 *Weight*—The weight within 0.005 % of specimen weight.

8.1.2 Characteristic dimensions of specimens may be measured as a function of immersion time to determine the amount of swelling induced by moisture absorption.

9. Visual Examination

9.1 Noticeable qualitative changes in surfaces, outline, and general appearance of the test specimen shall be recorded after each stage of the testing procedure. These changes include color, surface irregularities, odor, surface voids, delamination and cracking. The immersion liquid should also be observed for evidence of material that has leached from specimens or holders, and evidence of bacterial or fungal contamination. If bacterial or fungal contamination is found, specimens should be removed from the solution, washed with detergent and water, rinsed, and placed in fresh solution. If contamination is a recurring problem, antibacterial or antifungal agents must be added to the solution; minimal amounts should be used as they may affect specimen properties.

10. Procedures

10.1 *Procedure A—Moisture Saturation Determination at 37°C*:

10.1.1 *Specimen Preconditioning*—Bring the test specimens to a uniform 23 ± 2°C after manufacturing process.

10.1.2 *Moisture Absorption*:

10.1.2.1 Record the initial (baseline) weight, W_b.

10.1.2.2 Place the specimen in the conditioning bath, which has previously reached the specified temperature 37 ± 1°C. The pH value of immersion liquid used shall be maintained at 7.4 ± 0.2 throughout the conditioning process and monitored at least once a week. If the solution pH falls outside the designated range, the solution should be changed. The pH should not be maintained by repeatedly adding buffer to the same solution. This will change solution composition and may affect specimen properties. Evaporation losses should be made up with sterile deionized water if saline, serum, plasma, or other hydrous medium is used as the conditioning environment.

10.1.2.3 Monitor the weight gain of specimens over time. A suggested schedule is to weigh each specimen every 24 h for the first 120 h, then every 96 h.

10.1.2.4 At the end of each time interval, remove the specimens from the conditioning bath and place them in the specimen bag. Seal the bag and allow the specimens to come to laboratory standard temperature. Remove the specimens from the bag and wipe the specimens free of surface moisture with an absorbent lint-free cloth. Wait for 10 min and measure the weight of specimens to the required precision, and W_t, along with the corresponding total elapsed time and the time interval since the previous measurement.

10.1.2.5 Return the specimens to the conditioning bath. The specimens shall not be out of the conditioning bath for more than 30 min and shall not be out of the specimen bag for more than 15 min.

10.1.2.6 Calculate cumulative moisture content, M_t (%), using Eq 1 at each time interval and plot versus time.

10.1.2.7 The minimum time, t_{min}, required to reach nominal saturated moisture content, M_s, is the time at which the change in cumulative moisture content from the prior measurement is less than 0.010 % of specimen weight for three consecutive weighings with no less than 96 h of elapsed time between each consecutive weighing.

10.1.2.8 Following moisture saturation within the specified tolerance range, the specimen should be stored in a bath of the same fluid which is to be used for post-conditioning testing until the time the post-conditioning testing is conducted.

10.2 *Procedure B—Accelerated Moisture Saturation at Elevated Temperature*:

10.2.1 *Determination of Accelerated Temperature* (T_a) *Level*:

10.2.1.1 Specimens should be first saturated in the conditioning environment at 37°C and then evaluated by differential scanning calorimeter (DSC) evaluation over a temperature range of 37 to 120°C. The purpose of this is to determine if a material transition temperature (that is, glass transition or melting temperature), or a degradation temperature (such as an oxidation or thermal decomposition temperature), occurs within this temperature range. If the material is stable within this range, then accelerated conditioning may be conducted at T_a = 95°C in a conditioning environment containing water. If a transition or degradation temperature is found between 37 and 120°C, then the maximum acceleration temperature to be used should be at least 25°C below the lowest transition or decomposition temperature. If nonhydrous solutions are used as the conditioning environment (that is, pure lipid), then a similar procedure can be followed except the temperature would now be governed by the boiling or decomposition temperature of the given environment and specimen combination.

10.2.2 *Effect of Accelerated Temperature Conditioning*:

10.2.2.1 Once T_a is determined from 10.2.1.1, at least five samples representative of the specimen being evaluated should be conditioning at both T_a and 37°C and then tested to check for conditioning temperature induced differences. Because conditioning may influence different material properties of PMC specimens in different ways, the test implemented to check for differences between T_a and 37°C should closely match the intended post-conditioning test that the PMC specimen will be conditioned for. If T_a influences the properties in question, then a lower conditioning temperature must be identified by repeating this procedure at selected lower temperatures in which the property is not influenced by conditioning. If the property is determined to be not influenced by T_a, then T_a can be used to accelerate the conditioning process for subsequent specimens.

10.2.3 *Accelerated Conditioning*:

10.2.3.1 Follow the procedures outlined in 10.1.2 with the exception that the conditioning bath will be maintained at T_a ± 1.0°C. The same time-measurement sequence as described in 10.1.2 should be used to determine the minimum time, t_{min}, when saturation is reached. The bath should be adequately sealed to minimize evaporation loss and periodically monitored to ensure adequate bath depth is maintained for complete immersion of samples. If the bath is physically sealed, a safe mechanism of pressure relief (that is, pressure relief valve or releasable lid seal) must be provided to prevent pressure build-up if the oven is accidentally overheated. Evaporation losses should be made up with sterile deionized water if saline, serum, plasma, or other hydrous medium is used as the conditioning environment.

10.2.3.2 Following moisture saturation within the specified tolerance range, the specimen should be stored in a bath of the same fluid which is to be used for post-conditioning testing until the time the post-conditioning testing is conducted.

11. Selection of Conditioning Procedure

11.1 The choice between procedures should preferably be based on the one that gives the most reproducible results.

12. Report

12.1 Report the following information:

12.1.1 Description of the specimen or device being considered (that is, material name, dimensions, part number, model number, size designation).

12.1.2 The date of issue of this practice and the procedure used.

12.1.3 The date(s) and location(s) of the test.

12.1.4 The name(s) of the test operator(s).

12.1.5 Any variations to this practice, anomalies noticed during testing or equipment problems occurring during testing.

12.1.6 Description of the materials and fabrication method used in preparing the specimen including: cure cycle, consolidation method and a description of equipment used.

12.1.7 Method of preparing the test specimens.

12.1.8 Weight of the specimen following preconditioning prior to moisture conditioning and at the completion of the saturation procedure.

12.1.9 Type of conditioning bath used, liquid used for the test and its average pH value, the average actual test temperature, and measurement time interval.

12.1.10 Specimen weight at each interval.

12.1.11 Plots of percent weight changes versus time, calculated by (Eq 1).

12.1.12 Description of procedures, frequency and reasons for changing immersion liquid.

12.1.13 Any unusual observations described in 9.1.

12.1.14 Mean, standard deviation, number of specimens, coefficient of variation of specimen property measured, number of samples used in the verification test and T_a, if Procedure B is followed.

12.1.15 Any dimension changes during immersion due to swelling (if measured).

13. Keywords

13.1 accelerated conditioning; composite; diffusion; environmental conditioning; fiber; implant devices; moisture absorption; polymer

APPENDIX

(Nonmandatory Information)

X1. RATIONALE

X1.1 The primary reason for developing this practice is to establish methods for in vitro environmental conditioning of polymer matrix composite materials and implant devices (PMC specimens) prior to determining their properties and behavior. It is not the purpose of this practice to accurately determine actual percentages of moisture uptake at saturation or diffusion coefficients. Therefore, the PMC specimens do not need to be dried prior to environmental conditioning.

X1.2 On a molecular scale, PMC specimens are porous materials through which components of a surrounding environment, such as water and salt ions, can diffuse. Diffusion into a PMC specimen is a slow, temperature dependent process which may significantly influence material properties. Therefore, testing a PMC specimen in a simulated in vivo environment, without first conditioning the material to attain environmental saturation, may lead to erroneous test results regarding the performance of the material or device in the body. This practice presents test methods to condition PMC specimens.

X1.3 Theoretically, an infinite amount of time is necessary to allow a liquid diffusing into a solid to achieve full diffusion equilibrium. Therefore, some approximation to full saturation must be defined for practical use. Weight gain at diffusion equilibrium of water in most engineering thermoplastic polymers is less than 1.0 % by weight. In order to obtain the necessary sensitivity for weight gain measurement, a balance sensitivity is specified in this practice of at least 0.005 wt % of total specimen weight. This sensitivity was selected to provide a sufficient number of possible weight increments in between the baseline weight (W_b) and the approximate saturation weight (W_s) to adequately determine when the specimens are effectively saturated.

X1.4 In 9.1, the conditioning solution should be visually monitored on a periodic basis for evidence of bacterial or fungal contamination. Molecular species released from the bacteria or fungus, or both, may influence the properties of the test specimen. Therefore, the specimens should be removed and washed and the solution should be replenished if contamination is observed.

X1.5 In 10.1.2.2, the pH of the immersion solution is to be monitored at least once per week to ensure it is within the specified range of 7.4 ± 0.02. In buffer solutions, the pH may remain stable for a long period of time, and then abruptly change once all the buffer has been depleted. Also, solution pH may influence the properties of the PMC specimens that will be measured following environmental conditioning. It is therefore important that pH be monitored on a periodic basis throughout the conditioning process.

X1.6 In 10.1.2.2 and 10.2.3.1 it is stated that if hydrous solutions are utilized, then evaporation losses should be made up with deionized water. Evaporative losses from a physiologic solution will be due to loss of water only. The larger molecules and salt ions will remain, thus tending to concentrate the solution. It is therefore important to maintain a nearly constant volume of solution with evaporation losses being made up by adding water.

X1.7 A minimum of 96 h is suggested between consecutive weighings in 10.1.2.3. As the effective saturation level is approached, the rate of weight gain will become very slow well before reaching effective saturation. Time intervals less than 96 h between weighings may therefore lead to erroneous conclusions regarding whether or not effective saturation has been reached.

X1.8 Environmental conditioning of a material to saturation at a temperature above a given thermal transition temperature may influence specimen properties differently than if the material was conditioning to saturation below the transition temperature. Therefore, if accelerated conditioning is to be utilized, it is important to ensure that the material does not undergo a thermal transition within the temperature range between 37 and 25°C above the desired accelerated temperature. Thus, as indicated in 10.2.1.1, if accelerated conditioning is to be used, the specimen should be checked by differential scanning calorimetry (DSC) for the presence of any thermal transition within the range of 37 to 120°C. The upper limit of 120°C is specified as it is 25°C above 95°C, which is the upper temperature limit for accelerated conditioning in hydrous solutions at atmospheric pressure.

Designation: F 1635 – 95 (Reapproved 2000)

Standard Test Method for In Vitro Degradation Testing of Poly (L-lactic Acid) Resin and Fabricated Form for Surgical Implants[1]

This standard is issued under the fixed designation F 1635; the number immediately following the designation indicates the year of original adoption or, in the case of revision, the year of last revision. A number in parentheses indicates the year of last reapproval. A superscript epsilon (ϵ) indicates an editorial change since the last revision or reapproval.

1. Scope

1.1 This test method covers poly(L-lactic acid) resin intended for use in surgical implants.

1.2 The requirements of this test method apply to poly(L-lactic acid) in various forms:

1.2.1 Virgin polymer, or

1.2.2 Any form fabricated from virgin polymer such as a semi-finished component of a finished product, a finished product, which may include packaged and sterilized implants, or a specially fabricated test specimen.

2. Referenced Documents

2.1 *ASTM Standards:*

D 638 Test Method for Tensile Properties of Plastics[2]

D 671 Test Method for Flexural Fatigue of Plastics by Constant-Amplitude-of-Force[2]

D 695 Test Method for Compressive Properties of Rigid Plastics[2]

D 747 Test Method for Apparent Bending Modulus of Plastics by Means of a Cantilever Beam[2]

D 790 Test Method for Flexural Properties of Unreinforced and Reinforced Plastics and Electrical Insulating Materials[2]

D 882 Test Method for Tensile Properties of Thin Plastic Sheeting[2]

D 1708 Test Method for Tensile Properties of Plastics by Use of Microtensile Specimens[2]

D 1822 Test Method for Tensile-Impact Energy to Break Plastics and Electrical Insulating Materials[2]

D 2857 Test Method for Dilute Solution Viscosity of Polymers[3]

F 1251 Terminology Relating to Polymeric Biomaterials in Medical and Surgical Devices[4]

3. Summary of Test Method

3.1 Samples of poly(L-lactic acid) resin, semi-finished components, finished surgical implants, or specially designed test specimens fabricated from poly(L-lactic acid) resin are placed in buffered saline solution at physiologic temperatures. Samples are periodically removed and tested for various material or mechanical properties at specified intervals (typically 1, 3, 6, 12, 26, 52 and 104 weeks).

4. Significance and Use

4.1 This test method is intended to help assess the biodegradation rates and changes in material or structural properties, or both, of poly(L-lactic acid) materials used in surgical implants.

4.2 This test method may not be appropriate for all types of implant applications. The user is cautioned to consider the appropriateness of the test method in view of the materials being tested and their potential application.

4.3 The application of mechanical loading or other forms of energy to the specimens during aging may significantly alter (that is, increase) the rate at which properties change. This needs to be considered when comparing in vitro behavior with that expected/observed at an in vivo site.

5. Apparatus

5.1 *Physiologic Soaking Solution*—A phosphate-buffered saline (PBS) solution shall be used. The pH of the solution shall be maintained at 7.4 ± 0.2 (see X1.3). The ionic concentration should be in the physiological range (for example, a solution that contains 0.1 M phosphate buffer and 0.1 M NaCl would be appropriate). The solution:specimen mass ratio shall be as high as practical. Although there is some experience with ratios as low as 20:1, the experimenter is cautioned that at lower ratios (that is, less buffering capacity) the solution pH may change more quickly. In accordance with 9.1.3 and X1.4, aging/testing is to be terminated once solution temperature or pH are allowed to drift outside of the specified ranges. Higher solution:specimen ratios (that is, 100:1) will facilitate maintenance of stable aging conditions.

5.1.1 Over the course of the study it may be possible to adjust solution pH and ionic concentration through the addition of individual solution constituents; however, it is preferable to exchange the test solution completely when it nears the limits of acceptability. Refer to X1.5 for additional information.

5.1.2 Other physiologic solutions, such as bovine serum, may be substituted provided the solution is properly buffered. An anti-microbial additive should be used to inhibit the growth

[1] This test method is under the jurisdiction of ASTM Committee F04 on Medical and Surgical Materials and Devicesand is the direct responsibility of Subcommittee F04.15 on Material Test Methods.

Current edition approved Nov. 10, 1995. Published January 1996.

[2] *Annual Book of ASTM Standards*, Vol 08.01.

[3] *Annual Book of ASTM Standards*, Vol 08.02.

[4] *Annual Book of ASTM Standards*, Vol 13.01.

of microorganisms in the solution during the test period. Paragraph X1.6 provides additional information. The appropriate MSDS should always be consulted concerning toxicity, safe use, and disposal of such additives.

5.2 *Sample Container*— A self-contained, inert container (bottle, jar, vial, etc.) capable of holding the test sample and the required volume of physiologic soaking solution (see X1.7). Multiple samples may be stored in the same container provided that suitable sample separation is maintained to allow fluid access to each sample surface and to preclude sample-to-sample contact. Each container must be sealable against solution loss by evaporation.

5.3 *Constant Temperature Bath or Oven*—An aqueous bath or heated air oven capable of maintaining the samples and containers at physiologic temperatures, 37 ± 2°C, for the specified testing periods.

5.4 *pH Meter*—A pH metering device sensitive in the physiological range (pH 6 to pH 8).

5.5 *Balance*—A calibrated weighing device capable of measuring the weight of a sample to a precision of 0.1 % of its initial weight. A balance having precision to 0.05 % or 0.01 % will facilitate establishment of an appropriate specimen drying period.

5.6 *Other*—Additional equipment as deemed appropriate by the specific test method.

6. Sampling

6.1 *Weight Loss*— A minimum of three samples shall be tested per time period.

6.2 *Molecular Weight*— A minimum of three samples shall be tested per time period.

6.3 *Mechanical and Other Testing*—A minimum of three samples shall be tested per time period.

NOTE 1—Statistical significance may require more than the minimum number of samples to be tested.

6.4 *Solution Temperature and pH*—Soaking solutions shall be tested on a periodic basis throughout the test duration. The required test period is dependent on the solution:specimen mass ratio and the solution's buffering capacity; once per week is generally practical and suggested.

7. Sample and Test Specimen

7.1 All test samples shall be representative of the material under evaluation.

7.2 Samples for comparative tests shall be produced from the same material lot or batch and under the same fabricating conditions unless specifically noted.

8. Procedure

8.1 *Test A, Weight Loss*:

8.1.1 Test samples, in either resin or fabricated form, shall be weighed to a precision of 0.1 % of the total sample weight prior to placement in the physiological solution. Samples shall be dried to a constant weight before initial weighing (see Note 2 and Note X1.8). Drying conditions, including final relative humidity (if applicable), shall be reported and may include the use of a desiccator, partial vacuum or elevated temperatures (see Note 3).

8.1.2 Test samples shall be fully immersed in the physiological solution for a specified period of time (for example, 1 week, 2 weeks, etc.).

8.1.3 Upon completion of the specified time period, each sample shall be removed and dried to a constant weight (see Note 2 and Note X1.8). The weight shall be recorded to a precision of 0.1 % of the original total sample weight.

NOTE 2—Drying to a constant weight may be quantified as less than 0.1 % weight change over a period of 48 h, or less than 0.05 % change in 24 h if the balance used is capable of such precision. Paragraph X1.8 provides additional information.

NOTE 3—Elevated temperatures may be used to assist drying of the sample provided that the temperature used does not induce material or chemical changes in the sample. The drying conditions used for the samples prior to aging and for the samples retrieved at each test interval shall be identical. The actual drying conditions used are to be reported.

8.1.4 After weighing, the samples shall not be returned to the physiological solution and shall be retired from the study.

8.2 *Test B, Molecular Weight*:

8.2.1 Determine the inherent viscosity (logarithmic viscosity number) of representative samples in chloroform at 25°C using Test Method D 2857 prior to placement of samples in the physiological solution. Dilution ratio in g/mL shall be reported.

8.2.2 Test samples shall be fully immersed in the physiological solution for the specified period of time (for example, 1 week, 3 weeks, 52 weeks, etc.).

8.2.3 Samples shall be removed at each specified time period throughout the duration of the test, dried as in 8.1.1, and tested for inherent viscosity as above.

8.3 *Test C, Mechanical Testing*:

8.3.1 Determine the appropriate mechanical properties of representative samples of resin or fabricated forms using tensile, compressive, torque, bending or other appropriate mechanical tests prior to placement of the samples in the physiological solution (time zero). Relevant ASTM test methods may include one or more of the following:
Test Method D 638
Test Method D 671
Test Method D 695
Test Method D 747
Test Method D 790
Test Method D 882
Test Method D 1708
Test Method D 1822

8.3.2 Fully immerse test samples in the physiological solution at 37°C for the specified period of time (for example, 1 week, 2 weeks, etc.).

8.3.3 Remove samples at each specified time period throughout the duration of the test and retest using the originally selected mechanical test methods and conditions. Unless otherwise deemed relevant, samples should be tested in a non-dried or wet condition. Paragraph X1.9 provides additional information. Testing conditions, wet versus dry, testing temperature, etc., should be reported.

8.3.4 Unless specifically germane to the testing scheme, samples shall be retired after the completion of each test.

8.4 *Additional Testing*:

8.4.1 The characterization of other material properties and use of other test methods (that is, thermal properties measured using Differential Scanning Calorimetry) may also be performed at each test interval. Conditioning and testing parameters, as well as test results, should all be recorded and reported.

9. Test Termination

9.1 Testing of samples shall be terminated when one or more of the following has occurred:

9.1.1 A predetermined end point has been reached, that is, elapsed time (for example, 2 years), percent weight loss, minimum inherent viscosity, percent strength loss, etc.

9.1.2 Sample integrity has been compromised by the progression of degradation or by mechanical damage to the point that meaningful and reliable data may no longer be obtained.

9.1.3 The soaking solution temperature or pH has drifted outside of the ranges specified in Section 5. Any sample properties obtained since the last in-range temperature and pH measurements shall be considered invalid and so noted in the study report (see X1.4).

10. Report

10.1 Report the following information:

10.1.1 Test material description, batch or lot number and dimensions (as appropriate).

10.1.2 Solution composition and preparation procedures.

10.1.3 Measurements of solution temperature and pH with time, if applicable.

10.1.4 Sample weights expressed as an average percentage loss, initial and subsequent by time period.

10.1.5 Inherent viscosity, initial and subsequent by time period.

10.1.6 Mechanical properties (tensile strength, compressive strength, stiffness, elongation at break, etc.) appropriate for tests performed, at time zero and at each time period.

10.1.7 Other material properties measured.

10.1.8 Reason(s) for test termination.

11. Precision

11.1 Intralaboratory and interlaboratory reproducibility has not been systematically determined.

12. Keywords

12.1 bioabsorbable; degradation; in vitro; PLA, poly(L-lactic acid); polymer; surgical implant

APPENDIX

(Nonmandatory Information)

X1. RATIONALE

X1.1 With the development of absorbable polymers for use in implantable devices, there is a need to define standard testing methods that aid in characterizing material and mechanical properties with time in a simulated physiological environment. This method is intended only as a framework for assessing degradation of implant materials and devices.

X1.1.1 This method is written for use in characterizing poly(L-lactic acid) resin and devices. Many sections of this method may be applicable to other polymers. However, the wide variety of bioabsorbable polymers and copolymers of interest has precluded consensus on a list of specific compositions to include/exclude in this test method. It was therefore decided, following the second draft of this document, to focus first on the one composition of greatest interest. Once round robin testing is performed and reported, additional methods covering other specific individual or groups of polymer compositions should be developed.

X1.2 It is recognized that the use of test coupons or specimens in forms other than final implant configurations may be helpful in assessing relevant polymer properties. For example, rectangular or round rods may be necessary to measure flexural properties, while a screw geometry may be required to evaluate the performance of a specific implantable device. However, specimen size, surface area, and process considerations must be addressed in order to relate in vitro degradation of test specimens to in vivo behavior of implant devices.

X1.3 The pH level specified for the buffered saline solution (that is, 7.4 ± 0.2) was selected on the basis of information received from two consultants to the Task Group on that this range of pH values was representative of that found in human blood and extra-cellular fluid.

X1.4 Termination of testing, following a significant change in solution temperature or pH, is indicated in 9.1.3 in order to avoid the generation of invalid results once meaningful loss of control over soaking conditions has occurred.

X1.5 A wide variety of PBS compositions is available and in common use. The components are targeted to achieve final solutions that exert near-physiological osmotic pressures of ~280–300 mOsm. Common buffer concentrations range from ~0.01 M to 0.1 M with the higher concentrations providing greater buffering capacity. Additional information about the composition and preparation of pH proportioned monobasic-dibasic phosphate buffer solutions may be found in a handbook available from Calbiochem Inc.[5]

X1.6 Addition of sodium azide at a concentration of 0.1 % is common. However, this substance is highly toxic and all MSDS indicated cautions must be followed.

X1.7 The inert containers used to hold the samples and solution are usually glass or plastic. However, for some (short duration) tests, stainless steel containers may be appropriate.

[5] Available from Calbiochem, Inc.

X1.8 Revision or further specification of requirements for drying to a constant weight are intended to be developed from round robin testing to follow issuance of this test method. The requirements stated in Note 2 are based on experience with extruded 3.2-mm diameter rods dried under nominal full vacuum at room temperature. Constant weight was achieved after 3 to 4 days.

X1.9 Task Group members have observed the use of wet versus dry test conditions to result in significant differences in some mechanical property measurements. It is recommended that testing be performed on specimens that are immersed in water at 37°C at the time of testing. Report whichever conditions are actually used.

Standard Specification for Bores and Cones for Modular Femoral Heads[1]

ϵ^1 NOTE—Editorial changes were made throughout in December 1996.
ϵ^2 NOTE—Tables 1 and 2 were editorially corrected in May 2001.

1. Scope

1.1 This specification covers the functional dimensions and tolerances for tapered cones of proximal femoral stems and the bores of mating ceramic and metal heads.

1.2 This specification does not cover the dimensions of proximal femoral stems other than the cone portion, nor does it cover the dimensions of the ceramic/metal femoral heads, other than the inside tapers.

1.3 The dimensions stated in SI units are to be regarded as the standard.

1.4 The purpose of this specification is to codify matching bore and cone combinations for easy identification. Nonetheless, components from different manufacturers should not be mixed because the combinations of tolerances within the family, surface finish, and configuration from the different manufacturers may not have been validated through axial load strengths or fatigue strength. Information supplied by the manufacturer with the implants should include a precaution statement that informs the user (surgeon) that bores and cones with the same code letter from different manufacturers should not be used without first consulting the supplier of the femoral components.

1.5 The codification described in this specification represents the most current state of the art at the time of balloting. Future additions can be made but because of the time required to revise the specification, it is recommended that the manufacturer of new combinations label their components with at least the angles until such time that new code letters can be established in accordance with future revisions of this specification.

2. Referenced Documents

2.1 *ASTM Standards:*

F 75 Specification for Cast-Cobalt-ChromiumMolybdenum Alloy for Surgical Implant Applications[2]

F 136 Specification for Wrought Titanium 6A1, 4V ELI Alloy for Surgical Implant Applications[2]

F 138 Specification for Stainless Steel Bar and Wire for Surgical Implants (Special Quality)[2]

F 562 Specification for Wrought Cobalt-Nickel-Chromium-Molybdenum Alloy for Surgical Implant Applications[2]

F 563 Specification for Wrought Cobalt-Nickel-Chromium-Molybdenum-Tungsten-Iron Alloy for Surgical Implant Applications[2]

F 603 Specification for High-Purity Dense Aluminum Oxide for Surgical Implant Application[2]

F 620 Specification for Titanium 6Al, 4V ELI Alloy Forgings for Surgical Implants[2]

F 621 Specification for Stainless Steel Forgings for Surgical Implants[2]

F 799 Specification for Thermomechanically Processed Cobalt-Chromium-Molybdenum Alloy Forgings for Surgical Applications[2]

F 961 Specification for Cobalt-Nickel-Chromium-Molybdenum Alloy Forgings for Surgical Implant Applications[2]

F 1108 Specification for Ti-6Al, 4V Alloy Castings for Surgical Implants[2]

3. Terminology

3.1 *Definitions:*

3.1.1 *nominal neck length*—the distance, *K*, parallel to the taper axis, between the theoretical gage point and the horizontal plane through the center of the head; this distance does not include standard variants used to adjust for resection level, leg length, and so forth. The *K* dimension may be plus or minus (proximal or distal to the location of the theoretical gage Point *G*).

3.1.2 *residual or free length*—the distance, *A*, parallel to the cone axis, between the end of the cone and the theoretical gage point.

3.1.3 *theoretical gage point*—the diameter, *G*, at nominal tolerance, where the stem cone (external taper) theoretically engages the femoral head bore (internal taper).

4. Materials

4.1 The cones may be made from any of the implantable

[1] This specification is under the jurisdiction of ASTM Committee F04 on Medical and Surgical Materials and Devices and is under the direct responsibility of Subcommittee F04.22 on Arthroplasty.

Current edition approved Dec. 10, 1995. Published June 1996.

[2] *Annual Book of ASTM Standards*, Vol 13.01.

grade materials used for femoral stems including: Specifications F 75, F 136, F 138, F 562, F 563, F 620, F 621, F 799, F 961, and F 1108.

4.2 The ceramic heads may be made from Specification F 603 or a material determined to be substantially equivalent or superior in mechanical strength, wear properties, and biocompatibility. The metal heads may be made from any of the recognized materials used for femoral stems including: Specifications F 75, F 136, F 138, F 562, F 563, F 620, F 621, F 799, F 961, and F 1108.

5. Dimensions and Finish

5.1 The cone dimensions shall be as indicated in Fig. 1 and Table 1. A gaging system should be used to ensure that mating diameters of the cone will allow proper seating of the femoral head.

5.2 The inside taper of the femoral head shall have the dimensions as indicated in Fig. 2 and Table 2. It is important with ceramic heads that the tip of the cone reside in the relief of the head on final assembly.

5.3 The finish of the cone may be textured, machined, ground, or roughened surface. The adequacy of this surface finish shall be tested for the axial strength of the head and the pull-off load.

6. Marking

6.1 Each cone and head shall be marked with the appropriate size letter to designate matching bores and cones and, where possible, the manufacturer's code or logo.

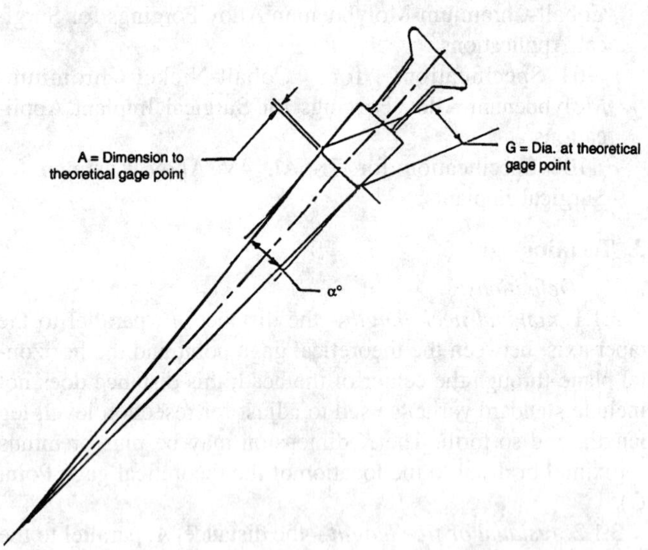

FIG. 1 Cones

TABLE 1 Cones

α°	Size	*G*—Diameter, mm	*A*—Dimension, mm
2° 50′ 30″, ±50″	A	12.8	1.0
3° 4′ 0″, ±6′	B	10.98	2.54
4° 0′ 0″, ±2.5′	C	11.5	1.0
4° 0′ 0″, ±1.6′	D	13.3	1.0
5° 0′ 0″, ±3′	E	12.7	2.34
5° 35′ 30″, ±2′	F	11.75	0.0
	G	9.6	1.4
	H	10.3	1.0
	J	11.1	1.0
5° 40′, +2.5′	K	11.87	5.75
	L	12.7	1.0
	M	12.7	1.4
	N	12.7	1.4
	P	14.3	1.0
	Q	14.3	1.4
	R	10.98	0.5
	S	11.082	1.5
5° 43′ 30″, ±2′	T	11.2	2.7
	U	11.082	3.0
	V	11.082	1.501
	W	11.082	1.502
6° 0′ 00″, +1′−0′	X	10.69	5.12
	Y	10.1	1.0
6° 0′ 00″, ±1′ 5″	Z	10.9	1.0
	AA	12.5	1.0
	BB	14.1	1.0
6° 0′ 00″, ±4′	CC	10.69	5.12
6° 21′ 34″, +0′−5′	DD	12.0	7.0
11° 25′ 00″, +1′−2′	EE	11.1	3.8

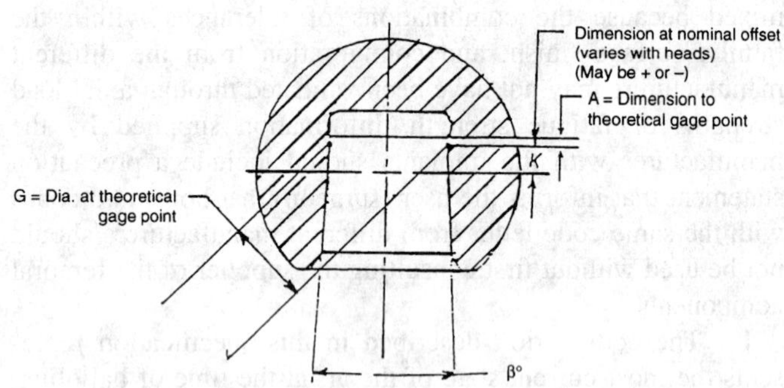

FIG. 2 Bores

7. Keywords

7.1 bores; ceramic; cones; dimensions; femoral heads; finish; marking; metal; sizes

TABLE 2 Bores

β°	Size	G—Diameter, mm	K = Nominal Neck, mm
2° 52′ 20″, +2′–0′	A	12.9	4.2
3° 2′ 00″, ±4′	B	10.98	3.38
4° 0′ 00″, +5.6′ –5.2′	C	11.5	1.5
4° 0′ 00″, ±4′	D	13.25	2.3
5° 0′ 00″, ±5′	E1	12.4	7.81
5° 8′ 00″, ±3′	E2	12.4	7.28
5° 43′ 30″, ±2′	F	11.8	4.0
	G1	9.6	1.7
5° 43′ 30″, +5′–0′	G2	9.6	3.7
	H	10.3	7.3
	J	11.1	5.4
5° 40′ 00″, +3′ 40″–0′	K	11.87	0.0
	L	12.7	2.8
	M	12.7	2.6
5° 43′ 30″ +5′ –0′	N	12.7	2.9
	P	14.3	7.3
	Q1	14.3	2.7
	Q2	14.3	3.0
	R	10.98	4.0
5° 51′ 30″, ±2′	S	11.082	1.0
	T	11.2	–1.8
	U	11.23	3.5
6° 0′ 00″, +2′	V	11.082	5.0
6° 8′ 30″, +2′	W	11.082	5.0
6° 0′ 00″, ±0′ –1′	X1	10.69	–4.5
	X2	10.69	–0.07
	Y	10.1	–7.5
6° 0′ 00″, ±1′ 5″	Z	10.9	3.6
	AA	12.5	3.6
	BB	14.1	7.5
6° 0′ 00″, +4′	CC1	10.69	–4.5
	CC2	10.69	–0.07
6° 21′ 34″, +5′ –0′	DD	12.0	0.0
11° 25′ 00″, +1′ –5′	EE	11.5	2.0

APPENDIX

(Nonmandatory Information)

X1. RATIONALE

X1.1 Ceramic aluminum oxide (Al2O3) heads have been successfully used on modular femoral stems since 1974. Their success has been the result of the high purity ceramic in conjunction with the mating characteristics of the inside taper of the head and those of the matching cones. When these characteristics are optimum, the axial fracture loads for the ceramic heads exceed 40 KN (45 times the body of a 200-lb person) and exceed the anatomical load carrying capabilities of femoral stems by at least a factor of two. Modular metal heads have been used successfully since 1982.

X1.2 The dimensional and surface characteristics of the cone are important to both the axial fracture loads of ceramic heads and the security of the seating of the head on the cone. Axial pull-off loads are used to evaluate the adequacy of the tenacity of the fit between the head and the cone.

X1.3 Angular and dimensional differences in cones can significantly affect the axial fracture load of ceramic modular heads. Therefore, it is necessary to classify the taper cone angles and dimensions and surface roughness to ensure proper function of modular heads and modular femoral stems.

Designation: F 1638 – 95 (Reapproved 1999)

Standard Terminology for Surgical Tissue/Dressing/Pick-Up Forceps (Thumb-Type)[1]

This standard is issued under the fixed designation F 1638; the number immediately following the designation indicates the year of original adoption or, in the case of revision, the year of last revision. A number in parentheses indicates the year of last reapproval. A superscript epsilon (ϵ) indicates an editorial change since the last revision or reapproval.

1. Scope

1.1 This terminology defines basic terms and considerations for components of thumb-type surgical forceps. Instruments with this terminology are limited to those fabricated from stainless steel and used for surgical procedures.

2. Referenced Documents

2.1 *ASTM Standards:*

F 899 Specification for Stainless Steel Billet, Bar, and Wire for Surgical Instruments[2]

F 921 Definitions of Terms Relating to Hemostatic Forceps[2]

3. Terminology

3.1 *Definitions:*

atraumatic—teeth that would interdigitate except for being spaced apart a predesigned distance so they will not stress, crush, or otherwise traumatize the tissue being grasped.

guide pin—a pin affixed to the inside of one of the forceps halves that aligns with a hole on the other tweezer half without protruding through when closed.

guide pin hole—the hole in one forceps half into which the guide pin fits without passing through when closed.

mesh—an alignment of opposing teeth. The teeth may be in-line or angled.

mouse teeth—distal tip teeth that interdigitate.

scissoring—lateral misalignment.

set—the at rest position of the instrument halves that will provide the intended closing relationship of fit and force.

stop pin—a pin of preset length affixed to the inside of one of the tweezer halves designed to limit teeth contact upon closure and prevent their damage.

teeth—serrations formed on the inside faces of the distal end of the tweezer halves.

tissue forceps—a device formed in two generally symmetrical halves with their proximal ends secured together and set so their distal ends will stay separated unless pressed together.

[1] This terminology is under the jurisdiction of ASTM Committee F-4 on Medical and Surgical Materials and Devices and is the direct responsibility of Subcommittee F04.33 on Medical/Surgical Instruments.

Current edition approved Oct. 10, 1995. Published December 1995.

[2] *Annual Book of ASTM Standards*, Vol 13.01.

APPENDIX

(Nonmandatory Information)

X1. RATIONALE

X1.1 Because there is a clinical need for a variety of instruments for surgical procedures, they are manufactured in various configurations and from various types of stainless steel. For practical purposes and patient safety, these devices supplied by different manufacturers necessitate a defined system of terms.

X1.2 The terms defined in this terminology are the most commonly used for this type of forceps. However, the intent is not to prohibit technological innovation or to exclude instruments manufactured with other types of features.

Designation: F 1651 – 95

Standard Guide for Training the Emergency Medical Technician (Paramedic)[1]

This standard is issued under the fixed designation F 1651; the number immediately following the designation indicates the year of original adoption or, in the case of revision, the year of last revision. A number in parentheses indicates the year of last reapproval. A superscript epsilon (ε) indicates an editorial change since the last revision or reapproval.

1. Scope

1.1 This guide covers the training standard for the emergency medical technician (paramedic) to deal with emergencies. Primary care and wilderness/delayed/prolonged context training for the emergency medical technician (paramedic) is not within the scope of this guide, but may be dealt with in other ASTM standards.

1.2 This guide identifies the knowledge and skills that all programs that train the emergency medical technician (paramedic) should include in their training program.

1.3 *This standard does not purport to address all of the safety concerns, if any, associated with its use. It is the responsibility of the user of this standard to establish appropriate safety and health practices and determine the applicability of regulatory limitations prior to use.*

2. Referenced Documents

2.1 *ASTM Standards:*

F 1149 Practice for Qualifications, Responsibilities, and Authority of Individuals and Institutions Providing Medical Direction of Emergency Medical Services[2]

F 1220 Guide for Emergency Medical Services Systems (EMSS) Telecommunications[2]

F 1254 Practice for Performance of Prehospital Manual Defibrillation[2]

F 1255 Practice for Performance of Prehospital Automated Defibrillation[2]

F 1258 Practice for Emergency Medical Dispatch[2]

F 1288 Guide for Planning for and Response to a Multiple Casualty Incident[2]

F 1489 Guide for Performance of Patient Assessment by the Emergency Medical Technician (Paramedic)[2]

F 1517 Guide for Scope of Performance of Emergency Medical Services Ambulance Operations[2]

3. Terminology

3.1 *Definitions of Terms Specific to This Standard:*

3.1.1 *auscultation*—examination by listening with a stethoscope.

3.1.2 *EMSS communications subsystem*—comprises those resource arrangements for notifying the EMS system of an emergency, for mobilizing and dispatching resources, for exchanging information, for remote monitoring of vital indicators, and for transmission of treatment procedures and directions (see Guide F 1220).

3.1.3 *human anatomy*—the branch of science dealing with the structure of the human organisms.

3.1.4 *human physiology*—the science dealing with the functions of the human living organism.

3.1.5 *incident command system*—the combination of facilities, equipment, personnel, procedures, and communications operating within a common organizational structure with responsibility for the management of assigned resources to effectively accomplish stated objectives pertaining to an incident.

3.1.6 *inspection*—examination by careful visualization of the body or a part of the body.

3.1.7 *management*—actions taken by the emergency medical technician (paramedic) for a patient in need of assistance due to a real or perceived traumatic or medical condition.

3.1.8 *palpation*—examination by touching with the hand(s).

3.1.9 *stress*—nonspecific response of the body to any demand made upon it.

3.1.10 *topographic anatomy*—a study of all the structures and their relationships in a given region.

3.1.11 *triage*—the process of sorting and making priorities for emergency medical care of the sick and injured on the basis of urgency and type of condition present, number of patients, and resources available.

4. Significance and Use

4.1 This guide establishes the national standard for training the emergency medical technician (paramedic).

4.2 This guide shall be used by those who develop the training curriculum to be used to train the emergency medical technician (paramedic).

4.3 Every person who is identified as an emergency medical technician (paramedic) shall have been trained to this guide.

4.4 It is understood that the scope of the medical practice is constantly evolving. Therefore, this guide does not contain recommendations for the management of illnesses and injuries. Furthermore, it is not intended to supersede the protocols and standing orders of the system medical director or the on-line medical physician (see Practice F 1149).

---

[1] This guide is under the jurisdiction of ASTM Committee F-30 on Emergency Medical Services and is the direct responsibility of Subcommittee F30.02 on Personnel, Training and Education.

Current edition approved Oct. 10, 1995. Published December 1995.

[2] *Annual Book of ASTM Standards*, Vol 13.01.

4.5 This guide does not standardize the scope of practice of the emergency medical technician (paramedic).

5. Anatomy and Physiology

5.1 The emergency medical technician (paramedic) shall describe the anatomy and physiology of the major body systems and the differences that exist because of age and gender to the extent needed to assess and manage patients with the illnesses and injuries in the following sections, using the techniques listed in this guide.

6. Communications and Medical Terminology

6.1 The emergency medical technician (paramedic) shall be able to communicate effectively, using standard medical terminology, about the illnesses and injuries, and the techniques, listed in this guide.

7. Pharmacology

7.1 The emergency medical technician (paramedic) shall be able to apply theory and principles of pharmacological intervention to manage patients with the illnesses and injuries in the following sections, using the techniques listed in this guide.

8. Universal Blood and Body Fluid Precautions

8.1 The emergency medical technician (paramedic) shall be taught the current local, state, Occupational Safety and Health Administration (OSHA), and Center for Disease Control (CDC) recommendations for preventing the transmission of communicable diseases. (See Refs (**1**, **2**, and **3**).)[3]

9. Examination Techniques

9.1 The emergency medical technician (paramedic) shall be trained to perform the following examination techniques and use appropriate modifications to accommodate the differences that exist because of age and sex:

9.1.1 Assess respirations for rate, rhythm, symmetry, and quality,

9.1.2 Auscultate for breath sounds,

9.1.3 Assess presence, rate, regularity, and quality of the following pulses: carotid, brachial, radial, femoral, temporal, dorsalis pedis, and posterior tibial,

9.1.4 Palpate blood pressure,

9.1.5 Auscultate blood pressure,

9.1.6 Assess capillary refill,

9.1.7 Assess mental status and level of consciousness,

9.1.8 Assess pupils,

9.1.9 Inspect the body,

9.1.10 Palpate the body,

9.1.11 Assess sensory perception,

9.1.12 Assess motor function,

9.1.13 Assess airway patency,

9.1.14 Assess electrical activity of the heart,

9.1.15 Assess blood glucose level,

9.1.16 Assess temperature,

9.1.17 Assess oxygen saturation level,

9.1.18 Assess the skin and mucous membranes for color, temperature, turgor, and dampness,

9.1.19 Assess the skin for basic primary skin rashes:

9.1.19.1 Macules and patches,

9.1.19.2 Papules and nodules,

9.1.19.3 Wheals (hives),

9.1.19.4 Bullae (blisters), vesicles, and pustules, and

9.1.19.5 Petechiae and purpura.

9.1.20 Assess the fontanelle in infants, and

9.1.21 Assess vision.

10. Examination Devices

10.1 The emergency medical technician (paramedic) shall be trained to use the following:

10.1.1 Blood glucose measurement devices,

10.1.2 Pulse oximeters,

10.1.3 Blood collection devices,

10.1.4 Sphygmomanometer,

10.1.5 Stethoscope,

10.1.6 Penlight,

10.1.7 Thermometer,

10.1.8 Cardiac rhythm monitor,

10.1.9 Twelve-lead ECG monitor,

10.1.10 Laryngoscope,

10.1.11 Amplified listening device, and

10.1.12 Exhaled CO_2 detection devices.

11. Patient Assessment

11.1 The emergency medical technician (paramedic) shall be educated to perform patient assessment in accordance with Guide F 1489.

12. Illnesses and Injuries

12.1 The emergency medical technician (paramedic) shall demonstrate understanding of both the pathophysiology necessary to recognize the clinical presentation and the management of the following in the prehospital context, including the differences that exist because of age and sex:

12.1.1 Airway obstruction or compromise,

12.1.2 Shock:

12.1.2.1 Hypovolemic,

12.1.2.2 Cardiogenic,

12.1.2.3 Distributive, and

12.1.2.4 Obstructive.

12.1.3 Wounds and impaled objects,

12.1.4 Contusions,

12.1.5 Orthopedic Injuries:

12.1.5.1 Extremity fractures, closed and open,

12.1.5.2 Extremity dislocations and subluxations, and

12.1.5.3 Extremity sprains and strains.

12.1.6 Head injuries,

12.1.7 Face fractures,

12.1.8 Eye injuries,

12.1.9 Spinal injuries:

12.1.9.1 Strains, sprains, and fractures, and

12.1.9.2 Back pain and herniated disks.

12.1.10 Chest injuries, including:

12.1.10.1 Pericardial tamponade,

12.1.10.2 Flail chest,

[3] The boldface numbers given in parentheses refer to a list of references at the end of the text.

12.1.10.3 Sucking chest wound,
12.1.10.4 Rib fractures,
12.1.10.5 Hemothorax, pneumothorax, and tension pneumothorax,
12.1.10.6 Lung and heart contusions, and
12.1.10.7 Great vessel injury.
12.1.11 Pelvic fractures,
12.1.12 Blunt or penetrating abdominal trauma,
12.1.13 Poisonings, drug overdoses, and substance abuse,
12.1.14 Environmental illness and injury:
12.1.14.1 Hypothermia and frostbite,
12.1.14.2 Heat-related illness,
12.1.14.3 Burns:
(1) Thermal,
(2) Electrical,
(3) Chemical,
12.1.14.4 Radiation exposure,
12.1.14.5 Electrical and lightning injuries,
12.1.14.6 Exposure to plant and animal toxins, both land and marine,
12.1.14.7 Near-drowning and cold-water submersion,
12.1.14.8 Altitude illness (acute mountain sickness, highaltitude pulmonary edema, high-altitude cerebral edema), and
12.1.14.9 Barotrauma and decompression sickness.
12.1.15 Obstetric and gynecological illness and injury:
12.1.15.1 Newborn infant,
12.1.15.2 Active labor,
12.1.15.3 Imminent delivery,
12.1.15.4 Uterine atony,
12.1.15.5 Vaginal bleeding,
12.1.15.6 Spontaneous abortion (miscarriage),
12.1.15.7 Pre-eclampsia and eclampsia,
12.1.15.8 Trauma in pregnancy,
12.1.15.9 Abnormal presentations,
12.1.15.10 Ectopic pregnancy,
12.1.15.11 Pelvic inflammatory disease (PID),
12.1.15.12 Abruptio placenta,
12.1.15.13 Placenta previa, and
12.1.15.14 Rape and sexual assault.
12.1.16 Endocrine disorders:
12.1.16.1 Diabetes mellitus,
12.1.16.2 Hyperthyroidism and hypothyroidism,
12.1.16.3 Adrenal insufficiency, and
12.1.16.4 Hypocalcemic tetany.
12.1.17 Respiratory disorders:
12.1.17.1 Respiratory failure and nonspecific respiratory distress,
12.1.17.2 Asthma,
12.1.17.3 Chronic obstructive pulmonary disease,
12.1.17.4 Pulmonary embolism,
12.1.17.5 Toxic inhalations,
12.1.17.6 Pneumonia, bronchitis, and active pulmonary tuberculosis,
12.1.17.7 Hyperventilation,
12.1.17.8 Spontaneous pneumothorax,
12.1.17.9 Bronchiolitis, and
12.1.17.10 Apnea of infancy.
12.1.18 Abdominal pain,
12.1.19 Cardiovascular illness:
12.1.19.1 Non-traumatic cardiac arrest,
12.1.19.2 Hypertension,
12.1.19.3 Angina and myocardial infarction,
12.1.19.4 Abdominal aortic aneurysm,
12.1.19.5 Aortic dissection,
12.1.19.6 Congestive heart failure and pulmonary edema,
12.1.19.7 Pre-excitation syndromes, for example, Wolff Parkinson White,
12.1.19.8 Cardiac rhythms:
(1) Normal sinus rhythm,
(2) Sinus tachycardia,
(3) Sinus arrhythmia,
(4) Sinus bradycardia,
(5) Atrial fibrillation,
(6) Atrial flutter,
(7) Atrial tachycardia,
(8) Premature supraventricular complexes,
(9) Supraventricular escape complexes,
(10) Wandering pacemaker,
(11) Paroxyxsmal supraventricular tachycardia (PSVT),
(12) Ventricular escape complexes,
(13) Premature ventricular complexes,
(14) Ventricular tachycardia/toursades de pointes,
(15) Ventricular fibrillation,
(16) Asystole,
(17) Supraventricular tachycardia,
(18) First-degree AV block,
(19) Second-degree AV block (Wenkebach/Mobitz Type I),
(20) Second-degree AV block (classical Mobitz Type II),
(21) Third-degree AV block,
(22) Bundle branch block/aberrant ventricular conduction,
(23) Junctional rhythms,
(24) Pacemaker rhythms,
(25) Electromechanical dissociation, and
(26) Arterial occlusion and deep venous thrombosis.
12.1.20 Neurological:
12.1.20.1 Headache, including subarachnoid hemorrhage,
12.1.20.2 Transient ischemic attack and cerebro-vascular accident (stroke),
12.1.20.3 Seizures,
12.1.20.4 Syncope and near sycnope,
12.1.20.5 Coma,
12.1.20.6 Meningitis,
12.1.20.7 Vertigo, and
12.1.20.8 Impaired level of consciousness.
12.1.21 Genitourinary illness:
12.1.21.1 Kidney stones,
12.1.21.2 Pyelonephritis,
12.1.21.3 End-stage renal disease,
12.1.21.4 Testicular torsion, and
12.1.21.5 Urinary retention.
12.1.22 Ear/nose/throat emergencies:
12.1.22.1 Epistaxis (nosebleed),
12.1.22.2 Dental fractures,
12.1.22.3 Epiglottis and croup,
12.1.22.4 Peritonsillar abscess,
12.1.22.5 Jaw dislocation,

12.1.22.6 Jaw fracture, and
12.1.22.7 Laryngeal injury.
12.1.23 Chest pain,
12.1.24 Gastrointestinal illness:
12.1.24.1 GI bleeding, and
12.1.24.2 Vomiting and diarrhea.
12.1.25 Allergic reactions:
12.1.25.1 Localized,
12.1.25.2 Generalized, and
12.1.25.3 Anaphylaxis.
12.1.26 Infectious disease,
12.1.27 Oncological illness (cancer):
12.1.27.1 Spinal cord compression, and
12.1.27.2 Airway compromise.
12.1.28 Terminal illness,
12.1.29 Psychiatric and behavioral illness (situational, organic, and primary psychiatric),
12.1.30 Sickle cell disease and crisis, and
12.1.31 Physical and emotional abuse in all age groups.

13. Patient Management Techniques

13.1 The emergency medical technician (paramedic) shall be trained in the use of the following patient management techniques and devices to the extent needed to manage the illnesses and injuries listed in this section:
13.1.1 Respiratory management techniques:
13.1.1.1 Techniques and devices to open and maintain the airway:
13.1.1.2 Head-tilt-chin-lift,
13.1.1.3 Finger sweeps,
13.1.1.4 Modified jaw thrust,
13.1.1.5 Jaw thrust,
13.1.1.6 Abdominal thrust,
13.1.1.7 Chest thrust,
13.1.1.8 Tongue-jaw-lift,
13.1.1.9 Sellick's maneuver (cricoid pressure),
13.1.1.10 Cricothyroidotomy,
13.1.1.11 Oropharyngeal/nasopharyngeal airways,
13.1.1.12 Orotracheal/nasotracheal intubation, and
13.1.1.13 Suction devices:
13.1.1.14 Mechanical suction,
13.1.1.15 Filtered small-bore trap suction (for example, modified DeLee),
13.1.1.16 Bulb syringe,
13.1.1.17 Suction catheters:
13.1.1.18 Rigid tonsillar suction catheter, and
13.1.1.19 Flexible suction catheter,
13.1.1.20 Techniques and devices to provide ventilatory assistance:
13.1.1.21 Mouth-to-mouth,[4]
13.1.1.22 Mouth-to-nose,[4]
13.1.1.23 Mouth-to-mouth and nose,[4]
13.1.1.24 Mouth-to-stoma,[4]
13.1.1.25 Mouth-to-mask[4], and
13.1.1.26 Positive pressure ventilatory devices,
13.1.1.27 Oxygen delivery devices:
13.1.1.28 Low-concentration oxygen delivery devices, and
13.1.1.29 High-concentration oxygen delivery devices,
13.1.1.30 Needle thoracostomy,
13.1.2 Techniques for management of the compromised circulatory system:
13.1.2.1 Direct pressure to the source of bleeding,
13.1.2.2 Pressure dressings,
13.1.2.3 Patient positioning,
13.1.2.4 The pneumatic antishock garment, and
13.1.2.5 Intraverenous (IV) fluid replacement therapy.
13.1.3 Use of spinal immobilization techniques and devices:
13.1.3.1 Manual immobilization,
13.1.3.2 Cervical spine immobilization devices,
13.1.3.3 Short-spine immobilization devices,
13.1.3.4 Long-spine immobilization devices, and
13.1.3.5 Helmet removal,
13.1.4 Techniques and devices for the management of musculoskeletal injuries (non-spine):
13.1.4.1 Manual stabilization,
13.1.4.2 External immobilization fixation techniques and devices:
13.1.4.3 Traction devices,
13.1.4.4 Rigid devices,
13.1.4.5 Pneumatic devices, and
13.1.4.6 Management of pulseless extremities,
13.1.5 Techniques for the management of soft tissue injuries:
13.1.5.1 Aseptic technique,
13.1.5.2 Management of amputations, and
13.1.5.3 Bandaging techniques.
13.1.6 Assisting with spontaneous newborn delivery:
13.1.6.1 Normal spontaneous vertex delivery,
13.1.6.2 Uterine massage, and
13.1.6.3 Abnormal presentations.
13.1.7 Techniques for restraining patients,
13.1.8 Patient positioning techniques for medical emergencies,
13.1.9 Techniques and routes for medication administration including:
13.1.9.1 Subcutaneous and intramuscular injections,
13.1.9.2 Intravenous bolus,
13.1.9.3 Intravenous drip,
13.1.9.4 Endotracheal route,
13.1.9.5 Intraosseous route,
13.1.9.6 Rectal route,
13.1.9.7 Sublingual route,
13.1.9.8 Transcutaneous route,
13.1.9.9 Medication nebulizer, and
13.1.9.10 Metered-dose inhaler, with and without spacer, and metered-dose sublingual spray,
13.1.10 Cardiac management techniques:
13.1.10.1 Electrical,
13.1.10.2 Defibrillation (automated/manual in accordance with Practice F 1254 and Practice F 1255),
13.1.10.3 Cardioversion,
13.1.10.4 Transcutaneous pacing,
13.1.10.5 External cardiac compression,

[4] The requirements of Refs **4**, **5**, and **6** should be taught with regard to the use of this procedure in the field.

13.1.10.6 Manual,
13.1.10.7 Mechanical, and
13.1.10.8 Vagal maneuvers.
13.1.11 Techniques to establish intravenous access:
13.1.11.1 Peripheral,
13.1.11.2 Central, and
13.1.11.3 Intraosseous.
13.1.12 Urinary catheterization devices,
13.1.13 Naso-gastric tubes,
13.1.14 Attached or emplaced medical devices—The emergency medical technician (paramedic) shall be able to recognize the following devices and describe the implications that their presence may have on the care of the patient:
13.1.14.1 Enteral tubes,
13.1.14.2 AV shunt/fistula/graft,
13.1.14.3 Chest drainage devices,
13.1.14.4 Ostomies:
13.1.14.5 Gastrointestinal,
13.1.14.6 Urologic, and
13.1.14.7 Airway,
13.1.14.8 Cervical traction fixation devices,
13.1.14.9 Urinary catheters,
13.1.14.10 Indwelling central lines,
13.1.14.11 Indwelling arterial lines,
13.1.14.12 Neonatal transport systems,
13.1.14.13 Peritoneal dialysis catheters,
13.1.14.14 Infusion pumps,
13.1.14.15 Intracranial pressure monitors,
13.1.14.16 Intra-aortic balloon pumps,
13.1.14.17 Fetal monitors,
13.1.14.18 External fixation devices,
13.1.14.19 Ventilators,
13.1.14.20 Pacemakers, and
13.1.15 Pain management.

14. Patient Lifting and Moving

14.1 Utilizing proper body mechanics, safely lift and move patients with the following methods:
14.1.1 Log rolls,
14.1.2 Straddle lifts,
14.1.3 Single and multiple rescuer lifts and carries, and
14.1.4 Patient drags.
14.2 Move patients utilizing the following mechanical devices:
14.2.1 Stair chair,
14.2.2 Scoop stretcher,
14.2.3 Short/long spinal immobilization devices,
14.2.4 Simple stretcher,
14.2.5 Standard ambulance cot,
14.2.6 Improvised devices, and
14.2.7 Basket litter.

15. Roles and Responsibilities

15.1 The emergency medical technician (paramedic) shall be trained to:
15.1.1 Provide scene evaluation and control,
15.1.2 Examine the patient for signs of illness or injury,
15.1.3 Obtain pertinent patient information,
15.1.4 Communicate with and provide emergency management for victims of sudden illnesses or injuries,
15.1.5 Ensure that the patient receives the available resources appropriate to his condition, for example, advanced life support, heavy rescue, specialized rescue situations, and so forth, in accordance with local protocol,
15.1.6 Communicate with the family of the patient and other involved individuals at the scene regarding the patient's status, needs, and recommended disposition,
15.1.6 Appropriately package and move the patient to an appropriate medical facility,
15.1.7 Communicate with medical facility for medical direction or to notify of patient's condition, or both,
15.1.8 Maintain accurate records,
15.1.9 Operate and maintain the emergency medical ground vehicle and its equipment and supplies.
15.1.10 Observe all safety precautions to protect self, patient, and others in all hazardous situations, and
15.1.11 Recognize the need for additional training when working with special vehicles such as aircraft, watercraft, and so forth.
15.2 The emergency medical technician (paramedic) shall be trained to act in a professional manner, to maintain an appropriate appearance and to consider the ethical implications of his roles and responsibilities.
15.3 The emergency medical technician (paramedic) shall perform the following functions in the event other emergency services are not available at the accident scene:
15.3.1 Use basic tools and procedures to gain access to and extricate the patient when safe, and
15.3.2 Control of the accident scene.
15.4 The emergency medical technician (paramedic) shall receive instruction in the organization of the emergency medical services system and the role of the emergency medical technician (paramedic) within the emergency medical services system.
15.5 The emergency medical technician (paramedic) shall be familiar with state and local EMS laws, codes, regulations, and policies.
15.6 The emergency medical technician (paramedic) shall be familiar with the role of medical direction in the delivery of pre-hospital emergency medical care including on-line and off-line medical control.

16. Legal Issues

16.1 The emergency medical technician (paramedic) shall receive instruction in the following legal concepts:
16.1.1 Standard of care,
16.1.2 Duty to act,
16.1.3 The emergency medical technician (paramedic) shall be trained to describe and report the following as required by law:
16.1.3.1 Child, adult, or elderly abuse,
16.1.3.2 Injury due to criminal act,
16.1.3.3 Drug-related injuries,
16.1.3.4 Childbirth,
16.1.3.5 Animal bites,
16.1.3.6 Attempted suicides,
16.1.3.7 Assaults and rape,
16.1.3.8 Scene of a crime,

16.1.3.9 The deceased, and

16.1.3.10 Communicable disease.

16.1.4 Patient Consent:

16.1.4.1 Implied consent,

16.1.4.2 Informed consent,

16.1.4.3 Actual/expressed consent,

16.1.4.4 Minor's consent,

16.1.4.5 Consent of the mentally ill/diminished mental capacity,

16.1.4.6 Patient's right to refuse treatment,

16.1.4.7 Use of restraint,

16.1.4.8 Do not resuscitate orders and living wills,

16.1.4.9 Medical power of attorney, and

16.1.4.10 Voluntary/involuntary committment and hold.

16.1.5 Legal liability:

16.1.5.1 Liability insurance,

16.1.5.2 Torts,

16.1.5.3 Abandonment,

16.1.5.4 Negligence,

16.1.5.5 Immunity from liability laws,

16.1.5.6 Libel,

16.1.5.7 Assault and battery, and

16.1.5.8 False imprisonment.

17. Certification and Licensure

17.1 Licensure, certification, and recertification shall be reviewed according to national, state, regional, and local requirements and shall include the following:

17.1.1 EMS statutes and regulations,

17.1.2 Medical practices act, and

17.1.3 EMS professional associations (for example, National Association of EMTs; National Registry of EMTs; National Association of State EMS Directors; National Association of EMS Physicians; and local, state, and regional organizations).

18. Stress Management/Critical Incident Stress

18.1 The occupation of an emergency medical technician (paramedic) is highly stressful and the training shall include the recognition and management of stress and stress reactions in self and family.

18.2 The emergency medical technician (paramedic) shall be taught the concept of critical incident stress, its long-term consequences, and how critical incident stress debriefing is used to mitigate its effects.

18.3 The emergency medical technician (paramedic) shall be taught techniques to assist the patient's family in recognizing and dealing with anxiety and stress related to acute incidents.

19. Patient Communication Problems

19.1 The emergency medical technician (paramedic) shall be trained to communicate effectively with the following types of patients and families, and in the following situations:

19.1.1 Geriatric,

19.1.2 Speech/hearing-impaired,

19.1.3 Blind,

19.1.4 Non-English speaking,

19.1.5 Confused,

19.1.6 Mentally disabled,

19.1.7 Sudden death crisis,

19.1.8 Terminal disease,

19.1.9 Abuse/assault,

19.1.10 Suicidal, and

19.1.11 Pediatric.

20. Records and Reports

20.1 The emergency medical technician (paramedic) shall be taught to prepare and maintain run reports and records on each patient, and the relation of such records to:

20.1.1 Continuity of care,

20.1.2 Patient's permanent medical record,

20.1.3 Evaluating the quality of care,

20.1.4 Legal evidence,

20.1.5 Administrative information, and

20.1.6 Research purposes.

20.2 The emergency medical technician (paramedic) shall be taught that essential patient care information for the record includes:

20.2.1 Patient's name, sex, age, and address,

20.2.2 Chief complaint and nature of illness or type and mechanism of injury,

20.2.3 Location of patient upon arrival at the scene,

20.2.4 Rescue and treatment measures provided by bystanders and first responders,

20.2.5 Findings of the primary and secondary surveys,

20.2.6 Care given at the site and during transport,

20.2.7 Vital signs, patient condition, and any changes of either during transport,

20.2.8 Source of on-line medical direction and disposition (receiving hospital or other),

20.2.9 Disposition of patient's valuables,

20.2.10 Signature of patient or legal guardian if patient care is refused, or notation and witnessed if patient refused to sign,

20.2.11 Circumstances involved in special situations identified in 16.1.3,

20.2.12 Unusual circumstances that affected patient care, and

20.2.13 Times of treatment interventions.

20.3 The emergency medical technician (paramedic) shall consider all patient information confidential and shall release it only to the proper authorities.

20.4 The emergency medical technician shall be taught the rationale and importance for recording other pertient information about each run including such things as the various response time intervals, other responder organizations, location information, and so forth.

21. Multiple-Casualty Incidents

21.1 The emergency medical technician (paramedic) shall be able to perform triage in a multiple-casualty incident in accordance with 9.3 of Guide F 1288.

21.2 The emergency medical technician (paramedic) shall be trained in the concept and application of the incident management system as described in Ref **(7)**.

22. Hazardous Materials

22.1 The emergency medical technician (paramedic) shall

be familiar with national and state standards or regulations regarding hazardous materials incidents.

22.2 The emergency medical technician (paramedic) shall be taught how to provide emergency care to patients who have been exposed to and decontaminated of hazardous materials including radiation.

23. Quality Improvement

23.1 The emergency medical technician (paramedic) shall be trained about the purpose and importance of quality improvement programs.

23.2 The emergency medical technician (paramedic) shall be taught how to participate in quality improvement activities.

24. Vehicle and Equipment Maintenance

24.1 The emergency medical technician (paramedic) will ensure routine vehicle and equipment preventive maintenance, regular inspections, and inspections after each run.

25. Ground Emergency Vehicle Driving

25.1 The emergency medical technician (paramedic) shall be trained to identify the risks associated with emergency medical ground vehicle operations.

25.2 The minimum training standard for ground emergency vehicle driving shall include a review of state, regional, and local laws, regulations, or ordinances or protocols that specifically addresses the following:

25.2.1 Vehicle parking or standing regulations.

25.2.2 When applicable, the emergency medical technician (paramedic) shall receive instruction in ambulance operations.

25.2.3 The emergency medical technician (paramedic) shall receive didactic instruction in defensive driving, accident avoidance, and principles of vehicle control.

25.3 The emergency medical technician (paramedic) shall receive instruction regarding the effects of vehicle operation on patient care, comfort, and safety.

26. EMSS Communications Subsystem Use

26.1 The emergency medical technician (paramedic) shall receive instruction about the EMSS communications subsystem. Such training shall include:

26.1.1 Relevant subparts of Part 90 of the FCC regulations,

26.1.2 The functions procedures and equipment used in the emergency medical dispatch process in accordance with Practice F 1258,

26.1.3 Notifying hospital emergency departments of incoming patients,

26.1.4 Typical communications equipment and protocol used for state, regional, or local areas,

26.1.5 Communicating pertinent patient information,

26.1.6 Receiving medical direction in accordance with local protocol,

26.1.7 Detection and reporting of accidents to dispatcher,

26.1.8 Alerting other emergency resources,

26.1.9 Maintaining contact between the vehicle, dispatcher, and hospital, and

26.1.10 Communicating with other emergency services, as needed.

27. Helicopter Operations

27.1 The emergency medical technician (paramedic) shall be educated about the basic concepts needed to work with aeromedical helicopters, including:

27.1.1 Landing zone selection and preparation,

27.1.2 Effect of barometric changes on patients and medical equipment (for example, air splints),

27.1.3 Safety around helicopters, and

27.1.4 Appropriate role of helicopter transportation in the EMS system.

28. Keywords

28.1 accidental poisoning: absorbed through the skin; accidental poisoning: exposure to radiation and other hazardous materials; accidental poisoning: inhaled poisons; accidental poisoning: substance ingestion; acute abdomen; acute mountain sickness; air embolism; airway management; airway management devices; burns; cardiac arrest—non traumatic; cardiac arrest—secondary to severe hypothermia; cardiac emergency; cerebrovascular accident; certification; chest injuries; closed soft tissue injuries; communication problems; decompression sickness; diabetic emergencies; dislocations; emergency ground vehicle operation; emergency medical technician (paramedic); EMT; EMT—P; examination techniques; fractures; frostbite; frostnip; hazardous materials; heat-related illness; head injuries; hypothermia; injuries; injuries to the eye; insect bites and stings; legal issues; licensure; management techniques; medical emergencies; multiple casualty incidents; non-traumatic chest pain; open soft tissue injuries; paramedic; pertinent patient information and scene evaluation; primary assessment; primary survey; preparation for medical transportation; quality assurance; radio communications; records; reports; respiratory medical emergencies; respiratory medical emergency in children; role; roles and responsibilities; secondary assessment; secondary shock; seizure; shock; skills; spinal column injuries; stress; training; unconscious patient; universal blood and body fluid precautions; venomous snake bites

REFERENCES

(1) Centers for Disease Control: *Recommendations for Prevention of HIV Transmission in Health-Care Settings*, MMWR 1987;36 (Suppl No 2S):3S–18S.

(2) Centers for Disease Control: Update: *Universal Precautions for Prevention of Transmission of Human Immunodeficiency Virus, Hepatitis B Virus, and Other Bloodborne Pathogens in Health-Care Settings*, MMWR 1988;37 No. 24:377–382.

(3) "Occupational Exposure to Bloodborne Pathogens: Final Rule," *Federal Register*, Vol 56, No. 235, Dec. 6, 1991, pp. 64175–64182.

(4) "Guidelines and Recommendations for Cardiopulmonary Resuscitation and Emergency Cardiac Care," *Journal of the American Medical Association*, Vol 268, No. 16, Oct. 28, 1992, pp. 2171–2302.

(5) Chameides, et al, *Textbook of Pediatric Advanced Life Support*, American Heart Association. Dallas, TX, 1988.

(6) Hackett, P., et al, *State of Alaska Cold Injury Guidelines*, Alaska Department of Health and Social Services. 1989.

(7) National Wildfire Coordinating Group, NFES-2426, *Incident Command System Curriculum Syllabus*, National Interagency Fire Center, Supply, 3833 South Development Ave., Boise, ID 83705, 1995.

Designation: F 1652 – 95

Standard Guide for Providing Essential Data Needed in Advance for Prehospital Emergency Medical Services[1]

This standard is issued under the fixed designation F 1652; the number immediately following the designation indicates the year of original adoption or, in the case of revision, the year of last revision. A number in parentheses indicates the year of last reapproval. A superscript epsilon (ϵ) indicates an editorial change since the last revision or reapproval.

1. Scope

1.1 This guide covers the functional elements and data records of prehospital Health Status Information Services (HSIS) needed to provide individual health status data for HSIS subscribers. When an HSIS subscriber experiences a medical emergency and becomes an EMS patient, a prehospital EMS care provider can rapidly access the individual's health status data by means of telecommunications. Access to this data will enable the EMS provider to improve patient assessment, and thereby render more appropriate treatments. This will improve the EMS provider's ability to stabilize trauma and other emergency medical conditions, and to restore and sustain vital functions, while avoiding treatments that may aggravate the severity of the medical emergency because of preexisting conditions.

1.2 In addition to improving on-site assessment, this guide will facilitate improved on-line medical direction of prehospital EMS care providers, particularly for persons experiencing life threatening medical emergencies.

1.3 Health status records provide a chronology of a person's health/medical data, including past diagnosis and treatments. The data in these records provide a vital link between the person experiencing a medical emergency, the EMS care provider, and subsequent emergency services. In order to provide the most informed care, EMS care providers and persons providing EMS medical direction need to be aware of the injured or ill person's health status.

1.4 This guide describes the minimum requirements for compiling, updating, computerizing, and storing individual's longitudinal health status data in authorized repositories, so as to protect patient privacy and confidentiality. This guide also describes requirements for providing authorized access and rapid transmittal of the data to attending EMS care providers in medical emergencies.

1.5 While this guide addresses data needed for prehospital EMS, there is also a recognized essential, but largely unmet need for similar patient health status records for emergency medical care of patients in hospital emergency departments and in definitive medical care facilities. Many development projects are in process to address this unmet need.[2] When available, such patient records are reviewed by attending physicians, in advance of hospital emergency medical care, to quickly access patient health status data that is needed for improved patient assessment and treatment and avoidance of treatments which may be contraindicated by preexisting conditions.

1.5.1 Future changes to this guide will result in health status information records for prehospital emergency medical care and analogous information systems for hospital emergency medical care, harmonized with each other and with future standards for computerized longitudinal health care patient records (see Guides E 1744 and F 1629) which are being developed by ASTM Committee E-31.

1.5.2 This guide describes requirements that are based on current ASTM medical informatics standards and will be updated to harmonize with future versions of these rapidly evolving standards.

1.6 The scope of this guide includes harmonization of the definitions of prehospital emergency medical services data element definitions used in this guide with definitions used in other ASTM standards. The definition of data elements in this guide will be the same as the definition of the data element in other ASTM standards. In cases where a data element used in this guide does not appear in another ASTM standard, the guide will use the definition specified for Federal health

---

[1] This guide is under the jurisdiction of ASTM Committee F-30 on Emergency Medical Services and is the direct responsibility of Subcommittee F30.03 on Organization/Management.

Current edition approved Oct. 10, 1995. Published December 1995.

[2] A number of projects are in process to develop such information systems. One Ref **(1)**1[3] is the Trauma Care Information Management System project funded under the Defense Technology Transfer Program that addresses health status data for both prehospital and hospital emergency medical care. Another companion development project **(2)**2, also funded under the Defense Technology Transfer Program, is the Development of Interoperability Platforms for the National Health Information System. In addition, in 1994 alone, the National Institute for Standards and Technology awarded sixteen cooperative agreements totaling over $100M for applied research in related medical informatics **(3)**3. It is expected that scheduled completion of these projects in three to five years will produce medical informatics products and processes that will enter competition in the next decade for adoption for national healthcare use.

Each of these major development projects will impact on the evolution of computerized patient health status information data bases for prehospital and hospital emergency medical care.

It is planned that testing and evaluation of the results of these projects will lead to the development of standards for such hospital information systems. Such standards will in turn be harmonized with the standards now used and being developed regarding information preparatory to patient hospital admission for non-emergent medical care. (See Specification E 1238, Guide E 1239, Guide E 1384, Specification E 1633, and Guides E 1744 and F 1629.)

services information systems (**4, 5**).[3]

2. Referenced Documents

2.1 *ASTM Standards:*

E 1238 Specification for Transferring Clinical Laboratory Data Messages Between Independent Computer Systems[4]

E 1239 Guide for Description of Reservation/Registration/ Admission Discharge, Transfer (R-ADT) Systems for Automated Patient Care Information Systems[4]

E 1384 Guide for Description of Content and Structure of an Automated Primary Record of Care[4]

E 1633 Specification for Coded Values in the Primary Record of Care[4]

E 1744 Guide for a View of Emergency Medical Care in the Computerized Patient Record[4]

F 1629 Guide for Establishing and/or Operating Emergency Medical Services Management Information Systems[5]

3. Terminology

3.1 *Definition:*

3.1.1 *health status information services (HSIS)*—a generic, non-proprietary term that describes the functional elements (data, resources, procedures, and processes) that constitute an information system designed, developed, and operated to provide individual health status data for subscribers in accordance with this guide.

4. Summary of Guide

4.1 This guide describes the standard functional elements that should exist to provide HSIS, namely:

4.1.1 An inventory of data elements that should be addressed in compiling individual health status records.

4.1.2 Uniform data element definitions for health status data. (See Guide F 1629 and Refs (**4, 5**, and **6**).)

4.1.3 Guidance for encoding of HSIS computerized data. (See Specifications E 1238 and E 1633.)

4.1.4 A computerized HSIS data base of the health status records of individuals who subscribe to a HSIS service.

4.1.5 A template and uniform format for on-site display or print out of an individual's health status data, for use by a prehospital EMS provider who has been authorized to access the record. (See Guide E 1744 and Ref (**6**).)

4.1.6 A confidential HSIS access password (or number) that can be made available by an individual or an authorized surrogate to an on-scene EMS provider or to an off-scene medical director to authorize access to an individual's health status record for a particular emergency medical episode. (See Guide E 1744.)

4.1.7 Provisions for updating and correcting an individual's health status record and for "refreshing" the individuals confidential HSIS access password (or number) after each use.

5. Significance and Use

5.1 This is a guide for recording, computerizing, storing, accessing, and transmitting data for an individual's uniform health status record so as to enable pre-hospital EMS providers to rapidly access the data for improved assessment and appropriate treatment of an individual experiencing a medical emergency.

5.2 Lack of health status information on an individual's preexisting medical conditions, such as data on allergies, diseases, medications being used, previous medical care, and so forth, may result in application of standard prehospital medical treatments that may be contraindicated and sometimes fatally incorrect.

5.3 At present, most people do not carry their health status data on their person. An individual's health status data may be distributed at various locations such as in hospital records, in physicians' files in various formats including hand-written paper forms. Some organizations, such as health maintenance organizations, schools, camps, and sports groups, attempt to maintain specific sets of health status data. Retrieval and transfer of selected information needed in emergencies from such records is usually slow and incomplete.

5.4 Currently, when a person suffers a medical emergency, pre-hospital EMS providers must rely on word-of-mouth information from the patient or from on-scene relatives or friends, for health status data that may be critical to selection and outcome of appropriate pre-hospital treatment. Often such data are not available because the patient is unconscious, otherwise unresponsive, or unaccompanied.

5.5 Increasingly, individuals with serious allergies, disease, or other health problems are being advised by their doctors to obtain and wear a tag (a durable bracelet or necklace) containing selected health status information so as to help ensure that in the case of a medical emergency, prehospital EMS providers will be alerted to preexisting conditions. Such tags may also contain the wearer's name, address, and phone number for identification purposes; and may indicate the presence on the wearer of a personal medical information card with further health status data as well as the name and telephone number of the wearer's doctor or health care organization, or both. This tag may also indicate the telephone number for accessing additional health status data for the wearer. Thus, this guide can be used by providers of such health status tags, to give their subscribers added safeguards from prehospital and hospital medical misadventure.

5.6 Use of this guide will lead to improved access by prehospital EMS providers to health status data needed to better assess a persons conditions and select the appropriate treatments while avoiding treatments that may be contraindicated because of the individual's preexisting health status. Information needed by a prehospital EMS provider to access this health status data may be provided by word of mouth by the person, through information provided on a health status tag worn by the person, on a patient's wallet card, or by interrogation of HSIS providers by means of the EMS communications system. (See 5.10.)

5.7 The lack of mobile communications and computer technology in ambulances, in some EMS systems, may make it impossible for prehospital emergency medical care providers to directly access the injured or ill person's health status

[3] The boldface numbers given in parentheses refers to a list of references at the end of the text.

[4] *Annual Book of ASTM Standards*, Vol 14.01.

[5] *Annual Book of ASTM Standards*, Vol 13.01.

records described in this guide. In such cases, the desired health status record may be accessed by the medical facility providing prehospital medical direction by means of wire-line computer modem connection, and used as a basis for providing improved on-line medical direction, particularly in instances of life threatening medical emergencies.

5.8 In addition to the primary use for EMS, existing HSIS are being adapted to other applications that reduce duplication of effort, help underwrite the costs of HSIS, and promote updating and accuracy of individuals' health status data.

5.8.1 For youth, HSIS record data may also serve as "ever green" immunization records, and as the health status data format for qualification for participation in school sports programs, extra school athletic activities, and for other youth programs where health status registration is required.

5.8.2 Organizations should meet these minimum requirements for a preexisting inventory and history form.

5.8.3 Adaptations of HSIS for applications other than EMS require development of appropriate data templates based on the needs of the HSIS users, the HSIS providers, and the informed prior consent of HSIS subscribers to the release of specific data to the HSIS users for specific predefined applications.

5.9 It is significant that different versions of HSIS are currently being marketed by companies interested in becoming HSIS providers. It is important that national voluntary consensus standards exist so as to help ensure that competitive HSIS meet minimum requirements as set forth in this guide.

5.10 Prehospital EMS providers and persons responsible for providing prehospital emergency medical direction should be aware of this guide and should be alert to look for and use HSIS for persons for whom it is available. HSIS providers should register with EMS systems and provide them with directions for interrogating their HSIS data base for an individual's health status records.

5.11 In the absence of necessary communications and computer technology, this guide may be used to develop paper-based, written health status information records that can be used for voice transmission.

6. HSIS Functional Elements

6.1 *Health Status Data Inventory*—HSIS providers should use the following inventory of data in compiling the health status record of subscribers:

6.1.1 *Subscriber Certification*—The data in the health status record should be certified as current, and correct by the individual or by the parent or legal guardian if the individual is a minor or has a legally designated guardian, or otherwise in conformance with state law. This certification should include:

6.1.1.1 Name (of individual),

6.1.1.2 Date of birth (of individual), and

6.1.1.3 Signature of individual, parent, or guardian.

6.1.2 *Physician's Certification*—A physician, licensed in accordance with state law, should certify that the data in the health status record are correct and are compiled from professional medical records. This certification should include:

6.1.2.1 Name (of certifying physician),

6.1.2.2 License number (physician's),

6.1.2.3 Address (physician's),

6.1.2.4 Telephone number (physician's),

6.1.2.5 Date (of physician's certification),

6.1.2.6 Date (of last professional medical record from which data is included), and

6.1.2.7 Signature (physician's).

6.1.3 *Individual Identification*—The health status record should include the following data that identify the individual and relates him/her to a particular record.

6.1.3.1 *Individual's Record Number*—This number is used by the HSIS provider for filing/locating the individual's record:

6.1.3.2 Name,

6.1.3.3 Address,

6.1.3.4 Date of birth,

6.1.3.5 Telephone number (home),

6.1.3.6 Telephone number (work),

6.1.3.7 Social security number,

6.1.3.8 Religion,

6.1.3.9 Medical insurance carrier name (primary),

6.1.3.10 Medical insurance policy number (primary),

6.1.3.11 Medical insurance carrier name (secondary),

6.1.3.12 Medical insurance carrier number (secondary),

6.1.3.13 Name of designated primary contact (for minors, usually a parent or guardian; for adult usually the spouse or other close associate),

6.1.3.14 Telephone numbers of primary contact,

6.1.3.15 Names of personal physicians (include all licensed professionals or providers such as psychiatrists, dentists, orthodontists, and so forth),

6.1.3.16 Telephone numbers of personal physicians,

6.1.3.17 Individual organ donor program participation (appropriate individual's donor card is necessary),

6.1.3.18 Sex,

6.1.3.19 Height,

6.1.3.20 Weight,

6.1.3.21 Color of eyes,

6.1.3.22 Color of skin, and

6.1.3.23 Color of hair.

6.1.4 *Subscriber Medical History*—The health status record should include the following data describing the medical history of the subject of this medical record.

6.1.4.1 *Previously Diagnosed Medical Problems*—Including "hidden diseases" and disabilities such as epilepsy, asthma, diabetes, blindness, deafness, AIDS, chromosomal abnormalities, congenital heart disease, anesthesia problems listed in order of severity by the individual's personal physician/s.

6.1.4.2 *Previously Diagnosed Allergies*—Such as animals, insect stings, house dust, foods, penicillin, pollen, chemicals, poison ivy, or other plants, listed in order of severity by the individual's personal physician/s.

6.1.4.3 *Prosthetic Devices and Devices Used or Implanted in Major Medical Procedures (Present or Previous)*—(Such as cardiac pacemaker, hearing aid, dentures, brain shunt, renal dialysis, colostomy, tracheotomy, lens implant, or other).

6.1.4.4 *Visual Prosthesis*—Contact lenses, regular glasses, artificial eye/s, and so forth.

6.1.4.5 *Immunizations*—Type, status, and date.

6.1.4.6 *Physiological Injuries or Growth Problems*—Most

recent to past (such as fractures, dislocations, soft tissue injuries).

6.1.4.7 *Psychological Disorders*—Most recent to past.

6.1.4.8 *Hospitalization*—Most recent to past (including name of hospital, address, reason for hospitalization, discharge date).

6.1.4.9 *Operations or Other Medical Procedures*—Most recent to past.

6.1.4.10 *Medical Conditions*—Current or past (such as arthritis, asthma, cancer, cardiac, diabetes, hypertension, and so forth).

6.1.4.11 *Allergies*—Current or past.

6.1.4.12 *Prescriptions Drugs*—Current or past.

6.1.4.13 *Radiation Treatment*—Current or past.

6.1.4.14 *Chemotherapy*—Current or past.

6.1.4.15 *Blood Test Results and Dates*—Most recent to past (including hemoglobin, white blood count, electrolytes, blood type, antibody screen, and so forth).

6.1.4.16 *Electrocardiogram Results and Dates*—Current or past.

6.1.4.17 *X-Ray Findings and Dates*—Most recent to past.

6.1.4.18 *Episodes of Prolonged Bleeding or Clotting*—Most recent to past including dates and circumstances.

6.1.5 Fig. 1Figs. 1- illustrates a sample paper form for inventorying and recording the above data for the individual health status record.

6.2 Fig. 2Figs. 2- lists definitions of the data that should be considered, if they exists, for recording in the inventory of the individual's health status record. Much of this data may not exist for young people or particularly healthful individuals.

6.3 Fig. 3Figs. 3-4 is a sample prehospital EMS health status data template of the "essential" and "desirable" data that should, if they exist, be extracted from an individual's health status data inventory for display/print out, in response to an authorized request by a prehospital EMS provider for use in assessment and prehospital care of medical emergencies. This minimum data set is based on guidelines in Guide E 1744 and Guide F 1629, and recommendations contained in Ref **(6)**.

6.3.1 The prehospital emergency medical care data template contained in Fig. 3 should be considered as a "minimum data set" since it includes only those health status data elements which are judged to be "essential" or "desirable" in the final report of the Uniform Pre-Hospital Emergency Medical Services (EMS) Data Element Consensus Development Conference, **(6)**, for defining "pre-existing" conditions.

6.3.2 HSIS providers may expand the list of data contained in their prehospital EMS health status data template, based on the expressed needs of participating EMS provider services, and with the prior consent of their subscribers. It should be emphasized that the HSIS providers have a responsibility to inform subscribers and obtain their consent regarding the specific data that will be made available in response to authorized requests from prehospital EMS providers.

6.4 *HSIS Database*—The HSIS providers should aggregate individuals' computerized health status records into a uniform HSIS database.

6.4.1 *Updating Individual Health Status Records*—Individuals who have a health status record should be provided with a manifold form for updating their records. The form should include copies for retention by the individual, for retention by health care providers or institutions submitting new or corrected information, and for submission to the HSIS provider. The form should include the individual's HSIS record number (see 6.1.3.1), should identify the data element/s to be changed, should specify the change/s, and should include individual subscriber and physician certification information in accordance with 6.1.1 and 6.1.2.

6.4.1.1 Individual subscribers are responsible for submitting changes and corrections to their HSIS providers. The HSIS providers should enter the certified changes and corrections in the individual's record, and if requested, provide individuals with an updated copy of their health status record.

6.4.2 *HSIS Database Confidentiality, Privacy, Access, and Security*—The HSIS operators should provide the following safeguards for health status information. These summarized safeguards have been extracted from the applicable ASTM draft standard (see Guide E 1744), and will, when the draft standard is approved, be incorporated by reference into this guide. Additional applicable information on this subject should be obtained from the referenced ASTM standard.

6.4.2.1 *Confidentiality*—Subject to exceptions provided by laws, physicians, nurses, midwives, secretaries, medical technicians, prehospital EMS providers, EMSS staff, social workers, hospital managers, computer staff, research investigators, social workers, and others with access to HSIS data should have a professional or contractual duty, or both, to safeguard the privacy of individuals' HSIS data, regardless of how it is acquired, collected, stored, processed, generated, retrieved, and transmitted. The HSIS providers should develop policies and procedures including penalties for inappropriate access and use of HSIS data.

6.4.3 *Privacy*—By reference, the following basic tenets outlined in the Privacy Act of 1974 apply to HSIS data:

6.4.3.1 Individuals have the right to know what specific identifiable personal data is available in their HSIS record and to know what those data are used for.

6.4.3.2 Individuals should have access to their records, have the right to have a copy made, and have the right to amend or correct the records.

6.4.3.3 The HSIS data should not be used for any application beyond that for which there is prior individual consent.

6.4.3.4 Prior consent of the individual must be obtained for all other uses of individual HSIS data.

6.4.3.5 Individual health status data should be collected and used only for necessary and lawful purposes.

6.4.3.6 *Access*—The HSIS provider shall provide each individual or individual's surrogate with his/her health status record number (see 6.1.3.1), and a password to be provided to prehospital EMS providers or to persons providing medical direction, to request authorized access and downloading EMS template data from the individual's health status record. The password should be changed after each use and after significant changes/corrections are made to an individual's record. Such changes in the password will help avoid unauthorized access to the individuals health status record and compromise of patient privacy and confidentiality and, will ensure that downloaded

1. INDIVIDUAL'S CERTIFICATION

1. **NAME**: ____
Last First MI

2. **DATE OF BIRTH**: ____________________
Year/Month/Day

3. As the subject of this record or the subject's parent or legal guardian, I hereby certify that these records are current and accurate.

SIGNATURE: ____
Subject, Parent, or Guardian)

2. PHYSICIAN'S CERTIFICATION

I hereby certify that this Health Status Record is compiled from professional medical records and is accurate as of the certification date cited below.

1. **NAME**: (Print) ____
(Signature) ____
Last First MI

2. **LICENSE NO**: ____________________ ____________
Number State

3. **PHYSICIAN'S ADDRESS**:
____
Street
____
City State Zip Code

4. **TELEPHONE NUMBER**: ______ __________

5. **DATE OF CERTIFICATION**: ____________________
Year/Month/Day

6. **MEDICAL RECORD SOURCE DATE**: ____________________
Year/Month/Day

3. INDIVIDUAL'S IDENTIFICATION

1. **INDIVIDUAL'S RECORD NUMBER**: ____________________

2. **NAME**: ____
Last First MI

3. **ADDRESS**:
____
Street
____
City State Zip Code

4. **DATE OF BIRTH**: ____________________
Year/Month/Day

5. **TELEPHONE NUMBER (HOME)**: ____________________

6. **TELEPHONE NUMBER (WORK)**: ____________________

7. **SOCIAL SECURITY NUMBER**: ____ ____ ______

8. **RELIGION**:
CATHOLIC ___ JEWISH ___
PROTESTANT ___ ISLAM ___
CHRISTIAN SCIENCE ___ JEHOVAH'S WITNESS ___
OTHER ____________________
Specify

FIG. 1 Individual's Health Status Record Data Inventory

health status data are current.

6.4.3.7 *Health Status Record Security*—The individual's health status record should be stored in a centralized HSIS database in an electronic format for rapid retrieval and transmission in an emergency situation on authorized request. The HSIS provider is responsible for the security and integrity of the database and for prevention of unauthorized access to or changes in the health status records. This includes provisions to safeguard records from occurrences and exposure to: (*1*) accidental or intentional disclosure to unauthorized persons,

5. **IMMUNIZATIONS:** **Fully Immunized** **Date - Year/Month/Day**

	Yes	No	Date - Year/Month/Day
Tetanus	_____	_____	__________
DP	_____	_____	__________
Polio	_____	_____	__________
MMR	_____	_____	__________
Chicken Pox	_____	_____	__________
Other - Specify	_____	_____	__________

6. **PHYSIOLOGICAL INJURIES OR GROWTH PROBLEMS:** List most recent to past including such conditions as fractures, dislocations, soft tissue damage, etc.

1. __________ 2. __________
3. __________ 4. __________

7. **PSYCHOLOGICAL DISORDERS:** List most recent to past including such conditions as panic disorder, depression, chronic phobias, etc.

1. __________ 2. __________
3. __________ 4. __________

8. **HOSPITALIZATIONS:** List most recent to past, including hospital name and address, reason for hospitalization, and discharge date.

1. ____________________
Name of Hospital
____
Address - (Street, City, State, Zip Code)
__________ __________
Reason for hospitalization **Discharge (Year/Month/Day)**

2. ____________________
Name of Hospital
____
Address - (Street, City, State, Zip Code)
__________ __________
Reason for hospitalization **Discharge (Year/Month/Day)**

3. ____________________
Name of Hospital
____
Address - (Street, City, State, Zip Code)
__________ __________
Reason for hospitalization **Discharge (Year/Month/Day)**

9. **OPERATIONS AND OTHER MEDICAL PROCEDURES:** List most recent to past, including such procedures as surgeries, radiation therapy, chemical therapies, etc.

1. __________ 2. __________
3. __________ 4. __________
5. __________ 6. __________

10. **MEDICAL CONDITIONS CURRENTLY UNDER TREATMENT:** List most recent to past, including such conditions as arthritis, asthma, cancer, cardiac, diabetes, and other conditions listed in 4.1 under "PREVIOUSLY DIAGNOSED MEDICAL PROBLEMS".

1. __________ 2. __________
3. __________ 4. __________
5. __________ 6. __________

11. **ALLERGIES CURRENTLY UNDER TREATMENT:** List most recent to past. (See "PREVIOUSLY DIAGNOSED ALLERGIES".)

1. __________ 2. __________
3. __________ 4. __________

FIG. 1 *(continued)*

(*2*) accidental or malicious alteration, (*3*) unauthorized copying, (*4*) loss or theft, or (*5*) destruction by hardware failures;

12. **PRESCRIPTION DRUGS:** List most recent to past, including periods of use (year/month/date to year/month/date), National Drug Code (NDC)/name/strength /and form of drug, daily dosage,and route of administration.

Period YY/MM/DD-YY/MM/DD	NDC,Name/Strength/Form	Dosage per Day	Route

13. **RADIATION TREATMENT:** List most recent to past including dates and purpose of radiation therapy.

Dates (YY/MM/DD-YY/MM/DD)	Purpose of Treatment/Therapy

14. **CHEMOTHERAPY:** List most recent to past including dates, chemical and reason for therapy.

Dates (YY/MM/DD-YY/MM/DD)	Chemical and Reason for Therapy

15. **BLOOD TEST RESULTS:** List most recent to past including date, blood type (A, B, AB, O), hemoglobin (g/DL), white blood count, Electrolytes (Including Glucose, BUN [Mg/DL], Na [ME G/L], K [ME G/L], CL [ME G/L], Antibody Screen (Positive/Negative).

Date	Type	Hemo	WBC	Electrolytes					Antibodies
				Glu	BUN	Na	K	CL	Pos/Neg

16. **ELECTROCARDIOGRAM DATES AND RESULTS:**

Date	Results

17. **X-RAY DATES AND FINDINGS:** List most recent to past.

Date	Findings

18. **EPISODES OF PROLONGED BLEEDING OR CLOTTING** - List most recent to past including date and circumstances.

Date	Circumstances

FIG. 1 *(continued)*

ITEM NUMBER. NAME: Definition: Coding

1. **INDIVIDUAL'S CERTIFICATION:** This block of data contains the individuals certification that the information contained herein is a current and accurate statement of his health status.: Coding not applicable.

1.1 **NAME:** Printed last name, first name, and middle initial, separated by commas, of the individual who is the subject of this health record: Alphabetic coding

1.2 **DATE OF BIRTH:** Date of birth of the subject of this health record.: Use numeric code (YY/MM/DD) to represent the year, month, and day of birth.

1.3 **SIGNATURE:** Handwritten signature of the subject. : Coding not applicable.

2. **PHYSICIAN'S CERTIFICATION:** This block of data contains a certification by a licensed physician's that the data being entered into the health status record is compiled from the individual's medical records and is accurate as of the date of certification.: Coding not applicable.

2.1 **NAME & SIGNATURE:** Printed last name, first name, and middle initial, separated by commas, of the certifying physician, followed by the physician's handwritten signature.: Alphabetic coding

2.2 **LICENSE NUMBER:** License number and issuing State of certifying physician: Use Alpha/numeric coding to represent the license number and two-letter abbreviation of State

2.3 **ADDRESS:** Street number and name plus apartment or suite number, followed by name of city, two-letter abbreviation of the State, followed by the nine number zip code of the certifying physician: Alpha/numeric coding.

2.4 **TELEPHONE NUMBER:** Three-digit area code followed by three-digit prefix and four-digit telephone numbers separated by spaces, plus extension number (if applicable) of certifying physician.: Numeric Coding

2.5 **DATE OF CERTIFICATION:** Year, month, and day of physician's certification of health status date being entered into the record.: Use numeric code (YY/MM/DD) to represent date of certification

2.6 **MEDICAL RECORD SOURCE DATE:** Year, month, and day of medical record which was the source of from which the health status record entry was taken.: Use numeric code (YY/MM/DD) to represent date of certification

FIG. 2 Individual's Health Status Record Data Element Definitions

software deficiencies; operating mistakes; physical damage by fire, water, smoke, excessive temperatures, electrical failure, or sabotage, or a combination thereof.

6.4.4 In EMS systems, where the existing telecommunications and computer technology do not permit access by means of computer modem, provisions should exist for accessing data in an individual's health status record by means of two-way voice communications, by telephone FAX transmission, or by means of other available telecommunications.

6.4.5 Hard copies of selected data from individuals' health status records may be authorized for specific applications such as for school or summer camp health files. Templates should be developed for each specific application and provisions should exist for the custodian(s) of such hard copy health status records to ensure the security and authorized use of the records.

6.5 *Health Status Record Data Transmission*—The HSIS data shall be transmitted from the HSIS provider to independent computers in accordance with Specification E 1238.

7. Keywords

7.1 health status information services; information services; prehospital emergency medical services

3. **INDIVIDUAL'S IDENTIFICATION:** This section contains data identifying the individual who is the subject of this health status record.: Coding not applicable.

3.1 **INDIVIDUAL'S RECORD NUMBER:** A number assigned by the HSIS provider to the individuals record and used for filing/locating the individual's record.

3.2 **NAME:** Printed last name, first name, and middle initial, separated by commas, of the individual who is the subject of this health record: Alphabetic coding

3.3 **ADDRESS:** Street number and name plus apartment or suite number, followed by name of city, two-letter abbreviation of the State, followed by the nine number zip code of the individual who is the subject of this health record: Alpha/numeric coding.

3.4 **DATE OF BIRTH:** Date of birth of the subject of this health record.: Use numeric code (YY/MM/DD) to represent the year, month, and day of birth. (Same as 1.2)

3.5 **TELEPHONE NUMBER (HOME):** Three-digit area code followed by three-digit prefix and four-digit telephone numbers separated by spaces, plus extension number (if applicable) of the subject of this health record.: Numeric Coding

3.6 **TELEPHONE NUMBER (WORK):** Three-digit area code followed by three-digit prefix and four-digit telephone numbers separated by spaces, plus extension number (if applicable) of the subject of this health record.: Numeric Coding

3.7 **SOCIAL SECURITY NUMBER:** Social Security Number of the subject of this health record consisting of 9 numbers represented by the numeric code (NN NNN NNNN)

3.8 **RELIGION:** The religious affiliation claimed by the subject of this health record expressed in a two-character alphabetic code as indicated in the following examples:

CATHOLIC	CA	JEWISH	JE
PROTESTANT	PR	ISLAM	IS
CHRISTIAN SCIENCE	CS	JEHOVAH'S WITNESS	JW

OTHER ________________________________
Specify

3.9 **PRIMARY MEDICAL INSURER:** The name of the primary health/medical insurance company of the subject of this health record: Alphabetic Coding:

3.10 **PRIMARY POLICY NUMBER:** The number of the primary health/medical insurance policy of the subject of this health record: Alpha/numeric coding:

FIG. 2 *(continued)*

3.11 **SECONDARY MEDICAL INSURER:** The name of the secondary health/medical insurance company of the subject of this health record: Alphabetic Coding:

3.12 **SECONDARY POLICY NUMBER:** The number of the secondary health/medical insurance policy of the subject of this health record: Alpha/numeric coding:

3.13 **DESIGNATED PRIMARY CONTACT:** Name of Designated Primary Contact (for minors, usually a parent or guardian; for adult usually the spouse or other close associate): Alphabetic coding:

3.14 **PRIMARY CONTACT TELEPHONE NUMBERS:** the letter "H" followed by ten-digits corresponding to the home telephone number followed by a space and the letter "W" followed by the ten digits corresponding to the work telephone number of the primary contact: Alpha/Numeric coding:

3.15 **PERSONAL PHYSICIANS' NAMES:** Names of physicians (include all licensed professionals or providers such as psychiatrists, dentists, orthodontists, etc.) who are currently providing medical care to the subject of this health record. Alphabetic coding:

3.16 **PERSONAL PHYSICIANS' TELEPHONE NUMBER/S:** Corresponding telephone number/s which can be used to contact the personal physicians. Numeric coding:

3.17 **ORGAN DONOR PROGRAM PARTICIPATION:** If the subject of this medical record has completed an organ donor statement, cite the form of the statement and where that statement can be found (drivers license, living will, donor card, etc.). Alphabetic coding:

3.18 **SEX:** The sex of the subject of this medical record expressed as M for Male or F for Female: Alphabetic Coding:

3.19 **HEIGHT:** Height of the subject of this medical record expressed in inches: Numeric coding:

3.20 **WEIGHT:** Current weight of the subject of this medical record expressed in pounds and tenths of pounds. Numeric coding:

3.21 **EYE COLOR:** Observed color of the eyes of the subject of this medical record (blue, brown, green, gray, etc.). Alphabetic coding:

3.22 **SKIN COLOR:** Observed color of skin of subject of this medical record (white, black, brown, yellow, etc.). Alphabetic coding:

3.23 **HAIR COLOR:** Observed color of hair of subject of this medical record (black, brown, red, blond, etc.). Alphabetic coding:

FIG. 2 *(continued)*

4. **INDIVIDUAL'S MEDICAL HISTORY:** This section contains data describing the medical history of the subject of this medical record.: Coding not applicable:

4.1 **PREVIOUSLY DIAGNOSED PROBLEMS:** A list, in order of severity based on certifying physician's judgment or assessment, of diagnosed problems of the subject of this medical record, including such "hidden diseases" and disabilities such as epilepsy, asthma, diabetes, blindness, deafness, AIDS, chromosomal abnormality, congenital heart disease, anesthesia problems, etc.: Alphabetic coding:

4.2 **PREVIOUSLY DIAGNOSED ALLERGIES:** A list, in order of severity, based on certifying physician's judgment or assessment of previously diagnosed allergies of the subject of this medical record, including such allergic substances such as animals, insect stings, house dust, pollen, chemicals, poison ivy or other plants, etc.: Alphabetic coding:

4.3 **PROSTHETIC DEVICES AND DEVICES USED IN MAJOR MEDICAL PROCEDURES:** A list of prosthetic devices & devices used in major medical procedures (present or previous) on the subject of this medical record(such as cardiac pacemaker, hearing aid, dentures, brain shunt, renal dialysis, colostomy, tracheotomy, lens implant, orother).: Alphabetic coding:

4.4 **VISUAL PROSTHESIS:** Visual prosthesis such as contact lenses, regular eye glasses, artificial eyes, etc. used by the subject of this medical record.: Alphabetic coding:

4.5 **IMMUNIZATIONS:** A list of the diseases (tetanus, diphtheria, polio, chicken pox, mumps/measles/rubella, etc) for which the subject of this medical record has been fully immunized followed by the date on which full immunization was administered.: Alpha/numeric coding:

4.6 **PHYSIOLOGICAL INJURIES OR GROWTH PROBLEMS:** A list of injuries or growth problems (fractures, dislocations, soft tissue injuries, etc.,) for which the subject of this health record has been diagnosed, from most recent to past.: Alphabetic coding:

4.7 **PSYCHOLOGICAL DISORDERS:** A listing of psychological problems (depression, chronic phobias, panic disorder, etc.) for which the subject of this health record has been diagnosed, from most recent to past.: Alphabetic coding:

4.8 **HOSPITALIZATIONS:** A listing of hospitalizations of the subject of this health record, from most recent to past, including the name and address of the hospital, reason for hospitalization, and date of discharge.: Alpha/numeric coding:

4.9 **OPERATIONS AND OTHER MEDICAL PROCEDURES:** A listing of medical procedures such as surgeries, radiation therapy, chemical therapies, etc., which the subject of this health record has received, from most recent to past.: Alphabetic coding:

FIG. 2 *(continued)*

4.10 MEDICAL CONDITIONS CURRENTLY UNDER TREATMENT: A listing from most recent to past, including previously diagnosed medical problems in 1.4 above, of such conditions as arthritis, asthma, cancer, cardiac, diabetes, and other conditions, for which the subject of this health record is currently being treated.: Alphabetic coding:

4.11 ALLERGIES CURRENTLY UNDER TREATMENT: A listing, from most recent to past of allergic conditions, such as are listed in 4.2 above, for which the subject of this health record is currently being treated.: Alphabetic coding:

4.12 PRESCRIPTION DRUGS: A listing, from most recent to past, including periods of use (year/month/date to year/month/date), National Drug Code(NDC)/name/strength/and form of drug, daily dosage, and route of administration of physician prescribed drugs used by the subject of this health record.: Alpha/numeric coding:

4.13 RADIATION TREATMENT: A listing, from most recent to past, including dates and purpose of radiation therapy administered to the subject of this health record.: Alpha/numeric coding:

4.14 CHEMOTHERAPY: A listing, from most recent to past, including dates, chemical and reason, of chemotherapy received by the subject of this health record.: Alpha/numeric coding:

4.15 BLOOD TEST RESULTS: A listing for the subject of this health record, from most recent to past including date, of blood test results including type (A, B, AB, O), hemoglobin (g/DL), white blood count, Electrolytes (Including Glucose, BUN [Mg/DL], Na [ME G/L], K [ME G/L], CL [ME G/L], Antibody Screen (Positive/Negative), etc.: Alpha/numeric coding:

4.16 ELECTROCARDIOGRAM DATES AND RESULTS: A listing of the dates and results of electrocardiograms administered to the subject of this health record.: Alpha/numeric coding:

4.17 X-RAY DATES AND FINDINGS: A listing, from most recent to past, of X-ray diagnostic exposures administered to the subject of this health record including dates and findings.: Alpha/numeric coding:

4.18 EPISODES OF PROLONGED BLEEDING OR CLOTTING: A listing, from most recent to past of episodes of prolonged bleeding or clotting of the subject of this health record, including dates and circumstances.: Alpha/numeric coding:

FIG. 2 *(continued)*

As a minimum, the following health status data should be downloaded for printout/display in response to an authorizeed request for access to an individual's health status data made by a prehospital EMS provider or by a person providing on-line medical dirction for a prehospital EMS response. This data is listed in two categories two categories as described in reference 2.1.6: Demographics of the Emergency Patient and Pre-existing Conditions.

Data number elements are those listed in Figure 1.

DEMOGRAPHICS OF THE EMERGENCY PATIENT

3.1 **INDIVIDUAL'S RECORD NUMBER:** ____________________

3.2 **NAME:** ____
Last First MI

3.3 **ADDRESS:**

____
Street

____
City State Zip Code

3.4 **DATE OF BIRTH:** ____________________
Year/Month/Day

3.5 **TELEPHONE NUMBER (HOME):** ____________________

3.7 **SOCIAL SECURITY NUMBER:** ____ ______ ______

3.8 **RELIGION:**

CATHOLIC	___	**JEWISH**	___
PROTESTANT	___	**ISLAM**	___
CHRISTIAN SCIENCE	___	**JEHOVAH'S WITNESS**	___

OTHER ____________________
Specify

3.9 Primary Insurance Carrier ____________ 3.10. **Policy No** ____________

3.11 **Secondary Insurance Carrier** ____________ 3.12 **Policy No** ____________

FIG. 3 Sample Prehospital EMS Health Status Data Template

3.13. DESIGNATED PRIMARY CONTACT: ______________________________
Name & Relationship

3.14. TELEPHONE NUMBERS OF DESIGNATED PRIMARY CONTACT:
HOME: ____ __________ **WORK:** ______ ___________

PERSONAL PHYSICIANS

Names		Telephone Numbers
3.15 ______________________	3.16	____________
______________________		____________
______________________		____________

3.17 ORGAN DONOR PROGRAM PARTICIPATION:
____
If yes, cite existence donor statement (driver's license, living will, donor card ,etc.)

3.18 SEX: ______ Male ______ Female **3.19 HEIGHT** ____________ Inches

3.20 WEIGHT: ____________ Pounds **3.21 EYE COLOR:** ____________ (State color)

3.22 SKIN COLOR: ____________ (State color) **3.23 HAIR COLOR:** ____________ (State color)

PRE-EXISTING CONDITIONS

4.1 PREVIOUSLY DIAGNOSED MEDICAL PROBLEMS: List in order of severity based on certifying physician's judgement or assessment. Include such "hidden diseases" and disabilities such as epliepsy, asthma, diabetes, blindness, deafness, AIDS, chromosomal abnormality, congenital heart disease, anesthesia problems, etc.
(1)____________ (2)____________ (3)____________
(4)____________ (5)____________ (6)____________
List additional problems in order of severity.

4.2 PREVIOUSLY DIAGNOSED ALLERGIES: List in order of severity based on certifying physician's judgement or assessment. Include such allergic substances such as animals, insect stings, house dust, pollen, chemicals, poison ivy or other plants, etc.
(1)____________ (2)____________ (3)____________
(4)____________ (5)____________ (6)____________
List additional allergies in order of severity.

4.3 PROSTHETIC DEVICES AND DEVICES USED IN MAJOR MEDICAL PROCEDURES - present or past:
cardiac pacemeker ________ **hearing aid** ________
dentures ________ **brain shunt** ________
renal dialysis ________ **colostomy** ________
tracheostomy ________ **lens implant** ________
other ________________(**Specify)**

FIG. 3 *(continued)*

4.4 **VISUAL PROSTHESIS:** **contact lenses** ____ **regular glasses** ____
artificial eye/s ____ other ____

4.6 **PHYSIOLOGICAL INJURIES OR GROWTH PROBLEMS:** List most recent to past including such conditions as fractures, dislocations, soft tissue damage, etc.

1. ____________________ **2.** ____________________
3. ____________________ **4.** ____________________

4.8 **MOST RECENT HOSPITALIZATION:**

____
Name of Hospital

____
Address - (Street, City, State, Zip Code)

____ ____________________
Reason for hospitalization **Discharge (Year/Month/Day)**

4.9 **OPERATIONS AND OTHER MEDICAL PROCEDURES:** List most recent to past, including such procedures as surgeries, radiation therapy, chemical therapies, etc.

1. ____________________ **2.** ____________________
3. ____________________ **4.** ____________________
5. ____________________ **6.** ____________________

4.10 **MEDICAL CONDITIONS CURRENTLY UNDER TREATMENT:** List most recent to past, including such conditions as arthritis, asthma, cancer, cardiac, diabetes, and other conditions listed in 4.1 under "PREVIOUSLY DIAGNOSED MEDICAL PROBLEMS".

1. ____________________ **2.** ____________________
3. ____________________ **4.** ____________________
5. ____________________ **6.** ____________________

4.11 **ALLERGIES CURRENTLY UNDER TREATMENT:** List most recent to past. (See "PREVIOUSLY DIAGNOSED ALLERGIES".)

1. ____________________ **2.** ____________________
3. ____________________ **4.** ____________________

4.12. **PRESCRIPTION DRUGS:** List drugs currently being used including periods of use (year/month/date to present), National Drug Code (NDC)/name/strength /and form of drug, daily dosage,and route of administration.

Period YY/MM/DD- PRESENT	NDC,Name/Strength/Form	Dosage per Day	Route

FIG. 3 *(continued)*

4.15 BLOOD TEST RESULTS: List most recent results, including date, blood type (A, B, AB, O), hemoglobin (g/DL), white blood count, Electrolytes (Including Glucose, BUN [Mg/DL], Na [ME G/L], K [ME G/L], CL [ME G/L], Antibody Screen (Positive/Negative).

Date	Type	Hemo	WBC	Electrolytes					Antibodies
				Glu	BUN	Na	K	CL	Pos/Neg
____	____	____	____	____	____	____	____	____	____

18. EPISODES OF PROLONGED BLEEDING OR CLOTTING - List most recent to past.

Date	Circumstances
____	____
____	____

NOTE 1—As a minimum, this health status data should be downloaded for printout/display in response to an authorized request for access to an individual's health status data made by a prehospital EMS provider or by a person providing on-line medical direction for a prehospital EMS response. This data is listed in two categories as described in Guide E1774 demographics of the emergency patient and preexisting conditions. Data number elements are those listed in

REFERENCES

(**1**) Rockwell International Corporation Project: Trauma Care Information Management System (TCIMS), funded under ARPA Agreement MDA972-94-200010.

(**2**) Rockwell International Corporation Project: National Information Infrastructure—Health Information Network (NII-HIN), funded under ARPA Agreement.

(**3**) *94-04 Program in Information Infrastructure for Healthcare*, U.S. Department of Commerce, Technology Administration, National Institute of Standards and Technology, 1994.

(**4**) *Uniform Ambulatory Care Data Set*, U.S. Department of Health and Human Services, 1994.

(**5**) *Uniform Hospital Discharge Data Set*, U.S. Department of Health and Human Services, 1994.

(**6**) Uniform Pre-Hospital Emergency Medical Services (EMS) Data Element Consensus Development Conference, *Final Report*, National Highway Traffic Safety Administration, June 1994.

Designation: F 1653 – 95

Standard Guide for
Scope of Performance of Triage in a Prehospital Environment[1]

This standard is issued under the fixed designation F 1653; the number immediately following the designation indicates the year of original adoption or, in the case of revision, the year of last revision. A number in parentheses indicates the year of last reapproval. A superscript epsilon (ϵ) indicates an editorial change since the last revision or reapproval.

INTRODUCTION

Triage is a word taken from the French verb *trier*, that means "to sort". During the time of the Napoleonic wars, a technique for assigning priorities to the treatment of battlefield casualties was established in order to maximize the use of limited resources. The basic principle of triage is to do the greatest good for the greatest number of casualties. Care is provided first to those with the most serious emergencies and to those who are most salvageable. This technique is identified as essential for good disaster medical care.

1. Scope

1.1 This guide covers minimum requirements for the scope of performance for individuals who perform triage at an emergency medical incident involving multiple casualties in a pre-hospital environment.

1.2 This guide acknowledges objectives based on an individual's required knowledge of signs and symptoms, patient assessment and basic life support.

1.3 Operating within the framework of this guide may expose personnel to hazardous materials, procedures, and equipment. For additional information see Practice F 1031, Guides F 1219, F 1253, F 1285, F 1287, F 1288, F 1489 and F 1651.

1.4 *This standard does not purport to address all of the safety concerns, if any, associated with its use. It is the responsibility of the user of this standard to establish appropriate safety and health practices and determine the applicability of regulatory limitations prior to use.* For specific precautionary statements, see Footnote 3. [2]

2. Referenced Documents

2.1 *ASTM Standards:*

F 1031 Practice for Training the Emergency Medical Technician (Basic)[3]

F 1177 Terminology Relating to Emergency Medical Services[3]

F 1219 Guide for Training the Emergency Medical Technician (Basic) to Perform Patient Primary Assessment[3]

F 1253 Guide for Training the Emergency Medical Technician (Basic) to Perform Patient Secondary Assessment[3]

F 1285 Guide for Training the Emergency Medical Technician (Basic) to Perform Patient Examination Techniques[3]

F 1287 Guide for the Scope of Performance of First Responders Who Provide Emergency Medical Care[3]

F 1288 Guide for Planning for and Response to a Multiple Casualty Incident[3]

F 1489 Guide for the Performance of Patient Assessment by the Emergency Medical Technician (Paramedic)[3]

F 1651 Guide for Training the Emergency Medical Technician (Paramedic)

3. Terminology

3.1 *Definitions of Terms Specific to This Standard:*

3.1.1 *ongoing triage, n*—the continuing process of patient assessment and prioritization in a multiple casualty incident. (Also known as *secondary* and *tertiary*).

3.1.2 *primary triage, n*—the initial process of rapid assessment, provision of life saving interventions and assignment of visual priority identification to each patient in a multiple casualty incident.

3.1.3 *triage, n*—the process of sorting and prioritizing care of the sick and injured on the basis of urgency and type of condition present, as well as the number of patients and resources available. The objective is to properly treat and transport patients to medical facilities appropriately situated and equipped for their care.

3.2 For definitions of other terms used in this guide, refer to Terminology F 1177.

---

[1] This guide is under the jurisdiction of ASTM Committee F-30 on Emergency Medical Services and is the direct responsibility of Subcommittee F30.02 on Personnel, Training and Education.

Current edition approved Oct. 10, 1995. Published December 1995.

[2] Most recent "Guidelines for Cardiopulmonary Resuscitation and Emergency Cardiac Care," as reprinted from the *Journal of the American Medical Association*, available from American Heart Association, 7320 Greenville Avenue, Dallas, TX 75231.

[3] *Annual Book of ASTM Standards*, Vol 13.01.

4. Significance and Use

4.1 This guide is not intended to be used by itself, but as a component of Guide F 1288. Merely conforming to the guidelines described herein will not ensure that adequate triage is carried out in a multiple casualty incident.

4.2 The purpose of this guide is to establish a methodology for performing triage.

4.3 Individuals responsible for performing triage must be proficient in triage methods and related life-saving techniques.

4.4 A basic concept of triage is to do the greatest good for the greatest number of casualties.

4.5 The assessment process must be focused so as to identify those most at risk of early death who are likely to be salvaged by rapid medical intervention.

4.6 Triage allows the most efficient use of available resources.

4.7 This guide acknowledges many types of individuals with varying levels of emergency medical training. It also establishes a minimum scope of performance and encourages the addition of optional knowledge, skills and attitudinal objectives.

4.8 A vital role in the development of and operational application of triage is that of medical control. This guide should be used by medical directors in the determination of operational and medical protocols for use during MCI's.

4.9 This guide is intended to assist those who are responsible for defining the scope of performance of individuals who perform triage.

4.10 For the purpose of this guide the word "injured" includes both sick or injured patients, or both.

5. Objectives

5.1 *Required Objectives*—These objectives are in an order suggesting a particular performance sequence although some may be performed concurrently. Some incidents may not require performance of all objectives. Individuals who perform triage shall be able to:

5.1.1 Identify health and safety hazards and initiate appropriate actions.

5.1.2 Recognize an incident that may require triage.

5.1.3 Determine the need for and request additional resources.

5.1.4 Initiate incident command Guide F 1288.

5.1.5 Identify conditions which may dictate a decision to treat patients at the scene or transfer them to a designated treatment area.

5.1.6 Initiate Primary Triage.

5.1.6.1 Identify victims who appear to be uninjured or minimally injured and able to help themselves, and direct them to a designated area of safety.

5.1.6.2 Perform a rapid assessment of the remaining victims. Check respiratory status, circulatory status and level of consciousness.

5.1.6.3 Immediate medical interventions should be limited to opening the airway and controlling gross hemorrhage. These interventions should not stop the process of triage.

5.1.6.4 Assign a triage priority to each victim, including the uninjured, and use a visual marker for individual identification. Patients are placed into the following categories in accordance with the assessment outcome and in accordance with the local standard of medical care.

5.1.6.4.1 *First Priority/Immediate (RED)*—Those patients with serious injuries that are life threatening but have a high probability of survival.

5.1.6.4.2 *Second Priority/Delayed (YELLOW)*—Those patients who are seriously injured and whose lives are not immediately threatened. The triage category of these patients may change to first priority based on medical resources at any time during an incident.

5.1.6.4.3 *Third Priority/Minor (GREEN)*—Those patients who are injured but do not require immediate medical attention and those apparently not physically injured.

5.1.6.4.4 *Fourth Priority/Dead/Mortally Wounded (BLACK)*—Those patients who are obviously dead as determined by medical protocol or those patients with severe injuries and a low probability of survival, despite immediate care. As this is a difficult field decision, actual practice may be to provide treatment and transportation.

5.1.6.5 Arrange for transfer of patients based on highest priority first, to a location where they can receive the appropriate level of care.

5.1.7 Initiate Ongoing Triage.

5.1.8 Document triage priority, assessment, treatment rendered and patient identification.

5.1.9 Continue transferring patients by highest priority as resources become available.

5.1.10 Triage is a dynamic process. It will be repeated and performed as necessary during an event and in other phases of the continuum of care.

5.2 *Optional Objectives*:

5.2.1 Demonstrate a knowledge of the principles of the Incident Command System (ICS).

5.2.2 Describe critical incident stress, its impact on rescuers and the availability of resources.

6. Keywords

6.1 emergency medical service (EMS); incident command system (ICS); triage

Standard Guide for Training and Evaluation of Individuals Who are Responsible for or Perform Triage in a Prehospital Environment[1]

This standard is issued under the fixed designation F 1654; the number immediately following the designation indicates the year of original adoption or, in the case of revision, the year of last revision. A number in parentheses indicates the year of last reapproval. A superscript epsilon (ε) indicates an editorial change since the last revision or reapproval.

1. Scope

1.1 This guide covers minimum requirements for the training and evaluation of individuals who perform triage at an emergency medical incident involving multiple casualties in a prehospital environment.

1.2 All training will be in accordance with Guide F 1653.

1.3 Included in this guide is a standard for knowledge and skill evaluation.

1.4 Operating within the framework of this guide may expose personnel to hazardous materials, procedures and equipment. For additional information see Practice F 1031 and Guides F 1219, F 1253, F 1285, F 1288, F 1453 and F 1489.

1.5 *This standard does not purport to address all of the safety concerns, if any, associated with its use. It is the responsibility of the user of this standard to establish appropriate safety and health practices and determine the applicability of regulatory limitations prior to use.* For specific precautionary statements, see the document cited in Footnote 3.

2. Referenced Documents

2.1 *ASTM Standards:*

F 1031 Practice for Training the Emergency Medical Technician (Basic)[2,3]

F 1177 Terminology Relating to Emergency Medical Services[2]

F 1219 Guide for Training the Emergency Medical Technician (Basic) to Perform Patient Primary Assessment[2]

F 1253 Guide for Training the Emergency Medical Technician (Basic) to Perform Patient Secondary Assessment[2]

F 1285 Guide for Training the Emergency Medical Technician (Basic) to Perform Patient Examination Techniques[2]

F 1288 Guide for Planning for and Response to a Multiple Casualty Incident[2]

F 1453 Guide for Training and Evaluation of First Responders Who Provide Emergency Medical Care[2]

F 1489 Guide for the Performance of Patient Assessment by the Emergency Medical Technician (Paramedic)[2]

F 1651 Guide for Training the Emergency Medical Technician (Paramedic)[2]

F 1653 Guide for Scope of Performance of Triage in Prehospital Environment[2]

3. Terminology

3.1 *Definitions of Terms Specific to This Standard:*

3.1.1 *first priority/immediate (RED)*—those patients with serious injuries that are life threatening but have a high probability of survival.

3.1.2 *fourth priority/dead/mortally wounded (BLACK)*—Those patients who are obviously dead as determined by local medical protocol or those patients with severe injuries and a low probability of survival, despite immediate care.

3.1.3 *injured, adj*—means both sick and injured patients.

3.1.4 *ongoing triage, n*—the continuing process of patient assessment and prioritization in a multiple casualty incident. (Also known as *secondary* and *tertiary.*)

3.1.5 *primary triage, n*—the initial process of rapid assessment, provision of life saving interventions and assignment of visual priority identification to each patient in a multiple casualty incident.

3.1.6 *second priority/delayed (YELLOW)*—those patients who are seriously injured and whose lives are not immediately threatened.

3.1.7 *third priority/minor (GREEN)*—those patients who are injured but do not require immediate medical attention and those apparently not physically injured.

3.1.8 *triage, n*—the process of sorting and prioritizing emergency medical care of the sick and injured on the basis of urgency and type of condition present as well as the number of patients and resources.

3.2 For definitions of other terms used in this guide, refer to Terminology F 1177.

4. Significance and Use

4.1 This guide is intended for use by those responsible for the development and implementation of training programs, that include competency evaluation, for triage in the prehospital environment.

4.2 This guide is not intended to be used by itself, but as a

---

[1] This guide is under the jurisdiction of ASTM Committee F-30 on Emergency Medical Services and is the direct responsibility of Subcommittee F30.02 on Personnel, Training and Education.

Current edition approved Oct. 10, 1995. Published December 1995.

[2] *Annual Book of ASTM Standards*, Vol 13.01.

[3] Most recent "Standards and Guidelines for Cardiopulmonary Resuscitation and Emergency Cardiac Care" as reprinted from the *Journal of the American Medical Association*, available from American Heart Association, 7320 Greenville Avenue, Dallas, TX 75231.

component of Guide F 1288.

4.3 This guide acknowledges many types of individuals with varying levels of emergency medical training. It also establishes a minimum training standard and encourages the addition of optional knowledge, skill, and attitudinal objectives.

4.4 A vital role in the development and operational application of triage is that of medical control. This guide should be used by medical directors in the determination of operational and medical protocols for use during MCIs and coordinated with those who are responsible for training.

4.5 At the beginning of the program, students shall be informed of the course objectives and requirements for successful completion.

5. Required Performance Objectives

5.1 Individuals who are responsible for, or perform triage in, the pre-hospital environment shall be trained in the following skills. These objectives are listed in a suggested instructional and performance order, although some may be performed concurrently. Some incidents may not require performance of all objectives.

5.1.1 *Health and Safety Hazards*—Describe the presence of conditions or situations and actions to be taken when there exists a potential hazard to rescuers, victims, or bystanders.

5.1.2 *Incident Recognition*—Describe the elements of a multiple-casualty incident that may require utilization of triage skills.

5.1.2.1 Describe a multiple casualty incident,

5.1.2.2 Describe why, when resources are limited, the greater may be served by obtaining additional resources, and managing existing resources, rather than providing patient care immediately,

5.1.2.3 Define triage, and

5.1.2.4 Describe the general principles of providing triage.

5.1.3 *Resources*:

5.1.3.1 Describe the concept of triage of doing the greatest good for the greatest number of casualties.

5.1.3.2 Describe existing and potential incident conditions and situations under which additional resources are needed but may or may not be available.

5.1.3.3 Describe methods for requesting needed resources.

5.1.4 *Incident Management*—Describe the methods for implementation of the local emergency incident management system as it relates to multi-casualty events.

5.1.5 *Medical Control*—Describe the role and responsibilities of medical control during an MCI, the application of protocols and the use of standing orders, on-scene, or on-line medical control.

5.1.6 *Primary Triage*:

5.1.6.1 Demonstrate the method(s) to identify victims who appear to be uninjured or minimally injured and able to help themselves.

5.1.6.2 Describe methods to identify safe areas for the placement of patients.

5.1.6.3 Demonstrate methods for directing uninjured or minimally injured victims to a designated area(s).

5.1.6.4 Describe the performance of a rapid assessment of remaining victim(s).

5.1.6.4.1 Demonstrate method(s) to assess respiratory status.

5.1.6.4.2 Demonstrate method(s) to assess circulatory status.

5.1.6.4.3 Demonstrate method(s) to assess level of consciousness.

5.1.6.5 Describe methods for performing immediate life saving aid without stopping the triage process.

5.1.6.5.1 Demonstrate method(s) for opening and maintaining an airway.

5.1.6.5.2 Demonstrate method(s) for controlling gross hemorrhage.

5.1.6.6 Describe methods for assigning a triage priority to each victim, including the uninjured.

5.1.6.6.1 Define triage priorities.

5.1.6.6.2 Demonstrate methods to visually identify each victim based on their individual triage priority.

5.1.6.7 Describe the categories of triage and their application in identifying patient priorities in an MCI.

5.1.6.8 Describe methods to transfer patients based upon triage priority and transport capability and availability. This may need to be accomplished several times on and off site until definitive care is provided.

5.1.7 *Ongoing Triage*:

5.1.7.1 Describe the purpose of ongoing triage.

5.1.7.2 Demonstrate methods for reassessing patients and revising triage priorities when required.

5.1.7.3 Describe conditions or situations which may dictate a decision to either treat patients at the scene, transfer them to a designated treatment area or a definitive care facility.

5.1.7.4 Describe the resources needed to provide patient care at the scene.

5.1.7.5 Describe the rationale for the continued assessment and treatment of patients.

5.1.7.6 Describe essential elements of patient information to be documented for maintaining incident status to include triage priority, assessment, treatment rendered, and patient identification.

5.1.7.7 Describe methods to transport patients based upon triage priority and transport capability.

5.1.7.8 Describe methods to communicate patient information.

5.2 *Optional Objectives*—Describe the principles of the Incident Command System (ICS).

6. Evaluation

6.1 A method to evaluate the student's knowledge and performance of these objectives shall be established.

6.2 There shall be a method for remediation.

7. Keywords

7.1 emergency medical service (EMS); incident command system (ICS); triage

Designation: F 1655 – 95

Standard Guide for Training First Responders Who Practice in Wilderness, Delayed, or Prolonged Transport Settings[1]

This standard is issued under the fixed designation F 1655; the number immediately following the designation indicates the year of original adoption or, in the case of revision, the year of last revision. A number in parentheses indicates the year of last reapproval. A superscript epsilon (ε) indicates an editorial change since the last revision or reapproval.

1. Scope

1.1 This guide covers minimum training standards for first responders who may care for sick or injured persons in the specialized pre-hospital situations of the wilderness, delayed, or prolonged transport settings, including catastrophic disasters.

1.2 This guide establishes supplemental or continuing education programs that will be taught to individuals trained to the first responder level by an appropriate authority.

1.3 This guide does not provide training to be used, ordinarily, in the traditional EMS or ambulance transportation environments.

1.4 Included in this guide is a standard for the evaluation of the knowledge and skills defined within this guide.

1.5 Successful completion of a course based on this guide neither constitutes nor implies certification or licensure.

1.6 This guide does not establish medical protocols, nor does it authorize invasive procedures without specific authorization and medical control.

1.7 The values stated in inch-pound units are to be regarded as the standard.

1.8 Operating within the framework of this guide may expose personnel to hazardous materials or environments, procedures, and equipment or all of these.

1.9 *This standard does not purport to address all of the safety concerns, if any, associated with its use. It is the responsibility of the user of this standard to establish appropriate safety and health practices and determine the applicability of regulatory limitations prior to use.*

2. Referenced Documents

2.1 *ASTM Standards:*

F 1177 Terminology Relating to Emergency Medical Services[2]

F 1287 Guide for Scope of Performance of First Responders Who Provide Medical Care[2]

F 1453 Guide for the Training and Evaluation of First Responders Who Provide Medical Care[2]

F 1490 Terminology Relating to Search and Rescue[2]

3. Terminology

3.1 *Definitions:*

3.1.1 *access, n*—the process of reaching the patient/subject and establishing physical contact.

3.1.2 *basic life support/cardiopulmonary resuscitation (BLS/CPR), n*—a set of skills that includes airway management, chest compressions, and others as defined by the American Heart Association.

3.1.3 *definitive care, n*—a level of therapeutic intervention capable of providing comprehensive health care services for a specific condition. (See Terminology F 1177.)

3.1.4 *evacuation, n*—the process used between the time of extraction and transportation. (See Terminology F 1490.)

3.1.5 *extraction, n*—the process of initial assessment, treatment, stabilization, and packaging of the patient as well as the removal of the patient/subject from the immediately hazardous environment. (See Terminology F 1490.)

3.1.6 *first responder, n*—an individual trained in accordance with Guide F 1453.

3.1.7 *transportation, n*—the use of a dedicated vehicle for the removal of the patient to a medical facility or definitive care facility.

3.2 *Definitions of Terms Specific to This Standard:*

3.2.1 *delayed or prolonged transport, n*—when time between patient injury and arrival to a definitive care facility is greater than 60 min.

3.2.2 *non-traditional EMS environment, n*—environments not readily accessible to a ground ambulance.

3.2.3 *wilderness first responder (WFR), n*—an individual trained to meet the requirements of this guide.

3.2.4 *wilderness setting, n*—situations in which EMS delivery is complicated by one or more of the following four factors: (*1*) remoteness as far as logistics and access; (*2*) a significant delay in the delivery of care to the patient; (*3*) an environment that is stressful to both patients and rescuers; and (*4*) a lack of equipment and supplies.

4. Significance and Use

4.1 Individuals will be initially or concurrently trained in accordance with U.S. D.O.T. Course Guide for First Responders[3] and Guide F 1453.

---

[1] This guide is under the jurisdiction of ASTM Committee F-30 on Emergency Medical Services and is the direct responsibility of Subcommittee F30.02 on Personnel, Training and Education.

Current edition approved Oct. 10, 1995. Published December 1995.

[2] *Annual Book of ASTM Standards*, Vol 13.01.

[3] U.S. D.O.T. HS 900-025, *Course Guide, Emergency Medical Services*, First Responder Training Course, March 1979.

4.2 This guide does not suggest a particular training sequence.

4.3 This guide may be used by individuals developing training programs for non-traditional EMS environments.

4.4 This guide acknowledges the need to provide additional specific training for first responders who will practice in the wilderness, delayed or prolonged transport settings.

4.5 Individuals responsible for training first responders should identify those who will practice in the wilderness, delayed or prolonged transport settings and must ensure that such personnel are competent in all skills needed for the unique settings.

5. Illustrative Examples

5.1 *Wilderness Settings*:

5.1.1 In May 1983, two climbers were at about 18 000 ft, near Denali Pass, on Mount McKinley, Alaska. These climbers took a tumbling 800 ft fall before coming to rest. One of the climbers was only responsive to pain, with a lacerated face and the pick end of his ice axe impaled in the right side of his chest, just below the nipple line. A nearby climbing party responded. They first attempted to stabilize the ice axe in place as per standard EMS protocols. They improvised a rescue toboggan using two plastic sleds, but moving the patient was very difficult with the ice axe still in his chest. And, with temperatures ranging from – 50 to – 70°F (in accordance with National Park Service reports), rescuers were unable to keep him from rapidly cooling. The danger of cold exposure and the difficulty with transportation created by the impaled ice axe led rescuers to remove it.

5.1.2 After removing the ice axe, the patient began to rewarm, the rescuers were able to evacuate him expeditiously, and he went on to make a full recovery.

5.2 *Rural (Delayed/Prolonged Settings)*—A man was driving along a gravel road in a remote rural area of Northern Idaho. He stooped to clear a fallen tree from the road, and in the attempt, he fell and dislocated his right shoulder. He managed to call for help with his CB radio. About 2 h later, an ambulance arrived. The EMTs on the ambulance checked the pulse and sensation in his right arm, and found them to be normal. The man pleaded with them to pull on his shoulder and relocate it; he had a similar dislocation of the left shoulder in the past, and he knew that it could be reduced with a little help. However the EMTs, mindful of their training, insisted on" splinting it in position" and drove him six hours to the nearest hospital, mostly along bumpy secondary roads. The patient was moaning and intermittently screaming the entire time, in severe pain. Later he wrote to various authorities critizing the care provided to him.

5.3 *Disaster (Delayed/Prolonged Settings)*:

5.3.1 It was rush hour, and the freeways were crowded, but otherwise the day was like any other. Suddenly the earth shook, and a freeway collapsed, entombing motorists in a mass of concrete and twisted metal.

5.3.2 For four days, rescuers attacked the mass of rubble with every tool available from pliers to massive construction equipment. They had given up hope of finding any one else alive when they found a 57 year old construction worker alive, his lower extremities being trapped and crushed.

5.3.3 No medical personnel were available to render care such as IV hydration, so the construction workers immediately extricated him. Despite later attempts at hydration, he later developed kidney failure and then sepsis; he died a few days later.

5.4 *Borderline Wilderness Settings*:

5.4.1 Several years ago, a light civil aircraft crashed near the top of Tinker Mountain in southwest Virginia. Atop Tinker Mountain's rugged, cliff-strewn ridgeline is the Appalachian Trail; the area is a favorite of hikers and climbers. The aircraft was located from the air, and a team responded to the site. The quickest way to reach the site was from a road near the bottom of the ridge. Those responding to the site fell into two groups: mountain rescue team members and "regular" fire/EMS personnel. Protocols for the fire/EMS personnel required them, when responding to an air crash, to wear full turnout gear and self-contained breathing apparatus, and to carry fire suppression equipment. The standard practice for the mountain rescue was to carry minimal lightweight equipment, to dress appropriately for the weather and brush, to drink plenty of fluids, and to pace themselves.

5.4.2 The Virginia summer weather was particularly hot and humid, and the mountainside very steep. Soon many of the fire/EMS personnel were disabled from heat exhaustion, and one even had to be evacuated. The mountain rescue personnel were able to handle all necessary extrication and fire suppression with what they had carried and whatever they could improvise at the scene.

5.4.3 Survivors were treated appropriately for burns and shock, evacuated and then transported to a local hospital.

6. Educational Objectives

6.1 Wilderness First Responders shall be trained to perform the following (these objectives do not suggest any specific training order):

6.1.1 Describe the specific differences between the training of First Responders who practice in the traditional EMS environment and those who practice in the wilderness, prolonged or delayed transport settings where traditional patient care is not sufficient or appropriate.

6.1.2 Recognize the differences in patient care required by practice in the wilderness, prolonged or delayed transport settings.

6.1.3 Describe any additional or specialized anatomy or physiology knowledge required.

6.1.4 Identify and demonstrate the management of the following medical problems in the wilderness, delayed or prolonged transport settings:

6.1.4.1 Abdominal pain,

6.1.4.2 Vomiting,

6.1.4.3 Diarrhea,

6.1.4.4 Diabetes,

6.1.4.5 Seizure disorders,

6.1.4.6 Respiratory distress (for example, asthma, altitude),

6.1.4.7 Allergies,

6.1.4.8 Hypertension,

6.1.4.9 Cardiac emergencies, and

6.1.4.10 Dental emergencies.

6.1.5 Identify and demonstrate the management of illness or

injury related to or caused by the environment in the wilderness, delayed or prolonged transport settings, including the following:

6.1.5.1 Altitude (for example, acute mountain sickness, high altitude pulmonary edema, high altitude cerebral edema, solar radiation),

6.1.5.2 Barotrauma,

6.1.5.3 Cold (for example, hypothermia, frostbite),

6.1.5.4 Heat (for example, heat stroke, heat exhaustion, burns),

6.1.5.5 Electrical and lightning,

6.1.5.6 Exposure to plant or animal (for example, insect, reptile, arachnid, marine) toxins,

6.1.5.7 Drowning, near-drowning, and cold water immersion, and

6.1.5.8 Dehydration.

6.1.6 Describe the proper disinfection of water and identify and manage illnesses associated with improper water disinfection.

6.1.7 Describe and demonstrate the skills needed to manage open wounds in the wilderness, delayed, or prolonged transport settings.

6.1.8 Describe and demonstrate the skills needed to manage orthopedic problems in the wilderness, delayed or prolonged transport settings, including dislocations, fractures, and open fractures.

6.1.9 Describe and demonstrate the skills needed to manage spinal injuries and associated problems in the wilderness, delayed, or prolonged transport settings.

6.1.10 Describe and demonstrate the skills needed to manage specific problems associated with cardiorespiratory arrest in the wilderness, delayed, or prolonged transport settings.

6.1.11 Describe the uses, side effects, administration concerns, and needed authorities for non-prescription and prescription medications in the wilderness, delayed, or prolonged transport settings.

6.1.12 Describe measures necessary to prevent illness or injury occurring in the wilderness, delayed, or prolonged transport settings, including management of immediate stress reactions.

6.1.13 Describe specific problems related to rendering care in severe weather, in environmental extremes, when equipment is not readily available, when access is limited, and when there is little or no additional assistance.

6.1.14 Describe and demonstrate as feasible, clothing, survival, emergency communications and bivouac skills necessary in environmental extremes.

6.1.15 Demonstrate patient packaging skills in the wilderness, delayed, or prolonged transport settings.

6.1.16 Describe and demonstrate documentation requirements for recording patient care.

6.1.17 Describe any unique or specialized requirements or obligations imposed by the EMS system or other legal principles.

6.1.18 Describe any medical control requirements and processes.

6.1.19 Describe the principles of disease transmission and body fluid isolation and demonstrate the use of personal protection techniques.

7. Evaluation

7.1 Policies for evaluation, grading, pass/fail criteria, remediation and re-education shall be established and distributed to all students.

7.2 End of course cognitive and psychomotor evaluations that measure the competency of the WFR in the objectives of this guide shall be given.

8. Keywords

8.1 delayed; first responder; pre-hospital; prolonged; wilderness

Last ASTM Designation: F 1658 – 95

Test Method for Shear Testing of Calcium Phosphate Coatings

This test method covers shear testing of continuous calcium phosphate coatings ahering to dense metal substrates at ambient temperatures.

Formerly under the jurisdiction of Committee F04 on Medical and Surgical Materials and Devices, this test method was withdrawn in November 2000 and replaced by Test Method F1044-99 for Shear Testing of Calcium Phosphate Coatings and Metallic Coatings.[1]

[1] Annual Book of ASTM Standards, Volume 13.01.

Designation: F 1659 – 95

Standard Test Method for Bending and Shear Fatigue Testing of Calcium Phosphate Coatings on Solid Metallic Substrates[1]

This standard is issued under the fixed designation F 1659; the number immediately following the designation indicates the year of original adoption or, in the case of revision, the year of last revision. A number in parentheses indicates the year of last reapproval. A superscript epsilon (ϵ) indicates an editorial change since the last revision or reapproval.

1. Scope

1.1 This test method covers the procedure for the performance of calcium phosphate ceramic coatings in shear and bending fatigue modes. In the shear fatigue mode this test method evaluates the adhesive and cohesive properties of the coating on a metallic substrate. In the bending fatigue mode, this test method evaluates both the adhesion of the coating as well as the effects that the coating may have on the substrate material. These test methods are limited to testing in air at ambient temperature. These test methods are not intended for application in fatigue tests of components or devices; however, the test method that most closely replicates the actual loading configuration is preferred.

1.2 The values stated in SI units are to be regarded as the standard. The inch-pound units given in parentheses are for information only.

1.3 *This standard does not purport to address all of the safety concerns, if any, associated with its use. It is the responsibility of the user of this standard to establish appropriate safety and health practices and determine the applicability of regulatory limitations prior to use.*

2. Referenced Documents

2.1 *ASTM Standards:*

E 6 Terminology Relating to Methods of Mechanical Testing[2]

E 206 Definitions of Terms Relating to Fatigue Testing and the Statistical Analysis of Fatigue Data[3]

E 466 Practice for Constant Amplitude Axial Fatigue Tests of Metallic Materials[2]

E 467 Practice for Verification of Constant Amplitude Dynamic Loads in an Axial Load Fatigue Testing Machine[2]

E 468 Practice for Presentation of Constant Amplitude Fatigue Test Results for Metallic Materials[2]

3. Terminology

3.1 *Definitions:*

3.1.1 The definitions of terms relating to shear and fatigue testing appearing in Terminology E 6 and Terminology E 206 shall be considered as applying to the terms used in this test method.

4. Summary of Test Methods

4.1 *Shear Fatigue Testing*:

4.1.1 The intent of the shear fatigue test is to determine the adhesive or cohesive strength of the coating, or both.

4.1.2 This test is designed to allow the coating to fail at either the coating/substrate interface, within the coating, or at the glue/coating interface.

4.2 *Bending Fatigue Testing*:

4.2.1 The intent of the bending fatigue test is to quantify the effect that the coating has on the substrate to which it is applied. It may also be used to provide a subjective evaluation of coating adhesion (that is, spalling resistance, cracking resistance, etc.).

4.2.2 This test method is designed to first provide a substrate fatigue strength to serve as a baseline to assess the effects of the coating on the resulting fatigue strength of the system.

5. Significance and Use

5.1 The shear and bending fatigue tests are used to determine the effect of variations in material, geometry, surface condition, stress, etc., on the fatigue resistance of calcium phosphate coated metallic materials subjected to direct stress for up to 10^7 cycles. These tests may be used as a relative guide to the selection of calcium phosphate coated materials for service under conditions of repeated stress.

5.2 In order that such basic fatigue data be comparable, reproducible, and can be correlated among laboratories, it is essential that uniform fatigue practices be established.

5.3 The results of the fatigue test may be used for basic material property design. Actual components should not be tested using these test methods.

6. Equipment Characteristics

6.1 Equipment characteristics shall be in accordance with Section 7 on Adhesive Bonding Materials of Practice E 466.

6.2 *Shear Fatigue Test Grips*:

6.2.1 *General*—Various types of grips may be used to transmit the load to the specimens by the testing machine. To ensure axial shear stress, it is important that the specimen axis coincide with the centerline of the heads of the testing machine

[1] This test method is under the jurisdiction of ASTM Committee F-4 on Medical and Surgical Materials and Devicesand is the direct responsibility of Subcommittee F04.13on Ceramic Materials.

Current edition approved Nov. 10, 1995. Published May 1996.

[2] *Annual Book of ASTM Standards*, Vol 03.01.

[3] Discontinued; see *1987 Annual Book of ASTM Standards*, Vol 03.01.

and that the coating test plane be parallel to the axial load. Any departure from this requirement (that is, any eccentric loading) will introduce bending stresses that are not included in the usual stress calculation (force/cross-sectional area).

6.2.2 A drawing of a typical gripping device for the test assembly is shown in Fig. 1.

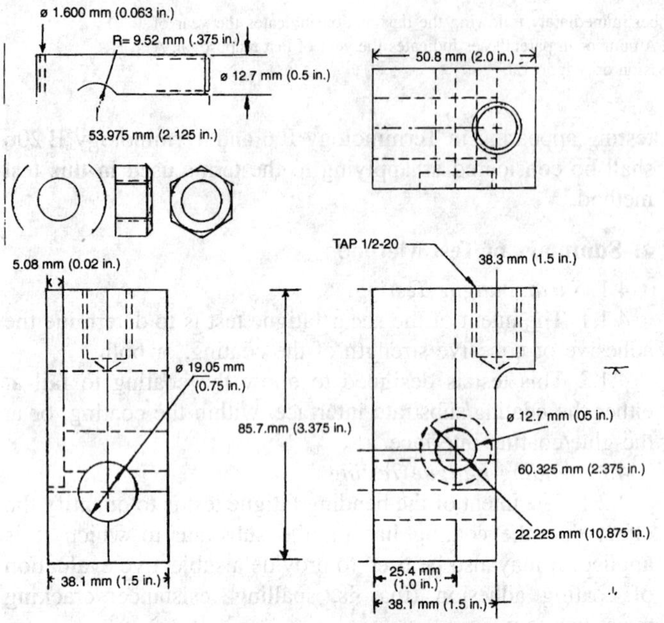

FIG. 1 Gripping Device for Shear Testing

6.2.3 Fig. 2 shows a drawing of the adaptor to mate the shear fixture to the tensile machine.

6.2.4 Fig. 3 shows a schematic of the test setup.

6.3 *Bending Fatigue Test Grips*—There are a variety of testing machines that may be employed for this test (that is, rotating beam fatigue machines and axial fatigue machines). The gripping method for each type of equipment shall be determined by either the manufacturer of that equipment (rotating beam machines) or the user.

7. Adhesive Bonding Materials

7.1 *Adhesive Bonding Agent*—A polymeric adhesive bonding agent in film form, or filled viscous adhesive cement, shall be identified and shall meet the following requirements.

7.1.1 The bonding agent shall be capable of bonding the coating on the test specimen components with an adhesive shear strength that is at least 34.5 MPa (5000 psi) or as great as the minimum required adhesion or cohesion strength of the coating.

7.1.2 In instances where coating porosity extends to the coating/substrate interface, the bonding agent shall be sufficiently viscous and application to the coating sufficiently detailed, to assure that it will not penetrate through the coating to the substrate. The FM 1000 Adhesive Film[4] with a thickness of 0.25 mm (0.01 in.) has proven satisfactory for this test.

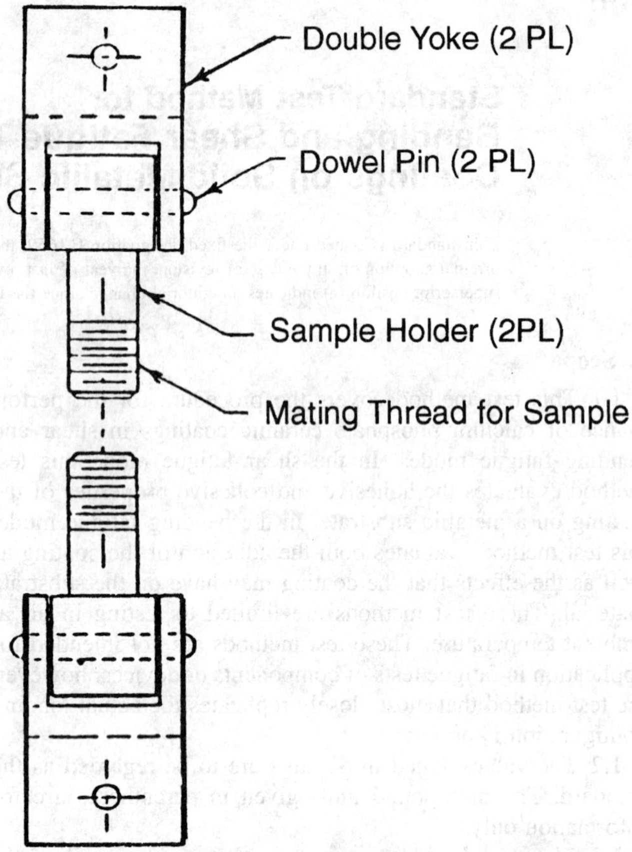

FIG. 2 Adaptor to Mate the Gripping Device to the Tensile Machine

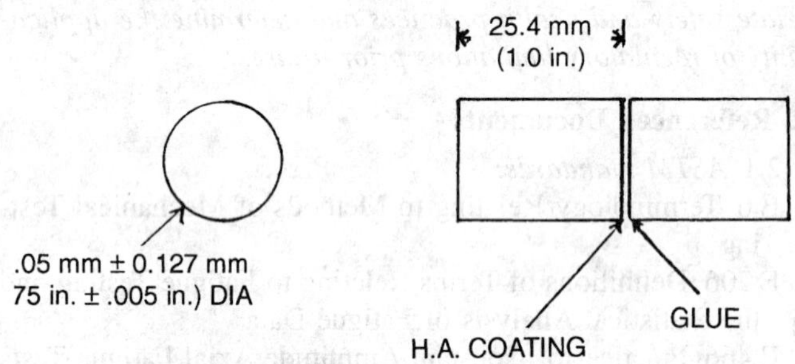

FIG. 3 Schematic of the Shear Test Set-up

7.1.3 If a material other than FM 1000[4] is used, or the condition of the FM 1000[4] is unknown, it must be tested to establish its equivalence fresh FM 1000.[4] Testing should be performed without the presence of the calcium phosphate coating to establish the performance of the adhesive.

8. Test Specimens

8.1 *Shear Fatigue Specimen*:

8.1.1 The recommended shear test specimen and setup is illustrated in Fig. 3 and Fig. 4, respectively. A complete, assembled test assembly, consists of two solid pieces: one with a coated surface and the other with an uncoated surface. The uncoated surface may be roughened to aid in the adhesion of the adhesive bonding agent.

8.1.2 The cross-sectional area of the substrate upon which the coating is applied shall be a nominal 2.85 cm^2 (0.44 in.^{2}).

[4] Available from American Cyanamid, Engineering Materials Division, Wayne, New Jersey.

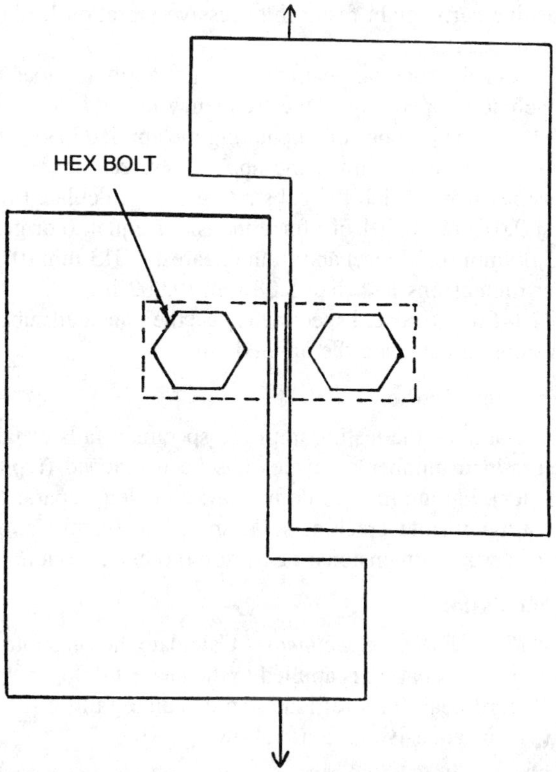

FIG. 4 Drawing of the Recommended Shear Test Specimen Assembly

When specimens of another cross-sectional area are used, the data must be demonstrated to be equivalent to the results produced using the 2.85 cm^2 standard cross-sectional area and the specimen size should be reported.

8.2 *Bending Fatigue Specimen*:

8.2.1 The type of specimen used will depend upon the objective of the test program, the type of equipment, the equipment capacity, and the form in which the material is available. The design, however, must meet certain general criteria as follows:

8.2.1.1 The design of the specimen should be such that if specimen failure should occur, it should occur in the test section (reduced area as shown in Figs. 5-8, and Fig. 9).

8.2.1.2 Specimens employing a flat tapered beam configuration should be designed such that a constant surface stress exists in the test section when the specimen is constrained at one end and point loaded perpendicular to the beam axis at the other end (that is, cantilever loading).

8.2.1.3 Rotating beam specimens may have unique dimensions, depending upon the type of machine used. Use appropriate manufacturers' specifications for these specimens.

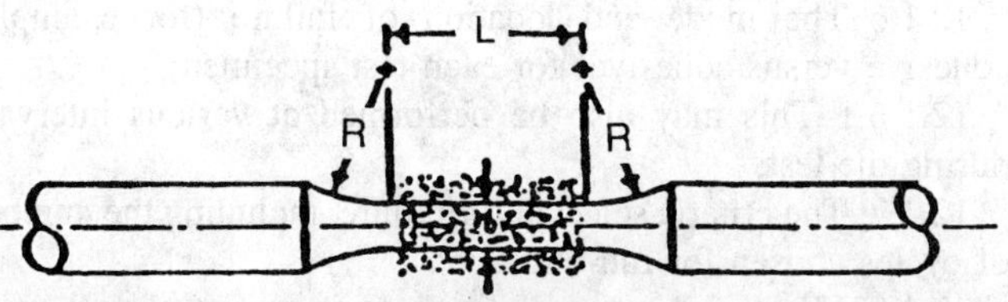

FIG. 5 Bending Fatigue Specimen With Tangentially Blending Fillets Between the Test Section and the Ends for Rotating Beam or Axial Loading

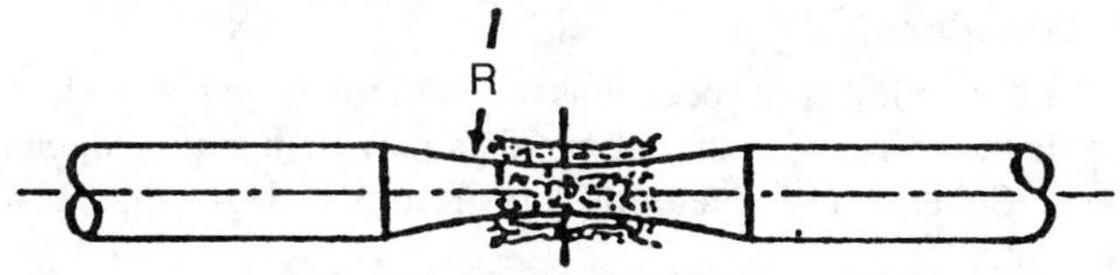

FIG. 6 Specimens With a Continuous Radius Between the Ends for Rotating Beam or Axial Loading

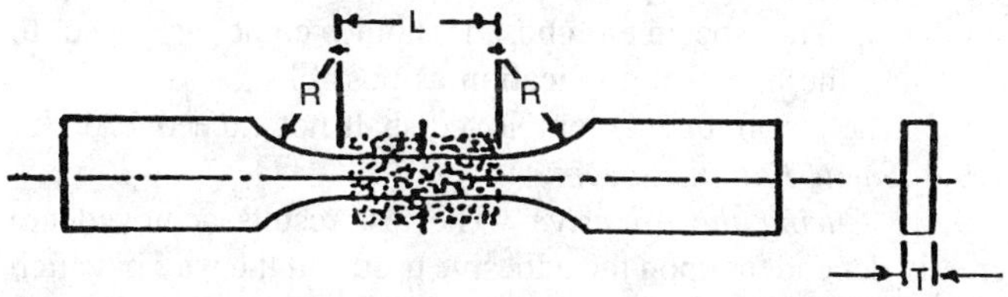

FIG. 7 Specimens With Tangentially Blending Fillets Between the Uniform Test Section and the Ends for Axial Loading

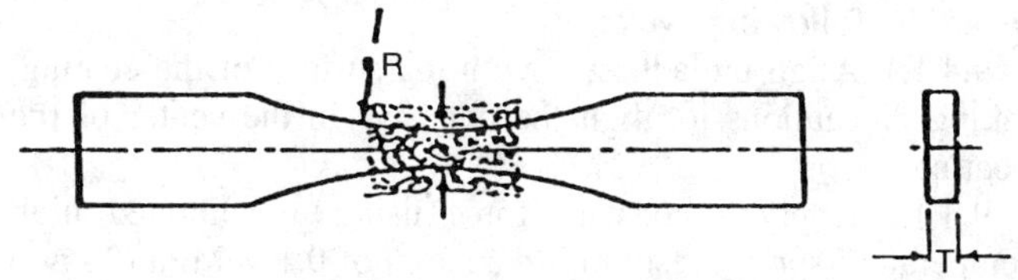

FIG. 8 Specimens With a Continuous Radius Between the Ends for Axial Loading

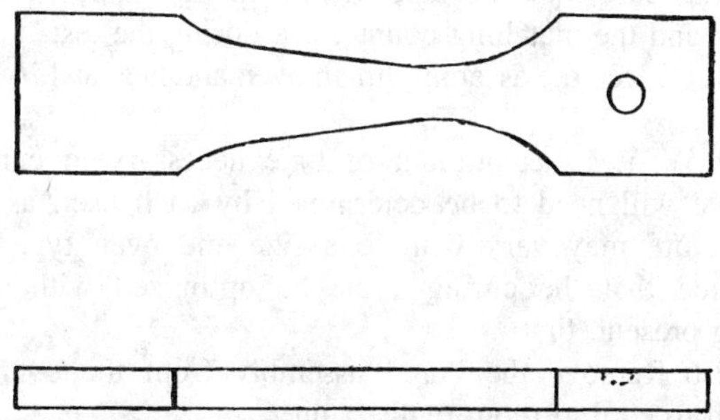

FIG. 9 A Tapered Beam Configuration for Bend Testing

8.3 *Specimen Coating Preparation*:

8.3.1 Calcium phosphate coatings may be applied by any one of a number of techniques. Apply the coating in the same manner as the actual device. The coating should consist of a layer that is mechanically or chemically attached and covers the surface.

8.3.2 Apply coatings as follows:

8.3.2.1 For the shear fatigue specimens apply the coating to the 19.05 mm (0.75 in.) diameter face only (see Fig. 4).

8.3.2.2 For the bending fatigue specimens, apply the coating to the reduced section only, with the exception of the constant stress specimen that should have coating in the entire region of constant stress (see Figs. 5-8, and Fig. 9).

8.3.3 Perform all thermal treatments normally performed on the devices on the test specimens.

8.3.4 If employed, passivation and sterilization techniques should be consistent with those used for actual devices.

8.3.5 *Inspection*—Before testing, perform visual inspections on 100 % of the test specimens. Lack of coating in highly stressed regions, as well as non-uniform coating density, shall be cause for specimen rejection.

9. Procedure

9.1 The number of specimens required for testing, as well as the methods in which the fatigue data may be interpreted, can vary. Several test methods are referenced in this test method.[5,6,7]

9.2 The type of specimen used will depend upon the objective of the test program, the type of equipment available, the equipment capacity, and the form in which the material is available. The specimen chosen should come as close to matching the intended application as possible.

9.3 The test frequency employed shall not exceed 170 Hz.

9.4 *Shear Fatigue Specimens*:

9.4.1 *Curing the Adhesive*—The test results achieved are greatly dependent upon the adhesive used and the way in which it is cured. One suggested adhesive commonly used with calcium phosphate coatings is FM-1000[4] having a thickness of 0.25 mm (0.01 in.). This material has successfully been cured using the following cycle:

9.4.1.1 Align the adhesive with the surface of the coating, taking precautions to align the adhesive in the center of the coating.

9.4.1.2 Apply a constant force using a calibrated high temperature spring, resulting in a stress of 0.138 MPa (20 psi) between the coating and the opposing device that will test the coating.

9.4.1.3 Care must be taken to maintain alignment of the coating and the matching counterface during the test.

9.4.1.4 Place the assembly in an oven and heat at 176°C for 2 to 3 h.

9.4.1.5 The exact amount of time necessary to cure the adhesive will need to be determined by each user, as oven temperature may vary with load size and oven type. It is suggested that the curing cycle be optimized without the coating present, first.

9.4.1.6 Remove the cured assembly from the oven and allow it to cool to room temperature.

9.4.1.7 Remove all excess glue that has protruded from the coated surface. This process must not compromise the integrity of the sample.

9.4.2 Place the specimen assembly in the grips so that the long axis of the specimen is perpendicular to the direction of the applied shear load through the centerline of the grip assembly (see Fig. 3).

9.5 *Bending Fatigue Specimens*:

9.5.1 Perform appropriate testing of the uncoated substrate material, upon which the coating will be applied, to establish a baseline from which to assess the effect of the coating.

9.5.1.1 The baseline test specimens may or may not be grit blasted depending upon the objective of the test. In either event, report the surface roughness.

9.5.2 When mounting the specimen, alignment is crucial. Factors such as poorly machined specimens and misalignment of machine parts might result in excessive vibration leading to erroneous results.

9.5.3 For the rotating beam test, do not apply the load until the machine is operating at the frequency desired for testing.

9.5.4 For the purpose of calculating the applied loads on the test specimen, to determine the applied stresses, measure the dimensions from which the substrate area is calculated to the nearest 0.03 mm (0.001 in.) for dimensions equal to or greater than 5.08 mm (0.200 in.) and to the nearest 0.013 mm (0.0005 in.) for dimensions less than 5.08 mm (0.002 in.).

9.5.4.1 For the coated specimens, use the uncoated substrate dimensions to calculate the applied stress.

10. Test Termination

10.1 Continue the testing until the specimen fails or until a predetermined number of cycles has been reached (typically 10^7 cycles). Failure may be defined as: complete separation of the coating; visible cracking at a specified magnification; a crack of certain dimensions; or by some other criterion.

11. Calculation

11.1 *Shear Fatigue Specimens*—Calculate the substrate area upon which the coating is applied to the nearest 0.06 cm^2 (0.01 $in.^2$). Record peak (failure) load and calculate failing stress in MPa (psi) of adhesive area as follows:

$$\textit{adhesion or cohesion strength} = \textit{maximum load/cross-section area} \tag{1}$$

11.2 *Bending Fatigue Specimens*—For the purpose of calculating the applied loads on the test specimen to determine the applied stresses, measure the dimensions from which the substrate adhesive area is calculated to the nearest 0.03 mm (0.001 in.) for dimensions equal to or greater than 5.08 mm (0.200 in.) and to the nearest 0.013 mm (0.0005 in.) for dimensions less than 5.08 mm (0.002 in.).

12. Report

12.1 The test report procedure and results shall be in accordance with Practice E 468, and include the following information:

12.1.1 Identification of the materials used in the specimen, including bonding agent used;

12.1.2 Identification of methods used to apply the coating including the coating method, heat-treatment, or other data, if available, including date, cycle number, and time and temperature of run;

12.1.3 Dimensional data including the bond cross-sectional area and the thickness of the coating;

12.1.4 Number of specimens tested;

12.1.5 All values for the applied stress and cycles to failure (or run-out);

12.1.6 The mode and location of failure (for example, cohesive versus adhesive) for each test specimen;

12.1.6.1 This may also be performed at various intervals during the test;

12.1.7 The criteria selected for failure, including the number of cycles chosen for run-out;

12.1.8 For the bending fatigue tests report the R ratio (minimum stress/maximum stress);

12.1.9 The test frequency;

---

[5] Collins, J. A., *Failure of Materials in Mechanical Design*, John Wiley & Sons, New York, 1981.

[6] *Handbook of Fatigue Testing, ASTM STP 566*, ASTM, 1974.

[7] Frost, N. C., Marsh, K. J., and Pook, C. P., *Metal Fatigue*, Oxford University Press, London, 1974.

12.1.10 The specimen size for the shear fatigue test if different than the standard size; and

12.1.11 The substrate surface roughness for the baseline bending fatigue test.

13. Precision and Bias

13.1 *Precision*—The precision of this test method is being established.[8]

[8] Test results that might allow statistical evaluation for this statement are herewith solicited.

13.2 *Bias*—The bias of this test method includes the quantitative estimates of the uncertainties of the dimensional measuring devices, the calibration of test equipment, and the skill of the operators. At this time, statements on bias should be limited to the documented performance of particular laboratories.

14. Keywords

14.1 ceramic materials; hydroxylapatite; fatigue testing; tribasic calcium phosphate

APPENDIX

(Nonmandatory Information)

X1. RATIONALE

X1.1 This test method is needed to aid in the development of a high quality material for use in load-bearing implant applications. The influence of calcium phosphate coatings on the resulting fatigue behavior of the system must be viewed as a combination of the surface roughening treatments required to apply the coating, the thermal effects of the coating process, and any other secondary treatments employed. The purpose of this test method is to provide the following information: the influence of the above processing steps and the integrity of the coating and the coating/substrate interface. Round robin testing of this test method is not available at this time.

Last ASTM Designation: F 1660 – 95 (Reapproved 1999)

Test Method for
Elastic Static Bending of Metallic Bone Staples

This test method covers a procedure for determining the rigidity of bone staples.

Formerly under the jurisdiction of Committee F04 on Medical and Surgical Materials and Devices, this test method was withdrawn in November 2000 and replaced by Specification F 564–00 for Metallic Bone Staples.[1]

[1] Annual Book of ASTM Standards, Volume 13.01.

Standard Specification for Adult Tracheostomy Tubes[1]

This standard is issued under the fixed designation F 1666; the number immediately following the designation indicates the year of original adoption or, in the case of revision, the year of last revision. A number in parentheses indicates the year of last reapproval. A superscript epsilon (ε) indicates an editorial change since the last revision or reapproval.

ϵ^1 NOTE—Editorial change was made to the title in October 1999.

1. Scope

1.1 This specification describes basic requirements for tracheostomy tubes made of plastic materials or rubber, or both; having inside diameters greater than 5.0 mm. Such tubes are primarily designed for adult patients who may require anesthesia, artificial ventilation, or other respiratory support, but need not be restricted to these uses. Specialized tubes are excluded from the scope of this specification.

2. Referenced Documents

2.1 The following standards contain provisions which, through reference in this text, constitute provisions of this standard. All standards are subject to revision, and parties to agreements based on this specification are encouraged to investigate the possibility of applying the most recent editions of the standards indicated below.

2.2 *ASTM Standards:*

F 640 Test Methods for Radiopacity of Plastics for Medical Use[2]

F 813 Practice for Direct Contact Cell Culture Evaluation of Materials for Medical Devices[2]

F 1054 Specification for Conical Fittings of 15 mm and 22 mm sizes[2]

F 1242 Specification for Cuffed and Uncuffed Tracheal Tubes[2]

2.3 *ISO Standards:*

ISO 4135 Anesthesiology—Vocabulary[3]

ISO 5366-1 Tracheostomy Tubes—Part 1: Connectors[3]

ISO 7000 Graphical Symbols for Use on Equipment—Index and Synopsis[3]

2.4 *ANSI Standard:*

ANSI/HIMA MD70.1 Medical Material—Leur Fittings—Performance[3]

3. Terminology

3.1 *Definitions:*

3.1.1 *angle of bevel*—acute angle between the plane of the bevel and the longitudinal axis of the tracheostomy tube at the patient end. (See Angle B in Fig. 1.)

3.1.2 *bevel*—slanted portion at the patient end of the tracheostomy tube.

3.1.3 *center-line length*—distance from the patient side of the neck-plate to the patient end of the outer tube along the center line.

3.1.4 *cuff*—inflatable balloon fitted near the patient end of the tracheostomy tube to provide a leak-resistant seal between the tube and the trachea.

3.1.5 *inflating tube*—tube through which the cuff is inflated.

3.1.6 *inner tube*—tube that fits closely to the inside contours of the outer tube (tracheostomy tube).

3.1.7 *introducer (obturator)*—specifically adapted stylet to facilitate the introduction of the outer tube into the trachea.

3.1.8 *machine end*—that end of the tracheostomy tube which is intended to project from the patient.

3.1.9 *neck-plate (shield)*—that part of the tracheostomy tube which approximates to the contour of the patient's neck and is used to secure the tube in position.

3.1.10 *outer tube*—that part of the tracheostomy tube which is normally in contact with the tissues.

3.1.11 *patient end*—that end of the tracheostomy tube which is intended to be inserted into the trachea.

3.1.12 *pilot balloon*—balloon fitted to the inflating tube to indicate inflation status of the cuff.

3.1.13 *tracheostomy (tracheotomy) tube*—tube designed for insertion into the trachea through a tracheostomy.

4. Materials and Manufacture

4.1 Tracheostomy tubes, including cuffs, in their ready-for-use state shall be compatible with the human tissues with which they are intended to be used. Compatibility shall be indicated by the implantation test given in Annex A1, a cell tissue culture test (see Practice F 813) or other tests that give an equivalent indication of freedom from biological hazard.

NOTE 1—See Annex A3 for guidance on materials and design.

5. Size and Dimensions

5.1 *Designation of Tube Size*:

5.1.1 The size designation of a single tracheostomy tube (no

---

[1] This specification is under the jurisdiction of ASTM Committee F-29 on Anesthetic and Respiratory Equipment and is under the direct responsibility of Subcommittee F29.12 on Airways.

Current edition approved Nov. 10, 1995. Published May 1996.

[2] *Annual Book of ASTM Standards*, Vol 13.01.

[3] Available from American National Standards Institute, 11 W. 42nd St., 13th Floor, New York, NY 10036.

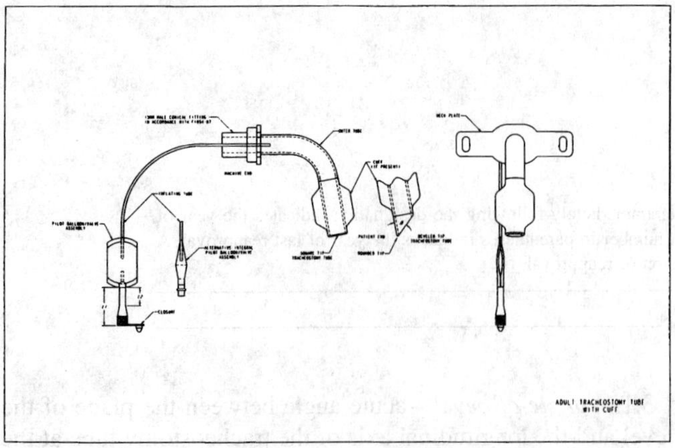

FIG. 1 Typical Tracheostomy Tube

inner cannula) shall be the nominal inside diameter (ID) of the tube expressed in millimetres, as measured at the minimum diameter, in accordance with Table 1, excluding any encroachment allowed by 6.5.1.

5.1.2 The size designation of a tracheostomy tube with inner cannula shall be indicated by both the nominal inner diameter (ID) of the outer tube and the inner diameter (ID) of the inner tube expressed in millimetres. The two numbers shall be juxtaposed by a slash or by a hyphen (*example:* 8/7 or 8–7).

5.2 *Outside Diameter*:

5.2.1 The outside diameter (OD) of sections A and B (see Fig. 2) of the outer tube, other than at the cuff, if provided, shall be expressed in millimetres, subject to a tolerance of ± 0.20 mm. Section "C" of the outer tube shall have a tolerance of ± 0.50 mm.

NOTE 2—The marked outside diameter relates to that portion of the tube intended to be within the wall and lumen of the trachea.

5.3 *Length*:

5.3.1 The center-line length (dimensions A + B + C in Fig. 2) shall extend from the patient side of the neck-plate (datum plane) to the patient end of the outer tube including to the tip of the bevel, if present (see Fig. 1), and shall be expressed in millimetres.

5.3.2 The actual center-line length shall not vary by more than 2.0 mm from the marked length.

5.3.3 Dimensions A, B and C shall be expressed in millimetres.

TABLE 1 Size Range of Single Tracheostomy Tubes

NOTE 1—Dimensions and tolerances are in millimetres.

Designed Size (Nominal Inside Diameter, (ID))	Inside Diameter and Tolerance
5.0	5.0 ± 0.20
5.5	5.5 ± 0.20
6.0	6.0 ± 0.20
6.5	6.5 ± 0.20
7.0	7.0 ± 0.20
7.5	7.5 ± 0.20
8.0	8.0 ± 0.20
8.5	8.5 ± 0.20
9.0	9.0 ± 0.20
9.5	9.5 ± 0.20
10.0	10.0 ± 0.20
11.0	11.0 ± 0.20

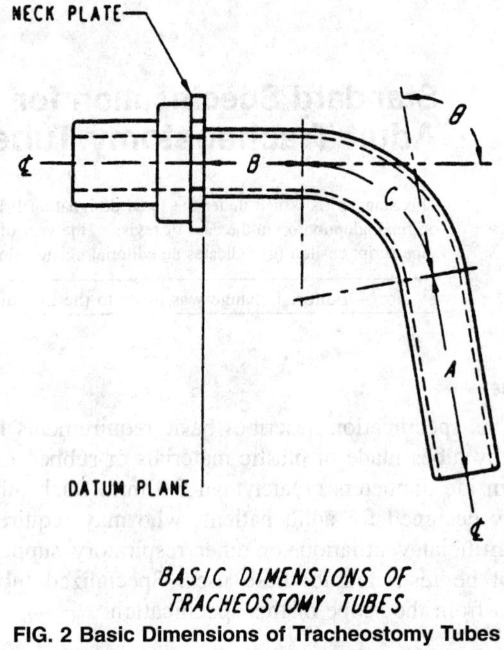

FIG. 2 Basic Dimensions of Tracheostomy Tubes

NOTE 3—Dimensions A or B, or both, may be, or approach, zero.

5.3.4 For tubes with an adjustable neck-plate, the range of center-line lengths shall be expressed in millimetres.

5.4 *Angle θ*—The angle θ (see Fig. 2) shall be expressed in degrees.

NOTE 4—Angle θ is the obtuse angle formed between the tangents to the longitudinal axes of the tube at the machine and the patient ends. As Dimensions A or B, or both, approach or equal zero, the angle θ shall be the obtuse angle formed between the tangents (planes perpendicular) to the longitudinal axes.

6. Design

6.1 *Machine End*— The machine end of tracheostomy tubes shall comply with the requirements specified in Specification F 1054.

6.2 *Neck-Plate*:

6.2.1 A tracheostomy tube shall have a neck-plate (see Fig. 1 and Fig. 2).

6.2.2 The neck-plate shall be provided with holes or other means to permit attachment to the patient.

6.2.3 If a tracheostomy tube has an adjustable neck-plate, it shall be securable to the tube, but not removable.

6.3 *Inner Tube*—The inner tube shall extend to within 1.0 mm of the patient end and not more than 3.0 mm beyond the patient end of the tracheostomy tube with which it is provided.

6.4 *Cuff*:

6.4.1 The cuff, if provided, shall be permanently attached to the tube.

6.4.2 Cuffs of tracheostomy tubes shall comply with the requirements specified in Specification F 1242.

6.5 *Inflating Tubes for Cuffs*:

6.5.1 *Inflating Tube*— The inflating tube, if fitted, shall have an outside diameter of not more than 2.5 mm. The secondary (inflation) lumen shall not encroach on the lumen of the tracheostomy tube by more than 10 % of the inside diameter of the tracheostomy tube.

NOTE 5—The wall around the secondary (inflation) lumen should not project substantially on the outside surface.

6.5.2 *Pilot Balloon*:

6.5.2.1 The inflating tube shall have a pilot balloon or other means to indicate inflation of the cuff, or both.

NOTE 6—This (these) device(s) may also serve as a pressure indicating or limiting device.

6.5.2.2 Neither the inflating tube nor any device shall act as a non-return valve to prevent the intentional evacuation of the cuff.

6.5.3 *Free End of Inflating Tubes for Cuffs*:

6.5.3.1 The end of the inflating tube may be open or sealed with a closure device or inflation valve, but in all instances it shall be capable of accepting a male conical fitting with a 6 % taper (Leur), complying with the requirements specified in ANSI/HIMA MD70.1. The length (see Fig. 1, Dimension 1_1) of the free end of the inflating tube shall be not less than 40 mm unless an inflation valve or closure device is provided.

If an inflation valve or closure device is provided, the length (see Fig. 1, Dimension 1_2) between the pilot balloon (or other device) and the 6 % conical fitting shall be not less than 10 mm unless the pilot balloon and valve or closure device are integral.

6.6 *Patient End*:

6.6.1 The patient end may be square, beveled, or of other configuration.

6.6.2 If a bevel is present, the angle of bevel β shall be not less than 45° (see Fig. 1).

6.7 *Introducer (Obturator)*:

6.7.1 Provision of an introducer is optional.

6.7.2 The introducer shall be smooth and facilitate rapid intubation.

6.7.3 The introducer shall be easy to insert and remove.

6.7.4 When correctly seated, the introducer should not fall out of the tracheostomy tube under its own weight when the tube is held by the neck-plate with the patient end uppermost.

7. Packaging and Package Marking

7.1 The following information shall be apparent on visual examination of the intact unit container:

7.1.1 The size and shape of the tube;

7.1.2 Whether a cuff is provided; and

7.1.3 Whether an introducer/obturator is provided.

NOTE 7—For example, the unit container may be transparent and the tube visible, or a drawing to scale, preferably full scale, may be used. If a drawing is provided, product dimensions may be included.

7.2 Each tracheostomy tube supplied and marked as "sterile" shall be contained in an individual pack. The pack shall serve as a microbiological barrier. The pack shall permit the aseptic extraction of the contents and shall not be capable of re-closure without clearly revealing that it has been opened.

7.3 *Marking of Tracheostomy Tubes*:

7.3.1 The neck-plate or tracheostomy tube, or both, shall be marked with the following:

7.3.1.1 The designated size expressed in millimetres in accordance with 5.1;

7.3.1.2 The outside diameter of the outer tube expressed in millimetres in accordance with 5.2; and

7.3.1.3 The name or trademark of the manufacturer, or both.

NOTE 8—The center line length (or maximum length for tubes having an adjustable neck plate) expressed in millimetres (see 5.3) may also be marked.

7.4 *Labelling of Unit Packs*:

7.4.1 Individual packs or a package insert shall be clearly labeled to indicate the following information:

7.4.1.1 A description of contents;

7.4.1.2 Designated size in mm in accordance with 5.1;

7.4.1.3 The nominal outside diameter of the outer tube expressed in mm (see 5.2);

7.4.1.4 The nominal centerline length expressed in mm (see 5.3);

7.4.1.5 The name or trademark, or both, of the manufacturer or supplier, or both;

7.4.1.6 The batch number;

7.4.1.7 The expiry date;

7.4.1.8 If relevant, instructions for cleaning and disinfection or sterilization;

7.4.1.9 The word "STERILE" or "NON-STERILE" as appropriate;

7.4.1.10 For tubes not intended for re-use, the words" For Single Patient Use Only" or equivalent.

NOTE 9—Symbol No. 1051 ("Do not re-use") given in ISO 7000 should also be used (see Fig. 3).

NOTE 10— For cuffed tubes, the resting diameter of the cuff, determined in accordance with Annex A2 and expressed in millimetres may be marked, or may be readily available from the manufacturer.

7.5 *Labeling of Inner Tube Unit Packs*:

7.5.1 Individual packs shall be clearly labelled to indicate the following:

7.5.1.1 The size designation of the tracheostomy tube (outer tube) into which it is designed to fit;

7.5.1.2 The inside diameter (ID) of the inner tube;

7.5.1.3 A description of the contents;

7.5.1.4 The name or trademark, or both, of the manufacturer or supplier, or both;

7.5.1.5 The batch number;

7.5.1.6 The expiry date;

7.5.1.7 The word "STERILE" or "NON-STERILE", as appropriate; and

7.5.1.8 For tubes not intended for re-use, the words" For Single Patient Use" or equivalent:

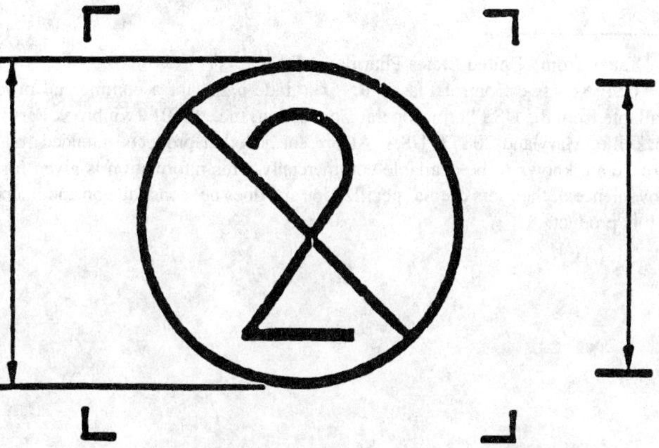

FIG. 3 ISO Symbol 7000/1051 "Do Not Re-Use"

NOTE 11—Symbol No. 1051 ("Do not re-use") given in ISO 7000 should also be used (see Fig. 3).

8. Keywords

8.1 anesthetic equipment; artificial breathing apparatus; dimensions; labelling; manufacturing requirements; marking; medical equipment; packaging; pipes (tubes); specifications; tests; tracheostomy tubes

ANNEXES

(Mandatory Information)

A1. IMPLANTATION TEST[4]

A1.1 General

A1.1.1 The implantation test is designed for the evaluation of a plastics material in direct contact with living tissue. Care shall be taken in the preparation of the implant strips and their proper implantation under aseptic conditions.

A1.2 Preparation of Test Samples

A1.2.1 Prepare for implantation eight strips of the sample and four strips of USP Negative Control Plastics RS[5]. Each strip shall measure not less than 10 by 1 mm. The edges of the strips should be as smooth as possible to avoid additional mechanical trauma upon implantation. Strips of the specified minimum size shall be implanted by means of a hypodermic needle such as a 15 gage needle with intravenous point and of 19 mm (0.75 in.) cannula length, and a sterile trocar. Use either presterilized needles into which the sterile plastics strips are aseptically inserted, or insert each strip into a needle, the cannula and hub of which are protected with an appropriate cover, and then subjected to the appropriate sterilization procedure.

NOTE A1.1—Allowance should be made for proper de-gassing if agents such as ethylene oxide are used.

A1.3 Test Animal

A1.3.1 Select healthy, adult rabbits weighing not less than 2.5 kg, and whose paravertebral muscles are sufficiently large in size to allow for implantation of the test strips. Do not use any muscular tissue other than the paravertebral site. The animals may be anaesthetized with a commonly used anaesthetic agent to a degree deep enough to prevent muscular movements, such as twitching.

A1.4 Procedure

A1.4.1 Perform the test in a clean area. On the day of the test or up to 20 h before testing, clip the fur of the animals on both sides of the spinal column. Remove loose hair by means of vacuum.

A1.4.1.1 Implant four strips of the sample into the paravertebral muscle on one side of the spine of each of two rabbits, 2.5 to 5 cm from the mid-line and parallel to the spinal column, and about 2.5 cm apart from each other. In a similar fashion, implant two strips of USP Negative Control Plastic RS in the opposite muscle of each animal. Insert a sterile stylet into the needle to hold the plastic strips in the tissue while withdrawing the needle. If excessive bleeding is observed after implantation of a strip, place a duplicate strip at another site. Close the incision after implantation is complete.

A1.4.1.2 Keep the animals for a period of not less than 72 h and sacrifice them at the end of the observation period by administering an overdose of an anaesthetic agent. Allow sufficient time to elapse for the tissue to be cut without bleeding. Examine macroscopically the area of the tissue surrounding the centre portion of each implant strip. Use a magnifying lens if necessary. The tissue immediately surrounding the USP Negative Control Plastic RS strips should appear normal and entirely free from hemorrhage, film, or encapsulation. The requirements of the test are met if, in each rabbit, the reaction to not more than one of the four sample strips is significantly greater than that to the strips of USP Negative Control Plastics RS.

NOTE A1.2—Another biocompatibility test recommended by the FDA is the *Tripartite Biocompatibility Guidance for Medical Devices*.[6]

[4] Taken from "United States Pharmacopeia."

[5] USP Negative Control Plastic RS is a trade name for a commercial product available from the US Pharmacopeial Convention, Inc., 12601 Twinbrook Parkway, Rockville, Maryland 20852, USA. At present no other products intended for this purpose are known to be available commercially. This information is given for the convenience of the users of this specification and does not constitute an endorsement of this product.

[6] Copies may be obtained from Food and Drug Administration, Center for Devices and Radiological Health, Office of Small Manufacturers Assistance (HF2 220), 1350 Piccard Drive, Rockville, MD 20850.

A2. METHOD FOR DETERMINING THE RESTING DIAMETER OF THE CUFF

A2.1 Principle

A2.1.1 The resting diameter of the cuff is measured when the cuff is inflated with a pressure that is intended to remove creases but minimize stretching of its walls.

A2.2 Apparatus

A2.2.1 Means to inflate the cuff with sufficient air to create an intracuff pressure of 2.0 kPa (20 cm H_2O) ± 5 %.

A2.3 Procedure

A2.3.1 Inflate the cuff with sufficient air to create an intracuff pressure of 2.0 kPa (20 cm H_2O) ± 5 % and leave to stabilize for 5 min at (23 ± 2)°C, maintaining that pressure.

A2.3.2 Measure the maximum cuff diameter in a plane perpendicular to the axis of the tube at intervals of 45°.

A2.4 Expression of Results

A2.4.1 Calculate the arithmetic mean of the measurements obtained in A2.3.2A2.3.2 and express the result in millimetres.

A3. GUIDANCE ON MATERIALS, DESIGN, AND FINISH

A3.1 Materials

A3.1.1 The material used for the manufacture of the tubes should have sufficient rigidity to allow the construction of a tube with the thinnest possible wall that, at the same time, maintains resistance to kinking. Tubes claimed by the manufacturer to be flexible and soft should conform to the patient's anatomy without exerting undue pressure on the body tissues.

A3.1.2 Unless intended and marked for single use, tracheostomy tubes should be reasonably resistant to deterioration by methods of cleaning, disinfection and sterilization as recommended by the manufacturer or the supplier.

A3.1.2.1 The recommended method(s) of sterilization should not produce changes in the tube material which will render the tracheotomy tube incompatible with human tissues with which it is intended to be used (see Annex A1).

A3.1.3 Tracheostomy tubes under normal conditions of use should be reasonably resistant to deterioration by anaesthetic vapors and gases.

A3.1.4 Tracheostomy tubes should be readily detectable by x-ray either by the nature of the material of which they are made or by the provision of a radiopaque marker at the patient end. The radiopaque marker shall have an optical density less than or equal to that of the aluminum comparison standard. The radiopaque marking shall be tested in accordance with Method B of Test Method F 640.

A3.1.5 Prior to use and in the case of tubes intended for re-use, between uses, the tube should maintain its intended shape when stored in accordance with the manufacturer's instructions.

A3.2 Design

A3.2.1 If provided, the introducer should be easily removable after introduction of the tracheostomy tube into the patient.

A3.2.2 The neck-plate or other means of attachment to the patient should be rounded at the edges and its shape should adapt to the contour of the patient.

A3.3 Finish

A3.3.1 Tracheostomy tubes, including the neck-plate or other means of attachment to the patient, should have smooth external and internal surfaces.

A3.3.2 The cuff should have a smooth surface.

Standard Specification for Resurfacing Patellar Prosthesis[1]

This standard is issued under the fixed designation F 1672; the number immediately following the designation indicates the year of original adoption or, in the case of revision, the year of last revision. A number in parentheses indicates the year of last reapproval. A superscript epsilon (ϵ) indicates an editorial change since the last revision or reapproval.

1. Scope

1.1 This specification covers patellar resurfacing devices used to provide a functioning articulation between the bones of the patella and the femur.

1.2 This specification is intended to provide basic descriptions of material and device geometry. Additionally, those characteristics determined to be important to in-vivo performance of the device are defined.

1.3 This specification does not cover the details for quality assurance, design control, and production control contained in 21 CFR 820 and ISO 9001.

NOTE 1—Devices for custom applications are not covered by this specification.

2. Referenced Documents

2.1 *ASTM Standards:*

F 75 Specification for Cast Cobalt-Chromium-Molybdenum Alloy for Surgical Implant Applications[2]

F 86 Practice for Surface Preparation and Marking of Metallic Surgical Implants[2]

F 90 Specification for Wrought Cobalt-Chromium-Nickel-Tungsten Alloy for Surgical Implant Applications[2]

F 136 Specification for Wrought Titanium 6Al-4V ELI Alloy for Surgical Implant Applications[2]

F 138 Specification for Stainless Steel Bar and Wire for Surgical Implants (Special Quality)[2]

F 451 Specification for Acrylic Bone Cement[2]

F 562 Specification for Wrought Cobalt-35 Nickel 20-Chromium 10-Molybdenum Alloy for Surgical Implant Applications[2]

F 563 Specification for Wrought Cobalt-Nickel-Chromium-Molybdenum-Tungsten-Iron Alloy for Surgical Implant Applications[2]

F 603 Specification for High-Purity Dense Aluminum Oxide for Surgical Implant Applications[2]

F 648 Specification for Ultra-High-Molecular-Weight Polyethylene Powder and Fabricated Form for Surgical Implants[3]

F 732 Practice for Reciprocating Pin-on-Flat Evaluation of Friction and Wear Properties of Polymeric Materials for Use in Total Joint Prostheses[2]

F 745 Specification for 18 Chromium-12.5 Nickel-2.5 Molybdenum Stainless Steel for Cast and Solution— Annealed Surgical Implant Applications[2]

F 746 Test Method for Pitting or Crevice Corrosion of Metallic Surgical Implant Materials[2]

F 748 Practice for Selecting Generic Biological Test Methods for Materials and Devices[2]

F 799 Specification for Cobalt-28 Chromium-6 Molybdenum Alloy Forgings for Surgical Implants[2]

F 981 Practice for Assessment of Compatibility of Biomaterials for Surgical Implants with Respect to Effect of Materials on Muscle and Bone[2]

F 983 Practice for Permanent Marking of Orthopaedic Implant Components[2]

F 1044 Test Method for Shear Testing of Porous Metal Coatings[2]

F 1108 Specification for Ti6Al4V Alloy Castings for Surgical Implants[2]

F 1147 Test Method for Tension Testing of Porous Metal Coatings[2]

2.2 *Government Document:*

21 CFR 820-Good Manufacturing Practice for Medical Devices[4]

2.3 *ISO Standard:*

ISO 9001-Quality Systems-Model for Quality Assurance in Design/Development, Production, Installation, and Servicing[5]

3. Terminology

3.1 *Definitions*—Dimensions defined as follows are measured in whole or in part in the sagittal, transverse, and coronal (or frontal) planes as appropriate. See Fig. 1 and Fig. 2.

3.1.1 T_1— total overall prosthetic thickness, for example, from the apex of the dome to the free end of pegs or other fixation geometry.

3.1.2 T_2— thickness of the patellar prosthesis from the plane of the bone-prosthesis interface (excluding pegs, keels, and so forth) to the apex of the articulating surface.

3.1.3 T_3— minimum polymer thickness of the patellar

[1] This specification is under the jurisdiction of ASTM Committee F04 on Medical and Surgical Materials and Devices and is under the direct responsibility of Subcommittee F04.22 on Arthroplasty.

Current edition approved Nov. 10, 1995. Published May 1996.

[2] *Annual Book of ASTM Standards*, Vol 13.01.

[3] Discontinued; see *1994 Annual Book of ASTM Standards,* Vol 13.01.

[4] Available from Superintendent of Documents, U.S. Government Printing Office, Washington, DC 20402.

[5] Available from American National Standards Institute, 11 W. 42nd St., 13th Floor, New York, NY 10036.

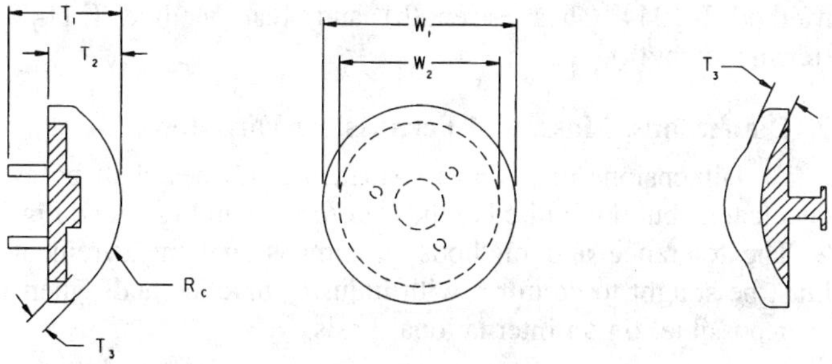

(a) (b) (c)

NOTE 1—Figure 1(*a*) and (*b*) show a dome style and Fig. 1(*c*) shows a sombrero style.

FIG. 1 Two Versions of Axisymmetric Patella Prostheses

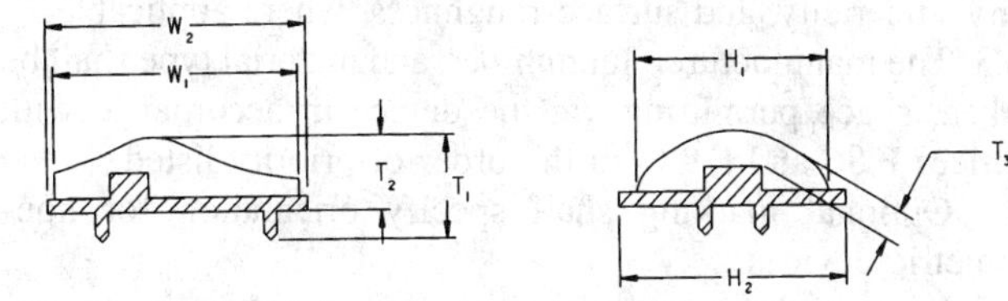

(*a*) Transverse Cross Section With Lateral to the Right

(*b*) Sagittal Cross Section

FIG. 2 Example of a Nonsymmetric Patella Prosthesis

prosthesis in direct contact with the femoral component that is "at risk" for wear; this is measured perpendicular to the tangent of the wear surface at the point of contact with the femoral component.

3.1.4 *Discussion*—The dimension T_3 is described in Fig. 1 and Fig. 2 to be a distance from a surface contact point to an internal peg or an edge of the metal back. The exact location of the minimum thickness at risk may be at a different site and will depend on the design of the patella prosthesis and the mating femoral component. For devices manufactured from a single material, T_3 should be measured from the wear surface to the back of the fixation surface.

3.1.5 W_1—maximum medial-lateral width of the articulating surface in the frontal plane.

3.1.6 W_2—maximum medial-lateral width of the metal back in the frontal plane.

3.1.7 H_1—articulating surface superior-inferior height in the frontal plane.

3.1.8 H_2—metal back superior-inferior height in the frontal plane.

3.1.9 *Rc*—radius of curvature for single radius axisymmetric domes only.

3.2 *Definitions of Terms Specific to This Standard:*

3.2.1 *dome*—a style of axisymmetric prosthesis that has a single uniform radius of curvature (that is, button).

3.2.2 *fixation element*—any peg, keel, or other protrusion from the nonarticulating side of the patellar component intended to increase the surface contact or mechanical interlock between the component, the bonding agent (bone cement) or the natural patella, or both.

3.2.3 *marker wire*—a nonstructural, generally thin metallic wire, designed to be apparent on X-rays taken after placement of implants that otherwise would be nonapparent on such X-rays.

3.2.4 *metal back*—a metal structure supporting the articulating surface material. This may be fixed rigidly to the articulating surface or it may be fixed such that it allows the articulating surface to rotate or translate.

3.2.5 *radii of curvature*—the geometry of the articular surface may be described by a list of appropriate radii of curvature.

3.2.6 *sombrero*—a style of axisymmetric prosthesis that has multiple radii of curvature. (See Fig. 1Fig. 1c.)

4. Classification

4.1 Patellar replacement devices may be classified according to geometry:

4.1.1 *Axisymmetric*— The articulating surface is symmetric on an axis perpendicular to the prepared bonding surface (for example, Dome patellas and sombrero-type patellas). See Fig. 1.

4.1.2 *Nonsymmetric*— The articulating surface is not axisymmetric but may be symmetric on a plane. Examples of this type are anatomical or oblong prosthesis. See Fig. 2.

4.2 It is important to define the type of fixation geometry so that the user can understand the degree of bone invasion:

4.2.1 *Peg*—Number, size (for example: length, width, diameter, and so forth), and location and

4.2.2 *Keel*—Width, length, thickness, geometry, and location.

5. Materials and Manufacture

5.1 The choice of materials is understood to be a necessary but not sufficient ensurance of function of the device made from them. All devices conforming to this specification shall be fabricated from materials, with adequate mechanical strength and durability, corrosion resistance and biocompatibility.

5.1.1 *Mechanical Strength*—Components of various prostheses have been successfully fabricated from the following materials. See Specifications F 75, F 90, F 136, F 138, F 562, F 563, F 603, F 648, F 745, F 799, and F 1108. The articulating surface should be fabricated from a material such as UHMWPE in accordance with Specification F 648.

5.1.2 *Corrosion Resistance*—Materials with limited or no history of successful use for orthopedic implant application must be determined to exhibit corrosion resistance equal to or better than one of the materials listed in 5.1.1 when tested in accordance with Test Method F 746.

5.1.3 *Biocompatibility*— Materials with limited or no history of successful use for orthopedic implant application must be determined to exhibit acceptable biological response equal to or better than one of the materials listed in 5.1.1 when tested in accordance with Practices F 748 and F 981.

6. Performance Requirements

6.1 The implant shall be capable of withstanding sustained static and dynamic physiologic loads without compromise of its function for the intended use and environment. At this time there are no device-specific test methods and there are no acceptable performance levels. Device testing shall be done in keeping with the implant's intended function.

6.2 There are relevant failure modes listed as follows which, at minimum, shall be considered in the evaluation of safety and efficacy of a patella prosthesis. Literature references **(1–8)** have been included in the rationale statement in support of these failure modes.

6.2.1 *Dislocation or Lateral Subluxation*—The subluxation over the lateral portion of the femoral articular surface. This has occurred in the past and is design and patient specific.

6.2.2 *Component Disassociation*—Devices made from multiple layers or components have disassociated under clinical use (for example, articulating surface from the metal back, porous coating from the metal back, and so forth). This disassociation may be evaluated through shear loading or compression loading, or a combination of the two.

6.2.3 *Fixation Failure*— Devices have loosened at the interface with bone. Attachment mechanisms such as pegs have sheared or failed. Components have become loose within the bone cement.

6.2.4 *Device Fracture*— Partial or complete fracture of either the articular surface or the metal back.

6.2.5 *Articular Surface Wear*—Patella prostheses have failed due to excessive wear of the articulating surface resulting in polymer debris and in some cases "wear through" of the articular surface with subsequent metal-on-metal wear debris. Thin UHMWPE may accelerate this wear but it is design dependent.

6.3 The failure modes may be addressed through relevant testing (for example, shear testing of device component interfaces) and analysis (for example, internal stress analysis due to loading). The testing may encompass some combination of static and dynamic loading environments.

6.4 Polymeric components as manufactured shall be made from materials demonstrating wear rates substantially equivalent to or less than UHMWPE as determined by Practice F 732.

NOTE 2—In situations where the pin-on-flat test may not be considered appropriate, other test methods may be considered.

6.5 Porous metal coatings shall be tested according to Test Method F 1044 (shear strength) and Test Method F 1147 (tensile strength).

7. Dimensions, Mass, and Permissible Variations

7.1 Dimensions of patellar resurfacing devices shall be as designated, but not limited to those described, in Fig. 1 and Fig. 2. The tolerance and methods of dimensional measurement must be sought to conform with industry practice and, whenever possible, on an international basis.

8. Finish and Product Marking

8.1 Items conforming to this specification shall be finished in accordance with Practice F 86, where applicable.

8.2 *Polymeric Bearing Surface Finish*—Shall conform to the manufacturer's documented standards concerning concentricity, sphericity, and surface roughness, where applicable.

8.3 The manufacturer, lot number, and material type shall be marked, space permitting, on the device in accordance with Practices F 86 and F 983 in the order of priority listed.

8.4 Optional marking shall specify orientation for nonsymmetric devices.

8.5 If one of the components is not radiographically opaque, it may be appropriately marked for radiographic evaluation. The marker wire is a noncritical element and may not be necessary. If a marker wire is used it should be placed in a noncritical area to avoid degrading the structural and functional properties of the device.

9. Packaging and Package Marking

9.1 Adequate dimensioning to describe overall size and shape (see Fig. 1 and Fig. 2 for examples) shall be included in the product labeling.

9.2 The material(s) used for the implant shall be specified on the package labels and inserts.

10. Keywords

10.1 arthroplasty; patella; prosthesis

APPENDIX

(Nonmandatory Information)

X1. RATIONALE STATEMENT

X1.1 The objectives of this specification are to establish guidelines for the manufacture and function of components for patellar replacement. Current prostheses include single material designs and multiple material/component designs all preassembled at the manufacturing site. Some multicomponent design allow a certain degree of mobility of the bearing surface over the fixation surface. Patellar replacement parts are intended for use in a patient who is skeletally mature. They will be subjected to considerable dynamic loads in a corrosive environment and virtually continuous motion at the bearing surfaces.

X1.2 This specification is designed to provide a standardization of device terminology, classification, dimensions, and labeling; alert designers to potential failure mechanisms such as disassociation, excessive wear, dislocation, and so forth (Refs **(1-8)**);[6] and provide guidance regarding suitable materials for fabrication based on current technology and clinical use.

X1.3 Laboratory tests to accurately simulate physiological loads, aggressive electrolytes, and complex constituents of body fluids cannot to date entirely simulate long-term in-vivo

[6] The boldface numbers given in parentheses refer to a list of references at the end of the text.

performance. It is recognized that failure of the arthroplasty can occur without failure of the device itself. Long-term projections of satisfactory performance can be suggested but not accurately predicted using available testing procedures. This specification identifies those factors felt to be important to ensure a satisfactory useful prosthetic life.

X1.4 Under applicable documents and materials, the lists reflect the current state of the art. It is recognized that should materials not now included appear and be proved acceptable, they shall be inserted in the process of revision. To date the vast majority of patella prostheses have been implanted using a bone bonding agent such as acrylic bone cement in accordance with Specification F 451. Although the bone bonding agent is not considered part of the patella prosthesis it may play an important role in the performance of the prosthesis and therefore should be considered during testing and evaluation.

X1.5 Marker wires have been used to make components radiographically detectable. They may not be necessary but when they are used, shall be located in a noncritical area to avoid any contribution to device failure. They shall not be located in critical wear areas nor regions that may see high stresses.

X1.6 *Performance Considerations*—Component performance can be predicted only indirectly at this stage, by referring to strength levels and other parameters. Reference to parameters applicable to materials may or may not adequately describe structures made from them. In a period of transition from device specifications standards to device performance standards, both methods of description may be appropriate. At this time there are no device specific standard test methods to evaluate the performance of resurfacing patella prostheses.

X1.7 The thickness of the UHMWPE may help in the distribution of contact stress, increase the resistance to bending under load, and provide sufficient material to resist normal wear, thus contributing to increased longevity of a device. Thin UHMWPE in some prosthetic designs may contribute to accelerated wear.

X1.8 For labeling of the implant, it is desirable to have complete information where space is available to do so, including manufacturer's trademark material, lot number, size, orientation, if any, and catalog number with date, in that order.

REFERENCES

(1) Brick, G. W., and Scott, R. D., "The Patellofemoral Component of Total Knee Arthroplasty," *Clinical Orthop. Rel. Res.*, No. 231, pp. 163–178, June 1988.

(2) Doolittle, K. H., and Turner, R. H., "Patellofemoral Problems Following Total Knee Arthroplasty," *Orthop. Rev., 17(7)*, pp. 696–702, July 1988.

(3) Leblanc, J. M., "Patellar Complications in Total Knee Arthroplasty, A Literature Review," *Orthop. Rev., 18(3)*, pp. 296–304, March 1989.

(4) Hsu, H. P., and Walker, P. S., "Wear and Deformation of Patellar Components in Total Knee Arthroplasty," *Clin. Orthop. Rel. Res.*, No. 246, pp. 260–265, September 1989.

(5) Berry, D. J., and Rand, J. A., "Isolated Patellar Component Revision of Total Knee Arthroplasty," *Clin. Orthop. Rel. Res.*, No. 286, pp. 110–116 January 1993.

(6) Firestone, T. P., Teany, S. M., Krackow, K. A., and Hungerford, D. S., "The Clinical and Roentgenographic Results of Cementless Porous-Coated Patellar Fixation," *Clin. Orthop. Rel. Res.*, No. 273, pp. 184–189, December 1991.

(7) Peters, J. D., Engh, G. A., and Corpe, R. S., "The Metal-Backed Patella. An Invitation For Failure?," *J. Arthroplasty, 6(3)*, pp. 221–228, September 1991.

(8) Andersen, H. N., Ernst, C., and Frandsen, P. A., "Polyethylene Failure of Metal-Backed Patellar Components," *Acta Orthop. Scand., 62(1)*, pp. 1–3, 1991.

Designation: F 1690 – 96

Standard Specification for Humidifiers for Medical Use—Part 1: General Requirements for Active Humidification Systems[1]

This standard is issued under the fixed designation F 1690; the number immediately following the designation indicates the year of original adoption or, in the case of revision, the year of last revision. A number in parentheses indicates the year of last reapproval. A superscript epsilon (ε) indicates an editorial change since the last revision or reapproval.

INTRODUCTION

Humidifiers are used to raise the water content of gases delivered to patients. Gases available for medical use do not contain sufficient moisture and may damage or irritate the respiratory tract of patients. Heat may be employed to increase the water output of the humidifier.

In addition, many humidifiers utilize heated breathing tubes in order to increase operating efficiency and reduce excessive water and heat loss. Ventilator and anesthesia breathing tubes in common use may not withstand the heat generated by humidifiers and heated breathing tube mechanisms.

Many humidifier manufacturers use off-the-shelf electrical connectors for their electrically heated breathing tubes. However, since different manufacturers have used the same electrical connector for different power outputs, electrically heated breathing tubes may be physically, but not electrically, interchangeable. Improper electrically heated breathing tube use has caused overheating, circuit melting, patient and care-giver burns, and fires. It was not found practical to specify the interface requirements for electrical connectors to ensure compatibility between humidifiers and breathing tubes produced by different manufactures.

Since the safe use of a humidifier is dependent on the interaction of the humidifier with its many accessories, this specification sets total system performance requirements, including accessories such as breathing tubes (both heated and non heated), temperature sensor, and devices intended to control the environment within these breathing tubes.

A rationale for the most important requirements is given in Appendix X1. It is considered that a knowledge of the reasons for the requirements will not only facilitate the proper application of this specification, but will expedite any subsequent revision.

This specification along with IEC (International Electrotechnical Committee) 601-1, henceforth known as the "General Standard," specify the minimum safety and performance requirements for humidification systems. This specification indicates which clauses of the General Standard apply and amends certain clauses with additions or modifications.

SECTION ONE—GENERAL

1. Scope

1.1 The requirements given in Clause 1 of the General Standard apply with the following additions and modifications:

1.1.1 Replace 1.1 with the following:

1.1.1.1 This specification includes requirements for the safety and performance of active vaporizing and nebulizing humidification systems, as defined in 3.63.1.6, suitable for inclusion in breathing systems (both intubated and non-intubated patients).

1.1.1.2 This specification also includes requirements for breathing tubes, including heated breathing tubes (heated-wire breathing circuits), and devices intended to control these heated breathing tubes, heated breathing tube controllers.

1.1.1.3 Heat and moisture exchangers (HMEs) are outside the scope of this specification. However, it is recognized that their safety and performance may affect that of humidification systems. Numerous studies have been published citing the benefits and risks of HMEs used in conjunction with humidification systems. It is advisable to review the instructions for use provided with the humidification systems and HMEs and the available literature for more details.

1.1.1.4 Devices commonly referred to as "room humidifiers," humidifiers used in heating, ventilation, and air-conditioning systems and humidifiers used to condition the environment within infant incubators are outside the scope of this specification.

1.1.1.5 It has not been found possible to include guidance

[1] This specification is under the jurisdiction of ASTM Committee F-29 on Anesthetic and Respiratory Equipment and is under the direct responsibility of Subcommittee F29.14 onVentilators.

Current edition approved Feb. 10, 1996. Published May 1996.

on the matter of droplet size in the case of nebulizing humidifiers.

1.1.1.6 Gas-powered nebulizers used for the delivery of drugs to patients through their respiratory system are outside the scope of this specification.

1.1.1.7 Appendices in this specification are not mandatory unless made so by an explicit statement in the main text.

1.2 The values stated in SI units are to be regarded as the standard.

2. Referenced Documents

2.1 The following standards contain provisions that, through reference in this text, constitute provisions of this specification. At the time of publication of this specification, the editions were current. All standards are subject to revision, and parties reading this specification are encouraged to investigate the possibility of applying the most recent editions of the following standards:

2.2 *ASTM Standards:*

F 1054 Specification for Conical Fittings of 15-mm and 22-mm Sizes[2]

F 1205 Specification for Anesthesia Breathing Tubes[2]

F 1463 Specification for Alarm Signals in Medical Equipment Used in Anesthesia and Respiratory Care[2]

2.3 *ANSI Standard:*

ANSI/CGA G7.1 Commodity Specification for Medical Grade Air[3]

2.4 *CGA Standard*

CGA Pamphlet G4.3 Commodity Specification for Medical Grade Oxygen[4]

2.5 *ISO Standards:*

ISO 3744 Acoustics—Determination of Sound Power Levels of Noise Sources—Engineering Methods for Free-Field Conditions Over a Reflecting Plane[3]

ISO 4135: 1979 Anesthesiology—Vocabulary[3]

ISO 8835-2: 1993(E) Inhalation Anesthesia Systems—Part 2: Anesthetic Circle Breathing Systems[3]

ISO 10651 Lung Ventilators for Medical Use—Part 3: Particular Requirements for Emergency and Transport Ventilators[3]

2.6 *IEC Standards*

IEC Publication 601-1—Safety of Medical Electrical Equipment—Part 1: 1988—General Safety Requirements[3]

IEC 601-2-19: 1990—Particular Requirements for the Safety of Baby Incubators[3]

IEC 601-1-2 Medical Electrical Equipment Part 1: General Requirements for Safety—Collateral Standard: Electromagnetic Compatibility[3]

IEC Publication 651: 1979 Sound Level Meters[3]

IEC Publication 801-2 Electromagnetic Compatibility for Industrial Process Measurement and Control Equipment—Part 2: 1990—Electrostatic Discharge Requirements[3]

[2] *Annual Book of ASTM Standards*, Vol 13.01.

[3] Available from American National Standards Institute, 11 W. 42nd St., 13th Floor, New York, NY 10036.

[4] Available from Compressed Gas Associoation, 1235 Jefferson Davis Highway, Arlington, VA 22202.

3. Terminology

3.1 *Definitions*—The definitions given in Clause 2 of the General Standard apply with the following additions:

3.1.1 *accessible surface temperature*—the temperature of any surface that can be touched by a hand or finger during normal use, that includes filling and refilling of the humidifier (see ISO 4135).

3.1.2 *breathing tube*—a tube used to convey gases or vapors, or both, to the patient. The breathing tube can be heated.

3.1.3 *delivered gas temperature*—the temperature of the gas or aerosol, or both, measured at the patient connection port (see ISO 4135).

3.1.4 *heated breathing tube controller*—the device which controls the heating of a breathing tube. It can either stand alone or be part of the humidifier.

3.1.5 *humidification chamber*—that part of the humidifier that vaporizes or nebulizers water or water-based medicament (see ISO 4135).

3.1.6 *humidification system*—the breathing tube, heated breathing tube controller (if applicable), and humidifier that together meet the requirements of this specification and are intended to be used together.

3.1.7 *humidifier*—a device to add water or water-based medicament in the form of droplets or vapor, or both, to the inspired gas (see ISO 4135).

3.1.8 *Discussion*—This term includes both nebulizing and vaporizing humidifiers.

3.1.9 *humidifier outlet*—the outlet port of the humidifier that delivers the humidified gases (see ISO 4135).

3.1.10 *humidifier output*—the total mass of water (in the form of liquid and vapor) per unit volume of gas normalized to body temperature, atmospheric pressure, and saturated (BTPS, that is, at 37°C, 101.3 kPa (760 mm Hg), saturated with water vapor) at the patient connection port.

3.1.11 *liquid container*—the portion of the humidifier that holds the liquid or the humidification chamber (see ISO 4135).

3.1.11.1 *Discussion*—The liquid container may be detachable for filling.

3.1.12 *liquid reservoir*—a portion of the humidifier that replenishes the liquid container (see ISO 4135).

3.1.13 *maximum operating pressure*—the maximum pressure in the humidification chamber.

3.1.14 *measured gas temperature*—the temperature of the gas or aerosol, or both, that the humidification system is measuring and, if applicable, displaying (see ISO 4135).

3.1.15 *nebulizing humidifier*—a type of humidifier that produces vapor and droplet output (see ISO 4135).

3.1.16 *operating volume*—the usable volume of the liquid container when operated between the maximum and minimum levels, if so marked (see ISO 4135).

3.1.17 *patient connection port*—that opening at the patient end of a breathing system intended for connection to a tracheal or tracheostomy tube connector or adapter, a face mask or a face mask angle-piece, or a laryngeal mask (see ISO 4135).

3.1.18 *relative humidity*—the water vapor pressure at a particular temperature expressed as a percentage of the saturation vapor pressure (see ISO 4135).

3.1.19 *set temperature*—the temperature at which the humidifier system attempts to maintain delivered gas temperature (may be operator adjustable).

3.1.20 *thermal hazard*—a hazard resulting from fire, excessive surface temperature of excessive delivered gas temperature (see ISO 4135).

3.1.20.1 *Discussion*—Any toxic materials resulting from abnormal temperatures also constitute a thermal hazard.

3.1.21 *vaporizing humidifier*—a type of humidifier intended to produce output in the vapor phase (see ISO 4135).

4. Relationship of This Specification to the General Standard

4.1 A = applies, NA = not applicable, AM/R = applies with an amendment, addition, or revision to the requirements in the General Standard.

	A	NA	AM/R
Section One—General:			
1. Scope and object,			X
2. Terminology and definitions,			X
3. General requirements,			X
4. General requirements for tests,			X
5. Classification,	X		
6. Identification, marking, and documents, and			X
7. Power input.	X		
Section Two—Environmental Condition:			
8. Basic safety categories,	X		
9. Removable protective means,	X		
10. Environmental conditions,	X		
11. Not used, and	X		
12. Not used.	X		
Section Three—Protection Against Electric Shock Hazards:			
13. General,	X		
14. Requirements related to classification,	X		
15. Limitation of voltage or energy, or both,	X		
16. Enclosures and protective covers,	X		
17. Separation,	X		
18. Protective earthing, functional earthing, and potential equalization,	X		
19. Continuous leakage currents and patient auxiliary currents, and			X
20. Dielectric strength.	X		
Section Four—Protection Against Mechanical Hazards:			
21. Mechanical strength,			X
22. Moving parts,	X		
23. Surfaces, corners, and edges,	X		
24. Stability in normal use,	X		
25. Expelled parts,	X		
26. Vibration and noise,	X		
27. Pneumatic and hydraulic power,	X		
28. Suspended masses,	X		
29. X-radiation,	X		
30. Alpha, beta, gamma, neutron radiation and other particle radiation,	X		
31. Microwave radiation,	X		
32. Light radiation (including lasers),	X		
33. Infrared radiation,	X		
34. Ultraviolet radiation,	X		
35. Acoustical energy (including ultrasonics), and	X		
36. Electromagnetic compatibility.			X
Section Six—Protective Against Hazards of Ignition of Flammable Anesthetic Mixtures:			
37. Locations and basic requirements,			X
38. Marking, accompanying documents,	X		
39. Common requirements for category AP and category APG equipment,	X		
	A	NA	AM/R
40. Requirements and tests for category AP equipment, parts and components thereof,	X		
41. Requirements and tests for category APG equipment, parts and components thereof,	X		
42. Excessive temperatures,			X
43. Fire prevention,			X
44. Overflow, spillage, leakage, humidity, ingress of liquids, cleaning, sterilization and disinfection,	X		
45. Pressure vessels and parts subject to pressure,	X		
46. Human errors,	X		
47. Electrostatic charges,	X		
48. Materials in applied parts in contact with the body of the patient, and	X		
49. Interruption of the power supply.	X		
Section Eight—Accuracy of Operating Data and Protection Against Hazardous Output:			
50. Accuracy of operating data, and			X
51. Protection against incorrect output.			X
Section Nine—Abnormal Operation and Fault Conditions; Environmental Test:			
52. Abnormal operation and fault conditions, and	X		
53. Environmental tests.	X		
Section Ten—Construction Requirements:			
54. General,	X		
55. Enclosures and covers,	X		
56. Components and general assembly,			X
57. Main parts, components, and layout,	X		
58. Protective earthing; terminals and connections, and	X		
59. Construction and layouts.	X		

5. Clauses Containing Amendments, Additions, or Replacements to the Text in IEC 601-1:1988, and Additional Clauses 60 Through 65

NOTE 1—The clause numbers used reference the specific section in the General Standard.

5.1 (3) *General Requirements*—The requirements given in Clause 3 of the General Standard apply with the following additions:

5.1.1 (k) Operation of the humidifier without any liquid.

5.1.2 (l) If the humidifier includes a temperature sensor; any single fault condition with the temperature sensor. For example:

5.1.2.1 Temperature sensor single open-circuit,

5.1.2.2 Temperature sensor single short-circuit, and

5.1.2.3 Temperature sensor disconnected from the temperature control system.

5.1.3 (m) A safety hazard (for example, thermal injury to the patient) resulting from software error.

5.2 (4) *General Requirements for Tests*—The requirements given in Clause 4 of the General Standard apply with the following additions and modifications:

5.2.1 (4.5) *Ambient Temperature, Humidity, Atmospheric Pressure*—Modify Clause 4.5(a) of the General Standard with the following:

5.2.1.1 (a) Unless otherwise specified, all tests shall be carried out at ambient condition "b": 23 ± 2°C, RH = 50 ± 5 % and an atmospheric pressure from 860 to 1060 hPa.

5.2.2 (4.6) *Other Conditions*—Amend Clause 4.6 of the General Standard with the follows:

5.2.2.1 (f) The test gas shall be medical-grade air, medical grade oxygen, or a mixture of the two.

5.2.2.2 (g) Unless otherwise specified, the liquid container shall be filled at the beginning of a test to the maximum operating volume with distilled water at the ambient test temperature. The liquid reservoir, if provided, shall also be filled with distilled water in accordance with the manufacturer's instructions.

5.2.2.3 (h) For the purpose of checking compliance the measured gas temperature shall be sensed no more than 50 mm from the patient connector port.

5.3 (5) *Classification*—The requirements given in Clause 5 of the General Standard apply.

5.4 (6) *Identification, Marking, and Documents*—The requirements given in Clause 6 of the General Standard apply with the following additions and modifications:

5.4.1 *Marking on the Outside of Equipment or Equipment Parts*—Amend Clause 6.1 as follows: (aa) The marking on the outside shall also include the following:

5.4.1.1 (1) The maximum and minimum liquid levels, if these are necessary for the correct operation of the humidifier.

5.4.1.2 (2) The direction of flow, in the case of flow-direction-sensitive humidifiers or humidification systems.

5.4.1.3 (3) If a pressure-relief mechanism is provided, the range of pressures over which it opens. This marking shall be on or near the relief device.

5.4.1.4 (4) If the humidifier is driven by compressed gas, the ranges of the supply flows and pressures that are required.

5.4.1.5 (5) If the humidifier is intended for use only with patients whose supraglottic airways have not been bypassed, a warning to indicate that the humidifier is not for use with patients whose supraglottic airways have been bypassed.

5.4.1.6 (6) If the manufacturer knows of the expected adverse effects on the performance of the humidifier when exposed to, for example: electrocautery, electrosurgery, defibrillation, X-ray (gamma radiation), infrared radiation, conducted transients, magnetic fields including magnetic resonance imaging (MRI), and radiofrequency interference, a warning to, for example, "See the accompanying documents" for information related to exposure of this device to, for example, electromagnetic fields.

5.4.2 (6.7) *Indicator Lights and Push Buttons*—The requirements of Clause 6.7 of the General Standard apply with the following modifications:

5.4.3 (6.7a) *Color of Indicator Lights*—Replace Clause 6.7(a) with the following:

5.4.3.1 Humidifiers and humidification systems for medical use shall meet the requirements of Specification 1463.

5.5 (6.8) *Accompanying Documents*—Amend Clause 6.8.2(a) as follows: The instructions for use shall also include the following information:

5.5.1 (1) For humidifiers, at least one breathing tube and other necessary accessories that, when used together with the humidifier, meet the requirements of this specification. In addition, a warning to the effect that it unsafe to configure this humidifier with any breathing tube or accessory that is not specified for use with this humidifier.

5.5.2 For breathing tubes or accessories, at least one humidifier that, when used with the breathing tube or accessories, will meet the requirements of this specification. In addition, a warning to the effect that it unsafe to configure this breathing tube or accessory with any humidifier that is not specified for use with this breathing tube or accessory.

5.5.3 (2) If the humidifier includes an integral venturi mechanism that entrains air for the purpose of diluting oxygen, the following shall be provided:

5.5.3.1 (a) A statement to the effect that the oxygen concentration may be affected by a partial obstruction downstream of the humidifier, for example, the use of accessory equipment.

5.5.3.2 (b) A recommendation that the oxygen concentration should be measured at the point of delivery to the patient.

5.5.4 (3) The intended use of the humidifier system:

5.5.4.1 (4) If the humidifier is intended for use with patients whose supraglottic airways are bypassed, the maximum flow and delivered gas temperature that permits a humidifier output of at least 33 mg/L, at a range of operator control settings.

5.5.4.2 (5) The operating volume and, if provided, the usable volume of the liquid reservoir.

5.5.4.3 (6) If the humidifier is powered by pressurized gas, the recommended ranges of flows or supply pressures and method(s) of connection.

5.5.4.4 (7) The maximum operating pressure of the humidifier.

5.5.4.5 (8) The pressure drop, as a function of flow, across the humidifier shall be stated, when tested in accordance with the test methods given in ISO 8835-2:1993(E).

5.5.4.6 (9) The gas leakage of the humidifier at the maximum operating pressure.

5.5.4.7 (10) The internal compliance of the humidifier, if the patient's tidal volume can be influenced by inclusion of the humidifier in the breathing system.

5.5.4.8 (11) The internal compliance of the humidifier at the maximum and minimum operating volumes if it can be affected by a change in the volume of liquid in the liquid container.

5.5.4.9 (12) The humidifier output over the humidifier's recommended operating range of gas flows and temperatures.

5.5.4.10 (13) The time required (warm-up time) for the delivered gas temperature to reach set temperature from a starting temperature of 23 ± 2°C when operated according to the manufactures instruction.

5.5.4.11 (14) The circumstances under which the A-weighted sound pressure level exceeds 50 db measured 1 m from the device (see Clause 63.2).

5.5.4.12 (15) The maximum delivered gas temperature if the humidification system is not provided with a means of continuously indicating the measured gas temperature (see Clause 56.1).

5.5.4.13 (16) Identification of all accessories, if the normal use of the humidifier requires specific accessory (for example, heated breathing tubes) in order to meet the requirements of this specification.

5.5.4.14 (17) The range of the measured gas temperature which will generate an alarm (accuracy alarm, see Clause 50.2.4.2).

5.5.4.15 (18) Appropriate warning about operation of the breathing tubes if they may be affected by normal clinical operation, for example, covering the tubes with a blanket.

5.5.4.16 (19) The temperature that, when exceeded by the delivered gas temperature, causes the humidification system to generate a medium priority alarm. This temperature shall not exceed 41°C (maximum temperature alarm, see Clause 51.6).

5.6 (6.8.2d) *Cleaning, Disinfection, and Sterilization of*

Parts in Contact With the Patient—Modify the beginning of Clause 6.8.2(d) as follows:

5.6.1 For reusable equipment parts which come into contact... .

5.7 (6.8.3) *Technical Description*—The requirements of Clause 6.8.3 of the General Standard apply with the following amendments:

5.7.1 Maximum operating potential:

5.7.2 The heated breathing tube controller shall state the maximum operating potential in terms of its mode of operation (for example, maximum steady-state voltage and current for electrically heated breathing tubes).

5.8 (7) *Power Input*—The requirements given in Clause 7 of the General Standard apply.

SECTION TWO—ENVIRONMENTAL CONDITIONS

6. (8) Basic Safety Requirements:

6.1 The requirements given in Clause 8 of the General Standard apply.

7. (9) Removable Protective Means:

7.1 The requirements given in Clause 8 of the General Standard apply.

8. (10) Environmental Conditions:

8.1 The requirements given in Clause 10 of the General Standard apply.

8.2 The requirements given in Clause 11 of the General Standard apply.

8.3 The requirements given in Clause 12 of the General Standard apply.

SECTION THREE—PROTECTION AGAINST ELECTRIC SHOCK HAZARDS

9. (13) General

9.1 The requirements given in Clause 13 of the General Standard apply.

10. (14) Requirements Related to Classification

10.1 The requirements given in Clause 14 of the General Standard apply.

11. (15) Limitation of Voltage or Energy, or Both

11.1 The requirements given in Clause 15 of the General Standard apply.

12. (16) Enclosures and Protective Covers

12.1 The requirements given in Clause 16 of the General Standard apply.

13. (17) Separation (Previous Title: Insulation and Protective Impedances)

13.1 The requirements given in Clause 17 of the General Standard apply.

14. (18) Protective Earthing, Functional Earthing, and Potential Equalization

14.1 The requirements given in Clause 18 of the General Standard apply.

15. (19) Continuous Leakage Currents and Patient Auxiliary Currents

15.1 The requirements given in Clause 19 of IEC 601-1:1988 apply with the following amendment: Amend 19.3 such that the enclosure leakage current for single-fault conditions is limited to 300 μA.

15.2 Amend 19.4 h) 9) as follows:

15.2.1 The humidifier connected to the breathing tube and other necessary accessories shall be tested using metal foil as described under Subclause 19.4g) 5). The metal foil is wrapped around the patient connection port.

15.2.2 See Fig. 25 of the General Standard.

16. (20) Dielectric Strength

16.1 The requirements given in Clause 20 of the General Standard apply.

SECTION FOUR—PROTECTION AGAINST MECHANICAL HAZARDS

17. (21) Mechanical Strength

17.1 The requirements given in Clause 21 of the General Standard apply.

18. (22) Moving Parts

18.1 The requirements given in Clause 22 of the General Standard apply.

19. (23) Surface, Corners, and Edges

19.1 The requirements given in Clause 23 of the General Standard apply.

20. (24) Stability in Normal Use

20.1 The requirements given in Clause 24 of the General Standard apply with the following addition:

20.1.1 (24.7) When the humidifier is tilted through 20° in any direction from its normal operating position, there shall be no spillage of water from the liquid container or liquid reservoir into the breathing system.

20.1.2 Compliance shall be checked by inspection.

21. (25) Expelled Parts

21.1 The requirements given in Clause 25 of the General Standard apply.

22. (26) Vibration and Noise

22.1 The requirements given in Clause 26 of the General Standard apply.

23. (27) Pneumatic and Hydraulic Power

23.1 The requirements given in Clause 27 of the General Standard apply.

24. (28) Suspended Masses

24.1 The requirements given in Clause 28 of the General Standard apply.

NOTE 2—The requirements given in Clauses 29 through 35 of the General Standard apply.

SECTION FIVE—PROTECTION AGAINST HAZARDS FROM UNWANTED OR EXCESSIVE RADIATION

25. (36) Electromagnetic Compatibility

25.1 The requirements given in Clause 36 of the General Standard apply with the following additions:

25.1.1 (36.1) Protection from electromagnetic disturbance.

25.1.1.1 The humidifier system shall continue to function and meet the requirements of this specification or shall fail without causing a safety hazard when tested in accordance with IEC 601-1-2:1993. If an anomally occurs, such as alarm activation, as loss of function without the integrity of the associated protective system being compromised, this shall not be considered a safety hazard, provided it is possible to restore normal operation within 30 s after cessation of the electromagnetic disturbance.

NOTE 3—Compliance should be checked by using a worst case system configuration, for example, temperature sensor having longest leads and electrically heated breathing tube of greatest length.

25.1.2 Discharges shall be applied only to accessible parts and coupling planes (as defined in 601-1-2 Clause 36.202.1). If an anomaly occurs, such as display interrupt or alarm activation, it should be possible to restore normal operation within 30 s after the electrostatic discharges have been applied.

NOTE 4—Silencing of an activated alarm shall not be considered a failure.

SECTION SIX—PROTECTION AGAINST THE HAZARDS OF IGNITION OF FLAMMABLE ANESTHETIC MIXTURES

26. (37) Locations and Basic Requirements

26.1 The requirements given in Clause 37 of the General Standard apply.

27. (38) Marking, Accompanying Documents

27.1 The requirements given in Clause 38 of the General Standard apply.

28. (39) Common Requirements for Category AP and Category APG Equipment

28.1 The requirements given in Clause 39 of the General Standard apply.

29. (40) Requirements and Tests for Category AP Equipment, Parts, and Components Thereof

29.1 The requirements given in Clause 40 of the General Standard apply.

30. (41) Requirements and Tests for Category APG Equipment, Parts, and Components Thereof

30.1 The requirements given in Clause 41 of the General Standard apply.

SECTION SEVEN—PROTECTION AGAINST EXCESSIVE TEMPERATURES AND OTHER SAFETY HAZARDS

31. (42) Excessive Temperatures

31.1 The requirements given in Clause 42 of the General Standard apply with the following additions:

31.1.1 (42.8) The accessible surface temperature within 25 cm of the patient connection port shall not exceed 44°C.

32. (43) Fire Prevention

32.1 The requirements given in Clause 43 of the General Standard apply, with the following additions:

32.1.1 In order to reduce the risk to patients, other persons or the surroundings due to fire or ignitable material, under normal and single-fault conditions, shall not, at the same time, be subjected to conditions in which:

32.1.2 The temperature of the material is raised to its minimum ignition temperature, and

32.1.3 An oxidant is present.

32.1.4 The minimum ignition temperature is determined in accordance with IEC 79-4 using the oxidizing conditions present under the normal and single-fault condition.

32.1.5 Compliance is checked by determining the temperature the material is raised to under the normal and singlefault condition.

32.1.6 If sparking can occur under normal or single-fault conditions, the material subjected to the energy dissipation of the spark shall not ignite under the oxidizing conditions present.

32.1.7 Compliance is checked by observing if ignition occurs under the most unfavorable combination of normal conditions with a single fault.

33. (44) Overflow, Spillage, Leakage, Humidity, Ingress of Liquids, Cleaning, Sterilization, and Disinfection

33.1 The requirements given in Clause 44 of the General Standard apply.

34. (45) Pressure Vessels and Parts Subject to Pressure

34.1 The requirements given in Clause 45 the General Standard apply.

35. (46) Human Error

35.1 The requirements given in Clause 46 the General Standard apply.

36. (47) Electrostatic Charges

36.1 The requirements given of Clause 47 of the General Standard apply.

37. (48) Materials in Applied Parts in Contact with the Body of the Patient

37.1 The requirements given in Clause 48 of the General Standard apply.

38. (49) Interruption of the Power Supply

38.1 The requirements given in Clause 49 of the General Standard apply.

SECTION EIGHT—ACCURACY OF OPERATING DATA AND PROTECTING AGAINST HAZARDOUS OUTPUT

39. (50) Accuracy of Operating Data

39.1 The requirements given in Clause 50 of the General

Standard apply with the following additions:

39.1.1 (50.1) *Marking of Controls and Instruments*—If the humidifier system includes a means of continuously indicating the measured gas temperature, then the displayed measured gas temperature shall have a temperature display range of at least 25 to 45°C.

39.1.2 (50.2) *Accuracy of Controls and Instruments:*

39.1.2.1 (50.2.1) All calibrated operator controls and graduated or digital indicators shall be accurate to ± 5 % of their full-scale value except temperature displays and controls.

39.1.2.2 (50.2.2) The displayed measured gas temperature shall be accurate to ± 2°C.

39.1.2.3 Compliance shall be checked by the test given in Annex A1.

39.1.2.4 (50.2.3) If the humidifier includes an integral venturi mechanism that entrains air for the purpose of diluting oxygen or other gas mixtures the nominal oxygen concentration value shall not differ by more than ± 10 % of the control setting.

39.1.2.5 (50.2.4) The following requirements do not apply during the period the system is in transition to a new state of thermal equilibrium following a change in gas flow or change in set temperature, or both; however, no thermal hazard shall exist during this period.

39.1.2.6 (50.2.4.1) Under normal conditions, the measured gas temperature averaged during any period of 5 min shall not differ by more than ± 2°C from the set temperature.

39.1.2.7 (50.2.4.2) If the measured gas temperature differs from the set gas temperature by more than the range that is specified by the manufacturer in the instructions for use (see Clause 6.8.2a), a medium priority (caution) alarm shall be generated.

40. (51) Protection Against Hazardous Output

40.1 The requirements given in Clause 51 of the General Standard apply with the following additions:

40.1.1 (51.5) Under normal conditions and single fault conditions, the volume of liquid-exiting the humidifier outlet shall not exceed 1 mL/min nor 20 mL/h for humidifiers intended for use with neonates or 5 mL/min nor 20 mL/h for all other humidifiers.

40.1.1.1 (51.6.1) If the delivered gas temperature is capable of exceeding 41°C under normal conditions or singlefault conditions, then the humidification system shall include a means of continuously indicating the measured gas temperature.

40.1.1.2 (51.6.2) The humidification system shall generate a medium priority alarm whenever the measured gas temperature exceeds a temperature specified by the manufacturer, which shall not exceed 41°C (see Clause 6.8.2 a) 19). If the operator is able to silence the auditory alarm, the duration of the cancellation shall not exceed 120 s.

40.1.2 (51.7) Under normal conditions and single-fault conditions, the humidification system shall interrupt heating when the measured gas temperature exceeds 41°C.

40.1.3 (51.8) Under normal conditions and single-fault conditions, a thermal overshoot at the patient connection port shall not exceed an energy equivalent to 43°C and 100 % relative humidity (a specific enthalpy not to exceed 194-kJ/kg dry gas) when averaged over any 30 s.

NOTE 5—Permissible combinations of temperature and relative humidity are for example:

Temperature	Relative Humidity, %
43	100
44	95
45	90
48	76
50	68

40.1.4 Compliance shall be checked by inspection and measurement of energy as specified in Annex A2 during normal use and under the following conditions:

40.1.4.1 Turn humidification system on, wait 30 min, and then run the minimum and maximum continuous flow as recommended by the manufacturer.

40.1.4.2 Operate humidification system, interrupt gas flow for 3 min, and then reinstate gas flow at minimum, maximum, and average continuous flow.

40.1.4.3 Operate the humidification system from a continuous minimum to maximum flow and from a continuous maximum to minimum flow.

NOTE 6—For the purpose of this test, the conditions above apply only under normal conditions.

SECTION NINE—ABNORMAL OPERATION AND FAULT CONDITIONS

41. (52) Abnormal Operation and Fault Conditions

41.1 The requirements given in Clause 52 of the General Standard apply.

42. (53) Environmental Tests

42.1 The requirements given in Clause 53 of the General Standard apply.

SECTION TEN—ABNORMAL OPERATION AND FAULT CONDITIONS

43. (54) General

43.1 The requirements given in Clause 54 of the General Standard apply.

44. (55) Enclosure and Covers

44.1 The requirements given in Clause 55 of the General Standard apply.

45. (56) Components and General Assembly

45.1 The requirements given in Clause 56 of the General Standard apply with the following additions and modifications:

45.1.1 (56.3) *Connector—General:*

45.1.1.1 If a humidifier is intended to be placed in a breathing system fitted with conical breathing system connectors, the conical connectors shall be in accordance with Specification F 1205. If intended for adult use, they shall be of 22-mm size; if intended for pediatric use or with neonates, the connectors shall be of 15-mm size.

45.1.1.2 If the humidifier is fitted with any other type of connector, these connectors shall mate with breathing tubes complying with Specification F 1205 and shall not accept or permit connection to the 15-mm or 22-mm conical connectors complying with Specification F 1205.

45.1.1.3 If the humidifier incorporates an independent filling or accessory orifice (for example, an air entrainment or a heater orifice), that orifice shall not accept any of the connectors specified in conical fitting of 18 122-mm sizes.

45.1.2 Compliance shall be checked by inspection and manipulation.

45.2 (56.12) *Breathing Tubes:*

45.2.1 (56.12.1.1) Breathing tubes intended for use in humidification systems shall meet the requirements of ISO 5367.

45.2.2 (56.12.1.2) The machine end of breathing tubes intended for use in humidification systems shall either:

45.2.2.1 Meet the requirements of ISO 5367, or

45.2.2.2 Be a proprietary fitting that shall not permit connection to breathing tubes complying with ISO 5367 or any of the conical connectors complying with ISO 5356-1.

45.2.2.3 Compliance is checked by inspection.

45.2.3 (56.12.2) Breathing tubes and associated connectors capable of being attached to humidifiers shall not kink, occlude, leak, or otherwise cause a safety hazard.

45.2.3.1 Compliance is checked by inspection and testing according to Clause 53.12.3 of ISO 10651.

45.2.4 (56.12.3) Breathing tubes that are capable of being attached to humidifiers shall not kink, occlude, leak or otherwise cause a safety hazard when the breathing tubes are subject to the constant maximum output potential of the heated breathing tube controller (see Clause 6.8.3.e).

45.2.4.1 Compliance is checked by inspection and testing according to Clause 56.12.3 of ISO 10651 while applying the constant maximum output potential of the heated breathing tube controller.

46. (57) Main Parts, Components, and Layout

46.1 The requirements given in Clause 57 of the General Standard apply.

47. (58) Protective Earthing—Terminals and Connections

47.1 The requirements given in Clause 58 of the General Standard apply.

48. (59) Construction and Layout

48.1 The requirements given in Clause 59 of the General Standard apply.

SECTION ELEVEN—ADDITIONAL REQUIREMENTS SPECIFICALLY RELATED TO HUMIDIFIERS

49. (60) Humidifier Output

49.1 All humidification systems shall be capable of producing a humidifier output of at least 10 mg H_2O/L; humidification systems intended for use with patients whose supraglottic airways have been bypassed shall also be capable of producing a humidifier output of at least 33 mg H_2O/L.

49.2 Compliance shall be checked by the test in Annex A3.

50. (61) Maximum Pressure Drop

50.1 The maximum pressure drop across the humidifier shall not exceed 2 kPa throughout the operating range of flows. Exclusive of nebulizing-type humidifiers, humidifiers intended for use with patients who's breathing is spontaneous or assisted, the pressure drop across the humidifier shall not exceed 0.2 kPa at a flow of 60 L/min.

50.2 Compliance shall be checked by functional test.

51. (62) Liquid Container

51.1 (62.1) *Filling*—Filling the liquid container, or liquid reservoir if provided, to the marked maximum liquid level if so marked, shall not allow more than 1 mL of liquid to enter any part of the breathing system if the humidifier is intended for use with neonates and nor more than 5 mL for all other humidifiers.

51.2 (62.2) *Liquid Level*—It shall be possible to determine the liquid level in the liquid container, and if fitted the liquid reservoir, without dismantling the humidifier.

51.3 (62.3) *Filling Cap*—If intended to be reused, the cap shall be attached to the humidifier.

52. (63) Noise Measurement

52.1 (63.1) If humidifiers within a humidification system are intended to be used in association with incubators, the humidifiers shall not cause the noise level requirements in IEC 601-2-19 to be exceeded.

52.2 (63.2) The steady state noise generated by the humidifier shall not exceed 50 dBA at any point 1 m from the humidifier.

52.3 Compliance is checked by testing in accordance with ISO 3744.

53. (64) Temperature Sensors and Temperature Sensor Ports

53.1 Temperature sensors and mating ports shall meet the following requirements:

53.1.1 (64.1) Temperature sensors shall meet the dimensional requirements in Annex A4, or shall meet the requirements in 53.1.3 (64.3).

53.1.2 (64.2) When the temperature sensors and mating ports are engaged according to the manufacturers recommendations, the following requirements shall be met:

53.1.2.1 (64.2.1) When tested as described in Annex A4, the engaged connection shall not become disconnected.

53.1.2.2 (64.2.2) When leak tested as described in Annex A4, the leakage from the engaged connector shall not exceed 5 mL/min.

53.1.3 (64.3) Temperature sensors that do not comply with the dimensional requirements of Annex A4 shall be sufficiently different that they cannot be interchanged with those that do.

54. (65) Humidifier Leakage

54.1 (65.1) The gas leakage from the humidifier shall not exceed 10 mL/min when tested in 54.2 (65.2).

54.2 (65.2) Seal off all parts but the humidifier inlet. Apply static pressure of 8.0 ± 0.5 kPa to the inlet port. Measure or calculate the leakage to atmosphere.

55. Annexes and Appendixes

55.1 Appendixes A to L of the General Standard and Annex A1-Annex A4, and Annex A5 apply.

ANNEXES

(Mandatory Information)

A1. TEMPERATURE DISPLAY ACCURACY

A1.1 Temperature display accuracy shall be confirmed by introducing two standard temperature sensors, as defined in Annex A5, into the humidifier system configured according to operating instructions and detailed in Fig. A1.1.

NOTE A1.1—If necessary add extension tubing so that no sensors are unduly influenced by ambient drafts and temperatures. The tubing shall be of equal diameter as the breathing tubes and long enough so that all sensors are at least located a distance from ambient equal to ten times the breathing tube diameter.

A1.2 The distances from the normal location of the humidification system's temperature sensor to the location of the standard temperature sensors ("dd" in Fig. A1.1) shall be equidistant, and shall be from 20 to 30 mm.

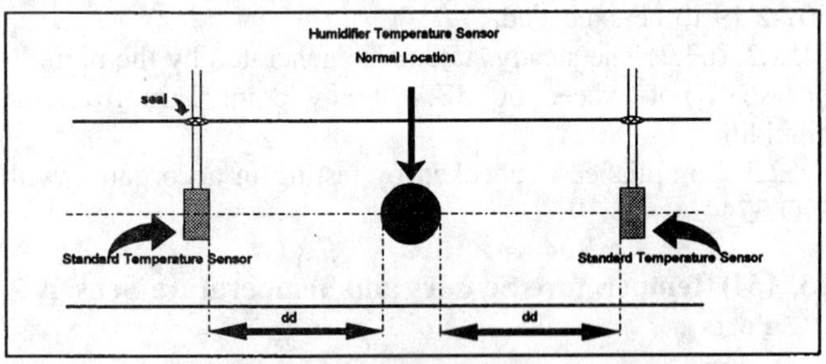

FIG. A1.1 Temperature Display Accuracy

A1.3 Temperatures shall be sampled at least every 2 s.

A1.4 Operate the humidification system over the manufacturer's recommended flow range.

A1.5 Set the minimum set temperature and confirm that the measured gas temperature equals the arithmetic mean ± 2°C of the two standard temperature sensors in a steady state condition.

A1.6 Quickly changing the set temperature from the minimum to maximum setting.

NOTE A1.2—This change should simulate a step function from minimum to maximum to the extent that it is practical.

A1.7 Confirm that the measured gas temperature equals the arithmetic mean ± 4°C of the two standard temperature sensors during the transition period from minimum to maximum set temperature.

A1.8 Confirm that the measured gas temperature equals the arithmetic mean ± 2°C of the two standard temperature sensors in a steady state condition for the maximum set temperature.

A2. SPECIFIC ENTHALPY CALCULATIONS

A2.1 Calculate specific enthalpy using the following formulas (see Refs (**and** , and **3**).[5] Measurements of the temperature at the humidifier outlet and the delivered gas temperature can be made with the standard temperature sensor, as defined in Annex A5, and should be sampled at least every 2 s.

t_d = delivered gas temperature, °C,
t_h = lower of delivered gas temperature and humidifier outlet temperature, °C

NOTE A2.1—$t_h = t_d$ when the humidifier outlet is the patient connection port.

A2.1.1 For each measurement calculate the p_v, g, and h as follows:

A2.1.2 *Absolute Temperature*:

$$Th = 273.16 + t_h \ [K] \quad (A2.1)$$

$$Td = 273.16 + t_d \ [K] \quad (A2.2)$$

A2.1.3 *Vapor Pressure*:

$$P_v = 10^{30.59051 - 8.2\log(Th) + 2.4804 \times 10^{-3} \times Th - \frac{3142.31}{T_h}} \ [\mathrm{kPa}] \quad (A2.3)$$

A2.1.4 *Moisture Content*:

$$g = 0.625 \times \frac{P_v}{101.325 - 1.005 p_v} \ [\mathrm{kg/kg}] \quad (A2.4)$$

A2.1.5 *Specific Enthalpy*:

$$h = 1.0067 \times t_d + gx(2501.82 + 1.8 \times t_d) \ [\mathrm{kJ/kg}] \quad (A2.5)$$

Then for any 30-s period, calculate the average specific enthalpy:

$$\bar{h} = \frac{1}{N\Delta t} \sum_{i=t'}^{i=t'+N\Delta t} h(t)\Delta \quad (A2.6)$$

where:
$h(t)$ = specific enthalpy h at time, t,
$\Delta t \leq 2$ s,
$N\Delta t$ = 30 s, and

[5] The boldface numbers given in parentheses refer to a list of references at the end of the text.

t' = any time after specified warm-up period.

A3. HUMIDIFIER OUTPUT CALCULATIONS

A3.1 Measurements shall be carried out between the minimum and maximum gas flows recommended by the manufacturer. If the humidifier incorporates an integral mechanism for the entrainment of air for the purpose of diluting oxygen, all entrainment orifices shall be occluded during the test.

A3.2 The following procedure should be performed at the specified test settings and with measurement equipment such that a total measurement accuracy of ± 1 mg/L is achieved:

A3.2.1 Configure the humidification system according to the operating instructions.

A3.2.2 The entire test setup should be mounted on a set of scales so that mass measurements can be made simply and accurately.

A3.2.3 If necessary, add extension tubing such that no sensors are unduly influenced by ambient drafts and temperatures. The tubing should be of equal diameter to the breathing tube and of length such that all sensors shall be displaced at least ten times the breathing tube diameter from ambient.

A3.2.4 Arrange relative elevations of the humidifier, breathing tube, and humidification chamber as applicable such that:

A3.2.4.1 Condensation that does not represent humidification reaching the patient does not leave the system and is included in m_1 (defined below).

A3.2.4.2 Condensation that represents humidification reaching the patient leaves the system and is not included in m_1(defined below).

A3.2.5 The humidifier output shall be expressed in milligrams per litre moist gas (normalized to 37°C).

A3.2.5.1 Install a temperature sensor as defined in Annex A5 in the air stream at a site representing the delivered gas temperature. Call this temperature T_2 (°C).

A3.2.5.2 Connect the humidifier to a medical-grade dry gas source. The temperature of this dry gas entering the humidification chamber should be ± m1°C of the ambient temperature. Call this temperature T_1 (°C).

A3.2.5.3 If the humidifier or its breathing tube is heated and the test is being carried out in the heated mode, allow the temperature to stabilize for the recommended warm-up time.

A3.2.5.4 Turn off the humidifier, disconnect all accessories, including the air supply, electrical connections, and any extension tubing to remove any extraneous influences on the weight measurement. Weigh only the humidifier, its contents and the recommended breathing tube; record this mass as m_0. This is the initial mass of the system.

A3.2.5.5 Reconnect all accessories. Turn the humidifier back on to begin the test (record time as t_0) and maintain operator control settings throughout the test. Monitor the dry gas flow rate and temperature to ensure compatibility with the objective of total measurement accuracy of 1 mg/L.

A3.3 The test may be stopped when the measurement error of the following quantities maintains a total measurement accuracy of ± 1 mg/L.

A3.3.1 The humidifier has used a sufficient quantity of the usable capacity of the liquid container; and

A3.3.2 The time of the test is of sufficient duration.

A3.3.2.1 Record the time as t_1, and record the duration of the test, $t_1 - t_0$.

NOTE A3.1—Special attention is drawn to the objective of a total measurement error of less than ±1 mg/L. Measurement of time, temperature, especially flow rate and mass-used should be sufficiently accurate relative to the value of the quantity to maintain that objective. In practice the mass and estimated output of the humidifier will give a guide as to the minimum duration of the test to maintain overall accuracy. An error analysis of the measurement equipment and estimated results is strongly recommended as a guide.

A3.3.2.2 Make a weight measurement as for A3.2.5.4; record this mass as m_1. The difference $m_0 - m_1$ represents the total moisture reaching the patient over the test duration.

A3.4 The humidifier output, expressed in milligrams per litre moist gas normalized to 37°C (that is, BTPS, body temperature, standard pressure, saturated) is given by the following formula:

$$\frac{1000\,m}{1.0658\,V(1 + 0.0034(37 - T_1))} \tag{A3.1}$$

where:

m = $(m_0 - m_1)$ is the mass, g, of water used,
m_0 = mass, g, at time t_0,
m_1 = mass, g, at time t_1,
V = volume of dry gas at ambient temperature (that is, the product of flow times the duration of test), and
T_1 = temperature of dry gas, °C.

A4. TEMPERATURE SENSORS AND MATING PORTS

A4.1 *Dimensional Requirements for Temperature Sensors:*

A4.1.1 The axial length of the taper of temperature sensors shall be at least 10.5 mm.Fig. A4.1

A4.1.2 When the temperature sensor is engaged with the ring gage shown below, by applying an axial force of 35.0 ± 3.5 *N* and while maintaining the same force rotating the sensor up to 20°, its leading edge shall be within the minimum and maximum steps of the gage. The temperature sensor and gage shall be maintained at ambient temperature.

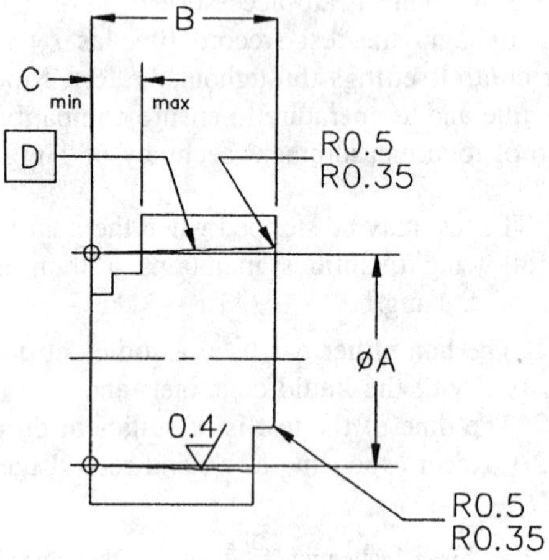

A = 7.550 ± 0.005
B = 9.000 ± 0.005
C = 2.50 ± 0.005
D = 1:40

FIG. A4.1 Temperature Sensor Engaged with Ring Gauge

A4.1.3 Dimensions in millimetres and surface roughness values in micrometres:

A4.2 *Test Method for Security of Engagement of the Temperature Sensors to Mating Ports*:

A4.2.1 Condition temperature sensors and mating ports at 41 ± 2°C and 95 ± 5 % RH for at least 1 h.

A4.2.2 Engage the temperature sensor with the mating port in accordance with the manufacturer's instructions for use.

A4.2.3 Condition the engaged components, without activation of any disengagement mechanism, for at least 1 h at the conditions specified in A4.2.1A4.2.1.

A4.2.4 Apply an axial separation force of 25 ± 2.5 *N* for 10 s at a rate not exceeding 20 Ns^{-1}.

A4.3 *Test Method for Leakage from Temperature Sensors Engaged in Mating Ports*:

A4.3.1 Apply a static pressure of 8.0 ± 0.5 kPa to the temperature sensor and mating port assembly.

A4.3.2 Measure or calculate the leakage to atmosphere from the sensor and mating port assembly.

A5. STANDARD TEMPERATURE SENSOR

A5.1 The standard temperature sensor can be constructed as indicated as follows:

A5.1.1 The standard temperature sensor shall have the following characteristics:

A5.1.1.1 Time constant ≥0.5 and ≤1.0 for a step change of 22 to 37°C in water at 1-m/s flow.

A5.1.1.2 Influence from changes in ambient temperature ≤0.01/1°C.

A5.1.2 An example for construction of such a sensor is indicated as follows:

A5.1.2.1 A sheath with thermal conductivity ≥386 W/(m°C) with the dimensions given in Fig. A5.1; for example, a piece of solid ⅛-in. copper rod with appropriate drilled spaces.

A5.1.2.2 A thermistor with an accuracy of ± 0.1°C from 25 to 45°C in isothermal stirred air or water.[6]

A5.1.2.3 The thermistor shall be epoxied into the copper sheath, as in Fig. A5.2. The epoxy shall have a thermal conductivity ≥0.183 W/(m°C).[7]

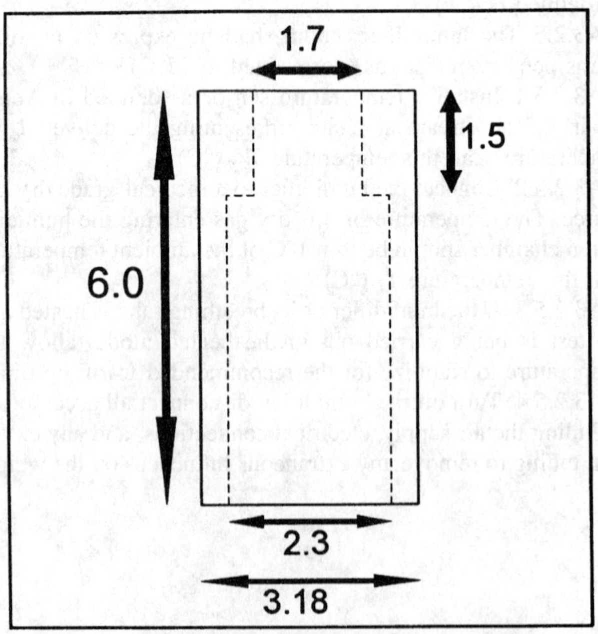

NOTE 1—All dimensions in millimetres.

FIG. A5.1 Temperature Sensor Construction

[6] The YSI Series 400 bead, Fenwal 192-222 LET-DO1, available from Yellow Springs Instruments, Inc., PO Box 279, Yellow Springs, OH 45387 has been found suitable for this purpose.

[7] For example, Creative Materials Inc. (CMI) 108-50 thermally conductive, low-stress epoxy, has been found suitable for this purpose.

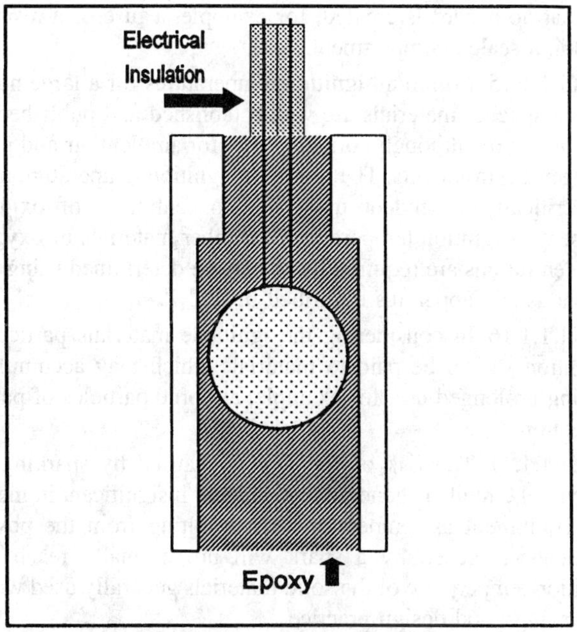

FIG. A5.2 Thermistor Epoxied Into the Copper Sheath

A5.1.3 Measure or calculate the leakage to atmosphere from the sensor and matting port assembly.

APPENDIX

(Nonmandatory Information)

X1. RATIONALE STATEMENT

X1.1 This appendix provides a rationale for certain requirements of this specification and is intended for those who are familiar with the design and use of humidifiers but who have not participated in its development. An understanding of the reasons for these requirements is provided to aid in the application of this specification. Furthermore, as clinical practice and technology change, it is believed that a rationale for the present requirements will facilitate a revision of this specification.

X1.1.1 The appropriate clause numbers are indicated.

X1.1.1.1 (6.1,aa),4 Gas supply pressures used in different parts of the world vary considerable, and it is important that the safe range of supply pressures are marked on the humidifier. Moreover, humidifiers of similar appearance may have different supply requirements. Fig. X1.1

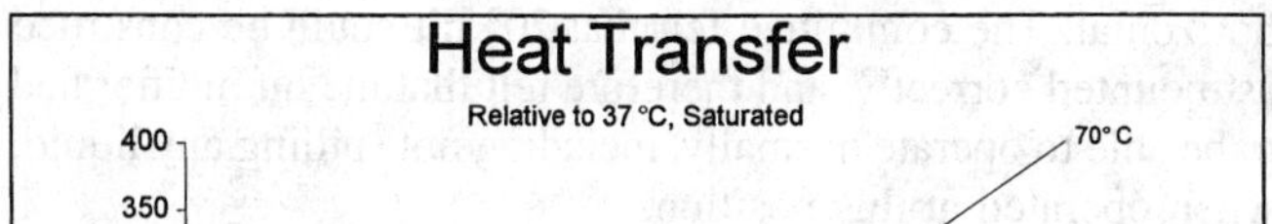

FIG. X1.1 Heat Transfer Calculations

X1.1.1.2 (6.8.2a) 1 The safe use of a humidifier is dependent on the interaction of the humidifier with its many accessories, such as breathing tubes (both heated and non heated), temperature sensors and heated breathing tube controllers. To that end, the committee felt that the best way to address the problems created by the proliferation of components which were physically, but not functionally, interchangeable was to consider the whole system in which all of the components operate, that is, the humidification system, and set total system performance requirements.

X1.1.1.3 The committee recognizes that there are many more breathing tube manufacturers than humidifier manufactures. It is the committee's intent for accessory manufactures, such as breathing tube manufactures, to test their accessories with a host of humidifiers so that users can configure the humidification system that is most appropriate.

X1.1.1.4 In addition, the user is warned that a humidification system that has not been tested together to meet the requirements of this specification may not be safe.

X1.1.1.5 (6.8.2a) 2 The amount of air entrained by a venturi for the dilution of oxygen is a function of gas velocity. Changes in gas velocity, for example, as a result of a partial obstruction of the ventilation circuit, will directly effect the oxygen concentration.

X1.1.1.6 (6.8.2a) 8 Resistance to flow may increase the work of breathing. It may also interfere with the effectiveness of intermittent mandatory ventilation (IMV) or triggering mechanisms in lung ventilators.

X1.1.1.7 (6.8.2a) 10 The internal compliance of the ventilator breathing system, that includes the humidifier, must be known in order to accurately determine the tidal volume settings of constant volume ventilators.

X1.1.1.8 (6.8.2a) 15 The noise levels generated by humidifiers may contribute significantly to ambient noise levels in hospitals. Humidifiers are often positioned close to the patient. In special environments, such as adjacent to infant incubators, the effect is more pronounced and may lead to permanent injury.

X1.1.1.9 (6.8.3e) So that manufactures of breathing tubes are able to completely test their components in order to meet the requirements of Clause 6.8.2 a) 1 and 56.12.3, the breathing tube controller manufacturer must disclose the maximum amount of energy that the breathing tube could ever experience. Since many of the breathing tube manufactures "reverse-engineer" the breathing tube, the worst-case, maximum energy output of the controller is not always known.

X1.1.1.10 (24.7) Humidifiers are often mounted on poles. However, these humidifiers are often not mounted perfectly horizontal. The committee felt that 20° tilt could be construed as mounted correctly, and therefore felt that the humidifier had to be able to operate normally, including not spilling any liquid, when operated at this position.

X1.1.1.11 (42.6) The objective of this clause is to protect the patient from skin burns due to contact with the external surface of the breathing tube. See reference section for rationale for selecting 44°C.

X1.1.1.12 (43) Reports of fire caused by medical devices are unusual. However, when such fires occur in the hospital environment they can have tragic consequences.

X1.1.1.13 The risk of a fire is fundamentally determined by the three elements that are necessary in order to start a fire: ignitable material (fuel), a temperature equal to or above the minimum ignition temperature of the material, or sparks with energy dissipation equal to or above the minimum ignition energy of the materials, and an oxidant.

X1.1.1.14 Therefore, following the basic safety concepts of the General Standard, the objective in the design of the equipment must be to ensure that under both normal and single-fault conditions the temperature of any material is not raised to its minimum ignition temperature or the spark energy does not exceed the material ignition energy level. Alternatively, contained ignition may occur provided it is self-limiting so that no hazard is created, for example, a fuse or a resistor within a sealed compartment.

X1.1.1.15 Minimum ignition temperatures for a large number of specific materials are well established and published in the literature, although normally only for ambient air and pure oxygen environments. The minimum ignition temperature may be critically dependent upon the concentration of oxidant present. If ignition temperatures for other materials or oxygen concentrations are required these may be determined using the methods and apparatus described in IEC 79-4.

X1.1.1.16 In considering the ignitable materials particular attention should be paid to materials which may accumulate during prolonged use, for example, airborne particles of paper or cotton.

X1.1.1.17 The risk of fire directly caused by sparking of electrical circuits is generally considered insignificant in medical equipment as temperature rise resulting from the power dissipation caused by a spark will not normally reach the ignition temperature of the solid materials generally used when following good design practice.

X1.1.1.18 However, if materials with a low ignition temperature and a very low thermal capacity, for example, cotton wool, paper or organic fibre accumulations, are present, then it may not be possible to determine the surface temperatures attained during exposure to spark energy and specific tests, for example, ignition tests, may be necessary to ensure safety under these conditions.

X1.1.1.19 In certain standards currently in use the requirements to minimize fire are based on a limitation on temperature and electrical energy and oxidant concentration to absolute values:

X1.1.1.20 The temperature value is based on the minimum hotplate ignition temperature for fire-retardant cotton in 100 % oxygen that is given in the American NFPA publication 53M as 310°C. The assumption was therefore made that 300°C was an acceptable temperature limit in medical equipment with oxygen-enriched atmospheres.

X1.1.1.21 The origin of the electrical energy values that have been used is less clear and it would seem that, in the absence of specific controlled tests, figures have been adopted from other published standards. However, simple tests and detailed analysis of the known factors involved in causing an oxygen fire show that these figures can be either over restrictive or potentially hazardous depending, in particular, on the manner in which the power may be dissipated and the proximity and type of any "fuel" present.

X1.1.1.22 It is now generally accepted that there are no single or universally applicable ranges of temperatures, energy, and concentration of oxidant which can ensure safety under all circumstances. Ultimately electrical energy is only significant in its ability to raise the temperature of ignitable materials, and this in turn depends upon the particular configuration and the proximity of any ignitable materials.

X1.1.1.23 Under single-fault conditions in a typical electrical circuit the possible number of failure modes is very high. In this case full ensurance of safety may only be possible by using appropriate hazard and safety analysis procedures taking into consideration the three basic elements, that is, material, temperature, and oxidant.

X1.1.1.24 An appropriate design might limit the electrical energy in the circuit to ensure that temperatures remain below the minimum air ignition temperature under normal conditions and seal compartments or add forced ventilation to ensure that the oxygen content does not exceed that of ambient air under a single-fault condition.

X1.1.1.25 Alternatively, it may be appropriate to limit the electric energy to ensure temperatures below the minimum ignition temperature for a pure oxygen environment, even under single-fault conditions.

X1.1.1.26 The particular combination of material, oxidant, and temperature determines whether a fire will occur, not a single value of any one of these variables.

X1.1.1.27 (50.1) For humidification systems that display the measured gas temperature, the committee concluded that a range from 25 to 45°C was the minimum that an operator needed to operate the humidification system. It should be very clear to the operator if the displayed measured gas temperature is higher than 45°C or lower than 25°C.

X1.1.1.28 (50.2.1) The committee concluded that ±5 % of full scale was an acceptable level for accuracy for this device.

X1.1.1.29 (50.2.2) In order to ensure patient safety, it is important that an operator is present with accurate information. The displayed measured gas temperature must be an accurate representation of the temperature sensors indicating actual delivered gas temperatures. An accuracy of ±2°C was believed by the committee to represent a practical and achievable level.

X1.1.1.30 (50.2.4) It was not found practical or necessary to apply the requirements of Clause 50.2 to control systems during transitioning.

X1.1.1.31 (50.2.4.1) Humidifier control systems, by their nature, continuously adjust the system components that effect the delivered gas temperature. The delivered gas temperature will tend to cycle about the set temperature. A good indication clinically of the performance of the humidification system is the average delivered gas temperature.

X1.1.1.32 (50.2.4.2) Since control circuits of humidifiers continuously adjust the system that effects the delivered gas temperature, this medium priority (caution) alarm will notify the clinician that the delivered gas temperature has exceeded the set temperature by more that an acceptable amount. It was agreed that this "acceptable amount" could be left to the manufacturer of the system to decide. Operators of these devices should take into account this information when purchasing and operating these devices.

X1.1.1.33 (51.5) Excessive liquid output could cause patient injury and water to accumulate in the breathing tube.

X1.1.1.34 (51.6) Sustained delivered gas temperatures above 41°C represents a potential thermal hazard to the patient. It is therefore important that the operator have a continuous display of the measured gas temperature and be alerted when the temperature exceeds 41°C.

X1.1.1.35 (51.7 and 51.8) Although it is rarely needed for patient care, a sustained delivered gas temperature of 41°C at any level of saturation is not a thermal hazard to the patient. Studies to measure the relative importance of exposure time and temperature in the causation of cutaneous burns determined that surface temperatures of at least 44°C and 6 h of exposure were required to cause irreversible damage to epidermal cells **(4)**. As the degree of perfusion to the tracheobronchial mucosa far exceeds that enjoyed by cutaneous tissue, it is permissible to use the results of these studies to establish a safe level of temperature exposure for the airway. This is confirmed by studies conducted by the U.S. Navy Medical Research and Development Command that concluded that fully saturated gas at 45°C can be inspired for up to 1 h without damaging the mucosa of the respiratory tract.

X1.1.1.36 Delivered gas temperatures above 41°C, depending on the combination of gas temperature, level of saturation, and the length of time the patient is exposed, may be hazardous. It is therefore important that the operator be provided with a continuous display of delivered gas temperature and that in the event that the gas temperature exceeds 41°C the humidifier automatically interrupt heating and an alarm be activated.

X1.1.1.37 Gas at body temperature and fully saturated (37°C and 100 % relative humidity (RH)) will not transfer thermal energy to or from the patient. Dry gas at body temperature (37°C and 0 % RH) will draw heat away through evaporation. Gas at 41°C and fully saturated has the capacity to deliver less than 130 kJ per kg of dry gas breathed by the patient.

X1.1.1.38 To protect the patient from thermal injury, heating of the humidification system is interrupted if the delivered gas temperature exceeds 41°C. A thermal overshoot not to exceed an energy equal to 43°C and 100 % RH averaged over 30 s (194 kJ per kg of dry gas) is inconsequential to the patient and is permitted to simplify construction of the humidifier.

X1.1.1.39 (56.12) Delivery tubes have been reported to kink, occlude, and perforate due to the heat generated by humidifiers and supplemental electrical heating. It is believed that a delivery tube that is tested to meet the requirements of this specification and that does not kink, occlude, and perforate during these tests, will not be a safety hazard in clinical use.

X1.1.1.40 (60.1) 10 mg H_2O/L is equivalent to approximately 60 % relative humidity at 22°C ambient conditions, that is the lowest recommended humidity level for non-intubated patients. Humidifiers may be used in patients whose supraglottic airway has been bypassed by a tracheostomy or tracheal tube. Normal nasal breathing delivers air just below the larynx with a water content of approximately 33 mg H_2O/L. Humidifiers should approximate performance of the nasal airway. (See Refs **5, 6**, and **7**.)

X1.1.1.41 (63) Excessive noise can hinder voice communications, mask audio signals, cause stress, and contribute to sociocusis (nearly loss caused by prolonged exposure to a noisy environment) in patients and attending clinical staff.

X1.1.2 (Annex A1)—It is difficult to measure temperature at the precisely the same location as the device temperature sensor without modifying the gas flow, hence thermal transfer characteristics from the gas to the sensor. The philosophy of the test is to measure temperature either side of the sensor and interpolate the temperature to the site under test. Temperature drop in the circuit may be non-linear hence the objective is to place the standard sensors as close as possible to the device under test, but with minimal disruption of gas flow patterns.

X1.1.3 (Annex A2)—Energy content or specific enthalpy is not directly measurable, however it is determinable from the temperature and water vapor content of the gas. The gas exiting the humidifier is assumed to be 100 % RH to give a worst case energy content by means of the maximum water vapor content. However, if it can be demonstrated or measured otherwise this would be a more appropriate figure to use. At the time of issue of this specification, no commercially available humidity measuring devices with adequate response time or appropriate thermal characteristics were known to exist.

X1.2 Temperature al one does not determine whether a humidified gas presents a thermal hazard to a patient. The degree of saturation must also be known in order to determine the thermal energy of the humidified gas (see chart following):

Q(total) = *Q(air)* + *Q(water vapor)* + *Q(latent heat of vaporization)*
Q(air) = *Cp(air)* × *mass(air)* × [*T(air)* – 37°C]
Q(water vapor) = *Cp(wv)* × *mass(wv)* × [*T(wv)* – 37°C]
Q(atent heat of vaporization) = 2257 J/g × *mas(water vapor)*

X1.2.1 *Example:*

TV = 1 L	
Temperature = 50°C	
Absolute Humidity:	
@37°C	= 44 mg H_2O/L
@50°C	= 83 mg H_2O/L
density (air)	= 1.293 g/L
Cp (dry air)	= 1.0067 J/g°C@37°C
Cp (water)	= 4.179 J/g°C@37°C
CP (wv)	= 1.884 J/g°C@37°C
Q(air)	= 1.0067 J/g°C × (1 L × 1.293 g/L) × (50-37)°C
	= 16.92
Q(water)	= 4.179 J/g°C × (1 L × (83-44) × 10^{-3} g/L) × (50-37)°C
	= 2.119 J
Q(wv)	= 1.884 J/g°C × (1 L × (83-44) × 10^{-3} g/L) × (50-37)°C
	= 1.08 J
Q(latht)	= 2257 J/g°C × (1 L × (83-44) × 10^{-3} g/L)
	= 88.02 J
Q(total)	= 16.92 + 2.119 + 1.08 + 88.02
	= 108.1 J

X1.2.2 The thermal energy of the humidified gas can be expressed in terms of its thermodynamic properties. Applying the first law of thermodynamics for the transfer of thermal energy under an isobaric (constant pressure) condition yields the following:

$$dQ = dU + dW \qquad \text{(X1.1)}$$

X1.2.3 Calculating work under an isobaric condition:

$$dW = PdV \qquad \text{(X1.2)}$$

Therefore:

$$dQ = dU + PdV \qquad \text{(X1.3)}$$

X1.2.4 From Ref **(8)** "We find that in this very restricted case (constant pressure), the heat transfer during the process is given in terms of the change in the quantity U + PV between initial and final states. Inasmuch as all of these quantities are thermodynamic properties, functions only of the state of the system, their combination must also have these same characteristics. Therefore, we find it convenient to define a new extensive property called enthalpy (H): H = U + PV".

X1.2.5 *Extensive Property*—That which can not be directly measured but must be calculated (for example, enthalpy). In contrast to an intensive property is one which can be directly measured (for example, temperature).

Differentiating:

$$dH = dU + PdV + VdP \qquad \text{(X1.4)}$$

Substituting:

$$dQ = dU + PdV \qquad \text{(X1.5)}$$

Therefore:

$$dH = dQ - PdV + PdV + VdP \qquad \text{(X1.6)}$$

$$dH = dQ + VdP \qquad \text{(X1.7)}$$

Under isobaric conditions, $dP = 0$, therefore:

$$dH = dQ \qquad \text{(X1.8)}$$

X1.2.6 The value of specific enthalpy of 194 kJ/jg (dry gas) represents a safe level delivered in any 30-s period. This specific enthalpy level is based on Refs **(4)** and **(9)**.

X1.2.7 (Annex A3) A gravimetric technique is selected as the simplest, most consistent method to give a measure of humidifier output. Hygrometers will not provide consistent and correct results when operated in the non-isothermal environment of the breathing circuit. Attention is drawn to the definition of humidifier output that is defined as milligram water vapor per unit moist gas at 37°C. This is physically and physiologically more appropriate than other definitions as, for example, milligram per litre of dry gas.

X1.2.7.1 *Derivation*— Humidifier output:

$$n = \frac{\textit{mass of water}}{\textit{volume of dry air at 37°C} + \textit{volume of water at 37°C (saturated)}} \qquad \text{(X1.9)}$$

$$n = \frac{m_w}{V_1(1 + y(37 - T_1)) + V_{water\ 37°C\ saturated}} \qquad \text{(X1.10)}$$

where: y = expansion coefficient for dry air from 23 to 37°C.

X1.2.7.2 *Derivation of y:*

$$y = \frac{\frac{(\textit{specific volume dry air, 37°C})}{(\textit{specific volume dry air, 23°C})} - 1}{37\text{–}23°C} = \frac{\frac{0.8784}{0.8387} - 1}{14} = \frac{0.04734}{14} = 0.00338 \qquad \text{(X1.11)}$$

$$V_{water\ 37°C,sat} = \textit{volume dry air 37°C} \times \frac{(\textit{specific volume water vapor, 37°C})}{(\textit{specific volume dry air, 37°C})} \qquad \text{(X1.12)}$$

$$V_{water\ 37°C} = V_1(1 + y(37 - T_1)) \times \frac{0.9362 - 0.8784}{0.8784} = 0.6580 \times V_1\,(1 + y(37 - T_1)) \qquad \text{(X1.13)}$$

X1.2.7.3 *Derivation of Water Vapor Volume*—Substituting Eq X1.13 and the value from Eq A2.3 into Eq A2.2, rationalizing units and rearranging:

$$humidifier\ output = \frac{1000\ \text{m}}{1.0658\ V(1 + 0.0034(37 - T_1))} \tag{X1.14}$$

X1.2.8 (Annex A5) The standard temperature sensor includes an additional copper thermal mass to effect an averaging of temperature across the circuit, to minimize effects of condensation forming on the sensor, to reduce effects of precise positioning of the sensor, to increase thermal transfer to the sensor, and to ensure a stable temperature measurement.

NOTE X1.1—The copper sleeve is most easily manufactured from standard copper tube, diameter 3.18 mm or ⅛ in. The temperature bead may be a YSI Series 400 bead or equivalent.[7] Dimensions are not critical within reason. The simplest dimension check on the copper sleeve is by weight. The sleeve is 0.23 g nominal; a tolerance of ± 0.05 mm on all dimensions equates to ± 0.03 g.

REFERENCES

(**1**) Goff, J. A., and Gratch, S., "Thermodynamic Properties of Mist Air," *Trans ASHVE*, Vol 51, 1945, pp. 125–164.

(**2**) Goff, J. A., and Gratch, S.," Thermodynamic Properties of Water From – 160 to 212°F," *Trans ASHVE*, Vol 52, 1946, pp. 92–122.

(**3**) Goff, J. A., "Standardization of Thermodynamic Properties of Moist Air," *Trans ASHVE*, Vol 55, 1949, pp. 459–484.

(**4**) Moritz, A. R., MD and Henriques, F. C., Jr, MD, "Studies of Thermal Injury II The Relative Importance of Time and Surface Temperature in the Causation of Cutaneous Burns," *The American Journal of Pathology*, Vol 23, 1947, pp. 695–720.

(**5**) Fonkalsrud, E., Sanchez, M., et al, "A Comparative Study of the Effects of Dry Versus Humidified Ventilation on Canine Lungs," *Surgery*, Vol 78, No. 3, September 1975, pp. 373–380.

(**6**) Dery, R., Pelletier, J., et al, "Humidity in Anesthesiology, III Heat and Moisture Patterns in the Respiratory Tract During Anesthesia with the Semi-Closed System," *Can Anes Soc J*, Vol 14, No. 4, July 1967.

(**7**) Dery, R., "The Evolution of Heat and Moisture in the Respiratory Tract During Anesthesia with a Non-Rebreathing System," *Can Anes Soc J*, Vol 20, No. 3, May 1973.

(**8**) Wylan, and Sonntag, *Fundamentals of Classical Thermodynamics*, John Wiley and Sons, 1985.

(**9**) Stoll, Alice M., and Greene, Leon C., "Relationship Between Pain and Tissue Damage Due to Thermal Radiation," *Journal of Applied Physiology*, Vol 14, 1959, pp. 373–382.

Last ASTM Designation: F 1691 – 96

Standard Test Method for Determining Axial Pull-Out Strength of Medical Bone Screws

This test method covers the test procedure for determining the axial pull-out strength of medical bone screws.

Formerly under the jurisdiction of Committee F04 on Medical and Surgical Materials and Devices, this test method was discontinued in 2001 and replaced by Specification and Test Methods F 543 for Metallic Medical Bones Screws[1] because the complete content of Test Method F 1691 is now contained in Specification and Test Methods F 543.

[1] *Annual Book of ASTM Standards*, Vol 13.01.

Standard Guide for Training Emergency Medical Services Ambulance Operations[1]

This standard is issued under the fixed designation F 1705; the number immediately following the designation indicates the year of original adoption or, in the case of revision, the year of last revision. A number in parentheses indicates the year of last reapproval. A superscript epsilon (ε) indicates an editorial change since the last revision or reapproval.

1. Scope

1.1 This guide provides minimum training standards for Emergency Medical Services (EMS) Ambulance Operators including legal aspects, operator qualifications and testing, history of EMS vehicle operations, vehicle types/equipment, safety, physical forces, mechanics, pre-run, operations, post-run, and special circumstances.

1.2 This training guide promotes the safe and efficient delivery of the ambulance, equipment, crew, passengers and patients, during all phases of the delivery of EMS involving the ambulance; at all times exercising the highest degree of care for the safety of the public. This standard may be applied to the driving of other EMS vehicles that do not necessarily provide patient transportation.

1.3 This guide shall be used as the basis for all programs relevant to the training of the emergency medical services operators.

1.4 *This standard does not purport to address all of the safety concerns, if any, associated with its use. It is the responsibility of the user of this standard to establish appropriate safety and health practices and determine the applicability of regulatory limitations prior to use* [2].

2. Referenced Documents

2.1 *ASTM Standards:*

F 1177 Terminology Relating to Emergency Medical Services[3]

F 1229 Guide for Establishing Qualifications, Education and Training of EMS Air-Medical Patient Care Providers[3]

F 1230 Specification for Minimum Performance Requirements for Emergency Medical Service (EMS) Ground Vehicles[3]

F 1258 Practice for Emergency Medical Dispatch[3]

F 1517 Guide for the Scope of Performance of Emergency Medical Services Ambulance Operations[3]

F 1651 Practice for Training the Emergency Medical Technician (Paramedic)

TABLE 1 Emergency Medical Services Ambulance Maintenance Guidelines for Checklist Completion

Runs per week (per vehicle)	Full check	Quick check
0 to 1	every 96 h	every 24 h
2 to 3	every 72 h	every 24 h
4 to 7	every 48 h	every 24 h
8 to 50	every 24 h	every 12 h
50 +	every 24 h	every 8 h

2.2 *KKK Standards:*

1822C Specifications

3. Terminology

3.1 For definitions of other emergency medical terms, refer to Terminology F 1177:

3.2 *Definitions of Terms Specific to This Standard:*

3.2.1 *ambulance operations*—the efficient delivery of the ambulance, equipment, crew, passengers and patients, during all phases of the delivery of EMS involving the ambulance at all times exercising the highest degree of care for the safety of the public.

3.2.2 *ambulance service provider*—as outlined in this guide, a person, company, corporation or political entity responsible for operation, maintenance or policy-making, or all three, regarding emergency medical vehicle operations.

3.2.3 *bona fide occupational qualification (BFOQ)*—the skills and knowledge relevant to the performance of a specific task.

3.2.4 *departure check*—the visual check of the vehicle and surrounding area ensuring that equipment and supplies have been retrieved and properly stored and that all compartment doors are secured.

3.2.5 *egress check*—the visual check of the vehicle and surrounding area prior to operating the ambulance.

3.2.6 *emergency mode*—as defined by individual state statutes that refer to emergency vehicles, equipment and operations.

3.2.7 *full check*—a comprehensive and systematic evaluation of the ambulance at specified intervals, including documentation of the inspection, deficiencies and their corrective actions.

3.2.8 *operator*—a person who operates or assists with the operation of an ambulance.

3.2.9 *driver*—the individual responsible for operating the

[1] This guide is under the jurisdiction of ASTM Committee F-30 on Emergency Medical Services and is the direct responsibility of Subcommittee F30.02 on Personnel, Training and Education.

Current edition approved June 10, 1996. Published September 1996.

[2] Available from Government Printing Office, Superintendent of Documents, Washington, DC 20402.

[3] *Annual Book of ASTM Standards*, Vol 13.01.

ambulance in a safe and efficient manner, exercising the highest degree of care.

3.2.10 *technician*—the individual responsible for patient care.

3.2.11 *post-run*—the managed return of the ambulance and operators to optimal pre-run readiness.

3.2.12 *pre-run*—all aspects of assuring response readiness.

3.2.13 *quick check*—an abbreviated version of the full check, focusing on the major operational functions of the vehicle.

3.2.14 *reaction time*—from the time the operator identifies the hazard until the appropriate action is taken.

3.2.15 *response mode management*—the response mode of the ambulance shall be determined by dispatch protocols based on (dispatch) determinants as approved by the medical director. The determinants shall be consistent with Practice F 1258.

3.2.16 *stopping distance*—the distance the vehicle travels until it comes to a stop after the brakes are applied.

4. Significance and Use

4.1 This guide provides minimum training guidelines for safe and efficient ambulance operations.

4.2 Ambulance providers and educators should follow this guide for the development of educational and training programs.

4.3 This training guide is intended to promote safe and efficient ambulance operations and to reduce morbidity, mortality and property loss associated with ambulance operations.

4.4 This training guide is intended to assist those who are responsible for the development and implementation of policies and procedures for ambulance operations.

4.5 Topics or concepts listed in this training guide are intended to serve as an outline of materials to be covered in the training of ambulance operators.

5. Legal Aspects

5.1 The training of the ambulance operator shall include all Federal and state laws, local ordinances including the provider's policies governing emergency medical vehicle operations. The operator/driver shall have a clear understanding of the impact of those laws on the operation of the vehicle.

5.1.1 *Constitutional Law*—Laws derived from the U.S. Constitution governing the patient's right before, during and after transport.

5.1.2 *Statutory Law*—Laws derived from legislative acts.

5.1.3 *Ordinances*—Laws or guidelines enacted by a governing municipal body or its agent.

5.1.4 *Rules and Regulations*—Guidelines enacted by an agency that have the force of law that are intended to provide greater specificity about statutory laws.

5.1.5 *Case Law*—Judicial interpretation of statutory law, rules or regulations that have been decided in a court of law.

5.1.6 *Consolidated Omnibus Reconciliation Act (COBRA)/ Omnibus Reconciliation Act (OBRA) Laws*.

5.2 Integration of state laws and local ordinances with company policies/procedures. Company policy should incorporate into guidelines, the principles of applicable state laws, local ordinances, rules and regulations.

5.3 *Highest Degree of Care (Law of Due Regard)*—A general principle, frequented in case law, that holds the ambulance operator responsible for his actions regardless of perceived exemptions from traffic laws governing the emergency vehicle operator.

5.4 *Legal Issues*:

5.4.1 *Negligence*—Any action that violates a standard of practice or care related to ambulance operation.

5.4.2 *Abandonment*—Terminating care or transportation prior to being relieved by other qualified health care providers. Once a patient provider relationship is established it must continue until responsibility for the patient is assumed by a provider of equal or higher qualifications.

5.4.3 *Emergency Medical Dispatch*—An organized system of emergency medical dispatching principles intended to provide guidelines for ambulance operations as delineated in Practice F 1258.

5.4.4 *Multiple Responding Units*:

5.4.4.1 *Vehicle Separation*—The operator shall be trained to maintain a minimum 300-ft buffer zone between the ambulance and other emergency vehicles on the same route of travel.

(*1*) Weather, traffic conditions or other factors may cause the operator to increase the length of the buffer zone for the safe operation of the ambulance.

5.4.4.2 *Escorts*—The operator shall be informed of the hazards involved in the use of emergency vehicle escorts and be trained to avoid such practices.

(*1*) The operator shall be trained to discourage private, non-emergency vehicles from following the ambulance during transport.

5.4.5 *Interacting with Public Safety Agencies*:

5.4.5.1 *Command*—Ambulance operations shall be consistent with operational guides delineated in Incident Command System (ICS).

5.4.5.2 *Communication*—Ambulance communication systems should allow the ambulance operator to communicate with other public safety agencies.

5.4.5.3 *Coordination*—Cooperative guidelines shall be established with other public safety agencies in order to provide a safe and adequate response.

5.4.6 *Motor Vehicle Accidents Involving the Ambulance*:

5.4.6.1 *Reporting*—The ambulance operator shall receive instructions regarding reporting guidelines for ambulance related accidents/incidents in accordance with state laws, local ordinances, rules or regulations, and organizational policies and procedures.

5.4.7 *Mitigation/Documentation Mechanical Failures*:

5.4.7.1 *Scheduled Maintenance*—The ambulance operator shall be trained in the importance of a scheduled maintenance program.

5.4.7.2 *Vehicle and Equipment Inspections*—The ambulance operator shall be trained in the fundamentals and application of vehicle and equipment inspections.

5.4.7.3 *Reporting of Deficiencies*—The ambulance operator shall understand the importance of inspecting the ambulance and equipment, and shall be familiar with the reporting procedures utilized by the provider. The ambulance operator shall be familiar with provider policies in regard to major deficiencies which have an affect on the serviceability of the vehicle.

6. Operator Qualifications to Drive

6.1 The training of the ambulance operator shall include the components of evaluation techniques which may be utilized in screening the operator candidate:

6.1.1 *Medical Fitness to Drive*—Operators shall be subject to periodic medical evaluations as determined by the ambulance service provider. The purpose of the physical examination is to determine whether the operator has the physical ability to adequately perform his or her duty as an operator of emergency vehicles. (See Guide F 1517.)

6.2 *Authorization*:

6.2.1 The authorization of ambulance operators must be based on Bona Fide Occupational Qualification (BFOQ) pursuant to the task of ambulance operations.

6.2.2 Authorization shall be based upon cognitive evaluation of the operator regarding laws, guidelines and policies relating to ambulance operation during emergency and non-emergency modes.

6.3 A periodic review of the operator's state motor vehicle record for the previous three years with specific attention to traffic convictions concerning:

6.3.1 Speed.

6.3.2 Careless and imprudent driving.

6.3.3 Driving under the influence of alcohol or other mind-altering substances.

6.3.4 Moving violations/other violations.

6.3.5 Suspension of driver's license.

6.4 A review of the operator's motor vehicle accidents for the previous three years.

6.5 The operator shall possess a valid motor vehicle license, and any other certification required by state or local laws or regulations.

6.6 The operator's qualifications and continuing education shall be reviewed annually.

7. Operator Testing

7.1 The training of the ambulance operator shall include the components of evaluation techniques which may be utilized in screening the operator candidate:

7.1.1 Psychological testing.

7.1.2 Physical agility.

7.1.3 Driving evaluation.

7.1.4 Cognitive evaluation.

8. History of EMS Vehicle Operation

8.1 The training of the emergency vehicle operator shall include the history of EMS vehicle operation:

8.1.1 Evolution of ambulance driving from high force pursuit driving to low G-force driving techniques.

8.1.2 Changes in vehicle design and dynamics.

8.1.3 Evolution of governmental regulation.

8.1.3.1 Specification F 1230, Minimum Performance Requirements for Emergency Medical Service Ground Vehicles.

8.1.3.2 KKK 1822 Standards: "A" through current specifications.

9. Vehicular Types and Equipment

9.1 The training of the ambulance operator shall include the different ambulance classifications (Type I, II, III, and specialty response vehicles) including maneuverability, handling, weight distribution, payload allowance, and GVWR.

10. Loss Control and Safety Issues in the Operations of Ambulances

10.1 *Preventive Maintenance*—The ambulance operator shall be trained in basic techniques, documentation and rationale for preventive maintenance.

10.1.1 The operator should follow provider policies or manufacturer's suggested maintenance schedule, or both, for the ambulance.

10.2 *Operator Fatigue*—The ambulance operator shall be trained in the recognition of the adverse affects of excessive fatigue. The provider/operator shall be familiar with methods and policies used to prevent fatigue related operator dysfunction.

10.3 *Interactive Crew Roles*—Operators shall receive instruction on the importance of interactive roles utilized to lessen risk exposure, such as the ground guide/driver relationship in backing the ambulance or the driver/technician relationship in approaching controlled intersections.

10.4 *Unsafe Thought Patterns*—The operator shall be made aware of the importance of concentration on the driving task at hand and should be aware of dangerous practices such as allowing the nature of the emergency to affect driving techniques or other high-risk behavior.

10.5 *Resolving Conflict*—The driver shall be trained to make determinations regarding the safe operation of the ambulance. The operator shall be aware that the senior medical crew member shall make determinations regarding transportation mode and patient destination.

10.6 *Patient Handling Equipment*—The ambulance operator shall be trained in the proper operation, storage, and handling of all equipment used in the treatment and transport of the patient.

10.7 *OSHA Guidelines*—The operator/provider shall be trained in the utilization of OSHA guidelines pertaining to factors affecting the operation of the emergency vehicle.

10.8 *Hazmat Guidelines*—The operator shall be trained to adhere to the regulations and guidelines regarding ambulance operations near a hazardous material environment.

11. Vehicular Dynamics

11.1 *Low Force Driving*—The operator shall be trained to utilize low force driving techniques in order to minimize fatigue, stress, mechanical degradation, and other risks associated with operation of the ambulance.

11.2 *Physical Forces*—The operator shall be trained regarding the impact of physical forces on the ambulance during various operational maneuvers.

11.3 *Weight Transfer*—The operator shall be trained regarding effects that weight transfer may have on the operation of the ambulance.

11.4 *Gross Vehicle Weight Rating (GVWR)*—The operator shall be trained regarding the payload capacity of the emergency vehicle, including the adverse effects of overloading.

11.5 *Adverse Driving Conditions*—The operator shall be trained to modify driving techniques to compensate for adverse driving conditions.

12. Major Mechanical Systems

12.1 The operator shall be trained in the basic concepts related to the proper use and function of the following systems:

12.1.1 Electrical.

12.1.2 Cooling.

12.1.3 Braking.

12.1.4 Engine/Drive train.

12.1.5 Fuel.

12.1.6 Chassis.

12.1.7 Environmental control.

12.1.8 Ancillary support equipment.

12.1.9 Auxillary power.

13. Pre-Run

13.1 *Geography*—The operator shall be trained regarding the geographical area served by the provider, as well as any locating systems used by the provider.

13.2 *Environmental Factors*—The operator shall be trained to be constantly aware of changing environmental factors and how they may affect ambulance operations.

13.3 *Traffic Patterns*—The operator shall be trained to be aware of traffic flow patterns and road conditions and how they may affect ambulance operations.

13.4 *Quick Check*—The operator shall be trained to perform the quick check as outlined below:

13.4.1 Visually checking for fluid leakage.

13.4.2 Conducting vehicle warm-up.

13.4.3 Checking fluid levels.

13.4.4 Condition of belts.

13.4.5 Condition of tires.

13.4.6 Proper function of emergency lighting.

13.4.7 Proper function of lighting system.

13.4.8 Proper function of audible warning devices.

13.4.9 Vehicle cleanliness.

13.4.10 Proper function of communications equipment.

13.4.11 Proper function of warning lights.

13.5 *Full Check*—The operator shall be trained to perform the full check as outlined below:

13.5.1 Body or glass damage.

13.5.2 Proper function of emergency lights.

13.5.3 Proper function of operating lights.

13.5.4 Condition of tires.

13.5.5 Loose or missing lugs on wheels.

13.5.6 Proper function and seal of compartment doors.

13.5.7 Fluid levels.

13.5.8 Fluid leakage.

13.5.9 Condition of hoses.

13.5.10 Condition of belts.

13.5.11 Cleanliness of exterior and interior.

13.5.12 Proper function of restraint devices.

13.5.13 Proper function of gages.

13.5.14 Proper function of windshield wipers/washer.

13.5.15 Proper function of communications equipment.

13.5.16 Proper adjustment of mirrors.

13.5.17 Proper function of audible warning devices.

13.5.18 Proper adjustment of seats.

13.5.19 Proper adjustment of steering wheel.

13.5.20 Condition of fire extinguishers.

13.5.21 Proper function of environmental control systems.

13.5.22 Inventory of equipment and supplies.

13.5.23 Level and alignment of chassis.

13.5.24 Proper function of warning indicator lights.

13.6 *Documentation of Problems*—The operator shall be trained in techniques of proper documentation and reporting of problems found through the quick or full check.

14. Operations

14.1 The operator shall be trained in all aspects of emergency vehicle operations as they pertain to the overall prehospital care within the response area. The following subjects shall be included in the training curriculum:

14.1.1 *Response Mode Management*:

14.1.1.1 The operator shall be informed of studies that indicate that 40 % of all ambulance calls are requested as an emergency and of those 20 % are true medical emergencies with less than 5 % being life-threatening.

14.1.1.2 The two response modes are:

(*1*) *Emergency*—Exercising emergency driving privileges and the utilization of all emergency warning lights and audible warning systems.

(*2*) *Non-emergency*—Operating the vehicle under all traffic laws which govern the general operation of motor vehicles.

14.2 *Route Selection*—The operator shall, on the basis of known information, and pre-run planning, determine the best route of travel.

14.2.1 If the location is unknown, the operator should communicate with the dispatcher or the on-scene personnel for the most direct route of travel.

14.3 *Egress Check*—Before beginning the response, the operator shall conduct a brief egress check consisting of the following:

14.3.1 Vehicle/compartment doors are closed and securely latched.

14.3.2 Vehicle hood is closed and securely latched.

14.3.3 Vehicle shore line is disconnected.

14.3.4 All equipment is secured.

14.3.5 Facility egress door is fully opened.

14.3.6 Patient stretcher is in place and secured.

14.4 *Operational Check*:

14.4.1 Utilize vehicle safety restraints.

14.4.2 Adjust the operator's seat.

14.4.3 Adjust the operator's mirrors.

14.4.4 Switch on the battery(-ies) (according to manufacturer's specifications).

14.4.5 Start the engine.

14.4.6 Review all gages.

14.4.7 Adjust environmental controls.

14.4.8 Activate communication system and contact dispatch.

14.4.9 Adjust tilt wheel (if applicable).

14.4.10 Activate headlights.

14.4.11 Activate the emergency warning lights (if applicable).

14.4.12 Activate the audible emergency warning devices (if applicable).

14.4.13 Partially open the driver's side window.

14.4.14 Evaluate brake pedal resistance.

14.4.15 Place the vehicle transmission in gear.

14.4.16 Activate the turn signal (if applicable).

14.5 *Operator (Crew) Roles*:

14.5.1 Operate the ambulance in a safe and efficient manner, exercising the highest degree of care.

14.5.2 Utilize eye sweep.

14.5.3 *Safe Following Distances*:

14.5.3.1 Maintain a 3 to 4-s following distance between the ambulance and the vehicle directly in front.

14.5.3.2 Operator reaction time will affect safe following distances.

14.5.3.3 Adverse and environmental conditions will affect safe following distances.

14.5.4 Operate the vehicle at a speed that is safe for conditions.

14.5.4.1 Under emergency response conditions, the speed shall not exceed that which is safe for road or environmental conditions. In no case shall the speed exceed 10 miles/h over the posted speed limit.

14.5.5 Operate all warning devices as appropriate for traffic conditions.

14.5.6 *Ambulance Communication System*:

14.5.6.1 Whenever possible, radio transmissions should be made by another crew member. This will enable the operator to devote full attention to the operation of the vehicle.

14.5.6.2 Whenever possible, the public address system operation should be done by another crew member. This will enable the operator to devote full attention to the operation of the vehicle.

14.5.6.3 The operator and crew members shall be trained in the proper operation of the vehicle communication system. In addition to general knowledge of the communication systems and protocols, the operator must have a total understanding of the emergency services' communication system within their service area.

14.5.6.4 The operator shall also be responsible for the understanding of all communications equipment used within the EMS and provider's system.

14.5.7 Adhere to the agency's policies and procedures in the driving of the emergency vehicle.

14.5.8 Utilize a smooth and constant rate of acceleration.

14.5.9 Use engine compression in slowing the emergency vehicle.

14.5.10 Utilize smooth braking and cornering of the emergency vehicle.

14.5.11 *Ensure Adequate Stopping Distance*:

14.5.11.1 When stopped in traffic, the operator must be able to see five feet of road, in addition to the bumper and both rear tires of the vehicle in front.

14.5.11.2 Exceeding the payload capacity will adversely affect the normal stopping distances.

14.5.11.3 Antilock braking systems (ABS) may affect stopping distances.

14.5.11.4 Operator reaction time will affect stopping distance.

14.5.11.5 Adverse and environmental conditions will affect the stopping distance.

14.5.12 Utilize the 10-s lane change procedure.

14.5.13 Maintain a rear and side space cushion.

14.5.14 *Backing with a Ground Guide*:

14.5.14.1 The operator is responsible for safely backing the emergency vehicle.

14.5.14.2 The operator shall never begin to back the vehicle before it has come to a complete stop.

14.5.14.3 A ground guide should be in place, 8 to 10 ft behind the left rear of the emergency vehicle.

14.5.14.4 Eye, hand and voice communications must be established between the operator and the ground guide.

14.5.15 Shall be trained in special transport procedures, (neonate, psychiatric, etc.).

14.5.15.1 Knowledge and use of specialized transport equipment.

14.5.16 Utilize special safety precautions with multiple personnel in the patient compartment.

14.5.16.1 Safety restraints.

14.5.16.2 Overloading.

14.5.16.3 Additional medical personnel.

14.5.16.4 Non-medical passengers.

14.5.17 Safely utilize patient handling equipment.

14.5.18 Utilize other crew members in the operation of the emergency vehicle.

14.5.18.1 Non-crew members operating the emergency vehicle.

14.6 *Warning Device Operation*:

14.6.1 The operator is responsible for utilization of appropriate warning devices to protect the scene and the vehicle.

14.7 *Passing Other Vehicles Safely*:

14.7.1 Verify that the oncoming lane is clear.

14.7.2 Check mirrors to find an opening in the adjacent lane.

14.7.3 Signal intentions by having the signal lever in the "on" position for at least 3 s before changing lanes.

14.7.4 Check blind spots.

14.7.5 Gradually turn the wheel for a smooth, accurate movement.

14.7.6 Increase speed slightly.

14.7.7 The operator should not reenter the lane of the passed vehicle until he has cleared it by a minimum of one vehicle length.

14.7.7.1 The operator shall use signaling devices prior to and during lane changes.

14.7.8 The operator shall time the vehicle's arrival into the other lane to avoid interfering with the flow of traffic.

14.8 *Oncoming Traffic Lane Operations*:

14.8.1 The operator shall not enter an opposing traffic lane until it is safe to do so and all other oncoming vehicle drivers are aware of the ambulance's presence.

14.9 *Controlled Intersection Management During an Emergency Response Mode*:

14.9.1 The operator shall ensure that the siren is in the wail mode 300 ft prior to the intersection.

14.9.2 The operator shall activate the yelp mode of the siren

150 ft prior to the intersection.

14.9.3 The operator shall remove his foot from the accelerator to cover the brake pedal and allow compression to slow the vehicle enabling the operator to start to apply the brake to bring the ambulance to a complete stop.

14.9.4 If the ambulance has an air-driven audible airhorn, give two short blasts on the airhorn.

14.9.5 Look to the left, look to the right, then again to the left. The operator may then proceed through the intersection at a speed of under 10 miles/h if traffic is stopped in all lanes to the left, in front of and to the right of the ambulance. After the operator has made eye contact with all stopped vehicle drivers, the ambulance may proceed through the intersection exercising the highest degree of care.

14.9.6 Continue the siren yelp mode activation and proceed through the intersection exercising the highest degree of care.

14.9.7 When there are vacant lanes to the left or right, the operator must complete the previous steps of clearing each lane of traffic prior to crossing that lane.

14.9.8 The operator should anticipate that any vacant lane to his left or right may become occupied by another vehicle which did not see or hear the ambulance's warning systems.

14.9.9 The operator should be aware that other emergency vehicles may be approaching the same intersection of which the operator has taken control. The ambulance should not enter the intersection until the other emergency vehicles have stopped or proceeded through the intersection.

14.9.10 The operator should avoid passing stopped vehicles on the right.

14.9.11 The operator should turn right at an intersection only after all vehicles have stopped and drivers on the right are aware of the ambulance.

14.9.12 The operator should anticipate that any vehicles in front may make an unexpected left turn in front of the ambulance after it has started to enter the intersection.

14.9.13 The operator must be aware of other hazards at the intersection, for example, pedestrians, road hazards, defective traffic control systems.

14.10 *U-turns*:

14.10.1 The operator shall not make U-turns in traffic until all traffic has stopped. When doing so, all warning devices must be activated prior to executing the U-turn.

14.11 *Defensive Driving Techniques*:

14.11.1 The operator is responsible for practicing defensive driving techniques under all conditions, exercising the highest degree of care.

14.12 *Scene Management*:

14.12.1 *Scene Approach and Size-Up*—The operator is responsible for overall evaluation and safe approach of the scene.

14.12.2 *Parking*—The operator shall not park the ambulance so as to create a traffic hazard unless warning or other traffic control devices, or both, are being utilized.

14.12.2.1 *Emergency Scene*:

(*1*) The operator is responsible for safely parking the ambulance at the scene to protect the ambulance, crew members, patients and the scene.

(*2*) The operator is responsible for setting the parking brake prior to placing the transmission in the park position.

(*3*) When there is a significant electrical load on the ambulance that is parked the automatic idle advance should be activated.

(*4*) When possible, the vehicle should be positioned so that it will not be required to back into traffic when leaving the scene.

15. Post-Run

15.1 *Decontamination*:

15.1.1 The operator shall be trained in infection control guidelines according to the Centers for Disease Control (CDC),[4] the Occupational Safety and Hazards Association (OSHA)[5] or applicable state laws for handling contaminated linen and cleaning the ambulance interior.

15.1.2 The operator shall be trained in the agency's exposure control plan, including biohazard disposal procedures.

15.1.3 Training shall include those procedures and activities required to make the ambulance ready for immediate service after the delivery of a patient.

15.1.3.1 *Cleaning the Patient Compartment*:

(*1*) Clean blood, vomitus and other body fluids.

(*2*) Remove and dispose of used or opened disposable items and dressings.

(*3*) Clean and disinfect the floor.

(*4*) Bag soiled linens appropriately.

(*5*) Use deodorizer to neutralize odors.

(*6*) Disinfect any equipment or surfaces that touched the patient or were otherwise contaminated.

15.1.3.2 *Make Up the Ambulance Cot*:

(*1*) Clean and disinfect the mattress surface.

(*2*) Clean and disinfect the cot.

(*3*) Remake the cot with clean linen per local protocols.

15.1.3.3 Air the ambulance by opening windows, using air conditioning or the ventilation system.

15.1.3.4 Crew members should wash their hands.

15.1.4 Training should include those procedures and activities necessary after returning to quarters.

15.1.4.1 Place contaminated items in biohazard containers.

15.1.4.2 Prepare the crew for service.

(*1*) Wash hands thoroughly.

(*2*) Change soiled clothes.

15.1.4.3 Clean vehicle exterior as needed.

15.2 *Resupply*:

15.2.1 The operator shall be trained in the local policies and procedures for restocking the ambulance to ensure that disposables and other equipment are replaced.

15.3 *Fuel*:

15.3.1 The operator shall be trained to ensure that the vehicle is replenished with fuel and other fluids. Refuel per local policy to maintain such a level that the ambulance can respond to the farthest point of coverage area and then to a medical facility without running out of fuel.

15.3.2 The operator shall be trained to ensure that the proper

[4] Centers for Disease Control, 4770 Buford Highway MS-46, Atlanta, GA 30341-3724.

[5] Occupational Safety and Health Administration, 200 Constitution Ave NW, Washington, DC 20277-2975.

quality and type of fuel is used in the ambulance pursuant to manufacturer's specifications.

15.4 *Documentation*:

15.4.1 The operator shall be trained to ensure that all documentation is completed in accordance with company policy and state or local regulation.

16. Special Circumstances

16.1 The training of the operator shall include special circumstances under which normal vehicle operation criteria may be altered.

16.1.1 *Aeromedical Scene Control*—The operator shall be trained in all aspects of scene control as it pertains to the safe approach, landing and take-off of fixed and rotary wing aircraft.

16.2 *Interfacility Transfers Under COBRA/OBRA Laws*—The operator shall be trained in all aspects including COBRA/OBRA laws.

16.3 *Multiple Casualty Incidents*—The operator shall be trained in accordance with local multiple casualty incidents/disaster plans.

16.4 *Unsecured Scene Approach*—The operator shall be trained to recognize and avoid any scene that may be unsafe.

APPENDIX

(Nonmandatory Information)

X1.

For additional information see the following sources:

X1.1 Department of Transportation (DOT)—Training Program for Operation of Emergency Vehicles

X1.2 National Safety Council—Coaching the Emergency Vehicle Driver

X1.3 American Ambulance Association (AAA) Clinical Standard for Operations

X1.4 The Brady Company—Emergency Ambulance Driving

X1.5 Life Link III—Emergency Vehicle Driving Program

X1.6 The Medical Commission on Accident Prevention, Medical Aspects of Fitness to Drive

X1.7 DOT/NHTSA Model Driver Screening and Evaluation Program (March 1, 1992, Draft)

X1.8 Federal Motor Carrier Safety Regulations (49 CFR 391 41 391 49)

X1.9 AzStar Center for Safety and Risk Management, Operator/Driver Training Program

X1.10 Occupational Safety and Health Administration (OSHA) Guidelines—Bloodborne Pathogens

X1.11 OSHA Guidelines—Hazardous Materials

X1.12 Americans with Disabilities Act (ADA)

X1.13 DOT, Functional Aspects of Driver Impairment

X1.14 Allsafe Driving System

X1.15 International Fire Service Training Association (IFSTA) Fire Department Pumping Apparatus, 7th Edition

X1.16 DOT Guidelines for the evaluation and structuring of a driver training process for law enforcement personnel

X1.17 Volunteer Insurance Services

X1.18 American Ambulance Association (AAA) Communicable and Infectious Disease Control

Standard Specification for Wrought Titanium-13Niobium-13Zirconium Alloy for Surgical Implant Applications[1]

This standard is issued under the fixed designation F 1713; the number immediately following the designation indicates the year of original adoption or, in the case of revision, the year of last revision. A number in parentheses indicates the year of last reapproval. A superscript epsilon (ϵ) indicates an editorial change since the last revision or reapproval.

1. Scope

1.1 This specification covers the chemical, mechanical, and metallurgical requirements for wrought titanium13niobium-13zirconium alloy to be used in the manufacture of surgical implants **(1)**.[2]

1.2 The values stated in inch pound units are to be regarded as the standard. The metric equivalents in parentheses are provided for information only.

2. Referenced Documents

2.1 *ASTM Standards:*

E 8 Methods of Tension Testing of Metallic Materials[3]

E 120 Test Methods for Chemical Analysis of Titanium and Titanium Alloys[4]

E 1409 Test Method for the Determination of Oxygen in Titanium and Titanium Alloys by the Inert Gas Fusion Technique[4]

E 1447 Test Method for the Determination of Hydrogen in Titanium and Titanium Alloys by the Inert Gas Fusion Thermal Conductivity Method[4]

F 748 Practice for Selecting Generic Biological Test Methods for Materials and Devices[5]

F 981 Practice for Assessment of Compatibility of Biomaterials for Surgical Implants with Respect to Effect of Materials on Muscle and Bone[5]

F 1472 Specification for Wrought TI-6AI-4V Alloy for Surgical Implant Applications[5]

2.2 *Other Standards:*

ASOC C1 Specification of General Requirements for a Quality Control Program[6]

AMS 2249 Chemical Check Analysis Limits, Titanium and Titanium Alloys[7]

3. Terminology

3.1 *Definitions of Terms Specific to This Standard:*

3.1.1 *capability aged, n*—the condition of the material that is obtained if, following solution treatment, a sample of the mill product is subjected to an aging treatment such as given below, for certification testing.

3.1.1.1 Ramp up from room temperature to 923 ± 25°F (495 ± 14°C) over 2.5 ± 1 h.

3.1.1.2 Age for 6 ± 0.25 h at 923 ± 25°F (495 ± 14°C).

3.1.1.3 Remove from furnace and air cool to room temperature.

3.1.2 *solution treated, n*—the condition of the material that is obtained if, following the final hot-working or cold-working operation, the mill product is rapidly quenched, for example, by water quenching, from a temperature above 1112°F (600°C).

3.1.3 *unannealed, n*—the condition of the material that is obtained after the normal hot-working or cold-working operation used for fabrication of the mill product. There are no subsequent heat treatment requirements.

4. Product Classification

4.1 *Strip*—Any product under 0.1875 in. (4.75 mm) in thickness and under 24 in. (610 mm) wide.

4.2 *Sheet*—Any product under 0.1875 in. (4.75 mm) in thickness and 24 in. (610 mm) or more in width.

4.3 *Plate*—Any product 0.1875 in. (4.75 mm) thick and over and 10 in. (254 mm) wide and over, with widths greater than five times thickness. Plate up to 4 in. (101.60 mm), thick inclusive is covered by this specification.

4.4 *Bar*—Rounds or flats from 3⁄16 in. (4.75 mm) to 4 in. (101.60 mm) in diameter or thickness. (Other sizes and shapes by special order.)

4.5 *Wire*—Rounds less than 3⁄16 in. (75 mm) in diameter.

5. Ordering Information

5.1 Include with inquiries and orders for material under this specification the following information.

5.1.1 Quantity (weight or number of pieces),

5.1.2 Applicable ASTM designation,

5.1.3 Form (sheet, strip, plate, wire, or bar),

5.1.4 Condition (see Section 3 and 6.1),

5.1.5 Mechanical properties (if applicable, for special conditions),

---

[1] This specification is under the jurisdiction of ASTM Committee F-4 on Medical and Surgical Materials and Devices and is the direct responsibility of Subcommittee F04.12 on Metallurgical Materials.

Current edition approved July 10, 1996. Published August 1996.

[2] The boldface numbers in parentheses refer to the list of references at the end of the text.

[3] *Annual Book of ASTM Standards*, Vol 03.01.

[4] *Annual Book of ASTM Standards*, Vol 03.05.

[5] *Annual Book of ASTM Standards*, Vol 13.01.

[6] Available from the American Society for Quality Control, 161 W. Wisconsin Ave., Milwaukee, WI 53203.

[7] Available from the Society of Automotive Engineers, 400 Commonwealth Drive, Warrendale, PA 15096.

5.1.6 Finish (see 6.2),

5.1.7 Applicable dimensions including size, thickness, width, or print number,

5.1.8 Special tests, and

5.1.9 Special requirements.

6. Materials and Manufacture

6.1 The various titanium mill products covered in this specification normally are formed with the conventional forging and rolling equipment found in primary ferrous and nonferrous plants. The ingot metal for such mill operations is usually multiple melted in arc furnaces (including furnaces such as plasma arc and electron beam) of a type conventionally used for reactive metals.

6.2 *Finish*—The mill product may be furnished to the implant manufacturer as descaled or pickled, sandblasted, ground, machined, or combinations of these operations.

7. Chemical Requirements

7.1 Ensure that the heat analysis conforms to the chemical composition of Table 1. Ingot analysis may be used for reporting all chemical requirements, except hydrogen. Take samples for hydrogen from the finished mill product.

7.1.1 Requirements for the major and minor elemental constituents are listed in Table 1. Also listed are important residual elements. Analysis for elements not listed in Table 1 is not required to verify compliance with this specification.

7.2 Product analysis tolerances do not broaden the specified heat analysis requirements but cover variations between laboratories in the measurement of chemical content. The manufacturer shall not ship material that is outside the limits specified in Table 1. Ensure that the product analysis tolerances conform to the check tolerances of Table 2.

7.3 For referee purposes, use Methods E 120 or other analytical methods agreed upon between the purchaser and the supplier.

7.4 Ensure that the samples for chemical analysis are representative of the material being tested. The utmost care must be used in sampling titanium for chemical analysis because of its affinity for elements such as oxygen, nitrogen, and hydrogen. In cutting samples for analysis, therefore, the operation should be carried out insofar as possible in a dust-free atmosphere. Chips should be clean and sharp. Samples for analysis should be stored in suitable containers.

8. Mechanical Requirements

8.1 Ensure that the material supplied under this specification conforms to the mechanical property requirements given in Table 3.

TABLE 1 Chemical Requirements

Element	Composition, %
Nitrogen, max	0.05
Carbon, max	0.08
Hydrogen, max	0.012[A]
Iron, max	0.25
Oxygen, max	0.15
Niobium	12.5–14.0
Zirconium	12.5–14.0
Titanium[B]	balance

[A] Material 0.032 in. (0.813 mm) and under may have hydrogen content up to 0.015 %.

[B] The percentage of titanium is determined by difference and need not be determined or certified.

TABLE 2 Product Analysis Tolerance[A]

Element	Tolerance Under the Minimum or Over the Maximum Limit[B]
Nitrogen	0.02
Carbon	0.02
Hydrogen	0.0020
Iron	0.10
Oxygen	0.02
Niobium	0.30
Zirconium	0.40

[A] Refer to AMS 2249.

[B] Under the minimum limit not applicable for elements where only a maximum percentage is indicated.

8.2 Specimens for tension tests shall be machined and tested in accordance with Test Methods E 8. Tensile properties shall be determined using a strain rate of 0.003 to 0.007 in./in./min (mm/mm/min) through the specified yield strength, and then the cross-head speed shall be increased so as to produce fracture in approximately one additional minute.

8.3 *Number of Tests*—Perform a minimum of two tension tests from each lot. A lot is defined as the total number of mill products produced under the same conditions at essentially the same time. Should either of the two test specimens not meet the specified requirements, test two additional test pieces representative of the same lot in the same manner. The lot will be considered in compliance only if both additional test pieces meet the specified requirements. If a specimen fails outside the gage, the test is null in accordance with Methods E 8, and a retest shall be performed.

9. Special Requirements

9.1 Ensure that the microstructure is martensitic with finely dispersed alpha or beta phases, or both. The alpha or beta phases, or both, may be too fine to be visible metallographically but must be present to ensure adequate strength. No continuous alpha network at prior beta grain boundaries will be present. The microstructure within the prior beta grain boundaries will be acicular. Perform metallographic evaluation in the aged condition.

9.2 Determine the beta transus temperature for each heat by a suitable method and reported on the materials certification, if required by the purchaser.

9.3 Products supplied with a machined or ground surface finish will have no alpha case. For other products, there will be

TABLE 3 Mechanical Properties[ABC]

Condition	Tensile Strength min, psi (MPa)	Yield Strength (0.2 % offset), min psi (MPa)	Elongation in 4d or 4w min, %[D]	Reduction of Area min, %[E]
Capability aged	125 000 (860)	105 000 (725)	8	15
Solution treated	80 000 (550)	50 000 (345)	15	30
Unannealed	80 000 (550)	50 000 (345)	8	15

[A] Up to 4 in. (101.60 mm) including thickness or diameter.

[B] Mechanical property requirements apply to both longitudinal and transverse directions in plate, sheet and strip only.

[C] Solution treated or unannealed material is not intended for use as a final product without subsequent hot working or heat treatment, or both.

[D] Measure elongation on material under 0.187 in. (4.75 mm) in thickness or diameter over a 2 in. gage length. Elongation on material under 0.032 in. (0.813 mm) in thickness may be obtained by negotiation.

[E] Applies to bar and plate only.

no continuous layer of alpha case, when examined at 100 ×.

10. Certification

10.1 The manufacturer will provide a certification of the material that the material was manufactured and tested in accordance with this specification. A report of test results will be furnished at the time of shipment.

11. Quality Program Requirements

11.1 The producer will maintain a quality program, such as is defined in Specification ASQC C1.

12. Keywords

12.1 metals (for surgical implants)–titanium alloys; orthopaedic medical devices—titanium/titanium alloy; titanium/titanium alloys (for surgical implants)

APPENDIXES

(Nonmandatory Information)

X1. RATIONALE

X1.1 The purpose of this specification is to characterize the chemical, physical, mechanical, and metallurgical properties of wrought titanium-13niobium-13zirconium alloy to be used in the manufacture of surgical implants.

X1.2 The microstructural requirements contained in this specification represent the current general consensus with respect to optimization of mechanical properties for implant applications.

X1.3 The minimum mechanical properties specified ensure a baseline of strength and ductility for the highly stressed devices for which this alloy is typically used.

X1.4 The stress corrosion cracking resistance of this alloy is similar to that of standard grade titanium-6aluminum4vanadium alloy **(2)**.

X2. BIOCOMPATIBILITY

X2.1 The suitability of this material from a human implant perspective is dependent on the specific application. The biologic tests appropriate for the specific site, such as recommended in Practice F 748 should be used as a guideline. A summary of the in vitro and animal testing that has been performed as of the approval date of this specification is provided in X2.3.

X2.2 No known surgical implant material has ever been shown to be completely free of adverse reactions in the human body. The alloy composition covered by this specification, however, has been subjected to testing in laboratory animals, and has been used clinically since June 1994. The results of these studies indicate a well-characterized level of local biological response that is equal to or less than that produced by the reference material titanium-6aluminum-4 vanadium alloy (see specification F 1472) that has a long history of successful clinical application in soft tissue and bone implants in humans.

X2.3 As of the time of the original approval of this specification, this titanium alloy material had a limited history of clinical use in humans. An extensive series of in vitro and animal studies had been performed **(3,4,5,6)**, as listed as follows, comparing the biological response to that of a reference material, titanium-6aluminum-4vanadium alloy. These tests were conducted to support the usage of this material in surgical implant devices **(6,7,8,9)**. In all cases, the results indicated that this material was no more reactive with the environment than the reference material.

X2.3.1 L929 MEM-Cytotoxicity (Mouse Fibroblasts),

X2.3.2 Sensitization Assay (Kligman Maximization Study),

X2.3.3 Rabbit Pyrogen Test,

X2.3.4 Mammalian Mutagenicity Test (Rodent Bone Marrow Micronucleus Test),

X2.3.5 Rabbit Intramuscular Implantation Test,

X2.3.6 Rabbit Blood Hemolysis Test,

X2.3.7 Ames Mutagenicity Assay, and

X2.3.8 Systemic Toxicity and Irritation Test (USP XXII Biological Test).

REFERENCES

(**1**) Mishra, A.K., Davidson, J.A., Kovacs, P., and Poggie, R.A., "Ti13Nb-13Zr: A New Low Modulus, High Strength, Corrosion Resistant, Near Beta Alloy for Orthopaedic Implants," Beta Titanium Alloys in the 1990's, D. Eylon, R.R. Boyer, and D.A. Koss, eds., The Minerals, Metals and Materials Society, Warrendale, PA, 1993, pp. 61–72.

(**2**) Mishra, A.K., and Davidson, J. A., "Stress Corrosion Cracking Resistance of Ti-13Nb-13Zr," *Annals of Biomedical Engineering*, Vol 21(1), 1993, pp. 67.

(**3**) Mishra, A.K., Davidson, J.A., Kovacs, P., and Poggie, R.A., "Mechanical, Tribological and Electrochemical Behavior of Ti13Nb-13Zr–A New, Low Modulus Titanium Alloy for Orthopaedic Implants," Proc. 12th S. Biomedical Eng. Conf., New Orleans, LA, April 2–4, 1993, IEEE, Piscataway, NJ, 1993, pp. 13–15.

(**4**) Goodman, S.B., Davidson, J.A., Fornasier, V.L., and Mishra, A.K., "Histological Response to Cylinders of a Low Modulus Titanium Alloy (Ti-13Nb-13Zr) and a Wear Resistant Zirconium Alloy (Zr-2.5Nb) Implanted in the Rabbit Tibia," *Journal of Applied Biomaterials*, Vol 4, 1993, pp. 331–339.

(**5**) Kovacs, P., and Davidson, J.A., "The Electrochemical Behavior of a New Titanium Alloy with Superior Biocompatibility," Titanium '92: Science and Technology, F.H. Froes and I. Caplan, eds., The Minerals, Metals and Materials Society, Warrendale, PA, 1993, pp. 2705–2712.

(**6**) FDA 510(k) No. K914343.

(**7**) FDA 510(k) No. K930480.

(**8**) FDA 510(k) No. K936233.

(**9**) FDA 510(k) No. K943523.

Designation: F 1714 – 96

Standard Guide for Gravimetric Wear Assessment of Prosthetic Hip-Designs in Simulator Devices[1]

This standard is issued under the fixed designation F 1714; the number immediately following the designation indicates the year of original adoption or, in the case of revision, the year of last revision. A number in parentheses indicates the year of last reapproval. A superscript epsilon (ε) indicates an editorial change since the last revision or reapproval.

1. Scope

1.1 This guide describes a laboratory method using a weight-loss technique for evaluating the wear properties of materials or devices, or both, which are being considered for use as bearing surfaces of human-hip-joint replacement prostheses. The hip prostheses are evaluated in a device intended to simulate the tribological conditions encountered in the human hip joint, for example, use of a fluid such as bovine serum, or equivalent pseudosynovial fluid shown to simulate similar wear mechanisms and debris generation as found in vivo, and test frequencies of 1 Hz or less.

1.2 Since the hip simulator method permits the use of actual implant designs, materials, and physiological load/motion combinations, it can represent a more physiological simulation than basic wear-screening tests, such as pin-on-disk (see Practice F 732) or ring-on-disk (see ISO-6474).

1.3 It is the intent of this guide to rank the combination of implant designs and materials with regard to material wear-rates, under simulated physiological conditions. It must be recognized, however, that there are many possible variations in the in vivo conditions, a single laboratory simulation with a fixed set of parameters may not be universally representative.

1.4 The reference materials for the comparative evaluation of candidate materials, new devices, or components, or a combination thereof, shall be the wear rate of extruded or compression-molded, ultra-high molecular weight (UHMW) polyethylene (see Specification F 648) bearing against standard counter faces [stainless steel (see Specification F 138); cobalt-chromium-molybdenum alloy (see Specification F 75); thermomechanically processed cobalt chrome (see Specification F 799); alumina ceramic (see Specification F 603)], having typical prosthetic quality, surface finish, and geometry similar to those with established clinical history. These reference materials will be tested under the same wear conditions as the candidate materials.

2. Referenced Documents

2.1 *ASTM Standards:*

D 883 Terminology Relating to Plastics[2]

F 75 Specification for Cast Cobalt-Chromium-Molybdenum Alloy for Surgical Implant Applications[3]

F 86 Practice for Surface Preparation and Marking of Metallic Surgical Implants[3]

F 136 Specification for Titanium 6A1-4V ELI Alloy for Surgical Implant Applications[3]

F 138 Specification for Stainless Steel Bar and Wire for Surgical Implants (Special Quality)[3]

F 370 Specification for Proximal Femoral Prosthesis[3]

F 565 Practice for Care and Handling of Orthopedic Implants and Instruments[3]

F 603 Specification for High-Purity Dense Aluminum Oxide for Surgical Implant Application[3]

F 648 Specification for Ultra-High-Molecular-Weight Polyethylene Powder and Fabricated Form for Surgical Implants[3]

F 732 Practice for Pin-on-Flat Evaluation of Friction and Wear Properties of Polymeric Materials for Use in Total Joint Prostheses[3]

F 799 Specification for Thermomechanically Processed Cobalt-Chrome-Molybdenum Alloy for Surgical Implants[3]

G 40 Terminology Relating to Erosion and Wear[4]

2.2 *ISO Standard:*

ISO 6474 Implants for Surgery–Ceramic Materials Based on Alumina[5]

3. Significance and Use

3.1 This guide uses a weight-loss method of wear determination for the polymeric components used with hip-joint prostheses, using serum or demonstrated equivalent fluid for lubrication, and running under a dynamic load profile representative of the human hip-joint forces during walking **(1,2)**.[6] The basis for this weight-loss method for wear measurement was originally developed **(3)** for pin-on-disk wear studies (see Practice F 732) and has been extended to total hip replacements **(4,5)** and to femoral-tibial knee prostheses **(6)**, and to femoropatellar knee prostheses **(6,7)**.

[1] This guide is under the jurisdiction of ASTM Committee F-4 on Medical and Surgical Materials and Devicesand is the direct responsibility of Subcommittee F04.22on Arthroplasty.

Current edition approved Sept. 10, 1996. Published October 1996.

[2] *Annual Book of ASTM Standards*, Vol 08.01.

[3] *Annual Book of ASTM Standards*, Vol 13.01.

[4] *Annual Book of ASTM Standards*, Vol 03.02.

[5] Available from American National Standards Institute, 11 W. 42nd St., 13th Floor, New York, NY 10036.

[6] The boldface numbers in parentheses refer to the list of references at the end of this standard.

3.2 While wear results in a change in the physical dimensions of the specimen, it is distinct from dimensional changes due to creep or plastic deformation, in that wear generally results in the removal of material in the form of polymeric debris particles, causing a loss in weight of the specimen.

3.3 This guide for measuring wear of the polymeric component is suitable for various simulator devices. These techniques can be used with metal, ceramic, carbon, polymeric, and composite counter faces bearing against a polymeric material (for example, polyethylene, polyacetal, and so forth). This weight-loss method, therefore, has universal application for wear studies of total-hip replacements that feature polymeric bearings. This weight-loss method has not been validated for high-density material bearing systems, such as metal-metal, carbon-carbon, or ceramic-ceramic. Progressive wear of such rigid bearing combinations generally has been monitored using a linear, variable-displacement transducers or by other profilometric techniques.

4. Apparatus and Materials

4.1 *Hip Prosthesis Components*—The hip-joint prosthesis comprises a ball-and-socket configuration in which materials such as polymers, composites, metal alloys, ceramics, and carbon have been used in various combinations and designs.

4.2 *Component Configurations*—The diameter of the prosthetic ball may vary from 22 to 54 mm or larger. The design may include ball-socket, trunnion, bipolar, or other configurations.

4.3 *Hip Simulator*:

4.3.1 *Test Chambers*—In the case of a multi-specimen machine, contain the components in individual, isolated chambers to prevent contamination of one set of components with debris from another test. Ensure that the chamber is made entirely of noncorrosive materials, such as acrylic plastic or stainless steel, and is easily removable from the machine for thorough cleaning between tests. Design the wear chambers such that the test bearing surfaces are immersed in the lubricant throughout the test **(3,7)**.

4.3.2 *Component Clamping Fixtures*—Since wear is to be determined from the weight loss of the components, the method for mounting the components in the test chamber should not compromise the accuracy of assessment of the weight-loss due to wear.

4.3.3 *Load*—Ensure that the test load profile is representative of that which occurs during the patients walking cycle, with peak hip-loads ≥2 kN **(2)**. The loading apparatus must be free to follow the specimen as wear occurs, such that the applied load is constant to within ±3 % for the duration of the test. Never allow the applied load to be below that required to keep the chambers seated (for example, 50 N) **(4)**.

4.3.4 *Motion*—Ensure that relative motion between the hip components oscillates and simulates the flexion-extension arc of walking. Addition of internal-external or abduction-adduction arcs is at the investigator's discretion. It is recommended that the orientations of the cup and ball relative to each other and to the load-axis be maintained by suitable specimen-holder keying.

4.3.5 *Oscillating Frequency*—Oscillate the hip prostheses at a rate of one cycle per second (1 Hz).

4.3.6 *Cycle Counter*—Include a counter with the hip-simulator to record the total number of wear cycles.

4.3.7 *Friction*—It is recommended that the machine include sensors capable of monitoring the friction forces transmitted across the bearing-surfaces during the wear test.

4.4 *Lubricant*:

4.4.1 It is recommended that the specimen be lubricated with bovine blood serum, however, another suitable lubrication medium may be used if validated.

4.4.2 If serum is used, then use filtered-sterilized serum rather than pooled serum since the former is less likely to contain hemolyzed blood material, which has been shown to adversely affect the lubricating properties of the serum **(3)**. Diluted solutions of serum also have been used for this purpose **(8)**. Filtration may remove hard, abrasive, particulate contaminants that might otherwise affect the wear properties of the specimens being tested.

4.4.3 Maintain the volume and concentration of the lubricant nearly constant throughout the test. This may be accomplished by sealing the chambers so that water does not evaporate, or periodically or continuously replacing evaporated water with distilled water.

4.4.4 To retard bacterial degradation, freeze and store the serum until needed for test. In addition, ensure that the fluid medium in the test contains 0.2 % sodium azide (or other suitable antibiotic) to minimize bacterial degradation. Other lubricants should be evaluated to determine appropriate storage conditions.

4.4.5 It is recommended that ethylene-diaminetetraacetic acid (EDTA) be added to the serum at a concentration of 20 mM to bind calcium in solution and minimize precipitation of calcium phosphate onto the bearing surfaces. The latter event has been shown to strongly affect the friction and wear properties, particularly of polyethylene/ceramic combinations. The addition of EDTA to other lubricant mediums should be evaluated.

4.4.6 A lubricant other than bovine serum may be used when it can be shown that its lubricating properties and, therefore, material wear properties are reasonably physiological **(8)**. In such a case, specify the lubricant in the test report.

4.5 Hold the bulk temperature of the lubricant at 37± 3°C or specified, if different.

5. Specimen Preparation

5.1 The governing rule for preparation of component counter faces is that the fabrication process parallels that used or intended for use in the production of actual prostheses, in order to produce a specimen with comparable bulk material properties and surface characteristics (see Practice F 86).

5.2 *Polymers and Composites*:

5.2.1 Obtain a fabrication history for each polymeric or composite component, including information such as grade, batch number, and processing variables, including method of forming (extruding, molding, and so forth), temperature, pressure, and forming time used, and any post-forming treatments, including sterilization.

5.2.2 Pretest characterization may include measurement of bulk material properties, such as molecular-weight range and distribution, percent crystallinity, density, or other. The surface finish of specimens may be characterized by profilometry, photomicrography, replication by various plastics, or other techniques.

5.2.3 *Sterilization*—Sterilize the components in a manner typical of that in clinical use for such devices, including total dose and dose rate, as these may affect the wear properties of the materials. Report these processing parameters with the aging time prior to each test when known. Sterilization of all test and control components within a specific test group should be done simultaneously (in a single container), when possible, to minimize variation among the specimens. This wear-simulation procedure makes no attempt to maintain the sterility of specimens during the wear test.

5.2.4 *Cleaning of Polymer Prostheses*—Prior to wear testing, careful cleaning of the polymer specimens is important to remove any contaminants that would not normally be present on the actual prosthesis. During the wear run, the components must be re-cleaned and dried before each weighing to remove any extraneous material that might affect the accuracy of the weighing. A suggested procedure for cleaning and drying of polymeric components is given in Annex A4. With some combinations of materials, wear may result in the transfer of particulate debris which may then become reimbedded or otherwise attached to polymeric, metal, or composite surfaces. Such an occurrence will render the weight-loss assessment of wear less reliable.

5.2.5 *Weighing of Polymeric Components*—Weigh the polymeric components on an analytical balance having an accuracy on the order of± 10 µg. This degree of sensitivity is necessary to detect the slight loss in weight of polymers, such as UHMW polyethylene, which may wear 30 mg or less per million cycles **(3,5)**. Always weight specimens in the clean, dry condition (see Annex A1). Keep the components in a dust-free container and handle with clean tools to prevent contamination that might affect the weight measurement. Weigh each wear and control component three times in rotation to detect random errors in the weighing process.

5.3 *Soaking of Polymeric and Composite Prostheses*:

5.3.1 Polymeric and composite components should be presoaked in the lubricant to minimize fluid-sorption during the wear run. Without presoaking, components of very low-wear polymers such as polyethylene may show a net increase in weight during the initial wear intervals, due to fluid sorption **(3,4)**. The error due to fluid sorption can be reduced through presoaking and the use of control soak specimens. The number of specimens required and the length of presoaking depends on the variability and magnitude of fluid sorption encountered **(4)**.

5.3.2 After fabrication and characterization, clean and dry the wear components and three soak-control components of each test material in accordance with Annex A4, and then weigh by precisely controlled and repeatable methods. Place the wear components and soak controls in a container of serum for a specified time interval. Then, remove, clean, dry, and reweigh the components, and calculate the weight (see Annex A4). Repeat the specimens until a steady rate of fluid-sorption has been established. The number of weighings will depend on the amount of fluid sorption exhibited by the specimens.

5.3.3 In general, the weight of the components will stabilize at an asymptotic value in a reasonable time period. With UHMW polyethylene, a presoak period of 30 days has been found adequate **(4,7)**. In any case, use the weight gain of the soak controls to correct for ongoing fluid sorption by the wear components during the wear test.

5.4 *Counterfaces of Metal Alloys, Ceramic, or Other Materials*:

5.4.1 *Characterization*—Include with the pretest characterization of metal, ceramic, or other materials, recording of fabrication variables, such as composition, forming method (forging, casting, and so forth) and any postforming processing, such as annealing. Obtain data on material properties relevant to wear (for example, grain structure, hardness, and percentage of contaminants).

5.4.2 *Surface Finish*—In tests that are intended to evaluate an alternate counter face material bearing against the standard UHMWPE, ensure that the counter face finish is appropriate for components intended for clinical use. In tests of alternate materials where a reference metal or ceramic is used, polish the counter face to the prosthesis quality.

5.4.3 Clean, degrease, and passivate components of referenced prosthetic metals or ceramics in accordance with Practice F 86. This practice may require modification for components of other materials. Ensure that cleaning of components produces a surface free of any particles, oils, greases, or other contaminants that might influence the wear process.

6. Measurement Procedure

6.1 At the completion of the presoak period, the wear components and soak controls should be removed from the soak bath, cleaned, dried, and weighed by precisely controlled and repeatable methods. Record these weights as the initial weights of the specimens for purposes of calculating the progressive weight loss during the wear test. Place the three soak control specimens in holders in a soak chamber of test lubricant, such that the total surface area exposed to the lubricant is equal to that of the wear components when mounted in the hip simulator. Maintain the soak chamber temperature at 37 ± 3°C, or specify if different. It is recommended that the soak chamber be attached to the simulator or otherwise agitate in the same manner as the actual wear chambers. In addition, it may be advantageous to apply a cyclic load to the soak control specimens (without tangential motion) comparable to that applied to the wear specimens, since this also can affect the rate of fluid sorption.

6.2 Frictional torque should be recorded for each specimen combination. This may be done in a preliminary test under a constant (static) load, or during the wear test under the cyclic, physiological load. These measurements may be repeated at various intervals during the wear test to determine changes in frictional properties with progressive wear.

6.3 Place the wear test components in the hip simulator, add the lubricant, apply the load, and commence the cyclic motion. Record the frictional force simultaneously with the wear cycling, where applicable.

6.4 Matching of components in each test set may be desirable to ensure optimum consistency of wear performance doing these tests.

6.5 As testing is commenced, monitor the components for

signs of erratic behavior that might require an early termination of the test.

6.6 Remove the wear and soak components at specified intervals, wash, rinse, and dry concurrently, in accordance with the procedure in Annex A4. It is important that both the wear and soak components be treated identically to ensure that they have the same exposure to the wash, rinse, and drying fluids. This will provide the most accurate correction for fluid sorption by the wear specimens.

6.7 After rinsing and drying, weigh the wear components and soak controls on the analytical balance as described in 5.2.5.

6.8 Thoroughly rinse the wear chambers and component surfaces with distilled water.

6.9 Inspect the bearing surfaces of the hip components and note the characteristics of the wear process. Visual, microscopic, profilometric, replication, or other inspection techniques can be used. Care must be taken, however, that the surfaces do not become contaminated or damaged by any substance or technique that might affect the subsequent wear properties. If contamination occurs, thoroughly reclean the specimens prior to restarting the wear test.

6.10 Replace the wear components and soak controls in fresh lubricant and continue wear cycling.

7. Determining Wear Rates

7.1 *Test Length*—The accuracy of the test method depends on the relative magnitudes of wear and fluid sorption. This is especially true when the fluctuations in the weight due to variation in the amount of surface drying are large in comparison to the incremental weight-loss due to wear. For high-wear low-sorption materials, the wear rate may be established clearly in as few as 50 000 wear cycles. With comparatively low-wearing materials, such as UHMWPE, several million cycles or more may be required to clearly establish the long-term wear properties.

7.2 *Number of Replicate Tests*—Perform tests intended to determine the relative wear rates of two materials with at lest three sets of specimens for each material to provide an indication of the repeatability of the results. As for any such experimental comparison, the total number of specimens eventually needed will depend on the magnitude of the difference to be established, the repeatability of the results (standard deviation), and the level of statistical significance desired.

7.3 *Correcting for Fluid Sorption*—Add to or subtract from the average weight gain (or loss) of the three soak control components the measured weight loss of each wear component (see Annex A6). This procedure corrects both for systematic sorption, as well as random differences in the amount of surface drying (of the entire set of test and control specimens) at each interval of weighing.

7.4 *Conversion to Volumetric Wear*—In tests where the wear rates of materials with different densities are evaluated, it may be preferable to compare these on the basis of volumetric wear, rather than weight loss. It is preferable that comparisons of the wear properties between components of polymeric materials having different densities be done on the basis of volumetric wear. The volumetric wear rate may be obtained by dividing the weight-loss data by the density of the material, in appropriate units. The accuracy of this calculation is dependent on the material being reasonably homogeneous, that is, having a constant density with wear depth. Report the density value used in this conversion.

8. Report

8.1 *Materials*:

8.1.1 Provide material traceability information from a raw material and fabrication or manufacturing standpoint for each material counter face. Examples of such information include material grade, batch number, and processing variables.

8.1.2 Pretest characterization for a plastic counter face may include measurement of bulk material properties, such as molecular-weight average, range and distribution, percent crystallinity, density, degree of oxidation, or others. The surface finish of both counter faces may be characterized by profilometry, photomicrography, replication, or other applicable techniques.

8.1.3 Report the method of sterilization, the sterilization and test dates, and the means of storage post-sterilization and pretest.

8.2 *Loading Conditions*—Describe the loading conditions used on the specimens. Report load curves and motions and timing relationships.

8.3 *Wear Rates*:

8.3.1 Graphically plot the weight loss of each specimen as a function of wear cycles. Wear may be reported as the weight loss of the bearing component as a function of the number of wear cycles, but it also may be converted to volumetric wear if the density of the material is known.

8.3.2 In tests where the wear rate is nearly constant over the test run, calculate the volumetric wear rate by the method of least squares in each regression.

8.3.3 If the wear rate changes during the test, as with a decrease due to wearing-in of the specimens or an increase due to the onset of fatigue wear, linear regression may be applied to separate intervals of the test to indicate the change in wear rate.

8.3.4 At the discretion of the investigator, more complex, nonlinear models may be fit to the wear-test data.

8.3.5 Report the test duration in cycles.

8.4 *Accuracy and Repeatability*:

8.4.1 In multiple tests where the wear rate is determined from the slope of the graph comparing wear versus test duration (cycles) for each specimen, report the individual rates, mean wear rate, and the 95 % confidence intervals for each rate.

8.4.2 In cases where the mean wear rate for two materials is different, evaluate and report the level of statistical significance of this difference.

8.5 Since the accumulation of wear debris in the lubricant may influence the wear rate, report any filtering of the lubricant during operation (continuously or periodically).

8.6 Record and report the room temperature and humidity during each weighing session.

8.7 Report the loading conditions on the soak control specimens. Load soaking, which is defined as a pulsing load profile equivalent to the wear profile without the tangential movement, has been shown to increase the fluid sorption rate.

8.8 In order that the simulator wear data be reproducible and comparable among laboratories, it is essential that uniform procedures be established. Sufficient data has not yet been produced using identical materials in different laboratories to permit determining the precision and bias of this recommended procedure. This guide is intended, in part, to facilitate uniform testing and reporting of data from hip joint simulator wear studies. It is anticipated that the references provided will permit validation of this methodology.

ANNEXES

(Mandatory Information)

A1. CHOICE OF WEAR-TEST LUBRICANT

A1.1 Comparative experiments have shown that distilled water or saline solutions do not duplicate the lubricating properties of fluids such as serum or synovial fluid that contain physiological concentrations of proteins (**1,3**). In particular, the heavy transfer of polyethylene to the surface of metal or ceramic implant that is typically observed with water or saline lubrication, is not typical of serum-lubricated specimens and is not typical of retrieved components after extended use in vivo. Care must be taken in the choice of lubricant to ensure that when used in simulated hip wear tests, it approximates the wear found clinically. Report the choice of lubricant along with the validation for its use.

A2. IMPLANT MATCHING FOR CONSISTENT WEAR PERFORMANCE

A2.1 The optimal clearance between the ball and socket of total hip prostheses is a matter of controversy with regard to its affect on the friction and wear properties, and this will vary for different combinations of materials and different designs of prostheses (**5,7,9**). It may be desirable to calculate the effects of design and installation procedures on frictional forces across the material components prior to performing an extended wear study.

A3. PRECAUTIONS IN PREPARING SPECIMEN SURFACES

A3.1 Do not polish or otherwise attempt to improve the polymer surfaces with abrasives, for example, aluminum oxide. Particles of the polishing compound may remain embedded in the polymeric material and could strongly affect the wear performance of the bearing materials.

A4. METHOD FOR CLEANING OF SPECIMENS

A4.1 Gently scrub cups with a nonabrasive material to remove all serum particles. Verify under a magnifying glass.

A4.2 Rinse under a stream of deionized water.

A4.3 Clean in an ultrasonic cleaner:

A4.3.1 Five minutes in deionized, particle-free water.
A4.3.2 Rinse in deionized water.
A4.3.3 Ten minutes in 10 mL of liquid ultrasonic cleaning detergent plus 500 mL of water.
A4.3.4 Rinse in deionized water.
A4.3.5 Ten minutes in deionized water.
A4.3.6 Rinse in deionized water.
A4.3.7 Three minutes in deionized water.
A4.3.8 Rinse in deionized water.

A4.4 Dry with a jet of nitrogen or suitable clean, dry gas.

A4.5 Soak in 95 % methyl alcohol for 5 min.

A4.6 Dry with a jet of nitrogen or suitable gas.

A4.7 Dry in a vacuum jar at a minimum vacuum 10^{-3} torr for 30 min.

A4.8 Weigh on a microbalance.

A4.9 To minimize weighing errors, weigh the entire set of specimens three times, in rotation, keeping the same specimen sequence each time. Polymeric cups typically gain or lose weight slightly between each weighing due to additional sorption or evaporation of fluid. The average of the three weights may be used for the wear calculations.

NOTE A4.1—This is a suggested cleaning procedure suitable for metals, ceramics, carbon, and UHMW polyethylene (**3**). Use methyl alcohol only for polymers that are essentially insoluble in this liquid. For polymers that dissolve or degrade in methyl alcohol, substitute a more appropriate volatile solvent. The purpose of this step is to remove the water from the surface layer of the specimen that otherwise tends to evaporate during the weighing process. Other aspects of this procedure might require modification for the particular polymer being tested.

A5. COMPONENT CLAMPING FIXTURES

A5.1 One technique that has proven practical has been to clamp each component in a mold (for example, polyurethane) that replicates the outer shape of the test component. The mounting mold is then press-fit into the stainless steel base of each chamber (**7**). The mounting method should permit the test components to be removed periodically for cleaning and weighing without damaging the test components or causing a separate loss of weight of the test components. If there is doubt, it is recommended that several specimens be mounted and removed from the machine several times each and weighted each time to detect any weight change caused by the mounting procedure.

A6. CALCULATION OF SPECIMEN WEAR

A6.1 The amount of fluid sorption over a wear interval is determined from the three soak controls, whereby the average weight gain, Sn, is calculated as follows:

$$Sn = 1/3\,(Sa + Sb + Sc) \tag{A6.1}$$

A6.2 Since fluid sorption by the wear specimens tends to mask the actual weight loss due to wear, increase the magnitude of the measured weight loss by the wear specimens by the magnitude of the weight-gain of the soak specimens. Where S1 equals initial average weight of the three soak specimens and S2 equals the final average weight of the three soak specimens.

A6.3 The actual net wear, then, is given as follows:

$$Wn = W1 - W3 \tag{A6.2}$$

A6.3.1 However, W3 is unknown. On the other hand, the apparent wear is given as follows:

$$Wa = W1 - W2 \tag{A6.3}$$

where:

$W1$ = initial weight of the wear specimen,
$W2$ = final weight of the wear specimen (including a gain due to fluid sorption), and
$W3$ = the actual final weight of the wear specimen if fluid sorption is subtracted out.

A6.3.2 The actual net wear (Wn) can be obtained by increasing the apparent wear (Wa) by an amount equal to the net soak gain.

$$Wn = Wa + Sn;\ \text{Where } Sn = S2 - S1 \tag{A6.4}$$

$$\text{Thus } Wn = (W1 - W2) + (S2 - S1) \tag{A6.5}$$

A6.4 Note that the four weights W1, W2, S1, and S2 are actual measured values. The sign convention in this equation for Wn takes into account occurrences, such as an apparent weight gain by the wear specimen (giving a negative value for Wa) or a net weight loss by the soak specimens (a negative value of Sn). In most cases the net wear, Wn, will be zero or positive.

A6.5 The net volumetric wear is then given as follows:

$$Vn = Wn/p \tag{A6.6}$$

where:

p = density of the polymer, expressed in appropriate units.

APPENDIX

(Nonmandatory Information)

X1. RATIONALE

X1.1 The hip simulator wear studies of materials may involve three types of evaluation:

X1.1.1 Comparing the wear rate of a candidate polymeric material to that of polyethylene, both bearing against one of the reference metal or ceramic counter faces.

X1.1.2 Comparing the polyethylene wear on the candidate counter face material to that of polyethylene wear on the reference metal or ceramic component.

X1.1.3 Comparing the wear rate of a new combination of candidate materials to the reference combinations.

X1.2 For the purpose of this guide, wear is defined as the progressive loss of material from a prosthetic component as a result of tangential motion against its mating component under load. For current designs of total hip prostheses, used since 1971 in the United States, the polymeric component bearing against metal, ceramic, composite, or carbon balls will be the sacrificial member, that is, the polymer will be the predominant source of wear debris. The metallic or other non-polymeric components, however, also may contribute either ionic or particulate debris. Depending on circumstances, therefore, wear may be generated by adhesion, two or three body abrasion, surface or subsurface fatigue, or some other process. Depending on the candidate materials and design combinations selected, it may be desirable in some instances to add additional techniques to identify the nature and magnitude of the wear process.

X1.3 While wear results in a change in the physical dimensions of the specimen, it is distinct from dimensional changes due to creep or plastic deformation in that wear generally results in the removal of material in the form of debris particles, causing a loss in weight of the specimen **(3, 7)**.

X1.4 Wear rate is the gravimetric or volumetric wear per million cycles of test.

X1.5 During wear testing in serum, calcium phosphate may precipitate on the surface of the test balls, particularly those of ceramic, and strongly affect the friction and wear properties. The addition of 20 mM EDTA in the lubricant may eliminate such precipitation.

REFERENCES

(1) Davy, D. T., Kotzar, G. M., Brown, R. H., Heiple, K. G., Goldberg, V. M., et al, "Telemetric Force Measurement Across the Hip After Total Arthroplasty,"*JBJS*, 70A(1):45, 1988.

(2) Paul, J. P., "Forces Transmitted by Joints in the Human Body. Lubrication and Wear in Living and Artificial Human Joints," *Proc. Instn. Mech. Engrs.*181 (3J):8, London 1966/67.

(3) McKellop, H. A., Clarke, I. C., Markolf, K., and Amstutz, H. C., "Wear Characteristics of UHMW Polyethylene: A Method for Accurately Measuring Extremely Low Wear Rates,"*J. Biomed. Mat. Res.*, 12:895, 1978.

(4) Clarke, I. C., Starkebaum, W., Hosseinian, A., McGuire, P., Okuda, R., Salovey, R., and Young, R. "Fluid-Sorption Phenomena in Sterilized Polyethylene Acetabular Prostheses," *J. Biomat.*, 6:184, 1985.

(5) McKellop, H. A., Lu, B., and Benya, P., "Friction, Lubrication and Wear of Cobalt-Chromium, Alumina and Zirconia Hip Prostheses Compared on a Joint Simulator," *Trans. Orthop. Res. Soc.*, 1992, p. 401.

(6) Treharne, R. W., Young, R. W., and Young, S. R.," Wear of Artificial Joint Materials III: Simulation of the Knee Joint Using a Computer Controlled System,"*Engineering in Medicine*, Vol 10, No. 3, 1981, pp. 137–142.

(7) McKellop, H. A., and Clarke, I. C., "Degradation and Wear of Ultra-High-Molecular-Weight Polyethylene," *ASTM Special Technical Publication 859*, ASTM, 1985.

(8) Streicher, R. M., "Ceramic Surfaces as Wear Partners for Polyethylene."*Bioceramics*, Vol 4, p. 9, W. Bonfield, G. W. Hastings, K. E. Tanner, eds., Butterworth-Heinemann Ltd., London, 1991.

(9) Rae, T., "Comparative Laboratory Studies on the Production of Soluble and Particulate Metal by Total Joint Prostheses,"*Arch. Orthop. Traumat. Surg.*, 95:71, 1979.

Designation: F 1715 – 00[ε1]

Standard Guide for Wear Assessment of Prosthetic Knee Designs in Simulator Devices[1]

This standard is issued under the fixed designation F 1715; the number immediately following the designation indicates the year of original adoption or, in the case of revision, the year of last revision. A number in parentheses indicates the year of last reapproval. A superscript epsilon (ε) indicates an editorial change since the last revision or reapproval.

ε[1] NOTE—Section 2 was editorially corrected in June 2001.

1. Scope

1.1 This guide covers a laboratory method for evaluating the wear properties of materials or devices, or both, that are being considered for use as the bearing surfaces of human knee joint replacement prostheses. The knee prostheses are evaluated in a device intended to simulate the tribological conditions encountered in the human knee joint.

1.2 The methods described in this guide are intended to apply to a number of fundamentally different types of knee wear simulators. These include apparatuses which are designed to apply some combination of axial load, flexion/extension angular motion, AP displacement or shear force, and tibial rotational displacement or torque to femoral and tibial wear test specimens.

1.3 Since the knee simulator method permits the use of actual implant designs, materials, and physiological load/motion combinations, it can represent a more physiological simulation than basic wear-screening tests, such as "pin-on-disc" (Test Method F 732) or "ring-on-disc" (ISO-6474).

1.4 It is the intent of this guide to rank the combination of implant designs and materials with regard to material wear rates under simulated physiological conditions. It must be recognized, however, since there are many possible variations in the in vivo conditions, a single-laboratory simulation with a fixed set of parameters may not be universally representative. **(1,2)**[2]

1.5 The reference materials for the comparative evaluation of candidate materials, designs, and processes shall be the wear rate of extruded or compression-molded ultra-high molecular weight (UHMW) polyethylene (Specification F 648) bearing against standard counter faces [cobalt-chromium-molybdenum alloy (Specification F 75); thermomechanically processed cobalt chrome (Specification F 799 or F 1537)], having typical prosthetic-quality surface finish and geometry similar to those with established clinical history. These reference materials will have been tested under the same wear conditions as the candidate materials.

2. Referenced Documents

2.1 *ASTM Standards:*

D 883 Terminology Relating to Plastics[3]

F 75 Specification for Cast Cobalt-Chromium-Molybdenum Alloy for Surgical Implant Applications[4]

F 86 Practice for Surface Preparation and Marking of Metallic Surgical Implants[5]

F 648 Specification for Ultra-High-Molecular-Weight Polyethylene Powder and Fabricated Form for Surgical Implants[5]

F 732 Test Method for Pin-on-Flat Wear Test for Polymeric Materials for Used in Total Joint Prostheses Which Experience Linear Reciprocating Wear Motion[5]

F 799 Specification for Thermomechanically Processed Cobalt-Chrome-Molybdenum Alloy for Surgical Implants[5]

F 1537 Specification for Wrought Cobalt-28-Chromium-6-Molybdenum Alloy for Surgical Implants[5]

F 2025 Practice for Gravimetric Measurement of Polymeric Components for Wear Assessment[5]

G 40 Terminology Relating to Erosion and Wear[5]

2.2 *ISO Standard:*

ISO 6474 Implants for Surgery–Ceramic Materials Based on Alumina[6]

3. Terminology

3.1 *Definitions*—For definitions of terms in this guide relating to plastics, refer to Definitions D 883. For definitions relating to erosion and wear, refer to Terminology G 40.

3.2 *Definitions of Terms Specific to This Standard:*

3.2.1 *wear, n*—the progressive loss of material from a prosthetic component as a result of tangential motion against

[1] This guide is under the jurisdiction of ASTM Committee F04 on Medical and Surgical Materials and Devicesand is the direct responsibility of Subcommittee F04.22on Arthroplasty.

Current edition approved May 10, 2000. Published August 2000. Originally published as F 1715 – 96. Last previous edition F 1715 – 96.

[2] The boldface numbers given in parentheses refer to the list of references at the end of the text.

[3] *Annual Book of ASTM Standards*, Vol 08.01.

[4] *Annual Book of ASTM Standards*, Vol 13.01.

[5] *Annual Book of ASTM Standards*, Vol 03.02.

[6] Available from American National Standards Institute, 25 W. 43rd St., 4th Floor, New York, NY 10036.

its mating component under load.

4. Significance and Use

4.1 This guide provides general guidelines for establishing test conditions, obtaining wear measurements, and determining the appropriateness of results for wear simulation of the femoro-tibial components of knee joint prostheses. Fundamental aspects of these methods include the use of bovine serum or demonstrated equivalent lubricant, and use of dynamic load and motion profiles representative of the human knee joint during activities of daily living. **(3)** The addition or substitution of other patient activities is at the discretion of the investigator.

4.2 While wear results in a change in the physical dimensions of the specimen, it is distinct from dimensional changes caused by creep or plastic deformation, in that wear results in the removal of material in the form of debris particles, causing a loss in weight of the specimen.

4.3 This guide for generating wear of the polymeric component is suitable for various simulator devices. These techniques can be used with metal, ceramic, carbon, polymeric, and composite counter faces bearing against a polymeric material (for example, polyethylene, polyacetal, and so forth). Thus, this method has universal application for wear studies of total-knee replacements which feature polymeric bearings. This method has not been validated for high-density material bearing systems, such as metal-metal, carbon-carbon, or ceramic-ceramic.

5. Apparatus and Materials

5.1 *Knee Prosthesis Components*:

5.1.1 The knee joint comprises femoral and tibial specimens in which materials such as metal alloys, ceramics, polymers, and carbon have been used in various combinations in different designs.

5.1.2 There shall be at least one control specimen, identical to the wear test specimens.

5.2 *Component Configurations*:

5.2.1 Polymeric tibial inserts used in some modular knee implants may contain geometrical features that either damage the polymer on removal or reduce the ability to clean the component satisfactorily. It may be necessary to modify the polymeric insert or the insert's immediate backing to a simple configuration to permit use of the weight-loss technique of wear assessment (Practice F 2025). Care must be taken to avoid altering knee design features that could affect the wear performance.

5.2.2 The knee joint components shall be assembled in a manner similar to that in which they would function in vivo. The exception to this would be if the intent of the wear test was to investigate the effect of improper assembly or implantation.

5.3 *Knee Simulator*:

5.3.1 *Test Chambers*—In the case of a multispecimen machine, contain the components in individual, isolated chambers to prevent contamination of one set of components with debris from another test. Design the chamber of entirely of noncorrosive materials, such as acrylic plastic or stainless steel, and ensure that it is easily removable from the machine for thorough cleaning between tests. Design the wear chambers such that the test bearing surfaces are immersed in the lubricant throughout the test **(3,6)**.

5.3.2 *Component Clamping Fixtures*—If wear is to be determined from the weight loss of the components, the method for mounting the components in the test chamber should not compromise the accuracy of assessment of weight loss as a result of wear.

5.3.3 *Load*—Ensure that the axial load profile is representative of that which occurs during the patient's walking cycle, with peak loads equal to or greater than 2 kN **(4)**. The loading apparatus must be free to follow the specimen as wear occurs, such that the applied peak load is constant to within ±3 % for the duration of the test. Never allow the applied load to be below that required to keep the chambers seated (for example, 50 N) **(6)**. If AP shear force or IE rotation torque profiles are used, these should also be representative of that which occurs during a patient's activity cycle **(7)** and the loading apparatus must be free to follow the specimen as wear occurs, maintaining a tolerance of ±3 % on the peak load for the duration of the test. Selection of these loading profiles should also be based on satisfaction of the criteria set forth the Annex A1.

5.3.4 *Motion*—Ensure that the flexion-extension motion between the knee components is oscillatory and simulates that of the targeted activity. Addition of internal-external rotation or AP displacement profiles is at the investigator's discretion. Selection of these motion profiles should also be based on satisfaction of the criteria set forth in Annex A1. It is recommended that the orientations of the knee components relative to each other and to the load axis be maintained by suitable specimen-holder keying.

5.3.5 *Oscillating Frequency*—Oscillate the knee prostheses at a nominal rate of 0.5 to 2.0 cycles per second (0.5 to 2.0 Hz). The selected frequency should maintain the criteria set forth in Annex A1.

5.3.6 *Cycle Counter*—Include with the knee simulator a counter to record the total number of wear cycles.

5.4 *Lubricant*:

5.4.1 It is recommended the specimen be lubricated with bovine blood serum; however, another suitable lubrication medium may be used if validated (see Annex A1 and Annex A2).

5.4.2 Since different bovine sera differ in composition (protein concentration, and so forth), dilution with deionized water of up to 75 % may be appropriate. The appropriate dilution shall be based on satisfaction of the criteria set forth in Annex A1.

5.4.3 If serum is used, then use filtered-sterilized serum since it is less likely to contain hemolyzed blood material, which has been shown to affect the lubricating properties of the serum adversely **(3)**. Diluted solutions of serum also have been used for this purpose **(9)**. Filtration may remove hard, abrasive, particulate contaminants or other impurities that might otherwise affect the wear properties of the specimens being tested.

5.4.4 Maintain the volume and concentration of the lubricant nearly constant throughout the test. This may be accomplished by sealing the chambers so that water does not evaporate, by periodically or continuously replacing evaporated water with deionized water, or by recirculating the lubricant.

5.4.5 To retard bacterial degradation, freeze and store the serum until needed for the test. In addition, it is recommended that the fluid medium in the test contains 0.2 to 0.3 % (weight fraction) sodium azide, or other suitable biocide, to minimize bacterial degradation. Other lubricants should be evaluated to determine appropriate storage conditions.

5.4.6 It is recommended that disodium dihydrogen ethylenediaminetetraacetate (EDTA) be added to the serum at a concentration of 20 mM (7.45 g/L) to bind calcium in solution and minimize precipitation of calcium phosphate onto the bearing surfaces. The latter event has been shown to strongly affect the friction and wear properties, particularly of polyethylene/ceramic combinations **(8)**. The addition of EDTA to other lubricant mediums should be evaluated.

5.4.7 Additives such as sodium azide and EDTA should be dissolved in deionized water and passed through a 0.2-μm filter before adding to the test lubricant.

5.4.8 The appropriate interval for replacing used serum depends on how the serum maintains its functional composition (that is, lubricating properties). This depends on factors such as the specific test conditions and materials being used and the additives present in the serum. There is no minimum replacement interval. The maximum recommended replacement interval is two weeks. The selected interval should again maintain the criteria set forth in Annex A1.

5.4.9 A lubricant other than bovine serum may be used when it can be shown that its lubricating properties and, therefore, the material wear properties are reasonably physiological **(7)** and the criteria set forth in Annex A1 can be met. In such a case, specify the lubricant in the test report.

5.5 The bulk temperature of the lubricant should be maintained at a given temperature, ±3°C, within the range of 21 to 39°C, or reported if different.

6. Specimen Preparation

6.1 The governing rule for preparation of component counterfaces is that the fabrication process parallels that used or intended for use in the production of actual prostheses to produce a specimen with comparable bulk material properties and surface characteristics (Practice F 86).

6.1.1 Because variations in geometrical tolerances between the total knee components may influence the friction and wear performance, check the overall dimensions of the knee components for consistency and record any differences.

6.1.2 In knee joint combinations in which polyethylene components are gripped directly, the clamping should not induce distortion of polyethylene components that could affect the friction and wear performance.

6.1.3 Obtain a fabrication history for each polymeric or composite component, including information such as grade, batch number and processing variables, method of forming (extruding, molding, and so forth), temperature, pressure and forming time used, articular surface preparation methods (see Annex A3), and any postforming treatments, including sterilization methods and parameters.

6.1.4 Pretest characterization may include measurement of bulk material properties, such as molecular-weight range and distribution, percent crystallinity, density, or other. The surface finish of specimens may be characterized by profilometry, photomicrography, and replication by various plastics or other techniques.

6.1.5 *Sterilization*—Sterilize the polymeric components in a manner typical of that in clinical use for such devices, as this may affect the wear properties of the materials. Report sterilization processing parameters with the aging time before each test. Sterilization of all test and control components within a specific test group should be done simultaneously (in a single container) when possible to minimize variation among the specimens. This wear-simulation procedure makes no attempt to maintain the sterility of specimens during the wear test.

6.1.6 *Cleaning of Polymer Prostheses*—Before wear testing, careful cleaning of the polymer specimens is important to remove any contaminants that normally would not be present on the actual prosthesis. During the wear test, the components must be recleaned and dried before each wear measurement to remove any extraneous material that might affect the accuracy of the measurement. The recommended procedure for cleaning and drying of polymeric components is given in Annex A4 (also, see Practice F 2025).

NOTE 1—With some combinations of materials, wear may result in the transfer of particulate debris that may then become reimbedded or otherwise attached to polymeric, metal, or composite surfaces. Such an occurrence will render the weight-loss assessment of wear less reliable.

6.2 *Soaking of Polymeric and Composite Prostheses*:

6.2.1 Polymeric and composite components should be presoaked in the test lubricant to minimize fluid sorption during the wear test. Without presoaking, components of very low-wear polymers, such as UHMWPE, may show a net increase in weight or volume during the initial wear intervals as a result of fluid sorption **(3,10)**. The error caused by fluid sorption can be reduced through presoaking and the use of control soak specimens. The number of specimens required and the length of presoaking depends on the variability and magnitude of fluid sorption encountered **(10)**.

6.3 *Counterfaces of Metal Alloys, Ceramic, or Other Materials*:

6.3.1 *Characterization*—Include with pretest characterization of metal, ceramic, or other materials recording of fabrication variables such as composition, forming method (forging, casting, and so forth), and any postforming processing, such as annealing. Obtain data on material properties relevant to wear, for example, grain structure, hardness, and percentage of contaminants.

6.3.2 *Surface Finish*—In tests that are intended to evaluate an alternate counterface material bearing against the standard, ensure that the counterface finish is appropriate for components intended for clinical use. In tests of alternate materials in which a reference metal or ceramic is used, polish the counterface to the prosthesis quality.

6.3.3 Clean, degrease, and passivate components of referenced prosthetic metals or ceramics according to Practice F 86. This practice may require modification for components of other materials. Clean components to produce a surface free of any particles, oils, greases, or other contaminants that might influence the wear process.

7. Procedure

7.1 Make any initial measurements required to determine

the subsequent amount of wear (refer to Practice F 2025 for gravimetric techniques).

7.2 Place the soak control specimen(s) in a soak chamber of test lubricant such that the total surface area exposed to the lubricant is similar to that of the wear components during testing. Maintain the soak chamber temperature at the wear test lubricant temperature. It is recommended that the soak chamber be attached to the simulator or otherwise agitated in the same manner as the actual wear chambers. In addition, it may be advantageous to apply a cyclic load to the soak control specimen(s) (without tangential motion) comparable to that applied to the wear specimens since this can also affect the rate of fluid sorption.

NOTE 2—Cyclic loading of the soak control specimen(s) is necessary if a dimensional wear measurement method is to be used.

7.3 Place the wear test components in the simulator, add the lubricant, apply the load, and commence cyclic loads and motions.

7.4 As testing is commenced, monitor the components for signs of erratic friction or wear behavior that might require an early termination of the test.

7.5 Remove the wear and soak components at specified intervals, wash, rinse, and dry concurrently, according to the procedure in the Annex A4. It is important that both the wear and soak components be treated identically to ensure that they have the same exposure to the wash, rinse, and drying fluids. This treatment will provide the most accurate correction for fluid sorption by the wear specimens.

7.6 After rinsing and drying, conduct wear measurements.

7.7 Thoroughly rinse all test assembly surfaces which have contacted the test lubricant using deionized water.

7.8 Inspect the bearing surfaces of the knee components and note the characteristics of the wear process. Visual, microscopic, profilometric, replication, or other inspection techniques can be used. Care must be taken, however, that the surfaces do not become contaminated or damaged by any substance or technique that might affect the subsequent wear properties. If contamination occurs, thoroughly clean the specimens before restarting the wear test.

7.9 Replace the wear components and soak controls in fresh lubricant and continue wear cycling.

7.10 *Test Length*—The accuracy of the test method depends on the relative magnitudes of wear and fluid sorption. This is especially true when the fluctuations in the weight as a result of variation in the amount of surface drying are large in comparison to the incremental weight loss caused by wear. For high-wear low-sorption materials, the wear rate may be clearly established in as few as 50 000 wear cycles. With comparatively low-wearing materials, such as UHMWPE, several million cycles or more may be required to clearly establish the long-term wear properties. In the latter case, the wear test should generally continue until one of the following events occurs:

7.10.1 Completion of 5×10^6 cycles;

7.10.2 Breaking up of articulating surfaces, detachment of particles greater than 1 mm^2, or delamination;

7.10.3 Failure of the test machine to maintain the force and displacement parameters within the given tolerances.

7.10.4 If the wear test involves a bearing surface with variable subsurface properties or one in which fatigue wear may potentially develop, it may be necessary to continue the wear test until 1×10^7 cycles or more.

7.11 *Number of Replicate Tests*—Perform tests intended to determine the relative wear rates of two conditions with at least three sets of specimens for each condition to provide an indication of the repeatability of the results. As for any such experimental comparison, the total number of specimens eventually needed will depend on the magnitude of the difference to be established, the repeatability of the results (standard deviation), and the level of statistical significance desired.

8. Reporting Results

8.1 *Materials*:

8.1.1 Provide material traceability information (raw material and fabrication or manufacturing methods and lots) for each material counterface. Examples of such information include material grade, batch number, and processing variables.

8.1.2 Pretest characterization for a plastic counterface may include measurement of bulk properties, such as molecular weight average, range, and distribution, percent crystallinity, density, degree of oxidation, or others. The surface finish of both counterfaces may be characterized by profilometry, photomicrography, replication, or other applicable techniques; these data should be reported.

8.1.3 The method of sterilization, the sterilization and test dates, and the means of storage poststerilization/pretest should be reported, if known. For irradiation-sterilized specimens, total dose and dose rate should be reported.

8.2 *Test Apparatus and Methodology*:

8.2.1 Report the number of stations on the machine and the number of stations used for this test. Report if replicate tests were conducted during more than one test series. Describe the mechanisms used to generate the motions and forces, the systems used to measure motions and forces, the arrangement for mounting specimens, a description of the lubricant used, the arrangement for lubricating the articular surfaces, the arrangement for lubricant temperature control, total lubricant volume per station, lubricant replacement interval, and arrangement for the exclusion of contaminant particles.

8.2.2 Since the accumulation of wear debris in the lubricant may influence the wear rate, report any filtering of the lubricant during operation (continuously or periodically) and the lubricant replacement intervals.

8.2.3 Record and report the room temperature and humidity during each weighing session.

8.2.4 Report the loading conditions, if any, on the soak control specimen(s). Load soaking that is defined as a pulsing load profile equivalent to the wear profile without the tangential movement may increase the fluid sorption rate.

8.3 *Wear Rates*:

8.3.1 Plot the wear of each specimen graphically as a function of wear cycles. Wear may be reported as the volumetric loss of the bearing component as a function of the number of wear cycles. If weight measurements are used, this will require knowing the density of the wear specimen material.

8.3.2 In tests in which the wear rate is nearly constant over the test run, calculate the volumetric wear rate by the method of linear regression.

8.3.3 If the wear rate changes during the test, as with a decrease caused by wearing-in of the specimens, or an increase as a result of the onset of fatigue wear, linear regression may be applied to separate intervals of the test to indicate the change in wear rate.

8.3.4 At the discretion of the investigator, more complex, nonlinear models may be fit to the wear test data.

8.3.5 Report the test duration in cycles. If this was less than 5×10^6 cycles, explain why.

8.3.6 Report the load and motion curves used.

8.3.7 Report how the wear mechanisms and wear rates resemble clinical wear behavior (in accordance with Annex A1). Provide a description of the articulating surfaces of all wear specimens.

8.4 *Accuracy and Repeatability*:

8.4.1 In multiple tests in which the wear rate is determined from the slope of the graph comparing wear versus test duration (cycles) for each specimen, report the individual wear rates, mean wear rate, and the 95 % confidence intervals for each rate.

8.4.2 In cases in which the mean wear rate for two materials is different, evaluate and report the level of statistical significance of this difference.

8.4.3 At the discretion of the investigator, other statistics methods may be used. All statistics methods and related assumptions should be reported.

8.5 Include a reference to this guide and to the standard used for the wear measurement method.

9. Precision and Bias

9.1 For knee simulator wear data to be reproducible and comparable among laboratories, uniform procedures should be established. Sufficient data has not yet been produced using identical materials in different laboratories to permit determining the precision and bias of this procedure. The publication of this guide is intended, in part, to facilitate uniform testing and reporting of data from knee joint simulator wear studies. Validation of this methodology may be achieved through round-robin testing.

10. Keywords

10.1 joint simulator; knee prosthesis; wear testing

ANNEXES

(Mandatory Information)

A1. GUIDELINES FOR DEMONSTRATING THAT KNEE SIMULATOR WEAR BEHAVIOR IS SIMILAR TO CLINICAL WEAR BEHAVIOR

A1.1 It is necessary to identify characteristics of test results that suggest that clinical wear behavior is being reproduced. It is suggested that a baseline result be established using the configuration with the most clinical history; a CoCr alloy femoral component articulating against a gamma-sterilized UHMWPE tibial component (unaged or aged less than five years). This combination should be evaluated in a baseline test series and demonstrate to meet the requirements below.

A1.2 Reproduction of In-Vivo Wear Quantities

A1.2.1 Clinical wear rates for tibial component materials in knee prostheses are very scarcely documented, mostly because of geometrical complexities. One study by Collier et al **(11)** found the average penetration rate of EtO-sterilized UHMWPE tibial components to be less than 0.1 mm/year, and for gamma-air-sterilized UHMWPE tibial components, greater than 0.5 mm/year. The latter group may have been influenced by postirradiation aging (and a subsequent fatigue wear mechanism). The many different wear mechanisms that have been reported in TKA **(12-15)** further complicates the target wear rate.

A1.2.2 A summary of reported knee simulator wear rates is listed in Table A1.1. As shown, there is a wide range of results, probably a reflection of the variability in machines and methods and, to some extent, different designs and materials. Wear rates ranging from imperceptible to catastrophic have been observed clinically; thus, it is different to provide guidelines unless the targeted clinical result is defined. Investigators who show convincing evidence that their simulator and clinical wear specimen surfaces look similar (A1.3) strengthen their argument that the wear rate they measure is appropriate. As such evidence is gathered, it will become more clear how narrow the range of wear rates, as shown in Table A1.1 should be.

A1.2.3 The appropriate duration of a laboratory wear test depends on the magnitude of wear, the linearity of wear rate as it is affected by the duration of a break-in period, predominating wear mechanism and wear transitions, the potential for long-term fatigue or other late failure mechanisms, and repeatability of results. It may be justifiable to run a test for as little as one million cycles based on these considerations, or it may be appropriate to extend the test to ten million cycles or more in some cases.

A1.3 Reproduction of In-Vivo Wear Mechanisms

A1.3.1 Because of the dearth of clinical data on wear rates, the appropriateness of knee simulator wear tests must rely on reproducing in vivo wear surfaces and debris characteristics. Many different wear mechanisms have been reported to predominate depending on UHMWPE sterilization method and shelf age, patient and surgical factors, device design, heat-pressed surfaces, presence of cement particles or other debris, and so forth. The clinical target becomes an issue in light of these numerous conditions. Based on the methods described in

TABLE A1.1 Reported UHMWPE Wear Rates from Knee Simulator Wear Tests

Study	Duration (10^6 Cycles)	Knee Design	Wear Rate ($mm^3/10^6$ Cycles)
Treharne et al[16]	1.0	RMC	1.59
		Total Condylar	3.71
		Townley	13.8
		Anametric	13.9
		UCI type	32.6
Dowson et al[17]	2.0	Geomedic	78.0
	1.5	Freeman-Swanson	79.5
	1.0	Polycentric	77.4
Dowson et al[18]	1.0	Leeds	55.5
		Freeman-Swanson	47.3
Walker[19]	2.1	Genesis (small)	3.8
Hastings[20]	4	AMK: gamma-N_2/aged	6
	2	AMK: gamma/aged	43-97
Polenini[20]	?	Howmedica	16
Burgess et al[21]	8.0	Kinemax	2.82
Sauer et al[22]	3.37	Genesis II, size 1-2	
		EtO/aged	14.5
		gamma-N_2/aged	8.4
Sauer et al[23,27]	2.6	Genesis II, size 5, group A	1.6
	5.6	Genesis II, size 5, group B	1.4
Kawanabe et al[24]	1.7	AGC (with AP translation)	34.1
	8.8	AGC (without AP translation)	9.9
Hastings[25]	10	AMK gas-plasma/aged	2.8
	10	AMK crosslinked/aged	0.7
Hastings[26]	10	AMK gamma/unaged	3.6
Gilbertson[27]	variable	MG-simulator A	1.9
		MG-simulator B	18.8
		MG-simulator B, no IE rotation	0.8
		MG-simulator B, no AP translation	1.9
Rieker[27]	...	Sulzer	2.2
Essner[27]	...	Howmedica, 13.5° rotation	14.2
		Howmedica, no IE rotation	3.5

this guide, one of two target wear mechanisms should be selected:

A1.3.1.1 Wear polishing (to include burnishing or microabrasive/microadhesive wear).

A1.3.1.2 *Delamination (fatigue wear mechanism)*

Wear polishing has been reported in the absence of aging and abrasion **(28)**. This mechanism may be accompanied by striations or ripples **(29,30)** as well as microcracks **(30)**. The delamination mechanism should be selected when the clinical target exhibits subsurface cracking **(12,31)**. This wear mechanism is considered a form of fatigue wear, typically requiring a certain latency period, but eventually overriding early wear mechanisms and resulting in the removal of relatively large amounts of material. Delamination wear has been successfully generated in knee simulator testing **(32)**.

A1.3.2 Wear debris particles may also be evaluated for assessing the appropriateness of the wear test method. If the size and morphology characteristics can be shown to be comparable to clinically retrieved debris for a comparable device, this may even substitute for the above validation criteria for wear mechanisms.

A1.4 Repeatability and reproducibility of results. A minimum of three and up to six replicate tests per condition should be conducted depending on repeatability. If the same specimen condition were tested in a separate series, there should be no significant difference in results.

A2. CHOICE OF WEAR-TEST LUBRICANT

A2.1 Comparative experiments have shown that distilled water or saline solutions do not duplicate the lubricating properties of fluids such as serum or synovial fluid that contain physiological concentrations of proteins **(3)**. In particular, the heavy transfer of polyethylene to the surface of a metal or ceramic implant that is typically observed with water or saline lubrication, but is not typical of serum-lubricated specimens and is not typical of retrieved components after extended use in-vivo. Care must be taken in the choice and dilution of bovine serum (or equivalent) to ensure that when used in simulated knee wear tests it approximates the wear found clinically (see Annex A1). Report the choice of lubricant along with the proof of validation for its use.

A3. PRECAUTIONS IN PREPARING SPECIMEN SURFACES

A3.1 Do not polish or otherwise attempt to improve the polymer surfaces with abrasives, for example, aluminum oxide. Particles of the polishing compound may remain embedded in the polymeric material and could strongly affect the wear performance of the bearing materials.

A4. METHOD FOR CLEANING OF SPECIMENS (FROM PRACTICE F 2025)

A4.1 Gently scrub specimens with a nonabrasive material to remove all serum particles. Verify under a magnifying glass.

A4.2 Rinse under a stream of deionized water.

A4.3 Clean in an ultrasonic cleaner:

A4.3.1 5 min in deionized, particle-free water,

A4.3.2 Rinse in deionized water,

A4.3.3 10 min in 10 mL of liquid ultrasonic cleaning detergent plus 500 mL of water,

A4.3.4 Rinse in deionized water,

A4.3.5 10 min in deionized water,

A4.3.6 Rinse in deionized water,

A4.3.7 3 min in deionized water, and

A4.3.8 Rinse in deionized water.

A4.4 Dry with a jet of nitrogen or suitable clean, dry gas.

A4.5 Soak in 95 % methyl alcohol, for 5 min (see Note A4.1).

A4.6 Dry with a jet of nitrogen or suitable gas.

A4.7 Dry in a vacuum jar at a minimum vacuum of 10^{-3} torr for 30 min.

A4.8 Powder-free gloves should be used during all specimen-handling procedures.

NOTE A4.1—This is a suggested cleaning procedure suitable for metals, ceramics, carbon, and UHMW polyethylene (**3**). Use methyl alcohol only for polymers that are essentially insoluble in such liquids. For polymers that dissolve or degrade in methyl alcohol, substitute a more appropriate volatile solvent. The purpose of this step is to remove the water from the surface layer of the specimen that otherwise tends to evaporate during the weighing process. Other aspects of this procedure might require modification for the particular polymer being tested.

A5. COMPONENT CLAMPING FIXTURES

A5.1 One technique that has proven practical is to clamp each component in a mold (for example, polyurethane) that replicates the outer shape of the test component. The mounting mold is then press-fit into the base of each chamber (**6**). The mounting method should permit the test components to be removed periodically for cleaning and wear measurement without this procedure damaging the test components or causing a separate loss of volume of the test components. If there is doubt, it is recommended that several specimens be mounted and removed from the machine several times each, and measured each time to detect any volumetric change caused by the mounting procedure.

APPENDIX

(Nonmandatory Information)

X1. RATIONALE

X1.1 For the purpose of the guide, wear is defined as the progressive loss of material from a prosthetic component as a result of tangential motion against its mating component under load. For current designs of total knee prostheses used since 1971 in the United States, the polymeric component bearing against metal, ceramic, composite, or carbon inserts will be the sacrificial member; that is, the polymer will be the predominant source of wear debris. The metallic or other nonpolymeric components, however, also may contribute either ionic or particulate debris. Depending on circumstances, therefore, wear may be generated by adhesion, two- or three-body abrasion, surface or subsurface fatigue, or some other process. Depending on the candidate materials and design combinations selected, it may be desirable in some instances to add additional techniques to identify the nature and magnitude of the wear process.

X1.2 While wear results in a change in the physical dimensions of the specimen, it is distinct from dimensional changes caused by creep or plastic deformation in that wear generally results in the removal of material in the form of debris particles, causing a loss in weight of the specimen (**3,6**).

X1.3 Wear rate is the gravimetric or volumetric wear per million cycles of test.

X1.4 During wear testing in serum, calcium phosphate may precipitate on the surface of the test balls, particularly those of ceramic, and strongly affect the friction and wear properties. The addition of 20-mM EDTA in the lubricant may eliminate such precipitation.

REFERENCES

(1) Rae, T., "Comparative Laboratory Studies on the Production of Soluble and Particulate Metal by Total Joint Prostheses," *Arch. Orthop. Traumat. Surg.*, 95:71, 1979.

(2) Treharne, R. W., Young, R. W., and Young, S. R., "Wear of Artificial Joint Materials III: Simulation of the Knee Joint Using a Computer Controlled System," *Engineering in Medicine*, Vol 10, No. 3, 1981, pp. 137–142.

(3) McKellop, H. A., Clarke, I. C., Markolf, K., and Amstutz, H. C., "Wear Characteristics of UHMW Polyethylene: A Method for Accurately Measuring Extremely Low Wear Rates," *J. Biomed. Mat. Res.*, 12:895, 1978.

(4) Paul, J. P., "Forces Transmitted by Joints in the Human Body. Lubrication and Wear in Living and Artificial Human Joints," *Proc. Instn. Mech. Engrs.* 181 (3J):8, London 1966/67.

(5) McKellop, H. A., Lu, B., and Benya, P., "Friction, Lubrication and Wear of Cobalt-Chromium, Alumina and Zirconia Hip Prostheses Compared on a Joint Simulator," *Trans. Orthop. Res. Soc.*, 1992.

(6) McKellop, H. A., and Clarke, I. C.," Degradation and Wear of Ultra-High-Molecular-Weight Polyethylene," *Special Technical Publication 859*, ASTM 1985.

(7) ISO/DIS 14243-1 Implants for Surgery - Wear of Total Knee Joint Prostheses, Part 1: Loading and Displacement Parameters for Wear Testing Machines with Load Control and Corresponding Environmental Conditions for Test, July 1999.

(8) McKellop, H., Lu, B., and Benya, P., "Friction, Lubrication, and Wear of Cobalt-Chromium, Alumina, and Zirconia Hip Prostheses Compared on a Joint Simulator," *Ceramors*, 92.

(9) Streicher, R. M., "Ceramic Surfaces as Wear Partners for Polyethylene," Bioceramics, Vol 4, Eds W. Bonfield, G. W. Hastings, K. F. Tanner, Butterworth-Heinemann Ltd, London, 1991.

(10) Clarke, I. C., Starkebaum, W., Hosseinian, A., McGuire P., Okuda, R., Salovey, R., and Young, R., "Fluid-Sorption Phenomena in Sterilized Polyethylene Acetabular Prostheses," *J. Biomat.*, 6:184, 1985.

(11) Collier et al., 64th *AAOS*, San Francisco, March 1997, #151.

(12) Engh, G.A., Dywer, K.D., and Hanes, C.K., "Polyethylene Wear of Metal-Backed Tibial Components in Total and Unicompartmental Knee Prostheses," *JBJS*, 74-B (1), 1992, pp. 9-17.

(13) Landy, M.M. and Walker, P.W., "Wear of Ultra-High-Molecular-Weight Polyethylene Components of 90 Retrieved Knee Prostheses," *J. Arthroplasty*, October 1988 Supplement: S73-S85.

(14) Hood, R.W., Wright, T.M., and Burstein, A.H., "Retrieval Analysis of Total Knee Prostheses: A Method and its Application to 48 Total Condylar Prostheses," *J. Bio. Mater. Res.*, 17, 1983, pp. 829-842.

(15) Sauer, W.L. and Tooms, R.W., "An Analysis of the Wear Characteristics and Property Changes in a Series of Explanted UHMWPE Tibial Components," *Trans. 11th Southern Biomedical Engineering Conference*, Memphis, TN, October 1992, pp. 70-71.

(16) Treharne, R.W., Young, R.W., and Young, S.R., "Simulation of the Knee Joint Using a Computer Controlled System," *J. Engineering in Medicine*, 10 (3) 1981, pp. 137-142.

(17) Dowson, D., Gillis, B.J., and Atkinson, J., "Penetration of Metallic Femoral Components into Polymeric Tibial Components Observed in a Knee Joint Simulator," American Chemical Society Symposium 287 on *Polymer Wear and its Control*, 1985, pp. 216-228.

(18) Dowson, D., McCullagh, P.J.J., and Wright, V., "An Assessment of the Relative Importance of Wear and Creep in the Overall Performance of Load Bearing Total Replacement Knee Joints," in "UHMWPE as Biomaterial in Orthopaedic Surgery," Eds. H.G. Willert, G.H. Buchhorn, and P. Eyerer, Hogrefe and Huber, Gottingen, 1990, pp. 32-40.

(19) Walker, P.W., "Wear of a Genesis TKR on a Knee Simulating Machine," Smith & Nephew Richards Research Report, January 1996.

(20) ASTM F04.22.11 Task Group Meeting on Knee Simulator Wear Test Methods, San Diego, November 1997.

(21) Burgess, I.C., Kolar, M., Cunning, J.L., and Unsworth, A., "Development of a Six-Station Knee Wear Simulator and Preliminary Wear Results," *IMechE-Proc.Instn.Mech.Eng.G.*, 211 (Part H), 1997, pp. 37-47.

(22) Sauer, W. and Hines, G., "Preliminary Comparison of EtO/Aged and Gamma-N_2/Aged UHMWPE Wear Using the AMTI 6-Station Knee Simulator," Smith & Nephew Research Report, October 1997.

(23) Sauer, W. and Anthony, M., "Knee Simulator Test GNR Results: Gen II Size-5, Normal vs. TKR Gait," Technical Memo TM343702, Smith & Nephew, Inc., January 1998.

(24) Kawanabe et al., Trans. 25th SFB, Providence, RI, May 1999, #462.

(25) Hastings, R.S., Huston, D.E., Reber, E.W., and DiMaio, W.G., "Knee Wear Testing of a Radiation Crosslinked and Remelted UHMWPE," *Trans. 25th SFB, 22*, 1999.

(26) Hastings, R.S., Huston, D.E., and Reber, E.W., "Knee Simulator Wear Testing: Comparison to Clinical Failures," ASTM F04 Workshop on Hip and Knee Simulator Testing, Seattle, May 18-19, 1999.

(27) ASTM F04 Workshop on Hip and Knee Simulator Testing, Seattle, May 18-19, 1999.

(28) Cornwall, G.B., Bryant, J.T., Hansson, C.M., Rudan, J., Kennedy, L.A., and Cooke, T.D.V.," A Quantitative Technique for Reporting Surface Degradation Patterns of UHMWPE Components of Retrieved Total Knee Replacements," *J. Applied Biomaterials*, 6, 1995, pp. 9-18.

(29) Wimmer, M.A., Loos, J., Andriacchi, T.P., and Schneider, E., "The Morphology of the Straited Wear Pattern in Total Knee Replacement." *Trans. 44th ORS*, New Orleans, March 1998: 354.

(30) Walker, P.S., Blunn, G.W., and Lilley, P.A., "Wear Testing of Materials and Surfaces for Total Knee Replacement," *J. Bio Mater. Res.*, 33, 1996, pp. 159-175.

(31) Blunn, G.W., Walker, P.S., Joshi, A., and Hardinge, K., "The Dominance of Cyclic Sliding in Producing Wear in Total Knee Replacements," *Clin. Orthop.*, 273, 1991, pp. 253-260.

(32) Walker, P.S., Blunn, G.W., Bell, C.J., Sathasivam, S., Andriacchi, T.P., Paul, J.P., and Campbell, P., "Methodology for Long-Term Wear Testing of Total Knee Replacement," *Trans 44th ORS*, New Orleans, March 1998.

Designation: F 1717 – 96

Standard Test Methods for Static and Fatigue for Spinal Implant Constructs in a Corpectomy Model[1]

This standard is issued under the fixed designation F 1717; the number immediately following the designation indicates the year of original adoption or, in the case of revision, the year of last revision. A number in parentheses indicates the year of last reapproval. A superscript epsilon (ε) indicates an editorial change since the last revision or reapproval.

1. Scope

1.1 This standard covers the materials and methods for the static and fatigue testing of spinal implant assemblies in a corpectomy model. The test materials for most combinations of spinal implant components can be specific depending on the intended spinal location and intended method of application to the spine.

1.2 This standard is intended to provide a basis for the mechanical comparison among past, present and future spinal implant assemblies. It allows comparison of spinal implant constructs with different intended spinal locations and methods of application to the spine. These test methods are not intended to define levels of performance, since sufficient knowledge is not available to predict the consequences of the use of a particular device.

1.3 The standard sets out guidelines for load types and methods of applying loads. Methods for three static load types and one fatigue test are defined for the comparative evaluation of spinal implant assemblies.

1.4 This standard establishes guidelines for measuring displacements, determining the yield load, evaluating the stiffness and strength of the spinal implant assembly.

1.5 Some spinal constructs may not be testable in all test configurations.

1.6 Values stated in SI units are to be regarded as standard.

1.7 *This standard does not purport to address all of the safety concerns, if any, associated with its use. It is the responsibility of the user of this standard to establish appropriate safety and health practices and determine the applicability of regulatory limitations prior to use.*

2. Referenced Documents

2.1 *ASTM Standards:*

D 638 Test Method for Tensile Properties of Plastic[2]

E 4 Practices for Force Verification of Testing Machines[3]

E 6 Terminology Relating to Methods of Mechanical Testing[3]

E 739 Practice for Statistical Analysis of Linear or Linearized Stress-Life (S-N) and Strain-Life (ε-N) Fatigue Data[3]

E 1150 Definitions of Terms Relating to Fatigue[3]

F 1582 Terminology Relating to Spinal Implants[4]

3. Terminology

3.1 *Definitions:*

3.1.1 For definitions of terms relating to the test method, see Terminology E 6, Terminology F 1582 and Definitions E 1150.

3.2 *Definitions of Terms Specific to This Standard:*

3.2.1 *active length of the longitudinal element*—the straight line distance between the center of attachment of the superior anchor and the center of attachment of the inferior anchor.

3.2.2 *angular displacement at 2 % offset yield (degrees)*—the angular displacement of a construct measured via the actuator that produces a permanent angular displacement in the *X-Y* plane equal to 0.020 times the torsional aspect ratio (see Point A in Fig. 1).

3.2.3 *block moment arm*—the perpendicular to the applied load between the insertion point of an anchor and the axis of the hidge pin.

3.2.4 *compressive or tensile bending stiffness (N/mm)*—the compressive or tensile bending yield force divided by elastic displacement (see the initial slope of line *BC* in Fig. 1).

3.2.5 *compressive or tensile bending ultimate load (N)*—the maximum compressive or tensile force in *X-Z* plane applied to a spinal implant assembly (see the force at Point E in Fig. 1). The ultimate load should be a function of the device and not of the load cell or testing machine.

3.2.6 *compressive or tensile bending yield load (N)*—the compressive or tensile bending force in *X-Z* plane necessary to produce a permanent deformation equal to 0.020 times the active length of the longitudinal element (see the force at Point D in Fig. 1).

3.2.7 *coordinate system/axes*—three orthogonal axes are defined in Fig. 2 and Fig. 3. The anterior-posterior axis is *X* with positive being anterior. The medial-lateral axis is *Y* with left being positive when viewed posteriorly. The superior-inferior axis is *Z* with superior being positive.

3.2.8 *displacement at 2 % offset yield (mm)*—the displacement of a construct measured via the actuator that produces a permanent deformation equal to 0.020 times the active length of the longitudinal element (see Point A in Fig. 1).

[1] These test methods are under the jurisdiction of ASTM Committee F-4 on Medical and Surgical Materials and Devices and are the direct responsibility of Subcommittee F04.25on Spinal Devices.

Current edition approved June 10, 1996. Published December 1996.

[2] *Annual Book of ASTM Standards*, Vol 08.01.

[3] *Annual Book of ASTM Standards*, Vol 03.01.

[4] *Annual Book of ASTM Standards*, Vol 13.01.

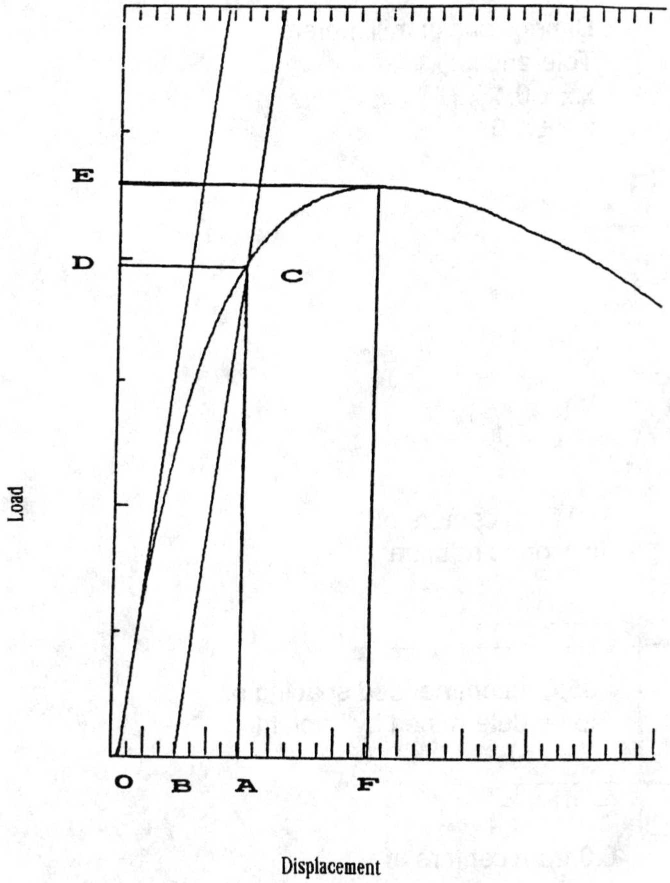

FIG. 1 Typical Load Displacement Curve or Torque Angulation Curve

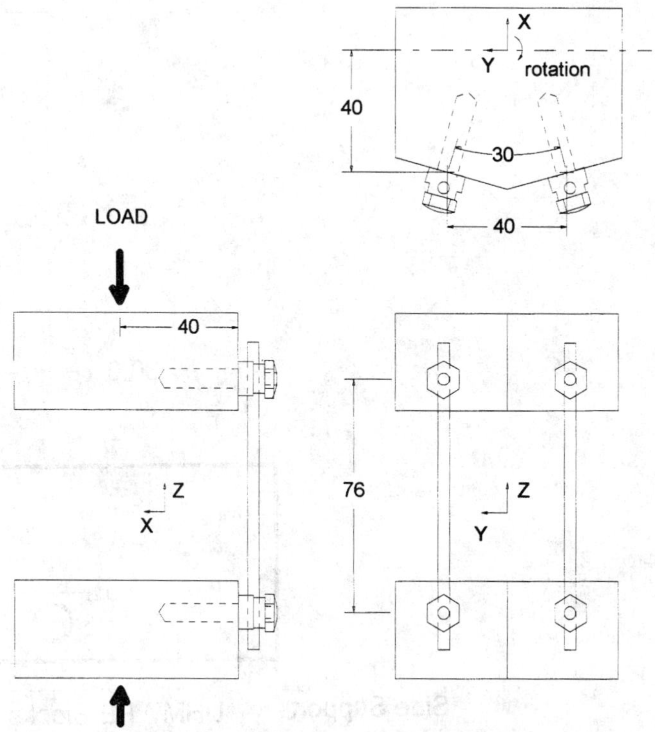

FIG. 2 A Standard Bilateral Construct Containing Screw, Rod and Screw

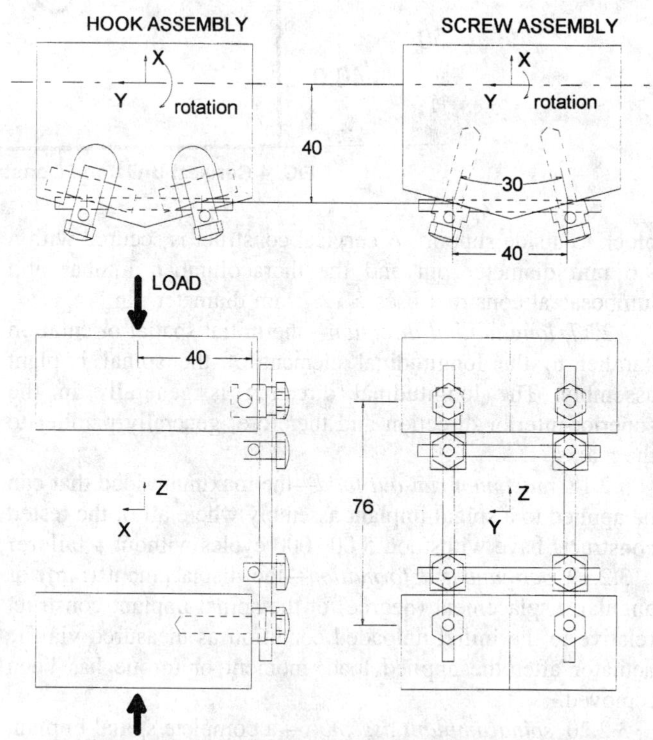

FIG. 3 A Bilateral Hook, Rod, Screw, and Transverse Element Construct

3.2.9 *elastic angular displacement (degrees)*—the angular displacement at 2 % offset yield (see Point A in Fig. 1) minus the 2 % offset angular displacement (see Point B in Fig. 1). (The distance between Point A and Point B in Fig. 1.)

3.2.10 *elastic displacement (mm)*—the displacement at 2 % offset yield (see Point A in Fig. 1) minus the 2 % offset displacement (see Point B in Fig. 1). (The distance between Point A and Point B in Fig. 1.)

3.2.11 *failure*—permanent deformation resulting from fracture, plastic deformation or loosening beyond the ultimate displacement or loosening that renders the spinal implant assembly ineffective or unable to adequately resist load.

3.2.12 *fatigue life*—the number of loading cycle, *N*, of a specified character that the spinal implant assembly sustains before failure of a specified nature occurs (see Definitions E 1150).

3.2.13 *insertion point of an anchor*—the location where the anchor is attached to the test block. The insertion points shown in Figs. 2-15 are to be adhered to if possible. In situations where the design of the spinal implant assembly or the manufacturer's surgical instructions for installation dictate otherwise, the attachment points may deviate from these dimensions.

3.2.14 *intended method of application*—spinal implant assemblies contain different types of anchors. Each type of anchor has an intended method of application to the spine.

3.2.15 *intended spinal location*—the anatomic region of the spine intended for the application of the spinal implant assembly. Spinal implant assemblies are developed for specific spinal locations such as the anterior cervical spine or the posterior thoracolumbar, lumbar and lumbosacral spine.

3.2.16 *hinge pin*—the cylindrical rod connecting a test

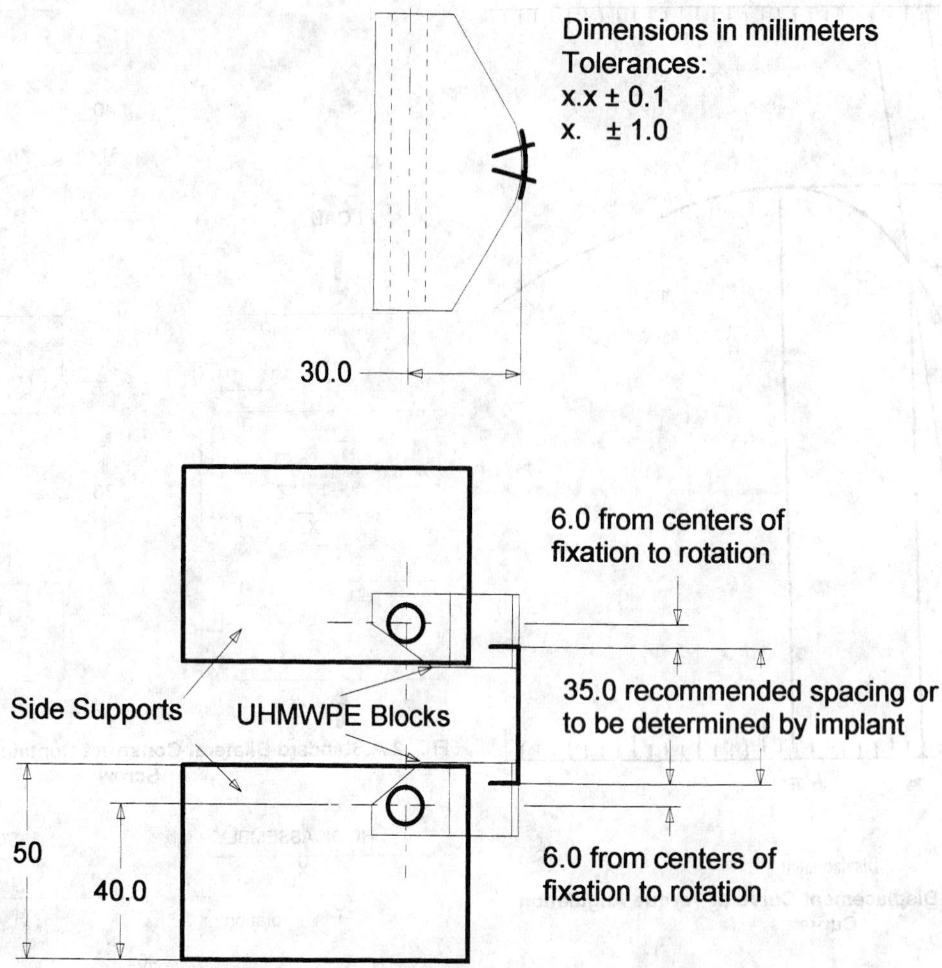

FIG. 4 Cervical Unilateral Construct Test Setup for Screws or Bolts

block to a side support. A cervical construct is secured with a 9.6 mm diameter pin and the thoracolumbar, lumbar and lumbosacral construct uses a 12.7 mm diameter pin.

3.2.17 *longitudinal direction*—the initial spatial orientation parallel to the longitudinal element of the spinal implant assembly. The longitudinal direction is generally in the superior-inferior direction and therefore, generally parallel to the *z* axis.

3.2.18 *maximum run out load*—the maximum load that can be applied to a spinal implant assembly where all of the tested constructs have withstood 5 000 000 cycles without a failure.

3.2.19 *permanent deformation*—the displacement (mm) or angular displacement (degree) of the spinal implant construct relative to the initial unloaded condition as measured via the actuator after the applied load, moment or torque has been removed.

3.2.20 *spinal implant assembly*—a complete spinal implant configuration as intended for surgical use. A spinal implant assembly will contain anchors, interconnections and longitudinal elements and may contain transverse elements (see Fig. 4, Fig. 6, Fig. 8, Fig. 10, Fig. 12 and Fig. 14).

3.2.21 *spinal implant construct*—a complete spinal implant assembly attached to the appropriate test blocks.

3.2.22 *test block*—the component of the test apparatus for mounting the spinal implant assembly. A specific design of test block is required for each intended spinal location and intended method of application. Fig. 5, Fig. 7, Fig. 9, Fig. 11, Fig. 13 and Fig. 15 describe the recommended designs for the test blocks; however alternate designs can be used as long as equivalence performance is demonstrated.

3.2.23 *test block load point*—the location on the test block at which the resultant load is transmitted from the test apparatus.

3.2.24 *tightening torque*—the specified torque that is applied to the various threaded fasteners of the spinal implant assembly.

3.2.25 *torsional aspect ratio*—the active length of the longitudinal element divided by the distance from the center of rotation to the insertion point of an anchor (for example: in Fig. 2 1.70 for a 76-mm active length, $X = 40$ mm and $Y = 40/2$ mm).

$$A = \frac{L}{D} = \frac{L}{(x^2 + y^2)^{1/2}} \quad (1)$$

where:

L = active length of longitudinal element,
D = distance to insertion point,
x = x distance to insertion point, and
y = y distance to insertion point.

3.2.26 *torsional stiffness (N-m/degree)*—the yield torque

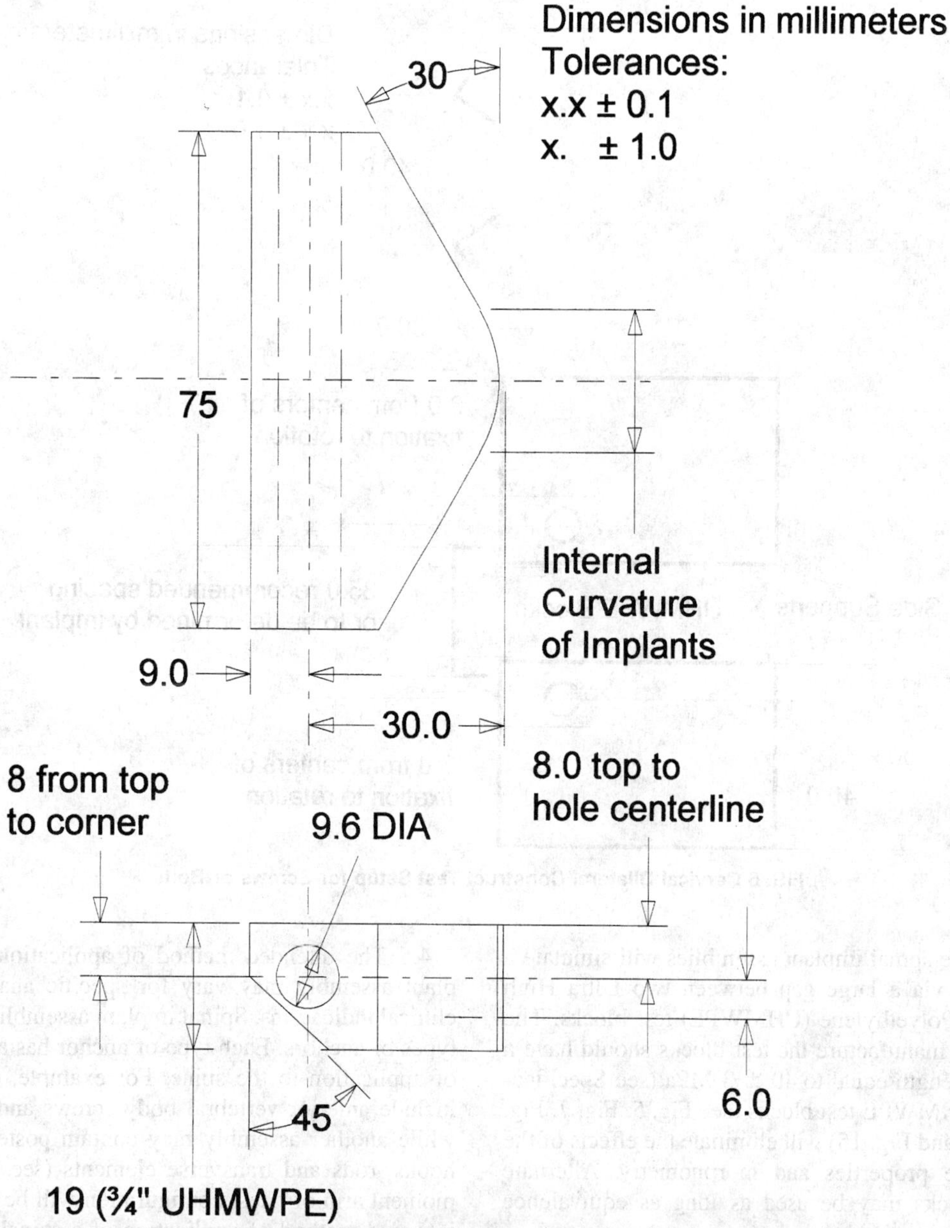

FIG. 5 Cervical Unilateral UHWMPE Block for Screws or Bolts

(N-m) divided by elastic angular displacement (degrees) (the initial slope of line BC in Fig. 1).

3.2.27 *torsional ultimate load (N-m)*—the maximum torque in *X-Y* plane applied to a spinal implant assembly (the torque at Point E in Fig. 1). The ultimate torque should be a function of the device and not of the load cell or testing machine.

3.2.28 *two percent (2 %) offset angular displacement (degrees)*—a permanent angular displacement in the *X-Y* plane measured via the actuator equal to 0.020 times the torsional aspect ratio (for example: 1.95° for 1.70 × 0.02 × 180°/pi) (see Point B in Fig. 1).

3.2.29 *two percent (2 %) offset displacement (mm)*—a permanent deformation measured via the actuator equal to 0.020 times the active length of the longitudinal element (for example: 1.52 mm for a 76 mm active length of the longitudinal element or 0.70 mm for 35 mm) (see Point B in Fig. 1).

3.2.30 *ultimate displacement (mm)*—the displacement associated with the ultimate load, ultimate bending load or ultimate torque (the displacement at Point F in Fig. 1).

3.2.31 *yield torque (N-m)*—the torque in *X-Y* plane required to produce a permanent displacement of 0.020 times the torsional aspect ratio (the torque at Point D in Fig. 1).

3.2.32 *zero displacement intercept (mm)*—the intersection of the straight line section of the load displacement curve and the zero load axis (the zero displacement reference Point 0 in Fig. 1).

4. Summary of Test Methods

4.1 Similar test methods are proposed for the mechanical evaluation of cervical spinal implant assemblies (see Fig. 4, Fig. 6 and Fig. 8) and thoracolumbar, lumbar and lumbosacral spinal implant assemblies (see Fig. 10, Fig. 12 and Fig. 14).

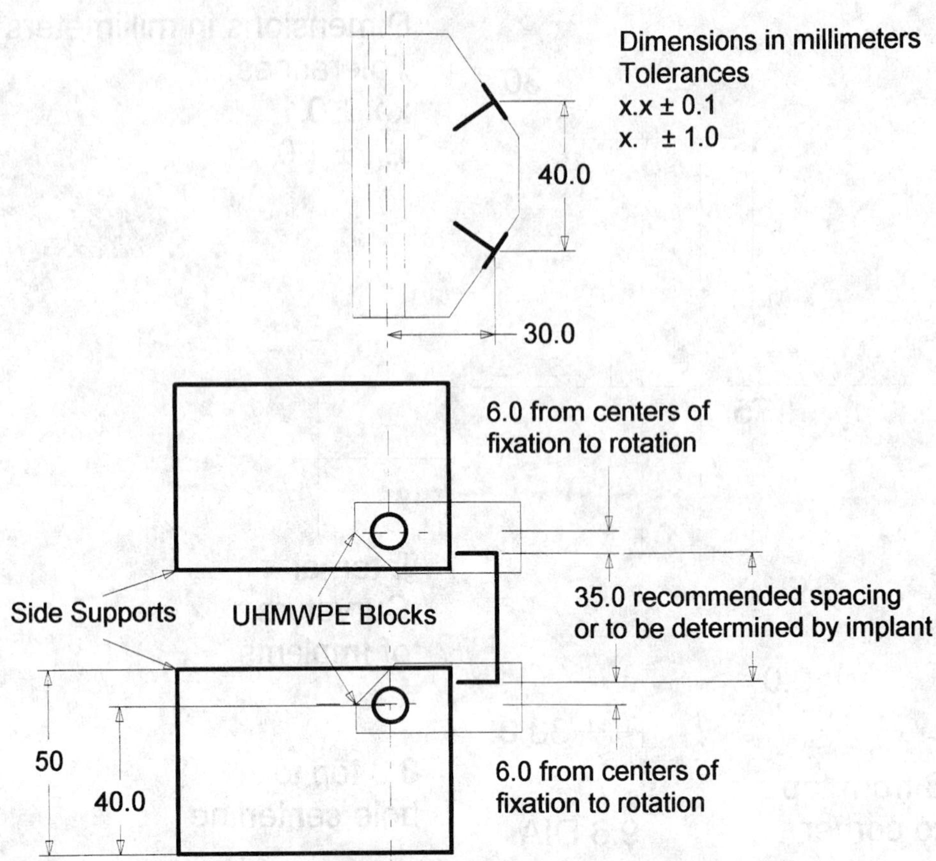

FIG. 6 Cervical Bilateral Construct Test Setup for Screws or Bolts

4.2 Testing of the spinal implant assemblies will simulate a corpectomy model via a large gap between two Ultra High Molecular Weight Polyethylene (UHMWPE) test blocks. The UHMWPE used to manufacture the test blocks should have a tensile breaking strength equal to 40 ± 3 MPa (see Specification F 638). The UHMWPE test blocks (see Fig. 5, Fig. 7, Fig. 9, Fig. 11, Fig. 13, and Fig. 15) will eliminate the effects of the variability of bone properties and morphometry. Alternate designs of test blocks may be used as long as equivalence performance is demonstrated.

4.3 Three static mechanical tests and one dynamic test will evaluate the spinal implant assemblies. The three static mechanical tests are compression bending, tensile bending and torsion. The dynamic test is a compression bending fatigue.

4.4 A specific clinical indication generally requires a specific spinal implant assembly. Spinal implant assemblies will be evaluated with test configurations which simulate the clinical requirements for the intended spinal location. The intended spinal locations are both anterior (see Fig. 4) and posterior (see Fig. 6 and Fig. 8) surfaces of the cervical spine or both anterior (see Fig. 10) and posterior (see Fig. 12 and Fig. 14) surfaces of the thoracolumbar, lumbar and lumbosacral spine. The block moment arm (see 6.6) for a test configuration depends on the intended spinal location. The cervical spine configuration (see Fig. 5, Fig. 7, and Fig. 9) specifies one block moment arm, while a larger block moment arm (see Fig. 11, Fig. 13, and Fig. 15) is specified for the thoracolumbar, lumbar and lumbosacral spine.

4.5 The intended method of application of the spinal implant assembly may vary for specific anatomic regions and clinical indications. Spinal implant assemblies contain different types of anchors. Each type of anchor has an intended method of application to the spine. For example, one assembly may include anterior vertebral body screws and rods (see Fig. 2), while another assembly may contain posterior sacral screws, hooks, rods and transverse elements (see Fig. 3). The block moment arm of a test configuration will be independent of the intended method of application of a spinal implant assembly, therefore the test data for different intended method of application may be compared.

5. Significance and Use

5.1 Spinal implants are generally composed of several components which, when connected together, form a spinal implant assembly. Spinal implant assemblies are designed to provide some stability to the spine while arthrodesis takes place. This standard outlines standard materials and methods for the evaluation of different spinal implant assemblies so that comparison between different designs may be facilitated.

5.2 This standard is used to quantify the static and dynamic mechanical characteristics of different designs of spinal implant assemblies. The mechanical tests are conducted *in vitro* using simplified load schemes and do not attempt to mimic the complex loads of the spine.

5.3 The loads applied to the spinal implant assemblies *in vivo* will, in general, differ from the loading configurations

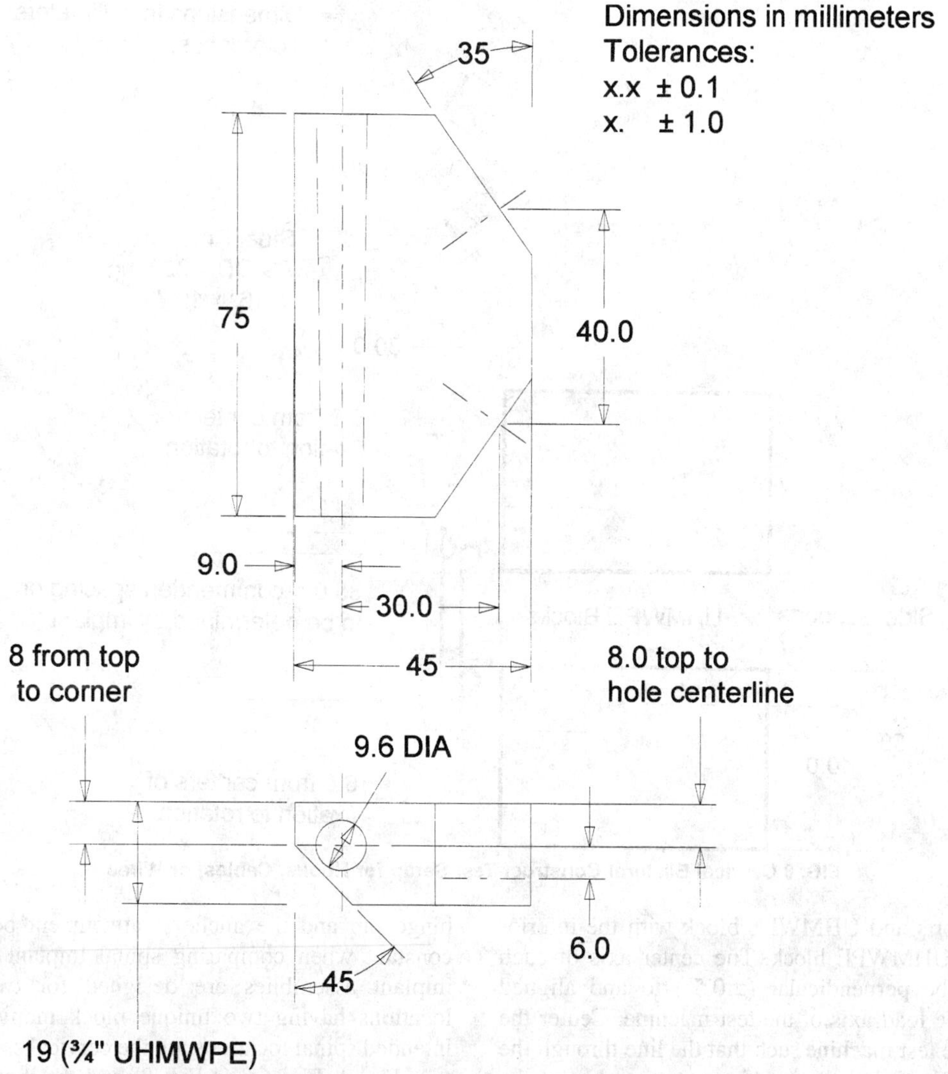

FIG. 7 Cervical Bilateral UHMWPE Block for Screws or Bolts

used in this standard. The results obtained here cannot be used directly to predict *in vivo* performance. The results can be used to compare different component designs in terms of the relative mechanical parameters.

5.4 Fatigue testing in a simulated body fluid or saline may cause fretting, corrosion or lubricate the interconnections and thereby affect the relative performance of tested devices. This test should be initially performed dry (ambient room conditions) for consistency. The effect of environment may be significant. Repeating all or part of these test methods in simulated body fluid, saline (9 g NaCl per 1000 mL water), a saline drip, water or a lubricant should be considered.

5.5 The location of the longitudinal elements is determined by where the anchors are clinically placed against bony structures. The perpendicular distance to the load direction (block moment arm) between the axis of a hinge pin and the anchor's attachment-points to a UHMWPE block is independent of anchor-type. The distance between the anchor's attachment point to the UHMWPE block and the center of the longitudinal element is a function of the interface design between the screw, hook, wire, cable, etc., and the rod, plate, etc.

6. Apparatus

6.1 Test machines will conform to the requirements of Practices E 4.

6.2 The test apparatus allows multiple loading regimes to be applied to all forms of spinal implant assemblies. Two pair of side supports are mounted on the test machine (see Fig. 4, Fig. 6, Fig. 8, Fig. 10, Fig. 12, and Fig. 14). One pair of side supports attach to the actuator and the second to the load cell. A mounting plate for one of the sets of side support plates should be free to rotate about the *Z* axis for the compression bending, tension bending and fatigue tests. UHMWPE blocks are connected to the side supports via hinge pins. All testing will simulate a corpectomy model via a large gap between the two UHMWPE blocks. Select the appropriate design of the UHMWPE blocks (see Fig. 5, Fig. 7, Fig. 9, Fig. 11, Fig. 13, and Fig. 15) to facilitate testing of the spinal implant assembly in a manner that simulates the specific clinical indication at the intended spinal location.

6.3 The design of the UHMWPE blocks causes the plane through the spinal implant assemblies to be parallel to the plane (the *Y-Z* plane) through the axes of the hinge pins. Align the

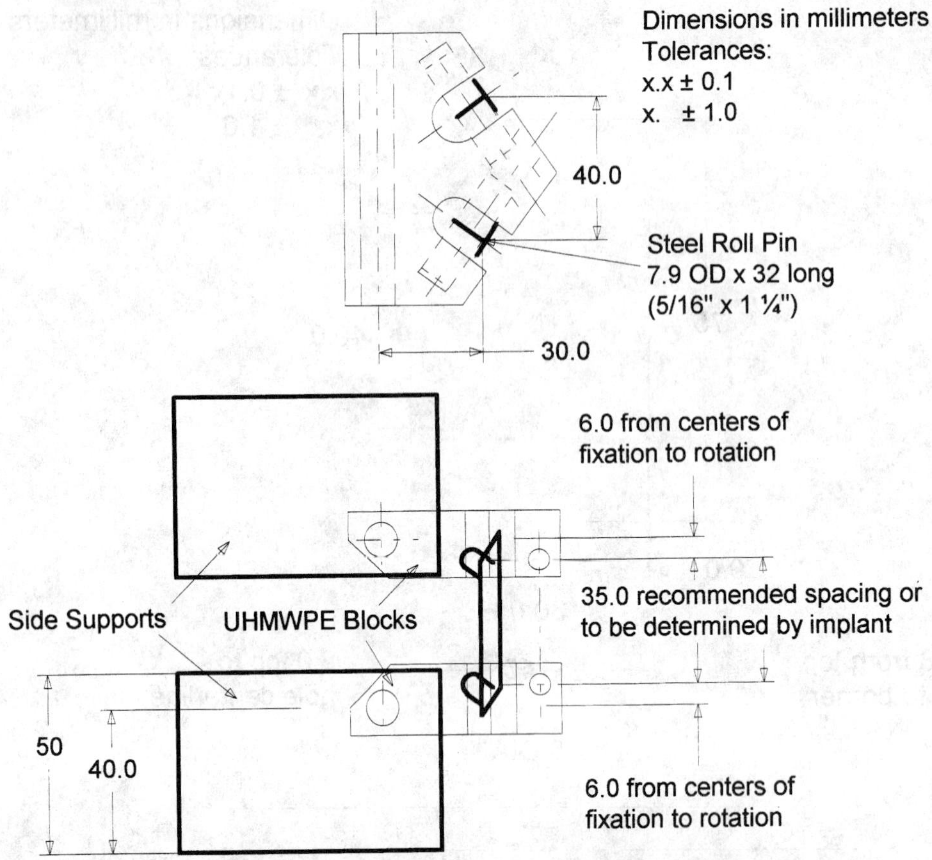

FIG. 8 Cervical Bilateral Construct Test Setup for Hooks, Cables, or Wires

superior side supports and UHMWPE block with the inferior side supports and UHMWPE block. The center axis of each hinge pin should be perpendicular (±0.5°) to and aligned (±0.5 mm) with the load axis of the test machine. Center the test apparatus in the test machine such that the line through the mid-point (0, 0, Z1) of the inferior hinge pin's axis and the mid-point (0, 0, Z2) of the superior hinge pin's axis is collinear within ±0.1 mm of the load and rotational axis of the test machine's actuator.

6.4 Alternate designs of test blocks may be used as long as equivalence is demonstrated. The solid UHMWPE test blocks may be replaced with metal blocks with UHMWPE inserts of appropriate size. Any surface or component of the spinal assembly which would contact the solid UHMWPE should also contact an appropriate thickness of the UHMWPE. If screws are used to mount the spinal construct to the test blocks (see Fig. 5, Fig. 7, Fig. 11 and Fig. 13), then the screws must be placed into UHMWPE inserts in the alternate design of test block. The diameter of the UHMWPE inserts must be equal to or greater than three times the diameter of the screws.

6.5 If the locations of the superior anchors, inferior anchors or both sets of anchors are dictated by the longitudinal element and are at different *Z* locations (a diagonal), then the set of anchors should be centered above and below the standard location such that they maintain the average *Z* location. If the anchors are secured into slots in the longitudinal element, then they should be centrally placed in the slots and not at either end to produce a worst case scenario.

6.6 The distance in the *X* direction between the axis of a hinge pin and the anchors' attachment point should remain constant when comparing spinal implant assemblies. Spinal implant assemblies are designed for two intended spinal locations having two unique block moment arms. The two intended spinal locations are the cervical spinal implant system (see Fig. 4, Fig. 6 and Fig. 8) and the thoracolumbar, lumbar and lumbosacral spinal implant system (see Fig. 10, Fig. 12 and Fig. 14). The test configurations for the cervical spinal implant system have a block moment arm equal to 30.0 mm. The thoracolumbar, lumbar and lumbosacral test configurations have a 40-mm block moment arm.

6.7 The UHMWPE blocks have been designed to provide similar block moment arms regardless of the anchor being tested. Different spinal implant assemblies have different intended methods of application to the UHMWPE blocks. The locations of the longitudinal elements are determined by the design of anchors and interconnections. The load capacity of the spinal construct would be a function of the designs of the interconnections, anchors and longitudinal elements but should not be a function of the test apparatus.

6.8 The hinge pin in the test configuration allows the same test apparatus to be used for the static compression bending test, static tensile bending test and static torsion test as well as the compression bending fatigue test. The UHMWPE blocks are allowed to rotate around the *Y*-axis of the hinge pin during the compression bending, tensile bending and fatigue tests.

6.9 Modified bilateral UHMWPE blocks (see Fig. 8, Fig. 9, Fig. 14 and Fig. 15) have been developed for testing hooks, wires or cables. Steel roll pins are placed into the modified

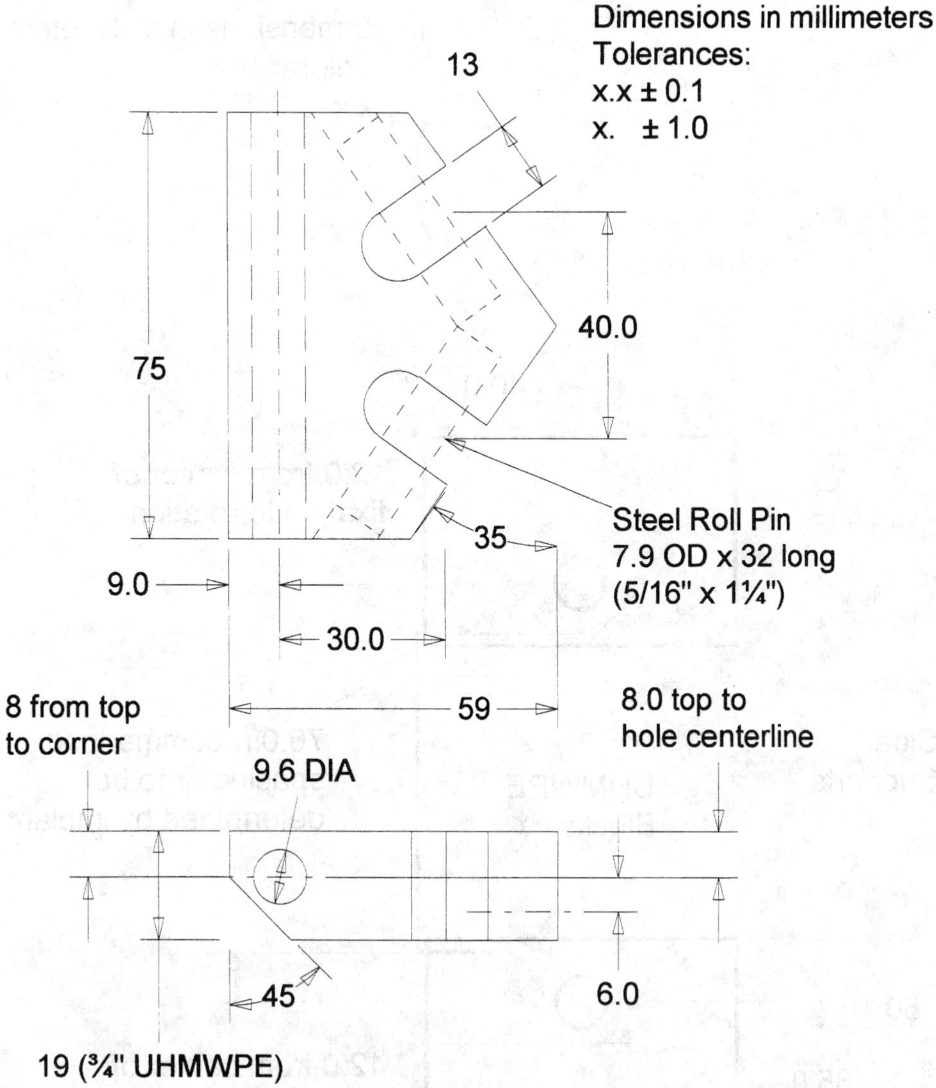

FIG. 9 Cervical Bilateral UHMWPE Block for Hooks, Cables, Wires

blocks such that the outer surfaces of the roll pins are parallel to the front surfaces of the standard bilateral UHMWPE block (see Fig. 6, Fig. 7, Fig. 12 and Fig. 13). Hooks, wires and cables are not fully constrained (semi-rigid) fixation devices because they cannot transfer bending moments in the three axes. The combination of the rotation of the modified UHMWPE block on the hinge pin and the rotation of the hooks, wires or cables around the steel roll pins means that the test configuration would be a mechanism. Therefore, the testing of hooks, wires and cables necessitates that the modified UHMWPE block must not rotate. Place an aluminum block between the modified UHMWPE block and the base plate to stop rotation around the hinge pin and eliminate a degree of freedom. The total clearance between an aluminum block, an UHMWPE block and a base plate will not exceed 0.10 mm.

6.10 The relative location (*X* direction versus *Z* direction) between the hinge pin and the insertion point of an anchor produces minimal variation in the block moment arm. The variation in the block moment arm is dependent on the direction of rotation of the UHMWPE blocks. The variation is minimized by having the hinge pins in the UHMWPE blocks rotate past the anchors as the test progresses. Position the hinge pins internal to the anchors during the tension bending test (not shown). Position the hinge pins external to the anchors during the compression bending, torsion and fatigue tests (see Fig. 4, Fig. 6, Fig. 8, Fig. 10, Fig. 12 and Fig. 14).

6.11 The thoracolumbar, lumbar and lumbosacral test apparatus have a recommended active length of the longitudinal element equal to 76.0 mm and based on the work of Cunningham, et al.[5] The recommended active length of the longitudinal element for the cervical spinal implant system is 35.0 mm. If the longitudinal element has fixed spacings and the recommended active length cannot be achieved, then select the longitudinal element that is nearest the recommended active length. The active length should be constant for all constructs used in comparative testing.

6.12 The testing machine and the apparatus used in the

[5] Cunningham, B. W., Sefter, J. O., Shono, Y., and McAfee, P. C.," Static and Cyclical Biomechanical Analysis of Pedicle Screw Spinal Constructs," Spine, Vol 18, No. 12, pp. 1677–1688.

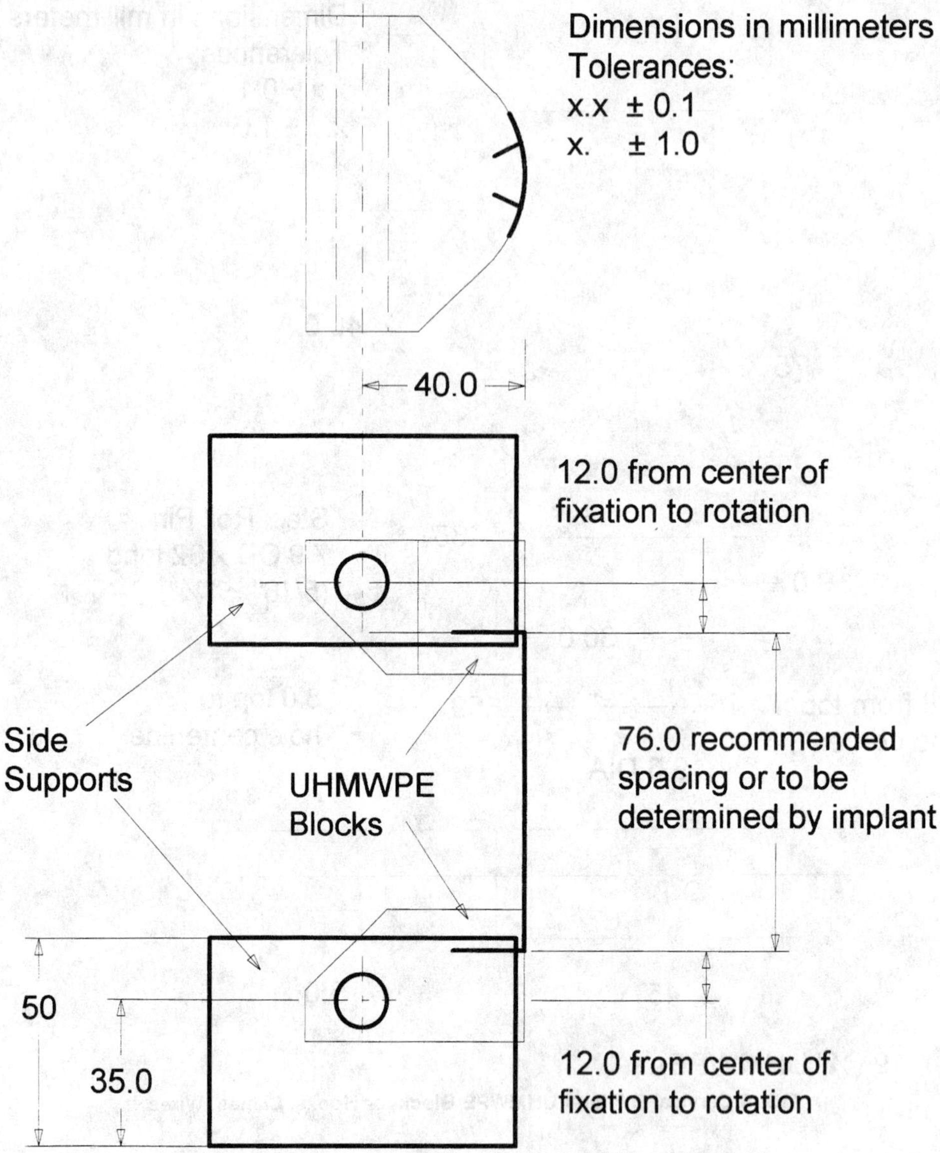

FIG. 10 Lumbar Unilateral UHMWPE Block for Screws or Bolts

static compression bending, static tension bending and compression bending fatigue tests applies load in the Z direction without constraining rotation in the X-Y plane. The hinge pin in the apparatus allows rotation in the X-Z plane during the static compression bending, static tension bending and compression bending fatigue tests. The compression bending fatigue test will use the same test configuration as static compressive bending.

6.13 The testing machine or the apparatus used in the static torsion test applies torque about the Z axis without constraining displacement in the Z direction. The aluminum blocks are placed in the apparatus to prevent rotation in the X-Z plane during the static torsion tests.

7. Sampling

7.1 All components in the spinal implant assembly shall be previously unused parts only. Implants shall not be retested.

7.2 Use the UHMWPE test blocks for only one test. The UHMWPE used to manufacture the test blocks should have a tensile breaking strength equal to 40 ± 3 MPa (see Test Method D 638). When alternate designs of test blocks are used, then all UHMWPE inserts should be replaced after each test. Alternate designs of test blocks which include steel roll pins (see Fig. 9 and Fig. 15) should replace the steel roll pins and UHMWPE inserts for the hinge after each test.

7.3 Label and maintain the test constructs according to good laboratory practice. Do not disassemble the test construct after testing unless disassembly is necessary to evaluate failure surfaces, interconnections, corrosion or loosening surfaces. Photograph the construct prior to disassembly.

7.4 All static tests should have a minimum of five samples. Examination of each load-displacement curve may reveal a laxity in the fixture. After the laxity has been removed, then the initial linear portion of the curve will define the straight line section of the load-displacement curves. The intersection of the straight line section and zero load axis is the zero load displacement (Point 0).

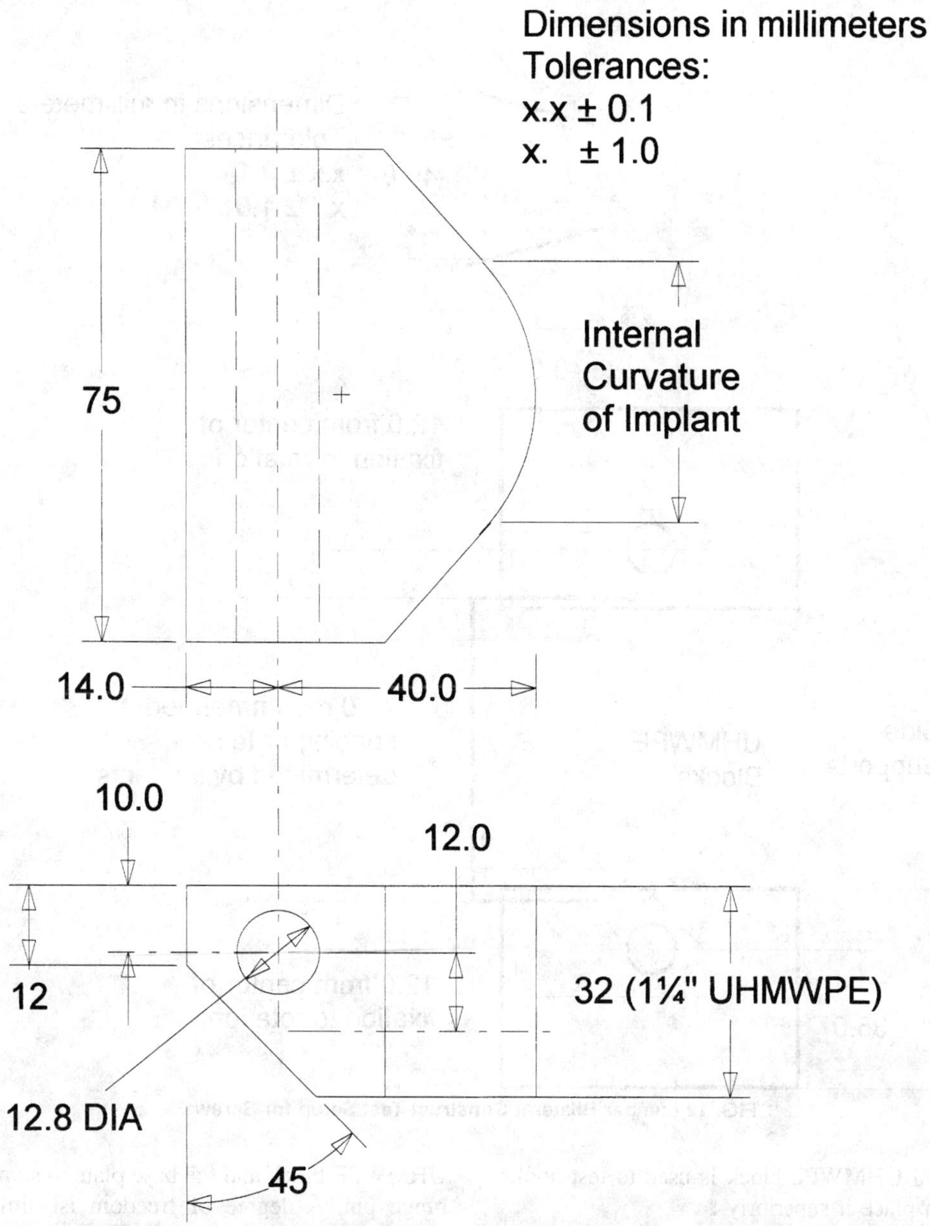

FIG. 11 Lumbar Unilateral UHMWPE Block for Screws or Bolts

7.5 The results of the fatigue testing will provide a curve of cyclical compression load or compression bending load versus the number of cycles to failure. The suggested initial fatigue loads should be 75, 50, and 25 % of the compression bending ultimate strength as determined in the static compression bending test. If a specimen does not fail by 5 000 000 cycles, then testing of that component should be considered run-out. The final sample size is recommended by Practice E 739. The differences between the maximum run out load and a load that results in a failed construct should be less than 10 % of the compression bending ultimate strength. Conduct a regression analysis on the load or moment versus number of cycles to failure data.

8. Procedure

8.1 *Procedure for Static Tests*—Evaluate only the load parameters in the relevant direction.

8.1.1 *Static Compression Bending Test*:

8.1.1.1 Select the appropriate UHMWPE blocks for the spinal implant assembly as previously described.

8.1.1.2 Install the anchors according to the manufacturer's instructions. If one modified bilateral UHMWPE block is used then place an aluminum spacer block between the modified UHMWPE block and the base plate to stop rotation around the hinge pin. A degree of freedom is eliminated in a similar manner to the axial compression test. If the spinal implant assembly requires two sets of modified bilateral UHMWPE blocks and aluminum spacer blocks, then it is equivalent to an axial compression test.

8.1.1.3 Place UHMWPE blocks into the test apparatus such that the position of the hinge pins are external to the anchors (the hinge pin in the superior block is more superior than the screw, hook, etc.). Secure UHMWPE blocks with hinge pins. If

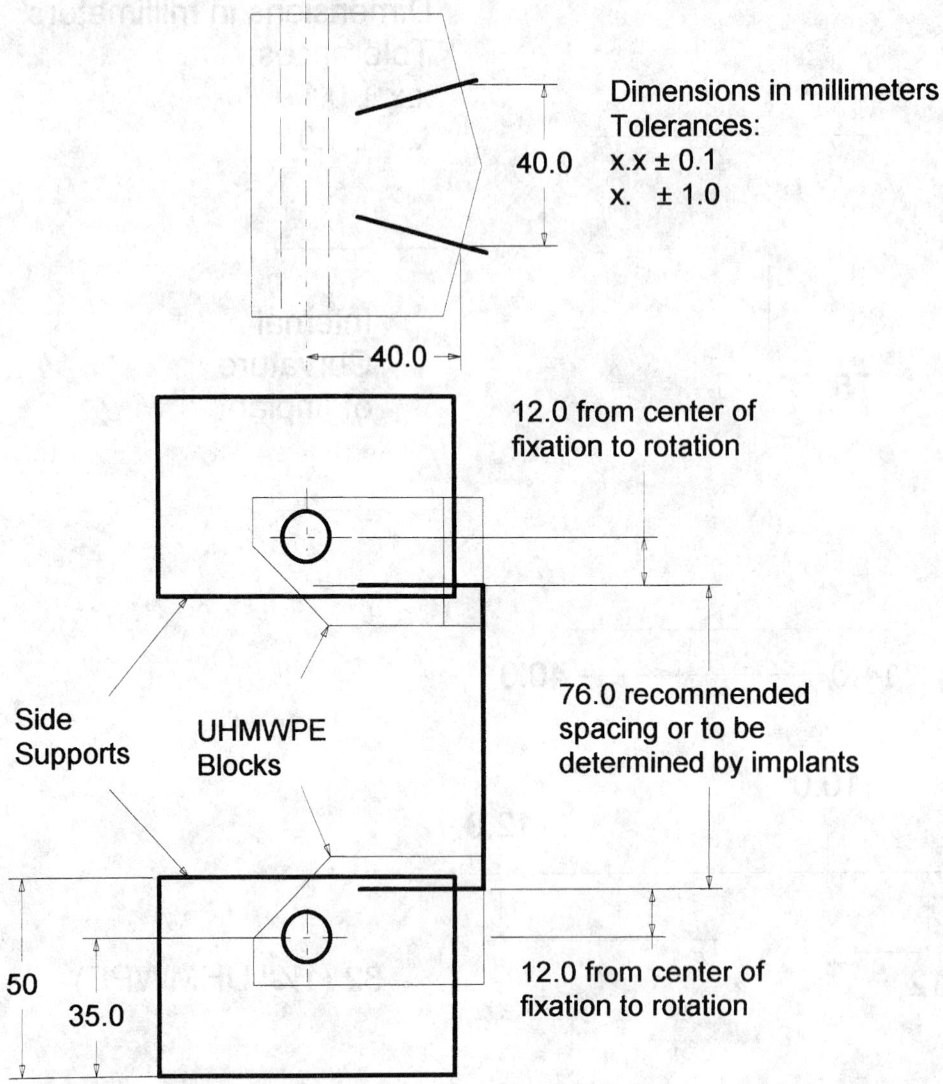

FIG. 12 Lumbar Bilateral Construct Test Setup for Screws

one modified bilateral UHMWPE block is used to test hooks, wires or cables, then place it superiorly.

8.1.1.4 Complete the spinal implant assembly in a standard construct (see Fig. 4, Fig. 6, Fig. 8, Fig. 10, Fig. 12 and Fig. 14) or a hybrid construct (see Fig. 3). Set the active length of the longitudinal element for the intended spinal location. Apply all tightening, crimping or locking mechanisms as specified by the manufacturer.

8.1.1.5 Load the test apparatus at a rate up to a maximum of 25 mm/min.

8.1.1.6 Record the load displacement curves. Establish the displacement at 2 % offset yield (mm), elastic displacement (mm), compressive bending yield load (N), compressive bending stiffness (N/mm), compressive bending ultimate displacement (mm) and compressive bending ultimate load (N).

8.1.2 *Static Tension Bending Test*:

8.1.2.1 Select the appropriate UHMWPE blocks for the spinal implant assembly as previously described.

8.1.2.2 Install the anchors according to the manufacturer's instructions. If one modified bilateral UHMWPE block is used, then place an aluminum spacer block between the modified UHMWPE block and the base plate to stop rotation around the hinge pin. A degree of freedom is eliminated in a similar manner to the axial compression test. If the spinal implant assembly requires two sets of modified bilateral UHMWPE blocks and aluminum spacer blocks, then it is equivalent to an axial tension test.

8.1.2.3 Place UHMWPE blocks into the test apparatus such that the position of the hinge pins are internal to the anchors (the hinge pin in the superior block is more inferior than the screw, hook, etc.). Secure UHMWPE blocks with hinge pins. If one modified bilateral UHMWPE block is used to test hooks, wires or cables, then place it superiorly.

8.1.2.4 Complete the spinal implant assembly in a standard construct (see Fig. 4, Fig. 6, Fig. 8, Fig. 10, Fig. 12 and Fig. 14 except the UHMWPE blocks are inverted) or a hybrid construct (see Fig. 3 except the UHMWPE block are inverted). Set the active length of the longitudinal element for the intended spinal location. Apply all tightening, crimping or locking mechanisms as specified by the manufacturer.

8.1.2.5 Load the test apparatus at a rate up to a maximum of 25 mm/min.

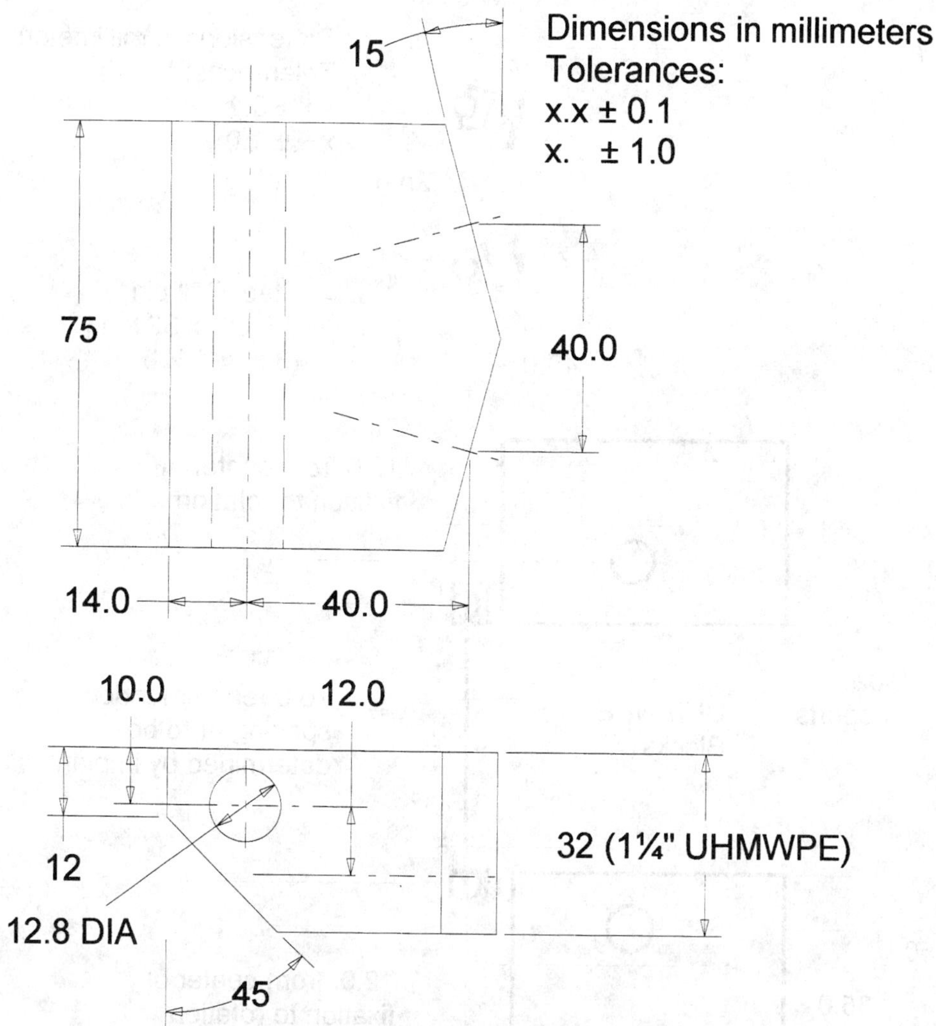

FIG. 13 Lumbar Bilateral UHMWPE Block for Screws or Bolts

8.1.2.6 Record the load displacement curves. Establish the displacement at 2 % offset yield (mm), elastic displacement (mm), tensile bending yield load (N), tensile bending stiffness (N/mm), tensile bending ultimate displacement (mm) and tensile bending ultimate load (N).

8.1.3 *Static Torsional Test*:

8.1.3.1 Select the appropriate UHMWPE blocks for the spinal implant assembly as previously described.

8.1.3.2 Install the anchors according to the manufacturer's instructions. If the spinal implant assembly contains only hooks, wires or cables then the system may not be able to resist torsional moments and need not be tested, however this should be verified by testing.

8.1.3.3 Place UHMWPE blocks in the test apparatus such that the positions of the hinge pins are external to the anchors. The hinge pin in the superior block is more superior than the screw, hook etc., and the hinge pin in the inferior block is more inferior than the screw, hook, etc. Secure UHMWPE blocks with hinge pins. If only one modified bilateral UHMWPE block is used to test hooks, wires or cables, then place it superiorly. Attach UHMWPE blocks to the side supports via hinge pins. Place the aluminum blocks between the UHMWPE blocks and the base plates to stop rotation around the hinge pin.

8.1.3.4 Complete the spinal implant assembly in a standard construct (Fig. 4, Fig. 6, Fig. 8, Fig. 10, Fig. 12 and Fig. 14) or a hybrid construct (Fig. 3). Set the active length of the longitudinal element for the intended spinal location. Apply all tightening, crimping or locking mechanisms as specified by the manufacturer.

8.1.3.5 Load the test apparatus at a maximum rate up to 60°/min.

8.1.3.6 Record the torque-angular displacement curves. Determine the angular displacement at 2 % offset yield (degrees), elastic angular displacement (degrees), yield torque (N-m), torsional stiffness (N-m/degree).

8.2 *Procedure for Fatigue Testing*:

8.2.1 Select the appropriate UHMWPE blocks for the spinal implant assembly as previously described. Use unilateral UHMWPE blocks (see Fig. 5 and Fig. 11) for singular longitudinal element constructs. Use bilateral UHMWPE block (see Fig. 7 and Fig. 13) for the testing of screws, bolts, etc. Use modified bilateral UHMWPE block (see Fig. 9 and Fig. 15) for the testing of hooks, wires or cables.

8.2.2 Install the anchors according to the manufacturer's instructions. If one modified bilateral UHMWPE block for hooks, wires, cables, etc. is used then place an aluminum

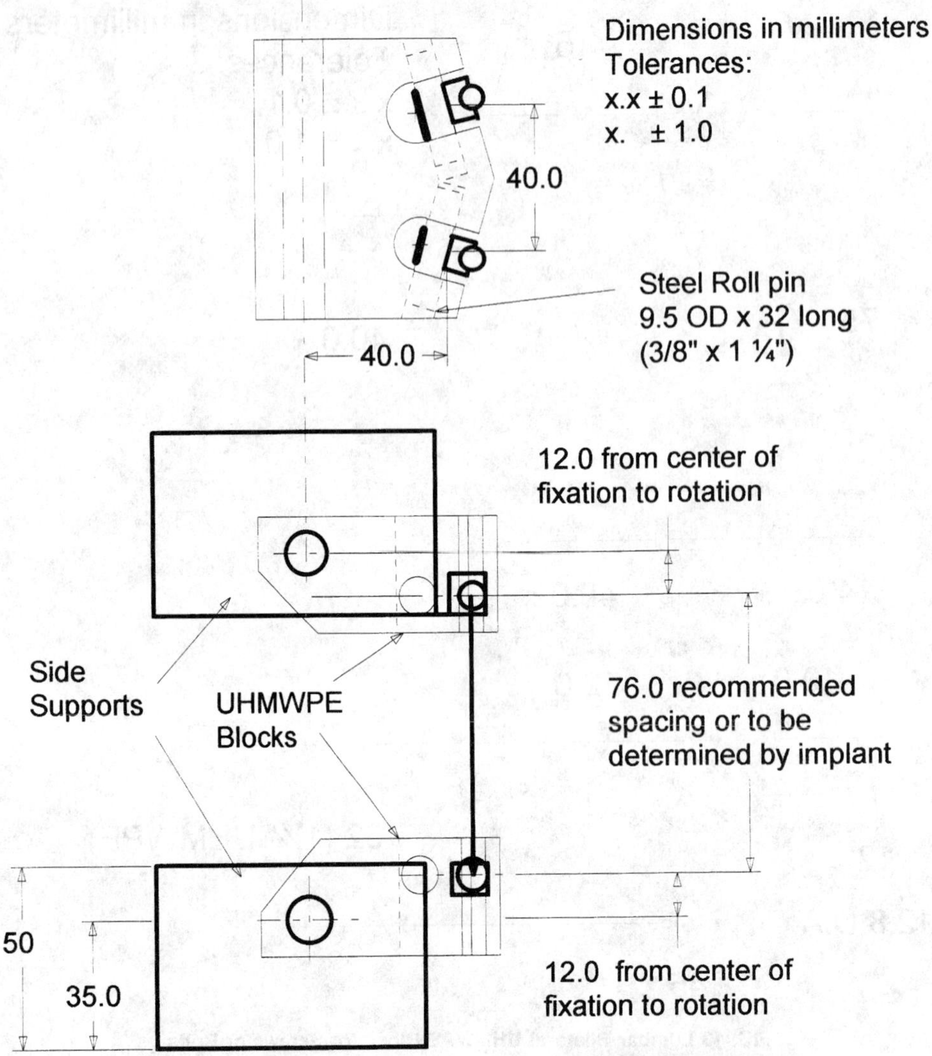

FIG. 14 Lumbar Bilateral Construct Test Setup for Hooks, Cables, or Wires

spacer block between the modified UHMWPE block and the base plate to stop rotation about the hinge pin. The extra degree of freedom is eliminated in a manner similar to the axial compression test. If the spinal implant assembly requires two sets of modified bilateral UHMWPE blocks and aluminum spacer blocks, then the testing mode becomes an axial compression fatigue test.

8.2.3 Place UHMWPE blocks in the test apparatus such that the positions of the hinge pins are external to the anchors. The hinge pin in the superior block is more superior than the anchor and the hinge pin in the inferior block is more inferior than the screw, hook, etc. Secure UHMWPE blocks with hinge pins. If only one modified bilateral UHMWPE block is used to test hooks, wires, cables, etc., then place it superiorly.

8.2.4 Complete the spinal implant assembly in a standard construct (Fig. 4, Fig. 6, Fig. 8, Fig. 10, Fig. 12 and Fig. 14) or a hybrid construct (Fig. 3). Set the active length of the longitudinal element for the intended spinal location. Apply all tightening, crimping or locking mechanisms as specified by the manufacturer.

8.2.5 The fatigue test applies a sinusoidal load to the spinal construct. The loading should be maintained via a constant sinusoidal load amplitude control. A constant load ratio (R) for all tests should be established and should be equal to or greater than 10

$$R = \frac{\textit{minimum load}}{\textit{maximum load}} \geq 10 \quad (2)$$

Example: if minimum load = −200 N and maximum load = −10 N then R = 20. The maximum cycle rate is five cycles per second for the fatigue test. The end of the test occurs when the spinal construct has a failure or reaches run-out.

8.2.6 Evaluate two specimens at the initial fatigue loads. Establish the maximum run out load (no specimens fail before 5 000 000 cycles). Continue fatigue testing pairs of specimens until the difference between a load in which a construct has failed and the maximum run-out load is no greater than 10 % of the compression bending ultimate load. A semi-log fatigue curve of the compression bending load versus number of cycles at failure will be plotted.

8.2.7 Note the initial and secondary failures, modes of failure and deformations of components prior to removing the spinal construct from the test apparatus. Evaluate all surface changes.

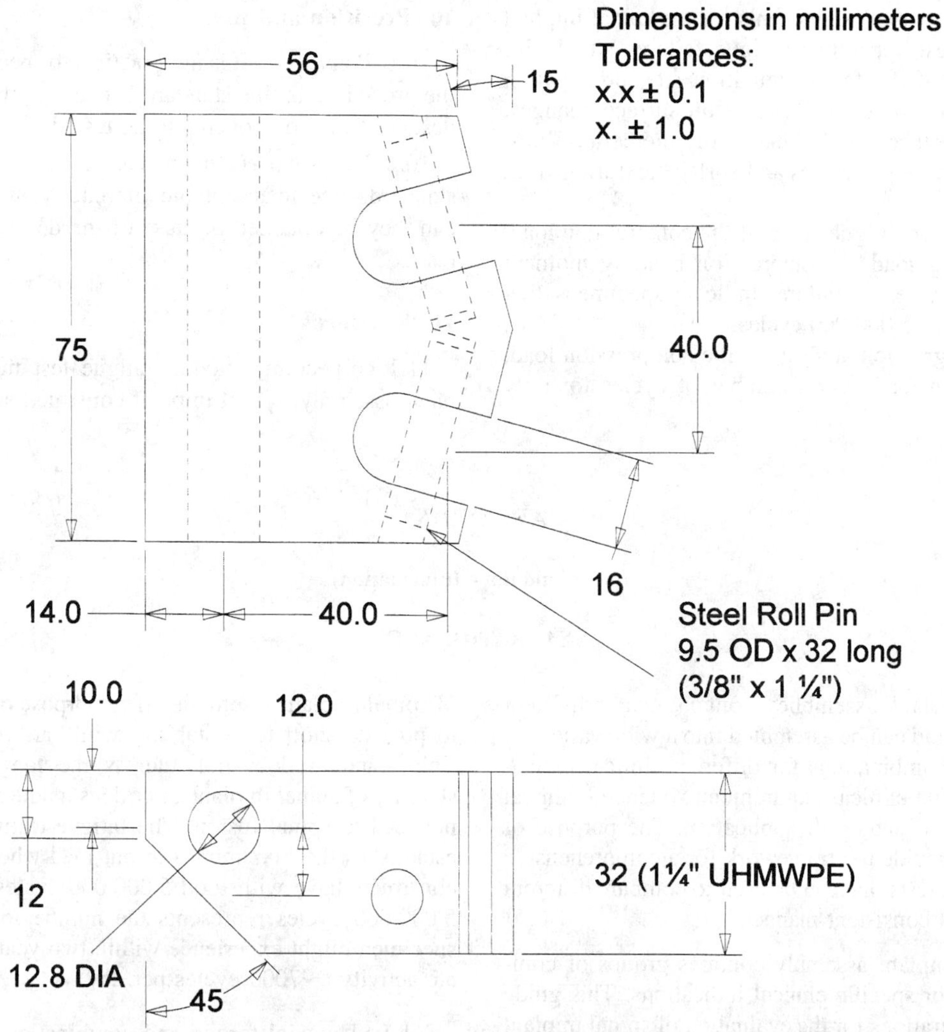

FIG. 15 Lumbar Bilateral UHMWPE Block for Hooks, Cables or Wires

9. Report

9.1 The report should specify the spinal implant components, the spinal implant assembly, the intended spinal location and the numbers of specimens tested. Describe all relevant information about the components including name, lot number, manufacturer, material, part number, etc. Also include any specific information necessary to produce the assembly including the tightening torque.

9.2 Include an illustration of the exact loading configurations. Describe the similarities and differences to relevant figures contained herein. Report the active length. Report the block moment arm and the distance in the *X* direction between the centerline of the longitudinal element and the insertion point of the anchors on the UHMWPE blocks. Note any deviations from the recommended test procedure. State the rate of loading.

9.3 The report of the static mechanical testing shall include a complete description of all failures, modes of failure, deformations of the spinal implant assembly or test apparatus. Include any noticeable fretting or surface texturing. The static mechanical test report shall:

9.3.1 Show the load-displacement curves for all static compression bending tests. Report all static compression bending test data, the mean and standard deviation for the displacement at 2 % offset yield (mm), elastic displacement (mm), compressive bending yield load (N), compressive bending stiffness (N/mm), compressive bending ultimate displacement (mm) and compressive bending ultimate load (N).

9.3.2 Show all load-displacement curves for the static tension bending test. Report all static tension bending test data, the mean and standard deviation for the displacement at 2 % offset yield (mm), elastic displacement (mm), tensile bending yield load (N), tensile bending stiffness (N/mm), tensile bending ultimate displacement (mm) and tensile bending ultimate load (N).

9.3.3 Show the torque-angular displacement curves for all static torsional test. Report all static torsional test data, the mean and standard deviation for the angular displacement at 2 % offset yield (degrees), elastic angular displacement (degrees), yield torque (N-m), torsional stiffness (N-m/degree).

9.4 The report of the dynamic mechanical testing shall:

9.4.1 State the final sample sizes and load versus number of cycles at failure for all fatigue tests. State the load levels for the specimens enduring 5 000 000 cycles and the maximum run out load. Report the constant load ratio (*R*).

9.4.2 Report all initial and secondary failures, modes of

failure and deformations of components for the spinal implant assembly and the test apparatus. Fatigue failures should include a description of the failure initiation site, propagation zone and ultimate failure zone. Describe all surface changes, any fretting of interfaces or loosening of interconnections. Include pictures of failure surfaces and surface texturing from fretting.

9.4.3 Plot a semi-log fatigue curve of the compression load, compression bending load or compression bending moment versus number of cycles at failure. Indicate specimens that have not failed before 5 000 000 cycles.

9.4.4 Report a regression analysis of the compression load, compression bending load versus number of cycles for only failed constructs.

10. Precision and Bias

10.1 *Precision*—It is not practical to specify the precision of the procedure in this standard because of the wide variance in design of the components to be tested.

10.2 *Bias*—No statement can be made as to bias of this standard since no acceptable reference values are available, nor can they be obtained because of the destructive nature of the tests.

11. Keywords

11.1 corpectomy model; fatigue test methods; spinal implant assembly; spinal implant construct; static test methods

APPENDIX

(Nonmandatory Information)

X1. RATIONALE

X1.1 Spinal implant assemblies contain many different component designs and can be assembled into a wide variety of configurations and combinations for different clinical indications dependent on the clinical requirements, intended clinical location and intended method of application. The purpose of this standard is to provide the framework for a comprehensive series of mechanical tests that can be used to compare different implant designs in a consistent manner.

X1.2 A spinal implant assembly contains groups of components necessary for specific clinical indications. This guide contains test configurations for the evaluation of spinal implant assemblies that simulate the clinical requirements for an intended clinical location and method of application. Some designs of thoracolumbar, lumbar and lumbosacral spine system are intended for both anterior and posterior attachment. These systems include anterior vertebral body/pedicle/sacral screws, hooks, rods and transverse interconnections. Fig. 2 is an example of a standard test configuration. Fig. 6 or Fig. 12 are constructs which simulating a common clinical group of components normally applied to the anterior surface of a vertebral body or posterior vertebral structures. The hybrid test configuration seen in Fig. 3 would normally be applied posteriorly and contains sacral screws, hooks, rods and transverse interconnections.

X1.3 A spinal implant construct installed in the test apparatus will simultaneously evaluate all components within the assembly in the worst case test configuration (corpectomy model). A corpectomy is assumed to be a worst case scenario because all loads are transferred from the fixture and are transmitted only through the implant assembly. All proposed test configurations are based on anatomical dimensions. Some asymmetric test assemblies may not be applicable to this standard. In these cases, the hinge pin might be replaced with a ball and socket.

X1.4 This standard covers the static and cyclic evaluation of spinal implant assemblies. The purpose of spinal implants is to provide short term stability while arthrodesis takes place. This standard does not address the long term mechanical stability of spinal implants, nor does it address implants that do not lead to spinal fusion. The fatigue testing in this standard establishes the maximum run out load where all of the tested constructs have withstood 5 000 000 cycles without a failure. 5 000 000 cycles represents the number of loading cycles a specimen might experience within two years based on moderate activity (~7000 cycles per day).

X1.5 Uniaxial torque and combination axial and bending loading are applied in this standard. Numerous combinations of multiaxial loading conditions *in vivo* have not yet been fully defined. This standard outlines a series of simplistic static and dynamic loading conditions and does not attempt to mimic the complex loading patterns in the spine.

X1.6 The influence of simulated body fluid or saline may affect the relative performance of tested devices. The tests outlined here should be performed dry (ambient room conditions) to eliminate unwanted complexity resulting from environmental factors. This will reduce the variability of the results. Individual investigators may consider additional evaluations in simulated body fluid, saline, water or lubricants to address environmental factors. It should be noted that corrosive fatigue testing may be influenced by the cycle rate, therefore the maximum cycle rate should be reduced.

X1.7 The variation in the block moment arm for the static and fatigue bending tests is a function of the relative location (*X*direction) between the hinge pin and the insertion point of the anchor. The variation in the relative location is dependent on the direction of rotation (tension or compression) and arrangement of the UHMWPE blocks. The variation in the block moment arm for the thoracolumbar, lumbar and lumbosacral test configuration ranges between ±4 % for a 57-mm displacement or 39° rotation of each block. The block moment arm variations for the cervical test configuration range between ±2 % for a 29-mm displacement or 27° rotation of each block.

X1.8 Reporting the compression or tensile bending moments and the bending moments versus numbers of cycles at failure are not recommended because confusion regarding the moment arm may exist. The block moment arms are constants per this standard. The block moment arm is 30.0 mm for cervical constructs (see Fig. 4, Fig. 6 and Fig. 8) and 40.0 mm for thoracolumbar, lumbar and lumbosacral constructs (see Fig. 10, Fig. 12 and Fig. 14). However, the moment arm at the longitudinal element can vary from one spinal assembly to another. The moment arm at the longitudinal element is the sum of the block moment arm and the Xdistance from the insertion point of an anchor to the longitudinal element.

X1.9 This standard is not intended to allow direct comparison between the *in-vitro* results and clinical results. This is due to a number of factors including, but not limited to, the test fixture materials, lack of physiologic fluids, applied loads, clinical assemblage of constructs, over tightening screws into the UHMWPE blocks such that they buttress tightly against the plastic, etc. In order to better mimic clinical failures seen with some devices, it is suggested that the researcher investigate means of testing which would create the type and locations of failures seen clinically. Several possible modifications to the methods and materials include inserting the screw such that its head does not tightly touch the UHMWPE block, counterboring the screw insertion holes 1 mm larger than the outer diameter of the screws for a depth equal to the screws' diameter or the addition of soft washers with oversized holes. Any modification to the methods and materials should maintain the specified block moment arm.

X1.10 This standard is not intended to define performance levels of spinal implants as insufficient knowledge is available to predict the consequence of the use of particular spinal implant design and assemblies.

Designation: F 1719 – 96

Standard Specification for Image-Interactive Stereotactic and Localization Systems[1]

This standard is issued under the fixed designation F 1719; the number immediately following the designation indicates the year of original adoption or, in the case of revision, the year of last revision. A number in parentheses indicates the year of last reapproval. A superscript epsilon (ε) indicates an editorial change since the last revision or reapproval.

1. Scope

1.1 This specification covers the combined use of stereotactic instruments or systems with imaging techniques, to direct a diagnostic or therapeutic modality into a specific target within the brain, based on localization information derived from such imaging techniques.

1.2 For the purpose of this specification, a stereotactic instrument or system is a guiding, aiming, or viewing device used in human neurosurgery for the purpose of manually directing a system or treating modality to a specific point within the brain by radiographic, imaging, or other visualization or identification of landmarks or targets or lesions.

1.3 *Definition of Stereotactic Imaging Systems*—Types of imaging-guided systems all require three components: an imaging system, a stereotactic frame, or other physical device to identify the position of a point in space, and a method to relate image-generated coordinates to frame or device coordinates. See Performance Specification F 1266. The imaging technique must reliably and reproducibly generate data concerning normal or abnormal anatomic structures, or both, that can interface with the coordinate system of the stereotactic frame or other stereotactic system. The imaging-guided systems must allow accurate direction of therapeutic, viewing or diagnostic modalities to a specific point or volume or along a specific trajectory within the brain or often accurate estimation of structure size and location allowing biopsy, resection, vaporization, implantation, aspiration, or other manipulation, or combination thereof. The standards of accuracy, reproducibility, and safety must be met for the imaging modality, the stereotactic system, and the method of interface between the two, and for the system as a whole. The mechanical parts of the imaging modality and the stereotactic system should be constructed to allow maximal interaction with minimal interference with each other, to minimize imaging artifact and distortion, and minimize potential contamination of the surgical field.

1.4 *General Types of Imaging that May Be Used With Stereotactic Systems*—Currently employed imaging modalities used in imaging-guided stereotactic systems include radiography, angiography, computed tomography, magnetic resonance imaging, ultrasound, biplane and multiplane digital subtraction angiography, and positron emission scanning. However, it is recognized that other modalities may be interfaced with currently available and future stereotactic systems and that new imaging modalities may evolve in the future. Standards for imaging devices will be dealt with in documents concerning such devices, and will not be addressed herein.

1.5 General types of diagnostic modalities include biopsy instruments, cannulas, endoscopes, electrodes, or other such instruments. Therapeutic modalities include, but are not limited to, heating, cooling, irradiation, laser, injection, tissue transplantation, mechanical or ultrasonic disruption, and any modality ordinarily used in cerebrospinal surgery.

1.6 *Probe*—Any system or modality directed by stereotactic techniques, including mechanical or other probe, a device that is inserted into the brain or points to a target, and stereotactically directed treatment or diagnostic modality.

NOTE 1—Examples presented throughout this specification are listed for clarity only; that does not imply that use should be restricted to the procedures or examples listed.

1.7 *Robot*—A power-driven servo-controlled system for controlling and advancing a probe according to a predetermined targeting program.

1.8 *Digitizer*—A device that is directed to indicate the position of a probe or point in stereotactic or other coordinates.

1.9 *Frameless System*—A system that does not require a stereotactic frame, that identifies and localizes a point or volume in space by means of data registration, and a method to relate that point or volume to its representation derived from an imaging system.

1.10 The values stated in SI units are to be regarded as the standard.

1.11 The following precautionary caveat pertains only to the test method portion, Section 3, of this specification: *This standard does not purport to address all of the safety concerns, if any, associated with its use. It is the responsibility of the user of this standard to establish appropriate safety and health practices and determine the applicability of regulatory limitations prior to use.*

2. Referenced Documents

2.1 *ASTM Standards:*

F 1266 Performance Specification for Cerebral Stereotactic Instruments[2]

---

[1] This specification is under the jurisdiction of ASTM Committee F-4 on Medical and Surgical Materials and Devices and is the direct responsibility of Subcommittee F04.31 on Neurosurgical Standards.

Current edition approved June 10, 1996. Published October 1996.

[2] *Annual Book of ASTM Standards*, Vol 13.01.

3. Types of Imaging-Guided Stereotactic Systems

3.1 Any type of stereotactic apparatus may be adapted to imaging-guided stereotactic surgery. A stereotactic system can be based on one or more of the following concepts:

3.1.1 *Arc-Centered Type*—A target centered arc with rectilinear adjustments is constructed according to the spherical radius principle so that the target point lies at the center of an arc along which the probe holder moves, so that when a probe is inserted into the probe holder perpendicular to a tangent of the arc and for a distance equal to the radius of the arc, the tip of the probe arrives at a single point in space, that is, the stereotactic target.

3.1.2 *Rectilinear Type*—The rectilinear type provides individually for the longitudinal, transverse, and vertical movements of the probe holder or the patient, or both, perpendicular to or at an angle to the planes along which the probe holder is moved.

3.1.3 *Aiming Type of Stereotactic Apparatus*—A device that is referenced to a specific entry point so the probe can be pointed to the desired target point and then advanced to it.

3.1.4 *Multiple-Arc Type*—An arc system that is not target centered and is a system of interlocking arcs, pivots, or joints arranged so that the orientation of the probe is controlled and can be directed to the target by independent movement of the elements. As the depth of each target may be different relative to the arc system, means for determining target depth must be provided.

3.1.5 An articulated arm that allows accurate determination of the position in space of a probe or other device held by the arm. Such a system ordinarily is coupled with computer graphics to allow identification of the location of the probe in relation to the position of the head in space. By relating the position of the head and the graphic image, the position of the probe relative to the head or structures within the head can be demonstrated.

3.1.6 A probe whose position and movement in space can be detected, calibrated, and related to the position on the patient's head or intracranial target by a nonmechanical modality, such as infrared, visual light, sound, or ultrasound.

3.1.7 The above represents a general classification of current systems and does not preclude future developments. Any given system may represent any of the above types of stereotactic device or may be a combination of two or more systems.

3.2 *Image Interactive Localization Systems*:

3.2.1 Any type of stereotactic apparatus may be adapted to function as an image interactive localization system. For such to occur, it is necessary for the stereotactic apparatus to be equipped with a means for relating its location in threedimensional space with the computerized image display system. These means of communication may include the following:

3.2.1.1 Optical encoders that record the amount of displacement on the set of coordinates axis and arcs that are used to position the probe of the stereotactic system.

3.2.1.2 Mechanical encoders that record the amount of displacement set on the coordinate axis and arcs that are used to position the probe of the stereotactic system.

3.2.1.3 Other means of recording the amount of displacement set on the coordinate axis and arcs that are used to position the probe of the stereotactic system.

3.2.2 Systems may be designed for image interactive localization that do not incorporate the stereotactic apparatus concepts discussed in 9.1.1. Regardless of whether these systems are framed-based, table-based or room-(space) based, they employ a means for generating a probe orientation in three-dimensional space that can be used by the computerized image display system. Intraoperative calibration of the system is desirable, and it should be incorporated where practical. Means for generating a probe orientation in three-dimensional space may include the following:

3.2.2.1 Multiple-degree-of-freedom "robotic" arms that use optical, mechanical, or other types of encoders to register the position/orientation of each joint. Calibration of the arm with respect to the known location of reference points in three-dimensional space is usually required.

3.2.2.2 Systems that use optical or sonic information to triangulate the location and orientation of the probe. Calibration of the system with respect to the known location of reference points in three-dimensional space is usually required.

3.2.2.3 Six-degree-of-freedom electromagnetic receiver/transmitters that may or may not require intraoperative calibration of the three-dimensional space.

3.2.2.4 Other alignment by means of generated information may be used by the computerized image display system, with or without three-dimensional space calibration.

3.2.3 The above represents a general classification of current systems or systems currently in development and does not preclude future development.

4. Applications of Imaging Techniques to Stereotactic Instruments

4.1 Some of the means used to relate an imaging system to stereotactic apparatus may be mated by:

4.1.1 Attaching the apparatus to the table during imaging and relating the position of the slice to fiducials on the apparatus,

4.1.2 Relating the height of the image to the stereotactic apparatus by attaching an indicator to the table, that can then be used as a phantom to adjust the apparatus,

4.1.3 Employing a translational imaging technique to relate the position of the image to the head or to the apparatus,

4.1.4 Including in the scanner plane markers or fiducials which can be used to calculate the position and inclination of the imaging slice,

4.1.5 Using three-dimensional computer reconstruction techniques to determine both the position of the target and the position of the apparatus, so these two positions might be correlated. Such techniques may make possible the visualization of the volume and shape of the target in space, so that each point in the entire target can be defined by stereotactic coordinates.

4.2 *Imaging Systems*:

4.2.1 The region of interest may either be constituted by abnormal structures (brain lesions) identified with imaging systems or normal anatomical structures (functional stereotaxis), or both, to which the sensitivity of the imaging technique should be addressed. In case of normal structures, the location may need the use of standard atlases or tables and the method of transposition and its accuracy should be addressed. Previously, the conversion of X-ray coordinates to stereotactic space was performed with manual triangulation. With the development of computed tomography and magnetic resonance imaging technology, most conversion is often now performed utilizing computer software.

4.2.2 The interface between imaging and stereotactic space may be performed by several methods; the identification of the location of normal structures within stereotactic space and then the use of standard atlases or other tables to define a given anatomical location, the identification of the relationship of normal and abnormal structures using an imaging technique with subsequent reconstruction of this relationship within the stereotactic system, digitization and conversion of analog imaging data to stereotactic space, and transformation of imaging data generated within the stereotactic system using manual transfer where indicated.

4.2.3 Imaging may be based on visualization in a slice, a reconstructed plane, or be represented by a volume, and the accuracy may vary depending of which system is used. The system should incorporate, wherever feasible, an alternate or back-up method to compensate for possible primary system failure or distortion. It is recognized that, in the future, changes are likely to occur in both imaging and technology and computer technology, and these standards should not be interpreted in such a manner as to impair development of new systems, as long as accuracy and safety requirements are met.

4.3 *Stereotactic Frame Requirements*—It should be possible to use the frame with an imaging system or systems for which it has been designed or adapted, as verified by the calibration considerations outlined in 4.3 and 4.4.

4.4 *Accuracy*—In addition to concerns of accuracy of each of the components of the stereotactic systems, enumerated in other sections of this specification, the components should interrelate in such a way that accuracy of the overall system is not compromised.

4.5 *Application Accuracy*:

4.5.1 Each system should include information from the manufacturer indicating the reproducible accuracy of the entire system in use for each imaging modality with which the system is to be used, how such accuracy was determined, and instructions so the surgeon might test the entire system to ensure that the indicated accuracy and degree of confidence has been preserved.

4.5.2 *MR-stereotactic Application Accuracy*—Since nonlinear distortion is an inherent property of magnetic resonance scanning, the surgeon should be aware of potential inaccuracies imposed in an individual case. Also, since accuracy of magnetic resonance imaging scanners varies from one scanner to another and from one technique to another, such user testing might demonstrate inaccuracies inherent in an individual MR-stereotactic system.

5. Anesthesia and Operating Room Safety

5.1 *Scope*—This specification is concerned with the definitions and standards that are required in the design of imaging-guided stereotactic systems to ensure patient and operating room personnel safety during the administration of anesthesia for imaging-guided stereotactic procedures.

5.2 *Definition*—For the purpose of this specification, general anesthesia may be defined as a state of altered consciousness occurring as a result of drug administration by intravenous, intramuscular, inhalational, or oral routes.

5.3 The choice of type of anesthesia (general versus monitored versus local) is the responsibility of the operating surgeon, with consultation with the anesthesiologist as indicated. The choice of anesthetic agent and means of administration is the responsibility of the anesthesiologist after consultation with the operating surgeon.

5.4 *General Requirements*—The standards for the use of anesthesthetics with imaging-guided stereotactic surgery are the same as indicated in Performance Specification F 1266.

5.5 *Specific Requirements*:

5.5.1 *Disconnect System*—The mechanism to connect or rapidly disconnect the patient from that part of the imaging-guided stereotactic apparatus as may be necessary in an emergency must be easily accessible, quickly operative, and independent of electrical supply, as may be necessary to manage any untoward drug reaction, excess secretions to cardiopulmonary failure during either the imaging or surgical part of the procedure.

5.5.2 *Airway Maintenance*—The apparatus shall allow reasonable access to the head and neck for maintenance of an airway either by endotracheal tube, laryngeal mask airway, or suctioning.

5.5.3 *Other Monitoring*—The apparatus shall also be constructed to allow monitoring of vital signs including, but not limited to, blood pressure, electrocardiogram, and pulse oximetry, during the operative portion of the procedure, or any part of the procedure during which sedation or general anesthesia is employed.

5.5.4 If there is a significant risk of pressure on or burns to any part of the patient, warnings and instructions to avoid this should be included.

5.5.5 The device should allow changing of the position of the patient's head as necessary to gain access to carry out the planned procedure safely and address any emergencies that may arise.

5.5.6 Attachment of the frame to the head should be possible by means which minimize infection and damage to the scalp, skull, brain, or other structures in the head.

5.5.7 The positioning of the frame should not interfere with free communication with the patient where this is necessary.

5.5.8 The localization method should be simple and straightforward enough to minimize errors of reading scales, interpretation of data, and calculation of coordinates.

6. Sterilizability

6.1 *Scope*—This specification establishes requirements for sterilizability of that part of the imaging-guided stereotactic system that must be sterilized because of its presence within the sterile operating field. Excluded from discussion are probes, as defined in 1.6.

6.2 *Requirements*:

6.2.1 The patient invasive components of the stereotactic apparatus must be sterilizable by an accepted procedure for sterilization of neurosurgical instruments (see also section 7.2.5).

6.2.2 If detached from the main apparatus during the sterilization procedure, it must be possible to reattach these patient invasive components to the apparatus with preservation of the sterility.

6.2.3 The probe and probe holder must satisfy the requirement of sterilizability by an accepted procedure for sterilization of surgical instruments.

6.2.4 If the design of the apparatus permits intraoperative adjustments of the probe holder, the apparatus design must reasonably permit the operator to make such adjustments while preserving the sterility of both the probe and the patient invasive components.

6.2.5 Instructions shall be included for the sterilization of the necessary parts of the stereotactic apparatus, using techniques that are ordinarily available within a hospital facility. These instructions shall include, but are not limited to, any special requirements for cleaning, disassembly and reassembly, packaging, or special handling of any parts of the apparatus if such a procedure does not conform to the usual techniques of sterilization of a surgical instrument. Instructions should include sterilization under special circumstances, such as with agents such as slow virus. Comments should be included about which sterilization techniques are not compatible with the system.

6.2.6 Advice concerning sterilization should deal both with avoidance of damage to the system by sterilization method and technique for prevention of cross-contamination, particularly with difficult organisms, such as slow viruses.

6.2.7 Any contraindication to sterilization of all or part of the stereotactic portion of the apparatus by the use of standard sterilization techniques shall be clearly noted. Any contraindication to steam autoclaving that may distort the parts shall be prominently labeled on the parts package.

6.2.8 Routine sterilization processes must not affect or impair the system so that numbers and markings become difficult to read.

6.2.9 Any items that are disposable should be clearly marked not to be resterilized, and the method of initial sterilization shall be made available upon request.

6.2.10 Labeling on the device package shall describe the recommended storing conditions to maintain sterility.

7. Instructions and Warnings

7.1 *General*—Instructions to be included with every apparatus to be used in imaging-guided stereotactic surgery sold by the manufacturer or his agent shall include the following information:

7.1.1 Clear instructions written in the official languages current in the country in which it is marketed.

7.1.2 Description of the apparatus and nomenclature for the component parts.

7.1.3 Instructions for assembling and disassembling, cleaning and sterilization, including warnings of damage to be anticipated from commonly used techniques.

7.1.4 Recommended means of checking for accuracy, malassembly, or other factors that would affect the use or accuracy of the equipment.

7.1.5 Recommendations for dimensions of probes to be used with the system.

7.1.6 Instructions or diagrams for recommended method of positioning the patient's head within the system or attachment of the apparatus to the patient's head, including advice about its application to cover special areas such as the cerebellum and suggestions to avoid unnecessary damage to tissues.

7.1.7 Instructions for performance of the imaging procedure in such a way that it is compatible with use in image-guided stereotactic surgery.

7.1.8 Instructions for performance of whatever calculations and computational procedures are necessary to utilize the imaging information with the operative part of the procedure, including methods for checking accuracy of a result. Whenever possible, the system should incorporate a technique to reconfirm the accuracy of the system intraoperatively.

7.1.9 The degree of accuracy required in various stereotactic applications varies greatly, depending on the nature of the surgery, the size of the target, and the proximity to functioning neurological and vascular structures. For instance, a great accuracy, within 1 to 2 mm, is required to insert an electrode into a physiological target that may be only a few millimetres in diameter and in the midst of other important neurological structures. Much less accuracy, perhaps 1 cm, may be required to guide a resection around the periphery of a mass with indistinct margins several centimetres in diameter. The manufacturer should provide with any stereotactic or localization system a documented statement of what application accuracy can be expected when the system is used properly with a prescribed imaging modality, in order to provide the surgeon the information necessary to decide whether that system is appropriate for the intended procedure.

7.1.10 Recommended procedure for positioning or changing position of the probe-holder indicating a technique that is compatible with the design of the apparatus.

7.1.11 Instructions for a recommended technique for insertion of the electrode or other probes into the probe-holder to minimize risk to straightness or insulation of the device.

7.1.12 Recommended procedure for repositioning the probe-holder or the patient's head in order to adjust the system properly to aim the insertion device to the target.

7.1.13 Warnings concerning any commonly encountered error with use of the system, such as determining lateral position when working on the back of the head when the part of the apparatus carrying the probe might be reversed.

7.1.14 Recommended procedure for rapidly disconnecting the patient from the apparatus for quick access to the head in the event of an emergency, if required.

7.1.15 Recommendations to follow in the event of system failure, recognizing that the computer systems are adjunct tools, and that the surgeon's judgment and experience should be used to decide how to complete the surgery by conventional means.

7.1.16 Procedures for which the frame is easily compatible and any special advice about other procedures for which it can be used but with certain cautions.

NOTE 2—It is recognized that there is no standard technique for the conduct of imaging-guided stereotactic surgery and that it is not appropriate for the manufacturer to dictate surgical procedures. Instructions should concern themselves primarily with matters regarding the design and use of the apparatus. It is recognized that the surgeon has the ultimate responsibility for the welfare of the patient and that surgeons have a variety of surgical approaches. The manufacturer cannot include all possible acceptable techniques in any instruction manual, but should include a recommended technique and sufficient detail so that a neurosurgeon schooled in the field of imaging-guided stereotactic surgery might know how to use the specific instrumentation, even if the operator has had no prior experience with it. It is recognized that the experience, training, and innovation of the operator may lead him to use or develop a technique other than the single technique outlined in the instruction manual.

7.1.17 A written description of an approved method for verifying that the instrument system is within the accepted tolerances for safe and effective use shall be provided by the manufacturer.

7.2 *Warnings*:

7.2.1 All stereotactic systems, whether frame-based or frameless should be viewed as adjuncts to the skills of the surgeon.

7.2.2 If the characteristics of the apparatus have been changed so there is any incompatibility between old and new versions, this should be clearly stated in the literature accompanying the system.

7.2.3 Parts of the system that can be used in only a single imaging modality should be clearly labeled as such, for example, "for use with CT scanning only."

8. Instruments and Manufacturers

8.1 *General*—Manufacturers of imaging compatible stereotactic devices and surgical instruments are responsible for the production of extremely precise intracranial guiding devices. Manufacturers have the responsibility to confirm adequate product testing and safety commensurate with standards established in this specification. Prior to marketing of any device, product safety documentation will include appropriate mechanical accuracy testing.

8.2 *Accessibility of Manufacturers*—Manufacturers of stereotactic instruments will provide as part of their product information current addresses and phone numbers so that buyers and users, whether actual or potential, can reach them for appropriate questions about the product.

8.3 *Product Information*—Manufacturers will have a description of the stereotactic device, including its usage, accuracy, and compatibility with imaging systems. Product information will also include associated instrumentation which can be sold together with or separately from the stereotactic system.

8.4 *Warranty*—Manufacturers of stereotactic instruments will provide a warranty certifying the function of the device for a fixed period of time. The length of warranty can be specified by the manufacturer.

8.5 *Replacement Parts*—Manufacturers will keep a current list of replacement parts available, including current prices and availability.

8.6 *Notification of Product Availability Changes, New Products or Replacement Parts, or Both*:

8.6.1 Manufacturers should retain as accurate a list as possible of all current and potential users or buyers of stereotactic instrumentation, or both, who may be notified of appropriate changes and product availability or discontinued products. Similarly, the manufacturer may wish to provide a list of new products or replacement products. This list should be kept current (validated once per year) so that purchasers and users may be notified of appropriate availability changes. This list will also be valuable in the event that timely warnings or changes can be communicated to users or buyers.

8.6.2 It is appropriate that if a company itself changes hands, is no longer operational, or has discontinued products, that buyers or purchasers be notified of these changes.

8.7 It is appropriate that manufacturers of stereotactic instruments provide timely notification of real or potential problems that are brought to their attention by either purchasers or users of their stereotactic systems.

8.8 *Documentation of Product Users; Results of Experimental or Clinical Trials*—It is appropriate that manufacturers maintain a current list of references published in both lay and scientific literature that details the current use and results of clinical trials using the products involved.

9. Uses and Significance of Imaging-Guided Stereotactic Neurosurgery

9.1 The following uses of imaging-guided stereotactic surgery have been documented in the literature, and are presented as examples. This list is not inclusive of all the techniques presently being used, and certainly does not reflect nor intend to impede the development of new techniques in the future:

9.1.1 Biopsy of intracranial tissue,

9.1.2 Implantation of radioisotopes by various techniques,

9.1.3 Aspiration of cysts,

9.1.4 Aspiration of abcesses,

9.1.5 Instillation of therapeutic agents, including antibiotics, chemotherapeutic agents, tissue, drugs, and neurotransmitters,

9.1.6 Insertion of electrodes for recording of electrical activity or impedance,

9.1.7 Insertion of probes for lesion production in functional neurosurgery,

9.1.8 Insertion of electrodes for stimulation,

9.1.9 Aspiration of hematomas,

9.1.10 Resection of mass lesions,

9.1.11 Laser vaporization or removal of intracranial tissue,

9.1.12 Guidance of externally delivered radiation therapy,

9.1.13 Adjunct to open surgical procedures,

9.1.14 Placement of catheters into ventricles, cysts, and so forth, and

9.1.15 Hyperthermia.

10. Calibration and Test Methods

10.1 The standards for the calibration and the test methods shall follow the same requirements as stated is Section 7 of Performance Specification F 1266.

10.2 As each of the imaging techniques produces its own problems relative to target determination, each of the presently known systems, as well as systems to be developed in the future, should be addressed separately. Some of the problems that relate to individual imaging techniques are listed as follows:

10.2.1 *Computerized Axial Tomographic Imaging*:

10.2.1.1 The presence of certain metals in the construction of the stereotactic system may cause the appearance of artifact or distortion on generated images. Such materials either should not be used or should be employed in such a manner that they do not interfere with the visualization of intracranial areas of interest or with fiducial markers.

10.2.1.2 The resolution of location of the AP and lateral coordinates within the plane of any image is determined by the resolution of the imaging system.

10.2.1.3 The resolution of the *Z* or vertical coordinate pertaining to location of any given image may be influenced by mechanical factors, however, such as slice thickness, accuracy of table travel, and accuracy of gantry angulation. Determination of this coordinate must utilize a method that is at least as accurate as the slice thickness for the imager. If table travel is used to determine this coordinate directly, then a means for verifying the accuracy of travel must be provided. If the stereotactic system requires that orthogonal slices be taken through the system for coordinate generation, then a means for aligning the gantry with the plane of the system must be provided.

10.2.2 *Magnetic Resonance Imaging*:

10.2.2.1 Stereotactic localization depends on the spatial accuracy of the images used. The MRI stereotaxis is potentially superior to other imaging techniques because MRI enables nonreformatted imaging in multiple planes, provides better anatomic resolution, can define the target using different pulse sequences or contrast enhancement, produces no ionizing radiation, and minimizes imaging artifacts caused by the frame itself.

10.2.2.2 A fundamental prerequisite for high-quality MRI is a stable magnetic field. The primary factors that introduce geometrical distortion are inhomogeneity in the magnetic field and nonlinear magnetic field gradients. Field homogeneity may be disrupted by imperfections in the manufacturer's magnet construction, temporal fluctuations in the power supply, thermal instability, internal or external ferromagnetic objects, or susceptibility artifacts at air-fat or air-water interfaces. The most common artifact is caused by patient movement. The lack of air-water or air-tissue interfaces in the brain should limit the occurrence of susceptibility artifacts that depend on the sequence method. Eddy currents are residual magnetic gradients that can result in more rapid dephasing of magnetization when noncylindrical or nonspherical shapes are imaged.

10.2.2.3 Optimal stereotactic MRI can be obtained by frequent calibration of the MRI unit to standard test phantoms, the use of nonferromagnetic frames and fiducial systems, and immobilization of the patient during image acquisition. The MRI stereotactic quality assurance program should include correction for inhomogeneous shimming of the magnet (suboptimal tuning of individual shim coils to achieve magnetic field homogeneity). Quality assurance measures designed to minimize magnet inhomogeneity and servicing of the magnet are recommended at two-week intervals, or according to individual MRI system manufacturers.

10.2.2.4 Because MRI data is usually acquired in a 256 by 256 matrix, individual MRI pixel size is approximately 1 mm. One-millimetre pixel selection differences can be anticipated when CT and MRI are compared in the same patient. A small field of view (FOV) and large matrix MRI technique reduce this potential discrepancy.

10.2.2.5 Users and manufacturers must understand the potential distortion effects of magnetic field inhomogeneity and provide techniques to reduce potential errors. Comprehensive quality assurance, machine calibration, proper frame alignment, and redundant systems for target selection and coordinate determination are desirable.

10.2.3 *Positron Emission Tomography*—Positron emission tomography (PET) is a diagnostic nuclear medicine clinical and research tool that can provide knowledge about biochemical processes of the brain, including regional tissue function and blood flow. Anatomic resolution is usually poorer with PET than with other imaging tools. Its plane resolution is approximately 2.5 mm or greater, and slice thicknesses are generally greater. Stereotactic PET imaging requires a commitment to quality assurance, immobilization of the patient and frame, and redundant systems to verity target coordinate calculations. Concurrent imaging with CT or MRI are recommended.

10.2.4 *Biplane Radiographic Techniques*:

10.2.4.1 *Magnification*—X rays are emitted from a point source in an X-ray tube, and the beams diverge radially from the point source. The beam divergence increases as a function of the distance from the central beam. The magnification depends on the distance of the object from the X-ray source, the distance of the object to the X-ray film, and the distance of the object from the central beam. The stereotactic system should correct for magnification distortion by using such maneuvers as teleradiography, collimation, calculation, or measurement of magnification.

10.2.4.2 *Parallax*—Stereotactic localization is optimal if the central beam of the X-ray source is perfectly orthogonal to and intersects the zero point of the coordinate axes of the stereotactic instrument both in lateral and in AP projections. Collimation reticules should be provided to indicate the proper alignment. Measurements on nonorthogonal radiographs are foreshortened by a factor related to the angle at which the midcoronal (on AP views) and midsagittal (on lateral views) planes of the patient's head lie with respect to the central X-ray beam. Parallax errors increase as tube-to-patient distances decrease, and should be compensated for mathematically, and should be addressed by the stereotactic system.

10.2.4.3 *Patient Orientation*—Patient orientation is related to the problems of collimation and parallax. When long tube-to-object distances are used, the system should provide collimation reticles and instructions to calculate the magnification factors. When short tube-to-object distances are used, the system should provide a radioopaque marker reference system in known positions that can be attached to the stereotactic head holder or the patient's head during stereotactic radiographs, such as angiography, X rays, and so forth. Mathematical methods accounting for magnification and parallax can be used, and software and instructions should be provided with the stereotactic system.

10.3 Calibrate each stereotactic device with the imaging device with which it is intended to be used, to ensure compatibility of materials with the imaging system, to ensure that no mechanical distortions occur when the apparatus is connected to the imaging device, and to ensure accuracy and reproducibility.

10.4 Since each imaging system has its own limits of resolution, the limit accuracy of the stereotactic system should be such that the accuracy of the entire system does not exceed the resolution of the imaging system by greater than 1 mm.

10.5 In those systems in which the arc fixation is integral with the head frame fixation, a method of determining that the system is within the design specification accuracy prior to being placed on the patient's head must be provided by the manufacturer. If this requires that a hardware device be used, such a device must be furnished with the instrument system.

10.6 In cases of frameless systems, if a hardware checking device, such as a phantom, is required to demonstrate that the system is not only within design tolerance specifications, but also within the limits of angular registration in all three rotational axes, the manufacturer shall furnish such a device with each system.

10.7 The accuracy of all measuring scales or devices should be traceable to the National Institute of Standards and Technology (NIST). The manufacturer's literature should make a statement that the accuracy of the company's manufacturing machines are also traceable to NIST.

Standard Practice for Multiple Persons Cold Water Survival/Rescue Technique: Huddle Position[1]

This standard is issued under the fixed designation F 1728; the number immediately following the designation indicates the year of original adoption or, in the case of revision, the year of last revision. A number in parentheses indicates the year of last reapproval. A superscript epsilon (ε) indicates an editorial change since the last revision or reapproval.

1. Scope

1.1 This practice covers the recommended water rescue procedure for performing the huddle position.

1.2 This practice is one in a set of self-rescue techniques for the water rescuer.

1.3 *This standard does not purport to address all of the safety concerns, if any, associated with its use. It is the responsibility of the user of this standard to establish appropriate safety and health practices and determine the applicability of regulatory limitations prior to use.*

2. Terminology

2.1 *huddle position, n*—a multiple person water rescue technique for heat conservation when immersed in cold water and the majority of the rescuers are wearing personal flotation devices. This technique conserves heat by using personal flotation devices and clothing, group body contact, and body posture to limit exposure of the body's major heat loss areas to the cold water.

2.2 *personal flotation device (PFD), n*—a buoyant device suitable for use by one person in water emergencies. These devices may be vests, ring buoys, life preservers, cushions, and other special purpose buoyant devices.

3. Significance and Use

3.1 This practice establishes a multiple person cold water survival/rescue procedure.

3.2 All persons who are identified as water rescuers shall meet the requirements of this practice.

3.3 This practice is intended to assist government agencies, state, local, or regional organizations; fire departments; and rescue teams and others who are responsible for establishing a minimum performance for personnel who respond to water emergencies.

3.4 The majority of the rescuers performing this technique must be wearing personal flotation devices. These devices should conform to standards set by the appropriate national regulatory authority, that is, the U.S. Coast Guard in the United States, and be in good and serviceable condition.

3.5 A water rescuer sometimes may be immersed in cold water for prolonged periods of time. They are unable to get to shore or shore is too far away, rescue is not imminent, no boat is available to get into or on top of, and no flotsam is available. The water rescuer needs to assume a defensive posture to conserve heat and increase survival time.

4. Procedure

4.1 Upon initial immersion in cold water, the rescuers should cover the mouth and nose to prevent the aspiration of water.

4.2 "Huddle" together, side by side, in a circle.

4.3 Float in a sitting position with the legs drawn up, knees together, and with the ankles crossed.

4.4 Place arms against the side of torso, bent at the elbows, joining the rescues together.

4.5 Place small children, injured people, and those without flotation in the center of the huddle.

4.6 Remain calm and think clearly.

4.7 Leave all clothing on.

4.8 Wait for rescue.

5. Keywords

5.1 cold water survival; huddle position; self-rescue technique; water rescue; water rescuers

[1] This practice is under the jurisdiction of ASTM Committee F32 on Search and Rescue and is the direct responsibility of Subcommittee F32.02 on Management and Operations.

Current edition approved Sept. 10, 1996. Published November 1996.

Standard Practice for Single Person Cold Water Survival/Rescue Technique: HELP Position[1]

This standard is issued under the fixed designation F 1729; the number immediately following the designation indicates the year of original adoption or, in the case of revision, the year of last revision. A number in parentheses indicates the year of last reapproval. A superscript epsilon (ε) indicates an editorial change since the last revision or reapproval.

1. Scope

1.1 This practice covers the recommended water rescue procedure for performing the heat escape lessening posture (HELP) position.

1.2 This practice is one in a set of self-rescue techniques for the water rescuer.

1.3 *This standard does not purport to address all of the safety concerns, if any, associated with its use. It is the responsibility of the user of this standard to establish appropriate safety and health practices and determine the applicability of regulatory limitations prior to use.*

2. Terminology

2.1 *HELP position, n*—heat escape lessening posture (HELP) is a single person water rescue technique for heat conservation when immersed in cold water. This technique conserves heat by using personal flotation devices, clothing, and body posture to limit exposure of the body's major heat loss areas to the cold water.

2.2 *personal flotation device (PFD), n*—a buoyant device suitable for use by one person in water emergencies. These devices may be vests, ring buoys, life preservers, cushions, and other special purpose buoyant devices.

3. Significance and Use

3.1 This practice establishes a single person cold water survival/rescue procedure.

3.2 All persons who are identified as water rescuers shall meet the requirements of this practice.

3.3 This practice is intended to assist government agencies, state, local, or regional organizations; fire departments; and rescue teams and others who are responsible for establishing a minimum performance for personnel who respond to water emergencies.

3.4 A rescuer needs to be wearing a personal flotation device to perform this technique. These devices should conform to standards set by the appropriate national regulatory authority, that is, the U.S. Coast Guard in the United States, and be in good and serviceable condition.

3.5 A water rescuer sometimes may be immersed in cold water for prolonged periods of time. They are unable to get to shore or shore is too far away, rescue is not imminent, no boat is available to get into or on top of, and no flotsam is available. The water rescuer needs to assume a defensive posture to conserve heat and increase survival time.

4. Procedure

4.1 Upon initial immersion in cold water, the rescuer should cover the mouth and nose to prevent the aspiration of water.

4.2 Float in a sitting position with the legs drawn up, knees together, and with the ankles crossed.

4.3 Place arms against the sides of the torso, bent at the elbows, and across the chest.

4.4 Remain calm and think clearly.

4.5 Leave all clothing on.

4.6 Wait for rescue.

5. Keywords

5.1 cold water survival; Heat Escape Lessening Posture (HELP) position; self-rescue technique; water rescue; water rescuers

---

[1] This practice is under the jurisdiction of ASTM Committee F32 on Search and Rescue and is the direct responsibility of Subcommittee F32.02 on Management and Operations.

Current edition approved Sept. 10, 1996. Published November 1996.

Standard Guide for Throwing a Water Rescue Throwbag[1]

This standard is issued under the fixed designation F 1730; the number immediately following the designation indicates the year of original adoption or, in the case of revision, the year of last revision. A number in parentheses indicates the year of last reapproval. A superscript epsilon (ε) indicates an editorial change since the last revision or reapproval.

1. Scope

1.1 This guide covers the recommended procedures for throwing a water rescue throwbag.

1.2 This guide is one in a series of water rescue techniques for the water rescuer.

1.3 *This standard does not purport to address all of the safety concerns, if any, associated with its use. It is the responsibility of the user of this standard to establish appropriate safety and health practices and determine the applicability of regulatory limitations prior to use.*

2. Terminology

2.1 *water rescue throwbag, n*—a rescue device comprised of a storage bag having a flotation element and a length of line attached.

2.1.1 *Discussion*—The line is randomly stuffed into the bag, which will allow the line to feed out freely when the bag is thrown. The line is held in one hand, while the bag is thrown with the other.

3. Significance and Use

3.1 This guide establishes a recommended procedure for a throwing rescue to ensure the safety of all water rescuers who may be involved in rescue techniques at a water rescue emergency.

3.2 This water rescue technique can be utilized from land, boat, or any stable platform.

3.3 All persons who are identified as water rescuers shall meet the requirements of this guide.

3.4 This guide is intended to assist government agencies, state, local, and regional organizations; fire departments; rescue teams and others who are responsible for establishing a minimum performance for personnel who respond to water emergencies.

3.5 The procedure outlined in the document may vary with the number and type of victims, and water conditions.

4. Procedure

4.1 The water rescuer shall make visual contact with the victim. Upon making visual contact the rescuer shall ready the rope to throw, and notify the victim by yelling, "rope."

4.1.1 To make the rope ready from the bag, the rescuer can remove a portion equal to two arms length from the bag and firmly grasp the free end of the rope above the knot. Do not place hand or fingers through the rope loop created by the knot in the end of the rope. Do not attach the rope to anything including the rescuer.

4.2 Before releasing the bag of rope in the direction of the victim, the rescuer may swing the bag underhand, overhand, or in a side arm fashion to establish clearance necessary for throwing the rope.

4.3 The rope bag should be thrown at or slightly beyond the victim, thereby placing the rope within arms reach.

4.4 The rescuer shall maintain a firm grasp on one end of the rope, preparing to belay if necessary, and await victim's contact.

4.5 As the victim grabs ahold of the line the rescuer shall direct the victim to roll into a supine position and place the rope over a shoulder, and to hold firmly.

4.6 The rescuer shall pull the victim slowly or allow the victim to pendulum to safety.

4.7 Multiple throws may be handled by pulling the rope in quickly, letting it collect between the feet without tangling. Pick up the bag with water in it. The water adds weight which enables the bag to be thrown again without restuffing the rope into the bag.

4.8 A second option for multiple throws is the coiled rope toss.

5. Keywords

5.1 throwbag; water rescue; water rescue throwbags

[1] This guide is under the jurisdiction of ASTM Committee F32 on Search and Rescue and is the direct responsibility of Subcommittee F32.02 on Management and Operations.

Current edition approved Sept. 10, 1996. Published November 1996.

Standard Guide for Performance of a Water Rescuer—Level I[1]

This standard is issued under the fixed designation F 1739; the number immediately following the designation indicates the year of original adoption or, in the case of revision, the year of last revision. A number in parentheses indicates the year of last reapproval. A superscript epsilon (ε) indicates an editorial change since the last revision or reapproval.

1. Scope

1.1 This guide covers minimum requirements for the scope of performance of a water rescuer I who may be responsible for the initial on scene evaluation, performing land based water rescues, and providing initial patient care at a water rescue incident.

1.2 This guide is one in a series; water rescuer I is only a beginning level designed for a water rescue responder. Duties and responsibilities at water rescue operations vary according to the water rescuer's skills and knowledge. As the water rescuer level I progresses and becomes more proficient, the individual will move from responder to in-water rescuer to rescue boat operator.

1.3 *This standard may involve hazardous materials, operations, and equipment. This standard does not purport to address all of the safety concerns, if any, associated with its use. It is the responsibility of the user of this standard to establish appropriate safety and health practices and determine the applicability of regulatory limitations prior to use.*

2. Referenced Documents

2.1 *American Red Cross Standards:*

Standards and Guidelines for Cardiopulmonary Resuscitation (CPR) and Emergency Cardiac Care

Standards and Guidelines for Standard First Aid

2.2 *American Heart Association:*

Basic Cardiac Life Support (BCLS)

3. Terminology

3.1 *Definitions of Terms Specific to This Standard:*

3.1.1 *water rescuer I, WRI, n*—an individual competent to perform on scene evaluations, water rescues only from land, and provide initial care for victims.

3.1.2 *basic life support cardiopulmonary resuscitation, BLS/CPR, n*—a set of skills which includes airway management, artificial respiration, and chest compressions.[2]

3.1.3 *drowning, n*—death due to submersion and usually suffocation in water or other fluid media.

3.1.4 *near drowning, n*—a resuscitated drowning victim who survives, at least temporarily, following a submersion injury.

3.1.5 *cold water near drowning, n*—a complex series of physiological reactions which occur as a result of being immersed in cold water (21°C or 70°F and below) which may allow a person to survive up to an hour, possibly more, under water.

3.1.6 *floating tether, tag line, n*—a water rescue technique which stretches a line across a body of water. This line has a flotation device attached to it to keep the rope on the surface of the water and to provide a buoyant object for the victim to grab and hold.

3.1.7 *heat-related illnesses, n*—conditions consisting of heat cramps, heat exhaustion, and heat stroke which develop from an overexposure to heat.

3.1.8 *hypothermia, n*—reduction of the body core temperature to 35°C (95°F) and below.

3.1.9 *h.e.l.p. position, n*—heat escape lessening posture is a single person water rescue technique for heat conservation when immersed in cold water. This technique conserves heat by using personal flotation devices, clothing, and body posture to limit exposure of the body's major heat loss areas to the cold water.

3.1.10 *huddle position, n*—a multiple person water rescue technique for heat conservation when immersed in cold water and the majority of the rescuers are wearing personal flotation devices. This technique conserves heat by using personal flotation devices and clothing, group body contact, and body posture to limit exposure of the body's major heat loss areas to the cold water.

3.1.11 *PFD, n*—a buoyant device suitable for use by one person in water emergencies. These devices may be vests, ring buoys, life preservers, cushions, and other special purpose buoyant devices.

3.1.12 *self rescue swim in moving water, n*—a defensive water survival/rescue technique for swimming swift rivers and rapids consisting of lying on the back (as horizontal and near to the surface as possible), feet first going downstream to fend off all obstacles including rocks, backstroking with arms, flutter kicking with feet, and angling body towards shore.

3.1.13 *sinking tether, snag line, n*—a water rescue technique which stretches a weighted line across a body of water to snag

[1] This document is under the jurisdiction of ASTM Committee F-32 on Search and Rescue and is the direct responsibility of Subcommittee F32.03 on Education.
Current edition approved Nov. 10, 1996. Published January 1997.

[2] Available from your local American Red Cross Chapter or your American Heart Association Chapter. Reprinted from the Journal of the American Medical Association (JAMA). Copies are available from the American Heart Association, 7320 Greenville Ave., Dallas, Texas 75231.

or support fully or partly submerged objects and people.

4. Significance and Use

4.1 The purpose of this guide is to establish a minimum level of knowledge and skills for the water rescue responder. The application will improve the quality of initial emergency response, the rescue of the water victims, and the safety of the rescuers.

4.2 All persons who are identified as water rescuers and water rescue responders shall meet the requirements of this guide.

4.3 This guide does not preclude the scope of performances for water rescuers needing more advanced or more specialized water rescue training.

4.4 This guide will assist government agencies, state, local, or regional organizations; fire departments; rescue teams, and others who are responsible for establishing a minimum performance for personnel who respond to water emergencies.

5. Requirements

5.1 *Knowledge Requirements*—These are not in any order and do not suggest a particular performance sequence. The water rescuer I shall be able to:

5.1.1 Identify potential water hazards,

5.1.2 Identify a drowning victim's behavior,

5.1.3 Identify treatment for a drowning victim and near drowning victim according to the standard of care to which the responder has been trained,

5.1.4 Identify heat-related illnesses and their treatments according to the standard of care to which the responder has been trained,

5.1.5 Identify hypothermia and its treatment according to the standard of care to which the responder has been trained,

5.1.6 Identify cold water near drowning and its treatment according to the standard of care to which the responder has been trained,

5.1.7 Identify the purpose and the important factors in selecting a personal flotation device (PFD) for basic water rescue work, that is, flotation for individual self, fit, freedom of movement, visibility, protection, and physical comfort. These devices should conform to standards set by the appropriate national regulatory, that is, the U.S. Coast Guard in the United States, and be in good and serviceable condition,

5.1.8 Identify other appropriate key pieces of personal safety equipment, that is, thermal protection, helmet, whistle, knife, lights, footwear,

5.1.9 Identify the elements of a water emergency, that is, extrication, medical, evacuation, communication, support,

5.1.10 Identify the water rescue sequence, that is, talk, reach, throw, row, go,

5.1.11 Identify the different types of lines (ropes) and their applications for basic water rescue, and

5.1.12 Identify the uses of a figure 8 knot (stopper), figure 8 on a bight, and the figure 8 bend knots, that is, to prevent the rope from slipping through equipment, to provide a reliable loop, to join two ropes together.

5.2 *Performance Requirements*—These are not in any order and do not suggest a particular performance sequence. The water rescuer I shall be able to:

5.2.1 Provide BLS/CPR in accordance with American Heart Association/American Red Cross (AHA/ARC) or other nationally accredited program,

5.2.2 Provide patient assessment and initial patient care according to the standard of care to which the responder has been trained,

5.2.3 Demonstrate the ability to continuously swim 30 metres (100 feet) while wearing a PFD,

5.2.4 Demonstrate the h.e.l.p. position,

5.2.5 Demonstrate the huddle position,

5.2.6 Demonstrate a self rescue swim in moving water,

5.2.7 Demonstrate a reach technique,

5.2.8 Demonstrate throwing rescues using a throw bag and using a coiled line,

5.2.9 Demonstrate the floating tether (tag line) rescue and the sinking tether (snag line) rescue as a shore based rescue,

5.2.10 Demonstrate by tying the figure 8 knot (stopper), figure 8 on a bight, and the figure 8 bend knot,

5.2.11 Evaluate a simulated rescue incident and initiate an appropriate shore based water rescue technique,

5.2.12 Evaluate the patient's current situation and condition,

5.2.13 Evaluate the current environmental conditions and take appropriate actions to protect rescuers, victims, and other persons, and

5.2.14 Evaluate the available flotation, reaching and throwing equipment, and use them properly.

6. Keywords

6.1 water rescue; water rescue responder; water rescue techniques; water rescuer I

Designation: F 1740 – 96

Standard Guide for Inspection of Nylon, Polyester, or Nylon/Polyester Blend, or Both Kernmantle Rope[1]

This standard is issued under the fixed designation F 1740; the number immediately following the designation indicates the year of original adoption or, in the case of revision, the year of last revision. A number in parentheses indicates the year of last reapproval. A superscript epsilon (ε) indicates an editorial change since the last revision or reapproval.

1. Scope

1.1 This guide covers procedures to assist in the management and care of kernmantle nylon, polyester, or nylon/polyester, or both kernmantle ropes by rescue personnel.

1.2 This guide provides information intended to assist qualified, experienced personnel in establishing procedures for determining whether a rope should be placed into or returned to service. Such procedures may be used to assist in determining serviceability of used rescue ropes. Other factors which may not be included in this guide may also need to be considered when evaluating ropes.

NOTE 1—Interpretation of the terms "qualified" and "experienced" when referring to individuals inspecting ropes may be debatable. Because rope evaluation is a subjective practice, it is in the best interest of the user to clearly define the needs of the user, and then to train personnel according to those needs. Needs and priorities may vary greatly between users.

1.2.1 A rope which has been used in any manner should not be returned to service without first undergoing a thorough inspection to include rope log review, visual inspection, and tactile inspection.

1.2.2 It is the responsibility of the user to understand that evaluation of a used rope is a subjective process. Due to the strength and longevity of kernmantle ropes presently used in rescue operations, it is perfectly reasonable, and even advisable, for these ropes to be reused on future operations unless the rope is physically compromised in some way. If the user chooses to reuse ropes, then the user should also establish specific guidelines, including and possibly in addition to those set forth in this guide, and provide training for personnel who will be responsible for examination of ropes.

1.3 *This standard does not imply approval of any specific type of rescue rope, nor does it purport to ensure the ability of any rope to function as desired. The information included here is not to be considered the only criteria for evaluating the serviceability of rescue rope.*

1.4 *This standard does not purport to address all of the safety concerns, if any, associated with its use. It is the responsibility of the user of this standard to establish appropriate safety and health practices and determine the applicability of regulatory limitations prior to use.*

2. Terminology

2.1 *core*—interior (kern) of a kernmantle rope. The core supports the major portion of the load on a kernmantle rope.

2.2 *in-service*—a rescue rope is considered to be "in service" if it is available for use in life safety applications.

2.3 *kernmantle*—a rope design consisting of two elements: an interior core (kern) and an outer sheath (mantle).

2.4 *rescue rope*—rope which is used for rescue purposes.

2.5 *retire*—permanent removal of a rope from service such that it is no longer used for life safety purposes.

NOTE 2—When a rope is retired it should be cut into short lengths which will discourage future use. It should not be stored, kept, or maintained in such a way that it could inadvertently be used as a lifeline. In some cases, when only a single point or a small area of a rope has been damaged and the rest of the rope is still in good condition, the user may elect to cut that section out of the rope and continue to use the shorter rope(s) in lifeline applications. This decision is left to the users' discretion.

2.6 *rope log*—a written reference kept separately for each rope. A rope log should contain pertinent information about the rope and conditions under which it was used.

2.7 *sheath*—outer cover (mantle) of a kernmantle rope. The sheath serves to protect the core of a kernmantle rope and may also support a portion of the load.

2.8 *use*—one or more individual applications during the course of an operation.

2.9 *user*—may be an individual, a department, a team, or any other entity using the products discussed herein.

3. Significance and Use

3.1 The purpose of this guide is to assist the user in developing procedures to determine the serviceability of rope based upon visual and tactile inspection of the rope and the rope history as documented in the rope log.

3.2 This guide is intended for use by experienced personnel deemed qualified by the user to assess the viability of rope, according to the specific needs of that user.

4. Procedure for Recording Rope History

4.1 Rope logs should be designed by the user according to the needs of the user and practices established by the user to ensure maintenance and monitoring of these records.

---

[1] This guide is under the jurisdiction of ASTM Committee F-32 on Search and Rescue and is the direct responsibility of Subcommittee F32.03 on Personnel, Training, and Education.

Current edition approved Nov. 10, 1996. Published January, 1997.

4.2 Rope logs should include, but not be limited to, the information outlined herein:

4.2.1 Rope Identification,

4.2.2 Date of rope purchase,

4.2.3 Date rope was put into service. (See 5.5.2 for information regarding use of dates.),

4.2.4 Dates and conditions under which rope is used, including weather, approximate load, unusual circumstances and any unusual shock loads, abrasion, or other abuse the rope sustains, and

4.2.5 Dates and actions taken, including inspection, cleaning, drying, storage, and return to service.

5. Procedure for Examining Ropes

5.1 Inspect all ropes for wear and damage prior to use. A rope which has not been inspected shall not be used again or placed into service until an inspection has been performed.

5.1.1 Inspect the entire length of the rope, whether or not the entire length was used.

5.1.2 Clean ropes which are dirty or wet and dried in accordance with manufacturer's recommendations before inspection.

5.2 Perform the complete inspection (visual, tactile, and rope log) by the same person for a given rope.

5.3 Visual inspection of a rope should be done by an experienced individual who is deemed qualified by his user to assess the serviceability of rope, according to the needs of the user. This inspection should take into consideration the current status of normal wear and tear as well as specific damages which may have occurred during use of the rope.

5.3.1 Any section of rope whose sheath appears to be glazed should receive additional scrutiny during the course of the tactile inspection to evaluate for further indication of damage. Significant damage may lead to retirement.

5.3.2 Discoloration may be an indication of rope damage. Retire the rope, if a part of a rope appears discolored and the cause of the discoloration is unknown or is suspected to be from a source harmful to the rope's fiber.

5.3.3 Retire a rope which shows any sign or smell to indicate that it may have been contaminated by an acid, alkaline, oxidizing agent, bleach, or other potentially hazardous chemical or substance.

5.3.4 Abrasion, cuts, or nicks in the outer sheath should indicate an area which should receive special consideration during the course of the tactile inspection to evaluate for indication of further damage.

5.3.5 Retire a rope whose sheath has been cut through or abraded to the extent that the core is visible.

5.3.6 If the diameter of a rope is smaller (or larger) in one area than throughout the rest of the rope, its condition shall be suspect.

NOTE 3—This refers to enough of a variation in the rope's diameter to suggest that the core of the rope has been damaged and closer inspection is needed. Holding the section of rope in question under constant tension aids in visualizing the extent of the change in diameter. A significant decrease in diameter, hour-glass appearance, is usually caused by separation of core fibers and the rope should be retired. A significant increase in the diameter may be caused by a bunching of the core or sheath, or some internal contamination of the core, and may require the rope to be retired.

5.3.7 When sections of rope are formed into approximate 30-cm (circumference) loops, the consistency of the loop should be uniform throughout. If it is not, retire the rope.

5.3.8 Establish additional criteria for visual rope inspection by the user in accordance with the specific needs of the user.

5.4 Tactile inspection of a rope shall be done by an experienced individual deemed qualified by the user to assess the viability of rope, according to the needs of the user. This inspection should take into consideration the current status of normal wear and tear as well as specific damages which may have occurred during use of the rope.

5.4.1 Inspect the entire length of the rope whether or not the entire length was used.

5.4.2 Tactile inspection should be performed in such a way that allows the inspector to feel for changes while maintaining a pressure on the rope.

5.4.3 Retire the rope if any inconsistencies in rope diameter are detected or suspected (if the rope seems to feel larger or smaller at any given point). (See Note 3.)

5.4.4 If a part of the rope feels "mushy" or soft in any area relative to the rest of the rope, the core of the rope may be damaged in that area and the rope shall be considered for retirement.

5.4.5 Retire the rope if the rope is extraordinarily stiff in any area, it has likely been overstressed in that area. If any area of the rope is more stiff or "brittle" feeling than the rest of the rope.

5.5 Rope examination shall include any analysis of the rope log.

5.5.1 Any rope which is noted to have experienced uncontrolled or excessive loading should be considered for retirement.

5.5.2 Retire any rope which is greater than ten years old, regardless of history and usage.

NOTE 4—There is at this writing no universally agreed upon "shelf life" for nylon, polyester, or nylon/polyester rope products. Shelf life will vary according to local atmosphere, storage conditions, heat, light, temperature, and other variables. The ten-year estimate cited in this guide should be considered carefully by any person(s) using this guide, with the understanding that depending on circumstances specific to each situation, rope strength may actually be reduced to unacceptable levels in a shorter period of time. While there is no conclusive data to show the precise effects of rope aging, users' experience as well as research such as that done by Smith, et al, 1984 and Mammut Ropes, 1979, may provide some subjective criteria for decision making about ropes based upon rope age and usage.

5.5.3 Retire any rope which is noted or suspected to have come into contact with harmful chemicals or other substance.

5.5.4 Any rope whose history is unknown shall not be used in lifeline or rescue applications.

5.6 Any doubt about the condition of the rope shall lead to its retirement.

Designation: F 1744 – 96

Standard Guide for Care and Handling of Stainless Steel Surgical Instruments[1]

This standard is issued under the fixed designation F 1744; the number immediately following the designation indicates the year of original adoption or, in the case of revision, the year of last revision. A number in parentheses indicates the year of last reapproval. A superscript epsilon (ϵ) indicates an editorial change since the last revision or reapproval.

1. Scope

1.1 This guide is intended to provide a better understanding of the care of stainless steel surgical instruments intended for reuse. This guide is not intended for use with electrical, pneumatic or other powered surgical instruments.

2. Referenced Documents

2.1 *ASTM Standards:*

F 899 Specification for Stainless Steel Billet, Bar, and Wire for Surgical Instruments[2]

F 921 Definitions of Terms Relating to Hemostatic Forceps[2]

F 1026 Specification for General Workmanship and Performance Measurements of Hemostatic Forceps[2]

F 1078 Terminology for Surgical Scissors—Inserted and Non-Inserted Blades[2]

F 1079 Specification for Inserted and Non-Inserted Surgical Scissors[2]

F 1089 Test Method for Corrosion of Surgical Instruments[2]

F 1325 Specification for Suture Needle Holders—General Workmanship Requirements and Corresponding Test Methods[2]

3. General

3.1 *Stainless Steel Types*—The stainless steels most used are martensitic and austenitic types such as those in Specification F 899. Martensitic stainless steel contains iron, chromium, and sufficient carbon so that when it is hardened by heat treatment, a substantial martensitic structure is the result. Austenitic stainless steel has better corrosion resistance and contains iron, chromium, and nickel. It has a substantial austenitic structure and a lower carbon content. Although it cannot be hardened by heat treatment, it can be work-hardened.

3.2 *Passivation*—Stainless steel can spot, stain, and corrode. This is minimized by passivation which is a process used to create a protective chromium oxide surface layer while removing surface carbon and iron. This is accomplished in the atmosphere slowly or through immersion in oxidizing solution or through an electro-polish process. Through repeated processing the passivation layer will thicken until a good protective film is formed.

3.2.1 Never expose instruments to strong acids such as hydrochloric, aqua regia, dilute sulphuric, carbonic, and tartaric.

3.2.2 Avoid contact with salt solutions such as aluminum chloride, mercury salts, stannous chloride. Also avoid contact with potassium thiocyanate and potassium permanganate and limit contact with iodine solutions to periods less than 1 h.

3.2.3 Chloride-bearing solutions such as blood and saline can cause localized corrosion. Avoid prolonged exposure to or rinsing in saline solutions or corrosion and pitting will occur. Use demineralized or distilled water instead. Place instruments into water, enzymatic solution, or disinfectant bath immediately after use so the blood or other material will not dry on them prior to transport to designated cleaning/reprocessing area.

4. General Care of Instruments

4.1 *General*—Use instruments only for their intended purpose, such as cutting, holding, clamping, retracting, etc. Avoid undue stress or strain when handling and cleaning. Standard terminology relating to Hemostatic Forceps and Surgical Scissors are found in Definitions F 921 and Specification F 1078.

4.1.1 *Hemostatic Forceps*—These forceps are designed to clamp blood vessels. They should not be used to clamp towels, suction tubing, or as needle holders or pliers. Misuse generally results in misalignment and even cracked box locks.

4.1.2 *Needle Holders*—Although designed to withstand some force, they are not to be used as pliers, jaw misalignments being the result. Select a needle holder matching the size needle being used.

4.1.3 *Scissors*—Do not use scissors for the wrong job, otherwise, the tips will become misaligned and the blades will dull or chip. Delicate scissors should be particularly guarded against misuses. Use tissue scissors for tissue dissections only, not for cutting suture material or wires.

4.1.4 *Microsurgical Instruments*—Microsurgical instruments are most susceptible to damage through misuse or rough handling. Consequently, extra care must be taken to avoid compromising their exacting performance. To minimize damage, the following should be done:

4.1.4.1 Inspect the instrument when purchased and after each use and cleaning, preferably under magnification.

4.1.4.2 Only use for its intended purpose.

4.1.4.3 After each use remove blood and debris from instrument. A non-fibrous sponge may be used to eliminate

---

[1] This practice is under the jurisdiction of ASTM Committee F-4 on Medical and Surgical Materials and Devicesand is the direct responsibility of Subcommittee F04.33 on Medical/Surgical Instruments.

Current edition approved Oct. 10, 1996. Published January 1997.

[2] *Annual Book of ASTM Standards*, Vol 13.01.

snagging and breakage. **When handling sharp instruments use extreme caution to avoid injury: consult with an infection control practitioner to develop and verify safety procedures appropriate for all levels of direct instrument contact.**

4.1.4.4 Clean and thoroughly dry before packaging or storing. Avoid using a washer decontaminator or an ultrasonic cleaner (see Appendix X.2).

4.1.4.5 Avoid metal-to-metal contact by using special racks designed to separate and protect.

4.1.4.6 Do routine preventive maintenance such as sharpening and realigning. Sterilization by dry heat or chemical vapor should be considered for these instruments.

4.1.5 *Instrument Kits*—Select an instrument tray which suits the size of the kit. Placing a large instrument kit in a small instrument tray may lead to broken instruments, bent tips, or dull scissors. Put heavier instruments such as retractors on the bottom and light weight instruments on the top. Ring-handled instruments should be kept open with a wire holder or pin. Curved clamps should all point in the same direction to protect the tips. Scissors should be kept separate. Cupped instruments should be placed so that water does not collect in them during sterilization. Separate instruments of dissimilar metals by separate processing, otherwise galvanic corrosion or electrolytic deposition may result.

4.1.6 *Other Sharp Instruments*—Rongeurs, bone cutting forceps, drill bits, reamers, etc. should be used to cut bone, not wire or pins. Sometimes it is necessary to use rongeurs or osteotomes to chip bone away from bone plates and screws, which may nick or dull the blades. An alternate approach is to keep an older set of rongeurs or osteotomes for such orthopedic procedures. Instruments that are recommended to be sharpened by the manufacturer should be processed and verified by the manufacturer's specific instruction. Instruments should be used only for their identified purpose. Careful planning is necessary for selection of the proper amount and type of instruments needed for each surgical procedure.

4.2 *Care During Use*:

4.2.1 Handle instruments gently.

4.2.2 Avoid dropping instruments or covering them with heavier instruments.

4.2.3 Handle instruments individually or in small numbers.

4.2.4 Protect instrument tips, especially sharp ones. Do not place instruments down on their tips.

4.2.5 Do not drop delicate or sharp instruments into any cleaning receptacle. Such practice may cause damage to the instruments.

4.2.6 After a surgical procedure, an instrument count should be made to avoid sending any instruments to the laundry with the soiled linen. Although they eventually may be returned, they create a injury hazard to laundry workers and many are damaged beyond economical repair.

4.3 *Marking*—Do not use a vibrating or impact type marking devices on the box lock portion. If marking is necessary, do it on the shanks, otherwise the box locks may fail.

5. Cleaning

5.1 *General*—Clean instruments as soon as possible after use. Do not allow blood and debris to dry on the instruments. If cleaning must be delayed, place groups of instruments in a covered container with appropriate detergent or enzymatic solution to delay drying. Wash all instruments whether or not they were used or were inadvertently contacted with blood or saline solution.

After surgery, open box locks and disassemble instruments with removable parts. Forceps and scissors should be cleaned and sterilized in the open position. This will limit blood drying on the instruments which may cause them to corrode. Delicate and sharp instruments should be cleaned separately. This is especially true for eye and microsurgery instruments. **When handling any sharp instruments use extreme caution to avoid injury: consult with an infection control practitioner to develop and verify safety procedures appropriate for all levels of direct instrument contact. Direct handling and cleaning of instruments should be done only when indirect methods, for example, tweezers, are not available or not possible.** Sort instruments by similar metal for subsequent processing so that electrolytic deposition due to contact between dissimilar metals will not occur.

Prior to regular cleaning, soak in enzyme solution or rinse instruments in demineralized or distilled water to remove blood and debris, especially those instruments with hollow tubes such as suction tubes and curettes.

Do not use abrasive pads or cleansers which will scratch the surface allowing dirt and water deposits to collect. Abrasive cleaning will remove the passive layer. Do not use chlorine bleach at a higher concentration than recommended by the manufacturer to clean or disinfect stainless steel instruments, as pitting will occur. High concentrations of chlorine-based solutions are not recommended as pitting and subsequent damage will occur. (See Appendix X3.)

5.2 *Detergents*—The detergent used should be in keeping with the cleaning equipment manufacturer's recommendations. Neutral pH detergents, between 7.0 and 8.5, which are low sudsing, free rinsing, and have good wetting are best over all for washer decontaminators and ultrasonic cleaners. High-sudsing detergents must be thoroughly rinsed or instruments will spot or stain. (See Appendix X2.)

5.3 *Washer Decontaminator*—Equipment of this type will wash and decontaminate instruments. Complete removal of soil from serrations and crevices depends on instrument construction, exposure time, pressure of delivered solution, and pH of the detergent solution, and thus may require prior brushing.

5.3.1 Be familiar with equipment manufacturers' use and operation instructions. Be aware that loading detergent water temperature and other external factors may change the effectiveness of the equipment. (See X4.5.)

5.3.2 Arrange heavier instruments on bottom, disassemble instruments with removable parts, open box locks, and protect cutting edges.

5.3.3 Follow equipment manufacturers' recommendations for detergent, preferably a liquid one. Solid detergents may not disperse as completely. Concentrated detergents placed on the instruments may cause corrosion.

5.3.4 Install a water softener if the water is hard and the water supply is not already treated. This will minimize scum formation. Deionized water is recommended for rinsing to prevent spotting.

5.3.5 If instruments are dirty after decontamination, the ejector may be fouled. If fouled, foreign matter remains to deposit on the instruments. The ejector must be cleaned and extraneous matter removed.

5.3.6 Regularly cleaning decontaminator walls will remove rust and mineral deposits and avoid transfer of this type of debris to the instruments being cleaned. Follow the equipment manufacturer's instructions or descaling detergent manufacturers' instructions to clean decontaminator walls.

5.4 *Ultrasonic Cleaner*—Ultrasonic cleaners, when used with hot water per manufacturer's recommended temperature and specially formulated detergents, are very effective and thorough. Debris of all sizes can be removed even from crevices and corners in five min. After ultrasonic cleaning, the instruments cleaned still need to be sterilized.

5.4.1 Follow manufacturer's instructions when using an ultrasonic cleaner. Be aware that loading patterns, instrument cassettes, water temperature, and other external factors may change the effectiveness of the equipment. (See X4.5.)

5.4.2 Arrange instruments with box locks open and cutting edges protected. Do not clean delicate instruments in an ultrasonic cleaner since the vibrations can cause the tips to wear if they come in contact with other metal surfaces.

5.4.3 It is not recommended to clean plated instruments in an ultrasonic cleaner since the ultrasonic vibration and the presence of other sharp instrument edges may crack or rupture the plating. When the plating is ruptured ultrasonic energy will accelerate flaking. Any plated instrument with ruptured plating should be removed from use and refurbished or discarded.

5.4.4 Use hot water per manufacturer's recommended temperature (usually 90–140°F or 30–75°C).

5.4.5 Follow manufacturer's recommendations for proper cleaning solution, or use cleaning solution formulated specifically for ultrasonic cleaners. Neutral detergents or products with less than 2 % available alkalinity are suitable for ultrasonic cleaning. Acidic or alkaline products with more than 2 % available alkalinity are not recommended for ultrasonic systems because they cannot be properly neutralized.

5.4.6 Rinse instruments thoroughly after cleaning.

5.4.7 Check screws of instruments after cleaning to ensure that they have not loosened through vibration.

5.4.8 Keep cleaning solution particulate-free by changing often or changing the filter per manufacturer's recommendations.

5.5 *Lubrication*—To protect instruments during sterilization and storage from staining and rusting, they should be lubricated with a water-soluble, preserved lubricant after each cleaning. Since effective ultrasonic cleaning removes all lubricant, re-lubrication of the instruments is important. The lubricant should contain a chemical preservative to prevent bacterial growth in the lubricant bath. The bath solution should be made with demineralized water. A lubricant containing a rust inhibitor helps prevent electrolytic corrosion of points and edges. Immediately after cleaning, instruments should be immersed completely for 30 s and allowed to drain off, not wiped off. A lubricant film will remain through sterilization to protect them during storage. "Frozen" box locks can be immersed overnight and the joint then worked free.

5.6 *Inspection*—After lubricating, instruments should be inspected. Incompletely cleaned instruments should be recleaned, and those that need repair set aside. For complex instruments, the manufacturer's inspection and testing recommendations should be followed.

5.6.1 For hinged instruments such as clamps and forceps, lock stiffness, jaw alignment, and teeth should be checked.

5.6.2 For sharp instruments such as scissors, rongeurs, and curettes, sharpness should be tested per manufacturer's instructions.

5.6.3 Check plated instruments for chipped plating. These defects can tear rubber gloves, or cause the instruments to rust. Any plated instrument with ruptured plating should be removed from use and refurbished or discarded.

5.6.4 Pins and screws should be checked to see if they are intact.

6. Testing

6.1 Forceps and hemostats shall conform to performance characteristics stated in Specification F 1026.

6.2 Scissors shall conform to performance characteristics stated in Specification F 1079.

6.3 Suture needle holders shall conform to performance characteristics stated in Specification F 1325.

6.4 Scalpel handles should be checked for fit when the blade is attached to the scalpel handle. If fit is not snug, discard the handle.

NOTE 1—Test Method F 1089 contains test methods for corrosion of surgical instruments.

7. Repair and Restoration

7.1 When instruments wear through repeated use and sterilization, they should be sent to the manufacturer or a repair service knowledgeable in the function of surgical instruments.

7.1.1 Some manufacturers offer preventive maintenance programs that can be a cost effective alternatives to a repair service by limiting repairs. Routine maintenance by people familiar with instrument manufacture will limit costly repairs.

8. Sterilization

8.1 *Steam Sterilization*:

8.1.1 Staining and spotting may result if residual chemicals are not completely rinsed from instruments that are subjected to steam sterilization. Following proper drying cycles and the equipment manufacturer's recommendations are vital to preventing formation of excess moisture and the resultant water spotting.

8.1.2 Routine care and equipment maintenance instructions provided by the manufacturer, if followed, will help ensure longer equipment life and minimize instrument processing difficulties. As a minimum, wiping the inner surfaces with the proper solution and servicing the traps regularly are two routine maintenance precautions to be taken.

8.1.3 High temperature steam filters may help reduce the incidence of staining and corrosion in cases where major systems changes may otherwise be needed to correct these problems.

8.2 *Dry Heat Sterilization*:

8.2.1 This sterilization method may be recommended for some heat stable microsurgical instruments as it is less prone to corrosion effects. Review manufacturer's specifications and recommendations before using this sterilization method.

8.3 *Chemical Vapor Sterilization (Alcohol, Formaldehyde, and anticorrosive with dry steam under pressure, made primarily for the dental industry)*:

8.3.1 This sterilization method may be recommended for some microsurgical instruments as it is less prone to corrosion effects. Review manufacturer's specifications and recommendations before using this sterilization method. **Caution**: After sterilization instruments must be kept dry otherwise corrosion may result.

9. Trouble Shooting

9.1 A fully detailed written procedure which includes steps, equipment, and supplies should be drafted to assure proper instrument care. Include other departments such as maintenance so there is information on boiler water additives and piping changes and any other related details. Do not use short cuts in caring for the instruments or rusting or staining may result.

9.2 Specific recommendation according to cause and corrective action to be taken is found in Appendix X1, Appendix X2, and Appendix X3.

10. New Hospitals

10.1 For new washer decontaminators and autoclaves there is a break-in period, especially for the water and steam lines. Have a qualified instrument or equipment expert present during start-up and initial processing to identify and correct problems.

11. Keywords

11.1 care and handling; stainless steel surgical instrument; sterilization; surgical instruments

APPENDIXES

(Nonmandatory Information)

X1. CORROSION ON BLADES AND BOX LOCKS

X1.1 Corrosion on blades and box locks is an indication of one or more of the following situations:

X1.1.1 Inadequate cleaning and drying after use.

X1.1.2 Either corrosive sterilizing solutions or excess exposure to the sterilizing solutions, especially the cold soak solution process, or both.

X1.1.3 Incorrect detergent.

X1.1.4 Autoclave contaminated (steam).

X1.1.5 Course surfaces.

X1.1.5.1 Knurled or grooved surfaces may rust while polished surfaces may not be affected.

X1.1.5.2 Satin or matte surfaces may behave similarly to grooved and knurled surfaces.

X1.1.6 Minerals in the water.

X1.1.6.1 If the water used is hard, spotting from minerals containing calcium or magnesium will result.

X1.1.6.2 Soft water may also be corrosive due to dissolved salts.

X1.1.6.3 Deionized, distilled, or otherwise demineralized water should be used.

X2. SPOTTING/STAINING

X2.1 Spotting/Staining maybe an indication of one or more of the following situations. The effect of a specific situations may be lessened by the application of the listed solution. (See Appendix X1.)

X2.1.1 Light-colored spot after autoclaving.

X2.1.1.1 *Cause*—Water droplets evaporating from the instrument slowly, the water containing calcium, or magnesium.

X2.1.1.2 *Solution*—Follow autoclave manufacturer's instructions. Do not open autoclave door until steam has been exhausted.

X2.1.2 Dark-colored spot.

X2.1.2.1 *Cause*—Generally same as for light-colored spot.

X2.1.2.2 *Solution*—Prepare all solutions with chloride-free demineralized or distilled water where pH is 7.0.

X2.1.3 Rust-colored film after autoclaving.

X2.1.3.1 *Cause*—Foreign matter left in new installed steam pipes or water supply containing iron.

X2.1.3.2 *Solution*—If new steam pipes, the problem should subside in two to three months. If iron is in the water, consult the engineering staff for treating the water to remove the iron.

X2.1.4 Bluish-Gray stain after sterilization.

X2.1.4.1 *Cause*—This condition may be caused by some liquid chemical disinfection; germicidal solutions.

X2.1.4.2 *Solutions*—(a) If a liquid chemical disinfectant solution is used, it should be rinsed from the instruments before they are sterilized by heat. (b) Change the solution more frequently; also use distilled water and a rust inhibitor. Follow manufacturer's directions.

X2.1.5 Brownish stain.

X2.1.5.1 *Causes*—(a) Chromium oxide film. This forms when stainless steel is excessively heated in the sterilizer. (b) Copper. Washing compounds containing polyphosphates can dissolve some copper from sterilizer components. The dissolved copper is deposited electrolytically on stainless steel.

X2.1.5.2 *Solutions*—(a) For chromium oxide, fill the sterilizer with the right amount of cold water. (b) For copper, use another instrument detergent which contains less polyphosphate or an instrument detergent that has been found to work.

X2.1.6 Purplish-Black stain.

X2.1.6.1 *Causes*—(a) Ammonia exposure. (b) Amines in steam lines. Amine chemicals are used to clean hard water scale from steam lines. This can contaminate the steam and react with stainless steel instruments.

X2.1.6.2 *Solutions*—(a) For ammonia exposure, identify and remove the source if possible or avoid exposure to these compounds. (b) For amines in steam lines, avoid descaling chemicals that use amines.

X2.1.7 Rust Deposit.

X2.1.7.1 *Causes*—(a) Sterilizing plated and stainless instruments together. If the plated instrument has plating missing, iron from where there is no plating will deposit on the stainless steel instrument. (b) Rinsing instruments in tap water with high concentrations of dissolved metals.

X2.1.7.2 *Solutions*—(a) For plated and stainless instruments, sterilize these instruments separately. When the plating on plated instruments starts to peel, replace them with stainless steel instruments or new plated instruments. (b) For dissolved metals in tap water, rinse with distilled or deionized water, especially in places where hard water is of concern.

X3. CORROSION/PITTING

X3.1 *Causes:*

X3.1.1 Ineffective rinsing of linens after washing with caustic chemicals by the laundry service.

X3.1.2 Dried blood in box locks, serrations, and ratchets which appears to be rust.

X3.1.3 Moisture left on instrument surfaces or crevices from end of autoclave cycle or from sterile warp packs.

X3.1.4 Hard water minerals deposited on the instruments.

X3.1.5 Chloride-bearing materials such as blood, saline, potassium chloride, chlorine based bleach solutions.

X3.1.6 Residue from acid-bearing detergents or detergents containing chloride.

X3.1.7 Unbuffered detergents that create a solution with a pH above 8.5 or detergents with more than 2 % available alkalinity can remove the chromic oxide passive layer.

X3.1.8 Dissimilar metals ultrasonically cleaned together.

X3.1.9 Exposure to chloride or halide containing solutions, or both, and high pressure steam from autoclaving in the presence of stress can promote stress corrosion cracking, which is difficult to detect until catastrophic failure occurs.

X3.2 *Solutions:*

X3.2.1 For ineffective rinsing of linens, rinse linens thoroughly with distilled or deionized water before using.

X3.2.2 For dried blood in box locks, clean instruments more thoroughly.

X3.2.3 For moisture left on surfaces, preheat autoclave. Do not rush drying time. Check valves for leakage.

X3.2.4 For hard water minerals, use distilled or deionized water during sterilization. To remove deposits on the autoclaving, wipe surfaces with acetic acid/water (50:50 mixture). If local water supply is used, wipe down weekly.

X3.2.5 For chloride-bearing materials, rinse instruments with running water as soon as possible after use and then clean as usual.

X3.2.6 For acid-bearing detergent residue, avoid acid-containing detergents capable of re-forming acid. For chloride containing residue, avoid detergents capable of leaving high concentrations of chloride in the residue.

X3.2.7 For high pH detergents, use a detergent that is buffered or creates a solution with pH ranging from neutral to 8.5. For cleaning solution with greater than 2 % alkalinity neutralize with mild acid rinse immediately after alkaline washing cycle is completed.

X3.2.8 Do not clean instruments made of dissimilar metals together: separate the instruments according to the metals for cleaning operations.

X3.2.9 Avoid exposure to chloride or halide containing solutions, or both, if possible. If instruments are sanitized in a solution containing chlorides or halides, or both, they should be rinsed thoroughly with distilled or deionized water before being autoclaved or sterilized by other methods.

X4. RATIONALE

X4.1 This guide was created to give a general understanding of the nature and concerns associated with the care and cleaning of surgical instruments. Attention has been paid to chemical and corrosion contacts that may inadvertently degrade, corrode, or otherwise shorten the expected useful life of hand held surgical instruments. This document is not meant to be complete or precise with regard to all the possible chemical contacts or reactions that may occur in a particular situation. The task group has attempted to identify those conditions that are most detrimental and pervasive.

X4.2 The term washer-sterilizer has been removed from this guide in favor of the term washer decontaminator. It is recognized that the term" washer sterilizer" is in common use to describe types of equipment used to clean/disinfect instruments before high level sterilization by other methods such as dry heat, gas, chemical vapor, or steam. It is the consensus opinion of this task group to use the term washer decontaminator in place of washer-sterilizer.

X4.3 It is the consensus opinion of this task group that

chloride ions in any concentration can be detrimental to the finish of hand held surgical instruments and should be avoided if and when possible. It is recognized that the use of bleach and other chlorine containing solutions are pervasive in current practice of care and handling of surgical instruments.

X4.4 Low foaming, free rinsing, detergents with good wetting ability and a neutral pH are compatible with most instrument metals including anodized aluminum. Detergents with greater than 2 % available alkalinity should not be utilized on stainless steel unless immediately neutralized with a mild acidic rinse after detergent cycles are completed.

X4.5 It is generally recognized that the best use of instruments and equipment fall within the guidance and specifications of the manufacturer. Please read and follow the manufacturer's instructions.

Last ASTM Designation: F1745 – 96

Test Method for External Fixator Connectors

This test method covers the procedures for determining the stiffness and strength of external fixator connecting elements (clamps) under axial loads and bending moments.

Formerly under the jurisdiction of Committee F04 on Medical and Surgical Materials and Devices, this test method was withdrawn in October 1999 and replaced by Specification F1541–99 for External Skeletal Fixation Devices[1].

[1] Annual Book of ASTM Standards, Volume 13.01.

Last ASTM Designation: F1746 – 96

Test Method for Determining In-Plane Compressive Properties of Circular Ring or Ring Segment Bridge Elements

This test method covers the test procedure for determining the in-plane compressive properties of circular or ring segment bridge elements of external skeletal fixators.

Formerly under the jurisdiction of Committee F04 on Medical and Surgical Materials and Devices, this test method was withdrawn in October 1999 and replaced by Specification F1541–99 for External Skeletal Fixation Devices .[1]

[1] Annual Book of ASTM Standards, Volume 13.01.

Last ASTM Designation: F1747 – 96

Test Method for External Fixator Joints

This test method covers the procedures for determining the stiffness and strength of external fixator joints under axial loads and bending moments.

Formerly under the jurisdiction of Committee F04 on Medical and Surgical Materials and Devices, this test method was withdrawn in October 1999 and replaced by Specification F1541–99 for External Skeletal Fixation Devices .[1]

---

[1] Annual Book of ASTM Standards, Volume 13.01.

Last ASTM Designation: F1748 – 96

Test Method for External Fixator Subassemblies

This test method covers the procedures for determining the stiffness and strength of external fixator subassemblies, under force loadings (axial, medial-lateral shear, anterior-posterior shear), or under moment loadings (torsion, medial-lateral bending, anterior-posterior bending), or both.

Formerly under the jurisdiction of Committee F04 on Medical and Surgical Materials and Devices, this test method was withdrawn in October 1999 and replaced by Specification F1541–99 for External Skeletal Fixation Devices .[1]

[1] Annual Book of ASTM Standards, Volume 13.01.

Designation: F 1764 – 97

Standard Guide for Selection of Hardline Communication Systems for Confined-Space Rescue[1]

This standard is issued under the fixed designation F 1764; the number immediately following the designation indicates the year of original adoption or, in the case of revision, the year of last revision. A number in parentheses indicates the year of last reapproval. A superscript epsilon (ε) indicates an editorial change since the last revision or reapproval.

1. Scope

1.1 This guide covers recommended criteria for the selection of hardwire communication systems for use in permit-required confined-space rescue operations.

1.2 *This standard does not purport to address all of the safety concerns, if any, associated with its use. It is the responsibility of the user of this standard to establish appropriate safety and health practices and determine the applicability of regulatory limitations prior to use.*

2. Referenced Documents

2.1 *ASTM Standards:*

F 1490 Terminology Relating to Search and Rescue[2]

2.2 *Federal Standards:*

29 Code of Federal Regulations 1910.146 Permit Required Confined Spaces[3]

29 Code of Federal Regulations 1910.7 Definition and Requirements for a National Recognized Testing Laboratory[3]

2.3 *National Code:*

National Electrical Code (NEC)/NFPA 70[4]

3. Terminology

3.1 *Definitions of Terms Specific to This Standard:*

3.1.1 *confined space rescue*—rescue operations within spaces that meet the definition of "permit-required confined space" in Fed. Std. 29 CFR 1910.146.

3.1.2 *hardline communication system*—any communication system where all users are connected to the system by a hardline or wire.

4. Significance and Use

4.1 Because of the many unique requirements of permit-required confined space rescue operations and the specific construction and composition of some confined spaces, hardline communications systems may be the only type that will meet the requirements for working within these spaces. Some of these requirements are set forth in Federal Regulation and some by safe operating procedures developed for working in confined spaces by industry.

4.2 This guide is not meant to preclude the use of other types of communication systems in confined-space rescue.

5. System Requirements

5.1 *System Safety*—The system must be safe for use in the atmosphere, or potential atmosphere, within the space.[5]

5.2 The system must have continuous, hands-free voice communications capability.[6]

5.3 The system must be dedicated and private so operations cannot be interfered with by outsiders not involved with the rescue.

5.4 The system shall not affect the readings of other safety equipment (that is, gas detectors).

5.5 Systems that are battery powered must have a low-battery warning or a backup power source that provides a minimum of 30 min before communications are lost.

5.6 The system must accommodate a minimum of three users.[7]

5.7 The system should allow for communication between all entrants as well as with the attendant.[8]

5.8 The system must work in conjunction with the personal protective equipment (PPE) necessary to work in the environment within the space.[9]

5.9 The system must be impervious to the chemicals within the space.

6. Keywords

6.1 confined space; hardline

---

[1] This guide is under the jurisdiction of ASTM Committee F-32 on Search and Rescue and is the direct responsibility of Subcommittee F32.01 on Equipment, Testing, and Maintenance.

Current edition approved February 10, 1997, Published April 1997.

[2] *Annual Book of ASTM Standards*, Vol 13.01.

[3] Available from Department of Labor, Occupational Safety and Health Administration, Office of Information and Consumer Affairs, Room N3647, 200 Constitution Ave., NW, Washington, DC 20210.

[4] National Electrical Code (NEC)/NFPA 70; Available from the National Fire Protection Association (NFPA), Battery March Park, PO Box 9101, Quincy, MA 02269-9959.

[5] See Annex A1.

[6] See X1.1.

[7] See X1.2.

[8] SeeX1.3.

[9] See X1.4.

ANNEX

(Mandatory Information)

A1. INHERENT SAFETY

A1.1 Equipment that requires electrical power to operate may be a source of ignition in the presence of flammable gases or vapors, combustible dusts, or ignitable fibers. Equipment that must operate in potentially flammable atmospheres must be unable to cause ignition (inherently safe) in those atmospheres. They can be certified as intrinsically safe or explosion-proof. Rescue teams that only work in known hazards, such as on-site rescue teams, may use equipment approved for only those hazards. Rescue teams that respond to unknown hazards, such as fire departments and other off-site rescue teams, must have equipment with the highest possible level of approval available, that is, equipment approved for atmospheres that are classified as: Class I Division 1 Groups A, B, C, D; Class II Division 1 Groups E, F, G; and Class III Division 1.[10,11] Division 1 locations are more hazardous than Division 2, therefore the test protocols for Division 1 are more stringent. As such, equipment certified for Division 1 is also approved for Division 2. Hardline systems that only have limited approval, when used only in atmospheres for which they are approved, meet this guide.[12] The NFPA does not certify equipment. Testing and certification must be done by a Nationally Recognized Test Laboratory (NRTL) that has been accredited by OSHA in accordance with 29 CFR 1910.7. All certified equipment must be clearly and permanently marked to show the class, division, and group it is approved for use in and the name or mark of the NRTL that granted the approval. It is insufficient to be simply labeled intrinsically safe.

[10] Classifications for hazardous locations are in the National Electrical Code (NEC).

[11] See X1.5.

[12] See Appendix X2.

APPENDIXES

(Nonmandatory Information)

X1. RATIONALE

X1.1 Continuous hands-free communication allows the rescue team to communicate with each other and with the attendant without stopping what they are doing to operate a push-to-talk switch. More importantly, it allows the attendant to monitor operations and entrant status inside the space. Slurred speech, out-of-character responses or irregular breathing patterns can all be signs of exposure to gases, vapors, or chemicals within the space. The attendant is required by Federal regulation to know the effects of exposure and be able to recognize if the entry team exhibits them.

X1.2 The system must accommodate a minimum of three users, the attendant, at least one person on the entry team, and one person on the backup or standby team.

X1.3 Most rescues are safer if the entry team consists of at least two members and the system should expand to include all members of both the entry and backup teams.

X1.4 The PPE used in confined-space rescue may include; breathing apparatus, protective clothing, and helmets or hardhats. Communication equipment must work in or under this equipment. Breathing apparatus may incorporate a microphone to overcome the problem of transmitting voice communication through the speaking diaphragm or the communication system may have a throat microphone which eliminates the need for a speaking diaphragm. Headphones that don't fit well under helmets may be replaced with earpieces or other listening devices that fit under the helmet. Earpieces that may fall out of the ear and are hard to replace under protective hoods while wearing gloves, may be replaced by small speakers held near the ear with a harness or attached to the breathing apparatus.

X1.5 Atmospheric hazards in confined spaces are the cause of a vast majority of confined-space incidents. Flammable or explosive atmospheres are just one type of hazardous atmosphere. The level of inherent safety approval of any electrically powered equipment that is used in confined spaces is of the utmost importance. Rescuers will not usually enter a space unless the atmosphere is at or below 10 % of the lower explosive limit (LEL) of the gas or vapor within the space. However, atmospheres in confined spaces are subject to rapid changes and what might have been acceptable upon entry may change dramatically in a very short period of time. Confined-space rescue teams must prepare for the worst possible scenario and have equipment that is safe in a wide variety of situations.

X2. EXAMPLES OF CLASSIFICATIONS AND CORRESPONDING RESCUE SITES

X2.1 *Class I, Division 1 and 2*—Examples include petroleum refineries, dry cleaning plants, petrochemical plants, hospitals, utilities, aircraft hangers, paint manufacturers, dip tanks containing flammable or combustible liquids, and spray finishing areas.

X2.2 *Class II, Division 1 and 2*—Examples include grain elevators, some coal handling or preparation plants, flour and feed mills, confectionary plants, fireworks manufacturing and storage, grain ships, areas for packaging and handling of pulverized sugar and cocoa, manufacturing and storage of magnesium, and spice grinding mills.

X2.3 *Class III, Division 1*—Examples include woodworking plants, textile mills, cotton gins, cotton seed mills, flax-producing plants, knitting mills, and weaving mills.

NOTE X2.1—Individual group classifications also apply to Appendix X2 and were omitted for brevity. Appendix X2 is meant as a guideline only. If you have specific sites you wish to categorize, please refer to the National Electrical Code.

Designation: F 1765 – 97a

Standard Guide for Ice Staff Self-Rescue Technique[1]

This standard is issued under the fixed designation F 1765; the number immediately following the designation indicates the year of original adoption or, in the case of revision, the year of last revision. A number in parentheses indicates the year of last reapproval. A superscript epsilon (ϵ) indicates an editorial change since the last revision or reapproval.

1. Scope

1.1 This guide describes the self-rescue technique on ice utilizing an ice staff.

1.2 This guide is one in a series of self-rescue techniques for the ice rescuer.

1.3 Individuals who will operate in the cold water or ice rescue setting need to be aware of the equipment and physical requirements necessary to be able to perform all identified objectives and necessary skills in the setting.

2. Terminology

2.1 *Definitions:*

2.1.1 *drysuit, n*—a protective suit that encompasses the wearer, prohibiting water from entering; a dry suit provides no buoyancy or thermal protection without insulative undergarments.

2.1.2 *ice awl, n*—a device, consisting of a sharp spike with a handle used for rescue on ice.

2.1.3 *ice staff, n*—a stick, pole, or rod with a sharp spike in one end used to traverse on ice or rescue on ice.

2.1.4 *immersion suit, n*—designed to provide cold water protection and buoyancy by one person in cold water emergencies.

2.1.4.1 *Discussion*—These devices should conform to standards set by the appropriate national regulatory authority, that is, the U.S. Coast Guard in the United States.

2.1.5 *personal flotation device (PFD), n*— a buoyant device suitable for use by one person in water emergencies.

2.1.5.1 *Discussion*—These devices should conform to standards set by the appropriate national regulatory authority, that is, the U.S. Coast Guard in the United States.

3. Significance and Use

3.1 This guide establishes a recommended procedure for utilizing an ice staff as a self-rescue technique on ice.

3.2 All persons who are identified as ice rescuers shall meet the requirements of this guide.

3.3 This guide will assist government agencies; state, local, or regional organizations; fire departments, rescue teams and others who are responsible for establishing a minimum performance for personnel who respond to ice emergencies.

3.4 This guide is not intended to be used in isolation, but as a component guide acknowledging many skills and techniques needed to respond at a cold water and ice emergency.

3.5 An ice rescuer shall be wearing an immersion suit, drysuit with PFD, or equivalent cold water protection and buoyancy to perform these rescues.

3.6 An ice rescuer shall carry a set of ice awls along with the ice staff as a backup technique.

4. Procedure

4.1 The ice rescuer should grasp the ice staff firmly near the spiked end.

4.2 Extend the staff in a downward slanting position tapping in a semicircle to test the ice.

4.3 Listen for a clear, hard resonating sound indicating good ice.

4.4 Move slowly onto the area of ice that has been tested.

4.5 Continue to traverse by sliding steps to lessen the impact of the footsteps while distributing body weight as evenly as possible.

4.6 When moving, continue listening for the clear, hard resonant sound; however, a dull sound or thud may indicate weaker ice.

4.7 The rescuer should use the spiked end of the staff to test those areas of ice by jabbing at the surface. If the ice breaks away or is deteriorative, select another path.

4.8 If the ice begins to break, lie down and roll to safety.

4.9 If the rescuer becomes immersed, cover the mouth and nose to prevent aspiration.

4.10 While immersed, remain calm and use the staff horizontally to lift up and onto the ice, rolling to safety.

4.11 The rescuer can utilize the staff while immersed in a vertical position by allowing feet and legs to float to the surface.

4.12 While stabbing the spiked end into the ice, pull and flutter kick, sliding forward if ice conditions allow.

4.13 If ice conditions do not allow, continue stabbing and kicking to reach stronger ice, then roll to safety.

5. Keywords

5.1 ice; ice rescue; ice rescuer; ice staff; water; water rescue; water rescuer

[1] This guide is under the jurisdiction of ASTM Committee F32 on Search and Rescue and is the direct responsibility of Subcommittee F32.02 on Search and Rescue Management.

Current edition approved Jan. 10, 1997. Published June 1997.

Standard Guide for Ice Awls Self-Rescue Technique[1]

This standard is issued under the fixed designation F 1766; the number immediately following the designation indicates the year of original adoption or, in the case of revision, the year of last revision. A number in parentheses indicates the year of last reapproval. A superscript epsilon (ε) indicates an editorial change since the last revision or reapproval.

1. Scope

1.1 This guide covers the self-rescue technique on ice utilizing the ice awl.

1.2 This guide is one of a series of self-rescue techniques for the ice rescuer.

1.3 *This standard does not purport to address all of the safety concerns, if any, associated with its use. It is the responsibility of the user of this standard to establish appropriate safety and health practices and determine the applicability of regulatory limitations prior to use.*

2. Terminology

2.1 *Definitions:*

2.1.1 *drysuit, n*—a protective suit that encompasses the wearer, prohibiting water from entering.

2.1.2 *ice awls, n*—a device used for rescue on ice consisting of a sharp spike with a handle.

2.1.3 *immersion suit, n*—a device designed to provide cold water protection and buoyancy by one person in cold water emergencies.

2.1.3.1 *Discussion*—These devices should conform to standards set by the appropriate national regulatory authority, that is, the U.S. Coast Guard in the United States.

2.1.4 *personal flotation device, PFD, n*—a buoyant device suitable for use by one person in water emergencies.

2.1.4.1 *Discussion*—These devices should conform to standards set by the appropriate national regulatory authority, that is, the U.S. Coast Guard in the United States.

3. Significance and Use

3.1 This guide establishes a recommended procedure for utilizing ice awls as a self rescue technique on ice.

3.2 All persons who are identified as ice rescuers shall meet the requirements of this guide.

3.3 This guide will assist government agencies; state, local or regional organizations; fire departments; rescue teams; and others who are responsible for establishing a minimum performance for personnel who respond to ice emergencies.

3.4 This guide is not intended to be used in isolation, but as a component guide acknowledging many skills and techniques needed to respond at a cold water and ice emergency.

3.5 An ice rescuer shall be wearing an immersion suit, drysuit with PFD, or equivalent cold-water protection and buoyancy to perform these rescues.

4. Procedure

4.1 Upon initial immersion in cold water, the rescuer should cover the mouth and nose to prevent the aspiration of water.

4.2 The rescuer should move to the edge of the opening in the ice.

4.3 Grasp the ice awls placing one in each hand.

4.4 Reach forward onto the ice and strike downward driving the point of the ice awl into the ice.

4.5 Allow feet and legs to float up behind you to the surface, so that you are floating horizontally on the surface of the water.

4.6 While pulling yourself forward onto the ice utilizing the ice awls, keep your horizontal position and add a strong flutter kick.

4.7 Ice conditions may not support the rescuer. It may be necessary to continue alternately stabbing and continuously kicking to reach stronger ice.

4.8 Once in a supportive ice, the rescuer should not stand up.

4.9 Roll to safety in the direction of shore or safer ice.

5. Keywords

5.1 ice; ice awls; ice rescue; ice rescuer; water; water rescue; water rescuer

[1] This guide is under the jurisdiction of ASTM Committee F32 on Search and Rescue and is the direct responsibility of Subcommittee F32.02 on Search and Rescue Management.

Current edition approved June 10, 1997. Published March 1998. Originally published as F 1766 – 97. Last previous edition F 1766 – 97.

Standard Guide for Forms Used for Search and Rescue[1]

This standard is issued under the fixed designation F 1767; the number immediately following the designation indicates the year of original adoption or, in the case of revision, the year of last revision. A number in parentheses indicates the year of last reapproval. A superscript epsilon (ϵ) indicates an editorial change since the last revision or reapproval.

ϵ[1] NOTE—Editorial changes were made to Sections 4.1 and Table 1 in October 1999.

INTRODUCTION

Many organizations have been working in the Search and Rescue (SAR) community using the Incident Command System (ICS) framework. In doing so, these organizations have adapted the existing ICS forms to fit their needs. They have also found that some new forms needed to be developed in order to address problems or areas not considered in the fire-oriented forms. Some of these organizations have developed their own standard packet of forms that will address the typical needs of that organization. By addressing the appropriate actions called for by the average mission, these forms can focus the team members' activities into a standard operating procedure. This guide will show examples of form packets used by some SAR organizations.

1. Scope

1.1 This guide gives examples of forms used in the SAR community.

1.2 It is not the intent of this guide to recommend one form over another, but to make the user aware of the many different types of forms used. This guide does not purport to contain every form used in SAR, only a few examples of forms in each category.

1.3 These forms cover a great variety of the many aspects involved in SAR. This guide will attempt to give a few versions of forms used for each aspect identified. The user may choose which form best fits his particular need.

1.4 *This standard does not purport to address all of the safety concerns, if any, associated with its use. It is the responsibility of the user of this standard to establish appropriate safety and health practices and determine the applicability of regulatory limitations prior to use.*

2. Referenced Documents

2.1 The forms in this guide have been submitted by members of various organizations who are presently using them. In some cases the organization logo will identify the source of the submitted form. Use of logos on forms in this guide does not constitute an endorsement by either ASTM or the contributing SAR organization. Use of these displays are for the convenience and information of the user.

2.2 ICS National Training Curriculum— *ICS Forms Catalog*[2]

3. Significance and Use

3.1 This guide will give SAR personnel options in choosing a form that will fit their specific need. These forms will assist in the organization, management, and documentation of a search or rescue incident.

3.2 Additional forms will be categorized by topics such as management, investigation, training documentation, equipment maintenance, and reports. This guide will compare the original ICS forms with samples of those developed to parallel them for SAR.

3.3 Once categorized, an explanation will be given for each type of form. Some examples of these forms will be shown. Some contributors have included detailed instruction for the use of their forms.

3.4 This guide may serve as the basis for new forms to be created using some information found here.

4. Summary of Guide

4.1 This guide has been arranged so that the user can locate an example of a form by identifying the way that it is used, or where it fits within the Incident Command System.

Section	Category
Section 5	Existing ICS Forms
Section 6	ICS forms Modified for SAR
Section 7	Additional Forms for SAR Management (these are listed by the four general staff functions)
7.2	Plans

[1] This guide is under the jurisdiction of ASTM Committee F-32 on Search and Rescueand is the direct responsibility of Subcommittee F32.02 on Management and Operations.

Current edition approved October 10, 1998. Published March 1999. Originally published as F 1767 – 97. Last previous edition F 1767 – 97.

[2] Available from the National Interagency Fire Center, 3833 S. Development Ave., Boise, ID 83705.

Section	Category
7.3	Operations
7.4	Logistics
7.5	Finance
Section 8	Additional Forms for SAR Investigation
Section 9	Additional Forms for SAR Training
Section 10	Additional forms for SAR Equipment Maintenance
Section 11	Additional Forms for SAR Reports & Critiques
Section 12	Additional Forms for Urban SAR
Section 13	Miscellaneous SAR Forms
Section 14	Form Packets
Section 15	Index

5. Existing ICS Forms

5.1 In adopting the incident command system as the preferred method for managing a search or rescue incident, we have also adopted the forms that go with that system. All the forms included in the ICS are shown for the reference of the user. It is up to the user to choose which form will fit the specific need of a given incident.

5.1.1 Appendix X1 is arranged as follows: (forms not included at this time):

201 Incident Briefing
202 Incident Objectives
203 Organization Assignment List
204 Division Assignment List
205 Incident Radio Communications Plan
206 Medical Plan
207 Chain of Command Flow Chart
209 Incident Status Summary
210 Status Change Card
211 Check In List
213 General Message
214 Unit Log
215 Operational Planning Work Sheet
216 Radio Requirements Worksheet
217 Radio Frequency Assignment Worksheet
218 Support Vehicle Inventory
219 Miscellaneous Equipment/Task Force (T-Card)
220 Air Operations Summary
221 Demobilization Checkout

6. ICS Forms Modified for SAR

6.1 These are forms that are based directly on the ICS but have been altered in some manner to fit specific needs of a particular organization. In many cases the forms show a parallel to ICS by using the number or the name that corresponds to the ICS system.

6.2 Forms included in SAR/ICS sections:

6.2.1 *201 Incident Briefing Forms*—This is a form to gather basic information, including but not limited to the situation, the subject, the overhead team, and initial response actions. It is used to brief incoming SAR personnel, and as a record of the initial response.

6.2.1.1 Examples found in Appendix X2:

(*1*) Incident Briefing (Fig. X2.1).

(*2*) General Briefing (Fig. X2.2).

(*3*) General Briefing—Missing Person with Instruction Sheets (Fig. X2.3).

(*4*) Daily Briefing (Fig. X2.4).

(*5*) Shift Briefing Format (Fig. X2.5).

6.2.2 *202 Incident Objectives Forms*— This form is the first sheet of the incident action plan. The objectives are developed by the incident commander at the planning meeting and then documented on this form.

6.2.2.1 Examples found in Appendix X2:

(*1*) Incident Objectives (Fig. X2.6).

6.2.3 *203 Organization Assignment List*— This form provides incident personnel with information as to which units have been established and the names of the individuals in each position. This form becomes part of the incident action plan and may be posted separately on information boards.

6.2.3.1 Examples found in Appendix X2:

(*1*) Organizational Assignment List (Fig. X2.7).

6.2.4 *204 Division Assignment List*—This form is used to detail the field assignment that is given to any particular resource. In many cases a segmented incident map will be given with this assignment sheet. (The maps may be copied on the back side).

6.2.4.1 The examples shown give a variety of additional information to the crew/team such as: debriefing, communications, subject profile, and equipment/transportation information.

6.2.4.2 Form instructions are included where available.

6.2.4.3 Examples found in Appendix X2:

(*1*) Task Assignment (Fig. X2.8).

(*2*) Field Team Assignments (Fig. X2.9).

(*3*) Crew Assignment (Fig. X2.10).

(*4*) Crew Assignment with Instructions (Fig. X2.11).

(*5*) Team Assignment with Instructions (Fig. X2.12).

6.2.5 *205 Incident Radio Communications Plan*—This plan provides information on all radio frequencies being used on the incident. It becomes part of the Incident Action Plan.

6.2.5.1 Examples found in Appendix X2:

(*1*) Incident Communications Plan (Fig. X2.13)

6.2.6 *206 Medical Plan*—This form provides information on incident medical aid stations, transportation services, hospitals, and medical emergency procedures. It becomes part of the Incident Action Plan.

6.2.6.1 Examples found in Appendix X2:

(*1*) Incident Medical/Evacuation Plan (Fig. X2.14).

6.2.7 *211 Check-In List*—This form is used to record the arrival of all incident personnel.

6.2.7.1 Examples found in Appendix X2:

(*1*) Daily Local Volunteer Personnel Register (Fig. X2.15).

(*2*) Daily SAR Unit/Government Personnel Register (Fig. X2.16).

(*3*) Personnel Check In/Out (Fig. X2.17).

(*4*) Registration of Search and Rescue Participants (Fig. X2.18).

6.2.8 *214 Unit Log*—This form is used to document any activity or events occurring in a particular unit.

6.2.8.1 Examples found in Appendix X2:

(*1*) Daily Unit Log (Fig. X2.19).

6.2.9 *215 Operational Planning Worksheet*— This form is used in planning which resources will be used for assignments. It is also used by logistics for ordering resources.

6.2.9.1 Examples found in Appendix X2:

(*1*) Daily SAR Resources Worksheet (Fig. X2.20).

6.2.10 *218 Support Vehicle Inventory*— This form provides

an inventory of vehicles assigned or available at the incident.

6.2.10.1 Example found in Appendix X2:

(*1*) Daily Vehicle Register (Fig. X2.21).

7. Additional Forms for SAR Management

7.1 These are forms that are not based on ICS forms but have been developed for use within the system because of the particular needs of the developing organization in managing an incident. These forms have been broken down into the four general staff functions.

7.2 *Forms Used Within the Plans Sections*:

7.2.1 *Debriefing Forms*—These forms are used to detail information coming from the field. This information is vital in planning strategy for future operational periods. This form also serves as a record of field activities.

7.2.1.1 Examples found in Appendix X2:

(*1*) Debriefing Form (Fig. X2.22).

(*2*) Team Debriefing with Supplement and Instructions (Fig. X2.23).

7.2.2 *Resource Forms*—These forms are used for ordering resources and can also be useful when planning assignments.

7.2.2.1 Examples found in Appendix X2:

(*1*) Search Capabilities Roster (Fig. X2.24).

(*2*) Resource Order Form (Fig. X2.25).

7.2.3 *Planning Worksheets/Checklist* — These are general forms used within the planning section.

7.2.3.1 Examples found in Appendix X2:

(*1*) Survival Time-frame Worksheet (Fig. X2.26).

(*2*) Planning Process Checklist (Fig. X2.27).

(*3*) Planning Cycle (Fig. X2.28).

7.2.4 *Aircraft Search Forms*—These forms are used when searching for downed aircraft.

7.2.4.1 Examples found in Appendix X2:

(*1*) Missing Aircraft Worksheet (Fig. X2.29).

(2) ELT Worksheet (Fig. X2.30).

7.2.5 *Situation Unit Forms*:

7.2.5.1 Examples found in Appendix X2.

(*1*) Situation Report (Fig. X2.31).

7.3 *Forms Used Within the Operations Section*:

7.3.1 *Assignment Record*—These forms are used for documenting tasks that have been assigned to particular resources.

7.3.1.1 Examples found in Appendix X2:

(*1*) Daily Task Log (Fig. X2.32).

(*2*) Crew Card with Instructions (Fig. X2.33).

7.3.2 *Field Forms*—These are forms used by resources in the field to document various activities.

7.3.2.1 Examples found in Appendix X2:

(*1*) ELT-DF Field Team Log (Fig. X2.34).

(*2*) Tracking Worksheet (Fig. X2.35).

(*3*) Track ID Form (Fig. X2.36).

7.4 *Forms Used Within the Logistics Section*:

7.4.1 *Supply Unit Form*—These forms are used in the supply unit for ordering, locating, and tracking supplies and equipment.

7.4.1.1 Examples found in Appendix X2:

(*1*) Equipment Roster (Fig. X2.37).

(*2*) Equipment Check (Fig. X2.38).

7.4.2 *Communications Unit Forms*—These forms are used within the communications unit.

7.4.2.1 Examples found in Appendix X2:

(*1*) Daily Communications Log (Fig. X2.39).

(*2*) Communications Log (Fig. X2.40).

7.4.3 *Medical Unit Forms*—These forms are used within the medical unit.

7.4.3.1 Examples found in Appendix X2:

(*1*) Medical Report (Fig. X2.41).

(*2*) Report of Injury (Fig. X2.42).

(*3*) Patient Referral (Fig. X2.43).

(*4*) Notice of Death Form (Fig. X2.44).

7.4.4 *Facilities Unit Forms*:

7.4.4.1 Examples found in Appendix X2.

(*1*) Operating Facilities (Fig. X2.45).

7.5 *Forms Used Within the Finance Section*:

7.5.1 *Time Unit Forms*—These are forms used within the time unit.

7.5.1.1 Examples found in Appendix X2:

(*1*) Monthly Time Report (Fig. X2.46).

(*2*) Time Record (Fig. X2.47).

7.5.2 *Cost Unit Forms*—These are forms used within the cost unit.

7.5.2.1 Examples found in Appendix X2:

(*1*) Search and Rescue Expenditure Report (Fig. X2.48).

(*2*) Cost Sheet (Fig. X2.49).

8. Additional Forms for SAR Investigation

8.1 Search investigation very often plays an important role in the planning and the operations of an incident. This is quite different than a fire. The investigation may deal with the subjects' history or with current events such as possible sightings. Some organizations have developed forms to assist them that have no connection to the ICS.

8.2 *Forms Used to Aid in the Investigation*:

8.2.1 *Subject Profile Forms*—These are forms that are used to gather information about the person or persons that is (are) the subject of the search. Some groups use short forms that only compile basic information used in the initial phases of the search, and get more detail later. Other groups have very detailed forms that serve as the foundation of their investigation.

8.2.1.1 Examples found in Appendix X3:

(*1*) Lost Person Questionnaire (Fig. X3.1).

(*2*) Search and Rescue Circumstance (Fig. X3.2).

(*3*) Incident Missing Person Questionnaire (Fig. X3.3).

(*4*) Lost Person Worksheet (Fig. X3.4).

(*5*) ML Quick Sheet (Fig. X3.5).

(*6*) Notification of Search and/or Rescue (Fig. X3.6).

8.2.2 *Information Compiling Forms*—These forms will assist the investigators in gathering and compiling information. They cover everything from the documentation of the initial source of the clue (whether it is physical or verbal) to the sorting and logging of the clue.

8.2.2.1 Examples found in Appendix X3:

(*1*) Urban Interview Log (Fig. X3.7).

(*2*) Daily Clue Log (Fig. X3.8).

(*3*) ELT-DF Reports (Fig. X3.9).

(*4*) Clue Card (Fig. X3.10).

8.2.3 *Miscellaneous Investigation Forms*:

8.2.3.1 Examples found in Appendix X3:

(*1*) Relative Search Urgency Rating Form (Fig. X3.11).

9. Additional Forms for SAR Training

9.1 These forms are used to document all phases of training from planning to implementation.

9.1.1 Examples found in Appendix X3:

9.1.1.1 Training Plan (Fig. X3.12).

9.1.1.2 Documented Training Form (Fig. X3.13).

9.1.1.3 Training Check-In (Fig. X3.14).

10. Additional Forms for SAR Equipment Maintenance

10.1 These are forms used to document information related to search and/or rescue equipment such as, serial numbers, age, use history, and maintenance.

10.1.1 Examples found in Appendix X3.

(*1*) PMI Usage and History (Fig. X3.15).

11. Additional Forms for SAR Reports & Critiques

11.1 These are forms used to report an incident. Some are formal reports used as a permanent record, while others are a general summary of information. Forms used in critiques are included here.

11.1.1 Examples found in Appendix X3:

(*1*) Mission Debriefing Form (Fig. X3.16).

(*2*) Mission Report (Fig. X3.17).

(*3*) Incident Report (Fig. X3.18).

(*4*) Incident After Action Report (Fig. X3.19).

(*5*) Mutual Aid Response Survey (Fig. X3.20).

12. Additional Forms for Urban SAR

12.1 These are forms intended to be used for an incident in an urban setting.

12.1.1 Examples found in Appendix X3.

12.1.1.1 Task Force Leader's Mission Assignment Checklist (Fig. X3.21).

12.1.1.2 Task Force Base Of Operations Location Checklist (Fig. X3.22).

12.1.1.3 Task Force Operations Report (Fig. X3.23).

12.1.1.4 Task Force Operations Site Sketch (Fig. X3.24).

12.1.1.5 Structure Triage (Fig. X3.25).

12.1.1.6 Urban Interview Log (Fig. X3.7).

13. Miscellaneous SAR Forms

13.1 It is recommended that SAR organizations develop a packet of forms that fits their particular needs. They should analyze how they respond to their typical incident. A preplan and a packet of forms could be made up to help guide them through the entire incident.

13.2 Examples found in Appendix X4:

(*1*) Public Information Summary—Incident Status (Fig. X4.1).

(*2*) Intra-Agency Registration Firm (Fig. X4.2).

(*3*) Call-out List (Fig. X4.3).

14. Form Packets

14.1 Included here is a form packet being used by the state of New Mexico. This packet is shown here to give an example of how an agency has developed a form packet to fit their specific needs. It is not the intention of this document to make this form packet a national standard. The purpose is to encourage SAR organizations to use the forms in this guide, or ones similar, to create their own form packet which will help to organize their SAR response more efficiently.

15. Alphabetical Index to Forms

15.1 Table 1 lists the forms in alphabetical order.

TABLE 1 Alphabetical Index to Forms

Title	Reference Number
Aircraft, Missing-Worksheet	2·29
Assignment list, Crew	2·10
Assignment list, Crew	2·11
Assignment list, Field Team	2·9
Assignment list, Organizational	2·7
Assignment list, task	2·8
Assignment list, team	2·12
Briefing General	2·2
Briefing, General-Missing Person	2·3
Briefing, Incident	2·1
Call Out List	4·3
Check-in List	X·X
Check List, Task Force Base of Operation Location	3·22
Check List, Task Force Leader Mission Assignment	3·21
Clue Card	3·10
Communications, Daily-log	2·39
Communications, log	2·40
Cost Sheet	2·49
Crew Card	2·33
Daily Briefing	2·4
Debriefing, Form	2·22
Debriefing Form, Mission	3·16
Debriefing Team	2·23
ELT-DF Reports	3·9
ELT Worksheet	2·30
ELT-DF field team log	2·34
Emergency Helicoptor Request Information Sheet	X·XX
Equipment Check In/Out	2·38
Equipment Roster	2·37
Expenditure Report, SAR	2·48
ICS Planning Guide	X·XX
Incident Briefing	X·XX
Incident Communications Plan	2·131
Incident Medical/Evacuation Plan	2·14
Incident Objectives	2·6
Incident Objectives	X·XX
Incident Organization Chart	X·XX
Incident Status Summary	X·XX
Injury, Report of	2·42
Liability Release	X·XX
Log, Daily Clues	3·8
Log, Daily Tasks	2·32
Log, Urban Interview	3·7
Lost Person Worksheet	3·4
Medical Report	2·41
Medical Plan	X·XX
ML Quicksheet	3·5
Non-segmented Areas	X·XX
Notification of Search and/or Rescue	3·6
Notice of Death Form	2·44
Operating Facilities	2·45
Operational Planning Worksheet	X·XX
Organization Assignment List	X·XX
Patient Referral	2·43
Planning Cycle	2·28
Planning Process Checklist	2·27
PMI Usage & History	3·15
"POD" End of Shift Report	X·XX
Public Information Summary-Incident Status	4·1
Questionaire, Incident Missing Person	3·3
Questionaire, Lost Persons	3·1
Radio Communications Plan	X·XX

TABLE 1 *Continued*

Title	Reference Number
Register-Personnel, Check In/Out	2·17
Register-Personnel, Daily SAR Unit/Gov't	2·16
Register-Personnel, Daily Local Volunteer	2·15
Registration Form, Intra-Agency	4·2
Registration of Search & Rescue Participants	2·18
Relevance of Clue	X·XX
Report, Incident	3·18
Report, Incident after Action	3·19
Report, Mission	3·17
Resource Order Form	2·25
Resources Worksheet, Daily SAR	2·20
Roster, Search Capabilities	2·24
SAR Incident Report	X·XX
SAR Injury Report	X·XX
SAR Questionnaire A & B	X·XX
Search & Rescue Circumstance	3·2
Search Clue Log	X·XX
Search Initiation Log	X·XX
Shift Briefing Format	2·5
Situation Report	2·31
Structure Triage	3·25
Survey, Mutual Aid Response	3·20
Survival Time Frame Worksheet	2·26
Task Assignment	X·XX
Task Force Operations Report	3·23
Task Force Operations Site Sketch	3·24
Time Record	2·47
Time Report, Monthly	2·46
Tracking ID Form	2·36
Tracking Worksheet	2·35
Training Check-In	3·14
Training Form, Documented	3·13
Training Plan	3·12
Unit Log	X·XX
Unit Log, Daily	2·19
Urgency Rating Form, Relative Search	3·11
Vehicle Register, Daily	2·21

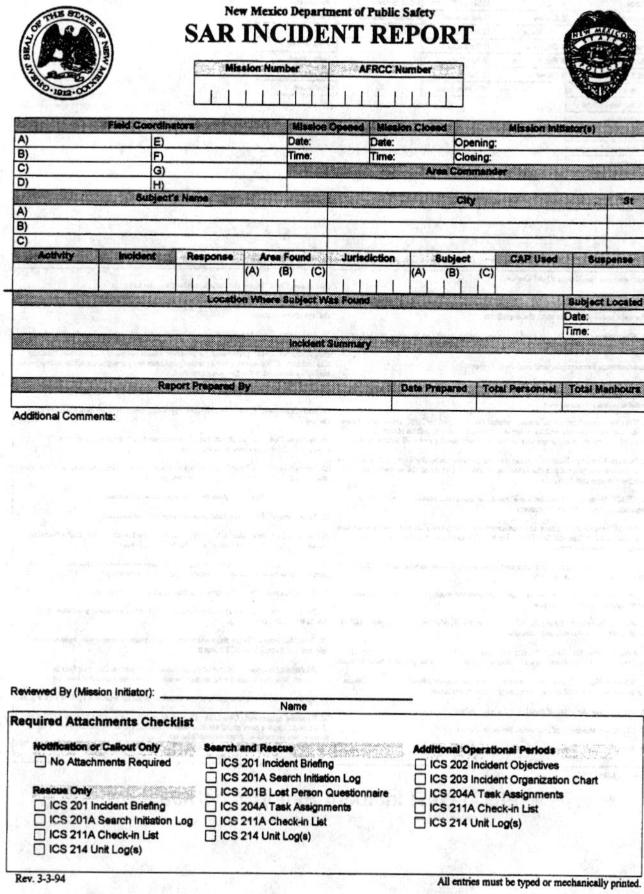

New Mexico Department of Public Safety

SAR INCIDENT REPORT

Mission Number	AFRCC Number

Field Coordinators		Mission Opened	Mission Closed	Mission Initiator(s)
A)	E)	Date:	Date:	Opening:
B)	F)	Time:	Time:	Closing:
C)	G)	Area Commander		
D)	H)			

Subject's Name	City	St
A)		
B)		
C)		

Activity	Incident	Response	Area Found (A) (B) (C)	Jurisdiction	Subject (A) (B) (C)	CAP Used	Suspense

Location Where Subject Was Found	Subject Located
	Date:
	Time:

Incident Summary

Report Prepared By	Date Prepared	Total Personnel	Total Manhours

Additional Comments:

Reviewed By (Mission Initiator): ______________________

Name

Required Attachments Checklist

Notification or Callout Only
- ☐ No Attachments Required

Rescue Only
- ☐ ICS 201 Incident Briefing
- ☐ ICS 201A Search Initiation Log
- ☐ ICS 211A Check-in List
- ☐ ICS 214 Unit Log(s)

Search and Rescue
- ☐ ICS 201 Incident Briefing
- ☐ ICS 201A Search Initiation Log
- ☐ ICS 201B Lost Person Questionnaire
- ☐ ICS 204A Task Assignments
- ☐ ICS 211A Check-in List
- ☐ ICS 214 Unit Log(s)

Additional Operational Periods
- ☐ ICS 202 Incident Objectives
- ☐ ICS 203 Incident Organization Chart
- ☐ ICS 204A Task Assignments
- ☐ ICS 211A Check-in List
- ☐ ICS 214 Unit Log(s)

Rev. 3-3-94

All entries must be typed or mechanically printed.

FIG. 1 SAR Incident Report

Activity	Incident	Response	Area Found	Jurisdiction	Subject	CAP Used	Suspense
1 Climber	1 Unknown	1 Standby	1 Primary Area	1 USFS	1 Uninjured	1 No	1 Closed
2 Hiker	2 Lost	2 Callout	2 Secondary Area	2 BLM	2 Injured	2 Yes	2 Suspended
3 Hunter	3 Stranded	3 Land Search	3 Previous Area	3 NPS	3 Fatality		3 Open
4 Skier	4 Injury	4 Water Search	4 Out of Area	4 Wilderness			
5 Snowmobile	5 Illness	5 Air Search	5 Bastard Search	5 State Land			
6 Vehicle	6 Runaway	6 Rescue	6 Other	6 Federal Land			
7 Aircraft	7 Overdue	7 Recovery		7 Private Land			
8 Boat / Raft	8 False Alarm	8 Self Evac.		8 Indian Land			
9 ELT	9 Other	9 Carry Out		9 Military Res.			
10 Caver		10 Other Evac.		10 Unknown			
11 Hospital Patient							
12 Motorbike							
13 Wood Cutter							
14 Gatherer-Forager							
15 Unknown							

General Instructions for Preparing SAR Incident Report

Instructions for Using Field Codes

1. The Field codes are printed on the reverse of the form. To use the codes, fold the bottom edge of the form along the bottom edge of the code fields and crease the form. The field codes will align with the code fields.

2. When typing the form, the field codes are visible above the top edge of the form when the form is positioned in the typewriter.

Instructions for completing Incident Report:

NOTE: Attachments are not required if resources were not used (other than MI and FC) or if mission was terminated prior to mobilization of resources.

1. This form satisfies the minimum information required by DPS. Incomplete forms or missing attachments will be returned to sender. Report will be electronically scanned, therefore it is mandatory to type or mechanically print all form entries.

2. Mission Number: Enter the state mission number using the form yy-dd-nn, where yy is the current year, dd is the state police district, and nn is the sequence number assigned to this incident.

3. AFRCC Number: Enter the Air Force Rescue mission number. Required for missions using Air Force resources.

4. Field Coordinators: Enter the last names of all certified FCs used on this mission in a Command or General Staff role. Up to 8 FCs can be listed. Use Additional Comments space for more.

5. Mission Opened: Enter the date and time that the mission was opened. Should agree with the opening teletype.

6. Mission Closed: Enter the date and time that the mission was closed. Should agree with the closing teletype.

7. Mission Initiators: Enter the last names of the MI who began the mission and the MI on duty when the mission was closed.

8. Area Commander: Enter the name on the On-call Area Commander during this incident. Area Commander must be notified on missions lasting longer than 4 hours.

9. Subject's Name: Enter the first and last names of each subject. Up to 3 subjects can be listed. Use Additional Comments space to list more.

10. City: Enter the town of residence for each subject.

11. ST: Enter the state of residence for each subject.

12. Activity Code: Enter the subject's activity from the key.

13. Incident Code: Enter the Incident type from the key.

14. Response Code: Enter the response codes for the incident. Multiple entries from the key are permitted.

15. Area Code: Enter the search area in which each subject was found using the key.

16. Jurisdiction Code: Enter each jurisdiction whose property was searched during this incident. If Wilderness was searched, indicate the jurisdiction of the wilderness. Multiple entries from the key are permitted.

17. Subject Code: Enter the status of each subject found from the key.

18. CAP Used Code: Enter whether CAP resources were used on this incident from the key.

19. Suspense Code: Enter the status of the incident at the time report was submitted. Select suspense code from key.

20. Where Subject was Found: Enter the common name of the area where the subject was located. Latitude and Longitude are acceptable.

21. Date Located: Enter the date that the subject was located.

22. Time Located: Enter the time that the subject was located.

23. Incident Summary: Give a brief description of the results of the SAR effort and rescue, i.e. "The subject was airlifted to BCMC by Lifeguard".

24. Report Prepared By: Enter the name of the person preparing this report. This information is needed in case a question arises at a later time.

25. Date Prepared: Enter the date that this report was submitted.

26. Total Personnel: Enter the total number of volunteers assisting on this incident (totals from ICS Form 211A).

27. Total Man-hours: Enter the total number of volunteer man-hours expended on this incident (totals from ICS Form 211A).

28. Additional Comments: Enter any additional information that you feel is important. Use this space for additional names, etc. as mentioned above.

29. Reviewed By: Enter the name of the Mission Initiator who will review this report.

30. Required Attachment Checklist: Be sure to attach the required forms for the type of incident. Make a note in Additional Comments field if no resources were used or mission was terminated prior to mobilization.

Rev. 3-3-94

FIG. 1 SAR Incident Report *(continued)*

NON-SEGMENTED AREAS

MISSION # ____________ PAGE ______ OF ________

(T)ype of (R)esource
H = Helicopter HA = Hasty Team DA = Air Scent Dog V = Vehicle HO = Horse
A = Fixed Wing FT = Foot Team DT = Trailing Dog P = Phone X = ________

SEG A-Z	ROAD, TRAIL, HOME CAMP, CAR, Etc.	TR	DATE/TIME CHECKED?	TR	DATE/TIME CHECKED?	TR	DATE/TIME CHECKED?

SEG A-Z	ROAD, TRAIL, HOME CAMP, CAR, Etc.	TR	DATE/TIME CHECKED?	TR	DATE/TIME CHECKED?	TR	DATE/TIME CHECKED?

SEG A-Z	ROAD, TRAIL, HOME CAMP, CAR, Etc.	TR	DATE/TIME CHECKED?	TR	DATE/TIME CHECKED?	TR	DATE/TIME CHECKED?

SEG A-Z	ROAD, TRAIL, HOME CAMP, CAR, Etc.	TR	DATE/TIME CHECKED?	TR	DATE/TIME CHECKED?	TR	DATE/TIME CHECKED?

SEG A-Z	ROAD, TRAIL, HOME CAMP, CAR, Etc.	TR	DATE/TIME CHECKED?	TR	DATE/TIME CHECKED?	TR	DATE/TIME CHECKED?

FIG. 2 Non-segmented Areas

SEARCH CLUE LOG

MISSION # ______________ PAGE ________ OF __________

ROC = RELEVANCE OF CLUE TO MISSION AT TIME CLUE WAS FOUND 0 - 100%

AREA	TYPE CLUE & LOCATION FOUND	ROC	DATE/TIME	ACTION TAKEN
		FOUND BY ?		
		FOUND BY?		
		FOUND BY?		
		FOUND BY?		

To figure relevancy of clue (ROC) you must subjectively select a number (0 - 100) that indicates your best guess as to how relevant the clue is to the mission at the time the clue is found. Information such as age of the clue, possibility of the clue belonging to victim, confidence in resource who found the clue etc., should be considered.

FIG. 3 Search Clue Log

RELEVANCE OF CLUE (ROC)

NEW POA = ROC x (1 - Old POA) + Old POA

ROC % \ Old POA %	10	20	30	40	50	60	70	80	90
10	19	28	37	46	55	64	73	82	91
20	28	36	44	52	60	68	76	84	92
30	37	44	51	58	65	72	79	86	93
40	46	52	58	64	70	76	82	88	94
50	55	60	65	70	75	80	85	90	95
60	64	68	72	76	80	84	88	92	96
70	73	76	79	82	85	88	91	94	98
80	82	84	86	88	90	92	94	96	99
90	91	92	93	94	95	96	97	98	99

To figure relevancy of clue (ROC) you must subjectively select a number (1% to 99%) that indicates your best guess as to how relevant that clue is to the mission. To adequately do this, you must use as much information about the circumstances surrounding the clue as possible. Such as; age of the clue, the possibility that the clue was left by the subject, confidence in the SAR resource which found the clue, etc.

FIG. 4 Relevance of Clue

"POD" END OF SHIFT REPORT

MISSION # __________ PAGE ____OF ______

Co-Ordinator ____________________

Date/Time Started ____/____ Date/Time Ended ____/____

RESPONSIVE

(T)ype of (R)esource

H = Helicopter T = Trackers DA = Air Scent Dogs HA = Hasty Team

A = Fixed Wing G = Grid Search DT = Trailing Dogs O = Other

AREA #	1st old	TR *	New POD	CUM	New POD	TR	CUM	New POD	TR	CUM	New POD	TR	CUM	(X) 90+	REMARKS

* = If 1st search of area include Type of Resource.
(X) = 90% POD or more

FIG. 5 "POD" End of Shift Report

UN-RESPONSIVE

(T)ype of (R)esource

H = Helicopter T = Trackers DA = Air Scent Dogs HA = Hasty Team

A = Fixed Wing G = Grid Search DT =Trailing Dogs O= Other

AREA #	1st old	TR *	New POD	CUM	New POD	TR	CUM	New POD	TR	CUM	New POD	TR	CUM	(X) 90+	REMARKS

* = If 1st search of area include Type of Resource.
(X) = 90% POD or more

FIG. 5 "POD" End of Shift Report *(continued)*

New Mexico Department of Public Safety
Search and Rescue Office

SAR Questionaire

(PART "A")

This is a Mandatory Form and MUST be filled out by a Mission Initiator (or FC if no MI Available)

Investigator MI/FC Assigned Call

Dist	Date Assigned	Time Assigned	Assigned Mission Initiator	Number of Subjects	Tracking Number
			#Name?		

Source of Information

Name of Reporting Party Number One	Address:	St	ZIP

Relationship to Subject	Phone Number	Call Back Number NOW	Call Back Number LATER

Name of Reporting Party Number Two	Address:	St	ZIP

Relationship to Subject	Phone Number	Call Back Number NOW	Call Back Number LATER

What is Believed to Have Happened

The above information ONLY has to be filled out on the FIRST Subject.

Subject _____ of _____ Subjects

Subject Information

Name	Age	Sex	Nickname(s)	Home Phone	Local Phone

Address	City	St	Zip

Local Address	Local City	St	Zip

Physical Description

Identification		Clothing/Style		Color	Health	
Height:		Shirt:			Physical Cond.:	
Weight:		Pants:			Medical Cond:	
Age:		Outer Wear:			Psychological:	
Build:		Head Wear:			Medication:	
Hair Color:		Gloves:			Amount Medications:	
Style:		Footwear:			Eyesight w/o Glasses:	
Glasses		Extra Clothing			What Might Subject do if Lost	
Mustache						
Beard						
Sideburns						

OVER

Page 1 of 3 - SAR Questionaire (PART "A")

FIG. 6 SAR Questionnaire A & B

Subject _____ of _____ Subjects

Place Last Seen

Subject Last Seen By	Date	Time

Subject Last Seen By	Date	Time

Location / Common Name / Description

Subject's Trip Plans

Itinerary		Transportation		
Starting Location:		Transported By:		
Start Date:		Veh Location:		
Start Time:		Make / Model / Color:		
Destination:		License:		

Additional Comments
#Name?

Actions Taken So Far By Family / Friends / Others

Action Taken by Family / Friends	Action Taken By Others

Contacts Upon Reaching Civilization

Name of Person Subject Would Contact	Relationship to Contact	Contact's Phone	Who is There Now

Notes

Page 2 of 3 - SAR Questionaire (PART "A")   MI "A" 2-4-95

FIG. 6 SAR Questionnaire A & B *(continued)*

New Mexico Department of Public Safety
Search and Rescue Office

SAR Questionaire
(Part "A")

Continued - Page 3

Tracking Number

This is a Mandatory Form and MUST be filled out by a Mission Initiator (or FC if no MI available)

SAR Priority Evaluation Chart

	3 - Low Urgency	2 - Medium Urgency	1 - High Urgency
Subject Profile			
Age		☐ Other	☐ Very Young ☐ Very Old
Medical Condition	☐ Healthy ☐ Known fatality		☐ Known/suspected injured, ill, Mental Problem
Number of Subjects	☐ More then one (unless separated)		☐ One alone
Subject Experience Profile	☐ Experienced, knows area	☐ Experienced, not familiar with area ☐ Not experienced, knows area	☐ Inexperienced, does not know area
Weather Profile	☐ No hazardous weather predicted	☐ Predicted hazardous weather, (>8 hrs.) ☐ Predicted Hazardous WX , (<8 hrs.)	☐ Past and/or existing hazardous weather
Equipment Profile	☐ Adequate for environment and weather	☐ Questionable for environment and weather	☐ Inadequate for environment and weather
Terrain/Hazards Profile	☐ Few or no hazards		☐ Known terrain or other hazards

Action Taken By Mission Initiator

Assigned to Field Coordinator

FC Assigned Mission (Name)	Phone Number	Mission Number	Date	Time
* FC on Standby (Name)	Phone Number (now)	Phone Number (later)	Date	Time
* Area Commander Contacted and Briefed	Phone Number (now)	Phone Number (later)	Date	Time

CHECKED?	Time	Discription of Other Action Taken
☐ Local Landowner(s)		
☐ Local Sheriff / Police		
☐ NM State Parks and Recreation		
☐ NM Game and Fish		
☐ Nat. Park Service		
☐ USFS ☐ BLM ☐ BIA		
☐ Other		

Mission Terminated before Assigning Mission to Field Coordinator - Explain:

Sign by (Mission Initiator)	Date

* *If Field Coodinator NOT Assigned Mission - Put one on STANDBY - (Dispatch has On-Call Field Coordinator Number)*

* *You MUST Brief Area Commander if no Field Coordinator Assigned - (Dispatch has On-Call Area Commander Number)*

Page 3 of 3 MI "A" 2.5.95

FIG. 6 SAR Questionnaire A & B *(continued)*

New Mexico Department of Public Safety
Search and Rescue Office

SAR Questionaire
(Part "B")

Subject ____ of ____ Subjects
(Fill Out One (1) Form For Each Subject)

Mission Number

This Form is Mandatory and MUST be filled out by the IC or General Staff

Incident Information

Subject Name	Address	City	ST	ZIP	Phone

Physical Description

Identification		Clothing/style		Color	Health	
Skin:		Rain Wear:			Health:	
Marks:		Snow Wear:				
Eyes:		Pack:				
Style:		Hunting Vest:				

Clues

☐ Sole Sample Available ☐ Candy
☐ Scent Articles Available ☐ Gum
☐ Scent Articles Secured ☐ Smoker
☐ Clothing Visible from Air ☐ Photo

Youth / Child	Equipment		
☐ Afraid of Dark	☐ Pack	☐ Fuel	☐ Snowshoes
☐ Afraid of Animals	☐ Tent	☐ Stove	☐ Skis
☐ Afraid of Strangers	☐ Sleeping Bag	☐ Compass	☐ Money
☐ Cries when hurt	☐ Ground Cloth	☐ Map	☐ Credit Cards
☐ Cries when scared	☐ Fishing Gear	☐ Food	☐ Other Docs
☐ Hides when afraid	☐ Climbing Gear	☐ Knife	☐ Rope
☐ HUG-A-TREE trained	☐ Liquid Container	☐ Camera	☐ Camp Tools
☐ Has a safe word	☐ Fire Starter	☐ Lens	☐ Gun

Subject Traits

☐ Alcohol	☐ Hitchiker
☐ Drugs	☐ Religous
☐ A Leader	☐ Educated
☐ A Survivor	☐ Local Hero
☐ Legal Problems	☐ Extravert
☐ Personal Probs	☐ Introvert
☐ Depressed	☐ Loner

Note	Other Equipment	Other Traits or Habits

Place Last Seen

Description		Additional Comments
Subject Last Seen By:		
Talked to Subject About:		
Weather at that Time:		
Weather Since:		
Direction of Travel:		
Subject's Attitude:		
Subjects Condition:		

Subject's Trip Plans

Itinerary		Transportation		Additional Comments
By Way Of:		Loc Cfm By:		
Purpose:		Time Cfm:		
Length of Stay:		Other Vehicles:		
Size of Group:		Alternates:		
Here Before?:		Discussed With:		

OVER

FIG. 6 SAR Questionnaire A & B *(continued)*

Mission Number

SAR Questionaire (PART "B")

Subject ____ of ____ Subjects

Subject's Outdoor Experience

General Experience		Additional Comments
☐ Familiar with Area	☐ Travels Alone	
☐ In Area Recently	☐ Stays on Route	
☐ Outdoors Training	☐ Travels X-C	
☐ Medical Training	☐ Lost Before	
☐ Scouting	☐ Will Stay Put	
☐ Military	☐ Keeps on Move	
☐ Overnight	☐ Climber	
☐ Other Training	☐ Athletic	

Overdue Groups

Kind of Group:		Personality Clashes:	
Group Leader:		Actions if Separated:	
Experience of Leader:		Competitive Spirit:	
Local Point of Contact:		Intragroup Dynamics:	

Photos, Notes, Etc:

Recording Official	Phone	Recording Official	Phone

IC "B" 2/6/95

FIG. 6 SAR Questionnaire A & B *(continued)*

SEARCH INITIATION LOG	Mission Initiator	Field Coordinator

Notifying Agency	Mission Initiator Notified (Date / Time)	Field Coordinator Notified (Date / Time)

Be Sure to Get	Person Reporting Incident
☐ Names ☐ Dates / Times ☐ Address ☐ Phone Numbers ☐ Place to Contact	

Be Sure to Get	Incident Description
☐ What Happened ☐ Where ☐ When ☐ Point Last Seen ☐ Number of Subjects Involved	

Be Sure to Get	Subject Information
☐ Subject(s) Name ☐ Physical Description ☐ Address ☐ Phone Number ☐ Planned Destination	

Search?	Determined By (Factors)
☐ Yes ☐ No	

District Mission Number	Date	Time	AFRCC Mission Number	Date	Time

ICS SAR 201A NMSAR Rev. 2-15-92	Page 1	

FIG. 7 Search Initiation Log

FIRST RESPONDER INFORMATION	

Items to Consider	Base Camp
☐ Accessibility to the Area ☐ Weather ☐ 4WD Access ☐ Communications Access ☐ Support Staff ☐ ETA & Enroute Delays	

Items to Consider	Communications
☐ Propagation over Terrain ☐ Commo Resources Available ☐ Repeaters Available in Area ☐ Commo Support Base ☐ Vehicular Communications ☐ Callback Plan if Cancelled	

Items to Consider	First Responders
☐ Special Equipment Needed ☐ Routing to Scene ☐ Subject Description ☐ Death Codes ☐ Checkpoints ☐ Support Needed	

Agencies to Notify	Agency Notification
☐ AFRCC ☐ National Guard ☐ USFS (Wilderness) ☐ BLM ☐ BIA ☐ State Parks & Recreation ☐ Local Sheriff / Police ☐ Local Landowner(s)	

Other Action Taken

ICS SAR 201A NMSAR Rev. 2-15-92	Page 2	

FIG. 7 Search Initiation Log *(continued)*

INCIDENT BRIEFING		Date Prepared	Time Prepared	Mission Number

Map Sketch

Current Organization

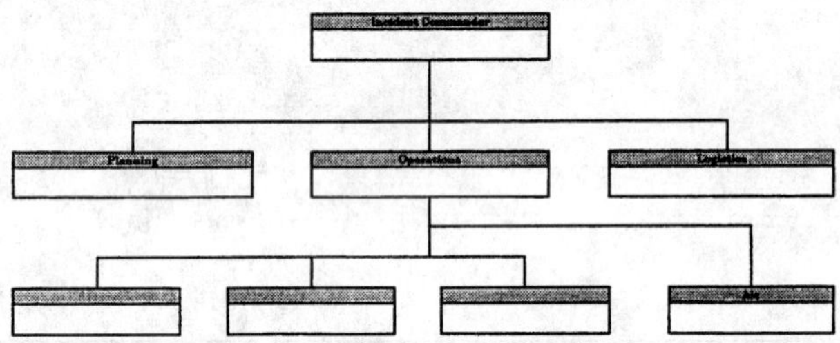

ICS 201 NMSAR Rev. 5-25-92	Page 1	Prepared By (Name and Position)

FIG. 8 Incident Briefing

Resources Summary				
Resources Ordered	Resource Name	ETA	On Scene	Location / Assignment

Summary of Current Actions

ICS 201 NMSAR Rev. 4-15-92	Page 2	

FIG. 8 Incident Briefing *(continued)*

INCIDENT OBJECTIVES		Date Prepared	Time Prepared	Mission Number
From: (Date)	From: (Time)	To: (Date)	To: (Time)	Operational Period

Objectives for Incident (Include Alternatives)

Weather Forecast for Operational Period

General Safety Message

Attachments (to Complete Incident Action Plan)		
☐ Organization Assignment List (ICS 203)	☐ Radio Communications Plan (ICS 205)	☐ ________
☐ Incident Map	☐ Traffic Plan (Internal & External)	☐ ________
☐ Task Assignment Forms (ICS SAR 204A)	☐ Medical Plan (ICS 206)	☐ ________

ICS 202	Prepared By (Planning Section Chief)	Approved By (Incident Commander)
NMSAR Rev. 5-25-92		

FIG. 9 Incident Objectives

ORGANIZATION ASSIGNMENT LIST	Date Prepared	Time Prepared	Mission Number	Operational Period

Incident Commander and Staff
Incident Commander:
Deputy:
Safety Officer:
Information Officer:
Liaison Officer:

Agency Representatives

Agency	Name

Planning Section
Chief:
Deputy:
Resources Unit:
Situation Unit:
Documentation Unit:
Demobilization Unit:
Technical Specialists:

Logistics Section
Chief:
Deputy

Support Branch
Director:
Supply Unit:
Facilities Unit:
Ground Support Unit:

Service Branch
Director:
Communications Unit:
Medical Unit:
Food Unit:

Operations Section
Chief:
Deputy

Branch I Division / Groups
Branch Director:
Deputy:
Division / Group:
Division / Group:
Division / Group:
Division / Group:
Division / Group:

Branch II Division / Groups
Director:
Deputy:
Division / Group:
Division / Group:
Division / Group:
Division / Group:
Division / Group:

Branch III Division / Groups
Branch Director:
Deputy:
Division / Group:
Division / Group:
Division / Group:
Division / Group:
Division / Group:

Air Operations Branch
Air Operations Director:
Air Ops. Supervisor:
Air Support Supervisor:

Finance Section
Chief:
Deputy:
Time Unit:
Procurement Unit:
Compensation / Claims:
Cost Unit:

ICS 203 NMSAR Rev. 5-25-92		Prepared By (Resources Unit)

FIG. 10 Organization Assignment List

TASK ASSIGNMENT	Team Name	Callsign	
		Mission Number	Operational Period

Planning Section

Type of Team	Name (Leader First)	Resource Name	Skill / Equipment	Briefing Summary
☐ Dog Team ☐ Hasty Team	1			☐ Overview ☐ Weather
☐ Foot Team ☐ Tracking Team	2			☐ Clues ☐ Subject Profile
☐ Grid Team ☐ Vehicle Team	3			☐ Time Frame ☐ Org. Chart
☐ Horse Team ☐ Mixed	4			☐ Family ☐ Media
☐ Fixed Wing A/C ☐ Helicopter	5			☐ Subject Info. ☐
☐ Boat / Amphib. ☐ Technical Rock	6			
☐ Communications ☐	7			

Operations Section

Assigment Date	Estimated Departure Time	Actual Departure Time	Estimated Time in Segment

Radio Frequency	Briefed By	Reviewed By

Resource Assignment & Map
Briefing Summary ☐ Tactics ☐ Terrain ☐ Maps ☐ Communications ☐ Rescue Plan ☐ Death Code ☐ Desired POD ______ % ☐ Pickup Time ☐ Safety ☐

ICS SAR 204A NMSAR Rev. 5-25-92	Page 1	

FIG. 11 Task Assignment

DEBRIEFING	Debriefed By		Mission Number	Operational Period
	Date Returned	Time Returned	Actual Time in Segment	

Explain What Your Team Actually Did

Estimate of PODs Responsive ______ % Not Responsive _____ %	Describe the Location of Any Clues Discovered

Current Status of These Clues

Describe Difficulties or Gaps in Coverage

Describe Any Hazards in Search Area

Suggestions, Ideas, Recommendations

ICS SAR 204A NMSAR Rev. 5-25-92	Page 2	

FIG. 11 Task Assignment *(continued)*

RADIO COMMUNICATIONS PLAN		Date Prepared	Time Prepared	Mission Number	Operational Period

Radio Channel Utilization

System	Channel	Function	Frequency	Assignment	Remarks

ICS 205 NMSAR Rev. 5-25-92		Prepared By (Communications Unit)

FIG. 12 Radio Communications Plan

MEDICAL PLAN	Date Prepared	Time Prepared	Mission Number	Operational Period

Incident Medical Stations

Medical Aid Stations	Location	Paramedics Yes	Paramedics No

Transporatation
Ambulance Services

Name	Address	Phone	Paramedics Yes	Paramedics No

Incident Ambulances

Name	Location	Paramedics Yes	Paramedics No

Hospitals

Name	Address	Travel Time Air	Travel Time Gnd	Phone	Helipad Yes	Helipad No	Burn Center Yes	Burn Center No

Medical Emergency Procedures

ICS 206 NMSAR Rev. 5-25-92	Prepared By (Medical Unit Leader)	Reviewed By (Safety Officer)

FIG. 13 Medical Plan

INCIDENT ORGANIZATION CHART	

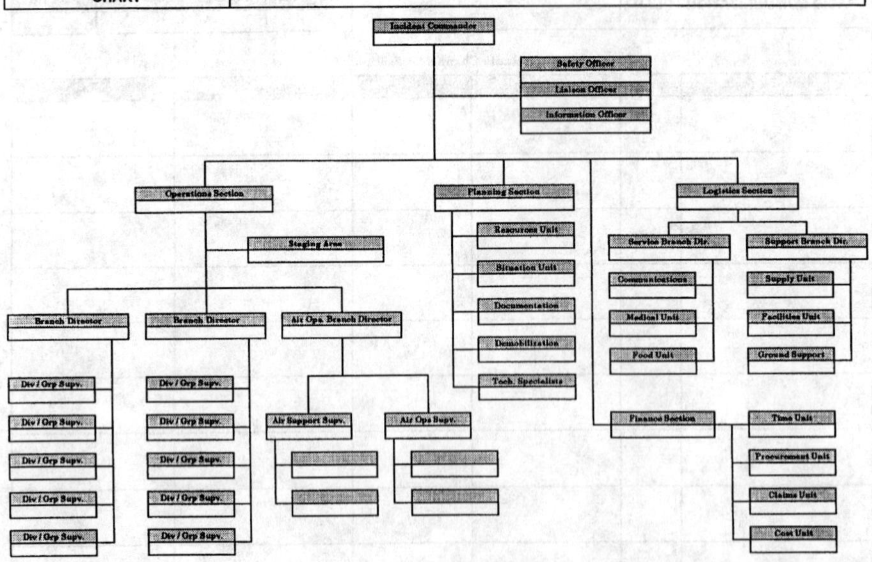

ICS 207 NMSAR Rev. 5-25-92		Mission Number	Operational Period	Prepared By

FIG. 14 Incident Organization Chart

INCIDENT STATUS SUMMARY	Period Covered by this Report	
	From (Date / Time)	To (Date / Time)
	Incident Name / Number	
	Incident Commander	
	Print:	
Future Considerations	Signature:	

Probable Leads That Require Checking

Proposed Overall Course Of Action

Weather Forecast For Next 24 Hours

Additional Comments

Resources Available Now

Team Name	Type of Resource	# of Personnel	Remarks

ICS 209 Rev. 7-12-92		Page 1

FIG. 15 Incident Status Summary

Resources Alerted for Use at a Later Time

Team Name	Type of Resource	# of Personnel	Remarks

Resources Used This Operational Period

Team Name	Type of Resource	# of Personnel	# of Hours
	Totals This Operational Period		

Totals for Other Types of Resources Used

Type of Resource	# of Hours	Type of Resource	# of Hours
		Total Used	

ICS 209 Rev. 7-12-92		Page 2

FIG. 15 Incident Status Summary *(continued)*

CHECK-IN LIST	Incident Name/Number:	CHECK-IN LOCATION ☐ BASE ☐ CAMP ☐ STAGING AREA ☐ HELIBASE	DATE:

	Single or Team (S/T)	Name (Print) (Check Box if NOT a SAR Volunteer)	Date/Time Check-in	Team Name Leader's Name	Home Base	Method of Travel	Availability & Other Qualifications	Date/Time Check-out	Hrs. (Nearest) 30 mins.
1		N.V. ☐					Will Stay ___ hrs. ☐ EMT ☐ FC		
2		N.V. ☐					Will Stay ___ hrs. ☐ EMT ☐ FC		
3		N.V. ☐					Will Stay ___ hrs. ☐ EMT ☐ FC		
4		N.V. ☐					Will Stay ___ hrs. ☐ EMT ☐ FC		
5		N.V. ☐					Will Stay ___ hrs. ☐ EMT ☐ FC		
6		N.V. ☐					Will Stay ___ hrs. ☐ EMT ☐ FC		
7		N.V. ☐					Will Stay ___ hrs. ☐ EMT ☐ FC		
8		N.V. ☐					Will Stay ___ hrs. ☐ EMT ☐ FC		
9		N.V. ☐					Will Stay ___ hrs. ☐ EMT ☐ FC		
10		N.V. ☐					Will Stay ___ hrs. ☐ EMT ☐ FC		
11		N.V. ☐					Will Stay ___ hrs. ☐ EMT ☐ FC		
12		N.V. ☐					Will Stay ___ hrs. ☐ EMT ☐ FC		

ICS 211A	Resources Unit:	Page _____ of _____	Total Hours (Volunteers only)	

Rev. 4-12-94

FIG. 16 Check-in List

SAR: CHECK-IN LIST (ICS FORM 211A)

Purpose. The Check-in List is used to keep track of all individuals that are participating on the incident. Personnel arriving at the incident can check in at various locations. Check-in consists of reporting specific information which is recorded on the check-in list. The check-in list is used for recording arrival and departure times for all incident personnel. Completion of this form is crucial for liability and insurance purposes. Information furnished on the standard Check-in List ~~(ICS Form 211)~~ is not satisfactory for SAR administrative purposes.

Preparation. The check-in list can be initiated at a number of locations including:

1. Staging areas, base, camps, helibase, and ICP. Managers at these locations record information and give it to the resources unit as soon as possible.

2. Communications unit radio operators located at communications center should record check-in information and forward it to the resources unit as soon as possible.

3. Check in at ICP should be done by a recorder from the resources unit.

Distribution. Check-in lists, which are completed by personnel at the various check-in locations, should be furnished by the resources unit. The resources unit maintains a master list of equipment and personnel that have reported to the incident.

ITEM TITLE - INSTRUCTIONS

***NOTE:** - Incident dispatchers, upon receipt of a check-in message by radio, record the information on the Check-in list and forward the information to the resources unit.

Incident Name/Number. Enter the SAR mission number assigned to this incident.

Check-in Location. Enter the location where this check-in list is being used. Space is provided for base, camp, staging area, or helibase.

Date. Enter the current date (month, day, year).

Single or Team. Enter S if this is a single resource, or T if a member of a team.

Name. Please print name. Everyone who is associated with this incident MUST CHECK IN! Check box if person is not a volunteer (such as paid emergency response or law enforcement personnel). Incident Commander and Staff must account for all who check in.

Date/Time. Enter the date and time that resource arrived on-scene. Do not include travel time from home base.

Team Name/Leader's Name. Enter the team name and team leader (for each entry).

Home Base. Enter the city for the team (should agree with SAR resource directory).

Method of Travel. Enter the transportation (bus, car, horse, foot) used by resource to arrive at scene.

Availability & Other Qualifications. Enter the approximate length of time resource is available for this incident. Leave blank for duration. Time is used only for planning purposes. The resource is not held to this number. Check the box if resource is a certified EMT, Paramedic, or Physician. Check the box if resource is a certified FC. Enter other specialty qualifications (such as ICS Staff, Technical Specialist, OMI, etc.) if resource has additional expertise that can by utilized, if needed.

Date/Time Check-out. Enter the date and time resource left the scene. Do not include travel time back to home base.

Hours. Enter the total hours rounded to nearest thirty (30) minutes. Show volunteer hours ONLY.

Resources Unit. Enter the name of the individual assigned by the Resources unit to record and maintain this check-in list.

Page Count. Enter the page number. At the end of the mission, enter the total number of pages submitted.

Total Hours. Enter the page total. Be sure hours listed are for volunteers ONLY.

FIG. 16 Check-in List *(continued)*

UNIT LOG

Mission Number	Operational Period	
		of

Unit Name/ Designator	Unit Leader	

Time	Activity / Event

ICS 214 NMSAR Rev. 5-25-92

Page 1

FIG. 17 Unit Log

Time	Activity / Event

ICS 214 Rev. 7-12-92

Page 2

FIG. 17 Unit Log *(continued)*

OPERATIONAL PLANNING WORK SHEET										Mission Number	Operational Period
Division Group or Other Location	Work Assignments		Resources by Type						Other	Reporting Location	Req. Arr. Time
		Req									
		Have									
		Need									
		Req									
		Have									
		Need									
		Req									
		Have									
		Need									
		Req									
		Have									
		Need									
		Req									
		Have									
		Need									
		Req									
		Have									
		Need									
		Req									
		Have									
		Need									
		Req									
		Have									
		Need									
		Req									
		Have									
		Need									
		Req									
		Have									
		Need									
		Req									
		Have									
		Need									
		Req									
		Have									
		Need									
		Req									
		Have									
		Need									
		Req									
		Have									
		Need									
		Req									
		Have									
		Need									
		Req									
		Have									
		Need									
ICS 215 NMSAR Rev. 5-25-92	Total Resources Required									Prepared By	
	Total Resources On Hand										
	Total Resources Needed										

FIG. 18 Operational Planning Worksheet

New Mexico Department of Public Safety
Search and Rescue Office

SAR Injury Report

Incident Number

This is a Mandatory Form and IF filled out MUST be done by a EMS provider and filed with Incident Report

Time Reported Lost / Injured	Time Patient Treated	Last Name	First Name	MI	Phone

Address	City	ST	ZIP	Sex	Age	Birthdate

Location of Incident

Resident Status
- ☐ Local ☐ State
- ☐ County ☐ Out of State

Primary Category - Code
- ☐ trauma ____
- ☐ cardiac ____
- ☐ burn ____
- ☐ ped/ob ____
- ☐ medical ____
- ☐ head / spinel ____
- ☐ poison ____
- ☐ behavioral ____

Severity
- ☐ MAJOR * LEVEL I
- ☐ MAJOR * LEVEL II
- ☐ MAJOR * LEVEL III

Prehospital Care Summary
- ☐ extrication
- ______ EST. MIN.
- ☐ assessment
- ☐ airway management
- ☐ oxygen
- ☐ pocket mask
- ☐ nasal / oral airway
- ☐ bag valve mask
- ☐ demand valve
- ☐ CPR
- ☐ control of bleeding
- ☐ wound care

- ☐ **BLS**
- ☐ spinal immobilzation
- ☐ limb splinting
- ☐ MAST
- ☐ OB delivery
- ☐ Other: (narrative)

- ☐ **IV level**
- ☐ IV
- ☐ EOA
- ☐ D 50 W
- ☐ Naloxone (Narcan)
- ☐ Blood sample
- ☐ other: (narrative

Disposition
- ☐ treatment not needed
- ☐ treatment refused
- ☐ transport refused
- ☐ transport not needed
- ☐ canceled
- ☐ false alarm
- ☐ trasported by POV
- ☐ other service trasport by

Name

Other Service Number

- ☐ Transported to

Facility

City

Destination Code

- ☐ dead at scene

Time				
Level of Consciousness (circle one)	A V P U	A V P U	A V P U	A V P U
Respiration				
Pulse Rate / Rhythm				
Blood Pressure	/	/	/	/

Medications:	Glascow Coma total
Alergies	Trauma Score Total

Narrative

Physican	Witness

Report Filled Out By	Date

See back side of this form if Patient refuses medical services.

SAR EMS 2/10/95

FIG. 19 SAR Injury Report

New Mexico Department of Public Safety, State Police Division
Search and Rescue Office
PO Box 1628
Santa Fe, New Mexico 87504

Liability Release

Date____________________ SAR Incident Number____________________
Location____________________ Incident Commander____________________

1. **REFUSAL OF CARE AGAINST MEDICAL ADVISE**
I have been informed that I have a potentially serious medical condition requiring assessment, treatment and transportation to a hospital. Of my own free will, without coercion or influence, I hereby REFUSE the care offered to me by the **New Mexico Department of Public Safety, State Police Division SAR Incident Commander** against the advice of attending personnel and their medical control physician. I understand that by my refusal I risk further illness, injury, disability or death. In the event that I later choose to accept treatment or transportation, I will call for emergency response.
INITIAL HERE ____________

2. **NON AMBULANCE TRANSPORT**
I have been assessed and treated as necessary by the personnel responding from the **New Mexico Department of Public Safety, State Police Division**. I will arrange condition promptly. I have been informed of signs and symptoms which could indicate that my condition is deteriorating. If I develop and additional signs or symptoms, or have any concerns about my health or safety, I will call for emergency response.
INITIAL HERE ____________

3. **NON - PATIENT**
I have no complaint, illness or injury and I do not consider myself to be a patient. If I develop any signs or symptoms, or if I have any concern about my health or safety, I will call my physician promptly or I will call for emergency response.
INITIAL HERE ____________

I have read and understand section ________ above. My condition has been explained to me and I have no questions. I knowingly and voluntarily release the **New Mexico Department of Public Safety, State Police Division** the ELMS director, the staff and physicians of the hospital having medical control from any liability for my decision regarding my medical care.

Patient Name and Signature ____________________ Date ____________

Address ____________ City ____________ State ____ ZIP ____

Date of Birth ________ Phone ________ Translator/Parent/Guardian ____________

EMS PROVIDER: This patient has indicated comprehension of the content and meaning of this form.
This patient is alert and oriented.

Name ____________ Signature ____________ Date/Time ________

Name ____________ Signature ____________ Date/Time ________

Name ____________ Signature ____________ Date/Time ________

FIG. 20 Liability Release

EMERGENCY HELICOPTER REQUEST INFORMATION SHEET

DATE: ________ TIME: ________ MISSION NO. ________ AFRCC NO.________

NAME OF REQUESTOR: ____________________ TITLE: ____________

AGENCY: ____________ CITY: ____________ PHONE: ________

FIELD COORDINATOR: ____________ BASE CAMP SITE: ____________

EMERGENCY & REASON FOR REQUEST (serious threat to life, transport searchers, etc)

____

____

TYPE OF ASSISTANCE NEEDED IN ADDITION TO HELICOPTER (medical personnel, rescue, gear, etc.)

____

NUMBER & NAMES OF PERSONS IN INCIDENT:____________________

____

EXTENT OF INJURIES & CONDITION, IF KNOWN:____________________

____

ESTIMATE WEIGHT OF PERSONS & EQUIPMENT BOARDING: ____________

NUMBER BOARDING: ________ TYPE OF EQUIPMENT BOARDING: ____________

____

OTHER PERSONS AT INCIDENT SITE: ____________________

____

WILL THEY NEED AIRLIFT OUT: ________ OTHER INFORMATION: ____________

____

LOCATION OF INCIDENT SITE. COORDINATES AND/OR ANY OTHER MEANS OF LOCATING THE AREA:

____

ARE PYROTECHNICS AVAILABLE AT SITE OR BASE: ____________

ELEVATION OF SITE/LANDING ZONE (LZ) ABOVE SEA LEVEL: ____________

IS SUITABLE LZ NEAR INCIDENT SITE? IF SO, HOW FAR AWAY, DESCRIBE TERRAIN, DEGREE OF SLOPE
TYPE OF SURFACT (snow, dirt, etc.) SIZE OF AREA: ____________

____

____

FIG. 21 Emergency Helicopter Landing Request Information Sheet

PAGE TWO

IF NO LZ NEARBY, CAN SUBJECTS BE HOISTED OUT SAFELY: __________ HAVE PEOPLE AT SITE WORKED WITH PENETRATORS: __________ HAVE PEOPLE AT SITE WORKED WITH HELICOPTERS: __________

DESCRIBE HAZARDS IN INCIDENT/LZ AREA (trees, power lines, cliffs, etc.): __________

WEATHER AT LZ: WIND DIRECTION & VELOCITY: __________

CLOUD COVER: __________ HEIGHT OF CLOUDS ABOVE GROUND AND/OR PEAKS: __________

VISIBILITY: __________ CURRENT PRECIPITATION: __________

APPROXIMATE TEMPERATURE __________ °F SNOW DEPTH: __________

WEATHER CONDITIONS IN DELIVERY AREA: __________

24-HOUR WEATHER FORECAST: __________

WHERE ARE SUBJECTS TO BE TRANSPORTED (hospital, base camp, etc.; if not closest hospital, why not): __________

HOW WILL LANDING AREA BE MARKED: (panels, pyrotechnics, mirrors, strobes, etc.): __________

ARE EMERGENCY MEDICAL PERSONNEL AT THE INCIDENT SITE: __________; IF NOT, WILL THEY BE THERE BY THE TIME HELICOPTER ARRIVES: __________ WILL EMERGENCY CARE PERSONNEL BE AT THE DELIVERY SITE TO RECEIVE PATIENTS: __________.

DETAILS OF ALTERNATE LZ (location and similar information as above): __________

RADIO COMMUNICATIONS ON THE GROUND (frequencies and call signs): __________

EN ROUTE RENDEZVOUS POINT WITH OTHER SAR PERSONNEL: __________

REQUESTED ETA AT INCIDENT SITE/LZ: __________

OTHER INFORMATION: __________

FIG. 21 Emergency Helicopter Landing Request Information Sheet *(continued)*

Mission Number:	
Time Period:	

ICS Planning Guide

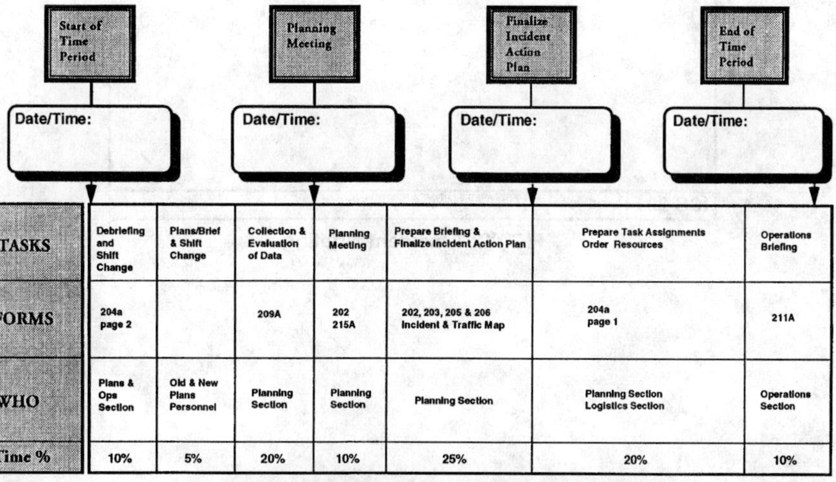

TASKS	Debriefing and Shift Change	Plans/Brief & Shift Change	Collection & Evaluation of Data	Planning Meeting	Prepare Briefing & Finalize Incident Action Plan	Prepare Task Assignments Order Resources	Operations Briefing
FORMS	204a page 2		209A	202 215A	202, 203, 205 & 206 Incident & Traffic Map	204a page 1	211A
WHO	Plans & Ops Section	Old & New Plans Personnel	Planning Section	Planning Section	Planning Section	Planning Section Logistics Section	Operations Section
Time %	10%	5%	20%	10%	25%	20%	10%

Time Period Planning Chart

FIG. 22 ICS Planning Guide

APPENDIXES

(Nonmandatory Information)

X1. EXISTING ICS FORMS

X1.1 See existing ICS Forms. Forms are not included in this appendix.

X2. ICS FORMS MODIFIED FOR SAR

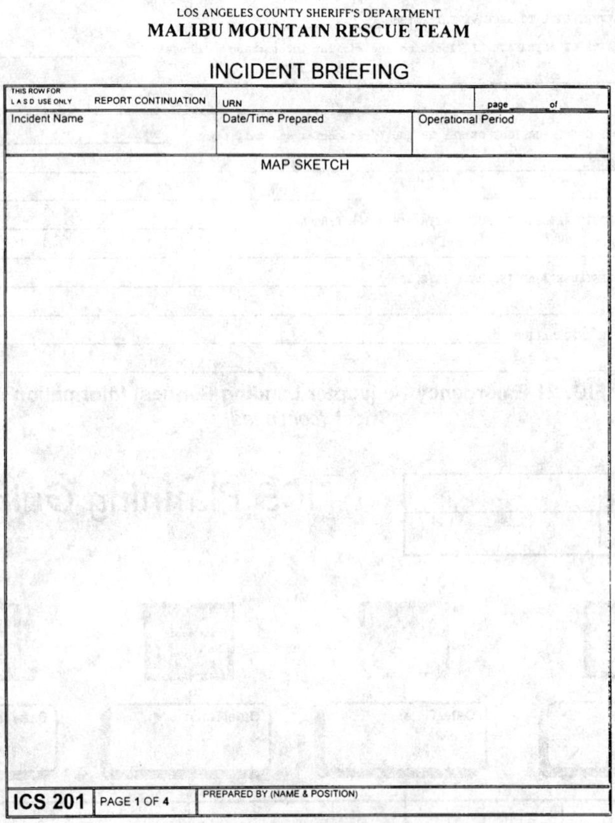
LOS ANGELES COUNTY SHERIFF'S DEPARTMENT

MALIBU MOUNTAIN RESCUE TEAM

INCIDENT BRIEFING

THIS ROW FOR L A S D USE ONLY REPORT CONTINUATION	URN		page ____ of ____
Incident Name	Date/Time Prepared	Operational Period	

MAP SKETCH

ICS 201	PAGE 1 OF 4	PREPARED BY (NAME & POSITION)

FIG. X2.1 Incident Briefing

LOS ANGELES COUNTY SHERIFF'S DEPARTMENT

MALIBU MOUNTAIN RESCUE TEAM

INCIDENT BRIEFING

THIS ROW FOR L.A.S.D. USE ONLY REPORT CONTINUATION	URN		page ___ of ___
Incident Name	Date/Time Prepared	Operational Period	

SUMMARY OF CURRENT ACTIONS

ICS 201 PAGE 2 OF 4

FIG. X2.1 Incident Briefing *(continued)*

LOS ANGELES COUNTY SHERIFF'S DEPARTMENT

MALIBU MOUNTAIN RESCUE TEAM

INCIDENT BRIEFING

THIS ROW FOR L.A.S.D. USE ONLY REPORT CONTINUATION	URN		page ___ of ___
Incident Name	Date/Time Prepared	Operational Period	

CURRENT ORGANIZATION

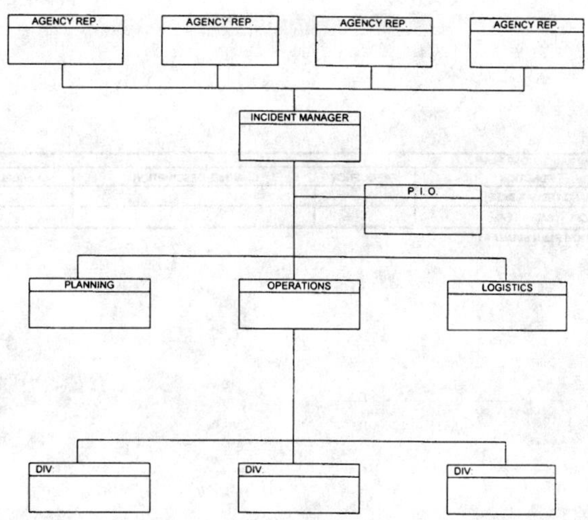

ICS 201 PAGE 3 OF 4

FIG. X2.1 Incident Briefing *(continued)*

LOS ANGELES COUNTY SHERIFF'S DEPARTMENT
MALIBU MOUNTAIN RESCUE TEAM

INCIDENT BRIEFING

THIS ROW FOR L.A.S.D. USE ONLY REPORT CONTINUATION	URN	page of
Incident Name	Date/Time Prepared	Operational Period

RESOURCES SUMMARY

RESOURCES ORDERED	RESOURCE IDENTIFICATION	E.T.A.	TIME ON SCENE	LOCATION / ASSIGNMENT

ICS 201 PAGE 4 OF 4

FIG. X2.1 Incident Briefing *(continued)*

GENERAL BRIEFING	1. INCIDENT NAME	2. OPERATIONAL PERIOD	3. INCIDENT NUMBER

4. INCIDENT SUMMARY

5. COMMUNICATIONS PLAN

FUNCTION	FREQUENCY	CHANNEL DESCRIPTION	CHANNEL
COMMAND (TEAM -- BASE)			
TACTICAL (TEAM -- TEAM)			

6. ACTION PLAN SUMMARY

SAR 100 BASARC 1/96	7. PREPARED BY	8. DATE PREPARED	9. TIME PREPARED

FIG. X2.2 General Briefing

GENERAL BRIEFING MISSING PERSON	1. INCIDENT NAME	2. OPERATIONAL PERIOD	3. INCIDENT NUMBER

4. INCIDENT SUMMARY

5. COMMUNICATIONS PLAN

FUNCTION	FREQUENCY	CHANNEL DESCRIPTION	CHANNEL
COMMAND (TEAM – BASE)			
TACTICAL (TEAM – TEAM)			

SUBJECT INFORMATION

6. NAME	7. SEX	8. AGE

9. NAME TO CALL	10. EXPECTED RESPONSE

11. SUBJECT'S PLANS OR INTENT

12. PHYSICAL DESCRIPTION	15. PHOTO
HEIGHT WEIGHT BUILD	
RACE COMPLEXION	
EYES HAIR	
13. CLOTHING DESCRIPTION	
14. FOOTWARE/TRACK DESCRIPTION	
SIZE	

SAR 100A BASARC 1/96	16. PREPARED BY	17. DATE PREPARED	18. TIME PREPARED

FIG. X2.3 General Briefing—Missing Person with Instruction Sheets

SAR 100A -- General Briefing -- Missing Person (1/96)

Overview

The General Briefing Form is intended to provide searchers with background information related to the incident. The form contains information that is not specific to any given assignment. This allows the form to be filled out once and photocopied. The intent is to reduce unnecessary duplication of information on Team Assignment Forms. The General Briefing Form should be included with each Team Assignment Form.

If more than one individual is missing, complete additional Subject Information portions of the General Briefing Form.

Instructions for Completing Form

1. Incident Name
The incident name should be established early in the operation. Be consistent and don't use several names, or change names in the middle. Good names often include either the last name of the subject ie. "Smith Search" or the name of the search location i.e. "Jones Gulch Search".

2. Operational Period
This is where the date goes. But it's more than just a date. An operational period has a beginning and an ending date and time. But the ending time may not be known at the time the forms is being filled out. It may be most useful to use the date followed by a word or two describing the time of day or phase of the search. For example

1/14/96 Initial Response	1/14/96 Night
1/15/96 Day 1	1/15/96 Daytime

1/14/96 2200 to 1/15/96 0600

3. Incident Number
The incident numbers assigned by the local responsible agency or a larger coordinating agency. Typically incident numbers are the last two digits of the year followed by a sequential number. If both the local agency and a larger coordinating entity have issued numbers, list them both, indicating who issued each number.

4. Incident Summary
After reading this short narrative, a searcher should have a good overview of the incident. Information in the summary may duplicate some of the subject information found later on the form. That's ok.

5. Communications Plan
For most small to medium sized operations it is sufficient to assign a single command (search base to teams) radio frequency along with a single tactical (team to team) radio frequency. If your incident requires more than this, refer readers to a more complete communications plan. There is space on the Team Assignment form for team specific communication plans.

It's important to note the frequency of the radio net. Different agencies may use different names and channel assignments.

The Channel Description can be used for the "Name" of the radio net. Sufficient room is provided to also include info about repeater offsets, and tone if required.

Remember the Channel number may be different on radios outside of your own agency, so use the space

FIG. X2.3 General Briefing—Missing Person with Instruction Sheets *(continued)*

with caution on a multiple agency operation.

6. Name
Name of the missing subject.

7. Sex
Sex of the missing subject.

8. Age
Age of the missing subject. Searchers don't need a precise age if one is not know, nor is the date of birth important to a ground searcher.

9. Name to Call
This is the name the searchers will call out, and listen for a response. It's usually a first name or nickname. For small children this would be a good place to also note their "safety word" if they have one.

10. Expected Response
How is the subject expected to respond to voice contact. Young children may be frightened by strangers or may have been taught not to talk to strangers. Older subjects may not respond to their name due to a number of conditions from poor hearing to alzhiemiers. When a subject has been missing for an extended period of time, the likelihood of their being responsive decreases.

11. Subject's Plans or Intent
A brief discussion of what the subject's intended to do. If known, mention the intended activity, as well as the planned location or route of travel.

12. Physical Description
This field contains the normal set of physical description information. Remember the level of detail required by searchers is typically less that of a police officer. A searcher is trying to identify a missing person in an area were there typically are not very many other people.This is opposed to the law enforcement need to pick a criminal out from a crowd.

13. Clothing Description
The clothing and equipment description helps the ground searcher in four ways. The colors of clothing will determine how visible the subject is in brush and trees. Knowing how the subject was equipped will help searchers think about what they may have done to survive the elements. When an Item of clothing or gear is found that matches this description it immediately becomes an important clue. Finally it helps identify the subject. Often the clothing descriptions provided by friends and family of the subject have proved to be incorrect. Searchers should not treat this description as absolute.

14. Footwear/Track Description
The tracks that a subject leaves are of such importance that there is a sperate space to describe them. If known, you should supply shoe size, track measurements of length, width at heal, and width at ball. In addition a short description of the sole or track. If one is available, a sperate picture should be provided to the searchers.

15. Photo
Remember that the photo selected for this space will be reproduced with a photocopier. Selecting a photo with good contrast and little background clutter will produce better results.

16. Prepared By
Knowing who prepared a form allows questions about the information to asked of the correct person.

FIG. X2.3 General Briefing—Missing Person with Instruction Sheets *(continued)*

17. Date Prepared
The date and time a form is completed allows users of the information to know how current it is. In addition it helps establish the chronology of events when the search paperwork is being examined after the face.

18. Time Prepared
See Date Prepared.

Notes

The Subject Information portion of this form is focused on the needs of a ground searcher. The Physical Description portion is not the full "Law Enforcement" set, but rather enough that a field searcher can identify the missing individual.

There is not a specific section of this form devoted to hazards and safety issues that are expected in the field. Most of the hazards I've seen noted before seemed obvious one that searchers should be expected to anticipate, such as heat, cold, cliffs, etc. It may be that we will find it necessary to add a second page to the form to deal with safety related issues. For now, don't hesitate to add hazard and safety information whenever they are not readily apparent to searchers.

Field 11. Subject's Plans or Intent may need to be bigger.

FIG. X2.3 General Briefing—Missing Person with Instruction Sheets *(continued)*

FEMA US&R RESPONSE SYSTEM
INCIDENT SUPPORT TEAM

DAILY BRIEFING	INCIDENT	OPERATIONAL PERIOD DATE TIMES	REPORTING UNIT ESF-9	FORM US&R—003 2/95

- MANAGEMENT COORDINATION
  - General Incident Objectives
  - Strategic Planning
- OPERATIONS/PLANNING
  - Accomplishments/Current Assessment
  - Personnel Status
  - Tactical Assignments
  - Safety/Health/Medical
  - Weather
  - Debriefing
- LOGISTICS
  - Comm Assignments/Freq.
  - Ordering Supplies/Support Facilities
  - Transportation
- MEDIA
  - Coverage/Field Involvement
- LIAISON
  - Assisting/Cooperating Agencies
- ADMIN/FINANCE
  - Accountability/Cost Issues
- DEMOBILIZATION
- ADDITIONAL COMMENTS

IST LEADER DATE TIME	DISTRIBUTION:

FIG. X2.4 Daily Briefing

FEMA US&R RESPONSE SYSTEM
INCIDENT SUPPORT TEAM

SHIFT BRIEFING FORMAT	INCIDENT	REPORTING UNIT ESF-9	FORM US&R—XXX 2/95
DISASTER #:	OPS PERIOD:	DATE/TIME PREPARED	UNIT LEADER

ACTION	RESPONSIBILITY
■ State strategic objectives	IST Leader
■ Update present incident situation	IST Operations Section Chief
■ Incident projection for the operational period	IST Planning Section Manager
■ Specific assignments	IST Operations Section Chief
■ Safety message	IST Safety Officer
■ Communications plan and other logistical issues	IST Logistics Section Chief
■ Questions and concerns	IST Leader

PREPARED BY	APPROVED BY	DATE

FIG. X2.5 Shift Briefing Format

Pennsylvania Search and Rescue Council

Incident Objectives

Incident Form 2 of 5

Incident Name:	Operational Period (Date/Time):	Date/Time Prepared:
Objectives — General Objectives for Incident:		
Weather — Weather Forecast for Operational Period:		
Safety — General or Safety Messages:		
List any Attachments:		
Prepared by (Plans Section Chief):	Approved by (Incident Commander):	
3/2/92	(similar to ICS 202)	Page 1 of 1

FIG. X2.6 Incident Objectives

New York State Department of Environmental Conservation
Forest Rangers
ORGANIZATION ASSIGNMENT LIST

INCIDENT COMMANDER AND STAFF	
Incident Commander	
Deputy	
Safety Officer	
Information Officer	
Liasion Officer	
AGENCY REPRESENTATIVES	
AGENCY	NAME
PLANNING SECTION	
Chief	
Deputy	
Restat Unit	
Sitstat Unit	
Documentation Unit	
Demobilization Unit	
Investigation	
TECHNICAL SPECIALISTS	
LOGISTICS SECTION	
Chief	
Deputy	
Support Branch	
Director	
Supply Unit	
Facilities Unit	
Ground Support Unit	
Service Branch	
Director	
Communications Unit	
Medical/Evac Unit	
Food Unit	
	Prepared by: (Resources Unit)
NYSAR 203 4/96	

Incident Name	Date Prepared	Time Prepared
Operational Period (date/time)		
OPERATIONS SECTION		
Chief		
Deputy		
Div. Supervisor A		
Crew Boss #		
Crew Boss #		
Crew Boss #		
Crew Boss #		
Div. Supervisor B		
Deputy		
Crew Boss #		
Crew Boss #		
Crew Boss #		
Crew Boss #		
Div. Supervisor C		
Deputy		
Crew Boss #		
Crew Boss #		
Crew Boss #		
Crew Boss #		
Air Operations Branch		
Air Ops Director		
Staging Area Manager		
FINANCE/ADMINISTRATION SECTION		
Chief		
Deputy		
Time Unit		
Procurement Unit		
Compensation/Claims Unit		
Cost Unit		

FIG. X2.7 Organizational Assignment List

Pennsylvania Search and Rescue Council	Task Assignment Form				
Task No.:	Team ID:	Team Type:	Date/ Time Out:	Task Assigned Base☐ Radio☐	Dispatcher:

Assignment

Task Map:	(Division):
Task Instructions:	
Transportation Instructions:	Special Equipment:

Personnel

Field Team Leader:	FTM:
Asst. FTL:	FTM:
Field Team Member:	FTM:
FTM:	**Medic:**
FTM:	**Radio Op:**
FTM:	**Rescue Spec:**

Commo

Team Callsign:	Channel/ Freq:	Base Callsign:	Channel/ Freq:
Phone Numbers:			
Instructions:			

3/2/92	**Debrief Information on Back**	Page 1 of 2

FIG. X2.8 Task Assignment

Task Assignment Form

Debriefing

Date/ Time In:	Debriefing Officer:	*(Vehicle Miles):*
Debriefing:		

3/2/92	Page 2 of 2

FIG. X2.8 Task Assignment *(continued)*

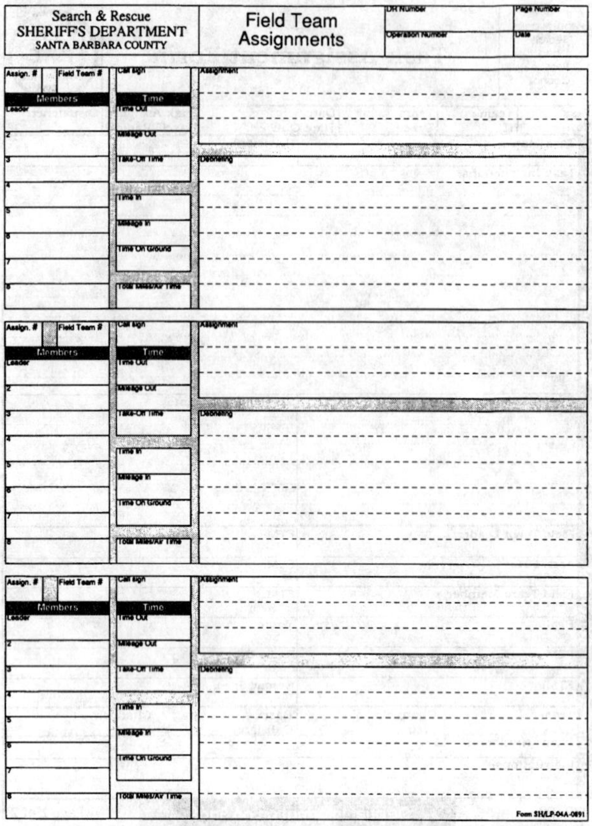
Search & Rescue
SHERIFF'S DEPARTMENT
SANTA BARBARA COUNTY

Field Team Assignments

DR Number | Page Number
Operation Number | Date

Assign. # | Field Team # | Call sign | Assignment
Members | Time
Leader | Time Out
2 | Mileage Out
3 | Take-Off Time | Debriefing
4 | Time In
5 | Mileage In
6 | Time On Ground
7
8 | Total Miles/Air Time

Assign. # | Field Team # | Call sign | Assignment
Members | Time
Leader | Time Out
2 | Mileage Out
3 | Take-Off Time | Debriefing
4 | Time In
5 | Mileage In
6 | Time On Ground
7
8 | Total Miles/Air Time

Assign. # | Field Team # | Call sign | Assignment
Members | Time
Leader | Time Out
2 | Mileage Out
3 | Take-Off Time | Debriefing
4 | Time In
5 | Mileage In
6 | Time On Ground
7
8 | Total Miles/Air Time

Form SH/LP-04A-0891

FIG. X2.9 Field Team Assignments

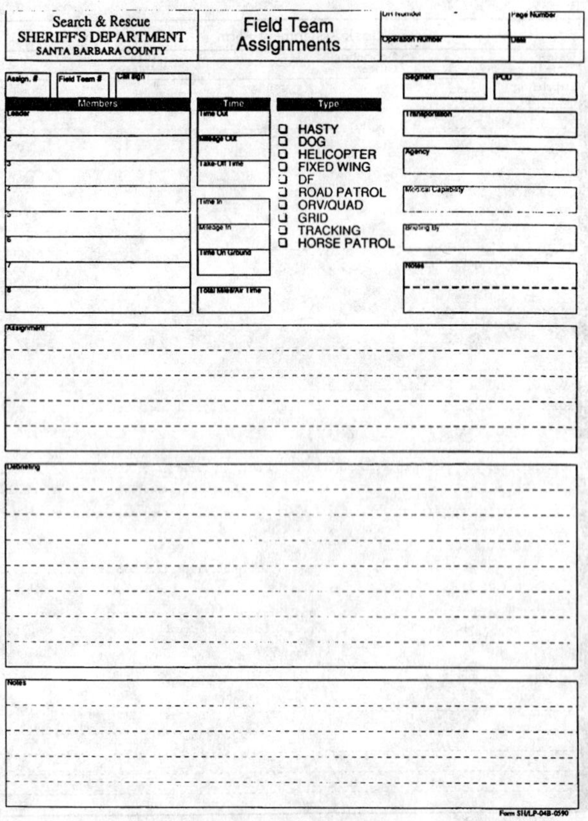
Search & Rescue
SHERIFF'S DEPARTMENT
SANTA BARBARA COUNTY

Field Team Assignments

DR Number | Page Number
Operation Number | Date

Assign. # | Field Team # | Call sign | Segment | POD
Members | Time | Type
Leader | Time Out
2 | Mileage Out
3 | Take-Off Time
4 | Time In
5 | Mileage In
6 | Time On Ground
7
8 | Total Miles/Air Time

Type:
❑ HASTY
❑ DOG
❑ HELICOPTER
❑ FIXED WING
❑ DF
❑ ROAD PATROL
❑ ORV/QUAD
❑ GRID
❑ TRACKING
❑ HORSE PATROL

Transportation
Agency
Medical Capability
Briefing By
Notes

Assignment

Debriefing

Notes

Form SH/LP-04B-0590

FIG. X2.9 Field Team Assignments *(continued)*

LOS ANGELES COUNTY SHERIFF'S DEPARTMENT
MALIBU MOUNTAIN RESCUE TEAM

Call Sign: ________ CREW ASSIGNMENT

THIS ROW FOR L.A.S.D. USE ONLY REPORT CONTINUATION	URN	page ___ of ___
Incident Name	Date/Time Prepared	Operational Period

Call Sign: ________ Freq: ________ T-Card Color: ________ By: ________
Assignment: ________________________________
Crew Leader: ________
Members: ________ ________ ________
Date/Time of Assignment: ________ Date/Time in Field: ________
Date/Time Assign. Complete ________ Date/Time in CP: ________

Call Sign: ________ Freq: ________ T-Card Color: ________ By: ________
Assignment: ________________________________
Crew Leader: ________
Members: ________ ________ ________
Date/Time of Assignment: ________ Date/Time in Field: ________
Date/Time Assign. Complete ________ Date/Time in CP: ________

Call Sign: ________ Freq: ________ T-Card Color: ________ By: ________
Assignment: ________________________________
Crew Leader: ________
Members: ________ ________ ________
Date/Time of Assignment: ________ Date/Time in Field: ________
Date/Time Assign. Complete ________ Date/Time in CP: ________

ICS 204 This form can be used for multiple crews, or a single crew with multiple assignments.

FIG. X2.10 Crew Assignment

81-14-67 (9/95)—10g

NEW YORK STATE DEPARTMENT OF ENVIRONMENTAL CONSERVATION
FOREST RANGERS

CREW ASSIGNMENT SHEET

CREW NUMBER	AFFILIATION	INCIDENT NAME	CREW BOSS
OPERATIONAL PERIOD (Date and Time) From: To:			

INCIDENT PERSONNEL (Name and Number)		CREW RADIO ID
INCIDENT COMMANDER	OPERATIONS	ICP PHONE
PLANS	STAGING AREA MANAGER	ICP TO FIELD FREQUENCY
LOGISTICS	DIVISION SUPERVISOR	FIELD TO FIELD FREQUENCY
INFORMATION OFFICER	STRIKE TEAM LEADER	REPEATER NAME / CHANNEL

CREW ASSIGNMENT	SPECIAL INSTRUCTIONS / EQUIPMENT / DROP POINT
	TRANSPORTATION

SUBJECT INFORMATION

NAME				NICKNAME		
SEX	RACE	AGE	HEIGHT	WEIGHT	HAIR	EYES

CLOTHING WORN	ITEMS CARRIED
TYPE OF EMPLOYMENT	FOOTWEAR

PERSONAL HABITS

EXPECTED WEATHER

SPECIAL INFORMATION

CREW BRIEFING CHECKLIST

☐ Summary to Date ☐ Subject Information ☐ Clues ☐ Time Frame (in field) ☐ Tactics ☐ Terrain
☐ Safety ☐ Family ☐ Media ☐ Weather ☐ Attitude

FIG. X2.11 Crew Assignment with Instructions

Crew Briefing Checklist
(Found on the bottom of the Crew Assignment Sheet)

Subject Info: can be read directly from the form.

Terrain: -nobody likes surprises
-advise the crew of what to expect
-remind them of safety

Tactics: -relate assignment both verbally and graphically (use map).
-define your assignment (ie, Type I, II, IIm, III)
-instruct/review how to execute search techniques.
-reiterate expected time needed to complete assignment.

Clues: -remind crew of the importance of looking for clues.
-emphasize that clues may include:
Items of clothing or items carried by the subject
Footprints, shelters, fires, matted vegetation, etc.
-emphasize the need to age the evidence.

Summary to date: relate information received in your briefing.
-keep it simple.
-answer two questions:
How long has the search been going on?
What areas have been searched?

Weather: can be read directly from the Crew Assignment Sheet

Safety: -identify known hazards.
-determine if crew members are prepared for weather and terrain.
-determine if crew members have adequate food, water, clothing, footwear, special gear (ie gloves, sun block, bug dope, flashlight, etc.)
-make sure each member understands serious nature of the assignment.
-complete an individual inspection
Crew is only as strong as it's weakest link.
Seek assistance from Operations section if not satisfied with an individual's equipment, clothing or conditioning.

Family: -advise your crew of family members present.
-may or may not be readily identifiable.
-advise crew to use discretion and act professionally at all times.
-DEC may identify family members with special badges.

Media: -all requests for information by the press should be politely referred to the Incident Commander or the Information Officer.

-press may be identified by special badges.

FIG. X2.11 Crew Assignment with Instructions *(continued)*

Time frame (in field): -crew members should advise crew boss of problems they may have
-crew should be informed of approximate timing of assignment.
Time crew expected to depart ICP
Anticipated duration of assignment
Time crew expected to return to ICP

Attitude: -reinforce values of positive attitude.
-establish sense of urgency and importance of your assignment.
-remind crew that finding nothing is as important as finding a clue.
-crew boss establishes rapport and sense of leadership.

FIG. X2.11 Crew Assignment with Instructions *(continued)*

TEAM ASSIGNMENT	1. INCIDENT NAME	2. OPERATIONAL PERIOD	3. ASGN. NUMBER

4. RESOURCE TYPE

5. PERSONNEL ASSIGNED   * L – TEAM LEADER M – MEDICAL

*	NAME	AGENCY	*	NAME	AGENCY
1			6		
2			7		
3			8		
4			9		
5			☐ ADDITIONAL NAMES ATTACHED		

6. ASSIGNMENT

☐ MAP(S) ATTACHED

7. PREVIOUS AND PRESENT SEARCH EFFORTS IN AREA

☐ (DE)BRIEFING INFO ATTACHED

8. TIME ALLOCATED	9. SIZE OF ASSIGNMENT	10. EXPECTED P.O.D.	H M L
			☐☐☐ RESPONSIVE SUBJECT ☐☐☐ UNRESPONSIVE SUBJECT ☐☐☐ CLUES

11. DROP OFF AND PICKUP INSTRUCTIONS

12. COMMUNICATIONS	RADIO CALL

FUNCTION	FREQUENCY	CHANNEL DESCRIPTION	CHANNEL
COMMAND (TEAM – BASE)			
TACTICAL (TEAM – TEAM)			

13. PREPARED BY	14. DATE PREPARED	15. TIME PREPARED

16. EQUIPMENT ISSUED

17. BRIEFER	18. TIME BRIEFED	19. TIME OUT	20. TIME RETURNED

SAR 104 BASARC 2/96	COPIES ☐ PLANS ☐ COMMUNICATIONS ☐ OPERATIONS ☐ TEAM	NOTES

FIG. X2.12 Team Assignment with Instructions

SAR 104 – Team Assignment (1/96)

Overview

The Team Assignment Form is intended to provide searchers with specific information related to their assignment. The form should be accompanied by a General Briefing Form that contains general information about the incident. A separate Team Assignment Form will be completed for each assignment made.

Instructions for Completing Form

1. Incident Name
The incident name should be established early in the operation. Be consistent and don't use several names, or change names in the middle. Good names often include either the last name of the subject ie. "Smith Search" or the name of the search location i.e. "Jones Gulch Search".

2. Operational Period
This is where the date goes. But it's more than just a date. An operational period has a beginning and an ending date and time. But the ending time may not be known at the time the forms is being filled out. It may be most useful to use the date followed by a word or two describing the time of day or phase of the search. For example

1/14/96 Initial Response   1/14/96 Night
1/15/96 Day 1   1/15/96 Daytime

1/14/96 2200 to 1/15/96 0600

3. Assignment Number
Assignments should be numbered sequentially for each incident. The ICS Plans function will number assignments as they are created.

4. Resource Type
What type of resource is this? Example include....
Hasty Search Team, Area Search Team, Dog Team, Mounted Team, Road Patrol, Communications Relay

5. Personnel Assigned
Who is on the team? List the name of each team member. To the left of their name there is room for a single letter note. "L" indicates Team Leader, "M" indicates highest medical training. Use additional symbols to fit your needs. There is room for 9 names on the form. That's more than enough for most assignments, but if you need more, check the additional names attached box.

6. Assignment
A written description of the teams assignment. This should describe the area or route to be searched. You should also give information about the search techniques to be used and the thoroughness with which to search.

Whenever possible you should attach a map marked with the area or route to be searched. Mark the map with a transparent highlighter so as not to obscure the details on the map. Good search maps include scale, contour, and north information.

7. Previous And Present Search Efforts In Area
A team that is looking for sign or tracks in their area needs to know if another search team has been through the area before. A dog handler needs to know if there is also a ground team working in the same area. A

FIG. X2.12 Team Assignment with Instructions *(continued)*

team researching an area needs to know how the previous team covered the area, what they focused on and areas they missed or glossed over. When you are trying to increase the cumulative POD for an area, attaching the debriefing notes from the previous search effort is a good idea.

8. Time Allocated
Search assignments shouldn't be open ended things. Planners should have an idea how long an assignment will take as well as when they want the team to return. This field can either be a length of time or a time to quit searching.

9. Size of Assignment
For area assignments this is the size of the area in square miles, square kilometers, or acres. For a route assignment it is the total length of the route in miles or kilometers.

10. Expected P.O.D.
This is were the planners give the searchers a clear idea of how thoroughly they should look for various things. The POD for a responsive subject relates to the team calling out for the subject, listening for, and being able to hear a response. The POD for an unresponsive subject relates to how thoroughly the team checks places that could conceal the subject. The POD for clues relates to how closely the entire assignment is examined for tracks, sign, and other small clues. If you need to map High ,Medium and Low to POD percentage values, use 80%, 50%, 20% respectively.

11. Drop Off and Pick Up Instructions
These are the transportation instructions. They should include the expected method of transport as well as the locations for pickup and drop off.

12. Communications
For most small to medium sized operations it is sufficient to assign a single command (search base to teams) radio frequency along with a single tactical (team to team) radio frequency. If your incident requires more than this, refer readers to a more complete communications plan. There is space on the Team Assignment form for team specific communication plans.

It's important to note the frequency of the radio net. Different agencies may use different names and channel assignments.

The Channel Description can be used for the "Name" of the radio net. Sufficient room is provided to also include info about repeater offsets, and tone if required.

Remember the Channel number may be different on radios outside of your own agency, so use the space with caution on a multiple agency operation.

13. Prepared By
Knowing who prepared a form allows questions about the information to asked of the correct person.

14. Date Prepared
The date and time a form is completed allows users of the information to know how current it is. In addition it helps establish the chronology of events when the search paperwork is being examined after the fact.

15. Time Prepared
See Date Prepared.

Fields 16 to 20 will not be filled in by Plans

16. Equipment Issued
By noting equipment that teams have been issued, such as radios and medical kits, both the team and the

FIG. X2.12 Team Assignment with Instructions *(continued)*

debriefed are reminded that they need to be sure the equipment is returned. This field will most likely be completed by logistics personnel.

17. Briefer
The name of the person who briefer the team on this assignment. To be completed by the briefer.

18. Time Briefed
The time at which the team was briefed. To be completed by the briefer.

19. Time Out
The time the team departed for the field. To be completed by the team and/or Operations.

20. Time Returned
The time the team returned from the field. To be completed by the team and/or Operations.

Copies
In a small search its may be good enough to give the team a copy and keep to keep a copy at the search base. In a larger incident, the distribution of copies of the assignment forms gets more complicated.

Notes
An empty space to be used for what ever need to be written there.

Notes

Team Number, Segment Number, Assignment Number, Individual Radio Call or SAR Number there seems to be some confusion in between these.

Segment Number -- How the search segment is identified on the overall search map and how it is identified in any POD tracking system. A single segment may have many search assignments in it.

Assignment Number -- How a given assignment is referred to. These are typically assigned sequentially as assignments are written. Sometimes there is a numeric sequence for each type of resource (i.e. Dog-5 and Ground-5) this has proved to be confusing.

Team Identifiers -- This is what you call the team when you want them on he radio. The first issue is should this identifier change when the team does an additional assignment or does it stick with the team? My position is this. The Team Identifiers should reflect the assignment they are working on. I think it should be prefixed with a name that id readily picked out by the team on the radio. (i.e. The agency or name of the team CARDA, BAMRU, CoCo, etc. or the type of the team (i.e. Dog) My position differs from the BASARC in that BASARC prefixes with the Agency Number (i.e. BAMRU-5 would be 1305, 13 is BAMRU's number)

Individual Radio Call -- Many teams assign a number to each of their members. Typically they're 3 digit numbers. Sometimes they are also used as radio calls. My experience is that these numbers should not be used as Team Identifiers, and that they should be avoided altogether on a multi agency search.

Expected POD. Will the expected POD for a responsive subject ever be anything but high? Perhaps it's a good thing to leave in to remind the team that they should be calling out and listening for a response.

Some of the most frequent complaints we get from teams are about the delay between their arrival, briefing and deployment into the field. By tracking time of briefing and deployment we can better examine this problem.

FIG. X2.12 Team Assignment with Instructions *(continued)*

Pennsylvania Search and Rescue Council	**Incident Communications Plan** Incident Form 4 of 5	PSARC
Incident Name:	Operational Period (Date/Time):	Date/Time Prepared:

Telephone		
Responsible Agency: ( ) -	State Coordinating Agency: ( ) -
Base Camp #1: ( ) -	Base Camp #2: ( ) -
( ) -	( ) -
( ) -	( ) -

Remarks									
Relays/ Repeaters									
Channel/ Frequency									
Net Name:									

Prepared by:	Approved by (IC or Logistics Chief):

3/2/92	(similar to ICS 205)	Page 1 of 1

FIG. X2.13 Incident Communications Plan

Pennsylvania Search and Rescue Council	**Incident Medical/Evacuation Plan** Incident Form 3 of 5	PSARC
Incident Name:	Operational Period (Date/Time):	Date/Time Prepared:

Base Camp

Base Camp Minor Injury/Illness to be Managed:

Additional Local Medical Resources (Minor Injury/Illness):

Evacuation

Resources and Plan for Field Evacuation:

Medical

Medical Resources and Response Plan for Field Medical Emergency:

EMS Transport

Name:	ALS? BLS? Ground? Air?	Response Time:	Contact Means:

Hospitals

Name:	Location:	Capabilities:	Travel Time (Ground/Air):	E.D. Phone #:
				( ) -
				( ) -
				( ) -

(List should include Level I Trauma Center, Burn Unit hospital, and local hospital(s).

Prepared by:	Approved by (IC or Safety Officer):

3/2/92	(similar to ICS 206)	Page 1 of 1

FIG. X2.14 Incident Medical/Evacuation Plan

Pennsylvania Search and Rescue Council	Daily SAR Unit/Government Personnel Register Daily Form 3 of 10	PENNSYLVANIA PSARC SEARCH & RESCUE COUNCIL

Incident Name:	Location:	Date*:	For this Date, Page: of:

Name (Last, First, MI)	Organization	Qualifications/ GSAR Level	Arrival Time	Estimated Departure Date/Time	**Actual Departure Date/Time**	Emergency Contact: Name and Phone

3/2/92	*Start new set of forms for each 24-hour period, midnight to midnight	(This is a 1-page form)

FIG. X2.15 Daily Local Volunteer Personnel Register

Pennsylvania Search and Rescue Council

Daily Local Volunteer Personnel Register

Daily Form 4 of 10

PSARC Pennsylvania Search & Rescue Council

Incident Name:	Location:	Date*:	For this Date, Page: of:

Name (Last, First, MI)	Address	Phone Number	Arrival Time	Estimated Departure Date/Time	**Actual Departure Date/Time**	Emergency Contact: Name and Phone

3/2/92 ***Start new set of forms for each 24-hour period, midnight to midnight** (This is a 1-page form)

FIG. X2.16 Daily SAR Unit/Government Personnel Register

LOS ANGELES COUNTY SHERIFF'S DEPARTMENT

MALIBU MOUNTAIN RESCUE TEAM

Agency Name ______________ Personnel Check In/Out

THIS ROW FOR L A S D USE ONLY REPORT CONTINUATION	URN	page____ of____
Incident Name	Date/Time Prepared	Operational Period

Name (Last, First)	Agency	Call Sign	Check-in Date	Check-in Time	Check-out Date	Check-out Time	Total Hours for Oper. Per.
1.							
2.							
3.							
4.							
5.							
6.							
7.							
8.							
9.							
10.							
11.							
12.							
13.							
14.							
15.							
16.							
17.							
18.							
19.							
20.							
21.							
22.							
						Totals for this Page:	

ICS 211-P Notes:

page ____ of____

FIG. X2.17 Personnel Check In/Out

42-14-20 (3/95)—10g

NEW YORK STATE DEPARTMENT OF ENVIRONMENTAL CONSERVATION
FOREST RANGERS

REGISTRATION OF SEARCH AND RESCUE PARTICIPANTS

AGENCY / GROUP AFFILIATION:	DATE:

NAME OF INCIDENT: ____________ REGION: ______ REGISTERED BY: ____________

NAME (Print)		ADDRESS	SPECIAL QUALIFICATIONS	SPECIAL SKILLS/EQUIPMENT	TIME
LAST, FIRST, MI		STREET	☐ DEC Certified ☐ EMT/1st Responder ☐ Crew Boss		IN
SOCIAL SECURITY NUMBER	TELEPHONE NUMBER ( )	CITY / STATE / ZIP			OUT
LAST, FIRST, MI		STREET	☐ DEC Certified ☐ EMT/1st Responder ☐ Crew Boss		IN
SOCIAL SECURITY NUMBER	TELEPHONE NUMBER ( )	CITY / STATE / ZIP			OUT
LAST, FIRST, MI		STREET	☐ DEC Certified ☐ EMT/1st Responder ☐ Crew Boss		IN
SOCIAL SECURITY NUMBER	TELEPHONE NUMBER ( )	CITY / STATE / ZIP			OUT
LAST, FIRST, MI		STREET	☐ DEC Certified ☐ EMT/1st Responder ☐ Crew Boss		IN
SOCIAL SECURITY NUMBER	TELEPHONE NUMBER ( )	CITY / STATE / ZIP			OUT
LAST, FIRST, MI		STREET	☐ DEC Certified ☐ EMT/1st Responder ☐ Crew Boss		IN
SOCIAL SECURITY NUMBER	TELEPHONE NUMBER ( )	CITY / STATE / ZIP			OUT
LAST, FIRST, MI		STREET	☐ DEC Certified ☐ EMT/1st Responder ☐ Crew Boss		IN
SOCIAL SECURITY NUMBER	TELEPHONE NUMBER ( )	CITY / STATE / ZIP			OUT
LAST, FIRST, MI		STREET	☐ DEC Certified ☐ EMT/1st Responder ☐ Crew Boss		IN
SOCIAL SECURITY NUMBER	TELEPHONE NUMBER ( )	CITY / STATE / ZIP			OUT
LAST, FIRST, MI		STREET	☐ DEC Certified ☐ EMT/1st Responder ☐ Crew Boss		IN
SOCIAL SECURITY NUMBER	TELEPHONE NUMBER ( )	CITY / STATE / ZIP			OUT
LAST, FIRST, MI		STREET	☐ DEC Certified ☐ EMT/1st Responder ☐ Crew Boss		IN
SOCIAL SECURITY NUMBER	TELEPHONE NUMBER ( )	CITY / STATE / ZIP			OUT

FIG. X2.18 Registration of Search and Rescue Participants

Pennsylvania Search and Rescue Council

Daily Unit Log

Daily Form 10 of 10

Incident Name:	Operational Period (Date/Time):	Unit:
ICS Position:	Name:	Period Serving (Date/Time to Date/Time):

24-hour Local Time:	Major Events:

3/2/92 — continue on reverse — Page 1 of 2

FIG. X2.19 Daily Unit Log

Daily Unit Log	
24-hour Local Time:	Major Events:
3/2/92	Check here if more pages for this log: ☐ Page 2 of 2

FIG. X2.19 Daily Unit Log *(continued)*

Pennsylvania Search and Rescue Council	Daily SAR Resources Worksheet Daily Form 9 of 10				
Incident Name:		Operational Period (Date/Time):		RESTAT Name(s):	
Name (Person or Team):	Type of Resource:	Status: A=Available R=Resting T=On Task X=Not Avail	(Team Identifier):	(Present Location):	(Time to be Available):
		A R T X			
		A R T X			
		A R T X			
		A R T X			
		A R T X			
		A R T X			
		A R T X			
		A R T X			
		A R T X			
		A R T X			
		A R T X			
		A R T X			
		A R T X			
		A R T X			
		A R T X			
		A R T X			
		A R T X			
		A R T X			
		A R T X			
		A R T X			
		A R T X			
		A R T X			
		A R T X			
		A R T X			
		A R T X			
		A R T X			
		A R T X			
		A R T X			
		A R T X			
		A R T X			
		A R T X			
3/2/92		incoming resources on reverse			Page 1 of 2

FIG. X2.20 Daily SAR Resources Worksheet

Daily SAR Resources Worksheet				
Type of Resource	Number:	Coming from:	ETA at Base:	Remarks:

Incoming Resources

3/2/92 — on-scene resources on front — Page 2 of 2

FIG. X2.20 Daily SAR Resources Worksheet *(continued)*

Pennsylvania Search and Rescue Council

Daily Vehicle Register

Daily Form 5 of 10

Incident Name:	Location:	Date*:	For this Date, Page:	of:

Driver's Name (Last, First, MI)	Make/Type of Vehicle	License Number and State	Point of Origin	Arrival Time	Estimated Departure Date/Time	**Actual Departure Date/Time**	*(Estimated Round-Trip Mileage)*

3/2/92 — *Start new set of forms for each 24-hour period, midnight to midnight — (This is a 1-page form)

FIG. X2.21 Daily Vehicle Register

LOS ANGELES COUNTY SHERIFF'S DEPARTMENT

MALIBU MOUNTAIN RESCUE TEAM

DEBRIEFING FORM

THIS ROW FOR L A S D USE ONLY REPORT CONTINUATION	URN	page ____ of ____
Incident Name	Date/Time Prepared	Operational Period
Crew:	Crew Leader:	Number in Crew:
Date/Time Start Assignment:	Date/Time End Assignment:	
Assignment:		
What You Actually Did:		
What would you estimate the PODs for your efforts to be? Define the types of subjects the PODs reference, (mobile, immobile, etc.)		
Describe the location of any clues you found. What is the current status of these clues?		
Describe any search difficulties or gaps in coverage.		
Describe any hazards observed in your assigned segment.		
Describe any problems encountered with communications.		
Any suggestions, ideas, or recommendations for future plans?		
MMRT 300	Use reverse side for additional notes and/or drawings.	

By:____________________

FIG. X2.22 Debriefing Form

THIS ROW FOR L A S D USE ONLY REPORT CONTINUATION	URN	page ____ of ____

FIG. X2.22 Debriefing Form *(continued)*

TEAM DEBRIEFING

1. INCIDENT NAME	2. OPERATIONAL PERIOD	3. ASGN.NUMBER

4. RESOURCE TYPE

5. ASSIGNMENT SUMMARY

6. DESCRIBE SEARCH EFFORTS IN ASSIGNMENT

7. DESCRIBE PORTIONS YOU WERE UNABLE TO SEARCH

8. DESCRIBE ANY CLUES, TRACKS, OR SIGN LOCATED, OR ANY PERTINENT TRAIL INTERVIEWS

9. DESCRIBE ANY HAZARDS OR PROBLEMS ENCOUNTERED

10. SUGGESTIONS FOR FURTHER SEARCH EFFORTS IN OR NEAR YOUR ASSIGNMENT

11. TIME ENTERED ASSIGNMENT	12. TIME EXITED ASSIGNMENT	13. TIME SPENT SEARCHING

15. DEBRIEFER	16. DATE & TIME

14. P.O.D. SUMMARY

H M L

____% ☐☐☐☐☐ RESPONSIVE SUBJECT
____% ☐☐☐☐☐ UNRESPONSIVE SUBJECT
____% ☐☐☐☐☐ CLUES

90% 50% 10%

SAR 110
BASARC 2/96

ATTACHMENTS
☐ DEBRIEFING MAP(S)
☐ ORIGINAL BRIEFING DOCUMENT
☐ SUPPLEMENTAL DEBRIEFING FORMS
☐ OTHER ____________

SUMMARY
NOTHING SIGNIFICANT LOCATED ☐
USEFUL INFORMATION, NEEDS REVIEW ☐
POTENTIAL CLUES, NEEDS URGENT REVIEW ☐
ASSIGNMENT COMPLETED ☐
ASSIGNMENT NOT COMPLETED ☐

FIG. X2.23 Team Debriefing with Supplement and Instructions

TEAM DEBRIEFING
SUPPLEMENT

1. INCIDENT NAME	2. OPERATIONAL PERIOD	3. ASGN.NUMBER

SAR 119
BASARC 1/96

FIG. X2.23 Team Debriefing with Supplement and Instructions *(continued)*

SAR 110 -- Team Debriefing (1/96)

Overview

The Team Debriefing Form is intended to provide plans with the results from the teams search effort.

This form will likely be reviewed as plans are being made for the next operational period. It's likely that both the debriefer and the team will not be available to answer questions at that time. (It usually happens in the wee hours of the morning.) Thus is very important that all of the information get written on the form and attached maps. Make sure there are not any bits of information that exist only as an understanding between the debriefer and the team. An example of this would be a shaded area on the map, with no notation as to its meaning. It was obvious what it meant when it was shaded, but at 3am it will be meaningless to the planner.

Instructions for Completing Form

1. Incident Name
The incident name should be established early in the operation. Be consistent and don't use several names, or change names in the middle. Good names often include either the last name of the subject ie. "Smith Search" or the name of the search location i.e. "Jones Gulch Search".

2. Operational Period
This is where the date goes. But it's more than just a date. An operational period has a beginning and an ending date and time. But the ending time may not be known at the time the forms is being filled out. It may be most useful to use the date followed by a word or two describing the time of day or phase of the search. For example

1/14/96 Initial Response	1/14/96 Night
1/15/96 Day 1	1/15/96 Daytime

1/14/96 2200 to 1/15/96 0600

3. Assignment Number
This should be the assignment number from the Team Assignment Form.

4. Resource Type
What type of resource is this? Example include....
Hasty Search Team, Area Search Team, Dog Team, Mounted Team, Road Patrol, Communications Relay

5. Assignment Summary
A short written summary of the assignment. It need not be as detailed as the description on the Team Assignment Form. By doing this summary the debriefer will get a chance to make sure both he and the team understand and agree on what the assignment was.

6. Describe Search Efforts in Assignment
Describe both where the team searched as well as the type of searching they did. Please don't just write see map. But on the other hand it's a great idea to also attach a map.

7. Describe Portions You Were Unable to Search
Describe the location of any areas not searched along with the reason why they were not searched. There may be specific areas not searched. And there may be categories of areas not searched. For example,"Found pockets of dense brush, which we did not penetrate." This is the information that is most needed by a team

FIG. X2.23 Team Debriefing with Supplement and Instructions *(continued)*

that is assigned to research an area. They will use it to determine if additional equipment is needed, where to search, and what techniques to use to get the pest overall coverage of the area.

8. Describe any Clues, Tracks, or Sign Located, or any Pertinent Trail Interviews
Note both what the clue is and its location. Note what was done with the clue (left in place, marked, recovered, etc.). In addition you should note how relevant the team thinks this clue is. Note if the clue has already be reported, and if so note any assigned identifier.

9. Describe any Hazards or Problems Encountered
Use your judgement here. There is no need to list hazards that are common to most of the search areas and already well known. For example on a winter operation cold and snow are a hazard that needn't be noted.

10. Suggestions for Further Search Efforts In or Near Your Assignment
The team has just been out to the search area and may have very good ideas for additional searching. Try to focus them on ideas related to what they found in the field rather that their overall theories about the search.

11. Time Entered Assignment
The time the team arrived at their search area.

12. Time Exited Assignment
The time the team left their search area.

13. Time Spent Searching
Time in hours that they actually spent searching. This doesn't include time spent eating lunch, resting, or trying to find themselves on the map.

14. P.O.D. Summary
Here is the final summary of how thoroughly the assignment was searched. Probability Of Detection (POD) is the likelihood that the subject or clues would have been located had they been in the search area.

The POD for a responsive subject relates to the team calling out for the subject, listening for, and being able to hear a response. The more frequently the team stopped, called out for the subject, and then listened for a response the higher a POD would be for a responsive subject. Wind and water noise will significantly reduce this POD.

The POD for an unresponsive subject relates to how thoroughly the team checks places that could conceal the subject.

The POD for clues relates to how closely the entire assignment is examined for tracks, sign, and other small clues.

The PODs you record apply only to the portion of the assignment that was completed. Do not reduce the POD because the assignment was not completed. Rather focus on evaluating the PODs for the completed portion.

The form has space for either a numeric value for POD or a High to Low scale.
If you need to map High ,Medium and Low to POD percentage values, use 80%, 70%, 50%, 30%,10%.

15. Debriefer
The Debriefers name, so we know who to wake up and question if things aren't clear.

16. Date & Time
Date and time the debriefing occurred. This information helps establish the chronology of events when the

FIG. X2.23 Team Debriefing with Supplement and Instructions *(continued)*

search paperwork is being examined after the fact.

Attachments
Note what paperwork goes with this form. Then we can tell if it's missing.

Summary
This is perhaps the most difficult portion of the form for the debriefer to complete. First of all decide if the team completed their assignment. In most cases this should be a clear cut call. Then prioritize the importance of these results. Debriefings marked for urgent review will get processed first. Forms marked needs review are next in line, followed by nothing significant located forms. Note that nothing significant located forms are stilled reviewed by the plans staff, only it's done last.

Notes

FIG. X2.23 Team Debriefing with Supplement and Instructions *(continued)*

LOS ANGELES COUNTY SHERIFF'S DEPARTMENT

MALIBU MOUNTAIN RESCUE TEAM

SEARCH CAPABILITIES ROSTER

THIS ROW FOR L A S D USE ONLY REPORT CONTINUATION	URN	page ____ of ____
Incident Name	Date / Time Prepared	Operational Period
Unit Name / Designator	Unit Leader	

#	CREW ASSIGN	NAME	RANK	TIME AVAIL	OVER NIGHT	MED QUAL	HELI QUAL	TRACK LEVEL	CLIMB LEVEL	ELT-DF	DIVE TEAM	OTHR
1												
2												
3												
4												
5												
6												
7												
8												
9												
10												
11												
12												
13												
14												
15												
16												
17												
18												
19												
20												

MMRT 303	Other Info:

SEE REVERSE SIDE FOR CODES 10/21/93

FIG. X2.24 Search Capabilities Roster

INFORMATION CODES
SEARCH CAPABILITIES ROSTER

CREW ASSIGNMENT Leave blank, a crew number will be assigned by Operations.

NAME

RANK Your rank within your organization

TIME AVAILABLE: If this member is not on scene, but will arrive at a later time, enter that time here.

OVER NIGHT: Do you have the experience and the equipment to spend the night in the field?
Answer with the number of nights you are prepared to spend in the field, ie. 0, 1, 2 etc..

MEDICAL QUALIFICATION: List only the **current** level of certification you possess.

MM	multimedia first aid qualification
ADV	Advanced First Aid and Emergency Care
FR	DOT First Responder Course
EMT-1	Emergency Medical Technician
EMT-P	Paramedic
MICN	Mobile Intensive Care Nurse
R.N.	Registered Nurse
P.A.	Physicians Assistant
M.D.	Physician

HELITAC QUALIFICATION: Check if you have undergone "in the air" helitactics training within the past year.

TRACKING LEVEL:

T-1	Can follow a very easy, perfect print.
T-2	Easy, complete print, imperfect.
T-3	Moderate, incomplete print.
T-4	Hard, partial print lacking positive I.D.
T-5	Severe, sign only. Tracking trained & monthly practice.
T-6	Very severe, obscure sign. High natural ability, practicing weekly.

CLIMBING ABILITY:

Class 3	Easy climbing; scrambling w/ use of hands, elementary use of climbing technique
Class 4	Moderate climbing using natural protection, short pitches.
Class 5	Roped climbing requiring artificial protection. 5.3- abundant handholds 5.7- obscure handholds
Direct Aid	A1 - A5

ELT - DF: Check here if you have been trained in the use of, and can operate an ELT direction finder.

DIVE TEAM: Check here if you are a member of an underwater dive rescue/recovery team.

FIG. X2.24 Search Capabilities Roster *(continued)*

FEMA US&R SPONSE SYSTEM
INCIDENT SUPPORT TEAM

RESOURCE ORDER FORM	INCIDENT	OPERATIONAL PERIOD DATE TIMES	REPORTING UNIT **ESF-9**	FORM 2/95 **US&R—005**
NAME:	POSITION TITLE:	MISSION ASSIGNMENT #:	TIME:	
LOCATION:	CALLBACK #:	PROCESSED AT DFO BY:		

ORDER CODES:
M — Miscellaneous; A — Aircraft; O — Overhead; TF — Task Force; C — Crews; T — Transportation; P — Personnel; S — Supplies; E — Equipment; F — Food; IST — Inc. Sppt Team; FC — Search Team; COM — Communications; FAsT — Field Assmnt

QUANTITY	CODE	ITEM ORDERED / COMMENTS (special instructions, names, etc.)	ETA	REQ. #	CONFIRMED

APPROVED BY DATE

DISTRIBUTION: Originial: Logistics/Copy: Finance Section/Copy: Planning Section

FIG. X2.25 Resource Order Form

LOS ANGELES COUNTY SHERIFF'S DEPARTMENT

MALIBU MOUNTAIN RESCUE TEAM

SURVIVAL TIME FRAME WORKSHEET

NOTE: This worksheet only provides guidelines to aid in the evaluation in survivability of an individual where no action is taken to seek protection. Add these quantifiable factors to other known circumstances to approximate time frames for survival.

Fill in the following information:

AIR TEMPERATURE (f).....................	LOW ______	HIGH ______	
WIND SPEED (mph)...........................	LOW ______	HIGH ______	See wind speed chart for estimate
PRECIPITATION..................................	YES / NO / UNK		Influencing factor?
WATER-BODY TEMPERATURE..........	LOW ______	HIGH ______	If immersion involved
IMMOBILE?	YES / NO / UNK		Influencing factor?
HUMIDITY (%)....................................	LOW ______	HIGH ______	

Follow these steps:

1. Is the subject immersed in water? If yes go to step # 10.
2. Is the air temperature less than 60 ° F? If no, go to step # 4.
3. Refer to WIND CHILL TEMPERATURE CHART, then go to step # 5.
4. Refer to HUMIDITY CHART, then go to step # 5.
5. Enter RELATIVE AIR TEMPERATURE: LOW______ HIGH ______
6. Is the subject in a hot desert climate? If yes, go to step # 11.
7. Is the subject wet? If yes, go to step # 8.
8. Refer to WET CHILL CHART using relative air temperature (step # 5).
9. Refer to HYPOTHERMIA CHART using relative air Temerature (step # 5).
10. Refer to IMMERSION CHART using water-body temperature information.
11. Refer to DESERT SURVIVAL CHART using the relative air temperature (step # 5).

Fill in the appropriate box(s):

	LOW	HIGH
WET CHILL SURVIVABILITY............ circle one (HOURS or DAYS)	MIN. ______ MAX. ______	MIN. ______ MAX. ______
HYPOTHERMIA SURVIVABILITY.... circle one (HOURS or DAYS)	MIN. ______ MAX. ______	MIN. ______ MAX. ______
IMMERSION SURVIVABILITY.......... circle one (HOURS or DAYS)	AVE. ______	
DEHYDRATION SURVIVABILITY..... circle one (HOURS or DAYS)	AVE. ______	

LIST OTHER INFLUENCING FACTORS BELOW (clothing, shelter, experience etc.)

1. ______
2. ______
3. ______
4. ______
5. ______

MMRT 304	PREPARED BY (NAME & POSITION)

FIG. X2.26 Survival Time-frame Worksheet

FEMA US&R RESPONSE SYSTEM
INCIDENT SUPPORT TEAM

PLANNING PROCESS CHECKLIST	INCIDENT	REPORTING UNIT ESF-9	FORM US&R—XXX 2/95
DISASTER #:	OPS PERIOD:	DATE/TIME PREPARED:	UNIT LEADER:

PLANNING STEP	RESPONSIBILITY
■ Give briefing on situation status	IST Planning Section Chief
■ Give briefing on resource status	IST Planning Section Chief
■ Review strategic objectives	IST Team Leader
■ Plot functional and geographic boundaries	IST Operations Section Chief
■ Recommend tactics for functional and geographic boundaries	IST Operations Section Chief
■ Determine resources needed	IST Operations Section Chief
■ Specify operations facilities and reporting locations. Plot on map.	IST Operations Section Chief
■ Discuss requirements for:	IST Logistics Section Chief
• communications	
• medical	
• traffic	
• other logistical issues	
■ Finalize Incident Action Plan	IST Planning Section Chief
Approve Incident Action Plan	IST Team Leader
PREPARED BY:	APPROVED BY: DATE

FIG. X2.27 Planning Process Checklist

FEMA US&R RESPONSE SYSTEM
INCIDENT SUPPORT TEAM

PLANNING CYCLE	INCIDENT	REPORTING UNIT ESF-9	FORM US&R—XXX 2/95
DISASTER #:	OPS PERIOD:	DATE/TIME PREPARED:	UNIT LEADER:

TIME	EVENT
	■ Shift change
	■ Prepare for Planning Meeting
	■ Planning Meetings (Command & General Staff, Agency Admin. Rep., Resource Status Officer, Situation Status Officer, Comm Support Officer, etc.)
	■ Prepare IAP
	■ Review and Finalize IAP
	■ Approve IAP
	■ Prepare for Operations Briefing
	■ Operations Briefing
	■ Finalize Reports
	■ Shift Change
PREPARED BY:	APPROVED BY: DATE:

FIG. X2.28 Planning Cycle

Los Padres Search & Rescue	Missing Aircraft WORKSHEET	Case No.
		SAR No.
		OES No. / AFRCC No.

AIRCRAFT DESCRIPTION

Registration Number	Manufacturer	Model	Color	
Remarks	Cruise Speed	Number of Engines	ELT Equipped	IFR Equipped
Pilot's Name: Last, First, MI	Age	D. O. B.		
Address: Street, City, State	Phone No.			
License	Rating	Hours	Other Flight Trained Crew Members	
Passengers	HAZARDOUS OR SENSITIVE CARGO			

LAST CONTACT

Location			
Reporting Party: Last, First, MI	Relation	Phone	Time

PLANNED ROUTE

Departure Point	Time	Date	IFR/VFR
Destination	ETA	Date	Alterante Airport
Route			
Source of Information	Flight Plan Filed With		

KNOWN ROUTE

Route
Weather Enroute
Source of Information

OTHER INFORMATION

Instrument Approach
Instrument Departure
Flight Service Station DF
Pilot/Witness Report

INFORMATION SOURCES

SBA Flight Service Station Contact	967-2305
SBA Tower Contact	967-9717
A/C Rental Agency Contact	Phone
Line Person/Gas Truck Contact	Phone
Civial Air Patrol Contact	Phone
Other	Phone

© Los Padres SAR 1989 Form LP-17-0990

FIG. X2.29 Missing Aircraft Worksheet

Los Padres Search & Rescue	ELT WORKSHEET	Case No.
		SAR No.

First Report

Reporting Party	Phone	Time
Report		
Source of Report		
Location of Reporting Party	Agency of Reporting Party	

AFRCC Data

Contact	Mission No.	1-800-851-3051	
Satellite Report: Latitude/Longitude	Time of Report	Time of Next Update	
Aircraft Report	Time	Type of A/C	Altitude of A/C

Civil Air Patrol Data

CAP Contact	Phone	Unit	Time
Report			
Source of Report			
Mission Coordinator	Base Location	Phone	
Ground Teams: Call Sign & Location			
Aircraft: Call Sign & Location			

Sheriff's Department Data

Contact	Phone	Location	Time
Report			
Source of Report	Time of Report		

FAA Data

Contact	Phone	Location/Office	Time	
Report				
Signal Received	Location of Receiver	Time Received	Direction	SBA FSS 967-2305
Pilot Report	Type of A/C / Altitude	Time Received	Location	SBA Tower 967-9717

Automatic Alert

Mesa	Airport/CMC	
Walnut Road	Cathedral Oaks	Direction
Comments		

ELT Report Data

Owner's Name: Last, First MI		
Location	Aircraft/Vessel Type	Registration No.
ELT Manufacturer	ELT Model No.	ELT Serial No.
Suspected Cause		
Time Off	Date Off	Distance From Satellite Plot

Form LP-14-0990 © Los Padres SAR 1990

FIG. X2.30 ELT Worksheet

FEMA US&R RESPONSE SYSTEM
INCIDENT SUPPORT TEAM

SITUATION REPORT	INCIDENT	OPERATIONAL PERIOD DATE TIMES	REPORTING UNIT ESF-9	FORM 2/95 US&R—004

The following reports on Urban Search & Rescue activities for the period shown:

- **CURRENT SITUATION**
- **CRITICAL ISSUES**
- **CASUALTY REPORT** (civilian/Federal)

ACCOMPLISHMENTS

- **RESOURCES ASSIGNED**
- **PLANNED ACTIVITIES** (next 24 - 72 hours)
- **ADDITIONAL INFORMATION**

IST LEADER DATE TIME	DISTRIBUTION: DFO: Information & Planning Section IST: *Command & General Staff	

FIG. X2.31 Situation Report

Pennsylvania Search and Rescue Council	**Daily Task Log** Daily Form 6 of 10	PSARC

Incident Name:	Location:	Date*:	For this Date, Page : of:

Task Number:	Team Identifier:	Team Type:	Number on Team:	Task:	Time Out:	Time In:	*(Total Hours)*

3/2/92 | *Start new set of forms for each 24-hour period, midnight to midnight | (1-page form)

FIG. X2.32 Daily Task Log

81 14-69 (11/93)—10g

NEW YORK STATE
DEPARTMENT OF ENVIRONMENTAL CONSERVATION

CREW CARD

CREW BOSS	DATE
CREW AFFILIATION	COLOR

CREW TYPE:
☐ 1 ☐ 2 ☐ 2M ☐ 3

AREA ASSIGNED

TIME OUT	TIME IN

CREW MEMBERS	BIB NO.

REMARKS

FRONT SIDE

FIG. X2.33 Crew Card with Instructions

UNIT LOG	
TIME	MAJOR EVENTS

BACK SIDE

FIG. X2.33 Crew Card with Instructions *(continued)*

Crew Card/Unit Log

Multi-copy form used to track resources/document crew activities

Original - Operations Section Chief
2nd Copy - Plans Section Chief &/or Communications Section Chief
3rd Copy - Crew Boss

Information found on Crew Card

Crew number: found on the Crew Assignment Sheet
Crew Boss: full name, first name first
Date: month/day/year
Crew Affiliation: (ie M.F. Whitney Fire Co., 3500 Club, etc.)
Bib Color: color of the assigned bibs
Crew type: check the search technique to be used (found on the Crew Assignment Sheet or obtained at briefing)
Area Assigned: found on the Crew Assignment Sheet
Time Out: time the assignment is started
Time In: time the assignment is completed or crew returns to the ICP
Crew Members/Bib number: print the names of all crew members; record their assigned bib numbers
Remarks: use as needed

Using the Unit Log

Found on the reverse side of the Crew Card

Crew boss maintains the Unit Log

Becomes permanent and integral part of the incident's records

Major events to note:
-time crew begins assignment
-time and place any clue found
-disposition of clues and/or instructions given by the ICP
-documentation of injuries
-time any crew member leaves the crew

FIG. X2.33 Crew Card with Instructions *(continued)*

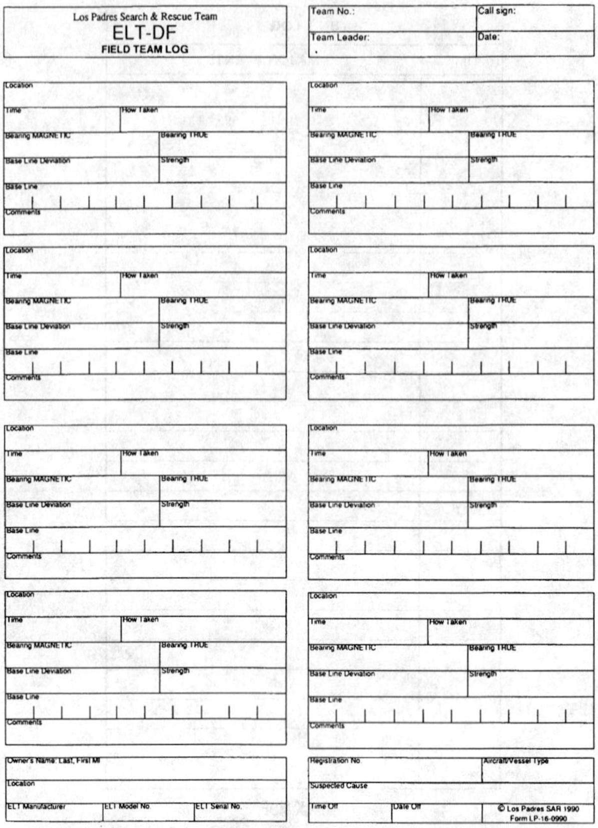

FIG. X2.34 ELT-DF Field Team Log

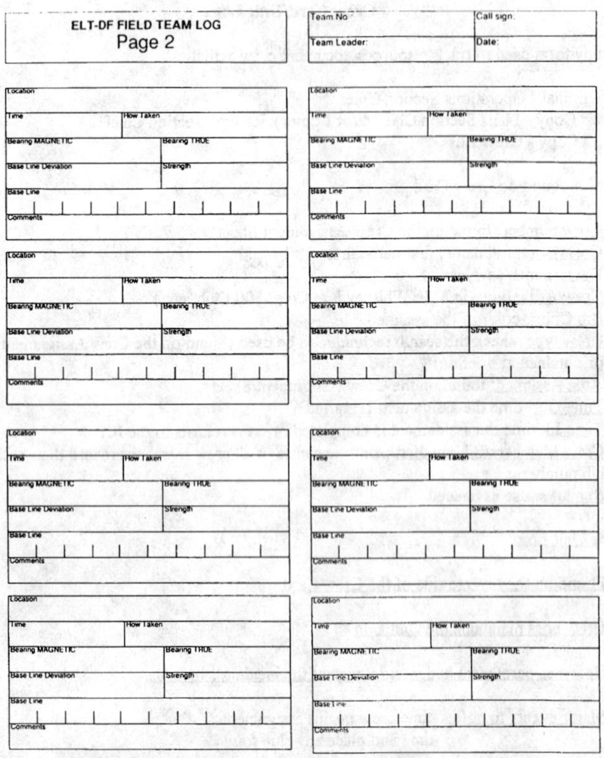

FIG. X2.34 ELT-DF Field Team Log *(continued)*

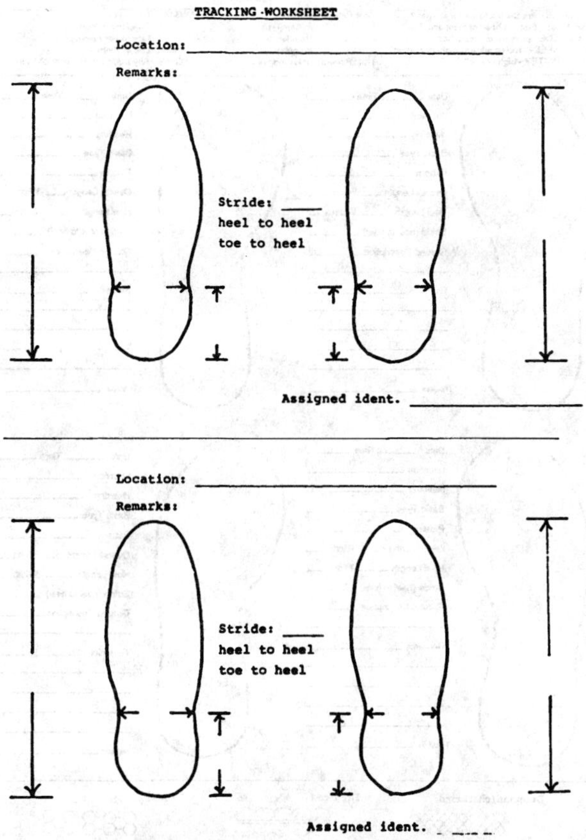

FIG. X2.35 Tracking Worksheet

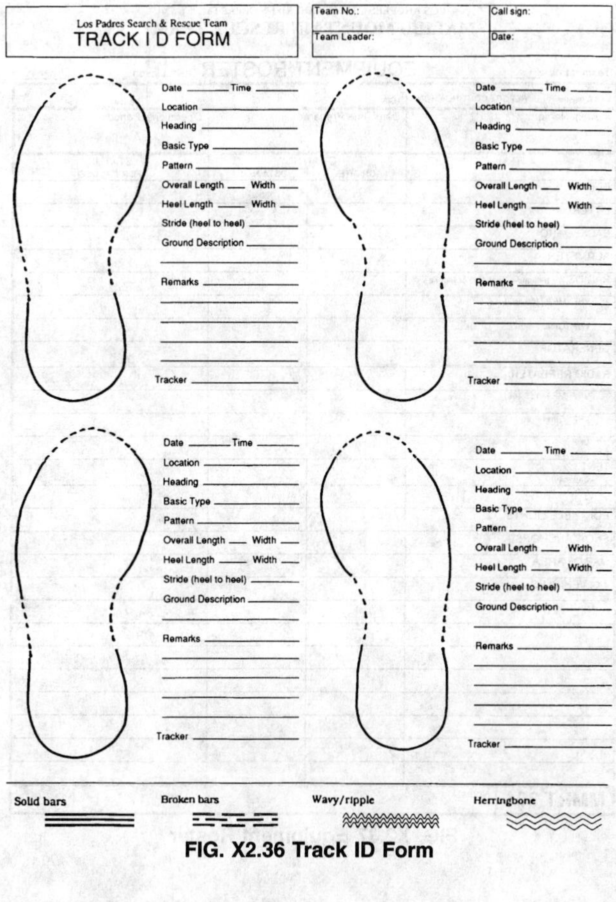

FIG. X2.36 Track ID Form

Right or Left: Are the tracks mirror images?
Basic Type: Flat (no heel) or Heel and Toe?
Shape: TOE - pointed, rounded, box square?
HEEL - leading edge straight or curved?
INSTEP - high or low?

Sole Pattern: General
PatternType
Regular
Irregular
Heel Pattern: holes, edges

Gait: Toes in or out?
Deep toe or heel dig?
Limping or running?
Mark: Left or Right
Circle: Any track detailed enough to ID.

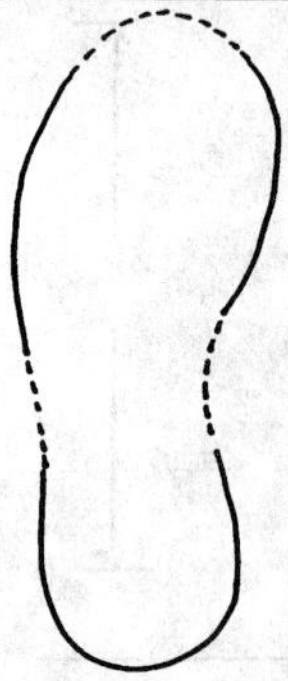

Date ______ Time ______
Location ______
Heading ______
Basic Type ______
Pattern ______
Overall Length ____ Width ____
Heel Length ____ Width ____
Stride (heel to heel) ______
Ground Description ______
Remarks ______
Tracker ______

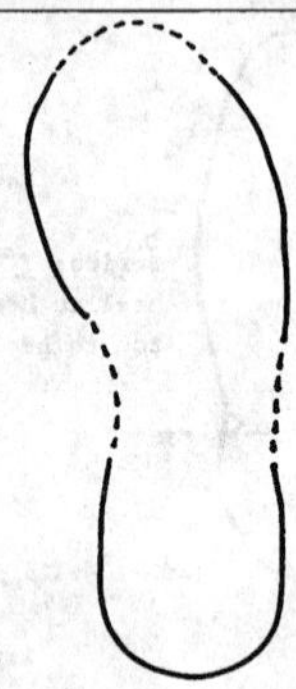

Date ______ Time ______
Location ______
Heading ______
Basic Type ______
Pattern ______
Overall Length ____ Width ____
Heel Length ____ Width ____
Stride (heel to heel) ______
Ground Description ______
Remarks ______
Tracker ______

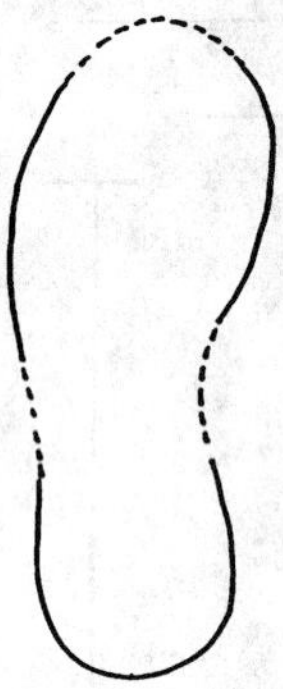

Date ______ Time ______
Location ______
Heading ______
Basic Type ______
Pattern ______
Overall Length ____ Width ____
Heel Length ____ Width ____
Stride (heel to heel) ______
Ground Description ______
Remarks ______
Tracker ______

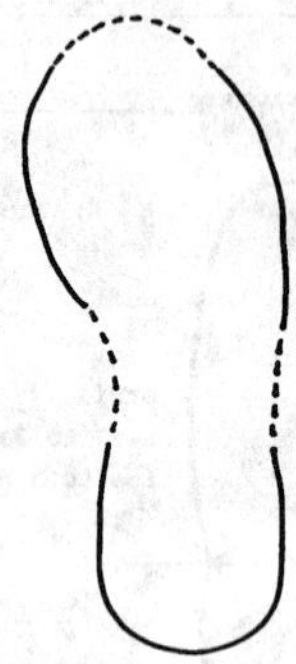

Date ______ Time ______
Location ______
Heading ______
Basic Type ______
Pattern ______
Overall Length ____ Width ____
Heel Length ____ Width ____
Stride (heel to heel) ______
Ground Description ______
Remarks ______
Tracker ______

Diamond/checkered

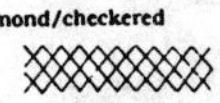

Tire tread

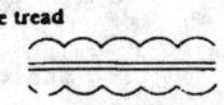

Honeycomb

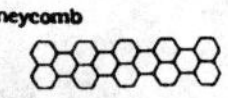

FIG. X2.36 Track ID Form *(continued)*

LOS ANGELES COUNTY SHERIFF'S DEPARTMENT
MALIBU MOUNTAIN RESCUE TEAM

Team Name: ______ **EQUIPMENT ROSTER** Team Liason: ______

THIS ROW FOR L.A.S.D. USE ONLY — REPORT CONTINUATION	URN		page ____ of ____
Incident Name	Date/Time Prepared		Operational Period
ITEM	QUANTITY ON SITE	QUANTITY OBTAINABLE	STATUS (FOR C.P. USE)
ELT - DF			
LITTER			
BACKBOARD			
ALTIMETER			
RADIOS: Indicate if Handheld or Mobile			
VHF (MRA 155.160)			
VHF (Other Freq.?)			
GENERATOR Watts ____			
RADIO REPEATER:			
VHF (MRA 155.160)			
VHF (Other Freq.)			
UHF			
TENT Capacity			
Capacity			
PORTABLE LIGHTS			
SNOW ANCHORS			
MAP OF AREA			
4X4 VEHICLES			
MMRT 301	Notes:		

FIG. X2.37 Equipment Roster

LOS ANGELES COUNTY SHERIFF'S DEPARTMENT

MALIBU MOUNTAIN RESCUE TEAM

Equipment Check In/Out

THIS ROW FOR L.A.S.D. USE ONLY REPORT CONTINUATION	URN		page ____ of ____
Incident Name	Date/Time Prepared	Operational Period	

Name (Last, First)	Agency	Equipment	SN / Unit #	Check Out Time	Check In Time

ICS 211-E Notes

page____ of____

FIG. X2.38 Equipment Check

Pennsylvania Search and Rescue Council	Daily Communications Log Daily Form 8 of 10		
Incident Name:	Location:	Date*:	For this Date, Page : of:

Local 24 Hr. Time:	Team or Station:	Message:	Location/ Grid Coords.:	Channel:

3/2/92 *Start new set of forms for each 24-hour period, midnight to midnight (1-page form)

FIG. X2.39 Daily Communications Log

ALPINE
RESCUE
TEAM, INC.

COMMUNICATIONS LOG

MISSION: ____________
M.L. ____________ CQ: ________
DATE: ________ PAGE ___ OF ___

TIME	TO	FROM	TRANSMISSION

COMMS LOG REVISED 1/96, MTH

FIG. X2.40 Communications Log

Search & Rescue SHERIFF'S DEPARTMENT SANTA BARBARA COUNTY	MEDICAL REPORT	DR Number	Date
		SAR Number	Location

Name (Last, First, Middle)	Age	D.O.B.	Dispact Time
Address	Sex	Weight	Arrived At Scene
City, State Zip	Phone		Release Time

Complaint/Injuries/Cause

Past History	Allergies
Medications	Private MD

Treatment

Mental Status	Pupils	Speech	Skin
❑ Alert	❑ PERL	❑ Normal	❑ Warm
❑ Concious	❑ Dilated	❑ Silent	❑ Hot
❑ Unconcious	❑ Constricted	❑ Coherent	❑ Cool
❑ Hysterical	❑ Unequal	❑ Incoherent	❑ Cold
❑ Combative	❑ Sluggish	❑ Slurred	❑ Dry
❑ Confused	❑ Eyes Fixed	Breathing	❑ Moist
❑ Oriented	Pulse	❑ Normal	Skin Color
❑ Name	❑ Regular	❑ Shallow	❑ Normal
❑ Place	❑ Irregular	❑ Absent	❑ Cyanotic
❑ Incident	❑ Bounding	❑ Wheezes	❑ Flushed
❑ Time	❑ Weak	❑ Rales	❑ Pale
	❑ None	❑ Rhonchi	❑ Jaundiced

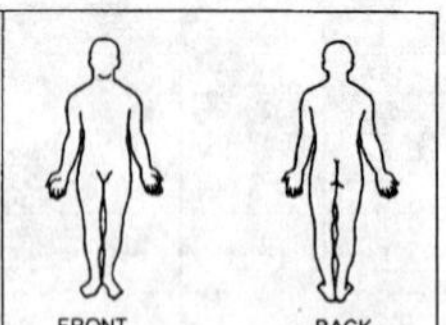

Time							
Pulse							
B.P.							
R.R.							
L.O.C.							

❑ Possible Contagious Disease CPR by ❑ Citizen ❑ EMS ❑ Other

REFUSAL OF SERVICE

I HEREBY RELEASE THE LOS PADRES SEARCH & RESCUE TEAM AND SANTA BARBARA SHERIFF'S DEPARTMENT OF ANY LIABILITY WHICH MAY BE INCURRED DUE TO ANY REFUSAL OF THEIR SERVICES. I HAVE BEEN ADVISED TO SEE A PHYSICIAN OF MY CHOICE.
VICTIM ____________ DATE ____________ WITNESS ____________

TRANSPORTED BY ❑ Ambulance ❑ Helicopter ❑ Private Vehicle ❑ Patient Refused Transport ❑ Cancelled Enroute

FIG. X2.41 Medical Report

Report of Injury	Search & Rescue **SHERIFF'S DEPARTMENT** SANTA BARBARA COUNTY	DR Number
		Operation Number

❑ Operation ❑ Training ❑ Other______	Date Occured

Name	Team

Assignment at Time of Injury

Description of the Incident and the Injury

Treatment at Time of Injury

Witnesses

INSTRUCTIONS
1. If injury results in a loss of work, any medical expenses, or hospitalization, contact the team's SAR Coordinator as soon as possible.
2. Copies of the Report of Injury Form should be sent to the Team's SAR Coordinator and included in the team's Operation Report or Training Report.

Form SH/LP-08-0590

FIG. X2.42 Report of Injury

FEMA US&R RESPONSE SYSTEM
INCIDENT SUPPORT TEAM

PATIENT REFERRAL	INCIDENT	REPORTING UNIT **ESF-9**	FORM **US&R—014** 2/95
DISASTER #:	OPS PERIOD:	DATE/TIME PREPARED:	PREPARED BY:

NAME:	TASK FORCE:
Patient Log #:	Time/Date of referral/admission:
Facility/Hospital:	Phone number:
Referral MD:	Phone & Pager numbers:
Complaint:	
Condition:	
Disposition:	
NAME:	TASK FORCE:
Patient Log #:	Time/Date of referral/admission:
Facility/Hospital:	Phone number:
Referral MD:	Phone & Pager numbers:
Complaint:	
Condition:	
Disposition:	
NAME:	TASK FORCE:
Patient Log #:	Time/Date of referral/admission:
Facility/Hospital:	Phone number:
Referral MD:	Phone & Pager numbers:
Complaint:	
Condition:	
Disposition:	
NAME:	TASK FORCE:
Patient Log #:	Time/Date of referral/admission:
Facility/Hospital:	Phone number:
Referral MD:	Phone & Pager numbers:
Complaint:	
Condition:	
Disposition:	
NAME:	TASK FORCE:
Patient Log #:	Time/Date of referral/admission:
Facility/Hospital:	Phone number:
Referral MD:	Phone & Pager numbers:
Complaint:	
Condition:	
Disposition:	

EMPLOYEE USE ONLY — NOT FOR CIVILIANS

FIG. X2.43 Patient Referral

FEMA US&R RESPONSE SYSTEM
INCIDENT SUPPORT TEAM

NOTICE OF DEATH FORM	INCIDENT	REPORTING UNIT **ESF-9**	FORM **US&R—013** 3/96
DISASTER #:	OPS PERIOD:	DATE/TIME PREPARED:	PREPARED BY:

TASK FORCE:
NAME OF DECEASED: DOB:
POSITION ON TASK FORCE: SS#:

CIRCUMSTANCES OF DEATH:

APPARENT CAUSE OF DEATH:

EXACT LOCATION OF DEATH:

NOTIFICATIONS:	FORMS COMPLETED:
[ ] EST Director	[ ] Local Worker's Comp
[ ] ESF-9 Leader	[ ] Jurisdiction Risk Management
[ ] IST Leader	[ ] Federal Worker's Comp
[ ] ESF-8	[ ] OSHA 200
[ ] Local Police (@ incident site)	[ ] As indicated by local jurisdiction
[ ] OSHA	
[ ] FEMA PIO	
[ ] Chaplain	
[ ] Deceased valuables secured by:	[ ] Location:

CORONER/MEDICAL EXAMINER:
Phone number: Pager number:
TF member assigned as body escort:
Funeral Home:
Phone number:
Location:
TASK FORCE NOTIFICATION PROTOCOLS COMPLETED:

TF ability to continue?

FIG. X2.44 Notice of Death Form

FEMA US&R RESPONSE SYSTEM
INCIDENT SUPPORT TEAM

OPERATING FACILITIES	INCIDENT	REPORTING UNIT ESF-9	FORM US&R—011 2/95
DISASTER #:	OPS PERIOD:	DATE/TIME PREPARED:	UNIT LEADER:
FACILITY NAME	LOCATION	PHONE #	COMMENTS
PREPARED BY:	APPROVED BY:	DATE:	

FIG. X2.45 Operating Facilities

FEMA US&R RESPONSE SYSTEM
INCIDENT SUPPORT TEAM

TIME RECORD	INCIDENT	MISSION NUMBER	REPORTING UNIT ESF-9	FORM US&R—007 2/95

- Employee Name
- Address
- Social Security #
- Position(s) Filled date(s) date(s)
- Sponsoring organization/TF

HOURS ON DUTY

Date	Start Time	Breaks	End Time	Daily Totals
				TOTAL:

IST LEADER DATE

FINANCE SECTION CHIEF DATE EMPLOYEE SIGNATURE DATE

FIG. X2.47 Time Record

Los Padres Search & Rescue	Monthly Time Report	Name: Month/Year:

Date	Start Time	End Time	Hours	Duty Type	Description of Activity

Special Duty Summary

Date	Description

Duty Types	Hours
O — Operations	
T — Training	
C — Committee	
P — Public Relations	
A — Administrative	
S — Special Duty	
TOTAL HOURS	

Monthly Time Reports Are Due At The Monthly Business Meeting Or By The 10th Day Of The Following Month.

Form LP-33-1190 © Los Padres SAR 1990

FIG. X2.46 Monthly Time Report

COUNTY OF LOS ANGELES — SHERIFF'S DEPARTMENT

SEARCH AND RESCUE EXPENDITURE REPORT

DATE   PAGE   OF

CLASSIFICATION	URN (FILE NO.)
CLASSIFICATION	
DATE, TIME, DAY OCCURRENCE STARTED	DATE, TIME, DAY OCCURRENCE ENDED

CODE: V — victim,   I — informant

CODE	NO. OF	LAST NAME	FIRST	MIDDLE	SEX	RACE	AGE	DOB
RESIDENCE ADDRESS			CITY	ZIP	RES. PHONE (AREA CODE)			
CODE	NO. OF	LAST NAME	FIRST	MIDDLE	SEX	RACE	AGE	DOB
RESIDENCE ADDRESS			CITY	ZIP	RES. PHONE (AREA CODE)			
CODE	NO. OF	LAST NAME	FIRST	MIDDLE	SEX	RACE	AGE	DOB
RESIDENCE ADDRESS			CITY	ZIP	RES. PHONE (AREA CODE)			

NOTE: FIELD PERSONNEL ARE TO COMPLETE ITEMIZED LIST OF EQUIPMENT AND PERSONNEL ON REVERSE

FOR BUSINESS OFFICE USE ONLY

PERSONNEL TOTALS

TOTAL PERSONNEL COST .... ______

(SEE REVERSE FOR ITEMIZED LIST)

EQUIPMENT TOTALS

LAND VEHICLE COST .... ______

AIRCRAFT COST .... ______

MISCELLANEOUS EQUIPMENT COST .... ______

TOTAL EQUIPMENT COST .... ______

(SEE REVERSE FOR ITEMIZED LIST)

SUB TOTAL ______

OVERHEAD @ ______ .... ______

TOTAL COST .... ______

LESS CREDIT ALLOWED .... ______

TOTAL NET COST .... ______

PRORATED COST PER VICTIM .... ______
(NET COST — # OF VICTIMS)

ATTACHMENTS:			
	BY DEPUTY		BADGE NO.
	DEPUTY		BADGE NO.
	STATION	UNIT/CAR NO.	SHIFT
	APPROVED	BADGE NO.	TIME
	ASSIGNMENT		

FIG. X2.48 Search and Rescue Expenditure Report

PAGE   OF

REPORT CONTINUATION	URN

ACTIVATED PERSONNEL ROSTER				BUSINESS OFFICE USE ONLY		
NAME	RANK	EMPLOYEE #	HRS.	UNIT CHARGE	COST	TOTAL

EQUIPMENT USAGE ROSTER				BUSINESS OFFICE USE ONLY		
GROUND EQUIPMENT	TYPE	CO. SER. #	HRS./MILES	UNIT CHARGE	COST	TOTAL
AIRCRAFT TYPE	REG. #	CO. SER. #	HRS.	UNIT CHARGE	COST	TOTAL
MISCELLANEOUS EQUIPMENT	TYPE	CO. SER. #	HRS.	UNIT CHARGE	COST	TOTAL

FIG. X2.48 Search and Rescue Expenditure Report *(continued)*

SAR COST REPORT
NEW YORK STATE DEPARTMENT OF ENVIRONMENTAL CONSERVATION
FOREST PROTECTION AND FIRE MANAGEMENT

Supervisor	Date	Regional Ranger	Date	Superintendent	Date

Region ______ Incident Number ______ Incident Name ____________________ Date ________

		NUMBER	HOURS	COST/HOUR	TOTAL COST
PERSONNEL	01 Incident Commander	____	____	$____	$____
	02 Volunteer Firemen	____	____	$____	$____
	03 Certified Members-SAR Team	____	____	$____	$____
	04 Uncertified Members-SAR Team	____	____	$____	$____
	05 DEC Certified Volunteers	____	____	$____	$____
	06 N.Y.S. Police Officers	____	____	$____	$____
	07 DEC Employees				
	.1 Forest Rangers (not I.C.)	____	____	$____	$____
	.2 Other Lands and Forests	____	____	$____	$____
	.3 Operations	____	____	$____	$____
	.4 Encon Police Officers	____	____	$____	$____
	.5 Fish and Game	____	____	$____	$____
	.6 DEC Dispatchers	____	____	$____	$____
	.9 Other	____	____	$____	$____
	08 Other Government Employees				
	.1 Village/City/Town	____	____	$____	$____
	.2 County	____	____	$____	$____
	.3 State	____	____	$____	$____
	.4 Federal	____	____	$____	$____
	09 Civil Air Patrol	____	____	$____	$____
	10 Military	____	____	$____	$____
	11 Volunteer Medical	____	____	$____	$____
	19 Other	____	____	$____	$____
ANIMAL	21 Search Dogs	____	____	$____	$____
	22 Riding Horses	____	____	$____	$____
	23 Draft Animals	____	____	$____	$____
	29 Other	____	____	$____	$____
VEHICLES	31 .1 Two-wheel Drive Pick-ups	____	____	$____	$____
	.2 Four-wheel Drive Pick-ups	____	____	$____	$____
	32 Automobiles	____	____	$____	$____
	33 ATV/Trail Bikes	____	____	$____	$____
	34 Snowmobiles	____	____	$____	$____
	35 .1 Motor driven boats	____	____	$____	$____
	.2 Non-motor driven boats	____	____	$____	$____
	36 Lrg Van/Small Bus (≤16 pass.)	____	____	$____	$____
	37 Large Bus (>16 pass.)	____	____	$____	$____
	39 Other	____	____	$____	$____
AIRCRAFT	41 .1 DEC Helicopters	____	____	$____	$____
	.2 Contract	____	____	$____	$____
	.3 N.Y.S. Police	____	____	$____	$____
	.4 Military	____	____	$____	$____
	.5 Civil Air Patrol	____	____	$____	$____
	.6 Private	____	____	$____	$____
	42 .1 DEC Fixed-wing Aircraft	____	____	$____	$____
	.2 Contract	____	____	$____	$____
	.3 N.Y.S. Police	____	____	$____	$____
	.4 Military	____	____	$____	$____
	.5 Civil Air Patrol	____	____	$____	$____
	.6 Private	____	____	$____	$____
OTHER	51 Food Costs (attach copy of bills)				$____
	52 Equipment Costs (attach copy of bills)				$____
	53 Phone Service (attach copy of bills)				$____

NYS DEC FP&FM 02/90

FIG. X2.49 Cost Sheet

X3. ADDITIONAL FORMS FOR SAR INVESTIGATION

LARIMER COUNTY SEARCH AND RESCUE

LOST PERSON QUESTIONNAIRE

SHORT FORM – OUTLINE FORMAT
based upon NASAR long form by Butch Farabee

INCIDENT:________________________________ DATE:________________

A – SOURCES OF INFORMATION (REPORTING PARTY)

B – LOST PERSON(S) – name, DOB, address, DOW license, etc.

C – PHYSICAL DESCRIPTION

D – TRIP PLANS OF SUBJECT

E – CLOTHING – (equipment on reverse, section J) – scent article ?___ – footprint ?___

F – LAST SEEN – where, when, direction of travel, weather, etc.

G – OUTDOOR EXPERIENCE

FIG. X3.1 Lost Person Questionnaire

H – HABITS / PERSONALITY

I – HEALTH / GENERAL CONDITION

J – EQUIPMENT – (clothing on obverse, section E)

K – CONTACTS SUBJECT WOULD MAKE UPON REACHING CIVILIZATION

L – CHILDRENs REACTIONS and ATTRACTIONS

M – GROUPs OVERDUE – personality interactions, etc.

N – ACTIONS TAKEN SO FAR – by RPs, other agencies

O – MEDIA / FAMILY RELATIONS

P – OTHER INFORMATION

FIG. X3.1 Lost Person Questionnaire *(continued)*

LOS ANGELES COUNTY SHERIFF'S DEPARTMENT
SEARCH AND RESCUE CIRCUMSTANCE

DATE AND TIME OF CALL ____________ FILE NO. ________

VICTIM ____________ NICKNAME (S) ________
(MAKE OUT SEPARATE SHEET FOR EACH VICTIM)

ADDRESS ____________ CITY ________ PHONE ________

SEX ____ RACE ______ AGE ____ HEIGHT ______ WEIGHT ______ BUILD ______ HAIR ______ EYES ______

MARKS/ SCARS ____________ PHOTO AVAIL ( ) SHOES ____________
TYPE COLOR SIZE DIMENSION SOLE AGE

CLOTHING WORN ____________

____________ MONEY CARRIED $ ________

PERSONALITY	ATTITUDE WHEN LAST SEEN	PHYSICAL COND.	SMOKER:	FAMILIARITY WITH AREA	ABILITY IN MTS.
CALM ( )	WORRIED ( )	VERY GOOD ( )	YES ( )	NONE ( )	NONE ( )
NERVOUS ( )	ANGRY ( )	GOOD ( )	NO ( )	SLIGHT ( )	AMATEUR ( )
CAUTIOUS ( )	FRIGHTENED ( )	SICK* ( )	TYPE FILTER ( )	GOOD ( )	GOOD ( )
CARELESS ( )	HAPPY ( )	TIRED ( )	CORK ( )		EXPERT ( )
		WEAK ( )	PLAIN ( )		
		*MEDICINE ______	BRAND ______		

ITEMS CARRIED:
FOOD & CANDY ____________

EQUIPMENT ____________

NUMBER IN PARTY ____ NO. LOST ____ PERSONS W/VICTIM ____________

LAST SEEN (PLACE/DATE) ____________ TIME ________ AM PM

SITUATION	AREA
LOST ( )	TRAIL ( )
FALL ( )	STREAM ( )
STRANDED ( )	RIDGE ( )
INJURED ( )	CANYON ( )
SICK ( )	
DEAD ( )	

DESTINATION ____________

ROUTE OF TRAVEL
FROM ____________ TIME ________ AM PM
TO ____________ TO ARR. ________ AM PM

WAS THERE A CHANGE OF PLANS ____ WHAT ____________

AREA/PLACES VICTIM FAMILIAR WITH ____________

KNOWN FRIENDS ____________

INFORMANT ____________ WAS INFORMANT MEMBER OF PARTY ______

ADDRESS ____________ CITY ________ PHONE ________

NEXT OF KIN ____________ RELATIONSHIP ________

ADDRESS ____________ CITY ________ PHONE ________

NOTE: IF VICTIM IS LOST, SECURE ARTICLE OF CLOTHING FOR TRACKING DOG. CLOTHING MUST HAVE BEEN WORN NEXT TO BODY AND MUST NOT HAVE BEEN LAUNDERED. DO NOT HANDLE, PICK UP WITH FORK OR STICK AND PLACE IN CLEAN PAPER BAG. USE REVERSE SIDE OF FORM FOR REMARKS.

DEPUTY ____________ BADGE ________

MOUNTAINEER ____________

CAR NUMBER ________ DESK ________ STATION ________

765346
SH-R-220 2/82

FIG. X3.2 Search and Rescue Circumstance

Pennsylvania Search and Rescue Council

Incident Missing Person Questionnaire
Incident Form 1 of 5

PENNSYLVANIA PSARC SEARCH & RESCUE COUNCIL

Incident Name: ________ Name of Interviewer: ________ Date/Time Prepared: ________

Interview

Source(s) of information (names and relationships):
(Use back page if needed)
____________ ( ) - (circle one): phone / in person
____________ ( ) - phone / in person

Subject I.D.

Name of missing person: ________ Age, Birthday, other: ________
Local Address: ________
Home Address, if different: ________
Nicknames/Aliases: ________

Description

Height: ____ Weight: ____ Build: ____ Hair Color: ____ Hair Length: ____
Sideburns? Beard? Moustache? Balding? ________
Facial Features/Shape: ________
Distinguishing Marks (scars, etc.): ________
Race/Skin Color and Complexion: ________
General Appearance: ________

Other

Other important information:
____

3/2/92 Page 1 of 6

FIG. X3.3 Incident Missing Person Questionnaire

Incident Missing Person Questionnaire

Clothing

Hat? Color/Style? ____________________
Shirt Color/Style: ____________________
Sweater? Jacket? Style/Color? ____________________
Pants/Skirt: ____________________
Raingear? Gloves or Mittens? ____________________
Sunglasses? Prescription Glasses? ____________________
Shoes: Style, Color, Sole Type? ____________________
Other Clothing? ____________________
Scent Articles Available? Where? ____________________

Equipment

Pack? Brand, Style, color? ____________________
Tent? Color, Type, Brand? ____________________
Sleeping Bag? Color, Type, Brand? ____________________
Water Bottle/Canteen? Color/Type? ____________________
Food? Brands, Amount? ____________________
Flashlight? Brand, Color, Battery Type? ____________________
Matches? Wooden? Paper? Describe: ____________________
Knife? Compass? ____________________
Fishing Equipment? ____________________
Money? Camera/Film/Accessories? ____________________
Firearms? Gauge? Ammunition? ____________________
Ice Axe/Skis/Snowshoes/Poles? ____________________
Other Equipment? ____________________

Trip Plans

Trip Destination and Purpose: ____________________
Planned Route and Alternate? ____________________
Planned Date/Time for Return: ____________________
Group Affiliation? Transportation? ____________________
Trip Starting Point and Time: ____________________
Car Description and Location: ____________________
Alternate Car or Alt. Pickup Plans: ____________________

3/2/92 — Page 2 of 6

FIG. X3.3 Incident Missing Person Questionnaire *(continued)*

Incident Missing Person Questionnaire

Last Seen Details

When? Where? ____________________
by Whom? (Name, Location, Phone): ____________________ ( )
going Which Way? ____________________
Weather? ____________________
Special Reason for Leaving? ____________________
Any Unusual Comments on Leaving? ____________________

Experience

Familiar with the Area? ____________________
Outdoor Experience Level? ____________________
First Aid/Scout/Military? ____________________
Hunting/Backpacking/Climbing? ____________________
Ever been lost before? Where? When? ____________________
Actions when lost before? ____________________
Ever go out alone? ____________________
Stay on trails or go cross-country? ____________________

Contacts

Who would subject contact ____________________ ( ) -
on reaching civilization? ____________________ ( ) -
(Name, Address, Phone) ____________________ ( ) -
Include friends, relatives, ____________________ ( ) -
habitual bars or restaurants ____________________ ( ) -
____________________ ( ) -
____________________ ( ) -

Health

General condition? ____________________
Any physical handicaps or limitations? ____________________
Psychological or psychiatric problems? ____________________
Any medications? Amount carried? ____________________
Consequences of loss? ____________________
Eyesight without glasses/contacts? ____________________
Carry spares? ____________________
Physician/psychiatrist/counselor: ____________________ ( ) -

3/2/92 — Page 3 of 6

FIG. X3.3 Incident Missing Person Questionnaire *(continued)*

Incident Missing Person Questionnaire

Personality

Recreational drugs: ____________________
What type/brand? How much? ____________________
Consequences of withdrawal? ____________________
(include tobacco, alcohol, ____________________
marijuana, cocaine, narcotics, ____________________
prescription drugs) ____________________
Particular outdoor interests? ____________________
(e.g., "likes to follow streams ____________________
because he's a fisherman") ____________________
Job history? ____________________
Recent problems at work ____________________
or school? (confirm with ____________________
co-workers or teachers) ____________________
Relationship with spouse, ____________________
family, or significant other(s)? ____________________
Any recent changes? ____________________
Closest relative? ____________________
Closest other friend/confidant? ____________________
Who had last significant conversation ____________________
with subject? What about? When? __________ ( ) -
Any recent mail that might be relevant? ____________________
Religious preference and beliefs? ____________________
Priest, minister, or other religious ____________________
leader who might provide information? __________ ( ) -
History of problems with law? When? ____________________
Locations where born/raised? ____________________
History of depression? ____________________
Ever run away from home? ____________________
Leader or follower? Give up easily? ____________________
Hole up and wait, or keep going? ____________________
Outgoing or quiet? ____________________
Like to be alone? ____________________
Likely response to searchers? ____________________
Hitch-hike often? ____________________

3/2/92 Page 4 of 6

FIG. X3.3 Incident Missing Person Questionnaire *(continued)*

Incident Missing Person Questionnaire

For Children

Fears: ____________________
Dogs? Horses? Farm animals? ____________________
Wild animals? Darkness? Being alone? ____________________
Training for what to do if lost? ____________________
Actions when hurt: Cry? ____________________
Quiet and withdrawn? ____________________
Temper tantrums? ____________________
Talk to strangers? ____________________
Accept rides? ____________________
Active or passive? ____________________

For Groups

Personality clashes? ____________________
Any leader-types other ____________________
than designated leader? ____________________
How strong were group ____________________
goals (making summit, ____________________
getting to next shelter, ____________________
etc.)? ____________________
What actions would members ____________________
take if separated? ____________________
Names, contact info., ____________________
and experience of ____________________
other members ____________________
(Indicate if need for ____________________
separate MPQ for ____________________
any other members) ____________________

3/2/92 Page 5 of 6

FIG. X3.3 Incident Missing Person Questionnaire *(continued)*

Incident Missing Person Questionnaire

Attach picture(s), boot/shoe prints, and scent articles as appropriate

3/2/92 | Page 6 of 6

FIG. X3.3 Incident Missing Person Questionnaire *(continued)*

Los Padres Search & Rescue Team

LOST PERSON WORKSHEET

Subject Number

INITIAL INFORMATION

Check One ❑ Adult ❑ Juvenile	Officer	Contact
Category ❑ At Risk ❑ Prior Missing ❑ Sexual Exploitation Suspected		
Reporting Agency	Date & Time SAR Called	Case No.

RECORD TYPE

- ❑ Runaway Juvenile
- ❑ Voluntary Missing Adult
- ❑ Parental/Family Abduction
- ❑ Non-Family Abduction
- ❑ Stranger Abduction
- ❑ Dependent Adult
- ❑ Lost
- ❑ Catastrophe
- ❑ Unknown Circumstances

SUBJECT INFORMATION

Name (Last, First, Middle)	Nickname/Alias	Phone
Residence	City	State/Zip
Time Last Seen	Location	
Last Seen By	Direction of Travel	
Destination		
Return Commitment		

TIME DONE

BOL/SO
BOL/PD & CHP
Hospitals
Jail

GENDER	RACE	HGT	WGT	EYE COLOR	HAIR COLOR	D.O.B. / AGE
❑ Male ❑ Female ❑ Unknown	❑ W ❑ C ❑ H ❑ J ❑ B ❑ F ❑ I ❑ O ❑ X			❑ BLK ❑ HAZ ❑ BLU ❑ MAR ❑ BRO ❑ PNK ❑ GRY ❑ MUL ❑ GRN ❑ XXX	❑ BLK ❑ RED ❑ BLN ❑ SDY ❑ BRO ❑ WHT ❑ GRY ❑ XXX Style	

Hat Type	Color	Medical Problem/Illness		Alchohol
Coat		Physical Condition		Drugs
Shirt		Vision	Glasses/Contacts?	Medications
Pants		Vision Without Eyewear		Next Dose?
Jewelry		Hearing	Hearing Aid?	How Long Without?
Shoes		Emotional State		Effects of Missing Dose
Size	Sole	Personality		

Type of Indentification Carried				Drivers License Number/State		SS#
Did Subject Have Money?	How Much?	Means to Get Money				
Vehicle License	State	Year	Make	Style	Color	Registered Owner

SOURCE OF INFORMATION

Name (Last, First, Middle)	Age/D.O.B.	Residence Address	Relation To Subject
Where To Contact	Phone	Interviewed By	Time

FIG. X3.4 Lost Person Worksheet

WILDERNESS TRIPS

Type of Activity	Purpose of Trip	Number Lost	Number In Party
Location of Point Last Seen or Last Known Point		Time	Date
Starting Point/Trailhead		Time	Date
Destination	Has Subject Been There Before?	Time	Date
Intended Route of Travel			
Alternate Plans		Other Vehicle(s) Involved (List)	
Exit Plan		Time	Date

CONTACT AT END OF TRIP

Name	Relation	Phone	Back Up Plan
Address			Contacts Current Location

EQUIPMENT

Maps	Pack	How Many Days Food?
Compass	Sleeping Bag	Type of Food (freeze dried, food bars)
Guidebook	Tent Or Shelter	Snack Foods
Flashlight	Stove	Gum/Candy
Water (How Much?, Container?)	Raingear	Smoker (Brand)
Knife	Climbing Equipment	Other Equipment
Firearm	Camera	

EXPERIENCE

Experience At Activity		Related Skills
Familiarity With Area		Last Time There
Previous Incident/Lost Before		When/Where?
Past Destinations		
Scouting Experience	Medical Training	Would Subject Leave Trail?
Military Experience	Outdoor Training Programs	How Far/Fast Does Subject Hike?

GROUPS

Name of Group/Organization	Type of Group	
Name of Leader	Experience of Leader	Phone Number
Actions if Separated (Planned or Suspected)		
Group Cohesiveness (Splinter Groups, Personality Clashes)		

FIG. X3.4 Lost Person Worksheet *(continued)*

CHILDREN

Afraid Of: ☐ Dark ☐ Animals ☐ Other:	
Feeling Toward Adults	Feeling Toward Strangers
Has Subject Ever Runaway? (When/Where)	Would Subject Get In A Car?
Reactions When Hurt	
Training When Lost	☐ Hug-A-Tree at Age:
Personality (Active, Lethargic, Anti-Social)	

WALKAWAY

Location Last Scene		Time	Date
Seen By Whom?	Location of Witness	Phone	Relation
Direction Going When Last Seen	Suspected Destination	Last Meal	
Knowledge Of Area	Previous Residence Or Address?		
Who Last Talked At Length With Subject?	Where/When?	Topic?	
Any Reason For Leaving?	Did Subject Have Any Complaints?		
Attitude At Time (confident, confused, normal, afraid)		Tired?	Hot/Cold?
Previous Event		Time	Date
Previous Event		Time	Date
Previous Event		Time	Date

ALZHEIMER / WALKER

Glasses/Contacts YES / NO	Description Of Glasses	Ability To See Without Eyewear
Right Or Left Handed	Walking Aids	Describe Walking Ability
Hearing Aid YES / NO	Description	Ability To Hear Without Hearing Aid

General Health	Normal Personality	Personality When Stressed or Upset	Current Medications: Name	Dosage	Frequency	Symptons If Not Taken
☐ Excellent	☐ Stable	☐ Stable				
☐ Good	☐ Changeable	☐ Confused				
☐ Fair	☐ Erratic	☐ Disoriented				
☐ Poor	☐ Violent	☐ Agitated				
	☐ Aggressive	☐ Compulsive				
☐ Weak	☐ Passive	☐ Other				
☐ Strong	☐ Friendly					
	☐ Other					

Familiar Object Subject May Recognize (Describe Photo, Clothing, Object)		
Can Subject Drive?	Describe Any Vehicle To Which Subject Has Access	Would Subject Use Taxi, Bus, Accept a Ride?
Would Subject Relate To A Certain Vehicle (Describe Make/Model/ Color)?		
Would Subject Talk To Strangers?	Would Subject Enter A Store?	Languages Spoken

FIG. X3.4 Lost Person Worksheet *(continued)*

CONFIDENTIAL INFORMATION
NOT FOR RELEASE BY SAR

KNOWN FRIENDS

Name(Last, First, Middle)	Relation To Subject	Age	Where To Contact	Phone ( )
Name(Last, First, Middle)	Relation To Subject	Age	Where To Contact	Phone ( )
Name(Last, First, Middle)	Relation To Subject	Age	Where To Contact	Phone ( )
Name(Last, First, Middle)	Relation To Subject	Age	Where To Contact	Phone
Name(Last, First, Middle)	Relation To Subject	Age	Where To Contact	Phone ( )
Name(Last, First, Middle)	Relation To Subject	Age	Where To Contact	Phone ( )

NEXT OF KIN

Name(Last, First, Middle)	Relation To Subject	Age	Where To Contact	Phone ( )
Name(Last, First, Middle)	Relation To Subject	Age	Where To Contact	Phone ( )
Name(Last, First, Middle)	Relation To Subject	Age	Where To Contact	Phone ( )

SCENT ARTICLE

Contact Name (Last, First, Middle)	Location	Phone ( )

SCENT ARTICLE: Clothing must have been worn next to the body. Bedding such as pillows if not touched by othersIt must not have been washed or handled by any other person. Pick up with a fork or other utensil and put in a clean bag.

DOJ ABBREVIATIONS

RACE		EYE COLOR		HAIR COLOR	
W	White	BLK	Black	BLK	Black
H	Hispanic/Mexican/Latin	BLU	Blue	BLN	Blond
B	Black	BRO	Brown	BRO	Brown
I	American Indian/Alaskan Native	GRY	Gray	GRY	Gray
C	Chinese	GRN	Green	RED	Red
J	Japanese	HAZ	Hazel	SDY	Sandy
F	Filipino	MAR	Maroon	WHT	White
O	All Other/Multi-Race	PNK	Pink	XXX	Unknown
X	Unknown	MUL	Multi-Color		
		XXX	Unknown		

FIG. X3.4 Lost Person Worksheet *(continued)*

ALPINE RESCUE TEAM, INC.

ML QUICK SHEET

MISSION #:______
DATE:______

TIMES	CODE	TYPE	SITUATION	
PAGED:____ ON:____ LOCATED:____ ____ CLEARED:____	☐ 2 ☐ 3	☐ RESCUE ☐ SEARCH ☐ RECOVERY ☐ STAND-BY ☐ OTHER	☐ LOST/OVERDUE ☐ STRANDED ☐ INJURY ☐ ILLNESS ☐ OTHER	ML: CO: COUNTY: MISSION CONTACT:

TEAM PAGE INFORMATION: (LOCATION, RESPONSE & DIRECTIONS)	MAP INFORMATION
	QUADS REQUIRED: COUNTY MAP: FOREST SERVICE MAP:

SUBJECT INFORMATION

NAME:______ AGE:____ SEX:____ D.O.B.____
ADDRESS:______ PHONE #: (H)______ (W)______
MEDICAL HISTORY:______
LAST SEEN POINT:______ OTHER INFORMATION:

REPORTING PARTY

NAME:______ LOCATION:______
PHONE#:______ RELATIONSHIP:______
OTHER INFORMATION:

WEATHER FORECAST

TIME OBTAINED:______ FOR TIME PERIOD:______
WIND:______ DIRECTION:______ PRECIPITATION:______
CLOUD COVER:______ CEILING______
PREDICTED LOW:______ @ PREDICTED HIGH:______ @
AVALANCHE HAZARD:______

QUICK SHEET REVISED

FIG. X3.5 ML Quick Sheet

NOTIFICATION OF SEARCH AND/OR RESCUE

CALLER'S NAME ______ DATE ______

CALLER'S PHONE # ______ TIME ______

INJURED/MISSING PERSON(S): AGE: ADDRESS: RACE:

(1) ______

(2) ______

(3) ______

(4) ______

DATE LAST SEEN ______ TIME LAST SEEN ______ SUBJECT MISSING SINCE ______

LOCATION LAST SEEN ______

INTENDED DESTINATION ______

TYPE OF INJURY (IF APPLICABLE)?

SUBJECT'S DESCRIPTION: Ht Wt Hair Eyes Distinguishing Features

CLOTHING WORN (shirt,pants,jacket,hat,boots/shoes,gloves,etc)?

EQUIPMENT (pack,canteen,rain gear,light,compass,map) INCLUDE COLOR & TYPE!

HIKING EXPERIENCE? HOW MUCH?

VEHICLE DESCRIPTION: LICENSE PLATE NO. ______ STATE ______

MAKE ______ MODEL ______ COLOR ______ YEAR ______

LOCATION OF VEHICLE ______

SUPERVISOR NOTIFIED: (who & time) | RANGERS NOTIFIED: (who & time)

FIG. X3.6 Notification of Search and/or Rescue

URBAN INTERVIEW LOG | 1. INCIDENT NAME | 2. OPERATIONAL PERIOD / DATE | 3.TEAM NUMBER

STREET ADDRESS	RESIDENT CONTACTED	RESIDENT'S NAME	OTHERS AT HOME	PHONE #	HOW LONG HOME	RESIDENT TO CHECK HOME/YARD	SAR CHECKED YARD?	PLACES TO HIDE IN THE AREA	COMMENTS	SUGGEST FOLLOWUP VISIT
	Y N		Y N			Y N	Y N			Y N
	Y N		Y N			Y N	Y N			Y N
	Y N		Y N			Y N	Y N			Y N
	Y N		Y N			Y N	Y N			Y N
	Y N		Y N			Y N	Y N			Y N
	Y N		Y N			Y N	Y N			Y N
	Y N		Y N			Y N	Y N			Y N
	Y N		Y N			Y N	Y N			Y N
	Y N		Y N			Y N	Y N			Y N
	Y N		Y N			Y N	Y N			Y N
	Y N		Y N			Y N	Y N			Y N
	Y N		Y N			Y N	Y N			Y N
	Y N		Y N			Y N	Y N			Y N
	Y N		Y N			Y N	Y N			Y N
	Y N		Y N			Y N	Y N			Y N
	Y N		Y N			Y N	Y N			Y N
	Y N		Y N			Y N	Y N			Y N
	Y N		Y N			Y N	Y N			Y N
	Y N		Y N			Y N	Y N			Y N
	Y N		Y N			Y N	Y N			Y N
	Y N		Y N			Y N	Y N			Y N

ICS ??? BASARC 8/95 | 4. COMPLETED BY

FIG. X3.7 Urban Interview Log

Pennsylvania Search and Rescue Council	**Daily Clue Log** Daily Form 7 of 10	Pennsylvania PSARC Search & Rescue Council

Incident Name:	Date*:	For this Date, Page: of:

Clue #:	Found by Task #:	Map Grid Coordinates:	Clue Description	Action Taken	IC Initials

3/2/92 ***Start new set of forms for each 24-hour period, midnight to midnight** (This is a 1-page form)

FIG. X3.8 Daily Clue Log

Los Padres Search & Rescue	ELT-DF Reports	Case No. / SAR No.

Time | Team | Location
Bearing MAGNETIC | Bearing TRUE | How Taken | Base Line Deviation | Strength
Comments

Time | Team | Location
Bearing MAGNETIC | Bearing TRUE | How Taken | Base Line Deviation | Strength
Comments

Time | Team | Location
Bearing MAGNETIC | Bearing TRUE | How Taken | Base Line Deviation | Strength
Comments

Time | Team | Location
Bearing MAGNETIC | Bearing TRUE | How Taken | Base Line Deviation | Strength
Comments

Time | Team | Location
Bearing MAGNETIC | Bearing TRUE | How Taken | Base Line Deviation | Strength
Comments

Time | Team | Location
Bearing MAGNETIC | Bearing TRUE | How Taken | Base Line Deviation | Strength
Comments

Time | Team | Location
Bearing MAGNETIC | Bearing TRUE | How Taken | Base Line Deviation | Strength
Comments

Time | Team | Location
Bearing MAGNETIC | Bearing TRUE | How Taken | Base Line Deviation | Strength
Comments

Time | Team | Location
Bearing MAGNETIC | Bearing TRUE | How Taken | Base Line Deviation | Strength
Comments

Time | Team | Location
Bearing MAGNETIC | Bearing TRUE | How Taken | Base Line Deviation | Strength
Comments

Page No.

Form LP-15-0990 © Los Padres SAR 1990

FIG. X3.9 ELT-DF Reports

Clue Card

Date________________ Time____________________ Recorded by:________________
Call-back Name & No.:____

Clue Type:____

Information:____

Article:____

Action Taken:____

(Returned to Plans - Date________________)

This form is a standard 3x5 card with the lined side left blank and the other side imprinted using a rubber stamp.

FIG. X3.10 Clue Card

New York State Department of Environmental Conservation
New York State Forest Rangers

Clue Card

Date: date the card was filled out.

Time: time that the card was filled out.

Recorded by: name of the person filling out this card.

Call back name and number: name and phone number of person giving you information or an article.

Clue type:

Information: Any information that has been given to you pertaining to the search, that you feel may be of some value. This would include sightings (include date and time of the sighting), personal habits of the subject, and/or known places where the subject might go.

Article: An article found during the course of your search.

Action Taken: present location and status of articles, and instructions given to the person providing the information.

Returned to Plans: the date/time the card was given to the Planning Section.

FIG. X3.10 Clue Card *(continued)*

LOS ANGELES COUNTY SHERIFF'S DEPARTMENT

MALIBU MOUNTAIN RESCUE TEAM

RELATIVE SEARCH URGENCY RATING FORM

NOTE: Use this form to aid in the justification of additional manpower and equipment requirements. This is not an absolute nor comprehensive system for estimating search urgency but may be helpful as a guideline.

SUBJECT PROFILE

Factor		Factor Value	
AGE	Very young	1	
	Very old	1	
	Other	2-3	____
MEDICAL COND.	Suspected injured/illness	1-2	
	Healthy	3	
	Known Fatality	3	____
NUMBER OF SUBECTS	One alone	1	
	Multiple unseparated	2-3	____
WEATHER	Existing hazardous	1	
	Predicted hazardous, with in 8 hrs. of less	1-2	
	Predicted hazardous, more that 8 hrs.	2	
	No hazardous weather predicted	3	____
EQUIPMENT	Inadequate for environment	1	
	Questionable for environment	1-2	
	Adequate for environment	3	____
SUBJECT EXPERIENCE	Not experienced, does not know area	1	
	Not experienced, knows area	1-2	
	Experienced, does not know area	2	
	Experienced, knows area	3	____
TERRAIN AND HAZARDS	Known hazardous terrain or other hazards	1	
	Few or no hazards	2-3	____
HISTORY OF INCIDENTS	In this area	1-3	____
BASTARD SEARCH		2-3	____

NOTES: The lower the value of each factor and of the sum of all factors, the more urgent the situation. Considerable elapsed time from when the subject was reported missing and the political sensitivity of the circumstances have the effect of increasing the relative urgency.

RESPONSE RATING

Emergency response	08-12	
Measured response	13-18	
Evaluative response	19-24	
Insufficient evidence	25-27	
TOTAL		____

MMRT 302 PREPARED BY (NAME & POSITION)

rev: 10/21/93

FIG. X3.11 Relative Search Urgency Rating Form

Santa Barbara Sheriffs Department

Los Padres Search & Rescue Team

Training Plan

Subject:

Date Submitted:

General Plan:

Skill Areas:

Instructor(s):

Planned Date:

Day of the Week:

Location:

Planned Start Time:

Estimated Finish Time:

Fiscal:

Training Leader:

Form LP-31A-0292 © Los Padres SAR 1992

FIG. X3.12 Training Plan

SANTA BARBARA COUNTY SHERIFF'S DEPARTMENT

DOCUMENTED TRAINING FORM

BUREAU/UNIT/TEAM Los Padres Search & Rescue Team

DATE OF TRAINING HOURS OF TRAINING

LOCATION TRAINED

MEMBERS PRESENT (List K-9 or horse with member if applicable)

FIG. X3.13 Documented Training Form

INSTRUCTOR OR PERSON SUPERVISING

ACTIVITIES TRAINED IN

PERSON COMPLETING FORM DATE

FIG. X3.13 Documented Training Form *(continued)*

LOS ANGELES COUNTY SHERIFF'S DEPARTMENT

MALIBU MOUNTAIN RESCUE TEAM

Training Check-In

Team Name: ______________________________

Team Contact: ______________________________

Phone: ____________________

Address: ____________________

____

(to be used for future updates or changes)

Total Number of Team Participants: __________

Field Personnel: __________

Support Personnel: __________

Expected Team Arrival Time ______________________________

Will you bring Snowmobiles / Snowcat? Number ________________

Any Problems or Concerns with the Training Plan? ________________

____

____

Any special requests to be added to the training?________________

____

____

____

Anything else:

FIG. X3.14 Training Check-in

PMI USAGE & HISTORY

SERIAL NUMBER | I.D. MARKING | LENGTH | DIAMETER

DATE OF MFG. | ISSUE DATE | DATE IN SERVICE

FIBER | COLOR | CONSTRUCTION | MFG'S LOT NUMBER

INSPECT ROPE FOR DAMAGE OR EXCESSIVE WEAR EACH TIME IT IS DEPLOYED AND AGAIN AFTER EACH USE.
IMMEDIATELY RETIRE ALL SUSPECT ROPES.

DATE USED	INCIDENT LOCATION	TYPE OF USE	ROPE EXPOSURE	DATE INSPEC-TED	INSPEC-TORS INITIALS	ROPE CONDITION & COMMENTS

FIG. X3.15 PMI Usage and History

Mission Debriefing Form
Larimer County Search and Rescue

ICS 2001A-1G925/Q.E

MISSION: ______________________ DATE: ______________

IC: ______________________

OPS: ______________________

Time of :

SAR MRG PAGE: ______________
TEAM PAGE: ______________
ON SCENE: ______________
TEAMS IN FIELD: ______________
SUBJECT FOUND: ______________
DEBRIEFING: ______________

Subject Status:

When Found: ______________
Last Reported: ______________

Number of :

LCSAR members responding: __________
Other resources: __________

Total :
Team hours: __________
man hours: __________

Equipment damaged:

Owner: ______________
What: ______________
How: ______________
Est Cost: ______________

FIG. X3.16 Mission Debriefing Form

Issues:

Response:

Field Assignments:

Safety:

Other:

For each issue identified

A) Will be discussed at next team meeting (SAR MGR/FIELD Coordinator)

or

B) Will be assigned to an individual team member, results/actions reviewed at team/sa manager/exec meeting.

FIG. X3.16 Mission Debriefing Form *(continued)*

Colorado Division of Wildlife

MISSION REPORT

Colorado Search & Rescue Board

County(where mission occur'd) LARIMER Co. Case #:______ AFRCC #:______
Unit Submitting Report: LARIMER COUNTY SEARCH AND RESCUE TEAM Unit Msn #:______ Other #:______
Primary unit (this mission): LCSAR Where incident occurred:______ Incident Commander:______
Mission started: Date:______ Time:______

SUBJECT INFORMATION

	Name	Sex	DOB	Street address	Town	State	CDOW lic.(atch'd)
A							
B							
C							

INCIDENT DATA

ACTIVITY: ○Climber ○Hiker ○Hunter ○Fisherman ○Skier ○Bicycle ○Boat ○OHV ○Snowmobile ○Aircraft ○Walkaway ○Evid. search ○Other

SITUATION: ○Lost/overdue ○Stranded ○Injury ○Illness ○Public service ○Other

DESCRIPTION OF INCIDENT

RESPONSE

RESPONSE TYPE: Standby, Responded, Search, Rescue, Recovery, Other; Land, Air, Water

(If lost) SEARCH TECHNIQUES USED: Confinement, Attraction, Hasty search, Visual tracking, Search dogs, Line search, Air search, Other

RESCUE/RECOVERY TECHNIQUES USED: Assist/own power, Carry-out by foot, Rock/scree evac., Evac. by animal, Watercraft evac., Vehicle evac., Aircraft evac., Other

DESCRIPTION OF RESPONSE

RESULTS

SUBJECT WAS FOUND/RESCUED Date:______ Time:______ ○By SAR effort ○By public (non-SAR) ○By self ○Never needed help ○Not found/rescued ○Other

REASON TERMINATED: Successful, Lack manpower, Lack equipment, Lack support, Lack clues, Hazardous terrain, Severe weather, Area too large, Authority decision, Family decision, Other______

(If lost)FOUND IN: Primary search area, Secondary search area, Area previously searched, Out of area, Home, bar, motel, etc, Other

CLUES FOUND BY / SUBJECT FOUND BY: Interrogation, Confinement, Attraction, Hasty search, Visual tracking, Search dogs, Line search, Helicopter, Fixed Wing, Subject's signal, Other

As a result of the SAR effort, Total number of persons: ___ Found, ___ Rescued, ___Saved

DESCRIPTION OF FIND/RESCUE:

MEDICAL

EXTENT OF INJURIES (A B C): ○○○Uninjured ○○○Slight/1st aid ○○○Moderate/Dr. ○○○Severe/Hospital ○○○Fatal

SUBJECT BEHAVIOR

CAUSE OF INCIDENT: Unknown, Human error(self), Another person, Darkness, Environment/wx, Falling object, Equipment failure, Other

(If lost) REASON(s): Unknown, Poor supervision, Accidental separation, Intentional separation, Took short cut, Poor/no map, Disoriented, Misjudge time/distance

(If injury) REASON(s): Unknown, Haste, Exceeded ability, Fatigue, Fall or slip, Inadeq. equip., Anchor/belay fail'd, Other

(If lost)-Travel Data: Air distance from last seen pt. (miles) ☐; Elevation change from last seen pt to where found (feet) ☐ ○Up ○Down ○Same elev; Time Moving(hrs): ☐ ○ Day ○ Night ○ Both

FIG. X3.17 Mission Report

Do you want to submit this mission/report for reimbursement from the Search and Rescue Fund? If so, please be sure to complete the license information on the front, fill in all relevant cost information and attach necessary receipts, etc. ○Yes ○No

RESOURCES

EQUIPMENT INVOLVED AND COSTS

No.		Mi/Hrs	Costs
___	Helicopters	___	___
___	Fixed Wing	___	___
___	Ambulances	___	___
___	2WD Vehicles	___	___
___	4WD Vehicles	___	___
___	Power Boats	___	___
___	Snowmobiles	___	___
___	Horses	___	___
___	Dogs	___	___

(Attach all receipts) (includes fuel, repairs, etc.)

Equipment Cost Subtotal ☐

MANHOURS SUMMARY

Total no. of your personnel involved ______
Total manhours expended by your unit ______
Total no. of ALL personnel involved ______
Total manhours expended by ALL personnel ______

MISCELLANEOUS COSTS (attach all receipts/documentation)

Motel(s) ______
Food/Meals ______
Personal Equipment ______ (Ropes, 1st aid, batteries, gloves, clothing, etc.)
Other misc costs: ______ (list on separate sheet)

Miscellaneous costs subtotal ☐

Total cost : ☐

OTHER SAR UNITS INVOLVED

	Unit Name	No.
1)		
2)		
3)		
4)		
5)		
6)		

AUTHORIZATION

I certify that the above report and listing of expenses is true and correct. I have attached all applicable receipts and understand that I am responsible for disbursement of monies to all agencies or groups that assisted in this search and rescue incident.

REQUEST/MISSION REPORT PREPARED BY: ______ Name Rank Telephone Date

REQUEST APPROVED BY: ______ (Sheriff's signature required for reimbursement) Date

MAKE CHECKS PAYABLE TO: ______ Name
______ Street address
______ City, State, Zip code

SAR FUND RECEIPT/APPROVAL

DO NOT USE
REQUEST RECEIVED: ______ Date BY: ______ Name
REQUEST APPROVED: ______ Date BY: ______ Name

FIG. X3.17 Mission Report *(continued)*

COUNTY OF LOS ANGELES
SHERIFF'S DEPARTMENT
MALIBU MOUNTAIN RESCUE TEAM

RECORDS AND STATISTICS BUREAU USE ONLY

INCIDENT REPORT DATE page of

ACTION ACTIVE ☐ INACTIVE ☐ | INDEX INFO YES ☐ NO ☐ | MMRT Operation # | URN (FILE No.)

CLASSIFICATION RESCUE: Vehicle Over ☐ Missing Person ☐ Injured Person ☐ Stranded Hiker ☐

CLASSIFICATION Disaster ☐ Recovery ☐ Other ☐

DATE, TIME, DAY BEGIN | DATE, TIME, DAY END | STATION COORDINATOR

LOCATION OF OCCURENCE | TYPE OF LOCATION | TAG #

CODE: V - victim, W - witness, I - informant P - patient list one victim (if named) and the informant on this page

CODE No OF | LAST NAME | FIRST | MIDDLE | SEX | RACE | DOB | CHECK DAY PHONE
RESIDENCE ADDRESS | CITY | ZIP | RES PHONE ( )
BUSINESS ADDRESS | CITY | ZIP | BUS PHONE ( )

CODE No OF | LAST NAME | FIRST | MIDDLE | SEX | RACE | DOB | CHECK DAY PHONE
RESIDENCE ADDRESS | CITY | ZIP | RES PHONE ( )
BUSINESS ADDRESS | CITY | ZIP | BUS PHONE ( )

CODE No OF | LAST NAME | FIRST | MIDDLE | SEX | RACE | DOB | CHECK DAY PHONE
RESIDENCE ADDRESS | CITY | ZIP | RES PHONE ( )
BUSINESS ADDRESS | CITY | ZIP | BUS PHONE ( )

NAME	EMP #	ASSIGNMENT	TIME IN	TIME OUT	HOURS
PAGER CALL-OUT CODE:				Total Hours:	

MODE	SEARCH	RESCUE	SYSTEM	ASSISTING UNITS	ASSISTED
Obs ☐	Missing person ☐	Injured Person ☐	Truck and Winch ☐	Other LASD Teams ☐	Other LASD Teams ☐
Detail ☐	Lost Person ☐	Vehicle Over ☐	Hike in / Hike out ☐	Outside Agencies ☐	Outside Agencies ☐
Call ☐	Evidence ☐	Cliffhanger ☐	Helicopter ☐	Fire ☐	Fire ☐
Patrol ☐	Homicide ☐	Medical Aid ☐	Technical ☐	State Parks ☐	State Parks ☐
Callout ☐	Aircraft ☐	Disaster ☐	Litter ☐	National Parks ☐	National Parks ☐
Cancelled ☐	Other ☐	Other ☐	Other ☐	Other ☐	Other ☐

VEHICLE USED IN CRIME YES ☐ NO ☐ UNKNOWN ☐ STORED ☐ IMPOUNDED ☐ | YR | MAKE | BODY TYPE | COLOR | BY DEPUTY | BADGE No

LICENSE (STATE & No) | V I N /FRAME No | DEPUTY | BADGE No

REGISTERED OWNER | STATION LOST HILLS/MALIBU | UNIT/CAR No 220R | SHIFT

IDENTIFYING CHARACTERSTICS | APPROVED | BADGE No | TIME

CHP 180 SUBMITTED YES ☐ NO ☐ | GARAGE NAME & PHONE | ASSIGNMENT LOST HILLS STATION RESERVE COORDINATOR

ATTACHMENTS ☐ ICS 201 ☐ ICS 202 ☐ ICS 204 ☐ ICS 211E ☐ ICS 211P ☐ ICS 211M ☐ ICS 214L ☐ ICS 209 | SPECIAL REQUEST DISTRIBUTION ESD RFB

☐ ____________ ☐ ____________ | TT B/C BY | DATE | TIME | SECTY

mmrt320 doc SAR-49 (11/26/93)

FIG. X3.18 Incident Report

COUNTY OF LOS ANGELES - SHERIFF'S DEPARTMENT
INCIDENT REPORT CONTINUATION | URN: | PAGE OF

STATISTICAL INFORMATION

CLASSIFICATION	# of Vict	# of Surv	# of Fatal	# of Miss or Unk	RESOURCES USED	# of Units or People	# of Hours of Work	MUTUAL AID REND # of Units or People	MUTUAL AID REND # of Hours of Work	MUTUAL AID REC'D # of Units or People	MUTUAL AID REC'D # of Hours of Work
HUNTERS					PAID DEPUTIES						
FISHERMAN					RESERVE DEPUTIES						
BACKPACKERS/HIKERS					CIVILIAN VOLUNTEERS						
CAMPERS					CO.OWNED HELICOPTERS						
CLIMBERS					CO. OWNED FIXED WING						
MOTORCYCLISTS					FEDERAL HELICOPTER						
MINES AND CAVES					FEDERAL FIXED WING						
SWIMMERS					STATE HELICOPTER						
SNOWSPORTS					STATE FIXED WING						
AIRCRAFT					PRIVATE HELICOPTER						
RAFTERS					PRIVATE FIXED WING						
VEHICLES					4X4 VEHICLE						
OTHERS					SNOW MOBILE						
TRAINING					SEARCH DOGS						
					HORSES						
					GROUND VEHICLES						

NARRATIVE

mmrt320s doc SAR-49 (10/21/93)

FIG. X3.18 Incident Report *(continued)*

Pennsylvania Search and Rescue Council	**Incident After Action Report** Incident Form 5 of 5	Pennsylvania PSARC Search & Rescue Council

Incident Name:		*Date/Time* Prepared:*
AFRCC Mission No.:	*State Mission No.:*	*Base Location:*

Mission Type/Extent

☐ *Missing Person* ☐ *Missing/Overdue Vessel* ☐ *Other:*
☐ *Missing/Overdue Aircraft* ☐ *Drowning*
☐ *ELT/EPIRB* ☐ *Cave Rescue*

Mission Started:	*Mission* ☐ *Closed or* ☐ *Suspended*
Date/ Time:*	*Date/ Time*:*

Locating and Medical Data

Objective Located by (Name/Organization):

Date/ Time:*		*Geographic Location:*	
Latitude/ Longitude:			
No. Subjects Involved:	*No. Subjects Found Alive:*	*No. Subjects Found Dead:*	*No. Subjects Still Missing:*

Remarks (include specific injury or illness and name of medical facility accepting any subjects):

Participating Organizations

Prepared by:	*Approved by (Incident Commander):*

3/2/92 *local time, 24 hour format Page 1 of 2

FIG. X3.19 Incident After Action Report

Incident After Action Report

Personnel/Equipment

Aircrew Personnel:*	*Ground Personnel*:*	*Non-SAR Tm. Volunteers*:*	*Other Personnel*:*
Staff Personnel:*	*Dogs:*	*Total Estimated Monhours:*	
Fixed-Wing Aircraft:	*Helicopters:*	*Ground Vehicles:*	*Boats:*
Other Equipment:			

Operational Summary - Air

No. of Air Sorties:	*Hours in Search Area:*	*Hours Enroute:*	*Total Flight Hrs.:*	*No. of Sq. Miles Searched:*

Summary of Grids/Areas Searched:

Operational Summary - Ground

No. of Ground Tasks:	*Vehicle Miles on Tasks:*	*Vehicle Miles Enroute:*	*Total Estimated Vehicle Miles:*

Summary of Areas Searched:

3/2/92 *For Personnel numbers, estimate total number of people involved in this role at any time during operation. Page 2 of 2

FIG. X3.19 Incident After Action Report *(continued)*

HMPART SRVY SAM 3/94

MOUNTAIN RESCUE

Mutual Aid Response Survey
A.R.T. HQ during missions: 526-2432

ALPINE RESCUE TEAM, INC.

POST OFFICE BOX 934
EVERGREEN, COLORADO 80439
(303) 526-2417

Mission: ____________________
Location: ____________________
Mission Leader: ____________________ ART #: ______________ Date: ______________

We are very happy we were recently able to provide mountain search and rescue assistance to your agency. How well we do in meeting the needs of the victim(s), and your agency, is important to us. It helps us learn what is needed to constantly improve our operations, and tells us what we are doing right. Please take two minutes right now to complete this survey, and mail back to us in the enclosed envelope. Thanks for your help.

(5 = excellent 4 = good 3 = average 2 = needs improvement 1 = let's talk! n/a = not applicable)

Pre-response						
Ease of contacting Clear Creek S.O.	5	4	3	2	1	n/a
General ease of dispatching team	5	4	3	2	1	n/a
Rapidness of S.O. dispatch	5	4	3	2	1	n/a
Pre-response mission review/briefing w/A.R.T.	5	4	3	2	1	n/a
Standing mutual aid protocols	5	4	3	2	1	n/a
Enroute						
Ease of radio communication with team	5	4	3	2	1	n/a
Updates passed back and forth	5	4	3	2	1	n/a
Rapidness of team response	5	4	3	2	1	n/a
Team and personal vehicle operations	5	4	3	2	1	n/a
Mission Operations						
Unified (or joint) Command operations	5	4	3	2	1	n/a
Turn over of command (if done)	5	4	3	2	1	n/a
Use of ICS	5	4	3	2	1	n/a
Number of A.R.T. personnel on scene	5	4	3	2	1	n/a
A.R.T.'s medical care of patient	5	4	3	2	1	n/a
Our acceptance of your assignments	5	4	3	2	1	n/a
Appropriateness of our overhead assignments of your personnel	5	4	3	2	1	n/a
Appropriateness of our field assignments of your personnel	5	4	3	2	1	n/a
Our direction of your personnel	5	4	3	2	1	n/a
Our overall use of your agency personnel & equipment	5	4	3	2	1	n/a
Overall cooperation of A.R.T. and your agency	5	4	3	2	1	n/a
Overall cooperation of all individuals	5	4	3	2	1	n/a
Post Mission						
Debriefing (on scene)	5	4	3	2	1	n/a
Mission follow-up (if needed)	5	4	3	2	1	n/a

☐ **Please contact me immediately regarding this mission.**

Name: ______________________________ Title: ______________
Agency: ____________________ Position/function during this mission: ______________
Day phone: ____________________ Night phone: ______________

Please use the back to offer any comments in regard to any portion of this mission.

A volunteer organization dedicated to saving lives through rescue and mountain safety education

FIG. X3.20 Mutual Aid Response Survey

FEMA US&R RESPONSE SYSTEM
URBAN SEARCH & RESCUE TASK FORCE 7/92

TASK FORCE LEADER'S MISSION ASSIGNMENT CHECKLIST

[ ] ASSIGNED LOCALITY/JURISDICTION: ____

[ ] TYPE OF ICS STRUCTURE IN PLACE: ____

[ ] TFL's IMMEDIATE SUPERVISOR (title/name): ____

[ ] ICP OR SUPERVISOR'S LOCATION: ____

[ ] PLNNG/BRFING MEETINGS SCHEDULE/LOCATION: ____

[ ] CURRENT SITUATION: ____

[ ] SEARCH & RESCUE ISSUES: ____
- [ ] TYPE OF AREA INVOLVED: ____
- [ ] PRIORITY BLDGs. (schools/hospitals/etc.): ____
- [ ] NUMBER/LOCATION OF KNOWN VICTIMS: ____

[ ] LOCAL MEDICAL SYSTEM: ____
- [ ] FUNCTIONING EMS/HOSPITALS?: ____
- [ ] MILITARY/DMAT TEAMS?: ____
- [ ] VICTIM HAND-OFF PROCEDURES: ____
- [ ] MEDEVAC OF INJURED TF MEMBER?: ____
- [ ] VETERINARY RESOURCES?: ____

[ ] COMMUNICATIONS PLAN: ____
- [ ] FREQUENCY ASSIGNMENT: ____
- [ ] REPORTING TYPE/SCHEDULE: ____
- [ ] LOCAL JURISDICTION's RADIO ASSIGNED TO TF?: ____

[ ] TRANSPORTATION: ____
- [ ] TRUCKS/BUSES: ____
- [ ] AIRCRAFT/HELICOPTERS: ____
- [ ] REQUESTING PROCEDURES: ____

[ ] TF SUPPORT: ____
- [ ] BASE OF OPS LOCATION?: ____
- [ ] SUPPLY AVAILABILITY (food/water/equip.): ____
- [ ] HEAVY EQUIPMENT/CRANES: ____
- [ ] LOCAL/MILITARY SECURITY SUPPORT: ____
- [ ] REQUEST PROCEDURES: ____

[ ] MEDIA ISSUES: ____
- [ ] LOCAL JURISDICTION PIO (title/name): ____
- [ ] PROCEDURES (info release/interviews/etc.) ____

FIG. X3.21 Task Force Leader's Mission Assignment Checklist

FEMA US&R RESPONSE SYSTEM
URBAN SEARCH & RESCUE TASK FORCE 7/92

TASK FORCE BASE OF OPERATIONS LOCATION CHECKLIST

[ ] SITE LOCATION/ADDRESS: ____

[ ] BEST ACCESS ROUTE(S): ____

[ ] DISTANCE TO ANTICIPATED WORK SITES: ____

[ ] ADEQUATE SPACE AVAILABLE? ____

[ ] PERSONNEL SHELTER CONSIDERATIONS: ____
- [ ] USEABLE STRUCTURES? [ ] TENTS REQUIRED?

[ ] CACHE SHELTER CONSIDERATIONS: ____
- [ ] USEABLE STRUCTURES? [ ] TENTS REQUIRED?

[ ] RADIO COMMUNICATIONS CONSIDERATIONS: ____
(high ground is usually more advantageous)

[ ] SITE SAFETY/SECURITY: ____
- [ ] Any tall adjacent buildings/utilities creating hazard?
- [ ] Terrain with regard to rain/water runoff?
- [ ] Site appropriately separated from rescue work sites?
- [ ] Security assistance request from military/local jurisdiction?
- [ ] Haz mat/exposure concerns

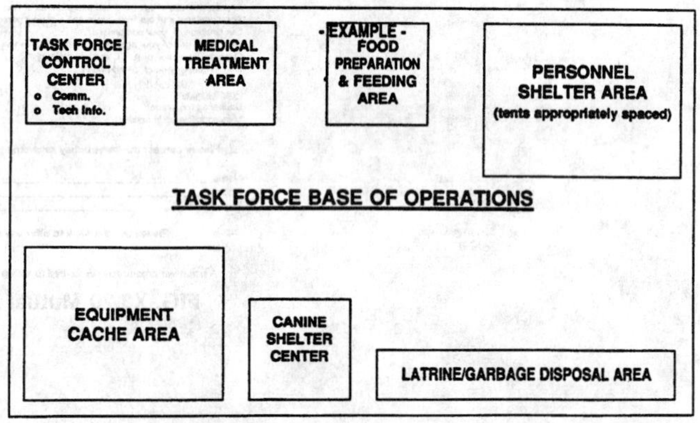

FIG. X3.22 Task Force Base of Operations Location Checklist

FEMA US&R RESPONSE SYSTEM
URBAN SEARCH & RESCUE TASK FORCE 7/92

TASK FORCE OPERATIONS REPORT

TASK FORCE DESIGNATION: ____________________

DATE: ____________________

START TIME: __________ COMPLETION TIME: __________

TF TEAM: __________ TEAM MANAGER: __________

TEAM/SQUAD MEMBERS:

1 __________ 2 __________
3 __________ 4 __________
5 __________ 6 __________
7 __________ 8 __________
9 __________ 10 __________

OPERATIONS SITE: ADDRESS: __________
SECTOR: __________

DESCRIPTION OF OPERATION: ____________________

COMMENTS/EVALUATIONS/RECOMMENDATIONS: ____________________

TEAM LEADER/SQUAD OFFICER: ____________________
Signature

FIG. X3.23 Task Force Operations Report

FEMA US&R RESPONSE SYSTEM
URBAN SEARCH & RESCUE TASK FORCE 7/92

TASK FORCE OPERATIONS SITE SKETCH

SIDE THREE

SIDE TWO

SIDE FOUR

SIDE ONE

TYPE OF OPERATION: ____________________

DEPICT:

[ ] BUILDING/STRUCTURE(s) [ ] SECTORS (team/squad assignments)
[ ] OPERATIONS POST [ ] MEDICAL TREATMENT AREA
[ ] EQUIPMENT STAGING AREA [ ] PERSONNEL STAGING AREA
[ ] ACCESS/ENTRY ROUTES [ ] CRIBBING/SHORING WORK AREA
[ ] CONTROL ZONES (Collapse/Hazard Zones, Work Zones, etc.)
[ ] PERSONNEL HAZARDS (Live Utilities, Haz Mat, Collapse Potentials, etc.)

EMERGENCY SIGNALLING

o EVACUATE THE AREA — 3 short blasts (one second each)
o CEASE OPERATIONS/ALL QUIET — 1 long blast (three seconds)
o RESUME OPERATIONS — 1 long and 1 short blast

FIG. X3.24 Task Force Operations Site Sketch

FEMA US&R RESPONSE SYSTEM
Appendix D
STRUCTURE TRIAGE, ASSESSMENT & MARKING SYSTEM

STRUCTURE TRIAGE

STRUCTURE TRIAGE EVALUATION • DATE/TIME PG of

MAP OF AREA
(PAGE 1 ONLY)

TEAM & S. SP.

UHR-2a

	TRIAGE CRITERIA	SCORE
BLDG I.D.	1. POTENTIAL NO. OF TRAPPED ÷ 5 (MIN = 1 MAX = 50)	
FLOOR AREA		
STORIES	2. CONDITION OF VOIDS 1 VERY COMPACT — SEPARATE LAYERS — PART COLLAPSE → 20	
OCCUPANCY	3. TIME GET TO VICTIM 1 ONE DAY — 2 HRS → 20	
MATERIAL (CIRCLE ONE) W C S URM PC	4. CHANCE OF COLLAPSE -1 LOW CHANCE — HI CHANCE → -20	
CACULATE AREA & NO. TRAPPED	5. SPECIAL INFO: SCHOOL / HOSPITAL = +25; KNOWN LIVE VICTIM = +5 EA	
	6. NO-GO: (CIRCLE ONE) FIRE HM ZERO VICTIMS OTHER (IF NO-GO PROBLEM IS FOUND, ENTER ZERO FOR BLDG TOTAL)	BLDG TOTAL

	TRIAGE CRITERIA	
BLDG I.D.	1. POTENTIAL NO. OF TRAPPED ÷ 5 (MIN = 1 MAX = 50)	
FLOOR AREA		
STORIES	2. CONDITION OF VOIDS 1 VERY COMPACT — SEPARATE LAYERS — PART COLLAPSE → 20	
OCCUPANCY	3. TIME GET TO VICTIM 1 ONE DAY — 2 HRS → 20	
MATERIAL (CIRCLE ONE) W C S URM PC	4. CHANCE OF COLLAPSE -1 LOW CHANCE — HI CHANCE → -20	
CACULATE AREA & NO. TRAPPED	5. SPECIAL INFO: SCHOOL / HOSPITAL = +25; KNOWN LIVE VICTIM = +5 EA	
	6. NO-GO: (CIRCLE ONE) FIRE HM ZERO VICTIMS OTHER (IF NO-GO PROBLEM IS FOUND, ENTER ZERO FOR BLDG TOTAL)	BLDG TOTAL

	TRIAGE CRITERIA	
BLDG I.D.	1. POTENTIAL NO. OF TRAPPED ÷ 5 (MIN = 1 MAX = 50)	
FLOOR AREA		
STORIES	2. CONDITION OF VOIDS 1 VERY COMPACT — SEPARATE LAYERS — PART COLLAPSE → 20	
OCCUPANCY	3. TIME GET TO VICTIM 1 ONE DAY — 2 HRS → 20	
MATERIAL (CIRCLE ONE) W C S URM PC	4. CHANCE OF COLLAPSE -1 LOW CHANCE — HI CHANCE → -20	
CACULATE AREA & NO. TRAPPED	5. SPECIAL INFO: SCHOOL / HOSPITAL = +25; KNOWN LIVE VICTIM = +5 EA	
	6. NO-GO: (CIRCLE ONE) FIRE HM ZERO VICTIMS OTHER (IF NO-GO PROBLEM IS FOUND, ENTER ZERO FOR BLDG TOTAL)	BLDG TOTAL

7/92

FIG. X3.25 Structure Triage

X4. MISCELLANEOUS SAR FORMS

LOS ANGELES COUNTY SHERIFF'S DEPARTMENT
MALIBU MOUNTAIN RESCUE TEAM

Public Information Summary - Incident Status

THIS ROW FOR L A S D USE ONLY REPORT CONTINUATION	URN	page ____ of ____
Incident Name	Date/Time Prepared	Operational Period

An Information Summary should be completed for Incident updates and Public Information.

1 Incident Name
2 Type
3 Cause
4 Location
5 Incident Manager
6 Start Time
7 Close Time
8 Areas Involved
9 Resorces Commited
10 Casualties
Personnel
Public
11 Damage Estimates
12 Warnings
Expected Hazards
Location
Type
Period
13 Weather
Current
Forecast
14 Areas Evacuated
15 Shelter Centers
16 Hospital Contact
17 Road Status
18 Misc
19 PIO
Phone Numbers
Location

ICS 209 Prepared by:

tpm\mmrt\forms\ics209.doc rev: 10/07/93

FIG. X4.1 Public Information Summary—Incident Status

Los Angeles County Sheriff's Department
MALIBU MOUNTAIN RESCUE TEAM

INTRA AGENCY REGISTRATION FORM

Rescue Member Name ____________________

Agency / Rank ____________________

Call Sign (if applicable) ____________________

Time frame that you are available ____________________

____

QUALIFICATIONS

Technical Rescue	____________	Heavy, Medium, Light, No Exposure
Medical 1st Aid	____________	MD, EMT-P, II, I, ARC, etc.
Climbing Skills	____________	Yosemite Rating, 5.4, 5.12d, etc.
Tracking Skills	____________	T1 - T7, or use words
Winter Training	____________	Heavy, Medium, Light, No Exposure
Operation Leader	____________	Heavy, Medium, Light, No Exposure
Snow Travel Ability	____________	Sno-Shoes, Skis, Crampons
Desert Operations	____________	Heavy, Medium, Light, No Exposure
Do you have gear for 48 hour stay in field	________	Yes, or No
Do you have gear for 24 hour stay in field	________	Yes, or No
Do you have a Personal Radio	________	Type and Frequencies
Are you Light Gear Ready (<20 lbs Search Only)	____	Yes or No
Are you familiar with search area (if applicable)	____	Yes or No

Point of contact for Emergency or Message ____________________

____

Do you have any Limitations or Restrictions ____________________

____

Size of your Shoe __________ Do you Smoke __________

FIG. X4.2 Intra-Agency Registration Form

SAR Call Out List: CURRENT DATE

AGENCY EMERGENCY COMMUNICATION TELEPHONE NUMBERS
PAGING TERMINAL TELEPHONE NUMBER/ SPECIAL RESCUE RESPONSE CALLBACK NUMBER
SEARCH DOG DISPATCH PAGER NUMBER

VEHICLE and EQUIPMENT CACHE Combination Lock/Access Numbers
EMERGENCY MANAGERS RADIO CALL SIGN

Time/ Date: ____________________

Incident Name: ____________________

Case #: ____________________

IC: ____________________

OPS: ____________________

PLANS/LOGS: ____________________

Vehicle Drivers: ____________________

Response Type: ____________________

Resources: ____________________

Directions: ____________________

Subject Info: ____________________

Scent Articles: ____________________

Track Age: ____________________

Weather: ____________________

Yes	No	NA	Nxt	Rating	Expt	Name	Home	Work	Page	Call	Medical	Special

OTHER COMMONLY USED EMERGENCY NUMBERS:
Air Force Rescue Coordination Center (AFRCC, Langley AFB): 1-800-xxx-xxxx

FIG. X4.3 Call-out List

X5. FORM PACKET

Figure	Forms
Fig. 1	SAR Incident Report
Fig. 2	Non-segmented Areas
Fig. 3	Search Clue Log
Fig. 4	Relevance of Clue
Fig. 5	"POD" End of Shift Report
Fig. 6	SAR Questionnaire A & B
Fig. 7	Search Initiation Log
Fig. 8	Incident Briefing
Fig. 9	Incident Objectives
Fig. 10	Organization Assignment List
Fig. 11	Task Assignment
Fig. 12	Radio Communications Plan
Fig. 13	Medical Plan
Fig. 14	Incident Organization Chart
Fig. 15	Incident Status Summary
Fig. 16	Check-in List
Fig. 17	Unit Log
Fig. 18	Operational Planning Worksheet
Fig. 19	SAR Injury Report
Fig. 20	Liability Release
Fig. 21	Emergency Helicoptor Request Information Sheet
Fig. 22	ICS Planning Guide

Standard Guide for
Using Whistle Signals During Rope Rescue Operations[1]

This standard is issued under the fixed designation F 1768; the number immediately following the designation indicates the year of original adoption or, in the case of revision, the year of last revision. A number in parentheses indicates the year of last reapproval. A superscript epsilon (ε) indicates an editorial change since the last revision or reapproval.

1. Scope

1.1 This guide covers the methodology for the use of whistles as a means of communication during rope rescue operations.

1.2 *This standard does not purport to address all of the safety concerns, if any, associated with its use. It is the responsibility of the user of this standard to establish appropriate safety and health practices and determine the applicability of regulatory limitations prior to use.*

2. Terminology

2.1 There are no terms in this guide that require new or other than dictionary definitions.

3. Significance and Use

3.1 Whistle signals are a simple and effective means of communication between rescuers and those operating a roperaising or rope-lowering system. They may be used as a primary means of communication or as a backup when radios fail or when ambient noise makes them unintelligible.

3.2 These same signals can be used in non-rescue situations, for example, by persons rappelling in caves.

4. Procedure

4.1 Using a whistle device, or method, with enough volume to be audible over ambient noise and for the distances involved, use the following pattern of whistle blasts to signal the required action:

4.1.1 **Stop,** *1 Long Whistle Blast*—Used to stop all movement until further instructions.

4.1.2 **Up,** *2 Short Whistle Blasts*—Means something or somebody is moving up or requires to be moved up. On horizontal systems it would indicate movement of the load towards the anchor or hauling system.

4.1.3 **Down,** *3 Short Whistle Blasts*—Means something or somebody is moving down or requires to be moved down. On horizontal systems it would indicate movement of the load away from the anchor or hauling system. It has an opposite field of use to **Up**.

4.1.4 **Rope Free,** *4 Short Whistle Blasts*—Used at the end of a climb, rappel, raise, or lower to communicate that one is off the rope, has found a safe position, and that the rope can be used by the next person or for the next operation.

4.1.5 **Help,** *Continuous Blast*—A general emergency call. Its use may indicate different actions depending upon the system in use at the time. For example, during a rappel, it would include the need for a bottom belay. The signal alerts others to come to the aid and, if necessary, work quickly and safely to effect a rescue.

4.2 A "Short Whistle Blast" is defined as 1 s in duration. Where the signal calls for multiple blasts there shall be a 1-s interval between each blast. A "Long Whistle Blast" is 3 s in duration. A "Continuous Blast" indicating the need for help should be long enough to attract attention and be differentiated from any other signal, at least 10 s if possible.

4.3 These same patterns could be used with any audible signaling device such as a compressed gas horn, vehicle horn, and so forth.

5. Keywords

5.1 signals; whistles

[1] This guide is under the jurisdiction of ASTM Committee F32 on Search and Rescue and is the direct responsibility of Subcommittee F32.02 on Search and Rescue Management.

Current edition approved Feb. 10, 1997. Published May 1997.

Designation: F 1781 – 97

Standard Specification for Elastomeric Flexible Hinge Finger Total Joint Implants[1]

This standard is issued under the fixed designation F 1781; the number immediately following the designation indicates the year of original adoption or, in the case of revision, the year of last revision. A number in parentheses indicates the year of last reapproval. A superscript epsilon (ε) indicates an editorial change since the last revision or reapproval.

1. Scope

1.1 This specification covers elastomeric flexible hinge finger total joint implants, used with and without metal grommets in the reconstruction of the metacarpophalangeal (MCP) and proximal interphalangeal (PIP) joints.

1.2 This specification excludes those implants that do not have an across-the-joint elastomeric linkage. The specification is limited to implants made from one material in a single one-step molding procedure.

1.3 The values stated in SI units are to be regarded as standard. The inch-pound units given in parentheses are for information only.

2. Referenced Documents

2.1 *ASTM Standards:*

D 412 Test Methods for Vulcanized Rubber and Thermoplastic Rubbers and Thermoplastic Elastomers—Tension[2]

D 624 Test Method for Tear Strength of Conventional Vulcanized Rubber and Thermoplastic Elastomers[2]

D 813 Test Method for Rubber-Deterioration—Crack Growth[2]

D 1052 Test Method for Measuring Rubber Deterioration—Cut Growth Using Ross Flexing Apparatus[2]

D 2240 Test Method for Rubber Property—Durometer Hardness[2]

F 67 Specification for an Unalloyed Titanium for Surgical Implant Application[3]

F 86 Practice for Surface Preparation and Marking of Metallic Surgical Implants[3]

F 601 Practice for Fluorescent Penetrant Inspection of Metallic Surgical Implants[3]

F 604 Specification for Silicone Elastomers Used in Medical Applications[3]

F 748 Practice for Selecting Generic Biological Test Methods for Materials and Devices[3]

F 981 Practice for Assessment of Compatibility of Biomaterials for Surgical Implants with Respect to Effect of Materials on Muscle and Bone[3]

F 983 Practice for Permanent Marking of Orthopaedic Implant Components[3]

2.2 *Government Standards:*

21 CFR Part 820 Good Manufacturing Practices for Medical Devices[4]

MIL STD 177A Rubber Products, Terms for Visible Defects[4]

2.3 *Other Standard:*

EN 30993-1 Biological Evaluations of Medical Devices Part 1: Guidance on Selection of Tests[5]

3. Significance and Use

3.1 The prostheses described in this specification are intended for use in the proximal interphalangeal (PIP) and metacarpophalangeal (MCP) joints.

4. Classification

4.1 *Constrained*—A constrained joint prosthesis is used for joint replacement and prevents dislocation of the prosthesis in more than one anatomical plane and consists of either a single, flexible, across-the-joint component, or more than one component linked together or affixed.

5. Materials and Manufacture

5.1 Proper material selection is necessary, but insufficient to ensure suitable function of a device. All devices conforming to this specification shall be fabricated from materials with adequate mechanical strength, durability and biocompatibility.

5.2 All elastomeric components shall conform to Specification F 604. Test and evaluation parameters that could be considered for the elastomeric implant materials are Specification F 604, Practice F 748, Test Methods D 813, D 1052, D 2240, D 412 and D 624. Before implants can be manufactured from other materials, 5.4 must be comply.

5.3 Titanium used as a material of construction for metal grommets shall conform to Specification F 67. Metal grommets must match the shape of the implant and not interfere with the flexible hinge implant function.

5.4 *Biocompatibility*—Flexible hinge implants shall be manufactured from the materials listed in 5.2 and 5.3. Before implants can be manufactured from other materials, their

---

[1] This specification is under the jurisdiction of ASTM Committee F04 on Medical and Surgical Material and Devices and is the direct responsibility of Subcommittee F04.22 on Arthroplasty.

Current edition approved February 10, 1997. Published June 1997.

[2] *Annual Book of ASTM Standards*, Vol 09.01.

[3] *Annual Book of ASTM Standards*, Vol 13.01.

[4] Available from Superintendent of Documents, U.S. Government Printing Office, Washington, DC 20402.

[5] Available from American National Standard Institute, 11 W. 42nd St., 13th Floor, New York, NY 10036.

biocompatibility must be demonstrated by producing an acceptable response after testing in accordance with Practices F 748 and F 981, and others (see EN 30993-1) as needed.

5.5 When appropriate for metallic grommets, fluorescent penetrant inspection shall be performed in accordance with Practice F 601.

5.6 Design and manufacture will follow 21 CFR Part 820.

6. Performance Requirements

6.1 *Fatigue Testing*—The fatigue characteristics of material from which the elastomeric components are fabricated must be evaluated according to Test Method D 813. Any test should be designed to measure fatigue rate (for example, crack growth length) as a function of a million(s) cycles.

6.2 *Range of Motion of the Device Before Implantation*—The implant shall be evaluated to determine the maximum flexion and extension possible before subluxation occurs or the motion is arrested by the implant (elastomer-to-elastomer contact within the hinge). These results shall be reported in the product labeling.

6.3 *Guidelines for In-Vitro Laboratory Testing*—No ASTM standards for testing finger implants have been developed. Laboratory testing that simulates the conditions of use, by a joint function simulator, is desirable to compare materials and designs and to provide an indication of clinical performance. Implant testing shall be done in keeping with the implants intended function, that is, implants intended to partially stabilize or stabilize a joint shall be subjected to the maximum destabilizing force or motion, or both, anticipated in clinical application during flexural testing.

6.4 *Durometer*—The hardness of elastomeric components shall be measured according to Test Method D 2240.

6.5 The mechanical properties (such as tensile strength, percentage elongation, modulus, and tear strength) of the elastomeric materials used in components shall be determined according to Test Methods D 412 and D 624.

7. Dimensions

7.1 Dimensions of finger and joint replacement components shall be reported in labeling (see Figs. 1 and 2):

7.1.1 Distal stem length,

7.1.2 Proximal stem length,

7.1.3 Hinge width in medial/lateral plane,

7.1.4 Hinge height in dorsal/palmar plane,

7.1.5 Distal stem width,

7.1.6 Proximal stem width, and

7.1.7 Distal-proximal hinge width.

7.2 Dimensions of finger implant with metal grommets shall be reported in labeling (see Fig. 3):

7.2.1 Distal stem length,

7.2.2 Proximal stem length,

7.2.3 Distal grommet length,

7.2.4 Proximal grommet length, and

7.2.5 Hinge height in dorsal/palmar plane.

8. Finish and Marking

8.1 Items conforming to this specification shall be finished and marked in accordance with Practice F 86 and F 983, where applicable.

8.2 *Polymeric Surface Finish*—Polymeric Surface Finish shall conform to manufacturer's documented standards concerning roughness, knit lines, void, bubbles, mold fill, color, inclusions, and dimensions, when applicable. Descriptions of these terms can be located in MIL STD 177A.

9. Labeling and Packaging

9.1 The maximum range of motion values as determined by 6.2 shall be included in the product labeling. The minimum limits for the mechanical properties of the elastomeric material(s) used in components shall be included in theproduct labeling.

9.2 The dimensions shall be included in the product labeling.

9.3 The material(s) used for the implant shall be specified in the package labeling.

9.4 The site, orientation (if any), and catalog number if space permits should be present on the component or within the labeling.

NOTE 1—If space permits the manufacturer's trademark must appear legibly on each of the components. If space does not permit such, the information must be written in the labeling.

10. Keywords

10.1 elastomer; finger; implant

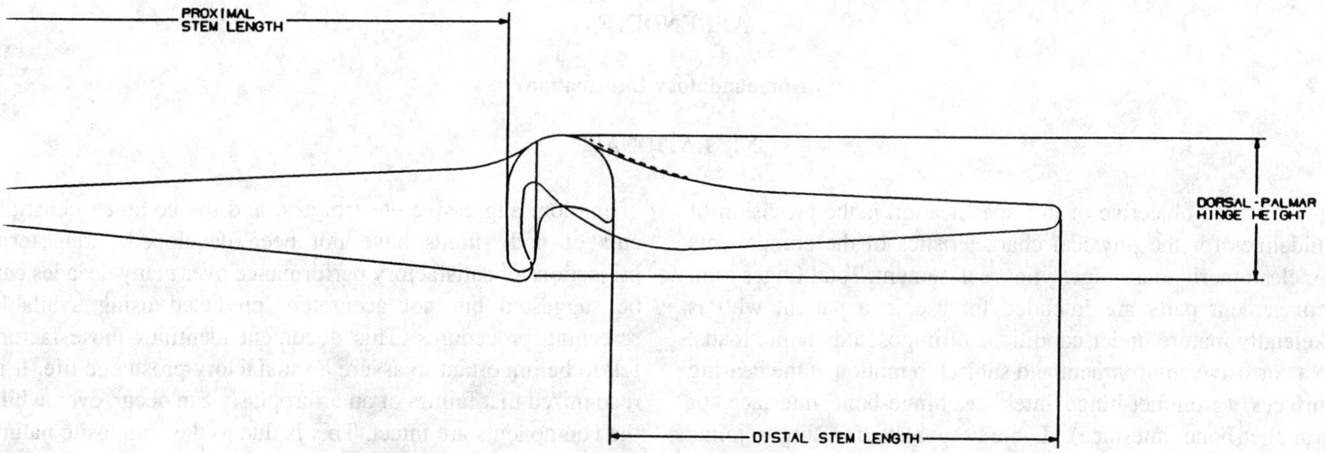

FIG. 1 Dimensions of Finger and Joint Replacement Components

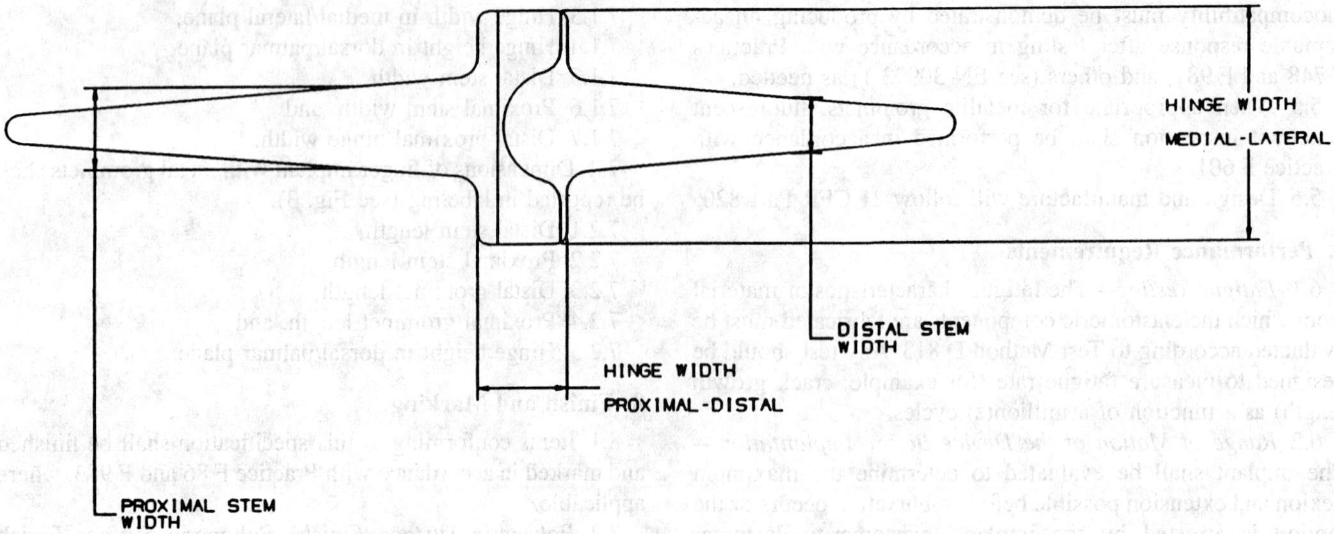

FIG. 2 Dimensions of Finger and Joint Replacement Components

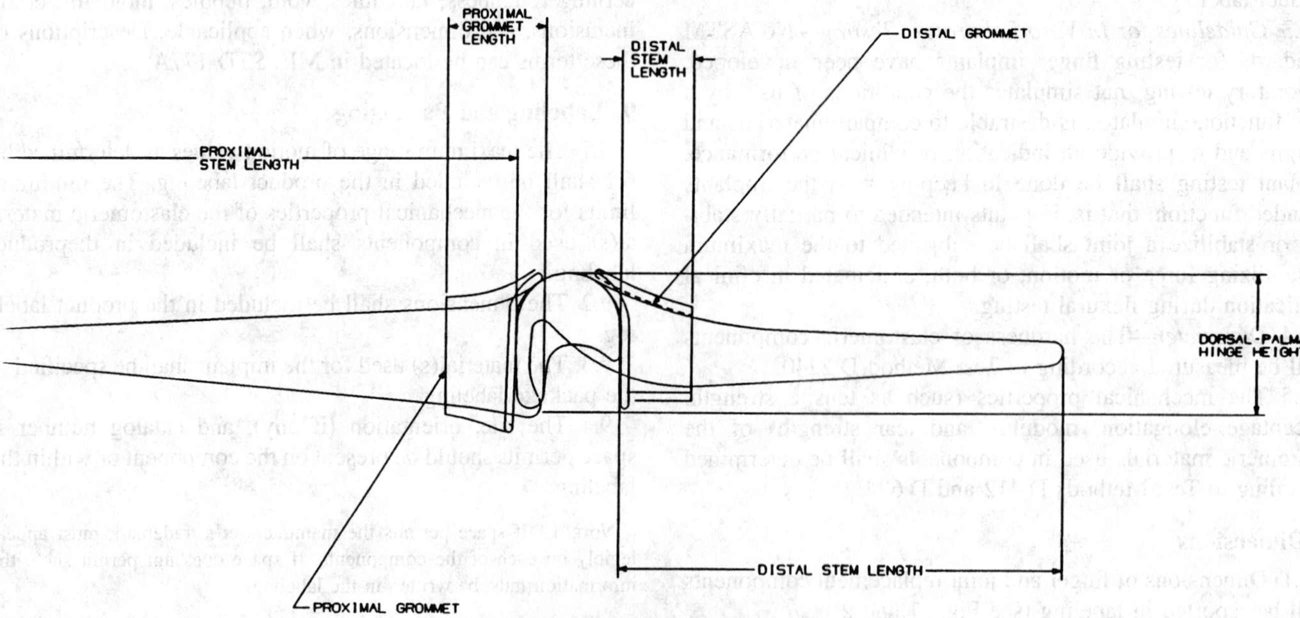

FIG. 3 Dimensions of Finger Implant

APPENDIXES

(Nonmandatory Information)

X1. RATIONALE

X1.1 The objective of this specification is the provision of guidelines for the physical characteristics of the components for elastomeric total finger joint replacement. Total finger joint replacement parts are intended for use in a patient who is skeletally mature under conditions of imposed dynamic loads, in a corrosive environment and subject to motion at the bearing surfaces, (grommet-hinge interface, hinge-bone interface, or grommet-bone interface). Laboratory tests for finger joints which accurately simulate imposed loads, appropriate ranges of motion, aggressive electrolytes, and the complex constituents of body fluids have not been developed. Long term projections of satisfactory performance over many decades can be suggested but not accurately predicted using available screening procedures. This document identifies those factors felt to be important to assure a satisfactory prosthetic life. It is recognized that failure of an arthroplasty can occur, even while the components are intact. This is due to the composite nature of the arthroplasty procedure, which includes the implants, the surgical procedure, post-operative care, patient use, and the physiological environment.

X1.1.1 This specification excludes those implants that do not have an across-the-joint elastomeric linkage and is limited to implants made from one material in a single, one-step molding procedure. It also excludes implants which utilize bone cement as affixation method, and implants defined as "partially constrained" or "non-constrained."

X1.1.2 Under applicable documents and materials, the list reflects the current state of the art. It is recognized that should materials not now included appear and be proved acceptable, they shall be inserted into this standard during the process of revision.

X1.2 *Performance Considerations*—Component performance can be predicted only indirectly at this stage by referring to fatigue performance, range of motion, and other parameters. Reference to parameters applicable to materials may or may not adequately describe a device made from the materials. In the future as new materials are developed, other material testing methods not described in the standard, such as Test Method D 1052, may be considered for screening possible materials for flexible hinge implants. If these materials are suitable, this standard will be revised to include them as potential candidate materials for total flexible finger implants. In a period of transition from materials specification standards to device performance standards, both methods of description may be appropriate.

X1.2.1 Component performance shall be considered with regard to patient anatomy. It is well recognized that physical stresses resulting from events or activities out of the ordinary range, as in accidents or especially vigorous sports, predictably exceed allowable stresses in levels in any component design. When mal-alignment, or dislocation/subluxation occurs in a MCP or PIP joint reconstructed with a constrained flexible hinge implant, the forces borne by the implant may cause premature destruction. It is also recognized that other forms of arthroplasty failure are known to occur, related primarily to patient factors, such as osteoporosis, aggressive rheumatoid disease misuse, and others.

X1.2.2 Specific criteria need to be established in assessing the biocompatibility of finger implants made of new materials. Practice F 748 will need to be used to determine which additional biocompatibility tests are required.

X1.2.3 In the course of evaluating new materials, it is recommended that if the material is used in an application that causes small particle formation from abrasion or normal wear processes that the biocompatibility of those particles be determined in addition to the bulk material.

X1.3 *Dimensions*—The methods of dimensional measurement must conform with the industry practice and whenever possible, on an international practice.

X1.4 *Finish and Markings*—Dimensions and tolerances are as described by manufacturers' standards. Material composition can be determined by referring to the manufacturers' information, instead of marking the material on each implant.

X2. ADDITIONAL PUBLICATIONS

Frisch, E. E., "High Performance Medical Grade Silicone Elastomer," *Advances in Biomaterials 1*, Stuart M. Lee ed., Technomic Publishing Co., Inc., Lancaster, PA, 1987, pp. 143–156.

Peimer, C. A., Meidige, J., Eckert, B. S., Wright, J. R., Howard, C. S., "Reactive Synovitis After Silicone Arthroplasty," *Journal of Hand Surgery, 11*, 1986, pp. 624–638.

Savory, K. M., Hutchinson, D. T., Bloebaum, R., "A Materials Testing Protocol for Small Joint Prostheses," *Transactions for Society for Biomaterials, 17:244*, 1994.

Schneider, L. H., M.D., and Kirschenbaum, D., M.D., "Arthroplasty at the Metacarpophalangeal Joints," *Operative Techniques in Orthopaedics*, *6*: 1996, pp. 110–116.

Swanson, A. B., Swanson, G. de Groot, Frisch, E. E., "Flexible (Silicone) Implant Arthroplasty in the Small Joint Extremities: Concepts, Physical and Biological Considerations, Experimental and Clinical Results," *Biomaterials in Reconstructive Surgery*, L. R. Rubin, M.D. ed., C. V. Mosby Company St. Louis, MO, Chapter 40, 1983.

Wilson, Y. G., Sykes, P. J., and Niranjan, N. S., "Long-Term Follow-Up of Swanson's Silastic Arthroplasty of the Metacarpophalangeal Joints in Rheumatoid Arthritis," *Journal of Hand Surgery*, 18B: 1993, pp. 81–91.

Standard Guide for Performance of an Ice Rescuer—Level II[1]

This standard is issued under the fixed designation F 1783; the number immediately following the designation indicates the year of original adoption or, in the case of revision, the year of last revision. A number in parentheses indicates the year of last reapproval. A superscript epsilon (ϵ) indicates an editorial change since the last revision or reapproval.

1. Scope

1.1 This guide covers minimum requirements for the scope of performance of an ice rescuer who performs cold water and ice rescues from the surface, assists with support for ice rescue divers, and provides initial patient care at a cold water or ice rescue incident.

1.2 This guide is one of a series that, together with Guide F 1739, describes the minimum performance requirements of an ice rescuer.

1.3 Individuals who will operate in the cold water or ice rescue setting need to be aware of the equipment and physical requirements necessary to be able to perform all identified objectives and necessary skills in the setting.

1.4 The values stated in both inch-pound and SI units are to be regarded separately as the standard. The values given in parentheses are for information only.

1.5 *This standard does not purport to address all of the safety concerns, if any, associated with its use. It is the responsibility of the user of this standard to establish appropriate safety and health practices and determine the applicability of regulatory limitations prior to use.*

2. Referenced Documents

2.1 *ASTM Standards:*

1739 Guide for Performance of a Water Rescuer—Level I[2]

3. Terminology

3.1 *Definitions of Terms Specific to This Standard:*

3.1.1 *drysuit, n*—a protective suit that encompasses the wearer, prohibiting water from entering. A dry suit may provide no buoyancy or thermal protection without insulation undergarments or a buoyancy compensating device.

3.1.2 *floating tether, tag line, n*—a water rescue technique which stretches a line across a body of water. This line has a flotation device attached to it to keep the rope on the surface of the water and to provide a buoyant object for the victim to grab hold.

3.1.3 *ice awls, n*—a device used for rescue on ice consisting of a sharp spike with a handle.

3.1.4 *ice staff, n*—a stick, pole, or rod with a sharp spike in one end used to traverse on ice or rescue on ice.

3.1.5 *immersion suit, n*—designed to provide cold water protection and buoyancy by one person in cold water emergencies. These devices should conform to standards set by the appropriate national regulatory authority, that is, the U.S. Coast Guard in the United States.

3.1.6 *personal flotation device, PFD, n*—a buoyant device suitable for use by one person in water emergencies. These devices should conform to standards set by the appropriate national regulatory authority, that is, the U.S. Coast Guard in the United States.

3.1.7 *sinking tether, snag line, n*—a water rescue technique that stretches a weighted line across a body of water to snag or support fully or partly submerged objects and people.

3.1.8 *vessel, n*—includes every description of watercraft, including nondisplacement craft and seaplanes, used or capable of being used as a means of transportation on water.

4. Significance and Use

4.1 This guide is to be used to expand the performance of water rescuers and improve the emergency response and patient care delivered to victims in the cold water and ice rescue environment.

4.2 All persons who are identified as ice rescuers shall meet the requirements of this guide.

4.3 This guide is not intended to be used in isolation, but as a component guide acknowledging many duties of response at a cold water and ice rescue emergency. It also establishes a minimum scope of performance and encourages the addition of optional knowledge, skills and attitudinal objectives.

4.4 This guide does not establish medical protocols, nor does it authorize invasive procedures without specific authorization and medical control.

4.5 This guide is intended to assist government agencies, state, local, or regional organizations, fire departments, rescue teams and others who are responsible for establishing a minimum performance for personnel who respond to cold water and ice emergencies.

4.6 An ice rescuer shall be wearing an immersion suit, drysuit with PFD, or equivalent cold water protection and buoyancy to perform these rescues.

---

[1] This guide is under the jurisdiction of ASTM Committee F-32 on Search and Rescue and is the direct responsibility of Subcommittee F32.03 on Personnel, Training, and Education.

Current edition approved April 10, 1997. Published June 1997.

[2] *Annual Book of ASTM Standards*, Vol 13.01.

5. Objectives

5.1 The ice rescuer shall be able to perform the objectives in Guide F 1739.

5.2 The ice rescuer shall be able to:

5.2.1 Swim continuously 274.32 meters (300 yards),

5.2.2 Escape from a water/ice victim's grasp or hold,

5.2.3 Turn a disabled, passive or unconscious water/ice victim's face up in such a manner that the chances of aggravating injuries or medical condition is minimized,

5.2.4 Identify ice characteristics, types of ice, and openings in the ice,

5.2.5 Identify factors which influence the strength of ice,

5.2.6 Identify the ice rescue sequence,

5.2.7 Perform a scene evaluation which includes evaluating ice conditions and assessing the scene for hazards, number of victims, victims' condition, need for additional personnel, need for additional equipment and then take appropriate action following the rescue sequence by utilizing risk benefit analysis,

5.2.8 Walk and traverse on ice,

5.2.9 Walk and traverse on ice utilizing the ice staff,

5.2.10 Perform the ice awls self rescue technique on ice,

5.2.11 Perform the ice staff self rescue technique on ice,

5.2.12 Identify the factors in selecting clothing for thermal protection of the ice, rescuer.

5.2.13 Demonstrate the technique utilized when ice starts to break, that is, lay down and roll to safety or stronger ice,

5.2.14 Perform reaching and extension rescue techniques on ice,

5.2.15 Perform throwing rescue techniques using a throw-bag and coiled rope throws on ice,

5.2.16 Perform the floating tether (tag line), weighted tether (snag line) and stabilization line techniques on ice,

5.2.17 Perform the boat rescue technique utilizing a 14 to 16 foot (4.26 to 4.87 m) jonboat, small inflatable, or other vessel which the agency owns or utilizes for ice rescue emergencies on ice,

5.2.18 Perform the tethered swimmer rescue technique utilizing an immersion suit, drysuit with PFD, or equivalent on ice,

5.2.19 Provide initial patient care, and

5.2.20 Move the victim(s) in conjunction with patient care activities in such a manner that the chance of aggravating injuries or medical condition is minimized.

5.3 *Optional Objectives*—The territory, bodies of water (ice), equipment, personnel and resources vary among ice rescuers in agencies. When emergency response capabilities are limited, the ability of an ice rescuer to perform the tasks in 5.1 and 5.2 may be sufficient to ensure satisfactory care. When an ice rescuer has a greater variety of responses, territory, and equipment demands, the scope of performance must be expanded accordingly.

6. Keywords

6.1 ice; ice rescue; ice rescuer; rescue; water rescue; water rescuer

Standard Guide for Evaluating the Static and Fatigue Properties of Interconnection Mechanisms and Subassemblies Used in Spinal Arthrodesis Implants[1]

This standard is issued under the fixed designation F 1798; the number immediately following the designation indicates the year of original adoption or, in the case of revision, the year of last revision. A number in parentheses indicates the year of last reapproval. A superscript epsilon (ε) indicates an editorial change since the last revision or reapproval.

1. Scope

1.1 This guide covers the measurement of uniaxial static and fatigue strength, and resistance to loosening of the component interconnection mechanisms of spinal arthrodesis implants.

1.2 The purpose of this guide is to provide a means of mechanically characterizing different designs of spinal implant interconnections. Ultimately, the various components and interconnections should be combined for static and fatigue testing of the spinal implant construct. It is not the intention of this guide to address the analysis of spinal implant constructs or subconstructs or to define levels of performance of spinal implants as insufficient knowledge is available to predict the consequences of the use of particular spinal implant designs.

1.3 This guide sets out definitions for use in measuring the strength of component interconnections of spinal implants, possible test methods themselves, and the reporting of test results.

1.4 The values stated in SI units are to be regarded as standard.

1.5 *This standard does not purport to address all of the safety concerns, if any, associated with its use. It is the responsibility of the user of this standard to establish appropriate safety and health practices and determine the applicability of regulatory limitations prior to use.*

2. Referenced Documents

2.1 *ASTM Standards:*

E 4 Practices for Force Verification of Testing Machines[2]

E 6 Terminology Relating to Methods of Mechanical Testing[2]

E 468 Practice for the Presentation of Constant Amplitude Fatigue Test Results from Metallic Materials[2]

E 739 Practice for Statistical Analysis of Linear or Linearized Stress - Life (*S-N*) and Strain - Life (e-N) Fatigue Data[2]

E 1150 Definitions of Terms Relating to Fatigue[2]

F 383 Practice for Static Bend and Torsion Testing of Intramedullary Rods[3]

F 1582 Terminology Relating to Spinal Implants[3]

3. Terminology

3.1 *Definitions of Terms Specific to This Standard:*

3.1.1 *active length of longitudinal element*—the span between rigid supports (for example, 50 mm is the active length in Fig. 1, Fig. 2, Fig. 3(*a*), Fig. 3(*b*), and Fig. 4.

3.1.2 *global coordinate system*—spinal column motion has six degrees of freedom, having translational motion along, and rotational motion about three axes. The axes are labeled anterior-posterior or a-p (X), medial-lateral or transverse (Y), and caudal-cranial or axial (Z). This coordinate system is right handed with +X in the anterior direction, +Y towards the left side of the body, and +Z in the cranial direction. Positive rotations are defined by the right hand rule (See Fig. 5(*a*)).

3.1.3 *gripping capacity*—the maximum applied load or moment across an interconnection mechanism within the first 1.5 mm of permanent displacement or 5° of permanent rotation between the connected components.

3.1.4 *local coordinate system*—the spine's global coordinate system shall be applied locally at the position of the interconnection. The local direction, z, shall be centered through the longitudinal element of the x-y plane. The local direction, x, shall be defined parallel to the axis of a screw or back of a hook. The local transverse axis, y, shall be parallel to a transverse element (See Fig. 5(*b*) and Fig. 5(*c*)).

3.1.5 *loosening torque*—the torque required to disconnect the various threaded fasteners that might comprise the implant's interconnection mechanism.

3.1.6 *major directions of loading*—directions of the predominant forces and moments (relative to the local axes) to which vertebral connection elements are subjected, (that is, axial load, Fz; A-P load, Fx; axial torsion, Mz; and flexion-extension moment, My).

3.1.7 *maximum run out load/moment*—the maximum load or moment that can be applied to a subassembly where all the tested constructs have withstood 2.5 × 106 cycles without a failure.

3.1.8 *relevant directions of loading*—those directions of

[1] This guide is under the jurisdiction of ASTM Committee F-4 onMedical and Surgical Materials and Devices and is the direct responsibility of Subcommittee F04.25on Spinal Devices

Current edition approved April 10, 1997. Published June 1998.

[2] *Annual Book of ASTM Standards*, Vol 03.01.

[3] *Annual Book of ASTM Standards*, Vol 13.01.

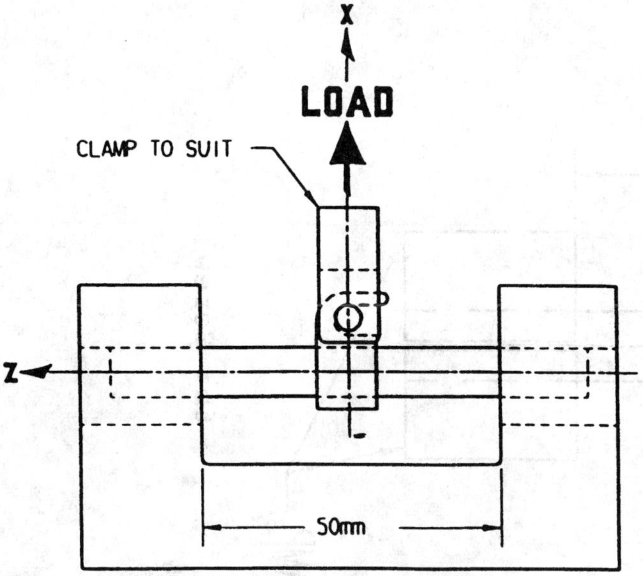

FIG. 1 A-P Test Apparatus for Subassembly

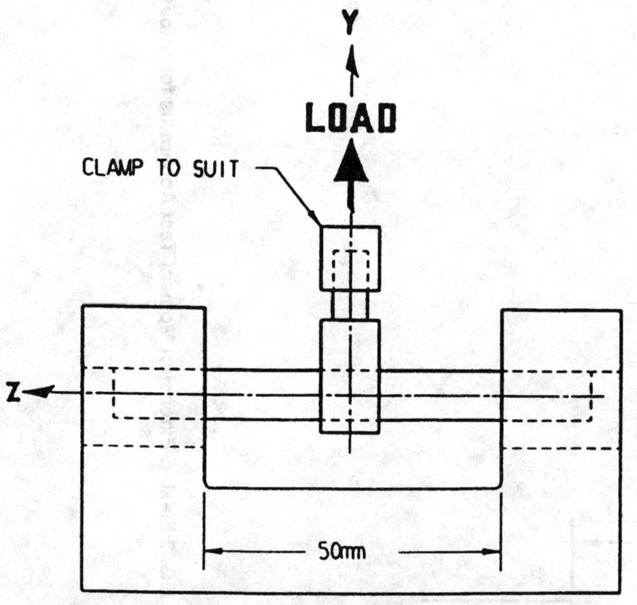

FIG. 2 Transverse Test Apparatus for Subassembly

loading in which a particular component interconnection is designed to provide resistance to loading. For example, a particular spinal hook may be designed to withstand a positive axial load, A-P load, and flexion-extension moment, but not a negative axial load or axial torsion. Hence, positive axial load, A-P load, and flexion-extension moment are relevant directions of loading.

3.1.9 *spinal arthrodesis implant*—an implant applied to the spine with the specific intention of providing temporary correction and stability to vertebrae while bony fusion occurs.

3.1.10 *subassembly failure*—permanent deformation resulting from fracture, plastic deformation, loosening or slippage that renders the subassembly ineffective or unable to adequately resist load.

3.1.11 *subassembly permanent deformation*—the displacement (mm) or angular displacement (degree of the subassembly relative to the unloaded condition remaining after the applied load moment or torque has been removed. Care must be taken to insure the loading fixtures are rigid and do not contribute to the measurement of deflection.

3.1.12 *tightening torque*—the specified torque that is applied to the various threaded fasteners that might comprise the implant's interconnection mechanism.

3.1.13 *ultimate load/moment of the subassembly*—maximum load or moment applied to a subassembly (see Point E in Fig. 6).

3.1.14 *yield load/moment of the subassembly*—the load or moment required to produce a permanent deformation equal to 0.020 times the active length of the longitudinal element (see Point D in Fig. 6).

4. Summary of Test Methods

4.1 Vertebral attachment components (for example, hook, screws, bands) and transverse elements must be attached to longitudinal elements (for example, rods, plates) to form spinal implant subassemblies.

4.2 The interconnections are tested only in the relevant directions of loading by applying loads at specific locations relative to the local coordinate system.

4.3 The interconnections and subassemblies are tested statically in a load to failure mode and also can be tested cyclically to estimate the maximum run out value at 2.5×10^6 cycles.

5. Significance and Use

5.1 Spinal implants are generally composed of several components that, when connected together, form a spinal implant construct. Spinal implant constructs are designed to provide some stability to the spine while arthrodesis takes place. This guide outlines standardized evaluations of different interconnection mechanisms so that comparison between different designs is facilitated. Comparisons must be made cautiously and with careful analysis, taking into account the effects that design differences can have on the loading configurations.

5.2 This guide is used to quantify the static and fatigue properties of different implant interconnection designs. The mechanical tests are conducted in vitro using simplified, unidirectional loads and moments. Fatigue testing in a simulated body fluid or saline may have a fretting, corrosive, or lubrication effect on the interconnection and thereby affect the relative performance of tested devices. Hence, the test environment, whether a simulated body fluid, saline (9g NaCl per 1000 mL H_2O), with a saline drip, or dry, is an important characteristic of the test and must be reported accurately.

5.3 The loading of spinal implant constructs in vivo will, in general, differ from the loading configurations used in this guide. The results obtained here cannot be used directly to predict in vivo performance. However, the results can be used to compare different component designs in terms of relative mechanical parameters.

6. Apparatus

6.1 Machines used for the test shall conform to the requirements of Practices E 4.

6.2 The apparatus for axial (z) gripping capacity measurements of an interconnection mechanism is depicted in Fig.

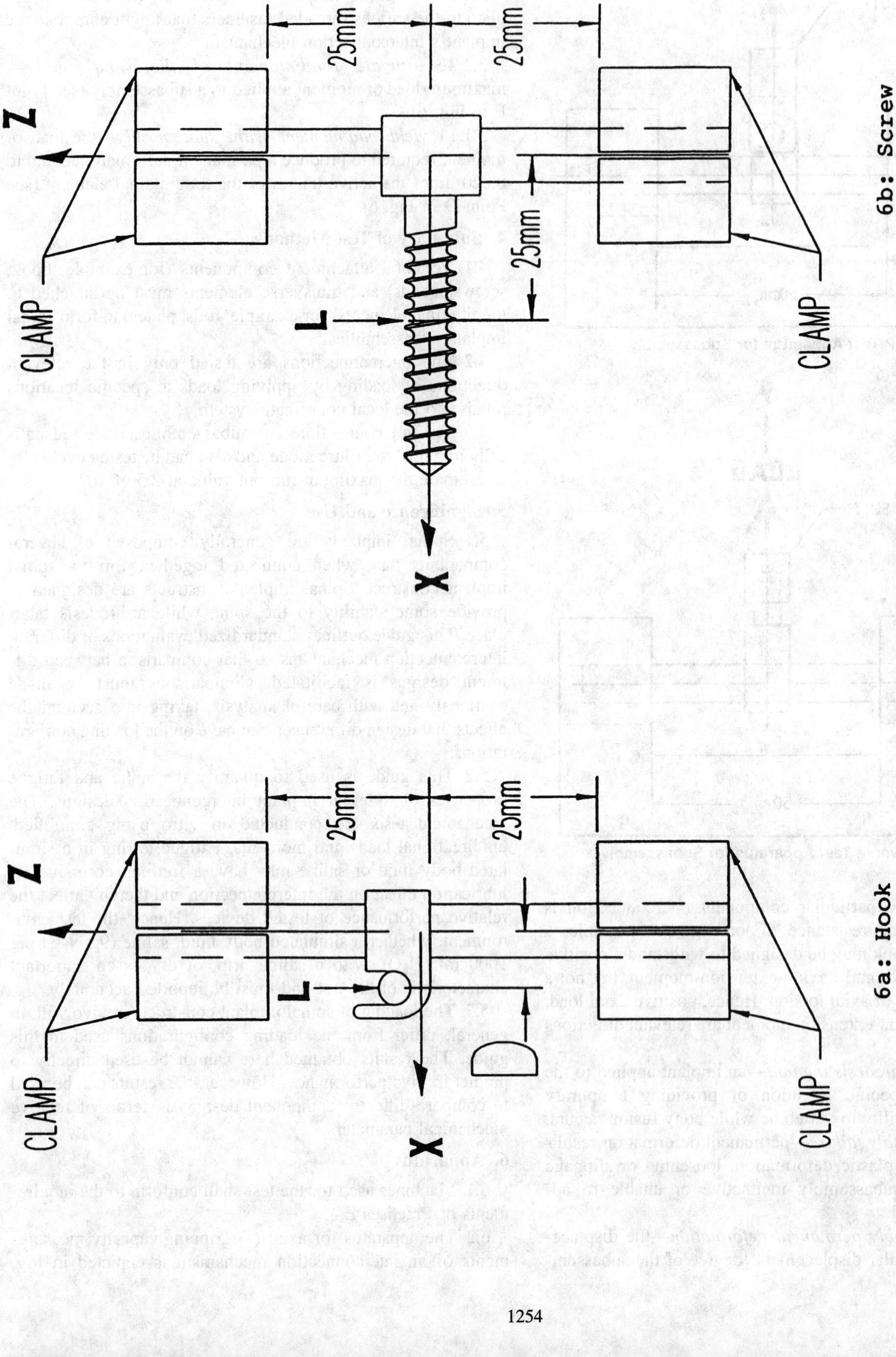

FIG. 3 Flexion-Extension Moment Test Apparatus for Subassembly

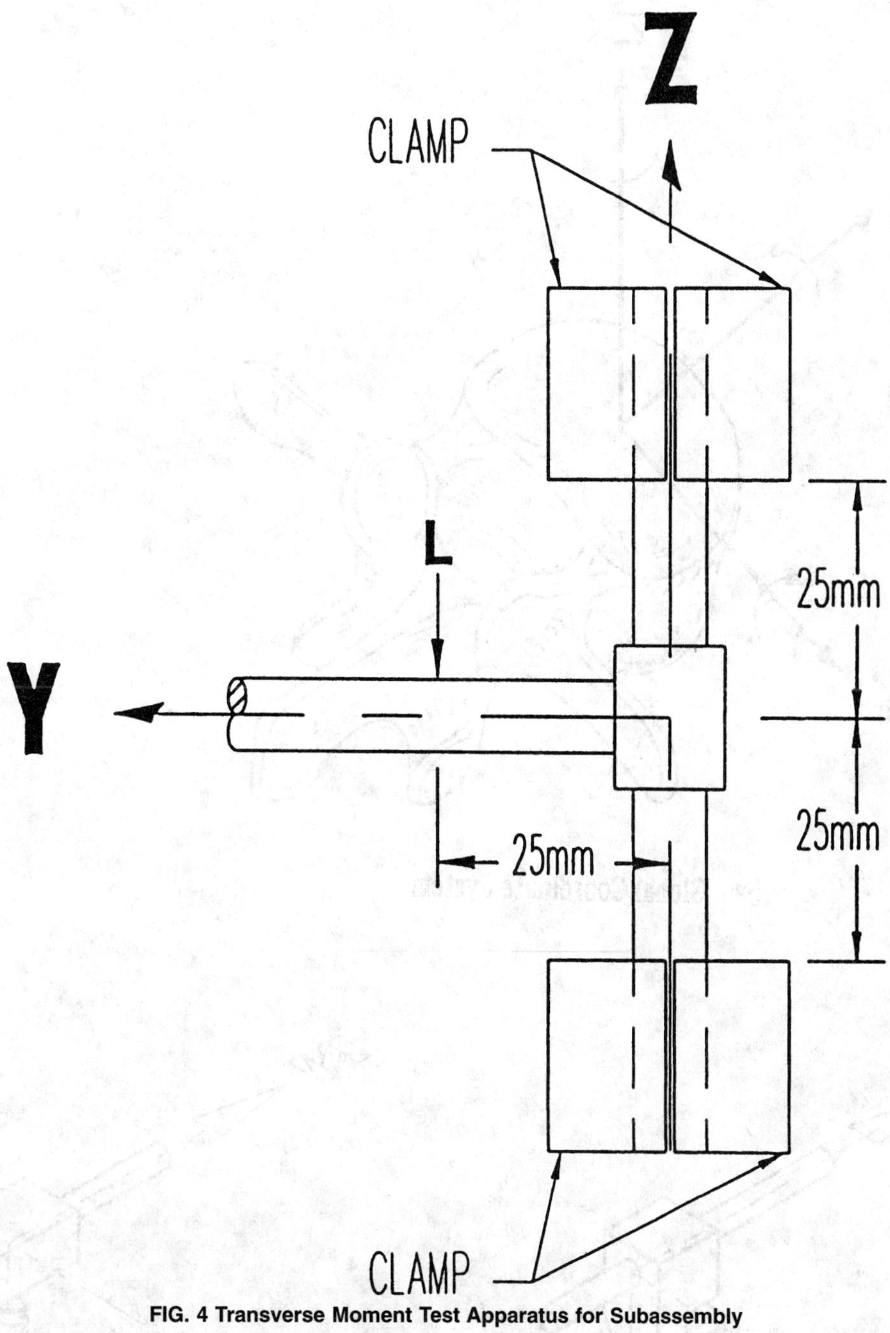

FIG. 4 Transverse Moment Test Apparatus for Subassembly

7(*a*). One end of the longitudinal element shall be clamped rigidly, leaving 5 mm exposed between the interconnection mechanism and the test machine base. A section of longitudinal element at least 5 mm shall extend beyond the interconnection linkage and remain unfixed. Axial loads are applied to the interconnection mechanism along the axis of the longitudinal element via a sleeve (collar) which freely surrounds the longitudinal element. The sleeve (collar) should evenly distribute the load around the interconnection. An alternate method, depicted in Fig. 7(*b*), applies the load to the longitudinal element and pushes it through the interconnection clamp.

6.3 The apparatus for A-P (x) mechanical property measurements of a subassembly is depicted in Fig. 1. Both ends of the longitudinal element shall be clamped rigidly, with the interconnection centered on a 50 mm section of the longitudinal element. The local origin of the interconnection mechanism shall be centered between the mounts. Loads are applied to the interconnection (perpendicular to the longitudinal element) via a clamp on the hook, screw, or band. The load should be centered through the local x coordinate axis.

6.4 The apparatus for transverse (y) mechanical property measurements of a subassembly is depicted in Fig. 2. Both ends of the longitudinal element shall be clamped rigidly, with the interconnection centered on a 50 mm section of the longitudinal element. The local origin of the interconnection mechanism shall be centered between the mounts. Loads are applied to the interconnection (perpendicular to the longitudinal element) via a clamp on the transverse connector. The load

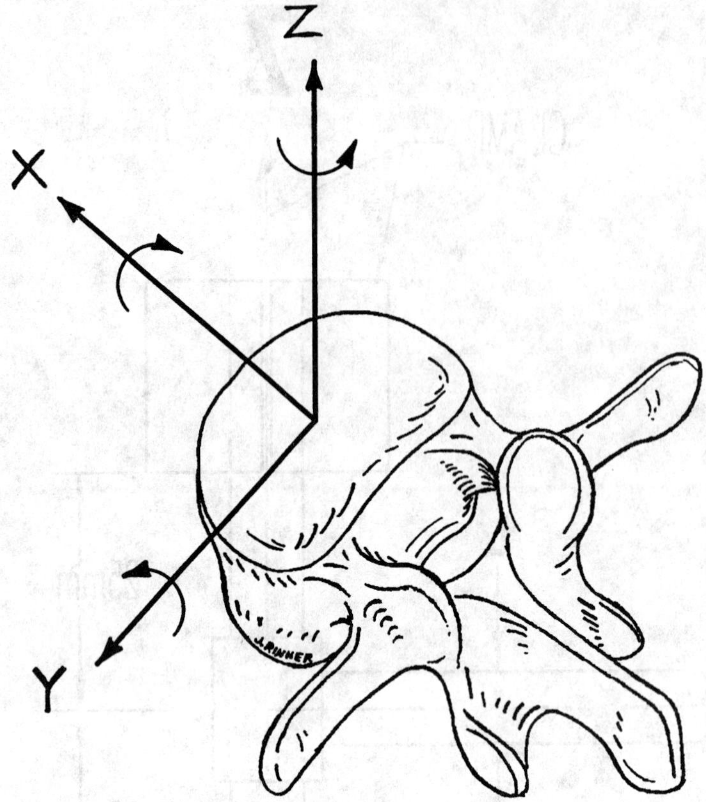

5a: Global Coordinate System

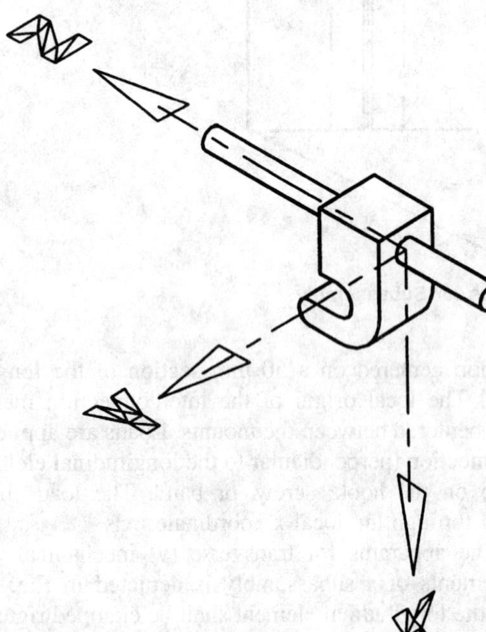

5b: Local Coordinate System- Hook

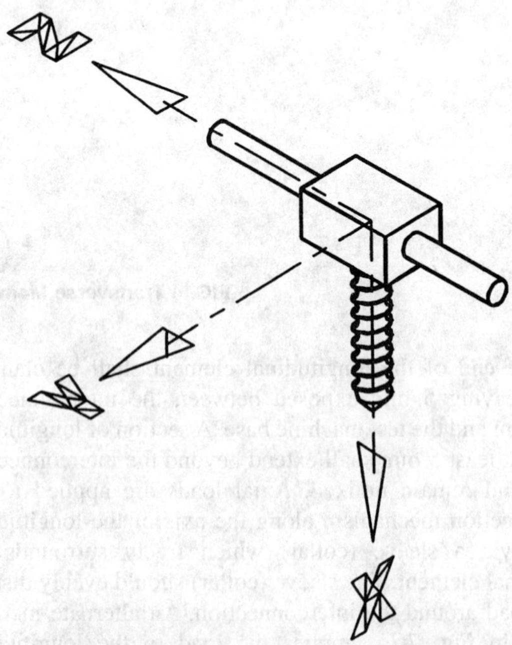

5c: Local Coordinate System -Screw

FIG. 5 Coordinate System

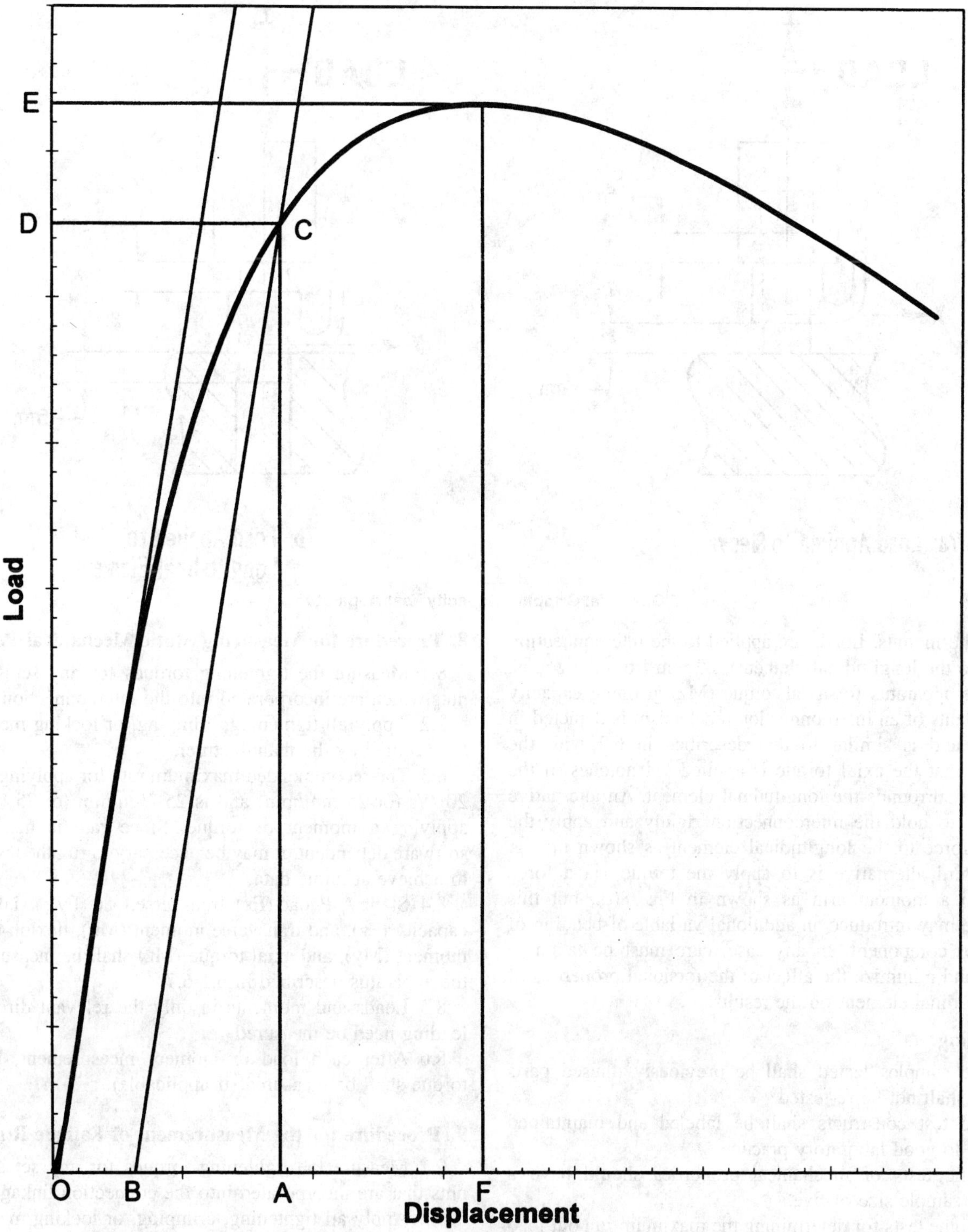

FIG. 6 Load/Displacement Curve

should be centered through the local y coordinate axis.

6.5 The apparatus for flexion-extension moment (My) mechanical property measurements of a subassembly is depicted in Fig. 3. Both ends of the longitudinal element shall be clamped rigidly, with the interconnection centered on a 50 mm section of the longitudinal element. The local origin of the interconnection mechanism shall be centered between the mounts. Loads are applied to the interconnection (parallel to the longitudinal element). For spinal hooks, the load shall be applied via a cylinder set in the hook notch, Fig. 3(*a*). For other elements (screws) the load shall be applied 25 mm from the local z axis, Fig. 3(*b*).

6.6 The apparatus for transverse moment (Mx) mechanical property measurements of a subassembly is depicted in Fig. 4. As in the previous test, 6.5, both ends of the longitudinal element shall be clamped rigidly, with the interconnection centered on a 50 mm section of the longitudinal element. The local origin of the interconnection mechanism shall be centered

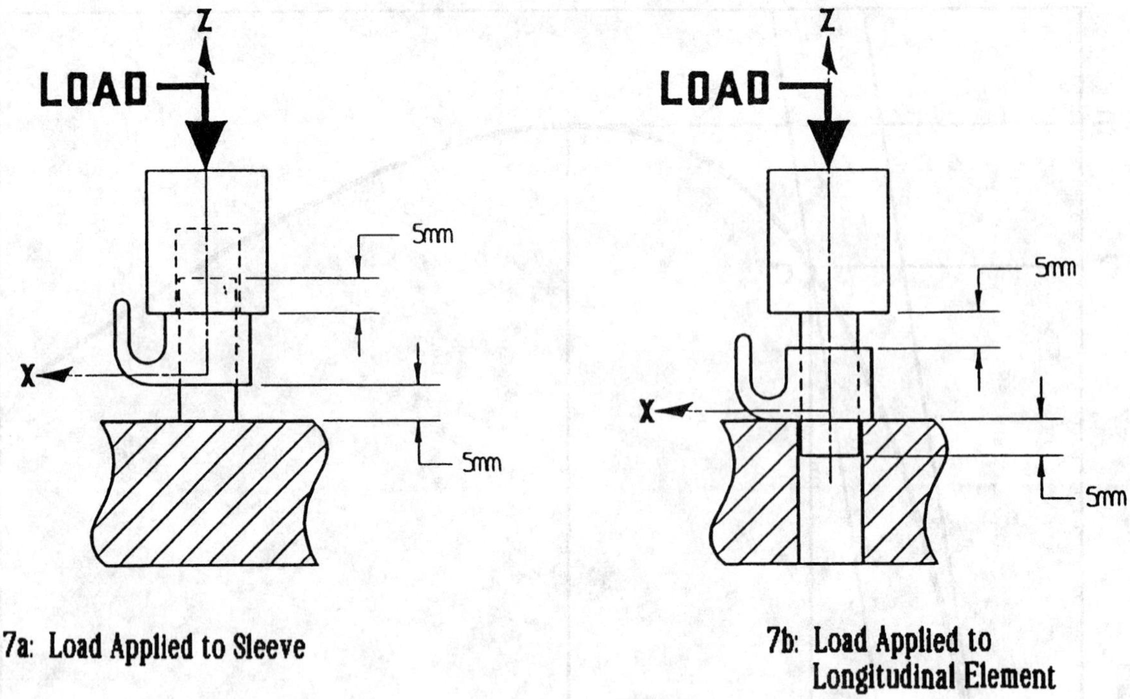

FIG. 7 Axial Gripping Capacity Test Apparatus

between the mounts. Loads are applied to the interconnection (parallel to the longitudinal element), 25 mm from the z axis.

6.7 The apparatus for axial torque (Mz) gripping capacity measurements of an interconnection mechanism is depicted in Fig. 8(*a*) and is similar to that described in 6.2 with the exception that the axial torque is applied via notches in the sleeve that surrounds the longitudinal element. An alternative method is to hold the interconnection rigidly and apply the torsional force to the longitudinal element as shown in Fig. 8(*b*). A third alternative is to apply the torque via a force applied to a moment arm as shown in Fig. 8(*c*), but this alternative may introduce an additional variable of bending of the anchor component. In any case, care must be taken to evaluate and minimize the affect of the torsional properties of the longitudinal element on the results.

7. Sampling

7.1 The samples tested shall be previously unused parts only, and shall not be re-tested.

7.2 The test constructs shall be labeled and maintained according to good laboratory practice.

7.3 Static tests of mechanical properties should have a minimum sample size of five.

7.4 Fatigue tests for determining the maximum run out load or moment of a subassembly at 2.5×10^6 cycles shall utilize a run down, half-interval approach[4] with one specimen per run down interval or half-interval and three consecutive specimens showing run out to 2.5×10^6 cycles. Alternative methods for determining the starting point of the fatigue curve are the run-up method or choosing 75 % of the ultimate static load or moment.

8. Procedure for Measuring Static Mechanical Properties

8.1 Measure the tightening torques for any set screws or nuts which are incorporated into the interconnection linkage.

8.2 Apply all tightening, crimping, or locking mechanisms as specified by the manufacturer.

8.3 The recommended maximum rate for applying a load is 20 *N*/s (or 25 mm/min) and is 25 *N*-m/min (or 25 °/min) for applying a moment or torque. Since rate is machine and software dependent, it may be necessary to run the tests slower to achieve accurate data.

8.4 Static A-P load (Fx), transverse load (Fy), axial gripping capacity (Fz), and transverse moment (Mx), flexion-extension moment (My), and axial torque (Mz) shall be measured using the apparatus described in 6.1-6.7.

8.5 Loads and moments in only the relevant directions of loading need be measured.

8.6 After each load or moment measurement, loosening torque shall be measured (if applicable).

9. Procedure for the Measurement of Fatigue Run Out

9.1 Measure the tightening torques for any set screws or nuts that are incorporated into the connection linkage.

9.2 Apply all tightening, crimping, or locking mechanisms as specified by the manufacturer.

9.3 The maximum frequency of cyclic loading is not specified but shall be measured and reported.

9.4 All fatigue loading should be sinusoidal, accomplished via continuous load amplitude control, rather than in a controlled deflection manner.

9.5 A-P fatigue run out (Fx), transverse fatigue run out (Fy), axial fatigue run out (Fz), transverse moment fatigue run out (Mx), flexion extension moment fatigue run out (My), axial torsional fatigue run out (Mz), if considered relevant, shall be determined using the apparatus described in 6.1-6.7.

[4] See "Optiminal Stress Amplitude Selection in Estimating Median Fatigue Limits Using Small Samples", Little, R.E., ed., *J. of Testing and Evaluation*, ASTM, 1990, pp. 115–122.

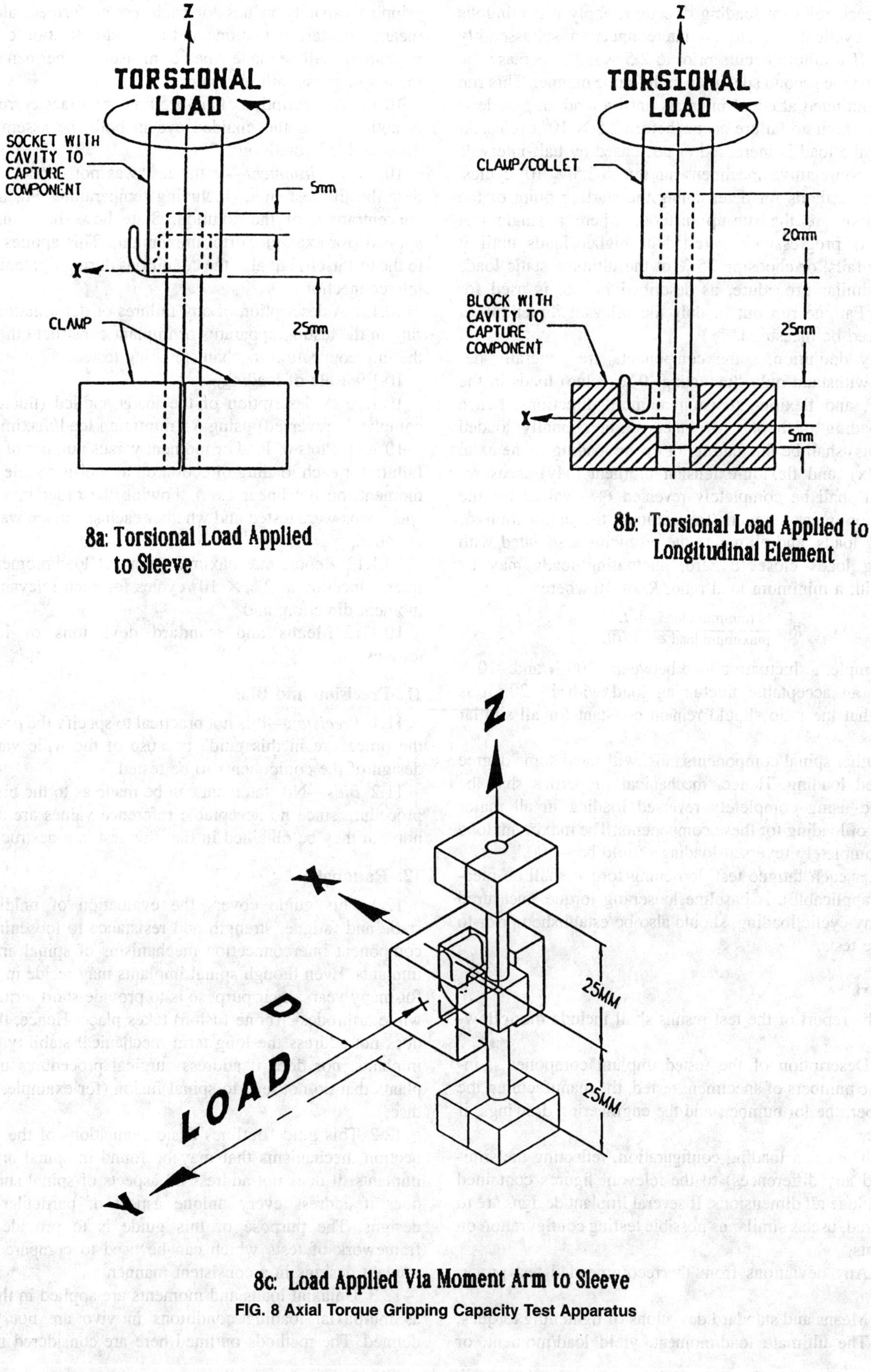

8a: Torsional Load Applied to Sleeve

8b: Torsional Load Applied to Longitudinal Element

8c: Load Applied Via Moment Arm to Sleeve

FIG. 8 Axial Torque Gripping Capacity Test Apparatus

9.6 In each relevant loading direction, apply a continuous amplitude cyclical load to an interconnection subassembly specimen. If a failure occurs prior to 2.5×10^6, decrease the load and test the second specimen in the same manner. This run down is continued at equal intervals until a load amplitude is reached at which no failure occurs before 2.5×10^6 cycles. At this point, the load is increased or decreased by half-intervals until three consecutive specimens run out to 2.5×10^6 cycles. Alternative methods for determining the starting point of the fatigue curve are the run-up method, where a single test specimen is progressively retested at higher loads until it eventually fails, or choosing 75 % of the ultimate static load.

9.7 A similar procedure, as described in 9.6, is used for moments. Fatigue run out in only the relevant directions of loading need be measured.

9.7.1 By definition, some components are generally designed to withstand only fluctuating (0 to value) loads in the axial, A-P, and flexion-extension moment directions, hence fatigue loading of hooks (or other unidirectionally loaded components) shall be fluctuating for cyclic loading in the axial (z), A-P (x), and flexion-extension moment (My) measurements, but shall be completely reversed (+/– value) for the axial torsion measurement. To facilitate the application of fluctuating loads, and eliminate the problems associated with controlling loads close to zero, fluctuating loads may be applied with a minimum load ratio, R, of 10 where:

$$R = \frac{\text{minimum load} = -L}{\text{maximum load} \geq -0.10L} \quad (1)$$

For example, a fluctuating load between –200 N and –10 N would be an acceptable fluctuating load with R=20. It is essential that the ratio should remain constant for all similar tests.

9.7.2 Other spinal components must withstand some degree of reversed loading. Hence, mechanical properties shall be determined using completely reversed loading in all major directions of loading for these components. The maximum load ratio in completely reversed loading should be –1.00.

9.8 After each fatigue test, loosening torque shall be measured (if applicable). A baseline loosening torque, measured prior to any cyclic loading, should also be established prior to the fatigue tests.

10. Report

10.1 The report of the test results shall include the following:

10.1.1 Description of the tested implant components, including the numbers of specimens tested, the manufacturer, the part number, the lot number, and the engineering drawings, if applicable,

10.1.2 The exact loading configuration, reflecting the similarity (and any differences) to the relevant figures contained herein. Include all dimensions. If several implant designs are to be compared, use as similar as possible testing configuration on all implants,

10.1.3 Any deviations from the recommended test procedures,

10.1.4 Means and standard deviations of tightening torques,

10.1.5 The ultimate load/moment, yield load/moment, or gripping capacity values for each test performed, along with means, standard deviations and all load-deflection curves. An indication shall be made whether measurable permanent deformation or gross failure occurred,

10.1.6 A description of any fretting or surface corrosion that is noticeable to the unaided eye in both the assembled and disassembled conditions,

10.1.7 *Environment*—If the test was not conducted in air, describe the test fluid, including temperature, Ph, and ionic concentration, of the solution. State how the solution was applied (for example, drip, immersion). This applies not only to the test itself, but also the conditions during tightening of the interconnections,

10.1.8 A description of any failures or deformations occurring in the testing apparatus or implant construct other than at the interconnection mechanism being tested,

10.1.9 Rate of loading,

10.1.10 A description of the loads applied (fluctuating or completely reversed) using R=minimum load/maximum load,

10.1.11 Plots of load or moment versus number of cycles to failure for each loading direction on a semi-log scale (load, or moment, on the linear axis) showing the order in which the specimens were tested and whether each specimen was run out or failed,

10.1.12 Report the maximum run out load/moment of the interconnection at 2.5×10^6 cycles for each relevant load or moment direction, and

10.1.13 Means and standard deviations of loosening torques.

11. Precision and Bias

11.1 *Precision*—It is not practical to specify the precision of the procedure in this guide because of the wide variance in design of the components to be tested.

11.2 *Bias*—No statement can be made as to the bias of this procedure since no acceptable reference values are available, nor can they be obtained in that this test is a destructive test.

12. Rationale

12.1 This guide covers the evaluation of unidirectional static and fatigue, strength and resistance to loosening of the component interconnection mechanisms of spinal arthrodesis implants. Even though spinal implants may reside in the body for many years, their purpose is to provide short term stability while arthrodesis (bone fusion) takes place. Hence, this guide does not address the long term mechanical stability of spinal implants, nor does it address surgical procedures using implants that do not lead to spinal fusion (for example, artificial discs).

12.2 This guide outlines basic evaluations of the interconnection mechanisms that may be found in spinal arthrodesis implants. It does not address all aspects of spinal surgery nor does it address every unique aspect of particular implant designs. The purpose of this guide is to provide a basic framework of tests which can be used to compare different implant designs in a consistent manner.

12.3 Uniaxial loads and moments are applied in this guide, as multiaxial loading conditions in vivo are not yet fully defined. The methods outlined here are considered minimum test conditions, and more sophisticated tests are encouraged.

12.4 The choice of 1.5 mm and 5° as the defined limits of gripping capacity are large compared to other standards (for example, Practice F 383; 0.13 mm and 1°). There are many ways to define failure. The choice of these arbitrary deflections are admittedly large to ensure ease of measurement from load-deflection curves.

12.5 In developing this guide, significant debate revolved around the question of whether to test in saline, in a simulated body fluid, or in air. Because it was impossible to define a fluid that exactly simulates the in vivo environment and because implants must be compared to one another until performance standards are defined, the test environment is left to the individual investigator.

12.6 In fatigue testing of spinal components (for example, pedicle screws), there is some history of researchers building bilevel constructs of two screws spanned by a rod or plate that is then cyclically loaded through plastic "pucks". From a practical standpoint, such a test should be considered similar to the loading configurations suggested here in Fig. 3. However, it should be noted that when testing bilevel constructs, the specified determination of measurable permanent deformation is altered by a factor of two. This guide describes tests that seek to determine performance of the interconnection mechanism alone. The bilevel test determines overall performance of the implant (for example, pedicle screw root fatigue strength). Based on various goals, individual investigators may seek to address both issues with a single test.

12.7 The question of the degree of fluctuating or completely reversed loading seen by various spinal implants is yet to be answered. Hence, the issue of whether to apply fluctuating or completely reversed loading is left to the investigator, until in vivo data can be generated.

12.8 In fatigue testing, load is the independent variable. The investigator is referred to Footnote 4 for a more complete description using small numbers of samples to estimate fatigue strength. Furthermore, the cycle rate is not specified since it is dependent on the test machine and the specimen. However, a recommended maximum is 16 Hz.

12.9 Depending on the intent of the investigator, different numbers of specimens may be necessary to establish a meaningful sample size. Hence, this guide does not set a specific number of specimens to be tested statistically.

12.10 It is not the intention of this guide to define levels of performance of spinal implants as insufficient knowledge is available to predict the consequences of the use of particular spinal implant designs.

12.11 The estimated number of cycles seen *in vivo* in a twelve month period, which can be considered the approximate average time until fusion, ranges from 1 to 2.5 million cycles. Doubling the 2.5 million cycles to 5 million provides a factor of safety, but substantially increases the cost of testing without providing additional meaningful data. Even if a failure is noted in the 2.5 to 5 million cycle range, it generally occurs in the horizontal run out portion of the curve, and does not significantly affect the curve itself. Therefore, 2.5 million cycles was chosen as the cyclic run out limit.

13. Keywords

13.1 gripping capacity; interconnection; run out; spinal arthrodesis implant; subassembly

Standard Test Method for Cyclic Fatigue Testing of Metal Tibial Tray Components of Total Knee Joint Replacements[1]

This standard is issued under the fixed designation F 1800; the number immediately following the designation indicates the year of original adoption or, in the case of revision, the year of last revision. A number in parentheses indicates the year of last reapproval. A superscript epsilon (ϵ) indicates an editorial change since the last revision or reapproval.

1. Scope

1.1 This test method covers a procedure for the fatigue testing of metallic tibial trays used in knee joint replacements. This standard covers the procedures for the performance of fatigue tests on metallic tibial components using a cyclic, constant-amplitude force. It applies to tibial trays which cover both the medial and lateral plateaus of the tibia. This test method may require modifications to accommodate other tibial tray designs.

1.2 This test method is intended to provide useful, consistent, and reproducible information about the fatigue performance of metallic tibial trays with one unsupported condyle.

1.3 The values stated in SI units are regarded as the standard. The inch-pound units given in parentheses are for information only.

1.4 *This standard does not purport to address all of the safety concerns, if any, associated with its use. It is the responsibility of the user of this standard to establish appropriate safety and health practices and determine the applicability of regulatory limitations prior to use.*

2. Referenced Documents

2.1 *ASTM Standards:*

E 4 Practices for Force Verification of Testing Machines[2]

E 467 Practice for Verification of Constant Amplitude Dynamic Loads in an Axial Load Fatigue Testing System[2]

E 468 Practice for the Presentation of Constant Amplitude Fatigue Results for Metallic Materials[2]

E 1150 Definitions of Terms Relating to Fatigue[2]

3. Terminology

3.1 *Definitions:*

3.1.1 *R value*—The R value is the ratio of the minimum load to the maximum load.

$$R = \frac{minimum\ load}{maximum\ load} \quad (1)$$

3.2 *Definitions of Terms Specific to This Standard:*

3.2.1 *anteroposterior centerline*—a line that passes through the center of the tibial tray, parallel to the sigittal plane and perpendicular to the line of load application. For asymmetric tibial tray designs, the appropriate center of the tibial tray shall be determined by the investigator and the rationale reported.

3.2.2 *fixture centerline*—a line that passes through the center of the fixture, parallel to the anteroposterior centerline. This line represents the separation between the supported and unsupported portions of the test fixture.

3.2.3 *mediolateral centerline*—a line that passes through the center of the tibial tray, parallel to the coronal, or frontal, plane and perpendicular to the line of load application. For asymmetric tibial tray designs, the appropriate center of the tibial tray shall be determined by the investigator and the rationale reported.

3.2.4 *moment arm "d_{ap}"*—the perpendicular distance between the mediolateral centerline of the tibia component and the line of load application.

3.2.5 *moment arm "d_{ml}"*—the perpendicular distance between the anteroposterior centerline of the tibia component and the line of load application.

4. Significance and Use

4.1 This test method can be used to describe the effects of materials, manufacturing, and design variables on the fatigue performance of metallic tibial trays subject to cyclic loading for relatively large numbers of cycles.

4.2 The loading of tibial tray designs *in vivo* will, in general, differ from the loading defined in this test method. The results obtained here cannot be used to directly predict *in vivo* performance. However, this test method is designed to allow for comparisons between the fatigue performance of different metallic tibial tray designs, when tested under similar conditions.

4.3 In order for fatigue data on tibial trays to be comparable, reproducible, and capable of being correlated among laboratories, it is essential that uniform procedures be established.

5. Specimen Selection

5.1 The test component selected shall have the same geometry as the final product, and shall be in finished condition.

6. Apparatus

6.1 The tibial tray shall be mounted as a cantilever beam (see Fig. 1 and Fig. 2). Care shall be taken to ensure that the

[1] This test method is under the jurisdiction of ASTM Committee F-4 on Medical and Surgical Materials and Devices and is the direct responsibility of Subcommittee F04.22 on Arthroplasty .

Current edition approved April 10, 1997. Published February 1998.

[2] *Annual Book of ASTM Standards*, Vol 03.01.

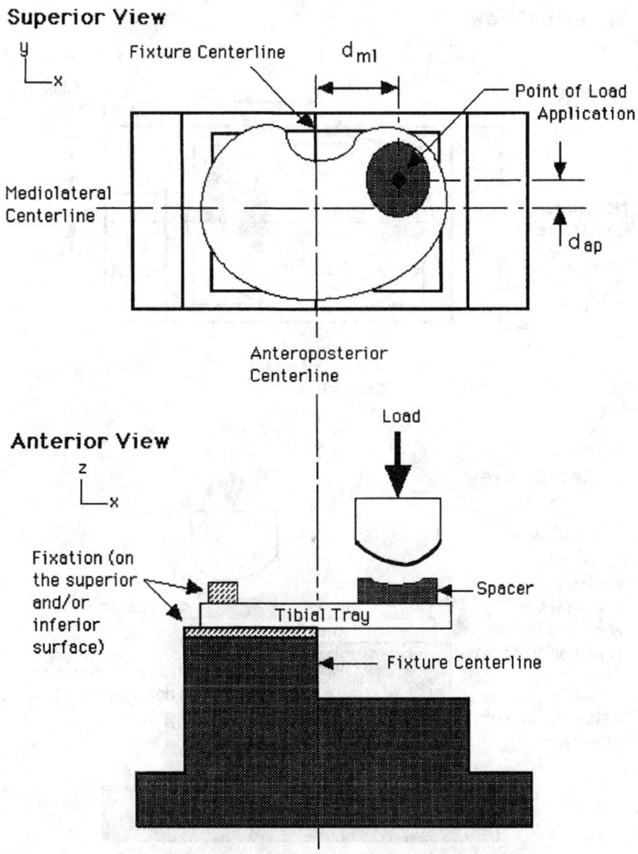

FIG. 1 Schematic of Test Setup Without a Central Keel

fixation of the tibial tray does not produce abnormal stress concentrations that could change the failure mode of the part. One possible setup involving fixation of the inferior surface or clamping of the superior surface is shown in Fig. 1 and Fig. 2. If necessary, bone cement or other high strength epoxy may be used on the supported aspect of the tibial tray to prevent loosening during the test.

6.2 The tibial tray shall be positioned such that the anteroposterior centerline and the fixture centerline are aligned with an accuracy of ± 1 mm in the *x* direction and± 2° in the *x–y* plane (see Fig. 1 and Fig. 2).

6.3 When the tibial tray design includes a central keel or other prominence, the proper method for support of the keel must be determined. Depending on the tibial tray design, it may be necessary to evaluate the design with or without support of the keel (see Fig. 2). The method of supporting (or not supporting) any such feature shall be reported.

6.4 A spacer of plastic possessing sufficient stiffness and creep resistance (for example, ultra high molecular weight polyethylene, acetal co-polymer) shall be placed between the tibial tray and the load applicator (see Fig. 3). The spacer shall contain a spherical indentation (or recess) for the spherical indenter. This recess shall be greater to or equal than the diameter of the spherical indenter and is included to minimize the chance of spacer fracture under load. The spacer shall have a minimum thickness of 6 mm (0.25 in.), measured at the dome of the sphere. It is recommended that the diameter of the spacer is 13 mm (0.5 in.).

NOTE 1—Actual dimensions of the spacer may vary as smaller tibial tray designs may require a smaller diameter disk.

6.4.1 The spacer shall be placed on the unsupported tibial condyle. The purpose of the spacer is to distribute load to the tibial tray condyle and to eliminate possible fretting fatigue initiated by contact between the metal indenter and the tibial tray.

6.5 The fixturing shall be constructed so that the load shall be applied perpendicular to the undeflected superior surface of the tibial tray.

6.6 The point of load application shall be located at a known distance from the anteroposterior centerline (d_{ml}) and from the mediolateral centerline (d_{ap}) .

6.7 The load shall be applied by means of a spherical indenter, a diameter of 32 mm (1.25 in.) is recommended.

7. Equipment Characteristics

7.1 Perform the tests on a fatigue test machine with adequate load capacity.

7.2 Analyze the action of the machine to ensure that the desired form and periodic force amplitude is maintained for the duration of the test (see Practice E 467 or use a validated strain gaged part).

7.3 The test machine shall have a load monitoring system such as the transducer mounted in line with the specimen. Monitor the test loads continuously in the early stages of the test and periodically thereafter to ensure the desired load cycle is maintained. Maintain the varying load as determined by suitable dynamic verification at all times to within ± 2 % of the largest compressive force being used.

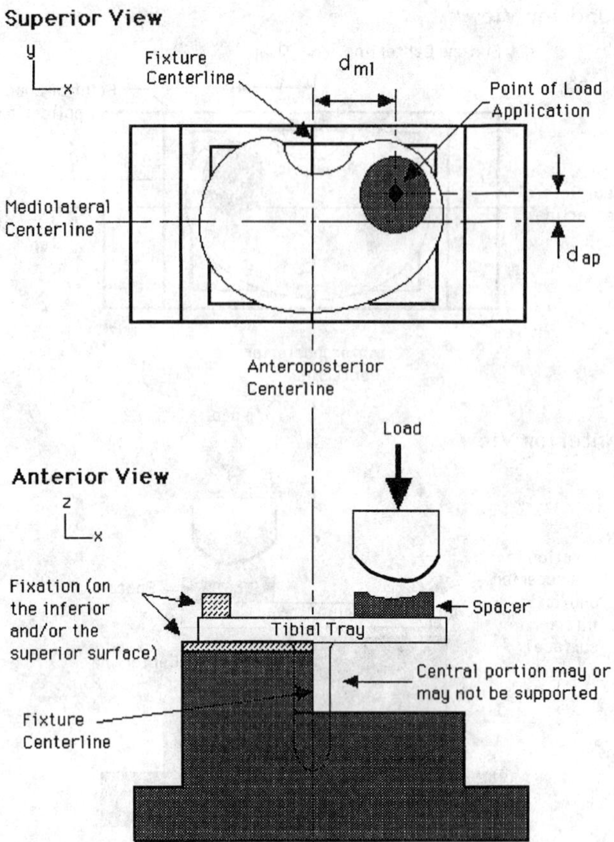

FIG. 2 Schematic or Test Setup With a Central Keel

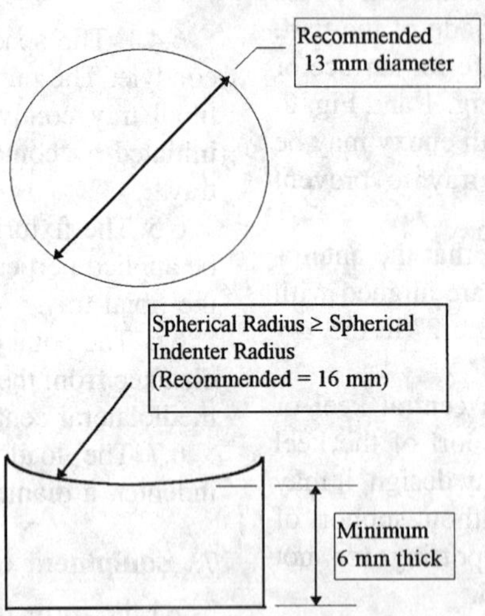

FIG. 3 Recommended Spacer Drawing

8. Procedure

8.1 Determine the size of the tibial tray component used by the investigator. Dimensions shall be reported.

8.2 Position the test specimen such that the load axis is perpendicular to the undeflected superior surface of the tray since the tray surface will not remain perpendicular to the load axis during loading.

8.3 Mount one side of a symmetric tibial component on the fixture (see Fig. 1 and Fig. 2). Use the centerline of the tray to distinguish between supported and non supported sides. If asymmetrical, fix the tibial component such that a worst case condition is tested. Report the criteria used to distinguish between supported and not supported sides.

8.4 Apply the load by means of a spherical indenter.

8.5 *Test frequency*—Run all tests at a frequency of 30 Hz or less. Take care to ensure that the test machine can maintain the applied load at the chosen frequency and that resonant conditions are not reached.

8.6 *R value*—Run all tests with an *R* value of 10.0

NOTE 2—In strict terms, since the force applied to the tray is compressive, the maximum force is the smallest negative amplitude. Consequently, the *R* value is ten when the negative signs cancel each other. In terms of applied bending moment at the cantilever plane, the *R* value would be 0.1. See Terminology E 1150 for the definition of the *R* value.)

8.7 Measure the vertical deflection of the tibial tray using a dial gage, displacement transducer, etc. Record the point at which the deflection is measured (that is, under the applied load, at the point of maximum deflection).

8.8 Report the test environment used.

9. Test Termination

9.1 Continue the test until the tibial tray fails or until a predetermined number of cycles has been applied to the implant. The suggested number of cycles is ten million. Failure may be defined as: a fracture of the tibial tray; formation of a crack detectable by eye, fluorescent dye penetrant, or other non-destructive means; or exceeding a predetermined deflection limit.

10. Report

10.1 Report the fatigue test specimens, procedures, and results in accordance with Practice E 468.

10.2 In addition, report the following parameters: tibial tray material, spacer diameter and thickness, indenter diameter, overall anteroposterior and mediolateral dimensions of the tray, location of anteroposterior and mediolateral centerlines (for asymmetric tibial trays), tibial condyle loaded (for asymmetric tibial trays), d_{ml}, d_{ap}, fixation method, largest compressive load, *R* value, cycles to failure, mode and location of failures, test environment, and test frequency. The rationale for determining the loading location on the tibial tray (that is, d_{ml}, and d_{ap}) shall be documented.

11. Precision and Bias

11.1 The precision and bias of this test method needs to be established. Test results that can be used to establish precision and bias are solicited.

12. Keywords

12.1 arthroplasty; orthopaedic medical devices; tibial components; total knee arthroplasty

APPENDIX

(Nonmandatory Information)

X1. RATIONALE

X1.1 Fractures of tibial trays in TKR have occurred in clinical applications **(1-5)**.[3] The tray design, quality of bone, and other features contribute to implant fracture. One recognizable mode of clinical failure occurs when the lateral portion of the tray is firmly anchored while bone support of the medial condyle is absent. As the body loads are applied through the tray of the prosthesis, significant stresses can result at the area where the tray is still firmly supported. Because it is believed that this lack of support is the primary reason behind fracture of the tibial trays, this test method was chosen as a simplified model to use in fatigue testing of actual implants.

X1.2 It is recognized that for some materials the environment may have an effect on the response to cyclic loading. The test environment used and the rationale for that choice shall be described in the test report.

X1.3 It is also recognized that actual *in vivo* loading conditions are not constant amplitude. However, there is insufficient information available to create standard load spectrums for metallic tibial components. Accordingly, a simple periodic constant amplitude force is recommended.

X1.4 Worst case loading of the tibial tray may vary depending on material, design, and clinical indications. The researcher shall evaluate the possible clinical and design related failure modes and attempt to determine a worst case situation. As stated above, loss of medial bone support has been clinically and is thus incorporated in this test method. Additional factor that may be of importance include wear that has been reported in the posterior medial region of the tibia **6**. Also, as the method of heat treatment can affect the strength of the tibial tray material, it shall be considered. For example, the high temperature sintering treatment used to apply a porous coating to a tibial tray may affect the fatigue strength of the tibial tray.

X1.5 The size of tibial tray to be tested shall be determined by the investigator. In general, the worst case size shall be chosen based on evaluation and/or experience. In a design with a constant tray thickness, maximizing the d_{ml} will result in the largest moment arm and therefore the highest stresses in the tray; however, a tray of non-uniform thickness may not adhere to this rule. There may also be a reason why an investigator wishes to test a size that is not worst case. This test method may also be used for this purpose.

X1.6 The tolerance chosen for the alignment of the tibial tray is based on finite element analysis of a tibial tray design with and without a central keel. The analysis represents one design under specific boundary conditions and is shown as one example of the variation that can occur due to tibial tray misalignment. The results of this analysis were as follows:

[3] The boldface numbers given in parentheses refer to a list of references at the end of the test.

Effect of Malignment (1 mm Shift)

Design	Change in Stress from Correct Alignment
no keel	4 % increase
keel	8 % increase

Effect of Malrotation (5° Rotation)

Design	Change in Stress form Correct Alignment
no keel	5.5 % increase
keel	10 % increase

The required tolerance limits (± 1 mm and ± 2°) were chosen to minimize the change in stress while ensuring a reasonable test setup.

X1.7 —It is recommended that testing be terminated at ten million cycles if failure of the tibial tray has not occurred. The tibial tray design addressed in this testing are designed to replace the knee joint and intended to carry load over the life of the implant. Ten million cycles represents the number of loading cycles a tibial tray might experience over ten years of clinical use (estimated at one million loading cycles per year). It is recognized that in this unsupported condition, the implant may not be required to withstand this number of loading cycles prior to revision.

X1.8 In developing this test method, it was recognized that alternative methods for testing tibial trays exist. One such test method would include placing a tibial insert in the metal tray and applying load through femoral component with a greater distribution on the medial condyle (at a ratio of 60/40 or 80/20). This test method attempts to simplify the loading conditions while addressing clinical failure modes of tibial tray designs. Based on various goals, investigators may seek to deviate from the test method defined here.

REFERENCES

(**1**) Gradisar, I. A., Hoffman, B. S., and Askew, M. S., "Fracture of a Fenestrated Metal Backing of a Total Knee Component", *Journal of Arthroplasty*, Vol. 4, No. 1, March 1989, pp. 27–30.

(**2**) Koeneman, J. B., Johnson, R. M., Weinstein, A. M., and Dupont, J. A., "Failure of Metal Tibial Trays", 12th *Annual Meeting of the Society for Biomaterials, 146,* 1986.

(**3**) Mendes, D. G., Brando, D., Galor, R. L., and Roffman, M., "Breakage of the Metal Tray in Tibial Knee Replacement", *Orthopedics*, Vol. 7, No. 5, May 1984, pp. 860–862.

(**4**) Morrey, B. F., and Chao, E. Y. S, "Fracture of the Porous-Coated Metal Tray of a Biologically Fixed Knee Prosthesis", *Clinical Orthopaedics and Related Research*, No. 228, March 1988, pp. 182–189.

(**5**) Scott, R. D., Ewald, F. C., and Walker, P. S., "Fracture of the Metallic Tibial Tray Following Total Knee Replacement: Report of Two Cases", *Journal of Bone and Joint Surgery*, Vol. 66A, 780, June 1984.

(**6**) Wasielewski, R. C., Galante, J. O., Leighty, R. M., Naterajan, R. N., and Rosenberg, A. G., "Wear Patterns on Retrieved Polyethylene Tibial Inserts and Their Relationship to Technical Consideration During Total Knee Arthroplasty," *Clinical Orthopaedics and Related Research*, No. 299, February 1994, pp. 31–43.

Designation: F 1801 – 97

Standard Practice for Corrosion Fatigue Testing of Metallic Implant Materials[1]

This standard is issued under the fixed designation F 1801; the number immediately following the designation indicates the year of original adoption or, in the case of revision, the year of last revision. A number in parentheses indicates the year of last reapproval. A superscript epsilon (ϵ) indicates an editorial change since the last revision or reapproval.

1. Scope

1.1 This practice covers the procedure for performing corrosion fatigue tests to obtain *S-N* fatigue curves or statistically derived fatigue strength values, or both, for metallic implant materials. This practice describes the testing of axially loaded fatigue specimens subjected to a constant amplitude, periodic forcing function in saline solution at 37°C and in air at room temperature. The environmental test method for implant materials may be adapted to other modes of fatigue loading such as bending or torsion. While this practice is not intended to apply to fatigue tests on implantable components or devices, it does provide guidelines for fatigue tests with standard specimens in an environment related to physiological conditions.

1.2 The values stated in SI units are to be regarded as the standard.

1.3 *This standard does not purport to address all of the safety concerns, if any, associated with its use. It is the responsibility of the user of this standard to establish appropriate safety and health practices and determine the applicability of regulatory limitations prior to use.*

2. Referenced Documents

2.1 *ASTM Standards:*

E 4 Practices for Force Verification of Testing Machines[2]

E 466 Practice for Conducting Force Controlled Constant Amplitude Axial Fatigue Tests of Metallic Materials[2]

E 467 Practice for Verification of Constant Amplitude Dynamic Loads on Displacements in an Axial Load Fatigue Testing Machine[2]

E 468 Practice for Presentation of Constant Amplitude Fatigue Test Results for Metallic Materials[2]

E 739 Practice for Statistical Analysis of Linear or Linearized Stress-Life (*S-N*) or Strain-Life (ϵ-*N*) Fatigue Data[2]

E 1012 Practice for Verification of Specimen Alignment Under Tensile Loading[2]

E 1150 Definitions of Terms Relating to Fatigue[2]

F 86 Practice for Surface Preparation and Marking of Metallic Surgical Implants[3]

F 601 Practice for Fluorescent Penetrant Inspection of Metallic Surgical Implants[3]

G 15 Terminology Relating to Corrosion and Corrosion Testing[4]

2.2 *ANSI Standard:*

ANSI B46.1 Surface Texture[5]

3. Terminology

3.1 *Definitions:*

3.1.1 The terminology used in conjunction with this practice complies to Terminology E 1150 and Terminology G 15.

3.2 *Definitions of Terms Specific to This Standard:*

3.2.1 *S-N curves*—*S-N* curves (also known as Wöhler-curves) show the correlation between the applied stress (*S*) and the counted number (*N*) of cycles to failure.

4. Significance and Use

4.1 Implants, particularly orthopedic devices, are usually exposed to dynamic forces. Thus, implant materials must have high fatigue resistance in the physiological environment.

4.1.1 This practice provides a procedure for fatigue testing in a simulated physiological environment. Axial tension-tension fatigue tests in an environmental test chamber are recommended as a standard procedure. The axial fatigue loading shall comply with Practice E 466 and Practice E 467.

4.1.1.1 Bending and rotating bending beam fatigue tests or torsion tests may be performed in a similar environmental cell.

4.1.2 This practice is intended to assess the fatigue and corrosion fatigue properties of materials that are employed or projected to be employed for implants. This practice is suitable for studying the effects of different material treatments and surface conditions on the fatigue behavior of implant materials. The loading mode of the actual implants may be different from that of this practice. Determining the fatigue behavior of implants and implant components may require separate tests that consider the specific design and loading mode.

4.1.3 As a substitute for body fluid, 0.9 % saline solution is recommended as a standard environment. One of the various Ringer's solutions or another substitute for body fluid may also be suitable for particular tests. However, these various solutions may not give equal fatigue endurance results. The chloride ions are the most critical constituent in these solutions in initiating corrosion fatigue.

---

[1] This practice is under the jurisdiction of ASTM Committee F-4 on Medical and Surgical Materials and Devices and is the direct responsibility of Subcommittee F04.15 on Material Test Methods.

Current edition approved April 10, 1997. Published April 1998.

[2] *Annual Book of ASTM Standards*, Vol 03.01.

[3] *Annual Book of ASTM Standards*, Vol 13.01.

[4] *Annual Book of ASTM Standards*, Vol 03.02.

[5] Available from American National Standards Institute, 11 W. 42nd St., 13th Floor, New York, NY 10036.

4.1.4 Because implants are manufactured from highly corrosion resistant materials, no visible corrosion may be detectable by optical or electron-optical (SEM) means. Only a decrease of fatigue strength in the high cyclic life range may be noticeable. Therefore, S-N curves covering a broad fatigue loading range should be generated in 0.9 % saline solution (Ringer's solutions) and air. Comparison of fatigue curves generated in air and saline solution may be the only way to assess the effect of the saline environment.

4.1.5 Where the fatigue behavior of a material system is already established, it may suffice to test modifications of the material properties or surface condition in only a selected stress range.

4.1.6 The recommended loading frequency of one Hertz corresponds to the frequency of weight-bearing during walking. For screening tests, higher test frequencies may be used; but it must be realized that higher frequencies may affect the results.

4.1.7 *Summary of Standard Conditions*—For interlaboratory comparisons the following conditions are considered as the standard test. Axial tension-tension tests with cylindrical specimens in 37°C 0.9 % saline solution and air under a loading frequency of 1Hz.

5. Testing Equipment

5.1 The mechanics of the testing machine should be analyzed to ensure that the machine is capable of maintaining the desired form and magnitude of loading for the duration of the test (compare Practice E 4).

5.2 *Axial Fatigue Testing*:

5.2.1 Tension-tension fatigue tests may be performed on one of the following types of axial fatigue testing machines:

5.2.1.1 Mechanical,

5.2.1.2 Electromechanical or magnetically driven, and

5.2.1.3 Hydraulic or electrohydraulic.

5.2.2 The machine shall have a load-monitoring system, such as a transducer mounted in series with the specimen. The test loads shall be monitored continuously in the early stage of the test and periodically thereafter, to ensure that the desired load is maintained. The magnitude of the varying loads, measured dynamically as described in Practice E 467 shall be maintained within an accuracy of less than or equal to 2 % of the extreme loads applied during testing.

5.3 *Non Axial Fatigue Testing*—Corrosion fatigue tests under loading conditions different from axial tension-tension may be requested. In such cases established experimental arrangements for bending, rotating bending beam, or torsional testing may replace the axial tension-tension mode. An environmental test chamber is attached to the equipment and the environmental tests are carried out under conditions as described in this standard. Except for the mechanical testing arrangements the conditions of this standard practice apply where possible. Reporting should follow Section 9 and should include all details where the testing deviates from the standard procedure.

5.4 *Environmental Chamber*:

5.4.1 For corrosion fatigue testing, the machine shall be fitted with an environmental test cell surrounding the specimen gauge section as shown in Fig. 1. A heated solution reservoir, a solution pump, and connecting lines for circulating the test solution to the specimen surface are required. The solution should be pumped from the reservoir through the system at a rate that will maintain the temperature at 37 ± 1°C in the test cell, but with flow rates low enough to avoid flow-dependent phenomena like erosion-corrosion. The reservoir should have a minimum capacity of 1000 mL per square centimeter of specimen surface exposed to the electrolyte. The reservoir shall be vented to the atmosphere. If the solution volume decreases, the reservoir shall be replenished with distilled water to maintain the saline concentration, or the solution should be exchanged. During long testing periods exchange of the solution is recommended. A typical environmental test cell for axial fatigue testing is shown in Fig. 1.

5.4.2 The test equipment should be manufactured of materials or should be protected in a manner that corrosion is avoided. In particular galvanic corrosion in conjunction with the test specimen and loosening of the specimen grips due to corrosion must be excluded.

6. Test Solution

6.1 To prepare the saline solution, dissolve 9 g of reagent-grade sodium chloride in distilled water and make up to 1000 mL. If other typical Ringer's solutions are used, note the solution in the report.

7. Test Specimen

7.1 *Specimen Design*:

7.1.1 *Axial Fatigue Testing*:

7.1.1.1 The design of the axial load fatigue test specimens should comply to Practice E 466 (see Fig. 2, Fig. 3, Fig. 4 and Fig. 5). For the dimensional proportions of flat specimens refer to the drawing in Practice E 468. The ratio of the test section area to end section area will depend on the specimen geometry and should comply to those standards. The test specimens specified in Practice E 466 and Practice E 468 are designed so that fatigue failure should occur in the section with reduced diameter and not at the grip section.

7.1.1.2 For bending tests one may refer to the specimen configuration suggested in Practice E 466.

7.1.1.3 To calculate the load necessary to obtain the required stress, the cross-sectional area of the specimen test-section must be measured accurately. The dimensions should be measured to the nearest 0.03 mm (0.001 in.) for specimens less than 5.00 mm thick (0.197 in.), and to the nearest 0.05 mm (0.002 in.) for specimens more than 5.00 mm thick (0.197 in.). Surfaces intended to be parallel and straight should be carefully aligned.

7.2 *Specimen Dimensions*—Consult Practice E 466 and Practice E 468 for the dimensions of fatigue specimens for axial tension-tension loading (Fig. 2, Fig. 3, Fig. 4, and Fig. 5). If bending specimens corresponding to the example of Practice F 466 are used, observe the suggested dimensions.

7.3 *Specimen Preparation*:

7.3.1 The method of surface preparation and the resulting surface condition of the test specimens are of great importance because they influence the test results strongly. Standard preparation shall consist of machining, grinding, or polishing, or all of these. A final mechanical polish is suggested to give a

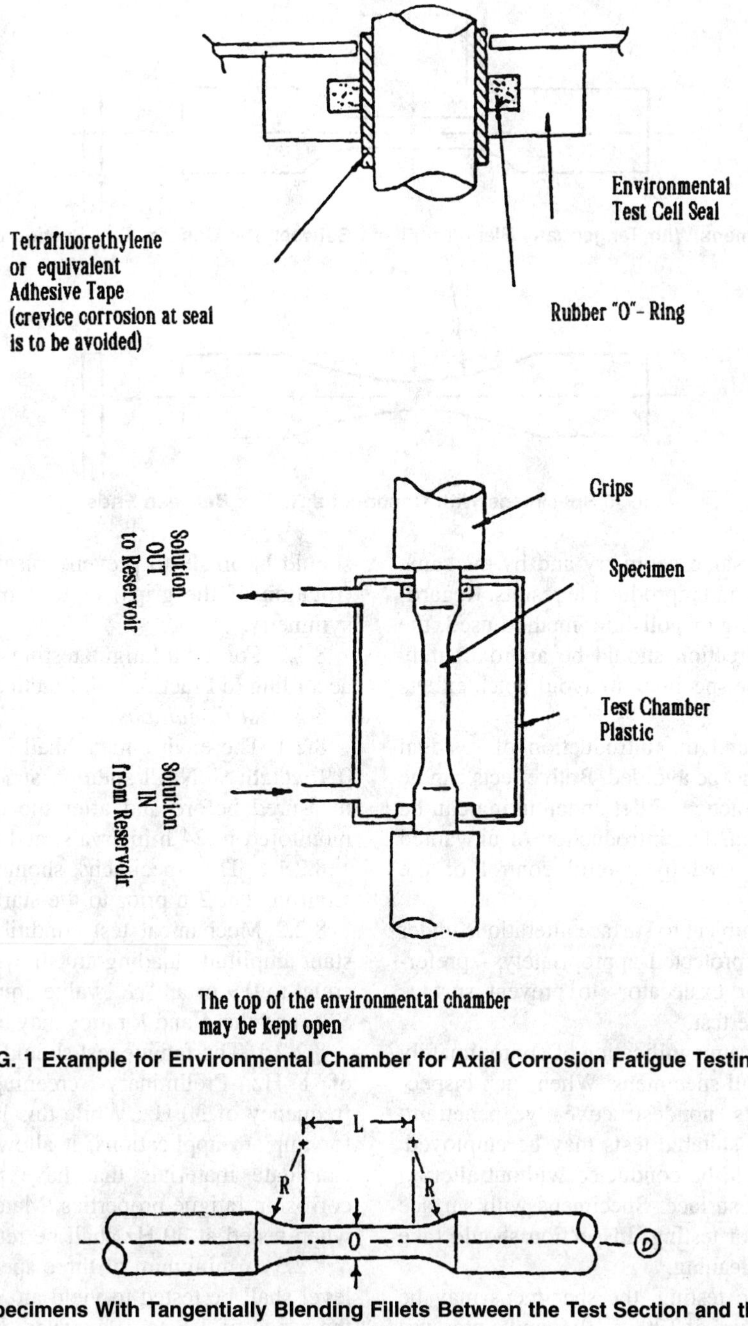

FIG. 1 Example for Environmental Chamber for Axial Corrosion Fatigue Testing

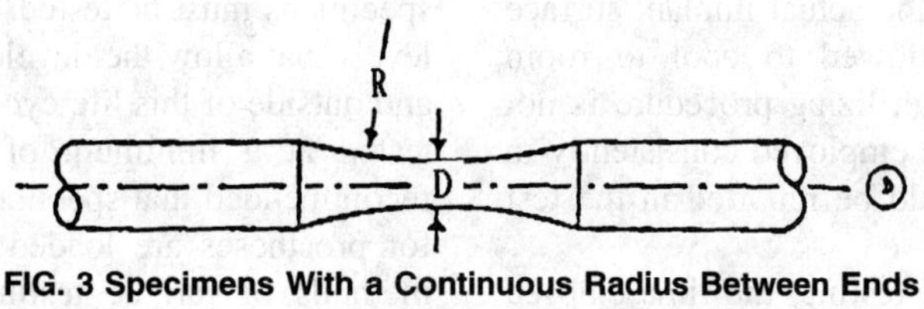

FIG. 2 Specimens With Tangentially Blending Fillets Between the Test Section and the Ends

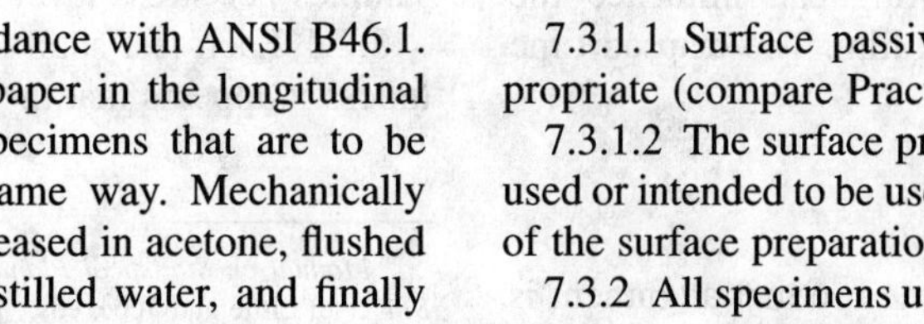

FIG. 3 Specimens With a Continuous Radius Between Ends

finish of 16 Min RA or less in accordance with ANSI B46.1. Alternatively a finish with 600 grit paper in the longitudinal direction may be used. However, specimens that are to be compared should be prepared the same way. Mechanically finished specimens must then be degreased in acetone, flushed first with ethyl alcohol, then with distilled water, and finally blown dry with warm air.

7.3.1.1 Surface passivation may be carried out where appropriate (compare Practice F 86).

7.3.1.2 The surface preparation may be also exactly such as used or intended to be used for surgical implants. A full account of the surface preparation should be given in the test protocol.

7.3.2 All specimens used in any given series of experiments, including comparison between air and liquid environment,

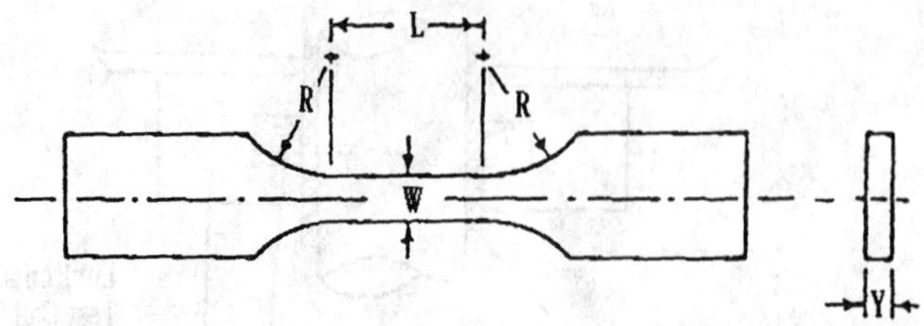

FIG. 4 Specimens With Tangentially Blending Fillets Between the Uniform Test Section and the Ends

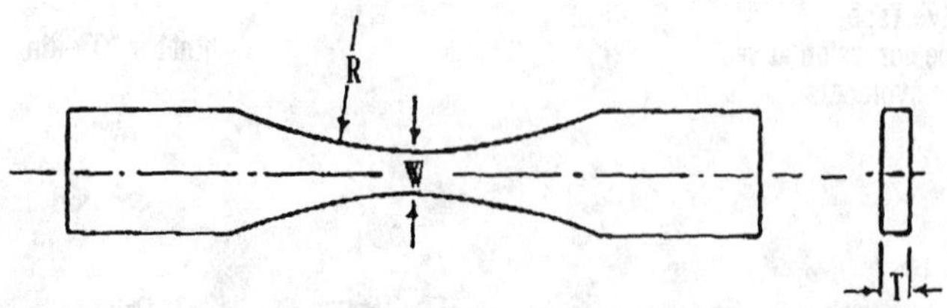

FIG. 5 Specimens With Continuous Radius Between Ends

should be prepared with the same geometry and by the same method to ensure comparable and reproducible results. Regardless of the machining, grinding or polishing method used, the final mechanical working direction should be approximately parallel to the long axis of the specimen to avoid notch effects of surface grooves.

7.3.3 Fillet undercutting and the introduction of residual stresses into the specimen must be avoided. Both effects can be caused by poor machining practice. Fillet undercutting can be identified by visual inspection. The introduction of unwanted residual stresses can be avoided by careful control of the machining process.

7.3.4 Specimens that are subject to surface alterations under ambient conditions shall be protected appropriately, - preferably in an inert medium or exsiccator- to prevent surface change until beginning of the test.

7.3.5 Visual inspections at a magnification of approximately 20× shall be performed on all specimens. When such inspections reveal potential defects, nondestructive dye penetrant, ultrasonic methods, or other suitable tests may be employed. Dimensional inspection should be conducted without altering or damaging the specimen's surface. Specimens with surface defects should not be used for testing. Inspection should take place prior to final surface cleaning.

7.3.6 Immediately prior to testing, the specimens may be steam sterilized at a temperature of 120 ± 10°C and a pressure of 0.10 MPa (14.5 psi) to simulate the actual implant surface conditions. Specimens shall be allowed to cool to room temperature prior to testing. This sterilizing procedure is not mandatory. If it is used, it should be employed consistently in test series that are related and should be reported in the test protocol.

7.3.7 In the liquid environmental testing, the time elapsed between surface preparation and testing can influence the results due to the growth of a passive film. The elapsed time should thus be reported.

8. Procedure

8.1 *Test Set-Up*:

8.1.1 Specimen grips must be designed so that alignment is consistently good from one specimen to the next. Every effort should be made to prevent misalignment, due either to twist (rotation of the grips) or to a displacement in their axes of symmetry.

8.1.2 For axial fatigue testing, alignment should be verified according to Practice E 4, Practice E 467, and Practice E 1012.

8.2 *Test Conditions*:

8.2.1 The environment shall be air at room temperature or 0.9 weight % NaCl solution at 37 ± 1°C. The pH should be measured before and after the test is begun and should be monitored in 24 h intervals, and at the end of the test.

8.2.1.1 The specimens should be exposed to the liquid environment 2 h prior to the start of the cyclic loading.

8.2.2 Mechanical test conditions for tension-tension, constant amplitude loading are shown in Fig. 6, with an "*A*" ratio equal to 0.9 or an "*R*" value equal to 0.053. Other values for S_{max} and the *A* and *R* ratios may be used, but must be reported.

8.2.2.1 The fatigue test should be carried out at a frequency of 1 Hz. Preliminary screening may be performed at a frequency of 30 Hz. While this is a relatively high frequency for implant applications, it allows rapid elimination of those candidate materials that have particularly poor fatigue or corrosion fatigue properties. Materials that appear satisfactory when tested at 30 Hz shall be retested at 1 Hz.

8.2.3 A minimum of three specimens at each chosen stress level shall be tested to yield an *S/N* curve that covers at least the range of 10^4 to 10^6 cycles, in case of uncertainties more specimens must be tested. Specimens shall be loaded to stress levels that allow the development of an *S/N* curve both within and outside of this life cycle range. Thus, specimens should be tested at a minimum of five different stress levels. It is recommended that specimens of materials intended to be used for prostheses are loaded up to 10^7 cycles. When statistical methods of fatigue testing are used[6,7], a minimum of six samples per stress level must be tested.

8.2.4 Each test shall be continued until the specimen fails, unless it appears that the stress is below the fatigue endurance

[6] *Manual on Statistical Planning and Analysis of Fatigue Experiments, ASTM STP 588*, Little and Tebe, eds.

[7] *Statistical Analysis of Fatigue Data, ASTM STP 744*, Little and Ekvall, eds.

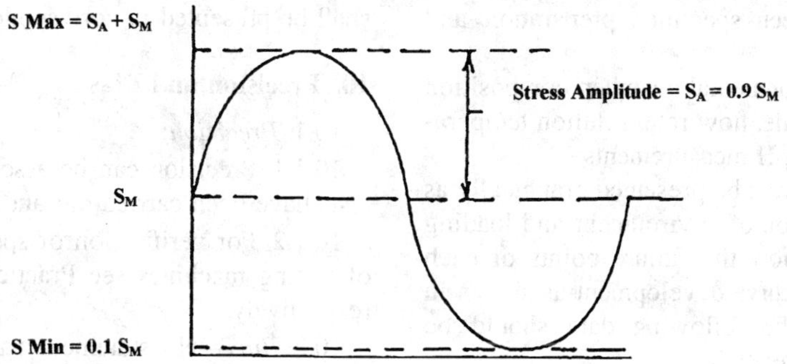

"A" Ratio = $\frac{S_A}{S_M}$ = 0.90

"R" Ratio = $\frac{S\ Min}{S\ Max}$ = 0.053

DEFINITIONS

SYMBOL	DESCRIPTION	FORMULA
S Min	Minimum Stress	S Min = 0.1 S_M
S Max	Maximum Stress	S Max = $S_A + S_M$
S_M	Mean Stress	$S_M = \frac{S\ Max + S\ Min}{2}$
S_R	Stress Range	S_R = S Max - S Min
S_A	Stress Amplitude	$S_A = \frac{S_R}{2} = \frac{S\ Max - S\ Min}{2}$
"R"	Stress Ratio	$R = \frac{S\ Min}{S\ Max}$
"A"	"A" Ratio	$A = \frac{S_A}{S_M}$

FIG. 6 Loading Conditions

limit. Failure is defined as complete separation. If this definition does not apply in cases where the axial tension-tension mode is not chosen, the failure criteria need to be reported.

9. Report

9.1 Specimen characteristics and preparation, fatigue test procedures, and results shall be reported in accordance with Practice E 468. The following minimum information and data shall be reported for each combination of environment and loading frequency:

9.1.1 *Material Indentification*:

9.1.1.1 Chemical composition,

9.1.1.2 Production process (casting, forging, extruded bar etc.),

9.1.1.3 Mechanical/thermal processing (cold worked, annealed, etc.),

9.1.1.4 Microstructure, and

9.1.1.5 Specification data (if appropriate).

9.1.2 *Material Properties*:

9.1.2.1 Ultimate tensile strength,

9.1.2.2 Yield strength,

9.1.2.3 Elongation at failure, and

9.1.2.4 Hardness.

9.1.3 *Type of Specimen*:

9.1.3.1 Shape of specimen and dimensions,

9.1.3.2 Machining method,

9.1.3.3 Surface condition and preparation, and

9.1.3.4 Sterilization (if used).

9.1.4 *Fatigue Test Program*:

9.1.4.1 Type of fatigue test,

9.1.4.2 Statistical approach and analysis,

9.1.4.3 Significant variations,

9.1.4.4 Type of machine,

9.1.4.5 Failure criterion, and

9.1.4.6 Wave form and frequency.

9.1.5 *Environmental Conditions*:

9.1.5.1 Ambient laboratory air temperature and humidity.

9.1.5.2 Time elapsed between specimen preparation and exposure to test solution.

9.1.5.3 Dimensions of environmental chamber, composition of test solution, reservoir volume, flow rate, solution temperature, pH values and timing of pH measurements.

9.2 The fatigue test results shall be presented graphically as *S/N* curves for each combination of environment and loading frequency; the curves shall show the failure points of each specimen, and the criteria for curve development as shown in Fig. 1 of Practice E 468. The following data should be obtainable from each S/N curve:

9.2.1 The fatigue strength at 10 000 and 100 000 cycles,

9.2.2 The fatigue strength at 1 000 000 cycles,

9.2.3 Indication of fatigue limit if possible, and

9.2.4 The report of fatigue strength at 10 000 000 cycles is suggested in cases where the material is intended to be used for prostheses.

9.3 If special statistical test methods are employed, the data shall be presented in correspondence to that method.

10. Precision and Bias

10.1 *Precision*:

10.1.1 Precision can be assessed only after interlaboratory tests have been carried out and the results are tabulated.

10.1.2 For verification of specimen alignment and loading of testing machines see Practice E 1012 and Practice E 467, respectively.

10.2 *Bias*—No statement can be made as to bias of this practice since no acceptable reference values are available, nor can they be obtained because of the destructive nature of the tests.

11. Keywords

11.1 corrosion fatigue; metallic implant materials; physiological environment

APPENDIX

(Nonmandatory Information)

X1. RATIONALE

X1.1 This practice provides a practice for the assessment of the corrosion fatigue behavior of metallic materials intended to be used in body environment.

X1.2 To evaluate the effect of the environment, fatigue tests must be performed in air and in the environment under otherwise exactly the same conditions. This may be achieved by testing in parallel in units with identical loading arrangements, or consecutively on the same testing unit.

X1.3 The physiological environment is simulated by 0.9 % saline solution at 37 ± 1°C temperature. Of significance in this test solution is the chlor ion concentration. Regarding metal corrosion, this is the most aggressive species which is contained in the body fluid in about the same concentration. Furthermore, the 0.9 % isotonic saline solution is used in surgery for irrigation.

X1.4 Other species of the physiological environment such as proteins can have inhibitory effects that counteract the chlor ion activity.

X1.5 The effect of the environment on the fatigue resistance may be very mild and without any morphological signs of corrosion. The environment may only influence the fatigue life by some effects on the growth or deterioration of the passive film on the metal surface.

X1.6 Environmental effects may be only observed in certain sections of the Wöhler curve.

Designation: F 1813 – 97$^{\epsilon 1}$

Standard Specification for Wrought Titanium - 12 Molybdenum - 6 Zirconium - 2 Iron Alloy For Surgical Implant Applications[1]

This standard is issued under the fixed designation F 1813; the number immediately following the designation indicates the year of original adoption or, in the case of revision, the year of last revision. A number in parentheses indicates the year of last reapproval. A superscript epsilon (ε) indicates an editorial change since the last revision or reapproval.

ϵ^1 NOTE—Footnote 1 was editorially revised June 2000.

1. Scope

1.1 This specification covers the chemical, mechanical and metallurgical requirements for wrought Ti-12 Mo-6 Zr-2 Fe alloy to be used in the manufacture of surgical implants[2].

1.2 The values stated in inch-pound units are to be regarded as the standard. The metric equivalents given in parentheses are provided for information only.

2. Referenced Documents

2.1 *ASTM Standards:*

B 348 Specification for Titanium and Titanium Alloy Bars and Billets[3]

E 8 Test Methods for Tension Testing of Metallic Materials[4]

E 112 Test Methods for Determining Average Grain Size[5]

E 120 Test Methods for Chemical Analysis of Titanium and Titanium Alloys[4]

E 1409 Test Method for the Determination of Oxygen in Titanium and Titanium Alloys by the Inert Gas Fusion Technique[4]

E 1447 Test Method for the Determination of Hydrogen in Titanium and Titanium Alloys by the Inert Gas Fusion Thermal Conductivity Method[4]

F 748 Practice for Selecting Generic Biological Test Methods for Materials and Devices[6]

F 750 Practice for Evaluating Material Extracts by Systematic Injection in the Mouse[6]

F 895 Test Method for Agar Diffusion Cell Culture Screening for Cytotoxicity[6]

F 981 Practice for Assessment of Compatibility of Biomaterials (Non-Porous) for Surgical Implants with Respect to Effect of Materials on Muscle and Bone[6]

2.2 *Aerospace Materials Specification:*

AMS 2249 Chemical Check Analysis Limits, Titanium and Titanium Alloys[7]

2.3 *American Society for Quality Standard:*

ASQ C1 Specification of General Requirements for a Quality Program[8]

3. Ordering Information

3.1 Inquiries and orders for material under this specification shall include the following information:

3.1.1 Quantity (weight or number of pieces),

3.1.2 ASTM Designation,

3.1.3 Dimensions,

3.1.4 Condition,

3.1.5 Finish (see 4.2), and

3.1.6 Special requirements.

4. Materials and Manufacture

4.1 The titanium mill products covered in this specification are normally formed with the conventional forging, rolling or other metal processing equipment found in primary ferrous and nonferrous plants. The ingot metal for such mill operations is usually multiple melted in arc furnaces (including furnaces such as plasma arc and electron beam) of a type conventionally used for reactive metals.

4.2 *Finish*—Annealed material may be furnished to the implant manufacturer as descaled or pickled, sandblasted, machined, ground, or combinations of these operations.

5. Chemical Requirements

5.1 The heat analysis shall conform to the chemical composition of Table 1. Ingot analysis may be used for reporting all chemical requirements, except hydrogen. Samples for hydrogen shall be taken from the finished mill product.

5.2 *Product Analysis*— Product analysis tolerances do not broaden the specified heat analysis requirements but cover variations between laboratories in the measurement of chemical content. The manufacturer shall not ship material that is outside the limits specified in Table 1. Product analysis limits

[1] This specification is under the jurisdiction of ASTM Committee F-4 on Medical and Surgical Materials and Devices and is the direct responsibility of Subcommittee F0.4.12 on Metallurgical Materials.

Current edition approved June 10, 1997. Published June 1998.

[2] Wang, K., Gustavson, L., Dumbleton, J., "The Characterization of Ti-12Mo-6Zr-2Fe - A New Biocompatible Alloy Developed for Surgical Implants", *Beta Titanium Alloys in the 1990's*, Proceedings of a Symposium on Beta Titanium Alloys held at the 1993 Annual TMS meeting in Denver, Colorado, February 22–24, 1993.

[3] *Annual Book of ASTM Standards*, Vol 02.04.

[4] *Annual Book of ASTM Standards*, Vol 03.01.

[5] *Annual Book of ASTM Standards*, Vol 03.05.

[6] *Annual Book of ASTM Standards*, Vol 13.01.

[7] Available from SAE; 400 Commonwealth Drive, Warrendale, PA 15096.

[8] Available from American Society for Quality; 161 West Wisconsin Avenue, Milwaukee, WI 53203.

TABLE 1 Chemical Requirements

Element	Composition, Weight %	
	Minimum	Maximum
Molybdenum	10.0	13.0
Zirconium	5.0	7.0
Iron	1.5	2.5
Oxygen	0.08	0.28
Nitrogen	—	0.05
Carbon	—	0.05
Hydrogen	—	0.020
Titanium[A]	Balance	Balance

[A]The percentage of titanium is determined by difference and need not be determined or certified.

shall be as specified in Table 2.

5.2.1 The product analysis is either for the purpose of verifying the composition of a heat or lot or to determine variations in the composition within the heat.

5.3 For referee purposes, Test Methods E 120, E 1409 and E 1447 or other analytical methods agreed upon by purchaser and supplier shall be used.

5.4 Samples for chemical analysis shall be representative of the material being tested. The utmost care must be used in sampling titanium for chemical analysis because of its affinity for elements such as oxygen, nitrogen, and hydrogen. Therefore, in cutting samples for analysis any contamination should be avoided. Chips should be clean, and sharp cutting tools should be used. Samples for analysis should be stored in suitable containers.

5.5 Requirements for the major and minor elemental constituents are listed in Table 1. Also listed are important residual elements. Analysis for elements not listed in Table 1 is not required to verify compliance with this specification.

6. Mechanical Requirements

6.1 Material supplied under this specification shall conform to the mechanical property requirements given in Table 3.

6.2 Perform tension testing in accordance with Test Methods E 8. Determine tensile properties using a strain rate of 0.003 to 0.007 in./in./min (mm/mm/min) through the specified yield strength, and then the cross-head speed shall be increased so as to produce fracture in approximately one additional minute.

6.3 *Number of Tests*— A minimum of two tension tests shall be made from each lot. A lot is defined as the total number of mill products produced under the same conditions at essentially the same time. Should either of the test specimens not meet the specific requirements two additional test pieces representative of the same lot shall be tested in the same manner. The lot shall be deemed to comply only if both additional test pieces meet the specific requirements. If a sample fails outside the gage section, the sample is void in accordance with Test Method E 8 and additional sample shall be tested.

TABLE 2 Permissible Variation in Product Analysis (Weight %)

Element	Tolerance Under Minimum or Over Maximum Limit
Molybdenum	0.25
Zirconium over 4 to 6 % inclusive	0.20
Zirconium over 6 to 10 % inclusive	0.30
Iron	0.20
Oxygen up to 0.2 %	0.02
Oxygen over 0.2 %	0.03
Nitrogen	0.02
Carbon	0.002
Hydrogen	0.0002

TABLE 3 Mechanical Properties of Ti-12Mo-6Zr-2Fe Bar and Wire[A]

Condition	Ultimate Tensile Strength, min, psi (MPa)	Yield Strength (0.2 %), min, psi (MPa)	Elongation[B] min, %	Reduction in Area min. (%)
Solution[C] Annealed	135 000 (931.5)	130 000 (897)	12	30

[A]Diameter 0.10 in. (2.54 mm) to 1½ in. (38.1 mm).

[B]Gage length = 4 × diameter.

[C]Solution annealing shall be performed at 1450 ± 25°F (788± 14°C) followed by a rapid quench to below 300°F (°C), for an appropriate time, as required to meet grain size and mechanical property requirements.

7. Microstructure

7.1 The microstructure shall be fully recrystallized single phase beta microstructure after solution annealing. There shall be no continuous alpha network at prior beta grain boundaries. There shall be no alpha precipitates.

7.2 Grain size of the solution annealed barstock shall be five or finer based upon Test Methods E 112.

7.3 Products supplied with a machined or ground surface finish shall have no alpha case. For other products, there shall be no continuous layer of alpha case when examined at 100X.

7.4 The beta transus temperature shall be determined by a suitable method and reported on the material certification for each heat.

8. Quality Program Requirements

8.1 The producer shall maintain a quality program, for example, such as defined in ASQ C1.

9. Certification

9.1 A certification shall be provided by the manufacturer of the material that the material was manufactured and tested in accordance with this specification. A report of the test results shall be furnished at the time of shipment.

10. Keywords

10.1 metals (for surgical implants); orthopaedic medical devices; titanium alloys; titanium/titanium alloy; titanium/titanium alloys (for surgical implants)

APPENDIXES

(Nonmandatory Information)

X1. RATIONALE

X1.1 The purpose of this specification is to characterize the composition and properties of wrought annealed Titanium-12Molybdenum-6Zirconium-2Iron titanium alloy to ensure consistency in the starting material used in the manufacture of medical devices, in particular of surgical implants.

X1.2 The microstructural requirements contained in this Specification represent the current general consensus with respect to optimization of mechanical properties for implant applications.

X1.3 The minimum mechanical properties specified assure a baseline of strength and ductility for the highly stressed devices which may be manufactured from this alloy.

X1.4 The stress corrosion cracking resistance of this alloy is similar to that of Titanium 6A1–4V ELI alloy.[9]

[9] FDA 510K application number K903630, submitted by Howmedica, Inc., Rutherford, NJ.

X2. BIOCOMPATIBILITY

X2.1 As of the time of the original approval of this specification, this titanium alloy material had a limited history of clinical use in humans. An extensive series of in-vitro and animal tests had been performed, as listed below, comparing the biological response to that of the control material, Titanium 6Aluminum-4Vanadium ELI alloy. These tests were conducted to support the usage of this material in specific surgical implant devices. In all cases, the results indicated that this material was no more bioreactive with the environment than that of the reference material.

X2.1.1 Acute systemic toxicity by mouse injection (See Practice F 750).

X2.1.2 Cytotoxicity by agar overlay (See Practice F 898).

X2.1.3 Hemolytic potential by direct exposure.

X2.1.4 Dermal sensitization by guinea pig maximization.

X2.1.5 Mutagenicity by the Ames test (saline and DMSO extracts).

X2.1.6 Response to particulate debris (release of IL-1, IL-6 and PGE_2 in cell culture and ex-vivo histology rabbits).

X2.2 The suitability of this material, from a biological performance perspective is dependent on the specific site. For new functional applications for this material it may be advisable to undertake some additional biologic tests appropriate for the specific site, such as recommended in Practice F 748.

X2.3 No known surgical implant material has ever been shown to be completely free of adverse reactions in the human body. However, the alloy composition covered by this standard has been subjected to testing in laboratory animals. The results of these studies indicate a well characterized level of biological response that is equal to or less than that produced by the reference material Titanium-6A1-4V ELI alloy which has a long history of successful clinical application in soft tissue and bone implants in humans.

Designation: F 1814 – 97a

Standard Guide for Evaluating Modular Hip and Knee Joint Components[1]

This standard is issued under the fixed designation F 1814; the number immediately following the designation indicates the year of original adoption or, in the case of revision, the year of last revision. A number in parentheses indicates the year of last reapproval. A superscript epsilon (ε) indicates an editorial change since the last revision or reapproval.

1. Scope

1.1 This guide covers a procedure to assist the developer of a modular joint replacement implant in the choice of appropriate tests and evaluations to determine device safety.

1.2 This guide does not attempt to define all test methods associated with modular device evaluation.

1.3 This guide does not cover intentional intraoperative disassembly but is meant only to suggest testing necessary to determine inadvertent disassembly loads.

1.4 *This standard does not purport to address all of the safety concerns, if any, associated with its use. It is the responsibility of the user of this standard to establish appropriate safety and health practices and determine the applicability of regulatory limitations prior to use.*

2. Referenced Documents

2.1 *ASTM Standards:*

F 648 Specification for Ultra-High-Molecular-Weight Polyethylene Powder and Fabricated Form for Surgical Implants[2]

F 897 Test Method for Measuring Fretting Corrosion of Osteosynthesis Plates and Screws[2]

F 1440 Practice for Cyclic Fatigue Testing of Metallic Stemmed Hip Arthroplasty Femoral Components Without Torsion[2]

F 1800 Test Method for Cyclic Fatigue Testing of Metal Tibial Components of Total Knee Joint Replacements[2]

2.2 *ISO Standard:*

ISO 7206 Implants for Surgery-Partial and Total Hip Joint Prosthesis[3]

Part 4 Determination of Endurance Properties of Stemmed Femoral Components With Application of Torsion[3]

Part 6 Determination of Endurance Properties of Head and Neck Region of Stemmed Femoral Components[3]

Part 8 Endurance Performance of Stemmed Femoral Components With Application of Torsion[3]

3. Terminology

3.1 *Definitions of Terms Specific to This Standard:*

3.1.1 *modular femoral hip implant*—any device, constructed of two or more mating parts intended for implantation into the femur for the purpose of replacing the femoral hip joint.

3.1.1.1 *bolts/screws*—a fastener used to secure modular pieces of a femoral component.

3.1.1.2 *bullets/distal sleeves*—modular accessories for increasing length or distal diameter of the femoral component.

3.1.1.3 *collars*—a medial platform located immediately distal to the femoral neck.

3.1.1.4 *femoral head*—a modular bearing, spherical in shape, that mates with the femoral component.

3.1.1.5 *neck extensions*—an intermediate modular couple between the femoral component and the femoral head. Attachment can vary (for example, threads, tapers).

3.1.1.6 *proximal sleeves/pads*—modular accessories for varying the geometry of the femoral component in the metaphyseal area.

3.1.2 *modular knee implant*—any device, constructed of two or more mating parts intended for implantation into the femur or tibia for the purpose of replacing the knee joint.

3.1.2.1 *metal backed patella*—a modular patellar replacement consisting of an articular piece which is secured to a metal backing by means of a locking mechanism.

3.1.2.2 *metal tibial tray*—a metal component secured to the proximal tibia which provides mechanical support to and couples directly with the modular tibial inserts.

3.1.2.3 *stem extensions or sleeve*—any modular extension to either a knee femoral or tibial component which extends into the medullary canal. Stem extensions may be attached to the femoral or tibial component by a variety of means including tapers, screws, etc.

3.1.2.4 *tibial insert*—a modular bearing member of a tibial component, usually made in accordance with Specification F 648, that is secured to a knee tibial tray by means of a locking mechanism.

3.1.2.5 *wedge*—a modular addition to a total knee replacement that serves the function of filling voids left by deficient or absent bone stock.

4. Significance and Use

4.1 The tests suggested within this guide cover many different, but not all possible, areas of research and concern with regard to modular hip stems and modular knee components.

[1] This guide is under the jurisdiction of ASTM Committee F-4 on Medical and Surgical Materials and Device and is the direct responsibility of Subcommittee F04.22 on Arthroplasty.

Current edition approved June 10 and Nov. 10,, 1997. Published June 1998.

[2] *Annual Book of ASTM Standards*, Vol 13.01.

[3] Available from American National Standards Institute, 11 W. 42nd St., 13th Floor, New York, NY 10036.

4.2 Due to the unlimited possible modular designs, this guide should be utilized as a guide for what should be considered with regard to device safety testing. There may be circumstances where alternative test methods may be useful. It is still the responsibility of the investigator to address all safety concerns that are inherent to individual modular designs.

4.3 The tests suggested herein should be utilized in such a way that the results reflect the effects of modularity, if any.

4.4 Tests that are checked in Fig. 1 or Fig. 2 or indicated in this guide as a possible test to consider may not be applicable to every implant design.

5. Testing

5.1 *Assembly*—Static assembly parameters should be evaluated to determine the minimum required loads (axial or torsional) that ensure adequate assembly strengths. This testing can be performed in conjunction with 5.2. Disassembly, to ascertain how various assembly loads affect disassembly

5.1.1 *Axial Engagement Force*—The force required to connect the components (for example, to engage a tapered connection consider the following:

5.1.1.1 The procedure for applying the engagement force (clinical relevance), and

5.1.1.2 The environment in which the components are connected (contamination).

5.1.2 *Torsional*—The torque required to connect the components (for example, Bolt or screw). This may only be applicable for threaded connections. Consider the following:

5.1.2.1 The procedure for applying the torsional force (clinical relevance).

5.2 *Disassembly*—Static disassembly parameters should be evaluated to assess minimum design requirements for preventing unintentional *in vivo* disassembly.

5.2.1 *Axial*—The axial force required to disassemble mating components (for example, force required to disassociate a tapered junction).

5.2.2 *Shear*—The shear force required to disassemble mating components (for example, force required to shear a wedge from a tray).

5.2.3 *Bending*—The possibility of static disassociation under combined loading. Consider the following:

5.2.3.1 Reporting a load versus deflection curve.

5.2.4 *Torsion*—The torque required to disconnect the components (for example, bolt or screw). This may only be applicable for threaded connections.

5.3 *Cyclic Fatigue Properties*—The nature of in vivo loading generates the need for cyclic fatigue evaluation. Tests should be designed to examine pre-cycle and post-cycle properties to gain an understanding of how the design withstands, and is affected by, cyclic loading.

5.3.1 *Fracture*—The possibility of fracture of either a modular construct or the connections under fatigue loading. Consider the following:

5.3.1.1 Loading that represents that applied to the component *in vivo*,

5.3.1.2 An P-N curve to determine the load levels at which the construct can withstand cyclic loading without fracture, and

5.3.1.3 Test Method F 1440, Test Method F 1800, and ISO 7206-4,6, 8.

5.3.2 *Disassembly*—The possibility of disassembly of the modular components under fatigue loading. Consider the following:

5.3.2.1 Loading that represents that applied to the component *in vivo*, and

5.3.2.2 Measuring the disassembly force after fatigue loading and comparing to static values.

5.3.3 *Sterilization*—The effects of sterilization on the fatigue integrity of the modular connection. Sterilization may cause material changes which could affect the performance of the modular connection. Sterilization should be performed according to manufacturer specifications. Consider the following:

5.3.3.1 The effect of sterilization of plastic components.

5.3.4 *Corrosion*—The environment in which the modular connection will be used may affect the ability of the connection to resist disassociation or fracture. Consider the following:

5.3.4.1 Corrosion of similar metal connections,

5.3.4.2 Corrosion of dissimilar metal connections,

5.3.4.3 The fluid environment,

5.3.4.4 The temperature,

5.3.4.5 The frequency, and

5.3.4.6 See Test Method F 897.

5.3.5 *Fretting*—Micromotion between two components of a modular connection may produce adverse effects (that is, wear debris, increased risk for disassociation). Consider the following:

5.3.5.1 Fretting of taper junctions

5.3.5.2 Fretting of mating, non articulating surfaces

5.3.5.3 Environmental test, and

5.3.5.4 See Test Method F 897.

6. Keywords

6.1 arthroplasty; disassembly; hip arthroplasty; knee arthroplasty; modular; orthopaedic medical devices

	ASSEMBLY		DISASSEMBLY				CYCLIC FATIGUE PROPERTIES				
	Axial	Torsional	Axial	Shear	Bending	**Torsional**	Fatigue	Disassembly Post-fatigue	**Effects of Sterilization**	Corrosion	Fretting
Proximal Modularity											
Femoral Heads	X		X				X	X	X	X	X
Neck Extensions	X		X				X	X	X	X	X
Collars	X		X	X			X	X	X	X	X
Bolts		X		X		**X**	X	X	X	X	X
Mid-Body Modularity											
Sleeves	X	X	X	X	X	**X**	X	X	X	X	X
Pads	X	X	X	X	X	**X**	X	X	X	X	X
Distal Modularity											
Bullets	X	X	X		X	**X**	X	X	X	X	X
Sleeves	X	X	X		X	**X**	X	X	X	X	X
Total Implant							X			**X**	**X**

Note: This document is intended to address modular connections of a femoral hip system. This list includes the majority of modular devices utilized today. This list is not all inclusive. Modular attachments not addressed in this document should be evaluated at the user's discretion.

FIG. 1 Total Hip Implants

	ASSEMBLY		DISASSEMBLY				CYCLIC FATIGUE PROPERTIES				
	Axial	Torsional	Axial	Shear	Bending	**Torsional**	Failure	Disassembly	Sterilization	Corrosion	Fretting
Stem Extensions	X	**X**	X		X	**X**	X	X	X	X	X
Wedge		**X**		X		**X**		X			X
Modular tibial insert (cruciate retaining)		**X**		X		**X**		X	X		
Modular tibial insert (posterior stabilized) or semi-constrained		**X**		X	X	**X**	X	X	X		
Metal backed patella			X	X	X		X	X	X		
Total Implant		~~X~~	X	X			X			X	X

Note: This document is intended to address modular connections of a total knee system. This list includes the majority of modular devices utilized today. This list is not all-inclusive. Modular attachments not addressed by this document should be evaluated at the user's discretion.

FIG. 2 Total Knee Implant

APPENDIX

(Nonmandatory Information)

X1. RATIONALE

X1.1 This guide is intended to be used to direct the reader to some of the most common areas of concern for modular hip and knee prosthetic implants. For each area of concern, there is a checklist of possible junctions to evaluate with appropriate topics to consider for each test. This guide is not intended to be all inclusive of the potential areas of concern or tests that can be performed for modular implants but is meant to cover some of the more common topics of modular implants. It is felt that this document will be particularly useful to the novice investigator in directing their efforts in the investigation of safety and efficacy of a modular hip or knee implant, or both.

X1.2 Assembly and disassembly may be useful to the investigator in determining the strength of a modular connection. The strength of the modular connection may be determined as a ratio if disassembly force to assembly force. This number may also provide information as to the strength of the modular connection over time.

Designation: F 1820 – 97

Standard Test Method for Determining the Axial Disassembly Force of a Modular Acetabular Device[1]

This standard is issued under the fixed designation F 1820; the number immediately following the designation indicates the year of original adoption or, in the case of revision, the year of last revision. A number in parentheses indicates the year of last reapproval. A superscript epsilon (ε) indicates an editorial change since the last revision or reapproval.

1. Scope

1.1 This test method covers a standard methodology by which to measure the attachment strength between the modular acetabular shell and liner. Although the methodology described does not replicate physiological loading conditions, it has been described as means of comparing integrity of various locking mechanisms.[2]

1.2 *This standard does not purport to address all of the safety concerns, if any, associated with its use. It is the responsibility of the user of this standard to establish appropriate safety and health practices and determine the applicability of regulatory limitations prior to use.*

2. Referenced Documents

2.1 *ASTM Standards:*

E 4 Practices for Force Verification of Testing Machines[3]

3. Terminology

3.1 *Definitions of Terms Specific to This Standard:*

3.1.1 *acetabular liner*—portion of the modular acetabular device with an internal hemispherical socket intended to articulate with the head of a femoral prosthesis. The external geometry of this component interfaces with the acetabular shell through a locking mechanism which may be integral to the design of the liner and shell or may rely upon additional components (for example, metal ring, screws, etc.)

3.1.2 *acetabular shell*—the external, hollow structure (usually metal) that provides additional mechanical support or reinforcement for an acetabular liner and whose external features interface directly with the bones of the pelvic socket (for example, through bone cement, intimate press-fit, porous ingrowth, integral screw threads, anchoring screws, pegs, etc.). The acetabular shell may be either solid or contain holes for fixation, or contain a hole for instrumentation, or all of these.

3.1.3 *locking mechanism*—any structure, design feature or combination thereof, that provides mechanical resistance to movement between the liner and shell.

4. Summary of Test Method

4.1 The axial disassembly of an acetabular device test method provides a means to measure the axial locking strength of the acetabular liner for modular acetabular devices.

4.2 Following proper assembly of the acetabular liner in an acetabular shell, the assembled device is attached to a fixture such that the cup opening is facing downward. The acetabular shell is supported and an axial force is applied to the acetabular liner until it disengages. The load required to disengage the acetabular liner from the acetabular shell is recorded. The acetabular liner should only be tested one time; however, the acetabular shell may used more than once if no damage to the locking mechanism has occurred.

5. Significance and Use

5.1 This test method is intended to help assess the axial locking strength of the acetabular liner in a modular shell when subjected to a tensile loading condition. Additional means of evaluating the locking mechanisms of modular acetabular devices may be appropriate depending upon the design of the device (that is, lever-out, torsional strength, fatigue, etc.).

5.2 This test method may not be appropriate for all implant applications. The user is cautioned to consider the appropriateness of the method in view of the materials and design being tested and their potential application.

5.3 While this test method may be used to measure the force required to disengage modular acetabular devices, comparison of such data for various device designs must take into consideration the size of the implant and the type of locking mechanism evaluated. The location of the locking mechanism relative to the load application may be dependent upon the size and design of the acetabular device. In addition, the locking mechanism itself may vary with size, particularly if the design is circumferential in nature (for example, larger diameter implants would have a greater area of acetabular shell/acetabular liner interface than a small diameter implant).

6. Apparatus

6.1 An apparatus capable of supporting only the acetabular shell while allowing the acetabular liner to be freely disassembled from the shell is required. The fixture shall be constructed so that the line of load application is through the

---

[1] This test method is under the jurisdiction of ASTM Committee F-4 on Medical and Surgical Materials and Devices and is the direct responsibility of Subcommittee F04.22on Arthroplasty.

Current edition approved Oct. 10, 1997. Published April 1998.

[2] Tradonsky M.D., Steve, et al, "A Comparison of the Disassociation Strength of Modular Acetabular Components," Clinical Orthopaedics and Related Research, Number 296, November 1993.

[3] *Annual Book of ASTM Standards*, Vol 03.01.

apex of the shell or is perpendicular to the face center of the acetabular shell.

6.2 The testing machine shall conform to the requirements of Practices E 4. The loads used to determine the attachment strength shall be within the range of the testing machine as defined in Practices E 4.

6.3 The test machine should be capable of delivering a compressive or tensile force at a constant displacement rate. The test machine should have a load monitoring and recording system.

7. Sampling

7.1 All acetabular liners shall be representative of implant quality products. This shall include any sterilization or thermal processes which may alter the material properties or geometry.

7.2 A partially finished acetabular shell or permanent fixture block may be substituted for a completed acetabular shell provided that the internal materials, finish, locking mechanism, and geometry are identical to the actual acetabular shell.

7.3 A minimum of five shells and liners shall be tested to determine the axial disassembly force of an acetabular device. Pairing of the acetabular shells and liners shall be at random unless otherwise reported. The appropriateness of performing multiple tests on the same acetabular shell will depend on the design of the device. The acetabular liner should only be tested one time; however, the acetabular shell may be used more than once if no damage has occurred to the locking mechanism.

8. Procedure

8.1 Assemble the liner and shell according to the surgical procedure guidelines. Once assembled, the liner shell construct should be placed in a fixture similar to that described in Fig. 1, that is, a fixture that will support the acetabular shell without distortion while allowing axial load to be applied to the liner. An axial load should be applied (coincident with the axes of the liner and shell) to the liner through a center hole in the shell at a rate of 5.1 cm/min. It may be necessary to create a hole in the shell at the apex in order to apply an axial load to the liner. A small diameter drill blank or plug could be used as a load applicator. The maximum load required to completely disengage the liner from the shell should be measured and recorded.

8.2 Record maximum disassembly force.

8.3 Testing of samples shall be terminated when one of the following has occurred:

8.3.1 The disengagement force becomes negligible.

8.3.2 Prior to disassembly, the liner suffers excessive damage (that is, puncture of the liner or severe liner deformation). Puncture of the liner should be considered an invalid test.

9. Report

9.1 Report the following information:

9.1.1 The device name, size, materials, and lot number, if applicable,

9.1.2 Maximum force required to disengage the liner from the shell from each of the test samples,

9.1.3 Mode of failure, and

9.1.4 Specify the orientation of the liner and outer shell if the axes are not coincident.

10. Precision and Bias

10.1 No information can be presented on the precision and bias of this test method for measuring the axial disassembly

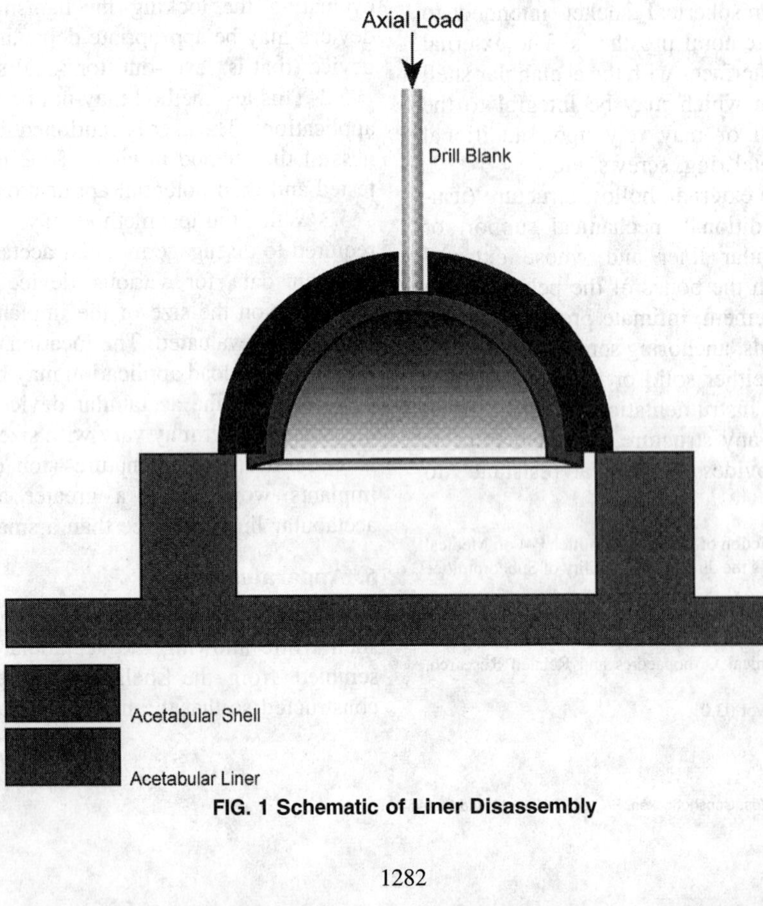

FIG. 1 Schematic of Liner Disassembly

force of modular acetabular devices, because no material having an accepted reference value is available.

11. Keywords

11.1 acetabular component; arthroplasty; disassembly

APPENDIX

(Nonmandatory Information)

X1. RATIONALE

X1.1 The intent of this test method is to establish a means of comparing various acetabular designs, not to set a minimum for the disassembly force of the acetabular prosthesis. In addition, this test method does not specifically address the locking mechanism's ability to maintain its integrity with sequential assemblies and disassemblies. However, if deemed appropriate by the user, the method could be considered for determining the ability of the locking mechanism to resist degradation after repeated assemblies.

X1.2 Prototype designs may be used with this test method and may be considered implant quality if the geometrical dimensions are within the tolerances of the final design and have been subjected to any processes that may effect the geometrical stability of the implant.

X1.3 Temperature and environment may effect the locking strength of the acetabular design. If the these factors are considered, then the environment and the temperature should be reported in the results.

X1.4 Occasionally shells without holes may need to be evaluated. For these designs it may become necessary to drill a hole in the apex of the shell for insertion of the drill blank or plug. Holes should not be made if the locking mechanism is compromised, and alternative methods should be considered to apply the load coincident with the acetabular liner and shell axis.

X1.5 Some designs may be susceptible to degradation in liner locking force after fatigue; therefore, consideration may be given to the effect of fatigue on the disengagement force of acetabular devices.[4]

[4] Fosco, D.R., and Buchanan, D.J., "The Importance of Fatigue Loading When Assessing Liner/Shell Distraction Resistance and Congruency for Modular Acetabular Components," *Modularity of Orthopaedic Implants, ASTM STP 1301*, Donald E. Marlowe and Michael B. Mayor, Eds., ASTM, 1997.

Designation: F 1823 – 97

Standard Guide for
Water Rescue Personal Flotation Device (PFD)[1]

This standard is issued under the fixed designation F 1823; the number immediately following the designation indicates the year of original adoption or, in the case of revision, the year of last revision. A number in parentheses indicates the year of last reapproval. A superscript epsilon (ϵ) indicates an editorial change since the last revision or reapproval.

1. Scope

1.1 This guide covers the minimum performance and safety requirements of a water rescue lifejacket/PFD (Personal Floatation Device).

1.2 In recognition of many broad and varied applications of such PFD's, many options are included.

1.3 *This standard does not purport to address all of the safety concerns, if any, associated with its use. It is the responsibility of the user of this standard to establish appropriate safety and health practices and determine the applicability of regulatory limitations prior to use.*

2. Referenced Documents

2.1 *Code of Federal Regulations:*
160.047 Buoyant Vests[2]
160.052 Buoyant Vests[2]
160.053 Work Vests[2]
160.060 Buoyant Vests[2]
160.064 Marine Buoyant Devices[2]
160.076 Inflatable Lifejackets[2]
160.077 Hybrid Inflatable Personal Flotation Device[2]
160.071 Immersion Suits[2]

3. Terminology

3.1 *Definitions:*

3.1.1 *Personal Flotation Device, PFD, n*—a buoyant device suitable for use by one person in water emergencies. These devices may be vests, ring buoys, life preservers, cushions, and other special purpose buoyant devices.

4. Significance and Use

4.1 This guide is applicable to all water rescue situations. The water situation, weather situation, and size of rescuer, will dictate what type of PFD to utilize.

4.2 This guide will assist government agencies, state, local, or regional organizations; fire departments; rescue teams and others who are responsible for purchasing and equipping personnel who respond to water emergencies.

4.3 This guide establishes criteria that shall be considered in the performance, specification, purchase, and acceptance testing of a water rescue PFD.

5. Classification

5.1 This guide includes the following types of PFD's:
5.1.1 *Type I*—Off Shore Life Preserver
5.1.2 *Type II*—Near Shore Buoyant Vest
5.1.3 *Type III*—Special Purpose Flotation Aid
5.1.4 *Type IV flotation devices*—Throwable Devices
5.1.5 *Type V flotation devices*—Special Use Devices

6. General Requirements

6.1 All PFD's should conform to standards set by the appropriate national regulatory authority, that is, the U.S. Coast Guard in the United States, and be in good and serviceable condition.

7. Performance Requirements

7.1 Highly visible.

7.2 Adequate flotation for individual and water rescue situation.

7.3 Proper size and fit for individual.

7.4 Offer unrestricted mobility.

7.5 Construction allows for impact protection for rescuer utilizing foam panels.

7.5.1 Design offers protection from hypothermia and heat illness associated with use.

7.5.2 Multiple closure devices for a secure fit.

8. Keywords

8.1 lifejacket; PFD; water rescue

---

[1] This practice is under the jurisdiction of ASTM Committee F-32 on Search and Rescue and is the direct responsibility of Subcommittee F32.01 on Equipment.
Current edition approved Dec. 10, 1997 . Published June 1998 .

[2] Title 33 and Title 46, Code of Federal Regulations. Copies available from the U.S. Government Printing Office.

Standard Guide for Performance of a Water Rescuer–Level II[1]

This standard is issued under the fixed designation F 1824; the number immediately following the designation indicates the year of original adoption or, in the case of revision, the year of last revision. A number in parentheses indicates the year of last reapproval. A superscript epsilon (ε) indicates an editorial change since the last revision or reapproval.

1. Scope

1.1 This guide covers minimum requirements for performance of a water rescuer who performs water rescues from the surface at lakes, ponds, quarries, and other similar bodies of water; assists with support for rescue divers; and provides initial patient care at a water emergency.

1.2 This guide is one of a series which together with Guide F 1739 Guide for the Performance of a Water Rescuer–Level I, describe the minimum performance requirements of a water rescuer.

1.3 Individuals who will operate in the water setting need to be aware of the equipment and physical requirements necessary to be able to perform all identified objectives and necessary skills in the setting.

1.4 *This standard does not purport to address all of the safety concerns, if any, associated with its use. It is the responsibility of the user of this standard to establish appropriate safety and health practices and determine the applicability of regulatory limitations prior to use.*

2. Referenced Documents

2.1 *ASTM Standards:*

F 1739 Guide for the Performance of a Water Rescuer – Level I[2]

3. Terminology

3.1 *Definitions:*

3.1.1 *drysuit, n*—a protective suit that encompasses the wearer, prohibiting water from entering.

3.1.2 *immersion suit, n*—designed to provide cold water protection and buoyancy by one person in cold water emergencies.

3.1.2.1 *Discussion*—These devices should conform to standards set by the appropriate national regulatory authority, that is, the U.S. Coast Guard in the United States.

3.1.3 *personal flotation device, PFD, n*—a buoyant device suitable for use by one person in water emergencies.

3.1.3.1 *Discussion*—These devices should conform to standards set by the appropriate national regulatory authority, that is, the U.S. Coast Guard in the United States.

4. Significance and Use

4.1 This guide is to be used to expand the performance of water rescuers and improve the emergency response and patient care delivered to victims in the water and cold water environment at lakes, ponds, quarries, and similar bodies of water.

4.2 All persons who are identified as water rescuers shall meet the requirements of this guide.

4.3 This guide is not intended to be used in isolation, but as a component guide, acknowledging various types/conditions at water emergencies and many duties of response at these incidents. It also establishes a minimum scope of performance and encourages the addition of optional knowledge, skills, and attitudinal objectives.

4.4 This guide is not for ice, coastal, or river/swiftwater rescues. There will be additional standards to cover the specifics for those water characteristics.

4.5 This guide does not establish water rescue protocols for the pool, beach, or other area lifeguards.

4.6 This guide does not establish medical protocols, nor does it authorize invasive procedures without specific authorization and medical control.

4.7 This guide is intended to assist government agencies, state, local, or regional organizations; fire departments; marine patrols; rescue teams and others who are responsible for establishing a minimum performance for personnel who respond to water emergencies.

4.8 A water rescuer shall be wearing a PFD, plus cold water protection when applicable.

5. Objectives

5.1 The water rescuer shall be able to perform the objectives in Guide F 1739.

5.2 The water rescuer shall be able to perform the following:

5.2.1 Swim continuously 274.32 m (300 yd),

5.2.2 perform a head first surface dive,

5.2.3 perform a feet first surface dive,

5.2.4 perform a stride jump entry,

5.2.5 perform a compact jump entry,

5.2.6 perform an unknown/hazard entry or ease in entry,

5.2.7 perform the approach to victim utilizing a modified crawl or breast stroke and initiate a quick reverse,

5.2.8 perform a swimming extension rescue with a rescue tube, type IV PFD, or other buoyant device,

---

[1] This practice is under the jurisdiction of ASTM Committee F-32 on Search and Rescue and is the direct responsibility of Subcommittee F32.03 on Personnel, Training and Education.

Current edition approved Oct. 10, 1997. Published December 1997.

[2] *Annual Book of ASTM Standards*, June 1988 Vol 13.01.

5.2.9 perform a double wrist grip escape,

5.2.10 perform a front head hold escape,

5.2.11 perform a rear head hold escape,

5.2.12 perform an unconscious one arm turn,

5.2.13 perform an unconscious two arm turn,

5.2.14 perform a collar tow,

5.2.15 perform an active and passive victim rear rescue,

5.2.16 perform a multiple victim rear rescue,

5.2.17 perform a submerged victim rescue,

5.2.18 perform the head splint spinal injury technique for both a face up and face down victim,

5.2.19 perform the head and chin support (vise grip) spinal injury technique for both a face up and face down victim,

5.2.20 immobilize and backboard the injured person in shallow and deep water; removing the person in such a manner that the chance of aggravating injuries is minimized,

5.2.21 perform the walking assist, the beach drag, and two person carry,

5.2.22 perform the double bounce, rope step assist, loop stirrup, blanket roll, and rope roll to extricate a person from the water into a boat,

5.2.23 identify the water rescue sequence,

5.2.24 perform a scene evaluation which includes evaluating water conditions, assessing the scene for hazards, number of victim(s), victim(s) condition, need for additional personnel, need for additional equipment, and take appropriate action following the rescue sequence by utilizing risk benefit analysis,

5.2.25 perform shore based reaching and extension rescues,

5.2.26 perform throwing rescue technique using a throwbag and coiled rope throws,

5.2.27 perform a tethered swimmer rescue technique utilizing immersion suit, drysuit with PFD, or equivalent,

5.2.28 perform a shallow water search,

5.2.29 perform a deep water line search,

5.2.30 perform a circular or semicircular search,

5.2.31 perform a parallel line search,

5.2.32 provide initial patient care, and

5.2.33 move the victim(s) in conjunction with patient care activities in such a manner that the chance of aggravating injuries or medical condition is minimized.

5.3 *Optional Objectives*—the territory, bodies of water, equipment, personnel, and resources vary among water rescuers in agencies. When emergency response capabilities are limited, the ability of a water rescuer to perform the tasks in 5.1 and 5.2 may be sufficient to ensure satisfactory care. When a water rescuer has a greater variety of responses, territory, and equipment demands, the scope of performance must be expanded accordingly.

6. Keywords

6.1 rescue; rescuer; water rescue; water rescuer

Standard Specification for Ureteral Stents[1]

This standard is issued under the fixed designation F 1828; the number immediately following the designation indicates the year of original adoption or, in the case of revision, the year of last revision. A number in parentheses indicates the year of last reapproval. A superscript epsilon (ϵ) indicates an editorial change since the last revision or reapproval.

INTRODUCTION

The objective of this specification is to describe the test methods used to evaluate the safety and effectiveness of an indwelling ureteral stent, having retention means at the kidney and bladder ends, used for urinary drainage of the kidney to the bladder via the ureter.

This specification includes referee test methods that can be used to evaluate the performance characteristics of ureteral stents. Note that the test methods are not to be construed as production methods, quality control techniques, or manufacturer's lot release criteria. The product parameters addressed by the standard include those determined by the ASTM task group to be pertinent to the product.

1. Scope

1.1 This specification covers the referee test methods for evaluating the performance characteristics of a single-use ureteral stent with retaining means at both ends, during short term use for drainage of urine from the kidney to the bladder. These stents are typically available in diameters of 3.7 Fr to 14.0 Fr, and lengths of 8 cm to 30 cm, and are made of silicone, polyurethane, and other polymers. They are provided non-sterile for sterilization and sterile for single-use.

1.2 *Exclusions*—Long-term indwelling usage (over 30 days) is encountered with this product, but not commonly, and is therefore considered an exception to this specification. Similarly, the use of ureteral stents for non-ureteral applications such as nephrostomy and ileostomy is excluded from the scope of this specification. Non-sterile ureteral stents are also excluded due to the variability of hospital sterilization equipment and processes and the resulting effects on ureteral stent characteristics.

1.3 The following precautionary statement pertains only to the test method portion, Section 5, of this specification:

1.4 *This standard does not purport to address all of the safety concerns, if any, associated with its use. It is the responsibility of the user of this standard to establish appropriate safety and health practices and determine the applicability of regulatory limitations prior to use.*

2. Referenced Documents

2.1 *ASTM Standards:*

D 412 Test Methods for Vulcanized Rubber and Thermoplastic Rubbers and Thermoplastic Elastomers — Tension[2]

F 640 Test Methods for Radiopacity of Plastics for Medical Use[3]

F 748 Practice for Selecting Generic Biological Test Methods for Materials and Devices[3]

3. Terminology

3.1 *Definitions of Terms Specific to This Standard:*

3.1.1 *artificial urine*—a solution of organic and inorganic compounds that closely simulates the chemical and physical properties of normal human urine. Artificial urine will be used as a substitute for human urine to simulate the effects of human urine on ureteral stents.

3.1.2 *bladder retention means*—physical feature of bladder end of stent the prevents movement of stent out of bladder.

3.1.3 *break strength*—peak tensile load required to break stent.

3.1.4 *cross section*—view of stent tube when cut in a plane perpendicular to length of stent.

3.1.5 *distal*—situated away from the point of origin. The distal end of a stent is the end that resides in the bladder, also known as the bladder end.

3.1.6 *drainage holes*—holes in wall of stent tubing that allow flow of urine into and out of lumen of stent.

3.1.7 *dynamic frictional force*—resistance to relative motion between two surfaces during motion. This force is defined as the coefficient of kinetic friction multiplied by the force acting on the surface of the material in a plane perpendicular to the surface.

3.1.8 *elongation*—expressed as a percent, is equal to the change in length of a sample of tubing at failure divided by its

[1] This specification is under the jurisdiction of ASTM Committee F-4 on Medical and Surgical Materials and Devices and is the direct responsibility of Subcommittee F04.34 on Urological Materials and Devices.

Current edition approved Nov. 10, 1997. Published May 1998.

[2] Annual Book of ASTM Standards, Vol 09.01.

[3] Annual Book of ASTM Standards, Vol 13.01.

original length. Stretching of the tubing is produced by tensile loading.

3.1.9 *French size*—Scale used to indicate size of tubular devices, each unit being approximately equal to 0.013 in. or 0.33 mm in diameter. Typical label French sizes are as follows:

French Size	Outside Diameter in. mm
3.7	0.050,1.23
4.5	0.060,1.50
4.7	0.061,1.57
6.0	0.079,2.00
7.0	0.092,2.33
8.0	0.105,2.67
8.5	0.112,2.83
10.0	0.131,3.33
14.0	0.183,4.66

3.1.10 *kidney retention means*—physical feature of kidney end of stent that prevents movement of stent out of the kidney.

3.1.11 *length*—length of stent is defined as the distance between the most proximal portion of the bladder retention means and the most distal portion of the kidney retention means when the stent is laying on a flat surface with the mainshaft straight. (See Fig. 1).

3.1.12 *lumen*—the channel within a tube.

3.1.13 *proximal*—situated toward the point of origin. In the urinary tract, the kidney is considered to be the point of origin. The proximal end of a stent is the end that resides in the renal pelvis, also known as the kidney end.

3.1.14 *radiopacity*—property indicating ability of device to absorb x-ray energy, allowing device to be seen in a radiograph or fluoroscopic screen.

3.1.15 *referee test method*—the method cited in the published specification for the device. This method will be used when the performance of the ureteral stent is to be evaluated. The manufacturer need not use this referee test method for inspection and quality control.

3.1.16 *retention strength*—force required to overcome the retaining means on a stent.

3.1.17 *sterility*—the state of being free of microorganisms. For purposes of this specification, sterility is defined as freedom from microorganisms when tested according to the methodology defined by the USP for nonparenteral devices.

3.1.18 *tolerances*—the allowable deviation from a standard size. The tolerance for the length of a ureteral stent is ± 0.5 cm (0.197 in). the tolerance for the specified French size of a ureteral stent is ± 0.01 mm (0.004 in), or approximately 1/3 French.

3.1.19 *ureteral stent*—an indwelling tubular device that resides in the kidney, ureter, and bladder containing means for retaining ends of tube in kidney and bladder.

4. Requirements

4.1 *Biocompatibility*— Ureteral stents shall be tested in accordance with the appropriate biological tests contained in Specification F 748 or similar guidance established by the U. S. Food and Drug Administration or International Organization for Standardization (ISO).

5. Special Precautions

5.1 The following cautionary comments recognize the sensitivity of the materials of construction to potential environmental conditions. These are outlined here to point out potential situations that could adversely affect the performance of the stent during testing.

5.1.1 Care should be taken during testing and use to prevent damage to the stents. Such damage can be caused by abrasion and contact with sharp objects or chemical products.

5.1.2 Stents should be kept away from generators, electric motors, diathermy machines, and fluorescent lights because the ozone produced may attack elastomeric materials. This applies to both storage and handling.

5.1.3 To help avoid contamination of the stents proper handling precautions should be observed.

6. Test Methods

6.1 *General Guidelines*:

6.1.1 Test samples should consist of actual ureteral stents, not material slabs.

6.1.2 Use statistically valid sample sizes in all tests.

6.1.3 Package all stent test samples and sterilize once using the method of sterilization intended to be used for product when it is sold.

6.1.4 Expose test samples to artificial urine at 37 ± 3° C for a period of 30 days. Use either of the two artificial urine formulations listed in Annex A1. In situations where testing in artificial urine is not practical, distilled water may be used.

6.1.5 Maintain artificial urine pH in the range of 5.5 to 6.5

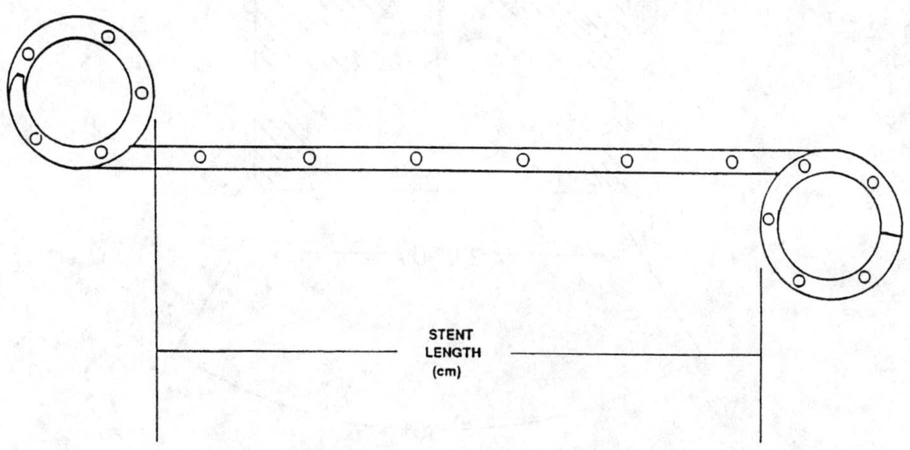

FIG. 1 Determine of Stent Length.

at all times. Replace urine should be weekly.

6.1.6 Perform tests prior to and after soaking for a minimum of 30 days. For products with intended chemical/mechanical changes such as softening, swelling, etc., do initial mechanical testing only after sufficient soaking time has elapsed that allow such chemical/mechanical changes to occur.

6.1.7 Dynamic frictional force test samples need only be soaked in distilled water for 1 min prior to testing. This test will not be repeated after 30 days.

6.2 *Retention Strength*:

6.2.1 *Scope*—This test method measured the ability of a ureteral stent to resist migration. It can be used for testing the proximal or distal ends of a ureteral stent.

6.2.2 *Summary of Test Method*:

6.2.2.1 The apparatus is set up as shown in Fig. 2. Clearance between the outside diameter of the stent and inside diameter of the funnel block hole must be present. (See Note 1 in Fig. 2 for a list of appropriate funnel block hole diameters to be used with stents of different French sizes.)

6.2.2.2 Maintain temperature in the water bath at 37± 3°C by whatever means is available to the test facility. Submerge the entire funnel block. Set the pull rate through the fixture at a constant 20 in.(mm)/min. Clean the test bath and fixture at the beginning of each testing day. The capacity of the load cell used with the tensile testing machine should not exceed 2 lb.

6.2.3 *Test Specimen Preparation*—The test specimen shall consist of actual sterilized product. The specimen shall be cut to allow a straight portion of the stent to be inserted upwards through the funnel fixture into the grip of the tensile test machine without loading the retention mechanism of the stent to be tested. Submerge the test specimen in the water bath for at least 1 min to allow it to reach thermal equilibrium. If the material is significantly affected by moisture, allow the specimen to equilibrate for a minimum of 24 h. Use distilled water, if possible.

NOTE 1—The portion of the stent held within the gripping mechanism of the tensile testing machine cannot be used for additional testing due to the potential destructive effects of the gripping mechanism.

6.2.4 *Test Procedure*:

6.2.4.1 Ensure test bath is at proper temperature and funnel is submerged. Monitor periodically.

6.2.4.2 When testing a new ureteral stent taken out of its sterile package, (*t*=0), straighten retention means with appropriate guidewire. Insert straight portion of stent through bottom of funnel and into grip. When testing at *t*=30 days, retention means is not to be straightened prior to testing.

6.2.4.3 Allow stent to reach thermal equilibrium.

6.2.4.4 Pull specimen up through funnel at 20 in./min. Record maximum force required to pull stent completely through funnel.

6.3 *Break Strength*:

6.3.1 Break strengths of test stents will be determined in accordance with Test Method D 412, with the following modifications:

6.3.1.1 Devices used to grip the test specimen in the tensile

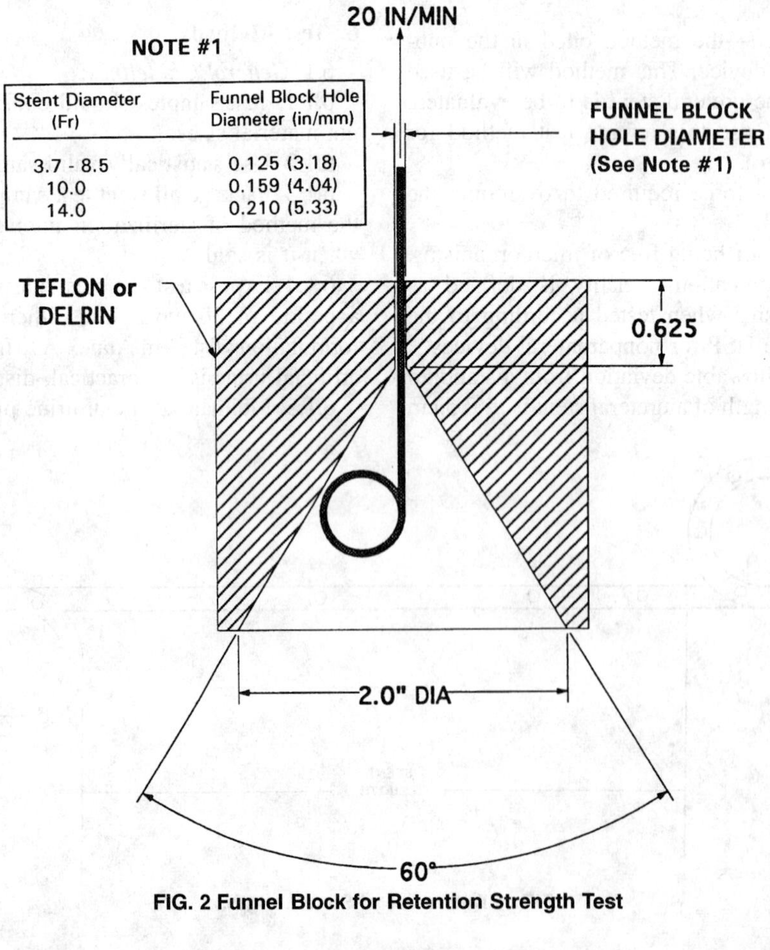

Stent Diameter (Fr)	Funnel Block Hole Diameter (in/mm)
3.7 - 8.5	0.125 (3.18)
10.0	0.159 (4.04)
14.0	0.210 (5.33)

FIG. 2 Funnel Block for Retention Strength Test

test machine should be chosen so that the test specimen does not break at the grip location.

6.3.1.2 Most stents contain drainage holes. Ideally, these stents should break at a drainage hole. This is how tensile failures typically occur in-vivo. However, stents may break in locations other than drainage holes. This type of failure may be indicative of potential design or process related problems. In stents without drainage holes, this type of failure is to be expected.

6.3.1.3 Only a segment of the test stent is used for the break strength test. The grippers should be separated by 1 in. This 1 in. segment must contain at least one drainage hole (if drainage holes are present) and should contain the section of the stent with the smallest cross sectional area or weakest point.

6.4 *Elongation*—The elongation of stent segments separated by 1 in. between the extensometer grips used to hold the segment in the tensile test machine or two marks placed on the surface of the stent will be determined in accordance with Test Method D 412.

6.5 *Dynamic Frictional Force — (Required for Support of Claims of Low Friction)*:

6.5.1 *Scope*—This test method measures the dynamic frictional force acting upon the outer surface of ureteral stent during placement through a small orifice. This test method is intended to simulate passage of a 6 Fr ureteral stent through an endoscope.

6.5.2 *Summary of Test Method*—Straighten the test stent using a wire mandrel and hydrated in a cylinder of distilled water. Then place it completely through the appropriate size grommet and into a water column. The mandrel is connected to a load cell that is pulled at constant rate of 20 in/min. Record the force values measured by the load cell on a chart recorder or minicomputer and average to determine the dynamic frictional force.

6.5.3 *Test Set-Up — (See* Fig. 3.*)*

6.5.3.1 *Cylinder*—capable of hydrating the full length of the ureteral stent sample.

6.5.3.2 *Water Column*— used to hydrate the full length of the test stent prior to passage through grommet.

6.5.3.3 *Distilled Water*— used to hydrate the test stent (and activate any hydrophilic coating present) at room temperature.

6.5.3.4 *Grommet*—A 0.040± 0.002 in. thick, 5/8 in. diameter disc, with a 0.079 ± 0.002 in. (± mm.) diameter hole in the center. The grommet is to be made of 55 Shore A Durometer silicone.

6.5.3.5 *Grommet Fixture*— The grommet is held in place by two aluminum plates containing relief holes approximately 1/8 in. larger is diameter than the hole in the grommet. When

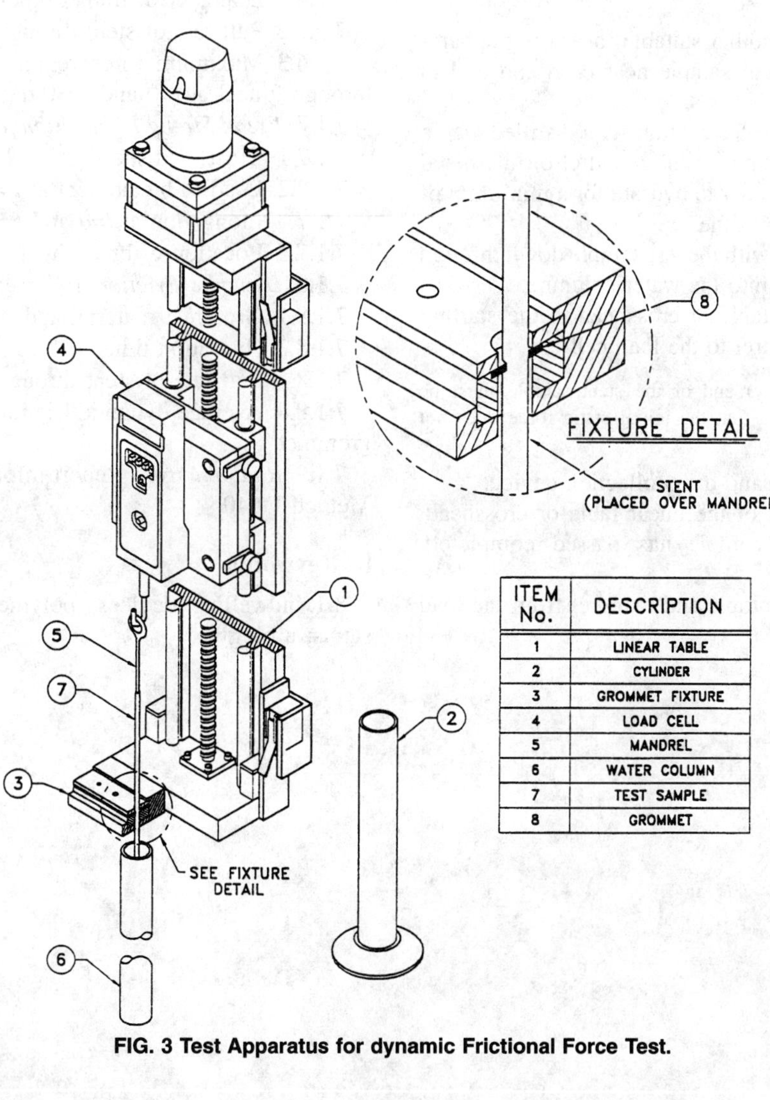

ITEM No.	DESCRIPTION
1	LINEAR TABLE
2	CYLINDER
3	GROMMET FIXTURE
4	LOAD CELL
5	MANDREL
6	WATER COLUMN
7	TEST SAMPLE
8	GROMMET

FIG. 3 Test Apparatus for dynamic Frictional Force Test.

mounted, the hole in the grommet should be centered about the relief hole in the aluminum plates.

6.5.3.6 *Load Cell*—Load cell capacity should not exceed 1 lb, and should be capable of measuring the frictional force within ± 5 % of its value.

6.5.3.7 *Linear Table*— used to pull the load cell at a constant rate. A linear table will not be necessary if a standard tensile test machine is used.

6.5.3.8 *Mandrel*—A mandrel large enough to straighten and hold the test stent during the test is used. An eyelet is used on one end to attach to the load cell.

6.5.4 *Precautions*:

6.5.4.1 Follow all proper safety precautions.

6.5.4.2 Take care prior to and during testing not to cause damage to the test stent or grommet. Avoid contact with sharp or abrasive objects and any solvents that may damage the materials.

6.5.4.3 Use fresh distilled water to limit the accumulation of bacteria and presence of any leached chemicals.

6.5.5 *Test Specimen*— The test specimen should consist of the manufacturer's new, finished, packaged, and sterilized untested product *without* drainage holes, if possible.

6.5.6 *Procedure*:

6.5.6.1 Inspect grommet for proper size and integrity (no splits) prior to testing.

6.5.6.2 Using calipers (or other suitable measuring apparatus) measure diameter of stent sample near each end and in center of sample.

6.5.6.3 Fill cylinder and water column with distilled water.

6.5.6.4 Load the stent sample of the mandrel on the distal end first and place in the cylinder to hydrate for a minimum of one minute. Record hydration time.

6.5.6.5 Place the mandrel with the test sample down through the top of the grommet and into the water column.

6.5.6.6 Return the linear table or crosshead to the starting position and attach the mandrel to the load cell.

NOTE 2—The proximal (kidney) end of the stent sample must be partially through the grommet so that the initial static force does not exceed the load cell range.

6.5.6.7 Zero the load cell and data collection device.

6.5.6.8 Initiate movement of the linear table or crosshead. Stop movement once the sample has passed completely through the grommet.

6.5.6.9 Remove the test sample and mandrel from the load cell.

6.5.7 *Interpretation of Results*:

6.5.7.1 The average value of the collected data should be calculated. This value (in grams) represents the average dynamic frictional force between the test stent material and the silicone grommet.

6.5.7.2 If a minicomputer is used to collect data, a minimum of 100 data points should be obtained per sample.

6.5.7.3 Calculate the average value of the stent sample diameter.

6.6 *Radiopacity*— Determine radiopacity of test stents in accordance with Test Method F 640. Actual stents will be used as the specimens required by Test Method F 640.

7. Report

7.1 Report the following information

7.1.1 Average diameter and material of stent tested,

7.1.2 Number of stents tested,

7.1.3 Method used to sterilize stents,

7.1.4 Length of initial exposure to artificial urine or distilled water, and

7.1.5 Artificial urine formulation used (if artificial urine used in tests).

7.1.6 *Retention Strength*:

7.1.6.1 Diameter of funnel block hole used,

7.1.6.2 Pull rate of stent through funnel, and

7.1.6.3 Maximum force required to pull stent completely through funnel at t=0 and t=30 days.

7.1.7 *Break Strength and Elongation*:

7.1.7.1 Crosshead speed,

7.1.7.2 Load to break stent at t=0 and t=30 days,

7.1.7.3 Elongation at t=0 and t=30 days, and

7.1.7.4 Location of break in stent.

7.1.8 *Dynamic Frictional Force*:

7.1.8.1 Grommet material and inside diameter,

7.1.8.2 Hydration time,

7.1.8.3 Pull rate of stent through grommet, and

7.1.8.4 Average dynamic frictional force between stent and grommet.

7.1.9 *Radiopacity*— Report information as specified in Test Method F 640.

8. Keywords

8.1 indwelling devices; polymers; test methods; ureteral stents; urology

ANNEX

(Mandatory Information)

A1. ARTIFICIAL URINE FORMULATIONS

A1.1 *Formulation Number 1*[4]:

A1.1.1 Components per liter of solution:

NaCl	6.17 g
NaH_2Po_4	4.59 g
Na_3Citrate	0.944g
$MgSo_4$	0.463g
Na_2SO_4	2.408g
KCl	4.75 g
$CaCl_2$	0.638g
Na_2Oxalate	0.043g
Distilled water	bring to 1 l volumetrically

NOTE A1.1—Add the above salts to a 1000 mL volumetric flask, then add the distilled water for a total volume of 1000 mL.

NOTE A1.2—Adjust pH to 5.5 to 6.5 range with a 1*N* solution of NH_4OH or 1*N* NH_4Cl.

A1.2 *Formulation Number 2*[5]:

A1.2.1 Components per liter of solution:

Urea	25.0g
NaCl	9.0g
Disodium hydrogen orthophosphate, anhydrous	2.5g
Potassium dihydrogen orthophosphate, anhydrous	2.5g
NH_4Cl	3.0g
Creatinine	2.0g
Sodium sulfite, hydrated	3.0g
Distilled water	bring to 1 L volumetrically

[4] Burns J.R., and Finlayson, B., "Proposal for a Standard Reference Artificial Urine in In-Vitro Urolithiasis Experiments," *Investigative Urology*, 18, 1980, pp. 167-169.

[5] British Standard 1695, *Urological Catheters, Part 2: Specification for Sterile, Single-Use Urethral Catheters of the Tiemann, Whistle-tip, 3-Way, and Haematuria Types*, Section D.2.4, BSI, September 1990.

APPENDIX

(Nonmandatory Information)

X1. RATIONALE

X1.1 Ureteral stents exhibit a range of physical properties that affect their clinical performance. These properties are affected by materials, manufacturing processes, and stent geometry. This specification is intended to describe standard test methods to be used to measure the important functional characteristics of ureteral stents such as retention strength, break strength, elongation, and dynamic friction.

X1.2 Minimum acceptable performance requirements are not presented in this specification for two reasons. First, different clinical situations may require the use of stents with different functional characteristics. In order to provide the required characteristics, some physical properties may be compromised. These tradeoffs between physical properties and functional characteristics make it difficult to establish absolute minimum performance requirements. Second, the experimental and anecdotal evidence existing at the time of writing of this specification is inadequate to support the establishment of specific absolute minimum acceptable performance requirements for ureteral stents.

Designation: F 1829 – 98

Standard Test Method for Static Evaluation of the Glenoid Locking Mechanism in Shear[1]

This standard is issued under the fixed designation F 1829; the number immediately following the designation indicates the year of original adoption or, in the case of revision, the year of last revision. A number in parentheses indicates the year of last reapproval. A superscript epsilon (ε) indicates an editorial change since the last revision or reapproval.

1. Scope

1.1 This practice covers a method for determining the static shear disassembly force of modular glenoid components used in shoulder prostheses. It is intended to be used as a design validation and for comparison with other prostheses.

1.2 This test method covers modular glenoid components comprised of a separate articular insert and backing. The insert and backing can be fabricated from any combination of the following materials: metal alloys, polymeric materials, composite materials.

1.3 The values stated in SI units are regarded as the standard.

1.4 *This standard does not purport to address all of the safety concerns, if any, associated with its use. It is the responsibility of the user of this standard to establish appropriate safety and health practices and determine the applicability of regulatory limitations prior to use.*

2. Referenced Documents

2.1 *ASTM Standards:*

E 4 Practices for Force Verification of Testing Machines[2]

F 1378 Specification for Shoulder Prosthesis[3]

3. Terminology

3.1 *Definitions:*

3.1.1 *articular insert*—the polymeric prosthetic portion of a multiple piece glenoid component that articulates with the humeral head.

3.1.2 *"d"*—offset distance from the edge of the glenoid backing locking mechanism to the centerline of the point of load application on the articular insert as shown in Fig. 1 and Fig. 2.

3.1.3 *glenoid backing*—the metallic or composite material prosthetic portion of a multiple piece glenoid component that attaches to the scapula.

3.1.4 *glenoid component*—the prosthetic portion that replaces the glenoid fossa of the scapula and articulates with the natural humeral head or a prosthetic replacement.

4. Significance and Use

4.1 This test method can be used to describe the effects of materials, manufacturing, and design variables on the performance of metal backed glenoid prostheses locking mechanisms to resist static shear loading.

4.2 The glenoid component is used in shoulder replacements and should conform to the criteria specified in Specification F 1378.

4.3 The loading of metal backed glenoid prostheses in vivo will, in general, differ from the loading defined in this test method. The results obtained here can not be used to directly predict in vivo performance. However, this test method is designed to allow for comparisons between different metal backed glenoid locking mechanism designs, when tested under similar circumstances.

4.4 This test method may not be appropriate for all types of implant applications. The user is cautioned to consider the appropriateness of the method in view of the materials being tested and their potential application.

4.5 In order for the test data on metal backed glenoid components to be comparable, reproducible, and capable of being correlated among laboratories, it is essential that uniform procedures be established.

5. Apparatus

5.1 The test fixture shall be constructed so that the line of load application is parallel to the intended axis of the implant (that is, inferior to superior or anterior to posterior).

6. Equipment

6.1 The tests will be performed on either mechanical or hydraulic load frames with adequate load capacity and that meet the criteria of Practices E 4.

7. Sampling

7.1 A minimum of five samples with the load oriented in the inferior to superior direction shall be tested per device.

7.2 A minimum of five samples with the load oriented in the

[1] This practice is under the jurisdiction of ASTM Committee F-4 on Medical and Surgical Materials and Devicesand is the direct responsibility of Subcommittee F04.22on Arthroplasty.

Current edition approved April 10, 1998. Published March 1999. Originally published as F 1829 - 97. Last previous edition F 1829 - 97.

[2] *Annual Book of ASTM Standards*, Vol 03.01.

[3] *Annual Book of ASTM Standards*, Vol 13.01.

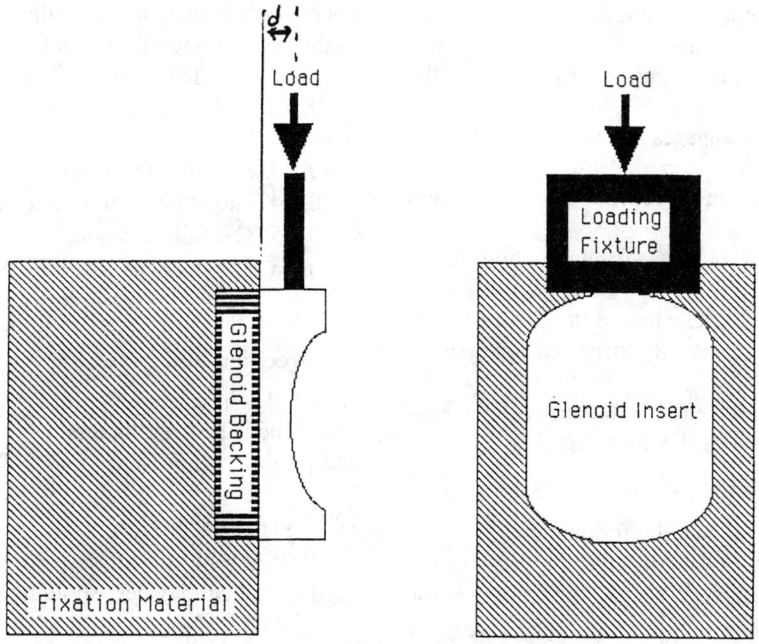

FIG. 1 Schematic of Static Glenoid Locking Strength Inferior to Superior Direction

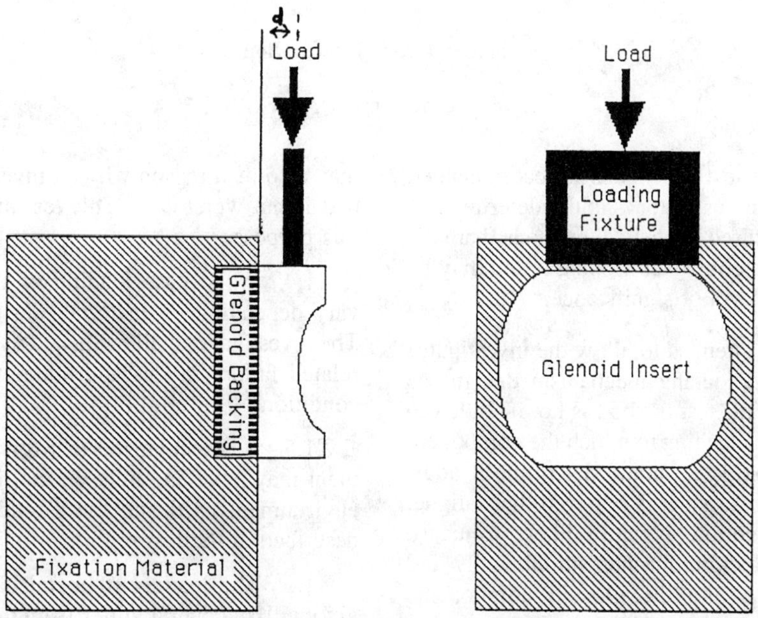

FIG. 2 Schematic of Static Glenoid Locking Strength Anterior to Posterior Direction

anterior to posterior direction shall be tested per device.

8. Sample and Test Specimen

8.1 All articular insert test components shall be representative of final manufactured implant quality products.

8.2 Glenoid backing test components may either be in the form of the final implant or may be a simplified model with the exact locking mechanism to be used on the final implant. The materials and surface shall be representative of implant quality products. All manufacturing processes (including heat treatment) should be followed.

8.3 All components should be sterilized according to manufacturer recommended specifications for clinical use, if this process could affect the results.

8.4 A new articular insert should be used for each test.

9. Procedure

9.1 Following proper assembly of an insert into a backing, the assembly is attached to the test machine such that the load is applied in an inferior to superior direction (see Fig. 1).

9.2 This test is to be performed in air at room temperature. It is permissible to perform this test in simulated physiological environment if the conditions of the test environment are recorded (that is, temperature, humidity, fluid).

9.3 Apply a vertical load to the assembly offset at a specified distance from the locking mechanism.

9.4 Load should be applied to the articular insert with a blunt edge loading applicator.

9.5 A constant displacement rate should be used and recorded (for example, 25.4 mm/min).

9.6 Testing of samples shall be terminated when one of the following occurs:

9.6.1 The articular insert disengages from the glenoid backing,

9.6.2 The disengagement force has reached a maximum and continues to decrease, and

9.6.3 Gross deformation of the insert occurs without dislocation of the insert.

9.7 Record load versus displacement and the failure mode. The glenoid backing should be visually inspected for damage after each test run.

9.8 Repeat the procedure with a new insert and with the load applied in an anterior to posterior direction (see Fig. 2).

10. Report

10.1 The test report shall include the following:

10.1.1 All details relevant to the particular implants tested (that is, size, thickness, materials). If the glenoid component is not symmetric then details of the non-symmetry and its relation to the test configuration should be specified,

10.1.2 The distance, *"d"*, between the top of the locking mechanism and the centerline of the point of load application (see Fig. 1),

10.1.3 The displacement rate,

10.1.4 The maximum load to failure,

10.1.5 The failure mode,

10.1.6 The indentor loading applicator configuration.

10.1.7 Number of glenoid backing test components used.

11. Precision and Bias

11.1 The precision and bias of this test method needs to be established. Test results that can be used to establish precision and bias are solicited.

12. Keywords

12.1 arthroplasty; disassembly; glenoid; modular; orthopaedic medical devices; shoulder arthroplasty

APPENDIX

(Nonmandatory Information)

X1. RATIONALE

X1.1 A minimum of five test specimens is recommended for this test method. The investigator should determine if additional specimens are required. Statistical methods that take into account variability in the components being tested may be used to achieve the desired level of significance.

X1.2 This test method is intended to allow the investigator to compare different glenoid locking mechanism designs as subjected to shear loading. This test method is not intended to test for all modes of failure or loading to which the component may be subjected. The investigator should determine if additional test conditions are necessary. It is believed that fatigue, particularly in a rocking motion, is more likely to cause disassembly of the glenoid locking mechanism clinically and will provide further insight into the glenoid components behavior.

X1.3 The size of the glenoid component shall be determined by the investigator. In general, the worst case size should be chosen based on evaluation or experience. There may also be a reason why an investigator wishes to test a size that is not worst case. This test method may also be used for this purpose.

X1.4 Worst case loading of the glenoid component may vary depending on material, design, and clinical indications. The investigator shall evaluate the possible clinical and design-related failure modes and attempt to determine a worst case condition.

X1.5 It is recognized that for some materials the environment may have an effect on the response to loading. The test environment used and the rationale for that choice shall be described in the test report.

X1.6 The loading of metal backed glenoid prostheses in vivo will, in general, differ from the loading defined in this test method. The results obtained here cannot be used to directly predict in vivo performance. The results obtained from this test method do not imply that the prosthesis will be clinically successful.

Designation: F 1830 – 97

Standard Practice for Selection of Blood for In Vitro Evaluation of Blood Pumps[1]

This standard is issued under the fixed designation F 1830; the number immediately following the designation indicates the year of original adoption or, in the case of revision, the year of last revision. A number in parentheses indicates the year of last reapproval. A superscript epsilon (ϵ) indicates an editorial change since the last revision or reapproval.

1. Scope

1.1 This practice covers blood that will be used for in vitro performance assessments of blood pumps. These assessments include the hemolytic properties of the devices.

1.2 This practice covers the utilization of blood for the in vitro evaluation of the following devices:

1.2.1 Continuous flow rotary blood pumps (roller pumps, centrifugal pumps, axial flow pumps, etc.) (see Practice F 1841).

1.2.2 Pulsatile blood pumps (pneumatically driven, electromechanically driven, etc.).

1.3 The source of blood utilized for in vitro evaluation of blood trauma (that is, hemolysis caused by the blood pumps, due to the pump design, construction, and materials used) substantially influences the results of the performance of these devices. Thus, a standardized blood source is required.

2. Referenced Documents

2.1 *ASTM Standards:*

F 1841 Practice for Assessment of Hemolysis in Continuous Flow Blood Pumps[2]

3. Terminology

3.1 *Definitions of Terms Specific to This Standard:*

3.1.1 *continuous flow pump*—a blood pump that produces continuous blood flow due to its rotary motion.

3.1.2 *hemolysis*—one of the parameters of blood damage caused by a blood pump. This can be observed by a change in the plasma color and can be measured as an increase of free plasma hemoglobin concentration.

3.1.3 *pulsatile pump*—a blood pump that produces blood flow to mimic a natural heart.

4. Summary of Practice

4.1 For the experimental evaluation of blood pump designs and materials, an in vitro hemolysis test is recommended using fresh bovine or porcine blood. The donor animals should have normal body temperature, no physical signs of disease, including diarrhea and rhinorrhea, and an acceptable normal range of hematological profiles. The blood from a slaughterhouse should not be used because it may be contaminated with other body fluids, unless obtained by controlled venipuncture. However, for the preclinical studies, fresh human blood is recommended for use (see Practice F 1841).

4.2 For the in vitro hemolysis test, fresh bovine or porcine blood is used within 48 h, including the time for transport. Fresh human blood should be used within 24 h after blood harvesting. The collected blood should be refrigerated at 2 to 8°C.

5. Significance and Use

5.1 The test results are substantially affected by donor species and age, the method of harvesting, the period of storage, the biochemical state of the blood, and the hemoglobin and hematocrit level of blood.[3,4] Therefore, standardization of proper blood usage for in vitro evaluation of blood pumps is essential, and this recommended practice will allow a universal comparison of test results.

5.2 Drawing several units of blood from healthy cattle does not affect them or their health. Therefore, bovine blood is strongly suggested for usage in experimental evaluation of blood damage. Mixing two donor sources of blood should be avoided in hemolysis tests because the mixture may induce added hemolysis or a change in red cell resistance against trauma.

6. Collection and Preparation of Blood

6.1 Blood will be drawn using a venipuncture technique through a large bore needle (14 G or larger) into a blood bag which contains anticoagulants such as citrate phosphate dextrose adenine (CPDA-1) anticoagulant solution (see Appendix X1) or heparin sulfate (see Appendix X2). The blood is obtained from human volunteers, cattle or pigs having normal body temperature, no physical signs of disease, including diarrhea, rhinorrhea, and whose hematological profiles are in an acceptable range. No negative pressure in excess of 100 mmHg should be applied during the drawing of the blood. Blood will be collected until the blood bag is full to obtain a total of 450 ± 45 mL of blood and with anticoagulants. A larger bag can also be used.

[1] This practice is under the jurisdiction of ASTM Committee F-4 on Medical and Surgical Materials and Devices and is the direct responsibility of Subcommittee F04.30 on Cardiovascular Standards.

Current edition approved Nov. 10, 1997. Published June 1998.

[2] *Annual Book of ASTM Standards*, Vol 13.01.

[3] Mueller NM, et al. In Vitro Hematological Testing of Rotary Blood Pumps: Remarks on Standardization and Data Interpretation. *Artif Organs*, 17 (2), 1993, pp. 103–110.

[4] Mizuguchi K, et al. Does Hematocrit Affect In Vitro Hemolysis Test Results?: Preliminary Studies with NASA Axial Flow Pump. *Artif Organs* 18 (9), 1994, pp. 650–656.

6.2 The blood should be refrigerated between 2 to 8° C temperature. For blood transportation, the temperature should be also within the range of 2 to 8° C.

6.3 Refrigerated blood should be warmed to the physiological temperature, using a water bath of 37 ± 1° C or other appropriate methods.

6.4 During warming of the blood, close attention should be given to micro air bubbles, and these air bubbles should be eliminated through the sampling port of the blood bag before starting the in vitro evaluation.

6.5 To accomplish the removal of particulate matter, microthrombus and aggregated platelets during priming of the test circuit, a transfusion kit with a micro filter, 80 μm pore size or less, should be used. As a quality control measure, any blood having free plasma hemoglobin of more than 20 mg/dL should not be used for the test. The inclusion of total blood hemoglobin and hematocrit data are recommended in addition to blood source screening. Proper physiological blood parameters should be maintained prior to and during testing (for example, pH, base excess, glucose concentration).[3]

7. Keywords

7.1 blood trauma; condition of test blood; index of hemolysis; source of blood donor

APPENDIXES

(Nonmandatory Information)

X1. CITRATE PHOSPHATE DEXTROSE ADENINE (CPDA1) SOLUTION USP

X1.1 63 mL CPDA1 solution USP is added for collection of 450 mL blood.

X1.2 Each 63 mL of CPDA1 contains 2 g of dextrose (monohydrate) USP, 1.66 g sodium citrate(dihydrate) USP, 188 mg citric acid (anhydrous) USP, 140 mg monobasic sodium phosphate (monohydrate) USP and 17.3 mg adenine USP. The pH of the solution may be adjusted with sodium hydroxide.

X2. HEPARIN

X2.1 500 mL of blood containing 2000 to 3000 USP units of heparin is utilized.

X3. RATIONALE

X3.1 The source of blood utilized for in viitro evaluation of blood trauma (that is, hemolysis caused by the blood pumps, due to the pump design, construction, and materials used) substantially influences the results of the performance of these devices. Thus, a standardized blood source is required.

Standard Specification for Cranial Traction Tongs and Halo External Spinal Immobilization Devices[1]

This standard is issued under the fixed designation F 1831; the number immediately following the designation indicates the year of original adoption or, in the case of revision, the year of last revision. A number in parentheses indicates the year of last reapproval. A superscript epsilon (ε) indicates an editorial change since the last revision or reapproval.

1. Scope

1.1 This specification covers standards a manufacturer shall meet in the designing, manufacturing, testing, labeling, and documenting of halo and tong external spinal immobilization devices, but it is not to be construed as production methods, quality control techniques, manufacturer's lot criteria, or clinical recommendations.

1.2 This specification represents the best currently available test procedures at this time and is a minimum safety and performance standard.

1.3 This specification covers only those halo and tong devices intended for use on humans for therapeutic purposes. This specification assumes the user is well-trained in the procedures and maintenance of halo and tong application and has the ability to determine if an abnormality is treatable by these procedures.

1.4 This specification describes those devices commonly known as halo external fixation devices and what is known as cranial traction tongs.

1.5 Cranial traction tongs and halo devices are used to achieve and maintain optimal spinal alignment, in order to enhance fusion and decrease neurological deficit.

1.6 Monitoring the progress of treatment after application of these devices is important, this should be done in accordance with the manufacturer's recommendation and guidelines pertaining to the specific device.

1.7 The values stated in both inch-pound and SI units are to be regarded separately as the standard. The values given in parentheses are for information only.

1.8 The following precautionary statement pertains only to the test method portions Sections 10-15 of this specification: *This standard does not purport to address all of the safety concerns, if any, associated with its use. It is the responsibility of the user of this standard to establish appropriate safety and health practices and determine the applicability of regulatory limitations prior to use.*

2. Referenced Documents

2.1 *IEC Standard:*

IEC 601-1 [2]

3. Terminology

3.1 *Definitions of Terms Specific to This Standard:*

3.1.1 *cranial traction tong*—a device providing weighted cervical traction to a patient through invasive attachment to the skull. This traction instrument is indicated for closed reduction of a cervical spine injury (that is, fracture or dislocation).

3.1.1.1 *adjustable tong*—a cranial traction tong that adjusts for size, pin positioning, or pin pressure.

3.1.1.2 *one-piece tong*—a rigid, single-piece, semicircular cranial traction tong designed to accommodate a minimum of two skull pins for mounting the device to the patients head below the equator.

3.1.2 *halo device*—an external fixator for cervical stabilization that fastens by invasive means to a patient's skull, and maintains the position of the skull in relation to the thoracic area of the patient.

3.1.3 *halo ring*—the portion of the halo device that fastens by invasive means to a patient's skull below the head equator.

3.1.3.1 *closed loop halo ring*—a halo ring incorporating a closed loop anywhere in the design for purposes of structural integrity when the ring is in use. This type of ring has multiple positioning options for the selection of pin sites and is mounted to the head with multiple skull pins.

3.1.3.2 *head equator*—the greatest circumference of the head in the coronal aspect

3.1.3.3 *open loop halo ring*—a halo ring with a posterior opening, such that the part does not incorporate a closed loop anywhere in the design for structural integrity. This ring has multiple position options for the selection of pin sites and is mounted to the head with multiple skull pins.

3.1.4 *halo superstructure*—a rigid external framework used to maintain positioning of the skull and cervical spine in relation to the thoracic and lumbar spine. Connects the halo ring to halo vest.

3.1.4.1 *halo superstructure adjustment mechanisms*— components that allow adjustment of angles and distances between ring and uprights or vest and uprights.

3.1.4.2 *transverse bar*—a rigid horizontal component of the halo superstructure.

---

[1] This specification is under the jurisdiction of ASTM Committee F-4 on Medical and Surgical Material and Devices and is the direct responsibility of Subcommittee F04.31 on Neurosurgical Standards.

Current edition approved Nov. 10, 1997. Published April 1998.

[2] Available from American National Standards Institute, 1430 Broadway, New York, NY 10018.

3.1.4.3 *upright bar*—a rigid vertical component of the halo superstructure.

3.1.4.4 *vest attachment mechanism*—attaches inferiorly to the halo superstructure and connects to vest shell, maintains positioning of the halo superstructure in relation to the vest shell.

3.1.4.5 *vest plate*—part of the superstructure attached to the vest shell to provide a stable mounting point for the vest attachment mechanisms.

3.1.5 *halo vest*—a body-orthosis that serves as a mounting point for the halo and superstructure.

3.1.5.1 *C.P.R. access*—mechanism in vest or superstructure to allow quick access to patient's chest for cardiopulmonary resuscitation (C.P.R.).

3.1.5.2 *vest liner*—padding worn inside of halo vest shell and against the skin which distributes the pressure of the vest shell against the skin.

3.1.5.3 *vest shell*—rigid portion of body orthosis.

3.1.6 *skull pin*—a rigid device used to invasively anchor the halo ring or cranial traction tongs to the skull at selected mounting points.

3.1.6.1 *adjustable skull pin*—(*1*) a pin that is force controlled by a mechanical mechanism, that is, spring-loaded pressure pin. (*2*) a solid threaded pin that maintains pressure and fixation against the skull through application of a calibrated torque.

3.1.6.2 *fixed skull pin*—a pin that is mounted directly to a tong structure requiring a drilled skull hole for positioning and fixation. Pressure is not adjusted directly through the pin.

3.1.7 *traction bail (traction hoop)*—a device that may be attached to the halo ring to facilitate the application of weighted longitudinal traction.

4. Conformance

4.1 Presently, this specification is voluntary and not by law. A manufacturer may label a product as conforming to this specification only if the product indeed meets all the requirements of this specification.

5. Classification

5.1 *Halo External Fixator*—Typically a complete system consisting of the halo ring, skull pins, vest and superstructure. The uniqueness of this system is its ability to provide self-contained cervical stabilization.

5.2 *Cranial Traction Tongs*—Either a rigid single-piece, semicircular device or an adjustable device. Both designs have accommodations for at least two skull pins to be mounted to the skull. Typically designed to be fitted over the top of the head and used for weighted cervical reduction or bed traction, or both, in the supine (bed restricted) patient.

6. Magnetic Resonance Imaging Compatibility Requirements

6.1 These halo external fixator and cranial traction tong magnetic resonance imaging (MRI) compatibility requirements are intended to protect the patient from harm during MRI imaging procedures.

6.2 Manufacturers shall be responsible for testing the MRI safety and efficacy of the device.

6.2.1 *Test Methods*— See Sections 13-15.

7. Mechanical Integrity

7.1 The purpose of this requirement is to ensure the user and the patient that the halo external fixator or cranial traction tongs, or both, are capable of withstanding the externally imposed conditions normally encountered during the useful life of the device.

7.2 *Cranial Traction Tongs Mechanical integrity*:

7.2.1 The cranial traction tongs and any of its components must be manufactured from a material that provides suitable rigid support to the skull pins and any other attached components including the traction weights.

7.2.2 Cranial traction tong pins shall be sufficiently strong to resist at least two times the normal maximum static loads that may be encountered during normal wear.

7.2.3 The cranial traction tongs and its components shall be resistant to deformation and sufficiently rigid such that pin position and pressure on the skull can be maintained at maximum manufacturer's specified pin pressures.

7.2.4 Adjustable skull pins shall be calibrated with force indicators.

7.2.5 *Test Method*— See Section 10.

7.3 *Halo Skull Pin Mechanical Integrity*:

7.3.1 Halo skull pins shall be sufficiently strong to resist at least two times the normal maximum static and dynamic loads that may be encountered during normal use.

7.3.2 *Test Method*— See Section 11.

7.4 *Halo Ring Mechanical Integrity*:

7.4.1 The halo ring shall be manufactured from a material that provides suitable rigid support to the attached skull pins and superstructure.

7.4.2 The halo ring shall be resistant to deformation and sufficiently rigid such that pin position and pressure on the skull can be maintained at maximum manufacturer's specified pin pressures.

7.4.3 *Test Method*— See Section 11.

7.5 *Halo Superstructure Assemblies Mechanical Integrity*:

7.5.1 A new halo external fixator device must be able to maintain structural integrity under normal physical loading when the system is fully assembled.

7.5.2 All mechanical components of the superstructure assembly must maintain rigidity and functional integrity throughout the useful life of the product.

7.5.3 *Test Method*— See Section 12.

7.6 *Halo Vest Assembly Mechanical Integrity*:

7.6.1 The halo vest assembly must provide a stable platform for rigid attachment of the superstructure.

7.6.2 The halo vest must provide an adjustable means of rigid fixation to the upper body of the patient.

8. Performance Requirements

8.1 The purpose of these requirements is to ensure that a halo external fixator or cranial tongs shall meet the minimum performance requirements as originally designed. The halo and tongs device requirements should not vary from procedure to procedure provided they are used and maintained according to the manufacturer's recommendation.

8.2 *Halo External Fixator Performance Requirements*:

8.2.1 All mechanical fixation components will be manufactured out of corrosion resistant materials.

8.2.2 All components shall be manufactured out of materials capable of providing functional integrity over the useful life of the device.

8.2.3 The manufacturer will be responsible to maintain adequate mechanical test data or equivalent clinical data in regard to the suitability of design, useful life and diagnostic imaging compatibility of the system.

8.2.4 The manufacturer will be responsible for supplying materials that are sterilizable by the manufacturer's recommended sterilization techniques.

8.3 *Halo Pin Performance Requirements*:

8.3.1 All portions of the skull pin that are in constant physical contact with the patient's skin shall be manufactured from biologically compatible material.

8.3.2 All halo skull pins shall be supplied with a method for locking the pin in place in the halo ring.

8.4 *Halo Ring Performance Requirements*—The manufacturer will be responsible for providing a ring assembly that allows for the following:

8.4.1 The halo ring shall be able to easily and rigidly attach to the superstructure.

8.4.2 The halo ring shall be able to easily accept a minimum of four halo skull pins.

8.5 *Halo Superstructure Assembly Performance Requirements*:

8.5.1 The halo vest and superstructure assemblies shall be able to be easily attached and detached from the halo ring with the appropriate tools.

8.6 *Halo Vest Performance Requirements*:

8.6.1 The vest material shall be trimmable and moldable with the appropriate tools to allow the medical personnel to provide suitable adaptability to the various anatomies encountered.

8.6.2 The manufacturer will provide suitable vest liner materials to maintain a substrate between the vest shell and the skin. These lining materials shall be free of any chemicals or toxins, or both, that could cause an allergic response in the average patient.

8.6.3 The halo vest shall have a vest attachment mechanism whereby the halo superstructure is suitably attached via the appropriate tools or mechanism.

8.6.4 The halo vest shall allow rapid and complete access to the chest in the event of a cardiac emergency to allow access to the chest for C.P.R.

8.7 *Halo Tools Performance Requirements*—All halo adjustment tools supplied by the manufacturer shall consistently perform in the manner to which they were designed throughout the useful life of the product or as indicated by the manufacturer's recommendations.

8.8 *Cranial Traction Tongs Performance Requirements*:

8.8.1 All mechanical fixation components will be manufactured out of corrosion resistant materials.

8.8.2 All components shall be manufactured out of materials capable of providing functional integrity over the useful life of the device.

8.8.3 The manufacturer will be responsible to maintain adequate mechanical test data or equivalent clinical data in regard to the suitability of design, useful life and diagnostic imaging compatibility of the system.

8.8.4 The manufacturer will be responsible for supplying materials that are sterilizable by the manufacturer's recommended sterilization techniques.

8.8.5 The cranial traction tongs must permit attachment of cables and other necessary hardware.

8.9 *Cranial Traction Tongs Pin Performance Requirements*:

8.9.1 All tong pins must be supplied by the manufacturer with a method of locking.

8.9.2 Any portion of the tong pin that is in direct contact with the patient's skin shall be manufactured from biologically compatible materials.

9. Disclosures, Labeling, and Documentation

9.1 These requirements are intended to ensure a manufacturer's written dissemination of all necessary information that allow a user to determine properly a halo external fixator or cranial traction tongs (and all of their related accessories) function, application and limitation. These disclosures, labeling and documentation requirements also ensure clear identification of the product and make available all pertinent data a user may require. A manufacturer may label his product as conforming to this standard only if the product fulfills all of the requirements listed in this specification.

9.2 *Disclosures*— A manufacturer shall disclose each specification listed where applicable.

9.2.1 *Single Patient Use Statement*—A manufacturer of halo external fixation systems or cranial traction tongs shall provide a warning statement to inform the user that the device is guaranteed for single patient use only.

9.2.2 *Sterilization*— A disclosure statement that states exactly which items of the halo external fixator and the cranial traction tongs and their accessories can be sterilized and the recommended sterilization procedures shall be included with each device.

9.2.3 *Presterilized Components*—A disclosure statement shall be included with each presterilized component of either the halo or the tongs. This statement shall include the following information: the device is sterile, the expiration date, notes of caution concerning means of shipping, storage and use of the instrument, and lot and batch information.

9.2.4 *Imaging Compatibility*—Manufactures shall be responsible for labeling the product according to imaging compatibility to avoid confusion by the end user.

9.3 *Labeling*:

9.3.1 All required labeling shall be legible in terms of size and color as dictated by FDA guidelines (21 CFR 820). The labeling must also be durable to last the life of the product and permanently attached so as not to be lost.

9.3.2 All halo external fixators and cranial traction tongs shall be labeled so as to contain the following information:

9.3.2.1 Model number and size,

9.3.2.2 Manufacturer or distributor name, or both,

9.3.2.3 Serial number or lot and batch number,

9.3.2.4 Diagnostic imaging compatibility indicators, and

9.3.2.5 C.P.R. access indicators.

9.3.3 If labeling is not conducive to direct attachment to the device then all information shall be provided in the manufacturer's instruction manual or on the final packaging.

9.4 *Documentation*:

9.4.1 All halos and tongs shall include instruction manuals.

9.4.2 All instruction manuals shall contain the following information when applicable:

9.4.2.1 Recommended sizing and application instructions

9.4.2.2 Recommended safe maximum traction loading information for the ring and traction bail or cranial traction tong as the composite system (ring and pins) excluding physiological parameters associated with the patient's skull.

9.4.2.3 CPR access instructions,

9.4.2.4 Recommended pin torque settings,

9.4.2.5 Cleaning instructions,

9.4.2.6 Patient care guidelines,

9.4.2.7 Diagnostic imaging compatibility guidelines, and

9.4.2.8 Manufacturer or distributor's name and address, or both.

10. Test Method for Mechanical Integrity of Cranial Traction Tongs

10.1 *Scope*—This test method covers the mechanical integrity of tongs with skull pins and their ability to withstand a loading without significant loss of function.

10.1.1 *Summary of Test Method*—The tongs are set up such that the loading is applied at the point on the tongs as it would be under normal use as recommended by the manufacturer. The tongs are supported as described in 10.1.3 and 10.1.3.1. The amount of deflection and ability of the device to withstand the loading is recorded.

10.1.2 *Significance and Use*—For safety reasons, the device shall be designed to withstand a minimum of twice the maximum load typically used during normal short-term clinical applications or as outlined by the manufacturer in the product's instruction manuals without adverse deflection of any components of the device.

10.1.3 *Apparatus*—Tongs shall be suspended, utilizing any attachment devices supplied with the product by the manufacturer as shown in Fig. 1. Skull pins shall be inserted into the unit and inserted into an aluminum mounting block such that any load applied to the tong will be carried equally by all skull pins and attachment points and so that the resultant load will be applied axially so as not to apply any angular force to the arms of the tongs and in such a way that any load applied to the tongs will be carried equally by all attachment points.

10.1.3.1 *Aluminum Skull Pin Mount*—An aluminum block shall be predrilled to a maximum depth of 2 mm to accommodate the tips of the skull pins.

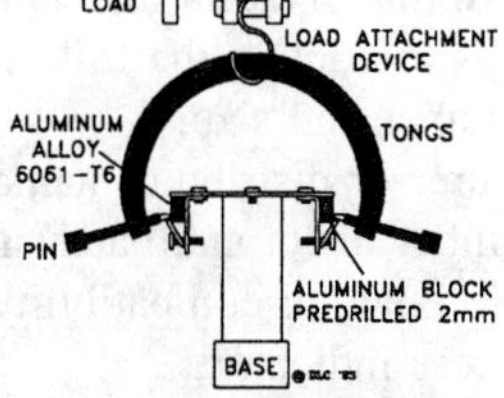

FIG. 1 Suspended Tongs

10.1.3.2 The test specimen shall consist of the manufacturer's new, finished, untested product.

10.1.4 *Procedure*:

10.1.4.1 If the tongs are adjustable, they shall be set in an average or typical position of use for a head with a lateral width of 17 cm, or to the median position within the range the device is designed to accommodate.

10.1.4.2 Insert the skull pins into the predrilled holes in the aluminum block and tighten them according to manufacturer's recommendations for optimum force.

10.1.4.3 Apply a load to the device where skeletal traction is applied in a clinical setting per the manufacturer's instructions. The load may be applied incrementally (maximum 10 lb (g) increments) or continuously at a maximum rate of 0.127 cm/min.

10.1.4.4 Load the device to either 100 kg or twice the maximum safe load recommended by the manufacturer.

10.1.4.5 After the necessary loading is achieved, leave the apparatus in place for a period of 20 min.

10.1.4.6 Document load versus displacement curves throughout the test.

10.1.4.7 After 20 min, unload the device and document the final displacement of the device in the unloaded state.

10.1.5 *Interpretation of Results*:

10.1.5.1 Any tong able to maintain the maximum load without signs of plastic deformation in any components of the device shall have passed the test.

10.1.5.2 Any tong demonstrating plastic deformation in any components of the device after unloading the maximum load shall have failed the test.

10.2 *Additional Test Method for Cranial Traction Tongs*:

10.2.1 *Scope*—This test method covers the mechanical integrity of tongs with skull pins and their ability to withstand loading without significant loss of function.

10.2.2 *Summary of Test Method*—The tongs are set up such that the loading is applied at the point on the tongs as it would be under normal use as recommended by the manufacturer. The tongs are supported as described in 10.2.3 and 10.2.3.1. The amount of deflection and ability of the device to withstand the loading is recorded.

10.2.3 *Significance and Use*—For safety reasons, the device shall be designed to withstand a minimum of twice the maximum load typically used during normal long-term clinical applications or as outlined by the manufacturer in the product's instruction manuals without plastic deformation of any component of the device. The rotational and dynamic loading component that occurs in a clinical setting as a result of turning the patient in bed must also be considered.

10.2.4 *Apparatus*—Tongs shall be suspended, utilizing any attachment devices supplied with the product by the manufacturer as shown in Fig. 1. Skull pins shall be inserted into the unit and inserted into an aluminum mounting block such that any load applied to the tong will be carried equally by all skull pins and attachment points and so that the resultant load will be applied axially so as not to apply any angular force to the arms of the tong and in such a way that any load applied to the tongs will be carried equally by all attachment points.

10.2.4.1 *Aluminum Skull Pin Mount*—An aluminum block

shall be predrilled to a maximum depth of 2 mm to accommodate the insertion of the tips of the skull pins.

10.2.4.2 The test specimen shall consist of the manufacturer's new, finished, untested product.

10.2.5 *Procedure*:

10.2.5.1 If the tongs are adjustable, they shall be set in an average or typical position of use for a head with a lateral width of 17 cm, or to the median position within the range the device is designed to accommodate.

10.2.5.2 Insert the skull pins into the predrilled holes in the aluminum block and tighten them according to manufacturer's recommendations for optimum force.

10.2.5.3 Apply a load to the device where skeletal traction is applied in a clinical setting in accordance with the manufacturer's instructions. The load may be applied incrementally (maximum 10 lb (g) increments) or continuously at a rate not to exceed 0.127 cm/min.

10.2.5.4 Load the device to 60 kgs.

10.2.5.5 After the necessary loading is achieved, leave the apparatus in place for a period of one week. During this time, alternate loading in increments of approximately 10° from center (+10°, 0°,– 10°) once every 24 h to simulate angular traction forces.

10.2.5.6 After one week, measure and document the change in displacement between the arms of the device from the unloaded state to the fully loaded state and back to the unloaded state.

10.2.6 *Interpretation of Results*:

10.2.6.1 Any tong able to maintain the 60 kg load for one week without signs of plastic deformation in any component of the device shall have passed the test.

10.2.6.2 Any tong demonstrating plastic deformation in any component of the device after unloading the 60 kg load shall have failed the test.

11. Test Method for Mechanical Integrity of Halo Rings and Attachment Bails

11.1 *Scope*—This protocol has been developed to test the mechanical integrity of halo rings and their corresponding bails, as well as their ability to withstand loading without significant loss of function. The equipment used for this test has been designed to accommodate all known sizes and shapes of halo rings.

11.1.1 *Summary of Test Method*—The halo rings and traction bails are configured to simulate normal use. Loads are applied at the points recommended by the manufacturer for normal traction application. The halo rings and traction bails are supported as described in 11.1.3.

11.1.2 *Significance and Use*—For safety reasons, the device shall be designed to withstand a minimum of twice the maximum load typically used during normal clinical applications or as outlined by the manufacturer in the product's instruction manuals without significant elastic deformation and without any plastic deformation. The traction bail must remain intact throughout testing.

11.1.3 *Apparatus*—The ring shall be suspended, utilizing any traction attachment components supplied with the product by the manufacturer as shown in Fig. 2. Skull pins shall be inserted into the ring and against an aluminum mounting block such that any load applied to the ring will be carried equally by all skull pins and attachment points and so that the resultant load will be applied axially so as not to apply any uneven distribution of load on the pins and in such a way that any load applied to the ring will be carried equally by all attachment points.

11.1.3.1 *Aluminum Skull Pin Mount*—An elliptical aluminum block shall be predrilled to a maximum depth of 1 mm to accommodate the tips of the skull pins. The locations of the predrilled holes should be chosen according to manufacturer's recommended pin placement and such that the applied load will be distributed equally by the skull pins.

11.1.3.2 The elliptical aluminum block shall be machined such that the minimum distance between the halo ring and the block is 1 cm. An assortment of aluminum blocks may be necessary to fit all halo ring sizes. If the ring is adjustable, it shall be set in an average or typical position of use for a head with a circumference of 51 cm, or to the median circumference within the range the device is designed to accommodate.

11.1.3.3 The thickness of the elliptical aluminum block may vary depending on whether or not all skull pins lie in the same plane. An example is detailed in Fig. 2.

11.1.3.4 The test specimen shall consist of the manufacturer's new, finished, untested product.

11.1.4 *Procedure*:

11.1.4.1 Make template of the halo ring prior to testing.

11.1.4.2 Insert the skull pins through the halo ring into the predrilled holes in the mounting block and tighten according to the manufacturer's recommendations for optimum torque.

11.1.4.3 Attach the traction bail to the halo ring such that the

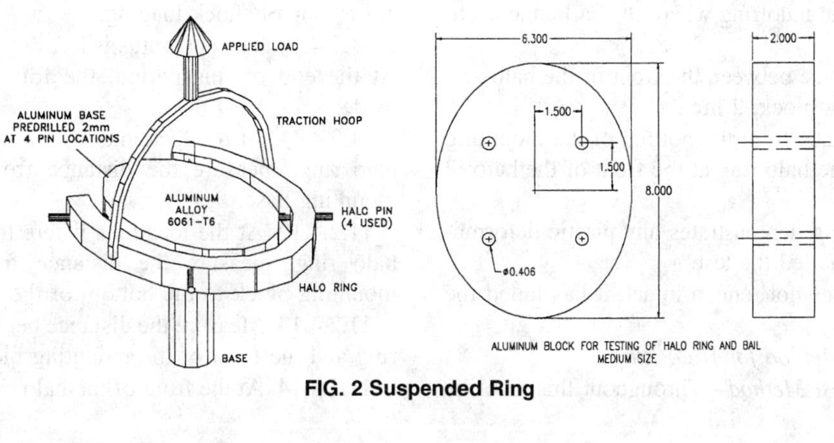

FIG. 2 Suspended Ring

applied load will be perpendicular to the halo ring (or as otherwise specified by the manufacturer) and carried equally by the skull pins.

11.1.4.4 Using calipers, make the following measurements before loading:

11.1.4.5 At the locations where the bail is attached to the halo ring, measure the distance from the halo ring to the mounting base.

11.1.4.6 At the locations where the bail is attached to the halo ring, measure the distance from the bottom of the mounting block to the bottom of the halo ring.

11.1.4.7 Measure the distance between the front of the halo ring and the front of the mounting block.

11.1.4.8 At the front of the halo ring, measure the distance from the bottom of the mounting block to the bottom of the halo ring.

11.1.4.9 Apply a 70 kg load to the bail in the position where skeletal traction would be applied for normal use in accordance with the manufacturer's instructions. Apply the load gradually so as not to impart shock loading.

11.1.4.10 Leave the apparatus in place for a period of 20 min. At the end of this period, make the following measurements.

11.1.4.11 At the locations where the bail is attached to the halo ring, measure the distance from the halo ring to the mounting base.

11.1.4.12 At the locations where the bail is attached to the halo ring, measure the distance from the bottom of the mounting block to the bottom of the halo ring.

11.1.4.13 Measure the distance between the front of the halo ring and the front of the aluminum mounting block.

11.1.4.14 At the front of the halo ring, measure the distance from the bottom of the mounting block to the bottom of the halo ring.

11.1.4.15 Remove the skull pins and check the free, unloaded halo ring with the template made in 11.1.4.1.

11.1.5 *Interpretation of Results*:

11.1.5.1 Compare the measurements from the unloaded halo ring (see 11.1.4.3) to those taken from the loaded halo ring (see 11.1.4.5). If the difference between any of the corresponding measurements exceeds the following, the halo ring has failed the test:

Difference in the distances from the halo ring to the mounting base where the bail attaches to the halo ring: 2 mm.

Difference in the distance from the bottom of the mounting block to the bottom of the halo ring where the bail attaches to the halo ring: 2 mm.

Difference in the distance between the front of the halo and the front of the mounting block: 2 mm.

Difference in the distance from the bottom of the mounting block to the bottom of the halo ring at the front of the halo: 2 mm.

11.1.5.2 If the halo ring demonstrates any plastic deformation in 11.1.4.15, it has failed the test.

11.1.5.3 If the bail does not remain intact, it has failed the test.

11.2 *Additional Test Method for Halo Rings*:

11.2.1 *Summary of Test Method*—Throughout this test, the halo rings and bails are configured to simulate normal use. The load is applied at the point which is recommended by the manufacturer for normal traction. The halo rings and traction bails are supported as described in 11.1.3.

11.2.2 *Significance and Use*—To test for creep of the halo ring, the ring must withstand 50 % of the load described in the previous test for a period of 24 h without significant elastic deformation and without any plastic deformation. The corresponding bail must remain intact throughout the testing.

11.2.3 *Apparatus*—The ring shall be suspended, utilizing any traction attachment components supplied with the product by the manufacturer as shown in Fig. 2. Skull pins shall be inserted into the ring and against an aluminum mounting block such that any load applied to the ring will be carried equally by all skull pins and attachment points and so that the resultant load will be applied axially so as not to apply any uneven distribution of load on the pins and in such a way that any load applied to the ring will be carried equally by all attachment points.

11.2.3.1 The test specimen shall consist of the manufacturer's new, finished, untested product.

11.2.4 *Procedure*:

11.2.4.1 Make a template of the halo ring prior to testing.

11.2.4.2 Insert the skull pins through the halo ring into the predrilled holes in the mounting block and tighten according to the manufacturer's recommendations for optimum torque.

11.2.4.3 Attach the bail to the halo ring such that the applied load will be perpendicular to the halo ring and carried equally by the skull pins.

11.2.4.4 Using calipers, make the following measurements prior to loading:

11.2.4.5 At the locations where the bail is attached to the halo ring, measure the distance from the halo ring to the mounting base.

11.2.4.6 At the locations where the bail is attached to the halo ring, measure the distance from the bottom of the mounting block to the bottom of the halo ring.

11.2.4.7 Measure the distance between the front of the halo ring at the front of the mounting block.

11.2.4.8 At the front of the halo ring, measure the distance from the bottom of the mounting block to the bottom of the halo ring.

11.2.4.9 A 35 kg load is applied to the bail in the position where skeletal traction would be applied for normal use per the manufacturer's instructions. The load is applied gradually so as not to impart shock loading.

11.2.4.10 The apparatus is left in place for a period of 24 h. At the end of this period, the following measurements are made:

11.2.4.11 At the locations where the bail is attached to the halo ring, measure the distance from the halo ring to the mounting base.

11.2.4.12 At the locations where the bail is attached to the halo ring, measure the distance from the bottom of the mounting block to the bottom of the halo ring.

11.2.4.13 Measure the distance between the front of the halo ring and the front of the mounting block.

11.2.4.14 At the front of the halo ring, measure the distance from the bottom of the mounting block to the bottom of the halo ring.

11.2.4.15 Remove the skull pins and check the free, unloaded halo ring with the template made in 11.1.4.1.

11.2.5 *Interpretation of Results*:

11.2.5.1 Compare the measurements from the unloaded halo ring (see 11.2.4.3) to those taken from the loaded halo ring (see 11.2.4.5). If the difference between any of the corresponding measurements exceeds the following, the halo ring has failed the test:

11.2.5.2 Difference in the distances from the halo ring to the mounting base where the bail attaches to the halo ring: 2 mm.

11.2.5.3 Differences in the distances from the bottom of the mounting block to the bottom of the halo ring where the bail attaches to the halo ring: 2 mm.

11.2.5.4 Difference in the distance between the front of the halo and the front of the mounting block: 2 mm.

11.2.5.5 Difference in the distance from the bottom of the mounting block to the bottom of the halo ring at the front of the halo: 2 mm.

11.2.5.6 If the halo ring demonstrates any plastic deformation in 11.2.4.15, it has failed the test.

11.2.5.7 If the bail does not remain intact, it has failed the test.

12. Test Method for Mechanical Integrity of Halo Superstructures

12.1 *Scope*—This test method covers the mechanical integrity of halo superstructures and their ability to withstand loading without significant loss of function.

12.1.1 *Summary of Test Method*—The halo superstructures and rings are anchored to a rigid support and loads are applied to the device that connects the halo superstructure to the skull. The halo superstructures are supported as described in 12.1.3. The amount of displacement and ability of the device to withstand the loading is recorded.

12.1.2 *Significance and Use*—or safety reasons, the device shall be designed to withstand a minimum of twice the average load typically used during normal clinical applications or as outlined by the manufacturer in the product's instruction manuals without significant deflection.

12.1.3 *Apparatus*—An individual rigid fixture shall be constructed for each model of halo superstructure. The fixture shall hold the superstructure in the same position as the superstructure would be held on an average patient. The fixture shall have a rigid rod originating from it's base and extend through the approximate center of the device that attaches the superstructure to the skull (see Fig. 3). All measurements of displacements of the superstructure shall be made in relation to this rod.

12.1.3.1 The test specimen shall consist of the manufacturer's new, finished, untested product.

12.1.4 *Procedure*:

12.1.4.1 Measure the pretest distance between the rigid rod and the device that connects the superstructure to the skull.

NOTE 1—Pretest measurements shall be taken prior to each separate loading condition.

12.1.4.2 *Loading Conditions:*

12.1.4.3 Apply the load to the device that connects the halo superstructure to the skull.

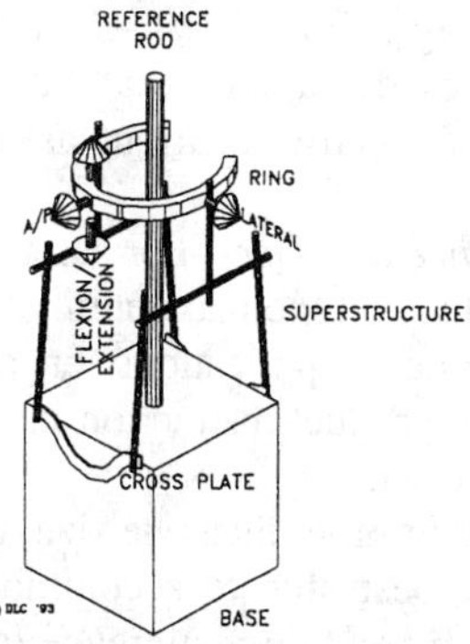

FIG. 3 Attachment of Halo Superstructure

12.1.4.4 In all cases, apply the load incrementally or all at once but not suddenly so as to impart shock loading.

12.1.4.5 If gravity is the loading mechanism then the weight of the cable, chain or other device should be considered into the total loading.

12.1.4.6 Apply loading separately and non-coincidentally.

12.1.4.7 Loads referenced below are in accordance clinically relevant maximum loads.[3,4]

12.1.4.8 *Anterior/Posterior Direction Loading*—Apply a 23 kg load to the device.

12.1.4.9 *Flexion/Extension Loading*—Apply an 18 kg load to the device.

12.1.4.10 *Lateral Direction Loading*—Apply an 18 kg load to the device.

12.1.4.11 Measure the deflection of the superstructure in relation to the rigid rod after each loading condition.

12.1.5 *Interpretation of Results*:

12.1.5.1 Any superstructure with a measured deflection from the reference rod to the point of load application of greater than 20 mm in the anterior, posterior or flexion/extension directions shall have failed the test. Any superstructure with a measured deflection of greater than 40 mm in the lateral direction shall have failed the test.

12.1.5.2 Any superstructure with a measured deflection from the reference rod to the point of load application less than or equal to 20 mm in the anterior-posterior or flexion/extension direction shall have passed the test. Any superstructure with a measured deflection of less than or equal to 40 mm in the lateral direction shall have passed the test.

13. Test Method for Calculation of Induced Current Flow of Halo External Fixators or Cranial Traction Tongs, or Both

13.1 *Scope*—This test method covers the calculation of electric current induced in halo external fixators and cranial traction tongs when exposed to the time-varying magnetic field in a magnetic resonance imaging machine and the ability of the product to prevent such a current from occurring during use.

---

[3] Lind, B. Sihlbom, H. and Nordwall, A., "Forces and Motions Across the Neck in Patients Treated With Halo-Vest," *Spine 13*, 1988, pp. 162–167.

[4] Walker, P.S., Lamser, D., Hussey, R.W., Rossier, A.B., Farberor, A., Dietz, J., "Forces in Halo-Vest Apparatus," *Spine 9*, 1984, pp. 773–777.

13.1.1 *Summary of Test Method*—Using Faraday's equation and Ohm's Law provide calculational data demonstrating that excessive values of electrical current are not induced in the device.

13.1.2 *Significance and Use*—For safety reasons the device shall be able to withstand the maximum voltage typically used during normal clinical applications or as outlined by the manufacturer in the product instruction manual without excessive current generation.

13.2 If available in more than one size, the test device shall consist of the size best able to accommodate a lateral head width of 17 cm or a head circumference of 51 cm.

13.3 *Procedure*:

13.3.1 Define the conductive loop between the two most distant pin sites along the perimeter of the device.

13.3.2 Calculate area (*A*) and perimeter (*L*) of conductive loop. (See Fig. 4.)

13.3.3 Using Faraday's law:

$$\int E\, dl = -db/dT \quad (1)$$

where:

E = the induced voltage,
B = the time-varying magnetic field strength, and
T = the time in seconds.

and Ohm's Law:

$$\text{Current} = E/\text{Resistance} \quad (2)$$

calculate E for the normal maximum clinically relevant voltage or as otherwise stated in the manufacturer's product literature.

13.4 *Interpretation of Results*:

13.4.1 Any device demonstrating an E value of less than or equal to 4 v between any two adjacent skull pin sites shall have passed the test.

13.4.2 Any device demonstrating an E value of greater than 4 v between any two adjacent skull pin sites shall have failed the test.

14. Test Method for Experimental Documentation of Current Induced Heating in Halo External Fixators or Cranial Traction Tongs, or Both, During Magnetic Resonance Imaging

14.1 *Scope*—This test method covers the experimental observation of electric current induced in halo external fixators and cranial traction tongs when exposed to the magnetic field in a magnetic resonance imaging machine and the ability of the product to prevent such a current from generating sufficient density within the tissue surrounding the pin to cause a health hazard (that is, burn) (see IEC 601–1).

14.1.1 *Summary of Test Method*—Through a system of sensitive measuring devices and imaging techniques demonstrate that excessive values of current density will not be produced in the tissue surrounding the pins.

14.1.2 *Significance and Use*—For safety reasons the device shall be able to withstand the maximum voltage typically used during normal clinical applications or as outlined by the manufacturer in the product instruction manual without excessive current/heat generation.

14.2 If available in more than one size, the test device shall consist of the size best able to accommodate a lateral head width of 17 cm or a head circumference of 51 cm.

14.3 *Procedural Set-Up*:

14.3.1 The difficulties associated with calculating current density in the device-patient-MR system can be avoided by a direct, experimental measurement of the current-generated time-temperature history of a simple biological model (that will ensure maximum current density) in the MR. A model system for tongs and conductive tissue is illustrated in Fig. 5.

14.3.2 The model in Fig. 5 is comprised of a flexible, ¾ in. (mm) OD polymer (vinyl) tube of ½ in. (mm) nominal ID filled with Ringer's lactate. The Ringer's solution serves as the analog of physiological electrolytes. The tube is packed with glass wool to minimize the formation of convective cells in the electrolyte around the pins. Convective cells would conduct heat away from the material immediately surrounding the tip. The ends of the tube are sealed with RTV sealant.

14.3.3 Insert skull pins through small punctures in the tube. The hole should close around the pins and provide a good seal. The pins should protrude approximately halfway into the tube.

14.3.4 Position a welded "K" type (nickel-chromium, nickel-aluminum) thermocouple near the tip (within 1 to 2 mm) of one pin. Solder thermocouple leads (11 in. (mm) long) to a BNC connector at approximately the same position to minimize temperature differences among the leads at the joints. This type thermocouple is minimally ferromagnetic and can, therefore, be used in the high magnetic field of the MRI.

14.3.5 Immerse the reference thermocouple in an ice bath that is insensitive to bulk heating (ice shavings must be present and well-distributed).

14.3.6 Measure the voltage produced by the thermocouple arrangement by a Fluke multimeter. Temperature may then be

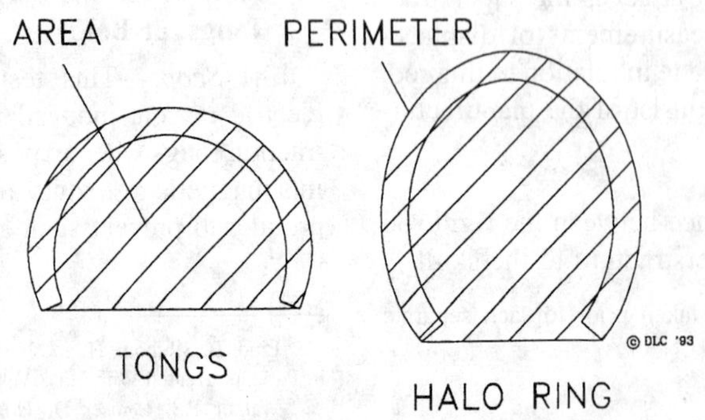

FIG. 4 Area and Perimeter of Conductive Loop

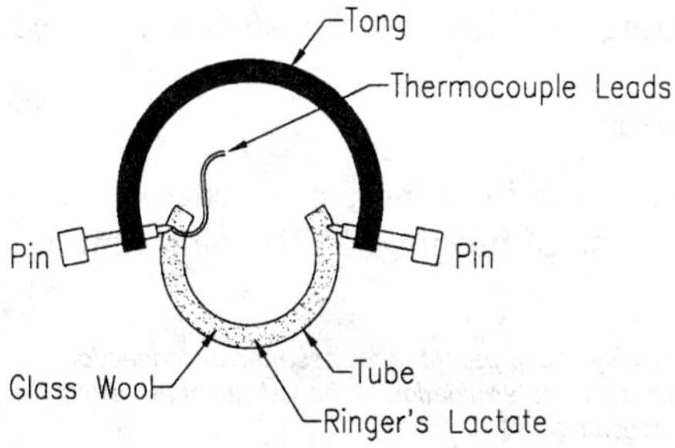

FIG. 5 Model Tong/Tissue System

determined from the measured voltage (using Omega Engineering conversion tables). Place the thermocouple immediately above the pin to detect convective heating if it occurs.

14.3.7 A typical temperature readout device would be overwhelmed by induced voltage transients created by an MRI unit, and therefore cannot be used to detect temperature increases in the model apparatus. A single pole low pass filter is used for this purpose in the following manner. The electrical signal from the thermocouple has two components: an intermittent 64 MHz component arising from the interaction of the MRI's radio frequency field with the thermocouple leads, and a much slower voltage rise produced by the thermocouple pair in response to a possible temperature rise of the sensor thermocouple. The high frequency signal is expected because the thermocouple leads are separated to assure that the temperature response is limited to the proximity of the pin. The separation introduces a small loop which will generate voltage.

14.3.8 The high frequency induced voltage from the rapid radio-frequency field of the MRI is many orders of magnitude faster than the time scale of temperature effects. This disparity in time rates is utilized by the low-pass filter temperature readout circuit used in this test method. The circuit employed is illustrated in Fig. 6. A low-pass filter circuit will block the high frequency component of a signal and respond to the near-DC component representing the temperature-driven voltage increase.

14.3.9 The filter circuit is housed in a grounded metal box and joints are sealed with conductive tape. A 75 Ohm coaxial cable of carries the thermocouple signal from the MRI to the electronic box in an adjacent room.

14.4 *Calibration Procedure*:

14.4.1 Calibration of the temperature readout circuit is conducted by placing the sensor thermocouple in an insulated

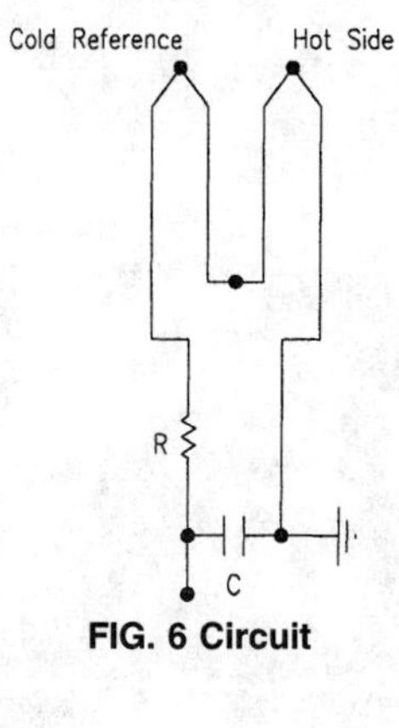

FIG. 6 Circuit

container of warm water and immersing the reference thermocouple in an insulated container filled with an ice-water mixture. Water temperatures are measured independently using a reliable device such as a "T" (copper-constant) thermocouple, an Omega Engineering model 661 temperature readout with electronic cold reference, or a glass immersion thermometer. An accuracy of ± 1°C with a resolution of approximately 0.5°C to temperature difference is required.

14.4.2 Repeat the calibration sequence with the apparatus placed in the MRI along with a phantom. The device is oriented horizontally. Allow the system to come to equilibrium.

14.4.3 Operate the MRI under prescan conditions to insure that the equilibrium temperature remains unchanged for a period of at least 90 s. When output readings coincide with the power-on period of the MRI, a high transient reading occurs, however, the baseline readings should remain otherwise unchanged throughout the test.

14.4.4 The calibration indicates that temperatures at the threshold of physiological damage from prolonged exposure can be readily sensed by the apparatus under separating conditions of the MRI.

14.5 *Test Procedure*— Image the device using MRI parameters that produce a duty cycle (long term average) of approximately 40 % peak power for a period of 20 min in a minimum 1.5 Tesla imaging system. One possible sequence is a fast spin echo or spin echo with Tr=100, Te=20, 4 echoes and 94 NEX. Power levels should exceed maximum levels commonly used in clinically relevant practice.

14.6 *Interpretation of Results*:

14.6.1 Equilibrium temperature should remain unchanged for the duration of the test. Any device for which the temperature do not increase by more than 2° Celsius shall have passed the test.

14.6.2 Any test during which the temperature readings vary more than 2° C shall have failed the test.

15. Optional Test Method for Clinical Evaluation of MR Compatibility of Halo External Fixators or Cranial Traction Tongs

15.1 *Scope*—This test method covers the clinical observation of the cervical spine anatomy after MR testing in halo external fixators and cranial traction tongs. This test demonstrates the diagnostic quality of images from a magnetic resonance imaging machine.

15.1.1 *Summary of Test Method*—Through a clinically relevant imaging technique used on a patient simulating wearing a test device, coronal and sagittal cervical images are taken to evaluate the diagnostic quality of the resulting images.

15.1.2 *Significance and Use*—For safety reasons the device shall be able to withstand the maximum voltage typically used during normal clinical applications or as outlined by the manufacturer in the product instruction manual without excessive current generation or imaging artifact.

15.2 The test shall be conducted on an adult subject and the device shall consist of the size best suited to the test subject.

15.3 *Procedure*:

15.3.1 Place the subject wearing the test device in the MR machine.

15.3.2 Image the subject using any standard diagnostic

technique utilizing power levels similar to maximum levels commonly used in clinically relevant practice.

15.4 *Interpretation of Results*:

15.4.1 Any device demonstrating coronal and sagittal images free from significant artifact shall have passed the test.

15.4.2 Any device demonstrating coronal and sagittal images indicating significant artifact shall have failed the test.

16. Keywords

16.1 cranial traction tongs; halo external fixation device; magnetic resonance imaging (MRI) compatibility

Standard Specification for Rigid Polyurethane Foam for Use as a Standard Material for Testing Orthopaedic Devices and Instruments[1]

This standard is issued under the fixed designation F 1839; the number immediately following the designation indicates the year of original adoption or, in the case of revision, the year of last revision. A number in parentheses indicates the year of last reapproval. A superscript epsilon (ε) indicates an editorial change since the last revision or reapproval.

1. Scope

1.1 This specification covers rigid unicellular polyurethane foam for use as a standard material for performing mechanical tests utilizing orthopaedic devices or instruments. The specification is applicable to sheets or blocks of foam, or foam that is made by the user using a two-part liquid mixture.

1.2 This specification covers polyurethane foam material that is used in the laboratory for mechanical testing, as described in 1.1. These materials are not intended for implantation into the human body.

1.3 The foam described herein possesses mechanical properties which are on the order of those reported for human cancellous bone. See Appendix X1 Rationale for further information regarding the appropriateness of using the specified foam as a model for human cancellous bone.

1.4 This specification covers compositional requirements, physical requirements, mechanical requirements, and test methods for rigid polyurethane foam in the solid final form.

1.5 This specification provides qualification criteria for vendor or end-user processes and acceptance criteria for individual material lots.

1.6 This specification provides mechanical properties of five different grades of foam in the solid final form.[2] A foam that does not meet the specified mechanical properties shall be identified as an ungraded foam.

1.7 Unless otherwise indicated, the values stated in SI units are to be regarded as standard. The values in parentheses are given for information only.

1.8 The following precautionary statement pertains to the test method portion only, Section 8, of this specification: *This standard does not purport to address all of the safety concerns, if any, associated with its use. It is the responsibility of the user of this standard to establish appropriate safety and health practices and determine the applicability of regulatory limitations prior to use.*

2. Referenced Documents

2.1 *ASTM Standards:*

C 273 Test Method for Shear Test in Flatwise Plane of Flat Sandwich Constructions or Sandwich Cores[3]

D 1621 Test Method for Compressive Properties of Rigid Cellular Plastics[4]

D 1622 Test Method for Apparent Density of Rigid Cellular Plastics[4]

E 4 Practices for Load Verification of Testing Machines[5]

F 117 Test Method for Driving Torque of Medical Bone Screws[6]

F 1691 Test Method for Determining the Axial Pullout of Medical Bone Screws[6]

2.2 *ISO Standards:*

5835-1 Implants for Surgery - Metal Bone Screws with Hexagonal Driver Connection, Spherical Under Surface of Head, Asymmetrical Thread - Dimensions[7]

3. Terminology

3.1 *Definitions:*

3.1.1 *final form*—the condition of the foam product when used by the end-user to perform tests of orthopaedic devices or instruments. The condition of the foam product of which all physical and mechanical tests required by this specification are performed.

3.1.1.1 *solid*—the foam is in a uniform solid form, such as a slab, plate or block.

3.1.2 *foam rise direction*—the nominal direction that the foam rises during the polymerization ("foaming") process, either at the suppliers production facilities for the solid supplied foam, or at the end-users facilities for foam produced from the liquid supplied form. The foam rise direction shall be marked on the foam block or indicated in the shipping documentation for foam that is supplied in the Solid form.

3.1.3 *grades*—The grade designation refers to the nominal density of the foam, in its Solid Final form, expressed in units of kg/m^3 (lbm/ft^3). Five grades of foam have been defined in this specification. Their nominal densities are given below:

---

[1] This test method is under the jurisdiction of ASTM Committee F-04 on Medical and Surgical Materials and Devices and is the direct responsibility of Subcommittee F04.21 on Osteosynthesis.

Current edition approved Dec. 10, 1997. Published May 1998.

[2] General Plastics Manufacturing Company, 4910 Burlington Way, Tacoma Washington, 98409, producers of Last-a-Foam® polyurethane foam, has been found to be a satisfactory supplier of this material. Other manufacturers of rigid polyurethane foam may also be available.

[3] *Annual Book of ASTM Standards*, Vol 15.03.

[4] *Annual Book of ASTM Standards*, Vol 08.01.

[5] *Annual Book of ASTM Standards*, Vol 03.01.

[6] *Annual Book of ASTM Standards*, Vol 13.01.

[7] Available from American National Standards Institute, 11 W. 42nd St., New York, NY 10036.

Grade 10:	160.2 kg/m^3(10.0 lbm/ft^3)
Grade 12:	192.2 kg/m^3(12.0 lbm/ft^3)
Grade 15:	240.3 kg/m^3(15.0 lbm/ft^3)
Grade 20:	320.4 kg/m^3(20.0 lbm/ft^3)
Grade 40:	640.7 kg/m^3(40.0 lbm/ft^3)

3.1.4 *supplied form*—the condition of the foam product when received from the supplier by the end-user.

3.1.4.1 *solid*—the foam is in a uniform solid form, such as a slab, plate or block.

3.1.4.2 *liquid*—two liquid components (base and activator) that can be mixed by the end-user to produce a rigid, unicellular foam slab.

3.1.5 *ungraded*—foam which does not fit into one of the five grades specified in 3.1, due to the foam not meeting one or more of the physical or mechanical requirements of Section 4.

4. Physical and Mechanical Requirements

4.1 *Composition*—The material shall be supplied either in solid or liquid form. The solid or combined liquid parts shall produce a foam consisting of polyether polyurethane.

4.2 *Appearance*:

4.2.1 *Solid Supplied Form*—The solid foam slab shall be free of obvious extraneous matter, and appear to the unaided eye to be uniform throughout the slab in color and porosity.

4.2.2 *Liquid Supplied Form*—The two liquid components shall appear to the unaided eye throughout its volume to be uniform and free from obvious extraneous matter or particulate debris.

4.2.3 *Solid Final Form*—The solid foam slab shall be free of obvious extraneous matter, and appear to the unaided eye to be uniform throughout the slab in color and porosity.

4.3 *Void Content*—The material in the Solid Final Form shall meet the requirements of Table 1 for voids, cracks and nonuniform areas, when examined using the procedures described in 8.1. All specimens shall meet this requirement.

TABLE 1 Requirements for Voids, Cracks and Nonuniform Areas

Defects	Requirements
Voids	
Void Depth (measured perpendicular to slab's transverse plane.)	Void depth shall be less than 50 % of the slab thickness, and less than 6.35 mm (0.250 inch)
Void Diameter (measured parallel to slab's transverse plane.)	
Larger than 6.35 mm (0.250 inch)	None allowed in any grade
Between 3.18 mm (0.125 inch) and 6.35 mm (0.250 inch)	No more than 1 allowed per 230 cm^2(36 in^2) surface area for grades 10, 12 and 15. None allowed in grades 20 and 40.
Between 1.57 mm (0.062 inch) and 3.18 mm (0.125 inch)	No more than 6 allowed per 230 cm^2(36 in^2) surface area for grades 10, 12 and 15. No more than 3 allowed in grades 20 and 40.
Cracks	None allowed
Nonuniform areas	Concentrated areas of poor construction, irregular cells, and hard and soft spots shall not exceed 10 % of the visible surface area

4.4 *Density*—The material in the solid final form shall have a density within the ranges specified in Table 2, according to the foam's grade specification. The density shall be determined using the method described in 8.2. All specimens shall meet this requirement.

4.5 *Dimensional Stability*—The material in the solid final form shall have an average percentage thickness of change less than 1.0 %, when tested according to the method described in 8.3.

4.6 *Compressive Strength*—The material in the solid final form shall meet the compressive strength requirements given in Table 3, when tested according to the method described in 8.4. All specimens shall meet this requirement. The values in Table 3 are stated at ± 16.0 kg/m^3 (± 1.0 lbm/ft^3) around each grade's nominal density.

4.7 *Compressive Modulus*—The material in the solid final form shall meet the compressive modulus requirements given in Table 4, when tested according to the method described in 8.4. All specimens shall meet this requirement. The values in Table 4 are stated at ± 16.0 kg/m^3 (± 1.0 lbm/ft^3) around each grade's nominal density.

4.8 *Shear Strength*—The material in the solid final form shall meet the shear strength requirements given in Table 5, when tested according to the method described in 8.5. All specimens shall meet this requirement. The values in Table 5 are stated at ± 16.0 kg/m^3 (± 1.0 lbm/ft^3) around each grade's nominal density.

4.9 *Shear Modulus*—The material in the solid final form shall meet the shear modulus requirements given in Table 6, when tested according to the method described in 8.5. All specimens shall meet this requirement. The values in Table 6 are stated at ± 16.0 kg/m^3 (± 1.0 lbm/ft^3) around each grade's nominal density.

4.10 *Screw Pullout*—The material in the solid final form shall meet the screw pullout requirements given in Table 7, when tested according to the method described in 8.6. All specimens shall meet this requirement.

5. Significance and Use

5.1 This standard describes the compositional requirements, physical requirements, mechanical requirements, and test methods for rigid unicellular polyurethane foam for use in testing orthopaedic devices or instruments.

5.2 This foam described in this standard is not intended to replicate the mechanical properties of human or animal bone. The requirements of this standard are intended to provide a consistent and uniform material with properties on the order of human cancellous bone to use as a test medium when testing various orthopaedic devices, such as bone screws.

6. Apparatus

6.1 *Analytical Balance or Scale*—capable of weighing foam

TABLE 2 Grade Designation and Density

Grade	Minimum Density kg/m^3(lbm/ft^3)	Maximum Density kg/m^3(lbm/ft^3)
10	144.2 (9.0)	176.2 (11.0)
12	176.2 (11.0)	208.2 (13.0)
15	224.3 (14.0)	256.3 (16.0)
20	304.4 (19.0)	336.4 (21.0)
40	624.7 (39.0)	656.8 (41.0)

TABLE 3 Requirements for Compressive Strength

Grade	Minimum Compressive Strength, kPa (psi)		Maximum Compressive Strength, kPa (psi)	
10	2095	(304)	2895	(420)
12	2895	(420)	3790	(550)
15	4280	(620)	5315	(770)
20	7000	(1015)	8245	(1195)
40	22 410	(3250)	24 300	(3525)

TABLE 4 Requirements for Compressive Modulus

Grade	Minimum Compressive Modulus, kPa (psi)		Maximum Compressive Modulus, kPa (psi)	
10	56 300	(8165)	76 700	(11 125)
12	76 700	(11 125)	99 200	(14 390)
15	111 200	(16 130)	136 650	(19 820)
20	178 100	(25 830)	207 800	(30 140)
40	539 600	(78 260)	582 800	(84 530)

TABLE 5 Requirements for Shear Strength

Grade	Minimum Shear Strength, kPa (psi)		Maximum Shear Strength, kPa (psi)	
10	1650	(240)	2170	(315)
12	2170	(315)	2725	(395)
15	3000	(435)	3620	(525)
20	4590	(665)	5275	(765)
40	12 340	(1790)	13 240	(1920)

TABLE 6 Requirements for Shear Modulus

Grade	Minimum Shear Modulus, kPa (psi)		Maximum Shear Modulus, kPa (psi)	
10	20 820	(3020)	27 680	(4015)
12	27 680	(4015)	35 100	(5090)
15	39 000	(5655)	47 130	(6835)
20	60 160	(8725)	69 400	(10 060)
40	167 170	(24 245)	179 470	(26 030)

TABLE 7 Requirements for Screw Pullout

Grade	Minimum Pullout, *N* (lb)		Maximum Pullout, *N* (lb)	
10	335	(75)	415	(95)
12	400	(90)	545	(125)
15	485	(110)	675	(150)
20	670	(150)	800	(180)
40	2455	(550)	2755	(620)

specimens to the nearest ± 0.1 %.

6.2 *Micrometer Dial Gage or Caliper*—capable of measuring dimensions of the foam specimens to ± 0.1 %.

6.3 *Conditioning Oven*—Forced-air circulating oven capable of maintaining 121 ± 2.8° C (250 ± 5°F) for 24 h.

6.4 *Desiccator*—containing desiccant with high affinity for water vapor (anhydrous calcium chloride or equivalent).

6.5 *Vacuum*—capable of applying a vacuum pressure of 508 mm (20 in.) of mercury to foam specimen for dimensional stability test.

6.6 A testing machine and load cell conforming to Practices E 4, and capable of applying tensile and compressive loads at a constant displacement rate.

7. Sampling and Test Specimens

7.1 The number of test specimens and the specimen sizes required for physical characterization and mechanical testing are described in 8.1-8.6. Test specimens are required for each grade and formulation.

7.2 Test specimens shall be solid foam blocks. The short-transverse direction of the specimens shall coincide with the foam rise direction of the original foam bun.

8. Procedure

8.1 *Determination of Void Content*:

8.1.1 Use the foam block specimens described and specified in 8.2-8.6.

8.1.2 Examine all of the surfaces and edges of test specimens for voids and nonuniform areas with the unaided eye. Measure the dimensions of the void or nonuniform areas using an instrument capable of measuring ± 0.025 mm (0.001 inch).

8.2 *Determination of Foam Density*:

8.2.1 Prepare three specimens, 25.4 by 25.4 by 25.4 mm (1 by 1 by 1 in.) from solid foam.

8.2.2 Determine the apparent density of the three foam specimens, in kg/m^3 (lbm/ft^3), in accordance with Test Method D 1622.

8.2.3 Calculate the average apparent density of the three foam specimens.

8.3 *Determination of Dimensional Stability*:

8.3.1 Prepare three specimens, 25.4 by 25.4 by 12.7 mm (1 by 1 by 0.5 in.) from solid foam.

8.3.2 Condition the specimen for 24 h at 21 ± 2.8° C (70 ± 5° F) and 50 ± 10 % relative humidity. Measure the specimen thickness near the center of the length to ± 0.025 mm (0.001 in.) and mark the location of the measurement.

8.3.3 Place the specimen on a 6.35 mm (0.25 in.) thick aluminum plate and apply a minimum vacuum pressure of 508 mm (20 in.) of mercury under a vacuum bag or diaphragm. Place this assembly in a circulating forced-air oven for 2 h minimum at 121 ± 2.8° C (250 ± 5° F). Remove the assembly and allow to cool to 49° C (120° F) or less while maintaining the vacuum.

8.3.4 Recondition and remeasure the thickness at the marked location in accordance with 8.3.2. Calculate the percent thickness change.

8.3.5 Calculate the average percent thickness change of the three specimens.

8.4 *Determination of Compressive Strength and Modulus*:

8.4.1 Prepare five specimens, 50.8 by 50.8 by 25.4 mm (2 by 2 by 1 in.), from solid foam, with the thickness of the specimen parallel to the foam rise direction. Measure the dimensions within ± 0.025 mm (± 0.001 in.). The specimens shall be conditioned at 24 ± 2.8° C (75 ± 5° F) for 3 h prior to testing.

8.4.2 Test in accordance with Test Method D 1621 at 24 ± 2.8° C (75 ± 5° F). The specimens shall be oriented such that the axis of the compressive load is applied parallel to the foam rise direction.

8.4.3 Determine the compressive strength using Procedure A of Test Method D 1621 and the maximum compressive modulus for each specimen.

8.4.4 Calculate the average compressive strength and modulus of the five specimens.

8.5 *Determination of Shear Strength and Modulus*:

8.5.1 Prepare five specimens, 76.2 by 25.4 by 6.35 mm (3

by 1 by 0.25 in.), from solid foam, with the thickness of the specimen parallel to the Foam Rise Direction. Measure the dimensions within ±0.025 mm (±0.001 inch). The specimens shall be conditioned at 24 ± 2.8° C (75 ± 5° F) for 3 hours prior to testing.

8.5.2 Bond the edges of the foam specimen directly to the shear plates with an appropriate adhesive, such as an epoxy, so that the Foam Rise Direction is perpendicular to the plane of maximum shear stress.

8.5.3 Test in accordance with Test Method C 273.

8.5.4 Determine the shear strength and shear modulus for each specimen.

8.5.5 Calculate the average shear strength and modulus of the five specimens.

8.6 *Determination of Screw Pullout Strength*

8.6.1 Prepare five specimens, 50.8 by 50.8 by 25.4 mm (2 by 2 by 1 in.), from solid foam, with the thickness of the specimen parallel to the foam rise direction.

8.6.2 Obtain five steel screws or threaded tools that meet the thread requirements given in ISO 5835-1. Grades 10, 12, and 15 shall utilize screws or threaded tools with the thread form of HB 6.5 screws (see Table 4 of ISO 5835-1), while Grades 20 and 40 shall utilize screws or threaded tools with the thread form of HA 4.5 screws (see Table 2 of ISO 5835-1).

8.6.3 Drill a 3.2 mm (0.126 in.) hole in the center of each foam specimen, parallel to the thickness direction. The hole shall be positioned a minimum of 10 mm (0.394 in.) from any void or nonuniform area. Tap the hole to a minimum depth of 25.4 mm (1 in.) using a tap that corresponds to HB 6.5 or HA 4.5, as appropriate.

8.6.4 Insert the screw or threaded tool into each foam specimen to a depth of 20 mm (0.787 in.).

8.6.5 Test in accordance with Test Method F 1691.

8.6.6 Determine the maximum force, in Newtons, required to remove the screw or threaded tool from the foam specimen.

8.6.7 Calculate the average pullout force for the five specimens.

9. Report

9.1 Include the following information in the test report of the mechanical properties of the foam:

9.1.1 The lot number, specified grade (if applicable), manufacturer, and date of manufacture of the foam or two-part liquid mixture.

9.1.2 For liquid supplied foams the report shall include the following:

9.1.2.1 Mixing ratio of the two liquid parts (expressed as a ratio of the base and activator based on either weight or volume).

9.1.2.2 Mixing and casting technique (for example, rate of stirring, pressurization, etc.).

9.1.2.3 Ambient temperature and humidity during mixing and casting.

9.1.2.4 Any other parameters which may affect the quality of the polyurethane foam in the solid final form.

9.1.3 Any test results that did not meet the requirements of Section 4.

9.1.4 The average and standard deviation of the foam density as determined in 8.2.

9.1.5 The average and standard deviation of the percent thickness change as determined in 8.3.

9.1.6 The average and standard deviation of the compressive strength and modulus as determined in 8.4.

9.1.7 The average and standard deviation of the shear strength and modulus as determined in 8.5.

9.1.8 The average and standard deviation of the screw or threaded tool pullout force as determined in 8.6.

10. Qualification and Acceptance Criteria

10.1 *Qualification Criteria*:

10.1.1 *Solid Supplied Form*—A supplier of foam in the solid supplied form shall demonstrate that its production process (for a lot of material in a particular grade) results in foam that meets all of the physical and mechanical requirements of Section 4, by providing a report described in Section 9. Once the supplier has demonstrated this, the supplier is qualified for that particular grade. Provided there are no changes made to the production process for the qualified grade, subsequent lots of material of the qualified grade are only required to meet the acceptance criteria described in 10.2.

10.1.2 *Liquid Supplied Form*—The end user of the foam provided in the liquid supplied form shall demonstrate that the solid final form produced meet all of the physical and mechanical requirements of Section 4, by providing a report described in Section 9. Once the end-user has demonstrated this, the user is qualified for that particular grade. Provided there are no changes made to the production process for the qualified grade (mixing ratio, humidity, temperature, mixing and pouring technique, etc.) subsequent lots of material of the qualified grade are only required to meet the acceptance criteria described in 10.2.

10.2 *Acceptance Criteria*—Provided the grade of foam is qualified according to the criteria described in 10.1, a lot of foam material is accepted as meeting the requirements of this standard provided the requirements of 10.2.2 and 10.2.3 are met, and reported in a manner consistent with 9.1.1-9.1.4 and 9.1.8.

10.2.1 *Test Specimens*—Five specimens, 50.8 by 50.8 by 25.4 mm (2 by 2 by 1 in.), as specified in 4.10, shall be used for the acceptance examination and testing.

10.2.2 *Physical Requirements*:

10.2.2.1 *Composition*—See 4.1,

10.2.2.2 *Appearance*—See 4.2.3,

10.2.2.3 *Void Content*—See 4.3, and

10.2.2.4 *Density*—See 4.4.

10.2.3 *Screw Pullout*—See 4.10.

11. Storage

11.1 The solid foam should be stored in a cool dry place between uses, and protected from exposure to light, especially direct sunlight. Exposure to ultraviolet light for an extended period of time may degrade the outer surface of the foam.

11.2 The supplier is responsible for storage of the solid foam until the time-of-delivery. Therefore, the supplier is responsible for ensuring that the requirements of this specification are met at time-of-delivery for any foam that had previously met the acceptance criteria of 10.2.

11.3 The end-user is responsible for storage of the solid

foam after delivery and until the time-of-use. Therefore, the end-user is responsible for ensuring that the requirements of this specification are met at time-of-use for any foam which had previously met the acceptance criteria of 10.2.

12. Precision and Bias

12.1 No information is presented about either the precision or bias of this test method for evaluating appearance or void content since these test results are nonquantitative.

12.2 The precision and bias of this test method for measuring Density are essentially as specified in Test Method D 1622.

12.3 Data establishing the precision and accuracy to be expected from this test method for determining dimensional stability have not yet been obtained.

12.4 The precision and bias of this test method for measuring compressive strength and compressive modulus are essentially as specified in Test Method D 1621.

12.5 The precision and bias of this test method for measuring shear strength and shear modulus are essentially as specified in Test Method C 273.

12.6 The precision and bias of this test method for measuring Screw Pullout are essentially as specified in Test Method F 1691.

13. Keywords

13.1 bone; cellular plastic; medical devices; polyurethane; rigid foam

APPENDIX

(Nonmandatory Information)

X1. RATIONALE

X1.1 This specification provides compositional, physical, and mechanical requirements for rigid polyurethane foam. These requirements ensure a consistent and uniform material that may be used as a test medium when testing various medical devices. These rigid polyurethane foam materials are not intended for implantation into the human body.

X1.2 Researchers have found that certain densities of rigid polyurethane foam exhibit similar closed-cell structure as human cancellous bone, and possess mechanical properties that are also in the range of those of human cancellous bone **(1-4)**[8]. The uniformity and consistent properties of rigid polyurethane foam make it an ideal material for comparative testing of bone screws and other medical devices and instruments **(5-7)**.

X1.3 The original purpose of this standard was to provide a consistent and uniform material for incorporation into the revision of Test Method F 117 for use as a standard medium for testing the driving torque of medical bone screws. Future applications may include: standard material for pullout tests of medical bone screws, standard material for measuring cutting diameter of intramedullary reamers, and standard material for measuring the cutting performance of medical drills.

X1.4 The mechanical properties of the foam that may be important for standardization or for comparison to human cancellous bone will likely depend on the particular test method that is being developed. It is suggested that a test method that references this specification foam material should also address the relative importance of the different mechanical properties of the foam and suggest foam grades which may provide similar performance as human cancellous bone.

X1.5 This specification provides five grades (densities) of rigid polyurethane foam to provide a range of mechanical properties. It also provides that the foam may be supplied either in a solid form, or as a two-part liquid that is mixed together by the end-user to produce a solid foam.

[8] The boldface numbers given in parentheses refer to a list of references at the end of the text.

REFERENCES

(**1**) Szivek, J.A., Thomas, M., and Benjamin, J.B., "Technical Note - Characterization of a Synthetic Foam as a Model for Human Cancellous Bone," *Journal of Applied Biomaterials*, Vol 4, 1993, pp. 269-272.

(**2**) Hein, T.J., Hotchkiss, R., Perissinotto, A., and Chao, E.Y.S., "Analysis of Bone Model Material for External Fracture Fixation Experiments," *Journal of Biomechanical Instrumentation*, Vol 22, 1987, pp. 43-48.

(**3**) Thompson, J.D., Szivek, J.A., and Benjamin, J.B., "Characterization of a Series of Closed Cell Foams to Simulate Trabecular Bone from Different Patient Populations," Presented at Society for Biomaterials 20th Annual Meeting, Boston, MA, April 5-9, 1994.

(**4**) Szivek, J.A., Thompson, J.D., and Benjamin, J.B., "Characterization of Three Formulations of a Synthetic Foam as Models for a Range of Human Cancellous Bone Types," *Journal of Applied Biomaterials*, Vol 6, 1995, pp. 125-128.

(**5**) Lee, R.W., Volz, R.G., and Sheridan, D.C., "The Role of Fixation and Bone Quality on the Stability of Tibial Knee Components," *Clinical Orthopaedics*, Vol 273, 1991, pp. 177-183.

(**6**) Chapman, J.R., Harrington, R.M., Lee, K.M., Anderson, P.A., Tencer, A.F., and Kowalski, D., "Factors Affecting the Pullout Strength of Cancellous Bone Screws," *Journal of Biomechanical Engineering*, Vol 118, 1996, pp. 391-398.

(**7**) Dawson, J.D., McNamara, M.J., Weld, K.J., and Spengler, D.M., "Effect of Crosslinking on Pedicle Screw Pull-Out Strength," Presented at American Academy of Orthopaedic Surgeons 61st Annual Meeting, New Orleans, LA, February 24-March 1, 1994.

Standard Terminology for Surgical Suture Needles[1]

This standard is issued under the fixed designation F 1840; the number immediately following the designation indicates the year of original adoption or, in the case of revision, the year of last revision. A number in parentheses indicates the year of last reapproval. A superscript epsilon (ε) indicates an editorial change since the last revision or reapproval.

1. Scope

1.1 This terminology covers general definitions for surgical needles.

2. Terminology

2.1 *Definitions of Terms Specific to the Instrument* (See Fig. 1):

attachment area, *n*—portion of the needle where the attachment of the suture takes place. For example, eyed, drilled, and channel.

body, *n*—central portion of the needle intended to be grasped by the needle holder.

chord length, *n*—the straight line distance between the two ends of a curved needle.

curvature, *n*—the shape of the needle viewed in profile. Some common shapes include, but are not limited to: straight, ½ curve or "ski", ⅛ circle, ¼ circle, ⅜ circle, ½ circle, ⅝ circle, and compound curvature (see Fig. 3).

cutting egde,, *n*—cutting edges are made of various goemetric shapes, that is, triangular, diamond, and hexagonal. The various edges may be sharpened by the manufacturer depending on the user performance.

needle length, *n*—the distance measured along the needle curvature from end to end.

needle radius, *n*—the radius of the uniformly curved portion or portions of the needle measured from the centerline of the needle body.

needle wire diameter, *n*—the gage or thickness of the needle wire, measured at a location between the needle body and the attachment area, where either no or minimal work has taken place.

point, *n*—portion of the needle intended to initiate tissue penetration.

point configuration, *n*—the shape of the point. Some common point configurations include, but are not limited to (see Fig. 2): taper, trocar, blunt, spatulated, conventional cutting edge, reverse cutting edge, cutting taper, and side cutting needle.

swage, *n*—the term used to describe any attachment method that uses mechanical force to crimp the end of the needle and firmly hold the suture in place

2.2 *Definitions of Terms Specific to Mechanical Properties of a Surgical Needle:*

bright or mirror finish—highly reflective surface.

finish—the final surface visual appearance of a needle, that may be classified as follows:

maximum bend moment—the greatest moment applied to a needle during a bend test.

needle ducility—a measure of the amount of plastic bending a needle can withstand.

satin, matte, or black finish—a reduced reflective surface varying from a dull appearance to a blackened surface.

yield bend angle—the angle at which the yield bend moment occurs.

yield bend moment—the amount of moment required to initiate plastic deformation during a bend test.

3. Keywords

3.1 needle; stainless steel- surgical applications; surgical; suture needle

---

[1] This specification is under the jurisdiction of ASTM Committee F-4 on Medical and Surgical Materials and Devices and is the direct responsibility of Subcommittee F04.65 on Medical/Surgical Instruments.

Current edition approved October 10, 1998. Published March 1999. Originally published as F 1840 - 97. Last previous edition F 1840 - 98.

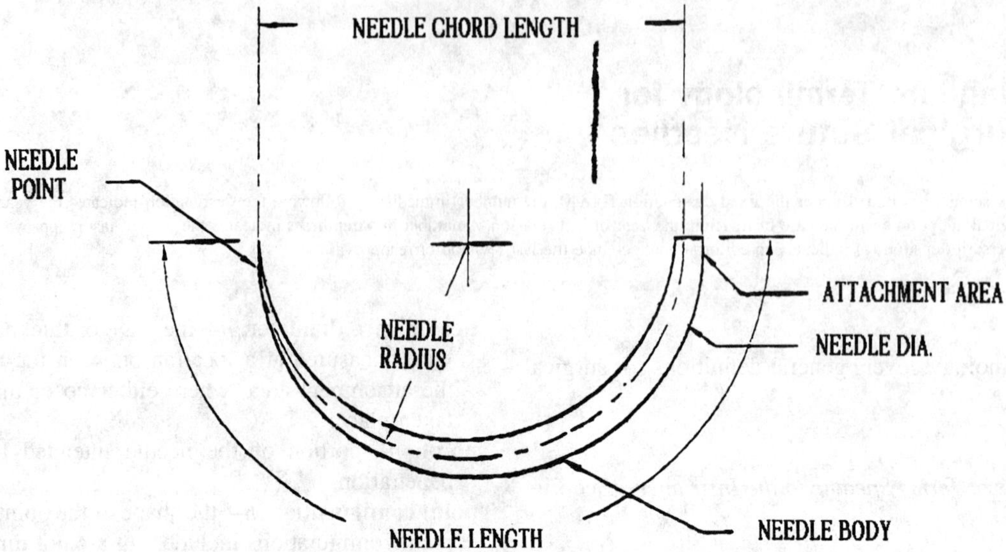

FIG. 1 Schematic of a Surgical Needle

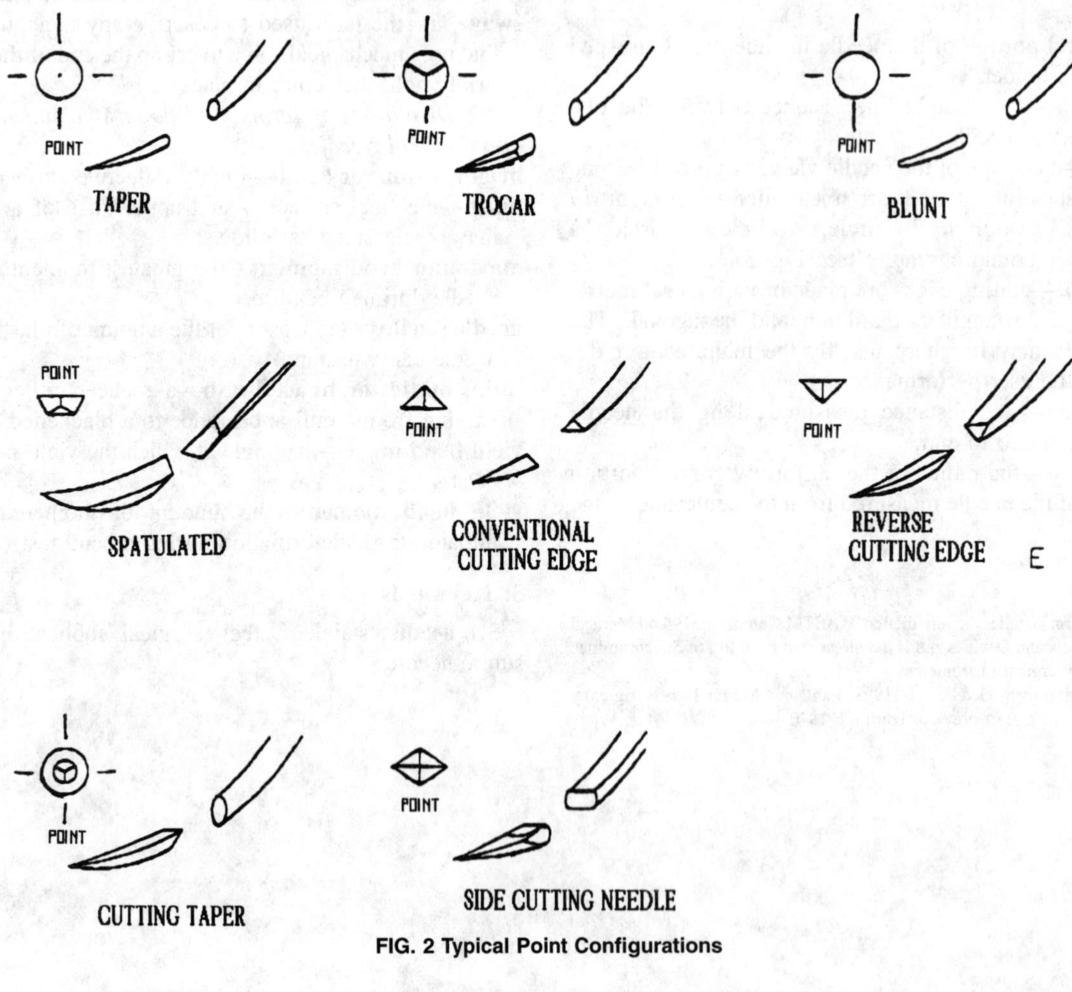

FIG. 2 Typical Point Configurations

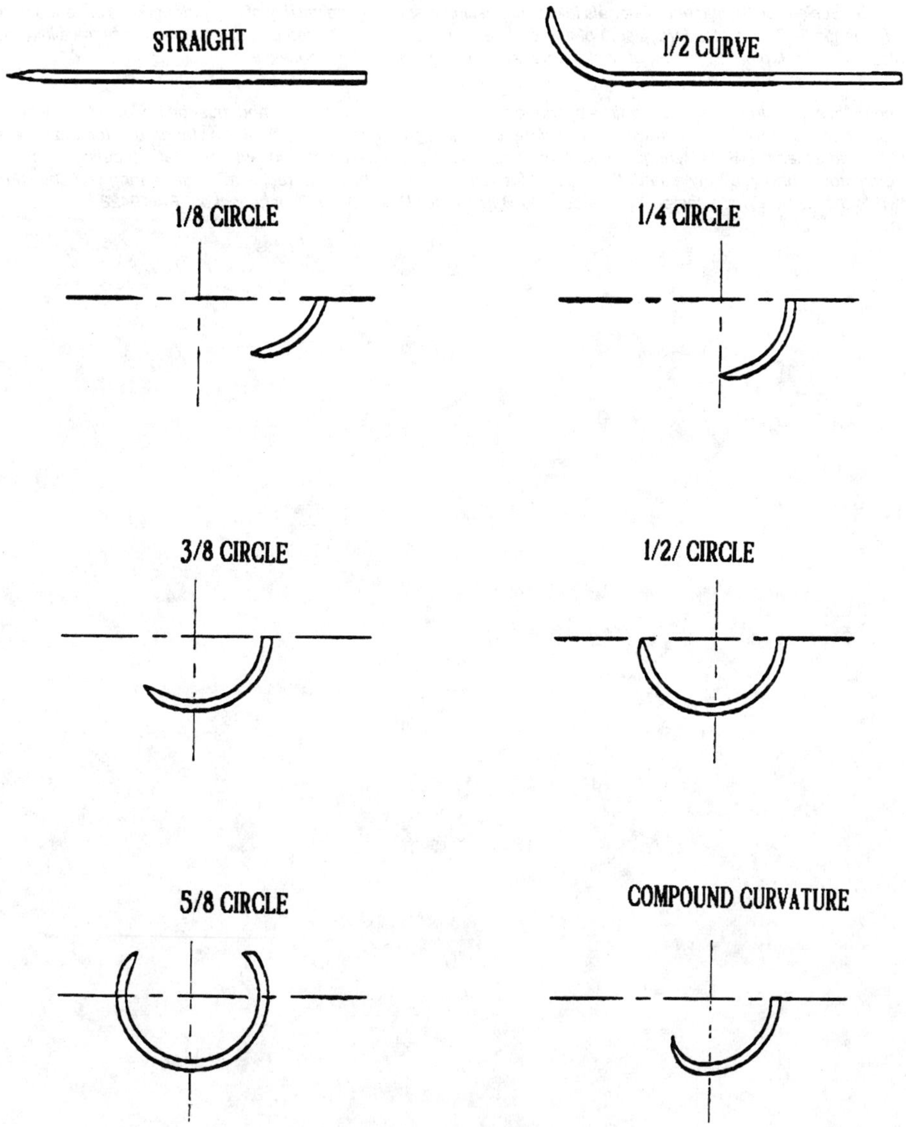

FIG. 3 Typical Curvatures

APPENDIX

(Nonmandatory Information)

X1. RATIONALE

X1.1 Because there is a clinical need for a variety of surgical suture needles for surgical procedures, they are manufactured in various configurations and from various materials. For practical purposes these devices supplied by different manufacturers necessitate a defined system of terms.

X1.2 The terms defined in this terminology are the most commonly used for surgical suture needles. However, the intent is not to prohibit technological innovation or to exclude surgical suture needles manufactured with other types of features.

Standard Practice for Assessment of Hemolysis in Continuous Flow Blood Pumps[1]

This standard is issued under the fixed designation F 1841; the number immediately following the designation indicates the year of original adoption or, in the case of revision, the year of last revision. A number in parentheses indicates the year of last reapproval. A superscript epsilon (ϵ) indicates an editorial change since the last revision or reapproval.

INTRODUCTION

The goal of blood pump development is to replace or supplement the function of the human heart. As a result, continuous flow blood pumps, including roller pumps and centrifugal pumps, are commonly used in clinical extracorporeal circulation. They are used not only for cardiopulmonary bypass in routine cardiac surgery but also for ventricular assist, percutaneous cardiopulmonary support, and extracorporeal membrane oxygenation.

Many investigators have attempted to develop an atraumatic blood pump. Hemolysis is one of the most important parameters of blood trauma induced by blood pumps. However, comparative in vitro evaluation of the reported results of hemolysis are difficult due to the lack of uniformity of the test methods employed. Thus, it is necessary to standardize the method of performing in vitro hemolysis tests for the evaluation of continuous flow blood pumps.

1. Scope

1.1 This recommended practice covers a protocol for the assessment of the hemolytic properties of continuous flow blood pumps used in extracorporeal or implantable circulatory assist. An assessment is made based on the pump's effects on the erythrocytes over a certain period of time. For this assessment, a recirculation test is performed with a pump for 6 h.

1.2 The values stated in both inch - pound and SI units are to be regarded as the standard. The SI units given in parentheses are for information only.

1.3 *This standard does not purport to address all of the safety concerns, if any, associated with its use. It is the responsibility of the user of this standard to establish appropriate safety and health practices and determine the applicability of regulatory limitations prior to use.*

2. Referenced Documents

2.1 *ASTM Standards:*

F 1830 Practice for Selection of Blood for In Vitro Evaluation of Blood Pumps[2]

3. Terminology

3.1 *Definitions:*

3.1.1 *continuous flow blood pump*—a blood pump that produces continuous blood flow due to its rotary motion.

3.1.2 *free plasma hemoglobin*—the amount of hemoglobin (iron or heme-containing protein) in plasma.

3.1.3 *hemolysis*—damage to erythrocytes resulting in the liberation of hemoglobin into the plasma.

3.1.4 *Index of Hemolysis*

3.1.4.1 *normalized index of hemolysis*—added grams of plasma free hemoglobin per 100 l of blood pumped, corrected for plasma volume using hematocrit and normalized by flow rate and circulation time.

3.1.4.2 *normalized milligram index of hemolysis*— normalized index of hemolysis expressed by milligram value of free plasma hemoglobin.

3.1.4.3 *modified index of hemolysis*—mass of hemoglobin released into plasma normalized by the total amount of hemoglobin pumped through the loop.

4. Formulas

4.1 *Normalized Index of Hemolysis (N.I.H.)* **(1,2,3,4)**[3]:

$$N.I.H.\ g/100l = \Delta freeHb \times V \times \frac{100 - Ht}{100} \times \frac{100}{Q \times T} \quad (1)$$

$\Delta free\ Hb$ = increase of plasma free hemoglobin concentration (g/L) over the sampling time interval,

where:

V = circuit volume (L),
Q = flow rate (L/min),

[1] This practice is under the jurisdiction of ASTM Committee F-4 on Medical and Surgical Materials and Devices and is the direct responsibility of Subcommittee F04.30 on Cardiovascular Standards.

Current edition approved Dec.10, 1997. Published June 1998.

[2] *Annual Book of ASTM Standards,* Vol 13.01.

[3] The boldface numbers given in parentheses refer to a list of references at the end of the text.

Ht = hematocrit (%), and
T = sampling time interval (min).

4.2 *Normalized Milligram Index of Hemolysis. (mg.N.I.H.)* **(2,3,4)**:

$$-mg.N.I.H.mg/100l = \Delta freeHb \times V \times \frac{100 - Ht}{100} \times \frac{100}{Q \times T} \quad (2)$$

4.3 *Modified Index of Hemolysis (M.I.H.)*:

4.3.1 Modified index of hemolysis (M.I.H.) **(5,6)** that can be written with no units or as (milligram of hemoglobin released into plasma/mg of total hemoglobin pumped through the loop):

$$M.I.H. = \Delta freeHb \times V \times \frac{100 - Ht}{100} \times \frac{10^6}{Q \times T \times Hb} \quad (3)$$

where:

Hb = total blood hemoglobin concentration at time zero (mg/L), and
$\Delta free\ Hb$ = increase of plasma free hemoglobin concentration (mg/L) over the sampling time interval.

4.3.2 Among these indices, M.I.H. is recommended as an index to express the degree of hemolysis caused by a blood pump in a recirculating system. N.I.H. was proposed to account for the plasma volume based on the hemotocrit. Recent development of less hemolytic blood pumps has since made it convenient to use mg. N.I.H. rather than N.I.H. However, both the N.I.H. and the mg N.I.H. vary with hematocrit of the blood **(6)**. M.I.H. is the recommended index to express the degree of hemolysis caused by a blood pump in a recirculating system. The M.I.H. equation corrects for differences in blood hemoglobin concentration and hematocrit directly **(5)**.

4.4 *Testing Blood*— Because the level of trauma-induced hemolysis is different based on the source of blood, it is necessary to identify the source of blood and its respective index of hemolysis. Human, bovine, or porcine blood are recommended as the primary sources of testing blood (see Practice F 1830). It is preferable that the blood collected at a standard slaughter house not be used due to the risk of being contaminated with fluids other than blood, unless the blood is obtained by controlled venipuncture. Although animal blood is used in the development stage of a pump, it is suggested that pre-clinical evaluation tests be repeated with human blood.

5. Summary of Practice

5.1 *Blood*—The blood is obtained from human volunteers, cattle or pigs having normal body temperatures, no physical signs of disease, including diarrhea or rhinorrhea, and an acceptable range of hemotological profiles. The blood should be collected by vascular puncture using a needle (14G or larger) and collected into the standard 500–2000 mL bags containing citrate phospate dextrose adenine (CPDA-1) anticoagulant solution (See Appendix X2) or heparin sulfate (See Appendix X3). The blood from a slaughterhouse can typically be used if it is obtained by controlled venipuncture.

5.2 *Test Loop* **(4)** *(See* Fig. 1*)*—The test loop consists of a total of 6.6 ft (2 m) of 3/8 in. (9.5 mm) ID polyvinylchloride tubing and a reservoir (typically, 13 by 13 cm) with a sampling port. The primed blood volume is 450 ± 45 mL. A screw clamp, that is positioned at the outlet side, is applied to produce the required conditions for the left heart assist application (5 L/min against 100 mm Hg pressure head (that is, with the pressure sampling ports at the same vertical height, the pressure in the outlet line of the pump is 100 mm Hg greater than in the inlet line)) and for the cardiopulmonary bypass application (5 L/min against 500 mm Hg pressure head). (Optional testing at 350 or 700 mm Hg is also advisable.) To monitor such pressure heads, the pressure monitoring lines are incorporated into the test loop both at the inlet and outlet tubes. An ultrasonic or electromagnetic flow probe is placed at the outlet side of the pump between the clamp and the reservoir to monitor the flow rate. A thermistor is connected to the loop, and the blood temperature is measured using a corresponding thermometer.

5.3 *Pump Conditions*— Pump flow rate is set at 5 ± 0.25 L/min at the circulating blood temperature of 37 ± 1°C. The total pressure head is set at 100 ± 3 mm Hg for the left heart assist application and 500 ± 15 mm Hg for cardiopulmonary bypass application. However, additional testing temperatures can be chosen from 0 to 42°C according to the intended clinical use of the pump (for example, cardiopulmonary bypass may include cooling and warming during surgery.)

5.4 *Evaluation*—The free plasma hemoglobin is determined by a clinically approved assay method (see 9.3). The free plasma hemoglobin is standardized by calculating the M.I.H.

6. Significance and Use

6.1 The objective of this practice is to standardize the evaluation method for detecting the hemolytic effect of a continuous flow blood pump used in extracorporeal circulation and circulatory assistance.

7. Preparation of Hemolysis Test

7.1 *Blood*—The blood is obtained from human volunteers having normal body temperature, exhibiting no physical signs of disease and having hematological profiles in the normal acceptable range. (Donors are subjected to standard blood donor screening procedures.) The donor should be fasted for 8 h or more to avoid additional hemolysis due to a high concentration of lipids in the blood. The delay in the collection of the blood and the hemolysis test should not exceed 48 h of refrigerated storage with the blood temperature kept between 2 and 8° C or more than 2 h at ambient condition. As an alternative source of blood, animal blood can be used, but it is necessary that the source of blood is identified. The preferred animal blood is bovine and porcine (See Practice F 1830). Since the use of completely fasted animals is impractical, it is recommended that the animals be subjected to a 12-h fasting. As a quality control measure, any blood having free plasma hemoglobin of more than 20 mg/dL should not be used for this test. In order to standardize the blood trauma testing, the blood subjected to the test should have the hematocrit value adjusted to be within the range 30 ± 2% by hemodilution (with phospate buffered saline) or hemoconcentration (via minimal centrifugation). Proper and acceptable ranges of the physiological blood parameters should be maintained prior to and during testing (for example, pH, base excess, glucose concentration).

7.2 *Test Loop (See* Fig. 1*)*—The closed test loop contains a total of 6.6 ft (2 m) of 3/8 in. (9.5 mm) ID polyvinylchloride

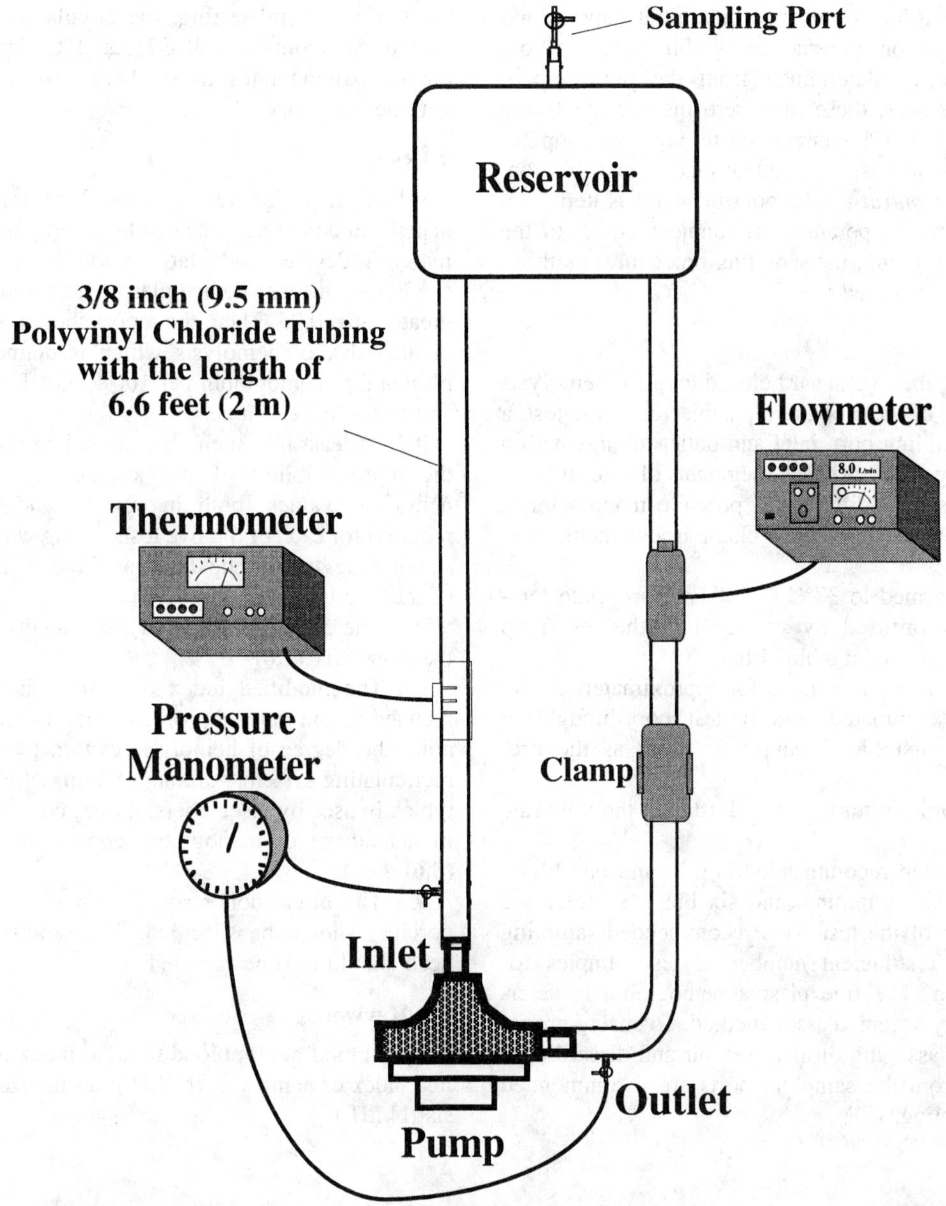

FIG. 1 Test Loop

tubing, a reservoir with a sampling port, an ultrasonic or electromagnetic flow probe and its corresponding flowmeter, a thermistor and its corresponding thermometer, and a blood pump. The loop should be filled with phosphate buffered saline that is recirculated for approximately 10 to 20 min to rinse and wet all of the blood-contacting surfaces. The phosphate buffered saline is drained completely from the loop prior to filling it with blood. After being washed with phosphate buffered saline, the circuit is primed with 450 ± 45 mL of fresh blood into the reservoir bag. Air collected in the reservoir should be eliminated and no air interface left in the reservoir. A screw clamp, that is applied to produce the required condition of pressure head, is positioned at the outlet side of the pump. The pressure monitoring lines are incorporated into the test loop both at the inlet and outlet tubes. An ultrasonic or electromagnetic flow probe is placed at the outlet side of the pump between the screw clamp and the reservoir to monitor the flow rate.

7.3 *Pump Conditions*— The flow meter should be calibrated using blood at the proper hematocrit and temperature. The pump revolution rate is adjusted to provide 5 ± 0.25 L/min flow rate as determined by the in-line flow meter, and all experiments are conducted at a 37 ± 1°C environment that is achieved through submerging portions of the loop into a water bath. However, additional tests conducted in temperatures ranging from 0 to 42°C can be performed according to the intended clinical use of the pump. Since all test runs are of a 6-h duration, sterility is generally considered not necessary.

7.4 *Evaluations*— Blood samples of 1 to 2 mL (preferably 1 mL) are drawn from the reservoir before pumping and at every hour of pumping. It would be preferable to withdraw at least two blood samples at each sample time. At each sampling, the first sample of 1 mL should be discarded because it may contain blood that was stagnant in the sampling port. The second sampling of 1 mL should be used for measurement of plasma free hemoglobin. If the saline is drained completely from the test loop prior to testing, the initial total blood hemoglobin concentration, plasma hemoglobin concentration, and hematocrit can be determined from the pre-pumping control blood. Preferably, these time zero measurements are obtained from blood that has circulated through the loop for approximately 5 min to ensure complete mixing and dilution.

7.5 *Static Blood Controls*—The control blood is kept in a blood bag at the same temperature environment as that of the testing blood. For sampling, the sampling procedures as those for testing blood are required (see 8.5).

8. Procedure

8.1 Figure 1 describes a standard closed loop for hemolysis testing, that consists of the blood pump subjected to the test, a reservoir with a sampling port, inlet and outlet tubings with a pressure monitoring port at each segment of the tubing, pressure transducers or a differencial pressure manometer, a thermistor, and a flow probe. A screw clamp is also included in this figure.

8.2 The blood warmed to 37°C (or other appropriate temperature) should be infused by gravity into the test loop through a sampling port of the blood bag.

8.3 After the test loop is operated for approximately 5 min and air bubbles are eliminated from the test loop through the sampling port, the first blood sample is taken as the pre-pumping control.

8.4 The blood pump is started and adjusted at the flow rate of 5 ± 0.25 L/min.

8.5 The test duration recommended is 6 h, and one blood sample is taken before pumping, and six blood samples are taken at every hour of the test. This recommended sampling schedule provides a sufficient number of test samples for statistical evaluation. The free plasma hemoglobin is determined by a clinically accepted assay method. To ensure proper samplings, gentle massaging of the reservoir and discarding 1 mL of the blood from the sampling ports are recommended prior to blood sampling.

8.6 For general testing, the circulating blood temperature should be maintained at 37° ± 1°C during the entire test duration, although testing at other appropriate use temperatures may be necessary.

9. Report

9.1 At first, the results should be reported as the time dependent hemolysis data displayed graphically for each of the five test devices and static blood controls. The regression coefficient of these device plasma hemoglobin plots should be greater than 0.95. Then, the report should be given in the form of an index of hemolysis which is defined as milligram of plasma free hemoglobin per 100 L blood pumped (mg N.I.H.) and as an M.I.H. value.

9.2 At least five such tests should be conducted to confirm the reproducibility of the tests. The individual index of hemolysis values (both mg N.I.H. and M.I.H.) should be reported for each of the five tests, along with the mean value ± standard deviation. The designated index should be the highest of the five tests.

9.3 The clinically accepted assay methods are referred to in the Appendix **(7,8)**.

9.4 The modified index of hemolysis (M.I.H.) is recommended as the most appropriate measurement index in evaluating the degree of hemolysis caused by a blood pump in a recirculating system. Although the mg NIH equation has been typically used by researchers, it does not correct for differences in hematocrit or hemoglobin content of the pumped blood **(5,6)**.

9.5 The blood donor source (for example human, bovine, porcine) should be specified. Test temperature and pressure head should also be reported.

10. Keywords

10.1 blood pump; blood trauma; index of hemolysis; modified index of hemolysis (M.I.H.); normalized index of hemolysis (N.I.H.)

APPENDIXES

(Nonmandatory Information)

X1. RATIONALE

X1.1 Even though blood trauma imposed on platelets and leukocytes by blood pumps should be studied, the hemolysis generated by a blood pump is the most significant blood trauma. Thus, this practice was generated.

X2. CITRATE PHOSPHATE DEXTROSE ADENINE (CPDA) SOLUTION USP

X2.1 A CPDAI solution USP of 63 mL is added for collection of 450 mL blood.

X2.2 Each 63 mL of CPDAI contains 2 g of dextrose (monohydrate) USP, 1.66 g sodium citrate (dihydrate) USP, 188 mg citric acid (anhydrous) USP, 140 mg monobasic sodium phosphate (monohydrate) USP, and 17.3 mg adenine USP.

X2.3 The pH of the solution may have been adjusted with sodium hydroxide.

X3. HEPARIN

X3.1 500 mL of blood containing 2000 to 3000 USP units of heparin is utilized.

X4. CLINICALLY ACCEPTED ASSAY METHODS (7,8)

X4.1 These are colorimetric assays, direct spectrophotometric assays, and, derivative spectrophotometric assays.

REFERENCES

(**1**) Allen J.G., *Extracorporeal Circulation*, Charles C Thomas, Springfield, IL, 1960.

(**2**) Keller T, Hawrylenko A., "Contribution to the In Vitro Testing of Pumps for Extracorporeal Circulation," *J Thoracic Cardiovasc Surg*, 1967;54:22-29.

(**3**) Naito K, Mizuguchi K, Nosè Y, The Need for Standardizing the Index of Hemolysis. *Artif Organs*, 1994, 18 pp.7-10.

(**4**) Noon G.P., Sekela M.E., Glueck J., Coleman C.L., Feldman L., "Comparison of Delphin and BioMedicus Pumps." *Trans Am Soc Artif Organs*, 1990;36: pp.616-619.

(**5**) Mueller MR, et al., "In Vitro Hematological Testing of Rotary Blood Pumps: Remarks on Standardization and Data Interpretation." *Artif Organs*, 1993; 17(2) pp.103-110.

(**6**) Mizuguchi K, Damm G.A., Aber G.S., et al. "Does Hematocrit Affect In Vitro Hemolysis Test Results-?" Preliminary study with Baylor/NASA prototype axial flow pump. *Artif Organs*, 1994;18(9) pp.650-656.

(**7**) Malinauskas R.A., "Plasma Hemoglobin Measurement Techniques for the In Vitro Evaluation of Blood Damage Caused by Medical Devices," *Artif Organs* Dec.1997 (in press).

(**8**) Fairbanks V.F., et al. "Methods for Measuring Plasma Hemoglobin in Micromolar Concentration Compared. *Clin Chem*, 1992;38 pp.132-140.

Designation: F 1846 – 98

Standard Practice for Symbols and Markings for Use With Land Search Maps[1]

This standard is issued under the fixed designation F 1846; the number immediately following the designation indicates the year of original adoption or, in the case of revision, the year of last revision. A number in parentheses indicates the year of last reapproval. A superscript epsilon (ϵ) indicates an editorial change since the last revision or reapproval.

1. Scope

1.1 This practice covers the symbols and markings to be used with land search maps to show resources, search coverage, status and results.

1.2 Operational usage of these symbols and markings, the resources they represent, and maps is not included in this practice.

1.3 *This standard does not purport to address all of the safety concerns, if any, associated with its use. It is the responsibility of the user of this standard to establish appropriate safety and health practices and determine the applicability of regulatory limitations prior to use.*

2. Referenced Documents

2.1 *Incident Command System Publications*:
Field Operations Guide ICS-420[2]

3. Terminology

3.1 *Definitions of Terms Specific to This Standard:*

3.1.1 *base map, n*—the master map or chart of the search area, normally maintained at the incident base or command post.

3.2 *base overlay, n*—the map overlay on which are placed the symbols and markings shown in Fig. 1 when it is desired to not mark on the base map.

3.3 *map overlay, n*—a transparent sheet placed over the base map on which markings and symbols are made. Overlays are used for symbols subject to change, to prevent marking the base map, or to avoid cluttering the base map.

4. Significance and Use

4.1 The base map and overlays are used in managing a search by graphically tracking progress, resource allocation and results. Standard symbols and markings allow a person to visually scan the map to obtain the status of the search without the need for a briefing or reading search documents.

4.2 Overlays are used for symbols which are likely to change during the search, that will cover other symbols or base map features, to prevent marking the base map and to avoid too many markings at one time.

4.3 The symbols and colors have been chosen to be compatible with the symbols defined in Incident Command System Field Operations Guide ICS-420. This compatibility is either exact (for example, incident command post) or functional (for example, search area boundaries).

5. Procedure

5.1 Symbols and markings for use on the base map or base overlay shall be made in accordance with Fig. 1 and Table 1.

5.2 Symbols and markings for use on overlays shall be made in accordance with Fig. 2 and Table 1.

5.3 Where words or letters are associated with a symbol, they shall be legible and as close to the symbol as possible. Size and placement may vary depending on map scale, the need for adjacent map features to remain visible and the writing instrument being used.

5.4 Locating marks shall be made on overlays so that they can be removed from the base map and reinstalled later with the proper alignment.

5.4.1 The base overlay shall have locating marks but should remain fixed with the base map throughout the search.

6. Keywords

6.1 management; maps; markings; search; symbols

---

[1] This practice is under the jurisdiction of ASTM Committee F-32 on Search and Rescue and is the direct responsibility of Subcommittee F32.02 on Search and Rescue Management.

Current edition approved Jan. 10, 1998. Published July 1998.

[2] Available from Fire Protection Publications, Oklahoma State University, Stillwater, Oklahoma, 74078.

SYMBOL	PURPOSE	COLOR
Date Time ⊗ (see note below)	**Point Last Seen (PLS) or Last Known Position (LKP)** Indicate date and time adjacent to symbol as shown	Red
Date Time Ⓒ (see note below)	**Clue or evidence** Indicate date and time found adjacent to symbol as shown	Red
Date Time Ⓔ (see note below)	**SARSAT hit (satellite ELT signal)** Indicate time and date of signal report adjacent to symbol as shown	Red
Date Time Ⓝ (see note below)	**NTAP (radar hit)** Indicate time and date of radar data adjacent to symbol as shown. If NTAP is also LKP, use LKP symbol with N next to it.	Red
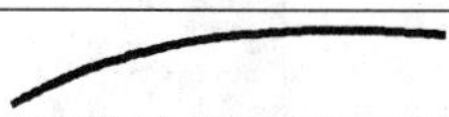	**Planned search area boundary**	Red
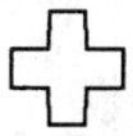 @	**Medical station or crew** Identify with station or crew designator adjacent to symbol as shown. Symbol may be drawn as solid cross.	Red
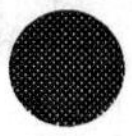 DF-@	**DF location** Indicate crew designator adjacent to DF as shown. Bearing line originates from this point. Bearing as reported, including true (T) or magnetic (M) is recorded along bearing line.	Color based on resource. See Table 1.
	**Incident Command Post**	Blue
Ⓑ (see note below)	**Incident Base** If collocated with CP, use CP symbol	Blue
Ⓗ (see note below)	**Helibase**	Blue
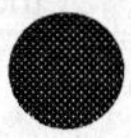 H-@	**Helispot** Identify with designator adjacent to symbol as shown.	Blue
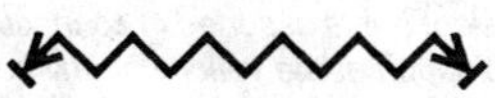	**Fixed confinement line** Use to indicate string lines, signs, fences, etc. which have been marked specifically for the search.	Black
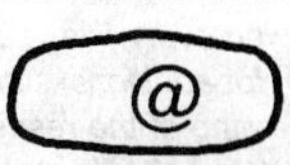	**Segment boundary** Identify with segment designator near center.	Black
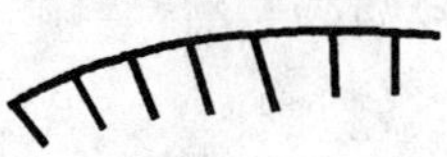	**Travel barriers** Existing natural or man-made barriers, use confinement symbol for search specific barriers.	Black

NOTE 1—Letter may be written next to circle rather than in it for clarity.
NOTE 2—@ - replace with designator number, letter, name, etc.

FIG. 1 Map Symbols and Markings for Base Map or Base Overlay

TABLE 1 Resource Colors

NOTE 1—Search crew are resources whose assignment will be carried out on foot. Search patrols' assignments are carried out by some other means, such as by vehicle, horseback, boat, etc.

Resource	Color
Search crew	Green
Search dog crew	Brown
Search patrol	Red
Helicopter	Blue
Fixed wing aircraft	Orange

SYMBOL	PURPOSE	COLOR
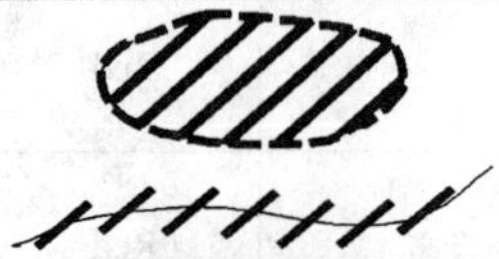	**First search coverage** Diagonal lines across segment, trail, road, etc. as shown. (Feature being searched is on base map.) See note 2 below.	Color is based on resource. See Table 1.
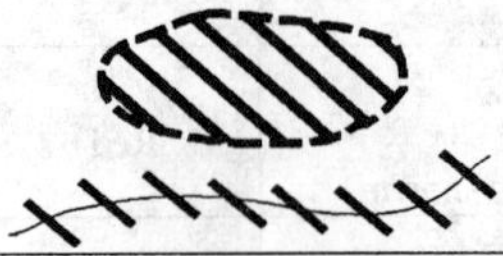	**Second search coverage** Diagonal lines across segment, trail, road, etc. as shown. Do not remove first coverage lines. See note 2 below.	
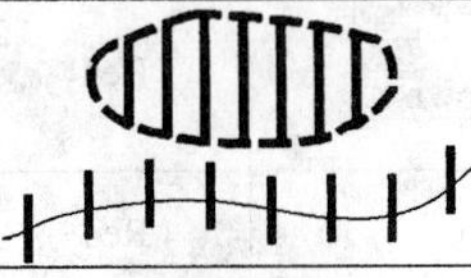	**Third search coverage** Vertical lines across segment, trail, road etc. as shown. Do not remove first and second coverage lines. See note 2 below.	
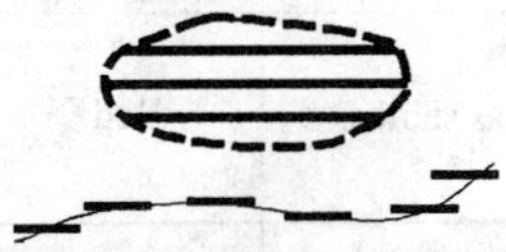	**Fourth search coverage** Horizontal lines across segment, trail, road, etc. as shown. Do not remove first, second and third coverage lines. See note 2 below.	
(see note 1 below) Ⓡ @	**Radio relay** Indicate relay designator adjacent to symbol as shown.	Black
Resource type - @ Date Time	**Resource designator** Indicate resource type (search crew, dog crew, etc.) and designator near assignment (segment, trail, etc.). Date and time are initially those of assignment. At completion of the assignment, the date and time shall be changed to those of completion.	Black

NOTE 1—Letter may be written next to circle rather then in it for clarity.

NOTE 2—The search coverage symbols are used to indicate the extent of actual coverage. If the task was not completed as assigned, then the symbols shall cover only those areas actually searched. Additional segment boundary lines shall be added to define the limits of the actual coverage.

NOTE 3—@ - replace with designator number, letter, name, etc.

FIG. 2 Map Symbols and Markings for Base Map or Base Overlay

Designation: F 1847 – 98

Standard Guide for Demonstrating Minimum Skills of Search and Rescue Dogs and Handlers[1]

This standard is issued under the fixed designation F 1847; the number immediately following the designation indicates the year of original adoption or, in the case of revision, the year of last revision. A number in parentheses indicates the year of last reapproval. A superscript epsilon (ε) indicates an editorial change since the last revision or reapproval.

1. Scope

1.1 This guide covers voluntary uniform training guidelines for dogs and handlers who engage in search and rescue (SAR) activities throughout the Unites States.

1.2 This guide provides a minimum set of training goals against which SAR dog teams and organizations may voluntarily evaluate their own training programs.

1.3 This guide provides a means of documenting a minimum standard for those agencies who request SAR dog resources for SAR operations and require such documentation.

1.4 Local SAR dog handlers and parent organizations are responsible for testing and verification that individual resources meet or exceed these guidelines.

1.5 *This standard does not purport to address all of the safety concerns, if any, associated with its use. It is the responsibility of the user of this standard to establish appropriate safety and health practices and determine the applicability of regulatory limitations prior to use.*

2. Referenced Documents

2.1 *ASTM Standards:*

F 1633 Standard Guide for Land Search Techniques[2]

F 1848 Classification for Search and Rescue Dog Crew/Teams[2]

F 1879 Standard Guide for Demonstrating Obedience and Agility in Search and Rescue Dogs[2]

3. Terminology

3.1 *Definitions of Terms Specific to This Standard:*

3.1.1 *alert*—an indication by a dog that signals the handler that the targeted scent has been found.

3.1.2 *bringsel*—an object carried by the dog or handler that is retrieved or tugged on by the dog when the dog finds its target.

3.1.3 *refind*—an action by a free-ranging dog that is initiated after the dog finds its target and results in the dog directing the handler back to the target.

3.1.4 *return*—an action of a free-ranging dog that brings the dog back to its handler after finding its target.

3.1.5 *scent article*—an object used by search personnel to familiarize a dog with the scent of a subject.

4. Summary of Guide

4.1 This guide provides dog handlers, units and organizations in differing locales with the ability to understand and replicate skills and training required to meet these minimum guidelines.

4.2 This guide identifies a minimum set of skills that will help establish the mission readiness of a search dog crew[3] for search and rescue operations.

4.3 The dog and handler skills demonstrate the crew's abilities to estimate probabilities of detection.

5. Significance and Use

5.1 This guide may be used by units, handlers, and requesting agencies when evaluating dog resources or as a basis for establishing local minimum performance guidelines or standards. All or a subst of this guide may be utilized.

5.2 Agencies and organizations who have responsibility for search and rescue operations may use this guide as a basis for developing standardized testing and certification of search dog resources.

5.3 This guide does not provide a theoretical basis for how a search dog crew works, rather it describes the minimum results desired. Definitions that are referenced are provided to develop consistency in interpretation.

5.4 Each dog team, unit or organization wishing to use this guide has the responsibility of managing and administering it. Units may wish to use evaluators from other units or organizations, or, request assistance in obtaining qualified evaluators from organizations such as the SAR Dog Section of the National Association of Search and Rescue (NASAR). This decision however, rests solely with the individual team or organization. The method of evaluation is also entirely at the discretion of each user of this guide.

6. Dog Skills

6.1 *Obedience and Agility Skills*:

6.1.1 Dogs used in SAR operations should posses an acceptable level of agility and obedience skills such as those listed in Guide F 1879.

---

[1] This guide is under the jurisdiction of ASTM Committee F-32 on Search and Rescue and is the direct responsibility of Subcommittee F32.02 on Management and Operations.

Current edition approved Jan. 10, 1998. Published July 1998.

[2] *Annual Book of ASTM Standards*, Vol 13.01.

[3] These Guides are currently under development

6.1.2 Obedience skills should ensure that the SAR dog will be under the control of the handler in a manner that allows the dog to participate in SAR operations without interfering with other search resources.

6.1.3 Agility skills should ensure the dog's ability to traverse obstacles and terrain that may be present during SAR operations.

6.1.4 The sufficiency of a dog's agility and obedience skills should be at the discretion of the agency having jurisdiction over search and rescue operations.

6.2 *Communication Skills*:

6.2.1 The dog should be able to indicate that it has detected the object of its search. This indication may be in the form of a classic physical alert such as a bark, whine, jump or capture of bringsel, or, in some other predetermined response that is known and can be described by the handler.

6.2.2 The dog, on command, should be able to leave a person found in order to search for additional subjects.

6.2.3 Upon finding the subject of a search, the dog should be able to execute a refind.

6.3 *Working Skills*:

6.3.1 Dogs should be able to work for a set duration of time without a break while maintaining optimum performance. An acceptable duration of work should be established jointly by the agency or organization utilizing these guidelines and the dog handler.

6.3.2 The dog must be able to work both during day and night and under weather and terrain conditions specified by the agency who will use the resource.

6.3.3 The dog should be under the control of the handler at all times and in a manner consistent with local conditions.

6.3.4 The dog should have the ability to be easily transported by means common to the working environment in which it will be used. This may include the back of a pick-up truck, aircraft, watercraft, snowmobile, ski-lift, ATV, or a raising or lowing system in harness. The applicable means of transportation should be determined by the agency or organization utilizing the resource.

7. Handler Skills

7.1 It is recommended that dog handlers acquire basic search and rescue skills when possible through a local and national or state affiliated, search and rescue organization. Affiliation with local SAR organizations ensures that handler skills are appropriate for local conditions and achieves a level of familiarity among all parties engaged in SAR operations.

7.2 *Basic SAR Skills*:

7.2.1 *First Aid/Survival/Safety Skills*:

7.2.1.1 The handler should demonstrate an acceptable level of training and performance of both human and canine first aid. Acceptable levels of performance should mimic the standard of care in the local community where the dog handler will work.

7.2.1.2 A handler should have the knowledge and ability to sustain themselves AND a lost person for at least 24 h with equipment they normally carry.

7.2.1.3 A handler should the knowledge and ability to evaluate hazards, select safe routes and follow safe procedures within their assigned working environment. This could include knowledge such as an awareness of avalanche potential, the use of flotation devices during water searches, the use of latex gloves in first aid or the preservation of evidence in cadaver searching, etc).

7.2.2 *Land Navigation*—The handler should with the aid of map and compass, be able to determine their location both during day and night, directing others to their location and find the best route of travel to a given location and for segmenting search areas.

7.2.3 *Communication Skills*—The handler should have the ability to use proper local agency radio protocols in radio communications and the ability to use available communications equipment properly.

7.3 *Search Management Skills*:

7.3.1 The handler should be able to work with each resource under the incident command system.

7.3.2 The handler should be able to demonstrate an understanding of the environmental conditions that affect the ability of the crew to locate lost people. These conditions include knowledge of scent transport, including the effect of terrain, vegetation, and weather conditions such as convection, wind and solar insolation; the dog's and handler's physical and mental energy applied to the search; the difficulty of the cover and terrain; and the length of time from the loss to the search. The handler should be able to give the planning section a report telling how well, in percentages the chance for detection was achieved. They must also be able to mark on a map their coverage, alerts, wind direction at the time of the alerts, clues, etc.

7.3.3 A handler should be able to analyze all factors that can affect probability of detection (POD)[3], for a given assignment; terrain, vegetation, slope, sun angle, cloud cover, wind, size of assignment, travel aids - and be able to adjust the dog crew's operating procedures to achieve the highest POD within the time allotted, by the planning section.

7.3.4 Handlers should be familiar with all of the typical strategies used by search and rescue teams including hasty searching, perimeter searching, track and sign cutting, contour grid searching, running ridges, running canyon bottoms, geometric gridding and combinations thereof.

7.3.5 The handler should have the ability to communicate the results of the dog crew's search efforts to search management. This should include the location of clues, the route followed, relevant meteorological conditions and an estimated POD.

7.4 *Physical Conditioning*—The handler should have the ability to effectively search in working environments requiring extended periods of strenuous and physically demanding activity and foot travel. The handler must have the ability to carry adequate survival, first aid, communications, and personnel equipment on their person for the duration of the search.

7.5 *Dog Handling Skills*:

7.5.1 A handler should understand and can tell others how to collect and preserve scent articles for search work.

7.5.2 A handler should be able to interpret the body language or trained responses of the search and rescue dog which indicate that the dog has detected human scent.

7.5.3 The handler should be able to communicate to the dog the end or conclusion of a search or operational period in a positive manner. This communication may be in the form of a reward such as play or food, or via some command or action, such as removal of a harness, coat, etc.

8. Keywords

8.1 dog training; handler skills; minimum training standards

Standard Classification for Search and Rescue Dog Crew/Teams[1]

This standard is issued under the fixed designation F 1848; the number immediately following the designation indicates the year of original adoption or, in the case of revision, the year of last revision. A number in parentheses indicates the year of last reapproval. A superscript epsilon (ϵ) indicates an editorial change since the last revision or reapproval.

1. Scope

1.1 This classification covers the aid of search and rescue managers in ordering resources for search and rescue incidents and to aid dog handlers in communicating the types of tasks for which they and their dogs have trained.

1.2 This classification is intended as a supplement to the resource typing specifications of the Incident Command System[2] and specifically as a means of typing search and rescue dog resources.

1.3 This classification is suitable for classifying dog resources for a wide variety of emergency management purposes including both search and rescue and law enforcement incidents.

1.4 This classification does not attempt to put forth standards of performance or training for dogs or their handlers. This is the responsibility of local agencies responsible for utilizing the resource.

2. Referenced Documents

2.1 *ASTM Standards:*

F 1633 Guide for Techniques in Land Search[3]

3. Terminology

3.1 *Definitions of Terms Specific to This Standard:*

3.1.1 *air-scenting, v*—a search dog action the dog to search for human scent within a defined search area

3.1.2 *kind, n*—a classification of a group of similar team/crew functions.

3.1.3 *scent discrimination, n*—the ability of a dog to distinguish between the scents of different individuals and to work an assigned scent to complete a SAR activity.

3.1.4 *tracking, v*—a search dog action that requires the dog to put its nose within 1 to 2 ft (or m) of the targets track as it moves towards the freshest scent.

3.1.5 *trailing, v*—a search dog action that allows the dog to range about a targets trail in proportion to the rafts of scent as it moves towards the freshest scent.

3.1.6 *type, n*—a classification that refers to resource capability.

3.1.7 *typing, v*—the classification of search and rescue resources by *type* and *kind.*

3.2 Terminology not defined in this guide but referenced in the text can be found in Terminology F 1633

4. Classification of Search and Rescue Dog Types

4.1 Typing of SAR dog resources is based upon the most basic methods of using working dogs engaged in search and rescue activities. These two basic types are based upon whether or not the dog can effectively discriminate between the human scent of different individuals.

4.2 *Type I*—Trained to discriminate human scent, and

4.3 *Type II*—Not trained to discriminate human scent.

5. Classification of Search and Rescue Dog Kinds

5.1 Kind classifications of SAR dog resources are based upon the specific tasks for which dogs are deployed.

5.2 *Kind A—Area Search Dog*—SAR dog teams trained to search moderately large unstructured areas of varied terrain.

5.3 *Kind B—Avalanche Search Dog*—SAR dog teams trained to search avalanche debris fields.

5.4 *Kind C—Cadaver Search Dog*—SAR dog teams trained to search for deceased human remains.

5.5 *Kind D—Disaster/Collapsed Structure Search Dog*—SAR dog teams trained to search for human scent in failed manmade structures, and natural debris fields.

5.6 *Kind E—Evidence Search Dog*—SAR dog teams trained to search for inanimate objects.

5.7 *Kind F—Trailing Search Dog*—SAR dog teams trained to search by trailing.

5.8 *Kind G—Tracking Search Dog*—SAR dog teams trained to search by tracking.

5.9 *Kind H—Water Search*—SAR dog teams trained to search for human scent in and along bodies of water.

6. Keywords

6.1 incident command system; resource typing; search dogs

[1] This classification is under the jurisdiction of ASTM Committee F32 on Search and Rescue and is the direct responsibility of Subcommittee F32.02 on Management and Operations.

Current edition approved Jan. 10, 1998. Published July 1998.

[2] International Fire Service Training Association, *Incident Command System Field Operations Guide, ICS 420* available from the International Fire Service Training Association, Fire Protection Publications, Oklahoma State University, Stillwater, OK 74078.

[3] *Annual Book of ASTM Standards*, Vol 14.01.

Designation: F 1850 – 00

Standard Specification for Particular Requirements for Anesthesia Workstations and Their Components[1]

This standard is issued under the fixed designation F 1850; the number immediately following the designation indicates the year of original adoption or, in the case of revision, the year of last revision. A number in parentheses indicates the year of last reapproval. A superscript epsilon (ε) indicates an editorial change since the last revision or reapproval.

INTRODUCTION

This specification covers minimum safety requirements for an ANESTHESIA WORKSTATION. It applies in addition to IEC Publication 601-1 (ed. 2 1988),[2] hereafter called the GENERAL STANDARD, and to IEC 601-1-1:1992[2] as amended, hereafter called the SYSTEMS STANDARD.

It is recognized that from time to time innovations and designs will appear that offer advantages and yet are not covered by specific safety related design or performance aspects of this specification; such innovations are not to be discouraged. If the techniques and technologies in these innovations advance beyond those described in this specification, then they must meet the safety objectives of this specification.

This specification also describes referee test methods necessary to ensure compliance with the performance and safety requirements described herein. While qualification test procedures to determine compliance are described and specified, equivalent or superior qualification test procedures to determine compliance with the requirements may be used.

SECTION ONE—GENERAL

1. Scope

This clause of the GENERAL STANDARD applies with the following amendment:

1.5 This specification presents particular requirements for an ANESTHESIA WORKSTATION when supplied as a complete unit, as well as particular requirements for individual devices which together make up a complete ANESTHESIA WORKSTATION.

It is the intent of this specification that both complete ANESTHESIA WORKSTATIONS and the individual devices be commercially available to allow USERS to configure an ANESTHESIA WORKSTATION to meet the needs of their clinical practice in conformance with their national regulations or guidelines, or both. To this end the standard has been structured in such a way as to clearly identify particular requirements pertinent to specific devices currently available.

NOTE 1—Although this specification does not mandate the use of a single communication protocol, the purpose of digital data communication in this standard is to facilitate transfer of data between devices. Possible uses of data from multiple sources include integrated data display and alarm annunciation, and aiding DECISION SUPPORT SYSTEMS. Centralized display integration and functional integration are the hallmarks differentiating this standard from previous anesthesia gas machine standards. Digital communication makes possible integration among workstation devices that may be modular, or interact only through communication interfaces. Documentation and disclosure requirements vary because of expected variations in implementation permitted by the specified standards. Additional documentation requirements are imposed when interface methods not included in the specified DIGITAL INTERFACE standards are encountered.

Equipment that can be used with flammable anesthetic agents, intermittent flow machines, that only deliver gas to the patient at varying rates in response to the patient's inspiratory efforts, and dental nitrous oxide - oxygen machines are not covered by this specification.

1.5.1 *This guide is arranged as follows:*

[1] This specification is under the jurisdiction of ASTM Committee F-29 on Anesthetic and Respiratory Equipment and is the direct responsibility of Subcommittee F29.10 on Anesthesia Workstations.

Current edition approved February 10, 2000. Published March 2000. Originally published as F 1850 – 98. Last previous edition F 1850 – 98.

[2] Available from American National Standards Institute, 11 W. 42nd St., 13th Floor, New York, NY 10036.

2. Terminology

2.1 Clause 2 of the GENERAL STANDARD applies together with ISO 4135[2] and the following:

2.13 Terminology and Definitions Related to ANESTHESIA WORKSTATIONS

2.13.1 *accuracy*—the quality that characterizes the ability of a device to give indications approximating to the true value of the quantity measured.

2.13.2 *alarm device*—a device that performs the task of annunciating visual or audible alarm signal(s), or both, when an alarm condition is present. Such devices are, for example, the power failure alarm, and oxygen supply failure alarm.

2.13.3 *anesthesia breathing system*—see ISO 4135 (Rev. 1995).

2.13.4 *anesthesia gas supply device*—an assembly of components that controls and delivers all gas flow and agent concentration in the fresh gas into the ANESTHESIA BREATHING SYSTEM. It may include a FLOW ADJUSTMENT CONTROL(s), a GAS MIXING SYSTEM and an ANESTHETIC VAPOR DELIVERY DEVICE(s)

2.13.5 *anesthesia gas supply piping*—all pipe work, including unions, from the UNIDIRECTIONAL VALVE(s) in the pipeline inlet(s), the piping connecting the high pressure supply to the GAS PRESSURE REDUCING DEVICE/SYSTEM, and from the GAS PRESSURE REDUCING DEVICE/SYSTEM outlet to the FLOW ADJUSTMENT CONTROL(s) and auxiliary gas outlets. It includes piping leading to and from pneumatic ALARM DEVICE(s), pressure indicator(s), oxygen flush, ANESTHETIC VAPOR DELIVERY DEVICE(s), and piping leading to the COMMON GAS OUTLET

2.13.6 *anesthetic vapor delivery device*— device where anesthetic agent is transformed from the liquid to the gaseous phase in a controllable concentration.

2.13.7 *anesthesia ventilator*—see ISO 4135 (Rev. 1995).[2]

2.13.8 *anesthesia workstation*— a system for administration of anesthesia to patients. It consists of the ANESTHESIA GAS SUPPLY DEVICE, ANESTHESIA VENTILATOR, MONITORING DEVICES and PROTECTION DEVICE(s).

2.13.9 *applied part*— for the purpose of this specification, the APPLIED PART is the COMMON GAS OUTLET (Fresh Gas Outlet) and other parts of the ANESTHESIA WORKSTATION intended to be connected with the patient or with the anesthesia breathing system.

2.13.10 *auxiliary oxygen flowmeter*—a self-contained oxygen flowmeter with its own FLOW ADJUSTMENT CONTROL, FLOW INDICATOR, and outlet, not ordinarily used during the administration of general anesthesia.

2.13.11 *bias*— a constant or systematic error as opposed to a random error. It manifests itself as a persistent positive or negative deviation of the method average from the accepted reference value.

2.13.12 *common gas outlet (fresh gas outlet)*—that port through which the dispensed mixture from the ANESTHESIA GAS SUPPLY DEVICE is delivered to the ANESTHESIA BREATHING SYSTEM.

2.13.13 *delivery system device*— a system/device used as part of an ANESTHESIA WORKSTATION that delivers energy or substances to the patient.

2.13.14 *flow adjustment control*—a device or assembly that controls the flow of gas(es), or gas mixtures.

2.13.15 *flow indicator*—a device that indicates the volume of a specific gas or gas mixture passing through it in a unit of time.

2.13.16 *gas mixing system*—a device or assembly that receives oxygen and other medical gas(es) and delivers a mixture of these gases in controllable concentrations.

2.13.17 *gas pressure reducing device/system*—a single device, or group of devices designed to provide a range of controlled delivery pressure over a specified range of inlet pressures.

2.13.18 *infusion device(s)*— mechanical and electromechanical devices intended to regulate the flow of liquids (parenteral fluids, drugs, and routine fluids) to the patient under positive pressure generated either by a pump, or by gravitational force.

2.13.19 *legible*—displayed qualitative or quantitative information, values, functions, and/or markings shall be discernible or identifiable to an OPERATOR with 6-6 (20/20) vision (corrected if necessary) from a distance of 1 m at a light level of 215 lux, when viewing the information, markings, etc. perpendicular to and including 15° above, below, left and right of the normal line of sight of the OPERATOR.

2.13.20 *medical gas pipeline system*—the complete system that comprises a central supply system with control equipment, a pipeline distribution system and terminal units at the points where non-flammable medical gases may be delivered.

2.13.21 *monitoring device*—a device that performs the task of indicating the value of a measured variable to the OPERATOR. Such devices are for example, the airway pressure monitor or the exhaled volume monitor.

2.13.22 *operator*—the clinician (for example anesthesiologist).

2.13.23 *peep (positive end expiratory pressure)*— the positive pressure within the airway at the end of expiratory flow.

2.13.24 *precision*— the quality that characterizes the ability of a device to give for the same value of the quantity measured, indications that agree amongst themselves, not taking into consideration the systematic errors associated with variations of the indications

2.13.25 *protection device(s)*—a device that, without intervention of the OPERATOR, performs the task of protecting the patient from hazardous output due to incorrect delivery of energy or substances. Such devices are for example, the oxygen supply failure device or the maximum pressure limitation device.

2.13.26 *reserve electrical power supply*—that portion of the equipment that supplies temporary power to the electrical system in the event of interruption of the normal electrical supply.

2.13.27 *user*-the owner of the ANESTHESIA WORKSTATION (for example, hospital).

2.14 Terminology and Definitions Related to Alarms (see Clause 51)

2.14.1 *disable*— to prevent an otherwise enabling condition from initiating a function.

2.14.1.1 *Discussion*-For the purpose of this specification, to DISABLE an alarm means to prevent the annunciation of the auditory alarm signal. Optionally, the visual component may be prevented.

2.14.2 *high priority alarm*—a signal that indicates a condition requiring immediate action.

2.14.3 *low priority alarm*—a signal that indicates a condition that requires OPERATOR awareness, but not necessarily action.

2.14.4 *medium priority alarm*—a signal that indicates a condition requiring prompt action.

2.14.5 *silencing*—to temporarily stop the annunciation of an audible alarm.

2.15 Terminology and Definitions Related to AARK's (Automated Anesthesia Record Keepers)

2.15.1 *artifact*—data that is not a true representation of the patient condition.

2.15.2 *back-up*—an electronic copy of an anesthetic record or collection of anesthetic records made for the purpose of securing the data for retrieval at a later time.

2.15.3 *editing*—changing a recorded value, comment, annotation, or event in the anesthetic record, whether stored automatically or entered manually, at any time after it has been made part of the record.

2.15.4 *input device*—a device connected to the AARK that is used to manually enter data or control the AARK. These may include, but are not limited to, keyboards, mice, trackballs, light-pens, bar code scanners, microphones, etc.

2.15.5 *network*—the connection between the AARK and another computer or another AARK, or both, for the purpose of transferring data.

2.15.6 *non-volatile*—stored electronically in such a way that the loss of all electric power (normal and reserve) to the system or storage device will not alter the data stored on the media.

2.15.7 *output devices*—a device that presents data from a computer system to an OPERATOR or USER for viewing or storage. Examples include printers and screens.

2.15.8 *recorded data*—captured data that is stored by the AARK.

2.16 Terminology and Definitions Related to Digital Communication and Information Systems

2.16.1 *control center (of an anesthesia workstation)*— the INFORMATION SYSTEM component of an ANESTHESIA WORKSTATION mediating the centralized alarm prioritization and management strategy, and possibly other functions.

2.16.2 *decision support system*— an INFORMATION SYSTEM intended to automatically process data from one or more sources, providing output information to assist the OPERATOR.

2.16.3 *digital interface*— hardware and protocol supporting bidirectional digital serial data communication complying with one of the following published data communication standards (see also Clause 85, Annex A, and Appendix B):

A. RS-232.[3]
B. IEEE 1073.[4]

2.16.4 *IEEE 1073*—Serial digital data communication complying with the signal characteristics, transport, protocol, and data formats defined by members of the IEEE 1073[4] family of standards. These standards are also widely known by the names MIB, or medical information bus.

2.16.5 *information system*— a digital system collecting, displaying, or processing information from other PRIMARY or SECONDARY DATA SOURCES. Digital data may be transferred through DIGITAL INTERFACES or NETWORKS. Examples include AARK's and DECISION SUPPORT SYSTEMS.

2.16.6 *network*— a connection between digital systems (computers or AARK's) for transmission of data over a communication medium using a common protocol.

2.16.7 *operator input*— data provided by various interactions of the OPERATOR with the ANESTHESIA WORKSTATION controls or record keeping components that can be stored and transmitted in digital form.

2.16.8 *primary data source*—a MONITORING DEVICE or DELIVERY DEVICE providing functional or measured data via DIGITAL INTERFACES or OPERATOR INPUT.

2.16.9 *RS-232*[3]—serial digital data communication complying with the electrical characteristics and cable connectors defined by EIA/TIA standard RS-232-C-1969[3] or its successors (EIA/TIA-232-D-1987, EIA/TIA-232-E-1991[3]).

2.16.10 *secondary data source*— an INFORMATION SYSTEM that re-transmits data collected from PRIMARY DATA SOURCES and other SECONDARY DATA SOURCES. A SECONDARY DATA SOURCE may have modular PRIMARY DATA SOURCES as components. Digital data may be primary or secondary due to origination either from within a MULTIPORT COMMUNICATION DEVICE or another digital source.

3. General Requirements

Clause 3 of the GENERAL STANDARD applies with the following additions:

Additions:

3.6j) Applicable single fault conditions are short and open circuits of components or wiring that can increase temperatures. (See SECTION SEVEN.)

3.6 k An oxidant leak which is not detected by an ALARM DEVICE or inspection procedures recommended by the manufacturer shall be considered a normal condition and not a single fault condition.

Test for compliance by simulation of a single fault condition.

4. General Requirements for Tests

Clause 4 of the GENERAL STANDARD applies with the following addition:

Addition:

---

[3] Available from EIA/TIA, Electronics Industries Association/ Telecommunications Industry Association, 2500 Wilson Blvd., Suite 300, Arlington, VA 22201–3834.

[4] Available from IEEE, Institute of Electrical and Electronics Engineers, 445 Hoes Lane, PO Box 1331, Piscataway, NJ 08855–1331.

4.12 Type testing of components of ANESTHESIA WORKSTATIONS

For type testing components of the ANESTHESIA WORKSTATION the requirements of the appropriate section(s), of this specification, including the referenced additional standards as stated in the appropriate section, apply. The manufacturer of components for ANESTHESIA WORKSTATIONS shall specify in the instructions for use the ANESTHESIA WORKSTATION(S) configuration(s) for which the compatibility and compliance with this specification have been established.

The manufacturer may use type tests different from those detailed within this specification, if an equivalent degree of safety is obtained.

5. Classification

Clause 5 of the GENERAL STANDARD applies.

6. Identification, Marking and Documents

Clause 6 of the GENERAL STANDARD applies with the following additions and amendments:

Amendment:

6.1j) *R* The input marking required in Sub-clause 6.1j of the GENERAL STANDARD shall be given in amperes for the ANESTHESIA WORKSTATION and for the sum of the allowed maximum current ratings for the ANESTHESIA WORKSTATION and the auxiliary mains socket outlets.

Amendment:

6.1k) *R* The requirement on marking of auxiliary mains socket outlets of Sub-clause 6.1k in the GENERAL STANDARD shall apply to each auxiliary mains socket outlet and shall be given in amperes.

NOTE 2—Marking should be provided to indicate the location of fuses or overcurrent release for the auxiliary mains socket outlet(s).

Auxiliary mains socket outlet(s) shall be marked with a warning to the effect that:

Equipment connected to auxiliary mains socket outlets must comply with IEC 601-1-1[2] and the total sum of the system leakage current shall not exceed 300 microamps (See Clause 19.4h). It is the USER'S responsibility to ensure compliance with the above standard and that the leakage current limits are not exceeded.

Additional Clauses:

6.1 aa) Device packaging or labeling, or both, shall distinguish between identical or similar products in both the sterile and non-sterile state from the same manufacturer.

6.1 bb) Each gas specific inlet shall be durably marked with either the gas name or chemical symbol in accordance with CGA V-5.[5] This marking shall be LEGIBLE, and if color coding is used, it shall be in accordance with CGA C-9.[5] (See Table 1.)

6.1 cc) The COMMON GAS OUTLET (Fresh Gas Outlet), if OPERATOR accessible, shall be durably marked. This marking shall be LEGIBLE.

6.1 dd) Controls for gas flow or agent output shall be durably marked with a LEGIBLE indication to inform the OPERATOR which action(s) is (are) required to increase/decrease the gas flow or agent output.

6.1 ee) For the ANESTHESIA VENTILATOR, all ports shall be durably marked. These markings shall be LEGIBLE. Symbols may be used, and when symbols are used, they shall be explained in the instructions for use.

6.1 ff) The ANESTHESIA WORKSTATION or its components, or both, shall be durably marked with the rated supply pressure(s) to which the equipment can be connected. These markings shall be LEGIBLE.

6.3g All OPERATOR interchangeable components, including ANESTHESIA VENTILATOR, ANESTHETIC AGENT DELIVERY SYSTEM(s), and recommended accessory components that are flow direction sensitive, and that can be misconnected, shall be durably marked with a LEGIBLE arrow showing the correct direction of flow.

6.3h The auxiliary gas outlet(s), if provided, shall be durably marked with either the gas-name or chemical symbol in accordance with CGA V-5.[5] This marking shall be LEGIBLE, and if color coding is used, it shall be in accordance with CGA C-9.[5] (See Table 1.)

6.3j *Pressure Indicators* All medical gas cylinder and pipeline pressure indicators shall be graduated and marked in units of kPa times 100. The markings and graduations shall be clearly identified with the pressure indicator(s) with which they are associated, and shall be LEGIBLE.

NOTE 3—Pressure indicators additionally may be marked in units of PSIG.

Each gas specific pressure indicator shall be identified by DURABLE and LEGIBLE marking using gas-name or chemical symbol in accordance with CGA V-5.[5] If color coding is used in addition, it shall be in accordance with CGA C-9.[5] (See Table 1.)

ANESTHESIA BREATHING SYSTEM pressure indicators shall be graduated and durably marked in units of kPa or cm H_2O, or both. These markings shall be LEGIBLE.

6.3.k FLOW ADJUSTMENT CONTROL(s)

Each FLOW ADJUSTMENT CONTROL or it surroundings shall be identified by a DURABLE and LEGIBLE marking using gas name or chemical symbol in accordance with CGA V-5.[5] If color coding is used in addition it shall be in accordance with CGA C-9.[5] (See Table 1.)

If applicable the point of reference for reading the FLOW INDICATOR shall be readily identifiable with the associated FLOW INDICATOR.

6.3.L ANESTHETIC AGENT DELIVERY DEVICE(s)

The maximum and minimum filling levels shall be marked on the liquid level indicator. These markings shall be DURABLE and LEGIBLE. As an alternative the actual usable volume and capacity shall be displayed.

Each OPERATOR-detachable ANESTHETIC AGENT DELIVERY DEVICE(s) shall be durably marked, either with the words "See Accompanying Documents" or symbol #14 from Table D1 of the GENERAL STANDARD.

If OPERATOR accessible, the agent reservoir or filling port, or both, shall be durably marked with the generic name of the anesthetic agent. The control(s) activating the delivery shall be durably marked, with the generic name in full spelling, or the

[5] Available from CGA, Compressed Gas Association, 1725 Jefferson Davis Highway, Suite 10004, Arlington, VA 22202–4102.

abbreviated form, of the anesthetic agent being administered, or the same information shall be displayed.

If color coding is used in addition, it shall be in accordance with Table 2.

The units for which the control of the ANESTHETIC AGENT DELIVERY DEVICE(s) is graduated shall be LEGIBLE and durably marked either on the control or shall be displayed continuously or on OPERATOR demand.

Graduated controls, if provided, shall be marked with "zero" or "off," or with both if the zero-position is not also the off-position.

6.3m The oxygen flush control shall be located on the front of the equipment, and shall be durably marked with one of the following:

OXYGEN FLUSH

O_2 FLUSH

O_2 +

These markings shall be LEGIBLE. If color coding is used in addition, it shall be in accordance with CGA C-9[5]. (See Table 1.)

6.8 Accompanying Documents

Clause 6.8 of the GENERAL STANDARD applies with the following additions and or amendments.

Amendment:

6.8.2a Manufacturers/suppliers of complete ANESTHESIA WORKSTATION(s) or ANESTHESIA GAS SUPPLY DEVICE(s) shall provide a listing of the applicable means for monitoring, alarm and protection against hazards from delivery of energy or substances to the patient. These are specified in Clause 51 of this specification and summarized in Table 3. The instructions for use shall state that the ANESTHESIA WORKSTATION or ANESTHESIA GAS SUPPLY DEVICE shall not be operated without the applicable MONITORING, ALARM and PROTECTION DEVICE(s).

Additional Clauses:

6.8.2j) The instructions for use shall describe methods of verifying alarm functions.

6.8.2k) If applicable, the instructions for use shall contain a warning to the effect that:

The connection of equipment to the auxiliary mains socket outlet(s) may increase the leakage currents to values exceeding the allowable limits in the event of a defective protective earth conductor. If multiple pieces of equipment are connected together, and one power cord supplies power, the leakage current of the whole assembled system should be measured.

6.8.2L) Instructions for use shall include testing for correct assembly and connection of each device supplying gas to the equipment and any ANESTHETIC VAPOR DELIVERY DEVICE(s) fitted to the equipment.

6.8.2m) The instructions for use shall include the operating characteristics of any pressure relieving device(s) fitted to the equipment.

6.8.2n) The instructions for use shall include the pressure and flow characteristics of any auxiliary gas outlet(s) when the pipeline supply pressure is 50 + 5 / – 0 psig. The manufacturer shall indicate the effects of variations in pipeline supply pressures on these pressure and flow characteristics.

6.8.2o) The instructions for use shall include the operating characteristics of the oxygen supply failure alarm system(s) and if provided, the associated cut-off devices.

6.8.2p) If the ANESTHESIA GAS SUPPLY DEVICE is fitted with a GAS MIXING SYSTEM, the instructions for use shall specify the leakage from one gas inlet to the other. The instructions for use shall also include the design pressure(s) and the recommended range of flows from the GAS MIXING SYSTEM.

6.8.2q) The instructions for use shall include the recommended service interval.

6.8.2r) If appropriate, the instructions for use shall include the operational characteristics of ANESTHESIA VENTILATOR(s) recommended for use with the ANESTHESIA WORKSTATION, including a pneumatic diagram.

6.8.2s) If appropriate, the instructions for use shall include the operational characteristics of ANESTHESIA BREATHING SYSTEM(s) and anesthetic gas scavenging system(s) recommended for use with the ANESTHESIA WORKSTATION.

6.8.2t) If the ANESTHESIA GAS SUPPLY DEVICE is fitted with an ANESTHETIC VAPOR DELIVERY DEVICE(s) by the manufacturer or it is intended that a recommended ANESTHETIC VAPOR DELIVERY DEVICE(s) is to be fitted according to the instructions for use, the following shall be provided in the instructions for use:

Details of the ANESTHETIC VAPOR DELIVERY DEVICE(s) performance, including the effects of variation in ambient temperature, ambient pressure, tilting, back pressure, input flow and gas mixture composition;

If applicable, a warning that the performance of the ANESTHESIA WORKSTATION or ANESTHETIC VAPOR DELIVERY DEVICE(s), or both, may be degraded if the two are mismatched;

Instructions for the use of any filling device(s) with which the ANESTHETIC VAPOR DELIVERY DEVICE(s) is fitted;

The carrier gas, gas flow(s) and analytical technique recommended for testing the ANESTHETIC VAPOR DELIVERY DEVICE(s).

A statement that the ANESTHETIC VAPOR DELIVERY DEVICE(s) should not be used between "off" and the first graduation above zero, if the ANESTHETIC VAPOR DELIVERY DEVICE(s) cannot be calibrated in this range.

If applicable, the volume of agent required to fill the agent reservoir from the minimum to the maximum filling level, and the total capacity.

6.8.2u) The instructions for use shall include information about disinfection or sterilization of reusable components, or both;

6.8.2v) The instructions for use shall include information about the cleanliness and sterility of respiratory gas conducting components upon delivery;

6.8.2w) The manufacturer shall disclose in the instructions for use the minimum detectable exhaled volume, the accuracy of the indicated exhaled volumes and the resolution of the exhaled volume monitor when tested according to method in Clause 51.6.4.2.

6.8.2x) The instructions for use shall include a statement that an alternative means of ventilation should be available whenever the ANESTHESIA WORKSTATION is in use.

6.8.2y) If alarm limits are preset by the manufacturer the limits shall be disclosed in the instructions for use.

6.8.2z) The instructions for use shall include a description of the functioning of the ANESTHESIA WORKSTATION or its individual devices, or both, after an interruption of the mains electrical power and/or a switch-over to a RESERVE ELECTRICAL POWER SUPPLY.

6.8.2aa) The instructions for use shall state the recommended applications (neonatal, pediatric, adult) for the ANESTHESIA VENTILATOR.

6.8.2bb) The manufacturer/supplier of the ANESTHESIA WORKSTATION shall disclose in the instructions for use the location of latex based components.

6.8.2cc) The location and instructions relevant to any filter elements recommended by the manufacturer shall be disclosed in the instructions for use.

6.8.2dd) The instructions for use shall state whether or not the ANESTHESIA WORKSTATION is suitable for use in a magnetic resonance imaging (MRI) environment.

6.8.3Technical Descriptions

Clause 6.8.3 of the GENERAL STANDARD applies with the following additions.

6.8.3a) Disclosure of accuracies (including BIAS and PRECISION), display resolutions and range of each calibrated control, and for each monitored variable that is displayed.

Disclosure of interdependence of controls, if applicable.

Disclosure of all information necessary to check that an ANESTHESIA WORKSTATION or its devices, or both, is/are installed correctly and is/are in safe and correct working order, and on the nature and frequency of maintenance operations necessary to ensure continuing safety and correct operation.

6.8.3b) The manufacturer of the ANESTHESIA VENTILATOR shall include:

A listing of the following:

(a) Maximum limited pressure, $P_{lim,max}$;
(b) Range of values to which the maximum working pressure can be set and the means by which the maximum is ensured (for example, pressure cycling, pressure limiting, pressure generation);
(c) A statement whether subatmospheric pressure is available in the expiratory phase,
(d) Minimum (most subatmospheric) limited pressure; and
(e) Range of values to which the minimum (most subatmospheric) working pressure can be set and the means by which the minimum is ensured.

A listing of the ranges of the following parameters:

(a) Cycling pressure,
(b) End-expiratory pressure, and
(c) The limiting pressure and generated pressure shall be listed if a facility for subatmospheric pressure in the expiratory phase is available,

A technical description of the means of triggering shall be provided.

The purpose, type, range and sensing position of all measuring and display devices either incorporated into the ventilator or recommended by the manufacturer.

The internal volume of any breathing attachments or other components or subassemblies recommended by the manufacturer to be placed between the patient connection port and the patient. The manufacturer shall disclose the test method on request.

Details of any restrictions on the location or sequence of components, or both, within the ventilator breathing system for example where such components are flow-direction-sensitive.

7. Power Input

Clause 7 of the GENERAL STANDARD applies.

SECTION TWO—ENVIRONMENTAL CONDITIONS

8. Basic Safety Categories

Appendix A1.2 of the GENERAL STANDARD applies.

9. Removable Protective Means

Not used, Replaced by subclause 6.1z).

10. Environmental Conditions

Clause 10 of the GENERAL STANDARD applies with the following additions:

10.2.3 Pneumatic Power—The ANESTHESIA GAS SUPPLY DEVICE and ANESTHESIA VENTILATOR shall continue to function within the specified tolerance throughout the specified range of pressure variation.

The time weighted average input flow required by the ANESTHESIA GAS SUPPLY DEVICE and ANESTHESIA VENTILATOR shall not exceed 60 L/min at a pressure of 50 +0/–5 psig measured at the gas inlet connector.

Test for compliance by simulating a pressure variation throughout the range specified by the manufacturer, while confirming that the ANESTHESIA GAS SUPPLY DEVICE and ANESTHESIA VENTILATOR continue to perform according to specification.

11. (Previous Title): Special Measures with Respect to Safety

Not used.

12. (Previous Title): Single Fault Condition

Not used. (Transferred to Sub-Clause 3.6).

SECTION THREE—PROTECTION AGAINST ELECTRICAL SHOCK HAZARDS

13. General

Clause 13 of the GENERAL STANDARD applies.

14. Requirements Related to Classification

Clause 14 of the GENERAL STANDARD applies.

15. Limitation of Voltage and/or Energy

Clause 15 of the GENERAL STANDARD applies.

16. ENCLOSURES and PROTECTIVE COVERS

Clause 16 of the GENERAL STANDARD applies.

17. Separation (Previous Title: Insulation and Protective Impedances)

Clause 17 of the GENERAL STANDARD applies.

18. Protective Earthing, Functional Earthing and Potential Equalization

Clause 18 of the GENERAL STANDARD applies.

19. Continuous Leakage Current and Patient Auxiliary Current

Clause 19 of the GENERAL STANDARD applies with the following amendment:

Amendment:

19.4 h) *R* Measurement of the patient leakage current.

The patient leakage current shall be measured from all APPLIED PARTS classified as the same type (See clause 14.6 of the GENERAL STANDARD). These parts shall be connected together electrically. Parts connected to the protective earth terminal shall be tested separately.

The leakage current limits specified in AAMI ES-1[6] apply.

20. Dielectric Strength

Clause 20 of the GENERAL STANDARD applies.

SECTION FOUR—PROTECTION AGAINST MECHANICAL HAZARDS

21. Mechanical Strength

Clause 21 of the GENERAL STANDARD applies.

22. Moving Parts

Clause 22 of the GENERAL STANDARD applies.

23. Surfaces, Corners, and Edges

Clause 23 of the GENERAL STANDARD applies.

24. Stability in NORMAL USE

Clause 24 of the GENERAL STANDARD applies with the following addition.

Addition:

The manufacturer shall specify any weight limits or placement restrictions, or both, under which Clause 24 of the GENERAL STANDARD is met.

25. Expelled Parts

Clause 25 of the GENERAL STANDARD applies.

26. Vibration and Noise

Not used.

27. Pneumatic and Hydraulic Power

Under consideration.

28. Suspended Masses

Clause 28 of the GENERAL STANDARD applies.

SECTION FIVE—PROTECTION AGAINST HAZARDS FROM UNWANTED OR EXCESSIVE RADIATION

29. X-Radiation

Clause 29 of the GENERAL STANDARD applies.

30. Alpha, Beta, Gamma, Neutron Radiation and Other Particle Radiation

Under consideration.

31. Microwave Radiation

Under consideration.

32. Light Radiation (Including Lasers)

Under consideration.

33. Infra-Red Radiation

Under consideration.

34. Ultra-Violet Radiation

Under consideration.

35. Acoustical Energy (Including Ultrasonics)

Under consideration.

36. Electromagnetic Compatibility

The requirements in Clause 36 of the GENERAL STANDARD apply with the following additions.

Additions:

36.1 IEC 601-1-2[2] applies with the following additions:

Addition:

36.2 Clause 36 of IEC 601-1-2[2] applies with the following addition:

If an anomaly occurs, such as display interrupt, alarm activation, etc., it shall be possible to restore normal operation within 30 s after the electrostatic discharges have been applied. (SILENCING of an activated alarm shall not be considered a failure.)

SECTION SIX — PROTECTION AGAINST HAZARDS OF IGNITION OF FLAMMABLE MIXTURES

37. Locations and Basic Requirements

R This clause of the GENERAL STANDARD does not apply.

38. Marking and Accompanying Documents

R This clause of the GENERAL STANDARD does not apply

39. Common Requirements for CATEGORY AP and CATEGORY EQUIPMENT

R This clause of the GENERAL STANDARD does not apply

40. Requirements and Tests for CATEGORY AP EQUIPMENT, Parts and Components Thereof

R This clause of the GENERAL STANDARD does not apply

41. Requirements and Test for CATEGORY APG EQUIPMENT, Parts and Components Thereof

R This clause of the GENERAL STANDARD does not apply

---

[6] Available from AAMI, Association for Advancement of Medical Instrumentations, 3330 Washington Blvd., Suite 400, Arlington, VA 22201–4598.

SECTION SEVEN—PROTECTION AGAINST EXCESSIVE TEMPERATURES, AND OTHER SAFETY HAZARDS

42. Excessive Temperatures

Clause 42 of the GENERAL STANDARD applies.

43. Fire Prevention

Clause 43 of the GENERAL STANDARD applies with the following additions:

Additions:

43.1 *R* In order to reduce the risk to patients, other persons or the surroundings due to fire, ignitable material, under normal and single fault condition, shall not at the same time be subjected to conditions in which:

The temperature of the material is raised to its minimum ignition temperature, and

An oxidant is present.

The minimum ignition temperature is determined in accordance with IEC 79-4[2] using the oxidizing conditions present under normal and single fault condition.

Compliance is checked by determining the temperature the material is raised to under normal and single fault condition.

If sparking can occur under normal or single fault condition(s), the material subjected to the energy dissipation of the spark shall not ignite under the oxidizing conditions present.

Compliance is checked by observing if ignition occurs under the most unfavorable combination of normal condition(s) with a single fault.

44. Overflow, spillage, leakage, humidity, ingress of liquids, cleaning, sterilization and disinfection

Clause 44 of the GENERAL STANDARD applies with the following additions:

Additions:

44.3 The ANESTHESIA WORKSTATION and its components shall be so constructed that spillage does not wet component parts which when wetted can cause a safety hazard.

Test for Compliance

Test in accordance with Clause 44.3 of the GENERAL STANDARD.

44.7 All components not specified by the manufacturer as single patient use, which come into contact with exhaled patient gas that may be rebreathed, shall be capable of being sterilized or disinfected unless means are provided for bacterial/viral filtration between the components and the patient.

Verify by visual inspection of the accompanying documents.

45. Pressure Vessels and Parts Subject to PRESSURE

Clause 45 of the GENERAL STANDARD applies.

46. Human Errors

Clause 46 of the General Standard applies with the following addition:

NOTE 4—In order to minimize OPERATOR errors and consider human factors in the design of ANESTHESIA WORKSTATIONS, monitors and controls that merit the OPERATOR's close attention should be arranged close to the OPERATOR's line of sight when observing the patient. It is also recommended that the contents of AAMI HE-48[6] be reviewed. While general guidance may be obtained from AAMI HE-48[6], the involvement in the device's design of individuals with human factors expertise is strongly urged.

47. Electrostatic Charges

Not used.

48. Materials in APPLIED PARTS in Contact with the Body of the Patient

Not used.

49. Interruption of the Power Supply

Clause 49 of the GENERAL STANDARD applies with the following additions:

Additions:

49.5*R* Means shall be provided to ensure continuous fresh gas flow and automatic ventilation during an interruption of the mains electrical power up to 30 min in duration.

49.6*R* There shall be at least a LOW PRIORITY ALARM when there is an automatic switch over to a RESERVE ELECTRICAL POWER SUPPLY. This alarm shall not be capable of being disabled.

49.7*R* When the RESERVE ELECTRICAL POWER SUPPLY reaches a level specified by the manufacturer to be such that failure of the RESERVE ELECTRICAL POWER SUPPLY is imminent, there shall be a MEDIUM PRIORITY ALARM. This alarm shall not be capable of being disabled.

49.8*R* There shall be a means for the OPERATOR to determine that the output of the RESERVE ELECTRICAL POWER SUPPLY is within the manufacturer's specified range.

Tests for Compliance:

49.5.1 *Verify by functional testing according to the manufacturer's instructions.*

49.6.1 *Verify that a LOW PRIORITY ALARM is activated upon the automatic switch over to the RESERVE ELECTRICAL POWER SUPPLY, and that this alarm cannot be disabled.*

49.7.1 *Verify by functional testing according to the manufacturer's instructions, that the MEDIUM PRIORITY ALARM is activated, and that this alarm cannot be disabled.*

49.8.1 *Verify by visual inspection.*

SECTION EIGHT—ACCURACY OF OPERATING DATA AND PROTECTION AGAINST INCORRECT OUTPUT

50. Accuracy of Operating Data

Clause 50 of the GENERAL STANDARD applies.

51. Protection Against Hazardous Output

Clause 51 of the GENERAL STANDARD applies with the following additions:

Additions:

51.5 The particular requirements of MONITORING, ALARM, and PROTECTION DEVICE(s) apply when the ANESTHESIA WORKSTATION is under normal power supply condition.

51.6 Each ANESTHESIA WORKSTATION or individual DELIVERY SYSTEM/DEVICE intended for use in a ANESTHESIA WORKSTATION shall either:

(*a*) Be provided with MONITORING, ALARM and PROTECTION DEVICE(s) specified in this specification, or,

(*b*) If such devices are not provided with the ANESTHESIA WORKSTATION, the manufacturer of the individual DELIVERY SYSTEM/DEVICE shall provide information about the MONITORING, ALARM and PROTECTION devices required.

Test for compliance by examination of the ANESTHESIA WORKSTATION, or by examination of the accompanying documents of the individual device(s) or system(s).

NOTE 5—The particular requirements for these PROTECTION DEVICE(s) are specified in Clause 51 of this specification. A tabulation of the different DELIVERY SYSTEM/DEVICE(s) and their associated MONITORING, ALARM and PROTECTION DEVICE(s) is summarized in Table 3.

NOTE 6—National or regional regulatory bodies may determine which PROTECTION DEVICE(s) shall be used with specific delivery devices in addition to the essential ones listed in this specification.

51.7 ALARM DEVICES

51.7.1 ALARM DEVICE(S) specified in this specification shall be grouped into one or more of three categories—HIGH PRIORITY, MEDIUM PRIORITY, LOW PRIORITY. These alarms shall comply with the requirements of Specification F 1463[7].

NOTE 7—The audible alarm signals should allow DISABLING by the OPERATOR during the administration of anesthesia, and should be capable of being disabled until the ANESTHESIA WORKSTATION is connected to the patient in order to prevent nuisance alarms unless otherwise specified by this standard.

51.7.2 If an alarm can be disabled by the OPERATOR, there shall be a visual indication that it has been disabled.

51.7.3 Audible alarm SILENCING by the OPERATOR shall not prevent the audible alarm from being activated by a new or different alarm condition.

51.7.4 The set points of adjustable alarms shall be indicated continuously, or on OPERATOR demand.

51.7.5 If either automatic change or OPERATOR adjustable change of alarm priority is provided it shall not be to a lower priority level than that specified in this specification.

51.7.6 If an interface for a remote alarm is provided, the interface shall be designed so that a failure in the remote alarm will not affect the correct functioning of the ANESTHESIA WORKSTATION.

51.7.7 R When a HIGH PRIORITY ALARM is activated and when the condition causing the alarm has cleared, the auditory signal shall reset automatically.

When an alarm that is specified as HIGH PRIORITY ALARM in this specification is activated and when the condition causing the alarm has cleared, it shall be possible for the OPERATOR to determine the alarm variable that caused the alarm, and that a HIGH PRIORITY ALARM had been activated.

The maximum time for which a HIGH PRIORITY ALARM can be silenced shall be 120 s.

Alarms specified as HIGH PRIORITY ALARM(s) in this specification shall not be capable of being disabled.

51.7.8 When a MEDIUM PRIORITY ALARM is activated and when the condition causing the alarm has cleared, the auditory signal shall reset automatically. The maximum time for which the MEDIUM PRIORITY ALARM can be silenced shall be 120 s.

51.8 Ventilatory Monitoring, Alarm, and Protection

51.8.1 The ANESTHESIA WORKSTATION shall be provided with the MONITORING, ALARM and PROTECTION DEVICE(s) as specified in Clause 51, or the manufacturer of the ANESTHESIA WORKSTATION shall state in the accompanying documents that such device(s) is/are required. The characteristics associated with each of these monitors and alarms are also specified in Clause 51.

NOTE 8—The displays of these monitors should be updated according to clinical needs and the risks associated with the variable being monitored.

Test for Compliance

Examine the ANESTHESIA WORKSTATION and the accompanying documents to verify compliance with Clause 51.

51.8.2 Operating Requirements

Means shall be provided to ensure that the specified monitors and alarms are enabled and functioning prior to use. (See Clause 72)

NOTE 9—These monitors and alarms may be automatically enabled and made to function by turning on the ANESTHESIA WORKSTATION, or the monitors and alarms can be manually enabled and made functional by following a pre-use check list.

Verify that all monitors and alarms are either enabled and functioning automatically, or by following the pre-use check list procedure in Clause 72.

51.8.2.1 Automatic Enabling

Means shall be provided that the monitor and alarms mentioned in clauses 51.9.3 (breathing system pressure), and 51.11 (oxygen concentration) shall be in the enabled condition and functioning automatically whenever the anesthesia gas supply device is in use. In addition, either the exhaled volume monitor (Clause 51.9.4) or the ventilatory Carbon Dioxide Monitor, or both, (Clause 51.10.5) shall be in the enabled condition and functioning automatically whenever the anesthesia gas supply device is in use.

51.8.2.2 For all other specified moniters, means shall be provided to ensure that the moniters and alarms are enabled and functioning prior to use.

NOTE 10—These additional monitors and alarms may be automatically enabled and made to function by turning on the anesthesia gas supply device, or the moniters and the alarms can be manually enabled and made functional by following a pre-use check list. (See Clause 72)

Test for Compliance

51.9.3 Breathing System Pressure (See also Clause 51.8.2)

51.9.3.1 Pressure Monitoring

The ANESTHESIA WORKSTATION shall be provided with a means to display continuously the pressure in the ANESTHESIA BREATHING SYSTEM, or the manufacturer(s) of the ANESTHESIA VENTILATOR and ANESTHESIA BREATHING SYSTEM shall state in the accompanying documents that such a means is required.

[7] *Annual Book of ASTM Standards*, Vol 13.01.

51.9.3.2 Pressure Alarm Device

51.9.3.2.1 The pressure monitor shall have associated ALARM DEVICES designed to activate a HIGH PRIORITY ALARM signal when the pressure in the ANESTHESIA BREATHING SYSTEM:

(*a*) Exceeds the OPERATOR adjustable limit for high pressure;

NOTE 11—This may be coupled to the OPERATOR adjustable pressure limitation device.

(*b*) Exceeds a OPERATOR adjustable limit for continuing positive pressure for 15 s ± 1.0 s. When PEEP is in use, this alarm shall be OPERATOR adjustable at a level no more than 30 cm H_2O above the set PEEP, or manufacturer preset at a level no more than 10 cm H_2O above the preset PEEP. The manufacturer's preset level above PEEP shall be stated in the accompanying documents:

(*c*) Is less than negative 10 cm H_2O for greater than 1.0 s.

Test for Compliance

After recommended calibration and warm up procedures have been completed, perform the following tests to ensure that the pressure monitoring and alarms comply with 51.6.3.2.1

Connect the ANESTHESIA BREATHING SYSTEM to a test lung, and induce a pressure rise in the ANESTHESIA BREATHING SYSTEM. Verify that the pressure monitor is functioning. Adjust continuing positive airway pressure alarm limits to the maximum value, if applicable. This alarm shall sound 15 ± 1s after airway pressure reaches this alarm limit. Permit the system pressure to continue to rise until the high pressure alarm limit is reached, at which time this alarm shall sound. Verify the activation of both visual and audible HIGH PRIORITY ALARM signal(s) in both conditions.

Compliance shall be determined by visual inspection, and functional testing by means of simulating the alarm condition in accordance with the accompanying documents.

51.9.3.2.3 When automatic ventilation is in use, there shall be at least a MEDIUM PRIORITY ALARM whenever the breathing system pressure falls below the alarm limit for more than 20 s. This alarm can be preset by the manufacturer, or can be OPERATOR adjustable. If OPERATOR adjustable, the alarm shall not be capable of being set lower than 5 ± 0.5 cm H_2O.

Compliance shall be determined by visual inspection, and functional testing by means of simulating the alarm condition in accordance with the accompanying documents.

51.9.3.3 Pressure Limitation

51.9.3.3.1 The ANESTHESIA WORKSTATION shall be provided with a breathing pressure limiting device which will ensure that the pressure in the ANESTHESIA BREATHING SYSTEM during intended use and under single fault condition shall not exceed 12.5 kPa (125 cm H_2O) or the manufacturer(s) of the ANESTHESIA VENTILATOR and ANESTHESIA BREATHING SYSTEM shall state in the accompanying documents that such a device is required.

An ANESTHESIA VENTILATOR shall be provided with an OPERATOR adjustable pressure limitation to prevent the pressure from exceeding the pressure limit by more than 3 cm H_2O or 15 % of the set value, whichever is the greater, or the manufacturer(s) of the ANESTHESIA VENTILATOR shall state in the accompanying documents that such a device is required.

The range within which the pressure limitation may be adjustable shall be stated by the manufacturer. This range shall include 20 cm H_2O.

NOTE 12—A reservoir bag complying with Specification F 1204[7] may be considered as a pressure limiting device for an ANESTHESIA WORKSTATION without a ventilator, or when the ventilator module is in the manual or spontaneous breathing mode.

Test for Compliance—Introduce a pressure rise in the ANESTHESIA BREATHING SYSTEM and verify compliance with Clause 51.9.3.3.1.

51.9.3.4 Anesthesia Breathing System Disconnect Alarm

51.9.3.4.1R The ANESTHESIA WORKSTATION shall be provided with at least a MEDIUM PRIORITY ALARM signal that activates in the event of a complete disconnection in the ANESTHESIA BREATHING SYSTEM.

NOTE 13—Alarms considered to comply with the above include, but are not limited to, low pressure, low or zero CO_2, and low volume.

NOTE 14—MONITORING DEVICES indicate specific alarm conditions and do not differentiate between possible causes.

Test for Compliance—Disconnect, in turn, each OPERATOR detachable connection of the ANESTHESIA VENTILATOR or ANESTHESIA BREATHING SYSTEM, or both, recommended by the manufacturer. Use the test method(s) specified by the manufacturer, and verify that the alarm(s) is/are activated.

51.9.4 Exhaled Volume (See also Clause 51.8.2)

51.9.4.1 The ANESTHESIA WORKSTATION shall be provided with a device to monitor the patient's exhaled tidal or minute volume, or both, or the manufacturer(s) of the ANESTHESIA VENTILATOR shall state in the accompanying documents that such a device is required. The accuracy of the displayed value shall be within ± 20 % of the actual value above 100 ml tidal volume, or ± 20 % of the actual value above 3 L/min minute volume. See Clause 6.8.2 w) for disclosure requirements below 100 mL tidal volume and 3 L/min minute volume.

51.9.4.2 *Test for compliance by visual and mechanical inspection. Connect an ANESTHESIA BREATHING SYSTEM to a test lung and adjust the parameters of the test lung and variables of ventilator performance as close as possible to values in Table 4 and in accordance with the intended use. Ventilate the test lung until measured exhaled volumes are stable. Verify compliance with 51.9.4.1.*

51.9.4.3 An alarm of at least MEDIUM PRIORITY shall be activated if the patient's exhaled volume falls below an OPERATOR adjustable minimum. If the MEDIUM PRIORITY ALARM can be delayed, the delay shall not exceed 90 s. The delay may be OPERATOR adjustable.

Test for Compliance—Connect the exhaled volume monitor to an ANESTHESIA BREATHING SYSTEM according to the manufacturer's instructions. Set the adjustable alarm delay, if provided, to its maximum setting. Ventilate a test lung until the monitor readings are stable. Reduce the volume of ventilation until the exhaled volume falls below the OPERATOR adjustable low volume alarm setting. Confirm that the MEDIUM PRIORITY ALARM is activated within 90 s.

51.10.5 Ventilatory Carbon Dioxide (See also Clause 51.8.2)

51.10.5.1 The ANESTHESIA WORKSTATION shall be provided with a device to monitor continuously the patient's ventilatory CO_2, or the manufacturer(s) of the ANESTHESIA BREATHING SYSTEM shall state in the accompanying documents that such a means is required.

Test for Compliance:
Verify by visual inspection.

51.10.5.2 The CO_2 monitor shall meet the requirements of Specification F 1456[7].

Test for Compliance:
Verify by visual inspection.

51.11 Inspiratory Oxygen Concentration Monitoring (See also Clause 51.8.2)

51.11.1 The ANESTHESIA WORKSTATION shall be provided with an oxygen monitor in compliance with Specification F 1462[7] for measurement of the O_2 concentration in the inspiratory limb or the Y-piece, or the manufacturer(s) of the ANESTHESIA GAS SUPPLY DEVICE and ANESTHESIA BREATHING SYSTEM shall state in the accompanying documents that such a means is required.

51.11.2 The oxygen monitor shall be provided with an adjustable low O_2 concentration alarm. A HIGH PRIORITY ALARM shall be activated within 30 s after the inspiratory oxygen concentration falls below the low oxygen concentration alarm limit. This 30 s time shall include the delay time of the oxygen monitor and the response time. The low oxygen concentration alarm shall not be adjustable below 18 % volume concentration.

Compliance Test
Compliance shall be tested by visual inspection and functional testing by means of generating an O_2 concentration below the set alarm limit.

NOTE 15—The monitoring of oxygen concentration in the fresh gas is also recommended.

51.12 Oxygen Supply Failure ALARM Protection

51.12.1 The ANESTHESIA GAS SUPPLY DEVICE shall be designed so that whenever the oxygen supply pressure is reduced to below the manufacturer-specified minimum the delivered oxygen concentration shall not decrease below 19 % at the COMMON GAS OUTLET. The performance of the ANESTHESIA GAS SUPPLY DEVICE under these conditions shall be stated in the accompanying documents.

51.12.2 Whenever the oxygen supply pressure falls below the manufacturer-specified threshold, at least a MEDIUM PRIORITY ALARM shall be activated within 5 s. This alarm shall not be capable of being disabled.

Test for Compliance:

51.12.1.1 *Test for compliance by visual inspection and by functional testing by simulating the conditions described in Clause 51.12.1 and according to the accompanying documents.*

51.12.2.1 *Attach a source of oxygen capable of being adjusted to pressures above and below the manufacturer's specified minimum oxygen pressure to the oxygen cylinder attachment of the ANESTHESIA GAS SUPPLY DEVICE,*

Adjust the oxygen pressure to below the manufacturer's specified minimum oxygen pressure. Verify that the auditory and visual alarms are activated.

51.13 Protection Against Accidental Delivery of Hypoxic Gas Mixtures

51.13.1 The ANESTHESIA WORKSTATION shall be provided with a device to protect against an OPERATOR selected delivery of a mixture of oxygen and nitrous oxide having an oxygen concentration below 21 % oxygen (V/V) in the fresh gas or in the inspiratory gas. If an override mechanism is provided to permit OPERATOR selection of oxygen concentration below 21 % (V/V), the activation of this mechanism shall be continuously indicated.

Test for Compliance:

Set the machine to deliver 30 % oxygen at the COMMON GAS OUTLET or at the patient connection port, and verify that 30 % oxygen is being delivered in the inspiratory gas or fresh gas.

Attempt to reduce the oxygen concentration below 21 % by any OPERATOR accessible means available on the ANESTHESIA WORKSTATION.

Verify that the oxygen concentration at the COMMON GAS OUTLET or at the patient connection port does not fall below 21 %.

51.14 Agent Concentration Monitor and Alarm

51.14.1 The ANESTHESIA WORKSTATION shall be provided with a device to monitor the concentration of anesthetic vapor in the inspiratory gas, or the manufacturer(s) of the ANESTHETIC VAPOR DELIVERY DEVICE(s) shall state in the accompanying documents that such a means is required. The monitor shall comply with the requirements of Specification F 1452[7].

NOTE 16—Monitoring of the anesthetic vapor concentration in the fresh gas and the expiratory gas is recommended.

Verify by visual inspection of the accompanying documents.

51.15 Other Monitors

To complete an ANESTHESIA WORKSTATION and comply with the ASA [8] and AANA[9] Monitoring Guidelines:

51.15.1 The ANESTHESIA WORKSTATION shall be provided with a device to monitor arterial hemoglobin oxygen saturation, or the manufacturer of the ANESTHESIA WORKSTATION shall state in the accompanying documents that such a means is required. If non-invasive, the monitor shall comply with the requirements of Specification F 1415.[7]

Verify by visual inspection of the accompanying documents.

51.15.2 The ANESTHESIA WORKSTATION shall be provided with a device to monitor the patient's blood pressure, or the manufacturer of the ANESTHESIA WORKSTATION shall state in the accompanying documents that such a means is required. The blood pressure monitor shall comply with the requirements of applicable standards for invasive or non-invasive blood pressure monitoring devices, AAMI BP22[6] and SP10[6] respectively.

Verify by visual inspection of the accompanying documents.

51.15.3 The ANESTHESIA WORKSTATION shall be provided with an electrocardiographic monitoring device, or the

[8] Available from American Society of Anesthesiologists, 520 N. Northwest Highway, Park Ridge, IL 60068–2573.

[9] Available from American Association of Nurse Anesthetists, 222 South Prospect Ave., Park Ridge, IL 60068.

manufacturer of the ANESTHESIA WORKSTATION shall state in the accompanying documents that such a device is required. This monitor shall comply with the requirements of AAMI EC13.[6]

Verify by visual inspection of the accompanying documents.

SECTION NINE—ABNORMAL OPERATION AND FAULT CONDITIONS; ENVIRONMENTAL TESTS

52. Abnormal Operation and Fault Conditions

Clause 52 of the GENERAL STANDARD applies.

53. Environmental Tests

Clause 53 of the GENERAL STANDARD applies

SECTION TEN—CONSTRUCTIONAL REQUIREMENTS

54. General

Clause 54 of the GENERAL STANDARD applies with the following additions.

Additions:

54.4 A single fault condition shall not cause a MONITORING DEVICE or ALARM DEVICE, or both, in accordance with Clause 51 of this standard and its corresponding ANESTHESIA WORKSTATION control function, to fail in such a way that the monitoring or alarm function, or both, becomes ineffective, simultaneous with its corresponding control function (that is, a failure of the ANESTHESIA WORKSTATION function cannot be detected by the corresponding monitoring or alarm function, or both.)

NOTE 17—All manually operated controls should be designed to minimize unintentional change from a set position.

55. Enclosures and Covers

Not Used

56. Components and General Assembly

Clause 56 of the GENERAL STANDARD applies with the following addition:

56.12 This ANESTHESIA WORKSTATION standard supersedes IEC 601-2-13[2].

57. Mains Parts, Components and Layout

Clause 57 of the GENERAL STANDARD applies with the following additions and amendments:

Amendment:

57.2e) *R* Auxiliary mains socket outlets on non- permanently installed equipment, intended for the provision of mains supply to other equipment, or to separated parts of equipment, shall be of a type complying with requirements of IEC 320.[2] (See Fig. 1.)

Such auxiliary mains socket outlets shall be marked in accordance with Clause 6.1k.

NOTE 18—Local codes and requirement may mandate the use of "hospital grade" outlets of NEMA[10] style 5-15.

[10] Available from National Electrical Manufacturers Association, NEMA, 1300 North 17th Street, Suite 1847, Rosslyn, VA 22209

Compliance is checked by inspection.

Addition

57.3a)*R*—The mains supply cord of an electrically powered ANESTHESIA WORKSTATION shall be a non-detachable cord or shall be protected against accidental disconnection.

Compliance is checked by inspection and, for equipment when provided with an appliance coupler, by the following test:

The detachable cord is subjected for 1 min to an axial pull of force as shown in Table 5.

During the test, the mains connector shall not become disconnected from the appliance inlet.

57.6 Main Fuses and Over Current Releases

Addition

R— The ANESTHESIA WORKSTATION and each auxiliary mains socket outlet shall be provided with separate fuses or over-current releases as required for a single equipment in sub-clause 57.6.

These fuses or overcurrent releases shall be designed such that the ANESTHESIA WORKSTATION, including the auxiliary mains socket outlets, shall maintain normal function with each auxiliary mains socket outlet, loaded to the maximum.

When each auxiliary mains socket in turn is additionally overloaded by a factor of 7.5 ± 2.5, all remaining auxiliary mains socket outlets and the ANESTHESIA WORKSTATION shall maintain normal function.

Test for compliance by visual inspection and functional testing.

58. Protective Earthing—Terminals and Connections

Clause 58 of the GENERAL STANDARD applies.

59. Construction and Layout

Clause 59 of the GENERAL STANDARD applies.

ADDITIONAL REQUIREMENTS FOR ANESTHESIA WORKSTATIONS

60. Medical Gas Cylinder Attachments

60.1 The ANESTHESIA WORKSTATION shall be provided with at least one attachment for an oxygen cylinder. All medical gas cylinder attachments shall be pin - indexed post - type valves complying with the requirements of CGA V-1-1987.[5]

60.2 All medical gas cylinder attachments shall be provided with a filter (100 μm maximum) for the entrapment of particulate matter prior to delivery of the gas to the GAS PRESSURE REDUCING DEVICE/SYSTEM or FLOW ADJUSTMENT CONTROL(s).

60.3 Each medical gas cylinder attachment shall incorporate a clamping device by which the valve of the cylinder can be adequately forced against a seal to provide a leak resistant gas conduit.

60.4 Each medical gas cylinder attachment shall be designed to prevent tightening of the clamping device until the pins of the pin-indexed safety system are correctly engaged with the appropriate pin-indexed safety system pin-receiving holes of the cylinder valve.

60.5 If two or more interconnected cylinder attachments are provided for the attachment of cylinders of the same gas, a means shall be provided to limit under normal conditions, the leakage from an attached cylinder to either an empty cylinder or to atmosphere, to less than 100 mL/min throughout the pressure range of 1380 kPa to the maximum pressure for the respective gas (that is, N_2O-5168 kPa, O_2 and AIR - 15 180 kPa).

Tests for Compliance:

60.1.1 *Verify by visual inspection.*

60.2.1 *Verify by visual inspection presence of the filter. Confirm that filter size does not exceed 100 μm.*

60.3.1 *Verify by visual inspection.*

60.4.1 *Verify by trying to clamp the post valve of the cylinder to the cylinder attachment without pins being aligned.*

60.5.1 *If two or more interconnected cylinder attachments are provided for the attachment of cylinders of the same gas, pressurize each cylinder attachment inlet with a gas source at varying pressures from 1380 kPa to the maximum pressure for the respective gas (that is, N_2O - 5168 kPa, O_2 and AIR 15 180 kPa). Measure the rate of leakage from the other cylinder attachment.*

If applicable, repeat the above procedure, but measure the rate of leakage to atmosphere.

61. Medical Gas Supply Pressure Indicator(s)

61.1 The ANESTHESIA WORKSTATION shall be equipped with a pressure indicator that indicates the cylinder pressure of each gas. The scale of the pressure indicator shall extend to a pressure at least 33 % greater than the maximum filling pressure of the cylinder, or the full indication position, at a temperature of 20 ± 3°C.

The pressure indicator shall be at least Grade B in accordance with ANSI/ASME B40.1[2] for indicating dial elastic element pressure gauges, and for other types of pressure indicators, the accuracy shall be at least ± (4 % of the full scale reading + 8 % of the actual reading).

This pressure indicator shall be LEGIBLE from the front of the ANESTHESIA WORKSTATION.

61.2 When only one pressure indicator is supplied for a specific gas where more than one medical gas cylinder attachment is provided for that gas, it shall be possible to determine the pressures in each of the separate cylinders.

NOTE 19—Pressure indicators cannot accurately indicate the quantitative contents of medical gas cylinders containing liquefied gas.

61.3 The ANESTHESIA WORKSTATION shall be equipped with a means to monitor the pressure for each gas supplied from a MEDICAL GAS PIPELINE SYSTEM. The monitoring point shall be upstream from the unidirectional valve.

This pressure indicator shall be LEGIBLE from the front of the ANESTHESIA WORKSTATION.

61.4 If in a single fault condition the pressure from the pressure sensing element can be conveyed to the gauge case or enclosure, the gauge shall be designed and constructed in such a manner that when a pressure equal to the maximum indicated on the dial or display is applied to a gauge having the pressure sensor removed, no parts shall be expelled free of the gauge enclosure. Gauge cases or enclosures shall have means of venting to prevent internal pressure buildup.

61.5 All elastic element type pressure indicators on the ANESTHESIA WORKSTATION shall be of cleanliness Class IV or higher as outlined for oxygen gauges in ANSI/ASME B40.1.[2]

61.6 The lowest pressure indication on all analog gauge scales or electronically displayed scales on a ANESTHESIA WORKSTATION shall be:

(a) (*a*) For dial type gauges, in the lower left quadrant of the dial face (that is, between 6 and 9 of a clock face),

(b) (*b*) For horizontal gauge faces, at the left of the scale, and

(c) (*c*) For vertical gauge faces, at the bottom of the scale.

61.7 Mechanical and electronic indicators shall be LEGIBLE.

Tests for Compliance:

61.1 *Verify by visual inspection.*

61.2.1 *Verify by visual inspection and sequential manipulation of cylinder valves.*

61.3.1 *Verify by visual inspection.*

61.4.1 *Verify presence of venting means by visual inspection.*

61.5.1 *Verify by inspection or evidence of certificate of compliance by the manufacturer.*

61.6.1 *Verify by visual inspection.*

61.7.1 *Verify by visual inspection.*

62. Gas Pressure Reducing Device/System

62.1 A GAS PRESSURE REDUCING DEVICE/SYSTEM shall be employed for each gas supplied from cylinders.

62.2 The gas flow from cylinders to the ANESTHESIA GAS SUPPLY DEVICE shall not exceed 10 mL/min when pressure in the MEDICAL GAS PIPELINE SYSTEM is 345 kPa (50 psig).

NOTE 20—Means should be provided to ensure that the ANESTHESIA GAS SUPPLY DEVICE uses gas from the MEDICAL GAS PIPELINE SYSTEM as long as the pressure is 345 kPa (50 psig) or greater.

62.3 An O_2 flow of 2 L/min shall be restored to 2 ± 0.1 L/min within a period of 2 s after operation of the oxygen flush.

62.4 To ensure safety of the ANESTHESIA WORKSTATION, adjacent structures, and personnel, a single GAS PRESSURE REDUCING DEVICE/SYSTEM, or the first of a series of GAS PRESSURE REDUCING DEVICE/SYSTEM in a series, shall meet either of the following requirements:

(a) (*a*) The GAS PRESSURE REDUCING DEVICE/SYSTEM shall be equipped with a pressure relieving device that opens at not more than four times the normal delivery pressure of that GAS PRESSURE REDUCING DEVICE/SYSTEM and at no more than two-thirds of the minimum burst pressure of the diaphragm. The pressure relieving device shall also be capable of venting the GAS PRESSURE REDUCING DEVICE/SYSTEM at the maximum relief pressure not exceeding the minimum burst pressure of the diaphragm when a pressure 50 % greater than the normal supply pressure of the corresponding gas is applied, or

(b) (*b*) The GAS PRESSURE REDUCING DEVICE/SYSTEM shall be designed to ensure rupture of its diaphragm, without hazard to its environment due to flying fragments, at a pressure not greater than 2760 kPa (400 psig). The diaphragm shall not rupture at pressures less than 1380 kPa (200 psig).

Tests for Compliance:

62.1.1 *Visually inspect the ANESTHESIA WORKSTATION to confirm that each gas circuit where the inlet pressure normally exceeds 345 ± 10 kPa (50 ± 1.5 psig) contains a GAS PRESSURE REDUCING DEVICE/SYSTEM.*

62.2.1 *Perform the following test to confirm that the GAS PRESSURE REDUCING DEVICE/SYSTEM complies with clause 62.2. These tests must be performed first with oxygen. After completing the test with oxygen, the oxygen supply must be left connected and the oxygen lines pressurized to 345 ± 10 kPa (50 ± 1.5 psig) before proceeding with the tests for other gases.*

Close all FLOW ADJUSTMENT CONTROL(s) and flush valves and shut "OFF" all other gases. Connect a compressed gas supply at a pressure of at least 90 % of the maximum cylinder pressure for the respective gas (that is, N_2O - 5168 kPa (750 psig), O_2 and AIR 15 180 kPa (2200 psig)) to one cylinder inlet connection; seal all other cylinder and pipeline inlet connectors for the gas. Verify that there is no leakage by opening the cylinder valve for a few seconds and then reclosing; adjust connections until the cylinder pressure indicator reading does not fall discernibly within 1 min after closing the cylinder valve.

Open the cylinder valve and open the FLOW ADJUSTMENT CONTROL to obtain a flowrate of 1.0 ± 0.05 L/min; record the cylinder pressure, (P_1).

Close the cylinder valve and measure the time (t_1) (in seconds) required for the cylinder pressure to fall to a value (P_2), that is between 10 and 20 % of (P_1).

Connect the pipeline inlet of the ANESTHESIA WORKSTATION to a supply of gas at 345 ± 10 kPa (50 psi) and reset the flowrate to 1.0 ± 0.05 L/min.

Open the cylinder valve and record the cylinder pressure, (P_3).

Close the cylinder valve and record the time (t_2) (in seconds) required for the cylinder pressure to decrease to a value (P_4), that is 75 to 84 % of P_3. Compute the forward flow, (Q), in mL/min according to the following:

$$Q = 16.67 [ml]P5 [(P_3 - P_4) / (P_1 - P_2)] [ml]P5 (t_1 / T_2) \quad (1)$$

This shall not exceed 10 mL/min.

62.3.1 *Using an indicated oxygen flow of 2.0 L/min, operate the oxygen flush for ten cycles of 10 s duration, with a pause of 5 s between each flush. Check that the flow is restored to 2.0 ± 0.1 L/min within 2 s after each flush.*

62.4.1 *For Option (a) Apply an ever increasing pressure at the outlet of the GAS PRESSURE REDUCING DEVICE/SYSTEM until the relief valve opens. Note this pressure. Continue to increase the pressure until the pressure stops increasing, and note this pressure. Verify that the opening pressure is not greater than four times the normal delivery pressure, and that the maximum pressure measured is less than two-thirds of the minimum burst pressure of the diaphragm.*

For Option (b)—Follow the manufacturer's recommended method for testing rupture of the diaphragm. Verify that the no safety hazard is created as a result of the diaphragm rupture, and that the diaphragm does not rupture at less than 1380 kPa (200 psig).

63. Anesthesia Gas Supply Piping

63.1 There shall be no hazard for patients, OPERATOR(s), or third person(s) arising if the ANESTHESIA GAS SUPPLY PIPING is subjected to the pressure which may occur during any single fault condition

63.2 Except for the venting of air or oxygen from fluidics or pneumatic elements, the leakage from the ANESTHESIA GAS SUPPLY PIPING:

(a) (a) For each gas service between the outlet of the GAS PRESSURE REDUCING DEVICE/SYSTEM and the inlet to the FLOW ADJUSTMENT CONTROL shall not exceed 25 mL/min at the manufacturer's specified normal working pressure, or

(b) (b) For each gas service between the cylinder attachment and/or pipeline inlet(s), including the GAS PRESSURE REDUCING DEVICE/SYSTEM and the inlet to the FLOW ADJUSTMENT CONTROL, this leakage shall not exceed 150 mL/min (corrected to 20 °C) when pressurized to the maximum and minimum inlet pressures for the respective gas service.

63.3 The leakage rate on each gas service between the FLOW ADJUSTMENT CONTROL and the COMMON GAS OUTLET shall not exceed 50 mL/min at a pressure of 3 kPa (30 cm H_2O). If applicable, this requirement shall be met under each of the following conditions:

(a) (a) With one ANESTHETIC VAPOR DELIVERY DEVICE installed and in the "ON" position;

(b) (b) With one ANESTHETIC VAPOR DELIVERY DEVICE installed and in the "OFF" position; and

(c) (c) With the ANESTHETIC VAPOR DELIVERY DEVICE removed if it is designated by the manufacturer as OPERATOR detachable.

Tests for Compliance

63.1.1 *Using oil free air, pressurize the ANESTHESIA GAS SUPPLY PIPING to the maximum pressure obtainable under a single fault condition, and verify that no safety hazard to OPERATOR or third person is created.*

63.2.1 *Compliance is met by completion of a test in accordance with manufacturer's instructions.*

63.3.1 *Compliance is met by completion of a test in accordance with manufacturer's instructions.*

64. Flow Adjustment Control(s)

64.1 When a GAS MIXER is not incorporated into the ANESTHESIA GAS SUPPLY DEVICE, a single FLOW ADJUSTMENT CONTROL shall be provided for each of the different gases supplied to the COMMON GAS OUTLET.

64.2 Each FLOW ADJUSTMENT CONTROL shall maintain for at least 30 min, any set rate of the allowable rates of flow within ± 10 % of the setting or ± 10 mL/min, whichever is the greater, whenever the supply pressures (pipeline or cylinder) and pressures at the COMMON GAS OUTLET vary within the limits specified by the manufacturer.

64.3 Each FLOW ADJUSTMENT CONTROL shall be adjacent to or identifiable with its associated FLOW INDICATOR.

64.4 FLOW ADJUSTMENT CONTROLS shall be located on the front of the ANESTHESIA WORKSTATION.

64.5 For rotary style FLOW ADJUSTMENT CONTROL(s), the oxygen knob shall have the physically distinguishable profile in accordance with Fig. 2. All other rotary style FLOW ADJUSTMENT CONTROL knobs shall be round. The oxygen knob diameter shall not be less than the diameter of any of the knobs controlling the other gases.

NOTE 21—The oxygen knob may project beyond the knobs controlling other gases when the knobs are grouped together.

Other types of FLOW ADJUSTMENT CONTROL(s) shall be designed so that the oxygen FLOW ADJUSTMENT CONTROL looks and feels different from the FLOW ADJUSTMENT CONTROL(s) for the other gases.

64.6 Where the FLOW ADJUSTMENT CONTROL requires a direct rotational motion by the OPERATOR for flowrate adjustment, the FLOW ADJUSTMENT CONTROL shall be designed so that either:

(1) Continuation of rotation will not cause "disassembly" of the FLOW ADJUSTMENT CONTROL, or

(2) Rotation is prevented prior to the point where "disassembly" would occur, or

(3) The stem of each rotary FLOW ADJUSTMENT CONTROL shall be captive so that it cannot be disengaged from its housing without the use of tools.

Tests for Compliance:

64.1.1 *Verify by visual inspection.*

64.2.1 *Attach a flowmeter to the COMMON GAS OUTLET of the ANESTHESIA WORKSTATION or follow the manufacturer's instructions for flow rate verification. Select a flow rate of the available flow rates for a specified gas. Vary the supply pressures and the outlet pressures to the extremes specified by the manufacturer, and verify compliance with Clause 64.2.*

64.3.1 *Verify by visual inspection.*

64.4.1 *Adjust lighting to a level of 215 lux. From a position 1 m in front of the ANESTHESIA WORKSTATION, verify that all FLOW ADJUSTMENT CONTROL(s) are LEGIBLE.*

64.5.1 *For rotary style FLOW ADJUSTMENT CONTROL(s), verify by visual inspection that the FLOW ADJUSTMENT CONTROL(s) comply with the requirements of Clause 64.6 and Fig. 2 for the oxygen-FLOW ADJUSTMENT CONTROL.*

For other types (non - rotary style) of FLOW ADJUSTMENT CONTROL(s) verify that the oxygen control is different from those of other gases.

64.6.1 *Where applicable, verify that when the required rotational motion is applied that the FLOW ADJUSTMENT CONTROL(s) comply with the requirements of Clause 64.6.*

65. Flow Indicators

65.1 When the ANESTHESIA WORKSTATION is equipped with FLOW ADJUSTMENT CONTROL(s), it shall be equipped with one or more FLOW INDICATOR(s) for each gas supplied to the ANESTHESIA WORKSTATION from either MEDICAL GAS PIPELINE SYSTEM(s) or cylinder(s).

65.2 If provided, each FLOW INDICATOR shall be graduated in units of liters per minute. For all flows less than 1 L/min, the flow may be expressed either in millilitres per minute or in decimal fractions of a litre per minute (with a zero before the decimal sign), but shall be consistent on any one ANESTHESIA WORKSTATION.

65.3 The manufacturer shall state in the accompanying documents of the ANESTHESIA WORKSTATION the limits of error for each of the FLOW INDICATORS when measured at ambient conditions of 20°C and 760 mm Hg.

65.4 If provided, the oxygen FLOW INDICATOR shall be on the right most extremity of a bank of FLOW INDICATORS as viewed from the front of the ANESTHESIA WORKSTATION.

65.5 FLOW INDICATORS of the tube type shall be separated or shall be designed to avoid confusion. The graduations shall be marked on the tube, or alternatively, a scale with the graduation markings shall be located immediately adjacent to the tube.

65.6 The name or chemical symbol in accordance with CGA V-5[5] for the gas shall be marked on or adjacent to the FLOW INDICATOR. This marking shall be LEGIBLE. If color coding is used it shall be in conformance with CGA C-9[5] (See Table 1).

NOTE 22—Where oxygen and other gases are delivered by their respective FLOW INDICATORS into a common manifold, the oxygen should be delivered downstream of all other gases.

Test for Compliance:

65.1.1 *Verify by visual inspection.*

65.2.1 *Verify by visual inspection.*

65.3.1 *Verify by reviewing the accompanying documents.*

65.4.1 *Verify by visual inspection.*

65.5.1 *Verify by visual inspection.*

65.6.1 *Verify by visual inspection and review of the accompanying documents.*

66. Gas Mixing System

66.1 When a GAS MIXING SYSTEM is used, there shall be an indication of the gases controlled, the concentration of oxygen (% V/V) in the mixture, and the minimum and maximum oxygen concentrations (% V/V). The range of oxygen concentrations shall be indicated continuously, or on OPERATOR demand.

66.2 At any flow and pressure given in the instructions for use, the oxygen concentration shall be within ± 5 % (V/V) of the set or indicated value.

66.3 Each GAS MIXING SYSTEM control(s) shall be adjacent to or identifiable with its associated indicator(s). The GAS MIXING SYSTEM control(s) or its surrounding shall be durably marked with the name or chemical formula in accordance with CGA V-5. These and the markings required in clause 66.1 shall be LEGIBLE from the front, and if color coding is used it shall be in accordance with CGA C-9[5] (See Table 1).

Test for Compliance:

66.1.1 *Test for compliance by visual inspection.*

66.2.1 *Test the GAS MIXING SYSTEM according to the instructions for use provided by the manufacturer. The accuracy of the indicated value shall be within ± 5 % of the actual value at the minimum indicated O_2 concentration, at 50 % of the maximum indicated O_2 concentration, and at the maximum indicated O_2 concentration for 5 min when tested under the following combinations, (see Table 6) of pressures and flows as* *specified by the manufacturer.*

66.3.1 *Test for compliance by visual inspection.*

67. Oxygen Flush

67.1 **R** The ANESTHESIA WORKSTATION shall be equipped with a manually operated single purpose flush for the delivery of a limited but unmetered flow of oxygen directly to the COMMON GAS OUTLET. The ANESTHESIA WORKSTATION shall not be provided with a flush for any other single gas.

67.2 The oxygen flush shall have only one "OFF" position, and should be designed to minimize unintentional operation.

67.3 The oxygen flush shall be operable with one hand, and be self - closing.

67.4 The oxygen flush shall deliver oxygen at a steady flow of not less than 35 L/min and not exceeding 75 L/min to the COMMON GAS OUTLET of the ANESTHESIA WORKSTATION, when oxygen is supplied to the flush at the manufacturer's specified operating pressure range.

67.5 The flow of oxygen from the oxygen flush shall be delivered to the COMMON GAS OUTLET of the ANESTHESIA WORKSTATION without passing through any ANESTHETIC VAPOR DELIVERY DEVICE(s). Pressure at the outlet of the ANESTHETIC VAPOR DELIVERY DEVICE shall either:

(a) (*a*) Not increase or decrease by more than 10 kPa (100 cm H_2O) during operation of the oxygen flush, when the COMMON GAS OUTLET is open to atmosphere, or

(b) (*b*) When tested as described in Annex A2, the output of anesthetic vapor shall not increase by more than 20 %

Tests for Compliance:

67.1.1 *Verify by visual inspection that the ANESTHESIA WORKSTATION is equipped with an oxygen flush and that no other single gas flush is provided.*

67.2.1 *Verify that the oxygen flush has only one "off" position, and that the possibility of accidental operation has been minimized.*

67.3.1 *Operate the oxygen flush to verify compliance.*

67.4.1 *Using a test flowmeter, verify that the flow delivered at the COMMON GAS OUTLET is between 35 L/min and 75 L/min when the pressure to the inlet of the oxygen flush is within the range specified by the manufacturer.*

67.5.1 *Verify by functional testing according to manufacturers instructions, or by following the test methods given in Annex A2.*

68. Anesthetic Vapor Delivery Device(s)

68.1 All ANESTHETIC VAPOR DELIVERY DEVICE(s) to be used with the ANESTHESIA WORKSTATION shall be concentration calibrated.

68.2 The calibrated control of the ANESTHETIC VAPOR DELIVERY DEVICE(s) shall be marked in such a way that it is LEGIBLE from the front of the ANESTHESIA WORKSTATION.

68.3 A system shall be provided that prevents gas from passing through the chamber or reservoir of one ANESTHETIC VAPOR DELIVERY DEVICE(s) to that of another.

68.4 ANESTHETIC VAPOR DELIVERY DEVICE(s) not intended for use in the ANESTHESIA BREATHING SYSTEM shall have non-interchangeable proprietary fittings or shall have 23 mm conical fittings in compliance with Fig. 3. In no case shall male or female 15 or 22 mm conical fittings be used. When 23 mm conical fittings are used, the inlet to the ANESTHETIC VAPOR DELIVERY DEVICE(s) shall be male and the outlet female.

68.5 The direction of gas flow through the ANESTHETIC VAPOR DELIVERY DEVICE shall be marked with arrows. ANESTHETIC VAPOR DELIVERY DEVICE(s) designed solely for use in the ANESTHESIA BREATHING SYSTEM shall be marked "for use only in the breathing system".

68.6 When tested in accordance with clause 68.6.1, the output of the ANESTHETIC VAPOR DELIVERY DEVICE(s) in the "Off" or "Zero" position, if the "Zero" is also the "Off" position, shall be less than 0.05 %. The control(s) of the ANESTHETIC VAPOR DELIVERY DEVICE(s) shall be designed to prevent unintentional operation from the "Off" position.

68.7 The ANESTHETIC VAPOR DELIVERY DEVICE(s) shall be equipped with a liquid level indicator visible from the front of the ANESTHESIA WORKSTATION. The ANESTHETIC VAPOR DELIVERY DEVICE(s) shall be designed so that it cannot be overfilled when in the normal operating position.

NOTE 23—If applicable, the ANESTHETIC VAPOR DELIVERY DEVICE(s) should be designed so that substantially all liquid but that contained in the wick (if present) can be drained when the ANESTHETIC VAPOR DELIVERY DEVICE(s) is emptied in accordance with the manufacturer's instructions. These requirements apply regardless of whether the agent bottle is being used as the agent reservoir.

NOTE 24—The filling mechanism(s) of the ANESTHETIC VAPOR DELIVERY DEVICE(s) should be fitted with a permanently attached AGENT SPECIFIC FILLING DEVICE to help prevent accidental filling with the wrong agent. It is recommended that this AGENT SPECIFIC FILLING DEVICE be either a manufacturer's proprietary device, or be in compliance with the requirements of ISO 5360[2].

68.8 When used, and mounted (if applicable), in accordance with the manufacturer's instructions, and filled to the maximum safe indicated level, the ANESTHETIC VAPOR DELIVERY DEVICE shall permit the use of maximum calibrated flows of O_2 and N_2O simultaneously in the "on" and in the "off" positions, without discharging liquid anesthetic through its outlet.

68.9 The average delivered concentration (volume percent or partial pressure) from the ANESTHETIC VAPOR DELIVERY DEVICE(s) shall not deviate from the set value by more than +30 % or −20 % or by more than +7.5 % or −5 % of the maximum setting, whichever is greater, under the following test conditions at an ambient temperature of 23°C ± 1°C at one standard atmosphere (1013 mbar):

(a) (*a*) The ANESTHETIC VAPOR DELIVERY DEVICE(s) is filled with the appropriate agent to approximately one quarter of the way between the minimum and maximum fill marks.

(b) (*b*) The pressure fluctuation is introduced at the COMMON GAS OUTLET of 15 ± 2 cycles per minute at an I:E ratio of 1:2 ± 20 %.

(c) (*c*) Condition 1: the pressure produced at the COMMON GAS OUTLET is 2 ± 0.3 kPa above ambient. The total gas

flow is 2 ± 0.2 L/min.

(d) (*d*) Condition 2: the pressure produced at the COMMON GAS OUTLET is 5 ± 0.4 kPa above ambient. The total gas flow is 8 ± 0.8 L/min.

(e) (*e*) The pressure falls from 100 % to 33 % in less than 0.6 seconds.

NOTE 25—When fresh gas flow is determined by ventilator settings, they are set for a minute volume of 2 L/min and 8 L/min.

Tests for Compliance:

68.1.1 *Verify by visual inspection.*

68.2.1 *Verify by visual inspection.*

68.3.1 *Verify by inspection of accompanying documents.*

68.4.1 *Verify by visual inspection and review of the accompanying documents. Details of a test to determine conformance to the requirement in clause 68.4 shall be furnished by the manufacturer upon request by the USER.*

68.5.1 *Test for compliance by visual inspection and functional testing.*

68.6.1 *Verify by visual inspection and functional testing using the carrier gas and analytic technique recommended by the manufacturer.*

68.7.1 *Verify by visual inspection and functional testing using the carrier gas and analytic technique recommended by the manufacturer.*

68.8.1 *Mount the ANESTHETIC VAPOR DELIVERY DEVICE(s) according to the manufacturers' instructions. Turn "On" the maximum calibrated flows of nitrous oxide and oxygen and inspect for liquid anesthetic at the ANESTHETIC VAPOR DELIVERY DEVICE(s) outlet.*

68.9.1 *Using the settings specified in Table 7, verify by functional testing by adhering to the temperature stabilization method, carrier gas, and analytic technique recommended by the manufacturer.*

68.10 Without back pressure produced at the COMMON GAS OUTLET, all other conditions being the same as specified in clause 68.9, the average delivered concentration (volume percent or partial pressure) from the ANESTHETIC VAPOR DELIVERY DEVICE shall not deviate form the set value by more than ± 20 % or ± 5 % of the maximum setting, whichever is greater, when the pressure at the COMMON GAS OUTLET is within the range of ± 0.5 kPa of ambient.

68.10.1 *Using the settings specified in Table 7, verify by functional testing by adhering to the temperature stabilization method, carrier gas, and analytic technique recommended by the manufacturer.*

69. Common Gas Outlet

69.1 If an OPERATOR accessible COMMON GAS OUTLET is provided, it shall be in compliance with one of the following: a 22 mm male conical fitting with a coaxial 15 mm female connector in accordance with Specification F 1054,[7] or a manufacturer's specific fitting.

There shall be only one functional COMMON GAS OUTLET at a time.

69.2 For manufacturer - specific fittings, the connector shall remain engaged after an axial pull of 35 *N* maintained for 30 s.

NOTE 26—The COMMON GAS OUTLET may also incorporate a load bearing fitting for secure attachment of accessory devices. If the COMMON GAS OUTLET is OPERATOR accessible, it should be provided with means to prevent unintentional disconnects.

69.3 For conical fittings, the supporting structure of the COMMON GAS OUTLET shall permit the simultaneous application of a bending moment of 3 Nm on, and a torque of 3 Nm around, the axis without permanent deformation or displacement of the mountings of the COMMON GAS OUTLET.

Tests for Compliance:

69.1.1 *Visually inspect the ANESTHESIA WORKSTATION and determine that if more than one OPERATOR accessible COMMON GAS OUTLET is provided, only one COMMON GAS OUTLET is functional at a time.*

69.2.1 *Verify that the COMMON GAS OUTLET is equipped with a retaining device, and that it is in compliance with the appropriate standard.*

69.3.1 *For manufacturer specific fittings, confirm that after an axial pull of 35 N maintained for 30 s the connector remains engaged, and then can be disengaged. Reconnect and disconnect the connector to ensure that its retaining ability remains.*

Test the structural integrity of the supporting structure of the COMMON GAS OUTLET with a torque wrench and special adapters to ensure compliance.

70. Pipeline Inlet Connections

70.1 The ANESTHESIA WORKSTATION shall be provided with pipeline inlet connectors for both oxygen and nitrous oxide. These connections as well as MEDICAL GAS PIPELINE SYSTEM connections for other gases (if provided) shall be DISS threaded body fittings in compliance with the applicable requirements of CGA V-5.[5] The attachment of these fittings to the ANESTHESIA WORKSTATION shall be such that they cannot be interchanged.

70.2 Each pipeline inlet shall be provided with a filter having a pore size not exceeding 100 micrometers.

70.3 When both pipeline inlet fittings and a medical gas cylinder attachment are present for the same gas, unidirectional valve(s) shall be provided to prevent the reverse flow of gas, from the ANESTHESIA GAS SUPPLY DEVICE to the MEDICAL GAS PIPELINE SYSTEM, or to atmosphere, from exceeding 50 mL/min at the manufacturer's specified working pressure.

Tests for Compliance:

70.1.1 *Verify by visual inspection that the ANESTHESIA WORKSTATION is equipped with pipeline inlet connections for both oxygen and nitrous oxide.*

Verify by inspection that all pipeline inlet connectors of the ANESTHESIA WORKSTATION are in compliance with the applicable requirements of CGA V-5.[5]

Verify that the pipeline inlet connectors are not interchangeable.

70.2.1 *Verify that a filter with a pore size less than 100 μm is present in all pipeline inlet connectors.*

70.3.1 *Attach a suitable test flowmeter to the pipeline inlet connector. Pressurize the system as specified by the manufacturer. The flow measured by the flowmeter is the leakage past the unidirectional valve and shall not exceed 50 mL/min.*

71. Gas Power Outlet(s)

71.1 Gas power outlet(s), if provided, shall be gas specific, and shall be durably marked with the name or symbol of the gas in accordance with CGA V-5[5], and the nominal output pressure. These markings shall be LEGIBLE. Where color coding is used, it shall be in accordance with CGA C-9.[5] (See Table 1.)

71.2 *Test for Compliance:*

71.2.1 *Verify by visual inspection, that if gas power outlet(s) are provided, that they are gas specific and marked in accordance with 71.1.*

72. Checklist

72.1 Each ANESTHESIA WORKSTATION shall be provided with a checklist(s) of the procedures recommended by the manufacturer to be performed prior to each use of the ANESTHESIA WORKSTATION.

Manufacturers of DELIVERY SYSTEM/DEVICE(s), MONITORING DEVICE(s), ALARM DEVICE(s) and PROTECTION DEVICE(s) intended for use in an ANESTHESIA WORKSTATION shall state in the instructions for use that whoever assembles an ANESTHESIA WORKSTATION from individual devices or systems shall provide the checklist for the ANESTHESIA WORKSTATION.

The USER who assembles an ANESTHESIA WORKSTATION from separate DELIVERY SYSTEM/DEVICE(s), MONITORING DEVICE(s), ALARM DEVICE(s) and PROTECTION DEVICE(s) shall provide a checklist comprising the procedures which shall be incorporated into the checklist for the ANESTHESIA WORKSTATION.

NOTE 27—These procedures may be performed automatically, in whole or in part, or by the OPERATOR. Attention is drawn to additional check lists established by regional or national medical associations, or government agencies. The use of electronic displays (for example, a CRT) integral to, or provided with the ANESTHESIA WORKSTATION or the module, to provide such a checklist is permitted.

SECTION ELEVEN—BREATHING SYSTEM, AND ANESTHETIC GAS SCAVENGING SYSTEM

73. Breathing Systems

NOTE 28—Different types of breathing systems may be used with the ANESTHESIA WORKSTATION. Attention is drawn to Specification F 1208[7] for requirements pertaining mainly to circle breathing systems.

74. Anesthetic Gas Scavenging Systems

74.1 The gas scavenging port and hoses shall comply with the requirements in Specification F 1343.[7]

SECTION TWELVE—AUXILIARY EQUIPMENT

75. Suction Equipment

75.1 Suction equipment provided as part of the ANESTHESIA WORKSTATION shall conform to the requirements of Specification F 960.[7]

76. Auxiliary Oxygen Flowmeter

NOTE 29—The presence of an AUXILIARY OXYGEN FLOWMETER is strongly recommended. Such a flowmeter is self contained usually with a maximum flow of 10 L/min and with a barbed fitting on the outlet (so that the oxygen that it delivers is not connected in any way to the COMMON GAS OUTLET of the ANESTHESIA WORKSTATION). It is usually mounted on the left side of the ANESTHESIA WORKSTATION, and may be used to provide supplemental inspired oxygenation (for example, via a nasal canula) to a patient under spinal, epidural, or other regional anesthesia. It may also be used to enrich the inspired gas mixture provided by a manually powered self-inflating resuscitator bag, which is called for on the pre-use checklist for emergency applications.

77. Other Auxiliary Equipment

All other auxiliary equipment provided with the ANESTHESIA WORKSTATION shall conform to the requirements of the appropriate ASTM Standard.

SECTION THIRTEEN—DATA INTERFACES

78. Data Interfaces

78.1 The ANESTHESIA WORKSTATION shall provide at least one DIGITAL INTERFACE.

78.2 DIGITAL INTERFACES of devices marketed as compatible with this ANESTHESIA WORKSTATION standard shall comply with one of the specified published communication standards. (See Clause 2.16.3)

NOTE 30—Some devices (for example, mechanical vaporizers, PROTECTION DEVICES) may not provide DIGITAL INTERFACES. Legacy devices with RS-232[3] interfaces may have only rudimentary communication capabilities inadequate for use as DIGITAL INTERFACES as defined in this standard.

NOTE 31—Devices having waveform output may offer an analog format (NTE ± 10 V) or a digital format. If digital, it may offer selectable output of one or more waveforms at a time (ideally, all waveforms should be available at all times). This waveform output feature may occur via the same DIGITAL INTERFACE used for parameter values and alarms. Optionally, a product may offer its waveform output via one or more additional DIGITAL INTERFACES. Transmitted waveform data should comply with suitable published standards (for example, Specification E 1467[11] or Guide E 1763[12]).

78.3 If a device has more that one DIGITAL INTERFACE, only one DIGITAL INTERFACE shall be used for control of the device's alarm parameters or annunciation.

78.4 f a DIGITAL INTERFACE employs the RS-232 standards[3], the manufacturer shall document the transmission protocol, data format, and hardware connector pinout as implemented to allow another party to implement a working DIGITAL INTERFACE. (See Appendix X1).

NOTE 32—RS-232 default parameters should include 9600 baud, 8 data bits, no parity, and 1 stop bit.

78.5 If a DIGITAL INTERFACE employing the RS-232 standards[4] operates at no more than 19.2 Kbaud, the product may operate in either a broadcast mode or a polling mode. If an RS-232[3] interface operates at more than 19.2 Kbaud, the product shall not operate in a broadcast mode.

NOTE 33—A polling protocol should minimally provide: a means of asking what data is available; selecting any component of that data for one time or continuing output; identifying when or if new data becomes available; and a means of stopping any portion or all outputs. Requests for

[11] *Annual Book of ASTM Standards*, Vol 14.01.

[12] *Annual Book of ASTM Standards*, Vol 03.06.

output of specific data should be available as both one time requests as well as continuing requests. The DIGITAL INTERFACE definition still requires bidirectional communication capability even if broadcast mode is employed (see Clause 79).

78.6 A SECONDARY DATA SOURCE shall provide an indication whether data originating from a PRIMARY DATA SOURCE have been modified before re-transmission.

79. Data Interface Requirements for Infusion Devices

79.1 INFUSION DEVICES marketed as compatible with this ANESTHESIA WORKSTATION standard shall comply with the requirements of ANSI/AAMI ID 26.[2]

79.2 INFUSION DEVICES shall accept a command from the ANESTHESIA WORKSTATION CONTROL CENTER to disable INFUSION DEVICE audible alarms.

79.3 INFUSION DEVICES shall respond to queries from the ANESTHESIA WORKSTATION CONTROL CENTER for identification and status. The INFUSION DEVICE shall be identified to the ANESTHESIA WORKSTATION CONTROL CENTER by one of the following: a unique identifier of the INFUSION DEVICE, a logical identifier, corresponding to the fluid being delivered, and the INFUSION DEVICE'S DIGITAL INTERFACE port location on the ANESTHESIA WORKSTATION.

NOTE 34—An INFUSION DEVICE should provide a minimum set of responses including: "not granted," "feature not available," and "unknown request."

79.4 Information transmitted to the ANESTHESIA WORKSTATION shall as a minimum include the information required for the anesthesia record.

79.5 Communication interfaces shall support a centralized alarm management strategy, accomplished in the following manner (also see Appendix X1):

The ANESTHESIA WORKSTATION CONTROL CENTER shall send a command to an INFUSION DEVICE instructing it to DISABLE its audible alarms. The command shall be transmitted using a predetermined rate and protocol. If an INFUSION DEVICE does not receive this command under the predetermined conditions, it shall enable audible alarms.

HIGH PRIORITY alarms shall be visually presented at the INFUSION DEVICE, periodically transmitted to the ANESTHESIA WORKSTATION CONTROL CENTER, and transmitted as a part of each query response until the condition is corrected at the INFUSION DEVICE.

MEDIUM PRIORITY and LOW PRIORITY ALARMS shall be visually presented at the INFUSION DEVICE and transmitted to the ANESTHESIA WORKSTATION CONTROL CENTER as part of each query response until the condition is corrected at the INFUSION DEVICE.

The ANESTHESIA WORKSTATION CONTROL CENTER shall present device alarm conditions to the OPERATOR in accordance with the centralized management prioritization scheme.

80. Data Interface Requirements for an Automated Anesthesia Record Keeper (AARK)

80.1 This section defines physical, functional, and electrical integration of an AARK with other components of an ANESTHESIA WORKSTATION.

NOTE 35—An AARK typically consists of a central processing unit, one or more data entry mechanisms, a MULTIPORT COMMUNICATION DEVICE, and a visual display. The AARK records data at defined intervals from other components of the ANESTHESIA WORKSTATION and may accept data from other sources. RECORDED DATA is typically displayed in a tabular or graphical format that emulates the traditional anesthesia record. The AARK also provides methods for entry of patient demographics, drugs, agents, and clinical notes and events. Data are saved on removable or non-removable storage media (for example, computer disks or paper).

The AARK may be part of a NETWORK that communicates with other INFORMATION SYSTEMS (for example, BACK-UP servers, other AARKs, hospital or laboratory information systems).

80.2 Requirements

80.2.1 The AARK shall be capable of automatically acquiring electronically monitored physiological parameters from patient monitoring components for the ANESTHESIA WORKSTATION. At a minimum the AARK shall provide a means of acquiring all mandatory patient parameters specified in the Standard for Basic Anesthetic Monitoring published by the American Society of Anesthesiologists[8] and the American Association of Nurse Anesthetists[9].

NOTE 36—Input data may include, but are not limited to, the following sources: ECG, pulse rate, temperature, blood pressure, end-tidal CO_2, pulse oximetry, cardiac output, airway gas, airway pressure and flow, other oxygen saturation, EMG, alarm status and combinations of these.

NOTE 37—In addition, the AARK should be capable of automatically acquiring data from the DELIVERY DEVICES that may be components of the ANESTHESIA WORKSTATION.

NOTE 38—The AARK may be capable of automatically generating, acquiring, or synchronizing additional data such as date, time, status, etc. among the ANESTHESIA WORKSTATION components.

NOTE 39—The AARK should be capable of communicating with other INFORMATION SYSTEMS that could contribute to the AUTOMATED ANESTHESIA RECORD. Interfaces should include but are not limited to, inputs from hospital information systems (for example, laboratory, pharmacy, DECISION SUPPORT, perioperative systems, or archived patient records).

NOTE 40—The AARK should be capable of sending the electronic anesthetic record to other medical record systems employing suitable standard methods.

80.2.2 The AARK shall have means for allowing OPERATOR INPUT of data that have not been acquired automatically.

NOTE 41—Data that may be entered manually include but are not limited to patient demographics, clinical notes, events, ARTIFACT indication, comments, personnel, equipment utilized, etc.

80.2.3 AARK devices marketed as compatible with the ANESTHESIA WORKSTATION shall provide DIGITAL INTERFACES capable of receiving measurement and status data from devices conforming to the data interface specification of Clause 78.

The AARK shall be capable of communicating via DIGITAL INTERFACES with patient monitoring and other digitally interfaced equipment configured as components of the ANESTHESIA WORKSTATION, utilizing applicable published standards whenever possible, and other means when necessary.

NOTE 42—The DIGITAL INTERFACES provided by the AARK may be configurable such that they can operate at different data rates, parity types, and framing types. Also, the AARK may employ other electronic interfaces to other types of non-medical electronic equipment such as various INPUT DEVICES, OUTPUT DEVICES, or a combination of both (for example, local area NETWORK, data storage media). Such additional electronic interface connections should not affect the operation of the data interfaces or the integrity of the data collected.

NOTE 43—The AARK may transform or process data from various sources.

NOTE 44—An AARK should be capable of transmitting and receiving data on a NETWORK. Data should comply with appropriate standards for health information exchange (for example, Specification E 1238[11], HL7 v2.3[13]). The data collected should be in a form that can be stored in a database or exported.

NOTE 45—The AARK should provide means to prevent loss of data, including: means to automatically and securely BACK-UP or archive all data stored by the AARK; an operational power supply even when the ANESTHESIA WORKSTATION power is "off"; and incorporation of an auxiliary RESERVE ELECTRICAL POWER SUPPLY enabling the AARK to continue to function in the event of low power or power interruptions or disturbances. (See Clause 80.4.2)

80.3 Specific Requirements

80.3.1 The AARK shall produce at least an acceptable perianesthetic record as defined by the ASA Standards, Guidelines and Statements (October 1996).[8]

80.3.2 The AARK shall provide means of EDITING the data that has been entered into the record.

80.3.3 A NON-VOLATILE audit trail of alterations (the original and modified) shall be generated, including the time of change and who made the change.

NOTE 46—If an AARK can place an electronic signature on the anesthetic record, it should comply with Guide E 1762.[11]

NOTE 47—The AARK should provide means to prevent unauthorized access to patient or provider data from the electronic record. The AARK may make data contained in the anesthesia record available to other INFORMATION SYSTEMS.

80.3.4 There shall be a means to display the data that comprises the anesthetic record. The AARK shall be capable of displaying this or other data as it is acquired.

NOTE 48—Not all of the data needs to be displayed simultaneously.

80.4 Physical & Technical Documentation

[13] Available from Health Level Headquarters, 3300 Washtenaw Avenue, Suite 227, Ann Arbor, MI 48104.

80.4.1 AARK devices marketed as compatible with the ANESTHESIA WORKSTATION shall have available technical documentation defining the physical dimensions and weight of the equipment as defined in 6.8 of this specification.

NOTE 49—Attachment of an AARK to an ANESTHESIA WORKSTATION should not cause the ANESTHESIA WORKSTATION to be out of compliance with the requirements of Section 4 of this specification.

NOTE 50—The ANESTHESIA WORKSTATION should accommodate the physical attachment of an AARK.

80.4.2 AARK devices marketed as compatible with the ANESTHESIA WORKSTATION shall have technical documentation defining the electrical specifications of the equipment. These specifications must at the minimum include voltage and current requirements of the equipment under operating conditions with applicable environmental specifications for the equipment under operating and non-operating conditions. This technical documentation shall be provided as part of the accompanying documents of the ANESTHESIA WORKSTATION as defined in 6.7 of this specification.

NOTE 51—Electrical power for the AARK may be provided by either an independent power outlet, or by the main power source within the ANESTHESIA WORKSTATION. If power for the AARK is provided by the main power source within the ANESTHESIA WORKSTATION, the AARK should be able to remain in an "ON" mode and not be affected by the ANESTHESIA WORKSTATION when the main power switch is in power "Off" mode. This will prevent possible loss of data should the operator accidentally switch off the power mains to the ANESTHESIA WORKSTATION prior to the complete writing of RECORDED DATA to a NON-VOLATILE storage media by the AARK.

NOTE 52—AARK devices should incorporate an auxiliary RESERVE ELECTRICAL POWER SUPPLY enabling the AARK to continue to function in the event of low power or power interruptions or disturbances. The inclusion of such a capability shall be documented in the appropriate accompanying documents as defined in 6.8 of this specification.

80.4.3 If the AARK transforms or processes data, the processes or transformations shall be described in the technical documentation.

80.4.4 If the AARK generates data elements, such as date, time, status, etc. the methods utilized shall be specified in the technical documentation.

ANNEXES

(Mandatory Information)

A1. REFERENCES

A1.1 *AAMI Documents*[6]:

AAMI HE-48 Human Factors Engineering Guidelines and Preferred Practices for the Design of Medical Devices

AAMI ES-1 Safe Current Limits for Electromedical Apparatus

AAMI EC-11 Electrocardiographic Devices

AAMI SP-10 Electronic or Automated Sphygmomanometers

A1.2 *ASME Standard*[14]:

ASME B40.1 Gauges - Pressure Indicating Dial Type - Elastic Element

A1.3 *ASTM Standards*:

D 3670 Guide for Determination of Precision and Bias of

[14] Available from American Society of Mechanical Engineers, ASME, 345 East 47th Street, New York, NY 10017.

Methods of Committee D-22[15]

E 1238 Specification for Transferring Clinical Observations Between Independent Computer Systems[11]

E 1467 Specification for Transferring Digital Neurophysiological Data Between Independent Computer Systems[9]

E 1713 Specification for Transferring Digital Waveform Data Between Independent Computer Systems[11]

E 1762 Guide for Electronic Authentication of Health Care Information[11]

F 960 Specification for Medical Surgical Suction and Drainage Systems[8]

F 1054 Specification for Conical Fittings of 15 mm and 22 mm Size

F 1161 Minimum Performance and Safety Requirements for Components and Systems of Anesthesia Gas Machines[7]

F 1204 Specification for Anesthesia Reservoir Bags[7]

F 1208 Specification for Performance and Safety Requirements for Anesthesia Breathing Systems[7]

F 1343 Specification for Scavenging Systems for Anesthetic Gases[7]

F 1415 Specification for Pulse Oximeters[7]

F 1456 Specification for Capnometers[7]

F 1452 Specification for Minimum Performance and Safety Requirements for Anesthetic Gas Monitors[7]

F 1462 Specification for Oxygen Analyzers[7]

F 1463 Specification for Alarm Signals in Medical Equipment Used in Anesthesia and Respiratory Care[7]

A1.4 *CGA Standards*[5]:

CGA C-9-1993 Standard Color Marking of Compressed Gas Cylinders Intended for Medical Use

CGA V-1-1994 Compressed Gas Cylinder Valve Outlet and Inlet Connections

CGA V-5-1989 Non-Interchangeable Low Pressure Connections for Medical Gas Applications

CGA G-7-1997 Commodity Specification for Air

A1.5 *EIA/TIA Documents*[3]:

[15] Annual Book of ASTM Standards, Vol 11.03.

EIA RS-232-C 1969 Interface between Data Terminal Equipment and Data Circuit-Terminating Equipment Employing Serial Binary Data Interchange

EIA/TIA-232-D 1987 Interface between Data Terminal Equipment and Data Circuit-Terminating Equipment Employing Serial Binary Data Interchange

EIA/TIA-232-E 1991 Interface between Data Terminal Equipment and Data Circuit-Terminating Equipment Employing Serial Binary Data

A1.6 *HL7 Document*[13]

HL7 An Application Protocol for Electronic Data Exchange in Healthcare Environments

A1.7 *IEC Standards*[2]:

IEC 601-1 Safety for Medical Electrical Equipment Part 1: General requirements (2nd Ed. - 1988)

IEC 601-1-1 Medical Electrical Equipment: General Requirements for Safety Collateral Standard: Safety Requirements for Medical Electrical Systems

IEC 601-1-2 Medical Electrical Equipment: General Requirements for Safety Collateral Standard: Electromagnetic Compatibility - Requirements and Tests

A1.8 *IEEE Standards*[4]:

IEEE STD 1073 IEEE Standard for Medical Device Communications—Transport Profile—Overview and Framework

IEEE STD 1073.3.1 IEEE Standard for Medical Device Communications—Transport Profile—Connection Mode (ANSI)

IEEE STD 1073.4.1 IEEE Standard for Medical Device Communications—Physical Layer Interface—Cable Connected (ANSI)

A1.9 *ISO Standards*[2]:

ISO/IEC 7498-1: Information Technology—Open Systems Interconnection—Basic Reference Model: The Basic Model (for many related references, see citations in IEEE STD 1073-1996)

ISO 4135 Anesthesiology Vocabulary

A2. METHOD OF TEST FOR THE ACCURACY OF DELIVERED VAPOR CONCENTRATION DURING OXYGEN FLUSH

A2.1 Test the ANESTHETIC VAPOR DELIVERY DEVICE on the ANESTHESIA WORKSTATION with a ANESTHESIA BREATHING SYSTEM recommended by the manufacturer or supplier (see 6.8.2).

A2.1.1 Connect an anesthetic vapor analyser to the COMMON GAS OUTLET of the ANESTHESIA WORKSTATION or, if applicable, to the inspiratory port of the ANESTHESIA VENTILATOR.

A2.1.2 Check to ensure that the components downstream of the ANESTHETIC VAPOR DELIVERY DEVICE will not affect the test results, for example by absorbing the volatile agents, by imposing time delays on response, or by leakage.

A2.2 Place the ANESTHESIA WORKSTATION with the specified test equipment and anesthetic agent in the test room for at least 3 h at 20 ± 3° C and maintain this temperature throughout the test procedure.

A2.3 Fill the ANESTHETIC VAPOR DELIVERY DEVICE with the appropriate anesthetic agent to approximately half of the maximum usable volume, and let it stand for at least 45 min.

NOTE A2.1—These 45 min may be within the 3 h period specified in A2.2.

A2.3.1 If the manufacturer recommends that when power is applied to the ANESTHETIC VAPOR DELIVERY DEVICE, a warm up period be allowed before use, power shall be applied for at least that period before testing. This period may be within the 45 min.

A2.4 Set the ANESTHETIC VAPOR DELIVERY DEVICE to the "on" position at the maximum concentration setting. Purge the ANESTHETIC VAPOR DELIVERY DEVICE for 3 min at a flow of 2 L/min.

A2.5 With the ANESTHETIC VAPOR DELIVERY DEVICE in the "off," "zero" or, if applicable, the "standby" position, set the gas flow through the ANESTHESIA WORKSTATION to 2 ± 0.2 L/min and adjust the ventilator to give 15 ± 2 breaths/min at an I:E ratio of 1:2 ± 20 % with the inspiratory flow control set to maximum.

NOTE A2.2—For an ANESTHESIA WORKSTATION in which the fresh gas flow is determined by the ventilator settings, set these to give a minute volume of 2 ± 0.2 L.

A2.6 Measure the output of anesthetic vapor (concentration of vapor × volume of gas) for 1 min before and then during a 10 s operation of the oxygen flush.

A2.6.1 Compare these two measurements expressed as volume of vapor per unit of time.

NOTE A2.3—The volume of gas may be determined for example, by integrating flow or by collecting the gas during the specified period.

APPENDIXES

(Nonmandatory Information)

X1. COMMUNICATION INTERFACE: DOCUMENTATION AND SUPPORT

X1.1 Devices marketed as compatible with this specification should provide the following:

X1.1.1 Documentation of the DIGITAL INTERFACE (that is, by including the protocol in the USER's Manual for the device). The seven-layer ISO communications model may be useful for this purpose. Some layers may have null implementations or cite appropriate published standards. Unique characteristics not defined by cited standards should be adequately disclosed by the manufacturer so that another party (for example, USER, manufacturer) may establish successful digital data transmission.

X1.1.1.1 Layer 1—Physical—Connector, pinouts, voltages, cable requirements, etc.,

X1.1.1.2 Layer 2—Data Link—Control information, frame length, etc.,

X1.1.1.3 Layer 3—Network—Address definition, etc.,

X1.1.1.4 Layer 4—Transport—Acknowledgment messages, sequence numbers, flow control, etc.,

X1.1.1.5 Layer 5—Session—Connection establishment and teardown, control mechanisms, remote procedure calls, etc.,

X1.1.1.6 Layer 6—Presentation—Transformation, formats, compression, expansion, encryption, decryption, etc., and

X1.1.1.7 Layer 7—Application—File access/transfer, virtual terminal information transfer, network management, directory services, etc.

X1.1.2 Appropriate supplemental support mechanisms for DIGITAL INTERFACES in addition to documentation (that is, technical support services, or provision of equipment by temporary arrangement).

X1.1.3 In cases where operation of special device options (for example, control) require a DIGITAL INTERFACE, manufacturers should/may negotiate appropriate agreements to ensure safe and predictable behavior of devices when integrated to function as parts of a system.

X2. COMMUNICATION INTERFACE: CONTROL OF ALARMS

X2.1 A product may allow another (controlling) product to remotely control its alarms. This control should at least affect the controlled product's visual and audible alarm notifications. Specific control of the controlled product's alarm "definitions" may also be provided.

X2.2 Devices that permit modification of their alarm state by another controlling device should revert to default behavior with auditory and visual alarms enabled when valid communication to verify continuation of a controlling relationship of one device over another is not periodically transmitted and acknowledged.

X2.3 If remote control over alarms is provided, it should be provided via a DIGITAL INTERFACE using a standard communication protocol. Ideally, this DIGITAL INTERFACE would also be used for communication of parameter values.

X2.4 An INFUSION PUMP should allow a potential controller to request control over the controlled product's alarm notification or definition functions, or both. Control of alarm functions may affect definitions and notification of alarm conditions. The controlled product should not grant this control request unless the request for control was preceded by a continuous output request for alarm and alert status information. It should allow the controlling product to request control over the controlled product's alarm notification or definition functions, or both.

X2.5 If control over alarm notification is provided, after

control is adequately requested and granted, the controlled device may initiate a visual alarm indication, but should not initiate any audible alarm indications, if so configured by the USER. The controlling device should visually and audibly indicate the alarm condition.

X2.6 If control over alarm "definition" (for example, alarm enabled (ON) or disabled (OFF), alarm limit value, etc.) is provided, the controlled device should identify which alarm definitions may be modified, which definitions are to be affected, and what values are acceptable. There should be a mechanism to permit the controlling device to verify that requested changes have been made or refused.

X3. RATIONALE

X3.1 Clause 6.1j—The marking of the ANESTHESIA WORKSTATION power input and the sum of the power input in amperes, gives information on the minimum mains fuses or OVER CURRENT RELEASES needed in different situations.

X3.2 Clause 6.1k—The marking of each auxiliary mains socket outlet with its output in amperes, gives information on the current ratings of the fuses or OVER CURRENT RELEASES of each auxiliary mains socket outlet.

X3.2.1 Note 2–Ideally, the fuses or OVER CURRENT RELEASES for these auxiliary mains socket outlet would always be immediately adjacent. However, this is not always the case; therefore this requirement that marking be provided to indicate the location of the fuses or OVER CURRENT RELEASES was felt to be justified.

X3.3 Clause 6.8.2k—The higher the leakage current the greater the risk for the patient or operator to suffer electrical shock. Leakage current of multiple devices connected together will be greater than that of any single device. Therefore, the connected devices should be tested for leakage current as a single assembled system.

X3.4 Clause19.4h—The definition of the APPLIED PART in this specification is the basis for, and clarification of, the requirements for and measurement of patient leakage current.

X3.4.1 It is not possible, however, to include any requirements in this Particular Standard for leakage currents from electrically operated attachments such as humidifiers and heating elements which may be connected in the ANESTHESIA BREATHING SYSTEM because the types of such attachments which will be used in clinical work with a specific type of ANESTHESIA WORKSTATION cannot be anticipated by the manufacturer or by a test house.

X3.4.2 However, parts integrated with the ANESTHESIA WORKSTATION such as temperature and carbon dioxide sensors that are intended to come into contact with the ANESTHESIA BREATHING SYSTEM and that are electrically connected to the ANESTHESIA WORKSTATION are considered as parts for which requirements for leakage currents can be specified in this specification. Such parts are therefore included in the definition of APPLIED PART. (See Fig. 1 of the General Standard.)

X3.4.3 The U.S. national standard, AAMI ES-1, states the allowable limits for leakage current.

X3.5 Clause 37—Equipment that can be used with flammable anesthetic agents is not covered by this specification.

X3.6 Clause 38—Equipment that can be used with flammable anesthetic agents is not covered by this specification.

X3.7 Clause 39—Equipment that can be used with flammable anesthetic agents is not covered by this specification.

X3.8 Clause 40—Equipment that can be used with flammable anesthetic agents is not covered by this specification.

X3.9 Clause 41—Equipment that can be used with flammable anesthetic agents is not covered by this specification.

X3.10 Clause 43—Reports of fire caused by medical devices are unusual. However, when such fires occur in the hospital environment they can have tragic consequences.

The risk of fire is fundamentally determined by the three elements that are necessary in order to start a fire:

Ignitable material (fuel),

Temperature equal to or above the minimum ignition temperature of the material or sparks with energy dissipation equal to or above the minimum ignition energy of the materials, and

An oxidant.

Therefore, following the basic safety concepts of the General Standard, the objective in the design of the equipment must be to ensure that under both normal and single fault conditions, and under the oxidizing conditions to which the material may be exposed, the temperature of any material is not raised to its minimum ignition temperature or the spark energy does not exceed the material ignition energy level. Alternatively, contained ignition may occur, provided it is self-limiting (e.g., a fuse or a resistor within a sealed compartment) so that no hazard is created.

Minimum ignition temperatures for a large number of specific materials are well established in published literature, although normally only in ambient air and 100 % oxygen environments. The minimum ignition temperature may be critically dependent upon the concentration of the oxidant present. If ignition temperatures for other materials or different oxygen concentrations are required these may be determined using the methods and apparatus described in IEC 79-4[2].

In considering the ignitable materials particular attention should be paid to materials that may accumulate during prolonged use, for example, airborne particles of paper or cotton.

The effect of sparks in environments containing oxidants is quite different from that in explosive gas mixtures. Spark energy is the most potent form of energy in igniting explosive gas mixtures whilst in environments containing oxidants thermal energy is more fundamental. It is possible that at higher power levels sufficient spark energy can be dissipated in the interface between sparking conductors or their surroundings so that sustained burning occurs; but there is at present no documented evidence as to the power level at which this might occur for different materials and environments. Where the potential spark power dissipations deviate from the well established safe practice, therefore, specific spark tests should be conducted simulating the most unfavorable environment which can be reasonably foreseen.

The accumulating materials mentioned above are particularly susceptible to ignition by spark energy because of their low ignition temperatures and very low thermal capacity coupled with poor conductance.

In certain standards currently in use the requirements to minimize fire risk are based on limitation of temperature and electrical energy and oxidant concentration to absolute values.

The temperature value is based on the minimum hotplate ignition temperature for fire retardant cotton in 100 % oxygen, which is given in the American NFPA Publication 53M[16] as 310°C. The assumption was therefore made that 300°C was an acceptable temperature limit in medical equipment with oxygen enriched atmospheres.

The origin of the electrical energy values that have been used is less clear and it would seem that, in the absence of specific controlled tests, figures have been adopted from accepted working practices or from tests performed in other environments. Simple tests and detailed analysis of the known factors involved in causing an oxygen fire show that these figures can be either over-restrictive or potentially hazardous depending, in particular, on the manner in which the power may be dissipated and the proximity and type of any "fuel" present.

It is therefore, now generally accepted that there are no single or universally applicable ranges of temperature, energy and concentration of oxidant which can ensure safety under all circumstances whilst not being unduly restrictive. Ultimately, electrical energy is only significant in respect of its ability to raise the temperature of ignitable materials and this in turn depends upon the particular configuration and the proximity of any ignitable materials.

Under single fault conditions in a typical electrical circuit the possible number of failure modes is very high. In this case full assurance of safety may only be possible with the use of appropriate hazard and safety analysis procedures, taking into consideration the three basic elements, that is, material, temperature, and oxidant.

An appropriate design might limit the electrical energy in the circuit to ensure that temperatures remain below the minimum air ignition temperature under normal conditions and seal compartments, or add forced ventilation, to ensure that the oxygen content does not exceed that of ambient air under single fault condition.

Alternatively, it may be appropriate to limit the electrical energy to ensure temperatures below the minimum ignition temperature for a pure oxygen environment, even under single fault conditions.

The particular combination of material, oxidant and temperature determines whether a fire will occur, not a single value of any one of these variables.

X3.11 Clause 49.5—During committee deliberations it was decided that fresh gas flow and automatic ventilation were the minimum performance characteristics that needed to be retained by the ANESTHESIA WORKSTATION, so as to permit the OPERATOR a period of at least 30 min to either correct the power failure or have the surgery completed and the patient moved to a safer location.

X3.12 Clause 49.6—The committee felt that going to reserve electrical power did not require an immediate OPERATOR response, but merely awareness. Accepting this premise, which is also based on a 30 min period during which the ANESTHESIA WORKSTATION will provide automatic ventilation and continuous fresh gas flow, a LOW PRIORITY ALARM which could not be disabled was provided for.

X3.13 Clause 49.7—The committee felt that the OPERATOR, having already been alerted by a LOW PRIORITY ALARM to the fact that the workstation was operating on RESERVE ELECTRICAL POWER SUPPLY, needed nothing more than a MEDIUM PRIORITY ALARM to indicate that the RESERVE ELECTRICAL POWER SUPPLY was approaching imminent failure. For obvious reasons they felt that this alarm should not be capable of being disabled.

X3.14 Clause 49.8—The committee after extensive deliberations felt that a means must be provided to the OPERATOR to determine the status of the RESERVE ELECTRICAL POWER SUPPLY and in some fashion to permit the OPERATOR to estimate how much time remained before complete failure of the RESERVE ELECTRICAL POWER SUPPLY.

X3.15 Clause 51.7.7—The first paragraph in this clause intends to avoid excessive noise in the operating room by having the HIGH PRIORITY ALARM stop as soon as possible, that is, as soon as the condition causing the alarm's activation stops. There are many alarm activating conditions that are frequently very brief, for example, as patient's cough during a ventilator inspiratory flow, a breathing tube compressed by a surgical assistant leaning on it, or more insidious still, an intermittent malfunction in a ventilator.

X3.15.1 For these, and similar situations that are very brief, or that occur while the anesthetist is otherwise occupied and not looking at the central display, or alarm panel, the committee felt that a "flight recorder" or more probably the AARK should store the event (not necessarily displaying or recording it on the anesthesia record). The practice of recording all events whether they are incorporated in the clinical record or not may assist detection and documentation of rare or intermittent events that are otherwise very resistant to diagnosis.

X3.16 Clause 51.9.3.4.1—The committee generally agreed that currently there is no way to indicate reliably the failure of breathing system integrity (for example, partial or even complete disconnection of the breathing system). Under certain

[16] Available from National Fire Protection Association, NFPA 7 Batterymarch Park, Quincy, MA 02209–9101.

specific circumstances, CO_2 monitoring, (low) pressure monitoring, (low) volume monitoring, anaesthetic vapor monitoring, or O_2 monitoring may indicate, or contribute to, the detection of loss of breathing system integrity. It is for these reasons that a medium priority alarm have been provided for the monitors mentioned. The manufacturer, in the accompanying documents, shall indicate which monitor, or combination of monitors, is most likely to indicate disconnection may have occurred.

X3.17 Clause 51.12.1—As defined in CGA standard G 7.1[6], "medical air" is permitted to have an oxygen concentration between 19.5 and 23.5 %. Allowing a minimum concentration of 19 % at the fresh gas outlet, permits the manufacturer to offer the OPERATOR to deliver air from the ANESTHESIA GAS SUPPLY DEVICE in the event of an oxygen supply failure.

X3.18 Clause 57.2e—In order to assist the USER/OPERATOR in managing total system leakage current, the committee agreed to require the auxiliary mains socket outlets, when provided, to be a specific type that will not accept a standard mains plug. The committee agreed that requiring these non-standard outlets will make it inconvenient to attach non-medical equipment (for example, vacuum cleaners), or inappropriate devices (for example, high current drawing devices such as a heating blanket) to the ANESTHESIA WORKSTATION.

X3.18.1 The committee also decided against limiting the number of these outlets to a small specific quantity (that is, four) since the number of outlets is by itself no guarantee that leakage current limits will not be exceeded.

X3.19 Clause 57.3a—Accidental disconnection of the mains supply cord could be hazardous to the patient.

X3.20 Clause 57.6aa—A short circuit of another equipment connected to the auxiliary mains socket outlet must not affect the normal function of the life support function of the ANESTHESIA WORKSTATION.

X3.21 Clause 64.2—This is a test for the stability of flow as adjusted by a flow control and is designed to determine the preset allowable flow shall be within ± 10 % of the setting chosen by the OPERATOR or within ± 10 mL/min for a 30 min period, whichever is greater; this to occur under normal operating conditions as described by the manufacturer. It is reasonable to expect that the ANESTHESIA WORKSTATION, once set, will not need checking every 10, 20, 30, 60 s or every 2 to 3 min. Traditionally, and commonly, anesthetists record blood pressure and pulse values at 5 min intervals. It is common to record the gas flows from the machine at 15 to 30 min intervals. Therefore, it was elected to use a 30 min period in which to assume that the OPERATOR would not have to pay close attention to the flows being delivered by the ANESTHESIA WORKSTATION. It was felt unreasonable, due to potential variations in piped gas pressures within a large hospital and operating room suite, or possible variations within the pressures of the gas machine piping due to power on, turn off, or change in settings of a gas powered ventilator, to demand beyond a 30 min period of stability.

X3.22 *Clause 78—Communication Interface: Rationale*

X3.22.1 *Prologue*:

X3.22.1.1 Digital technologies open new design alternatives for anesthetic delivery systems, while digital communication technologies may facilitate better integration of traditionally independent monitors and delivery devices used for monitoring and administration of anesthesia to patients. Integration of formerly independent devices into systems opens opportunities that were formerly unachievable. A relatively simple example is prioritization and presentation of alarms at a central location, dealing with one of the critical human factors and safety issues during anesthetics. Clinical DECISION SUPPORT and apparatus fault diagnosis are more sophisticated examples drawing on information from multiple sources.

X3.22.1.2 Many considerations pertaining to the use of digital communications as a core technology have arisen during the development of this ANESTHESIA WORKSTATION standard. This appendix attempts to distill the most important rationales and issues from many discussions. Different issues and significance depend on whether one is considering passive data collection and display, centralized management of alarms, modification of alarm annunciation, or feedback control of delivery systems.

X3.22.1.3 Other issues arise when considering the flow of data and its availability according to need. In systems using serial digital interfaces to transmit information, one device may potentially intercept data destined for another. In such cases a mechanism to pass the data to the needful recipient should exist. In contrast, on a data network broadcast data can be collected by any able recipient. However data transmission within this standard for an ANESTHESIA WORKSTATION does not employ a broadcast NETWORK model.

X3.22.2 *Necessity*:

X3.22.2.1 It is one of the intentions of this specification to enable assembly of well-integrated ANESTHESIA WORKSTATIONS employing modular components that may originate from different manufacturers.

X3.22.2.2 This specification on one hand recognizes changes in ANESTHESIA DELIVERY SYSTEM technology that may provide alternatives to previously standardized anesthesia gas delivery systems based on mechanical technology (Specification F1161[8]). An additional motivation for the creation of this standard is the rapid advance of information technologies in the last several years. Successful communication, presentation, and storage of digital data is essential to developing a systematically integrated ANESTHESIA WORKSTATION that improves upon prevailing haphazard associations of independent ANESTHESIA DELIVERY SYSTEMS, MONITORS, and recordkeeping devices (AARKs). Poor integration and harmonization create a confusing working environment for the OPERATOR, especially regarding alarms; that is a widely recognized factor degrading human performance. Therefore it is a significant patient safety issue.

X3.22.3 *Framework*:

X3.22.3.1 The perioperative period has a uniquely high information density that is rarely integrated with other evolving medical INFORMATION SYSTEMS. This specification attempts to define a suitable framework for acquisition, use, and storage of the perianesthetic portion of that information.

X3.22.3.2 The remainder of this appendix will focus on important considerations too diverse to standardize affecting integration of ANESTHESIA WORKSTATIONS. Restrictions imposed by this standard are explained, and pivotal issues are identified to assist manufacturers and USERS.

X3.22.4 *Safety*:

X3.22.4.1 Not all types of data that may be transmitted have the same implications for patient safety. For instance, failed transmission of monitor data or alarm status information is unlikely to be a critical problem if the primary monitors are still functioning properly and independently. However, improperly managed control of alarms, indication of alarms in a centralized alarm management scheme, or control of AGENT DELIVERY SYSTEMS could produce critical or life-threatening situations.

X3.22.4.2 When pertinent standards are mute, and because of the potentially critical safety considerations involved when one device exerts control over another, vendors may choose to negotiate agreements regarding control functions mediated by digital interfaces.

X3.22.5 *Digital Interfaces*:

X3.22.5.1 Communication interfaces should be defined by published, public digital communication standards whenever possible. All control functions, if implemented, should be transmitted through a compliant digital serial interface. Types of data that may be transmitted using a DIGITAL INTERFACE include: device connection and status, protocol negotiation, parameter values, alarm status and current limits, and control signals, for example, to alter alarm settings, delivery device control, etc.

X3.22.5.2 Numerous standard and proprietary data communication mechanisms are possible. The committee resolved after many discussions that the number of acceptable communication standards should be restricted to improve the likelihood of successful integration of modular components possibly provided by several manufacturers. EIA RS-232-C[4] and its successors (EIA/TIA-232-D and E)[4] are permitted because of the widespread use of these interfaces in clinical devices, computers, and computer peripherals. Because many elements of protocol, data format, assured connection, etc. are not specified by the RS-232[4] standards, a burden of documentation is placed on the manufacturer to facilitate coherent communication between devices employed in an ANESTHESIA WORKSTATION system. Since RS-232[4] does not provide a "reliable" transport protocol, precautions should be taken to ensure robust and reliable communication when using RS-232[4] interfaces, especially detection of lost connections and corruption of data (for example, checksums, connection queries).

X3.22.5.3 Other related serial communication standards were considered (for example, RS-422, RS-423, RS-449, RS-485[4]). While these have specific advantages, none holds a dominant position or special suitability for medical purposes, and all suffer significant limitations since they were not designed with clinically motivated design requirements.

X3.22.5.4 IEEE-1073 (MIB, Medical Information Bus) standards are cited because they are designed for the unusual requirements of the clinical arena. The requirements include patient safety, electrical suitability, robust interface reliability, timing synchronization, and consistency of DIGITAL INTERFACES across the spectrum of medical devices. A primary purpose is that connection and configuration of a bedside data network be no more difficult for a primary clinician than plugging the devices into their mains power supplies. Manufacturers should document which members of the IEEE 1073[5] family of standards are employed. Deviations from the published standards should be noted as necessary.

X3.22.5.5 Not all modular components of an integrated anesthesia workstation system will have DIGITAL INTERFACES. For instance, ANESTHETIC AGENT DELIVERY DEVICES (vaporizers) do not now routinely have DIGITAL INTERFACES, while future electronic vapor delivery devices may be designed with DIGITAL INTERFACES.

X3.22.5.6 Access to unmodified data from PRIMARY DATA SOURCES should be unrestricted since it is not possible to completely anticipate all purposes for which ANESTHESIA WORKSTATION INFORMATION SYSTEMS may need to employ digitally transmitted data. When it is necessary for digital data to pass through another device's DIGITAL INTERFACES it should be made available by retransmission. Retransmitted data should be annotated if the original data or format were modified. A possible solution to this dilemma is provision of a MULTIPORT COMMUNICATION DEVICE to accumulate digital data from all available PRIMARY DATA SOURCES, making all data available to any number of potential INFORMATION SYSTEM consumers. A MULTIPORT COMMUNICATION DEVICE may also need to be able to "patch" digital communication between specific ports (for example, between a central alarm controller and alarm-controlled devices).

X3.22.6 *Non-Serial Data Interfaces*:

X3.22.6.1 Use of other communication mechanisms in addition to acceptable standard DIGITAL INTERFACES in the context of this standard are permitted. Use of alternate communication mechanisms (for example, analog voltages, SCSI (Small Computer System Interface), IEEE-488)[5] should be disclosed by the manufacturer.

X3.22.6.2 More advanced interfaces, protocols, and formats may be used as technology advances.

X3.22.7 *Centralized Alarm Strategy*:

X3.22.7.1 Control over alarms is necessary for implementation of a centralized alarm strategy. Centralization of alarm management is one of the least complex INFORMATION SYSTEMS contemplated by this standard, yet it still requires a thorough analysis of the ramifications of centralized alarm management. The analysis should include possible information requirements of the INFORMATION SYSTEMS that might communicate with the AARK, yet also need data, alarm status or limit settings from devices communicating primarily with the alarm centralization or AARK modules of the anesthetic workstation. Examples of systems potentially needing access to primary data passed through by another intermediate system include clinical data repositories and DECISION SUPPORT SYSTEMS. Time limits for annunciation of specified conditions may constrain the tolerable delay for data being received from an intermediate system.

X3.22.8 *Control, Main Power*:

X3.22.8.1 A product may allow another (controlling) product to remotely control its main power state. The controlling product may exercise this control as means of ensuring that the controlled product is operational when the controlling device is turned on. Alternatively, a controlled product may allow remote control of "standby" versus "active" modes using commands from the controlling device transmitted via a DIGITAL INTERFACE.

X3.22.9 *Multiple Device Digital Interfaces*:

There is a potential hazard that requests for control of alarms or other device features via DIGITAL INTERFACES may be received from more than one potential controller over different interfaces. Should multiple control be granted, none of the controllers would actually know the state of the controlled device, since its state may have been changed by a different controller on another interface. Therefore, if a device has more than one DIGITAL INTERFACE and control is granted via a DIGITAL INTERFACE between a controller and device accepting external control instructions, such control should only be granted over the first interface where it is granted.

X3.22.9.1 This feature, if provided, should be hardware selectable, so that it may be DISABLED at the discretion of the USER. A controlled device should not be required to respond in such a manner as to grant control to more than one potential controller at any time.

X3.22.9.2 The USER or OPERATOR should ensure that the controlled device is set up correctly and that requests for control will only originate at one device DIGITAL INTERFACE.

X3.22.10 *Control of Power or Standby Status*:

X3.22.10.1 This type of control requires that the product include special hardware if it cannot be or is not plugged directly into the controlling product to obtain its main electrical power. This type of control may require a product to support a special "shut-down" mode of operation. In this mode, the controlled product may appear to be "off," but still accepts specific commands received through its DIGITAL INTERFACE. This control should occur after the complete system (for example, controlling product with controlled product) has been configured by the USER or OPERATOR to enable this special operational mode of the controlled product.

TABLE 1 Assigned Color Codes and Gas Symbols (See Clauses 6.1.b.b: 6.3.h: 6.3.J: 6.3.k: 6.3.m: 65.6: 66.3: 71)

Intended Gases	CGA Color Code	Pantone Color Numbers	Munsell Color Designations	Federal Std 595a Color Numbers	Gas Symbol
Oxygen	Green	363	10G5/10	14187	O_2
Nitrous Oxide	Blue	292	2.5PB 4/8	Not specified	N_2O
Medical Air	Yellow	Yellow	6.25Y 8.5/12	23655	MED AIR
Carbon Dioxide	Grey	428	7.5GY 6/1	26492	CO_2
Helium	Brown	470	7.5YR 3/4	Not Specified	He
Nitrogen	Black	Black	5 Y 1/0	37038 (Lusterless) 27038 (Semigloss)	N_2
Mixtures - Except mixtures of Oxygen and Nitrogen	Color markings of mixtures shall be a combination of colors corresponding to each component gas.	Combinations of the above	Combinations of the above	Combinations of the above	$He-O_2$ (He > 80 %) O_2-He (He < 80 %) CO_2-O_2 (CO_2> 7 %) O_2-CO_2 (CO_2< 7 %) O_2-AIR
Mixtures - Oxygen and Nitrogen					
- 19.5 % - 23.5 % Oxygen	Yellow	Yellow	6.25Y 8.5/12		O_2- N_2
- All other Oxygen concentrations	Black and Green	Black & 363	5 Y 1/0& 10G5/10		O_2 - N_2

TABLE 2 Recommended Colors for Color Coding of Vaporizers[A,B] (See Clause 6.3.L)

Agent	Color	USA Federal Standard	Pantone	Munsell
Desflurane	Blue	N.A[C]	3015C	10B4/10
Enflurane	Orange	22510	151C	2.5YR 6/16
Halothane	Red	11105	200C	5R4/14
Isoflurane	Purple	N.A.[C]	254C	7.5P 4/12
Methoxyflurane	Green	14187	334C	10G 5/10
Sevoflurane	Yellow	13655	108C	6.25Y 8.5/12

[A] Colors for color coding of vaporizers and appropriate color samples extracted from the following documents or standards: Munsell Book of Color[12]; USA Federal Standard 594a[13]; and Pantone Color Standard. [14]

[B] Recommended abbreviations for anesthetic agents:
Desflurane – DES or D
Enflurane– ENF or E
Halothane – HAL or H
Isoflurane– ISO or I
Methoxyflurane– MET or M
Sevoflurane – SEV or S

[C] N.A. = Not Available

TABLE 3 Summary of ALARM, MONITORING, and PROTECTION DEVICES(S)

Delivery System/Device	Alarm Device	Monitoring Device	Protection Device
Electric power supply:			
a)Mains power supply	Clause 49.6	N/A[A]	Clause 49.5
b)Reserve power supply	Clause 49.6 and 49.7	Clause 49.8	N/A[A]
Pneumatic power supply:			
a)Cylinder pressure	N/A[A]	Clause 61.1	N/A[A]
b)Pipeline pressure	N/A[A]	Clause 61.1 and 61.3	N/A[A]
Gas delivery device:			
a) Oxygen supply failure	Clause 51.12.2	Clause 61.1 and 61.3	Clause 51.12.1
b) Other gases supply failure	N/A[A]	Clause 61.1 and 61.3	N/A[A]
c) Hypoxic mixture	N/A[A]	Clause 61.1 and 61.3	Clause 51.13.1
Agent Delivery Device	Clause 51.14.1	Clause 51.14.1	N/A[A]
Anesthesia Ventilator			
- VBS pressure[B]	Clause 51.9.3.2.1	Clause 51.9.3.1	Clause 51.9.3.1
- Exhaled volume	Clause 51.9.4.3	Clause 51.9.4.1	N/A[A]
Anesthesia Breathing System			
- VBS pressure[B]	Clause 51.9.3.2.1	Clause 51.9.3.1	51.9.3.1
- Carbon Dioxide	Clause 51.10.5.2	Clause 51.10.5.1	N/A
- Oxygen concentration	Clause 51.11.1	Clause 51.11.1	N/A
- Exhaled volume	Clause 51.9.4.3	Clause 51.9.4.1	N/A
	Clause 51.15.1 SpO2	Clause 51.15.1 SpO2	N/A
	Clause 51.15.2 BP	Clause 51.15.2 BP	N/A
	Clause 51.15.3 ECG	Clause 51.15.3 ECG	N/A

[A]N/A = Not Applicable
[B]VBS = Ventilator Breathing System

TABLE 4 Test Conditions for Determining Compliance of an Exhaled Volumeter in accordance with Clause 51.9.4.2

Variables or Parameters	Test Conditions		
	Adult Use	Pediatric Use	Neonatal Use
Tidal Volume V_T (mL) derived from pressure sensor on test lung ($V_T = C$ multiplied by P_{max})	500	300	30
Frequency	10	20	30
I/E Ratio	1:1.5 to 1:2.5	1:1.0 to 1:1.5	1:1.0 to 1:1.5
Resistance (R) kPa/L/s	0.5 ± 10 %	2.0 ± 10 %	5.0 ± 10 %
Isothermal Compliance (C) (mL/kPa)	500 ± 10 %	200 ± 10 %	10 ± 10 %

TABLE 5 Axial Pull Force Test (In Accordance with Clause 57.3.a)

Mass of Equipment (kg)	Pull(N)
Up to and including 1	30
Over 1 up to and including 4	60
Over 4	100

TABLE 6 Gas Mixing System Test (In Accordance with Clause 66.2.1)

		Oxygen		2nd Gas	
		Inlet Pressure minimum	Inlet Pressure Maximum	Inlet Pressure minimum	Inlet Pressure Maximum
Total Flow	Minimum	X	...	X	...
		...	X	...	X
		X	...	...	X
		...	X	X	...
	Maximum	X	...	X	...
		...	X	...	X
		X	...	...	X
		...	X	X	...

TABLE 7 Settings to be Used for Testing Accuracy of Delivered Concentration

Order of Test	Setting (% v/v of Anesthetic Vapor)
1	off, standby, and zero, if separately marked
2[A]	lowest graduation above zero
3[B]	10 % FS
4[B]	20 % FS
5[B]	50 % FS
6[B]	75 % FS
7	maximum graduation (full scale)

[A]If 10 % of Full Scale (FS) is the lowest graduation, step 2 is omitted.
[B]If the percentages of Full Scale (FS) do not coincide with a marked setting, use the nearest lower marked setting.

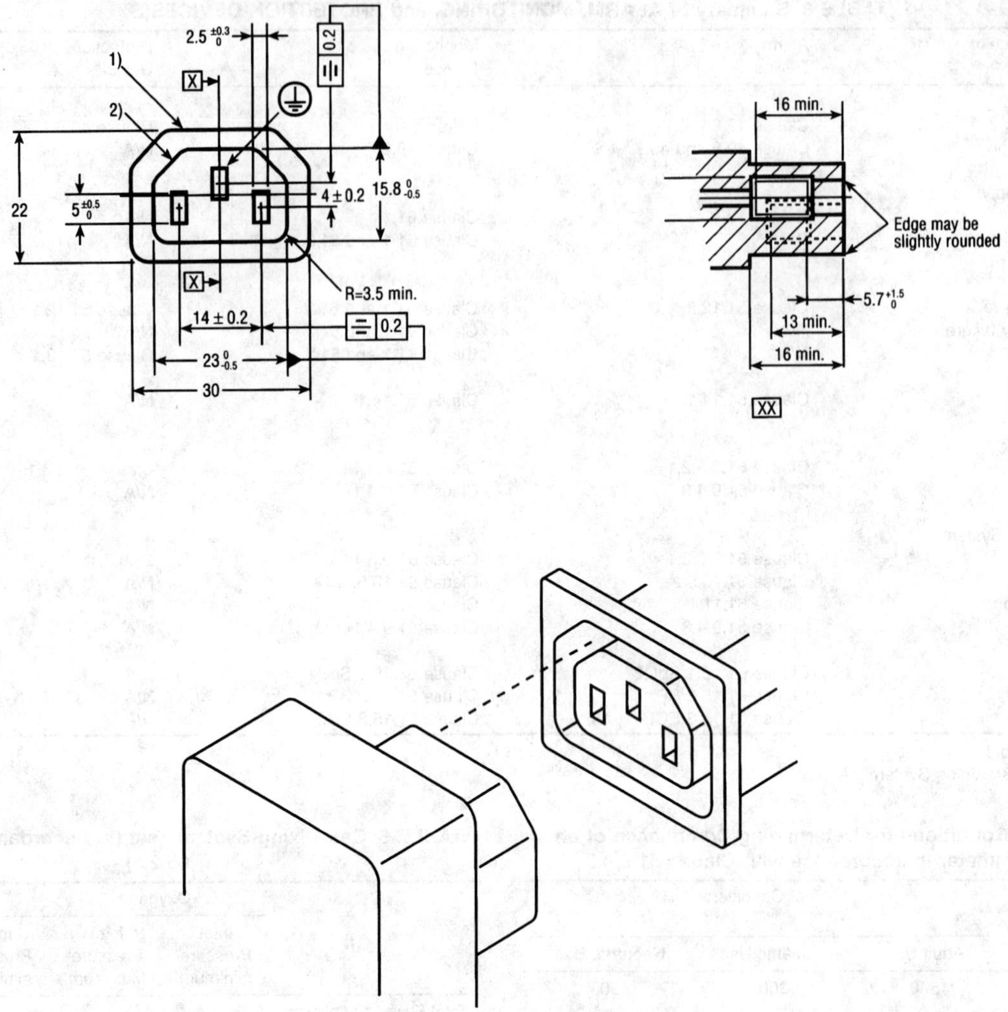

FIG. 1 IEC 320—Appliance Couplers

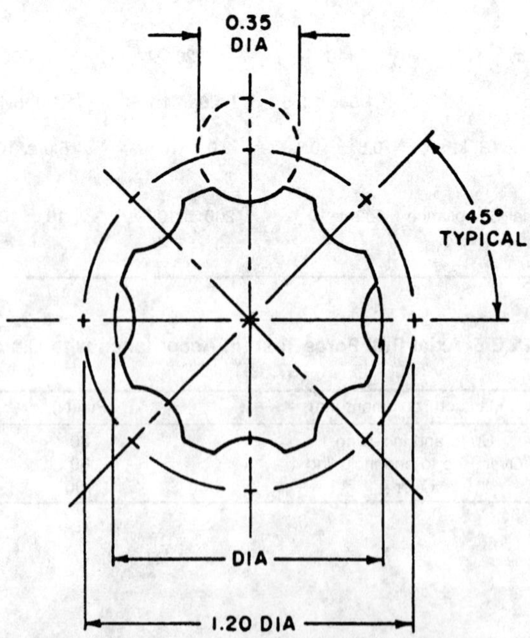

FIG. 2 Oxygen FLOW ADJUSTMENT CONTROL

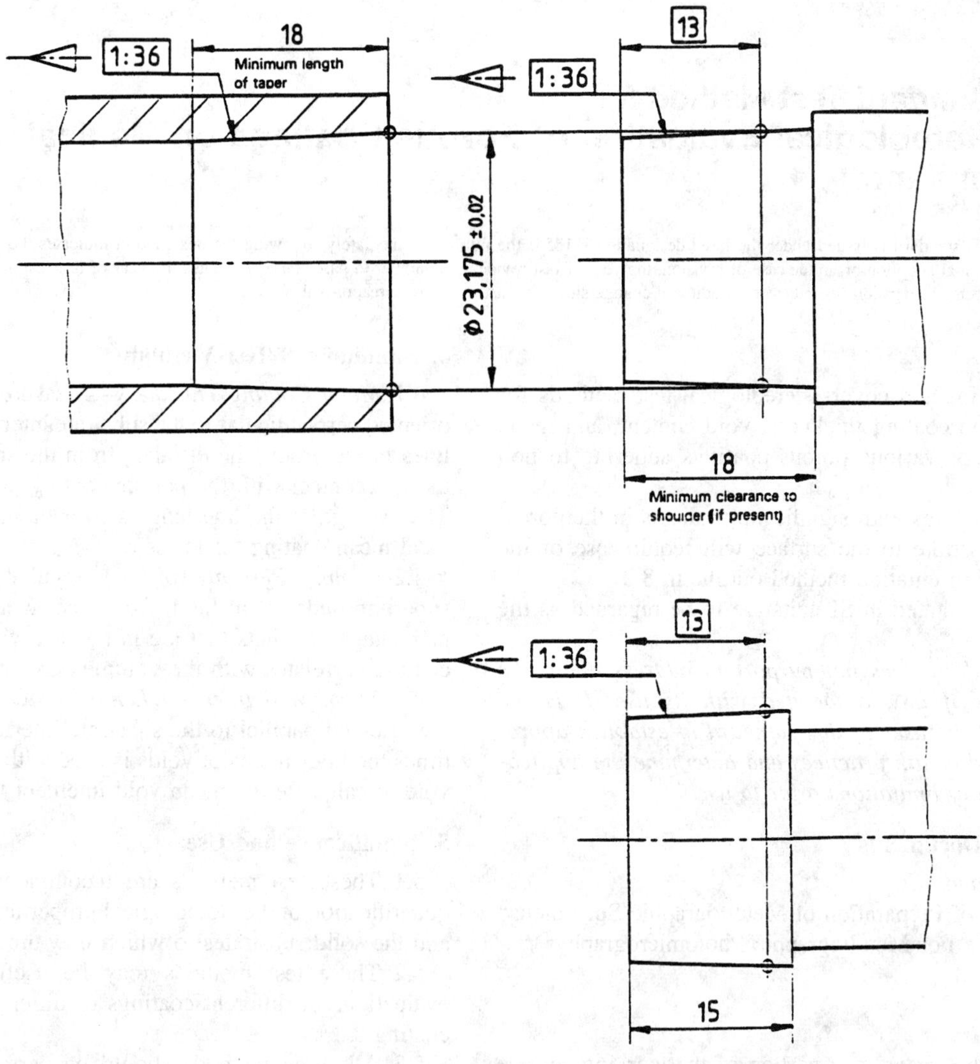

NOTE 1—Maximum radius on the entrance to the female connector and on the leading edge of the male cone should be not less than 0.5 mm and not more than 0.8 mm.

NOTE 2—All dimensions in millmetres.

FIG. 3 Conical Fittings of 23 mm Size

Designation: F 1854 – 98

Standard Test Method for Stereological Evaluation of Porous Coatings on Medical Implants[1]

This standard is issued under the fixed designation F 1854; the number immediately following the designation indicates the year of original adoption or, in the case of revision, the year of last revision. A number in parentheses indicates the year of last reapproval. A superscript epsilon (ε) indicates an editorial change since the last revision or reapproval.

1. Scope

1.1 This test method covers stereological test methods for characterizing the coating thickness, void content, and mean intercept length of various porous coatings adhering to non porous substrates.

1.2 Porous coatings with significant gradients in the porosity from the substrate to the surface will require use of the alternate sample orientation method outline in 8.2.

1.3 The values stated in SI units are to be regarded as the standard.

1.4 *This standard does not purport to address all of the safety concerns, if any, associated with its use. It is the responsibility of the user of this standard to establish appropriate safety and health practices and determine the applicability of regulatory limitations prior to use.*

2. Referenced Documents

2.1 *ASTM Standards:*

E 3 Methods of Preparation of Metallographic Specimens[2]

E 883 Practice For Metallographic Photomicrography[2]

3. Terminology

3.1 *Definitions:*

3.1.1 *field*—the image of a portion of the working surface upon which measurements are performed.

3.1.2 *intercept*—the point on a measurement grid line projected on a field where the line crosses from solid to void or vice versa.

3.1.3 *measurement grid lines*—a evenly spaced grid of parallel lines all of the same length

3.1.4 *porous coating*—coating on an implant deliberately applied to contain void regions with the intent of enhancing the fixation of the implant.

3.1.5 *substrate*—the solid material to which the porous coating is attached.

3.1.6 *substrate interface*—the region where the porous coating is attached to the substrate.

3.1.7 *working surface*—the ground and polished face of the metallographic mount where the measurements are made.

4. Summary of Test Method

4.1 *Mean Coating Thickness*—Measurement grid lines are oriented perpendicular to the substrate interface. On each of the lines in the group, the distance from the substrate interface to the last contact with the porous coating material is measured. The average of the line lengths over the group of lines is the local mean coating thickness.

4.2 *Volume Percent Void*—A regular grid of points is superimposed on a field from the working surface. The percentage of points that are in contact with void areas in the coating correlates with the volume percent of void present.

4.3 *Mean Void Intercept Length*—Measurement grid lines are oriented parallel to the substrate interface. The number of times the lines intercept voids is used with the volume percent void to calculate the mean void intercept length.

5. Significance and Use

5.1 These test methods are recommended for elementary quantification of the stereological properties of porous coatings and the solid substrates to which they are bonded.

5.2 These test methods may be useful for comparative evaluations of different coatings or different lots of the same coating.

5.3 All three methods should be performed on the same working surface.

5.4 A statistical estimate can be made of the distributions of the mean coating thickness and the volume percent void. No estimate can be made of the distribution of intercept lengths unless the void is a regular geometric shape that can be defined mathematically.

6. Apparatus

6.1 The procedures outlined in this test method can be performed manually or by an automated procedure. The following apparatus are necessary for manual calculations.

6.2 *Microscope*, or other suitable device with a viewing screen or photomicrographic capability of at least 125 by 175 mm should be used to image the working surface.

6.3 *Transparent Sheet*, with measurement grid lines or points is superimposed on the viewing screen or photomicrograph for the measurements. The grid lines grids of points should be uniformly spaced and parallel with at least five parallel lines.

---

[1] This test method is under the jurisdiction of ASTM Committee F-4 on Medical and Surgical Materials and Devices and is the direct responsibility of Subcommittee F04.15 on Material Test Methods.

Current edition approved February 10, 1998. Published June 1998.

[2] *Annual Book of ASTM Standards*, Vol 03.01.

7. Metallography

7.1 The procedures outlined in this test method for characterizing porous coatings require the preparation of metallographic sections through the entire coating thickness into the solid substrate. Good metallographic preparation techniques, in accordance with Test Methods E 3 and Practice E 883 must be used to prevent deformation of the surface of the section or creation of any other artifacts that will alter the stereological properties of the metallographic section. An example of an unacceptable artifact would be the absence of a portion of the porous coating, caused by its removal, thereby creating an artificial void area.

7.2 Care must be taken to ensure that the working surface is perpendicular to the interface between the porous coating and the solid substrate. In the case of the alternate mounting method shown in 8.4, extreme care must be taken to keep the substrate interface parallel to the final working surface.

8. Sample Selection

8.1 *Normal Section Orientation*:

8.1.1 A description of type of sample from which the sample metallographic sections are removed and the location of those sample metallographic sections should be included as part of the results.

8.1.2 For accurate coating thickness measurements, the orientation of sample working surfaces should be approximately perpendicular to the substrate.

8.2 *Alternative Orientation Method*:

8.2.1 An alternate orientation is required for the volume percent void and mean intercept length measurements of coatings with a varying amount of porosity in the coating. The porous material and substrate should be mounted with the substrate interface parallel to the metallographic mount surface. The mount is ground parallel to the substrate interface and the measurements are taken at a fixed distance from the substrate interface. It is recommended that the measurements be made at 50 % of the mean coating thickness

8.2.2 At least one surface must also be ground on the same mount at 90° to the measurement surface. These will confirm that the interface surface is parallel to the working surface and allow measurement of the distance from the working surface to the substrate. The working surface must be parallel within ± 5° of the substrate.

8.2.3 This test method is not suitable for substrate interfaces with a radius of curvature less than 1 in. (25 mm)

8.2.4 Since this test method also requires more aggressive porous surface removal to reach 50 % of the mean coating thickness, it may be more susceptible to creation of metallographic artifacts. Care should be exercised to assure that the metallographic sections that are used are free of artifacts.

9. Procedure

9.1 *Mean Coating Thickness*:

9.1.1 Appendix X2 includes two sets of typical measurement grids. Each with ten measurement lines, one set separated by a distance of 1 cm and one set separated by a distance of 0.5 cm.

9.1.2 The magnification should be chosen such that the thickness of the coating in the image is at least 4 cm.

9.1.3 The transparency of the measurement grid lines is superimposed on the field in an orientation approximately perpendicular to the substrate interface. The length of each line between the substrate interface to the last contact with the porous coating is measured on each line.

9.1.4 If the angle between the substrate interface and any individual line of the group of parallel lines is not between 80 and 100°, the individual measurement is invalid.

9.1.5 The procedure is repeated on a minimum of ten unique fields on each working surface.

9.1.6 The average of all the measurements is the mean coating thickness for that working surface. The standard deviation estimator and the 95 % confidence interval should be calculated for each working surface. The equations for calculating these values are as follows:

$$\bar{T} = \frac{1}{Mxn} \sum_{i=1}^{n} t_i \quad (1)$$

where:

t_i = the individual magnified thickness line length,
M = the magnification, and
T = the mean coating thickness.

$$\hat{S} = \sqrt{\frac{1}{n-1} \sum_{i=1}^{n} \left[\frac{t_i}{M_i} - \bar{T}\right]^2} \quad (2)$$

where:

S = the standard deviation estimator.

$$CI = 2 \times \frac{\hat{S}}{\sqrt{n}} \quad (3)$$

where:

CI = the confidence interval.

9.2 *Volume Percent Void*:

9.2.1 X2.1 includes three different typical sets of 100 point grids. Two of the grids are spaced 10 by 10 (1.0 by 1.0 and 0.5 by 1.0 cm separation) and the other is a 20 by 5 grid (0.5 by 1.0 cm separation).

9.2.2 If the void areas form a regular or periodic pattern on the working surface, the use of a grid having a similar pattern should be avoided.

9.2.3 The transparency is superimposed randomly on a fields. The magnification of the field is chosen such that one of the available grids can fit completely within the porous coating in the working surface.

9.2.4 Grid height must be greater than 50 % of the mean coating thickness. For coatings consisting of regularly shaped particles, or those having porosity gradients, care must be taken not to influence results by non random grid placement.

9.2.5 The number of points in contact with void areas in the working surface will be counted and recorded.

9.2.6 Count any points falling on a boundary between void area and solid area as one half. Any doubtful point should be counted as one half.

9.2.7 The number of contact points, divided by the total number of points on the grid times 100 gives the percentage of grid points on the void for that field. This should be calculated for each grid application.

$$P_v = \frac{P_\alpha}{P_T} \times 100 \quad (4)$$

where:
$P(\alpha)$ = the total number of counted points,
$P(T)$ = the total number of grid points, and
$P(v)$ = the volume percent void.

9.2.8 A minimum of 30 fields should be measured per working surface.

9.2.9 Fields to be analyzed should include as much of the coating thickness as possible. When there are porosity gradients are present, the accuracy of the measurement is related to the amount and repeatability of gradient in the portion of the coating section analyzed in each field.

9.2.10 The average percentage of the grid points on the voids provides an unbiased statistical estimator for the void volume percentage in the three dimensional structure. The mean void percentage (P_v) for that working surface, the standard deviation estimator (S) and the 95 % confidence interval (CI) should be calculated for each working surface. The equations for calculating these values are as follows:

$$\bar{P}_v = \frac{1}{n} \sum_{i=1}^{n} P_{v_i} \quad (5)$$

$$\hat{S} = \sqrt{\frac{1}{n-1} \sum_{i=1}^{n} [P_{v_i} - \bar{P}_v]^2} \quad (6)$$

$$CI = 2 \times \frac{\hat{S}}{\sqrt{n}} \quad (7)$$

9.2.11 The volume percent void estimate is given by the following relationship:

$$V_v = P_v \quad (8)$$

9.3 *Mean Intercept Length*

9.3.1 Appendix X2 includes two sets of ten measurement lines, one set separated by a distance of 1 cm and one set separated by a distance of 0.5 cm. A transparency can be made of a group for manual work.

9.3.2 The transparency is superimposed on each of the fields. The measurement line grid should fit completely within the porous coating cross section.

9.3.3 The magnification will be chosen such that the number of counted intercepts per line should average five or more.

9.3.4 The number of times that a void region is intercepted by the test lines (N_v) is counted and recorded. There are two methods that can be used for counting.

9.3.4.1 The first method counts the number of intersections along the grid lines. Each time the grid line goes from either solid to void or void to solid is counted as one intersection. The number of intersections (n_i) is twice the number of intercepts (N_v).

$$N_v = \frac{n_1}{2} \quad (9)$$

9.3.4.2 In the second method the crossing direction of any intersection on any line determines if it is counted as an intercept. If the beginning of the line starts on a void, count the transitions from void to solid. If that same line ends on a void, count that as a one more intercept. If the beginning of a line starts on solid, count the transitions from solid to void. If the same line ends on a solid, there is no additional count.

9.3.5 At least ten different fields should be counted on each working surface.

9.3.6 For the alternative method, the orientation of the grid should be random.

9.3.7 The mean intercept length (L_v) can be calculated from the total length of lines (L_T), the number of intercepts (N_v), the magnification M, and the previously calculated volume percent void (V_v). The calculation is as follows:

$$L_v = \frac{V_v \times \frac{L_t}{M}}{N_v} \quad (10)$$

10. Report

10.1 Report the chemical composition of the substrate structure and the coated material.

10.2 The original morphological form of the coated material (that is, powder, wire, etc.) and the method of application will be reported.

10.3 The number of fields of view for each measurement, the magnifications used, and the grids and lines used shall be reported.

10.4 The mean coating thickness and confidence interval, the volume percent void and confidence interval, and the mean linear intercept will be reported.

10.5 If curved substrates are used, that information must be included in the report, along with an estimate of the local radius of curvature.

10.6 If the alternative orientation method is used, that information must be reported together with the distance from the substrate for each set of measurements.

10.7 For image analysis systems that measure on digitized video images, the minimum measurement value (i.e. the dimension of a single pixel) must be reported at all magnifications used in the measurements.

11. Precision and Bias

11.1 The presence of structural gradients or inhomogeneities in the section can influence the precision and accuracy of the measurements. If the amount of void in the porous coating changes with thickness, the alternative mounting method and serial grinding may be used to characterize the gradient.

11.2 The quality of sample preparation can influence precision and bias.

11.3 The counting of grid points and line ends at void boundaries, presents an opportunity for bias in the measurements. The method outlined in 9.3.4.1 and 9.3.4.2 must be used.

11.4 The number of fields measured, the method of field selection, and their spacing can influence the precision and accuracy. Random selection of fields and except where noted random orientation of grids within the field can help eliminate bias.

12. Keywords

12.1 metallography; porosity; porous coatings; stereology; thickness

APPENDIXES

(Nonmandatory Information)

X1. RATIONALE

X1.1 Porous coatings are applied to the surface of medical implants. Standardized techniques should be available to characterize the structure of the porous coatings. These techniques can be used to estimate the uniformity and repeatability of these porous structures.

X1.2 Porous coatings with significant gradients in the porosity from the substrate to the surface may not be accurately measurable using these test methods.

X2. SAMPLE ARRAYS OF LINES FOR LINE INTERCEPT WORK

X2.1 See Fig. X2.1

X3. ARRAYS OF POINTS FOR POINT COUNTING METHODS

X3.1 See Fig. X3.1

REFERENCES

(1) Underwood, Ervin E., *Quantitative Stereology*, Addison-Wesley Publishing Company, 1970.

(2) Vandervoort, George, *Metallography, Principles and Practice*, McGraw-Hill, N.Y., 1984.

(3) *Stereology and Quantitative Metallography*, ASTM STP 504, 1972.

(4) *Practical Applications of Quantitative Metallography*, ASTM STP 839, 1984.

Sample Arrays of Lines
for Line Intercept Work

1.0 cm line spacing

0.5 cm line spacing

FIG. X2.1 Sample Arrays of Lines for Line Intercept Work

Arrays of Points
for Point Counting Methods

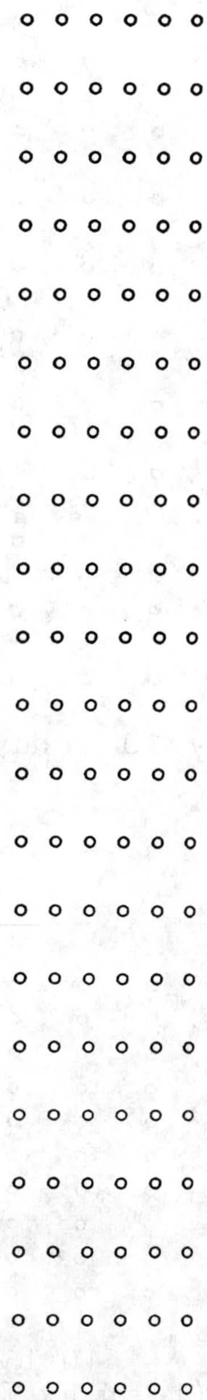

5 by 20 array
(1 cm by 0.5 cm separation)

FIG. X3.1 Array of Points for Point Counting Methods

Arrays of Points for Point Counting Methods

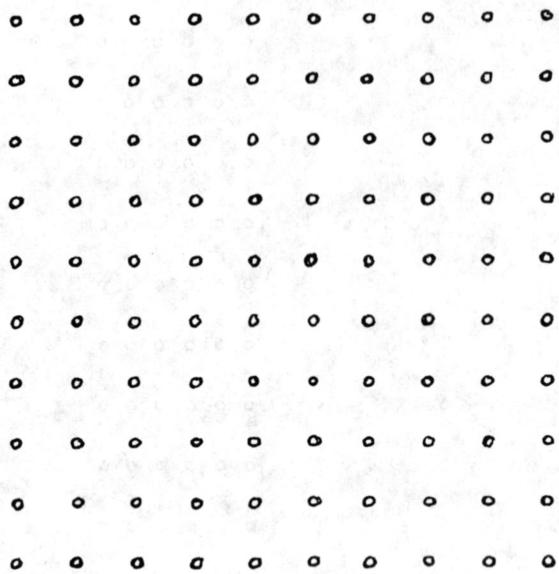

10 by 10 array (1 cm separation)

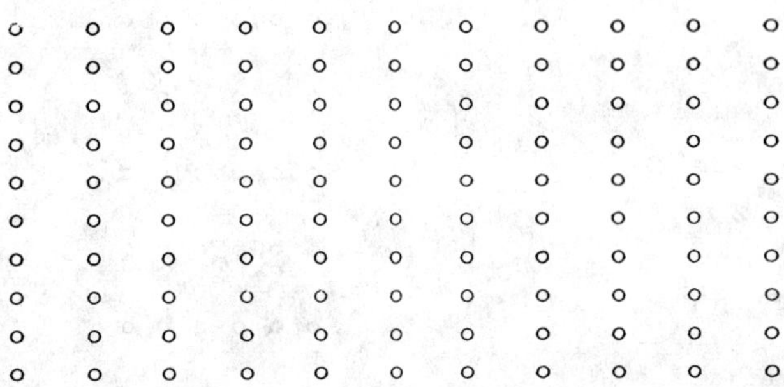

10 by 10 array
(1 cm by 0.5 cm separation)

FIG. X3.1 Array of Points for Point Counting Methods *(continued)*

Standard Specification for Polyoxymethylene (Acetal) for Medical Applications[1]

This standard is issued under the fixed designation F 1855; the number immediately following the designation indicates the year of original adoption or, in the case of revision, the year of last revision. A number in parentheses indicates the year of last reapproval. A superscript epsilon (ε) indicates an editorial change since the last revision or reapproval.

1. Scope

1.1 This specification covers polyoxymethylene (acetal) resin for medical applications. This specification provides requirements and associated test methods for a form of this thermoplastic which is intended for use in manufacturing medical devices, instrumentation or components there of.

1.2 As will any material, some characteristics may be altered by the processing techniques (such as molding, extrusion, machining, sterilization, etc.) required for a specific application. Therefore properties of fabricated forms of this resin should be evaluated using appropriate test methods to assure safety and efficacy.

1.3 Although this resin has been used and for specific implant applications in the United States, the use of this resin in medical devices should be restricted to non-implant applications until biocompatibility evaluations appropriate for the intended applications are successfully completed.

1.4 The biocompatibility of plastic compounds made up of polyoxymethylene (acetal) resin containing colorants, fillers, processing aids, or other additives as well as polymer blends which contain polyacetal should not be assumed on the basis of resin biocompatibility alone. Their biocompatibility must be established by testing the final (end-use) compositions using evaluation methods appropriate for the intended applications. It should be noted that the types, test levels and biological effects of extractives yielded by the additives contained in a compound or blend may also have to be evaluated for some end-use applications.

1.5 *This standard does not purport to address all of the safety concerns, if any, associated with its use. It is the responsibility of the user of this standard to establish appropriate safety and health practices and determine the applicability of regulatory limitations prior to use.*

2. Referenced Documents

2.1 *ASTM Standards:*

D 4181 Specification for Acetal (POM) Molding and Extrusion Materials[2]

D 883 Terminology Relating to Plastics[3]

D 1600 Terminology for Abbreviated Terms Relating to Plastics

F 748 Practices for Selecting Generic Biological Test Methods for Materials and Devices[4]

3. Chemical Composition

3.1 The chemical composition of the material shall conform to Specification D 4181. The FTIR spectrum of the material must be consistent with a reference or standard piece of the appropriate grade of the polymer. It may be helpful for the reader to review standards D 883 and D 1600 for clarification of terminology.

3.2 Class 1, Grade 1 of polyoxymethylene of Group 1, 2, or 3 (as described in ASTM D 4181), is recommended for use in medical applications, however other grades of this polymer may be found to be acceptable through appropriate testing.

4. Physical Properties

4.1 The mechanical properties of the material shall conform to those listed in Specification D 4181 for the appropriate grade and class of polymer being evaluated. Table 1 provides typical values for both physical and mechanical properties of medical grade polyoxymethylene (Acetal) for medical applications.

5. Inspection and Certification

5.1 The following information shall be reported in the material certification: Grade and color identification (that is, color number).

NOTE 1—Some coloring agents have the potential to elicit an adverse biological response, therefore any grades containing pigments, dyes, or additives should be separately evaluated for biocompatibility as appropriate for the particular application.

6. Biocompatibility

6.1 Biocompatibility of acetal resins and implant devices made using these materials shall be determined in accordance with Practice F 748, unless otherwise agreed upon by packager and consumer, and regulating bodies.**(1-5)**[5] Any potential filler colorants, processing aids, or sterilization processes, or all of

[1] This specification is under the jurisdiction of ASTM Committee F-4 on Medical and Surgical Materials and Devices and is the direct responsibility of Subcommittee F04.11 on Polymeric Materials.

Current edition approved May 10, 2000. Published August 2000. Originally published as F1855–98. Last previous edition F1855–98.

[2] *Annual Book of ASTM Standards*, Vol 08.02.

[3] *Annual Book of ASTM Standards*, Vol 08.01.

[4] *Annual Book of ASTM Standards*, Vol 03.03.

[5] The boldface numbers given in parentheses refer to a list of references at the end of the text.

TABLE 1 Physical and Mechanical Properties of Medical Grade Polyoxymethylene (Acetal) for Medical Applications

	Temperature	Units	ASTM Test Method	Results
Physical:				
Specific Gravity	73°	gms/cc	D 792	1.41
Water Absorption	73°	%	D 570	0.22
Equilibrium	73°	%	D 570	0.8
Mechanical:				
Tensile Yeild Strength	73°	10^3 psi	D 638	8.8
Tensile Elongation Break	73°	%	D 638	75
Tensile Modulus	73°	10^3 psi	D 638	380–390
Tensile Impact Strength		ft-lb/in.	D 1822	90
Compressive Strength				
1% deflection		10^3psi	D 695	4.5
10% deflection		10^3psi	D 695	16.0
Sheer Strength	73°	10^3psi	D 732	7.7

these, anticipated for the end product should be incorporated in these tests.

7. Keywords

7.1 acetal; copolymer; homopolymer; polyoxymethylene; thermoplastic resin

APPENDIX

(Nonmandatory Information)

X1. RATIONALE

X1.1 The intent of this specification is to guide the user in selection of an appropriate grade of polyoxymethylene when considering the use of this polymer in a medically related application. This specification does not attempt to cover all tests that may be applicable to the specific application, but is meant to aid the user in the selection process.

References

(1) Autian, J., Toxicological Evaluation of Biomaterials: "Primary Acute Toxicity Screening Program," *Journal of Artificial Organs,* Vol 1, No. 1, 1977.

(2) Autian, J. "The New Field of Plastic Toxicological Methods and Results," *CRC Critics Review in Toxicology,* 1973.

(3) Homsy, C.A., Ansevin, K.D., O'Brannon, W., Thompson, S.H., Hodge, R., and Estrella, M.E., "Rapid in Vitro Screening of Polymers for Biocompatibility," *Journal of Macromolecular Science, Chemistry,* Vol A4, No. 3, May 1970, pp 615-634.

(4) *Biological Evaluation of Medical Devices-Part 1: Guidance on Selection of Tests,"* American National Standard, ANSI/AAMI 10993-1: 1994.

(5) Alpert, Susan, "Use of International Standard ISO-10993, 'Biological Evaluation of Medical Devices Part 1: Evaluation and Testing' ", *General Program Memorandum #95-1,* May 1, 1995. Online: http://www.fda.gov/cdrh/g951.html

Designation: F 1873 – 98

Standard Specification for High-Purity Dense Yttria Tetragonal Zirconium Oxide Polycrystal (Y-TZP) for Surgical Implant Applications[1]

This standard is issued under the fixed designation F 1873; the number immediately following the designation indicates the year of original adoption or, in the case of revision, the year of last revision. A number in parentheses indicates the year of last reapproval. A superscript epsilon (ε) indicates an editorial change since the last revision or reapproval.

1. Scope

1.1 This specification covers material requirements for high-purity dense yttria tetragonal zirconium oxide polycrystal (Y-TZP) for surgical implant applications.

1.2 The values stated in SI units are to be regarded as the standard.

2. Referenced Documents

2.1 *ASTM Standards:*

C 373 Test Method for Water Absorption, Bulk Density, Apparent Porosity, and Apparent Specific Gravity of Fired Whiteware Products[2]

C 1161 Test Method for Flexural Strength of Advanced Ceramics at Ambient Temperature[3]

C 1198 Test Method for Dynamic Young's Modulus, Shear Modulus, and Poisson's Ratio for Advanced Ceramics by Sonic Resonance[3]

C 1239 Practice for Reporting Uniaxial Strength Data and Estimating Weibull Distribution Parameters for Advanced Ceramics[3]

C 1259 Test Method for Dynamic Young's Modulus, Shear Modulus, and Poisson's Ratio for Advanced Ceramic by Impulse Excitation of Vibration[3]

C 1327 Test Method for Vickers Identation Hardness of Advanced Ceramics[4]

E 112 Test Method for Determining Average Grain Size[4]

F 748 Practice for Selecting Generic Biological Test Methods for Materials and Devices[5]

F 981 Practice for Assessment of Compatibility of Biomaterials for Surgical Implants with respect to Effects of Materials on Muscle and Bone[5]

2.2 *American Society for Quality Control Document:*

C 1 Specification of General Requirements for a Quality Program[6]

3. Chemical Composition

3.1 The chemical composition shall be as follows, measured by X-ray fluorescence (XRF) or mass spectroscopy:

	Weight %
ZrO_2 HfO_2+ Y_2O_3	≥ 99
Y_2O_3	4.5 to 5.4
HfO_2	≤ 5
Al_2O_3	≤ 0.5
Other Total Oxides	≤ 0.5
TiO_2	
SiO_2	
CaO	
Fe_2O_3	
Na_2O	
K_2O	

NOTE 1—The radioactivity, defined as the sum of the massic activity of U^{238}, Ra^{226}, Th^{232} and determined by γ-spectroscopy on the ready to use powder, should be less than 200 Bq/kg. This value will be reviewed at the next revision of this standard and will be based upon the radioactivity data from ceramic implant manufacturers.

4. Physical Properties

4.1 The minimum bulk density of yttrium oxide stabilized zirconium oxide shall be 6.00 g/cm³ or greater as determined by Test Method C 373 as applied with the following modifications:

4.1.1 Weight determination in 3.1 and 5.1 of Test Method C 373 shall be made to the nearest 0.5 mg.

4.1.2 The calculation of bulk density in 12.1 of Test Method C 373 shall be calculated as follows:

$$B=(D\cdot d)/M-S) \quad (1)$$

where:

B = bulk density, g/cm³,
D = dry weight, g,
M = saturated weight, g,
S = suspended weight, g, and
d = density of water at the temperature when measurement is taken.

4.2 The total porosity shall be no greater than 1.0 vol % and open porosity shall be no greater than 0.1 vol % as determined by Test Method C 373.

4.3 *Grain Size*—The mean linear intercept distance shall be 0.6 μm or less, in accordance with Section 10 of Test Method E 112.

[1] This specification is under the jurisdiction of ASTM Committee F-4 on Medical and Surgical Materials and Devices and is the direct responsibility of Subcommittee F04.13 on Ceramic Materials.

Current edition approved June 10, 1998. Published August 1998.

[2] *Annual Book of ASTM Standards*, Vol 15.02.

[3] *Annual Book of ASTM Standards*, Vol 15.01.

[4] *Annual Book of ASTM Standards*, Vol 03.01.

[5] *Annual Book of ASTM Standards*, Vol 13.01.

[6] Available from the American National Standards Institute, 11 W. 42nd St., 13th Floor, New York, NY 10036.

4.4 The monoclinic phase shall be 5 % or less on a polished surface with surface finish equivalent to 0.05 µm Ra (0.8 µm cutoff). Peak height of tetragonal phase, T(111) at $2\theta=30.2°$, and monoclinic phase, $M(\bar{1}11)$ at $2\theta=28.2°$ and M(111) at $2\theta=31.3°$ shall be identified by X-ray diffraction (Copper K Alpha radiation) analysis to calculate percent of monoclinic phase by the following equation (**1**)[7]:

$$\text{monoclinic phase } \% = M(\bar{1}11)+M(111)/M(\bar{1}11)+T(111)+M(111) \quad (2)$$

5. Mechanical Properties

5.1 The average room temperature flexural strength shall be 800 MPa (116 ksi) or greater by four point bend in accordance with Test Method C 1161. A minimum of ten samples (sample size "B") are to be tested.

5.2 A Weibull modulus value is not considered mandatory for general acceptance and use of this material. For certain applications, the manufacturer and end user may agree that Weibull modulus testing is mandatory. If Weibull modulus is tested it shall be tested in accordance with Practice C 1239. The minimum number of specimens tested shall be 30 and the minimum acceptable Weibull modulus shall be 10.

5.3 The minimum room temperature elastic modulus shall be 200 GPa (29×10^6 psi) in accordance with Test Method C 1198. A rectangular specimen with dimensions of 60 mm by 10 by 3 mm is recommended. An acceptable alternative test method for elastic modulus is Test Method C 1259.

5.4 The minimum Vickers hardness value shall be 1200 HV in accordance with Test Method C 1327. The load shall be 1 kg and the dwell time shall be 15 s.

6. Test Specimen Fabrication

6.1 Specific test specimens shall be prepared from the same batch of material and by the same processes as those employed in fabricating ceramic implant devices.

7. Quality Program Requirements

7.1 The producer shall maintain a quality program, such as the program defined in ASQC C1 to maintain quality consistency of test specimens.

8. Keywords

8.1 advanced ceramics; surgical implant; Y-TZP; yttria stabilized zirconia; zirconium oxide

[7] The boldface numbers given in parentheses refer to a list of references at the end of the text.

APPENDIXES

(Nonmandatory Information)

X1. RATIONALE

X1.1 The purpose of this specification is to characterize the composition and properties of high purity dense yyttria tetragonal zirconium oxide polycrystal (Y-TZP) to assure consistency in the starting material used in the manufacture of medical devices, in particular surgical implants.

X2. BIOCOMPATIBILITY

X2.1 This specification is needed to ensure a high-quality material for use in biological applications. Yttria stabilized tetragonal zirconia polycrystal (Y-TZP) has been demonstrated (**2, 3**) to exhibit a well-characterized biological response that is equivalent to or better than that exhibited by the reference materials cited and tested in Practice F 981 and Practice F 748 or equivalent. The chemical, physical and mechanical requirements contained in this specification serve as criteria for a high-purity, consistent product that can be implanted in the body. The suitability of this material from a human implant perspective is dependent on the specific application. The biological test appropriate for the specific site, such as recommended in method Practice F 748 should be used as a guideline. Further testing (roughness, static/fatigue strength, aging effects, etc.) may be required for specific applications.

X3. STERILIZATION OF Y-TZP

X3.1 Immersion of Y-TZP in water at elevated temperature and pressure has been shown to cause changes in the material structure and properties (**4**). These property changes are affected by the processing of the basic material.

X3.2 Post processing, including any type of sterilization, should be cautiously considered only after consultation with the manufacturer of the material or device.

X4. RADIOACTIVITY OF Y-TZP

X4.1 Biomedical materials are known to contain radioactivity. This does not, however mean that these materials pose an unacceptable risk to human health or even that they pose any net risk. Zirconia materials rank well below the dose limit of 1mSv/Year defined for the general public (**5**). This limit recommended by the International Commission on Radiological Protection (ICRP) is oriented to the average natural dose (1.5 to 3.5 mSv/Year) caused by naturally occurring radionuclides and cosmic radiation.

REFERENCES

(**1**) Garvie, Ronald C. and Nicholson, Patrick S. "Phase Analysis in Zirconia Systems," *J. Amer. Ceram. Soc.*, 55 [6], 1972, pp. 303–305.

(**2**) Ohashi, T. et al, "Studies on Mechanical Strength, Tissue Affinity and Cytoxicity of UTZ-30 Zirconia," *The World Biomaterials Congress*, 1988.

(**3**) Christel, P. et al, "Mechanical Properties and Short Term in Vivo Evaluation of Yttrium-Oxide-Partially-Stabilized Zirconia," *J. Biomed. Mater. Res.*, Vol 23, Jan. 1989, pp.45-61.

(**4**) Lilley, E., "Review of Low Temperature Degradation in Y-TZPs," in *Corrosion and Corrosive Degradation of Ceramics, Ceramics Transactions*, Vol 10 Ed. R. Tressler and N. McNallan, 1990.

(**5**) Porstendorfer, J., Reineking, A., and Willert, H.G., "Radiation Risk Estimation Based on Activity Measurements of Zirconium Oxide Implants," *Journal of Biomedical Materials Research*, Vol 32, 1996, pp. 663-667.

Standard Test Method for Bend Testing of Needles Used in Surgical Sutures[1]

This standard is issued under the fixed designation F 1874; the number immediately following the designation indicates the year of original adoption or, in the case of revision, the year of last revision. A number in parentheses indicates the year of last reapproval. A superscript epsilon (ε) indicates an editorial change since the last revision or reapproval.

1. Scope

1.1 This test method describes the procedure for bend testing needles used for the placement of surgical sutures.

1.2 *This standard does not purport to address all of the safety concerns, if any, associated with its use. It is the responsibility of the user of this standard to establish appropriate safety and health practices and determine the applicability of regulatory limitations prior to use.*

2. Referenced Documents

2.1 *ASTM Standards:*

F 1840 Terminology for Surgical Suture Needles[2]

3. Terminology

3.1 *Definitions*— Definitions of terms used in this test method are in accordance with Terminology F 1840.

3.2 *Definitions of Terms Specific to This Standard:*

3.2.1 *needle test gripping location, n*— for test methods, the needle will be clamped two-thirds of the distance back from the point of the needle. Since the needle will deform during the bend test, the needle test gripping location only applies to an unbent needle.

3.2.2 *test chord length, n*—the straight line distance from the center of rotation of the needle in the test fixture to the initial point of contact with the bending platform or knife edge.

4. Summary of Test Method

4.1 Surgical needles are grasped approximately two-thirds of the distance from the point of the needle, then bent against a knife edge or platform. The force deflection data obtained from the test will be used to calculate the yield bend moment and the maximum bend moment.

4.2 The decision to use a knife edge or a platform for the bending surface will be determined by the equipment available.

5. Significance and Use

5.1 This test method provides a means of assessing the yield moment and maximum moment of a surgical needle.

5.2 The needle is bent against a platform or knife edge, and it is bent at the approximate location where a pair of needle holders would grip it. This simulates the actual bending of a needle while in surgical use.

6. Apparatus

6.1 *Clamping Fixture*— A device to firmly clamp and rotate the needle.

6.2 *Bending Platform*— The surface on which the curved needle will exert force during the test. The bending platform will have its top surface located along the horizontal axis of the center of rotation of the clamping fixture.

6.3 *Knife Edge*—The knife edge will be placed parallel to the centerline of rotation to provide a single point contact for reading the torque generated by the needle.

6.4 *Data Collection System*—The data will be collected as a function of rotational angle.

6.5 *Rotation Speed*— The clamping fixture must be rotated at a continuous and constant speed. This speed will be less than 30°/s.

7. Sampling

7.1 A sample size of no less than five needles shall be used.

8. Procedure (see Fig. 1)

8.1 Securely clamp the needle into the clamping fixture at a position approximately two-thirds of the distance back from the tip of the needle.

8.2 Rotate the clamping fixture forward until the needle touches the bending platform or knife edge. Continue rotating the clamping fixture through a sufficient angle to generate the required data. While the needle is bending, collect the bending force data as a function of the bend angle.

9. Calculation (see Fig. 2)

9.1 Data will be reported as a moment versus degrees of rotation. Units will be reported.

9.2 *Yield Bend Moment*—Using the graph obtained during the needle bend test, calculate the initial slope of the graph. Draw a line with the same slope through the 2° offset on the degree axis. Read the bending moment at the point where the 2° offset slope crosses the data line. This is the yield bend moment.

9.3 *Yield Bend Angle*— Read the angle at the point where the 2° offset slope line crosses the data line.

9.4 *Maximum Bend Moment*—The maximum bend moment is the largest bending moment achieved by the needle during the bend test.

[1] This test method is under the jurisdiction of ASTM Committee F-04 on Medical and Surgical Materials and Devices and is the direct responsibility of Subcommittee F04.33 on Medical/Surgical Instruments.

Current edition approved April 10, 1998. Published March 1999.

[2] *Annual Book of ASTM Standards*, Vol 13.01.

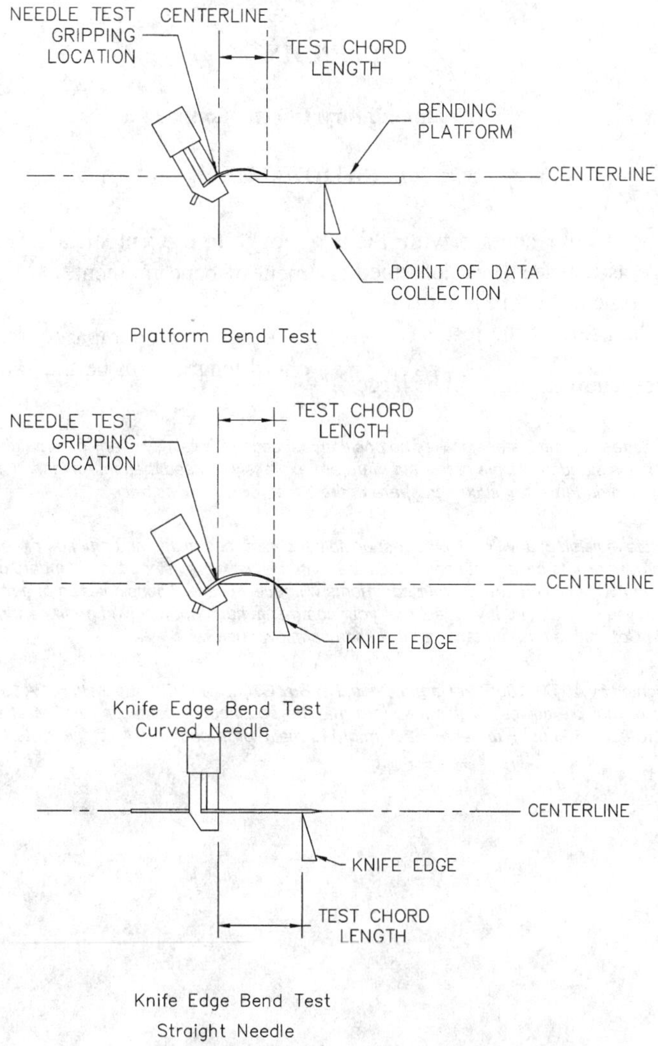

FIG. 1 Sample Bend Tests

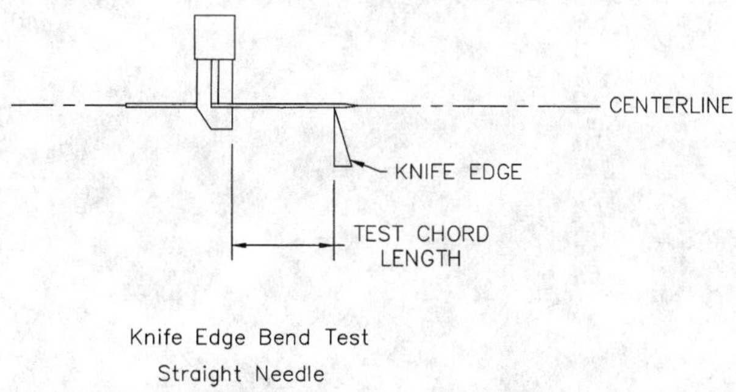

FIG. 2 Bend Test Data Curve

10. Report

10.1 Include the following information:

10.1.1 Sample identification, test conditions, and apparatus.

10.1.2 Test chord length.

10.1.3 Yield bend moment.

10.1.4 Yield bend angle.

10.1.5 Maximum bend moment (angle at which it was achieved should be reported).

11. Precision and Bias

11.1 *Precision*—The precision of the results of this test method are dependent on the equipment selected.

11.2 *Bias*—No standard material has been selected for reference; therefore, bias for this test method cannot be determined.

12. Keywords

12.1 bend test; needle; strength; surgical; suture

APPENDIX

(Nonmandatory Information)

X1. RATIONALE

X1.1 It is understood that the needle contact with the platform or knife edge will change as the needle is deformed during the test, effecting the value of the test chord length. This is an agreed upon convention by the users of the test.

X1.2 It is understood that the test chord length will be large enough to prevent shear effect on the test and allow measurement of bend moment.

X1.3 When comparing results, it is understood that the test chord lengths will be the same.

The American Society for Testing and Materials takes no position respecting the validity of any patent rights asserted in connection with any item mentioned in this standard. Users of this standard are expressly advised that determination of the validity of any such patent rights, and the risk of infringement of such rights, are entirely their own responsibility.

This standard is subject to revision at any time by the responsible technical committee and must be reviewed every five years and if not revised, either reapproved or withdrawn. Your comments are invited either for revision of this standard or for additional standards and should be addressed to ASTM Headquarters. Your comments will receive careful consideration at a meeting of the responsible technical committee, which you may attend. If you feel that your comments have not received a fair hearing you should make your views known to the ASTM Committee on Standards, at the address shown below.

Standard Practice for Fretting Corrosion Testing of Modular Implant Interfaces: Hip Femoral Head-Bore and Cone Taper Interface[1]

This standard is issued under the fixed designation F 1875; the number immediately following the designation indicates the year of original adoption or, in the case of revision, the year of last revision. A number in parentheses indicates the year of last reapproval. A superscript epsilon (ϵ) indicates an editorial change since the last revision or reapproval.

1. Scope

1.1 This practice describes the testing, analytical, and characterization methods for evaluating the mechanical stability of the bore and cone interface of the head and stem junction of modular hip implants subjected to cyclic loading by measurements of fretting corrosion. **(1-5)** Two test methods described are as follows:

1.1.1 *Method I*—The primary purpose of this method is to provide a uniform set of guidelines for long-term testing to determine the amount of damage by measurement of the production of corrosion products and particulate debris from fretting and fretting corrosion. Damage also is assessed by characterization of the damage to the bore and cone surfaces.**(4, 5)**

1.1.2 *Methods II*—This method provides for short-term electrochemical evaluation of the fretting corrosion of the modular interface. It is not the intent of this method to produce damage nor particulate debris but rather to provide a rapid method for qualitative assessment of design changes which do not include material changes.**(1-4)**

1.2 This practice does not provide for judgment or prediction of in vivo implant performance, but rather, provides for a uniform set of guidelines for evaluating relative differences in performance between differing implant designs, constructs, or materials with performance defined in the context of the amount of fretting and fretting corrosion. Also, this practice should permit direct comparison of fretting corrosion data between independent research groups, and thus, provide for building of a data base on modular implant performance.

1.3 This practice provides for comparative testing of manufactured hip femoral heads and stems and for coupon type specimen testing where the male taper portion of the modular junction does not include the entire hip implant, with the taper portion of the coupon identical in design, manufacturing, and materials to the taper of the final hip implant.**(4,5)**

1.4 Method I of this practice has been provided in a manner to permit simultaneous evaluation of the fatigue strength of a femoral hip stem (in accordance with Practice F 1440) and the mechanical stability and debris generated by fretting and fretting corrosion of the modular interface.

1.5 The general concepts and methodologies described in this practice could be applied to the study of other modular interfaces in total joint prostheses.

1.6 *This standard may involve hazardous materials, operations, and equipment. This standard does not purport to address all of the safety concerns, if any, associated with its use. It is the responsibility of the user of this standard to establish appropriate safety and health practices and determine the applicability of regulatory limitations prior to use.*

2. Referenced Documents

2.1 *ASTM Standards:*

E 4 Practices for Force Verification of Testing Machines[2]
E 466 Practice for Conducting Force Controlled Constant Amplitude Axial Fatigue Tests of Metallic Materials[2]
E 467 Practice for Verification of Constant Amplitude Dynamic Loads in an Axial Load Fatigue Testing Machine[2]
F 561 Practice for Retrieval and Analysis of Implanted Medical Devices and Associated Tissues[3]
F 746 Test Method for Pitting or Crevice Corrosion of Metallic Surgical Implant Materials[3]
F 897 Test Method for Measuring Fretting Corrosion of Osteosynthesis Plates and Screws[3]
F 1440 Practice for Cyclic Fatigue Testing of Metallic Stemmed Hip Arthroplasty Femoral Components Without Torsion[3]
F 1636 Specification for Bores and Cones for Modular Femoral Heads[3]
G 3 Practice for Conventions Applicable to Electrochemical Measurements in Corrosion Testing[4]
G 5 Reference Test Method for Making Potentiostatic and Potentiodynamic Anodic Polarization Measurements[4]
G 15 Terminology Relating to Corrosion and Corrosion Testing[4]
G 40 Terminology Relating to Wear and Erosion[4]
G 61 Test Method for Conducting Cyclic Potentiodynamic Polarization Measurements for Localized Corrosion Susceptibility of Iron-, Nickel-, or Cobalt-Based Alloys[4]
G 102 Practice for Calculation of Corrosion Rates and Related Information from Electrochemical Measurements[4]

[1] This practice is under the jurisdiction of ASTM Committee F-04 on Medical and Surgical Materials and Devices and is the direct responsibility of Subcommittee F04.15 on Material Test Methods.

Current edition approved April 10, 1998. Published June 1998.

[2] *Annual Book of ASTM Standards*, Vol 03.01.
[3] *Annual Book of ASTM Standards*, Vol 13.01.
[4] *Annual Book of ASTM Standards*, Vol 03.02.

2.2 *ISO Standards:*

ISO 7206-7 Endurance Performance of Stemmed Femoral Components Without Application of Torsion[5,6]

3. Terminology

3.1 *Definitions:*

3.1.1 *corrosive wear, n*—wear in which chemical or electrochemical reaction with the environment is significant.

3.1.2 *coverage, n*—the length, parallel to the taper surface, that the bore and cone interfaces are in contact.

3.1.3 *crevice corrosion, n*—localized corrosion of a metal surface at, or immediately adjacent to, an area that is shielded from full exposure to the environment because of close proximity between the metal and the surface of another material.

3.1.4 *external circuit, n*—the wires, connectors, measuring devices, current sources, etc., that are used to bring about or measure the desired electrical conditions within the test cell.

3.1.5 *femoral head neck extension, n*—a distance parallel to the taper axis, from the nominal neck offset length (*k*) as defined in Specification F 1636, and the center of the head. Such variants from the nominal length are used to adjust for resection level, leg length, and so forth. A positive neck extension equates to the center of the head being located further away from the stem.

3.1.6 *fretting, n*—small amplitude oscillatory motion, usually tangential, between two solid surfaces in contact.

3.1.7 *fretting corrosion, n*—the deterioration at the interface between contacting surfaces as the result of corrosion and slight oscillatory slip between the two surfaces.

3.1.8 *fretting wear, n*—wear arising as a result of fretting.

3.1.9 *total elemental level, n*—the total weight of particulate matter and corrosion ions generated by fretting wear and fretting corrosion. Most analytical techniques are unable to accurately differentiate between ions and particulates, and therefore, total elemental level refers to all matter and corrosion products released by fretting wear and corrosion.

3.1.10 *wear, n*—damage to a solid surface, generally involving progressive loss of material, due to relative motion between that surface and a contacting substance or substances.

4. Summary of Test Method

4.1 *Method I*—The femoral stem and head components, or coupons to simulate head-taper-neck geometry, are loaded cyclically in a manner similar to that described in Practice F 1440. The head neck junction is exposed to a saline or proteinaceous solution, either by immersion of the entire device, or with a fluid containing envelope. The cyclic load is applied for a minimum of 10 million cycles. At the conclusion of testing, the isolated fluid is withdrawn for chemical analysis for total elemental level, and characterization of particulate debris. The taper interface is subsequently disengaged and the surfaces inspected for fretting wear and corrosion using optical microscopy and scanning electron microscopy. The output of these methods is a quantitative measure of total elemental level and a qualitative evaluation of damage of the modular interface caused by fretting wear and corrosion.

4.2 *Method II*—A coupon similar to that used in Method I, or an entire femoral stem and head construct may be mounted in an inverted position in a test chamber. The chamber is filled with an electrolyte solution to a level sufficient to submerge the bore and cone interface, and a small portion of the exposed neck. The area of contact and articulation between the ball and the test apparatus is isolated from the electrolyte, either by being above the fill level, or with an elastomeric seal used to isolate the bottom of the test chamber.

4.2.1 *Procedure A*— A saturated calomel electrode with a luggin probe is used as a reference electrode to measure changes in the corrosion potential with an electrometer. A counter electrode also may be employed and the polarization characteristics measured with a potentiostat.

4.2.2 *Procedure B*— A large surface area counter electrode is immersed in the solution to simulate the area of the stem. A zero resistance ammeter is connected between the test device and the counter electrode. The difference in current, thus measured prior to and during cyclic loading represents the fretting corrosion current flowing between the modular interface (anode) and the metal sheet (cathode).

5. Significance and Use

5.1 The modular interfaces of total joint prostheses are subjected to micromotion that could result in fretting and corrosion. The release of corrosion products and particulate debris could stimulate adverse biological reactions, as well as lead to accelerated wear at the articulation interface. Methods to assess the stability and corrosion resistance of the modular interfaces, therefore, are an essential component of device testing.

5.2 Long-term in vitro testing is essential to produce damage and debris from fretting of a modular interface. **(4,5)** The use of proteinaceous solutions is recommended to best simulate the in vivo environment.

5.3 Short-term tests often can be useful in evaluations of differences in design during device development.**(1-4)** The electrochemical methods provide semiquantitative measures of fretting corrosion rates. The relative contributions of mechanical and electrochemical processes to the total corrosion and particulate release phenomena, however, have not been established; therefore, these tests should not be utilized to compare the effects of changes in material combinations, but rather be utilized to evaluate design changes of bore (head) and cone (stem) components.

5.4 These tests are recommended for evaluating the fretting wear and corrosion of modular interfaces of hip femoral head and stem components. Similar methods may be applied to other modular interfaces where fretting corrosion is of concern.

5.5 These methods are recommended for comparative evaluation of the fretting wear and corrosion of new materials, coatings, or designs, or a combination thereof, under consideration for hip femoral head and neck modular interfaces. Components for testing may be those of a manufactured modular hip device (finished product) or sample coupons,

[5] Available from American National Standards Institute, 11 W. 42nd St., 13th Floor, New York, NY 10036.

[6] The bold face numbers in parentheses refers to the list of references at the end of this standard.

which are designed and manufactured for simulation of the head, taper, and neck region of a modular hip device.

6. Apparatus

6.1 *Testing Machines*— The action of the machine should be analyzed to ensure that the desired form and periodic force amplitude is maintained for the duration of the test (see Practice E 467). The test machine should have a load monitoring system, such as the transducer mounted in line with the specimen. The loads should be monitored continuously in the early stages of the test and periodically thereafter to ensure the desired load cycle is maintained. The varying load as determined by suitable dynamic verification should be maintained at all times to within ±2 % of the maximum force being used in accordance with Practices E 4 and E 466.

6.2 *Specimen Mounting Devices, Method I*—Modular hip and stem components shall be set-up as described in Practices F 1440. Coupon samples shall be set-up as shown in Fig. 1. The set-up must provide for identical loading geometry as that in Practice F 1440.

6.3 *Specimen Mounting Devices, Method II*—Modular hip and stem components shall be set-up in an inverted position, as shown in Fig. 2. Coupon samples may be set up as shown in Fig. 1, or in an inverted orientation.

6.4 *Environmental Containment, Method I*—The prosthesis may be placed in an environmental chamber, which is filled with the appropriate fluid. Care should be taken to ensure that the contact area between the head and the low friction thrust bearing is not exposed to the electrolyte solution. The modular interface of the prostheses or coupon samples also may be enclosed in an elastomeric sleeve, which contains the electrolyte. The materials used for such isolation must be nonreactive and capable of retaining the fluid environment, (that is, prevent leakage), throughout the course of testing. The volume of the chamber shall be between 5 and 100 mL.

NOTE 1—The use of small fluid volumes with the sleeve containment method may not produce as much fretting corrosion as full prosthesis exposure, due to the reduced surface area of the cathodic metal exposed.

6.5 *Environmental Chamber, Method II*—The chamber shall be filled with electrolyte so as to submerge the modular interface. An elastomeric seal is used to isolate the contact area between the head and the load application surface. Similar seals should be employed for coupon sample testing. For coupons orientated shown in Fig. 1, the chamber fill level shall be kept below the articulation between the head and the loading apparatus.

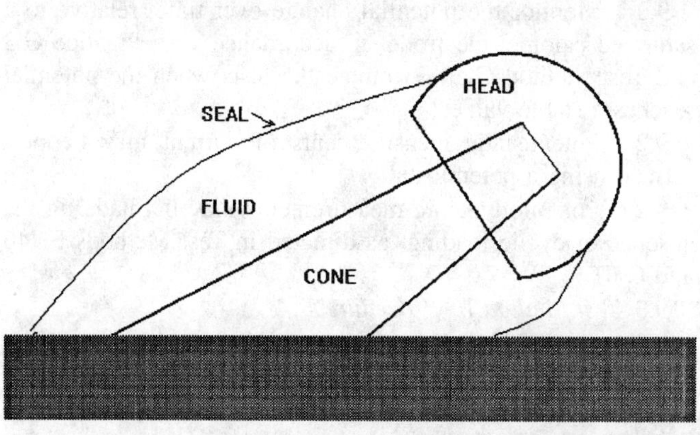

NOTE 1—For Method I, the fluid is contained within the sleeve. For Method II, the device should be submerged in an electrolyte while the contact area between the top of the head and the loading apparatus is not exposed to the fluid. A counter electrode is placed in the same bath.

FIG. 1 Sketch of a Coupon Style of Test Specimen

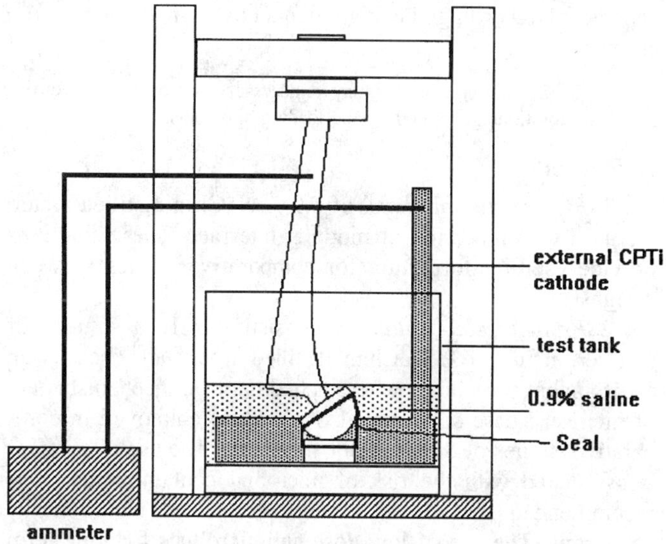

NOTE 1—The cathode sheet surrounds, but does not make contact with the device being tested. For Procedure A, the counter electrode is not utilized, and is substituted with a luggin probe and calomel electrode.

FIG. 2 Suggested Set Up for Method II Procedure B, Measurements of Fretting Corrosion Currents of a Complete THR

6.6 *Counter and Reference Electrodes, Method II*—A counter electrode is included in the external circuit of Method II to act as a cathode for measurement of corrosion currents. A reference electrode is employed for measurement of the corrosion potential of the specimen.

6.6.1 *Method II, Procedure A*—The counter electrode and saturated calomel electrode (SCE) shall be employed in accordance with Test Methods G 5 and G 61.

6.6.2 *Method II, Procedure B*—The counter electrode is used to simulate the surface area of the femoral stem. It should be made of the same alloy as the stem material being tested. A surface area at least equal to the stem and any porous coating should be employed. An area of 400 cm^2 is recommended. The counter electrode should not be in contact with the test specimen, but rather is connected to it via the zero resistance ammeter.

6.7 *Potential and Current Measuring Equipment, Method II, Procedure A*—The potential shall be measured by a high impedance voltmeter. This could either be a free standing electrometer with an impedance > 10^{10} Ω, or the electrometer in a potentiostat in accordance with Test Methods G 5 and G 61. The potentiostat is used to measure current in potentiostatic or cyclic polarization tests, using the sign conventions of Practice G 3. The use of a printer provides a permanent record.

6.8 *Current Measurement Equipment, Method II, Procedure B*—A zero resistance ammeter is used to measure current in Procedure B. The output of the ammeter should be connected to a recording oscilloscope, strip chart recorder, or computer capable of recording the high frequency components of the current signal.

NOTE 2—Special precautions may be necessary to protect the electronics from vibrations generated by the loading apparatus.

7. Reagents

7.1 *Electrolyte Solutions*, of 0.9 % NaCl in distilled water, are used for immersion of modular interface. These solutions provide useful information for comparative studies between designs.

7.2 *Protienaceous Solutions*, consisting of 10 % solution of calf serum in 0.9 % NaCl in distilled water, are used as an environment for studies where actual damage mechanisms are of interest. These solutions also would be employed in comparative studies of different alloy systems. The use of proteins is associated with the risk of microbial contamination. It is recommended that these tests be conducted under sterile conditions. The use of low dose antimicrobials for long term tests is indicated, as well.

8. Test Specimen

8.1 *Modular Hip Devices*—The hip components shall be representative of typical manufactured components; no extraordinary procedures for manufacturing, quality control and assurance, and inspection shall be used. Whenever possible, the size of the hip shall conform to the medium size of a given range of sizes. The length of the femoral head offset shall be the maximum, typical of the hip stem being offered, or the maximum length offered within the product catalogue for the tested stem-taper component. In the case of hip products manufactured by different sources where availability of specific components is limited, (for example, hip stem size, femoral head off-set, etc; comparative testing shall be performed so as to identically match total head off-set, neck angle and extension. In other words, if two different hip components are to be tested, every effort shall be made to test components that would fulfill the specific needs of a given patient. This is due to the fact that there are many different systems for sizing femoral stem and head components, and they are specific to the manufacturer and design of the hip implant device.

8.2 *Sample Coupons*— Sample coupons shall be designed and manufactured to replicate the taper-head-neck region of a hip prosthesis. An example of such sample coupons is given in Fig. 1. Taper angles and dimensions, with specific references to the critical areas of design, shall be in accordance with Specification F 1636. The methods of machining and finishing of the taper surfaces shall be the same as that used for production prostheses.

8.3 *Number of Test Specimens*—Except in the case of product testing, in which component availability may be limited, at least five samples shall be tested for each configuration under evaluation.

9. Procedure

9.1 *Test Method*:

9.1.1 The head-taper components shall be assembled in accordance with Practice F 1440, or using standard interoperative surgical protocol for assembly of modular hip devices.

9.1.2 The modular components shall be assembled dry. Apply a single static load to 2000 N, as per head pull off test.

9.1.3 The modular interface shall be exposed to the test solution in accordance with 6.4.

9.1.4 Cyclic testing of modular interface shall be carried out as prescribed by Practice F 1440.

9.1.5 Apply a cyclic load of 3 kN with a minimum load of 300 N and a maximum load of 3.3 kN (67 to 740 lbs), in accordance with ISO 7206-7. Tests should be conducted at a frequency of 5 Hz, and be terminated after 10 million cycles.

9.1.6 At the completion of the test, collect the fluid for analysis of total metal content and particle characterization. The procedures for chemical analysis and particle harvesting given in Practice F 561 can be used as guide. The fluid shall be reserved in a clean container suitable for subsequent dilution and digestion.

9.1.7 The taper-head components which shall be disassembled in a manner so as to reserve any entrapped fluids and particulate debris, which may include flushing of the interface region with DI water. All collected fluids and debris shall be collected in a common container for subsequent analysis or subsequent digestion prior to chemical analysis. Particles generated in protienaceous solutions may need protein digestion as described in Practice F 561 to prevent agglomeration of particulate debris.

9.1.8 Analyze for all major elements in the alloys, using Practice F 561 as a guide. Qualitative evaluation of taper surfaces should done by optical microscopy and scanning electron microscopy. In cases where the weight of the coupon specimens is small enough, weight loss of the specimens may be made by microbalance in accordance with Test Method F 897.

9.2 *Test Method II, Procedure A*:

9.2.1 Mount the specimen and apply a cyclic load as described above.

9.2.2 Load ranges as directed in 9.1.5 may be used. Since this is not a simulation test, lower load ranges are recommended. Apply cyclic loads of 2000 N, with a minimum of 40 N and a maximum of 2040 N.

9.2.3 To best characterize the electrochemical components of fretting corrosion, a frequency of 1 Hz is recommended.

9.2.4 Monitor the potential change over time, relative to a saturated calomel electrode, in accordance with Practice G 3 and Test Method G 5. Terminate the tests when the potential reaches a stable value.

9.2.5 Potentistatic measurements of current may be performed using a potentiostat.

9.2.6 Potentiodynamic measurements may be made, in the absence of cyclic loading, as directed in Test Methods F 746 and G 61.

9.3 *Test Method II, Procedure B*:

9.3.1 Assemble the components and apply a cyclic load, as above described in 9.2.1-9.2.6

9.3.2 Load ranges as directed in 9.1.5 may be used. Since this is not a simulation test, lower load ranges are recommended. Apply cyclic loads of 2000 N, with a minimum of 40 N and a maximum of 2040 N.

9.3.3 To best characterize the electrochemical components of fretting corrosion, a frequency of 1 Hz is recommended.

9.3.4 Measure the fretting corrosion current with a zero resistance ammeter. Record the currents as directed in 6.8.

9.3.5 Periodic measurement of the peak to peak currents can be utilized to quantitate the amount of fretting corrosion. Measurements taken at 3, 8.3, 15, and 30 min, at a loading frequency of 2 Hz, to produce data points at 360, 1000, 1800, and 3600 cycles are recommended.

9.3.6 Simultaneous measurement of potential also may be made, but the connection to the ammeter and counter electrode will result in different values than those observed with Procedure A.

9.4 *Optional Test Procedures*—Additional measurements, such as relative micromotion between the interfaces may provide useful information.

10. Calculation

10.1 *Test Method I*— The total amount of metal release can be calculated by multiplying the concentration of measured species times the total fluid volume.

10.1.1 The test results shall be reported for each of the elements potentially present in the collected solutions.

10.1.2 Total weight loss would be the sum of the amount of each of the major elements.

10.2 *Test Method II, Procedure B*—These electrochemical methods only provide a qualitative measure of the amount of damage produced. The amount of metal released due to electrochemical corrosion can be calculated using Faraday's law, as provided in Practice G 102. These calculations, however, will need validation by elemental analysis in tests of mixed metal devices.

11. Report

11.1 Report the following information:

11.1.1 *Modular Hip Components*—When available, the materials, manufacturer, catalogue number, size, head off-set length, taper dimensions in accordance with Specification F 1636.

11.1.2 *Coupons or Simulated Head-Taper Neck*—The materials, head off-set length, extension, and geometry and dimensions, degree of coverage, and surface finish.

11.1.3 The details of the test protocols, test solutions, length of testing, and methods of disassembly.

11.1.4 The type and quantities of fluids used for dilution, flushing of disengaged components, and digestion of elemental particles.

11.1.5 Representative scanning electron or optical photographs of the taper interfaces for the untested and tested components.

12. Precision and Bias

12.1 The precision and bias of this practice has not yet been established.

13. Keywords

13.1 bore and cone; debris; fretting corrosion; modular total hips

APPENDIX

(Nonmandatory Information)

X1. RATIONALE

X1.1 The use of modular designs for total joint replacement provides many advantages; however, the modular interfaces are subjected to micromotion that could result in fretting and corrosion. The release of corrosion products and particulate debris could stimulate adverse biological reactions, as well as lead to accelerated wear of the articulation; therefore, methods to assess the stability and corrosion resistance of the modular interfaces are an essential component of device testing.

X1.2 Short-term comparative tests of the effects of design variables can be conducted in physiological saline solutions, such as 0.9 % NaCl. Long term in vitro testing is essential to produce damage and debris from fretting of a modular interface. In order to simulate the in vivo conditions as close as possible, these tests should be conducted in electrolyte solutions containing proteins.

X1.3 Chemical analysis of the test solutions from long-term tests are recommended as a method to determine total amount of corrosion.**(4,5)** Determination of damage by measurements of weight loss is impracticable due to the large mass of the total joint prosthesis. Analysis of particles can produce information regarding the fretting process, but quantification by this practice is imprecise, since some particles may have corroded during the test. Chemical analysis also can be useful in determinations of the contributions of the two components in mixed alloy systems.

X1.4 Short-term tests often can be useful in evaluations of differences in design during device development.**(1,2,4)** The electrochemical methods provide semiquantitative measures of fretting corrosion rates; however, the relative contributions of mechanical and electrochemical processes to the total corrosion and particulate release phenomena have not been established.

REFERENCES

(1) Flemming, C.A.C., Brown, S.A., and Payer, J.H., "Mechanical Testing for Fretting Corrosion of Modular Total Hip Tapers," *Symposium on Biomaterials, Mechanical Properties, ASTM STP 1173*, ASTM, 1994, p. 156.

(2) Brown, S.A., Abera, A., D'Onofrio, M., and Flemming, C., "Effects of Neck Extension and Coverage, and Frequency on Fretting Corrosion of Modular THR Bores and Cone Interface," *Symposium on Modularity of Orthopedic Implants, ASTM STP 1301,* ASTM, 1997, p. 189.

(3) Winkler-Gniewek, W, and Ungethum, M., "Untersuchung der Reibkorrosion an mehreteiligen Spezialendoprosthesen unter Berucksichtigung der Werkstoffkombination" (An Investigation of Frictional Corrosion Concerning Special Multiple Component Prostheses With Regard to the Material Combination) *Biomed. Technik 28*, 160-167, 1993.

(4) Goldberg, J.R., Buckley, C.A., Jacobs, J.J., and Gilbert, J.L., "Corrosion Testing of Modular Hip Implants," *Symposium on Modularity of Orthopedic Implants, ASTM STP 1301,* ASTM, 1997, p. 157.

(5) Jani, S. C., Sauer, W. L., McLean, T. W., Lambert, R. D., Kovacs, P., "Fretting Corrosion Mechanisms at Modular Implant Interfaces," *Symposium on Modularity of Orthopedic Implants, ASTM STP 1301,* ASTM, 1997, p. 261.

Designation: F 1876 – 98

Standard Specification for Polyetherketoneetherketoneketone (PEKEKK) Resins for Surgical Implant Applications[1]

This standard is issued under the fixed designation F 1876; the number immediately following the designation indicates the year of original adoption or, in the case of revision, the year of last revision. A number in parentheses indicates the year of last reapproval. A superscript epsilon (ε) indicates an editorial change since the last revision or reapproval.

1. Scope

1.1 This specification covers polyetherketoneetherketoneketone (PEKEKK) resins in virgin forms as supplied by a vendor, such as flakes, pellets, blocks, etc. It provides requirements and associated test methods for these thermoplastics when they are to be used in the manufacturing of intracorporeal devices, such as surgical implants or components of surgical or dental devices.

1.2 As with any material, some characteristics may be altered by the processing techniques, such as molding, extrusion, machining, assembly, sterilization, etc. required for the production of a specific part or device; therefore, properties of fabricated forms of these resins should be evaluated using test methods that are appropriate to assure safety and efficacy as agreed upon by the vendor, purchaser, and regulating bodies.

1.3 The properties included in this specification are those applicable for PEKEKK resins only. Fabricated forms, material or forms containing colorants, fillers, processing aids, or other additives, as well as polymer blends that contain PEKEKK, are not covered by this specification.

1.4 This specification is designed to recommend physical, chemical, and biological test methods to establish a reasonable level of confidence concerning the performance of virgin PEKEKK resins for use in medical devices. The properties listed should be considered in selecting material according to the specific end-use requirements.

1.5 *This standard does not purport to address all of the safety concerns, if any, associated with its use. It is the responsibility of the user of this standard to establish appropriate safety and health practices and determine the applicability of regulatory limitations prior to use.*

2. Referenced Documents

2.1 *ASTM Standards:*

D 149 Test Method for Dielectric Breakdown Voltage and Dielectric Strength of Solid Electrical Insulating Materials at Commercial Power Frequencies[2]

D 256 Test Methods for Determining the Impact Resistance of Plastics and Electrical Insulating Materials[3]

D 570 Test Method for Water Absorption of Plastics[3]

D 638 Test Method for Tensile Properties of Plastics[3]

D 648 Test Method for Deflection Temperature of Plastics Under Flexural Load[3]

D 695 Test Method for Compressive Properties of Rigid Plastics[3]

D 696 Test Method for Coefficient of Linear Thermal Expansion of Plastics[3]

D 790 Test Methods for Flexural Properties of Unreinforced and Reinforced Plastics and Electrical Insulating Materials[3]

D 792 Test Methods for Relative Density, Density of Plastics and Specific Gravity by Displacement[3]

D 955 Test Method for Measuring Shrinkage from Mold Dimensions of Molded Plastics[3]

D 1238 Test Method for Flow Rates of Thermoplastics by Extrusion Plastometer[3]

D 1505 Test Method for Density of Plastics by the Density-Gradient Technique[3]

D 1898 Practice for Sampling of Plastics[3]

D 3417 Test Method for Heats of Fusion and Crystallization of Polymers by Thermal Analysis[4]

D 3418 Test Methods for Transition Temperatures of Polymers by Thermal Analysis[4]

D 4000 Classification System for Specifying Plastic Materials[4]

F 748 Practice for Selecting Generic Biological Test Methods for Materials and Devices[5]

2.2 *ISO Standards:*

ISO 1628/1 Plastics–Guidelines for the Standardization of Methods for Determination of Viscosity Number and Limiting Viscosity Number of Polymers in Dilute Solution–Part 1: General Conditions[6]

ISO 1133 Plastics–Determination of the Melt Mass-Flow Rate (MFR) and the Melt Volume-Flow Rate (MVR) of Thermoplastics[6]

---

[1] This specification is under the jurisdiction of ASTM Committee F-4 on Medical and Surgical Materials and Devices and is the direct responsibility of Subcommittee F04.11 on Polymeric Materials.

Current edition approved April 10, 1998. Published June 1998.

[2] *Annual Book of ASTM Standards*, Vol 10.01.

[3] *Annual Book of ASTM Standards*, Vol 08.01.

[4] *Annual Book of ASTM Standards*, Vol 08.02.

[5] *Annual Book of ASTM Standards*, Vol 13.01.

ISO 10993 Biological Evaluation of Medical Devices, Parts 1–12[6]

2.3 *Other Documents:*

FDA Regulation CFR 177.1580[7]

United States Pharmacopeia, Vol XXI, or latest edition[8]

3. Terminology

3.1 *Definitions of Terms Specific to This Standard:*

3.1.1 *fabricated forms, n*—those items into which the virgin forms may be converted. These forms include shapes and forms produced by means of machining, extruding, and compression molding virgin forms into a subsequent entity, for example, rods, slabs, sheets, film, complex shaped parts and devices.

3.1.2 *formulated compound, n*—PEKEKK materials, parts, or devices fabricated from virgin forms in such a way as to contain intentional or unintentional adjuvant substances.

3.1.3 *virgin forms, n*—that form of the PEKEKK resin as obtained by the synthesizer after removal of residual monomers, solvents, catalysts, etc. It typically will be in the form of pellets, chips, or blocks. It is the material from which rods, slabs, sheets, films, or specific parts and devices are fabricated.

4. Classification

4.1 PEKEKK resins in the scope of this specification are pure semicrystalline homopolymers consisting of phenylene rings connected by either (E) and carbonyl (or ketone, K) groups along the polymer chain (see Fig. 1). Their polymeric structures are defined by the repeating unit EKEKK.

4.2 Types of PEKEKK plastics, molding, and extrusion grades are described in Classification D 4000.

5. Properties

5.1 PEKEKK resins used in medical applications may comply with the Food and Drug Administration (FDA) Regulation 21 CFR 177.1580, which covers both wet and dry food contact applications.

[6] Available from American National Standards Institute, 11 W. 42nd St., 13th Floor, New York, NY 10036.

[7] Available from the Food and Drug Administration, Pittsburgh, PA.

[8] Available from U.S. Pharmacopeial Convention, Inc., Easton, PA.

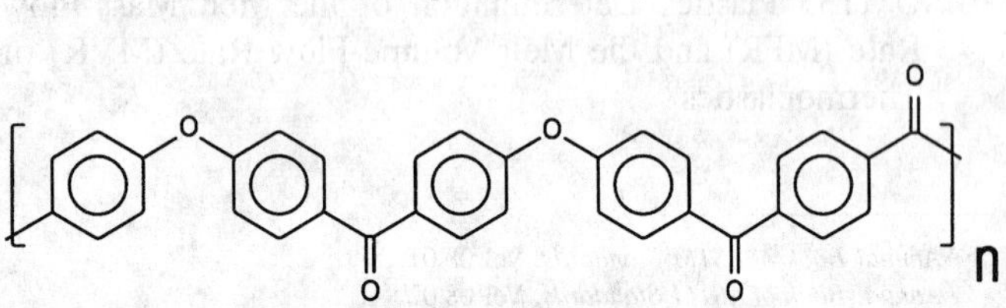

FIG. 1 Chemical Structure of PEKEKK

5.2 The infrared spectrum (**1**)[9] of these materials is characteristic of their molecular repeating units. A representative spectrum is provided in Fig. 2. The PEKEKK resin shall yield an infrared transmittance spectrum that exhibits major bands only at the wavelengths listed for a standard reference spectrum of that material.

5.2.1 The infrared spectrum, as used herein, is to identify the specific type of PAEK present and does not necessarily indicate an acceptable degree of material purity.

5.2.2 The presence of additional bands in the sample's infrared spectrum compared to that of the reference material may indicate a different PAEK, impurities, or both.

5.3 The physical and chemical property requirements for the virgin resin are listed in Table 1. If additional characteristics are necessary because of a specific application, the procedures referenced in 5.7 are recommended, or as agreed upon by vendor and purchaser.

5.4 The solution viscosity requirements listed in Table 1 may be supplemented, or replaced, by rheological or complex viscosity data as agreed upon by vendor and purchaser.

5.5 The chemical, physical, and mechanical properties of fabricated forms are related to the processes utilized in producing the fabricated form, for example, molding, machining, sterilization, etc. Additionally, the properties necessary for a particular device to perform properly will vary from one device type to another. Table 2 lists some typical properties of nonsterilized injection molded material.

5.6 Test specimens shall be fabricated (machined, injection molded, etc.) from the virgin resin, or finished part, in such a way to effectively represent the material characteristics of the nonsterilized finished part.

5.7 Tests and test procedures shall be such as to assure a high level of control and characterization of the virgin resin as received from the supplier (see Test Methods D 149, D 256, D 570, D 638, D 648, D 695, D 696, D 790, D 792, D 955, D 1238, D 1505, D 3417, D 3418, and D 4000).

6. Sampling

6.1 The material should be sampled in accordance with standard sampling procedures, such as those described in Practice D 1898, or other sampling techniques unless otherwise agreed upon between consumer and supplier.

7. Biocompatibility

7.1 Biocompatibility of PEKEKK resins and implant devices made using these materials shall be determined in accordance with Practice F 748 or the ISO 10993 series, unless otherwise agreed upon by packager and consumer, and regulating bodies (**2-5**).

8. Keywords

8.1 PEKEKK; polyetherketoneetherketoneketone

[9] The boldface numbers in parentheses refer to the list of references at the end of this standard.

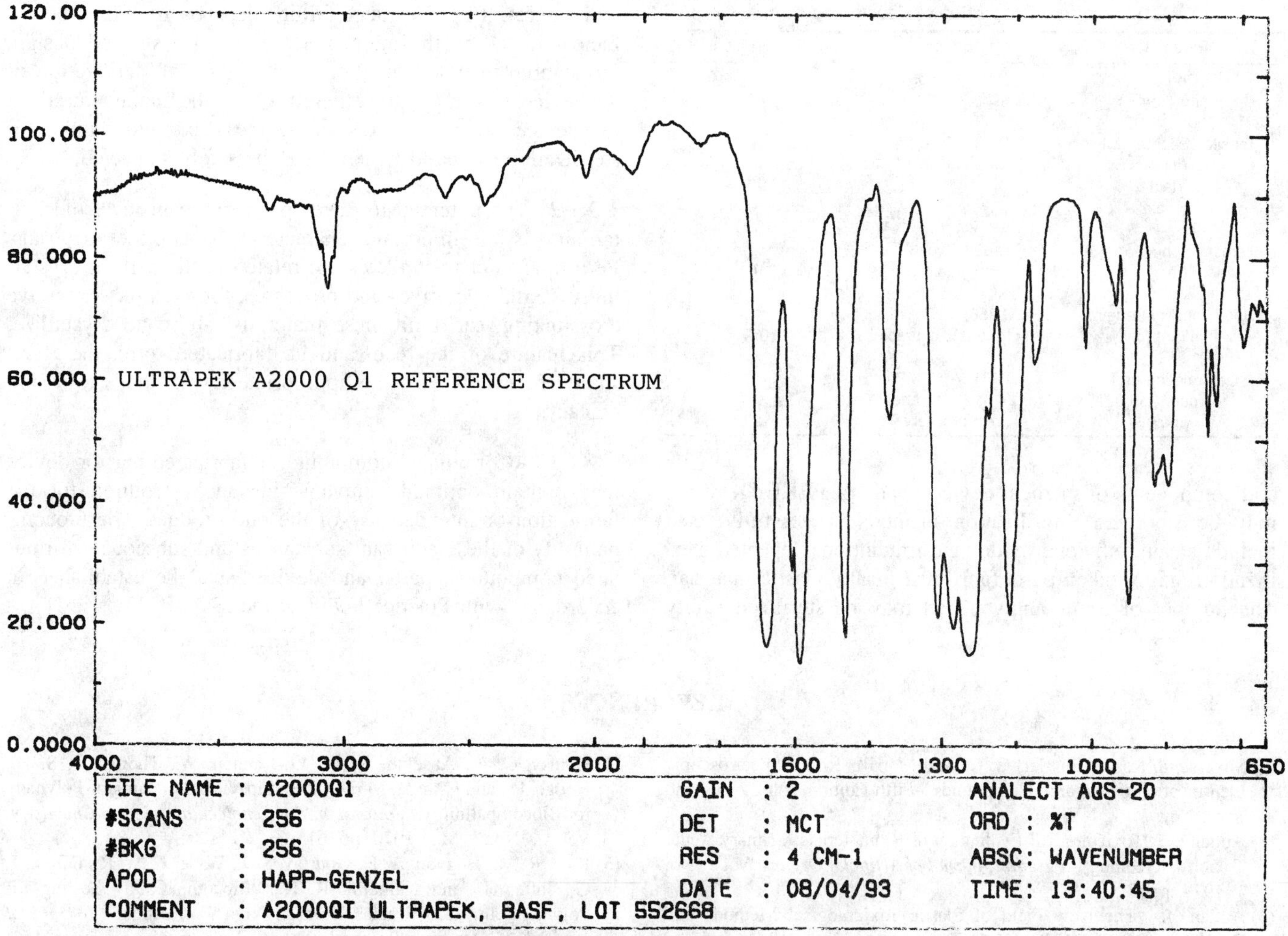

FIG. 2 Representative Infrared Spectra of PEKEKK

TABLE 1 Required Properties of Virgin Resin

Parameter	Method	Requirement
T_g, (°C)	DSC, 20 °C/min, sealed sample	160-200
T_m, (°C)	DSC, 20 °C/min, sealed sample	360-400
Viscosity number, (min) (mL/g)	ISO 1628, conc. sulfuric acid, 0.5 % w/v, 25 °C	55
Melt volume flow rate, (cm^3/10 min)	ISO 1133, 400° C, 10 Kg	25-120
Total heavy metals as Pb, (max) (%)	U.S. Phamacopeia, Test 231	0.1

APPENDIX

(Nonmandatory Information)

X1. RATIONALE

X1.1 PEKEKK resins may be processed by most techniques available for thermoplastic polymers. Medical devices

TABLE 2 Typical Properties of Fabricated Forms

Parameter	Method	Requirement
Density, (min) (kg/m^3)	ISO D 1505	1.2
Tensile strength, (MPa) (min)	D 638, Type IV, 5.08 cm/min	
Yield		90
break		70
Percent elongation, (%) (min)	D 638, Type IV, 5.08 cm/min	10
Izod impact strength, (ft-lbf/in), (min)	D 256, 0.254 cm depth, 0.025 cm radius	0.7
Deformation under load, (%) (max)	D 621 (A), 7 MPa for 24 h, 23 °C, after 90 min recovery	2

and components of medical devices made of PEKEKK resins may be sterilized. Sterilization methods successfully used include steam, ethylene oxide, and irradiation. Repeated sterilization may weaken parts fabricated of any plastic material. The number of times a given part may be sterilized safely without fear of subsequent failure depends on a number of factors including the molecular weight of resin and design, fabrication, intended function, and method of sterilization of the device. It is imperative, therefore, that the manufacturer test the device in order to determine the maximum number of sterilization cycles to which it can be safely subjected.

X1.2 The potential to develop a significant level of crystallinity is an important characteristic of these materials. Performance characteristics are related to the percent crystallinity. Certain additives and processes, for example, excessive crosslinking, can limit these materials' ability to crystallize. This feature of the resin and its fabricated form, therefore, should be evaluated using appropriate test methods to assure efficacy.

X1.3 A formulated compound or fabricated part or device may contain optional adjuvant substances required for the fabrication or intended use of the end product. The biocompatibility of these adjuvant substances and subsequent formulated compounds, parts, and devices shall be established in accordance with Practice F 748 or the ISO 10933 series.

REFERENCES

(**1**) Silverstein, R. M., Bassler, G. C., and Morrill, T. C., "Spectroscopic Identification of Organic Compounds," Fifth Edition, John Wiley and Sons, New York, NY.

(**2**) Autian, J., "Toxicological Evaluation of Biomaterials: Primary Acute Toxicity Screening Program," *Journal of Artificial Organs*, Vol 1, No. 1, 1977, p. 53.

(**3**) Autian, J., "The New Field of Plastic Toxicological Methods and Results," *CRC Critics Review in Toxicology*, 1973, p. 18.

(**4**) Homsy, C. A., Ansevin, K. D., O'Brannon, W., Thompson, S. H., Hodge, R., and Estrella, M. E., "Rapid in Vitro Screening of Polymers for Biocompatibility," *Journal of Macromolecular Science, Chemistry*, Vol A4, No. 3, May 1970, pp. 615-634.

(**5**) Rice, R. M., Hegyeli, A. F., Gourlay, S. J., Wade, C. W. R., Dillon, J. G., Jaffe, H., and Kulkarni, R. K., "Biocompatibility Testing for Polymers: In Vitro Studies With In Vivo Correlation," *Journal of Biomedical Materials Research*, Vol 12, 1978, p. 43.

Designation: F 1877 – 98

Standard Practice for Characterization of Particles[1]

This standard is issued under the fixed designation F 1877; the number immediately following the designation indicates the year of original adoption or, in the case of revision, the year of last revision. A number in parentheses indicates the year of last reapproval. A superscript epsilon (ε) indicates an editorial change since the last revision or reapproval.

1. Scope

1.1 This practice outlines a series of procedures for characterization of the morphology, number, size, and size distribution of particles. The methods utilized include sieves, optical, SEM, and electrooptical.

1.2 These methods are appropriate for particles produced by a number of different methods. These include wear test machines, total joint simulation systems, abrasion testing, methods for producing particulates, such as shatter boxes or pulverizors, commercially available particles, and particles harvested from tissues in animal or clinical studies.

1.3 The debris may include metallic, polymeric, ceramic, or any combination of these.

1.4 The digestion procedures to be used and issues of sterilization of retrieved particles are not the subject of this practice.

1.5 A classification scheme for description of particle morphology are included in Appendix X3.

1.6 As a precautionary measure, removed debris from implant tissues should be sterilized or minimally disinfected by an appropriate means that does not adversely affect the particulate material. *This standard does not purport to address all of the safety concerns, if any, associated with its use. It is the responsibility of the user of this standard to establish appropriate safety and health practices and determine the applicability of regulatory limitations prior to use.*

2. Referenced Documents

2.1 *ASTM Standards:*

E 11 Specification for Wire-Cloth Sieves for Testing Purposes[2]

E 20 Practice for Particle Size Analysis of Particulate Substances in the Range of 0.2 to 75 μm by Optical Microscopy[3]

E 161 Specification for Precision Electroformed Sieves (Square Opening Series)[2]

E 1617 Practice for Reporting Particle Size Characterization Data[2]

E 766 Practice for Calibrating the Magnification of Scanning Electron Microscopes (SEMs)

F 561 Practice for Retrieval and Analysis of Implanted Medical Devices, and Associated Tissues[4]

F 660 Practice for Comparing Particle Size in the Use of Alternative Types of Particle Counters[2]

F 661 Practice for Particle Count and Size Distribution Measurement in Batch Samples for Filter Evaluation Using an Optical Particle Counter[2]

F 662 Method for Particle Count and Size Distribution in Batch Samples for Filter Evaluation Using an Electrical Resistance Particle Counter[2]

F 690 Particle Size Distribution of Alumina or Quartz by Electric Sensing Technique[2]

F 732 Practice for Reciprocating Pin-on-Flat Evaluation of Friction and Wear Properties of Polymeric Materials for Use in Total Joint Prostheses[4]

F 1714 Guide for Gravimetric Wear Assessment of Prosthetic Hip Designs in Simulator Devices[4]

F 1715 Guide for Gravimetric Wear Assessment of Prosthetic Knee Designs in Simulator Devices[4]

3. Terminology

3.1 *Definitions of Terms Specific to This Standard:*

3.1.1 *agglomerate, n*—a mass formed by the cementation of individual particles, probably by chemical forces.

3.1.2 *aggregate, n*—a mass formed of mixtures of particulate and agglomerate particles having a binding force intermediate between agglomerates and flocculates. Formation of aggregates can occur after sampling if the samples are improperly kept or treated.

3.1.3 *aspect ratio (AR), n*—a ratio of the major to the minor diameter of a particle, which can be used when the major axis does not cross a particle outline (see 11.3.3).

3.1.4 *elongation (E), n*—ratio of the particle length to the average particle width (see 11.3.4).

3.1.5 *equivalent circle diameter (ECD), n*—a measure of the size of a particle (see 11.3.2 and Appendix X1).

3.1.6 *Feret diameter, n*—the mean value of the distance between pairs of parallel tangents to a projected outline of a particle.

3.1.7 *flocculate, n*—a group of two or more attached particles held together by physical forces, such as surface tension, adsorption, or similar forces.

[1] This practice is under the jurisdiction of ASTM Committee F04 on Medical and Surgical Materials and Devices and is the direct responsibility of Subcommittee F04.16 on Biocompatibility.

Current edition approved April 10, 1998. Published March 1999.

[2] *Annual Book of ASTM Standards*, Vol 14.02.

[3] *Discontinued 1994*—Vol 14.02.

[4] *Annual Book of ASTM Standards*, Vol 13.01.

3.1.8 *form factor (FF), n*—a dimensionless number relating area and perimeter of a particle, as directed in 11.3.6.

3.1.9 *irregular, adj*—a particle that cannot be described as round or spherical. A set of standard nomenclature and reference figures are given in Appendix X2.

3.1.10 *particle, n*—the smallest discrete unit detectable as determined in Test Methods.

3.1.11 *particle breadth, n*—distance between touch points of the shortest Feret pair, orthogonal to length.

3.1.12 *particle length, n*—distance between touch points of maximum Feret pair. This value will be greater than or equal to the maximum Feret diameter.

3.1.13 *rectangular, adj*—a particle that approximates a square or rectangle in shape.

3.1.14 *roundness (R), n*—a measure of how closely an object represents a circle as determined in 11.3.5.

3.1.15 *spherical, adj*—a particle with a generally spherical shape that appears round in a photograph.

4. Summary of Practice

4.1 Particles produced by implant wear in vivo in animal or clinical studies are harvested from tissues after digestion utilizing methods, such as those in Practice F 561. Particles generated in vitro, or obtained from commercial sources, are used as received, or after digestion, if they were generated in protein solutions, and further separation if there are signs of aggregation. A two level analysis is provided. For routine analysis, the particles are characterized by the terms of morphology and by size using Feret diameters. For more detailed studies, several methods are described that may be utilized for numerically characterizing their dimensions, size distribution, and number.

5. Significance and Use

5.1 The biological response to materials in the form of small particles, as from wear debris, often is different significantly from that to the same materials as larger implant components. The size and shape (morphology) of the particles may have a major effect on the biological response; therefore, this practice provides a standardized nomenclature for describing particles. Such a unified nomenclature will be of value in interpretation of biological tests of responses to particles, in that it will facilitate separation of biological responses associated with shape from those associated with the chemical composition of debris.

5.2 The quantity, size, and morphology of particles released as wear debris from implants in vivo may produce an adverse biological response which will affect the long term survival of the device. Characterization of such debris will provide valuable information regarding the effectiveness of device designs or methods of processing components and the mechanisms of wear.

5.3 The morphology of particles produced in laboratory tests of wear and abrasion often is affected by the test conditions, such as the magnitude and rate of load application, device configuration, and test environment. Comparison of the morphology and size of particles produced in vitro with those produced in vivo will provide valuable information regarding the degree to which the method simulates the in vivo condition being modeled.

6. Interferences

6.1 Particles may form aggregates or agglomerates during preparation and storage. These would result in an increase in measured particle size and decrease in particle number. It is essential that care be taken to resuspend particles prior to analysis and to note any effects of the dispersant used.

6.2 Debris from wear tests or harvested from tissues may contain a mixture of materials. Care should be taken to separate the particles and methods utilized to determine the chemical composition of the particles.

6.3 Many automated particle counters operate on the assumption that the particles are spherical. These methods may not be appropriate for nonspherical debris. Additional methods should be used to verify size using methods that take aspect ratio into consideration, for example, SEM image analysis.

7. Apparatus

7.1 *Scanning Electron Microscope (SEM)*:

7.1.1 Standard SEM equipment can be utilized for many studies. In special instances, such as with polymeric particles, a low acceleration voltage (1-2 kV) machine with a high brightness electron source, such as a field emission tip may be utilized.

7.1.2 Elemental analysis may be accomplished with an energy dispersive spectrometer (EDS) for energy dispersive X-ray analysis (EDXA).

7.2 *Optical Microscope*—An optical microscope operating in the transmission mode may be utilized. Dark field illumination may enhance visualization of some particles. Polarized light will facilitate identification of semicrystalline polymeric materials.

7.3 *Automatic Particle Counters (see Practice F 660)*:

7.3.1 *Image Analyzer*—This instrument counts particles by size as those particles lie on a microscope slide.

7.3.2 *Optical Counter*—This instrument measures the area of a shadow cast by a particle as it passes a window. From this area the instrument reports the diameter of a circle of equal area (see Practice F 661).

7.3.3 *Electrical Resistance Counter*—This instrument measures the volume of an individual particle. From that volume the instrument reports the diameter of a sphere of equal volume (see Method F 662).

8. Reagents

8.1 *Particle-Free (0.2 μm Filtered) Deionized Water*, for nonpolymeric particles.

8.2 *Particle-Free (0.2 μm Filtered) Methanol or Ethanol*, for polymeric or mixed debris.

8.3 *Ultra-Cleaning Reagent*, for apparatus or labware cleaning.

9. Specimen Preparation

9.1 Specimens from explanted tissues from animal or clinical studies may need to be harvested and digested using methods, such as those described in Practice F 561.

9.2 Particles from in vitro cell culture tests also may need to be digested and harvested.

9.3 Particles from wear tests should be centrifuged at atleast 400 g for 10 min, and resuspended in water or methanol. Resuspended particles may be filtered in accordance with Practice F 561 prior to examination by SEM.

10. Particle Imaging by Light or Scanning Electron Microscopy

10.1 Images may either be captured electronically or photographically for subsequent analysis.

10.2 For the characterization and measurements to be accurate, it is essential that the particles be imaged at the largest magnification as possible. The magnifications in Table 1 are recommended.

10.3 For particle size distribution measurements, divide each of the size ranges specified in Table 1, into 10 bins.

11. Particle Characterization

11.1 *Particle Shape (Morphology)*—Refer to the photographs and classify the morphology of the particles using the nomenclature in Appendix X2.

11.2 *Routine Particle Size Determination Using Feret Diameters*:

11.2.1 The use of multiple Feret diameters especially is useful for spherical and rectangular particles.

11.2.2 Determine the particle size and aspect ratio as the mean of two Feret diameters.

11.2.3 Calculate the particle size distribution based on the volume of solution used and the size of the filters.

11.3 *Detailed Particle Shape Analysis for Irregular Shaped Particles*:

11.3.1 Five particle dimensional measurements are provided using examples shown in Appendix X1.[5] One is a measure of particle size while the other four are shape descriptors.

11.3.2 *The Equivalent Circle Diameter (ECD) as a Measure of Particle Size*:

11.3.2.1 The ECD is defined as the diameter of a circle with an area equivalent to the area (*A*) of the particle and has the units of length:

$$\mathrm{ECD} = (4*A/\pi)^{\frac{1}{2}} \tag{1}$$

11.3.3 *The Aspect Ratio (AR) is a Common Measure of Shape*:

11.3.3.1 The *AR* is the ratio of the major diameter (d_{max}) to the minor diameter (d_{min}). The major diameter is the longest straight line that can be drawn between any two points on the outline. The minor diameter is the longest line perpendicular to the major diameter:

$$AR = d_{max}/d_{min} \tag{2}$$

11.3.4 The elongation (*E*), is similar to the *AR* except it is more suited for the measurement of much longer particles, especially fibrilar particles, where the major axis line does not stay within the particle boundaries. Refer to particle types *A* and *C* in Appendix X1.

11.3.4.1 The *E* is the ratio of the length (*FL*) to the breadth (*FW*):

$$E = FL/FW \tag{3}$$

11.3.5 The roundness (*R*) is a measure of how closely a particle resembles a circle. The *R* varies from zero to one in magnitude with a perfect circle having a value of one.

$$R = (4A)/(\pi\, d_{max}^{\ 2}) \tag{4}$$

where:
A = area, and
d_{max} = the maximum diameter.

11.3.6 The form factor (*FF*) is similar to *R* but is based on the perimeter (*p*) of the particle outline rather than the major diameter. The *FF* is more sensitive to the variations in roughness of the particle outline.

$$FF = 4\pi A/p^2 \tag{5}$$

where:
p = perimeter of the particle outline.

11.4 *Other Particles Size Determination Methods*:

11.4.1 Particles larger than 20 µm may be determined by sieves described in Specifications E 11 and E 161.

11.4.2 Particles in liquid suspension may be sized as directed in Practice F 661 or Method F 662.

12. Elemental Analysis

12.1 SEM-EDS analysis should be conducted at a magnification suggested in 10.2.

12.2 Elemental analysis should be conducted for at least 10 s for each particle. Since detailed compositional analysis is of questionable meaning for micron and submicron sized particles, it is recommended that composition be determined based on identification of key elemental peaks for the major elements likely to be present in the sample.

13. Report

13.1 Report the following information:

13.1.1 The source of the particles and materials and methods for generation.

13.1.2 Methods utilized to digest and separate the particles.

13.1.3 Morphological description of the particles.

13.1.4 Results of particle size and shape analysis.

14. Precision and Bias

14.1 The precision and bias of this practice has not been determined.

15. Keywords

15.1 biocompatibility; morphology; particles; SEM; wear debris

[5] The examples provided were analyzed with the NIH Image Program by Landry and Agarwal. A set of macros is available from the Department of Orthopaedics, University of Texas Health Science Center at San Antonio.

TABLE 1

Magnification	Particle Size Range (µm)
10000	0.1 to 1.0
1000	1 to 10
100	10 to 100

APPENDIXES

(Nonmandatory Information)

X1. SAMPLE FIGURES FOR CALCULATION OF PARTICLE SIZE AND SHAPE

X1.1 See Fig. X1.1.

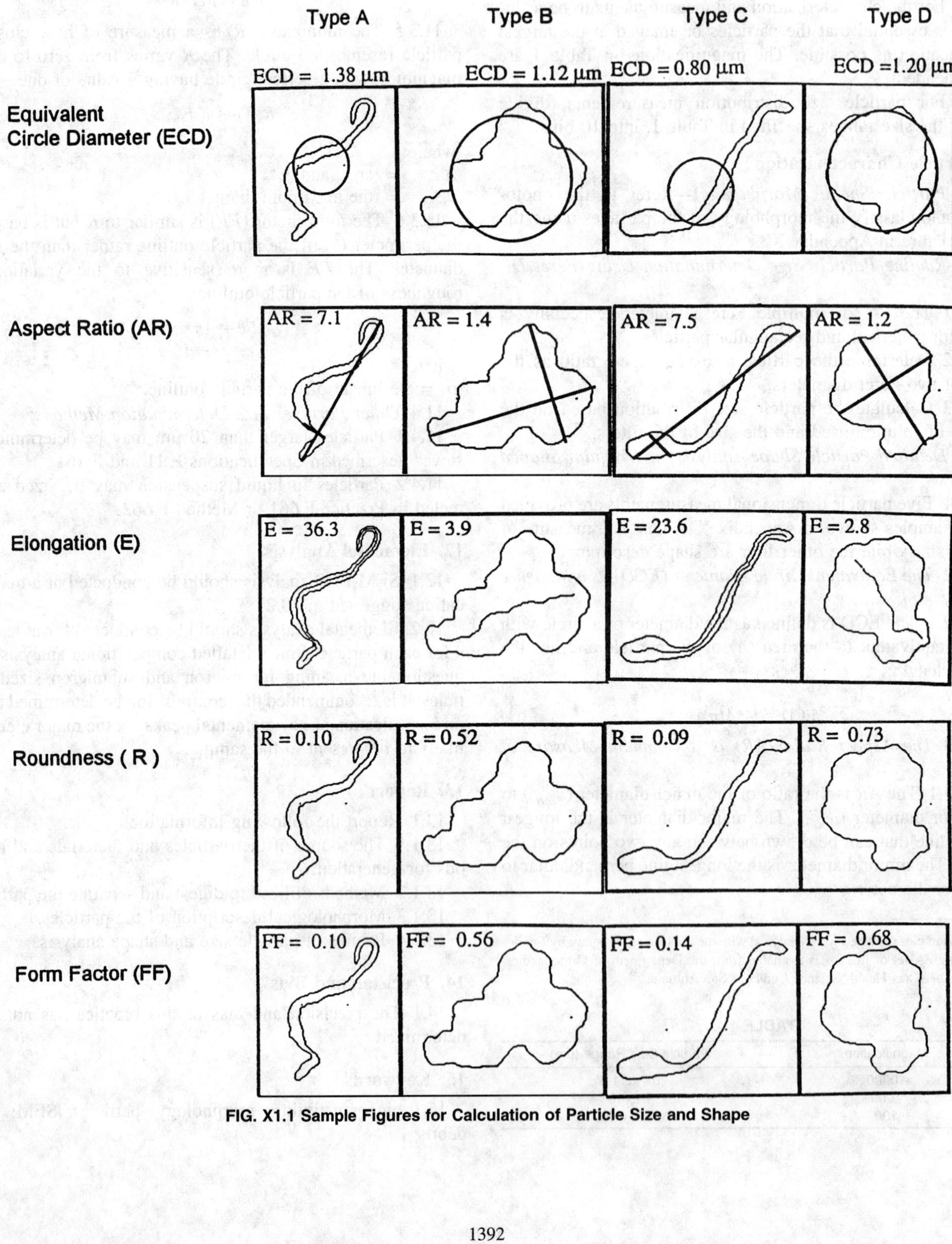

FIG. X1.1 Sample Figures for Calculation of Particle Size and Shape

X2. NOMENCLATURE FOR PARTICLE MORPHOLOGY DESCRIPTION

X2.1 This collection is not intended to be all inclusive, but rather to provide a frame work for describing the morphology of particles.

NOTE X2.1—These figures are used as illustrative examples. Sources are indicated in parentheses (used with permission).

X2.1.1 *Spherical or Spheroidal*:

X2.1.1.1 Smooth, round (Fig. X2.1).[6]

X2.1.1.2 Smooth, oblong (Fig. X2.1).[6]

X2.1.1.3 Agglomerated, red blood cell - like (Fig. X2.2).[7]

X2.1.1.4 Rough (Fig. X2.3).[6]

X2.1.1.5 Spongy, porous (Fig. X2.4).[8]

X2.1.2 *Granular, Irregular*:

X2.1.2.1 Smooth (Fig. X2.5).[9]

X2.1.2.2 Rough (Fig. X2.6).[10]

X2.1.2.3 Porous (Fig. X2.7).[10]

X2.1.2.4 Angulated (Fig. X2.8).[11]

X2.1.2.5 Fines, too small to characterize accurately (Fig. X2.9).[6]

X2.1.3 *Globular*:

X2.1.3.1 Clumped, florets, cauliflower (Fig. X2.10).[12]

[6] Lalor, P., donated photographs from Howmedica R and D laboratories.

[7] Szivek J.A., donated sample set.

[8] Jacobs J.J., and Urban R.M., donated photograph.

[9] Margevicius K.J., Bauer T.W., McMahon J.T., Brown S.A., Merritt K.," Isolation and Characterization of Debris in Membranes Around Total Joint Prostheses," *J Bone Joint Surg*, 76A:1664-1675, 1994.

[10] Kieswetter K., Bauer T.W., Brown S.A., Van Lente F., Merritt K, "Characterization of Calcium Phosphate Powders by ESCA and EDXA," *Biomaterials*, 15:183-188, 1994.

[11] Lerouge S., Huk O., Yahia L.H., Sedel L., "Characterization of In Vivo Wear Debris from Ceramic-Ceramic Total Hip Arhroplasties," *J Biomed Mater Res*, 32:627-633, 1996.

[12] Hailey J.L., Ingham E., Stone M., Wroblewski B.M., Fisher J., "Ultra-High Molecular Weight Polyethylene Wear Debris Generated *In Vivo* and in Laboratory Tests: the Influence of Counterface Roughness," *Proc Inst Mech Eng*, 210:3-10, 1996.

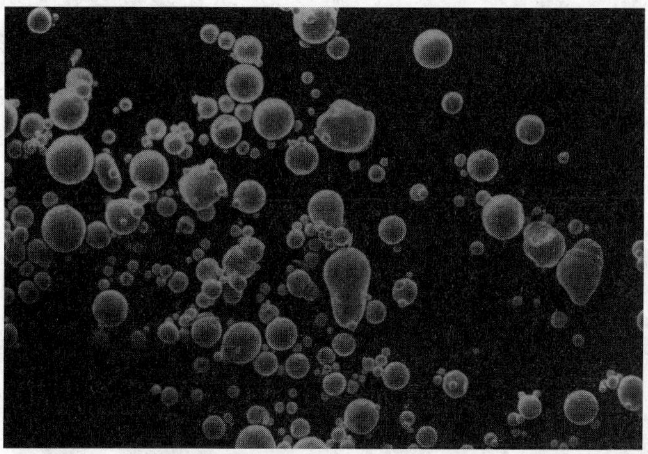

FIG. X2.1 Spherical or Spheroidal—Smooth, Round or Oblong

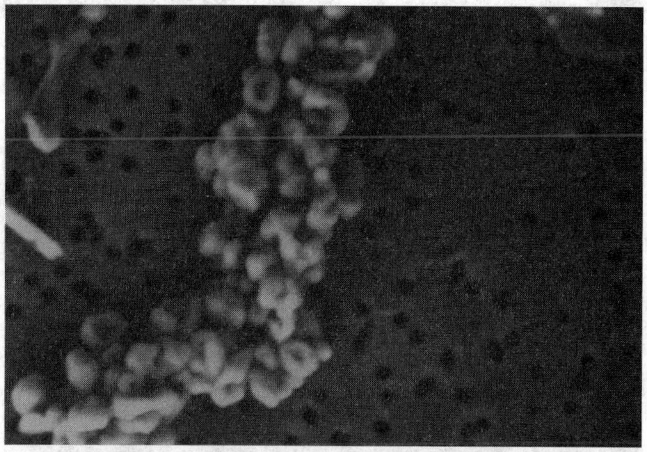

FIG. X2.2 Spherical or Spheroidal—Agglomerated Red Blood Cell-Like

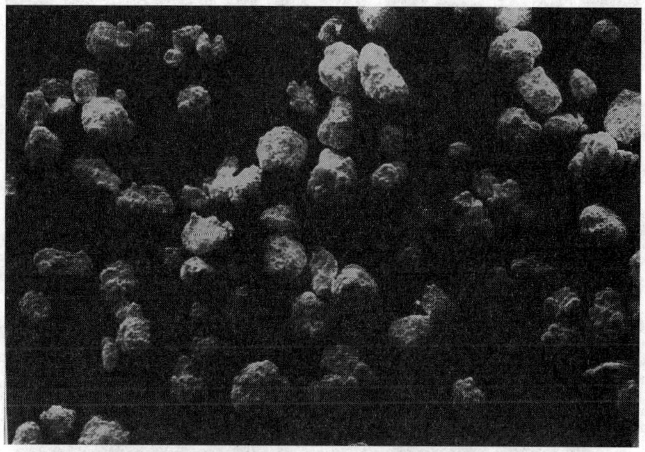

FIG. X2.3 Spherical or Spheroidal—Rough

X2.1.3.2 Agglomerated, diffuse (Fig. X2.11).[13]

X2.1.4 *Flakes*:

X2.1.4.1 Smooth (Fig. X2.12).[12]

X2.1.4.2 Roughened (Fig. X2.13).[12]

X2.1.4.3 Irregular (Fig. X2.14).[13]

X2.1.4.4 Shards (probably thin cross sections of flakes) (Fig. X2.15).[6]

X2.1.5 *Fibrillar*:

X2.1.5.1 Straight (Fig. X2.16).[7]

X2.1.5.2 Twisted (Fig. X2.17 and Fig. X2.18).[7]

X2.1.5.3 Hammer head (Fig. X2.19 and Fig. X2.18).[13]

X2.1.5.4 Tadpole (Fig. X2.19).[13]

X2.1.5.5 Seahorse (Fig. X2.18).[13]

X2.1.6 *Sharps or Shards*:

X2.1.6.1 Flakes, stacked sheets (Fig. X2.20).[14]

[13] Campbell, P., donated photographs.

[14] Shanbhag A.S., donated photograph.

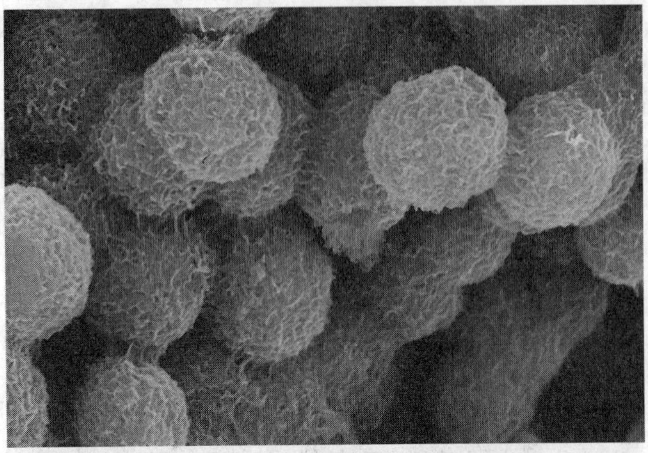

FIG. X2.4 Spherical or Spheroidal—Spongy, Porous

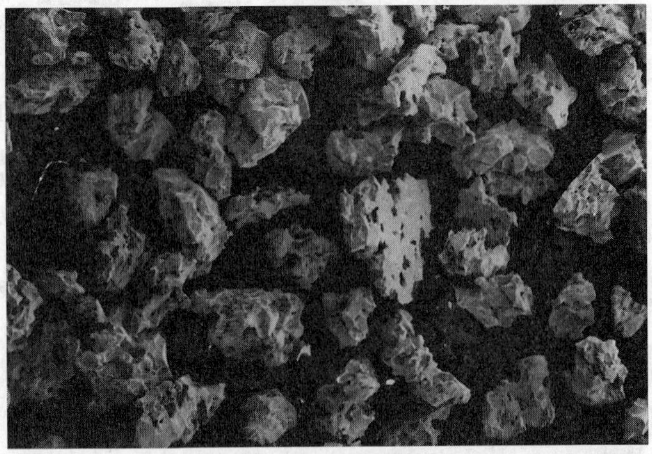

FIG. X2.7 Granular, Irregular—Porouss

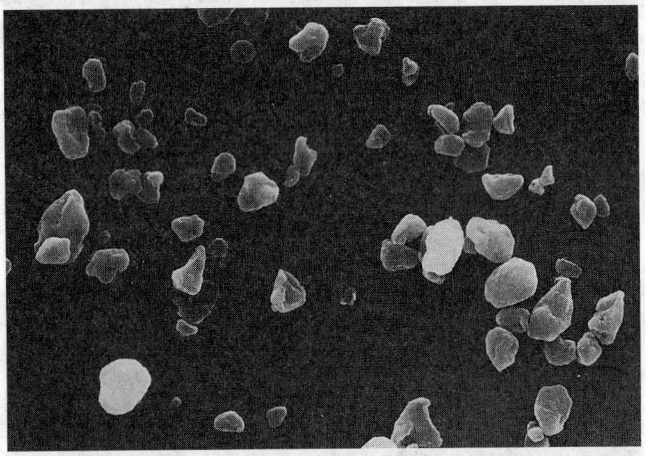

FIG. X2.5 Granular, Irregular—Smooth

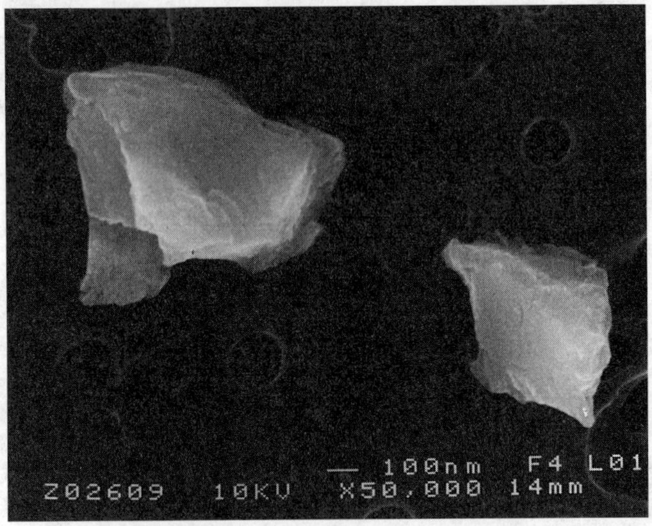

FIG. X2.8 Granular, Irregular—Angulated

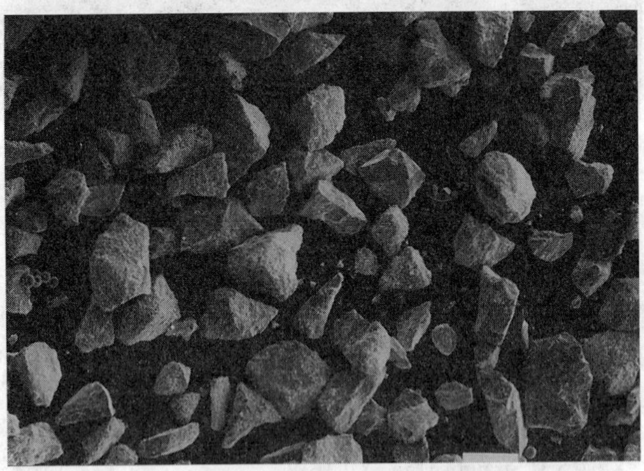

FIG. X2.6 Granular, Irregular—Rough

X2.1.6.2 Rectangular, fibers (Fig. X2.21).[15]
X2.1.6.3 Lathe-like (Fig. X2.22).[10]
X2.1.6.4 Cuttle fish (Fig. X2.23).[12]

---

[15] Bauer T.W., donated photograph.

FIG. X2.9 Granular, Irregular—Fines Too Small to Characterize Accurately

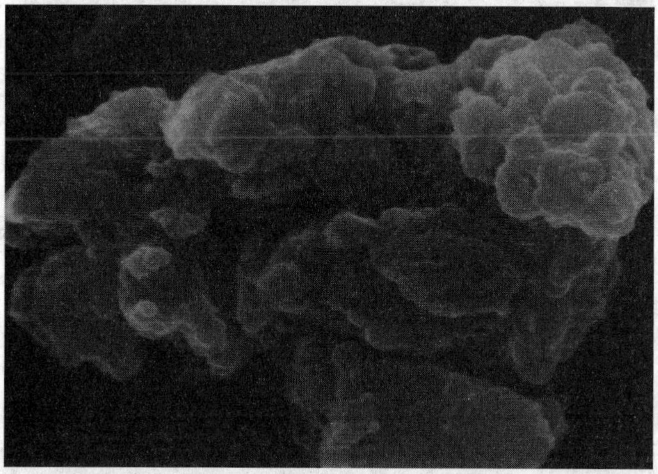

FIG. X2.10 Globular—Clumped, Florets, Cauliflower

FIG. X2.11 Globular—Agglomerated, Diffuse

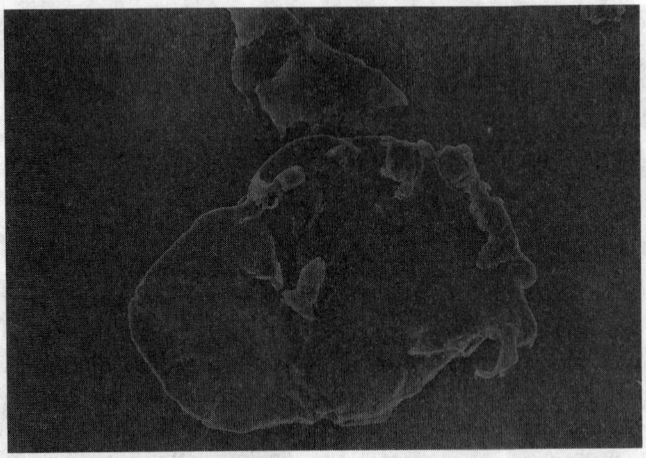

FIG. X2.12 Flakes—Smooth

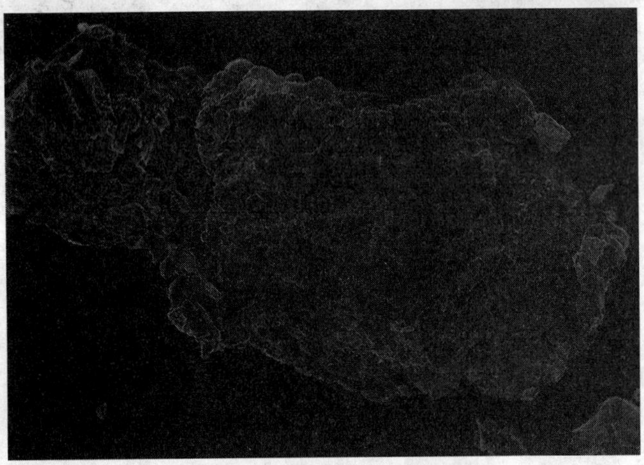

FIG. X2.13 Flakes—Roughened

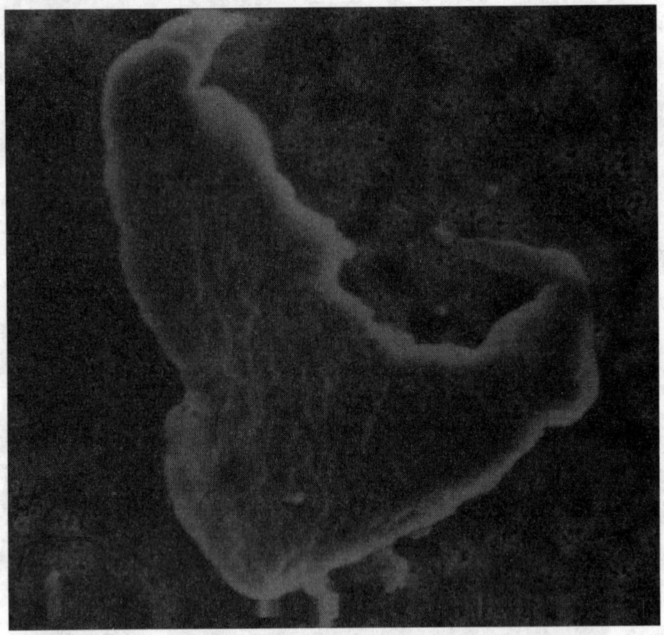

FIG. X2.14 Flakes—Irregular

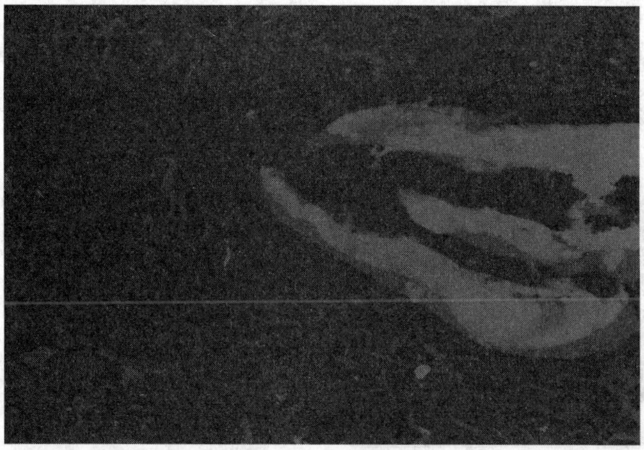

FIG. X2.15 Flakes—Shards

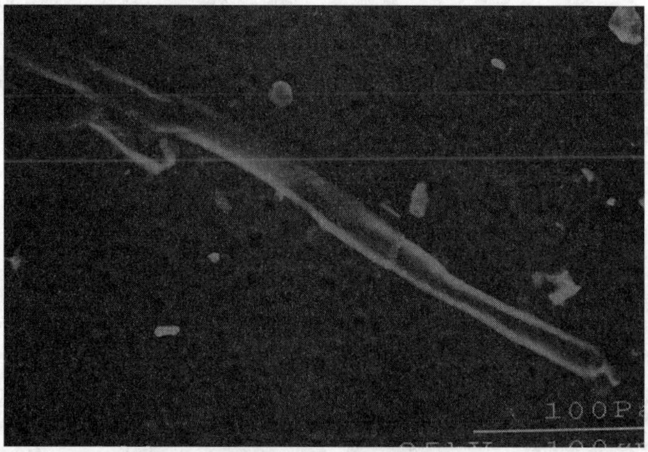

FIG. X2.16 Fibrillar—Straight

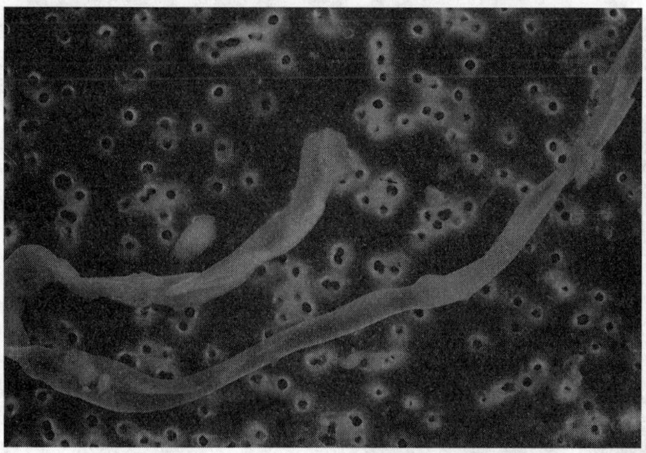

FIG. X2.17 Fibrillar—Twisted

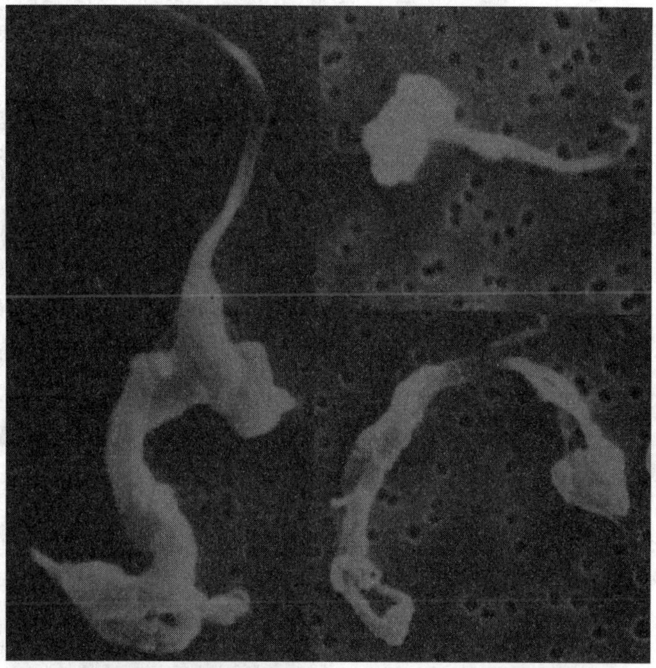

FIG. X2.18 Fibrillar—Seahorse / Hammerhead / Twisted

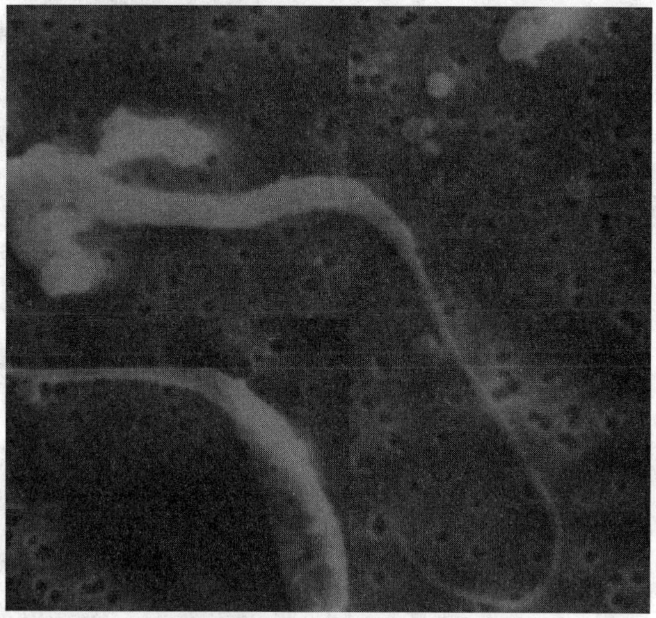

FIG. X2.19 Fibrillar—Humerhead / Tadpole

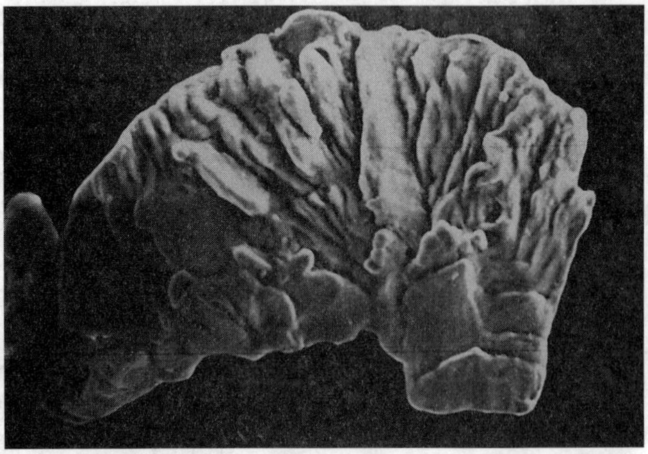

FIG. X2.20 Sharps or Shards—Flakes, Stacked Sheets

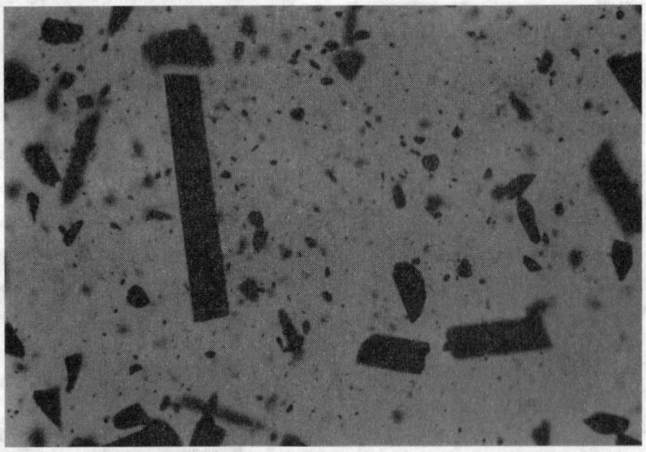

FIG. X2.21 Sharps or Shards—Rectangular Fibers

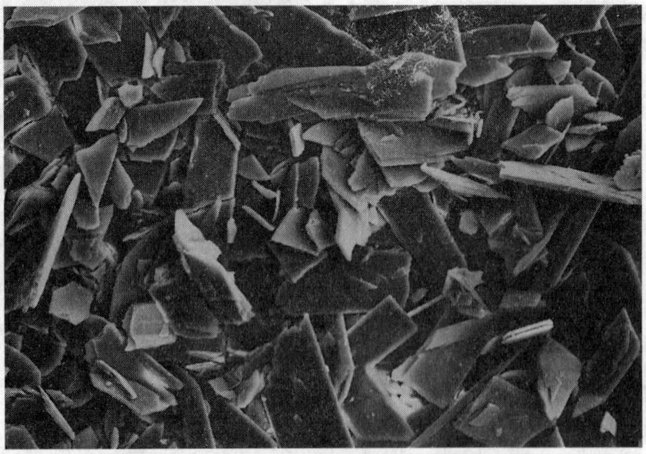

FIG. X2.22 Sharps or Shards—Lathe-Like

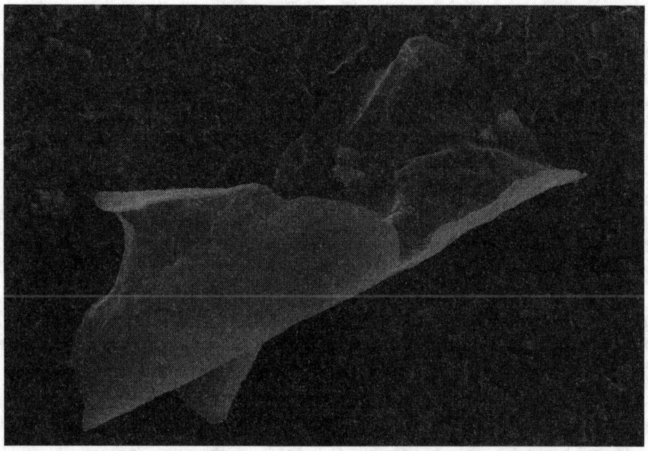

FIG. X2.23 Sharps or Shards—Cuttlefish

X3. RATIONALE

X3.1 Establishment and use of a standardized nomenclature for describing particulate debris is critical for a wide range of studies regarding implants and devices. By using a common vocabulary for particle description, biological responses to different shapes of debris can separated from other factors such as chemistry. Matching morphology of debris produced in the laboratory with that produced in vivo will better refine the accuracy of laboratory test methods. Characterization of debris produced in vivo will help in assessment of device performance.

The sample morphologies provided are not intended to be all inclusive of those published in the literature. The intent is to provide illustrative examples of morphologies and to assign names to each type. Thus, communication between investigators should be more precise.

The detailed methods of calculating particle shape have been developed by M. E. Landry and C. M. Agrawal at the University of Texas Health Science Center at San Antonio and are the basis for a Masters of Science in Engineering thesis by M. E. Landry at the University of Texas at Austin. These methods are provided as a way to numerically describe complicated particle shapes. While not all measurements need to be made, standardization of these methods should provide an additional data set for description of the wide variety of particle morphologies generated in vivo and in vitro.

Standard Guide for Demonstrating Obedience and Agility in Search and Rescue Dogs[1]

This standard is issued under the fixed designation F 1879; the number immediately following the designation indicates the year of original adoption or, in the case of revision, the year of last revision. A number in parentheses indicates the year of last reapproval. A superscript epsilon (ε) indicates an editorial change since the last revision or reapproval.

1. Scope

1.1 This guide is intended to provide voluntary uniform guidelines for obedience and agility training for Search and Rescue (SAR) dogs throughout the United States.

1.2 This guide provides a minimum set of training goals against which SAR dog teams and organizations may voluntarily evaluate their own training programs.

1.3 This guide provides a means of documenting a minimum standard for those agencies who request SAR dog resources for SAR operations and require such documentation.

1.4 Local SAR dog handlers and parent organizations are responsible for testing and verifying that individual resources meet or exceed these guidelines.

2. Referenced Documents

2.1 *ASTM Standards:*

F 1633 Guide for Techniques in Land Search[2]

F 1848 Classification of Search and Rescue Dog Crew/Teams[2]

3. Terminology

3.1 *Definitions of Terms Specific to This Standard:*

3.1.1 *agility, n*—an aspect of a dog's physical condition that characterizes the dog's dexterity and ease of movement.

3.1.2 *obedience, n*—an aspect of a dog's behavior that characterizes the dog's ability to follow instructions.

3.1.3 *off-lead, n*—a working mode for a dog where the dog and handler are not connected physically and the control of the dog is established through audible commands or visual signals.

3.1.4 *on-lead, n*—a working mode for a dog and handler attached physically by a leash and the dog may be controlled by the leash.

3.2 Definitions of terms not defined in this standard can be found in Guide F 1633 and Classification F 1848.

4. Summary of the Practice

4.1 This guide provides dog handlers, units and organizations in differing locales with the ability to understand and replicate skills and training required to meet these minimum guidelines.

4.2 The obedience skills ensure the dog is under the control of the handler sufficiently to participate in a search operation without interfering with other search resources, individuals, and dogs.

4.3 The agility skills demonstrate the team's abilities to traverse the obstacles which may be present in a search situation.

4.4 Dogs that work incidents involving natural disaster and collapsed structures require all of these basic skills, as well as special techniques, and so are designated as having additional minimum requirements.

5. Significance and Use

5.1 This guide may be used by units, handlers, and requesting agencies when evaluating dog resources or as a basis for establishing local minimum performance guidelines or standards. It is suggested, however, that units and teams not train to these guidelines, but rather train and work in conditions requiring obedience and agility skills, then use these guidelines as a uniform method of evaluating progress.

5.2 This guide does not provide a theoretical basis for how a search dog works, rather it describes the minimum results desired.

5.3 Each dog team, unit, or organization wishing to use this guide has the responsibility of managing and administering it. Units may wish to use evaluators from other units or organizations, or request assistance in obtaining qualified evaluators from organizations, such as the SAR Dog Section of the National Association of Search and Rescue (NASAR)[3] or the American Kennel Club (AKC)[4]. This decision, however, rests solely with the individual team or organization. The method of evaluation also is entirely at the discretion of each user of this guide.

6. Obedience Skills

6.1 Obedience skills are recommended to ensure that the dog can be worked and transported without interference from other dogs and personnel, is under the control of the handler,

[1] This guide is under the jurisdiction of ASTM Committee F-32 on Search and Rescue and is the direct responsibility of Subcommittee F32.02 on Management and Operations.

Current edition approved April 10, 1998. Published June 1998.

[2] *Annual Book of ASTM Standards*, Vol 13.01.

[3] National Associatio for Search and Rescue, 4500 Southgate Place, Suite 100, Chantilly, VA 20151-1714.

[4] The American Kennel Club, 5580 Centerview Drive, Suite 200, Raleigh, NC 27606-3390.

can be left safely and, if necessary, be evacuated by someone other than the handler in an emergency. Both on-lead and off-lead obedience skills should be demonstrated around a group of strangers and other dogs with accompanying noise and confusion common to search and rescue operations. This demonstration might follow a fixed format, such as outlined in the AKC Canine Good Citizen[4] test or a free format with the following elements.

6.2 *Recommended On-Lead Skills*:

6.2.1 On-lead obedience skills should include the ability to "heel" with stops and the ability to make right, left, and about-turns with both the handler and an alternate handler. The ability to sit, stand, and down are optional on-lead commands.

NOTE 1—The actual command used to achieve a desired action from the dog is at the discretion of the handler. Commands may be audible, visual, or both.

6.2.2 While on-lead, the handler should be able to place the dog in a vehicle with other dogs and strangers without the dog displaying aggressive behavior towards the stranger or other dogs. The dog should demonstrate the ability to remain there until released.

6.3 *Recommended Off-Lead Skills*:

6.3.1 Off-lead obedience skills to be demonstrated should include right, left, and about-turns, with the dog following the handler and a come directly to the handler on demand from at least 50 ft. Additionally, the dog should demonstrate the ability to stop during a come. A "heel" with stops also is recommended for dogs engaged in collapsed structure/disaster work.

6.3.2 The dog also should demonstrate that is can be left unattended for 3 min with the handler out of sight and scent. The dog may change positions but must remain within 5 ft of its original location even when distractions include other dogs and strangers moving close by. For dogs engaged in collapsed building/disaster work, it is recommended that this area be reduced to the body length of the dog. The demonstration should include a minimum of three other dogs that are within 20 ft of the demonstrating dog.

6.3.3 Dogs engaged in collapsed structure/disaster work additionally should demonstrate the ability to change their pace at the request of the handler and to be directed to more than two distinct areas, which have different elevations and are separated by at least 25 yds.

7. Agility Skills

7.1 Agility skills ensure that a dog will be controlled and confident in stressful or unusual physical surroundings, such as unstable, slippery, or uneven surfaces.

7.2 For dogs engaged in collapsed structure and disaster activities, it is recommended that additional skills be demonstrated (see 7.5), and that they have the ability to execute their movement with minimal disturbance to obstacles. These additional skills should demonstrate the dogs' ability to work in an environment where things are unusual and where footings are loose and often move under the dogs' weight. Dogs engaged in these activities should further demonstrate an ability to independently avoid dangerous objects and avoid causing any further injury to trapped individuals.

7.3 For safety reasons, it is recommended that spotters be available when dogs are demonstrating agility skills. The use of spotters, however, should neither enhance nor diminish dogs ability to demonstrate agility.

7.4 *Recommended Agility Skills for All Dogs*:

7.4.1 All dogs should be able to jump at least 2.5 ft up into a specified area, such as four-wheel drive pick-up truck.

7.4.2 All dogs should be able to crawl under an obstacle that is not higher than three-quarters the dog's height.

7.4.3 All dogs should be able to climb onto and walk along a log or other narrow obstacle without jumping off. It is recommended that the log or obstacle be taller and wider than the dog.

7.4.4 All dogs should be able to walk through a culvert or small tunnel that has at least one right or left turn. Ideally, some portion of the culvert or tunnel will be of a size that requires the dog to crawl on its belly.

7.4.5 The dog should be able to long jump over a ditch, which is as wide as the height of the dog's withers.

7.4.6 The dog should be able to swim 50 ft.

7.5 *Additional Agility Skills Recommended for Dogs Engaged in Collapsed Structure/Disaster Work*:

7.5.1 The dog should be able to climb a flat-runged ladder at least 6-ft long, which is set at a 45° angle.

7.5.2 The dog should be able to walk from one end of a teeter-totter (no more than 12-in. wide) to the other without jumping off.

7.5.3 The dog should be able to maneuver over 1 22-in. high log or barrel on its side after checking the other side for safety.

7.5.4 The dogs should be able to climb a ramp, or ladder, then proceed to the end of a second plank and return without jumping off. The ramps and planks should no more than 12 in. wide, at least 10 ft long, and at least 3 ft above the ground.

7.5.5 The dog should be able to climb onto and cross a slippery surface.

7.5.6 The dog should be able to climb onto and cross a wobbly surface, for example, warped plywood, which is at least 12 ft long, 12 in. wide, and 3 ft above the ground.

7.5.7 The dog should be able to climb onto and cross a nonstationary plank, (supported by two barrels on their side), which is no more than 12 ft long by 12 in. wide.

8. Keywords

8.1 agility; canine training; conditioning; obedience; obstacle course

The American Society for Testing and Materials takes no position respecting the validity of any patent rights asserted in connection with any item mentioned in this standard. Users of this standard are expressly advised that determination of the validity of any such patent rights, and the risk of infringement of such rights, are entirely their own responsibility.

This standard is subject to revision at any time by the responsible technical committee and must be reviewed every five years and if not revised, either reapproved or withdrawn. Your comments are invited either for revision of this standard or for additional standards and should be addressed to ASTM Headquarters. Your comments will receive careful consideration at a meeting of the responsible technical committee, which you may attend. If you feel that your comments have not received a fair hearing you should make your views known to the ASTM Committee on Standards, 100 Barr Harbor Drive, West Conshohocken, PA 19428.

Standard Practice for Testing For Biological Responses to Particles *In Vitro*[1]

This standard is issued under the fixed designation F 1903; the number immediately following the designation indicates the year of original adoption or, in the case of revision, the year of last revision. A number in parentheses indicates the year of last reapproval. A superscript epsilon (ϵ) indicates an editorial change since the last revision or reapproval.

1. Scope

1.1 This practice covers the production of wear debris and degradation products from implanted materials that may lead to a cascade of biological responses resulting in damage to adjacent and remote tissues. In order to ascertain the role of particles in stimulating such responses, the nature of the responses, and the consequences of the responses, established protocols are needed. This is an emerging, rapidly developing area and the information gained from standard protocols is necessary to interpret responses and to determine if there is correlation with the *in vivo* responses. Since there are many possible and established ways of determining responses, a single standard protocol is not stated. However, well described protocols are needed to compare results from different investigators using the same materials and to compare biological responses for evaluating (ranking) different materials. For laboratories without established protocols, recommendations are given and indicated with an *.

1.2 Since the purpose of these studies is to predict the response in humans, the use of human cells would provide much information. However in the interest of safety in laboratory protocols, the use of non-human and non-primate cells is described.

1.3 The values stated in SI units are to be regarded as the standard.

1.4 *This standard does not purport to address all of the safety concerns, if any, associated with its use. It is the responsibility of the user of this standard to establish appropriate safety and health practices and determine the applicability of regulatory limitations prior to use.*

2. Referenced Documents

2.1 *ASTM Standards:*

F 619 Practice for Extraction of Medical Plastics[2]

F 748 Practice for Selecting Generic Biological Test Methods for Materials and Devices[2]

3. Summary of Practice

3.1 Biological responses to particles may be evaluated using specimens from animals being tested according to the Practice F 748 matrix for irritation and sensitivity, or for implantation. Blood, organs, or tissues from the animals may be used.

3.2 Biological responses to particles may be evaluated using materials or extracts according to Practice F 619. These materials or extracts may be used for *in vivo* tests or for the *in vitro* tests. Particles generated by other methods may also be used.

4. Significance and Use

4.1 This practice is to be used to help assess the biocompatibility of materials used in medical devices. It is designed to test the effect of particles from the materials on macrophages. For safety reasons, the use of non human, non primate cells is recommended in this practice. For laboratories equipped and approved to work with human blood and tissue, the use of these same protocols would be advantageous for development of understanding of the interaction of cells and particles.

4.2 The appropriateness of the methods should be carefully considered by the user since not all materials or applications need be tested by this practice.

4.3 *Abbreviations*:

4.3.1 *LPS*—lipopolysaccharide (endotoxin).

4.3.2 *LAL*—Limulus Amebocyte Lysate.

4.3.3 *ATCC*—American Type Culture Collection.

4.3.4 *FCS (FBS)*—Fetal Calf Serum.

4.3.5 *NCS*—Newborn Calf Serum.

4.3.6 *PBS*—Phosphate Buffered Saline.

4.3.7 *HANKS*—A balanced salt solution.

4.3.8 *MMPS*—Matrix Metallo Proteases.

4.3.9 *RPMI* 1640—Specific Growth Medium (Roswell Park Memorial Institute).

4.3.10 *PBS*—Phosphate Buffered Saline.

4.3.11 *HEPES*—A buffering salt.

5. Responses from Cells Grown *In Vitro*

5.1 *Particles*—Define the nature of the particles used:

5.1.1 Source,

5.1.2 Chemistry,

5.1.3 Size (mean and range),

5.1.4 Shape,

5.1.5 Method of sterilization,

5.1.6 If the presence of bacterial lipopolysaccharide (LPS) was determined, specify how this was done and the sensitivity of the method. (LAL testing with a sensitivity of at least 0.06 EU is recommended),

5.1.7 Concentration of particles used as weight or number or

---

[1] This practice is under the jurisdiction of ASTM Committee F-4 on Medical and Surgical Devicesand is the direct responsibility of Subcommittee F04.16on Biocompatibility Test Methods.

Current edition approved June 10, 1998. Published August 1998.

[2] *Annual Book of ASTM Standards*, Vol 13.01.

surface area/10^6 cells, and

5.1.8 Surface charge (if known).

5.2 *Cells*—Define the nature of the cells used:

5.2.1 *Established Cell Line* (if not, go to 5.2.2)—The use of established cell lines provides a known cell type with a reproducible response. Although the correlation with the *in vivo* system may not be known at this time, careful studies with established cell lines could eventually allow determination of correlation between *in vivo* and *in vitro* systems.

5.2.1.1 Source of cell and identifying number or code,

5.2.1.2 Nature of the cell (for example, macrophage), and

5.2.1.3 Special attributes of the cell line (for example, nonphagocytic),

5.2.1.4 *ATCC murine macrophages such as RAW 264.7, J774A, P388D1, or IC-21 are recommended.

5.2.2 *Primary Isolate* (if not, go to 1.2.1):

5.2.2.1 Source of cell including species and location (for example, murine, alveolar),

5.2.2.2 Nature of the cell (for example, macrophage),

5.2.2.3 Mechanism of isolation (for example, lavage), and

5.2.2.4 Specify if stimulant used and if so which one (for example, mineral oil).

5.2.2.5 *Mouse (specify strain, age, and sex used) peritoneal exudate cells are recommended with a mild stimulant such as nutrient broth.

5.3 *Culture Conditions*:

5.3.1 Specify source and type of medium. If not a commercial source, list ingredients and sources of ingredients.

5.3.2 Specify source and type of serum, and whether it was heat inactivated. If the presence of LPS was determined, specify method and sensitivity of the method.

5.3.3 Specify culture conditions (for example, 37°C, humidified, 5 % CO_2 incubator).

5.3.4 Specify time of termination of culture or sampling of culture medium.

5.3.5 If cell counts were determined specify as to when and how. If estimates of cell number/mL specify when and how.

5.3.5.1 *Medium and serum specified by the supplier of the cells are recommended. Generally RPMI 1640 with heat inactivated 10 % newborn or fetal calf serum are recommended. LPS levels are generally provided or available from the distributor. Recommended culture conditions are 37°C, with 5 % CO_2, in a humidified incubator. Cell counts at the time of initial plating and at the termination of the culture are recommended using a hemocytometer with monolayer cells resuspended by trypsin solution (not recommended for macrophages), washing with Ca and Mg free PBS or Hanks, or scraping in 1 mL of Ca and Mg free PBS or Hanks. The addition of trypan blue is helpful. The supernatant of the medium from macrophages exposed to particles for specified time periods is assayed.

5.3.6 *Controls*:

5.3.6.1 Cells not stimulated with particles should be maintained at the same time under the same conditions.

5.3.6.2 Polystyrene particles, spherical, size range 1 to 5 µm, should be used as a reference control.

5.3.6.3 LPS is a known stimulant and is a good positive control. A concentration between 0.25 and 1 ng/mL of culture medium is sufficient.

5.3.6.4 Culture medium is a recommended diluent for the assays.

5.4 *Products or Response Determined*—One or more of the following:

5.4.1 Cell viability can be determined by any of several methods:

5.4.1.1 From the total cell counts and viable cell count with trypan blue dye exclusion,

5.4.1.2 From flow cytometry with vital stains,

5.4.1.3 From uptake of DNA precursors, and

5.4.1.4 From total DNA or RNA in the culture.

5.4.2 *Soluble Cell Products Elaborated*:

5.4.2.1 Reliable reagents or kits are available to detect products. The products are classified into three classes: growth factors such as TNFα, TGF beta, and PGE2, interleukins such as IL-1, IL-1 receptor antagonist, IL-1 beta, and IL-6, and reactive oxygen species such as superoxide or nitric oxide (NO) (usually measured as nitrite produced using the Griess reagent). The release of at least two products, which are from different classes, should be determined.

5.4.2.2 The time in culture should be specified since these products peak at different times (for example, TNFα peaks by 24 h, NO peaks around 72 h, the others generally peak at 48 to 72 h). The detection of NO and TNFα are strongly recommended and the assay procedures are described in some detail in this recommended practice.

5.4.3 *Assay for Nitric Oxide*:

5.4.3.1 The production of NO is most conveniently measured by detection of the stable endproduct nitrite. This reflects the action of NO on arginine. The technique is simple, inexpensive and quantitative. The reagent used to quantitate nitrite is the Griess reagent. This is prepared by dissolving 100 mg of Sulfanilamide and 10 mg of N-(1-naphthyl)ethylenediamine in 2.5 % phosphoric acid. Assay of culture medium: 100 uL of the culture medium is placed in a 96-well microtiter plate and then 100 uL of the Griess reagent is added. This is incubated at room temperature for 10 min and the optical density determined at 540 nm wavelength. A standard curve is prepared with sodium nitrite in water. It is recommended that two-fold serial dilutions be prepared encompassing the range of 32 to 0.125 nmoles/mL. The standard curve is prepared using 100 uL of the dilutions of sodium nitrite and 100 uL of the Griess reagent.

5.4.4 *Assay for TNFα*:

5.4.4.1 Kits for assay of TNFα using immunological assays are available from supply houses including, but not limited to, R&D Systems and Endogen. Instructions are provided with the kits. These are sensitive and reliable.

5.4.4.2 There is a bioassay for TNFα using L929 cells which may be more convenient for some laboratories. There are several methods available, and a recommended method is described here.

5.4.4.3 L929 cells (available from ATCC and other sources) are seeded at 10^5 cells/mL of RPMI 1640 with 10 % RBS using 100 uL per well in a 96 well culture plate leaving one column empty as a blank. These are grown for 24 h at 37°C in 5 % CO_2.

5.4.4.4 Assay media is RPMI 1640 with 10 % FBS, 2 ug/mL of actinomycin D, and 20 µmolar HEPES buffer.

5.4.4.5 Prepare TNFα standard curve (TNFα standards are available from supply houses including R&D Systems) of 0.1, 0.25, 0.5, 1, 2.5, and 5 units/mL. A 96-well plate is dedicated to the standards and the unknowns are done in other 96-well plates and the concentration of TNFα is determined from the standard curve. Each standard is run in eight replicates. The recommendation is that 6 of the eight well columns are used for the standards, one column is used for the blank, and three columns are used for cells and media control. The unknowns to be assayed are diluted at least ½ in the assay medium.

5.4.4.6 The media in the plates with the 24 h L929 cell cultures are poured off or pipetted off. Then 100 uL of the assay media, the standards in the assay media, or the unknowns in the assay media is added to the appropriate wells. These are incubated for 24 h at 37°C with 5 % CO_2. At the end of the 24-h incubation, pour off the media, shake the remaining media off, invert the plates onto absorbent paper for a few minutes to drain.

5.4.4.7 *Stain*—500 mg crystal violet, 8mL of 40 % formaldehyde, 170 mg NaCl, and 22.3 mL ethanol made to 100 mL with water. Dissolve the crystal violet and filter the solution. Add 100 uL of the stain to each well. Leave at room temperature for 10 min with occasional gentle shaking. Pour off the stain, wash with distilled water, invert the plates onto absorbent paper for 10 min. There should be no stain dripping off. If there is, wash with water again. Place the plates in the upright position and leave to dry. Add 100 uL of 33 % acetic acid/well, swirl the plate, read the optical density at 595 to 600 nm.

5.4.4.8 Other products detected should be specified and the method used specified. Suggested products would be other reactive oxygen species such as superoxide, other interleukins (IL-2, IL-4, IL-10), collagenase, MMPS.

5.4.5 *Effects of the Culture Media on Other Systems*:

5.4.5.1 Bone resorption using bone slices or calvaria cultures, and

5.4.5.2 Effect on chondrocyte cultures.

5.4.6 Methods should be clearly described and results compared to a standard that is readily available to other laboratories for validation.

6. Data Collection and Analysis

6.1 Cell viability should be reported as cell number, or percent survival, or DNA or RNA concentrations, or estimated survival and these results compared to the results with the cell control without particles and the results with the polystyrene reference particles. (PS particles are available from commercial suppliers.)

6.2 Soluble products elaborated should be reported as µg or ng or units/mL, or µg or ng or units/cell number, or concentration such as mM. Alternatively, the report of the optical density of the solution will suffice. The results with the particles should be compared to the results with the cell control without particles and the results with the cells and the polystyrene reference particles.

7. Keywords

7.1 biocompatibility; growth factors; interleukins; macrophages; nitric oxide; particles; TNFα

APPENDIXES

(Nonmandatory Information)

X1. RATIONALE

X1.1 The primary purpose of this practice is to describe methodology to determine the biological response to particles using *in vitro* cellular responses.

X1.2 It is well recognized that the biological responses to particles could be different from those to solid materials. The interaction of the particles with phagocytic cells, notably macrophages, is a key to the final biological response.

X1.3 The interaction of macrophages with particles has been an active research area for many years. Many investigators have developed procedures for doing these studies. This document is intended to delineate the information necessary so that the results from these various studies can be interpreted and to describe methodology appropriate for those investigators developing such studies.

X1.4 The interaction of phagocytic cells with particles will lead to the production of various soluble mediators which may influence the progression of the biological response and the immune response. It is unknown at this time which of these responses are favorable and which are unfavorable to the host. Similarly it is unknown whether quantitative evaluation of these factors is predictive of the biological response. Studies such as the ones described here are needed to determine the importance of these responses in biocompatibility and biocompatibility testing of materials.

X1.5 The level of LAL for device evaluation is commonly 0.5 EU/m/L . LAL testing with a sensitivity of 0.06 EU/mL is recommended in this practice for evaluating in vitro responses to particles since levels of LPS above 0.06 EU/mL may be stimulatory to macrophages. This will permit distinguishing cellular responses to particles from cellular responses to LPS.

X1.6 Polystyrene (PS) particles were chosen as a reference control for this standard practice so that testing results from different laboratories of from different cell lines or assay systems could be compared and normalized to PS. The anticipated responses of the cells to these particles and production of various cytokines and other growth factors are unknown. They may stimulate some factors and not others. These particles are not device material applicable and serve as a neutral territory, commercially available, well characterized particulate material for normalization of results.

X2. ADDITIONAL REFERENCES

Green, L.C., DA Wagner, J Glowoski, PL Skipper, JS Wishnok, SR Tannenbaum, "Analysis of Nitrate, Nitrite, and [15N] Nitrate in Biological Fluids," *Anal. Biochem. 126:131*, 1982.

Flick DA, GE Gifford, "Comparison of *In Vitro* Cell Cytotoxicity Assays for Tumor Necrosis Factor," *J. Immunol Methods 68: 167*, 1984.

Chapekar, MS, TG Zaremba, RK Kuester, VM Hitchins, "Synergistic Industion of Tumor Necrosis Factor α by Bacterial Lipopolysaccharide and Lipoteichoic Acid in Combination with Polytetrafluoroethylene Particles in a Murine Macrophage Cell Line RAW 264.7," *J. Biomed. Mater. Res. 31:* 1996, pp 251-256.

St. John K.R., (ed), *Particulate Debris from Medical Implants: Mechanisms of Formation and Biological Consequences, STP 1144*, ASTM, Philadelphia, PA 1992.

Wright, T.M., Goodman, S.B., (eds), *Implant Wear: The Future of Total Joint Replacement*, American Academy of Orthopaedic Surgeons, Rosemont, IL 1996.

Ruff, M.R., Gifford, G.E., "Tumor Necrosis Factor," *Lymphokines 2:* 1991, pp. 235-272.

Bonfield, T.L., Anderson, J.M., "Functional Versus Quantitative Comparison of IL-1 Beta from Monocytes/Macrophages on Biomedical Polymers," *J. Biomed. Mater. Res. 27:*, 1993, pp. 1195-1199.

Standard Practice for Testing the Biological Responses to Particles *In Vivo*[1]

This standard is issued under the fixed designation F 1904; the number immediately following the designation indicates the year of original adoption or, in the case of revision, the year of last revision. A number in parentheses indicates the year of last reapproval. A superscript epsilon (ε) indicates an editorial change since the last revision or reapproval.

ε1 NOTE—Section 1.1 was editorially revised in June 2000.

1. Scope

1.1 This practice covers the production of wear debris and degradation products from implanted materials that may lead to a cascade of biological responses resulting in damage to adjacent and remote tissues. In order to ascertain the role of particles in stimulating such responses, the nature of the responses, and the consequences of the responses, established protocols are needed. This is an emerging, rapidly developing area and the information gained from standard protocols is necessary to interpret responses. Some of the procedures listed here may, on further testing, not prove to be predictive of clinical responses to particulate debris. However, only the use of standard protocols will establish which are useful techniques. Since there are many possible and established ways of determining responses, a single standard protocol is not stated. However, this recommended practice indicates which necessary information should be supplied with test results. For laboratories without established protocols, recommendations are given and indicated with an *.

1.2 *This standard does not purport to address all of the safety concerns, if any, associated with its use. It is the responsibility of the user of this standard to establish appropriate safety and health practices and determine the applicability of regulatory limitations prior to use.*

2. Referenced Documents

2.1 *ASTM Standards:*

F 561 Practice for Analysis of Retrieved Metallic Orthopaedic Implants[2]

F 619 Practice for Extraction of Medical Plastics[2]

F 748 Practice for Selecting Generic Biological Test Methods for Materials and Devices[2]

F 1877 Recommended Practice for Characterization of Particles[2]

3. Summary of Practice

3.1 Biological responses to particles testing may be done using specimens from animals being tested according to the Practice F 748 matrix for irritation and sensitivity, or for implantation. Blood, organs, or tissues from the animals may be used. Procedures according to F 561 may be used to assess the cellular response.

3.2 Biological responses to particles may be tested using materials or extracts according to Practice F 619. These materials or extracts may be used in *in vivo* tests or for the *in vitro* tests. Particles generated by other methods may also be used. The method of generation must be described.

4. Significance and Use

4.1 This practice is to be used to help assess the biocompatibility of materials used in medical devices. It is designed to test the effect of particles from the materials on the host tissues.

4.2 The appropriateness of the methods should be carefully considered by the user since not all materials or applications need be tested by this practice. The validity of these studies in predicting the human response is not known at this time and studies such as described here are needed.

4.3 *Abbreviation Used*:

4.3.1 *LPS*—Lipopolysaccharide (endotoxin).

4.3.2 *LAL*—Limulus amebocyte lysate.

4.3.3 *PCR*—Polymerase chain reaction.

4.3.4 *CD*—Cluster differentiation.

4.3.5 *HLA*—Human leukocyte antigens.

5. Responses from In Vivo Systems

5.1 *Particles*—Define the nature of the particles used:

5.1.1 Source,

5.1.2 Chemistry,

5.1.3 Size (mean and range),

5.1.4 Shape,

5.1.5 Surface charge (if known),

5.1.6 Method of sterilization,

5.1.7 If the presence of bacterial lipopolysaccharide (LPS) was determined, specify how this was done and the sensitivity of the method. (LAL testing with a sensitivity of at least 0.06 EU is recommended),

5.1.8 Concentration of particles used as weight, or number, or surface area/implant, and

5.1.9 Polystyrene particles, spherical, 1 to 5 μm in size should be used as a reference particle.

5.2 *Biological System*—One or more of these sites should be used:

[1] This practice is under the jurisdiction of ASTM Committee F-4 on Medical and Surgical Devicesand is the direct responsibility of Subcommittee F04.16on Biocompatibility Test Methods.

Current edition approved June 10, 1998. Published August 1998.

[2] *Annual Book of ASTM Standards*, Vol 13.01.

5.2.1 *Air Pouch Model*— This is an emerging model to simulate synovial tissue. The volume of air and the time allowed before introduction of the particles should be specified. This model needs to be validated for length of time of implantation and relevance to other *in vivo* systems.

5.2.2 *Cages*—Cages made of porous materials such as stainless steel mesh or porous teflon can be implanted with a test material inside the cage. These may be implanted subcutaneously or intraperitoneally. The material and the implant location chosen should be specified. The fluid accumulating in the cage can be sampled at various time intervals. The time intervals must be specified. The cage and contained material is removed at the termination of the experiment (specify time chosen) and evaluated for cell adhesion, cell type, and products. Fluid containing large number of red blood cells should be discarded since it represents blood, not cage fluid.

5.2.3 *Bone Implant Chamber*—This is a modification of the cage system and allows determination of the effect of particles and the resulting biological response on bone remodeling

5.2.4 *Direct Injection*— Intraperitoneal, intravenous, intramuscular, subcutaneous are the favored routes. The end use application should govern the route of injection and the organ or tissue utilized in this test. Inhalation may be suitable for some end use applications.

5.2.5 Examination of tissue at implant retrieval from animal models or clinical conditions is dealt with in F 1877. Some of the procedures defined here are also applicable to these tissues.

5.2.6 All sites used in these studies should be carefully evaluated for infection at the termination of the study. The presence of infection will have a major impact on the outcome since it stimulates many responses.

5.3 *Biological Response Determined*—One or more of the following:

5.3.1 Cell accumulation at the site of the particles should be evaluated for relative number and type of cells. Standard paraffin or plastic embedded sections are usually sufficient to identify acute inflammatory cells, lymphocytes, macrophages, foreign body giant cells, osteoclasts, osteoblasts, osteocytes, eosinophils, etc. But in some cases special histological procedures, or immunohistochemical stains such as those described in F 561, or flow cytometry may be needed to confirm the identity of lymphocytes and macrophages. An evaluation scale of 0 to 5 with 0 being no cell response, 1 being accumulation of a few cells, 2 being a mild response with some cell accumulation, 3 being a moderate response, 4 being a large response, and 5 being a severe response is recommended. It should also be noted whether the response is focal or diffuse.

5.3.1.1 Transport of particles to relevant draining organs and histologic responses in these organs should be determined, especially when direct injection is used. The relevant organs would be spleen, liver, kidney, and some cases the lung. The draining nodes should be harvested if identifiable. Some types of debris are distinctive (for example, carbon fibers), but lymph nodes and lung commonly contain particles and bits of birefringent stuff that may be confused with particles used in the experiment. Light microscopy with and without polarized light can be suggestive of particle migration, but other methods, (for example, EDAX, may be necessary to confirm the composition of the migrating particles. Organs from control animals should also be evaluated.

5.3.2 *Soluble Cell Products Elaborated*—This is a rapidly emerging area of technology. Histochemical and immunohistochemical techniques can be used to great advantage in these studies. Reliable reagents, kits, or hybridization protocols are available to detect the following products IL- 1β, IL-2, IL-4, IL-6, IL-10, PGE2, TNFα, immunoglobulins, as well as the lymphocyte CD markers and some HLA markers. It is not necessary to measure all of these and the selection should be based on whether there is emphasis on the macrophage response or the specific immune response.

5.3.3 Where other products from the cellular response are being detected, they should be specified and the method used specified.

5.4 Effects of the particles on other systems such as bone remodeling, chondrocyte function, cartilage repair, and synovial tissue function and repair are also important studies. The methods used should be fully described.

6. Report Section and Data Analysis

6.1 The histologic response should be compared to that of normal tissues with no particles and to that of tissues receiving the polystyrene reference particle. This may be done by counting, by digitization, by cell analyzer, or by estimation in the field of view. In some circumstances presence or absence of marker or response will suffice. In some circumstances quantitation of the response may be obtained with data on responses such as Ca++ released, enyzyme levels. DNA or RNA levels, etc.

7. Keywords

7.1 biocompatibility; biological response; *in vivo*; interleukins; particles

APPENDIX

(Nonmandatory Information)

X1. RATIONALE

X1.1 The primary purpose of this practice is to describe methodologies to determine the biological response to particles using *in vivo* responses.

X1.2 It is well recognized that the biological responses to particles could be different from those to solid materials. The interaction of the particles with cells in the tissue, notably macrophages and other phagocytic cells, is a key to the final biological response.

X1.3 The interaction of particles with host tissue has been an active research area for many years. Many investigators have developed procedures for doing these studies. This practice is intended to delineate the information necessary for interpretation of the results from these various studies and to describe methodology appropriate for those investigators developing such studies.

X1.4 The interaction of the biological system with particles will lead to the accumulation of various cells which may produce soluble mediators which influence the progression of the biological response and the immune response. It is unknown at this time which of these responses are favorable and which are unfavorable to the host. Studies such as the ones described here are needed to determine the importance of these responses in biocompatibility and biocompatibility testing of materials.

Designation: F 1905 – 98

Standard Practice For Selecting Tests for Determining The Propensity Of Materials To Cause Immunotoxicity[1]

This standard is issued under the fixed designation F 1905; the number immediately following the designation indicates the year of original adoption or, in the case of revision, the year of last revision. A number in parentheses indicates the year of last reapproval. A superscript epsilon (ϵ) indicates an editorial change since the last revision or reapproval.

1. Scope

1.1 This practice covers the introduction of foreign materials into the body that may have an impact on the immune system. One possible effect is that the immune system will be depressed or certain cell types may be affected. Immunotoxicity may be determined with blood and tissue samples from the animals used in the other biocompatibility test procedures such as implantation and blood contact test protocols. It is also possible to use these techniques with blood samples from human patients in a clinical trial. Any procedures with human subjects should follow the appropriate rules of the local institutional review board and the appropriate regulatory agencies. This document may serve as an annex to Practice F 748.

1.2 The material may affect the humoral immune response, the cell mediated response, or both.

1.3 *This standard does not purport to address all of the safety concerns, if any, associated with its use. It is the responsibility of the user of this standard to establish appropriate safety and health practices and determine the applicability of regulatory limitations prior to use.*

2. Referenced Documents

2.1 *ASTM Standards:*

F 619 Practice for Extraction of Medical Plastics[2]

F 748 Practice for Selecting Generic Biological Test Methods for Materials and Devices[2]

3. Terminology

3.1 *Definitions:*

3.1.1 *antigens*—these are substances that stimulate the host to produce an immune response

3.1.2 *cell mediated immunity (CMI)*—some antigens stimulate the production of lymphocytes that react specifically with the antigen. These cells do not circulate widely in the host and are generally located at the site of antigen deposition. The use of living lymphocytes is required to test for CMI to an antigen.

3.1.3 *complement*—this is a complex system of circulating proteins (enzymes, pro-enzymes, and co-factors) found in the blood. This system is usually activated by antigen-antibody reactions and is a reflection of humoral immunity. However it is apparent that other factors can activate the complement system. These include large polysaccharides and various materials and tissues. Activation of complement can affect the immune system, inflammation, and vascular activity with fever and shock as a consequence of complement activation in the host.

3.1.4 *humoral immunity*—some antigens stimulate the host to produce antibodies (immunoglobulins) which are specific for the antigen and react with the antigen. Antibodies circulate in the blood and tissue fluids. The antibodies produced can be detected using blood from the host.

3.1.5 *inflammatory factors*—various soluble substances may be produced by lymphocytes in response to an antigen. This may occur in humoral immune responses or in CMI. These substances may influence the function of other cells and are called cytokines. Many of these act on various white cells and are called interleukins. They are reflection of antigenic stimulation of the host.

4. Summary of Practice

4.1 Immunotoxicity testing is done using specimens from animals being tested according to the Practice F 748 matrix for irritation and sensitivity, or for implantation. Blood, organs, or tissues from the animals may be used. In predicting biocompatibility, tests using animals are recommended even though the material will eventually be used in humans. The use of human material is also feasible in this testing protocol for those laboratories having approval for such studies.

4.2 Immunologic testing is done using materials or extracts according to Practice F 619. These materials or extracts may be used for *in vivo* tests or for the *in vitro* tests.

5. Significance and Use

5.1 This practice is to be used to help assess the biocompatibility of materials used in medical devices. It is designed to test the immunotoxicity of such materials.

5.2 The appropriateness of the methods should be carefully considered by the user since not all materials or applications need be tested by this practice.

5.3 The testing suggestions in Practice F 748 and in the matrices of recommended tests issued by regulatory agencies such as the FDA Immunotoxicity Testing Guide may be considered before proceeding with these tests.

---

[1] This practice is under the jurisdiction of ASTM Committee F-4 on Medical and Surgical Materials and Devices and is the direct responsibility of Subcommittee F.16 on Biocompatibility Test Methods.

Current edition approved June 10, 1998. Published August 1998.

[2] *Annual Book of ASTM Standards*, Vol 13.01.

5.4 *Abbreviations*:

5.4.1 *BSA*—Bovine Serum Albumin.

5.4.2 *IgG, IgA, IgM, IgE, IgD*—Immunoglobulin Class G, Class A, Class M, Class E, Class D.

5.4.3 *ELISA*—Enzyme Linked Immunosorbent Assays

5.4.4 *EIA*—Enzyme Immunoassays.

5.4.5 *RIA*—Radio Immunoassays.

5.4.6 *PHA*—Phytohemagglutinin.

5.4.7 *ConA*—Concanavalin A.

5.4.8 *IL*—Interleukin (identified by numbers).

5.4.9 *C*—Complement (components are numbered or lettered).

5.4.10 *SRBC*—Sheep Red Blood Cells.

5.4.11 *CD*—Cluster of Differentiation (antigenic markers on cells).

5.4.12 *CNS*—Central Nervous System.

6. In Vitro Tests for Immunotoxicity

6.1 *Effects on the Humoral Response*—The following determinations are important in assessing the ability of a material to depress the immune response.

6.1.1 *Total Immunoglobulins*—Commercially available kits are recommended for measuring immunoglobulin Class specific (IgG, IgM, IgA, IgD, IgE) immunoglobulins may also be measured and commercially available kits are recommended.

NOTE 1—Changes in total immunoglobulins are seen only after major disturbance of the immune system.

6.1.2 *Effect on Specific Immune Response*:

6.1.2.1 The use of BSA as the antigen is recommended in animal studies. Tetanus toxoid or another approved vaccine is recommended in human clinical trials. The immune response in those receiving the material and the antigen and the immune response in those receiving only the antigen should be determined and compared. A standard ELISA or RIA assay for the immune response is recommended.

6.1.2.2 The use of SRBC is also recommended in animal studies. The assay for plaque forming cells using single cell suspensions from spleens harvested four days after immunization is a sensitive test for IgM antibody.

6.1.2.3 The use of a known adjuvant such as Complete Freund's Adjuvant or Titer Max is recommended. The use of physiologic saline or phosphate buffered saline as a negative control is recommended.

6.1.3 *Effect on B Cell Numbers*—This provides direct information on the effect of the material on the B cell proliferation and killing. This should be done with commercially available, labeled anti-species IgM or IgD, or with an appropriate anti CD antibody and with the use of a cell sorter for enumeration.

6.2 *Effects on the cell Mediated System*:

6.2.1 *Enumeration of Lymphocytes*:

6.2.1.1 *Total T Cell Counts*—This should be done using species specific labeled anti T cell CD antigens, preferably anti CD2 or anti CD3 and a cell sorter.

6.2.2 *Enumeration of T Cell Types*—This should be done using species specific labeled anti CD4 and anti CD8.

6.2.3 *Responses of T Cells*—T cells have receptors on their surfaces for plant lectins such as PHA, ConA and they will divide and proliferate in response. T cells are incubated with PHA or ConA in tissue culture for four days. The level of response can be determined by cell counts or by the uptake of tritiated thymidine.

6.3 *Effects on Inflammatory Factors*:

6.3.1 *Interleukins*—The incubation of lymphocytes in culture with the material may lead to the stimulation of the production of cytokines. The most common, and the ones that are readily detectable and quantifiable, are the interleukins, IL-1 and IL-2 are the recommended ones.

6.4 *Complement*—Materials, especially those in devices that are blood contacting, or in contact with the CNS or large extracorporeal circuits, may affect complement which is a series of proteins important in inflammation and the immune response. The usual method is to determine levels of a component of complement. Commercially available kits are recommended. It is essential to follow the instructions since serum and plasma may not be interchangeable in these tests. The use of a known nonstimulatory biomaterial and a known stimulant such as cobra venom factor are recommended as controls. (NB: measurable effects on the complement system generally occur only after major alterations in the immune system.)

6.4.1 To determine the effect on the Classical Pathway, measurement of C2 is recommended or the split products of C4.

6.4.2 To determine the effect on the Alternate Pathway, measurement of factor B, Bb, or D are recommended.

6.4.3 To determine the effect on the total complement system, measurement of C3 is recommended. Measurement of the split products of C3 or C5 is highly recommended.

6.4.4 The activity of the complement system is best determined with a hemolysis assay or by assay for the terminal complex (Sc5b-9). The standard 50 % hemolytic assay (CH 50) is still a method of choice and is described in the cited "other documents".

7. Data Analysis and Report

7.1 The data obtained should be compared to the results in control animals not receiving the material. In tests where actual numbers are obtained these should be reported as mean and standard deviation or standard error. In some cases, the report of presence or absence of response or estimation of the magnitude of the responses will suffice.

8. Keywords

8.1 B cells; biocompatibility; cell mediated immunity; complement; humoral immunity; immunotoxicity; T cells

APPENDIXES

(Nonmandatory Information)

X1. RATIONALE

X1.1 The primary purpose of this practice is to describe methodologies to determine the propensity of materials to affect the immune response.

X1.2 It is well recognized that the immune response is an important defense mechanism of the host. The interaction of materials with host tissue might alter this response and it is important to understand what materials affect which parts of the immune system.

X1.3 The nature of the immune response and features of immunotoxicity have been an active research area for many years. However, not many studies have been done with medical materials. Many investigators have developed procedures for doing immunotoxicity studies. This document is intended to delineate the information necessary for selection of tests to be done.

X1.4 The interaction of the immunological system with materials could lead to the production of various responses. It is unknown at this time whether immunotoxicity which may be caused by the materials is unfavorable to the host. Immunotoxicity studies using medical materials are important so that this information can be obtained.

X2. ADDITIONAL REFERENCES

Burleson, GR, Dean JH, Munson AE., *Methods in Immunotoxicology*, Wiley-Liss, New York, 1995.

Coligan JE, Kruisbeek AM, Margulies DH, Shevach EM, Strober W. *Current Protocols in Immunology*, N.Y., John Wiley, 1992 (appended frequently).

Price, CP, Newman, DJ., *Principles and Practice of Immunoassay*, Stockton Press, NY, NY 1991.

Rose NR, Friedman H., *Manual of Clinical Immunology*, Washington DC, American Society for Microbiology, 1992.

Wild, D., *The Immunoassay Handbook*, Stockton Press, 1994.

Designation: F 1906 – 98

Standard Practice for Evaluation of Immune Responses In Biocompatibility Testing Using ELISA Tests, Lymphocyte Proliferation, and Cell Migration[1]

This standard is issued under the fixed designation F 1906; the number immediately following the designation indicates the year of original adoption or, in the case of revision, the year of last revision. A number in parentheses indicates the year of last reapproval. A superscript epsilon (ε) indicates an editorial change since the last revision or reapproval.

1. Scope

1.1 This practice covers the introduction of a foreign substance into mammalian body that may induce the formation of an immune response. The immune response may lead to inadvertent tissue damage and be an undesirable event. In the standard protocols for biocompatibility testing, various studies in animals are done. These animals or their blood and tissues could be used to determine if immune responses have occurred and what types have occurred. At the current time, the immunologic testing in biocompatibility protocols is very limited. Techniques can be developed in the future which are simple, reliable, and sensitive.

1.2 It is the purpose of this practice to delineate some possible test methods. It must be remembered that these are protocols for use in biocompatibility testing, they are not diagnostic tests for evaluation of human conditions. Diagnostic tests for use on humans must go through evaluation at the regulatory agencies. The tests described here are clearly adaptable for use in humans and can be used for research purposes and provide data in clinical trials, but are not necessarily cleared for diagnostic purposes. This practice present selected methods. Other validated methods may be equally applicable.

1.3 The values stated in SI units are to be regarded as the standard.

1.4 *This standard does not purport to address all of the safety concerns, if any, associated with its use. It is the responsibility of the user of this standard to establish appropriate safety and health practices and determine the applicability of regulatory limitations prior to use.*

2. Referenced Documents

2.1 *ASTM Standards:*

F 619 Practice for Extraction of Medical Plastics[2]

F 719 Practice for Testing Biomaterials in Rabbits for Primary Skin Irritation[2]

F 720 Practice for Testing Guinea Pigs for Contact Allergens: Guinea Pig Maximization Test[2]

F 748 Practice for Selecting Generic Biological Test Methods for Materials and Devices[2]

F 763 Practice for Short-Term Screening of Implant Materials[2]

F 981 Practice for Assessment of Compatibility of Biomaterials for Surgical Implants with Respect to Effect of Materials on Muscle and Bone[2]

3. Summary of Practice

3.1 Immunologic testing is done using specimens from animals being tested according to the Practice F 748 matrix for irritation and sensitivity, or for implantation. Blood, organs, or tissues from the animals may be used. Blood or biopsies from patients in a clinical trial may also be used. Animals (rabbits or mice) are also immunized with various antigens in this practice. Humans may be immunized with an approved vaccine.

3.2 Immunologic testing is done using materials, known components of the materials, or extracts prepared according to Practice F 619. These materials, components, or extracts may be used for *in vivo* tests or for the *in vitro* tests.

4. Significance and Use

4.1 This practice is to be used to help evaluate the biocompatibility of materials used in medical devices in terms of the immune response.

4.2 The appropriateness of the methods should be carefully considered since not all materials or applications need to be tested by this practice.

4.3 The testing suggestions in Practice F 748 and in the matrices of recommended tests issued by regulatory agencies may be considered before proceeding with these tests.

4.4 These tests require the use of blood. Procedures for obtaining whole blood or serum should follow the recommendations of the animal research committee of the institution responsible for the animals. In general serum and plasma behave the same in these tests, but it should be noted which was used.

4.5 *The Testing Protocols*—These will be divided into the two specific areas of humoral immunity and cell mediated immunity, and subdivided from there. The tests for the humoral

---

[1] This practice is under the jurisdiction of ASTM Committee F-4 on Medical and Surgical Materials and Devices and is the direct responsibility of Subcommittee F04.16 on Biocompatibility Test Methods.

Current edition approved June 10, 1998. Published August 1998.

[2] *Annual Book of ASTM Standards*, Vol 13.01.

immune responses will be based on solid phase immunoassays for use with enzyme linked immunoassays (ELISA) techniques.

4.6 *Abbreviations*:

4.6.1 *RPMI 1640*—Specific growth medium (Roswell Park Memorial Institute).

4.6.2 *FCS (FBS)*—Fetal Calf Serum (Fetal Bovine Serum).

4.6.3 *NCS*—Newborn Calf Serum.

4.6.4 *MTT*—(3-[4,5-Dimethylthiazol-2-yL]-2,5-diphenyltetrazolium bromide: Thiazolyl blue.

4.6.5 *LIF*—Leukocyte Migration Inhibition Factor.

4.6.6 *Ig*—Immunoglobulin.

4.6.7 *MIF*—Macrophage Migration Inhibition Factor.

4.6.8 *PEC*—Peritoneal Exudate Cells.

4.6.9 *PMNS (POLYS)*—Polymorphonuclear Leukocytes.

4.6.10 *PHA*—Phytohemagglutinin.

4.6.11 *ConA*—Conconavalin A.

4.6.12 *PBS*—Phosphate Buffered Saline.

4.6.13 *PBS/T*—Phosphate Buffered Saline with Tween 20.

4.6.14 *MW*—Molecular Weight.

4.6.15 *MED 199*—Medium 199, a specfic growth medium.

5. Tests for Production of Humoral Immune Responses

5.1 These tests are generally done with serum or plasma. The use of peritoneal or ascites fluid is also permissible.

5.1.1 *Response to Immunogenic Substances*—Proteins and most carbohydrates will adhere to polystyrene, especially when dissolved in buffer at pH 8 to 9. Other materials also usually will adhere. Solid materials may be used as the solid support substrate with appropriate controls for nonspecific binding.

5.1.2 The use of polystyrene 96-well microtiter plates is recommended. There are several manufacturers (for example, Costar, Falcon, Nunc) and they are available from standard supply houses (for example, Fisher, VWR, Thomas). No specific source is recommended, however the choice should be documented in the report.

5.1.2.1 The configuration of the testing protocol is up to the evaluator but control wells must be included in the matrix. It is recommended that 8 wells receive no antigen and serve as reagent controls. A negative control using serum from matched animals not receiving the material should be used in at least four wells. If known positive antisera is available, this should be used in at least four wells. If quantitation is desired, standard solutions of at least three different concentrations should be run in triplicate and a buffer control run in triplicate. Each specimen to be tested should be run at two different dilutions and each in triplicate.

5.1.3 Dissolve the substance in an aqueous based solution. Adjust the pH to between 8.5 and 9.5 or as high as possible before it precipitates. A phosphate buffer is recommended. The final concentration of the substance should be 0.5 mg/mL. (Any extract prepared according to Practice F 619 may be used in this protocol. The pH should be adjusted to pH 8.5 to 9.5 where possible without precipitation of the extract.

5.1.4 Add 100 uL of this to each of the wells except the control wells. Incubate the plates in a humid environment at room temperature (18 to 22°C) or 37°C for 1 h, place in the cold (4 to 8°C) overnight. Wash the plates with phosphate buffered saline with Tween 20 (PBS/T) at least three times. Wash at least twice with coating buffer that is the PBS/T with a protein source such as 1 % gelatin, egg albumin, or serum. This blocks other combining sites on the plates and reduces the background. The plates may be used immediately or stored in the cold until used.

5.1.5 Add 100 uL of the appropriate serum samples or buffer control to the wells. The test serum samples should be run in at least two dilutions. It is recommended that eight wells receive only buffer and serve as an antigen-second antibody control. Incubate at room temperature or 37°C for 1 to 2 h. Wash well with PBS/T.

5.1.6 Add 100 uL of the appropriate antiserum to all of the wells. This second antibody should be labeled with an enzyme (horse radish peroxidase or alkaline phosphatase are recommended). These antisera can be purchased from scientific supply houses and should be used at the dilution recommended by the manufacturer. It is recommended that polyvalent antisera directed against IgG, IgM, IgA of the appropriate species of the animal be used and that IgE specific antisera be used separately. The plates should be incubated at room temperature or 37°C for 1 to 2 h. They should then be washed well with PBS/T.

5.1.7 Add 100 uL of the appropriate substrate to all wells. The substrate specific for the enzyme label and at the correct concentration should be used. This information should be supplied by the supplier of the antisera. Incubate at room temperature (usually in the dark) for the recommended time (usually 20 to 30 min). Read the optical density at the appropriate wave length for the substrate.

5.1.8 *Analysis of the Data*—The results of the optical density achieved with the test serum samples should be compared to the control samples. Significant elevations or depressions would be signified by values outside two standard deviations of the control. If known standards were included, the results can be expressed from comparison with the standard curve.

6. Response to Haptenic Substances

6.1 The immune response to haptens (low molecular weight materials) is similar to the immune response already described. However, this response will be dealt with separately here since there are substantial differences in testing methodologies.

6.1.1 The production of an immune response to low molecular weight degradation, wear, or elution products from materials is an important issue in biocompatibility. These low molecular weight substances may bind to host tissue or protein and become immunogenic. It is not apparent that determination of responses to haptenic materials can be determined using a simple modification of the procedure in Section 5. It is necessary to first coat the plates with a carrier to bind the hapten. For most haptens, albumin serves as an appropriate carrier.

6.2 Step one is to add 100uL of carrier (0.5mg/mL) bovine serum albumin is recommended) to the wells in the plate. Incubate for 1 to 2 h at room temperature or 37°C and then overnight in the cold (4-8°C). Wash the plates well with PBS/T.

6.3 Add 100 uL of the solution containing the hapten. PBS alone should be used as a negative control. Incubate for 1 to 2 h at room temperature. Wash well with the blocking wash

(PBS/T containing gelatin).

6.4 Proceed as described in 5.1.5-5.1.7.

6.5 *Analysis of the Data*—The results of the optical density achieved with the test serum samples should be compared to the control samples. Significant elevations or depressions would be signified by values outside two standard deviations of the control. If known standards were included, the results can be expressed from comparison with the standard curve.

7. Stimulation of Immune Responses to Unrelated Antigens

7.1 It is now known that various substances, especially oils, gels, and colloidal suspensions, can stimulate the immune response to unrelated antigens. This is not necessarily a harmful situation, and may be beneficial. The ability of the material or extract to do this needs to be documented.

7.1.1 For this procedure animals should be given an unrelated antigen (such as bovine serum albumin) with and without the material. The antibody levels should be measured at 7 to 10 days, 21 days, and 8 weeks. The antibody levels should be measured using the techniques in 5.1.

7.1.2 *Protocol*:

7.1.2.1 Control animals receiving only the antigen,

7.1.2.2 Test animals receiving the antigen mixed with the material or extract, and

7.1.2.3 Test animals receiving the antigen in one site and the material or extract in another site.

7.1.3 The following controls are recommended but not required:

7.1.3.1 Animals receiving only saline and no material, extract, or antigen,

7.1.3.2 Animals receiving only the material or extract and not antigen, and

7.1.3.3 Animals receiving the antigen and a known adjuvant such as Complete Freunds's Adjuvant or Titer Max.

7.2 An alternative or additional procedure is to use sheep red blood cells (SRBC) as the unrelated antigen. The plaque forming assay can be used with minced spleen cells obtained four days after immunization with SRBC.

7.3 *Analysis of Results*—The antibody responses in groups 7.1.2.2 through 7.1.2.4 should be compared to the results of group 7.1.2.1 to detect enhancement or suppression.

8. Tests for Production of Cell Mediated Immune Responses

8.1 These tests require the use of living cells. These cells may be obtained from peripheral blood, peritoneal exudates, alveolar washes, or minced lymphoid organs. These tests are based on the stimulation of lymphocytes by antigen with the release of various substances (cytokines and interleukins) that affect other cells. The polyclonal T cell stimulants (mitogen) such as PHA or ConA serve as positive controls. It is essential for these tests that strict aseptic precautions be used. The use of antibiotics other than penicillin/streptomycin or gentamicin is not advised because their mode of action may interfere with the cell responses.

8.1.1 *Lymphocyte Transformation Tests*—This detects the production of a cytokine that stimulates other lymphocytes to divide. Thus one lymphocyte responding specifically to an antigen or nonspecifically to a mitrogen will be activated and stimulate other cells to divide, thus amplifying the response.

8.1.1.1 Isolate lymphocytes by differential sedimentation and suspend in growth medium (RPMI 1640 with 10 % fetal or newborn calf serum (FCS or NCS)) at a concentration of 10^6 cells/ mL.

8.1.2 Dispense 1 mL of lymphocyte suspension into test tubes for each of four tests. It is recommended that each be run in triplicate.

8.1.2.1 Cell control,

8.1.2.2 Cells plus mitogen (PHA or ConA),

8.1.2.3 Cells plus antigen (material or extract) at first concentration, and

8.1.2.4 Cells plus antigen (material or extract) at second concentration.

8.1.3 The tests should be incubated at 37°C in 5 % CO_2 for seven days. The response to mitogen peaks at four days, the response to antigen peaks at seven days. After seven days of incubation add tritiated thymidine or I-125 thymidine to the cultures. Incubate for 4 to 6 h. Collect the cells (usually by filter wash) and determine the uptake of radioisotope. MTT is being used increasingly as a simple dye marker for proliferation assays. Alamar Blue may also be used.

8.1.4 The use of antigen and mitogen together will detect immunosuppression.

8.1.5 *Data Analysis*—The uptake of radioisotope in the presence of antigen should be compared to that of the cell control. The use of the mitogen confirms the test system was working. However comparison of the response to antigen to the response to the mitogen is permissible.

8.2 *Leukocyte Migration Inhibition (LIF)*—This test is limited to human and rabbit peripheral blood. It does not work with peritoneal exudate cells and may not work with dog blood. Blood must be used within 24 h of drawing. The PMNS are the indicator cell.

8.2.1 *Preparation of Detection Plates*—Prepare 0.75 mg SeaKem agarose in 80 mL distilled water. Autoclave and cool to 45 to 55°C. Add 10 mL newborn calf serum or horse serum and 10 mL of Med 199 10X. Mix and pipette 5 mL into 60 × 15 mm petri dishes. Allow to solidify and leave at room temperature overnight. Place the dishes into a sealed plastic bag and store in the refrigerator until used. The shelf life is 2 to 3 months. Be sure they are stored upright and level.

8.2.2 *Preparation of Antigens*—Prepare suspension of antigens at the appropriate concentration. The use of PHA or ConA is recommended as a control. The cell control is saline or PBS. These may be stored in the refrigerator until use. Shelf life varies but should be several months. Assays should be done to check for purely and activity before using the test protocol.

8.2.3 *Test Procedure*—Obtain 10 mL of peripheral blood that is anticoagulated with sodium or lithium heparin. Mix the blood 2 volumes to 1 volume of 2 % 500 000 MW dextran in PBS or saline. Allow to settle at room temperature for 1 h. Draw off the top layer (buffy coat) and place in a centrifuge tube. Centrifuge at 400 g for 15 to 20 min. Discard the supernatant. Resuspend the cells in 100 uL of PBS.

8.2.4 Place 20 uL of control and antigen solutions in test tubes. Add 20 uL of cell suspension and incubate 15 min at room temperature. Cut wells approximately 2 mm in diameter and 3 to 4 mm apart in the agarose plate. A cork borer or immunodiffusion punch is recommended. Remove the agarose plug if it did not come out with the punch. The use of a 20 gage hypodermic needle is recommended.

8.2.4.1 Pipette 10 uL of the cell-solution mixtures into each of two wells cut into the agarose plate. Incubate overnight at 37°C with 5 % CO_2. Examine the plate with a microscope (inverted scope with 4X lens and 10X eyepiece is recommended) for migration of cells from the well. The amount of migration may determined by area of migration, maximum distance from the well, or estimated as none, very little, some, or good.

8.2.5 *Data Analysis*—Compare the cell migration to that of the control. The cell control should be good and if there is a cell mediated response, the migration from the wells containing cells with material or extract will be none to very little.

8.3 *Macrophage Migration Inhibition (MIF)*—(Cells isolated from the peritoneal cavity (best animals: mouse or hamster), lung (best animals: mouse, hamster, rabbit), or lymphoid organs (any animal) are used. The macrophage is the indicator cell.

8.3.1 *Direct Test*—Collect cells that include macrophages and lymphocytes from desired site.

8.3.1.1 Wash and resuspend to a dense concentration in medium (RPMI 1640 with 10 % FCS is the recommended medium).

8.3.1.2 Place the cell suspension in capillary tubes (use a syringe and needle to place into sealed tubes or draw up by capillary action into unsealed tubes and gently heat seal one end) Centrifuge at 400 g for 10 to 15 min. Cut the tube at the cell fluid interface.

8.3.1.3 Place the tube into culture wells (six well plates or 35X10 mm petri dishes) using vacuum grease to hold the tube onto the bottom of the dish.

8.3.1.4 Add the medium (same as used above) with and without material extract or mitogen and incubate overnight at 37°C in 5 % CO_2.

8.3.1.5 The recommended test materials are: medium only, medium plus material or extract, medium plus material or extract at a different concentration, and medium plus mitogen.

8.3.1.6 Measure the area of migration from the capillary tube or estimate none, very little, some, good. Compare the response to the material or extract to that of the control or mitogen.

8.3.2 *Indirect Test*—This takes advantage of the accessibility of PEC from the mouse and uses the lymphocytes from another test animal of the same or different species.

8.3.2.1 For this procedure, lymphocytes are obtained (usually peripheral blood) from the test animal. They are isolated and incubated with the material or extract in a manner similar to that in 8.3.1. At the end of 24 h incubation, the media is withdrawn. This medium is then used as one of the tests described in the direct test. Thus the macrophages are obtained from normal mice, prepared as above in capillary tubes and placed into dishes. The test preparations are medium alone, medium from the lymphocyte incubation, and medium with mitogen.

8.3.2.2 Measure the area of migration from the capillary tube or estimate none, very little, some, good.

8.3.3 *Data Analysis*—Compare the cell migration in the culture containing the medium from the lymphocyte stimulation with material or extract to that of the medium only control and the medium with mitogens (PHA or ConA). A decrease in cell migration compared to medium alone will indicate that a cell mediated response was stimulated.

9. Keywords

9.1 biocompatibility; cell migration; ELISA; haptens; immune response; lymphocyte proliferation

APPENDIXES

(Nonmandatory Information)

X1. RATIONALE

X1.1 The primary purpose of this test method is to describe methodologies to determine the propensity of materials to stimulate the immune response specifically or nonspecifically.

X1.2 It is well recognized that the immune response is an important defense mechanism of the host. The interaction of materials with host tissue might alter this response and it is important to understand what materials affect which parts of the immune system. The production of an immune response directed against components of the material (specific immunity) may be favorable to the host. On the other hand, in some circumstances such responses may be harmful.

X1.3 The nature of the immune response has been an active research area for many years. However, not many studies have been done with medical materials. Many investigators have developed procedures for doing immunological studies. This document is intended to delineate some methods for such testing. However, there are many validated test methods that could be substituted for the ones described here as long as their modifications for use with materials, components, or extracts are fully described.

X1.4 The interaction of the immunological system with materials will lead to the production of various responses. It is unknown at this time whether the immune responses which may be stimulated by the materials are favorable or unfavorable to the host. Immune response studies using medical materials, components, or extracts are important so that this information can be obtained.

X2. ADDITIONAL REFERENCES

Burleson, GR, Dean JH, and Munson AE., *Methods in Immunotoxicology*, Wiley-Liss, New York, 1995.

Coligan JE, Kruisbeek AM, Margulies DH, Shevach EM, and Strober W. *Current Protocols in Immunology*, N.Y., John Wiley, 1992 (appended frequently).

Price, CP, and Newman, DJ., *Principles and Practice of Immunoassay*, Stockton Press, NY, NY 1991.

Rose NR, and Friedman H., *Manual of Clinical Immunology*, Washington DC, American Society for Microbiology, 1992.

Wild, D., *The Immunoassay Handbook*, Stockton Press, 1994.

Designation: F 1925 – 99[ε1]

Standard Specification for Virgin Poly(L-Lactic Acid) Resin for Surgical Implants[1]

This standard is issued under the fixed designation F 1925; the number immediately following the designation indicates the year of original adoption or, in the case of revision, the year of last revision. A number in parentheses indicates the year of last reapproval. A superscript epsilon (ε) indicates an editorial change since the last revision or reapproval.

ε[1] NOTE—Figure 2 was editorially added in July 2001 because it had been inadvertently left out of the previous edition.

1. Scope

1.1 This specification covers virgin poly(L-lactic acid) resin (or abbreviated as PLLA resin) intended for use in surgical implants. This specification does not cover stereoisomeric compositions based on various D, L, or DL copolymer ratios.

1.2 This specification addresses material characteristics of virgin poly(L-lactic acid) resin and does not apply to packaged and sterilized finished implants fabricated from this material.

1.3 As with any material, some characteristics may be altered by processing techniques (such as molding, extrusion, machining, assembly, sterilization, and so forth) required for the production of a specific part or device. Therefore, properties of fabricated forms of this resin should be evaluated using those test methods which are appropriate to assure safety and efficacy.

1.4 The values stated in SI units are to be regarded as the standard.

1.5 *This standard does not purport to address all of the safety concerns, if any, associated with its use. It is the responsibility of the user of this standard to establish appropriate safety and health practices and determine the applicability of regulatory limitations prior to use.*

2. Referenced Documents

2.1 *ASTM Standards:*

D 1505 Test Method for Density of Plastics by the Density-Gradient Technique[2]

D 1898 Practice for Sampling of Plastics[3]

D 2857 Practice for Dilute Solution Viscosity of Polymers[3]

D 3536 Test Method for Molecular Weight Averages and Molecular Weight Distribution by Liquid Exclusion Chromatography (Gel Permeation Chromatography - GPC)[4]

D 3593 Test Method for Molecular Weight Averages and Molecular Weight Distribution of Certain Polymers by Liquid Size-Exclusion Chromatography (Gel Permeation Chromatography - GPC) Using Universal Calibration[4]

D 3892 Practice for Packaging of Plastics[4]

F 748 Practice for Selecting Generic Biological Test Methods for Materials and Devices[5]

2.2 *ISO Standard:*

ISO/DIS 10993-9, Biological Evaluation of Medical Devices, Part 9 Degradation of Materials Related to Biological Testing, Annex A[6]

3. Terminology

3.1 *Definitions of Terms Specific to This Standard:*

3.1.1 *generic property*—that property which is determined solely by the chemical composition and structure of the virgin polymer

3.1.2 *virgin polymer*—the form of poly(L-lactic acid) as obtained from the manufacturer and before fabrication into a medical device.

4. Virgin Poly(L-Lactic Acid) Resin Requirements

4.1 *Generic Properties*:

4.1.1 The virgin polymer shall be a homopolymer of L-lactide with a density between 1.20 and 1.28 g/cm^3 (see 6.5 for evaluation method).

4.1.2 The molecular mass of the virgin polymer shall be indicated by relative solution viscosity in accordance with 6.2. In addition to solution viscosity (but not in place of), weight average molecular mass and molecular mass distributions may be determined by gel permeation chromatography (GPC) according to Test Methods D 3536 or D 3593.

4.1.3 The virgin polymer shall be identified as a polylactide by infrared or ^{1}H-NMR spectroscopy.

4.1.3.1 The virgin polymer shall yield an infrared spectrum which exhibits major absorption bands only at the wavelengths that appear in a suitable reference spectrum. A typical infrared transmission spectrum is shown in Fig. 1.

4.1.3.2 Additional absorption bands may be indicative of known, or unknown, impurities including residual solvents and catalysts (refer to residual solvent limits specified in Table 1).

4.1.3.3 An infrared spectrum cannot distinguish between the different available stereoisomeric polylactic acids. It is used

[1] This specification is under the jurisdiction of ASTM Committee F04 on Medical Surgical Materials and Devices and is the direct responsibility of Subcommittee F04.11 on Polymeric Materials.

Current edition approved Nov. 10, 1999. Published January 2000. Originally published as F 1925 – 98. Last previous edition F 1925 – 98.

[2] *Annual Book of ASTM Standards*, Vol 08.01.

[3] *Annual Book of ASTM Standards*, Vol 08.02.

[4] *Annual Book of ASTM Standards*, Vol 08.03.

[5] *Annual Book of ASTM Standards*, Vol 13.01.

[6] Available from American National Standards Institute, 25 W. 43rd St., 4th Floor, New York, NY 10036.

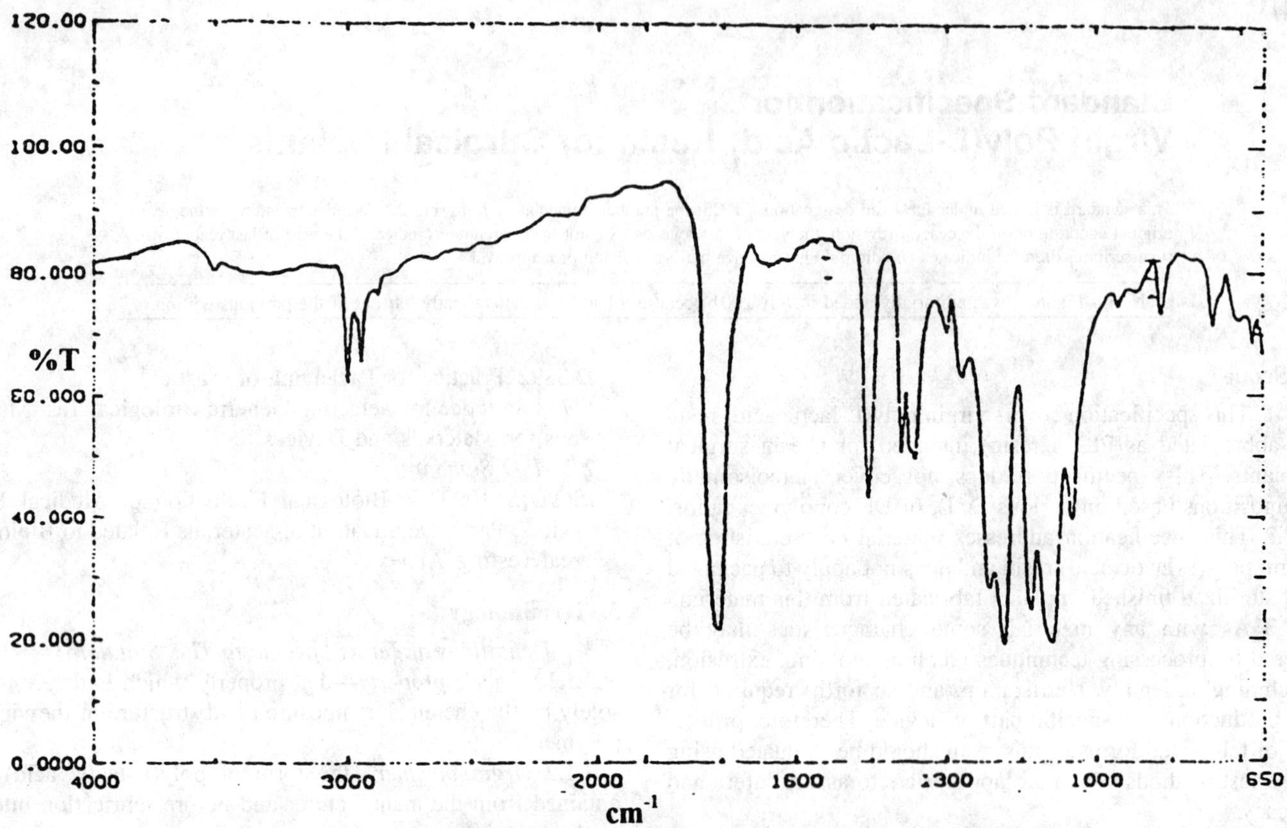

FIG. 1 Poly(L-Lactic Acid) Resin Infrared Spectrum

TABLE 1 Physical/Chemical Property Requirements of Virgin Poly(L-Lactic Acid) Resins

Analyte	Residual Solvent(s), (Total, %)	Residual Water, %	Residual Tin (Sn), ppm	Heavy Metals, (as Lead), ppm	Sulfated Ash, %
Requirement	≤0.01	≤0.5	≤200	≤300	≤0.1

here only as a means of identifying the material as a polylactide.

4.1.3.4 The virgin polymer shall yield a ^{1}H-NMR spectrum which exhibits major absorption bands only at the frequencies that appear in a suitable reference spectrum. A typical ^{1}H-NMR spectrum is shown in Fig. 2.

4.1.3.5 Additional absorption bands may be indicative of known, or unknown, impurities including residual solvents and monomers, and catalysts (refer to residual solvent, monomer, and tin (catalyst) limits specified in Table 1) and 4.1.5.

4.1.3.6 A ^{1}H-NMR spectrum cannot distinguish between the different available stereoisomeric polylactic acids. It is used here only as a means of identifying the material as a polylactide.

4.1.4 The virgin polymer shall have a specific optical rotation between −155 and −160° when measured as specified in 6.3.

4.1.5 The virgin polymer shall have a residual monomer content less than or equal to 2.0 % when assayed in accordance with 6.4. Virgin polymers having inherent viscosities greater than 2 dL/g and intended for injection molding or load-bearing applications shall not have a residual monomer content greater than 0.1 % when assayed in accordance with 6.3.

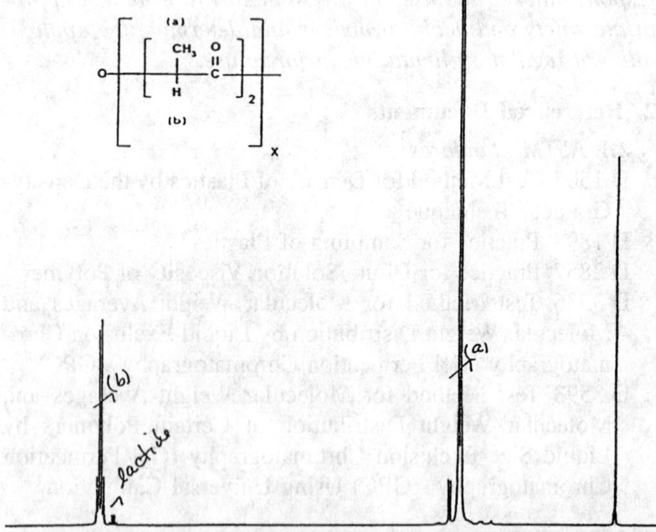

FIG. 2 Poly(L-Lactic Acid) Resin ^{1}H-NMR Spectrum

4.1.6 The virgin polymer shall have the chemical and physical properties as listed in Table 1 as determined by the methods listed in Section 6.

5. Sampling

5.1 Where applicable, the requirements of this specification

allow for the placement of the stirrer propeller[5] immediately above the test specimen (see Fig. 3).

7.3.1 *Stirrer Propeller*[5]—(2.5 in. (63.50 mm) diameter, 0.875 in. (22.22 mm) blades, three blades, 45° pitch, stainless steel).

7.3.2 A different type of stirrer design and stirring rate may be used provided equivalence in experimental results can be demonstrated. Any modification must be reported in 10.1.1.

7.4 The dissolution vessel shall be thermostatically controlled at 37 ± 0.5 °C.

7.5 The dissolution apparatus may include various data recording and storage devices, strip chart recorders, computers, etc., to facilitate continuous monitoring throughout the duration of the experiment.

8. Preparation of Test Specimens

8.1 The standard test specimen for coating evaluation is defined in Fig. 2.

8.2 The test specimen shall be manufactured from the same materials and processes as substrates produced for sale.

8.3 The test specimen shall have the upper shank threaded so as to mate with the stirrer shaft described in Fig. 3.

8.4 By appropriate masking, or other techniques, the coating shall be applied only to the central 0.5 ± 0.005 in. of the test specimen.

8.5 The coating shall be applied to the test specimen, and receive all processing steps as the actual product.

9. Procedure for Monitoring Changes in pH, Calcium, and Phosphorus Concentrations

9.1 Prepare the test specimen as described in Section 8.

9.2 Procure the appropriate volume of dissolution media needed for the experiment and equilibrate at 37 ± 0.5 °C.

9.3 Calibrate the pH probe, the ion-selective probes, and any other analytical instrumentation to be used immediately before starting the experiment as recommended by the manufacturers.

9.4 Adjust the stirrer-test specimen assembly to at least 80 rpm.

9.5 Assemble the dissolution apparatus (see Fig. 1). The dissolution media, all calibrated sensing electrodes, and the stirrer should be in place and operating. However, do not include the test specimen. Then equilibrate this assembly at 37 ± 0.5 °C.

9.6 Set the experiment timing device to zero.

9.7 When ready to begin the experiment, add the test specimen to the stirrer and dissolution vessel. Start the timer and stirrer, and make any necessary adjustments to the equipment.

9.8 As soon as practical after the introduction of the test specimen to the dissolution media, record the initial pH and the dissolved Ca++ and phosphorus concentrations.

9.9 Repeat the measurement of the pH, dissolved Ca++, and dissolved phosphorus concentrations at appropriate time intervals to define their dissolution rate curves.

9.9.1 A typical initial sampling rate shall be at least every 15 min for the first 2 h. More frequent sampling may be necessary for some materials in order to accurately determine the slope of the initial linear portion of the dissolution curve.

9.9.2 A typical final sampling rate shall be at least every hour for the last 8 h of the experiment.

9.9.3 The total volume of all aliquots taken during the course of the experiment shall not comprise more than 5 % of the initial volume.

9.9.4 The duration of a typical experiment shall be at least 48 h. Longer times may be needed for some materials if their measured pH or concentrations of dissolved Ca^{++} or phosphorous continue to change by more than 10 % over a 3 h period.

10. Report

10.1 Report the following results for each of the media systems used:

10.1.1 All procedural details that differ from those described in this test method.

10.1.2 The identity of the dissolution media, the substrate material, and the mass to volume ratio used.

10.1.3 The pH and concentrations of dissolved Ca++ and phosphorus recorded at the start of the experiment (see 9.8).

10.1.4 The pH and concentrations of dissolved Ca^{++} and phosphorus at the end of the experiment.

10.1.5 Plots of the pH and concentrations of total dissolved Ca^{++} and phosphorus versus time data for the duration of the experiment.

10.1.6 The calculated initial dissolution rates (R_i) as follows:

10.1.6.1 Calcium phosphate coatings typically display two quasi-linear regions in their dissolution rate curves. The initial dissolution rate is usually distinguished from the final dissolution rate by a significantly higher rate of increase in the concentrations of dissolved Ca^{++} and phosphorus. The final dissolution rate occurs later in the experiment.

10.1.6.2 The initial dissolution rate (R_i) of a coating is expressed in terms of the initial changes in total Ca^{++} or phosphorus concentrations with time:

$(R_i)_{Ca}$ = Initial slope of the Ca^{++} concentration versus time curve expressed in terms of the total milligrams of Ca^{++} dissolved per milligram of coating per millilitre of media per hour.

$(R_i)_P$= Initial slope of the phosphorus concentration versus time curve expressed in terms of the total milligrams of phosphorus dissolved per milligram of coating per millilitre of media per hour.

10.1.7 The calculated final dissolution rates (R_f) as follows:

10.1.7.1 The final dissolution rate of a coating expressed in terms of the final changes in Ca^{++} and phosphorus concentrations:

$(R_f)_{Ca}$ = Final slope of the Ca^{++} concentration versus time curve expressed in terms of the total milligrams of Ca^{++} dissolved per milligram of coating per millilitre of media per hour.

$(R_f)_P$= Final slope of the phosphorus concentration versus time curve expressed in terms of the total milligrams of phosphorus dissolved per milligram of coating per millilitre of media per hour.

[5] The sole source of supply of the apparatus known to the committee at this time is VWR Scientific, Item 58957-116, P.O. Box 66929, O'Hare AMF, Chicago, IL 60666. If you are aware of alternative suppliers, please provide this information to ASTM Headquarters. Your comments will receive careful consideration at a meeting of the responsible technical committee, which you may attend.

11. Precision and Bias

11.1 Precision and bias of this test method will be determined after interlaboratory tests are carried out and the results tabulated. The interlaboratory tests will be carried out following Practice E 691.

12. Keywords

12.1 calcium-phosphate ceramic; coating; dissolution rate; environmental stability

REFERENCES

(1) Cranin, A. N., Tobin, G., Gelbman, J., and Varjan, R., *Trans. Soc. Biomaterials*, 1986.

(2) Kent, J. N., Quinn, J. H., Zide, M. F., Guerra, L. R., and Boyne, P., J. *Oral and Maxillofacial Surg.*, Vol 41 (10), 1983.

(3) Yukna, R. A., Mayer, E. T., and Brite, D. V., *J. Periodontology*, Vol 55 (11), 1984.

(4) Jarcho, M. P., Kay, J. F., Gumaer, K. I., Doremus, R. H., and Drobeck, H. P., *J. Bioengineering*, Vol 1, 1977.

(5) Drobeck, H. P., Rothstein, S. S., Gumaer, K. I., Sherer, A. D., and Slighter, R. G., *J. Oral and Maxillofacial Surg.*, Vol 42, 1984.

(6) Tracy, B. M. and Doremus, R. H., *J. Biomedical Materials Research*, Vol 18, 1984.

(7) Cook, S. D., Kay, J. F., Thomas, K. A., and Jarcho, M., *Clin. Orthop.*, Vol 230, 1988.

(8) Kay, J. F., Golec, T. S., and Riley, R. L., *J. Prosthet. Dent.*, Vol 58, 1987.

(9) Jarcho, M., *Clin. Orthop.*, Vol 157, 1981.

(10) Sendax, V., *Dent. Clin. N. Am.*, Vol 36, 1992.

(11) Hergenrother, P. J., and Martin, S. F., *Anal. Biochem.*, Vol 251, p. 45, 1997.

Standard Specification for Medical Oxygen Delivery Systems for EMS Ground Vehicles[1]

This standard is issued under the fixed designation F 1949; the number immediately following the designation indicates the year of original adoption or, in the case of revision, the year of last revision. A number in parentheses indicates the year of last reapproval. A superscript epsilon (ε) indicates an editorial change since the last revision or reapproval.

INTRODUCTION

Within the United States, there are several widely recognized national and international standards organizations that have established standards and guidelines for oxygen delivery systems. These standards and guidelines were largely developed for intra-facility use. This standard, developed by ASTM Subcommittee F30.01, addresses the requirements for oxygen systems, both liquid and gaseous, for emergency medical services (EMS) ground vehicles.

1. Scope

1.1 This standard covers minimum requirements for primary medical oxygen delivery systems for EMS ground vehicles used in the following applications:

1.1.1 The transportation of the sick and injured to or from an appropriate medical facility while basic, advanced, or specialized life support services are being provided,

1.1.2 The delivery of interhospital critical transport care,

1.1.3 The delivery of nonemergency, medically required, transport services, and

1.1.4 The transportation and delivery of personnel and supplies essential for proper care of an emergent patient.

1.2 This standard establishes criteria to be considered in the performance, specification, purchase, and acceptance testing of ground vehicles for EMS use.

1.3 This entire standard should be read before ordering an ambulance in order to be knowledgeable of the types of equipment that are available and their performance requirements. Due to the variety of ambulance equipment or features, some options may be incompatible with all chassis manufacturers' models. Detailed technical information is available from the chassis manufacturers.

1.4 The sections in this standard appear in the following sequence:

2. Referenced Documents

2.1 The following documents, of the issue currently in effect, form a part of this standard to the extent specified herein.

2.2 *ASTM Standards:*

F 1177 Terminology Relating to Emergency Medical Services[2]

2.3 *Military Standards:*[3]

MIL-STD-461 Requirements for the Control of Electromagnetic Interference Emissions and Susceptibility

MS 33584 Standard Dimensions for Flared Tubing End

MS 33611 End Bend Radii

2.4 *Federal Specifications:*[3]

RR-C-901 Cylinders, Compressed Gas: High Pressure, Steel DOT3AA, and Aluminum Applications, General Specification for

2.5 *ASME Standard:*[4]

B31.3 Chemical Plant and Petroleum Refinery Piping

2.6 *CGA Standards:*[5]

E-7 Standard for Medical Gas Regulators and Flowmeters

V-1 Compressed Gas Cylinder Valve Outlet and Inlet Connections

S-1.1 Pressure Relief Device Standards Part 1 - Cylinders for Compressed Gases

[1] This specification is under the jurisdiction of ASTM Committee F30 on Emergency Medical Services and is the direct responsibility of Subcommittee F30.01 on EMS Equipment.

Current edition approved January 10, 1999. Published March 1999.

[2] *Annual Book of ASTM Standards*, Vol 13.01.

[3] Available from Standardization Document Order Desk, 700 Robbins Ave., Building #4, Section D, Philadelphia, PA 19111-5094.

[4] Available from the American Society of Mechanical Engineers, United Engineering Center, 345 East 47th St., New York, NY 10017.

[5] Available from the Compressed Gas Association, Inc., 1725 Jefferson Davis Highway, Suite 1004, Arlington, VA 22202-4102.

3. Terminology

3.1 *Definitions*—Specific terms used throughout this specification are defined in 3.2. Other applicable terms are contained in Terminology F 1177.

3.2 *Definitions of Terms Specific to This Standard:*

3.2.1 *design operating pressure, n*—the nominal pressure at which the oxygen equipment or container is designed to operate during normal use.

3.2.2 *LOX container, n*—a vessel used to store or transport liquid oxygen.

3.2.3 *maximum allowable working pressure, n*—the maximum gage pressure to which the equipment or container can be subjected without exceeding the allowable design stress.

3.2.4 *maximum filling volume, n*—the maximum filling volume of liquid at its maximum permissible level.

3.2.5 *pressure relief device, n*—a device designed to open in order to prevent a rise of internal fluid pressure in excess of a specified value.

3.3 *Symbol*:

g = the normal or standard constant of gravity at sea level; approximately 32.2 ft/s/s (9.81 m/s/s)

3.4 *Acronyms:*

3.4.1 *GOX, n*—gaseous oxygen.

3.4.2 *LOX, n*—liquid oxygen.

4. Significance and Use

4.1 The intent of this standard is to establish minimum requirements, test parameters, and other criteria essential for oxygen system design, performance, and appearance, and to provide for a practical degree of standardization. The object is to provide oxygen systems that are properly constructed, and which, when properly serviced and maintained, will reliably function on an EMS ground vehicle.

5. Design Requirements

5.1 The medical oxygen delivery system may be either a gaseous oxygen (GOX) system, or a liquid oxygen (LOX) system.

5.2 The oxygen delivery system shall be a piped oxygen system designed and installed as follows:

5.2.1 *Capacity*—The oxygen system shall be capable of storing and supplying a minimum of 3000 L of gaseous medical oxygen.

5.2.2 *Components*—All oxygen delivery system components shall be approved by the manufacturer of the component for the intended service. The system shall include the following:

5.2.2.1 *Oxygen Piping System*, designed and sized to deliver the required flow rates at the utilization pressures. Piping and tubing shall be of non-ferrous or corrosion-resistant steel material and shall comply with the design requirements of ASME B31.3. Hose shall be electrically conductive and approved by the manufacturer for oxygen service at the pressure and temperatures the hose will be subjected to in service. Fittings shall be of non-ferrous or corrosion-resistant steel material and shall comply with the design requirements of ASME B31.3. Cast fittings shall not be used.

5.2.2.2 *Flow Control Device*, of a pressure-compensated type that includes a means to display and monitor delivered flow rate. It shall be continuously adjustable over a minimum range of 0 to 15 L/min, with a calibrated display resolution of at least 0.5 L/min. The flow control device shall be calibrated for 50 psig inlet pressure and be able to withstand a minimum inlet pressure of 200 psig without damage or failure. It shall incorporate an inlet filter and be electrically conductive from inlet to outlet. Flow control device accuracy shall be within ±10 % of the indicated flow, or 0.25 L, whichever is greater.

5.2.2.3 *Oxygen Outlet*, piped to a self-sealing duplex oxygen outlet station. One of the outlets shall be for a flow control device or humidifier and the second oxygen outlet shall be for gas-specific, noninterchangeable, quick disconnect plug-in devices not requiring humidification. Outlets shall be marked and identified in accordance with CGA E-7.

5.2.2.4 *Shutoff Valve*, when specified, furnished in the 50-psig line and controlled and identified from the EMT panel. If a solenoid valve is utilized, a readily accessible, emergency bypass valve shall be furnished and identified.

5.2.2.5 *Secondary Oxygen Outlet*, when specified, of the self sealing, duplex wall outlet type. Additional outlets may also be specified. The outlets shall be marked and identified in accordance with CGA E-7 (see 6.1).

5.2.3 *Oxygen Compartment*—The oxygen compartment shall be provided with at least a 9-in.[2] cover device which will dissipate or vent leaking oxygen to the outside of the vehicle. The oxygen compartment shall not be utilized for the storage of any other equipment. No wiring or components shall terminate in the oxygen compartment except for the oxygen control solenoid, compartment light, switch plunger or trigger device, or other equipment that is integral to the oxygen system. Wiring passing through the oxygen compartment shall be routed in a metallic conduit.

6. Performance Requirements

6.1 *Delivery Flowrate*—The oxygen system shall be capable of delivering a minimum continuous gas flow of 100 L/min of gaseous oxygen, per patient, simultaneously, down to the 10 percent tank content level.

6.2 *Delivery Pressure*—The oxygen system shall provide a delivery pressure of 50 ± 5 psig, at the specified flowrate at each medical oxygen gas outlet.

6.3 *Delivery Temperature*—The temperature of the gaseous oxygen supplied from each medical oxygen gas outlet shall be within +10 or –20°F (+6 or –11°C) of ambient temperature when the oxygen delivery system is subjected to the continuous flow described in 7.1.

6.4 *Temperature Conditions*

6.4.1 *Storage Temperatures*—The oxygen system, when serviced and maintained in accordance with the manufacturer's recommendations, shall be capable of being stored without damage or deterioration in ambient temperatures of –30°F (–34°C) to 125°F (52°C).

6.4.2 *Cold Soak*—The oxygen system shall operate at a temperature of 0°F (–18°C) after being cold soaked for 6 h at –30°F (–34°C) followed by a 1 h cold soak at 0°F (–18°C).

6.4.3 *Heat Soak*—The oxygen system shall operate at a temperature of 110°F (43°C) after being heat soaked for 6 h at 125°F (52°C) followed by a 1 h heat soak at 100°F (43°C).

6.5 *Electromagnetic Interference*—Electrical or electronic

componentry, or both, of the oxygen system shall meet the electromagnetic interference emissions and susceptibility requirements of MIL-STD-461 for ground vehicles.

6.6 *Structural Integrity*—Each oxygen system component, when mounted by its normal means of attachment and fitted with the equipment item(s) that are normally attached to it, shall have the structural integrity to withstand the vibration, acceleration, and shock environments described in 6.6.1-6.6.3.2. Pneumatic components may be non-operating but shall be pressurized to their maximum allowable working pressure when subjected to these environments. Electrical components may be non-operating but shall be "powered-up" when subjected to these environments. The vibration, acceleration, and shock environments shall produce no out-of-specification performance degradation or malfunctions except that allowed in 6.6.3.2.

6.6.1 *Vibration*—The component shall withstand sinusoidal vibration applied along each of three mutually perpendicular axes with the frequency range varying from 5 to 200 Hz with an amplitude of 1.0 in. from 5 to 5.5 Hz and an applied acceleration of 1.5 *g* from 5.5 to 200 Hz. The duration of applied vibration shall be 5.5 h per axis (a total time of 16.5 h). The frequency of applied vibration shall be swept over the specified range logarithmically with a sweep time of 12 min. The sweep time is that of an ascending plus a descending sweep.

6.6.2 *Acceleration*—The component shall withstand steady state acceleration loads applied along three mutually perpendicular axes in two opposite directions along each axis. The duration of applied acceleration in each direction shall be at least 1 min. The applied acceleration levels shall be 4 *g* laterally in all four directions, 9 *g* vertically downward, and 3 *g* vertically upward.

6.6.3 *Shock*—The component shall withstand the basic design and crash worthiness shock loads defined in 6.6.3.1 and 6.6.3.2 The applied shock pulse shall be of the amplitude specified, a half sine wave configuration, and 11 ms duration.

6.6.3.1 *Basic Design Shock Load*—The component shall withstand three shocks in each direction along three mutually perpendicular axes of the container (a total of 18 shocks). The peak value of the shock loads shall be 20 *g*.

6.6.3.2 *Crash Worthiness Shock Load*—The component shall withstand two shocks in each direction along three mutually perpendicular axes (a total of 12 shocks). The peak value of the shock loads shall be 60 *g*. The crash worthiness shock loads shall produce no failure of the mounting attachments. The component shall not break free from its mounting provisions or otherwise create a hazard. Permanent bending and distortion shall be permitted. The component need not be functional following application of the crash worthiness shock loads.

7. Installation Requirements

7.1 The installation of the oxygen system shall be in accordance with the following requirements:

7.1.1 *Oxygen Piping*—Oxygen piping shall be concealed and not exposed to the elements. The piping shall be accessible for inspection and replacement.

7.1.1.1 *Piping Routing and Mounting*—In routing the piping, the general policy shall be to keep total length to a minimum. Allowances shall be made for expansion, contraction, vibration, and component replacement. All piping shall be mounted to prevent vibration and chafing. This shall be accomplished by the proper use of rubberized or cushion clips installed at no greater than 20-in. intervals as close to the bends as possible. The piping, where passing through or supported by the vehicle structure, shall have adequate protection against chafing by the use of flexible grommets. The piping shall not strike against the vehicle during vibration and shock encountered during normal use of the vehicle.

7.1.1.2 *Flaring and Bending*—Tubing shall be single flared to conform with MS 33584. As an alternative, tubing may be welded, brazed or swaged using methods and quality controls that produce leakproof joints, provided there is no undue degradation of tubing strength, corrosion resistance, or fatigue life. Tubing systems having these permanent type of joints shall be designed for ease of fabrication, inspection, and installation in the vehicle. The system layout shall provide for rapid in-service repair and component replacement. Tubing bends shall be uniform, without kinks, and fit the span between fittings without tension. The minimum bend radius to tube center lines shall be in accordance with MS 33611.

7.1.2 *Flow Control Device*—Flow control devices shall be installed so that they are readable from the EMT seat and squad bench. Flowmeters shall be installed vertically.

7.1.3 *Oxygen Outlet Stations*—Oxygen outlet stations shall be provided with sufficient vertical space to permit connection of a humidifier or nebulizer, or both, directly to the oxygen flow control device.

7.1.3.1 *Primary Patient Oxygen Outlet*—The primary patient oxygen outlet shall be located within 35 in. from the center of the patient's head when in the normal supine position.

7.1.3.2 *Optional Oxygen Outlets*—When optional oxygen outlets are provided they shall be located at the patient's head area. (See 6.1).

8. GOX System Design Requirements

8.1 In addition to the design requirements and components listed in Section 5 of this specification, GOX systems shall also meet the following design requirements and include the following components:

8.1.1 *Cylinders*, conforming to Federal Specification RR-C-901.

8.1.2 *Cylinder Changing Wrenches*, made of a non-sparking material.

8.1.3 *Cylinder Outlet Valve*, conforming to CGA V-1.

8.1.4 *Cylinder Pressure Gage*, having a range of 0 to 2500 psi with the gage scale graduated in no more than 100-psi increments.

8.1.5 *Pressure Regulator*, conforming to CGA E-7. The pressure regulator shall be preset to provide a line pressure of 50 ± 5 psig. The regulator shall supply a minimum flowrate of 100 L/min from the oxygen station outlet with a pressure of 150 psig applied to its inlet. The pressure regulator shall limit the line pressure to a maximum of 62 psig at lock-up with a pressure of 2000 psig applied to the regulator inlet. The pressure regulator shall be easy to connect and shall incorporate an inlet filter and a line relief valve set at 200 psig maximum. The pressure regulator shall be electrically conductive from inlet to outlet.

8.1.6 *Alternative or Optional Components*—When required or when specified, the GOX system shall also include the following components:

8.1.6.1 *Remote Cylinder Pressure Indicator*, such as a multi-light indicator showing "Full","¾" , "½", "¼", and "Empty" or a digital or analog indicator, displaying cylinder contents in increments of at least 25 %. Pressure-driven remote pressure indicators shall not exceed 200 psig.

8.1.6.2 *Low Level Alarm*, actuating when the content of the oxygen system is down to between 10 and 25 %.

9. GOX System Installation Requirements

9.1 In addition to the requirements of Section 7, GOX systems shall comply with the following installation requirements:

9.1.1 *Cylinder*—Cylinders shall be installed such that the cylinder controls are accessible from both the inside and outside of the vehicle. The cylinder shall be accessible for changing from the exterior of the body and, on Type II vehicles, through a sealed door. Access to the cylinder, when located under the squad bench, shall be through the rear half of a two section squad bench cover. The oxygen cylinder shall be located in an area that provides for proper balance and weight distribution of the vehicle.

9.1.2 *Cylinder Retention Systems*—The cylinder retention system shall be mounted to the vehicle as required to comply with the requirements of 6.6.

9.1.3 *Cylinder Changing Wrench*—The cylinder changing wrench shall be chained and clipped within the oxygen cylinder compartment.

9.1.4 *Cylinder Outlet Valve*—The cylinder outlet valve shall be installed directly into the cylinder outlet port.

9.1.5 *Cylinder Pressure Gage*—The cylinder pressure gage shall be visible from the EMT's seat or the squad bench, or both.

9.1.6 *Pressure Regulator*—The pressure regulator shall be mounted directly to the main oxygen cylinder at the outlet of the cylinder outlet valve and shall be accessible from both the inside and the outside of the vehicle.

9.1.7 *Remote Cylinder Pressure Indicator*—The remote cylinder pressure indicator shall be mounted to the EMT panel.

10. GOX System Test Requirements

10.1 *Pressure Test*—The installed oxygen piping and outlet system shall be leak tested at 200-psig pressure for 4 h. The system shall be tested with dry air or nitrogen gas, or equal, and kept decontaminated. After the successful completion of the test, the system shall be capped then tagged with the date and signature of the person and the firm performing the test.

11. LOX System Design Requirements

11.1 In addition to the design requirements and components listed in Section 5, LOX systems shall also meet the following design requirements and include the following components:

11.1.1 *LOX Container*:

11.1.1.1 *Design*—Containers shall be designed, fabricated, tested, and marked (or stamped) in accordance with the Regulations of the U.S. Department of Transportation (DOT) Specification 4L[6] or the ASME rules for the construction of unfired pressure vessels applicable on the date of manufacture.[7]

11.1.1.2 *Reuse*—Containers complying with 11.1.1.1 shall be permitted to be reused, reinstalled, or continued in use. The user of the container shall be responsible for its suitability for continued service.

11.1.1.3 *Repair*—Repair or alteration of containers shall be in accordance with the code under which the container was fabricated.

11.1.1.4 *Maximum Filling Volume*—Containers shall be equipped to provide a signal to prevent them from becoming liquid full and to prevent liquid from covering the inlet of the relief devices when the pressure in the container reaches the set pressure of the pressure relief device.

11.1.1.5 *Pressure Control Valves and Pressure Relief Devices*—Containers shall be equipped with pressure control valves and pressure relief devices sized and selected as to type, location, and quantity and tested in accordance with CGA S-1.1. The pressure relief devices and pressure control valves shall communicate directly with the vapor space of the container. Pressure relief devices and pressure control valves shall be designed to minimize the possibility of tampering.

11.1.1.6 *Container Shutoff Valves*—A shutoff valve shall be installed directly on the tank at the vapor outlet nozzle with no intervening fittings, other than pressure relief devices, and shall be marked with the words "VAPOR SHUTOFF VALVE". Another shutoff valve shall be installed directly on the tank at the liquid outlet nozzle and shall be marked with the words "LIQUID SHUTOFF VALVE". (Decals or stencils are acceptable.) Normally closed automatic shutoff valves that are held open by electric current, pneumatic or hydraulic pressure, or a combination thereof, or manually operated shutoff valves shall be permitted to be used to meet this requirement.

11.1.2 *Quantity Gaging System*—The quantity gaging system shall provide an indication of the amount of oxygen remaining in the liquid oxygen container within an accuracy of ±10 % of the capacity of the container. The gaging system shall display container contents in at least 25 % increments such as by a multi-light display showing "Full," "¾,""½," "¼" and "Empty" or a digital or analog display.

11.1.3 *Pressure Gage*—The system shall include a pressure gage designed for the pressure and temperature conditions to which it will be subjected with a minimum burst pressure safety factor of 4. The dial shall be graduated to indicate at least 1.2 times the marked set pressure of the container pressure relief device. The opening at the inlet connection shall not exceed 0.055 in.

11.1.4 *Fill Valve*—The fill valve shall be a quick disconnect device which shall open automatically when fully engaged with its mating filling connector and shall automatically and instantaneously close upon disengagement from its mating connector. The connection shall be leak-tight and shall not

[6] Available from Government Institutes, Inc., 4 Research Place, Suite 200, Rockville, MD 20850.

[7] "Rules for the Construction of Unfired Pressure Vessels," ASME Boiler and Pressure Vessel Code, available from ASME.[4]

become disconnected by shocks or jars.

11.1.5 *Supply Heat Exchanger*—The supply heat exchanger shall have the capacity to completely vaporize the liquid oxygen supply and warm the vapor to the temperature required to comply with 6.3.

12. LOX System Installation Requirements

12.1 In addition to the requirements of Section 7, LOX systems shall also comply to the following installation requirements:

12.1.1 *LOX Container*—The LOX container shall be mounted to the vehicle as required to comply with the structural integrity requirements of 6.6 when filled to its maximum filling volume with LOX.

12.1.2 *LOX Contents Indicator*—The LOX contents indicator shall be mounted on the EMT Panel.

13. LOX System Test Requirements

13.1 *Pressure Tests*—The installed LOX system shall be leak tested at a pressure equivalent to the maximum allowable working pressure of the system for 4 h. The system shall be tested with dry air or nitrogen gas, or equal, and kept decontaminated. After the successful completion of the test, the system shall be tagged with the date and signature of the person and the firm performing the test.

14. Keywords

14.1 ambulance liquid oxygen delivery system; ambulance oxygen delivery system; medical gaseous oxygen delivery system; medical liquid oxygen delivery system; medical oxygen delivery system

Designation: F 1956 – 99

Standard Specification for Rescue Carabiners[1]

This standard is issued under the fixed designation F 1956; the number immediately following the designation indicates the year of original adoption or, in the case of revision, the year of last revision. A number in parentheses indicates the year of last reapproval. A superscript epsilon (ε) indicates an editorial change since the last revision or reapproval.

1. Scope

1.1 This specification covers six mechanical tests, one corrosion resistance test, and the minimum performance requirements for these tests. This specification applies to carabiners designed specifically for use by rescue personnel during both training exercises and actual rescue operations. This specification does not apply to recreational use carabiners.

1.2 Two different types of carabiners are defined in this specification, a heavy-duty rescue carabiner and a light-duty rescue carabiner.

1.3 The values stated in SI units are to be regarded as the standard.

1.4 Tests contained herein are destructive in nature. Carabiners subjected to any of these tests shall not be used in any way after testing except in evaluation the results of such testing.

1.5 This specification does not imply approval of any method of use of rescue carabiners. In addition, the tests described are laboratory tests and do not duplicate field conditions. Furthermore, the test load values contained herein are not to be interpreted as the forces which a rescue carabiner may be subjected to, or may be expected to sustain, in actual field use.

1.6 This standard may involve hazardous materials, operations, and equipment. *This standard does not purport to address all of the safety concerns, if any, associated with its use. It is the responsibility of the user of this standard to establish appropriate safety and health practices and determine the applicability of regulatory limitations prior to use.*

2. Referenced Documents

2.1 *ASTM Standards:*

B 117 Practice for Operating Salt Spray (Fog) Apparatus[2]

E 4 Practices for Force Verification of Testing Machines[3]

3. Terminology

3.1 *Definitions:*

3.1.1 *carabiner*—a load-bearing, connective device with a self-closing gate.

3.1.2 *heavy-duty rescue carabiner*—a carabiner that meets the specifications for a heavy-duty rescue carabiner as defined in Section 8.

3.1.3 *light-duty rescue carabiner*—a carabiner that meets the specifications for a light-duty rescue carabiner as defined in Section 8.

3.1.4 *locking carabiner*—a carabiner with a locking mechanism which reduces the possibility of a gate being opened inadvertently. A locking mechanism requires at least two different consecutive manual actions to open the gate (see appendix).

3.1.5 *non-locking carabiner*—any carabiner that does not have a locking mechanism that reduces the possibility of a gate being opened inadvertently.

3.1.6 *rescue carabiner*—a carabiner intended for life support in rescue systems. It may be classified as heavy-type or light duty.

3.1.7 *ultimate strength*—the maximum force sustained by a carabiner during an ultimate force test, prior to failure.

3.1.7.1 *failure*—the point at which some part of the carabiner physically breaks or distorts to an extent that the test members are released.

4. Significance and Use

4.1 *Gate Function Load Test*—This test verifies that the gate can be opened (with the gate locking mechanism in the unlocked position) and that the gate can not be opened (with the gate locking mechanism in the locked position) while loaded with Function Test Force #1 along the major axis.

4.2 *Gate Locking Mechanism Function Load Test*—This test verifies that the gate locking mechanism can be unlocked, after Function Test Force #2 has been applied along the major axis and released.

4.3 *Major Axis Gate Closed Function Load Test*—This test verifies that the gate functions as originally intended, after Function Test Force #3 has been applied and released.

4.4 *Major Axis Gate Closed Ultimate Strength Test*—This test is intended to show the ultimate strength of the carabiner in the major axis with the gate closed.

4.5 *Major Axis Gate Open Ultimate Strength Test*—This test is intended to show the ultimate strength of the carabiner in the major axis with the gate open.

4.6 *Minor Axis Gate Closed Ultimate Strength Test*—This test is intended to show the ultimate strength of the carabiner in the minor axis with the gate closed.

---

[1] This specification is under the jurisdiction of ASTM Committee F–32 on Search and Rescue, and is the direct responsibility of Subcommittee F32.01 on Equipment, Testing, and Maintenance.

Current edition approved March 10, 1999. Published June 10, 1999.

[2] *Annual Book of ASTM Standards,* Vol. 03.02.

[3] *Annual Book of ASTM Standards,* Vol 03.01.

4.7 *Corrosion Test*—This test is intended to verify that the carabiner is produced from a corrosion-resistant material, or adequately covered with a protective coating.

5. Apparatus and Conditions

5.1 *Tensile Test Machine*—The tension testing machine shall be maintained in good operation condition, used only in the proper loading range, and calibrated periodically in accordance with the latest revision of Practices E 4.

5.2 *Test Fixtures and Supplies*:

5.2.1 There are four test pins required, two test pins with 6 ± 0.05-mm radii and two test pins with 5 ± 0.05-mm radii. Test pins must be AISI SAE Type 01 Tool Steel (commonly purchased as 01 Drill Rod) heat treated to a minimum Rockwell hardness, C scale 60. The mean surface roughness, *Ra* must not exceed 0.8 μm and the peak to valley height. *R*max, must not exceed 6.3 μm. The fixture must be designed to prevent the test pins from rotating and so that the carabiner is free to locate itself on the test pins when force is applied. See Figs. 1 and 2.

NOTE 1—Test pin cross section is not required to be round. Any cross section necessary to prevent test pin failure or any design to prevent test pin rotation is acceptable, as long as the contact point (between test pin and carabiner) of the test pin has the specified radius, material type, hardness, and surface roughness.

5.2.2 *Molybdenum-Based Grease*.

5.3 *Test Conditions*:

5.3.1 The ambient temperature, test samples, test fixture, and supplies shall be between 15 and 23°C (59 and 73°F).

5.3.2 All six mechanical tests must be conducted with the force applied parallel to the gravitational pull of the earth.

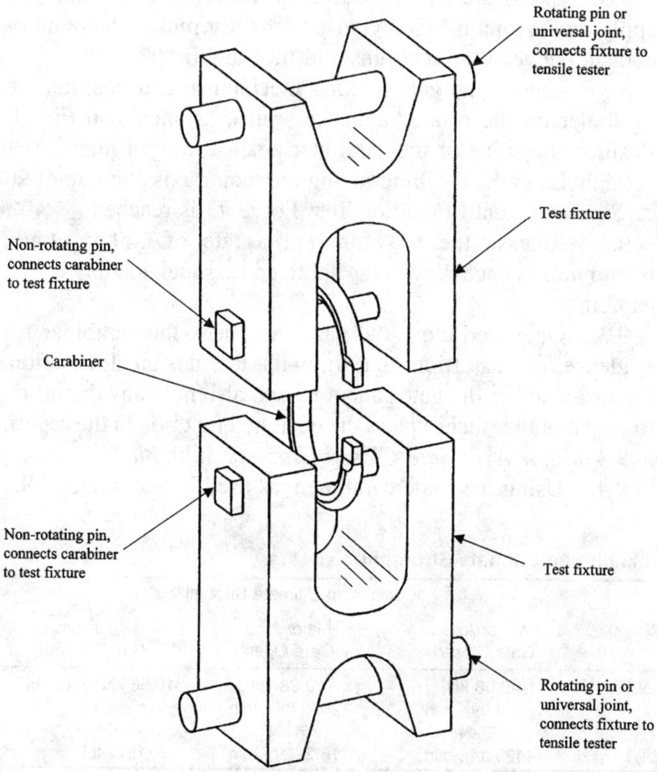

FIG. 1 Major Axis Test Setup

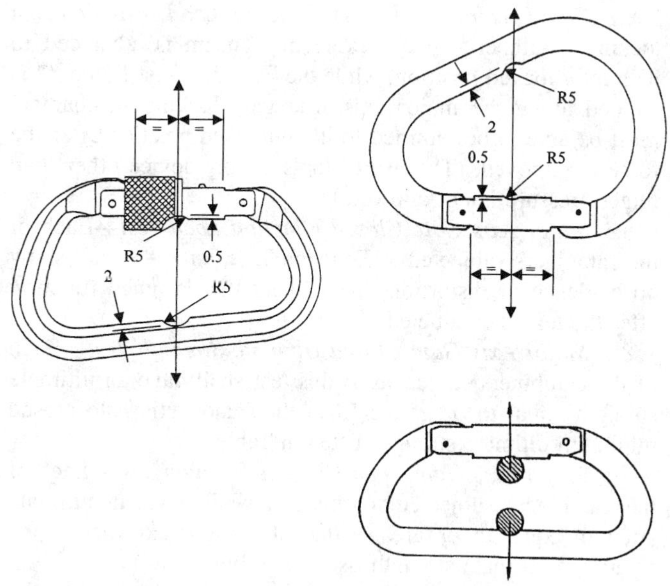

FIG. 2 Test Fixture

6. Hazards

Carabiners may disengage or eject parts from the test fixture. Use a safety screen and wear safety glasses while testing. Do not perform these tests alone.

7. Sampling

7.1 *Sample Selection*—Randomly select the carabiners in accordance with 7.2.2. Each user of this test method may specify the lot size from which the carabiners are to be selected.

7.2 *Number of Samples*:

7.2.1 The same number of carabiners must be used for each of the tests in this specification.

7.2.2 A minimum of five carabiners will be used, in sequence, for the Gate Function Load Test, Gate Locking Mechanism Function Load Test, Major Axis Gate Closed Function Load Test, and Major Axis Gate Closed Ultimate Strength Test. A minimum of five carabiners will be used for the Major Axis Gate Open Ultimate Strength Test. A minimum of five carabiners will be used for the Minor Axis Gate Closed Ultimate Strength Test. A minimum of five carabiners will be used for the Corrosion Test.

7.2.3 Label the randomly selected carabiners 1 through X (X being the total number of carabiners selected).

8. Performance Specifications

8.1 *Gate Function Load Test*:

8.1.1 With the gate locking mechanism in the unlocked position and Function Test Force #1 applied along the major axis, each carabiner gate shall open and close as designed and with the same quality and performance as before the test. The use of tools or any device other than finger pressure is not allowed.

8.1.2 With the gate locking mechanism in the locked position and Function Test Force #1 applied along the major axis, the gate must not open. (The use of tools or any device other than finger pressure is not allowed.)

8.2 *Gate Locking Mechanism Function Load Test*—When a locking carabiner's gate locking mechanism is advanced to its's fully locked position, while the Function Test Force #2 is applied along the major axis. The gate locking mechanism must be able to be returned to it's unlocked position after the force is removed. (The use of tools or any device other than finger pressure is not allowed.)

8.3 *Major Axis Gate Closed Function Load Test*—Each of the carabiners subjected to Function Test Force #3 shall show no evidence of distortion that impairs the designed function after the test is conducted.

8.4 *Major Axis Gate Closed Ultimate Strength Test*—Each of the carabiners subjected to this test shall have an ultimate strength equal to or greater than the major axis gate closed minimum ultimate strength listed in Table 1.

8.5 *Major Axis Gate Open Ultimate Strength Test*—Each of the carabiners subjected to this test shall have an ultimate strength equal to or greater than the major axis gate open minimum ultimate strength listed in Table 1.

8.6 *Minor Axis Gate Closed Ultimate Strength*—Each of the carabiners subjected to this test shall have an ultimate strength equal to or greater than the minor axis gate closed minimum ultimate strength listed in Table 1

8.7 *Corrosion Test*—Each of the carabiners subjected to the corrosion test shall not have more than light-surface corrosion following the test. In addition, each carabiner gate shall open and close with the same quality and performance as before the test. (The use of tools or any device other than finger pressure is not allowed.) Furthermore, each gate locking mechanism must be able to move through its full range of travel with the same quality and performance as before the test. (The use of tools or any device other than finger pressure is not allowed.)

9. Procedure

9.1 *Gate Function Load Test*:

9.1.1 Open and close the gate and gate locking mechanism to feel the action of each carabiner prior to conducting this test. Record any interferences in the report.

9.1.2 Apply molybdenum-based grease to the test pins at the point of contact between the test pins and the carabiner.

9.1.3 Unlock the gate locking mechanism and position the carabiner on the 6-mm radius test pins, as shown in Fig. 1. Position the spine of the carabiner against the test pins.

9.1.4 Load the carabiner along the major axis at a rate of 5 ± 1 mm/min until Function Test Force #1 is reached.

9.1.5 While maintaining the force, open and close the gate and check that the gate functions as it did prior to the application of Test Force #1 (The use of tools or any device other than finger pressure is not allowed). Record whether the gate opens or close, or both, and the actual test force applied to the carabiner in the report.

9.1.6 While maintaining the force, lock the gate locking mechanism. (The use of tools or any device other than finger pressure is not allowed.) Verify that with the gate locking mechanism in the locked position, the gate does not open. (The use of tools or any device other than finger pressure is not allowed.) Record whether the gate opens in the report.

9.1.7 Release the test force at a rate of 120 mm/min maximum, as necessary, so as not to cause shock loading on the carabiner.

9.2 *Gate Locking Mechanism Function Load Test*:

9.2.1 Using the same carabiners as used in 9.1. Apply molybdenum-based grease to the test pins at the point of contact between the test pins and the carabiner.

9.2.2 Unlock the gate locking mechanism and position the carabiner on the 6-mm radius test pins, as shown in Fig. 1. Position the spine of the carabiner against the test pins.

9.2.3 Load the carabiner along the major axis at a rate of 10 ± 5 mm/min until Function Test Force #2 is reached.

9.2.4 While maintaining the force, lock the gate mechanism. (The use of tools or any device other than finger pressure is not allowed.) Record the actual test force applied to the carabiner in the report.

9.2.5 Release the test force at a rate of 120 mm/min, maximum, as necessary, so as not to cause shock loading on the carabiner.

9.2.6 Unlock the gate locking mechanism. (The use of tools of any device other than finger pressure is not allowed.) Record whether the gate locking mechanism can be returned to it's unlocked position in the report.

9.3 *Major Axis Gate Closed Function Load Test*:

9.3.1 Using the same carabiners as used in 9.1 and 9.2, apply molybdenum-based grease to the test pins at the point of contact between the test pins and the carabiner.

9.3.2 Unlock the gate locking mechanism and position the carabiner on the 6-mm radius test pins, as shown in Fig. 1. Position the spine of the carabiner against the test pins.

9.3.3 Load the carabiner along the major axis at a rate of 20 ± 5 mm/min until Function Test Force #3 is reached.

9.3.4 Release the test force at a rate of 120 mm/min, maximum, as necessary, so as not to cause shock loading on the carabiner.

9.3.5 Open and close the gate and check the carabiner for evidence of distortion that impairs the designed function. Record whether the gate functions and also note any distortion to the carabiner that impairs the designed function in the report.

9.4 *Major Axis Gate Closed Ultimate Strength Test*:

9.4.1 Using the same carabiners as used in 9.1, 9.2, and 9.3

TABLE 1 Function Test Forces and Minimum Ultimate Strengths

Carabiner Type	Function Test Forces[A]			Minimum Ultimate Strength		
	#1	#2	#3	Major Axis Gate Closed	Major Axis Gate Open	Minor Axis Gate Closed
Heavy-Duty Rescue carabiner	1.33 kN (300 lbf)	10.68 kN (2400 lbf)	26.69 kN (6000 lbf)	40.03 kN (9000 lbf), min	10.68 kN (2400 lbf), min	10.68 kN (2400 lbf), min
Light-Duty rescue carabiner	0.8 kN (180 lbf)	7 kN (1575 lbf)	14 kN (3145 lbf)	20 kN (4495 lbf), min	7 kN (1575 lbf), min	7 kN (1575 lbf), min

[A] ± 5 %.

apply molybdenum-based grease to the test pins at the point of contact between the test pins and the carabiner.

9.4.2 Lock the gate locking mechanism and position the carabiner on the 6-mm radius test pins, as shown in Fig. 1. Position the spine of the carabiner against the test pins.

9.4.3 Load the carabiner along the major axis at a rate of 30 ± 5 mm/min until failure.

9.4.4 On the test report, record the maximum force sustained.

9.5 *Major Axis Gate Open Ultimate Strength Test*:

9.5.1 Secure the gate in the open position.

9.5.2 Apply molybdenum-based grease to the test pins at the point of contact between the test pins and the carabiner.

9.5.3 Position the carabiner on the 6-mm radius test pins, as shown in Fig. 1. Position the spine of the carabiner against the test pins.

9.5.4 Load the carabiner along the major axis at a rate of 30 ± 5 mm/min until failure.

9.5.5 On the test report, record the maximum force sustained.

9.6 *Minor Axis Gate Closed Ultimate Strength Test*:

9.6.1 Apply molybdenum-based grease to the test pins at the point of contact between the test pins and the carabiner.

9.6.2 Position the carabiner on the 5-mm radius test pins as shown in Fig. 2. Verify that the gate locking mechanism is in the locked position. In order to avoid movement of the carabiner with respect to the test pins, machine notches in the body and the gate as shown in Fig. 2. If the internal clearance between the gate and the spine does not accommodate two 5-mm radius test pins, modify the pins so that they can be positioned as shown in Fig. 2.

9.6.3 Load the carabiner along the minor axis at a rate of 30 ± 5 mm/min until failure.

9.6.4 On the test report, record the maximum force sustained.

9.7 *Corrosion Test*:

9.7.1 Verify that the gate locking mechanism is in the locked position. Conduct a 50-h salt spray test in accordance with Practice B 117.

9.7.2 After the test, visually inspect the carabiner for signs of corrosion. Open and close the gate and check that the gate functions as it did prior to the salt spray test. Move the gate locking mechanism from it's locked position to its fully unlocked position and check that the gate locking mechanism functions as it did prior to the sale spray test.

9.7.3 Record whether there is light surface-type corrosion, whether the gate functions as it did prior to the salt spray test, and whether the gate locking mechanism functions as it did prior to the salt spray test in the report.

10. Certification

10.1 When specified in the purchase order or contract, the purchaser shall be furnished certification that samples representing the purchased lot have met the requirements of this specification. Certifications may be written by the contracted laboratory or the company who manufactured the carabiners. When specified in the purchase order or contract, a report of the test results shall be furnished.

11. Report

11.1 Report the following information:

11.1.1 Name of the laboratory or agency that performed the mechanical test.

11.1.2 Date of testing.

11.1.3 Manufacturer or brand and model of carabiners tested.

11.1.4 Information required by Practices E 4 for test machine.

11.1.5 Name of test administrator

11.1.6 Identification of lot and size of lot tested.

11.2 *Results of Gate Function Load Test*:

11.2.1 Actual function test force applied.

11.2.2 Gate opens / gate does not open.

11.2.3 Gate closes / gate does not close.

11.2.4 With gate locking mechanism locked, gate opens / gate does not open.

11.3 *Results of Gate Locking Mechanism Load Test*:

11.3.1 Actual function test force applied.

11.3.2 Gate locking mechanism can / can not be moved to the unlocked position.

11.4 *Results of Major Axis Gate Closed Function Load Test*:

11.4.1 Actual function test force applied.

11.4.2 Gate opens / gate does not open.

11.4.3 Distortion to carabiner that impairs designed function.

11.5 *Major Axis Gate Closed Ultimate Strength Test*:

11.5.1 Maximum force sustained.

11.6 *Major Axis Gate Open Ultimate Strength Test*:

11.6.1 Maximum force sustained.

11.7 *Minor Axis Gate Closed Ultimate Strength Test*:

11.7.1 Maximum force sustained.

11.8 *Corrosion Test*:

11.8.1 Light surface-type corrosion.

11.8.2 Gate opens/closes.

11.8.3 Gate locking mechanism moves through it's full range of travel.

12. Precision and Bias

12.1 It is not practical to specify the precision of the procedure in this specification for measuring the ultimate strengths of carabiners because insufficient laboratory or interlaboratory test data exists at this time.

APPENDIXES

(Nonmandatory Information)

X1. RESPONSIBILITY FOR QUALITY ASSURANCE

X1.1 Quality assurance is solely the responsibility of the manufacturer and is not addressed by this specification.

X2. GATE LOCKING MECHANISM

X2.1 A locking mechanism requires at least two different consecutive manual actions open the carabiner gate. One manual action to release the gate locking mechanism and one different manual action to open the carabiner gate.

X3. HEAVY-DUTY AND LIGHT-DUTY CARABINERS

X3.1 All mechanical tests, the corrosion test, performance requirements, and procedures contained in this specification apply to heavy-duty and light-duty carabiners. Users of this specification must specify which type of carabiner is being submitted before testing begins.

X4. LOCKING AND NON-LOCKING CARABINERS

X4.1 For simplification this specification has been written in the context for testing of locking carabiners. However, this specification can be used for non-locking carabiners as well. For testing of non-locking carabiners, disregard all test procedures and performance specifications which require a gate locking mechanism.

X5. UNANTICIPATED FAILURE

X5.1 If any of the carabiners used in the sequence testing for 9.1-9.3, or 9.4 fail prior to completion of all four tests. It is up to the discretion of the user of this specification as to whether they want to continue testing.

X6. CORROSION TEST

X6.1 Practice B 117 was chosen as the standard test method for corrosion, because it is an established, widely used, accepted, and repeatable test. It is applicable to the testing of ferrous and nonferrous metals and is also used to test inorganic and organic coatings, especially where the tests are the basis for material or product specifications.

X6.2 The 50-h time duration for Practice B 117 was adopted from NFPA 1983 and has been used for a number of years. Representative hardware samples, which have been tested in accordance with Practice B 117 for 50 h, have proven to be adequately coated for severe field service applications.

X7. PARTS OF A CARABINER

X7.1 See Fig. X7.1.

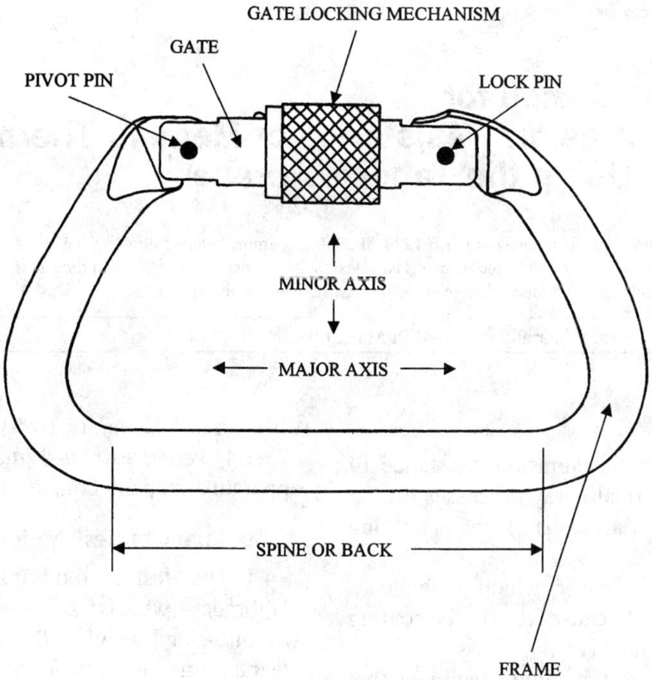

FIG. X7.1 Parts of a Carabiner

The American Society for Testing and Materials takes no position respecting the validity of any patent rights asserted in connection with any item mentioned in this standard. Users of this standard are expressly advised that determination of the validity of any such patent rights, and the risk of infringement of such rights, are entirely their own responsibility.

This standard is subject to revision at any time by the responsible technical committee and must be reviewed every five years and if not revised, either reapproved or withdrawn. Your comments are invited either for revision of this standard or for additional standards and should be addressed to ASTM Headquarters. Your comments will receive careful consideration at a meeting of the responsible technical committee, which you may attend. If you feel that your comments have not received a fair hearing you should make your views known to the ASTM Committee on Standards, 100 Barr Harbor Drive, West Conshohocken, PA 19428.

Standard Test Method for Measuring Abrasion Resistance of Metallic Thermal Spray Coatings by Using the Taber™ Abraser[1]

This standard is issued under the fixed designation F 1978; the number immediately following the designation indicates the year of original adoption or, in the case of revision, the year of last revision. A number in parentheses indicates the year of last reapproval. A superscript epsilon (ε) indicates an editorial change since the last revision or reapproval.

ε[1] NOTE—Tables 1 and 2 were editorially corrected in May 2001.

1. Scope

1.1 This test method quantifies the abrasion resistance of metallic coatings produced by thermal spray processes on flat metallic surfaces. It is intended as a means of characterizing coatings used on surgical implants.

1.2 This test uses the Taber™[2] abraser, which generates a combination of rolling and rubbing to cause wear to the coating surface. Wear is quantified as cumulative mass loss.

1.3 This test method is limited to flat, rigid specimens that do not react significantly with water and do not undergo a phase transformation or chemical reaction between room temperature and 100°C in air.

1.4 *This standard does not purport to address all of the safety concerns, if any, associated with its use. It is the responsibility of the user of this standard to establish appropriate safety and health practices and determine the applicable regulatory limitations prior to use.*

2. Referenced Documents

2.1 *ASTM Standards:*

E 691 Practice for Conducting an Interlaboratory Study to Determine the Precision of a Test Method[3]

3. Terminology

3.1 *Definitions of Terms Specific to This Standard:*

3.1.1 *abraser, n*—an instrument that is designed to determine the resistance of surfaces to composite rolling and rubbing action.

3.1.2 *particle shedding, n*—the loss of surface particles and fragments from a coating.

3.1.3 *thermal spray coating, n*—coating produced by spraying melted or softened powder or wire by means of combustible gases, plasma, or two-wire arc.

3.1.4 *weight loss, n*—amount of mass removed by the test apparatus over the course of testing.

4. Summary of Test Method

4.1 This test method uses a Taber™ abraser with H-22 Calibrade™ wheels[2] and the 250-g mass of the abrading head without added weights. Specimens are abraded repeatedly and cleaned ultrasonically for a set number of rotational cycles (2 to 100 cycles). The specimens are weighed after each cleaning, and the mass loss is the measure of abrasive wear to the specimen.

5. Significance and Use

5.1 This test method provides a means to evaluate the resistance to particle shedding of a thermal sprayed coating. Such particle shedding might occur during surgical insertion of an implant or as the result of micromotion of the implant after surgical insertion.

5.2 This abrasion test method may be useful for quality control analysis of a coating, and it can be used to evaluate the effects of processing variables, such as substrate preparation before coating, surface texture, coating technique variables, or postcoating treatments, any of which may influence the susceptibility of the coating to particle shedding.

5.3 This abrasion test method is for flat plate-shaped specimens of a size sufficient that the wheels of the abrader do not leave the surface of the specimen. It is not recommended, however, for devices with other shapes or sizes.

6. Apparatus

6.1 *Taber™ Abraser Model 5150*, or equivalent.

6.2 *Two H-22 Taber™ Calibrade™ Wheels*, or equivalent, with abrading head of 250-g mass and no added weights.

6.3 *Taber™ Vacuum Unit*, made by Shop-Vac™,[2] 7.4 amps, or equivalent.

6.4 *Taber™ Wheel Refacer Model 200*[2].

6.5 *Ultrasonic Cleaning Unit*, for cleaning specimens after abrading.

6.6 *Drying Oven*, capable of operation at 100 ± 2°C, for drying specimens.

6.7 *Analytical Balance*, capable of weighing specimens to

[1] This test method is under the jurisdiction of ASTM Committee F04 on Medical and Surgical Materials and Devices and is the direct responsibility of Subcommittee F04.15 on Material Test Methods.

Current edition approved Nov. 10, 2000. Published February 2001. Originally published as F 1978 – 99. Last previous edition F 1978 – 99.

[2] The sole source of supply of the apparatus known to the committee at this time is Taber Industries, North Tonawanda, NY 14120 USA. If you are aware of alternative suppliers, please provide this information to ASTM Headquarters. Your comments will receive careful consideration at a meeting of the responsible technical committee, which you may attend.

[3] *Annual Book of ASTM Standards*, Vol 14.02.

an accuracy of 0.0001 g.

7. Test Specimen

7.1 Abrasion test specimens shall be 10-cm (4-in.) squares or 10-cm diameter circles of at least 0.16-cm (0.0625-in.) thickness with a 0.64-cm (0.25-in.) diameter hole through the center to allow the specimen to fit on the pin of the Taber™ abraser. For substrates other than titanium, consideration shall be given to the weight of the test specimen relative to the capacity of the analytical balance.

7.2 The coating shall be applied in a manner representative of that used on the finished surgical implant.

7.3 A minimum of six samples for each coating shall be tested. At least one set shall contain seven samples.

7.4 One specimen, randomly selected, from each group of six specimens shall be reserved to measure weight loss caused by ultrasonic cleaning. This specimen shall be called the "blank" specimen and shall be weighed, cleaned, and re-weighed for an equal number of times to the cleaning and weighing of the abraded specimen

7.5 Of the seven sample set, one sample shall be selected to determine the time required for ultrasonic cleaning.

8. Procedure

8.1 *General Test Conditions*:

8.1.1 Prepare a fresh cleaning solution for the ultrasonic cleaner by adding 0.1 ± 0.005 g of reagent grade NaCl to each litre of deionized water.

8.1.2 Resurface the abrading wheels using Taber™ Wheel Refacer Model 200 for each new specimen. Check the radius of the wheel, it is essential that the radius of the abrading wheels not fall below the marked minimum level over the course of the test. Should the wheel radius fall below the labeled mark, the test run shall be discarded and a new specimen shall be run in its place.

8.1.3 Mount the wheels by placing the wheel marked "Left Hand This Side" on the left hand abrading head and the wheel marked" Right Hand This Side" on the right hand abrading head.

8.1.4 Before running the battery of tests, the ultrasonic cleaner shall be evaluated. This shall be done by by selecting the coated extra coated sample from Step 7.3, 7.5, and abrading.

8.1.4.1 Using the analytical balance, weigh the sample no fewer than three times and record the average weight of these measurements.

8.1.4.2 Place the sample on the Taber Abraser, as described in 8.2.5

8.1.4.3 Set the Taber abraser for ten cumulative cycles and start the turntable.

8.1.4.4 Clean the sample for ten minutes with a fresh saline solution, using the ultrasonic cleaner to be used for the coating analysis.

8.1.4.5 Place the cleaned sample in a 100°C oven and dry for 10 min.

8.1.4.6 Allow the sample to cool to room temperature before weighing

8.1.4.7 Using the analytical balance, weigh the sample no fewer than three times and record the average weight of these measurements.

8.1.4.8 Repeat Steps 8.1.4.4-8.1.4.7 until the same mass (within balance error) is recorded for two consecutive cleanings.

8.1.4.9 Record the total number of cleanings used in 8.1.4.4-8.1.4.8.

8.1.4.10 Determine the required cleaning time necessary to obtain a stable mass, as $(10*(n-1))$ min, where n is the total number of cleanings determined in 8.1.4.9.

8.1.5 Abrasion shall be done with only the 250-g mass of the abrading head assembly. No extra weights shall be added to the abrading head.

8.1.6 If there is more than one set of specimens to test, the specimens shall be tested in a random sequence.

8.1.7 A single complete specimen run shall consist of a series of partial runs, commencing with an initial two-cycle partial run and continuing until 100 cycles have been completed. Once a specimen run is initiated, no other specimens shall be tested using the same wheel until the specimen run is finished.

8.1.8 At the start of each new complete specimen run, the display indicating the number of cycles run shall be reset. This is done by pressing the "reset cycles completed" button. The Taber™ abraser counts cumulative cycles (cycles completed) and so the number of cycles set for each partial run shall be the cumulative number of cycles (2, 5, 10, or 100) designated as the end of that partial run.

8.1.9 *Reference Standards*—Each group of six specimens shall include one unabraded "blank" specimen, as specified in 7.4. Once in every six tests, an unabraded specimen shall be used as a control to determine the weight loss caused by the ultrasonic cleaning. This specimen shall be weighed, cleaned, and reweighed for as many cycles as would normally be used if abrasion testing were being performed. These values shall be logged as "blank" weight loss values.

8.2 *Operation*:

8.2.1 Clean the specimen for the time determined in 8.1.4.10 using an ultrasonic cleaner with saline solution. This solution shall be changed to a fresh solution before the first cleaning done that day.

8.2.2 Place the cleaned specimen in a 100°C oven for 10 min to dry.

8.2.3 Allow the specimen to cool to room temperature before weighing.

8.2.4 Using the analytical balance, weigh the specimen no fewer than three times, and record the average of these weight measurements on a data sheet.

8.2.5 Place the specimen on the Taber™ abraser, coating side up and the turntable pin through the hole in the center of the specimen. Place the metal flange over the specimen, and secure the specimen and flange to the turntable with the screw fastener. Lower the abrading heads gently so that abrading wheels rest on the surface of the specimen. Lower the vacuum pick up after the abrading heads are resting on the coating surface.

8.2.6 Set the Taber™ abraser to reach the appropriate number of cumulative cycles (2, 5, 10, or 100). With the vacuum set at 100 % power, start the Taber™ abraser in "vacuum only" mode. Let it run for no less than 5 s to allow vacuum to reach full power, then start the turntable rotation. When the turntable rotation for that partial run is completed, turn the vacuum off.

8.2.7 Clean, dry, cool, and weigh the specimen as before (see 8.2.1-8.2.4).

8.2.8 Repeat Steps 8.2.5-8.2.7 for 5, 10, and 100 cumulative cycles.

8.2.9 Repeat the steps specified in 8.2.1-8.2.8 for all specimens not reserved as blanks for the test.

8.2.10 Run each blank through the steps specified in 8.2.1-8.2.8 skipping the steps specified in 8.2.5 and 8.2.6.

9. Calculation

9.1 Calculate the cumulative mass loss for each specimen for the number of revolutions used with the following equation:

$$\Delta w_n = <w_o> - <w_n> \tag{1}$$

where:

n = number of cumulative cycles to which specimen has been exposed (2, 5, 10, 100),
Δw_n = cumulative mass loss for n cycles,
$<w_o>$ = average of three mass measurements at start the start of the test, and
$<w_n>$ = average of three mass measurements after n cumulative cycles.

10. Report

10.1 The report shall include the following information:

10.1.1 Identification of the test coupon materials including traceability information, such as coating process lot and raw material lot numbers.

10.1.2 Dimensional data including coupon dimensions and coating thickness dimensions.

10.1.3 The number of specimens tested.

10.1.4 Nominal laboratory temperature and humidity during the test.

10.1.5 The number of minutes needed for ultrasonic cleaning, as determined in 8.1.4.10.

10.1.6 All cumulative mass losses associated with each specimen or blank following abrasion.

10.1.7 The mean cumulative mass loss and its standard of deviation for 2, 5, 10, and 100 cycles.

10.1.8 Observations made during the course of the study, including but not limited to, observation of wear tracks and when they occur, appearance of discoloration of specimen, removal of large sections of coating, and evidence of corrosion.

11. Precision and Bias

11.1 An interlaboratory study (ILS) was conducted to establish the precision and bias of this test method. The number of laboratories, materials, and determinations in this study meet the minimum requirements for determining precision as prescribed in Practice E 691 (see Table 1). These tests were done for 2, 5, 10, and 100 cycles for a total of 12 material and cycle combinations.

11.2 *Precision*—Precision, characterized by repeatability, S_r, and reproducibility, S_R, have been determined for the materials and cycle combinations provided in Table 2.

12. Keywords

12.1 abrasion; particle shedding; porous coatings; Taber™ abraser; thermal spray coatings; wear

TABLE 1 ILS Study Parameters

	This Study	Practice E 691 min
Laboratories	6	6
Materials	3	3
Determinations	5	2

TABLE 2 Precision and Bias Data for the Full Study

Coating	Cycles	Average Weight Loss (g)	S_r (g)	S_R (g)	r (g)	R (g)
a	2	0.008 52	0.004 09	0.004 37	0.011 45	0.0122
b	2	0.011 66	0.003 92	0.006 24	0.010 97	0.0175
c	2	0.049 55	0.015 16	0.016 86	0.042 45	0.0472
a	5	0.014 83	0.005 44	0.006 08	0.015 23	0.017
b	5	0.020 77	0.006 34	0.007 53	0.017 76	0.0211
c	5	0.097 64	0.025 18	0.034 27	0.0705	0.0959
a	10	0.021 12	0.006 43	0.007 08	0.018	0.0198
b	10	0.030 2	0.007 92	0.000 06	0.022 17	0.0248
c	10	0.136 71	0.034 02	0.045 38	0.095 27	0.1271
a	100	0.054 06	0.012 22	0.017 17	0.034 22	0.0481
b	100	0.077 22	0.020 34	0.025 53	0.056 94	0.0715
c	100	0.274 51	0.063 06	0.066 52	0.176 57	0.1862

APPENDIX

(Nonmandatory Information)

X1. Rationale

X1.1 Abrasion may occur in implantable devices with metallic coatings produced by thermal spray processes. Excessive weight loss, however, is undesirable, as it may lead to third body wear of articulating surfaces.

X1.2 Although the use of sprayed flat specimens and the Taber™ abraser do not mimic the effect of bone and daily usage, this test method has been shown to be a reliable measure of the average wear/abrasion resistance of a thermal spray coating.

X1.3 Measurements are taken at 2, 5, 10, and 100 cycles. A minimum of two cycles was chosen to ensure that the turntable of the Taber™ abraser makes at least one complete rotation before any abrasion weight loss values are determined. After 100 cycles, which is the set maximum number of cycles, the mechanism of wear is no longer related to particle shedding.

X1.4 The ultrasonic cleaning solution used, as of yet, has had no corrosive effect on the coupons tested. Deionized water is used because it is both readily available and has a minimal amount of contaminants. A small amount of sodium chloride is added to the deionized water to neutralize the corrosiveness of the water. The amount of salt is well below the amount used for a physiologic saline solution and does not require that the specimens be rinsed with water after ultrasonic cleaning.

Standard Specification for Suction Catheters for Use in the Respiratory Tract[1]

This standard is issued under the fixed designation F 1981; the number immediately following the designation indicates the year of original adoption or, in the case of revision, the year of last revision. A number in parentheses indicates the year of last reapproval. A superscript epsilon (ϵ) indicates an editorial change since the last revision or reapproval.

INTRODUCTION

This specification provides dimensions and requirements for suction catheters for use in the respiratory tract. The basis of this specification is ISO 8836: 1997. There are major differences in the addition of mandatory suction catheter "eyes," removal of color coding, and inclusion of closed circuit suction catheters.

Size is designated by outside diameter, which is important when selecting catheters, because of its relationship to the ease with which the catheter can be passed through a tracheal or tracheostomy tube (see Specifications F 927, F 1242, F 1627, and F 1666 for details of requirements for tracheal tubes and tracheostomy tubes). Requirements for suction catheters made of rubber have been deleted because they are no longer in general use.

1. Scope

1.1 This specification provides requirements for suction catheters intended for use in suction of the respiratory tract.

1.2 Angled-tip suction catheters, for example, Coudé catheters, and closed circuit suction catheters are not considered to be specialized, and therefore, are included in this specification. Specialized suction devices are excluded from this specification.

1.3 Flammability of suction catheters, for example if flammable anesthetics, electrosurgical units, or lasers are used, is a well-recognized hazard that is addressed by appropriate clinical management and is outside the scope of this specification.

2. Referenced Documents

2.1 *ASTM Standards:*

F 813 Practice for Direct Contact Cell Culture Evaluation of Materials for Medical Devices[2]

F 927 Specification for Pediatric Tracheostomy Tubes[2]

F 1205 Specification for Anesthesia Breathing Tubes[2]

F 1242 Specification for Cuffed and Uncuffed Tracheal Tubes[2]

F 1627 Specification for Tracheostomy Tubes—Pediatric Tracheostomy Tubes[2]

F 1666 Specification for Adult Tracheostomy Tubes[2]

2.2 *ISO Standards:*

ISO 7000 Graphical Symbols for Use on Equipment—Index and Synopsis[3]

ISO 8836–1997 Suction Catheters for Use in the Respiratory Tract[3]

3. Terminology

3.1 *Definitions of Terms Specific to This Standard:*

3.1.1 *adapter, n*—specialized connector to establish functional continuity between otherwise disparate or incompatible components.

3.1.2 *closed circuit suction catheter, n*—a suction catheter that is encased in a flexible, collapsible sleeve attached to a breathing circuit connector and intended to permit airway suctioning while maintaining the integrity of the breathing circuit.

3.1.3 *connector, n*—fitting to join together two or more components.

3.1.4 *eye, n*—lateral aperture near the patient end of the catheter.

3.1.5 *machine end, n*—end of the catheter intended to be connected to a source of vacuum.

3.1.6 *patient end, n*—end of the catheter intended to be inserted into the patient.

3.1.7 *residual vacuum, n*—negative pressure at the patient end of the suction catheter when the vacuum control device is in the relief position.

3.1.8 *shaft, n*—main part of the catheter, which is of uniform outside diameter.

3.1.9 *suction catheter, n*—flexible tube designed for introduction into a patient airway to remove material by suction.

3.1.10 *terminal orifice, n*—central opening at the patient end of the suction catheter.

---

[1] This specification is under the jurisdiction of ASTM Committee F-29 on Anesthetic and Respiratory Equipment and is the direct responsibility of Subcommittee F29.12 on Airways.

Current edition approved May 10, 1999. Published September 1999.

[2] *Annual Book of ASTM Standards*, Vol 13.01.

[3] Available from American National Standards Institute, 11 W. 42nd St., New York, NY 10036.

3.1.11 *tip, n*—the patient end of a suction catheter.

3.1.12 *vacuum control device, n*—means provided at or near the machine end of a suction catheter to control the flow of gases and entrained material.

4. Material

4.1 Suction catheters for use in the respiratory tract, in their ready-to-use state after any preparation for use recommended by the manufacturer, shall satisfy appropriate biological safety testing, as indicated in Specification F 813.

NOTE 1—It is recommended that the shaft be colorless and either transparent or translucent.

NOTE 2—The outside surface of the suction catheter should have characteristics, which would facilitate insertion through all types of plastic, rubber, and metal oro- and naso-tracheal tubes, tracheostomy tubes, and appropriate connectors.

NOTE 3—Suction catheters, under normal conditions of use, should be reasonably resistant to deterioration by anesthetic vapors and gases in clinical concentrations.

5. Size Designation and Dimensions

5.1 *Size Designation*—The size of suction catheters shall be designated by the following:

5.1.1 The nominal outside diameter of the shaft, expressed in mm. Additionally, it may be expressed in French (Charrière)-gage size;

NOTE 4—For the purposes of this specification, the French (Charrière)-gage system of size (F) is based on the outside diameter of the shaft gaged in steps of thirds of 1 mm. For example, 1 mm corresponds to 3F. The French (Charrière)-gage size is not an SI unit.

5.1.2 The nominal shaft length, expressed in mm.

5.2 *Dimensions*:

5.2.1 The outside diameter and the minimum inside diameter of suction catheters, excluding the tip, shall be in accordance with Table 1.

5.2.2 The diameter of the terminal orifice shall not be less that 90 % of the minimum inside diameter specified in Table 1.

5.2.3 The actual shaft length shall be the marked shaft length ± 5 %. For closed circuit catheters, the marked length shall be the length that can be inserted into the patient's airway.

6. Design

6.1 *Lumen*—The inside diameter of the shaft at any point between the machine end and the eye nearest to the machine end shall be not less than the inside diameter of the shaft at that eye.

6.2 *Patient End*:

6.2.1 The suction catheter shall have a terminal orifice and one or more eyes.

NOTE 5—The use of a catheter with eye(s) reduces the likelihood of mucosal trauma during suctioning[4,5] (see Appendix X1).

NOTE 6—The dimensions of the eye(s) should be such that they do not cause the suction catheter to kink or collapse in use.

NOTE 7—The edges of eye(s) and the terminal orifice of the suction catheter should be smooth and free from sharp edges.

NOTE 8—The tip should be well-rounded.

6.2.2 The axis of the patient end may be at an angle to the long axis of the shaft (see Coudé catheter tips in Fig. 1).

6.3 *Machine End*:

6.3.1 The machine end of the suction catheter shall be one of the following:

6.3.1.1 *Female*—Designed to receive a male-to-male adapter suitable for connection to a vacuum source that terminates in a female end;

6.3.1.2 *Male*—Designed for connection to a vacuum source that terminates in a female end; or,

6.3.1.3 A permanently-attached vacuum control device that terminates in either a male or female end.

6.3.2 Female ends shall be semi-rigid or elastomeric and shall be either conical or cylindrical (see Fig. 1) over a length of not less than 20 mm.

NOTE 9—Where a suction catheter with a female machine end is provided for use with a vacuum source with a female end, a male-to-male adapter is needed. The minimum inside diameter of the adapter should be not less than the minimum inside diameter of the suction catheter with which it is provided. The adapter should fit inside elastomeric tubing having an inside diameter of 6 mm.

6.3.3 Male ends shall be rigid or semi-rigid and shall fit inside elastomeric tubing having an inside diameter of 6 mm (see Fig. 1). The inside diameter of the male end shall not be less than the minimum inside diameter of the suction catheter with which it is provided.

NOTE 10—It is advantageous if the male end fits inside elastomeric tubing with a larger inside diameter, which may be used in an emergency to clear the airway.

6.3.4 The machine end of a suction catheter having an angled patient end, by a mark or other means, shall indicate the direction in which the tip points.

7. Performance Requirements

7.1 *Security of Construction*—When tested in accordance with Annex A1, the force required to detach any component permanently attached to the shaft shall be not less than that specified in Table 2.

7.2 *Shaft*—When the machine end of the suction catheter is connected to a vacuum source at 40 kPa below ambient

TABLE 1 Basic Dimensions of Suction Catheters-Metric Sizes

Designated Size: Nominal Outside Diameter, mm	Designated Size: French (Charrière) Size Equivalent, F or Ch	Outside Diameter Tolerance, mm	Minimum Inside Diameter, mm
1.33	4	±0.1	0.55
1.5	4.5	±0.1	0.7
1.67	5	±0.1	0.8
2	6	±0.1	1.05
2.5	7.5	±0.1	1.45
2.67	8	±0.1	1.5
3	9	±0.15	1.75
3.33	10	±0.15	2
4	12	±0.15	2.45
4.67	14	±0.2	2.95
5	15	±0.2	3.2
5.33	16	±0.2	3.4
6	18	±0.2	3.9
6.67	20	±0.2	4.3

[4] Link, W. J., Spaeth, E. E., Wahle, W. M., Penny, W., and Glover, J. L., "The Influence of Suction Catheter Design on Tracheobronchial Trauma and Fluid Aspiration Efficiency," *Anesthesia and Analgesia*, Vol 55, pp. 290–97, 1976.

[5] Lomholt, N., "Design and Function of Tracheal Suction Catheters," *Acta Anaesthesiologica Scand*. Vol 29, pp. 1–3, 1982.

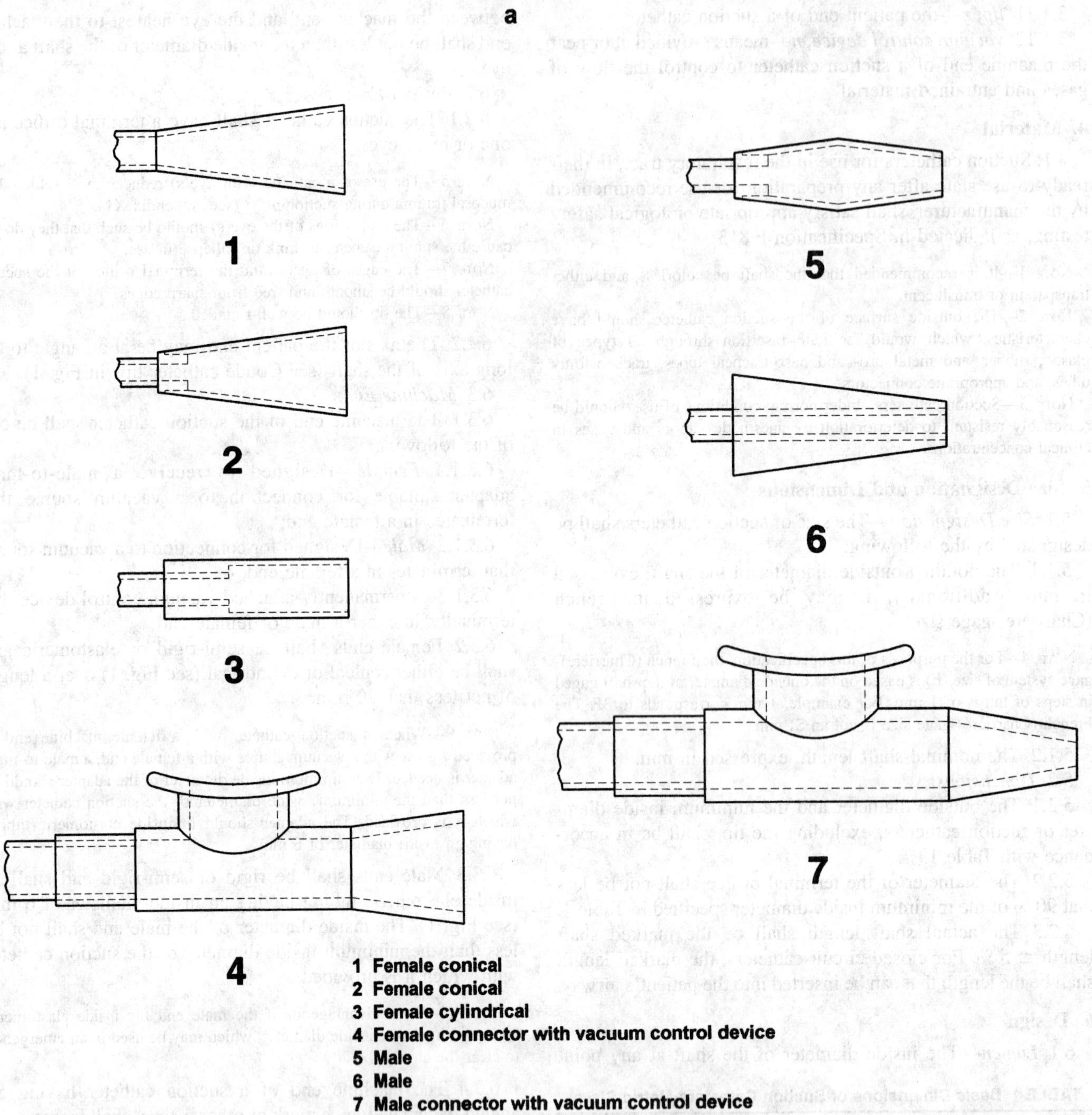

FIG. 1 Examples of Different Designs for a) Machine Ends, and b) Patient Ends of Suction Catheters for Use in the Respiratory Tract

pressure for 15 s at a temperature of 23 ± 2°C with the patient end openings occluded and the vacuum control device, if present, occluded, the shaft shall not collapse.

NOTE 11—Occlusion of the vacuum control device is intended for control devices that normally are open to atmosphere and require occlusion to apply the vacuum. Catheters that have vacuum control devices, which normally are closed and require opening to apply the vacuum, should be placed in the fully open position for this test.

7.3 *Residual Vacuum*—When a suction catheter fitted with a permanently-attached vacuum control device is tested in accordance with Annex A2, the residual vacuum shall not exceed 0.33 kPa.

7.4 *Leakage for Closed Circuit Suction Catheter Systems*—Closed circuit systems must meet the leakage requirements for breathing tubes (see Specification F 1205) when tested with the suction catheter fully retracted, vacuum applied to the catheter sleeve as specified in Annex A2, and with the relief control device in the suction relief/cutoff position (see Appendix X1.2).

8. Packaging and Labeling

8.1 *Marking of Suction Catheters*:

8.1.1 Suction catheters that are not individually packaged

b

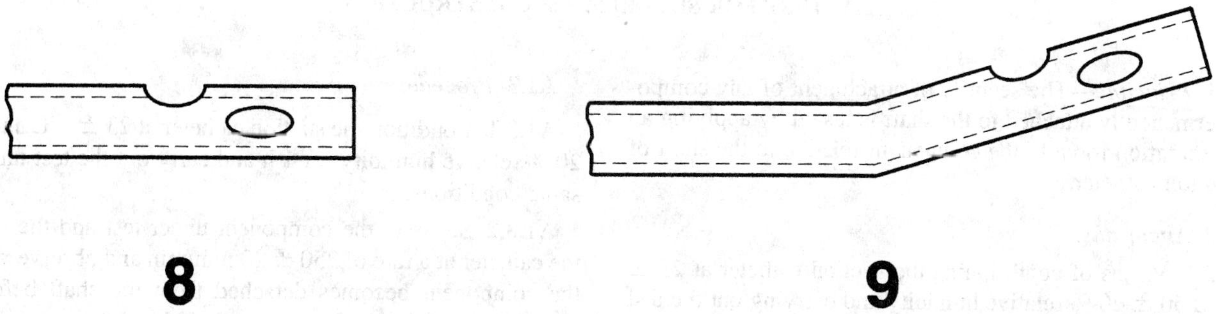

8 Catheter tip with eyes
9 Coudé catheter tip with eyes

FIG. 1 Examples of Different Designs for a) Machine Ends, and b) Patient Ends of Suction Catheters for Use in the Respiratory Tract *(continued)*

TABLE 2 Minimum Force Needed to Detach Any Component Permanently Attached to Shaft

Designated Size (Outside Diameter), mm	Minimum Force, *N*
1.33 to 2.67	5
3 to 4.67	15
≥5	20

shall be marked with the nominal outside diameter in accordance with 5.1.

8.1.2 Suction catheters that are individually packaged may be marked with the nominal outside diameter, expressed as millimeters or French (Charriére)-gage (see 5.1).

NOTE 12—Manufacturers of the smaller sizes of suction catheters for pediatric use are encouraged also to mark the distance, in cm or parts thereof, from the patient end.

8.2 *Marking of Individual Packs*—The marking of individual packs shall include the following:

8.2.1 A description of contents;

8.2.2 The designated size in accordance with 5.1.1, expressed in accordance with one or both of the following examples:

8.2.2.1 6 mm (18 F) × 500 mm; or,

8.2.2.2 6 mm (18 Ch) × 500 mm;

8.2.3 The name or trademark, or both, of the manufacturer or supplier, or both;

8.2.4 The batch number;

NOTE 13—It is strongly recommended that the "use by" date be given.

8.2.5 The word "STERILE," if appropriate;

8.2.6 For suction catheters not intended for reuse, the words "single use," or the equivalent.

8.3 *Marking of Shelf or Multi-Unit Packs*—The marking of shelf or multi-unit packs shall include the following:

8.3.1 A description of contents; and

8.3.2 The designated size in accordance with 5.1.1, expressed in accordance with one or both of the following examples:

8.3.2.1 6 mm (18 F) × 500 mm; or,

8.3.2.2 6 mm (18 Ch) × 500 mm;

8.3.3 The name or trademark, or both, and the address of the manufacturer or supplier, or both;

8.3.4 The batch number;

NOTE 14—It is strongly recommended that the "use by" date be given.

8.3.5 The word "STERILE," if appropriate;

8.3.6 For suction catheters intended for reuse, instructions for cleaning and sterilization shall be given. For suction catheters supplied nonsterile, appropriate instruction on preparation for use shall be provided.

8.3.7 For suction catheters not intended for reuse, the words "single use," or the equivalent.

8.4 *Use of Symbols*—The requirements of 8.2 and 8.3 may be met by the use of appropriate symbols as given in ISO 7000.

ANNEXES

(Mandatory Information)

A1. TEST FOR SECURITY OF CONSTRUCTION

A1.1 *Principle*—The security of attachment of any component permanently attached to the shaft is tested by applying an axial separation force to the component relative to the shaft of the suction catheter.

A1.2 *Apparatus*:

A1.2.1 Means of conditioning the suction catheter at 23 ± 2°C and 50 ± 20 % relative humidity and carrying out the test under the same conditions.

A1.2.2 Means of separately securing the component under test and the shaft of the suction catheter and separating the two at a rate of 250 ± 20 mm/min and measuring and recording the axial separation force applied.

A1.3 *Procedure*:

A1.3.1 Condition the suction catheter at 23 ± 2°C and 50 ± 20 % relative humidity for 1 h and carry out the test under the same conditions.

A1.3.2 Separate the component under test and the shaft of the catheter at a rate of 250 ± 20 mm/min and observe whether the component becomes detached from the shaft before the appropriate minimum force given in Table 2 has been reached.

A1.4 *Expression of Results*—Record whether the component becomes detached from the shaft before the appropriate minimum force given in Table 2 has been reached.

A2. MEASUREMENT OF RESIDUAL VACUUM

A2.1 *Principle*—The effectiveness of the vacuum control device as a means of relieving vacuum at the patient end is tested by measuring the residual vacuum at the tip of the catheter with the vacuum control device in the relief position and with suction being applied to the machine end of the catheter. Vacuum control devices, which rely on cutoff mechanisms, cannot be tested effectively by this test method; therefore, these devices are excluded from this test method.

NOTE A2.1—More stringent requirements are provided in 7.4 regarding leakage for closed circuit suction catheter systems.

A2.2 *Apparatus*:

A2.2.1 *Flowmeter*, capable of measuring a flow of 30 L/min with an accuracy of ± 5 % and a resistance to flow of less than 0.1 kPa at 30 L/min.

A2.2.2 *Adjustable Vacuum Pump*.

A2.2.3 *Manometer*, with an accuracy of ± 0.01 kPa.

A2.3 *Procedure*:

A2.3.1 Assemble the apparatus, as shown in Fig. A2.1, with the flowmeter fitted to the exit of the vacuum pump, ensuring an airtight fit between the catheter and the manometer.

A2.3.2 Place the catheter vacuum control device in the relief position.

A2.3.3 Switch on the vacuum pump and adjust the applied vacuum until a flow of 30 L/min is indicated on the flowmeter.

A2.4 *Expression of Results*—Express the residual vacuum, in kilopascals, as indicated by the reading on the manometer.

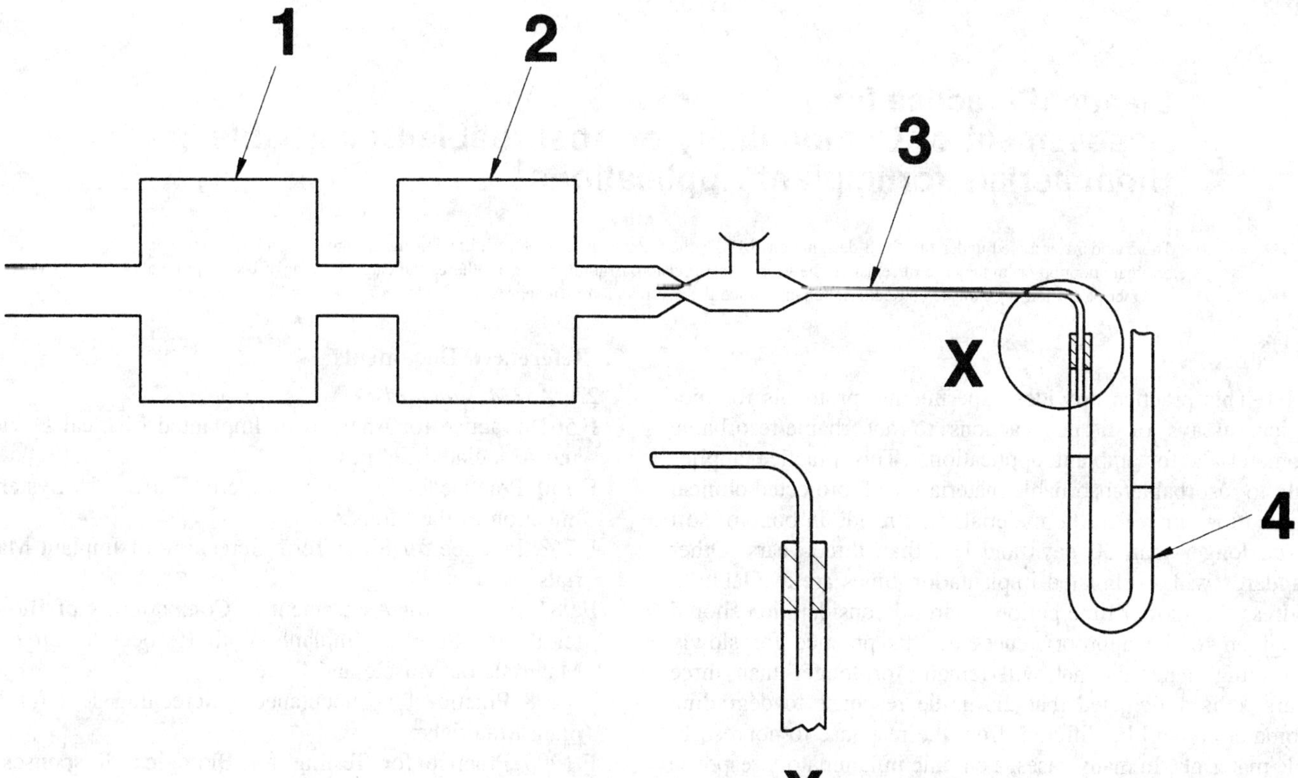

1 Flowmeter
2 Vacuum pump
3 Suction catheter with vacuum control device
4 Manometer

FIG. A2.1 Apparatus for Residual Vacuum Test

APPENDIX

(Nonmandatory Information)

X1. RATIONALE FOR REQUIREMENTS

X1.1 The requirement for a minimum of one eye, in addition to the terminal orifice, is included because suction catheters with only a terminal orifice have been shown to cause more mucosal damage than those with eyes.

X1.2 The rationale for the requirements provided in 7.4 is that closed circuit suction catheters are intended to remain a part of the breathing circuit; therefore, a cross-reference to the breathing tube standard, Specification F 1205, is included.

Standard Practice for Assessment of Compatibility of Absorbable/Resorbable Biomaterials for Implant Applications[1]

This standard is issued under the fixed designation F 1983; the number immediately following the designation indicates the year of original adoption or, in the case of revision, the year of last revision. A number in parentheses indicates the year of last reapproval. A superscript epsilon (ε) indicates an editorial change since the last revision or reapproval.

1. Scope

1.1 This practice provides experimental protocols for biological assays of tissue reactions to absorbable/resorbable biomaterials for implant applications. This practice applies only to resorbable/absorbable materials with projected clinical applications in which the materials will reside in bone or soft tissue longer than 30 days and less than three years. Other standards with designated implantation times are available to address the shorter time periods. Careful consideration should be given to the appropriateness of this practice for slowly degrading materials that will remain for longer than three years. It is anticipated that the tissue response to degrading biomaterials will be different from the response to nonresorbable materials. In many cases, a chronic inflammatory response may be observed during the degradation phase, but the local histology should return to normal after degradation; therefore, the minimal tissue response usually equated with "biocompatibility" may require long implantations.

1.2 The time period for implant degradation will vary depending on chemical composition and implant size; therefore, the implantation times for examination of tissue response will be linked to the rate of resorption. No single implantation time is indicated in this practice.

1.3 These protocols assess the effects of the material on the animal tissue in which it is implanted. The experimental protocols do not fully assess systemic toxicity, carcinogenicity, teratogenicity, or mutagenicity of the material. Other standards are available to address these issues.

1.4 To maximize use of the animals in the study protocol, all toxicological findings should be recorded. There are some aspects of systemic toxicity, including effects of degradation products on the target organs, that can be addressed with this practice, and these effects should be documented fully.

1.5 *This standard does not purport to address all of the safety concerns, if any, associated with its use. It is the responsibility of the user of this standard to establish appropriate safety and health practices and determine the applicability of regulatory limitations prior to use.*

2. Referenced Documents

2.1 *ASTM Standards:*

F 561 Practice for Analysis of Implanted Medical Devices and Associated Tissues[2]

F 750 Practice for Evaluating Material Extracts by Systemic Injection in the Mouse[2]

F 763 Practice for Short-Term Screening of Implant Materials[2]

F 981 Practice for Assessment of Compatibility of Biomaterials for Surgical Implants With Respect to Effect of Materials on Muscle and Bone[2]

F 1408 Practice for Subcutaneous Screening Test for Implant Materials[2]

F 1903 Practice for Testing for Biological Responses to Particles[2]

F 1904 Practice for Testing the Biological Responses to Particles[2]

F 1905 Practice for Selecting Tests for Determining the Propensity of Materials to Cause Immunotoxicity[2]

F 1906 Practice for Evaluation of Immune Responses in Biocompatibility Testing Using ELISA Tests, Lymphocyte Proliferation, and Cell Migration[2]

3. Summary of Practice

3.1 Under strict aseptic conditions, specimens of the final implant form candidate material are implanted into the most relevant anatomical tissue site in small laboratory animals, preferably mice, rats, hamsters, or rabbits.

3.2 The use of larger animals, such as the dog, goat, or sheep may be justified based upon special considerations of the particular study. Choice of species also should consider the availability of historical data on biological responses of these animals to similar devices to aid in analysis and comparison of data obtained.

3.3 All animal studies must be done in a facility approved by a nationally recognized organization and in accordance with all appropriate regulations.

4. Significance and Use

4.1 This practice is a guideline for a screening test for the evaluation of the local tissue response to materials that may be selected for implantation into the human body and which are

[1] This practice is under the jurisdiction of ASTM Committee F-04 on Medical and Surgical Material and Devices and is the direct responsibility of Subcommittee F04.16 on Biocompatibility Test Methods.

Current edition approved June 10, 1999. Published September 1999.

[2] *Annual Book of ASTM Standards*, Vol 13.01.

expected to undergo degradation by absorption or resorption within three years.

4.2 This practice is similar to that for studies on candidate materials that are not resorbable, such as those specified in Practices F 763, F 981, and F 1408; however, analysis of the host response must take into account the effect of degradation and degradation products on the inflammatory response at the local tissue site and on subsequent healing of the implantation site.

4.3 The material to be tested should be in the final finished form as for intended use, including sterilization. Material/body ratios should be relevant to that of intended device use. Material surface area or mass to body mass ratios of 1X, 10X, and 50X if applicable, are recommended.

4.4 Materials that are designed for use in devices with in situ polymerization shall be introduced in a manner such that in situ polymerization occurs. Testing of individual precursor components is not recommended.

5. Test Animals and Sites

5.1 Choice of test animal shall take into consideration the normal life span of the animal and the length of the implantation study. Small laboratory animals are preferred. The strain, sex, age, and origin of the animals used should be noted. If larger animals are used, justification for their use should be provided. The source of the animals, species/strain, weight, age (where known or approximate if not known), general health, and boarding conditions should be recorded. Animal use and care regulations must be followed.

5.2 The number of implant sites shall depend on the size of the implant and the animal. The distance between implants shall be sufficient so that separate tissue blocks are prepared easily for each implant and sufficient that the biological reactions do not overlap or interfere with each other. Implants may be placed bilaterally in soft tissue, including muscle. Bilateral implantation into bone should be considered carefully and justification given. In general, mice, rats, hamsters, and other similarly sized rodents should receive no more than one implant on each side. Larger animals, including rabbits, may receive up to five implants on each side. When the implant is composed of a collection of particles, pellets, etc., each collection is considered one implant site.

5.3 Before embarking on studies in large animals, it is recommended that a pilot study in rodents be undertaken to determine expected rate of degradation and the distribution and metabolism of the degradation products. When feasible, initial prediction may be done by radio-labeling the material and following the loss of radioactivity; however, radioactive specimens shall not be used for biocompatibility testing. Other methods of following the degradation are acceptable. The target organs of the metabolism and excretion of the products should be identified. It is recommended that acute systemic studies with material extracts according to Practice F 750 be completed prior to the initiation of the implantation study.

6. Implant Specimens

6.1 *Design of the Implant*—Specimens may be made from the final finished form candidate material in configurations specific for the animal study. As described in 4.3, the material/host ratio should be available and referrable to ultimate use in the human with material/body mass ratios of 1X, 10X, and 50X, if applicable, recommended. Relevant configurations of implant specimens, such as cylinders, flat cloth, amorphous gels, and polymerizable liquids may be used.

6.2 The use of positive and negative controls is not required in this practice; however, the implantation of the candidate material must be accompanied by the use of an implanted marker or other permanent method, such as a template, to mark the implant site to allow identification of the implant site at the various time periods. A sham surgical site, or a sham surgical animal, is necessary.

6.3 The material used shall be in its final finished form and sterilized as indicated for its ultimate use. It shall be handled for implantation in a manner analogous to that for intended final use, for example, special forceps, special cannulas or needles, special syringes, etc.

6.4 The candidate material shall be described thoroughly to facilitate development of a suitable implant application protocol. The absorption, distribution, metabolism, and excretion of the material and its degradation products should be described. The information shall include, but is not limited to, the following:

6.4.1 Expected method of degradation, for example, hydrolysis, enzymatic, phagocytosis, etc.

6.4.2 Expected nonresorbable degradation products, for example, fibrils, particles from composites.

6.4.3 Expected rate of degradation.

6.4.4 Expected target organ effects where known or expected, for example, eliminated in kidney, stored in liver, stored in spleen or lymph nodes.

6.5 For each time period, at least six rodents shall be used with either single or bilateral implants. For the larger animals, at least four animals shall be used per time period. It is recommended that additional animals be included in the initial protocol to accommodate any unexpected changes in degradation rates of the material.

7. Procedure

7.1 *Implantation:*

7.1.1 Implant the specimen under sterile conditions in anesthetized animals. Where possible, implant the specimen using a trochar method to avoid the need for an incision. If an incision is needed, insert the implant as far from the incision site as possible. Close the insertion site with a suitable suture material.

7.1.1.1 A sham site or sham animal with the identical implantation procedure, but not the test material, should be included in the protocol. If animals are to be used as part of systemic toxicity study, the sham must be a separate animal.

7.1.2 The implantation site must be marked in manner suitable for identification of the site at the designated time periods. The use of a permanent skin marker and a template marking the placement of the specimen and the sham site is recommended. Specimens that are radiopaque may have serial radiographs to identify the location. The implantation of a nonabsorbable marker material such as a monofilament, nonabsorbable suture attached to the specimen or embedded in the gel or liquid also is acceptable. If an implanted marker material is used with the specimen, this marker material shall be included in the sham site. The test specimen site and the sham site shall be marked.

7.1.3 Keep the animals in standard housing according to current animal protection requirements. The individual animals should be marked for identification.

7.2 *Post-Operative Care*:

7.2.1 Care of the animals shall be in accordance with accepted standards as outlined in Guide for Care and Use of Laboratory Animals according to the local and national government ordinances in an approved facility.

7.2.2 Carefully observe each animal during the specified time period and record any abnormal clinical findings.

7.2.3 If infection or accidental injury of the test implant site occurs, record the information and process the implant site and tissues and organs as described in 7.3 and 8.1. Record the data in the results, but do not use the data in the final analysis of results from the other animals. A replacement animal may be added, if desired.

7.2.4 If an animal dies before the scheduled termination, record the information and process the implant site and tissues and organs as described in 7.3 and 8.1. Record the data, but do not use the data in the final analysis of results from the other animals. If the death is related to anesthesia, a replacement animal may be selected.

7.3 *Euthanasia and Implant Retrieval*:

7.3.1 Euthanasia method shall be according to the recommended method for the particular animal species according to local and government regulations. Euthanasia times shall be based on expected degradation rate of the material. The initial euthanasia interval shall be when there is expected to be a 50 % loss of mass or release of 50 % of the degradation products. Additional euthanasia times shall include expected 100 % loss of mass, and when complete healing and return to normal histology is anticipated. It is permissible to establish euthanasia times during the study period if at the established time period expected loss has not occurred, for example, if 50 % loss has not occurred when expected, then the euthanasia time for 50 % loss shall again be estimated. Euthanasia at this additional time period is needed. The additional time frames should be advanced to accommodate this slower than expected degradation. The additional animals recommended in 6.5 may be used for this purpose of additional euthanasia times.

7.3.2 At euthanasia, record the general appearance of the skin at the implantation site; then, carefully expose the region of the initial implantation. This is facilitated by the use of a template and skin marker at surgery. If a marker suture is used, the site of the marker suture shall be noted. Record the color and consistency of the tissues in the region of the original site of the material. The use of gross photography should be considered carefully since it may aid in maintaining an adequate permanent record. Remove the intact tissue envelope around the marker or template and extend beyond any identifiable remaining candidate material. If the candidate material is not evident at the site, extend the explanation site to include several mm of normal tissue on all sides of the marker material or template mark. If any abnormal tissue is observed elsewhere, this shall be removed for further examination. Transfer the tissue specimen as soon as possible into a fixing agent suitable for further histologic processing. The use of alcohol, formaldehyde, or glutaraldehyde is recommended, but other agents, such as freezing, may be considered. Reference to Practices F 561, F 981, and F 1408 is encouraged for processing procedures.

7.3.3 Although systemic toxicity is not addressed specifically in this practice, examination of target organs should be conducted to maximize use of the animal. After the implantation site is harvested, the abdominal and thoracic viscera should be examined. The liver, spleen, kidney, local lymph nodes, gonads, and lung should be retained in fixative in case of future need. If any abnormalities are noted, the specimen should be subjected to histologic examination. If the release of particles is anticipated, then the target organs shall be processed in an appropriate manner to preserve the particles as discussed in Practices F 1903 and F 1904.

7.3.4 It is recommended that tissues from the target organs listed in 7.3.3 be processed for histologic analysis since the data may be useful in evaluation of systemic toxicity. Although this practice does not substitute for systemic toxicity studies (see Practice F 750), remote organs should be collected and assessed for toxicological findings to maximize use of the animals. Similarly, blood chemistry and hematology, as well as urine studies, may be done on these animals for inclusion in systemic toxicity analysis. The use of these animals for immunotoxicity studies, as discussed in Practices F 1905 and F 1906, also may be considered.

8. Histologic Evaluation

8.1 *Histological Preparation*:

8.1.1 In general, the standard methods according to Practices F 561, F 981, and F 1408 should be followed. Standard laboratory practices for histological preparation of the implant/tissue specimens and staining are used **(1-5)**.[3] The tissue and histologic sections should be examined by qualified personnel.

8.1.2 Preservation of the implant material and the tissue reaction are essential, and therefore, the entire explant shall be processed without removal of the candidate material. Solvents that dissolve the candidate material before embedding should be avoided where possible. If the material is such that its hardness precludes sectioning with standard microtomes, then cutting and grinding techniques shall be employed. Conventional embedding in paraffin with standard microtomy is not recommended unless it is shown that the candidate material and surrounding tissue are preserved in the specimen. If it is not possible to avoid dissolving the material during fixation and embedding, then care should be taken to mark the location of the material in the tissue.

8.1.3 Tissue response should be characterized in regard to acute inflammation, chronic inflammation, granulation tissue formation, foreign body reaction, and foreign body giant cell formation. Special attention should be given to any change in the integrity of the form of the material, such as solid or mesh changing to particulate and to corresponding changes in tissue response to the altered form of the specimen. Focal tissue loss,

[3] The boldface numbers in parentheses refer to the list at the end of this text.

necrosis, and granulomas shall be noted. The tissue reaction to the nonabsorbable marker material also should be noted but analyzed separately. Cell numbers may be determined on a histologic evaluation scale of 0 to +4 with 0 being no cellular reaction and +4 being an extensive or severe reaction.

8.1.4 As the material degrades, it can be anticipated that the form of the material may change, and this may result in an altered cellular response. It is important that both the material form and the tissue response be recorded at each time interval.

9. Report

9.1 The report shall include the following information:

9.1.1 *Implants*—Describe the implant material, its size, weight, shape and form at implantation, mode of degradation, the material characteristics at degradation, for example, free particles, long fibers, amorphous gel, changes in crystallinity, and difficulty in implantation or explantation.

9.1.2 The sterilization method and the method of handling for implantation shall be recorded.

9.1.3 Describe the animal host used, the age, sex, strain, and weight of the animal. Implantation method used shall be described. The records of examination revealing abnormal clinical signs, infection, or death shall be indicated. The cause of death prior to scheduled euthanasia shall be reported.

9.1.4 The length of implantation time, euthanasia method, retrieval technique, gross observation of tissues and organs, and identification of marker suture should be recorded.

9.1.5 The methods of histologic evaluation and the results of histologic evaluation of the implant site and the target organs shall be described. Histologic analysis shall include evaluation scales for acute inflammation, chronic inflammation, foreign body giant cell formation, and other evidence of foreign body reactions including necrosis.

9.1.6 The material form at explantation shall be recorded.

10. Keywords

10.1 absorbables; biocompatibility; degradables; implantation; resorbables

APPENDIX

(Nonmandatory Information)

X1. RATIONALE

X1.1 This practice modifies existing ASTM standards on in vivo assessment of tissue responses to implanted solid and porous materials, such as, Practices F 763, F 981, F 1408, in order to evaluate the local tissue response to resorbable, absorbable, and degradable materials. The test procedures for solid and dense materials have a long history of reproducible and meaningful results.

X1.2 The tissue response to resorbable, absorbable, or degradable materials is expected to be different from that of nonresorbable materials, and there is not a long history of reproducible and meaningful evaluation. A fibrous capsule is unlikely to be formed, and the presence of cells actively degrading the material or phagocytizing the degradation products may be noted. In many cases, this may have the appearance of a chronic inflammatory response.

X1.3 It is necessary to extend the implantation time in these studies to assess the tissue response during active degradation of the material, when the material has been degraded entirely, and when the tissue has healed and returned to normal histology. This time period will vary greatly for various types of materials and may extend to more than a year.

X1.4 Some materials may stimulate lengthy remodeling of bone and other tissues and some may be resorbed so slowly that considerable material may remain at the three years designated in 1.1. Materials that are designed for tissue remodeling and slow degradation, may be studied in a similar manner as described herein; however, the endpoint for this evaluation should be the formation of the expected normal tissue at the site rather than complete degradation. For those materials, in which tissue remodeling is expected, the time periods should include at least two time periods. The first is when approximately 50 % integration/remodeling has been achieved and the second when the anticipated final histologic response of remodeling and healing is achieved. For slowly degrading materials, the time periods should include at least two time periods. The first is when approximately 50 % loss of mass or release of 50 % of the degradation products has occurred, and the second when the biological response indicates return to the normal tissue histology, such as, the histologic response of the sham site. For example, calcium phosphate ceramics for bone apposition and remodeling should be considered at 100 % endpoint when remodeling bone of normal appearance is observed at the remaining material.

X1.5 This practice does not address all of the issues of subchronic or chronic systemic toxicity; however, it is recommended that the information obtainable from this study that relates to systemic toxicity be analyzed as such. The number of animals suggested in systemic toxicity studies exceeds the number that are needed for local tissue responses. In some cases, therefore, the animals being evaluated for local tissue responses may be a subset of the chronic systemic toxicity study. Each animal in these studies should be used for the maximum obtainable information.

X1.6 It is recognized that it may be difficult to adequately predict the degradation rate and determine when the 50 % degradation has occurred. Imaging techniques, radiopaque markers, or surgical observation may be permitted, as long as they do not impact on the animal welfare or the anticipated biological response.

REFERENCES

(**1**) Cohen, J., "Assay of Foreign Body Reaction," *J. Bone Jt. Surg.*, 41A:152–166, 1959.

(**2**) Laing, P. G., Ferguson, A. B., and Hodhe, E. S., "Tissue Reaction in Rabbit Muscle Exposed to Metallic Implants," *J. Biomed. Mater. Res.*, 1:135–149, 1967.

(**3**) Ferguson, A. B. Jr., Laing, P. G., and Hodge, E. S., "The Ionization of Metal Implants in Living Tissues," *J. Bone Jt. Surg.*, 42A: 77–90, 1960.

(**4**) Hooper, K. A., Macon, N. D., and Kohn, J, "Comparative Histological Evaluation of New Tyrosine-Derived Polymers and Poly (L-Lactid Acid) as a Function of Polymer Degradation," *J. Biomed. Mater. Res.*, 41:443–454, 1998.

(**5**) Gogolewski, S., Jovanovic, M., Perren, S. M., Dillon, J. G., Hughes, M. K., "Tissue Response and *In Vivo* Degradation of Selected Polyhydroxyacids: Polylactides (PLA), Poly(3–hydroxybutyrate (PHB), and Poly(3–hydroxybutyrate-co-3–hydroxyvalerate) (PHB/VA)," *J. Biomed. Mater. Res.* 27:1135–1148, 1993.

Standard Practice for Testing for Whole Complement Activation in Serum by Solid Materials[1]

This standard is issued under the fixed designation F 1984; the number immediately following the designation indicates the year of original adoption or, in the case of revision, the year of last revision. A number in parentheses indicates the year of last reapproval. A superscript epsilon (ε) indicates an editorial change since the last revision or reapproval.

1. Scope

1.1 This practice provides a protocol for rapid, in vitro screening for whole complement activating properties of solid materials used in the fabrication of medical devices that will contact blood.

1.2 This practice is intended to evaluate the acute in vitro whole complement activating properties of solid materials intended for use in contact with blood. For this practice, the words "serum" and "complement" are used interchangeably (most biological supply houses use these words synonymously in reference to serum used as a source of complement).

1.3 This practice consists of two procedural parts. Procedure A describes exposure of solid materials to a standard lot of human serum, using a 0.1-mL serum/13 x 100-mm disposable test tube. Cellulose acetate powders and fibers are used as examples of test materials. Procedure B describes assaying the exposed serum for significant functional whole complement depletion as compared to control samples.

1.4 This practice does not address function, elaboration, or depletion of individual complement components, nor does it address the use of plasma as a source of complement.

1.5 This practice is one of several developed for the assessment of the biocompatibility of materials. Practice F 748 may provide guidance for the selection of appropriate methods for testing materials for other aspects of biocompatibility.

2. Referenced Documents

2.1 *ASTM Standards:*

F 748 Practice for Selecting Generic Biological Test Methods for Materials and Devices[2]

2.2 *ISO Document:*

ISO 10993-4: Biological Evaluation of Medical Devices, Part 4: Selection of Tests for Interactions with Blood[3]

3. Terminology

3.1 *Abbreviations:*

3.1.1 *Ab*—antibody (hemolysin).

3.1.2 *BBS*—barbital buffered saline.

3.1.3 *BBS-G*—barbital buffered saline—gelatin.

3.1.4 *BBS-GM*—barbital buffered saline—gelatin metals.

3.1.5 *C′*—complement.

3.1.6 *EDTA*—ethylenediaminetetraacetic acid, disodium salt: dihydrate.

3.1.7 *HS*—human serum.

3.1.8 *PVDF*—polyvinylidene fluoride.

3.1.9 *RBC*—red blood cell(s).

4. Summary of Practice

4.1 Solid material specimens are exposed to contact with a standard lot of complement under defined conditions (Procedure A). Exposed serum then is tested for significant functional complement depletion compared to controls under identical conditions (Procedure B).

5. Significance and Use

5.1 Inappropriate activation of complement by blood-contacting medical devices may have serious acute or chronic effects on the host. This practice is useful as a simple, inexpensive screening method for determining functional whole complement activation by solid materials in vitro.

5.2 This practice is composed of two parts. In Part A (Section 11), human serum is exposed to a solid material. Complement may be depleted by the classical or alternative pathways. In principle, nonspecific binding of certain complement components also may occur. The alternative pathway can deplete later acting components common to both pathways, that is components other than C1, C4, and C3 (**1**).[4] In Part B (Section 12), complement activity remaining in the serum after exposure to the test material is assayed by classical pathway-mediated lysis of sensitized RBC.

5.3 Assessment of in vitro whole complement activation, as described here, provides one method for predicting potential complement activation by medical materials intended for clinical application in humans when the material contacts the blood. Other test methods for complement activation are available, including assays for specific complement components and their split products (see X1.3 and X1.4).

5.4 This in vitro test method is suitable for adoption in

[1] This practice is under the jurisdiction of ASTM Committee F-04 on Medical and Surgical Materials and Devices and is the direct responsibility of Subcommittee F04.16 on Biocompatibility Test Methods.

Current edition approved June 10, 1999. Published September 1999.

[2] *Annual Book of ASTM Standards*, Vol 13.01.

[3] Available from American National Standards Institute, 11 W. 42nd St., New York, NY 10036.

[4] The boldface numbers in parentheses refer to the list of references at the end of this specification.

specifications and standards for screening solid materials for use in the construction of medical devices intended to be implanted in the human body or placed in contact with human blood.

6. Preparation of Buffers

6.1 *Buffers*, are prepared according to detailed protocol **(2)**. "Water" refers throughout to distilled, endotoxin-free water. The use of barbital (veronal) buffer is recommended. Barbital is a class IV regulated substance and requires a DEA **(3)** license for purchase. The use of other buffer systems, such as, TRIS, is permissible if they have been demonstrated not to activate complement**(4)**.

6.2 *5X Stock BBS (barbital-buffered saline)*, is prepared by adding 20.75 g NaCl plus 2.545 g sodium barbital (sodium-5,5-diethyl barbiturate) to about 400 mL water. The pH is adjusted to 7.35 with 1 N HCl, then brought to a final volume of 500 mL in a volumetric flask.

6.3 *Metals Solution*, is prepared by making a 2.0 M solution of $MgCl_2$ (40.66 g $MgCl_2 \cdot 6\ H_2O$ into 100 mL distilled endotoxin-free water), and a 0.3 M solution of $CaCl_2$ (4.41 g $CaCl_2 \cdot 2\ H_2O$ into 100 mL distilled endotoxin-free water), and combining the two solutions 1:1 (v:v). These solutions are stable one month at 4°C.

6.4 *BBS-GM Working Solution*, is prepared daily, by dissolving 0.25 g gelatin in 50 mL endotoxin-free distilled water that is gently heated and stirred. The gelatin solution is added to 50 mL 5X stock BBS plus 0.25 mL metals solution, brought up to about 200 mL, then adjusted to pH 7.35 (with 1 N HCl or 1 N NaOH) before bringing the final volume to 250 mL in a volumetric flask.

6.5 *BBS-G Working Solution*, is prepared the same way, but the addition of the metals solution is omitted.

6.6 *10X Stock EDTA (0.1 M disodium dihydrate EDTA)*, is prepared by adding 7.44 g disodium $EDTA \cdot 2\ H_2O$ to about 160 mL water, adjusting the pH to 7.65 (with 1 N NaOH or 1 N HCl), then bringing the volume to 200 mL in a volumetric flask.

6.7 *BBS-G-EDTA (to be used in preparing RBC before being washed out)*, is prepared by adding 10 mL of stock 10X EDTA to 90 mL of BBS-G in a volumetric flask.

7. Preparation of Sheep RBC

7.1 Commercially-obtained sheep red blood cells (RBC) preserved in Alsever's solution are stored at 4°C. The cells are discarded after eight weeks or when the supernatant from the second wash contains hemoglobin by visual inspection.

NOTE 1—All centrifugations are at 4°C. Except where indicated, all reagents, tubes, and cell preparations are kept on ice.

7.2 Five mL of sheep RBC are centrifuged at 1 000 x g for 10 min.

7.3 The cell pellet is resuspended in 10 mL of cold BBS-G-EDTA and incubated for 10 min at 37°C. The cells are centrifuged, and the pellet resuspended in 10 mL of BBS-G-EDTA.

7.4 The cells are centrifuged, the supernatant discarded (first wash), and the pellet resuspended in 10 mL of cold BBS-GM. Repeat twice (total of three washes).

7.5 Adjust cell count spectrophotometrically (where an absorbance of 0.56 corresponds to 1.5×10^8 sheep RBC/mL, at a wavelength of 412 nm and a 1.0-cm light path for 1 volume of cells in BBS-GM plus 24 volumes of water) or count with a hemocytometer, preparing 10 mL of 1.5×10^8 cells/mL in cold BBS-GM.

7.6 The washed, diluted RBC can be held on ice and used for at least 12 h.

8. Absorption of Serum (Complement)

8.1 The use of human complement is required since there are species differences in the efficiency of complement activation and the test materials are to be used in humans. Human serum suitable as a source of complement may be purchased from biological supply houses, and generally, is labeled as reagent-grade complement.

8.2 Human serum may be absorbed with sheep RBC in order to remove naturally-occurring anti-sheep RBC hemolytic antibodies, though for most purposes, the amount of heterophile antibody in human serum is not enough to influence the reaction assuming the cells are optimally sensitized with hemolysin. The procedure is detailed in 8.3-8.8.

8.3 Fresh human serum or a commercial lot of human serum is obtained and stored at −70°C. Fresh serum is preferred as lyophilized complement often is not as active as fresh serum.

8.4 The serum is thawed on ice or reconstituted (if lyophilized) with ice-cold (4°C) distilled endotoxin-free water.

8.5 All manipulations are done on ice, with ice cold reagents and cells; centrifugations are carried out at 1000 x g at 4°C. It is critical that this entire procedure be done in the cold to avoid activation of complement in this step.

8.6 Cold serum and cold, packed, washed sheep RBC are mixed, 0.1 mL RBC/2.5 mL serum, incubated for 10 min on ice, then centrifuged at 1 000 x g for 10 min at 4°C. The supernatant is transferred carefully to a new container on ice.

8.7 The procedure in 8.6 is repeated twice.

8.8 The absorbed human serum is stored in 0.5–1.0-mL aliquots (convenient for one-experiment use), in cold snap-cap microfuge tubes and kept at −70°C until used. Aliquots should be thawed on ice, used on the day of thawing, and not be refrozen.

9. Determination of Optimal Hemolysin Concentration

9.1 Determination of optimal hemolysin concentration is necessary in order to conserve expensive reagents and to avoid prozone effects. Commercial rabbit anti-sheep RBC serum (Hemolysin) is obtained, thawed, or, if lyophilized, reconstituted with distilled endotoxin-free water), heat-inactivated at 56°C for 30 min to inactivate the rabbit complement, aliquoted in convenient volumes, and stored at −70°C until used.

9.2 To cold 13 x 100 mm disposable glass tubes, placed in a rack in an ice-bath, 0.1 mL of washed sheep RBC at 1.5×10^8 cells/mL is added. If statistical evaluation of the results is desired, three replicate tubes for each condition should be used. Otherwise, duplicates or even single dilution tubes are sufficient. One set of three replicate tubes receives only 0.1 mL of cold BBS-GM/tube (no RBC control, for complement color).

9.3 To the RBC-containing tubes, one set of three tubes gets 1.1 mL cold distilled H_2O/tube (total lysis control), another gets 0.1 mL BBS-GM (no hemolysin control), and the other sets get 0.1 mL each of 1:2 serial dilutions of hemolysin (tests). Dilutions between 1:400 to 1:25 600 antibody are recommended, with two sets of 1:400. The no RBC control receives 0.1 mL of additional BBS-GM.

9.4 Each tube is mixed quickly by gentle shaking to resuspend cells, the rack is placed in a 37°C water bath, incubated 10 min, then returned to the ice bath.

9.5 One of the two sets of 1:400 antibody gets 1.0 mL of cold BBS-GM (no-complement control). All other tubes besides the total lysis control set get 0.5 mL cold BBS-GM, then 0.5 mL of absorbed human serum (complement) diluted 1:100 or 1:200.

NOTE 2—For a particular lot of human serum, a 1:100 or 1:200 dilution should provide sufficient complement activity. Also, percent lysis in the no-hemolysin (complement only) control should not exceed 10 %. If lysis with the 1:100 dilution of complement exceeds 10 %, use 1:200. If the no-hemolysin control still exceeds 10 %, a different lot of serum will need to be tested.

9.6 Tubes are shaken manually to suspend cells, then the rack is incubated in a 37°C water bath for 1h, and intermittently shaken to keep cells in suspension.

9.7 At the end of 1h, the rack is placed on ice. The cold tubes then are centrifuged at 1 000 x g for 10 min at 4°C, and the supernatants decanted to correspondingly numbered 13 x 100-mm glass tubes.

9.8 Absorbance of the supernatants is measured at 412 nm. Percent lysis is calculated for each test and control tube by subtracting from the 412 nm absorbance the no RBC control (mean of the three replicate tubes), dividing by the total lysis control value (mean of the three replicate tubes), and multiplying by 100.

$$\% \text{ lysis} = \frac{\text{test absorbance} - \text{no RBC control absorbance}}{\text{total lysis absorbance}} \times 100 \tag{1}$$

9.9 Final % lysis for each condition is expressed as mean ± standard deviation of the three % lysis values for each three-replicate set.

9.10 A titration curve is obtained by plotting the inverse of the hemolysin concentration versus % specific lysis. Twice the concentration of hemolysin that is just on the plateau of the titration curve is used for sensitizing RBC for subsequent assays (optimal hemolysin concentration). Hemolysin is freshly diluted from stock each day of use.

10. Whole Complement Titration to Determine Optimal Serum Dilution

10.1 If statistical evaluation of results is desired, all conditions should be assayed in triplicate, using three 13 x 100 disposable glass test tubes per condition. Otherwise, duplicates or single tubes are sufficient. Tubes are numbered in advance. Conditions include total lysis, no complement (no C'), tests (dilutions of human serum—HS) with and without hemolysin, and no RBC (complement color control, at highest concentration of serum used). All reagents, tubes, and manipulations are done ice-cold, with tubes held in a rack in an ice slurry.

10.2 Washed RBC are added to all tubes except no RBC tubes (0.1 mL/tube of a 1.5 x 10^8 cells/mL suspension). No RBC tubes get 0.1 mL cold buffer.

10.3 Total lysis tubes get 1.1 mL distilled H_2O. The no C' and test with hemolysin tubes get 0.1 mL optimal hemolysin (see 9.10), and no RBC tubes get 0.1 mL cold BBS-GM. All tubes are shaken to resuspend cells, incubated in a 37°C water bath for 10 min, and placed back on ice.

NOTE 3—Another acceptable procedure is to make up one large batch of hemolysin-sensitized erythrocytes to cover all the tests planned within one week's time. These cells are made up at 5 x 10^8/mL and are stored at 4°C. They are washed each time they are used, and if hemolysis occurs, new sensitized cells are prepared. These sensitized cells are ready to use, making the addition of hemolysin to each tube unnecessary, which simplifies the experiment. Unsensitized RBC can be used as controls for nonspecific lysis.

10.4 To all but the total lysis tubes, a maximum volume of 1.0 mL of cold BBS-GM is added, reduced by the amount of diluted serum (see 10.5), which will be added at a maximum 0.5 mL volume. The no C' tubes get 1.0 mL BBS-GM.

10.5 The cold serum is diluted in cold BBS-GM to the desired concentration (with minimal agitation). It is recommended to test the HS initially at 1:50 to 1:300. The diluted serum is added to each test tube in a 0.5 mL volume. Final volume in each tube should be made up to 1.2 mL with BBS-GM.

10.6 The tubes then are treated as detailed in 9.6-9.9.

10.7 The optimal human serum dilution of a particular lot of human serum is defined as that in which the nonspecific lysis (HS + RBC, in absence of hemolysin antibody) is ≤ 10 %, while specific lysis (total lysis [RBC + Ab + HS] minus nonspecific lysis) is at least 20 % but not greater than 80 %, that is, the specific lysis is on the linear part of the complement titration curve. A typical optimal dilution for a lot of absorbed human serum is 1:200 added as a 0.5 mL volume in the assay.

11. Procedure A—Exposure of Material to Human Serum

11.1 *Powder*:

NOTE 4—An example of a powder is cellulose acetate. Centrifugation in a typical table-top clinical centrifuge is insufficient to pellet the powder following incubation with complement. Hence a filtration step, with appropriate control, is required.

11.1.1 Cold, absorbed human complement is placed onto the bottom of cold 13 x 100 disposable glass tubes on ice, 0.1 mL/tube. A minimal assay requires four tubes, labeled M (material), NM (no material control), I_1 (Ice-one, the filtration control), and I_2 (Ice-two, maximal complement activity control).

NOTE 5—Other controls might include a comparison to another material with same unit surface area or other appropriate measurable parameter, or a positive control for complement activation, such as zymosan or heat-aggregated gamma globulin, HAGG, or both.

11.1.2 The upper portions of the M and NM tubes are warmed briefly by hand, to prevent powder from adhering to moisture on the sides. A defined quantity of powder is dropped onto the 0.1 mL serum at the bottom of the tube, such that the liquid is just covered, for example, 6 mg, by the powder. With no mixing, the two tubes are placed in a 37°C water bath and incubated for 1h. I_1 and I_2 are kept on ice.

11.1.3 Three syringe filters are prepared as follows. Recommended filters are low proteinbinding, such as hydrophilic PVDF membranes, with 0.22-μm pore size. Each filter is flushed with 2.0 mL cold BBS-GM, excess liquid expelled with air, and placed in holder on ice until needed.

11.1.4 At the end of 1h incubation, the M and NM tubes are put back on ice. Immediately, 4.9 mL of cold BBS-GM is added to each tube (a 1:50 dilution of the exposed serum). Using separate Pasteur glass pipettes, the contents of each tube are slowly drawn up and back down into the tube, insuring mixture of the serum and buffer.

11.1.5 The tubes then are centrifuged at 4°C, 2 000 x g, for 10 min. Place the pipette at midheight in the liquid, draw 3 mL, and transfer to another tube from which the contents are filtered through separate, prepared 0.22-μm syringe filters into fresh, cold tubes.

11.1.6 The contents of each tube then are diluted to the optimal human serum dilution (see 10.7) in cold tubes and kept on ice. Serum should be assayed within 1h for complement activity (see Section 12).

11.2 *Fibers or Solid Pieces*:

11.2.1 Assay for whole complement activation by solid fibers or pieces of material is similar to that detailed in 11.1 for powders, except that a defined amount of fiber or material (mg amounts, just enough to be covered fully by 0.1 mL serum) is put first into room temperature 13 x 100 tubes. Then 0.1 mL of serum is added to the M, NM, I_1, and I_2 tubes. Immediately the M and NM tubes are placed in a 37°C water bath while I_1 and I_2 are put on ice. At the end of 1h, the M and NM tubes are taken out of the 37°C water bath and also put on ice.

11.2.2 If the materials tested do not float, or if they form a firm pellet following the 2 000 x g centrifugation, the filtration step and the I_1 control may not be needed.

11.3 *Assay Size and Conditions Tested*:

11.3.1 The preceding general format can be used to test differing amounts of material to yield dose-response curves, the same quantity exposed to 37°C for various periods of time (time course), or to compare C' activation by various materials.

NOTE 6—This procedure does not preclude exposure of volumes of serum other than 100 μL to materials where the size or shape could not be tested in 13 x 100 disposable glass tubes.

11.3.2 Since each condition should be assayed for % specific hemolysis, which requires determination of % total hemolysis (Ab + RBC + HS) and % nonspecific hemolysis (RBC + HS), and each condition is assayed in triplicate, it is recommended that the total number of test samples to be assayed not exceed ten/experiment/technician (so as to not exceed final assay size of around 100 tubes.)

12. Procedure B—Assay of Serum for Complement Depletion

12.1 Procedure B is used to assay serum, which previously has been exposed to a material (Procedure A) for possible depletion of whole complement activity.

12.2 All conditions are assayed in triplicate, using three 13×100 disposable glass test tubes/condition. Tubes are numbered in advance. Conditions include total lysis, no complement (no C'), tests (dilutions of human serum—HS) with and without hemolysin (three tubes each), and no RBC (at highest concentration of serum used). All reagents, tubes, and manipulations are done ice-cold, with tubes held in a rack on ice.

12.3 Addition of washed RBC, and then hemolysin is conducted as directed in 10.2 and 10.3.

12.4 To the no-C' tubes, 1.0 mL of BBS-GM is added. To all except the "total lysis" tubes, 0.5 mL of cold BBS-GM is added. Then, 0.5 mL from each of the test or control condition tubes from the material exposure step, which are being held on ice and already are diluted to the optimal human serum concentration (see 10.7), is added to each of three tubes containing hemolysin-sensitized RBC and each of three tubes containing nonsensitized RBC.

12.5 The tubes then are treated as detailed in 9.6-9.9.

13. Report Section and Data Analysis

13.1 Incubation of serum not exposed to materials at 37°C (tube NM) may result in reduction in complement hemolytic activity compared to serum kept on ice (I_2). If a filtration step is needed (controlled for by the ice-1 tube, I_1), significant reduction from I_2 also may be seen in I_1.

13.2 At a minimum, materials should be tested in triplicate in Procedure A, with each of the three exposure tubes from Procedure A being assayed in triplicate in Procedure B. This allows demonstration of significant differences between the means of different conditions despite intertube assay variation. If small differences are being studied, the number of replicate tubes for each condition in Procedure A may need to be increased to five or more.

13.3 Significant depletion of control hemolytic activity in Procedure B denotes whole complement activation by test materials in Procedure A.

13.4 Differences in hemolysis are considered significant at $p \leq 0.05$, as calculated by an appropriate statistical test, such as ANOVA. Results may be presented as a bar graph displaying each condition as a mean and standard deviation.

14. Keywords

14.1 biocompatibility; blood compatibility; whole complement testing

APPENDIX

(Nonmandatory Information)

X1. RATIONALE

X1.1 The primary purpose of this practice is to describe a simple, inexpensive functional test to screen serum for complement activation by blood-contacting materials. Though serum is not the same as the plasma to which a material is exposed in vivo, artificially collected plasma, that is, with anticoagulant, is a poor choice because of the interference of these anticoagulants with the complement activation process.

X1.2 It is well recognized that complement activation is an important defense mechanism of the host; however, complement activation by material components of blood-contacting devices may be harmful to the host.

X1.3 Complementology has been an active research area for many years; however, the importance of chronic local complement activation on material/device function and actual impact on patient health is largely unknown. Many investigators have developed tests for whole complement functional activity, depletion of specific complement components, or generation of specific complement split products. Other validated test methods may be substituted for the functional whole complement-depletion assay described here. If immunological assays for individual complement pathway components are used, consideration should be given as to whether component depletion is by nonspecific binding to a material or by pathway activation.

X1.4 The procedure as presented is intended as a routine screening procedure. It is not to be represented as being the most sensitive nor the most specific procedure for assessing the complement-activation potential of all materials in all applications. Substances that activate weakly might still generate enough relevant split products (C3a, C5a, etc.) to cause a local inflammatory response but not be reflected by significant change in whole complement activity. The results obtained with this practice are intended to be used in conjunction with the results of other tests in assessing the blood compatibility of the test material.

REFERENCES

(1) Giclas, P.C., "Complement Tests," *Manual of Clinical Laboratory Immunology*, fifth edition, eds N.R. Rose, E.C. de Macario, J.D. Folds, H.C. Lane, and R.M. Nakamura, ASM Press, 1997, pp. 181–186.

(2) Gee, A.P., "Molecular Titration of Components of the Classical Complement Pathway," *Methods in Enzymology*, Vol 93, Immunochemical Techniques, eds J.J. Langone, H.V. Vunakis, Academic Press, 1983, pp. 339–375.

(3) United States Drug Enforcement Agency, Washington, DC.

(4) Lin, W-Q., White, Jr., K.L., "Complement Assays to Assess Immunotoxicity," *Methods in Immunotoxicology*, Vol I, eds G.R. Burleson, J.H. Dean, and A.E. Munson, Wiley-Liss, 1995, pp. 357–375.

Designation: F 1992 – 99

Standard Practice for Reprocessing of Reusable, Heat-Stable Endoscopic Accessory Instruments (EAI) Used with Flexible Endoscopes[1]

This standard is issued under the fixed designation F 1992; the number immediately following the designation indicates the year of original adoption or, in the case of revision, the year of last revision. A number in parentheses indicates the year of last reapproval. A superscript epsilon (ϵ) indicates an editorial change since the last revision or reapproval.

1. Scope

1.1 This practice covers reusable, heat-stable endoscopic accessory instruments (EAI) designed to be inserted into flexible endoscopes and clearly defined in the user instructions as devices intended for reuse among patients. The EAIs covered by this practice may or may not have lumens or loosely joined surfaces, may or may not have access ports for flushing, and may or may not be capable of being completely disassembled prior to reprocessing.

1.2 This practice is not intended to be applied to the reprocessing of single-use, disposable EAIs specifically designed and labeled as such by their manufacturers.

1.3 This practice is not intended to address reprocessing of heat-sensitive EAIs, for example, those not capable of withstanding heat sterilization. Reprocessing of each heat-sensitive EAI must be considered on an individual basis according to specific instructions from the manufacturers of the EAI and the low-temperature sterilization device.

1.4 This practice is intended to complement, not replace, the instructions provided by product manufacturers. EAI manufacturers should provide properly validated instruction and labeling necessary for users to understand the basic design, specifications, nomenclature, and components of specific accessories and to properly inspect, prepare, use, reprocess, and store these instruments.

1.5 Endoscopic technique and the medical aspects of endoscopy are not covered in this practice.

1.6 This practice details the basic steps necessary to reprocess a heat-stable EAI and render it patient-ready.

1.7 A patient-ready EAI is one that has been thoroughly cleaned using a validated cleaning procedure, rinsed with water to remove residual detergent, lubricated (if necessary) and drained to remove excess lubricant, dried, packaged, heat sterilized and stored to prevent from being compromised sterility before use.

1.8 This practice describes only manual reprocessing and does not address cleaning of an EAI by an automated reprocessing device.

1.9 To ensure the proper adherence to this practice, reprocessing personnel should meet certain requirements as specified in 5.5 to 5.7.

1.10 This practice does not address the steps necessary for the reprocessing of flexible endoscopes (see Practice F 1518).

1.11 *This standard does not purport to address all of the safety concerns, if any, associated with its use. It is the responsibility of the user of this standard to establish appropriate safety and health practices and to determine the applicability of regulatory limitations prior to use.*

2. Referenced Documents

2.1 *ASTM Standards:*

F 1518 Practice for Cleaning and Disinfection of Flexible Fiberoptic and Video Endoscopes Used in the Examination of the Hollow Viscera[2]

3. Terminology

3.1 *Definitions of Terms Specific to this Standard:*

3.1.1 *clean, adj*—visibly free from external debris after a thorough, manufacturer-validated regimen.

3.1.2 *critical medical device, n*—an instrument that may be introduced directly into the bloodstream or into other normally sterile areas of the body, that is, an invasive device.

3.1.3 *endoscopic accessory instrument, EAI, n*—medical instrument designed to be inserted into a flexible endoscope.

3.1.3.1 *Discussion*—EAIs may be critical- or semi-critical devices. EAIs may or may not have lumens, porous or loosely joined surfaces, or access ports for flushing and may or may not be capable of being completely disassembled during reprocessing.

3.1.4 *flexible endoscope, n*—a flexible tubular instrument that utilizes fiberoptic or video imaging technology to examine the interior of a canal or hollow viscus.

3.1.5 *heat-stable medical device, n*—an instrument capable of withstanding sterilization using a heat-based process.

3.1.6 *lubrication, n*—the application of a substance used to reduce friction or wear.

3.1.7 *manual cleaning, n*—removal of debris from an instrument by hand using detergent solution, cleaning devices

---

[1] This practice is under the jurisdiction of ASTM Committee F-4 on Medical and Surgical Materials and Devices and is the direct responsibility of Subcommittee F 04.35 on GI Endoscopes.

Current edition approved October 10, 1999. Published January 2000.

[2] *Annual Book of ASTM Standards*, Vol 13.01.

such as brushes, cloths, and irrigating devices, and water for rinsing.

3.1.8 *patient-ready, adj*—term used to describe endoscopic accessory instrument that, following prior patient use, has undergone an appropriate reprocessing protocol, including heat sterilization, to render it safe, as established by contemporary professional standards, for use on a subsequent patient; an operational check to ensure proper functionality is an essential component of preparing the EAI for reuse.

3.1.9 *reprocessing, n*—the precise sequence of cleaning, lubricating (if necessary), and sterilizing steps that, when performed properly and completely, will assure an endoscopic accessory instrument is patient-ready.

3.1.10 *reusable, adj*—instrument designed and validated by the manufacturer to be used more than once, provided that after each use, an appropriate reprocessing protocol and functionality check is performed.

3.1.11 *semi-critical medical device, n*—an instrument intended to contact only mucous membranes or non-intact skin during use.

3.1.12 *sterilization, n*—the complete elimination or destruction of all forms of microbial life, including high numbers of bacterial spores.

3.1.12.1 *Discussion*—In this standard, the only methods of sterilization considered are heat-based, for example, saturated steam under pressure (a steam autoclave) or a forced-air dry heat oven certified for medical use.

3.1.13 *ultrasonic cleaning, n*—a process in which ultra-high frequency sound waves are converted into mechanical vibrations capable of cleaning via a process called cavitation.

3.1.13.1 *Discussion*—During cavitation, microscopic bubbles in the cleaning solution implode (burst inward), resulting in a vacuum action that pulls soil and debris away from the surface of items being cleaned.

4. Summary of Practice

4.1 Each brand, type, and model of EAI has unique specifications, nomenclature, interior design, function, and components.

4.2 Most EAIs are critical medical devices because they come into direct contact with the bloodstream, enter normally sterile areas of the body, or break normally intact mucosal surfaces.

4.3 To prevent patient-to-patient transmission of infection, heat-stable EAIs should be thoroughly cleaned, rinsed, lubricated if necessary, dried, packaged, and sterilized using a heat-based process, for example, a steam autoclave or a forced-air dry heat oven.

4.4 After sterilization, a packaged EAI should be stored in a limited-access, well-ventilated area that provides protection from dust, moisture, and extremes of temperature and humidity so as not to compromise sterility before use.

4.5 Before use, the EAI should be tested for functionality.

5. Significance and Use

5.1 EAIs may have design features such as coiled metal sheaths, pivoting joints, opposed surfaces, and internal lumens or wires which make visual inspection for cleanliness difficult if not impossible.

5.2 By nature of their design requirements, EAIs are more difficult to reprocess than many other types of medical instruments.

5.3 Because EAIs are used to diagnose and treat disease in both immunocompetent and immunocompromised individuals, care must be taken to ensure that only patient-ready devices are used for examination.

5.4 The use of EAIs in patients having diagnosed or suspected infections such as hepatitis B, hepatitis C, or human immunodeficiency virus (HIV) is not contraindicated. Further, EAIs need not be dedicated for use only in these patients.

5.5 Persons responsible for reprocessing must understand the specifications, nomenclature, function of component parts, and interior design of EAIs in order to render them patient-ready.

5.6 Persons responsible for reprocessing EAIs should follow this practice and associated labeling and instructions from manufacturers after each endoscopic procedure to ensure that the EAI will be patient-ready.

5.7 Reprocessing of EAIs should be the specific responsibility of appropriately trained personnel. Temporary employees without the requisite training should not be given these responsibilities.

5.7.1 The responsibility for reprocessing of EAIs should not be delegated from person to person unless each has the appropriate training for the position.

5.7.2 Reprocessing personnel should have the ability to read, understand, and implement instructions from manufacturers and regulatory agencies as they relate to EAI reprocessing.

5.7.3 Reprocessing personnel should have the opportunity to become completely familiar with the mechanical aspects of the devices. They may gain this knowledge through study of the manufacturer's information and demonstration by representatives.

5.7.4 Reprocessing personnel should be made fully aware of the potential chemical and infectious hazards for patients and health care personnel associated with the reprocessing of EAIs. Training should include:

5.7.4.1 A thorough background in infection control principles and concepts based on written in-house infection control procedures.

5.7.4.2 A thorough background regarding the potential for negative patient outcomes resulting from lapses in compliance with written reprocessing guidelines,

5.7.4.3 Familiarization with OSHA regulations and in-house policies regarding the appropriate and safe handling of chemical reprocessing agents and equipment used during reprocessing of EAIs, and

5.7.4.4 Information on the safe handling of EAIs contaminated with patient tissue and fluids after use, including familiarization with principles and practices of standard (universal) precautions.

NOTE 1—Although healthcare workers and patients may benefit from adhering to the regulatory guidelines issued by federal and state Occupational Safety and Health Administration (OSHA) agencies, these guidelines are directed only toward healthcare worker safety and health. They may not be sufficiently inclusive for optimum safety and health of patients. Therefore, contemporary infection control guidelines should be consulted in addition to OSHA guidelines.

5.8 This practice is not intended to replace the reprocessing instruction provided by the manufacturers of EAIs or suggest specific equipment or chemical reagents to be used for reprocessing. Rather, it is to be used together with manufacturers' instructions that provide specific instructions for specific products. See Appendix X1.1.

5.9 This practice is not intended to cover endoscopic techniques, patient care, or other medical aspects of flexible endoscopy.

5.10 This practice does not include instruction for reprocessing flexible endoscopes.

6. Reagents

6.1 *Air*—Air flow provided by a syringe or compressed air source. (Refer to the EAI manufacturer's instruction to avoid the use of excessively high air pressure)

6.2 *Detergent*—A low foaming, neutral pH detergent, with or without enzymes, used for initial soaking and manual cleaning that is compatible with EAIs and is specifically formulated for use with medical devices.

6.3 *Ultrasonic Cleaning Detergent*—A detergent that is compatible with EAIs and specifically formulated for use in an ultrasonic cleaner.

6.4 *Water*—Fresh, potable water.

NOTE 2—In areas where water hardness may result in scaling or corrosion of metal instruments, the use of distilled, deionized, or softened water should be considered as appropriate for rinsing and preparation of cleaning reagent dilutions.

6.5 *Lubricant*—A lubricant that is compatible with EAIs that require lubrication before sterilization and is specifically formulated for use with medical devices.

7. Equipment and Supplies

7.1 *Basins*—Must be large enough to totally immerse the EAIs without coiling too tightly. See the EAI manufacturer's instruction for minimum radius of coiling of specific accessories. Basins needed are:

7.1.1 Cleaning basin, and

7.1.2 Lubrication basin.

7.2 *Cleaning Tools*—Soft, lint-free cloth, brushes, adapters, sponges, syringes, and other manufacturer-recommended cleaning items.

7.3 *Personal Protective Equipment*:

7.3.1 *Gloves*—High-quality latex, butyl, or nitrile rubber gloves that fit properly and are of adequate length to prevent skin exposure to liquids.

7.3.1.1 Gloves must be changed at appropriate times to limit cross contamination and must be removed prior to leaving the designated reprocessing area. They must be discarded if they are cracked, peeling, punctured, or when their ability to function as a barrier has been otherwise compromised. Hands must be washed thoroughly with soap and water before each donning and after removal of gloves.

7.3.2 *Gowns*—Fluid impervious protective clothing must be worn when handling contaminated EAIs and when working with reprocessing chemicals.

7.3.2.1 Gowns used during EAI reprocessing must be removed prior to leaving the designated reprocessing area.

7.3.3 *Protective Eye Wear*—Face masks and protective eyewear or face shields should be worn to protect the face and eyes from contact with reprocessing chemicals and potentially infectious material.

7.4 *Ultrasonic Cleaner*—Must be large enough to totally immerse the EAIs without coiling them too tightly, and must be able to operate within a frequency and power range that will not damage the instruments. See the EAI manufacturer's instructions for specifications regarding the minimum radius of coiling of specific models, the required frequency range of the ultrasonic cleaner, and the maximum power of ultrasonic transducers.

7.5 *Sterilizer*—Must be a heat-based process (for example, a steam autoclave or forced-air dry heat oven) and capable of meeting the conditions for the sterilization cycle validated by the EAI manufacturer.

7.5.1 The sterilizer also should be used to dry the packaged EAIs at the conclusion of a moist heat sterilization cycle.

7.5.2 Biological and chemical (temperature/color change) monitoring of the sterilizer should be done routinely according to the facility's protocol or national standards, or both.

7.5.3 General operation, maintenance, and calibration of the sterilizer should be done according to the sterilizer manufacturer's instructions.

7.6 *Air Ventilation*—A well-ventilated area with between 8 and 10 air exchanges per hour to protect personnel from potentially hazardous fumes or chemical or biological aerosols.

8. Procedure

8.1 *Cleaning*:

8.1.1 *Manual Cleaning*:

8.1.1.1 Don all necessary personal protective equipment.

8.1.1.2 Prepare fresh aqueous detergent solutions for manual cleaning in accordance with the manufacturer's specifications, at the dilution strength recommended by the detergent manufacturer.

8.1.1.3 Immediately after removal of the EAI from the endoscope, completely submerge the EAI in the detergent solution. Do not permit the EAI to dry while contaminated with patient material.

8.1.1.4 Brush or wipe, or both, all debris from all assessable surfaces of the EAI using a clean, detergent-soaked, lint-free cloth or brush, or both.

8.1.1.5 If the EAI is equipped with a port that permits flushing of its internal lumen, inject fresh detergent solution into the port with a syringe until it exits the distal end and the solution is clear and free from visible patient material. Discard this solution after a single use.

8.1.1.6 If required, disassemble the EAI according to the manufacturer's instructions.

8.1.1.7 Activate the EAI through normal motions and working mechanisms to help expose all surfaces for manual cleaning and to dislodge residual patient material. Carefully clean all accessible surfaces and moving parts of the submerged EAI, taking care not to stress or damage those components.

8.1.1.8 Allow the EAI (and component parts) to soak in the detergent solution for the time and temperature specified by the detergent manufacturer. Soaking times may range in duration from a few minutes to several hours. Discard this solution after a single use.

8.1.1.9 Rinse the instrument (and component parts) under fresh running water.

8.1.1.10 If the EAI is equipped with a port that permits flushing of its internal lumen, inject water into the port with a syringe until it exits the distal end, until the solution is clear and free from visible foam or patient debris, or both.

8.1.2 *Ultrasonic Cleaning*:

8.1.2.1 Transfer the EAI (and component parts) to an ultrasonic cleaner containing an ultrasonic cleaning detergent solution recommended by the EAI manufacturer as being compatible with the instrument. If required, dilute the ultrasonic cleaning detergent solution in accordance with the recommendations of the detergent manufacturer.

8.1.2.2 Prepare fresh detergent solutions for ultrasonic cleaning in accordance with the manufacturer's specifications, at the dilution strength recommended by the detergent manufacturer. Change the solution at the end of the day or when visibly soiled.

8.1.2.3 If the EAI is equipped with a port that permits flushing of its internal lumen, inject detergent solution into the port with a syringe until it exits the distal end to ensure that the solution contacts all internal parts.

8.1.2.4 Ultrasonically clean the EAI (and component parts) at the frequency, power, and time recommended by the EAI manufacturer.

8.2 *Rinse After Cleaning*:

8.2.1 Remove the EAI (and component parts) from the ultrasonic cleaner and submerge in a basin for rinsing.

8.2.2 For an EAI equipped with a port that permits flushing of its internal lumen, inject three syringe volumes of fresh water into the port to ensure that residual detergent is removed. Discard this solution after a single use.

8.2.3 Purge excess water from the lumen with air.

8.2.4 Remove excess water from the exterior surfaces with a clean, lint-free cloth.

8.2.5 For an EAI requiring disassembly and for which the manufacturer's instructions indicate that the instrument can be sterilized in an assembled configuration, reassemble the component parts. If an instrument requiring disassembly cannot be reassembled prior to sterilization, then reassemble the sterilized parts immediately prior to use (see 8.8.1).

8.3 *Lubrication*:

8.3.1 Consult the reprocessing instruction of the EAI manufacturer to determine whether or not lubrication is required prior to sterilization. If lubrication is not required, proceed to 8.4.

8.3.2 If lubrication is required, refer to the lubricating agent's labeling for preparation and use instructions of the agent.

8.3.3 Immerse the instrument in the lubricant solution in the manner and time specified by the EAI manufacturer.

8.3.4 If the instrument is equipped with a port permitting flushing of its internal lumen, inject lubricant into the port with a syringe until it exits the distal end. Purge excess lubricant from the lumen using air.

8.3.5 Remove excess lubricant and dry the exterior surfaces with a clean, lint-free cloth.

8.4 *Inspection and Operational Check*—Closely inspect the EAI for damage and, if feasible, perform appropriate functional checks as indicated by the manufacturer to ensure instrument integrity and smooth operation (see 8.8.2).

8.5 *Heat-Based Sterilization*:

8.5.1 Consult the EAI manufacturer's instruction regarding the recommended sterilization methodology (that is, gravity displacement or prevacuum steam sterilization, forced-air dry heat oven). It is necessary to employ a heat sterilization methodology that is properly maintained, biologically monitored according to institution protocol or national standards, or both, and for which quality assurance logs of operational parameters (for example, time and temperature charts) are kept.

8.5.2 Place the EAI in the type of packaging material and package configuration recommended by the manufacturer of the sterilizer. Refer to the EAI manufacturer's instructions regarding the minimum radius of curvature, as coiling a flexible EAI too tightly will damage the device.

8.5.3 Place a fresh color change heat process indicator strip inside each package, or place a strip of process indicator tape on the external surface of the package. Seal the packaging and label it appropriately for subsequent identification and record keeping.

8.5.4 Place the sealed packaging into the sterilizer in the manner specified by the sterilizer manufacturer.

8.5.5 Sterilize the EAI using a cycle recommended by the EAI manufacturer. A steam sterilization cycle should include a drying phase that permits complete drying of the sterile packaging prior to handling. This drying may be accomplished either by using a distinct phase of the sterilization cycle or by leaving the packages for the necessary time at the end of the cycle with the autoclave door slightly ajar.

8.6 *Inspection Before Storage*—Confirm that the sterile packaging is free from tears and is sealed. If tears or inadequate sealing, or both, are detected, remove the EAI from the package, repackage and resterilize appropriately.

8.7 *Storage*—After removal of the packaged instruments from the sterilizers, store in a limited-access, well-ventilated area that provides protection from dust, moisture, and extremes of temperature and humidity.

8.8 *Assembly, Inspection and Operational Check*:

8.8.1 If an instrument requiring disassembly could not be reassembled prior to sterilization, reassemble in a hygienic manner on a clean work surface with fresh gloves immediately prior to use.

8.8.2 If not done during reprocessing, perform appropriate functional checks as indicated by the manufacturer to ensure instrument integrity and smooth operation.

9. Keywords

9.1 cleaning; endoscopic accessory instrument (EAI); flexible endoscope; heat stable instrument; heat sterilization; reprocessing; reusable; ultrasonic cleaning

APPENDIX

(Nonmandatory Information)

X1. RATIONALE

X1.1 Manufacturers of heat-stable EAIs provide reprocessing instruction for each type/model produced. These have not been standardized in the past. Although certain professional organizations have also produced guidelines that address reprocessing of EAIs, these guidelines also have not been standardized. This has led to confusion among users of the devices as to how to properly care for the instrumentation. Table X1.1 gives examples of these types of devices.

X1.2 Virtually all cases of patient infection or cross-contamination reported in the medical literature are the result of short cuts in reprocessing or other breaks in proper reprocessing procedure (user non-compliance), use of inappropriate chemicals, or a misunderstanding of the consequences of eliminating important steps of the overall reprocessing protocol.

X1.3 Other important information:

X1.3.1 *Low-Sudsing Detergents*—The presence of excessive sudsing can prevent good fluid contact with the EAI being reprocessed.

X1.3.2 *Basin Size*—Coiling a flexible EAI too tightly will damage the device. Refer to the EAI manufacturer's instructions regarding the minimum radius of curvature.

X1.3.3 *Fume and Aerosol Controls*—Airborne material from basins containing cleaning solutions and from ultrasonic cleaners may contain toxic fumes or potentially infectious agents. Using proper physical barriers and engineering controls should minimize exposure of patients and medical staff to chemical fumes, splashes or aerosols.

X1.3.4 *Soft, Lint-Free Cloth*—Abrasive materials will damage EAIs. Lint may collect in and occlude internal lumens or moving parts, or both, of the instruments.

X1.3.5 *Personal Protective Equipment*:

X1.3.5.1 Gloves and gowns help prevent the healthcare worker from contact with contaminated instruments, patient secretions, blood, stool, and any reprocessing chemicals that may be irritating to the skin.

X1.3.5.2 Face masks and protective eye gear help prevent reprocessing chemicals and potentially infectious material from contaminating the face, mouth, or eyes.

X1.3.6 *Immediate Cleaning After Use*—Meticulous cleaning of EAIs immediately after use prevents drying of organic material on interior and exterior surfaces, removes large numbers of micoorganisms, and is a necessary prerequisite to any sterilization or other decontamination procedure.

X1.3.7 *Disassembly*—EAIs designed to be disassembled and then reassembled during reprocessing should be disassembled during preliminary cleaning in order to ensure complete removal of debris. Disassembly will permit contact of cleaning agents with formerly inaccessible regions of the assembled EAI. Residual patient material or other debris that is not removed from the instrument may cause a sterilization cycle to fail and may contain endotoxic or immunogenic substances and other material potentially harmful to the next patient.

X1.3.8 *Internal Lumens*—If an EAI has an internal lumen, it is important that the lumen be adequately contacted with detergent solution, rinsed to remove residual detergent, and dried to remove water used for rinsing prior to sterilization. EAIs that have lumens may have special fittings to permit the connection of cleaning adapters, for example, luer-lock syringes. Refer to the EAI manufacturer's instructions for specifics regarding the cleaning of EAI lumens.

X1.3.9 *Dilution of Solutions*—Dilution of reprocessing solutions such as detergents and ultrasonic cleaning solutions to the recommended strength should be performed very carefully, since excessive dilution may render the solution ineffective, while inadequate dilution may corrode EAIs or increase the difficulty of performing adequate rinsing.

X1.3.10 *Functional Checks*—Users should refer to manufacturers' instructions for reusable EAIs. Manufacturers must provide adequate instructions for functional checks to allow the user to confirm that its performance is acceptable for reuse.

X1.4 This practice represents current standard practice and is generic in nature. The steps in this practice may be modified should an alternative reprocessing procedure be developed and properly validated.

TABLE X1.1 Reusable, Heat-Stable Endoscopic Accessory Instruments (EAI) for Use with Flexible Fiberoptic and Video Gastrointestinal Endoscopes[A]

Description	Type
Biopsy forceps	Standard fenestrated
	Standard fenestrated with needle
	Fenestrated ellipsoid with needle
	Non-fenestrated with needle (large cup)
	Fenestrated with needle (large cup)
	Standard ellipsoid
	Fenestrated ellipsoid
	Fenestrated with side teeth
	Standard fenestrated for ultrasound
	Fenestrated V-shaped
	Alligator type
	Alligator jaws
	Rat tooth
	Oval static cup
	Oval rat tooth static cup
	Oval fenestrated rat tooth swing jaw
Rotatable biopsy forceps	Fenestrated
	Fenestrated with needle
	Rat tooth with alligator jaws (swinging type)
Hot biopsy forceps	Hot biopsy forceps
Grasping forceps	Alligator jaws
	Rat tooth
	Tripod type (for polyps)
	Pentapod (for polyps)
	Shark tooth
	W/V-shape jaw (for coins)
	Pelican type (for food obstruction)
	Basket type (for marbles, stones, seeds)
	Rubber tips (for needles, nails)
	Magnetic extractor (for metallic objects)
	Rat tooth with alligator jaws
	Rotatable rat tooth with alligator jaws
Cytology brushes	Reusable standard cytology brush
Aspiration biopsy needles	Reusable sheath for standard type needle
	Reusable sheath for side port type needle
Curette	Double-joint curette
Injector needles	Reusable sheath for injector needles
Measuring devices	Straight type
	Bendable tip
ERCP cannulae	Standard beveled tip
	Standard beveled stiff tip
	Long tapered tip
	Short tapered tip
	Metal tip
	Metal ball tip
	Indwelling type
Sphincterotomes	Push type
	Pull type
	Push and pull type
Mechanical lithotriptor	Mechanical lithotriptor
Stone retrieval baskets	Soft wire basket
	Hard wire basket
Suture cutters	Suture cutters
Surgical scissors	Surgical scissors
Washing pipes	Standard type
	Spray type
	Back flushing type
Electrosurgical snare	Crescent
	Hexagonal
	Oval
	Mini oval
	Oval with spike (thorn)
	Mini oval with spike (thorn)
Coagulation electrode	Ball point type
	Irrigation type
	Suction type
Clip fixing device for marking or hemostasis, or both	Clip fixing device for marking or hemostasis, or both
Diathermic pre-cutting knives	Needle type
	Flat type
Guideware	Guideware
Heat probe	Heat probe

[A]The descriptions and/or specific types of accessories listed in this appendix are only examples for reference purposes. The application of this standard practice includes, but is not limited to the instruments identified in this section of the appendix.

Designation: F 1993 – 99

Standard Classification of Human Search and Rescue Resources[1]

This standard is issued under the fixed designation F 1993; the number immediately following the designation indicates the year of original adoption or, in the case of revision, the year of last revision. A number in parentheses indicates the year of last reapproval. A superscript epsilon (ε) indicates an editorial change since the last revision or reapproval.

1. Scope

1.1 This classification is intended to aid search and rescue (SAR) managers in ordering resources for search and rescue incidents and to aid in communicating the types of tasks for which search and rescue crews have been trained.

1.2 This classification is intended as a supplement to the resource typing specifications of the Incident Command System and specifically as a means of typing human resources used in search and rescue activities.

1.3 This classification is suitable for classfying search and rescue crews for a wide variety of emergency management purposes.

1.4 This classification does not attempt to classify individuals or put forth standards of performance or training for individuals, nor is it meant to convey certification, skill proficiency or other measures of the level of performance of the resource. These qualifications are the responsibility of the local agencies responsible for utilizing the resource.

2. Referenced Documents

2.1 *ASTM Standards:*

F 1633 Guide for Techniques in Land Search[2]

F 1848 Classification of Search and Rescue Dog Crews/Teams[2]

2.2 *NFPA Standard:*

NFPA 1670 Operation and Training for Technical Rescue Incidents[3]

2.3 *International Fire Service Training Association Standard:*

ICS 420 Incident Command System Field Operations Guide[4]

3. Terminology

3.1 *Definitions*—Terminology not defined in this guide but referenced in the text can be found in Guide F 1633 and Classification F 1848.

3.1.1 *wilderness, n*—an uncultivated, uninhabited and natural area, usually but not necessarily, far from human civilizations and trappings.

3.1.1.1 *Discussion*—Wilderness areas often include collections of various environments such as forests, mountains, deserts, natural parks, animal refuges, rain forests and so forth. Depending upon terrain and environmental factors, a wilderness can be as little as a few minutes into the backcountry or less than a few feet off the roadway. **(NFPA 1670)**

4. Significance and Use

4.1 Typing of human resources in SAR is based upon the building and deployment of crews and teams for specific tasks. Because of the wide variety of tasks which are performed during SAR incidents, three common types of resources are acknowledged: search; rescue; and untrained resources.

4.2 The nature of typical search and rescue incidents in local jurisdictions and the financial resources of the local jurisdiction will dictate which types and kinds of resources will be maintained by the jurisdictions. Not all types or kinds of resources are expected to be available in all jurisdictions.

4.3 Kind classifications of human resources are based upon the specific environments in which SAR crews are asked to work. Specialties, of which there are many, within each of the kind classifications are not acknowledged by this classification. It is up to the jurisdiction ordering resources to ascertain whether additional subcategories of kind classifications are appropriate for the task at hand. These categories might include special capabilities for weather or terrain extremes, or for any other unusual circumstances or requirements.

4.4 SAR crews may be classified as more than one kind but not as more than one type.

5. Classification of Human Search and Rescue Resource Types

5.1 There are four types of human search and rescue resources, as follows:

5.1.1 *Type I*—Crews trained in both search and rescue techniques,

5.1.2 *Type II*—Crews trained in search techniques,

5.1.3 *Type III*—Crews trained in rescue techniques, and

5.1.4 *Type IV*—Crews untrained in either search or rescue techniques.

---

[1] This guide is under the jurisdiction of ASTM Committee F-32 on Search and Rescue and is the direct responsibility of Subcommittee F32.02 on Management and Operations.

Current edition approved October 10, 1999. Published December 1999.

[2] *Annual Book of ASTM Standards*, Vol 13.01.

[3] Available from National Fire Protection Association, 1 Batterymarch Park, PO Box, 9101, Quincy, MA 02269–9101.

[4] Available from the International Fire Service Training Association, Fire Protection Publications, Oklahoma State University, Stillwater, OK 74078.

6. Classification of Human Search and Rescue Resource Kinds

6.1 There are twelve kinds of human search and rescue resources, as follows:

6.1.1 *Kind A*—Wilderness; crew/team trained to work in wilderness areas of varied terrain,

6.1.2 *Kind B*—Urban; crew/team trained to work in urban areas,

6.1.3 *Kind C*—Mountainous; crew/team trained to work in mountainous and alpine terrain and with both high and low angle rescue systems,

6.1.4 *Kind D*—Disaster/collapsed structure; crew/team trained to work in failed manmade structures and natural debris fields (including confined spaces),

6.1.5 *Kind E*—Inland water; crew/team trained to work in and along bodies of water including swift-water and ice,

6.1.6 *Kind F*—Marine water; crew/team trained to work in and along oceans,

6.1.7 *Kind G*—Cave; crew/team trained to work in the confined spaces of caves,

6.1.8 *Kind H*—Mine; crew/team trained to work in mines,

6.1.9 *Kind I*—Avalanche; crew/team trained to work in and around avalanche debris fields,

6.1.10 *Kind J*—Evidence/cadaver; crew/team trained to search for inanimate objects and human remains,

6.1.11 *Kind K*—Aircraft; crew/team trained to search for missing aircraft, and

6.1.12 *Kind L*—Unclassified; a search or rescue crew that does not have any of the above specialties.

7. Keywords

7.1 incident command system; resource typing

The American Society for Testing and Materials takes no position respecting the validity of any patent rights asserted in connection with any item mentioned in this standard. Users of this standard are expressly advised that determination of the validity of any such patent rights, and the risk of infringement of such rights, are entirely their own responsibility.

This standard is subject to revision at any time by the responsible technical committee and must be reviewed every five years and if not revised, either reapproved or withdrawn. Your comments are invited either for revision of this standard or for additional standards and should be addressed to ASTM Headquarters. Your comments will receive careful consideration at a meeting of the responsible technical committee, which you may attend. If you feel that your comments have not received a fair hearing you should make your views known to the ASTM Committee on Standards, at the address shown below.

Designation: F 2002 – 01a

Standard Terminology Relating to Anesthesia and Respiratory Equipment[1]

This standard is issued under the fixed designation F 2002; the number immediately following the designation indicates the year of original adoption or, in the case of revision, the year of last revision. A number in parentheses indicates the year of last reapproval. A superscript epsilon (ε) indicates an editorial change since the last revision or reapproval.

INTRODUCTION

Consistent use of terminology contributes to improved safety and performance of anesthetic and respiratory care equipment by helping manufacturers, operators, and users communicate more effectively. It is expected that this terminology will be used on labels and markings on equipment and documents that accompany equipment. If other terminology is used on labels or markings on equipment or documents that accompany equipment, or both, that terminology should be defined in the accompanying documents.

1. Scope

1.1 This terminology covers terms, symbols, and abbreviations associated with anesthesia and respiratory care equipment.

2. Referenced Documents

2.1 *ASTM Standards:*

F 896 Specification for Flexible Fiberoptic Bronchoscopes[2]

F 920 Specification for Minimum Performance and Safety Requirements for Resuscitators Intended for Use with Humans[2]

F 927 Specification for Pediatric Tracheostomy Tubes[2]

F 960 Specification for Medical and Surgical Suction and Drainage Systems[2]

F 965 Specification for Rigid Laryngoscopes for Tracheal Intubation—Hook-on Fittings for Laryngoscope Handles and Blades with Lamps[2]

F 984 Specification for Cutaneous Gas Monitoring Devices for Oxygen and Carbon Dioxide[2]

F 1054 Specification for Conical Fittings of 15-mm and 22-mm Sizes[2]

F 1100 Specification for Ventilators Intended for Use in Critical Care[2]

F 1101 Specification for Ventilators Intended for Use During Anesthesia[2]

F 1161 Specification for Minimum Performance and Safety Requirements for Components and Systems of Anesthesia Gas Machines[2]

F 1195 Specification for Rigid Laryngoscopes for Tracheal Intubation—Hook-on Fittings for Fiberilluminated Blades and Handles[2]

F 1204 Specification for Anesthesia Reservoir Bags[2]

F 1205 Specification for Anesthesia Breathing Tubes[2]

F 1208 Specification for Minimum Performance and Safety Requirements for Anesthesia Breathing Systems[2]

F 1218 Specification for Bronchoscopes (Rigid)[2]

F 1242 Specification for Cuffed and Uncuffed Tracheal Tubes[2]

F 1243 Specification for Tracheal Tube Connectors[2]

F 1343 Specification for Anesthetic Equipment—Scavenging Systems for Anesthetic Gases[2]

F 1415 Specification for Pulse Oximeters[2]

F 1452 Specification for Minimum Performance and Safety Requirements for Components and Systems of Anesthetic Gas Monitors[2]

F 1456 Specification for Capnometers[2]

F 1462 Specification for Oxygen Analyzers[2]

F 1463 Specification for Alarm Signals in Medical Equipment Used in Anesthesia and Respiratory Care[2]

F 1464 Specification for Oxygen Concentrators for Domiciliary Use[2]

F 1573 Specification for Anesthetic Equipment—Oropharyngeal and Nasopharyngeal Airways[2]

F 1590 Specification for Tracheostomy Tube Connectors[2]

F 1627 Specification for Tracheostomy Tubes—Pediatric Tracheostomy Tubes[2]

F 1628 Specification for Labeling and Marking of Cuffed and Uncuffed Tracheal Tubes and Related Treatments Intended for Use During Laser Surgery[2]

F 1666 Specification for Adult Tracheostomy Tubes[2]

2.2 *Other Documents:*

ISO 8835-2:1993 Inhalational anaesthesia systems—Part 2: Anaesthetic circle breathing systems[3]

---

[1] This terminology is under the jurisdiction of ASTM Committee F29 on Anesthetic and Respiratory Equipment and is the direct responsibility of Subcommittee F29.16 on Terminology.

Current edition approved March 10, 2001. Published April 2001. Originally published as F2002–00. Last previous edition F2002–01.

[2] *Annual Book of ASTM Standards*, Vol 13.01.

[3] Available from American National Standards Institute, 11 W. 42nd St., 13th Floor, New York, NY 10036.

ISO 9703-1:1992 Anaesthetic and respiratory alarm signals—Part 1: Visual alarm signals[3]

ISO 9360:1992 Anaesthetic and respiratory equipment—Heat and moisture exchangers for use in humidifying respired gases in humans[3]

ISO /FDIS 9170-2 Terminal units for medical gas pipeline systems—Part 2: Terminal units for anaesthetic gas scavenging systems[3]

ISO Standards from TC 210 Quality Management and Corresponding General Aspects for Medical Devices[3]

ISO 4135:1995 Anaesthesiology—Vocabulary[3]

3. Terminology

3.1 *Definitions:*

adjustable pressure limiting valve (APL), *n*—operator-adjustable device intended to limit the maximum pressure in an anesthesia breathing system when it is part of the flow pathway of the breathing system, by controlling the rate of escape of gases from the system.

anesthesia breathing system, *n*—those inspiratory and expiratory pathways through which gas flows at respiratory pressures between the fresh gas inlet, the patient connection port, and the exhaust valve or port.

anesthesia gas supply device, *n*—assembly of components that controls and delivers all gas flows and agent concentrations in the fresh gas into the anesthesia breathing system. Note: it may include a flow adjustment control(s), a gas mixing system, and an anesthetic vapor delivery device(s).

anesthesia gas supply piping, *n*—all pipe work, including unions, from the unidirectional valve(s) in the pipeline inlet(s), the piping connecting the high pressure supply to the gas pressure-reducing device/system, and from the gas pressure-reducing device/system outlet to the flow adjustment control(s) and auxiliary gas outlet. It includes piping leading to and from pneumatic alarm device(s), pressure indicator(s), oxygen flush, anesthetic vapor delivery device(s), and piping leading to the common gas outlet.

anesthesia ventilator, *n*—ventilator designed to be used with or integral to an anesthesia breathing system. **F 1101**

anesthesia workstation, *n*—system for administration of anesthesia to patients. It consists of the anesthesia gas supply device, anesthesia ventilator, and associated monitoring, alarm, and protection device(s).

anesthetic-gas scavenging systems, *n*—complete systems that collect and remove the excess gases released from equipment used in administering anesthesia or exhaled by the patient during anesthesia for the purpose of conveying these gases to an appropriate place of discharge.

anesthetic vapor delivery device, *n*—device in which anesthetic agent is transformed from the liquid to the gaseous phase of controllable concentration.

circle breathing system, *n*—breathing system in which the direction of gas flow is through separate inspiratory and expiratory pathways that form a circle.

common gas outlet (fresh gas outlet), *n*—that port through which the dispensed mixture from the anesthesia gas supply device is delivered to the anesthesia breathing system.

control center, *n*—information system component of an anesthesia workstation mediating the centralized alarm prioritization and management strategy(ies).

decision support system, *n*—information system that provides output information intended to facilitate decision making by the operator.

editing, *v*—changing a recorded value, comment, annotation, event, or other information at any time after it has been made part of the record.

flow adjustment control, *n*—device or assembly that controls the flow of gas(es) or gas mixtures. Note: the flow adjustment control is often called the flow control valve.

flow indicator, *n*—device that indicates the volume of a specific gas or gas mixture passing through it in a unit of time. Note: the flow indicator is sometimes called a flowmeter.

gas mixing system, *n*—device or assembly that receives oxygen and other medical gas(es) and delivers a mixture of these gases in concentrations controllable by the operator.

information system, *n*—digital system collecting, displaying, or processing information from primary or secondary data sources or both. Note: examples includes AARKs and decision support systems.

infusion device, *n*—mechanical or electromechanical device regulating the flow of liquids to the patient under positive pressure. Note: the positive pressure may be generated either by a pump or by gravitational force.

legible, *adj*—discernible or identifiable to an operator with 6–6 (20/20) vision (corrected if necessary) from a distance of 1 m at a light level of 215 lux when viewing displayed qualitative or quantitative information, values, functions, or markings perpendicular to and including 15° above, below, left, and right of the normal line of sight of the operator.

lung ventilator, *n*—automatic device designed to augment or provide ventilation to a patient when connected to the patient's airway.

medical gas pipeline system, *n*—complete system that comprises a supply system, a monitoring and alarm system, a pipeline distribution system, and terminal units at the points where medical gases or vacuum may be required.

medium priority alarm, *n*—signal(s) indicating that prompt operator action is required.

monitoring device, *n*—device that measures and indicates the value of a variable. Note: examples of such devices are the airway pressure monitor and the exhaled volume monitor.

network, *n*—connection between two or more computers for the purpose of transferring data.

nonvolatile, *adj*—stored electronically in such a way that loss of all electrical power (normal and reserve) to the system or storage device will not alter the stored data.

operator, *n*—person handling the equipment.

positive end expiratory pressure (PEEP), *n*—positive airway pressure at the end of expiratory flow.

primary data source, *n*—monitoring device, delivery device, or operator input providing function or measured data via digital interfaces.

protection device, *n*—device that, without intervention of the operator, protects the patient from incorrect delivery of energy or substances. Note: such devices include the oxygen supply failure device and maximum pressure limitation device.

recorded data, *n*—captured data that is stored by a computer.

reserve electrical power supply, *n*—that portion of the equipment that supplies temporary electrical power in the event of interruption of the normal electrical supply.

secondary data source, *n*—information system that transmits data collected from primary data sources and other secondary data sources. Note 1: a secondary data source may have modular primary data sources as components. Note 2: digital data may be primary or secondary depending on whether it originates from within a multiport communication device or another digital source.

selector valve, *n*—device that permits the switching of the route taken by a fluid.

selector valve, *n*—*in anesthesia breathing systems,* device that is used to direct gases to an anesthesia reservoir bag or a ventilator intended for use during anesthesia.

selector valve, *n*—device that permits the switching of the route taken by a fluid.

sensor, *n*—part of the monitor that is sensitive to the variable being measured.

transducer, *n*—device for converting energy from one form to another. In measurements applications, a transducer senses energy related to a property of a substance and transforms it into a form that can be observed and interpreted as information about the substance, for example into an electrical signal for monitoring or recording.

user, *n*—authority responsible for the use and maintenance of equipment.

4. Keywords

4.1 anesthesia; anesthesia delivery; breathing systems; monitors; respiratory care equipment; respiratory equipment

Standard Guide for Accelerated Aging of Ultra-High Molecular Weight Polyethylene[1]

This standard is issued under the fixed designation F 2003; the number immediately following the designation indicates the year of original adoption or, in the case of revision, the year of last revision. A number in parentheses indicates the year of last reapproval. A superscript epsilon (ε) indicates an editorial change since the last revision or reapproval.

1. Scope

1.1 It is the intent of this guide to permit an investigator to investigate the oxidative stability of ultra-high molecular weight polyethylene (UHMWPE) materials as a function of processing and sterilization method. This guide describes a laboratory test method for accelerated aging of UHMWPE specimens and components for total joint prostheses. The UHMWPE is aged at elevated temperatures and, alternatively, at elevated partial pressures of oxygen, to accelerate oxidation of the material and thereby allow for the evaluation of its long-term chemical and mechanical stability.

1.2 Although the accelerated-aging test methods described by this guide will permit an investigator to compare the oxidative stability of UHMWPE, it is recognized that these test methods may not precisely simulate the degradative mechanisms for an implant during real-time shelf aging and implantation. However, these accelerated oxidation methods have been successfully used to rank UHMWPE materials for their long-term oxidative stability.

1.3 The accelerated aging test methods specified herein have been validated based on oxidation levels exhibited by certain shelf-aged UHMWPE components packaged in air and sterilized with gamma radiation. The methods have not been shown to be representative of shelf aging when the UHMWPE is packaged in an environment other than air. For example, these test methods have not been directly correlated with the shelf life of components that have been sealed in a low-oxygen package, such as nitrogen.

1.4 *This standard does not purport to address all of the safety concerns, if any, associated with its use. It is the responsibility of the user of this standard to establish appropriate safety and health practices and determine the applicability of regulatory limitations prior to use.*

2. Referenced Documents

2.1 *ASTM Standards:*

D 883 Terminology Relating to Plastics[2]

F 648 Specification of Ultra-High Molecular-Weight Polyethylene Powder and Fabricated Form Surgical Implants[3]

F 1714 Guide for Gravimetric Wear Assessment of Prosthetic Hip-Designs in Simulator Devices[3]

F 1715 Guide for Gravimetric Wear Assessment of Prosthetic Knee-Designs in Simulator Devices[3]

2.2 *ISO Standards:*

ISO 5834 Implants for surgery—Ultra-high molecular weight polyethylene[4]

ISO 14242 Implants for surgery—Wear of total hip joint prostheses[4]

ISO 14243 Implants for surgery—Wear of total knee joint prostheses[4]

3. Terminology

3.1 *Definitions*—For definitions of terms in this guide relating to plastics, refer to Terminology D 883. For definitions of terms in this guide relating to UHMWPE, refer to Specification F 648 and ISO 5834.

3.2 *Definitions of Terms Specific to This Standard:*

3.2.1 *oxidation, n*—the incorporation of oxygen into another molecule (for example, UHMWPE) by means of a chemical covalent bond.

3.2.2 *oxygen bomb, n*—a pressure vessel suitable for preconditioning of UHMWPE at an elevated temperature and partial pressure of oxygen.

4. Significance and Use

4.1 This guide summarizes test methods that may be used to accelerate the oxidation of UHMWPE components using elevated temperatures and, alternatively, elevated partial pressures of oxygen. Under real-time conditions, such as shelf aging and implantation, oxidative changes to UHMWPE after sterilization using high energy radiation may take months or years to produce changes that may result in deleterious mechanical performance. The test methods outlined in this guide permit the evaluation of oxidative stability in a relatively short period of time (for example, weeks).

4.2 This guide may also be used to precondition UHMWPE test specimens and joint replacement components prior to characterization of their physical, chemical, and mechanical

[1] This guide is under the jurisdiction of ASTM Committee F-4 on Medical and Surgical Materials and Devices and is the direct responsibility of Subcommittee F04.15 on Test Material Methods.

Current edition approved Jan. 10, 2000. Published April 2000.

[2] *Annual Book of ASTM Standards*, Vol 08.01.

[3] *Annual Book of ASTM Standards*, Vol 13.01.

[4] Available from American National Standards Institute, 11 W. 42nd St., 13th Floor, New York, NY 10036.

properties. In particular, this guide may be used for preconditioning of UHMWPE components prior to evaluation in a hip or knee joint wear simulator as outlined in Guide F 1714 (hip wear), Guide F 1715 (knee wear), ISO 14242 (hip wear), or ISO 14243 (knee wear), or combination thereof.

5. Apparatus and Materials

5.1 *UHMWPE Test Specimens*—The test specimens shall be prepared in final form in accordance with the requirements of any subsequent physical, chemical, or mechanical tests to be performed after preconditioning. For example, if the specimens will ultimately be subjected to hip joint simulation, they should be prepared in final form in accordance with Guide F 1714 and ISO 14242. Because the accelerated oxidation methods outlined in this guide result in inhomogeneous distribution of chemical, physical, and hence mechanical properties through the thickness of a preconditioned part, it is not recommended that finished test specimens be machined after preconditioning of (bulk) stock materials. Because this guide is not intended to reproduce the aging of UHMWPE that is stored in a low-oxygen environment, test specimens should be removed from their packaging prior to preconditioning.

5.2 *Preconditioning Chamber*—Accelerated oxidation (preconditioning) of the UHMWPE shall be conducted in a convection, air circulating oven that can maintain the desired temperature with an accuracy of ±2°C. The spatial variation of temperature within the oven shall be measured using thermocouples and verified to be less than ±1°C. The chamber will need to be sufficiently large to accommodate a pressure vessel, if it is desired to precondition the UHMWPE at an elevated partial pressure of oxygen. An oxygen bomb (pressure vessel) that is capable of maintaining the desired temperature with an accuracy of ±2°C by itself may be used.

NOTE 1—It may be desirable to use an oven with the capability of heating the test specimen at a controlled heating rate with an accuracy of ±0.1°C/min.

5.3 *Pressure Vessel*—When preconditioning UHMWPE at elevated partial pressures of oxygen, it will be necessary to enclose the specimens within a pressure vessel, also known as an oxygen bomb, capable of withstanding a static pressure of 690 kPa (100 psi). The pressure vessel shall be manufactured from stainless steel or aluminum. The pressure vessel shall be equipped with either a regulator or a safety release valve to maintain the internal pressure to the desired value, when at equilibrium, to an accuracy of ±7 kPa (±1 psi). Because oxygen-air mixtures will be maintained at elevated temperatures for weeks at a time, it is recommended that appropriate safety precautions be taken by a laboratory performing preconditioning at elevated partial pressures. For this reason, the use of a commercially available and properly validated oxygen bomb is recommended.

6. Preconditioning Test Methods

6.1 *Test Method A (Ambient Air Preconditioning)*—Conduct Test Method A in a suitable thermal chamber. Precondition test specimens at a constant temperature of 80°C for 3 weeks prior to subsequent testing.

NOTE 2—To maximize the extent and penetration of oxidative degradation into bulk hip or knee components using Test Method A, it is recommended that specimens be inserted into the thermal chamber while at room temperature, and that the chamber be elevated to the constant preconditioning temperature at a slow constant heating rate, ranging from 0.1 to 0.6°C/min (**1**).[5]

6.2 *Test Method B (Preconditioning at Elevated Partial Pressures of Oxygen)*—Conduct Test Method B using an oxygen bomb placed inside a suitable thermal chamber. Precondition test specimens at a constant temperature of 70°C and at an equilibrium pressure of 503 kPa (73 psi, 5 atmospheres) of pure oxygen for 2 weeks prior to subsequent testing.

6.3 Regardless of the preconditioning test method used (Test Method A or B), array the test specimens within the test chamber or oxygen bomb such that all relevant surfaces have equivalent access to oxygen during the test. For example, with hip and knee components, the articulating surface which may subsequently be subjected to wear simulation shall not be obstructed or covered by other parts or materials that might interfere with uniform access of the surface to oxygen.

6.4 For both Test Methods A and B, maintain the test chamber or oxygen bomb, or both, at ambient humidity. The user should be aware that adding water to the test chamber may affect the oxidation mechanism during the preconditioning process.

7. Report of Specimen Preparation and Test Conditions

7.1 It is important that details regarding the preparation of the test samples, the chronology of the preconditioning, the storage conditions for the test samples, and the test method used be recorded in a report.

7.2 *Test Sample Preparation*—Report the size, shape, and method of manufacture of the test samples. Report the type of resin used, the manufacturer/supplier of the UHMWPE, and any subsequent processes that were performed on the test articles after manufacture, such as sterilization or high-energy irradiation.

7.3 *Chronology*—Report the time at which the test specimens were manufactured, subsequently sterilized, and later preconditioned. Report the time that any subsequent analysis or testing was performed on the preconditioning items.

7.4 *Test Sample Storage Conditions*—It is important to document the storage conditions of the test samples before and after preconditioning. Report the environmental conditions (that is, storage in air versus nitrogen) and temperature under which the specimens were stored.

7.5 *Test Method*—Report the preconditioning test method that was used (A or B), the heating rate, the test temperature, and the test duration.

8. Keywords

8.1 aging; oxidation; preconditioning; stability; UHMWPE; UHMW PE; ultra-high molecular weight polyethylene

[5] The boldface numbers in parentheses refer to the list of references at the end of this standard.

APPENDIX

(Nonmandatory Information)

X1. Rationale

X1.1 Post-irradiation aging results in degradative changes to the physical, chemical, and mechanical properties of UHMWPE **(2, 3)**. Even under ambient conditions, oxidation of irradiated UHMWPE evolves at a slow pace, with a degradation rate measured in years **(2)**. As a result, preconditioning test methods have been developed in the past four years to accelerate the oxidation process in UHMWPE and thereby assess oxidative stability during a comparatively short time period.

X1.2 Oxidation of UHMWPE proceeds in a complex cascade of chemical reactions which may be accelerated by increasing the temperature or by increasing the concentration of available oxygen, or both **(4)**. Consequently, in several studies, post-irradiation aging has been simulated using a combination of thermal preconditioning and elevated oxygen partial pressures **(1, 5, 6)**. Despite the variation in test conditions reported by these studies, accelerated oxidation protocols have increasingly been employed not only to characterize the effects of gamma sterilization in air, but also to evaluate the oxidation resistance of UHMWPE sterilized by alternative methods.

X1.3 Accelerated oxidation test methods for UHMWPE are not without their limitations. Even though the protocols outlined in this guide are now widely used for preconditioning UHMWPE specimens prior to mechanical testing, the question remains as to whether or not the thermal techniques precisely recreate the morphology and mechanical properties of shelf-aged UHMWPE **(7, 8)**. Although research is still needed to elucidate the differences between thermal conditioning and long-term shelf-aging, this guide is intended to provide information about established test methods for evaluating the oxidative stability of UHMWPE specimens.

REFERENCES

(1) Sun, D.C., Stark, C., and Dumbleton, J.H., "Development of an Accelerated Aging Method for Evaluation of Long-Term Irradiation Effects on UHMWPE Implants," *Polymer Reprints*, Vol 35, 1994, pp. 969-970.

(2) Kurtz, S.M., Rimnac, C.M., and Bartel, D.L., "Degradation Rate of Ultra-High Molecular Weight Polyethylene," *Journal of Orthopaedic Research*, Vol 15, 1997, pp. 57-61.

(3) Currier, B.H., Currier, J.H., Collier, J.P., Mayor, M.B., and Scott, R.D., "Shelf Life and In Vivo Duration: Impacts on Performance of Tibial Bearings." *Clinical Orthopaedics and Related Research* Vol 342, 1997, pp. 111-22.

(4) Premnath, V., Harris, W.H., Jasty, M., and Merrill, E.W., "Gamma Sterilization of UHMWPE Articular Implants: An Analysis of the Oxidation Problem," *Biomaterials*, Vol 17, 1996, pp. 1741-1753.

(5) McKellop, H., Yeom, B., Sun, D.C., and Sanford, W.M., "Accelerated Aging of Irradiated UHMW Polyethylene for Wear Evaluations," *42nd Orthopedic Research Society*, Vol 21, 1996, p. 483.

(6) Sanford, W.M., and Saum, K.A., "Accelerated Oxidative Aging Testing of UHMWPE," *Transactions of the 41st Orthopedic Research Society*, Vol 20, 1995, p. 119.

(7) Greer, K.W., Schmidt, M.B., and Hamilton, J.V., "The Hip Simulator Wear of Gamma-Vacuum, Gamma-Air, and Ethylene Oxide Sterilized UHMWPE Following a Severe Oxidative Challenge," *Transactions of the 44th Orthopedic Research Society*, Vol 23, 1998, p. 52.

(8) Kurtz, S.M., Pruitt, L.A., Crane, D.J., and Edidin, A.A., "Evolution of Morphology in UHMWPE Following Accelerated Aging: The Effect of Heating Rates," *Journal of Biomedical Materials Research*, Vol 46, 1999, pp. 112-120.

Designation: F 2004 – 00

Standard Test Method for Transformation Temperature of Nickel-Titanium Alloys by Thermal Analysis[1]

This standard is issued under the fixed designation F 2004; the number immediately following the designation indicates the year of original adoption or, in the case of revision, the year of last revision. A number in parentheses indicates the year of last reapproval. A superscript epsilon (ε) indicates an editorial change since the last revision or reapproval.

1. Scope

1.1 This test method defines procedures for determining the transformation temperatures of nickel-titanium shape memory alloys.

1.2 The values stated in SI units are to be regarded as the standard.

1.3 *This standard does not purport to address all of the safety concerns, if any, associated with its use. It is the responsibility of the user of this standard to establish appropriate safety and health practices and to determine the applicability of regulatory limitations prior to use.*

2. Referenced Documents

2.1 *ASTM Standards:*

E 473 Terminology Relating to Thermal Analysis[2]

E 967 Practice for Temperature Calibration of Differential Scanning Calorimeters and Differential Thermal Analyzers[2]

E 1142 Terminology Relating to Thermophysical Properties[2]

F 2005 Terminology for Nickel-Titanium Shape Memory Alloys[3]

3. Terminology

3.1 Specific technical terms used in this test method are found in Terminologies E 473, E 1142, and F 2005.

4. Summary of Test Method

4.1 This test method involves heating and cooling a test specimen at a controlled rate in a controlled environment through the temperature interval of the phase transformation. The difference in heat flow between the test material and a reference material due to energy changes is continuously monitored and recorded. Absorption of energy due to a phase transformation in the specimen results in an endothermic peak on heating. Release of energy due to a phase transformation in the specimen results in an exothermic peak on cooling.

5. Significance and Use

5.1 Differential scanning calorimetry provides a rapid method for determining the transformation temperature(s) of nickel-titanium shape memory alloys.

5.2 This test method uses small, stress-free, annealed samples to determine whether a sample of nickel-titanium alloy containing nominally 54.5 to 56.5 % nickel by weight is austenitic or martensitic at a particular temperature. Since chemical analysis of these alloys does not have sufficient precision to determine the transformation temperature by measuring the nickel to titanium ratio of the alloy, direct measurement of the transformation temperature of an annealed sample of known thermal history is recommended.

5.3 This test method is useful for quality control, specification acceptance, and research.

5.4 Transformation temperatures derived from differential scanning calorimetry (DSC) may not agree with those obtained by other test methods due to the effects of strain and load on the transformation.

6. Interferences

6.1 Make sure the material to be tested is homogeneous since milligram sample quantities are used.

6.2 Take care in preparing the sample. Cutting and grinding can cause cold work, which affects the transformation temperature. Oxidation during heat treatment can change the thermal conductance of the sample.

6.3 Set the gas flow to provide adequate thermal conductivity in the test cell.

7. Apparatus

7.1 Use a differential scanning calorimeter capable of heating and cooling at rates up to 10°C/min and of automatically recording the differential energy input between the specimen and the reference to the required sensitivity and precision.

7.2 Use sample capsules or pans composed of aluminum or other inert material of high thermal conductivity.

7.3 Use nitrogen or helium gas purge supply. See 10.3.1.

7.4 Use an analytical balance with a capacity of 100 mg capable of weighing to the nearest 0.1 mg.

8. Sampling

8.1 Use a sample size of 20 to 50 mg. Cut the sample to

[1] This test method is under the jurisdiction of ASTM Committee F04 on Medical and Surgical Materials and Devices and is the direct responsibility of Subcommittee F04.15 on Material Test Methods.

Current edition approved Jan. 10, 2000. Published April 2000.

[2] *Annual Book of ASTM Standards*, Vol 14.02.

[3] *Annual Book of ASTM Standards*, Vol 03.01.

maximize surface contact with the (DSC) sample pan.

8.2 Anneal the sample at 800°C minimum, for a 15-min minimum in vacuum of inert atmosphere, or in air with adequate protection from oxidation. Rapidly cool the sample to prevent precipitation of phases which may change transformation temperature of the alloy.

8.3 Clean the sample of all foreign materials such as cutting fluid. If the sample is oxidized in heat treatment, grind, polish, or etch the sample to remove the oxide. Take care to avoid cold working the sample as this will change its thermal response. Slight oxidation is permissible but remove all heavy oxide scale.

9. Calibration

9.1 Calibrate the temperature axis of the instrument using the same heating rate, purge gas, and flow rate as those used for analyzing the specimen in accordance with Practice E 967.

10. Procedure

10.1 Place the sample on the sample pan and place the pan on the test pedestal.

10.2 Place an empty pan on the reference pedestal.

10.3 Turn on the purge gas at a flow rate of 10 to 50 mL/min.

10.3.1 Use helium or nitrogen as the purge gas for the sample chamber.

10.3.2 Use a dry air, helium, nitrogen, or oxygen cover gas. The dry gas shall have a dew point below the lowest temperature of the cooling cycle.

10.4 Run the cooling and heating program.

10.4.1 Use the heating and cooling rates of 10 ± 0.5°C/min.

10.4.2 Heat the sample from room temperature to a temperature of at least A_f + 30°C; hold at temperature for a time sufficient to equilibrate the sample with the furnace.

10.4.3 Cool the sample to a temperature of below M_f – 30°C; hold for a time sufficient to equilibrate the sample with the furnace. Then, heat the sample to a temperature of at least A_f + 30°C.

10.5 *Data Acquisition*—Record the resulting curve from the heating and cooling program from A_f + 30°C to M_f – 30°C.

11. Graphical Data Reduction

11.1 Draw the baselines for the cooling and heating portions of the curve as shown in Fig. 1.

11.2 Draw the tangents to the cooling and heating spikes through the inflection points as shown in Fig. 1. If a computer program is used to construct the tangents, care must be taken in locating the tangent points.

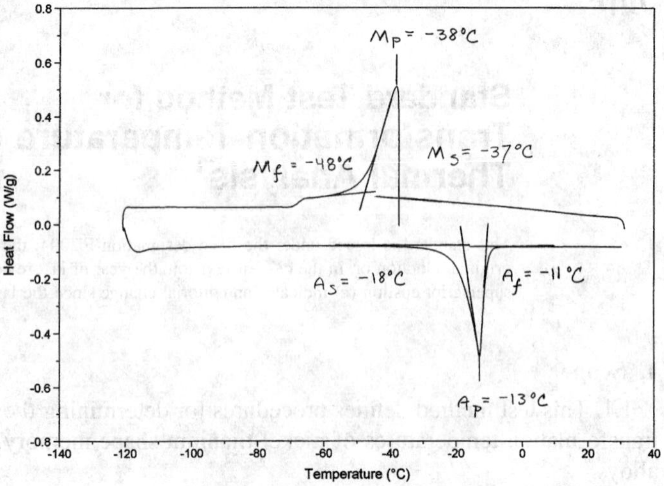

FIG. 1 DSC Curve for NiTi

11.3 Obtain M_s, M_f, A_s, and A_f as the graphical intersection of the baseline with the extension of the line of maximum inclination of the appropriate peak of the curve as shown in Fig. 1. A_p is the peak minimum of the endothermic curve, and M_p is the peak maximum of the exothermic curve. Read A_p and M_p directly from the graph as shown in Fig. 1.

12. Report

12.1 Report the following information with the test results:

12.1.1 Complete identification and description of the material tested including the specification and lot number.

12.1.2 Description of the instrument used for the test.

12.1.3 Statement of mass, dimensions, and geometry.

12.1.4 Material for the specimen pan and temperature program.

12.1.5 Description of the temperature calibration procedure.

12.1.6 Identification of the specimen environment by gas, flow rate, purity and composition.

12.1.7 Results of the transformation measurements using the nomenclature in accordance with Terminology F 2005. Temperature results should be reported to the nearest 1°C.

13. Precision and Bias

13.1 Precision and bias will be the subject of a future test program.

14. Keywords

14.1 differential scanning calorimeter; DSC; nickel-titanium alloy; NiTi; Nitinol; shape memory alloy; TiNi; transformation temperature

Standard Terminology for Nickel-Titanium Shape Memory Alloys[1]

This standard is issued under the fixed designation F 2005; the number immediately following the designation indicates the year of original adoption or, in the case of revision, the year of last revision. A number in parentheses indicates the year of last reapproval. A superscript epsilon (ε) indicates an editorial change since the last revision or reapproval.

1. Scope

1.1 This terminology is a compilation of definitions of terms used in ASTM documents relating to nickel-titanium shape memory alloys used for medical devices. This terminology includes only those terms for which ASTM either has standards or which are used in ASTM standards for nickel-titanium shape memory alloys. It is not intended to be an all-inclusive list of terms related to shape memory alloys.

1.2 Definitions that are similar to those published by another standards body are identified with abbreviations of the name of that organization, for example, ICTAC is the International Confederation for Thermal Analysis and Calorimetry.

1.3 A definition is a single sentence with additional information included in a discussion. This standard is reviewed every five years, and the year of the last revision is appended.

2. Referenced Documents

2.1 *ASTM Standards:*

E 7 Terminology Relating to Metallography[2]

E 473 Terminology Relating to Thermal Analysis[3]

3. Terminology

alloy phase, *n*—*in a shape memory alloy*, the crystal structure stable at a particular temperature and stress.

anneal, *v*—to heat treat in order to remove the effects of cold-working or aging heat treatments, or both.

DISCUSSION—Annealing shall be at a minimum temperature of 800°C for a minimum time of 15 min followed by rapid cooling by water quenching, gas quenching, or air cooling.

austenite, *n*—the highest temperature phase in Ni-Ti shape memory alloys.

DISCUSSION—In Ni-Ti the high-temperature phase has the B2 body-centered cubic crystal structure.

austenite finish temperature (A_f), *n*—the temperature at which the martensite to austenite transformation is completed on heating in a single-stage transformation (Fig. 1) or the temperature at which the R-phase to austenite transformation is completed on heating in a two-stage transformation (Fig. 2).

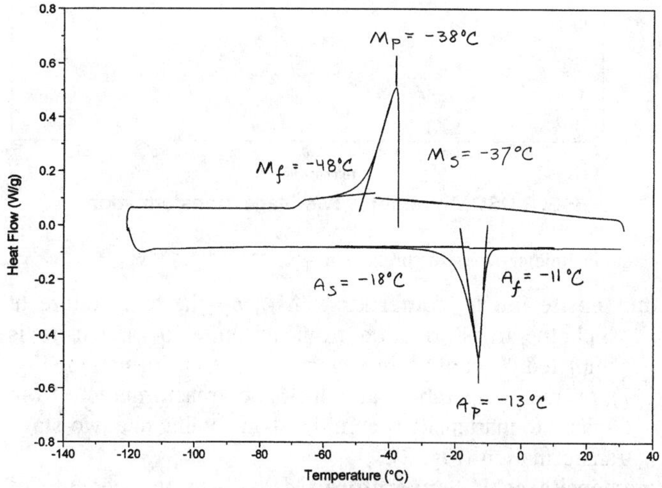

FIG. 1 DSC Graph for Single-Stage Transformation

austenite peak temperature (A_p), *n*—the temperature of the endothermic peak position on the differential scanning calorimeter (DSC) curve upon heating for the martensite to austenite transformation in a single-stage transformation (Fig. 1) or the temperature of the endothermic peak position on the DSC curve upon heating for the R-phase to austenite transformation in a two-stage transformation (Fig. 2).

austenite start temperature (A_s), *n*—the temperature at which the martensite to austenite transformation begins on heating in a single-stage transformation (Fig. 1) or the temperature at which the R-phase to austenite transformation begins on heating in a two-stage transformation (Fig. 2).

differential scanning calorimeter (DSC), *n*—a device which is capable of heating a test specimen and a reference at a controlled rate and of automatically measuring the difference in heat flow between the specimen and the reference both to the required sensitivity and precision.

differential scanning calorimetry (DSC), *n*—a technique in which the difference in heat flow into or out of a substance and an inert reference is measured as a function of temperature while the substance and the reference material are subjected to a controlled temperature program.
(E 473) (ICTAC) (1993)

martensite, *n*—the lowest temperature phase in Ni-Ti shape memory alloys.

DISCUSSION—In Ni-Ti the lowest temperature phase has the B19

[1] This terminology is under the jurisdiction of ASTM Committee F-4 on Medical and Surgical Devices and is the direct responsibility of Subcommittee F04.12 on Metallurgical Materials.

Current edition approved Jan 10, 2000. Published April 2000.

[2] *Annual Book of ASTM Standards*, Vol 03.01.

[3] *Annual Book of ASTM Standards*, Vol 14.02.

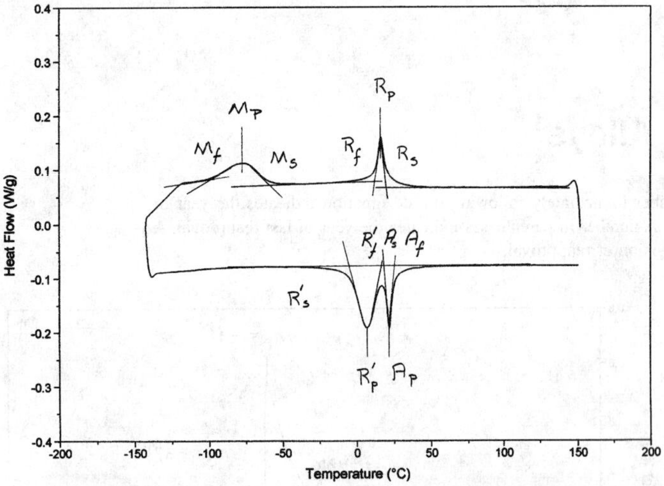

FIG. 2 DSC Graph for a Two-Stage Transformation

monoclinic crystal structure.

martensite finish temperature (M_f), *n*—the temperature at which the transformation from austenite to martensite is completed on cooling in a single-stage transformation (Fig. 1) or the temperature at which the transformation from R-phase to martensite is completed on cooling in a two-stage transformation (Fig. 2).

martensite peak temperature (M_p), *n*—the temperature of the exothermic peak position on the DSC curve upon cooling for the austenite to martensite transformation (Fig. 1) or the R-phase to martensite transformation (Fig. 2).

martensite start temperature (M_s), *n*—the temperature at which the transformation from austenite to martensite begins on cooling in a single-stage transformation (see Fig. 1) or the temperature at which the transformation from R-phase to martensite begins on cooling in a two-stage transformation (Fig. 2).

Nitinol—a generic trade name for a Ni-Ti alloy.

pseudoelasticity, *n*—See **superelasticity**.

R-phase, *n*—the intermediate phase which forms from austenite prior to martensite formation.

DISCUSSION—This occurs in Ni-Ti shape memory alloys under certain conditions. The crystal lattice of the R-Phase is a rhombohedral distortion of the cubic austenite crystal lattice structure, hence the name "R-phase."

R-phase finish temperature (R_f), *n*—the temperature at which the transformation from austenite to R-phase is completed on cooling in a two-stage transformation (Fig. 2).

R-phase peak temperature (R_p), *n*—the temperature of the exothermic peak position on the DSC curve upon cooling for the austenite to R-phase transformation (Fig. 2).

R-phase start temperature (R_s), *n*—the temperature at which the transformation from austenite to R-phase begins on cooling in a two-stage transformation (Fig. 2).

R′-phase finish temperature (R'_f), *n*—the temperature at which the martensite to R-phase transformation is completed on heating in a two-stage transformation (Fig. 2).

R′-phase peak temperature (R'_p), *n*—the temperature of the endothermic peak position on the DSC curve upon heating, for the martensite to R-phase transformation in a two-stage transformation (Fig. 2).

R′-phase start temperature (R'_s), *n*—temperature at which the martensite to R-phase transformation begins on heating in a two-stage transformation (Fig. 2).

shape memory alloy, *n*—a metal which, after an apparent plastic deformation in the martensitic phase, undergoes a thermoelastic change in crystal structure when heated through its transformation temperature range resulting in a recovery of the deformation.

superelasticity, *n*—nonlinear recoverable deformation behavior of Ni-Ti shape memory alloys at temperatures above the austenite finish temperature (A_f).

DISCUSSION—The nonlinear deformation arises from the stress-induced formation of martensite on loading and the spontaneous reversion of this crystal structure to austenite upon unloading.

thermoelastic martensitic transformation, *n*—a diffusionless thermally reversible phase change characterized by a change in crystal structure.

DISCUSSION—This is a process in which an incremental change in temperature produces a proportionate increase or decrease in the amount of phase change.

transformation temperature range, *n*—*in a shape memory alloy*, the temperature range in which a change of phase occurs. **(E 7) (1988)**

The American Society for Testing and Materials takes no position respecting the validity of any patent rights asserted in connection with any item mentioned in this standard. Users of this standard are expressly advised that determination of the validity of any such patent rights, and the risk of infringement of such rights, are entirely their own responsibility.

This standard is subject to revision at any time by the responsible technical committee and must be reviewed every five years and if not revised, either reapproved or withdrawn. Your comments are invited either for revision of this standard or for additional standards and should be addressed to ASTM Headquarters. Your comments will receive careful consideration at a meeting of the responsible technical committee, which you may attend. If you feel that your comments have not received a fair hearing you should make your views known to the ASTM Committee on Standards, at the address shown below.

Designation: F 2009 – 00

Standard Test Method for Determining the Axial Disassembly Force of Taper Connections of Modular Prostheses[1]

This standard is issued under the fixed designation F 2009; the number immediately following the designation indicates the year of original adoption or, in the case of revision, the year of last revision. A number in parentheses indicates the year of last reapproval. A superscript epsilon (ε) indicates an editorial change since the last revision or reapproval.

1. Scope

1.1 This test method establishes a standard methodology for determining the force required, under laboratory conditions, to disassemble tapers of implants that are otherwise not intended to release. Some examples are the femoral components of a total or partial hip replacement or shoulder in which the head and base component are secured together by a self-locking taper.

1.2 This test method has been developed primarily for evaluation of metal and ceramic head designs on metal tapers but may have application to other materials and designs.

1.3 *This standard does not purport to address all of the safety concerns, if any, associated with its use. It is the responsibility of the user of this standard to establish appropriate safety and health practices and determine the applicability of regulatory limitations prior to use.*

2. Referenced Documents

2.1 *ASTM Standards:*

E 4 Practices for Force Verification of Testing Machines[2]

F 1636 Specification for Bores and Cones for Modular Femoral Heads[3]

3. Summary of Test Method

3.1 The axial disassembly test method provides a means to measure the axial locking strength of the taper connection for modular prostheses.

3.2 Following assembly, an axial tensile force is applied to disassemble the taper connection and the maximum force is recorded.

4. Significance and Use

4.1 This test method helps to assess the axial locking force of a modular taper. Examples of these devices are described in Specification F 1636. Some types of devices that may utilize this type of connection are the modular shoulder and modular hip prostheses. Additional means of evaluating the locking mechanisms of tapers may be appropriate, depending upon the design of the device.

4.2 This test method may not be appropriate for all implant applications. The user is cautioned to consider the appropriateness of the practice in view of the materials and design being tested and their potential application.

4.3 While this practice may be used to measure the force required to disengage tapers, any comparison of such data for various component designs must take into consideration the size of the implant and the type of locking mechanism evaluated.

5. Apparatus

5.1 The cone portion of the assembly shall be constrained by suitable fixtures that can sustain high loads.

5.2 The fixtures shall be constructed so that the line of load application is aligned with the axes of the male and female taper components within ±1°.

5.2.1 For example, modular heads may be assembled by a solid metal 100° cone as shown in Fig. 1. The cone should provide line contact around the diameter of the head.

5.2.2 For example, modular heads may be disassembled with a metal cage that surrounds the head and provides even contact around the inferior edge of the head as shown in Fig. 2.

5.3 The testing machine shall conform to the requirements of Practices E 4. The loads used to determine the attachment strength shall be within the range of the testing machine as defined in Practices E 4.

5.4 The test machine should be capable of delivering a compressive and tensile force at a constant displacement rate. The test machine should have a load monitoring and recording system.

6. Sampling and Test Specimens

6.1 The male and female taper components can be finished implants or they can be simplified test specimens. The test specimens must have tapers manufactured to the specifications of a finished implant including material and preferably manufactured with the same equipment.

6.2 The supporting material around the female taper must be similar in size and shape to the finished implant.

6.3 A minimum of five taper assemblies shall be tested to determine the axial disassembly force between the tapered

[1] This test method is under the jurisdiction of ASTM Committee F-04 on Medical and Surgical Materials and Devices and is the direct responsibility of Subcommittee F04.22 on Arthroplasty.

Current edition approved March 10, 2000. Published May 2000.

[2] *Annual Book of ASTM Standards*, Vol 03.01.

[3] *Annual Book of ASTM Standards*, Vol 13.01.

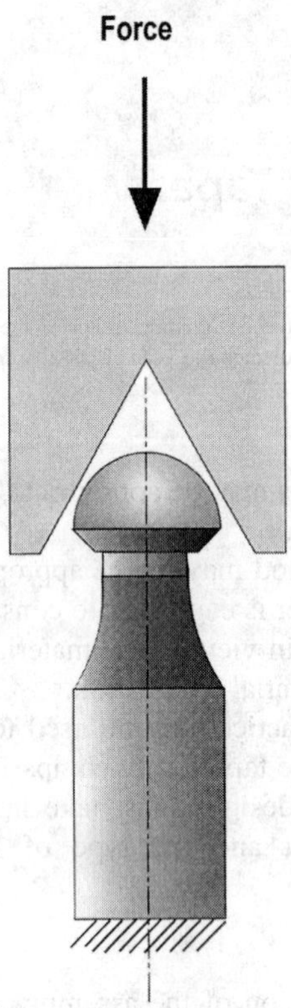

FIG. 1 Modular Head Assembly

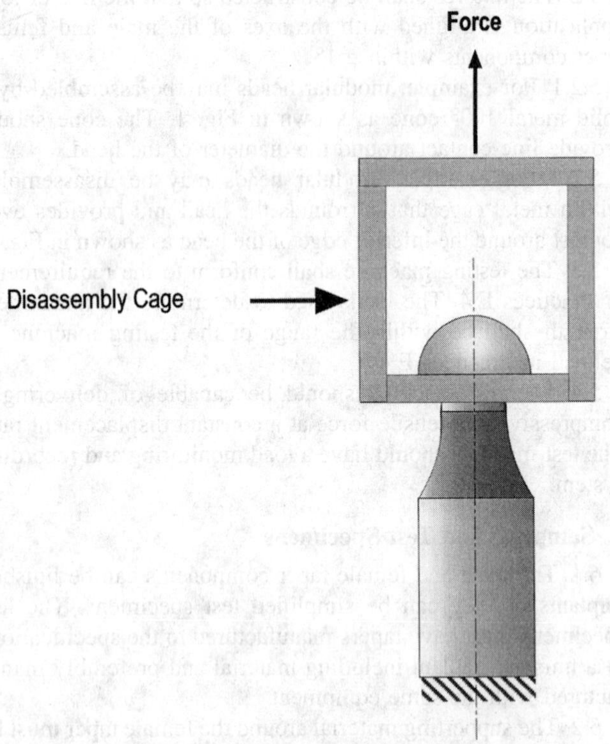

FIG. 2 Modular Head Disassembly

components. Pairing of the components shall be random unless otherwise reported. The appropriateness of performing multiple tests on the same taper connection will depend on the design and application of the device.

6.4 Sterilization of test components is not required unless it has known effects on the parts being evaluated. Generally, sterilization does not have an effect on metallic materials.

7. Procedure

7.1 Following normal laboratory cleaning procedures to remove any debris or other surface contaminants, the taper components are assembled on a suitable test machine. A suggested procedure for cleaning and drying of the specimens is given in Appendix X1.

7.2 Each specimen should be characterized prior to testing. This information may include, but is not limited to the following: material, hardness, bore and taper diameters, concentricity, surface roughness, taper angle, and length of engagement.

7.3 Tapers can be assembled using two methods. Depending on the intended use, the user may use the assembly method that best suits the taper application.

7.3.1 *Constant Rate Assembly Method*—A 2 kN peak static load is applied to the taper component along the long axis of the taper within ± 1°; the load may be applied using a constant displacement rate until the maximum load (2 kN) is achieved. A suggested displacement rate is 0.05 mm/s.

7.3.2 *Drop Weight Assembly Method*—The two components may be assembled with an impact load, that is, a 907-g weight dropped from a 254-mm height.

7.4 *Disassembly Procedure*—The taper assembly should be placed in appropriate fixtures in a qualified test machine. The fixture should be capable of maintaining the load axis angle to within ±1°. Special care should be taken to ensure that no artificial hoop stresses or bending moments are placed on the taper assembly while disassembling the tapers. A displacement rate of 0.05 mm/s may be used. The load and displacement should be recorded continuously until the test is terminated.

7.5 Testing of each specimen shall be terminated when the disassembly load drops by at least 90 % of the peak load.

8. Report

8.1 The test report shall include the following:

8.1.1 The device name, materials, assembly method, load versus displacement graph, sample size, and manufacturer and lot number, if applicable. Additional information pertaining to the drop weight method is desirable and may include, but is not limited to the following: description of the drop weight apparatus, drop weight mass, drop height.

8.1.2 Maximum load required to disassemble the tapers.

8.1.3 The displacement rate if the constant rate method is used.

8.1.4 Additional information characterizing each test specimen prior to testing is desirable to better interpret the test results. This information may include, but is not limited to the following: material, hardness, bore and taper diameters, concentricity, surface roughness, taper angle, and length of engagement.

9. Precision and Bias

9.1 No information can be presented on the precision and bias of this test method for measuring the axial disassembly force of tapers because no material having an accepted reference value is available.

10. Keywords

10.1 arthroplasty; disassembly; heads; hip prosthesis; modular; shoulder prosthesis; tapers

APPENDIXES

(Nonmandatory Information)

X1. METHOD FOR CLEANING SPECIMENS

X1.1 Rinse with tap water to remove bulk contaminants.

X1.2 Wash in ultrasonic cleaner in a solution of 1 % detergent for 15 minutes.

X1.3 Rinse in a stream of diluted water.

X1.4 Rinse in an ultrasonic cleaner of distilled water for 5 minutes.

X1.5 Rinse in a stream of distilled water.

X1.6 Allow to air dry at room temperature.

X2. RATIONALE

X2.1 It is not the intent of this method to specifically address the locking mechanism's ability to maintain its integrity with sequential assemblies and disassemblies. If deemed appropriate by the user, the method could be considered for determining the ability of the locking mechanism to resist degradation after repeated assemblies.

X2.2 Modular femoral heads have been used in various THR designs since approximately 1970. This concept provides features to suit the patient as planned preoperatively, or selected intraoperatively by the surgeon such as component material, neck length, and head diameter, or both.

X2.3 Modular heads typically are installed in surgery using manual impact loads; however, because there can be large variations due to individual strength, impact rate, hammer mass, off-axis loading, soft tissue damping, etc., and because impact and dissociation forces are directly related[4, 5] a repeatable assembly method is recommended in order to compare dissociation forces.

X2.3.1 Other assembly methods, however, could be desirable. Two other methods have been discussed: the dropped-weight impact method and manufacturer's recommendation. Some manufacturers may provide a tool that delivers the recommended force to assemble the modular components. These methods could be justified, but because of the potential variation in assembly loads and limited access to instruments, these methods are not recommended within the scope of this test method. For the instances that necessitate these assembly methods, proper documentation detailing the procedure should be required.

X2.4 An aspect of modular junction integrity to consider may be the affect of fatigue. Fatigue is known to affect the mechanical stability of materials and components that fit together. It may be necessary to determine the post fatigue disengagement force of modular junctions.

[4] Loch, K.A. Gleason, R.F. Kyle, and J.E. Bechtold, "Axial Pull-Off Strength of Dry and Wet Taper Head Connections on a Modular Shoulder Prosthesis," *Trans Orthopaedic Research Society*, p. 826, 1994.

[5] Blevens, X. Deng, P.A. Torzilli, D. Dines, and R.F. Warren, "Disassociation of Modular Humeral Head Components: A Biomechanical and Implant Retrieval Study," *Shoulder and Elbow Surgery*, Vol 6, No. 2, p. 113–124.

Designation: F 2020 – 00

Standard Practice for Design, Construction, and Procurement of Emergency Medical Services Systems (EMSS) Ambulances[1]

This standard is issued under the fixed designation F 2020; the number immediately following the designation indicates the year of original adoption or, in the case of revision, the year of last revision. A number in parentheses indicates the year of last reapproval. A superscript epsilon (ϵ) indicates an editorial change since the last revision or reapproval.

1. Scope

1.1 This practice covers certified, tested, commercial type, EMSS ambulances built on chassis that are suitable for the intended application and meet the requirements herein. The ambulances are front or rear wheel driven (4x2) or four wheel driven (4x4) and warranted as specified in Section 9.

1.1.1 *Definition of Ambulance*—An ambulance is a vehicle for emergency medical care which provides: a driver's compartment; a patient compartment to accommodate an emergency medical technician (EMT)/paramedic and two litter patients (one patient located on the primary cot and a secondary patient on a folding litter located on the squad bench) so positioned that the primary patient can be given intensive life-support during transit; equipment and supplies for emergency care at the scene as well as during transport; two-way radio communication; and, when necessary, equipment for light rescue/extrication procedures. The ambulance shall be designed and constructed to afford safety, comfort, and avoid aggravation of the patient's injury or illness.

1.1.2 This standard may be used to procure an ambulance and the applicable additional systems and equipment.

1.1.3 Purchasers should follow the ordering data in 9.2 to aid them with the preparation of their procurement specification, requisition, and contract. The purpose of this practice is to describe minimum requirements for design, construction, performance, equipment, testing, and appearance of EMSS ambulances which are authorized to display the "Star of Life" symbol so as to provide a practical degree of standardization. The reasons for such standardization are to provide ambulances that are easily detected, nationally recognizable, properly constructed, easily maintained, and, when appropriately equipped, will enable Emergency Medical Technicians (EMTs) to safely and reliably perform their functions as basic and advanced pre-hospital life support providers as set forth in national EMSS standard training guidelines. These functions include:

1.1.3.1 Responding to, providing appropriate basic or advanced life support, on-site, to persons reported experiencing acute injury or illness in a pre-hospital setting, and transporting them, while continuing such life support care, to an appropriate medical facility for definitive care.

1.1.3.2 Providing interhospital critical transport care.

1.1.3.3 Transporting essential personnel and equipment to and from the site of a multiple medical emergency or a triage site and transporting appropriately triaged patients to designated medical facilities.

1.1.3.4 Other functions deemed appropriate by EMSS ambulance service managers and approved by designated EMSS medical directors.

1.2 *"Star of Life" Certification*—Ambulance manufacturer/contractor shall furnish the purchaser(s) citing this standard an authenticated certification and label (See 6.19) that certifies a "Star of Life" ambulance and equipment complying with this standard and applicable amendments (if any) in effect on the date of manufacture (See 7.3). Ambulance vehicles so certified may display the registered "Star of Life" symbol, as defined by the U.S. Department of Transportation (DOT) and the National Highway Traffic Safety Administration (NHTSA), see Fig. 1.

1.3 *Classification*— "Star of Life" ambulance designs included in this standard may be described in terms of their body type (I, II, or III), class of drive ("1" for two rear wheel drive or "2" for four wheel drive), and floor configuration (A for Advanced Life Support or B for Basic Life Support). Such descriptions may be used to define a variety of ambulance designs which are eligible for certification as "Star of Life" ambulances. (To specify, see 9.2.2 and 9.2.3).

NOTE 1—For optional advanced life support (ALS) applications, users should consider specifying a modular (Type I or III) ambulance. Modular ambulances provide additional space and compartmentation for cardiac monitors, drug cases, etc. The basic life support (BLS) configuration is standard on all types.

1.3.1 *Type I*—Conventional truck, cab-chassis with modular ambulance body.

Class	Configuration
Two rear wheel driven (4x2)	A or B
Four wheel driven (4x4)	A or B

NOTE—Configuration A: Elevating cot and squad bench for ALS (See 6.1.5.1 and 6.11.4).

Configuration B: Elevating cot and squad bench for BLS (See 6.1.5.2).

1.3.1.1 *Type I -AD (Additional Duty)*—A or B or Neonatal, Critical Patient Transport, or A or B with Rescue and Fire

---

[1] This practice is under the jurisdiction of ASTM Committee F-30 on Emergency Medical Services and is the direct responsibility of Subcommittee E30.01 on EMS Equipment.

Current edition approved June 10, 2000. Published August 2000.

"Star of Life Symbol"

The "Star of Life" is a six-barred cross upon which is superimposed the Staff of Aesculapius (es"cu-la'pi-us) who, in both Greek and Roman Mythology, was the god of medicine and healing.

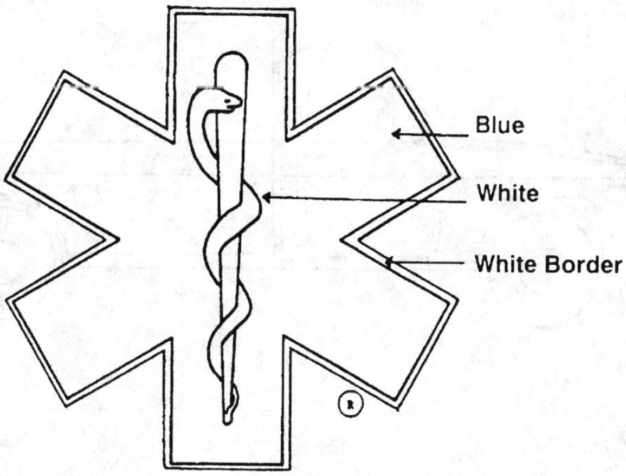

DIMENSIONS

Dimensions (min.):	Size A		Size B		Size C		Size D	
Length of bar	76 mm	(3")	30.5 cm	(12")	40.6 cm	(16")	81.3 cm	(32")
Width of bar	25 mm	(.75")	76 mm	(3")	10.2 cm	(4")	20.3 cm	(8")
Length of staff	63 mm	(2.5")	24.1 cm	(9.5")	31.7 cm	(12.5")	63.5 cm	(25")
White border		(.25')		(.375')		(.5')	-	-

All angles 60°

Deviations must be proportionate.

FIG. 1 "Star of Life Symbol"

Suppression Package or a combination thereof. (See 6.1.2.1)

Class	Configuration
Two rear wheel driven (4x2)	A or B or*
Four wheel driven (4x4)	A or B or*

NOTE—* As specified by purchaser. The configuration shall provide for a neonatal, critical patient transport, configuration A or B with fire suppression package and rescue capability when specified.

1.3.2 *Type II*—Standard van, integral cab-body ambulance (See 6.1.3 and Fig. 3.)

Class	Configuration
Two rear wheel driven (4x2)	A** or B
Four wheel driven (4x4)*	A** or B

NOTE—** On a Type II, ALS features are limited, (see 9.2.3)

*Requires conversion of chassis to four wheel drive (4x4), (see 6.1.6).

1.3.3 *Type III*—Cutaway van, cab-chassis with integral or containerized modular body ambulance (See 6.1.4 and Fig. 4).

Class	Configuration
Two rear wheel driven (4x2)	A or B
Four wheel driven (4x4)*	A or B

NOTE—*Requires conversion of chassis to four wheel drive (4x4), (See 6.1.6).

Configuration A: Elevating cot and squad bench for ALS (See 6.1.5.1 and 6.11.4).

Configuration B: Elevating cot and squad bench for BLS (See 6.1.5.2).

1.4 *Order of Precedence*—In the event of a conflict between the text of this specification and the references cited herein, the text of this specification shall take precedence, except where required by law including Federal, State, and local laws and regulations.

1.5 *This standard does not purport to address all of the safety concerns, if any, associated with its use. It is the responsibility of the user of this standard to establish appropriate safety and health practices and determine the applicability of regulatory limitations prior to use.*

Type I Ambulance
Conventional Cab-Chassis with Modular Body

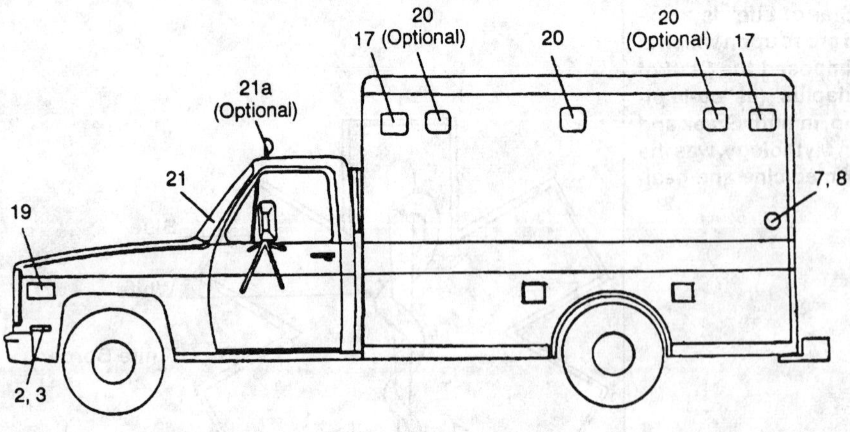

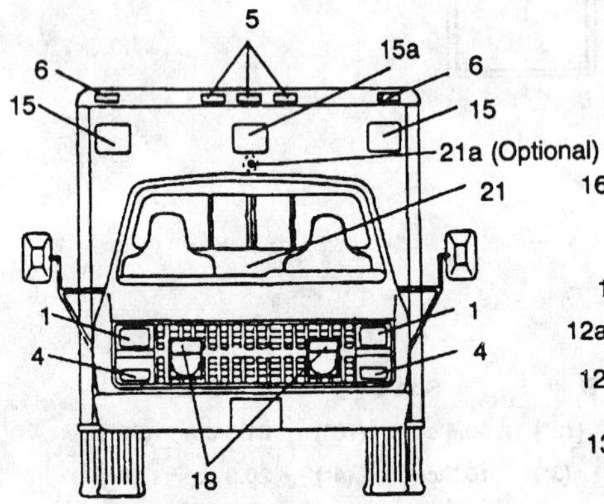

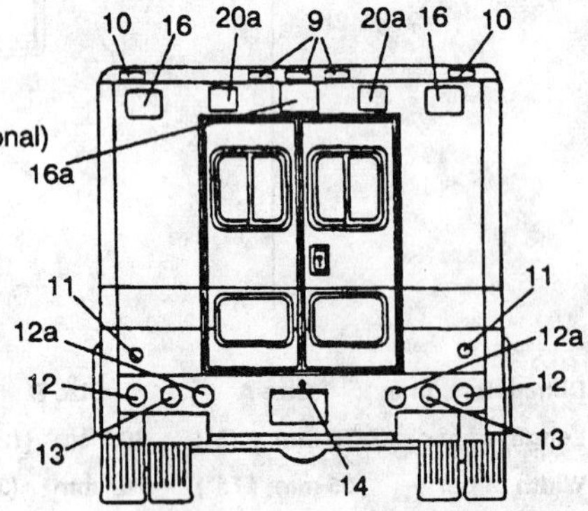

1. Headlamp, (2) white [(4) white optional]
2. Front side marker lamp, (2) amber
3. Front side reflector, (2) amber
4. Front turn signal, (2) amber, (includes vehicular hazard warning signal flasher)
5. Front identification lamps, (3) amber
6. Front clearance lamp, (2) amber
7. Rear side marker lamp, (2) red
8. Rear side reflector, (2) red
9. Rear identification lamps, (3) red
10. Rear clearance lamp, (2) red
11. Rear reflector, (2) red
12. Rear, stop, tail, lamp, (2) red

12a. Rear turn signal, (2) amber. Includes vehicular hazard warning signal flasher. (optional location)

13. Rear backup lamp, (1) white
14. Rear license plate lamp, (1) white
15. Front warning light, (2) red

15a. Front warning light, (1) white

16. Rear warning light, (2) red

16a. Rear warning light. (1) amber

17. Side warning light, (2) red per side
18. Grille light, (2) red
19. Intersection lights, (1) red per side
20. Side floodlight, (2) white

20a. Rear floodlight, (1) white

21. Spotlight, (white) hand held

21a. Spotlight, (white), (optional location)

Lamps and reflectors may be mounted at other practicable locations provided locations and visibility requirements of Federal Motor Vehicle Safety Standard No. 108 are met. The warning lights shown are for the standard warning light systems. The number of devices and their locations may be different in alternative warning light systems

FIG. 2 Type I Ambulance

Type II Ambulance

Standard Van, Forward Control, Integral Cab-Body Ambulance

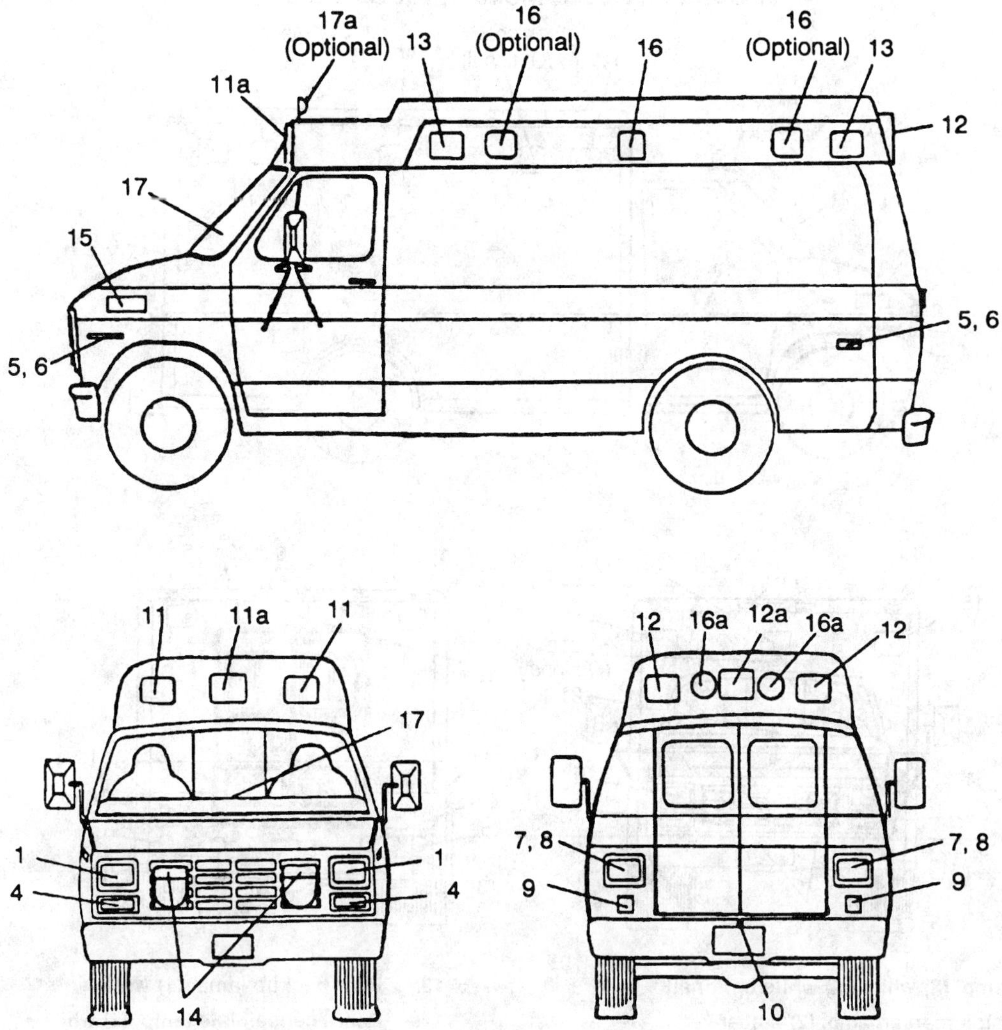

1. Headlamp, (2) white (4 white optional)
***2. Front side marker lamp, (2) amber**
3. Front side reflector, (2) amber
4. Front turn signal, (2) amber (includes vehicular hazard warning signal flasher)
5. Rear side marker lamp, (2) red
6. Rear side reflector, (2) red
7. Rear reflector, (2) red
8. Rear stop, tail & turn signal lamp, (2) red, (turn signal section may be amber, includes vehicular hazard warning signal flasher)
9. Rear backup lamp, (1) white
10. Rear license plate lamp, (1) white

11. Front warning light, (2) red
11a. Front warning light, (1) white
12. Rear warning light, (2) red
12a. Rear warning light, (1) amber
13. Side warning light, (2) red per side
14. Grille light, (2) red
15. Intersection lights, (l) red per side
16. Side floodlight, (2) white
16a. Rear floodlight, (1)
17. Spotlight, hand held, white
17a. Spotlight (white, optional location)
***Flashes with front/rear turn signal & vehicular hazard warning signal flasher.**

Lamps and reflectors may be mounted in other practicable locations provided location and visibility requirements of Federal Motor Vehicle Safety Standard No. 108 are met. The warning lights shown are for the standard warning light systems. The number of devices and their locations may be different in alternative warning light systems.

FIG. 3 Type II Ambulance

TYPE III AMBULANCE

Specialty Van, Forward Control and Control Integral Cab-Body or Containerizeed Modular Ambulance

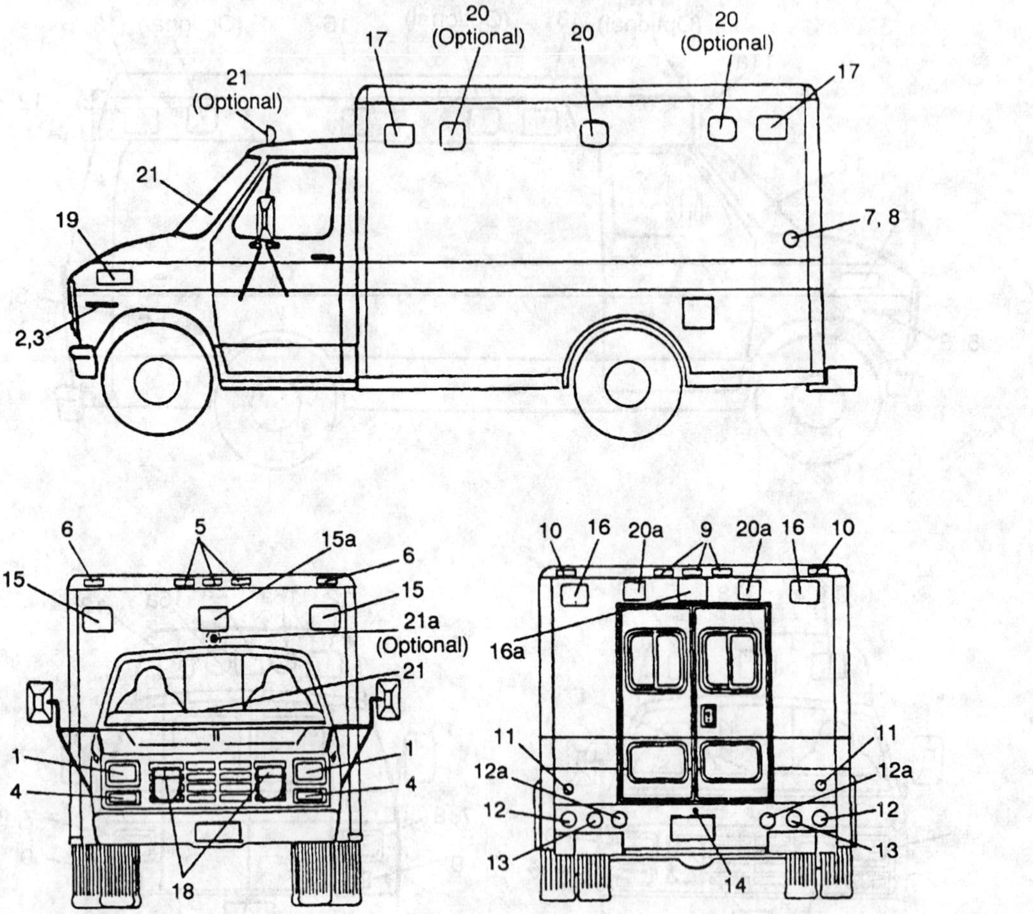

1. Headlamp, (2) white [(4) white optional]
*2. Front side marker lamp, (2) amber
3. Front side reflector, (2) amber
4. Front turn signal, (2) amber, (includes vehicular hazard warning signal flasher)
5. Front identification lamps, (3) amber
6. Front clearance lamp, (2) amber
*7. Rear side marker lamp, (2) red
8. Rear side reflector, (2) red
9. Rear identification lamps, (3) red
10. Rear clearance lamp, (2) red
11. Rear reflector, (2) red
12. Rear, stop, tail, lamp, (2) red
12a. Rear turn signal, (2) amber (includes vehicular hazard warning signal flasher) (optional location)
13. Rear backup lamp, (1) white
14. Rear license plate lamp, (1) white
15. Front warning light, (2) red
15a. Front warning light, (1) white
16. Rear warning light, (2) red
16a. Rear warning light, (1) amber
17. Side warning light, (2) red per side
18. Grille light, (2) red
19. Intersection lights, (1) per side
20. Side floodlight, (2)
20a. Rear floodlight, (1)
21. Spotlight (white) (hand held)
21a. Spotlight (white) (optional location)

*Flashes with front/rear turn signal & vehicular hazard warning signal flasher.

Lamps and reflectors may be mounted in other practicable locations provided location and visibility requirements of Federal Motor Vehicle Safety Standard No. 108 are met. The warning lights shown are for the standard warning light systems. The number of devices and their locations may be different in alternative warning light systems.

FIG. 4 Type III Ambulance

2. Referenced Documents

2.1 *ASTM Standards:*

B 117 Practice for Operating Salt Spray Apparatus[2]

F 920 Specification for Minimum Performance and Safety Requirements for Resuscitators Intended for Use With Humans[3]

F 960 Specification for Medical and Surgical Suction and Drainage Systems[3]

F 1177 Terminology Relating To Emergency Medical Services[3]

F 1328 Guide for Training the Emergency Medical Technician (Basic) to Prepare Patients for Medical Transportation[3]

F 1517 Guide for Scope of Performance of Emergency Medical Services Ambulance Operations[3]

2.2 *Federal Specifications:*[4]

L-S-300 Sheeting and Tape, Reflective, Nonexposed Lens, Adhesive Backing

RR-C-901/3 Cylinders Compressed Gas: With Valve or Plug and Cap; ICC3aa

2.3 *Federal Standards:*[4]

Federal Standard No. 297, Rustproofing of Automotive Vehicles

2.4 *Military Standards:*[5]

MIL-STD-461 Requirements for the Control of Electromagnetic Interference Characteristics of Subsystems and Equipment

MIL-STD-1223 Nontactical Wheeled Vehicles, Painting, Identification Marking and Data Plate Standards

2.5 *Laws and Regulations:*[6]

21 CFR 820 Quality System Regulation (QSR) (FDA)

40 CFR 86 Control of Air Pollution from New Motor Vehicles and New Motor Vehicle Engines

47 CFR, PART 90 Private and Land Mobile Radio Services; Sub Part B: Public Safety Radio Pool

49 CFR 393 Federal Motor Carrier Safety Regulations (FMCSR)

49 CFR 571 Federal Motor Vehicle Safety Standards (FMVSS)

2.6 *Other Publications*—The following documents form a part of this standard to the extent specified. Unless a specific issue is identified, the issue in effect on date of invitation for bids or request for proposal shall apply.

State of California Motor Vehicle Code[7]

The Tire and Rim Association Inc. Yearbook[8]

Society of Automotive Engineers (SAE), Inc., Standards and Recommended Practices:[9]

J163 Low Tension Wiring and Cable Terminals and Splice Clips

1537 Storage Batteries

J541 Voltage Drop for Starting Motor Circuits

J551 Measurement of Electromagnetic Radiation from Motor Vehicles and Devices

J553 Circuit Breakers

J561 Electrical Terminals, Eyelet and Spade Type

J575 Tests for Motor Vehicle Lighting Devices & Components

J576 Plastic Materials, For Use In Optical Parts Such As Lenses and Reflectors of Motor Vehicle Lighting Devices

J578 Color Specification for Electric Signal Lighting Devices

J595 Flashing Warning Lamps for Authorized Emergency, Maintenance, and Service Vehicles

J638 Test Procedure and Ratings for Hot Water Heaters for Motor Vehicles

J639 Safety Practices for Mechanical Vapor Compression Refrigeration Equipment or Systems Used To Cool Passenger Compartment of Motor Vehicles

J682 Rear Wheel Splash and Stone Throw Protection

J683 Tire Chain Clearance

J689 Approach, Departure, and Ramp Breakover Angles

J771 Automotive Printed Circuits

J845 Method for Determining the Flash Energy of a Light

J858 Electrical Terminals, Blade Type

J928 Electrical Terminals, Pin and Receptacle Type

J994 Backup Alarms, Performance Test and Application

J1054 Warning Lamp, Alternating Flashers

J1127 Battery Cable

J1128 Low Tension Primary Cable

J1292 Automobile, Truck, Truck-Tractor, Trailer, and Motor Coach Wiring

J1318 Strobe Warning Lights

J1349 Engine Power Test Code, Spark Ignition and Diesel

J2498 Minimum Performance of the Warning Light System Used on Emergency Vehicles

National Truck Equipment Association/AMD:[10]

AMD Standard 001 Static Load for Ambulance Body Structure Test

AMD Standard 002 Body Door Retention Components Test

AMD Standard 003 Oxygen Tank Retention System Test (Main and Portable Cylinders)

AMD Standard 004 Litter Retention System Test

AMD Standard 005 Ambulance 12 Volt DC Electrical Systems Test

AMD Standard 006 Sound Level Test Code

---

[2] *Annual Book of ASTM Standards*, Vol 03.02

[3] *Annual Book of ASTM Standards*, Vol 13.01.

[4] Copies of Federal Standards and Specifications are available from Federal Standards and Specifications, Superintendent of Documents, U.S. Government Printing Office, Washington, DC 20402.

[5] Copies of Military Specifications and Standards required by suppliers in connection with specific procurement functions should be obtained from the procuring activity or as directed by the contracting officer.

[6] Available from the Superintendent of Documents, U.S. Government Printing Office, Washington, DC 20402. When indicated, reprints of certain regulations may be obtained from the Federal agency responsible for issuance thereof.

[7] Available from Department of Motor Vehicles, 2570 24th Street, Sacramento, California 95809.

[8] Application for copies should be addressed to The Tire and Rim Association, Inc., 175 Montrose W. Ave., Suite 150, Copley, Ohio 44321. Phone (216) 666-8121.

[9] Available from Technical Division, SAE, 400 Commonwealth Dr., Warrendale, PA 15096.

[10] Available from the Ambulance Manufacturer's Division (AMD) of the National Truck Equipment Association, 37400 Hills Tech Drive, Farmington Hills, MI 48331, (810) 489–7090.

AMD Standard 007 Carbon Monoxide Levels For Patient Compartment Interiors
AMD Standard 008 Ambulance Patient Compartment Grab Rail (Load Test)
AMD Standard 010 Water Spray Test
AMD Standard 011 Ambulance Equipment Temperature Test
AMD Standard 012 Temperature Tests
AMD Standard 013 Weight Distribution Test
AMD Standard 014 Cooling System Test
AMD Standard 015 Ambulance Oxygen System Test

3. Terminology

3.1 *Definitions:*

3.1.1 *ambulance, n*—See 1.1.1.

3.2 For definitions of terms used in this practice, refer to ASTM F 1177, Terminology Relating to Emergency Medical Services.

4. Summary of Practice

4.1 The principle of this practice is to define the range of designs, features, performance characteristics for manufacturers, purchasers, and users, of "Star of Life" ambulances recommended for EMSS ambulance services.

5. Significance and Use

5.1 This standard describes the practices for commercial ambulance manufacturers/venders for:

5.1.1 Design and construction, and outfitting of a variety of EMSS ambulances designs using commercially available light truck vehicle chassis, fabricated vehicle bodies, and commercially available components and equipment.

5.1.2 Testing the performance of ambulances and equipment in accordance with nationally accepted ambulance manufacturers (AMD) test standards.

5.1.3 Outfitting and equipping ambulances with medical equipment as recommended by appropriate medical associations to meet needs specified by purchasers.

5.1.4 Certification of ambulances m accordance with "Star of Life" criteria.

5.1.5 Painting coloring and marking EMS ambulances in accordance with "Star of Life" standards preparatory to delivery to purchasers.

5.2 This standard describes practices for ambulance purchasers for:

5.2.1 Preparation of a purchase description for the procurement of an EMSS ambulance in accordance with this standard, using guidance contained in Section 9.

5.2.2 Specifying ambulance inspections, tests and documentation preparatory to acceptance of delivery.

5.3 This standard describes practices for ambulance users for:

5.3.1 Acquainting ambulance service medical directors with features of various ambulance designs and capabilities for planning purposes.

5.3.2 Acquainting ambulance service managers and operators (EMTs) with ambulance designs, equipment, and expected performance characteristics to enable them to safely operate EMS ambulances in accordance with Guide F 1517, and effectively prepare patients for medical transport in accordance with Guide F 1328.

5.4 *Standard Coverage*—This Practice does not include all the varieties of medical service vehicles commercially available. This Practice covers only the ambulances approved to display the "Star of Life" symbols and purchased to provide pre hospital emergency medical services in accordance with provisions of other ASTM F-30 Standards for Emergency Medical Services Systems.

5.5 *Precautions and Observations*—Purchasers should read the entire document before requisitioning an ambulance, in order to be knowledgeable of just what equipment is standard, and which options need to be exercised. Due to the variety of ambulance equipment or features, some options may be incompatible with the model desired (reference chassis and ambulance manufacturer's data books).

6. Requirements

6.1 *General Vehicular Design, Types, and Floor Plan:*

6.1.1 *Design*—The ambulance and the allied equipment furnished under this practice shall be the manufacturer's current commercial vehicle of the Type, Class, and Configuration specified. The ambulance shall be complete with the operating accessories, as specified herein, and furnished with such modifications and attachments as may be necessary to enable the vehicle to function reliably and efficiently in sustained operation. The design of the vehicle and the specified equipment shall permit accessibility for servicing, replacement, and adjustment of component parts and accessories with minimum disturbance to other components and systems. The term "heavy-duty", as used to describe an item, shall mean in excess of the standard quantity, quality, or capacity and represents the best, most durable, strongest, etc., part, component, system, etc., that is commercially available on the Original Equipment Manufacturer's (OEM) chassis.

NOTE 2—Ambulance crash tests and analysis are being conducted to identify ambulance occupant crash injury mechanisms. Problems identified in these tests should lead to ambulance design changes in 6.4.1, 6.10.5, 6.10.6, 6.10.7, 6.10.8.1, and 6.11.3 which will prevent or reduce the severity of ambulance crash injuries. Appropriate changes, based on automotive crashworthiness principles will be incorporated in future changes to this standard.

6.1.2 *Type I Ambulance*— Type I vehicle, Class 1 or 2, Configuration A or B, shall be a chassis furnished with a 2-door enclosed cab. The chassis-cab shall be suitable for subsequent mounting of a transferable, modular, ambulance body conforming to the requirements specified herein. (See Fig. 2.)

6.1.2.1 *Type I - AD (Additional Duty) Ambulance*—Type I-AD, Class 1 or 2, Configuration A, B, or other user specified configurations such as for critical patient or neonatal transport, shall be a conventional truck, cab-chassis with modular body. Additionally, other on board systems or equipment may be specified for rescue or fire suppression or combination of applications. The chassis shall be suitable for mounting of a transferable modular ambulance body conforming to the requirements herein.

6.1.3 *Type II Ambulance*—Type II vehicle, Class 1 or 2, Configuration A or B, shall be OEM chassis manufacturer's commercial, long wheel base, integral van. This vehicle shall be suitable for subsequent ambulance conversion/modification in compliance with the requirements herein. (See Fig. 3.)

6.1.4 *Type III Ambulance*—Type III, Class 1 or 2, Configuration A or B shall be a "cutaway" van with a transferable, modular, ambulance body or unitized cab-body mounted on a chassis. The chassis with unitized cab-body or front section cab-chassis shall be suitable for the subsequent fabrication, conversion, or modification into an ambulance incorporating the requirements and the equipment specified herein. (See Fig. 4.)

6.1.5 *Configuration of Patient Compartment*—Unless otherwise specified (See 9.2.3), Configuration "B", Basic Life Support (BLS) shall be provided in the patient compartment. All litters shall be loaded to position the patient's head forward in the vehicle.

6.1.5.1 *Configuration "A" (ALS)*—When specified for Types I or III (See 9.2.2), Advanced Life Support (ALS) applications, one primary patient shall be on a wheeled elevating cot and a secondary patient lying on a folding stretcher or combination stretcher chair on the squad bench, or one primary patient and three secondary seated patients on the squad bench (See 6.11.4) and one seated EMT/paramedic. The primary cot shall be center mounted or, when specified (See Table 10, Item 21), a dual position mount shall be furnished. Unless otherwise specified (See Table 9, Item 28), a CPR seat conforming to all specification requirements shall be furnished on the left (street) side of the body facing the patient's thoracic region and include a seat belt and padding at the EMT's head region. Space shall also be furnished in the action wall/counter area for placement of a cardiac monitor/defibrillator. When specified (See Table 10, Item 25), a crash stable mounting bracket for securing the cardiac monitor/defibrillator shall be furnished. A locking drug kit compartment per Table 9, Item 14 and high intensity light per Table 9, Item 8 shall also be furnished. Two I.V. hangers, per 6.11.9, shall be provided for the primary patient, one at the patient's head and one at the patient's lower extremities.

6.1.5.2 *Configuration "B" (BLS)*—Unless otherwise specified (See 9.2.3), Configuration "B" shall provide for one primary patient on a wheeled elevating cot and one secondary patient on a folding stretcher or combination stretcher/chair on a squad bench, which is also capable of accommodating three seated patients (See 6.11.5) and one seated EMT (See 6.10.3).

NOTE 3—It is preferable that the primary patient's cot be positioned on the left (street) side or centered in the ambulance patient compartment. The anatomy of the tracheal bronchial tree is such that an unconscious patient will be less likely to aspirate fluids into the trachea if placed on their left side with the right side up.

6.1.6 *Four Wheel Drive, Class 2, 4x4*—When a 4x4 chassis is specified (See 9.2.2), the additional curb weight of the 4x4 chassis above the 4x2 chassis will reduce the payload proportionally. When available, a Class 2 ambulance shall be an original chassis manufacturer's (OEM) 4x4 chassis for Type 1 ambulances, or an OEM 4x2 model with a professionally engineered conversion to a four wheel drive (4x4) conforming to all applicable requirements herein. All workmanship, welding, mechanical fit grade, and quality of components and materials used in conversions shall be equal to or greater than OEM manufacturer's production 4x4 units. Conversion components shall not interfere with other body, chassis, or mechanical parts through the complete range of suspension and wheel angle travel and allow proper alignment of axles. The tracking of the front/rear axles shall be identical on both sides of the vehicle and wheelbase. When available, the chassis manufacturer's OEM components shall be furnished, including but not limited to: spring hangers, shackles, drive axle, integral transmission/transfer case, universal joints, steering linkage, stabilizer bars, radius and torque rods, transfer case shaft linkage, brake calipers, pads, rotors, shock absorbers and springs. When available, the chassis manufacturer's guidelines/requirements for 4x4 conversions shall be followed. The design of the 4x4 conversion shall minimize the height of the vehicle's chassis. The 4x4 converter shall include a complete chassis modifier FMVSS certification and sticker.

The 4x4 converter shall provide to the purchaser a full parts and labor warranty covering all added 4x4 parts and materials, including workmanship and design. The warranty shall also cover all OEM components affected or modified by the conversion process. This warranty shall be at least equivalent, in mileage and time, to the OEM chassis manufacturer's warranty, including any extended warranties required or furnished.

Accompanying each conversion shall be complete manuals showing operation, maintenance, and repair procedures, chassis manufacturer's part numbers, drawings for components used in the conversion, and dimensioned drawings for manufactured parts, alignment procedures, and specifications.

6.2 *Vehicle Ambulance Components, Equipment, and Accessories*—The emergency medical care vehicles, including chassis, ambulance body, equipment, device, medical accessories, and electronic equipment shall be standard commercial products, tested and certified to meet or exceed the requirements of this specification. The ambulance shall comply with all Federal Motor Vehicle Safety Standards (FMVSS) and other Federal and state regulations applicable or specified for the year of manufacture. The chassis, components, and optional items shall be as represented in the chassis manufacturers current technical data. The ambulance body, equipment, and accessories shall be as represented in their respective manufacturer's current technical data. Data shall be limited to specifications and technical materials identical to that furnished to the authorized company representatives and shall be furnished to the engineering/technical offices of the procuring activity and the suppliers (contractor's) offices prior to acceptance of the ambulance. The supplier shall provide total standardization and interchangeability between similar vehicles, equipment, items, and accessories specified for all ambulance units under each contract.

TABLE 1 Wiring Criteria

Circuit Breaker Rating (Amps)	Minimum Wire Size For Circuit Rating & Voltage Drop
10 Amps	16
15 Amps	14
20 Amps	12
30 Amps	10

6.3 *Recovered Materials*—All equipment, material, and articles required under this specification are to be new or fabricated from new materials produced from recovered materials. The term "recovered materials" means materials, which have been collected or recovered from solid waste and reprocessed to become a source of raw materials, as opposed to virgin raw materials. None of the above shall be interpreted to mean that the use of used or rebuilt products is allowed under this document.

6.4 *Vehicle Operation, Performance, and Physical Characteristics:*

6.4.1 *Operation and Performance*—Unless otherwise specified by the purchaser, all requirements in 6.4 shall be met with the ambulance loaded to meet or exceed the minimum specified payload including all specified equipment and devices installed and operating at the maximum power-consuming condition, for example, air conditioning, lights, radio(s), etc., with the chassis performing in accordance with the specified chassis manufacturer's technical data. The vehicle shall be capable of operating safely and efficiently under environmental conditions outlined herein or as specified in the invitation for bid, contract, or order. When specified by the purchaser for ambulances requiring higher GVWR's to carry additional specialty equipment, for example, medical; rescue; neonatal; (See 9.2.4), lower performance levels are acceptable in 6.4.6-6.4.8.2.

6.4.2 *Temperature Conditions*—The ambulance, including all required systems, equipment, and medical devices (except when medical devices are regulated by another agency) furnished inside the ambulance, when serviced and maintained in accordance with the OEM manufacturer's recommendations (7.4), shall be capable of being stored without damage or deterioration in ambient temperatures of -34°C to 52°C (-30°F to 125°F). Testing shall be in accordance with AMD Standard 011 (Ambulance Equipment Temperature Test). Medical devices, such as resuscitation and suctioning apparatus, shall be cold tested for the required flow performance on 12 V DC vehicle power and 115 V AC power modes (See 6.12.1.1). Type certification from medical and other equipment manufacturers is acceptable.

6.4.3 *Noise and Sound Level Limits, Exterior*—Unless more stringent sound levels are regulated by the states and municipalities where the ambulance will be based, the exterior noise level produced by the vehicle, except siren, shall not exceed Federal regulations.

6.4.4 *Vehicle Performance*—The ambulance shall provide a smooth, stable ride with minimum noise and vibration. Test under 7.4.4.

6.4.5 *Brakes*—The ambulance braking system as delivered to the user shall comply to performance values required by Federal Motor Vehicle Safety Standards (FMVSS), and when available from the chassis manufacturer shall include ABS.

6.4.6 *Speed*—The vehicles shall be capable of a sustained speed of not less than 105 km/hr (65 mph) over dry, hard surfaced, level roads, at sea level, and passing speeds of 113 km/hr (70 mph) when tested under normal ambient conditions.

6.4.7 *Acceleration*— Vehicle shall have a minimum average acceleration, at sea level, of 0-88 km/hr (0-55 mph) within 25 s. Test shall be performed under normal ambient conditions. Test under 7.4.4.

6.4.8 *Gradeability*— At full payload, the vehicle shall be capable of meeting the following requirements. The determination shall be made by actual test or chassis manufacturer's certified computer prediction or chassis manufacturer's certification.

6.4.8.1 *Gradeability at Speed*—Minimum gradeability at speed shall be 89 km/hr (55 mph) on a 3% (1.72 degrees) grade.

6.4.8.2 *Minimum Low Speed Gradeability*—The minimum low speed gradeability of 8 km/hr (5 mph) on a 35% (19.3 degrees) grade is required for Class I (4x2) vehicles and 45% (24.2 degrees) grade for Class 2 (4x4) vehicles in the low 4x4 range.

6.4.9 *Fuel Range*—Unless otherwise specified (See 9.2.5), the ambulance shall be capable of being driven for at least 402 km (250 miles) without refueling under the conditions in 7.4.4.

6.4.10 *Fording*—The vehicle shall be capable of three fordings, without water entering patient and equipment compartments while being driven through a minimum of 20 cm (8 in.) of water, at speeds of 8 km/hr (5 mph), for a distance of at least 30.5 m (100 feet). Test under 7.4.4.

6.4.11 *Vehicle Physical Dimensional Requirements:*

6.4.11.1 *Length* —Overall length of the ambulance shall not exceed 671 cm (22 ft), including bumpers, but excluding rear step and bumper guards. Purchaser may specify (See 9.2.6) additional length if necessary to accommodate special equipment or larger bodies but should consult with the manufacturer to determine that other safety/handling characteristics are not compromised.

6.4.11.2 *Width*—Unless otherwise specified (See 9.2.7), the overall (OA) width of ambulance bodies having single rear wheels shall be between 200 and 213 cm (79 and 84 in.), excluding mirrors and lights. The ambulance body sides, on a chassis with dual rear wheels, shall be within ± 5 cm (± 2 in.) of the overall width of the tires (outside sidewalls) (See 6.5.6, 6.6.5.6, and 6.9.7). Tires shall not extend beyond the fenders. Unless approved by the purchaser and permitted by state laws, the maximum ambulance body width shall not exceed 244 cm (96 in.), excluding mirrors, lights, and other safety appurtenances. The wide track axle shall be furnished on dual rear wheeled vehicles, unless a narrow ambulance body is specified by the purchaser (See 9.2.7).

6.4.11.3 *Height*—Unless otherwise specified (See 9.2.8), overall height of the ambulance at curb weight (See 6.5.1) shall not exceed 279 cm (110 m.), including roof mounted equipment, but excluding two-way radio antenna(s).

6.4.11.4 *Ground Clearance*— With the exception of the chassis manufacturer's furnished and installed components, the lowest part of the vehicle, when loaded to the Gross Vehicle Weight Rating (GVWR), shall have a minimum of 20 cm (8 in.) of ground clearance.

6.4.11.5 *Angle of Approach, Ramp Breakover, and Departure*—The ambulance, loaded to the GVWR, including payload, (See 6.5.2) with bumpers and rear step (down if folding style), shall provide not less than the following clearance, measured in accordance with SAE J689.

Approach angle = 20 °
Ramp breakover = 10 °
Departure angle = 10 °

6.4.11.6 *Turning Radius*— Shall not be greater than chassis OEM standard.

6.4.11.7 *Floor Height*— The finished floor (loading) heights shall not exceed 84 cm (33 in.) on Class I (4x2) vehicles and 97 cm (38 in.) for Class 2 (4x4) vehicles. The height shall be measured at curb weight plus full payload but minus patients and personnel. The use of an automotive "dump valve" on air suspension vehicles is acceptable to achieve the loading height requirement. The system shall include an interlock that permits vehicle lowering only when the vehicle is in neutral or park, the parking brake is set, and the rear door(s) are open. Removing any one of the above criteria shall re-inflate the air bags. The above interlocks shall not conflict with the chassis manufacturer's requirements.

6.5 *Vehicle Weight Ratings and Payload:*

6.5.1 *Curb Weight*— Curb weight is the total weight of the complete ambulance and is defined as: chassis (including batteries, spare tire, jack tire changing tools), cab, body, minimum required equipment per this specification, and a full complement of fuel, lubricants, and coolant, excluding optional equipment in 6.15.3 and 6.15.4, and any non-portable vehicle mounted rescue (extrication) equipment, permanently mounted fire suppression system and equipment including nozzles, hoses, tanks, pumps, etc. and including a full complement of water and related foam, chemicals, etc.

6.5.2 *Payload Allowance*—Each vehicle's payload allowance shall be determined and displayed in accordance with the weight/payload certification form (sticker) (See Fig. 5). Sticker shall be located in a conspicuous location in the vehicle. Payload shall be over and above the specified curb weight (See 6.5.1) of the vehicle and include specified options, miscellaneous medical equipment, and communications equipment that is appropriately distributed within the vehicle. The usable payload for additional duty modular Type I or Type III ambulances shall be specified by the customer.

NOTE 4—**Warning:** Due to potential hazards and damage to vehicle's chassis, the ambulance shall not be overloaded. The purchaser should consult with the ambulance and chassis manufacturer(s) or both to determine actual reserve capacity above the specified minimum required herein.

Unless additional payload is specified (See 9.2.9) by the purchaser, the required minimum payload per vehicle shall be as follows:

6.5.2.1 Single, rear wheeled, modular (Type I or III)—680 kg (1500 lbs.)

6.5.2.2 Single, rear wheeled, van ambulances (Type II)—771.11kg (1700 lbs.)

6.5.2.3 Dual, rear wheeled, modular ambulances (Type I or III)—793.79 kg (1750 lbs.)

6.5.2.4 Additional Duty Modular Ambulances (Type I)—payload as specified by customer. The payload shall be evenly distributed throughout the vehicle and shall consist of the following:

6.5.2.4.1 Driver and EMT at 79 kg (175 lbs.) each. See Fig. 5.

6.5.2.4.2 Two patients at 79 kg (175 lbs.) each.

6.5.2.4.3 Main and portable oxygen cylinders, stretchers, cots, and patient handling equipment.

6.5.2.4.4 Portable, removable, medical devices.

6.5.2.4.5 Durable and disposable medical items.

6.5.2.4.6 Optional vehicle equipment such as battery charger, inverter, or any other optional items or equipment not supplied as a base vehicle requirement.

6.5.2.4.7 Communications equipment.

6.5.2.4.8 Extrication and rescue equipment.

6.5.2.4.9 Portable fire extinguishers in addition to units required in 6.15.2 as specified by purchaser.

6.5.3 *Gross Vehicle Weight Rating (GVWR)*—The ambulance gross vehicle weight rating shall equal or exceed the combination of the vehicle's curb weight and payload weight. The chassis manufacturer's rating label shall show the actual gross vehicle weight rating (GVWR) and the gross axle weight rating (GAWR) of the vehicle (See 6.19).

6.5.4 *Weight Distribution*—To provide for maximum safety, purchasers and manufacturers shall locate vehicle mounted components, equipment, and supplies to provide a vehicle that is laterally balanced and has front/rear loading that is proportional to axle ratings. The weight distribution of a properly loaded ambulance on a level surface shall permit conformance to the braking requirements in FMVSS 105 and for air brake vehicles FMVSS 121. The right and left wheel of each axle, at curb weight, (See 6.5.1) of a completed ambulance, shall be weighed to determine weight distribution. The weight between the right and left side of a given axle, when on a level surface, shall be within 5 percent when calculated in accordance with 7.4.3.1 and tested in accordance with AMD Standard 013 (Weight Distribution Test). The ambulance manufacturer shall locate the center of gravity (CG) of the ambulance/ambulance body to determine and assure the purchaser that the CG of the completed ambulance does not exceed the maximum limits set by the chassis manufacturer. Consideration shall be given by the purchaser and manufacturer to locate equipment and components to permit inherently proper lateral balance, front/rear axle loading, and center of gravity. Ballasting (dead weight) shall not be used for proper weight distribution, counter balance, leveling, or lowering the center of gravity.

NOTE 5—**Warning:** Ambulance purchasers and manufacturers should pay particular attention to the front/rear weight distribution of the completed vehicle in order to maximize handling characteristics, traction, and braking performance. Weight distribution should be proportional to the front and rear GAWRS.

6.5.5 *Ratings*—Vehicle and component ratings shall be the chassis manufacturer's published ratings and shall not be raised above the chassis manufacturer's rating. When ratings are not published or chassis has been modified, the verification data of the component manufacturer's rating shall be made available to the appropriate offices of the procuring activity.

6.5.6 *Cab to Axle (CA), Type I and III Vehicles*—Cab to axle (CA) dimension of the vehicle chassis shall permit a minimum of 50 percent of the outside body length forward of the rear axle centerline, pins cab to body clearance. Bodies designed with wheel openings shall have the rear wheels centered, ± 5

PAYLOAD ALLOWANCE CERTIFICATION

NOTICE: THIS VEHICLE, AS MANUFACTURED, CONFORMS TO THE PAYLOAD REQUIREMENTS OF THE ASTM STANDARD PRACTICE FOR EMSS AMBULANCES. USERS SHALL NOT LOAD VEHICLE ABOVE THE GVWR. USERS SHOULD DETERMINE THAT THE ACTUAL LOAD TO BE PLACED ON THE VEHICLE DOES NOT EXCEED THE USABLE PAYLOAD.

Ambulance Manufacturer's Name ____________________

Chassis Model, Year of Manufacture ____________________

1 Vehicle Type and Class ____________________

2. Chassis Manufacturer GAWR-Front ____________________ kg.(lbs.)

3.Chassis Manufacturer GAWR Rear ____________________ kg.(lbs.)

4. Chassis Manufacturer GAWR ____________________ kg. (lbs.)

5. Minimum Payload As Specified. (Section 3.5 2) ____________________ kg.(lbs.)

6. Curb Weight-Front Base Vehicle ____________________ kg.(lbs.)

7. Curb Weight-Rear Base Vehicle ____________________ kg.(lbs.)

8. Curb Weight Base Vehicle
(Item 6 Plus Item 7) (Section 3.5.1) ____________________ kg.(lbs.)

9. Payload of Basic Vehicle
(Item 4 Minus Item 8)
Must Meet Or Exceed item 5. ____________________ kg.(lbs.)

10. Total Weight of Options as Specified on Vehicle ____________________ kg.(lbs.)

11. REMAINING USABLE PAYLOAD
(ACTUAL WEIGHT USER MAY ADD)
(Item 9 Minus item 10) ____________________ kg.(lbs.)

CAUTION:
THIS STICKER/PLATE SHALL BE MOUNTED ON THE BODY (MODULE) IN A CONSPICUOUS LOCATION.

The certification sticker is shown here as a suggested format. Deviations In dimensions are acceptable. All text must be included in manufacturer's sticker.

FIG. 5 Payload Allowance Certification

cm (2 in.) longitudinally, within the opening, and ± 13 mm (0.5 in.) laterally.

6.6 *Chassis Power Unit, and Components:*

6.6.1 *Chassis Frame*— The chassis shall include the chassis manufacturer's ambulance component package or, if not available, chassis manufacturers heavy duty components that will enhance vehicle's reliability, durability, safety, and comfort. The chassis frame and components shall be constructed to withstand the strains of on-off road service and any special service and equipment requirements specified herein. All chassis (including cab) components shall be as represented in the chassis manufacturer's technical data.

6.6.2 *Vehicle Lubrication*—The chassis components, devices, accessories, and added equipment requiring lubrication shall be fully equipped with lubrication fittings, as provided by the chassis or equipment manufacturer.

6.6.3 *Power Unit, Engines:*

6.6.3.1 *Power Unit*—The power unit shall meet or exceed the required vehicle performance specified herein (see 6.4), at not more than the engine manufacturer's recommended operating engine speed. It shall be of such design and construction that it will provide a smooth flow of power, at all rpm's, without undue vibration, strain, or overheating of engine parts.

6.6.3.2 *Engine Low Temperature Starting*—The engine shall start satisfactorily without the aid of preheating devices (except glow plugs) at -12°C (10°F), for the diesel engine, and -28.9°C (-20°F) when a gasoline engine is specified (see 9.2.10). When specified by the purchaser, auxiliary engine/battery heating and starting devices, or both, (see) shall be provided to meet other starting requirements. Verification test to be performed during environmental test.

6.6.3.2.1 Power Plant Heaters, Minimum -34°C (-30°F) Startability—In addition to the chassis manufacturers standard block heater on diesel engines, when specified (See Table 9, Item 16), the manufacturer's standard power plant heater(s) (coolant or immersion type crankcase heaters and battery heaters) shall be furnished for the gasoline engine, which limits starting an engine at -34°C (-30°F).

6.6.3.3 *Diesel Engine*— The chassis manufacturer's highest horsepower/displacement diesel engine and power train shall be provided, complying with requirements of 6.4. Net horsepower rating shall conform to SAE J1349. Additionally, the chassis manufacturer's block heater shall also be furnished. For type AD vehicles the power train shall meet the performance requirements specified herein or as specified or approved by the purchaser.

6.6.3.4 *Gasoline Engine*— When specified (See 9.2.10), a gasoline engine shall be furnished which permits warranted operation on unleaded gasoline, when operated in accordance with OEM's manual. When specified (See 9.2.50) or required for export, the vehicle shall be capable of warranted operation on either leaded or unleaded gasoline. Engine horsepower end torque requirements shall be sufficient to comply with the requirements specified in 6.4. Net horsepower ratings shall conform to SAE J1349. Vehicle(s) being offered/supplied with catalytic converters shall be identified to all purchasers.

NOTE 6—Purchasers should be aware that, because of the severe operating conditions to which an ambulance is exposed, the use of a gasoline engine results in substantially higher underhood and under vehicle temperatures which could seriously impact vehicle reliability, dependability, safety, and may result in some manufacturer's chassis warranty being voided.

6.6.4 *Power Unit Components:*

6.6.4.1 *Oil Filter*—The oil filter shall be the chassis manufacturer's standard for the engine offered.

6.6.4.2 *Air Filter*—The air filter shall be the chassis manufacturer's standard for the engine offered.

6.6.4.3 *Air Pollution Control (See* 9.2.11*)*—Vehicles destined for the 50 states, the District of Columbia, Puerto Rico, the Virgin Islands, Guam and American Samoa shall comply with the Environmental Protection Agency (EPA) regulations governing Control of Air Pollution from New Motor Vehicles and New Motor Vehicle Engines in effect on date of manufacture of the chassis/engine. In addition, vehicles destined for California shall comply with State of California regulations governing air pollution control in effect the date of manufacture. When specified (See Table 9, Item 17), the vehicle shall comply with the EPA high altitude regulations. For export vehicles, the chassis/engine manufacturer's export vehicle emission package shall be furnished that complies with destination requirements.

6.6.4.4 *Fuel System*— The fuel system shall conform to FMCSR Subpart E, 393.65 and 6.4.9 herein. Unless otherwise specified (See 9.2.5), fuel tank(s) capacity shall be the maximum available from the chassis manufacturer. When more than one tank is furnished, tanks shall be interconnected and, when available from the chassis manufacturer, separately controlled and shall have a dash-mounted fuel gauge controlled by a selector switch which will permit separate fuel level readings for each tank. When available from the chassis manufacturer, the Class 2 ambulance shall have the fuel tank(s) protected by a metal shield (skid-plate) and shall be located in an area which will be free from hazards encountered in off-road, cross-country operation. A permanent plate at the fuel filler opening shall be specifying type of fuel required.

6.6.4.5 *Cooling System*— The engine cooling system shall be a closed, air free, liquid state type with a coolant overflow recovery tank. The supplier shall provide the heaviest duty components and maximum size cooling system available from the chassis manufacturer. The cooling system design shall maintain the engine at safe operating temperatures at all driveable altitudes and grades encountered during on and off road vehicle use. Verification test: the cooling system shall be capable of maintaining a safe stabilized engine operating temperature for a minimum of one hour, at a minimum ambient temperature of 38°C (100°F), at all altitudes up to 3048 m (10,000 ft). For gasoline engines, the cooling system shall be capable of maintaining a safe operating temperature for not less than 40 min, at sea level, in a minimum ambient temperature of 35°C (95°F). Testing shall be at the engine speed required to maintain the generating systems specified in 6.7.6 and shall be in accordance with AMD Standard 014 (Cooling System Test).

6.6.4.5.1 Antifreeze—The cooling system shall be protected with a 50/50 solution of permanent type antifreeze.

6.6.4.6 *Exhaust System*— Vehicle shall be equipped with an exhaust system in accordance with Federal Motor Carrier Safety Regulations, Part 393.83. The exhaust system shall be suspended using not less than three hangers, excluding the manifold attachment. The exhaust shall discharge at the vertical side(s) of the ambulance at a maximum distance of 25 mm (1 in) beyond the side of the module away from the door(s) to minimize fumes and contaminants entering the interior. On modular vehicles, the tailpipe outlet shall not terminate within 15 mm (6 in.) of the vertical axis of the fuel tank filler opening(s). Modifications or extensions made to the OEM exhaust system shall meet or exceed chassis manufacturer's requirements in terms of backpressure, components, design, and workmanship.

6.6.5 *Drive Train:*

6.6.5.1 *Drive Train Components*—The drive train and component's torque capacity shall meet or exceed the maximum torque developed in the lowest gear ratio by the engine. Transmission and controls shall comply with FMVSS 101 and 102.

6.6.5.2 *Automatic Transmission*—Unless otherwise specified (See), the chassis manufacturer's automatic transmission shall be provided. The transmission shall provide not less than three speeds forward and one reverse and shall be equipped with the chassis manufacturer's heaviest duty oil cooler.

6.6.5.2.1 Automatic Transmission Auxiliary Heavy-Duty Oil Cooler—When specified (See Table 9, Item 20), a heavy-duty fin type auxiliary transmission oil cooler in addition to the OEM manufacturer's basic cooler (See 6.6.5.2) shall be provided and installed, in series, in a suitable location except behind the radiator.

6.6.5.3 *Transfer Case for Class 2 Ambulance*—Unless otherwise specified (See 9.2.12), a part-time four wheel drive system shall be provided for Class 2 vehicles. These vehicles shall be furnished with 2-speed transfer case that is integral with the main transmission. A shift pattern located on the shift knob or decal, within the cab shall be provided. Front-wheel drive hubs (See 6.6.5.9) and special traction rear-end differential (See 6.6.5.8), shall also be furnished on 4x4 vehicles. When furnished as part of a Class 2 conversion, the differential shall be identical to or heavier duty than the unit furnished on the OEM's original 4x4 Type I, Class 2 chassis.

6.6.5.3.1 Heavy Duty Skid Plate (Class 2, (4x4))—Unless otherwise required (See 9.2.12) and when available from the chassis manufacturer, a heavy-duty skid plate shall be installed protecting engine, transmission, and transfer case from ground contact if there is less than 38 cm (15 in.) of clearance to the ground. Skid plate shall be demountable for servicing the engine and transmission. Openings shall be provided to enable draining of transmission and servicing the underside of the engine. For fuel tank protection, see 6.6.4.4.

6.6.5.4 *Clutch*—Vehicles with manual transmissions shall be furnished with the manufacturer's largest, heavy-duty clutch available for the engine and model offered.

6.6.5.5 *Drive Line*—The drive-line (driveshaft, U-joints, etc.) shall be balanced and supported to perform throughout the design range without whipping or vibrating. Modifications resulting from lengthening the wheelbase or from 4x4 conversion shall be of chassis manufacturer's approved design.

6.6.5.6 *Axle Ratings, Ratios*—Axle ratings shall exceed the load imposed on each axle, measured at the ground, when vehicle is loaded. When specified (See 9.2.12) that the vehicle is used in mountainous terrain, manufacturer shall provide the highest numerical axle ratio. The chassis OEM "wide dual" rear axle shall be furnished on dual rear wheel chassis, unless otherwise specified (See 9.2.12) for a narrow modular body.

6.6.5.7 *Brake System Service and Parking*—Chassis manufacturer's heaviest duty, power assisted brakes, linings, and parking brake shall be furnished on the chassis model offered. ABS brakes shall be furnished when available. When air brakes are furnished, the system shall be designed to provide braking proportional to the front-rear weight distribution of the fully loaded vehicle. Additionally an air drier with moisture ejector shall be furnished and shall include a heater to prevent icing.

6.6.5.8 *Special Traction (Rear End) Differential*—Unless otherwise specified (See 9.2.12) or if not available from chassis manufacturer, all vehicles shall have a positive traction, limited slip differential or automatic, locking type differential.

6.6.5.9 *Drive Hubs, Front Wheel, (4x4, Class2)*—Unless otherwise specified (See 9.2.12), and when available from the chassis manufacturer, automatic type front wheel locking hubs shall be provided. Additionally, when a 4x4 conversion is furnished, the heaviest duty front hubs available from the axle manufacturer shall be furnished.

6.6.5.10 *Suspension*—Vehicle shall be equipped with matched sets (front and rear) of spring, torsion, or air suspension system components. Components shall have a rated capacity in excess of the load imposed on each member. For better riding quality, vehicle springs shall have chassis manufacturer's lowest clamped deflection rating (smoothest riding suspension) for the model offered. Suspension stabilizer bar(s) shall be furnished for front and rear, when available from chassis manufacturer for the model chassis furnished. Only corrections permitted by the chassis manufacturer to compensate for lean due to normal spring tolerance variations are permitted. Correction of lean due to imbalance is not permitted. Vehicle shall be balanced.

6.6.5.11 *Spring Stops*— The chassis manufacturer's standard spring bumpers and axle stops shall be furnished. The stops/bumpers shall prevent the wheel and axles from striking the engine, oil pan, fenders, and body under all conditions of operation. Additionally, when a 4x4 conversion is furnished, spring stops/bumpers shall be provided and, at a minimum, be of OEM quality.

6.6.5.12 *Shock Absorbers*— Shock absorbers, double-acting type, heaviest duty available from chassis manufacturer for model offered, shall be furnished on the front and rear axles. Class 2 (4x4) vehicles shall additionally be furnished with quad front shocks when available from chassis manufacturer.

6.6.6 *Steering*—The OE chassis manufacturer's standard, power assisted steering shall be furnished.

6.6.7 *Wheels*—Unless otherwise specified (See 9.2.13), Types I and III vehicles shall be equipped with dual metal wheels. Type II vehicles shall be equipped with single, front and rear wheels. Wheels shall conform to the recommendations of the Tire and Rim Association, Inc., and shall be identical in type, size, and load rating for all wheels on the vehicle, including the spare.

6.6.8 *Tires* —Unless otherwise specified or permitted by purchaser (See 9.2.14), tires shall be OEM tubeless, steel belted radials with "All Season Type Tread" for the GVWR of the vehicle. All tires furnished shall be identical and comply to FMVSS 120. To provide a softer ride for a loaded ambulance, the tires shall be inflated only to the tire manufacturers cold inflation air pressure absolutely necessary to support the load on each tire measured at the ground. The manufacturer shall provide instruction for the correct front and rear tire pressures required for the ambulance GVWR.

6.6.9 *Inner Tubes*— When tube type tires are furnished, inner tubes shall conform with the recommendations of the Tire and Rim Association, Inc.

6.6.10 *Spare Tire and Storage*—Unless otherwise specified by the purchaser (See 9.2.15), one inflated spare wheel/tire assembly identical to those on the vehicle shall be furnished. The spare assembly shall be stored in an accessible weather protected compartment or area. When available from the chassis manufacturer, the spare tire shall be located under the rear of the vehicle. The spare tire assembly shall be accessed by the chassis manufacturer's winch type carrier. An equivalent winch carrier assembly may be retrofitted on other chassis. When locating spare tire assembly under the vehicle, all other specification requirements (for example, departure angle, ground clearance, weight distribution) shall be in compliance. Access door shall be fitted with suitable latch and lock when accessible from outside the vehicle. Loose or removable panel(s)/door(s) shall not be acceptable. The spare tire assembly shall be accessible without removal of the patients from the compartment. The spare assembly and tools shall have restraining devices to eliminate rattling and dislocation in case of an accident. The carrier design shall enable removal and mounting of the spare assembly using only the tools specified in 6.6.13 (See 6.11.3).

6.6.11 *Tire Chain Clearance*—Tire chain clearance on the furnished body shall be provided for all driving wheels per SAE J683. Additionally, sufficient chain clearance shall be provided to permit off road operation with the ambulance loaded to the maximum payload.

6.6.12 *Wheel Tire Balancing*—Wheel/tire, hubs, and brake drum assemblies of the vehicle shall be in balance to a minimum of 112 km/hr (70 mph).

6.6.13 *Tools (Tire Changing)*—Vehicle shall be furnished with tools for exchanging mounted tire assembly with the spare assembly and shall include at least a jack, jack handle, and wheel nut wrench. The jack height, when closed, shall permit its location under the axle or other satisfactory lift point at any wheel with the tire flat. The jack, without having to block the jack shall be capable of raising any wheel of the loaded vehicle to a height adequate to permit removal and replacement of the wheel and tire assembly. Tools shall be stored in accordance with 6.6.10.

6.6.14 *Hub Caps*—Manufacturer's (OEM) standard hubcap or wheel cover shall be fitted on each wheel except the spare. Vehicles with dual wheels and Class 2 modular vehicles (See 6.16.2.1) do not require hubcaps.

6.7 *Electrical System and Components*

6.7.1 *Electrical System*—(See Fig. 7). The ambulance electrical system shall be equipped with but not limited to, the following: dual chassis manufacturer's 12 V batteries; generating, starting, lighting, visual and audible warning systems; specified electronics equipment and devices (including master consoles located in the cab and patient compartment); and other specified accessory wiring. The electrical systems and equipment shall comply with all applicable FMVSS, Federal Motor Carrier Safety Regulations (FMCSR), and shall also conform to all the applicable SAE recommended standards and practices, whether or not specifically referenced in this document, while complying with the subparagraphs herein. All electrical and electronic components shall be selected to minimize electrical loads thereby not exceeding the vehicle's generating system capacity. All electrical system components and wiring shall be readily accessible through access panels for checking and maintenance. All switches, indicators, and controls shall be located and installed in a manner that facilitates easy removal and servicing. All exterior housings of lamps, switches, electronic devices, and fixtures shall be corrosion resistant and weatherproofed.

All electrical devices and equipment installed, which produce RFI, shall include filters, suppressors, or shielding to prevent electromagnetic radiation and the resultant interference

PORTABLE EQUIPMENT BATTERY CHARGING CIRCUIT (See Section 6.7.7.2)

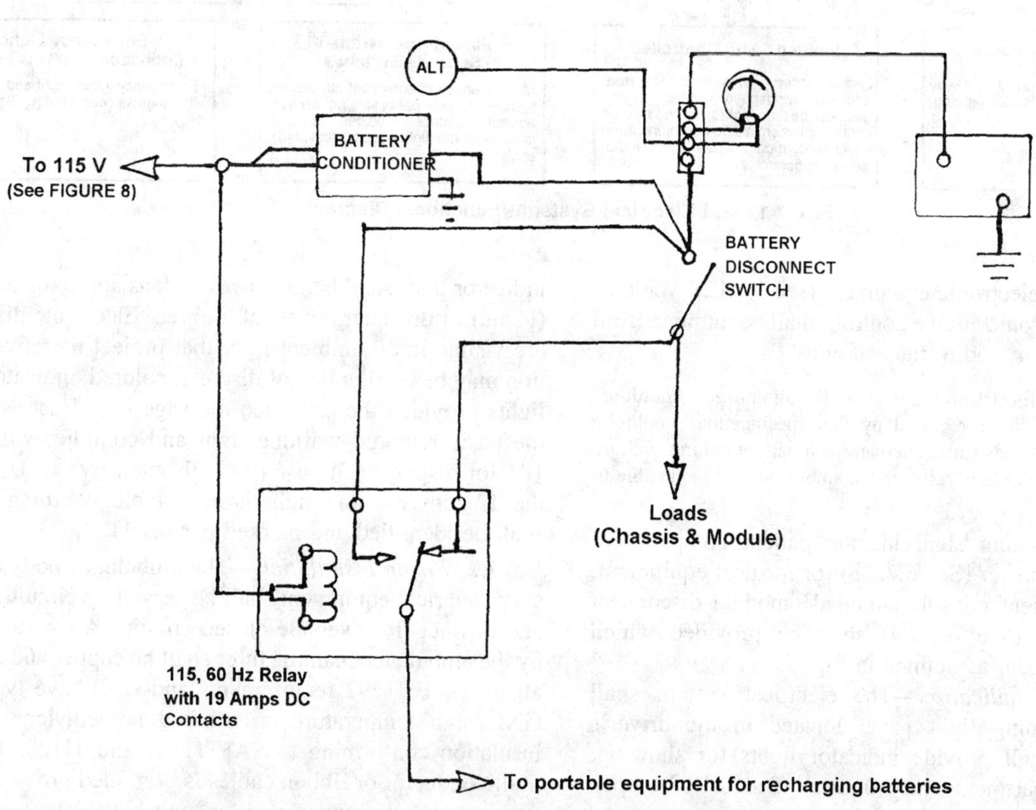

Permits recharge of portable equipment batteries only when vehicle is running or vehicle is plugged into 115 VAC sore power and the battery conditioner is energized.

FIG. 6 Portable Equipment Battery Charging Circuit (See 6.7.7.2)

12 VOLT ELECTRICAL SYSTEM – FUNCTIONAL DIAGRAM

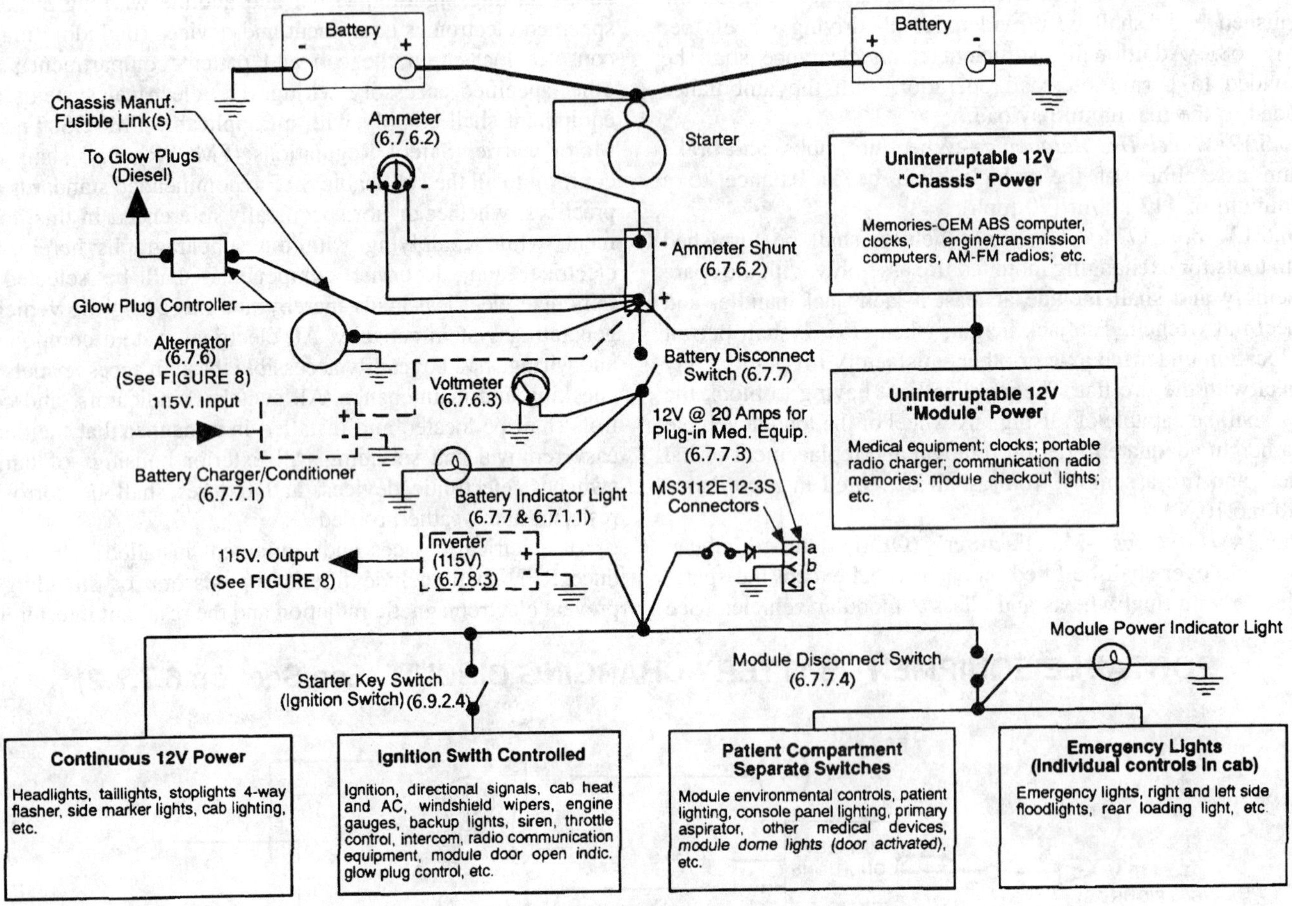

FIG. 7 12 Volt Electrical System - Functional Diagram

to radios and other electronic equipment (see 6.7.12). Vehicles equipped with electronic engine controls shall be immune from interference caused by radio transmissions.

NOTE 7—**Warning:** Electrical loads shall be minimized. Additional electrical loads above those required by this specification should be avoided because heavy loads cause alternator and battery failures. Failure of these components will likely result in the ambulance not being able to complete its mission.

The electrical system shall include patient compartment outlets for 12 volt power (See 6.7.7.3) for medical equipment. A driver compartment console-mounted "module disconnect switch or device" (See 6.7.7.4) shall be provided which controls the equipment as defined in Fig. 7.

6.7.1.1 *Warning Indicators*—The electrical system shall incorporate a warning light panel located in the driver's compartment. It shall provide indicator lights for showing: open patient compartment entry door(s) (See 6.10.8); open equipment compartment door(s); and when batteries are turned on by the battery disconnect switch (See 6.7.7). The "Door Open" warning lights shall be red, flash battery and approximately 13 mm (½ in) in diameter, or equal, in area. The hazard indicator light shall be green with a lens approximately 13 mm (½ in.) in diameter, or equal, in area. Electronic displays that are visible in all ambient light that project narrative information may be used in lieu of discrete, colored, indicator/warning lights provided the projected message is at least as visible as the basic required warning light and complies with FMVSS 101 for displays. The use of "high intensity" LEDs in lieu of the 13 mm warning light is acceptable. Warning indicators shall be identified and marked per 6.7.11.

6.7.2 *Wiring Installation*—The ambulance body and accessory electrical equipment shall be served by circuit(s) separate and distinct from vehicle closed circuits. All wiring provided by the ambulance manufacturer shall be copper and conform to all the SAE J1292 requirements and shall have type SXL or GXL high temperature crosslinked polyethylene, or better, insulation conforming to SAE J1127 and J1128. The use of multiconductor or ribbon cables is permitted provided they are not exposed to underhood or under vehicle temperatures/conditions. The wiring shall be permanently color coded or marked the entire length of the wire for identification with easily read numbers and letters, or both, and routed in conduit or high temperature looms with a rating of 149°C (300°F). When cables are supplied by a component manufacturer to interconnect system components, these cables need not be continuously color coded/identified. They shall be coded/identified at the termination or interconnection points. All added wiring shall be located in accessible, enclosed, protected locations and kept at least 15 cm (6 in.) away from exhaust system components. Electrical wiring and components shall not terminate in the oxygen storage compartment except for the oxygen controlled solenoid, compartment light, and switch plunger or trigger device. Wiring necessarily passing through an oxygen compartment shall be routed in a metallic conduit (See 6.11.3). All conduits, looms, and wiring shall be secured to the body or frame with insulated metal cable straps in order to prevent sagging and movement which results in chafing, pinching, sagging, or any other damage. All apertures on the vehicle shall be properly grommeted for passing wiring and conform to SAE 1292. All items used for protecting or securing the wiring shall be appropriate for the specific application and be standard automotive, aircraft, marine, or electronic hardware. Cable ties shall not be used to support harnesses but may be used for bundling purposes. Electrical panels that are accessible to accidental contact shall have a protective cover, shield, etc. to prevent shorts that can result in injury, fire, or damage to the electrical system.

6.7.2.1 *Wiring Criteria*— All wiring (including grounds), devices, switches, outlets, etc., except circuit breakers, shall be rated to carry at least 125 percent of the maximum ampere load for which the circuit is protected. A service loop of wire or harness shall be provided at all electrical components, terminals, and connection points that permits at least two replacements of the wire(s) termination. All splices and terminals provided shall comply with SAE J163, J561, or J928 as applicable. All wiring between the cab/chassis and module in Type I and III ambulances shall be connected to a terminal strip(s), block(s), or multi-pin connector(s) near the point of entry to the patient module. All terminals shall be permanently numbered or coded. Terminal strip(s), block(s), or multi-pin connector(s) shall be readily accessible for checking and service. All exterior wiring to lights or any other component shall utilize sealed connectors or splices.

The ambulance electrical system shall incorporate a master circuit breaker panel with circuit breakers or other electronic, non-disposable, current protection devices, in each circuit, which comply with SAE J553 Type I or Type III, if circuit breaker is readily accessible for resetting by the driver or EMT. When multiconductor cables/ribbon cables are used for low current (self limiting) circuits, additional fuses/circuit breakers are not required. Additionally, one 15 ampere circuit breaker shall be provided for future use. For high current circuits, where SAE Type I breakers are not commercially produced, protection for these circuits may be provided with other types of circuit breakers. All circuit breakers shall be securely mounted, easily removable, and readily accessible for inspection and service. All electrical and electronic components, switches, connectors, circuit breakers, lamps, and indicators, including the vehicle batteries, shall be marked with an easily read identification code number and letter, or both. Complete, highly legible, wiring diagrams and schematics, including identification codes and parts list for the ambulance's standard and optional equipment furnished, shall be included in the service manual and be supplied with each ambulance in accordance with 9.8.

6.7.2.2 *Printed Circuits*— When printed circuits utilized, they shall conform to SAE J771. Printed circuit boards shall be securely mounted and protected from physical damage and accidental shorts. Printed circuit board connections and components shall conform to all other specification requirements.

6.7.3 *Grounding:*

6.7.3.1 Dedicated grounds for all appliances, circuits, etc. shall be furnished. The use of appliance mounting screws/hardware shall not be used for grounding purposes unless specifically designed for such use by the appliance manufacturer.

6.7.3.2 To provide RF grounding and minimize potential interference with chassis manufacturer's computers, the module and chassis cab shall be connected to the chassis frame with a separate dedicated minimum 19 mm (¾ in.), braided ground strap with soldered ends that are secured to cleaned metal surfaces on the body and frame with star washers, etc. To prevent corrosion, both ends of the attached ground strap shall then be sealed with either rustproofing compounds or non-hardening battery terminal sealer.

NOTE 8—Regular stranded copper wire, while providing a DC ground, does not provide RF grounding.

6.7.4 *Windshield Wipers and Washers*—Vehicle shall be equipped with dual, electric, multi-speed, windshield wipers and washer complying with FMVSS 104. When specified (See 9.2.16), the OEM intermittent wipers shall be furnished.

6.7.5 *Horns*—The chassis manufacturer's dual electric horns shall be furnished. See 6.14.6 for switching arrangements.

6.7.6 *Electrical Generating System*—(See Fig. 7) Unless otherwise specified (See 9.2.17), the ambulance shall be equipped with a generating system rated at not less than 135 amperes, at 14 volts, with an underhood temperature of 93°C (200°F). As a minimum, the generating system shall be capable of supplying at its regulated voltage, at 93°C (200°F), the continuous electrical load which consists of the following electrical equipment and systems: engine/transmission control system; headlights (low beam); all FMVSS 108 lights; windshield wipers (low speed); cab air conditioning (at coldest setting with highest blower speed); radio in receiving mode (or equal load, if not equipped); patient module dome lighting (in the high intensity setting); patient module air conditioning (at coldest setting with highest blower speed); emergency warning lighting system (in the daytime "primary" mode) (See 6.8.2); and 20 amp medical load or equal.

NOTE 9—**Warning:** Additional (optional), continuous load, electrical devices or systems, (additional warning lights, on board 115 V AC supply, etc.), are permitted, providing reserve or additional generating capacity is available or added.

NOTE 10—**Warning:** Manufacturers/purchasers should note that the "cold", maximum rpm, output rating of the alternator may be substantially higher than the hot 93°C (200°F) operational speed ratings. For example, the cold, high speed rating may be 165 amps while the hot operational speed rating may be approximately 135 amps.

The generating system shall supply the maximum electrical load, at the regulated voltage, at 93°C (200°F) underhood temperature, and with an engine speed not exceeding 40 percent of the furnished engine's SAE net HP, RPM rating. The throttle control device, specified in 6.7.6.1, shall control the engine RPM necessary to maintain the heating and air conditioning systems, at full operating capacity, and to maintain the generating system's required output when the vehicle is stationary. The 12 V electrical system shall incorporate an ammeter (see 6.7.6.2) and a voltmeter or voltage warning device (See 6.7.6.3) which are functionally connected as shown in Fig. 7. The final stage manufacturer/supplier shall test each ambulance prior to delivery and provide, to the purchaser, a written certification (tag) indicating the amount of generating capacity remaining, at the regulated voltage, at 93°C (200°F), after supplying the total electrical load as manufactured (including the purchaser options). Testing and tagging shall be in accordance with AMD Standard 005 (Ambulance Electrical System).

6.7.6.1 *Engine High-Idle Speed Control, Automatic*—An engine high-idle speed control shall be furnished on all vehicles which automatically increases the engine speed (RPM) to sustain the ambulance's total continuous electrical load and maximum heating/air conditioning output. The device shall be preset so that, when activated, it will operate the engine at the appropriate RPM (See 6.7.6). The device shall operate only when switched to the "ON" position and the transmission is in "NEUTRAL", "PARK" and the parking brake is applied (when required by the chassis manufacturer). For transmissions without a "PARK" position, the device shall function only with the transmission in "NEUTRAL" and with the parking brake applied. The device shall disengage when the operator depresses the service brake pedal or the transmission is placed in gear, and automatically re-engage when the service brake is released or when the transmission is placed in neutral or park. The device shall be furnished by the chassis manufacturer when available.

NOTE 11—Diesel engine manufacturers state that their engines should be set at an elevated speed during extended idle periods. Additionally, the elevated idle speed reduces torsional vibration which causes alternator belt slippage.

6.7.6.2 *Ammeter*—The electrical system (See Fig. 7) shall incorporate a center scale ammeter or equivalent electronic digital display which is capable of indicating a current of ± 150 amperes to or from (charging or discharging) the vehicle's batteries. The ammeter, or equivalent electronic, digital display shall incorporate an external shunt or current monitoring device which does not exceed 150 millivolts at maximum current. The ammeter and shunt, or equivalent device, shall have a combined accuracy of ± 10 percent of the full scale reading. The meter shall be mounted in a location highly visible to the vehicle operator and shall be illuminated for night operation. The shunt or monitoring device shall be protected against physical damage, weather, road spray, and shall be mounted in an easily accessible location which shall minimize the length of the power cables.

6.7.6.3 *Voltmeter of Voltage Monitor*—A voltmeter, or equivalent electronic device, illuminated for nighttime operation, which constantly monitors the 12 V electrical system or a warning device and indicates abnormally high or low electrical system voltages shall be furnished. The device furnished must be mounted so it is clearly visible to the driver at all times.

6.7.7 *Battery System*— Two 12 V batteries (or additional batteries as required by the chassis manufacturer), with a labeled "Battery Disconnect Switch", shall be furnished. A switch operated solenoid may be employed to provide the battery disconnect function. Unless otherwise specified (See Table 9, Item 5), the batteries shall be equivalent to the chassis OEM batteries. When high cycle batteries are specified, performance ratings for each battery shall not be less than 625 cold cranking amps and 180 min reserve capacity.

Battery ratings shall conform to SAE J537. Batteries shall be located in a ventilated area, sealed off from occupant compartments, and shall be readily accessible for servicing and removal. When batteries are mounted in the engine compartment, they shall be provided with a heat shield as a safeguard against high underhood temperatures.

Unless the "Battery Disconnect Switch" is clearly visible to the driver, in the seated position, a green indicator light, indicating the batteries are "ON" (See 6.7.1.1), shall be furnished. Battery selector device wiring and added/modified starting motor requirements shall meet or exceed the SAE J1127 for high temperature SGX wire and SAE J541 for maximum voltage drop requirements for 12 V heavy-duty applications. The "Battery Disconnect Switch" shall be wired per Fig. 7, and shall select both batteries simultaneously.

When specified (See 9.2.18), the batteries, on Types I & III vehicles, shall be located in the module, sealed from the interior, or on Type II vehicles, in a compartment or lower skirt. Batteries shall be on a slide out tray or be readily available for service. When relocating batteries, the method of relocation shall be approved by the chassis manufacturer.

NOTE 12—Module battery locations can provide for improved front/rear and lateral weight distribution and for a lower center of gravity.

6.7.7.1 *Battery Charger or Conditioner*—When specified (See Table 9, Item 7), either a 12 V DC taper type battery charger or automatic conditioner shall be provided. The charger/conditioner shall be listed by an organization meeting the requirements in 6.7.8, and connected to the 12 V DC battery system as shown in Fig. 7. The charger shall be capable of supplying a minimum of 10 amperes charging current. The charger/conditioner shall be permanently mounted, in the vehicle, in a properly ventilated, accessible location and wired to the 115 V AC utility power as specified in 6.7.8 and Fig. 7. Battery charger controls shall include an "ON/OFF" switch and a charging indicator. When a battery conditioner is provided, it shall monitor the battery state of charge and, as necessary, automatically charge or maintain the batteries without gassing, depleting fluid level, overheating, or overcharging

6.7.7.2 *Portable Equipment Charging Circuit*—(See Fig. 6) A circuit shall be furnished for the module and the cab for charging all portable battery powered devices, for example, suction units, hand lights, defibrillators, portable radios, etc. This circuit shall prevent discharge of chassis batteries by only permitting the charging of portable devices when the vehicle is either running or the battery conditioner is operational. Circuit breaker protection shall be provided and shall have a minimum of 10 amp capacity. Additional tagged, identified leads shall be furnished in both the cab and module for connection of additional equipment that requires recharging. A decal shall be furnished in a conspicuous location in the cab stating, "This vehicle is equipped with a battery conditioner to maintain batteries in a full state of charge, and a dedicated 12 V recharging circuit for portable battery powered equipment." For operation, vehicle shall be plugged into 115 V AC shore power during periods of non-use.

6.7.7.3 *Internal 12 V DC Power*—(See Fig. 7). Unless otherwise specified by the purchaser (See 9.2.19), the patient compartment shall be furnished with a 12 V DC, 20 ampere capacity, separately protected circuit, with two outlet receptacles. The circuit shall include a (low voltage drop) "Schottky" diode to isolate medical equipment batteries from any electrical loads that the remainder of the ambulance electrical system may impose. The "Schottky" diode shall be heat-sink mounted, have an inverse voltage rating of at least 45 V and also be rated to carry the maximum short circuit current, until the circuit breaker opens. The diode shall be physically located in an accessible location and be electrically connected between the circuit breaker and the "action wall" mounted receptacle. Unless otherwise specified (See 9.2.19), the receptacles shall be a military type connector of the following generic configuration, MS3112E12-3S or its interchangeable commercial equivalent. The polarity of the connector shall be as follows: Pin A (+12V), Pin B (Ground), Pin C (not used). The receptacles shall be located on a vertical surface of the "action wall" or other location specified by the purchaser. The mating plug attached to the medical equipment shall be an MS3116FI2-3P or its interchangeable commercial equivalent. The polarity for the plug shall be the same as above. Two of these unwired plugs shall be furnished and tagged with polarity requirements and shall be connected to the receptacles.

NOTE 13—These connectors are widely available directly from most major industrial electronics distributors.

When required or specified (See 9.2.19) for constant power source for medical equipment battery charging a 12V protected circuit shall be furnished that connects directly to the battery side of the load disconnect switch.

6.7.7.4 *Master Module Disconnect Switch or Device*—This switch (See Fig. 7) shall be located in the driver's compartment, be legibly marked, illuminated when "ON", and rated to carry at least 125 percent of the circuit's maximum current.

6.7.8 *115 V or 115/230AC Utility Power*—(See Fig. 8). Unless otherwise specified, the ambulance shall be furnished with a 2–wire plus ground 115 V AC wiring system that is separate and distinct from the vehicle's 12 V DC wiring system(s). The AC electrical system, including wiring and associated equipment, shall comply with AMD Standard 009. Listing shall be by a nationally recognized testing laboratory, recognized by OSHA under Appendix A to 29 CFR 1910.7. The AC system is to be utilized while the vehicle is stationary for powering maintenance devices, medical equipment battery chargers, and when specified (See 6.15.3 and 9.2), vehicle battery conditioner/charger, and any other device(s) deemed necessary by the purchaser. The AC system shall incorporate a ground fault circuit interrupter (GFCI) device and a minimum 15 ampere circuit breaker which can be used as a master AC disconnect switch. The GFCI and circuit breaker may be an integral unit. The AC wiring shall utilize stranded wire in armored cable, nonmetallic sheathed cable, "Type SO" or better flexible cable rated at 600V and 90°C, covered with a minimum 149°C (300°F), flame retardant wire loom, or approved wire in conduit.

When an onboard AC 9 supply is specified (see 6.7.8.3), an automatic transfer switch shall be furnished which turns off this onboard AC supply (interlock) and disconnects its output, when the AC utility power is applied.

115 VOLT ELECTRICAL SYSTEM – FUNCTIONAL DIAGRAM

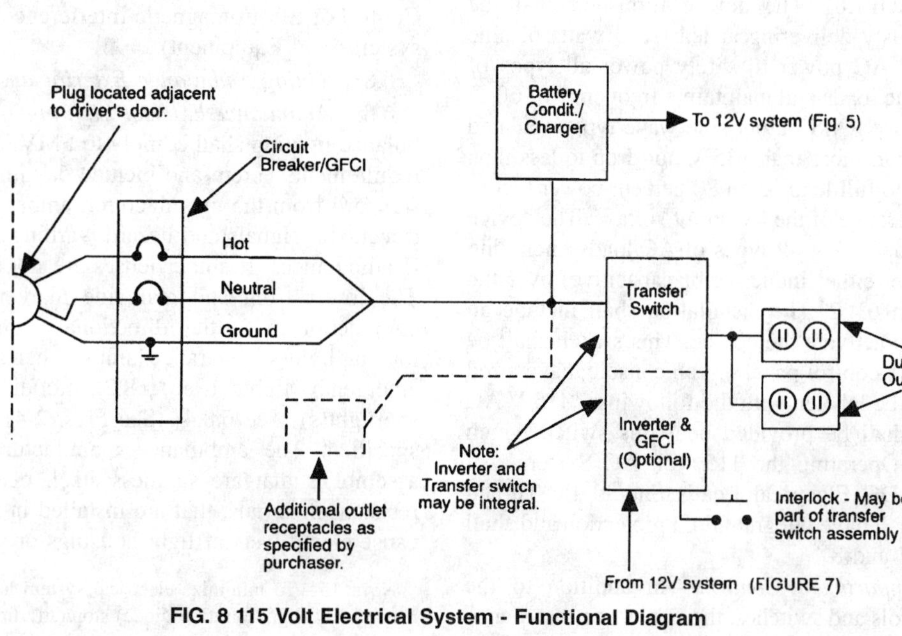

FIG. 8 115 Volt Electrical System - Functional Diagram

When the 12 VDC battery charger (see Table 9, Item 7) and any power plant heater(s) (see Table 9, Item 16) are furnished and connected to this system, they shall be wired so that they can be energized only from the utility power, and not the onboard AC supply. The onboard AC system shall not be utilized for operational ambulance interior lighting, such as dome and cot lights.

6.7.8.1 *Utility Power Connector*—Unless additional capacity is required, a 115 V AC (male) plug (NEMA 5-15P), rated at 15 amps with spring loaded cover assembly suitable for wet locations, shall be installed on the driver's side of the ambulance body in close proximity to driver's door. The connection shall be permanently labeled with the following: "This Connection is for [115] Volt AC, 60 Hz, 15 Ampere Supply."

NOTE 14—The above label shall reflect actual voltage and current connections if other than shown.

This receptacle shall energize the vehicle's internal AC circuit(s) from an exterior power source (utility power). The purchaser's stationary utility power circuit supplying the ambulance's 115 V AC power should incorporate ground fault protection. A proper mating weatherproof, 15 ampere or more when required, female receptacle (NEMA 5- 15R) shall also be furnished without cable and tagged specifying the size, type of wire necessary, and the polarity of the future hookup.

6.7.8.2 *Electrical 115 V, A/C Receptacles*—The patient compartment shall be furnished with a pair of 2-wire plus ground duplex 115 V AC receptacles. Receptacles shall be near flush mounted with one outlet located on the vertical, primary patient, action wall and the other vertically located at the torso area of the secondary patient (squad bench). Both outlets shall be at least 31 cm (12 in.) from any oxygen outlet. An indicator shall be located within each 115 V AC receptacle as a line monitor indicating a live (hot) circuit. The receptacles shall be labeled with the following: "115 V AC."

6.7.8.3 *Solid State Inverter for Onboard 115 V A/C Power*—When specified under Table 9, Item 6, a DC to AC inverter shall be provided in conjunction with the onboard 115 V AC wiring system (See 6.7.8). The device furnished shall be capable of continuously delivering at least 750 watts of sine wave type regulated AC power to safely power all types of electrical or electronic loads and maintain a frequency of 60 ± 4 Hz. The single phase RMS output sine wave type regulated voltage shall not rise to more than 135 V nor drop to less than 105 V from no load to full load, at an 80 percent power factor, over the 12.8 to 14.8 range of the DC input voltage. The device shall be capable of operating all types of AC loads, including resistive and reactive (either inductive or capacitive) over the temperature range in 6.4.2. The installation shall include an "ON-OFF" switch to activate the device. This switch shall be located on the EMT's control panel or cab console, have a red "ON" indicator, and be labeled with the following: "115 V AC Inverter." A decal shall be provided near this switch which states that: "When Operating the 115 Volt AC System, All Unnecessary 12 V DC Electrical Loads Should Be Turned Off." The inverter shall have integral GFCI protection and shall be wired per Figs. 7 and 8.

6.7.9 *Driver Compartment Controls*—In addition to the left-hand drive controls and switches, the final stage ambulance manufacturer shall provide and locate, within easy normal reach of the driver, the specified controls and instruments. The battery and module disconnect switches or devices (see 6.7.7.4) shall be different in feel from each other and be supplied with a handle or knob which feels different to the touch than the other switches or be physically isolated from them.

6.7.10 *Patient Compartment Controls*—Unless otherwise specified by the purchaser (See 9.2.20), the patient compartment controls, switches, and instruments shall be panel mounted and located within normal reach of the seated EMT (See 6.10.3).

6.7.11 *Marking of Switches, Indicators, and Control Devices*—All switches, indicators, and control devices supplied by the end product manufacturer of the ambulance shall be clearly visible to the ambulance personnel. They shall be perceptively and permanently identified with at least 12 point letters for the noun or function and 8 point for the remainder of the legend. The identifications shall be contrasting colors etched or engraved in plastic or metal, or printed and laminated in see through plastic, and grouped according to function, mounted in illuminated or backlit panel(s) or console.

6.7.12 *Electromagnetic Radiation and Suppression*—In addition to OEM chassis, all added electrically operated or electrical generating devices, including alternators, air conditioning warning light systems, and medical equipment including portable medical equipment that can be operated from its own internal power source, shall be electromagnetic radiation suppressed, filtered, or shielded to prevent interference to radios, telemetry equipment, and other medical devices operated aboard the vehicle and the surrounding area and shall not exceed SAE J551 limits. Type certification for these devices is acceptable. When specified by the purchaser (see 9.2.21), the completed ambulance vehicle shall be tested and certified to demonstrate that the RFI does not exceed the maximum limits of SAE J551. When electrically operated medical equipment is specified, such equipment shall be in compliance with and tested in accordance with MIL-STD-461 (Requirements for the Control of Electromagnetic Interference Charateristics of Subsystems and Equipment)..

6.8 *Lighting Ambulance Exterior and Interior:*

6.8.1 *Ambulance Exterior Lighting*—The basic exterior ambulance lighting shall comply to FMVSS Std. No. 108 and the requirements herein and include daytime running lights when standard from the manufacturer, amber colored front and rear directional signals and hazard warning lights (except on Type II ambulances, if amber lenses are not available from OEM). The lower front and rear side marker lights shall flash in conjunction with the directional signals. Backup light(s)/ loading light(s), clearance lamps (when applicable), ambulance emergency lights (See 6.8.2), floodlights (See 6.8.3), and spotlight(s) (See 6.8.4) (See Figs. 2-4), shall be furnished as specified. The ambulance manufacturer shall furnish light assemblies that are stainless steel, plastic, or other weather resistant materials, that are installed in a manner that will not cause electrolysis of light housings or vehicle body.

NOTE 15—To minimize electrical system loading and reduce maintenance LED (light emitting diode) stop/tail, directional and marker lights shall be furnished when specified by the purchaser, (See 9.2.58) on modular bodies.

6.8.2 *Ambulance Emergency Lighting*—As specified (See 9.2.22), a strobe, halogen, HID, or any other source of light for the emergency lighting system shall provide the ambulance with 360° of conspicuity for safety during its missions. The system must display highly perceptible and attention-getting signals that function in a modal system and convey the message in the Primary Mode - "Clear the Right-of-Way" and in the Secondary Mode - "Hazard, Vehicle Stopped on Right-of-Way." The ambulance warning light system shall not impose a continuous average electrical load exceeding 40 amperes at 14.2 volts and 42 amperes with the optional second amber rear light.

NOTE 16—**Warning:** Purchasers should not specify warning lights beyond those required herein. Additional lighting will utilize reserve alternator capacity and could result in overloaded electrical systems. (See Warnings in 6.7.1 and 6.7.6).

Additional warning lights are not required but if specified (See 9.2.22), shall not obscure the light output of the warning light system. Additional warning light systems furnished shall be separately switched. Any warning devices furnished, in addition to the specified system, shall be compensated for with reserve or additional generating capacity as required in 6.7.6.

6.8.2.1 *Standard Emergency Lighting System Configuration*—The ambulance standard emergency warning light system shall contain twelve fixed red tights, one fixed clear light and one or two fixed amber or SAE "selective yellow" light(s). These lights shall function in a dual mode system as shown in Table 2 and meet the physical and photometric requirements of 6.8.2.2 and Table 3. The upper body warning lights shall be mounted at the extreme upper corner areas of the ambulance body, below the horizontal roofline. The single clear light shall be centered between the two front facing, red upper corner lights or in a dedicated housing mounted forward of the body on the cab roof (see Fig. 2, Fig. 3, Fig. 4, and Fig. 9). The lights may also be mounted in dedicated housings on the cab roof if necessary due to limited body dimensions and the physical size of the outboard forward facing lights. The standard warning lights shall not be obstructed by doors or other ancillary equipment. The amber light(s) shall be symmetrically located between the two rear facing red lights. The red "grille" lights shall be located at least 76 cm (30 in.) above the ground and below the bottom edge of the windshield and be laterally separated by at least 46 cm (18 in.), measured from centerline to centerline of each lamp. The lateral facing intersection lights shall be mounted as close as possible to the front upper edge of each front fender and may be angled forward a maximum of 30°. All warning lights furnished shall be mounted to project their highest intensity beams on the horizontal axis, (See 6.8.2.4).

6.8.2.2 *Standard Emergency Warning Lighting System Photometric and Physical Requirements*—Each emergency light shall flash 75 to 125 times per minute. All warning lights shall project a beam spread of at least 5° up and 5° down and at least 45° left and right of H-V. Each light shall produce a decreasing flash energy per flash, measured from the H-V to all the extreme test point coordinates and shall be tested at all 5° increments. At no point shall the flash energy values drop to less than the minimum values as shown in Table 3, when tested at 14.2 volts. Flash energy shall be determined in accordance with SAE J845 method for determining the flash energy of a light. Testing shall be conducted on the devices as manufactured including use of the actual light source and all other related system components.

6.8.2.3 *Switching Arrangements*—The emergency light switches shall be wired and arranged to provide the warning

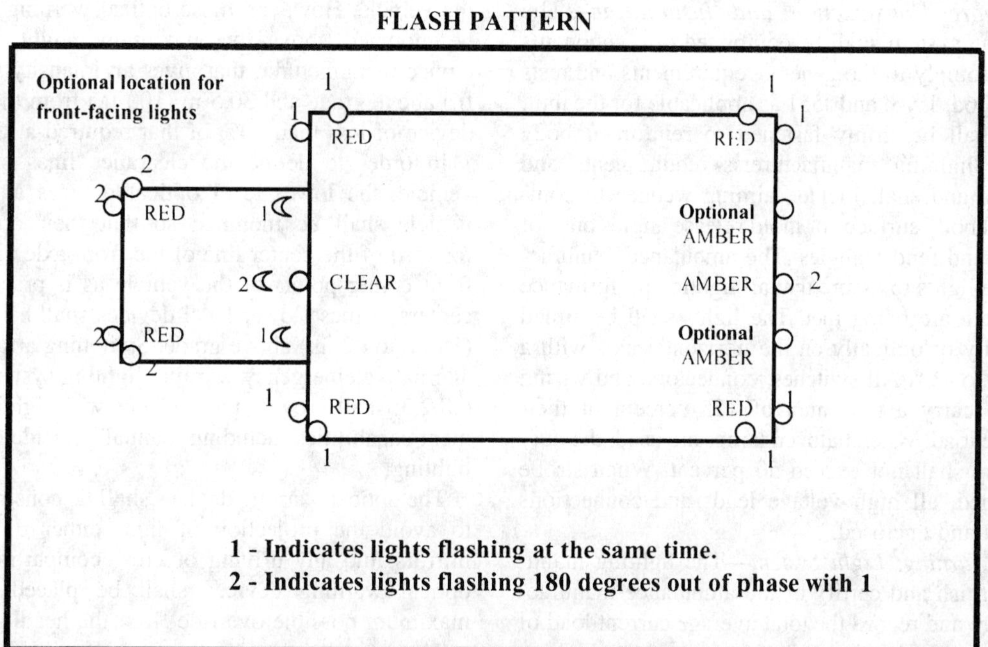

FIG. 9 Flash Pattern

TABLE 2 Modal Emergency Lighting System

Mode of Operation	Color & Location Red Front and Rear Corners	Clear Front Upper Center	Amber Rear Center	Red Grille and Fender
Primary "Clear the Right-of-Way"	On	On	On	On
Secondary "Hazard-Vehicle Stopped on Right-of-Way"	On	Off	On	Off

TABLE 3 Minimum Flash Energy, (cd.s) Per Flash, Per Fixture

Color Location	Red Grill & Fenders	Red Upper Body Corners	Clear Front Center	Amber Rear Center
Day	160 cd.s @ HV 80 cd.s @ ± 5° 12 cd.s @ All 5° V-45° H Points[A]	240 cd.s @ HV 120 cd.s @ ± 5° H Points 32 cd.s @ All 5° V-45° H Points[A]	900 cd.s @ HV 450 cd.s @ ± 5° H Points 96 cd.s @ All 5° V-45° H Points[A]	600 cd.s @ HV 300 cd.s @ ± 5° H Points 72 cd.s @ All 5° V-45° H Points[A]
Night		10–30 % of the above		

[A]Single center rear or dual rear (optional).
Flash Energy reduced 20% per flash per fixture for optional dual amber lights.

light signal modes and combinations as specified. All emergency light switches shall be labeled (see 6.7.11) and each primary/secondary mode switch shall have an amber or red indicator light to show the driver which mode is activated. When strobe lights are furnished or, when specified (See 9.2.22) for incandescent lights, a day-night switch shall be provided. When specified (See 9.2.23) from the lighting system manufacturer, an automatic switch to secondary mode in "Park" with manual override to "Primary Mode" shall be furnished. Additionally, when specified (See 9.2.22) from the lighting system manufacturer, the lighting system shall provide an ambient light sensing circuit to automatically switch to the night position while in the secondary mode. A manual override to the daytime (bright) mode shall be provided. Operator's manual (See 6.20) shall include suggestive management instructions for the warning systems.

6.8.2.4 *Hardware Construction and Installation*—The emergency lighting system shall be comprised of components and devices that comply to the general requirements and tests of SAE J575g, J576d, J578, and J551 as applicable for the unit. Warning lights shall be firmly fastened to reinforced body surfaces per the lighting manufacturer's requirements and recommendations, and shall include aiming wedges to compensate for sloped body surfaces or mold release angles on roof caps, grill, hood, and fender angles. The ambulance manufacturer shall aim the lights to assure that all lighting performance requirements herein are being met. The lights shall be aimed either mechanically or optically on the horizontal axis with a tolerance of +0 ° to -2 °. All switches, connectors, and wiring shall be rated to carry a minimum of 125 percent of their maximum ampere load. When halogen lamps are used, the duty cycle of any lamp shall not exceed 50 percent. When strobe lights are furnished, all high voltage leads and connections shall be insulated and enclosed.

6.8.2.5 *Tests, Warning, Light System*—The lighting manufacturers shall furnish and certify or the ambulance manufacturer shall measure and record the total average current load of the standard emergency warning light system on the vehicle as manufactured at the regulated voltage of 14.2 V, when operated in the mode which draws maximum current. This load current test shall be conducted in accordance with AMD Standard 005 (Ambulance DC Electrical Systems Test). The warning light system and related components and devices shall conform to temperature conditions in 6.4.2 and be tested and approved by an accredited laboratory for compliance with the requirements in this standard.

6.8.2.6 *Alternative Emergency Warning Light System*—A warning light system that complies with the requirements of 6.8.2, 6.8.2.3, 6.8.2.4, 6.8.2.5, 6.8.2.7, 6.8.2.8and may be used as an alternative to the standard emergency warning light system (See 9.2.22).

6.8.2.7 *Alternative Emergency Warning Light System Configuration*—The upper level optical warning devices shall be mounted as high and as close to the corner points of the vehicle as is practical in order to define the clearance lines of the vehicle. However, these optical warning devices shall not be mounted above the maximum height, specified by the device manufacturer, that gives an intensity value at 1.2 m (4 ft.) above grade and 30.5 m (100 ft.) from the optical warning device of less than 50% of that required at the optical center.

In order to define the clearance lines of the emergency vehicle, the lower level optical devices at the front of the vehicle shall be mounted so that their optical centers are forward of the center line of the front axle and as close to the front comer points of the vehicle as is practical. The optical centers of these lower level devices shall be 46 cm to 157 cm (18 in. to 62 in.) above grade. Switching arrangements for the alternative emergency warning lighting system as described in 6.8.2.3, shall provide the operator with lighting load management capabilities including manual override of the lower level lighting.

The optical warning devices shall be constructed or arranged to avoid the projection of light either directly or through mirrors into any driving or crew compartment(s). The front optical warning devices shall be placed to maintain the maximum possible override from the headlights.

The optical sources in the optical warning devices mounted on the upper level shall be of sufficient number and arranged so that failure of a single optical source does not create a measurement point in any zone, on the same level as the failed optical source, without a warning signal at a distance of 30.5 m. (100 ft) from the geometric center of the emergency vehicle.

6.8.2.8 *Alternative Emergency Warning Light System Photometric and Physical Requirements*—For the purpose of defining and measuring the required optical performance, the upper and lower warning levels shall each be divided into four warning zones. The four zones shall be by drawing lines through the geometric center of the emergency vehicle at 45 degrees to a line lengthwise of the emergency vehicle through the geometric center. The four zones shall be designated A, B, C, and D in a clockwise direction with zone A to the front of the emergency vehicle. Zones BF and DF comprise the front half of zones B and D which are adjacent to Zone A, (See Fig. 10).

The Zone Totals reflect the combined performance of the individual optical warning devices oriented as intended on the vehicle when viewed along the perimeter of a circle of 30.5 m (100 ft.) radius from the geometric center of the vehicle.

The Zone Total is the sum of the optical power of all optical sources projecting signals of permissible color into the zone as measured at 5 degree increments along H. There are 19 measurement points in Zones A, B, C, and D and 10 measurement points in Zones BF and DF. The calculation of zone totals assumes that all optical sources are mounted at the geometric center of the vehicle.

With the H-V point of each optical source oriented as installed, the optical power contributed by every optical source at a given point is taken from the test reports and added together to determine the total optical power at that point. The Zone Total is the sum of the optical power at the measurement points in the zone. The upper and lower level optical sources are calculated independently.

For each operating mode, the combined optical power of all the optical sources shall meet or exceed the Zone Total optical power requirement shown in Table 4. No individual measurement point shall be less than that described in 6.8.2.8 and shown in Table 4.

Permissible colors or combination of colors in each zone, within the constraints imposed by applicable laws and regulations, shall be as shown in Table 5. All colors shall be as specified in SAE J578, Color Specification, for white, red, yellow, or blue.

6.8.3 *Flood and Loading Light (Exterior)*—Flood and loading lights shall be not less than 191 cm (75 in.) above the ground and unobstructed by open doors. Floodlights shall be located on the left, right, and rear sides of the ambulance and firmly fastened to reinforced body surfaces, below the roofline. When specified by the purchaser (See 9.2.23) two flood lights shall be furnished on each side and rear. These flood lights shall have the maximum possible spacing between them. The lamp(s) H-V shall be projected downward, either mechanically or optically, at an angle of 12 to 18 degrees from the horizontal plane and the lighting on each side of the ambulance shall provide a minimum of 800 beam candle power with a trapezoidal beam pattern. Floodlight switches shall be located on the cab console and control each side independently. Loading light(s) shall provide a minimum of 500 candle power with an 80° horizontal by 30° vertical beam spread, and shall illuminate the area surrounding the back loading doors. Loading light(s) shall automatically be activated when rear doors are opened and may be incorporated with the FMVSS backup lighting system.

6.8.4 *Spotlight*—A hand held spotlight shall be provided with a lamp that produces a minimum of 100,000 CP. It shall have a corrosion-proof housing with momentary switch, and minimum 244 cm (8 ft.) heavy-duty coiled cord. It shall be hard wired to the vehicle 12 V DC system (for anti-theft reasons) and stowed in a holder in a compartment/area, accessible to the driver and passenger. When specified (See Table 9, Item 25), a remote controlled spotlight shall be

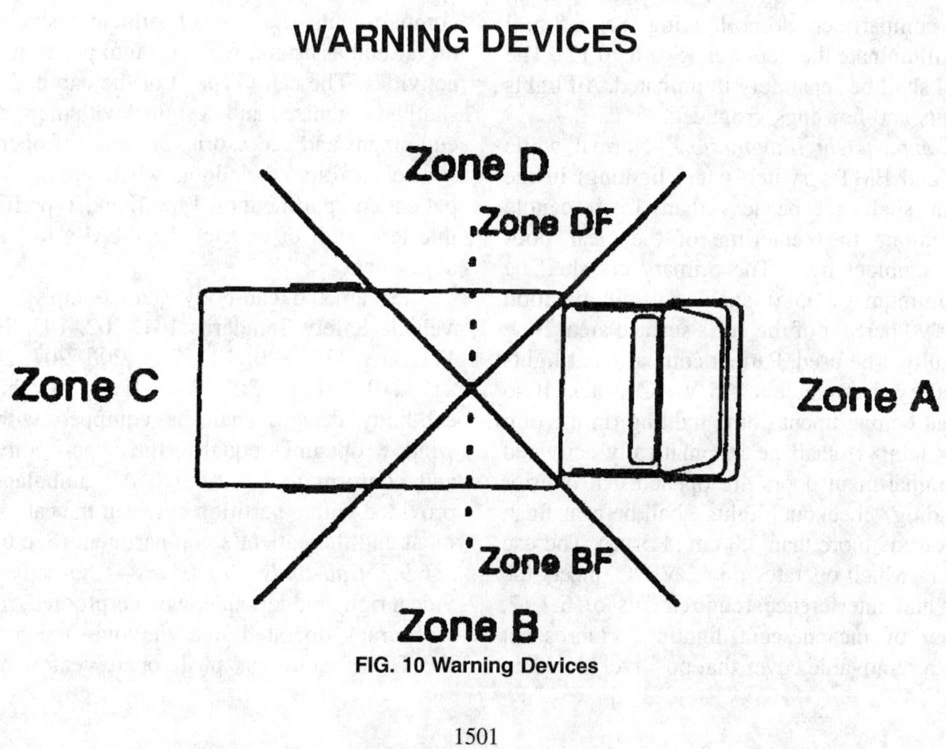

FIG. 10 Warning Devices

TABLE 4 Minimum Optical Power Requirements

Mode of Operations									
Clearing the Right of Way					Blocking the Right of Way				
Zones	Level	Zone Total at H	Min. Value at any H Point	Min. Value at any ± 5° H Point	Zones	Level	Zone Total at H	Min. Value at any H Point	Min. Value at any ± 5° H Point
A	Upper	1,000,000	10,000	3,500	A	Upper	400,000	10,000	3,500
B	Upper	400,000	10,000	3,500	B	Upper	400,000	10,000	3,500
C	Upper	400,000	10,000	3,500	C	Upper	400,000	10,000	3,500
D	Upper	400,000	10,000	3,500	D	Upper	400,000	10,000	3,500
A	Lower	150,000	3,750	1,300	A	Lower	150,000	3,750	1,300
BF	Lower	75,000	3,750	1,300	BF	Lower	75,000	3,750	1,300
C	Lower	None	None	None	C	Lower	None	None	None
DF	Lower	75,000	3,750	1,300	DF	Lower	75,000	3,750	1,300

NOTE 1—All values are in candela-seconds/minute. H = Horizontal plane passing through the optical center. The minimum number of flashes from all of the optical sources visible at each measurement point shall be 150 flashes per minute.

TABLE 5 Zone Colors

Color	Call for Right-of-Way	Blocking Right-of-Way
Red	Any Zone	Any Zone
Blue	Any Zone	Any Zone
Yellow	Any Zone Except A	Any Zone
White	Any Zone Except C	Not Permitted

furnished, having an "ON/OFF" panel switch and variable speed fingertip control. The spotlight shall be a minimum 13 cm (5 in.) in diameter and shall be capable of producing a beam of 100,000 CP. Lights shall be operable over 360 degrees horizontal sweep and approximately 90 degrees vertical range.

6.8.5 *Ambulance Interior Lighting*—The basic interior ambulance lighting configuration shall be designed to minimize electrical loads and include: A driver's compartment dome light; instrument panel lights; master switch panel; and console light(s). When specified (See Table 9, Item 33), a map light for the front seat passenger shall be furnished. Lighting shall be designed and located so that no glare is reflected into the driver's eyes or his line of vision, from switch, control panels or other areas that are illuminated while the vehicle is in motion. The patient compartment dome lighting (See 6.8.5.1) shall be sufficient to illuminate the step-well (See 6.10.12). The EMT's control panel shall be separately illuminated. All lights shall have lamp shells and housings grounded.

6.8.5.1 *Patient Compartment Illumination*—Normal while illumination (dome and EMT's switch panel lighting) in the patient compartment shall not be less than 15 ft candle intensity, measured along the centerline of the clear floor without any outside ambient light. The primary cot shall be provided with a minimum of 35 ft candles of illumination measured on at least 90 percent of the cot's surface area. Blue light(s) or lenses shall not be used. Patient compartment lights shall not be powered by the vehicle's 115 V AC system if so equipped. The patient compartment dome lighting (in the dim setting) and loading lamp(s) shall be automatically activated when the patient compartment doors are opened. All interior dome lighting, including "checkout" lights, shall be near flush mounted and not protrude more than 3.8 cm (1.5 in.). The use of fluorescent lighting which operates on 12 V DC, meets the above performance and interference requirements of 6.7.12, can be used in lieu of incandescent lighting. Fluorescent fixture(s) shall have a removable cover that positively locks in place. The fluorescent tube shall be positively locked in place to preclude loosening due to vehicle movement or vibration.

Dome lighting shall not consume more than 15 amps in the bright setting and shall have two separately protected and controlled circuits. Switches, electronic controls, or fireproofed rheostats may be used to control lighting.

6.8.5.2 *Patient Compartment "Checkout Lights"*—When specified (See Table 9, Item 9). two "patient compartment checkout lights" shall be furnished with 6 candle power lamps, or equal, and 5 minute timer switch that is wired directly to the ammeter shunt (battery side of load disconnect switch), (See Fig. 7). One of the light fixtures shall be located towards the front of the patient compartment and one towards the rear. The checkout lights may be integrated into the standard patient compartment lighting by activating two of the lamps in the "dim" circuit.

NOTE 17—Use of checkout lights minimizes battery cycling, precludes the necessity for turning on batteries, and use of higher power compartment lighting.

6.9 *Cab-Body Driver Compartment and Equipment:*

6.9.1 *Driver's Compartment, Cab-Body Structure*—All cab compartments shall be of sufficient size to accommodate a driver and assistant, with space to perform driving and control activities. The cab (Type I) or the cab-body (Types II and III) shall be organized and designed with the specified and required equipment and accessories for ease of operation and safety.

The partition and door, when provided between cab and patient compartment on Type II and Type III vehicles, shall not interfere with or restrict the OEM's full range of front seat adjustment.

The cab and cab-body shall comply with Federal Motor Vehicle Safety Standards 101, 102, 103, 104, 105, 107, 108. 111, 113, 115, 120, 124, 205, 206, 207, 208, 209, 210, 211, 212, 219, 301, and 302. Types II and III vehicles, of the integral cab-body design, shall be equipped with front doors and window openings equal to the Type I conventional truck cab and conform to 6.9.2-6.9.8. All ambulance Types shall be provided with a partition between the cab or driver's compartment and the patient's compartment (See 6.10.2 and 6.10.15).

6.9.2 *Cab-Body Provisions*—Cab-body section shall provide a right and left side, weatherproofed, forward hinged door with crank operated side windows and, when available from the OEM: crank or push open vent windows; door stops;

external key operated door locks with two sets of keys; trim or closed panels and headliner (washable vinyl upholstery, or flooring type materials); floor covering (OEM's heat, noise and appearance trim packages); panel mounted instrument; and seat(s). All exposed interior surfaces shall be painted. Hardware and other exterior other exposed metal shall be chrome plated, stainless steel, or anodized aluminum. When specified by the purchaser (See 6.10.15.2 and Table 9, Item 29), a console shall be furnished that will contain a map book, clip board, radio control head(s) speaker(s), etc. The console shall be furnished per purchaser's specifications. Additionally, the vehicle shall be furnished with at least the following equipment:

6.9.2.1 Dual sun visors (padded)

6.9.2.2 Armrests, mounted on each side door.

6.9.2.3 Compartment ventilation, other than windows.

6.9.2.4 Key operated ignition/starter switch.

6.9.2.5 Ammeter and voltmeter (see 6.7.6.2 and 6.7.6.3).

6.9.2.6 Fuel gauge(s).

6.9.2.7 Oil pressure gauge.

6.9.2.8 Engine temperature gauge.

6.9.2.9 Speedometer with odometer.

6.9.2.10 Environmental controls (heater-defroster/air conditioner, etc.).

6.9.2.11 Seatbelts and shoulder harness for driver and passenger, when available from chassis manufacturer.

6.9.2.12 Dual outside mirrors (See 6.9.5).

6.9.2.13 Cab lighting and controls.

6.9.2.14 Tinted windshield.

6.9.2.15 Dual electric horn(s).

6.9.2.16 Throttle control (See 6.7.6.1).

6.9.3 *Cab Compartment Driver and Assistant Seat*—Unless otherwise specified (See 9.2.24), the driver's compartment shall be furnished with at least two individual bucket-type seats (driver and assistant) or, when specified (See 9.2.24), bench style seating for three. The seats shall be frame constructed with cushioned springs or foam rubber, padded and upholstered to provide maximum riding comfort. Unless otherwise specified (See 9.2.24), the seats shall be covered with fire-retardant, washable, nonabsorbent material. Driver's seat shall have the OEM's full, unobstructed range of adjustment.

6.9.4 *Controls and Operating Mechanism*—All controls and operating mechanisms shall be located for left-hand drive. Lever controls, equipment, items, and devices shall be installed, located, and stowed for the convenience of the purpose intended and shall not interfere with the ambulance personnel or patient's ingress or egress of respective compartments.

6.9.5 *Outside Rearview Mirrors*—Unless otherwise specified (See 9.2.25), dual, firmly secured, vibrationless, rearview mirrors, having a combination flat/convex mirror system, shall be furnished. Convex shall be a minimum 13 cm (5 in.) diameter. Mirrors shall have the largest usable reflective area practical for the designed ambulance, totaling at least 806 square centimeters (125 square in.) per vehicle. Unless the mirror assembly is manufactured as an integral assembly, all four mirror head faces shall be independently adjustable. Hardware and mirror heads shall be chromed, polished stainless steel, or polished aluminum.

6.9.6 *Bumpers and Steps*—Chassis manufacturer's standard chrome bumper shall be furnished in the front of the chassis. The rear of the ambulance shall be furnished with a sturdy, full-width, rear bumper, with step secured to the vehicle's chassis-frame. The rear bumper and step shall be adequate to support a test weight of 227 kg (500 pounds) without flexing. A step shall be furnished at the back (loading) door opening, if the patient compartment floor is more than 46 cm (18 in.) above the ground. Unless otherwise specified by the purchaser for Class 2 vehicles (See 9.2.26), the step installation shall be equal distance ± 5 cm (2 in.) between the ground and the floor. The bumper-step shall be designed to prevent the accumulation of mud, ice, or snow and made of anti-skid open grating metal (a folding style step if specified in Table 9, Item 21). These steps shall not be located or exposed to the interior of the ambulance when the door(s) are closed. All necessary steps shall be at least the width of the door opening for which they are provided. The step's tread shall have a maximum depth of 13 cm (5 in.) and a maximum depth of 25 cm (10 in.). If the step protrudes more than 18 cm (7 in.) from the rear of the vehicle, a foldup step shall be furnished.

6.9.6.1 *Override Front Grille Guard*—When specified and permitted by the chassis manufacturer (See Table 9, Item 22), an override protection (high-rise heavy-duty grille guard) shall be furnished to protect the vehicle grille, siren speakers, grill lights, radiator, and air conditioner condenser. The heavy-duty grille guard shall be custom fit to the front bumper and bolted to the vehicle frame. The grille guard shall be of all steel construction with not less than 9.5 mm–10 mm (3⁄8 in.) thick side plates and two horizontal 5.0 cm (2 in.) diameter tube crossmembers. The grille guard shall be of a height to extend from the bottom edge of the front bumper to not less than 20.3 cm (8 in.) above the top edge. Unless otherwise stated in ordering data the grille guard shall be chrome plated or painted to match the vehicle exterior color.

NOTE 18—**Warning:** Purchasers should be aware that grille guards add additional front end weight and should not be ordered unless absolutely necessary.

6.9.6.2 *Bumper Guards*— When specified and permitted by the chassis manufacturer (See Table 9, Item 22) or required for protection of grille mount siren speakers which extend beyond the face of the bumper, a set of bumper guards shall be furnished. Bumper guards shall be rubber faced, 30 cm (12 in.) to 36 cm (14 in.) high, polished aluminum, chromed steel, or polished stainless steel. They shall bolt or clamp to the bumper or chassis, and shall protect the bumper, siren speakers, grill lights, etc.

6.9.7 *Body Protection:*

6.9.7.1 *Fenders*—Fenders and wheelhousings (See 6.10.13) shall be provided to cover all tires. Fender extension(s) over dual rear tires are permitted on ambulance bodies to cover tires, providing they are less than 20 cm (8 in.) wide, reinforced, secured, and may be painted black, unless polished metal is specified (See 6.4.11.2 and 9.2.27).

6.9.7.2 *Running Boards*— When specified (See Table 9, Item 30), bright finish aluminum running boards shall be provided from the rear of the front wheel opening to the rear of the cab (Type I); to the front of the rear wheel opening (Type

II); and to the front of the modular body (Type III). All running boards shall be securely attached to the cab and body, or both, as required, and include nonmetallic spacers to prevent contact of dissimilar metals and prevent trapping of dirt and water between the running board and the cab body. All running boards shall be gusseted and provide brackets to prevent flexing, sagging, and damage. Design of the running boards may incorporate mud flaps. Running board installation shall conform to the manufacturer's recommendation.

6.9.7.3 *Mud Flaps*—When specified (See Table 9, Item 31), mud flaps, at least as wide as the tire(s), shall be provided per SAE J682 behind the front and rear wheels and shall be reinforced at the point of attachment to the vehicle. Mud flaps may be incorporated into the running boards.

6.9.7.4 *Mud/Stone Guards*— When specified (See Table 9, Item 15), bright finished aluminum diamond plate shall be provided to protect the lower part of Type I and Type III ambulances.

6.9.7.5 *Rub Rail*—When specified on Type I and III bodies (See Table 9, Item 19), a body rub rail, minimum 25.4 mm (1 in.) thick x 50.8 mm (2 in.) wide, shall be provided that extends the full length of the right and left sides of the lower third section of the module. The rub rail shall be firmly attached to the body.

6.9.7.6 *Fuel Fill Splash Plates*—The painted surface of the ambulance body shall be protected from discoloration due to spilled fuel during refueling. Protection shall be provided by a drain in the fuel fill housing(s) or by splash plate(s) under the fuel fill opening.

6.9.8 *Engine Hood*— Engine hood and cowl shall be fitted to prevent precipitation, heat, odors, and noise from entering the interior of the cab and body. Cab compartment engine covers, on Types II and III ambulances, shall be removable for easy access to engine and components.

6.9.9 *Cab Connecting Bellows for Type 1 Vehicle*—A flexible, weather-tight bellows, fabricated from EPDM, Hypalon, sheet or molded rubber, or other durable materials that meet the temperature requirements herein and resist ozone, sunlight, oil, fungus, and will not crack or deteriorate, shall be provided between the Type I cab and the modular body. Bellows shall be designed for proper fit and finish and be able to absorb lateral, vertical, and torsional displacement due to body/cab movement. Window in the cab or body shall be of the sliding type, shall be aligned, and connect with the modular body window opening (See 6.10.2, 6.10.14, and 6.10.15) and shall conform to requirements of the partition.

6.10 *Ambulance Body and Patient Area:*

6.10.1 *Body Accommodations*—The ambulance body and patient compartment shall be sufficient in size to transport occupants, as specified in Configuration A or B (see 6.1.5), and accommodate and store all the stretchers, cots, and litters through the range of dimensions as specified in Table 6. There shall be space around the patients to permit a technician to administer life support treatment to at least one patient during transit (see dimensional parameters in 6.10.4).

6.10.2 *Cab/Patient Compartment Access Window*—The ambulance and body bulkheads shall have an aligned window opening of at least 968 square cm (150 square in.), for visual checking and voice communications between the cab and the patient's compartment for Type I vehicles and, when specified (see 6.10.15.2). in lieu of walkthru door on Types II & III. The window shall be latchable from the cab side and shall be an adjustable, transparent, shatterproof panel (See 6.9.9 and 6.10.14).

6.10.3 *Emergency Medical Technician (EMT) Seating*—The EMT shall be provided with a seat conforming to FMVSS 207 and equipped with a safety belt and a padded back and a padded headrest. Unless otherwise specified (See 9.2.28), the seat shall be not less than 46 cm (18 in.) deep by 46 cm (18 in.) wide and 38 to 46 cm (15 to 18 in.) high, measured to the top of the seat cushion (See 6.11.1.1) and adjustable a minimum of 10 cm (4 in.) (front to rear) when a bucket type seat is furnished. The EMT shall be seated at the head of the primary patient, near the bulkhead or position behind cab compartment facing rearward (See 6.1.5). The space under the seat may be designed as a storage compartment or utilized for other equipment. The EMT seat shall be upholstered per 6.11.4. When an ambulance manufacturer's fabricated seat is furnished, the padded backrest shall be the maximum practical width and height. When specified and available (See 9.2.28), an EMT seat with integral infant/child safety seat shall be furnished and conform with all requirements including FMVSS 213.

6.10.4 *Patient Compartment Interior Dimensional Parameters*—The patient compartment shall provide, but not be limited to, a minimum of 9.2 cubic meters (325 cubic feet) of space, less 1 cubic meter (35 cubic feet) for cabinets, while complying with the following:

6.10.4.1 *Length*—Unless otherwise specified or permitted by the purchaser (See 9.2.29), length, measured from the partition to the inside edge of the rear loading doors at the floor, shall be at least 310 cm (122 in.). This length in the compartment shall provide at least 64 cm (25 in.) and not more than 76 cm (30 in.) of unobstructed space at the head of the primary patient measured from the face of the backrest of the EMT seat to the forward edge of the Style I cot. A minimum of 25 cm (10 m.) shall be provided, from the end of the cot to the rear loading doors, to permit clearance for traction or long board splints.

6.10.4.2 *Width*—The width of the compartment, after installation of the cabinets, shall provide 46 cm (18 m.) ±15 cm (6 in.) of clear aisle walkway between cot and base of squad bench, with the cot located in the street side (non-centered) position.

6.10.4.3 *Height*—Unless otherwise specified by the purchaser (See 9.2.30), the patient compartment shall provide at least 152 cm (60 in.) height, over the primary patient area, measured from floor to ceiling panels.

6.10.5 *Body, General Construction*—For modular construction, the body shall be all welded aluminum or, when specified or approved by the purchaser (See 9.2.31), other lightweight, inherently corrosion resistant materials of equal, or greater, strength. The exterior of the body shall be finished smooth with symmetrically radiused corners and edges, including rub-rails when specified (See Table 9, Item 19), and shall include doors and windows specified herein. Ambulance body, as a unit, shall

TABLE 6 Ambulance Stretchers, Cots, and Litters

Stretchers, Cots, and Litters	Dimensions cm/in. Length Minimum	Width Minimum	Bed Height Maximum (Collapsed)
Style 1– Wheeled Cot (Elevating)	191/75	56/22	38/15[A]
Style 2– Wheeled Cot (Elevating with Additional Front Roll-in Casters)	203/80	56/22	25/10
Style 3– Folding Stretcher or Combination Stretcher Chair	189/73.5	48/19	21/8.25
Style 4– Navy Stokes Litter (Resting on Floor)	215/84.75	60/23.5	19/7.5
Style 5– Standard Army and NATO Litters (With Poles)[B]	90 (+0, -¼)	23 (+⁹⁄₁₀, -¾)	17/6.75

[A]Measured to top of positioned 7.6 cm (3 in.) thick mattress.
[B]Dimensions of Army and NATO litters are in accordance with North Atlantic Treaty Organization Standardization agreement STANAG No. 2040.

be designed and built to provide impact and patient compartment penetration resistance and shall be of sufficient strength to support the entire weight of the fully loaded vehicle on its top or side, if overturned, without separation of joints or permanently deforming roof bow or reinforcements, body posts, doors, stringers, floor, inner linings, outer panels, rub-rails, and other reinforcements. Wood, or wood products, shall not he used for structural framing. As evidence that the ambulance body meets the above criteria, the manufacturer's body (fabricated, modified, or converted), excluding the conventional cab, shall furnish for each body model (Type) a certification that the ambulance body meets AMD Standard 001 (Static Load Test for Ambulance Body Structure).

Additionally, the roof structure, liner, and outer skin or cap shall be designed and constructed to prevent separation and the possible ejection of patients or crew in the event of an accident and shall include welded and, if necessary, reinforced attachments to the body.

NOTE 19—**Warning:** Any absorbent material such as carpeting, fabric, or inside/outside plastic type carpeting, etc. that resists cleaning and decontamination shall not he used in any storage or patient compartment.

6.10.6 *Ambulance Body Structure*—All parts of the ambulance body and attachments shall be fastened with rust-resistant fasteners in a manner which will preclude loosening. Cabinets, benches, partitions, oxygen cylinder holders, guide rails, and cot holders shall he attached to metal tapping plates and flaming welded to the body structure, or both. These components shall he fastened by welding, bolting, or self-tapping machine screws, on at least 46 cm (18 in.) centers or less, as applicable to the component being installed. Sheet metal, self-tapping wood/metal screws, nails, staples, etc. shall not be used in assembling the ambulance structure, except for self-threading sheet metal screws used for light trim panels and for retention of wood flooring. Vehicles furnished with fiberglass/plastic, exterior roof panel shall have the center section embedded with metal wire screening (See 6.14.3) for a radio antenna ground plane. Ambulance bodies with an extended roof shall have the roof structural members permanently fastened to structural members of the body (welded, bolted, and sealed) to prevent separation in an accident. Body structure shall, as necessary, include gusseting to provide diagonal strength. Drip rail(s) shall be provided around the entire modular body and have drain points at each corner. Drip rails shall also be furnished over each entry, and compartment door. When structure permits, drip rail shall extend 2.5 cm (l in.) beyond the edge of the doors.

Body skirt(s) shall not extend more than 8 cm (3 in.) below the vehicle cab/body. The body, roof and panel joints shall be watertight. All openings between the chassis-body and occupant carrying compartments, including the bulkhead between cab and body of Type I and III (See 6.9.9), shall be sealed to prevent intrusion of water, dust, and exhaust gases.

6.10.7 *Body Mounting*— On Types I and III ambulance bodies, to reduce stress on body and frame, minimize height above the frame, and isolate the patient compartment from noise and vibration, full floating, automotive style, rubber body mounts or other chassis manufacturer's approved body mounting systems shall be furnished with a minimum four per side on bodies up to 371 cm (146 in.) and five per side on bodies over 371 cm (146 in.). Reinforcements or filler blocks shall be used where mounting device(s) may deform frame flanges. Mounting devices shall be locked units which will minimize loosening, but which may be re-tightened, if necessary. Modular bodies shall be interchangeable with other chassis of the same manufacturer having the same cab to axle (CA) dimension (reference 6.5.6).

6.10.8 *Doors*—Two patient compartment door openings shall be provided. There shall be a door opening on the right forward side and at the rear of the body for loading a patient on a cot. The side opening shall have a single forward hinged door for Types I and III, double hinged doors for Type II, or if specified (See 9.2.32) a sliding type door for Type II vehicles shall be furnished. Door(s) shall provide a minimum right-side clear opening of 76 cm (30 in.) wide and of 160 cm (63 in.) high for Types I and III and the chassis manufacturers standard opening for Type II vehicles. Unless otherwise specified (See 9.2.32), for example, wide offset doors, rear loading door(s) shall cover a clear opening of not less than 117 cm (46 in.) in height for Type II and a minimum height of 117 cm (46 in.) for Types I & III and 112 cm (44 in.) in width for Types I and III and the chassis manufacturer's standard opening for Type II vehicles. All ambulance body doors shall be equipped with not less than 1613 cm^2 (250 square in.) of safety glass area per door. Doors shall be designed for easy release and meet the requirements of 6.10.9. A "Door-Open" warning device shall signal (indicate in the cab) when doors are not closed (See 6.7.1.1). Each door shall have effective compression or overlapping seals to prevent leakage of exhaust fumes, dust, water, and air. Doors may contain and be equipped with recessed compartments as applicable to the interior for storage of supplies and devices.

Patient compartment doors, on Types I & III, shall be flush or near flush style, full box type construction with removable inner panel. Inner panel shall be finished with a durable, washable type material and include trim moldings around all unfinished exposed edges.

A red light or reflector, minimum 7.6 cm (3 in.) diameter, shall be installed, one on the interior surface of each side or rear door. The reflectors shall be so positioned as to provide maximum visibility when the doors are in the fully open position. At the manufacturer's option, red reflective tape, conforming to L-S-300, Type L Class 3, reflectively 1, may be furnished. The tape shall be 10 cm (4 in.) wide and shall extend the full width of each rear door panel.

6.10.8.1 *Protection of Patients and Crew*—Upholstered padding/cushions shall be provided at the upper interior areas of the door frames. Similar padding/cushions shall also be furnished at other areas that may be capable of causing injury.

6.10.9 *Door Latches, Hinges, and Hardware*—Door latches, hinges, and hardware furnished by chassis and ambulance manufacturers shall comply with FMVSS 206. When doors are open, the hinges, latches, and doorchecks shall not protrude into the access area. All doors shall have hardware or devices to prevent inadvertent opening and closing. To facilitate entry and exit from the vehicle, a minimum 15 cm (6 in.), tubular or semi-oval, minimum 19 mm (3/4 in.) wide (diameter), grab handle shall be provided on the inside of each door or the adjacent body structure (in addition to a door operating handle). Door stops, to prevent damage to body sides, and a handle with latches, operable from inside (even if key locked externally) and from outside of the body after unlocking, shall be furnished. One external operated lock, with one key per door opening, shall be provided. All patient compartment door locks shall be identically keyed. Hardware shall be chrome plated bright finish, stainless steel, or anodized aluminum. Inside door latch handles shall be designed and placed so they cannot be operated when accidentally hit or used as a grab handle. Ambulance body side and rear door hardware, installed by the ambulance body manufacturer, shall be tested to ensure installation meets or exceeds the requirements of AMD Standard 002 (Body and Door Retention Components Tests).

6.10.10 *Floor*—Floor shall be at the lowest level permitted by the chassis/body, but not exceed the height permitted in 6.4.11.7. It shall be flat, except when the area near the rear entrance door is sloped for a lower entering height, and with the exception of cot related hardware, shall be unencumbered in the door(s) access and work area. All floor areas shall withstand a distributed load of 73 kg/1000 cm^2(150 lbs./ft^2). Metal floors shall be reinforced to eliminate "oil canning" and insulated against outside heat and cold. The subfloor of the Types I and III patient compartment shall be water resistant. When plywood is utilized, it shall be water resistant, not less than 13 mm (1/2 in.) thick, 5 ply minimum, supported by body framework. Under the subfloor of the Type I and III vehicles shall be a aluminum heatshield/splash pan, minimum 1.3 mm (0.050 in.), with silicone or other non-hardening sealant evenly distributed around its perimeter. The subfloor of the Type II patient compartment shall be not less than 13 mm (1/2 in.) thick density, marine or exterior grade plywood. Fiberglass, aluminum, or other non-hydroscopic composites with at least the equivalent strength of plywood may be used as the subfloor. Particle board or equivalent type materials are not acceptable. Additionally, noise/thermal insulation shall be provided under the floor as necessary.

Voids or pockets, where water or moisture can become trapped to cause rotting and unsanitary conditions, are not acceptable. Voids and pockets shall be filled with sealer or caulking compound. Flooring shall extend the full length and width of the patient compartment or body (including space under the cabinets, unless otherwise insulated).

6.10.11 *Floor Coverings and Color*—Floor covering shall be easily cleaned, sanitized, and harmonize with the interior color and decor of the patient compartment. The floor covering shall be seamless, one piece, no wax type, solid linoleum, vinyl or poured epoxy not less than 1.6 mm (1/16m.) thick and permanently applied to the subfloor. The floor material shall cover the entire length and width of the compartment's working area. The covering of joints (corners, etc.), where the sidewalls and covering meet, shall be sealed and bordered with corrosion resistant cove molding or the covering shall extend at least 7.6 cm (3 in.) up the sidewalls. Cabinets at floor level shall be finished with floor covering material. Floor covering shall comply with FMVSS 302.

6.10.12 *Stepwell (Side Door)*—Steps shall be provided in the door openings, if the floor is more than 46 cm (18 in.) above the ground. Stepwell, when applicable, shall be the enclosed two-step type. Height of the bottom step shall not exceed 46 cm ± 5 cm (18 ± 2 in.) (Types I and III vehicles), and 56 cm (22 in.) (Type II) with the exception of Class 2 vehicles. Stepwells shall be lighted by interior lights and all step surfaces shall be fabricated from reinforced, bright finish, aluminum diamond plate or covered with anti-slip material.

6.10.13 *Wheelhousings*— Wheelhousings of Type I and III vehicles shall include metal or plastic splash shields between the body wheelhousing and the wheel(s) (See 6.9.7) extending over the top of the tires to the bottom of the body side skirting. Wheelhouse openings shall allow for tire chain usage and easy tire removal and service. Chassis manufacturer's standard wheelhousings will be acceptable. Wheelhousings shall be undercoated or rustproofed.

6.10.14 *Windows*—Glazing shall comply to FMVSS 205 and unless otherwise specified (See Table 9, Item 12), the patient's compartment shall not have windows, except the viewing panel in the partition or bulkhead(s) (See 6.10.15) and in the side and rear doors (see 6.10.8). All windows shall be tinted and when specified (See 9.2.33), upper windows shall open and, when vertical windows are furnished, shall have provisions to prevent accidental closure.

6.10.15 *Bulkhead/Partition for Type II and III Vehicles*—A full height and width partition or bulkhead (with or without compartments), having rollbar characteristics and a walkthru opening with a door shall be placed between the driver and patient's compartment. This partition shall be located directly behind the driver and companion seats when in the rearmost position. The partition shall be secured on the sides, ceiling, and floor by welding or bolting to tapping plates.

6.10.15.1 *Door/Walkthru*— Unless otherwise specified to delete walkthru or to specify door opening dimension (See 9.2.34), the door opening shall be at least 43 cm (17 in.) wide and 117 cm (46 m.) high and shall provide an aisle between the compartments. The door shall have at least a 968 cm^2(150 square in.), transparent, shatterproof viewing panel in the center section at the driver's eye level. The door shall be secured with a driver's side self-latching device in the open and closed positions. (See 6.10.2).

6.10.15.2 *Walkthru Deletion*—When specified (See 9.2.34), the partition door shall be deleted and a window, as specified in 6.10.2, shall be furnished. When specified (See 9.2.34), additional compartments shall also be furnished in the space normally occupied by the door opening, including the area above the required pass thru window. Further, a console (See Table 9, Item 29) may be specified between the driver and passenger seat.

NOTE 20—Purchaser should consider deleting the walkthru because, in addition to providing increased space for compartments and the capability of adding a radio control head/map book console (See 6.9.2 and Table 9, Item 29) between the front seats, the deletion of the door also provides for isolation of the driver from violent patients and the separation of individuals that may be accompanying the patient who could interfere with patient care.

6.10.16 *Insulation*—The entire body, sides, ends, and roof of the patients compartment shall be completely insulated to enhance the performance of the environmental systems, specified in 6.4.2 and 6.13, and prevent external noise from entering the vehicle interior. The insulation shall be a non-settling type, vermin-proof, mildew-proof, fire retardant, non-toxic, and non-hygroscopic, If fiberglass insulation is used, it shall not be exposed to water, for example door, panels.

6.10.17 *Interior Surfaces*—The interior of the body shall be free of all sharp projections. All hangers or supports for equipment and devices shall be mounted as flush as possible with the surrounding surface. The finish of the entire patient compartment, including interiors of storage cabinets, shall be impervious to soap and water, disinfectants and mildew, fire resistance, in compliance with FMVSS 302, and be easily cleaned/disinfected (carpeting, cloth, and fabrics are not acceptable). Interior body lining and cabinetry materials, excluding the cab compartment (See 6.9), shall be selected to minimize dead weight and shall be plastic laminated or painted aluminum panels or plastic laminated wood or other lightweight, equivalent strength materials such as fiberglass, composites, and fiberglass reinforced plastics. Panels shall be installed in a manner that prevents sagging, deflection, warpage, or vibration. The ceiling/headliner shall be of similar lightweight materials. For interior colors, see 6.16.2.

6.11 *Storage Compartments*—Storage compartments shall be furnished for all items required by this specification and specified by the purchaser , or both, and include storage for, but not be limited to, backboards, portable cots/litters, stair chairs, and any other specified patient handling devices. Any absorbent material such as carpeting, fabric, or inside/outside plastic type carpeting, etc. that resists cleaning and decontamination shall not be used in any storage or patient compartment.

6.11.1 *Interior Stowage Accommodations*—Unless otherwise specified by the purchaser (See 9.2.35). the interior of the patient compartment shall provide a minimum volume of 1 cubic meter (35 cubic feet) of enclosed stowage cabinetry, compartment space, and shelf space which shall be conveniently located for medical supplies, devices, and installed systems as applicable for the service intended. Enclosed compartments and spaces shall be located at, in, or on the partition, sidewalls, overhead, squad bench, technician seat, and doors. Compartment(s) under the floor, with opening panel(s) inside the patient compartment, shall not be acceptable.

At a minimum stowage shall be required for the following items as shown in Table 7.

TABLE 7 Minimum Interior Storage Requirements

Item	Minimum Volume Cubic Meters	Cubic Feet
Medicine dispensary cabinet(s)	0.17	6
Medical supplies cabinet	0.25	9
Linen supplies	0.11	4
Trash receptacle compartment and sharps disposal container	0.06	2
Oxygen installation (main) (see 6.12)	0.17	6
Oxygen unit (portable)	0.06	2
Telemetry equipment	0.06	2
Radio equipment & antenna	0.03	1
Storage, miscellaneous	0.06	2
Vacuum aspirator unit	0.03	1
Air conditioning unit	As required	
Heating system	As required	

6.11.1.1 *Location of Medical Equipment and Supplies*—Location of medical supplies and equipment shall be dictated by their relative importance and shall be readily accessible to the Emergency Medical Technician (EMT). Priority shall be given to items necessary to cope with life threatening conditions at the scene and in transit. The equipment and supplies necessary for airway maintenance, ventilation, oxygenation, and suction shall be at the head of the primary litter (action area). When items for cardiac monitoring/defibrillation, mechanized CPR, administration of intravenous fluids/medications, and the monitoring of blood pressure are furnished, they shall also be readily available to the EMT at the action area. Supplies, devices, tools, etc., shall be stored in enclosed compartments and drawers designed to accommodate the respective items. All medical devices and equipment shall be stowed or properly fastened in/on the action area or in cabinets or to the rail system(s) brackets' when specified (See Table 10, Item 1), to prevent items from becoming projectiles in the patient compartment that can cause injury while the vehicle is in motion or involved in an accident.

6.11.1.2 *Interior Compartment with Exterior Access*—When specified by the purchaser, on Types I and III vehicles (See Table 9, Item 32), an interior/exterior compartment with 2 shelves shall be provided in the front, right comer of the body or other location as specified. This compartment shall also have an exterior door and, unless otherwise specified (See Table 9, Item 32) or permitted by the purchaser, a roll-up, inside door with an enclosed, roller assembly. When viewed from the vehicle's interior, this compartment shall have the following minimum dimensions: W 76 cm (30 in.), D 46 cm (18 in.), and H 102 cm (40 in.). The rollup door shall be equipped with the necessary gaskets, seals or other vibration and noise silencing devices, a positive mechanical latch and a grab handle to facilitate opening and closing. The shelves shall be adjustable and have an approximate ¾ in. lip covered with automotive edge molding.

6.11.1.3 *Waste and Sharps Disposal:*

6.11.1.3.1 A trash receptacle compartment for general waste, with closure over the opening, shall be furnished with a full size plastic/rubber trash can and disposable plastic liners, with 12 spare liners. The trash compartment shall be accessible to the EMT seat and to the head of the squad bench. The consignee shall furnish bags/liners that meet OSHA requirements, for disposing regulated medical waste (as defined by OSHA).

6.11.1.3.2 A sharps receptacle compartment/storage or a commercially available container mounted in a convenient area shall be furnished for retention of a sharps container that meets OSHA requirements.

6.11.2 *Exterior Storage Accommodations*—On Types I & III and when specified (See 9.2.25) on Type II vehicles, outside entered, weatherproof, storage compartments shall be provided in the ambulance body for extrication, spare tire, oxygen, and miscellaneous equipment. When specified, (See 9.2.35), additional exterior storage compartments shall be furnished. Exterior compartment doors and hardware shall be flush or near flush style construction. All doors shall have spring or gas tube type, hold open devices that permit one hand closure. Hardware (hinges, locks, latches, etc.) shall be rust resistant. All exterior compartments shall have latches with locks and shall be keyed alike. All exterior compartments, except the long narrow backboard storage compartment, shall be automatically lighted when opened. When top and vertically hinged doors are furnished, they shall employ ratchet or spring loaded or gas tube hold open device.

6.11.2.1 *Extrication Equipment and Storage*—The extrication equipment compartments, maximum of two, shall provide at least 28 cu meters (10 cu feet) of storage accommodations. Small hand-tools shall be contained in a single pouch type carrying device. An example of items and other miscellaneous extrication equipment which shall be stored in the extrication storage compartment(s) follows. The contractor shall furnish specific items as specified under Table 9, Item 18.

6.11.3 *Storage Compartments and Cabinet Design*—Storage cabinets, drawers, and kits shall be easily opened but shall not come open in transit. For rapid identification of contents, medical supply cabinets above the litter patients shall have shatterproof, transparent or lightly tinted, sliding doors provided with two recessed metal finger cups, near flush grip, or low profile handles. Storage compartments shall be divided into sections, shelves shall be adjustable, drawers shall be marine style slide or tilt and all shall be removable. Sliding doors for cabinets designed to carry light weight items such as dressings, bandages, etc. shall automatically latch or be fitted with friction holding devices when in a closed position. Other compartments designed to carry heavier items such as first aid and drug kits, portable and spare oxygen cylinders, suction units, etc. shall have positively locked latches that are bolted to the door and the door frame structure and are designed to remain closed in an accident, including rollovers. Use of sheet metal or wood screws is not acceptable. Side cabinet shelves shall be no more than 51 cm (20 in.) in depth, when located above the vehicle belt level. Storage compartments, cabinets, and support equipment area interior surfaces shall be finished in accordance with 6.10.17. To preclude injury, in the event of an accident, all cabinets shall be firmly anchored (bolted or welded) to tapping plates of the body structure (See 6.10.6). Tops of the cabinets and shelves shall be surrounded by a lip of not less than 13 mm (½ in.) in height covered in a soft, pliable molding. All shelves shall be continuously adjustable. Storage for the main oxygen cylinder (See 6.12.1) shall be accessible for replacement from an outside position. The oxygen compartment shall be provided with at least a 58 cm^2(9 $in.^2$) louvered device to dissipate/vent leaking oxygen to the outside of the ambulance. Oxygen cylinder compartment shall not be utilized for storage of any other equipment. Any wiring and electrical devices within this compartment shall comply with 6.7.2. Oxygen cylinder(s) shall be mounted with a restraining device(s), as required for the crashworthiness tests of AMD Standard 003 (Oxygen Tank Retention System).

TABLE 8 Miscellaneous Extrication Equipment

1. One wrench; 30 cm (12 in.), adjustable, open end.
2. One screwdriver, 30 cm (12 in.), regular blade (slot).
3. One screwdriver; 30 cm (12 in.), Phillips type.
4. One hacksaw; with 12, wire blades (carbide).
5. One pliers; 25 cm (10 in.), vise grip and one pair, channel lock pliers.
6. One hammer; 1.4 kg (3 lb.), 38 cm (15 in.) handle (engineer style).
7. One fire ax; flat head.
8. One crowbar; 130 cm (51 in.), pinch point.
9. One wrecking bar; 61 cm (24 in.), combination tool.
10. One bolt cutter; 91 cm (36 in.), jaw opening of 32 mm (1¼ in.) or greater.
11. One power jack; portable, hydraulic and spreader tool kit, hand powered, minimum 4,064 kg (4 ton) capacity.
12. One shovel; pointed blade (folding type).
13. One tin snip; double action, minimum 20 cm (8 in.).
14. Two ropes; synthetic, kernmantle, 15 m (50 ft) x 19 mm (¾ in.) diameter each.
15. Three pairs gloves; leather (gauntlets).
16. Three pairs goggles; clear eye protective.
17. One cold chisel; and one center punch; 13 mm (½ in.) x 305 mm (12 in.).
18. One cold chisel; 25 mm (1 in.) x 305 mm (12 in.).
19. One seatbelt cutter.
20. Two utility knives; curved blade.
21. One rope; weighted, polypropylene, 30 m (100 ft.), 13 cm (½ in.) diameter.
22. One pair lineman's rubber gloves with leather shells.
23. Two lights; portable, battery operated.
24. One fire blanket and case (min. 152 cm (5 ft.) x 183 cm (6 ft.)).
25. Two baling hooks.
26. Three hard-hats with face and eye protection device.
27. One spring loaded, window punch.
28. Twelve (12) hardwood, shoring blocks, 51 mm (2 in.) x 102 mm (4 in.) x 254 mm (10 in.) with rope handles.
29. Four blocks; hardwood, cribbing, 102 mm (4 in.) x 102 mm (4 in.) x 304 mm (12 in.) with rope handles.
30. Four blocks; hardwood, cribbing, wedge shaped, with rope handles.
31. One come-along, 1814 kg (2 ton), chain type with hooks.
32. Two alloy steel, rescue, pull chains, 3 m (10 ft.) minimum, with grab hooks and rings.
33. One gun kit; air cutting, 1722 kPa (250 psi), with cylinder and chisels.
34. One truck jack, hydraulic, 2722 kg (3 ton).
35. Two extrication straps, synthetic fabric, 2.7 m (9 feet), with quick release buckles.
36. One extrication, loop sling, 2.5 cm (1 in.) wide nylon, or equal, 183 cm (6 ft.) circumference with closure ring.

6.11.4 *Squad Bench, Seats, and Backrests*—The squad bench shall have post cups and wheel cups, or both, to prevent lateral and longitudinal movement and support the Style 3 folding stretcher, combination stretcher chair specified (see

6.10.1 and 6.11.5), or other purchaser specified stretcher Table 10, Item 16, or Style 5). The squad bench top shall be between 48 cm (19 in.) and 56 cm (22 in.) wide, a minimum of 183 cm (72 in.) long, and a height of between 43 cm (17 in.) and 51 cm (20 in.) measured from the floor to the top of the padded seat. Top opening squad bench platform(s) shall be fitted with an automatic hold open and closed latching device for safety. All seats in the patient compartment shall be padded, at least 46 cm (18 in.) wide, and have the largest practical padded backrest. Padding furnished shall be rubber or polyester urethane foam of a medium to firm density, in covered, finish thickness of at least 6.3 cm (2.5 in.) for seats, and approximately 5.1 cm (2 in.) for head and backrests. All padding and upholstery shall be fire retardant and meet FMVSS 302. Additionally, the upholstery shall be non-absorbent, washable and impervious to disinfectants. Non OEM seats shall have 40 oz. reinforced vinyl upholstery. To facilitate cleaning and disinfecting, all seats furnished and installed by the ambulance manufacturer shall be seamless and all exposed surfaces shall be free of perforating decorative stitching or vent devices that would permit the entrapment of biological contaminates.

Squad bench shall be furnished with at least three sets of lap (Type I) safety belts for seated occupants and for retention of a cot/stretcher when positioned on the squad bench. The belts shall be positioned at the patients chest, hips, and legs. Seatbelts shall comply to FMVSS 209. The anchorages for the side facing seatbelt assembly shall withstand a minimum of 1134 kg (2,500 lbs.) force when tested in accordance with FMVSS 210–S5.1. Other side facing seats shall have a Type I lap safety belt.

Sealed storage shall be provided for the specified oxygen cylinder, when located under the rear of the squad bench, with separate compartment under the front of the bench, and the maximum possible volume. The squad bench cover latching device(s) shall be a quick release, slam type latch similar to a Cleveland Model 3300 TL with 3400–15 striker pin. For configuration A (ALS) or, when specified (See Table 9, Item 28), a side facing "CPR" seat located on the street side of the vehicle at the patients thoracic region shall be furnished. This seat shall also be furnished with a seat belt meeting the above requirements and shall have rear and lateral padding at the head areas.

6.11.5 *Stretchers, Cots, and Litters*—When specified (See Table 10, Item 10 and 9.2.36), the ambulance supplier shall provide the following: a Style 1 (Ferno Washington Model 30 or equal) or Style 2 (Ferno Washington Model 93 ES or equal, with roll-in feature) cot for the primary patient and a Style 3 folding stretcher or a combination stretcher chair, each with legs and two wheels designed to permit a patient to be carted (or wheeled) on stairways and through other narrow areas (See 6.11.5.1), or equivalent. Stretchers, cots, and litters shall conform to the dimensions of Table II (See 6.10.1). Length and width measurements shall be taken at the metal framing, excluding joint fittings. Wheeled cots shall include foot and head pulls, when available from the cot manufacturer, and a polyester foam mattress at least 8 cm (3 in.) thick or an equivalent mattress covering with vinyl coated, nylon fabric or other non-porous fabric conforming to FMVSS 302, or equivalent, and restraint straps per 6.11.8.1.

6.11.5.1 *Combination Stretcher Chair*—When specified in Table 10, Item 16, a Ferno Washington Model 107B Combination Stretcher Chair, or equivalent, shall be furnished, in lieu of the stored stairway stretcher specified in 6.11.5. The stretcher shall conform to the dimensions of Style 3 in Table II (See 6.10.3). Stretcher shall have posts, wheels, folding handles at foot-end, straps, and convert to a stair chair or stretcher.

6.11.6 *Seat Safety Belts and Anchorages*—All seats shall comply with FMVSS 207. Safety belts and anchorages shall comply with FMVSS 208, 209, and 210, except as otherwise specified (See 6.11.4). Seatbelts shall have retractor devices for all seat positions in the vehicle, including the squad bench.

6.11.7 *Litter Fasteners and Anchorages*—A crash stable side or center mounting Ferno-Washington Model 175 type cot fastener assembly with quick release latch shall be furnished. It shall secure the Style 1 or Style 2 wheeled cot or infant transporter to the ambulance body. Style 4 and Style 5 litters need not be provided with fastening devices unless otherwise specified (See 9.2.36). The installed cot fastener device(s) for wheeled cots shall he tested to comply with AMD Standard 004 (Litter Retention System). Additional cot related hardware is permitted, provided the patient compartment exit/entry is not encumbered with the cot in place. The furnished devices shall have a bright colored finish, if the device presents a tripping hazard in the entry/exit area when the cot is removed.

6.11.8 *Patient Restraints:*

6.11.8.1 *Cot Straps*—At least three strap type restraining devices (chest. hip, and knee) shall be provided per stretcher, cot, and litter to prevent longitudinal or transverse dislodgment of the patient during transit. Additionally, the head of the cot shall be furnished with upper torso (over shoulder) restraints that mitigate forward motion of the patient during severe braking or in a frontal impact accident. Restraining straps shall incorporate metal-to-metal quick release buckles, be not less than 51 mm (2 in.) wide, and fabricated from nylon or other materials easily cleaned and disinfected.

6.11.8.2 *Infant/Child Carrier*—When specified (See Table 10, Item 26) an infant/child spinal immobilization/carrier device shall he furnished that safely secures those patients to the cot.

6.11.9 *Holders for Intravenous Fluid Containers*—Two near flush style, I.V. ceiling holders specifically designed for holding I.V.'s, with a velcro type strap to hold and control I.V. bags/bottles, shall be provided. The ceiling holders shall not protrude more than 2.5 cm (1 in.) and shall be located on or adjacent to the side wall, one at the head of the primary patient and one at the head of the secondary patient's cot (squad bench). When an ALS configuration (See 6.1.5.1) is specified, one additional I.V. hanger shall be furnished for each patient, at the lower extremities. When specified (See Table 10, Item 2), a folddown, rigid, telescoping I.V. pole and holder, with a 107 cm (42 in.) minimum height (when extended), shall be provided on the left side of the Style I cot.

NOTE 21—**Warning:** Swing down I.V. hangers that can cause injury shall not be specified or furnished.

6.12 *Oxygen and Suction Systems and Equipment*—The

ambulance manufacturer, as required, shall furnish devices/equipment under 6.12-6.12.4 complying to this specification or to other Medical Associations approved standard(s) (for example, ASTM). The specified device shall be tested and certified by an independent, medical testing laboratory for EMS use.

6.12.1 *Oxygen, Main Supply and Installation*—The ambulance shall have a hospital type piped medical oxygen system capable of storing and supplying a minimum of 3,000 liters (see cylinder data 9.7) of medical oxygen. Unless otherwise specified (See 9.2.37), the main oxygen supply shall be from a single "M" size cylinder which consignee will provide and install at the time the vehicle is placed in service. Cylinder(s), when furnished, shall conform to Federal Specification RR-C-901, DOT Specification 3AA2015 and MS-39226-8. Unless otherwise specified by the purchaser (See 9.2.37), the oxygen cylinder shall be located in an area that provides for proper balance and weight distribution (See 6.5.4).

The cylinder controls shall be accessible from the inside and outside of the vehicle. The cylinder pressure gauge or equivalent device shall he visible from the EMT's seat and the squad bench or both. The oxygen cylinder shall be accessible for changing from the exterior of the body and, on Type II vehicles, through a sealed door. Access to the cylinder, when located under the squad bench, shall also be through the rear half of a two section squad bench cover.

If necessary, or when specified (See Table 10, Item 8), a remote cylinder pressure indicator, such as a multilight indicator showing "Full", "¾", "½" and "¼", and "Empty" or a digital indicator or other analog type that displays cylinder capacity, in at least 25% increments, shall be furnished and mounted on the EMT panel. Systems with audible alarms shall have a resetable, audible alarm that sounds when the capacity is down to 20-25%. A shutoff valve or solenoid, when specified, shall be furnished in the 344 kPa (50 psi) line, and shall be located on the EMT panel. If a solenoid is utilized, a readily accessible, emergency bypass valve shall be furnished and identified. The purchaser shall specify the type of quick disconnect, for example, DISS, NCG, or Ohio Diamond (See 9.2.38) to be used to interface the flow meter and oxygen powered, manually triggered (resuscitator) valve (See Table 10, Items 7 and 20).

A cylinder changing wrench shall be furnished, chained and clipped within the oxygen cylinder compartment. The contractor shall install all other components and accessories required for the piped oxygen system which shall include, but not be limited to: a pressure regulator preset to 344 ± 34 kPa (50 ± 5 psi) line pressure, nonferrous piping and low pressure, electrically conductive hose approved for medical oxygen at the flow rate specified in 6.12.1.1 or a combination thereof.

NOTE 22—Industrial or welding type oxygen hose shall not be used.

Oxygen piping shall be: concealed and not exposed to the elements, securely supported to prevent damage, and readily accessible for inspection and replacement. Oxygen shall be piped to a self-sealing duplex oxygen outlet station for the primary patient and, when specified (See Table 10, Item 9), for the secondary patient. An oxygen outlet shall be located within 89 cm (35 in.) from the center of the patient's head when the patient is in the supine position with the cot located in the position closest to the action wall. One of the outlets shall be for a flow meter/humidifier, and the second oxygen outlet shall be used for quick disconnect plug-in devices not requiring humidification. Outlets shall be adequately marked and identified (See 6.7.11) and not interfere with the suction outlet. The entire system shall be leak tested in accordance with AMD Standard 015 (Ambulance Oxygen System Test).

6.12.1.1 *Oxygen Pressure Regulator and Flowmeter*—The medical, oxygen pressure reducing and regulating valve with inlet filter at the cylinder shall have line relief valve set at 1378 kPa (200 psi) maximum, and a gauge range of 0 to 17,225 kPa (0 to 2,500 psi) [27,560 kPa (4,000 psi) tested] with the gauge scale graduated in not more than 100 PSI increments. The regulator shall be easy to connect and preset, with a locking adjustment, at 344 ± 34 kPa (50 ± 5 per line pressure, permitting a minimum 100 LPM flow rate at a cylinder pressure of 689 kPa (150 psi) (empty). In order to show actual oxygen flow rate, the flow meter (See Table 10, Item 7), shall be a pressure compensated type (with floating ball indicator-Thorpe type). It shall have calibrations and be continuously adjustable over a minimum range of 0 to 15 liters per minute (LPM). The flowmeter shall withstand a minimum 1378 KPa (200 psi) inlet pressure without failure or damage. Flowmeter(s) shall be installed vertically and shall be readable from the EMT seat and squad bench. Both the oxygen regulator and flowmeter, when specified (See Table 10, Item 7), shall have standardized connections, be electrically conductive from inlet to outlets (rated hose), and incorporate an inlet filter. These devices shall maintain accurate readings and calibrations under ambulance operation and shall be unaffected by temperature conditions of 6.4.2. All settings, calibrations, safety valves, limiters for pressure, and flowmeters shall maintain accuracy to within ± 10 percent. Servicing, parts, and instructional manuals shall be provided and included in 6.20. Each device shall be color coded green and also be approved for use by recognized national medical associations and societies. The oxygen regulator and flowmeter shall each be permanently identified with the manufacturer's name, model number, calibrated conditions, and specific markings including warning/caution information.

6.12.2 *Portable Oxygen Unit*—When specified (See Table 10, Item 17), a portable oxygen unit of at least 300 liters ("D" size cylinder, see 9.7) shall be provided having a yoke regulator with pressure gauge, dual 344 kPa (50 psi) ports, regulator/dial type flowmeter, delivery tube, and oxygen mask(s). The unit shall be capable of delivering an oxygen flow of at least 15 liters per minute through the flowmeter and 40 L per minute to the manually triggered, oxygen (resuscitator) valve in 6.12.2.2. A full spate cylinder of oxygen for this unit shall be furnished and stored. Portable cylinder(s) and kit shall be secured and, when located in patient compartment, shall include a crash stable, quick release bracket that meets the test requirements in the AMD Standard 003 (Oxygen Tank Retention System Test - Main and Portable Cylinders). A quick release mounting bracket(s) shall also be included for the portable oxygen unit and spare cylinder(s) when located in a secure compartment (See 6.11.1.2) or other purchaser specified

(See 9.2.39) location not requiring a crash stable mounting system.

6.12.2.1 *Self-inflating Bag-Valve-Mask Systems*—When specified (See Table 10, Item 6), portable self-inflating bag-valve-mask systems shall be furnished. (Also see Table 11 for infant-specific size bag-valve-mask system). The bag-valve-mask systems shall comply with the following:

6.12.2.1.1 Two self-inflating bags without sponge rubber inside. One bag of at least 1,300 mL for adults, one bag of not more than 750 mL volume for children.

6.12.2.1.2 Three see-through face-masks one each in adult, child, and infant sizes. Two masks covering the full range of adult through pediatric sizes may be furnished in lieu of three masks.

6.12.2.1.3 Standard 15 mm/22 mm fittings.

6.12.2.1.4 A true non-breathing valve.

6.12.2.1.5 An oxygen reservoir system for delivery of 80-100 percent oxygen through an ancillary oxygen inlet. The system shall be capable of accepting at least 15 liters/min. of oxygen without valve jam.

6.12.2.2 *Oxygen Powered, Manually Triggered (Resuscitator) Valve*—When specified (See Table 10, Item 20), an oxygen powered manually triggered (resuscitator) valve shall be provided. This device shall have a see through inflatable face mask, interface with the action wall outlet via the specified quick disconnect device, and the dual port regulator/flowmeter of the portable oxygen system, or both, and meet the following requirements of F 920.

6.12.2.3 *Automatic Resuscitator*—When specified (See Table 10, Item 29), an automatic resuscitator/volume ventilator shall be furnished. The device's features and performance shall conform to AHA or other medical standards organization requirements. The device shall be furnished with a connection hose and ambulance and portable oxygen system compatible quick disconnect fittings, or both.

6.12.3 *Suction Aspirator, Primary Patient*—An electrically powered suction aspirator system shall be furnished with an illuminated switch and a panel mounted, labeled, quick disconnect inlet device on the EMT panel. The system shall meet the minimum safety and performance requirements of Specification F 960. The suction pump shall be located in an area that is accessible but sound and vibration insulated from the patient compartment. The pump shall be vented to the vehicle's exterior. All components, electrical, pressure and vacuum or both, and other lines and accessories, shall be securely mounted yet readily accessible. The electric type aspirator system shall be connected per Fig. 7. The aspirator system shall provide a free air flow of at least 30 LPM and achieve a minimum of 300 mm (11.81 in.) Hg vacuum within four seconds after the suction tube is closed. A vacuum control and a shut-off valve, or combination thereof, shall be provided to adjust vacuum levels and to discontinue aspiration instantly. A vacuum indicator gauge of 76 mm ± 13 mm (3 ± 0.5 in.) in diameter, with numerical markers at least every/100 mm Hg and a total range of 0 to 760 mm Hg, shall be provided. The collection bottle or bag shall be nonbreakable and transparent with a minimum 1,000 ml capacity. The following accessories shall be furnished: one suction rinsing water bottle; one semi-rigid pharyngeal suction tip, with thumb suction control port, (nonmetallic) of sufficient diameter to allow aspiration of semi-solid gastric contents; a 3 m (10 ft) length of transparent or translucent, non-kinking suction tubing which shall not collapse under high suction; and a minimum of ten spare collection bags when the bag type system is furnished. To assure high air flows and free passage of aspirate, minimum inside diameter for the suction tubing and tubing connectors shall be at least 6.4 mm (¼ in.). The user shall provide any additional suction catheters. An operator's manual containing clearly illustrated instructions for operation, cleaning, assembly/disassembly, decontamination/sterilization, trouble-shooting, parts list, etc., shall be provided. The apparatus shall be clearly marked with manufacturer's name, address, and any applicable standards ratings (See 6.20).

6.12.4 *Portable Suction Aspirator*—When specified (See Table 10, Item 18), a portable suction aspirator meeting the minimum safety and performance requirements of Specification F 960 and having the following characteristics shall be provided. The unit shall be capable of operation from the vehicle's 12 V DC electrical system. It shall also operate from an integral battery supply which will allow the unit to meet the air flow and suction requirements of this Section for at least 20 minutes of continuous operation. The portable suction aspirator shall provide an air flow of at least 30 L per minute at the end of the suction tube and a vacuum level of at least 300 mm Hg to be reached within 4 s after the tube is clamped. A vacuum control and a shut-off valve, or combination thereof, shall be provided to adjust vacuum levels and to discontinue aspiration instantly. A true vacuum indicator with numerical markers at least every 100 mm Hg and having a total range of 0 to 760 mm Hg, shall be provided. The portable aspirator shall be provided with the following accessories: one suction rinsing water bottle, one semirigid pharyngeal suction tip with thumb suction control port (nonmetallic) of sufficient diameter to allow aspiration of semi-solid gastric contents; and one 2 m (6 ft) length of transparent or translucent non-kinking suction tubing which shall not collapse under high suction. The inside diameter of the tubing shall be at least 6.4 mm (¼in.). The user shall provide any additional suction catheters. If the integral battery supply is rechargeable, it shall be rechargeable from the vehicle's 12 V DC electrical system and from 115 V AC. The 115 V AC charging system need not be integral to the portable suction unit. The unit shall be provided with applicable power cords and plugs (MS 3116F12-3P). The polarity of the DC plug shall be as follows: Pin A (+12 V), Pin B (ground), Pin C (not used). An operator's manual containing clearly illustrated instructions for operation, cleaning assembly/disassembly, decontamination/sterilization and troubleshooting, parts list, etc., shall be provided. The apparatus shall be clearly marked with manufacturer's name, address, and any applicable standards ratings (See 6.20).

6.13 *Environmental: Climatic and Noise Parameters:*

6.13.1 *Environmental Systems*—All ambulances shall be equipped with a complete climate environmental system(s) to supply and maintain clean air conditions and specified level of inside temperature in both driver and patient compartments.

The various systems for heating, ventilating, and air conditioning may be separate or combination systems which shall permit independent control of the environment within each compartment. All ambulances shall be equipped with heating, ventilating, and air conditioning systems that can be made to collectively operate using recirculated air and outside ambient air and shall be capable of maintaining interior temperature of 20°C to 26°C (68°F to 78°F) when operated between -18°C to 35°C (0°F to 95°F) outside ambient temperature. Ambulance shall be tested in accordance with AMD Standard 012 (Ambient Temperature Test). The air systems shall be high volume capacity with low velocity delivery, for minimum draft circulation while providing a positive pressure within each closed compartment (positive pressure may be attained through the fresh air ventilation system either apart from or as an integral part of the heating/air conditioning system). Environmental system components shall be readily accessible for servicing at the installed location(s). Connecting hoses for heating and the air conditioning system shall be supported by rubber insulated metal clamping devices at least every 30 cm (12 in.). The driver and patient compartment environments shall not in any way be dependent upon each other.

6.13.2 *Driver's Compartment Environmental Equipment*—The driver's compartment shall be furnished with the chassis manufacturer's hot water, fresh air, high capacity, heater, defroster, and air conditioning system. The patient compartment heater shall be installed in a manner that does not adversely affect the chassis manufacturer's FMVSS 103 performance certification for windshield defrosting.

6.13.3 *Patient Compartment Environmental Equipment*—The patient compartment shall be heated, ventilated, and air conditioned in accordance with the criteria specified hereto. During the performance testing (See 7.4.2) of the heating and air conditioning systems, the use of fans or motors within the test chamber is permitted only to provide air circulation to help maintain the required ambient test temperature. The use of these fans or blowers to direct air through the vehicle's radiator and condenser(s) is not permitted, or both.

6.13.4 *Heating Criteria*— The heating system(s) shall have sufficient capacity to simultaneously raise the temperature at the midpoints in each compartment to a minimum dry bulb temperature of 20°C (68°F) at all twelve test points (9 patient compartment and 3 cab) within 30 min. Test conditions: the ambulance (with doors open) shall be cold soaked for three hours in an ambient temperature of (0°F), then the engine started and allowed to run at the high-idle setting (See 6.7.6) while the transmission is in park or neutral. Three verification readings shall be made (start, middle, and final) by nine equally spaced test thermocouples in the patient compartment, and three in the cab compartment. Heating equipment may be in the recirculating mode and all compartment openings, including partition doors/windows and exhaust vents, shall be closed. Heater(s) furnished shall comply to applicable Motor Carrier Safety Regulation 393.77. Heater(s) shall, to the maximum extent possible, be connected to the chassis manufacturer's furnished interconnection points. When interconnection points are not furnished, chassis manufacturers unused engine water pump supply ports shall be utilized. All added heater hose shall meet or exceed chassis manufacturers requirements and when specified silicone hoses shall be furnished.

6.13.5 *Air Conditioning Criteria*—The air conditioning system(s) shall have sufficient capacity to simultaneously lower the temperature at the midpoints in each compartment to a maximum dry bulb temperature of 26°C (78°F), at all twelve (9 patient compartment plus 3 cab) test points within 30 min. Test conditions: the ambulance (with doors open) shall be heat soaked for three h in an ambient temperatures of 35°C (95°F), then the engine started and allowed to run at high-idle setting (See 6.7.6), while the transmission is in park or neutral, with test verification and thermocouples placement as specified in 6.13.4. Air conditioning equipment may be in the recirculating mode and all compartment openings, including partition doors/windows shall be closed. When available, chassis manufacturers interconnection points shall be utilized.

6.13.5.1 *Auxiliary Air Conditioning Condenser*—When specified by the purchaser (See 9.2.41) or required for high temperature geographic areas or furnished as standard equipment, an auxiliary condenser shall be provided which will allow for maximum system performance, based on the air conditioning and ambulance manufacturer's recommendations. If the condenser is located above the cab, it shall not block the emergency lights. All added refrigeration lines and fittings shall be mechanical fittings compatible with OEM components furnished by the chassis manufacturer. An auxiliary condenser may be furnished or specified to function in lieu of the chassis manufacturers condenser provided it meets or exceeds all other system performance requirements.

6.13.6 *Ventilation Criteria*—Ventilation system(s) of the driver and patient compartments shall provide a complete change of ambient air within each compartment at least every two minutes with the vehicle stationary. Ventilation shall be separately controlled within each compartment. Fresh air intakes shall be located towards the front of the vehicle and exhaust vents shall be located on the upper rear of the vehicle. Exhaust vents may be located on the rear lower half of the module/body, provided the vent/device incorporates a reverse flow damper to prevent backdraft and intrusion of vehicle engine exhaust, dust, dirt, or road spray. The patient compartment shall be ventilated by the air delivery system of the environmental equipment (heater-air conditioner) or by separate system(s), such as power intake, exhaust ventilator(s).

6.13.7 *Environmental Controls*—Adjustable, manual or thermostatically operative controls shall permit heating and air conditioning and ventilation, or a combination thereof, in either compartment without affecting the other compartment. Switches and controls shall be located in EMT's panel and remote panel or both, and identified for function and operating position (See 6.7.9-6.7.11). Switches, wiring and control components shall be rated at a minimum of 125 percent of the maximum electrical load of the blower(s) and other components (See 6.7.2). Blower or fan system shall have at least three speeds (excluding "OFF"). Separate noncorroding brass, bronze, stainless steel, plastic or other inherently corrosion proof shutoff valves, for the patient compartment hot water heating system, shall be provided to allow servicing and shutoff. The use of vacuum operated shutoff valves are acceptable provided the above criteria is met and the valve provides inherent sealing when vacuum is removed. This sealing shall prevent engine cooling system pressure and water pump pressure from causing any leakage when vacuum is removed. Air systems shall have adjustable louvers to direct the flow of air.

6.13.8 *Patient Compartment Sound Level Criteria*—Unless otherwise specified (See 9.2.42) by Federal or State regulations, the patient compartment decibel level shall not exceed 80 dB and shall be tested in accordance with AMD Standard 006 (Sound Level Test Code).

6.14 *Communications:*

6.14.1 *Communications and Electronic Equipment*—The ambulance, driver compartment console, and patient compartment console shall be configured for convenient installation of two-way radio control(s), electronic siren, public address amplifiers/speakers and microphones, front/rear compartment intercom, radio telemetry, cellular telephone, computer and other electronic equipment, or both, as specified herein or as required or specified by the purchaser (See 9.2.43). Switches and controls shall be panel mounted and conform to 6.7.9-6.7.11. When electronic or communications equipment is specified and installed, all technical manuals and installation diagrams shall be provided to the purchaser as part of the delivery documentation. All electronic equipment shall be installed in conformance with the requirements and specifications of the manufacturer of the equipment. All communications equipment shall be type accepted and licensed by the Federal Communications Commission.

6.14.2 *Mobile Radio Provisions*—The ambulance shall be provided with a locked ventilated compartment designed for the convenient installation of two-way radio communications equipment. The area shall be provided with fused 12 V battery electrical power sufficient to provide 50 amp service to the installed radios. Fuses shall be identified and installed as close to the battery as possible. Electrical power in the radio compartment shall be terminated in an appropriate insulated barrier strip or insulated connector of sufficient size and current capacity to handle the required power. Both Negative and Positive battery leads shall be provided. The wiring shall be color coded and identified by marking. An additional switched electrical lead shall be provided to the radio installation compartment that becomes energized when the ignition switch of the ambulance is activated. The switched ignition lead shall be fused and identified.

6.14.3 *Antenna, Cable Conduit, and Antenna Mounting*—The ambulance shall be provided with a ground plane, antenna opening and conduit from the roof antenna opening to the ventilated radio installation compartment. An additional conduit shall extend from the radio installation compartment to the driver compartment console area and from the driver compartment console to the patient compartment radio control console location. The conduits shall be sufficient to permit antenna, intercom or control cable wiring to be conveniently installed between these locations.

6.14.3.1 Antenna mounting locations shall be on the centerline of the patient compartment roof. An antenna inspection/access port shall be provided in the patient compartment directly under the antenna mounting area. The port shall provide at least a 10 cm. x 10 cm. (4 in. x 4 in.) opening and be marked as specified in 6.7.11. The inspection port shall provide access to the conduit that connects between the antenna and the ventilated radio installation compartment. The conduit is intended to permit RF coaxial transmission cables to be installed from the antenna to the radio installation compartment. A fish lead shall be provided to pull the cables from the antenna port to the radio installation compartment.

6.14.3.2 Any nonmetallic patient compartment roof shall be provided with a metal radio antenna ground plane molded into the roof. The metal antenna ground plane shall be grounded to the vehicle chassis and electrical system. The ground plane shall be a minimum 102 cm x 102 cm (40" x 40").

6.14.3.3 All antennas shall be installed with due consideration given to the radio and antenna manufacturer's instructions, requirements, and specifications. Antennas shall be designed and installed to minimize the risk of damage to the antenna by garage doors, low underpasses, trees or porticos.

6.14.3.4 All radio equipment and antennas shall be installed so as to minimize the electromagnetic energy present in the vehicle or patient compartment. All Federal Communications Commission requirements regarding EMI (electromagnetic interference) shall be complied with.

6.14.4 *Intercom System*— When specified (See Table 9, Item 4), solid state intercom equipment shall be provided between the driver and patient compartments. The driver shall have the capability to place the patient compartment in standby "talk" mode and to control any necessary talk/listen switching. The intercom system shall be independent of the two-way radio equipment. Cab compartment intercom shall be mounted in accordance with 6.7.9 and patient compartment intercom in accordance with 6.7.10, and comply to 6.7.11.

6.14.5 *Siren-Public Address System*—A combination electronic siren with integral public address system and other upgrading features, including radio interface capability, shall be provided. Dual speakers shall be installed, outside the vehicle, in the bumper/hood area. Speakers shall not protrude beyond the face of the bumper or bumper guards. The microphone shall be a noise canceling type. The siren's control shall permit the following sounds: Manual, Wail, and Yelp. Other applicable sounds such as "Rapid Yelp", "Air Horn" or composite type sounds may be specified (See 9.2.44) or furnished. The system shall provide plug-in connections and connecting cables with control capability from the passenger seat and driver's horn ring by means of a siren/horn switch or, when specified (See 9.2.44), by a foot switch, and all other necessary hardware for the siren/public address operation. The public address amplifier shall be independent of the two-way radio, except that a common microphone and control housing group may be employed. The illuminated (in siren mode) "Horn/Siren" switch shall be provided on the driver's console.

The siren, with the exception of cancellation effects due to dual speakers, when tested in a full anechoic chamber that conforms to ANSI Standard S1.13-1971, with test equipment and methods conforming to California Administrative Code, Title 13, Article 8, shall be capable of producing a continuous warning sound at a minimum level of 123 dB, A-weighted, at 3 m (10 ft) on axis in the "Wail mode" with "Yelp" falling within 1 dba with 13.6 V ± 1% input, at a fundamental frequency in the range of 500 to 2,000 Hz maximum.

The output over the sweep range shall not drop to less than 116 dBa. The speakers shall be located in the configuration that is representative of the vehicle on which they will be mounted.

In the "Wail" mode the siren shall have a sweep rate of 10-18 cycles per minute and in the "Yelp" mode, a sweep rate of 150 to 250 cycles per minute. All sweep modes shall cover a range of at least one octave.

In voice (P.A.) operation, the unclipped sine wave output shall be at least 55 watts RMS into a resistive load matching the nominal speaker system impedance at 1000 Hz. The frequency response of the amplifier shall be from 500 to 3,000 Hz ± 3 dB, when measured from 1,000 Hz reference. Total harmonic distortion shall not exceed 10 percent, at 20 watts RMS, over the specified frequency range when measured with the load shown above.

In addition, the electronic siren furnished with the exception of cancellation effects attributable to dual speakers shall comply to all the other requirements included in the State of California Vehicle Code Section 1020 thru 1029, Title 13, Article 8, the latest issue for Class A sirens. The electronic system shall be tested and approved by an accredited laboratory for compliance with the requirements of this standard.

6.14.6 *Air Horns*—When specified by the purchaser, air horn(s) shall be furnished. Horns shall be activated as specified by the purchaser. Horn(s) shall be mounted forward of the cab compartment.

6.15 *Additional Systems, Equipment, Accessories, and Supplies:*

6.15.1 *Additional And Optional Equipment*—When specified (See 9.2.45), additional or optional system(s), equipment, accessories, and supplies shall be furnished, in addition to the standard ambulance component systems and devices specified herein. These items shall be selected by the purchasers. Optional items may be further described in authoritative procurement documents. In no event shall the specified or furnished optional item(s) reduce the quality and intent of the ambulance but shall enhance its design and purpose. The materials, devices, items, and fabrication, if not specifically described, shall be not less in quality, strength, performance, and service than those normally provided by the most reputable manufacturers.

6.15.2 *Standard Mandatory Miscellaneous Equipment*—Unless otherwise precluded in the contract, each ambulance shall he equipped with, but not limited to the following:

6.15.2.1 *Fire Extinguishers*—Two, ABC dry chemical, minimum 2.3 kg (5 lb.) units, in a quick-release bracket, one mounted in the driver/cab compartment or in the body reachable from outside the vehicle and one in the patient compartment. When located in either the driver or patient compartments, the mounting bracket shall be a stable design.

6.15.2.2 "No Smoking Oxygen Equipped" and "Fasten Seat Belts" signs: Conspicuously placed in the cab and patient compartment.

6.15.2.3 Overhead grabrail, minimum 152 cm (60 in.) long, maximum 10.2 cm (4 in.) depth on the ceiling over the primary patient. Grabrail shall be stainless steel, aluminum, or other corrosion resistant material, and have padded or curved up ends, and rounded corners. Mounting brackets shall be chromed, stainless steel, polished cast aluminum or other corrosion resistant materials. The grabrail(s) shall he installed in a manner that precludes loosening and shall meet a 136 kg (300 lb.) pull test in all three axes. The grabrail shall be tested in accordance with AMD Standard 008 (Ambulance Patient Compartment Grab Rail-Load Test).

6.15.2.4 Backup alert alarm, (audible warning device) activated when the vehicle is shifted into reverse. Device must meet OSHA and SAE J994 requirements, and shall be rated (SAE) for Type C or B (97 or 107 dba at 122 cm (4 feet)) or purchaser may specify (See 9.2.45) alarms that automatically adjust to ambient noise levels.

6.15.3 *Optional Equipment* —When specified (See 9.2.45), the ambulance shall be equipped with but not limited to the equipment listed in Table 9. Additional weight resulting from specified options, shall be deducted from the specified payload allowance (See 6.5.2).

6.15.4 *Medical, Surgical, and Biomedical Equipment*—When specified (See 9.2.45), the ambulance shall be equipped with the following:

6.15.4.1 *Pediatric Medical Equipment and Supplies*—In addition to the items in Table 10, ambulances should carry appropriate equipment and supplies to enable EMTs and Paramedics to care for ill and injured infants and children. Guidelines for such equipment have been prepared by a Committee on Ambulance Equipment and Supplies convened by the National EMSC Resource Alliance. These guidelines consist of two minimum lists of equipment and supplies: one for BLS and one for ALS ambulances as shown in Table 11. Each list has two categories, Essential and Desirable. For purposes of these lists, Essential means that the item is necessary and should be carried. A Desirable item is worth having and may improve care; however, its use will depend on local policy, cost and scope of practice of the providers. A number of items on these lists are also listed in Table 10 and need not be duplicated on board an ambulance so as to conserve space and weight. Intentionally excluded from these lists are specific drugs and fluids useful for pediatric care. The use of such drugs and fluids by prehospital care providers is subject to local medical direction, and their availability and use on ambulances should be approved by Ambulance Service Medical Directors.

6.15.4.1.1 Organization and Storage of Pediatric Equipment and Supplies—Equipment and supplies used primarily for treatment of infants and children should be organized separately so as to be easily retrievable, either in a specific pediatric pack such as a Pediatric Emergency Medical Jump Kit/Drug Kit, or a special compartment in the ambulance. Fluids and drugs locally approved for pediatric use on ambulances by prehospital care providers should also be packaged and stored separately, so to avoid confusion with drugs and fluids intended for use for adults.

6.16 *Preparation far Painting, Color, and Markings:*

6.16.1 *Preparation for Painting*—Ambulance body and all

TABLE 9 Optional Ambulance Equipment

1. Reserved.
2. Tachograph; 145 km/hour (90 mph), with 24-hour chart, warning light, and siren recording.
3. Intercom, Silent; The system shall consist of amber, red, and green lights in the driver's compartment controlled by the EMT. It shall include an alerting buzzer in the driver's compartment.
4. Intercom; voice intercommunication system between driver and technician compartments as per 6.14.5.
5. Batteries, 12VDC, heavy-duty "high cycle life," maintenance-free automotive type per 6.7.7.
6. 115 VAC onboard electric power supply, Inverter (specify brand or equal) per 6.7.8.3.
7. 12 VDC battery charger or conditioner onboard, per 6.7.7.1 and 6.7.8.
8. High intensity cot light[A]; with flexible or adjustable shaft located near head of primary cot.
9. "Checkout light" for patient compartment (See 6.8.5.2).
10. Patient fan; located near primary cot, minimum 250 CFM rating, 12VDC.
11. Rear step storage compartment for Type I and III when available on specified chassis.
12. Window; tinted, right side panel of patient compartment, minimum 2774 sq. cm (430 sq. in.) per 6.10.14.
13. Reserved.
14. Drug kit compartment[A]; locking, security compartment located near primary patient with piano hinge and non–exposed fasteners, door with key lock, minimum size 56 cm (22 in.)W x 36 cm (14″)D x 46 cm (18″)H per 6.1.5.1.
15. Stone/mud guard; to protect lower front end of body (for Type I and III) (See 6.9.7.4).
16. Power plant heaters; minimum -34°C (-30°F) startability per for severely cold areas only per .
17. High altitude operations; engine adjustments and emission control(s), or both, and test if available and applicable per 6.6.4.3.
18. Extrication equipment, specified in 6.11.2.1. (This equipment may normally be carried on the ambulance unless it is routinely accompanied by a rescue vehicle. Select which items, (1 through 36) and fully detail specific items wanted by brand, model, size, quantity, as required.
19. Body rubrails; for Types I and III as specified in 6.9.7.5.
20. Automatic transmission heavy-duty oil cooler, additional unit (for very hot areas only), per when not furnished from the chassis manufacturer.
21. Folding style step; at ambulance body rear loading doors, per 6.9.6.
22. Front bumper override, grille, and radiator protection, per 6.9.6.1 (grille guard) and 6.9.6.2 (bumper guards).
23. Emergency safety kit; in sturdy metal/plastic carrying case containing: 3 bi-directional reflective triangles (approved FMVSS 125) 6 fuses, 15 minutes each with holders, 2 sets of chassis circuit electrical system spare fuses.
24. Towing devices (if permitted by chassis manufacturer), not less than 2 towing devices on the front of the vehicle.
25. Spotlight, 360° horizontal and 90° vertical controlled per 6.8.4.
26. Radio-Chassis manufacturers, AM/FM, as specified. Additional speakers shall be furnished as specified.
27. Reserved.
28. CPR seat[A] on left, street side of vehicle (right side of patient) (See 6.1.5.1 and 6.11.4)
29. Cab Console between driver and passenger seat. Purchaser shall specify layout and dimensions (See 6.9.2 and 6.10.15.2).
30. Running boards (See 6.9.7.2).
31. Mud flaps (See 6.9.7.3).
32. Interior/exterior compartment, two shelves, at the front right corner of the body with exterior access per 6.11.1.2 (for Types I & III).
33. Map light, dash or ceiling mounted as required by the purchaser and shall be separately switched. Purchaser shall specify type or model required (see 6.8.5).
34. Siren system. Specify features, for example, foot switch or other requirements (See 6.14.5)
35. Audible warning indicator, in the cab, that sounds only when the patient or equipment compartment(s) are open and when the vehicle is placed in forward or reverse gear.
36. Air horns, bumper/grill mounted (See 6.14.6)

[A]Items furnished as standard equipment when Configuration 'A' (ALS) is specified (See Section 6.1.5.1).

TABLE 10 Medical, Surgical, and Biomedical Equipment[A]

1. Rail system; a medical device(s) attaching aluminum rail, with quick release mounting mechanisms, fastened securely in the action area at the side of the primary cot. Rail length 152 cm to 229 cm (60 to 90 in.) long. Medical devices shall be rail mounted, and 3 spare mounting devices supplied per 6.11.1.1.
2. I.V. telescoping pole for primary cot (See 6.11.9).
3. Electric clock, 12 volt DC chassis powered, with sweep second hand, illuminated (when module is turned on), 10 cm (4 in.) minimum dial. Clock shall be located on the action wall and shall be visible to the EMT from both the EMT seat and squad bench. Other types of clocks as specified or approved by the purchaser may be furnished.
4. Suction jar (clear plastic) for secondary patient with 20 disposable inserts or spare bottle (clear plastic) with holder (See 6.12.3).
5. Sphygmomanometer; 15 cm (6 in.) dial type, wall mounted or rail mounted, when Item 1 is specified, cuff, stethoscope, inflating bulb and mounting. Specify size, obese, adult, child, or pediatric.
6. Self-inflating bag-valve-mask system, portable, for artificial ventilation (See 6.12.2.1).
7. Oxygen flowmeter (pressure compensated) and humidifier (See 6.12.1.1), with specified disconnect fittings. Specify quantity.
8. Remote oxygen indicator for main cylinder. Specify type (See 6.12.1).
9. Oxygen outlet. A second, self-sealing, duplex oxygen outlet for the secondary patient to be located at patients head area (See 6.12.1). Additional outlets may also be specified.
10. Cot for primary and secondary patients (per 6.11.5). Specify desired models. Cot straps per 6.11.8.1.
11. A lower-extremity traction splint with all necessary straps, attachments, and case. Specify type and adult, pediatric size or universal type.
12. Emergency medical jump kit or drug kit, specify model (case only).
13. Scoop stretcher, specify model.
14. Backboards; wood, aluminum, or plastic, one long- minimum size 183 x 41 cm (72 x 16 in.), one short- minimum size 81 cm x 41 cm (32 x 16 in.) with three straps. Boards shall be X-ray translucent. Specify type and quantity.
15. Reserved.
16. Combination stretcher, in lieu of folding stretcher (See 6.11.5.1 and 6.11.4).
17. Oxygen, portable unit (See 6.12.2).
18. Suction aspirator, portable (See 6.12.4).
19. Mast, compartmentalized individually inflatable sections, pneumatic trouser kit, complete with carrying case. Specify adult, pediatric and model.
20. Oxygen-powered, manually triggered, positive pressure valve with mask (See 6.12.2.2). Specify type of valve and quick disconnect fitting required.
21. Dual position cot fastener mounting assembly (quick detachable type for center and side positions). Specify type (See 6.1.5 and 6.11.7).
22. Vest type (wrap around) extrication device to provide spinal immobilization for seated patient, complete with all necessary belts, head straps, padding, etc., and case. Specify type.
23. Extrication collar, specify type and size (pediatric, extra small, short, medium, tall, etc.).
24. Automatic external defibrillator or monitor defibrillator (specify desired model).
25. Cardiac Monitor/defibrillator mounting bracket. Specify type of bracket.
26. Pediatric, spinal immobilization/transport device with cot interface capability. Device shall be complete with all straps, attachment devices, and case. Specify desired model (See 6.11.8.2).
27. Reserved.
28. Infant/child carrier per 6.11.8.2.
29. Automatic Resuscitation/ventilator (See 6.12.2.3). Specify type desired and type oxygen system interface device (See 9.2.38).

[A]Items furnished as standard equipment when Configuration "A" (ALS) is specified (See 6.1.5.1).

attached equipment exterior surfaces, except polished metal parts, shall be thoroughly cleaned, treated, and coated with a firm primer and preservative with rust inhibiting properties, and painted in the finish color as specified (See 9.2.46). Ferrous metal interior surfaces shall be painted or, when not exposed for painting, shall be treated or coated to resist corrosion. Chassis and chassis frame components shall be preserved and finished in accordance to industry's standard practice.

6.16.2 *Color, Paint, and Finish*—Unless otherwise specified, (See 9.2.46), the exterior color of the ambulance shall be gloss white in combination with a solid uninterrupted orange stripe and blue lettering and emblems. The stripe should be as close to parallel as possible with the road but a stripe transition angle is acceptable to connect the module beltline stripe with the chassis stripe. The exterior finish on painted metal modular bodies and metal roofs on Type II ambulances shall be an acrylic composition urethane or polyurethane paint. The final

TABLE 11 Pediatric Medical Equipment and Supplies

Basic Life Support
Essential
Oropharyngeal airways infant, child, adult (sizes 00–5)
Self-inflating resuscitation bag, infant, child and adult sizes
Masks for bag-valve-mask device: child, adult sizes
Oxygen masks: infant, child and adult sizes
Nonrebreathing mask: pediatric and adult sizes
Stethoscope
Backboard
Cervical immobilization devices: infant, child, and adult sizes
Blood pressure cuff: infant, child, adult sizes
Portable suction unit with a regulator
Suction catheters: tonsil-tip and 6F-14F
Extremity splints: pediatric sizes
Bulb syringe
Obstetric pack
Thermal blanket
Water soluble lubricant
Desirable
Infant car seat
Nasopharyngeal airways (sizes 18F-34F, or 4.5–8.5 mm)
Glasgow Coma Scale reference
Pediatric Trauma Score reference
Small stuffed toy
Advanced Life Support
ALS ambulances should carry everything on the BLS List plus the following:
Essential
Transport monitor
Defibrillator for pediatric and adult use with adult and pediatric paddles and with discharge range of 5 to 360 J
Monitoring electrodes: pediatric sizes
Laryngoscope with straight blades 0–2, curved blades 2–4
Endotracheal tube stylets: pediatric and adult size
Endotracheal tubes: uncuffed sizes 2.5–6.0, cuffed sizes 6.0–8.0
Magill forceps: pediatric and adult
Nasogastric tubes: 8F-16F
Nebulizer
Intravenous catheters: 16–24 gauge
Intraosseous needles
Length/weight-based drug dose chart or tape
Needles: 20–25 gauge
Resuscitation drugs and intravenous fluids that meet the local standard of practice
Desirable
CO2 detection device (disposable)
Blood glucose analysis systems

NOTE—Guidelines for the selection and use of the above equipment have been prepared by the Committee on Ambulance Equipment and Supplies of the National EMS for Children Resource Alliance and are contained in Guidelines for Pediatric Equipment and Supplies for Basic and Advanced Life Support Ambulances published in the Annals of Emergency Medicine, Vol 28, No. 6 pp 699–701.

stage manufacturer's painted components shall have a paint film not less than 1.25 mils. thick and a minimum total thickness of 4 mils., including primers. The orange stripe shall not be less than 15 cm (6 in.) wide, nor more than 36 cm (14 in.) wide and shall encircle the entire ambulance body at the belt line below the bottom edge of cab windows but may exclude the front of the hood panel. The orange stripe, as specified by the purchaser (See 9.2.46) may be reflective tape conforming to 6.16.4 or be painted and may be edged/pin striped in black or blue. This single, solid band (except when interrupted by windows, locks, etc.), when viewed horizontally, shall appear as a stripe near parallel to the road. The interior finish shall be the manufacturer's standard light color harmonizing with the color of upholstery. The final film of painted surfaces shall be smooth and uniform, free of grit, streaks, blushing, runs, sagging, blisters, "fish-eyes", "orange peel", pinholes, or other surface irregularities. Exterior finish paint shall not be required on the underbody and inside surface of the body skirting.

NOTE 23—Users should avoid specifying darker or alternate colors because of the adverse effect on vehicle visibility, and increased heat load that the darker colors impose on the air conditioning system. Specifically, the white/orange combination provides the most visible vehicle under different light conditions, (for example, mercury and sodium vapor lights), as well as providing, on an international basis, the most easily recognized color configuration.

6.16.2.1 *Color Standards and Tolerances*—The exterior surface including the wheels shall be manufacturer's standard gloss white. The ambulance colors, orange stripe or band and blue markings shall be the same as specified Orange and Blue in American National Standard Z53.1-1974, Safety Color Code for Marking Physical Hazards. They shall comply with the tolerances expressed in terms of Munsel hue, value (lightness), and chroma (saturation).

Color tolerance charts containing the color standards and tolerances for Ambulance Orange and Ambulance Blue are available from the Department of Transportation, Research and Special Program Administration, Information Services Division (DMT-11), 400 7th Street, SW, Washington, DC 20590.

6.16.3 *Salt Spray Resistance*—Treated exterior sheet metal of the ambulance body (except OEM Type II van) shall be capable of withstanding 250 hours of salt spray tested in accordance with Practice B 117. The specimen used for the salt spray test shall be run through all steps of the cleaning and treating process, including priming. The primed specimen shall be scored from corner to corner using a sharp knife. After the test, the specimen panels shall exhibit no failure and not more than 3 mm (⅛ in.) rust or blister creapage from the scored lines.

6.16.4 *Emblems, and Markings*—The material for the emblems and markings shall be applied using reflectorized material conforming to Federal Specification L-S-300, Type 1, Class 1 or 3 reflectivity 1. The reflective color used shall be blue (color a) and white (color i) when applicable. The emblems and markings shall be of the type, size, color, and location as follows:

6.16.4.1 *Front Markings*

6.16.4.1.1 The word "AMBULANCE", mirror imaged, shall be in block, blue, die cut style letters, not less than 10 cm (4 in.) high, centered above the grille, on the orange or white background. The placement of the word ambulance on the curved surface of the hood or on a flat plastic type bugscreen is permitted.

6.16.4.1.2 A "Star of Life" in 7.6 cm (3 in.), blue, die cut style, with a white border, conforming to Fig. 1 (size A) shall be located both to the right and left of the word "AMBULANCE."

6.16.4.2 *Side and Rear Markings:*

6.16.4.2.1 The word "AMBULANCE" shall be block, blue, die cut style letters of not less than 15 cm (6 in.) in height, centered, with a white border, alongside or under the "Star of Life" on each side and rear of the vehicle body.

6.16.4.2.2 A "Star of Life", not less than 40.6 cm (16 in.), in blue, die cut style, with a white border, conforming to Fig. 1

(size C), on the right and left side panels. A "Star of Life" emblem, size B, shall be provided on each rear door.

6.16.4.2.3 All additional lettering and markings (required by the purchaser) should be below the word "AMBULANCE", except the units abbreviated identification lettering/number, which may be located on the uppermost white space of the front, rear, and sides.

6.16.4.3 *Top Markings:*

6.16.4.3.1 A "Star of Life", of not less than 81 cm (32 in.) (Size D) in blue, die cut style, conforming to Fig. 1 (may be without the white Staff of Aesculapius), shall be provided on the ambulance rooftop.

6.17 *Undercoating*— Unless the ambulance is rustproofed, the vehicle shall be undercoated for sound deadening, corrosion, and stone damage protection. A commercial, sandless, petroleum base undercoating or other materials providing equivalent protection, shall be applied to the underbody and under chassis sheet metal surfaces to a thickness of 1.6 mm to 3.2 mm (1/16to 1/8 in.), except to the drive shafts, drain holes, lubrication points, engine/transmission oil pans, fuel tanks, heavy castings, suspension components, heat shields, heat diffusing devices, catalytic converters, and areas 30.5 cm (12 in.) or less from the exhaust system(s) as well as other areas specifically excluded by the chassis manufacturer. These areas shall be kept free of coating material. Chassis frame, underside of engine compartment hood, and underbody surfaces in excess of 3.2 mm (1/8 in.) thickness, or that are inaccessible without removing vehicle fuel tank(s) or other major components shall not require undercoating.

6.18 *Rustproofing*— When specified (See 9.2.47), ambulance shall be rustproofed in accordance with Fed. Std. No. 297.

6.19 *Markings, Data Plates, Warranty Notice, Etc.*—Unless otherwise specified (See 9.2.48), final stage manufacturer's caution plates and identification plates shall be conspicuously installed for all equipment, etc., furnished requiring such notices. Other than the manufacturer's trademark(s) names, no identification other than that authoritatively specified shall be shown on exterior of the vehicle. The ambulance/vehicle manufacturer's "Star of Life" certification shall be provided on a placard or label as shown in Fig. 11 below, permanently affixed and easily visible in the ambulance oxygen compartment (See 7.3). All ambulances shall display a decal or sticker providing at least the following information: contract number, purchaser order number, date of delivery, month and year, and the warranty time, in months and miles (GSA Form 1398 or equal). Apply these data to the right or left front door lock face or door jam after final inspection and acceptance by the purchaser. As specified (See 9.2.48) by the procuring activity for the appropriate military service, identification markings and data plates, shall be provided conforming with MIL-STD-1223.

6.20 *Manuals, and Handbook of Instruction*—The supplier shall furnish with each ambulance, at the time of ambulance's acceptance, one copy of the reference as specified in 9.8 and herein. This reference handbook shall provide instructions for the operation, care, and repair for all ambulance related accessory, component equipment, and system(s) furnished as part of the emergency medical care vehicle. This handbook shall also contain all installation instructions, drawings, schematics wiring diagrams, illustrations, and safety precautions to insure proper management, operation and maintenance. The chassis manufacturer's repair manual and parts book shall be furnished when specified (See 9.2.49).

STAR OF LIFE CERTIFICATION LABEL

MFG BY____________________ DATE OF MANUFACTURE MO, YR________

ADDRESS____________________________

CITY__________________ STATE______ ZIP______

This Ambulance conforms to ASTM Standard _______ in effect on the date of manufacture shown above.

AMBULANCE IDENTIFICATION NUMBER____________________________

TYPE - CLASS - FLOOR PLAN - SERIAL NO.

CURB WEIGHT	PAYLOAD MAX	GROSS WT. MAX
________	________	________
kg/lbs	kg/lbs	kg.lbs

CERTIFIED "STAR OF LIFE" AMBULANCE.

SAMPLE LABEL

FIG. 11 "Star of Life" Certification Label

6.21 *Predelivery Inspection and Servicing*—The supplier prior to acceptance and inspection of the ambulance(s) shall service and inspect each vehicle in accordance with the chassis manufacturer's approved predelivery form, and the ambulance manufacturer's predelivery (test, inspection, and road test) form. A signed copy of these forms (check sheets) shall be furnished with the vehicle (See 9.8). Servicing shall comply to ambient temperatures and conditions applicable with the route of transport to the consignee's ultimate destination (See 8.1). Servicing shall include all tank(s) full of fuel; checking to determine satisfactory and complete operation of all mechanical and electrical features, equipment and system; elimination of rattles, noises, and squeaks; cleaning the interior and exterior. Thus the vehicle shall be delivered ready to use.

6.22 *Special Requirements*—Purchaser shall specify (See 9.2.50) additional requirements and state unusual operating conditions, miscellaneous items, permissible exceptions, marking, etc., not specified herein. If in conflict with the manufacturer's standards and options, those specified shall take precedence. Contractor shall comply to the requirements of 9.3.

6.22.1 *Overseas Vehicle Requirements*—When specified (See 9.2.51), the following equipment changes, items, devices, and adjustments to systems shall be furnished:

6.22.1.1 Left dip headlights (as used on right-hand drive vehicles) adjusted for driving on the left side of the road (prior to shipment).

6.22.1.2 Speedometer-odometer, calibrated in kilometers.

6.22.2 *Export Vehicle Safety, Emissions, and Fuel*—Unless otherwise specified (See 9.2.51), export vehicle(s) shall conform to applicable safety standards of U.S.A. Vehicles exported to countries marketing only leaded gasoline fuel shall be capable of accepting (refueling nozzles), and operating on leaded gasoline. Vehicle modifications needed for leaded fuel operation shall be made prior to shipment. Vehicle(s) being offered/supplied with catalytic converters shall be identified in each bid.

6.22.3 *Tiedown Points*— When specified (See 9.2.51), hard points (tow hooks, bumpers, axles, or other component points) suitable for use as tiedown points for the vehicle shall be identified. Identification of the points shall be provided by stenciling instructions and applying data plates to the vehicle or by, supplementary instructions included with each copy of the owner's-operator's manual. Each identified tiedown or hard point shall be capable of withstanding its proportionate share of the GVWR.

6.22.3.1 *Lift Points*— When specified (See 9.2.51), a minimum of four hard points for use as lift-points shall be identified. Identification of the points shall be provided by stenciling instructions and applying data plates to the vehicle or by supplementary instructions included with each copy of the owner's-operator's manual. Each identified hard point shall withstand without permanent deformation a working load equal to its proportionate share of the GVW and shall have an ultimate strength of at least 1.5 times the GVW. In addition, slinging provisions shall be located so that:

6.22.3.1.1 Attached sling legs shall converge over the center of gravity of the vehicle when at its GVW.

6.22.3.1.2 The attached sling apex does not exceed a height of 7.3 m (24 ft) above the lowest extremity of the equipment when suspended with each sling leg at a 45° maximum true angle.

6.23 *Workmanship*— Defective components shall not be furnished. Parts, equipment, and assemblies, which have been repaired or modified to overcome deficiencies shall not be furnished without the approval of the purchaser. Welded, bolted, and riveted construction utilized shall be in accordance with the highest standards of industry. Component parts and units shall be manufactured to definite standard dimensions with proper fits, clearances, and uniformity. General appearance of the vehicle shall not show any evidence of poor workmanship.

The following shall be reason for rejection:

6.23.1 Rough, sharp or unfinished edges, burrs, seams, sharp corners, joints, cracks, and dents.

6.23.2 Non-uniform panels. Edges that are not radiused, beveled, etc.

6.23.3 Paint runs, sags, orange peel, "fish eyes", etc., in addition to 6.16.2 and any other imperfection or lack of complete coverage.

6.23.4 Body panels that are uneven, unsealed, or have voids.

6.23.5 Misalignment of body fasteners, glass, viewing panels, light housings, other items with large or uneven gaps, spacing etc. such us door, body panels, and hinged panels.

6.23.6 Improper body design or interface with the chassis that could cause injury during normal use or maintenance.

6.23.7 Improperly fabricated and routed wiring or harnesses.

6.23.8 Improperly supported or secured hoses, wires, wiring harnesses, mechanical controls.

6.23.9 Loose, vibrating, abrading body parts, components, subassemblies, hoses, wiring harnesses, or trim.

6.23.10 Interference of chassis components, body parts, doors, etc.

6.23.11 Leaks of any gas or fluid lines, (AC, coolant, oil, oxygen, etc.)

6.23.12 Noise, panel vibrations, etc.

6.23.13 Sagging, non-form fitting upholstery or padding.

6.23.14 Incomplete or incorrect application of rustproofing.

6.23.15 Inappropriate or incorrect use of hardware, fasteners, components, or methods of construction.

6.23.16 Incomplete or improper welding, riveting.

6.23.17 Visual deformities.

6.23.18 Lack of uniformity and symmetry where applicable.

6.23.19 Unsealed appurtenances or other body components, gaskets, etc.

In addition, any deviation from specification requirements or any other item stipulated herein, that affects form, fit, function, durability, reliability, safety, performance or appearance shall be cause for rejection.

7. Quality Assurance Provisions

7.1 *Responsibility for Inspection and Tests*—The contractor is responsible for the performance of all inspections and test requirements specified herein. The supplier may use his own or any other facilities suitable for the predelivery and acceptance inspections unless disapproved by the purchaser. The purchaser reserves the right to perform any of the inspections and tests set forth in the specification where such actions are deemed necessary to assure supplies and service conform to the specification and contract. The contractor shall provide the purchaser's inspection representatives with the manufacturer's readily available instruments and all such assistance as they may find necessary.

7.1.1 *Purchaser Verification*—Quality assurance operations performed by the supplier will be subject to purchaser verification at unscheduled intervals. Verification will consist of observation of the operations to determine that practices, methods, and procedures of the supplier's inspection are being properly applied. Failure of the supplier to promptly correct observed deficiencies shall be cause for suspension of acceptance of the ambulance(s) until conformance to specification criteria has been demonstrated.

7.2 *Classification of Inspection (For Purchaser's Acceptance)*—Purchasers should select either or both of the following methods of inspections: Source Inspection and Destination Inspection, or both. (To specify see 9.2.51.)

7.2.1 *Source Inspection*—Ambulance(s) shall be inspected upon completion by the purchaser prior to shipment from manufacturer's factory, or assembly plant and may consist of the following:

7.2.1.1 Workmanship inspection (See 6.23).

7.2.1.2 Quality conformance inspection (See 7.2.3).

7.2.1.3 First production ambulance inspection (See 7.2.5).

7.2.2 *Destination Examination*—When specified (See 9.2.51), the contracted ambulance shall be examined at the destination. The vehicle(s) shall be visually examined to determine compliance to the contract requirements and the quality conformance inspection of 7.2.3. Vehicle component chassis failures and other minor defects may be accepted subject to correction by the contractor/manufacturer of those points.

7.2.3 *Quality Conformance Inspection*—Quality conformance inspection applies to all ambulance(s) offered for acceptance under the contract. Quality conformance inspection shall be as follows:

7.2.3.1 Workmanship inspection (See 6.23).

7.2.3.2 Operational checks (See 7.2.4).

7.2.3.3 Water spray test (See 7.4.5).

7.2.3.4 Examine ambulance handbook (See 6.20).

7.2.4 *Operation Checks*— Operational checks of the ambulance shall cover all controls, electrical systems, and devices, doors, windows, cabinets, accessories, in and outside the ambulance. Ambulance shall be driven at highway speeds, turns made at minimum radii, brakes tested for dependability, checked for rattles and squeaks, and compliance to 6.21. All controls and mechanisms shall function and operate as intended.

7.2.5 *First Production Ambulance Inspection*—When specified (See 9.2.53), the first production ambulance of each Type and Class specified under contract shall be inspected. This first ambulance shall be completely representative of the balance of the vehicles to be delivered under the contract. The purpose of the inspection shall determine vehicle conformity to the contract. The ambulance shall be inspected by the contractor at his plant under the direction of and in the presence of the purchasers' representative(s). Inspections shall be conducted during normal weekday working hours. The cost of inspections, examination, all tests, and vehicle support exclusive of personal expenses incurred by participating purchaser's representatives, shall be borne by the contractor. Acceptance of the first production vehicle shall not constitute a waiver by the purchaser of any rights under the provisions of the contract.

7.2.6 *Inspection Failure of Ambulance(s)*—Failure of a production ambulance to have the certifications required or successfully complete the examinations and tests shall be cause for non-acceptance of any of the contract quantity until deficiencies and evidence of the corrective action preclude recurrence of similar deficiencies. Failure of the vehicle to successfully complete inspection shall not constitute an excusable delay in meeting scheduled deliveries.

7.2.7 *Production Sample*—The first production ambulance, once it has been accepted by the purchaser, shall remain at the manufacturing facility as a production sample and shall be the last vehicle shipped on the contract. The contractor shall maintain the vehicle in a serviceable condition for the duration of the contract. Vehicle shall be then cleaned, serviced, and refurbished to the extent required for delivery of a new vehicle to the purchaser.

7.3 *"Star of Life" Certification Requirements:*

7.3.1 *Qualifying Provisions*—The manufacturer/supplier is obligated to certify, to the purchasers that the ambulance bearing the "Star of Life," its components, and equipment meet or exceed all the requirements and tests set forth in this specification. The certification and "Star of Life" label (See 6.19), verify that the ambulance conforms to this standard on the date of manufacture. Compliance for a "Star of Life" label is defined as certification backed by confirmed verifications of inspections and tests. The verifications shall be in possession of the issuer and presented if and when challenged. For the benefit of purchaser's procuring activity evaluation and review, prior to or with each proposed bid (solicitation), the bidder/supplier shall provide and forward representative material of their "Star of Life" ambulance(s). This material shall include: a letter certified by a company officer, stating that the delivered ambulance(s) shall comply with 7.3.2-7.3.5. Failure to provide certification, at the time the vehicle is presented for inspection, will deem the vehicle unacceptable and shall constitute grounds for termination in accordance with the terms of the contract. Also included shall be: general specification data. exterior and interior pictures, dimensional drawings/data, etc., and other information as requested.

7.3.2 *Documentation of "Star of Life" Certification*—The ambulance manufacturer shall compile complete certified documentation of verifications for all the tests required under 7.4 conforming to 7.3.3 and 7.3.5 in a booklet similar to that described in 9.8, for each Type and Class ambulance intended to be marketed to the Emergency Medical Care industry, as a "Star of Life" ambulance.

7.3.3 *Criteria of Certifications*—The testing and inspection(s) required for certification shall be performed by either an independent testing facility or the ambulance manufacturer's own testing facility. In-plant tests shall be supervised by a staff registered professional engineer, or consulting registered professional engineer. The individual certifications will remain valid so long as they are applicable to the vehicle model, component(s) and equipment offered as tested under this specification, and are furnished without alterations for five years; the ambulance shall then be recertified. Certifications that appear on the vehicle need not be re-submitted (i.e., Department of Transportation, (DOT); Environmental Protection Agency, (EPA), etc.). Certification(s) will be acceptable in lieu of actual verification test during inspections (See 7.2) providing supporting verifying data complying to 7.3.5 is on file for examination. Certifications from the chassis manufacturer and individual equipment manufacturers are acceptable providing the equipment in not part of a system or altered and in accordance with 7.3.4. Type certifications of individual components and equipment products are acceptable.

7.3.4 *Certification Letter Format*—Certification letters submitted for the ambulance model, components, and equipment being certified shall contain the following information on supplier's letterhead stationery: to whom certifying, date, units or items, manufacturer and address, date product tested, model number, and specification data, applicable specification references and test requirement, summary of the test report, a certifying statement, and official signature.

7.3.5 *Certification Verification Data Reports*—The testing facility (See 7.3.3) for each certification shall supply supportive verification data and information on letterhead stationary, for whom tested, report date, name of sample product or device, manufacturer's address, serial and model number(s), specification referral and amendment number(s), test requirement(s), test facilities used and location, test equipment used, test procedure, test results, verifying test data, photographs, test conclusion(s), witness(es), and authorized signature.

7.4 *Tests:*

7.4.1 *Test Criteria*— The ambulance shall be prepared for operation in accordance with chassis manufacturer's recommendations and 6.21. The ambulance shall be manned and loaded when applicable, to simulate the maximum payload required for the Type, Class, and plan being tested. Road tests and test course(s) shall be documented with pictures and route map. Test room(s) designed and equipped to simulate ambient temperature environments shall be used to perform tests.

7.4.2 *Performance Tests*—The following ambulance items, systems, and equipment shall be inspected, tested, and verified for conformance to the specification:

7.4.2.1 Ambulance physical dimensions (See 6.4.11-6.4.11.6 and 6.10-6.11.4).

7.4.2.2 Vehicle weight distribution (See 7.4.3 and 7.4.3.1).

7.4.2.3 Road test and performance tests (See 7.4.4).

7.4.2.4 Exterior mounted devices tested for temperature conditions (See 6.4.2).

7.4.2.5 Cooling system (See 6.6.4.5).

7.4.2.6 Electrical systems and components (See 6.7-6.8.5.2).

7.4.2.7 Electrical generating system (See 6.7.6-6.7.6.3).

7.4.2.8 Electromagnetic radiation and suppression (See 6.7.12), type approval acceptable.

7.4.2.9 Warning light and siren system(s) (See 6.8.2-6.8.2.3, and 6.14.6).

7.4.2.10 Ambulance body structure (See 6.10.5 and 6.10.9).

7.4.2.11 Patient compartment interior surfaces, FMVSS 302 (See 6.10.17).

7.4.2.12 Oxygen system (See 6.11.3, 6.12.1, 6.12.1.1).

7.4.2.13 Litter fastener and anchorage (See 6.11.7).

7.4.2.14 Suction aspiration system (See 6.12.3 and 6.12.4).

7.4.2.15 Environmental systems (See 6.13.1-6.13.7, and 6.6.3.2).

7.4.2.16 Patient compartment sound level (See 6.13.8).

7.4.2.17 Painting, color, and marking (See 6.16-6.16.4).

7.4.2.18 Manuals and handbook (See 6.20 and 9.8).

7.4.3 *Vehicle Weights*— The vehicle shall be weighed to determine curb weight and distribution of curb weight on front and rear axle. The imposed loading on front and rear axle will be computed using the curb weight and the payload as specified in 6.5-6.5.6. Calculated imposed loads on front and rear axle will be utilized to ascertain that suspension, axles, and tires furnished are of adequate capacity to meet contract requirements.

7.4.3.1 *Weight Distribution Tolerance*—The mathematical method to calculate the weight distribution shall be in accordance with AMD Standard 013 (Weight Distribution Test).

7.4.4 *Road Test*—The vehicle shall be subjected to a minimum 241 km (150 mile) road test of which 121 km (75 miles) shall be continuous miles on paved highways at highway speeds up to 113 km/hr (70 mph); 48 km (30 miles) on city streets; 24 km (15 miles) on gravel or dirt roads at speeds up to at least 56 km/hr (35 mph); and not less than 8 km (5 miles) in simulated or actual cross-country operation at speeds applicable to the terrain. Cross-country operation is defined as travel over open fields, rolling and side-sloping hills, rough and muddy terrain. Class 2 vehicles shall demonstrate cross-country operation in 4-wheel drive for an additional 32 km (20 miles). Ambulances shall meet performance requirements specified in 6.4.4-6.4.10 during road tests or by certification. Balance of the 241 km (150 miles) road test may be accumulated during other tests and checks requiring vehicle movements. After completion of the road test, vehicle shall be subjected to the water spray test (See 7.4.5). Road test may be performed at any ambient temperature.

7.4.4.1 *Test Failure of First Ambulance*—Vehicle utilized for the road test shall successfully complete 241 km (150 miles) of test. Rejection of the test vehicle shall be for deficiencies, including but not limited to the following:

7.4.4.1.1 Damage caused by collision.

7.4.4.1.2 Failure of any major component.

7.4.4.1.3 Vibration due to misalignment of wheels, frame, driveshaft, or defective tires, etc.

7.4.4.1.4 Vibration due to type of body construction or mounting.

7.4.4.1.5 Evidence of abnormal tire wear due to misalignment or unbalanced wheels/tires.

7.4.4.1.6 Failure of any vehicular safety device such as brakes, steering assembly, windshield washers and wipers or electrical circuits.

7.4.4.1.7 Evidence of structural weakness in any part of the vehicle, vehicle components, or accessories.

7.4.4.1.8 Loose mountings of parts or accessories due to workmanship or vehicular operation.

7.4.4.1.9 Failure of any vehicular performance requirements.

7.4.5 *Water Spray Test*— The ambulance shall be subjected to a water spray test in accordance with AMD Standard 010 (Water Spray Test) for a minimum of 15 minutes. The spray shall be delivered by nozzles operating at 172 kPa (25 psi) water pressure, sufficient in number and placed approximately 91 cm (3 ft) from the body to afford full coverage of sides, roof, front, rear, and undercarriage of the vehicle. Ambulance undergoing quality conformance inspection (See 7.2.3) shall be subjected to water spray test for not less than 2 minutes duration. Evidence of water leakage shall be cause for rejection until leaks are corrected.

7.4.6 *Oxygen System Test*—The installed medical oxygen piping and outlet system (See 6.12.1) shall be leak tested at 1033 kPa (150 psi) pressure, for a time period of four hours. The system shall be tested in accordance with AMD Standard 015 (Ambulance Oxygen System Test) with dry air or nitrogen gas or equal and kept decontaminated. After the successful completion of tests, the system shall be capped then tagged with date and signature of person and firm performing the tests.

8. Preparation for Delivery

8.1 *Preparation*— Unless otherwise specified (See 9.2.54). the ambulance(s) shall be preserved and packaged for mobile delivery, in accordance with the supplier's standard commercial practice, insuring carrier acceptance and safe delivery to destination in compliance with regulations applicable to the mode of transportation.

9. Application of Standard

9.1 *Intended Use of Standard*—This specification may be used as described below to procure a certified "Star of Life" ambulance.

9.2 *Ordering Data*— Purchasers should prepare their procurement document(s) (specification, requisition, contract) in the following sequence. Select the preferred options and provide the necessary information requested:

9.2.1 Title, number, and date of this specification and amendment number, if any.

9.2.2 Quantity, Type (I, II or III), and Class (1 or 2) of the ambulance required (See 1.3) and chassis brand if desired. (See 6.1.2-6.1.4).

9.2.3 Patient compartment configuration A (ALS) or B (BLS). B (BLS is standard on all types). If ALS is required (on Types I & III), specify Configuration A (See 6.1.5).

NOTE 24—Type II vehicles may be ordered with some ALS features depending on manufacturer.

9.2.4 Special performance requirements and other chassis, or both, that may be needed for special use applications such as carrying additional rescue/extrication equipment or heavily equipped patient/neonatal transport ambulances (See 6.4.1).

9.2.5 *Fuel Range*—OEM manufacturers maximum fuel tanks shall be standard. Specify if reduced fuel capacity required (See 6.4.9 and 6.6.4.4).

9.2.6 *Length*—Standard length is 671 cm (22 ft.). Specify if additional length is required for specific applications (See 6.4.11.1).

9.2.7 *Width*—For modular units, wide bodies on wide track axles are standard. Specify if a narrower body on a dual or single rear wheel chassis is required (See 6.4.11.2).

9.2.8 *Height*—279 cm (110 in.) is the maximum standard height. Specify if other heights are required, for example,for air transportability. (See 6.4.11.3).

9.2.9 *Payload* Purchaser may specify additional payload if available from manufacturer for a specific model or a medium-duty chassis when available (See 6.5.2).

9.2.10 *Engine Power Unit (diesel is standard)*—Only if absolutely necessary should gasoline engine be specified (See 6.6.3-6.6.3.4).

9.2.11 *Air Pollution Controls*—Cite where ambulance will operate. State and county, and if for export, name country, or both.(See 6.6.4.3 and 6.22.2).

9.2.12 *Drivetrain and Transmission*—Automatic transmission is standard for all models. Specify if a manual transmission or other drivetrain options are required, other than that specified. Check manufacturer's data (See 6.6.5-6.6.5.9).

9.2.13 *Wheels*—Wide, dual rear wheels are standard equipment on all Type I and III units (See 6.6.7). Specify if narrow dual or single rear wheels are specifically desired.

NOTE 25—Ambulance body widths are established in 6.4.11.2. Specify if narrow, modular type bodies with single or dual rear wheels are required.

9.2.14 *Tires*—"All Season" steel belted radials are standard for all models. Mud and snow, or all purpose type tires may be desirable and specified on 4x4 vehicles. (See 6.6.8-6.6.12).

9.2.15 *Spare*—Purchaser may state specific location of spare/wheel, when furnished, or delete requirement for spare tire.

NOTE 26—Purchaser should consult with ambulance manufacturer since moving spare can affect weight distribution of the vehicle (See 6.6.10).

9.2.16 *Intermittent Wipers*—Specify if required (See 6.7.4).

9.2.17 *Electrical Generating System*—Suppliers are required to provide adequate generating capacity in ambulances as manufactured. If reserve generating capacity is desired for owner installed electrical devices beyond that already provided, specify minimum additional generating capacity required (See 6.7.6).

9.2.18 *Battery Location*—Specify other locations (See 6.7.7).

9.2.19 *12 V DC Power*—Specify if other than standard 12 V DC outlets or higher current level required to power medical equipment, portable radio chargers, etc. (See 6.7.7.3).

9.2.20 *Patient Compartment Controls*—Specify if other than standard EMT panel/controls, instruments, etc. are required (See 6.7.10).

9.2.21 Electromagnetic Radiation Type Certification by equipment and ambulance manufacturers is standard. Specify if entire vehicle shall be tested. (See 6.7.12).

9.2.22 *Warning Lights*—Red, clear, and amber lights are standard. Specify other color(s) only if required by State or local regulations. If a standard vehicle warning light system is desired, specify whether strobe or quartz halogen. If an alternative emergency warning light system is desired, specify additional parameters, brand, model numbers and equal and details, or a combination thereof. Specify if other automatic switching arrangements are required (See 6.8-6.8.2.5). Specify if automatic primary to secondary mode and automatic day/night switching arrangements are required. Standard system includes manual "Primary" and "Secondary" mode switch and, on strobe systems, a day/night dimming switch (See 6.8.2.3).

NOTE 27—Additional warning lights are not necessary and should not be specified in order to avoid overloading the electrical system, and reducing usable payload.

9.2.23 *Flood Lights*—Specify if two flood lights per side and rear are required. (See 6.8.3).

9.2.24 *Seats*—Specify if bench type seat is desired or permitted on Type I vehicles. Specify if high back bucket type seats are required and specify if other than vinyl type upholstery is desired or acceptable (See 6.9.3).

9.2.25 *Mirrors*—Specify if other than standard mirrors are required, for example, West Coast, integral convex, heated mirrors, etc. (see 6.9.5).

9.2.26 *Bumpers and Steps*—On Class 2 vehicles, specify if other than standard step height is necessary for increased departure angles, for example, severe off road use, air transportability (See 6.9.6).

9.2.27 *Fenders*—Required per specification. Specify type (See 6.9.7.1).

9.2.28 *EMT Seating*—Specify other than standard requirements. Specify if integral EMT/child safety seat is required (See 6.10.3).

9.2.29 *Patient Compartment Length*—310 cm (122 in.) is minimum required. Specify additional requirements (See 6.10.4).

NOTE 28—Lengths less than 310 cm (122 in.) could result in rear door interference with traction splints on tall patients.

9.2.30 *Patient Compartment Height*—Minimum height of 152 cm (60 in.) required, specify additional requirements (See 6.10.4).

9.2.31 *Body Construction*—Aluminum is standard for modular ambulances. Specify if other materials are required or permitted (See 6.10.5 and 6.10.6).

9.2.32 Dual hinged doors are standard on Type II. Specify if sliding door is required (See 6.10.8). Specify if other door opening widths/configurations are required for specific applications.

9.2.33 *Windows*—Specify if other than standard, tinted, or when opening windows are required or permitted (See 6.10.14).

9.2.34 Walkthru on Type II & III is standard. Specify if walkthru deletion is required (See 6.10.15-6.10.15.2). When walkthru is deleted, a pass thru window shall be furnished and additional compartments above and below the window can be furnished as specified by the purchaser.

9.2.35 *Interior and Exterior Storage Accommodations*—Specify any specific additional requirements (See 6.11.1-6.11.4).

9.2.36 *Stretchers, Cots, and Litters*— Specify specific cot fastening device, item(s) required, and any upgrading features preferred (See 6.11.5-6.11.7, and Table 10, Items 10, 16, and 21). Cots are optional and not standard with vehicle. Cot fastener is standard. Specify specific model.

9.2.37 *Oxygen System (on board)*—Specify if other than "M" size cylinder and other than manufacturer's standard location (See 6.12.1).

9.2.38 *Oxygen*—Quick disconnect fitting for action wall and specified accessories. Specify type (See 6.12.1)

9.2.39 *Portable Oxygen Unit*—Specify location of portable oxygen unit and spare cylinder if other than location in 6.12.2.

9.2.40 *Suction Aspirator System*—Electrically powered type, is standard. (See 6.12.3 and 6.12.4).

9.2.41 *Air Conditioning, Auxiliary Condenser*—Specify if auxiliary condenser is required (See 6.13.5.1).

9.2.42 *Patient Compartment Sound Level Criteria*—Specify if more stringent patient compartment sound level limits are required (See 6.13.8).

9.2.43 *Communication Equipment*—Two-way radio, telemetry, modulator (local purchase of radio equipment and installations is recommended). Specify if contractor is to furnish and install the radio(s), and cite brand(s) acceptable, power output, frequencies needed, etc. Be aware of bid requirements if equipment brands are specified. Also be aware of pre-installation requirements to obtain FCC radio license and to coordinate such licensing through the local FCC designated radio frequency coordinator. Give complete details and provide the FCC designated radio frequency coordinator's name, address, and telephone number (See 6.14-6.14.4). One antenna lead is standard. Specify additional antenna leads and locations. Specify that the radio remote control head be so installed as to not interfere with airbag or other safety equipment installation, be convenient for operation by the driver, and be equipped with indicators and controls that are easy to view and operate.

9.2.44 *Siren*—Specify if foot switch or other siren upgrading features are required (See 6.14.6).

9.2.45 *Additional Systems, Equipment, Accessories, and Supplies*—(See 6.15-6.15.4). Cite additional parameters, brand, model numbers, and equal, and details, or both. User should be aware that additional equipment reduces usable payload capacity and if electrically operated reduces spare or reserve capacity that may be available and requires additional generating capacity (See 6.15.1).

9.2.45.1 Specify if automatically adjustable backup alarm is required. (Fixed sound level is standard) (See 6.15.2.4.)

9.2.45.2 Select optional vehicle equipment desired (See 6.15.3).

9.2.45.3 Select optional medical equipment desired (See 6.15.4).

9.2.46 *Paint*—White-Orange is standard. Only if absolutely necessary, specify other requirements. Reflective tape may be specified for the orange band (See 6.16.2).

9.2.47 *Rustproofing*—If required. Undercoating is standard. (See 6.18).

9.2.48 *Markings, Data Plates, and Warranty Notices*—Specify if additional or military markings are required (See 6.19).

9.2.49 *Manuals and Handbooks*—State if chassis manufacturer's complete repair manual and parts book(s), or both, are required (See 6.20).

9.2.50 *Special Requirements*—State any other additions and permitted changes or deletions in the specification (See 6.22).

9.2.51 *Overseas Vehicle Requirements*— Select requirements (See 6.6.3.4 and 6.22.1-6.22.3.1), include tiedown points, liftpoint requirements, additional safety requirements and fuel requirements for the consignees location.

9.2.52 *Quality Assurance Provisions*—Specify classification of inspection desired (See 7-7.2.7).

9.2.52.1 *Source inspection*—(See 7.2.1).

9.2.52.2 *Destination Examination*—(See 7.2.2).

9.2.53 *First Production Ambulance Inspection*—State if required. If quantity contract see 7.2.5.

9.2.54 *Preparation for Delivery*—Specify if different (See 8.1). State mode of delivery preferred.

9.2.55 *Procurement Requirements*—(See 9.3). Specify other purchaser's contractual requirements.

9.2.56 *Foreign Use*—State any additional or different warranty, requirements for foreign use applications (See 9.4.3).

9.2.57 *Statement of Origin*—Specify if other ownership documents are required and locations to which they shall be forwarded.

9.2.58 *Light Emitting Diodes (LED); Stop, Tail, Directional, and Marker Lights*—(See 6.8.1). Specify LED lighting for reduced current draw and lifetime durability

9.3 *Procurement Requirements*—Unless otherwise specified (See 9.2.55) in the invitation for bids, contract, or orders, the following are contractual requirements (See 9.4-9.6), except in those instances where it is determined by the purchaser that inclusion thereof would not be to the best interests of the Government or purchaser.

9.4 *Warranty:*

9.4.1 *Warranty Coverage*—The contractor shall warrant the vehicle and furnished equipment against parts failure or malfunction due to design, construction, or installation errors, defective workmanship, and missing or incorrect parts (See 9.4.4 for warranty exceptions) for a minimum period of 12 months, and 15 months for vehicles outside the contiguous (48) United States and District of Columbia from date of acceptance,(The warranty begins when the purchaser accepts the vehicle from the contractor FOB point of origin/destination. (See 6.19)) or 12,000 miles of operation, exclusive of any authorized accumulated driveway mileage, whichever occurs first. However, if the contractor received from any supplier or subcontractor additional warranty on the whole or any component of the vehicle, in the form of time and mileage, or both, including any prorata arrangements, or the contractor generally extends to his commercial customers a greater or extended warranty, coverage, the Government/purchaser shall receive corresponding warranty benefits.

9.4.2 *Domestic Use*— When vehicles are used within the 50 States of the United States, the District of Columbia, Puerto Rico, and the Virgin Islands, the warranty shall include the furnishing, without cost to the purchaser (FOB contractor's nearest dealer or branch to vehicle's location or station) new parts and assemblies to replace any that failed or malfunctioned within the warranty period. In addition, when the purchaser elects to have the work performed at the contractor's plant, branch, dealer, or with the contractor's approval, (1) to correct the defect itself or (2) to have it corrected by a commercial facility, the cost of the labor involved in the replacement of the failed or malfunctioned parts or assemblies shall be borne by the contractor

9.4.3 *Foreign Use*— Unless otherwise specified (See 9.2.56), when vehicles are used outside the 50 States, the District of Columbia, Puerto Rico, and the Virgin Islands, the warranty shall include the furnishing of new parts or assemblies to replace any returned to the contractor which failed or malfunctioned within the warranty period. The replacement parts or assemblies shall be delivered by the contractor to the port of embarkation in the United States designated by the purchaser. The contractor shall not be required to bear the cost of the labor involved in correcting defects in vehicles operated in foreign countries.

9.4.4 *Warranty Exclusions*—Unless within the additional coverage under 9.4.1, the following items are considered normal maintenance and repair for which the contractor need not assume liability for reimbursing the Government/purchaser regardless of the vehicle age or mileage:

9.4.4.1 Abuse, negligence, or an approved alteration of original parts;

9.4.4.2 Damage from accidents;

9.4.4.3 Standard brake and clutch adjustments;

9.4.4.4 General tightening, headlamp adjustments;

9.4.4.5 Wheel alignment or tire balancing;

9.4.4.6 Tires, batteries, medical supplies and equipment, and radio(s) (if warranted by their manufacturers);

9.4.4.7 Miscellaneous expense such as fuel, towing, telephone, travel, lodging, or loss of personal property.

9.4.5 *Warranty Extension*—In addition to the warranty provisions specified, the following shall also apply:

9.4.5.1 The ambulance chassis, chassis components (powertrain, etc.) and applicable body and cab shall be warranted and implemented in accordance with the original chassis manufacturer's standard warranty.

9.4.5.2 For vehicle(s) located within a country which has branch, dealer, or approved contractor service facilities, the cost of labor, parts, and materials involved in correcting warranted defects shall be borne by the contractor (See 9.4.3).

9.4.5.3 If action to effect repairs under warranty (except for chassis as specified in 9.4.5.1) is not initiated within seven (7) working days by a dealer or supplier and completed within a reasonable length of time, or if the contractor does not have regular facilities in the city or county in which the vehicle operates, and in the event of emergency, or dire need for the vehicle, the purchaser reserves the right to make such repair, and be reimbursed the contractor as follows:

If work is performed at a purchaser facility, the per hour rate for labor based on the manufacturer's flat rate time schedule, and full cost of expenditures for parts and material; or actual labor time and materials, for repairs of nonscheduled operations, or when warranty services are performed at a commercial facility because no contractor facility is available, the new cost of the correction will be billed to the contractor.

9.5 *Repair Parts and Service*—As a continuous operation of the vehicle described by this specification is of utmost importance for the successful bidder to be in a position to render prompt service and to furnish replacement parts.

Accordingly, bidders shall indicate the extent of their ability to render prompt service by furnishing a list of branch offices or agencies where complete stocks of repair parts are maintained and can be secured within a reasonable time after ordering by part number from the manufacturer's part book and at such discount as may be quoted from year to year by the manufacturer of the vehicle purchased under this specification.

9.6 *Statement of Origin or Bill of Sale*—A manufacturer's Statement of Origin or Bill of Sale showing the applicable purchase order number is required for each vehicle procured under this specification. Unless otherwise specified (See 9.2.57), such documents shall be forwarded to the consignee.

9.7 *Oxygen Tanks*— Following are the approximate dimensions, weights, and capacities of the various size oxygen cylinders referenced in this specification:

TABLE 12 Oxygen Tank Dimensions, Weights and Capacities

Oxygen Cylinders	D	M	H
Outside diameter (cm/inch)	11/4.5	18/7	23/9
Outside heights, without valve (cm/inch)	51/20	119/47	142/56
Capacity (gallons)	95	800	1825
Capacity (liters)	360	3,000	6,900
Capacity, flow @ 10 liters/minute (minutes)	30	325	700
Capacity (cubic feet)	13	106	244
Weight, empty (kg/lbs)	5.9/13	34/75	54/119
Weight, full (kg/lbs)	6.3/14	37.6/83	61.3/135

9.8 *Reference Handbook*—The handbook and all the material referenced in this specification (See 6.20) for the model ambulance furnished shall be provided in an 21.6 x 28 cm (8½ x 11 in.), 3-ring. hard cover, loose-leaf binder, inscribed with the complete address and telephone number of the manufacturer and shall contain the following:

9.8.1 Table of contents.

9.8.2 Copy of supplier's invoice/date of delivery, including chassis.

9.8.3 Manufacturer's "Star of Life" certification of compliance statement.

9.8.4 Ambulance manufacturer's illustrative, pictorial literature and a copy of predelivery inspection/test form signed by inspector.

9.8.5 Complete copy of this Standard and all amendments including purchaser's specifications and modifications in effect for date of manufacture.

9.8.6 Conditions of sale and contract (unless otherwise specified).

9.8.7 Shipping papers.

9.8.8 List of ambulance manufacturers service points (See 9.5).

9.8.9 Copy of chassis manufacturer's warranty and owner manual.

9.8.10 Final stage manufacturer's components and equipment information (hardware, fixture, etc.) including supplier's part numbers.

9.8.11 Complete wiring diagrams and schematics (See 6.7.2).

9.8.12 Manufacturer's operating and servicing instructions for the entire ambulance, electrical system(s) of the ambulance, components, devices, and equipment aboard, etc., including each equipment manufacturer's data.

All contents of the handbook that cannot be punched with three holes shall be secured in plastic leaves.

Designation: F 2024 – 00

Standard Practice for X-ray Diffraction Determination of Phase Content of Plasma-Sprayed Hydroxyapatite Coatings[1]

This standard is issued under the fixed designation F 2024; the number immediately following the designation indicates the year of original adoption or, in the case of revision, the year of last revision. A number in parentheses indicates the year of last reapproval. A superscript epsilon (ε) indicates an editorial change since the last revision or reapproval.

1. Scope

1.1 This practice is for the determination, by the Reference Intensity Ratio External Standard Method, of the percent by weight of the crystalline phases, hydroxyapatite (HA), beta-(whitlockite) tricalcium phosphate (β-TCP), and calcium oxide (CaO) in coatings deposited upon metallic substrates by plasma-spraying hydroxyapatite.

1.2 A major component in plasma-sprayed HA coatings other than HA is expected to be amorphous calcium phosphate (ACP). Crystalline components other than HA that may be present include alpha- and beta- (whitlockite) tricalcium phosphates, tetracalcium phosphate (TTCP), calcium oxide, and calcium pyrophosphates. Quantification of the minor crystalline components has proven to be very unreliable due to extreme overlap and confounding of X-ray diffraction peaks. Therefore, this practice addresses the quantification of only HA, β-TCP, and CaO.

1.3 This practice was developed for plasma-sprayed HA coatings with HA contents of at least 50 % of the total coating. It is recognized that the analysis of the crystalline components uses diffraction from regions of the pattern that also includes a small contribution from the amorphous component. However, within the limits of applicability of this practice, the effect of such interference is believed to be negligible.

1.4 The coating analyzed shall be produced and processed under equivalent manufacturing conditions to that on the device of interest.

1.5 This practice requires the use of monochromated copper Kα radiation and flat samples.

1.6 *This standard does not purport to address all of the safety concerns, if any, associated with its use. It is the responsibility of the user of this standard to establish appropriate safety and health practices and determine the applicability of regulatory limitations prior to use.*

2. Referenced Documents

2.1 *ASTM Standards:*

F 1185 Specification for Composition of Ceramic Hydroxylapatite for Surgical Implants[2]

F 1609 Specification for Calcium Phosphate Coatings for Implantable Materials[2]

3. Terminology

3.1 *Definitions*:

3.1.1 *crystalline phases*:

Chemical and Mineral Names	Formula	PDF Card No.[3]
whitlockite beta-tricalcium phosphate	β-$Ca_3(PO_4)_2$	9-169
calcium phosphate alpha-tricalcium phosphate	α-$Ca_3(PO_4)_2$	9-348
lime calcium oxide	CaO	37-1497
hydroxyapatite (hydroxylapatite)	$Ca_5(PO_4)_3OH$	9-432

3.2 *plasma-sprayed hydroxyapatite coating*—a coating, consisting of at least 50 % hydroxyapatite by weight, prepared by plasma-spraying hydroxyapatite on a substrate.

4. Significance and Use

4.1 Calcium phosphate coatings have been shown in animal and clinical studies to be biocompatible and to enhance the early attachment of bone to implant surfaces (see Refs. **1-5**)[4]

4.2 It is believed that the form of calcium phosphate ceramic and its purity with respect to secondary crystalline phases and amorphous material have an effect on its physical, mechanical, and biological properties. However, no definitive studies of effects on biological properties have been completed. To achieve reproducible clinical results and to permit the determination of the effects of properties of the coating on biological performance, it is essential that the properties of both clinical and experimental materials be well-characterized and consistent.

4.3 This practice provides procedures for determination of the percentage by weight of the crystalline phases identified as

[1] This practice is under the jurisdiction of ASTM Committee F-4 on Medical and Surgical Materials and Devices and is the direct responsibility of Subcommittee F04.13 on Ceramic Materials.

Current edition approved May 10, 2000. Published Aug. 2000.

[2] *Annual Book of ASTM Standards*, Vol 13.01.

[3] Joint Committee on Powder Diffraction Standards, Swarthmore, PA.

[4] The boldface numbers in parentheses refer to the list of references at the end of this standard.

hydroxyapatite, β-TCP and CaO in plasma-sprayed hydroxyapatite coatings.

5. Quantitative Phase Analysis by the External Standard Technique

5.1 The external standard technique allows the determination of weight fractions of individual phases in a mixture containing an amorphous fraction by comparison of the integrated intensity of one or more peaks from the phase(s) of interest to the external standard under identical instrumental conditions **(6)**. The sample analyzed may be a solid such as a plasma-sprayed coating or may be a powder. The mass absorption coefficients of the sample and standard must be known.

5.2 The weight fraction of the analyte phase in the mixture is given by Equation 11 of Ref **(6)**, as follows:

$$W_i = \left(\frac{I_i^{hkl}}{I_i^{REL}}\right) \cdot \left(\frac{\chi_m}{\chi_s}\right) \cdot \left(\frac{1}{I_s^{Pure} \cdot RIR_i}\right) \quad (1)$$

where:

I_i^{hkl} = integrated intensity of the analyte phase (hkl) peak or sum of peaks,

I_i^{REL} = relative intensity of the analyte phase (hkl) peak or sum of peaks,

χ_m = mass absorption coefficient of the mixture,

χ_s = mass absorption coefficient of the standard,

I_s^{Pure} = integrated intensity of the most intense peak of the pure standard measured under identical conditions, and

RIR_i = reference intensity ratio of the analyte phase to the standard.

Values of the relative intensities, mass absorption coefficients, and reference intensity ratios which have been measured for HA, β-TCP, and CaO are given in Appendix X1.

6. Procedure

6.1 *Sample Preparation*:

6.1.1 Plasma sprayed coating samples in the form of flat coupons of nominal dimensions 2.5 by 2.5 by 0.6 cm (1 by 1 by 0.125 in.) may be analyzed directly on the coated surface. The coating must be at least 44 μm thick to provide a sample opaque to the X-ray beam. Thinner samples must be removed from the substrate and either deposited in a layer of at least 44-μm thickness and area sufficient to exceed the dimensions of the irradiated area.

6.1.2 Reliable quantitative analysis cannot be performed by X-ray diffraction on curved surfaces because of errors caused by absorption and defocusing.

6.1.3 Microabsorption caused by variations in either particle size or surface roughness will produce errors in the measured diffracted intensity. The effective particle size and variation in surface roughness of the alpha-corundum external standard must be less than 5 μm.

6.2 *X-ray Equipment*:

6.2.1 A standard Bragg-Brentano focusing diffractometer equipped with a pyrolytic graphite monochromator is recommended. Because of the need to resolve closely spaced and overlapping peaks, a diffracted beam monochromator is required unless a solid-state detector is used. Linearity of the instrument and associated electronics must be verified daily prior to utilizing this method. Use of NIST silicon powder standard, SRM 640 is suggested.[5]

6.2.2 An X-ray source with a copper target is required. Characteristic copper radiation provides the needed X-ray diffraction peak resolution and allows for separation of peaks from contaminant phases at a suitable range of diffraction angles from nominally 20 to 60° 2θ. A 1.0° incident beam divergence, a 0.2° receiving slit, and soller slits in either incident or diffracted beam, or both, are suitable.

6.3 *X-ray Method and Data Reduction Strategy*:

6.3.1 Collect a diffraction pattern from 20 to 60 ° 2θ at 0.02° increments for a minimum of 1s/point.

6.3.2 X-ray diffraction peaks (or peak groups) from the crystalline phases must be separated in order to quantify the HA content. The following outline provides a data reduction strategy in order to provide the integrated intensities necessary to determine the HA, β-TCP, and CaO content of mixtures of amorphous calcium phosphate, α-TCP, β-TCP, CaO, β-$Ca_2P_2O_7$, tetracalcium phosphate, and hydroxyapatite. Accomplish the determination of integrated intensities using computer techniques, with least-squares fitting of the selected peak shape to the experimental data. Manual fitting of peak and background is not permitted under this standard practice.

6.3.2.1 Obtain the β-TCP content by integration from 30.5 to 31.5° 2θ. The β-TCP peak being used for quantification is the (0 2 10) peak. This region is integrated by assuming a linear background and a Pearson VII functional form of the peaks surrounding the region.

6.3.2.2 Determine the calcium oxide content by integration from 37.0 to 38.5° 2θ and correct for the β-TCP (1 2 11) and (315) peaks. This region contains the 100 % (200) calcium oxide peak, and is integrated by assuming a linear form to the background.

6.3.2.3 Finally, determine by integration the region from 38.5 to 59.0° 2θ HA and correct for interference by β-TCP and calcium oxide. A large angular range is used in order to use as many peaks as possible and to reduce the effects of preferred orientation. Again, this region is integrated assuming a linear form of the background.

6.3.3 Perform the analysis as an external standard technique with reference to an alpha-corundum standard, using the relative intensities, mass absorption coefficients, and reference intensity ratios shown in Appendix X1. Reference intensity ratios determined experimentally using the equipment and conditions used for analysis of unknown samples may be substituted for those shown, provided that their validity under the experimental conditions used for analysis has been verified using known standards. An example calculation is shown as Appendix X2.

6.3.4 Verify the validity of the analytical procedures applied using known mixtures of powders ranging from nominally 50 to 95 % hydroxyapatite. Conduct periodic revalidation (at least annually) of instrument conditions and analytical technique using retained plasma-sprayed hydroxyapatite samples.

[5] National Institute of Standards and Technology, Gaithersburg, MD 20899.

7. Report

7.1 Report following information:

7.1.1 Sample identification,

7.1.2 Condition of analyzed sample, as-sprayed coating on coupon or powder spalled from sample,

7.1.3 Analytical results expressed as percent hydroxyapatite, percent β-TCP, and percent CaO relative to the entire sample,

7.1.4 Balance expressed as balance-amorphous calcium phosphate (ACP) and other minor phases, and

7.1.5 Statistical variability of the results based on the variability in the RIR values (shown in Table X1.1) and instrumental conditions.

7.2 Further reporting by the device manufacturer shall include any treatment applied to the coating after plasma-spraying.

8. Precision and Bias

8.1 The precision and bias of this practice are currently being determined in an interlaboratory test program. Individual experience indicates that reproducibility is on the order of ±3 % for determination of the HA content of plasma-sprayed coatings.

9. Keywords

9.1 amorphous calcium phosphate (ACP); hydroxyapatite coatings; hydroxyapatite (HAP); hydroxylapatite coatings; phase analysis; tricalcium phosphate; whitlockite

APPENDIXES

(Nonmandatory Information)

X1. REFERENCE VALUES FOR ANALYSIS

TABLE X1.1 Experimentally Determined Reference Intensity Ratios (RIR) Relative to Alpha-Corundum, αAl_2O_3

Phase	RIR
Hydroxyapatite (commercial powder)	1.276 ± 0.001
β-TCP	1.146 ± 0.004
CaO	3.375 ± 0.004

TABLE X1.3 Combined Relative Intensities for the Integration Regions Indicated (6)

Phase	Range 2θ,°	I^{Rel}
Hydroxyapatite	38.5 - 59.0	2.16 ± 0.02
β-TCP	30.5 - 31.6	1.00 ± 0.00
	37.0 - 38.5	0.145 ± 0.001
	38.5 - 59.0	2.35 ± 0.01
CaO	37.0 - 38.5	1.00 ± 0.00
	38.5 - 59.0	1.32 ± 0.007

TABLE X1.5 Mass Absorption Coefficients

Phases(s)	Mass Absorption Coefficient
Ca-P from hydroxyapatite (all phases)	$\chi_m = 87.23$
Alpha-corundum, αAl_2O_3	$\chi_s = 31.78$

X2. EXAMPLE CALCULATION

X2.1

Phase	Net Intensity (after correction), counts · s/°
β-TCP	23.9
CaO	12.4
HA	603.2
Standard	989.0

X2.2 The weight percentages are determined from Equation 11 of Ref **(6)** with the RIR, I_{rel}, and mass absorption coefficients from Appendix X1.

$$W_{\beta-TCP} = \left(\frac{23.9}{1}\right)\cdot\left(\frac{87.23}{31.78}\right)\cdot\left(\frac{1}{989.0\cdot 1.146}\right) = 0.058 = 5.8\ \% \quad (X2.1)$$

$$W_{CaO} = \left(\frac{12.4}{1}\right)\cdot\left(\frac{87.23}{31.78}\right)\cdot\left(\frac{1}{989.0\cdot 3.375}\right) = 0.010 = 1.0\ \% \quad (X2.2)$$

$$W_{HA} = \left(\frac{603.2}{2.16}\right)\cdot\left(\frac{87.23}{31.78}\right)\cdot\left(\frac{1}{989.0\cdot 1.276}\right) = 0.607 = 60.7\ \% \quad (X2.3)$$

REFERENCES

(1) Cook, S.D., Thomas, K.A., Kay, J.F., and Jarcho, M., "Hydroxylapatite-Coated Titanium for Orthopedic Implant Applications," *Clinical Orthopaedics*, Vol 232, 1988, p. 225.

(2) Cook, S.D., Kay, J.F., Thomas, K.A., and Jarcho, M., "Interface Mechanics and Histology of Titanium and Hydroxylapatite-Coated Titanium for Dental Implant Applications," *International Journal of Oral and Maxillofacial Implants*, Vol 2, 1987, p. 15.

(3) Kent, J.N., Block, M.S., Finger, I.M., Guerra, L.S., Larsen, H., and Misiek, D.J., "Biointegrated Hydroxylapatite-Coated Dental Implants: 5-Year Clinical Observations," *Journal of the American Dental Association*, Vol 121, 1990, p. 138.

(4) D'Antonio, J.A., Capello, W.N., and Jaffe, W.L., "Hydroxylapatite-Coated Hip Implants: Multicenter Three-Year Clinical and Roentgenographic Results," *Clinical Orthopaedics*, Vol 285, 1992, p. 102.

(5) Thomas, K.A., "Hydroxyapatite Coatings," *Orthopedics*, Vol 17, 1994, p. 267.

(6) Prevey, P.S., and Rothwell, R.J., "X-ray Diffraction Characterization of Percent Crystallinity and Contaminants in Plasma-Sprayed Hydroxylapatite Coatings," *Characterization and Performance of Calcium Phosphate Coatings for Implants, ASTM STP 1196*, Emanuel Horowitz and Jack E. Parr, eds., American Society for Testing and Materials, Philadelphia, PA, 1994, p. 63.

Standard Practice for Gravimetric Measurement of Polymeric Components for Wear Assessment[1]

This standard is issued under the fixed designation F 2025; the number immediately following the designation indicates the year of original adoption or, in the case of revision, the year of last revision. A number in parentheses indicates the year of last reapproval. A superscript epsilon (ε) indicates an editorial change since the last revision or reapproval.

1. Scope

1.1 This practice describes a laboratory method using a weight-loss (that is, mass-loss; see X1.4) technique for evaluating the wear properties of polymeric materials or devices which are being considered for use as bearing surfaces of human joint replacement prostheses, or both. The test specimens are evaluated in a device intended to simulate the tribological conditions encountered in the human joint; for example, use of a fluid such as bovine serum, or equivalent pseudosynovial fluid shown to simulate similar wear mechanisms and debris generation as found in vivo.

2. Referenced Documents

2.1 *ASTM Standards:*

D 792 Test Methods for Density and Specific Gravity (Relative Density) of Plastics by Displacement[2]

D 1505 Test Method for Density of Plastics by the Density-Gradient Technique[2]

F 732 Practice for Pin-on-Flat Evaluation of Friction and Wear Properties of Polymeric Materials for Use in Total Joint Prostheses

F 1714 Guide for Gravimetric Wear Assessment of Prosthetic Hip-Designs in Simulator Devices[3]

F 1715 Guide for Gravimetric Wear Assessment of Prosthetic Knee-Designs in Simulator Devices[3]

3. Significance and Use

3.1 This practice uses a weight-loss method of wear determination for the polymeric components or materials used in human joint prostheses, using serum or demonstrated equivalent fluid for lubrication, and running under a load profile representative of the appropriate human joint application **(1,2)**.[4] The basis for this weight-loss method for wear measurement was originally developed **(3)** for pin-on-disk wear studies (Practice F 732) and has been extended to total hip replacements (**4,5**, and Guide F 1714) and to femoro-tibial knee prostheses (**6** and Guide F 1715), and to femoro-patellar knee prostheses (**6,7**).

3.2 While wear results in a change in the physical dimensions of the specimen, it is distinct from dimensional changes due to creep or plastic deformation, in that wear results in the removal of material in the form of polymeric debris particles, causing a loss in weight of the specimen.

3.3 This practice for measuring wear of the polymeric component is suitable for various simulator devices. These techniques can be used with metal, ceramic, carbon, polymeric, and composite counter faces bearing against a polymeric material (for example, polyethylene, polyacetal, and so forth). Thus, this weight-loss method has universal application for wear studies of human joint replacements which feature polymeric bearings. This weight-loss method has not been validated for non-polymeric material bearing systems, such as metal-metal, carbon-carbon, or ceramic-ceramic. Progressive wear of such rigid bearing combinations has generally been monitored using a linear, variable-displacement transducers, or by other profilometric techniques.

4. Components and Materials

4.1 *Hip Prosthesis Components*—The hip joint prosthesis comprises a ball-and-socket configuration in which materials such as polymers, composites, metal alloys, ceramics, and carbon have been used in various combinations and designs.

4.1.1 *Component Configurations*—The diameter of the prosthetic ball may vary from 22 to 54 mm or larger. The design may include ball-socket, trunnion, bipolar, or other configurations. If applicable, the normal metal backing for the polymeric component shall be used provided disassembly and reassembly of these components for the measurement does not have an unrepresentative effect on the weight measurements or wear behavior. Otherwise, a modified backing may be used, again provided this has no unrepresentative effect on the weight measurements or wear behavior (see X1.5).

4.2 *Knee Prosthesis Components*—The knee joint comprises femoral, tibial, and patellar configurations in which materials such as metal alloys, ceramics, polymers, and carbon materials have been used in various combinations in different designs.

4.2.1 *Component Configurations*—The polymeric components may be backed by either metal, ceramic, or composite reinforcements. If applicable, the normal metal backing shall

---

[1] This practice is under the jurisdiction of ASTM Committee F-4 on Medical and Surgical Materials and Devices and is the direct responsibility of Subcommittee F04.22 on Arthroplasty.

Current edition approved May 10, 2000. Published Aug. 2000.

[2] *Annual Book of ASTM Standards*, Vol 08.01.

[3] *Annual Book of ASTM Standards*, Vol 13.01.

[4] The numbers in parentheses refer to the list of references at the end of this standard.

be used provided disassembly and reassembly of these components for the measurement does not have an unrepresentative effect on the weight measurements or wear behavior. Otherwise, a modified backing may be used, again provided this has no unrepresentative effect on the weight measurements or wear behavior (see X1.5).

4.3 Other prosthesis components and test coupons may be used to represent other human joint replacement applications.

5. Specimen Preparation

5.1 *Polymers and Composites*—Material Condition:

5.1.1 A fabrication history shall be obtained for each polymeric or composite component, including information such as grade, batch number and processing variables, method of forming (extruding, molding, and so forth), temperature, pressure and forming time used, and any post-forming treatments, including sterilization method and parameters.

5.1.2 Pretest characterization may include measurement of bulk material properties such as molecular-weight range and distribution, percent crystallinity, or other. Density is a particularly important property because of the conversion of weight measurements to volumetric wear (see 7.4). Density measurements shall be obtained in accordance with Test Methods or Test Method D 792 or D 1505. If it can be justified that previous density measurements are representative of the material used in the current wear test, reference to these previous measurements and suitable justification shall be provided (see also X1.6). The surface finish of specimens may be characterized by profilometry, photomicrography, and replication by various plastics or other techniques.

5.1.3 *Sterilization*—The components shall be sterilized in a manner typical of that in clinical use for such devices, as this may affect the wear properties of the materials. Sterilization of all test and control components within a specific test group should be done simultaneously (in a single container) when possible to minimize variation among the specimens. The wear testing procedure makes no attempt to maintain the sterility of specimens during the wear test.

5.2 *Polymer Specimen Cleaning Procedure*—Prior to weighing and wear testing, careful cleaning of the polymer specimens is important to remove any contaminants that would not normally be present on the actual prosthesis. During the wear test, the components must be re-cleaned and dried before each weighing to remove any extraneous material that might affect the accuracy of the weighing. The procedure for cleaning and drying of polymeric components is given in Annex A1. With some combinations of materials, wear may result in the transfer of particulate debris which may then become re-imbedded or otherwise attached to polymeric, metal, or composite surfaces. Such an occurrence will render the weight-loss assessment of wear less reliable.

5.3 *Polymer Specimen Weighing Procedure*—The polymeric components shall be weighed on an analytical balance having a sensitivity on the order of 10 μg. This degree of sensitivity is necessary to detect the slight loss in weight of polymers such as UHMW polyethylene, which may wear 1 mg or less per million cycles. Specimens shall always be weighed in the clean, dry condition (Annex A1). The components shall be kept in a dust-free container and handled with clean tools to prevent contamination which might affect the weight measurement. Each wear and control component shall be weighed three times in rotation to detect random errors in the weighing process.

5.4 *Pre-soaking of Test Specimens*:

5.4.1 Polymeric and composite components made from materials which absorb fluid initially, but saturate within a few weeks, should be presoaked in the test lubricant to reduce the error due to fluid sorption during the wear run. If the fluid sorption behavior of a particular material is unknown, the investigator shall conduct a preliminary study to determine whether or not the material is exempt from presoaking.

5.4.2 *Preliminary Study*—A minimum of three soak specimens (these can be test coupons or actual devices) per material shall be cleaned and dried in accordance with the procedure in Annex A1, and then weighed by precisely controlled and repeatable methods (Annex A1). The specimens shall then be placed in a container of test lubricant and removed, cleaned, dried, and weighed (in accordance with Annex A1) once or twice a week. The weight change shall be calculated in accordance with Annex A1. The procedure shall be repeated until the specimens have soaked for five weeks. Specimen weight change shall be averaged at each interval and plotted versus time. Data points shall be fit using a second or third order polynomial or hyperbolic function, connecting through zero. The fit of this curve should have an R^2 value of 0.8 or greater. If the slope of this curve at five weeks is ten or more times less than the slope of the curve at zero (see X1.7), then this material must be subjected to presoaking before wear testing (if gravimetric wear measurement is to be used). Otherwise, it is exempt.

NOTE 1—Even if presoaking is not required, one to three soak control components are still necessary per material condition to account for fluid sorption by the wear components during the wear test.

5.4.3 *Pre-soaking Procedure (if Required)*—After fabrication and characterization, the wear components and one to three soak-control components of each test material shall be cleaned in accordance with the procedure in Annex A1. The wear components and soak control(s) shall then be placed in a container of test lubricant for a minimum of five weeks (35 days).

6. Measurement Procedure

6.1 After fabrication, characterization, and the completion of the presoak period (if required), the wear components and soak control(s) should be cleaned, dried, and weighed by precisely controlled and repeatable methods (Annex A1). These weights shall be recorded as the initial weights of the specimens for purposes of calculating the progressive weight loss during the wear test. The soak control specimen(s) shall be placed in holders in a soak chamber of test lubricant, such that the total surface area exposed to the lubricant is equal to that of the wear components when mounted in the test chamber. The soak chamber temperature shall be maintained at the same temperature as the bulk lubricant in the wear test, or specified if different. It is recommended that the soak chamber be attached to the test machine or otherwise agitated in the same manner as the actual wear chambers. In addition, it may be advantageous to apply a cyclic load to the soak control specimen(s) (without tangential motion) comparable to that applied to the wear specimens, since this can also affect the rate of fluid sorption.

6.2 The wear and soak component(s) shall be removed at specified intervals, washed, rinsed, and dried concurrently, in accordance with the procedure in Annex A1. It is important that both the wear and soak component(s) be treated identically to ensure that they have the same exposure to the wash, rinse, and drying fluids. This will provide the most accurate correction for fluid sorption by the wear specimens.

6.3 After rinsing and drying, the wear components and soak controls shall be weighed on an analytical balance in accordance with 5.3.

6.4 The wear chambers and component surfaces shall be thoroughly rinsed with distilled or deionized water.

6.5 The bearing surfaces of the components shall be inspected, and the characteristics of the wear process noted. Visual, microscopic, profilometric, replication, or other inspection techniques can be used. However, care must be taken that the surfaces do not become contaminated or damaged by any substance or technique which might affect the subsequent wear properties. If contamination occurs, the specimens shall be thoroughly re-cleaned prior to restarting the wear test.

6.6 The wear components and soak control(s) shall be replaced in fresh lubricant and wear cycling continued.

7. Determination of Wear Rates

7.1 *Test Length*—The accuracy of the test method depends on the relative magnitudes of wear and fluid sorption. This is especially true when the fluctuations in the weight due to variation in the amount of surface drying are large in comparison to the incremental weight-loss due to wear. For high-wear low-sorption materials, the wear rate may be clearly established in as few as 50 000 wear cycles. With comparatively low-wearing materials, such as UHMWPE, several million cycles or more may be required to clearly establish the long-term wear properties.

7.2 *Number of Measurements per Test*—When specimens can be removed for intermediate weight measurement, at least three measurements per test series shall be made.

7.3 *Correcting for Fluid Sorption*—The average gain (or loss) of the soak control component(s) shall be added to (or subtracted from) the measured weight loss of each wear component (Annex A2.6); this procedure corrects both for systematic sorption as well as random differences in the amount of surface drying (of the entire set of test and control specimens) and balance fluctuations due to environmental or other variables at each interval of weighing.

7.4 *Conversion to Volumetric Wear*—In tests where the wear rates of materials with different densities are evaluated, it may be preferable to compare these on the basis of volumetric wear, rather than weight loss. The volumetric wear rate may be obtained by dividing the weight loss data by the density of the material, in appropriate units. The accuracy of this calculation is dependent on the material being reasonably homogeneous (that is, having a constant density with wear depth). The density value used in this conversion shall be reported.

8. Report

8.1 *Materials*:

8.1.1 Material traceability information shall be provided for each material counter face and shall include pertinent details related to raw material and fabrication or manufacturing history. Examples of such information include material grade, batch number, and processing variables.

8.1.2 Pretest characterization for a plastic counter face may include measurement of bulk material properties such as molecular-weight average, range and distribution, percent crystallinity, density, degree of oxidation, or others. The surface finish of both counter faces may be characterized by profilometry, photomicrography, replication, or other applicable techniques.

8.1.3 The method of sterilization, the sterilization date and test date, and the means of storage post-sterilization and pretest shall be reported. For irradiation-sterilized specimens, total dose and dose rate shall be reported.

8.1.4 If presoaking was not conducted, justification shall be provided.

8.2 *Wear Rates*:

8.2.1 The weight loss of each specimen shall be plotted graphically as a function of wear cycles. Wear may be reported as the weight loss of the bearing component as a function of the number of wear cycles, but is preferentially converted to volumetric wear if the density of the material is known (see X1.6 and X1.8)

8.2.2 In tests where the wear rate is nearly constant, the volumetric (or gravimetric) wear rate shall be calculated by the method of least-squares regression.

8.2.3 If the wear rate changes during the test as with a decrease due to wearing in of the specimens or an increase due to the onset of fatigue wear, linear regression may be applied to separate intervals of the test to indicate the change in wear rate.

8.2.4 At the discretion of the investigator, more complex, nonlinear models may be fit to the wear test data.

8.2.5 The test duration in cycles shall be reported.

8.2.6 Sliding distance per wear cycle shall be reported, if known.

8.3 *Accuracy and Repeatability*:

8.3.1 In multiple tests, where the wear rate is determined from the slope of the graph comparing wear versus test duration (cycles) for each specimen, the individual rates, mean wear rate, and the 95 % confidence intervals for each rate shall be reported.

8.3.2 In cases where the mean wear rate for two materials is different, the level of statistical significance of this difference shall be evaluated and reported.

8.3.3 At the discretion of the investigator, other statistics methods may be used. All statistics methods and related assumptions shall be reported.

8.4 Since the accumulation of wear debris in the lubricant may influence the wear rate, any filtering of the lubricant during operation (continuously or periodically) shall be reported.

8.5 The room temperature and humidity during each weighing session shall be recorded and reported (see X1.9).

8.6 The loading conditions on the soak control specimen(s)

shall be reported. Load soaking which is defined as a pulsing load profile equivalent to the wear profile without the tangential movement may increase the fluid sorption rate.

ANNEXES

(Mandatory Information)

A1. METHOD FOR CLEANING OF SPECIMENS

A1.1 Gently scrub components with a nonabrasive material to remove all serum particles. Verify under a magnifying glass.

A1.2 Rinse under a stream of deionized water.

A1.3 Clean in an ultrasonic cleaner.

A1.3.1 Five minutes in deionized, particle-free water.

A1.3.2 Rinse in deionized water.

A1.3.3 Ten minutes in 10 mL of liquid ultrasonic cleaning detergent plus 500 mL of water.

A1.3.4 Rinse in deionized water.

A1.3.5 Ten minutes in deionized water.

A1.3.6 Rinse in deionized water.

A1.3.7 Three minutes in deionized water.

A1.3.8 Rinse in deionized water.

A1.4 Dry with a jet of nitrogen or suitable clean, dry gas.

A1.5 Soak in 95 % methyl alcohol for 5 min (see Note A1.1).

A1.6 Dry with a jet of nitrogen or suitable gas.

A1.7 Dry in a vacuum jar at a minimum vacuum 10^{-3} torr for 30 min.

A1.8 Weigh on a micro-balance.

A1.9 To minimize weighing errors, weigh the entire set of specimens three times, in rotation, keeping the same specimen sequence each time. Polymeric cups typically gain or loss weight slightly between each weighing due to additional sorption or evaporation of fluid. The average of the three weights may be used for the wear calculations.

NOTE A1.1—This is a suggested cleaning procedure suitable for metals, ceramics, carbon, and UHMW polyethylene (**3**). Methyl alcohol shall be used only for polymers that are essentially insoluble in this liquid. For polymers which dissolve or degrade in methyl alcohol, a more appropriate volatile solvent shall be substituted. The purpose of this step is to remove the water from the surface layer of the specimen that otherwise tends to evaporate during the weighing process. Other aspects of this procedure might require modification for the particular polymer being tested.

A2. CALCULATION OF SPECIMEN WEAR

A2.1 *Definitions*—For the sake of clarity, the terms used in the calculation of specimen wear are defined as follows:

A2.1.1 *Measured Values* ("weight" values should be in milligrams):

n = number of soak control specimens,
i = one of a series of soak control specimens,
$W1$ = initial weight of a wear specimen,
$W2$ = final weight of a wear specimen, not adjusted for fluid sorption, and
ρ = polymer density (g/mm^3).

A2.1.2 *Calculated Values* ("weight" values should be in milligrams):

$S1$ = average initial weight of the soak control specimen(s),
$S2$ = average final weight of the soak control specimen(s),
S_i = weight gain of a soak control specimen for a wear interval,
Sn = average weight gain of all soak control specimens for a wear interval (S2 − S1),
$W3$ = final weight of a wear specimen, adjusted for fluid sorption ($W2 + Sn$),
Wa = apparent gravimetric wear (W1 − W2),
Wn = net gravimetric wear (W1 − W3), and
Vn = net volumetric wear (mm^3).

A2.2 The amount of fluid sorption over a wear interval is determined from the soak control specimen(s), whereby the average weight gain, *Sn*, is calculated as follows:

$$Sn = (1/n) \sum_i^n S_i \tag{A2.1}$$

A2.3 Since fluid sorption by the wear specimens tends to mask the actual weight loss due to wear, the magnitude of the measured weight loss by the wear specimens shall be increased by the magnitude of the weight-gain of the soak control specimen(s). Where *S*1 equals initial average weight of the soak specimen(s); and *S*2 equals the final average weight of the soak specimen(s).

A2.4 Thus the actual net wear is given as follows:

$$Wn = W1 - W3 \tag{A2.2}$$

However, *W*3 is unknown. On the other hand, the apparent wear is given as follows:

$$Wa = W1 - W2 \tag{A2.3}$$

where:

$W1$ = initial weight of the wear specimen,
$W2$ = final weight of the wear specimen (including a gain due to fluid sorption), and
$W3$ = actual final weight of the wear specimen if fluid sorption is subtracted out.

Therefore the net wear (Wn) can be obtained by increasing the apparent wear (Wa) by an amount equal to the net soak gain as follows:

$$Wn = Wa + Sn \tag{A2.4}$$

where $Sn = S2 - S1$,

Thus $Wn = (W1 - W2) + (S2 - S1)$

A2.5 Note that the four weights W1, W2, S1, and S2 are actual measured values (S1 and S2 may be averages of measured values). The sign convention in this equation for *Wn* takes into account occurrences such as an apparent weight gain by the wear specimen (giving a negative value for *Wa*) or a net weight loss by the soak specimens (a negative value of *Sn*). In most cases the net wear, *Wn*, will be zero or positive.

A2.6 The net volumetric wear is then given as follows:

$$Vn = Wn/\rho \tag{A2.5}$$

where ρ = density of the polymer, expressed in appropriate units.

APPENDIX

(Nonmandatory Information)

X1. RATIONALE

X1.1 For the purpose of this practice, wear is defined as the progressive loss of material from a prosthetic component as a result of tangential motion against its mating component under load. For current designs of total joint prostheses, the polymeric component bearing against a metal, ceramic, composite, or carbon component will be the sacrificial member; that is, polymer will be the predominant source of wear debris. However, the metallic or other non-polymeric components may also contribute either ionic or particulate debris. Thus, depending on the circumstances, wear may be generated by adhesion, two or three body abrasion, surface or subsurface fatigue, or some other process. Depending on the candidate materials and design combinations selected, it may be desirable in some instances to add additional techniques (that is, non-gravimetric) to identify the nature and magnitude of the wear process.

X1.2 While wear results in a change in the physical dimensions of the specimen, it is distinct from dimensional changes due to creep or plastic deformation in that wear generally results in the removal of material in the form of debris particles, causing a loss in weight of the specimen **(3,7)**.

X1.3 Wear rate is the gravimetric or volumetric wear per million cycles of test.

X1.4 While it is understood that the loss of material caused by wear is technically "mass-loss," the term "weight-loss" is commonly used and appears in existing standards and, for the purpose of this practice, is considered to be synonymous.

X1.5 For many joint replacement devices, a polymeric specimen is normally fit into a metal backing using some type of locking mechanism. In order to make periodic weight measurements during a wear test, the polymeric specimen must be removed. Some locking mechanisms, however, disallow this removal without causing damage to the specimen or the locking mechanism, thus, subjecting the accuracy and relevance of the test to question. Provided it can be justified that the wear at this secondary interface is negligible or not relevant to the test objectives, a modified backing may be fabricated to facilitate disassembly and reassembly. Adequate justification should be provided that the modified backing maintains clinically relevant wear behavior and accurate weight measurements. Likewise, if the normal backing is to be used, adequate justification should be provided to show that repeated disassembly and reassembly does not change wear behavior or affect weight measurements.

X1.6 It is understood that for some material conditions, such as gamma-irradiated and aged UHMWPE, density can vary with depth into the surface. In general, the error related to such variation is small compared to other factors or to the magnitude of wear (which generally increases when large density gradients are present) and can be ignored. There may, however, be unusual cases where the density gradient in a representative specimen should be measured and accounted for in determining volumetric wear. It should also be noted that the density of a polymer may change under loading.

X1.7 There is no known study that has been conducted specifically to differentiate polymeric materials that quickly saturate in wear test lubricants from those that do not. Relevant studies such as that by Clarke et al **(4)** suggest that commonly used materials, such as UHMWPE (irradiated and nonirradiated) may exhibit different levels of fluid absorption but do not exhibit a rapid saturation or other unusual absorption behavior. Recent discussions (such as at ASTM F04.22.10, 5/99) have led to agreement that presoaking of such common materials has not improved the accuracy of weight measurements during testing and may even have a nonrepresentative effect on the specimen surface at the start of a wear test. The cutoff specified in 5.4.2 designating a quickly saturating material is indeed arbitrary but selected to allow materials with known absorption and wear behaviors to be exempt from this presoaking procedure.

X1.8 The suggestion of reporting wear in terms of volumetric wear is done for means of standardization. Some wear tests are configured such that only volumetric measurements can be taken. In some cases, volumetric wear measurements may be more accurate than gravimetric measurements. Volumetric wear rates should be reported as cubic millimetres per million cycles, and the sliding distance per cycle should be reported, if possible, to facilitate conversion to wear volume per unit sliding distance.

X1.9 Minimizing fluctuations in laboratory temperature and humidity may be helpful in avoiding additional variables that can influence results. The use of untested control specimens, however, will theoretically account for the effects of such fluctuations.

REFERENCES

(**1**) Davy, D.T., Kotzar, G.M., Brown, R.H., Heiple, K.G., and Goldberg, V.M., et al, Telemetric force measurement across the hip after total arthroplasty," *JBJS*, 7OA(1):45, 1988.

(**2**) Paul, J.P., "Forces Transmitted by Joints in the Human Body. Lubrication and Wear in Living and Artificial Human Joints," *Proceedings Inst. Mech. Engrs.*, Vol 181(35), London, 1996-1967, p. 8-15.

(**3**) McKellop, H.A., Clarke, I.C., Markolf, K., and Amstutz, H.C., "Wear Characteristics of UHMW Polyethylene: A Method for Accurately Measuring Extremely Low Wear Rates," *Journal of Biomed.* Mat. Res., 12:895, 1978.

(**4**) Clarke, I.C., Starkebbaum, W., Hosseinian, A., McGuire, P., Okuda, R., Salovey, R., and Young, R., "Fluid-sorption Phenomena in Sterilized Polyethylene Acetabular Prostheses," *Journal of Biomat.*, 6:184, 1985.

(**5**) McKellop, H.A., Lu, B., and Benya, P., "Friction, Lubrication and Wear of Cobalt-chromium, Alumina and Zirconia Hip Prostheses Compared on a Joint Simulator," Trans. Orthop. Res. Soc., 1992, p. 401.

(**6**) Treharne, R.W., Young, R.W., and Young, S.R., "Wear of Artificial Joint Materials III: Simulation of the Knee Joint Using a Computer Controlled System," *Engineering in Medicine*, Vol 10, No. 3, 1981, pp. 137142.

(**7**) McKellop, H.A., and Clarke, I.C., "Degradation and Wear of Ultra-High-Molecular-Weight Polyethylene," *Special Technical Publication 859*, ASTM, 1985.

Standard Specification for Polyetheretherketone (PEEK) Resins for Surgical Implant Applications[1]

This standard is issued under the fixed designation F 2026; the number immediately following the designation indicates the year of original adoption or, in the case of revision, the year of last revision. A number in parentheses indicates the year of last reapproval. A superscript epsilon (ε) indicates an editorial change since the last revision or reapproval.

1. Scope

1.1 This specification covers polyetheretherketone (PEEK) resins in virgin forms as supplied by a vendor (flakes, pellets, blocks, and so forth). It provides requirements and associated test methods for these thermoplastics when they are to be used in the manufacture of intracorporal devices such as surgical implants or components of surgical or dental devices.

1.2 As with any material, some characteristics may be altered by the processing techniques (molding, extrusion, machining, assembly, sterilization, and so forth) required for the production of a specific part or device. Therefore, properties of fabricated forms of these resins should be evaluated using test methods which are appropriate to ensure safety and efficacy as agreed upon by the vendor, purchaser, and regulating bodies.

1.3 The properties included in this specification are those applicable for PEEK resins only. Fabricated forms, material or forms containing colorants, fillers, processing aids, or other additives, as well as polymer blends which contain PEEK, are not covered by this specification.

1.4 This specification is designed to recommend physical, chemical, and biological test methods to establish a reasonable level of confidence concerning the performance of virgin PEEK resins for use in medical devices. The properties listed should be considered in selecting material in accordance with the specific end-use requirements.

1.5 When evaluating material in accordance with this specification, hazardous materials, operations, and equipment may be involved. *This standard does not purport to address all of the safety concerns, if any, associated with its use. It is the responsibility of the user of this standard to establish appropriate safety and health practices and determine the applicability of regulatory limitations prior to use.*

2. Referenced Documents

2.1 *ASTM Standards:*

D 149 Test Method for Dielectric Breakdown Voltage and Dielectric Strength of Solid Electrical Insulating Materials at Commercial Power Frequencies[2]

D 256 Test Method for Determining the Pendulum Impact Resistance of Notched Specimens of Plastics[3]

D 570 Test Method for Water Absorption of Plastics[3]

D 621 Test Methods for Deformation of Plastics Under Load[4]

D 638 Test Method for Tensile Properties of Plastics[3]

D 648 Test Method for Deflection Temperature of Plastics Under Flexural Load[3]

D 695 Test Method for Compressive Properties of Rigid Plastics[3]

D 696 Test Method for Coefficient of Linear Thermal Expansion of Plastics Between –30C and 30C[3]

D 790 Test Methods for Flexural Properties of Unreinforced and Reinforced Plastics and Electrical Insulating Materials[3]

D 792 Test Methods for Density and Specific Gravity Relative Density) of Plastics by Displacement[3]

D 955 Test Method for Measuring Shrinkage from Mold Dimensions of Molded Plastics[3]

D 1238 Test Method for Flow Rates of Thermoplastics by Extrusion Plastometer[3]

D 1505 Test Method for Density of Plastics by the Density-Gradient Technique[3]

D 1898 Practice for Sampling of Plastics[5]

D 3417 Test Method for Enthalpies of Fusion and Crystallization of Polymers by Differential Scanning Calorimetry (DSC)[6]

D 3418 Test Method for Transition Temperatures of Polymers by Thermal Analysis[6]

D 4000 Classification System for Specifying Plastic Materials[6]

F 748 Practice for Selecting Generic Biological Test Methods for Materials and Devices[7]

2.2 *ISO Standards:*

ISO 1628/1 Plastics—Guidelines for the Standardization of Methods for Determination of Viscosity Number and

[1] This specification is under the jurisdiction of ASTM Committee F-4 on Medical and Surgical Materials and Devices and is the direct responsibility of Subcommittee F04.11 on Polymeric Materials.

Current edition approved May 10, 2000. Published August 2000.

[2] *Annual Book of ASTM Standards*, Vol 10.01.

[3] *Annual Book of ASTM Standards*, Vol 08.01.

[4] Discontinued; see *1993 Annual Book of ASTM Standards*, Vol 08.01.

[5] Discontinued; see *1997 Annual Book of ASTM Standards*, Vol 08.02.

[6] *Annual Book of ASTM Standards*, Vol 08.02.

[7] *Annual Book of ASTM Standards*, Vol 13.01.

Limiting Viscosity Number of Polymers in Dilute Solution—Part 1: General Conditions[8]

ISO 1133 Plastics—Determination of the Melt Mass-Flow Rate (MFR) and the Melt Volume-Flow Rate (MVR) of Thermoplastics[8]

ISO 10993 Biological Evaluation of Medical Devices, Parts 1-12[8]

2.3 *Other Document:*

United States Pharmacopeia, Vol. XXI, or latest edition[9]

Food and Drug Administration, Regulation 21 CFR 177.1580[10]

3. Terminology

3.1 *Definitions of Terms Specific to This Standard:*

3.1.1 *fabricated forms*—those items into which the virgin forms may be converted. These include shapes and forms produced by means of machining, extruding, and compression molding virgin forms into a subsequent entity (for example, rods, slabs, sheets, film, or complex shaped parts and devices).

3.1.2 *formulated compound*—the PEEK materials, parts, or devices fabricated from virgin forms in such a way as to contain intentional or unintentional adjuvant substances.

3.1.3 *virgin forms*—that form of the PEEK resin as obtained by the synthesizer. It typically will be in the form of pellets, chips, or blocks. It is the material from which rods, slabs, sheets, films, or specific parts and devices are fabricated.

4. Classification

4.1 The PEEK resins in the scope of this specification are pure semicrystalline homopolymers consisting of phenylene rings connected by ether (E) and carbonyl (or ketone, K) groups along the polymer chain (see Appendix X2). Their polymeric structures are defined by the repeating unit EEK.

4.2 Types of PEEK plastics, molding, and extrusion grades are described in Classification System D 4000.

5. Properties

5.1 The PEEK resins used in medical applications may comply with the Food and Drug Administration (FDA) regulation 21 CFR 177.1580 which covers both wet and dry food contact applications.

[8] Available from American National Standards Institute, 11 W. 42nd St., 13th Floor, New York, NY 10036.

[9] Available from U.S. Pharmacopeial Convention, Inc., Easton, PA.

[10] Available from the Food and Drug Administration.

TABLE 1 Required Properties of Virgin Resin

Parameter	Method	Requirement
T_g, ° C	DSC, 20°C/min, sealed sample	125 - 165
T_m, ° C	DSC, 20°C/min, sealed sample	320 - 360
Viscosity number, min, mL/g	ISO 1628, concentrated sulfuric acid, 0.5 % w/v, 25°C	77
Melt volume flow rate, cm^3/10 min	ISO 1133, 400°C, 10 Kg	25 - 60
Total heavy metals as lead, max, %	US Pharmacopeia, Test 231	0.1

TABLE 2 Typical Properties of Fabricated Forms

Parameter	Method	Requirement
Density, kg/m^3	ISO D 1505	1280 - 1320
Tensile Strength, min, MPA, Yield Break	Test Method D 638, Type IV, 5.08 cm/min	90 70
Percent elongation, min, %	Test Method D 638, Type IV, 5.08 cm/min	40
Izod Impact Strength, min, ft-lbf/in.	Test Method D 256, 0.254-cm depth, 0.025-cm radius	1.1
Deformation Under Load, max , %	Test Methods D 621 (A), 7 MPa for 24 h, 23°C, after 90-min recovery	2

5.2 The infrared spectrum[11] of these materials is characteristic of their molecular repeating units. A representative spectrum is listed in Appendix X3. The PEEK resin shall yield an infrared transmittance spectrum which exhibits major bands only at the wavelengths listed for a standard reference spectrum of that material.

5.2.1 The infrared spectrum, as used in this specification, is to identify the specific type of poly aryl ether ketone (PAEK) present and does not necessarily indicate an acceptable degree of material purity.

5.2.2 The presence of additional bands in the sample's infrared spectrum compared to that of the reference material may indicate a different PAEK or impurities, or both.

5.3 The physical and chemical property requirements for the virgin resin are listed in Table 1. If additional characteristics are necessary because of a specific application, the procedures referenced in 5.7 are recommended, or as agreed upon between the vendor and the purchaser.

5.4 The viscosity requirements listed in Table 1 may be supplemented, or replaced, by rheological or complex viscosity data as agreed upon between the vendor and the purchaser.

5.5 The chemical, physical, and mechanical properties of fabricated forms are related to the processes utilized in producing the fabricated form (for example, molding, machining, sterilization, and so forth). Additionally, the properties necessary for a particular device to perform properly will vary from one device type to another. Table 2 lists some typical properties of non-sterilized injection molded material.

5.6 Test specimens shall be fabricated (machined, injection molded, and so forth) from the virgin resin, or finished part, in such a way to effectively represent the material characteristics of the non-sterilized finished part.

5.7 Tests and test procedures shall be such as to ensure a high level of control and characterization of the virgin resin as received from the supplier. The following are some test methods that may be appropriate: Test Method D 149, Test Method D 256, Test Method D 570, Test Method D 638, Test Method D 648, Test Method D 695, Test method D 696, Test Methods D 790, Test Methods D 792, Test Method D 955, Test Method D 1238, Test Method D 1505, Test Method D 3417, Test Method D 3418, and Classification System D 4000.

6. Sampling

6.1 The material should be sampled in accordance with the

[11] Silverstein, R. M., Bassler, G. C., and Morrill, T. C., "Spectroscopic Identification of Organic Compounds," 5th ed., John Wiley & Sons, New York, NY.

standard sampling procedures, such as those described in Practice D 1898, or other sampling techniques unless otherwise agreed upon between the consumer and the supplier.

7. Biocompatibility

7.1 Biocompatibility of PEEK resins and implant devices made using these materials shall be determined in accordance with Practice F 748 or the ISO 10993 series, unless otherwise agreed upon between the packager and the consumer and regulating bodies.[12]

8. Keywords

8.1 PEEK; polyetheretherketone

[12] Other useful references for testing biocompatibility of materials include:

Autian, J., "Toxicological Evaluation of Biomaterials: Primary Acute Toxicity Screening Program," *Journal of Artificial Organs*, Vol 1, No. 1, 1977, p. 53.

Autian, J., "The New Field of Plastic Toxicological Methods and Results," *CRC Critics Review in Toxicology*, 1973, p. 18.

Homsy, C. A., Ansevin, K. D., O'Brannon, W., Thompson, S. H., Hodge, R., and Estrella, M. E., "Rapid In Vitro Screening of Polymers for Biocompatibility," *Journal of Macromolecular Science Chemistry*, Vol A4, No. 3, May 1970, pp. 615-631.

Rice, R. M., Hegyeli, A. F., Gourlay, S. J., Wade, C. W. R., Dillon, J. G., Jaffe, H., and Kulkarni, R. K., "Biocompatibility Testing for Polymers: In Vitro Studies With In Vivo Correlation," *Journal of Biomedical Materials Research*, Vol 12, 1978, p. 43.

APPENDIXES

(Nonmandatory Information)

X1. RATIONALE

X1.1 The PEEK resins may be processed by most techniques available for thermoplastic polymers. Medical devices and components of medical devices made of PEEK resins may be sterilized. Sterilization methods successfully used include steam, ethylene oxide, and irradiation. Repeated sterilization may weaken parts fabricated of any plastic material. The number of times a given part may be sterilized safely without fear of subsequent failure depends on a number of factors including the molecular weight of resin and design, fabrication, intended function, and method of sterilization of the device. Therefore, it is imperative that the manufacturer test the device in order to determine the maximum number of sterilization cycles to which it can be safely subjected.

X1.2 The potential to develop a significant level of crystallinity is an important characteristic of these materials. Performance characteristics are related to the percent crystallinity. Certain additives and processes (for example, excessive cross linking) can limit these materials' ability to crystallize. Therefore, this feature of the resin and its fabricated form should be evaluated, using appropriate test methods, to ensure efficacy.

X1.3 A formulated compound or fabricated part or device may contain optional adjuvant substances required for the fabrication or intended use of the end product. The biocompatibility of these adjuvant substances, and subsequent formulated compounds, parts, and devices shall be established in accordance with Practice F 748 or the ISO 10993 series.

X2. CHEMICAL STRUCTURE OF PEEK

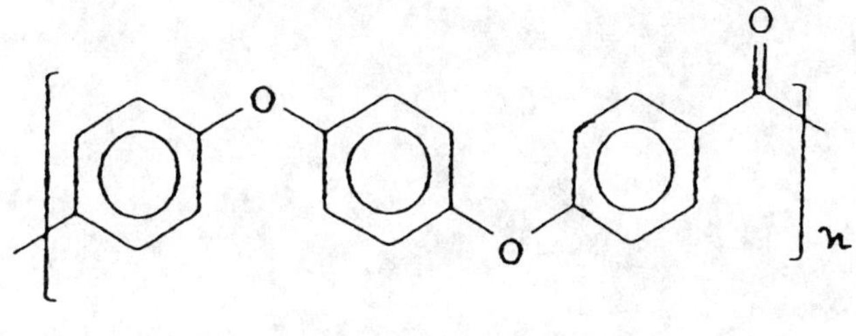

X3. REPRESENTATIVE INFRARED SPECTRA OF PEEK

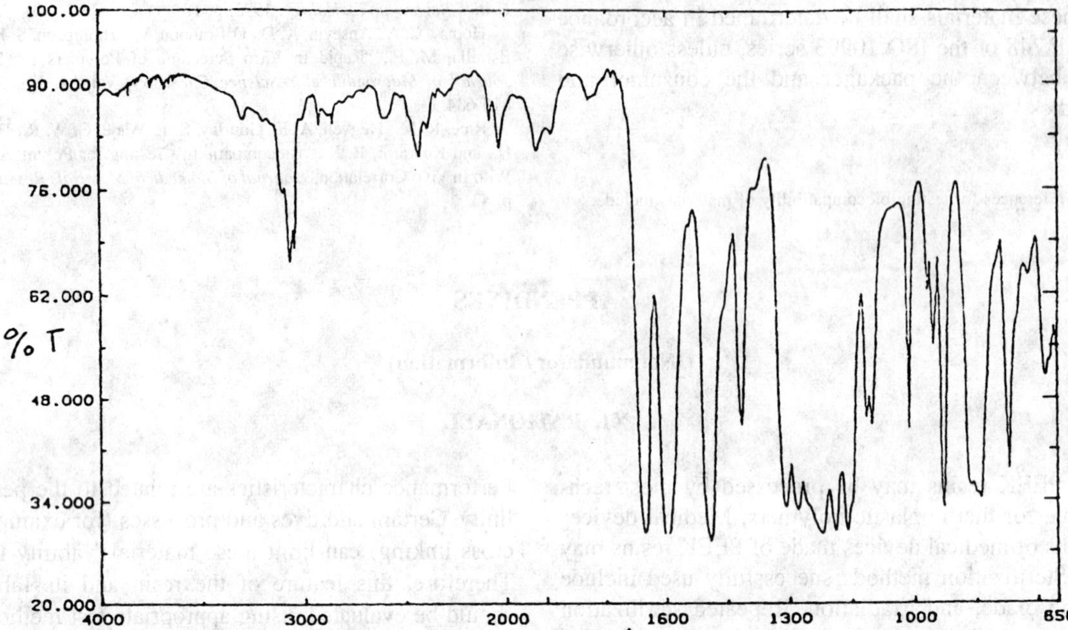

Designation: F 2027 – 00$^{\epsilon 1}$

Standard Guide for Characterization and Testing of Substrate Materials for Tissue-Engineered Medical Products[1]

This standard is issued under the fixed designation F 2027; the number immediately following the designation indicates the year of original adoption or, in the case of revision, the year of last revision. A number in parentheses indicates the year of last reapproval. A superscript epsilon (ε) indicates an editorial change since the last revision or reapproval.

ϵ^1 NOTE—Table 1 was editorially corrected in June 2001.

1. Scope

1.1 This guide addresses material characteristics of raw or virgin materials in a nonfabricated form that will ultimately undergo additional processing into growth, support, or delivery vehicles for cells or biomolecules. This guide does not apply to packaged, sterilized, and finished tissue-engineered medical products.

1.2 The purpose of the guide is to assist the developer of tissue-engineered medical products to locate relevant existing standards and test methods and to provide guidance for interim use of materials for which a standard does not exist.

2. Referenced Documents

2.1 *ASTM Standards:*

D 1763 Specification for Epoxy Resins[2]
D 1898 Practice for Sampling of Plastics[3]
E 1298 Guide for Determination of Purity, Impurities, and Contaminants in Biological Drug Products[4]
F 67 Specification for Unalloyed Titanium for Surgical Implant Applications[5]
F 451 Specification for Acrylic Bone Cement[5]
F 560 Specification for Unalloyed Tantalum for Surgical Implant Applications[5]
F 603 Specification for High-Purity Dense Aluminum Oxide for Surgical Implant Application[5]
F 604 Specification for Silicone Elastomers Used in Medical Applications[5]
F 624 Guide for Evaluation of Thermoplastic Polyurethane Solids and Solutions for Biomedical Applications[5]
F 641 Specification for Implantable Epoxy Electronic Encapsulants[5]
F 665 Classification for Vinyl Chloride Plastics Used in Biomedical Application[5]
F 702 Specification for Polysulfone Resin for Medical Applications[5]
F 748 Practice for Selecting Generic Biological Test Methods for Materials and Devices[5]
F 749 Practice for Evaluating Material Extracts by Intracutaneous Injection in the Rabbit[5]
F 755 Specification for Selection of Porous Polyethylene for Use in Surgical Implants[5]
F 756 Practice for Assessment of Hemolytic Properties of Materials[5]
F 763 Practice for Short-Term Screening of Implant Materials[5]
F 813 Practice for Direct Contact Cell Culture Evaluation of Materials for Medical Devices[5]
F 895 Test Method for Agar Diffusion Cell Culture Screening for Cytotoxicity[5]
F 981 Practice for Assessment of Compatibility of Biomaterials for Surgical Implants with Respect to Effect of Materials on Muscle and Bone[5]
F 997 Specification for Polycarbonate Resin for Medical Applications[3]
F 1088 Specification for Beta-Tricalcium Phosphate for Surgical Implantation[5]
F 1185 Specification for Composition of Ceramic Hydroxylapatite for Surgical Implants[5]
F 1251 Terminology Relating to Polymeric Biomaterials in Medical and Surgical Devices[5]
F 1425 Specification for Virgin Poly (L-lactic Acid) Resin for Surgical Implants[3]
F 1439 Guide for Performance of Lifetime Bioassay for the Tumorigenic Potential of Implant Materials[5]
F 1472 Specification for Wrought Ti-6Al-4V Alloy for Surgical Implant Applications[5]
F 1579 Specification for Polyaryletherketone (PAEK) Resins for Surgical Implant Applications[5]
F 1581 Specification for Composition of Anorganic Bone for Surgical Implants[5]
F 1634 Practice for In Vitro Environmental Conditioning of Polymer Matrix Composite Materials and Implant Devices[5]
F 1635 Test Method for In Vitro Degradation testing of Poly (L-Lactic Acid) Resin and Fabricated Forms for Surgical Implants[5]
F 1855 Specification for Polyoxymethylene Acetal for

[1] This guide is under the jurisdiction of ASTM Committee F04 on Medical and Surgical Materials and Devicesand is the direct responsibility of Subcommittee F04.43on Tissue Engineered Biomaterials.

Current edition approved May 10, 2000. Published August 2000.

[2] *Annual Book of ASTM Standards*, Vol 08.01.

[3] Discontinued; see *1997 Annual Book of ASTM Standards*, Vol 08.01.

[4] *Annual Book of ASTM Standards*, Vol 11.05.

[5] *Annual Book of ASTM Standards*, Vol 13.01.

Medical Applications[5]

F 1876 Standard Specification for Polyetherketoneetherketoneketone (PEKEKK) Resins for Surgical Implant Applications[5]

F 1926 Test Method for Evaluation of the Environmental Stability of Calcium Phosphate Coatings[5]

2.2 *Other Document:*

U.S. Pharmacopeia, Edition XXIII[6]

2.3 *ISO Standards:*[7]

ISO 6474:1994 Implants for Surgery - Ceramic Materials Based on Alumina

ISO 10993-1, Biological Evaluation of Medical Devices—Part 1: Evaluation and testing

ISO 10993-9—Part 9: Framework for identification and quantification of potential degradation products

ISO 10993-12 - Part 12: Sample preparation and reference materials

ISO/DIS 10993-13 - Part 13: Identification and quantification of potential degradation products from polymeric medical devices

ISO/DIS 10993-14 - Part 14: Identification and quantification of potential degradation products from ceramics

ISO/DIS 10993-15—Part 15: Identification and quantification of potential degradation products from metals and alloys

ISO/DIS 10993-17—Part 17: Methods for the establishment of allowable limits for leachable substances using health-based risk assessment

ISO/CD 10993-18—Part 18: Chemical characterization of materials

ISO/NWI 10993-19—Part 19: Physico-chemical, mechanical and morphological characterization of materials

prEN 12442-1 Animal tissues and their derivatives utilized in the manufacture of medical devices—Part 1: Analysis and management of risk

prEN 12442-2—Part 2: Controls on sourcing, collection and handling

prEN 12442-3—Part 3: Validation of the elimination and/or inactivation of virus and transmissible agents

ISO 111607 Product packaging

2.4 Code of Federal Regulations, Title 21, Part 820. Federal Register Vol. 43, No 141. July 21, 1978[8]

3. Terminology

3.1 *Definitions:*

3.1.1 *natural materials*, *n*—synthesized or produced by living cells.

3.1.2 *substrates*, *n*—raw or virgin materials that will ultimately be used in tissue-engineered medical products for growth, support, or delivery of cells or biomolecules.

[6] Available from US Pharmacopia, Vol. 23 Mack Publishing Co., Easton, PA, 1995.

[7] Available from the American National Standards Institute, 25 W. 43rd St., 4th Floor, New York, NY 10036.

[8] National Archives and Records Administration, 700 Pennsylvania Ave, NW, Washington, DC 20408.

4. Descriptive Chemical and Physical Information

4.1 The substrate material shall have specifications for an extensive set of chemical and physical properties such as, but not limited to, those listed in Table 1.

4.2 The necessary chemical and physical tests are a function of the class of material (for example, ceramic, polymer, metal, composite, or natural material). Each type of material has specific sets of properties to be specified. Natural polymers such as collagen or demineralized bone, and natural ceramics such as anorganic bone, are considered a subset of the polymers and ceramics categories respectively. The following AAMI, ISO, ASTM, and other recognized voluntary standards committee standards, include specific techniques for determining the chemical and physical properties listed in Table 1 and are suggested as guides for new standards development or for interim use for those materials without existing standards.

4.2.1 *Metals*—Specification F 1472, Specification F 560, Specification F 67, and ISO/DIS 10993-15 - Part 15.

4.2.2 *Ceramics*, (for example, calcium phosphate, calcium carbonate, aluminum oxide, glasses) Specification F 603, Specification F 1088, Specification F 1185, Specification F 1581, Test Method F 1926, ISO 6474:1994, and ISO/DIS 10993-14 - Part 14.

4.2.3 *Polymers*—Specification D 1763, Practice D 1898, Specification F 451, Specification F 604, Guide F 624, Specification F 641, Classification F 665, Specification F 702, Specification F 755, Specification F 997, Terminology F 1251, Specification F 1425, Specification F 1579, Practice F 1634, Test Method F 1635, Specification F 1855, Specification F 1876, and ISO/DIS 10993-13 - Part 13.

4.2.4 Other General Test Methods—ISO/CD 10993-18—Part 18, ISO/NWI 10993-19—Part 19.

4.3 The following web site is suggested as an additional resource for relevant existing standards: www.fda.gov/cdrh/modact/recstand.html.

5. Sampling

5.1 It is suggested that the requirements shall be determined for each lot of the substrate material by sampling sizes and procedures in accordance with Practice D 1898 or some other equivalent.

6. Handling, Packaging, and Labeling

6.1 The product should be handled and packaged as specified in USP 661 or ISO 111607 and prEN 12442-2 — Part 2, and ISO 111607.

TABLE 1

Chemical	Physical
Composition	density
Purity	molecular weight
Stability during storage	viscosity
Additives	compresseion strength
Trace elements	tension strength
Extractables (metals or solvents)	elastic modulus
Degradation kinetics	fatigue strength
Resorption kinetics	yield strength
Resorption kinetics	hardness
Degradation products	foreign particles
	structure - long range
	- short range

7. Quality Program Requirements

7.1 The manufacturer should conform to Quality Systems Regulations (see CFR 21, Part 820) or its equivalent.

8. Biocompatibility

8.1 Many materials have been shown to produce a well-characterized level of biological response following long-term clinical use in laboratory animals. When new applications of a material, or modifications to the material or physical forms of the material, are being considered, then the recommendations and test methods of the following standards should be considered: Practice F 748, F 619, Practice F 749, Practice F 756, Practice F 763, Practice F 813, Practice F 981, and Guide F 1439-92 as well as Test Method F 895, ISO 10993-1, ISO/DIS 10993-9, Part 9, ISO/DIS 10993-17 - Part 17, prEN 12442-1 – Part 1, and prEN 12442-3– Part 3.

9. Keywords

9.1 biomaterials; ceramics; composites; materials; metals; polymers; substrates; tissue-engineered medical products

Standard Test Methods for the Dynamic Evaluation of Glenoid Loosening or Disassociation[1]

This standard is issued under the fixed designation F 2028; the number immediately following the designation indicates the year of original adoption or, in the case of revision, the year of last revision. A number in parentheses indicates the year of last reapproval. A superscript epsilon (ε) indicates an editorial change since the last revision or reapproval.

1. Scope

1.1 These test methods measure how much a prosthetic glenoid component rocks or pivots following cyclic displacement of the humeral head to opposing glenoid rims (for example, superior-inferior or anterior-posterior). Performance is judged by the tensile displacement opposite each loaded rim after dynamic rocking.

1.2 The same setup can be used to test the locking mechanism of modular glenoid components, for example, for disassociation.

1.3 The test method covers shoulder replacement designs with both monolithic and modular humeral and glenoid components with either cemented or noncemented fixation.

1.4 The values stated in SI units are to be regarded as the standard. The values given in parentheses are provided for information purposes only.

2. Referenced Documents

2.1 *ASTM Standards:*

E 4 Practices for Force Verification of Testing Machines[2]

F 1378 Specification for Shoulder Prostheses[3]

F 1839 Specification for Rigid Polyurethane Foam for Use as a Standard Material for Testing Orthopaedic Devices and Instruments[3]

3. Terminology

3.1 *Definitions:*

3.1.1 *glenoid*—the prosthetic portion that replaces the glenoid fossa of the scapula and articulates with a prosthetic replacement of the humeral head. It may consist of one or more components from one or more materials, for example, either all-polyethylene or a metal baseplate with a polymeric insert.

3.1.2 *humeral head*—the prosthetic portion that replaces the proximal humerus or humeral head and articulates with the natural glenoid fossa or a prosthetic replacement.

3.1.3 *glenoid plane*—see Fig. 1. In symmetric glenoids, the plane is defined by joining the two articular edges; in planar and asymmetric glenoids, it is defined by the back surface.

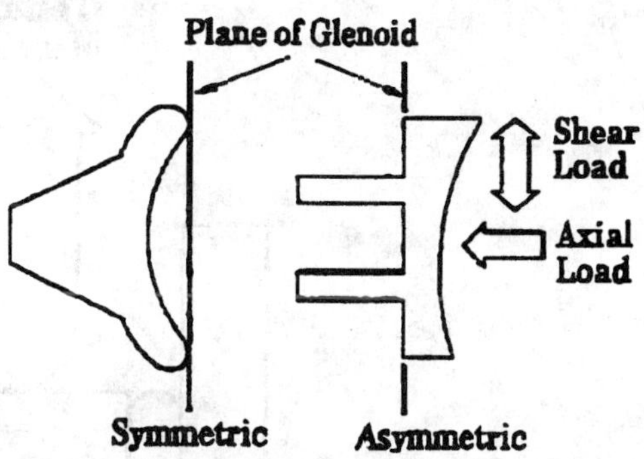

FIG. 1 Glenoid Plane and Load Directions

3.1.4 *axial load; axial translation*—the force and displacement, respectively, perpendicular to the glenoid plane; the axial load simulates the net compressive external and muscle forces (see Fig. 1).

3.1.5 *shear load; shear translation*—the force and displacement, respectively, parallel to the glenoid plane, applied, for example, in the superior/inferior or anterior/posterior direction (see Figs. 1 and 2); the shear load simulates the net shear external and active and passive soft tissue forces.

3.1.6 *subluxation load*—the peak shear load required for subluxation, for example, the peak resistive force at the glenoid articular rim opposing movement of the humeral head.

3.1.7 *subluxation translation*—the distance from the glenoid origin (see Fig. 2), parallel to the glenoid plane, to the point at which the subluxation load occurs.

3.1.8 *superior/inferior (SI), anterior/posterior (AP)*—the SI axis is the longest dimension and the AP axis the widest dimension of the glenoid (see Fig. 2).

3.1.9 *edge displacements*—the translation, perpendicular to the glenoid plane, of a specific point on the outside edge of the glenoid, when subjected to loading (see Fig. 3).

---

[1] This test method is under the jurisdiction of ASTM Committee F04 on Medical and Surgical Materials and Devices and is the direct responsibility of Subcommittee F04.22 on Arthroplasty.

Current edition approved May 10, 2000. Published August 2000.

[2] *Annual Book of ASTM Standards*, Vol 03.01.

[3] *Annual Book of ASTM Standards*, Vol 13.01.

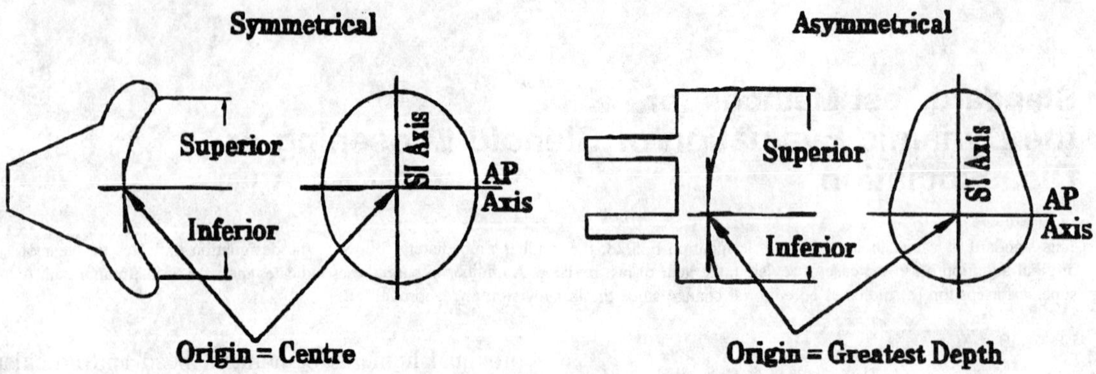

FIG. 2 Glenoid Axes and Origin

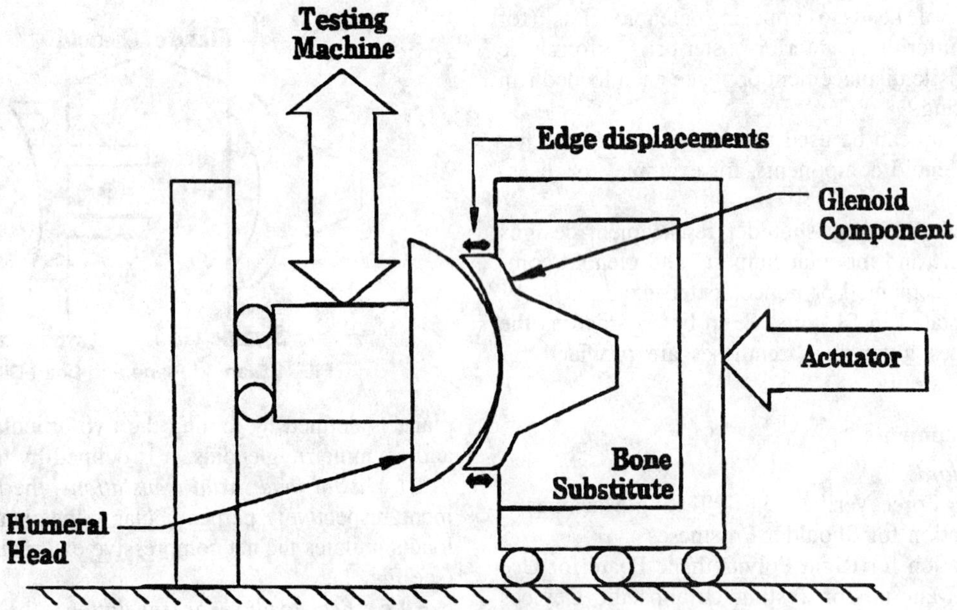

FIG. 3 Biaxial Testing Apparatus

GLENOID LOOSENING TEST METHOD

4. Summary of Test Method

4.1 The prosthetic glenoid component is fixed into a bone substitute using the normal surgical technique.

4.2 The subluxation translation is determined experimentally on additional components. This is accomplished, using a biaxial apparatus (see Fig. 3). by applying an axial load perpendicular to the glenoid, then translating the humeral head parallel to the glenoid plane until encountering a peak shear load. This is performed in both directions, corresponding to the direction of intended rocking (for example, superior-inferior, anterior-posterior, or an alternative angle).

4.3 The edge displacements of the glenoid are measured before cycling: a given axial load is first applied perpendicular to the glenoid, then the edge displacements are measured with the humeral head in three positions: at the glenoid origin, and positioned to 90 % of the subluxation translation (see X1.2), in both directions, as defined in 4.2. (Cycling to 90 % of the subluxation load would be acceptable, but is not practically feasible as a result of the large displacements, quick speeds, and deformable polyethylene.)

4.4 The humeral head is cycled to 90 % of the subluxation distance for a fixed number of cycles.

4.5 The edge displacements (4.3) are either repeated following the cycling or measured continuously during the cycling.

5. Significance and Use

5.1 This test method is intended to investigate the resistance of a glenoid component to loosening. Glenoid loosening is the most common clinical complication in total shoulder arthroplasty (see X1.1). The method assumes that loosening occurs because of edge loading, often called the rocking-horse phenomenon.

5.2 The test method can be used both to detect potential problems and to compare design features. Factors affecting loosening performance include articular geometry, flange geometry, materials, fixation design, bone quality, and surgical technique.

6. Apparatus and Equipment

6.1 The test apparatus shall be constructed such that an axial load is applied perpendicular to the glenoid plane and a shear load is applied parallel to the glenoid plane (see Fig. 1). Fig. 3 shows the axial load to be horizontal and the shear load to be vertical; however, this arrangement may be reversed.

6.2 A bone substitute representing the strength or glenoid cancellous bone (see X1.5) shall be used. If a polyurethane foam is used, it shall conform to Specification F 1839.

6.3 The glenoid and humeral head shall be enclosed in a chamber with water heated to 37°C (98.6°F) ± 2°C (3.6°F), at least for the dynamic portion of the test (see X1.6). A buffer may be added, if the tester deems this necessary.

6.4 A means to measure the axial load, shear load, shear translation, and glenoid edge displacements is required. A means to measure the axial translation is desirable.

6.5 The tests win be performed on either mechanical or hydraulic load frames with adequate load capacity and shall meet the criteria of Practices E 4.

7. Sampling and Test Specimens

7.1 A minimum of three samples shall be tested. At least two additional components should be used to determine the subluxation translation. The test may be conducted along the superior-inferior axis, the anterior-posterior axis, or another axis of interest to the user.

7.2 All glenoid components shall be in the final manufactured condition. All plastic components shall be sterilized according to the manufacturer-recommended specifications for clinical use.

7.3 The humeral head shall include the identical radius or radii and material as the actual implant. Other features of the humeral component such as the shaft may be omitted. The same head may be used for all tests unless the surface becomes damaged.

7.4 Glenoid and humeral components axe used in total shoulder arthroplasty and should conform to the criteria specified in Specification F 1378.

8. Procedure

8.1 The following steps are common to both the subluxation (4.2) and rocking (4.3-4.5) tests:

8.1.1 Secure the glenoid component in a bone substitute using the normal surgical procedure and instrumentation using bone cement for cemented components and mechanical fixation for noncemented components. Do not perform tests until the cement has properly cured.

8.1.2 Position the path of the humeral head on the glenoid within ±0.5 mm (sideways) of the desired path, for example, by using a dye to locate the contact point of the humeral head; a dye is unnecessary for congruent prostheses. Locate the center of the path (for the subluxation test, this need not be exact; for the rocking test, the peak loads at each rim during cycling should be within ±10 % of each other for symmetrical designs).

8.1.3 Perform the static measurements (subluxation and edge displacements) either in air at room temperature or in water at 37°C. The cyclic testing must be performed in 37°C water (see 6.3, X1.3, and X1.6).

8.1.4 Apply a given axial load to the glenoid, for example, 750 N (169 lb) ± 7.5 N (see X1.4).

8.2 Determine the subluxation translation experimentally on separate components (see X1.2):

8.2.1 After applying the axial load, displace the humeral head at a constant rate to a given displacement ensuring that a peak load is achieved in both directions. A rate of 50 mm/min (2 in./min) is recommended to avoid polyethylene creep.

8.2.2 Yielding is expected at the recommended load and does not constitute a failure. The test shall be terminated if the insert of a modular glenoid disassociates.

8.2.3 Record the axial load, subluxation load, and subluxation translation.

8.3 Measure the edge displacements before rocking:

8.3.1 Create a foundation for measurements at both ends of the glenoid at a similar distance from the back surface of the glenoid for all prostheses. One possibility is to insert 2-mm-diameter screws into the outside edge at each end of the glenoid prosthesis, parallel to the articular surface (to avoid exiting either into the articular surface or into the bone substitute); flatten the screw head parallel to the glenoid plane. Alternative methods are acceptable.

8.3.2 Rest a displacement measuring device, for example, an LVDT, DVRT, or dial gauge, on each foundation to measure the displacements perpendicular to the glenoid plane. Continuous measurement is desirable, but measurement at the beginning and end of the rocking is sufficient.

8.3.3 Condition the prosthesis/bone substitute system, for example, for ten cycles at 0.25 Hz.

8.3.4 Measure the edge displacements with the humeral head located at the glenoid origin (see Fig. 2).

8.3.5 Translate the humeral head parallel to the glenoid plane to 90 % of the subluxation translation determined previously (8.2) in one direction. Measure both edge displacements.

8.3.6 Translate the humeral head to 90 % of the subluxation translation in the opposite direction and measure both edge displacements.

8.3.7 Repeat the three readings at least once to ensure repeatability.

8.4 Cyclically translate the humeral head to 90 % of the subluxation translation to cause a rocking motion of the glenoid at a given frequency (for example, 2 Hz as a result of the large translations, or up to a maximum of 6 Hz) to a maximum number of cycles (for example, 100 000, see X1.7). Maintain the axial load and specified displacement.

8.5 Terminate the test when either the maximum number of cycles has been reached or a modular glenoid insert disassociates.

8.6 Repeat the glenoid edge displacement measurements (8.3) if measurements were not taken continuously.

8.7 Testing may be continued to a higher number of cycles if desired.

9. Report

9.1 The test report shall include the following:

9.1.1 All details relevant to the particular implants tested including type, size, and lot number as well as the glenoid radius, humeral head radius or radii, and the prosthesis material.

9.1.2 The axis and direction of testing, for example, central-superior-inferior.

9.1.3 *Subluxation Test*—The subluxation load and translation for each specimen, as well as the axial load and displacement rate. A chart plotting the load versus displacement with the 90 and 100 % subluxation loads clearly marked should be included.

9.1.4 *Rocking Test*—The axial load, cyclic displacement, maximum number of cycles, testing frequency, and cause of test termination. Testing parameters that differ from those recommended shall be justified.

9.1.5 *Displacement Test*—The edge displacements before and following cycling, highlighting the tensile displacement on the unloaded side following rocking (for example, the displacement opposite the loaded side minus the value with the head at the glenoid origin).

9.1.6 If the amplitude of the axial translation decreases suddenly during the test (indicating a tilt of the glenoid and the probable onset of loosening), the number of cycles at which this occurred should be recorded.

10. Precision and Bias

10.1 The precision and bias of this test method has not been established. Test results that could be used to establish precision and bias are solicited.

11. Keywords

11.1 arthroplasty; glenoid; loosening; subluxation; total shoulder replacement

MODULAR DISASSOCIATION TEST METHOD

12. Summary of Test Method

12.1 The prosthetic glenoid component is fixed in to a bone substitute or grouting agent using the normal surgical technique.

12.2 The subluxation translation is determined experimentally on the intended test samples or additional components. This is accomplished, using a biaxial apparatus (see Fig. 3), by first applying an axial load perpendicular to the glenoid, then translating the humeral head parallel to the glenoid plane until encountering a peak shear load. This is performed in both directions, corresponding to the direction of intended rocking (for example, superior-inferior, anterior-posterior, or an alternative angle).

12.3 The humeral head is cycled to 90 % of the subluxation distance for a fixed number of cycles (see X1.2). (Cycling to 90 % of the subluxation load would be acceptable, but is not practically feasible because of the large displacements, quick speeds, and deformable polyethylene.)

13. Significance and Use

13.1 This test method is intended to investigate the locking mechanism of a modular glenoid. Disassociation of the insert is the greatest issue in modular glenoid components. The test method can be used either to detect potential problems or to compare design features.

14. Apparatus and Equipment

14.1 The test apparatus shall be constructed such that an axial load is applied perpendicular to the glenoid plane and a shear load is applied parallel to the glenoid plane (see Fig. 1). Fig. 3 shows the axial load to be horizontal and the shear load to be vertical; however, this arrangement may be reversed.

14.2 The glenoid and humeral head shall be enclosed in a chamber with water heated to 37°C (98.6°F) ± 2°C (3.6°F), at least for the dynamic portion of the test (see X1.6). A buffer may be added, if the tester deems this necessary.

14.3 A means to measure the axial load and shear translation is required.

14.4 The tests will be performed on either mechanical or hydraulic load frames with adequate load capacity and shall meet the criteria of Practices E 4.

15. Sampling and Test Specimens

15.1 A minimum of three samples shall be tested. The test may be conducted along the superior-inferior axis, the anterior-posterior axis, or another axis of interest to the user. The initial shear displacement or load should be set just below the subluxation displacement or load. Each test will result either in a failure or, if no disassociation occurs within the set number of cycles, a runout. The load should be progressively stepped down until at least one runout occurs.

15.2 All glenoid components shall be in the final manufactured condition. All plastic components shall be sterilized according to the manufacturer-recommended specifications for clinical use.

15.3 The humeral head shall include the identical radius or radii and material as the actual implant. Other features of the humeral component such as the shaft may be omitted. The same head may be used for all tests unless the surface becomes damaged.

15.4 Glenoid and humeral components are used in total shoulder arthroplasty and should conform to the criteria specified in Specification F 1378.

16. Procedure

16.1 The following steps are common to both the subluxation (12.2) and rocking (12.3) tests:

16.1.1 Secure the glenoid component in a bone substitute using the normal surgical procedure and instrumentation, using bone cement for cemented components and mechanical fixation for noncemented components. Do not perform tests until the cement has properly cured.

16.1.2 Position the path of the humeral head on the glenoid within ±0.5 mm (sideways) of the desired path, for example, by using a dye to locate the contact point of the humeral head; a dye is unnecessary for congruent prostheses. Locate the center of the path (for the subluxation test, this need not be exact; for the rocking test, the peak loads at each run during cycling should be within ±10 % of each other for symmetrical designs).

16.1.3 Perform the measurements in 37°C water (see 14.2, X1.3 and X1.6).

16.1.4 Apply a given axial load to the glenoid, for example, 750 N (169 lb) ± 7.5 N (see X1.4).

16.2 Determine the subluxation translation experimentally on the intended test specimens or separate components (see X1.2):

16.2.1 After applying the axial load, displace the humeral head at a constant rate to a given displacement ensuring that a peak load is achieved in both directions. A rate of 50 mm/min (2 in./min) is recommended to avoid polyethylene creep.

16.2.2 Yielding is expected at the recommended load and does not constitute a failure. The test shall be terminated if the modular insert disassociates.

16.2.3 Record the axial load and subluxation translation. The subluxation load is not required for the rocking test, but may be of interest to characterize the prosthesis.

16.3 Cyclically translate the humeral head to 90 % of the subluxation translation to cause a rocking motion of the glenoid at a given frequency (for example, 2 Hz as a result of the large translations, or up to a maximum of 6 Hz) to a maximum number of cycles (for example, 100 000 or higher, see X1.7). Maintain the axial load and specified displacement.

16.4 Terminate the test when either the maximum number of cycles has been reached or the glenoid insert disassociates. The load should be set high enough to produce a failure, then reduced to produce at least one runout.

16.5 Testing may be continued to a higher number of cycles if desired.

17. Report

17.1 The test report shall include the following:

17.1.1 All details relevant to the particular implants tested including type, size, and lot number as well as the glenoid radius, humeral head radius or radii, and the prosthesis materials.

17.1.2 The axis and direction of testing, for example, central-superior-inferior.

17.1.3 *Subluxation Test*—The subluxation load and translation for each specimen, as well as the axial load and displacement rate. A chart plotting the load versus displacement with the 90 and 100 % subluxation loads clearly marked should be included.

17.1.4 *Rocking Test*—The axial load, cyclic displacement, maximum number of cycles, testing frequency, and cause of test termination. Testing parameters that differ from those recommended shall be justified.

18. Precision and Bias

18.1 The precision and bias of this test method has not been established. Test results that could be used to establish precision and bias are solicited.

19. Keywords

19.1 arthroplasty; disassociation; glenoid; subluxation; total shoulder replacement

APPENDIX

(Nonmandatory Information)

X1. RATIONALE

X1.1 This test method characterizes the dynamic loosening of a glenoid component or the locking mechanism of a modular glenoid component. Glenoid loosening is the most common clinical complication in total shoulder arthroplasty **(1, 2)**, and modular disassociations have been reported clinically. Many surgeons consequently limit the indications for implanting a glenoid prosthesis **(2)** despite improvements in pain relief, range of motion, and patient satisfaction associated with glenoid replacement **(3)**. Although glenoid loosening is multifactorial **(2, 4)**, some designs showed high failure rates **(1, 2)**. Thus, a test that can compare the physical performance of different glenoid prostheses is valuable.

X1.2 The cyclic displacement was chosen to be close to (for example, 90 %) the subluxation translation because loosening is suggested to be due to eccentric loading on the glenoid rim **(1, 2, 4)**. Neither testing to a fixed translation nor testing to a fixed load would lead to rim loading for all shapes and sizes (imagine the very smallest, very largest, most constrained, and least constrained prostheses), thus a translation relative to the subluxation distance was chosen as the consistent criterion. Highly constrained prostheses have shown higher loosening rates **(2)** because all shoulder loads were transferred via the prosthesis to the bone. In less constrained designs, active and passive soft tissues carry a greater load. Thus higher loads for a more constrained design are justified. Cycling relative to the subluxation load would be justifiable, but is not practically feasible because of the large displacements, quick speeds, and deformable polyethylene. The subluxation translation must be determined experimentally because, as a result of polyethylene deformation, it cannot be predicted from rigid-body theory **(5)**. For example, the vertical rigid-body-predicted subluxation translation for a conforming prosthesis would be zero.

X1.3 Dynamic testing is necessary because the ranking of all-polyethylene prostheses cannot be predicted from the initial static prerocking measurements **(6)**.

X1.4 Although normal loading on the glenohumeral joint is low, even daily-living activities can exert several times body weight across the joint. An axial load of 750 N, as recommended in this test method, leads to resultant loads of between about 800 and 1000 N depending on the glenoid geometry or about one to one-and-a-half times body weight. This represents carrying a 5- to 8-kg object at the side or lifting a 2- to 4-kg load to shoulder height and is even less than that exerted while getting out of a chair or walking with a cane (**7**). Higher loads could be justified for component strength testing but do not represent typical performance.

X1.5 Glenoid loosening normally occurs at the bone-cement interface. Since this represents a system failure rather than component failure, the mechanical properties of the bone substitute are important (**8**). Although it is advantageous to use a consistent bone substitute, and cancellous bone represents the worst-case condition, the user is permitted to use a different bone model. At the load and cycle numbers used in this method, a gap does not typically occur between the prosthesis and bone substitute. The substrate is not important when testing for modular disassociation.

X1.6 The dynamic tests must be performed in water because testing in air resulted in disintegration of the bone substitute, extrusion of the cement, and component breakage. The water acts both as a lubricant and a temperature controller. A modular locking mechanism should be tested at 37°C since the properties of polyethylene change with temperature. Circulation of the water is recommended, but not required because of the relatively short duration of the test.

X1.7 The number of cycles is currently suggested to be 100 000 because the test does not investigate component strength; activities causing higher loads at the shoulder occur much less frequently than in the lower limb; and people with shoulder prostheses would be expected to load their arms even less frequently. This number of cycles would represent approximately 25 higher-load activities a day for 10 years. Testing may be continued to a higher number of cycles if desired, especially when testing a modular locking mechanism.

REFERENCES

(**1**) Cofield, R.H. and Edgerton, B.C., "Total shoulder arthroplasty: complications and revision surgery," *Inst. Course Lect.*, 39:(1990)449-462.

(**2**) Wirth, M.A. and Rockwood, C.A., Jr., "Current concepts review: complications of total shoulder replacement arthroplasty," *J. Bone Joint Surg [Am.]*, 78A(4):(1996)603-616.

(**3**) Boyd, A.D., Thomas, W.H., Scott, R.D., et al, "Total shoulder arthroplasty versus hemiarthroplasty," *J. Arthroplasty*, 5(4):(1990)329-336.

(**4**) Franklin, J.L., Barrett, W.P., Jackins, S.E., and Matsen, F.A. III, "Glenoid loosening in total shoulder arthroplasty: association with rotator cuff deficiency," *J. Arthroplasty*, 3(1):(1988)39-46.

(**5**) Anglin, C., Wyss, U.P., and Pichora, D.R., "Shoulder prosthesis subluxation: theory and experiment," *J. Shoulder Elbow Surgery* (2000).

(**6**) Anglin, C., Wyss, U.P., and Pichora, D.R., "Mechanical testing of shoulder prostheses and recommendations for glenoid design," *J. Shoulder Elbow Surgery* (2000).

(**7**) Anglin, C., Wyss, U.P., and Pichora, D.R., "Glenohumeral contact forces," *Proc. Instn. Mech. Engrs. [H]* (2000).

(**8**) Anglin, C., Tolhurst, P., Wyss, U.P., and Pichora, D.R., "Glenoid cancellous bone strength and modulus," *J. Biomechanics*, 32(10):(1999)1091-1097.

Standard Specification for Total Hip Joint Prosthesis and Hip Endoprosthesis Bearing Surfaces Made of Metallic, Ceramic, and Polymeric Materials[1]

This standard is issued under the fixed designation F 2033; the number immediately following the designation indicates the year of original adoption or, in the case of revision, the year of last revision. A number in parentheses indicates the year of last reapproval. A superscript epsilon (ε) indicates an editorial change since the last revision or reapproval.

1. Scope

1.1 This specification covers the requirements for the mating bearing surfaces of total hip prostheses and hip endoprostheses. More specifically, this specification covers hip joint replacement of the ball-and-socket configuration. This specification does not address the tolerance match between the mating bearing surfaces.

1.2 This specification covers the sphericity, surface finish requirements, and dimensional tolerances for the spherical articulating metallic or ceramic femoral heads of total hip joint prostheses.

1.3 This specification covers the sphericity, surface finish requirements, and dimensional tolerances for the spherical concave mating surface of metallic and ceramic acetabular components, including the inner polymeric bearing surface of bipolar heads, and the surface finish requirements and dimensional tolerances for the spherical concave mating surface of polymeric acetabular components.

1.4 This specification covers the sphericity and surface finish requirements for the spherical metallic or ceramic femoral heads of hip endoprostheses, and the outer bearing surface of bipolar heads.

1.5 The values stated in SI units are to be regarded as the standard.

1.6 This specification is intended for standard practice regarding the design of total hip joint bearing surfaces. Additionally, the tolerances imposed on the polymeric portion of the bearing surface are intentionally large due to temperature-induced size changes and other manufacturing concerns. Some manufacturing methods or designs may intentionally reduce the diameter of the polymeric bearing to more closely mate with the diameter of the head.

2. Referenced Documents

2.1 *ASTM Standards:*

F 370 Specification for Proximal Femoral Endoprostheses[2]

2.2 *ISO Documents:*

ISO 468 Surface Roughness-Parameters, Their Values, and General Rules for Specifying Requirements[3]

ISO 4287/1 Surface Roughness - Terminology[3]

ISO 4291 Methods for the Assessment of Departure from Roundness, Measurement of Variations, and Radius[3]

ISO 5436 Surface Texture of Products – Calibration Specimens for Stylus Instruments[3]

ISO 6318-1985 Measurement of Roundness—Terms, Definitions, and Parameters of Roundness (Equivalent to BS 3730 Part 1: 1987)[3]

ISO 7206-1 Implants for Surgery—Partial and Total Hip Joint Prosthesis—Part I: Classification, Designation of Dimensions, and Requirements[3]

ISO 7206-2 Implants for Surgery—Partial and Total Hip Joint Prosthesis—Part II: Bearing Surfaces Made of Metallic and Plastics Materials[3]

2.3 *ANSI/ASME Document:*

ANSI/ASME B46.1-1995 Surface Texture[3]

3. Dimensions and Characteristics

3.1 *Definition:*

3.1.1 *Pole of the Articulating Surface*—The pole of an articulating surface is defined by a point at the intercept of the revolution axis of the component and the spherical articulation surface.

3.1.2 *Equator of the Articulating Surface*—The equator of the articulating surface is the circle normal to the revolution axis of the component, the center of which is the center of the spherical articulating surface.

3.1.3 *Cutoff Length*—The cutoff length defines the maximal value of the mean twist of profile irregularities that shall be considered in the roughness measurement, that is, with a cutoff length of 0.8 mm, the profile irregularities with a mean twist higher than 0.8 mm shall not be considered.

3.1.3.1 Precise definitions of roughness parameters, cutoff length, and roundness are given in ISO 4287/1, ISO 5436, ISO 4291, and ISO 6318:1985.

3.1.4 *Stylus Tip*—The stylus tip is the tip of the measuring device (diamond or Focodyn) which measures the surface

---

[1] This specification is under the jurisdiction of ASTM Committee F04 on Medical and Surgical Materials and Devices and is the direct responsibility of Subcommittee F04.22 on Arthroplasty.

Current edition approved Nov. 10, 2000. Published January 2001.

Originally published as F2033-00. Last previous edition F2033–00.

[2] *Annual Book of ASTM Standards*, Vol 13.01.

[3] Available from American National Standards Institute, 11 W. 42nd St., 13th Floor, New York, NY 10036.

roughness. A stylus has a pseudoconical shape with a hemispherical tip. Typical sizes for the tip are 2, 5, or 10 μm. The selection of the stylus tip is dependent on the range of the roughness measured.

3.2 *Total Hip Joint Prosthesis*:

3.2.1 *Femoral Head*:

3.2.1.1 When inspected visually under 5-diopter magnification, the bearing surface shall be free from particles, scratches, and score marks other than those arising from the finishing process.

3.2.1.2 *Sphericity*—The metal or ceramic spherical bearing surface of a femoral hip component shall have a departure from roundness of not greater than 10 μm (390 μin.) This shall be measured as ΔZ_z in accordance with the Minimum Zone Center Method in ISO 4291 measuring the roundness in more than two planes, or by the method in Appendix X2. For metallic femoral heads used in conjunction with metallic acetabular components and ceramic femoral heads used in conjunction with ceramic acetabular components, the departure from roundness values shall not be greater than 5 μm (200 μin.).

3.2.1.3 *Surface Finish*—When measured in accordance with ISO 468 or ANSI/ASME B46.1, the spherical bearing surface of a femoral component shall have a R_a value not greater than 0.05 μm (2 μin.). The measurements shall be taken at the location of the pole and 30° from the pole.

3.2.1.4 *Dimensional Tolerances*—The spherical bearing surface shall have a diameter equal to the nominal diameter with a tolerance of +0.0, −0.2 mm (+0.000, −0.008 in.)

3.2.1.5 For metallic femoral heads used in conjunction with metallic acetabular components, or ceramic femoral heads used in conjunction with ceramic acetabular components, the manufacturer should report the diameters and tolerances of the heads, if different from the tolerance values in 3.2.1.4.

3.2.2 *Polymeric Acetabular Components*:

3.2.2.1 When inspected visually under 5-diopter magnification, the bearing surface shall be free from particles, scratches, and score marks other than those arising from the finishing process.

3.2.2.2 *Surface Finish*—When measured in accordance ISO 468 or ANSI/ASME B46.1, the spherical bearing surface of the acetabular component shall have a R_a value not greater than 2 μm (80 μin.)

3.2.2.3 *Dimensional Tolerances*—The spherical socket shall have a diameter equal to the nominal diameter within a tolerance of +0.3, −0.0 mm (+0.012, −0.0 in) at a temperature of 20 ± 2°C (68 ± 4°F). The socket should be oversized to the nominal within the given tolerance range.

3.2.3 *Metallic Acetabular Components*:

3.2.3.1 When inspected visually under 5-diopter magnification, the bearing surface shall be free from particles, scratches, and score marks other than those arising from the finishing process.

3.2.3.2 *Sphericity*—The spherical bearing surface of the metal acetabular component shall have a departure from roundness of not greater than 5 μm (200 μin.). This shall be measured as ΔZ_z in accordance with the Minimum Zone Center Method in ISO 4291 measuring the roundness in more than two places, or as determined by the method in Appendix X2.

3.2.3.3 *Surface Finish*—When measured in accordance with ISO 468 or ANSI/ASME B46.1, the spherical bearing surface of the acetabular component shall have a R_a value of not greater than 0.05 μm (2 μin.).

3.2.3.4 Under maximum material condition (MMC), the articulating part of the socket and metallic head, there should be clearance and both components never produce an interference fit.

3.2.3.5 Metallic heads and sockets from different manufacturers should not be mated because the combinations of tolerances within the family, surface finish, and configuration for the different manufacturers may not have been validated through appropriate testing.

3.2.4 *Ceramic Acetabular Components*:

3.2.4.1 When inspected visually under 5-diopter magnification, the bearing surface shall be free from particles, scratches, and score marks other than those arising from the finishing process.

3.2.4.2 *Sphericity*—The ceramic spherical bearing surface of a acetabular component shall have a departure from roundness of not greater than 5 μm (200 μin.). This shall be measured as ΔZ_z in accordance with the Minimum Zone Center Method in ISO 4291 measuring the roundness in more than two planes, or as determined by the method in Appendix X2.

3.2.4.3 *Surface Finish*—When measured in accordance with ISO 468 or ANSI/ASME B46.1, the spherical bearing surface of the acetabular component shall have a R_a value of not greater than 0.05 μm (2 μin.).

3.2.4.4 Under MMC, the articulating part of the socket and ceramic head, there should be clearance and both components never produce an interference fit.

3.2.4.5 Ceramic heads and sockets from different manufacturers should not be mated because the combinations of tolerances within the family, surface finish, and configuration for the different manufacturers may not have been validated through appropriate testing.

3.3 *Hip Endoprostheses*, in accordance with Specification F 370:

3.3.1 *Sphericity*—The metal or ceramic spherical bearing surface of a femoral hip component shall have a departure from roundness of not greater than 100 μm (3940 μin.). This shall be measured as ΔZ_z in accordance with the Minimum Zone Center Method in ISO 4291 measuring the roundness in more than two planes, or as determined by the method in Appendix X2.

3.3.2 *Surface Finish*—When measured in accordance with ISO 468 or ANSI/ASME B46.1, the spherical bearing surface of femoral endoprostheses components shall have a R_a value not greater than 0.5 μm (20 μin.).

3.4 *Bipolar Heads*:

3.4.1 *Inner Surface*—The inner surface of bipolar heads shall comply with the specification in 3.1.2.

3.4.2 *Outer Surface*—The outer surface of bipolar heads shall comply with the specifications in 3.2.

4. Report

4.1 When reporting results of tests to evaluate total hip joint and hip endoprosthesis components for conformance to this specification, deviations from the specified stylus tip radius, cutoff length of the measuring instrument, and locations of the measurements shall be included.

5. Keywords

5.1 acetabular cup; arthroplasty; femoral head; roundness

APPENDIXES

(Nonmandatory Information)

X1. RATIONALE

NOTE X1.1—Individual designs may vary from this if there is good engineering rationale supporting the design modifications.

X1.1 The primary reasons for this specification are:

X1.1.1 To define common parameters for characterization of the roundness and surface finish requirements, and establish dimensional relationships for articulating metallic and ceramic femoral heads of total hip joint prosthesis.

X1.1.2 To characterize the surface finish requirements and dimensional relationships for the spherical concave mating surfaces of articulating components, such that the concave surfaces are always oversized compared to the mating femoral head.

X1.1.3 To characterize the roundness and surface finish requirements for the spherical femoral heads of hip endoprosthesis, the tolerance requirements being specified in Specification F 370

X1.1.4 To provide for interchangeability of femoral heads and acetabular cups.

X1.1.5 To provide for minimum dimensions based on acceptable clinical usage.

X1.2 This specification is based in ISO 7206-2.

X1.3 Tolerance mismatches between mating articulating surfaces are part of the design of the device. These mismatches tend to vary with design concepts and manufacturing philosophies. Consequently, they are not addressed in this specification.

X1.4 The specification of standardized nominal dimensions for femoral head diameters or acetabular cup inside diameters is beyond the scope of this specification.

X1.5 Roundness measured in more than one plane provides a measure of sphericity. The MZC method of measuring roundness is much more precise than the appended method of measuring sphericity. The MZC method of measuring roundness takes a large number of points around a section of the sphere and determines the roundness of that circle. By checking two or more nonparallel sections, sphericity can be assumed to be the maximum out-of-roundness. Where the appended method only uses 25 points over the whole surface and is allowed to ignore the pole as long as it is a negative feature. The appended method is not a preferred method to determine the sphericity of a femoral head and should only be used if no other method is available to measure roundness.

X1.6 The specification of standardized dimensions for femoral head diameters or acetabular socket diameters is beyond the scope of this specification.

X2. DETERMINATION OF THE GEOMETRIC PROPERTIES OF THE FEMORAL HEAD AND ACETABULAR COMPONENTS

X2.1 *Femoral Head*:

X2.1.1 Using a three-dimensional measuring machine, with a measuring stylus in accordance with the device to be tested, 25 points situated as shown in Fig. X2.1 shall be measured. The 25 points shall consist of 8 points spaced equally about the circumference of the planes AA, BB, and CC, and a measurement at the pole. If the articulating surface extends below the equator, then AA shall be coincident with the equator of the femoral ball. Otherwise, AA shall be a diametral plane, located within 1 mm of the border or the articulating surface. The angles a, b, and c are measured relative to the neck axis and shall be as follows:

$$c = a/3$$
$$b = 2a/3$$

NOTE X2.1—If AA is coincident with the equator, a = 90°, b = 60°, and c = 30°.

X2.1.2 Determine the average diameter by the least squares method as well as the coordinates of the center 0 of the sphere of average diameter.

X2.1.3 Determine the departure from roundness as the difference between the smaller and the larger measured distances from this 0 center.

X2.1.4 Determine the measured imprecision due to both the machine and the method. Imprecision on the average diameter shall include the factor departure from roundness.

X2.1.5 The same measures may be repeated on 24 points, excluding the polar point, in order to determine whether the polar point is in a depression (and thus does not significantly affect function) or is projecting.

X2.2 *Acetabular Component*:

X2.2.1 Using a three-dimensional measuring machine, with a measuring stylus in accordance with the device to be tested,

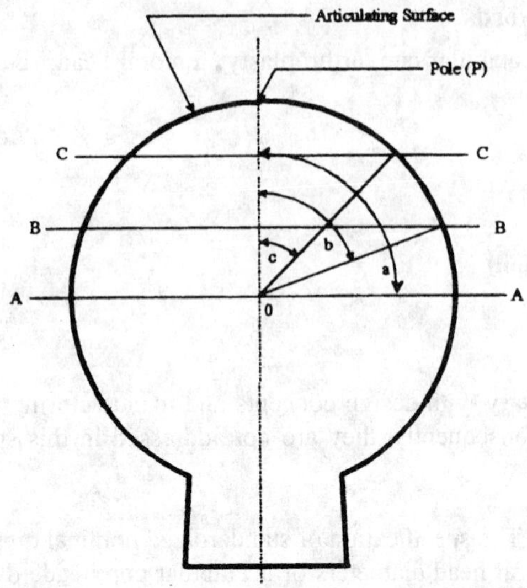

FIG. X2.1 Locations of Measurement Points on the Surface of the Femoral Head

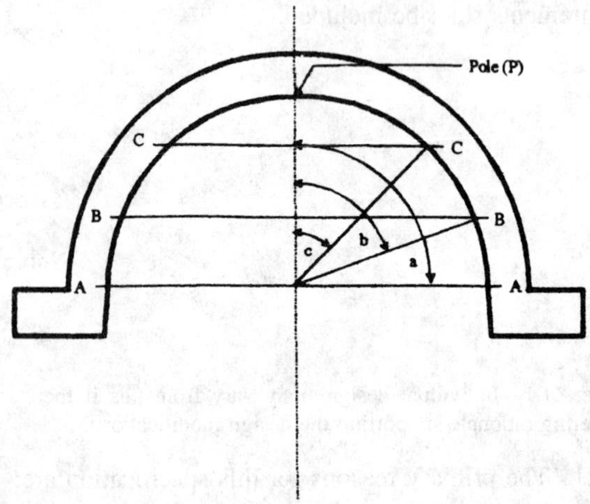

FIG. X2.2 Location of Measurement Points on the Acetabulum

25 points situated as shown in Fig. X2.2 shall be measured. The 25 points shall consist of 8 points spaced equally about the circumference of the planes AA, BB, and CC, and a measurement at the pole. If the articulating surface extends below the equator, then AA shall be coincident with the equator of the femoral ball. Otherwise, AA shall be a diametral plane, located within 1 mm of border or the articulating surface. The angles a, b, and c are measured relative to the neck axis and shall be as follows:

$$c = a/3$$
$$b = 2a/3$$

See Note X2.1.

X2.2.2 Determine the average diameter by the least squares method as well as the coordinates of the center 0 of the sphere of average diameter.

X2.2.3 Determine the departure from roundness as the difference between the smaller and the larger measured distances from this 0 center.

X2.2.4 Determine the measured imprecision due to both the machine and the method. Imprecision on the average diameter shall include the factor departure from roundness.

X3. ROUGHNESS MEASURES

X3.1 The roughness measurement R_a is used in this specification because it is a widely recognized parameter of roughness; it has a long history of use in literature regarding prosthetic joints; and it is specified in ISO 7606-2 (Rev 1996). A number of other surface roughness parameters may be calculated such as R_z, R_p, R_{max}, R_{tm}, R_p, R_{pm}, and others. However, the complex, three-dimensional topography of the surface of a femoral ball cannot be completely described by any single numerical parameter, and the relative influence of these roughness parameters on the friction and wear of the bearing surfaces has not yet been established. For this reason, it is recommended that a full characterization of the roughness characteristics of a given ball include several roughness parameters, as well as qualitative imaging, such as scanning electron microscopy.

Standard Guide for Silicone Elastomers, Gels and Foams Used in Medical Applications Part I — Formulations and Uncured Materials[1]

This standard is issued under the fixed designation F 2038; the number immediately following the designation indicates the year of original adoption or, in the case of revision, the year of last revision. A number in parentheses indicates the year of last reapproval. A superscript epsilon (ε) indicates an editorial change since the last revision or reapproval.

ε[1] NOTE—Fig. 2 was editorially revised in June 2001.

1. Scope

1.1 This guide is intended to educate potential users of silicone elastomers, gels and foams relative to their formulation and use. It does not provide information relative to silicone powders, fluids, and other silicones. The information provided is offered to guide users in the selection of appropriate materials, after consideration of the chemical, physical and toxicological properties of individual ingredients or by-products. This standard offers general information about silicone materials typically used for medical applications. Detail on the crosslinking and fabrication of silicone materials is found in Part II of this standard.

1.2 Fabrication and properties of elastomers is covered in the companion document, F 604, Part II. This monograph addresses only components of uncured elastomers, gels and foams.

1.3 Silicone biocompatibility issues can be addressed at several levels, but ultimately the device manufacturer must assess biological suitability relative to intended use.

1.4 *This standard does not purport to address all of the safety concerns, if any, associated with its use. It is the responsibility of the user of this standard to establish appropriate safety and health practices and determine the applicability of regulatory limitations prior to use.* Users are also advised to refer to Material Safety Data Sheets provided with uncured silicone components.

1.5 Biological and physical properties tend to be more reproducible when materials are manufactured in accordance with accepted quality standards such as ANSI ISO 9001 and current FDA Quality System Regulations/Good Manufacturing Practice Regulations.

2. Referenced Documents

2.1 *ASTM Standards:*

D 1566 Standard Terminology Relating to Rubber[2]

F 813 Standard Practice for Direct Contact Cell Culture Evaluation of Materials for Medical Devices [3]

2.2 *Sterility Standards:*[4]

ANSI/AAMI ST41 Good Hospital Practice: Ethylene Oxide Sterilization and Sterility Assurance

ANSI/AAMI ST50 Dry Heat (Heated Air) Sterilizers

ANSI/AAMI ST29 Recommended Practice for Determining Ethylene Oxide in Medical Devices

ANSI/AAM1 ST30 Determining Residual Ethylene Chlorohydrin and Ethylene Glycol in Medical Devices

AAMI 13409-251 Sterilization of Health Care Products—Radiation Sterilization—Substantiation of 25kGy as a Sterilization Dose for Small or Infrequent Production Batches

AAMI TIRS-251 Microbiological Methods for Gamma Irradiation Sterilization of Medical Devices

2.3 *Quality Standards*[5]*:*

ANSI/ASQC Q9001 Quality Systems—Model for Quality Assurance in Design, Development Production, Installation, and Servicing

21 CFR 820 Quality System Regulation (current revision)

21 CFR 210 Current Good Manufacturing Practice in Manufacturing, Processing, Packing or Holding of Drugs; General (current revision)

21 CFR 211 Current Good Manufacturing Practice for Finished Pharmaceuticals (current revision)

3. Terminology

3.1 Additional pertinent definitions can be found in standard D 1566.

3.2 *Definitions:*

3.2.1 *silicone polymer*—polymer chains having a backbone consisting of repeating silicon-oxygen atoms where each silicon atom bears two organic groups. The organic groups are typically methyl, but can be vinyl, phenyl, fluorine, or other organic groups.

3.2.2 *cyclics and linears*—low molecular weight volatile

[1] This specification is under the jurisdiction of ASTM Committee F04 on Medical and Surgical Materials and Devicesand is the direct responsibility of Subcommittee F04.11on Polymeric Materials.

Current edition approved June 10, 2000. Published September 2000.

[2] *Annual Book of ASTM Standards,* Vol. 09.01

[3] *Annual Book of ASTM Standards,* Vol. 13.01

[4] Available from the American National Standards Institute, 11 West 42nd St., 13th Floor, New York NY 10036.

[5] Available from the Superintendent of Documents, U.S. government Printing Office, Washington, DC 20402.

cyclic siloxane species are referred to using the "D" nomenclature which designates the number of Si-O linkages in the material (usually D_4-D_{20}); species from D_7 to D $_{40}$(or more) may be called "macrocyclics". Linears are straight chain oligomers that may be volatile or of higher molecular weight, depending on chain length; they are designated by "M" and "D" combinations, where "M" is R_3Si-O, and D is as explained above; "R" is usually methyl. (For example, MDM is $(CH_3)_3SiOSiOSi(CH_3)_3$). Low molecular weight species are present in silicone components to varying degrees depending on process and storage. The levels of macrocyclics that can be removed from silicone polymers by vacuum, high temperature stripping, or oven post-cure is dependent on the conditions used.

3.2.3 *catalyst*—a component of a silicone elastomer formulation that initiates the crosslinking reaction when the material is vulcanized.

3.2.4 *crosslinker or crosslinking agent*—a component of a silicone elastomer that is a reactant in the crosslinking reaction that occurs when an elastomer is vulcanized.

3.2.5 *inhibitor*—a component of a silicone elastomer added to moderate the rate of the crosslinking reaction.

3.2.6 *filler*—a finely divided solid that is intimately mixed with silicone polymers during manufacture to achieve specific properties. The fillers used in silicone elastomers are one of two types:

3.2.6.1 *reinforcing fillers*— usually have high surface areas and are amorphous in nature such as fumed or precipitated silica. Such fillers impart high strength and elastomeric physical properties to the elastomer.

3.2.6.2 *extending fillers*— typically have lower surface area and lower cost than reinforcing fillers. They include crystalline forms of silica and diatomaceous earths. While they provide some reinforcement, because they are relatively inexpensive, they are used primarily to extend the bulk of the silicone.

3.2.7 *additives*—a component of a silicone elastomer used in relatively small amounts to perform functions such as marking, coloring, or providing opacity to the elastomer.

3.2.8 *silicone base*—a uniformly blended mixture of silicone polymers, fillers, and additives which does not contain crosslinkers or catalyst.

3.2.9 *uncured elastomer*—a silicone base which contains crosslinker and/or catalyst but has not been vulcanized.

3.2.10 *silicone elastomer*—an uncured elastomer that has been subjected to conditions which cause it to become crosslinked. Elastomers may be either high consistency rubbers, low consistency rubbers, or RTVs. (see below)

3.2.10.1 *high consistency rubbers (HCRS)*—are materials which cannot be pumped by conventional pumping equipment. They normally must be processed using high shear equipment such as a two-roll mill and parts are typically fabricated using compression or transfer molding techniques.

3.2.10.2 *low consistency rubbers or liquid silicone rubbers (LSRS)*—are normally flowable materials which can be readily pumped. They can be mixed by pumping through static mixers and parts can be fabricated using injection molding techniques.

3.2.10.3 *RTVs (room temperature vulcanization)*— are one-part elastomers which cure in the presence of atmospheric moisture. Little, if any, acceleration of cure rate is realized by increasing temperature. Because cure is dependent upon diffusion of water into the elastomer, cure in depths greater than 0.25 inches (0.635 cm) is not recommended.

3.2.10.4 *gels*—are lightly crosslinked materials having no or relatively low levels of reinforcement beyond that provided by the crosslinked polymer. They are usually two-part formulations utilizing a platinum catalyzed addition cure system. The hardness of the gel can be adjusted within wide limits. The material is not usually designed to bear heavy loads but rather to conform to an irregular surface providing intimate contact. As a result, loads are distributed over a wider area. These materials may also be used to provide protection from environmental contaminants.

3.2.10.5 *foams*—are crosslinked materials which have a component added to them that generates a volatile gas as the material is being vulcanized. This results in a material with a very low density. These are usually two-part formulations utilizing a platinum catalyzed addition cure system. They conform to an irregular surface as they expand to provide intimate contact and protection from the environment but are more rigid and provide more strength than gels. Since foams are expanded elastomers, on a weight basis they are highly crosslinked relative to gels. Most cure conditions will result in a closed cell foam.

3.2.11 *lot or batch*—a quantity of material made with a fixed, specified formulation in a single, manufacturing run carried out under specific processing techniques and conditions.

3.2.12 *vulcanization*—an irreversible process in which covalent chemical bonds are formed between silicone polymer chains. During vulcanization, the material changes from a flowable or moldable compound to an elastomeric material which cannot be reshaped except by its physical destruction.

3.2.13 *types of cure*—based upon the cure chemistry employed, silicone elastomers used in medical applications fall into one of three categories: condensation cure, peroxide cure, and addition cure.

3.2.13.1 *condensation cure*—these materials liberate an organic leaving group during curing and are normally catalyzed by an organometallic compound.

one-part—material supplied ready to use in an air tight container which cures upon exposure to atmospheric moisture. The material cures from the surface down and cure depths of greater than about 0.25 inches (0.635 cm) are not practical.

two-part—material supplied in two separate containers which must be intimately mixed in the prescribed proportions shortly before use. Because they do not rely upon dispersion of atmospheric moisture into the silicone, the cure depth is not limited.

3.2.13.2 *peroxide cure*—one-part formulations vulcanized by free radicals generated by the decomposition of an organic peroxide.

3.2.13.3 *addition cure*—two-part elastomers which must first be mixed together and then cure by addition of a silylhydride to a vinyl silane in the presence of a platinum catalyst.

3.2.14 *dispersion*—an uncured silicone elastomer dispersed

in a suitable solvent to allow application of a thin layer of elastomer to a substrate by either dipping or spraying.

4. Significance and Use

4.1 This standard is intended to provide guidance for the specification and selection of silicone materials for medical device applications.

4.2 Silicone manufacturers supplying materials to the medical device industry should readily provide information regarding non-proprietary product formulation to their customers either directly, or through the US FDA master file program.

5. Formulation

5.1 Elastomers, gels, and foams shall be manufactured using formulations containing combinations of the following raw materials.

5.1.1 *silicone polymer*—any polymer of medium or high molecular weight of the structure shown in Fig. 1 where R is a methyl, an unsaturated alkyl group or a hydroxy group, R is generally a methyl or an unsaturated alkyl group but may also be a phenyl, trifuoropropyl, or other hydrocarbon radical, and x and y are integers greater than or equal to zero. At least 2.0 alkenyl groups must exist per chain if R is not a hydroxy group.

5.1.2 *catalyst*—an organometallic complex of platinum or tin bonded to ligands made of any suitable combination of elements such as carbon, hydrogen, oxygen, fluorine and silicon.

5.1.2.1 *platinum*—this catalyst may be dispersed in a silicone polymer of the structure shown in Fig. 1 having a viscosity low enough that the resulting dispersion is easily pourable. Platinum catalysts can be used in the range of 5 to 20 ppm of active platinum but typically are present at about 7.5 ppm.

5.1.2.2 *tin*—one-part condensation cure formulations will typically contain from 0.1 to 0.5 wt percent of an organotin compound. Two-part condensation cure formulations will typically contain from 0.5 to 2.0 weight percent organotin compound. The ligands attached to tin will be some combination of alkyl groups, alkoxy groups, or the anions of a carboxylic acid.

5.1.3 *Crosslinker or crosslinking agent*—

5.1.3.1 *Two-part, addition cure formulation*—the crosslinker is a polymer of the structure shown in Fig. 2 where R is generally a methyl or a hydrogen group such as to provide at least 2.0 SiH groups per chain and x and y are integers greater than or equal to zero. In order to avoid chain extension, the functionality of either the vinyl-containing polymer or the SiH-containing crosslinker must be at least 3.0.

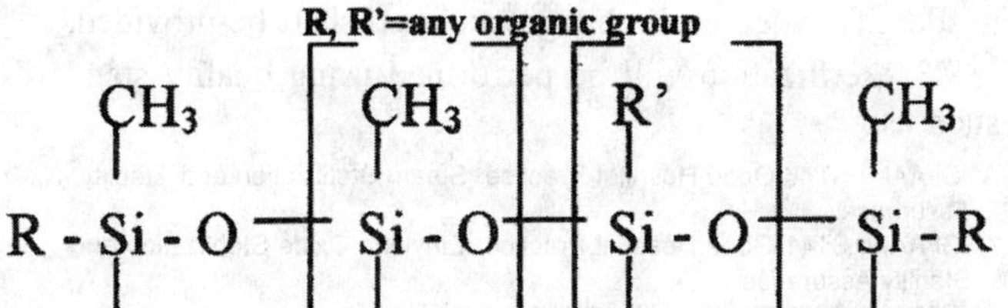

FIG. 1

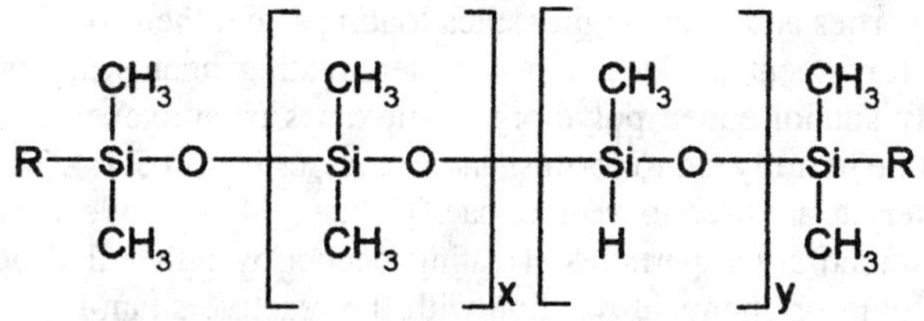

FIG. 2

Because of the limitless possibilities for the structure of both the crosslinker and the functional (vinyl containing) polymer, it would be meaningless to define a weight range for the level of crosslinker in a formulation. However, the amount of crosslinker will typically be sufficient to provide a stoichiometric excess of SiH groups over the amount of unsaturated alkyl groups when the 2 components (parts) of the addition cure silicone elastomer are mixed together in the manufacturer's recommended ratio.

5.1.3.2 *One-part RTVs and two-part addition cure formulations*—the crosslinker may be an organosilane monomer of the general formula:

$$R_xSi(OR')_{4-x} \quad (1)$$

where:

R = organic group excluding phenyl
OR' = hydrolyzable group such as alkoxy, acetoxy, ketoximo, etc.

5.1.3.3 *Peroxide vulcanized elastomers*— organic peroxides comprise a third type of crosslinking agent which participates in the crosslinking reaction that does not become directly incorporated into the crosslinked network. Peroxide levels range from less than a percent to as high as a couple of weight percent in the total formulation. These peroxides decompose, at a rate which is dependent upon the temperature, to form radicals which then abstract hydrogen atoms from some of the alkyl groups attached to the silicone backbone. Recombination of these radicals results in the formation of a crosslinked silicone network. One commonly used peroxide is 2,4,-dichlorobenzoyl peroxide. Decomposition of this peroxide results in the formation of small amounts of polychlorinated biphenyls and other catalyst decomposition by-products which must be, and are, removed from the cured elastomer during post-curing.

5.1.4 *Filler*—a high purity amorphous silica commercially known as fumed or precipitated silica. This silica can be treated with a silane of the formula Me_3SiX or Me_2SiX_2 where X is a hydrolyzable group or treated with one or more polysiloxane oligomers of the formula $HOMe_2SiO(SiMe_2O)_x$ $(SiMeRO)_ySiMe_2OH$ where R is a methyl or an unsaturated alkyl group. Filler will be added at an appropriate level to provide the desired physical property profile. This level will be dependent upon the type of treatment, level of treatment, and surface area of the fumed silica. Alternatively the filler may be a crystalline quartz compound such as sand which has been ground to a fine powder. Diatomaceous earths which contain approximately 88% silica are also sometimes used.

5.1.4.1 *plasticizers/filler treating agents*—materials added during compounding of an elastomer formulation to pacify the surface of fumed silica. These materials stabilize elastomer properties and allow higher silica loadings, and therefore better reinforcement, to be attained. Filler treating agents are typically silanol ended polydiorganosiloxanes or siloxanes which can be hydrolyzed to form silanols as described in 5.1.4. These materials are used to treat, or pacify, the highly reactive surface of fumed silica particles. Treating occurs by either hydrogen bonding or chemical reaction with the reactive silanol groups on the surface of the silica to form covalent bonds. By preferentially reacting filler treating agents with the silica surface, similar interactions with the higher molecular weight base polymer are avoided, thereby minimizing creping of the uncured elastomer and changes in hardness of the cured elastomer that would otherwise occur.

5.1.5 *Additives*—any of a class of materials usually comprised of salts or oxides of metals such as barium, titanium, or calcium.

5.1.6 *Inhibitor*—a substance or mixture of substances capable of reducing the rate of crosslinking. It typically contains an unsaturated alkyl group, capable of reacting with the crosslinker via a hydrosilylation (addition) reaction. It is composed of any suitable combination of elements such as carbon, hydrogen, oxygen and silicon.

5.1.7 *Solvent*—a liquid used to form a dispersion by mixing with an uncured elastomer. It typically is toluene or xylene but may be composed of any suitable combination of the following elements: carbon, hydrogen, oxygen and possibly silicon.

6. Packaging, Labeling, and Storage

6.1 Uncured silicone elastomer components for use in medical applications shall be supplied in proper packaging to prevent their contamination during typical conditions of shipment and storage, as well as their adulteration from the package itself.

6.2 All packages shall be labeled so as to identify the manufacturer, specific product name, and lot or batch number.

6.3 The material supplier shall provide information regarding recommended material storage conditions and product warranties.

7. Health and Safety

7.1 Because this standard applies only to uncured silicone elastomers, and most silicone elastomers are cured at the time of end use, most health and safety concerns related to the use of these materials are those encountered during handling; namely eye, skin, and respiratory exposure.

7.2 Each type of filler has its own associated hazards. Potential respiratory effects are typically of no concern, since fillers cannot easily become airborne from compounded materials.

7.3 Catalysts may have some toxicological effects, depending on concentration, form and type. Inhibitors are usually volatilized or incorporated into the elastomeric network during cure, or are at levels generally considered to have negligible toxicological effects.

7.4 Suitability for intended use (i.e. biocompatibility) must be determined on final devices tested in their intended applications. Information about the biocompatibility of cured silicone elastomers is most relevant to the selection of device constituents, and is specific to preparation, sterilization and testing conditions.

7.5 Where uncured silicone elastomers are applied to the body directly and cured *in situ*, consideration must be given to formulation components and cure by-products. Some of these elastomers utilize cure systems which generate organic compounds which can cause local tissue irritation.

7.6 Toxicological test data on uncured materials applies only when all formulating and manufacturing starts with specified ingredients, and is accomplished in accordance with accepted quality standards such as ISO 9001 and current Quality System Regulations/Good Manufacturing Practices (GMP) regulations promulgated by the FDA.

8. Sterilization

8.1 Manufacturers of uncured silicone elastomers may supply such materials sterile or may want to advise fabricators on sterilization methods. These methods should be validated before use.

8.2 Ethylene oxide is highly soluble in silicone. Those users sterilizing with ethylene oxide must do testing to ensure acceptable levels of residues if such sterilized material is used as is (See references). Cell culture tests, such as Practice F 813, may be used to show absence of sterilant residues.

8.3 Autoclave sterilization of uncured elastomers, gels, and foams is not typically used and is not recommended because it may result in fabrication difficulties. Specific details relating to autoclaving will not be discussed here because it is more typically performed on devices made from fabricated elastomers.

8.4 Radiation sterilization of uncured elastomers, gels and foams is not typically used and is not recommended. Additional information about radiation sterilization is available in Part II.

9. Quality Control Provisions

9.1 Silicone elastomers should be designed and manufactured utilizing quality control programs such as that discussed in ANSI/ASQC CI (Specification of General Requirements for a Quality Program), preferably in accordance with ISO 9001 and ISO 9002 standards. Batch-to-batch consistency/acceptability can also be monitored by matching product performance to lot acceptance requirements, providing these are specific and reasonably narrow.

9.2 Manufacturers of uncured silicone elastomers will inform customers of changes in formulation, test methods, specifications or packaging. Details of the changes and a means to identify when each change occurred shall be provided.

9.3 Sterilization will be performed using quality standards such as:

ANSI/AAMI ST46 Good Hospital Practice: Steam Sterilization and Sterility Assurance
ANSI/AAMI ST41 Good Hospital Practice: Ethylene Oxide Sterilization and Sterility Assurance
ANSI/AAMI ST50 Dry Heat (Heated Air) Sterilizers
ANSI/AAMI ST29 Recommended Practice for Determining Ethylene Oxide in Medical Devices
ANSI/AAMI ST30 Determining Residual Ethylene Chlorohydrin and Ethylene Glycol in Medical Devices

AAMI 13409-251 Sterilization of Health Care Products—Radiation Sterilization—Substantiation of 25kGy as a Sterilization Dose for Small or Infrequent Production Batches
AAMI TIR8-251 Microbiological Methods for Gamma Irradiation Sterilization of Medical Devices

10. Keywords

10.1 elastomer; foam; gel; HCR; high consistency rubber; liquid silicone rubber; LSR; moisture cure; medical device material; peroxide cure; platinum cure; RTV

APPENDIX

(Nonmandatory Information)

X1. RATIONALE

X1.1 Medical devices made from silicone elastomer are widely used in the care of public health and have a history of biocompatibility in many applications. This standard educates the user as to the formulation of such elastomers, the first level at which biocompatibility of the ultimate device is affected. Also impacting the biocompatibility of the finished device is the fabrication of the silicone elastomer; fabrication is addressed in the companion standard.

X1.2 The previous version of this standard has now been split into two parts, one addressing formulation, and one, fabrication. The codes previously used in this standard were not widely accepted by manufacturers, and therefore the monograph had minimal utility. The information provided here (and some suggestions for further investigation) at least provide a starting point from which the user can seek guidance on the biological impact of silicone formulations. Manufacturers' responsibilities as defined here are now or are expected to be practiced in the industry; manufacturers can be differentiated on the basis of the information they provide on the topics introduced herein.

Designation: F 2042 – 00$^{\epsilon 1}$

Standard Guide for Silicone Elastomers, Gels, and Foams Used in Medical Applications Part II — Crosslinking and Fabrication[1]

This standard is issued under the fixed designation F 2042; the number immediately following the designation indicates the year of original adoption or, in the case of revision, the year of last revision. A number in parentheses indicates the year of last reapproval. A superscript epsilon (ε) indicates an editorial change since the last revision or reapproval.

ϵ^1 NOTE—Figs. 1-3 and Figs. 5-9 were editorially revised in June 2001.

1. Scope

1.1 This guide is intended to educate potential users of silicone elastomers, gels and foams relative to their fabrication and processing. It does not provide information relative to silicone powders, fluids, pressure sensitive adhesives, or other types of silicone products.

1.2 The information provided is offered to guide users in the selection of appropriate processing conditions for specific medical device applications.

1.3 Formulation and selection of appropriate starting materials is covered in the companion document, F 2038 Part I. This monograph addresses only the curing, post-curing, and processing of elastomers, gels and foams as well as how the resulting product is evaluated.

1.4 Silicone biocompatibility issues can be addressed at several levels, but ultimately the device manufacturer must assess biological suitability relative to intended use. Biocompatibility testing may be done on cured elastomers prior to final fabrication, but the most relevant data are those obtained on the finished device. Data on selected lots of material are only representative when compounding, and fabrication are performed under accepted quality systems such as ISO 9001 and current Good Manufacturing Practice Regulations. Extractables analyses may also be of interest for investigation of biocompatibility, and the procedures for obtaining such data depend on the goal of the study (see F 619, the HIMA Memorandum 7/14/93, and USP 23, for examples of extraction methods).

2. Referenced Documents

2.1 *ASTM Standards:*

D 395 Test Methods for Rubber Property—Compression Set[2]

D 412 Test Methods for Rubber Properties in Tension[2]

D 430 Test Methods for Rubber Deterioration—Dynamic Fatigue[2]

D 624 Test Method for Tear Strength of Conventional Vulcanized Rubber and Thermoplastic Elastomers [2]

D 792 Test Methods for Specific Gravity (Relative Density) and Density of Plastics by Displacement [3]

D 813 Test Method for Rubber Deterioration—Crack Growth[2]

D 814 Test Method for Rubber Property—Vapor Transmission of Volatile Liquids[2]

D 926 Test Method for Rubber Property—Plasticity and Recovery (Parallel Plate Method) [2]

D 955 Test Method of Measuring Shrinkage from Mold Dimensions of Molded Plastics[3]

D 1349 Practice for Rubber—Standard Temperatures for Testing[2]

D 1566 Terminology Relating to Rubber[2]

D 2240 Test Method for Rubber Property—Durometer Hardness[2]

F 619 Practice for Extraction of Medical Plastics[4]

F 719 Practice for Testing Biomaterials in Rabbits for Primary Skin Irritation[4]

F 720 Practice for Testing Guinea Pigs for Contact Allergens—Guinea Pig Maximization Test[4]

F 748 Practice for Selecting Generic Biological Test Methods for Materials and Devices[4]

F 813 Practice for Direct Contact Cell Culture Evaluation of Materials for Medical Devices[4]

F 981 Practice for Assessment of Compatibility of Biomaterials for Surgical Implantation With Respect to Effect of Materials on Muscle and Bone[4]

F 1905 Practice for Selecting Tests for Determining the Propensity of Materials to Cause Immunotoxicity [4]

F 1906 Practice for Evaluation of Immunological Responses in Biocompatibility Testing Using ELISA Tests, Lymphocyte Proliferation, and Cell Migration[4]

F 1984 Practice for Testing Whole Complement Activation in Scrum by Solid Materials[4]

F 2038 Guide for Silicone Elastomers, Gels and Foams Used in Medical applications Part I: Formulations and Uncured Materials[4]

2.2 *Other Biocompatibility Standards:*

[1] This specification is under the jurisdiction of ASTM Committee F04 on Medical and Surgical Materials and Devices and is the direct responsibility of Subcommittee F4.11 on Polymeric Materials.

Current edition approved July 10, 2000. Published October 2000.

[2] *Annual Book of ASTM Standards,* Vol 09.01.

[3] *Annual Book of ASTM Standards,* Vol 08.01.

[4] *Annual Book of ASTM Standards,* Vol 13.01.

United States Pharmacopeia, current edition (appropriate monographs may include: <87>, <88>, <151>, <381>) [5]

FDA Department of Health and Human Services General Program Memorandum #G95–1, May 1, 1995: Use of International Standard ISO-10993, Biological Evaluation of Medical Devices Part I: Evaluation and Testing[6]

ANSI/AAMI 10993–1 Biological Evaluation of Medical Devices, Part I: Guidance on Selection of Tests[7]

HIMA Memorandum Guidance for Manufacturers of Silicone Devices Affected by Withdrawal of Dow Corning Silastic Materials, 7/14/93[8]

2.3 *Sterilization Standards:*

ANSI/AAMI ST46 Good Hospital Practice: Steam Sterilization and Sterility Assurance[7]

ANSI/AAMI ST41 Good Hospital Practice: Ethylene Oxide Sterilization and Sterility Assurance[7]

ANSI/AAMI ST50 Dry Heat (Heated Air) Sterilizers[7]

ANSI/AAMI ST29 Recommended Practice for Determining Ethylene Oxide in Medical Devices[7]

ANSI/AAMI ST30 Determining Residual Ethylene Chlorohydrin and Ethylene Glycol in Medical Devices[7]

AAMI 13409–251 Sterilization of Health Care Products—Radiation Sterilization—Substantiation of 25kGy as a Sterilization Dose for Small or Infrequent Production Batches[9]

AAMI TIR8–251 Microbiological Methods for Gamma Irradiation Sterilization of Medical Devices[9]

2.4 *Quality Standards:*

ANSI/ASQC Q9001 Quality Systems—Model for Quality Assurance in Design, Development, Production, Installation and Servicing[7]

21 CFR 820 Quality System Regulation (current revision)[10]

21 CFR 210 Current Good Manufacturing Practice in Manufacturing, Processing, Packing or Holding of Drugs: General (current revision)[10]

21 CFR 211 Current Good Manufacturing Practice for Finished Pharmaceuticals (current revision)[10]

2.5 *Other Standards:*

Dow Corning CTM 0155 (Gel-Like Materials With Modified Penetrometer)

Dow Corning CTM 0813 (Gel-Like Materials With One Inch Diameter Head Penetrometer)

PCB Test Methods such as those used for MRI project No. 4473, 1/24/97, [11]

Biological Performance of Materials: J. Black, Marcel Dekker, NY 1992

[5] Available from United States Pharmacopeia 12601 Twinbrook Parkway Rockville, MD 20852.

[6] Available from Food and Drug Administration HFI-40, Rockville, MD 20857.

[7] Available from American National Standards Institute, 11 West 42nd Street, 13th Floor, New York, NY 10036.

[8] Available from Advanced Medical Technology Association, 1200 G St. N.W. Suite 400 Washington, D.C. 20005–3814.

[9] Available from Association for the Advancement of Medical Devices, 1110 North Glebe Rd., Suite 220, Arlington, VA 22201–4795.

[10] Available from Standardization Documents Order Desk, Bldg. 4 Section D, 700 Robins Ave., Philadelphia PA 19111–5094, Attn: NPODS

[11] Available from Midwest Research Institute, 425 Volker Blvd., Kansas City, MO 64110–2299

3. Terminology

3.1 The classification of silicone elastomers is based upon a number of interrelated factors which include the chemical system used to crosslink the elastomer, the physical characteristics of the uncured elastomer, and the methods used to fabricate the elastomers. Additional pertinent terms are defined in standard D 1566.

3.2 *Definitions:*

3.2.1 *manufacture*—the process which occurs in the supplier's facility in which the various components of the elastomer are brought together, allowed to interact, and are packaged to provide the uncured elastomer for sale.

3.2.2 *fabrication*—the process by which the uncured elastomer is converted into a fully vulcanized elastomer of the desired size and shape. This process may occur in the same facility as the manufacture of the uncured elastomer but is more typically performed at the facility of a customer of the silicone manufacturer.

3.2.2.1 *injection molding*—fabrication of elastomers into forms defined by molds constructed so that the uncured elastomer can be transferred by pumping into the closed mold. This method requires venting of the mold in some manner. The elastomer may be vulcanized by heating the mold after it is filled but more typically the molding conditions (temperature and filling rate) are adjusted so that uncured elastomer can be added to a pre-heated mold in which it will then cure. The mold is than opened and the part removed and post-cured, if necessary.

3.2.2.2 *compression molding*—a process in which the uncured elastomer is placed in an open mold. The mold is closed and pressure applied to the mold to fill the cavity. Heat is applied to vulcanize the elstomer, the mold is than opened and the fabricated part is removed.

3.2.2.3 *freshening*—because of the interaction that can occur between the fumed silica and silicone polymers, thick uncured high consistency elastomers can become so stiff over time that they are very difficult to process. To overcome this problem, a 2–roll mill is used to disrupt this interaction, resulting in a material which is easier to fabricate. This process is called freshening and is typically done immediately before catalyzation.

3.2.2.4 *transfer molding*—a process in which the mixed, uncured elastomer is placed in a compartment connected to the mold. The compartment is then closed, pressure is applied to transfer the uncured elastomer to the mold, filling the cavity. Heat and pressure are applied to the mold to vulcanize the elastomer, the mold is then opened, and the fabricated part is removed.

3.2.2.5 *extrusion*—a continuous process in which the mixed, uncured elastomer is forced through an orifice having the desired cross-sectional profile. The elastomer is then vulcanized by passing it through either a hot air or radiant heat oven. The most common application of extrusion processing is the fabrication of tubing but it can be used to produce other items as well.

3.2.2.6 *post-cure*—the process of subjecting a vulcanized elastomer to elevated temperature, usually in a hot-air oven, after its initial fabrication. This process step is done to complete cross-linking of the object, remove peroxide by-products, and eliminate changes in its physical properties. Post-cure is often necessary when the component is only partially cross-liked by molding; it is performed in an attempt to accelerate molding process, and increase its output.

3.2.2.7 *calendaring*—the process of forming an uncured, mixed elastomer into a thin sheet or film by passing it between two rolls.

3.2.2.8 *dispersion*—the process of placing an uncured elastomer in a solvent. This lowers the viscosity of the material and is usually done to allow the fabrication of thinner films that can be obtained by calendaring or to form coatings. Following dispersion use, the solvent must be removed either before or during the vulcanization process. Care must be taken to assure that the solvent is compatible with the elastomer, to prevent preferential settling of the components of the formulation by excessive dilution of the elastomer.

3.2.3 *one-part elastomer*—an elastomer supplied in the uncured form in one package containing all of the formulation components. It does not require mixing before fabrication.

3.2.4 *two-part elastomer*—an elastomer supplied in two packages which must be mixed in specified proportions before fabrication.

3.2.5 *liquid silicone rubber or low consistency silicone rubber (LSR)*—an elastomer having a viscosity such that it can be moved or transferred by readily available pumping equipment. LSRs are typically used in injection molding operations.

3.2.6 *high consistency rubber (HCR)*—an elastomer having a viscosity such that it cannot be moved or transferred by readily available pumping equipment. These elastomers are fabricated using high shear equipment such as a two-roll mill and cannot be injection molded. They are typically used in compression or transfer molding and extrusion processes.

3.2.7 *RTV (room temperature vulcanization)*—a one-part elastomer which cures in the presence of atmospheric moisture. Little, if any, acceleration of cure rate is realized by increasing temperature. Because cure is dependent upon diffusion of water into the elastomer, cure in depths of greater than 0.64 cm is not recommended.

3.2.8 *gel*—a lightly crosslinked material having no or relatively low levels of reinforcement beyond that provided by the crosslinked polymer. Gels are usually two-part formulations utilizing a platinum catalyzed addition cure system. The hardness of the gel can be adjusted within wide limits. The material is not usually designed to bear a heavy load but rather to conform to an irregular surface providing intimate contact. As a result, loads are distributed over a wider area. These materials may also be used to provide protection from environmental contaminants.

3.2.9 *foam*—a crosslinked material which has a component added to it which generates a volatile gas as the material is being vulcanized. This vulcanization process results in a material with a relatively low density. Foams are usually two-part formulations utilizing a platinum catalyzed addition cure system. They conform as they expand to irregular surfaces just as gels do to provide intimate contact and protection from the environment but are more rigid and provide more strength than gels. Since foams are expanded elastomers, on a weight basis, they are highly crosslinked relative to gels. Most cure conditions will result in a closed cell foam.

4. Significance and Use

4.1 This standard is intended to provide guidance for the specification and selection of fabrication methods for silicones used in medical devices. It also provides guidance relative to testing that might be done to qualify lots of acceptable material, based on desired performance properties.

4.2 Silicone manufacturers supplying material to the medical device industry should readily provide information regarding non-proprietary product formulation to their customers either directly or through the US FDA Master File program.

5. Crosslinking Chemistry

5.1 Silicone elastomers used in medical applications are typically crosslinked by one of three commonly used cure systems. These involve the platinum catalyzed addition of a silylhydride to an unsaturated site, the generation of free radicals by a peroxide or the reaction of an easily hydrolyzable group of silicon.

5.1.1 *addition cure*—this cure system utilizes the addition of a silylhydride to a site of unsaturation, usually a vinyl group. As shown in Fig. 1, this reaction is catalyzed by a platinum complex. The catalyst will be present at a level such that the concentration of platinum is in the range of 5 to 20 ppm but is more typically present at a level of about 7.5 ppm. When multiple silylhydrides are present in the same molecule, for example, in a crosslinker molecule, and they react with vinyl groups attached to a silicon in a silicone polymer, a crosslinked network results.

Elastomers using this cure system are two-part elastomers and are utilized in both LSRs and HCRs. In practice, the platinum catalyst, an inhibitor, and vinyl functionality on the silicone backbone are present in one part of the formulation and the crosslinker in the presence of vinyl functionality on the silicone backbone is present in the other. These two parts are intimately mixed shortly before they are intended to be used. At room temperature a certain amount of working time (time before the crosslink network builds to unacceptable levels) is provided to allow time to fabricate the silicone part. Heat is then applied to activate the platinum, the crosslinking reaction occurs, and the elastomer is vulcanized. The amount of working time and rate of cure are determined by the amount of crosslinker, catalyst, and inhibitors used in the formulation.

Mixing of LSRs of this type is usually accomplished by pumping the material in the prescribed ratios through a static mixer. HCRs are usually mixed by placing the prescribed ratios of the two parts on a two-roll mill and crossblending until adequately mixed. Mixing of the two components of the formulation at other than the ratio prescribed by the vendor is

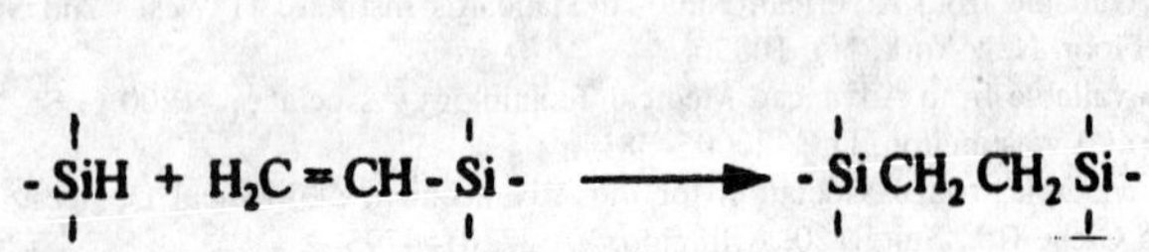

NOTE—Si=Silicon
Pt=Platinum

FIG. 1

likely to result in changes in the cure characteristics, cured physical properties, or both, and may result in changes in the extractables profile.

5.1.2 *peroxide cure*—this cure system utilizes the decomposition of an organic peroxide, as shown in Fig. 2.

Radicals A and B then form organic radicals on the alkyl groups attached to silicon atoms along the polymer chain by abstracting hydrogen atoms as shown in Fig. 3.

These elastomers may be provided as two part materials but are more commonly supplied as one-part materials where the peroxide is already present in the elastomer. Alternatively, only a base material may be supplied to which the fabricator can add the peroxide of his choice. The elastomers will usually be HCRs but some LSRs also employ this cure system.

The peroxide used will determine the shelf-life and cure rate of the elastomer at a particular temperature. Because peroxides are used at levels of 0.5–2 wt % and decomposition products form as the organic peroxide breaks down, these elastomers must be post-cured to remove those materials from the elastomer before use in medical applications.

Peroxides are classified as either non-vinyl specific, depending upon the type of radical reaction they promote.

5.1.2.1 *non-vinyl specific peroxides*—these peroxides promote the combination of two radicals on adjacent chains as shown in Fig. 4, resulting in an ethylene linkage between the polymer chains.

5.1.2.2 *vinyl-specific peroxides*—these peroxides promote the addition of the radical to a vinyl group attached to silicon on a polymer chain as shown in Fig. 5, resulting in a propylene linkage between the polymer chains. As these reactions are repeated, the crosslink network results.

5.1.3 *condensation cure*—elastomers of those type may be either one-part or two-part RTVs and contain hydroyzable groups on the crosslinker and on the polymer ends.

5.1.3.1 *one-part RTV*—elastomers of this type must be packaged in containers that are impermeable to moisture. When extruded from the container, they react with moisture from the atmosphere which diffuses through the elastomer. This results in the hydrolysis of the reactive groups on a crosslinker molecule as shown in Fig. 6.

The silanol species formed can then react with a hydrolyzable group attached to the end of a polymer chain as shown in Fig. 7. As this reaction is repeated on the same crosslinker molecule, the crosslink network results.

RTV formulations normally contain an organometallic compound to facilitate the reaction. Because they rely on the permeation of moisture through the elastomer to cure, use in applications where thicknesses of greater than 0.64 cm are desired are not normally recommended because of the long cure times necessary. RTVs are normally used in adhesive applications where two silicones, or other substrates, are being bonded together.

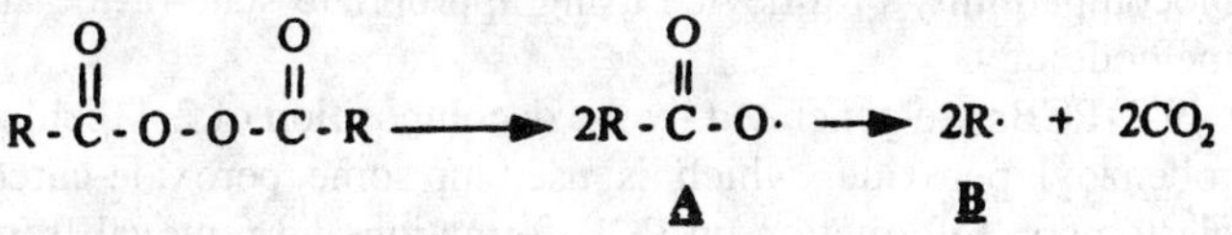

NOTE—R=any organic group

FIG. 2

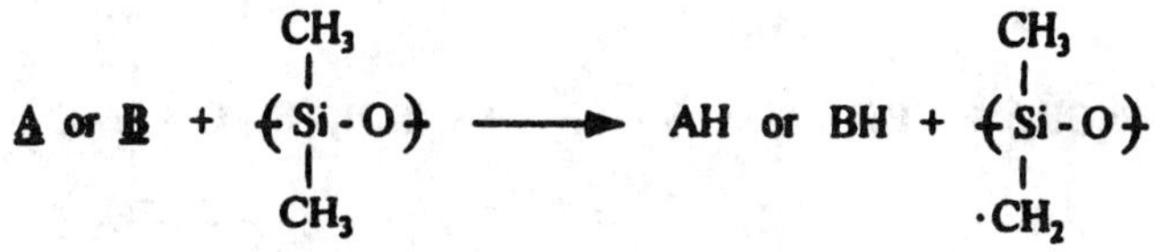

FIG. 3

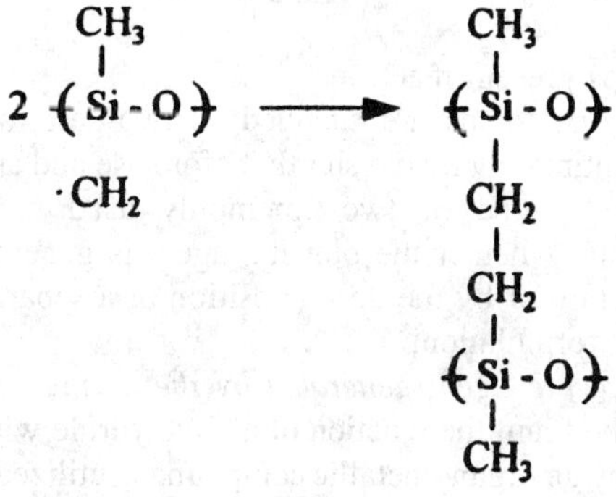

FIG. 4

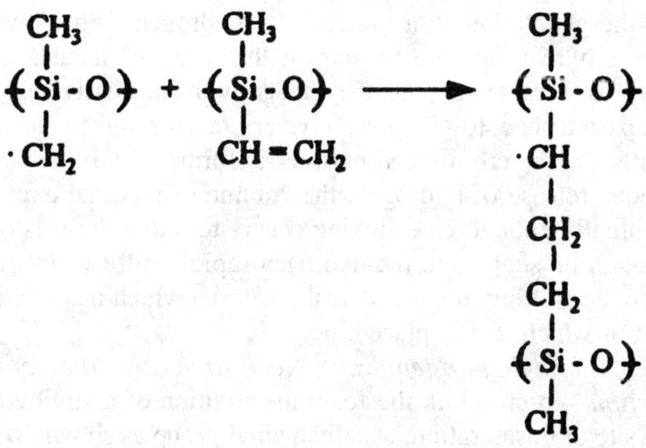

FIG. 5

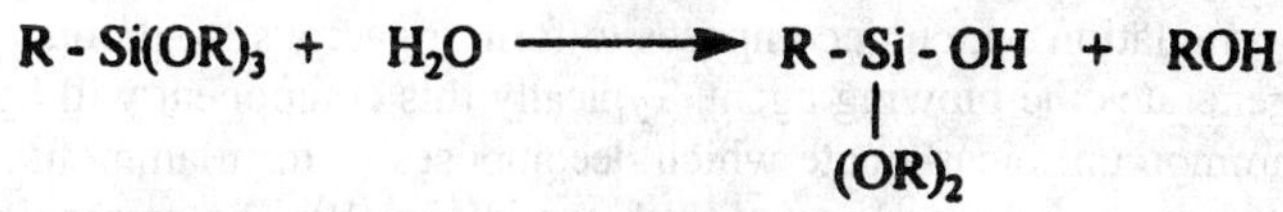

FIG. 6

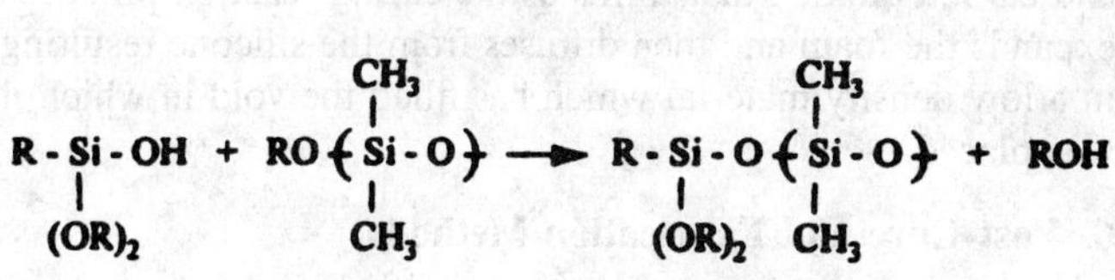

FIG. 7

5.1.3.2 *two-part RTVs (deep section condensation cure)*—another cure system which has found some utility in medical applications involves the reaction of an alkoxy crosslinker with a silanol ended polymer in the presence of an organometallic compound as shown in Fig. 8. The system results in rapid cures in deep-section because it does not rely upon the diffusion of water through the silicone. The organometalic compound is usually a tin compound.

5.2 Silicone gels are supplied as two-part formulations which are intimately mixed shortly before use and are cured using the chemistry shown in Fig. 1. However the relative ratio of SiH to SiVi is adjusted so that only a fraction of the total

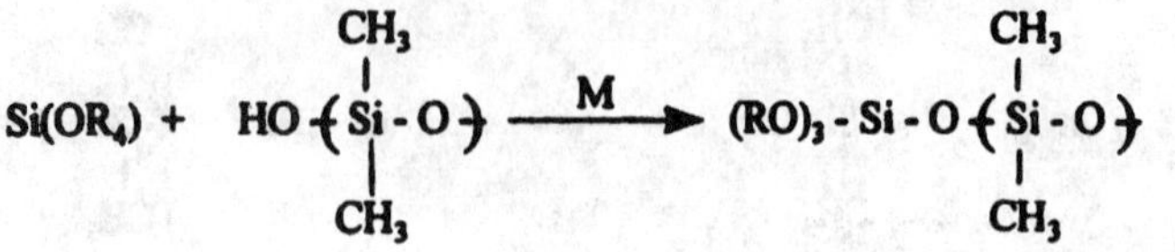

NOTE—M=Metal

FIG. 8

vinyl groups present react.

5.3 Silicone foams are supplied as two-part formulations which are intimately mixed shortly before use and are typically vulcanized by one of two commonly used cure systems depending on whether the blowing agent is generated by the curing reaction or by the decomposition of a separate component of the formulation.

5.3.1 *blowing agent generated by the curing reaction*—to crosslink the foam the reaction of a silylhydride with a silanol catalyzed by an organometallic compound is utilized. Typically the catalyst will be an organotin compound. This reaction is shown in Fig. 9 and results in the formation of a siloxane bond and the generation of a molecule of hydrogen. When two or more silylhydrides are present in the same molecule, i.e. a crosslinker molecule, as they react with successive silanol groups attached to silicone polymers, a crosslinked network results. As the crosslinked network is formed, with the simultaneous release of hydrogen, the volume of material expands. Eventually enough crosslinking occurs to allow the elastomer to retain its shape and the hydrogen rapidly diffuses from the silicone resulting in a low density material which has filled the void in which it was placed.

5.3.2 *blowing agent not generated by the curing reaction*—to crosslink the foam the addition of a silylhydride to a site of unsaturation, usually a vinyl group as shown in Fig. 1, is utilized. During the vulcanization process, as the crosslinked network is being built up, a component of the formulation which decomposes to form a gaseous by-product, generates the blowing agent. Typically this component will be ammonium bicarbonate which decomposes to form ammonia, carbon dioxide, and water as shown in Fig. 10. The ammonia and carbon dioxide that forms as the curing reaction proceeds expands the foam and then diffuses from the silicone resulting in a low density material which has filled the void in which it was placed.

$$(NH_4)HCO_3 \longrightarrow NH_3 + CO_2 + H_2O$$

FIG. 10

6. Post-Cure and Fabrication Methods

6.1 Fabrication methods will be determined by the type of elastomer being used for the application. High consistency elastomers are generally fabricated using two-roll mills in conjunction with compression and transfer molding or extrusion techniques. Liquid silicone rubber elastomers are generally fabricated by using injection molding processes.

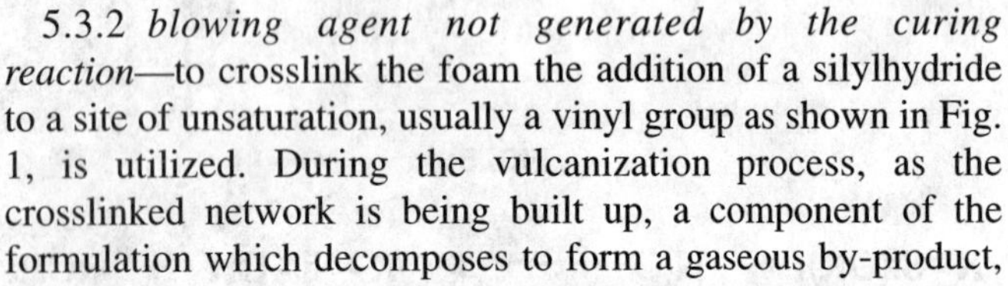

NOTE—Me=Methyl

FIG. 9

6.2 Vulcanization and post-curing guidelines are usually recommended by the manufacturer but may vary depending upon the detail, configuration and size of the object being fabricated. Peroxide cured elastomers must be post-cured. Platinum catalyzed elastomers may or may not require post-curing, depending on the particular application and/or object being made.

7. Physical Properties

7.1 Physical properties of elastomers are used by manufacturers to insure that the elastomer has been properly formulated and processed and by the fabricator to determine that the elastomer will perform as intended in the application. Properties of both uncured and vulcanized elastomers may be determined. While customer specific testing may be done, the following ASTM methods describe tests that are of general utility and are commonly used in the industry. In addition, standard D 1349 addresses temperatures at which such testing occurs.

D 395 Test Methods for Rubber Property—Compression Set
D 412 Test Methods for Rubber Properties in Tension
D 430 Test Methods for Rubber Deterioration—Dynamic Fatigue
D 624 Test Methods for Tear Strength of Conventional Vulcanized Rubber and Thermoplastic Elastomers
D 792 Test Methods for Specific Gravity (Relative Density) and Density of Plastics by Displacement
D 813 Test Methods for Rubber Deterioration—Crack Growth
D 926 Test Method for Rubber Property—Plasticity and Recovery (Parallel Plate Method)
D 955 Test Method of Measuring Shrinkage from Mold Dimensions of Molded Plastics
D 2240 Test Method for Rubber Property—Durometer Hardness
Dow Corning CTM 0155 (Gel-Like Materials With Modified Penetrometer)
Dow Corning CTM 0813 (Gel-Like Materials With One Inch Diameter Head Penetrometer)

8. Packaging, Labeling and Storage

8.1 Cured silicone elastomers or components for use in medical applications shall be supplied in proper packaging to prevent their contamination during typical conditions of shipment and storage, as well as their adulteration from the package shelf.

8.2 All packages shall be labeled so as to identify the manufacturer, specific product name, and lot or batch number.

8.3 The material supplier shall provide information regarding recommended storage conditions and product warranties.

9. Biocompatibility

9.1 The biocompatibility of silicone elastomers as a class of materials cannot be categorically established; it depends on formulation, processing conditions and ultimate use. Device manufacturers are ultimately responsible for ensuring the biocompatibility of a device using appropriate state-of-the-art methodology.

9.2 PCBs are generated by the decomposition of 2,4 dichlorobenzoyl peroxide, which is used in some peroxide-cured elastomers. Information on PCB formation and removal from elastomers catalyzed with this peroxide should be available from the manufacturer, or may be obtained by direct testing

(MRI Project No. 4473, Jan 24, 1997; Midwest Research Institute, 425 Volker Boulevard, Kansas City, Missouri 64110–2299; Ph. (816) 753–7600. This method is useful for the determination of PCB levels in cured elastomers only). The user is ultimately responsible for determining acceptable levels of PCBs for their application.

9.3 Biocompatibility testing may be conducted on the silicone materials that are used to manufacture a medical device to guide in the selection of material or manufacturer.

9.4 Biological Test Methods for obtaining information on the biocompatibility of silicone elastomers as part of medical devices can be found in Practices such as F 748, F 813, F 719, F 720, F 981, F 1905, F 1906, and F 1984 and ISO 10993–1 and USP documents (<87>, <88>, <151>, <381>). Considerations for sample preparation and presentation that may impact biological test results are provided in references such as Biological Performance of Materials by J. Black (1992).

9.5 Toxicological test data on cured silicone materials applies only when all formulating and processing utilizes specified ingredients, and is accomplished in accordance with accepted quality systems such as ISO 9001 and current Quality System Regulations/Good Manufacturing Practices (GMPs) promulgated by the FDA.

9.6 Extraction is a part of most biological screening tests on cured elastomers and on finished medical devices. Typical extraction methods designed for this purpose are described in USP 23 (<88>) and F 619. Other methods may be directed towards specific goals, and should be chosen based on the question addressed, and the selectivity and sensitivity of the methods available for extract analysis. The HIMA Memorandum of 7/14/93 addresses extraction study methods intended to establish equivalency between silicone materials. Extract results will be influenced by sample, extraction, and analysis parameters.

10. Sterilization

10.1 Manufacturers of fabricated silicones elastomers may supply such materials sterile or may want to advise end users (hospitals, clinics and physicians, for example) on sterilization methods. These methods should be validated before use.

10.2 Ethylene oxide is highly soluble in silicone. Those users sterilizing with ethylene oxide must do testing to ensure acceptable levels of harmful residues if sterilized material is used as is (See References). Cell culture tests, such as Practice D 813, may be used to show absence of sterilant residues. Material characteristics may also change as a result of ethylene oxide sterilization.

10.3 Autoclave sterilization is permissible for most silicone elastomers because material characteristics are not significantly altered during autoclave sterilization.

10.4 Radiation sterilization of silicone elastomers results in a dose-related increase in crosslink density that may increase durometer and modulus of elasticity and reduce elongation and flexural durability. When silicone elastomer devices are sterilized by radiation, qualifying performance testing on finished medical devices or reasonable near-finished components subjected to the maximum radiation dosage shall be conducted to ensure that radiation sterilization has not adversely affected expected performance.

11. Quality Control Provisions

11.1 Silicone elastomers should be processed and tested utilizing quality control programs such as that discussed in ANSI/ASQC C1 (Specification of General Requirements for a Quality Program), preferably in consistency/acceptability can also be monitored by matching product performance to lot acceptance requirements, providing these are specific and reasonably narrow.

11.2 Fabricators of silicone elastomer components will inform customers of changes in formulation, test methods, specifications or packaging. Details of the changes with a means to identify when each change occurred shall be provided.

11.3 Sterilization will be performed using quality standards such as:

ANSI/AAMI ST46 Good Hospital Practice: Steam Sterilization and Sterility Assurance
ANSI/AAMI ST 41 Good Hospital Practice: Ethylene Oxide Sterilization and Sterility Assurance
ANSI/AAMI ST50 Dry Heat (Heated Air) Sterilizers
ANSI/AAMI ST29 Recommended Practice for Determining Ethylene Oxide in Medical Devices
ANSI/AAMI ST30 Determining Residual Ethylene Chlorohydrin and Ethylene Glycol in Medical Devices
AAMI 13049–251 Sterilization of Health Care Products—Radiation Sterilization—Substantiation of 25kGy as a Sterilization Dose for Small or Infrequent Production Batches
AAMI TIR8–251 Microbiological Methods for Gamma Irradiation Sterilization of Medical Devices

11.4 Material suppliers shall provide certification to specified product requirements.

12. Keywords

12.1 foam; gel; high consistency rubber; liquid silicone rubber; medical device material; moisture cure; peroxide cure; platinum cure; RTV

APPENDIX

(Nonmandatory Information)

X1. RATIONALE

X1.1 Medical devices made from silicone elastomer are widely used in the care of public health and have a history of biocompatibility in many applications. This standard educates the user as to the fabrication of such elastomers, and tests which can be used to characterize and compare performance of processed materials. Formulation, the first level at which biocompatibilty of the ultimate device is affected, is covered in Part I of this monograph.

X1.2 The previous version of this standard has now been split into two parts, one addressing formulation, and one, fabrication. The codes previously used in this standard were not widely accepted by manufacturers, and therefore the monograph had minimal utility. The information provided here at least provides a starting point from which the user can seek guidance on the biological impact of various processing conditions on silicone devices. Manufacturers' responsibilities as defined here are now or are expected to be practiced in the industry; manufacturers can be differentiated on the basis of the information they provide on the topics discussed herein.

Standard Practice for Workers' Compensation Coverage of Emergency Services Volunteers[1]

This standard is issued under the fixed designation F 2047; the number immediately following the designation indicates the year of original adoption or, in the case of revision, the year of last revision. A number in parentheses indicates the year of last reapproval. A superscript epsilon (ε) indicates an editorial change since the last revision or reapproval.

1. Scope

1.1 This standard defines the application of insurance benefits for Emergency Services Volunteers and Units in the manner and extent as provided for under the Workers' Compensation statutes of the state in which the Volunteer or Unit provides services.

1.2 This standard identifies the basic types of Emergency Service Volunteer, and the types of activities that should be covered by workers' compensation insurance.

1.3 This standard includes both Emergency Service Units who operate as organized resources to a public authority legally responsible for the provision of search and rescue and other emergency services, as well as those volunteers who respond to a general request to the Public for their services.

2. Terminology

2.1 *Workers' Compensation Insurance*— insurance required by law of employers for the medical expenses and loss of wages incurred by an employee by reason of a job-related injury, illness or death.

2.2 *Legal Authority (Agency)*—the individual or government agency given responsibility and authority for search, rescue, fire, and other emergency or disaster services by statute. Where multiple, concurrent or overlapping authorities exist, the term is used to refer to the legal authority ultimately empowering and accepting responsibility for the volunteer unit. For the purposes of this Standard, the terms Legal Authority and Agency shall bear the same definition of terminology and meaning.

2.3 *Emergency Services Volunteer (ESV)*— an individual who volunteers his/her services to, and whose services are accepted by, an Agency in response to a request for an emergency function for which no substantive monetary benefit is expected or received. The Legal Authority incurs Workers' Compensation Insurance responsibility for Emergency Services Volunteers (ESVs) while the ESV is actively providing services to the Agency as defined in Section 5 of this Standard. This period of activity shall be considered to be employment as defined by the Workers' Compensation Statutes in the State in which the Agency exists.

Emergency Services Volunteers are presumed to be requested irregularly to provide special skills or assistance on behalf of the Agency. As such, these volunteers act as part-time employees of the Agency and are empowered to act to provide these services when specifically requested to do so, or pursuant to an approved plan or schedule, or under the supervision of a full-time employee.

2.3.1 *Search and Rescue Volunteer*—an individual who volunteers his/her services in the performance of searches and/or rescues, with the accompanying training proficiency. In addition to those specifically described in this Standard, this definition may be applied to air, ground or water search volunteers, search dog specialists and emergency managers, and others not included by specific reference.

2.3.2 *Volunteer Firefighter*—an individual who volunteers his/her services in the performance of fire suppression activities, with the accompanying training proficiency.

2.3.3 *Emergency Medical Services (EMS) Volunteer*—an individual who volunteers his/her services in the performance of emergency medical services, with the accompanying training proficiency.

2.3.4 *Disaster Services Volunteer*—an individual who volunteers his/her services to an agency upon a request for services upon the occurrence of an emergency or disaster, under the direct supervision of the agency, and with the appropriate training activity.

2.4 *Emergency Services Unit (ESU)*— an individual, or a collection of individuals forming an association, organization, group, team or similar resource organized or volunteering to provide search and/or rescue, fire or other emergency service activity for a responsible Agency. An individual or other single resource may be considered a unit if the service can be appropriately rendered (e.g. a dog handler or tracker, air search volunteer or emergency manager).

An Emergency Services Unit operates within a formal division of the legal authority as a recognized unit of the legal authority or agency, and is organized and recognized by that agency as a resource of its emergency and disaster services general plan.

. Such a unit is expected to adopt a training program sufficient to maintain a skill level equal to or greater than recognized national standards or as acceptable to the Agency requesting their services, and will typically engage in community education programs.

[1] This practice is under the jurisdiction of ASTM Committee F32 on Search and Rescue and is the direct responsibility of F32.02 on Management and Operations.

Current edition approved July 10, 2000.

Other examples of an ESU include, but are not limited to, volunteer search and rescue units, volunteer emergency medical squads, volunteer fire fighters or designated civilian volunteers who have formed organized and trained groups and who serve their city, county or state agency in the performance of their services.

2.5 *Auxiliary Unit (AU)*—an individual, or a collection of individuals forming a unit called to respond by a legal authority responsible for an emergency response function, which otherwise has no standing as a formal division or resource of that authority. For the purposes of this standard, the auxiliary status of an ESU means it has no legal responsibility for the services itself within the jurisdiction of the Agency, and no authority to provide them without acting under that of the Agency.

The Auxiliary Unit is typically organized as a division of an Agency (as defined in 2.2), or as a non-profit corporation as defined in IRS Section 501(c)3, and which has a command structure that enables it to fit within the Incident Command System of a requesting Agency.

Such a unit is expected to adopt a training program sufficient to maintain a skill level equal to or greater than recognized national standards or as acceptable to the Agency requesting their services, and will typically engage in community education programs.

Some examples of an AU are volunteer search and rescue resources, air search squads, emergency managers, search dog specialists, ambulance squads, fire fighters, disaster service workers and communication specialists who are asked to respond to assist another state, county or national park to provide their services to augment those available to the authorized requesting agency in that other state or jurisdiction.

2.6 *General Public Emergency Volunteer (GPEV)*—an individual who volunteers his/her services, and whose services are accepted, in response to a request to the Public for emergency assistance.

A GPEV is typically not a member of an organized emergency services unit, nor responding to a call for such organized units.

An example of a GPEV is an individual who is contacted pursuant to a radio or television broadcast for the assistance of the general public with instructions to respond to a search base to assist in a search operation.

2.7 *Training*—a curriculum of classroom education and field exercises designed to create a level of competence meeting national standards for such activity, or as acceptable to the agency requesting the services of such a volunteer.

Training will typically include equipment familiarity and maintenance, both at the storage and readiness facility, at areas removed from the facility, and as further defined in 3.8 of this document.

2.8 *Community Education*—activities generated by the ESU to contact the Public to increase the awareness and preparedness of the Public in areas of preventative search and rescue (PSAR), fire prevention, medical and disaster preparedness and survival.

2.9 *Call-Out*—the notice and request to activate an ESU or ESV by an Agency for the purpose of providing emergency services on behalf of the requesting agency.

If members are requested to respond directly, through radio paging, for example, then each member is considered to be called-out and responding as of that time.

2.10 *Mobilization*—the activity of an ESU or ESV as required to respond to the call-out in an equipped and prepared manner.

Mobilization typically includes travel to an equipment cache or vehicle readiness area to obtain equipment or to unite the ESU for responding as a unit, and the travel of the unit to the incident site or search base.

2.11 *De-mobilization*—the activity of an ESU or ESV as required to return from a call-out to the point of origin or to a non service-related stop enroute home or to the point of origin of the ESU or ESV after having been relieved of duty by the requesting legal authority.

De-mobilization typically includes equipment retrieval, mission debriefing, personnel review, and travel from the incident site or search base to an equipment cache, station or vehicle readiness area to return the vehicles and equipment to a condition of readiness for the next call-out.

2.12 *Emergency Services*—any activity requiring an increased level of urgency in the rendering of assistance to the entity requesting such assistance.

For the purposes of this Standard, emergency services are defined as those related to search and rescue, fire suppression, medical and disaster services.

2.13 *Check-In*—the process by which one party notifies a second of being in-service or responding to a request for services, and the second party acknowledges, typically by voice and entry in a formal log.

Check-in occurs when an individual ESV contacts the responding ESU, or when the ESU or ESV contacts the requesting legal authority.

Members of an ESU will typically be checked-in by the ESU upon first verification of their response to the call-out, either in person at a rendezvous point or search base, by radio, or other means dictated by the type of response.

The ESU will typically check-in with the legal authority either at the incident site or search base, or by radio once it is mobilized appropriately to establish itself as ready for deployment to the incident.

A GPEV is required to check-in at the response place designated for such volunteers, and to be marked as in service on the personnel log.

2.14 *Check-out*—the process by which one party notifies a second that it is concluding its on-site services, and the second party acknowledges, typically by voice and entry in a formal log.

Check-out occurs when contact is made between the on-site Agency and the ESV or ESU to notify either entity that their services are being withdrawn from the activity.

Members of an ESU will typically be checked-out by the ESU upon the termination of the individual's service pursuant to their response to the call-out, either in person at the point of de-mobilization, at a rendezvous point or search base, by radio, or other means dictated by the type of response.

The ESU will typically check-out with the legal authority either at the incident site or search base, or by radio once it is prepared appropriately to establish itself as ready for check-out and de-mobilization from the incident.

A GPEV is required to check-out at the same check-in place for designated for such volunteers, and to be marked as out of service on the incident personnel log.

2.15 *Activity Period*—The period during which the Emergency Services Volunteer, Unit or Auxiliary is exercising the skills for which it has been requested.

This activity period may include a wide variety of functions, including but not limited to: a search and rescue team member searching or climbing a cliff, a dog team handler following a scent; a firefighter engaged in suppressing a fire or rescuing a person from a burning building; an ambulance driver or medic providing medical assistance; a tracker leading a tracking team; a disaster worker in a collapsed building; a pilot engaged in an air search flight; or emergency communications personnel providing communications during a time of need.

3. Significance and Use

3.1 It is presumed for the purposes of this Standard that the Legal Authority (Agency) having responsibility for emergency services in a given jurisdiction also has a legal responsibility to provide Workers' Compensation Insurance coverage for regular paid employees.

3.2 Emergency Services Volunteers are presumed to be requested irregularly to provide special skills or assistance on behalf of the Agency. As such, these volunteers act as part-time employees of the Agency and are empowered to act to provide these services when specifically requested to do so, or pursuant to an approved plan or schedule, or under the supervision of a full-time employee.

3.3 The Legal Authority incurs Workers' Compensation Insurance responsibility for Emergency Services Volunteers (ESVs) while the ESV is actively providing services to the Agency as defined in Section 5 of this Standard. This period of activity shall be considered to be employment as defined by the State Workers' Compensation Statutes of the Agency.

3.4 When a Legal Authority (Agency) requests the services of Emergency Services Volunteers as defined by this Standard to provide services, the Agency shall assume responsibility for the injuries, medical treatment, loss of wages and death of those Emergency Services Volunteers while providing services as described in this Standard.

3.5 Responsibility for the injuries, medical treatment, loss of wages and death of those Emergency Services Volunteers while providing services as described in this Standard shall be at the statutory limits of the Workers' Compensation laws of the state of the agency requesting the services of the Emergency Services Volunteer, and shall be administered in accordance with that Agency's State Workers' Compensation laws and regulations.

3.6 Responsibility for Workers' Compensation for members of Emergency Services Units shall be the same as outlined in 3.1, and shall be provided by the Agency normally directing the activities of the ESU.

3.7 Responsibility for Workers' Compensation for members of Emergency Services Auxiliary Units shall be the same as outlined in 3.1, and, unless provided for by other statute or agreement, shall be provided by the Agency requesting the services and directing the activities of the AU.

3.8 To provide an agency with trained personnel who are able to work in a safe and effective manner, it is generally required that the Emergency Service Volunteer engage in training activity with the Emergency Service Unit.

A training plan is considered essential in establishing the basis for workers' compensation insurance coverage during training. The plan serves as both prior notice to the Responsible Legal Authority and documentation of training done to support the level of service provided. The training plan is considered to be a dynamic document, reflecting necessary changes due to weather, unit participation, newly identified skills, and rearranged priorities. As changes are made to the training plan, the revised plan is to be submitted to the Agency.

The training plan may be required by the Agency, municipality or government entity providing coverage and benefits in accordance with its contract for services or merely as a convenience to define activity periods.

The training plan should establish goals and list measurable objectives. These goals provide a basis for a relationship between training and the incident response services provided. The plan should list all planned activity of the unit and who is expected to participate. This will delineate where insurance coverage is needed and expected. The plan should detail what supervision of activities and resources of the legal authority is expected. The plan should establish a means of accountability to the responsible legal authority for the unit's training activities, such as by check-in with a central dispatch, and listing on a formal activity roster.

The training plan will contain the following elements to qualify for inclusion in workers' compensation coverage.

(*a*) Identification of the Emergency Services Unit.

(*b*) Definition of the period of time covered by the plan, usually a year.

(*c*) Establishment of the relationship of the ESU with the legal authority.

(*d*) Establishment of the overall plan goals.

(*e*) Broad outline of training plan (ie: field and classroom, equipment maintenance, training outside of the jurisdiction of the Agency, etc.).

(*f*) Specific outline of training plan (such as rappelling, nighttime field navigation, search and fire fighting techniques, medical applications, etc.).

(*g*) Establishment of criteria for objective satisfaction.

This training plan and activity must address techniques, skills and safety, and must be designed to enable the individual and the unit to meet recognized national standards or other standards as acceptable to the requesting agency.

It is recognized that training for hazardous activity is often hazardous in and of itself, by the nature of the skills that the ESV is required to master.

Since the Agency is the beneficiary of this training, the ESV is said to be employed by the Agency for the purposes of Workers' Compensation benefits while engaging in training as a member of an Emergency Services Unit. Covered training activities are those activities defined as official activities in a memorandum of understanding or other agreement between the ESU and the Agency, where the Agency is providing workers' compensation benefits.

3.9 An Emergency Services Volunteer or unit may be requested by an Agency to provide public education services. These services may include public appearances, preventative search and rescue (PSAR) programs, air search familiarization for ground search operations, first aid and CPR education, fire prevention education and others.

When engaged in such activities authorized by the Agency, the ESV or ESU is considered to be employed by the Agency for the purposes of Workers' Compensation Insurance.

4. Classification of Emergency Services Volunteers

4.1 *Emergency Services Volunteer (ESV)*— an individual who volunteers his/her services to, and whose services are accepted by, an Agency in response to a request for an emergency function. Typically, the ESV will be a member of a Emergency Services Unit (ESU) or Auxiliary Unit (AU), or will function as such, and will be covered by Workers Compensation Insurance to the same extent as of the ESU and AU.

4.2 *Emergency Services Unit (ESU)*— as defined in 2.4, is often organized as a division of an Agency (as defined in 2.2), or as a non-profit corporation as defined in IRS Section 501(c)3, and which has a command structure that enables it to fit within the Incident Command System.

The ESU typically provides services to a single Agency. The ESU may provide services to other Agencies upon request and approval of the ESU's local Agency pursuant to a Memorandum Of Understanding or Mutual Aid Agreement between the Agencies.

As defined by this Standard, Workers' Compensation Insurance benefits will be provided to the members of the ESU by the Agency to which the ESU normally provides services.

4.3 *Auxiliary Unit (AU)*—as defined in 2.5, is often organized as a division of an Agency (as defined in 2.2), or as a non-profit corporation as defined in IRS Section 501(c)3, and which has a command structure that enables it to fit within the Incident Command System.

The Auxiliary Unit typically provides services as an Emergency Services Unit to a single Agency, its "home" agency as it were, and operates as an Auxiliary Unit when providing services to, and under the direction of, another Agency. When providing such services to other Agencies upon request and approval of the other Agency, the Unit is said to by an Auxiliary Unit of the requesting Legal Authority for the purposes of the incident for which the Unit is being requested.

As defined by this Standard, Workers' Compensation Insurance benefits will be provided to the members of the AU by the Agency requesting and directing the services of the Auxiliary Unit.

4.4 *General Public Emergency Volunteer (GPEV)*—is an individual, as defined in 2.6, and is typically not a member of a trained and organized Unit as defined in 2.4 or 2.5. The GPEV generally requires significant supervision to enable it to fit within the Incident Command System.

The GPEV typically provides services to a single Agency, upon a specific request, for a specific incident, and for a specific length of time.

As defined by this Standard, Workers' Compensation Insurance benefits will be provided to the GPEV by the Agency which requests the services of the General Purpose Emergency Volunteer.

5. Required Workers Compensation Coverage

Any Agency or Legal Authority which utilizes the services of Emergency Services Volunteers as defined in this Standard bears the responsibility to provide Workers' Compensation Insurance benefits for the individuals providing these services.

It is recognized that employment of volunteers to provide services which qualify the volunteer for benefits such as Workers' Compensation Insurance creates a risk that must be appropriately managed by the Agency.

In recognition of the nature of the services performed by Emergency Services Volunteers and Units, it is acknowledged that these Volunteers will at certain times work in a semi-autonomous manner under the general direction of the Agency pursuant to a call-out.

The period of coverage for Workers' Compensation Insurance shall commence upon the start of the activity as listed below and continue until the volunteer has returned home or stopped enroute at a non mission-related stop. Such non mission-related stops would not include stops to fuel the volunteer's vehicle enroute or such safety related stops as rest breaks.

However, General Purpose Emergency Volunteers (volunteers who are not members of an organized response agency or unit) shall end their service when they have checked out and cease their activity period.

To enable the Agency to manage, control and limit the exposure to such risk, the levels at which coverage is extended to such volunteers during the performance of services is subject to the activity limits as defined in Section 3 of this document and as listed herein.

5.1 The Emergency Services Unit (ESU) is said to be on-duty and actively providing services to the Agency during:

(*a*) Call-out
(*b*) Mobilization
(*c*) Check-in
(*d*) Activity Period
(*e*) Check-out
(*f*) De-mobilization
(*g*) Training
(*h*) Public Education

5.2 The Auxiliary Unit (AU) is said to be on-duty and actively providing services to the Agency during:

(*a*) Call-out
(*b*) Mobilization
(*c*) Check-in
(*d*) Activity Period
(*e*) Check-out
(*f*) De-mobilization

5.3 The Emergency Service Volunteer (ESV) is said to be on-duty and actively providing services to the Agency when functioning as an ESU or AU, and will be subject to the covered activity limits applying to an ESU or AU.

5.4 The General Public Emergency Volunteer (GPEV) is said to be on-duty and actively providing services to the Agency during:

(*a*) Check-in at the designated incident meeting place and listing on an in-service log as noted in 2.13.

(*b*) Activity Period

(*c*) Check-out at the designated incident meeting place and listing as out-of- service as noted in 2.14.

Standard Specification for Implantable Saline Filled Breast Prosthesis[1]

This standard is issued under the fixed designation F 2051; the number immediately following the designation indicates the year of original adoption or, in the case of revision, the year of last revision. A number in parentheses indicates the year of last reapproval. A superscript epsilon (ϵ) indicates an editorial change since the last revision or reapproval.

1. Scope

1.1 This specification covers the requirements for single use saline inflatable, smooth and textured silicone shell implantable breast prostheses, intended for use in surgical reconstruction, augmentation, or replacement of the breast.

1.2 *Limitations*

1.2.1 This specification does not cover custom fabricated implantable breast prostheses.

1.2.2 This specification does not cover gel/saline type implants, which are within the scope of F 703 (Standard Specification for Implantable Breast Prostheses).

1.3 *This standard does not purport to address all of the safety concerns, if any, associated with its use. It is the responsibility of the user of this standard to establish appropriate safety and health practices and determine the applicability of regulatory limitations prior to use.*

2. Referenced Documents

2.1 *ASTM Standards:*

D 412 Test Methods For Rubber Properties in Tension[2]

D 1349 Recommended Practices for Rubber-Standard Temperatures and Atmospheres for Testing and Conditioning[2]

D 3389 Standard Test Method for Coated Fabrics Abrasion Resistance (Rotary Platform, Double-Head Abrader)[3]

F 604 Specification for Silicone Elastomers Used in Medical Applications[4]

F 748 Practice for Selecting Generic Biological Test Methods for Materials and Devices[4]

F 1251 Standard Terminology Relating to Polymeric Biomaterials in Medical and Surgical Devices[4]

2.2 *Other Documents:*

USP (United States Pharmacopeia)[5]

Federal Register, Title 21, Part 820

Association for the Advance of Medical Instrumentation

ANSI/AAMI/ISO 10993-1, Biological Testing of Medical and Dental Materials and Devices – Part 1: Guidance on Selection of Tests

ANSI/AAMI/ST50-1995, Dry Heat (Heated Air) Sterilizers

ANSI/AAMI/ISO 111355-1994, Medical Devices – Validation and Routine Control of Ethylene Oxide Sterilization

ANSI/AAMI/ISO 11137-1994, Sterilization of Health Care Products – Requirements for Validation and Routine and Routine Control – Radiation Sterilization

ANSI/AAMI/ISO 11134-1993, Sterilization of Health Care Products – Requirements for Validation and Routine Control – Industrial Moist Heat Sterilization

Parenteral Drug Association, 1981 Technical Report No. 3, Validation of Dry Heat Processes Used for Sterilization and Depyrogenation

3. Terminology

3.1 *Definitions:*

3.1.1 *fused or adhered joints (seams)*—sites in the shell or other parts of implantable breast prosthesis where materials have been joined (fused or bonded) together, with or without adhesive, as part of the manufacturing process.

3.1.2 *inflatable breast prosthesis*—implantable breast prostheses not containing silicone gel – implantable breast prostheses designed and provided prefilled with saline or empty and to be filled with saline at the time of use to adjust the volume of the prosthesis.

3.1.2.1 *type 1*—fixed volume inflatable breast prosthesis – an implantable breast prosthesis composed of a single lumen, empty when supplied and having a valve to facilitate filling the lumen with saline at the time of use.

3.1.2.2 *type 2*—variable volume inflatable breast prosthesis – an implantable breast prosthesis composed of a single lumen, empty when supplied and having a valve to facilitate filling the lumen with a portion of the volume of saline at the time of use. The valve system is designed to facilitate further post-operative adjustment with saline as instructed in product literature.

3.1.2.3 *type 3*—fixed volume inflatable breast prosthesis – an implantable breast prosthesis composed of a single lumen, prefilled with saline by the manufacturer prior to time of use.

3.1.3 *lumen*—a cavity within a shell of an implantable breast prosthesis. Inflatable lumens are accessible by valve to facilitate the addition of saline to adjust the volume of the prosthesis at the time of use.

3.1.4 *orientation means*—any mark or palpable portion of

---

[1] This specification is under the jurisdiction of ASTM Committee F04 on Medical and Surgical Materials and Devices and is the direct responsibility of Subcommittee F04.32 on Plastic and Reconstructive Surgery.

Current edition approved July 10, 2000. Published April 2001.

[2] *Annual Book of ASTM Standards*, Vol 09.01.

[3] *Annual Book of ASTM Standards*, Vol 09.02.

[4] *Annual Book of ASTM Standards*, Vol 13.01.

[5] United States Pharmacopeia, Vol XXI, Mack Publishing Company, Easton, PA 1989. Available from Pharmacopeia Convention, Inc., 12601 Twinbrook Parkway, Rockville, NC 00852.

an implantable breast prosthesis to assist the surgeon in positioning the implant.

3.1.5 *saline*—only sodium chloride for injection (USP) is recommended for filling lumens of inflatable breast prosthesis.

3.1.6 *shell*—a silicone elastomer continuous layer or membrane container (sac) which encloses a lumen of an implantable breast prosthesis.

3.1.7 *silicone elastomer*—an elastomer containing cross-linked silicone polymer and fumed amorphous (non-crystalline) silica as a reinforcing filler.

3.1.8 *valve*—sealable or self sealing opening in an inflatable prosthesis, extending from the exterior surface of the shell into a lumen, designed to facilitate addition of saline at the time of use or postoperatively to adjust prosthesis volume.

3.1.9 *patch*—a piece of silicone elastomer which covers and seals the hole which results from the manufacturing process of shell fabrication.

4. Significance and Use

4.1 This specification contains requirements based on state-of-art science and technology as applicable to various considerations that have been identified as important to assure reasonable safety and efficacy as it relates to the biocompatibility and the mechanical integrity of the device components in implantable breast prostheses.

4.1.1 This standard specification is not intended to limit the science and technology that may be considered and applied to assure performance characteristics of subject breast prostheses in intended applications. When new information becomes available or changes in state-of-art science and technology occur and relevance to subject prostheses has been established by valid science, it is intended that this specification will be revised in accordance with ASTM guidelines.

5. Materials

5.1 *Silicone Elastomer*—Select and specify elastomers for use in implantable breast prostheses in keeping with F 604.

5.1.1 *Shell*—The following describes suitable silicone elastomer compositions for use as the primary material of construction of the shell including the exterior (tissue contact) surface:

polymer types	MQ or VMQ
fillers	A, B or C
additive	J (for radiopacity)
catalysts	B, G, J or K

NOTE 1—The composition listed in this section are not intended to limit the compositions that may be used providing all other requirements of this specification are satisfied.

5.1.2 *Fabrication*—Fabrication techniques must necessarily be dependent on the type of elastomer, the portion of an implantable breast prosthesis fabricated, its shape, location and function on the prosthesis.

5.1.3 *Vulcanization and Postcure*—Time and temperature of vulcanization and postcure must be adjusted with consideration of the elastomer type and the multi-step fabrication requirements of specific prostheses. Final postcure is typically done only after the shell or shells and all other portions have been completely assembled. Time and temperature of final postcure shall be adequate to drive the chemistry of vulcanization of all elastomer to completion and remove by-products of the cure in keeping with the chemical stoichiometry of the specific cure system (e.g., after postcure no additional vulcanization should occur when heated additionally at recommended cure temperature).

5.1.4 *Physical Property Testing and Requirements*—Silicone elastomer shells shall demonstrate an acceptable response in physical property tests. Prostheses for testing should be selected from standard production batches which have gone through all manufacturing processes, including sterilization.

5.1.4.1 *Specimen Preparation*—Cut required tests specimens from shells with D 412 Dies. Devices or specimens shall be conditioned before testing for at least 1 h at 23 ± 2°C (73.4 ± 3.6°F).

5.1.4.2 *Dimension*—The individual shape, range of volume (displacement), base size, and anterior projection are determined by the manufacturer.

6. Volume and Dimensions

6.1 *Volumes of Prostheses*:

6.1.1 *Saline Inflatable Prostheses*—The designed or minimum and maximum recommended volume of saline fill shall be listed in instructions for use.

6.2 *Dimensions*—The ranges of shapes, volumes, base sizes, and anterior projections are determined by the manufacturer. Pertinent information shall be contained in the package insert.

7. Fixation Sites

7.1 The presence of fixation sites on any type of implantable breast prosthesis is optional. When used, the size and locations of fixation sites shall be clearly stated in instructions for use.

8. Orientation Means

8.1 Orientation means are optional features of subject prostheses. When orientation means are claimed, the location and recommended techniques for use shall be clearly described in instructions for use.

9. Test Methods and Requirements

9.1 *Biocompatibility*:

9.1.1 *Standard Practice F 748*—New or existing materials shall be in compliance with Standard Practice F 748 or other accepted standards such as ISO/AAMI/ANSI 10993-1. Assays recommended by Standard Practice F 748 include Cell Culture Cytotoxicity Assays, Short-Term Intramuscular Implantation Assay, Short-Term Subcutaneous Assay, Carcinogenicity, Long-Term Implant Test, Systemic Injection (Acute Toxicity) Assay, Sensitization Assay, Mutagenicity, and Pyrogenicity.

9.1.2 *Silicone Saline Filled Prostheses*— Test specimens for chronic implantation assays (carcnogenciity and long term implant tests) shall be fabricated from the same combination of silicone elastomer and by the same or similar procedures and conditions used in fabricating prostheses. The thickness of shell in specimens shall be typical of thickness used in prostheses.

9.1.3 *Prior Biocompatibility Assays*— When prior biocompatibility data are available for silicone elastomer in clinical use in breast implants, even if not done by the exact protocols described in more standards, such data may satisfy all or part of the specific biocompatibility requirements of F 748 or equivalent methodology.

9.2 *Physical Properties*:

9.2.1 Unless otherwise specified, the standard temperature for testing shall be 23 ± 2°C (73.4 ± 3.6°F). When testing at any other temperature is required, use one of temperatures specified in Recommended Practice D 1349. Tests are as follows:

9.2.2 *Shell Leakage Testing*—Fill a 5 to 8 qt. stainless steel bowl with 70 % isopropyl alcohol. Submerge patched shell in bowl and gently apply pressure to the shell assembly. Visually inspect for any bubbles. Reposition shell in hand until entire surface of shell has been tested while exposed. Reject shells whenever any bubbles are seen.

9.2.3 *Shell*—Cut the test specimens from units made by standard production processes including sterilization. Clean with appropriate (polar, for example, 2-propanol, or non polar, for example, 1,1,1-trichloroethane) solvent if necessary.

9.2.3.1 *Percent Elongation*—Three thickness measurements shall be taken prior to test, percentage elongation shall be 350 % minimum when tested in accordance with D 412, Die C.

9.2.3.2 *Breaking Strength*—Ultimate Breaking Force in Tension shall be no less when 2.5 pounds (11.12 Newtons) when tested in accordance with test method D 412, Die C.

9.2.3.3 *Tensile Set*—The tensile set shall be < 10%, determine in accordance with Test Method D 412. Determine tensile at 300 % elongation, stress the specimen for 3 min. then allow 3 min. for relaxation.

9.2.3.4 *Fused or Adhered Joined*—Requirements for adhered or fused silicone rubber materials shall be critical to their integrity.

9.2.3.4.1 Critical Fused or Adhered Joints— Joints or seams that are critical to the integrity of the prostheses envelope shall not fail when the shell adjacent to the joint stressed to 200 % elongation for 10 s (see Fig. 1).

9.2.3.4.2 Non-Critical Fused or Adhered Joints—Fused joints or seams that are bonded to the prosthesis envelope but are not critical to the envelope integrity (fixation sites, orientation means, valve covers, etc.) shall not fail when the shell adjacent to the joint is stressed to 100 % elongation for 10s (see Fig. 1).

9.3 *Shell Rupture/Failure Testing*— No standard test for assessing shell rupture has yet been developed. When such test method has been developed it will be added to this standard.

9.4 *Valve Competence*:

9.4.1 *Test Method*—Prior to testing, manipulate valve to duplicate its use for filling and inflate prosthesis with saline as described in instructions for use. Test such manipulated valve at both high and low retrograde pressures. Use air or other suitable gas, distilled water or isotonic saline as test media. Pressures, in order to be tested, are 30 cm and 3 cm H_2O pressure respectively. Maintain each test pressure for 5 min. When air or other suitable gases are tested, immediately immerse valve opening in water to check for leakage (bubbles). With water or isotonic saline check for droplets at the valve opening.

9.4.2 *Test Requirements*—No observable or detectable leakage.

9.5 *Abrasion Testing*—The criteria for shell abrasion in this testing have not been established.

9.5.1 *Abrasion Testing*—Wet method – See A1.1.

9.5.2 *Abrasion Testing*—Dry method – See A1.2.

9.5.3 Particle sizes generated by these test methods may not be able to be correlated with particulates resulting from clinical use, and therefore, has questionable meaning.

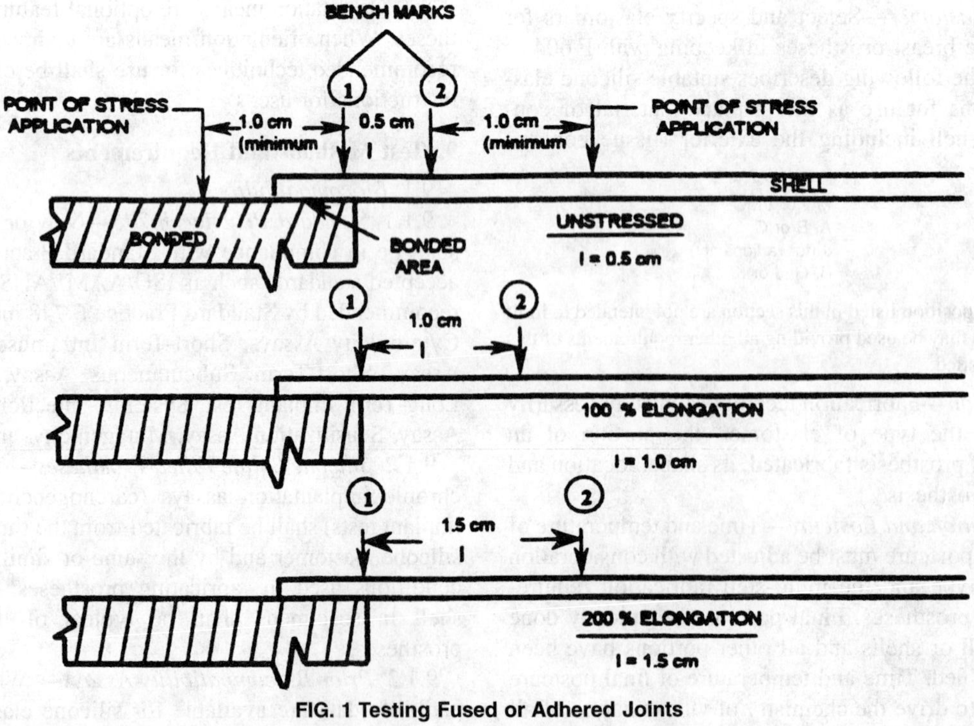

FIG. 1 Testing Fused or Adhered Joints

10. Sterilization

10.1 Implantable breast prostheses may be supplied pre-sterilized in accordance with current AMI and PDA procedures and good manufacturing practices (GMP) established by FDA.[6]

10.2 If user sterilization or re-sterilization of prostheses are intended, validated instructions for cleaning and sterilization shall be supplied with package insert.

11. Packaging, Labelling, and Package Inserts

11.1 *Packaging*—Prostheses shall be packaged to protect against damage and maintain cleanliness and sterility during the customary conditions of processing, storage, handling and distribution.

11.2 *Labeling*—Each package shall be labelled in a manner that ensures the labelling arrives at the point of use with the prostheses. The package labelling shall include the following information:

11.2.1 Manufacturer's name and address.

11.2.2 Product name, shape, type and lot number.

11.2.3 Minimum and maximum volume and relevant dimension information.

11.2.4 Date (month and year) of sterilization or packaging and method of sterilization.

11.2.5 Special storage requirements, if any.

11.2.6 Self-adhering label suitable for application to the patient's medical records containing following information:

11.2.6.1 Prosthesis name and manufacturer.

11.2.6.2 Lot number.

11.2.6.3 Type and volume.

11.3 *Implant Marking*—Each implant unit shall be clearly and permanently marked with a manufacturer's unique identifying mark and the nominal volume of the device in milliliters (ml), or cubic centimeters (cc). The marking method shall not compromise the strength or integrity of the device.

11.4 *Package Insert*—Shall contain information: *1)* to identify the manufacturer; *2)* to describe the prosthesis; *3)* on storage, handling, cleaning, sterilization and re-sterilization; *4)* to provide directions for use to the surgeon, and; *5)* warnings and precautions concerning known and potential patient adverse reactions and risks.

12. Keywords

12.1 breast prosthesis; gel saline prosthesis; implant; saline inflatable prosthesis; silicone elastomer; soft tissue implant

[6] Federal Register, Vol. 43, No. 141, Friday, July 21, 1978 Part II.

ANNEX

A1. TEST METHODS FOR ABRASION TESTING

A1.1 Abrasion Test – Wet Method

A1.1.1 *Criteria*—The criteria for shell abrasion in this testing have not been established.

A1.1.2 *Test Limitations*—The conditions of this test method do not replicate physiological conditions. This test method is designed to accelerate the abrasion process in order to evaluate various implant designs/materials comparatively, in a reasonable time frame.

Validation of the repeatability and accuracy of this test method have not been demonstrated. Typically a Round Robin test battery at different laboratories at different locations around the country is done for this validation.

A1.1.3 *Testing and Requirements*:

Test equipment and fixtures:

- Teledyne Taber® Abraser Model 5130 or 5150.
- Aluminum wheels 2.062″ O.D. × 0.625″ I.D. × 0.500″ W.
- 140-57 Auxiliary Weights (1000 gram load).
- Taber S-31 glass mounting plates.
- 6″ Aluminum specimen holder.
- 1.417″ Dia cylinder mandrel for silicone wheel cover fabrication (approx. 6″ length).
- RTV adhesive.

A1.1.3.1 *Test Sample*— Adhere approx. 5″ Dia silicone test specimen on glass mounting plate. Weigh the specimen plus glass mounting plate on analytical balance to determine its initial equilibrated mass. Cover aluminum wheel with silicone band made by dipping from cylinder mandrel, fill air gaps between silicone cover and aluminum wheel with RTV adhesive.

A1.1.3.2 Place glass mounting plate with test specimen on specimen holder. Secure test sample to holder by tightening the finger nut. Place silicone covered wheel onto abrading arm. Tighten in place. Place 1,000 gram weight onto arm. Lower arm until the silicone covered wheels contact with test surface.

A1.1.3.3 *Testing*—Add 40-50 ml's of physiological saline to specimen holder. Press ON key to energize the Taber abrader. Set the number cycles for the abrasion testing to 10,000. Press start key to initiate testing. Testing will cease after 10,000 cycles have been completed. Ensure saline is covering test area during the testing.

A1.1.3.4 After 10,000 cycles, remove specimen from the tester and gently wipe away any loose abraded material from the surface of the sample. Saline may be used to flush any loose abraded particles. Be careful to avoid contacting the abraded area of the test specimen while cleaning. Using microscope, examine specimen for failure. Look for worn areas or tears on surface of test specimen. Repeat testing and examining specimens every 10,000 cycles or until specimen fails.

A1.1.3.5 If failure has occurred, carefully remove the specimen and record number of cycles. Place sample on metal tray in an oven for 1 hour at 115°C (239°F ± 9°F). Using tweezers, remove specimen from the oven and let cool to room temperature at least 1 hour. Record specimen weight, and cumulative weight change.

A1.1.4 *Calculation*:

A1.1.4.1 Calculate the loss in mass as follows:

Mass loss per revolution, g = original mass (before test) – final mass (after test)/number of revolutions.

A1.2 Abrasion Test – Dry Method

A1.2.1 *Criteria*—The criteria for shell abrasion in this testing have not been established.

A1.2.2 *Test Limitation*— The conditions of this test method do not replicate physiological conditions. This test method is designed to accelerate the abrasion process in order to evaluate various implant designs/materials comparatively, in a reasonable time frame.

Validation of the repeatability and accuracy of this test method have not been demonstrated. Typically a Round Robin test battery at different laboratories at different locations around the country is done for this validation.

A1.2.3 *Testing and Requirements*:

Test Equipment and Fixtures:

- Taber 5-12 Long Handle Brush
- Aluminum Wheels 2.026″ OD × 0.625 ID × 0.50 W
- RTV adhesive
- Taber S-16 Steel Mounting Plates
- Teledyne Taber Abraser Model 5130 or 5150
- Hexane, greater than 95 %
- 140-57 Auxiliary Weights (1,000 gram load)
- Analytical Balance, Accurate to 0.1 mg or equivalent
- 1.417″ DIA cylinder mandrel for silicone wheel cover fabrication (approx. 6″ length)
- Temperature Humidity Chamber (to contain Taber Abraser)

A1.2.3.1 *Test Sample*— S-16 Specimen plates and aluminum wheels are soaked in Hexane for the removal of oil and contaminants and dried.

NOTE A1.1—**Caution:** Exercise Caution while using Hexane. Using RTV adhesive adhere approximately 5″ diameter silicone test specimen on S-16 mounting plate removing all air bubbles before curing. Weigh the specimen plus mounting plate on an analytical balance to determine its initial equilibrated mass. Cover aluminum wheels with silicone band made by dipping from cylinder mandrel; fill air gaps between silicone cover and aluminum wheel with RTV adhesive.

A1.2.3.2 Place specimen plate with test specimen on specimen holder. Secure test sample to holder by tightening the finger nut. Place silicone covered wheels on to abrading arms and tighten in place. Place 1,000 gram weight on to each arm. Lower arms until the silicone wheels contact with test surface.

A1.2.3.3 *Testing*—Press ON key to energize the Taber abrader. Set the number of cycles for the abrasion testing to 6,000. Press start key to initiate testing. Testing will cease after 6,000 cycles have been completed.

A1.2.3.4 After completion of 6,000 cycles, the specimen plate shall be removed and gently brushed with the Taber-512 long handled brush to remove particles. The specimen weight shall be recorded. Repeat testing and examining specimen every 6,000 cycles for a total of 30,000 cycles.

A1.2.3.5 For relative comparisons, samples having higher weight loss after 30,000 cycles are considered "less abrasion resistant".

A1.2.4 *Calculation*:

A1.2.4.1 Calculate the loss in mass as follows:

Total mass loss; g = original mass (before test)-final mass (after test).

Mass loss per revolution; g = original mass (before test) – final mass (after test)/number of revolutions.

APPENDIX

(Nonmandatory Information)

X1. RATIONALE

X1.1 Implantable saline filled breast prostheses are soft tissue implants used to simulate breast tissue in surgical procedures for breast augmentation, reconstruction, or replacement.

X1.2 Implantable breast prostheses are constructed with continuous, closed outer shells of silicone elastomer in various shapes, sizes, and combinations. Lumen is the space enclosed by the shell. The lumen of saline inflatable prostheses may be prefilled or empty as supplied and filled through a valve at the time of use with isotonic, injection grade saline in fixed or variable volume.

X1.2.1 Saline filled breast implants are known to fail from abrasion occurring in shell folds. To minimize the occurrence of shell folds these implants should be filled to the proper volume. Proper fill volume is determined at surgery and must not be less than the nominal implant volume or exceed the manufacturers recommended maximum.

X1.3 The only material currently acceptable as material of construction for implantable saline filled breast prostheses is silicone elastomer. This specification addresses the composition and vulcanization/cure of silicone elastomer and the physical properties of materials as determined from specimens obtained from final prostheses. These requirements include bonded (fused, adhered or joined) areas of the shells.

X1.3.1 There are a variety of other tests and considerations that have been proposed for incorporation into this specification including total energy to rupture, cyclic compression testing, specific chemical characterization of all silicone species, and others as such contained in FDA's *Draft Guidance for Preparation of PMA Applications for Silicone Inflatable (Saline) Breast Prostheses*. These proposals merit consideration, and the current content of this standard is not intended to limit its revision and updating to appropriately reflect changes and advancements in the state-of-the-art and the availability of relevant consensus test methods. The current content of this standard is believed to accurately represent currently available technology where there has been consensus on test methods and requirements.

X1.4 To ensure integrity of subject prostheses, this specification contains provisions for testing shells and any associated inflation valves for leakage.

Designation: F 2052 – 00

Standard Test Method for Measurement of Magnetically Induced Displacement Force on Passive Implants in the Magnetic Resonance Environment[1]

This standard is issued under the fixed designation F 2052; the number immediately following the designation indicates the year of original adoption or, in the case of revision, the year of last revision. A number in parentheses indicates the year of last reapproval. A superscript epsilon (ε) indicates an editorial change since the last revision or reapproval.

1. Scope

1.1 This standard test method covers the measurement of the magnetically induced displacement force produced by the spatial gradients of a magnetic field on passive implants (implants that function without the supply of electrical power) and the comparison of that force to the weight of the implant.

1.2 This method does not address the issues of magnetically induced torque or RF heating.

1.3 This method is intended for devices that can be suspended from a thin string. Devices which cannot be suspended from a thin string are not covered by this test method.

1.4 The weight of the thin string from which the device is suspended during the test must be less than 1% of the weight of the tested device.

1.5 This method is applicable only to magnet systems in which the direction of the magnetic field (and the direction of the magnetically induced deflection force) is horizontal.

2. Referenced Documents

2.1 *ASTM Standards:*

A 340 Standard Terminology of Symbols and Definitions Relating to Magnetic Testing

F 1542 Standard Specification for the Requirements and Disclosure of Self-Closing Aneurysm Clips

3. Terminology

3.1 *Definitions:*

3.1.1 *diamagnetic material*—a material whose relative permeability is less than unity.

3.1.2 *ferromagnetic material*—a material whose magnetic moments are ordered and parallel producing magnetization in one direction.

3.1.3 *magnetic field strength* (H in A/m)—strength of the applied magnetic field.

3.1.4 *magnetic induction or magnetic flux density* (B in T)—that magnetic vector quantity which at any point in a magnetic field is measured either by the mechanical force experienced by an element of electric current at the point, or by the electromotive force induced in an elementary loop during any change in flux linkages with the loop at the point. The magnetic induction is frequently referred to as the magnetic field. B_o is the static field in an MR scanner.

3.1.5 *magnetic resonance diagnostic device*—a device intended for general diagnostic use to present images which reflect the spatial distribution and/or magnetic resonance spectra which reflect frequency and distribution of nuclei exhibiting nuclear magnetic resonance. Other physical parameters derived from the images and/or spectra may also be produced.

3.1.6 *magnetic resonance (MR) environment*—refers to the electromagnetic environment present in the vicinity of an MR scanner within the 5 gauss line.

3.1.7 *magnetic resonance imaging* (MRI)—imaging technique that uses static and time varying magnetic fields to provide images of tissue by the magnetic resonance of nuclei.

3.1.8 *magnetically induced displacement force*— force produced when a magnetic object is exposed to the spatial gradient of a magnetic field. This force will tend to cause the object to translate in the gradient field.

3.1.9 *paramagnetic material*—a material having a relative permeability which is slightly greater than unity, and which is practically independent of the magnetizing force.

3.1.10 *passive implant*—an implant that serves its function without the supply of electrical power.

3.1.11 *tesla, (T)*—the SI unit of magnetic induction equal to 10^4 gauss.

4. Summary of Test Method

4.1 An implant is suspended by a fine string at the point in a magnetic field that will produce the greatest magnetically induced deflection. The angular deflection of the string from the vertical is measured. If the implant deflects less than 45°, then the magnetically induced deflection force is less than the force on the implant due to gravity (its weight).

5. Significance and Use

5.1 This test is one of those required to determine if the presence of a passive implant may cause injury to the person with the implant during an MRI scan and in the vicinity of the MRI scanner. Other safety issues which should be addressed

[1] This test method is under the jurisdiction of ASTM Committee F04 on Medical & Surgical Materials & Devices and is the direct responsibility of Subcommittee F04.15 on Materials Test Methods.

Current edition approved July 10, 2000. Published September 2000.

include magnetically induced torque and RF heating.

5.2 If the implant deflects less than 45°, then the magnetically induced deflection force is less than the force on the implant due to gravity (its weight). For this condition, it is assumed that any risk imposed by the application of the magnetically induced force is no greater than any risk imposed by normal daily activity in the Earth's gravitational field.

5.3 A deflection of less than 45° at the location of the maximum spatial gradient in one MRI scanner does not preclude a deflection exceeding 45° in a scanner with a higher field strength or larger spatial gradients.

5.4 This test alone is not sufficient for determining if an implant is safe in the MR environment.

6. Apparatus

6.1 The test fixture consists of a sturdy structure capable of holding the test device in the proper position without deflection of the test fixture and containing a protractor with 1° graduated markings, rigidly mounted to the structure. The 0° indicator on the protractor is oriented vertically. The test device is suspended from a thin string that is attached to the 0° indicator on the protractor. In order for the weight of the string to be considered negligible when compared to the weight of the device, the weight of the string should be less than 1% of the weight of the device. The string should be long enough so that the device may be suspended from the test fixture and hang freely in space. Motion of the string should not be constrained by the support structure or the protractor. The string may be attached to the device at any convenient location.

7. Test Specimens

7.1 For purposes of device qualification, the device evaluated according to this standard test method should be representative of manufactured implant devices that are in the finished sterilized condition.

7.2 For purposes of device qualification, implant devices should not be altered in any manner prior to testing.

7.3 This standard test method may be used on prototype devices during product development.

8. Procedure

8.1 Any magnet with a horizontal magnetic field that produces a large spatial gradient may be used for the test. Fig. 1 shows the test fixture mounted on the patient table of an MRI scanner. The test device is suspended from a thin string attached to the 0° indicator on the test fixture protractor. Position the test fixture so that the center of mass of the device is at the location where the deflection is a maximum. Hold the device so that the string is vertical and then release it. Record α, the deflection of the device from the vertical direction to the nearest 0.5° (Fig. 2).

8.2 Repeat the process in 8.1 three times for each device tested.

NOTE 1—For a paramagnetic, diamagnetic or ferromagnetic device below saturation, the location of maximum deflection is at the point where $|B|\,|\nabla B|$ is a maximum. For a ferromagnetic device above the magnetic saturation point, the maximum deflection will occur at the location where ∇B is a maximum. If it is not known whether the device is paramagnetic, diamagnetic or ferromagnetic, perform the test at both locations.

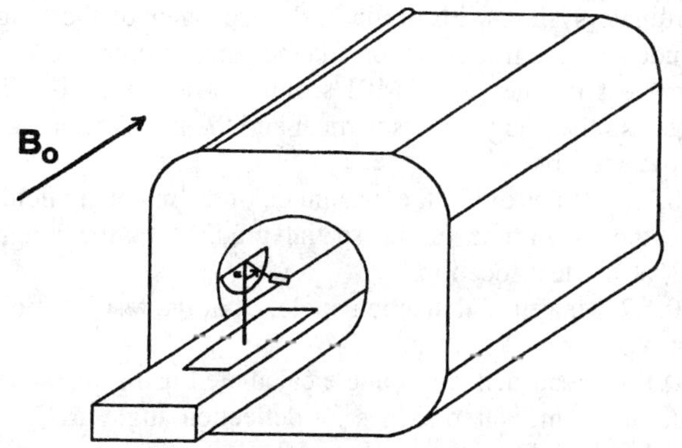

FIG. 1 Test Fixture Mounted on the Patient Table of an MRI Scanner

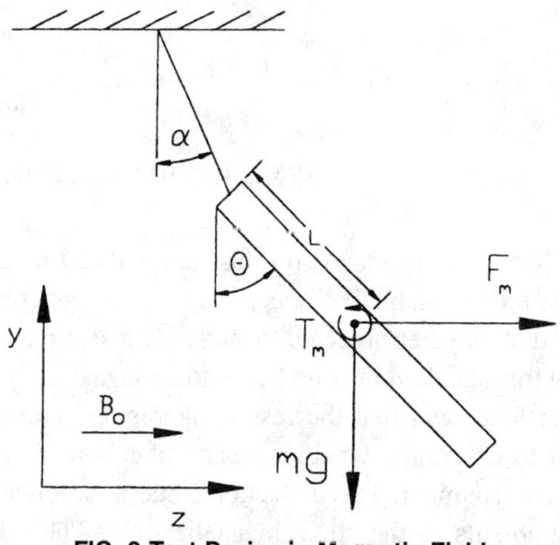

FIG. 2 Test Device in Magnetic Field

9. Calculations

9.1 Calculate the mean deflection angle using the absolute values of the 3 values for deflection angle, α, measured in Section 8. (It is possible that instead of being attracted to the magnet, the device might be repelled by the magnet. Therefore, the absolute value of the deflection angle should be used when calculating the mean deflection angle.)

9.2 Calculate the mean magnetically induced deflection force for the device using the mean value for the deflection angle α determined in 9.1 and the following relation (derived in Appendix X2): $F_m = mg \tan\alpha$, where m is the mass of the implant and g is the acceleration due to gravity. If the mean value for α is less than 45°, F_m, the magnetically induced deflection force, is less than the force on the device due to gravity (its weight).

10. Report

10.1 The report shall include the following for each specimen tested:

10.1.1 Device product description.

10.1.2 Device product number.

10.1.3 Materials of construction (ASTM designation or other).

10.1.4 Number of specimens tested with explanation for the sample size used.

10.1.5 Cartesian coordinate (x, y, z) location of the center of mass of the device during the test using a right handed coordinate system with origin at the isocenter of the magnet. Include a diagram showing the magnet and the coordinate axes. If the test magnet is an MRI scanner, orient the coordinate system so that the y-axis is vertical and the z-axis is parallel to the patient table.

10.1.6 Values of |B|, the magnitude of the magnetic field and |∇B|, the magnitude of the spatial gradient of the magnetic field, at the test location.

10.1.7 Measured deflection angle, α, at the test location for each repetition of the test.

10.1.8 Mean deflection angle calculated using the absolute value of the measured values for deflection angle, α.

10.1.9 Weight of the implant.

10.1.10 Weight of the string used to suspend the implant from the test fixture.

10.1.11 Mean magnetically induced displacement force, F_m, calculated from measured test data for each device tested.

11. Precision and Bias

11.1 The precision and bias of this test method has not been established.

12. Keywords

12.1 implant; metals (for surgical implants); MRI (magnetic resonance imaging); MR safety

APPENDIXES

(Nonmandatory Information)

X1. RATIONALE FOR DEVELOPMENT OF THE TEST METHOD

X1.1 The primary reason for this standard test method is to determine the magnetically induced deflection force on passive implants that may be subjected to magnetic resonance imaging. Note that this standard only addresses the magnetically induced deflection force and that the results of this test alone are not sufficient to determine whether a particular implant is safe in the MR environment. The deflection force is produced by the spatial gradients in the static magnetic field. The static field also produces a torque on an implant that acts to align the object with the magnetic field (like a compass needle aligns itself with the Earth's magnetic field). For a device to be safe in the MR environment, the magnetically induced deflection force and torque should be less than forces and torques to which the implant would be subjected if it were not in a large magnetic field, e.g. a force less than the weight of the device and a torque less than that produced by normal daily activities (which might include rapidly accelerating vehicles or amusement park rides). In addition, for a device to be safe in the MR environment, it must be shown to produce negligible levels of RF induced heating and gradient induced voltages. The terms MR safe and MR compatible are defined below.

*MR safe** —The device, when used in the MR environment, has been demonstrated to present no additional risk to the patient or other individuals, but may affect the quality of the diagnostic information.

*MR compatible** —The device, when used in the MR environment, is MR Safe and has been demonstrated to neither significantly affect the quality of the diagnostic information nor have its operations affected by the MR device.

* The MR conditions in which the device was tested should be specified in conjunction with the terms MR safe and MR compatible since a device which is safe or compatible under one set of conditions may not be found to be so under more extreme MR conditions.

A device which produces a deflection of less than 45° using this standard test method, passes a torque test and demonstrates negligible levels of RF heating and gradient induced voltages may be designated MR Safe for the MR environment in which it was tested.

Currently, a commercial 1.5 T MRI scanner produces the conditions that would most commonly be encountered by an implant.

X2. DERIVATION OF FORCE RELATION

X2.1

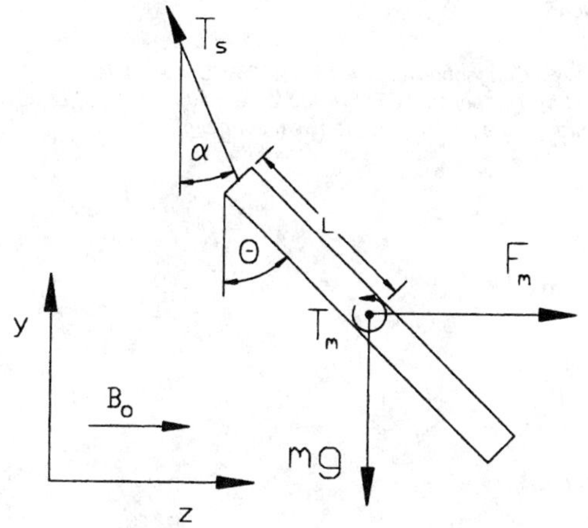

FIG. X2.1 Free Body Diagram of Implant in Magnetic Field

Definitions of symbols:

T_s = tension in string
T_m = torque due to magnetic field
F_m = magnetically induced deflection force due to magnetic field spatial gradient
L = distance from string attachment to center of mass of device
m = mass of device
α = angular deflection of string measured with protractor
θ = angular rotation of device
g = acceleration due to gravity

Assumptions:

1. Magnetism is a body force like gravity.
2. The center of magnetic force is not required to coincide with the center of mass, though the two locations are shown to be coincident in Fig. X2.1. The force equations written below are independent of the point of application of the magnetically induced force and torque.
3. The device is oriented in the magnetic field so that F_m and T_m are the only components of magnetically induced force and torque.

Summing forces in the free body diagram in Fig. X2.1:

$$\Sigma F_z = 0 = F_m - T_s sin\alpha \quad (X2.1)$$

$$\Sigma F_y = 0 = T_s cos\alpha - mg \quad (X2.2)$$

Solving the two equations gives $F_m = mg tan\alpha$.

Note that the solution is independent of the point of attachment of the string. Also note that because the derivation of the relation for F_m uses only the force equilibrium equations, the relation for F_m also holds if the center of magnetic force does not coincide with the center of mass, as might be the case for an implant composed of more than one material.

REFERENCES

(1) Gegauff, A. G., Laurell, K. A., Thavendrarajah, A., and Rosenstiel, S. F., "A Potential MRI Hazard: Forces on Dental Magnet Keepers," *Journal of Oral Rehabilitation*, vol. 17, 1990, pp. 403-410.

(2) Kagetsu, N. J., and Litt, A. W., "Important Considerations in Measurement of Attractive Force on Metallic Implants in MR Imagers," *Radiology*, vol. 179, 1991, pp. 505-508.

(3) Kanal, E., and Shellock, F. G., "Aneurysm Clips: Effects of Long-term and Multiple Exposures to a 1.5-T MR System," *Radiology*, vol. 210, 1999, pp. 563-565.

(4) New, P. F., Rosen, B. R., Brady, T., J., Buonarmo, F. S., Kistler, J. P., Burt, C. T., Hinshaw, W. S., Newhouse, J. H., Pohost, G. M., and Taveras, J. M., "Potential Hazards and Artifacts of Ferromagnetic and Nonferromagnetic Surgical and Dental Materials and Devices in Nuclear Magnetic Resonance Imaging," *Radiology*, vol. 147, 1983, pp. 139–148.

(5) Planert, J., Modler, H., and Vosshenrich, R., "Measurements of Magnetism-Related Forces and Torque Moments Affecting Medical Instruments, Implants, and Foreign Objects During Magnetic Resonance Imaging at all Degrees of Freedom," *Medical Physics*, vol. 23, 1996, pp. 851-856.

(6) Planert, J., Modler, H., Lüjdecke, and Eger, M., "A Miniaturised Force-Torque Sensor with Six Degrees of Freedom for Dental Measurements," *Clin. Phys. Physiol. Meas.*, vol. 13, 1992, pp. 241-248.

(7) Schenck, J. F., "The Role of Magnetic Susceptibility in Magnetic Resonance Imaging: MRI Magnetic Compatibility of the First and Second Kinds," *Medical Physics*, vol. 23, 1996, pp. 815-850.

(8) Shellock, F. G., and Kanal, E., "Yasargil Aneurysm Clips: Evaluation of Interactions with a 1.5-T MR System," *Radiology*, vol. 207, 1998, pp. 587-591.

(9) Shellock, F. G., and Shellock, V. J., "Cardiovascular Catheters and Accessories: Ex Vivo Testing of Ferromagnetism, Heating, and Artifacts Associated with MRI," *JMRI*, vol. 8, 1998, pp. 1338-1342.

(10) Shellock, F. G., and Shellock, V. J., "Cranial Bone Flap Fixation Clamps: Compatibility at MR Imaging," *Radiology*, vol. 207, 1998, pp. 822-825.

(11) Teitelbaum, G.P., Lin, M.C.W., Watanabe, A.T., Nogray, J.F., Young, T.I., and Bradley, W. G., Jr., "Ferromagnetism and MR Imaging: Safety of Carotid Vascular Clamps," *American Journal of Neuroradiology*, vol. 11, 1990, pp. 267-272.

(12) Teitelbaum, G. P., Yee, C. A., Van Horn, D. D., Kim, H. S., and Colletti, P. M., "Metallic Ballistic Fragments: MR Imaging Safety and Artifacts," *Radiology*, vol. 175, 1990, pp. 885-859.

Standard Specification for Square Drive Interconnections on Surgical Instruments[1]

This standard is issued under the fixed designation F 2062; the number immediately following the designation indicates the year of original adoption or, in the case of revision, the year of last revision. A number in parentheses indicates the year of last reapproval. A superscript epsilon (ε) indicates an editorial change since the last revision or reapproval.

1. Scope

1.1 This specification applies to interconnections of surgical instruments used for drilling, tapping, driving, or placing of medical devices during surgery.

1.2 This specification includes dimensions and tolerances for both driving and driven elements.

1.3 The values stated in SI units are to be regarded as the standard. Inch-pound values are in separate tables.

1.4 The specifications given in ASME B107.4M-1995 are designed for industrial applications and are considered to loose for surgical applications. Springs used for industrial applications are generally made from carbon steel and are capable of higher loads than their stainless steel counterparts. The specifications given in this standard have been written to lessen the chance of accidental disengagement of surgical instruments. This accidental disengagement could injure the patient or end user, or damage or contaminate the instrument.

2. Referenced Documents

2.1 *ASTM Standards:*

F 899 Specification for Stainless Steel Billet, Bar, and Wire for Surgical Instruments[2]

2.2 *Other Standard:*

ASME B107.4M-1995 (Revision of ANSI B107.4-1982), Driving and Spindle Ends for Portable Hand, Impact, Air, and Electric Tools Percussion Tools Excluded[3]

3. Terminology

3.1 *Definitions of Terms Specific to This Standard:*

3.1.1 *drilling*—the act of forming a hole.

3.1.2 *driving*—the act of turning, pushing, or pulling a surgical instrument to place a medical device during surgery.

3.1.3 *square drive*—a male or female interconnection with four driving surfaces that are of equal width and perpendicular to each other.

3.1.4 *tapping*—the act of forming threads.

4. Material

4.1 This specification is intended to apply only to stainless steel instruments that conform to Specification F 899. If other types of materials are used to interconnect with stainless steel instruments, then they should adhere to this specification.

5. Gage Use and Design

5.1 Tables 1-8 are descriptive and not restrictive, and are not intended to preclude the manufacture of product or gages which are otherwise in accordance with this specification.

5.2 Manufacturers may use gages with tighter dimensions or tolerances than shown herein to ensure device acceptance.

5.3 The extreme size for all limit (GO and NO-GO) gages shall not exceed the extreme limits of interconnections specified within this specification. All variations (manufacturing tolerance, calibration error, wear allowance, and so forth) in the gages, whatever their cause or purpose, shall bring these gages within the extreme limits of the gage size specified in this specification. Thus, a gage representing a minimum limit may be larger, but never smaller, than the minimum size specified for the interconnection in this specification; likewise, a gage representing a maximum limit may be smaller, but never larger, than the maximum size specified for the interconnection in this specification.

6. Keywords

6.1 instrument; interconnection; square drive; surgical

[1] This specification is under the jurisdiction of ASTM Committee F04 on Medical and Surgical Materials and Devices and is the direct responsibility of Subcommittee F04.33 on Medical/Surgical Instruments.

Current edition approved Nov. 10, 2000. Published February 2001.

[2] *Annual Book of ASTM Standards*, Vol 13.01.

[3] Available from American Society of Mechanical Engineers, 345 E. 47th St. New York, NY 10017

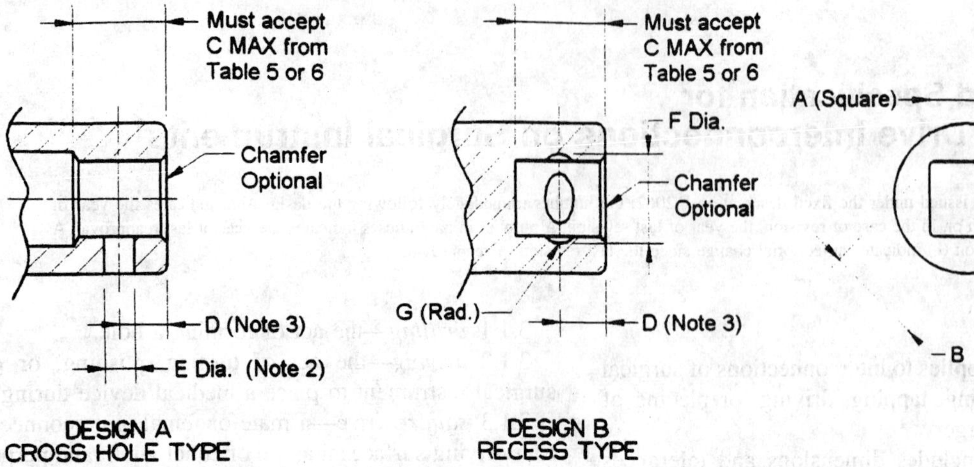

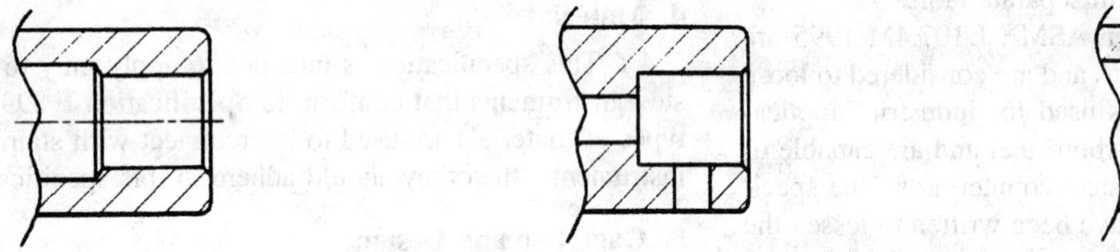

OPTIONAL CROSS SECTIONS

NOTES:

(1) Square tolerances shall be such as to insure acceptance when gauged with gages conforming to Table 2.

(2) Design A requires cross hole to be on one, two, or four sides. Recess Design B must require radius G to be on all four sides.

(3) D MAX (Tables 1 & 2) doesn't equal D MIN (Tables 5 & 6); however, due to edge radius, plunger diameter, and square dimension interactions, no interference or interchangeability problem exists.

TABLE 1 Square Drive Specifications – Female End, mm

Drive Size		A (square)		B	D (Note 3)		E (Note 2)	F (diameter)		G (radius)	
mm	in.	max	min	min	max	min	min	max	min	max	min
4.76	0.1875	4.88	4.80	6.68	3.30	3.05	1.98	6.25	6.15	1.32	1.07
6.35	0.2500	6.48	6.38	8.51	3.94	3.43	2.29	7.75	7.49	1.73	1.47
9.53	0.3750	9.70	9.60	13.13	5.84	5.33	4.32	10.92	10.41	2.41	2.16

TABLE 2 Square Drive Specifications – Female End, in.

Drive Size		A (square)		B	D (Note 3)		E (Note 2)	F (diameter)		G (radius)	
in.	mm	max	min	min	max	min	min	max	min	max	min
0.1875	4.76	0.192	0.189	0.263	0.130	0.120	0.078	0.246	0.242	0.052	0.042
0.2500	6.35	0.255	0.251	0.335	0.155	0.135	0.090	0.305	0.295	0.068	0.058
0.3750	9.53	0.382	0.378	0.517	0.230	0.210	0.170	0.430	0.410	0.095	0.085

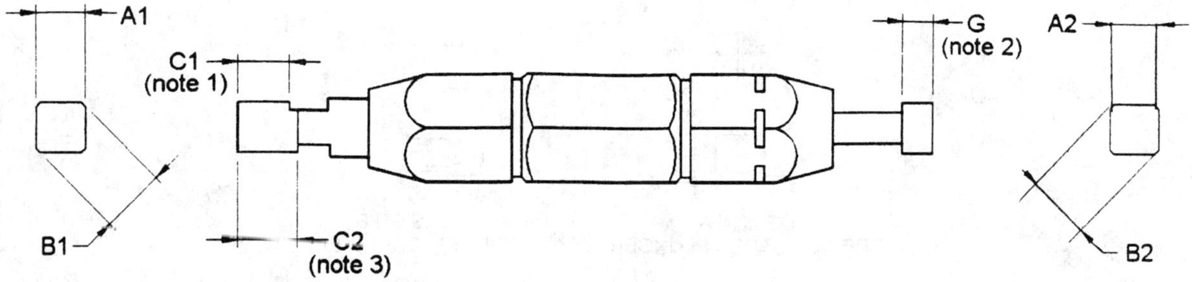

NOTES:
(1) Minimum length requirement from table 5 or 6.
(2) Minimum length for NO GO gage.
(3) Optional maximum length gage from table 5 or 6.

TABLE 3 Square Drive Gage Specifications – Female End, mm

Drive Size		A1	A2	B1	B2	C1	C2	G
mm	in.	+0.005 −0.000	+0.000 −0.005	+0.005 −0.005	+0.038 −0.038	+0.005 −0.000	+0.000 −0.005	min
4.76	0.1875	4.801	4.877	6.680	6.553	6.350	6.604	1.981
6.35	0.2500	6.375	6.477	8.509	8.331	7.366	7.874	2.286
9.53	0.3750	9.601	9.703	13.132	13.005	10.592	11.100	4.318

TABLE 4 Square Drive Gage Specifications – Female End, in.

Drive Size		A1	A2	B1	B2	C1	C2	G
mm	in.	+0.0002 −0.0000	+0.0000 −0.0002	+0.0002 −0.0002	+0.0015 −0.0015	+0.0002 −0.0000	+0.0000 −0.0002	min
0.1875	4.76	0.1890	0.1920	0.2630	0.2580	0.2500	0.2600	0.0780
0.2500	6.35	0.2510	0.2550	0.3350	0.3280	0.2900	0.3100	0.900
0.3750	9.53	0.3780	0.3820	0.5170	0.5120	0.4170	0.4370	0.1700

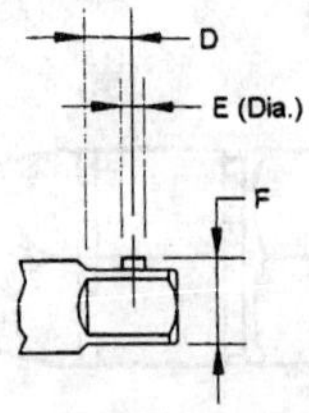

DESIGN A
SPRING LOADED PLUNGER

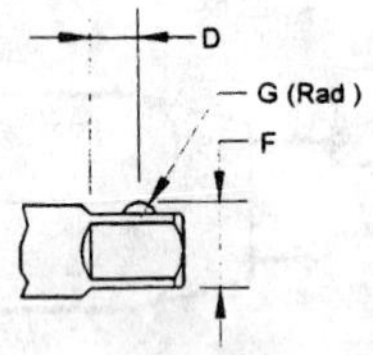

DESIGN B
SPRING LOADED BALL

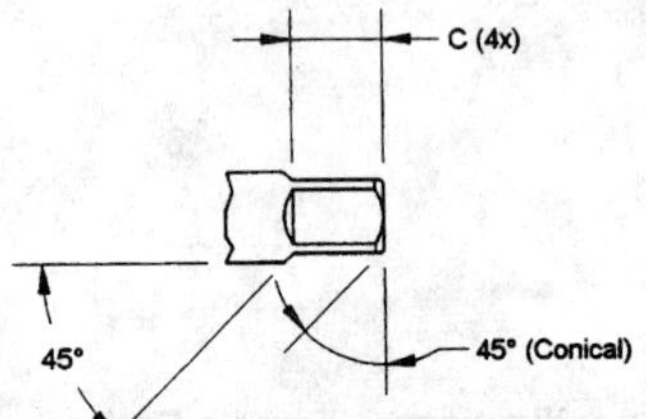

DESIGN C
APPLICABLE TO ALL TYPES

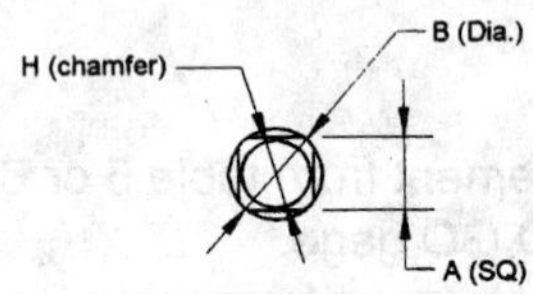

END VIEW
APPLICABLE TO ALL TYPES

TABLE 5 Square Drive Specifications – Male End, mm

Drive Size		A (square)		B (dia)	C		D (Note 1)		E	F (lock height)		G (radius)		H
mm	in.	max	min	±0.002	max	min	max	min	min	max	min	max	min	max
4.76	0.1875	4.75	4.70	6.35	6.60	6.35	3.43	3.18	5.33	5.59	5.33	1.30	1.17	4.50
6.35	0.2500	6.35	6.30	7.92	7.87	7.37	4.19	3.81	6.86	7.36	6.86	1.70	1.57	6.10
9.53	0.3750	9.53	9.45	12.70	11.10	10.59	5.56	5.44	10.34	10.97	10.34	2.49	2.36	9.27

TABLE 6 Square Drive Specifications – Male End, in.

Drive Size		A (square)		B (dia)	C		D (Note 1)		E	F (lock height)		G (radius)		H
in.	mm	max	min	±0.002	max	min	max	min	min	max	min	max	min	max
0.1875	4.76	0.187	0.185	0.250	0.260	0.250	0.135	0.125	0.210	0.220	0.210	0.051	0.046	0.177
0.2500	6.35	0.250	0.248	0.312	0.310	0.290	0.165	0.150	0.270	0.290	0.270	0.067	0.062	0.240
0.3750	9.53	0.375	0.372	0.500	0.437	0.417	0.219	0.214	0.407	0.432	0.407	0.098	0.093	0.365

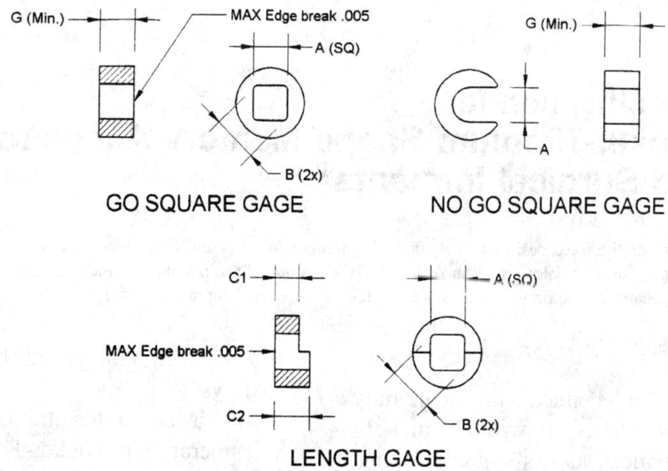

TABLE 7 Square Drive Gage Specifications – Male End, mm

Drive Size		A1	A2	B1	C1	C2	G
mm	in.	+0.005 –0.000	+0.000 –0.005	min	+0.005 –0.000	+0.000 –0.005	min
4.76	0.1875	4.750	4.699	6.680	6.350	6.604	1.981
6.35	0.2500	6.350	6.299	8.509	7.366	7.874	2.286
9.53	0.3750	9.525	9.449	13.132	10.592	11.100	4.318

TABLE 8 Square Drive Gage Specifications – Male End, in.

Drive Size		A1	A2	B	C1	C2	G
mm	in.	+0.0002 –0.0000	+0.0000 –0.0002	min	+0.0002 –0.0000	+0.0000 –0.0002	min
0.1875	4.76	0.1870	0.1850	0.2630	0.2500	0.2600	0.0780
0.2500	6.35	0.2500	0.2480	0.3350	0.2900	0.3100	0.0900
0.3750	9.53	0.3750	0.3720	0.5170	0.4170	0.4370	0.1700

APPENDIX

(Nonmandatory Information)

X1. RATIONALE

X1.1 The objective of this specification is the provision of guidelines for the physical characteristics of square drive interconnections specifically used for medical device applications. This specification identifies those factors felt to be important to ensure compatibility of square drive interconnections made by various manufacturers.

X1.2 Not all stainless steels listed in Specification F 899 may be appropriate for this application.

Designation: F 2063 – 00

Standard Specification for Wrought Nickel-Titanium Shape Memory Alloys for Medical Devices and Surgical Implants[1]

This standard is issued under the fixed designation F 2063; the number immediately following the designation indicates the year of original adoption or, in the case of revision, the year of last revision. A number in parentheses indicates the year of last reapproval. A superscript epsilon (ε) indicates an editorial change since the last revision or reapproval.

1. Scope

1.1 This specification covers the chemical, physical, mechanical, and metallurgical requirements for wrought nickel-titanium bar, wire, flat rolled products, and tubing containing nominally 54.5 % to 57.0 % nickel and used for the manufacture of medical devices and surgical implants.

1.2 The values stated in SI units are to be regarded as the standard. The values given in inch-pound units are for information only.

2. Referenced Documents

2.1 *ASTM Standards:*

E 8 Test Methods for Tension Testing of Metallic Materials[2]

E 112 Test Method for Determining Average Grain Size[2]

E 120 Test Method for Chemical Analysis of Titanium and Titanium Alloys[3]

E 1019 Test Method for Determination of Carbon, Sulfur, Nitrogen and Oxygen in Steel and in Iron, Nickel, and Cobalt Alloys[4]

E 1097 Guide for Direct Current Plasma Emission Spectrometry Analysis[4]

E 1172 Practice for Describing and Specifying a Wavelength-Dispersive X-Ray Spectrometer[4]

E 1245 Practice for Determining the Inclusion or Second-Phase Constituent Content of Metals by Automatic Image Analysis[2]

E 1409 Test Method for Determination of Oxygen in Titanium and Titanium Alloys by the Inert Gas Fusion Technique[4]

E 1447 Test Method for Determination of Hydrogen in Titanium and Titanium Alloys by the Inert Gas Fusion Thermal Conductivity Method[4]

E 1479 Practice for Describing and Specifying Inductively-Coupled Plasma Optical Emission Spectrometers[4]

F 2004 Test Method for Transformation Temperature of Nickel-Titanium Alloys by Thermal Analysis[5]

F 2005 Terminology for Nickel-Titanium Shape Memory Alloys[5]

F 2082 Method for the Determination of Transformation Temperature of Nickel-Titanium Shape Memory Alloys by Bend and Free Recovery[5]

2.2 *ASQ Standard:*

C1 General Requirements for a Quality Program[6]

3. Terminology

3.1 The terminology describing the physical and thermal properties of these alloys shall be as defined in Terminology F 2005.

3.2 E4: General Terminology

4. Product Classification

4.1 *bar*—Round bars and flats from 5 mm (0.196 inches) to 130 mm (5.1 inches) in diameter or thickness (other sizes or shapes by special order).

4.2 *plate*—Any product 5 mm (0.196 inches) thick and over and 250 mm (9.8 inches) wide and over, with width equal to or greater than five times the thickness.

4.3 *strip*—Any product under 5 mm (0.196 inches) thick and under 600 mm (23.6 inches) wide.

4.4 *sheet*—Any product under 5 mm (0.196 inches) thick and 600 mm (23.6 inches) or more wide.

4.5 *wire*—Rounds less than 5 mm (0.196 inches) in diameter.

4.6 *tubing*—Hollow cylindrical shapes up to 50 mm (1.96 inches) in outside diameter.

5. Ordering Information

5.1 Inquiries and orders for material under this specification shall include the following information:

5.1.1 *Quantity:* weight, length, or number of pieces.

5.1.2 *Alloy formulation*, in terms of transformation temperature parameter (see Section 8).

5.1.3 *Form:* bar, plate, strip, sheet, wire, or tubing (see Section 4).

5.1.4 *Condition* (see Sections 6.3 and 10.1).

5.1.5 *Mechanical Properties*, if applicable for special conditions (see Section 10).

[1] This specification is under the jurisdiction of ASTM Committee F04 on Medical and Surgical Materials and Devices and is the direct responsibility of Subcommittee F04.12 on Metallurgical Materials.

Current edition approved Nov. 10, 2000. Published February 2001.

[2] *Annual Book of ASTM Standards*, Vol 03.01.

[3] *Annual Book of ASTM Standards*, Vol 03.05.

[4] *Annual Book of ASTM Standards*, Vol 03.06.

[5] *Annual Book of ASTM Standards*, Vol 13.01.

[6] Available from the American Society for Quality, 611 East Wisconsin Ave., Milwaukee, WI 53203.

5.1.6 *Surface Condition* (see Sections 6.4).

5.1.7 *Applicable Dimensions*, including diameter, thickness, width, spool size, coil diameter, and length (exact, random, multiples) or print number.

5.1.8 *Special Tests*, for example, chemical analysis on the finished mill product.

5.1.9 *Special Requirements* (see section 11).

6. Manufacture

6.1 The material shall be made from ingot made from nickel and titanium with no other intentional alloy additions.

6.2 The material shall be vacuum or inert atmosphere melted to control metallurgical cleanliness and alloy chemistry.

6.3 Bar, plate, tubing, wire, and flat rolled products shall be supplied as hot finished or cold finished and annealed or heat treated as specified in the purchase order.

6.4 Surface condition may be oxidized, descaled, pickled, blasted, machined, ground, mechanically polished, or electropolished.

7. Chemical Composition

7.1 The heat analysis shall conform to the requirements of Table 1. Ingot analysis may be used for reporting all chemical requirements except hydrogen. Samples for hydrogen analysis shall be taken from the finished mill product see Section 4 or as agreed upon between the customer and supplier. The supplier shall not ship material that is outside the limits specified in Table 1

7.1.1 Requirements for major and minor elements are listed in Table 1. Important residual elements are also listed. Analysis for elements not listed in Table 1 is not required to verify compliance with this specification.

7.2 *Analytical Methods*—Major elements shall be analyzed by direct current plasma spectrometry according to Guide E 1097; atomic absorption, inductively coupled plasma spectrometry according to Practice E 1479; X-ray spectrometer according to Practice E 1172 or an equivalent method. Carbon shall be measured by combustion according to Test Method E 1019. Hydrogen shall be measured by inert gas fusion or vacuum hot extraction according to Test Methods E 120 or E 1447. Nitrogen and oxygen shall be measured by inert gas fusion according to Test Method E 1409.

7.3 The titanium content of these alloys shall be determined by difference and need not be analyzed.

7.4 Product analysis limits shall be as specified in Table 2. Product analysis tolerances do not broaden the specification heat analysis requirements, but cover variation between laboratories in the measurement of chemical content. The manufacturer shall not ship material that is outside the limits specified in Table 1.

TABLE 1 Chemical Requirements

Element	Weight Percent
Nickel	54.5 to 57.0
Carbon, maximum	0.070
Cobalt, maximum	0.050
Copper, maximum	0.010
Chromium, maximum	0.010
Hydrogen, maximum	0.005
Iron, maximum	0.050
Niobium, maximum	0.025
Oxygen, maximum	0.050
Titanium	Balance

TABLE 2 Product Analysis Tolerance[A]

Element	Tolerance Under the Minimum or Over the Maximum, (wt. %)
Nickel	0.2
Element	**Tolerance Over the Maximum, (wt. %)**
Carbon	0.002
Cobalt	0.001
Copper	0.001
Chromium	0.001
Hydrogen	0.0005
Iron	0.01
Niobium	0.004
Oxygen	0.004

[A]Product analysis tolerance limits are based on analytical capabilities that have been demonstrated for this composition.

8. Transformation Temperature

8.1 The nickel and titanium contents of nickel-titanium shape memory alloys cannot be measured to a precision required to guarantee shape memory or superelastic properties. Calorimetry or an equivalent thermomechanical test method must be used to assure the alloy formulation in terms of transformation temperature.

8.2 Alloy formulation shall be specified in terms of the transformation temperature parameter(s) required by the purchase order. This parameter shall be one of the following: M_f, M_p, M_s, A_s, A_p, A_f as defined in Terminology F 2005 and as measured in accordance with Method F 2004, Method F 2082 or as measured in accordance with another appropriate thermomechanical test method.

8.3 When measured in accordance with Method F 2004 for transformation temperature by thermal analysis, the A_s shall be uniform to within ±10°C on the purchased product or as agreed upon by the customer and supplier.

8.4 Transformation temperature parameters are normally specified in the wrought product in the annealed condition as defined in F 2005. Other conditions for the certification of alloy transformation temperature shall be considered a special requirement.

9. Metallurgical Structure

9.1 *Microstructure*:

9.1.1 Annealed product 6 mm (0.236 in.) to 50 mm (1.96 in.) in section shall have a grain size of ASTM 4 or finer as measured by Test Method E 112.

9.2 *Non-metallic Inclusions and Porosity*:

9.2.1 For all mill products, porosity and nonmetallic inclusions such as $Ti_4Ni_2O_x$ and TiC particles shall be no larger than 12.5 μm (0.0005 in.). Furthermore, porosity and nonmetallic inclusions shall not constitute more than 1.0 % (area percent) of the structure as viewed at 400X to 500X in any field of view. Porosity and nonmetallic inclusions shall be evaluated in mill product at a section size not larger than 94.0 mm (3.70 in.) and not smaller than 6.3 mm (¼ in.) in any direction except for the mill product length (that is, diameter, thickness, width, height, wall thickness, etc.). Measurements shall be made in accordance with Practice E 1245 or an equivalent method, except that the plane-of-polish shall be either transverse or parallel to the working direction as agreed upon by the customer and the supplier. The supplier and purchaser shall agree upon the number and location of samples in the product, the sample preparation, the number of fields of view and the measurement technique.

10. Mechanical Property Requirements

10.1 Samples from the final product annealed as specified in F 2005 shall conform to the mechanical properties found in Table 3.

10.2 Material may be ordered in the cold worked or heat treated condition to higher ultimate tensile strength and lower elongation or other physical and mechanical properties as agreed upon between the supplier and purchaser.

10.3 Specimens for product above 50 mm (1.96 in.) in diameter or thickness may be taken from plate or strip rolled from the product. For product 50 mm (1.96 in.) or less in diameter or thickness, specimens shall be made from the product.

10.4 Tensile properties shall be measured in the longitudinal direction with respect to the final fabrication of the sample. Transverse tensile properties for wide flat products shall be as agreed upon between the customer and the supplier.

10.5 Tensile testing shall be performed in accordance with Test Method E 8. Tensile properties shall be those listed in Table 3 using the appropriate gage length for the product size being tested.

TABLE 3 Annealed Mechanical Properties[A]

Diameter or Distance Between Parallel Sides, mm	Tensile Strength MPa, Minimum	Elongation in 50 mm (2 in.) or 4 D, % Minimum[B]
Up to 50 (1.96 in.)	551 (79.9 KSI)	10
Over 50	551 (79.9 KSI)	5

[A]Tested at ambient temperature of 20 to 25C (68 to 77°F).
[B]4D indicates 4 times diameter.

10.6 Other special mechanical tests shall be as specified on the purchase order.

11. Special Requirements

11.1 Size variation and out-of-round tolerance shall be specified in the purchase order.

11.2 Special transformation temperature requirements in terms of product form, test location or heat treatment shall be specified on the purchase order.

11.3 Surface roughness shall be specified on the purchase order.

12. Certification

12.1 The supplier shall provide at the time of shipment a certification that the material was manufactured and tested in accordance with this specification. The certification shall include a summary of the test results for chemical composition, transformation temperature, metallurgical structure and mechanical properties as agreed upon by the customer and supplier (see Sections 7, 8, 9, and 10).

13. Quality Program

13.1 The supplier shall maintain a quality program such as defined in Requirements C1.

14. Keywords

14.1 cardiac devices; metals; NiTi; TiNi; nitinol; nickel-titanium alloys; titanium-nickel alloys; orthopaedic medical devices; vascular devices; shape memory alloys; stents; superelastic alloys; surgical implants

APPENDIXES

(Nonmandatory Information)

X1. RATIONALE

X1.1 The purpose of this specification is to characterize the chemical, physical, thermomechanical and metallurgical properties of wrought nominally 54.5 to 57.0 % nickel-titanium alloys to be used in the manufacture of medical devices and surgical implants.

X1.2 The purchaser's choice of shape memory alloy transformation temperature and mechanical properties is dependent upon the design and application of the medical device.

X1.3 Thermo-mechanical process history particularly cold work and heat treatment affect the transformation temperature and other physical and mechanical properties of nickel-titanium shape memory alloys. The annealed condition stipulated in Sections 8.4 and 10.1 are for the test samples only. Finished product is normally purchased in the cold worked or cold worked and heat treated condition.

X1.4 Ingot chemical analysis can be affected by subsequent thermo-mechanical and chemical processing. For example, pickling can result in hydrogen pick up. Therefore, hydrogen is specified for the finished mill product (see Section 7.2).

X1.5 The nickel-titanium alloys covered by this standard are commonly called nitinol alloys. Nitinol is not a single alloy, It is a family of alloys each designated by a transformation temperature measured under controlled conditions and after a specified thermo-mechanical history.

X1.6 Transformation temperature uniformity refers to the range of As measured on an alloy formulation tested by a single laboratory working to Test Method F 2004..

X1.7 The elements C, Co, Cu, H, Fe, Nb and O are residual elements in these alloys (see Table 1). They are controlled to special limits in order to ensure good shape memory physical and mechanical properties. The product analysis tolerance limits are based upon the analytical capabilities that have been demonstrated for these compositions.

X2. BIOCOMPATIBILITY

X2.1 The material compositions covered by this specification have been employed successfully in human implants, exhibiting a well-characterized level of local biological response for over 10 years. References are as follows:

Castleman, L. S., and Motzkin, S. M., "Biocompatability of Nitinol," *Biocompatability of Clinical Implant Materials*, Williams, D. F. (ed.), CRC Press, Boca Raton, Fl, 1981.

Castleman, L. S., et al., "Biocompatability of Nitinol Alloy as an Implant Material," *J. Biomed. Materials Research*, Vol 10, 1976, pp. 695–731.

Oshida, Y., and Miyazaki, S., "Corrosion and Biocompatability of Shape Memory Alloys," *Corrosion Engineering*, Vol 40, 1991, pp. 1009–1025.

Shabalovskaya, S. A., "On the Nature of the Biocompatability and Medical Applications NiTi Shape Memory and Superelastic Alloys," *Bio-Medical Materials and Engineering*, Vol 6, No 4, 1996, pp. 267–289.

Ryhanen, J., et al., "The Biocompatability and Corrosion Behavior of Nitinol in Human Oseto- and Fibroblast Cell Cultures," in *SMST-97 Proceedings of the Second International Conference on Shape Memory and Superelastic Technologies*, Pelton, A., et al., (eds), SMST, Santa Clara, CA, 1997, pp. 407–410.

Armitage, D. A., et al., "Haemocompatability of Surface Modified NiTi," *SMST-97 Proceedings of the Second International Conference on Shape Memory and Superelastic Technologies*, Pelton, A., et al., (eds.), SMST, Santa Clara, CA, 1997, pp. 411–416.

Villermaux, F. et al., "Cytocompatability of Niti Shape Memory Alloy Biomaterials," *SMST-97 Proceedings of the Second International Conference on Shape Memory and Superelastic Technologies*, Pelton, A et al., (eds.), SMST, Santa Clara, CA, 1997, pp. 417–422.

Trepanier, C. et al., "In Vivo Biocompatability Study of NiTi Stents," *SMST-97 Proceedings of the Second International Conference on Shape Memory and Superelastic Technologies*, Pelton, A et al., (eds.), SMST, Santa Clara, CA, 1997, pp. 423–428.

Ryhanen, J., "Biocompatibility Evaluation of Nickel-Titanium Shape Memory Alloy," ACTA UNIVERSITATIS OULUENSIS, *D Medica*, 518, Oulu University Press, April, 1999.

X2.2 No known surgical implant has ever been shown to be completely free of adverse reaction in the human body. Long term clinical experience in the use of the materials referred to in this specification, however, has shown that an acceptable level of biological response can be expected, if the material is used in an appropriate application.

Designation: F 2064 – 00

Standard Guide for Characterization and Testing of Alginates as Starting Materials Intended for Use in Biomedical and Tissue–Engineered Medical Products Application[1]

This standard is issued under the fixed designation F 2064; the number immediately following the designation indicates the year of original adoption or, in the case of revision, the year of last revision. A number in parentheses indicates the year of last reapproval. A superscript epsilon (ε) indicates an editorial change since the last revision or reapproval.

INTRODUCTION

Alginate has found uses in a variety of products ranging from simple technical applications such as viscosifiers to advanced biomedical matrices providing controlled drug delivery from immobilized living cells. As for most hydrocolloids, the functionality of alginate is related to its chemical and structural composition. The aim of this guide is to identify key parameters relevant for the functionality and characterization of alginates for the development of new commercial applications of alginates for the biomedical and pharmaceutical industries.

1. Scope

1.1 This guide covers the evaluation of alginates suitable for use in biomedical or pharmaceutical applications, or both, including, but not limited to, tissue-engineered medical products (TEMPS).

1.2 This guide addresses key parameters relevant for the functionality, characterization, and purity of alginates.

1.3 As with any material, some characteristics of alginates may be altered by processing techniques (such as molding, extrusion, machining, assembly, sterilization, and so forth) required for the production of a specific part or device. Therefore, properties of fabricated forms of this polymer should be evaluated using test methods that are appropriate to ensure safety and efficacy and are not addressed in this guide.

1.4 *This standard does not purport to address all of the safety concerns, if any, associated with its use. It is the responsibility of the user of this standard to establish appropriate safety and health practices and determine the applicability of regulatory limitations prior to use.*

2. Referenced Documents

2.1 *ASTM Standards:*

D 2196 Test Methods for Rheological Properties of Non-Newtonian Materials by Rotational (Brookfield) Viscometer[2]

F 619 Practice for Extraction of Medical Plastics[3]

F 748 Practice for Selecting Generic Biological Test Methods for Materials and Devices[3]

F 749 Practice for Evaluating Material Extracts by Intracutaneous Injection in the Rabbit[3]

F 756 Practice for Assessment of Hemolytic Properties of Materials[3]

F 763 Practice for Short-Term Screening of Implant Materials[3]

F 813 Practice for Direct Contact Cell Culture Evaluation of Materials for Medical Devices[3]

F 895 Test Method for Agar Diffusion Cell Culture Screening for Cytotoxicity[3]

F 981 Practice for Assessment of Compatibility of Biomaterials for Surgical Implants with Respect to Effect of Materials on Muscle and Bone[3]

F 1251 Terminology Relating to Polymeric Biomaterials in Medical and Surgical Devices[3]

F 1439 Guide for Performance of Lifetime Bioassay for the Tumorigenic Potential of Implant Materials[3]

F 1903 Practice for Testing for Biological Responses to Particles In Vitro[3]

F 1904 Practice for Testing the Biological Responses to Particles In Vivo[3]

F 1905 Practice for Selecting Tests for Determining the Propensity of Materials to Cause Immunotoxicity[3]

F 1906 Practice for Evaluation of Immune Responses in Biocompatibility Testing Using ELISA Tests, Lymphocyte Proliferation, and Cell Migration[3]

2.2 *USP Document:*

USP Monograph USP 24/NF 19<719> Sodium Alginate[4]

2.3 *ISO Documents*[5]*:*

[1] This guide is under the jurisdiction of ASTM Committee F04 on Medical and Surgical Materials and Devices and is the direct responsibility of Subcommittee F04.43 on Tissue-Engineered Biomaterials.

Current edition approved Nov. 10, 2000. Published February 2001.

[2] *Annual Book of ASTM Standards*, Vol 06.01.

[3] *Annual Book of ASTM Standards*, Vol 13.01.

[4] Available from United States Pharmacopeia and National Formulary, U.S. Pharmaceutical Convention, Inc. (USPC), Rockville, MD.

[5] Available from American National Standards Institute, 11 W. 42nd St., 13th Floor, New York, NY 10036.

ISO 10993 Biological Evaluation of Medical Devices:
ISO 10993-1 Biological Evaluation of Medical Devices—Part 1: Evaluation and Testing
ISO 10993-3 Part 3: Tests for Genotoxicity, Carcinogenicity and Reproductive Toxicity
ISO 10993-9—Part 9: Framework for identification and quantification of potential degradation products
ISO/DIS 10993-17—Part 17: Methods for establishment of allowable limits for leachable substances using health-based risk assessment
ISO 13408-1: 1998: Aseptic processing of health care products—Part 1: General requirements.

2.4 *ICH Documents*[6]:
International Conference on Harmonization (ICH) S2B Genotoxicity: A Standard Battery for Genotoxicity Testing of Pharmaceuticals (July 1997)[6]
International Conference on Harmonization (ICH) Q1A ICH Harmonized Tripartite Guidance for Stability Testing of New Drug Substances and Products (September 23, 1994)

2.5 *FDA Documents*[7]:
FDA Guideline on validation of the Limulus amebocyte test as an end-product endotoxin test for human and animal parenteral drugs, biological products and healthcare products. DHHS, December 1987.
FDA. Interim guidance for human and veterinary drug products and Biologicals. Kinetic LAL techniques. DHHS, July 15, 1991.

2.6 *ANSI Documents*[5]:
ANSI/AAMI/ISO 11737-1: 1995: Sterilization of medical devices—microbiological methods—Part 1: Estimation of bioburden on product.
ANSI/AAMI/ISO 11737-2: 1998: Sterilization of medical devices—microbiological methods—Part 2: Tests of sterility performed in the validation of a sterilization process.

2.7 *AAMI Documents*[8]:
AAMI/ISO 14160—1998: Sterilization of single-use medical devices incorporating materials of animal origin—Validation and routine control of sterilization by liquid chemical sterilants.
AAMI ST67/CDV-2: 1999: Sterilization of medical devices—requirements for products labeled "sterile".
AAMI TIR No. 19—1998: Guidance for ANSI/AAMI/ISO 10993-7: 1995, Biological evaluation of medical devices—Part 7: Ethylene oxide sterilization residuals.

2.8 *prEN Documents*[9]:
prEN 12442-1 Animal tissues and their derivative utilized in the manufacture of medical devices—Part 1: Analysis and management of risk
prEN –12442 Part 3:Validation of the elimination and/or inactivation of virus and transmissible agents.

2.9 *Other Documents:*
21CFR184.1724 Listing of Specific Substances Affirmed as GRAS–Sodium Alginate[10]
Williams, DF. The Williams Dictionary of Biomaterials. Liverpool University Press, 1999.

3. Terminology

3.1 *Definitions of Terms Specific to This Standard:* (see also Terminology F 1251):

3.1.1 *alginate, n*—a polysaccharide substance containing calcium, magnesium, sodium, and potassium salts obtained from some of the more common species of marine algae. Alginate exists in brown algae as the most abundant polysaccharide, mainly occurring in the cell walls and intercellular spaces of brown seaweed and kelp. Its main function is to contribute to the strength and flexibility of the seaweed plant. Alginate is classified as a hydrocolloid. The most commonly used alginate is sodium alginate.

3.1.2 *decomposition, n*—structural changes of alginates due to exposure to environmental, chemical or thermal factors, such as temperatures greater than 180°C. Decomposition can result in deleterious changes to the alginate.

3.1.3 *degradation, n*—change in the chemical structure, physical properties, or appearance of a material. Degradation of polysaccharides occurs by means of cleavage of the glycosidic bonds, usually by acid catalyzed hydrolysis. Degradation can also occur thermally. It is important to note that degradation is not synonymous with decomposition. Degradation is often used as a synonym for depolymerization when referring to polymers.

3.1.4 *depolymerization, n*—reduction in length of a polymer chain to form shorter polymeric units. Depolymerization may reduce the polymer chain to oligomeric or monomeric units, or both. In alginates, hydrolysis of the glycosidic bonds is the primary mechanism.

3.1.5 *Endotoxin, n*—a high-molecular weight lipopolysaccharide (LPS) complex associated with the cell wall of gram-negative bacteria that is pyrogenic in humans. Though endotoxins are pyrogens, not all pyrogens are endotoxins.

3.1.6 *hydrocolloid, n*—a water-soluble polymer of colloidal nature when hydrated.

3.1.7 *molecular mass average (molecular weight average), n*—the given molecular weight (Mw) of an alginate will always represent an average of all of the molecules in the population. The most common ways to express the Mw are as the number average ($\bar{M}_n$) and the weight average ($\bar{M}_w$). The two averages are defined by the following equations:

$$\bar{M}_n = \frac{\sum_i N_i M_i}{\sum_i N_i} \quad \text{and} \quad \bar{M}_w = \frac{\sum_i w_i M_i}{\sum_i w_i} = \frac{\sum_i N_i M_i^2}{\sum_i N_i M_i} \qquad (1)$$

where:

[6] Available from ICH Secretariat, c/o IFPMA, 30 rue de St-Jean, P.O. Box 758, 1211 Geneva 13, Switzerland

[7] Available from U. S. Food and Drug Administration 5600 Fishers Lane, Rockville MD 20857-0001

[8] Association for the Advancement of Medical Instrumentation 1110 North Glebe Rd., Suite 220, Arlington, VA 22201–4795.

[9] Available from European committee for Standardization CEN Management Centre 36, rue de Stassart B-1050 Brussels, Belgium

[10] Available from Superintendent of Documents, U.S. Government Printing Office, Washington, DC 20402

N_i = number of molecules having a specific molecular weight, M_i, and

w_i = weight of molecules having a specific molecular weight M_i

In a polydisperse molecular population the relation $\bar{M}_w > \bar{M}_n$ is always valid. The coefficient $\bar{M}_w/\bar{M}_n$ is referred to as the polydispersity index, and will typically be in the range from 1.5 to 3.0 for commercial alginates.

3.1.8 *pyrogen, n*—any substance that produces fever when administered parenterally.

4. Significance and Use

4.1 This guide contains a listing of those characterization parameters that are directly related to the functionality of alginate. This guide can be used as an aid in the selection and characterization of the appropriate alginate for a particular application. This guide is intended to give guidance in the methods and types of testing necessary to properly characterize, assess, and ensure consistency in the performance of a particular alginate. It may have use in the regulation of these devices by appropriate authorities.

4.2 The alginate covered by this guide may be gelled, extruded, or otherwise formulated into biomedical devices for use in tissue-engineered medical products or drug delivery devices for implantation as determined to be appropriate, based on supporting biocompatibility and physical test data. Recommendations in this guide should not be interpreted as a guarantee of clinical success in any tissue engineered medical product or drug delivery application.

4.3 To ensure that the material supplied satisfies requirements for use in TEMPS, several general areas of characterization should be considered. These are: identity of alginate, physical and chemical characterization and testing, impurities profile, and performance-related tests.

5. Chemical and Physical Test Methods

5.1 *Identity of Alginate*—The identity of alginates can be established by several methods including, but not limited to the following:

5.1.1 Sodium alginate monograph USP 24/NF19.

5.1.2 *Fourier Transform Infrared Spectroscopy (FT-IR)*—Almost all organic chemical compounds absorb infrared radiation at frequencies characteristic for the functional groups in the compound. A FT-IR spectrum will show absorption bands relating to bond stretching and bending and can therefore serve as a unique fingerprint of a specific compound. Cast an alginate film from a 0.25 % (w/v) solution of sodium alginate by drying approximately 500 μL of the sample onto a disposable IR card for 3 to 4 h at 60°C. Record a background spectrum between 4000 and 400 cm^{-1} using 128 scans at a resolution of 4 cm^{-1}. Record the IR spectrum of a dried blank IR card, then record the IR spectrum of the sample using 128 scans at a resolution of 4 cm^{-1}, % transmission mode. Label the peaks. Typical frequencies (cm^{-1}) for sodium alginate are 3375-3390 (b), 1613 (s), 1416 (s), 1320 (w), 1125, 1089, 1031 (s), 948 (m), 903 (m), and 811 (m). The peak designators are: sh: sharp; s: strong; m: medium; w: weak; and b: broad.

5.2 *Physical and chemical characterization of alginate*:

5.2.1 The composition and sequential structure of alginate can be a key functional attribute of any alginate. Variations in the composition or the sequential structure, or both, may, but not necessarily, cause differences in performance of an alginate in a particular end use. This information may be determined by the following method: High-resolution ^1H and ^{13}C-nuclear magnetic resonance spectroscopy (NMR). Sodium alginate should be dissolved in D_2O and partially degraded to a degree of depolymerization of 20 to 30 using mild acid hydrolysis before recording proton or carbon NMR spectra (Grasdalen, H., Larsen, B., and Smidsrød, O., Carbohydr. Res., 68, 23-31, 1979). Techniques have been developed to determine the monad frequencies F_G (fraction of guluronate residues) and F_M (fraction of mannuronate residues), the four nearest neighboring (diad) frequencies (F_{GG}, F_{GM}, F_{MG}, and F_{MM}) and the eight next nearest neighboring (triad) frequencies (F_{GGG}, F_{GGM}, F_{GMM}, F_{GMG}, F_{MGM}, F_{MGG}, F_{MMG}, and F_{MMM}). A typical ^1H-NMR spectrum of alginate is shown as follows. Alginate is characterized by calculating parameters such as M/G ratio, G-content, consecutive number of G monomers (that is, G>1), and average length of blocks of consecutive G monomers.

5.2.2 Molecular mass (molecular weight) of an alginate will define certain performance characteristics such as viscosity or gel strength, or both. As such and depending on the sensitivity of a particular end use to these variations, determination of molecular mass directly or indirectly may be necessary. Commercial alginates are polydisperse with respect to molecular weight (M_w). Molecular weight may be expressed as the number average (M_N) or the weight average (M_W). Molecular weights may be determined by methods such as, but not limited, to the following

5.2.2.1 *Molecular Weight Determination Based on Intrinsic Viscosity*—The intrinsic viscosity describes a polymer's ability to form viscous solutions in water and is directly proportional to the average molecular weight of the polymer. The intrinsic viscosity is a characteristic of the polymer under specified solvent and temperature conditions; it is independent of concentration. The intrinsic viscosity (η) is directly related to the molecular weight of a polymer through the Mark-Houwink-Sakurada (MHS) equation: $[\eta] = KM^a$, where K is a constant, M is the viscosity derived average molecular weight, and a is an empirical constant describing the conformation of the polymer. For alginate, the exponent (a) is close to unity at an ionic strength of 0.1 (for example, 0.1 M NaCl). By measuring the intrinsic viscosity, the viscosity average molecular weight can be determined if K and a are accurately known for the sample: $\log [\eta] = \log K + a(\log M)$, where M is the molecular weight. The intrinsic viscosity is determined by measuring the relative viscosity in a Ubbelohde capillary viscometer. The measurements should be performed in a solvent containing 0.1 M NaCl (a non-gelling, monovalent salt) at a constant temperature of 20°C, and at a sufficiently low alginate concentration. Automatic operation and data acquisition are preferred.

5.2.2.2 *Molecular Weight and Polydispersity Determination by Size Exclusion Chromatography With Multiple Angle Laser Light Scattering Detection (SEC-MALLS)*—As there are no alginate standards currently available, refractive index detectors can not be adequately calibrated. It is not sufficient to only use pullulan standards as a calibration material. Therefore, the

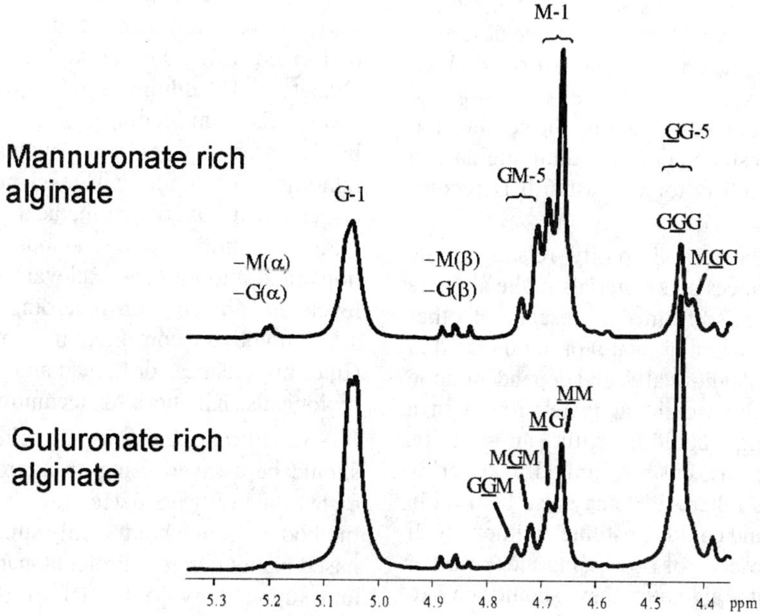

FIG. 1 Typical ^{1}H NMR of Sodium Alginate

method of choice is to use refractive index coupled to multiple angle laser light scattering detection (MALLS). For separation of the alginate into different molecular weight fractions a hydrophilic column with the appropriate pore size is required. Such columns include, but are not limited to, those mentioned in the techniques as follows: The precision of these techniques must be determined as results can vary by 10 to 20 %. Typical methods using these techniques include, but are not limited to the following:

(*1*) Using 0.01 *M* sodium EDTA/0.05 *M* sodium sulfate, pH 6.0 as the mobile phase with separation using TSK 3000, TSK 4000, and TSK 5000 columns.

(*2*) Using 0.1 *M* $NaNO_3$ (sodium nitrate) as an eluant in combination with a Waters Ultrahydrogel 2000 column in series with an Ultrahydrogel Linear column.

5.2.2.3 *Polydispersity*—Depending on the end use and the sensitivity of the application to the molecular mass, the presence of a wide range of alginate fractions may be an issue. In such cases, calculation of the polydispersity will be important. Typically, this is between 1.5 and 3.0 for commercial alginates.

5.2.2.4 Depending on the final use and the required performance control, other characterization assays can include, but are not limited to the following:

5.2.2.5 *Viscosity in Aqueous Solution*—Viscosity is defined as a liquid's resistance to flow. The molecular mass of an alginate will determine the extent to which it will thicken an aqueous solution. Therefore, a simple viscosity test may yield information on the relative differences in molecular mass among alginate samples. To allow comparison between laboratories, the viscometer used must be calibrated with traceable standards (see Test Methods D 2196). The viscosity measured will depend on several parameters related to how the testing is conducted. Important parameters to control include, but are not limited to the following:

(*1*) *Temperature*—The temperature at which the measurement is performed is critical. An increase in temperature will, in almost every case, result in a decrease in the viscosity. Consistent and controlled temperature (that is, with a standard temperature bath) is critical to achieving reproducible results. Typically, the temperature used to measure viscosity can be 20, 25, or 37°C, or a combination thereof.

(*2*) *Alginate Concentration*—The moisture content of the alginate must be known in order to prepare correct concentrations of alginate.

(*3*) *Ionic strength*—The viscosity of an alginate solution is very sensitive to the ionic environment in which the measurement is made. Although any ion can have an impact, multivalent ions other than magnesium will have the most effect. The most important aspect is to keep the ionic content consistent. Typically viscosity measurements are made in deionized water or a standardized ionic environment such as isotonic saline.

(*4*) *Molecular Mass*—Viscosity measurements are sensitive to the molecular mass of the alginate. The following is one suggestion concerning the measurement of alginate viscosity, but any appropriate method would apply. To measure the apparent viscosity of sodium alginate, prepare a solution in deionized water with a concentration (w/w, corrected for dry matter content) appropriate for the end use. For example, if the sample has a suspected molecular weight above about 50 000 g/mol prepare a 1 % (w/w) solution; if the suspected molecular weight is less than about 50 000 g/mol, then prepare a 10 % (w/w) solution. The viscosity is measured using a rotational viscometer (for example, Brookfield type) at 20 ± 0.2°C (or other controlled temperature) using the appropriate spindle, spindle rotation speed, and a temperature-controlled water bath.

5.2.2.6 *Dry Matter Content*—Various alginates are supplied with different moisture contents. The dry matter content determination is based upon the removal of water from the sample. Normally with alginate, gravimetric techniques are used. They are adapted directly from <731> USP 24/NF19,

Loss on Drying, and utilize a calibrated drying oven at 105°C.

5.2.2.7 *Ash Content*—The ash content of a sample describes the total amount of inorganic material present. After combustion, the sample contains a mixture of salts. The composition of the ash depends on the temperature used during the combustion of the organic material. For ash content of sodium alginate, a combustion temperature of 800°C for at least 6 h is recommended.

5.3 *Impurities Profile*—The term impurity relates to the presence of extraneous substances and materials in the alginate powder. Impurities can also arise from the presence of other alginate salts (for example, calcium alginate) or alginic acid in the sodium alginate material. Additionally, and dependent upon the end use, a high molecular weight alginate present in a sample of low molecular weight could constitute an impurity. Various processing aids, such as, but not limited to, filtering and clarifying agents such as Filter Aid(TM) may also be used in the manufacture of alginate and could constitute an impurity. If there is a concern for the presence of processing aids or other contaminants associated with alginate, they should be addressed with the supplier. The major impurities of concern include, but are not limited to the following:

5.3.1 *Endotoxin Content*—Endotoxin contamination is difficult to prevent because it is ubiquitous in nature, stable, and small enough to pass through sterilizing filters. There are several tests to determine the presence of endotoxin in the alginate powder. These are the gel clot, endpoint assay and the kinetic assay. The gel clot test is the simplest and easiest of the limulus amebocyte lysate (LAL) test methods, although much less sensitive than the kinetic assay. A firm gel that maintains its integrity upon inverting the tube is scored as a positive test. Anything other than a firm gel is scored as a negative test. The endpoint assay is based on the linear relationship between the endotoxin concentration and the formation of color (chromogenic assay) over a relatively short range of standard dilutions. A standard curve is then constructed by plotting the optical densities of a series of endotoxin standards as a function of the endotoxin concentration.

5.3.1.1 Using linear regression analysis, the standard curve covers an endotoxin range of approximately 1 log (usually 1.0 to 0.1 EU/mL). The most sensitive means of determining the endotoxin content is with a quantitative, kinetic assay. This test utilizes a LAL and a synthetic color producing substrate to detect endotoxin chromogenically (such as, but not limited to, BioWhittakers Kinetic-QCL(TM) methodology, or other equivalent assay). The kinetic assay measures the amount of time required to reach a predetermined optical density (kinetic turbidimetric) or color intensity (kinetic chromogenic), sometimes called the onset optical density or reaction optical density. The FDA currently defines linearity as a correlation coefficient of ≥0.980 (Food and Drug Administration. Guideline on validation of the Limulus amebocyte test as an end-product endotoxin test for human and animal parenteral drugs, biological products, and healthcare products. DHHS, December 1987). It is important that operators of the LAL method are qualified and that each new lot of reagents is validated. Positive product controls (PPC) must be added to test inhibition in the sample. Recovery of the known added amount of endotoxin standard must be obtained for a valid assay. It is recommended that endotoxin measurements be performed using an initial 0.1 % concentration of sodium alginate and 3 dilution ranges (for example, 20×, 50×, and 100×). Calcium binding by alginate may produce interference in the assay. Magnesium may be added to reverse this inhibition. The endotoxin level in alginate will ultimately be critical to its use in biomedical applications where they are regulatory limits to the amount of endotoxin that can be implanted into humans. Relevant FDA guidance for allowable levels and information regarding validation of endotoxin assays should be consulted if human trials are contemplated (Interim guidance for human and veterinary drug products and biologicals. Kinetic LAL techniques. DHHS. July 15, 1991).

5.3.2 *Protein Content*—Protein content in sodium alginate should be assayed using an appropriate method having sufficient sensitivity to detect low levels of contamination. One method, although not the only suitable one, is the fluorescence-based NanoOrange(TM) Protein Quantification method developed and supplied by Molecular Probes. This method is able to quantitate protein content as low as 10 ng/mL. The protein content should be assayed using a 1 % (w/w) alginate solution corrected for moisture. It is important to confirm that the method chosen is insensitive to materials present in the sample and to validate it against a reference method on a one-time basis. It is the responsibility of the end user to evaluate the alginate product for the presence of specific proteins that could cause undesirable immunological or tissue reactions.

5.3.3 *Heavy Metal Content by the USP Method*—This test is provided to demonstrate that the content of heavy metal impurities does not exceed a limit in the individual product specification in terms of ppm lead in the test substance. Under the specified test conditions, the limit is determined by a concomitant visual comparison of metals that are colored by sulfide ion with a control prepared from a standard lead solution. Substances that typically respond to this test are lead, mercury, bismuth, arsenic, antimony, tin, cadmium, silver, copper, and molybdenum. This method is based on <231> Heavy Metals, USP 24/NF 19.

5.3.4 *Microbiological Safety*—The presence of bacteria, yeast, and mold are also impurities that can arise in an alginate sample. The presence of bacteria may also contribute to the presence of endotoxins. The following Microbiological Tests in USP 24 are of particular relevance: Microbial Limit Tests <61>, Sterility Tests <71>, Sterilization and Sterility Assurance of Compendial Articles <12211>, and the Biological Tests and Assays: Bacterial Endotoxins Tests <85>. The user should also consider other relevant standards, such as, but not limited to, Association for the Advancement of Medical Instrumentation (AAMI) standards and international standards, of which the following are examples: ANSI/AAMI/ISO 11737-1: 1995: Sterilization of Medical Devices-Microbiological Methods—Part 1: Estimation of bioburden on product; ANSI/AAMI/ISO 11737-2: 1998: Sterilization of Medical Devices—Microbiological Methods—Part 2: Tests of sterility performed in the validation of a sterilization process; ISO 13408-1: 1998: Aseptic processing of health care products—Part 1: general requirements. Membrane filtration can be used for the determination of bacteria, yeast, and mold in alginate samples. The alginate salt is first dissolved in sterile, deionized water, then filtered using sterile techniques through a 0.45-μm membrane filter. The filters are subsequently incubated on Tryptic Soya Agar to determine the presence of bacteria, and on sabouraud dextrose agar to determine the presence of yeast and mold. If alginate products are intended to serve as a barrier to microorganisms, this function will need to be validated with specific experiments.

6. Product Development Considerations

6.1 *Type of Solvent (for example, Medium or Water)*—The conformation of the alginate molecule will vary with changes in the ionic strength of the solute. Therefore, the apparent viscosity of an alginate solution may change depending upon whether the alginate is dissolved in water or in a salt-containing medium.

6.2 *Stability of Alginate*—For alginate, the most relevant stability-indicating parameters are those related to the functionality of the polymer. Dependent upon what function the alginate will have in the final formulation, parameters such as viscosity (apparent and intrinsic), and molecular weight should be evaluated during a stability study. Storage conditions are of importance, especially for alginate solutions. International Conference on Harmonization (ICH) guidance documents should be consulted for information on stability testing of pharmaceuticals (that is, ICH Q1A ICH Harmonized Tripartite Guideline for Stability testing of New Drug Substances and Products, September 23, 1994).

6.3 *Methods of Sterilization*—Sterilization is intended for the final application or formulation. If sterilization of the alginate is required, then there are several alternative methods available. However, the listing of alternative sterilization methods does not imply that commercial suppliers of alginate need provide a sterile product. Alginate powder can be sterilized by gamma irradiation (with subsequent degradation of the alginate chain resulting in a reduction in molecular weight) or by ethylene oxide. Solutions of alginate may be (*1*) filter sterilized if the viscosity of the alginate solution permits, (*2*) gamma-irradiated with a resulting loss in viscosity (molecular weight), and (*3*) autoclaved (which also reduced the viscosity of the solution). Selection of the method of sterilization will depend upon the viscosity or molecular weight needs of the final application. Use of ethylene oxide will also require testing for residuals. The reader should refer to the relevant standards regarding the sterilization of healthcare products by radiation, steam, and ethylene oxide gas, such as AAMI TIR No. 19—1998: Guidance for ANSI/AAMI/ISO 10993-7: 1995, Biological evaluation of medical devices—Part 7: Ethylene oxide sterilization residues; AAMI/ISO 14160—1998: Sterilization of single-use medical devices incorporating materials of animal origin—Validation and routine control of sterilization by liquid chemical sterilants; AAMI ST67/CDV-2: 1999: Sterilization of medical devices—requirements for products labeled "sterile."

7. Safety and Toxicology Aspects of Alginate

7.1 Sodium alginate is listed on the list of materials affirmed generally recognized as safe (GRAS) by the US Food and Drug Administration (FDA) (21CFR184.1724). This permits sodium alginate (but not other salts such as magnesium) to be used in foods as a thickener or gelling agent, but does not indicate approval for the use of alginate in pharmaceutical or biomedical applications, or both.

7.2 The safety of alginate in biomedical and pharmaceutical applications and in tissue-engineered medical products (TEMPS) should be established in accordance with current guidelines such as ISO 10993 and Practice F 748. Suppliers of alginate may have such documentation on file. Preclinical safety studies specific to the clinical application under consideration must also be in accordance with 21CFR312.

7.3 *Biocompatibility*:

7.3.1 Biomaterials are materials of natural or manmade origin that are used to direct, supplement, or replace the functions of living tissues. These materials may be considered biocompatible if the materials perform with an appropriate host response in a specific application (Williams 1999).

7.3.2 Many materials have been shown to produce a well-characterized level of biological response following long-term clinical use in laboratory animals. When new applications of a material, or modifications to the material or physical forms of the material are being considered, then the recommendations and test methods of the following standards should be considered: Practices F 748, F 619, F 749, F 756, F 763, F 813, F 981, F1903, F1904, F1905, and F1906; Guide F 1439 as well as Test Method F 895 and ISO 10993-1, ISO/DIS 10993-9, Part 9, ISO/DIS 10993-17—Part 17, prEN 12442-1—Part 1, prEN 12442-3—Part 3. Additional guidance can be obtained in ICH S2B Genotoxicity: A Standard Battery for Genotoxicity Testing of Pharmaceuticals, July 1997, as well as ISO 10993–3—Part 3: Tests for Genotoxicity, Carcinogenicity and Reproductive Toxicity.

7.4 Alginate for use in biomedical and pharmaceutical applications and in tissue-engineered medical products (TEMPS) should ideally be documented in a device or drug master file to which end users may obtain a letter of cross reference from suppliers of alginate. Such a master file should be submitted to the US FDA and to other regulatory authorities, both national and international.

8. Keywords

8.1 alginates; biomedically engineered; tissue-engineered medical products

APPENDIXES

(Nonmandatory Information)

X1. RATIONALE

X1.1 The use of naturally occurring biopolymers for biomedical and pharmaceutical applications and in TEMPS is increasing. This guide is designed to give guidance in the characterization and testing parameters for sodium alginate used in such applications. Knowledge of the physical and chemical properties of the alginate, such as guluronate to mannuronate ratio, G-block size, molecular weight (or viscosity), and so forth, will assist end users in choosing the correct alginate for their particular application. Knowledge of these parameters will also ensure that users can request and obtain similar material from suppliers on reordering. Molecular characterization of alginate will also assist end users in documentation of their formulation or device. Finally, characterization of the alginate will allow the functionality of the alginate to fit the application or end product. Tests outlined in this guide are sufficient for release of alginate to the end user. Other validated tests that would accomplish the same purposes as those set forth in this guide may be substituted. The tests may not be suitable for characterization and functionality of the final product.

X2. BACKGROUND

X2.1 "Alginate" refers to a family of non-branched binary copolymers of 1-4 glycosidically linked β-D-mannuronic acid (M) and α-L-guluronic acid (G) residues. The relative amount of the two uronic acid monomers and their sequential arrangement along the polymer chain vary widely, depending on the origin of the alginate. The uronic acid residues are distributed along the polymer chain in a pattern of blocks, where homopolymeric blocks of G residues (G-blocks), homopolymeric blocks of M residues (M-blocks), and blocks with alternating sequence of M and G units (MG-blocks) co-exist. Thus, the alginate molecule can not be described by the monomer composition alone. The NMR characterization of the sequence of M and G residues in the alginate chain is needed in order to calculate average block lengths. It has also been shown by NMR spectroscopy that alginate has no regular repeating unit. The length of the polymer chain is rather long in native form, but will decrease during the manufacturing process. Depolymerization is a natural process for alginate. The molecular weight of commercial alginates will seldom be higher that 500 000 g/mol, similar to a degree of polymerization (DP) of approximately 2500.

X2.2 *Raw Materials for Alginate Production*:

X2.2.1 All current industrial manufacture of alginate is based on the extraction of the polymer from brown algae. Alginate may also be synthesized as an exocellular material by some bacteria. It has been found feasible to manufacture certain specialty grades of alginate by fermentation.

X2.2.2 The seaweed grows naturally mainly in the temperate zone, but large amounts are also cultivated in the Far East, off the coast of China, and near Japan, in particular.

X2.2.3 The stiffness of the plant reflects the content of guluronic acid, and in particular, the content of G-blocks. An increase in the G-block length results in an increase in gel strength due to increased cross-linking of alginate molecules by calcium.

X2.3 *Variability in Chemical Composition and Sequential Structure of Alginate*—The variability in chemical composition and sequential structure of alginate is related to the seaweed and kelp species from which the alginate is extracted. Table X2.1 represents some of the differences in alginate composition from various seaweed sources. Table X2.1 indicates that

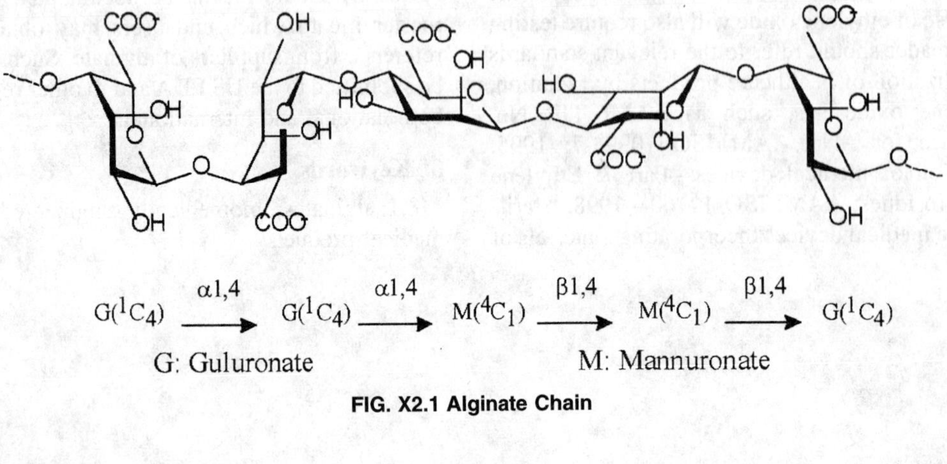

FIG. X2.1 Alginate Chain

TABLE X2.1 Differences in Alginate Composition from Various Seaweed Sources

Seaweed	M/G	%M	%G	%MM	%GG
Laminaria hyperborea (stem)	0.45	30	70	18	58
Laminaria hyperborea (leaf)	1.22	55	45	36	26
Laminaria digitata	1.22	55	45	39	29
Macrocystis pyrifera	1.50	60	40	40	20
Lessonia nigrescens	1.50	60	40	43	23
Ascophyllum nodosum	1.86	65	35	56	26
Laminaria japonica	1.86	65	35	48	18
Durvillea antarcitica	2.45	71	29	58	16
Durvillea potarum	3.33	77	23	69	13

there is a range of compositions that must be defined and described for alginate utilized in biomedical and pharmaceutical applications. The range in chemical composition and sequential structure can be broad or narrow depending upon the end use.

X2.4 *Functional Properties and Applications of Alginate*:

X2.4.1 The functional properties of alginate of primary importance for most biomedical applications are the viscoelastic ones. Solubility, swellability, and film-forming properties are other characteristics exploited in biomedical and pharmaceutical applications.

X2.4.2 Gelling properties are a function of the M/G composition and the sequential structure of M and G along the alginate chain. Consecutive guluronic monomers form a G-block, which represents areas within the alginate molecule able to cross-link with multivalent cations. In practice, calcium is most often used as the cross-linking cation.

X2.4.3 Thickening (viscosifying) properties of alginate are a function of the molecular weight and the conformation of the alginate molecule in solution. Interaction with other molecules in the solution as well as competition for water at high alginate concentrations affect the flow properties of alginate solutions. Calcium or other cross-linking materials present in small quantities artificially increase the measured viscosity because of aggregate formation. This results in solutions with thixotropic flow properties. A sequestrant that binds the cross-linking agent can be added to avoid measuring an artificially high viscosity.

X2.4.4 Both gelling and thickening properties of alginate are dependent upon the order in which the different materials are added.

X2.4.5 Solubility of alginate is related to the rate of dissociation of the alginate molecule. At pH <3, both M- and G-structures will precipitate as alginic acid, while alternating structures will still remain in solution even when fully protonated.

X2.4.6 Sellability of alginate is related to the rate of hydration, and it will depend strongly on the form in which alginate interacts with the solute (water). Cross-linked alginates will, for instance, swell slower than pure sodium alginate.

X2.4.7 Films can be formed from alginate solutions simply by evaporation of the solvent. The molecular weight of alginate needs to be above a certain lower limit in order to achieve film formation and avoid brittleness. Films can be formed easily in situ by spraying an alginate solution onto a binding surface.

X2.4.8 *Degradation*—As described in 3.1.3, degradation of alginate occurs by means of cleavage of the glycosidic bond. Compared with other sugars, glycosidic bonds involving uronic acids such as M and G are quite resistant to hydrolysis in very strong acids, (that is, conditions normally used to convert polysaccharides into monosaccharides). The degradation rate is directly proportional to the concentration of protons below about pH 1. However, at pH values near the pK of alginates (pH 1-4), the degradation rate is less dependent on pH. In this range, the protonated (-COOH) form of M and G contributes to the hydrolysis by intramolecular catalysis in addition to that caused by the free H ions. For this reason, alginate is less stable than some other polymers (for example, methylcellulose) between pH 1-5. Optimum stability is normally obtained at pH 7-8. For higher pH values, other degradation processes come into play. In most cases, degradation results in a decrease in the solution viscosity (η). The polymer concentration and the viscosifying power of the molecules involved determine the viscosity.

Standard Practice for Testing for Alternative Pathway Complement Activation in Serum by Solid Materials[1]

This standard is issued under the fixed designation F 2065; the number immediately following the designation indicates the year of original adoption or, in the case of revision, the year of last revision. A number in parentheses indicates the year of last reapproval. A superscript epsilon (ε) indicates an editorial change since the last revision or reapproval.

ε[1] NOTE—Editorial corrections were made throughout this standard in June 2001.

1. Scope

1.1 This practice provides a protocol for rapid, in vitro screening for alternative pathway complement activating properties of solid materials used in the fabrication of medical devices that will contact blood.

1.2 This practice is intended to evaluate the acute in vitro alternative pathway complement activating properties of solid materials intended for use in contact with blood. For this practice, "serum" is synonymous with "complement."

1.3 This practice consists of two procedural parts. Procedure A describes exposure of solid materials to a standard lot of C4-deficient guinea pig serum [C4(-)GPS], using 0.1-mL serum per 13 × 100-mm disposable glass test tubes. Sepharose™[2] CL-4B is used as an example of test materials. Procedure B describes assaying the exposed serum for significant functional alternative pathway complement depletion as compared to control samples. The endpoint in procedure B is lysis of rabbit RBC in buffer containing EGTA and excess Mg^{++}.

1.4 This practice does not address function, elaboration, or depletion of individual complement components except as optional additional confirmatory information that can be acquired using human serum as the complement source. This practice does not address the use of plasma as a source of complement.

1.5 This practice is one of several developed for the assessment of the biocompatibility of materials. Practice F 748 may provide guidance for the selection of appropriate methods for testing materials for other aspects of biocompatibility. Practice F 1984 provides guidance for testing solid materials for whole complement activation in human serum, but does not discriminate between the classical or alternative pathway of activation.

2. Referenced Documents

2.1 *ASTM Standards:*

F 748 Practice for Selecting Generic Biological Test Methods for Materials and Devices[3]

F 1984 Practice for Testing for Whole Complement Activation in Serum by Solid Materials[3]

2.2 *Other Document:*

ISO 10993-4: Biological Evaluation of Medical Devices. Part 4: Selection of Tests for Interactions with Blood[4]

3. Terminology

3.1 *Definitions of Terms Specific to This Standard:*

3.1.1 *water*—distilled, endotoxin-free.

3.2 *Abbreviations:* Abbreviations:

3.2.1 *Ab*—antibody (hemolysin)

3.2.2 *BBS*—barbital buffered saline

3.2.3 *BBS-G*—barbital buffered saline – gelatin

3.2.4 *BBS-G-EGTA/Mg (Mg Buffer)*—barbital buffered saline – gelatin EGTA Mg^{++}

3.2.5 *BBS-GM (Ca Buffer)*—barbital buffered saline – gelatin metals

3.2.6 *C′*—complement

3.2.7 *C4(-)GPS*—C4-deficient guinea pig serum [serum from guinea pigs genetically incapable of producing C4, the fourth component of complement]

3.2.8 *EDTA*—ethylenediaminetetraacetic acid, disodium salt: dihydrate

3.2.9 *EGTA*—ethylene glyco-bis(β-aminoethyl ether)-N,N,N′,N′-tetraacetic acid, tetrasodium salt

3.2.10 *HAGG*—heat aggregated gamma globulin

3.2.11 *HS*—human serum

3.2.12 *I*—control tube with serum but no material, kept on ice.

3.2.13 *M*—tube containing serum plus a test material

3.2.14 *NM*—tube containing serum but no material

3.2.15 *PVDF*—polyvinylidene fluoride

3.2.16 *RBC*—red blood cell(s)

4. Summary of Practice

4.1 Solid material specimens are exposed to a standard lot of C4(-)GPS complement under defined conditions, in parallel to appropriate controls (Procedure A). If the alternative

[1] This practice is under the jurisdiction of ASTM Committee F04 on Medical and Surgical Materials and Devices and is the direct responsibility of Subcommittee F04.16 on Biocompatibility Test Methods.

Current edition approved Nov. 10, 2000. Published February 2001.

[2] Sepharose™ is a registered trademark of Pharmacia, Inc.

[3] *Annual Book of ASTM Standards*, Vol 13.01.

[4] Available from American National Standards Institute, 11 W. 42nd St., 13th Floor, New York, NY 10036.

complement pathway is activated by the material, complement components will be depleted from the serum. Exposed serum is then tested for remaining functional complement activity, by determining complement mediated lysis of rabbit RBC in buffer containing EGTA and excess Mg^{++}(Procedure B).

5. Significance and Use

5.1 Inappropriate activation of complement by blood-contacting medical devices may have serious acute or chronic effects on the host. Solid medical device materials may activate the complement directly by the alternative pathway. Unlike the classical complement activation pathway (see Practice F 1984), antibodies are not required for alternative pathway activation. This practice is useful as a simple, inexpensive screening method for determining alternative whole complement activation by solid materials in vitro.

5.2 This practice is composed of two parts. In Part A (Section 10) C4(-)GPS is exposed to a solid material. Since C4 is required for classical pathway activation, activation of complement in C4(-)GPS can only occur by the alternative pathway **(1)**.[5] In principle, nonspecific binding of certain complement components to the materials may also occur. In Part B (Section 11), complement activity remaining in the serum after exposure to the test material is assayed by alternative pathway-mediated lysis of rabbit RBC.

5.3 Assessment of in vitro whole complement activation as described here provides one method for predicting potential complement activation by solid medical device materials intended for clinical application in humans when the material contacts the blood. Other test methods for complement activation are available, including assays for specific complement components and their split products in human serum (X1.3 and X1.4).

5.4 This in vitro test method is suitable for adoption in specifications and standards for screening solid materials for use in the construction of medical devices intended to be implanted in the human body or placed in contact with human blood outside the body.

6. Preparation of Buffers

6.1 Buffers are prepared in accordance with established protocols **(1, 2)**. "Water" refers throughout to distilled, endotoxin-free H_2O. The use of barbital (veronal) buffer is recommended. In the United States, barbital is a class IV regulated substance and requires a DEA **(3)** license for purchase. The use of other buffer systems (such as TRIS) is permissible if they have been demonstrated not to activate complement **(4)**. These solutions are stable for one month at 4°C unless otherwise indicated.

6.2 The 5X stock BBS (barbital-buffered saline) is prepared by adding 20.75 g of NaCl plus 2.545 g of sodium barbital (sodium-5,5-diethyl barbiturate) to about 400 mL water. The pH is adjusted to 7.35 with 1 *N* HCl, then brought to a final volume of 500 mL in a volumetric flask.

6.3 Metals solution is prepared by making a 2.0-*M* solution of $MgCl_2$ (40.66 g $MgCl_2 \cdot 6\ H_2O$ up to a final volume of 100 mL water), and a 0.3-*M* solution of $CaCl_2$(4.41 g $CaCl_2 \cdot 2H_2O$ up to a final volume of 100 mL of water), and combining the two solutions 1:1 (v:v).

6.4 The Ca buffer (BBS-GM working solution) is prepared daily, by dissolving 0.25 g of gelatin (type A: Porcine Skin, Approx. 300 Bloom, such as available from Sigma [G-1890]) in 50 mL of water that is gently heated and stirred. The gelatin solution is added to 50 mL 5X Stock BBS plus 0.25 mL metals solution, brought up to about 200 mL then adjusted to pH 7.35 (with 1 *N* HCl or 1 *N* NaOH) before bringing the final volume to 250 mL in a volumetric flask. The Ca buffer contains both Mg^{++} and Ca^{++}, which allows both classical and alternative pathway complement. activation to occur.

6.5 The BBS-G working solution is prepared the same way, but omitting addition of the metals solution.

6.6 10X Stock EDTA (0.1-*M* disodium dihydrate EDTA) is prepared by adding 7.44 g disodium EDTA·2 H_2O to about 160 mL of water, adjusting the pH to 7.65 (with 1 *N* NaOH or 1 *N* HCl), then bringing the volume to 200 mL in a volumetric flask.

6.7 The 0.1 *M* EGTA (tetrasodium salt, EGTA·4.5 H_2O) is prepared by adding 4.683 g tetrasodium EGTA to about 80 mL of water, adjusting the pH to 7.35 (with 1 *N* NaOH or 1 *N* HCl), then bringing the volume to 100 mL in a volumetric flask.

6.8 BBS-G-EDTA (to be used in preparing RBC before being washed out) is prepared by adding 10 mL of stock 10X EDTA to 90 mL of BBS-G in a volumetric flask.

6.9 The Mg Buffer (BBS-G-EGTA/Mg working solution) is prepared daily, by dissolving 0.25 g gelatin in 50 mL water that is gently heated and stirred. The gelatin solution is added to 50 mL 5X stock BBS, plus 0.625 mL 2.0 *M* $MgCl_2$, plus 4 mL of 0.1 *M* EGTA, brought up to about 200 mL, then adjusted to pH 7.35 (with 1 *N* HCl or 1 *N* NaOH) before bringing the final volume to 250 mL in a volumetric flask. The Mg buffer has EGTA to bind Ca^{++}. The presence of Mg^{++} allows the alternative pathway activation to proceed, while the absence of Ca^{++} prevents activation of the classical pathway.

7. Preparation of Sheep and Rabbit RBC

7.1 Commercially obtained sheep RBC preserved in Alsever's solution and defibrinated rabbit RBC are stored at 4°C. The sheep cells are discarded after eight weeks or when the supernatant from the second wash contains hemoglobin (red color) by visual inspection (as lots of RBCs age, they are more sensitive to complement lysis in parallel with increased spontaneous lysis). The rabbit cells are more fragile than the sheep cells, and should be discarded after four weeks or when the supernatant from the second wash contains hemoglobin by visual inspection.

NOTE 1—All centrifugations are at 4°C. Except when indicated, all reagents, tubes, and cell preparations are kept cold in chipped ice or an ice slurry.

7.2 Five millilitres of sheep or rabbit RBC are centrifuged at 1000 × g, at 4°C, for 10 min.

7.3 The cell pellet is resuspended in 10 mL of cold BBS-G-EDTA and incubated for 10 min at 37°C. The cells are centrifuged, and the pellet resuspended in 10 mL of 4°C BBS-G-EDTA.

[5] The boldface numbers in parentheses refer to the list of references at the end of this specification.

7.4 The cells are centrifuged, the supernatant discarded (first wash), and the pellet resuspended in 10 mL of cold BBS-GM (Ca buffer) or BBS-G-EGTA/Mg (Mg buffer) (cells to be used in absorbing serum are washed in Ca buffer; cells to be used for detecting alternative pathway C′ depletion, Procedure B, are washed and suspended in Mg buffer). Repeat twice (total of three washes.)

7.5 Adjust cell count spectrophotometrically (where an absorbance of 0.75 for sheep RBC and 1.30 for rabbit RBC corresponds to 2.0×10^8 RBC/mL, at a wavelength of 412 nm and a 1.0-cm light path for 1 volume of cells in BBS-GM or BBS-G-EGTA/Mg plus 24 volumes of water) or count with a hemocytometer. Prepare 10 mL of 2.0×10^8 cells/mL in 4°C BBS-GM.

7.6 The washed, diluted RBC can be held on ice and used for at least 12 h.

8. Absorption of Serum (Complement)

8.1 Although human serum would be preferable to guinea pig serum for alternative pathway complement activation by materials to be used in medical devices intended to contact patient blood, genetically deficient human sera are not routinely available. Human sera depleted of components by antibody absorption on columns are unsuitable for this purpose for the following two reasons: (*1*) specific component depletion is incomplete, so significant classical pathway activation remains; and (*2*) column material may activate the alternative pathway, depleting functional activity. Serum from guinea pigs genetically deficient in C4 [C4(-)GPS] has no classical pathway complement activity but is fully competent for alternative pathway complement activation. Although the titers are different (a greater concentration of C4(-)GPS is required to produce the same lysis of rabbit RBC as human serum)(5)C4(-)GPS gives equivalent results to human serum in detecting biomaterial complement activation (see Sepharose™ example in Table 1). Thus, C4(-)GPS is suitable as a screen for subsequent confirmatory immunoassays that detect complement components and split-products indicative of alternative pathway activation in whole human serum. The C4(-)GPS suitable as a source of complement may be purchased from biological supply houses, and is generally labeled as reagent-grade complement.

8.2 Serum may be absorbed with sheep RBC and rabbit RBC in order to remove naturally occurring anti-sheep and anti-rabbit RBC hemolytic antibodies. The procedure is as follows:

8.3 Commercially available C4(-)GPS is stored at –70°C.

8.4 The serum is thawed on chipped ice or reconstituted (if lyophilized) with ice-cold water.

8.5 All manipulations are done in chipped ice or in an ice slurry, with ice cold (4°C) reagents and cells. Centrifugations are carried out at 1000 × g at 4°C. It is critical that this entire procedure be done in the cold to avoid activation of complement in this step.

8.6 Cold serum and 4°C, Ca buffer-washed RBC (a 1:1 mixed volume of sheep and rabbit packed RBC) are gently mixed (by slow rocking), 0.1 mL of packed RBC/2.5 mL of serum, incubated for 10 min on ice, then centrifuged at 1000 × g for 10 min at 4°C. The supernatant liquid is carefully transferred to a new container on ice.

8.7 The procedure in 8.6 is repeated twice.

8.8 The absorbed C4(-)GPS is stored in 0.5–1.0-mL aliquots (convenient for one-experiment use), in cold snap-cap microfuge tubes and kept at –70°C until used. Aliquots should be thawed in chipped ice or an ice slurry, used on the day of thawing, and not refrozen.

9. Whole Complement Titration to Determine Optimal Serum Dilution

9.1 If statistical evaluation of results is desired, all conditions should be assayed in triplicate, using three 13 × 100 mm round-bottomed, disposable glass test tubes per condition. Otherwise, single or duplicate tubes are sufficient. Tubes are numbered in advance. Conditions include "total lysis," "no complement (RBC only)" (no C′), "tests" (dilutions of C4(-)GPS) with and without hemolysin, and "no RBC (serum color)" (complement color control, at highest concentration of serum used). All reagents, tubes, and manipulations are done at 4°C, with tubes held in a rack in an ice slurry.

9.2 Two sets of tubes are prepared in accordance with 9.3–9.4. One set contains diluted sera placed on Mg buffer-washed sheep RBC, and one set contains diluted sera placed on Mg buffer-washed rabbit RBC.

9.3 The Mg buffer-washed rabbit RBC are added to all tubes except "no RBC (serum color)" tubes (0.05 mL/tube of a 2.0×10^8 cells/mL suspension.) Since this is a small volume for the tube area, care should be taken to deliver the accurate volume to the center of the bottom of each tube. "No RBC (serum color)" tubes get 0.05 mL 4°C Mg buffer.

9.4 HS and C4(-)GPS at 4°C are diluted in 4°C Mg buffer to the desired concentrations (with minimal agitation.) It is recommended to test the sera initially at 1:2 to 1:20 dilutions. Diluted serum is added directly to the bottom of each test tube in a 0.05-mL volume. The "RBC only (serum color)" tubes get 0.05 mL of Mg buffer containing no serum. "Total lysis" tubes get 0.05 mL of distilled water in place of buffer.

9.5 Tubes are shaken manually to suspend cells, then the rack is incubated in a 37°C water bath for 1 h, and intermittently shaken (every 15 min) to keep cells in suspension.

9.6 At the end of 1 h, the rack is placed in an ice slurry. All tubes receive the same volume of additional 4°C Mg buffer (if supernatants following centrifugation are to be removed to a

TABLE 1 Percent Lysis[A] of Rabbit RBC in Mg Buffer by Human Serum or C4(-)GPS Pre-exposed 1 h at 37 °C, in 100-µL volumes, to Different Amounts of Sepharose™ CL-4B

µL Sepharose, ™ CL-4B[B] [HS/C4(-)GPS]	HS prep. 1[C]	HS prep. 2[D]	C4(-)GPS[E]
50/12.5	3.3 ± 1.2	3.4 ± 1.7	6.5 ± 2.6
25/6.25	14.2 ± 0.6	11.8 ± 0.8	21.3 ± 3.3
12.5/3.13	23.6 ± 5.2	19.6 ± 2.8	20.1 ± 0.9
6.25/1.57	33.2 ± 2.8	29.4 ± 3.8	27.3 ± 1.4
0/0 [37°C control]	49.9 ± 0.2	45.3 ± 4.6	41.3 ± 0.7
0/0 [Ice control]	51.4 ± 1.6	52.9 ± 0.7	58.4 ± 0.5

[A]Mean plus or minus standard deviation of three replicate tubes.
[B]The indicated volume of Sepharose™ CL-4B was added to 100 µL of HS or C4(-)GPS.
[C]Whole human serum [Quidel (NHSC)], diluted 1:8 in Mg buffer.
[D]Reconstituted lyophilized human serum [Sigma (S1764)], diluted 1:4 in Mg buffer.
[E]Whole guinea pig serum, C4-deficient [Sigma (C1038)], 1:3 in Mg buffer.

microtiter well plate for reading, an additional 0.4 mL/tube is sufficient; if readings will be done on a flow-through spectrophotometer, then 1.1 mL/tube should be added). The cold tubes are then centrifuged at 1000 × g for 10 min at 4°C, and the supernatants decanted to correspondingly numbered 13 × 100-mm glass tubes (or placed directly in microtiter wells for plate reader scanning).

NOTE 2—Although supernatant liquids can be placed in microtiter plate wells for reading in a plate reader, the alternative C′ pathway test itself can not be carried out in microtiter plates because the plastic may directly activate the alternative pathway.

9.7 Absorbance of the supernatants is measured at 412 nm, the percent of lysis is calculated for each test and control tube by subtracting from the 412-nm absorbance of the "no-RBC serum color" control (mean of the three replicate tubes) or proportional value for greater dilutions dividing by the total lysis control value (mean of the three replicate tubes), and multiplying by 100.

$$\%\ \text{lysis} = \frac{\text{test absorbance} - \text{"no}-\text{RBC" control absorbance}}{\text{total lysis absorbance}} \times 100 \qquad (1)$$

9.8 The final percent of lysis for each condition is expressed as mean ± 1 standard deviation of the three "percent" lysis values for each three-replicate set.

9.9 The optimal dilution of a particular lot of serum, for example, the dilution at which serum exposed to a material will be assayed for rabbit cell lysis in Procedure B, can now be determined. The optimal dilution is defined as that in which the percent of lysis for sheep RBC is ≤5 % while the percent of lysis for rabbit RBC is at least 40 % but not greater than 80 % (that is, lysis is on the linear part of the complement titration curve.) A typical optimal dilution for a lot of absorbed, lyophilized HS is 1:4 (used to conform that C4(-)GPS is a good surrogate for human serum) (see Table 1) added as a 0.05-mL volume in the assay. A typical optimal dilution for a lot of absorbed, whole HS is 1:8. A typical optimal dilution for a lot of absorbed, whole C4(-)GPS is 1:3.

10. Procedure A—Exposure of Material to C4(-)GPS

10.1 *Preparation of Material*:

10.1.1 Sepharose™ CL-4B (cross-linked 4 % beaded agarose) is presented here as an example of a solid material used in medical devices that contact patient blood (such as antibody-depleting columns). Sepharose™ CL-4B has a fractionation range (molecular weight) from 60 000 to 20 000 000 daltons for globular proteins and from 30 000 to 5 000 000 daltons for dextrans, with a wet bead diameter of 40 to 165 µm. It is stored as a suspension containing 20 % ethanol between 2 to 8°C, and not frozen. Sepharose™ CL-4B, which is a moderate activator of the alternative C′ pathway, can be used as a positive control material, and is presented here as an example. Other materials shown to activate the alternative pathway may also be used (see Section 12).

NOTE 3—Sepharose™ CL-4B forms a discrete pellet upon centrifugation. For materials where centrifugation in a typical tabletop clinical centrifuge is insufficient to pellet the material following incubation with complement, a filtration step, with appropriate control, is required. The procedure presented in 10.1.2-10.2.5 is specifically designed for Sepharose™CL-4B, although other materials can be assayed in the same way. The main objective is to expose a known quantity of material to a minimum volume of 100 µL serum in a way that allows for the following: (*1*) exposure of the maximum surface area of the material to the serum and (*2*) easy separation of the material from the serum following exposure, for subsequent assay of remaining alternative complement activity against rabbit RBC. Any configuration of material/serum that meets these objects is suitable. For instance, for materials that can easily be weighed and transferred, round-bottomed upright 13 × 100 glass tubes may be more suitable than tilted glass centrifuge tubes needed for the Sepharose™ CL-4B in this example.

10.1.2 Sepharose™ CL-4B is prepared for assay by washing five times with Ca buffer. Put a defined quantity of stock, suspended Sepharose™ CL-4B (enough for the proposed assay, such as 1.4 mL) previously determined to yield a set volume after five washes in a plastic centrifuge tube, on ice. Ten mL of 4°C Ca buffer is added by pipette, squirted down with sufficient force such that the Sepharose™ is well-suspended. The suspension is centrifuged at 4°C, 1000 × g, for 10 min, then the supernatant is drawn out to near the pellet. This is reapeated four times more. At the last wash, all remaining fluid is carefully removed from above the pellet, and a volume of Ca buffer equal to the total volume of the pellet is added (in this case, 800 µL). The suspension of Sepharose™ CL-4B is held in chipped ice until needed.

10.1.3 Mix well the 1:2 dilution of Sepharose™ suspension and place an appropriate volume into the bottom of 15-mL disposable glass centrifuge tubes such that the desired volume of particles is delivered to each tube (for example, 25µL, 12.5µL, 6.25µL, and 3.17-µL beads). (The pointed tips of the glass centrifuge tubes allow for more complete removal of liquid without disturbing or aspirating any pelleted Sepharose™ CL-4B following centrifugation, even when very small volumes are present.) All material (M) tubes, no material (NM) 37°C control tubes, and Ice (I) control tubes receive 1.0-mL Ca buffer, necessary to ensure that none of the Sepharose™ CL-4B in the small volumes dispensed remains adhered to the sides of the tubes. All tubes are centrifuged at 4°C, 1 000 x g, for 10 min, and all fluid cafefully removed from the top of the pellets. The tubes are capped and left at 4°C in chipped ice until serum is added.

10.2 *Incubation of Material with Undiluted C4(-)GPS*:

10.2.1 200 µL of absorbed, undiluted C4(-)GPS at 4°C is placed onto the pelletted Sepharose™ CL–4B at the bottom of the cold 15-mL conical disposable glass centrifuge M tubes in chipped ice, into the NM tubes, and into the Ice control tubes. In this example, 200 µL is needed instead of the minimum 100 µL of serum in order to provide sufficient volume after dilution for assay in Procedure B. Sufficient surface area is provided by tilting the tubes (see 10.2.3) for good exposure of material to serum. This might not be the case if 13 × 100 glass tubes were being used for another type of material (in which case replicates would be needed to provide sufficient pooled exposed serum).

NOTE 4—A minimum assay requires three tubes, labeled M (material), NM (no material, 37°C control), and I (Ice, maximal complement activity control). For statistical evaluation, a minimum of three replicate tubes/condition should be used. In addition, other controls besides I and NM could include a comparison to another alternative-pathway activating material (with the same unit surface area or other appropriate measurable parameter), a positive reagent control for alternative pathway complement activation (such as zymosan or inulin), or a negative reagent control for alternative pathway complement activation (such as heat-aggregated human gamma globulin (HAGG) which activates complement by the classical pathway), or a combination thereof. (See Section 12 for a more detailed discussion of how to use Zymosan and HAGG as controls.)

10.2.2 Using a 100-µL pippeter and tips with ends that have been cut back to provide larger apertures (to allow for rapid mixing of the Sepharose™ CL-4B particles), quickly and carefully mix the volumes by pipetting the suspension up and down 4X/tube, starting with I, then going to NM, then going on up the range of concentrations of M tubes from lowest to highest concentration.

10.2.3 All tubes except the I tubes are immediately capped, placed in a rack, tilted at an angle (10–15°), and place in a 37°C circulating water bath such that the tips are submerged but the tops are supported on the rim of the bath. In this fashion, the Sepharose™ CL-4B does not form a compact pellet away from the serum, but instead settles onto a large surface area for maximum contact with the serum. The I tubes are left in chipped ice.

10.2.4 At the end of 1-h incubation, put the M and NM tubes back on ice. Immediately dilute the 100 µL of C4(-)GPS in each tube to its optimal assay concentration (see Section 9) by addition of 4°C BBS-G-EGTA/Mg [Mg buffer]. (For instance, if to be used for assay at a 1:3 dilution, 400 µL of Mg buffer is added to all tubes.) Using separate Pasteur glass pipets, the contents of each tube are slowly drawn up and back down into the tube, insuring that the serum and buffer are mixed well.

10.2.5 The tubes are then centrifuged at 4°C, 1000 × g, for 10 min. 400 µL, drawn by placing a pipet tip at mid height in the liquid, is transferred to another labeled glass tube in chipped ice. Serum should be assayed within 1 h for complement activity (Section 11).

10.3 *Fibers or Solid Pieces*—Assay for whole complement activation by solid fibers or pieces of material is similar to that detailed in 10.2 for Sepharose™ CL-4B, except that a defined amount of fiber or material (milligram amounts, just enough to be fully covered by a minimum of 0.1 mL of serum) is put first into room temperature 13 × 100-mm glass tubes. Then 0.1 mL of 4°C serum is added to the M, NM, and I tubes. Immediately place the M and NM tubes in a 37°C water bath while the I tube is put in chipped ice. At the end of 1 h, take the M and NM tubes out of the 37°C water bath and put them also in chipped ice.

10.4 *Assay Size and Conditions Tested*:

10.4.1 The preceding general format can be used to test differing amounts of material to yield dose-response curves, the same quantity exposed to 37°C for various periods of time (time course), or to compare C′ activation by various materials.

10.4.2 It is recommended that the total number of test samples to be assayed not exceed a number requiring a final assay size of around 100 tubes.

11. Procedure B—Assay of Serum for Alternative Pathway Complement Activation in Procedure A

11.1 Procedure B is used to assay serum which has previously been exposed to a material (Procedure A) for possible activation of complement by the alternative pathway. Alternative pathway complement activation in Procedure A (in which complement components are depleted from the serum) is detected in Procedure B as decreased lysis of rabbit RBCs in Mg buffer when the material-exposed serum M is compared to a no-material 37°C control NM.

11.2 All conditions are assayed in triplicate, using three 13 × 100 disposable glass test tubes per condition. Tubes are numbered in advance. Conditions include "total lysis," "no complement (RBC only)" (no C′), tests, and "no RBC (serum only)" (a color-control.) All reagents, tubes, and manipulations are done ice-cold, with tubes held in a rack in chipped ice or in an ice-slurry.

11.3 Rabbit RBC previously washed in Mg buffer and adjusted to 2 × 10^8/mL (Section 7) are added to all tubes except, "no RBC (serum color)" tubes (0.05 mL/tube). "No RBC (serum color)" tubes get 0.05mL 4°C Mg buffer.

11.4 To the "no C (RBC only)" tubes, 0.05 mL of Mg buffer is added. The total lysis tubes receive 0.05 mL of water. Then, add 0.05 mL from each of the test or control condition tubes from the material exposure step (Section 10), which are being held on ice and are already diluted to the optimal serum concentration for assay on rabbit cells (Section 9), to each of the three correspondingly marked tubes containing rabbit RBC.

11.5 The tubes are then treated as detailed in Sections 9.5-9.8.

12. Necessary Controls

12.1 Controls needed in each Procedure B assay (Section 11) are: "total lysis," "no complement (RBC only)" (background lysis from RBC in buffer, in the absence of serum), "no RBCs (serum color)", and "no material" ("37°C only" or NM, with no material exposure in part A). In addition, at some point sheep cells should be tested in parallel to rabbit cells to demonstrate lack of nonspecific lysis by the standard serum lot in use, under Procedure B conditions in Mg buffer.

12.2 Controls other than "no material" used in Procedure A (Section 10) may include: (*1*) a known positive material such as Sepharose™ CL-4B (Section 10), (*2*) a known negative material (for which the glass of a test tube without test material can suffice), (*3*) a positive reagent (such as Zymosan or Inulin), and (*4*) a negative reagent (such as heat-aggregated human gamma globulin HAGG)**(6)**.

12.3 Zymosan A (a yeast cell wall component from *Saccharomyces cerevisiae*) may be used as a standard positive control for activation of the alternative pathway. It is stored at 4°C. Ten milligrams of Zymosan is added to 1.0 mL of Ca buffer, then serially diluted to give 1/10 and 1/100 dilutions. Ten microlitres of each of these three solutions will deliver 100, 10, and 1 µg of Zymosan into 100 µL of serum per glass tube for comparison to test materials. The other tubes should receive 10 µL of Mg buffer containing no Zymosan. These amounts of Zymosan should produce complete, partial, and little alternative pathway depletion of complement activity (though percent depletion may vary depending on the lot of serum). Zymosan centrifuges into a tight pellet from which the overlying serum is easily separated following procedure A. Zymosan suspensions should be prepared fresh for each experiment. When final dilution of the serum is done for assay in Procedure B, compensation with buffer should be made for the 10-μL additional volume.

12.4 Preparation of HAGG: Human γ-globulins (from Cohn Fraction II, III) are stored at 4°C. 10 mg is added to 1.0–mL room temperature BBS in a glass tube. After gentle mixing and setting at room temperature for 10 min, there should be a clear liquid with no precipitate. This preparation is then placed in a 63°C water bath for 20 min. Following incubation, the solution is placed on ice, then aliquoted in 0.1-mL volumes and frozen at −70°C, providing a stock solution of 100 μg/10 μL. For use as a negative control substance (not activating the alternative pathway, only the classical pathway) the heat aggregated human gamma globulin (HAGG) is thawed and 10-μL volumes are added to serum in parallel with tested materials. Although this amount of HAGG will deplete complement by the classical pathway (which can be observed using the whole-complement assay of Practice F 1984, no depletion should occur in C4(-)GPS.

13. Report and Data Analysis

13.1 The 37°C serum-only control (tube NM) should have less rabbit cell lysis than a serum-only control kept in chipped ice (I) because some complement proteins are temperature sensitive (see example in Table 1). If a filtration step is needed to completely remove the material after Procedure A, controlled for by a second ice tube—in which the same procedure was carried out on serum without material, I_2—significant reduction in complement activity from I may also be seen in I_2.

13.2 In Procedure B, each tube from Procedure A is assayed in triplicate to allow detection of significant differences ($p \leq 0.05$ by an appropriate statistical test such as ANOVA) between Procedure A tubes. Also, especially when only small differences are present between conditions, each condition in Procedure A may need to be set up as a minimum of three replicates. Thus, in order to obtain statistical significance, materials may need to be tested in triplicate in Procedure A, with each of the three exposure tubes being assayed in triplicate in Procedure B.

13.3 Significant reduction of hemolytic activity in the M tubes as compared to the NM tubes in Procedure B denotes complement activation (with depletion of complement components) by test materials in Procedure A by the alternative pathway.

13.4 Differences in hemolysis are considered significant at $p \leq 0.05$, as calculated by an appropriate statistical test (such as ANOVA.) Results may be presented as a bar graph displaying each condition as a mean and standard deviation.

14. Keywords

14.1 alternative pathway; biocompatibility; blood compatibility; complement testing; materials; medical devices

APPENDIX

(Nonmandatory Information)

X1. RATIONALE

X1.1 The primary purpose of this practice is to describe a simple, inexpensive functional test to screen serum for alternative pathway complement activation by blood-contacting solid materials. Practice F 1984 provides guidance for testing solid materials for whole complement activation, but does not discriminate between the classical or alternative pathways. This practice tests specifically for the complement activation pathway preferred by blood-contacting solid biomaterials, the alternative pathway **(7)**. Confirmation that a material activates complement in vitro by the alternative pathway suggests that in vivo complement activation by this material is a potential concern. Although serum is not the same as the plasma to which a material is exposed in vivo, blood collected with an anticoagulant to give plasma should not be used in this practice because anticoagulants may interfere with complement activation.

X1.2 C4 genetically deficient guinea pig serum can not support complement activation by the classical pathway. Thus, if a material depletes complement activity in C4(-) GPS, it must have occurred via activation of the alternative complement pathway. Rabbit RBC in buffer containing EGTA and excess Mg^{++} are used to assay C4(-)GPS exposed to a material for C′ depletion, because rabbit cells, unlike sheep cells used in classical pathway assays, lack membrane-bound alternative pathway inhibitor molecules **(7)**. Also, the classical pathway requires Ca^{++} and Mg^{++}, whereas the alternative pathway can proceed when only Mg^{++} is present. Therefore, using buffer with EGTA to preferentially bind Ca^{++} in the presence of excess Mg^{++} also ensures that the rabbit cell lysis is only due to alternative pathway activation. (Adding EGTA plus excess $Mg^{++}$to whole human serum in Procedure A can not be used to exclude the classical pathway in this step because this gives substantially different results than when the reagents are used in a buffer-diluted serum.)

X1.3 It is well-recognized that complement activation is an important defense mechanism of the host **(8, 9)**. However, complement activation by material components of blood-contacting devices may be harmful to the host or potentially contribute to failure of devices **(6, 10,11)**. Although complementology has been an active research area for many years, the importance of chronic local complement activation on material/device function and actual impact on patient health is not completely understood.

X1.4 Many investigators have developed tests for whole complement functional activity, depletion of specific complement components, or generation of specific complement split products **(1, 2,4,12,13,14)**. Other validated test methods may be substituted for the functional alternative pathway complement-depletion assay described in this practice. If immunologic assays for individual complement pathway components are used, consideration should be given as to whether component depletion is by nonspecific binding to a material or by pathway activation.

X1.5 The procedure as presented is intended as a routine screening procedure. It is not represented as being the most sensitive or the most specific procedure for assessing the complement-activation potential of all materials in all applications. Further analysis of materials found to activate the alternative pathway might involve the use of human serum and immunoassays that detect reduction of complement pathway components or elaboration of complement pathway-specific split products (such as Bb and C4d). Complement component-depleted human serum is unsuitable because, (in contrast to genetically deficient C4(-)GPS), depletion by immunoadsorption may result in the following: (*1*) incomplete reduction in the level of classical pathway activity and (*2*) direct activation of the alternative pathway resulting in a reduction in alternative pathway complement titer.

X1.6 Substances that are weak alternative pathway activators might still generate enough relevant split products (C3a, C5a, and so forth) to cause a local inflammatory response in vivo, that may not be reflected by significant changes in whole complement activity. The results obtained with this procedure may be used in conjunction with the results of other tests in assessing the blood compatibility of the test material.

REFERENCES

(**1**) Giclas, P.C., "Complement Tests," *Manual of Clinical Laboratory Immunology*, 5th ed, N.R. Rose, E.C. de Macario, J.D. Folds, H.C. Lane, and R.M. Nakamura, eds., ASM Press, 1997, pp. 181-186.

(**2**) Gee, A.P., "Molecular Titration of Components of the Classical Complement Pathway," *Methods in Enzymology*, Vol 93, Immunochemical Techniques, J.J. Langone, and H.V. Vunakis, eds., Academic Press, 1983, pp. 339-375.

(**3**) United States Drug Enforcement Agency, Washington, DC.

(**4**) Lin, W-Q., and White, Jr., K.L., "Complement Assays to Assess Immunotoxicity," *Methods in Immunotoxicology*, Vol I, G.R. Burleson, J.H. Dean, and A.E. Munson, eds., Wiley-Liss, 1995, pp. 357-375.

(**5**) Tanaka, S., Kitamura, F., and Suzuki, T., "Studies on the Hemolytic Activity of the Classical and Alternative Pathway of Complement in Various Animal Species," 1987, Complement 4:33-41.

(**6**) Chenoweth, D.E., "Complement Activation Produced by Biomaterials," 1986, Trans. Am. Soc. Artif. Intern. Organs 32:226-232.

(**7**) Platts-Mills, T.A.E., and Ishizaka, K., "Activation of the Alternative Pathway of Human Complement by Rabbit Cells," *Journal of Immunology*, 1974, 113:348-358.

(**8**) Sakamoto, M., Fujisawa, Y., Nishioka, K., "Physiologic Role of the Complement System in Host Defense, Disease, and Malnutrition," Nutrition 14:391–398, 1998.

(**9**) Law, S.K.A., Reid, K.B.M., Complement, second edition, Oxford University Press, 1995

(**10**) Kazatchkine, M.D., Carreno, M.P., "Activation of the Complement System at the Interface Between Blood and Artificial Surfaces," Biomaterials, 9:30–36, 1998

(**11**) Hakim, R.M., "Complement Activation by Biomaterials," Cardiovasc. Pathol. 2:187S-197S,1993

(**12**) McLean, R.H., Welch, T.R., "Complement" Handbook of Human Immunology, eds M.S. Leffell, A.D. Donnerburg, and N.R. Rose, CRC Press, pp. 267–318, 1997

(**13**) Labarre,D., Montdargent,B., Carreno,M-P., Maillet,F., "Strategy for In Vitro Evaluation of the Interactions between Biomaterials and Complement System," J. Applied Biomat. 4: 231–240, 1993.

(**14**) Complement Methods and Protocols, ed B.P. Morgan, Humana Press, 2000

Designation: F 2066 – 01

Standard Specification for Wrought Titanium-15 Molybdenum Alloy for Surgical Implant Applications (UNS R58150)[1]

This standard is issued under the fixed designation F 2066; the number immediately following the designation indicates the year of original adoption or, in the case of revision, the year of last revision. A number in parentheses indicates the year of last reapproval. A superscript epsilon (ε) indicates an editorial change since the last revision or reapproval.

1. Scope

1.1 This specification covers the chemical, mechanical, and metallurgical requirements for wrought titanium-15 molybdenum alloy to be used in the manufacture of surgical implants (**1**).[2]

1.2 The values stated in inch-pound units are to be regarded as the standard. The SI equivalents in parentheses are for information only.

2. Referenced Documents

2.1 *ASTM Standards:*

E 8 Test Methods for Tension Testing of Metallic Materials[3]

E 112 Test Methods for Determining Average Grain Size[3]

E 120 Test Methods for Chemical Analysis of Titanium and Titanium Alloys[4]

E 290 Test Methods for Bend Testing of Material for Ductility[3]

E 1409 Test Method for Determination of Oxygen in Titanium and Titanium Alloys by the Inert Gas Fusion Technique[5]

E 1447 Test Method for Determination of Hydrogen in Titanium and Titanium Alloys by the Inert Gas Fusion Thermal Conductivity Method[5]

F 67 Specification for Unalloyed Titanium for Surgical Implant Applications[6]

F 748 Practice for Selecting Generic Biological Test Methods for Materials and Devices[6]

F 981 Practice for Assessment of Compatibility of Biomaterials for Surgical Implants with Respect to Effect of Materials on Muscle and Bone[6]

F 1408 Practice for Subcutaneous Screening Test for Implant Materials[6]

2.2 *Aerospace Material Specification:*

AMS 2249 Chemical Check Analysis Limits, Titanium and Titanium Alloys[7]

2.3 *American Society for Quality Standard:*

ASQ C1 Specification of General Requirements for a Quality Program[8]

2.4 *ISO Standard:*

ISO 6892 Metallic Materials — Tensile Testing[9]

3. Terminology

3.1 *Definitions of Terms Specific to This Standard:*

3.1.1 *beta annealed, n*—the condition of the material that is obtained if, following the final hot-working or cold-working operation, the mill product is rapidly quenched, for example, by water quenching or pressurized helium gas quench, from a temperature above the beta transus of approximately 1382°F (750°C).

3.1.2 *beta transus, n*—the minimum temperature at which the alpha plus beta phase can transform to 100 % beta phase.

4. Product Classification

4.1 *Strip*—Any product under 0.1875 in. (4.76 mm) in thickness and under 24 in. (610 mm) wide.

4.2 *Sheet*—Any product under 0.1875 in. (4.76 mm) in thickness and 24 in. (610 mm) or more in width.

4.3 *Plate*—Any product 0.1875 in. (4.76 mm) thick and over and 10 in. (254 mm) wide and over, with widths greater than five times the thickness. Plate up to 4 in. (101.60 mm), thick inclusive, is covered by this specification.

4.4 *Bar*—Rounds or flats from 0.1875 in. (4.76 mm) to 4 in. (101.60 mm) in diameter or thickness. (Other sizes and shapes by special order.)

4.5 *Wire*—Rounds or flats less than 0.1875 in. (4.76 mm) in diameter or thickness.

5. Ordering Information

5.1 Include with inquiries and orders for material under this specification the following information.

5.1.1 Quantity,

---

[1] This specification is under the jurisdiction of ASTM Committee F04 on Medical and Surgical Materials and Devices and is the direct responsibility of Subcommittee F04.12 on Metallurgical Materials.

Current edition approved May 10, 2001. Published May 2001. Orinially published as F 2066 - 00. Last previous edition F 2066 - 00.

[2] The boldface numbers in parentheses refer to the list of references at the end of this standard.

[3] *Annual Book of ASTM Standards*, Vol 03.01.

[4] *Annual Book of ASTM Standards*, Vol 03.05.

[5] *Annual Book of ASTM Standards*, Vol 03.06.

[6] *Annual Book of ASTM Standards*, Vol 13.01.

[7] Available from the American Society of Automotive Engineers, 400 Commonwealth Dr., Warrendale, PA 15096.

[8] Available from the American Society for Quality, 600 N. Plankinton Ave., Milwaukee, WI 53203.

[9] Available from the American National Standards Institute, 25 W. 43rd St., 4th Floor, New York, NY 10036.

5.1.2 Applicable ASTM designation,

5.1.3 Form (strip, sheet, plate, bar, or wire),

5.1.4 Condition (see Section 3 and 6.1),

5.1.5 Mechanical properties (if applicable for special conditions),

5.1.6 Finish (see 6.2),

5.1.7 Applicable dimension including size, thickness, width, or drawing number,

5.1.8 Special tests, if any, and

5.1.9 Special requirements.

6. Materials and Manufacture

6.1 The various titanium mill products covered in this specification normally are formed with the conventional forging and rolling equipment found in primary ferrous and nonferrous plants. The alloy is usually multiple melted in arc furnaces (including furnaces such as plasma arc and electron beam) of a type conventionally used for reactive metals.

6.2 *Finish*—The mill product may be furnished to the implant manufacturer as descaled or pickled, sandblasted, chemically milled, ground, machined, peeled, polished, or combinations of these operations.

7. Chemical Requirements

7.1 The heat analysis shall conform to the chemical composition of Table 1. Ingot analysis may be used for reporting all chemical requirements, except hydrogen. Samples for hydrogen shall be taken from the finished mill product.

7.1.1 Requirements for the major and minor elemental constituents are listed in Table 1. Also listed are important residual elements. Analysis for elements not listed in Table 1 is not required to verify compliance with this specification.

7.2 *Product Analysis*—Product analysis tolerances do not broaden the specified heat analysis requirements but cover variations between laboratories in the measurement of chemical content. The manufacturer shall not ship material that is outside the limits specified in Table 1. The product analysis tolerances shall conform to the check tolerances in Table 2.

7.2.1 The product analysis is either for the purpose of verifying the composition of a heat or manufacturing lot or to determine variations in the composition within the heat.

7.2.2 Acceptance or rejection of a heat or manufacturing lot of material may be made by the purchaser on the basis of this check analysis.

7.3 For referee purposes, use Test Methods E 120, E 1409, and E 1447 or other analytical methods agreed upon between the purchaser and the supplier.

7.4 Ensure that the samples for chemical analysis are representative of the material being tested. The utmost care must be used in sampling titanium for chemical analysis because of its affinity for elements such as oxygen, nitrogen, and hydrogen. In cutting samples for analysis, therefore, the operation should be carried out insofar as possible in a dust-free atmosphere. Cutting tools should be clean and sharp. Samples for analysis should be stored in suitable containers.

TABLE 1 Chemical Requirements

Element	Composition, %, (Mass/Mass)
Nitrogen, max	0.05
Carbon, max	0.10
Hydrogen, max	0.015
Iron, max	0.10
Oxygen, max	0.20
Molybdenum	14.00-16.00
Titanium[A]	balance

[A]The percentage of titanium is determined by difference and need not be determined or certified.

TABLE 2 Product Analysis Tolerances[A]

Element	Tolerance Under the Minimum or Over the Maximum Limit[B], %, (Mass/Mass)
Nitrogen	0.02
Carbon	0.02
Hydrogen	0.0020
Iron	0.10
Oxygen	0.02
Molybdenum	0.25

[A]Refer to AMS 2249.

[B]Under the minimum limit not applicable for elements in which only a maximum percentage is indicated.

8. Mechanical Requirements

8.1 The material supplied under this specification shall conform to the mechanical property requirements in Table 3 or Table 4.

8.2 Specimens for tension tests shall be machined and tested in accordance with Test Methods E 8. Tensile properties shall be determined using a strain rate of 0.003 to 0.007 in./in./min (mm/mm/min) through the specified yield and then the cross-head speed shall be increased so as to produce fracture in approximately one additional minute.

8.3 *Number of Tests*—Perform a minimum of two tension tests from each lot. A lot is defined as the total number of mill products produced under the same conditions at essentially the same time. If either of the two test specimens does not meet the specified requirements, test two additional test pieces representative of the same lot in the same manner. The lot will be considered in compliance only if both additional test pieces meet the specified requirements. If a specimen fails outside the gage, the test is null in accordance with Test Methods E 8, and a retest shall be performed.

8.4 For sheet and strip, the bend test specimen shall withstand being bent cold through an angle of 105° without fracture in the outside surface of the bend portion. The bend shall be made over a mandrel with a diameter equal to that shown in Table 4. Test conditions shall conform to Test Method E 290.

9. Special Requirements

9.1 The microstructure shall consist of a fully recrystallized beta phase structure. Primary alpha and alpha prime (also known as martensitic alpha) are not permitted in the microstructure when viewed at 100× magnification.

9.2 The grain size in the annealed condition shall be 5 or finer, in accordance with Test Methods E 112.

9.3 Determine the beta transus temperature for each heat by a suitable method and report on the material certification if required by the purchaser.

9.4 Alpha case is not permitted for products supplied with a machined, ground, or chemically milled surface finish. For other products, there will be no continuous layer of alpha case when examined at 100× magnification.

TABLE 3 Mechanical Properties—Bar and Wire

Condition	Ultimate Tensile Strength, min, psi (MPa)	Yield Strength (0.2 % Offset), min, psi (MPa)	Elongation[A] in 4D or 4W, min, %	Reduction of Area, min, %
Beta annealed	100 000 (690)	70 000 (483)	20	60

[A] 4D = 4X diameter; 4W = 4X width. Alternately, a gage length corresponding to ISO 6892 may be used when agreed upon between supplier and purchaser.

TABLE 4 Mechanical Properties—Sheet, Strip, and Plate[A]

Condition	Ultimate Tensile Strength, min, psi (MPa)	Yield Strength (0.2 % Offset), min, psi (MPa)	Elongation in 2 in. (50 mm), min, %	Bend Test Mandrel Diameter[B]	
				Under 0.070 in. (1.78 mm) in Thickness	0.070 to 0.1875 in. (1.78 to 4.76 mm) in Thickness
Beta annealed	105 000 (724)	80 000 (552)	12	5T	6T

[A] Limits apply to tests taken both longitudinal and transverse to the direction of rolling.
[B] T equals the thickness of the bend test specimen. Bend tests are not applicable to material over 0.1875 in. (4.76 mm) in thickness.

10. Certification

10.1 The supplier's certification that the material was manufactured in accordance with this specification together with a report of the test results shall be furnished to the implant manufacturer at the time of shipment.

11. Quality Program Requirements

11.1 The producer shall maintain a quality program in accordance with ASQ C1.

12. Keywords

12.1 metals (for surgical implants); orthopaedic medical devices; titanium alloys; titanium alloys (for surgical implants)

APPENDIXES

(Nonmandatory Information)

X1. RATIONALE

X1.1 The purpose of this specification is to characterize the chemical, mechanical, and metallurgical properties of wrought titanium-15 molybdenum alloy to be used in the manufacture of surgical implants **(1-4)**.

X1.2 The microstructural requirements contained in this specification represent current general consensus with respect to optimization of mechanical properties for implant applications.

X1.3 The minimum mechanical properties specified ensure a baseline of strength and ductility for the highly stressed devices for which this alloy is typically used.

X1.4 The stress corrosion cracking resistance of this alloy is similar to that of titanium-6 aluminum-4 vanadium ELI alloy **(5)**.

X2. BIOCOMPATIBILITY

X2.1 The suitability of this material from a human implant perspective is dependent on the specific application. The biological tests appropriate for the specific site, such as recommended in Practice F 748 should be used as a guideline. A summary of the in vitro and animal testing that has been performed as of the approval date of this specification is provided in X2.3.

X2.2 No known surgical implant material has ever been shown to be completely free of adverse reactions in the human body. The alloy composition covered by this specification, however, has been subjected to testing in laboratory animals, and has been used clinically since Feb. 6, 1998. The results of these studies indicate a well-characterized level of local biological response that is equal to or less than that produced by the reference material unalloyed titanium (see Specification F 67) that has a long history of successful clinical application in soft tissue and bone implants in humans.

X2.3 As of the time of the original approval of this specification, this titanium alloy material had a limited history of clinical use in humans. An extensive series of in vitro and animal studies had been performed as follows, comparing the biological response to that of a reference material. These tests were conducted to support the usage of this material in surgical implant devices **(6-10)**. In all cases, the results indicated that this material was no more reactive with the environment than the reference material.

X2.3.1 L929 MEM-Cytotoxicity (**11**).

X2.3.2 Molybdenum Sensitization Study (**12**).

X2.3.3 Molybdenum In-Vitro Organ Culture (**13**).

X2.3.4 Rabbit Pyrogen Test (**6**).

X2.3.5 Acute Systemic Toxicity (Albino Swiss mice) (**6**).

X2.3.6 Practice F 1408 Subcutaneous Implantation in Mice (**1**).

X2.3.7 Practice F 981 Implantation in Dogs (**1**).

X2.3.8 Ames Mutagenicity Assay (**14**).

REFERENCES

(**1**) Zardiackas, L., Mitchell, D., and Disegi, J., "Characterization of Ti-15Mo Beta Titanium Alloy for Orthopaedic Implant Applications," *Medical Applications of Titanium and Its Alloys: The Material and Biological Issues, ASTM STP 1272*, S. Brown and J. Lemons, Eds., American Soceity for Testing and Materials, W. Conshohocken, PA, 1996, pp. 60-75.

(**2**) Disegi, J. and Fairer, R., "Torsional Properties of Ti-15Mo Bone Screws," *Transactions*, 21st Annual Meeting, Society for Biomaterials, 18-22 March 1995, p. 351.

(**3**) Meusli, P., et al., "Properties of Surface Oxides on Titanium and Some Titanium Alloys," *Proceedings*, Sixth World Conference on Titanium, 6-9 June 1988, pp. 1759-1764.

(**4**) Khan, M.A., Williams, R.L., and Williams, D.F., "In-Vitro Corrosion and Wear of Titanium Alloys in the Biological Environment," *Biomaterials*, Vol 17, No 22, 1996, pp. 2117-2126.

(**5**) Bogan, J., Zardiackas, L., Disegi, J., "Stress Corrosion Cracking Resistance of Titanium Implant Materials," *Transactions*, 27th Annual Meeting, Society for Biomaterials, 24–29 April 2001, p. 438.

(**6**) FDA 510(k) No. K952272.

(**7**) FDA 510(k) No. K962616.

(**8**) FDA 510(k) No. K963798.

(**9**) FDA 510(k) No. K974555.

(**10**) FDA 510(k) No. K982732.

(**11**) Disegi, J. and Paika, I., "Cytotoxicity Evaluation of Ti-15Mo Alloy," *Transactions*, 20th Annual Meeting, Society for Biomaterials, 1994, p. 202.

(**12**) Hierholzer, S., and Hierholzer, G., *Internal Fixation and Metal Allergie: Clinical Investigations, Immunology, and Histology of the Implant Tissue Interface*, Thieme Medical Publishers, New York, 1992.

(**13**) Gerber, H., and Perren, S., "Evaluation of Tissue Compatibility of in vitro Cultures of Embryonic Bone," *Evaluation of Biomaterials*, John Wiley & Sons, 1980, pp. 307-314.

(**14**) Disegi, J., and Prezioso, J., "Mutagenicity Evaluation of Ti-15Mo Alloy," *Transactions*, 5th World Biomaterials Congress, 29 May–2 June 1996, p. 675.

SUMMARY OF CHANGES

Committee F04 has identified the location of selected changes to this standard since the last issue F 2066 - 00 that may impact the use of this standard.

(*1*) Test Methods E 290 was added to the Referenced Documents section.

(*2*) 8.4 was added to cover the bend test requirement.

(*3*) Table 4, Footnote B was clarified.

(*4*) Reference (**5**) citation was changed from an internal report to a peer-reviewed publication in the 2001 edition of this standard.

Designation: F 2068 – 00

Standard Specification for Femoral Prostheses—Metallic Implants[1]

This standard is issued under the fixed designation F 2068; the number immediately following the designation indicates the year of original adoption or, in the case of revision, the year of last revision. A number in parentheses indicates the year of last reapproval. A superscript epsilon (ε) indicates an editorial change since the last revision or reapproval.

1. Scope

1.1 This specification covers metallic stemmed femoral prostheses used to replace the natural hop joint by means of hemi-arthroplasty or total hip surgical procedures. Prostheses for hemi-arthroplasty are intended to articulate with the natural acetabulum of the patient. Prostheses for total hip replacement are intended to articulate with prosthetic acetabular cups. Prostheses may have integral femoral heads or cones designed to accept modular heads.

1.2 Modular femoral heads, which may be affixed to cones on implants covered by this specification, are not covered by this specification. The mechanical strength, corrosion resistance, and biocompatibility of the head portions of one-piece integral implants are covered by this specification.

1.3 Femoral prostheses included within the scope of this specification are intended for fixation by press fit between the prosthesis and host bone, the use of bone cement, or through the ingrowth of host bone into a porous coating.

1.4 Custom femoral prostheses, designed explicitly for a single patient, are not covered within the scope of this specification.

1.5 Prostheses incorporating nonmetallic (for example, polymer composite) implants, nonporous bioactive ceramic coatings, or porous-polymer coatings, are specifically excluded from the scope of this specification.

1.6 The requirements for modular connections of multicomponent modular femoral hip prostheses are not covered by this specification.

1.7 The values stated in SI units are to be regarded as the standard.

2. Referenced Documents

2.1 *ASTM Standards:*

F 67 Specification for Unalloyed Titanium for Surgical Implant Applications[2]

F 75 Specification for Cast Cobalt—Chromium-Molybdenum Alloy for Surgical Implant Applications[2]

F 86 Practice for Surface Preparation and Marking of Metallic Surgical Implants[2]

F 90 Specification for Wrought Cobalt-Chromium-Tungsten-Nickel Alloy for Surgical Implant Applications[2]

F 136 Specification for Wrought Titanium-6 Aluminum-4 Vanadium ELI (Extra-Low Interstitial) Alloy (R56401) for Surgical Implant Applications[2]

F 138 Specification for Wrought 18 Chromium-14 Nickel-2.5 Molybdenum Stainless Steel Bar and Wire for Surgical Implants (UNS S31673)[2]

F 562 Specification for Wrought Cobalt-35 Nickel-20 Chromium-10 Molybdenum Alloy for Surgical Implant Applications[2]

F 563 Specification for Wrought Cobalt-Nickel-Chromium-Molybdenum-Tungsten-Iron Alloy for Surgical Implant Applications[2]

F 620 Specification for Titanium 6Al-4V ELI Alloy Forgings for Surgical Implants[2]

F 745 Specification for 18 Chromium-12.5 Nickel-2.5 Molybdenum Stainless Steel for Cast and Solution-Annealed Surgical Implant Applications[2]

F 746 Test Method for Pitting or Crevice Corrosion of Metallic Surgical Implant Materials[2]

F 748 Practice for Selecting Generic Biological Test Methods for Materials and Devices[2]

F 799 Specification for Cobalt-28 Chromium-6 Molybdenum Alloy Forgings for Surgical Implants[2]

F 981 Practice for Assessment of Compatibility of Biomaterials for Surgical Implants with Respect to Effect of Materials on Muscle and Bone[2]

F 983 Practice for Permanent Marking of Orthopedic Implant Components[2]

F 1044 Test Method for Shear Testing of Porous Metal Coatings[2]

F 1108 Specification for TI6Al4V Alloy Castings for Surgical Implants[2]

F 1147 Test Method for Tension Testing of Porous Metal Coatings[2]

F 1440 Practice for Cyclic Fatigue Testing of Metallic Stemmed Hip Arthroplasty Femoral Components Without Torsion[2]

F 1472 Specification for Wrought Ti-6Al-4V Alloy for Surgical Implant Applications[2]

F 1537 Specification for Wrought Cobalt-28 Chromium-6 Molybdenum Alloy for Surgical Implants[2]

F 1580 Specification for Titanium and Titanium-6 % Aluminum-4 % Vanadium Alloy Powders for Coatings of Surgical Implants[2]

[1] This specification is under the jurisdiction of ASTM Committee F04 on Medical and Surgical Materials and Devices and is the direct responsibility of Subcommittee F04.22 on Arthroplasty.

Current edition approved Nov. 10, 2000. Published January 2001.

[2] *Annual Book of ASTM Standards*, Vol 13.01.

F 1612 Practice for Cyclic Fatigue Testing of Metallic Stemmed Hip Arthroplasty Femoral Components with Torsion[2]

F 1636 Specification for Bores and Cones for Modular Femoral Heads[2]

F 1814 Specification for Evaluating Module Hip and Knee Joint Components[2]

F 1854 Test Method for Stereological Evaluation of Porous Coatings on Medical Implants[2]

F 1978 Test Method for Measuring Abrasion Resistance of Metallic Thermal Spray Coatings by Using the Taber® Abraser[2]

2.2 *ISO Documents:*

ISO 5832-1:1997 Implants for Surgery—Metallic Materials—Part 1: Wrought Stainless Steel[3]

ISO 5832-3:1996 Implants for Surgery—Metallic Materials—Part 3: Wrought Titanium 6-Aluminum 4-Vanadium Alloy[3]

ISO 5832-4:1996 Implants for Surgery—Metallic Materials—Part 4: Cobalt-Chromium-Molybdenum Casting Alloy[3]

ISO 5832-9:1992 Implants for Surgery—Metallic Materials—Part 9: Wrought High Nitrogen Stainless Steel[3]

ISO 7206-2:1996 Implants for Surgery—Partial and Total Hip Joint Prostheses—Part 2: Articulating Surfaces Made of Metallic, Ceramic and Plastics materials[3]

ISO 7206-4:1989 Implants for Surgery—Partial and Total Hip Joint Prostheses—Part 4: Determination of Endurance Properties of Stemmed Femoral Components with Application of Torsion[3]

ISO 7206-8:1995 Implants for Surgery—Partial and Total Hip Joint Prostheses—Part 8: Endurance Performance of Stemmed Femoral Components with Application of Torsion[3]

3. Terminology

3.1 *Definitions of Terms Specific to This Standard:*

3.1.1 *bore, n*—an internal cavity, in the form of a truncated right cone, used to engage with the cone of a femoral neck.

3.1.2 *collar, n*—flange at the junction of the neck and proximal body.

3.1.3 *cone, n*—the truncated conic geometry on a femoral hip prosthesis used to engage with the bore of a femoral head.

3.1.4 *distal stem, n*—region of the implant that extends distally from the proximal body. This part of the implant is intended for insertion within the femoral medullary canal. The distal stem may be in direct apposition with bone or may be fixed in the femoral medullary canal using bone cement.

3.1.5 *head, n*—convex spherical bearing member for articulation with the natural acetabulum or prosthetic acetabulum.

3.1.6 *hemi-arthroplasty, n*—replacement of the natural femoral head with a prosthetic femoral head held in place by an implant extending into the shaft of the femur. The natural acetabulum is not altered.

3.1.7 *modular (Type II) head, n*—a femoral head that is not integral with the neck and proximal body. It is a convex bearing member for articulation with either natural acetabulum or the prosthetic acetabulum. It possesses an integrally machined bore for fitting the cone of a modular (Type II) implant.

3.1.8 *modular (Type II) implant, n*—a femoral hip component of which the head is not integral with the neck and proximal body of the implant. The modular implant is intended for insertion within the femoral medullary canal. It possesses a cone that provides a stable connection for the modular (Type II) head.

3.1.9 *mono-block (Type I) implant, n*—a femoral hip component in which the head is integral with the neck and proximal body of the implant.

3.1.10 *neck, n*—the portion of the femoral prosthesis connecting the proximal body and the prosthetic femoral head. The neck is integral with the proximal body, and is either permanently attached to the head (Type I devices) or to a cone designed to accept a modular head (Type II devices).

3.1.11 *porous surface, n*—an outermost layer(s) of all or part of the femoral implant characterized by interconnecting subsurface pores, generally with the volume porosity between 30 and 70 %, average pore size between 50 and 1000 μm, and a thickness between 250 and 1500 μm (in accordance with Test Method F 1854). This porous layer may be manufactured directly into the metallic implant by casting or by various electro/chemical/thermal/mechanical means, or applied as a coating of particles, beads, or mesh by processes such as sintering or plasma spray.

3.1.12 *proximal body, n*—region of the implant which extends distally from the trochanteric region to the diaphyseal region of the femur. This portion of the implant may be in direct apposition with bone or may be fixed in the femoral medullary canal using bone cement.

3.1.13 *total hip arthroplasty, n*—replacement of the natural femoral head with a prosthetic femoral head held in place by an implant extending into the shaft of the femur and replacement of the natural acetabulum with a prosthetic acetabulum. The prosthetic femoral head articulates with the bearing surface of the prosthetic acetabulum.

4. Classification of Implant Type

4.1 Femoral prostheses falling within the scope of this specification are of four types as defined as follows. There are not distinguishing features (for example, collars or lack thereof, fenestrations, and so forth) that would exempt any device from any requirement of this specification.

4.1.1 *Type IA*—Single-piece (mono-block), metallic femoral total hip or hemi-arthroplasty hip prosthesis with an integral stem, neck and head. The stem is designed such that the center of the head, the axis of the neck, and proximal body, and the distal stem all lie in the same medial/lateral plane.

4.1.2 *Type IB*—Single-piece (mono-block), metallic, femoral total hip or hemi-arthroplasty his prostheses with an integral stem, neck, and head. The stem is designed such that the center of the head, the axis of the neck, the proximal body, and the distal stem dot not lie in the same medial/lateral plane. This would include anteverted necks, proximally curved stems, distally bowed stems and so forth.

[3] Available from American National Standards Institute, 11 W. 42nd St., 13th Floor, New York, NY 10036.

4.1.3 *Type IIA*—Modular metallic femoral hip prostheses that could include a modular (Type II) head or other modular components, or both. Such "modular" designs allow for more flexible inventory management and provide a means for adjusting prosthesis neck length and, therefore, leg length at surgery. The stem is designed such that the center of the head, the axis of the neck, the proximal body, and the distal stem all lie in the same medial/lateral plane.

4.1.4 *Type IIB*—Modular metallic femoral hip prosthesis that could include a modular (Type II) head or other modular components, or both. Such "modular" designs allow for more flexible inventory management and provide a means for adjusting prosthesis neck length and, therefore, leg length at surgery. The stem is designed such that the center of the head, the axis of the neck, the proximal body, and the distal stem do not lie in the same medial/lateral plane. This would include anteverted necks, proximally curved stems, distally bowed stems, and so forth.

5. Materials

5.1 All devices conforming to this specification shall be fabricated form materials with adequate mechanical strength and durability, corrosion resistance, and biocompatibility. Some examples of materials from which femoral hip prostheses have been successfully fabricated include Specifications F 67, F 75, F 90, F 136, F 138, F 562, F 563, F 620, F 745, F 799, F 1108, F 1472, F 1537 and F 1580 and ISO Standards 5832/1:1997/3:1996/4:1996/9:1992.

5.1.1 *Mechanical Strength*—Not all of the materials listed in 5.1 possess sufficient mechanical strength for critical highly stressed components. Conformance of a selected material to its standard and successful clinical usage of the material in a previous implant design are not sufficient to ensure the strength of an implant. Manufacturing processes and implant design can strongly influence material properties. Therefore, regardless of the material selected, the femoral hip implant must meet the performance requirements of Section 6.

5.1.2 *Corrosion Resistance*—Materials with limited or not history of successful use for orthopedic implant application must be determined to exhibit corrosion resistance equal to or better than one of the materials listed in 5.1 when tested in accordance with Test Method F 746.

5.1.3 *Biocompatibility*—Materials with limited or no history of successful use for orthopedic implant application must be determined to exhibit acceptable biological response equal to or better than on of the materials listed in 5.1 when tested in accordance with Practices F 748 and F 981.

5.1.4 The selection, strength, and processing of implant materials shall be consistent with the performance requirements contained in Section 6, corrosion resistance of 5.1.2, and the biocompatilibity requirements of 5.1.3.

6. Performance Considerations

6.1 *Structural Requirements*—Femoral prostheses conforming to this specification shall be capable of withstanding normal static and dynamic loading in the physiological range without overload fracture, plastic deformation, or fatigue fracture.

NOTE 1—Consult the rationale in Appendix X2 for comments regarding the application of 6.1.

6.1.1 Fatigue performance of the femoral hip components may be characterized by testing in accordance with ISO 7206-4:1989, Practice F 1612, or Practice F 1440. Representative samples shall be able to withstand cyclic loading with a minimum load of 300 N and a maximum load of 2.3 kN in accordance with ISO 7206-8:1995 when tested in accordance with ISO 7206-4:1989 or Practice F 1612, or cyclic loading with a minimum load of 300 N and a maximum load of 3.3 kN when tested in accordance with Practice F 1440. For ASTM test methods, use an unsupported implant length of 50 mm in accordance with the ASTM definition. The representative test samples should be selected from the standard (average patient) size range and which presents the worse case stress conditions for the design series. To meet the worse case stress recommendation, implants should be tested with the worst-case offset head.

6.1.2 Alternatively, the demonstrated fatigue strength of the implant size with the highest stresses, when tested with the worst-case offset head and in accordance with ISO 7206-4:1989, Practice F 1612, or Practice F 1440, shall be equivalent to or exceed the demonstrated fatigue strength of a comparable, clinically successful femoral implant design.

NOTE 2—While ISO 7206-4:1989 specifies testing in a saline environment, some researches test in saline and some researchers test in ambient laboratory air. Consideration should always be given to corrosion effects on fatigue and fretting behavior in establishing a test protocol. Materials which are suspected to environmental sensitivity or which the sensitivity level is not know, should be tested in a simulated physiological environment as recommended in ISO 7602-4:1989 and suggested in Practices F 1440 and F 1612.

6.2 *Coating Integrity Metal Coating* (for example, plasma spray, porous, and fiber metal)— The porous surface morphology shall be capable of accepting tissue (soft or hard) ingrowth to accomplish firm fixation of the device. The porosity may be uniform, or may be graded from surface to substrate in a manner to maximize both the interfacial strength and ingrowth potential.

6.2.1 *Shear Strength*—When tested in accordance with Test Method F 1044, the average shear strength of the surface/substrate interface shall equal or exceed 20 MPa (2900 psi).

6.2.2 *Tensile Strength*—When tested in accordance with Test Method F 1147, the average tensile strength of the surface/substrate interface shall equal or exceed 20 MPa (2900 psi).

6.2.3 *Abrasion Resistance of Plasma Spray Thermal Coatings*—When tested in accordance with Test Method F 1978, samples fabricated and coated using this process shall not have an average mass of liberated porous coating material in excess of 65 mg/100 cycles.

7. Dimensions and Permissible Variations

7.1 *Cone Requirements*—Type II designs, incorporating a modular head concept, should either conform to the dimensional requirements or be dimensionally defined in terms of the parameters in accordance with Specification F 1636.

8. Surface Condition and Marking

8.1 *Surface Condition*—Femoral prostheses conforming to

this specification shall be processed in accordance with Practice F 86 and ISO 7206-2:1996.

8.2 *Marking*:

8.2.1 Femoral implants conforming to this specification shall be marked in accordance with Practice F 86 and Practice F 983, where space permits. Marking shall specify the manufacturer's logo and lot number and material.

8.2.2 Implant marking shall be carried out in such a way as to minimize the effects on the performance of the implant in regards to strength or biocompatibility.

8.3 *Femoral Head*—The femoral head bearing surface of Type I femoral prostheses shall be in accordance with ISO 7206-2:1996.

APPENDIXES

(Nonmandatory Information)

X1. RATIONALE STATEMENT

X1.1 The objectives of this specification are to augment common terminology, identify currently acceptable materials, set forth dimensional requirements, and provide guidelines for the mechanical performance of femoral components used for partial and total hip replacement. The investigator should also review Specification F 1814 which outlines additional parameters recommended for consideration in the design and fabrication of modular hip implants.

X1.2 Partial hip replacement parts are used in hemi-arthroplasty and are intended for use in patients who are skeletally mature and have joint degradation of only their femoral head or who have fractured the neck of their femur. Total hip replacement parts are intended for use in patients who are skeletally mature and have joint degeneration on both femoral head and acetabulum. The requirements of this specification are based upon more than forty years of successful clinical experience with these types of implant. They identify those factors recognized to effect prosthesis performance and longevity. It is recognized, however, that failure of an arthroplasty can occur due to factor completely unrelated to the characteristics of the prostheses.

X1.3 It is also recognized that failures of a total hip arthroplasty of hemi-arthroplasty can occur even though the components are intact. This is true owing to the goal of the surgical procedure, which is a composite construction comprised of implant components, hose bone, surrounding tissue, and body fluids. Failure of the procedure may occur due solely to host factors not at all influenced by properties of the device components.

X2. PERFORMANCE REQUIREMENTS

X2.1 It should be recognized that laboratory testing, even with accurately simulated imposed loading and a corrosive environment of electrolytes and complex constituents of body fluids, cannot accurately predict performance over many decades of use in vivo. In vivo performance is influenced by many factory including surgical technique, patient weight, canal size, activity, and so forth. The recommended test practices described in ISO 7206-4:1989, Practice F 1440 and Practice F 1612 are based on the correlation of clinical fractures with laboratory simulations and should be considered guidelines useful for characterizing fatigue performance.

X2.2 The general requirements provide for generally good workmanship and design. Fatigue strength requirements are primarily based on the work of Semlitsch et. al (**4**), with allowances for alternative test methodology that provide simulation of specific functional aspects.

X2.3 Implant fatigue requirements, specified in 6.1, are derived from this specification and first specified in ISO 7206-7:1993 (obsolete) and ISO 7206-8:1995. The 3.3-kN requirement for Practice F 1440 is based on ISO 7206-7:1993 which defined the requirements for implant strength when tested without torsion. ISO 7206-7:1993 has been withdrawn and is no longer current, but the recommended value is still generally accepted in the industry.

X2.4 The femoral stem fatigue strength performance criterion outlined in ISO 7206-7:1993 (obsolete) and ISO 7206-8:1995 has a relatively vague definition regarding the range of application. Both ISO 7206-8:1995 and ISO 7206-7:1993 indicate that the performance criterion is appropriate for "an average size patient" (in Europe) with a caveat regarding small sizes. This criterion has been successfully utilized by many manufacturers, resulting in a low incidence of clinical implant fractures. Because the defined range of application is so broad, further refinement may be useful. There is general consensus that the performance criterion is particularly appropriate when applied to the "average" patient whose body size, weight, and lifestyle are consistent with the patents described by Semlitsch. It is also consensus that implants designed for distal canal diameters of 11 mm or larger generally represent the "average" patient population. Anatomic data gathered by Noble (**15**) and coworkers may help manufacturers determine an "average" patient population based on specific femoral prosthesis design and intended use.

X2.5 Implant designs targeted at patient population groups

significantly different from the Semlitsch group (such as small canal size or unusual geometries) may not be capable of meeting this broad performance requirement. Our recommendation is that the performance criterion be applied to the "average" population as described in this specification. For those designs which fall outside of the average patient population it may be appropriate to consider alternative design requirements which reflect device loading conditions specific to the target patient group. The best alternative measure is one based on the historical clinical evidence of a comparable device (in accordance with the guidelines in 6.1.2).

X2.6 In execution of 6.1.1 and 6.1.2, selection of the implant assembly with the worst case stress condition should not be assumed to be configured with the longest offset femoral head. The worse case stress condition depends on the combined effect of the head offset and the cross-sectional properties of the cross section near the cantilever plane. The ISO test method specifies the location to be 80 mm from the center of the head. Longer offset heads naturally produce greater height and a resulting change in the location of the cantilever cross section. In distally tapered implants, the change in cross section may be greater than the increase in offset, decreasing the maximum stress condition. With this effect in mind, the representative samples should produce the worse case stress condition for the possible combinations of head and implant size.

X2.7 The specific requirements on tensile and shear strengths of porous materials are derived from recommendations in FDA guidance documents and are generally accepted in the industry as reasonable lower bound strength limits. FDA guidance documents are living documents and, as such, are not consistent referenceable resources. The investigator is encouraged to review these documents for additional information related to femoral hip testing.

X3. MATERIALS

X3.1 The materials listed in 5.1 represent some of the materials from which femoral hip prostheses have been successfully fabricated. Use of these materials does not, in and of itself, guarantee a successful design, and use of the materials may be equally successful. The necessary corrosion-resistance and biocompatibility requirements provide baseline assurance for the acceptance of new materials by the body.

X3.2 The investigator should also be aware of the galvanic corrosion potential of the materials intended for multicomponent femoral hip prostheses. Evaluation of the galvanic corrosion potential should be conducted as is recommended in 5.3.4 of Specification F 1814.

X4. DIMENSIONS

X4.1 Because of the modularity of designs and the potential for partial revisions of this type of surgery, standard nomenclature and critical dimensions of mating parts must be ensured to assist the surgeons in selecting appropriate matching components.

REFERENCES

(1) Lorenz, M., Semlitsch, M., Panic, B., Weber, H.G., "Fatigue Strength of Cobalt-base Alloys with High Corrosion Resistance for Artificial Hip Joints"; Engineering in Medicine, Vol 7, No 4: pp. 241-250, Oct. 1978.

(2) Semlitsch, M., Panic, B., "Corrosion Fatigue Testing of Femoral Head Prostheses Made of Implant Alloys of Different Fatigue Resistance," Mechanical Properties of Biomaterials, ed. Hastings, G.W., Williams, D.E., Wiley & Sons, Ltd., 1980.

(3) Semlitsch, M., Willert, H.G., "Properties of Implant Alloys for Artificial Hip Joints, Mechanical and Biological Engineering and Computing," 18: pp. 511-520, July 1980.

(4) Semlitsch, M., Panic, B., "Fracture Proof Anchorage Stems of Artificial Hip Joints, Ten Years of Experience with Test Criteria," Engineering In Medicine, Vol.12, No. 4, pp. 185-198.

(5) Anon, "Joint Motion – Method of Measuring and Recording," American Academy of Orthopedic Surgeons, 1965, pp. 56-64.

(6) ANSI B46.1-1962 (ISO 468), Surface Texture – Surface Roughness, Waviness, and Lay, ANSI, 1430 Broadway, NY, NY. Reaffirmed 1971.

(7) English, T.A. and Kilvington, M., "In Vivo Records of Hip Loads Using a Femoral Implant with Telemetric Output (A Prelimary Report)," J. Biomed. Engr., Vol 1, No. 2, Apr., 1979, pp. 111-115.

(8) Hodge, W.A., Fijan, R., Mann, R.W., and Harris, W. H., "Preliminary In Vivo Pressure Measurements in a Human Acetablum," 31st Ann., ORS, Las Vegas, Nev., Jan. 1985.

(9) Brown, R. H., Davy, D.T., Heiple, K.G. Sr., Kotzar, G.M., Heiple, K.G. Jr., Berilla, J., Goldberg, V. M., Burstein, A. H., "In-Vivo Load Measurements on a Total Hip Prosthesis," 31st Ann., ORS, Las Vegas, Nev., Jan. 1985.

(10) Kilvington, M., and Goodman, R.M.F., "Engr. In Vivo Hip Joint Forces Recorded on a Strain Gauged "English" Prosthesis Using and Implanted Transmitter," Engineering in Medicine, Vol. 10, No. 4, Oct 1981, pp. 175-187.

(11) Rybicki, E. F., "The Role of Finite Element Models in Orthopaedics," Finite Elements in Biomechanics, Ed. R.H. Gallagher, et al, J. Wiley & Sons, Ltd. 1982.

(12) Fatigue strength of ceramic hip endoprostheses (author's transl) Dauerfestigkeit keramischer Huftendoprothesen. Dorre E., Dawihl W., Altmeyer G., Biomed Tech (Berl) (GERMANY, WEST), Jan-Feb 1977, 22 (1-2) pp. 3-7.

(13) Davy, D.T., et al, "Telemetric Force Measurements Across the Hip

After Total Arthroplasty," J. Bone Joint Surgery, 70A:45-50 (1988).

(14) Humphrey, S.M., and Gilbertson L.N., "Fatigue Testing of Femoral Hip Prostheses with a Two-Beam Simulated Femoral Bone Support Fixture," in *Composite Materials for Implant Applications in the Human Body*, Jamison/Gilbertson, eds., ASTM STP 1178, ASTM (Philadelphia), 1993.

(15) Noble, P. C., Alexander, J. W., Lindahl, L. J., Yew, D.T., Granberry, W. M., Tullos, H.S., "The Anatomic Basis of Femoral Component Design", Clinical Orthopaedics & Related Research, 1998, pp. 148-165.

Standard Practice for Communicating an EMS Patient Report to Receiving Medical Facilities[1]

This standard is issued under the fixed designation F 2076; the number immediately following the designation indicates the year of original adoption or, in the case of revision, the year of last revision. A number in parentheses indicates the year of last reapproval. A superscript epsilon (ε) indicates an editorial change since the last revision or reapproval.

INTRODUCTION

Throughout all areas of emergency medical services (EMS), there exists a need for the EMS provider to consult with medical direction and receiving medical facilities. These consultations can be purely for patient arrival notification, medical consultation, or to request additional medical intervention orders. Within the EMS community, no "standard" reporting scheme exists. Hundreds of verbal reporting formats are currently used. Some agencies divide these further for those assessments involving medical from trauma. Failure to use a standard reporting scheme makes initial student education difficult, makes recording of information cumbersome, and can lead to time delays in patient care or worse yet an error.

This consensus format was developed from a survey sent to over 100 emergency physicians, nurses, and field providers. The 25 that were returned were analyzed to construct the initial draft. One clear theme was present. **Receiving medical facilities want to know the most important information first** . . . medical information that affects the logistics of running a busy emergency department (ED). With the increased use of standing orders, the traditional detailed report to the ED was often not seen as time effective or making any change in the patient's outcome.

This practice uses the acronym **PISA** to describe the information to be presented in a generic patient report. **P** is priority information that is considered absolutely critical if only 15 s of transmission (or reception) is accomplished; **I** is important information that needs to be communicated if an additional 16 to 30 s is available; **S** is significant information that would be transmitted if an additional 31 to 60 s were available; **A** is additional information that should be transmitted if 61+ s are available.

1. Scope

1.1 This practice establishes the EMS standard for communications entailing a patient radio (phone) report to a receiving medical facility.

1.1.1 This report is based on receiving facility needs and is generic for medical, traumatic, (ALS), and (BLS) patients.

1.1.2 This report standard is based on the hierarchical information needs of an average medical receiving facility.

2. Referenced Documents

2.1 *ASTM Standards:*

F 1418 Guide for Training the Emergency Medical Technician (Basic) in Roles and Responsibilities[2]

F 1629 Guide for Establishing and/or Operating Emergency Medical Services Management Information Systems[2]

F 1651 Guide for Training the Emergency Medical Technician (Paramedic)[2]

2.2 *Other Documents:*

USDOT National Standard Curriculum for EMT-B[3]

USDOT National Standard Curriculum for EMT-P[3]

3. Terminology

3.1 *Definitions of Terms Specific to This Standard:*

3.1.1 *AVPU*—a brief neurological examination to determine a baseline level of consciousness and to assess central nervous system function. This assessment is universally taught as part of the initial assessment for EMS providers.

3.1.2 **A**lert

3.1.3 responds to **V**erbal stimuli

3.1.4 responds to **P**ainful stimuli

3.1.5 **U**nresponsive—no gag or cough

3.1.6 *Glasgow Coma Scale (GCS)*—standard neurological evaluation that uses eye opening, motor response, and verbal response. This assessment is universally taught as part of the detailed assessment for EMS providers.

3.1.7 *LOC*—level of consciousness.

[1] This practice is under the jurisdiction of ASTM Committee F30 on Emergency Medical Services and is the direct responsibility of Subcommittee F30.04 on Communications.

Current edition approved Jan. 10, 2001. Published April 2001.

[2] *Annual Book of ASTM Standards*, Vol 13.01.

[3] Available from the Superintendent of Documents, U.S. Government Printing Office, Washington, DC 20402.

3.1.8 *PMS*—neurological evaluation checking pulses, motor, sensory status of the four extremities.

3.1.9 *trauma score*—numerical injury rating system based on several parameters that may include patient body region injured, type of injury, central nervous system assessment, and vital sign evaluation.

4. Significance and Use

4.1 This practice establishes the national standard for training the EMT in communicating pertinent patient information to the receiving medical facility.

4.2 Appropriate physiological data and patient assessment information should be collected from the scene or while en route to the receiving medical facility or medical command site.

4.3 This practice is based on the information needs of a receiving medical facility to assist them in medical triage, ED resource management, and the provision of medical direction.

4.4 This practice should be used by those who develop curricula, provide continuing medical education, or desire a needs-based reporting approach.

4.5 This practice should be used to develop documentation aids such as EMS note pads and medical command documentation sheets.

4.6 The communication format in each **PISA** subsection in the practice are not necessary in sequential order. The report may vary dependent upon patient presentation.

5. Communication of Pertinent Patient Information

5.1 After establishing communications with the receiving medical facility, patient information will be reported in the following format:

5.1.1 Organization of patient medical information into the categories of **P**riority, **I**mportant, **S**ignificant, **A**dditional.

5.1.1.1 **Priority** = "Need to know" or critical information to be transmitted in the 0- to 15-s time frame.

5.1.1.2 **Important** = Additional important information transmitted in the 16- to 30-s time frame.

5.1.1.3 **Significant** = Additional information that supports the critical information; transmitted in the 31- to 60-s time frame.

5.1.1.4 **Additional** = "Nice to know" information transmitted in the 61+-s time frame.

5.1.2 **P—Priority** information items to be communicated:

5.1.2.1 Unit's name or call sign,

5.1.2.2 EMS provider identification,

5.1.2.3 Patient age and gender,

5.1.2.4 AVPU/LOC,

5.1.2.5 Chief complaint, and

5.1.2.6 Mechanism of injury/nature of illness.

5.1.3 **I—Important** information items to be communicated:

5.1.3.1 Respiratory status,

5.1.3.2 Level of distress,

5.1.3.3 Skin color and condition, and

5.1.3.4 Vital signs.

5.1.4 **S—Significant** information items to be communicated:

5.1.4.1 Scene description if pertinent,

5.1.4.2 History of the present illness,

5.1.4.3 Medications taken by patient,

5.1.4.4 Pertinent technical findings,

(*a*) Pulse oximetry,

(*b*) Glucometer,

(*c*) Three-lead/twelve-lead EKG, and

(*d*) Other.

5.1.4.5 Head/neck assessment, and

5.1.4.6 Glasgow Coma Scale/Trauma Score.

5.1.5 **A—Additional** information items to be added if up to 61+ s were available:

5.1.5.1 Further neurological assessment (if needed),

5.1.5.2 Abdominal assessment/pelvic stabilization,

5.1.5.3 Extremity assessment (PMS),

5.1.5.4 Allergies (if pertinent),

5.1.5.5 Field treatment provided,

5.1.5.6 Response to field treatment,

5.1.5.7 Destination, and

5.1.5.8 Estimated time of arrival.

6. Documentation Template

6.1 Fig. 1 is a sample receiving medical facility form.

7. Keywords

7.1 emergency medical services; patient report form

Anytown Medical Center
EMS Call Report

Date: __________ Time:__________ Unit________ EMS Provider__________

Age_____ Male Female Chief Complaint_________________________

Mechanism: Illness / Medical_______________________________________
Injury / Trauma_______________________________________

Scene Description____

A - V - P - U LOC_______________

Skin Color_____________ Pulse______ Respirations______ BP_____/_____

Respiratory Status_________________ Level of Distress_______________

History of Present Illness____

Patient Medications____

Technical Findings: Pulse oximetry_________ Glucometer__________

EKG / 12 Lead_________ Other_____________

Head / Neck____

GCS______________________________ Trauma Score____________

Further Neuro Exam________________ Abdominal:_______________

Extremities_______________________ Allergies_________________

Field Treatment____

Response to Field Treatment______________________________________

Additional Orders____

Destination_______________________ ETA_________________________

Report taker:___________________________

FIG. 1 Sample Receiving Medical Facility Form

Designation: F 2077 – 01

Test Methods For Intervertebral Body Fusion Devices[1]

This standard is issued under the fixed designation F 2077; the number immediately following the designation indicates the year of original adoption or, in the case of revision, the year of last revision. A number in parentheses indicates the year of last reapproval. A superscript epsilon (ε) indicates an editorial change since the last revision or reapproval.

1. Scope

1.1 This test method covers the materials and methods for the static and dynamic testing of intervertebral body fusion device assemblies, spinal implants designed to promote arthrodesis at a given spinal motion segment.

1.2 This test method is intended to provide a basis for the mechanical comparison among past, present, and future non-biologic intervertebral body fusion device assemblies. This test method allows comparison of intervertebral body fusion device assemblies with different intended spinal locations and methods of application to the intradiscal spaces. This test method is intended to enable the user to compare intervertebral body fusion device assemblies mechanically and does not purport to provide performance standards for intervertebral body fusion device assemblies.

1.3 The test method describes static and dynamic tests by specifying load types and specific methods of applying these loads. These tests are designed to allow for the comparative evaluation of intervertebral body fusion device assemblies.

1.4 This test method does not purport to address expulsion testing of intervertebral body fusion device assemblies. However, since expulsion is a potential clinical failure mode, the user should address the implant's resistance to expulsion.

1.5 Guidelines are established for measuring displacements, determining the yield load or moment, evaluating the stiffness, and strength of the intervertebral body fusion device assemblies.

1.6 Some intervertebral body fusion device assemblies may not be testable in all test configurations.

1.7 The values stated in SI units are to be regarded as the standard with the exception of angular measurements, which may be reported in terms of either degrees or radians.

1.8 *This standard does not purport to address all of the safety concerns, if any, associated with its use. It is the responsibility of the user of this standard to establish appropriate safety and health practices and determine the applicability of regulatory limitations prior to use.*

2. Referenced Documents

2.1 *ASTM Standards:*

E 4 Practices for Force Verification of Testing Machines[2]

E 6 Terminology Relating to Methods of Mechanical Testing[2]

E 1823 Terminology Relating to Fatigue and Fracture Testing[2]

F 1582 Terminology Relating to Spinal Implants[3]

3. Terminology

3.1 For definition of terms refer to Terminology E 6, E 1823, and F 1582.

3.2 *Definitions of Terms Specific to This Standard:*

3.2.1 *coordinate system/axes, n*—Three orthogonal axes are defined by Terminology F 1582. The center of the coordinate system is located at the geometric center of the intervertebral body fusion device assembly. The *XY* plane is to bisect the sagittal plane angle between superior and inferior lines (surfaces) that are intended to simulate the adjacent vertebral end plates. The positive *Z* axis is to be directed superiorly. Force components parallel to the *XY* plane are shear components of loading. The compressive axial force is defined to be the component in the negative *Z* direction. Torsional load is defined to be the component of moment parallel to the *Z* axis.

3.2.2 *fatigue life, n*—The number of cycles, *N*, that the intervertebral body fusion device assembly can sustain at a particular load or moment before mechanical or functional failure occurs.

3.2.3 *functional failure, n*—Permanent deformation that renders the intervertebral body fusion device assembly ineffective or unable to resist load and/or maintain attachment adequately.

3.2.4 *ideal insertion location, n*—The implant location with respect to the simulated inferior and superior vertebral bodies (polyacetal or metal blocks) dictated by the type, design, and manufacturer's surgical installation instructions.

3.2.5 *intended method of application, n*—Intervertebral body fusion device assemblies may contain different types of stabilizing anchors such as threads, spikes, and knurled surfaces. Each type of anchor has an intended method of application or attachment to the spine.

3.2.6 *intended spinal location, n*—The anatomic region of the spine intended for the intervertebral body fusion device assembly. Intervertebral body fusion device assemblies may be

[1] This test method is under the jurisdiction of ASTM Committee F04 on Medical and Surgical Materials and Devices and is the direct responsibility of Subcommittee F04.25 on Spinal Devices.

Current edition approved May, 10 2001. Published June 2001. Originally published as F 2077 - 00. Last previous edition F 2077 - 00.

[2] *Annual Book of ASTM Standards*, Vol 03.01.

[3] *Annual Book of ASTM Standards*, Vol 13.01.

designed and developed for specific regions of the spine such as the lumbar, thoracic, and cervical spine. Also, there exists different anatomical potential surgical approaches, which will result in different implant orientation at different levels of the spine.

3.2.7 *intervertebral body fusion device, n*—A structure (biologic or synthetic) that is placed in the disc space between two adjacent vertebral bodies to provide support for eventual arthrodesis of the two adjacent vertebral bodies.

3.2.8 *intradiscal height, n*—The straight-line distance along the Z axis between the unaltered simulated vertebral bodies—minimum height of 4 mm and a maximum height of 18 mm. See Fig. 1.

3.2.9 *load point, n*—The point through which the resultant force on the intervertebral device passes (that is, the geometric center of the superior fixture's sphere) (Figs. 2-5).

3.2.10 *maximum run out load or moment, n*—The maximum load or moment for a given test that can be applied to an intervertebral body fusion device assembly in which all of the tested constructs have withstood 5 000 000 cycles without functional or mechanical failure.

3.2.11 *mechanical failure, n*—That associated with the onset of a defect in the material (that is, initiation of fatigue crack or surface wear).

3.2.12 *offset angular displacement, n*—(Distance OB—Fig. 6)—Offset on the angular displacement axis equal to 10 % of the intradiscal height, *H*, divided by the outside diameter or height of the implant (maximum dimension of implant in *XZ* plane if not cylindrical) (for example, for a 10-mm intradiscal height and 16-mm intervertebral body fusion device assembly, distance OB = 10 mm/16 mm (0.10)(180°)/π = 3.6°).

3.2.13 *offset displacement, n*—(Distance OB—Fig. 6)—Offset on the displacement axis equal to 2 % of the intradiscal height (that is, 0.2 mm for a 10-mm intradiscal height).

3.2.14 *permanent deformation, n*—The remaining displacement (mm or degrees or radians) relative to the initial unloaded condition of the intervertebral body fusion device assembly after the applied load has been removed.

3.2.15 *stiffness (N/mm or N*mm/Degree (Radian)) (The Slope of Line OG—Fig. 6), n*—The slope of the initial linear portion of the load-displacement curve or the slope of the initial linear portion of the moment—angular displacement curve.

3.2.16 *test block, n*—The component of the test apparatus for mounting the intervertebral body fusion device assembly for the intended test configuration.

3.2.17 *ultimate displacement (millimetres or degrees or radians) (Displacement OF—Fig. 6), n*—The displacement associated with the ultimate load or ultimate moment.

3.2.18 *ultimate load or moment (N or N*mm) (Point E—Fig. 6), n*—The maximum applied load, *F*, transmitted by the pushrod (assumed equal to force component parallel to and indicated by load cell), or the applied moment about the *Z* axis that can be applied to an intervertebral body fusion device assembly.

3.2.19 *yield displacement (Distance OA—Fig. 6), n*—The displacement (mm) or angular displacement (deg) when an interbody fusion device asembly has a permanent deformation equal to the offset displacement or the offset angular displacement.

3.2.20 *yield load or moment (Point D—Fig. 6), n*—The applied load, *F*, transmitted by the pushrod (assumed equal to force component parallel to and indicated by load cell), or the applied moment about the *Z* axis required to produce a permanent deformation equal to the offset displacement or the offset angular displacement.

4. Summary of Test Method

4.1 These test methods are proposed for the mechanical testing of intervertebral body fusion device assemblies specific to the lumbar, thoracic, and cervical spine.

4.2 Fatigue testing of the intervertebral body fusion device assemblies will simulate a motion segment via a gap between two polyacetal test blocks. The polyacetal will eliminate the effects of the variability of bone properties and morphology for the fatigue tests. The minimum ultimate tensile strength of the polyacetal blocks shall be no less than 61 MPa.

4.3 Static testing of the intervertebral body fusion device assemblies will simulate a motion segment via a gap between two stainless steel blocks. The minimum ultimate tensile strength of the blocks shall be no less than 1310 MPa.

4.4 The pushrod shall also be manufactured from stainless steel, which shall also have a minimum ultimate tensile strength no less than 1310 MPa.

4.5 Static and dynamic tests will evaluate the intervertebral body fusion device assembly. The user of this test method must decide which series of tests are applicable to the intervertebral body fusion device assembly in question. The user of this test

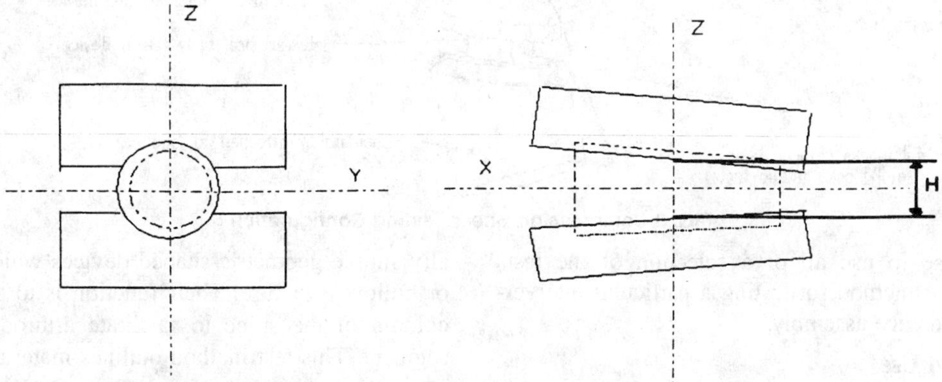

FIG. 1 Intradiscal Height Diagram

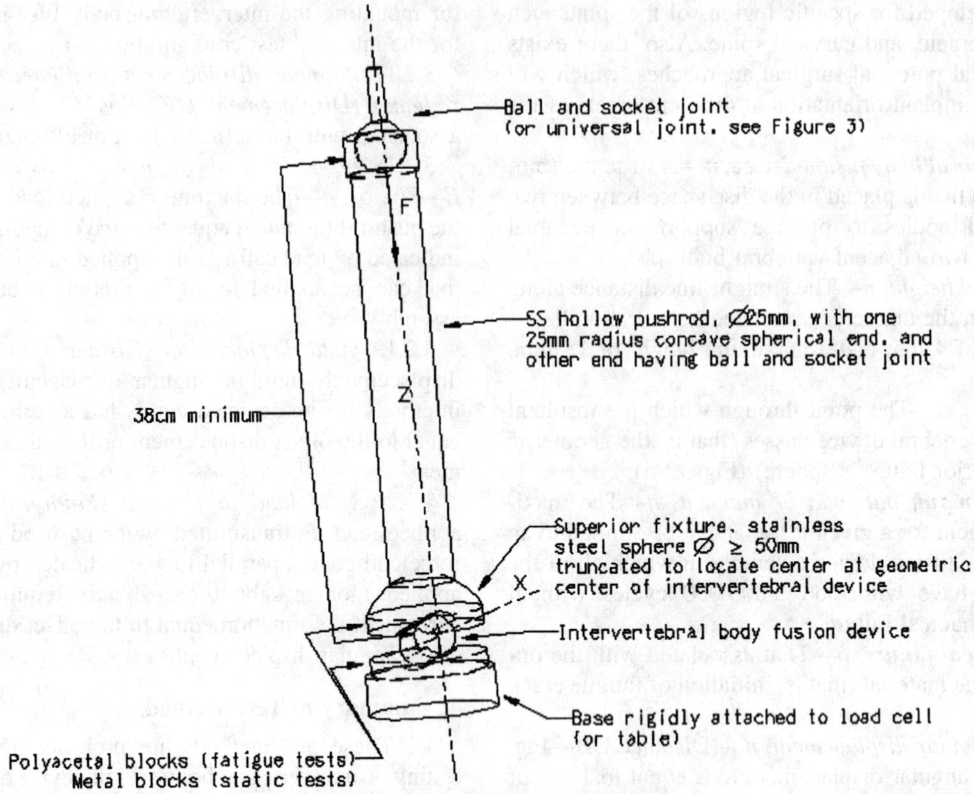

FIG. 2 Compression Testing Configuration

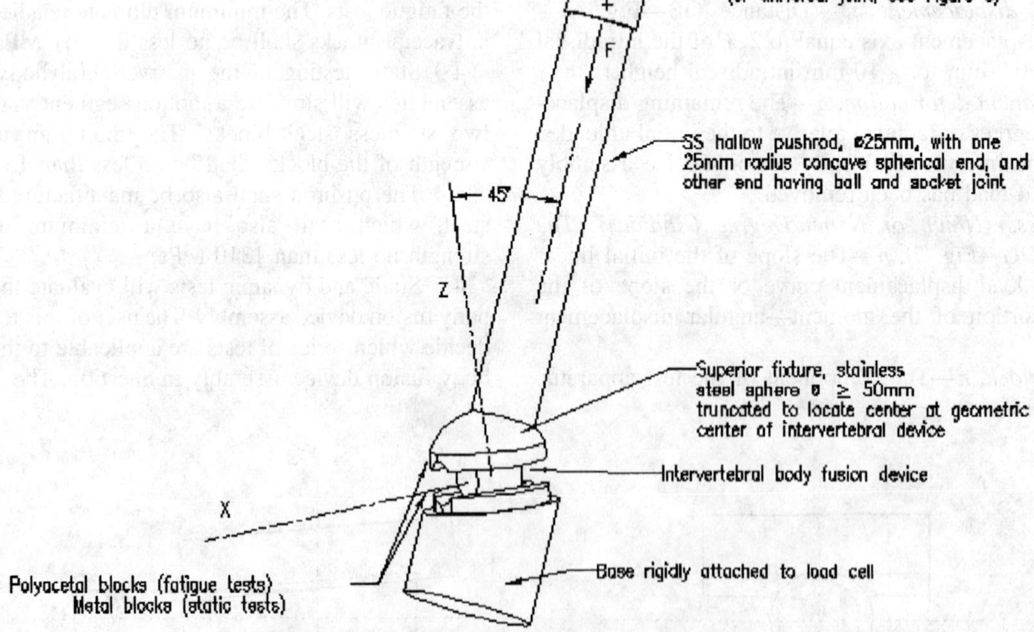

FIG. 3 Compression-Shear Testing Configuration

method may choose to use all or a selection of the tests described in this test method for testing a particular intervertebral body fusion device assembly.

5. Significance and Use

5.1 Intervertebral body fusion device assemblies are generally simple geometric-shaped devices which are often porous or hollow in nature. Their function is to support the anterior column of the spine to facilitate arthrodesis of the motion segment. This test method outlines materials and methods for

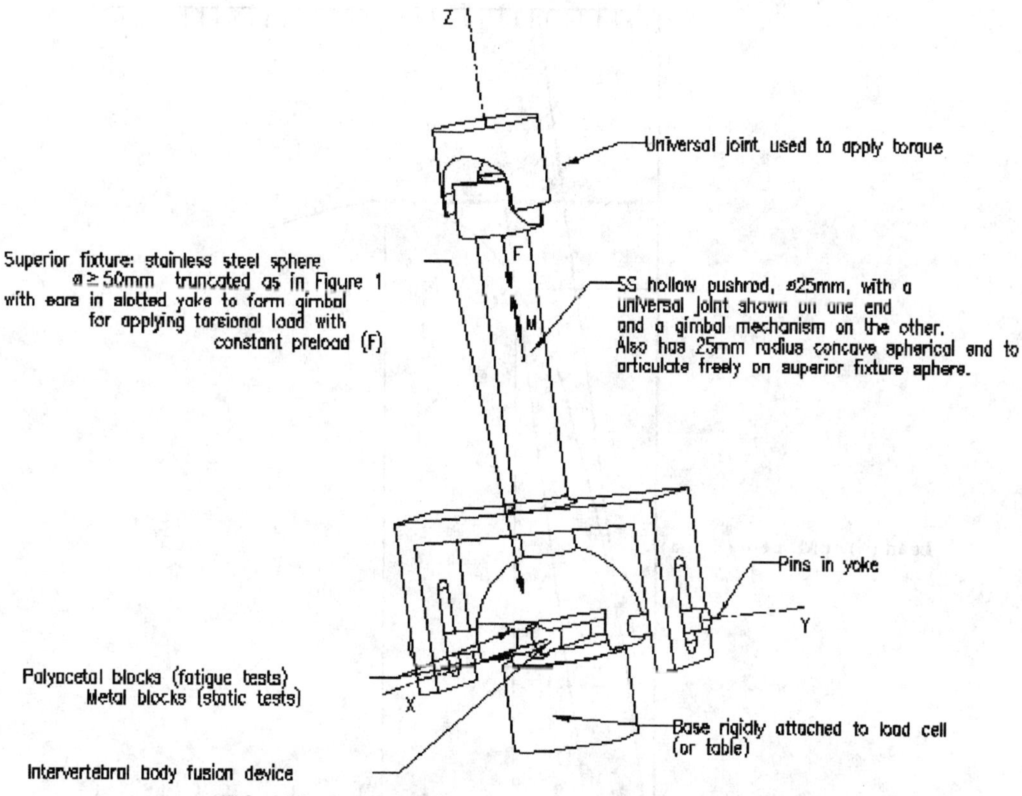

FIG. 4 Torsion Testing Configuration With Pin-Slot Gimbal

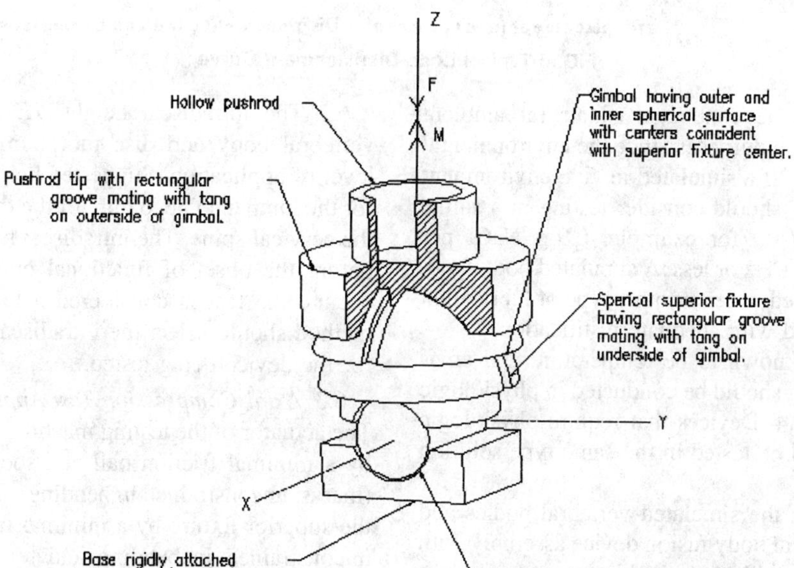

FIG. 5 Spherical Gimbal (Cross Section) for Torsion Testing Apparatus

the characterization and evaluation of the mechanical performance of different intervertebral body fusion device assemblies so that comparisons can be made between different designs.

5.2 This standard is designed to quantify the static and dynamic characteristics of different designs of intervertebral body fusion device assemblies. These tests are conducted in vitro to allow for analysis and comparison of the mechanical performance of intervertebral body fusion device assemblies to specific load modalities.

5.3 The loads applied to the intervertebral body fusion assemblies may differ from the complex loading seen in vivo, and therefore, the results from these tests may not directly predict in vivo performance. The results, however, can be used to compare mechanical performance of different intervertebral body fusion device assemblies.

5.4 Since the environment may affect the dynamic performance of intervertebral body fusion device assemblies, dynamic testing in a saline environment may be considered.

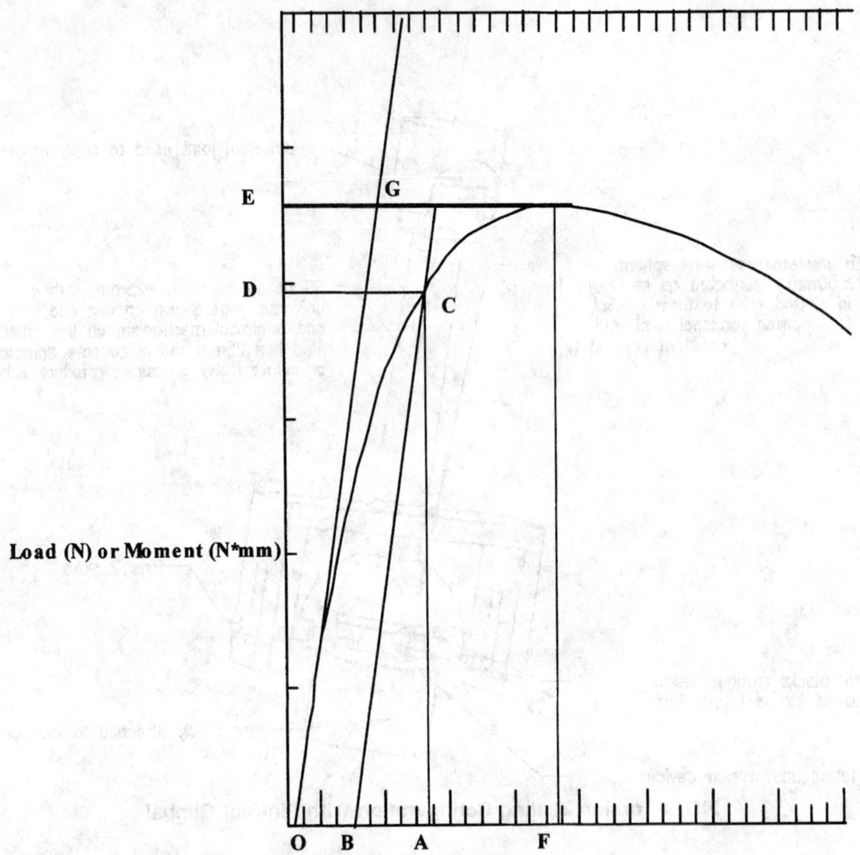

FIG. 6 Typical Load Displacement Curve

Fatigue tests should first be conducted in air (at ambient temperature) for comparison purposes since the environmental effects could be significant. If a simulated in vivo environment is desired, the investigator should consider testing in a saline environmental bath at 37°C (for example, 0.9-g NaCl per 100-mL water) at a rate of 1 Hz or less. A simulated body fluid, a saline drip or mist, distilled water, or other type of lubrication at 37°C could also be used with adequate justification.

5.5 If the devices are known to be temperature and environment dependent, testing should be conducted in physiologic solution as described in 5.4. Devices that require physiologic solution for testing should be tested in the same type solution for comparison purposes.

5.6 The location within the simulated vertebral bodies and position of the intervertebral body fusion device assembly with respect to the loading axis will be dependent upon the design, the manufacturer's recommendation, or the surgeon's preferred method for implant placement.

5.7 It is well known that the failure of materials is dependent upon stress, test frequency, surface treatments, and environmental factors. Therefore, when determining the effect of changing one of these parameters (for example, frequency, material, or environment), all others must be kept constant to facilitate interpretation of the results.

6. Apparatus

6.1 Test machines will conform to the requirements of Practices E 4.

6.2 The intradiscal height, *H*, shall be determined from vertebral body and disc morphometric data at the intended level of application. Suggested heights are as follows: 10 mm for the lumbar spine, 6 mm for the thoracic spine, and 4 mm for the cervical spine. The intradiscal height should not reach zero before the onset of functional or mechanical failure. If this occurs, the test is considered a failure. The user of the test method should select the intradiscal height that is appropriate for the device being tested.

6.3 *Axial Compression Test Apparatus*

The actuator of the testing machine is connected to the pushrod by a minimal friction ball and socket joint or universal joint (that is, unconstrained in bending). The pushrod is connected to the superior fixture by a minimal friction sphere joint (that is, unconstrained in bending and torsion). The hollow pushrod should be of minimal weight so as to be considered a "two-force" member. It thus applies to the intervertebral body fusion device assembly a resultant force directed along the pushrod's axes and located at the center of the superior fixture's sphere joint (the geometric center of the device being tested). For the fatigue tests, the device is placed between two polyacetal blocks, which are rigidly attached to the metal blocks (Fig. 2). For the static tests, metal blocks are to be used, which could be incorporated as an integral part of the superior and inferior fixtures. The blocks are to have surfaces that mate geometrically with the intervertebral device similar to how the device is intended to mate with vertebral end plates. The test apparatus will be assembled such that the Z axis of the intervertebral device is initially coincident with the pushrod's axis and collinear with the axis of the testing machine's actuator and load cell. The length of the pushrod between the center of the ball-and-socket joint to the center of the spherical surface is to be a minimum of 38 cm. This is required to minimize deviation of the pushrod's axis (direction of applied force, F) from that of the test machine's load cell axis. In other words, this is to minimize the error in using and reporting that the force indicated by the load cell "F_{ind}" is the applied load, F, and is equal to the compressive force, F_z, on the intervertebral body fusion device assembly. For example, a 1-mm displacement of the spherical surfaces center in the XY plane would produce an angle between axes of 0.15°, (10 mm producing 1.5°). Fig. 2 is a schematic of this test set up.

6.4 *Compression-Shear Testing Apparatus*—The compression-shear test apparatus (Fig. 3) with exception of the inferior fixture is identical to the axial compression apparatus (Fig. 2). The inferior fixture is to be designed to orient the initial position of the intervertebral device's Z axis at 45° flexion relative to the pushrod's axis. The resultant force, F, being applied to the intervertebral body fusion device assembly passes through the center of the superior fixture's spherical surface and is coincident with the pushrod's axis. Thus a combined compressive load F_z and an anterior shear load F_x is created, which initially are equal in magnitude and pass through the geometric center of the intervertebral body fusion device assembly.

6.5 *Torsion Testing Apparatus*—The torsion test apparatus (Fig. 4) is similar to the axial compression test apparatus (Fig. 2) with exception of the pushrod interconnections. The actuator of the testing machine must be connected to the pushrod by a minimal friction (that is, unconstrained in bending) universal joint to be able to transmit torsional moment in addition to axial load. The pushrod is connected to the superior fixture by a spherical gimbal mechanism to apply combined compressive force, F, and moment, M, with negligible bending moment to the intervertebral body fusion device assembly. Two examples of a gimbal mechanism are: (*1*) a sphere with pegs engaged in a slotted yoke attached to the pushrod (Fig. 4) and (*2*) a pair of spherical surfaces with interdigitating tongue and grooves located 90° to each other (Fig. 5). The test apparatus is to be assembled so that the Z axis of the intervertebral body fusion device assembly is initially coincident with the pushrod's axis and collinear with the axis of the testing machine's actuator and load cell. This setup is designed so that the initially applied load, F, and moment, M, are equal to the compression force, F, and torsional moment, M, on the intervertebral body fusion device assembly.

7. Sampling

7.1 All components in the intervertebral body fusion device assembly shall be previously unused parts only; no implants shall be retested.

7.2 Each pair of polyacetal blocks shall be used for one test only. Metal blocks may be reused if undamaged.

7.3 The test assemblies (that is, intervertebral body fusion device assembly and polyacetal blocks) shall be labeled and shall be maintained according to good laboratory practice. The test assembly can be disassembled to facilitate examination of surface conditions.

7.4 All static tests should have a minimum of five test samples.

7.5 The user of the test method should select the necessary loads to plot a well-defined max load-cycle to failure trend and to establish the maximum run out load. This trend must be comprised of at least six data points. The precision in establishing the value for the maximum run out load should be less than 10 % of the ultimate load or moment for a given test. A regression analysis will be conducted on the load or moment versus number of cycles to failure data.

8. Procedure for Static Tests

8.1 The intervertebral body fusion device assembly is to be inserted between two prepared metal blocks having the appropriate matching geometry of the intervertebral body fusion device assembly (Fig. 7). The intradiscal height, H, shall be constant for all tests for an intervertebral body fusion device assembly of a given size.

8.2 The load, F, and moment, M_z, are to be applied as described in Section 6 of this test method in position control at a rate no greater than 25mm/min or 60°/min (radians/minute) until functional or mechanical failure of the intervertebral body fusion device assembly is obtained.

8.3 Physiological compressive preloads of 100, 300, and 500 N for cervical, thoracic and lumbar intervertebral body fusion device assemblies, respectively, are required for the static torsion test to avoid separation of the blocks during testing. Other loads may be used with adequate justification.

8.4 The load displacement curve shall be recorded. The yield displacement (mm or degrees or radians), stiffness (N/mm or N*mm/degree (radian)), yield load or moment (N or N*mm), ultimate displacement (millimetres or degrees or radians), and ultimate load or moment (N or N*mm) are to be established.

9. Procedure for Dynamic Tests

9.1 An intervertebral body fusion device assembly is to be inserted between two prepared polyacetal blocks having the appropriate matching geometry of the intervertebral body fusion device assembly (Fig. 7). The intradiscal height, H, shall be constant for all tests for an intervertebral body fusion device assembly of a given size.

9.2 Load, F, and moment, M_z, are to be applied as described in Section 6 of this test method in load control. The user of this standard should select the necessary loads to develop a well-defined load-cycle to failure trend comprised of a minimum of six data points. Suggested maximum loads for initial dynamic tests are 25, 50, and 75 % of the ultimate static load. A semi-log fatigue graph of maximum applied load, F, or moment, M_z, versus the number of cycles to failure is to be plotted. The end of the test is defined as functional failure of the construct or attainment of 5 000 000 cycles without functional failure. However, any mechanical failure should be noted at the 5 000 000 cycle point (for example, surface wear, crack initiation, crack propagation, and so forth). The maximum runout load is to be determined. The precision in establishing the maximum runout load should not deviate more

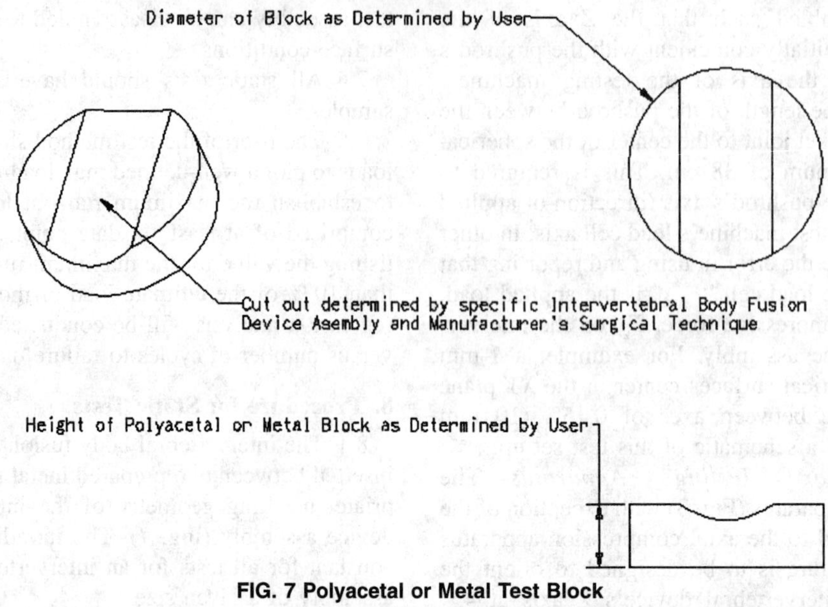

FIG. 7 Polyacetal or Metal Test Block

than 10 % of the static strength of the intervertebral body fusion device assembly.

9.3 An R value of 10 shall be used for the axial compression and compression-shear tests, and an R value of –1 shall be used for the torsional testing.

9.4 The frequency of the dynamic test shall be determined by the user of this test method and recorded (see X1.9).

10. Report

10.1 The report shall specify the intervertebral body fusion device assembly components, the intervertebral body fusion device assembly, the intended spinal location, and the numbers of specimens tested. Any pertinent information about the components such as name, design, manufacturer, material, part number, lot number, and size shall also be reported. All information necessary to reproduce the assembly shall also be included.

10.2 Exact loading configurations for the testing apparatus shall be included. All deviations (with adequate justification) from the recommended test procedures shall be reported, and all relevant testing parameters shall be reported. Rationale for testing configurations not used shall also be reported.

10.3 The report of the static mechanical testing shall include a complete description of all failures (functional and mechanical), modes of failure, and deformation of the intervertebral body fusion device assembly or test apparatus. The static mechanical test report shall include the following:

10.3.1 All load-displacement curves are to be included in an appendix. These curves should illustrate the pertinent static data. All static test data, including the mean and standard deviation will be reported for yield displacement (mm or degrees or radians), yield load or moment (N or N*mm), stiffness (N/mm or N*mm/degree (radian)), ultimate displacement (mm or degrees or radians), and ultimate load or moment (N or N*mm).

10.4 The report on the dynamic testing shall include the following:

10.4.1 Final sample sizes, test frequencies, and semi-log load versus number of cycles to failure are to be listed for each type of fatigue test conducted. The highest load level for the specimen enduring 5 000 000 cycles without functional or mechanical failure should be stated as the maximum runout load or moment. Specimens that have not mechanically or functionally failed before 5 000 000 cycles should be indicated.

10.4.2 All initial and secondary failures, modes of failure, and deformations of components should be reported for the intervertebral body fusion device assembly. Fatigue failures should be described completely with the following information: failure or crack initiation site, propagation zone, and ultimate failure zone. Any wear or loosening of the assembly must be described. In addition, the testing environment should be described. Any other noteworthy observations should be included.

10.4.3 A regression analysis of the load or moment versus number of cycles to failure data should be reported.

11. Precision and Bias

11.1 *Precision*—Data establishing the precision of this test method have not yet been obtained.

11.2 *Bias*—No statement can be made as to bias of this test method since no acceptable reference values are available nor can they be obtained because of the destructive nature of the tests.

12. Keywords

12.1 dynamic test methods; intervertebral body fusion device; spinal implants; static test methods

APPENDIX

(Nonmandatory Information)

X1. STATEMENT OF RATIONALE FOR TEST METHODS

X1.1 Intervertebral body fusion device assemblies are manufactured in a variety of sizes, materials, and shapes with various design features. The purpose of this test method is to allow for a consistent, repeatable comparison of different intervertebral body fusion device assemblies through a comprehensive series of mechanical tests.

X1.2 All of the spinal implants that fall into the category of intervertebral body fusion device assemblies are intended for the purpose of arthrodesis, and therefore, all of the implants will reside in the disc space with varied orientations and methods of fixation to the adjacent vertebral bodies. This test method will allow for comparison of these devices since the methods and loading configuration remains consistent regardless of method of application.

X1.3 The proposed test configurations are based on anatomical dimensions.

X1.4 This standard covers the static and dynamic evaluation of intervertebral body fusion device assemblies. The purpose of an intervertebral body fusion device assembly is to provide short-term stabilization of the spine to facilitate fusion; it is for this relatively short functional life duration that these dynamic tests seek to simulate. This standard does not attempt to address the questions related to long-term performance in the absence of a successful arthrodesis.

X1.5 The influence of saline or other simulated or actual body fluids may have an effect on the performance of the assemblies and therefore should be considered as an adjunct to testing in an ambient environment (dry) as described in this test method. The individual investigator may wish to investigate different environmental testing agents to simulate body fluid for subsequent testing such as saline or other lubricants.

X1.6 If the devices are known to be temperature and environment dependent, testing should be conducted in physiologic solution. Devices that require physiologic solution for testing should be tested in the same type solution for comparison purposes.

X1.7 Polyacetal blocks are used to simulate the vertebral bodies in dynamic testing to avoid introducing wear associated variables to the test. However, metallic blocks are used for the static testing of intervertebral body fusion device assemblies so that the stiffness measurements reflect that of the intervertebral device itself.

X1.8 Since the main purpose of an intervertebral body fusion device assembly is fusion, the maximum runout load or moment is defined from a clinical standpoint. Since fusion should occur well within one year of implantation, the device should withstand normal intervertebral spinal loading until fusion occurs. If one uses a factor of safety of 2.5, the intervertebral fusion device assembly should withstand 2.5 years of loading, which corresponds to 5 million cycles[4].

X1.9 Frequencies over 10 Hz may result in heating and subsequent melting of the test blocks. Since this phenomenon is device and environment specific, the user of this test method is left to discern an appropriate cyclic frequency.

X1.10 The purpose of this test method is to allow for the comparison of different intervertebral body fusion device assemblies and does not attempt to dictate performance standards for these types of devices since in vivo spinal loading is very complex, highly variable, and not yet fully understood.

[4] Hedman, T.P., Kostuick, J.P., Fernie, G.R., Hellier, W.G., "Design of an Intervertebral Disc Prosthesis," *Spine*, 16: 65, 1991, pp. S 256-260.

Designation: F 2079 – 01

Standard Test Method for Measuring Recoil of Balloon-Expandable Stents[1]

This standard is issued under the fixed designation F 2079; the number immediately following the designation indicates the year of original adoption or, in the case of revision, the year of last revision. A number in parentheses indicates the year of last reapproval. A superscript epsilon (ε) indicates an editorial change since the last revision or reapproval.

1. Scope

1.1 The purpose of this test is to quantify the percentage by which the diameter of a stent decreases from its expanded diameter while still on the delivery balloon to its relaxed diameter after deflating the balloon. This test is appropriate for stents manufactured from a material that is plastically deformed when the stent's diameter is increased from its predeployed size to its postdeployed size by mechanical means. This test may be performed in air at room temperature unless there is a known temperature dependence of the material, in which case, the temperature at which the test is conducted shall be stated in the report.

1.2 *This standard does not purport to address all of the safety concerns, if any, associated with its use. It is the responsibility of the user of this standard to establish appropriate safety and health practices and determine the applicability of regulatory limitations prior to use.*

2. Terminology

2.1 *Definitions:*

2.1.1 *labeled diameter, n*—desired final stent (inner/outer) diameter after deflation of the delivery balloon.

2.1.2 *stent recoil, n*—the amount, expressed as a percentage, by which the diameter of a stent changes from the expanded diameter measured with the stent on the inflated delivery balloon to the final value measured after deflating the balloon.

3. Summary of Test Method

3.1 The delivery balloon bearing a sample device representative of product that will be marketed either premounted, or mounted on the delivery balloon at the time of use, is inflated to expand the stent to slightly greater than its labeled diameter. The outer diameter of the stent is measured in a minimum of two approximately orthogonal projections while the stent is still on the inflated delivery balloon. The balloon is deflated and the outer diameter of the stent is remeasured in the same projections at approximately the same location.

4. Significance and Use

4.1 Minimal stent recoil is a desirable feature of a stent because it minimizes the maximum diameter to which a stent must be expanded to achieve its final relaxed diameter. A stent having a high recoil must be expanded to a greater diameter to achieve its final relaxed diameter than a stent having low recoil. Practically, excessive expansion of the vessel into which the stent is to be implanted may cause tissue damage resulting in a poor immediate result or poor long-term outcome. Stent recoil is affected by intrinsic properties of the material used to construct the stent and the specific geometric design of the stent; therefore, measuring stent recoil is an essential part of evaluating the design.

5. Apparatus

5.1 A means to inflate with noncompressible fluid, typically water, the delivery balloon on which the stent is mounted. The means used must be capable of achieving the pressure required to maintain the expanded diameter of the stent until it can be measured and may include a device to monitor pressure.

5.2 A means to measure the outer diameter of the stent without deforming the stent. Typically, a calibrated optical system, which does not require contact with the stent, is used. The resolution of the measurement system shall be 0.01 mm or better. The accuracy of the system shall be 2 % of reading or better.

6. Sampling, Test Specimens, and Test Units

6.1 Unless otherwise justified, all samples selected for testing should be taken from fully processed, clinical quality product. It is not required that these devices undergo terminal sterilization. Cosmetic rejects or other nonclinical samples may be used if the cause for rejection has been shown not to affect stent recoil.

6.2 The number of specimens tested for each unique stent geometry should be sufficient to meet sampling requirements for desired specification limits. If a single stent geometry is intended to be used for more than one labeled diameter, recoil shall be evaluated for test specimens expanded to the smallest and largest diameters intended for that geometry.

6.3 Most stents are comprised of a repetitious continuous pattern or of repeating subunits. If stents are made longer by additional repetition of the basic geometric pattern or by adding identical subunits, then recoil need be measured on only a single length of each diameter stent. If, however, dimensions of the substructure of the repeating pattern or of the subunits is altered to change the length, then recoil must be measured for each unique geometry.

[1] This test method is under the jurisdiction of ASTM Committee F04 on Medical and Surgical Materials and Devicesand is the direct responsibility of Subcommittee F04.30on Cardiovascular Standards.

Current edition approved Jan. 10, 2001. Published March 2001.

7. Procedure

7.1 Corresponding paired outer diameter measurements, (that is, $Diameter_{inflated}$ and $Diameter_{final}$) shall be obtained with the stent in approximately the same rotational position with respect to the measurement system.

7.2 The number of locations along the length of the stent at which recoil is measured should be determined by initial assessment of the stent geometry. For example, if the stent is specifically designed to recoil less at the ends than in the middle, recoil should be measured at both locations.

7.3 Pressurize the balloon to expand the stent to slightly greater than its labeled diameter.

7.4 Measure the outer diameter of the stent in a minimum of two approximately orthogonal projections.

7.5 Deflate the balloon.

7.6 Measure the outer diameter of the stent at the same location(s) and in the same rotational positions with respect to the measurement system as in 7.4. These measurements should be taken no sooner than 10 s after deflating the balloon.

8. Calculation

8.1 Calculate the stent recoil for the location(s) measured in 7.4 for each stent using the following equation:

$$\text{Stent Recoil (\%)} = \left(1 - \left(\frac{Diameter_{final}}{Diameter_{inflated}}\right)\right) * 100 \tag{1}$$

where:

$Diameter_{inflated}$ = outer diameter of stent while on inflated delivery balloon and

$Diameter_{final}$ = outer diameter of stent after deflating delivery balloon.

8.2 Calculate the average and standard deviation of stent recoil for each location at which recoil is measured.

9. Report

9.1 Report the following information for each labeled diameter of each unique stent geometry:

9.1.1 Labeled stent diameter.

9.1.2 Labeled stent length.

9.1.3 Number of samples measured.

9.1.4 $Diameter_{\text{inflated}}$ (mean ± standard deviation).

9.1.5 $Diameter_{\text{final}}$ (mean ± standard deviation).

9.1.6 Stent recoil average (mean ± standard deviation) for each location measured.

9.1.7 Temperature at which test is performed.

10. Precision and Bias

10.1 *Precision*—The precision of this test method has not yet been established. An interlaboratory comparison to determine the precision is being planned.

10.2 *Bias*—No information can be presented on the bias of this test method because no material having an acceptable reference value is available.

11. Keywords

11.1 recoil; stent

APPENDIX

(Nonmandatory Information)

X1. RATIONALE

X1.1 Balloon-expandable stents typically are deployed for permanent implant by plastically deforming the material of construction. Upon release of the balloon pressure, the diameter will decrease, the exact amount of which depends on the material used to construct the stent and the specific design of the stent. For optimal clinical results, it is critical that the final deployed diameter be appropriate for the exact location of deployment. Moreover, a stent with excessive recoil must be inflated to a larger diameter to achieve the desired final diameter. This larger required initial inflation diameter may cause more damage to the vessel than would the lower inflation diameter required for a stent with a lower recoil. The implanting physician must have guidance as to how much any given stent design will recoil so that the balloon may be inflated to the expanded diameter required to achieve the desired final diameter. This test method provides a standardized procedure to determine the recoil characteristics of stents so that consistent labeling can be written. Note that this test method measures the intrinsic recoil of the stent and may not predict how the stent will perform when implanted in a vessel in which stent recoil, stent stiffness, and vessel stiffness interact to determine the final diameter.

Standard Guide for Characterization and Presentation of the Dimensional Attributes of Vascular Stents[1]

1. Scope

1.1 This guide covers the identification of and recommended measurement methods for those dimensional attributes of vascular stents that are deemed relevant to successful clinical performance. The delivery system packaged with and labeled specifically for use during the placement of the stent is also included within the scope of this guide.

1.2 This guide addresses only the *dimensional* characteristics of stents. Material property and stent functional characteristics are not addressed herein. All dimensional characteristics described in this guide refer to in-vitro ("bench-top") characterization. Because of variable patient factors, for example, vessel compliance, the actual in-vivo characteristics may be slightly different.

1.3 This guide includes recommendations generally applicable to balloon-expandable and self-expanding stents fabricated from metals and metal alloys. It does not specifically address any attributes unique to coated stents or polymeric or biodegradable stents, although the application of this guide to those products is not precluded.

1.4 While they are not specifically included within the scope of this guide, stents indicated for placement in nonvascular locations, such as the esophagus or bile duct, also might be characterized by the methods contained herein. Likewise, this guide does not include recommendations for endovascular grafts ("stent-grafts") or other conduit devices commonly used to treat aneurysmal disease or peripheral vessel trauma or to provide vascular access, although some information included herein may be applicable to those devices.

1.5 This guide does not include recommendations for balloon catheters sold as stand-alone angioplasty catheters, even though some of those catheters may be used for the delivery of unmounted stents supplied without a delivery system. Requirements for angioplasty catheters are contained in standards ISO 10555-1 and ISO 10555-4.

1.6 The units of measurements used throughout this guide reflect the hybrid system in common clinical use in the United States as of the time of the original approval of this guide. Since a primary purpose of this guide is to promote uniformity of labeling to facilitate the selection of devices by clinical users, the units most preferred by users were selected for this guide. Where those units are not SI units, or derivatives thereof, SI units are provided in parentheses.

2. Referenced Documents

2.1 *ISO Standards:*

ISO 10555-1, Sterile, Single-Use Intravascular Catheters, General Requirements[2]

ISO 10555-4, Sterile, Single-Use Intravascular Catheters—Balloon Dilation Catheters[2]

3. Terminology

3.1 *Definitions of Terms Specific to This Standard:*

3.1.1 *balloon-expandable stent, n*—a stent that is expanded at the treatment site by a balloon catheter. The stent is altered permanently by the balloon expansion such that the stent remains expanded after deflation of the balloon.

3.1.2 *bridge, n*—a connecting element between the radial support aspects of a stent. A bridge may have unique design features, as compared to a strut, to enhance longitudinal flexibility and minimize shortening.

3.1.3 *crimp, v*—to secure the stent on the delivery system by compressing the stent onto the balloon. Stents sold unmounted must be crimped manually by the clinical staff before use.

3.1.4 *crossing profile, n*—a linear measure of the maximum breadth of the stent/delivery system over the distal-most region of the delivery system.

3.1.5 *delivery system, n*—a system that is used to deliver and deploy a stent at the target site. A delivery system may be similar to a balloon dilatation catheter; a delivery system for a self-expanding stent might not have a balloon.

3.1.6 *diameter, n*—refers to the outside diameter of the stent unless otherwise noted.

3.1.7 *percent metal area, n*—that percentage of the projected cylindrical side surface area (π times outside diameter times length at labeled diameter) that is covered by stent material, when the stent is expanded to its labeled diameter.

3.1.8 *premounted stent, n*—a stent supplied by a manufacturer already mounted on a delivery system.

3.1.9 *self-expanding stent, n*—a stent that expands without

[1] This guide is under the jurisdiction of ASTM Committee F04 on Medical and Surgical Materials and Devicesand is the direct responsibility of Subcommittee F04.30on Cardiovascular Devices.

Current edition approved Jan. 10, 2001. Published April 2001.

[2] Available from American National Standards Institute, 11 W. 42nd St., 13th Floor, New York, NY 10036.

extrinsic force or pressure, to a size and shape close to the desired final size and shape, when released from the delivery system. The self-expanding nature of some stents is a design feature resulting from the materials of construction or the structural geometry, or both.

3.1.10 *sheath, n*—a movable cover that constrains a self-expanding stent on the delivery system until its desired release or protects a balloon-expandable stent during delivery before deployment.

3.1.11 *shortening/lengthening, n*—the percentage change in length between the undeployed mounted condition and the expanded labeled-diameter condition.

3.1.12 *stent, vascular, n*—a synthetic tubular structure that is permanently implanted in the native or grafted vasculature and that is intended to provide mechanical radial support to enhance vessel patency. For the purposes of this guide, a stent is metallic and not covered by synthetic textile or tissue graft material.

3.1.13 *strut, n*—the smallest individual element of the radial support aspect of a stent that has a solid cross section in both the radial and circumferential directions.

3.1.14 *unmounted stent, n*—a stent that is not crimped on a delivery system as supplied by the manufacturer. Before use, the clinical staff must manually crimp unmounted stents onto a delivery device.

4. Significance and Use

4.1 Vascular stents are intended for permanent implant in the human vasculature (native or graft) for the purposes of maintaining vessel patency. The dimensional attributes of vascular stents are critical parameters that aid clinicians in the selection of devices for individual patients. This guide contains a listing of those attributes that are directly related to the clinical utility and performance of these devices, along with recommendations for consistent methods of measuring these attributes and presenting the information for use in clinical decision making. This guide can be used by the manufacturers and researchers of stents to provide consistency of measurement and labeling of these dimensional characteristics. It may have use in the regulation of these devices by appropriate authorities.

4.2 The dimensional attributes included in this guide are those that are deemed related to or possibly predictive of successful clinical performance of the stent, based on prior clinical experience; however, because of the myriad patient and medical factors that influence the clinical outcome of any individual treatment, conformance of a stent and delivery system with the recommendations in this guide should not be interpreted as a guarantee of clinical success in any individual patient or group of patients.

5. Classification

5.1 Stents may be classified by the following characteristics, as defined in Section 3.

5.1.1 *Mounting*—Premounted or unmounted.

5.1.2 *Expansion*—Balloon expandable or self-expanding.

6. Test Devices and General Procedures

6.1 Unless otherwise justified, all samples selected for testing or measuring the attributes described in this guide should be taken from finished, clinical-quality product. Cosmetic rejects or other nonclinical samples may be used if the cause for rejection is not related to the attribute being assessed. Sterilization can be omitted if it can be demonstrated that sterilization has no affect on the attribute being assessed.

6.2 When specimen preparation (for example, manual crimping onto a delivery system, balloon expansion), is required before testing, this should be done in accordance with the Instructions for Use (IFU).

6.3 The preconditioning and test environments must be appropriately selected for each design and attribute. Temperature and fluid immersion may have a significant effect on some attributes but a negligible affect on others. For example, fluid sorption may swell catheters and affect the measurement of crossing profile. Temperature may affect the final deployed diameter for stents made from shape memory materials. For measurements for which deployment, or measurement, or both, is to be made in a controlled environment, the stent or delivery system, or both, should be immersed in a water bath maintained at 37 ± 2°C and allowed to equilibrate.

6.4 The number of specimens evaluated for each diameter for each stent design should be sufficient to meet the sampling requirements for the desired labeling. In general, a minimum of ten test devices is recommended. If a single stent design is intended to be deployed over a broad range of diameters by use on different size delivery systems, the dimensional attributes should be evaluated for each stent/delivery system combination.

7. Dimensions and Measurement Methods

7.1 *Deployed Diameter*—Unless otherwise specified, all deployed diameters refer to the outside diameter, reported in millimetres to the nearest 0.1 mm, after balloon deflation (for balloon-expandable stents).

7.1.1 *Measurement*—The outside diameter of deployed stents should be measured by noncontacting instruments (profile projection, laser micrometer, and so forth) with a resolution of 0.05 mm or better.

7.1.2 *Labeled Diameter*—The labeled diameter is that typically used to identify the nominal deployed size of a particular device, for example, 3 mm, 3.5 mm, and must be clearly identified as inside or outside diameter (ID or OD).

7.1.3 *Stent System Compliance*—For balloon-expandable stents, a table or graph of inflation pressure versus expanded diameter should be developed and included in the labeling. A minimum of ten devices should be measured at each labeled inflation pressure. The expanded stent outside diameter at each inflation pressure, reported to the nearest 0.1 mm, should be the mean of all measurements taken on all stents at that pressure. The inflation pressure should be expressed in atmospheres. This attribute does not apply to self-expanding stents.

7.1.4 *Uniformity of Expansion*—The uniformity of expansion refers to the difference between the largest and smallest diameter measurement on a single stent deployed to its labeled diameter. Uniformity of expansion is not intended to characterize deliberate deviations from cylindricity, such as tapered construction, end flares, antimigration barbs, and so forth. Measurements for the uniformity of expansion should be taken at three axial locations (midlength and close to each end) at each of two circumferential orientations at about 90° separation. The uniformity of expansion reflects both the deviation from circularity of the stent cross section and unintended differences in diameter along the stent length.

7.2 *Stent Length*:

7.2.1 *Measurement*—The length of mounted or expanded stents should be measured by noncontacting instruments (profile projection, laser micrometer, and so forth) with a resolution of 0.1 mm or better. Measurements should be taken on each stent in the mounted state and at the labeled diameter. Lengths should reflect measurements on a minimum of ten devices and should be reported to the nearest 1 mm.

7.2.2 *Labeled Expanded Length*—The labeled expanded length is that typically used to identify the nominal size of a particular device, for example, 20 mm.

7.2.3 *Mounted (Undeployed) Length*—This attribute has no significance in and of itself. It provides a baseline for the determination of shortening. Direct measurement of the mounted length may not be possible for sheathed systems. Other appropriate methods may be used.

7.2.4 *Shortening/Lengthening*—Refers to the percentage change in length between the undeployed mounted condition and the expanded labeled-diameter condition. Shortening/lengthening should be reported as a percentage of the mounted (undeployed) length to the nearest 1 %.

7.3 *Crossing Profile*:

7.3.1 *Measurement*—With the stent premounted or hand-crimped on the delivery system in accordance with the instructions for use, and the sheath (if any) in place, measure the maximum diameter over the length from the proximal end of the mounted stent to the distal tip of the delivery system. A minimum of ten test articles should be measured. The measurement instrument should be either noncontacting (optical profilometer, laser micrometer, and so forth) or a ring/hole gage, and should have a resolution of 0.001 in. (0.025 mm) or better. The crossing profile should be reported as the mean measurement result to the nearest 0.001 in. (0.025 mm).

7.4 *Strut and Bridge Thickness*:

7.4.1 *Measurement*—Strut and bridge thickness of the expanded stent may be measured by subtraction of measured inside and outside diameters, by direct measurement with specialized instrumentation, by scanning electron microscopy, by profile projection, or destructively by cutting, or flattening, or both, a stent for access by standard micrometers. Since polishing or other manufacturing processes may change strut and bridge thickness from that of raw material, measurements from other-than-finished product should be used judiciously. Strut and bridge thickness should be measured at the stent midlength and near each end, at two circumferential locations at each axial location. If strut thickness and bridge thicknesses are systematically different by design, they should be measured and reported separately. Strut and bridge thickness should be reported in inches to the nearest 0.0005 in. (0.013 mm).

7.5 *Percent Metal Area*:

7.5.1 *Measurement*—The reference area is the full cylindrical side surface area for the stent expanded to the labeled diameter (π • diameter • length at labeled diameter). The metal area may be estimated by stereology or image analysis of suitably magnified photographs, by calculation based on stent mass, material density, and strut thickness, by CAD software, or by other suitable means. The metal area may be determined on unexpanded stents and assumed not to change significantly during expansion. The percent metal area is the ratio of the metal area to the reference area and should be reported as a percentage to the nearest 1 %.

7.6 *Delivery System Dimensions*—The requirements for delivery system dimensions are detailed in ISO 10555, Parts 1 and 4. These include the following:

7.6.1 The effective length of the catheter.

7.6.2 The catheter outside diameter.

7.6.3 The maximum guidewire diameter (if applicable).

7.6.4 The effective length of the balloon (if applicable).

8. Keywords

8.1 angioplasty; coronary artery; dimensional characteristics; dimensions; vascular stent

APPENDIX

(Nonmandatory Information)

X1. RATIONALE

X1.1 This guide contains a listing of and methods for characterizing those dimensional attributes deemed necessary or prudent to demonstrate successful performance of vascular stents in humans. As of the time of adoption of this guide, there is adequate clinical evidence to support that the dimensional characteristics addressed herein are at least somewhat predictive of clinical utility and success in most patients.

X1.2 *Expanded Diameter (Nominal and Uniformity)*—It is desirable to achieve the maximum vessel lumen diameter with a minimum of injury to the vessel. Too small a minimum lumen diameter (MLD) has been shown to correlate with a higher restenosis rate, while too large an MLD may be accompanied with increased vessel injury, which also may result in increased restenosis. Proper sizing of the stent in vivo requires a thorough knowledge of the expansion characteristics of the stent when used in accordance with the Instructions for Use (IFU), including the delivery system pressure required to achieve the desired stent diameter (for balloon-expandable stents).

X1.3 *Expanded Length (Nominal, Lengthening/Shortening)*—Accurately placing the expanded stent in the lesion minimizes restenosis and dissections. It is desirable to use a stent that is no longer than necessary because longer stents might compromise side branches and may relate to a higher incidence of restenosis. Shortening of the stent during expansion makes placement of the stent more difficult and sometimes forces the clinician to choose a stent that is longer than desirable to ensure full lesion coverage. Devices deemed clinically useful as of the time of adoption of this guide have reported length changes (shortening) during expansion in the range 0 to 20 %.[3]

X1.4 *Crossing Profile*—The ability of a mounted stent to be delivered across a lesion depends in part on the diameter of the mounted stent relative to the size of the lumen. A smaller crossing profile is beneficial for crossing tight lesions, especially for direct stenting. Devices deemed clinically useful as of the time of adoption of this guide had crossing profiles in the range <1.0 to 2.0 mm.

NOTE X1.1—Crossing profile is not the same as compatibility with a guiding catheter.

X1.5 *Strut and Bridge Thicknesses*—Strut and bridge thicknesses indirectly affect several other stent attributes and are important primarily because of this indirect effect. Knowledge of strut and bridge thickness allows one to estimate the stent internal diameter from the outside diameter, and vice versa. Strut thickness is one of several factors that influence radial strength, radiopacity, flexibility, and crossing profile. It directly influences the amount of the lumen diameter occupied by the stent. Bridge thickness is one of several factors that may influence predeployment flexibility and postdeployment conformability. Devices deemed clinically useful[3] as of the time of adoption of this guide had strut thicknesses in the range 0.025 to 0.177 mm.

X1.6 *Percent Metal Area*—The percent metal area is an indicator of the overall amount of vessel wall area covered by metal. This is important in evaluating the response of the body to a foreign material. This parameter also has been used as a crude measure of vessel wall coverage related to tissue prolapse; however, tissue prolapse is also strongly dependent on the distribution of metal rather than simply the gross percentage area. Devices deemed clinically useful as of the time of adoption of this guide have percent metal area values in the range 7 to 20 %.

X1.7 *Delivery System Dimensions*—The delivery system dimensions that are clinically important are the same as those for balloon angioplasty catheters. These dimensions help assure the suitability of a particular device for a specific application and the dimensional compatibility of mating devices.

[3] Serruys, Patrick, W., and Kutryk, Michael, J. B., Eds., *Handbook of Coronary Stents, Second Edition*, Martin Dunitz Ltd., London, 1998.

Designation: F 2082 – 01

Standard Test Method for Determination of Transformation Temperature of Nickel-Titanium Shape Memory Alloys by Bend and Free Recovery[1]

This standard is issued under the fixed designation F 2082; the number immediately following the designation indicates the year of original adoption or, in the case of revision, the year of last revision. A number in parentheses indicates the year of last reapproval. A superscript epsilon (ϵ) indicates an editorial change since the last revision or reapproval.

1. Scope

1.1 This test method describes a procedure for determining the martensite-to-austenite transformation temperatures of nickel titanium alloys by measuring the deformation recovered during the thermal transformation.

1.2 The values in SI units are to be regarded as the standard. The values given in inch-pound units are provided for information only.

1.3 *This standard does not purport to address all of the safety concerns, if any, associated with its use. It is the responsibility of the user of this standard to establish appropriate safety and health practices and determine the applicability of regulatory limitations prior to use.*

2. Referenced Documents

2.1 *ASTM Standards:*

E 220 Test Method for Calibration of Thermocouples by Comparison Techniques[2]

F 2005 Terminology for Nickel-Titanium Shape Memory Alloys[3]

3. Terminology

3.1 *Definitions*—Specific technical terms used in this test method are found in Terminology F 2005.

3.2 *Abbreviations:*

3.2.1 *LVDT*—linear variable differential transducer.

3.2.2 *RVDT*—rotary variable differential transducer.

4. Summary of Test Method

4.1 This test method involves cooling a test specimen to its nominally fully martensitic phase, deforming the specimen, and heating the specimen to its fully austenitic phase. During heating, the motion of the specimen is measured and plotted versus the specimen temperature. For a two-stage transformation, the R'_s, R'_f, A_s, and A_f, as defined in Terminology F 2005, are determined. For a single-stage transformation, the A_s and A_f are determined.

5. Significance and Use

5.1 This test method provides a rapid, economical method for determination of transformation temperatures.

5.2 Measurement of the specimen motion closely parallels many shape memory applications and provides a result that is applicable to the function of the material.

5.3 This test method uses wire, tube, or strip samples; thus, it is able to provide an assessment of the product in its semifinished form.

5.4 This test method may be used on annealed samples to determine the transformation temperatures and assure the alloy formulation, since chemical analysis is not precise enough to determine adequately the nickel-to-titanium ratio of shape memory alloys.

5.5 Transformation temperatures derived from this test method may differ from those derived from other methods as a result of effects of strain and load on the transformation temperature.

5.6 The test method is applicable to shape memory alloys with A_f temperatures in the range of approximately –25 to +90°C.

6. Apparatus

6.1 *LVDT*, with range greater than half the mandrel diameter (see 9.2), with power supply, mounted in an appropriate fixture with counterbalanced probe (see Fig. 1); or RVDT with range greater than 45°, with power supply, mounted in an appropriate fixture (see Fig. 2).

6.2 *Thermocouple and Indicator*, with resolution of 0.1°C (0.2°F) or better.

6.3 *XY Chart Recorder*, or equivalent manual or automated data acquisition system.

6.4 *Hot Plate and Stirrer.*

6.5 *Denatured Alcohol Bath*, or water bath.

6.6 *Mandrel*, for deforming the sample in the martensitic state.

6.7 *Fixture*, for holding the sample during recovery.

6.8 *Probe or Needle*, for contacting and moving with the sample during recovery.

6.9 *Liquid Nitrogen*, or dry ice.

7. Sampling

7.1 Test specimen can be a wire, tube, or strip with diameter

[1] This test method is under the jurisdiction of ASTM Committee F04 on Medical and Surgical Materials and Devices and is the direct responsibility of Subcommittee F04.15 on Material Test Methods.

Current edition approved Jan. 10, 2001. Published April 2001.

[2] *Annual Book of ASTM Standards*, Vol 14.03.

[3] *Annual Book of ASTM Standards*, Vol 13.01.

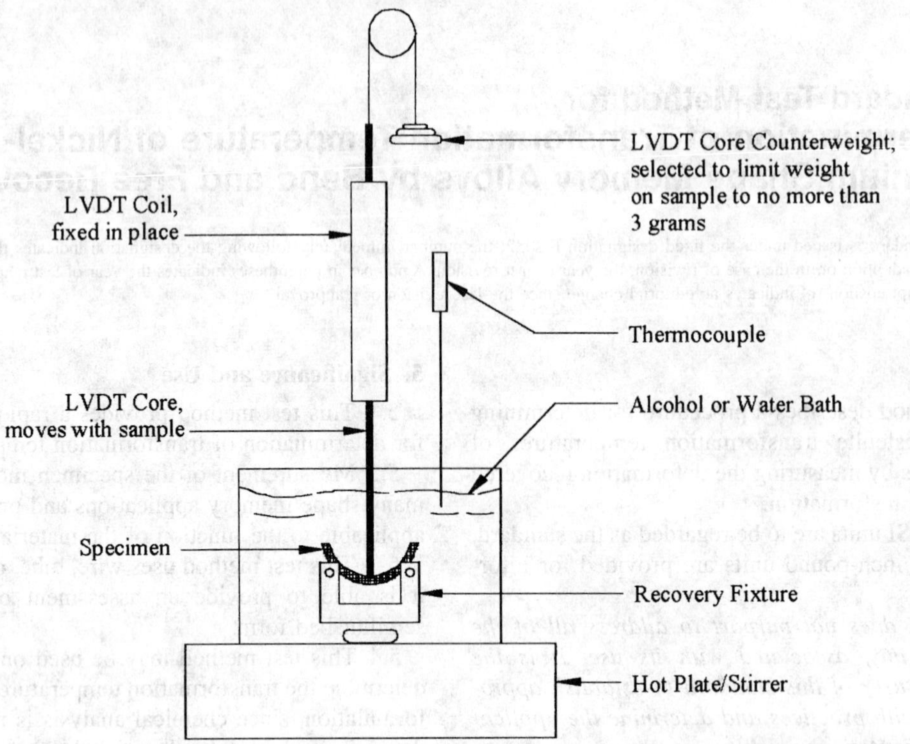

FIG. 1 Schematic Showing Side View of Test Apparatus Using a Vertically Mounted and Counterbalanced LVDT (LVDT Power Supply, Thermocouple Indicator, and Data Acquisition System Are Not Shown)

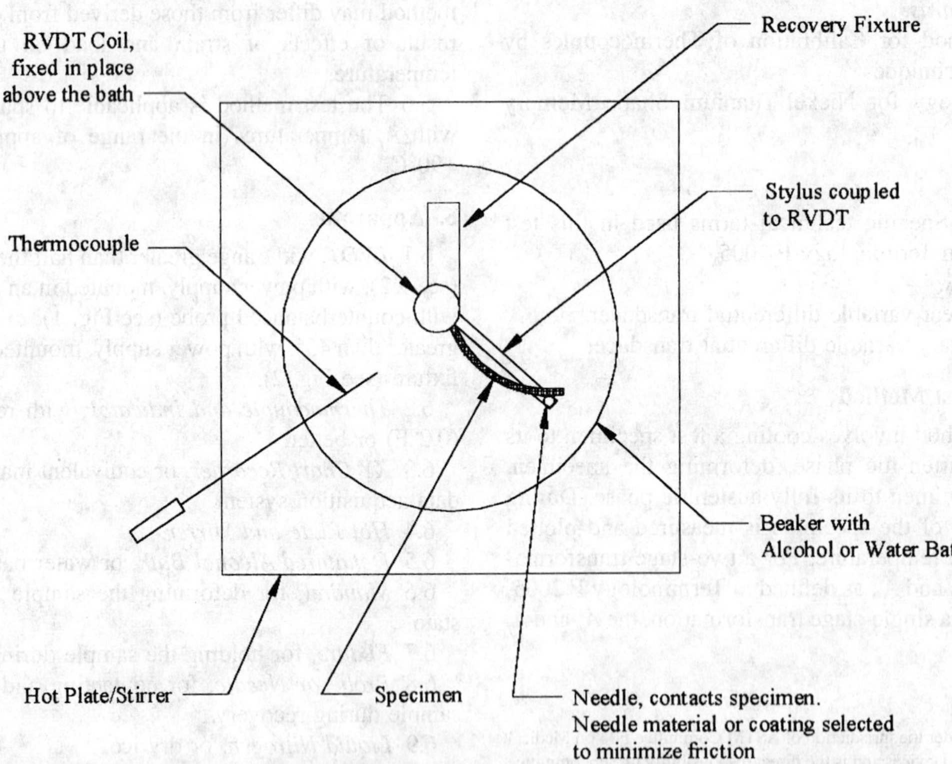

FIG. 2 Schematic Showing Top View of Test Apparatus Using an RVDT (RVDT Power Supply, Thermocouple Indicator, and Data Acquisition System Are Not Shown)

or thickness in the range of 0.3 to 3.0 mm (0.012 to 0.12 in.).

7.2 Specimens may be tested in the semifinished (heat-treated) or annealed condition. Anneal is defined in Terminology F 2005.

8. Calibration

8.1 The thermocouple and indicator shall be kept in a calibrated condition, traceable to the National Institute for

Standards and Technology.

8.2 The thermocouple shall be calibrated using Test Method E 220.

9. LVDT Procedure

9.1 For alloys that are superelastic at room temperature, cool the alcohol bath to –40°C (–40°F) or lower using liquid nitrogen or dry ice. For alloys that are martensitic at room temperature, cool the water bath to 10°C (50°F) or lower.

9.2 Select a mandrel according to the sample diameter or thickness to give an outer fiber strain of 2 to 4 %. For these strains, mandrel diameter shall be between 24 and 49 times specimen diameter or thickness.

9.3 Cut a test specimen long enough to wrap 180° around the mandrel.

9.4 Place the recovery fixture and the mandrel, along with the test specimen, in the bath and wait a minimum of 2 min for the fixtures to equilibrate to the bath temperature.

9.5 Deform the specimen in the bath by wrapping it 180° around the mandrel.

9.6 Remove the mandrel from the bath.

9.7 Place the deformed specimen on the recovery fixture. For best results, the recovery fixture should support the deformed specimen on two pins spaced at a distance equal to 80 to 95 % of the diameter of the mandrel.

9.8 Set the device to measure the motion of the sample. Lower the LVDT core onto the specimen as shown in Fig. 3. The weight of the LVDT core must be counterbalanced such that the weight on the specimen is no more than 3 g.

9.9 Place the thermocouple in the bath as close to the specimen as is practical.

9.10 Set the *XY* chart or data acquisition system to record the temperature on the *X* axis and sample motion on the *Y* axis.

9.11 Stir and heat the bath on the hot plate to a temperature above the A_f. Limit the heating rate to no more than 4°C/min during the recovery.

9.12 Stop the test once the temperature is at least 10°C above the A_f, as determined by noting that the sample is straight and the displacement versus temperature curve has flattened. Turn off the hot plate and stop recording.

10. RVDT Procedure

10.1 For alloys that are superelastic at room temperature, cool the alcohol bath to –40°C (–40°F) or lower using liquid nitrogen or dry ice. For alloys that are martensitic at room temperature, cool the water bath to 10°C (50°F) or lower.

10.2 Select a mandrel according to the sample diameter or thickness to give a strain of 2 to 4 %. For these strains, mandrel diameter shall be between 24 and 49 times specimen diameter or thickness.

10.3 Cut a test specimen long enough to wrap 90° around the mandrel, plus a tail for clamping.

10.4 Place the recovery fixture and the mandrel, along with the test specimen, in the bath and wait a minimum of 2 min for the fixtures to equilibrate to the bath temperature.

10.5 Clamp the specimen in the recovery fixture. The fixture shall hold the sample in the horizontal plane.

10.6 Deform the specimen in the bath by wrapping it 90° around the mandrel.

10.7 Remove the mandrel from the bath. Alternately, for the RVDT method, the mandrel can be attached to the recovery fixture and left in the bath. In this case, the thermal mass of the mandrel and fixture must be such that the temperature of the fixture and the bath is uniform throughout the test.

10.8 Set the device to measure the motion of the sample. Make sure the needle is in contact with the test specimen (Fig. 4). To minimize friction effects, the needle shall be encased in a PTFE sheath, or the needle shall be constructed from or coated with an equivalent material.

10.9 Place the thermocouple in the bath as close to the specimen as is practical.

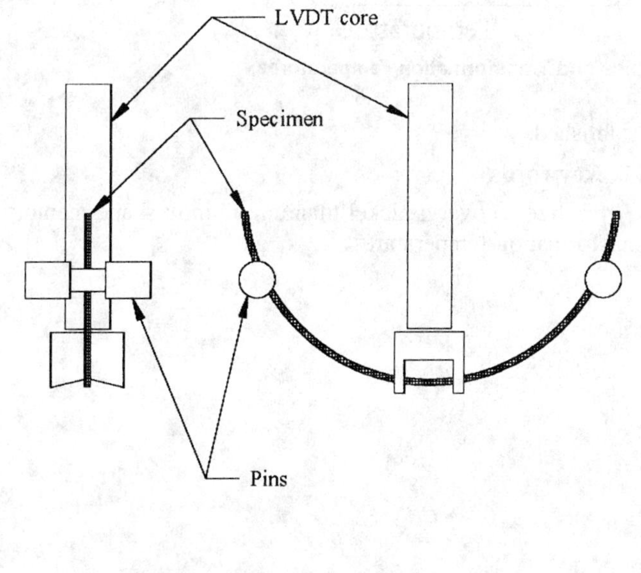

FIG. 3 Placement of LVDT Core on Deformed Specimen, Which Is Resting on Recovery Fixture Pins

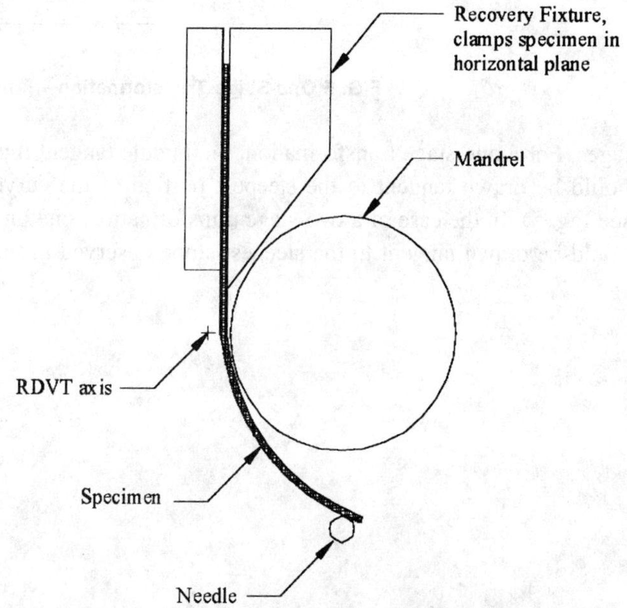

FIG. 4 Placement of Needle on Deformed Specimen, Which Is Clamped to the Recovery Fixture. Top View Shown with Stylus and RVDT Removed. Note the Recommended RVDT Axis Location Is Offset from the Mandrel by the Radius of the Needle

10.10 Set the *XY* chart or data acquisition system to record the temperature on the *X* axis and sample motion on the *Y* axis.

10.11 Stir and heat the bath on the hot plate to a temperature above the A_f. Limit the heating rate to no more than 4°C/min during the recovery.

10.12 Stop the test once the temperature is at least 10°C above the A_f, as determined by noting that the sample is straight and the displacement versus temperature curve has flattened. Turn off the hot plate and stop recording.

11. Determination of Transformation Temperature

11.1 Determine the transformation temperatures according to Fig. 5 or Fig. 6. The transformation may occur in one or two stages. For a one-stage transformation, the middle tangent line should be drawn tangent to the steepest portion of the curve (see Fig. 5). In the case of a two-stage transformation, one line should be drawn tangent to the steepest slope observed in the first stage of the transformation, and a second line should be drawn tangent to the steepest slope in the second stage of the transformation (see Fig. 6).

12. Report

12.1 The report shall include the following information:

12.1.1 Complete identification of the material tested including specification, lot number, and heat treatment.

12.1.2 Results of the transformation measurements, reported to the nearest 1°C.

13. Precision and Bias

13.1 The precision and bias of this test method is to be established.

14. Keywords

14.1 free recovery; nickel titanium; nitinol; shape memory; transformation temperature

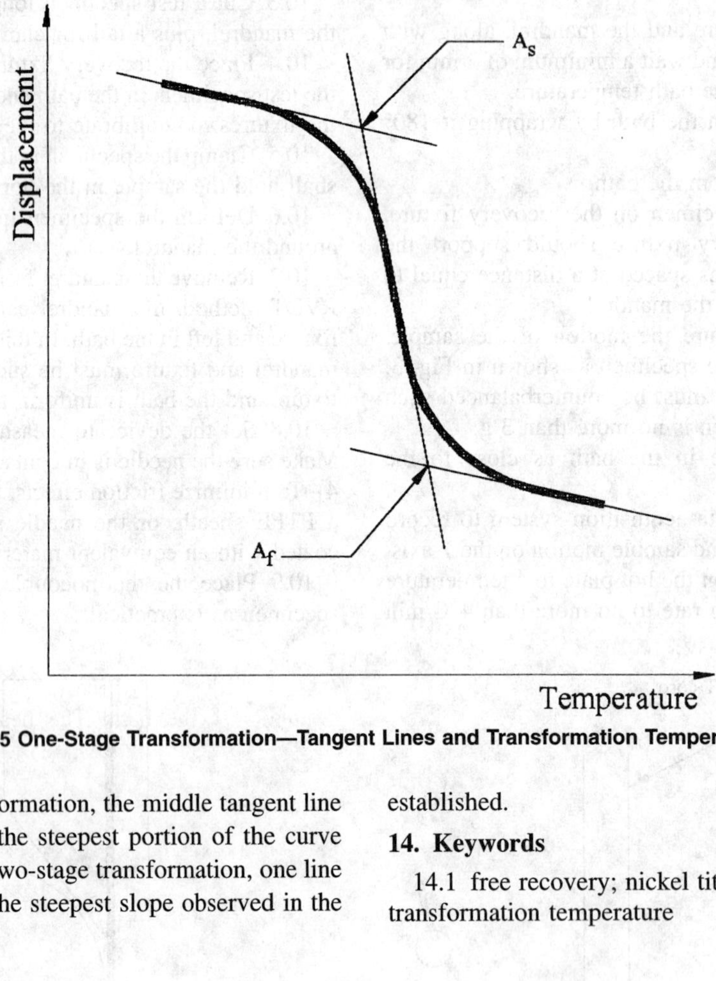

FIG. 5 One-Stage Transformation—Tangent Lines and Transformation Temperatures

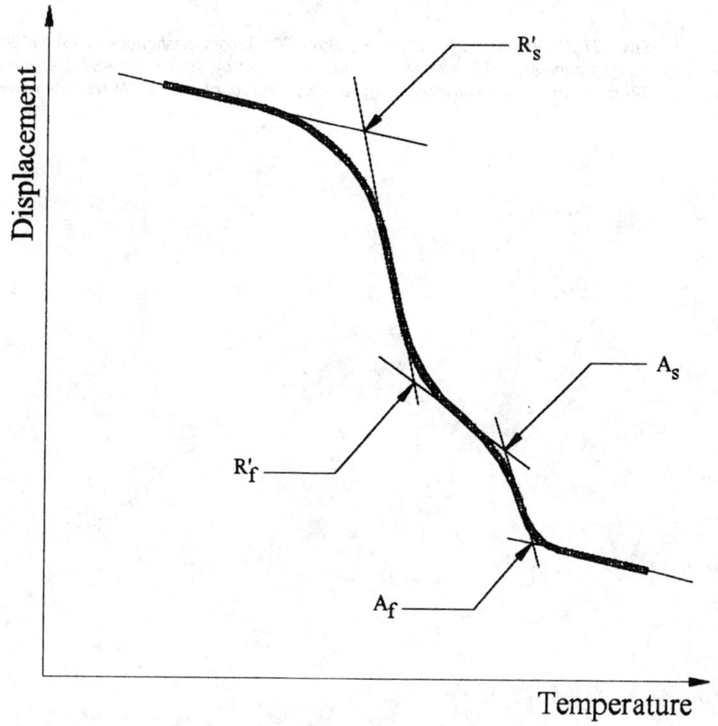

FIG. 6 Two-Stage Transformation—Tangent Lines and Transformation Temperatures

APPENDIX

(Nonmandatory Information)

X1. RATIONALE

X1.1 Transformation temperature is used to characterize nickel-titanium alloys in the form of raw material, semifinished material, and finished product. In the case of raw material, transformation testing is necessary because chemical analysis is not precise enough to predict the desired shape memory and superelastic properties.

X1.2 This test method provides a rapid, economic means of determining the martensitic-to-austenitic transformation temperatures by recording the motion of the samples as it exhibits the shape memory effect. In the case of finished products, this test method often is used to determine the shape memory behavior of the product in its final application.

X1.3 Transformation temperatures measured by this test method will differ from those measured by thermal analysis or other techniques as a result of the effects of strain and load.

X1.4 A strain level of 2 to 4 % is selected to minimize the effect of strain on the transformation temperatures.

X1.5 The heating rate is limited to minimize the thermal gradients in the bath. The heating rate may be controlled manually or through the use of a temperature controller.

X1.6 The thermal mass of the fixture inside the bath should be minimized so that the fixture and the bath are uniform.

X1.7 Sample size is limited to diameter or thickness in the range of 0.3 to 3.0 mm. Larger samples can be tested with this test method with the addition of a fixture to aid in the deformation of the sample. Smaller samples cannot be easily tested with this test method because of friction in the motion-recording system. Smaller samples, however, can be tested using a similar approach in which the motion is recorded with a vision system.

Standard Specification for Total Knee Prosthesis[1]

This standard is issued under the fixed designation F 2083; the number immediately following the designation indicates the year of original adoption or, in the case of revision, the year of last revision. A number in parentheses indicates the year of last reapproval. A superscript epsilon (ϵ) indicates an editorial change since the last revision or reapproval.

1. Scope

1.1 This specification covers total knee replacement (TKR) prostheses used to provide functioning articulation by employing femoral and tibial components. Although a patellar component may be considered an integral part of a TKR, the detailed description of this component is excluded here since it is provided in Specification F 1672.

1.2 Included within the scope of this specification are replaceable components of modular designs, for example, tibial articulating surfaces and all components labeled for or capable of being used with cement, regardless of whether the same components can also be used without cement. This includes primary and revision prostheses and also covers fixed and mobile bearing knee designs.

1.3 This standard is intended to provide basic descriptions of material and prosthesis geometry. Additionally, those characteristics determined to be important to in-vivo performance of the prosthesis are defined.

1.4 Excluded from the scope are hemiarthroplasty devices that replace only the femoral or tibial surface, but not both; unicompartmental designs, which replace the articulating surfaces of only one condyle; and patellofemoral prostheses. Also excluded are devices designed for custom applications.

2. Referenced Documents

2.1 *ASTM Standards:*

F 67 Specification for Unalloyed Titanium (UNS R50250, UNS R50400, UNS R50550, UNS R50700) for Surgical Implant Applications

F 75 Specification for Cobalt-28 Chromium-6 Molybdenum Casting Alloy and Cast Products for Surgical Implants (UNS R30075)[2]

F 86 Practice for Surface Preparation and Marking of Metallic Surgical Implants

F 90 Specification for Wrought Cobalt-20 Chromium-15 Tungsten-10 Nickel Alloy for Surgical Implant Applications (R30605)[2]

F 136 Specification for Wrought Titanium-6 Aluminum-4 Vanadium ELI (Extra Low Interstitial) Alloy (UNS R56401) for Surgical Implant Applications[2]

F 138 Specification for Wrought 18 Chromium-14 Nickel-2.5 Molybdenum Stainless Steel Bar and Wire for Surgical Implants (UNS S31673)[2]

F 451 Specification for Acrylic Bone Cement[2]

F 562 Specification for Wrought Cobalt-35 Nickel-20 Chromium-10 Molybdenum Alloy for Surgical Implant Applications UNS R30035[2]

F 563 Specification for Wrought Cobalt-20Nickel-20Chromium-3.5Molybdenum-3.5Tungsten-5Iron Alloy for Surgical Implant Applications (UNS R30563)[2]

F 565 Practice for Care and Handling of Orthopedic Implants and Instruments[2]

F 648 Specification for Ultra-High-Molecular-Weight Polyethylene Powder and Fabricated Form for Surgical Implants[2]

F 732 Test Method for Wear Testing for Polymeric Materials Used in Total Joint Prostheses[2]

F 745 Specification for 18 Chromium-12.5 Nickel-2.5 Molybdenum Stainless Steel for Cast and Solution-Annealed Surgical Implant Applications[2]

F 746 Test Method for Pitting or Crevice Corrosion of Metallic Surgical Implant Materials[2]

F 748 Practice for Selecting Generic Biological Test Methods for Materials and Devices[2]

F 799 Specification for Cobalt-28 Chromium-6 Molybdenum Alloy for Surgical Implants (UNS R31537, R31538, R31539)[2]

F 981 Practice for Assessment of Compatibility of Biomaterials for Surgical Implants with Respect to Effect of Material on Muscle and Bone[2]

F 983 Practice for Permanent Marking of Orthopaedic Implant Components[2]

F 1044 Test Method for Shear Testing of Calcium Phosphate Coatings and Metallic Coatings[2]

F 1108 Specification for Titanium-6 Aluminum-4 Vanadium Alloy Castings for Surgical Implants (UNS R56406)[2]

F 1147 Test Method for Tension Testing of Calcium Phosphate and Metallic Coatings[2]

F 1160 Test Method for Shear and Bending Fatigue Testing of Calcium Phosphate and Metallic Medical and Composite Calcium Phosphate/Metallic Coatings[2]

[1] This specification is under the jurisdiction of ASTM Committee F04 on Medical and Surgical Materials and Devices and is the direct responsibility of Subcommittee F04.22 on Arthroplasty.

Current edition approved June 10, 2001. Published June 2001. Originally published as F 2083 - 01. Last previous edition F 2083 - 01.

[2] *Annual Book of ASTM Standards*, Vol 13.01.

F 1223 Test Method for Determination of Total Knee Replacement Constraint[2]

F 1377 Specification for Cobalt-28 Chromium-6 Molybdenum Powder for Coating of Orthopedic Implants (UNS-R30075)[2]

F 1472 Specification for Wrought Titanium-6 Aluminum-4 Vanadium Alloy (UNS R56400) for Surgical Implant Applications[2]

F 1537 Specification for Wrought Cobalt-28 Chromium-6 Molybdenum Alloy for Surgical Implants (UNS R31537, UNS R31538, and UNS R31529)[2]

F 1580 Specification for Titanium and Titanium-6 % Aluminum-4 % Vanadium Alloy Powders for Coatings of Surgical Implants[2]

F 1672 Specification for Resurfacing Patellar Prosthesis[2]

F 1715 Guide for Wear Assessment of Prosthetic Knee Designs in Simulator Devices[2]

F 1800 Test Method for Cyclic Fatigue Testing of Metal Tibial Tray Components of Total Knee Joint Replacements[2]

F 1814 Guide for Evaluating Modular Hip and Knee Joint Replacement Components[2]

2.2 *ISO Standard:*

ISO 6474 Implants for Surgery—Ceramic Materials Based on Alumina[3]

2.3 *FDA Document:*

US FDA 21 CFR 888.6 Degree of Constraint[4]

2.4 *ANSI/ASME Standard:*

ANSI/ASME B46.1-1995, Surface Texture (Surface Roughness, Waviness, and Lay)[3]

3. Terminology

3.1 *Definitions of Terms Specific to This Standard:*

3.1.1 *constraint, n*—the relative inability of a TKR to be further displaced in a specific direction under a given set of loading conditions as dictated by the TKR's geometric design.

3.1.2 *extension, n*—motion of the tibia toward bringing it into axial alignment with the femur.

3.1.3 *femoral component, n*—bearing member fixed to the femur for articulation with the tibial component and the patellar component or natural patella.

3.1.4 *flexion, n*—motion of the tibia toward bringing it into contact with the posterior femoral surface.

3.1.5 *interlock, n*—the mechanical design feature used to increase capture of one component within another and to restrict unwanted displacement between components, that is, component locking mechanism for modular components.

3.1.6 *patella component, n*—bearing member fixed to the natural patella for articulation with the femoral component, which is described in Specification F 1672.

3.1.7 *radiographic marker, n*—a nonstructural, generally thin wire, designed to be apparent on X-rays taken after implantation for those components that would otherwise be nonapparent on such X-rays.

3.1.8 *tibial component, n*—bearing member fixed to the tibia for articulation with the femoral component, typically either monoblock UHMWPE or consisting of two major components, a metallic tibial tray and a UHMWPE bearing surface.

3.1.9 *total knee replacement (TKR), n*—prosthetic parts that substitute for the natural opposing tibial, patellar, and femoral articulating surfaces.

4. Classification

4.1 The following classification by degree of constraint is suggested based on the concepts adopted by the U.S. Food and Drug Administration (see 2.3).

4.1.1 *Constrained*—A constrained joint prosthesis prevents dislocation of the prosthesis in more than one anatomic plane and consists of either a single, flexible, across-the-joint component or more than one component linked together or affined.

4.1.2 *Semiconstrained*—A semiconstrained joint prosthesis limits translation and/or rotation of the prosthesis in one or more planes via the geometry of its articulating surfaces. It has no across-the-joint linkages.

4.1.3 *Nonconstrained*—A nonconstrained joint prosthesis minimally restricts prosthesis movement in one or more planes. Its components have no across-the-joint linkages.

5. Material

5.1 The choice of materials is understood to be a necessary but not sufficient assurance of function of the device made from them. All devices conforming to this specification shall be fabricated from materials with adequate mechanical strength and durability, corrosion resistance, and biocompatibility.

5.1.1 *Mechanical Strength*—Various components of total knee replacement devices have been successfully fabricated from the following materials. See Specifications F 75, F 90, F 136, F 138, F 562, F 563, F 745, F 799, F 1108, F 1377, F 1472, F 1537, and F 1580. Polymeric bearing components have been fabricated from UHMWPE as specified in Specification F 648. Porous coatings have been fabricated from the materials specified in Specifications F 67 and F 75. Not all of these materials may possess sufficient mechanical strength for critical highly stressed components nor for articulating surfaces.

5.1.2 *Corrosion Resistance*—Materials with limited or no history of successful use for orthopaedic implant application must be determined to exhibit corrosion resistance equal to or better than one of the materials listed in 5.1.1 when tested in accordance to Test Method F 746.

5.1.3 *Biocompatibility*—Materials with limited or no history of successful use for orthopaedic implant application must be determined to exhibit acceptable biological response equal to or better than one of the materials listed in 5.1.1 when tested in accordance with Practices F 748 and F 981 for a given application.

6. Performance Requirements

6.1 *Component Function*—Each component for total knee arthroplasty is expected to function as intended when manufactured in accordance with good manufacturing practices and to the requirements of this specification. The components shall

[3] Available from American National Standards Institute, 25 W. 43rd St., 4th Floor, New York, NY 10036.

[4] Available from the Food and Drug Administration, Center for Devices and Radiological Health, 1350 Piccard Dr., Rockville, MD 20850.

be capable of withstanding static and dynamic physiologic loads without compromise to their function for the intended use and environment. All components used for experimental measures of performance shall be equivalent to the finished product in form and material. Components shall be sterilized if it will affect their performance.

NOTE 1—Computer models may be used to evaluate many of the functional characteristics if appropriate material properties and functional constraints are included and the computer models have been validated with experimental tests.

6.1.1 Individual tibial and femoral components may be fatigue tested using relevant test methods under appropriate loading conditions to address loss of supporting foundation (see Test Method F 1800).

6.1.2 Contact area and contact pressure distributions may be determined at various flexion angles using one of several published methods[5,6,7] to provide a representation of stresses applied to the bearing surfaces and to the components. Flexion angles of 0, 15, 30, 60, and 90° are recommended. If these tests are performed, it is important to maintain consistent test parameters and to evaluate other TKR prostheses under the same conditions.

6.1.3 Range of motion in flexion/extension shall be greater than or equal to 0°, flexion shall be greater than or equal to 110°. These measurements apply to components mounted in neutral alignment in bone or in an anatomically representative substitute. It is critical to define the location of the neutral alignment position, for example, center of contact areas or patches, in terms of dimensions from outside edges of the components. The initial positioning or location of the neutral alignment point will affect the range of motion values for certain TKR prostheses.

6.1.4 Total knee replacement constraint data for internal-external rotation, anterior-posterior displacement, and medial-lateral displacement may be determined in accordance with Test Method F 1223. Testing implants at 0 and 90° of flexion at a minimum is recommended.

6.2 All modular components must be evaluated for the integrity of their connecting mechanisms. As suggested in Guide F 1814, static and dynamic shear tests, bending tests, and tensile tests or any combination may be necessary to determine the performance characteristics. The connection mechanisms must show sufficient integrity for the range of loads anticipated for the application.

6.3 It is important to understand the wear performance for articulating surfaces. Any new or different material couple must not exceed the wear rates of the following material couple when tested under physiological conditions. The current standard wear couple is CoCrMo alloy (see Specification F 75) against UHMWPE (see Specification F 648) both having prosthetic-quality surface finishes as described in 8.2 and 8.3.

6.3.1 Materials may be tested in a pin-on-flat or pin-on-disk test apparatus such as described in Test Method F 732 with adequate controls for comparison. A number of different load levels may be used to cover the range of anticipated stresses between articulating components.

NOTE 2—In situations in which the pin-on-flat test may not be considered appropriate, other tests may be considered, that is, knee simulation modes of prosthesis wear performance testing or those described in ISO 6474 or other published documents.

6.3.2 Functional wear tests also may be performed to evaluate material and design performance. Since it is unlikely that one set of test conditions can simulate all aspects of knee function, it is recommended that various test conditions be used. Among the simulated conditions, there should be consideration of the effect of third-body abrasive interaction.

6.3.3 Evaluation of wear may be done gravimetrically in accordance with Guide F 1715. Consideration should also be given to other evaluation methods such as volumetric measurements through the use of contact and noncontact profilometry and three dimensional scanning techniques, semiquantitative measures of damage assessment, and measurement of friction factors.

6.3.4 It may be important to understand the characteristics of debris generated during the wear tests. Wear debris generated from specific wear tests of new materials may be characterized for morphology and size distribution and compared to wear debris from standard controls or to wear debris collected from in-vivo clinical service or animal studies. The wear debris also may be characterized for biological response in accordance with Practice F 748.

6.4 Porous metal coatings shall be tested in accordance with Test Method F 1044 (shear strength) and Test Method F 1147 (tensile strength) and the average for each test should exceed 20 MPa. The fatigue properties may be evaluated in accordance with Test Method F 1160.

7. Dimensions

7.1 Dimensions of total knee replacement components may be designated in accordance with Fig. 1 and the items specified in the glossary. The tolerance and methods of dimensional measurement must be sought to conform with industry practice and, whenever possible, on an international basis.

8. Finishing and Marking

8.1 Metallic components conforming to this specification shall be finished and marked in accordance with Practice F 86, where applicable.

8.2 *Metallic Bearing Surface*—The main bearing surfaces shall have a surface finish no rougher than 0.10-μm (4-μin.) roughness average, R_a, when measured in accordance with the principles given in ANSI/ASME B46.1-1995. The following details should be documented: stylus tip radius, cutoff length of measuring instrument (0.25 mm recommended), and position of measurement on specimen. When inspected visually, the component shall be free from embedded particles, defects with raised edges, and scratches and score marks.

8.3 *Polymeric Bearing Surface*—The main bearing surface

[5] McNamara, J.L., Collier, J.P., Mayor, M.B., Jensen, R.E., "A Comparison of Contact Pressures in Tibial and Patellar Total Knee Components Before and After Service In-Vivo," *Clin. Orthop. Rel. Res.*, No. 299, pp. 104–113, February 1994.

[6] Szivek, J.A., Cutignola, L., Volz, R.G., "Tibiofemoral Contact Stress and Stress Distribution Evaluation of Total Knee Arthroplasties," *J. Arthroplasty*, 10(4), pp. 480–491, August 1995.

[7] Hara, T., Horii, E., An, K.N., Cooney, W.P., Linscheid, R.L., Chao, E.Y.S., "Force Distribution Across Wrist Joint: Application of Pressure-Sensitive Conductive Rubber," *J. Hand Surg. [Am]*, 17(2), pp. 339–347, March 1992.

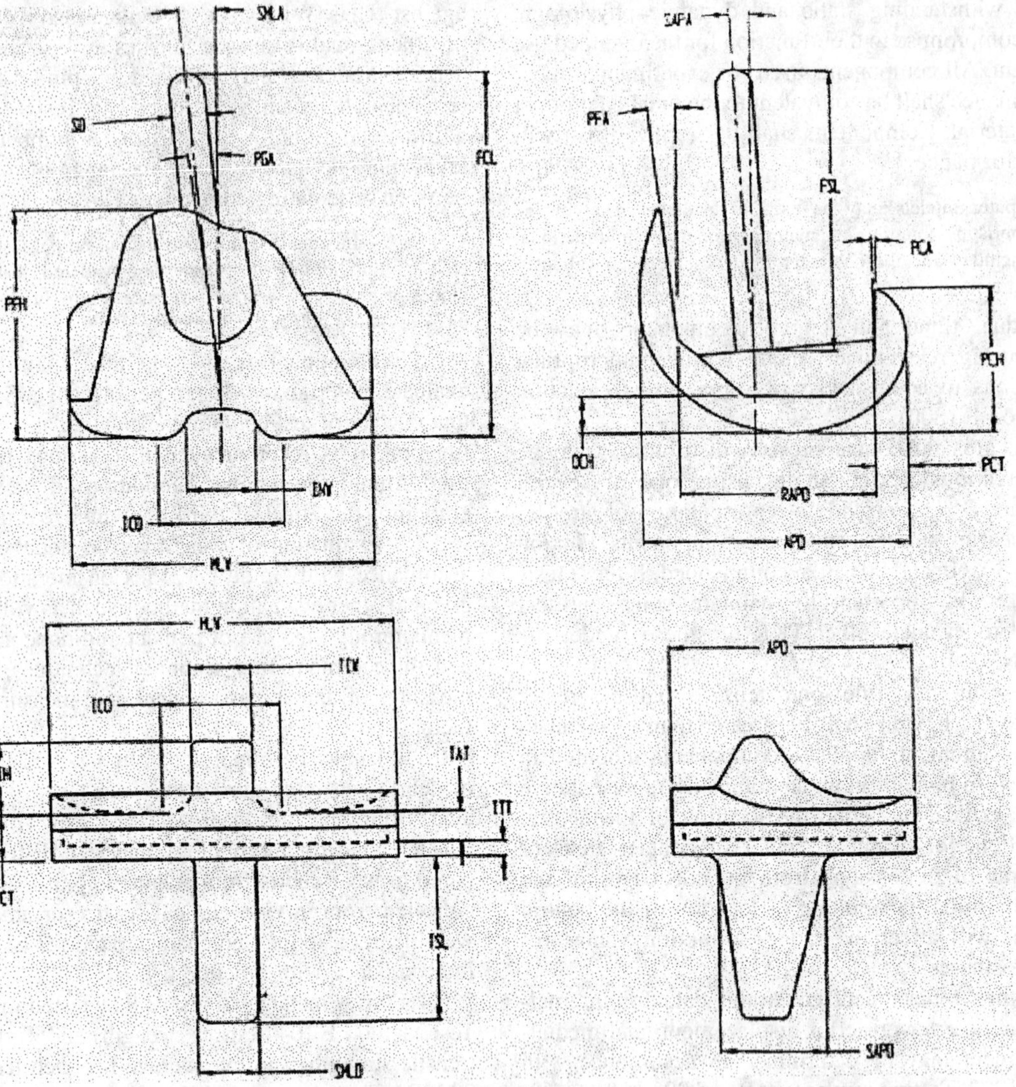

FIG. 1 General Depiction of Important Attributes of Total Knee Arthroplasty Components

of a UHMWPE component shall have a surface roughness no greater than 2–μm (80–μin.) roughness average, R_a, when measured in accordance with the principles given in ANSI/ASME B46.1-1995. The following details should be documented: stylus tip radius, cutoff length of measuring instrument (0.80 mm recommended), and position of measurement on specimen. When inspected with normal or corrected vision, the bearing surface shall be free from scale, embedded particles, and scratches and score marks other than those arising from the finishing process.

NOTE 3—Measurements should be taken in at least two orthogonal directions.

8.4 In accordance with Practices F 86 and F 983, items conforming to this specification shall be marked as follows in order of priority where space permits: manufacturer, material, lot number, catalog number, and size. Additional markings may be included, that is, left, right, front, and so forth.

8.5 If one of the components is not radiographic opaque, it may be appropriately marked for radiographic evaluation. Radiographic markers have been used in the past and are considered noncritical and may not be necessary. If a radiographic marker is used, it should be placed in a noncritical area to avoid degrading the structural and functional properties of the device.

9. Packaging and Package Marking

9.1 Adequate description of overall size and shape shall be included in the packaging. Dimensions, when used, shall conform to the convention as described in the glossary and Fig. 1.

9.2 The end user shall be able to determine the minimum thickness (TAT) of the UHMWPE in the main bearing area for either integral or modular systems from the package material. This may be achieved by directly specifying the TAT dimension or by providing a means to calculate the TAT dimension (see X2.12).

9.3 Packaging material for the TKR prosthesis system (femoral and tibial components) may include information developed from Test Method F 1223.

10. Keywords

10.1 arthroplasty; contact area; contact pressure; fatigue; knee; knee constraint; knee prosthesis; knee wear; particles; surface roughness; total knee replacement; TKR; UHMWPE

APPENDIXES

(Nonmandatory Information)

X1. GLOSSARY (Refer to Fig. 1)

X1.1 *anteroposterior distance (APD), n*—for both femoral and tibial components, the maximum A-P distance in a sagittal plane.

X1.2 *distal condylar height (DCH), n*—thickness of the femoral component from the transverse resection plane to the functional surface.

X1.3 *effective bone resection distance or overall thickness (OT), n*—the minimum distance that must exist between the femur and tibia to enable implantation of the device. Numerically equal to the distal condylar height (DCH), plus, the tibial component thickness (TCT).

X1.4 *femoral stem length (FSL), n*—that portion of the prosthesis intended for intramedullary fixation measured from stem origin, if this is the superior surface of the intercondylar box, to the tip of the stem. The length of a modular stem attachment shall also be described this way.

X1.5 *intercondylar dimension (ICD), n*—mediolateral distance between most distal point of each condyle of the femoral and the tibial components, respectively. Not applicable to hinged joints.

X1.6 *intercondylar notch width (INW), n*—the mediolateral width of the notch between the femoral condyles.

X1.7 *mediolateral distance width (MLW), n*—for both femoral and tibial components, the maximum width of the components in the frontal elevation.

X1.8 *overall femoral component length (FCL), n*—the overall length of the femoral component from the most distal articular surface to the most proximal surface. This may be equivalent to PFH in many cases.

X1.9 *patellar flange angle (PFA), n*—the angle formed by the anterior patellar articulating surface of the femoral component with respect to the distal articular surface in the neutral position in the saggital plane.

X1.10 *patellar flange height (PFH), n*—the distance from the most superior tip of the anterior patellar articulating surface of the femoral component to the distal articular surface in the neutral position.

X1.11 *patellar groove angle (PGA), n*—the angle formed by the patellar articulating depression in the patellar flange and the neutral axis of the femoral component in the frontal plane.

X1.12 *posterior condylar angle (PCA), n*—the angle formed by the posterior condylar flange with respect to the distal articular surface of the femoral component in the neutral position.

X1.13 *posterior condylar height (PCH), n*—the distance from the most superior tip of the posterior condylar flange to the distal articular surface of the femoral component in the neutral position.

X1.14 *posterior condylar thickness (PCT), n*—thickness of the femoral component from the posterior plane to the posterior articular surface.

X1.15 *resected anteroposterior distance (RAPD), n*—the minimum distance from the posterior condylar resection surface to the anterior condylar resection surface.

X1.16 *stem anteroposterior angle (SAPA), n*—the angle formed by the femoral stem relative to the neutral axis of the femoral component in the saggital plane.

X1.17 *stem mediolateral angle (SMLA), n*—the angle formed by the femoral stem relative to the neutral axis of the femoral component in the frontal plane.

X1.18 *stem diameter (SD), n*—the stem diameter for either femoral or tibial components. If the stems are not uniform diameters, such as wedge shaped tibial stems, then specify the mediolateral and anteroposterior dimensions.

X1.19 *stem mediolateral dimension (SMLD), n*—the cross-sectional mediolateral width of a nonsymmetric stem at its midpoint on the frontal plane.

X1.20 *stem anterioposterior dimension (SAPD), n*—the cross-sectional anterioposterior distance of a nonsymmetric stem at its midpoint on the saggital plane.

X1.21 *tibial component thickness (TCT), n*—the thickness from the functional articular surface to the distal inferior surface of the plateau. This is equal to TAT plus TPT for any multicomponent system. This is equal to TAT for all single material systems.

X1.22 *tibial articular surface thickness (TAT), n*—the minimum distance from the articular surface of the tibial component to the superior surface of the supporting plateau.

X1.23 *tibial tray thickness (TTT), n*—the minimum thickness of the tibial tray when measured from the superior surface to the inferior surface. In the case of a single component, this dimension is TAT.

X1.24 *tibial stem length (TSL), n*—that portion of the tibial component intended for intramedullary fixation. Measured from stem origin at the inferior surface of the plateau to the distal tip of the stem.

X1.25 *tibial intercondylar spine width (TIW), n*—the mediolateral width of the posterior stabilization spine.

X1.26 *tibial intercondylar spine height (TIH), n*—the distance from the superior condylar articulating surface to the top of the posterior stabilization spine.

X2. RATIONALE

X2.1 The objectives of this specification are to establish guidelines for the manufacture and function of components for total knee replacement. This specification describes the femoral and tibial components and relies on Specification F 1672 to describe the patella component for a total knee replacement. These total knee replacement parts are intended for use in a patient who is skeletally mature under conditions of imposed dynamic loads in a corrosive environment and virtually continuous motion at the bearing surfaces. Laboratory tests to simulate accurately imposed loads, aggressive electrolytes, and complex constituents of body fluids cannot be usefully accelerated. Long-term projections of satisfactory performances over many decades can be suggested but not accurately predicted using currently available screening procedures.

X2.2 This specification identifies those factors felt to be important to assure a satisfactory useful prosthesis life. It is here recognized that failure of an arthroplasty can occur even while the components are intact. This specification is expected to provide reasonable assurance that devices in compliance with the standard will not experience mechanical failure of the device or undesirable tissue reaction to the materials of the device or its design. Other factors affecting outcome of the arthroplasty not addressed by this standard include infection, surgical technique, misuse by the patient, and unpredicted tissue response.

X2.3 Under applicable documents and materials, the list reflects the current state of the art. It is recognized that should materials not now included appear and be proved acceptable, they shall be inserted in the process of revisions. To date, a majority of knee prosthesis components have been implanted using a bone bonding agent, such as acrylic bone cement in accordance with Specification F 451. Although the bone bonding agent is not considered part of the knee prosthesis, it may play an important role in the performance of the prosthesis and, therefore, should be considered during testing and evaluation.

X2.4 *Constraint Classification*—Total knee prosthetic components in common use comprise three recognized classes of prosthetic pairs: constrained, partially or semiconstrained, and nonconstrained. No general consensus has emerged to establish clearly the most widely acceptable classification; however, the qualitative descriptors included herein have been adopted by the U.S. Food and Drug Administration for the purposes of evaluating new device applications. It is also anticipated that through the application of Test Method F 1223 appropriate categorization may be achieved and data sufficient to allow proper selection of a device for a particular patient will be available. Note that devices within a particular classification may allow significantly different degrees of freedom, that is, translation, rotation, or flexion ranges or limits, from other devices within the same classification, depending on device geometry and the means and relative amount of constraint. Conversely, devices in different classifications may allow similar degrees of freedom and provide comparable motion and clinical results.

X2.5 In the course of evaluating new materials, it is recommended that if the material is used in an application that causes small particle formation from abrasion or normal wear processes then the biocompatibility of these particles be determined in addition to that of the bulk material.

X2.6 *Performance Considerations*—Component performance can be predicted only indirectly at this stage by referring to strength levels and other parameters. Reference to parameters applicable to materials may or may not adequately describe structures made from them. In a period of transition from device specification standards to device performance standards, both methods of description may be appropriate. Mechanical values derived from materials testing and cited as minimum allowable levels must be applicable to the structures described in the specifications. Usual and customary sampling procedures shall be considered adequate assurance of compliance. Exemption from sampling is justified where no degradation in mechanical properties is to be expected during fabrication of components.

X2.7 It is anticipated that as new performance data becomes available, such as that developed by the task force on standard practice for the cyclic fatigue testing of metal backed tibial tray components of knee joint replacement designs, it will be incorporated into the body of this document.

X2.8 Component performance should be considered with regard to body weight, with unusually small patients being served well by small components. It is well recognized that physical stresses resulting from events or activities out of the ordinary range, as in accidents or especially vigorous sports, predictably exceed allowable stress levels in any component design. It is also recognized here that other forms of arthroplasty failure are known to occur, related primarily to patient factors, such as osteoporosis, Paget's disease, misuse and disuse, and others.

X2.9 Radiographic markers have been used to make components radiographically detectable. They may not be necessary, but when they are used, shall be located in a noncritical area to avoid any contribution to device failure. They shall not be located in critical wear areas nor regions that may see high stresses since this could reduce the service life of the component.

X2.10 For marking of the components, it is desirable to have complete information, where space is available to do so, including manufacturer's trademark, material, lot number, size, orientation, if any, and date in that order.

X2.11 For the purposes of this specification, packaging may include product brochures and associated literature.

X2.12 It is important to allow the end user to determine the minimum thickness of a bearing material in the areas that may undergo high loading. One common region, as described in Fig. 1, is the minimum amount of UHMWPE in the tibial component under the femoral condyle at full extension. Although the thickness does not necessarily determine clinical performance, it may be helpful to the end user.

Standard Guide for Use of Universal Transverse Mercator (UTM) Grids When Preparing and Using a Field Map for Land Search[1]

This standard is issued under the fixed designation F 2099; the number immediately following the designation indicates the year of original adoption or, in the case of revision, the year of last revision. A number in parentheses indicates the year of last reapproval. A superscript epsilon (ϵ) indicates an editorial change since the last revision or reapproval.

1. Scope

1.1 This guide describes one method of setting up a Universal Transverse Mercator (UTM) grid system on a base map for transfer to a field map.

1.2 This guide provides a uniform way of communicating UTM coordinates.

1.3 This guide is intended to be used with United States Geological Survey (USGS) 7.5-min quadrangle topographical maps with a scale of 1:24 000, with or without UTM grid lines.

1.4 The values stated in SI units are to be regarded as standard. No other units of measurement are included in this standard.

1.5 *This standard does not purport to address all of the safety concerns, if any, associated with its use. It is the responsibility of the user of this standard to establish appropriate safety and health practices and determine the applicability of regulatory requirements prior to use.*

2. Referenced Documents

2.1 *ASTM Standards:*

F 1846 Practice for Symbols and Markings for Use with Land Search Maps[2]

3. Terminology

3.1 *Definitions of Terms Specific to This Standard:*

3.1.1 *field map, n*—a copy of a base map or portion thereof provided to search and rescue field teams or crews.

3.1.2 *grid overlay, n*—a transparent piece of material used for interpolating UTM coordinates on a USGS topographical map. For a 1:24 000 scale map, the overlay contains, as a minimum, lines representing at least two adjacent sides of a 1000-m square, with the lines subdivided into tenths.

3.1.3 *Universal Transverse Mercator (UTM), n*—a rectangular grid system that covers the earth between latitude 80° South and latitude 84° North.

3.1.4 *UTM grid lines, n*—a series of straight lines that connect the UTM tick marks having identical numbers on the top and bottom of the map, as well as a series of lines that similarly connect the left and right side UTM tick marks.

3.1.5 *UTM tick marks, n*—small vertical or horizontal lines on 1:24 000 USGS maps, light blue in color, approximately 0.3 cm (⅛ in.) in length spaced 1000 m (1 km) (scale) apart.

4. Significance and Use

4.1 The base map, field maps, and the UTM grid lines are used during search operations to ensure that field personnel and the command post can accurately communicate specific position information in the search area.

4.2 Section 5 verifies if the UTM grid lines are on the base map or not. If the UTM grid lines are not on the base map, Section 5 describes how to draw them on the map.

4.3 Section 6 establishes how to set up and prepare field maps for personnel to use in the field.

4.4 Section 7 describes the uniform way of determining and communicating UTM coordinates.

5. Verifying and Drawing UTM Grid Lines

5.1 Obtain the USGS quadrangle map (7.5 min or 1:24 000) with the area that is to be copied. Review the map to see if UTM grid lines are marked on the map. If so, proceed to Section 6, otherwise continue with 5.2.

5.2 Obtain a straightedge long enough to connect opposite UTM tick marks and which can be used to draw full-length straight lines in a single stroke, and a pen or pencil. Continue with 5.3.

5.3 *Drawing Horizontal and Vertical UTM Grid Lines*:

5.3.1 Starting at the top or bottom of the map, align the straightedge on the UTM tick marks at the left and right sides of the map, ensuring the numbers are the same. In a single stroke, draw a line connecting the tick marks. Move the straightedge to the next set of UTM tick marks and again draw a single line connecting them. Continue this process until all horizontal lines are drawn.

5.3.2 Starting at either side of the map, align the straightedge on the UTM tick marks at the top and bottom of the map, ensuring the numbers are the same. In a single stroke, draw a line connecting the tick marks. Move the straightedge to the next set of UTM tick marks and again draw a single line connecting them. Continue this process until all vertical lines are drawn.

5.4 When possible, maps should be reviewed and grid lines drawn on the maps before being used on a search so that the

---

[1] This guide is under the jurisdiction of ASTM Committee F32 on Search and Rescue and is the direct responsibility of Subcommittee F32.02 on Management and Operations.

Current edition approved April 10, 2001. Published May 2001.

[2] *Annual Book of ASTM Standards*, Vol 13.01.

procedure in 5.3 does not have to be performed during the search.

6. Preparing UTM Coordinates on a Base Map for Copying to a Field Map

6.1 Position a sheet of paper, the same size as the paper onto which the map will be copied, over the area of the base map which is to be copied.

6.1.1 When placing the paper, consider that succeeding steps of this procedure will shift the copy area down and to the left and that the copy machine may not be able to copy to the edges of the desired area.

6.2 Place a piece of removable, nondestructive tape, such as white copy or correction tape or transparent tape, on the base map along the entire bottom edge of the paper.

6.3 Place a piece of removable, nondestructive tape, such as white copy or correction tape or transparent tape, on the base map along the entire left edge of the paper.

6.4 Remove the sheet of paper from the base map.

6.5 Wherever the tape along the bottom edge of the copy area crosses a vertical line connecting UTM tick marks, transfer the last two (large) digits of the corresponding UTM coordinates from the top or bottom of the map to the tape.

6.6 Wherever the tape along the left edge of the copy area crosses a horizontal line connecting UTM tick marks, transfer the last two (large) digits of the corresponding UTM coordinates from the left or right side of the map to the tape.

6.7 Place the marked area of the map on the copy machine, with the lower left corner of the tape being the reference corner. Ensure that the information transferred to the tape appears within the copy area, considering that the copy machine may not copy completely to the edges of the original.

6.8 Make copies as needed for the anticipated size of the incident.

7. Reading the UTM Coordinates for Search and Rescue Operations

7.1 Reading the UTM coordinates using eight digits provides a 10-m (32.8-ft) accuracy. All numbers are read right, then up. Reading four digits to the right and four digits up provides the eight digits.

7.2 The four digits read to the right and the four digits read up are the ten-thousands, thousands, hundreds, and tens of metres.

7.3 The ten-thousands and thousands of metres digits are read directly from the map and are the digits transferred to the tape in 6.3. The hundreds of metres digit is the first interpolation from the grid overlay and the tens of metres is the second interpolation.

8. Keywords

8.1 management; map; search; topographical; universal transverse; USGS; UTM

APPENDIX

(Nonmandatory Information)

X1. METHOD FOR FINDING THE UTM COORDINATES OF A POINT ON A 1:24 000 SCALE USGS TOPOGRAPHIC MAP

X1.1 On a 1:24 000 scale USGS topographic map (7½ min), the UTM values are shown at tick marks along the edges of the map. At each tick mark there is a three- or four-digit number. The first one or two numbers will be printed smaller than the third and fourth. One of the numbers along each edge may have small trailing zeroes and the letter "m" with a larger "E" or "N." See Fig. X1.1. Position is reported using these numbers.

X1.2 The intersections of the UTM tick marks form squares 1000 m to a side.

X1.3 To find the UTM coordinates of a point, the 1000-m square containing the point is divided into ten equal parts in each direction and the position is reported in tenths reading right, then up. Dividing the grid into tenths can be done by estimating or with a transparent overlay. Each UTM grid for a given map scale is the same size and is a true square (height equals width; sides are at right angles), which is why an overlay can be used.

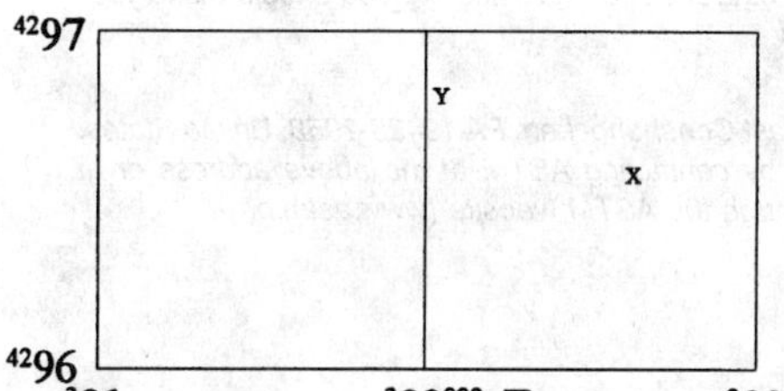

FIG. X1.1 1000-m UTM Grids Representation

X1.4 As an example of determining UTM coordinates, the position of "X" in Fig. X1.2 will be found.

X1.4.1 First, the "X" is to the right of the large digits "92" (ignore the letters and small numbers). Then, counting to the right, the "X" is between Lines 6 and 7. Since it is closer to Line 6, its position is noted as 926.

X1.4.2 Next, find the large digits that the "X" is above or up from, in this case, "96." Then counting up, the "X" is between Lines 5 and 6. Since it is closer to Line 5, its position is noted as 965.

X1.4.3 The location of the "X" would be reported as "926965." The coordinates are read right and up.

X1.4.4 This set of six numbers locates the position of "X" to within 100 m.

X1.5 To find the position of "X" within 10 m, the 100-m

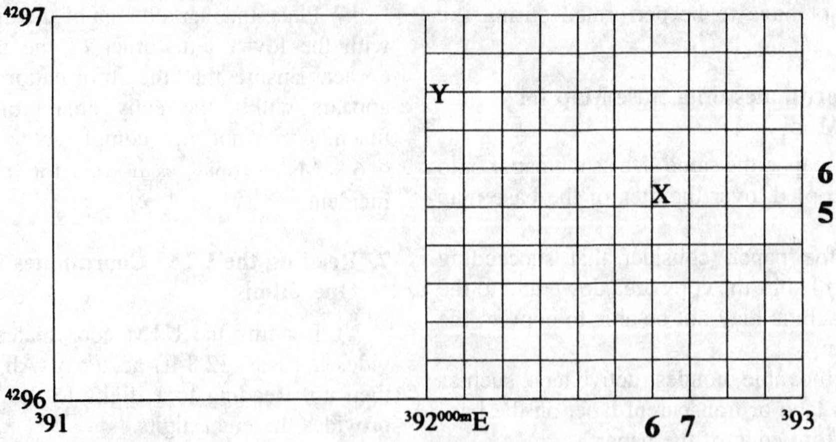

FIG. X1.2 UTM Grids of Fig. X1.1 Showing Divided Grid for Determining Position

square containing "X" is divided into tenths in a similar fashion.

X1.5.1 The center of the "X" is to the right of Line 6 and approximately one quarter of the way across the 100-m grid towards Line 7. This coordinate would be 9262 (or 9263 depending on how the position is interpolated.)

X1.5.2 In the vertical or up direction, the center of the "X" is three or four tenths of the way up from Line 5. This coordinate would be 9653 (or 9654).

X1.5.3 The position of "X" would be reported as 92629653. This locates "X" to within 10 m.

X1.6 Always report the right then up coordinates, but do not use those words in the position report and do not leave a space between the numbers. A pause may be inserted between the two sets of digits when reading them aloud.

X1.7 There must always be an even number of digits in the location coordinates so a leading or trailing zero (0) must be used when necessary.

X1.8 The number of digits in the right and up coordinates must be equal.

X1.9 As a second example, the location of "Y" is 920968 to within 100 m and 92049679 to within 10 m.

X1.10 A grid, drawn to 1:24 000 scale is shown in Fig. X1.3. When copied onto transparent material, it can be used as an overlay for determining UTM position.

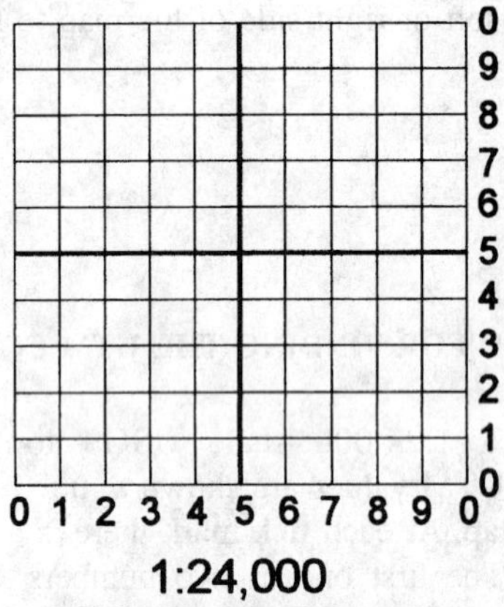

FIG. X1.3 Grid for Making a UTM Overlay

The American Society for Testing and Materials takes no position respecting the validity of any patent rights asserted in connection with any item mentioned in this standard. Users of this standard are expressly advised that determination of the validity of any such patent rights, and the risk of infringement of such rights, are entirely their own responsibility.

This standard is subject to revision at any time by the responsible technical committee and must be reviewed every five years and if not revised, either reapproved or withdrawn. Your comments are invited either for revision of this standard or for additional standards and should be addressed to ASTM Headquarters. Your comments will receive careful consideration at a meeting of the responsible technical committee, which you may attend. If you feel that your comments have not received a fair hearing you should make your views known to the ASTM Committee on Standards, at the address shown below.

Standard Guide for Evaluating the Extent of Oxidation in Ultra-High-Molecular-Weight Polyethylene Fabricated Forms Intended for Surgical Implants[1]

This standard is issued under the fixed designation F 2102; the number immediately following the designation indicates the year of original adoption or, in the case of revision, the year of last revision. A number in parentheses indicates the year of last reapproval. A superscript epsilon (ε) indicates an editorial change since the last revision or reapproval.

1. Scope

1.1 This guide describes a method for the measurement of the relative extent of oxidation present in ultra-high-molecular-weight polyethylene (UHMWPE) intended for use in medical implants. The material is analyzed by infrared spectroscopy. The intensity (area) of the carbonyl absorptions (>C=O) centered near 1720 cm^{-1} is related to the amount of chemically bound oxygen present in the material. Other forms of chemically bound oxygen (C-O C, C O O C, C-O-H, and so forth) are not captured by this method.

1.2 Although this method may give the investigator a means to compare the relative extent of carbonyl oxidation present in various UHMWPE samples, it is recognized that other forms of chemically bound oxygen may be important contributors to these materials' characteristics.

1.3 The applicability of the infrared method has been demonstrated by many literature reports. This particular method, using the intensity (area) of the C-H absorption centered near 1370 cm^{-1} to normalize for the sample's thickness, has been validated by an Interlaboratory Study (ILS) conducted according to Practice E 691.

1.4 The following precautionary caveat pertains only to the test method portion, Section 5, of this specification: *This standard may involve hazardous materials, operations, and equipment. This standard does not purport to address all of the safety concerns, if any, associated with its use. It is the responsibility of the user of this standard to establish appropriate safety and health practices and determine the applicability of regulatory requirements prior to use.*

2. Referenced Documents

2.1 *ASTM Standards:*

E 691 Practice for Conducting an Interlaboratory Study to Determine the Precision of a Test Method[2]

3. Terminology

3.1 *Definitions:*

3.1.1 *bulk oxidation index (BOI)*—a sample's bulk oxidation index (BOI) is the average of the oxidation indices collected over a 500-μm section at the center of the sample.

3.1.1.1 *Discussion*—Typically, this is a plateau region with the smallest oxidation indices.

3.1.1.2 *Discussion*—For samples less than about 8 to 10 mm thick, this central region may display the sample's highest oxidation indices, depending on its state of oxidation.

3.1.2 *depth locator (DL)*—a measurement of the distance from the articular surface, or surface of interest, that a spectrum was collected and a corresponding OI calculated.

3.1.3 *oxidation index (OI)*—an oxidation index (OI) is defined as the ratio of the area of the absorption peak(s) between 1650 and 1850 cm^{-1} to the area of the absorption peak(s) between 1330 and 1396 cm^{-1}, as shown in Fig. 1.

3.1.4 *oxidation index profile*—an oxidation index profile is the graphical representation of variation of the sample's oxidation index with distance from its articular surface or the surface of interest. This is a plot of an OI versus DL. Typically, the graph will show the profile through the entire thickness of the sample.

3.1.5 *surface oxidation index (SOI)*—a sample's surface oxidation index (SOI) is the average of the oxidation indices from the sample's articular surface, or the surface of interest, to a depth of 3-mm subsurface.

4. Apparatus

4.1 *Infrared Spectrometer*:

4.1.1 A calibrated infrared spectrometer capable of recording a transmission absorption spectrum over the range of about 1200 to about 2000 cm^{-1} using about 200-mm-thick films at a resolution of 4 cm^{-1} and an aperture of about 200 by 200 μm.

4.1.1.1 Other modes of collection (that is, percent reflection, attenuated total reflection (ATR), and so forth) and aperture and increment sizes may be used to generate the sample's absorption spectrum provided they can be demonstrated to produce equivalent results. Too large an aperture can result in a loss of profile accuracy.

4.1.1.2 When a Fourier Transform Infrared (FTIR) spectrometer is used, a minimum of 32 scans shall be collected per spectrum.

4.1.1.3 The FTIR instrument and sample compartment

[1] This guide is under the jurisdiction of ASTM Committee F04 on Medical and Surgical Materials and Devicesand is the direct responsibility of Subcommittee F04.15on Material Test Methods.

Current edition approved May 10, 2001. Published June 2001.

[2] *Annual Book of ASTM Standards*, Vol 14.02.

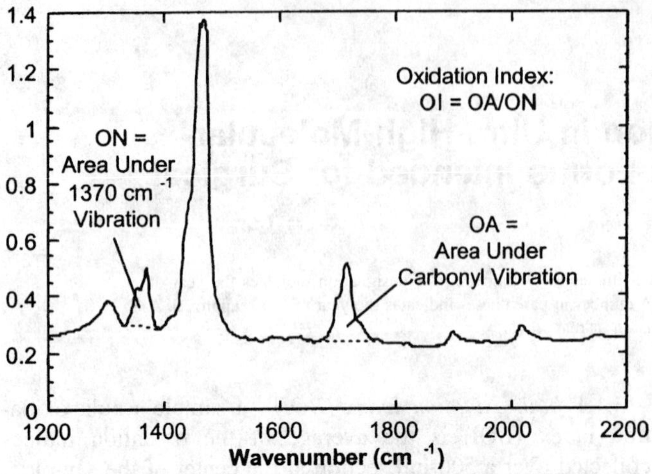

FIG. 1 Typical FTIR Spectra of Oxidized UHMWPE, Showing the Definition of an Area-Based Oxidation Index Based on Normalization Using the 1370-cm^{-1} Peak

should be purged with a moisture- and carbon-dioxide-free inert gas (for example, nitrogen, helium, or argon) to minimize spectral interference from these components.

4.2 *Specimen Holder*:

4.2.1 Equipment capable of accurately positioning the sample under the orifice in increments at the scale of the aperture dimensions.

4.3 *Microtome*:

4.3.1 Equipment capable of producing about 200-μm-thick slices (films) of a sample perpendicular to the articular surface or the surface of interest.

5. Procedure

5.1 *Preparation of the Infrared Spectrometer*:

5.1.1 Prepare the infrared spectrometer for collection of a transmission absorption spectrum from a thin film of the UHMWPE sample according to the manufacturer's recommendations and the conditions described in Section 4 above.

5.1.2 Collect the sequence of spectra per 5.2 and 5.3.

5.2 *Preparation of Test Specimen*:

5.2.1 Using a microtome, or other appropriate device, prepare a thin slice of the sample about 200 μm thick.

5.2.2 The slice shall typically be taken near the center of the sample's articular surface or the surface of interest.

5.2.3 The orientation of the slice shall typically be perpendicular to the articular surface or the surface of interest.

5.3 *Configuration of the Test Specimen in the Spectrometer*:

5.3.1 The test film (slice) shall be first configured in the spectrometer (after an appropriate background spectrum has been collected) such that the aperture is positioned over the first 200 μm of the film starting at the surface of interest.

5.3.2 Subsequent spectra shall be collected sequentially at increments matching the aperture size (that is, about 200 μm) from the articular surface, or surface of interest, across the width of the film to the opposite surface.

5.3.2.1 Larger increments may be used; however, too large an increment size may result in a loss of profile accuracy.

6. Calculations

6.1 *Oxidation Peak Area*:

6.1.1 For each absorbance spectrum calculate the total area of the peak absorptions between 1650 and 1850 cm^{-1} (see Fig. 1).

6.1.1.1 This is the area below the sample's absorption curve and above the straight line baseline drawn between the same starting and ending points, namely, 1650 and 1850 cm^{-1}.

6.2 *Normalization Peak Area*:

6.2.1 For each absorbance spectrum, calculate the total area of the peak absorptions between 1330 and 1396 cm^{-1} (see Fig. 1).

6.2.1.1 This is the area below the sample's absorption curve and above the straight line baseline drawn between the same starting and ending points, namely, 1330 and 1396 cm^{-1}.

6.3 *Oxidation Index (OI)*:

6.3.1 For each absorbance spectrum, calculate its OI by dividing the area of its oxidation peak (6.1) by the area of its normalization peak (6.2), as shown in Fig. 1.

6.4 *Oxidation Index Depth Locator (DL)*:

6.4.1 Calculate the distance from the articular surface, or surface of interest (DL), for each spectrum and its corresponding OI from the following equation.

$$DL = 0.5(A) + n(S)$$

where:

A = the size of the aperture in micrometres in the step direction,

n = the number of steps (increments) the aperture had been moved from its initial location at the articular surface or surface of interest, and

S = the step (increment) size in micrometres.

6.5 *Sample's Oxidation Index Profile*:

6.5.1 Construct a plot of a sample's oxidation indices (OI) versus their corresponding depth locators (DL).

6.6 *Surface Oxidation Index (SOI)*:

6.6.1 Calculate a sample's SOI by calculating the average of the sample's oxidation indices (OI) with depth locator (DL) values between 0 and 3000.

6.7 *Bulk Oxidation Index (BOI)*:

6.7.1 Calculate a sample's BOI by calculating the average of the sample's oxidation indices (OI) corresponding to the center 500 mm of material.

7. Report

7.1 The report shall contain at least the following experimental details and results:

7.1.1 *Material Information*:

7.1.1.1 Resin type and resin lot number.

7.1.1.2 Consolidation method and manufacturer and manufacturer lot number.

7.1.1.3 Any special postconsolidation treatments, for example, HIPing, annealing, sterilization, cross-linking, stabilization, accelerated aging, and storage conditions.

7.1.2 *Sample Information*:

7.1.2.1 Orthopedic implant or laboratory test specimen.

7.1.2.2 Articular surface or nonarticulator surface.

7.1.2.3 Test sample's original dimensions.

7.1.2.4 Any special posttreatments of the original test sample, for example, annealing, sterilization, cross-linking, stabilization, accelerated aging, and storage conditions.

7.1.2.5 Test film thickness and total width.

7.1.2.6 Any special posttreatments of the test films, for example, annealing, sterilization, cross-linking, stabilization, accelerated aging, and storage condition.

7.1.3 *Spectrometer Information*:

7.1.3.1 Manufacturer and model number.

7.1.3.2 Analogue or Fourier Transform spectrometer.

7.1.3.3 Aperture dimensions, profile step size, spectral resolution, and number of scans per spectrum.

7.1.4 *Data Analysis Information*:

7.1.4.1 Manual or by spectrometer's software algorithms.

7.1.4.2 Calculated SOI and BOI.

8. Precision and Bias

8.1 *Precision*—The data in Table 1 is based on a series of international interlaboratory studies using this method which were conducted in 1999 and 2000, in accordance with Practice E 691, involving up to twelve institutions across the United States and Europe. Metrics of repeatability and reproducibility between different institutions were calculated as outlined in Practice E 691 and normalized with respect to the mean oxidation index to estimate relative uncertainty. The data for the GUR 4150 HP rod stock were collected on as-irradiated microtomed samples. For the long-term shelf-aged tibial implants, the data were collected below the surface at the location of maximum oxidation. All samples were 200-mm-thick microtomed films gamma irradiated in air.

8.2 *Bias*—No statement may be made about the bias of this test method, as there is no standard reference material or reference test method that is applicable.

9. Keywords

9.1 FTIR; implant; oxidation; oxidation index; UHMWPE

TABLE 1 International Interlaboratory Study Test Results

UHMWPE Resin, Component Type	Shelf Age,	Average Oxidation Index (OI),	Absolute Uncertainty			Standard Relative Uncertainty	
	years	$\bar{x}$	s_x	s_r	s_R	s_r, %	s_R, %
GUR 4150 HP, rod stock	0.0	0.232	0.077	0.017	0.078	7.2	33.8
GUR 1120, tibial insert	5.3	1.28	0.138	0.040	0.142	3.1	11.1
GUR 1120, tibial insert	7.5	4.51	0.823	0.168	0.834	3.7	18.5
GUR 1120, tibial insert	11.5	4.53	0.823	0.483	0.912	10.7	20.2

APPENDIX

(Nonmandatory Information)

X1. RATIONALE

X1.1 The extent of overall oxidation and specifically certain oxidation index profiles present in orthopaedic implant components made of UHMWPE have been shown to degrade their mechanical properties and thus potentially adversely affect their in vivo performance. It is, therefore, important to have standard methods for assessing the oxidative characteristics of such materials.

X1.2 The method described herein is an adaptation of several similar methods described in the literature. The particular technique used to calculate an oxidation index used here has been validated by interlaboratory studies per Practice E 691.

X1.3 Although the method described herein has been shown to be useful for comparing the oxidation states of different UHMWPE samples, it is clear that this method does not account for all the different types of oxidative products present or potentially important in a sample.

X1.4 This method is useful for comparing the oxidation state of real-time shelf-aged UHMWPE components and UHMWPE materials assumed to have undergone oxidation via the same mechanisms.

X1.5 This method is also useful for comparing the oxidation state of retrieved components. It is, however, complicated by the effects of biological residues potentially present in retrieved samples. Common methods used to reduce such residuals (for example, extraction with hexane) may improve the comparative power of this technique.

X1.6 Use of this method to make comparisons between real-time shelf-aged components, accelerated aged components, and retrieved components is less useful because of the potential for different, and other, modes of oxidizing the UHMWPE in vivo compared to shelf or accelerating aging.

X1.7 At the present time, there is no clear correlation between the extent of oxidation or the oxidation profile present in a sample of UHMWPE and its functional characteristics. For this reason, no maximum SOI or BOI has been specified in this document.

REFERENCES

(**1**) Kurtz, S. M., Muratoglu, O. K., Mounib, L., Buchanan, F., Currier, B., et al, "Confirmed Interlaboratory Validation Studies of a Standard Method for Determining the Oxidation Index of UHMWPE," *Transactions of the 25th Society for Biomaterials*, 22, 46, 1999.

(**2**) Kurtz, S. M., Muratoglu, O. K., Buchanan, F., Currier, B., Gsell, R., et al, "Interlaboratory Reproducibility of Standard Accelerated Aging Methods for Oxidation of UHMWPE," *Biomaterials*, 2001.

(**3**) Collier, J. P., Sperling, D. K., Currier, J. H., Sutula, L. C., Saum, K. A., et al, "Impact of Gamma Sterilization on Clinical Performance of Polyethylene in the Knee," *J Arthroplasty*, 11, 377-89, 1996.

(**4**) Currier, B. H., Currier, J. H., Collier, J. P., Mayor, M. B., Scott, R. D., "Shelf Life and In Vivo Duration. Impacts on Performance of Tibial Bearings," *Clin Orthop*, 342, 111-22, 1997.

(**5**) Sutula, L. C., Collier, J. P., Saum, K. A., Currier, B. H., Currier, J. H., et al, "Impact of Gamma Sterilization on Clinical Performance of Polyethylene in the Hip," *Clin Orthop*, 319, 28-40, 1995.

(**6**) Kurtz, S. M., Bartel, D. L., Rimnac, C. M., "Post-Irradiation Aging Affects the Stresses and Strains in UHMWPE Components for Total Joint Replacement," *Clin Orthop*, 350, 209-220, 1998.

(**7**) Edidin, A. A., Jewett, C. W., Kwarteng, K., Kalinowski, A., Kurtz, S. M., "Degradation of Mechanical Behavior in UHMWPE After Natural and Accelerated Aging," *Biomaterials*, 21, 1451-1460, 2000.

(**8**) Kurtz, S. M., Muratoglu, O. K., Evans, M., Edidin, A. A., "Advances in the Processing, Sterilization, and Crosslinking of Ultra-High Molecular Weight Polyethylene for Total Joint Arthroplasty," *Biomaterials*, 20, 1659-88, 1999.

(**9**) Collier, J. P., Sutula, L. C, Currier, B. H., Currier, J. H., Wooding, R. E., et al, "Overview of Polyethylene as a Bearing Material: Comparison of Sterilization Methods," *Clin Orthop*, 333, 76-86, 1996.

(**10**) Gillis, A. M., Furman, B. D., Li, S., "Variations in the Determination of Oxidation in UHMWPE by 10 Different FTIR Protocols and a Proposed Standard Protocol," *Transactions of the 44th Orthopedic Research Society*, 23, 359, 1998.

(**11**) Di Maio, W. G., Lilly, W. B., Moore, W. C., Saum, K. A., "Low Wear, Low Oxidation Radiation Crosslinked UHMWPE," *Transactions of the 44th Orthopedic Research Society*, 23, 363, 1998.

(**12**) Sanford, W. M., and Saum, K. A., "Accelerated Oxidative Aging Testing of UHMWPE," *Transactions of the 41st Orthopedic Research Society*, 20, 119, 1995.

(**13**) McKellop, H., Yeom, B., Sun, D. C., Sanford, W. M., "Accelerated Aging of Irradiated UHMW Polyethylene for Wear Evaluations," *42nd Orthopedic Research Society*, 21, 483, 1996.

(**14**) McKellop, H., Shen, F. W., Ota, T., Lu, B., Wiser, H., et al, "Wear of UHMWPE Acetabular Cups after Gamma, Sterilization in Nitrogen, Thermal Stabilization, and Artificial Aging," *Transactions of the 23rd Annual Meeting of the Society for Biomaterials*, 20, 45, 1997.

(**15**) Sun, D. C., Stark, C., Dumbleton, J. H., "Development of an Accelerated Aging Method for Evaluation of Long-Term Irradiation Effects on UHMWPE Implants," *Polymer Reprints*, 35, 969-970, 1994.

(**16**) Shen, F. W., Yu, Y. J., McKellop, H., "Potential Errors in FTIR Measurement of Oxidation in Ultrahigh Molecular Weight Polyethylene Implants [In Process Citation]," *J Biomed Mater Res*, 48, 203-10, 1999.

(**17**) Sun, D. C., Scmidig, G., Stark, C., Dumbleton, J. H., "A Simple Accelerated Aging Method for Simulations of Long-Term Oxidative Aging Effects in UHMWPE Implants," *Transactions of the 42nd Orthopedic Research Society*, 21, 493, 1996.

(**18**) Greer, K. W., Schmidt, M. B., Hamilton, J. V., "The Hip Simulator Wear of Gamma-Vacuum, Gamma-Air, and Ethylene Oxide Sterilized UHMWPE Following a Severe Oxidative Challenge," *Transactions of the 44th Orthopedic Research Society*, 23, 52, 1998.

(**19**) Taylor, G., King, R., Devanathan, D., Lin, S., "Stability of N2 Packaged Gamma Irradiated UHMWPE," *Transactions of the 43rd Orthopedic Research Society*, 22, 776, 1997.

(**20**) Costa, L. and Brach Del Prever, E. M., *UHMWPE for Arthroplasty*, Edizioni Minerva Medica, S.p.A., Turin, 2000.

(**21**) James, S. P., Blazka, S., Merrill, E. W., Jasty, M., Lee, K. R., et al, "Challenge to the Concept that UHMWPE Acetabular Components Oxidize In Vivo," *Biomaterials*, 14, 643-7, 1993.

Designation: F 2103 – 01

Standard Guide for Characterization and Testing of Chitosan Salts as Starting Materials Intended for Use in Biomedical and Tissue-Engineered Medical Product Applications[1]

This standard is issued under the fixed designation F 2103; the number immediately following the designation indicates the year of original adoption or, in the case of revision, the year of last revision. A number in parentheses indicates the year of last reapproval. A superscript epsilon (ε) indicates an editorial change since the last revision or reapproval.

INTRODUCTION

Biopolymers from marine sources have been studied and used in commercial applications and product development for a number of years. Chitosan, a linear polysaccharide consisting of glucosamine and *N*-acetyl glucosamine derived mainly from crustacean shells, has been used in many technical applications such as water purification (as a flocculant), in cosmetics, and recently as a proposed fat-binding weight control product. In solution, the cationic nature of chitosan gives this polymer a mucoadhesive property. Chitosan salts can be used as a matrix or scaffold material as well as in nonparenteral delivery systems for challenging drugs. Chitosan salts have been shown to increase the transport of polar drugs across the nasal epithelial surface. The purpose of this guide is to identify key parameters relevant for the functionality and characterization of chitosan salts for the development of new commercial applications of chitosan salts for the biomedical and pharmaceutical industries.

1. Scope

1.1 This guide covers the evaluation of chitosan salts suitable for use in biomedical or pharmaceutical applications, or both, including, but not limited to, tissue-engineered medical products (TEMPS).

1.2 This guide addresses key parameters relevant for the functionality, characterization, and purity of chitosan salts.

1.3 As with any material, some characteristics of chitosan may be altered by processing techniques (such as molding, extrusion, machining, assembly, sterilization, and so forth) required for the production of a specific part or device. Therefore, properties of fabricated forms of this polymer should be evaluated using test methods that are appropriate to ensure safety and efficacy.

1.4 *This standard does not purport to address all of the safety concerns, if any, associated with its use. It is the responsibility of the user of this standard to establish appropriate safety and health practices and determine the applicability of regulatory limitations prior to use.*

2. Referenced Documents

2.1 *ASTM Standards:*

D 2196 Test Methods for Rheological Properties of Non-Newtonian Materials by Rotational (Brookfield) Viscometer[2]

F 619 Practice for Extraction of Medical Plastics[3]

F 748 Practice for Selecting Generic Biological Test Methods for Materials and Devices[3]

F 749 Practice for Evaluating Material Extracts by Intracutaneous Injection in the Rabbit[3]

F 756 Practice for Assessment of Hemolytic Properties of Materials[3]

F 763 Practice for Short-Term Screening of Implant Materials[3]

F 813 Practice for Direct Contact Cell Culture Evaluation of Materials for Medical Devices[3]

F 895 Test Method for Agar Diffusion Cell Culture Screening for Cytotoxicity[3]

F 981 Practice for Assessment of Compatibility of Biomaterials for Surgical Implants with Respect to Effect of Materials on Muscle and Bone[3]

F 1251 Terminology Relating to Polymeric Biomaterials in Medical and Surgical Devices[3]

F 1439 Guide for Performance of Lifetime Bioassay for the Tumorigenic Potential of Implant Materials[3]

F 1903 Practice for Testing for Biological Responses to Particles *In Vitro*[3]

F 1904 Practice for Testing the Biological Responses to Particles *In Vivo*[3]

F 1905 Practice for Selecting Tests for Determining the

[1] This guide is under the jurisdiction of ASTM Committee F04 on Medical and Surgical Materials and Devices and is the direct responsibility of Subcommittee F04.43 on Tissue Engineered Biomaterials.

Current edition approved May 10, 2001. Published June 2001.

[2] *Annual Book of ASTM Standards*, Vol 06.01.

[3] *Annual Book of ASTM Standards*, Vol 13.01.

Propensity of Materials to Cause Immunotoxicity[3]

F 1906 Practice for Evaluation of Immune Responses in Biocompatibility Testing Using ELISA Tests, Lymphocyte Proliferation, and Cell Migration[3]

2.2 *Ph. Eur. Document:*

Ph. Eur. Monograph Chitosan Chloride, Nov. 2000[4]

2.3 *ISO Documents:*

ISO 10993 Biological Evaluation of Medical Devices[5]

ISO 10993-1 Biological Evaluation of Medical Devices—Part 1: Evaluation and Testing[5]

ISO 10993-3—Part 3: Tests for Genotoxicity, Carcinogenicity and Reproductive Toxicity[5]

ISO 10993-9—Part 9: Framework for Identification and Quantification of Potential Degradation Products[5]

ISO 10993-17—Part 17: Methods for Establishment of Allowable Limits for Leachable Substances Using Health-Based Risk Assessment[5]

ISO 13408-1: 1998: Aseptic Processing of Health Care Products—Part 1: General Requirements[5]

2.4 *ICH Documents:*

International Conference on Harmonization (1997) Guidance for Industry M3 Nonclinical Safety Studies for the Conduct of Human Clinical Trials for Pharmaceuticals 62 FR 62922[6]

International Conference on Harmonization (1996) Guideline for Industry S2A Specific Aspects of Regulatory Genotoxicity Tests for Pharmaceuticals 61 FR 18199[6]

International Conference on Harmonization (1997) Guidance for Industry S2B Genotoxicity: A Standard Battery for Genotoxicity Testing of Pharmaceuticals 62 FR 62472[6]

International Conference on Harmonization (1994) Guideline for Industry S5A Detection of Toxicity to Reproduction for Medicinal Products 59 FR 48746[6]

International Conference on Harmonization (1996) Guidance for Industry S5B Detection of Toxicity to Reproduction for Medicinal Products: Addendum on Toxicity to Male Fertility 61 FR 15360[6]

International Conference on Harmonization (1996) Guideline for Industry S1A The Need for Long-term Rodent Carcinogenicity Studies of Pharmaceuticals 61 FR 8153[6]

International Conference on Harmonization (1998) Guidance for Industry S1B Testing for Carcinogenicity of Pharmaceuticals 63 FR 8983[6]

International Conference on Harmonization (1995) Guideline for Industry S1C Dose Selection for Carcinogenicity Studies of Pharmaceuticals 60 FR 11278[6]

International Conference on Harmonization (1997) S1C[R] Guidance for Industry Addendum to Dose Selection for Carcinogenicity Studies of Pharmaceuticals: Addition of a Limit Dose and Related Notes 62 FR 64259[6]

International Conference on Harmonization (ICH) Q1A ICH Harmonized Tripartite Guidance for Stability Testing of New Drug Substances and Products (September 23, 1994)[6]

2.5 *FDA Documents:*

FDA Guideline on Validation of the Limulus Amebocyte Test as an End-Product Endotoxin Test for Human and Animal Parenteral Drugs, Biological Products and Healthcare Products DHHS, December 1987[7]

FDA Interim Guidance for Human and Veterinary Drug Products and Biologicals. Kinetic LAL Techniques-DHHS, July 15, 1991[7]

2.6 *ANSI Documents:*

ANSI/AAMI/ISO 11737-1: 1995 Sterilization of Medical Devices—Microbiological Methods—Part 1: Estimation of Bioburden on Product[5]

ANSI/AAMI/ISO 11737-2: 1998 Sterilization of Medical Devices—Microbiological Methods—Part 2: Tests of Sterility Performed in the Validation of a Sterilization Process[5]

2.7 *AAMI Documents:*

AAMI TIR No. 19—1998: Guidance for ANSI/AAMI/ISO 10993–7: 1995, Biological Evaluation of Medical Devices—Part 7: Ethylene Oxide Sterilization Residuals[8]

AAMI/ISO 14160—1998: Sterilization of Single-Use Medical Devices Incorporating Materials of Animal Origin—Validation and Routine Control of Sterilization by Liquid Chemical Sterilants[8]

AAMI ST67/CDV-2: 1999: Sterilization of Medical Devices—Requirements for Products Labeled "Sterile"[8]

2.8 *EN Documents:*

EN 12442-1 Animal Tissues and Their Derivative Utilized in the Manufacture of Medical Devices—Part 1: Analysis and Management of Risk[9]

EN 12442-Part 3: Validation of the Elimination and/or Inactivation of Virus and Transmissible Agents[9]

3. Terminology

3.1 *Definitions:*

3.1.1 *chitosan, n*—a linear polysaccharide consisting of $\beta(1\rightarrow4)$ linked 2-acetamido-2-deoxy-D-glucopyranose (GlcNAc) and 2-amino-2-deoxy-D-glucopyranose (GlcN). Chitosan is a polysaccharide derived by *N*-deacetylation of chitin.

3.1.2 *decomposition, n*—structural changes of chitosans as a result of exposure to environmental, chemical, or thermal factors, such as temperatures greater than 200°C. Decomposition can result in deleterious changes to the chitosan.

3.1.3 *degradation, n*—change in the chemical structure, physical properties, or appearance of a material. Degradation of polysaccharides occurs by means of cleavage of the glycosidic bonds, usually by acid catalyzed hydrolysis. Degradation

[4] Available from EDQM, Publications and Services European Pharmacopoeia, BP 907 226, avenue de Colmar, F-67029 Strasbourg Cedex 1, France.

[5] Available from American National Standards Institute, 25 W. 43rd St., 4th Floor, New York, NY 10036.

[6] Available from ICH Secretariat, c/o IFPMA, 30 rue de St-Jean, PO Box 758, 1211 Geneva 13, Switzerland.

[7] Available from U.S. Food and DrugAdministration, 5600 Fishers Lane, Rockville, MD 20857–0001.

[8] Association for the Advancement of Medical Instrumentation, 111 N. Glebe Rd., Suite 220, Arlington, VA 22201–4795.

[9] Available from European Committee for Standardization, CEN Management Centre, 36 rue de Stassart, B-1050 Brussels, Belgium.

can also occur thermally. Note that degradation is not synonymous with decomposition. Degradation is often used as a synonym for depolymerization when referring to polymers.

3.1.4 *degree of deacetylation, n*—the fraction or percentage of glucosamine units (deacetylated monomers) in a chitosan polymer molecule.

3.1.5 *depolymerization, n*—reduction in length of a polymer chain to form shorter polymeric units. Depolymerization may reduce the polymer chain to oligomeric or monomeric units, or both. In chitosan, hydrolysis of the glycosidic bonds is the primary mechanism.

3.1.6 *endotoxin, n*—a high molecular weight lipopolysaccharide (LPS) complex associated with the cell wall of gram-negative bacteria that is pyrogenic in humans. Though endotoxins are pyrogens, not all pyrogens are endotoxins.

3.1.7 *molecular mass average (molecular weight average), n*—the given molecular weight (Mw) of a chitosan will always represent an average of all of the molecules in the population. The most common ways to express the Mw are as the number average ($\bar{M}_n$) and the weight average ($\bar{M}_w$). The two averages are defined by the following equations:

$$\bar{M}_n = \frac{\sum_i N_i M_i}{\sum_i N_i}$$

and

$$\bar{M}_w = \frac{\sum_i W_i M_i}{\sum_i W_i} = \frac{\sum_i N_i M_i^2}{\sum_i N_i M_i}$$

where:

N_i = number of molecules having a specific molecular weight M_i and

w_i = weight of molecules having a specific molecular weight M_i. In a polydisperse molecular population the relation $\bar{M}_w > \bar{M}_n$ is always valid. The coefficient $\bar{M}_w / \bar{M}_n$ is referred to as the polydispersity index, and will typically be in the range 1.5 to 3.0 for commercial chitosans.

3.1.8 *pyrogen, n*—any substance that produces fever when administered parenterally.

4. Significance and Use

4.1 This guide contains a listing of those characterization parameters that are directly related to the functionality of chitosan. This guide can be used as an aid in the selection and characterization of the appropriate chitosan or chitosan salt for a particular application. This standard is intended to give guidance in the methods and types of testing necessary to properly characterize, assess, and ensure consistency in the performance of a particular chitosan. It may have use in the regulation of devices containing chitosan by appropriate authorities.

4.2 The chitosan salts covered by this guide may be gelled, extruded, or otherwise formulated into biomedical devices for use as tissue-engineered medical products or drug delivery devices for implantation as determined to be appropriate, based on supporting biocompatibility and physical test data. Recommendations in this guide should not be interpreted as a guarantee of clinical success in any tissue-engineered medical product or drug delivery application.

4.3 To ensure that the material supplied satisfies requirements for use in TEMPS, several general areas of characterization should be considered. These are: identity of chitosan, physical and chemical characterization and testing, impurities profile, and performance-related tests.

5. Chemical and Physical Test Methods

5.1 *Identity of Chitosan*—The identity of chitosan and chitosan salts can be established by several methods including, but not limited to the following:

5.1.1 Chitosan chloride monograph Ph. Eur.

5.1.2 *Fourier Transform Infrared Spectroscopy (FT-IR)*—Almost all organic chemical compounds absorb infrared radiation at frequencies characteristic for the functional groups in the compound. A FT-IR spectrum will show absorption bands relating to bond stretching and bending and can therefore serve as a unique fingerprint of a specific compound. Cast a chitosan film from a 0.25 % (w/v) solution of chitosan (in 1 % acetic acid) or chitosan salt (dissolved in water) by drying approximately 500 μL of the sample onto a disposable IR card[10] for 3 to 4 h at 60°C. Record a background spectrum between 4000 and 400 cm-1 using 128 scans at a resolution of 4 cm^{-1}. Record the IR spectrum of a dried blank IR card, then record the IR spectrum of the sample using 128 scans at a resolution of 4 cm^{-1}, percent transmission mode. Label the peaks. Typical frequencies (cm^{-1}) for chitosan are as follows:

Chitosan Base (as Acetate)	Chitosan Chloride	Chitosan Glutamate
3362b	3344b	1555b
1556	1605	1396
1406	1513	1154
1153	1379	1085s
1083s	1154	
	1086s	

The peak designators are: sh: sharp; s: strong; m: medium; w: weak; and b: broad.

5.2 *Physical and Chemical Characterization of Chitosan*:

5.2.1 The composition and sequential structure of chitosan can be a key functional attribute of any chitosan or chitosan salt. Variations in the composition or the sequential structure, or both, may, but not necessarily, cause differences in performance of a chitosan in a particular end use. This information may be determined by the following method: High-resolution ^{1}H- and ^{13}C-nuclear magnetic resonance spectroscopy (NMR).

5.2.2 The degree of deacetylation of chitosan can be established using a number of techniques including, but not limited to, the following:

5.2.2.1 *High-resolution ^{1}H- and ^{13}C-Nuclear Magnetic Resonance Spectroscopy (NMR)*—Chitosan salts should be dissolved in D_2O and partially degraded to a degree of depolymerization of 20 to 30 using sodium nitrite before recording proton or carbon NMR spectra.[11]

[10] No suitable commercially available IR cards are available for the IR analysis of chitosan glutamate salt. Alternative methods are under investigation.

[11] Vårum, K. M., Anthonsen, M. W., Grasdalen, H., and Smidsrod, O., *Carbohydrate Research*, Vol 211, 1991, pp. 17–23.

5.2.2.2 *Determination of the Degree of Deacetylation by UV Spectroscopy*—This method is based upon that reported by Muzzarelli et al.[12] The method is actually a quantitative measure of the number of amine functional groups in the polymer. The method uses a standard curve produced from varying concentrations of *N*-acetyl glucosamine. The degree of deacetylation is calculated from recordings of the first derivative of the UV spectra of *N*-acetyl glucosamine and of chitosan samples at 202 nm.

5.2.3 Molecular mass (molecular weight) of a chitosan will define certain performance characteristics such as viscosity. As such and depending on the sensitivity of a particular end use to these variations, determination of molecular mass directly or indirectly may be necessary. Commercial chitosans are polydisperse with respect to molecular weight (M_W). Molecular weight may be expressed as the number average (M_N) or the weight average (M_W). Molecular weights may be determined by methods such as, but not limited to the following:

5.2.3.1 *Molecular Weight Determination Based on Intrinsic Viscosity*—The intrinsic viscosity describes a polymer's ability to form viscous solutions in water and is directly proportional to the average molecular weight of the polymer. The intrinsic viscosity is a characteristic of the polymer under specified solvent and temperature conditions. It is independent of concentration. The intrinsic viscosity (η) is directly related to the molecular weight of a polymer through the Mark-Houwink-Sakurada (MHS) equation:

$$[\eta] = KM^a$$

where:
K = a constant,
M = viscosity derived average molecular weight, and
a = an empirical constant describing the conformation of the polymer.

By measuring the intrinsic viscosity, the viscosity average molecular weight can be determined if K and a are accurately known for the sample: $\log [\eta] = \log K + a (\log M)$, where M is the molecular weight. The intrinsic viscosity is determined by measuring the relative viscosity in a Ubbelohde capillary viscometer. The measurements should be performed in a solvent containing 0.1M NaCl (a nongelling, monovalent salt) at a constant temperature of 20°C, and at a sufficiently low chitosan concentration. Automatic operation and data acquisition are preferred.

5.2.3.2 *Molecular Weight and Polydispersity Determination by Size Exclusion Chromatography with Multiple Angle Laser Light Scattering Detection (SEC-MALLS)*—As there are no chitosan standards currently available, refractive index detectors can not be adequately calibrated. It is not sufficient to only use pullulan standards as a calibration material. Therefore, the method of choice is to use refractive index coupled to MALLS. For separation of the chitosan into different molecular weight fractions, a hydrophilic column with the appropriate pore size is required. Such columns include, but are not limited to those mentioned in the following techniques. The precision of these techniques must be determined as results can vary by 10 to 20 %. Typical methods using these techniques include, but are not limited to: using 0.01M sodium acetate/acetic acid buffer, pH 5.5 as the mobile phase with separation using TSK 3000, TSK 4000, and TSK 5000 columns.

5.2.3.3 *Polydispersity*—Depending on the end use and the sensitivity of the application to the molecular mass, the presence of a wide range of chitosan fractions may be an issue. In such cases, calculation of the polydispersity will be important. Typically, this is between 1.5 and 3.0 for commercial chitosans.

5.2.4 Depending on the final use and the required performance control, other characterization assays can include, but are not limited to the following:

5.2.4.1 *Viscosity in Aqueous Solution*—Viscosity is defined as a liquid's resistance to flow. The molecular mass of a chitosan will determine the extent to which it will thicken an aqueous solution. Therefore, a simple viscosity test may yield information on the relative differences in molecular mass among chitosan samples. To allow comparison between laboratories, the viscometer used must be calibrated with traceable standards (see Test Methods D 2196). The viscosity measured will depend on several parameters related to how the testing is conducted. Important parameters to control include, but are not limited to the following:

(*1*) *Temperature*—The temperature at which the measurement is performed is critical. An increase in temperature will, in almost every case, result in a decrease in the viscosity. Consistent and controlled temperature (that is, with a standard temperature bath) is critical to achieving reproducible results. Typically, the temperature used to measure viscosity can be 20°, 25°, or 37°C, or combination thereof.

(*2*) *Chitosan Concentration*—The moisture content of the chitosan must be known to prepare correct concentrations of chitosan or chitosan salts.

(*3*) *Ionic Strength*—The viscosity of a chitosan solution is very sensitive to the ionic environment in which the measurement is made. The most important aspect is to keep the ionic content consistent. Typically, viscosity measurements are made either in deionized water or a standardized ionic environment such as isotonic saline.

(*4*) *Molecular Mass*—Viscosity measurements are sensitive to the molecular mass of the chitosan. The following is one suggestion concerning the measurement of chitosan viscosity, but any appropriate method would apply. To measure the apparent viscosity of chitosan or chitosan salts, prepare a solution in deionized water (for chitosan salts) or 1 % acetic acid (for chitosan) with a concentration (w/w, corrected for dry matter content) appropriate for the end use. For example, if the sample has a suspected molecular weight above approximately 50 000 g/mol, prepare a 1 % (w/w) solution; if the suspected molecular weight is less than about 50 000 g/mol, then prepare a 10 % (w/w) solution. The viscosity is measured using a rotational viscometer (for example, Brookfield type) at 20 ± 0.2°C (or other controlled temperature) using the appropriate spindle, spindle rotation speed and a temperature-controlled water bath.

5.2.4.2 *Dry Matter Content*—Various chitosan and chitosan

[12] Muzzarelli, R. A. A., Rochetti, R., Stanic, V., and Weckx, M., *Chitin Handbook*, R. A. A. Muzzarelli and M. T. Peters, Ed., Atec Grottammare, 1997.

salts are supplied with different moisture contents. The dry matter content determination is based upon the removal of water from the sample. Normally with chitosan, gravimetric techniques are used. They are adapted directly from <731> USP 24/NF19 and use a calibrated drying oven at 105°C.

5.2.4.3 *Ash Content*—The ash content of a sample describes the total amount of inorganic material present. After combustion, the sample contains a mixture of salts. The composition of the ash depends on the temperature used during the combustion of the organic material. For ash content of chitosan, a combustion temperature of 800°C for at least 6 h is recommended. Chitosan or chitosan salts intended to be used in biomedical applications should have a very low ash content.

5.2.4.4 *Insolubles*—The percentage of insolubles describes the total amount of insoluble impurities (insoluble salts, chitosan, or other contaminants) in a chitosan/chitosan salt sample. The determination of insolubles content is based upon dissolving the chitosan in acetic acid, or chitosan salt in water, and filtering the chitosan solution. Then, the insolubles are calculated form the weight of chitosan dissolved and the weight of insoluble particles obtained on a filter. While no specific limits are suggested, chitosan/chitosan salts used in biomedical and tissue-engineered medical products should have as low an insolubles content as possible.

5.3 *Impurities Profile*—The term impurity relates to the presence of extraneous substances and materials in the chitosan powder. Additionally, and dependent upon the end use, a high molecular weight chitosan present in a sample of low molecular weight could constitute an impurity. Various processing aids may also be used in the manufacture of chitosan and could constitute an impurity. If there is a concern for the presence of processing aids or other contaminants associated with chitosan, they should be addressed with the supplier. The major impurities of concern include, but are not limited to the following:

5.3.1 *Endotoxin Content*—Endotoxin contamination is difficult to prevent because it is ubiquitous in nature, stable, and small enough to pass through sterilizing filters. There are several tests to determine the presence of endotoxin in the chitosan salts. These are the gel clot, end point assay, and the kinetic assay. The gel clot test is the simplest and easiest of the Limulus amebocyte lysate (LAL) test methods, although much less sensitive than the kinetic assay. A firm gel that maintains its integrity upon inverting the tube is scored as a positive test. Anything other than a firm gel is scored as a negative test. The end point assay is based on the linear relationship between the endotoxin concentration and the formation of color (chromogenic assay) over a relatively short range of standard dilutions. A standard curve is then constructed by plotting the optical densities of a series of endotoxin standards as a function of the endotoxin concentration. Using linear regression analysis, the standard curve covers an endotoxin range of approximately 1 log (usually 1.0 to 0.1 EU/mL). The most sensitive means of determining the endotoxin content is with a quantitative, kinetic assay. This test uses a LAL and a synthetic color producing substrate to detect endotoxin chromogenically (such as, but not limited to, BioWhittaker's Kinetic-QCL™ methodology, or other equivalent assay). The kinetic assay measures the amount of time required to reach a predetermined optical density (kinetic turbidimetric) or color intensity (kinetic chromogenic), sometimes called the onset optical density or reaction optical density. The Food and Drug Administration (FDA) currently defines linearity as a correlation coefficient of ≥ 0.980. See FDA Guideline DHHS, December 1987. It is important that operators of the LAL method are qualified and that each new lot of reagents is validated. Positive product controls (PPC) must be added to test inhibition in the sample. Recovery of the known added amount of endotoxin standard must be obtained for a valid assay. It is recommended that endotoxin measurements be performed using an initial 0.1 % concentration of chitosan and 3 dilution ranges (for example, 20, 50, and 100x). The endotoxin level in chitosan will ultimately be critical to its use in biomedical applications where there are regulatory limits to the amount of endotoxin that can be implanted into humans. Relevant FDA guidance for allowable levels and information regarding validation of endotoxin assays should be consulted if human trials are contemplated. See FDA Guideline DHHS, July 15, 1991.

5.3.2 *Protein Content*—Protein content in chitosan or chitosan salts should be assayed using an appropriate method having sufficient sensitivity to detect low levels of contamination. One method, although not the only suitable one, is the Coomassie brilliant blue G dye binding assay as described by Read and Northcote.[13] This method is able to quantitate protein content as low as 3 µg/mL. The protein content should be assayed using a 1 % (w/w) chitosan solution corrected for dry matter content. It is important to confirm that the method chosen is insensitive to materials present in the sample and to validate it against a reference method on a one-time basis. It is the responsibility of the end user to evaluate the chitosan product for the presence of specific proteins that could cause undesirable tissue reactions.

5.3.3 *Heavy Metal Content by the USP Method*—This test is provided to demonstrate that the content of heavy metal impurities does not exceed a limit in the individual product specification in terms of parts per million lead in the test substance. Under the specified test conditions, the limit is determined by a concomitant visual comparison of metals that are colored by sulfide ion with a control prepared from a standard lead solution. Substances that typically respond to this test are lead, mercury, bismuth, arsenic, antimony, tin, cadmium, silver, copper, and molybdenum. This method is based on (231) heavy metals, USP24/NF19. The presence of specific heavy metals may be detected by methods such as atomic absorption spectroscopy using flame or graphite furnace techniques; or by inductively coupled plasma techniques.

5.3.4 *Microbiological Safety*—Bacteria, yeast, and mold are also impurities that can arise in a chitosan sample. The presence of bacteria may also contribute to the presence of endotoxins. The following Microbiological Tests in USP 24 are of particular relevance: Microbial Limit Tests <61>, Sterility Tests <71>, Sterilization and sterility assurance of compendial articles <12211> and the Biological Tests and Assays: Bacterial Endotoxins Tests <85>. The user should also consider other relevant standards, such as, but not limited to, Association for

[13] Read and Northcote, *Analytical Biochemistry*, Vol 116, 1981, pp. 53–64.

the Advancement of Medical Instrumentation (AAMI) standards and international standards, of which the following are examples: ANSI/AAMI/ISO 11737-1: 1995, ANSI/AAMI/ISO 11737-2: 1998, and ISO 13408-1: 1998. Membrane filtration can be used for the determination of bacteria, yeast and mold in chitosan samples. The chitosan salt is first dissolved in sterile, deionized water, then filtered using sterile techniques through a 0.45-μm membrane filter. The filters are subsequently incubated on tryptic soya agar to determine the presence of bacteria, and on sabouraud dextrose agar to determine the presence of yeast and mold. If chitosan products are intended to serve as a barrier to microorganisms, this function will need to be validated with specific experiments.

6. Product Development Considerations

6.1 *Type of Solvent (that is, acid, medium, or water)*—The conformation of the chitosan molecule will vary with changes in the pH and ionic strength of the solute. Therefore, the apparent viscosity of a chitosan solution may change depending upon whether the chitosan is dissolved in water, acid, or in a salt-containing medium.

6.2 *Stability of Chitosan*—For chitosan, the most relevant stability-indicating parameters are those related to the functionality of the polymer. Dependent upon what function the chitosan will have in the final formulation, parameters such as viscosity (apparent and intrinsic) and molecular weight should be evaluated during a stability study. Storage conditions are of importance, especially for chitosan solutions. The following ICH guidance documents should be consulted for information on stability testing of pharmaceuticals: 62 FR 62922, 61 FR 18199, 62 FR 62472, 59 FR 48746, 61 FR 15360, 61 FR 8153, 63 FR 8983, 60 FR 11278, 62 FR 64259, and Q1A.

6.3 *Methods of Sterilization*—Chitosan powder can be sterilized by gamma irradiation or *E*-beam (with subsequent degradation of the chitosan polymer chain resulting in a reduction in molecular weight) or by ethylene oxide. Solutions of chitosan may be (*1*) filter sterilized if the viscosity of the chitosan solution permits; (*2*) gamma-irradiated with a resulting loss in viscosity (molecular weight); and (*3*) autoclaved (which also reduced the viscosity of the solution). Selection of the method of sterilization will depend upon the viscosity or molecular weight needs of the final application. Use of ethylene oxide will also require testing for residuals. The reader should refer to the relevant standards regarding the sterilization of healthcare products by radiation, steam, and ethylene oxide gas, such as AAMI TIR No. 19—1998, AAMI/ISO 14160—1998, and AAMI ST67/CDV-2: 1999.

7. Safety and Toxicology Aspects of Chitosan

7.1 Chitosan has been included in the Codex Alimentarius Inventory of Processing Aids (ALINORM 91/12, para 104), effective by the 22nd Session of the Codex Committee on Food Additives and Contaminants, Hague, March 20, 1990. This listing, however, does not indicate approval for the use of chitosan in pharmaceutical or biomedical applications, or both.

7.2 The safety of chitosan in biomedical and pharmaceutical applications and in TEMPS should be established according to current guidelines such as ISO 10993 and Practice F 748. Suppliers of chitosan or chitosan salts may have such documentation on file. Preclinical safety studies specific to the clinical application under consideration must also be done in accordance with 21CFR312.

7.2.1 A database generated to support the safety of chitosan-containing pharmaceuticals should reflect consideration of the proposed clinical route of administration and product formulation, although it may be appropriate for certain studies to involve a route of administration or formulation which differ from the clinical situation. Guidance on the need for, timing, and conduct of the nonclinical toxicology studies is available in the ICH (International Conference on Harmonization) guidelines on the respective topics. Such studies may include, but are not limited to: acute toxicology testing, repeated dose toxicology testing with a treatment regimen and duration that is relevant to the proposed clinical use (ICH guidance M3), hypersensitivity testing, and genetic toxicology testing (ICH guidances S2A and S2B). Additional studies that may be relevant to a proposed pharmaceutical use include reproductive/developmental toxicology testing (ICH guidances S5A and S5B) and carcinogenicity testing (ICH guidances S1A, S1B, S1C, and S1C[R]). Additional testing may be specific to the route of administration, for example, application or injection site irritation, ocular irritation, dermal carcinogenicity testing, or studies of photoirritation and photo co-carcinogenicity potential. Other testing may be appropriate, depending on the results of early studies and the intended clinical use of the product. Specific guidance on the development or marketing of drug products, biologics, or biomedical devices in the United States may be obtained by contacting the Center for Drug Evaluation and Research, Center for Biologics Evaluation and Research, or the Center for Devices and Radiological Health, respectively, of the U.S. Food and Drug Administration.

7.3 *Biocompatibility*

7.3.1 Biomaterials are materials of natural or man-made origin that are used to direct, supplement, or replace the functions of living tissues. These materials may be considered biocompatible if the materials perform with an appropriate host response in a specific application.[14]

7.3.2 Many materials have been shown to produce a well-characterized level of biological response following long term clinical use in laboratory animals. When new applications of a material, or modifications to the material or physical forms of the material are being considered, then the recommendations and test methods of the following standards should be considered: Practices F 748, F 619, F 749, F 756, F 763, F 813, F 981, F 1903, F 1904, F 1905, and F 1906; Guide F 1439; Test Method F 895; Terminology F 1251; and ISO 10993-1, ISO/DIS 10993-9—Part 9, ISO/DIS 10993-17—Part 17, EN 12442-1—Part 1, EN 12442-3—Part 3.

7.4 Chitosan or chitosan salts for use in biomedical and pharmaceutical applications and in TEMPS should ideally be documented in a device or drug master file to which end users may obtain a letter of cross reference from suppliers of chitosan or chitosan salts. Such a master file should be

[14] Williams, D. F., *The Williams Dictionary of Biomaterials*, Liverpool University Press, 1999.

submitted to the U.S. FDA and to other regulatory authorities, both national and international.

8. Keywords

8.1 biomedical; chitosan salts; tissue-engineered medical product applications (TEMPS)

APPENDIXES

(Nonmandatory Information)

X1. RATIONALE

X1.1 The use of naturally occurring biopolymers for biomedical and pharmaceutical applications and in TEMPS is increasing. This guide is designed to give guidance in the characterization and testing parameters for chitosan and chitosan salts used in such applications. Knowledge of the physical and chemical properties of the chitosan, such as degree of deacetylation, molecular weight (or viscosity), counterion, and so forth, will assist end users in choosing the correct chitosan for their particular application. Knowledge of these parameters will also ensure that users can request and obtain similar material from suppliers on reordering. Molecular characterization of chitosan will also assist end users in documentation of their formulation or device. Finally, characterization of the chitosan will allow the functionality of the chitosan to fit the application or end product. Tests outlined in this guide are sufficient for release of chitosan or chitosan salts to the end user. Other validated tests that would accomplish the same purposes as those set forth in this guide may be substituted. The tests may not be suitable for characterization and functionality of the final product.

X2. BACKGROUND

X2.1 Chitosan is a linear polymer that is composed of glucosamine (GlcN) and *N*-acetyl glucosamine (GlcNAc) units linked in a β(1→4) manner. The glucosamine and *N*-acetyl glucosamine are randomly distributed along the polymer chain. Chitosan as such is not soluble in aqueous solution, but can be solubilized using acids such as acetic acid, hydrochloric acid, and solutions of organic acids. In solution, chitosan salts will carry a positive charge through protonization of the free amino group on glucosamine. Reactivity with negatively charged surfaces is a direct function of the positive charge density of chitosan. The cationic nature of chitosan gives this polymer a mucoadhesive property (see Fig. X2.1).

X2.2 *Raw Materials for Chitosan Production*—All current industrial manufacture of chitosan is based on the extraction of the polymer from crustacean shells. Chitosan has also been processed from the pens of squid. Since chitosan is also synthesized as an exocellular material by some mold and yeast, this polymer can be obtained through fermentation.

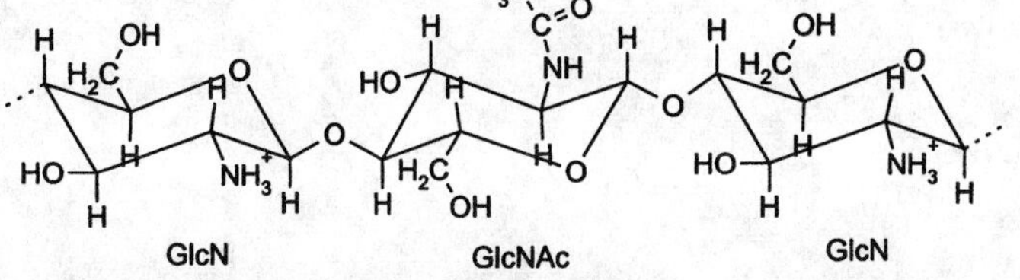

FIG. X2.1 Chitosan

X2.3 *Functional Properties and Applications of Chitosan:*

X2.3.1 The functional properties of chitosan of primary importance for most biomedical applications are the bioadhesive ones. Solubility, swellability, and film-forming properties are other characteristics exploited in biomedical and pharmaceutical applications.

X2.3.2 Gelling properties are a function of the degree of deacetylation.

X2.3.3 Thickening (viscosifying) properties of chitosan are a function of the molecular weight and the conformation of the chitosan molecule in solution. Interactions with other molecules in the solution as well as competition for water at high chitosan concentrations affect the flow properties of chitosan solutions.

X2.3.4 Both gelling and thickening properties of chitosan are dependent upon the order in which the different materials are added.

X2.3.5 Solubility of chitosan is related to the rate of dissociation of the chitosan molecule.

X2.3.6 Films can be formed from chitosan solutions simply by evaporation of the solvent. The molecular weight of chitosan needs to be above a certain lower limit to achieve film formation and avoid brittleness. Films can be formed easily in situ by spraying a chitosan solution onto a binding surface.

RELATED MATERIAL

Any documents included in this section that are marked "proposed" are published for information only. They have received the approval of the sponsoring technical committee for publication as "proposed" but have not been officially accepted by the Society. Comments are solicited and should be addressed to ASTM, 100 Barr Harbor Drive, PO Box C700, West Conshohocken, PA 19428-2959.

SI QUICK REFERENCE GUIDE:
International System of Units (SI)
*The Modernized Metric System**

UNITS

The International System of Units (SI) is based on seven fundamental (base) units:

Base Units

Quantity	*Name*	*Symbol*
length	metre	m
mass	kilogram	kg
time	second	s
electric current	ampere	A
thermodynamic temperature	kelvin	K
amount of substance	mole	mol
luminous intensity	candela	cd

and a number of derived units which are combinations of base units and which may have special names and symbols:

Examples of Derived Units

Quantity	*Expression*	*Name*	*Symbol*
acceleration			
angular	rad/s²		
linear	m/s²		
angle			
plane	dimensionless	radian	rad
solid	dimensionless	steradian	sr
area	m²		
Celsius temperature	K	degree Celsius	°C
density			
heat flux	W/m²		
mass	kg/m³		
current	A/m²		
energy, enthalpy			
work, heat	N·m	joule	J
specific	J/kg		
entropy			
heat capacity	J/K		
specific	J/(kg·K)		
flow, mass	kg/s		
flow, volume	m³/s		
force	kg·m/s²	newton	N
frequency			
periodic	1/s	hertz	Hz
rotating	rev/s		
inductance	Wb/A	henry	H
magnetic flux	V·s	weber	Wb
mass flow	kg/s		
moment of a force	N·m		
potential,electric	W/A	volt	V
power, radiant flux	J/s	watt	W
pressure, stress	N/m²	pascal	Pa
resistance, electric	V/A	ohm	Ω
thermal conductivity	W/(m·K)		
velocity			
angular	rad/s		
linear	m/s		
viscosity			
dynamic (absolute)(μ)	Pa·s		
kinematic (ν)	m²/s		
volume	m³		
volume, specific	m³/kg		

*For complete information see *IEEE/ASTM SI-10*.

SYMBOLS

Symbol	*Name*	*Quantity*	*Formula*
A	ampere	electric current	base unit
Bq	becquerel	activity (of a radio nuclide)	1/s
C	coulomb	electric charge	A·s
°C	degree Celsius	temperature interval	°C = K
cd	candela	luminous intensity	base unit
F	farad	electric capacitance	C/V
Gy	gray	absorbed dose	J/kg
g	gram	mass	kg/1000
H	henry	inductance	Wb/A
Hz	hertz	frequency	1/s
ha	hectare*	area	10 000 m^2
J	joule	energy, work, heat	N·m
K	kelvin	temperature	base unit
kg	kilogram	mass	base unit
L	litre	volume	m^3/1000
lm	lumen	luminous flux	cd·sr
lx	lux	illuminance	lm/m^2
m	metre	length	base unit
mol	mole	amount of substance	base unit
N	newton	force	kg·m/s^2
Ω	ohm	electric resistance	V/A
Pa	pascal	pressure, stress	N/m^2
rad	radian	plane angle	m/m (dimensionless)
S	siemens	electric conductance	A/V
Sv	sievert	dose equivalent	J/kg
s	second	time	base unit
sr	steradian	solid angle	m^2/m^2 (dimensionless)
T	tesla	magnetic flux density	Wb/m^2
t	tonne, metric ton	mass	1000 kg; Mg
V	volt	electric potential	W/A
W	watt	power, radiant flux	J/s
Wb	weber	magnetic flux	V·s

*allowed with SI

Use of Symbols

The correct use of symbols is important because an incorrect symbol may change the meaning of a quantity. Some SI symbols are listed in the Symbol table.

SI has no abbreviations—only symbols. Therefore, no periods follow a symbol except at the end of a sentence.

Examples: A, *not* amp; s, *not* sec; SI, *not* S.I.

Symbols appear in lower case unless the unit name has been taken from a proper name. In this case the first letter of the symbol is capitalized.

Examples: m, metre; Pa, pascal; W, watt

Exception: L, litre

Symbols and prefixes are printed in upright (roman) type regardless of the type style in surrounding text.

Example: . . . *a distance of* 73 km *between* . . .

Unit symbols are the same whether singular or plural.

Examples: 1 mm, 100 mm; 1 kg, 65 kg

Leave a space between the value and the symbol.

Examples: 115 W, *not* 115W; 0.75 L, *not* 0.75L
88 °C, not 88°C or 88° C

Exception: No space is left between the numerical value and symbol for degree of plane angle.

Examples: 73°, not 73 °

Note: Symbol for coulomb is C; for degree Celsius it is °C

Do not mix symbols and names in the same expression.

Examples: radians per second or rad/s
not radians/second; not radians/s
m/s or metres per second,
not metres/second; *not* metres/s
J/kg or joules per kilogram,
not joules/kilogram; *not* joules/kg

Symbol for product—use the raised dot (·)

Examples: N·m; mPa·s; W/(m^2·K)

Symbol for quotient—use one of the following forms:

Examples: m/s or $\frac{m}{s}$ or use negative exponent

Note: Use only one solidus (/) per expression and parentheses to avoid any ambiguity.

Do not use modifying terms such as electrical, alternating current, etc.

Examples: kPa (gage); MW (e); V (ac)

PREFIXES

Most prefixes indicate orders of magnitude in steps of 1000 and provide a convenient way to express large and small numbers and to eliminate nonsignificant digits and leading zeros in decimal fractions.

Examples: 64 000 watts is the same as 64 kilowatts*
0.057 metre is the same as 57 millimetres
16 000 metres is the same as 16 kilometres*
*except for intended accuracy

Prefix	*Symbol*	*Represents*
yotta	Y	10^{24}
zetta	Z	10^{21}
exa	E	10^{18}
peta	P	10^{15}
tera	T	10^{12}
giga	G	10^{9}
mega	M	10^{6}
kilo	k	10^{3}
hecto	h*	10^{2}
deka	da*	10^{1}
deci	d*	10^{-1}
centi	c*	10^{-2}
milli	m	10^{-3}
micro	µ	10^{-6}
nano	n	10^{-9}
pico	p	10^{-12}
femto	f	10^{-15}
atto	a	10^{-18}
zepto	z	10^{-21}
yocto	y	10^{-24}

To realize the full benefit of the prefixes when expressing a quantity by numerical value, choose a prefix so that the number lies between 0.1 and 1000. For simplicity, give preference to prefixes representing 1000 raised to an integral power (i.e., µm, mm, km).

**Exceptions*:

In expressing area and volume, the prefixes hecto, deka, deci, and centi may by required; for example, cubic decimetre (L), square hectometre (hectare), cubic centimetre.

Tables of values of the same quantity.

Comparison of values.

For certain quantities in particular applications. For example, the millimetre is used for linear dimensions in architectural and engineering drawings even when the values lie far outside the range of 0.1 mm to 1000 mm; the centimetre is usually used for anatomical measurements and clothing sizes.

Compound units. A compound unit is a derived unit expressed with two or more units. The prefix is attached to a unit in the numerator.

Examples: V/m *not* mV/mm
MJ/kg *not* kJ/g

Compound prefixes formed by a combination of two or more prefixes are not used. Use only one prefix.

Examples: 2 nm *not* 2 mµm
6 m^3 *not* 6 kL
6 MPa *not* 6 kkPa

Exponential Powers. An exponent attached to a symbol containing a prefix indicates that the multiple (of the unit with its prefix) is raised to the power of 10 expressed by the exponent.

Examples: 1 $mm^3 = (10^{-3}\ m)^3 = 10^{-9}\ m^3$
1 $ns^{-1} = (10^{-9}\ s)^{-1} = 10^{9}\ s^{-1}$
1 $mm^2/s = (10^{-3}\ m)^2/s = 10^{-6}\ m^2/s$

NUMBERS

International practice separates the digits of large numbers into groups of three, counting from the decimal to the left and to the right, and inserts a space to separate the groups. In numbers of four digits, the space is not necessary except for uniformity in tables.

Examples: 6.358 568; 85 365; 51 845 953; 88 000;
0.246 113 562; 7 258

Small Numbers. When writing numbers less than one, always put a zero before the decimal marker.

Example: 0.046

Decimal Marker. The recommended decimal marker is a dot on the line (period). (In some countries, a comma is used as the decimal marker.)

Because **billion** means a million million in most countries but a thousand million in the United States, avoid using billion in technical writing.

DO'S AND DON'TS

The units in the international system of units are called SI units—*not* Metric Units and *not* SI Metric Units.

Non-SI units in the US are called Inch-Pound units (I-P units)—*not* conventional units, *not* U.S. customary units, *not* English units, and *not* Imperial units.)

Treat all spelled out names as nouns. Therefore, do not capitalize the first letter of a unit except at the beginning of a sentence or in capitalized material such as a title.

Examples: watt; pascal; ampere; volt; newton; kelvin
Exception: Always capitalize the first letter of Celsius.

Do not begin a sentence with a unit symbol—either rearrange the words or write the unit name in full.

Use plurals for spelled out words when required by the rules of grammar.

Examples: metre—metres; henry—henries;
kilogram—kilograms; kelvin—kelvins
Irregular: hertz—hertz; lux—lux; siemens—siemens

Do not put a space or hyphen between the prefix and unit name.

Examples: kilometre *not* kilo metre or kilo-metre;
milliwatt *not* milli watt or milli-watt

When a prefix ends with a vowel and the unit name begins with a vowel, retain and pronounce both vowels.

Example: kiloampere
Exceptions: hectare; kilohm; megohm

When compound units are formed by multiplication, leave a space between units that are multiplied.

Examples: newton metre, *not* newton-metre; volt ampere, *not* volt-ampere

Use the modifier squared or cubed after the unit name.

Example: metre per second squared
Exception: For area or volume the modifier may be placed before the units.
Example: square millimetre; cubic metre

When compound units are formed by division, use the word *per,* not a solidus (/).

Examples: metre per second, *not* metre / second; watt per square metre, *not* watt / square meter

Do not use modifying terms such as electrical, alternating current, etc. after the symbol.

Examples: kPa (gage); MW (e); V (ac)

SELECTED CONVERSION FACTORS

CAUTION: These conversion values are rounded to three or four significant figures, which is sufficiently accurate for most applications. When making conversions, remember that a converted value is no more precise than the original value. Round off the final value to the same number of significant figures as those in the original value. See ANSI SI 10 for additional conversions with more significant figures.

Multiply	*By*	*To Obtain*
acre	0.4047	ha
atmosphere, standard	*101.325	kPa
bar	*100	kPa
barrel (42 US gal, petroleum)	159	L
Btu, (International Table)	1.055	kJ
Btu / lb·°F (specific heat, c^p)	4.184	kJ/(kg·K)
bushel	0.03524	m³
calorie, kilogram (kilocalorie)	4.187	kJ
candle, candlepower	*1.0	cd
centipoise, dynamic vicosity, μ	*1.00	mPa·s
centistokes, kinematic viscosity, ν	*1.00	mm²/s
ft	*0.3048	m
ft	*304.8	mm
ft / min, fpm	*0.00508	m/s
ft / s, fps	*0.3048	m/s
ft of water	2.99	kPa
ft²	0.09290	m²
ft²/s, kinematic viscosity, ν	92 900	mm²/s
ft³	28.32	L
ft³	0.02832	m³
ft³/h, cfh	7.866	mL/s
ft³/min, cfm	0.4719	L/s
ft³/s, cfs	28.32	L/s
footcandle	10.76	lx
ft·lb$_f$ (torque or moment)	1.36	N·m
ft·lb$_f$ (work)	1.36	J
ft·lb$_f$ / lb (specific energy)	2.99	J/kg
ft·lb$_f$ / min (power)	0.0226	W
gallon, US (*231 in³)	3.785	L
gph	1.05	mL/s
gpm	0.0631	L/s
gpm / ft²	0.6791	L/(s·m²)
gr / gal	17.1	g/m³
horsepower (550 ft·lb$_f$/s)	0.746	kW
inch	*25.4	mm
in of mercury (60°F)	3.377	kPa
in of water (60°F)	248.8	Pa
in·lb$_f$ (torque or moment)	113	mN·m
in²	645	mm²
in³ (volume)	16.4	mL
in³ (section modulus)	16 400	mm³
in⁴ (section moment)	416 200	mm⁴
km / h	0.278	m/s
kWh	*3.60	MJ
kip / in² (ksi)	6.895	MPa
litre	*0.001	m³
micron (μm) of mercury (60°F)	133	mPa
mil (0.001 in.)	*25.4	μm
mile	1.61	km
mile, nautical	1.85	km
mph	1.61	km/h
mph	0.447	m/s
millibar	*0.100	kPa
mm of mercury (60°F)	0.133	kPa
mm of water (60°F)	9.80	Pa
ounce (mass, avoirdupois)	28.35	g
ounce (force of thrust)	0.278	N
ounce (liquid, US)	29.6	mL
ounce (avoirdupois) per gallon	7.49	kg/m³
pint (liquid, US)	473	mL
pound		
lb$_m$ (mass)	0.4536	kg
lb$_m$ (mass)	453.6	g
lb$_f$ (force or thrust)	4.45	N
lb$_m$ / ft (uniform load)	1.49	kg/m
lb$_m$ / (ft·h) (dynamic viscosity, μ)	0.413	mPa·s
lb$_m$ / (ft·s) (dynamic viscosity, μ)	1490	mPa·s
lb$_f$·s / ft² (dynamic viscosity, μ)	47 880	mPa·s
lb$_m$ / min	0.00756	kg/s
lb$_m$ / h	0.126	g/s
lb$_f$ / ft²	47.9	Pa
lb$_m$ / ft²	4.88	kg/m²
lb$_m$ / ft³ (density, ρ)	16.0	kg/m³
lb$_m$ / gallon	120	kg/m³
ppm (by mass)	*1.00	mg/kg
psi	6.895	kPa
quad (10¹⁵ Btu)	1.06	EJ
quart (liquid, US)	0.946	L
rpm	0.105	rad/s
tablespoon (approx.)	15	mL
teaspoon (approx.)	5	mL
therm (100,000 Btu)	105.5	MJ
ton, short (2000 lb)	0.907	Mg; t (tonne)
yd	*0.9144	m
yd²	0.836	m²
yd³	0.7646	m³

*Conversion factor is exact.

Note: In this list the kelvin (K) expresses temperature intervals. The degree Celsius symbol (°C) may be used for this purpose as well.

ANNUAL BOOK of ASTM STANDARDS

Index

Volume 13.01

Medical Devices; Emergency Medical Services

This index covers the standards and related material appearing in this volume(s) or section only. The boldface references represent the ASTM designations. For multiple volume or section indexes, the volume in which the standard appears is included in parentheses. A triangle (Δ) preceding the ASTM designation denotes that Adjunct Material for the standard is available separately; the Adjunct No. is given in the standard. A Combined Index, covering the standards appearing in all volumes of the *2001 Annual Book of ASTM Standards*, is issued as Volume 00.01.

Alphabetization in the index is letter-for-letter, with no consideration to punctuation or word division. Initial prepositions of (indented) subentries are ignored for alphabetization.

In the preparation of indexes, every attempt has been made to index standards on three levels: (1) by main subject, using general and specific search terms; (2) by tests or other significant sections of ASTM standards; and (3) by cross-references to locate main subject entry terms. *(See also* references are abbreviated as *Sa* and appear under main entry terms.) The following examples illustrate ASTM's method of indexing.

INDEX TERMS FOR SPECIFICATIONS

Steel pipe—carbon steel
Seamless and Welded Steel Pipe for Low-Temperature Service, Specification for, **A 333/A333M (01.01)**

Steel tube—ferritic stainless steel
Seamless and Welded Ferritic/Austenitic Stainless Steel Tubing for General Service, Specification for, **A 789/A789M (01.01)**

INDEX TERMS FOR TESTS

Gold—electrodeposited coating
Installing Corrugated Aluminum Structural Plate Pipe for Culverts and Sewers, Practice for, **B 789/B789M (02.02)**

Effective elastic parameter (E_{eff})
Determining the Effective Elastic Parameter for X-Ray Diffraction Measurements of Residual Stress, Test Method for, **E 1426 (03.01)**

CROSS-REFERENCES

Water—drinking
See **Drinking water**

PDB (pressure design basis)
See **Pressure design basis (PDB)**
Sa **Pressure testing**

A

C

D

E

F

M

P

V